CONTENTS—cont'd

MEDICAL-SURGICAL NURSING

CONCEPTS AND CLINICAL PRACTICE

EDITED BY

WILMA J. PHIPPS, PH.D., R.N., F.A.A.N.

Professor Emeritus of Medical-Surgical Nursing
Frances Payne Bolton School of Nursing
Case Western Reserve University
Cleveland, Ohio

BARBARA C. LONG M.S.N., R.N.

Associate Professor Emeritus of Medical-Surgical Nursing
Frances Payne Bolton School of Nursing
Case Western Reserve University
Cleveland, Ohio

NANCY FUGATE WOODS, PH.D., R.N., F.A.A.N.

Professor and Chair, Parent and Child Nursing
University of Washington, Seattle, Washington

VIRGINIA L. CASSMEYER, PH.D., R.N.

Associate Professor of Medical-Surgical Nursing
University of Kansas, Kansas City, Kansas

GAIL OSTERFIELD, MSN, RN

Assistant Professor of Nursing,
Kent State University,
Kent, Ohio

JUDITH HILL OZUNA, MN, RN

Clincal Lecturer, Physiological Nursing,
University of Washington;
Clinical Nurse Specialist, Neurology,
Veterans' Administration Medical Center,
Seattle, Washington

KYLE M. PASKERT, MSN, RN

Clinical Nurse Specialist,
University Hospitals of Cleveland;
Clinical Instructor in Medical-Surgical Nursing,
Frances Payne Bolton School of Nursing,
Case Western Reserve University,
Cleveland, Ohio

DEBORAH POWER, MN, RN

Formerly Lecturer, Physiological Nursing,
University of Washington, Seattle, Washington

JANET PRIMOMO, PhD, RN

Senior Research Fellow,
University of Washington School of Nursing,
Seattle, Washington

ANTOINETTE T. RAGUCCI, PhD, RN

Associate Professor Emerita of Medical-Surgical
Nursing, Frances Payne Bolton School
of Nursing,
Case Western Reserve University,
Cleveland, Ohio

CAROL SUN REDFIELD, MN, RN

Northwest Cancer Clinic,
Seattle, Washington

REBECCA ANNE ROBERTS, MSN, RN, ET

Clinical Nurse Specialist,
University Hospitals of Cleveland;
Clinical Instructor in Medical-Surgical Nursing,
Frances Payne Bolton School of Nursing,
Case Western Reserve University,
Cleveland, Ohio

DORA RICE, MSN, RN

Infection Control Nurse,
Cleveland Veterans Administration Medical Center,
Cleveland, Ohio

GRACE A. ROTTER, MSN, RN

Infection Control Nurse,
Cleveland Veterans Administration Medical Center;
Clinical Instructor in Community Health Nursing,
Frances Payne Bolton School of Nursing,
Case Western Reserve University,
Cleveland, Ohio

ELIZABETH ANNE SCHENK, MSN, RNC, CRRN

Vice President of Nursing,
Healther Hill, Inc,
Munson, Ohio

LINDA TRAXLER SCHURING, MSN, RN

Doctoral Student, Case Western Reserve University,
Cleveland, Ohio;
Director of the Balance Disorder Clinic,
Warren Otologic Group,
Warren, Ohio

MARY ELLEN SHANDS, MN, RN

Research Associate, Community Health Care Systems,
University of Washington School of Nursing;
Bereavement Specialist,
Community Home Health Care,
Seattle, Washington

CAROL E. SMITH, PhD, RN

Professor, School of Nursing,
University of Kansas Medical Center,
Lenexa, Kansas

BARBARA SOLTIS, MSN, RN

Nurse Consultant,
Soltis Associates,
Ponte Vedra Beach, Florida

KATHRYN SABO THOMPSON, MSN, RN

Project Leader, Special Care Unit,
University Hospitals of Cleveland,
Cleveland, Ohio

M. EILEEN WALSH, MSN, RN, CCRN

Assistant Professor, School of Nursing,
Medical College of Ohio;
Coordinator, Cardiovascular Risk Intervention Programs,
Henry L. Morse Physical Health Research Center,
Toledo, Ohio

E. RONALD WRIGHT, PhD

Associate Professor of Nursing and Biology,
Case Western Reserve University,
Cleveland, Ohio

ELLEN H. ZAHLIS, MN, RN

Research Associate, Community Health Care Systems,
University of Washington School of Nursing;
Consultant to Families, Cancer Lifeline,
Seattle, Washington

To **our students,** past and present, who have inspired us to develop a textbook
that will assist them to provide intelligent, thoughtful, and skillful nursing care to patients.
And to **our family and friends** for their support during this revision.

Preface

The social environments in which nursing is practiced continue to change as we move toward the twenty-first century. Changes in society and in the delivery of health care in the United States are reflected in this fourth edition. Several new chapters have been added, some chapters have been deleted, and some chapters have been combined in an attempt to provide information that is relevant to the practice of medical-surgical nursing today. We continue to believe, as we did when the first edition was published, that nurses need a textbook that is up-to-date and that incorporates information from nursing and a wide variety of other disciplines.

Although it has been suggested that we add "caring" to the title of the book, we have not done so because we have always believed that one cannot practice nursing without "caring," which is an essential part of the nurse's role. We trust that the text reflects our commitment to caring.

Throughout this book the recipients of the services of nurses are referred to as *patients* rather than *clients*. Although client is widely used in the nursing community, the article "Complexities and clarity in nurse-client and nurse-patient relationships" by L. Nowakowski, which appeared in the July-August 1985 issue of the *Journal of Professional Nursing*, makes a distinction between who is a client and who is a patient. Using her framework, we decided that patient was a better term for use in this book. We found Nowakowski's criteria for differentiating between clients and patients to be thought provoking and helpful, and we recommend the article to the reader.

ORGANIZATION

The eighty-one chapters in this edition are divided into four major parts (see Table of Contents):

PART I   Overview
PART II   Stressors, Stress, and Coping
PART III Alterations in Human Functioning
PART IV Special Environments of Care

Part I contains two units, *Perspectives for Nursing Practice with Ill Adults* and *Illness: Developmental and Sociocultural Perspectives*. Chapter 1 now includes material on health care delivery systems and quality assurance, which were presented previously in separate chapters. The other three chapters in Unit I have been revised to reflect newer knowledge about theoretic perspectives of the nursing care of ill adults, health and illness, and epidemiology. Chapter 6, in Unit II, is a new chapter that should assist the reader's understanding of families in relationship to the ill adult. Other topics in this unit include adult development and culture as related to illness.

Part II, *Stressors, Stress, and Coping*, contains three units: *Stress and Stress Management, Common Psychophysiologic Stressors*, and *Surgery: Perioperative Nursing*. Chapter 8, *Biologic defense mechanisms* in the first unit (Unit III), has been moved to this unit because it provides a basis for understanding the concepts of infection and immunity found in subsequent chapters. Chapter 9, *Neuroendocrine Response to Stressors*, is a new chapter that lays the ground work for a better understanding of the following two chapters on stress and coping and stress management. Unit IV contains common physiologic stressors experienced by the ill adult. Chapter 12, *Stressors in Care Environments*, is a new chapter that incorporates material presented in other chapters in previous editions. Chapter 19, *Addictive Behaviors*, is a new title for the chapter on substance abuse that appeared in the third edition. We believe the new chapter title better reflects today's thinking on the subject of addiction.

Part III, *Alterations in Human Functioning*, contains six units that discuss the care of patients with alterations within body systems. Unit VI, *Alterations of Fluid/Gas Transport*, has three sections: *Fluid and Electrolytes, Cardiovascular System*, and *Respiratory System*. The material on fluids and electrolytes has been divided into two chapters, fluid and electrolyte imbalance and acid-base imbalance. Shock is also included in this section. Beginning with Section 2, *Cardiovascular System*, each subsequent unit in Part III is initiated by an assessment chapter. Content in cardiovascular nursing has been expanded. New content in cystic fibrosis has been added to Chapter 33, *Management of Persons with Problems of the Lower Airway*, because of the number of persons with this disorder now living into adulthood.

Unit VII, *Alterations in Metabolism and Energy Balance*, contains two sections, *Endocrine system* and *Liver*. Unit VIII, *Alteration in Nutrition and Elimination*, is divided into four sections: nutrition, the gastrointestinal system, gallbladder and exocrine pancreas, and urinary system. Readers of the third edition will note that content pertinent to the gallbladder and exocrine pancreas has been separated from the endocrine system and placed in this section because of functions related to digestion. We believe this placement will be helpful to the reader.

Unit IX, *Alterations in Sexuality and Reproduction*, has been divided into two sections: *Sexuality* and *Reproductive system and breast*. Management of persons with reproductive problems includes separate chapters for women and for men. Chapter 58, *Management of Persons with Sexually Transmitted Diseases*, is a new chapter. Although STDs were discussed in previous editions, we believe that the content merits being placed in a separate chapter.

Unit X, *Alterations in Cognition, Sensation, and Motion*, contains three sections: nervous system, eye and ear, and musculoskeletal system, as appeared in the last edition. Chapter 61, *Sleep Disorders*, is a new chapter that discusses current information on these disorders that we feel is pertinent for health care teaching.

Unit XI, *Alterations in Defense and Protection*, has two sections: skin (including burns) and immune system. Chapter 75, *Assessment of the Immune System*, is a new chapter and includes a brief review of the immune system (also discussed in Chapter 8) as a point of reference before the subsequent chapters of this section. Chapter 77, *Management of Persons with HIV Infection and AIDS*, is a new chapter. Although material on AIDs had been included in the previous edition, this new chapter concisely presents the current information and care of these persons.

The final part, Part IV, *Special Environments of Care*, has been divided into two units. Unit XII, *Community*, contains new material in Chapter 78, *Home Care of the Ill Adult*. Because patients spend fewer days in the hospital, more persons with complex medical-surgical problems are being cared for in the home. Early discharge presents a special challenge to the nurse in the hospital who has only a short time to prepare the patient and family for care at home. This chapter addresses the home care of patients that may require the use of complex technology. The concluding unit of the text, *Critical Care Units*, includes concepts pertaining to the care of the acutely ill patient in a CCU and a case study of a critically ill patient.

FEATURES

Nursing diagnoses and their *possible etiologies* are included in the management chapters. The nursing diagnoses used in this edition are those adopted at the Ninth NANDA Conference (1990). In most instances, the nursing diagnoses are presented in alphabetical order. This was an arbitrary decision of the editors for easy retrieval by the student and we would suggest that, as the practitioner uses the diagnoses, thought be given to their order of priority when implementing care. Additional *nursing care plans* have been added to this edition. The plans are *sample* nursing care plans and pertain to the care of *specific* patients, thus only selected nursing diagnoses have been described. Lists of other possible nursing diagnoses are located in the text. All plans include the rationale for nursing interventions.

Chapter objectives, a *chapter summary*, and *questions to consider* have been added to each chapter. It is our hope that these items will assist the reader to make the best possible use of the content of each chapter.

As in previous editions, the emphasis of this revised edition is on assisting the nurse to provide the physical care, emotional and social support, and teaching necessary to assist the patient to attain, maintain, or regain health. We believe that the patient's significant others, be they family or friends, provide essential support to the person, and therefore we make reference to involving them as appropriate in the care of the individual. These elements, we believe, represent not only the elements necessary to the "cure" of the patient, but also those that reflect the art of nursing that is involved in "caring" for the patient.

Many new figures and tables have been added to this edition and much material has been set in boxes so that important points are stressed in summary format. All chapters contain appropriate new material.

TEACHING-LEARNING PACKAGE

With the fourth edition of our text, we are pleased to offer an extensive group of ancillary products to assist both instructors and students in the classroom and clinical settings.

The Instructor's Manual includes overviews of each chapter and suggested ways to present content. The extensive Testbank with answer key and page references assists instructors in formulating test questions and referring students to the text for rationales.

Microtest III, a computerized Testbank for use with IBM PC and Apple IIe, II+, and IIe, includes multiple-choice questions and a user's manual so that instructors can add, delete, or rearrange test items from any part of the text.

The second edition of the CLINICAL MANUAL OF MEDICAL-SURGICAL NURSING, prepared by Judith Sands, is a practical spiral-bound reference that presents strong clinical information in an easily accessible format. A useful adjunct to our text, it features nursing responsibilities for nearly 300 common medical-surgical conditions.

One hundred two-color overhead transparencies provide visual reinforcement of key illustrations and concepts from the text.

It is our hope that this revision meets the needs of nursing students and practicing nurses to assist them in providing the best possible care to their patients.

ACKNOWLEDGMENTS

With this edition we welcome Virginia Cassmeyer as a new editor. Dr. Cassmeyer has been a contributor to this book since the first edition. Her background in physiology and her wide experience in nursing make her an ideal addition as an editor of this text.

Many experts have contributed to this fourth edition. For some, this is their first appearance as an author or co-author of a chapter(s) in this text. Many others have been involved since the first edition and have assisted us to make the changes deemed necessary so that this edition is as current as possible. We are indebted to each of our contributors for the knowledge, interest, and skill that they brought to their chapter(s). We also wish to thank all the readers and reviewers who made comments and suggestions about the last edition. We trust that they will be pleased with the changes made in this edition.

The new illustrations for this edition are the work of Nancy Burgard of Cleveland. The preparation of parts of the manuscript was by Sondra Patrizi of Cleveland, and we thank her for her assistance.

We are grateful to Linda Duncan, Joanna May, and Celeste Clingan of Mosby–Year Book, Inc. for their support and guidance during the preparation of this fourth edition.

Wilma J. Phipps
Barbara C. Long
Nancy Fugate Woods
Virginia L. Cassmeyer

Contents

14 Loss, Dying, and Death, 245

Benita C. Martocchio, Sr. Karin Dufault

15 Infection, 273

Grace A. Rotter, Dora Rice

16 Pain, 297

Virginia Burke Karb

17 Cancer, 327

Rosemarie Hogan

PART THREE

ALTERATIONS IN HUMAN FUNCTIONING

UNIT VI
ALTERATIONS OF FLUID/GAS TRANSPORT

SECTION ONE   Fluid and electrolytes

SECTION THREE **Respiratory system**

31 **Assessment of the Respiratory System, 813**
Josephine Brucia

32 **Management of Persons with Problems of
the Upper Airway, 841**
Wilma J. Phipps, Linda Anne Broseman

44 Management of Persons with Problems of Intestinal Elimination, 1303
Barbara C. Long, Rebecca Anne Roberts

SECTION THREE **Gallbladder and exocrine pancreas**

45 Assessment of the Gallbladder and Exocrine Pancreas, 1353
Virginia L. Cassmeyer

46 Management of Persons with Problems of the Gallbladder and Exocrine Pancreas, 1363
Virginia L. Cassmeyer

PART IV
SPECIAL ENVIRONMENTS OF CARE

UNIT XII
COMMUNITY

OVERVIEW OF NURSING PRACTICE

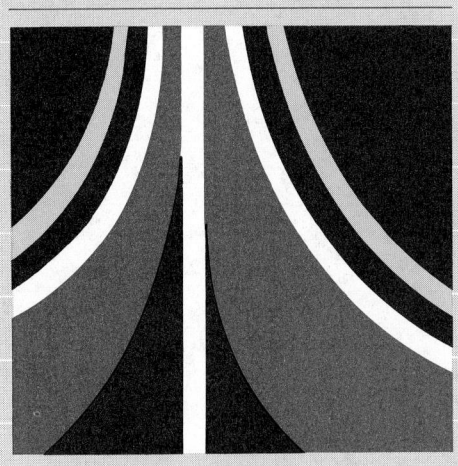

PERSPECTIVES FOR NURSING PRACTICE WITH ILL ADULTS

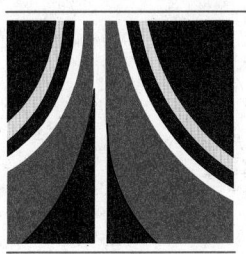

CHAPTER 1

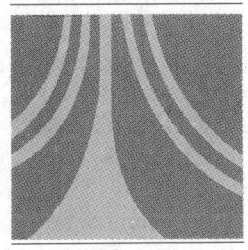

Nursing Practice with Ill Adults

CONTEXT, STRUCTURE, PROCESS, AND OUTCOMES

WILMA J. PHIPPS
KATHERINE SCHENK

CHAPTER OBJECTIVES

After studying this chapter, the student should be able to:
1. Identify changing characteristics of American society and implications for nursing.
2. Recognize the impact of technologic advances and changes in health care costs on the health care delivery system, nursing practice settings, nursing roles, and nursing education.
3. Identify factors that have affected the evolution of the health care system in the United States.
4. Define health care from a systems approach.
5. Discuss the evolution and purpose of diagnostic related groups and their affect on health care agencies and nursing practice.
6. Discuss the reasons for the proliferation of ambulatory care centers, home care, and hospice care.
7. Discuss the differences between functional, team, and primary nursing care.
8. Identify characteristics of potential nursing students and factors that will influence their choice of nursing as a profession.
9. Describe characteristics of nursing schools and nursing practitioners in the year 2000.
10. Define quality assurance.
11. Identify three reasons why quality assurance is an important aspect of the practice of nursing.
12. Describe the steps of the American Nurses Association (ANA) model of quality assurance.
13. Describe the use of quality indicators as a means for monitoring quality of care.

Rapid changes in our society affect the way nurses practice today and how they will practice in the future. Several factors are responsible for these changes; this chapter will concentrate on six major ones. These are: (1) social changes in America, (2) technologic advances influencing medical and nursing practice, (3) the effect of pressures to reduce health care costs on the health care delivery system, (4) changes in the characteristics of nursing students, (5) coming changes in nursing education in the 21st century, and (6) evaluating the outcomes of nursing care using the quality assurance process.

CHANGES IN AMERICAN SOCIETY

Today, for the first time in the history of the United States, there are more persons 65 years of age and over in the population than ever before. This increase in longevity and a simultaneous decline in the birth rate is being experienced by all Western societies. Between 2001 and 2027, persons born during the World War II baby boom will reach age 65. This means that by 2030 there will be only three active workers for every retired worker as compared with five workers today. Even earlier than that however, by 1993, there will be 2.5 million more persons over the age of 85 than there are today. This segment of the population, called the "old old," is the most rapidly increasing portion of the population in the United States. Between now and 2010 this segment of our population will increase by 111%. During the same period, the percentage of "young elderly," persons 74 to 84 years of age, will increase by 52%.

The "old-old" use 10 times the health care resources than persons under 85 years of age, and 22% of these persons require institutionalization of some kind. More of the elderly, especially women, are living alone rather than with other family members. As a result, they may require some type of assisted living. The amount of assistance ranges from "Meals on Wheels" for persons in their own homes, to apartments for the elderly with special services like one or more meals a day, to group living homes, to nursing homes for those unable to meet their own daily needs.

Many of the elderly could not survive without Social Security and yet the financial viability of the Social Security program is being questioned. Will a proportionally smaller working population be able to support Social Security for an increasingly older population?

The financial implications of an aging society and advances in health care raise questions about how health care for the elderly will be financed in the future. Medicare reimbursement for persons over age 65 has been reduced several times since it was established in 1965. Presently Part A of Medicare (which covers the cost of hospitalization) requires the individual to pay a deductible of $592 for each spell of illness. Medicare then pays for up to 60 days of hospital care. Patients requiring longer hospitalization pay $148 per day in coinsurance for days 61 to 90. Part B of Medicare (which pays for physician fees and other *defined* services) reimburses for 80% of costs after the individual pays a deductible of $75. For these reasons, persons over age 65 are urged to carry supplemental insurance to help with the payment of their hospital and medical bills.

TECHNOLOGIC ADVANCES AND HEALTH CARE COSTS

Technologic advances have changed medical care and driven up health care costs dramatically. Increasingly, questions are being raised about how health care monies will be allocated. Many of these questions are ethical and will require hard decisions. For example, will money be allocated to treat chronic illnesses such as end-stage renal disease, which now costs the United States billions of dollars yearly? Or will the United States decide on allocation of resources as has been done in Great Britain, where only persons under the age of 40 are eligible for hemodialysis and renal transplantation?

Other issues include prolongation of life. Presently billions of dollars are spent on neonatal intensive care units that keep extremely small babies alive. If they do survive, many of these babies will have lifetime physical problems that will require long-term medical care. At the other end of the life span, prolongation of life, especially for those persons not wishing to be kept alive by artificial means, is a common problem. The issue of the "Living Will" and its validity under a variety of circumstances is being addressed in several forums, including state legislatures. Nurses cannot escape being involved in these issues, and most of them, need support in clarifying their own values, especially when they may differ from those of the persons for whom they are caring.

Other technologic advances in terms of joint replace-

ments and organ transplants are widely discussed issues. These advances are costly and organ transplantation raises questions about who will receive an organ when the demand for them always exceeds the supply.

Will better informed consumers continue to demand the latest in health care technology, despite its cost? Currently, evidence indicates that the demand for technology will continue to increase, and, in turn, will continue to drive up medical costs. For this reason the federal government and other third-party payers have begun to exert controls to keep health care costs from further escalation. These controls are having and will continue to have a major impact on the health care delivery system.[17] This, in turn, will affect nurses especially in hospitals, because this is where the greatest number of nurses are employed.

HEALTH CARE IN THE UNITED STATES

The tremendous diversity in this country is well exemplified by the beliefs, expectations, and traditions related to health and health care. The words *health* and *illness* mean different things to different people. On a health-illness continuum, a person's own concept often defines his or her state of wellness. The term *health,* as in health care and health insurance widely used in our society, in reality usually means "illness."

HISTORICAL PERSPECTIVE

Because social systems exist for the protection and enhancement of the members, it would seem that planning for and providing health care would be of very great importance, but the Constitution of the United States makes no provision for the health care of its citizens. In the late eighteenth century health and illness were considered to be individual concerns, taken care of within the family or community. For many years thereafter waves of immigrants brought their own ways of maintaining health and coping with illness.

Despite this, government at several levels soon became involved in health care out of necessity. In the early years, the federal government established a hospital for merchant seamen, which became the nucleus of the United States Public Health Service.

Individual states within the United States have been semiautonomous from the beginning of the nation. They soon found it essential to establish rules and regulations for the public health in such areas as safe drinking water and food, protection from communicable diseases, and so on. Some cities, especially those on the eastern seaboard, established hospitals to care for homeless immigrants and others who became public charges because of communicable diseases or mental or other illnesses. For example, New York City has a complex publicly supported hospital system that began in that way.

Over time all of these institutions grew, diversified, and changed, dealing with far more varied and complex problems. The federal government now has a cabinet-level agency, the Department of Health and Human Services. The Social Security Administration, which has overall responsibility for Medicare and Medicaid, is within this department. The Department of Veteran's Affairs, whose administrator operates one of the largest hospital and ambulatory care services in the world, was made a cabinet level position under the Bush administration. The legal responsibility for all of these services lies within the domain of the United States Congress.

Another factor in the evolution of health care in this country is the philosophy of individual initiative and private enterprise. Except for those conditions that affect the health of large segments of the population and, thus, come under the aegis of public health, the delivery of health care has been traditionally on a fee-for-service basis.

Every industrialized country in the world today, except the United States, has some kind of national health system that guarantees a basic level of care to all of its citizens. In developing countries, the provision of basic health care is generally one of their early goals. These systems begin with the premises that (1) there should be a minimum of health care services for all citizens, (2) that whatever health care is available should be equally available to all, and (3) that resources above the minimum should be distributed according to need; with any deviation being permitted only if those worse off would be made better off.

SYSTEMS APPROACH TO HEALTH CARE

A systems model (Figure 1-1) illustrates how one would proceed to plan for health care provision within a social system of any size. In Great Britain today, for example, under the National Health Service, this kind of planning goes on at the national level and also at area and local levels. Changes in implementation occur frequently based on evaluation of changing needs, newer technology, economic resources, and other factors. The system is not perfect, but there seems to be little question that the British people value their health care system and would not readily give it up. Most complaints about the system come from providers who do not believe that they are adequately compensated. For the more affluent British citizens, a parallel fee-for-service system that providers have developed is available. The most important concern, however, is addressed: that there is a basic level of care for every citizen.[76]

In the United States a large aggregate of illness care systems, often poorly articulated with each other, continue to exist. There have been many attempts to estab-

lish some kind of an organized system, at least to the extent that everyone would be entitled to basic care. In 1965 Medicare, a form of health insurance for persons over 65 years of age and receiving Social Security, was established under Title XVIII of the Social Security Act. Medicaid, a health insurance plan for welfare recipients that is administered by individual states, was established under Title XIX of the same act. This still left large segments of the citizenry without assurance that they could afford to receive essential care when ill or in need.

During the 1970s some form of national health insurance for U.S. citizens seemed inevitable, even though it was not determined "how soon" or "how broad" such a plan would be.[5,43] However, countervailing forces—most of them economic concerns of physicians, hospitals, and other providers—prevailed, and no national plan was developed. At the same time health care costs increased dramatically for a variety of reasons, including inflation and the introduction of more sophisticated technology. As new technology became available, everyone expected to benefit from it no matter what the cost.

ILLNESS CARE

Most illness care is provided by physicians in private practice, operating on a fee-for-service basis. Relatively few physicians are employed by public health services (federal, state, and local), the Veterans Administration, and the armed services. All physicians are licensed by the states to practice medicine and thus become the "gatekeepers" of the health care systems.

Health care is generally thought of as being delivered in physician's offices, in clinics, and in hospitals. Admission to hospitals is normally through one's personal physician. It is also possible to be admitted through a hospital emergency room, where a physician will be assigned if necessary. Most hospitals in the United States were built during the first decades of this century when scientific medicine was developing rapidly and physicians and surgeons needed a work place for their activities. Even the smallest communities believed that they must have a hospital and worked hard to obtain one. Fund drives, private philanthropy, and taxes were used in varying ways to build, maintain, and add to hospitals to meet community needs. The federal Hill-Burton Act provided large amounts of tax money to communities to build or improve hospitals throughout the country.

After World War II, great medical complexes burgeoned, sometimes several in one large city. Medical care became more and more concentrated in large cities while rural areas were underserved. Within these large medical complexes, which are often associated with schools of medicine, research and technology were producing the miracles of modern medical science. At the same time many of the medically indigent were receiv-

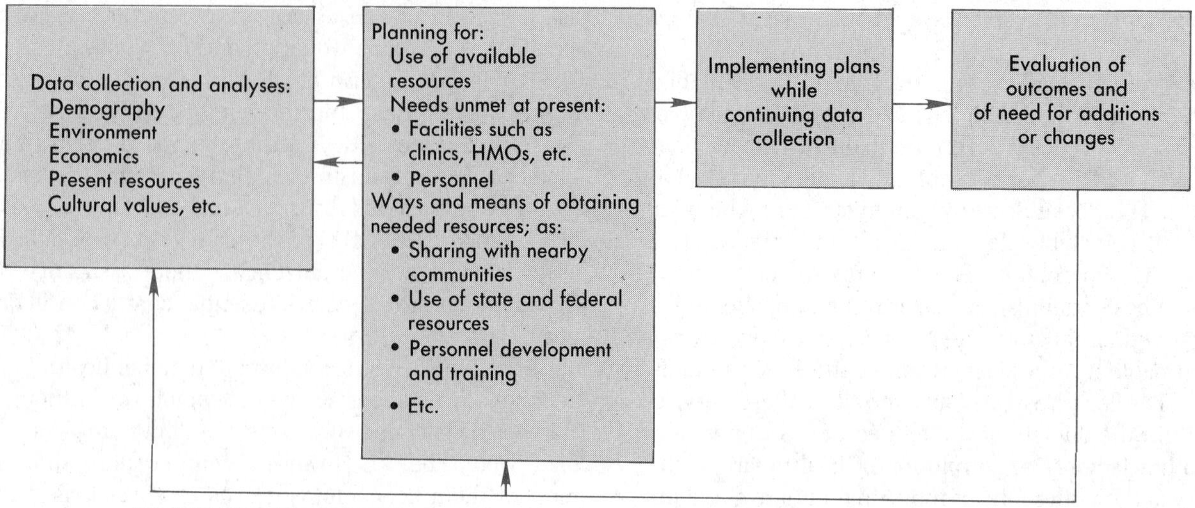

FIGURE 1-1 Model for developing health care delivery systems.

ing no medical care at all. They were either unable to afford the cost or to figure out how to negotiate the health care delivery system to get the care they needed. Today this continues to be a serious concern. During the 1960s the appearance of alternative, nontraditional agencies, such as store front clinics and neighborhood health care centers, began to appear in response to the obvious need.[52,63]

Hospitals continue to be a major setting for medical technology, growing larger and more complex each year. Many hospitals have consolidated into multihospital complexes, which allow for sharing of costs, facilities, and expertise.[20] Only very recently has some effort to restrain hospital proliferation been enforced; this will be discussed later in the chapter.

CHANGES IN HEALTH CARE DELIVERY
HEALTH MAINTENANCE ORGANIZATIONS

A relatively new development on the health care scene in the United States is the *health maintenance organization* (HMO). Congress appropriated funds in 1974 to encourage the start-up of medical group practice financed on a prepayment basis. The focus of an HMO is health promotion and illness prevention, at least to the point at which the financial advantage to both provider and client is *wellness*. Some group health plans that were precursors of the present HMO movement have been in existence since the 1940s and 1950s. These include the Health Insurance Plan of New York (HIP), the Ross-Loos Plan in California, and the Kaiser-Permanente Foundation. Employees of the Kaiser Corporation in California, for example, were provided with preventive and health maintenance facilities and ambulatory care clinics as fringe benefits of their employment. This

model has been adopted by other industries and also by some private medical practices, many of which include nurse practitioners as care givers.[34]

In these systems clients pay a set fee for regular preventive and screening services as well as for illness care. Fees are prepaid, usually on a yearly basis similar to an insurance plan. The HMO fares best financially when clients are kept well and out of hospitals. An additional feature, accountability to the public, was built into the HMOs that were financed in their beginning stages by the federal government. Peer review of the quality of care provided was required as a condition of funding.[32,76] Physicians and medical societies in the past often opposed the establishment of HMOs, seeing them as a form of "socialized medicine." More recently, however, cost containment has led to the development of many more of these organizations. Employers looking to cut their health insurance costs, wide public acceptance, and an increasing supply of physicians willing to meet the public demand as competition among them increases have encouraged the growth of HMOs. Quality assurance becomes an important issue in HMOs, since there may be a decrease in quality in favor of cost saving.

Some adaptations of the HMO have been the *preferred provider organization* (PPO), in which clients may choose their own physician, and the *independent practice association* (IPA), structured on the general model of the HMO, in which physicians render care out of their own offices instead of a central clinic. Nationally the IPA is said to be the fastest growing form of HMO. The problems of quality control, however, are seen to be greater, because health records are not available in a central location.

PREPAID HEALTH INSURANCE

So-called health insurance has been a very large factor in the interplay of health and illness care in the United States. At one time prepaid health insurance was a very small segment of the insurance industry. It began to assume more and more importance as health care costs, both in and out of hospitals, rose sharply. In its early days insurance by private companies, then by the "nonprofit" complex termed Blue Cross—Blue Shield, was purchased by individuals for themselves or their families. Then it was purchased by groups in order to share cost and spread liability. Today such insurance is part of the fringe benefits of nearly every type of employment, and the self-employed purchase their own. Medicare, as has been noted, is also a form of insurance for physician and hospital expenses and is administered through the Social Security Act.

Although all of these provisions for payment removed the burden of concern for paying for hospitalization from the average citizen, there was no evaluative control over the use of this resource. Health care costs escalated to the point that in 1989 health care accounted for 12% of the gross national product (GNP). Inflation was a major national concern, and in the health care field inflation was greater than that in many other industries.

Cost and cost control now dominate the health care scene; all other concerns, such as a national health policy and health insurance coverage for all citizens, have been pushed into the background.[40,86] Emphasis on business-oriented cost accounting and encouragement of competition among health care providers is the order of the day. Recently the federal government instituted a revolutionary plan for payment of Medicare benefits to hospitals. Up to this time, hospitals were paid for the costs they incurred in caring for a patient. This change from *retrospective* to *prospective* reimbursement based on certain criteria has had a major impact on hospitals, physicians, and other health care providers.

DIAGNOSTIC RELATED GROUPS

In the 1980s Medicare developed a list of 467 illnesses based on diagnostic related groups (DRGs). Hospitals were notified how much they will be reimbursed for patients in each of the 467 groups based on a specified number of days of hospitalization. If a hospital can provide treatment and care for the patient for the specified reimbursement, they will break even. If they can treat and discharge the patient earlier than the predetermined number of days, they will make money that they can keep. On the other hand, if they cannot treat and discharge the patient in the allotted time, they will lose money, since they will not be reimbursed for the additional days of care. Although this plan has been in existence for a relatively short time, it is evident that hospitals are becoming more and more competitive as they seek to attract the patients on whom they can make money and avoid admitting those patients on whom they will lose money. This has already resulted in a phenomenon known as "dumping," in which some hospitals triage the more ill patients to other hospitals when they believe that they will lose money on them.

At present DRGs are used only for patients on Medicare; however, other third-party payers (Blue Cross—Blue Shield and other insurance carriers), as well as employers who are paying more and more for insurance coverage for their employees, are looking at the concept with great interest. It appears to be only a matter of time before the DRG, or prospective payment concept, is applied to physician fees and all of ambulatory care, at least by federally financed systems.

The outcome of the DRGs is inevitably shorter hospital stays, with patients being discharged before recovery is completed. This means that the population within hospitals is more acutely ill; it also means that a much greater burden is placed on the community to provide some kind of posthospital care for these patients, many of whom are not able to assume full self-care when discharged.

This factor, plus others, is decreasing the demand for hospital beds, and many communities have a surplus of hospital beds. It is predicted that acute care beds in the United States will be reduced dramatically from 1250 to 450 beds per 100,000 population. One major factor in the decrease in hospital admissions is the rapid proliferation of same-day surgeries. Some of these procedures are performed in Ambulatory Surgery Centers, within hospitals, while others take place in free-standing Surgi-Centers located in the community. More and more surgery is being performed in these centers, and many of the patients being treated at these centers need follow-up care of some type after discharge.

Most hospitals are "leaning down" by closing unnecessary beds and laying off personnel. Some smaller hospitals have already closed, and it can be predicted that other hospitals will be forced to close if their occupancy rates are not high enough to keep them viable.

Because of these changes, proportionally fewer nurses will be employed in hospitals. Today, two thirds of the nearly 2 million nurses practicing in the United States work in hospitals. This represents a decrease from only a few years ago, when three-quarters of all practicing nurses were employed in hospitals.

As hospital admissions are decreasing, outpatient visits are increasing (Figure 1-2). All of these trends are having and will continue to have considerable impact on nursing care within the hospital and the community. Stringent cost control measures within hospitals with more acutely ill patients means that nurses are being asked to be even more productive than in the past.

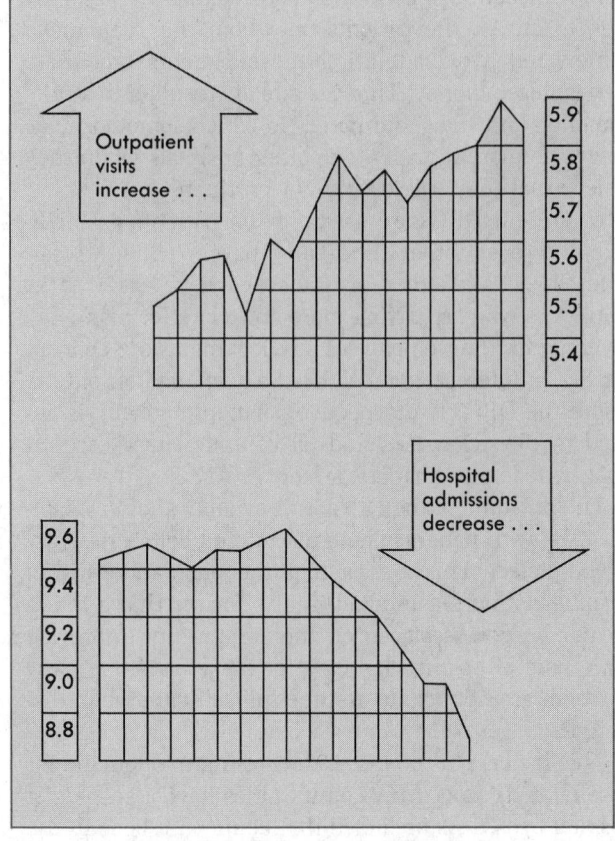

FIGURE 1-2 How hospital use is changing. (Based on data from *Boston Globe,* June 30, 1985.)

Many hospitals have moved to a predominantly all registered nurse (RN) staff, since the RN has a larger repertoire of skills and abilities than do less well-prepared care givers, thus making the hospital more productive and cost effective.

FOR PROFIT HOSPITALS

Before discussing the large topic of ambulatory care, we must look at one more important aspect of the inpatient hospital scene: the for-profit hospital corporations (such as Humana and Hospital Corporation of America), which, unlike the community hospital or medical center, are operated for the purpose of making a profit. Although some of these hospitals have existed for a long time, in recent years they have proliferated and have become an important segment of the competitive scene in health care provision. They vary in type from the provision of up-to-the-minute acute technical facilities (organ transplantation, for example) to chronic and mental illness care and nursing home care. Many have demonstrated the ability to make a profit for their investors and have become very large corporations. They have concentrated on providing medical and surgical services to those patients who are able to finance their care, either because they are well insured or financially able to pay for their care. These corporations provide no care to the medically indigent. They have attracted well-qualified physicians by providing them with the latest technology and equipment, attached office space at little or no cost to the physician, and so on. They also have the resources to build modern, up-to-date hospitals with amenities that are aimed at attracting the paying consumer. Because of their ability to buy supplies and equipment in volume and because of their centralized accounting and billing services, they have been able to control costs and provide a profit for their investors. It appears that these corporations will continue to proliferate and prosper, often at the expense of those hospitals that until now have provided care to all segments of society, regardless of the patients' ability to pay for their care.

AMBULATORY CARE AND HOME CARE SERVICES

The areas of health care delivery that are experiencing a very heavy demand (as a result of the DRGs as well as other cost control measures) are ambulatory care and home health care. For this reason, we have added a chapter on home care of ill adults to this edition. See Chapter 78 for a detailed discussion of home health care.

Until the early decades of this century, and before the great boom in hospital construction and use, nearly all illness care fell into these categories. Physicians saw patients in their offices or in the patient's own home. People were born and died at home. Several types of agencies for the care of ill people at home developed from the early days of this nation. Many Visiting Nurse Associations (VNAs) began with the custom of helping people who were ill at home. Many tax-supported public health agencies also provided some care for the ill in their homes, although their first mission was controlling and preventing communicable disease and protecting the health of the public. The term *community health agency* is an overall designation, with the added "home health agency" used to indicate that many expanded services, such as physical therapy and homemaker care, are also available. Many of these agencies began or expanded their services in recent years since Medicare pays for the delivery of certain kinds of care to the homebound.

In their early days the focus of most home care agencies was on the care of infants and children and their mothers. The Children's Bureau of the federal government was established based on concerns of leaders of these agencies. Since in the early years of our nation most people did not live to be as old as persons today, those who did were usually cared for by their own families. Today, however, people are living longer, and the care of the elderly has become a national concern as more and more people are living into the seventh, eighth, and ninth decades of life. Although less than 5% of those persons over 65 are now institutionalized, it is clear that health problems increase as one ages and that persons over 65 need a larger share of the health care resources. As mentioned previously, the number of "old old", those 85 years and older, is now the fastest growing age group in the United States; in other words, the elderly group is itself aging. Not enough is known about this group; it is a new phenomenon in our world. In the past only the occasional person lived to such a great age. Although many of the elderly, even the very old, function effectively with some assistance with certain tasks, a larger proportion inevitably suffer from one or more chronic illnesses and may need institutional care.[91]

HEALTH CARE FOR THE ELDERLY

For the aging who remain in their own homes or elsewhere in the community, it is evident that additional facilities for their care and well-being, including health care, must be provided. In addition to home health care services, a comparatively new development, the day care center for the chronically ill and the elderly adult, shows evidence of becoming an important part of the health care scene. Also, there are a large number of nursing homes for care of the chronically ill, especially the elderly. It is perhaps unfortunate that many of these day care centers and nursing homes have developed as private profit-making enterprises similar to the private practice of medicine and that they often are not closely associated with other health and illness care facilities.

In 1982, HMOs that had formerly been reluctant to enroll older clients were encouraged to do so by an amendment to the Social Security Act that provided payment by way of Medicare at 95% of the average per capita cost, leaving only a small amount to be covered by the client. Recently several demonstration projects termed *social health maintenance organizations* (SHMOs) have been federally funded to test the potential for delivering expanded health services as well as other services needed by the elderly to Medicare and Medicaid recipients on a prepaid basis. These SHMOs will attempt to meet the problems of long-term community-based care and should be followed with great interest by all concerned with the health care of older Americans.[19]

It is becoming increasingly evident that the present health care delivery system, especially with its cost control restrictions, will not be able to do all that needs to be done. Many sectors are concerned about the development of a two-tier system of health care—one for the have's and the other for the have not's—with some people receiving no care at all. The magnitude of the problem is reflected in recent figures that indicate that 35 million Americans (15% of the population) have no medical insurance. Forty percent of the uninsured are children, because less than one third of indigent children are covered under Medicaid.[58] It may be that the economic forces of competition and cost control will finally impose some kind of systematic organization on the delivery of health/illness care in the United States, although it may be many years before we see actual evidence of this. In our health delivery systems model (see Figure 1-1), it is only the economic segment that is being addressed at the moment. Questions of what happens to the poor and needy have not been fully examined by society. This and other questions about what we value in the society will need to be addressed before change in the health care delivery system can occur.

NURSING CARE IN THE UNITED STATES

HISTORICAL PERSPECTIVE

Professional nursing in the United States is about 100 years old. It has assumed an indispensable place in every aspect of health care delivery. Nursing is the largest professional group on the health care scene. Within institutional settings it is essential in acute and chronic care hospitals, in long-term care facilities, and in community nursing agencies.

PRIVATE DUTY NURSING

In the early part of this century, most nurses were employed in patients' homes. In this model of practice, nurses were private entrepreneurs. Even though they often depended on the favor and recommendations of a physician for employment, they provided service for a fee and were paid directly by the clients they served. Some of these private duty nurses became skilled in caring for patients with a specific illness and were known as experts in that particular care. Before the turn of the century private duty nursing was provided mostly in the homes of the affluent; but as the care of the ill moved into hospitals, so did this service. It was total patient care, although more an art than a science in those early days.

Private duty nursing was greatly affected by the great depression of the 1930s. Many of these nurses were unable to find employment in homes and were forced into hospital nursing. In some instances nurses employed by hospitals worked for only room and board and perhaps a small monthly stipend.

Prepaid hospital insurance plans became more prevalent in the early 1940s, resulting in more patients being able to afford hospitalization. Thus private duty nurses were employed by affluent patients in the hospital and very few of them were employed in patients' homes unless they went home with these patients after discharge.

HOSPITAL NURSING

Even when employed by the hospital, the registered nurse before World War II usually did everything prescribed for and needed by her several patients, since there were few other health care providers. By far the greatest amount of care to those in hospitals then was provided by nursing students.

During World War II many nurses entered the Army and Navy Nurse Corps. This resulted in a severe shortage of staff nurses in hospitals, and hospitals were staffed primarily by nursing students under the guidance of a few RNs. Sometimes the only RNs in hospitals were head nurses and supervisors, and it is from them that students sought guidance. To increase the number of nursing students, the Cadet Nurse Corps was established by Congress in 1942. Students who belonged to the Corps were issued uniforms for street wear, received full tuition assistance, and were paid a small monthly stipend.

NURSING CARE DELIVERY SYSTEMS WITHIN HOSPITALS
FUNCTIONAL METHOD

With the shortage of registered nurses during the years of World War II, total patient care gave way to the *functional method* of practicing, in which each nurse or nursing student, in the interest of time and efficiency, did a particular task, for example, administering medications to every patient on a unit. This was the beginning of the wide support for and the increasing preparation of licensed practical (vocational) nurses. Although continued long after the war and even into the present, the functional model of nursing care is generally considered both by health care providers and by patients to be unsatisfactory because the care provided is so fragmented.

TEAM NURSING

Functional nursing was succeeded by team nursing, in which a group of health care providers with a variety of preparation (registered nurse, licensed practical [vocational] nurse, and the nursing assistant or aide) cared for a designated group of patients, using the skills of each to best advantage. Theoretically, this was the ideal way to care for patients with a variety of needs in the presence of a shortage of RNs. In practice it often did not work as well as conceptualized. One of the main problems seemed to be finding time for the needed team planning and conferences essential for good team nursing. The guidance and coordination of the team by the professional nurse, an essential component of the method, was often sketchy or completely lacking. There were and still are places in which team nursing is practiced, both within acute and chronic hospital settings and in community settings where the basic concepts and plans can be better implemented.

PRIMARY NURSING

A more recent development in the care of clients in organizational settings (which includes the community health agency) is *primary nursing*. This term must be distinguished from *primary care*, which will be discussed later. In the primary nursing model, one professional nurse is totally responsible for planning, implementing, and evaluating the nursing care given to a relatively small number of clients. To those who were active in nursing before World War II this does not appear to be a new method but a coming of full circle. The model was demonstrated early at the Loeb Center for Nursing and Rehabilitation in New York, where for many years nurses have been providing care through the primary nursing model.[18] Many agencies have since moved to primary nursing because studies indicate that it is more satisfying both to patients and to nurses and it is more cost effective than team nursing. It also makes the RNs accountable for the care the patient receives, and this is most important with the emphasis on quality assurance. In other nursing care delivery systems, accountability is hard to determine and sometimes it is as "if everyone who cares for the patient is equally accountable, then no one is really accountable." Studies have clearly demonstrated that in addition to the satisfaction of patients and nurses, physicians and other health care providers are also better satisfied with primary nursing, because it is clear with whom they should communicate their questions and suggestions about the patient. Primary nursing has changed markedly the role of the head nurse, who in the past in some institutions was the only person who gave and received all communications in regard to patients.

With the complexity of patient care today, especially in larger hospitals and medical centers, it is clear that it is impossible for one person to know all that is necessary to know about 30 or more patients. One facet of primary nursing that is under study now is matching patient needs with the abilities of individual nurses. This movement, along with not overburdening the RN with more primary patients than he or she can adequately care for, is essential to providing the best possible quality of care in this age of cost containment.

There have been many attempts to find the ideal way of providing nursing care to groups of clients designated as ill or in need of care. It is likely that all of these will be used in one way or another, even coexisting within the same organization, in accordance with the philosophy of the organization.

Individual nursing practice, advanced beyond the skills learned in basic programs leading to state registration, has probably always existed, as was noted previously in regard to private duty nurses, and as anyone observing skilled professional nurses can see. But skilled clinical practice was seldom recognized or rewarded financially; until very recently the nurse looking to advancement had to move to administrative or academic positions.

With a perceived critical shortage of medical care in the 1960s coinciding with the development of scientific and theoretically based nursing, several distinctive models of advanced professional practice that fit clients' identified health care needs have been developed and tested. Such terms as *extended* and *expanded roles* have been used. The question has been raised: Are these terms accurate, or are client needs expanding and is nursing moving to provide for these needs?[65] The much-used terms *clinician* and *practitioner* have also been critically questioned by nursing leaders. If professional nurses are prepared and licensed to practice nursing, are they not all in fact nurse practitioners? And if nurses must practice in a clinical setting in order to be practicing at all, must they not all be nurse clinicians?

SPECIALIZED ROLES FOR NURSES
CLINICAL NURSE SPECIALISTS

From the maze of titles that appeared through the 1960s and 1970s, two seem to be viable at present and sufficiently able to be defined and recognized. These are the clinical nurse specialist and the nurse practitioner. The *clinical nurse specialist* (CNS) is a registered nurse who has completed a master's degree program in a clinical specialty (usually with a specified population of patients such as maternity or psychiatric patient or with a population of patients with specific system problems such as renal, cardiovascular, and so on). Clinical specialists may give direct patient care, provide consultation to nursing staff, teach nursing staff about the special care required by patients, and coordinate nursing care services for patients under their jurisdiction. The function of the CNS varies and is determined by the employing agency. Some clinical nurse specialists are unit based and work most closely with the nursing staff on that unit; others provide consultation to several units; some give much direct care while others may provide mainly consultation, teaching, and supervision of the staff who are giving direct care. Some clinical nurse specialists are in administrative line positions because they are in charge of units, such as intensive care.

Clinical nurse specialists also consult with other health care providers to plan the best possible care for patients and their families both during and after hospitalization. Although most clinical nurse specialists are employed in the hospital setting, many may be found in ambulatory care agencies. An example is an ostomy nurse specialist and an oncology nurse specialist, both practicing in a community home health agency.

Although some hospitals and other agencies employ nurses who are called clinical nurse specialists regardless of their educational background, the American Nurses Association (ANA) standards for CNS states that the title of clinical nurse specialists be limited to nurses with master's degrees in nursing.

Several specialty organizations offer certification for nurses practicing in their specialty. Each of these organizations set their own criteria. At the present time the ANA is the only organization requiring master's preparation in nursing to sit for the certification examination for clinical nurse specialist. Some of the nurses certified by organizations such as the American Association of Critical Care Nurses (AACN) hold master's degrees, but the majority of nurses certified by the AACN do not. In the future, it can be predicted that the increasing sophistication of nursing and health care will demand better preparation of clinical nurse specialists. As a result, more specialty organizations will require a master's degree in nursing for those wishing to become certified in that specialty.

NURSE PRACTITIONERS

The title *nurse practitioner* (NP) first appeared in 1965 when the Pediatric Nurse Practitioners were prepared to work in rural areas of Colorado to provide primary health care to children in areas seriously underserved by physicians. *Primary health care* is a term used to describe the kind of care needed by most of the people most of the time. It generally denotes the first contact of a person needing care with the health care system. It may be preventive, including identification of health problems at an early stage, or the care of minor, noncritical, and chronic illnesses. Most primary care is for those who are ambulatory (not requiring care in inpatient settings), and most but not all ambulatory care is primary care. Several studies have shown that primary care provided by nurses is at least as good as and sometimes better than care provided by physicians. It is highly valued by clients and equally positive results have been found when nurse practitioners work with clients who have chronic and long-term health problems.[90,87] Although in the past NPs have been prepared in a great variety of ways, from very short certificate-awarding programs to a master's degree program, the trend now is toward the latter, as a broad background of knowledge with specialization in the care of a particular population at risk is needed by the practitioner. The American Nurses Association offers certification in several such areas: family, school, pediatric, adult, and gerontologic nurse practitioner.

The issues of responsibility and accountability for one's own professional actions are vital in this type of practice. To some extent it is governed by individual state laws related to medical and nursing practice, although most state laws allow the nurse to practice *nursing* independently. A more telling restriction has been the payment of fees for service. Most third-party payers (Blue Cross—Blue Shield, Medicare, Medicaid, and other insurers) have been unwilling to reimburse nurses directly for independent nursing services. Recently there has been some progress in this area as some states and some insurers have permitted direct reimbursement of nurses for their practice without going through the screen of paying a "supervising" physician. Observers believe that it is only a question of time before third-party payment for nursing services becomes widely accepted, as practice and research demonstrate public acceptance, quality care, and cost effectiveness.[34,45]

Until recently, mainly because of the fee-for-service problem, it was more common to find the nurse practitioner in a group practice with physicians and other professional health care providers. This is changing and many NPs are practicing alone or in groups with other NPs.[34] Many are employed by agencies such as mental health centers, schools, nursing homes, and HMOs. The practice is in collegial relationship with other health care providers within the work setting; the NP is a team member in terms of professional expertise in practice, consultation, referral, and planning.

Although the distinctions between the CNS and the NP may sound fairly clear, the situation is in fact not always so. Some individuals combine the CNS and the NP qualifications and roles. Because graduates of baccalaureate programs in nursing are prepared to obtain health histories and to perform routine physical assessment, combining these roles will become even easier. Some states have established an additional licensing examination through the state board of nursing registration to set qualifications for "advanced practice." New Hampshire, for example, licenses by special examination the Advanced Registered Nurse Practitioner (ARNP) who may be either a CNS or an NP. Some authorities believe that there will be a merging of the two titles over time.[85]

NURSING CARE FOR SPECIFIC POPULATIONS AT RISK

Traditionally nursing has identified populations at risk and set up systems of health care delivery to serve them. The educational focus and the broad humanistic approach of caring for individuals and families, with emphasis on primary prevention of illness and disease, led to the establishment of agencies such as the _Frontier Nursing Service_ and the _Henry Street Settlement_ in New York, which was the first community nursing service in the United States. These were systems developed by nurses in response to identified needs of clients. Much of the focus in those early days was on children and on the neonatal period. Nurses in those systems expanded their activities to meet the needs of the clients; nurses in the Frontier Nursing Service delivered babies in areas accessible only by horseback. Although the needs of mothers, infants, and children remain critically

important, nurses now also identify additional groups of vulnerable persons, notably those with long-term and chronic illness, and the aged. Health care for such identified populations at risk has become the concern of a specific group of nurses who practice in the area of gerontology.

Hospice care is a rapidly growing segment of health care. The concept was pioneered by a nurse-physician in England who deplored the inhumane care received by dying patients in busy, acute care hospitals. From its beginnings in a small, homelike institutional setting, it has developed, especially in the United States, almost entirely into a home care service. The hospice movement has spread rapidly and widely throughout the United States; most communities have some facilities to make it possible for people with a terminal illness to remain in their own homes. Much planning is necessary for this to occur, and nursing is the logical professional group to provide hospice care. Great personal and family satisfaction is reported by those who have been through the hospice experience.[39] It is incidentally significant in a cost control climate in reducing hospital occupancy.

A population at risk that has always been of concern to nurses is the poor. As discussed earlier, we are seeing a greater distance between the "haves" and the "have nots" of our society. Ability to pay for increasingly expensive health care is growing ever more difficult. Many who work at low-paying jobs, or who may be unemployed for variable periods, have no "health" insurance. Many others are homeless, often as a result of discharge from mental institutions without proper follow-up care. Nurses have been and continue to be concerned with these problems.[1] One example of such concern is a clinic established in Atlanta by three nurses, two of them nurse practitioners, for care of the homeless of that city.[80]

HEALTH PROMOTION

Although it is evident that until recently our national concern has been more with curing illness than with preventing it, the concept of self care and of people assuming more responsibility for their own health is not a new one. A goal of public health and of community nursing services has been to prevent illness and maintain the highest level of health and well-being for individuals, families, and the community. In recent years a broad segment of the American public is demonstrating acceptance of the concept and moving toward greater independence from unquestioning reliance on the medical establishment for health maintenance. Americans are more aware of such factors as the need for proper diet and exercise, the use of seat belts, the negative aspects of smoking, and the importance of early warning signals for cancer detection.

A philosophy of promoting and facilitating clients' self-help care has been extensively developed by Orem[64] and has been used as a basis of practice by many nurses. Such concepts are a part of basic nursing curricula and are importantly related to all aspects of ambulatory nursing care. Health promotion and health maintenance are frequently the philosophical basis for nurses in private practice such as nurse practitioners.

Thus, along the continuum from maintaining high-level wellness to care of the seriously ill and dying, nursing is playing a significant part in high-quality, cost-conscious health care. The need for technically skilled nurses in the critical care of hospitalized patients is, if anything, even greater now than in the past; such nurses are desperately needed. Technology that was provided only in hospitals has been added to the traditionally provided home services of community nursing. This not only demands great technical skill on the part of the community-based nurse but also an understanding of the interpersonal dynamics of client with family members and significant others, and the ability to teach, help, and support those involved in often frightening, wearying responsibility.

The concept that nursing has a unique service to offer the health care consumer has been held by nurses throughout history. The reality of that concept is evident both in nursing practice and research.

CHALLENGES TO NURSES AND NURSING

IMPACT ON HEALTH CARE DELIVERY

Other factors to be considered by nurses and the nursing profession in this changing health care scene are ways in which nurses can have the greatest impact on the health care delivery system, since the United States is rapidly approaching an oversupply of physicians. Not all of these physicians will be accommodated in specialty fields and will result in many of them providing primary care—a field that until now has not been considered very attractive. Thus they will be in direct competition with those nurses who are presently supplying primary care.

Nurses will have to be risk takers in identifying areas where nursing input can affect the health care delivery system. This includes entrepreneurship and incorporation by groups of nurses to provide a variety of services in a wide variety of settings.

COLLABORATION BETWEEN NURSING PRACTICE AND NURSING EDUCATION

The many changes in the health care delivery system and pressures on educational institutions are forcing the issue of increased collaboration between education and practice.[62] There has been some movement toward such collaboration for at least the past 20 years, but today's pressures are causing both nursing service directors and nurse educators to examine the issue even more seriously.

There are several good reasons for this. Some of these reasons are: (1) both groups of nurses have the patient as their focus, (2) nursing education requires a practice laboratory for students, and (3) health care agencies must rely on nursing schools to produce practitioners to work in their agencies. Also, nurses engaged in practice may not have the preparation or time to carry out their own nursing research but they can work closely with nursing faculty engaged in research to identify phenomena encountered in practice that should be systematically studied.

An increasing number of nurses are receiving PhD degrees in nursing. This is accelerating the amount of research in areas germane to nursing practice. The findings of nursing research will form a knowledge base for the science of nursing. Nursing scholars are examining the results of this research, identifying theories, and organizing the knowledge derived from research. These results will be incorporated into nursing education and practice as nursing moves toward the future.

Presently, nurses are examining the use of conceptual frameworks for nursing practice and will be expected to use a conceptual framework to guide their practice. Classification systems and nursing diagnoses will be used to help describe the nursing care delivered to patients. This will be essential if the impact of nursing care on a patient's recovery is to be delineated and documented.

As Naisbitt[59] has pointed out, the increase in "high tech" demands a concomitant increase in "high touch." There is no setting in which this is more evident than in intensive care units where some nurses have asked whether they are nursing patients or machines.

MEETING THE DEMAND FOR NURSES

The supply of nurses and the demand for them has fluctuated since the middle 1940s. The supply of nurses is closely related to wages. When hospitals and other health care agencies experience a nursing shortage, the typical response is to increase wages. Then when the supply is increased, wages tend to become depressed. This cycle has been repeating itself since the 1960s.

Although more nurses are working now than ever before the need for nurses has continued to increase. Several factors mentioned previously in this chapter account for this need. First, patients in hospitals are more acutely ill, and many of them are attached to complex machinery. Often the care of these complicated patients requires a ratio of one nurse per patient per shift. In some intensive care units two nurses may be assigned to one patient, which some nurses say, "one nurse is nursing the machines and the other is nursing the patient." Second, patients are being discharged from hospitals less recovered than in the past. They go either to a nursing home or to their own home where nursing services must be supplied. Third, the population is living longer, and the older age-groups require more nursing services.

When nurses are in short supply, the increase in wages is highest at the entry level as hospitals vie with each other to attract staff nurses. As a result, less money is budgeted for other nursing positions. Thus in comparison with other occupations nursing salaries are very compressed with only a small difference between minimum and maximum salary ranges. Although nursing salaries may be competitive with other occupations at the entry level, they do not remain so. See Table 1-1 for comparison of starting and average maximum salaries.[70]

Prescott suggests that the solution to the supply and demand question can be found in reframing the problem. She suggests that it may be useful to reframe the problem from too few nurses to too little professional nursing practice.[70] She lists the following reasons for this reframing: (1) the work of nurses has changed, (2) nurses are misused in hospitals, (3) nurses are underused as patient care givers, (4) nurses are considered interchangeable units, and (5) nurses are constrained by physicians and hospital policy from making decisions and taking action, which their education and experience have prepared them to do.

Most experienced nurses would agree with Prescott's observations. We have discussed how the work has changed, but a brief explanation of the other points seems in order. Often nurses are *misused* because they pick up the slack in the health care system. When there is an all RN staff, nurses must do all tasks for patients even though some of these tasks could safely be performed by less-skilled workers. If nursing assistants were assigned to nurses instead of to patients, as in the past, then the nurse would provide the professional care and have the nursing assistant help with other tasks.

Nurses are *underused* when they spend more time on indirect patient care activities than they do on direct patient care. Nurses often refer to this as "nursing the system." Nurses are used to make sure that patients have the supplies, medications, and so on that they need; that they reach scheduled appointments on time; and that obstacles to patient care are resolved.

Although nursing care has become more sophisticated and requires considerable knowledge and skill to care for a specific population of patients, some administrators still view all nurses as being the same and therefore *interchangeable* from one population of patients to another. Floating nurses from one unit to another has always been one of the factors that causes dissatisfaction.

A major complaint of nurses is lack of autonomy. This is closely related to the *constraints placed on nurses in decision making*. Nurses are more satisfied with the practice environment when they are allowed to make decisions about patient care and are not constrained by policies that require a physician's order for such activities as shampooing a patient's hair and so on.

If these problems are addressed, nursing may become a more attractive profession to prospective stu-

TABLE 1-1 Salary progression in various occupations, 1986

Occupation	Average Starting Salary ($)	Average Maximum Salary ($)	Salary Progression in Field (%)
Accountants	21,024	61,546	192.7
Attorneys	31,014	101,169	226.2
Buyers	21,242	41,304	94.4
Computer programmers	20,832	42,934	106.1
Personnel directors	39,917	75,710	88.8
Chemists	22,539	74,607	231.0
Engineers	27,866	79,021	183.6
Accounting clerks	12,517	21,872	74.7
Personnel clerks/ assistants	14,193	23,702	67.0
Purchasing clerks/ assistants	13,994	29,834	110.0
Secretaries	16,326	28,051	71.8
General clerks	10,478	19,744	84.5
Staff registered nurses	20,340	27,744	36.4

Data from National survey of professional, administrative, technical and clerical pay. Washington, DC: US Department of Labor, Bureau of Labor Statistics (Bulletin 2271). Oct 1986:11-3. Staff nurse salaries from University of Texas Medical Branch at Galveston. National survey of hospital and medical schools salaries. Galveston, Texas: University of Texas Medical Branch, 1986:29. Reproduced with permission of The CV Mosby Co. Prescott PA: Shortage of professional nursing practice: a reframing of the shortage problem, Heart Lung 18(5):436-443, Sept, 1989. Salary progression figures represent differences between national average starting and maximum salaries in a given profession or occupation for a certain year, in this case 1986.

TABLE 1-2 Nursing school enrollments

Year	Change (%)	No. Enrolled
1983	+3.5	250,553
1984	−5.3	237,232
1985	−8.1	217,955
1986	−11.1	193,712
1987	−5.6	182,947

From Rosenfeld P: Nursing student census with policy implications: 1988, New York, Division of Research, National League for Nursing, 1989. Reproduced with permission of The CV Mosby Co. Prescott PA: Shortage of professional nursing practice: a reframing of the shortage problem, Heart Lung 18(5):436-443, Sept, 1989.

dents. This is especially important because nursing school enrollments have been decreasing since 1984 (see Table 1-2). Data collected in 1989 indicates that enrollments in nursing schools are increasing. It is too early to tell whether this trend will continue in the 1990s.

ISSUES IN NURSING EDUCATION
NURSING SCHOOLS IN THE YEAR 2000

It seems clear that by the year 2000 the education of nursing students will take place in institutions of higher education. The nursing profession has been grappling with this issue for more than 25 years, and the action by the 1985 ANA House of Delegates, which is being supported by the National League for Nursing, should assure that this comes to pass.

Because of the social changes discussed earlier in this chapter the following seems clear. All nursing students will have less experience in acute care hospitals and more in alternative sites, such as primary care facilities, wellness centers, and facilities that assist the chronically ill. Because of changes in how information is processed, it can be expected that all nursing students will be computer literate. Much of the basic information that nurses need to know will be transmitted by computer assisted instruction (CAI) and less by textbooks, lectures, and so on. Currently, many nursing programs use several CAI materials and new materials continue to be developed. In addition, several researchers are studying how nurses make clinical decisions.[10,66] This knowledge will help nursing students to acquire the vast amount of knowledge they must master before entering practice. There is no doubt that all nursing programs will need to address the question of how nurses can assist those they serve to attain, maintain, or regain the highest level of health possible. Although nursing students will gain experience working with patients of all ages in a variety of settings, emphasis needs to be placed on the health care of the rapidly increasing number of elderly and on what nurses can do to assist them.

While the question of entry into practice is being addressed, there is a movement within the profession to move preparation of nursing to the postbaccalaureate level.[75] Case Western Reserve University opened the first N.D. (doctorate of nursing) program in 1979,[48] the second program opened at Rush University in 1989, and a third program will open at the University of Colorado in 1990. In addition, several other schools are now considering offering N.D. degrees. Other schools (Yale, Pace) offer a generic master's degree.

The N.D. Degree

The basis for the N.D. degree is the belief that preservice preparation for nursing should be built on a strong undergraduate base as is true in other professions such as medicine, dentistry, pharmacy, or law.[79] In this respect, the establishment of the N.D. degree is an evolutionary process similar to that which has occurred in other comparable professions.

For example, there has been a remarkable increase in the number of Pharm. D. degree programs in the last 15 years and although some universities continue to offer both bachelor's in pharmacy degree and the Pharm. D., others have phased out their undergraduate program completely.

It can be predicted that the number of N.D. programs will increase by the end of this century. Some of the reasons for this projected increase are listed below:

1. The recognition that current nursing education is too vocational and narrow as it tries to encompass both liberal and professional education in one program[75]
2. The move to have nursing recognized as an autonomous health profession
3. The need to prepare nurses who will be able to function better and compete for positions in a much more competitive health care system
4. The need to provide nurses with more parity with other health professionals, especially physicians; symbols such as degrees and titles of address (Dr.) are becoming even more important in today's society.

CHARACTERISTICS OF NURSING STUDENTS

The population of nursing students is more heterogeneous today than it was 20 years ago and this will continue. It can be hoped that an increasing number of men will be attracted to nursing, as will both women and men who are selecting nursing as a midcareer change. Future students will be more concerned with what the nursing profession has to offer them. Some of the factors that will determine whether potential students will be interested in nursing as a profession are listed in the box below.

NURSING EDUCATION IN THE FUTURE

All the changes discussed previously will affect nursing education now and in the future. Many questions are being addressed by nurse educators as they prepare for the year 2000. These questions include the following:

1. What is the fundamental knowledge that students need to master before they enter nursing practice?

FACTORS INFLUENCING CHOICE OF NURSING AS A PROFESSION

1. Status and image of nursing
2. Remuneration when compared with other professions
3. Autonomy
4. Opportunities for practice

---

2. What parts of the nurse's role require professional education and what parts require technical education?

3. How should professional nurses be educated? How should technical nurses be educated?

4. How does nursing achieve equity with other health professions?

Several recent projects have studied the content essential for nursing practice. These include: (1) the National Commission on Nursing Implementation Project (NC-NIP[27]), (2) the Midwest Alliance in Nursing projects on differentiating ADN and BSN competencies[71]; and (3) the American Association of Colleges of Nursing (AACN) project on essentials of college and university education for nursing.[2]

The findings of these projects will help to define what will be expected of technical nurses (associate degree prepared) and professional nurses (baccalaureate degree prepared) as nursing moves forward with implementing the 1985 ANA House of Delegates recommendations for two levels of entry into nursing practice.

EVALUATION OF THE OUTCOMES OF NURSING CARE — QUALITY ASSURANCE IN NURSING

IMPETUS FOR QUALITY ASSURANCE

Nursing is committed to professional excellence by providing the highest quality of care possible. Implicit in this commitment is the responsibility to evaluate the quality and appropriateness of that care. However, during the past 20 years attempts have been made to develop an extrinsic, systematic approach to monitor and improve care. The impetus for this change has come from a variety of sources: (1) health care legislation, (2) changes in third-party reimbursement, (3) economic factors, and (4) the nursing profession.

HEALTH CARE LEGISLATION

Since the passage of Medicare/Medicaid legislation in 1965, the federal government has become the largest source of third-party health care payment. Because of this increasing financial commitment, Congress and government officials at all levels are under pressure to ensure that the services rendered are necessary, that they meet professionally recognized standards of care, and that they contain costs.

THIRD-PARTY REIMBURSEMENT

To establish some system of accountability for third-party reimbursement, Congress created a system for reviewing these expenses as part of Public Law 92-603, the Social Security Amendments of 1972. This legislation established a nationwide network of professional standards review organizations (PSROs) for review of patient care financed by the federal government. Private insurance carriers such as Blue Cross also established standards for review of the care for which they have been asked to make payment.

These efforts were essentially ineffectual, and by 1981 more stringent fiscal measures were passed by Congress in the Onmibus Reconciliation Act, which imposed cost-sharing requirements on Medicare beneficiaries and made substantial reductions in federal contributions to Medicaid. Changes in the Social Security Act in 1982 mandated prospective Medicare payments using the 467 Diagnosis Related Groups (DRGs) categories. Both of these later legislative changes have resulted in cost-containment strategies, increasing questions of whether the quality of health care has diminished because of increased emphasis on reducing costs.

ECONOMIC FACTORS

Because health care costs continue to assume an increasing share of the gross national product (GNP), there has been increased scrutiny of the components of this cost by consumers, as well as by legislators. Reviewing the cost of illness raises vital questions about the relationship of quality of care to cost. For example, the principle of "high cost/low benefit" is defined as poor quality of health care in terms of overdiagnosis or overtreatment, which can lead to excessive health care expenditures even in the absence of any iatogenic or untoward consequences. Poor quality of health care in the form of misdiagnosis, mistreatment, or inadequate nursing care can increase mortality or morbidity, increase length of hospital stay, increase loss of earnings, and therefore increase the costs of health care to individuals and to society.

The current economic situation of growing health care costs at an unacceptable rate, budgetary cutbacks, and the DRG reimbursement scheme has serious implications for nursing. More than ever before, the nursing profession must demonstrate the value and benefits of its service if it wishes to retain government and consumer support.

PROFESSIONAL STANDARDS

Last but certainly not least is the professional and ethical concern that the nursing profession places on itself for quality care. In 1973 the American Nurses Association (ANA) published generic *Standards of Nursing Practice* for the purpose of ensuring quality nursing care to the public (see box , p. 19). The primary responsibility for implementing these standards, however, rests with the individual nurse, who bears the responsibility of ensuring that these criteria are met in his or her own practice setting. To fulfill this responsibility, professional nurses must be familiar with both the generic (general) and the specific standards pertinent to the

AMERICAN NURSES ASSOCIATION STANDARDS OF NURSING PRACTICE

Standard I
The collection of data about the health status of the client/patient is systematic and continuous. The data are accessible, communicated, and recorded.

Standard II
Nursing diagnoses are derived from health status data.

Standard III
The plan of nursing care includes goals derived from the nursing diagnoses.

Standard IV
The plan of nursing care includes priorities and the prescribed nursing approaches or measures to achieve the goals derived from the nursing diagnoses.

Standard V
Nursing actions provide for client/patient participation in health promotion, maintenance, and restoration.

Standard VI
Nursing actions assist the client/patient to maximize his health capabilities.

Standard VII
The client's/patient's progress or lack of progress toward goal achievement is determined by the client/patient and the nurse.

Standard VIII
The client's/patient's progress or lack of progress toward goal achievement directs reassessment, reordering of priorities, new goal setting, and revision of the plan of nursing care.

From American Nurses Association. Reprinted by permission of the American Nurses Association, Standards of Nursing Practice, Kansas City, Mo, 1973, The Association.

care of the patient population for whom the nurse is responsible. These standards identify the elements of nursing care that must be met to ensure quality care and to provide a baseline for measuring that quality.

Three other sets of professional standards must also be considered: the nurse practice acts, the medical practice acts, and the standards set by the Joint Commission on Accreditation of Health Care Organizations (JCAHO). Presently, almost every state has a nurse practice act and a medical practice act. Both of these constitute external sources of standards for nursing practice. Taken together they define and delineate the content and practice of nursing from a legal standpoint.

Nurse practice acts define nursing practice and identify those activities that fall within the province of nursing. *Medical practice acts* further delineate nursing practice by outlining those areas that constitute the exclusive province of the physician. Such exclusions restrict the activities in which nurses may engage. Neither type of act sets actual standards for practice; rather the acts designate general areas of activity for both pro-

fessions, and they establish the legal relationship of the nurse to society and to other related professions.

The *Joint Commission on Accreditation of Health Care Organizations* (JCAHO), formerly the Joint Commission on Accreditation of Hospitals, is another highly influential external source of nursing standards. In 1976 the Joint Commission added a section on quality of professional services to their *Accreditation Manual for Hospitals*. The standard delineates the characteristics of patient care evaluation programs. It includes an effective review and evaluation of the quality and appropriateness of patient care. The following quality assurance activities are prescribed by the JCAH (1985)[42]:

1. A planned and systematic process for monitoring and evaluating patient care
2. Regular data collection to accomplish monitoring and periodic assessment to evaluate it
3. Action plans and evaluation of action plans to assess whether they have improved care
4. Documented reports of findings
5. Documented reports of actions
6. Annual appraisal of the nursing quality assurance program

The JCAHO is a voluntary, nongovernmental organization that establishes standards for operation of hospitals and other health-related facilities. It conducts surveys and accreditation programs to promote high-quality care in all respects, to ensure that patients receive the optimal benefits that medical science has to offer. It emphasizes organization and administration of functions for efficient care of the patient. Compliance with the JCAHO standards is recognized by issuance of certificates of accreditation.

JCAHO accreditation is a voluntary process and it is not the same as licensure or certification by the state or local authorities. However, accreditation has come to be recognized as a benchmark of quality and is used by some regulatory agencies as one criterion for licensure or certification and by some insurance agencies as a condition for honoring reimbursement claims.

DEFINITION OF QUALITY ASSURANCE

The definition of *quality* when applied to nursing care is complex and multidimensional. Wandelt and Stewart[98] define quality as "a characteristic or attribute of something." Phaneut[68] defines quality as "the essential character of care considered within the context of degree or merit." Zimmer[102] postulates that quality of care is "the observable characteristics that describe a desired and valued degree of excellence and the expected, observed variations." *Assurance* is defined as "safeguarding a quality by instituting a systematic evaluation to be sure that the care that is delivered meets the standard that is set."

Quality assurance therefore is defined as a *process*

that involves evaluating the degree of excellence of the observable and measurable characteristics of delivered nursing care. Quality assurance can be described on two levels: in its strictest sense it is described as a set of techniques for assuring the maintenance and improvement of standards and the efficiency and effectiveness of nursing care. More broadly, it is an effort to control nursing practice. As such, it involves relationships between nurses and consumers and between nurses and governmental bodies.

In health care delivery the purpose of quality assurance evaluation is always twofold. The first part determines the extent to which the predetermined standards are being met by a particular nursing program. Second, these findings are used to make decisions about changes that are to be implemented by the persons carrying out the program of care. These two parts must be in place if nursing is to ensure its accountability to the consumer. Although the specific target of each evaluation may differ depending on what information about quality is desired, the purpose of the evaluation is always the same.

Nurses who are engaged in the delivery of health care cannot escape inclusion of quality assurance reviews in their practice responsibilities. Indeed, some proficiency in evaluation must become part of a modern nurse's basic repertoire of skills. Corresponding to this responsibility on the part of the individual nurse is also a responsibility on the part of nurse educators to ensure that this skill is an ongoing part of nursing education and practice.

Fortunately the process is not a mysterious one. Indeed, most nurses are more than halfway toward expertise in this area by virtue of their basic education and experience. Nurses who are expert in the care of a specific patient population, by definition, possess the knowledge necessary to determine desired *health* and *wellness outcomes* for that population. These nurses already know what direct care processes to employ in assisting patients toward health and wellness. They also know what observable changes in patient's problems should occur at certain intervals.

Unfortunately, most nurses are not expert in the methods that are needed to conduct these evaluation reviews. This is the one remaining critical piece that nurses can learn from staff development programs in employing agencies or from other continuing education programs in the community.

QUALITY ASSURANCE REVIEW

A variety of models have been proposed to describe the quality assurance review process. The model devised by the American Nurses Association (ANA) will be presented here.[4] This model is a problem-solving process that utilizes *structure, process,* and *outcome criteria* as

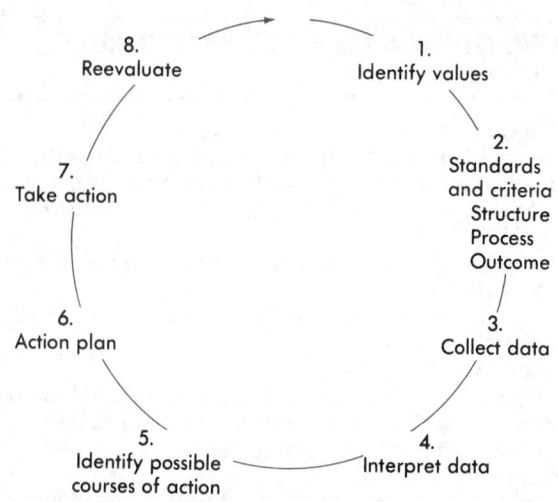

FIGURE 1-3 American Nurses Association model for quality assurance review. (From American Nurses Association: Quality assurance for nursing care, Kansas City, Mo, 1976, The Association. Reprinted by permission of the American Nurses Association.)

the primary tools of inquiry. As illustrated in Figure 1-3, the model contains the following eight steps:
1. Identification of values
2. Identification of structure, process, outcome standards, and criteria
3. Collection of data necessary to measure degree of attainment of standards and criteria
4. Interpretation of the data in terms of the strengths and weaknesses of the program
5. Identification of possible courses of action
6. Choosing a course of action
7. Taking action
8. Reevaluation

Each of these steps is discussed below, then illustrated by means of a clinical example. Note that the model is circular, suggesting that the process is continuous (Figure 1-3).

The priority of topics for a quality assurance review is usually determined by its real or potential impact on patient care. The review may have impact on either the *effectiveness* of care or the *efficiency* with which care is delivered or both. If a nursing care problem has been identified with some frequency, it is, of course, given a higher priority.

IDENTIFICATION OF THE FOCUS OF THE REVIEW

The focus of the evaluation can be the institution, the nurses, the patient, or a combination of these. Selection of the exact focus will vary depending on individual and institutional values.

If the quality assurance review focuses on the *institution,* it may examine the types of services delivered, the administrative structure, or features of the health care setting such as the physical plant, equipment, organization, or staffing. A quality assurance review could also be employed if one wanted to measure the institution's adherence to external standards, selected personnel policies, or the qualifications of nursing staff assigned to special care areas, such as intensive care units.

If the focus of the review is *the nurse,* an area of nursing practice will be selected for review. The review could examine almost any aspect of nursing activity. It might be utilized if the objective of the evaluation is to measure adherence to nursing department policies and procedures or it might be employed if the objective were to evaluate whether the most appropriate nursing care methods were being used.

Specific examples of measures that focus on the nurse might include criteria that assess frequency of vital sign monitoring in the immediate postoperative period, criteria that establish content and time frames for completion of the nursing assessment form, or criteria that the nurse uses to assess the patient's intravenous needle puncture site. Measures that focus on nursing can therefore include activities of a single nurse, of all nurses assigned to a specific unit, or of all nurses in the department of nursing.

If the purpose of the review is to examine the care of *patients,* the review might be limited to certain categories of patients or expanded to include a specific number of patients. Variables that might be used for selecting the patient population to be studied include age, ethnicity, nursing problems, disease, or degree of illness.

It must be emphasized here, however, that the perspective of the consumer must be considered in any evaluation. If the focus is on patient outcomes or the results of nursing care, for example, then the patient and/ or the family must have input regarding the quality of the nursing care.

Quality assurance nursing review committees should be formed from the committee structure that already exists within a health care agency and should carry administrative sanction. Membership on any quality assurance committee will depend on the focus and activity of that committee. The purpose of the review will dictate whether the committee should be composed of nurses from one specialty or of nurses from multiple specialties. A committee that is composed only of surgical nurses, for example, would review nursing care only for surgical patients. On the other hand, a committee composed of nurses from multiple specialties might review the nursing care of an entire institution.

Multidisciplinary committees might also be formed. These would be composed of representatives from several health professions, such as medicine, nursing, die-

tetics, social work, occupational therapy, physical therapy, and pharmacy. A multidisciplinary committee would have as its focus the total care that a patient or population of patients received during hospitalization. In these circumstances, committee members would develop jointly the criteria to be used in the patient care review.

Step 1. Identify Values

Before the implementation of this or any other quality assurance review model, there must be an examination of the *societal, professional,* and *individual values* that guide the activities of the health care agency. Such a process is unavoidably inherent in the use of the word *quality.* The very word *quality* implies that somewhere, someone has determined that certain outcomes have more value than other outcomes. As the term *value* applies to nursing care, it means that the individual nursing department, hospital, or health care agency, as well as the surrounding community, will interact to influence the development of criteria that will be used in the review process.

To cite some obvious examples, in most Catholic hospitals a high value is placed on human life from the moment of conception; therefore in Catholic institutions no abortions will be performed. In another hospital a prevailing societal or cultural value may have influenced it to favor a youth orientation. The emphasis in health care at that institution may therefore be oriented toward teen and young adult programs as opposed to geriatric programs. In whatever setting the nurse happens to be, that setting operates under a set of values that must be identified and understood if the quality assurance review is to be fair and accurate.

Step 2. Identify Structure, Process, Outcome Standards, and Criteria

After selecting the focus of the review, the next step in the ANA model is to specify the criteria and standards that are appropriate to evaluating care.

A *standard* is defined as the desired or achievable level or range of performance of a certain criterion, or as a framework against which performance is compared.[42] A *criterion measure* is defined as the variable that is believed to be an indicator of the quality of care.[42] Thus the statement that "every patient will have a plan of care recorded on the nursing care plan" would be a standard, whereas the statement that "a nursing care plan will be developed by a registered nurse within 12 hours of admission" would be a criterion measure.

The task of the *quality assurance review committee* is to develop *criteria* that will be used in the actual evaluation. The *standards* for nursing practice are usually developed by clinical nursing experts and are written in a form that can be operationalized at the practice level.

In effect, these criteria are developed by professionals, for professionals, by relying on professional expertise and professional literature. The criteria that are developed can be statements of either structure, process, or outcome.

Structure criteria are statements that describe the environmental elements, setting, and conditions under which the nurse-patient relationship occurs. It includes the philosophy and objectives of the health care agency, its fiscal resources, legal responsibilities, equipment, physical facilities, management structure, licensure, and accreditation as well as the quality and characteristics of professional nonprofessional, and technical employees.

Structure criteria can be written for the institution, for the nurse, or for the patient. The statement that "patient beds must be 3 feet from one another" is an institutional statement. "Any nurse assigned to the intensive care unit must have satisfactorily completed the 4-week intensive care orientation course" is a nurse-oriented statement. And, "all patients are to sign a written consent form before any surgical or invasive radiological procedure" is a patient-oriented statement.

Process criteria focus on the nature and sequence of health care activities. They focus on the activities that the nurse engages in to respond to the patient's illness. For example, process criteria might describe the communication patterns that a nurse has with a dying patient or the preoperative teaching plan for the cardiac patient scheduled for surgery.

Outcome criteria focus on the results of the processes of health care. They are considered by many to be the ultimate indicators of the quality of patient care. For the patient *the measurable outcome could be a change in health, knowledge, or functional status.* In addition, these outcomes can be either positive or negative. Examples of outcome measures are presented in the box above right.

After the criteria have been developed, they need to be validated before being used in a quality review process. This *validation* process is usually performed by a "consensus among peers." The rationale for this validation step is to be certain that the selected criteria are accurate and relevant and that they reflect the realities of nursing practice at that particular institution. The nurses who work daily with the topic chosen for the review are usually in the best position to make these determinations.

Following criteria development and validation, the next step is for the committee to establish a specific observable and measurable level of performance for each criteria; for example, "At discharge 100% of the patients should be afebrile" or "By the time of discharge, 75% of all ostomy patients should be able to apply their own bags."

OUTCOME CRITERIA FOR A PERSON WITH A COLOSTOMY OR ILEOSTOMY

The patient or significant other can:
1. Demonstrate how to measure the stoma for an appliance
   (The stoma shrinks as healing occurs. Measure the stoma before purchasing new appliances.)
2. Demonstrate proper application of the appliance
   (Application includes appliance removal, skin care, and reapplying an appliance.)
3. State plans for follow-up care
4. State community resources available for obtaining permanent appliances and financial assistance, and list support groups
   (Include the name of one surgical supply house and the telephone number of the Ostomy Association, the Visiting Nurses Association, or some other home care support group.)
5. State need to observe stoma and skin around it for redness, bleeding, or excoriation

The patient or significant other has:
6. An information packet, which has been reviewed with the nurse

---

Not all criteria, however, necessarily carry a 100% level of performance. In the second example mentioned above, a 75% compliance level was selected because many of the patients may be discharged to extended care facilities for further care and are not expected to be fully independent by the time of discharge.

Step 3. Measure Degree of Attainment of Standards and Criteria

A wide variety of methods can be used to gather data on nursing performance. The degree to which actual practice meets or exceeds the validated criteria in turn provides the data necessary to evaluate the strengths and weaknesses of the nursing care program. These data gathering methods might include *self-assessment, supervisor evaluation, performance observation, utilization review, audits, review of patient records, staff surveys, or patient/medical staff/employee complaints.*

Whatever method of review is chosen, the data should be easily accessible and retrievable. The review may be looking at activities that happened in the past, or it may be examining current nursing activities. A review that examines past happenings is called a *retrospective review.* A *concurrent review* looks at what is happening in the present, while the patient is receiving care.

Specific questions that the quality assurance review committee needs to answer at this point include:
- Who will collect the data?
- What will be the source of the data?
- Where will the data be collected?

TABLE 1-3 Criteria tracking form

Outcome Criteria for Person With Colostomy	Expected Level of Performance (Percent Compliance)*	Identified Problems, Strengths, and Weaknesses
Patient or significant others can:		
Demonstrate how to measure the stoma for an appliance	85%	One patient was blind; no documentation on two patients
Demonstrate proper application of the appliance	85%	Two patients stated it would have been helpful to have a mirror provided; one patient was blind
State plans for follow-up care	60%	Forty percent of patients were being transferred to an extended care facility
State community resources available for purchase of permanent appliances, for financial assistance, and support groups	75%	No documentation of this being done on 25% of charts
Patient or significant others have ostomy informational booklet, which has been reviewed with nurse	100%	

*Expected compliance in these areas is 100%.

- When will the data be collected?
- How will the data be collected?

The answers to these questions will assist the committee in deciding whether the review can be accomplished as planned given the inherent requirements for efficiency and accuracy. As a final check, the committee should be certain that each criterion measure is written so that a decision can be easily made as to whether the standard has been met.

Once the data collection has occurred, the results are tabulated and it is determined whether the percent of yes and no answers corresponds to the previously established level of performance (that is, percent compliance) for each criterion. If the level of performance does not achieve the expectations, the criterion for this evaluation item has not been met.

Table 1-3 illustrates one method of keeping track of a multicriterion evaluation process.

Step 4. Interpret Strengths and Weaknesses

The degree to which the levels of performance have been met serves as a basis for describing the strengths and weaknesses of the nursing care program or practice. But in addition to this obvious analysis there are other factors that are frequently overlooked. These include factors that might be related to the degree of success in achieving certain outcomes. Consider the following case:

On Nursing Unit A there was 100% compliance with the criterion that all ostomy patients would be able to apply their own ostomy bag by the time of discharge. However, on Unit B the compliance was only 65%. A comparison of the procedures and practices on the two units revealed that the ages of the patients on Unit B were significantly higher than those on Unit A and that the majority of Unit B patients were discharged to extended care facilities instead of to their homes.

This comparison provides insight into reasons for the differences in these two units and would have been missed had not the evaluator been careful to look for extenuating factors.

In some instances the cause of the identified problem may lie outside the control of nursing and fall within the purview of medicine or hospital administration. For example, an evaluation of the nursing management of postoperative pain at one hospital revealed that the physician staff was ordering almost identical pain relief medication for all patients. The consequence of this lack of individualized patient assessment regarding pain relief measures by the physicians caused frequent patient complaints as well as frequent calls to the physicians by the nursing staff. These results were shared with the physician staff who agreed that an educational program for physicians and corrective measures were needed in this area.

Step 5. Identify Possible Courses of Action

After identification of strengths and weaknesses, possible courses of action are developed. They will have as their primary focus the *reduction* or *elimination* of the *weaknesses* and *reinforcement* of the *strengths* of the existing program and practices. Consideration must also be given to the best means of *motivating the nursing staff* to accomplish the needed changes. Indeed, the best results are usually obtained when the persons most affected by the quality assurance review are involved in the process of planning the subsequent course of action. The eventual attainment of the preset levels of performance coupled with appropriate availability of resources and cooperative relationships between evaluators and those affected by the evaluation generally serve as the basis for most successful changes in nursing practice.

QUALITY ASSURANCE REVIEW TOPIC: LEARNING NEEDS OF THE OSTOMY PATIENT

Patient and family education and patient's involvement in their care were high priorities at this institution. Nurses on the surgical units were concerned that ostomy patients in particular were not receiving adequate discharge information.

STEP 2. IDENTIFY CRITERIA

The outcome criteria for the ostomy patient were selected as the evaluation criteria.

STEP 3. DATA COLLECTION

Thirty patients' charts with the discharge diagnosis of some type of ostomy were selected at random from the previous 6 months. Reviews of the patient charts using the Ostomy Outcome Criteria revealed incomplete teaching plans and no record of the patient receiving any type of information booklets. (The rule is: if it isn't documented, it hasn't been done.)

STEP 4. INTERPRET DATA

The quality assurance committee was certain that the patients had received more information than had been documented in the record. But where was the information to be found? It was also apparent to the committee that some of the criterion elements required updating.

STEP 5. IDENTIFY POSSIBLE COURSES OF ACTION

It was observed that the documentation system for discharge planning for these patients needed to be more efficient, yet at the same time more thorough. The surgical nursing staff suggested that the outcome criteria sheet be printed on a nurse's note form. Another suggestion was to use a large stamp that would contain elements of the teaching plan that could be checked off as completed. A group of experienced nurses was formed and, with the assistance of the clinical nurse specialist, rewrote and assisted in the validation process for the outcome criteria.

STEP 6. WRITE THE ACTION PLAN

The quality assurance committee met with the surgical nursing staff and concluded that the best choice was to have the outcome criteria overprinted on the nurse's note sheet. The appropriate administration approval was obtained.

STEP 7. IMPLEMENT THE ACTION PLAN

One member of the quality assurance committee was assigned to oversee the production of the new forms. After they were obtained, the unit nursing staff took the responsibility for introducing them and explaining their purpose to the remaining staff members. An evaluation was planned for 4 months later.

STEP 8. REEVALUATE

Four months after the implementation, the surgical staff conducted a repeat review using the revised outcome criteria. There was 100% compliance to each criterion element.

Solutions to an identified problem can be numerous. Frequently, these actions include administrative changes, further clinical research into the problem, continuing education, changes in practice, environmental changes, a reward system for improved compliance, or even the organization of peer pressure.

Each of the above alternatives has advantages and disadvantages and each must be weighed by the peer group in terms of how efficiently and effectively the problem can be solved. At times the involvement of nurses in the development of criteria is all that is needed to bring about changes in practice.

Step 6. Select Course of Action

After examination of the alternatives, the best course of action is selected by the nurse peer group. The specific course of action will generally depend on the identified problem, the availability of resources, and the inherent organizational structure of the institution. In certain cases there may be multiple causes for an identified problem, and many possible solutions may have to be explored.

After a decision is made, the individual institution will vary as to how the plan for change is presented to the administration and in how the change is to be implemented. In the case of a nursing practice change, the director of nursing may wish to make the final decision. At other institutions the director of nursing may only wish to be informed of the findings, and the committee will be charged with making appropriate changes.

Step 7. Take Action

Attempting to improve the quality of nursing care implies change. This in turn implies that the persons making decisions about changes will somehow find a way to execute their decisions. If it is felt that the information has been inadequate, the action taken may be to gather more information systematically. Sooner or later, however, *action must be taken*. This is a critical point. Without this step the entire quality assurance review process becomes a hollow, futile exercise.

Step 8. Reevaluate the Process

We have added this step to the original ANA model. The rationale for its addition is to illustrate that once a corrective or other type of action has been taken, the action must be monitored to ascertain if it has been effective in solving the problem. Therefore, once an action has been taken, the cycle begins over again. (See the box on the left for a clinical example of a quality assurance review.)

MONITORING ACTIVITIES AND INSTRUMENTS

In addition to the problem-focused quality assurance reviews, a variety of methods have been devised to assess the nursing care program on an ongoing basis. A brief description follows of some of the more frequently used methods.

INCIDENT REPORTS

Whenever an untoward event occurs to patients, personnel, or visitors, an incident report should be completed. A statistical analysis of these reports comparing year-to-date and monthly statistics is generally compiled

by a hospital or by the hospital's liability insurance carrier. Increases in certain types of incidents, such as medication errors, would be a signal to the quality assurance committee that it should begin a review of the entire medication delivery system.

Additionally, there are a variety of other instruments that have been developed by nurses to assess various aspects of nursing practice. Table 1-4 contains a brief description of a number of these instruments.

TABLE 1-4 Comparison of eight nursing instruments

Name of Assessment Tool	Therapeutic Basis for Tool	Focus	Type/Number of Criteria/Items	Time Frame for Review	Data Collection	Use of Tools
JCAHO's *Pep Patient Care Evaluation*	Problem-solving process	Nursing process and/or patient outcomes	Varies by study	Concurrent and/or retrospective	Usually medical record review	Review of quality of nursing care in any setting
ANA's *Guidelines for Review of Nursing Care at Local Level*	Problem-solving process	Patient outcomes	Sample sets of outcome criteria (15 topics)	Retrospective	Usually medical record review	PSRO screening of quality, necessity, appropriateness of nursing care in variety of settings
HEW's *Methodology for Monitoring Quality of Nursing Care*	Nursing process plus patient classification	Nursing process	Master list of 216 process criteria/subset of 56 criteria per study	Concurrent	Nurse observer completes work sheet	Review of medical, surgical, pediatric, intensive care nursing in acute care setting
Slater Nursing Competencies Rating Scale	Six primary scientific and cultural bases for nursing care actions	Nursing performance	84 process items	Concurrent	Nurse observer completes scale	Evaluation of nursing personnel, review of care as it relates to performance
Quality Patient Care Scale (QualPacs)	Six primary scientific and cultural bases for nursing care actions	Nursing process	68 process items (subset of Slater)	Concurrent	Nurse observer completes scale	Measure of quality of nursing care in any setting
Phaneuf Nursing Audit	Seven functions of professional nursing	Nursing process	50 process items	Retrospective (portions could be concurrent)	Medical record review	Review of quality of nursing care in hospitals, nursing homes, home health agencies
Rush-Medicus Nursing Process Instrument	Process model of patient care	Nursing process	Master list of 220 process criteria/subsets of 30-50 criteria per study	Concurrent	Nurse observer completes work sheet based on observations plus documentation review	Review of quality of medical, surgical, pediatric nursing care in acute care settings
Horn-Swain Criteria/ Measures of Nursing Care Quality	Orem's care theory of nursing	Patient outcomes	Master list of 539 outcome criteria/subsets available for individual study	Concurrent	Nurse observer/ interviewer completes work sheet	Research on models for delivery of nursing care, subsets assess quality of care

From InterQual: Quality assurance in nursing seminar manual, Chicago, 1980, Interqual, Inc.

QUALITY INDICATORS (MONITORS OR SCREENS)

More recently the JCAHO has mandated that quality indicators be monitored on an on-going basis. Each department in an institution determines its own quality indicators.

Quality indicators are those items that a health care agency believes are indicators of quality patient care. For example, quality indicators used by a nursing service would depend on the patient population being served and on high-risk, high-volume events that need to be monitored. In medical-surgical nursing, quality indicators might include number of patient falls, ratio of medication errors to the total doses administered, and the number of pressures sores (decubiti). For each of the quality indicators a threshold of acceptance is set. In the case of falls it might be not more than one patient fall per nursing unit each month.

By setting the threshold for acceptance, a determination can be made as to how well the quality indicator is being met. It is important to establish in advance how data will be collected and at what intervals for each quality indicator. The appropriateness of a quality indicator should be assessed on a regular basis. If a particular indicator is no longer of high risk or high volume, consideration should be given to deleting it. The quality indicators should change as circumstances change.

NURSING AUDIT/EVALUATION STUDY

The term *nursing audit* or evaluation study is generally used when one wishes to compare predetermined criteria with the documentation found in the patient record. There are basically two types of audit, *retrospective* and *concurrent*. A retrospective audit is a critical examination of nursing actions with a view toward improvement in practice. A retrospective review is done after the patients' discharge. The reviewer has the advantage of using data for the full continuum of the patient's stay, from admission to discharge, and of evaluating the results for a large series of comparable cases. One advantage of a retrospective audit is that at times practitioners gain impressions from single cases in which they are personally involved. These impressions, however, may or may not be borne out by later systematic study of a large number of cases.

A *concurrent audit* is a critical examination of the patient's progress toward a desired health status (*outcome*) and patient care management activities (*processes*) while the care is still in progress. Patient questionnaires, interviews, observation, and review of the patient record are possible sources of data for a concurrent review. Concurrent review has the advantage of providing opportunities for making changes in the ongoing care program. Retrospective and concurrent reviews each have their own advantages and they may be used singly or together in a quality assurance review. The term *nursing audit* is being used less frequently; it is being supplanted by the term *evaluation study*.

PEER REVIEW

Nursing peer review occurs when the nurses establish the standards and criteria and evaluate the quality of care among themselves. When development of specific criteria is difficult it is often useful to break down the care components into smaller units for which specific criteria can be written. For example, instead of reviewing care of the surgical patient or a specific operative procedure, a type of preoperative teaching could be reviewed. When feasible, patient care evaluation should go beyond patient record review to include direct observation of patients, direct observation of nurses giving care, and interviews with patients and/or staff.

Many aspects of care do not lend themselves to the development of objective criteria, and reviewer variability may be introduced into the evaluation. In this case, reviewers respected for their expertise in the specific care can be used. When an aspect is complex or controversial, two reviewers might review a case. If two reviewers disagree, a third expert should be consulted. An alternative to individual experts is a committee of reviewers, which can review cases and compare opinions as to whether certain review criteria have been met.

Mechanisms for a peer review process include reviews within a single patient care unit or by specialty, such as orthopedic nurses coming together for peer review. Clinical nurse specialists frequently have a peer review group where they monitor their own practice.

PATIENT SATISFACTION QUESTIONNAIRES

Patient satisfaction questionnaires are frequently employed if written data are desired regarding patient's perceptions of their hospitalization experience. Many health care agencies distribute such questionnaires to patients as part of the admission procedure and request that the patients complete and return the forms at the end of their hospitalizations. Some hospitals have initiated patient ombudsman programs. In these programs the ombudsman visits the majority of inpatients, questions them regarding their perceptions of their hospitalization experiences, and intervenes in their behalf when it is appropriate.

PATIENT FOCUS GROUPS

The primary purpose of a focus group is to relate patient and family concerns to the professional staff quality assurance activities. The focus group consists of 10 to 12 consumers who meet informally under the guidance of a moderator trained in group dynamics. The information obtained from these groups is not quantifiable but identifies areas of reasonable concern. Inappropriate or unreasonable patient concerns can be addressed through public service announcements or health workshops. Patient concerns that are realistic and reasonable can form the basis for future quality assurance activities. This approach has been used successfully by business and industry for many years.

STAFF SATISFACTION SURVEYS

A staff satisfaction questionnaire or interview is generally employed by administration to assess organizational changes, policies, or the general satisfaction that might be experienced in a specific work setting.

UTILIZATION REVIEW

The utilization review program was mandated by the JCAH in 1978. It has as its primary goal the appropriate allocation of a hospital's resources. Although a utilization review program is not oriented specifically toward nursing, the monitoring activities of this program occasionally identify nursing areas that may need to be evaluated further.

INFECTION CONTROL REPORT

Because of their direct contact with patients, the nursing staff is frequently involved in programs to monitor and control infection rates. An infection control report provides monthly data on the number and types of nosocomial infections on a given hospital unit. Questions can then be raised about nursing procedures or practices that may influence the number or types of infections. See Chapter 15 for details about infection control studies.

CONFIDENTIALITY AND THE QUALITY ASSURANCE PROCESS

Confidentiality of data is an issue frequently associated with quality assurance. The availability and use of evaluative data about a patient or groups of patients has always been of concern to health professionals. The increasing use of *computerized data* has generated enormous concern for the potential threats to privacy. Most quality assurance studies can be conducted without recording patients' names and are reported in terms of *aggregate data*. Review of care provided to an individually identified patient requires constant vigilance to ensure the protection of the patient identity.

ETHICS AND QUALITY ASSURANCE

Ethical problems can and do influence the quality assurance concerns of nurses. Certainly there are traditional areas of mutual interest: patient education, informed consent, and unnecessary surgery or procedures. But ethical problems probably occur much more frequently than is apparent through patient care evaluation, particularly because quality assurance has focused primarily on technical aspects of care—whether appro-

priate tests are ordered, whether surgical complications were prevented or managed, and whether patient records list the steps taken in treatment.

For several reasons, quality assurance needs to focus more on *ethical decision making in the future*. First, the rapidly increasing opportunities in patient care will provide more options for patients and providers. A heart transplant for one patient, for example, may mean that a heart must be sacrificed in a comatose patient who is on a ventilator. *Balancing individual rights* with social good will become more frequent and more difficult in the future. Second, as resources continue to diminish, problems of *distributive justice* will arise. It is quite possible that in the future some type of *health care rationing could exist*. Who should receive this service? How much? Who should pay? As public policy makers attempt to reduce all care choices to cost-benefit analyses, nurses must see the limitations of these calculations and the inability to account for human pain and suffering mathematically. Third, nurses as well as other health professionals must participate in these ethical decisions or risk loosing their unique influence entirely. For example, in cases of the comatose, terminally ill patient, peer review would focus not only on the clinical aspects of death but also on the human dimension. Did the health care provider confer with the patient and/or family to keep them totally informed? Were the providers guided by the wishes of the patient and family? Did provider seek competent, objective, and relevant third-party opinions?

None of the decisions can be made irrespective of federal or state laws. But there are questions of quality that lie within the realm of quality assurance activity. Besides questions of nontreatment, other *ethical dilemmas* must be recognized, analyzed, and resolved within a quality assurance framework. One approach suggests that decisions themselves are less important than the approach taken by the participants. In analyzing problems did they use accurate and necessary information? Was the reasoning logical? Did the decision maker account for the values and rights of the individual? Use of the systematic quality assurance process has much to offer in this area in the future.

FUTURE CONCERNS

Changes in the health care sector and its financing mechanisms will undoubtedly continue to affect quality assurance activities in the future. There is increasing concern that quality of health care may come second to the concern about the cost of that care. Properly designed and executed quality assurance activities are irreplaceable feedback devices needed to allow nursing to define and describe for physicians, consumers, and other health professionals the efficacy and importance of nursing care in bringing about desired patient outcomes.

CHAPTER SUMMARY

- American society is aging, and the greatest increase is in persons over age 85, called the "old-old."

- Questions are being raised about the ability of a proportionately smaller working population supporting Social Security for the elderly.

- Technologic advances have dramatically changed medical care and driven up costs.

- Ethical problems arise in the use of technologic advances such as organ transplants.

- There has been no decision in the United States how health care is to be financed, especially for those not covered by prepaid hospital insurance.

- The United States is the only industrial society that does not have some form of national health insurance.

- There are many changes in health care delivery. These include Health Maintenance Organizations (HMOs), Diagnostic Related Groups (DRGs), and ambulatory surgery centers.

- For-profit hospitals are increasing in many areas of this country. These hospitals do not provide health care for the medically indigent, whose burden of care falls on public and teaching hospitals.

- Patients are being discharged sooner from the hospital as the result of DRGs and other cost containment measures resulting in an increase need for ambulatory care and home care services.

- Several methods have been used to deliver nursing care in the hospital, including functional, team, and primary nursing.

- Primary nursing, which clearly defines accountability for the care of each primary patient to the assigned primary nurse, requires a greater proportion of RNs.

- Clinical nurse specialists and nurse practitioners are specialized positions in nursing.

- Alternate health care settings such as hospice care are rapidly growing in the United States.

- Health promotion is becoming a major focus of nursing care with individuals expected to assume more responsibility for their own health.

- A major concern to nurses is that the United States is rapidly moving toward two-tier health care system—one for the "haves" and another for the "have nots."

- Collaboration, viewed as a positive move, is increasing between nursing practice and nursing education.

- The increase in "high tech" in hospitals demands an increase in high touch. Nurses are being challenged to provide high touch to patients who are attached to highly complex equipment.

- The demand for nurses continues to increase even though more nurses are employed now than ever before.

- Supply, demand, and wages of nurses are closely interrelated.

- Nursing salaries are competitive at the entry level but do not remain so.

- Prescott suggests that the answer to the supply and demand question can be found in reframing the problem from too few nurses to too little professional nursing practice.

- She suggests that work of nurses has changed, that nurses are misused, that nurses are underused as patient care givers, that nurses are viewed as being interchangeable units, and that nurses are constrained by physicians and hospital policy from making decisions and taking action.

- Nursing schools are changing to reflect the changes in society. This includes assurance that all students are computer literate.

- Some nursing schools are moving the preparation of nursing to the post-baccalaureate level, which is what other professions are (such as pharmacy) choosing to do.

- More attention should be paid to factors that influence the choice of nursing as a profession.

- Nursing's commitment to professional excellence includes monitoring the quality of care given.

- Four factors that have influenced quality assurance in nursing: (1) health care legislation, (2) changes in third-party reimbursement, (3) economic factors, and (4) professional standards.

- The ANA Standards of Nursing Practice include eight standards to be followed by all nurses who provide health care.

- The Joint Commission on the Accreditation of Health Care Organizations (JCAHO) is a voluntary organization that accredits hospitals and other health care organizations. It publishes an Accreditation Manual that includes a standard for quality of professional services. This standard provides the basis for evaluating patient care.

- Outcome criteria pertinent to a specific patient population must be developed as part of the quality assurance process and before an evaluation of the quality of nursing care can be made. Outcome criteria should be measurable in terms of change in health, knowledge, or functional status of the patient.

✔ *Structure criteria* describe the setting and conditions under which the nurse-patient relationship occurs.

✔ *Process criteria* describe the nature and sequence of nursing care activities.

✔ Quality assurance is an ongoing process in which the results of the evaluation of patient care are transmitted to care givers so that needed improvements can be made.

✔ Quality indicators are items that a health care agency believes indicate quality care.

QUESTIONS TO CONSIDER

■ What changes in American society have you seen reflected in the persons you cared for or are caring for?

■ Discuss how you believe money should be allocated for health care in the United States.

■ List some of the positive and negative factors about nursing as a profession that you would discuss with prospective nursing students.

■ Discuss the reasons for the increase in the number of alternative care settings such as ambulatory surgical centers, hospices, and so on.

■ Explain the difference between primary care and primary nursing.

■ Develop a teaching plan for adults who are interested in promoting their own health.

■ List four reasons why a quality assurance program is essential to professional nursing practice.

■ Describe the steps in the ANA quality assurance model.

■ What effect does cost containment have on the quality of health care?

REFERENCES AND SELECTED READINGS

1. *Aiken L: Am Nurs 17:4,18, 1985 (editorial).
2. American Association of Colleges of Nursing: Essentials of college and university education for nursing: a working document, February, 1986, Washington, DC.
3. *American Nurses Association: Standards of nursing practice, Kansas City, Mo, 1973, The Association.
4. American Nurses Association: Quality assurance for nursing care, Kansas City, Mo, 1976, The Association.
5. American Nurses Association: A national policy for health care: principles and positions, Pub no G-130, Kansas City, Mo, 1977, The Association.
6. American Nurses Association: A social policy statement, Kansas City, Mo, 1981, The Association.
7. Anderson EH: Are we giving away the store to home health care agencies? J Prof Nurs 1:319-320, 1985 (editorial).
8. *Andrews LB: Health care providers: the future marketplace and regulations, J Prof Nurs 2:51-63, 1986.
9. *Annas, GJ: Your money or your life: "dumping" uninsured patients from hospital emergency wards, Am J Public Health 76:74-77, 1986.
10. *Benner P: From novice to expert, Menlo Park, Calif, 1984, Addison-Wesley Publishing Co Inc.
11. Betz M: Some hidden costs of primary nursing, Nurs Health Care, 2:150-154, 1981.
12. Bezold C and Carlson R: Nursing in the 21st century: an introduction, J Prof Nurs 2:2-9, 1986.
13. Bezold C and Carlson R: Nursing in the 21st century: conclusion, J Prof Nurs 2:69-71, 1986.
14. *Blake B: Quality assurance: an ethical responsibility, Supervisor Nurs 12:32-38, 1981.
15. *Blendon RJ, Aiken LH, Freeman HE, and Corey CR: Access to medical care for black and white Americans, JAMA 261(2):278-281, Jan 13, 1989.
16. *Booth RZ: Financing mechanisms for health care: impact on nursing services, J Prof Nurs 1:34-40, 1985.
17. *Boufford JI: Public hospital in the changing health system, Am J Public Health 76:12-13, 1986.
18. *Bower-Ferres S: Loeb Center and its philosophy of nursing, Am J Nurs 75:810-815, 1975.
19. *Bradshaw R: The SHMO, Am Nurs 17:5, 16, 1985.
20. Brown M: Multihospital systems in the 80's: the new shape of health care industry, Hospitals 56:71, 1982.
21. *Brown BJ: Quality assurance update. Nurs Admin Quarterly 7(3):1-93, 1983.
22. Bulman T: Ambulatory care: a practical way to quality assurance, Nurs Management 16(12):19-24, 1985.
23. Chapman CB and Talmage JM: The evolution of the right to health concept in th United States, Pharos 34:31-33, 1971.
24. *Chavigny K and Lewis R: Team or primary nursing care? Nurs Outlook 32:322-327, 1984.
25. *Curtin L: Editorial opinion: where will all the money go? Nurs Management 16:7-9, 1985.
26. *Curtis B and Simpson L: Auditing: a method for evaluating quality of care, J Nurs Admin 15(10):14-21, 1985.
27. Deback V: Nursing today and tomorrow: the role of the NC-NIP, Nurs Health Care 7:131-132, 1986.
28. Detmer SS: The future of health care delivery systems and settings, J Prof Nurs 2:20-27, 1986.
29. Donley Sr R: Nursing: 2000, an essay, Image 16:4-6, 1984.
30. *Evans RG et al: Controlling health expenditures—the Canadian reality, N Engl J Med 320(9):571-577, March 2, 1989.
31. Fries JF: The future of disease and treatment: changing health conditions, changing behaviors, and new medical technology, J Prof Nurs 2:10-19, 1986.
32. Ginsberg E: Cost containment—imaginary and real, N Engl J Med 308:1220-1223, 1983.
33. *Ginsberg E: The economics of health care and the future of nursing, J Nurs Adm 11:28-32, 1981.
34. *Griffith H: Who will become the preferred providers? Am J Nurs 85:539-542, 1985.
35. *Harris SH, Krieger SM, and Davis MZ: A problem focused quality assurance program, Nurs Management 20(2):54-60, 1989.
36. Howe M: Developing instruments for measurement of criteria: a clinical nursing perspective, Nurs Res 29:100-103, 1980.

_____

*References preceded by an asterisk are particularly well suited for student reading.

37. Inglehart JK: Health policy report, N Engl J Med 308:976-980, 1983.

38. Inzinga M: Legislative issues and health care trends—quality assurance, Nurs Admin Quarterly—Legislative Update 8:80-85, 1984.

39. *Jaret P: Nurses—the final guardians, Newsweek 104:16, 1984.

40. Jennett B: High technology medicine: how defined and how regarded, Milbank Mem Fund Q 63:141-145, 1985.

41. Joel LA: The economics of health care: trends and problems in the economics of health care and nursing, Am Acad Nurs 7-18, 1985 (keynote address).

42. Joint Commission on Accreditation of Health Care Organizations: Accreditation manual for hospitals, Chicago, 1989, The Commission.

43. Kennedy EM: Congress and the national health policy, Rosenhause lecture, Am J Public Health 68:241-244, 1978.

44. *Kinlein ML: Independent nursing practice with clients, Philadelphia, 1977, JB Lippincott Co.

45. Kotthoff E: Current trends and issues in nursing in the U.S.: the primary health care nurse practitioner, Int Nurs Rev 28:24-28, 1981.

46. *Lane G, Cronin K, and Peirce A: Teaching diploma students how to utilize the ANA quality assurance model, J Nurs Educ 21(9):42-44, 1982.

47. LeRoy L: Continuity in change: power and gender in nursing, J Prof Nurs 2:28-38, 1986.

48. *Lutz EM and Schlotfeldt RM: Pioneering a new approach to professional education, Nurs Outlook 33:139-143, 1985.

49. *Maciorowski L, Larson E, and Keane A: Quality assurance evaluate thyself, J Nurs Admin 15:38-42, 1985.

50. Marram GB, Barrett NW, and Bevis EO: Primary nursing: a model for individualized care, ed 2, St Louis, 1979, The CV Mosby Co.

51. Marriner A: The research process in quality assurance, Am J Nurs 79:2158-2161, 1979.

52. Milio N: The storefront that didn't burn, Ann Arbor, 1970, University of Michigan Press.

53. *Milio N: Telematics in the future of health care delivery: implications for nursing, J Prof Nurs 2:39-50, 1986.

54. *Moccia P and Mason D: Poverty trends: implications for nursing, Nurs Outlook 34:20-24, 1986.

55. Moody LE and Henry BM: Futurist approaches in nursing education, Nurs Economics 4:134-137, 1986.

56. Mullane MK: Classics from our heritage: the nature of the university or college and the mission of the school of nursing, J Prof Nurs 1:315-316, 1985.

57. *Muller C: A window on the past: the position of the client in 20th century public health thought and practice, Am J Public Health 75:470-576, 1985.

58. *Mundinger MO: Health service funding cuts and the declining health of the poor, N Engl J Med 313:113-115, 1985.

59. Naisbitt J: Megatrends, New York, 1982, Warner Books.

60. *National League for Nursing: Developing a national health plan—why now? why nurses? Public Policy Bulletin, Fall 1989.

61. *New NA and New JR: Quality assurance that works, Nurs Management 20(6):21-24, 1989.

62. *O'Koren ML: Reflections on facilitating collaboration between nursing service and nursing education, J Prof Nurs 2:73-74, 1986 (editorial).

63. Olendski MC: Cautionary tales, Wakefield, Mass, 1973, Contemporary Publications.

64. Orem DE: Nursing: concepts of practice, ed 2, New York, 1981, McGraw-Hill Book Co.

65. Ozimek D and Yura H: Who is the nurse practitioner? New York, 1975, National League for Nursing.

66. Paulen A: A time for reassessment, Cancer Nurs 9:2, 1986 (editorial).

67. Perlich LJM: catalyzing educational change, J Nurs Adm 16:6, 1986 (guest editorial).

68. Phaneuf M: The nursing audit, ed 2, New York, 1976, Appleton-Century-Crofts.

69. *Porter P: The changing role of the independent nurse practitioner, Nurs Clin North Am 15:419-428, 1980.

70. *Prescott PA: Shortage of professional nursing practice: a reframing of the shortage problem, Heart Lung 18(5):436-443, Sept, 1989.

71. *Primm PL: Entry into practice: competency statements for BSNs and ADNs, Nurs Outlook, 34:135-137, 1986.

72. Reschak GLC et al: Accounting for nursing costs by DRG, J Nurs Adm 15:15-20, 1985.

73. Rogers ME: Classics from our heritage: the nature and characteristics of professional education for nursing, J Prof Nurs 1:381-383, 1985.

74. Rukeyser L: Home health care booms, Syndicated column, May, 1985.

75. *Sakalys JA and Watson J: Professional education: post-baccalaureate education for professional nursing, J Prof Nurs 2:91-97, 1986.

76. Saltus R: Soaring expenses change the face of the medical care, Boston Globe, special report, June 30, 1985, pp 1,32.

77. Schenk K: Nursing abroad in an undergraduate program, Int Nurs Rev 27:108-111, 1980.

78. *Schlotfeldt RM: Classics from our heritage: a brave, new nursing world: exercising options for the future, J Prof Nurs 1:244-251, 1985.

79. *Schlotfeldt RM: The professional doctorate: rationale and characteristics, Nurs Outlook 26:302-311, 1978.

80. Selby T: Nurses establish clinic for the homeless, Am Nurs 17:1, 20, 1985.

81. Sellick K et al: Primary nursing: an evaluation of its effects on patient perception of care and staff satisfaction, Int J Nurs Stud 20:265-273, 1983.

82. Silver JK, Ford LC, and Stearly SG: A program to increase the care for children: the pediatric nurse practitioner program, Pediatrics 39:756-760, 1967.

83. Smeltzer C, Fettman B, and Rajki K: Nursing quality assurance: a process, not a tool, J Nurs Admin 13(1):5-9, 1983.

84. *Sovie MD et al: Amalgam of nursing acuity, DRGs and costs, Nurs Mgmt 16:22-42, 1985.

85. *Spross J and Hamrick AB: A model for future clinical specialist practice. In Hamrick AG and Spross J, editors: The clinical nurse specialist in theory and practice, New York, 1983, Grune & Stratton Inc.

86. Starr P: Public health, then and now, Am J Public Health 72:77-88, 1982.

87. Stoeckle JD et al: Medical nursing clinic for the chronically ill, Am J Nurs 63:87-89, 1963.

88. *Stull MK: Entry skills for BSNs, Nurs Outlook 34:136, 153, 1986.

89. *Styles MM and Holzemer WL: Educational remapping for a responsible future, J Prof Nurs 2:64-68, 1986.

90. Sultz H, Zielman M, and Matthews J: Highlights, phase 2, longitudinal study of nurse practitioners. In Millman N, editor: Nursing personnel and the changing health care system, Cambridge, Mass, 1978, Ballinger Publishing Co.

91. Suzman R and Riley NW: Introducing the oldest old, Health and society, Milbank Mem Fund Q 63:177-86, 1985.

92. Tanner CA: Research on clinical judgment. In Holzemer W, editor: Review of research in nursing education, Thorofare, NJ, 1983, Slack, Inc.

93. Tarlov AR: The changing structure of the health services system and the future practice of medicine, N Engl J Med 308:1235-1244, 1985.

94. *Thorpe KE, Siegel JE, and Dailey T: Including the poor: the fiscal impacts of Medicaid expansion, JAMA 261(7):1003-1007, Feb 17, 1989.

95. *Thurow LC: Medicine versus economics, N Engl J Med 313:611-614, Sept, 1985.

96. *Tribulski JA: How you can use that federal report on nursing, RN 52:61-67, Feb, 1989.

97. *Vanservellan GN: Primary nursing: variation in practice, J Nurs Adm 11:40-46, 1981.

98. Wandelt M and Slater Stewart D: Slater Nursing Competencies Rating Scale, New York, 1975, Appleton-Century-Crofts.

99. Wellington M: Decentralization: how it affects nurses, Nurs Outlook, 34:36-39, 1986.

100. Westfall UE: Nursing diagnosis: its use in quality assurance, Topics in Clin Nurs 78-87, 1983.

101. Williams CA: The nursing shortage and research opportunities, J Prof Nurs 5(1):5, Jan-Feb, 1989.

102. Zimmer M: Quality assurance for outcomes of patient care, Nurs Clin North Am 9:305-315, 1974.

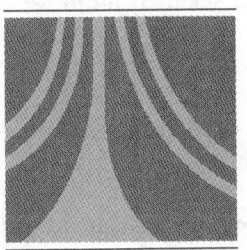

CHAPTER 2

Nursing Care of Ill Adults: Theoretic Perspectives

MARIE L. LOBO

CHAPTER OBJECTIVES

After studying this chapter, the student should be able to:
1. Analyze historical and current conceptual foundations for nursing practice.
2. Compare definitions of nursing, health, person, and environment proposed by contemporary nurse theorists.
3. Examine underlying theoretic assumptions about nursing ill adults.

The practice of modern nursing is based on knowledge of nursing, as well as that of other disciplines such as psychology, biology, physiology, sociology, and philosophy. Within each of these disciplines, including nursing, many different perspectives help predict and explain the phenomena of concern. The discipline of nursing is concerned with human health, including its physical and mental components, and the environments that promote or interfere with health. This chapter will focus on human-environment interactions and the theoretic perspectives that provide structure to examine those interactions that promote an optimum state of well-being in the ill adult.

Through the development of theoretic perspectives, nurse theorists have attempted to provide a structure for guiding the science of nursing care. These perspectives have been presented in a number of books and articles, some of which are referenced at the end of this chapter. The authors of these nursing perspectives provide a developing nursing science some suggestions for organizing the way nurses solve patient care problems. These theoretic perspectives provide a variety of foundations for organizing nursing care, although most reflect core concern for person, environment, nursing, and health. None of the current nursing perspectives accounts for every aspect of the person and the environment in a manner that is useful to the practice of nursing. Therefore it is important for the caregiver to integrate various theoretic perspectives and select the one perspective or combination of perspectives most appropriate for the patient.

The following literature has been developed for several purposes. George's *Nursing Theories: The Base for Professional Nursing Practice*[12] was written to provide beginning students with ready access to information about the theories influencing current nursing practice. Fitzpatrick and Whall,[11] Fawcett,[10] Parse,[42] and Riehl-Sisca[47] take the next step in the presentation of conceptual models of nursing by analyzing the concepts using criteria found in the theory development literature. These texts provide nurses an opportunity to explore in more depth the theories and concepts cited in this chapter.

Since the late 1970s there have been a number of works by nurses to assist nurse researchers, nurse educators, and practicing nurses in understanding the meaning of theory, theory construction, and the use of theoretic perspectives in nursing practice.* Thought-stimulating discussion of concepts and application of theoretic perspectives assist the nurse in providing care to ill adults from a holistic perspective.

HOLISM

According to Webster, holism is a theory that the universe and especially living nature consists of interacting wholes that are more than the mere sum of elementary particles.[64] Murray and Zentner[33] define holism as the view that the individual is a part of all that is within and around him or her and that the individual is more than the sum of the parts. In nursing, holistic care implies nurses consider all aspects of the person, including the family and community, as well as the cells and organ systems, when planning care. For example, when the ill adult is worried about paying the rent to keep the family

---

*References 1-3, 6, 9-24, 26-32, 34-58, 60-63, 66.

housed, it may be difficult to concentrate on learning how to manage a diet for diabetes. The holistic view always considers the individual to be more than the sum of the parts. In providing nursing care from a holistic perspective, the impact of the nurse as a part of the ill person's environment must also be considered.

MAJOR DOMAINS OF NURSING

The major domains of concern in nursing have been identified as person, environment, nursing, and health. These areas of concern cross all patient classification schemes, as well as all environments of care. Major consideration must be given to the treatment of ill adults in a holistic manner, which allows for the impact of the caregiver and environment on ill adults, as well as the impact of the patient on the caregiver and the environment.

As the concepts of person, environment, nursing, and health are reviewed in this chapter, the importance of Nightingale's suggestions for creating a supportive, nurturing environment for the provision of total patient care will become more apparent.[36] The major theorists have based their writings on assumptions about person, environment, nursing, and health. The assumptions made by nurse theorists may be related to assumptions made in other practice disciplines; however, Meleis[32] believes assumptions made by nurse theorists are uniquely interrelated and provide direction for research, practice, theory, and education in the discipline of nursing. Different theorists have different assumptions about the four main concepts, but there are common threads among their writings that assist in guiding nursing practice in a holistic manner.

The concepts most frequently used as the foundation for organizing nursing theories are person, environment, nursing, and health. These concepts are traditionally discussed in the order presented in the previous sentence. However, it is essential that a definition of nursing be identified and agreed upon before addressing the other concepts. Therefore this chapter will address the definition of nursing and how that definition influences nursing care before identifying the information related to person, environment, and health.

NURSING

Nursing is a practice discipline that contains elements of both science and art. According to Donaldson and Crowley[8], a discipline has a unique perspective that defines the limits and nature of its inquiry. To state that nursing is a science implies that nursing has a knowledge base gained through systematic study and practice. Webster[64] defines art as the faculty of carrying out expertly what is planned or devised, the conscious use of skill and creative imagination especially in the pro-

duction of aesthetic objects. Nursing requires the integration of the knowledge from the science and the skill in the expert implementation of the art of nursing therapies. According to Webster[64], therapy is defined as the remedial treatment of a bodily disorder. Therefore nursing therapies can be defined as remedial treatment of human responses to health and illness.

Understanding the current definition of the nursing discipline and the evolution of that definition is needed to practice the art and science of nursing successfully. Two major nursing leaders of the past have defined nursing in ways that are still cited and remain useful in organizing and providing nursing care. First is Nightingale's 1859 definition: nursing is "to put the patient in the best condition for nature to act upon him."[36] Perhaps more important to consider in the high-technology twentieth century are the rarely cited next sentences: "Generally, just the contrary is done. You think fresh air, and quiet and cleanliness extravagant, perhaps dangerous, luxuries, which should be given to the patient only when quite convenient, and medicine the sine qua non, the panacea."[36] As nursing care is provided to ill adults in high-technology environments where windows cannot be opened and noisy alarms abound, consider the quality of the environment provided these patients. Nurses have the power and knowledge to structure the environment in such a manner that it is supportive to their patients, enhancing the ill adult's ability to achieve optimum wellness.

Virginia Henderson also developed a definition of nursing that profoundly affected the practice of nursing. Early in her career Henderson recognized that nursing was different from medicine, and that a clear definition of nursing was needed. By 1960 Henderson had proposed that the "unique function of the nurse is to assist the individual, sick or well, in the performance of those activities contributing to health or its recovery (or to peaceful death) that he would perform unaided if he had the necessary strength, will or knowledge. And to do this in such a way as to help him gain independence as rapidly as possible."[13] This definition assists in identifying the area of practice where nurses can make independent decisions and prescriptions of nursing therapies. The importance of Henderson's perspective of considering the individual's biologic, emotional, social, and spiritual well-being at a time when nursing was often focused on only the biologic response becomes more evident to nurses the longer they are in practice.

Definitions of nursing by Nightingale and Henderson were influential in the development of the American Nurses Association (ANA) definition of nursing published in the pamphlet *Nursing: A Social Policy Statement*.[4] The *Social Policy Statement* defines nursing as "the diagnosis and treatment of human responses to actual or potential health problems."[4] This definition provides nurses the opportunity to consistently define nursing to society, patients, and other health care providers. It is often difficult for nurses to explain what nursing is and what nurses do. The popular image of nursing includes giving baths, measuring vital signs, administering medications, and so forth. The more subtle aspects of nursing are the thinking and decision-making activities that guide nursing therapies. Although critical for patients' well-being, the cognitive aspects of nursing are rarely acknowledged by the patient or other professionals. As nurses explain what the "diagnosis and treatment of human responses" means to patients and families, society will gain a better understanding of the complex nature of nursing care. The explanations of nursing care need to include information about the decision-making process that occurs in the assessment, planning, implementation, and evaluation aspects of nursing therapies.

Meleis[32] has expanded the definition of nursing to "a human science that deals with human and environmental responses or potential responses to health and illness situations."[32] She states the goals of nursing include the mobilization of "human and environmental resources to promote healing, maintain well-being, prevent illness, and promote health." The focus on the human and environmental responses affords the opportunity for a holistic approach to providing nursing care for ill adults. Broadening the focus to the environment allows the nurse to respond to the needs of the patient's family or significant others, as well as the individual patient.

Meleis also reminds the caregiver to consider the therapeutic aspects of nursing care. Nursing therapies are those acts by nurses to intervene with human responses during health or illness. Nursing care has often been provided on an intuitive basis, without considering the scientific rationale behind the nursing action. Because nurses believe that each individual responds in a unique way to an episode of illness, there has been resistance to the use of scientific generalizations to support nursing care. The base of knowledge generated by nursing research is rapidly expanding, and nurses must begin integrating their experiences with the scientific base of knowledge in nursing and related disciplines.

The integration of the environment with the major concepts of nursing is not new. The critical nature of the patient's environment has been noted since Nightingale's *Notes on Nursing* was published in 1859. Nightingale believed the observational power of the nurse was critical in providing optimal levels of nursing care. She also believed the nurse needed to maintain the environment at an optimal level to allow the patient to become well. Today environment remains a central concern to nurses. The environment includes the people, staff, and family, as well as the inanimate or physical aspects surrounding the patient.

PERSON

Among the phenomena of concern to nurses are human responses to actual or potential health problems.[4] To understand human responses implies an understanding of the characteristics of the person who receives nursing care.

The person or client or patient has been described by most of the major nursing theorists. There are essential components of the definitions that bridge the various perspectives. Each person is viewed as unique, with individual responses to actual or potential health problems. In viewing each person as unique, nurses can interpret their therapeutic activities in one of two ways. First, the person is so unique that nursing care must be individualized at the time of contact, without reliance on previous experience or empiric findings. Second, the nurse can view the person as responding to actual or potential health problems and acknowledge that some aspects of those responses will be consistent with experiences of other individuals whose responses have been studied. Knowledge about how individuals have responded to those health problems in the past can influence the therapeutic actions of the nurse. The art of nursing is in the integration of knowledge about the individual patient with the knowledge gained from the scientific study of groups of individuals with the same problem.

Another characteristic of the person that is reflected in nursing literature is the concept of unitary human, or a holistic perspective that embraces the person as a bio-psycho-social being.* Acceptance of these characteristics as an integral component of the person influences the nursing therapies used with the patients. It means nurses must look beyond the organ system or systems that are affected by pathophysiology when developing nursing care strategies for ill adults. Consideration of the psychologic impact of the illness must be given, along with the social implications, such as a decrease in financial resources or inability to manage the stairs in a two-story home.

Although some nursing authors[43,62,63] have attempted to address the issues related to spirituality, the spiritual meaning of an illness to the patient and family is difficult for many nurses to grasp. The meaning of life and death, quality of life, and quality of death relate to the religious upbringing, culture, and past life experiences of each person. Spirituality is more than religion; it embraces other experiences in the individual's life and gives meaning and purpose to that life. Spirituality, then, is an important component in providing nursing care that is sensitive to human responses of the individual who struggles to find answers about the health or illness experience.

---

*References 34, 41, 44, 45, 48, 53-57, 61-63.

Nurses are interested in persons interacting with the environment and in their responses to the environment.* The unique ability of humans to attach meanings to situations and communicate those thoughts is important to consider in providing holistic nursing care. Communication during interactions is the foundation of the nurse-patient relationship. The ability to interact is dynamic, consisting of actions and reactions by both the nurse and the patient.

How nurses view persons interacting with the environment has been discussed in two ways.[42] First is the totality paradigm in which the environment can be manipulated to maintain or promote equilibrium. In this paradigm, reflected in the works of King,[20-24] Orem,[38] and Roy,[54-57] the person is viewed as adapting to the environment. Second is the simultaneity paradigm in which humans and environment are continuously interacting, influencing each other. The whole is always considered as greater than the sum of the parts. The person in the interaction is viewed as being in control of the situation, defining it in a manner most appropriate for himself or herself. In the simultaneity paradigm ill adults ascribe meaning to their illnesses and determine how they will respond to meet the challenge of the illness. The simultaneity paradigm is reflected in the work of Newman,[35] Parse,[41,42] Paterson and Zedrad,[43] Rogers,[48-53] and Watson.[61,62]

The ANA *Social Policy Statement*[4] further defines person to include family and groups. This is particularly important in the care of ill adults. Assumptions are often made that ill adults can adequately make all necessary decisions related to their care. Responses may be blunted by medication, environmental deprivation or overstimulation, and psychologic response to the information about a health problem. Ill adults are a part of a larger system, usually a family, on whom the illness also has an effect. In considering nursing therapies for ill adults, the family's response must also be considered.

The definition of family is also an issue. The traditional view of family as a mother, a father, and 1.8 children does not accurately reflect North American society. In the late twentieth century there are families that include three or four generations, single parents, same-sex partners, or multiple unrelated adults sharing the same home, both with and without children. In the holistic care of ill adults these individuals, whether family or significant others, must be considered important adjuncts in providing nursing therapies that enhance the individual's opportunity for attaining the maximal levels of wellness possible.

Some nurses may question whether they are providing adequate nursing care to families, particularly to families of ill adults. In some environments families are

well integrated into the nursing care of the patient. The reciprocal nature of the ill adult and the family's well-being is acknowledged. Many hospice units are excellent examples of adult care facilities that assist the family in dealing with the approaching death of a family member. Contrast this with an ill adult in an intensive care unit (ICU) where family members are restricted to visits once every 2 or 3 hours for 10 or 15 minutes, the first visit of the day occurring at noon. More information is needed about the effectiveness of nursing therapies that are family centered, versus nursing therapies that are individual focused. Integration of the family into the care of the ill adult may help the ill adult reach an optimum level of wellness. Reaching an optimal level of wellness may mean facilitating a comfortable death.

ENVIRONMENT

Environment is a concept that is well developed in the general systems literature and the nursing literature. Environment is all that surrounds an individual. Yarrow[67] described the environment as containing both animate and inanimate components. Animate components of the environment are the people or animals in the environment who can respond to or initiate interaction with the ill adult. The nurse, the physician, the family, and other visitors are all a part of the ill adult's animate environment. The inanimate components of the environment include the physical aspects of the environment that cannot initiate interaction, such as the bed, the physical surroundings or rooms and halls, and the equipment.

The critical nature of the ill adult's environment was first presented in Nightingale's classic *Notes on Nursing*.[36] Nightingale viewed the environment as those factors exterior to the patient that affect life and development. She focused on noise, light, ventilation, effluvia or odor, and warmth. Although much of her work emphasized the inanimate environment, she also included a chapter entitled "Chattering Hopes and Advices." In this chapter she discussed the impact that comments from visitors and staff can have on the ill person. She described "whispered conversations" by the staff in the patient's room as "absolutely cruel."[36] Nightingale thought this type of noise was stressful to patients as they strained to hear what was being said and that the patient would presume something important was being said about him or her. The importance of whispered and overheard conversations becomes even more critical when a patient's level of consciousness has been altered by pharmacologic agents. Drugs used for sedation may alter a patient's perception of the meaning of a statement.

Although Nightingale uses very tangible examples of the environment, Martha Rogers was very abstract in her conceptualization of the environment. Nonetheless,

_____
*References 23, 34, 36, 38, 39, 41, 43, 45, 48.

she viewed the environment as critical to the patient's well-being. Rogers examines the patterns and rhythms in the environment in the context of a four-dimensional energy field and as a part of the overall system in which the patient exists. For Rogers energy fields signify the dynamic nature of the interaction between person and environment. Four dimensionality characterizes the human environment fields as nonlinear, without spatial or temporal attributes, but representative of the "relative present."[51]

Rogers sees the environment as contiguous and mutually influential with the patient. Parse describes this as the man-environment simultaneity paradigm. Patterns and rhythms that can be addressed in practice include day/night cycling, work patterns, visiting patterns, meal patterns, noise patterns, sleep patterns, and rhythms of the hospital. For example, in teaching hospitals when an influx of residents and medical students makes rounds, the noise and confusion levels on the unit greatly increase. On a unit where the lights are dimmed at a certain time of the evening, the noise level may decrease as the staff uses lower tones of voice and is more careful not to make noise with use of equipment.

The environment can be either supportive or nonsupportive to the well-being of the patient. It is within the domain of nursing to moderate the environment to enhance patients' well-being. Noise, noxious odors, frequently changing caregivers, lack of day/night cycling, denying access to family and friends, and other factors can all be a part of an environment that is nonsupportive to the ill adult. Lack of predictability in the provision of care can also be a part of a nonsupportive environment. It is important for patients to know what to expect in terms of caregiver and treatment patterns and that their needs will be met without undo stress. Fear of the unknown is stressful and can often be alleviated by sharing information about the care environment with the patient.

HEALTH

The concept of health has been defined in many ways. The most basic definition was proposed by Nightingale, who saw health as the state of being free of disease. Others have viewed health as the highest level of functioning possible given the physiologic constraints present,[13] whereas others see it as defined by each individual person as the life experience.* The more complex definitions have been proposed by theorists who emphasize human-environment interaction. Roy views health as a part of a continuum with illness and as adaptation to the bio-psycho-social state.[57] Newman views health as a part of the life process.[35] Others view health as a

part of a dynamic or active life process.[20-24] Use of the term *dynamic* implies that health is an active force in human responses to illness conditions.

The United Nations World Health Organization defines health as a "state of complete physical, mental, and social well-being and not merely the absence of disease." Murray and Zentner define health in a more dynamic manner as "a state of well-being in which the person is able to use purposeful, adaptive responses and processes, physically, mentally, emotionally, spiritually, and socially, in response to internal and external stimuli (stressors) in order to maintain relative stability and comfort and to strive for personal objectives and cultural goals."[33] A major strength of Murray and Zentner's definition of health is that it guides nurses to develop appropriate nursing therapies aimed at the human responses to health and illness.

Health may also be defined as well-being. Woods and associates found that women defined health as an "exuberant well-being."[65] Women included in their aspects of "exuberant well-being" such characteristics as actively reaching one's optimum while feeling good about all aspects of oneself, including being in balance. The terms used by these women are rarely found in professional definitions of health but were critical components of health from the "person" perspective. These findings are supported by the work of Thurkettle[59] who found that men and women defined health as a balance or being in control, having the ability to self-actualize, knowing the risks in their lives, and having a sense of well-being, freedom, and sharing. Nurses working with ill adults can facilitate nursing care by assessing the ill adult's conception of health and using that information to plan care.

HOLISTIC PERSPECTIVE—HISTORICAL

The consideration of the ill individual from a holistic perspective is not a new concept. Both Nightingale and Henderson advocated a holistic perspective of nursing. Other nursing theorists who have supported a holistic perspective of providing nursing care to patients include Orem,[38] Peplau,[45] Rogers,[48] King,[23] Roy,[57] Parse,[41] and Watson.[63] Each of these authors encourages the nurse to consider the patient from a slightly different perspective.

Nightingale[36] observed that symptoms are often the result of impairments in the environment, such as want of fresh air, light, warmth, quiet, or cleanliness in human care. She believed that in a nurturing environment the body could repair itself. Nightingale advocated manipulating the basic environment: providing fresh, odor-free air, pure water, efficient drainage, and cleanliness; eliminating unnecessary noise; and providing variety in colors and forms as a means of stimulating recovery.

---

*References 35, 41-43, 59, 61-63, 65.

She proposed the practice of gathering data about the person by observation. From her point of view, nursing ought to signify the proper use of these factors and the proper selection and administration of diet in which the least amount of energy is expended by the patient.

Henderson[13] advocated holistic care through her 14 components of basic nursing care to help the client perform the tasks that contribute to health or recovery. These include breathing normally, eating and drinking adequately, eliminating body wastes, moving and maintaining desirable posture, and sleeping and resting. In addition, Henderson emphasized selecting suitable clothing, maintaining body temperature within a normal range by adjusting clothing and modifying the environment, keeping the body clean and well groomed and protecting the integument, avoiding dangers in the environment, avoiding injuring others, and communicating with others to express emotions, needs, fears, or opinions. Henderson also emphasized the importance of worshiping according to one's faith; working in such a way that there is a sense of accomplishment; playing or participating in various forms of recreation; learning, discovering, or satisfying the curiosity that leads to normal development and health; and using the available health facilities.[13]

Henderson's perspective on nursing reflects concern for the person's biologic as well as emotional, social, and spiritual well-being. Like Nightingale, she recognized the important influence of the environment on health. Because of the diversity of the components of nursing care, Henderson advocated a solid knowledge base for nurses in the biologic sciences, as well as the social sciences, so that they might assess, plan, implement, and evaluate care. Her framework can guide nursing care with clients at any point on the continuum from health to illness and is particularly useful when the goal for the client is achieving maximal independence or attaining a peaceful death.

HOLISTIC PERSPECTIVE IN MEDICAL SURGICAL NURSING

A holistic perspective in the care of medically or surgically ill adults goes beyond a focus on the body systems involved in the illness. It means taking a bio-psycho-social approach to the individual. It means considering the spiritual meaning of the illness, as well as the impact of cultural and past experiences. It also means considering the family and the physical environment of ill adults as the nursing therapies are developed.

The high-technology environment for nursing practice at the end of the twentieth century can seduce nurses into focusing on the machines and technology in the environment rather than the patient or focusing on the technologic indicators of patient response rather than the actual human responses to the illness experience. Considering ill adults from a holistic perspective means considering their understanding of their illness and their understanding of the complex and often chaotic environments in which they find themselves. As Nightingale advocated, observation of the patient is one of the nurse's most important actions. In the 1800s nurses did not have electronic equipment to observe; they watched the patient. Although watching a monitor can provide valuable information on heart and respiratory rate and central venous pressure, monitors do not provide nurses with the information about the ill adult's emotional response to the illness. The technology cannot substitute for the reassurance given ill adults by the touch of the nurse's hand during assessment and care. If monitors become the primary measure of patient response, a nurse's identification of subtle physiologic changes that precede a major shift in physiologic status, such as the restlessness at the beginning of loss of blood that precedes a drop in blood pressure and increase in heart rate, may not occur until the loss is physiologically significant and the patient's life is in danger. At times, however, the focus on the technology in the environment can be so compelling that it is easy to forget that it is important to also assess the skin and the bedding to make certain the sheets are smooth under the patient's back and a decubitus is not being formed.

In her work on defining the expert practitioner Benner[5] has developed a taxonomy that includes the domains of nursing practice. The roles nurses practice include helping, teaching-coaching, diagnostic and patient-monitoring, effectively managing rapidly changing situations, administering and monitoring therapeutic interventions and regimens, monitoring and ensuring the quality of health care practices, and organizational and work-role competencies. In providing holistic care for ill adults, nurses must execute all of these areas of practice while considering the patient, the family, the influence of the environment, and the impact the nurse has on them. In the exemplars used by Benner,[5] the expert nurse always considered the situation beyond the simple physiologic data available. The ill adult's concerns and behaviors and the physiologic data were integrated with the scientific knowledge base and experience in caring for similar patients to provide holistic care that had the potential for optimal results.

A nurse caring for ill adults must attend to all aspects of the patients' environment. This includes not only the equipment but the family members. Family interaction patterns are established long before the individual becomes ill. Attending to the family's responses to the illness situation will improve the ill adult's response to the illness. Health care institutions are the domain of the nurse and other health care professionals. The strange environment of the hospital with a maze of hallways, complicated equipment, new people, perceived loss of control, and fear of the consequences of the illness can be intimidating to the patient and the family. Their responses to this environment are sometimes overlooked by nurses who are familiar with the hospital environment. In providing holistic care to ill adults, nurses must consider how the patient and environment interact to affect the patient's ability to reach an optimal state of health.

In addition, nurses must interact with the patient and family and consider the impact of the interaction. The focus on the patient's physiologic response to a health condition is critical, particularly in life-threatening situations. However, some of the interventions used with ill children may also be appropriate. Nurses who work with children have long recognized the influence of the environment on the child's well-being. Environments of care have been modified to support optimum well-being in the ill child. Families of children in intensive care are permitted to visit their children on a 24-hour basis. Parents and grandparents are urged to touch and comfort their child or grandchild. Familiar objects from home decrease the stress of being in a strange environment. The positive impact of family members on the child has been well documented. It is not clear, however, that younger family members have a negative impact on the ill adult. If it is helpful for parents to visit a critically ill child, it is probably helpful for children or spouses to visit with their ill adult loved ones. There are no data to support the institutional rules that separate ill patients from their most important supporters, their families. Institutional rules that separate ill adults from their families and care environments structured for the benefit of health care professionals may be providing one-dimensional care that is good for the physiologic condition of the patient but fails to consider the person from a holistic perspective.

One nursing leader, Rogers,[48] has focused on the human-environment interaction in her holistic approach to providing nursing care. One aspect of Rogers' work that is critical is the inclusion of time with the three dimensions of space to create a four-dimensional energy field. Adding the concept of time is particularly meaningful in nursing because human responses to health and illness, nursing therapies, and the human response to nursing therapies occur through time. That is, the effects of nursing therapies on human responses to health and illness states may take some time to become evident. When providing holistic care to ill adults, nurses may not always know when their therapeutic actions will take effect. That is, nurses do not always have a clear understanding of when they will see the outcomes of their therapies. If ill adults are in intensive care unit (ICU) environments where day-night cycling is not practiced and no attempt is made to orient the patients

to day, place, and time, intensive care psychosis or confusion is likely to develop. Nurses using orientation to person, place, and time as a therapy may not know when or if the therapy was effective because the patients are moved out of ICU before they become confused. Nurses who allow family members to visit ill adults, participate in care when appropriate, talk with them about familiar events, and touch them for comfort may not be able to measure the anxiety that was alleviated in patients. At other times, nurses witness immediate results such as sleep after a back rub or a pulse decreasing to normal range after the administration of pain medication. It is important for nurses caring for ill adults to consider the consequences, both short-term and long-term, of the therapies they apply.

CHAPTER SUMMARY

✔ Providing hoslistic care to ill adults is a challenge to nurses.

✔ A major consideration in the provision of holistic care to ill adults is the human-environment interaction.

✔ The interface of patients with the environment is one area in which nursing therapies can influence adults to reach their optimal state of wellness.

✔ Nurses must consider both the animate and inanimate environments.

✔ Nurses control many dimensions of the environment for ill adults and can make it positive by providing care that is sensitive to the whole human being.

✔ The tradition of nursing from the time of Nightingale has been to care for the whole person, a concept that can get lost in the high-technology of the late twentieth century.

✔ Nurses can use aspects of many theoretic perspectives, putting together an eclectic framework that is most appropriate for client-environment situations.

✔ Although there is no theory that applies uniformly in a given situation, there is a base of knowledge in nursing and related disciplines that guides nurses in providing holistic care to ill adults.

QUESTIONS TO CONSIDER

- How do you define nursing? How do you describe the person who is a recipient of nursing care? What is health? What aspects of health receive the most emphasis in hospitals?

- What does the concept *holistic* mean? How could you provide holistic care to an ill person?

- How can the family and friends of ill adults be integrated into the nursing care plan?

- What modifications in the inanimate environment can be made to facilitate holistic care of ill adults?

- How can you assess the ill adult's need for psychosocial interventions in a care environment that emphasizes the physiologic interventions?

REFERENCES AND SELECTED READINGS

1. Abdellah FG et al: New directions in patient-centered nursing, New York, 1973, Macmillan Publishing Co.
2. Abdellah FG and Levine E: Better patient care through nursing research, New York, 1965, Macmillan Publishing Co.
3. Abdellah FG et al: Patient-centered approaches to nursing, New York, 1960, Macmillan Publishing Co.
4. American Nurses Association: Nursing: a social policy statement, Kansas City, Mo, 1980, The Association.
5. *Benner P: From novice to expert: excellence and power in clinical nursing practice, Menlo Park, Calif, 1984, Addison-Wesley Publishing Co Inc.
6. Chinn PL and Jacobs MK: Theory and nursing: a systematic approach, ed 2, St Louis, Mo, 1987, The CV Mosby Co.
7. Clements IW and Roberts FB, editors: Family health: a theoretical approach to nursing care, New York, 1983, John Wiley & Sons Inc.
8. *Donaldson S and Crowley D: The discipline of nursing, Nurs Outlook, 26, 113-120, 1978.
9. Duldt BW and Giffin K: Theoretical perspectives for nursing, Boston, 1985, Little, Brown & Co Inc.
10. *Fawcett J: Analysis and evaluation of conceptual models of nursing, Philadelphia, 1984, FA Davis Co.
11. *Fitzpatrick J, Whall A, and Bowie MD: Conceptual models of nursing: analysis and application, Bowie, MD, 1983, Robert J Brady Co.
12. *George JB, editor: Nursing theories: the base for professional nursing practice, ed 3, Norwalk, CT, 1990, Appleton & Lange.
13. Henderson V and Nite G: Principles and practice of nursing, ed 6, New York, 1978, Macmillan Publishing Co.
14. Henderson V: Basic principles of nursing care, Geneva, 1960, International Council of Nurses.
15. Henderson V: Excellence in nursing, Am J Nurs 69, 2133-2137, 1969.
16. Henderson V: The nature of nursing, Am J Nurs 69, 64-68, 1964.
17. Henderson V: The nature of nursing, New York, 1966, Macmillan Publishing Co.
18. Henderson V: We've come a long way, but what of direction? Nurs Res, 26:163, 1977.
19. Johnson DE: The behavioral system model for nursing. In Riehl JP and Roy C, editors: Conceptual models for nursing practice, ed 2, New York, 1980, Appleton-Century-Crofts.
20. King I: A conceptual frame of reference for nursing, Nurs Res 17:27-31, 1968.
21. King I: Nursing theory—problems and prospect, Nurs Sci 2:394-403, 1964.
22. King IM: A theory for nursing: systems, concepts and processes, New York, 1981, John Wiley & Sons Inc.
23. King IM: King's general systems framework and theory. In Riehl-Sisca JP, editor: Conceptual models for nursing practice, ed 3, Norwalk, Conn, 1989, Appleton & Lange.
24. King IM: Toward a theory for nursing, New York, 1971, John Wiley & Sons Inc.
25. Kopf EW: Florence Nightingale as statistician, Am Stat Assoc, pp. 338-405, 1916.
26. Levine ME: Holistic nursing, Nurs Clin North Am 6:253-264, 1971.
27. Levine ME: Introduction to clinical nursing, ed 2, Philadelphia, 1973, FA Davis Co.
28. Levine ME: The conservation principles: twenty years later. In Riehl-Sisca JP, editor: Conceptual models for nursing practice, ed 3, Norwalk, Conn, 1989, Appleton & Lange.
29. Levine ME: The four conservation principles of nursing, Nurs Forum, 6:45-59, 1967.
30. Levine ME: The pursuit of wholeness, Am J Nurs 69:93-98, 1969.
31. Meleis AI: Theoretical nursing: development and progress, Philadelphia, 1985, JB Lippincott Co.
32. Meleis AI: Theory development and domain concepts. In Moccia P, editor: New approaches to theory development, New York, 1986, National League for Nursing.
33. Murray RB and Zentner JP: Nursing concepts for health promotion, ed 3, Englewood Cliffs, NJ, 1985, Prentice Hall.
34. Neuman B: The Neuman systems model: application to nursing education and practice, New York, 1982, Appleton-Century-Crofts.
35. Newman M: Theory development in nursing, Philadelphia, 1979, FA Davis Co.
36. *Nightingale F: Notes on nursing, Philadelphia, 1859, JB Lippincott Co.
37. The Nursing Development Conference Group: Concept formalization in nursing: process and product, ed 2, Boston, 1979, Little, Brown & Co Inc.
38. Orem DE: Nursing: concepts of practice, ed 2, New York, 1980, McGraw-Hill Inc.
39. Orlando IJ: Behind the theory of nursing practice, Am J Nurs 63:54-55, 1963.
40. Orlando IJ: The dynamic nurse-patient relationship, New York, 1961, GP Putnam's Sons.
41. *Parse RR: Man-living-health: a theory of nursing, New York, 1981, John Wiley & Sons Inc.
42. *Parse RR: Nursing science: major paradigms, theories, and critiques, Philadelphia, 1987, WB Saunders Co.
43. Paterson JG and Zderad LT: Humanistic nursing, New York, 1976, John Wiley & Sons Inc.
44. Peplau HE: Interpersonal relations and the process of adaptation, Nurs Sci, 272-279, 1963.
45. Peplau HE: Interpersonal relations in nursing, New York, 1952, GP Putnam's Sons.
46. Riehl JP and Roy C: Conceptual models for nursing practice, ed 2, New York, 1980, Appleton-Century-Crofts.

*References preceded by an asterisk are particularly well suited for student reading.

47. *Riehl-Sisca JP, editor: Conceptual models for nursing practice, ed 3, Norwalk, Conn, 1989, Appleton & Lange.

48. Rogers ME: An introduction to the theoretical basis of nursing. Philadelphia, 1970, FA Davis Co.

49. Rogers ME: Educational revolution in nursing, New York, 1969, Macmillan Publishing Co.

50. Rogers ME: Nursing: a science of unitary human beings. In Riehl-Sisca JP, editor: Conceptual models for nursing practice, ed 3, Norwalk, Conn, 1989, Appleton & Lange.

51. Rogers ME: Nursing: A science of unitary man. In Riehl JP and Roy C, editors: Conceptual models for nursing practice, ed 2, New York, 1980, Appleton-Century-Crofts.

52. Rogers ME: Reveille in nursing, New York, 1965, FA Davis Co.

53. Rogers ME: Science of unitary human beings. In Malinski V, editor: Explorations in Martha Rogers' science of unitary human beings, New York, 1986, Appleton-Century-Crofts.

54. Roy C and Roberts SL: Theory construction in nursing: an adaptational model, Englewood Cliffs, NJ, 1981, Prentice-Hall.

55. Roy C: Adaptation: a basis for nursing practice, Nurs Outlook, 19:254-257, 1971.

56. Roy C: Introduction to nursing: an adaptation model, Englewood Cliffs, NJ, 1976, Prentice-Hall.

57. Roy C: The Roy adaptation model. In Riehl-Sisca, JP, editor: Conceptual models for nursing practice, ed 3, Norwalk, Conn, 1989, Appleton & Lange.

58. Steven BJ: Nursing theory: analysis, application, evaluation, ed 2, Boston, 1984, Little Brown & Co.

59. Thurkettle MA: Health conceptions among lay persons: a descriptive study. Unpublished dissertation, Cleveland, 1987, Case Western Reserve University.

60. Torres G: The place of concepts and theories within nursing. In George JB, editor: Nursing theories: the base for professional nursing practice, ed 3, Norwalk, CT, 1990, Appleton & Lange.

61. Watson J: Nursing: human science and human care, East Norwalk, Conn, 1985, Appleton-Century-Crofts.

62. Watson J: Nursing: The philosophy and science of caring. Boston, 1979, Little, Brown & Co.

63. Watson J: Watson's philosophy and theory of human caring in nursing. In Riehl-Sisca JP, editor: Conceptual models for nursing practice, ed 3, Norwalk, Conn, 1989, Appleton & Lange.

64. Webster's New Collegiate Dictionary, Springfield, Mass, 1974, G & C Miriam Company.

65. Woods NF et al: Being healthy: women's images, ANS, 11:36-44, 1988.

66. Wooldridge PJ et al: Behavioral science and nursing theory, St Louis, 1983, The CV Mosby Co.

67. Yarrow L: Conceptualizing the early environment. In Dittman L, editor: Early child care, New York, 1968, Atherton Press.

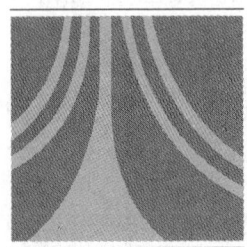

CHAPTER 3

Health and Illness: The Human Experience

GRETCHEN KRAMER DERY LONGENECKER
NANCY FUGATE WOODS

CHAPTER OBJECTIVES

After studying this chapter, the student should be able to:
1. Analyze conceptions of health, illness, and disease from the perspectives of patients and health professionals.
2. Analyze health-related behavior using models of health behavior, illness behavior, and sick role behavior.
3. Critically appraise the utility of the health belief model, health promotion model, at-risk behavior, sick role, and illness behavior on the basis of clinical experience.

PERSPECTIVES OF HEALTH, DISEASE, AND ILLNESS

Lay persons and health professionals alike have notions of health, illness, and disease that guide their behavior.[58] In some instances, the lay and professional definitions vary significantly, which leads to difficulty in communication between the professional who desires to deliver acceptable health care and the lay person who desires to receive health care.[68,94]

HEALTH

Professionals dealing with health and illness care have chosen varying ways of describing health and illness, and these definitions are now guiding these professionals' practice. Health can be defined and categorized according to four basic models: the clinical model, the adaptive model, the role performance model, and the eudaemonistic model.[106]

The clinical model defines health as the absence of disease or of aberrant functioning. Health or normality is identified by the absence of abnormal signs and symptoms as delineated by medical science. Thus health becomes a negative concept, the absence of disease.

The adaptive model of health defines the healthy state as one of stability. The stable and therefore healthy individual is one who can react, accommodate, and adjust to the various stressors in the internal and external environment. The stability-based model derives from the physiologic concepts of homeostasis and adaptation and assumes an environment that is hostile to human existence.

The role performance model describes health as individuals' ability to effectively perform the roles and tasks for which they have been socialized.[87] Health according to this model is a relativistic concept, based on current descriptions of social norms. Norms of health are constructed ranges of variation that fluctuate according to current social approval.[10]

The eudaemonistic model defines health as exuberant well-being, fulfillment, enthusiasm, meaningful interaction with the living and nonliving environment, and self-determined growth. Explanations of health that could be classified according to this model are process oriented, since the ultimate goal of perfect health is ideal.[106]

Each of the above models of health have served in the past as useful paradigms on which nursing and other health and illness care professionals have based their practice. The four models are not mutually exclusive, and each contains within its formulation limitations of description and measurement.

Lay definitions of health reflect both positive and negative aspects. Three orientations to health include:
1. The feeling-state orientation, described as "feeling good"
2. The symptom orientation, characterized by lack of general or specific symptoms of disease
3. The performance orientation, defined as activities that a person who is healthy should be able to perform

Recent evidence suggests that women who were not health professionals provided descriptors of health that spanned the four models of health described earlier. In

RESEARCH

Woods N et al: Being healthy: women's images, Adv Nurs Sci 11(1):36-46, 1988.

Over 500 women residing in a large metropolitan area participated in a women's health survey and responded to the question, "What does being healthy mean to you?" They identified over 100 different meanings that confirmed the importance of the clinical, role performance, adaptive, and eudaemonistic dimensions of health. In addition, they identified several different categories of the eudaemonistic model:

actualization of the self—reaching one's optimum, achieving one's goals

practicing healthy lifeways —taking action to promote health or to prevent disease

positive self-concept—feeling good about oneself; having a positive sense of one's worth

positive body image—feeling good about one's body and appearance

social involvement—ability to interact, love, care, and enjoy relationship through both giving and receiving pleasure

fitness—feeling strong, energetic, and in good shape and having stamina

cognitive function—thinking rationally, being creative, having many interests, feeling alert and inquisitive

positive mood—feeling positive affect, such as happiness, joy, affection, excitement, and exhilaration

harmony—feeling spiritually whole, centered, in balance, and content ∎

addition to the clinical, role performance, and adaptive models of health, women described multiple dimensions of a eudaemonistic conception of health.[121] (See the box above.)

DISEASE AND ILLNESS

The medical-clinical orientation defines disease as objective, observable, and quantifiable. Disease involves change in the structure or function of the body or mind of the human organism. A knowledge of anatomy and physiology is essential for studying disease. Objective changes in structure and function are called *signs* of disease. Although the medical profession also looks at subjective information concerning disease, this type of data is often considered as a secondary source for diagnosis. Subjective information about disease is called *symptoms* and includes reports such as perception of pain, anxiety, and nausea. Such perceptions are difficult to quantify and tend to be influenced by a variety of factors, which are not necessarily directly related to the disease process. Thus some professionals believe that subjective reports provide less reliable diagnostic information than objective signs. The signs and symptoms of certain diseases tend to recur among geographic, cul-

tural, social, and socioeconomic populations. The frequent recurrence of combinations of signs and symptoms is labeled a clinical *syndrome*. There are, in addition to signs and symptoms, other characteristics of disease, including incidence, onset, course, prognosis, duration, and communicability.[122] *Incidence,* or frequency with which the disease occurs (or more accurately, is diagnosed), results in such labels as "common childhood diseases" and the "common cold" versus such entities as "rare blood dyscrasias." The *onset,* or beginning appearance of signs and symptoms, can be insidious, obvious, gradual, or rapid. The *course,* or path, may be smooth, rough, predictable, or unpredictable. The *prognosis,* or ultimate outcome, can be hopeful or guarded or can range from poor to excellent. The *duration,* or length, can be short, long, or permanent. *Acute* and *chronic* are words frequently used to describe duration but have such a diversity of interpretation that there is little universal agreement on their precise meaning. "Chronic" is generally applied to diseases of a long-term nature. *Communicability* refers to the contagious or transmissible quality of a disease. Contrasting examples of communicability are gastric ulcer and sexually transmitted diseases (STD), the former being noncommunicable and the latter considered highly communicable.

The terms *disease* and *illness* are commonly used interchangeably by the medical profession, which adds confusion to the attempts to clarify the concepts. The medical definition of disease remains inadequate and essentially conceptually undefined, because there exists a comfortable delusion that everyone knows what it is.[9]

The person experiencing a disease regards it from a completely different framework than does the professional treating the disease. Whereas the medical diagnostician considers disease in terms of medical knowledge and objectively evaluates the meaning of signs and symptoms, the lay person generally tends to perceive disease from a subjective, personalized, and *phenomenologic* framework. That is, the lay person perceives the illness in terms of its meaning to that particular individual.

In a study of lay perceptions of illness, researchers have tried to determine at what point health problems are considered illness by lay persons. The findings suggested that for middle-class Americans, being ill meant *having an ailment of recent origin that interfered with one's usual activities.* Interference with usual activities seemed to be the most important criterion lay persons applied to the definition of illness.[6] Another study revealed that lay persons often perceived disease as *an object or thing that invaded the body.* These individuals regularly referred to a wide spectrum of diseases as objects, that is, invading and foreign "its." They impersonalized both the symptoms and organs involved through the use of depersonalized language.[24]

Illness has been viewed by the lay person at times as a metaphor, especially illness caused by diseases that are overlaid with mystification and wrapped in an aura of inescapable fatality.[107] Persons afflicted with such illnesses provoke dread and social ostracism. Today cancer qualifies as a metaphorical disease, possessing both mythology and mystique. The lay person views cancer as the supreme body insult because the body devours itself through the metastatic process.

Disease can occur in an individual without the person's awareness of illness and without others perceiving illness. On the other hand, a person can feel very ill even though no pathologic processes can be identified.[29]

RELATIONSHIPS BETWEEN HEALTH AND ILLNESS

The most pervasively held definitions of health and disease view them in relationship as two parts of the same phenomenon. Health and disease are presented as opposite ends of a single linear continuum, with death t one end and health at the opposite end.[45,56,115] As refinements have developed in the description of the health-illness continuum, new areas have been defined along the continuum to further describe and clarify where an individual might be placed.[119]

Currently, there are descriptions of this linear continuum that progress from the negative end with death, to disease/illness, toward an area described as neutral health, toward an area of wellness and ending with an area of high-level wellness. Although this view has provided guidance for all professionals, it contains inherent contradictions. It has been suggested that there is health even in illness and death.

One approach that has been suggested to avoid the continuum of death and wellness is to view health as the synthesis of disease and nondisease. In this view health encompasses conditions previously categorized as illness or disease. Health is a totality of life processes, and disease becomes one meaningful aspect of life.[84]

Recently there have been suggestions that confusion will continue to proliferate if health and illness are seen as one phenomenon. It has been suggested that health and illness are qualitatively different and should be studied as separate but related phenomena.[62,84,93] Health and illness can be viewed as falling on separate continua. This approach fosters clearer operational definitions of health and illness and permits nurses to promote health in individuals who are very ill.

CONCEPTS OF HEALTH

Although much of the nursing and medical literature describes disease and illness, increased attention is being devoted to health. Two contemporary concepts of health are Maslow's hierarchy of needs and Dunn's concept of high-level wellness.

MASLOW'S HIERARCHY OF NEEDS

Maslow[69] describes a hierarchy of needs in which the physiologic needs are considered as most basic, followed by safety, love, esteem, and self-actualization needs. A need that is not satisfied constitutes a motivating factor for an individual.

Needs are generally more unconscious than conscious. Basic needs are not seen as being exclusive determinants of behavior(s), since almost all behaviors have social, cultural, and biologic motivations. Any particular behavioral incident is more likely to be influenced by all the needs in varying degrees than by a single need.

It is necessary to recognize that for most people the needs in the hierarchy exist simultaneously and in differing degrees and that new needs emerge not suddenly but very gradually. At varying times an individual will have different amounts of various needs being met. Lower-level needs do not need to be met *completely* before higher level needs can emerge. Maslow suggests that the degree of need satisfaction is positively related to mental health and that, theoretically, total need gratification and ideal health are synonymous.

PHYSIOLOGIC NEEDS

Physiologic needs include hunger, thirst, sleep, and rest. Totally deprived human beings would generally find the physiologic needs to be their major motivating force. All other needs would be pushed into the background or cease to exist for those persons. However, once physiologic needs are satisfied, the higher-level needs begin to emerge; and when they are satisfied, new and still higher-level needs are manifested.

SAFETY NEEDS

Safety needs are the second level of needs. For the majority of citizens of developed countries, these are not the prime motivators of human behavior. Societies usually succeed in protecting their members from extremes in temperature and from such forms of aggression as assault, murder, and tyranny. In the lower socioeconomic groups of these same societies it is possible that safety needs may not be met and that these safety needs may become the prime motivators of behavior within these segments of the society. In general, however, safety needs are seen as prime motivators only in times of national, natural, or personal crises (for example, war, natural disasters, and illness). When safety needs are satisfied, the need for love and belonging emerges.

LOVE AND BELONGING NEEDS

Love is associated not only with sexual behavior, but also with a desire for affectionate relationships with people in general. Deprivation of love and belonging needs is believed to cause the basic maladjustment seen in the more severe psychopathologies, whereas less severe thwarting of these needs is seen among those who are lonely.

ESTEEM NEEDS

The need for esteem consists of two subsets. The first includes a desire for strength, achievement, adequacy, mastery, competence, and independence. The second subset is geared toward reputation or prestige entities received from others such as status dominance, recognition, attention, importance, and appreciation. Thwarting of these needs produces negative feelings such as inferiority, weakness, and helplessness. Satisfaction of self-esteem needs leads to positive feelings of being useful and necessary in the world.

SELF-ACTUALIZATION NEED

The need for self-actualization is the highest need and describes persons continually moving toward achieving their potential. Few persons achieve self-actualization, a need more commonly met during the mature years.

Although there is generally a progression in the hierarchy of needs, it is not a rigid scheme of classification. A person who has had basic needs satisfied for a consistent period throughout life demonstrates ability to withstand the thwarting of needs. However, a person's aspiration level may be permanently lowered by consistent deprivation; for example, chronically unemployed persons may be totally satisfied as long as they have enough food, and they may cease to strive for more than that. When a need has been long satisfied and then is deprived, its importance may be underevaluated. For example, many people who have met their physiologic and higher needs throughout life may find the fact that

RESEARCH

Laffrey S: Health behavior choice as related to self-actualization and health conception, W J Nurs Res 7:297-300, 1985.

The relationship between self-actualization, health conception, and health behavior choice was examined in 95 white adults 18 to 69 years of age. The Health Conception Measure was based on four health concepts: clinical, role performance/functional, adaptive, and eudaemonistic views of health. The Health Behavior Choice Scale required participants to select a response describing their reason for participating in a health behavior that could include promotion/prevention, promotion/maintenance, or prevention/maintenance. Self-actualization was related to neither health conceptions nor health behavior choice. Health conceptions and health behavior choice were significantly related, so that persons with a more complex health conception selected more health-promoting behavior choices than persons with less complex health conceptions. Conceptions of health appear to be important in determining individuals' reasons for performing health behaviors. ■

they presently have only one meal a day *not* a potent motivator. Such a situation can frequently be observed among our aged population today.

DUNN'S HIGH-LEVEL WELLNESS

Dunn[43] describes high-level wellness in relation to the individual, family, community, environment, and society. Individual high-level wellness is described as integrated functioning oriented toward maximizing individual potential while maintaining balance and purposeful direction in the environment. It includes three components: an upward and forward direction toward higher functional potential; an open-ended future containing challenges to achieve higher potential; and an integrated being, that is, body-mind-spirit participating in the functioning process.[43] Wellness is differentiated from good health. "Good health" is viewed as a relatively passive state of freedom from illness.[7] In fact, in the United States, "normal health" is seen as a sorry state of existence.[45]

NATURE OF PEOPLE

Dunn's view of wellness is based on a philosophy of the nature of people that includes the following five aspects. First, each individual functions as a *total personality*. Next, each person possesses enormous *dynamic energy*. Third, each person has and must maintain *peace with inner and outer worlds*. Fourth, each person has a *relationship* between *energy use* and *self-integration,* when self-integration is defined as the interweaving of all the known aspects of life. Finally, each individual possesses an *inner* and an *outer world*. The inner world can be described as each and every body cell composing an organized whole. The outer world refers simply to the individual's environment with all its components. A person must find his or her being and belonging in both worlds. Questions to be explored are: "What and why am I?" and "Where am I going?"

Dunn maintains that humans have the capacity to recognize certain *processes* that help provide them with the answers to the above questions. These processes are being, belonging, becoming, and befitting. In *being,* one can recognize oneself after the neonatal period as something separate and distinct from the rest of the world. Additionally, if one is a separate part, there must be a whole to which one *belongs*. People grow and develop in all spheres of their being; that is, they are *becoming*. As people grow and become, they individually and selectively make choices; that is, they *befit* themselves for the future.

CELLULAR COMMONWEALTH

From a physiologic standpoint, a person is composed of a cellular commonwealth organized into systems. The optimal functioning of the cellular commonwealth is an essential component of wellness. Each of the body's cells is seen as a unique totality, is made of energy, has an inner and outer world, and is an open system. Protoplasm, the main constituent of cells, has six qualities, which then become qualities of each cell. These qualities or functions are:

Irritability: the ability to attract or repel

Mobility: the ability to move about, sacrificed by some cells in the name of organization and cooperation

Metabolism: the ability to perform chemically

Growth and reproduction: the abilities to expand and replicate

Adaptability: the ability to be interdependent and to maintain an organized whole

Systems have several functions to perform if the cellular needs are to be met, including keeping ports of entry and exit open, transforming energy and waste, growing, reproducing, and problem solving (including the storage, integration, and use of information). The overall function served by the commonwealth of cells is maintenance of unity.

THE MIND AND PROBLEM SOLVING

The *mind,* called the emergent mind because of its developing state, is characterized by its potential for problem solving in daily living. The mind's total functioning is not yet fully understood. Problem solving, its chief function, involves eight components: communication, storage, values, imagination, concept of self, integration of self, maturity in wholeness, and purpose.

High-level wellness cannot exist without *communication* and freedom to pick and choose solutions. One of society's greatest crimes against a person is constriction of channels of communication so that the individual cannot problem solve.

Three types of *storage mechanisms* exist for people: memory stored in the nervous system, memory stored in muscles as tension patterns, and chemical memory of cells. Dunn believes that pain and fear can be locked into body tissues and can constitute an ongoing source of increasing tension. Trapped physical pain can raise tension and prevent tissue healing; trapped emotional pain can prolong grieving. For the storage mechanism to function, access to data must be maintained. Blocked accesses must be cleared. Long-standing barriers may require psychotherapy or other therapeutic measures. New blocks caused by recent physical or emotional pain can be diminished or dispersed through discussion and sharing.

Values are essential problem-solving components because they provide a means for selection of options and decision making. The ultimate goal of people can be seen as seeking enhancement of the value attributes or experiences.

Imagination refers to mental synthesis of new ideas from elements experienced separately and appears to be a uniquely human phenomenon. Imagination helps people see alternatives; for example, when problems arise, the mind perceives similarity to situations previously encountered, and possible solutions are postulated with freedom of choice. Creative imagination is one part of the problem-solving process whereby people can explore their futures and maximize their potential to reach high-level wellness.

The "self" in the problem-solving process provides the reason for choosing. Although the *self-concept,* or how we see ourselves, tends to be rigid, every "self" is continually changing. If one does not periodically bring the "self" and the self-concept into the focus, the "self" idea of oneself may become less and less reality oriented. Self-fulfillment and satisfaction come from what one is, not what one was. Health requires that one be capable of facing the facts about one's self.

Integration of self is the sixth component of problem solving. Integration of body-mind-spirit is more feasible when body and mind are in balance. Rest, sleep, relaxation, and leisure are necessary for body-mind-spirit balance. Mental health, physical health, spiritual health, and social health are possible only when there is balance between the interacting and integrated energy fields of the body-mind-spirit and the environment.

Maturity in wholeness is related to how the body-mind-spirit grows. It is not an end point but varies at different points in the life cycle. The principal expressions of maturity in wholeness lie in the development of conceptual thought, formation of knowledge, self-integration, group integration, and development of purpose. Maturity in wholeness involves understanding of and harmony between the individual and others.

The final component of the problem-solving mechanism is *purpose.* It is in the pursuit of purpose that humans boldly attempt to solve complex problems.

FAMILY, COMMUNITY, AND SOCIAL HIGH-LEVEL WELLNESS

To this point high-level wellness has been discussed in relation to the individual. The concept is easily applied to groups. The family is an essential group in our society that fulfills several functions: reproduction, rearing of children, and provision of an emotional setting for the stabilization of the adult personality. Family wellness is reflected in the degree to which the family unit succeeds in providing security for all members; love characterized by caring, responsibility, knowledge of other family members, and shared values; a future with the opportunity to develop to full potential; and integration so that problem solving can be done in unity.

Community wellness does not involve only good sanitation, water supply, living space, lack of crime, or sound businesses but might include concern for beauty and wildlife, an environment conducive to interchange between generations, and decentralization of industry to decrease long commuting hours. *High-level environmental wellness* includes more than absence of air, water, and noise pollution; it assumes people's cooperation with nature.

Social wellness involves a forward direction in *progress,* an open-ended expanding future, and the integration of the society into a total personality. Dunn maintains that societies would benefit from learning to fight *for* things and not against them and that problems must be dealt with on a world basis, for there is no possible unilateral human survival.

Other authors have elaborated on Dunn's concept of high-level wellness.[15,91,96] The concept of high-level wellness can be applied by health professionals, especially nurses, as they begin to focus attention on the wellness of people rather than focusing exclusively on sickness.[40,55,87] To shift the emphasis in this fashion, wellness needs to be viewed not as a simple category or static entity but as a dynamic process.

Dunn[44] suggested the following nine specific areas for future wellness research:

1. Methods for improving family and community living
2. Methods for teaching wisdom as well as knowledge
3. Methods for developing and adjusting in human relationships
4. Methods for cultivating high-level wellness in those having leadership positions
5. Methods for developing and maintaining open communication and access to knowledge
6. Methods to enhance the importance of creative expression
7. Methods to continue to make clear the importance of altruistic expression
8. Methods for continued development of the concept of maturity
9. Methods for extending the current life span coupled with opportunities for fully matured persons who have achieved high-level wellness to contribute to society

An acceptance of the holistic approach outlined in this chapter will not allow the nurse-patient relationship to be superficial. It will not be sufficient to know only the name and health care need of the person to be served. A functional relationship will be replaced by one of care and concern for the total person, incorporating full consideration of both inner and outer worlds.[18,51,48]

BEHAVIOR IN HEALTH AND ILLNESS

Health and illness are usually considered from their clinical perspectives, but it is the social system perspective that has provided practitioners with a wealth of insight into the behavioral aspects of health and illness. Social scientists have examined health and illness in terms of the statuses and roles involved. *Status* refers to the position that could be occupied by members of a society, and *roles* are behaviors of persons who fill a particular status. The individuals of a particular social system share certain common expectations about how people of a specific status should behave in the performance of their roles. These expectations, called *role expectations,* are different for each status. All of these expectations together form the normative framework of a social system. The *norms* outline the expected behaviors for a status. These norms may impose a behavior as obligatory, may prohibit a behavior, or may allow the individual a choice about certain optional behaviors.[61,74] A summary of the models of human behavior in health and illness roles follows.

HEALTH BEHAVIOR

Health behavior has been generally defined as any activity undertaken by well persons to promote health or to prevent or detect disease.

Recent attempts have been made to clarify definitions by separating health-promoting behavior from disease-preventing behavior.[23] Health-promoting behaviors are defined as those behaviors that are geared toward sustaining or increasing the level of well-being, self-actualization, or personal fulfillment of the person or group. Health-protecting behaviors are defined as behaviors directed toward decreasing the probability of encountering illness by actively protecting the body against unnecessary stressors or detecting illness at an early stage.[93]

CATEGORIES OF HEALTH BEHAVIOR

Health behaviors can be classified into three general categories: behavior geared toward the individual's health, health behavior related to the source and utilization of health care, and individual health behavior in relation to the larger community and health care system as a whole. Each of the three categories describes behaviors geared toward health protection and health promotion.

The first category, *behaviors geared toward the individual's health,* is admittedly very broad and in need of further research.[17] Promotive behaviors include eating a well-balanced diet, obtaining proper rest, participating in a daily exercise program, and avoiding risk-taking behaviors, such as smoking. Some protective behaviors in this category could include monthly self-examination of the breasts by women, taking one's temperature, and a host of other activities.

The second category, *health behavior related to the source and utilization of health care,* has received a great deal of study.[57] Protective behaviors in this category include such activities as receiving immunizations, seeking information about health problems such as warning signals of cancer, getting fluoride treatment for teeth, seeking routine screening of vision and hearing, Pap smears, physical examinations, and chest x-ray film studies.

The third category, *individual health behavior in relation to the larger community and health care system as a whole,* has received comparatively little attention. These behaviors might include individual involvement in health legislation, service as a volunteer in health programs, financial support of health organizations, and voting on health proposals. Understanding that health-promoting and health-protecting behaviors can influence health status and influencing such behaviors are appropriate goals for nursing and other health care professionals.[18,56,115]

HEALTH BELIEF MODEL

One widely used model for explaining health behavior is the health belief model (Figure 3-1). The health belief model was designed to explain the widespread failure of people to accept low-cost or free health screening and detection measures for asymptomatic disease.

Health behavior, viewed from the perspective of this model, includes health-protecting as well as health-promoting behaviors, and these behaviors are influenced by individual perceptions about the threat of the disease; modifying factors, including demographic variables and cues to action; and the likelihood of action. Recently self-efficacy has been added to the health belief model. Self-efficacy refers to the belief that one is personally capable of adopting the new behavior.[101]

Individual Perceptions

The perceived threat of disease results from two factors: perceived susceptibility and perceived seriousness. *Perceived susceptibility* is the extent to which individuals feel threatened with contraction of a disease. The perceived threat, or the person's sense of vulnerability, has been demonstrated to be the single best predictor of health utilization behaviors in selected settings.[64] Since this is a phenomenologic or subjective assessment, the individual's perception of risk may be similar to or vary widely from the perception of a health professional. Perceived susceptibility could conceivably range from being very afraid one will contract a certain condition to complete denial of any risk and feelings of invulnerability. Persons who smoke two packages of cigarettes each day may see themselves as highly susceptible to lung cancer or they may deny the risk of contracting the disease.

Perceived *seriousness,* the second factor making up the perceived threat, can be viewed from two perspectives: inherent seriousness and impact on one's lifestyle. A disease such as a brain tumor may be seen as

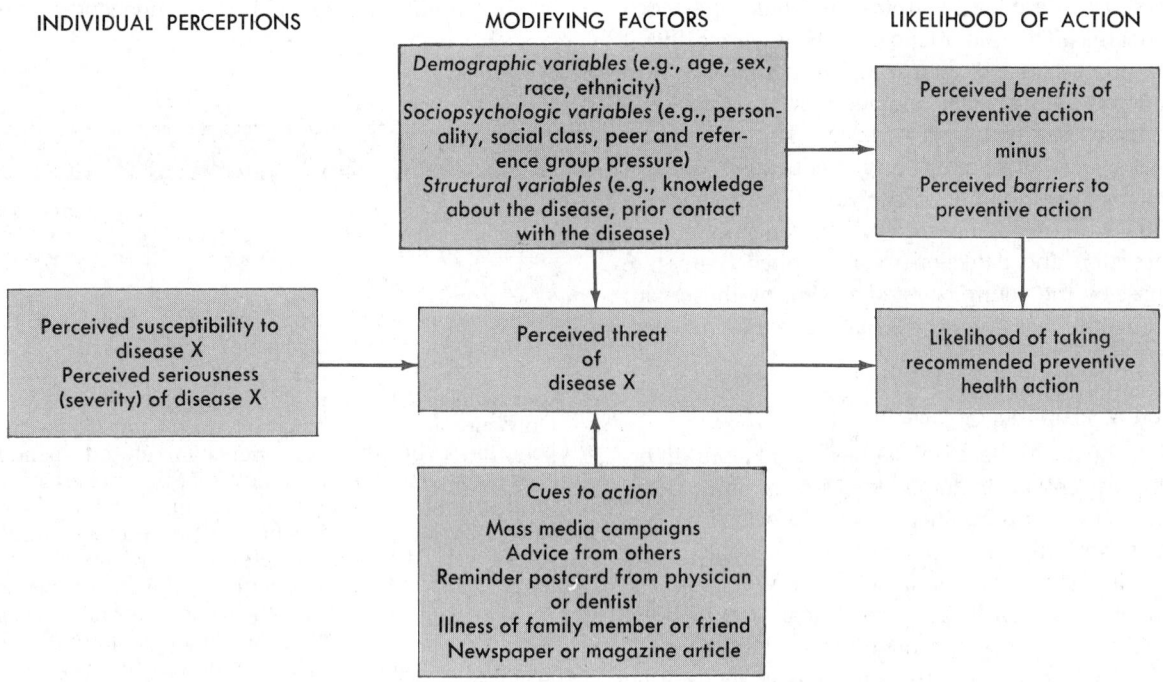

FIGURE 3-1 Health belief model. (From Becker MH, Drachman RH, and Kirscht J: Am J Public Health 64:205-216, 1974.)

inherently serious inasmuch as the disease process could lead to extensive physical disability or death. The impact of this disease on the person's life-style may also be judged as quite serious inasmuch as it can necessitate drastic adjustments in employment, function, and ability to care for oneself. Perceived seriousness is calculated on the basis of knowledge about a particular condition and constitutes a force leading to action. The actual performance of a particular recommended action is further influenced by two factors: the individual's conviction that performing the health behavior will prevent or modify the disease, and the person's perception of the unpleasantness or cost of performing the health behavior as compared with taking no action. These two factors can be combined in several ways, providing a large range of resultant behaviors.

Modifying Factors and Likelihood of Action

Even though the *perceived threat of the disease* and the *perceived value of the action* are both high, it is possible that the individual involved may elect to engage in no health behavior at all. Cues seem to be necessary to initiate health behavior. These cues are most likely to be external and may take a wide variety of forms such as a discussion with a friend, a television or newspaper message, or a postcard reminder from the dentist.

People are thought to vary in their susceptibility to cues.[100] In a situation where the perceived value of action and the perceived threat are high, a weak cue may be effective in eliciting health behavior. In another situation where the perceived value of the action and the perceived threat are low, a strong cue would be needed to be effective. The role of cues has been very difficult to determine because of their transient nature.

Other modifying factors include demographic, sociopsychologic, and structural variables. Thus such variables as sex, age, race, ethnic origin, education, occupation, income, and amount of knowledge are considered influential in health behavior.[1,22,96] In general, services for prevention and detection in the United States are used most by the young or middle aged, by those with higher income and greater formal education, and by whites.[99]

Appraisal of Health Belief Model

Although the health belief model has been helpful in organizing prevention programs, it has some limitations. First, it focuses on preventive services provided by professionals, yet only 6% to 30% of health problems receive medical attention, with the majority of problems being handled by self or home treatment, lay consultation, or consultation with a nonorthodox health practitioner.[37] Because the health belief model focuses on perceived threat of disease, it is more applicable for the study of preventative or health-protecting behavior than

for that of health-promoting behavior. It does not attempt to account for achieving higher levels of health.

The model is supposedly applied in situations where the behavior is purely voluntary and the individuals are symptom free, yet much of health behavior is a result of social pressure, legal compulsion, and job requirements.[98] It is conceivable that only a small proportion of the population presently takes voluntary health action to detect or prevent disease in the absence of symptoms. Careful study of those who do could lead to a broader understanding of health behavior. Looking at how people utilize preventive or detection health services does not explain *why* they use such services. Little is known about the stability of health beliefs over time or about the acquisition of health beliefs. There may be different patterns of behavior for beliefs established early in life versus those established later in life.[14,65,75]

Other research has suggested that health behaviors, no matter how well described and analyzed, might in fact *not* be predictably related to the impetus to seek preventive or diagnostic services.[41] Several items are thought to be significant other than as modifying factors for preventive and promotive health behaviors. Gender, socioeconomic status, and life-style are factors known to influence health behaviors.[19,83] Questions are being asked relative to the interrelationships among preventive and promotive behaviors. Is health behavior unidimensional; that is, are people consistent across health behaviors? Are people who use seat belts the same ones who obtain medical checkups, get preventive dental care, and engage in regular exercise? Or are health behaviors multidimensional; that is, independent and to-

RESEARCH

Murdaugh C and Hinshaw A: Theoretical model testing to identify personality variables effecting preventive behaviors, Nurs Res 35:19-23, 1986.

The impact of perceived barriers and benefits to preventive behaviors and health value orientations were tested on two health behaviors—smoking and exercise—in 76 persons who had taken part in a health screening program. Only one variable was important in accounting for smoking behavior, a health value orientation toward spontaneous expression of impulses and desires. Six variables accounted for the number of miles exercised, including several health values, barriers, and benefits. People who perceived barriers as well as benefits to preventive behavior were more likely to have a future orientation and were inclined toward spontaneous expression of their impulses and desires. People who were collateral or group oriented, present oriented, and whose health values focused on being-in-becoming (a developmental orientation) were also more likely to have exercised more. ■

tally unrelated to each other? Or are there differing patterns of behavior; that is, are some people consistent in a variety of health behaviors whereas other people are inconsistent? Or are some behaviors performed consistently and others inconsistently; that is, preventive versus promotive behaviors? In response to these and other questions, additional suggestions for the revision of the health belief model continue to appear.[63,77,78,92,93]

HEALTH PROMOTION MODEL

Pender[92,93] has proposed a health promotion model to provide a framework for the study of health-promoting behavior in adults.[73] The health promotion model is based on previous work done with the health belief model, but the central orientation of the model is health promotion.

The health promotion model contains three major categories: cognitive/perceptual factors, modifying factors, and participation in health-promoting behaviors. (Figure 3-2).

Pender[93] has identified seven *cognitive/perceptual factors* believed to influence health-promoting behavior. These factors are importance of health, perceived control of health, perceived self-efficacy, definition of health, perceived health status, perceived benefits of health-promoting behavior, and perceived barriers to

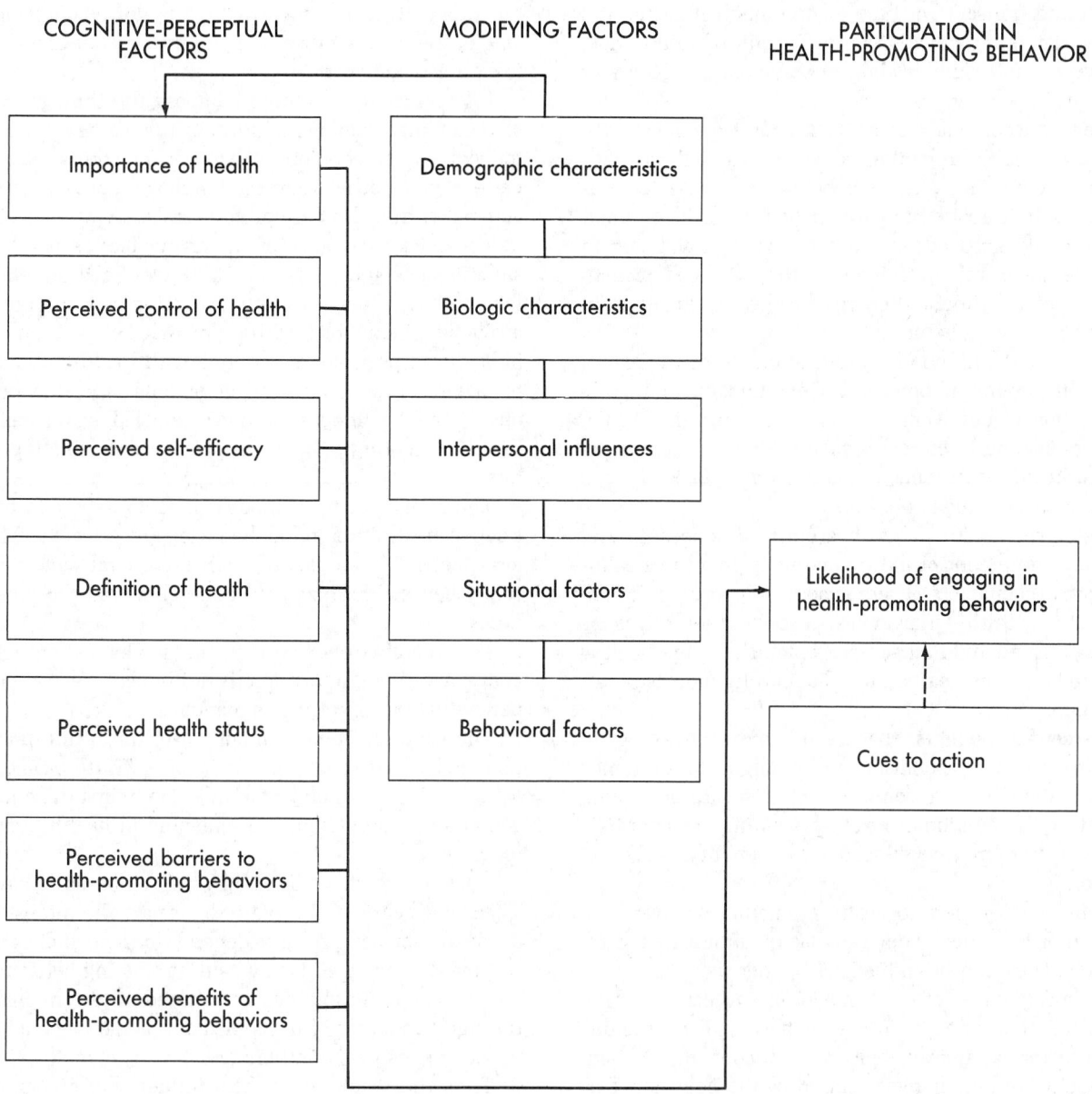

FIGURE 3-2 Health promotion model. (From Pender NJ: Health promotion in nursing practice, Norwalk, Conn, 1987, Appleton-Century-Crofts.)

health-promoting behavior. These factors, influenced by the modifying factors, are thought to result in either participation or nonparticipation in health promoting behaviors.

The importance of health to the individual is included in the model, because health is known to be valued differently. People who value health may seek additional knowledge about improving and maintaining health.

Individual perceptions of control of health include personal belief of control over health status and desire to exert control over health status. Perceived control is thought to influence the initiation as well as the continuation of health promotion practices.

Perceived self-efficacy is the ability to effectively interact and transact with the environment. It is thought to be related to motivation toward acquiring knowledge, resources, and skills leading to self-initiated activity or self-care.

Self-awareness is seen as having motivational significance in health-promoting behaviors, as well as influencing continuance of such behaviors. Self-esteem is believed to be related to participation in health-promoting behaviors, based on the assumption that belief in high personal worth will increase the likelihood of justification of the time and energy needed for engaging in health-promoting behavior.

Personal definition of health can influence the extent of health-promoting behaviors. Definitions including actualization would seem to lead toward engaging in behaviors leading to increased healthfulness, whereas defining health as absence of disease might logically lead to disease-avoidance behaviors.

Perceived health status apparently influences the frequency and extent of individual engagement in health-promoting behaviors. There is some support for the notion that healthy individuals perceive themselves as more satisfied and that self-perceptions of being healthy lead to behaviors geared toward achieving increased satisfaction.

Perceived benefits that result from engaging in health-promoting behaviors are thought to influence participation in and continuation of health-promoting behaviors. Repetition of health-promoting behaviors appears to reinforce beliefs about the benefits of the behavior.

Perceived barriers to health-promoting behavior can be real or imagined. They can also be diminished or removed. They can be influenced by increasing the positive consequences of the behavior or by decreasing the negative consequences of the behavior. They include such factors as unavailability, cost, inconvenience, and the extent of life change required by the behavior. Perceived barriers to health-promoting behavior are thought to be influential in the decision to engage in health-promoting behavior.

The second major section of the model, the *modifying factors* section, includes five areas: demographic characteristics, biologic characteristics, interpersonal influences, situational factors, and behavioral factors.

Demographic factors include such characteristics as age, race, ethnicity, gender, education, and income. These variables might possibly account for selected variation in health-promoting behaviors, and further study of these variables should elicit their individual and cumulative effect on such behavior.

Biologic characteristics are the second group of modifying factors that could conceivably influence health-promoting behavior. One example of such biologic factors currently under investigation is the relationship, if any, of the resting pulse rate and the percent of body fat to exercise behavior.

Interpersonal influences compose the third category of modifying factors. Included in this category are the individual's expectations of significant others, existing patterns of health care in the family, and previous interactions with health care professionals.

The fourth category of modifying factors is labeled situational factors. Two currently identified situational factors that influence health-promoting behavior are the available options for health-promoting behavior and the individual's previous experience with health-promoting behaviors. A range of available options as well as previously gained confidence of one's knowledge and skills of health-promoting behavior appear to be facilitating factors.

The final category of modifying factors thought to influence health-promoting behavior are selected behavioral factors. Examples of such behavioral factors currently being scrutinized are adherence and self-motivation.

The modifying factors of the model as presented above are thought to directly influence the cognitive/perceptual factors of the individual.

The third and final component of the health-promotion model consists of *participation in health-promoting behavior*. This section of the model contains the cues to action and the likelihood of engaging in health-promoting behavior.

Cues to action trigger health-promoting behavior. These cues can be internal or external. The intensity of a cue to act as a trigger depends on the individual's readiness to engage in the health-promoting behavior. A cue to action might be transmitted to an individual through some type of mass media or could be contained in the suggestions of others.

Thus the modifying factors influence the cognitive/perceptual factors, which increase the likelihood of engaging in health-promoting behavior. This likelihood may also be influenced by selected cues to action.

APPRAISAL OF THE HEALTH PROMOTION MODEL

The importance of the various components of the health-promotion model is beginning to receive support from research. Pender's model has clarified the concept of health promotion, allowing it to be differentiated from disease prevention and health maintenance. It is a much needed organizing framework for research and practice in the rapidly expanding area of health promotion.

Concern is being voiced in the areas of both health protection and health promotion that a strong trend toward a victim-blaming ideology is developing concurrently with an increasing focus on self-care and self-responsibility.[34,86,102] Although individual self-responsibility does appear to influence health or illness status, it is a gross oversimplification to say that, if individuals would behave more responsibly, they could attain high-level wellness and avoid disease. Proposing a unicausal relationship between health and self-responsibility without also considering the political, social, economic, environmental, and occupational influence upon health and illness is simplistic and prejudicial.

There is beginning evidence to support the concept that health behaviors, both protective and promotive, are a part of a complex life-style and in part will be influenced by an individual's ability to anticipate problems and formulate goals, mobilize resources to meet them, and cope actively.[77,63] The cumulative research data presently available provide nursing and other health care professionals with a beginning framework for analyzing and encouraging health-protecting and health-promoting behavior.[30]

AT-RISK ROLE

There are four states in which individuals can find themselves while fluctuating between various states of health and illness: healthy, at risk, ill, or convalescent. The term *healthy,* as applied by this study, is reserved for those persons who pursue no dangerous habits such as smoking, who do not engage in certain activities that directly involve some health hazard, and who are not in an age range in which there is a high risk from some designated health threat. Those persons who participate in activities that elevate their risk to a significant degree but who are neither convalescent nor ill are termed *at risk. Ill* persons are defined as persons under medical treatment or who must perform certain activities in addition to receiving medical treatment. *Convalescents* are those who need treatment or rehabilitation before regaining their full working capacity. Thus those individuals who according to the study are not healthy, ill, or

convalescent constitute a group whose health status warrants their behaving in a way that will reduce their risk of illness—that is, assuming the at-risk role.[12]

PHASES OF THE AT-RISK ROLE

There are four phases of the at-risk role. The first phase involves acquiring information related to a threat through mass media or through participating in screening procedures and applying that data to one's specific situation. The second phase involves validating the credibility of and attitudes toward both the threat and the recommended preventive action in the social milieu—that is, the lay system. The third phase involves pursuing medical validation of the threat and its applicability to the individual. The fourth phase is acceptance of the high-risk status and is accompanied by compliance with behaviors recommended to reduce the threat.[12]

APPRAISAL OF THE AT-RISK ROLE

The tendency of healthy persons to accept the at-risk role is limited by several factors. First, the at-risk role possesses no rights, only responsibilities. The person at risk is expected to maintain the usual healthy-role responsibilities, to change or modify present behavior, and to do this with no right to social recognition for any achievements. Besides these disadvantages, the at-risk role is not time-limited. Its appropriate behaviors could be required over a long period. Results of behaviors are not immediately evident, although they may have a positive outcome that is likely to be manifested in the remote future.[98] Further, the at-risk role is *noninstitutionalized,* and the assumption of it depends solely on the individual. That is, the person at risk must take action to reduce the risk status without the benefits of social reinforcement.

Many times the social environment will negatively reinforce the behaviors necessary for the at-risk role by tempting individuals to deviate from those necessary behaviors. Positive reinforcement, if there is any, could come in the form of additional information concerning the health threat.

Two final disadvantages of the at-risk role exist. First, the at-risk role is based on a statistical probability (as opposed to cause and effect) between certain behaviors and the health threat and often relates to diseases for which no cure exists.[5] The role allows for no transfer of responsibility for cure to the medical profession, since the individual can be considered to be responsible for his or her own illness.

Three criteria need to be met before the at-risk role can promote increased levels of wellness in our society. The first involves recognition and acceptance of the at-risk role by individuals. The second involves institutionalization of the at-risk role. All medical practitioners, since they are considered to be the legitimizing agents, would need to confirm the at-risk status and reinforce it periodically. The third criterion is the development of norms related to the at-risk role; that is, society would need to begin to regulate the demands and expectations related to this role. This would provide a basis for the social network of the person at risk to exert pressure to conform to those expectations, for example, social pressure not to smoke.

Nursing could become involved in the acceptance of the at-risk role by focusing on the value system of nursing. The validity of the nursing profession could become a significant part of the legitimizing force. Nurse practitioners, community health nurses, and others are presently discovering and validating the existence of the at-risk role in individuals and providing reinforcement to persons who have assumed the at-risk role. The concept of the at-risk role is presently used by many nurses teaching in clinics for birth control, hypertension, smoking, and obesity. It could easily become an integral part of every nurse's function to assess clients for their at-risk status and to follow through by reinforcing appropriate behaviors.

ILLNESS BEHAVIOR

Behavior during illness can be viewed as a five-stage model that facilitates consideration of social, cultural, and psychologic implications of the illness experience.

The five stages are symptom experience, assumption of the sick role, medical care contact, dependent patient role, and recovery or rehabilitation. The decisions, behaviors, and outcomes associated with each phase are summarized in Figure 3-3.[110]

Symptom experience begins as the person makes a *decision* that something is wrong. This decision has three components: physical, cognitive, and emotional. The *physical* aspects include the presence of signs or symptoms such as nausea, vomiting, or a rash. The *cognitive* aspects include the personal meaning that the signs and symptoms have for the individual. The *emotional* responses to the physical experience and cognitive interpretation constitute the third aspect.

A community survey based on this model demonstrates that pain was the most significant symptom experienced during the first phase, followed by fever and chills and shortness of breath. The initial signs and symptoms were extremely difficult to ignore, were usually severe, were continuous, and could not be alleviated by lay interventions. Most of the individuals, when faced with frightening and serious symptoms, thought immediately of seeking professional health care. This observation supports the premise that the severity of the symptoms determines the rapidity with which the ill individual seeks care from professionals.

Aspects of symptom experience that have meaning to health care professionals include the results of symptom denial, delay in seeking treatment, and possibly the use

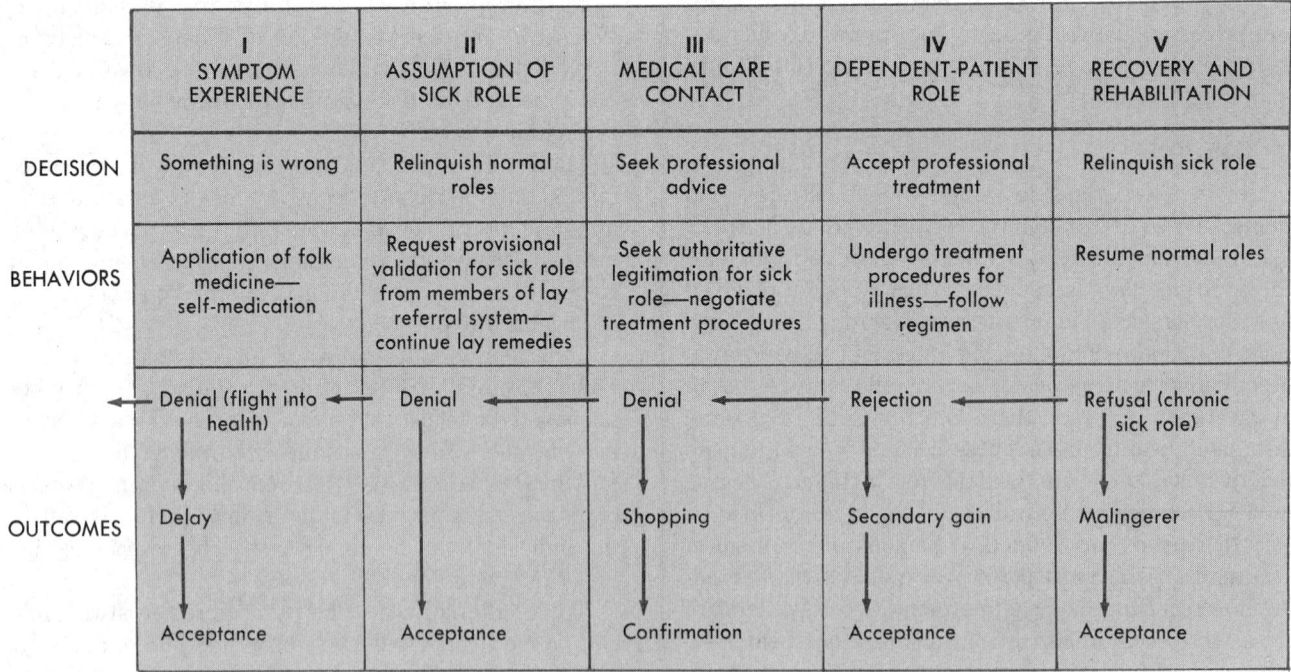

	I SYMPTOM EXPERIENCE	II ASSUMPTION OF SICK ROLE	III MEDICAL CARE CONTACT	IV DEPENDENT-PATIENT ROLE	V RECOVERY AND REHABILITATION
DECISION	Something is wrong	Relinquish normal roles	Seek professional advice	Accept professional treatment	Relinquish sick role
BEHAVIORS	Application of folk medicine—self-medication	Request provisional validation for sick role from members of lay referral system—continue lay remedies	Seek authoritative legitimation for sick role—negotiate treatment procedures	Undergo treatment procedures for illness—follow regimen	Resume normal roles
OUTCOMES	Denial (flight into health) ↓ Delay ↓ Acceptance	Denial ↓ ↓ Acceptance	Denial ↓ Shopping ↓ Confirmation	Rejection ↓ Secondary gain ↓ Acceptance	Refusal (chronic sick role) ↓ Malingerer ↓ Acceptance

FIGURE 3-3 Stages of illness experience. (From Coe R: Sociology of medicine, New York, 1970, McGraw-Hill Book Co. Used with permission of McGraw-Hill Book Co.)

of illness for unusual purposes as in hypochondriasis. It becomes a problem to establish a suitable balance between denial of symptoms and overreaction to symptoms (hypochondriasis) at this stage. Because chronic illness is insidious in its onset and not immediately productive of serious or incapacitating effects, some persons may need to be encouraged to seek early health care for symptoms that they do not view as being acute.

The second stage of illness, the *assumption of the sick role,* involves a decision that one is ill and needs competent care. The ill individual now consults with selected respected lay persons. This serves two purposes. Validation is provided (or not provided) by the friend or relative consulted that the person really is sick. If validation is given, there is a *provisional excuse* for nonperformance of usual role obligations. It is provisional because American society requires that a health professional legitimize one's entrance into the sick role.

The ill person seeks *advice* as well as validation. The majority of people in the survey did discuss their illnesses, usually with one other person, most often their spouse. This discussion occurred before seeking medical help, and almost all discussion took place as soon as the signs and symptoms were noticed.

The majority of the persons consulted by the sick individual also interpreted the signs and symptoms as illness, and most of them recommended seeking professional assistance. Sick persons tended to follow the options suggested by the lay consultant, whether the advice was to seek medical assistance, begin self-treatment, or await further developments. On the whole the discussion process provided a necessary and usually positive impetus toward seeking adequate care.

The *medical care contact stage* involves the decision to seek medical care, that is, to obtain a diagnosis, prognosis, and treatment plan from a medical source. It is here that the person receives authoritative permission to assume the sick role. If such validation is not forthcoming, the sick individual either returns to normal role and status obligations or continues seeking professional opinions until an acceptable diagnosis is found. During this stage most of the individuals in the survey did in fact receive diagnoses, prognoses, and plans of care that they were able to accept.

The fourth stage, the *dependent patient role stage,* includes the ill individual's decision to delegate control to the health care provider and to cooperate with the prescribed therapy. Now the sick person becomes a patient and tends to look on this role with ambivalence because of the dependency component of the role. Although the role in itself is almost always deemed undesirable, it is often looked on as the only means to the desired end—that is, a cure. Patients expressed difficulty with the assumption of this role. While they were willing to follow the provider's recommendations, they displayed concern and expressed a desire to be kept informed.

It remains unclear how much of the dependency and regression imposed on the person during this phase is essential to the patient and how much fulfills the needs of the patient's significant others and health professionals. Issues that await further research include:

1. Why much of the decision making tends to be delegated to the medical profession
2. What benefits could derive from leaving more decision making and autonomy with the patient
3. How helpful it would be to offer the well-informed patient the choice of feasible, promising treatments rather than leave the selection entirely to the professional

The fifth and final stage, *recovery and rehabilitation,* involves the decision to relinquish the sick role. During this phase the individual resumes normal roles and tasks and rejoins the world of the well. In acute limited illness, there are generally no major problems encountered in resuming normal roles. In chronic illness, however, the return to normal roles can be more difficult.

During this phase the majority of persons were being cared for at home and reported satisfaction with their care. It was concluded that most patients are either satisfied with their care or reluctant to complain. Patients who do not successfully accomplish the tasks of this final stage are identified as malingerers.

The major and recurrent concerns of persons during the entire illness experience were variations of questions about chances of full recovery, residual effects of the illness, ability to carry on usual activities, and method of payment for services.

Variations of this model are being developed to further define and analyze illness behavior in specific situations such as emergency or life-threatening conditions.[2]

TYPES OF ILLNESS BEHAVIOR

Illness behavior can be of various types. The individual can take action for symptom relief, take no action, vacillate, or take counteraction.[122]

Illness behavior involves symptom perception, evaluation, and response. The individual reacts or does not react to such cues or symptoms as pain, discomfort, or malfunction. Not only is the form of illness extremely variable, but the individual's definition and recognition of and response to the illness are highly complex, interrelated, and diverse. Persons who decide to *take action* can seek help from either health care professionals or nonhealth-oriented professionals, such as a minister or some identifiably significant person in the community whom people consult for guidance in various sorts of problems. When one decides to *take no action,* there are several possible reasons. Perhaps the appearance of symptoms is just not that important to the individual. In this instance the person recognizes the symptom but does not feel that it is significant enough to warrant action. On the other hand, it could be that fear, lack of resources (or knowledge about the resources), or dislike of entering the health care system leads the individual to delay initiation of help-seeking behavior. Should the symptom subside, the person will usually consider the procrastination effective and adequate. Should the symptom continue and intensify, most people will then take action. Inability to decide either way can cause one to *vacillate*. The desire to take action may be present, but some type of cost to the individual remains a significant deterrent. *Taking counteraction* is a form of denial. It consists of attempting to demonstrate that no illness exists. This behavior opposes definition and assessment of the symptoms and resists action to alleviate or correct them. This type of response to illness sometimes is labeled *deviant illness behavior,* or "pathological health."[81] The term does not apply, however, to the behaviors demonstrated by persons who, perhaps because of lack of knowledge of the situation, do not realize that the symptoms could be illness related.[122]

The type of illness behavior demonstrated by the individual is probably determined by a number of variables:

1. Visibility and importance of the symptoms
2. Perceived seriousness of the situation
3. Degree of discomfort caused by the symptoms
4. Tolerance threshold of the individual experiencing the symptoms
5. Interpretation of the symptoms
6. Availability and accessibility of treatment resources[76]

APPRAISAL OF ILLNESS BEHAVIOR

Since almost all health care is delivered on the initiative of individuals who choose to seek professional help, the study of illness behavior is very important. If we are to understand how persons select themselves for professional health care, then we must learn more about how they define themselves as ill and decide to take action.[73,82] Attention needs to be focused on the nonusers of health care.

Attempts have been made to define illness behavior by determining the prevalence of signs and symptoms that do *not* receive medical attention but are socially and medically significant and consequential. Illness or some type of health status deviation is almost an everyday occurrence and only results in contact with a health professional in highly selected situations.[3]

If too much attention is devoted to examining the characteristics of those who do seek professional care, whereas relatively little attention is turned to those who do not seek care, an unbalanced, or biased, understanding of illness behavior could result. Once the motivating factors influencing both use and nonuse of professional health care are understood, improved educational programs geared toward increasing options for those experiencing illness can be developed. The study of illness behavior can also increase the accuracy of history taking. Response tendencies that are a part of a person's illness behavior pattern, such as denial, adversely influence the diagnostic process. Illness behavior patterns could influence the patient's response to varying treatment modalities; an awareness of these response patterns could improve compliance with therapy regimens.

SELF-CARE

The importance of illness behavior and health-promoting efforts that people assume for themselves without seeking care from a professional has been recognized since the time of Florence Nightingale. Indeed, Nightingale wrote *Notes on Nursing: What it is and What it is not*[85] as a manual to teach women how to nurse their families. She based her recommendations on her observations of bedside care of ill persons and care of healthy persons in families. Over the last two decades Orem[88] has proposed a theory of nursing that differentiates the professional and lay roles in self-care. She proposed that humans required three types of self-care: universal, developmental, and health deviation self-care. *Universal self-care,* which is common to all humans during all stages of life, is associated with life processes and maintenance of the integrity of human structure, function, and general well-being. Universal self-care requisites include maintenance of intakes of air, food, and water; maintenance of waste elimination; a balance of rest with activity and solitude with social interaction; avoidance of hazards to life, functioning, and well-being; and promotion of human functioning and development within social groups. *Developmental self-care* requisites are associated with human developmental processes, conditions, and events that occur during various life-cycle stages, including those which adversely affect development. Developmental self-care includes bringing about and maintaining living conditions that support life processes and promote processes of development. It also includes prevention of deleterious effects of conditions affecting human development or mitigating or overcoming the effects of such conditions as educational deprivation or oppressive living conditions. *Health deviation self-care* requisites include seeking and securing appropriate medical assistance; being aware of and attending to effects of pathologic conditions and states; carrying out medically prescribed diagnostic, therapeutic, and rehabilitative measures; being aware of and attending to or regulating the uncomfortable or deleterious effects of medical care measures; modifying the self-concept; and learning to accomodate the effects of pathologic conditions and of diagnostic and treatment measures within one's life-style in such a way as to promote personal development. *Self-care agency* reflects the individual's ability to provide the self-care requisites. One's self-care agency, along with self-care requisites and deficits, influence the type of nursing care needed.

Self-care spans a person's efforts to promote optimum health, prevent illness, detect symptoms at an early date, and manage chronic illness. Self-care also involves self-monitoring and assessment; symptom perception and labeling, evaluation of the severity of illness; and evaluation and selection of treatment alternatives, including self-help efforts, lay resources, over-the-counter drugs and curatives, and professional health care.

A recent analysis of published self-care literature reveals that people's self-care efforts reflect various models of health. Symptom perception and monitoring, evaluation, and response to symptoms, including discretionary nonaction, use of prescription and nonprescription medications, lay consultation, and use of formal health services, are usually undertaken to limit morbidity or prevent death, reflecting a clinical model of health. Self-care strategies aim to enhance functional capacity or role performance; these include strategies to deal with chronic illness or rehabilitation strategies to promote performance of activities of daily living. Stress management and self-management efforts aimed at promoting behavioral change, enhancing self-efficacy, or reducing stress-related symptoms reflect the adaptive model of health. Health promotion programs, such as exercising, meditating, or practicing optimum nutritional intake, are aimed at enhancing well-being, harmony, and fitness, and reflect a eudaemonistic conception of health.[120]

SICK ROLE

Being sick may result in the person's inability to perform normally expected roles and tasks. Our society has institutionalized a set of expectations and sanctions regarding the behavior of persons unable to perform their usual roles because of illness: the sick role.

COMPONENTS OF THE SICK ROLE

On assuming the sick role the person is exempted from normal social roles and responsibilities as necessitated by the kind and severity of the illness. Being exempted from normal social roles requires that the illness be legitimized, usually by a physician. The sick person is not considered responsible for an acquired illness; that is, the individual cannot be expected to get well by personal volition. "He can't help it." Being ill is seen as undesirable; the sick person is expected to want to get well and to seek technically competent help.[90]

Three factors produce variations in the sick role: the unique background and experience of the individual, the specific disease process and its severity, and the interactional context in which the person seeks to assume the role. It has been suggested that the demands placed on the individual by roles other than the sick role may cause the greatest variation in assumption of the sick role.[72]

The necessity for legitimizing the illness and seeking competent help confers on the therapeutic agency a method for social control. These agencies are allowed to regulate and define the individual illness process as well as facilitate recovery from the illness state.[90] *Negative control* is exerted through isolating the sick person, both from other sick persons and from the healthy. This accomplishes two goals: the sick cannot reinforce the illness behavior of others, and thus a subculture of sick people does not develop; and the visibility of the sick role and thus the likelihood that healthy people will choose to imitate it are decreased.

Society exerts *positive control* by having sick persons place themselves under the control of therapeutic agencies. This places the ill persons in a situation of dependency on health professionals rather than on others who are ill.

APPRAISAL OF THE SICK ROLE PARADIGM

Questions have been raised about the applicability of the sick role paradigm to all types of illnesses.[72] It could be argued that the sick role paradigm is less applicable to the person with a mental illness than to the person with a physical illness, since the mentally ill are seen as more responsible for their illness, mental illness is less acceptable than physical illness as legitimized illness, and those who are mentally ill often maintain the ability to perform their normal social roles.[26,70]

Similar concerns have been raised regarding the applicability of the sick role paradigm to the chronically ill. Health professionals do not encourage the chronically ill to define their states as undesirable but to accept and learn to live with their limitations. The chronically ill often are able to perform some of their social roles and thus are not exempted from total responsibility to society. The maintenance care required by the chronically ill person requires that the individual rather than the health care professional assume a great deal of responsibility for his or her own condition. The utility of the sick role paradigm has also been questioned for those who are aging, abusing drugs or alcohol, suicidal, or pregnant.[97]

The legitimized sick role requires the seeking of technically competent help, yet most persons do not consult a health professional when ill. Often their illnesses are legitimized by family members or friends. Some individuals simply exempt themselves from their usual roles by going to bed. Individuals with some acute illnesses, such as venereal disease, may desire to get well, seek technically competent help, but continue to perform their usual roles.

Several aspects of the sick role require further research:

1. Whether different groups of people have different expectations of the sick role
2. Which specific role and task exemptions are permissible with which types of illnesses
3. How significant others influence sick role expectations
4. Whether different illnesses elicit different types of sick role behavior
5. Whether people accept responsibility for contracting certain illnesses
6. Whether there are changing behavioral expectations over time while one is experiencing the sick role[53,103]

RESPONSES TO CHRONIC AND CRITICAL ILLNESS

In response to the concepts of illness behavior and the sick role, investigators have studied people's experiences of being chronically or critically ill. The resultant literature reveals that illness is a multidimensional experience, some aspects of which are common to many different diseases. Strauss and colleagues[108] identified several tasks common to a variety of chronic illnesses, such as diabetes, arthritis, and pulmonary disease. These tasks included preventing and managing medical crises, managing regimens, controlling symptoms, restructuring time, managing the trajectory of the illness, living with the social isolation imposed by the illness, normalizing life, and funding the necessary costs to maintain health. Moos and Tsu[80] identified major adaptive tasks for individuals and families adjusting to critical illnesses. These included adjusting to pain and incapacitation, dealing with hospital environments and special treatment procedures, developing adequate relationships with the professional staff, preserving a reasonable emotional balance, maintaining a satisfactory self-image, preserving relationships with family and friends, and preparing for an uncertain future. Although this orientation provides understanding of experiences common to a variety of illnesses, it does not account for the unique ways in which different individuals and their families respond to the same illness. Understanding the unique as well as the common aspects of the experience is essential to provide a basis for caring for patients and families experiencing chronic and critical illness.

Studies of individuals' illness experiences have demonstrated that people encounter several different types of demands. Some are related to the disease itself, such as fatigue, pain, dyspnea, nausea, and weakness. Others are personal disruptions, changes in the status quo as a result of the illness. Personal disruptions include a de-

pletion of personal integrity, such as altered body image or self-concept; disruptions in one's sense of continuity in daily living, such as preoccupation with the meaning of the illness and attributions about the illness; and disruptions in normalcy, such as the necessity of monitoring changes in body sensations and functions. Demands linked to environmental transactions include challenges in relationships with family members, one's broader social network, and health care providers.[89]

DEVIANCE, HEALTH, AND ILLNESS

Deviance implies the violation of the norms of a group or society.[61] Persons who are ill might be considered deviant if they are no longer able to meet the expectations associated with their roles.[67]

Deviant behaviors violate norms; nondeviant behaviors do not. Variant behaviors depart from specified norms but are still within a permissible or acceptable range.[113] In this context primary deviance occurs when a person defined as normal commits a deviant act; for example, a nondrug-user experiments once with drugs. Secondary deviance occurs when a person defined as deviant commits a deviant act; for example, a "drug abuser" habitually uses drugs.

Labeling a person as deviant alters the expectations that the person will behave normally and may perpetuate the deviance. Labeling the chronically ill or physically handicapped as deviant results in stereotypic expectations that they will not be able to perform adequately in certain situations. Employers and others may consequently deny the chronically ill or physically handicapped the opportunity to demonstrate their abilities.

Illness can be differentiated from other forms of deviance (for example, crime and sin). The criminal and the sinner commit their acts volitionally, whereas ill persons lack voluntary control over their health state. The social response to sin and crime is punishment in hopes of eliciting conformity. The social response to the sick person is to use some form of therapy to change the factors that prevent that person from conforming. In all situations there are role changes inasmuch as the sinner, criminal, and ill person are pronounced incapable of accepting full responsibility for their behavior; others must intervene to control their behavior.

Several investigators have criticized the *deviance model* of illness,[9,113] yet others believe that the deviance model has utility for the health field.[11] The deviance model allows labeling of populations as deviant rather than labeling individuals. The labeling of populations such as smokers as deviant would then allow health professionals the right and give them the responsibility to change unhealthful situations. This change would be accomplished by social sanctions and pressures and education to change the deviants into conformists. However effective it might be, this approach does little to foster individual autonomy and responsibility for health.[12]

Medicine as an institution is increasingly assuming more responsibility for controlling deviant behaviors.[90,113] Some behaviors that in previous eras would have been defined as sin or crime and would have been controlled by religious or legal institutions are now being defined as illness and being controlled through medical institutions.

Simultaneously, legal and religious institutions are increasingly adopting medical approaches to control deviance. Churches utilize the mental health model of deviance to provide pastoral counseling similar to psychotherapy. The legal profession often chooses confinement to mental institutions rather than imprisonment, and prisons now frequently define rehabilitation rather than punishment as their goal.

Szasz,[111] a psychiatrist and well-known crusader for the rights of individuals, warns against this medicalization of social deviance. In his view medicine, sociology, psychiatry, and psychology should have nothing to say about whether a person ought to be free to use drugs, commit suicide, engage in homosexual acts, or have delusions. The potential ability to injure or destroy oneself is a basic freedom and there are no grounds for regarding self-injury as a crime to be controlled by police power. Szasz warns of the "therapeutic state," a society in which government, advised by health professionals, increasingly makes individuals' decisions for them. Self-determination is replaced by a powerful medicopsychiatric complex, a subtle and yet real threat to individual liberty. The medicopsychiatric complex has grown in the last decades to a government monopoly that has a strong voice in public policy and legislative decisions. It is armed with federal funds to provide therapy when people get out of line.

Maslow asks for studies of the *positive effects* of deviance, a much neglected area of study. Culture can never be advanced without persons who are not afraid to be different. He asks why these persons are usually seen as pathologic and if deviance can be healthy.[69]

The labeling of behavior as deviant can be confined to those areas that impinge on the rights of others. Certain behaviors that have been labeled deviant are presently being reconsidered. Nursing could be a force in preventing the labeling of behaviors as deviant when in fact they are only variant, thus increasing individual freedom and the number of acceptable options available to people.

CHAPTER SUMMARY

✔ There are multiple conceptions of health, disease, and illness. Moreover, conceptions of patients and health professionals vary.

✔ Clinical, role performance, adaptive, and eudaemon-

istic conceptions of health guide people's health-related behavior.

✔ Behavior in health and illness has been studied by investigators from the social and health sciences. The health belief model, health promotion model, at-risk role, illness behavior, and sick role can help health professionals understand patients' behaviors.

✔ Limitations of the models from the social sciences have prompted nurses to develop additional models, such as Pender's model of health promotion and Orem's model of self-care.

QUESTIONS TO CONSIDER

■ In what ways does your own personal definition of health resemble those described by patients? professionals?

■ What does being ill mean to you? Your family members?

■ Where would you rank yourself on Maslow's hierarchy of needs? Why? How does your ranking affect what you do to promote your health?

■ Describe your own behavior in relation to using preventive services or performing a self-care effort to reduce your risk of illness, such as a breast self-examination. Use the health belief model to analyze your own situation.

■ Using Pender's health promotion model, analyze your own efforts to promote your health, for example, by exercising or eating healthfully.

■ How does the model of illness behavior presented in the chapter help you understand your patients' experiences?

■ Describe the process of surgery and recovery for one of your patients. Do any of the models presented in the chapter enhance your understanding of their experiences? Which one?

REFERENCES AND SELECTED READINGS

1. Alan DK and Boldt J: A study of preventive health attitudes and behaviors in a family practice setting, J Fam Pract 11:77-84, 1980.
2. Alonzo AA: Acute illness behavior: a conceptual exploration and specification, Soc Sci Med 14A:515-526, 1980.
3. Alonzo AA: Everyday illness: a situational approach to health status deviations, Soc Sci Med 13A:397-404, 1979.
4. Antonovsky A: Health, stress, and coping, San Francisco, 1979, Jossey-Bass.
5. *Antonovsky A: Unraveling the mystery of health, San Francisco, 1987, Jossey-Bass.

*References preceded by an asterisk are particularly well suited for student reading.

6. Apple D: How laymen define illness, J Health Soc Behav 1:219-225, 1960.

7. Ardell DB: Fourteen days to a wellness lifestyle, Mill Valley, Calif, 1985, Whatever Publishing Company.

8. Ardell DB: The nature and implications of high level wellness, or why "normal health" is a rather sorry state of existence, Health Values: Achieving High Level Wellness 3:17-24, 1979.

9. Armstrong D: The structure of medical education, Med Educ 11:244-248, 1977.

10. Balog JE: The concepts of health and disease: a relativistic perspective, Health Values: Achieving High Level Wellness 6:7-13, 1982.

11. Baric L: Conformity and deviance in health and illness, Int J Health Educ 12:2-12, 1969.

12. *Baric L: Recognition of the at-risk role: a means to influence behavior, Int J Health Educ 12:24-34, 1969.

13. Bauman B: Diversities in conceptions of health and physical fitness, J Health Soc Behav 2:39-46, 1961.

14. *Becker MH, Drachman RH, and Kirschit J: A new approach to explaining sick-role behavior in low income populations, Am J Public Health 64:205-216, 1974.

15. Bell JM: Stressful life events and coping methods in mental-illness and -wellness behaviors, Nurs Res 26:136-141, 1977.

16. Belloc NB: Relationship of health practices and mortality, Prev Med 2:67-81, 1973.

17. Belloc NB and Breslow L: Relationship of physical health status and health practices, Prev Med 1:409-421, 1972.

18. Blair SN et al: Health promotion for educators: impact on health behaviors, satisfaction and general well-being, Am J Public Health 74:147-149, 1984.

19. Blattner B: Holistic nursing, Englewood Cliffs, New Jersey, 1981, Prentice-Hall, Inc.

20. Breslow L and Enstrom JE: Persistence of health habits and their relationship to mortality, Prev Med 9:469-483, 1980.

21. Brown J and Rawlinson M: Relinquishing the sick-role following open heart surgery, J Health Soc Behav 16:12-27, 1975.

22. Bullough B: Poverty, ethnic identity and preventive health care, J Health Soc Behav 13:347-359, 1972.

23. Carlyon WH: Reflections: disease prevention and health promotion—bridging the gap to wellness, Health Values: Achieving High Level Wellness 8:27-30, 1984.

24. Cassel EJ: Disease as an "it": concepts of disease revealed by patients' presentation of symptoms, Soc Sci Med 10:143-146, 1976.

25. Champion VL: Instrument development for health belief model constructs, Adv Nurs Sci 6:73-85, 1984.

26. Cheetham RW and Rzadkowolski A: Crosscultural psychiatry and the concept of mental illness, S Afr Med J 58:320-325, 1975.

27. *Clarke H and Driever M: Vulnerability: the development of a construct for nursing. In Chinn P, editor: Advances in nursing theory development, Rockville Md, 1983, Aspen Systems. 1983.

28. Coburn D and Pope CR: Socioeconomic status and preventive health behavior, J Health Soc Behav 15:67-78, 1974.

29. Coe R: Sociology of medicine, New York, 1970, McGraw-Hill Book Co.

30. Coulton C: Factors related to preventive health behavior: implications for social work intervention, Soc Work Health Care 3:297-310, 1978.

31. Cox C: The interaction model of client health behavior: application to the study of community based elders, Adv Nurs Sci 9(1)40-57, 1986.

32. Cox C, Miller E, and Mull C: Motivation in health behavior: measurement, antecedents, and correlates, Adv Nurs Sci 10(4)1-15, 1987.

33. Cox C, Sullivan J, and Roghmann K: A conceptual explanation of risk reduction behavior and intervention development, Nurs Res 33(3)168-173, 1984.

34. Crawford R: You are dangerous to your health: the ideology and politics of victim blaming, Int J Health Serv 7:663-680, 1977.

35. Dean K: Lay care in illness, Soc Sci Med 22:275-284, 1986.

36. Dean K: Self care responses to illness: a selected review, Soc Sci Med 15a:673-687, 1981.

37. Demers RW et al: An explanation of the dimensions of illness behavior, J Fam Pract 11:1085-1092, 1980.

38. Diekelmann N: Wellness: approaches and resources, Nurse Pract 5:41-44, 1980.

39. Dolfman M: Toward an operational definition of health, J Sch Health 43:206-209, 1974.

40. Dougherty CJ and Walker VR: Scientific medicine, technology, and the concept of health, Ethics Sci Med 5:75-81, 1978.

41. Dowie J: The portfolio approach to health behavior, Soc Sci Med 9:619-631, 1975.

42. Dubos R: Man overadapting, Psychology Today 4:50-53, 1971.

43. Dunn H: High-level wellness, Arlington, Va, 1961, RW Beatty, Ltd.

44. Dunn HL: Points of attack for raising the levels of wellness, J Natl Med Assoc 49:225-235, 1957.

45. Dunn HL: What high level wellness means, Health Values: Achieving High Level Wellness 1:9-16, 1977.

46. Fabrega H: The position of psychiatric illness in biomedical theory: a cultural analysis, J Med Philos 5:145-168, 1980.

47. Fabrega H: Toward a model of illness behavior, Med Care 11:470-484, 1973.

48. Fink DL: Holistic health: implications for health planning, Am J Health Planning 1:23-31, 1976.

49. Flynn PR: Holistic health: the art and science of care, Bowie, Md, 1980, Robert J Brady Co.

50. Fredric D and Wolinsky SR: Background attitudinal and behavioral patterns of individuals occupying eight discrete health states, Sociol Health Illness 3:31-48, 1981.

51. Fry PW: The scientific method and its impact on holistic health, Sociol Health Illness 2:1-7, 1980.

52. Hochbaum G: Health behavior, Belmont, Calif, 1966 Wadsworth Inc.

53. Hover J and Juelsgaard N: The sick role reconceptualized, Nurs Forum 17:407-416, 1978.

54. Hyner MC and Melby CL: Health risk appraisals: use and misuse, Fam Commun Health 7(4):13-25, 1985.

55. Jeffers J: Wellness: teaching students to assess, Health Values: Achieving High Level Wellness 4:119-123, 1980.

56. Johnson J and Parsons M, editors: Symposium on health promotion, Nurs Clin North Am 19:193-281, 1984.

57. *Kasl SV and Cobb S: Health behavior, illness behavior, and sick role behavior, Arch Environ Health 12:246-266, 1966.

58. Keller MJ: Toward a definition of health, Adv Nurs Sci 4:43-64, 1980.

59. Kelman S: Social organization and the meaning of health, J Med Philos 5:133-144, 1980.

60. *Kogan H and Betrus P: Self management: a nursing mode of therapeutic influence, Adv Nurs Sci 6:55-73, 1984.

61. Koltow M: Defining health, Med Hypotheses 6:1097-1104, 1980.

62. Lambertson MM: Health and illness: a co-existence hypothesis, Nurse Pract 8:47-49, 1983.

63. Langlie JK: Interrelationships among preventive health behaviors: a test of competing hypotheses, Public Health Rep 94:216-225, 1979.

64. Leavitt F: The health belief model and utilization of ambulatory care services, Soc Sci Med 13A:105-112, 1979.

65. Leventhal H and Cameron L: Behavioral theories and the problem of compliance, Patient Educ Couns 10:117-138, 1987.
66. Lewis CE and Lewis MA: Child-initiated health care, J Sch Health 49:144-148, 1980.
67. Macleod A: Illness as a deviant role: a clue to the rejection of symptoms, Nurs Times 74:1400-1401, 1978.
68. Magi M and Allander E: Toward a theory of perceived and medically defined need, Sociol Health Illness 3:49-71, 1981.
69. Maslow AH: Motivation and personality, New York, 1954, Harper & Row, Publishers.
70. Mayou R: Comments: sick role, illness behavior and coping, Br J Psychiatry 144:320-322, 1984.
71. McGinnis JM: Trends in disease prevention: assessing the benefits of prevention, Bull NY Acad Med 56:38-44, 1980.
72. *McKinlay J: The sick role: illness and pregnancy, Soc Sci Med 6:561-572, 1972.
73. *Mechanic D: The concept of illness behavior, J Chronic Dis 15:189-194, 1962.
74. Mechanic D: Illness behavior and medical diagnosis, J Health Soc Behav 1:86-94, 1960.
75. Mechanic D: Medical sociology: a selective view, New York, 1968, The Free Press.
76. Mechanic D: The stability of health and illness behavior: results from a sixteen year follow up, Am J Public Health 69:1142-1145, 1979.
77. Mechanic D and Cleary P: Factors associated with the maintenance of positive health behavior, Prev Med 9:805-814, 1980.
78. Mikhail B: The health belief model: a review and critical evaluation of the model, research and practice, Adv Nurs Sci 4:65-82, 1981.
79. Moore PV and Williamson GC: Health promotion: evolution of a concept, Nurs Clin North Am 19:195-206, 1984.
80. *Moos R and Tsu V: The crisis of physical illness: an overview. In Moos R, editor: Coping with physical illness, New York, 1977, Plenum Publishing Co.
81. Musaph H: The right of falling ill: on pathological health behavior, Psychother Psychosom 31:19-23, 1979.
82. Najam JM: Theories of disease causation and the concept of a general susceptibility: a review, Soc Sci Med 14A:231-237, 1980.
83. Nathanson CA: Sex roles as variables in preventive health behavior, J Community Health 3:142-155, 1977.
84. Newman M: Theory development in nursing, Philadelphia, 1979, FA Davis Co.
85. *Nightingale F: Notes on nursing: what it is and what it is not, New York, 1969, Dover Publications, Inc. (Unabridged republication of the first American edition as published in 1860 by D. Appleton & Co.)
86. O'Connell JK and Price JH: Ethical theories for promoting health through behavioral change, J Sch Health 53:476-479, 1983.
87. Oelbaum CH: Hallmarks of adult wellness, Am J Nurs 74:1623-1625, 1974.
88. *Orem D: Nursing: concepts of practice, New York, 1985, McGraw Hill Book Co.
89. Packard N, Haberman M, and Woods: Demands of illness: exploration of the concept among chronically ill women, Western Journal of Nursing Research (in press).
90. Parsons T: Definitions of health and illness in the light of American values and social structure. In Jaco EG: Patients, physicians and illness, New York, 1958, The Free Press.
91. Pelletier KR: In search of optimal health, Med Self-Care, pp. 48-50, Winter 1980.
92. Pender NJ: Health promotion and illness prevention, Annu Rev Nurs Res 2:83-105, 1984.
93. *Pender NJ: Health promotion in nursing practice, Norwalk, Conn, Appleton-Century-Crofts, 1987.
94. Peters BM: School-aged children's beliefs about causality of illness: a review of the literature, Matern Child Nurs J 7:143-154, 1978.
95. Rankin WR: Concepts of illness and care of the ill, Ethics Sci Med 6:239-243, 1979.
96. Reif AE: High level wellness and low level wellness: an overview, Health Values: Achieving High Level Wellness 2:198-210, 1978.
97. Ries JK: Public acceptance of the disease concept of alcoholism, J Health Soc Behav 18:338-344, 1977.
98. Robbins LC and Hall JH: Perspective medicine, ed 2, Indianapolis, 1979, Methodist Hospital of Indiana.
99. Rosenstock I: The health belief model and preventive health behavior, Health Educ Monogr 2:354-386, 1974.
100. Rosenstock I: Historical origins of the health belief model, Health Educ Monogr 2:328-335, 1974.
101. *Rosenstock I, Strecher V, and Becker M: Social learning theory and the health belief model, Health Educ Q 15(2):175-183, 1988.
102. Sechrist W: Causal attribution and personal responsibility for health and disease, Health Educ Q 10:51-54, 1983.
103. Segall A: The sick role concept: understanding illness behavior, J Health Soc Behav 17:163-170, 1976.
104. Segall A: Sociocultural variation in sick role behavioral expectations, Soc Sci Med 10:47-51, 1976.
105. Shortridge LM and McLain BR: Levels of intervention for a coexistence model, Nurse Pract 8:74-80, 1983.
106. *Smith JA: The idea of health: a philosophical inquiry, Adv Nurs Sci 3:43-50, 1981.
107. Sontag S: Illness as a metaphor, New York, 1979, Vintage Books.
108. Strauss A et al: Chronic illness and the quality of life, ed 2, St Louis, 1985, The CV Mosby Co.
109. Suchman EA: Health attitudes and behavior, Arch Environ Health 20:105-110, 1970.
110. Suchman EA: Stages of illness and medical care, J Health Soc Behav 6:114-128, 1965.
111. Szasz T: Our despotic laws destroy the right to self-control, Psychology Today 8:19-127, 1974.
112. Tatro S and Gleit CJ: A wellness model for nursing: promoting high level wellness in any setting through independent nursing functions, Nurs Leadership 6:5-9, 1983.
113. Twaddle AC: Illness and deviance, Soc Sci Med 7:751-762, 1973.
114. Verbrugge L and Ascione F: Exploring the iceberg: common symptoms and how people care for them, Med Care 25:965-978, 1987.
115. Webster JA: The wellness model: feeling good about you, AORN J 41:713-718, 1985.
116. Weinstein N: The precaution adoption process, Health psychol 7(4):355-386, 1988.
117. Williams JS: Disease as deviance, Soc Sci Med 5:219-226, 1971.
118. Wilson R: The sociology of health: an introduction, New York, 1979, Random House, Inc.
119. Wolinsky FD and Wolinsky SR: Background, attitudinal and behavioral patterns of individuals occupying eight discrete health states, Sociol Health Illness 3:31-48, 1981.
120. *Woods N: Conceptualizations of self care: toward health-oriented models, Adv Nurs Sci 12(1):1-13, 1989.
121. Woods N et al: Being healthy: women's images, Adv Nurs Sci 11(1):36-46, 1988.
122. Wu R: Behavior and illness, Englewood Cliffs, NJ, 1973, Prentice-Hall, Inc.

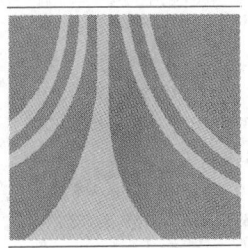

CHAPTER 4

Patterns of Health and Illness: Epidemiologic Approach

NANCY FUGATE WOODS

CHAPTER OBJECTIVES

After studying this chapter, the student should be able to:
1 Analyze contemporary patterns of health and illness for adults in the United States' population across the life span, including longevity, mortality, morbidity, illness consequences, health practices, and perceptions of health.
2 Apply concepts from epidemiology to understand patterns of health and illness for adults.

People's health experiences change across the life span. Although some experiences are unpredictable, some health and illness experiences occur in patterns. Awareness of these patterns enables clinicians to help people promote health, prevent illness, and control the spread of disease. Major health problems and people's concerns about their health have changed over the course of history. Raging pandemics of infectious diseases that claimed the lives of a large portion of a population have given way to contemporary health problems that are largely the product of life-style and environment. The purpose of this chapter is to describe contemporary patterns of health and illness among adults living in the United States from an epidemiologic perspective.

Epidemiology, named for its original focus on studies of epidemics, is the discipline that studies a variety of health-related phenomena and the people affected by them. The phenomena of interest to epidemiologists include health states, disease, and death; health-related behavior; and population dynamics, as well as the outcomes of intervention programs for each of these. The characteristics of people studied might include age, gender, behavior, risk factors in certain population groups, and environmental settings in which people live. An epidemiologist's perspective focuses on populations or aggregates of people rather than on individuals, whereas a clinician's perspective usually focuses on individuals or families. The epidemiologist's perspective is useful to clinicians, however, because it allows a clinician to compare an individual's situation with the experience of an entire population and to use knowledge about the population's health experiences to guide care for individuals.

Epidemiologists describe and analyze health-related conditions. One common focus is the description of the natural history of disease, how the course differs in people having different characteristics or environments, and how the disease course may be altered in response to prevention or therapy. Another focus includes the description of patterns of health and disease in communities, often referred to as "community diagnosis." Commonly used descriptive measures of health status are the incidence or prevalence rates of a disease or the mortality associated with it. Description of population dynamics is another important concern of epidemiologists, as is the development of descriptive indices such as the rates and ratios used in describing morbidity and mortality.

Epidemiology has contributed significantly to the understanding of the etiology of disease. These contributions have included the documentation of causal relationships between risk factors and disease, as well as the study of epidemics to identify their origin.

Increasingly, epidemiologic methods are used in experimentation, such as in the clinical trials of new therapies or preventive measures, and even experiments with animal models. Studies of program acceptance and evaluation of health programs commonly use epidemiologic methods.

With this overview of the scope of epidemiology in mind, we shall explore the patterns of health and illness for the United States' adult population using concepts from epidemiology. Descriptive epidemiologic approaches yield important information concerning the etiology of various health problems. The traditional descriptive variables explored by epidemiologists are person, place, and time. By studying the number and distribution of various health conditions within a population according to these three variables, epidemiologists have been able to generate hypotheses to guide more focused investigations.

DESCRIPTIONS OF HEALTH AND ILLNESS PATTERNS

VARIATIONS BY PERSONAL CHARACTERISTICS

Although there are numerous characteristics of individuals that may be explored, it is customary for epidemiologists to explore the frequency of disease for various age, gender, and ethnic or racial groups. In addition, such variables as religion, social class, occupation, income, education, marital status, family variables (for example, family size and type, birth order, parental characteristics) and the individual's general health status are explored.

MORTALITY RATES

Table 4-1 displays the most prevalent causes of death for women and men and for Whites, Blacks, and persons of other races throughout the adult years. Rates in line 1 of the table for each disease group are for all persons, men, and women respectively, and rates in line 2 of the table are for Whites, Blacks, and people of other races, respectively. Notice that death rates increase for most causes as the age-groups become higher. In addition, the nature of leading causes of death changes throughout the life span, with accidents, homocides, and suicides accounting for high death rates during the period from 15 to 34 years of age. In contrast, diseases of the heart claim more lives for the 35- to 44-year agegroup, and this statistic continues to climb throughout the remaining decades of life. Likewise, cerebrovascu-

lar diseases, malignant neoplasms, chronic obstructive pulmonary diseases, pneumonia and influenza, chronic liver disease and cirrhosis, and diabetes mellitus account for more deaths in the middle and late years of life. In addition to differences in death rates for different age-groups, there are differences in death rates for various causes according to gender and race. Death rates for women are lower than those for men for all categories at most points across the life span. These rates reflect the significant advantage in length of life span for women. Of concern are the death rates for people of color than for Whites from homocide and legal intervention, accidents and adverse consequences, and major chronic disease such as diseases of the heart, cerebrovascular diseases, malignant neoplasms, chronic obstructive pulmonary diseases, pneumonia and influenza, and diabetes mellitus throughout the middle and later years of life.[13]

Investigation of the frequency with which certain health problems are seen among populations with varying personal characteristics is important for several reasons. First, high-risk groups can be identified, and close surveillance can be planned so that health problems can be detected and treated early in their course. Next, trends in incidence and mortality among high-risk groups can be systematically studied. Third, identification of characteristics associated with these problems can provide a basis for generation of hypotheses regarding their etiology and further etiologic studies. For ex-

TABLE 4-1 Death rates for selected causes of death for adults by 10-year age groups, race, and gender: United States, 1986*

Causes of Death	15-24 Years	25-34 Years	35-44 Years	45-54 Years
Diseases of the heart	2.8, 3.5, 2.1	8.6, 11.8, 5.5	37.5, 58.0, 17.7	144.6, 221.4, 72.1
	2.3, 5.6, 5.0	6.8, 21.9, 18.4	32.7, 83.5, 67.7	132.9, 218.6, 258.8
Cerebrovascular diseases	.7, .7, .6	2.2, 2.3, 2.2	7.1, 7.7, 6.5	20.4, 21.7, 19.1
	.6, 1.1, 1.0	1.7, 6.1, 5.0	5.3, 22.4, 18.3	16.0, 48.1, 56.2
Malignant neoplasms	5.4, 6.6, 4.2	13.1, 13.4, 12.8	45.3, 40.8, 49.7	165.7, 171.0, 160.7
	5.5, 5.5, 5.0	12.8, 16.1, 14.8	42.5, 71.8, 62.6	157.0, 254.8, 220.4
Chronic obstructive pulmonary disease	.5, .6, .4	.6, .6, .6	1.6, 1.8, 1.5	9.8, 11.0, 8.7
	.3, 1.4, 1.2	.4, 1.6, 1.4	1.3, 4.3, 3.5	9.3, 15.1, 12.8
Pneumonia and influenza	.7, .8, .6	1.7, 2.1, 1.3	3.6, 4.8, 2.5	7.0, 9.2, 5.0
	.6, 1.2, 1.0	1.3, 4.8, 3.9	2.5, 13.2, 10.6	5.7, 18.5, 15.5
Chronic liver disease and cirrhosis	.2, .2, .1	2.8, 3.7, 1.8	9.6, 14.0, 5.4	20.3, 28.9, 12.2
	.1, .3, .3	2.0, 7.6, 6.7	7.8, 25.4, 21.2	18.3, 36.4, 32.8
Diabetes mellitus	.4, .4, .4	1.5, 1.7, 1.3	3.6, 4.2, 2.9	9.5, 10.2, 8.7
	.3, .5, .4	1.4, 2.1, 1.8	3.0, 8.4, 6.9	7.7, 24.4, 20.7
Accidents and adverse effects	51.2, 78.5, 23.3	39.5, 63.2, 15.9	31.1, 48.7, 14.1	30.7, 47.2, 15.1
	54.4, 34.8, 36.4	38.6, 47.0, 44.3	29.2, 47.6, 43.0	28.8, 46.3, 42.7
Suicide	13.1, 21.7, 4.4	15.7, 25.5, 5.9	15.2, 23.0, 7.6	16.4, 24.4, 8.8
	14.3, 6.8, 7.7	16.4, 12.0, 11.8	16.1, 9.5, 9.3	17.8, 7.5, 7.5
Homicide and legal interventions	14.2, 22.0, 6.1	16.1, 25.5, 6.7	11.4, 18.3, 4.8	8.3, 13.5, 3.5
	8.4, 47.2, 40.8	9.6, 62.4, 51.4	7.5, 44.2, 35.8	5.6, 29.9, 25.2

From the US Department of Health and Human Services: Vital statistics of the United States, Vol II. Mortality, Part A, 1988, Hyattsville Md, Centers for Disease Control, National Center for Health Statistics.
*For all persons: men, women, Whites, Blacks, and other ethnic groups.

ample, the data demonstrating health disadvantages of people of color warrant further exploration of social conditions that may account for these differences.

Mortality rates provide only one index of ill health in a population. Ill health resulting from serious but nonfatal conditions is termed morbidity. In recent years, morbidity has been defined as the result of disease or injury that has an impact on an individual's life through the person's awareness of the departure from health and the restrictions or disabilities that accompany the disease or injury. Estimates from a recent National Health Interview Survey[11] show that in addition to their favorable mortality rates, women in the United States report more illness than do men and also use health services at higher rates. The following estimates are based on data from the Health Interview Survey of a stratified random sample of households drawn from the civilian, noninstitutionalized population of the United States, which measured several factors affecting morbidity and use of health services.

ACUTE CONDITIONS

Illnesses and injuries that last less than three months and involve 1 or more days of restricted activity or medical attention are termed acute. The annual incidence of acute conditions is estimated by including only those conditions that began during the 2 weeks before the interview for the National Health Interview Survey. Table 4-2 shows the incidence of acute conditions for women and men and for Whites and Blacks. Acute conditions

for women exceeded those for men for nearly every condition, except injuries. Rates for Whites exceed those for Blacks, with the exception of digestive system conditions and all other acute conditions not included in the table.

CHRONIC ILLNESS

A chronic condition refers to one that was noticed at least 3 months or more before the interview or that belongs to a group of conditions (including heart disease, diabetes, and others) that persist for a long period of time, regardless of when the condition began. As seen in Table 4-3, women experienced higher rates of arthritis, cataracts, orthopedic impairments, diabetes, hemorrhoids, hypertension, chronic bronchitis, asthma, and chronic sinusitis than did men in 1985. Men experienced higher rates of visual impairment, hearing impairment, ulcer and abdominal hernia, heart disease, and emphysema than did women. Table 4-4 demonstrates that Blacks experienced higher rates of arthritis, diabetes, and hypertension than did Whites, who had higher rates of hearing impairment, orthopedic impairment, abdominal hernia, heart disease, hemorrhoids, chronic bronchitis, and asthma than did Blacks, especially during the later decades of life. Rates of some chronic conditions differ across income categories, with people in lower income brackets being at greater risk for diabetes, heart disease, hypertension, emphysema, arthritis, visual impairment, cataracts, and hearing impairment (Table 4-5).

55-64 Years	65-74 Years	75-84 Years	85 Years and Older
424.2, 627.1, 244.1	1043.0, 1446.7, 724.2	2637.5, 3375.8, 2196.9	7178.7, 7911.5, 6889.3
405.4, 653.3, 567.2	1024.5, 1348.1, 1202.6	2636.4, 2920.2, 2651.6	7332.9, 5906.6, 5585.7
53.0, 59.9, 46.8	164.1, 185.0, 147.6	573.8, 629.2, 540.7	1762.6, 1656.4, 1804.6
45.4, 125.1, 110.3	151.8, 297.9, 270.2	563.0, 748.3, 680.9	1798.1, 1462.6, 1395.9
444.4, 524.2, 373.6	847.0, 1086.9, 657.6	1287.3, 1845.6, 954.2	1612.0, 2459.5, 1277.2
433.2, 598.1, 529.4	837.7, 1030.7, 927.1	1280.5, 1484.1, 1356.0	1612.4, 1694.3, 1607.8
47.2, 59.3, 36.4	149.2, 211.0, 100.5	294.8, 501.9, 171.2	362.9, 745.3, 211.9
47.9, 47.0, 41.4	155.3, 105.8, 96.7	308.4, 164.0, 160.1	379.1, 189.6, 195.9
18.6, 25.5, 12.6	58.6, 81.7, 40.3	242.8, 342.2, 183.4	1032.1, 1360.9, 902.3
16.8, 37.5, 32.3	56.6, 83.5, 75.5	243.8, 244.1, 232.5	1064.5, 679.1, 697.6
32.2, 45.2, 20.7	37.2, 51.9, 25.6	31.5, 44.2, 23.9	20.8, 33.6, 15.8
31.6, 40.6, 37.0	37.8, 34.1, 32.0	32.3, 22.5, 23.4	21.7, 7.6, 11.4
26.0, 26.6, 25.5	59.2, 59.7, 58.9	121.9, 121.9, 122.0	213.9, 208.7, 216.0
22.0, 63.0, 56.1	53.5, 120.5, 109.2	114.3, 214.0, 197.8	206.2, 312.3, 294.3
34.8, 51.1, 20.2	49.0, 66.6, 35.2	106.3, 144.9, 83.3	252.2, 354.5, 211.9
32.5, 56.6, 52.0	47.5, 67.3, 62.6	104.8, 127.2, 121.6	254.6, 226.1, 227.3
17.0, 26.7, 8.4	19.7, 35.5, 7.2	25.2, 54.8, 7.5	20.8, 61.6, 4.7
18.3, 6.7, 7.2	20.9, 8.5, 9.2	26.9, 7.7, 8.3	22.1, 5.7, 7.8
5.4, 8.7, 2.4	4.4, 6.4, 2.8	4.6, 6.5, 3.5	4.7, 6.4, 4.0
3.8, 19.7, 16.9	3.1, 17.8, 15.1	3.6, 15.9, 14.2	3.6, 17.1, 15.9

TABLE 4-2 Number of acute conditions per 100 persons per year, by race, gender, age, and type of condition: United States, 1985*

	White		Black		Female		Male	
	18-44 Yr	45+ Yr	18-44 Yr	45+ Yr	18-44 Yr	45+ Yr	18-44 Yr	45+ Yr
All acute conditions	173.6	109.4	130.4	98.4	193.0	117.1	140.7	95.7
Infective and parasitic diseases	18.9	6.1	8.9	3.3	21.6	5.9	12.8	5.4
Respiratory conditions	88.4	55.8	53.7	51.5	96.4	59.0	69.5	49.8
Common cold	26.4	19.6	23.9	20.4	30.7	21.1	21.4	17.7
Other acute upper respiratory infections	9.0	4.5	4.0	1.7	10.5	4.6	5.9	3.6
Influenza	47.1	28.0	23.5	21.7	49.7	29.1	37.0	24.8
Digestive system conditions	5.9	5.3	10.1	7.2	8.0	6.2	4.8	4.5
Injuries	31.0	18.3	29.1	12.3	23.7	19.5	38.2	15.4
Selected other acute conditions	21.2	14.2	18.4	9.6	32.3	15.7	9.4	11.3
All other acute conditions	8.2	9.7	10.2	14.5	11.0	10.7	6.0	9.3

From National Center for Health Statistics: Current estimates from the national health interview survey, United States, 1985, US Public Health Service Pub No 86-1588, Washington, DC, 1986, US Government Printing Office.
*Data are based on household interviews of the civilian noninstitutionalized population.

TABLE 4-3 Number of selected reported chronic conditions per 1000 persons, by gender and age: United States, 1985*

	Men				Women			
Type of Chronic Condition	Under 45 Yr	45-64 Yr	65-74 Yr	75 Yr and over	Under 45 Yr	45-64 Yr	65-74 Yr	75 Yr and over
Arthritis	21.6	205.9	342.2	398.5	43.9	325.4	550.5	550.5
Visual impairment	36.1	62.1	87.9	133.6	12.7	27.0	67.4	126.0
Cataracts	1.7	26.5	63.9	181.9	2.1	22.5	140.8	298.3
Hearing impairment	45.5	208.0	323.2	443.1	30.5	114.3	214.2	291.4
Deformity or orthopedic impairment	90.4	162.6	144.4	126.0	89.0	158.8	186.2	204.2
Ulcer	12.6	36.1	48.3	35.3	12.9	37.1	21.3	35.2
Hernia of abdominal cavity	10.3	44.1	69.3	79.3	5.1	35.0	74.9	44.8
Diabetes	5.9	52.4	104.0	95.7	6.6	51.4	112.7	95.5
Heart disease	28.4	137.8	302.1	377.7	37.1	120.9	256.9	332.7
High blood pressure (hypertension)	45.5	253.8	382.0	292.3	34.9	263.5	461.7	453.8
Hemorrhoids	29.2	69.9	61.0	67.2	38.9	72.0	71.2	46.1
Chronic bronchitis	37.8	35.9	47.6	44.3	54.6	71.0	82.1	62.7
Asthma	35.9	27.4	42.4	21.9	42.0	28.9	52.9	22.4
Chronic sinusitis	106.1	162.3	147.0	142.1	141.4	205.4	154.4	170.3
Emphysema	0.8	23.5	81.5	77.2	1.2	7.6	25.5	16.8

From National Center for Health Statistics: Current estimates from the national health interview survey, United States, 1985, US Public Health Service Pub No 86-1588, Washington, DC, 1986, US Government Printing Office.
*Data are based on household interviews of the civilian noninstitutionalized population.

CONSEQUENCES OF ILLNESS

There are several consequences of illness. People may treat themselves, perhaps spending a day away from work or in bed. In the National Health Interview Survey, four types of disability days are reported: restricted activity days, bed-disability days, work-loss days, and school-loss days. A restricted activity day is one on which an individual reduces his or her normal activity for the entire day because of an illness or injury. By def-

inition, bed-disability days are ones in which the person spends all or most of the day in bed; these are counted as days of restricted activity. Each day lost from work or school is also counted as a day of restricted activity. Table 4-6 shows that all types of restriction for acute and chronic conditions increase with age. Moreover, men have higher rates of bed-disability days, but women have higher rates of work- or school-loss days. Blacks have higher rates of bed-disability or work- or school-

TABLE 4-4 Number of selected reported chronic conditions per 1000 persons, by race and age: United States, 1985*

Type of Chronic Condition	White				Black			
	Under 45 Yr	45-64 Yr	65-74 Yr	75 Yr and over	Under 45 Yr	45-64 Yr	65-74 Yr	75 Yr and over
Arthritis	34.6	264.4	452.8	492.6	28.0	331.9	581.1	577.8
Visual impairment	25.1	43.6	74.1	131.0	21.6	44.9	103.5	78.4
Cataracts	1.5	24.6	105.4	256.9	3.7	26.6	111.2	253.3
Hearing impairment	41.3	163.3	265.9	353.4	18.1	128.4	237.8	277.4
Deformity or orthopedic impairment	93.4	163.8	170.6	177.9	73.5	120.9	144.8	147.2
Ulcer	12.2	35.6	34.2	33.0	16.7	36.6	27.3	51.9
Hernia of abdominal cavity	7.9	41.7	79.0	63.1	8.1	26.6	16.8	—
Diabetes	6.5	45.6	102.0	89.7	6.5	112.1	172.0	153.2
Heart disease	34.6	131.0	276.9	376.4	23.0	137.0	266.4	80.8
High blood pressure (hypertension)	38.0	247.2	415.8	393.6	58.8	368.5	537.1	427.0
Hemorrhoids	36.8	71.7	70.1	57.3	21.3	70.4	35.0	21.7
Chronic bronchitis	48.8	55.0	71.5	60.9	36.4	59.3	30.8	4.8
Asthma	39.6	28.7	47.9	22.6	42.5	27.5	54.5	7.2
Chronic sinusitis	131.9	189.6	154.7	159.6	95.3	174.4	139.2	170.1
Emphysema	1.0	16.0	52.5	41.7	0.4	11.3	32.2	12.1

From National Center for Health Statistics: Current estimates from the national health interview survey, United States, 1985, US Public Health Service Pub No 86-1588, Washington, DC, 1986, US Government Printing Office.
*Data are based on household interviews of the civilian noninstitutionalized population.

loss days than do Whites, and people in low-income brackets have higher rates of restriction than those who have a higher income during middle and later life.

UTILIZATION OF HEALTH SERVICES

Another response to illness is using health services. People commonly contact physicians and other health care providers via the telephone, in their offices, or in hospitals. The use of telephone calls and office visits tends to increase with age. Men tend to make more hospital visits than do women, and women make more telephone calls and office visits than do men. Whites tend to make more telephone calls and office visits than do Blacks, whereas Blacks make more hospital visits than do Whites. People in low-income brackets tend to make more hospital contacts than their socially advantaged counterparts. (Table 4-7) In 1985 there was an average of 5.3 physician contacts per person per year, and 75% of the persons interviewed had one or more contacts in the past year. Approximately 12 persons per 100 were hospitalized in the past year. The average length of stay per hospitalization, however, was 6.7 days.

HEALTH PERCEPTIONS

In addition to asking about morbidity experiences, the National Health Interview Survey requests that people rate their own health or that of family members living in the same household as excellent, very good, good, fair, or poor. Only about 3% of the population rated their health as poor, with nearly 40% rating their health as excellent. Table 4-8 demonstrates that people's perceptions of their health vary with age, gender, race, and income. In general, older adults are more likely to rate their health as poor than younger adults, older men are more likely to rate their health as poor than older women, and older Blacks are more likely to rate their health as poor than older Whites. People in a low-income bracket are more likely to rate their health as poor than people who are wealthier.

VARIATIONS BY PLACE

The frequency of occurrence of various health problems and practices can also be related to the geographic area in which they occur. Place can be described in terms of natural boundaries, political subdivisions, international scope, or rural versus urban comparisons. In addition, the comparison of rates for people who migrate from one area to another is of assistance in separating the role of genetic from environmental factors in disease incidence.

Recently investigators compared adult health practices of people living in the United States and Canada in the following areas: smoking; drinking status and average daily alcohol consumption; physical activity; eating breakfast; use of seatbelts and child safety restraints; ownership of smoke detectors; recentness of blood pressure checks, Pap tests, and breast exams; and practice of breast self-examination.[10] Based on 1985 data, three health-promoting practices (not smoking, not drinking alcohol, and not skipping breakfast) were more common

TABLE 4-5 Number of selected reported chronic conditions per 1000 persons, by income and age: United States, 1985*

Type of Chronic Condition	Less Than $10,000			$10,000-19,999			$20,000-$34,999			$35,000 or more		
	Under 45 Yr	45-64 Yr	65 Yr and over	Under 45 Yr	45-64 Yr	65 Yr and over	Under 45 Yr	45-64 Yr	65 Yr and over	Under 45 Yr	45-64 Yr	65 Yr and over
Arthritis	48.2	408.5	545.9	38.7	349.5	448.9	34.3	279.1	457.3	23.6	186.4	433.3
Visual impairment	32.2	93.8	115.6	26.0	47.7	89.2	23.1	49.4	88.6	23.7	29.5	50.8
Cataracts	2.8	39.7	198.6	2.3	25.8	125.6	1.9	31.2	115.3	1.8	11.8	152.8
Hearing impairment	41.4	288.6	315.1	38.0	172.0	279.2	37.9	141.5	255.4	39.2	133.9	288.1
Deformity or orthopedic impairment	106.7	213.4	212.5	100.3	192.6	167.7	81.7	160.1	155.5	82.1	133.2	137.7
Ulcer	21.7	64.3	28.6	19.5	32.2	34.7	10.8	33.7	36.9	6.9	32.5	40.5
Hernia of abdominal cavity	10.0	65.3	55.9	9.4	39.2	82.9	8.7	28.0	76.4	5.3	48.3	58.3
Diabetes	7.1	82.4	117.2	6.2	71.7	110.4	6.8	45.5	101.8	4.1	28.9	84.9
Heart disease	43.4	202.9	357.3	31.6	176.5	315.1	33.4	153.2	242.3	33.2	70.5	288.1
High blood pressure (hypertension)	47.5	361.0	460.5	41.8	294.9	393.4	42.5	286.9	346.6	35.5	197.5	437.7
Hemorrhoids	26.7	96.1	81.8	37.5	73.5	69.6	52.5	78.0	51.2	32.3	66.1	61.9
Chronic bronchitis	47.6	76.7	63.6	46.2	76.5	72.2	47.2	50.7	68.8	47.2	41.0	51.6
Asthma	49.6	26.4	44.5	32.5	19.1	57.0	39.9	30.5	27.4	39.7	40.0	19.4
Chronic sinusitis	112.4	242.6	192.3	114.5	208.7	168.0	128.4	166.5	140.3	138.5	195.4	116.7
Emphysema	1.8	33.9	55.1	1.9	29.3	48.8	0.6	10.6	33.9	0.8	7.0	44.4

From National Center for Health Statistics: Current estimates from the national health interview survey, United States, 1985, US Public Health Service Pub No 86-1588, Washington, DC, 1986, US Government Printing Office.
*Data are based on household interviews of the civilian noninstitutionalized population.

TABLE 4-6 Number of days per person per year of activity restriction resulting from acute and chronic conditions, by type of restriction and sociodemographic characteristics: United States, 1985

Age and Characteristic	All Types	Type of Restriction Bed Disability	Work or School Loss*
ALL PERSONS†	14.8	6.1	5.2
18-24 yr	9.4	3.7	4.4
25-44 yr	11.9	4.8	5.0
45-64 yr	20.3	8.3	6.5
65 yr and over	33.1	13.7	7.0
MALE			
18-24 yr	7.0	2.6	3.5
25-44 yr	10.2	3.7	4.3
45-64 yr	18.8	7.2	6.1
65 yr and over	29.8	13.4	8.4
FEMALE			
18-24 yr	11.7	4.8	5.4
25-44 yr	13.6	5.8	5.9
45-64 yr	21.6	9.3	6.9
65 yr and over	35.4	13.9	5.1
WHITE			
18-24 yr	9.7	3.7	4.5
25-44 yr	11.3	4.4	4.7
45-64 yr	19.1	7.5	6.4
65 yr and over	32.0	13.1	7.2
BLACK			
18-24 yr	8.2	3.8	4.4
25-44 yr	17.0	7.4	7.7
45-64 yr	31.8	15.0	7.7
65 yr and over	47.2	20.6	5.5
UNDER $10,000 PER YR			
18-24 yr	11.9	5.1	4.8
25-44 yr	23.2	11.1	8.5
45-64 yr	45.4	20.5	8.5
65 yr and over	45.8	17.7	6.4
$10,000-$19,999 PER YR			
18-24 yr	11.0	4.5	4.9
25-44 yr	13.4	5.4	5.6
45-64 yr	25.2	10.7	8.4
65 yr and over	30.2	12.4	6.9
$20,000-$34,999 PER YR			
18-24 yr	9.3	3.2	5.1
25-44 yr	10.9	4.0	5.3
45-64 yr	16.9	5.6	6.9
65 yr and over	26.1	11.1	8.6
$35,000 OR MORE PER YR			
18-24 yr	6.5	2.7	3.7
25-44 yr	9.3	3.3	4.0
45-64 yr	11.9	4.7	5.3
65 yr and over	25.2	9.7	8.1

From National Center for Health Statistics: Current estimates from the national health interview survey, United States, 1985, US Public Health Service Pub No 86-1588, Washington, DC, 1986, US Government Printing Office.
*Sum of work-loss days for currently employed persons 18 years of age and over. Work-loss days are shown for persons aged 18 years and older.
†Includes other races and unknown family income.

TABLE 4-7 Number per person per year and number of physician contacts, by place of contact and sociodemographic characteristics: United States, 1985*

Characteristic	Telephone	Office	Hospital
ALL PERSONS†	0.7	3.0	0.8
18-24 yr	0.5	2.2	0.7
25-44 yr	0.7	2.8	0.7
45-64 yr	0.8	3.6	1.0
65-74 yr	0.8	4.6	1.1
75 yr and over	1.0	5.3	0.9
MALE			
18-44 yr	0.3	1.8	0.6
45-64 yr	0.5	3.0	1.1
65 yr and over	0.8	4.6	1.2
FEMALE			
18-44 yr	0.9	3.4	0.8
45-64 yr	1.0	4.1	0.9
65 yr and over	0.9	5.1	0.9
WHITE			
18-44 yr	0.7	2.7	0.6
45-64 yr	0.8	3.6	0.9
65 yr and over	0.9	5.0	1.0
BLACK			
18-44 yr	0.3	2.2	1.1
45-64 yr	0.4	3.5	1.8
65 yr and over	0.5	3.8	1.4
UNDER $10,000			
18-44 yr	0.5	2.5	1.1
45-64 yr	1.0	3.9	2.0
65 yr and over	0.8	4.9	1.1
$10,000-$19,999 PER YR			
18-24 yr	0.6	2.5	0.7
25-44 yr	0.7	3.9	0.9
65 yr and over	0.9	4.7	1.1
$20,000-$34,999 PER YR			
18-24 yr	0.7	2.7	0.7
45-64 yr	0.8	3.6	1.0
65 yr and over	1.1	5.2	1.3
$35,000 OR MORE PER YR			
18-44 yr	0.7	2.9	0.6
45-64 yr	0.8	3.5	0.8
65 yr and over	1.0	5.8	0.7

From National Center for Health Statistics: Current estimates from the national health interview survey, United States, 1985, US Public Health Service Pub No 86-1588, Washington, DC, 1986, US Government Printing Office.
*Does not include physician contacts if contact occurred when person was an overnight patient in a hospital.
†Includes other races and unknown family income.

TABLE 4-8 Number of persons and percent distribution by respondent-assessed health status, according to sociodemographic characteristics: United States, 1985

Characteristic	Excellent	Very Good	Good	Fair	Poor
18-24 yr	45.1	31.2	19.7	3.4	0.5
25-44 yr	42.4	30.2	21.1	4.9	1.4
45-64 yr	27.0	25.3	29.2	12.4	6.1
65 yr and over	15.9	20.2	32.5	21.5	9.9
MALE					
18-24 yr	50.4	28.5	17.9	2.7	0.5
25-44 yr	46.3	29.5	18.6	4.3	1.3
45-64 yr	29.5	25.4	27.1	11.4	6.6
65 yr and over	16.5	19.7	31.4	21.3	11.1
FEMALE					
18-24 yr	40.1	33.8	21.4	4.0	0.6
25-44 yr	38.6	30.9	23.4	5.6	1.5
45-64 yr	24.6	25.2	31.1	13.4	5.7
65 yr and over	15.4	20.6	33.3	21.7	9.0
WHITE					
18-24 yr	46.4	32.3	17.9	2.9	0.6
25-44 yr	44.0	30.9	19.7	4.2	1.2
45-64 yr	28.3	26.0	28.7	11.3	5.6
65 yr and over	16.6	20.5	33.0	20.9	9.1
BLACK					
18-24 yr	37.2	26.3	29.7	6.3	0.5
25-44 yr	29.9	26.8	30.1	10.3	2.8
45-64 yr	15.1	18.8	32.9	21.6	11.5
65 yr and over	8.3	16.8	27.8	28.3	18.8
UNDER $10,000 PER YR					
18-24 yr	38.0	32.8	23.4	5.0	0.9
25-44 yr	26.5	25.2	30.3	12.9	5.2
45-64 yr	12.7	13.8	26.5	26.0	20.9
65 yr and over	11.6	17.9	30.4	26.5	13.7
$10,000-$19,999 PER YR					
18-24 yr	40.2	33.9	21.6	3.8	0.6
25-44 yr	35.8	30.2	25.5	6.8	1.7
45-64 yr	18.8	22.5	32.5	17.6	8.6
65 yr and over	14.6	20.3	33.8	21.7	9.6
$20,000-$34,999 PER YR					
18-24 yr	48.2	30.8	17.7	2.9	0.4
25-44 yr	43.0	32.6	19.7	3.9	0.8
45-64 yr	27.2	26.2	31.5	11.0	4.1
65 yr and over	20.0	22.7	33.8	17.5	6.0
$35,000 OR MORE PER YR					
18-24 yr	56.1	28.7	13.9	0.9	0.4
25-44 yr	51.9	30.0	15.5	2.3	0.4
45-64 yr	37.8	30.8	24.5	5.5	1.4
65 yr and over	27.7	24.8	27.9	14.4	5.2

From National Center for Health Statistics: Current estimates from the national health interview survey, United States, 1985, US Public Health Service Pub No 86-1588, Washington, DC, 1986, US Government Printing Office.

TABLE 4-9 Summary of health practices in the United States and Canada, 1985

Practice	United States	Canada
Regularly smoke	30	35
Currently drink	65	82
2 drinks or more daily average	12	14
Regularly active physically	40	53
Rarely eat breakfast	24	29
Usually wear seatbelts	36	79
Children usually wear restraints	52	91
Own 1 smoke detector or more	69	77
Blood pressure checked within 1 year	74	76
Breast examination within 1 year	50	69
Pap smear within 3 years	78	76
Perform breast self-examination at least monthly	32	41

From National Center for Health Statistics: Current estimates from the national health interview survey, United States, 1985, US Public Health Service Pub No 86-1588, Washington, DC, 1986, US Government Printing Office.

in the United States, but six practices were more common in Canada (regular physical activity, using seatbelts and child restraints, owning smoke detectors, having a breast examination in the past year, and performing breast self-exam at least monthly). Three health-related practices were equal in both countries (having a recent blood pressure checkup, having a recent Pap smear, and drinking two or more alcoholic beverages per day). (Table 4-9). These findings warrant an investigation of differences in the social structure and cultural characteristics of both countries that influence health practices.

VARIATIONS BY TIME

The occurrence of various health conditions and their distribution by personal characteristics and place are important. Nonetheless, changes in patterns of occurrence of health conditions over time are also important to consider. Time variations can be described in several ways. First one can differentiate endemic and epidemic disease. *Endemic* conditions are always present in an area in some form, whereas an *epidemic* is a temporary rise in the incidence of a disease to a level greater than that usually expected. Next, one can examine the *periodicity* of a disease to determine if it is seasonal or cyclic. Finally, *secular trends* in disease or mortality can be described. Such a trend has been noted in the incidence of lung cancer among women, and examination of secular trends in the incidence of smoking women has suggested a relationship between smoking and lung cancer.

TABLE 4-10 Life expectancy at birth, according to sex: selected countries, selected periods*

Country	Period	Life Expectancy in Years	Period	Life Expectancy in Years
MALE				
Japan	1976	72.2	1983	74.2
Sweden	1974-78	72.2	1983	73.6
Netherlands	1977	72.0	1982-83	72.8
Switzerland	1968-73	70.3	1981-82	72.7
Norway	1977-78	72.3	1982-83	72.7
Israel	1978	71.5	1983	72.5
Australia	1965-67	67.6	1983	72.1
Canada	1970-72	69.3	1980-82	71.9
Denmark	1977-78	71.5	1982-83	71.5
England and Wales	1974-76	69.6	1981-83	71.3
Cuba	1970	68.5	1977-78	71.2
United States	1979	70.0	1984	71.2
New Zealand	1970-72	68.6	1983	70.8
Federal Republic of Germany	1976-78	69.0	1981-83	70.5
France	1977	69.7	1981	70.4
Spain	1970	69.7	1975	70.4
Finland	1978	68.5	1983	70.2
Greece	1970	70.1	1970	70.1
Italy	1970-72	69.0	1974-77	69.7
Austria	1977	68.5	1983	69.5
Ireland	1970-72	68.8	1978-80	69.5
German Democratic Republic	1978	68.8	1983	69.5
Scotland	1971-73	67.2	1981-83	69.3
Northern Ireland	1975-77	67.5	1983	69.3
Panama	1970	64.3	1980-85	69.2
FEMALE				
Japan	1976	77.4	1983	79.8
Sweden	1974-78	78.1	1983	79.6
Switzerland	1968-73	76.2	1981-82	79.6
Norway	1977-78	78.7	1982-83	79.5
Netherlands	1977	78.4	1982-83	79.5
Canada	1970-72	76.4	1980-82	78.9
Australia	1965-67	74.2	1983	78.7
France	1977	77.9	1981	78.5
United States	1979	77.8	1984	78.2
Finland	1978	77.1	1983	78.0
Denmark	1977-78	77.5	1982-83	77.5
England and Wales	1974-76	75.8	1981-83	77.4
Federal Republic of Germany	1976-78	75.6	1981-83	77.1
New Zealand	1970-72	74.6	1983	76.9
Austria	1977	75.6	1983	76.8
Spain	1970	75.0	1975	76.2
Israel	1978	75.0	1983	75.9
Italy	1970-72	74.9	1974-77	75.9
Northern Ireland	1975-77	73.8	1983	75.7
Scotland	1971-73	73.6	1981-83	75.5
German Democratic Republic	1978	74.4	1983	75.4
Poland	1975-76	75.0	1983	75.2
Belgium	1968-72	74.2	1972-76	75.1
Ireland	1970-72	73.5	1978-80	75.0
Cuba	1970	71.8	1977-78	74.6

*Data are based on reporting by countries.
NOTE: Rankings are from highest to lowest life expectancy based on the latest available data for countries or geographic areas with at least 1 million population and most recent data for 1970 or later. This table is based only on data from the official life tables of the country concerned, consistent with the data presented in the United Nations, Demographic Yearbook, 1984.
(Data from United Nations Demographic Yearbook, 1979, 1984; Pub Nos ST/ESA/STAT/SER.R/9 and ST/ESA/STAT/SER.R/14, New York, United Nations, 1980, 1986; National Center for Health Statistics: Vital statistics of the United States, 1979, Vol II, Mortality, Part A, Pub No 84-1101, 1984, Washington, DC, US Government Printing Office; Public Health Service: Advance report of final mortality statistics, 1984, Pub No 86-1120, Hyattsville, Md, Sept 26, 1986.)

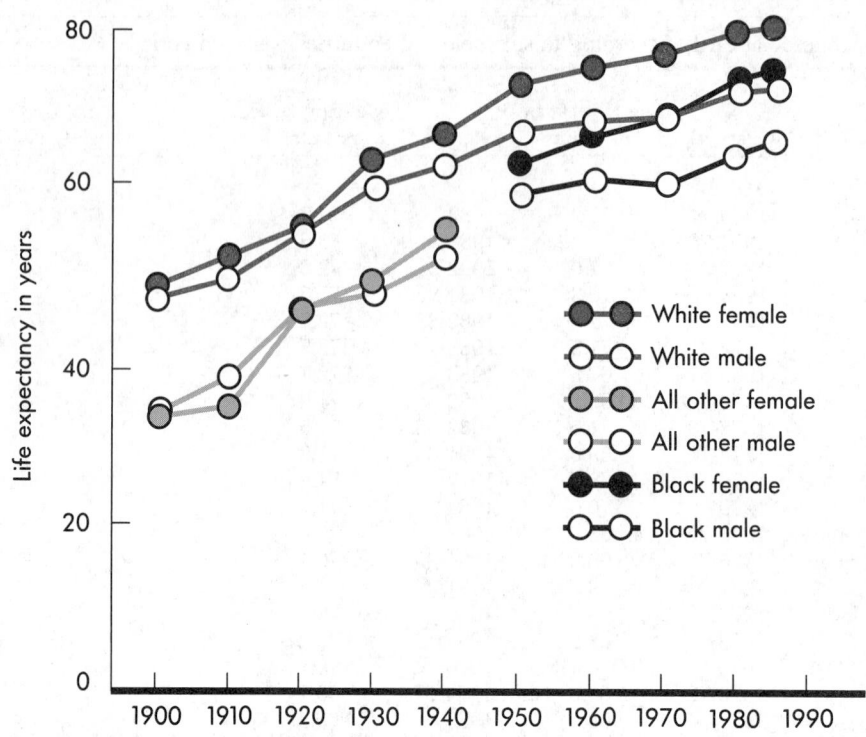

FIGURE 4-1 Life expectancy at birth, according to race and sex: United States, selected years 1900-1985. (From National Center for Health Statistics, Division of Vital Statistics: National Vital Statistics System, USPHS, Washington, DC, 1987.)

Life expectancy at birth (Table 4-10) has increased significantly since 1900 for all American men and women, regardless of race (see Figure 4-1). During the first half of the century, increases in life expectancy were attributable to reductions in infant and childhood mortality, but in contrast, recent increases in longevity are attributable to decreasing mortality from chronic disease among middle-aged and elderly persons. Throughout the entire period studied, White women had the longest life expectancy, with Black women surpassing White men in life expectancy around 1970. Racial differences in life expectancy have narrowed, with White women living 5.2 years longer than Black women and White men living 6.1 years longer than Black men. Although differences in longevity between races remain in 1985, they have narrowed considerably when compared with the 14-year difference in life expectancy for White men and Black men and the 15-year difference for White women and Black women that existed in 1900.[12] When life expectancy for men and women in the United States is compared to that of other selected countries, it is evident that the populations of several countries with a national health plan have greater longevity than United States' residents.[12]

Leading causes of death in the United States have changed since 1900, when such infectious diseases as

tuberculosis claimed the greatest number of lives. In 1985 the leading cause of death was heart disease, with cancer and cerebrovascular disease the second and third leading causes of death. People now survive infectious diseases to live to middle and old age, in which they develop chronic diseases.[12]

QUANTIFICATION OF HEALTH AND ILLNESS EXPERIENCES

One means of describing health and illness patterns for a population is using rates and ratios. Table 4-11 defines some of the most commonly used approaches to quantifying health and illness experiences, including prevalence rate, incidence rate, *mortality rate,* and *age-specific mortality rate.* These rates are proportions; that is, they are calculated by determining the number in the total population who have the disease or who die from it compared with the total number in the population or those at risk of the disease.

Prevalence rates summarize the proportion of a population affected by the health condition at any point in time. This includes the total number of cases, whether they were newly diagnosed or had been diagnosed several years earlier. If one considers the prevalence of colon cancer in men in the United States for 1990, then one must consider in the numerator the men who were

TABLE 4-11 Rates commonly employed in epidemiologic studies

	Definition

Prevalence rate = $\dfrac{\text{Number of persons with a disease}}{\text{Total number in group}}$

Period prevalence rate = $\dfrac{\text{Number of persons with a disease during a period of time}}{\text{Total number in group}}$

Incidence rate = $\dfrac{\text{Number of persons developing a disease}}{\text{Total number at risk}}$ per unit of time

Mortality rate = $\dfrac{\text{Number of persons dying from a particular cause}}{\text{Total number in group}}$ per unit of time

Age-specific mortality rate = $\dfrac{\text{Number of persons dying in a particular age group}}{\text{Total number in that age group}}$ per unit of time

diagnosed in 1971 and are still surviving as well as the men who were diagnosed in 1990. The denominator would include these same men, as well as all other men at risk for colon cancer. A variation of this rate, termed *period prevalence*, describes the number of persons with a disease during a period of time, such as from 1985 to 1990, per the total number of persons in the group.

Incidence rates describe the occurrence of *new* cases of disease over a specified period of time. Incidence rates imply the rate of development of a disease over time. When calculating incidence rates, epidemiologists consider that persons who have already developed diseases of lifelong duration cannot be counted as new cases more than once. Therefore the denominator for incidence rates includes only the population at risk of developing the disease, rather than the total population. In the case of cancer, we find that the estimated incidence for 1980 was about 785,000 new cases, whereas the prevalence of cancer was estimated to be 3 million cases. Thus the incidence rate would be calculated as follows:

Cancer incidence rate
= 785,000 (total U.S. population − 3,000,000)

Mortality rates are commonly used to reflect the number of deaths from certain causes as compared with the total population. For example, the death rate per 100,000 population for heart disease in 1986 was 317.5. Rates may refer to special subgroups of the population as well as to the total population. The *age-specific mortality* refers to the number of persons dying in a particular age group, compared with the total number of persons in that same age group per unit of time. For example, the age-specific mortality for lung cancer for women 35 to 54 years old for 1990 could be calculated by counting all women who died from lung cancer in that age group and dividing that number by the total

number of women who were 35 to 54 years of age in 1990.

Rates allow for comparison of groups and comparison of phenomena over time. For example, one might compare the rate of lung cancer among smokers to the rate of lung cancer in nonsmokers. One might also compare the incidence rate of lung cancer for a population during one period of time to the same rate for another period.

UNDERSTANDING CAUSES OF HEALTH AND ILLNESS

In addition to being able to describe patterns of health and illness, it is important for clinicians to understand what produces health and illness. The search for causes of health and disease, with the ultimate goal of prevention of disease and death and promotion of health, motivates much health-related research.

CRITERIA FOR CAUSAL ASSOCIATIONS

A hypothesis of causation asserts that X is a factor that determines Y. In other words, whenever X occurs, Y will follow. It is recognized, however, that conditions often occur in which a single factor is a partial or contributory cause. Furthermore, in epidemiologic studies, events are usually viewed in a probabilistic rather than a deterministic way. Our current frameworks for causation of disease recognize that usually a web of causation exists in which multiple variables are involved. Where it was once believed that one could find a single cause that was both necessary and sufficient to produce disease, it is now recognized that most health problems are determined by multiple factors.

There are generally accepted criteria for causal associations: *covariation, causal direction,* and *nonspuriousness.* Covariation means that the dependent variable varies with the independent variable, or that a change in X results in a change in Y. A dose-response relationship implies that for a range of X there is a gradient in the degree of Y. Causal direction implies that the cause must precede the effect in time: X → Y (antecedent-consequent relationship). Nonspuriousness means that we must be able to observe that there are no other variables that cause changes in the dependent variable and are associated with the independent variable.

There are two basic approaches to testing causal hypotheses: observational and experimental. In the *observational* study, the investigator can only perceive and report the natural variation of two variables, whereas in an *experimental* study the investigator can manipulate the causal variable under controlled conditions. The observational study will undoubtedly continue to provide a major contribution to the understanding of causes of disease, although experimentation can establish a causal relationship between a factor and a disease more conclusively than observation. Sometimes groups may be similar in every characteristic except in exposure to a specific factor. In this instance, the conditions for making a causal inference are so favorable that a "natural experiment" may be said to occur. An example of a natural (but unfortunate) experiment was that afforded by the bombing of Japan during World War II. Observation of people who had been exposed to varying amounts of radiation led to the discovery of an increased risk of certain cancers, for example, leukemia.

Because of the need to rely on observational methods in epidemiologic studies, additional considerations in establishing a causal relationship are appropriate. Once the noncausal explanations for the association have been excluded, the following additional criteria can be used to explore the likelihood of a causal association:

1. *Strength of the association.* The stronger the association, the less likely it is that it might be produced by unknown confounding factors.
2. *Consistency of the association.* The relationship is repeatedly observed by different investigators, in different samples, and in different places and times by different research designs.
3. *Coherence.* The relationship does not contradict current knowledge about the phenomenon. The finding is coherent with the body of knowledge.
4. *Experimental confirmation.* Confirming an association in an experiment is a powerful way to establish a causal relationship.

When considering the relationship between two variables, it is important to recognize that they may be one of the following types:

1. Independent (not statistically associated)
2. Statistically associated
   a. Noncausally associated
   b. Causally associated
      (1) Indirectly causal
      (2) Directly causal

Independence between two variables, for example, a characteristic and a type of cancer, can be established by means of statistical tests of significance. If the two variables are statistically associated, that is, associated not simply by chance, the investigator must then proceed to determine whether the relationship is a noncausal or a causal one.

NONCAUSAL ASSOCIATIONS
ARTIFACT

Two variables can be statistically but noncausally related simply because of artifact. Such an association would be spurious. It is well known that in a certain proportion of statistical tests, an association will be declared statistically significant when in fact it is not (type I error). In this instance the association may simply be a result of random fluctuation, or *chance*.

A second source of artifact is *bias*, that is, the false labeling of either the characteristic or the condition under study. Bias can occur as a result of lack of reliability or validity in measurement, selective recall of the person being studied, or the reverse bias of the investigator. Selective recall may occur when the person either exaggerates part of a history or fails to recall some characteristic such as exposure. For example, a mother whose child is born with a congenital anomaly will probably remember her behavior during pregnancy more clearly than a mother whose child is born without any problems. Sometimes characteristics or conditions are falsely labeled in a study. For example, statistics may indicate that a disease rate has changed when in reality all that has changed is the ability to diagnose it. Sometimes investigators have strong preconceived notions about the relationship between a characteristic and a condition. This may result in their being more attentive to these characteristics in persons who have the condition. Sometimes reverse bias occurs when the investigator makes a conscious effort to avoid bias; this leads to underdetection; for example, the person with a mild version of the disease is not labeled as a case. Bias can be prevented by measuring concordance between observers or diagnosticians whenever possible and establishing the validity, sensitivity, and specificity of measuring instruments.

Another source of artifact is *selection bias*. This occurs when by some fault in the research design or sampling, it has become easier for people in whom there is an association between the characteristic and disease to be selected into the study or excluded from it. The former results in an inflation of the strength of the association, and the latter leads to an underestimation of the association.

SECONDARY ASSOCIATION

Secondary association occurs when the association between two factors is produced by a third factor, termed a *confounding* factor. Confounding factors are associated with both the characteristic and the condition. An example of a secondary association is that seen between race and birth weight. The incidence of low-birth weight infants is much higher among Blacks than Whites. Race is associated with both socioeconomic status and birth weight, such that Blacks as a group have lower incomes, and lower income is associated with low birth weight. When one controls for the effect of socioeconomic status on birth weight, the effect of race disappears, thus indicating this was a *secondary association*. Fortunately, confounding factors can usually be controlled both in the study design and in analytic approaches.

CAUSAL ASSOCIATIONS

Causal associations may be classified as indirect or direct. An association is said to be *indirect* when the characteristic and condition are related only because they both are encompassed by the actual case. In other words, if X is causally related to Y, and Y is causally related to Z, there will be a causal relationship between X and Z, but the association is indirect. An example of an indirect association was related to the notion of miasma popular in the early nineteenth century. People believed that foul emanations from the soil and water caused disease. It was not until the germ theory had been popularized and the existence of microorganisms was discovered that the indirect association became evident. The soil and water contained bacteria that caused the disease: soil → microorganisms → disease.

The *direct* causal association occurs when the characteristic can be associated with the condition with some specificity. Usually, however, the distinction between indirect and direct causal associations is a relative one, and assertion of a direct relationship depends on our current level of knowledge.

A final type of causal relationship is known as *configurational association*. This means that one factor is capable of producing a condition only in the presence of another factor. For example, we know that co-carcinogens are involved in the development of certain cancers; certain malignancies are caused by more than one co-carcinogen, and one of these may be capable of producing cancer only in the presence of the other.

TESTING CAUSAL HYPOTHESES

Studies designed to test causal hypotheses involve searching for not only a single cause, but a web of factors that together produce a specific health condition. To investigate causes of disease and other health conditions, researchers use epidemiologic methods to study data sources, including persons with a given disease or condition and persons who are disease-free, clinical records, and laboratory data. Generally, hypothesis-testing studies take one of two forms: prospective or retrospective.

PROSPECTIVE STUDIES

Prospective studies are a very important form of epidemiologic investigation for testing hypotheses about disease causation. The study population for a prospective study consists of people who initially do not have the disease to be studied. From the reference population, people who are free from the disease are selected. They are subsequently classified according to presence or absence of the characteristic or characteristics thought to be related to the disease. The sample (usually termed a *cohort*) is then studied prospectively for a specified period of time (often for several years) to determine what proportion of the comparison groups under study develop the disease. Figure 4-2 includes an example of a prospective study of the relationship between social networks and mortality. In 1965, 4452 occupied housing units were selected from Alameda County; 6928 adults returned questionnaires.[2] Participants were asked a series of questions regarding the number of social ties they had and their relative importance. In 1974, a follow-up survey was conducted of death records of those people who died within the state and, where records were obtainable, out of state. In addition, all but 302 of the original participants were located. The mortality from all causes was computed for four groups of people who ranged from having the least to the most social connections. As the number of social connections decreased, the mortality increased. With this introduction in mind, let us consider in more detail the process of conducting a prospective study.

Selecting the Cohort

The initial cohort can be selected for a number of reasons: (1) they may have been exposed to the particular factor under study, (2) they may belong to a group where follow-up is facilitated, or (3) they may be as appropriate as any other cohort for the study. In this study the cohort was originally selected to participate in a large-scale study of health in Alameda County. They were subsequently observed in 1974 to assess mortality outcomes. Other cohorts frequently studied might include special occupational groups exposed to disease-producing agents, such as workers, persons enrolled in prepaid medical plans who will receive most of their care through a single source of care, persons taking out life insurance policies, obstetric populations (for neonatal or prenatal experiences), and volunteer groups of subjects, such as persons who volunteer for screening or who are identified by other volunteers. Other cohorts

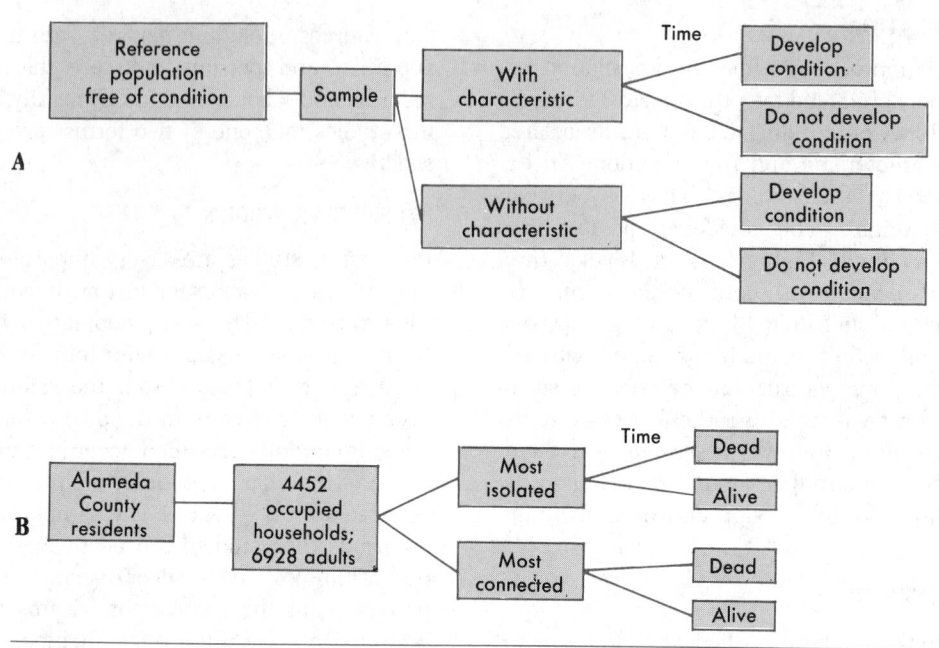

FIGURE 4-2 An illustration of a prospective study. **A,** Basic approach. **B,** Example.

might be selected on the basis of their presence in a single geographic location to either facilitate continued study of the cohort over time or to facilitate quantification of exposure, for example, with air pollution studies.

Exposure

Once the cohort has been identified, the investigator must collect data that allow classification of the subjects as exposed or not exposed. As we have seen earlier, it is frequently possible to define several different levels of exposure, for example, the use of four categories of social contacts. This procedure provides the investigator with an opportunity to assess the effects of a gradient of exposure, sometimes referred to as a dose-response effect. In other words, the investigator can ascertain whether the incidence of disease increases with the grade of exposure.

Data regarding exposure can be obtained from records, from individual members of the cohort, through testing or examining members of the cohort, or from assessing the environment in which they live. Berkman and Syme[2] used questionnaires to assess the number of personal ties.

One of the difficult aspects of obtaining data from individual members of a cohort is that there is frequently nonresponse. When a certain proportion does not provide data regarding exposure, it is possible that the loss of the respondents is biased with respect to either exposure, disease outcome, or both. The effects of bias in exposure or bias in disease or outcome differ from the effects of bias in *both* exposure and disease. When persons with high exposure levels fail to respond, the impression of the distribution of the exposure factor in the population will be inaccurate, but the association between the exposure and the disease will probably be accurate. When the nonresponse is biased with respect to disease (for example, the most ill do not respond), the disease rates for the cohort will be underestimated, but the ratio of disease rates among the exposed to disease rates among the nonexposed will probably be similar to that in the population as a whole. When persons who do not respond to the study are biased with respect to both the exposure factor and the disease, the true relationship between the factor and the disease will be biased.

It is often difficult to ascertain which type of bias is operative. Some approaches include more intense efforts to obtain data about exposure from nonrespondents, such as sending out a second questionnaire. Comparing the nonrespondents to the respondents on other variables, monitoring outcomes in the nonrespondents, and assessing the disease rates in the cohort over time (normally the effects of selection bias would be most apparent early in the study) may also help.

Another concern in assessing exposure is that people may be exposed to different experiences over time. For example, a person may change jobs and alter industrial exposure to toxic substances. Thus it is often important to verify the exposure categories periodically during the study.

Comparisons

Comparison groups in the prospective study are entered into the study at its inception. For example, in the Berkman and Syme study[2] all participants, regardless of their social contacts, were entered into the study at the same time. Often, however, other comparison groups are needed. In the case of a study of a special population selected for its exposure experience, for example, rubber workers, an appropriate nonexposed comparison group must be found. Often the experience of the general population at the time the cohort is being observed provides an appropriate comparison. Sometimes comparison cohorts or multiple groups are selected.

Follow-Up

The appearance of disease or death is usually the outcome to be ascertained. Procedures may include examination of members of the cohort or the surveillance of other data sources such as death certificates. Berkman and Syme used death registry data in ascertaining mortality. There are many difficulties associated with the use of these procedures to assess outcome, not the least of which is migration of members of the cohort, misclassification of disease on death certificates, or changes in diagnostic procedures. When cohort members are examined, there is also the possibility of bias in diagnosis when the examiner is aware of the individual's exposure status. This can be limited by use of objective measures and by keeping information regarding the exposure status from the examiner.

Analysis

Rates. The primary focus of analysis of data from prospective studies is the derivation of rates of an outcome (disease or mortality) for the cohorts studied. The rates are then usually compared across exposure groups.

Because of variability in the number of years during which each person in the cohort is observed, a commonly used denominator for calculating rates is personyears. The concept of person-years considers the number of persons observed and the duration of each observation. For example, let us consider the following distribution:

Years of Observation	Number of Persons
5	30
10	20
15	10

The person-years denominator for this study would be computed as follows:

$$(5 \times 30) + (10 \times 20) + (15 \times 10) = 500 \text{ person-years}$$

This denominator allows for the variation in entrance dates into the study (for example, often persons in the cohort are enrolled over several years), as well as for loss of certain individuals from the cohort.

The age distribution of the cohort also changes over time. For this reason, separate calculations of rates are usually made for persons in certain age groups.

When persons are lost to follow-up, a situation ana-

TABLE 4-12 Social isolation and age-adjusted mortality

Social Network Index	Men	Women
I (fewest connections)	15.6	12.1
II	12.2	7.2
III	8.6	4.9
IV (most connections)	6.4	4.3

logous to failure to obtain exposure information occurs. Losses that are biased with respect to both exposure and outcome will affect the relative rates of disease or death for exposure categories. When losses are large, there may be considerable distortion of estimates of risk. Often investigators compute several estimates based on different sets of assumptions regarding possible biases. For example, the investigator might assume that persons lost to follow-up were lost immediately after entry into the cohort. The investigator then may use only the number of persons examined on each occasion (beginning and end of the study) to compute rates. Another possibility is to make varying assumptions regarding the number of years persons lost to follow-up were actually observed. This may be a useful technique when multiple measures are made of the outcome at varying intervals during the study. Yet another approach might be to calculate a range of rates possible in each exposure category. In this instance the investigator might first assume that none of the persons lost developed the outcome and second, that all of them developed the outcome. The usefulness of the latter option, however, is limited inasmuch as the frequency of the outcome measured is often smaller than the proportion lost to follow-up.

Risk estimates. In addition to calculating rates of disease or death, an estimate of the association between exposure to certain factors and the risk of a particular outcome can be made. Two commonly used measures are the relative risk and the attributable risk. The *relative risk* (RR) is the ratio of the incidence rate in those exposed to the risk factor (or characteristic) to the incidence rate in the population not exposed. One can use as an example the relative risk of death for those who were the most isolated, compared with those with the most connections. The age-adjusted mortality associated with each group is given in Table 4-12. Taking the ratio of $RR = I_e/I_o$, where I_e is the incidence in the exposed, or here the least connected to a social network (15.6 for men), and where I_o is the incidence in the nonexposed, or here those with many connections (6.4 for men), we find that $RR = 15.6/6.4 = 2.5$. The relative risk of mortality for those men with few connections compared with those with many is 2.5. *Attributable risk* (AR_e) is another measure of association between risk factors and outcome. AR_e is the rate of the disease in exposed persons that can be attributed to the exposure: $AR_e = I_e - I_o$. With the use of the Berkman and Syme data, the attributable risk for those with few connections would be $15.6 - 6.4 = 9.2$. In addition, the attributable risk percent ($AR_e\%$) can be computed, where $AR_e\% = (I_e - I_o)/I_e$. The attributable risk percent, also referred to as the etiologic fraction among the exposed, is the proportion of disease in the exposed population that is attributable to the risk factor.

The population-attributable risk (AR_p) is the rate of the disease in the entire population that can be attributed to the risk factor. The population-attributable risk percent ($AR_p\%$), sometimes referred to as the etiologic fraction in the population, is the proportion of the disease rate in the total population that is attributable to exposure to the risk factor: $AR_p\% = (I_t - I_o)/I_t$.

The comparison of rates can also be achieved for a number of risk factors. Often it is found that two risk factors act synergistically. That is, the joint effect of the two risk factors results in a rate that exceeds the sum of the risks of those exposed to either risk factor individually. Recently, synergistic effects have been observed in workers exposed both to asbestos and smoking.

Interpretation

Results of a cohort study are interpreted in relation to two primary questions: (1) Are there alternative explanations for the association (or lack of association) between risk factors and outcome? (2) Is the association likely to be a causal relationship? To answer question 1, the investigator must meticulously review all previous steps in the study. The second question can be answered by considering the criteria for causal relationships discussed earlier in this chapter.

Advantages and Disadvantages

The fact that the cohort is drawn from a reference population enables the investigator to generalize from the sample to the reference population with some degree of certainty. In addition, it is clear that the characteristic precedes the development of the condition, one of the necessary conditions for a causal relationship. The investigator can directly quantify the risk of developing a condition in the presence of a risk factor. The likelihood of bias in reporting the relationship between the characteristic and the condition is reduced, since the characteristic is described before the outcome is measured. Selective survival, the survival of only special groups until the study in initiated, is not a problem here as it is for retrospective studies.

Prospective studies are very costly in time, personnel, and follow-up. They are not feasible when the condition

being studied is rare. Attrition of persons in the cohort constitutes a considerable problem in interpretation of results. Likewise, there may be attrition among investigators. Finally, other changes may occur over time in the environment, individuals, or treatment of the condition, and these may affect the outcomes.

RETROSPECTIVE STUDIES

Retrospective studies involve comparisons between groups of individuals who have the disease (cases) and groups who do not have the disease. The cases and comparison groups (commonly referred to as controls or referent group) are then compared with respect to current or past characteristics that the investigator believes have relevance to the particular disease being studied.*

Figure 4-3 illustrates the approach used in a recent study of smoking and nonfatal myocardial infarction (MI) in women.[16] All married female registered nurses 30 to 55 years of age residing in 11 of the larger states in the United States were polled in 1976. They were asked questions regarding many health-related variables, as well as smoking history and whether they had been hospitalized for an MI. All who had MIs were asked for permission to review their hospital records; 173 records were reviewed, and 128 diagnoses of acute MI were confirmed. For each woman who had had an MI (case), 20 women who had not had an MI (controls) and were born in the same year as the index case were chosen. The investigators then compared the relative proportion of smokers among the cases and controls.

Selection of Cases

In selecting the cases for a case-control study, the criteria for the definition of the disease, the source of cases, and the inclusion of incident or prevalent cases are extremely important considerations. Valid and reliable definitions of the disease are essential. Often the investigator must decide whether to include borderline cases or how to cope with differences in pathologists' use of diagnostic categories. One investigator[16] attempted to use a medical record review as the criterion for whether an MI had actually occurred. Other studies might include criteria such as electrocardiogram documentation, enzyme elevation, symptoms, or autopsy results to confirm the diagnosis.

Cases may be obtained from persons being treated for the disease at a certain facility or from persons with the disease from a more general population. Willett and associates[16] tried to identify all the cases of MI from a large study of nurses in 11 states. This approach allows the investigator to avoid problems of bias associated

---

*This approach is also commonly referred to as a case-control study. It is apparent, however, that the "controls" in this case are not equivalent to the controls in an experimental study.

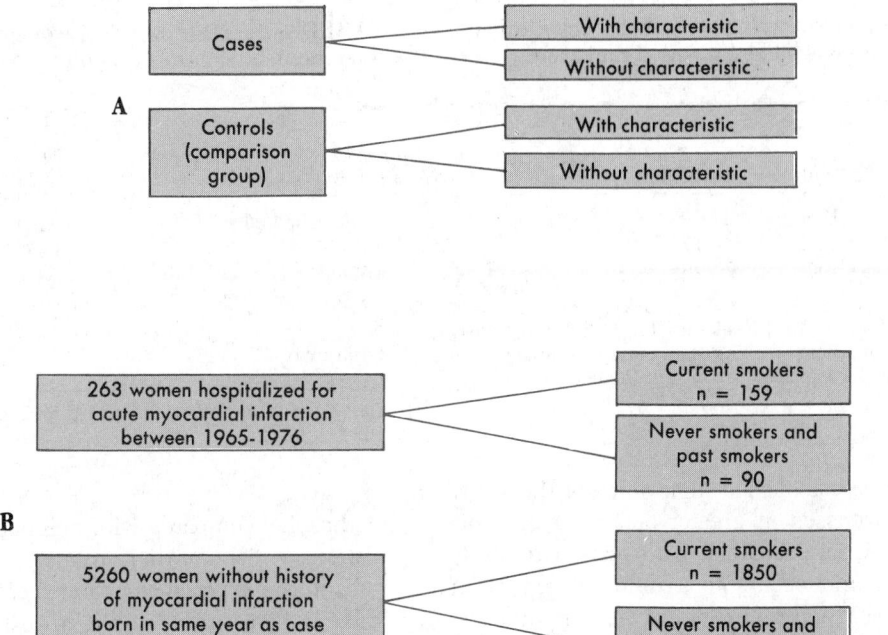

FIGURE 4-3 An illustration of a retrospective study. **A,** Basic approach. **B,** Example.

with use of a certain source of medical care, as would have been the case had the cases been selected from a hospital or clinic.

Inclusion of incident or prevalent cases is also an important consideration. Willett and co-workers studied only those cases occurring from 1965 to 1976.

Selection of Controls

Decisions about the source of controls are also important in the conduct of case-control studies. Controls may be obtained from the general population, hospitalized patients, or relatives or associates of the cases. In general, if the cases represent all the affected persons in a defined population, then controls should be selected from that same population. Some of the concerns in the selection of controls relate to whether information on the study factors can be obtained from the control group in a manner similar to that by which it was obtained from the cases, whether to match the controls with the cases to control for a certain confounding factor, whether the controls are similar to the cases in general, and practical and financial considerations. Willett and colleagues studied 20 women who were the same age as each case. Matching women on age was done to control for the confounding effects of age; that is, age is likely to be associated with both smoking history and MI. If age were not controlled, the proportion of women smoking among the cases might be greater than that among the controls, simply because the cases were older. The

data were obtained by the same questionnaire for cases and controls.

Sampling

Once the source of controls is identified, the investigator must decide whether to study the entire population or a sample from the population. Because of the difficulty encountered in enumeration of everyone in order to draw a random sample from a large population, paired sampling is often used. This means that for each case, one or more controls is selected. This may be accomplished, for example, by asking the cases to identify someone in the same neighborhood of the same age. In this study, controls were obtained from the nurses who had not had an MI.

Information about Exposure

Sources of data on exposure include the individual being studied or a relative and records such as hospital charts, birth certificates, and employment records. If the data on exposure differ systematically in completeness or accuracy between cases and controls, the association between exposure and disease will be spurious. The validity of exposure data is extremely important; where possible, information about exposure recorded before the discovery of the disease is desirable to reduce bias in reporting. Further efforts to ensure validity are the use of similar procedures for cases and controls. Finally, the sensitivity and specificity of classification

TABLE 4-13 Number of women who had a myocardial infarction and controls who had reported they were currently smoking*

Currently Smoking	Cases	Controls	Totals
Yes	159 (a)†	1850 (b)	2009
No	90 (c)	3127 (d)	3217
TOTALS	249	4977	5226

Data from Willett W et al: Am J Epidemiol 113(5):572-582, 1981.
*Excludes women for whom smoking status was unknown.
†Letters refer to further explanation given in the text.

TABLE 4-14 Distribution of women with a myocardial infarction and controls according to cigarettes smoked per day

Cigarettes per Day	Cases (n = 220)	Controls (n = 3991)	Relative Risk
Never smoked	61	2141	1.0
1-14	37	473	2.7
15-24	68	836	2.9
25-34	21	319	2.3
35+	32	216	5.2
Unknown	1	6	—

Data from Willett W et al: Am J Edpidemiol 113(5):572-582, 1981.

schemes should be established in advance of the study (these will be discussed in greater detail later in this chapter). When misclassification with respect to study variables occurs, and occurs to a different extent in cases and controls, then a problem of lack of comparability exists. In some cases, misclassification can lead the investigator to conclude that no difference exists when, in fact, it does exist. Willett and associates used a series of questions on smoking history to document exposure.

Analysis

The analysis of a case-control study consists of a comparison between cases and controls of the frequency of the characteristic believed to be related to the condition.

It can be seen from Figure 4-3 that the proportion of current smokers was much greater among the cases than among the controls. The number of women who had an MI and the number of controls who smoked are given in Table 4-13. Another approach to analysis in retrospective studies involves comparison of the intensity and duration of exposure for the cases and controls (Table 4-14). Such a display offers the advantage of observing dose-response relationships and estimation of risk for a variety of levels of exposure.

In addition to assessing the significance of observed differences between cases and controls, investigators can also estimate the risk of developing the disease associated with the exposure and determine to what extent differences in the two groups might be attributable to a confounding variable.

When cases are referable to a population and controls are also representative of the same population, it is possible to estimate rates of the disease in exposed and nonexposed groups and also to derive relative and attributable risks from these estimates.[7] Procedures similar to those described for calculating relative risk for prospective studies would be appropriate.

Many retrospective studies, however, cannot be related to a defined population, such as cases from a sin-

gle hospital compared with neighbors. Because the populations at risk are then unknown, one cannot estimate rates in the exposed and nonexposed. Using the data in Table 4-12 as an example, an estimate of the relative risk of the disease given exposure to the characteristic can be made for retrospective studies in the following manner:

1. The rate in exposed persons is calculated. In Table 4-13, the rate in the nonexposed persons is $a/(a + b)$ or $159/2009 = .079$.
2. The rate in the nonexposed persons is also calculated. In Table 4-13, the rate in the nonexposed persons is $c/(c + d)$ or $90/3127 = .029$.
3. The rate in the exposed is then divided by the rate in the nonexposed, $[a/(a + b)]/[c/(c + d)] = .079/.029$, to give 2.38.

The result is an estimate of the relative risk of developing an MI given the exposure to smoking. (A more correct name, the relative odds, is usually given this estimate inasmuch as it is the ratio of affected to unaffected individuals in one group relative to the same ratio for the other group.)

The relative risk of developing the disease can also be calculated for each level of exposure. Referring to the data in Table 4-14, it was determined that the relative risk of developing MI for the group who smoked 1 to 14 cigarettes a day was 2.7; for those who smoked 15 to 20 per day, 2.9; 25 to 34 per day, 2.3; and 35 or more, 5.2. Thus women who smoked 35 or more cigarettes per day had a fivefold increase in the risk of developing an MI when compared with nonsmokers.

The investigators noted that age was related both to having an MI and smoking. It was therefore necessary to take age into account in analyses to prevent any distortion of the association between smoking and age.

Adjustment can be made for confounding variables in the study design or in analysis. One way of controlling for the effects of age was used in this study. Each case was matched with one or more controls of the same or similar age. Although this is a useful technique, it is cumbersome and often an appropriate match cannot be found for the cases, or the data for many controls must be ignored. Another approach to controlling for confounding is *stratification analysis*. This implies examining the relationships between the exposure and disease for each of several strata. In the analysis of relative risk, the investigators then would standardize for age. (For further information about stratification analysis, see Mausner and Bahn[8]; for further information about matching see MacMahon and Pugh.[7])

Advantages and Disadvantages

There are several advantages associated with retrospective studies. They are short term and relatively inexpensive when compared with cohort studies. The retrospective study is feasible, particularly when the disease occurs only rarely. The problem of attrition often associated with cohort studies is less marked in the retrospective study, although people may refuse to participate in the study. As earlier illustrated, these studies can support the estimation of a dose-response relationship, and they are particularly powerful when the cases and controls were both obtained from a referent population. When a number of retrospective studies conducted by different investigators on different populations confirm one another, confidence can be attached to the conclusions.

There are, however, some major disadvantages associated with retrospective studies. First, the reference population for the cases and controls is often unknown, whereas the sample drawn for a cohort study is based on a reference population. Therefore generalization to a reference is usually not possible. Because there is often not much information about the population from which those with the disease come, it is difficult to give precise estimates of risk, although such estimates as the relative odds are commonly used. Because of the retrospective nature of the study, it is often impossible to know whether the exposure characteristic is antecedent to the disease or consequent to it.

Often the investigator must be concerned with bias, which may take the form of *selective recall, selection, false labeling,* or *reverse bias* (see earlier discussion). A final problem associated with retrospective studies is selective survival. When this type of study is initiated, only persons who have survived the disease are available for the investigation. Survival may be associated with a variable such as income, which in turn influences access to treatment and survival. Thus it is easy to see how the representation of certain groups, such as the wealthy, might be artificially inflated. This in turn might give the impression that the wealthy are at greater risk of developing the disease, when in fact it is only that the wealthy who have the disease survive.

Interpretation

MacMahon and Pugh[7] suggest that two important questions to consider in interpreting findings from a case-control study are (1) Do the findings reflect the true situation with respect to the presence or absence of association between the disease and the study factor? and, (2) If an association *is* observed, is it a causal one? In considering the first question, the investigator must refer again to all previous steps of the study, attempting to find alternative explanations for the observed association. In addition, the investigator is concerned with the findings as a whole. In considering the differences between cases and controls, one or only a few sharp differences are more compelling than many differences. The second question can be considered in relation to the earlier discussion on causality.

CROSS-SECTIONAL STUDIES

Another approach used in epidemiologic investigations is the cross-sectional study. A reference population is identified, and for a sample of that population, both the characteristic and the condition are ascertained simultaneously. Because these studies begin with a reference population, rates such as prevalence can be computed, as well as risk estimates. These studies enable the investigator to generalize to the reference population. Although bias and attrition can present problems, they can be minimized with careful designs. These are short-term, relatively inexpensive studies in comparison with prospective studies. The cross-sectional study does, however, have some disadvantages—it is sometimes impossible to disentangle antecedent-consequent relationships, and selective survival or migration may occur.

EXPERIMENTAL APPROACHES TO STUDYING EFFECTIVENESS OF INTERVENTIONS

Prevention and treatment programs are often conducted with enthusiasm but without careful assessment of their effectiveness and possible undesirable outcomes. Clinical therapy is often chosen based on assumptions about effectiveness and outcomes, rather than the results of carefully conducted clinical trials.

An important intervention trial of early hospital discharge and home follow-up of very low birth weight infants illustrates the power of clinical trials in assessment of new therapies. Brooten and her colleagues[3] conducted a trial to determine the safety, efficacy, and cost savings of early hospital discharge of very low birth weight infants (<1500 g). They randomly assigned infants to one of two groups: an early discharge group and a control group. Those in the early discharge group ($n = 39$) were discharged before they reached 2200 g if they met a standard set of conditions, including being clinically well and bottle fed or breast fed every 4 hours; able to maintain their body temperature in an open crib

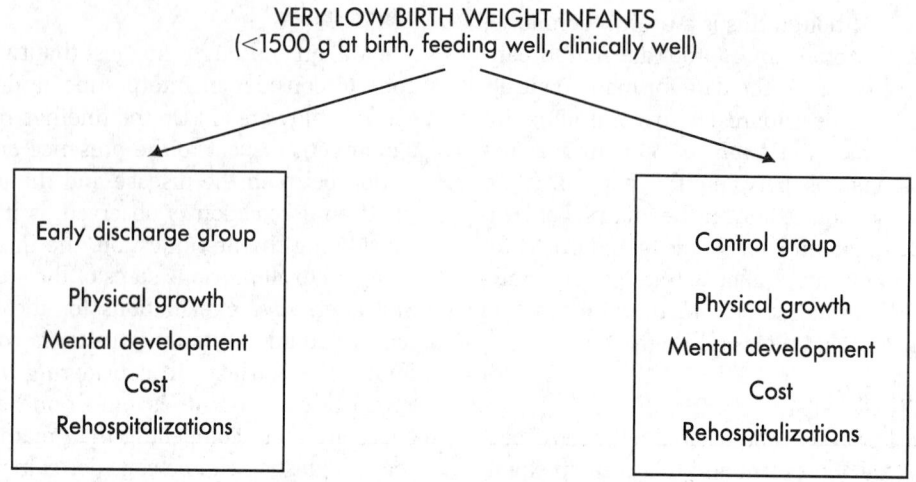

FIGURE 4-4 Design for a randomized clinical trial of early hospital discharge and home follow-up of very low birth weight infants. (From Brooten D et al: N Engl J Med 315:934-939, 1986.)

in room air; having no evidence of serious apnea or bradycardia in a 12-hour recording of heart rate and respiration; having a mother or other caretaker demonstrating satisfactory care-taking skills, and having an adequate physical home environment and facilities for care. Families of infants in the early-discharge group received instruction, counseling, home visits, and daily on-call availability of a hospital-based nurse specialist for 18 months. Infants in the control group ($n = 40$) were discharged according to routine nursery criteria, which included a weight of about 2200 g, being clinically well, and feeding well (Figure 4-4).

The Intervention Trial

In an intervention trial, the investigator manipulates the treatment, which becomes the independent variable, and measures the effect, the dependent variable. The basic strategy involves an application of the experimental method, with some special modifications necessary in view of the concern for the human population being studied.

Study Groups

In some studies it is possible to enroll a study group that receives the treatment and a control group or groups that are not given the treatment but perhaps a placebo. In other instances, it would be considered unethical to withhold any treatment at all, such as in the study of breast cancer treatment. The reference population for the study is the group to which the investigator can ideally generalize results of the study.

In the trial of early discharge, the reference population would be very low birth weight infants (1500 g) who met the inclusion criteria for the trial, such as being clinically well and feeding well. The experimental population is the actual population being studied—in this example, the infants and their families who actually participated in the study. It is ideal when the experimental population is as similar as possible to the reference population. Convenience and accessibility, incidence of the disease to be prevented (in prophylactic trials), and size of the population needed to detect statistically significant differences are all important considerations in selecting the experimental group. Because humans have the right to refuse involvement in an experiment, the final composition of the experimental population is not in the control of the investigator. Careful assessment of systematic differences between volunteers and refusals should be made when possible. Usually, allocation to the experimental or control group is done *after* the person consents to participate. In an attempt to attain equivalence or similarity of the experimental and control groups, the investigator can randomly allocate participants to one or more treatment or control groups. It is best that a system of randomization be developed in advance of the study to limit the noncomparability between the groups.

The Double-Blind Trial

The double-blind trial includes two safeguards to prevent bias in the ascertainment of the outcome as a result of knowledge of the group to which the participant was assigned: blind assignment is made of the participants to the study groups, and a blind assessment of outcome is achieved. First, neither the study personnel nor the participants know to which group the participants are assigned. While this is feasible in studies of medications, it is clearly impossible in the study of surgical or other procedures where both the staff and the patients are obviously aware of the treatment. The second component involves blind ascertainment of outcome. This might be achieved by keeping knowledge of the treatment group from a pathologist or interviewer measuring disease, survival, or other outcomes and from the statistician or epidemiologist analyzing the data.

Protocols

To ensure that each participant in the experimental and control groups receives the same treatment, study protocols are usually developed that describe in detail the types of procedures to be used in both groups. This is particularly important when several investigators from different areas participate in a collaborative trial. In our example a single protocol was used for the home and follow-up care provided by a clinical specialist in perinatal and neonatal nursing. The nurse specialist contacted one or both parents shortly after the infant's birth and at least weekly during the infant's hospitalization to promote parent interactions with the infant; to evaluate their perceptions and concerns about the infant; to teach them to bathe, handle, and soothe their infant, to take its temperature, and to prevent infection; and to provide information to the parents about the infant's sleeping patterns, variations in temperature, reportable signs and symptoms, and when the infant should have routine medical care. Before discharge, parents demonstrated satisfactory basic caregiving skills and a basic knowledge of medications or special procedures required in the infant's care. About 1 week before discharge, the nurse specialist made a home visit to coordinate planning for the discharge and to evaluate the adequacy of heat in the home, safety of the environment, and adequacy of facilities for care of the infant. Problems encountered in the home setting were referred to appropriate medical and social agencies. After the infant was discharged, the nurse made home visits during the first week and at 1, 9, 12, and 18 months. Visits in-

cluded a physical examination of the infant; developmental screening; confirmation of appointments for medical follow-up care; assessment of the parents' coping ability, caregiving skills, and support systems; and instructions and counseling regarding infant care and stimulation. In addition, the nurse specialist contacted parents by telephone three times a week for the first 2 weeks after discharge and weekly thereafter, for a period of 8 weeks. The nurse specialist was on call daily to respond to families' telephone calls regarding their concerns and special problems.

Ascertaining Outcomes

Ascertaining outcome in cases in which the outcome does not occur for several years presents the same problems that were discussed in conjunction with prospective studies, namely, migration and selective survival. Measures are usually taken to ensure as complete a follow-up as possible, and blind assessment is desirable. A very important concern is the type of outcome measure most appropriate to the study. In the trial of early discharge and home follow-up of very low birth weight infants, infants in the early discharge group left the hospital an average of 11 days earlier, weighed 200 g less, and were 2 weeks younger at discharge than infants in the control condition. Mean hospital costs for infants discharged early were 27% less than those for the control group, and the average physician's charge was 22% less. The average cost of the home follow-up care in the early discharge group was $576, providing a net savings of about $18,500 per infant. The two groups of infants did not differ in the number of rehospitalizations and acute care visits or in measures of physical and mental growth.

Sequential designs are sometimes employed in intervention studies. This means that data are continuously analyzed during the trial, and as soon as statistically significant differences appear the trial is stopped. It is possible to maintain double-blind procedures and incorporate sequential designs by having investigators not involved in the clinical work analyze the data submitted to them.

TABLE 4-15 Rates and risk estimates associated with specific study approaches

	Cohort Study	Case-Control Study	Cross-Sectional Study
Rates	Incidence	Proportion of the cases with the characteristic, unless the cases are from an identifiable reference population; then incidence can be estimated directly.	Prevalence
Risk estimate	Relative and attributable risk	Relative odds; when cases and controls are from an identifiable reference population, then relative risk is appropriate	Relative and attributable risk

Analysis

The analysis of an intervention trial is similar to that for a cohort study (Table 4-15). Special attention, however, must be given to those who did not participate in the control group or study group and any systematic differences between those who participated and those who did not. This can be attained by attempting to measure outcome for at least a sample of the nonparticipants.

SCREENING

Screening is an extremely important approach to detecting various health conditions. It is assumed that, by selecting from apparently healthy volunteers, treatment of those who are predisposed to a certain disease will be easier and more effective. An instrument used for screening a population is not intended to be diagnostic; instead, it is intended only to separate those persons with a high probability of having a health condition from those with a low probability. In turn, the former are subjected to further diagnostic tests and to treatment, if appropriate.

Screening tests must meet several criteria. First, they must be valid and reliable. The *validity* of the test refers to whether it is able to separate those with the condition from those without the condition. In epidemiology the validity of a test is commonly assessed by determining its sensitivity and specificity. *Sensitivity* refers to the test's capacity to identify correctly those with the condition, whereas *specificity* refers to its ability to identify correctly those who do not have the condition. Such values are determined by comparing results on the screening tool to those derived from a definitive diagnostic procedure. Usually, the sensitivity and specificity can be varied by raising or lowering the level at which the test is considered positive.

The Cornell Medical Index (CMI) is a commonly used measurement of general health status, with the M-R subscales reflecting mental health status. Using the data in the boxes above, we can see that the sensitivity of the CMI, using a cutoff point of a total score over 30, correctly identifies those women who physicians rate as in poor health 78% of the time. The specificity, those who are not ill and have CMI scores less than 30, is only 57%. When the value of the screening tool's results is continuous (for example, the level in units of an enzyme), the sensitivity and specificity can be adjusted by changing the cutoff point for "positives" on the test. In some instances, multiple tests can be used to increase the sensitivity of the screening.

Reliability (precision) of a screening test refers to the reproducibility of its results. Variation in the method and observer error can be sources of inconsistent results. Standardizing procedures and training observers improve reliability.

The *yield* of a screening tool refers to the amount of a previously undiagnosed condition that can be diagnosed and treated as a result of the screening. The yield depends not only on the sensitivity of the test, but also on the prevalence of unrecognized conditions, the extent of previous screening in the population, and the degree to which people will participate in the screening.

There are varying opinions regarding what criteria should be used to judge whether to implement a screening program. The following criteria suggested by Wilson and Jungner[17] are often applied:

1. The condition to be screened should constitute an important health problem.
2. For patients with recognized disease, there should be an accepted treatment.
3. Facilities for diagnosis and treatment should be available.
4. The disease should have a recognizable latent or early symptomatic stage.
5. A suitable test or examination should exist.
6. The test should be acceptable to the population to whom it is applied.
7. The natural history of the disease, including development from latent to declared disease, should be adequately understood.
8. There should be a policy on whom to treat as patients after they are identified as possible cases.

PHYSICIANS' GENERAL HEALTH RATINGS FOR WOMEN

SCREENING RESULTS	I	II	III	IV
Cornell Medical Index ≥30	23	26	21	8
Cornell Medical Index <30	54	10	7	1
TOTALS	77	36	28	9

$$\text{Sensitivity}^* = \frac{21 + 8}{28 + 9} = 0.78$$

$$\text{Specificity}^* = \frac{54 + 10}{77 + 36} = 0.57$$

Data are interpolated from Abramson J et al: Br J Prev Med 19:103-110, 1965.
*Using grades III and IV as an indicator of ill health.

DISEASE BY DIAGNOSIS

SCREENING RESULTS	PRESENT	ABSENT
Positive	True positive (TP)	False positive (FP)
Negative	False negative (FN)	True negative (TN)

$$\text{Sensitivity} = \frac{\text{TP}}{\text{TP} + \text{FN}} \qquad \text{Specificity} = \frac{\text{TN}}{\text{TN} + \text{FP}}$$

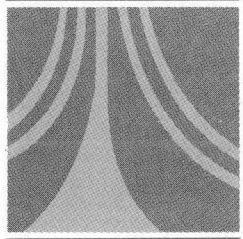

CHAPTER 5

Adult Development and Illness

JANET PRIMOMO

CHAPTER OBJECTIVES

After studying this chapter, the student should be able to:
1 Analyze physical, psychosocial, cognitive, sexual, and spiritual aspects of development during young, middle, and late adulthood in selected clients.
2 Describe potential effects of illness on adult development.
3 Propose health promotion plans appropriate to adult developmental requirements for selected clients.

Human growth and development occur throughout the life span, from the time of conception to the time of death. This lifelong process of growth and development encompasses biologic, psychosocial, cognitive, sexual, and spiritual spheres (Figure 5-1). Changes in physical development such as mobility and neurologic status are important in helping nurses evaluate the patient's self-care potential. The sphere of psychosocial development includes family, social, and occupational tasks that normally accompany a specific period in the life span. Cognitive changes in adulthood such as problem solving ability and intellectual capacity have implications for

how nurses teach patients about health care. Sexuality differs across the life span and may be threatened by certain illness situations. Spiritual changes over the years include the ability to find meaning in life and accept the inevitable end of life. Development in each of the spheres does not happen independently, but rather the changes are linked together and can influence each other. A developmental perspective gives nurses a road map to help them understand the many physical and psychosocial changes that occur during the adult years. In this chapter, development during the adult years is reviewed, and implications for nursing care are identified.

Adulthood is not a static period of life. The subtle intrinsic and adaptive sequence of changes that evolves over the adult years must be understood in order to provide optimum nursing care. Indeed, there is a great deal of variation in the ways people cope and adapt to illness situations. A developmental perspective helps highlight the salient issues that people are faced with at specific points in the life span. A person's development may in-

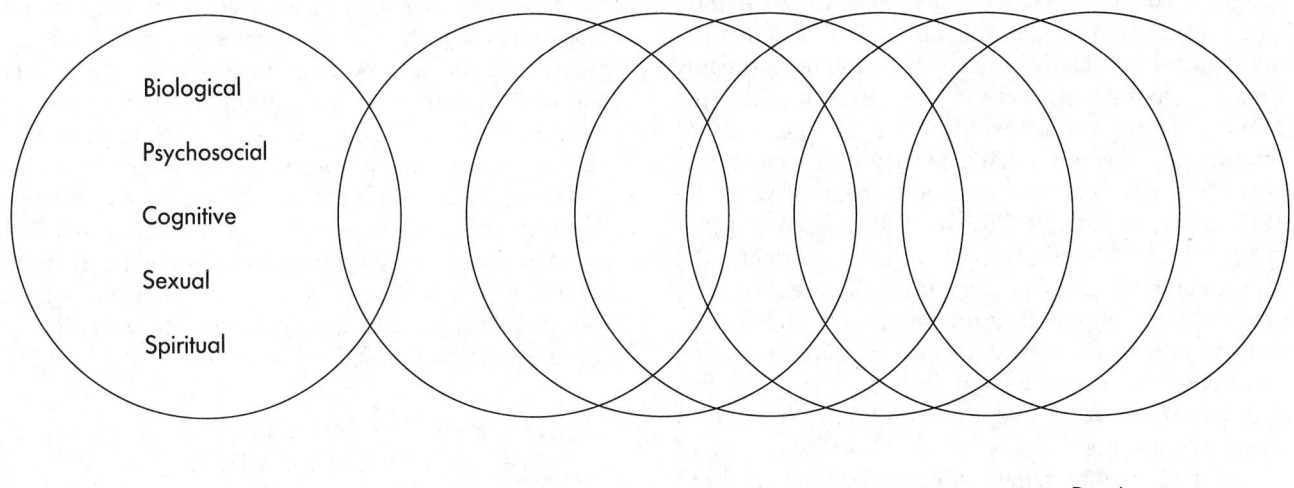

FIGURE 5-1 Interrelated aspects of human development through the life span.

fluence how the person copes with an illness situation. For example, a woman in her mid-thirties who has young children and an elderly ill parent to care for may find it very difficult to find the time to take care of her own chronic health needs. Rather than identify the woman as "noncompliant," nurses must consider the developmental processes and needs of adults as they experience health and illness situations in order to plan and provide sensitive and appropriate nursing care.

DEMOGRAPHIC TRENDS

Although most of society's attention to growth and development has been on children or the elderly, increasing attention is being given to the growth and development issues of adults in their early and middle years. Societal changes partly account for the interest in adulthood. Adults in the middle years may find themselves "sandwiched" between members of the older and younger generations who depend on them for care. Adults in the middle years experience chronic and short-term illness at a time when they are supposed to contribute to society by raising a family, caring for the older generation, and maintaining occupational productivity. The more we understand about adults in their middle years, the better we can help them cope with the challenges they face when illness is experienced.

Demographic changes that have occurred over the past few decades also account for the interest in adulthood (Table 5-1). A major trend is the increasing growth rate of the population over age 65.[82] In fact, at present, the number of persons 75 years of age or older is increasing proportionately faster than the total group over age 65. In 1986, 12% of the U.S. population, or 29.1 million people, were over 65 years of age. By the year 2000, it is estimated that 34.8 million people or 13% of the population will be made up of people over age 65.[82] There will be more older adults to be cared for by the young and middle adults in society. The increasing number of elderly persons has resulted primarily from the dramatic increase in the life expectancy (the number of years we can expect to live) of Americans. At the turn of the century, life expectancy for women was about 48 years, and for men it was about 46 years. By 1986, it had increased to 78.3 years for women and 71.3 years for men.[82] The decrease in infant mortality, the prevention and control of communicable disease during childhood, the improved treatment of acute and chronic disease, and improvements in medical care in general contributed to the increased life expectancy in this country. At the same time, the birth rate in the United States is declining.

Other dramatic demographic trends include the lower rates of life expectancy for non-Whites versus Whites and the higher number of elderly women than

TABLE 5-1 Adult population by age and sex (in millions)

Age (Years) and Sex	Actual 1986	Projected 1990	Projected 2000
TOTAL			
18-24	27.7	26.1	25.2
25-34	42.8	43.9	37.1
35-44	33.1	37.9	43.9
45-54	22.8	25.5	37.2
55-64	22.2	21.4	24.2
65-74	17.3	18.4	18.2
≥75	11.8	13.2	16.6
MALE			
18-24	14.1	13.2	12.8
25-34	21.6	22.1	18.7
35-44	16.4	18.8	21.9
45-54	11.1	12.4	18.3
55-64	10.5	10.1	11.6
65-74	7.6	8.2	8.2
≥75	4.2	4.7	6.0
FEMALE			
18-24	13.8	12.9	12.5
25-34	21.4	21.8	18.5
35-44	16.8	19.1	22.0
45-54	11.7	13.1	18.9
55-64	11.8	11.3	12.6
65-74	9.7	10.2	10.0
≥75	7.7	8.5	10.6

U.S. Bureau of the Census: Statistical abstracts of the United States, 1988, annual ed 108, Washington, DC, 1987, US Government Printing Office.

men. In 1986 life expectancy was 73.6 years for Black women and 78.9 years for White women. Black men had a life expectancy of 65.5 years, compared with 72.0 years for White men in 1986. Table 5-1 shows the number of women and men in each group.[82] Although the proportions of both men and women in the over 65 age-groups will increase over the next decade, the population of women over age 65 outnumbers that of men by about 6.1 million. In the year 2000, 59% of those over 65 years of age will be women.[82] These trends have important implications for the health care system. Because the main source of income for most women in this age-group is Social Security, more older women will probably be living in poverty than are today. Many women are widowed, live alone, and have limited resources to purchase needed health and social services.

CYCLES OF HUMAN GROWTH AND DEVELOPMENT IN ADULTHOOD

Growth and development are processes that occur throughout the life span. Physical growth, caused by the development and integration of differentiated cells, is a continuous process from the moment of conception until maturity. *Growth* results in a change in body structure or size. *Development* denotes increases in functional capacity evolving from physical and mental maturation and learning. Development implies expansion in detail and growth into an advanced state.

Adulthood is characterized as a period of stability, growth potential, and decline. Dramatic physical changes are few, but various changes do occur. Psychologic changes occur during the adult years, but there is relative stability in values, attitudes, and feelings about self and others. As people grow older, the personality, though basically the same, may become increasingly mature, and there is increased integration and interdependence with others. Adolescents, in contrast, may focus primarily on their own independence and achievements. Because psychosocial development is greatly influenced by interpersonal and social elements, psychologic changes may be in part responses to changing life events.

Adulthood covers a long period of life. Life circumstances and developmental tasks differ across the wide range of the adult years. The adult years are separated into three general stages: young adulthood, middle adulthood, and older adulthood. In this chapter the young adult period is considered to be the years between 18 and 40. Middle adulthood refers to the years between 40 and 65. Older adulthood is the period beginning at age 65. For each general stage, physical and psychosocial development is discussed. Nursing interventions appropriate for the health promotion needs of each age-group are reviewed.

YOUNG ADULTHOOD

Young adulthood, extending approximately from age 18 to age 40, is a complex period of life in which the achievement of personal goals is the primary focus. The young adult years are referred to as the expansion years, during which energies are directed toward family building and maintenance, career fulfillment, and social involvement.[6,78] In the following section, physical and psychosocial development during the early adult years is reviewed, and the health needs and concerns of young adults are discussed.

PHYSICAL DEVELOPMENT

Full growth and development are completed by the midtwenties, and most body systems are functioning at maximum levels.[30,57] Of the physical changes that occur in adulthood, some begin early and others begin in middle age; some are abrupt and some are gradual. Cardiac output and stroke volume begin to decrease. Vital capacity of the respiratory system decreases. As an individual grows older, the gastrointestinal system slows down so that digesting, absorbing, and eliminating food takes longer. Changes in weight and muscle mass occur primarily because of alterations in diet and exercise. Thinning and graying of hair and wrinkling of skin occur as the young adult years progress. After age 25, visual acuity begins to decline. Finally, fertility in women declines as the years progress.[30]

PSYCHOSOCIAL DEVELOPMENT

Adulthood is often equated with maturity; it is characterized by a sense of responsibility, the maintenance of appropriate impulse control, the ability to plan and implement realistic goals, the development of a career, and the capacity to enter into intimate relationships. Everyone does not arrive at young adulthood with the same level of maturity; therefore age-related norms may be misleading. Psychosocial development, emotional maturity, intellectual ability, and physical characteristics may vary from person to person, men to women, and culture to culture. In addition, psychosocial development in young adults who experience illness, especially chronic illness, may be altered. Conversely, the experience of illness may be shaped by the person's development. Theories of psychosocial development and their implications for nursing are reviewed in the following section.

Table 5-2 shows selected theories of psychosocial development especially relevant to nursing practice. Most of the theories include sequential stages and developmental tasks, but they vary in the number of stages and types of processes involved. Erikson emphasized the conflicts or turning points that the individual must cope with at different stages throughout the life span. Failure to successfully resolve the tasks at one stage would preclude development in the next higher stage. Erikson identified an alternative to each stage that would occur if the person did not successfully complete the tasks relevant to that stage.[25]

In Erikson's *eight ages of man,* the first adult stage is characterized by *intimacy versus isolation*[25] (Table 5-2). Intimacy implies sharing the self to form a commitment to an intense lasting relationship with another person, a cause, or a creative effort without fearing the loss of identity. Intimacy requires responsibility, impulse control, the ability to plan, and also the ability to trust. The inability to develop some form of intimacy draws the person into increasing feelings of isolation, alienation, and self-absorption.

Stevenson, a nurse theorist, identified young adulthood as the time for achieving independence from parents, assuming adult responsibility, and beginning a family.[78] The tasks of new parenthood add another dimension to the adult's life. Similarly, Levinson emphasized the life structures or tasks and the transitions that occur in the adult years.[48] The Early Adult Transition is

TABLE 5-2 Summary of selected theories on psychosocial development in adulthood

Age	Erikson[25]	Levinson[48]	Loevinger[49]	Stevenson[78]
Young adulthood	Intimacy versus isolation Significant objects— persons, causes	Early adult transition (17-22) Entering adult world (22-28)	Conformist Identification with group Conscientious Increased sense of personal responsibility	Young adulthood (18-30) Achieving independence
Adulthood	Generativity versus stagnation Significant persons— spouse, family, friends	Age 30 transition (28-33) Settling down (33-40) Midlife transition (40-45) Entering middle adulthood (45-50) Age 50 transition (50-55) Culmination of middle adulthood (55-60)	Autonomous Mutual interdependence, coping with conflict Integrated Cherishing individual difference	Core middle years (30-50) Assist older and younger generations New middle years (50-70) Assume primary responsibility for cultural and social survival
Maturity	Integrity versus disgust, despair Significant persons— spouse, family	Late adult transition (60-65) Late adulthood (65 +)		Late 70s Responsible to review life, share wisdom, put affairs in order

the bridge between preadulthood and early adulthood when a person leaves home and establishes independence. In Early Adulthood the person explores adult roles, makes interpersonal commitments, and builds and maintains an adult life-style. The early adult years are a time of great energy when people try to find their niche in society. There are many rewards during this period of life, including satisfaction with love, family, work, and life-style. However, the competing demands for a person's time, creativity, and energy may have a cost.

Loevinger presented a somewhat different view of psychosocial development. Rather than identifying developmental stages according to social tasks, her theory emphasizes how a person's overall perception of the world varies across the life span and influences behavior and attitudes. The development of the "ego" or self is the focus.[49] Loevinger described milestones of ego development that can be considered stages. The stages are marked by sources of conflict, and each successive stage is more complex. At each stage the person's frame of reference and attitudes about life vary. In other words, a person's behavior and perception of the world reflect the developmental stage of the individual. Loevinger's theory differs from other theories in that age norms are not specified, and all individuals may not reach the highest stage.

DEVELOPMENTAL TASKS

Psychologic and social aspects of the young adult's development can be gleaned from the developmental tasks common to this period (see the box). The developmental tasks of early adulthood, most concretely seen in the choice of a vocation and a marriage partner, clearly involve a certain choice of lifestyle. Although fairly clear boundaries have been established between self and parents by this time, parental attitudes and value systems have been internalized in young adults to become a salient part of their identity, thus affecting future life choices. Inherent in these choices is the quest for freedom from family, social, and economic dependence.[48,78]

Occupational Choice

An occupation represents much more than a set of skills and functions or a way to earn a living. It is a way of life that determines much of the environment, both physical and social, in which a person lives. Occupational choice plays a significant part in further shaping the person by providing a social system, status, roles, and a life-style. The choice of an occupation often requires consideration of appropriate educational preparation, and thus educational goals and achievements become a very important part of this choice.

During the young adult years when involvement in an occupation is of prime importance, unemployment

TASKS OF YOUNG ADULTHOOD

Achieving relative independence from parents
Developing a sense of responsibility for one's own life
Developing a sense of social, civic, and economic responsibility
Choosing a life-style
Choosing and starting an occupation or vocation
Choosing a marriage partner and raising children
Managing a home

---

may cause the individual to feel unneeded or unwanted, thus fostering feelings of inadequacy and failure. Furthermore, unemployment has dire consequences for the individual and the family, including poverty, homelessness, and limited access to health care. When working with an individual, the nurse must be sensitive to concerns and anxieties regarding unemployment or changes in employment due to illness, accidents, and altered ability to conduct former work. Vocational counseling or rehabilitation may be recommended for people with disabilities who need to restructure their vocation following illness or injury[24]; for example, a construction worker who sustained a spinal cord injury in an industrial accident may need to learn new skills to maintain the life-style of a productive adult. When individuals are temporarily or permanently unable to work, they should be referred to social service agencies that can help them obtain public assistance, housing, and access to health care.

Over the past few decades, social and economic forces have changed the composition of the work force in this country. In fact, well over 50% of women are in the labor force today.[82] The feminist movement exerted a significant influence on women's occupational choices. Indeed, it is now socially acceptable for a woman to choose a career as an alternative or supplement to the traditional housewife-mother role of the 1950s. In addition, it is an economic reality that many women, especially single parents, must work outside the home and provide for the economic needs of their families. Among young adults, there is a growing tendency to delay having children until career goals are solidified. Overall, employment outside the home has a positive influence on women's lives.[64] However, employed women who are responsible for dependent children or aging parents may be burdened with additional demands such as child care or adult day care. Therefore, during a time of illness, a woman may have concerns about the welfare of her family as well as employment-related concerns.

Marital Choice

Another major decision of early adulthood is whether or not to marry. Our society continues to strongly support marriage among young adults. However, some people are choosing not to marry, enjoying the independence and freedom of single living. Although there may be many reasons for entering into the marital relationship, marriage is generally recognized as a close and loving partnership between two people where intimacy and affection exist in a free and equal relationship as opposed to only a social institution where the man is the undisputed head of the house and the wife is the childbearer.[57]

The arrival of the first child transforms the spouses into parents, and they take on the roles and parenting behavior learned from parents.[52] Parenthood is experienced as a joy as well as a crisis: a joy because a child is the product of their common bond and fulfillment of goals; a crisis because the child necessitates adjustments in daily routine and life-style, which are often seen as a burden. Preparation for parenthood has not been widespread in our society. It is therefore difficult for individuals to anticipate many of the stresses of being parents and the changes required in themselves and their marital relationship. If the nurse assesses that an individual is experiencing undue stress and an inability to cope, resources for assistance can be made available.

Although personality characteristics and interpersonal problems are primary sources of difficulties in adjustment to marriage and parenthood, cultural and societal variables often make these adjustments difficult. For instance, the mobility of our society results in a dispersal of family members and close relatives, with less available help from these significant others in times of need and stress.

While the institutions of marriage and family are the most socially acceptable, there is an increasing tolerance for diversity in living patterns. Alternatives to traditional family life that are increasingly common include cohabitation with members of the same or opposite sex, living alone, becoming a single parent, remaining a childless couple, and communal living. Other alternative family structures include homosexual couples who sometimes make a lifelong commitment and choose to raise a family. Divorce, a common occurrence today, is a highly stressful event that often creates a crisis. In 1984 almost half of all marriages ended in divorce.[82] The young adult may perceive divorce as a failure to achieve intimacy, one of the normal developmental tasks. However, most adults who are divorced go on to marry again, and the result is another type of family called the "blended family." In fact, in over 45% of all marriages, one or both partners were married previously.[82] Blended families are made up of a married couple with either or both spouses having children from previous marriages. These couples may also have children of their own. Role adjustment for all family members may occur. Nurses should be in touch with their attitudes about varying life-styles and choices and remain nonjudgmental when caring for patients.

Developmental theory is useful in exploring the possible effects that chronic or life-threatening health conditions may have at different points in the life span. During the intimacy versus isolation stage of young adulthood, a chronic condition may be viewed as a limiting factor in finding a mate.[24,45,64] In one study, Primomo found that some young women with diabetes mellitus were concerned about disclosing their illness to prospective partners for fear that they would "frighten them away."[64] When faced with a chronic illness, people may question their ability to provide for and raise children.[2] Having a health condition that can be passed on to children can influence a person's decision to have a family. An altered body image may be perceived as affecting relationships with peers. Young adults with physical disabilities and chronic conditions that are stigmatized by society may have limited opportunities to achieve intimacy and sexual and vocational fulfillment.[20] A young adult who experiences an illness may need parental assistance at a time when freedom and independence are desired. Family roles may have to be adjusted and redefined.[24] Theories of psychosocial development that focus on developmental tasks are useful in helping nurses to recognize the "normal" activities that young adults engage in. When an individual is faced with a long-term threat to health that requires emotional, physical, vocational, and social adaptation on the part of the person and family, the nurse can listen carefully to the concerns expressed and acknowledge that distress is a normal reaction. Information can be provided, and referrals to counseling can be made.

Loevinger's theory provides an alternative developmental framework for considering how people adapt to illness and the intervention strategies used. Rigid treatment approaches may be less effective than strategies that take into account the unique characteristics of the individual. For example, at higher stages of development the needs of others, as well as the individual's own needs are considered, even when the needs are conflicting. Therefore nurses must find out how patients think an illness situation affects those around them so that treatment strategies can include concern for others. In recent years researchers have studied how development in women is different from that in men. Interdependence with others and interpersonal relationships are especially significant for women in their early adult years.[33,34] Again, the importance of taking women's concerns into account and including family members when planning treatment strategies may increase the nurse's effectiveness in caring for patients with chronic conditions.

The successful resolution of the young adult phase of the life cycle depends on a positive self-concept. How people feel about themselves affects relationships as well as the choices made during this period. A person who feels adequate and competent in setting and achieving goals tends to experience more positive outcomes than one whose self-concept is that of inadequacy and incompetency. These negative feelings tend to foster withdrawal and inability to mobilize resources for positive gains.[77] When caring for the young adult it is therefore important to assess the individual's self-perception. These data not only provide information as to motivation potential but are also a basis for nursing interventions that help to increase the individual's self-esteem.

Body image, an important aspect of self-concept, is a mental picture of the body's appearance as well as the attitudes, emotions, and personality of the individual. At a period of life when acceptance by others is most important, and with society's emphasis on youth, beauty, and physical fitness, any alteration in body function or structure poses a threat to a positive body image. Adaptation to these alterations depends on the nature and meaning of the threat, coping mechanisms, and available support systems.

Therefore nursing intervention to help someone deal with a threat to or change of body image involves (1) careful assessment of the individual's perception of the condition, (2) assistance in helping the individual maintain a realistic perception of the threat in relation to the person's total self-image, (3) assistance in identifying useful coping mechanisms, and (4) identification of support systems (see Chapter 18).

INTELLECTUAL DEVELOPMENT

Cross-sectional studies have shown that the highest overall intelligence test performance occurs at some time between the late teens and late twenties. People in their thirties, forties, and fifties tend to score somewhat lower. Longitudinal evidence has shown, however, that general intelligence either remains the same or increases slightly during the adult years.[76] Certain factors, such as education and other sociocultural advantages, may influence intellectual development and performance.

SEXUALITY IN YOUNG ADULTHOOD

Sexuality is an integral part of self-concept. Competence in the area of one's sexuality is of prime importance during the adult years. Sexuality may be defined as a "deep pervasive aspect of the total person, the sum total of one's feelings and behavior as a male or female, the expression of which goes beyond genital response."[57] Young adulthood is normally the time when the body's sexual response is powerful, and there is a need to find adequate and satisfactory expression. It is known that a man reaches his peak sexual capacity at about 18 years of age. Women, however, reach their peak of sexual capacity in their early thirties.

If the expression of sexual feelings is restricted, perhaps because of illness or injury, causing a felt or imagined change in body image, sexual concerns may become paramount. Nurses frequently are asked by young adults for assistance with marital or sexual concerns. Unless the nurse is secure in his or her own sexual identity and has had adequate preparation to deal with such matters, the person should be referred to appropriate persons who can deal with these concerns (see Chapters 51 and 52).

HEALTH PROMOTION NEEDS

The cessation of physical growth, changes in life-style, the experience of a chronic or life-threatening illness, or the potential risk of experiencing illness can necessitate certain alterations in physical and psychosocial needs. Aspects of nutrition, exercise, and rest and sleep are discussed here. Health concerns of young adults are addressed as well.

NUTRITION

Nutrition needs of the young adult are somewhat different from those of the growing adolescent due to the cessation of physical maturation.[30,57] Young men should increase their consumption of foods high in Vitamins C, E, B_6, and riboflavin. Men need only 10 mg of iron in their daily diets, whereas women require 18 mg. In young women the need for protein and Vitamins A, E, B_6, B_{12}, and riboflavin remains about the same, but the need for Vitamin C and calcium increases. For example, women need 1000 mg of calcium daily along with vitamin D to prevent osteoporosis. Furthermore, women who are childbearing or breast-feeding have added nutritional requirements.

Dietary modification may be indicated, depending on whether the young adult has a chronic illness. For example, diabetes mellitus is partially controlled by diet. Modifications in diet are recommended for those at risk for illnesses that are considered to be diet-related, such as cancer, heart disease, atherosclerosis, hypertension, and Type II diabetes. In fact, the Surgeon General recommended that all Americans eat a balanced diet of the minimum number of calories needed to maintain desirable weight; lower their intake of saturated fat, cholesterol, sugar, and salt; and increase consumption of complex carbohydrates (whole grains, fruits, and vegetables), fish, poultry, and legumes.

Nutritional problems of young adults may result from their life-styles; for example, busy schedules, limited income, and increased family, job, or educational demands may contribute to poor nutritional choices and habits. Eating disorders such as anorexia (extreme self-imposed food restriction and exercise) and bulemia (recurrent episodes of binge eating followed by self-induced vomiting or laxative abuse) that primarily affect adolescent girls may be identified in young women and men as well. Nurses can be alert to signs and symptoms of nutritional deficits and help the young adult understand the importance of adequate nutrition for maintaining well-being, preventing illness, and recovering from illness. Nurses and dieticians can assist young adults in developing nutritionally balanced meal plans that are tailored to their health status, income, life-styles and preferences.

EXERCISE

Exercise serves several functions in the young adult. It helps to regulate appetite, burn calories, control fat accumulation, improve or maintain muscle tone, enhance cardiac function, release tension, aid sleep, and improve overall well-being. To be most beneficial, exercise should be regularly scheduled three or four times weekly for at least 30 minutes. The type of exercise should be appropriate to the individual's overall health status. For example, a woman with diabetic neuropathy may find swimming to be a safer form of exercise than running since she would be less likely to encounter problems with shoes that rub and cause potentially serious ulcerations.

Many activities such as walking, jogging, bicycling, swimming, tennis, rowing, and jumping rope provide exertion that benefits the cardiopulmonary system. However, intermittent exercise is not as effective as a regular, planned exercise program because sporadic exertion produces sudden demands on the body system

---

RESEARCH

Jenny J: A comparison of four age-groups' adaptation to diabetes, Can J Public Health, 75(3), 237-244, 1984.

In this exploratory study the variations in adaptation to diabetes were studied across four age-groups. Different profiles of self-care were found among the different age-groups based on a questionnaire that explored diabetes compliance and the health belief model. The young group (ages 16-24) reported a great deal of frustration related to the impact that diabetes had on their life-styles. For those in the middle age-group (ages 25-45), family problems and special concerns contributed to the barriers in adhering to the diabetes regimen. Diabetes was viewed as a burden because of the difficulties associated with the regimen. The middle to older group (ages 46-65) had the highest level of health motivation, but diet and exercise presented the greatest problems. The oldest group (ages 66 and older) had more health problems and functional deficits and less social support than the other groups. This research is useful in identifying developmental and age-related differences in adaptation to chronic illness. ▪

without allowing the body to adequately adjust. When an individual begins an exercise program, a gradual increase in the intensity of exertion is recommended to allow the body to adapt to the physical demands. Continued and regular exercise contributes to the sustained maintenance and optimal functioning of body systems.[57]

REST AND SLEEP

Sleep is a basic requirement for all human beings. Sufficient sleep is needed to maintain energy levels, physical appearance, and well-being. For adults, approximately 6 to 8 hours of uninterrupted sleep per day is considered adequate.[30] Although an individual can adjust to a lack of sleep for a short time, prolonged periods of decreased sleep and rest can contribute to anxiety, fatigue, irritability, lack of concentration, reduced alertness, and slowed recovery from illness. The sleep patterns of young adults may be altered due to family responsibilities such as caring for growing children, work roles including jobs that require night and rotating shifts, social activities, and career development such as further education.

HEALTH CONCERNS OF YOUNG ADULTHOOD

The health of adults depends on a complex set of social and environmental circumstances, including life-style and health practices. There is increasing recognition that social and economic conditions can influence health status. Research has shown that the death rates from cancer, diabetes, tuberculosis, heart disease, and multiple sclerosis in urban populations are higher for those of lower income than for the more economically advantaged, suggesting that environmental conditions such as poverty may be important determinants in these diseases.

During young adulthood, threats to health include accidents, drug and alcohol abuse, stress-related disorders, and preexisting chronic conditions such as heart disease, epilepsy, and diabetes. Sexual concerns include sexually transmitted diseases (including *Chlamydia trachomatis* and AIDS), contraception, unwanted pregnancy, sexual identity conflicts, and guilt related to parental and societal values about sexual practices. Accidents (including motor vehicle accidents), suicide, homicide, and malignant neoplasms are the leading causes of death among young adults between 25 and 34 years of age.[82] Death rates for accidents are three times higher for males than for females, in part because of greater risk-taking behaviors more commonly associated with young men. The accident death rates for Blacks are higher than for Whites.[82] Injuries and illnesses that restrict normal activity may create social and economic problems for the young adult. As stated previously, dependence on others, especially parents, during injury or

illness may create conflict for the young adult's quest for independence.

According to the National Center for Health Statistics, the most common chronic conditions in young adults are chronic sinusitis, hay fever or allergic rhinitis, and deformities or orthopaedic impairments.[58] The most effective nursing interventions might be to assist young adults in managing these chronic conditions through self-care. Upper respiratory tract infections are common among young adults; environmental pollutants, occupational exposure to agents, smoking, and child rearing may contribute to the problem. The nurse's primary responsibility lies in teaching preventive measures. Prevention is directed at supporting the body's own defenses through basic health practices (adequate rest and sleep, exercise, and a balanced diet). Reducing the susceptibility to and risk of illness can be accomplished by encouraging health-promoting behaviors, maintaining weight, limiting alcohol intake, reducing smoking, practicing safe sex to reduce sexually transmitted diseases, managing stress, maintaining safety measures at work and leisure, using seat belts, and practicing self-care such as breast self-examination.

Physiologic and psychologic changes resulting in unusual or disturbed adaptive behavior patterns may occur when the young adult has difficulty coping with newly acquired tasks and responsibilities. Mate selection, marriage, childbearing, college, job demands, social expectations, and independent decision making are all stressors, carrying the threats of insecurity and some degree of failure. Some stress reactions take the form of physical illness. Related to the stresses of achievement in the young adult years is the occurrence of gastric and duodenal ulcers. Prevention here is directed at reinforcement of appropriate diet, exercise, and rest. When stressors are perceived as overwhelming, the result may be self-destructive behavior such as drug abuse and addiction, alcoholism, excessive smoking, and suicide (ranked as one of the leading causes of death among this age group).

Sensitivity to the many pressures and responsibilities facing the young adult is vital to good nursing care. The patient's major concern often is not about himself or herself. He or she may be the breadwinner of a family. How is the family being supported during the illness? How are the medical bills to be paid? The patient may be a parent of small children. Who will care for them? When hospitalized, the patient is often concerned about how the family is getting along at home. The patient may have no family nearby. Who will look in on the patient if he or she is ill at home? Who will provide care during convalescence? These are only a few of the problems frequently facing the young adult patient. Some problems of hospitalized patients may be alleviated by providing the use of a telephone or by arranging a visit

RESEARCH

Primomo J: Patterns of chronic illness management, psychosocial development, family and social environment, and adaptation among women with diabetes. Unpublished doctoral dissertation, Seattle, 1989, University of Washington.

The purpose of this study was to explore psychosocial development in women with chronic illness. The measurement of psychosocial development was based on Loevinger's theory. Forty women in their early to middle adult years who had diabetes mellitus were studied. Overall, women's level of psychosocial development was between the conformist and conscientious stages during which heightened self-awareness is common. The average developmental level for women in the study was similar to the average level for adults in other studies. There was variation in women's scores across the last five stages of development. Women who had higher levels of psychosocial development were less depressed than women who scored lower on the development measure. Developmental stage was not related to chronologic age or diabetes health status. Women at lower stages of psychosocial development had a more difficult time adjusting to diabetes than did women with higher levels of development. Results from this study show that adult women may have different levels of psychosocial development and ways of thinking about their experiences that may not necessarily be age-related. ■

with a family member, friend, or business associate. Help needed by the patient may be available through other support systems such as social services in the hospital or through family service or community health agencies. The nurse in a physician's office or clinic also should be alert for persons who need this kind of assistance.

MIDDLE ADULTHOOD

In recent years, scientists have become increasingly interested in the unique psychosocial and physiologic phases of adulthood. Although there is no consensus about the exact stages of adulthood and the timing of those stages, there is general agreement that during the middle adult years (between ages 40 and 65), human beings continue to develop. Middle adulthood is characterized as a time of few physical changes unless an illness, which may create profound changes in every aspect of the person's life, is experienced. Middle adulthood is a time rich in psychosocial alterations. The middle years are approached with a sharpened sense of awareness as adults begin to evaluate their lives. Ideally, there is a sense of self-acceptance and a willingness to revise aspirations based on the reality of the current life situation. In the following sections, some of the physical and psychosocial changes that take place during middle adulthood are discussed. Factors that influence how people adapt to this stage of life are reviewed.

PHYSICAL DEVELOPMENT

Physically, the adult usually enters this phase of life functioning at near-peak efficiency.[30] As the middle years progress, physiologic changes occur gradually. If a chronic condition or illness is experienced, the resulting physical changes must be taken into account since they may influence how a person adapts during this period of life.

Some of the physical changes during the middle adult years are a continuation of changes that began during the end of the young adult period.[69] The loss of elasticity and the changes in arterial structure may contribute to cardiovascular problems. As activity and metabolism slow down, the weight gain that often results may have detrimental effects on other body systems. These factors put adults at risk for cardiovascular disease, hypertension, atherosclerosis, diabetes, kidney disease, cancer, and gallstones. The decreased elasticity of the lungs contributes to certain chronic respiratory diseases. A redistribution of fatty tissue occurs, regardless of any change in diet or exercise patterns. A loss of muscle strength, especially in the back and legs, is noted, and muscle and joint stiffness can occur. The individual may become aware of the appearance of gray hairs, little creases or lines in the face, and dry skin that begins to show signs of decreasing elasticity.[30]

The sense organs undergo change in the middle years. One of the most noticeable conditions affects the eyes. Presbyopia, a reduction in elasticity of the lens of the eye, results in decreased accommodation for near points of vision and acuity in darkness.[30] Many adults need to wear bifocals, trifocals, or reading glasses to correct this. During the middle years, there is a gradual deterioration and hardening of the auditory cells and nerves, resulting in some loss of hearing.

In women, menopausal changes that affect hormonal levels take place between 40 and 55 years of age. Some women may experience mood swings, nervousness, headaches, heart palpitations, insomnia, fatigue, and mild depression.[86] As ovarian function gradually diminishes, decreased amounts of estrogen and progesterone are produced by the ovaries. Small amounts of estrogen continue to be produced by other tissues for several years after ovarian function ceases. Some of the symptoms associated with "the change of life" are hot flashes, night sweats, and atrophic vaginitis in which the vaginal mucosa becomes thin and dry, contributing to itching, burning, and possible discharge.[86] Osteoporosis is not necessarily a result of menopause, but it often accompanies or follows menopause as bone demineralization accelerates in the absence of estrogens.

The psychologic changes that sometimes accompany

menopause may not be precipitated by the hormonal deficiency but may be more appropriately related to the personal and life-style adjustments that occur in the middle years. For example, the loss of fertility or the experience of a chronic or life-threatening illness may be a significant cause for grief. Changes in the family system such as children leaving home, divorce, illness or death of a spouse, and the illness or death of parents may contribute to the emotional difficulties women experience during this phase of life.

Physical changes in the male reproductive organs are minimal. Hypertrophy of the prostate gland can cause urinary frequency, dribbling, and urinary retention. Controversy exists over whether a male climacteric occurs. Although there are some emotional changes in men during the middle adult years, they are not believed to be the result of hormonal changes because androgen levels decline very slowly.[86] In fact, reproductive capabilities continue into the later years. Any loss of sexual desire or potency may be the result of psychologic changes, stress, illness (particularly diabetes), disability, or medications (especially hypertensive drugs), rather than physiologic changes of aging.

PSYCHOSOCIAL DEVELOPMENT

Numerous theories of adulthood have furthered the notion that middle adulthood is a distinct phase of life with specific inner growth and developmental tasks. Many of the changes during middle adulthood involve role transitions that may alter self-image, life-style, values, and attitudes. The ability to give up roles and adapt to new roles may contribute to a creative and productive life during the middle years and beyond.

Erikson, one of the first theorists to study the universal dilemmas faced during adulthood, described this stage in terms of resolving the generativity versus stagnation crisis (See Table 5-2). Generativity involves the creation and guidance of children, products, or ideas; it includes productivity, creativity, and concern for others in the broadest sense.[25] Similarly, Stevenson described this as a stage of social productivity in which the individual focuses on bringing up a family and contributing to society to ensure its survival.[78] According to Erikson, when this enrichment and fulfillment is not experienced, stagnation and personal impoverishment occur, causing isolation and preoccupation with the self. If a person fails to be a productive adult who tries to improve society or influence future generations, life may be tedious and void of further development. However, the mobilization of inner resources generates the creativity and productivity that encourage continued growth throughout the remaining years.

In Levinson's description of the "seasons of life" or the life course, the Midlife Transition is the period when adults become more compassionate, more evaluative,

more tolerant and loving of themselves and others, and less driven by external demands and conflicts than in previous stages.[48] This external orientation to the world contrasts the internal orientation of young adults when the individual is more preoccupied with achieving goals, obtaining independence, and gaining approval from the outside world. Midlife is a time when renewal and full development of relationships can occur. Once children are grown, child-centered patterns are altered and the intimate relationship between husband and wife can be nurtured. However, mutual support, open communication, and an awareness of each other's needs are necessary ingredients for an enriching relationship. While the person may be enjoying the enrichment of a new and renewed relationship, there is the inevitable experience of loss of significant others. Death may take friends, parents, family, or spouse, necessitating alterations in relationships and life-styles.

Middle Adulthood is thought to be a time of continued social influence, prosperity, economic success, and stability. Because work is an important part of the middle adult years, job loss or change at this point may threaten the self-concept and can result in altered health status. Unless illness or injury hampers a person's life, most individuals become the "senior member" in their particular world niche. This means that middle adults must be responsible for their own work, the work of others, and the mentorship of younger adults. For many adults the middle years are approached with a sense of frustration and failure if goals and expectations set in earlier years have not been reached and are not realistically attainable. The realization that the time has passed for achieving status and success is often a crisis-producing situation. Reevaluation often results in ambivalence and uncertainty regarding everyday tasks, reflecting a change in values and attitudes. The adult who once considered daily responsibilities to be fulfilling and enjoyable may begin to complain about being trapped. It is likely that the job or situation has not changed, but the person has.

Stevenson described the Core Middle Years (between ages 30 and 50) as years concerned with assisting both the younger and older generations.[78] The term "sandwich generation" is used to refer to adults who are caught between the needs of their growing children and aging parents. For adults who delayed childbearing, parenting roles must be learned. Families with children experience predictable stages such as the preschool years, school-age years, teen years, and the launching period, each with its own unique challenges.[23] With the maturation of children comes the need to let go of parenting roles so that children can achieve independence and establish adult relationships. In situations where life revolved solely around the children, parents may experience a profound sense of loss upon the children's departure. Often referred to as the "empty nest syndrome," this sudden loss of the parenting role sometimes leads to depression in women.

This may also be a time when the health status of the adult's parents is changing. Illness and perhaps impending death often necessitate assuming the role of parent to one's own parent(s). Middle-age adults are faced with difficult decisions regarding their parent's care. If the parent(s) is no longer able to continue living independently, the family must consider options such as intermittent or live-in care at the parent's home, having the parents live with the family, or institutionalization. These decisions may have profound emotional, lifestyle, and economic effects on the entire family.[24]

Although Loevinger's theory of psychosocial development does not provide age norms, the stages are consistent with those of some other theories. Younger adults and people in Loevinger's Conscientious stage tend to strive for independence, mastery, and achievement of goals.[49] However, as human beings get older, characteristics of higher stages of development, such as interdependence with others and the ability to cope with conflicting demands in relationships, are present.

The developmental milestones or achievements described are generalizations and do not occur for every adult according to the age-related guidelines. For example, the timing of developmental tasks may be altered depending on when the childbearing years begin. If a chronic or life-threatening illness strikes a person in the middle adult years, limitations posed by the illness or its treatment may alter the developmental schedule and require the person and family to adapt.[24] Although an illness situation could make it difficult for the person to achieve the "expected" tasks, knowledge of developmental theory helps nurses to assist patients. For example, a man who develops cardiac disease may decide to make a vocational change to reduce the stress of the corporate work environment. His marital partner may adjust, too, by increasing her employment from part-time to full-time to supplement the family income. She might join him in an exercise routine, and they may seek joint counseling to help them work through the changes they experience. By recognizing norms, the nurse can assist families experiencing an illness situation as they strive to maintain a fulfilling family life and community involvements.

Patients and their families often adjust to the challenges of illness situations and reformulate goals and roles so that generativity can be achieved. The grown family of a woman in her middle years who develops metastatic breast cancer may find that the traditional roles played by the father in the family have changed. Over the course of the mother's illness, the father learns to run a household, grocery shop, and do laundry, in addition to being a caregiver. Together, the family may struggle with the mother's limited life span and may plan special family events and celebrations that take into account the mother's limited physical functioning so that she has the opportunity to pass along family history and the wisdom she has acquired with age.

INTELLECTUAL DEVELOPMENT IN MIDDLE ADULTHOOD

Creativity, productivity, and cognitive capacity remain stable in the middle years, contrary to some popular beliefs.[81] Researchers who have studied intellectual functioning in middle adults suggest that there is little or no decline in learning capability and memory function.[5,76] Active use of mental capacity throughout life contributes to mental productivity in the later years. Encouraging adults to maintain activities that are intellectually stimulating is an important aspect of health promotion for middle adulthood.

SEXUALITY IN MIDDLE ADULTHOOD

Sexuality in the middle years is affected by numerous factors, including the physical aspects of aging, general health status, preexisting illness, the family and work pressures common to this phase of the life span, and attitudes about sexuality and sexual functioning. However, it is a myth that with middle age comes the end of physical attractiveness and a decline in sexual interest and capacity for competent sexual functioning.[86] Youth-oriented sociocultural influences have perpetuated the notion that aging brings sexual decline. The middle adult who approaches these years with self-acceptance, an understanding about normal changes in sexuality, and alternatives to traditional ways of expressing sexuality is apt to have a satisfying and fulfilling sexual life in later years.

Some of the physical changes that accompany menopause may affect the pleasure of sexual intercourse. For example, delay in the production of vaginal lubrication caused by the decrease in steroids may result in some discomfort during intercourse, and on occasion the irritation may cause cystitis. There may be a tendency to refrain from sexual activity because of discomfort. If such problems exist, the nurse can explain their causes, suggest use of a water-soluble lubricant during inter-

---

TASKS OF MIDDLE ADULTHOOD

Assisting children to become responsible adults
Coping with role transition
Renewing and redeveloping earlier relationships
Maintaining involvement in occupational, social, and civic spheres
Assisting in the care of aging parents
Reevaluating life's goals
Developing adult leisure-time activities

course, and advise the woman to consult her health care practitioner.

As men age, certain social and psychologic factors have an influence on their sexual responsiveness. Masters and Johnson noted several recurrent themes in interviews concerned with waning of sexual responsiveness: monotony in the sexual relationship or a feeling of being taken for granted, concerns with economic or career pursuits, mental and physical fatigue, physical or mental illness of the individual or spouse, overindulgence in food or drink, and fear of failure. They suggest that practice of sexual activity contributes to the quality of the sexual relationship as well as to the continuation of sexual activity into the later years.[86] In another study of individuals aged 45 to 69 years, previous satisfaction with sexual experience was the most significant contributing factor to current sexual functioning, including interest in, frequency of, and enjoyment of sexual relations.[21]

Because of prevailing cultural attitudes about waning sexual interest in the middle years, sexual concerns are often ignored in the care and rehabilitation of the middle-aged adult. It is very important that health care providers become knowledgeable about and sensitive to the sexual needs of patients, particularly those who experience injury or illness that restricts physical activity. Also, the nurse must recognize that certain illnesses and medications can interfere with sexual functioning.[86] Patients can be monitored, and alterations in treatment regimens can be made so that patients do not experience undesirable side effects. Nurses can help the patient cope with anxieties regarding sexual functioning by providing the opportunity to discuss these concerns with a urologist, gynecologist, or nurse trained in sexual counseling.

Finally, with the recognition that sexual functioning continues throughout the adult years, all women and men who are sexually active and not in a long-term monogamous relationship should be instructed to practice safe sex to help prevent the spread of sexually transmitted diseases, including the AIDS virus.

HEALTH PROMOTION NEEDS

As people develop and change through the life span, so do their health needs. A developmental perspective is helpful for understanding the physical and psychosocial factors that influence health at various points in the life span. During middle adulthood, adults may experience increased disability due to illness, chronic conditions, occupational factors, stress, and life-style. However, health promotion and maintenance in the middle adult years can be very important in promoting optimal functioning and recovery from illness. Specific health-promoting behaviors—proper nutrition, exercise, and sleep and rest—during the middle adult years are reviewed

here. Health concerns and nursing assessment and intervention for middle adults are addressed.

NUTRITION

For the adult in the middle years, fewer calories are required because of reduced energy requirements. Excessive caloric intake relative to physical demands may contribute to obesity and atherosclerosis, which are risk factors for coronary artery disease, hypertension, renal failure, and diabetes.[30,57] Adults in their middle years need to be aware of the fact that biologic changes necessitate a reduction in calories, saturated fats, and cholesterol. The diet should contain the four basic food groups, and the caloric intake should be based on age, body build, size, and activity patterns. Diet counseling should include specific examples of polyunsaturated oils, dairy products, and meats that can be substituted for those high in saturated fats and cholesterol. Adequate fluid intake will help prevent constipation, and a balanced diet will maintain weight control.

The calcium needs of middle adults, especially women, increase because of bone reabsorption. To prevent osteoporosis, daily calcium requirements for premenopausal women are 1000 to 1200 mg/dl, and 1500 to 2000 mg/dl for postmenopausal women. Because chronic disease is more prevalent in the middle years than among younger adults, diets may need to be tailored to the individual's specific health conditions.

EXERCISE

Consistent exercise may minimize some of the physical changes associated with aging. Throughout the adult years, exercise helps to maintain and improve muscle tone, strength, coordination, and weight. It improves work performance, reduces chronic fatigue, increases the efficiency of the cardiopulmonary system, and promotes relaxation. The regularity of exercise is important; sporadic exercise is not as effective. Exercise activities that are performed incorrectly and cause overexertion can be detrimental to a person's health. Middle adults should increase exercise gradually, exercise consistently, and avoid overexertion.[57] Heart and respiratory rates should return to their normal status 10 minutes after the exercise is stopped.

Before beginning any exercise program, a thorough health assessment including preexisting health conditions should be conducted. An assessment of daily activity patterns and a discussion about exercise preferences are useful to establish the specific kind and amount of exercise program desired. Consultation with specialists is recommended if the person is overweight, has a personal or family history of cardiovascular or respiratory illness, or has lead a physically inactive life.

Exercise programs are an important part of treatment in many chronic diseases. For some people with Type II diabetes, the illness is managed with diet and exercise. Following cardiac illness, monitored exercise is prescribed as part of the treatment regimen. Nurses can play an important role as part of the health care team involved in the management of people with chronic conditions by assisting people with exercise regimens.

REST AND SLEEP

Rest and sleep must be balanced with physical activity to keep the body functioning at its best. Sleep requirements remain the same for the middle adult as for the young adult—between 6 and 8 hours daily.[30] After 40 years of age, middle adults experience some differences in sleep cycles and patterns, such as less deep sleep and frequent awakening during the night.[30] Subsequently, they may feel less rested. As with younger adults, sleep patterns may be altered if a person's work requires rotating or night shifts. If a person experiences sleep difficulties, nurses can recommend naps, decreased caffeine intake, reduction of stress, and warm baths to promote sleep.

HEALTH ASSESSMENT

Middle adults should have a thorough yearly health examination that includes a detailed medical history, occupational history, physical assessment of body systems, blood and urine tests, electrocardiogram, chest x-ray examination, and rectal or proctoscopic examination. Men should have testicular exams, and women should have Pap smear tests, breast examinations, and mammography as indicated. Routine dental, vision, and hearing examinations should be done because periodontal disease, glaucoma, and hearing loss may be prevented or treated if detected early.[85]

HEALTH CONCERNS

The health of middle-age adults is influenced in part by health practices, diet, environmental exposure to hazards, and the demands of daily living, such as family responsibility, job-related stress, and social obligations. The leading causes of death for this age-group are malignant neoplasms, heart disease, accidents, and strokes.[82] Smoking is a major identified risk factor in the development of lung cancer, heart disease, chronic obstructive pulmonary disease, and peptic ulcer. Certain dietary patterns are thought to contribute to the incidence of heart disease, some types of cancer, diabetes, and hypertension. Work-related hazards including dust and chemicals, radiation, and environmental pollutants are thought to contribute to the risk of cancer development.

The most common chronic conditions that affect middle adults are arthritis, hypertension, and chronic sinusitis.[58] Obesity, alcoholism, substance abuse, anxiety, and depression may create serious problems for people

and their families during the middle adult years. Gum disease or periodonitis, which is caused by bacterial plaque, is the leading cause of tooth loss for people over age 35. Loss of teeth can lead to altered self-image and nutritional deficits. Accidents and injuries are common acute health problems of this period of life. Fractures and dislocations (often occupation-related) are leading causes of injury to both sexes.

Prevention of illness and injury is the most effective means of dealing with these problems. Education tailored to the person's level of understanding, unique psychosocial circumstances, and cultural background should include information on diet, exercise, the need for routine health examinations and screening, and proper dental care. Moderate use of alcohol, not smoking, and safety-related practices such as using seat belts are very effective means of preventing illness and injury for adults.

NURSING ASSESSMENT AND INTERVENTION

When working with an adult who is experiencing physical or emotional stress, the nurse must assess the medical problems at hand, as well as the physical, psychosocial, and situational factors relative to the person's developmental status. These data provide guidance in understanding those factors that may be affecting the individual's response to stress, feelings and attitudes about recovery, and potential to adapt.

Middle adulthood is a time when productivity, achievement, and responsibilities are dominant concerns in the individual's life.[24] When goals and expectations are thwarted by illness or disability, a crisis may result. This crisis affects members of the family, as well as the individual, and may require adaptation on their part, also. The nurse should demonstrate acceptance of the person's behaviors and attitudes, realizing that this may be the individual's unique manner of coping with stress. When stress is intense, problem-solving abilities may be diminished. The nurse can help the individual and family make decisions by offering options and referral to resources. In this way, their needs can be met, while the nurse fosters and maintains their independence by facilitating participation in the care planning and decision making.

LATE ADULTHOOD

The later adult years are viewed as a time of growing up and growing down. Decline occurs as the adult continues the process of moving toward old age and dissolution. However, recent research has shown that older adults continue to experience personal growth and development throughout life. An analogy may help to explain the systematic differences between younger and older adults. When faced with climbing a hill, a young adult may select a direct, steep route. The older adult may choose a longer, less demanding route. Both get to the top of the hill, but the elderly person uses alternative strategies and different techniques to reach the goal. Although 65 years of age is usually considered the beginning of late adulthood or old age, tremendous individual variation exists. A group of individuals who are the same chronological age (for example, 70 years) will have had very different lifelong experiences in the development of social relationships, wide variations in environmental exposures (for example, climates and toxins), and divergent patterns of both physical growth and development and health status as affected by genetic tendencies and life-styles. Therefore although late adulthood is a period of growth and development that can be described with general developmental trends, it is also a period of life that may span more than 35 years and is reflective of individuals who tend to be less like each other and more like themselves. Some people may be "old" at 45 years of age, whereas others are not "old" at 80.

The study of older adults has become increasingly more popular with scientists, including nurses, over the past few decades. Many factors have contributed to the growing interest in gerontology, the study of normal aging. A major stimulus for this research is the fact the that the elderly population is growing more rapidly in proportion to other age segments, with persons age 85 and over constituting the most rapidly growing portion of the American population (Figure 5-2). Also, in 1974 the National Institute of Aging (NIA) was formed, and additional federal funds have been channeled toward gerontologic research. Because more Americans are living longer, societal change is necessary to meet the unique social and health needs of this growing group. A developmental perspective is extremely useful in planning this change and caring for older adults.

GENERAL RESPONSES TO AGING

Many of the physical changes that begin gradually during adulthood continue through the older adult years. Biologic aging leads to some general responses in the older person. First, there is a gradual decline in functional ability, particularly where multisystem coordination is required. These age decrements are greater in performances that require more complex functioning than in those involving individual system functions.

The research on biologic aging has generated a body

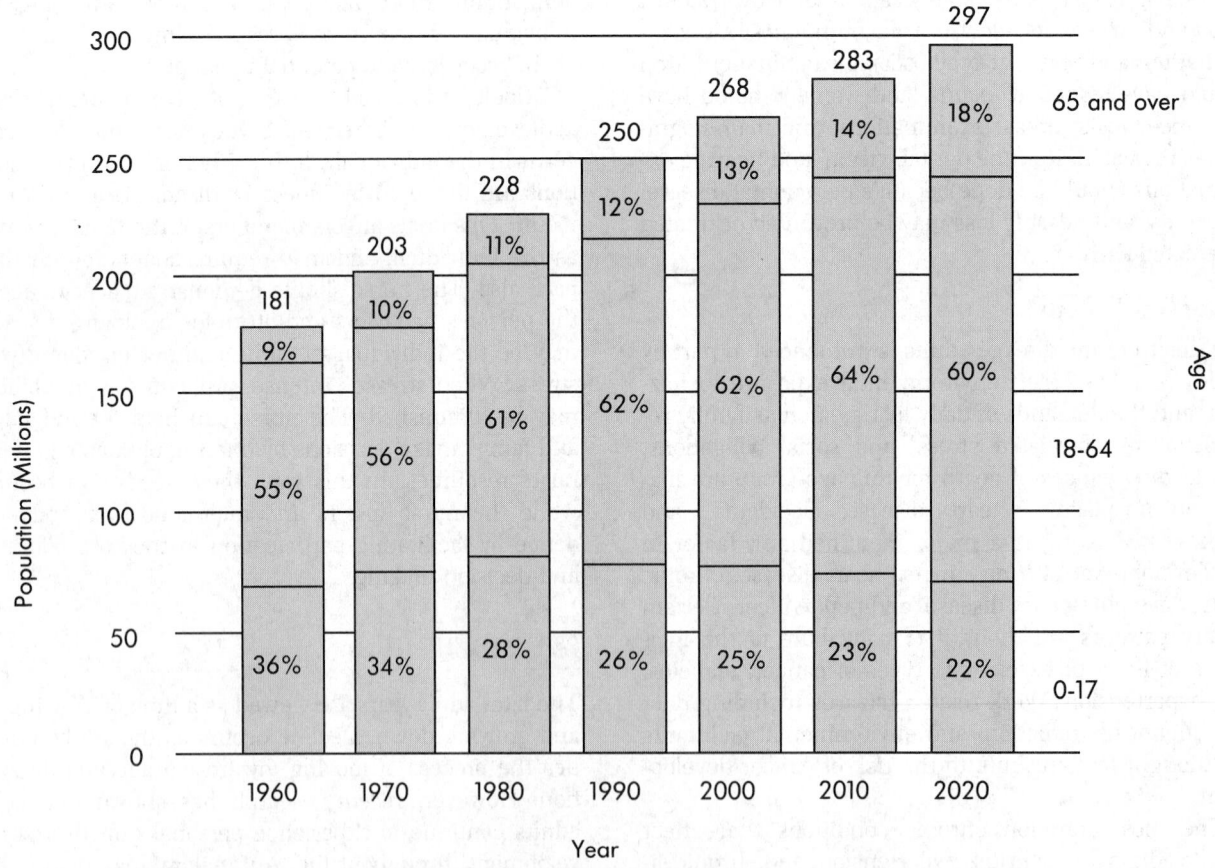

FIGURE 5-2 U. S. population by age group (1960-2020). (From the U.S. Census Bureau.)

of knowledge regarding the normal and abnormal changes associated with the aging process. Normal aging changes are those that are (1) universal to all members of the species, (2) intrinsic to the organism, (3) progressive and cumulative, and (4) deleterious to the organism as a whole and associated with an increased mortality.

These normal aging changes are called *primary changes*. Such effects of aging—for example, thinning hair and decreased pulmonary capacity—have been demonstrated through research to occur universally. As more knowledge is generated, it becomes evident that many changes once thought to be associated with aging, such as arthritis and senility, are actually *secondary changes* and do not occur universally as a part of aging. For example, the muscle atrophy and weakened joints seen in many elderly have been discovered to be more related to a sedentary life-style than to a primary change of aging. Primary changes of aging are summarized in Table 5-3.

In addition to the primary changes of aging listed in Table 5-3, some other variations in organ function bear mentioning. First, the variation in organ function between individuals is much greater in the elderly than in younger persons. For example, glucose tolerance values of young adults cluster around a norm, whereas those of the elderly have a much wider range.

Second, the rate of decline from one function to another varies. Basal metabolic rate and total body water of

the elderly decrease only minimally to about 80% of that of young adults. On the other hand, renal blood flow and maximum breathing capacity show a significant decline in most elderly persons.

A third major change related to the aging process occurs in response to stress. Although an aged person may have an adequate cardiac output at rest, stress in the form of an infection, exertion, or emotional shock will decrease cardiac output, and it will take much longer for it to return to the person's baseline level. In addition, there is a loss of reserve capacity related to a decline in hormonal and neural regulation, leading to poorer coordination of brain interactions. This decline causes a slowing of reaction time and a greater susceptibility to infection and accidents.

PSYCHOSOCIAL DEVELOPMENT IN LATE ADULTHOOD

Human beings have a tremendous potential to grow and change during every phase of life. Psychosocial development is a life-long process that is reflected in how human beings perceive the nature of the world.[6,66] Knowledge of developmental changes and events that occur in the older adult years is useful in understanding how people adapt to health and illness situations. Basic knowledge about developmental processes is vital to understanding behavior changes throughout the life span, interpreting behaviors of older adults, and assisting them with their health and developmental needs.

TABLE 5-3 Primary changes of aging

Body System	Change	Body System	Change
Skin	Loss of subcutaneous supportive tissue	Liver	Minimal change
	Decreased sebaceous secretions	Bowel	Minimal change
	Thinning and graying hair	Gastrointestinal	Minimal loss of digestive enzymes
Muscular	Increased fat substitution for muscle		Decreased absorption
	Muscle atrophy	Endocrine	Decreased utilization of insulin
Skeletal	Loss of calcium from bones		Cessation of progesterone
	Shrinkage of vertebral disks		Decline, then plateau of estrogen
	Deterioration of cartilage		Gradual decline in testosterone
Pulmonary	Reduced chest wall compliance	Vision	Deterioration in ability of lens to focus
	Decreased breathing capacity		Loss of color sensitivity
	Decreased vital capacity		Decreased dark adaptation
	Increased residual volume		Decreased peripheral vision
	Reduced cough reflex		Decreased sensitivity to glare
	Reduced ciliary activity	Hearing	Increased threshold for high frequencies
Cardiac	Endocardial thickening		Difficulty in speech discrimination
	Thickened heart valves		Degeneration of cochlea and auditory pathways
	Decreased cardiac output (under stress)	Sexual	Minimal change in amount of sexual response
Vascular	Progressive stiffening of arteries		Increase in time for full sexual response
	Atherosclerotic plaques		Decreased vaginal lubrication
Renal	Decreased blood flow		Increased refractory period for males
	Decreased glomerular filtration rate		
	Reduced nephrons		
	Decreased creatinine clearance		

From Rossman I: Clinical geriatrics, ed 3, Philadelphia, 1986, JB Lippincott Co.[69]

Emotional development is reflected in Erikson's description of the mature years, integrity versus disgust or despair.[25] The individual who looks back and perceives life to have been rich and fulfilling, with purpose and meaning, will feel a sense of satisfaction and contentment in the remaining years. If one does not evaluate his or her life as such, the final years of late adulthood may be faced with despair.[25] The manifestations of despair might include regrets about one's life or the fear of death.[25]

In other theories of psychosocial development, Levinson[48] and Stevenson[78] (see Table 5-2) described some of the issues faced in old age. For example, reviewing life, sharing wisdom with others, and putting personal affairs in order were identified by Stevenson as responsibilities of the older adult. A list of developmental tasks associated with late adulthood is listed in the box below. Many of these tasks are associated with loss. Older adults must face multiple losses when they retire or experience the death of their spouse, family, and friends. They may change their life-styles dramatically to care for an ill spouse, or they may have to move out of their homes because they can no longer manage independently. Independence may be lost if a person can no longer drive a car or if physical disability prevents use of public transportation. Failing health constitutes a major loss as well.

Loevinger's theory of ego development is consistent with these general ideas. At higher stages of development, people are better able to cope with inner conflict and tolerate the diversity of thinking among human beings.[49] Mutual interdependence is characteristic of human relationships. At the highest stage, the Integrated stage, people cherish rather than just tolerate individual differences, and they actually reconcile conflicting demands rather than just cope with them. Loevinger suggests that the highest stage is primarily a theoretic one because only about 1% of all people fall into this stage.

TASKS OF THE OLDER ADULT

Assuming responsibility for sharing the wisdom of age
Reminiscing and participating in life review
Putting affairs in order
Accepting life with serenity
Adjusting to new limitations of declining physical strength and declining health
Adjusting to reorganized family patterns
Adjusting to a new pattern of social and civic responsibilities
Adjusting to death of spouse and other loved ones
Establishing affiliation with one's age group
Maintaining satisfactory living arrangements
Accepting death with serenity and assisting others to accept death

Loevinger's description of the higher stages of development gives us a better understanding of how people might adjust to the later years of life. As people age and increasingly depend on others for assistance, they may also provide assistance to those who help them. There are many examples of this mutual interdependence. When grandparents provide child care assistance to the childrearing family, all three generations benefit mutually. The grandparents have an opportunity to share their wisdom, the parents have tangible assistance while they pursue their vocational roles, and the children receive love and nurturance. Some older adults who want to maintain their independence as long as possible choose to live in retirement complexes where assistance is available if needed. The decision to enter a residential facility may result in inner conflict concerning giving up and moving out of one home, establishing a new home, and accepting the possibility of dependence in the future.

Emotional and psychologic responses to aging have been explored by numerous researchers. In one survey elderly persons were asked what they considered essential for happiness. They mentioned good health, a place to live, enough money to live comfortably, recognition by others, and the opportunity for a variety of experiences.[36] Reed, a nurse scientist, identified four dimensions of development in older adults: (1) transcendence, the orientation toward purposes greater than the self, (2) temporal awareness, the awareness of time and that a person's time is limited, (3) plasticity, the ability to make changes, and (4) the maintenance of physical integrity.[66,67] Cummings described the elderly's response to the reality of death as one of release, characterized by "a mutual withdrawal or disengagement."[17] Either the individual or the social system might initiate the withdrawal. The outcome of this response might be a movement away from involvement, achievement, and productivity on the part of the older adult.

Many younger people falsely assume that older people have no interest in sex and lack the ability to perform sexually. Men and women of all ages are capable of sexual arousal and orgasm. Masters and Johnson emphasize that one of the primary factors in maintaining sexual activity in old age is the frequency of sexual performance.[86] Studies conducted at the Duke University Center for the Study of Aging revealed sexual activity in the eighth and ninth decades. Often the aged person becomes sexually inactive because of lack of an acceptable partner or the presence of symptoms associated with chronic disease (pain, dyspnea, chronic fatigue), especially in those over 80 years old.

The primary nursing focus of meeting the psychosocial needs of elderly persons is to help them make the adjustments necessary to achieve the desired goals. A first step is to understand the needs of the person. The desires of the elderly and the difficulties that must be overcome to obtain them should both be considered in planning the nursing care of elderly people. Success in meeting this objective will depend on the nurse developing a plan that reflects the following concepts of normal aging and individual variations: (1) emotional development continues in the older adult years and is associated with new tasks of living, (2) each elderly individual has different expectations of a life that is worth living, (3) each will react differently to the limitations and frustrations that are imposed on achieving and maintaining this worthwhile existence, and (4) elderly persons will often react (cope) essentially as they have reacted to other stresses throughout their lives.

ILLNESS PATTERNS IN THE ELDERLY

In assessing the health and illness patterns of the elderly, some general factors must be recognized. First, age-related decline in immune function results in a less rapid and less effective response to infections and in an increased incidence of autoimmunity and malignancy.[11] Second, stress situations (either physiologic or psychosocial) produce more pronounced reactions in the aged and require a longer period of time for readjustment. Third, complex functions that require multisystem coordination show the most obvious decline and require the greatest compensation and support. Fourth, the elderly frequently have an atypical presentation of an illness. Pain may be *less pronounced,* and some typical symptoms may be either missing or the opposite of what is expected (as compared to what is seen in other age groups). Confusion, restlessness, or other altered mentation is a common occurrence in the presence of illness. Obscure or unexplained deterioration of health or function should not be accepted as normal aging and must be carefully evaluated.

Multiplicity and chronicity of diseases are common among the elderly, and many patients have several chronic ailments. Most have developed slowly. Heart disease, cancer, renal disease, vascular disease such as cerebrovascular accident, chronic obstructive pulmonary disease such as emphysema, and accidents are the most common problems that bring older patients to the hospital. Other common chronic ailments such as arthritis, skin disorders, mild neuromuscular conditions, and hearing impairments are usually cared for while the person is ambulatory. The most common morbidities are arthritis, heart disease, hypertension, and diabetes.[15] The three most common causes of death for older adults are heart disease, malignant neoplasms, and cerebrovascular accidents.[82]

NURSING INTERVENTION

The goal of health care is to keep people functioning at the highest possible level for their age. This includes helping them to live with chronic ailments and continuing degenerative changes while maximizing the unique strengths and resources each elderly person possesses. The nurse who views aging as a normal, inevitable process that requires adjustments in living patterns but not a withdrawal from life is best prepared to work with the aging patient.

The nursing care plan depends on the physiologic and anatomic changes that have taken place, the diseases that are present, the person's own emotional makeup and apparent adjustment to the particular situ-

---

RESEARCH

Reed P: Mental health of older adults, West J Nurs Res 11(2), 143-157, 1989.

In this study, a sample of clinically depressed older adults was studied to determine the relationship between developmental resources and depression. Development was viewed as a process of trading away old psychosocial resources (behaviors, skills, and perspectives) for new ones that are relevant as the context of the person's life changes. The Developmental Resources of Later Adulthood scale used in the study included items such as "sharing my wisdom and experiences with others, adjusting to changes in my physical abilities, [and] having interests I can enjoy." Higher levels of developmental resources were related to less depression. The ability to transcend, or expand beyond personal boundaries and consider purposes greater than the self, was associated with better mental health. Although the results are preliminary, the well-being and mental health of older adults appears to be related to the developmental resources available. ■

RESEARCH

Ryden M: Environmental support for autonomy in the institutionalized elderly, Res Nurs Health 8:363-371, 1985.

The climate for autonomy was studied in four urban proprietary nursing homes. Data for 113 residents, 137 caregivers, and 10 administrative personnel demonstrated that caregivers perceive themselves as the predominant decision-makers. Although the caregivers indicate they preferred a slightly higher level of self-determination for their clients, only in one-to-one and solitary activities did they prefer giving residents the primary decision-making role. Residents saw themselves as having more control than did their caregivers. Grooming and eating were identified by both groups as areas in which residents had the least control. Caregivers estimated a lower percentage of residents were capable of autonomy in making decisions about their daily activities and care than did administrative staff. ■

ation, and the support available from others. In planning nursing care for elderly patients, consideration is given to the unique physical, social, economic, and psychologic capacities and limitations of each patient. Many elderly persons have visual and auditory impairments. The nurse should optimize the patient's vision and hearing by restructuring or adapting the interviewing environment to facilitate obtaining accurate information relative to past health and personal history. Eyeglasses and hearing aids should be used. If the elderly patient is ill and has a number of chronic diseases, the same questions will be asked many times by various health professionals. As a result, the elderly person may be reluctant to tell his or her own story yet another time. If instead, the nurse encourages the patient to tell his or her own story, allowing a reminiscent quality but deliberately guiding the conversation, the result will most likely be an excellent history and an established base of trust and confidence. The long-term nursing goal should be to maximize and maintain function and independence within the person's preferred life-style.

Many different resources are available to augment the older person's existing capabilities and resources

TYPES OF COMMUNITY SUPPORT SERVICES FOR OLDER PERSONS

Senior citizen centers	Social, nutritional, and educational counseling, health screening (for example, blood pressure and weight), and often foot care services
Adult day centers	Assistive daytime nursing care; social, recreational, nutritional, and rehabilitative services (physical, occupational, and speech therapy); often function as respite care centers for caregivers of elderly participants
Adult foster home care	Care in another private home when older person unable to live alone; may or may not be licensed by state
Meals on wheels	Meals delivered to person's home
Homemaking service	Includes household chores and shopping
Transportation service	Arranged pickup by transportation system (may be private enterprise with a fee, or local church groups or other community agency at low or no cost)
Home health service	Skilled intermittent home nursing care; visits on an intermittent basis by a nurse or occupational, physical, or speech therapist for skilled care; home health aide also available for personal care and/or homemaker for shopping and cleaning

(see the box). Hospital discharge planners should be contacted to assist the patient and family in arranging for home care services or institutional care if needed. Information and referral services for the elderly are often available in communities through home health agencies. In recent years many local governments have established offices that provide telephone information and referral to community resources for the elderly. They are an excellent clearinghouse for the nurse who is trying to match a resource to a need of their elderly patient. Since many community resources may blossom or vanish literally overnight, it is often helpful to contact this service if you believe there is even a remote chance of finding help for some problem.

COGNITIVE CHANGES

Intellectual development in older adults can be characterized by the coexistence of stability, growth, and decline.[5] In order to develop strategies to help older adults function at optimum levels, nurses must recognize that different aspects of cognitive functioning stay the same, improve, or decline during the later adult years. This perspective reflects a positive view of aging.

Very little research is available that documents intellectual decline.[5,76] The prevailing attitude is that no general decline in intellectual capacity occurs until adults reach their sixties and seventies. If cognitive changes do occur, it is possible that they are measurable only at the maximum level of difficulty. In fact, adults can improve their performance in some intellectual tasks when learning material is divided into smaller units and practice is encouraged. Although there is tremendous variation from person to person, older adults are thought to have the capacity to learn and profit from experience, think or reason abstractly, adapt to change and uncertainty in the environment, and self-motivate to accomplish goals.

Older adults can continue to adapt and meet challenges (or climb hills) if we take into account how they optimize their current capacities and compensate for deficits. When teaching older adults, it is helpful to adapt teaching strategies.[35] Some simple measures that help older adults to learn include the following:

1. allowing some time for socialization at the beginning
2. modifying instructions for hearing, visual, mobility, and cognitive status
3. shortening learning periods
4. providing less information per session
5. slowing the pace of instruction
6. providing more repetition
7. using memory aids
8. using large black print for printed materials

Although mental functioning can remain stable and can sometimes be enhanced in older adults, cognitive impairments do occur. Cognitive impairments have many causes, and some are reversible. Cognitive functioning may be impaired by acute delerium or chronic dementias or by depression. Acute delerium or confusion states, which are potentially reversible, may be caused by fluid and electrolyte imbalances, malnutrition, metabolic imbalances, toxic states, trauma, infections, decreased cardiac or renal function, drugs, or overwhelming stress. The person is physically ill, confused, and experiences hallucinations.

Alzheimer's disease and multi-infarct dementia are the most common dementias. Alzheimer's disease accounts for 50% to 60% of dementias and multi-infarct dementia for 6% to 12%.

Depression is often confused with dementia and can be superimposed on true dementia; therefore many elderly persons with treatable depression are not recognized. Depression is a dysphoric mood causing loss of interest in usual activities. It is characterized by at least four of the following symptoms present for a period of at least 2 weeks: (1) altered appetite or weight; (2) altered sleep patterns; (3) expressions of self-reproach, guilt, and hopelessness; (4) lack of energy; (5) psychomotor retardation or agitation; (6) loss of interest or pleasure in usual activities; and (7) recurrent thoughts of suicide. Depressed elderly may or may not be disoriented to time, place, or person. If there is any possibility of the existence of depression, the older person should receive treatment. Suicide rates in the United States continue to be high in old age. Whenever an elderly person demonstrates changes in cognitive functioning, a diagnostic workup by a physician is the first step in ruling out reversible causes of the problem.

Nursing interventions for the person with only mild cognitive loss should focus on the individual's strengths. This conveys a message of belief in the individual's overall competence. The mildly confused are often fearful of "losing control"; recognizing their abilities and avoiding patronizing overtones will minimize this underlying fear and enhance a more honest line of communication about the real problems the confusion is causing in life. The mildly confused often have difficulty processing new information quickly. A slower pace is recommended, with shorter periods of teaching, less information, and more repetition than is needed for other age-groups. Most elderly people will benefit from methods that enhance or support short-term memory. For example, the use of appointment calendars, reminder calls about appointments, prefilled medication boxes, and instructions written in large black print serve as memory aids.[35] Instructions may also be modified according to the person's hearing, visual acuity, and mobility. Nursing interventions for the moderately to severely demented elderly should focus on establishing a predictable, safe environment; reducing the number

RESEARCH

Williams MA et al.: Nursing activities and acute confusional states in elderly hip-fractured patients, Nurs Res 28:25-35, 1979.

This often-quoted study looked at hip fracture patients over the age of 60 to determine what activities and other variables were related to confusion. The best predictor of postoperative confusion was confusion on admission. Other significant variables were postoperative urinary retention or incontinence, limited mobility, and the absence of clocks and television. ■

and complexity of sensory stimuli while providing basic sensory stimulation; and supporting family and/or caretakers so that they do not develop ill health or the premature desire to relinquish the care of the elder because of frustration or fatigue. All interactions with the demented elder should be aimed at reducing the complexity of cognitive processing to the level the confused person can understand (that is, keep sentences simple, use one-level instructions, demonstrate tasks along with verbal instruction, exaggerate facial expressions to provide the visual sensory input that will be more readily interpreted than the verbal input).

PROMOTING SELF-CARE IN HOSPITALIZED ELDERLY

One of the primary nursing goals when working with the elderly is to promote and maintain self-care.

Placing equipment conveniently so that assistance need not be requested will increase independence and a sense of control, especially for the hospitalized person who loses significant control just by being a "patient." Self-help devices will help maintain and promote some degree of independence. For example, an overbed trapeze or side rails on the bed may facilitate movement in bed. Handrails along hallways and in the bathroom or a walker may make it possible to walk alone. Sturdy chairs with arms and seats that are 18 to 20 inches from the floor make it easier for many elderly patients to get into and out of chairs themselves (low chairs and chairs without arms require increased quadriceps strengths and make it difficult to use arm strength to supplement leg strength. Electric beds allow for more independence. If the patient uses a walker or cane, glasses, hearing aid, or dentures, these devices should be readily available. Showers or bathtubs equipped with handrails and with nonskid strips may make it possible for some patients to bathe independently and safely.

Many adjustments can be made to help the patient who is confined to a wheelchair retain some measure of independence. If the patient is able to transfer onto the toilet, arranging a bathroom to facilitate this maneuver is desirable. Some patients, especially if they have urinary frequency or incontinence, appreciate their wheel-chair or chair being adapted to serve as a commode. Removal of door sills may make it possible for an elderly patient confined to a wheelchair to move about the house. If elderly patients are unable to propel the chair manually, they may be able to use a motorized wheel-chair.

Elderly patients may appreciate help with personal care such as arranging the hair, applying cosmetics, shaving, and dressing. Personal appearance is important to everyone's morale.

Many elderly patients can give most or all necessary physical care to themselves. Some may need encouragement to do so; others resent not being allowed to care for themselves. The nurse or the family member giving care must be patient and allow adequate time. The older, hospitalized, ill patient often is exceptionally slow and fatigues easily. It is helpful to negotiate a daily program of activities with the hospitalized elderly that includes rest periods. The nurse should always ascertain which individuals are physically able to give their own care and be alert to changes in baseline patterns of vital signs and general health that indicate need for treatment and a temporarily lowered level of activity.

When possible, many hospital routines can be adjusted for elderly patients. For instance, they may prefer to bathe and shave in the afternoon or early evening. The nursing care plan for physical care of each elderly patient should include what self-care is possible, what assistance is needed, the method used, and the schedule the patient follows. Most elderly patients find comfort in familiar things and processes. Therefore it is important to maintain routine as much as possible. The patient should participate in planning the schedule, and whenever possible it should parallel the pattern of care at home.

PROMOTING SKIN INTEGRITY

Usually one or two baths a week are sufficient, although the patient who is incontinent needs local cleansing at frequent intervals and perhaps more frequent baths. Because regular soaps can be irritating, mild superfatted soaps are preferred. Bath oils may be used, or lanolin or body lotions can be applied after bathing to promote water retention in the skin.

If the patient is confined to bed, an alternating pressure mattress, flotation pad, or flotation mattress may be extremely helpful in maintaining the skin in good condition. Above all, the patient's position should be changed frequently, and bony prominences and weight-bearing areas should be massaged at least every 2 hours. Sheepskin pads placed under bony prominences are also used to relieve pressure and to prevent irritation of the skin. Every effort should be made to get the elderly out of bed as much as possible. This not only helps

RESEARCH

Magilvy J: Experiencing hearing loss in later life: a comparison of deaf and hearing-impaired older women, Res Nurs and Health 8:347-353, 1985.

Effects of hearing loss on lives of two groups of older women, including those who were deaf before beginning a vocation ($n = 27$) and those who became deaf with aging ($n = 39$) were studied. Women 54 to 96 years of age were interviewed, using their preferred mode of communication. Both groups of women experienced a high degree of handicap but experienced their problems differently. Women with later onset of hearing loss emphasized emotional situation problems related to their deafness, whereas those who had an early onset of deafness expressed communication difficulties. ■

to redistribute pressure over the body and improve circulation but can also give patients a psychologic boost.

Because of dryness, poor circulation, and low resistance to infection, the skin of elderly persons readily becomes infected, particularly in the lower extremities. Elderly persons often need assistance in drying their feet after bathing and in cutting and caring for their toenails. Nails are often hard and scaly; soaking the feet in warm water or applying oil to the nails before cutting softens them and makes cutting easier and safer. A podiatrist should be asked to care for very hard nails and other conditions such as calluses, corns, and bunions.

As the tissue age and circulation becomes sluggish, the hair becomes thin, dry, and colorless. Massage of the scalp and daily brushing with a soft-bristled brush help to preserve its integrity. Frequent shampooing should be avoided, since the shampoo will dry the hair and scalp. Dry shampoos may be used intermittently or regularly for individuals in the home or hospital setting who are unable or too ill to be positioned for a wet shampoo.

PROMOTING EYE CARE

Changes occur in the eyes with aging. There is a decrease in the conjunctival secretions, and sometimes the lower lid droops (ectropion), causing the moistening fluid of the eye to be lost.[11,15] Therefore irritation of the conjunctivae and tearing are common complaints of the aged. Smoke also may be more irritating to their eyes than to those of younger persons. Isotonic solution eyedrops are frequently ordered as a comfort measure.

An accumulation of secretions at the inner canthus of the eye may be present, particularly on awakening, and may be a prodromal of infection. A sterile cotton sponge moistened with a physiologic solution of sodium chloride can be used to cleanse the eyes. Care must be taken not to press on the eyeballs or to irritate any exposed conjunctiva. Cataracts, failing vision, and actual blindness are common in the aged. The lens of the eye loses its ability to accommodate effectively as aging progresses. Most people over 50 years of age need glasses, at least for reading. In the hospital or nursing home setting, care of glasses is important. Glasses should be labeled with the patient's name, and they should be kept clean and accessible to the elderly person. If glasses are worn by the hospital patient, but were lost, broken, or left at home at the time of hospital admission, arrangements should be made to have new glasses made or the existing ones brought to the hospital. No patient education, rehabilitation (such as ambulation activities), or increased self-care measures can be initiated in the treatment plan until the person is using his or her maximum visual skill with the aid of the glasses. The eyes of older people adapt more slowly to changes in light and are increasingly sensitive to glare. Therefore bright lights or sunlight may be almost unbearable to some elderly people, and vision is often poor in the dark; nightlights should be used to increase illumination and prevent falls and possible confusion.

PROMOTING CARE OF MOUTH AND TEETH

Oral health in the elderly is important for several reasons. First, the mouth is the portal for nutritional intake, and any problems here could affect overall ability to meet the nutritional needs of cells and tissues throughout the body. Second, lesions or disorders of the mucous membranes, gums, or teeth may lead to severe discomfort, affecting both the emotional and social status (for example, inability to partake in usual activities including dining with others) of the individual. Third, debilitated individuals who are unable to regularly perform mouth care and have a poor cough reflex are at increased risk for pneumonia caused by aspiration of bacteria-laden oral secretions.

With increasing age there is a recession of the gums (gingiva) and exposure of the root surface, which results in an increase in the prevalence of root (cervical) caries. The occurrence of caries can be a source of discomfort and expensive to repair; if it affects the anterior teeth, it poses an aesthetic problem. Since over 65% of the elderly have an edentulous jaw; dental caries is not a concern of the majority of older persons.[69] However, future generations are more likely to retain their teeth throughout late adulthood because of the current emphasis on preventive dental care and with advances in disease prevention and dental technology. Teaching preventive care to minimize caries in the elderly must be considered a priority in dental care.

Lesions of the oral mucosa may result from a number of causes (for example, infections, drug reactions, cancer). Especially noteworthy are oral neoplasms and lesions caused by dentures. Because cancerous and benign lesions look similar, any lesion of the oral mucosa that is not directly attributable to irritation from dentures or another identifiable source should be referred to a specialist for diagnosis.[69] Care of dentures, prevention of denture-associated problems, and prevention of denture loss is part of the general care of the elderly. Poorly fitting dentures may cause chronic irritation to areas on the gums or oral mucosa and cause ulcerations or hyperkeratosis. Denture use and fit should be a part of the general nursing assessment. Persons with recent significant weight loss that may alter the oral-facial tissue contour, or disease (anemia) or drugs (chemotherapy) that may affect oral tissue integrity are at risk for denture-associated lesions.[11]

Persons with loose-fitting dentures are also at risk for airway obstruction during sleep and should be instructed to wear dentures only when awake. General care and teaching should include (1) cleaning dentures after each meal, (2) soaking dental plates in tap water or a denture solution when not in use, and (3) strategies to avoid loss or mix-ups, including placing dental plates in a safe, convenient place and putting the name or other identification marking on the dentures.

There is some recent evidence that older people, particularly those without teeth, may normally experience changes in the muscles used to masticate food.[15] These changes may prevent the elderly person from chewing food adequately prior to swallowing. Additionally, the older person is more willing to swallow larger-size particles than the younger person and may be less aware of this functional change. Complaints such as "slow chewing" or "hard to chew" or avoiding certain foods may suggest oral muscular weakness or difficulties. Oral motor dysfunction may occur because of pathologic conditions such as paresis associated with a cerebrovascular accident or tardive dyskinesia associated with phenothiazine use. The consequences of such motor dysfunction can include choking, apnea, or regurgitation.[15] The nursing assessment should include an evaluation of oral muscle function and development of a plan of care if a problem exists. This individualized plan might include patient education regarding selection and preparation of foods that require less chewing without sacrificing essential nutrients or a pleasing taste and appearance. The individual should maintain a sitting position when eating, avoid talking while eating, and avoid eating in stressful situations. Finally, when possible, the individual should be encouraged to eat when others are present to assist if choking does occur.

PROMOTING ACTIVITY

The benefits of physical fitness are the same at any age: maintenance of aerobic capacity of the cardiovascular system, flexibility, strength, balance, kinesthetic sense, and relaxation. For the elderly who are experiencing normal aging changes and chronic health problems contributing to diminished physical capacity, fitness will be more critical to maintenance of their independent function and ability to pursue enriching leisure activities. In one study, elders reported a problem with physical ability three times more often than other problems (that is, lack of transportation, no money) as the main factor deterring their pursuit of leisure activities (walking, gardening, fishing, or driving).[75]

As with, and perhaps more than, other age groups, the elderly vary considerably in their physical abilities and overall physical fitness. One may distinguish between the (1) "active" elderly (those persons who seem little affected by their age and continue with lifelong activity habits), (2) the "inactive" elderly (those persons who are hindered by a variety of age-related problems that mentally or physically limit their physical ability) and, (3) the "very active" elderly (those individuals who have maintained a high degree of fitness and still participate in competitive sports events).[75]

Because fitness levels vary among the elderly, nursing care will take focus in one of two general ways: (1) to promote continued activity in those already engaged in moderate to high levels of activity, or (2) to motivate and assist the less active elderly to engage in physical activities that are appropriate for their abilities and needs and are of interest to them. For the group of moderately to highly active individuals, the nurse's responsibility is to promote and support their preferred activities.

In local communities there are often groups or organizations that provide opportunities for elderly exercise in the form of protected and appropriately challenging hiking trails, swimming facilities, or other group exercise programs at YMCAs or senior centers. By becoming familiar with the local exercise resources, the nurse is readily able to direct elderly individuals to appropriate resources. If the active individual becomes hospitalized or admitted to an extended-care facility for rehabilitation, all members of the interdisciplinary team (for example, occupational and physical therapists, physiatrists) will be involved in assessing with the individual a prescribed plan of activity that will help restore the individual's physical abilities and overall health. This prescribed plan will most likely consist of formal physical or occupational therapy sessions with the specialists in these areas as well as a more informal plan that outlines the individual's participation in self-care activities and mobilization. The latter area requires considerable input from the nurse who is in the best position to assess, implement, and evaluate individual activity patterns on a sustained basis.

For the less active elderly who may be in the nursing home or at home and using home care resources (for example, skilled nursing service, homemaker), prescribed rehabilitation activities often will be needed. However, there are additional general nursing measures to be considered in planning activity for individuals who are partially or fully immobilized. When the individual is confined to bed, proper body alignment, frequent repositioning, and range-of-motion exercises will aid in maintaining comfort and maximum range of motion at the joints. Unless there is some particular contraindication, exercises for the arms and legs, exercises to keep abdominal and gluteal muscles in good tone, and exercises to strengthen the extensor muscles of the spine should be performed several times each day by every bed patient. The patient is taught to flex, abduct, adduct, and extend each leg separately and both legs simultaneously. The heel of one foot can be placed on the knee of the opposite leg and then the heel passed slowly down the leg to the ankle. This can then be repeated, alternating the legs. Arms, hand, neck, and shoulder movements can be encouraged by having the patient first raise and lower the head, neck, and shoulders from a flat supine position without a pillow and then by having the patient extend the arms in front of the chest, followed by raising them above the head. The person should be encouraged to do as many of the exercises as possible and to take deep breaths and exhale fully in coordination with the exercises. Daily exercises should be supervised by the nurse or caregiver. The regular performance of exercises helps to prevent the loss of muscle tone that occurs in all bed patients, regardless of age. If the person is unable to do active range-of-motion exercises independently, the nurse should help with them or do passive range-of-motion exercises.

Because the immobile elderly are at high risk for orthostatic hypotension, osteoporosis, venous stasis and thrombus formation, respiratory infections, and sensory deprivation, the nursing care plan should include regular daily intervals out of bed spent walking with assistance or sitting in a chair.

PROMOTING SLEEP

There are certain changes in sleep and sleep patterns that seem to occur as part of normal aging. These include a prolonged sleep latency (time it takes to fall asleep), an increase in the number of awakenings during the sleep period, a decrease in slow-wave sleep (thought to be associated with physical restoration), and a decrease in rapid eye movement (REM) sleep that occurs in advanced old age (thought to be associated with mental restoration).[15] These changes often result in more fragmented sleep than that experienced in earlier years. Although many elderly adapt to these normal sleep changes, there are others who experience acute or chronic insomnia. Physical problems that cause pain, shortness of breath, frequency of urination, incontinence, impairment of mobility, or confusion may disrupt sleep. Other contributing factors include certain drugs (for example, some antihypertensives) and environmental factors such as temperature, light, noise, and type of bed and its location.

Since quality of sleep can have far-reaching effects on the individual's general well-being, an essential component of the nurse's health assessment of the elderly must include an evaluation of sleep. If a sleep problem is identified, it should be analyzed as to its onset, subjective complaint (how the problem is described by the patient), previous treatments and effectiveness, and sleep patterns prior to the onset of the problem.

Promotion of sleep in the elderly includes identification and treatment of the specific sleep problem when one exists. Health care settings (hospital, nursing home, retirement home) should be planned so that individual sleep needs can be preserved. Flexibility such as providing areas for night persons to enjoy activities is a prerequisite to planning.

Nursing interventions that teach manipulation of the environment may be part of the treatment plan for acute insomnia or chronic insomnia. The goal of this strategy is to promote restoration of the sleep-wake cycle by identifying the specific factors that are disrupting sleep, and minimizing or eliminating them. If the individual has pain, the pain must be controlled; if there is nocturia, the cause should be found and treated; if there is a disruptive partner, beds or rooms should be changed. Warm milk or a snack at bedtime will aid in inducing sleep naturally. The elderly person should be allowed nap times during the day. In addition, mind-stimulating activities and exercise should not be engaged in before bedtime.[4]

Sedatives are indicated with acute insomnia only and must be prescribed with caution in the elderly. Sedatives can widely depress the central nervous system and result in coordination impairment and decreased mental alertness.

PROMOTING NUTRITION

Nutritional requirements of the elderly are essentially the same as for other adults, except that calorie needs diminish because of a decrease in lean body mass relative to fat (which burns fewer calories).[13] Fiber (that is, fruits, vegetables, whole grain bread, cereals), although undigestible, is an important constituent in the diet. Fiber holds water in the fecal mass, which softens the stools and enhances regular evacuation. The incidence of diverticulitis, colon cancer, or gallstones is thought to be influenced by diets chronically low in fiber. Although one might argue that low dietary fiber as a risk factor for these diseases is more relevant to those in their middle and earlier years, individuals at or near age 65 may still have a life expectancy of 15 or more years during which dietary fiber deficiencies might play a role in develop-

ment of colon cancer, diverticulitis, or gallstones. Because the latter disorders and constipation are common problems in the elderly, it is important that moderate amounts of fiber be regularly included in the diet.[30]

Water is vital for function and temperature regulation. There are a number of situations that may predispose the elderly to a deficiency in body water. Approximately 50% of the body's water supply is obtained from solid foods; therefore a reduction in calorie intake by the elderly may mean that water intake from food sources is not adequate. Some elderly, especially those who are chronically ill, may have a defective thirst sensation mechanism resulting in a diminished awareness of the body's signal to increase fluid intake. Finally, the elderly individual may lose water from commonly occurring conditions such as the use of diuretics, diarrhea, excessive perspiration, or polyuria. In the event of a water deficit, elderly people should be encouraged to consume more fluids, particularly water (minimum of 1500 to 2000 ml/day unless contraindicated by conditions such as congestive heart failure).

Many elderly, especially those who are ill, are frequently malnourished and have inadequate levels of energy expenditure through regular activity or exercise. Diets are often deficient in calcium, vitamins A and C, iron, and zinc. A vitamin-mineral supplement may be indicated.[87] Other than acute and chronic illnesses, possible causes of malnutrition are changes in taste, vision, smell, or dentition; limited financial resources; psychologic factors such as boredom and lack of companionship when eating; edentia; lifelong faulty eating patterns; fads and misconceptions regarding certain foods; lack of energy to prepare food; inability to feed oneself; and lack of sufficient knowledge of the essentials of a well-balanced diet. Living arrangements may affect dietary patterns; elderly men who live alone were found to have less adequate diets than older women living alone.[19]

Because malnutrition may be related to a number of coexisting factors, promotion of optimal nutrition will depend heavily on accurate identification of the involved factors. Improved nutritional states will be more likely to occur if (1) the elderly individual has participated in the development of a plan to resolve the problems, and (2) there are regularly scheduled intervals for evaluation and modification of these plans. Nursing interventions should be focused on resolving the specific problem. Interventions may include (1) experimentation with varying types of foods and seasonings to improve the range of food group options that are palatable and suitable to the individual's food preparation and serving capabilities, (2) referral to a dentist for dental problems (in many communities there are low income or mobile dental units available for the poor and homebound elderly that may be identified by contacting the state Dental Association or a local senior information center), (3) educational sessions and literature to improve the individual's understanding of the relationship between nutrition and health (involvement of family, friends, or others who live with the individual or help in food preparation will increase the likelihood of a sustained change in nutritional intake), (4) referral to Meals on Wheels or another similar program in the community, (5) referral to hot lunch programs at senior centers for those who are not homebound and desire the opportunity for companionship and social interaction at meals, or (6) referral to or consultation with an occupational therapist specializing in the elderly who can provide suggestions or specific adaptive devices for individuals who have difficulty with food handling or feeding caused by functional deficits (that is, decreased vision, impaired joint mobility associated with arthritis, hemiparesis associated with cerebrovascular accidents).

Some elderly persons are obese even though they may be undernourished. Excess weight burdens the heart, liver, kidneys, and musculoskeletal system and should be avoided. Weight reduction for the aged person, however, should be gradual. The weight loss program should be coordinated by the nurse through the physician and the nutritionist (if one is available). Sudden loss of weight is poorly tolerated by many elderly persons whose vascular system has become adjusted to the excess weight. Sudden weight reduction may lead to serious consequences, including confusion associated with lowered blood pressure, exhaustion, and vasomotor collapse.

Elderly persons often enter the hospital in a poorly nourished state because of chronic illness or other factors previously described. Trauma, surgery, or sepsis may increase nutritional demands and cause further nutritional deficiencies, particularly in protein and calories, to develop rapidly. Often, the poor state of nutrition upon admission, increased nutritional needs, and decreased appetite coexist in the hospitalized elderly. A nutritional assessment, including a record of food intake over several days and weight on admission with regular weight checks thereafter, should be a priority in nursing to detect deficiencies early.

General nursing care should include planning diagnostic tests between meals when possible; helping with tray setup and feeding when needed; encouraging the consumption of variety and quantity in the various food groups, and providing between-meal, high-protein, high-calorie snacks, especially if the individual becomes easily satiated and consumes only small quantities at meals. Family members can be consulted about the patient's favorite foods and encouraged to bring special foods from home unless contraindicated by medical treatment.

"Liquid meals" are available (the type may vary de-

pending on changes in market products and hospital and nutrition department preference) that are usually very palatable. These liquid drinks are often successful forms of supplemental nourishment if the individual has difficulty chewing or has a poor appetite.

The nurse should consult the physician if there is a sustained poor intake of food over several days and/or greatly increased nutritional demands on the body. On the basis of a full evaluation, the physician may consider intervention in the form of parenteral or enteral nutritional supplementation. The placement of a nasogastric feeding tube is an invasive procedure that may cause the patient discomfort at the time of insertion and while in place. Despite these concerns, other measures often fail, and the elderly individual simply cannot eat enough to keep up with bodily demands, in many cases because of extreme fatigue. Therefore the risks and benefits of nasogastric feeding must be carefully considered in the early phases of nutritional deficits in the elderly patient if prompt resolution of nutritional problems is to occur.

PROMOTING ELIMINATION

A common concern for many elderly is bowel function. Many factors contribute to constipation. The absence of routines, a different environment, decreased physical activity, reduced dietary roughage, decreased fluid intake, and the routine use of enemas may result in reduced bowel function and contribute to constipation.[30] Any marked change in bowel habits, however, and any unusual reactions to normal doses of laxatives should be reported, since malignancies of the large bowel and diverticulitis are fairly common among this age group.

Nursing intervention to manage constipation in the elderly includes increasing dietary fiber, fluids, and activity. Antacids that can cause constipation and laxatives should be avoided. Frequency in elimination is important since it provides regular stimulus to evacuate the bowel. Therefore attempts should be made to establish regular toileting patterns.[30] The very elderly and somewhat confused patient should be reminded to go to the bathroom following meals. The addition of bran to a person's daily food intake has been found to be helpful in preventing constipation and resultant impaction. If the patient is constipated, it may be necessary occasionally to carefully insert a gloved finger into the rectum to be certain impaction has not occurred.

Frequency of voiding is common with aging (caused in part by a smaller bladder capacity) and becomes a problem during illness. It may be necessary to catheterize the patient to check for residual urine. One of the first signs of diminishing or failing kidney function is frequency of micturition during the night. Frequency, urgency, and slight burning on urination are symptoms of bladder infection.

Unless there is a definite contraindication to high fluid intake, the elderly patient should be urged to take sufficient fluids to dilute urine and decrease its irritating properties. Fluids may be limited in the evening if nocturia is interfering with sleep. If the patient is weak or has mobility problems, a urinal or bedpan should be offered during the night.

Elderly women have relaxation of perineal structures, which may interfere with complete emptying of the bladder and predispose to bladder infection. Some elderly patients have decreased sensation and do not realize when the bladder must be emptied.[15] Periodic dribbling of urine suggests that the bladder is not being emptied completely. The nurse should observe the very elderly patient for distention of the bladder and consult the physician.

Incontinence is common in the elderly, especially among elderly women. This problem is embarrassing to the woman and should be brought to the health care provider's attention. Incontinence is never normal. It may be sign of an infection or another easily reversible condition. The nurse can assist the patient by assessing voiding patterns, instituting regular toileting regimens, and suggesting that women perform Kegel's exercise to strengthen the muscles in the pelvic floor.[86] Involutional changes in the lining of the vagina lead to lessened resistance to invasion of organisms. Mild infections with troublesome symptoms and discharge are not unusual in elderly women. This condition should be reported to the physician, who may order specific therapy for it. Frequent bathing of the perineum may be helpful in allaying itching. Embarrassment may prevent the elderly patient from reporting symptoms. The nurse should be aware of the symptoms of this condition and watch for them.

Almost all elderly men have hypertrophy of the prostate gland, which makes urination difficult. The nurse must report or must urge the patient to report such complaints to his physician, because specific treatment is often necessary and can be safely administered even when the patient is far advanced in years.

MEETING PSYCHOSOCIAL NEEDS

Psychosocial development in older adults is centered around integrating life experiences, sense of identity, and realistic perspectives of future opportunities and events.[25,66,78] Ideally, the goal of aging for each person is the congruence of life experiences and self-identification with the environment.[67] In order to meet patient needs, the combination of environmental resources and inner strengths that has helped the patient become a "survivor" should be considered.

Resources include the wisdom that comes from a lifetime of effective coping, a realistic perspective of time, religion (spirituality), and the process of reminis-

cence.[67,78] Effective movement through developmental crises and challenges during the first half of life as well as during middle age provides a variety of effective approaches to new challenges and experiences. In essence, elderly men and women are survivors; they have proven their stamina for adaptation by virtue of having attained old age.

In order to develop nursing interventions to promote psychologic health, nurses must understand what is needed from the patient's perspective. Meeting the needs of older adults is enhanced by an understanding of the general developmental processes and changes of aging. What losses has the person experienced? What is the person's health status? Who does the person consider to be available for emotional support and assistance with day-to-day living? When planning care for the elderly, the available personal, family, and social resources that can be mobilized to assist the patient should be considered. By providing the patient with a range of choices, it is often possible to negotiate care plans in such a way that minimal or acceptable life pattern change is required. Nursing interventions should focus on facilitating the use of previous coping styles; promoting the preferred, established life-style; and supporting maximum independence, particularly when this is threatened by hospitalization or the probability of nursing home placement.[80] Emotional stress and maladaptation may result with problems of stimulation, self-image, socialization, life review, self-control, losses, dying, and death.

Nursing intervention should be aimed at avoiding overstimulation or understimulation, both of which can lead to confusion, depression, or anxiety. The basic level of stimulation must include *regular* daily activation of each of the special senses (sight, hearing, touch, smell, taste). The nurse should identify interventions that will both stimulate the senses and provide variety. Understimulation is most likely to occur when the individual's ability to move independently in the environment is restricted and sensory input becomes limited, nonvaried, or both. Fractured hips, strokes, widespread arthritis, and generalized weakness associated with severe malnutrition or chronic illness are but a few of the health problems that may result in a loss of independent movement..

Overstimulation often occurs when the elder is hospitalized or institutionalized and is being cared for by many new people in a strange environment with high levels of activities and noises. The nurse can explore possible ways to more evenly distribute activities to avoid or minimize days of tightly scheduled tests and therapies.

Self-image is a basic element for emotional health. Threats to self-image occur as a result of perceived losses in physical powers, emotional or financial security, and roles. Nursing care should be designed to maintain or enhance the elderly person's perceived needs for a healthy self-image. Perceived needs for physical appearance may include aspects such as makeup, jewelry, hair style, or clothing styles; body integrity and shape (threatened by procedures that invade such as mastectomy, amputation, fluctuations in weight); and physical agility. Perceived needs for emotional comfort may include physical contact, privacy, communication with loved ones (including pets), productivity, opportunities to help others, and participation in pleasurable activities.

Because socialization needs are individualized, they vary in older persons just as they do in those who are younger. Some persons have always been extroverts while others are more introverted. Unfortunately, what happens in many health care settings is that the extroverted person's life-style is usually considered as the normal, healthy pattern, while the person who prefers less socialization is suddenly and obtrusively encouraged or required to adopt a pattern of socialization that is emotionally uncomfortable. This phenomena (of encouraging increased socialization) may occur because of the myth that all older people are lonely because they have lost family or friends and/or the ability to "connect" with others because of illness or immobility. This is often true for the extroverted person who is at greater risk for loss of social opportunities. The nurse must be aware of previous social patterns of the person and should foster surroundings (socialization) that approximate preferred patterns.

Life review is a healthy activity in achieving emotional integrity in the later years.[78] Nursing interventions can include providing the opportunity to verbalize past achievements and experience. Volunteers and clergy can assist the person in a life review. The opportunity for life review may occur naturally in the nurse's process of gathering assessment data and in the provision of day-to-day nursing care. Tasks that do not require focused attention can be done while engaging in conversation that allows the person to talk about his or her past. Life review may trigger unexpected feelings of loss (for example, of career, family, or social contacts). If this occurs, it is important to allow the person to discuss the loss and express emotion if desired.

Death and the process of dying are life events that elicit a multitude of emotional responses. Elderly patients are usually aware of death as an imminent possibility, and some see this as a welcome natural event. Others who may not have achieved a sense of wholeness and closure to their lives in later years may anticipate their death with concern and fear. Nursing interventions should include the opportunity to discuss death and dying with one or more persons—the nurse, a clergyman, or family members. Often the opportunity

to talk about death and putting life in order (estates, etc.) is more important to the elderly than their medical treatment.

PROMOTING SAFETY IN THE USE OF MEDICATIONS

The most common treatment modality for illness, especially chronic illness, is the use of prescribed medications.[62] The use of both prescribed and nonprescribed medications increases with age. The elderly consume disproportionately more of all kinds of drugs than do middle adults, partly because older adults experience more chronic illness. Medications provide tremendous benefits to older adults, but they can also create problems for the patient, family, and health care provider. The medication regimen may be complex and troublesome for the patient or family to administer. Some medications may be difficult to tolerate and can cause unpleasant side effects; others may produce adverse reactions and interactions or unpredictable responses in the elderly.[62]

Numerous age-related physical changes in older adults affect the response to medications. The *absorption* of drugs may be influenced by the presence or absence of nutrients, or because of the decrease of hydrochloric acid that normally occurs with aging; drugs that depend on an acid medium may be absorbed less effectively. Absorption may also be altered because the rate of transit through the gastrointestinal system tends to slow with age.

The *distribution* of drugs within the body is affected by the loss of lean body mass and the increased proportion of body fat. Fat-soluble drugs tend to be stored in fat, thereby decreasing the intensity of the reaction while increasing the duration. Within the bloodstream the distribution of drugs is affected by the amount of serum protein, specifically the albumin, available as binding sites for drugs. In aging persons, the serum albumin levels tend to be lower, resulting in altered concentrations of bound (inactive) and unbound (active) drugs. Unbound drugs in the circulation are active in producing the effects of the drug. The unbound drug can be excreted by the kidneys or metabolized by the liver. A principal mechanism of drug interaction seems to be the displacement of one drug by another from these protein-binding sites. For example, warfarin may be displaced by aspirin, indomethacin, and other drugs, causing increased anticoagulation activity.

The *metabolism* of drugs in the elderly may be altered by lower levels of enzyme activity in the liver. The result of prolonged or incomplete metabolism is an increase in the half-life of some drugs, which allows the drug to exert its effect over a longer period of time.

The kidney is the primary route of excretion of drugs. *Aging* changes such as decreased renal plasma flow to the kidney, the decreased glomerular filtration rate, and the decreased number of functional tubules combine to result in inefficient excretion of active drug. This increases the risk of accumulation of drugs to potentially toxic levels because of decreased renal clearance. The decreased rate of excretion and the changes in binding sites in the blood unite to prolong the elevated blood level and activity of many drugs. Digoxin has a narrow margin of safety and is an example of a drug that is critically affected by the change in renal excretion.

Medications have a definite place in the therapeutic regimen for the older adult, but they must be handled carefully. One general principle in medication therapy is that the drug level should be built up gradually, and the lowest dose and fewest possible number of drugs should be used. In prescribing medications for the elderly, it is wise to "start low and go slow" because standard doses typically have been developed for younger groups.[32] Nurses should check for untoward reactions to medications and report them to the health care provider. If a patient is emaciated or elderly, medication should be prescribed with caution and the use of a full adult dose of any drug should be questioned.

As part of the health care team, nurses can assist patients and families in developing strategies to improve medication-taking behaviors. In a recent study of home care clients, nurses identified medication-taking behavior as the number one problem with clients.[62] Some of the common problems with medication administration experienced by the elderly include forgetfulness, regulation of dosages, poor storage, sharing medications, outdated prescriptions, difficulty in reading and understanding labels, and inability to open child-proof containers. Nursing assessment to determine the patient's ability to independently administer medications involves observation and interviews with the patient and family. Elderly persons should understand the purpose for the medications they are taking. Because the elderly are more susceptible to drug reaction, they should be cautioned against taking extra doses of medication or "trying out" someone else's prescribed medication. Simple information written in large black print about the purpose of each medication can be helpful. Other interventions to assist patients and families with medications include the following:

1. Determining the easiest time for the person to remember to take the medication (arising or with meals)
2. Using medication check sheets
3. Keeping the medication visible so that seeing it will be a reminder
4. Being careful to keep it out of the reach of small children
5. Using medication sets (egg cartons may be used) with the day and time for the medication marked to help the individual remember if the medication was taken

CARE DURING DIAGNOSTIC TESTS

Diagnostic testing can create a stressful situation for the elderly patient and the family. Because the patient and family may experience a number of fears regarding the tests, the actual procedures for testing should be explained and patients and families should have ample opportunities to ask questions. Both patient and family may experience distress caused by the uncertainty of the test results and the patient's future. If the patient desires, the family should be allowed to be with the patient for as much of the testing as possible.

Elderly patients who are undergoing diagnostic tests requiring withholding of meals or the use of enemas or cathartics should be attended unless they are in their beds, because they often become quite weak and dizzy. No elderly patient should ever be left unattended on a treatment table, and such patients should be helped on and off the table. Since the person may be dizzy, it is advisable for him or her to arise slowly and sit on the edge of the table for a few moments before standing. The dizziness may be caused by the slow compensation of inelastic blood vessels. Older patients with cardiovascular disease may also be orthopneic and cannot tolerate lying flat for examinations.

Because of the rapidity with which they develop pressure ulcers, elderly patients who must lie on x-ray, treatment, or operating room tables for lengthy periods of time need pads placed under the normal curves of their backs and a pad of material such as sponge rubber placed under bony prominences. Skin over bony prominences should be rubbed occasionally to improve the circulation to the area. On return to the unit, the patient's skin should always be checked for pressure areas, and, if any signs of pressure are evident, these areas should be massaged frequently until the tissue appears normal in color.

If the patient is placed in lithotomy position, care must be taken to place both legs in the stirrups at the same time to prevent undue pull on unresilient muscles. The same applies when removing the legs from the stirrups. Care must also be taken to prevent hyperextension and hyperflexion of the joints, since many elderly patients have arthritis and reduced flexibility.

CASE STUDY

Ms. T. is a 31-year-old woman who lives alone. She has had insulin-dependent diabetes for 8 years. She is divorced and has no children. Ms. T. works full-time in medical research and is in graduate school part-time. Her diabetes is treated with two injections of insulin per day. Her most recent self-monitored blood glucose was 240 mg/dl fasting. She says her normal blood glucose is between 180 and 240 mg/dl. She prefers to run her blood glucose high to avoid an insulin reaction. Fluctuations in blood glucose are normal for her because she diets on occasion, even though according to standards, she is underweight. She has irregular menstrual periods. She talks about her desire to minimize the impact of diabetes on her social interactions. She say she is not open about her diabetes and tries to conceal it from other people. Ms. T. would like to get married and have a family but feels socially isolated and is depressed about that. Dating is a problem because she does not want to reveal her diabetes. She admits she has not accepted her diabetes.

A nursing diagnosis of *altered growth and development* is appropriate as evidenced by Ms. T.'s stated desire to achieve developmental tasks (marriage and family) of young adulthood.

Ms. T. will work toward accepting her diabetes and becoming more comfortable in social situations so that she can overcome the social isolation she finds distressing.

Nursing interventions include:
1. Discussing Ms. T.'s perceptions of herself, how she thinks others see her, and her concerns
2. Assessing her support network; consider referral to a support group or counseling
3. Discussing with Ms. T. ways she would feel comfortable mobilizing a support system
4. Assisting Ms. T. in problem solving through role playing social situations so that she can attend to her diabetes needs comfortably when with people
5. Recommending assertiveness training so that Ms. T. can learn to better communicate her needs to others
6. Monitoring Ms. T.'s diabetic control and management
7. Involving Ms. T. in strategies to improve her diabetes management

Over time, Ms. T. will report having attended more social situations in which she can meet people and date. A decrease in social isolation might occur when Ms. T. turns to a larger number of people for help and demonstrates more openness about her diabetes.

CHAPTER SUMMARY

✔ Every human being grows and develops physically and psychosocially in a unique way during the adult years.

✔ Psychosocial stages in young adults can be characterized by an emphasis on gaining and maintaining individual goals and independence. In contrast, older adults place greater emphasis on mutual interdependence with others.

✔ Physiologically, young adults are functioning at peak efficiency. As the adult years progress, normal changes occur very gradually. In the older adult, natural physical changes are sometimes difficult to distinguish from illness processes.

✔ Older adults have the capacity to improve their intellectual functioning in some areas. Slightly altered teaching methods may be effective.

✔ Human behavior is extremely complex, and it is very difficult to predict how patients might respond to illness situations. Theories of life-span development combine physical, psychosocial, sexual, cognitive, and spiritual aspects of the growth process; they provide nurses with general guidelines about specific periods of the life span that are useful in planning nursing care for adults of all ages.

✔ Although implications for nursing care of young, middle, and older adults can be suggested, it is critical to include the patient in the decision-making process to individualize the plan of care to each person's unique personal, family, and social situation.

QUESTIONS TO CONSIDER

■ Using the theories and stages identified in Figure 5-2, choose the developmental stage that best describes you at this point in your life. What are the typical developmental tasks associated with your present stage?

■ Think about a young adult patient with whom you have recently worked. How did the patient's illness situation affect the achievement of developmental tasks (or how might have the illness affected developmental tasks)?

■ Describe some measures you can take to assist older adults who have experienced cognitive decline to improve memory.

■ Describe some of the primary changes of aging.

■ Think about an elderly adult you know. Describe the person's behavior using the theories of Erikson and Stevenson.

REFERENCES AND SELECTED READINGS

1. Adams M: Aging: gerontological nursing research. In Werley H, Fitzpatrick J, and Taunton R, editors: Annual Review of Nursing Research, vol 4, New York, 1986, Springer Publishing Co Inc.
2. Ahlfield J, Soler N, and Marcus S: The young adult with diabetes: impact of the disease on marriage and having children, Diabetes Care 8(1):52-56, 1985.
3. Andreason M: Making a safe environment by design, J Gerontol Nurs 11(6):18-22, 1985.
4. Bahr T and Gross L: The 24-hour cycle, J Gerontol Nurs 11(4):14-18, 1985.
5. Baltes P: Theoretical propositions of life-span developmental psychology: on the dynamics between growth and decline, Dev Psychol 23(5):611-626, 1987.
6. *Bee H and Mitchell S: The developing person: a life-span approach, ed 2, New York, 1984, Harper & Row, Publishers Inc.

*References preceded by an asterisk are particularly well suited for student reading.

7. Bee H: The journey of adulthood, New York, 1987, MacMillan Publishing Co.[1]

8. Belenky M, Clinchy B, Goldberger N, and Tarule J: Women's ways of knowing, New York, 1986, Basic Books Inc, Publishers.

9. Binstock E and Shanas E, editors: Handbook of aging and the social sciences, New York, 1984, Van Nostrand Reinhold Co Inc.

10. Birren JE and Schaie KW, editors: Psychology of aging, ed 2, New York, 1985, Van Nostrand Reinhold Co Inc.

11. Brocklehurst JC: Textbook of geriatric medicine and gerontology, New York, 1985, Churchill Livingstone Inc.

12. *Burggraf V and Stanley M: Nursing the elderly: a care plan approach, Philadelphia, 1989, JB Lippincott Co.

13. *Burnside I: Nursing and the aged: a self-care approach, ed 3, New York, 1988, McGraw-Hill Inc.

14. *Carnevali DL and Patrick M: Nursing management for the elderly, ed 2, Philadelphia, 1986, JB Lippincott Co.

15. Cassel CK and Walsh JR, editors: Geriatric medicine, vols I and II, New York, 1984, Springer-Verlag New York Inc.

16. Comfort A: Biology of senescence, New York, 1979, Elsevier Science Publishing Co Inc.

17. Cummings E and Henry WE: Growing old, New York, 1955, Basic Books Inc, Publishers

18. Darling-Fisher C and Leidy N: Measuring Eriksonian development in the adult: the modified Erikson psychosocial stage inventory, Psychol Rep 62:747-754, 1988.

19. Davis MA et al: Living arrangements and dietary patterns of older adults, J Gerontol 40(4):434-442, 1985.

20. *Dimond M and Jones S: Chronic illness across the life span, Norwalk, Conn, 1983, Appleton-Century-Crofts.

21. *Dresen SE: The middle years: the sexually active middle adult, Am J Nurs 75:1001-1005, 1975.

22. Duffy M: Determinants of health promotion in midlife women, Nurs Res 37(6):358-362, 1988.

23. *Duvall EM: Marriage and family development, ed 5, Philadelphia, 1977, JB Lippincott Co.

24. *Eisenberg M, Sutkin L, and Jansen M, editors: Chronic illness and disability through the life span, New York, 1984, Springer Publishing Co Inc.

25. Erikson EH: Childhood and society, ed 2, New York, 1963, WW Norton Co Inc.

26. Esberger KK and Hughes ST Jr: Nursing care of the aged, Norwalk Conn, 1989, Appleton & Lange.

27. FallCreek S and Mettler M: A healthy old age: a sourcebook for health promotion with older adults, New York, 1984, The Haworth Press Inc.

28. Franz M: Nutritional requirements of the elderly, Am J Elderly 1(2):39-53, 1981.

29. Frieberg KL: Human development, a life-span approach, ed 3, Boston, 1987, Jones & Bartlett Publishers Inc.

30. *Gallagher L and Kreidler MC: Nursing and health: maximizing human potential throughout the life cycle, Norwalk, Conn, 1987, Appleton & Lange.

31. Geokas MC, editor: The aging process, Clin Geriatr Med vol 1, no 1, Philadelphia, 1985, WB Saunders Co.

32. Gibaldi M: Drug dosage and the elderly, Perspect Clin Pharmacol 5(2):9-16, 1987.

33. Giele JZ: Women in the middle years, New York, 1982, John Wiley & Sons Inc.

34. Gilligan C: In a different voice: psychological theory and women's development, Cambridge, 1982, Harvard University Press.

35. Hallburg JC: The teaching of aged adults, J Gerontol Nurs 2(3):13-19, 1976.

36. Havinghurst RJ: Perspectives on health care for the elderly, J Gerontol Nurs 3(2):21-24, 1977.

37. Havinghurst RJ et al: Psychology of aging, Bethesda conference, Public Health Rep 70:837-856, 1955.

38. *Hogstel M: Nursing care of the older adult, ed 2, New York, 1988, John Wiley & Sons Inc.

39. Howells JG, editor: Modern perspectives in the psychology of middle age, New York, 1981, Brunner/Mazel Inc.

40. Jenny J: A comparison of four age groups' adaptation to diabetes, Can J Public Health 75(3):237-244, 1984.

41. Kane RL, Kane RA, and Arnold SB: Prevention and the elderly. II. Risk factors, Health Serv Res 19(6):945-1005, 1985.

42. Kegan R: The evolving self: problems and process in human development, Cambridge, 1982, Harvard University Press.

43. Knox AB: Adult development and learning, San Francisco, 1977, Jossey-Bass Inc, Publishers.

44. *Lambert V and Lambert C Jr: The family with the middlescent 45-65 years. In Bradshaw M: Nursing of the family in health and illness, Norwalk, Conn, 1988, Appleton and Lange.

45. *Lancaster L: Impact of chronic illness over the life span, ANNA J 15(3):164-198, 193, 1988.

46. Lawton MP et al: Community planning for an aging society, Stroudsburg, Pa, 1976, Dowden, Huchinson & Ross, Inc.

47. Levinson D: A conception of adult development, Am Psychol 41(1):3-13, 1986.

48. Levinson D: The seasons of a man's life, New York, 1978, Ballantine/Del Rey/Fawcett Books.

49. Loevinger J: Ego development: conceptions and theories, San Francisco, 1976, Jossey-Bass Inc, Publishers.

50. Lowenthal M, Thurner M, and Chiroboga D: Four stages of life, San Francisco, 1977, Jossey-Bass Inc, Publishers.

51. Maslow A: Motivation and personality, ed 2, New York, 1970, Harper & Row, Publishers Inc.

52. McBride A: The experience of being a parent. In Werley H, Fitzpatrick J, and Taunton R, editors: Annual Review of Nursing Research, vol 2, New York, 1984, Springer Publishing Co Inc.

53. McIntosh JL: Suicide among the elderly: levels and trends, Am J Orthopsychiatry, 55(2):288-293, 1985.

54. *McWeeny M: Life span growth and development: a review and application to nursing diagnosis, J Enterostomal Ther 15(2):81-86, 1988.

55. Mercer R: The relationship of developmental variables to maternal behavior, Res Nurs Health 9:25-33, 1986.

56. Mercer R, Nichols E, and Doyle G: Transitions over the life cycle: a comparison of mothers and nonmothers, Nurs Res 37(3):144-151, 1988.

57. *Murray R and Zentner J: Nursing assessment and health promotion through the life span, ed 4, Englewood Cliffs, NJ, 1989, Prentice-Hall.

58. National Center for Health Statistics, Collins J: Prevalence of selected chronic conditions, United States, 1983-1985, Advance Data From Vital and Health Statistics, No 155, Department of Health and Human Services Pub no (PHS) 88-1250, 1988, Hyattsville, Md, US Public Health Service.

59. Neugarten BL, editor: Middle age and aging, Chicago, 1968, The University of Chicago Press.

60. Neugarten BL: Personality in middle and late life, New York, 1964, Atherton Press.

61. Norman WH and Scaramella TJ, editors: Mid-life: developmental and clinical issues, New York, 1980, Brunner/Mazel Inc.

62. *Patsdaugher C and Pesznecker B: Medication regimens and the elderly home care client, J Gerontol Nurs 14(10):30-34, 1988.

63. *Peplau H: Life in the middle years: mid-life crises, Am J Nurs 75:1761-1765, 1975.

64. Primomo J: Patterns of chronic illness management, psychso-

cial development, family and social environment, and adaptation among diabetic women, unpublished doctoral dissertation, Seattle, 1989, University of Washington.

65. Rankin S and Weekes D: Life-span development: a review of theory and practice for families with chronically ill members, Scholarly Inquiry for Nursing Practice, 3(1):3-27, 1989.

66. Reed P: Implications for life-span developmental framework for well-being in adulthood and aging, ANS 6:18-25, 1983.

67. Reed P: Mental health of older adults, West J Nurs Res 11(2):143-163, 1989.

68. *Rendon D et al: The right to know the right to be taught, J Gerontol Nurs 12:33-38, 1986.

69. Rossman I: Clinical geriatrics, ed 3, Philadelphia, 1986, JB Lippincott Co.

70. Schaie KW: Adult development and aging, ed 2, Boston, 1986, Little, Brown & Co, Inc.

71. Schaie KW and Willis S: Can decline in intellectual functioning be reversed? Developmental Psychology, 22(2):223-232, 1986.

72. Schuster CS and Ashburn S: The process of human development, Boston, 1986, Little, Brown & Co, Inc.

73. Siegfried K: Aging myths, reversible causes of mind and memory loss, New York, 1986, McGraw-Hill, Inc.

74. Smelser N and Erikson E, editors: Themes of love and work in adulthood, Cambridge, 1980, Harvard University Press.

75. Smith E and Sergass RC: Exercise and aging: the scientific basis, Hillside, NJ, 1981, Enslow Publishers.

76. Sorensen A, Weinert F, and Sherrod L, editors: Human development and the life course: multidisciplinary perspectives, Hillsdale, NJ, 1987, Erlbaum Associates, Publishers.

77. Stanwyck D: Self-esteem through the life span, Fam Community Health 6(2):11-28, 1983.

78. Stevenson J: Adulthood: a promising direction for future research. In Werley H, Fitzpatrick J, and Taunton R, editors: Annual Review of Nursing Research, vol 1, New York, 1983, Springer Publishing Co Inc.

79. *Stevenson J: Issues and crisis during middlescence, New York, 1977, Appleton-Century-Crofts.

80. Thorson JA and Thorson JR: How accurate are stress scales? J Gerontol Nurs 12(1):21-24, 1986.

81. Troll LE: Early and middle adulthood, Monterey, Calif, 1975, Brooks/Cole Publishing Co.

82. US Bureau of the Census: Statistical abstracts of the United States, 1988, annual ed 108, Washington, DC, 1988, US Government Printing Office.

83. Voda A and George T: Menopause. In Werley H, Fitzpatrick J, and Taunton R, editors: Annual Review of Nursing Research, vol 4, New York, 1986, Springer Publishing Co Inc.

84. Wolanin M: Clinical geriatric nursing research. In Werley H, Fitzpatrick J, and Taunton R, editors: Annual Review of Nursing Research, vol 1, New York, 1983, Springer Publishing Co Inc.

85. Wolanin MD and Philips LRF: Confusion, prevention, and care, St Louis, 1981, The CV Mosby Co.

86. *Woods NF: Human sexuality in health and illness, ed 3, St Louis, 1984, The CV Mosby Co.

87. Young E: Nutrition, aging and the aged, Med Clin North Am 67(2):295-313, 1983.

88. *Yurick A, Spier B, Robb S, and Ebert N: The aged person and the nursing process, ed 3, Norwalk, Conn, 1989, Appleton & Lange.

RESOURCES ON OLDER ADULTS

American Association of Retired Persons (AARP)
Program Resources Department
1909 K Street, N.W.
Washington, DC 20049
(202) 872-4700
Provides information, including a list of reading materials, educational programs, and numerous booklets for patient teaching on many topics. (AARP is the nation's largest and oldest organization of over-50 Americans, retired or not.)

Children of Aging Parents
2761 Trenton Road
Levittown, PA 19056
Offers lists of support groups for some states, information about case-management workers, and caregiving booklets.

National Council on the Aging
NCOA Publications
P.O. Box 7227
Ben Franklin Station
Washington, DC 20044
(202) 479-1200
Write for listing of books and pamphlets.

National Institute on Aging (NIA)
NIA Information Center
2209 Distribution Circle
Silver Spring, MD 20910
(301) 495-3455
Publication list and information on health topics of interest to older people are available. (NIA is part of U.S. Department of Health and Human Services, Public Health Service, National Institutes of Health)

Audiovisual Resources

Aging: 54 minute color VHS videocassette, 1988.
PBS Video
1320 Braddock Place
Alexandria, VA 22314-1698
PBS Video
475 L'Enfant Plaza, S.W.
Washington, DC 20024
1-800-344-3337 or
1-800-424-7963

Aging: 16mm color film.
CRM educational films
1104 Camino Del Mar
Del Mar, CA 92014
PBS Video
475 L'Enfant Plaza, S.W.
Washington, DC 20024
1-800-344-3337 or
1-800-424-7963

Be well: Health in the later years, 24 minute 16mm color film, 1983.
Churchill Films
662 North Robertson Blvd.
Los Angeles, CA 90069
1-800-334-7830 or
(213)657-5110

Development of the adult: 29 minute 16mm color film, 1977.
Motorola Teleprograms
c/o Simon and Schuster Communications
108 Wilmot Road
Deerfield, IL 60015
1-800-621-2131

Everybody rides the carousel, Part 3: 29 minute 16mm color film.
Pyramid Film and Video
P. O. Box 1048
2801 Colorado Ave.
Santa Monica, CA 90406
1-800-421-2304 or
(213)828-7577

Exploring aging: 10 minute color videocassette.
University of Washington Press
1416 N. E. 41st (JI-50)
Seattle, WA 98105
(206)543-4050

Geriatric patient, 22 minute color videocassette, 1977.
University of Washington Press
1416 N. E. 41st (JI-50)
Seattle, WA 98105
(206)543-4050

Growing Old in America, Part 1: The Retirement Years Dilemma, 58 minutes; Part 2: Crisis in health care, 51 minutes; Part 3: The search for care, 59 minutes, 1985, ¾ ″ videocassette, contact local ABC affiliated station.

Last of life: Aging as a natural process: 28 minute 16mm color film, 1977.
Filmakers Library, Inc.
133 East 58th St., Suite 703A
New York, NY 10002
(212)355-6545

Patient mental health, psychological growth and adjustment: Color filmstrip and audiotape.
Westinghouse Learning Corporation
Oakland, IL 60453.

Perspectives on aging, Costa Mesa, California, Concept media.

What shall we do about mother?: 49 minute 16mm color film.
Carousel Films, Inc.
241 East 34th St., Room 304
New York, NY 10016
(212)683-1660

What you don't know CAN hurt you (Health care and the elderly patient): 19 minute 16mm color film, 1982.
Grandview Hospital
P. O. Box 45132
Westlake, OH 44145

General Resources

Local Chapters of:

Alzheimer's Disease and Related Disorders Association
800-621-0379
American Cancer Society
(404)320-3333
American Heart Association
(214) 373-6300
American Lung Association
(212) 315-8700
National Association for Hearing and Speech Action
(301) 897-8682
National Stroke Association
(303) 762-9922

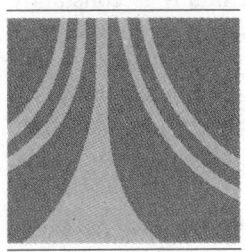

CHAPTER 6

Families and Illness

MARY ELLEN SHANDS
ELLEN H. ZAHLIS

CHAPTER OBJECTIVES

After studying this chapter, the student should be able to:
1. Describe the theoretic frameworks that explain how families function when a stressor such as illness is present.
2. Describe the impact on family members when caring for an ill family member during the early diagnostic, treatment, chronic, and terminal stages of illness.
3. Identify ways that nurses can support families caring for an ill family member.

Serious illness of a family member can pose one of the most challenging situations facing families. Each member of the family may be affected as routines are altered, family members' responsibilities change, and heightened concern and anxiety occur. The impact that illness has on families may depend on whether the illness is short-lived (acute) or long-term (chronic). Although acute illness may demand rapid, intense mobilization of family resources, chronic illness may allow families to adjust more slowly but may require a long-term commitment of family resources. Many chronic illnesses may begin with an acute episode, such as a heart attack, which may be the first indication of longstanding cardiac disease. Although the impact of acute illness on the family is discussed, much of this chapter focuses on the family experience with chronic illness.

With advances in medical technology, people are living longer than ever before. Longer life in turn increases the probability of developing chronic illness. Chronic illness may include arthritic conditions, Parkinson's disease, emphysema, multiple sclerosis, heart disease, stroke, diabetes, and cancer. In all industrialized countries, chronic illness has become a salient health care issue. According to 1982 statistics from the U.S. Bureau of the Census, 31.5 million persons in the

United States have chronic health problems.[72] Despite the common belief that our societal norms foster less reliance on family members for assistance in crisis situations, it has been well documented that families do play a vital role in providing physical, emotional, social, and economic support to ill relatives.[4,11,17]

DEFINITION OF FAMILY CONSIDERED

The definition of family has been changing over time. In the past the concept of family as extended family was considered the societal norm. With the advent of urbanization, the norm became the nuclear family (mother, father, and children). Today, the concept of family includes the single-parent family, the reconstituted family, and the gay or lesbian couple, among others. Family may be defined according to geographic proximity, as in shared households or residential retirement homes. Family also may be defined by shared emotional bonds between individuals or by one's support network. For this reason, throughout this chapter family is regarded as those people whom the ill individual identifies as family.

THEORETIC MODELS OF FAMILY FUNCTIONING

Theoretic models of family functioning provide ways of thinking about the family that allow one to understand and predict behavior. Models are useful because they suggest ways that families can be helped. The two models described here are useful to nurses when thinking about how families cope with illness.

FAMILY SYSTEMS THEORY

The family systems perspective is derived from general systems theory (GST), as described by the work of Ludwig von Bertalanffy.[73] Family systems theory conceptualizes the family as an open system that functions within the broader context of the environment. The more open the family system, the greater is the exchange of information with the environment. Within

This chapter was supported in part from a grant from the National Center for Nursing Research, No 01000, Family functioning in chronic illness.

the boundary of the family, dynamic interactions between the members, or subsystems (such as the subsystem of parents or children), are governed by the family's organization. The organization of the family system is characterized by roles, relationships, expectations, and rules.

The terms *roles, relationships, expectations,* and *rules* are used to define organization in the family systems literature. Family members occupy and function in roles in relationship to one another.[54] They seem to function in these roles according to the expectations of the whole family. Thus, one family member may take on the role of breadwinner, whereas another may take on the role of homemaker. One family member may be the decision maker, and another may be the primary caregiver for the small children.

The term *rules* applies to the family expectations about how each person in his or her role relates to other family members; this becomes a standard for behavior over time. Whether spoken or implicit, these rules result in patterns of relating that characterize the family's interpersonal relationships and attempts to maintain equilibrium.[7,30,53]

The dynamic interactions that take place within the family are governed by the family's organization. According to family systems theory, the interactions are directed toward achieving and maintaining equilibrium within the system.[7,29,54] *Homeostasis* reflects the family's striving to maintain equilibrium in the face of internal or external changes. More recently, family theorists have refined the thinking on homeostasis with development of the concepts of morphogenesis and morphostasis.[16,65] Whereas *morphostasis* describes maintenance of the status quo within the family system, *morphogenesis* reflects the ability of the family to change its basic structure and organization in order to survive and remain viable.[5] Morphogenesis and morphostasis describe the family system as being in a dynamic balance between change and stability in response to the environment.[16]

Certain principles describe the characteristics of a system. The principle of *circular causality* describes a family as a group of individuals who are interrelated such that changes in one member evoke changes in another, which in turn affects the first individual. Individuals living in a family do not exist in a vacuum. They are constantly affected by the behavior of others in the family, which in turn affects their own behavior.

The principle of *nonsummativity* holds that the family as a whole is more than the sum of the individuals who make up that family. A family cannot be described by the characteristics of its individuals alone because this does not allow for the interaction between them. Thus one cannot look at each member of a family individually and have an appreciation of the characteristics of the family as a whole.

Understood within the framework of family systems theory is that the organism of the family is constantly moving toward goals.[36] The principle of *equifinality* states that different outcomes may have the same beginnings and that the same origins may lead to different outcomes.[74] Because families are open systems, they are constantly exchanging information with the larger environment. Thus the outcome of the system is affected by more than just its initial conditions.[75]

FAMILY STRESS THEORY

Family stress theory stems from the work of Hill,[27] who described families' responses to dealing with the loss of the father-husband following being drafted into the armed services. Hill's ABC = X conceptualization of the family's response to stress serves as the foundation for investigation and theory building in the area of family stress research. Although researchers have made some modifications over the years to provide clarity and empiric support to the framework,[6,25,28,52] it has remained essentially unchanged. The family crisis framework can be stated as follows:

> A (the event) + Interacting with B (the family's crisis-meeting resources) + Interacting with C (how the family defines the event) = X (the crisis)

The *A* factor represents the stressor event, which can be either external or internal to the family. It can result from normative changes or catastrophic events. In the case of an illness, the illness itself is the stressor event to the family.

The *B* factor represents family resources, which may be two types. Resources may be (1) those already available to the family or (2) coping resources strengthened or developed in response to the crisis event. Resources already available to the family might include a family member who is a health care professional or who has had previous experience in caring for an ill person.

The *C* factor represents the family's perception of the crisis. This is related to the family's view of the event's seriousness as well as what the event means to the family. If a family has experienced the death of a member from a stroke, the family might view a stroke in a second family member more seriously than would another family.

The *X* factor represents the crisis as experienced by the family. It is the outcome of the stressor event for the family after it is interacted on by family resources and perception.[43]

The family's resources, the *B* factor, represent the area of the family stress framework that has received the most attention by researchers. Family resources may include the family member's personal resources and the family system's internal resources, social support, and coping skills. Two of the most important internal resources are the adaptability and cohesion of the family unit.

ADAPTABILITY AND COHESION

Family adaptability is the family's ability to reorganize and change roles, rules, and patterns of interaction in response to either situational or developmental stress.[53] Adaptability refers to how flexible family members are in changing roles to accommodate changes in the family. Is the wife-mother able to move in and take over her husband's role of breadwinner and family disciplinarian if he is no longer able to fulfill that role? Can the children accept the mother as the new family disciplinarian? To the extent that family members can be flexible in their roles, rules, and patterns of interaction, the family can successfully manage changes brought about by having a chronically ill member. Families who cannot make the necessary changes in their role structure and who have difficulty changing family rules are described as being *rigid*. Families at the opposite end of the adaptability continuum are described as being *chaotic;* they experience dramatic role shifts and dramatic changes in rules. Family members often do not know what rules apply.[53]

Family cohesion describes the extent to which family members feel bonded to each other and concerned and committed to the family.[46] As with adaptability, cohesion is conceptualized as being on a continuum. Extreme cases of cohesion are *enmeshment,* an overinvolvement of family members in each other's lives, and *disengagement,* when family members are detached from the family and have little commitment to it. Healthy families lie somewhere between these two extremes. A sense of commitment in family members is vital if the ill member is to be cared for and the family is to continue.

CHARACTERISTICS OF FAMILIES

Particular qualities either increase the family's resources or add to the *pileup,*[43] a term used to describe the family experience of having additional stressors at the time of a stressor event. An awareness of a family's characteristics can give insight into the amount of burden families experience or the resources families have in caring for an ill member. These characteristics include, but are not limited to, the following:

Family-life cycle—does the family have the additional burden of caring for young children or elderly parents, and can older children or young adults share in the caregiving?

Socioeconomic status—can the family afford to hire extra help to compensate for the loss of the ill member's job, or does the cost of the illness place an added strain on the family?

Family composition—is it a large family, with several people who can share in the caregiving, or is it a single-parent household already pressed to care for its members?

Problem solving—do family members have the knowledge and the ability to do the necessary problem solving required to care for an ill member and meet the family's demands?

Family health—does the caregiver have a chronic illness as well, as often occurs in an elderly family?

Support network—are there people external to the family who can help the members carry out their tasks and give them emotional support?

These are just a few of the characteristics intrinsic to families that impact on their experience as caregivers to a chronically ill member. As positive attributes, they can be indicators of family resources. As negative attributes, they may be predictors of deficits in family coping.

ILLNESS TRAJECTORY

The course an illness takes has been termed the illness trajectory.[10] The trajectory involves not only the physical manifestations of the illness, but also the work involved in managing it, its impact, and the changes it demands in the lives of the ill individual and other family members. Thinking of it as a line on paper, an illness trajectory takes on different shapes depending on the phases the illness passes through or the overall trend of the illness (Figure 6-1).

The *acute phase* is characterized by a line turning sharply downward and then upward. Depending on the extent of recovery, the upward line may be the same length (if health returns to preillness status), shorter (if a health deficit exists when compared to the preillness status), or longer (if health status exceeds the preillness level). During this phase work is directed at obtaining and receiving immediate medical attention, stabilizing the illness, and promoting recovery. It may coincide with the diagnosis of a chronic illness characterized by an acute episode, such as a heart attack.

The *comeback phase* is marked by a line angling upward. This phase is characterized by the recovery that may occur after an acute phase. Work is directed at regaining functional ability and reconciling any residual disability. This occurs in, although is not limited to, the treatment stage, as when an individual is treated immediately following a heart attack.

The *stable* phase is depicted by a straight line, which describes a period when changes occur gradually over years. Work by family members is directed at maintaining stability. This is the chronic stage of an illness.

The *unstable* phase can occur at any time during the course of an illness. During this time the illness is continuously out of control, and work is directed at finding the source of instability. Examples of an unstable phase of an illness are when cancer recurs or when an infection exacerbates an already existing health problem. During this time planning daily activities may be difficult because the illness is unpredictable.

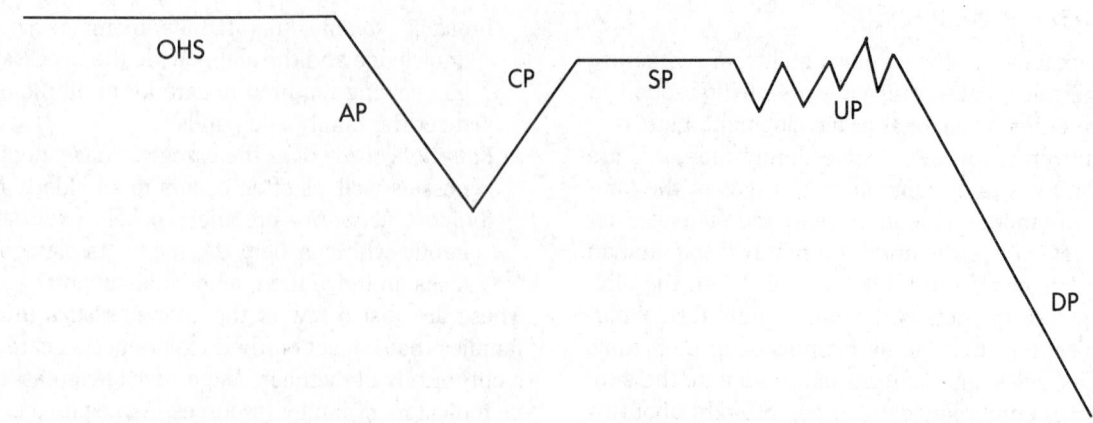

FIGURE 6-1 Illness trajectories. *OHS,* Original health status; *AP,* acute phase; *CP,* comeback phase; *SP,* stable phase; *UP,* unstable phase; *DP,* downward phase.

The *downward* phase is marked by a steady descent on a line; points at which acute phases begin are never really regained, and an overall downward trend to the trajectory occurs. This happens with progressive disability or terminal stages of illness. During this time work is directed at controlling the rate and extent of descent. Each phase may have subphases, and each may combine or alternate with one or more other major phases.[10]

EARLY DIAGNOSTIC STAGE

The early diagnostic period of an illness may be triggered by a sudden event, such as when a heart attack or accident victim is rushed to the emergency room. Another scenario might involve someone visiting a physician's office to confirm or discount the meaning of symptoms. A third situation might result from a routine physical examination that points to serious illness. Although we are aware that the ill individual is experiencing and reacting to the events, we are often less aware that the family members are also experiencing their own set of reactions.

Corbin and Strauss[10] described the early diagnostic period as a "diagnostic quest" involving a prediagnostic phase, announcement phase, and postdiagnostic phase. Each phase may be long or short; each requires an expenditure of physical and emotional energy from family members. The whole process may need to be repeated many times as new symptoms appear throughout the course of the illness.

The onset of chronic illness is often insidious. Small discomforts are explained away or adapted to over time without the individual being fully aware of making life changes. As symptoms become harder to ignore, they may become visible to family members or a greater concern to the individual. Family members' initial responses may be to read about the symptoms and compare them to symptoms friends have experienced. Depending on the severity of the symptoms, reactions may range from feeling that nothing is wrong to fear of death. At some point, when the symptoms can no longer be ignored, a visit is made to the physician and the diagnostic work begins.[56]

Frustrations are inherent to the diagnostic process. Having tests scheduled in a timely manner, undergoing multiple diagnostic tests, and receiving inconclusive findings and false-positive results can all add to the emotional strain for family members as well as the patient. Family members have said that their greatest concerns during this period are (1) problems created by the symptoms of the disease, (2) fear of the future, (3) waiting, and (4) difficulty obtaining information.[79] Some family members have described the waiting period between the testing and the announcement from the physician as the most difficult. As one stated, "The most difficult part for me was when she was under the knife and I was waiting for word from the pathologist to say if it had infiltrated or metastasized."[80]

Family members' involvement in this prediagnostic phase may require them to rearrange their lives. For instance, they may need to take time off from work, schedule child care, or juggle other tasks. A financial burden may result from loss of work, cost of child care, and expense of testing and may have a significant impact on family resources. All these stressors place an additional emotional and physical strain on family members.

Many factors influence how the diagnosis is relayed and received. Depending on the results and the physician's style, the information may be given compassionately or bluntly. The diagnosis may be certain or tentative, and a prognosis may or may not be given. Some physicians may be selective about what information is given to the patient and what information is given to the family. This can sometimes be difficult for family members because it makes communication with the patient more problematic.[20] Hoping to protect the patient, some family members may ask the physician to withhold information. Sometimes the same information may be given but heard differently by various members of the family.[10]

Shock and disbelief are often reported on hearing the diagnosis.[19,60] One person said, "I threw my arms around Connie, crying bitterly. I had always found it difficult to cry. That night I could not seem to stop. 'CJ, it isn't true; the doctor's wrong. It isn't happening.' "[59] Some members may feel relief because the ambiguity of the diagnostic period has ended.[38]

Family members may have numerous questions. Is surgery necessary before a diagnosis can be confirmed? Should a second opinion be sought to either validate or disprove it? (This may result in additional diagnostic procedures, and the process starts again.) What are the treatment options? What will be the extent of disability? What changes in day-to-day living will have to be made? What will life be like for the family in 6 months, a year, 5 years? All these unanswered questions and concerns create a tremendous amount of uncertainty for the patient and family members.

In an effort to preserve family life as it was before the illness and to close off uncertainty, some family members may deny that the patient has a serious illness.[76] They may persist in the notion that the illness has been misdiagnosed or that the situation is not as serious as portrayed. They may choose not to hear what they have been told. Some argue that denial of the problem's seriousness can be a valuable first response to a situation and can provide the individual with time to pull resources together before dealing with the problem.[37]

Hearing the diagnosis may be accompanied by feelings of guilt, fear, and remorse. Family members may wonder if they could have detected the illness earlier or what they might have done to contribute to its onset.[13,22,55,67] One man stated, "The uncertainty of Martha's future filled me with stone-cold fear. Mingled with it was an aching remorse: I should have insisted that she have the biopsy when the lump was first discovered. Failing that, I should have insisted on a biopsy when the tumor couldn't be aspirated just a few weeks before."[47]

For some family members a sense of fear accompanies the diagnosis, particularly the diagnosis of cancer. Often, a diagnosis of a cancer may trigger terror from memories of others who had suffered with cancer.[19]

In addition to trying to gain an understanding of the illness and how it will affect family life, family members often attempt to find meaning in the illness and understand why this has happened to them. They may spend energy researching the illness in an effort to understand how the illness developed and what behaviors or characteristics of the patient led to it. Family members not only attempt to find meaning for the illness event, but

also wish to assure themselves that the same condition will not strike another member of the family.[18]

Family members may employ various strategies when coping with the diagnosis. They may cope by taking some form of action, such as providing support, providing assistance, or obtaining information. They also seek out an empathic listener,[44] seek direction from such authority as the physician, or find something favorable about the situation.[19]

In addition to coping with the diagnosis, family members are faced with how to share the information with others. They must decide how much to tell, when, and with whom to share the information of the diagnosis.[18]

The role family members play in making a decision about treatment may vary. Some family members may be very involved in helping the patient make a decision about treatment. Family members may become active participants, researching options and alternatives for treatment and accompanying the patient for second opinions. Some family members may choose to be passive, assuming that they have no right to voice their opinions, since it is not their body or their illness. Passive approaches may also be taken by those who believe "the doctor knows best what to do." In disengaged families, reactions may include unconcern or disinterest. Wellisch, Jamison, and Pasnau[78] reported that men who had been highly involved in the decision-making process regarding their partners' mastectomies thought that their relationships were sound and rewarding, whereas those who were relatively uninvolved identified the decision-making time as the point at which emotional disruption began in the relationship. In addition, most of these men wished in retrospect that they had been more involved in the decision-making process.

A major challenge for the family is to decide how to continue on with their lives while accommodating the illness. The response to this ongoing uncertainty is often to continue researching, reading, and talking with others.

TREATMENT STAGE

Depending on the illness and the regimen prescribed, treatment may take place in a hospital, outpatient clinic, rehabilitation center, or at home. Technical advances in treatment protocols and the economic impact of diagnosis-related groups (DRGs) are resulting in shorter hospital stays, necessitating that family members become increasingly more involved in providing care during the treatment phase.[8,51]

When illnesses require the person to be hospitalized for treatment, this period can be a particularly distressing time for family members. The time during and immediately after surgery was reported by partners of mastectomy patients as very stressful.[69,77] Stolar[69] speculated that these men confronted the possibility of their spouse's death during this time. In addition to spending time visiting and offering support to the patient, family members may need to manage home and child care, as well as work responsibilities.[49,50,80]

Family members' participation in the delivery of treatment may extend from being a supportive presence to actually providing care. Treatment regimens may be simple or complex, may be quickly accomplished, or may take hours to complete, as in dialysis. Family members may have to spend considerable time learning specialized procedures. In the critical care setting, family participation is limited, and families may often feel excluded from the focus of care.[64]

In situations where patients do not experience many side effects and are otherwise feeling well enough to carry on with regular activities, the impact of treatment may be minimal. For other caregivers, however, providing transportation to treatment,[51] following through on protocols at home, and managing side effects of treatment can be an emotionally and physically demanding time. Attempting to provide this care to the ill individual while continuing with already existing responsibilities may be difficult at best. Often families need to redefine their roles, rules, and responsibilities to accommodate the illness. Also, while all this is taking place, uncertainty regarding treatment outcomes remains a major concern for all.

CHRONIC STAGE

The chronic stage is characterized by a relatively stable trajectory. The ill family member may experience a gradual decline in health, which may be interrupted occasionally with acute episodes. Family members adapt to this period by making changes in their day-to-day living to accommodate caring for the ill member and taking over role responsibilities as needed. As the chronic period continues, sometimes for years, the physical and emotional demands of caregiving may take their toll on the family.

The caregiving role is frequently assumed by the spouse of the ill individual. If the couple is elderly, the caregiving spouse is not only aged but may have chronic health problems as well. When an ill person is divorced or a widow or widower, the caregiving role often falls to an adult daughter. Many women work full time in addition to raising young children. Therefore, assuming a caregiving role for a chronically ill relative while contending with health problems or while working and raising children can create significant stress and strain. Stressors can include fatigue, financial hardship, uncertainty, role overload, family conflict, a sense of loss, and a feeling of being trapped by the illness, as evidenced by the following:

Here's the image. You and the man or woman you chose out of all the world because you loved and trusted and admired that

one are walking in the woods. The one you love steps in a bear trap. He lies there bleeding and in pain. You both work on the trap, but this is long, long ago and far off in the woods and neither rocks nor fingernails are strong enough to open the trap. He's cold. He's hungry. You build a shelter and look for berries. That's one day. The leg rots. His pain increases. It snows. That's one year. It snows again. You plant a few pumpkin seeds and slap a little mud on the shelter. At what point, exactly, do you say "So Long, Charlie"?[70]

The family caregiver may experience a constant drain on physical energies. The patient may be incapable of self-care and may require total physical care. Often, the patient's dependency needs allow the caregiver little time for self.[22,26] In addition, caregiving responsibilities may continue throughout the night, leaving the caregiver constantly deprived of much-needed sleep.

Depending on the family's financial situation, considerable stress may be generated by loss of income.[3,13,22] Because of a family member's illness, the caregiver may no longer be able to work. In addition, home responsibilities and fatigue may make outside employment an impractical possibility for the family member caregiver. Even when the household does not lose income, financial hardship may result from incurred medical expenses.[13,22]

Family members may experience a range of stresses resulting from increased or changed responsibilities. The roles of family members may be radically altered. They may need to learn new skills. They may find that an increase in caregiving responsibilities leaves less time to accomplish other role responsibilities.[3,13,14,34] If the caregiver is an older daughter, caregiving responsibilities may leave her less time for her own family and her role as a mother. A caregiver may be required to undergo a reversal in roles with the ill family member or a role change, perhaps becoming head of the household for the first time in a long-term marriage.[22,55] The role changes undergone are likely to require additional decision making on the part of the caregivers, often without the benefit of input from the ill family member. Thus, in addition to the increased role responsibilities inherent to caregiving, family members may be required to take on additional role responsibilities once belonging to the patient.[13,14,34]

Additional stresses within the family context may be caused by conflicts stemming from care issues related to the ill family member. Family members may differ in their goals for the patient and the best way to meet these goals. Interfamilial conflict may arise around such issues as need for institutionalization versus home care.[22] Another area of interfamilial conflict surfaces when a family member looks to other relatives for assistance or respite. When help is not forthcoming, the caregiver may perceive this as a lack of support in coping with the increased responsibilities of caregiving.[3]

Finally, the losses experienced by family members may impose a tremendous emotional strain. These losses are largely dictated by the nature of the patient's illness. For some families the loss may include the mental as well as the physical capabilities of the patient,[12,13] and with those, the loss of a best friend and confidant.[22] Some family members report their interactions with the ill person are no longer mutually satisfying and supportive because the patient is more dependent on them for emotional and physical care and they have to depend less on the patient in these areas.[3,55] One family member stated, "All that stuff that we shared before is now my responsibility. Being emotionally strong and not falling apart is also my responsibility. If I'm home and I cry, Joel asks me not to because it gets him upset. So I either have to go out to the sidewalk and cry, wait until he is out, or not cry at all."[58] Another potential loss experienced by partners of chronically ill individuals is that of a sexual partner.[33,41,66]

As a result of increased responsibilities, family members may find they have less time for relationships outside of the home.[14,22,62] Many family members will almost certainly experience a loss of time for self.[14,22] Many families may lose their financial security and may need to put aside plans made for the future.[13] Living without the ill family member may be yet another loss the caregiver anticipates if the illness is life threatening.[3] Living with the uncertainty of treatment outcomes can cause ongoing stress in dealing with many chronic illnesses, especially life-threatening ones.[3,40] For the family the losses may affect every aspect of life.

For some family members these losses lead to increased feelings of resentfulness, anger, anxiety, impatience, frustration, guilt, and ambivalence. Resentfulness may arise as an outgrowth of increased worries and responsibilities. Some may express anger at the illness and the situation in which the family now finds itself. This anger comes from crushed expectations and the loss of quality time that could have been spent together.[13] Guilt may arise as family members continue to blame themselves for the patient's illness[13,55] or for their inability to prevent the illness.[13,22] Many family members express the concern that they are not doing enough for the patient.[3,13,26] Ambivalence may surface as family members feel anger at the situation created by the illness and the desire for it to end, and yet they do not want the ill member to die. This ambivalence may be a source of tension and guilt.[40]

The consequences of long-term caregiving can result in a health risk for the family members. Because of the time involved in the caregiving role, they may experience social isolation. An intact social support system has been demonstrated to be of prime importance in helping individuals cope with stress.[23,31,32] A lack of supportive relationships, particularly in times of crisis and transition, place family members at risk for developing physical and emotional illness and even increased mortality.[2,9,32] In addition to the health risk created by a lack of support, caregivers are also at risk from the stress and strains inherent in caregiving role.[1,13,34,61]

Family members of chronically ill people have a tremendous need for information regarding the course, duration, outcome, and potential impact of the illness.[15] Studies of caregiving demands during advanced disease often show that problems arise in regard to information exchange with health care professionals.[68,79] As previously described, many factors influence the course of chronic illnesses, and concrete answers may not be possible. However, needs such as being informed of patient's condition, being assured that the patient is comfortable, and being informed of any changes have been identified as important information needs by family members of individuals with advanced disease.[79]

For the adolescent members of the family, adjusting to the changes in responsibility imposed by the illness may be difficult. Developmentally, adolescence is a time for emotionally and physically moving away from the home and family. These activities run counter to the demands placed on the adolescent as a result of the illness, which include helping with chores, being increasingly involved with family, and providing emotional support.[40,77] When a parent is ill, the inherent role modeling that usually occurs for children may be compromised.[55] A parent who is tired, is always in bed, or is depressed may be sending unintended messages. Lastly, children of all ages may be sensitive and fearful about their parent's health, harboring worries and concerns about death and its implications.

TERMINAL STAGE

One of the greatest challenges families face is caring for a dying family member. For many family members this may be their first intimate experience with death. Members are forced to face issues that they may have long avoided, even in the face of a long-term illness. Suddenly, their relationship with the health care system may seem more problematic as the focus of care moves from prolonging life to controlling symptoms and enhancing the quality of life that remains.

When a family member is dying, other family members need information so that they can make decisions and plan and provide care. However, in a complex health care setting when multiple physicians are involved, family members may not even be able to identify the primary physician.[35]

As the family confronts the reality of losing a loved one, they are asked to make major decisions about care and perhaps to take on more of that care. Families may be asked to decide where their family member will die. Can the patient's symptoms be managed at home by family members with the help of home health nurses, or is home care not a feasible option? Sometimes a nursing home is the appropriate choice, particularly if the terminal period is prolonged. Admission to an inpatient hospice for symptom control or imminent terminal care may be desirable. Each choice has its advantages and costs to family members. Some evidence suggests that if communication between the patient and family is poor, the family is more apt to choose for the patient to die in the hospital rather than at home.[35] If the family member is to remain at home, who will do the caregiving, and what assistance will that person need? All this is further complicated because often these decisions are not clear-cut, and family members continue to wrestle with the question of ongoing treatment or exactly how much will be done to prolong the patient's life.

At a time when family members need most to share their feelings and concerns, communication between them may become most troublesome. They may find themselves responding differently to the situation, and tension may arise as they find their feelings and concerns at odds with others in the family and with the ill member. One family member may still want to explore treatment as a possibility, whereas another may be trying to accept the finality of the illness. Another family member may feel angry with the physicians or nurses for their handling of the care, and another family member may be working hard to keep peace within the family. The dying person may have strong feelings about remaining home to die, but family members may not be able to provide the care. Family members may not have previously talked about their feelings with each other. Many do not talk about death, even with the patient.[35]

The final stages of an illness may come after a long period of family members giving physical care and expending much emotional energy. Somehow family members must find the reserves to carry on with even greater intensity.

When an ill person is in the terminal stage of an illness, family members often begin to anticipate what lies ahead. The term *anticipatory grief* has been used to describe this experience. This allows family members to absorb the reality of the loss over time, attend to unfinished business with the dying person (express feelings, resolve past conflicts), begin to change assumptions about life and identity, and make plans for the future so that they will not feel they betrayed their loved one once he or she has died.[57] Multiple losses, including what the individual's death will mean to each person as well as to the family, may surface as these aspects of the terminal period are addressed.

SUPPORT FOR FAMILIES

More than ever before, families are being asked to care for family members at home using sophisticated technology. Nurses are often in a position to bridge the gap for families between the home and hospital settings. An important role of the nurse working with the chronically ill patient is to see how the family manages with the illness on a day-to-day basis. This knowledge, along with an understanding of the illness, creates the foundation for nursing intervention.

Before nursing interventions can be defined to assist those experiencing illness in a family member, an assessment should be made of the family's resources using the family characteristics described at the beginning of this chapter. Assessment includes not only asking pertinent questions, but also actively listening to what is said.[57] The nurse should be aware of the family's understanding and perception of the illness. The assessment should include how adaptable, or flexible, family members are in dealing with the illness. From this assessment a picture of family strengths and weaknesses will emerge, thus helping in the identification of effective interventions for a particular family.

One of the major needs identified by family members across all illness periods is for information. In the critical care setting, family members want their questions answered honestly and want facts regarding the patient's progress, treatment changes, and prognosis. Families also want explanations that are understandable.[39,44,45] When a family member is being treated for cancer, the family members need to know what symptoms the disease or treatment can cause and when to expect symptoms to occur.[71]

If the family is to care for the patient at home, they will need the help of nurses in learning new skills related to caregiving. Family members report that they need learning assistance with helping the patient walk, managing the patient's bowels and dietary needs, managing pain, and increasing comfort for the patient.[21] In addition, family members may have to learn how to care for wounds, to suction, or to manage parenteral narcotics.

Information should be given in a compassionate and caring manner rather than abruptly and matter-of-factly. The way information is relayed can be problematic for families. For instance, a health care professional may inadvertently remark about a test result, giving the false impression that a serious health problem exists.

For some families, being given special knowledge not shared with with the patient can be harmful. Some family members report that receiving such information creates difficulties in how they communicate as a family.[20] Nurses need to be sensitive to how information is shared within the family and to respect the family's choices.

In complex health care settings, such as teaching hospitals, family members may not know who the primary health care professionals are or how to access them. Helping families to understand the roles of different health care professionals and how to access them is a necessary step if families are to function more comfortably and effectively in the health care setting.

Hospitalization during the course of a chronic illness can be a difficult time for family members. They are used to providing care and making day-to-day decisions about that care. When the patient is hospitalized, this role is taken over by the health care system. Providing family members with maximal opportunity to be involved in treatment and care helps foster a sense of control.[42] Nurses should encourage family members to maintain physical closeness to the patient, despite the presence of equipment and machines, and to give as much of the physical care as they wish.

The need to ensure that the ill family member is comfortable and receiving the best possible care is an important aspect of the hospital experience for family members.[24,39,44,45,63] Family members feel reassured when they are certain that the patient is comfortable. Nurses must be open with family members about the care being provided and how the patient's needs are being met.

One of the most useful interventions nurses may provide is to act as an interpreter in helping families understand information given by other health care professionals. The nurse can then help families identify what information they still need to make appropriate decisions. Families may have to make many decisions about care and treatment in the course of a chronic illness, and they must have an accurate understanding of the information they receive.

Families may need referral to other sources of information to assist them with decision making or in managing the illness and resulting strains on the family. For instance, nurses can make a referral to a social worker to assist with handling the financial burden of the illness or to a home health agency to acquire the services of a home care nurse or home health aide.

Effective communication between family members is an important family strength. Open discussions allow family members to share concerns and feelings, which assists with problem solving and decision making. The nurse can facilitate this type of communication by helping to clarify issues and by encouraging discussion. This type of intervention is essential when treatment goals are being determined. During the terminal period of an illness, when the decision to prolong or terminate treatment must be made, the nurse may play a key role in helping family members understand each other's wishes.

For family members, being able to share openly concerns experienced throughout illness prevents misunderstandings and builds family cohesion. The nurse can be instrumental in facilitating this communication. Family cohesion can act as a buffer for families during the illness by building the family's sense of competence and self-worth. A strong sense of family cohesion can help family members find meaning in the illness experience and some positive outcomes.

The nurse can be a valuable resource to families as an empathic listener. Family members need to talk about what is happening with someone whom they feel understands their plight. Even when the family has an open pattern of communication among members, the nurse can listen to thoughts and feelings too sensitive to share with the patient.

The need for a sense of hope is an important aspect of coping with illness.[48] Hope allows one to envision the idea of a future. Fostering hope within a family is another aspect of the nurse's role. Hope, at different stages of the illness, takes on different meanings for the family. The nurse who can be with the family and help them cultivate a sense of hope also helps them deal with feelings of despair.[18,42]

The stress and strains of caregiving over time are extensive for family members. Often they may feel uncomfortable leaving the ill member in the care of others or may feel guilty about wanting time for themselves. Nurses can teach family members to pace themselves and share the caregiving burden with others. Also important is the nurse's acknowledgment that "time away" is an important and legitimate activity for caregivers.[13,57] Nurses can inform families about such important resources as caregiver support groups and respite care.

Nurses are in a key position to help families manage illness. Assessing family strengths and weaknesses, identifying knowledge deficits, providing information, and teaching caregiving skills are important activities for nurses. Nurses can refer families to available resources to help meet their needs. In addition, nurses help families deal with their concerns by being available to listen and by facilitating family communication and problem solving.

CHAPTER SUMMARY

- Family systems theory and family stress theory provide a basis for understanding the impact of a family member's illness on family functioning.

- The way families respond to illness is a function of the family's characteristics and the illness trajectory.

- Each stage of the illness—early diagnostic, treatment, chronic, and terminal—presents the family with emotional and physical challenges.

- As a family moves through the illness experience, the nurse plays an important role in supporting them by assessing their resources, providing information, and facilitating family coping.

QUESTIONS TO CONSIDER

- How does the stress of illness affect other family members? What resources do families have to help them cope with illness?

- What effects can a family's past have on how they respond to illness in a member?

- What characteristics of families are most relevant to consider when a member has a chronic illness?

- What is the difference in families' experiences when they care for an ill member during the diagnostic, treatment, and chronic states versus terminal states?

- How does the illness trajectory affect families' abilities to cope with the illness?

- Have you experienced an illness in a family member? What did people do for you that was helpful? Not helpful? Based on your experiences, would you agree or disagree with the Family Stress Model presented in this chapter? Justify your position.

REFERENCES AND SELECTED READINGS

1. Archbold P: Impact of parent caring on middle age offspring, J Gerontol Nurs 6:79-85, 1980.
2. Berkman L and Syme S: Social networks, host resistance, and mortality: a nine-year follow-up study of Alameda County residents, Am J Epidemiol 109(2):80-85, 1977.
3. *Blank J et al: Perceived home care needs of cancer patients and their caregivers, Cancer Nurs 12(2):78-84, 1989.
4. Brody S, Poulshock S, and Masciocchi C: The family caring unit: a major consideration in the long-term support system, Gerontologist 18(6):556-561, 1978.
5. Buckley W: Society as a complex adaptive system. In Buckley W, editor: Modern systems research for the behavioral scientist, Chicago, 1968, Aldine Publishing Co.
6. Burr W: Families under stress. In McCubbin H, Cauble A, and Patterson J, editors: Family stress, coping, and social support, Springfield, Ill, 1973, Charles C Thomas, Publisher.
7. Cassileth B and Hamilton J: The family with cancer. In Cassileth B, editor: The cancer patient, Philadelphia, 1979, Lea & Febiger.
8. *Cawley M and Gerdts E: Establishing a cancer caregivers program, Canc Nurs 11(5):267-273, 1988.
9. Cobb S: Social support as a moderator of life stresss, Psychosom Med 38(5):300-314, 1976.
10. *Corbin J and Strauss A: Unending work and care: managing chronic illness at home, San Francisco, 1988, Jossey-Bass, Inc, Publishers.
11. Croog S, Lipson A, and Levine S: Help patterns in severe illness: the roles of kin network, nonfamily resources, and institutions, J Marriage Fam, February 1972, pp 32-41.
12. Elipoulos C: Chronic care and the elderly: impact on the client, the family, and the nurse, Top Clin Nurs 3(1):71-83, 1981.
13. Farkas S: Impact of chronic illness on the patient's spouse, Health Soc Work 5:39-46, 1980.
14. Fengler A and Goodrich N: Wives of elderly disabled men: the hidden patients, Gerontologist 19(2):175-183, 1979.
15. Finlayson A and McEwen J: Coronary heart disease and patterns of living, New York, 1977, Prodist.
16. Fisher B and Sprenkle D: Therapists' perceptions of healthy family functioning, Int J Fam Counseling 6:9-18, 1978.
17. *Foxall F, Eckberg J, and Griffith N: Spousal adjustment to chronic illness, Rehabil Nurs 11(2):13-16, 1986.
18. *Giacquinta B: Helping families face the crises of cancer, Am J Nurs October 1977, pp 1585-1588.
19. *Gotay C: The experience of cancer during early and advanced stages: the views of patients and their mates, Soc Sci Med 7:605-613, 1984.
20. Gould A and Toghill P: How should we talk about acute leukaemia to adult patients and their families? Br Med J 282:210-212, 1981.
21. *Grobe M, Ilstrup D, and Ahmann D: Skills needed by family members to maintain the care of an advanced cancer patient, Cancer Nurs 4(5):371-375, 1981.
22. *Gwyther L and Matteson M: Care for the caregivers, J Gerontol Nurs 9(2):72-95, 110, 116, 1983.
23. Hamburg D and Killilea M: Relation of social support, stress, illness, and the use of health services. In US Department of Health, Education, and Welfare: Healthy people: the surgeon general's report on health promotion and disease prevention, Washington DC, 1979, US Government Printing Office.
24. *Hampe S: Needs of the grieving spouse in a hospital setting, Nurs Res 24(2):113-119, 1975.
25. Hansen D and Hill R: Families under stress. In Christensen H, editor: Handbook of marriage and the family, Chicago, 1964, Rand McNally & Co.
26. Hartford M and Parson R: Groups with relatives of dependent older adults, Gerontologist 22(3):394-398, 1982.
27. Hill R: Families under stress, New York, 1949, Harper and Bros.
28. Hill R: Generic features of families under stress, Soc Casework 39:139-150, 1958.
29. Jackson D: The question of homeostasis, Psychiatr Q Suppl 31:79-90, 1954.
30. Jackson D: The study of the family, Fam Process 4:1-20, 1965.
31. Kahn R and Antonucci T: Convoys over the life course: attachment, roles, and social support, Life Span Dev Behav 3:253-286, 1980.
32. Kaplan B, Cassel J, and Gore S: Social support and health, Med Care 15(suppl):47-58, 1977.
33. Kavanagh T and Shephard R: Sexual activity after myocardial infarction, Can Med Assoc J 116:1250-1253, 1977.
34. Klein R, Dean A, and Bogdonoff M: The impact of illness upon the spouse, J Chronic Dis 20:241-248, 1967.
35. Krant M and Johnston L: Family perceptions of communications in late stage cancer, Int J Psychiatry Med 8(2):203-217, 1977-1978.
36. L'Abate L, Ganahl G, and Hansen J: Methods of family therapy, Englewood Cliffs, NJ, 1986, Prentice-Hall, Inc.
37. Lazarus R: The costs and benefits of denial. In Monat A and Lazarus R, editors: Stress and coping: an anthology, New York, 1985, Columbia University Press.
38. *Leahy M and Wright L: Families & life-threatening illness, Springhouse, Pa, 1987, Springhouse Corp.
39. *Leske J: Needs of relatives of critically ill patients: a follow-up, Heart Lung 15(2):189-193, 1986.

*References preceded by an asterisk are particularly well suited for student reading.

40. Lewis F, Ellison E, and Woods N: The impact of breast cancer on the family, Semin Oncol Nurs 1(3):206-213, 1985.

41. *Lilius H, Valtonen E, and Wikstrom J: Sexual problems in patients suffering from multiple sclerosis, J Chronic Dis 29:643-647, 1976.

42. *Martocchio B: Family coping: helping families help themselves, Semin Oncol Nurs 1(4):292-297, 1985.

43. McCubbin I and Patterson J: Family adaptation to crisis. In McCubbin H, Cauble A, and Patterson J, editors: Family stress, coping, and social support, Springfield, Ill, 1982, Charles C Thomas, Publisher.

44. Millar B: Critical support in critical care, Nurs Times 85(16):31-33, 1989.

45. *Molter N: Needs of relatives of critically ill patients: a descriptive study, Heart Lung 8(2):332-339, 1979.

46. Moos R and Moos B: A typology of family social environments, Fam Process 15(4):357-371, 1976.

47. Murcia A and Stewart B: Man to man: when the woman you love has breast cancer, New York, 1989, St Martin's Press.

48. Murdaugh C: Coping responses of spouses of M.I. patients and of hemodialysis patients as measured by the Jalowiec Coping Scale, J Cardiovasc Nurs 2(1):67-74, 1987.

49. *Northouse L and Swain M: Adjustment of patients and husbands to the initial impact of breast cancer, Nurs Res 36(4):221-225, 1987.

50. *Oberst M and James R: Going home: patient and spouse adjustment following cancer surgery, Top Clin Nurs April 1985, pp 46-57.

51. *Oberst M et al: Caregiving demands and appraisal of stress among family caregivers, Cancer Nurs 12(4):209-215, 1989.

52. Olsen D and McCubbin H: Circumplex model of marital and family systems. V. Application to family stress and crisis intervention. In McCubbin H, Cauble A, and Patterson J, editors: Family stress, coping, and social support, Springfield, Ill, 1982, Charles C Thomas, Publisher.

53. Olsen D, Sprenkle D, and Russell C: Circumplex model of marital and family systems. I. Cohesion and adaptability dimensions, family types and clinical applications, Fam Process 18:3-28, 1979.

54. *Olson E: The impact of serious illness on the family system, Postgrad Med 47(2):169-174, 1970.

55. Piening S: Family stress in diabetic renal failure, Health Soc Work 9(2):134-141, 1984.

56. Pitzele S: We are not alone: learning to live with chronic illness, Minneapolis, Thompson & Co, Inc.

57. Rando T: Grief, dying, and death: clinical interventions for caregivers, Champaign, Ill, 1984, Research Press.

58. Rosenberg M: Patients: the experience of illness. Philadelphia, 1980, WB Saunders Co.

59. Ryan C and Ryan K: A private battle, New York, 1979, Fawcett Popular Library.

60. Sabo D, Brown J, and Smith C: The male role and mastectomy: support groups and men's adjustment, J Psychosoc Oncol 4(1/2):19-31, 1986.

61. Sexton D and Munro B: Impact of a husband's chronic illness (COPD) on the spouse's life, Res Nurs Health 8:83-90, 1985.

62. Skippe J, Fink S, and Hallenbeck P: Physical disability among married women: problems in the husband-wife relationship, J Rehabil, September-October 1968, pp 16-19.

63. *Skorupka P and Bohnet N: Primary caregivers' perceptions of nursing behaviors that best meet their needs in a home care hospice setting, Cancer Nurs 5:371-374, 1982.

64. Speedling E: Social structure and social behavior in an intensive care unit: patient-family perspectives, Soc Work Health Care 6:1-15, 1980.

65. Speer D: Family systems: morphostasis and morphogenesis, or "Is homeostasis enough?" Fam Process 9(3):259-278, 1970.

66. Steele T, Finkelstein S, and Finkelstein F: Hemodialysis patients and spouses, J Nerv Ment Dis 162(4):225-237, 1976.

67. Stern J and Pascale L: Psychosocial adaptation postmyocardial infarction: the spouse's dilemma, J Psychosom Res 23:83-87, 1979.

68. *Stetz K: Caregiving demands during advanced cancer: the spouse's needs, Cancer Nurs 10(5):260-268, 1987.

69. Stolar E: Coping with mastectomy: issues for social work, Health Soc Work 7:26-34, 1982.

70. Strong M: Mainstay: for the well spouse of the chronically ill, Boston, 1988, Little, Brown & Co.

71. Tringali C: The needs of family members of cancer patients, Oncol Nurs Forum 13(4):65-70, 1986.

72. US Bureau of the Census: Statistical abstract of the United States, 1981, annual ed 102, Washington, DC, 1982, US Government Printing Office.

73. von Bertalanffy L: General systems theory and psychiatry. In Arieti S, editor: American handbook of psychiatry, ed 2, New York, 1974, Basic Books.

74. Walsh F: Conceptualizations of normal family functioning. In Walsh F, editor: Normal family processes, New York, 1982, The Guilford Press.

75. Watzlawick P, Bavelas J, and Jackson D: Pragmatics of human communication, New York, 1967, WW Norton & Co, Inc.

76. Weisman A: The coping capacity, New York, 1984, Human Services Press, Inc.

77. *Wellisch D: Family relationships of the mastectomy patient: interactions with the spouse and children, Isr J Med Sci 17(9-10):993-996, 1981.

78. *Wellisch D, Jamison K, and Pasnau R: Psychosocial aspects of mastectomy. II. The man's perspective, Am J Psychiatry 135(5):543-546, 1978.

79. *Wright K and Dyck S: Expressed concerns of adult cancer patients' family members, Cancer Nurs 7(5):371-374, 1984.

80. *Zahlis E and Shands ME: Breast cancer: illness demands experienced by the partner, Manuscript submitted for publication, 1989.

CHAPTER 7

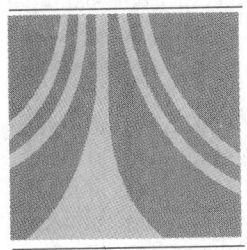

Culture and Illness

KAREN K. ALLMAN
ANTOINETTE T. RAGUCCI

CHAPTER OBJECTIVES

After studying this chapter, the student should be able to:
1. Analyze experiences of nurses and persons from social and cultural perspectives.
2. Apply strategies of cultural assessment to selected nursing care situations.
3. Develop necessary dimensions to provide culture-sensitive care: knowledge, mutual respect, and negotiation.

Health, sickness, and death are universal human experiences and yet are perceived, defined, and experienced differently within divergent sociocultural contexts and historic time periods. Preventive, diagnostic, curing, and caregiving behaviors are examples of attempts to cope with and adapt to not only threats to the physiologic integrity of ill individuals but also rifts in the social and symbolic integrity of the sociocultural group. Knowledge of and sensitivity to the social and cultural contexts of all patients provides a basis for mutual understanding that enhances nurses' efforts to plan and provide effective, compassionate, and holistic care. This chapter examines the effects of culture and social factors on the patient's experience of illness and introduces principles of *culture-sensitive care*.

SOCIAL AND CULTURAL DIMENSIONS OF HEALTH AND HEALTH CARE

SOCIAL DIMENSIONS

Social phenomena are conceptualized as those human actions and interactions that involve two or more persons. Subsumed under the category *social* are the constructs of social structure, social system, and social organization. In general, *social structure* refers to ongoing, recurring, or patterned relationships. The concept is applied to small groups (for example, the nuclear family) as well as to large organizations or aggregates (for example, the community and society). A social structure consists of arrangements of positions or statuses variously created and maintained or a network of relationships among persons.

A *social system* is made up of the interactions of a number of individuals whose relationships to each other are defined and mediated by a system of culturally structured and shared expectations. Thus the analytic unit of the social system is the role (or role sets) that serves to link or relate the individual to one or more others. A role, which may be interpreted as a unit of society, is differentiated from a status, which defines a persons's place or position within a social group or society.

Rules underlying social behavior are often unspoken and unwritten but are understood by persons within the group or society. Feelings of discomfort, confusion, and even anger may result when persons who are from different sociocultural backgrounds and expectations for appropriate behavior interact with others. One example is that of an Argentinian undergraduate student who felt rejected and disliked because Anglo-American students persistently backed away when he tried to talk to them. The Argentinian student is comfortable standing quite close to others while engaging in casual conversations, whereas the Anglo-American students find his standing so close intrusive. Both the Argentinian and the Anglo-American students are following cultural guidelines for social-spatial distance appropriate to casual conversation with a relatively unfamiliar person. The clash of cultural "norms" for this situation may be experienced as a vague sense of discomfort and the feeling that one or the other person is somehow behaving incorrectly. Power imbalances, such as those present when persons belonging to the majority culture interact with members of a minority group, often determine whose cultural "norms" will prevail or of which conflicting groups is labeled deviant.

CULTURAL DIMENSIONS

Culture has been defined as a *learned, shared, and symbolically transmitted design for living.*[4] *Culture* has also been described as *shared and learned assumptions, beliefs, symbols,* and *ways of behaving that characterize a human society;*[18, 37] as explicit and implicit rules for living;[25] and as a shared way of life. Chrisman[4a] describes *culture* as a set of *perspectives that influences how we view the world*: ourselves, those close to and distant from us, and the nature of life around us. Primarily, culture helps us make sense out of life. Culture may be seen as shared, both stable and dynamic, pervasive, and mostly unconscious.[20] Culture also may be seen as providing the range of possibility of action, meaning, and interpretation. Although culture is universal to humans and some aspects of particular cultures may be shared, no two cultures are identical.

Culture is sometimes misunderstood as belonging only to someone different than oneself or having an attribute of foreign or racial/ethnic minority peoples.[4a,4d] Having culture is part of being human and thus influences all human activities, including nursing the sick, and doing scientific and other types of scholarly research.

Societies, particularly heterogenous societies like the United States, *contain many subcultural groups. A subculture may be defined as a recognized social group that maintains a distinctive set of beliefs and behaviors but shares some cultural traits with the mainstream society.*[4a]

An example of a type of American subculture is the ethnic group. *Ethinic groups are collectives of persons sharing a common* (often foreign) *ancestry.* Specific beliefs of particular ethnic groups varies both within and between groups. Having "Irish blood" or facial features that appear Swedish or Chinese does not necessarily determine one's membership in or affiliation with an ethnic group; social relations and personal identification with such a group determine ethnic group membership.[4b] Other types of subcultures may be regional (New Englanders), religious (the Amish or Evangelical Christians), ones of location (urban, suburban, rural), age-related, or based on sexual preference (the gay or lesbian community).

Race is another important social subgroup among North Americans. Races are often described as biologic rather than social categories, though little evidence supports the notion of racial groups.[5a] *Genetic differences* between two individuals of the same racial group may range in the tens of thousands, whereas genetic differences between different races are relatively small, under two dozen. Pure racial types are also problematic. People considered "white" in one sociocultural setting may be considered "black" in another. This is also true for racially mixed persons.

The notion of what is a *biologic race* may differ from century to century as well. In the early part of this century, Irish-Americans were considered racially (biologically) distinct from white Americans of English descent and hypothesized as being genetically more susceptible to rheumatic fever. As work and living conditions for Irish-Americans improved, this susceptibility was reduced. Similarly, poor and working class African-Americans inherited not only the substandard working and living conditions of the Irish-American but also the "genetic susceptibility" to rheumatic fever.[5a] This example illustrates the danger of confusing social groups and social phenomena with nature. (See reference 14 for further discussion).

The names by which various ethnic and racial groups identify themselves also change with sociohistoric context. The majority of North Americans who were formerly known as Orientals now prefer the terms Asian or Asian-American, or prefer a more specific term, for example, Japanese-American. Similarly, persons formerly described as Negro now prefer African-American or Black American. Patients' rights to choose and name themselves should be respected, regardless of whether the patients' appearances or races/ethnicities coincide with the nurse's preconceptions.

SOCIAL AND BIOCULTURAL DIMENSIONS OF HEALTH AND ILLNESS

The existence of ethnicity and race as social rather than biologic groupings, does not rule out differences in morbidity, mortality, and some physical traits among (as well as within) different ethnic and racial groups. The construct *adaptation* relates to a particular environment or the possession of traits or attributes that make it possible for individuals to function effectively and to reproduce in this environment.[9] Adaptation, however, may be bought at a high price, and certain peculiarities that are assets in some geographic areas may be handicaps in others. The sickle cell hemoglobin condition, which may have evolved as a protection against malaria, is an example of such a change. Cancer, heart disease, and diabetes have all been referred to as diseases of civilization. Many types of *neoplastic disease* have been traced to environmental factors. The incidence of cancer has been shown to vary according to culture and social class.[9] Lung cancer is a common cause of death in the United States, England, Wales, and several other Western countries where cigarette smoking is common. Stomach cancers account for 50% of cancer among men in Iceland and Japan but only 10% in the United States. Liver cancer accounts for half of all causes of death among the Bantu in Africa and less than 4% in Europe. Breast cancer is eight times more common in Israel than in Japan.[9] Regional variations have been found for skin and lip cancer in the United States and Russia. There are more cases in the south than in the north for both countries.

The etiologic factors in *diabetes* are still poorly understood. Some epidemiologic and genetic evidence suggests that a virus may be involved in causing at least one type of diabetes.[26] Both genetic and environmental factors are believed to play an important role in the high incidence of diabetes in some cultural groups, such as among some native American tribes. The high incidence of obesity among some populations is also correlated with the prevalence of diabetes. Changes in the specific components of a cultural group's diet and activity patterns have been identified as leading to an increased expression of diabetes.[29,38] The data accumulating about geographic and cultural differentials in the incidence of diabetes and pathologic complications raise questions relative to the nature of human adaptation to culture change and cultural domination. The increased incidence of diabetes reported for rural migrants to urban centers in Israel,[5,36] South Africa,[36] and Canada[38,39] has led some to label diabetes a disease of civilization.

The relationship between increasing urbanization and diabetes morbidity reinforces Neel's hypothesis[31] of diabetes as a "thrifty" genotype. The theory holds that in prehistoric times the prediabetic individual was better equipped to adapt to the environment. The gene or genes responsible for diabetes mellitus permitted gaining extra weight during times of relative plenty and thus enhanced survival during times of famine. Once these factors no longer existed, the diabetic gene once considered functional for survival became a liability.

Studies of the differences in population frequencies of *lactose intolerance* suggest a genetic, as well as an acquired, basis.[16,17] Adults of cultures as diverse as the Thai, Japanese, Andean Indians, and Chinese have reduced levels of lactase. In the United States the rate for lactose intolerance among adults of predominantly European ancestry is between 10% and 20%. This contrasts with 70% lactose intolerance among adults of African descent.[16] The geographic distribution of the trait supports the hypothesis that primary adult lactose intolerance arose after the cultural practice of the domestication of milk-producing animals and large-scale milk production.

Given the high nutritional value placed on milk in the United States and its inclusion in special diets, a reassessment of milk consumption is indicated. Individuals with the enzyme deficiency suffer discomforts such as flatulence, bloating, severe abdominal cramping, and diarrhea after ingesting milk; thus, contrary to the popular slogan, some people especially those of African and Asian origin, do outgrow their need for milk. There is evidence that many lactose-intolerant adults in the milk-drinking culture of the United States simply restrict the amount of milk they drink at any one time to an amount that does not provoke symptoms. In this way they derive some benefits without suffering adverse effects.[17] In addition, cheese, yogurt, sour milk, and other milk products with a lower lactose content may be substituted.

Differences in mortality and morbidity for whites, blacks, and other minorities continue to the present decade.

Much attention has been paid to sickle cell anemia, a genetically transmitted condition found primarily in African-Americans. Deaths from sickle cell anemia account for about .17% of the excess total mortality rate of African-Americans as compared with the total mortality rate of white-Americans.[5a] A study by the Task Force on Black and Minority Health, reported by the Department of Health and Human Services in 1985, revealed that blacks have the highest overall cancer rates for both incidence and mortality of any population group. Cancer incidence is 25% higher among black males than white males; black females have a 4% higher incidence rate for cancer than white females; the prevalence of diabetes is significantly greater among blacks, Hispanics, American Indians, and Asian and Pacific Islanders than among whites; coronary heart disease rate for black women is twice that for white women; and stroke deaths among black males are nearly double those of white males. Although minorities generally have poorer health rates than whites, in some areas they actually do better. The overall cancer rate for Asian-Americans— Chinese, Japanese, and Filipinos—is lower than that for whites. American Indians have the lowest mortality for all cancers combined.

THE "SICK ROLE"—A SOCIAL AND CULTURAL CONSTRUCT

Parsons[32] analyzed the expectations of the role functions of physician and patients during episodes of acute illness. The focus of the analysis was on definition of somatic and mental health and illness in light of dominant (that is, white American middle-class) values. In addition, he attempted a tentative and sketchy impression of differences between white-American, Soviet, and British definitions of health and illness and in the role of patient and "therapeutic agencies," that is, physicians, within societies having different political and social ideologies.

Butler[3] reported the findings of a cross-cultural comparative study of three communities (each with a rural and urban component) in England, Yugoslavia, and the United States that tested empirically the notion of cultural relativity in the definition of illness and the assumption of the sick role. The study showed that in the English and American communities fewer than one third sought professional advice or reported limitation of usual activities. On the other hand, the proportion reporting limitation of usual work activities in the Yugoslavian community was 59%. In Yugoslavia over half of those who reported limitation of activities failed to seek medical treatment. In a summary of the international cooperative effort to study the cultural dimensions of the sick role, it was concluded that to define people as being ill solely in terms of social adjustment is to disregard a number of people who, using a different set of nonclinical criteria, also define themselves as ill and in some cases as seriously ill.

The concept of "patient work" explicated by Strauss and colleagues[41,42] extends and enhances the understanding of the normative aspects of the "sick role." The concept of "patient work" within the context of the high technology of the intensive care unit considers the two-way sharing of knowledge with the patient viewed as teacher as well as recipient of health professionals' teaching. On the basis of several years of observation and interviews, the study illuminates the complexities of chronic disease and medical (and nursing) care organization. By focusing on the *work itself*, insights are gained into how complicated, varied, and frequently unrecognized the actual "work" is, especially that of patient and kin.

A classic example of patient work in the specific role as teacher is the study of Gassow and Tracy[12] of *impression management* by patients with leprosy that describes patients' attempts to alter and control the negative social responses of others to this stigmatized disease. Impression management refers to efforts people make to create a desired image about themselves and to control the conduct of others by controlling what they say and hear. Patients have developed theories that redefine the disease so that it may be removed from its position as the "idealized maximal horrible illness." Patients function in the role of educators in the attempt to change the public image of the leper. The development of these "educational specialists" has led to a new concept that is descriptive of their function: the career patient status.

The destigmatizing ideology and the concept of a career patient status may be applied to other disease entities. Social organizations such as the "ostomy clubs," (Chapter 44), the Lost Chord Club for laryngectomees (Chapter 32), and Alcoholics Anonymous (Chapter 12) are among those groups that use career patients who employ their own theories and concepts to facilitate adaptation, as well as to bring about changes in society's attitudes.

ILLNESS REFERRAL SYSTEM

A concept or construct that may be useful for analysis and comparison of people's social systems is that of illness referral system. An *illness referral system* is conceptualized as a subsystem of the medical system and includes all health actors and their actual or expected behavior in illness situations. Summarizing the definitions of a number of investigators and theorists, Weaver[44] has defined a *medical system* as comprising the "whole complex of a people's beliefs, attitudes, practices, and roles associated with concepts of health and disease and with patterns of diagnosis and treatment." The patterns

and modes of treatment have meaning only when the totality of social, structural, and group actions is taken into account. This construct of an illness referral system is similar to Friedson's conceptualization[11] that a *lay referral system* consists of a "variable lay culture and a network of personal influence along which the patient travels on his way to the physician."

THE HEALTH CARE SYSTEM

Kleinman has developed a three-part model of the health care system: professional, folk, and popular sectors. The *professional sector* includes formally educated, state-licensed practitioners of western-style scientific medicine, also referred to as *biomedicine*. Professional sector practitioners include physicians, nurses, and physical therapists. The *folk sector* of the health care system includes healers, whose education is often obtained through apprenticeship and whose practice is based on a traditional medical system. These healers often display inborn or spirit-given talent. The third sector, the *popular sector*, includes the sharing of health and illness information among family members, friends, and other knowledgeable, informal helpers.[24] Lock further makes the distinction between *folk medical systems*, which are derived from a nonbiomedical, scholarly medical tradition and require formal education of practitioners (such as traditional Chinese medicine or the East Indian Ayurvedic medicine), and *local folk medical systems*, which are less sophisticated and organized (such as the local Japanese folk practitioners who practice moxibustion, which is the burning of an herb on specific, strategic sites on the body).[27]

Knowledge and practice of medicine from each of the sectors mutually influence each other, and many health beliefs and practices are not limited to one sector. Knowledge from scientific medicine is readily available to many lay persons through health teaching, television, and print media. Alcoholics Anonymous 12-step recovery programs, which may be considered "folk" practice, are used within hospitals, which are biomedical institutions. Physicians and nurses who believe in and practice scientific medicine may also use home remedies learned from parents and grandparents.

DISEASE, ILLNESS, AND DISORDER

The experience of sickness has been described as both a personal and a collective experience.[27] Determination of the presence and manifestations of sickness is itself influenced by and a part of culture.[27] Hahn has introduced the concept of suffering as a universal human experience, usually considered unfortunate. Suffering includes three dimensions:

1. *Illness*—the experience and perspective of the patient

2. *Disease*—the perspective of the professional biomedical practitioners (nurses, physicians, physiologists, etc)
3. *Disorder*—the perspectives of folk or other than biomedical health practitioners (curanderas, practitioners of Chinese medicine, etc).[15]

Chrisman[4d] notes that biomedically trained physicians and nurses often regard sickness as some form of organic pathology and may view sickness as not explainable in traditional physiologic terms as malingering or as superstition. Kleinman similarly notes that many biomedical practitioners regard patients' illness narratives, or stories about the courses and experiences of illness, as filled with superfluous details unrelated to real diseases. Perspectives of folk practitioners or alternative healers are often ridiculed or ignored.[24]

Hahn uses the three dimensions of suffering to describe and explain sickness. He questions the validity and appropriateness of one best explanatory system. Considerable variation occurs even within the various systems. Professional sector biomedical beliefs and practices are influenced by cultural factors, varying considerably among the United States, England, West Germany, and France, for example.[15]

Further, not all sickness can be classified under the biomedical system. Susto, roughly defined as soul loss and present as part of the folk belief systems of many Latin cultures, may have physical, biomedically recognized symptoms. Yet it is incompletely described and treated outside the cultural belief system in which it occurs. Ignoring, devaluing, or ridiculing the patient's beliefs are all examples of poor nursing care in which patients are given labels (hypochondriac, malingerer, or hysterical) instead of appropriate treatment. The respectful consideration of the patient's perspective of the illness leads the health care team, instead, to consult family, community resources, and a folk healer. Thus, the health care team learns that suffering from susto is a shared cultural belief, not an idiosyncratically held one. The biomedical health team provides necessary care in the area of its expertise and, additionally, provides emotional support and validation for the patient and family. The folk healer may then be called in as a "specialist" to take care of the susto.

CROSS-CULTURAL COMPARATIVE APPROACHES

Planning health care for various subcultural groups in American society requires identification of traditional beliefs and practices and determination of the extent of practice of these traditions within a group. Information may then be used to deliver culturally sensitive health care. One way to facilitate identification of the universal features of human rsponses to illness as well as responses unique to a group or subculture is by means of a cross-cultural comparative approach.

A comparative approach is developing within nursing. One nurse-anthropologist advocates a transcultural nursing approach, which offers a frame of reference that "can offer insight, new relationships, new foci, and new dimensions of caring about one's own culture in relation to another.[25] Transcultural health care is defined as an evolving body of knowledge and practices regarding health-illness caring patterns from a comparative perspective of two or more cultures to determine major care features and the health services of cultures.[25]

The comparison of illness referral systems discussed above offer one approach for the comparison and contrast of the social processes by which people make initial diagnosis and seek therapy. Cultural categories and criteria for defining illness may also be studied and compared by use of ethnographic or ethnoscientific strategies or techniques. Culture is uniquely human. All human groups have a culture, but it is in the analysis of detailed differences and similarities within and between groups that subtle relationships and understanding emerge.

The ethnographic approach is a naturalistic comparative method aimed at studying human behavior, beliefs, and attitudes through observation and interviews in the natural setting. Ethnoscience or ethnoscientific analysis comprises one aspect of the ethnographic approach. The suffix "science" is not used in the usual sense. It refers to classification or taxonomy. Ethnoscience refers to a system of cognition or classification typical of a given culture. The terms *emic* and *etic* are used for arriving at a cultural group's classification system. Emic categories are culturally specific; etic categories are universal, that is, common to more than one culture. Emic analysis seeks to discover significant distinctions made by members of a particular culture and avoids the use of priori definitions or categories.[42a] The etic perspective concerns observations and definitions of the situation by the observer and not the member of a cultural group. Etic analysis composed of externally derived criteria permit the observer to compare and theorize across several cultures. Etic features are considered culture free, since they can be applied across cultures; emic features are culturally unique. Categories derived from Western biomedicine use etic clasification or explanatory systems.

Ethnographies or ethnographic descriptions take into account the perspective of members of a social or cultural group and include the beliefs, behaviors, and values that underlie and organize the activities related to health maintenance and restoration. They rely on observations and formal and informal interviews to elicit peoples' interpretations and responses to health-threatening or health-enhancing situations. There are an increasing number of ethnographic studies initiated by nurses[14a,35,42b,14b] that would facilitate a comparative study of lay person's responses (emic) with those of the health professional (etic) for a number of illness entities or phenomena.

In addition to differentiation of lay persons and professional perspectives by an emic-etic analysis, there are a number of constructs that are similar in analytic and interpretive power. These include: folk-modern, little tradition—great tradition, common sense models—biomedical, lay explanatory models—biomedical. The constructs enable nurses to make distinctions between popular or lay persons' and the orthodox or professional perspective. Comparison and contrasts are facilitated and nursing interventions may then be planned to decrease the gap or culture lag between lay perons or professionals. Nurses may then frame questions about the consequences of beliefs and behaviors that differ tfrom the modern, biomedical, or professional criteria.

Tables 7-1 and 7-2 depict the hot/cold classificatory system used by urban Puerto Ricans and interventions appropriate for professionals working within the hot/cold framework.[19]

BELIEFS ABOUT CAUSE OF ILLNESS

Beliefs about causation of illness reveal variations across cultural groups. Americans in general attribute sickness to physiologic and psychologic causes. People as diverse as the Gadsup of New Guinea and the Azande of Africa stress the social and cultural causes of a number of illnesses. Many ethnic groups attribute sickness to fate, destiny, or God's will. This is common in the United States where biomedicine is a dominant force in explaining sickness: biomedicine can predict, identify, and treat proximal or immediate causes, not ultimate ones. In other words, biomedical science can identify the virus that causes a particular leukemia or a particular constellation of biologic, environmental, and social factors that may lead to a disease, but not why one person is stricken and a neighbor or family member is not.

Health care and health care information are also not equally accessible to many persons. Obstacles to seeking health care include inadequate financial resources, illiteracy, inability to read or converse in the health practitioner's language (including overuse of jargon or scientific terms), insensitive or uninformed health care

TABLE 7-1 Puerto Rican hot/cold classifications

Category	*Frío* (Cold)	*Fresco* (Cool)	*Caliente* (Hot)
Illnesses and bodily conditions	Arthritis Colds and upper respiratory symptoms (including asthma) *Empacho** Menstrual period Muscular spasm (*pasmo*) Pain in the joints Upset stomach (*frialdad del estómago or frío en el estómago*)	None	Constipation Diarrhea Rashes Tenesmus (*pujo*) Ulcers
Medicines and herbs	None	Bicarbonate of soda Linden flowers (*flor de tilo*) Mannitol (*maná de manito*) Mastic bark (*almácigo*) $MgCO_3$ (*magnesia boba*) Milk of magnesia Nightshade (*yerba mora*) Orange-flower water (*agua de azahar*) Sage	Anise Aspirin Castor oil Cinnamon Cod-liver oil Iron tablets Penicillin Rue (*ruda*) Vitamins
Foods	Avocado Bananas Coconut Lima beans Sugar cane White beans	Barley water Bottled milk Chicken Fruits Honey Raisins Salt cod (*bacalao*) Watercress	Alcoholic beverages Chili peppers Chocolate Coffee Corn meal Evaporated milk Garlic Kidney beans Onions Peas Tobacco

Reprinted by permission from Harwood A: Ethnicity and medical care, Cambridge, Mass, 1981, Harvard University Press.
*Characterized by nausea, vomiting, and/or diarrhea, mainly in children, *empacho* is attributed to an obstruction in the stomach or intestines caused by either a bolus of undigested food or saliva swallowed by a teething baby.

providers, lack of health education or access to health information, or lack of support from family and peers to seek health care. Information and care received may also conflict with patients' health or illness beliefs.

Cultural themes pertaining to curing and healing, particularly in regard to nutrition or foods, have been identified. A study of Puerto Rican families in New York revealed that hot-cold notions associated with the Hippocratic humoral theories continued to find expression.[19] Health, according to the humoral theoretic orientation, was defined as a state of balance among four *bodily humors, namely, blood, phlegm, black bile, and bile. An imbalance in these humors results in illness, which causes the body to become excessively dry, cold, hot, wet, or a combination of these qualities.* Foods and medicinal herbs are classified as having hot or cold qualities and are prescribed to return the body to its proper balance.

Vestiges of theories directed toward correcting body imbalance form the basis for treatment within a number of ethnic and cultural groups. Some New England Yankees, for example, used apple cider and honey to maintain proper acid-base balance.[22] In a Guatemalan community two concepts, *fresco* (fresh or cool) and *alimento* (highly nutritive substance), were used to accommodate and reinterpret modern health and nutritional beliefs.[6] Fresh or cool substances (carrot juice, tea, chicken, rice) rather than cold were considered the best treatment for "hot" illnesses. Many of the health professionals working with the Guatemalans were not aware of the distinctions people made between highly nutritive substances *(alimentos)* and other foods. The wet-dry polarity forms the basis of the therapeutic beliefs about foods of several eastern and western European groups.[35,43] A balance in the wet and dry foods is believed to be important in maintaining a healthy state. Meals or prescribed diets lacking soups and green leafy vegetables are perceived as "too dry" and detrimental to maintaining the body in its proper state.

The identification by nurses of cultural themes associated with caring and curing behaviors is facilitated within settings such as the hospital, where these behaviors would be more likely to be manifested. Acknowledgement and respectful recognition by nurses of the functional nature of folk or lay persons' beliefs aid in decreasing the social and cultural distance between patient and professional. Beliefs and practices that reinforce or interfere with the physicians' and nurses' pre-

TABLE 7-2 Management issues with Puerto Rican patients who follow hot/cold theory

General Problem	Example	Recommended Solution Within Hot/Cold Framework
Patient fails to take prescribed medication or eat recommended foods because they directly contradict notions of good therapy within hot/cold framework.	Pregnant women avoid "hot" foods and medications to prevent their babies from being born with a rash or red skin. As a result, they do not take prescribed iron or vitamin supplements.	When patient rejects "hot" substances, use neutralization principle. When patient rejects "cool" medication, use an alternative drug not classified in the hot/cold system.
Patient on maintenance dose of a "hot" medication stops therapy when he experiences a "hot" symptom Patient on maintenance dose of a "cool" medication stops therapy when a "cold" symptom develops.	Patient on prophylactic program of penicillin stops therapy when he experiences diarrhea or constipation and may discontinue therapy entirely to prevent a recurrence.	With "hot" medications, follow neutralization principle and advise patients to take them with a "cool" substance. With "cool" medications, use a drug not classified in the hot/cold system or prescribe an equivalent "hot" drug until the "cold" symptom subsides.
Patient discontinues "hot" or "cold" foods in a dietary regimen if symptoms within the same category develop.	Patients on diuretics who are told to eat dried fruits, oranges, and bananas (all "cold" or "cool" foods) as sources of potassium will stop these foods should "cold" symptoms develop. Since these symptoms include menstruation, women are most at risk.	For any dietary recommendation, provide options from all three categories of the hot/cold system. (For example, "hot" cocoa or peas might also be suggested as sources of potassium.)
Substances traditionally used to "refresh" the stomach (that is, to neutralize "hot" foods) may be harmful in themselves.	To protect babies from developing rashes or other "hot" symptoms from formula made with evaporated milk, some mothers add "cool" $MgCO_3$ or mannitol to the bottle, often in quantities sufficient to cause diarrhea.	Stress use of harmless "cool" additives (barley water, fruit juice) in place of potentially harmful ones.

Reprinted by permission from Harwood A: Ethnicity and medical care, Cambridge, Mass, 1981, Harvard University Press.

scriptions require identification. Nurses may then be able to develop therapeutic plans of care working within the patient's belief system. For example, it was found that Puerto Rican patients receiving diuretics discontinued use of orange juice, a source of potassium, when they had a cold because of its "cold" quality.[19] In such cases nurses can suggest alternate potassium-rich foods that do not fall into the "cold" category (Table 7-2).

Different views of health maintenance and modes of healing are not limited to urban poor and ethnic minorities. Many middle-class, educated Americans of diverse ethnic origins define illness and its causes in ways that differ from the health professional's definition. These views comprise distinctive cognitive and classificatory systems—that is, common sense models—that differ considerably from the biomedical in analytic and interpretive power.[13] Popular and folk notions based on causal observations and unsystematic inferences are found in a number of publications purchased predominantly by persons of the middle class. These include the magazine *Prevention* and the published works of Norman Cousins[2] and Adele Davis.

Cousins,[7] for example, attributed development of an illness to "lowered resistance" and exhaustion during a trip to Moscow that made him vulnerable to hydrocarbons from diesel exhaust at the airport and the Moscow construction sites near his hotel. Davis[8] explained the harmful effects of vitamin deficiency on the body by the principle of oxidation and applied the metaphor of rust forming on iron to the process of oxidation that "pits and corrodes the cell membrane." In her view, the process of oxidation facilitates entry of bacteria or viruses into the cell and therefore leads to cell changes.

Chrisman[4a] has described four common illness belief systems:

1. Germ theory
2. Equilibrium
3. Sorcery and witchcraft
4. God- or spirit-caused

Germ theory involves the incorporation and reformulation by lay persons of certain biomedically based information related to disease. Technical terms may be used, but understood differently than by biomedical practitioners. Although biomedical practitioners may assume that patients understand hypertension as a condition that is measured with a sphygmomanometer and related to obesity, sodium intake, and narrowed blood vessels, Blumhagen found that over 80% of his sample of clinic patients understood "hyper-tension" to be related to stress and being tense.[1] Patients then decided to stop taking medicines and follow prescribed diets because they "no longer felt tense." Hypertension, described as high blood pressure, may also be confused with a rural Southern folk illness called "high blood," in which excess blood accumulates in the body, possibly leading to stroke, and is treated with pickle juice.[40] This example demonstrates the need for clear communication between health practitioners and patients.

High blood is an example of Chrisman's[4a] second type of illness beliefs: those related to equilibrium. *Balance and harmony are thought to relate to the promotion of health.* Humoral pathology systems, including both hot/cold beliefs as well as the blood, phlegm, black bile and yellow bile of pre-twentieth century medical practice, are other examples. Equilibrium beliefs may also involve the maintenance of equilibrium with the universe, with the social/spiritual worlds, or in one's vital energy force.

God or spirits may also be seen as the *source of both illness and cures.* "God's will" may be considered the ultimate cause of illness by patients and practitioners. Illness and cures may be regarded as either gifts, challenges, or punishments, depending on the circumstance or particular frame of reference of the patient, or may be regarded as unrelated in a particular instance to God. Similarly, traditional Asian and Native American patients may regard the spirits of ancestors, places, nature, and objects as having a role in illness causation, cure, or comfort.

Finally, *witchcraft*, which is often defined as *inherent possession of evil supernatural power,*[4a] and *sorcery, intentional supernatural activity* in order to promote harm, are sometimes considered to be causes of illness. Such beliefs are not uncommon in many ethnic and other subcultural groups and are often very frightening. The perpetrator of the witchcraft or sorcery is usually a member of the family, friend, or acquaintance who is envious of the patient. Leininger has demonstrated similarities between witchcraft beliefs and white middle-class beliefs about stress[25] in that both seem related to strained social relations.

Dual-use[34] or relying on several or all of the illness belief systems described previously to explain or treat one or more sicknesses is not uncommon nor is reliance on popular, professional, and folk practitioners in one or a variety of illness episodes. For example, a white middle-class woman, who is a health professional, has adenocarcinoma of the lung and is receiving radiation treatments. Uncertain as to the effectiveness of radiation treatments for her cancer, she followed a macrobiotic diet, received psychotherapy, had acupuncture and massage, ingested herbal treatments and purifiers, participated in native American "sweat lodge" ceremonies, and did a type of breath therapy. The biomedical practitioners were unable to identify a proximal cause, and she considered the many proximal and ultimate causes delineated by the various popular and folk systems with which she had engaged. Since her biomedical practitioners were unsympathetic to her multiple use of illness belief systems, she stopped mentioning them and eventually ceased visiting her physician.

PROVIDING CULTURALLY SENSITIVE HEALTH CARE

CULTURAL ASSESSMENT

Cultural assessments are made to identify patterns or regularly recurring behaviors and beliefs that may assist or interfere with nursing interventions and treatment regimens. It is important to realize that cultural assessment does not require information on every aspect of a specific culture. In collecting data the nurse considers the client as the chief informant about customary actions. During the assessment interview no judgments or conclusions are made. Data are collected and recorded in the client's own words as much as possible. Observations during the initial encounter would include content that may influence interaction between nurse and client (for example, language, styles of communication, and norms of etiquette).[43] Data should elicit ethnic identity including generation in America (that is, first, second generation), religious affiliation, identification of sect (for example, Roman Catholic, Orthodox Greek, Baptist, Jehovah's Witnesses), determination of social class with education and occupation as major determinants, and specific neighborhood or location of residence to facilitate identification of demographic factors that may have relevance for health.

The patient's explanatory models[4a,24] for his or her present health problem will yield the *emic* perspective. The following set of questions may be helpful for assessment of the client's perspective and the definition of his situation:

1. What do you call your illness?
2. When did it start? Why do you think it started then?
3. What do you think caused it?
4. How does the illness work in your body?
5. How have you been taking care of yourself? Who made those suggestions?
6. How long will it last? Is it serious? What problems has it caused you?
7. Is there anything you would like to add?

BEHAVIORS ASSOCIATED WITH PAIN

The pain experience is a universal component of the human condition, and the phenomena associated with pain have been encountered by all nurses. Health professionals tend to be aware of the psychologic, social, and cultural components of patient pain responses (see Chapter 16). Differences in responses to pain in relation to the variables of ethnicity, religious affiliation, and race have been the subject of several studies.[28,46,47] Zborowski's study was one of the earliest to focus on differentials in cultural responses to pain. The findings of this study are still applied without question by some nurses. However, the study has been criticized for its failure to distinguish between pain as a basically physi-

ologic phenomenon and the *pain experience*, which has cognitive and emotional components.[47] Social classes and generation variables were not adequately controlled in the study, and subsequent studies revealed that immigrant and other groups (for example, religious and racial) will follow the patterns of the majority group in the society if the subjects are made aware of the ethnic or religious differences.[47] A comprehensive review of research of cultural factors and pain responses concluded that there is a paucity of adequately controlled experimental studies of the pain experience; that any attempt to delineate cultural factors in human responses should be made in the wider context of cultural attitudes toward sickness and health; and that religious attitudes, insofar as they "influence perception of the physical self," may be an important variable for study.[47]

The beliefs and attitudes about social and cultural differences in the pain experience are not the only examples of conflicting viewpoints. For example, the adoption of anesthesia in the nineteenth century was not universally accepted. Not only did physicians' ideas about pain influence their responses to the medical innovation—the introduction of anesthesia—but also their beliefs about variability in response according to gender, social class, and ethnicity. For example, women were supposedly more sensitive to pain than men and required surgical anesthesia more often than men. Blacks and American Indians were believed to have a higher pain threshold than whites and therefore surgical anesthesia was withheld. Wealthy, educated, native-born Americans could endure less pain than the uneducated and poor immigrants. Upon the basis of the survey of prevalent attitudes and practices, Pernick[33] concluded that hidden behind the physicians' approach to pain and anesthesia use were value judgments about women, ethnic groups, and the poor that were an expression of the values of elitism and moralism prevalent in Victorian American culture and that were held by highly educated wealthy men.

Similar beliefs continue to find expression in the modern environments of health and nursing care. Nurses functioning within tertiary environments of care have an excellent opportunity for observation and development of heightened awareness of the expression of these beliefs among medical and nursing professionals and ancillary workers who have contact and responsibility for direct patient care. Nurses then must ask the question: What are the consequences of these beliefs and attitudes in providing comfort and alleviation of suffering of hospitalized patients?

CULTURE-SENSITIVE CARE

Culture-sensitive nursing care[4a,4d] reflects both the history of *nursing's attention to issues of cultural diversity in patients and nursing's goal of providing effective, compassionate, and holistic patient care.*[4] The elaboration of such a model is intended to provide guidance by which cultural sensitivity may be incorporated within nursing practice not only in providing care to people of color and people of foreign origin but also to all patients. The three aspects of culture-sensitive care are *knowledge, mutual respect,* and *negotiation.*

KNOWLEDGE

The first step in building knowledge is to *increase self-awareness* and to *reduce ethnocentrism.* An evaluation of values and beliefs and their relationship to one's own sociocultural context and to one's enculturation in the subculture of nursing increases self-awareness. Nursing students may remember feeling confused and uncomfortable after encountering unfamiliar language, practices, and value systems upon entering nursing school. Using the concepts provided earlier to analyze one's own sickness beliefs and practices and their shift over time may prove a useful exercise.

Ethnocentrism is a belief that one's own culture provides the only correct ways of believing or behaving.[4a] Although some degree of ethnocentrism is inevitable and probably necessary to interact in the world, adopting *an attitude of cultural relativism,* in which *multiple perspectives and explanations are possible and acceptable, helps the health care provider understand and communicate with persons from different sociocultural backgrounds.* Though a particular belief or value may seem irrational to a particular nurse from a particular sociocultural context, it is better understood when interpreted within its own context.[4c] This information may become critical if it is necessary to halt or substitute a cultural practice. Stopping the behavior or initiating a new one must be explained in a way that makes sense to the patient.

Chrisman[4d] also describes *medical ethnocentrism as the belief that scientific medicine provides the only correct information about sickness,* which inhibits the possibility of receiving any information to the contrary and interferes with accurate information gathering. However, many health beliefs attributed to scientific medicine reflect the values of dominant white middle-class values[4] and are supported by little empirical scientific research.[30] The *power behind this type of ethnocentrism* is from *claiming to be universal* (relegating different beliefs to the abnormal or unhealthy), *sanctioning by professionals* (many of whom are from the dominant white middle class), and *using scientific terminology.*

The nurse's knowledge of the patient's and family's illness beliefs may be derived from the patients and families, possibly with an explanatory model interview. Personal experiences, including successes and failures, provide valuable information in building a knowledge base on *culture-sensitive care.* Other sources of information include faculty, nurses, and other health providers; hospital staff; students; community leaders; and

friends who are either members of or well-acquainted with the particular cultural/subcultural group. If language barriers exist, using translators and learning a few key terms, such as the words for "pain" or "water," are important. Finally, the health/sickness-related literature on various cultural groups provides information essential to providing culture-sensitive care. Whenever possible, read not only the literature by biomedical practitioners but also that from the perspective of the people.[45] If this seems overwhelming, specialization in one or two subcultures common to the geographic location can be combined with a general knowledge of the principles of culture-sensitive care.

MUTUAL RESPECT

Knowledge and self-awareness help prepare the culture-sensitive nurse to respect the beliefs and values of patients different from themselves. *Remaining nonjudgemental, listening, and showing some level of knowledge and sensitivity toward patients enhances trust and is important in developing a therapeutic relationship.* Relationships of mutual respect are not possible in the presence of prejudice against others of dissimilar national origin than one's own or against others on the basis of gender, social class, race, ethnicity, religion, and sexual preference. *Racism,* for example, may be described as related to ethnocentrism in that the lifeways of the "other" people are seen as wrong and as somehow "naturally" inferior. *Racism is different from ethnocentrism in that it is socially sanctioned and enforced through economic inequities, practices of institutions, (including that of health care and educational systems), and is expressed through stereotyping and oppressing some races while allowing privileges to others.*[10] Racism has been and is present within the health care system in the differential allocation of health resources and choices available to ethnic minority persons, particularly poor, African-American women and children who are then sometimes hypothesized to have inherently poorer health than white middle-class Americans.[45] Racism has also been institutionalized in differences with standards of care in health care research[23] and in access to nursing education, professional association membership, and employment.[21] Boyd, in describing effective psychotherapy with African-American women when the therapist is not an African-American, notes that understanding the cultural framework of African-American women is essential:

For to ignore the meaning of the client's identity is to ignore the person. If that occurs, treatment cannot take place. Only through recognizing that the client has a history and identity that is completely different from one's own, can one take an effective look at the symptoms presented.[2]

Part of developing a relationship with an ethnic or racial minority patient is the awareness of the effects of racism, which may discourage the patient from seeking health care and from trusting health care professionals.

NEGOTIATION

Mutual respect and the information gathered and analyzed provide the basis for negotiation of treatment. Often, patients refuse or simply neglect ordered treatments nor accept ordered medications. When no opportunities for discussion are presented and the patient does not feel comfortable communicating with the nurse, reasons for noncompliance may seem mysterious or unreasonable. Chrisman[4a,4d] advocates a negotiation process in which the nurse carefully listens to the patient's perspective in which the nursing perspective fits both the nurse's and the patient's, compares and contrasts the nurse's and the patient perspectives, and arrives at a mutually agreeable compromise. Giving in on less important issues or instituting mutually aggreeable substitutions helps provide for greater future cooperation and is a sign of respect for the patient. If having family visitors is important to the patient, but all of the family visiting at once is overwhelming and disruptive to the staff and other patients, perhaps the nurse can negotiate a visitation schedule with a representative of the family. Further examples of possible negotiation are presented in Table 7-2.

CHAPTER SUMMARY

✔ Social class differences and cultural beliefs and values affect health-caring behaviors and actions directed at the prevention, treatment, and amelioration of sickness.

✔ Beliefs about the causation of illness vary according to cultural groups (ethnic or subcultural) and social class. The consideration of similarities and differences within and between groups aids in the identification of health beliefs and actions that are apply to many people or are specific and unique for a group or social class or are idosyncratic, that is, applicable only to an individual.

✔ Culture-sensitive care emphasises knowledge-seeking, mutual respect, and negotiation.

QUESTIONS TO CONSIDER

- How has your own cultural background influenced your beliefs as a nurse? How are your personal beliefs different from biomedical beliefs?

- In what ways has racism influenced your personal development? Your professional practice?

- Analyze a nursing care situation you have experienced recently. How could you have provided culture-sensitive care?

- Complete a cultural assessment with a selected patient. Analyze how the information you gained will affect your nursing care.

REFERENCES AND SELECTED READINGS

1. Blumhagen D: The meaning of hyper-tension. In Chrisman NJ and Maretzki TJ, editors: Clinically Applied Anthropology, Dordrecht, Holland, 1982, D. Reidel.
2. Boyd JA: Ethnic and cultural diversity in feminist therapy: keys to power. In White E, editor: The black women's health book, Seattle, 1990, Seal Press.
3. Butler JR: Illness and the sick role: an evaluation in three communities, Br J Sociol 21:241-261, 1970.
4a. Chrisman NJ: Culture-sensitive nursing care, In Patrick M et al, editors: Medical surgical nursing. In press.
4b. Chrisman NJ: Ethnic persistence in an urban setting; Ethnicity 8:256-292, 1981.
4c. Chrisman NJ: The health-seeking process: an approach to the natural history of illness, Culture, Medicine & Psychiatry 1:351-377, 1977.
4d. Chrisman NJ: Antrothopology in nursing: an exploration of adaption. In Chrisman NJ and Maretzki TJ, editors: Clinically applied Anthropology, Dordrecht, Holland, 1982, D. Reidel.
5. Cohen AM: Prevalence of diabetes among different ethnic Jewish groups in Israel, Metabolism 10:50, 1961.
5a. Cooper R: The biological concept of race and its applications to public health and epidemiology; J Health Politics, Policy and Law 11:97-116, 1986.
6. Cosminski S: Alimento and fresca: nutrtional concepts and implications for health care, Hum Org 36:203-207, 1977.
7. Cousins N: The healing heart: antidotes to panic and helplessness, New York, 1983, WW Norton and Co Inc.
8. Davis A: Let's eat right to keep fit, New York, 1954, Harcourt Brace Jovanovich Inc.
9. Dubos R: Man, medicine and evvironment, New York, 1968, Mentor Books.
10. Frankenberg R: Growing up white: feminism, racism and the social geography of childhood. In Alarcon N et al, editors: The third wave: feminist perspectives on racism, New York, Kitchen Table Women of Color Press.
11. Friedson E: Patient's view of medical practice, New York, 1961, Russell Sage Foundation.
12. Gassow Z and Tracy GC: Status, ideology and adaptation to stigmatized illness: a study of leprosy, Hum Org 27:316-325, 1968.
13. Gillick MR: Commonsense models of health and illness, N Engl J Med 313:700-703,1985.
14. Guillaumin C: Race and nature: The system of marks. The

idea of a natural group and social relationships, Fem Issues 25-43, (Fall) 1988.

14a. German C: The cancer unit: an ethnographic study, Wakefield, Mass, 1979, Nursing Resources.

14b. Hagey R: Drumming and dancing, Canadian Nurs 79:28-31, 1983.

15. Hahn RA: Rethinking "illness" and "disease." In Daniel EV and Pugh JF, editors: Contributions to Asian studies, vol 18: South Asian systems of healing, Leiden, Netherlands, 1984, EJ Brill.

16. Harris M: One man's food is another man's whitewash, Nat Hist 81:12-13, 1972.

17. Harrison GG: Primary adult lactase deficiency: a problem in anthropologic genetics, Am Anthropol 77:812-835, 1975.

18. Harrison and Rittenbaugh

19. Harwood A, editor: Ethnicity and medical care, Cambridge, Mass, 1981, Harvard University Press.

20. Herskovits MJ: Cultural anthropology, New York, 1955, Alfred A Knopf.

21. Hine DC: Black women in white: racial conflict and cooperation in the nursing profession, 1890-1950, Bloomington, Ind, 1989, Indiana University Press.

22. Jarvis DC: Folk Medicine, Greenwich, Conn, 1958, Crest Books.

23. Jones JH: Bad blood: the Tuskegee syphilis experiment—a tragedy of race and medicine, New York, 1981, Free Press.

24. Kleinman A, Eisenberg L, and Good B: Culture, illness and care: clinical lessons from anthropologic and cross-cultural research, Ann Intern Med 88:251-258, 1978.

25. *Leininger M: Transcultural health care: issues and conditions, Philadelphia, 1976, FA Davis Co.

26. Livingstone FB: Anthropological implications of sickle cell gene distribution in West Africa, Am Anthropol 60:533-562, 1958.

27. Lock M: East Asian medicine in urban Japan: varieties of medical experience, Berkeley, Calif, 1980, University of California Press.

28. Meehan JP, Stoll AM, and Hardy JP: Cutaneous pain threshold in native Alaskan, Indian and Eskimo, J Appl Physiol 6:397-400, 1954.

29. Miller FJW: The epidemiological approach to the family as a unit in health statistics and the measurement of community health, Soc Sci Med 8:479-482, 1974.

30. Navarro V: Crisis, health and medicine: a social critique, New York, 1986, Tavistock.

31. Neel JV: Diabetes mellitus: a "thrifty" genotype rendered detrimental by progress, Am J Hum Genet 14:353-362, 1962.

32. Parsons T: Definitions of health and illness in the light of American values and social structure. In Jaco GE, editor: Patients, physicians and illness, New York, 1957, Free Press.

33. Pernick MS: A calculus of suffering: pain, professionalism, and anesthesia in nineteenth-century America, New York, 1985, Columbia University Press.

34. Press I: Urban illness: physicians, curers and dual use in Bogota, J Health Soc Behavior 10:209-218, 1969.

35. Ragucci AT: Ethnographic approach and nursing research, Nurs Res 21: 485-490, 1972.

36. Remoin DL: Ethnic variability in glucose tolerance and insulin secretion, Arch Intern Med 124:695-700, 1969.

37. Ritenbaugh C: New approaches to old problems: interactions of culture and nutrition. In Chrisman NJ and Maretzki TJ, editors: Clinically applied anthropology, Dordrecht, Holland, 1982, D. Reidel.

38. Schaefer O: The changing health picture in the Canadian North, Can J Ophthalmol 8:196-204, 1973.

39. Schaefer O: When the Eskimo come to town, Nutr Today 6:8-16, 1971.

40. Snow LF: Folk medical beliefs and their implications for care of patients, Ann Intern Med 81:82-96, 1974.

41. Strauss A, et al: Social organizations of medical work, Chicago, 1985, University of Chicago Press.

42. Strauss A, et al: Patient's work in the technologized hospital, Nurs Outlook 29:404-412, 1981.

42a. Tripp RT: Reconceptualizing the construct of health: integration of emic and etic perspectives, Res Nurs Health 6:101-109, 1984.

42b. Tripp-Reimer T: Retention of folk healing practice (Matiasma) among four generations of urban Greek immigrants, Nurs Res 32:97-101, 1983.

43. Tripp-Reimer T, Brink PJ, and Saunders JM: Cultural assessment: content and process, Nurs Outlook 32:79-82, 1984.

44. Weaver T: use of hypothetical situations in a study of Spanish-American illness referral system, Hum Org 29:140-154, 1970.

45. White E, editor: The black women's health book, Seattle, 1990, Seal Press.

46. *Wolff BB and Langley S: Cultural factors and the response to pain: a review, Am Anthropol 70:494-501, 1968.

47. Zborowski M: Cultural components in response to pain, J Soc Issues 8:16-30, 1952.

STRESSORS, STRESS, AND COPING

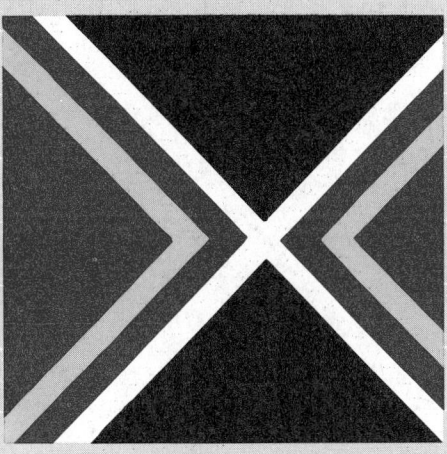

STRESS AND STRESS MANAGEMENT

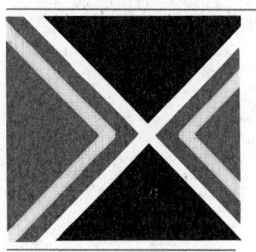

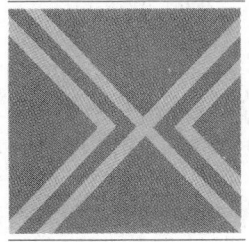

CHAPTER 8

Biologic Defense Mechanisms

E. RONALD WRIGHT

CHAPTER OBJECTIVES

After studying this chapter, the student should be able to:
1. Differentiate between the concepts of self and non-self.
2. Identify the external and internal nonspecific biologic defense mechanisms.
3. Describe the mechanism and function of the complement cascade.
4. Describe the steps of the inflammatory process and biologic basis of symptoms.
5. Define immunogens and immunoglobulins, and identify the site, structure, and function of each immunoglobulin.
6. Identify the cells involved in the provision of specific immune responses and their genesis, location, and function.
7. Describe the humoral and cell-mediated immune responses, and differentiate between primary and secondary immune responses.
8. Explain the immunologic bases for passive and active immunizations, cancer, human immunodeficiency virus (HIV) infection, tissue transplantation, and monoclonal antibodies.

CONCEPT OF BIOLOGIC DEFENSE

The human body exists within a milieu of antagonistic environmental forces that are constantly attacking and threatening the integrity of the individual. In response to these onslaughts, the body exhibits a wide array of adaptations (structures, mechanisms, responses) designed to provide a defense against these encroachments. These mechanisms serve to protect the body from both external and internal deleterious agents. This chapter deals with those anatomic and biologic mechanisms that provide protection against environmental factors that physically threaten the client's body. The implications and applications of the functions of these systems are also discussed.

Knowledge of the basic structures and mechanisms that provide this protection helps in the understanding of (1) resistance to infectious disease, (2) diagnosis of disease and physiologic state, (3) rejection of tissue transplants, (4) prevention of the development of malig-

nancies, (5) adaptations in the aging process, (6) immunization against infectious disease, (7) expression of disease of autoimmunity or immunodeficiency, (8) development of allergic reaction, and (9) significance of the localized or systemic inflammatory response. Much of preventive and restorative nursing practice is built on the maintenance or restoration of the cells, systems, and mechanisms that provide defenses against harmful factors in the external and internal environment.

SELF VERSUS NONSELF

Each human being can be regarded as a genetically and immunologically unique collection of cells and molecules that make up a biologic unit of *self*. It is the function of the biologic defense mechanisms of the body to protect the integrity of self from encroachment by *nonself* (or foreign) materials. These mechanisms (Figure 8-1) serve to protect self from both external and internal destructive agents in the following ways:
1. *Exclusion* of harmful agents from the body
2. *Recognition* of harmful agents within the body
3. *Response* designed to rid the body of the harmful agents that do gain access

The sources of these harmful nonself materials are generally external. These external agents include nonliving materials of the environment such as potentially harmful inorganic chemicals and compounds produced by other living organisms. The most serious external threats to biologic integrity, however, come from the living organisms that constantly surround the body. Some of these organisms pose no real threat because the mechanical, biochemical, and metabolic processes of the human body will not support them or offer them shelter. There are a myriad of living forms, on the other hand, for which the human body is an ideal haven for growth and survival. Most of these organisms, if allowed to penetrate the body, would wreak havoc on the normal functionings of the body. The living forms that come to mind in this regard are the organisms classified as *pathogenic* (disease causing). Although the progress of these organisms in the body can be altered by external agents such

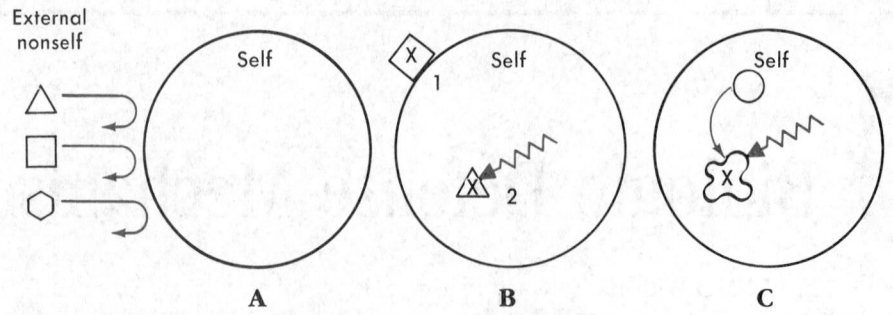

FIGURE 8-1 Mechanisms of biologic defense in the human body. **A,** Exclusion of external nonself. **B,** Destruction of external nonself by *(1)* nonspecific external mechanisms and *(2)* nonspecific or specific internal mechanisms. **C,** Destruction of altered self. X indicates nonspecific mechanisms; → indicates specific mechanisms.

as antibiotics, the eradication of the offending organism from the body must be accomplished by the host's own adaptive mechanisms.

In addition to protection against external agents, the defense mechanisms also offer protection against the accumulation of damaged or dysfunctional self material. Without these processes to carry out the systematic, specific removal of damaged or worn out cellular material, the body would become clogged with debris. An-

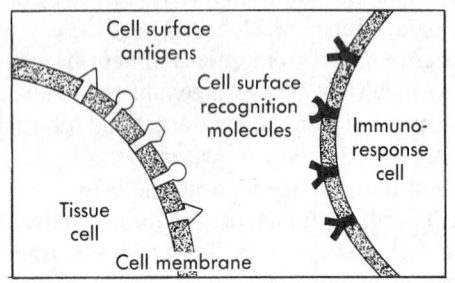

A. CELL SURFACE MARKERS

B. CELL SURFACE MARKER RECOGNITION OF SELF vs. NONSELF

FIGURE 8-2 Cell surface markers for recognition of self versus nonself.

other general function of these systems is recognition of a self's alteration to a potentially dangerous state. When this defense function falters, the tragedy of malignancy (cancer) may result.

RECOGNITION OF SELF FROM NONSELF

The previous discussion shows that a critical feature of the protective mechanisms of the human body's immune response system is the ability to discriminate between self and nonself materials. This is accomplished by certain specific protein molecules embedded in the cell membrane of all human body cells (Figure 8-2). The recognition process then occurs at the cell membrane surface. Immunoresponsive cells (lymphocytes) have specific protein molecules embedded in their membranes that recognize foreign (nonself) proteins. A person's own immunoresponsive cells recognize nonself proteins on cells that are genetically different, and this triggers a sequence of cellular reactions within the immune response system. This sequence of cellular reactions leads to the elaboration of materials and cells that attack the nonself materials. Contact with self proteins (markers) does not produce an immune attack. This explains why cells from different species or genetically dissimilar members of the same species cannot be transplanted from one host to another without triggering an immunologic attack and rejection of the tissue.

SCOPE OF DEFENSE MECHANISMS

The array of defense mechanisms that have been adapted to protect the normal human body is formidable and complex. For the sake of orderly presentation, they may be divided into *nonspecific* and *specific* mechanisms (Table 8-1). The specific and nonspecific mechanisms can be further divided on the basis of where the lines of defense are formed; that is, *external* for the mechanisms of mechanical exclusion, biochemical destruction, and microbial competition and *internal* for the physiologic reactions. The nonspecific mechanisms

TABLE 8-1 Biologic defense mechanisms

	Nonspecific Mechanisms	Specific Mechanisms

External	Mechanical exclusion
	  Physical structures
	    Skin
	    Mucous membranes
	    Specialized structures
	  Physical actions
	Biochemical factors
	  Body secretions
	  pH
	  Lysozyme
	Microbial antagonism
		Immunoglobulin A
		  In mucosal secretions
		  In mucosal cells

Internal	Reticuloendothelial system
	Blood
	  Cellular components
	  Fluid components
	    Complement
	    Acute-phase proteins
	  Phagocytosis
	Inflammatory response
	Interferons
		Antigen processing by macrophage
		Primary immune response
		  Humoral immune response
		    Synthesis of circulating immunoglobulins by B cells
		    Interaction of immunoglobulins with antigen
		  Cell-mediated immune response
		    Activation of T cell response
		    Lymphokines
		  Combined immune response
		Secondary immune response

are nonselectively directed against *any* foreign substance. The specific mechanisms are specifically elicited by *unique* substances to which the body has *acquired* the ability to respond.

EXTERNAL NONSPECIFIC DEFENSE MECHANISMS

ANATOMIC STRUCTURES AND MECHANICAL ACTIONS

SKIN AND MUCOUS MEMBRANES

The first line of defense against penetration by foreign materials, including pathogenic microorganisms, is the skin. When the skin is intact, it serves as an extremely efficient physical barrier to harmful agents and environmental forces such as heat, cold, and trauma. This protection is afforded by the keratinized surface cells, which provide a tough, dense, waterproof covering. Beneath this outermost layer is a dense layer of highly vascularized connective tissue (see Figure 71-1).

Even though some of the fatty acids derived from sebaceous gland secretions have antimicrobial activity, the environment provided by the skin does allow the growth of microorganisms on its upper layers and within hair follicles and sweat glands. These resident microorganisms mainly are nonpathogenic; however, when these organisms gain entrance to the tissues of a host exhibiting reduced resistance, they may cause significant problems. Because even thorough scrubbing with soap and water removes only the surface organisms, the skin can never be considered sterile.

Any time the physical integrity of the skin is broken, such as with surgery, indwelling venous catheterization, or physical irritation or trauma, there is significant risk of microorganisms gaining entrance to the body. The skin must be kept relatively dry, since the continued presence of moisture tends to cause maceration of the skin. Further, when essential oils are lost from the skin surfaces, they should be supplemented by lotions to maintain the resilience and unbroken texture of the surface cells. Adequate care of the skin of the hospitalized patient is not just a luxury but a necessity for the provision of an extremely important aspect of biologic defense.

Mucous membranes protect the eye and line all body tracts that have external openings. When intact, the mucous membranes, as with the skin, are basically impervious to foreign materials and microorganisms. The surfaces are covered by a viscous secretion that tends to trap and inactivate microorganisms. The mucous membrane of the respiratory tract is further protected by the surface activity of the ciliated epithelial cells, which sweep foreign material out of the tract. The mucous membranes are highly vascularized so that the internal defense mechanisms are readily available to attack any microorganisms that do gain access to the surface of these cells.

Also found in the mucosal secretions and in high concentration within the secretory mucosal cells of the respiratory and intestinal tracts are a specific class of immunoglobulins (antibodies) known as immunoglobulin A (IgA) (see p. 163). These specific antibodies are secreted from the mucosal cells and have antibacterial, antiviral, and antitoxic properties. These antibodies serve to prevent microbial adherence and colonization of these tracts by pathogens.

SPECIALIZED STRUCTURES AND MECHANICAL FUNCTIONS

Other structures and functions of the human body that are generally taken for granted actually serve extremely important roles in defense. The filtration action of the nasal hairs serves to trap particles and microorganisms. The flushing action of saliva and urine prevents the buildup of organisms. The eyes are protected from dirt particles and organisms by the lids and lashes. Foreign material that does gain entrance to the eye tends to be washed out by tears. The constant movement of foods through the stomach and intestines prevents the buildup of organisms or toxic waste products. Even the action of vomiting and the watery stools of diarrhea are active mechanisms of removal of harmful products from the gastrointestinal (GI) tract. Dysfunction or blockage of any of these processes means that special measures must be taken to protect against the establishment of pathogenic organisms and the buildup of toxic materials.

BIOCHEMICAL FACTORS

Many areas of the body are protected not only by mechanical barriers but also by specific antimicrobial chemicals that provide added protection.

SKIN

The acetic acid and salt concentration of perspiration is toxic to many pathogenic microorganisms. Some of the fatty acids released to the skin surface by the sebaceous glands also serve to inhibit the growth of some microorganisms.

GASTROINTESTINAL TRACT

In the stomach the acidity (approximately pH 2) of the gastric juice kills many organisms and detoxifies certain potentially toxic substances. For this reason, when gastric pH is increased, special precautions must be taken to avoid introduction of organisms through the nose and mouth. A higher gastric pH is characteristically encountered in neonates; therefore special care should be taken in feeding and handling babies to prevent exposure to pathogens by the oral route. The upper intestine is generally freed of organisms by the action of bile and proteolytic enzymes.

VAGINA

Vaginal secretions allow certain harmless acid-producing bacteria to colonize the vagina and create an acidic environment. This reduces the chance of pathogens colonizing the vagina. When either the amount or the acidity of the vaginal secretions is reduced, a much greater chance exists that a vaginal infection will develop. Since vaginal secretions are not present before puberty and are greatly reduced after menopause, both young girls and older women are more prone to vaginitis. The use of certain types of oral contraceptives may cause a shift in the composition and pH of the vaginal secretions, which increases the possibility of colonization of the vagina, especially by the causative agent of gonorrhea, *Neisseria gonorrhoeae*.

LYSOZYME

The most ubiquitous antimicrobial factor in the body is the enzyme lysozyme. It is capable of lysing (splitting) the bacterial cell wall of many gram-positive organisms and causing their destruction. The enzyme is present in mucus, tears, saliva, and skin secretions and is also found in many of the internal fluids and cells of the body. Within the body lysozyme tends to work in combination with complement and other blood factors to destroy bacteria directly.

MICROBIAL ANTAGONISM

The skin and mucosal surfaces offer varying nutritional and environmental conditions for the growth and multiplication of certain microbial cells. Although the surfaces of the body are constantly exposed to temporary contamination by organisms from the environment, most of these organisms, known as *transient flora*, do not find conditions suitable for the colonization of the body; however, many microorganisms do colonize the

TABLE 8-2 Distribution of normal microbic flora

Region of Body	Sterile Areas	Nonsterile Areas	Microorganisms
Skin	None	All skin	*Staphylococcus, Bacillus, Corynebacterium, Mycobacterium, Streptococcus,* transient environmental organisms
Respiratory tract	Larynx, trachea, bronchi, bronchioles, alveoli, sinuses	Nose, throat, mouth	*Staphylococcus, Candida, Streptococcus, Neisseria, Pneumococcus,* oral organisms
GI tract	Esophagus, stomach, upper small intestine	Esophagus and stomach (transiently), large intestine	Gram-negative rods, *Streptococcus, Bacteroides, Proteus, Clostridium, Lactobacillus*
Genitourinary tract	Cervix, uterus, fallopian tubes, ovaries, prostate gland, epididymis, testes, bladder, kidney	External genitalia, anterior urethra, vagina	Skin organisms, *Lactobacillus, Bacteroides*
Body fluids and cavities	Blood, pleural fluid, synovial fluid, spinal fluid, lymph, etc.	None	

skin and mucosal surfaces. These organisms make up what is known as the *normal microbic flora*. Although this normal flora varies from site to site within the body and may vary in response to environmental, hygienic, and physiologic changes, it is capable of reestablishment and reflects a fairly predictable pattern. Table 8-2 provides an overview of the body areas normally colonized and shows which organisms most often make up the normal flora of the various areas.

The maintenance of this balanced microbic flora makes it difficult for pathogenic organisms to establish themselves on the body surfaces. Since the normal flora have a selective advantage in their environmental niche, they compete for nutrients and space. Some release antimicrobial substances to retard the growth of transient organisms seeking to occupy the same site. These microbial interferences are known as *microbial antagonism*.

Most of the normal microbic flora are basically non-pathogenic; however, some overtly pathogenic organisms such as *Staphylococcus aureus* and *Streptococcus pyogenes* can be part of the normal flora. The individual who harbors such organisms without demonstrating any symptoms of disease is known as a *carrier*. This carrier state is significant because the carrier may be unknowingly shedding organisms into the environment and infecting others.

The protective effects of the normal microbic flora become most apparent when something upsets the microbic balance within the body. The extended use of broad-spectrum antibiotics sometimes creates such an effect. The imbalance may allow a segment of the normal flora to gain ascendency, causing adverse reactions. An example of this phenomenon is seen when certain oral antibiotics induce marked shifts in the normal intestinal flora, allowing organisms generally suppressed by the growth of competitors to thrive to an unusual degree. This imbalance may induce uncomfortable GI tract problems or even allow gastroenteritis to develop.

INTERNAL NONSPECIFIC DEFENSE MECHANISMS

Once a foreign agent (living or nonliving) penetrates the external resistance barriers, it is met by an even more complex array of defense mechanisms, which provides for the recognition, capture, and disposal of the foreign material. The key to this process is the specific recognition and vigorous action taken against the foreign material and at the same time the protection of the host tissues from extensive damage. The physiologic reactions that serve to contain and inactivate the foreign agent are carried out through interactions of cells and molecules of the reticuloendothelial system (RES), blood, vascular system, and body tissues.

RETICULOENDOTHELIAL SYSTEM

The RES is a widespread system of phagocytic cells (devouring cells) scattered throughout various body tissues (Figure 8-3). The role of these cells is to ingest foreign particulate matter and damaged host tissues. Some of

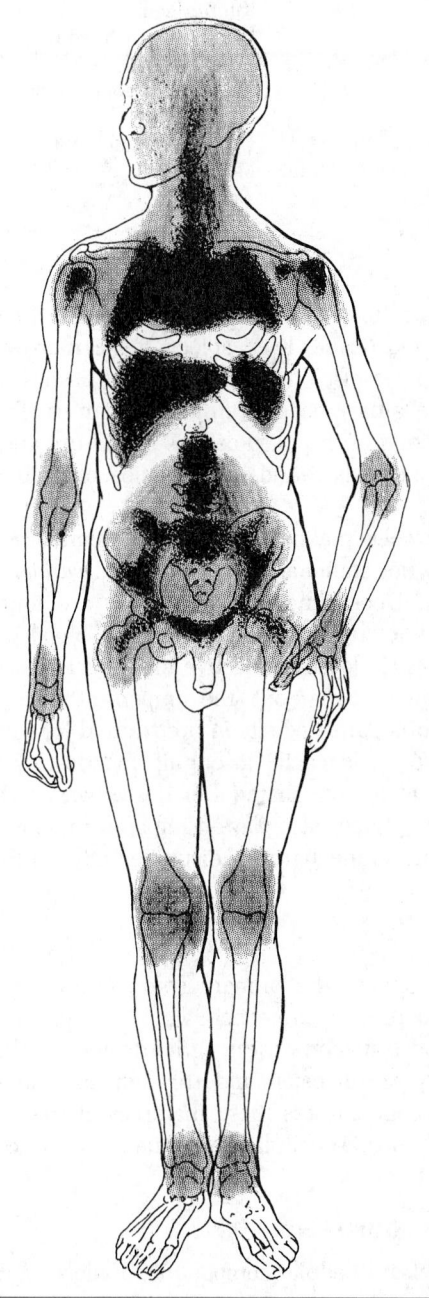

FIGURE 8-3 Reticuloendothelial system. Note anatomic distribution of maximal activity in system, as indicated by black areas over body. To produce such an image, certain radioactive colloidal particles are given to the subject, and radiation detection techniques delineate tissue uptake. Note definition of liver, spleen, and active bone marrow in axial skeleton and proximal parts of long bones. (From Smith AL: Microbiology and pathology, ed 12, St Louis, 1980, The CV Mosby Co.)

TABLE 8-3 Distribution and names of macrophages in various tissue sites

Tissue	Name
Peripheral blood	Monocyte
Loose connective tissue	Histiocyte
Liver	Kupffer cells
Spleen, RES	Wandering or fixed macrophage
Lung	Alveolar macrophage or dust cell
Granulomatous tissue	Epithelioid and giant cells
Peritoneal cavity, pleural cavity, bone	Macrophages

the phagocytic cells are *fixed* in a variety of tissues such as lymphoid tissue, liver, spleen, bone marrow, lungs, and blood vessels. Within the different tissues these anchored cells have been given unique names (Table 8-3). The function of the fixed cells is to capture and destroy foreign materials found in the fluids of their environment.

Other cells making up the reticuloendothelial network are not stationary and are called *wandering macrophages*. Depending on where they are found, they may be known as *monocytes* (in the bloodstream) or *histiocytes* (in loose connective tissues). The wandering macrophages carry out the important role of final cleanup of a damaged site in preparation for repair. The cells have the capacity to engulf and destroy virtually any type of foreign material or debris within the body. The macrophages also play an important role in the specific response mechanisms discussed later in this chapter.

BLOOD

Blood is one of the primary sources of elements designed to provide protection against injurious agents. The blood transports these active factors to the site of an injury or intrusion and through specific vascular changes concentrates these materials at the site. Both the fluid and the cellular constituents of blood contain these factors.

CELLULAR COMPONENTS

The important cellular components of blood in this nonspecific response include granulocytes, lymphocytes, monocytes, and thrombocytes (platelets) (see Figure 8-11). The granulocytes, also referred to as polymorphonuclear leukocytes (PMNs), and the monocytes are the most important because of their phagocytic activity.

One of the key methods of nonspecific defense is the ingestion of microorganisms and other particulate matter by the phagocytic white blood cells (WBCs). The ph-

agocytes carry out the process of *phagocytosis* in several discrete steps (Figure 8-4). Most infecting microbes are quickly and efficiently destroyed by phagocytosis; however, some pathogens can escape this destruction. Some bacteria, such as strains of the streptococci and staphylococci and *Bacillus anthracis* (anthrax), actually produce factors that will kill the phagocyte. Other organisms resist ingestion or digestion. Some organisms may survive within the phagocytes or reticuloendothelial cells and multiply there. This may lead to the transport of the organism to other sites in the body or serve as a chronic focus of continued infection.

The granulocytes can be divided on the basis of their structure and function into neutrophils, eosinophils, and basophils. The "granules" found within these cells represent discrete packets of degradative enzymes used to digest the ingested materials. The neutrophils are the most numerous in circulation and are the most efficient and responsive phagocytic cells involved in the inflammatory process. Where there is adequate blood supply to a region, the phagocytes are constantly available to move from the blood vessels to the site of injury or infection. The neutrophils and monocytes are actually attracted to the scene by chemicals released during infection or injury. This cellular response to chemical attractants is known as *chemotaxis*, and the substances released are called *chemotactic substances*.

FLUID FACTORS

The fluid portion of uncoagulated blood is called *plasma*. Some of the components of plasma provide important constituents for the internal defense mechanisms. Plasma transports the *circulating immunoglobulins* produced in specific response to antigen stimulation. These immunoglobulins bind to the specific antigens against which they are formed. The antigens become coated with these immunoglobulins. The phagocytotic cells can recognize the immunoglobulin bound to the antigen through receptors on the surface of the phagocyte, thereby greatly enhancing the ability of the cell to engulf the antigen. This process of enhanced phagocytosis is known as *opsonization*. Through this process the specific immune response mechanism contributes to the nonspecific mechanism and makes it significantly more efficient.

Another plasma constituent, *fibrin*, may create a meshwork around the injured area, sealing it off. Microorganisms may also become trapped within this meshwork, where they are more easily captured by the phagocytic cells.

Complement

One of the most important constituents of plasma is a complex series of 11 proteins known by the singular name of *complement*. The primary role of complement is

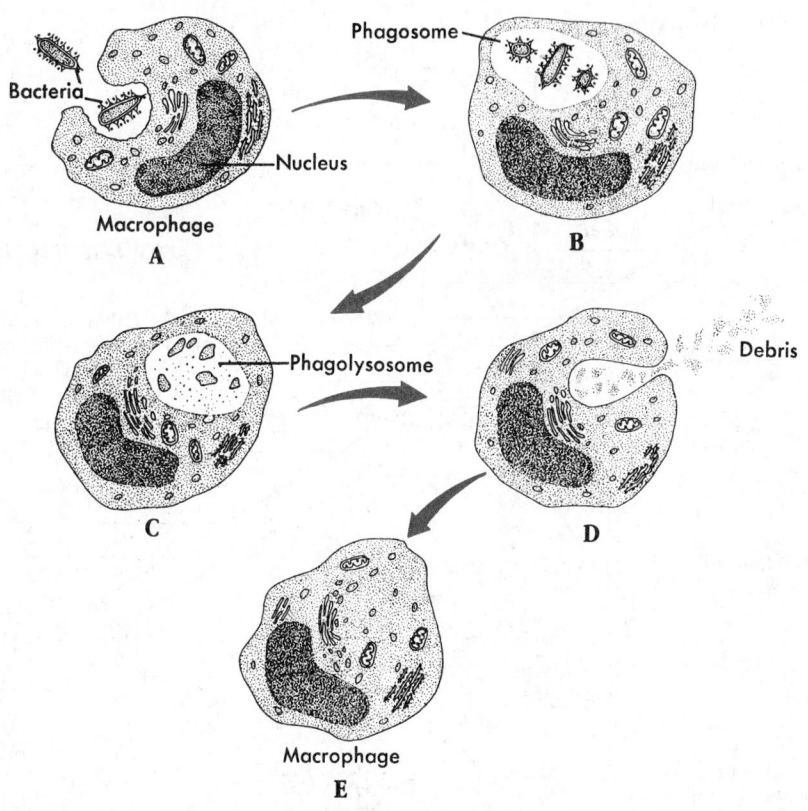

FIGURE 8-4 Phagocytosis sketched in macrophage. **A,** Opsonized bacteria engulfed by phagocyte (macrophage). **B,** Phagosome formed. **C,** Phagosome becomes phagolysosome; bacteria digested. (To this point the process of phagocytosis is comparable to either macrophage or neutrophil, not shown.) **D,** Debris is egested. (Neutrophil would succumb here.) **E,** Macrophage returns to resting state. (From Smith AL: Microbiology and pathology, ed 12, St Louis, 1980, The CV Mosby Co.)

to provide specific lysis (rupturing) of cell membranes. The initiation of the *complement cascade* is most often triggered by the binding of the first complement protein to complement-binding immunoglobulins that have already bound to their antigens. Thus complement serves to accentuate or complete the action of an immunoglobulin. The immunoglobulin by itself cannot produce cell lysis, but with the recruitment of complement in the reaction, the cell may be ruptured. However, other nonimmune substances can also activate complement. Complement is considered a nonspecific component of the plasma because it is not increased by immunization. In addition to its cytolytic effects, complement is involved in leukocyte chemotaxis, release of histamines, enhancement of phagocytosis by PMNs, viral neutralization, and bactericidal activity.

The classical activities ascribed to complement depend on the sequential interaction of nine protein subunits (C1 to C9), the first component of which consists of three subfractions termed C1q, C1r, and C1s (thereby accounting for the 11 separate proteins). When the first component, C1, is bound by an antigen-immu-

noglobulin complex on the surface of a cell, it acquires the enzymatic ability to activate many molecules of the next components in the sequence, C4 and C2, to form an active C42 complex (Figure 8-5). (Unfortunately, the numbering system of the complement components reflects their order of discovery and not their sequential additive pattern.) Each of the activated C42 complexes is then able to act on multiple molecules of the next components and so on, both producing a cascade effect and greatly amplifying the reaction. As each component is added, new enzymatic activity is created to initiate the next step. This cascade effect is similar to that of blood coagulation. The final component, C89, has the ability to create a lesion in the cell membrane, and if enough lesions are created on the membrane, cell death results. The intermediate stages in the complement sequence also give rise to complexes and fragments with other significant biologic activities. Figure 8-5 depicts the generation of some of these activities. These include the following:

1. *Histamine release.* Histamines cause an extreme increase in vascular permeability and contraction

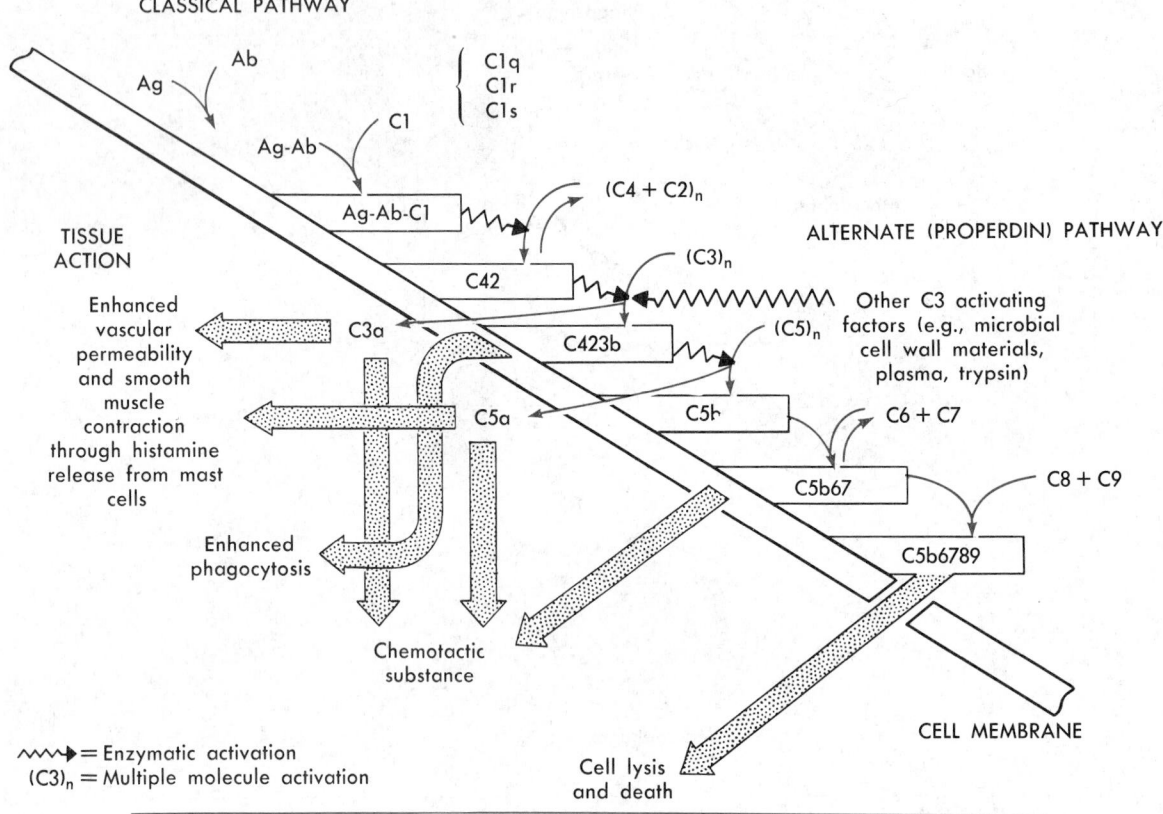

FIGURE 8-5 Classical and alternate complement cascade. Sequence of complement activation generates multiple biologically active intermediate molecules, which are active in the inflammatory response.

of smooth muscle. A fragment (C3a) split off during the activation of C3 and another fragment (C5a) created by the activation of C5 are released into the surrounding tissues, where they cause the release of histamine from mast cells. The histamines in turn exert their physiologic effects on the smooth muscle tissues and vascular system. Because these histamine-mediated reactions are the same as those created during anaphylactic shock (see Chapter 76), these fragments are called *anaphylatoxins*.

2. *Enhanced phagocytosis*. Neutrophils and macrophages have receptors for C3b on their cell surfaces, which adds to the opsonization effect. Complement activation at the site of infection labels foreign materials with the C3b fragments and makes them more subject to phagocytosis. The contribution of the process to protection is most apparent in individuals who are genetically deficient in the synthesis of the C3 protein. Such individuals suffer from recurrent bacterial infections and septicemia.

3. *Chemotactic substance formation*. Several of the fragments and intermediate factors serve as chemotactic substances to attract phagocytes to the site of the reaction.

All these activities are central to the inflammatory response.

The plasma fraction contains several proteins that inhibit the action of the activated components of complement in the fluid phase; that is, off the membrane surface. Such inhibitors serve to localize the effects of the membrane surface and thereby protect the "innocent bystander" membranes.

In addition to the activated C42 complement complex, several other enzymes exhibit *C3 convertase* activity. These include trypsin, plasmin, and thrombin as well as bacterial endotoxins and a factor derived from cobra venom. Each leads to alterations in C3, which are similar, if not identical, to those produced by the complement cascade–derived C3 convertase. These activations are mediated through a plasma component known as *properdin* and are referred to as the *alternate*, or *properdin, pathway*.

Acute-Phase Proteins

Acute-phase proteins are serum proteins with concentrations that increase dramatically in the serum of individuals suffering from any type of severe inflammatory response. Both infectious and noninfectious inflammations trigger an increase of these proteins in plasma. These proteins include liver-synthesized haptoglobin, fibrinogen, complement proteins, ceruloplasmin, and C-reactive protein. Because C-reactive protein is more prevalent and is easily measured, it is often used interchangeably with acute-phase proteins. C-reactive protein derives its name from its ability to bind to the C protein of the cell walls of *Streptococcus pneumoniae*. C-reactive protein binds to a variety of bacteria and fungi and has the property of activating the complement C3 protein to initiate the subsequent steps in the complement cascade on the surface of the foreign cells, leading to their destruction.

The amount of acute-phase proteins found in the serum is roughly proportional to the severity of the inflammation; therefore a test for these proteins is useful in the diagnosis and management of diseases that are difficult to differentiate and have a hidden inflammatory aspect, such as bacterial endocarditis, cryptic abscesses, rheumatic fever, and certain types of cancer.

INTERFERONS

Interferons are a group of proteins produced by various human cells, usually in response to the viral infection of the cell. When a cell is infected by a virus, the infected cell begins to make interferon almost immediately (Figure 8-6). The interferon is released into its surrounding environment, where it induces uninfected cells to pro-

duce alterations that protect those cells from viral multiplication. This antiviral action is exerted before the synthesis of immunoglobulins specific for the virus reach protective levels. The elaboration of interferons from virally infected cells continues for a few hours (up to about 24 hours) following infection, thereby playing a significant role in isolating the infective foci in many, but not all, viral infections.

Although viruses seem to be the most potent agents for the induction of interferon, production is not restricted to virus infection of cells. Other intracellular parasites such as rickettsia, bacteria, and parasites may also trigger the formation of interferon. Even bacterial and fungal extracts, as well as such other materials as double-stranded ribonucleic acid (RNA), synthetic polymers, and plant extracts, may serve as signals.

Three distinct types of interferons are produced by different cell types in the human body, and each type seems to exert different protective effects. *Alpha-interferon* is produced by lymphocytes and seems to have antiviral activity. *Beta-interferon* is formed by fibroblasts, epithelial cells, and macrophages; it is definitely antiviral. *Gamma-interferon* is produced by T cell lymphocytes of the specific immune response system and has an immunoregulatory effect. In addition to their antiviral activities, the interferons are capable of inhibiting cell growth; therefore they are being used widely in clinical trials as an *antitumor agent*.

In general the production of interferon occurs regardless of the viral agent that initiated its formation; thus interferon is said to be *virus nonspecific*. It does not inhibit all viruses equally. Among the viruses that seem to be especially sensitive are the arboviruses, in-

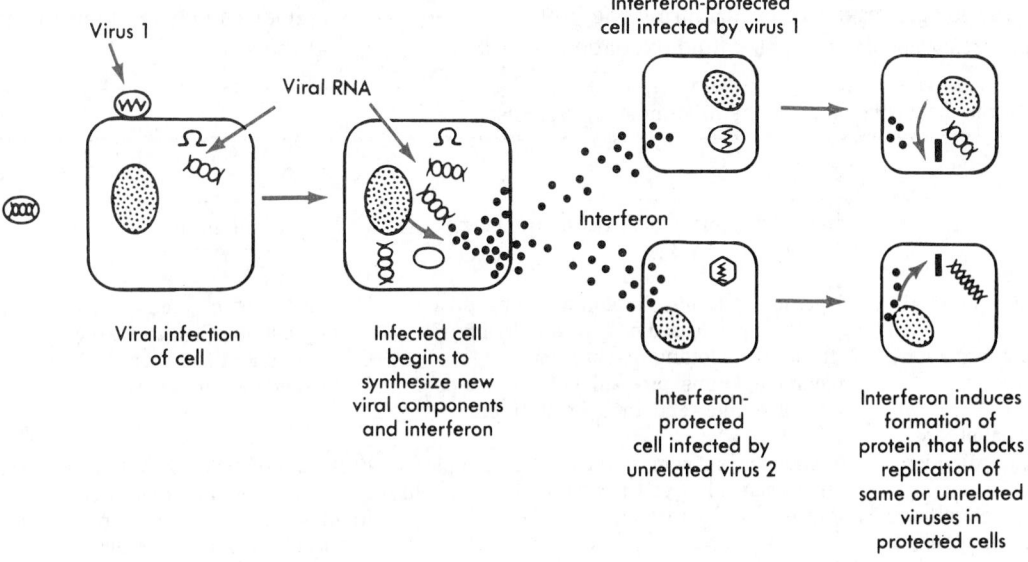

FIGURE 8-6 Mechanism of interferon action.

fluenza virus, and smallpox virus. Most vertebrate species seemingly are capable of producing interferons; however, each animal species interferon is protective against viral infection only in that species. This means the bovine (cow) interferon has only limited protective value in the human, and vice versa. The term *species specificity* is used to describe this quality. This characteristic limited early research into the effects of interferon, since it was difficult to obtain enough human interferon to conduct clinical trials. Through the use of recombinant deoxyribonucleic acid (DNA) technology, the human interferon gene has been introduced into bacterial cells. By growing such bacteria in culture, large amounts of specific types (alpha [α], beta [β], and gamma [γ]) of interferon can be harvested, purified, and used in clinical studies. The other benefit of this application of genetic engineering is to greatly reduce the cost of the purified interferon.

INFLAMMATORY RESPONSE

When injury occurs in the body, all the nonspecific and to some degree the specific defense mechanisms are directed toward localizing the effects of the injury, protecting against microbial invasion at the site, and preparing the site for repair. This process is called *inflammation*.

The inflammatory response can be initiated by any type of injury: heat, cold, irradiation, chemicals, trauma, infection, immunologic injury, or neoplasia. Whatever the stimulus, the response of the body is the same, but the extent of the involvement of the nonspecific response system's various facets depends on the degree and severity of the injury.

STEPS IN THE RESPONSE

Three major physiologic responses occur during the inflammatory process: vascular response, fluid exudation,

and cellular exudation (Table 8-4). The *vascular response* consists of a transitory vasoconstriction (stress response) followed immediately by vasodilation. This occurs as a result of chemical substances such as histamine or kinins released at the site of injury or invasion. The amount of blood flow to the area is thus increased (*hyperemia*), causing redness and heat. Blood flow slows as the capillaries dilate. Increased permeability of the capillary walls facilitates fluid and cellular exudation.

Fluid exudation from the capillaries into the interstitial spaces begins immediately and is most active during the first 24 hours after injury or invasion. Initially the fluid exudate is primarily serous fluid, but as the capillary wall becomes more permeable, protein (albumin) is lost into the interstitial spaces. This increases the colloid osmotic pressure in these spaces, which encourages more fluid exudation. The swelling of the tissue from the fluid in the interstitial spaces is called *edema*.

Cellular exudation refers to the migration of WBCs (leukocytes) through the capillary walls into the affected tissue. An increased number of WBCs are attracted to the vessels in the affected area as a result of chemotactic substances being released from the tissues by cell injury and complement activation. The WBCs adhere to the capillary wall and then pass in ameboid fashion through the widened endothelial junctions of the capillary wall. Neutrophils (PMNs), which make up about 60% of the circulating WBCs, are the first leukocytes to respond, usually within the first few hours. The neutrophils ingest the bacteria and dead tissue cells (phagocytosis); then they die, releasing proteolytic enzymes that liquefy the dead neutrophils, dead bacteria, and other dead cells (pus). Monocytes and lymphocytes appear later. The macrophages continue the phagocytosis, and the lymphocytes play a role in the antigen-antibody response at the site.

TABLE 8-4 Summary of the steps in the inflammatory response

Steps	Mediators	Outcome
1. Injury	Physical, chemical, biologic, immunologic stimulus	Cell and tissue injury
2. Vascular response		
a. Vascular dilation	Histamine, plasmin, serotonin, kinins, prostaglandins released or activated by injury	Dilation of vessels, causing stasis of blood and margination of leukocytes
b. Fibrin clot formation	Activation of clotting mechanism	Containment of irritants
3. Fluid exudation	Histamine, kinins, prostaglandins cause opening of venule–endothelial cell junction	Fluid exudation into tissues
4. Cellular exudation		
a. Leukocyte exudation	Chemotactic substances released by complement activation, clot formation, injured cells	Passage of leukocytes from blood to site of injury and accumulation there
b. Attack and engulfment of foreign materials	Neutrophils, macrophages	Removal and digestion of bacteria, foreign particles, damaged tissues
5. Healing	Fibroblasts produce collagen fibers, tissue regeneration	Resolution of inflammation, formation of scar tissue

LOCAL MANIFESTATIONS OF INFLAMMATION

The five cardinal symptoms of inflammation were identified many centuries ago. These are redness (*rubor*) and heat (*calor*) caused by the hyperemia, swelling (*tumor*) caused by the fluid exudate, pain (*dolor*) caused by the pressure of the fluid exudate and by chemical (bradykinin, prostaglandins) irritation of the nerve endings, and *loss of function* of the affected part caused by the swelling and pain.

The inflammatory response prepares the tissue for healing and contains the spread of bacterial invasion. To prevent the spread of bacteria, fibroblasts are attracted to the area and secrete fibrin, a threadlike substance that encircles the affected area to wall it off from healthy tissue. If interference occurs with this walling-off process, bacteria can spread into the surrounding tissue. This explains why an abscess should not be incised and drained until it has "come to a head" or until the walling-off process is completed.

REGIONAL LYMPH NODE MANIFESTATIONS

Bacteria may fail to be contained locally and may spread to other parts of the body by means of the lymph system or bloodstream. If picked up by the lymph stream, the bacteria will be carried to the nearest lymph node. These nodes are located along the course of all lymph channels, and bacteria can be ingested and destroyed here as well. If the bacteria are virulent enough to resist the action of the lymph nodes, leukocytes are brought in by the bloodstream to attack and engulf the bacteria in the node. The node then becomes swollen and tender because of the accumulation of phagocytes, bacteria, and destroyed lymphoid tissue. This is known as *lymphadenitis*. Swollen lymph nodes can be palpated primarily in the neck, axilla, and groin.

SYSTEMIC MANIFESTATIONS

Moderate to severe inflammatory responses can produce generalized systemic manifestations. The three major manifestations are (1) increase in body temperature (*fever*), (2) increase in WBCs in peripheral circulation (*leukocytosis*), and (3) increased *erythrocyte sedimentation rate* (ESR).

Fever is produced by the release of substances known as *endogenous pyrogens* at the inflammatory site. These pyrogens come from injured cells, materials released by WBCs that accumulate at the site, and components of the bacterial cell wall. The pyrogens include prostaglandins, leukotrienes, and bacterial endotoxins. The substances are carried to the temperature-regulating center in the hypothalamic region of the brain, where they signal a resetting of the body temperature set point. The body responds by increasing heat production and decreasing heat loss. As long as the pyrogens remain in circulation, the set point will be elevated. The fever response is designed as part of the defense mechanism and helps increase production of antimicrobial agents such as interferon. It also tends to support increased phagocytic activity of some cells, including fixed and wandering macrophages.

Leukocytosis develops when agents released from damaged cells and WBCs accumulating at the inflammatory site are carried by the circulation to the bone marrow, where WBCs are produced. These agents are known as *leukopoietins*. When these agents reach the bone marrow, they signal the release of mature neutrophils held in reserve there. This leads to an immediate rise in the WBC count in the peripheral circulation to greater than 10,000/mm^3. The chemotactic agents draw these cells to the inflammatory site. Leukopoietins also increase the production of WBCs in the bone marrow. With prolonged inflammation the bone marrow stores of WBCs are depleted, and the synthesis of mature WBCs may not be able to keep pace with the needs of the inflammatory site; thus the marrow releases more immature neutrophils as the inflammation continues. These immature cells, known as *bands,* become more prevalent in the peripheral circulation and indicate a significant ongoing inflammation. The condition is sometimes referred to as a "shift to the left." This clinical phrase was derived from the past clinical laboratory method of counting the immature cells and tabulating them in the left-hand columns of differential count forms.

With inflammation an increased blood sedimentation rate also occurs; that is, when an anticoagulant is added to the blood in the laboratory, the red blood cells (RBCs) settle to the bottom of a test tube more rapidly than normal. This increase in the ESR is believed to be caused by an increase in fibrinogen, a blood protein essential to the healing process. The ESR is elevated during the acute inflammatory stage of infection, which indicates that the body's defense mechanisms for the repair of damaged tissue are operating.

Inflammations can be classified as acute or chronic. *Acute* inflammations are characterized by a sudden onset and an increase in the fluid exudative response. *Chronic* inflammations have a slower, more insidious onset and are characterized by increased cellular exudation.

Knowledge of the physiologic changes that occur during the inflammatory process helps the nurse to understand the changes that occur in a variety of diseases. For example, whenever cells die as a result of injury or disease (*necrosis*), such as during a myocardial infarction, the inflammatory process occurs. Fat deposits (*atheromas*) on blood vessel walls cause injury to the lining of the vessel wall and initiate an inflammatory response. Irritation of the peritoneum by trauma or bacterial invasion can cause inflammation of the peritoneum (*peritonitis*).

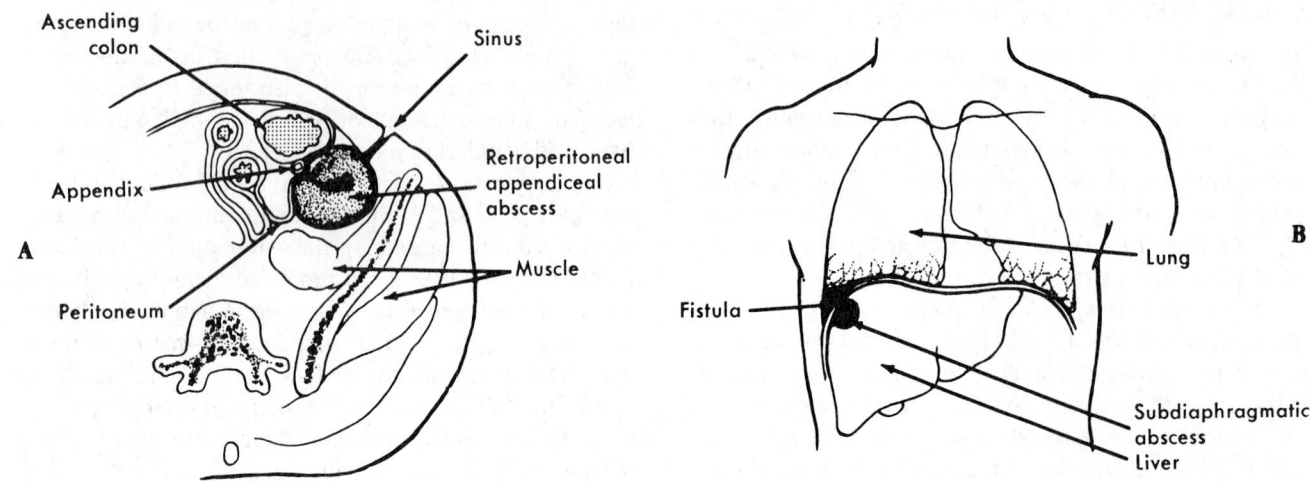

FIGURE 8-7 A, Cross section of torso showing appendiceal abscess with sinus that has developed through abdominal wall. **B,** Subdiaphragmatic abscess that has developed fistula opening into pleural cavity.

REPAIR AND HEALING

No healing will occur until inflammation has subsided and pus and dead tissue have been removed. Pus is a local accumulation of dead phagocytes, dead bacteria, and dead tissue. The bacteria most frequently causing this reaction are the staphylococci, streptococci, *Neisseria,* and *Pseudomonas aeruginosa* (*P. pyocyanea*). A collection of pus that is localized by a zone of inflamed tissue is called an *abscess* (Figure 8-7). An inflammation that involves cellular or connective tissue is called *cellulitis,* whereas an inflammation in which pus collects in a preexisting cavity such as the pleura or gallbladder is called *empyema.* When infection forms an abscess within the body, develops a suppurating channel, and ruptures onto the surface or into a body cavity, it is called a *sinus.* If the infection forms a tubelike passage from an epithelium-lined organ or normal body cavity to the surface or to another organ or cavity, it is called a *fistula.*

After the infected area is clean, new cells are produced to fill in the space left by the injury. They may be the normal structural cells, or they may be fibrotic tissue cells known as *scar tissue.* If they are fibrotic cells, they will not function as the cells functioned formerly but only serve to fill in the injured area. Some body cells readily regenerate; for instance, after the bowel has healed, it is almost impossible to find the injured area. The respiratory tract also regenerates its tissues readily. Liver tissue has the capacity to regenerate its tissue, but over a longer period. Some nerve cells are always replaced with fibrous tissue. If a large amount of tissue is destroyed, structural cells may not be replaced, regardless of the type of tissue. (See Chapter 22 for discussion of wound healing.)

Some people, especially those with brown or black skin, are prone to excessive scar formation. Such tissue formation, known as a *keloid,* is hard and shiny in appearance and may enlarge to a surprising degree. It may cause disfigurement or undergo malignant degeneration and thus is usually excised surgically. Serous membranes sometimes become adherent during inflammatory and healing processes, and as the inflammation subsides, fibrous tissue forms, holding the membranes together. This fibrous tissue is called an *adhesion.* Adhesions may occur in the pleura, in the pericardium, about the pelvic organs, and in many other parts of the body. They often occur in and around the intestinal tract, where they may cause an obstruction.

Instead of healing, necrosis, or death of the tissue, may occur. Bacteria, both pathogens and nonpathogens, often invade the necrotic tissue and cause decomposition, which is called *gangrene.* The body defenses are useless in preventing or curing gangrene because no blood can get to the area. Gangrenous tissue must be completely removed before healing can occur.

SPECIFIC DEFENSE MECHANISMS
CONCEPT OF AN ADAPTIVE SPECIFIC IMMUNE SYSTEM

Specific defense mechanisms within the body provide specific protection against a particular microorganism or molecular entity. This mechanism of protection leads to what is termed *specific immunity.* Depending on the relative levels of protection, the body may be able to defend itself totally or only partially from damage by the agent. The *immune system* is composed of many of the same organs, cells, and molecular entities operating to provide nonspecific defense. It works with the nonspecific mechanisms to focus and amplify the general mechanisms of defense against specifically recognized foreign materials.

The fundamental nature of the specific immune response is characterized by diversity, specificity, recognition, memory, and action. Among the most intriguing aspects of immune response is its *diversity of ability to respond* while at the same time responding with *specificity of action*. Almost any conceivable organic molecular array on the surface of a molecule has been shown to be able to induce a series of cellular events culminating in the production of *antibodies* (immunoglobulins).* These antibodies combine with the inducing *antigen (immunogen)* by virtue of combining sites on the immunoglobulin molecule that exhibit an extremely narrow specificity. The remainder of the immunoglobulin molecule is chemically and structurally similar to all other antibody molecules with distinctly different combining-site specificities.

Recognition and *memory* are two other aspects of this system that make it unique. The normal organism recognizes its own antigenic makeup and will not produce antibodies against its own antigens. This is known as *recognition of self*. At the same time this intricate system of self-recognition must be able to recognize extremely subtle changes in its own cells when incipient tumors that differ only slightly in antigenic constitution are forming. Further, once the immune system has responded to an antigen, subsequent encounters with that antigen produce an even more vigorous and rapid response. This response includes a wide variety of mechanisms designed to take *action* against the offending agent. Many of these actions are among the most potent biochemical and cellular reactions that the body can produce, yet they are focused so discretely that the foreign agent is rapidly destroyed with a minimum of damage to the host.

BASIC DESIGN OF THE SYSTEM

The basic design of the specific immune response system is such that the body provides itself with cells and molecules that can respond to and thwart encroachment by nonself materials rapidly and efficiently. The

system has two major interactive divisions: (1) a humorally mediated system of specifically designed proteins known as *antibodies* or *immunoglobulins* and (2) a cell-mediated system of specifically reactive WBCs known as *activated lymphocytes* or *T cells*. Both arms of the system are usually triggered to respond to encroachment; however, only one of the systems may provide the most protection against certain types of encroachment.

The *humorally mediated system* provides major immunity against (1) bacteria that produce acute infection (*Staphylococcus, Streptococcus, Hemophilus*, etc.), (2) bacterial exotoxins (diphtheria, botulinus, and tetanus toxins), (3) viruses that must enter the bloodstream to reach their target tissues (poliomyelitis, hepatitis virus, etc.), and (4) organisms that enter the body from the mucosal tissues (cold viruses, enteroviruses, influenza viruses, etc.). Even though circulating antibodies may be produced against other organisms (tuberculosis, HIV, fungi, etc.) these antibodies do not protect the body from infection.

The *cell-mediated system*, on the other hand, offers protection from: (1) chronic bacterial infections (syphilis, tuberculosis, leprosy, etc.), (2) many viral infections (measles, herpesvirus infections, chickenpox, etc.), (3) fungal infections (candidiasis, histoplasmosis, cryptococcosis, etc.), (4) parasitic infections (leishmaniasis, toxoplasmosis, *Pneumocystis* pneumonia, etc.), and (5) transplanted or transformed cells (tissue transplants, some transformed cells of cancer, etc.).

An individual can be immunodeficient (see Chapter 76) in one or both of these systems. When one system is not functioning properly, the individual becomes susceptible to infection or encroachment by the agents against which that system provided primary protection. For example, human immunodeficiency virus (HIV) infection and acquired immunodeficiency syndrome (AIDS) reduce the protection afforded by the cell-mediated system, making the individual susceptible to fungal infections (candidiasis), protozoan infections (*Pneumocystis* pneumonia), viral infections (herpesvirus infection), and cancers (Kaposi's sarcoma, lymphoma). Alternatively, the loss of the humorally mediated system that occurs in Bruton type agammaglobulinemia is accompanied by increased incidence of acute bacterial infections, respiratory tract infections, and GI tract problems. If both systems are lost or compromised, the individual is fully susceptible to infectious agents and cannot survive in an unprotected, nonsterile environment.

IMMUNE RESPONSE SYSTEM
IMMUNOGENS AND IMMUNOGLOBULINS
Immunogens (Antigens)

An immunogen is defined as a substance that, when introduced into an animal, elicits the formation of antibodies, or specifically sensitized cells. The antigen must be

---

*The terms *antibody* and *immunoglobulin* can be used more or less interchangeably and are used that way throughout this chapter. Specifically, antibody is the original, more general term describing serum agents that inactivate foreign substances in the body. It was coined in the early part of this century before the specific proteins of the serum had been identified as the globulin proteins of the γ-globulin fraction. The term *immunoglobulin* more specifically identifies the molecules of the serum that have antibody activity. In the same way, *antigen* is the original, more general term for foreign materials that elicit the immune response reaction; the newer, more accurate and interchangeable term for such materials is *immunogen*.

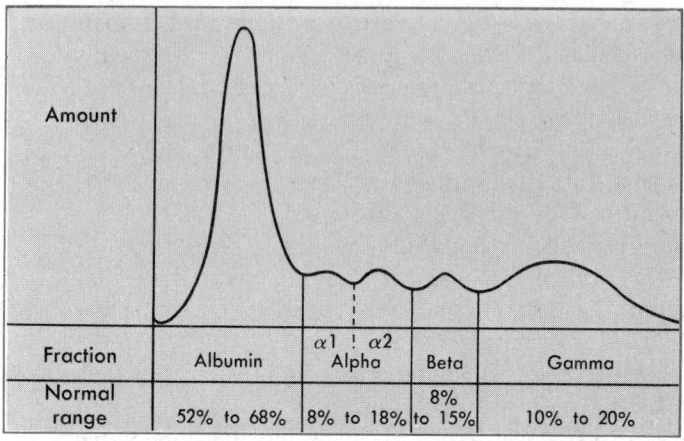

FIGURE 8-8 Electrophoretic separation of major serum proteins. Most antibody activity lies within the γ-globulin fraction. This fraction will rise with active synthesis of antibodies in response to antigenic stimulation.

recognized as nonself or foreign material within the body. Although most antigens are naturally occurring proteins of at least 10,000 molecular weight, other substances, such as polysaccharides, nucleoproteins, lipoproteins, and glycoproteins, may also serve as antigens. The bulk of the antigen consists of subsurface molecular structures that do not elicit an immune response but do serve as carriers for the multiple *antigenic determinants* on the surface. Most antigens have many antigenic determinants and are termed *multivalent antigens;* however, some molecules may be monovalent.

Because of their small size, certain molecules cannot induce the synthesis of antibodies; however, when cou-

FIGURE 8-9 Basic structure of IgG immunoglobulin monomer. All immunoglobulin classes are composed of variations of this basic structure with combinations to form dimers (IgA) or pentamers (IgM).

pled with a high-molecular-weight carrier, they can serve as antigenic determinants. These molecules are *incomplete antigens,* or *haptens.* They take on specific significance in the consideration of hypersensitivities, which are allergies to low-molecular-weight compounds such as certain drugs and antibiotics (see Chapter 76).

Immunoglobulins (Antibodies)

The body's response to the introduction of an immunogenic substance is the production of a specific, soluble immunoglobulin or a sensitized (antigen-reactive) lymphocyte population. The type of antigen introduced determines the immune response: antibody synthesis, antigen-reactive lymphocyte, or a combination of both.

The circulating antibodies represent modified (for example, antigen-specific) globulin proteins found in blood serum. The serum contains several distinct protein fractions, which are separable on the basis of their net electrical charge, molecular size, and molecular conformation into several fractions: albumin, α-globulins, β-globulins, and γ-globulins (Figure 8-8). The antibody activity of the serum is characteristically associated with the γ-globulin and β-globulin fractions. Those γ-globulins with the ability to bind antigens are called *immunoglobulins.* The immunoglobulins can be further subdivided into different *classes* on the basis of structure and function of the molecules. The generic symbol for immunoglobulins is Ig, and each of the classes is designated by a letter of the alphabet: IgA, IgD, IgE, IgG, and IgM (Table 8-5).

The basic pattern of structure for all immunoglobulins is based on a four-peptide chain monomeric unit (Figure 8-9). Two of the chains are of higher molecular weight and are termed *heavy* (H) *chains;* two are of lower molecular weight and are called *light* (L) *chains.*

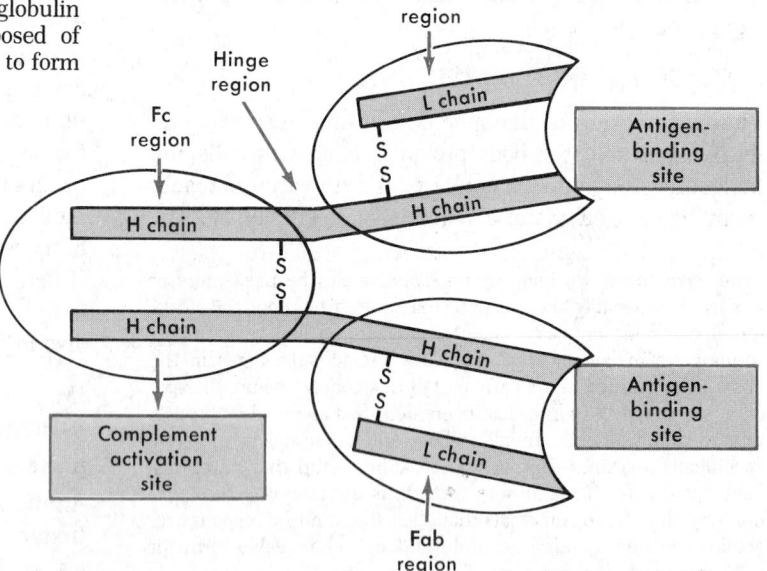

Each L chain is linked by disulfide (—ss—) bonds to an H chain, and in turn the H chains are linked to each other by disulfide bonds. When immunoglobulin monomers are visualized by electron microscopy, they are seen to have a Y-shaped structure. At the ends of the two arms of the Y are the sites where antigen is bound. Both the H and L chains participate in the formation of these *antigen-binding sites*. Thus most monomers of immunoglobulin have two antigen-binding sites and are termed *bivalent*. The two arms of the Y are designated the *Fab* (for fragment, antigen-binding) *regions*. The base of the Y is called the *Fc region* (for fragment, crystallizable). In the region of the disulfide bond joining the H chains, the molecule seems to be flexible, and this region is known as the *hinge region*.

The predominant class of immunoglobulins in normal adult serum is *IgG*. It makes up about 75% to 85% of the immunoglobulin fraction. Because of its structure and biologic activity, it is also found in the extravascular fluids of the body (Table 8-5). IgG is capable of crossing the placenta to provide the newborn with temporary natural passive immunity to those diseases against which the mother has circulating antibodies. It functions primarily in the processes of toxin neutralization and virus and bacterial inactivation and in the formation of antigen-antibody-complement immune complexes associated with certain types of hypersensitivity (see Chapter 76). IgG is the immunoglobulin class primarily responsible for the rise in serum antibodies during a secondary (anamnestic, booster) response (see p. 169).

IgM structurally is composed of five monomeric units attached to each other at the Fc region. Thus the star-shaped molecule with the antigen-binding sites pointed outward that results from this macromolecular arrangement is termed a *pentamer*. Sometimes this immunoglobulin class, which constitutes about 7% of the immunoglobulin in serum, is called the *macroglobulin* because of its molecular size. As a result of its size, it is confined primarily to the intravascular fluids. IgM, as with IgG, is capable of binding the C1 component of complement and initiating the complement cascade. In each antigenic stimulation, IgM antibodies are the first to appear, but they neither reach the levels of IgG nor exhibit an anamnestic response on subsequent antigen contact. They are primarily involved in providing protection against viral and bacterial invaders in the blood. Because of their ability to bind complement, they too are responsible for certain immune complex hypersensitivities and autoimmune diseases, such as rheumatoid arthritis.

IgA constitutes about 10% of the total immunoglobulin in serum. It can be found in a variety of polymeric forms (primarily monomer in serum and dimer in exocrine secretions). IgA is also termed the *secretory immunoglobulin* because it is found in the exocrine secretions of the body (milk, mucin, saliva, tears). Within these secretions IgA provides specific protection of the mucosal surfaces of the respiratory, digestive, and genital tracts from pathogenic invasion.

IgD makes up only about 1% of the immunoglobulin fraction of serum. Its biologic functions are unknown. Most of the IgD is found on the surface of some lymphocytes, where it probably plays a role in the activation and suppression of lymphocyte function.

TABLE 8-5 Properties of immunoglobulin classes

Property	Immunoglobulin Class				
	IgG	IgM	IgA	IgE	IgD
Physiochemical					
Percentage of Ig	82	7	10	0.002	1
Configuration	Monomer	Pentamer	Monomer, dimer	Monomer	Monomer
Half-life in serum (days)	23	5	6	2	3
Functional antigen-binding sites	2	5	2	2	2
Biologic					
Principal site found	Internal body fluids	Serum	Serum and exocrine secretions	Tissue bound	Bound to lymphocyte surface
Fixed complement	Yes	Yes	No	No	No
Crosses placenta	Yes	No	No	No	No
Principal functions	Agglutination, detoxification, virus neutralization; enhances phagocytosis	Agglutination, cytolysis, enhances phagocytosis	Protection of mucosal surfaces	Mediates immediate type of hypersensitivity	Control of lymphocytic activation and suppression

IgE is present in the serum in extremely small amounts (0.002%). This is the result of this immunoglobulin's predilection for attachment to the surface of mast cells and basophils. Once bound by the Fc region of the monomer to the surface of these cells, which are rich in the potent, physiologically active substances histamine, kinins, and serotonin, IgE serves to mediate the severe and occasionally fatal anaphylactic type of hypersensitivities. These include anaphylactic shock, allergic asthma, and hay fever (see Chapter 76). The protective role of these immunoglobulins is not clear, but they may be effective in providing protection against certain parasitic worms.

Immunogen-Immunoglobulin Interactions

When an immunoglobulin comes in contact with its specific antigen, a physical interaction occurs between the two, causing a reversible binding of the antibody to the antigen. The antibody's affinity for the antigen and the avidity, or tightness, of the binding depend on the location and spatial arrangement of the antigenic determinants on the antigen's surface and how well the antigen-combining site on the antibody molecule "fits" the antigenic determinant. Since the antigen is usually multivalent and the antibody is generally at least bivalent, the antigen molecules may be cross-bound and clumped (agglutinated, precipitated) by antibody molecules (Figure 8-10).

Within the body the binding of antibody to the antigen can have direct beneficial effects, such as detoxification of toxins, inactivation of viruses, or, coupled with complement, the direct lysis of cells. However, in most cases the antigen-antibody combination initiates and facilitates the nonspecific defense mechanisms (phagocytosis, complement, inflammatory response, and so forth).

CELLS INVOLVED

The cells involved in the specific immune response are all derived from the original undifferentiated stem cells of the bone marrow. The stem cell may develop into any of the blood cells of the body, depending on various signals and influences. The primary cells of the immune response system develop from the lymphocytic cell population (Figure 8-11). One population of lymphocytic cells undergoes differentiation under the influence of the thymus gland and becomes *thymus-dependent lymphocytes,* or *T cells.* These cells become responsible for mediating the *cell-mediated immune* (CMI) *response.* Another population of lymphocytes matures in a site other than the thymus and is known as *thymus-independent lymphocytes,* or *B cells.* The designation B cell comes from the fact that in the chicken, where this process was first detected, a single site exists where this differentiation occurs, that is, the *bursa of Fabricius.* No such singular lymphoid organ is found in humans, but it is believed that the process occurs in the bone marrow or possibly the gut-associated lymphoid tissues (tonsils, Peyer's patches of the intestines, appendix). The exact site in the human has not been unequivocably identified, so it is often referred to as the *bursa equivalent.* The B cells are responsible for production of the immunoglobulins and provision of the *humoral immune response.*

The role of the lymphocytes (B or T cells) is to recognize the presence of an antigen and to initiate specific mechanisms of disposal. Just as important, the lymphocyte must recognize a component of host tissues as *self* and protect that tissue from immunologic response reactions.

B cell and T cell lymphocytes can be differentiated from each other on the basis of specific *markers* (membrane-bound proteins) on the surface of the cells. For instance, T cells have a marker that causes the binding of sheep RBCs, whereas B cells are lacking such protein. B cells, on the other hand, usually have immunoglobulins displayed on their cell surface. By the identification of the specific markers on the cell surface, cells can be divided into B cell or T cell type and even further subdivided into subtypes (see later discussion on helper and suppressor T cells).

A third type of cell is directly involved in the immune response, the *antigen-presenting cell* (APC). These cells are found primarily in lymph nodes (follicular dendritic cells), spleen, thymus, and skin (Langerhans' cells). The macrophage of the bloodstream and lymphoid tissues may also function as APCs as well. The main role of these cells is to capture antigens introduced into the tissues or draining to regional lymphoid tissues, process the antigen within the cell, concentrate the antigenic determinant, and present the antigen to antigen-sensitive lymphoid cells. The processed antigenic signal is displayed on the surface membrane of the APC. Antigen presented to lymphocytes by cell-to-cell contact triggers the series of events within the lymphocytes that leads to full immunologic response.

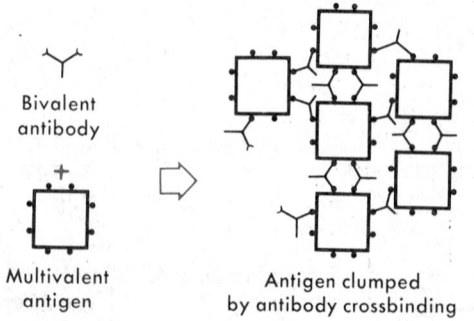

Bivalent antibody

+

Multivalent antigen

Antigen clumped by antibody crossbinding

FIGURE 8-10 Clumping of multivalent antigen by its specific antibody.

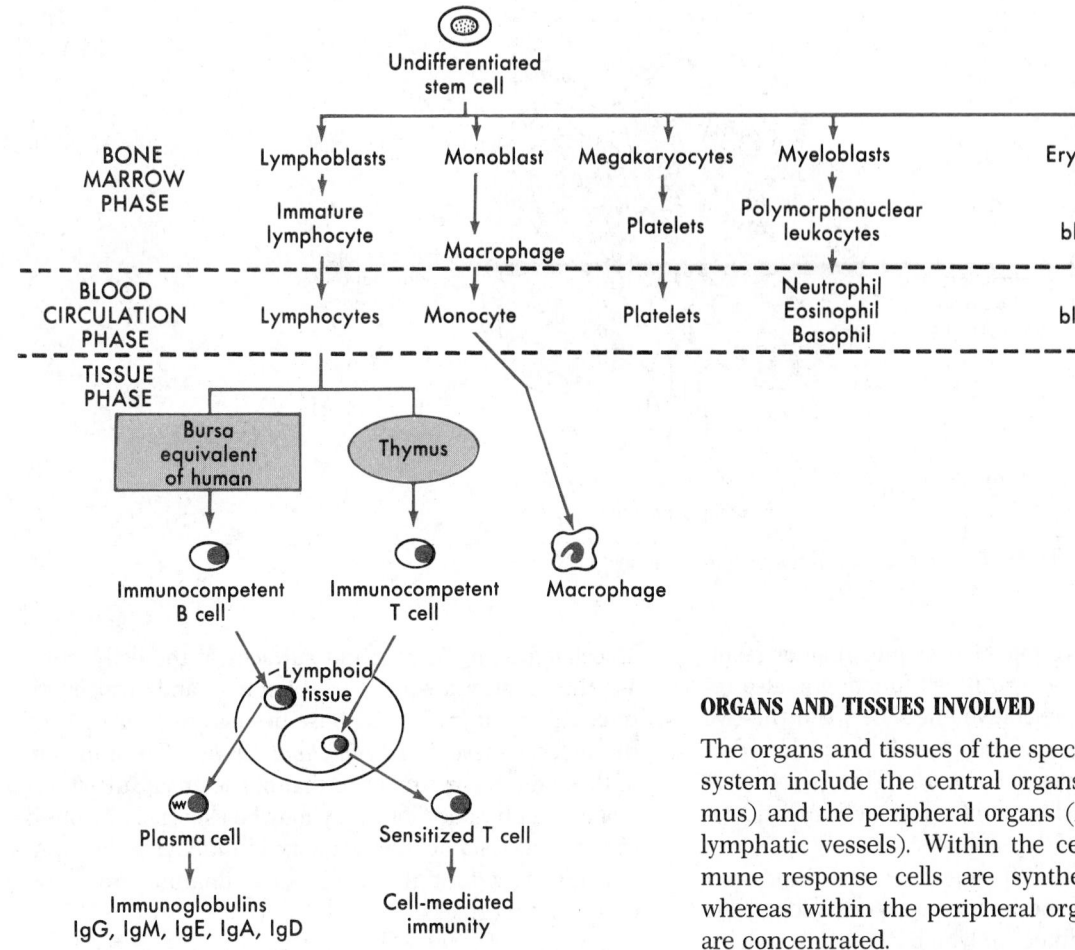

FIGURE 8-11 Development of B and T cell lymphocytes.

At the other end of the immune response, the macrophage is activated by activated lymphocytes to its maximum of phagocytic efficiency by the release of stimulatory, soluble substances known as *lymphokines* (Table 8-6). In this way the macrophage is stimulated at the site of an immune reaction. Other soluble lymphokines serve to attract the macrophages to the site by chemotaxis. In addition, activated macrophages, sometimes called "angry" macrophages, produce complement components, prostaglandins, and interferon.

Another type of lymphoid cell, called the *null cell,* has characteristics of B lymphocytes, T lymphocytes, and macrophages. Currently it is thought that these cells are not programmed to respond to specific antigens but are rather recruited by immune response reactions to nonspecifically attack and kill tumor cells and virally infected cells. When activated and directed against foreign cells, these are referred to as *natural killer* (NK) *cells.*

ORGANS AND TISSUES INVOLVED

The organs and tissues of the specific immune response system include the central organs (bone marrow, thymus) and the peripheral organs (lymph nodes, spleen, lymphatic vessels). Within the central organs the immune response cells are synthesized and matured, whereas within the peripheral organs the mature cells are concentrated.

The *thymus* serves as the control organ of the immune system. It is the differentiation site of the T cell lymphocytic populations and, through certain soluble thymic hormones, serves to regulate the overall immune system. The activity of the thymus reaches its peak in childhood, and the organ begins to shrink in size after puberty. If the thymus is removed (thymectomy) very early in an animal's life, a severe state of immunodeficiency is induced and T cell–mediated immunity never develops. The thymectomized animal develops a wasting disease characterized by stunted growth, diarrhea,

TABLE 8-6 Lymphokines liberated by activated T cell lymphocytes

Lymphokine	Function
Lymphocyte-derived chemotactic factors	Chemotactic for macrophages
Lymphocytotoxins	Nonspecific lysis of cells
Macrophage inhibition-activation factors	Maintains macrophage at site and activates it
Interferon	Inhibits replication of viruses
Lymphocyte-activating factors	Activates nonsensitized lymphocytes

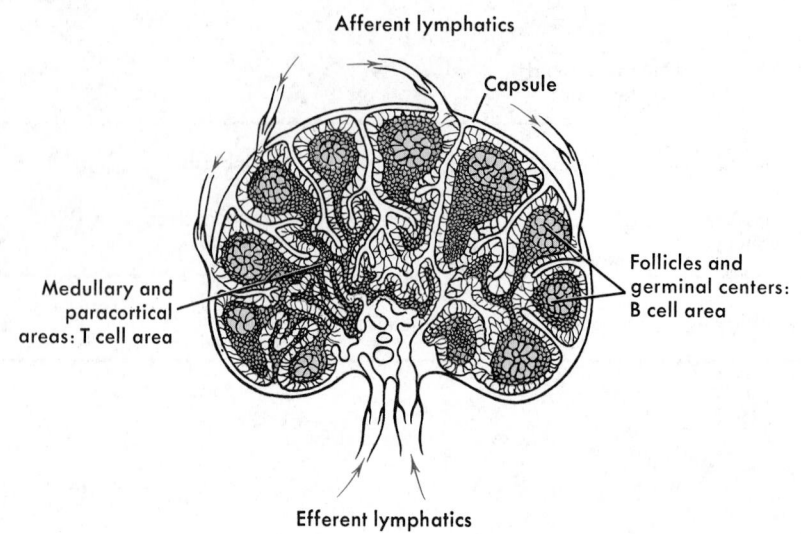

FIGURE 8-12 B and T cell areas of lymph node.

and death from massive infection by intestinal or respiratory tract normal flora. The B cell function is also reduced, pointing to a cooperative effect between the two basic systems. The loss of the thymus from the adult animal creates less severe reactions. This is probably caused by the establishment of an already functional, long-lived population of T cells.

The *lymph nodes* and *spleen* serve as the primary sites of localization of the immune response cells. The lymph node serves to filter the lymph drained from a region of tissue. The structure of the lymph node (Figure 8-12) consists of an inner medullary and paracortical region made up primarily of T cells and an outer cortex composed of clusters, or germinal centers, of B cells known as follicles. The spleen is structured on somewhat the same pattern with diffusely packed T cell areas and germinal centers of tightly packed B cells. In certain types of antigenic stimulation, either the T cell or the B cell areas show tissue proliferation, whereas the other area remains quiescent. By the same principle, if a person is suffering a basic primary immunodeficiency of one system, the corresponding area of lymph nodes and spleen may not be populated by its normal contingent of cells (hypoplastic).

During the course of the immune response reaction, within the lymph nodes there is significant proliferation of specific cells and migration of phagocytic cells to the site, which may lead to lymph node enlargement. Enlargement of the lymph nodes in a region may be the result of (1) infections, (2) immune diseases, (3) intrinsic neoplasms of the lymph node itself, or (4) metastatic spread of malignant cells to the node. The presence of an enlarged spleen or enlarged lymph nodes is almost always an important clinical finding.

Other nonencapsulated lymphoid tissues are found associated with the mucosal surfaces of the body, such as the gastrointestinal, respiratory, and urogenital tracts. These immune response tissues are referred to as the *mucosal-associated lymphoid tissues*. The function of these tissues is similar to that of the encapsulated regional lymph nodes, but they may be especially involved in the synthesis of the secretory immunoglobulin, IgA, which is important in providing total immune protection of mucosal surfaces.

PRIMARY IMMUNE RESPONSE

Antigenic Challenge

When an antigen is introduced into the body, it can trigger a wide or narrow spectrum of response mechanisms. The specific pattern of response depends on (1) the amount of antigen introduced, (2) the site of introduction, and (3) the type of antigen introduced.

Small amounts of a noninvasive, large, particulate antigen introduced at a single body site are quickly and efficiently handled at a local site with little or no systemic involvement beyond the local lymph node. Since the inflammatory response and local lymph node can localize the spread of the antigen, the immune response may go completely unnoticed by the host organism. Larger, particulate antigens are readily cleared, but small, soluble antigens are more difficult to clear from the circulation.

Large amounts of an antigen may allow the antigen to escape from the local site by simply overwhelming the local defense mechanisms. Even though the lymph nodes and reticuloendothelial organs can clear 80% to 90% of an antigen on a single pass, if the amount of the antigen is extremely large, some antigen may escape the local site. An excessively large, sustained antigen dose can exhaust not only the local site but the entire

RES as well. This greatly reduces the body's ability to respond to even minor invasive challenges and renders the host vulnerable to secondary infections.

Highly invasive antigens (for example, bacteria such as *S. aureus* or *S. pyogenes*) or those introduced directly into the bloodstream by blood transfusion, intravenous catheterization, or injection can immediately establish a systemic type of immune response. This is why extreme care must be exercised in the use of any type of medical procedure that would allow the introduction of antigens into the general circulation. The localization action of the immune response is critical to efficient functioning of the response.

Antigenic Processing and Presentation

When an antigenic substance is introduced into the body, it is either carried directly by lymphocytic circulation to a regional lymphoid tissue, where it is engulfed by an APC, or an APC engulfs the antigen at the site of introduction and carries the antigen to the lymphoid tis-

sues. In the APC the complex antigen is degraded, and the antigenic determinants are attached to one of the cell membrane proteins on the APC known as a *major histocompatability complex* (MHC) antigen on its surface. These same MHC antigens are the markers on the surface of the cell that allow recognition of self versus nonself cells (see Figure 8-2). The APC, with the concentrated antigenic determinants, then *presents* this antigenic signal to specifically reactive B cells or T cells in the regional lymph node. This is accomplished by a cell-to-cell contact. With this interaction the specific B cell or T cell is stimulated to undergo proliferation (cell division) and differentiation (change in structure and function). A soluble material known as *interleukin 1* (IL-1) released from the APC signals the lymphocyte to divide and differentiate.

Humoral Response

When the antigen is introduced for the first time, one of three basic mechanisms of response is elicited: (1) a re-

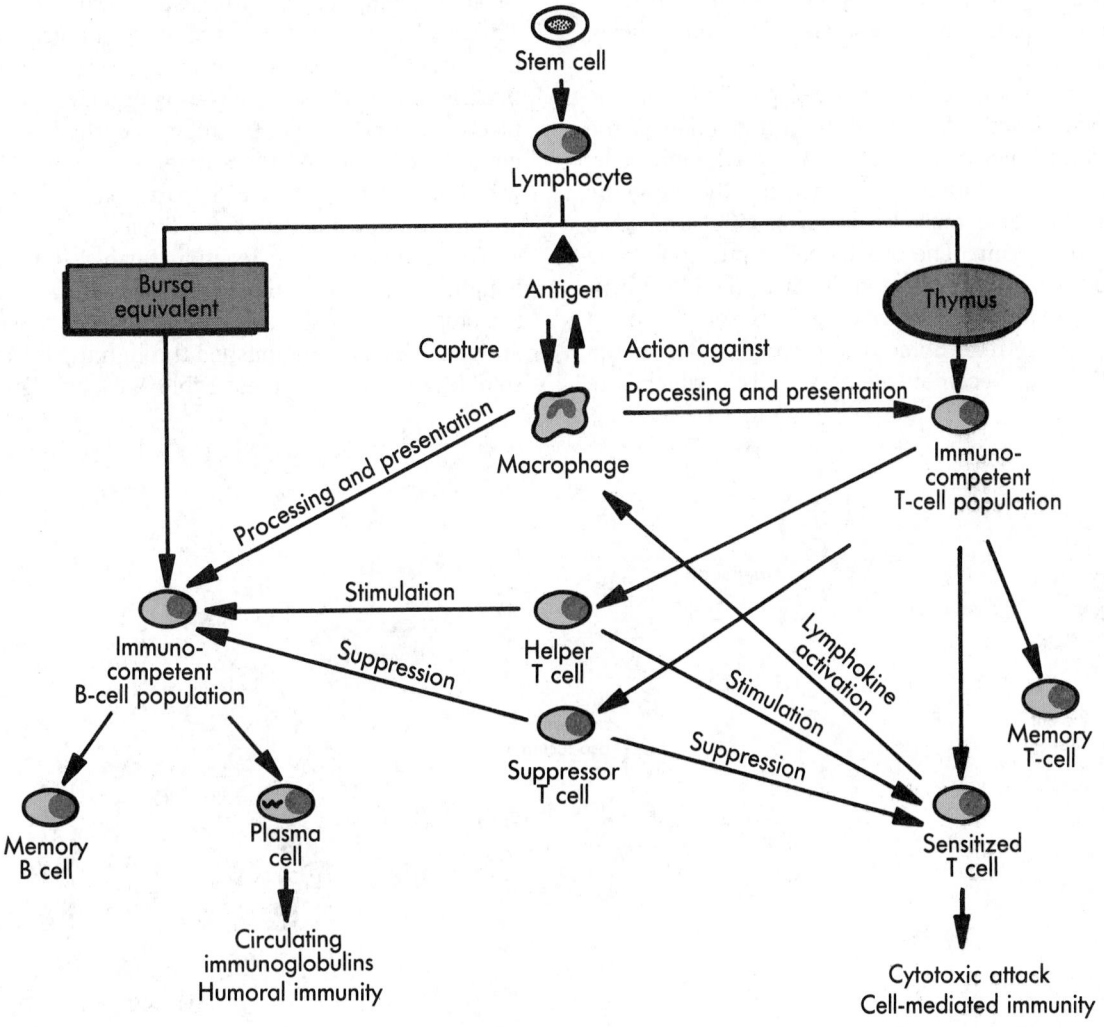

FIGURE 8-13 Combined response of B and T cell systems.

sponse mediated primarily by B cells, the humoral response; (2) a response in which the T cells are primarily involved, the CMI; or (3) a combined type of response.

If the antigen is the type that triggers a humoral response, the first time the body is exposed to the antigen the B cell system responds with the synthesis of circulating immunoglobulins (Figure 8-13).

Antigen-specific B cells bear receptors on their surface, which allow them to recognize their antigenic stimulant. These receptors are the antigen-specific immunoglobulin molecules that the cell is programmed to produce. They are embedded in the membrane by the Fc region of the monomer with their antigen-binding sites extended out. Seemingly only a few lymphocytes within a lymph node have the ability to respond to the antigen. The stimulated B cell then begins a process of proliferation and differentiation. The progeny of the stimulated cell increases in number within the lymph node, forming *clones* of specifically adapted lymphocytes. With each generation of new cells within the clone, the lymphocytes become more differentiated toward a cell population ideally suited for the synthesis and release of immunoglobulin. These cells are known as *plasma cells*.

With the development of this cell population in the lymph node (several days after the introduction of the antigen), antibodies can be detected in the lymph node. However, it is not until about 7 days after the antigenic challenge that detectable levels of specific antibodies appear in the serum. The plasma cell population of the lymph node and the levels of antibody in the blood continue to increase for another 2 to 3 weeks, and then both begin to retreat. Some of the lymphocytes of the activated clone become "memory cells," which are

much more responsive, both in time of reaction and efficiency of antibody synthesis, to subsequent contact with the antigen (Figure 8-14).

The humoral response serves to protect the body from such agents as microbial toxins, bacteria within the extravascular spaces in the blood and on mucosal surfaces, and viruses that must pass through the circulatory system to reach their site of infection (for example, poliomyelitis virus).

Cell-Mediated Immune Response

Certain antigens trigger a response mediated by T cell proliferation and reaction. A T cell that has received its antigenic stimulus is referred to as a *sensitized T cell lymphocyte* (see Figure 8-13).

The initial steps of the CMI response, those involving the antigen processing by the macrophage, or APC, seem to be the same as in the humoral response. Following the presentation of the antigenic stimulus to lymph node T cells, proliferation in the T cell domain occurs. Circulating antibodies are not released; rather, sensitized lymphocytes are released into the circulation. These cells migrate to the site of the antigen's entrance into the body, where the invading agent or residual antigen is found. These activated lymphocytes, along with macrophages, infiltrate the regions of the tissue and begin a direct attack on the antigen or tissue cells labeled with the antigen. The T cells participating in this direct attack are known as *cytotoxic T cells*.

To amplify the site reaction further, the sensitized lymphocytes activate the nonspecific phagocytotic cells (macrophages, PMNs, null cells) in the region of the antigen. This is accomplished through the release of the soluble lymphokines (see Table 8-6), which marshal

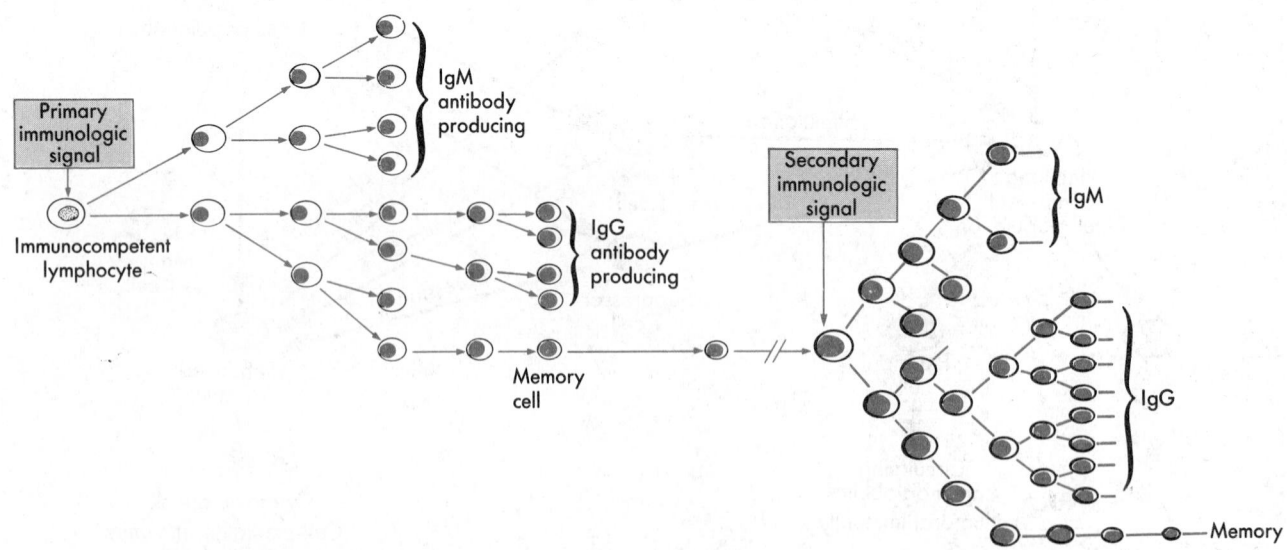

FIGURE 8-14 Response of memory cells to antigen signal.

this additional cellular involvement to attack the antigenic materials.

The observable results of this attack of antigen-labeled tissues is classically illustrated by a positive tuberculin test reaction. In this case the inflammation (erythema, induration) observed at the site of the intradermal injection of a small amount of cell wall extract of *Mycobacterium tuberculosis* represents a T cell attack on the antigen-labeled cells. The positive test is actually mediated by a secondary immune response (see following discussion) produced by prior exposure to *M. tuberculosis*. With the introduction of the antigen, it is engulfed, processed, and presented by the APC to responsive clones of T cells in the regional lymph node. That clone of cells is stimulated to undergo proliferation, and activated T cells are released into circulation. The activated T cells seek out the antigen (at the site of injection) and begin to accumulate at the site, where they release lymphokines that stimulate null cells and macrophages to attack the tissues at the focal site. The lag time (24 to 48 hours) required for the development of the inflammation at the site is consistent with the time needed to trigger the release of the responsive cells from the regional lymph node and their accumulation at the site of the antigen-labeled tissues.

The CMI response is especially effective in protection against diseases that grow and do their damage intracellularly, where the circulating immunoglobulins cannot reach them. Diseases of this type include viral and rickettsial diseases and those produced by certain chronic types of infective agents, the most outstanding of which are fungal pathogens and tubercle bacillus. One other important function of this system is the provision of *cancer cell surveillance* (see p. 175).

Combined Immune Response

Most antigens do not cause a purely humoral or purely CMI response; rather, both types of response are evoked. Likewise, our protection against most harmful antigens is the result of both these specific response systems being brought to bear on the antigen involved. In the combined type of response an initial perturbation occurs within the T cell areas of the lymph node. This becomes obvious within about 2 days after the introduction of the antigen. About 3 to 5 days later the B cell areas begin to proliferate.

Control of Immune Response

The production of a full immune response is, of necessity, under control systems. One type of control is a nonspecific mechanism known as *antibody feedback*, by which the increasing level of circulating immunoglobulins serves as a negative force on the further synthesis of antibodies. In other words, if circulating immunoglobulin levels are elevated, it is more difficult to stimu-

late antibody production with further antigenic challenge. This has clinical significance in the case of abnormal antibody production by individuals suffering from gammopathies, such as multiple myeloma or macroglobulinemia, (see Chapter 76). These diseases are marked by significant elevation of the γ-globulin fraction of the blood and a seemingly paradoxical increased susceptibility to infection. The high levels of nonspecific γ-globulin exert an immunosuppressive effect on further specific antibody synthesis when the host is challenged by a pathogen.

The immune response system is also controlled by the presence of specific regulator T cells. A subset of the T cell population of the body is known as *helper T cells* (designated T_H or T_4 cells). The function of these cells is to cooperate with the B cells and T cells to allow the full expression of a B cell or T cell response. If a B cell clone required the aid of a helper T cell clone and the T_H cell clone is missing, the B cell clone will not undergo proliferation and differentiation to form plasma cells that produce the specific immunoglobulin. On the other hand, the presence of *suppressor T cell* clones (designated T_S or T_8 cells) prevents or suppresses the full development of the immunoresponsive clones (see Figure 8-13).

If for some reason the normal balance between immunoresponsive T or B cells and T_S and T_H cells is disrupted, control over proper immune response reactions may be lost. The classical example of this problem can be observed in AIDS, where a disproportionate rise occurs in the number of T_S (T_8) cells compared to T_H (T_4) cells in peripheral circulation; this results from destruction of the T_H cells caused by HIV infection. In other conditions, such as some autoimmune diseases, the loss of certain T_S clones may allow the production of antibodies against self antigens.

SECONDARY IMMUNE RESPONSE

As emphasized at the outset of this section, one of the touchstone characteristics of the specific response system is its ability to remember prior contact with an antigen and to provide a more rapid and efficient protective reaction on subsequent contact. The first contact between the immune response system and an antigen leads to the primary response, as just described. When antibody synthesis is measured in a primary response, there is a significant lag time to the appearance of antibodies in the circulation (Figure 8-15). Immunoglobulins of the IgM class are the first to appear, but they maintain protective levels for only a short period. Specific IgG antibodies follow and reach protective levels within 12 to 14 days, but they also fall off fairly quickly with only this initial exposure. When the "primed" immune response system encounters the antigen again, a secondary response ensues, which is more rapid, of

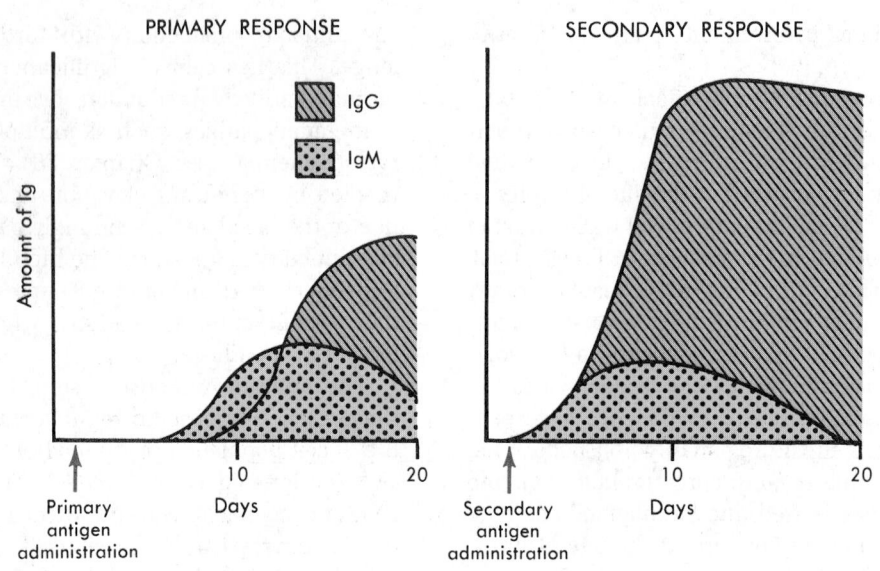

FIGURE 8-15 Primary and secondary humoral responses.

greater intensity, and longer lasting than the primary response. This secondary response is also termed an *anamnestic response*. This "remembered" response is a characteristic of both the B and the T cell systems. The prior contact with the antigen is stored in special memory cells of both cell lines. As illustrated in Figure 8-14, the memory cells respond immediately to the antigenic signal, so the lag time between exposure to the antigen and production of protective antibody levels is greatly reduced. This phenomenon provides the basis for active immunization and "booster" doses to maintain the protective levels of immunity. In an immunized individual the memory cells elicit the rapid response in time for the immune system to overwhelm the pathogen or toxin before it can produce its damage. These memory cells are long-living lymphocytes, surviving and able to respond for years following their development.

IMMUNE TOLERANCE

Immune tolerance is defined as the state of immunologic nonresponsiveness. By some mechanisms the body becomes tolerant to self while maintaining responsiveness to foreign materials. Evidence establishes that self-tolerance is acquired primarily during embryonic development; however, the exact mechanisms by which it develops remain an issue. During fetal development the immune system is presented with antigens from the developing tissues. These become identified as self antigens; thus, when exposed to these antigens postnatally, the individual is tolerant of them.

One proposed mechanism by which this state could be induced is known as the *clonal selection theory*. This theory states that when potentially responsive clones of

B or T cells come into contact with an antigen prenatally, the responsive cell line is killed or controlled, thus eliminating the responsiveness to that antigen from the body. This produces a state of *natural tolerance*. This theory is supported by experimental data that show that, by exposing experimental animals to foreign antigens in utero, a tolerance to that antigen is developed; however, some antigens introduced in this manner are found to be more *tolerogenic* (capable of inducing tolerance) than others. Further, the clonal selection theory does not explain how it is possible to break tolerance in adults, as indicated in certain experimental studies or with certain autoimmune diseases (see Chapter 76). In some cases at least, tolerance is not caused by the total elimination of specifically reactive cells but by the blocking of expression or temporary inactivation of the responsive cells. The action of suppressor T cells or the failure of mobilization by helper T cells has been shown to play a significant role in maintaining the state of self-tolerance.

DEVELOPMENTAL ASPECTS OF IMMUNE RESPONSE

Lymphoid cells first appear in the fetus as stem cells in the fetal liver at about the end of the first trimester. The lymphoid tissues of the thymus also develop fairly early in the fetus. At birth, however, the lymph nodes and spleen are still underdeveloped, but T and B cell responsiveness is fully functional. The fetus is capable of some immune response if challenged by an in utero (within the uterus) infection, such as congenital syphilis or rubella. Unless the fetus has been exposed to a congenital infection, at birth the neonate-synthesized immunoglobulin levels are low (Figure 8-16). The child does

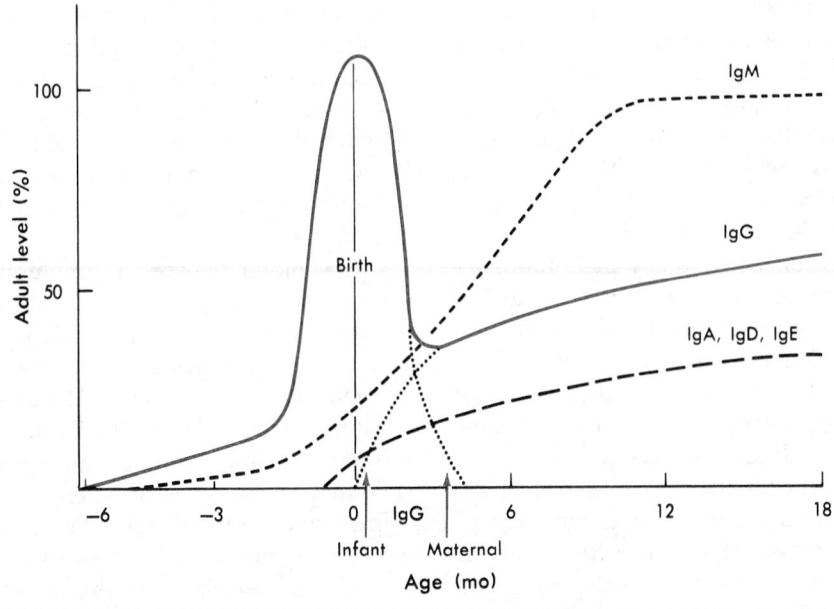

FIGURE 8-16 Immunoglobulin levels in fetus and neonate.

have high levels of transplacentally acquired maternal IgG antibodies. These maternal antibodies have a half-life of about 30 days in the child; this, coupled with the increase in blood volume in the growing infant, leads to a drop in the IgG levels of the blood over the first 3 months. Thereafter the rate of the child's own synthesis of IgG provides for a steady increase in the immunoglobulin concentration within the serum. IgM levels reach adult concentrations by about age 9 months.

Numerous studies in both animals and humans have shown that during the aging process a progressive loss of immunologic vigor occurs. The prime immunologic age probably is achieved during the late adolescent years, when virtually the full complement of immunities has been developed and the responsiveness of the system peaks. The middle years are characterized by a plateau and slowly falling curve until the later years of life, when a sharp decline becomes evident. This decline is seen in both CMI and humoral response systems. This loss in immunologic sensitivity is associated with an increasingly less effective and more misdirected immune response. There is an increasing frequency of autoimmune disease, susceptibility to pathogenic and opportunistic microorganisms, and incidence of cancer.

NEUROENDOCRINE FACTORS INFLUENCING IMMUNE RESPONSE

The cells of the immune response system are influenced by and in turn influence the other regulatory communication systems in the body, that is, the endocrine and neural systems. The immune response cells have receptors on their surface to receive modifying inputs from the full array of hormones: insulin, growth hormone, glucocorticoids, estrogen, testosterone, and so on. Some of these hormone signals (glucocorticosteroids, testosterone, estrogen, progesterone) have been shown to depress immune function. Other hormones (growth hormone, thyroxine, insulin) tend to improve immune function. Other neurotransmitters and hormones found in lower doses in the body also influence immune response cell function. The negative effects of the corticosteroids are so great that they are widely used as pharmacologic agents to suppress immune function (see Chapter 76).

The thymus gland functions as an endocrine organ, releasing hormones that influence not only immunoresponsive cells and lymphoid tissues but other body cells that have receptors for these hormones. Interleukin 1 and other lymphokines have been shown to stimulate glucocorticosteroid synthesis by influencing the pituitary gland to release adrenocorticotropic hormone (ACTH). The thymus and lymphoid tissues receive direct innervation from autonomic and sensory neurons that control blood circulation to these organs and also seem to exercise more direct control over the immune response cells themselves.

The physiologic control of the neuroendocrine function has long been recognized in the immunosuppressive effects produced by the stress response. Growing evidence suggests that this immunosuppression is also produced indirectly through neural signals to the immunoresponsive tissues.

These interconnections between the three major communication systems of the body has led to the development of the following concept: although many aspects of each system can be considered to stand alone, a broader, more holistic perspective views them as functioning as an interrelated complex. The term *psychoimmunoendocrine system* has been developed to reflect this more inclusive conceptualization. With this perspective in mind, the increasing use of psychotherapeutic methods and cognitive visualization has been increasingly used as adjunctive therapy in immune-related diseases and cancer. However, because most of the connections between these systems are fairly indirect and because our understanding of the control functions of each is still tenuous, these therapies should never be relied on as a primary approach. Also, some potential danger exists in leading clients to believe that they can exercise direct cognitive control over their pathologies. When they are not successful, clients may become disillusioned and lose hope, which then removes whatever positive aspects might be derived from the indirect betterment of their overall improved immune state. The emphasis should be on the general and broad improvement of their general immune state.

APPLICATIONS AND IMPLICATIONS OF IMMUNE RESPONSE

CONCEPT OF SUSCEPTIBILITY AND IMMUNITY

The objective of the biologic defense mechanisms is to provide the host with protection. The ultimate protection would be total resistance to encroachment or damage by an organism or agent; this is usually termed *absolute immunity*. Absence of such protective barriers is called *susceptibility*. Although these terms are generally applied to immunity from infectious organisms, they can be used to describe the relative susceptibility to encroachment by an external agent. As described earlier, nonspecific immunity, or innate immunity, is provided when the external and internal nonspecific defense mechanisms serve as the barrier excluding or destroying the invading agent. Specific immunity protects against a single, unique agent through the development of specific antibodies or responsive cells in the body. It is acquired from prior contact with the agent (antigen) or through the introduction of specifically protective antibodies or cells into the body.

The acquisition of specific immunity may result from a natural encounter or artificial introduction. Immunity acquired *naturally* means under such natural conditions as recovery from a disease. Immunity acquired *artificially* means the antigen or protective antibodies were purposely introduced into the body by vaccination. The immunity may be active or passive. When an individual is producing the antibodies within the body, the immunity is termed *active*. When an individual receives the protective antibodies from some other source, the

immunity is termed *passive*. Thus, when antibodies are transferred from the mother across the placenta, the child is said to have a natural passive immunity. When a vaccine is given so that antibodies are produced within the body, the immunized individual is characterized as having an artificial active immunity. Table 8-7 summarizes the different types of acquired specific immunities.

Specific or nonspecific immunity to harmful agents is a relative state. The effects of different dosages of an infectious organism or the toxic products of such organisms in experimental studies clearly demonstrate that administration of sufficiently large numbers of an organism or high dosages of a toxin can overwhelm even the most highly immunized animal. Further, when the normal mechanisms of defense are breached, even in the highly resistant host, disease can result. Thus acquired immunity to infection is not always an absolute condition but depends on many complex variables. These include not only the defense mechanisms of the host but also the dosage, route of contact, and virulence of the harmful agent.

IMMUNIZATION

Long before the mechanisms of immune response were worked out, it was recognized that recovery from certain diseases conferred protection against subsequent exposure to that disease. Dating from the days of Jenner's vaccination with cowpox exudate to protect against smallpox (1798), through the success of Pasteur with anthrax and rabies (1880s), and up to the present, the specific protective mechanisms of the immune system have been used to protect against serious infectious diseases.

PASSIVE IMMUNIZATION

Temporary protection, usually measured in days or at most weeks, is afforded by the acquisition of preformed antibody from another host. As the acquired antibodies are used up through binding with antigen or by being catabolized, the protection is lost.

Transplacental passive immunization occurs through the transfer of IgG antibodies from the maternal circulation across the placenta to the fetal blood. Some acquisition of immunoglobulins also occurs through the colostrum of the mother's milk. A common misconception is that infants acquire large amounts of circulating antibodies from breast milk that are added to their own. Most of the protective immunoglobulins passed in maternal milk are of the IgA class and offer some protection to the infant's GI tract. Antimicrobial factors other than immunoglobulins are also present in the milk and probably account for most of the decreased incidence of infections observed in breast-fed versus bottle-fed infants.

TABLE 8-7 Types of acquired specific immunity

Type of Immunity	Acquisition of Immunity	Protection	Examples
ACTIVE			
Antibodies synthesized by body in response to antigenic stimulation	*Natural:* natural contact with antigen through clinical or subclinical case	*Development:* develops slowly; protective levels reached in a few weeks. *Duration:* long term; often lifetime. *Spectrum:* specific to antigen contacted	Recovery from childhood diseases (for example, chickenpox, measles, mumps)
	Artificial: immunization with antigen	*Development:* develops slowly; protective levels reached in a few weeks. *Duration:* several years; extended protection with "booster" doses. *Spectrum:* specific to antigen immunized against	Immunization with live or killed vaccines; toxoid immunization
PASSIVE			
Antibodies produced in one individual transferred to another	*Natural:* transplacental and colostrum transfer from mother to child	*Development:* immediate. *Duration:* temporary; several months. *Spectrum:* to all antigens that mother has immunity	Maternal immunoglobulins in neonate
	Artificial: injection of serum from immune human or animal	*Development:* immediate. *Duration:* temporary; several weeks. *Spectrum:* to all antigens that source has immunity	Injection of pooled human γ-globulin; injection of animal hyperimmune sera

Artificial passive immunization may be necessary if the individual to be immunized has suffered exposure to a serious infectious agent to which he or she has no immunity or if the individual's own immune system is impaired or deficient. The sources of these preformed antibodies are pooled human adult γ-globulin or heterologous (from another species) globulin fractions. Pooled human γ-globulin has been used to modify the effects of measles, particularly in premature infants, in children with primary immunodeficiencies, and in patients undergoing immunosuppressive therapies. Individuals who have contact with persons with hepatitis and smallpox may also be protected by this method. It should be noted, however, that isolated γ-globulin preparations tend to form small protein aggregates; if injected intravenously, these could lead to severe anaphylactic reactions (see Chapter 76). For this reason the material is always administered *intramuscularly.*

The most frequently used heterologous antibody fractions are antitetanus and antidiphtheria antisera derived from horse globulins. Since these are foreign proteins, they can lead to the development of serum sickness (see Chapter 76). Serum sickness is more likely to occur in subjects already primed by previous contact with horse globulin; thus multiple use of heterologous sera is to be avoided.

ACTIVE IMMUNIZATION

The objective of active immunization is to provide effective long-term immunity by establishing within the individual's own body the capacity (1) to produce effective levels of immune response and (2) to establish a population of sensitive cells that can respond to a subsequent antigenic contact.

Immunizing agents ideally should be noninjurious to the individual being immunized. To accomplish this, the pathogenic effects must be modified, and at the same time the antigenicity of the agent must be maintained. Bacteria exotoxins such as those produced by diphtheria and tetanus bacteria can be successfully detoxified by formaldehyde treatment without destroying the major antigenic determinants on the protein molecule. Such detoxified antigenic materials are called *toxoids.* The use of *killed vaccines* of viruses and bacteria can also provide a safe antigen for immunization. Killed vaccines include those for pertussis (whooping cough), typhoid and cholera, and the Salk poliomyelitis vaccine. The protection conferred by these vaccines is generally inferior to that produced by live vaccines. Some of the most successful vaccines consist of living organisms that have been modified so that they are non-virulent. The *attenuated live vaccines* provide excellent protection, but some risk exists in their use because of the possibility of reversion to the virulent form of the organism. Live vaccines of importance are those for measles, mumps, and tuberculosis (BCG) and the Sabin poliomyelitis vaccine.

The provision of protective levels of residual immunity depends on the inducement of (1) the right type of response (that is, cell mediated or humoral), (2) in sufficient amounts, (3) at the right place (that is, where the immune response can contact the antigen), and (4) against the right antigenic determinants (that is, the antibodies formed produce an inactivating effect). Simply inducing an immune response is not sufficient to provide protection. For example, the early killed virus measles vaccines elicited a splendid production of circulating antibodies against the measles virus, but protection against measles is most effectively mediated by cellular immune responses. The humoral protection did not prevent infection.

Another problem of immunization for which provision must be made is the *interference* that one antigen may have with another if the two are given simultaneously. The live virus vaccines occasionally interfere with each other; when measles and smallpox vaccines are administered at the same time, they each interfere with the development of immunity by the other. This is probably the result of interferon production. Some live virus vaccines contain more than one strain of the virus, and these can cross-inhibit. In the case of the Sabin oral polio vaccine, three separate doses are required because there are three strains within the same vaccine. With the initial dose, immunity to only one strain may develop if the strain interferes with the other two.

COMPLICATIONS OF IMMUNIZATION

Although immunization is the most successful approach to control many infectious diseases, minimal but potentially serious risks are involved. The development of postvaccination encephalitis or other neural autoimmune complications is a serious risk with such vaccines as those for smallpox or rabies. Children with immunodeficiencies may be overwhelmed by vaccination with live vaccine. With viral vaccines, which are produced in monkey kidney of human cell culture, a slight risk exists of introducing oncogenic (cancer-causing) viruses. A fetus may be significantly at risk if the mother receives a live virus vaccine during pregnancy. Such live vaccines should never be administered to a pregnant woman.

Besides these rather serious risks, general discomfort is to be expected from some forms of immunization.

The typhoid vaccine, for instance, is composed of large numbers of killed *Salmonella* bacteria; since the endotoxic cell wall materials of these cells is a pyrogenic (fever-producing) substance, fever and malaise are possible sequelae. The influenza vaccines often produce febrile reactions in children.

TISSUE TRANSPLANTS

The transfer of healthy tissues and organs from one individual to replace damaged or diseased tissues in another has been surgically possible for many years. Early attempts failed because the body rejected the foreign cells and tissues. With the growing knowledge of the immune response, the mechanisms of this rejection process became more apparent. It is now possible to make judgments and predictions concerning the likelihood of transplantation success. The course of the graft transfer process now can be controlled to favor the acceptance of the transplanted tissue.

The antigenic determinants of the tissues that lead to graft rejection are primarily found on the surface of the cells within the transplanted tissues. These antigens are known as *histocompatibility antigens* and are controlled by independently segregating genes on chromosome 6 within the chromosomal structure of the human. They are also called *human leukocyte antigens* (HLA). Some of the histocompatibility antigens are more antigenic than others; thus some antigens are referred to as major and others as minor. The major transplantation antigens are those of the ABO and Rh blood groups and the HLA (see Chapter 76).

Graft rejection can be minimized by use of chemical (drug) or physical (radiation) agents that nonspecifically or specifically interfere with the development of an immune response reaction against the foreign tissue. Clinically, four types of chemical immunosuppressive agents are effective in providing the transitional protection needed to promote establishment of the graft (Table 8-8).

Glucocorticoids, especially prednisone, are significantly antiinflammatory and impair lymphocyte (B and T cell) activation and function. Prednisone exerts a wide spectrum of activity against all immune response and inflammatory response mechanisms. Although it suppresses the cell-mediated system more than the humoral system, the continued high dosage needed to maintain cell-mediated suppression creates significant risks in reducing the responsiveness of the humoral system. Often lower dosages of prednisone and azathioprine are used together because they seem to act synergistically.

Antimetabolites and *alkylating agents,* such as azathioprine and cyclophosphamide, act nonspecifically against rapidly dividing cells within the body, and thus they are also used for cancer chemotherapy. They inter-

TABLE 8-8 Effect of selected drugs on the immune system

Drug	Immune System Impairment	Indications for Immunosuppressive Therapy
Corticosteroids	Impairment of T cell function Catabolism of immunoglobulins (decreased IgG) Lymphocytopenia Type 1 hypersensitivity: vasoconstriction, eosinopenia Type 3 hypersensitivity: decreased vascular permeability Type 4 hypersensitivity: decreased macrophage function	Diseases for which immune disorder is unknown Tissue and organ transplantation Autoimmune diseases
Antimetabolites (azathioprine)	Interference with RNA, DNA, and protein synthesis Depression of bone marrow and antibody reproduction Decreased primary immune response	Autoimmune diseases Tissue transplantation Dermatologic disease (pemphigus, psoriasis) Neoplasia
Alkylating agents (cyclophosphamide)	Interference with DNA, RNA, and protein synthesis Lymphocytolytic effect Suppression of primary immune response	Autoimmune disease Tissue transplantation Inflammatory disease of unknown cause
Antilymphocytic serum (ALS, ALG)	Inhibition of lymphocyte stimulation by specific antigens Inhibition of lymphocyte mobility Agglutination and lysis of lymphocytes in the presence of complement	Renal transplantation Bone marrow transplantation Autoimmune diseases
Antibiotics (actinomycin D, chloramphenicol, tetracycline, cyclosporine)	Interference with DNA-directed RNA synthesis Suppression of primary immune response Inhibition of protein synthesis	Cyclosporine for tissue transplantation

fere with DNA synthesis and with the B and T cell systems.

A more specific immunosuppression of the T cell system is achieved with *antilymphocytic serum* (ALS). ALS blocks the action of the sensitized cells in circulation while leaving the lymph node B cell system only slightly suppressed. This leaves the host with protection against the humorally protected infectious agents while guarding against the most active rejection system.

Cyclosporine (cyclosporin A), is an antibiotic derived from fungi that exerts its action on the T lymphocytes. Success with this drug has greatly improved the prognosis after transplantation.

CANCER IMMUNOLOGY

One of the primary functions of the CMI system seems to be the recognition and destruction of cancer cells within the body. By the same mechanisms operative in allograft rejection, it is postulated that the immune system continually protects against the establishment of tumor growths. The recognition of these cells as nonself is based on the appearance of "new" surface antigens that allow identification. A growing body of evidence supports the view that this is a vital function of the immune system. Patients in whom the cellular immune system is impaired (immunosuppressed) or defective (immunodeficient) for significant periods are at especially high risk of developing certain neoplastic diseases. To these data is coupled the observation that cancers are most prone to appear early in life, before the immune system is fully functional, or in later life as the system becomes less effective.

Cancers may become established in the body by escaping the surveillance mechanisms or by growing so rapidly that they outdistance the immune system's ability to respond. Experimentally, if a few thousand tumor cells are transferred from a cancerous animal to a noncancerous animal, the latter is capable of responding and destroying the tumor; however, if the tumor cell load is increased to several billion cells, the tumor may become established. The humoral immune system may actually serve to protect the developing cancer by producing noncytotoxic antibodies (*enhancing antibodies*) that coat the tumor cell surfaces and mask the surface from recognition by sensitized lymphocytes. As a tumor grows, it is capable of both specific and nonspecific suppression of the immune system. This further reduces the effectiveness of a response.

Some of the new surface antigens, known as *tumor-specific transplantation antigens* (TSTA), appearing on the cancerous cell are shed into the circulation and can be immunologically detected there. Some of these antigens, such as carcinoembryonic antigen (CEA) and α-fetoprotein (α-FP), are present during fetal development but are not expressed in the adult. Their reappearance lends support to the theory that cancer represents a dedifferentiation to a more primitive cell. These antigens, termed *oncofetal antigens* (OFA), are of some significance in early detection, diagnostic confirmation, and determination of malignant disease progress.

Some very early progress has been made in stimulating, both specifically and nonspecifically, the body's immunologic response to cancers in the hope of preventing further growth of the tumors. With further knowledge of both the cancer process and the immune response mechanisms, the possibility of using immunotherapy, immunoprophylaxis, and immunodiagnosis as specific tools against malignancies seems realistic.

MONOCLONAL ANTIBODIES

A recent technologic breakthrough in tissue culture technique has made it possible to develop and isolate antibodies of great specificity for single antigenic determinants. Normally, immunoglobulins that are produced in the body in response to antigenic challenge bind to various antigenic determinants introduced on the multivalent antigen. The antibodies themselves are produced by a variety of B cells responding to the antigen signal;

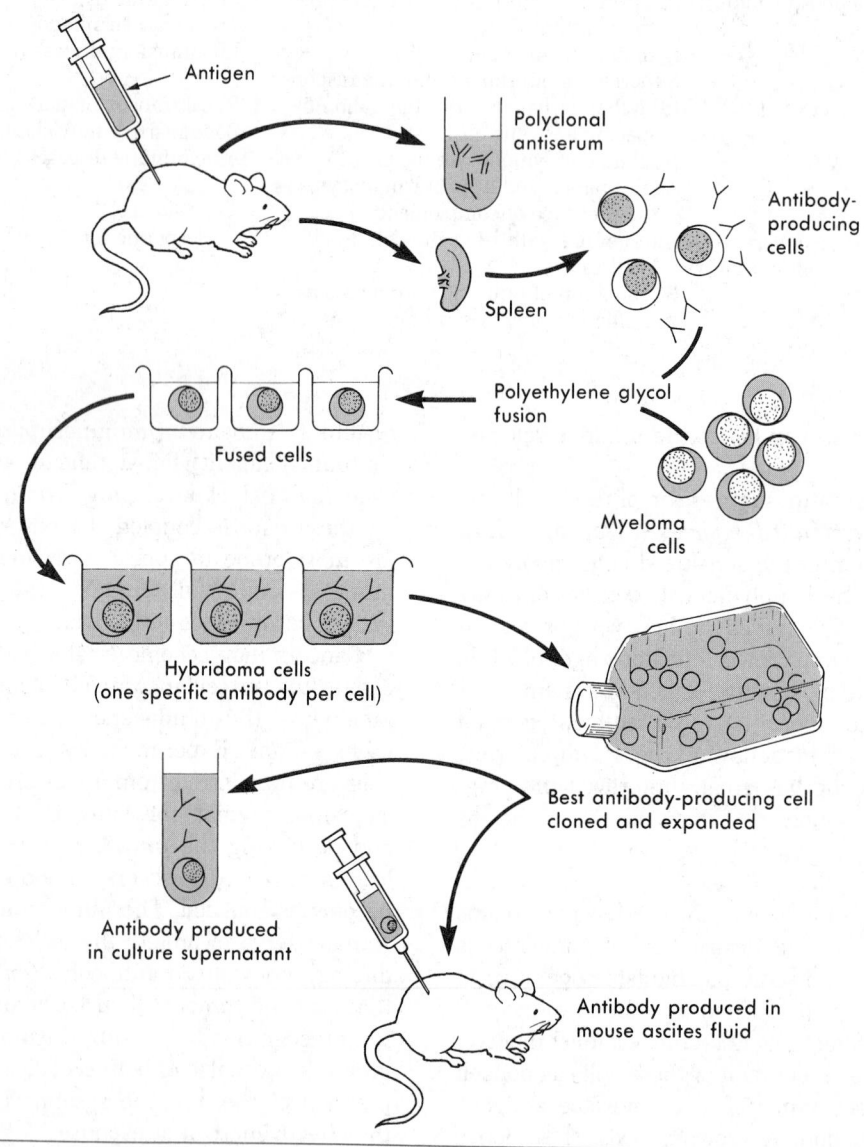

FIGURE 8-17 Production of a monoclonal antibody. (From Baron ES and Finegold SM: Bailey and Scott's diagnostic microbiology, ed 8, St Louis, 1989, The CV Mosby Co.)

thus 90% of the antibodies produced have little or no avidity for specific antigenic determinants. By a technique for the production of immortal clones of *hybridoma* cells (made by the fusion of normal antibody-producing B cells with an appropriate B cell tumor line) and selection of single clones of cells producing only a single, highly specific antibody, large quantities of highly antigen-specific antibodies can be isolated (Figure 8-17). These immunoglobulins are known as *monoclonal antibodies*.

The clinical and diagnostic implications for the use of monoclonal antibodies are enormous. It is now possible to identify individual cell types (such as T_H versus T_S lymphocytes, partially differentiated versus mature cells) with very specific cell markers, to diagnose malignant transformed cells, or to type tissue using monoclonal antibodies for each HLA subtype. Therapeutically, it is possible to bind a toxic molecule or radioactive isotope to the monoclonal antibody and have it delivered specifically to a tumor cell bearing a specific tumor cell marker, thus sparing all nontumor cells of the body. Monoclonal antibodies will dramatically alter our ability to identify, characterize, and treat many of the most significant pathologies.

CHAPTER SUMMARY

✔ The human body is protected from encroachment by foreign materials and cells by a system of protective structural and biochemical barriers.

✔ If foreign materials or cells gain access to internal body tissues, they are recognized and attacked by a system of specifically and nonspecifically responding mechanisms.

✔ The humorally mediated immune response is mediated by B cell lymphocytes, which produce circulating antibodies that bind antigens.

✔ The cell-mediated immune response is mediated by T cell lymphocytes, which produce activated T cells that seek out and attack antigen-labeled cells.

✔ The secondary immune response provides a faster and more efficient response on contact with the specific antigen a second time.

✔ Immunization provides the body with protection against tissue-damaging infections and toxic substances.

✔ The immune response system plays a direct role in rejection of tissue transplants and in recognition of and protection against neoplastic transformation.

QUESTIONS TO CONSIDER

- What would happen if the immune response system did not properly distinguish "self" cells and inappropriately labeled them as "nonself"?

- We have come to regard fever and leukocytosis as negative pathologic responses that call for intervention, such as antipyretic therapy. Why may this be an inappropriate perspective?

- Several years ago, David, the child who had been raised throughout his entire life in a germ-free, controlled environment in Houston, died following an attempt to transplant bone marrow taken from his sister. He represented a most severe case of altered immune response.
  a. What is the usual fate of children born with the same alteration as David?
  b. The decision to place David in the controlled environment was made in 1973, when it was considered just a matter of time before theoretic and technical breakthroughs would reverse his condition. What were some of the expected breakthroughs?
  c. Why was a bone marrow transplant attempted? What was the medical team hoping would happen?
  d. Why was David's sister chosen to be the donor?
  e. After David's death, his body was autopsied and revealed a cancer caused by the Epstein-Barr virus, which normally does not produce cancer. Explain the probable reason for the cancerous response in David.
  f. What similarities seem to exist between David and AIDS patients?

REFERENCES AND SELECTED READINGS

1. *Ada GL and Nossal G: The clonal selection theory, Sci Am 257:52-69, 1987.
2. Alt FW et al: Development of primary antibody repertoire, Science 238:1079-1087, 1987.
3. *Baradana EJ: A conceptual approach to immunodeficiency, Med Clin North Am 65:959-962, 1983.
4. Barrett JT: Textbook of immunology, ed 5, St Louis, 1987, The CV Mosby Co.
5. *Besedovsky HO, Del Ray AE, and Sorkin E: What do the immune system and brain know about each other? Immunol Today 4:342-347, 1986.
6. *Beverly PC: Antibodies and cancer therapy, Nature 297:358-359, 1982.
7. Bloom BR: Natural killer cells to rescue immune surveillance? Nature 300:214-217, 1982.

*References preceded by an asterisk are particularly well suited for student reading.

8. Bolognesi D, editor: Human retroviruses: cancer and AIDS, New York, 1988, Alan R Liss, Inc.

9. Bornstein DL: Leukocytic pyrogen: a major mediator of the acute phase reaction, Ann NY Acad Sci 389:323-326, 1982.

10. *Cassileth, B: Mind over body, Cancer News, Winter 1986, pp 6-20.

11. *Cohen IR: The self, the world and autoimmunity, Sci Am 258:52-60, 1988.

12. *Cohn ZA, editor: Innate immunity, Current opinion in immunology, vol I, London, 1988, Current Science Ltd.

13. Colter HR, Alper CA, and Rosen FS: Genetics and biosynthesis of complement proteins, N Engl J Med 304:653-655, 1981.

14. *Fauci AS: Activation and regulation of human immune responses: implications in normal and disease states (NIG conference), Ann Intern Med 99:61-65, 1983.

15. Gewurz H et al: C-reactive protein and the acute phase response, Ann Intern Med 27:345-348, 1982.

16. Goodwin JS, Searles RP, and Tung SK: Immunological responses of a healthy elderly population, Clin Exp Immunol 48:403-407, 1982.

17. *Grey HM, Sette A, and Baus S: How T cells see antigens, Sci Am 261:56-64, 1989.

18. *Hall NR and Goldstein AL: Thinking well: the chemical links between emotions and health, Ann NY Acad Sci 34:40-45, 1986.

19. Herberman RB: Natural killer cells, Hosp Pract 17:93-97, 1982.

20. Herberman RB, editor: Basic and clinical tumor immunology, Boston, 1983, Martinus Nijhoff Publishing.

21. *Jaroff L: Stop that germ, Time 131:56-64, 1988.

22. *Jett MF and Lancaster LE: The inflammatory-immune response: the body's defense against invasion, Crit Care Nurs 5:64-66, 1983.

23. Joiner KA, Brown EJ, and Frank MM: Complement and bacteria, Annu Rev Immunol 2:461-472, 1984.

24. Law SKA and Reid KBM: Complement, Oxford, 1988, IRL Press.

25. *Lind M: The immunologic assessment: a nursing focus, Heart Lung 9:658-660, 1980.

26. LoBuglio AF, editor: Clinical immunotherapy, New York, 1980, Marcel Dekker, Inc.

27. *Lydyard DM, editor: Immune response, Current opinion in immunology, vol II, London, 1988, Current Science Ltd.

28. Marrack P and Kappler J: The T cell receptor, Science 238:1073-1078, 1987.

29. *Matje D: Stress and cancer: a review of the literature, Cancer Nurs 9:339-401, 1984.

30. McMichael AJ and Fabre JW, editors: Monoclonal antibodies of clinical medicine, New York, 1982, Academic Press, Inc.

31. *Merigan TC: Human interferon as a therapeutic agent—current status, Science 308:1530-1535, 1983.

32. Mims CA and White DW: Viral pathogenesis and immunology, Oxford, 1984, Blackwell Scientific Publications, Ltd.

33. *National Institute of Health: Understanding the immune system, No 84-529, Washington, DC, 1983, US Department of Health and Human Services.

34. Playfair JHL: Immunology at a glance, ed 2, Oxford, 1984, Blackwell Scientific Publications, Ltd.

35. *Porth CM: Pathophysiology, ed 2, Philadelphia, 1986, JB Lippincott Co.

36. *Riley V: Psychoneuroendocrine influences on immunocompetence and neoplasia, Science 212:1100-1103, 1981.

37. Roitt I: Essential immunology, ed 6, London, 1988, Blackwell Scientific Publications, Ltd.

38. Roitt I, Brostoff J, and Male D: Immunology, ed 2, St Louis, 1989, The CV Mosby Co.

39. *Seeley RR, Stephens TD, and Tate P: Lymphatic system and immunity: anatomy and physiology, St Louis, 1989, Times Mirror/Mosby College Publishing.

40. Stites DP et al: Basic and clinical immunology, ed 6, Los Angeles, 1987, Lange Medical Publications.

41. Truitt RL, Gale RT, and Bortin MM, editors: Cellular immunotherapy of cancer, New York, 1987, Alan R Liss, Inc.

42. Unane ER: Antigen-presenting function of the macrophage, Annu Rev Immunol 2:395-397, 1984.

43. Underdown BJ and Schiff JM: Immunoglobulin A, Annu Rev Immunol 4:389-417, 1986.

44. Vitetta ES et al: Redesigning nature's poisons to create antitumor reagents, Science 238:1098-1104, 1987.

45. *Weksler ME: The senescence of the immune response, Hosp Pract 16:55-58, 1981.

46. Young JD and Cohn ZA: How killer cells kill, Sci Am 258:38-44, 1988.

47. Young JD and Doherty PC: Multiple mechanisms of lymphocyte-mediated killing, Immunol Today 9:140-144, 1988.

CHAPTER 9

Neuroendocrine Response to Stressors

VIRGINIA L. CASSMEYER

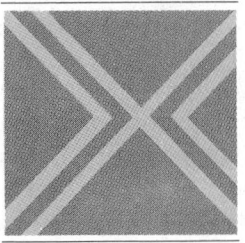

CHAPTER OBJECTIVES

After studying this chapter, the student should be able to:
1. Define stressor and stress.
2. Describe the general adaptation syndrome.
3. List three criticisms of the stress response as identified by Seyle.
4. List major stressors common to adult hospitalized patients.
5. Diagram the neuroendocrine response to stressors.
6. Describe the major functions of epinephrine, norephinephrine, cortisol, aldosterone, ADH, beta-endorphins, and growth hormone in response to stressors.
7. Describe three situations in which an impaired or compromised neuroendocrine response to stressors may occur.

The ability of the human body to initiate and sustain a response to noxious stimuli is one of the major protective mechanisms that allows individuals to exist in a hostile environment. Both the healthy and ill—those in the hospital, in extended care facilities, or in their own homes—are exposed to noxious stimuli. Because noxious stimuli are so ubiquitous, the individual must possess some mechanism to deal with them. One such mechanism is the stress response.

STRESS/STRESSORS DEFINED

Every reader will have some concept of the word stress. But for the purpose of this chapter *stress is defined* as:

An integrated body response, including intellectual, behavioral, emotional, and physiologic components, to a stimuli that is perceived on a conscious or unconscious level as noxious or threatening. The response serves as a protective mechanism. It is elicited to allow the individual to adapt to or adjust to noxious or threatening stimuli and is graded; varies depending on the type, strength, and duration of the stimuli; and is modified by characteristics of the person.

Stressor is defined as

A noxious or threatening stimulus that can elicit the stress response. A stressor may be actual or potential, biophysical-

chemical, or psychosocial-cultural. Although most of the stressors that are seen in patients in the hospital are negative stimuli and severe in nature, stressors can be positive stimuli, such as marriage, physical exercise, or the birth of a child. They can be nonsevere, everyday hassles. Also important in the definition of stressors is that, although some of the more severe stimuli would probably be stressors for anyone, there is great individualization of stressors, with individuals differing as to which stimuli are perceived as stressors.

Before preceding with a discussion of the stress response, mention must be made of one scientist whose work provided a basis for our current knowledge about the stress response.

HANS SELYE

The scientist with whom the concepts of stress and stressor are most closely associated is Hans Selye. Selye, while a medical student, observed in diverse persons with various diseases similar signs and symptoms that he labeled as the *syndrome of just being sick*.[27] When he first observed this syndrome, he questioned whether the underlying mechanism could be identified. Years later, while involved in experimental studies designed to discover a new hormone, he noted that injections of a tissue extract, which supposedly contained the hormone, resulted in enlargement of the adrenal cortex, ulcers of the gastrointestinal tract, and atrophy of the lymph nodes and thymus gland.[26] Although, Selye[27] at first ascribed these changes to the hypothetical hormone supposedly in the tissue extract, he later found that injections of any extracts, as well as other stimuli, such as cold and x-rays, caused the same response.

GENERAL ADAPTATION SYNDROME

Selye labeled this nonspecific response to various agents the general adaptation syndrome (GAS).[26,27] GAS became known as the stress syndrome and was viewed by Selye as having three stages:
1. *The alarm reaction,* during which protective resources are mobilized

2. *The stage of resistance* that occurs when the full syndrome is in place and the stressor is being controlled

3. *The stage of exhaustion* that occurs when the body is not able to control the stressor.

Selye[26] also proposed that the hormones produced during GAS were responsible for the diseases of adaptation. The stress response or GAS involves the sympathetic branch of the autonomic nervous system and the pituitary and adrenal glands. Selye also described the *local adaptation syndrome* (LAS), which is the response to a locally applied stimulus. The inflammatory process is an example of LAS.

Selye's work built on the work of Walter Cannon, who in 1935 described the stresses and strains of homeostasis. Cannon was most interested in the mechanisms by which the body maintained a relatively constant composition. Although we now know that the body composition is in a dynamic state, Cannon's idea that the body had to make adjustments to internal changes to remain healthy was a building block for understanding the body's response to noxious stimuli.

Some major criticisms of Selye's work must also be noted. First, in his early work, Selye did not acknowledge that psychological events could serve as stressors. It is important to note that his later writings did acknowledge this fact.[25] The work of various persons as early as the 1950s[12] revealed that the GAS could be elicited in response to psychological stimuli.

Another criticism of Selye's work was the idea that stimuli that serve as stressors were stressors for everyone. The work of Lazarus[16] and Cox[7] pointed out that a stimulus must be preceived as a stressor before the GAS response is elicited. Important in this perception process is the analysis of the stimulus in terms of the person's resources and the perception of the stimulus as controllable or uncontrollable.

Another important factor in relation to psychological and emotional influences on physiologic stressors is that in some experiments[19-21] where physical stressors were induced while controlling or minimizing the discomfort, suddeness, or unpleasantness of the stimuli, the GAS was not elicited. This may mean that all stressor stimuli must have a psychosocial-cultural component.

One last criticism of Selye's work relates to his description of the stress response as nonspecific. This characteristic meant that the same response occurred regardless of the stressor. Current data do not support this assumption. In animal studies,[17] it has been shown that different hormonal and neurochemical responses occur in response to different stressors. Despite these criticisms, Selye's work still provides the basis of the physiologic response that can be elicited by stressors and an appreciation of the various stimuli that may serve as stressors in many persons.

STRESSORS

Many different studies have shown that stressors can be biologic, physical, chemical, social, developmental, cultural, or psychological stimuli.[2,8,13,23,29] Stressors can range from the daily hassles of an alarm clock that doesn't go off on time, to an approaching deadline, to the onset of the common cold in a relatively healthy person, to major burns over 50% of the body. The stressors that the nurse deals with vary depending on the patient population. The nurse in an outpatient setting, in home health care, or in discharge planning may focus more on the daily hassles and primary health care problems. The nurse working with patients during the acute or critical stages of illness may deal with more severe stressors.

The box below lists some common stimuli affecting hospitalized adults that may be perceived as stressors. This list is not inclusive, but does contain stressors that might be more universally found in acute and critical care settings. The list can be used by the nurse as assessment of a patient is being implemented. One of the first steps in providing quality care to control stressors is to be able to identify potential stressors.

COMMON STIMULI AFFECTING HOSPITALIZED ADULTS THAT MAY BE PERCEIVED AS STRESSORS

BIOPHYSICAL-CHEMICAL

Hypoxia	Infections
Hypercapnia	Trauma
Hypoglycemia	Pain
Hypovolemia	Any illness
Hypotension	Surgery
Decreased cardiac output	Immobilization
Alcohol	Restraints
Caffeine	Constant light
All drugs	Noise
X-ray contrast media	Sleep deprivation
Anesthesia	Discomfort
Blood transfusions	Fatigue
Weakness	Burns

PSYCHOSOCIOCULTURAL

Anger	Anxiety
Fear	Uncertainty
Loss	Dependency
Isolation	Invasion of privacy
Sensory overload	Sensory deprivation
Role changes	Financial burdens
Guilt	Language barriers
Loss of control	Exposure of body
Stigma of diagnosis	Unpleasant sights and sounds
Unfamiliar sounds	Change in body image

STRESS RESPONSE

Although the stress response includes intellectual, behavioral, and emotional components, such as decision-making activities, withdrawal, and anger, a major part of the response is the psysiologic components.

The physiologic components involved in the stress response include the central nervous system, the hypothalamus, the sympathetic nervous system, the anterior and posterior pituitary gland, the adrenal medulla, and the adrenal cortex. The physiologic components and their secretions (hormones and catecholamines) are responsible for the neuroendocrine response to stressors. As discussed earlier in this chapter, not all of these components will necessarily be involved in the response to every stressor; but to provide wholistic nursing care, the nurse must know the effects of stimulation of each of these components of the neuroendocrine response to stressors. Understanding the response is critical to (1) identify persons at high risk for impaired ability to deal with stressors, (2) understand how prolonged or repeated stressors can result in disease, and (3) understand how the neuroendocrine component of the stress response can eventually become a threat to health.

The physiologic components of the neuroendocrine response to stress are diagrammed in Figure 9-1. Stressors, either perceived at the level of the central nervous system or on an unconscious level by baroreceptors, chemoreceptors, or glucoreceptors, which transfer information to the medulla oblongata, serve as the afferent input. This information is eventually forwarded to the hypothalamus, which coordinates the response. The hypothalamus activates the sympathetic nervous system and the anterior and posterior pituitary glands. The adrenal medulla is an extension of the sympathetic nervous system and thus is activated when the sympathetic nervous system is stimulated.

The hypothalamus stimulates the anterior pituitary gland by releasing hormones such as corticotropin-releasing hormone (CRH), growth hormone-releasing

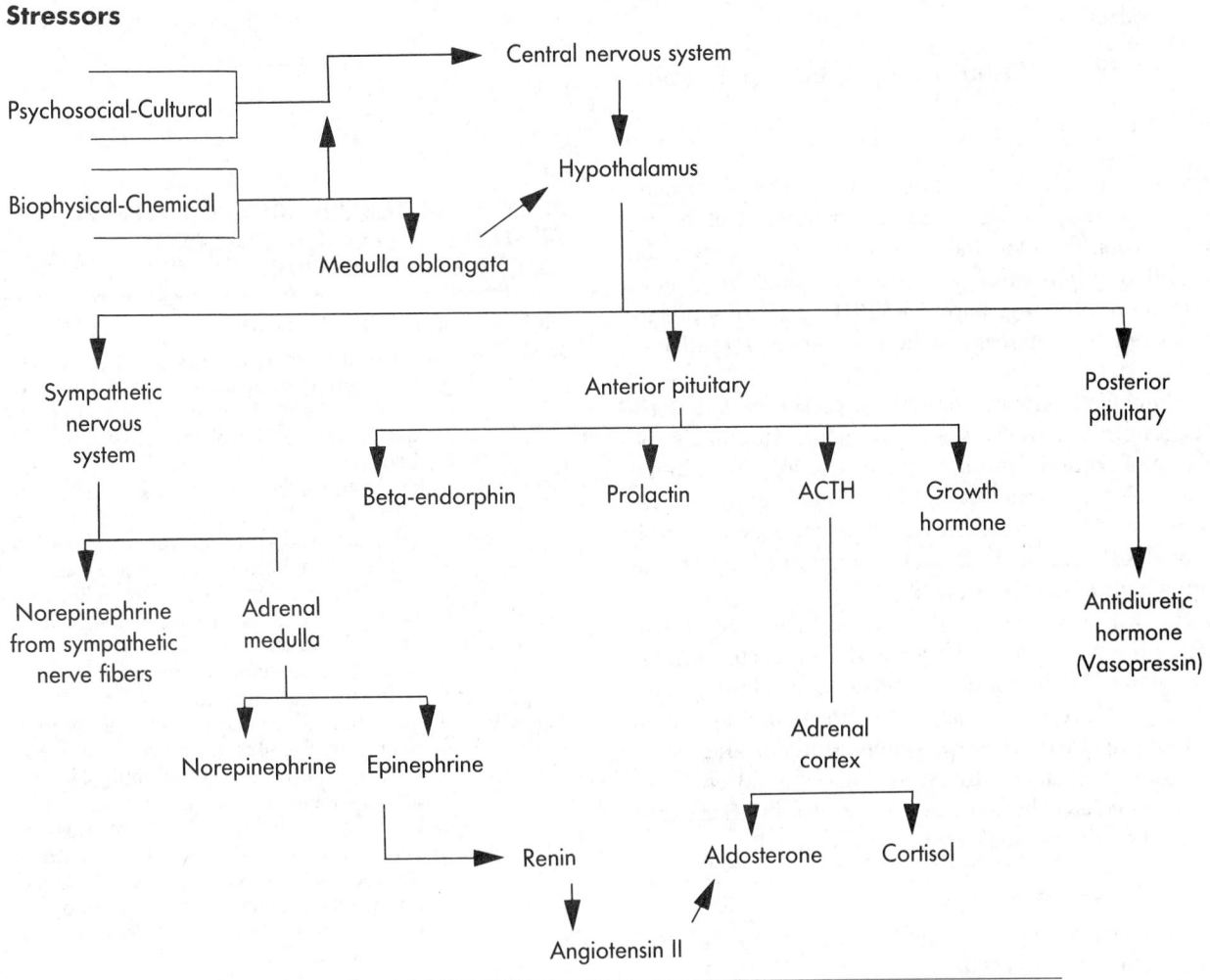

FIGURE 9-1 Physiologic components involved in the neuroendocrine response to stressors.

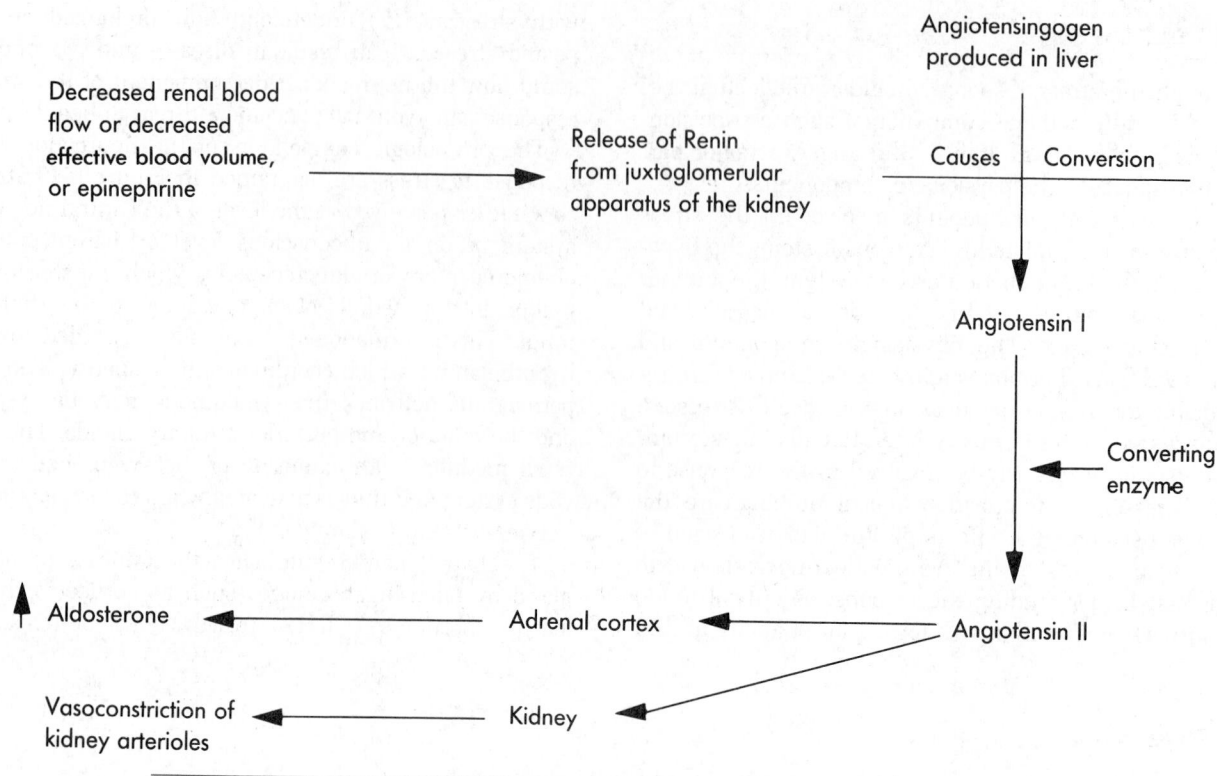

FIGURE 9-2 Renin-angiotensin-aldosterone system.

hormone (GHRH), or prolactin-releasing hormone (PRH). Some anterior pituitary hormones will be released when the hypothalamus diminishes its secretion of inhibiting hormones. For example, dopamine acts as a prolactin-inhibiting hormone (PIH), and thus prolactin secretion is increased when dopamine secretion is decreased.

Adrenocorticotropin hormone (ACTH), which is released from the anterior pituitary gland, stimulates the release of cortisol from the adrenal cortex. The adrenal cortex also releases the hormone aldosterone in response to ACTH secretion. However, the major controller of aldosterone secretion is the renin-angiotensin system, which is shown in Figure 9-2.

The last endocrine gland activated by the hypothalamus is the posterior pituitary gland. The posterior pituitary gland, when stimulated, releases antidiuretic hormone (ADH) or vasopressin. The effects of stimulation of the sympathetic nervous system, anterior and posterior pituitary glands, adrenal medulla, and adrenal cortex are mediated by the catecholamines and hormones released by the nervous system or the glands.

CATECHOLAMINES

The catecholamines, epinephrine and norepiniphrine, act by stimulating receptors unique for them. The receptors are located on various cells throughout the body.

SUMMARY OF THE PHYSIOLOGICAL EFFECTS OF STIMULATION OF THE DIFFERENT CATECHOLAMINE RECEPTORS[10,21,28]

RECEPTOR	EFFECT OF STIMULATION
Beta 1	Increased heart rate (chronotropic), increased contractility of atria and ventricles (ionotropic), increase in automaticity and conduction of ventricular electrical system; lipolysis
Beta 2	Dilation of the smooth muscles of the coronary, skin, skeletal muscle, and pulmonary arterioles and systemic veins; relaxation of bronchial smooth muscle; decreased motility of stomach and intestines; relaxation of bladder muscle; secretion of renin; increased gluconeogenesis and hepatic and muscle glycogenolysis; increased secretion of insulin and glucagon
Alpha 1	Contraction of smooth muscles of coronary, skin, mucosa, skeletal muscle, cerebral, pulmonary, mesenteric, renal, and salivary gland arterioles and systemic veins; Contraction of radial muscle of eye (mydriasis); contraction of sphincters of gastrointestinal tract; contraction of sphincter of bladder and urethra; ejaculation; contraction of pilomotor muscles; increased secretion of localized sweat glands
Alpha 2	Decreased motility of gastrointestinal tract; decreased insulin secretion; platelet aggregation; possibly decreased secretion of intestinal tract

TABLE 9-1 Systemic effects of epinephrine and norepinephrine release during the neuroendocrine response to stressors

Organ	Effects
Brain	Dilated blood vessels resulting in increased blood flow; increased metabolism; patient may seem more alert or restless
Eyes	Pupilary dilation; patient appears startled
Heart	Dilated coronary blood vessels with increased blood flow; increased heart rate and contractility; patient's cardiac output and stroke volume may increase if the heart is able to keep up with increased demand
Vascular system	Constriction of arterioles to skin, mucosa, renal, and abdominal viscera, with decreased blood flow; increased constriction of veins with increased venous return; skin is cool and pale; urine output may be decreased; ischemia with resultant tissue death and failure of kidneys and abdominal viscera may occur; toe temperature may be decreased
Lungs	Dilation of pulmonary vascular bed; bronchodilation; increased rate and depth of respiration; oxygen uptake and excretion of CO_2 will be increased; and the patient may show respiratory alkalosis ($\downarrow$ pCO_2 and $\uparrow$ pH).
Gastrointestinal tract (GI)	Decreased motility and secretion; Production of mucus is decreased and with decreased blood flow patient may have irritation of GI tract and GI bleeding
Exocrine pancreas	Decreased enzyme and fluid and electrolyte secretions
Endocrine pancreas	Decreased insulin secretion
Liver	Increased gluconeogenesis and glycogenolysis; decreased glycogen synthesis; these processes along with decreased insulin and decreased glucose uptake may result in hyperglycemia
Adipose tissue	Increased lipolysis and fatty acid production; serum may show increased triglycerides and lipoproteins
Skeletal muscle	Increased muscle glycogenolysis; decreased glucose uptake, increased contractility; generalized muscle tension may be evident
Skin, sweat glands	Decreased blood flow, increased localized secretion of sweat; piloerection; skin is cool, pale, moist, and often has goose bumps

The catecholamine receptors are divided into two major classes, alpha (α) and beta (β), with two subclasses of each major class. The activation of these receptors by endogeous or exogenous catecholamines results in selected physiologic actions.

Stimulation of α_1 receptors is primarily associated with excitation or stimulation, and stimulation of α_2 receptors is primarily associated with relaxation or inhibition. Stimulation of β_1 receptors is primarily associated with stimulation of cardiac activity, and stimulation of β_2 receptors is associated with all other effects associated with beta receptors such as bronchial dilation. See the accompanying box on p. 184 for a more detailed description of functions associated with stimulation of specific receptor types.

During the neuroendocrine response to stressors, both norepinephrine and epinephrine are released. Norepinephrine binds primarily to α receptors, whereas epinephrine activates both α and β receptors. The effects of catecholamines during the stress response then is due to a combination of the actions of both catecholamines and activation of several different receptors. The effects seen with the release of catecholamines during the stress response are summarized in Table 9-1.

CORTISOL

Cortisol is released from the adrenal cortex under the control of ACTH and CRH. Cortisol has major effects on glucose, protein, and fat metabolism and on fluid and electrolyte balance and has anti-inflammatory and immunosuppressant effects. It enhances the activity of other hormones and works with epinephrine, glucagon, and growth hormone in elevating the blood glucose. Cortisol also augments the effects of other hormones and catecholamines in maintaining cardiac output and blood pressure. Detailed information of the effects of cortisol on the body are presented in the box on p. 184.

Cortisol's effect on metabolism and fluid and electrolytes, and its permissive effect on other hormones seem logical in response to the body's needs in the presence of stressors; however, the anti-inflammatory and immunosuppressant effects seem illogical in that they would seem to be more detrimental than helpful. Munck et al.[24] and associates have suggested that the major beneficial effect of cortisol release during the neuroendocrine response to stressors is to inhibit, or turn off, the body's protective response to stressors so that the response does not damage the body.

ALDOSTERONE

Aldosterone primarily is released from the adrenal cortex in response to activation of the renin-angiotensin system as diagramed in Figure 9-2. Some aldosterone is released in response to ACTH from the anterior pituitary gland. Aldosterone acts on the distal kidney tubule cells and causes reabsorption of sodium and water and

SYSTEMIC EFFECTS OF CORTISOL RELEASE DURING THE NEUROENDOCRINE RESPONSE TO STRESSORS

METABOLIC EFFECTS

1. Maintains blood glucose by:
   Increasing gluconeogenesis
   Decreasing glucose uptake by many body cells, particularly muscle
2. Increases protein catabolism, which provides substrate for glucose formation
3. Promotes lipolysis to provide alternative nutrient sources

FLUID AND ELECTROLYTE EFFECTS

1. Promotes sodium and water retention
2. Promotes potassium excretion

ANTI-INFLAMMATORY/IMMUNOSUPPRESSIVE EFFECTS

1. Decreases eosinophils, basophils, monocytes, and lymphocytes in the circulation
2. Increases neutrophil (polymorphonuclear leukocytes) by movement from bone marrow and circulatory pools
3. Decreases leukocyte accumulation at inflammatory sites
4. Inhibits release of inflammatory substances (kinins, prostaglandins, leukotrienes)
5. Degrades collagen
6. Decreases scar tissue formation
7. Decreases lymphoid tissue mass, participation of T-lymphocytes in cellular-mediated immunity, and production of interleukin 1 and 2

MISCELLANEOUS EFFECTS

1. Maintains emotional stability
2. Increases red blood cell formation
3. Possibly increases platelet formation
4. Increases gastric acid and pepsin production
5. Is permissive for other hormones and catecholamines (i.e., cortisol is necessary for the full functioning of some other hormones and catecholamines), particularily in relation to effects of epinephrine and norepinephrine on blood pressure control, cardiac output, and metabolism.

excretion of potassium and hydrogen ions. Aldosterone helps to maintain vascular volume and blood pressure.

ANTIDIURETIC HORMONE

Antidiuretic hormone (ADH) or vasopressin is released during the neuroendocrine response to stressors from the ends of axons of hypothalamic neurons that terminate in the posterior pituitary gland. ADH acts on the distal tubules and collecting ducts of the kidneys and causes an increase in the size of pores within the cell membrane so that water can be reabsorbed. Water is reabsorbed in response to the osmotic gradient established by the difference in osmolality of the tubular fluid and the medullary interstitial fluid. ADH controls the osmolality of body fluid. ADH in high concentration can result in arteriole vasoconstriction and can help to in-

crease blood pressure. Vasopressin also stimulates the release of ACTH and thus influences the pituitary-adrenal-cortical response to stressors.[9]

OTHER PITUITARY HORMONES

Endogenous opiates (B-endorphins) are released as part of the neuroendocrine response to stressors. These endogenous opiates may be involved in the pituitary-adrenal-cortical response to stressors.[9] The endogenous opiates are known to increase tolerance to painful stimuli. Release of endogenous opiates in stressful situations may account for the analgesic effect experienced by persons who have major trauma experience.

Growth hormone is released from the anterior pituitary during the neuroendocrine response to stressors. Hypoglycemia and strenuous exercise are two stressors associated with an increase in growth hormone. Growth hormone helps to provide nutrients for the energy needs of various cells and tissues during the stress response. Growth hormone decreases glucose use and is an insulin antagonist; thus it helps to maintain the blood glucose level, which provides glucose for the nervous tissue. Growth hormone increases lipolysis, free fatty acid levels, and ketone formation, which provides nutrients for various tissues, such as skeletal and cardiac muscles.

Prolactin[21] is also released in the presence of certain stressors. The function of prolactin in relation to dealing with stressors is unknown.

EFFECTS OF STRESS RESPONSE

The catecholamines, ACTH, cortisol, ADH, endogenous opiates, and growth hormone released during the neuroendocrine response to stressors provide through their various actions a total body response that allows the individual to cope with stressors or to withdraw from the stressors (fight or flight response). The total body response includes the following:

1. Increase in blood levels of substrates necessary for energy:glucose for nervous tissue, and fatty acid substrates for other tissues.
2. Increase in oxygen uptake to provide O_2 for metabolic processes.
3. Maintenance of vascular volume and increase in cardiac function for transport of nutrients and O_2 to tissues and for removal of waste products.
4. Increase in respiratory activity allows for the elimination of excessive carbon dioxide that will be produced while the person is coping with the stressor.
5. Increase in muscle activity that might allow for flight from the stressor.
6. Increase in blood flow to brain that might allow for critical decision making, activation of psychological defense mechanisms, or problem solving.

STRESS RESPONSE PROBLEMS

Although the neuroendocrine response to stressors is protective, nurses need to be aware that the stress response may place demands on the body that can lead to damage to various organs. Nurses also need to be aware that not every person is able to mount an adequate stress response.

The actions initiated by the neuroendocrine response to stressors such as increased blood flow to the brain, heart, and lungs and increased gluconeogenesis are initiated at the expense of other body systems that are not necessary for immediate coping with the stressor, including the gastrointestinal system, the pancreas, the kidneys, protein stores, and so forth. A prolonged stress response to stressors can lead to damage to these later systems. For example, a person with some underlying renal insufficiency may develop worsening insufficiency because of the vasoconstriction to the kidney during the stress response.

A second reason for problems induced by the stress response is that it will place great strain on many body systems. If a person has some underlying pathophysiologic process of a system that will be called into demand, the stress response can cause insufficiency in functioning of the diseased system. For example, if a patient has coronary artery disease, ischemia with resultant chest pain or arrhythmias can occur when a stressor places increased demand on the heart.

Inability to mount an adequate stress response will be seen in some patients. Persons with diseases of the hypothalamic pituitary-adrenal axis will have a diminished ability to respond to stressors. Also persons with impaired autonomic nervous system response will have a diminished ability to handle stressors. The presence of diminished physiologic functioning of the total body as is seen in the very young, very old, and persons exposed to multiple stressors also will result in compromised response to stressors.

CHAPTER SUMMARY

- The stress response is an integrated body response involving various components.
- The stress response is a protective response that is graded and varies with stimuli and is initiated when a stressor is perceived.
- Hans Selye is one of the major scientist whose work provides a basis for our current knowledge about the stress response.
- Selye labeled the response to stressors as the general adaptation syndrome, which has three phases: the alarm reaction, stage of resistance, and stage of exhaustion.
- Stressors can be biophysical-chemical or psychosocial-cultural in nature.
- Stressors show great individualization and range from daily hassles to severe burns.
- The physiologic stress response consists of stimulation of the sympathetic nervous system, adrenal medulla, anterior and posterior pituitary glands, and the adrenal cortex.
- The neuroendocrine response to stress is integrated by the hypothalamus.
- Norepinephrine released by the sympathetic nervous system and the adrenal medulla primarily causes vasoconstriction of blood vessels of the skin; mucous membrane, and abdominal and pelvic organs shifting blood to blood vessels of the heart, lung, and brain, which were dilated by the action of epinephrine.
- In addition to dilating selected blood vessels, epinephrine increases cardiac function, dilates bronchial smooth muscles, and alters metabolism to provide substrates for energy needs.
- Cortisol, acting in concert with catecholamines, growth hormone, and glucagon, helps to mobilize substrates for energy.
- Cortisol may also serve a major function by its anti-inflammatory and immunosuppressive actions by dampening the stress response to prevent overactivity.
- Water and sodium balance, osmolality, and blood volume are protected by the action of aldosterone and ADH, which are released during the neuroendocrine response to stressors.
- Overall the neuroendocrine response to stressors helps the person maintain stability while the stressor is present and to fight the stressor or to withdraw from the stressor (fight-or-flight response).
- Persons with diseases or insufficiency of the physiologic systems that are placed in demand during the stress response can experience worsening of the system's functioning.
- Persons with dysfunction of the hypothalamic-pituitary-adrenal axis, sympathetic nervous system, or adrenal medulla or diminished physiologic reserves will have a compromised neuroendocrine response to stressors.

QUESTIONS TO CONSIDER

- What historical and physical assessment data would be critical to assess to determine a person's ability to deal with stressors?

- What patients would have difficulty dealing with stressors? (You should be able to identify at least ten examples.)

- What clinical manifestations of the neuroendocrine response to stressors would you expect to see in a patient experiencing a major psychophysiologic stressor, such as second-degree burns over 50% of the body?

REFERENCES AND SELECTED READINGS

1. Axelrod J and Reisine T: Stress hormones: their interaction and regulation, Science 224:452-453, 1984.
2. Ballard KS: Identification of environmental stress for patients in the surgical intensive care unit, Unpublished master's thesis, University of Kansas School of Nursing, Kansas City, 1979.
3. Berne RM and Levy MN, editors: Physiology, ed 2, St Louis, 1988, The CV Mosby Co.
4. Cannon WB: Stresses and strains of homeostasis, Am J Med Sci 189:1-14, 1935.
5. Cannon WB: The wisdom of the body, New York, 1963, WW Norton Co.
6. *Clarke M: Stress and coping: constructs for nursing. J Adv Nurs, 9:3-13, 1984.
7. Cox T: Stress, New York, 1978, Macmillan Press.
8. *Frain M and Valiga T: The multiple dimensions of stress. Top Clin Nurs 1(1):43-57, 1979.
9. Gaillard RC, and Al-DamLeiji S: Stress and the pituitary-adrenal axis. Baillieres Clini Endocrinol Metab 1:319-354, 1987.
10. Granner D: Hormones of the adrenal medulla, In Murray RK, et al, editors: Harper's biochemistry, ed 21, New York, 1988, Lange Medical Books.
11. Groeï MW and Shekleton ME: Basic pathophysiology: a holistic approach, ed 3, St Louis, 1989, The CV Mosby Co.

12. Hetzel BS, et al: Changes in urinary 17-hydroxy-corticosteroid excretion during stressful life situations in man, J Clin Endocrinol 15:1057-1068, 1955.
13. Hornberger CA: Perceived stressors, perceived stress response, and level of cardiac reactivity in wellness sample, Unpublished master's thesis, University of Kansas School of Nursing, Kansas City, 1989.
14. Johnson D: Metabolic and endocrine alterations in the multiple injured patient, Crit Care Nurs Q 11(2):35-41, 1988.
15. Lazarus R: Patterns of adjustment, New York, 1976, McGraw Hill.
16. Lazarus R: Psychological stress and the coping process, New York, McGraw Hill, 1966.
17. Lenox RH, et al: Specific hormonal and neurochemical responses to different stressors, Neuroendocrinology 30:300-308, 1980.
18. *Lindsay AM and Carrieri VK: Stress response, In Linday AM, Carrieri VK, West CM, editors: Pathophysiological phenomenon in nursing: human responses to illness, Philadelphia, 1985, WB Saunders.
19. Mason JW: A re-evaluation of the concept of nonspecificity in stress theory, J Psyciatr Res 8:323-333, 1971.
20. Mason J: Specificity in the organization of neuroendocrine response profiles, In Seeman P, Brown GM, editors: Frontiers in neurology and neuroscience research. First International Symposium of the Neuroscience Institute, University of Toronto, 1974, pp 68-80.
21. McCance K and Huether SE: Pathophysiology: the biologic base for disease in adults and children, St Louis, 1990, The CV Mosby Co.
22. McEwen B and Brinton RE: Neuroendocrine aspects of adaptation, Prog Brain Res 72:11-26, 1987.
23. Meyer D: Development of an instrument to measure perceived environmental stressors of surgical intensive care patients, Unpublished master's thesis, University of Kansas School of Nursing, Kansas City, 1985.
24. *Munck A, Guyre PM, and Holbrook NJ: Physiological functions of glucocorticoids in stress and their relation to pharmacological actions, Endocr Rev 5:25-44, 1984.
25. *Selye H: Stress in health and disease, Sevenoaks, 1976, Butterworth.
26. Selye H: The general adaptation syndrome and the diseases of adaptation, J Clin Endocrinol 6:117-230, 1946.
27. Selye H: The stress syndrome, Am J Nurs 65:97-99, 1965.
28. Shoemaker W et al, editors: Textbook of critical care, ed 2, Philadelphia, 1989, WB Saunders.
29. *Sutterley DC: Stress and health: a survey of self-regulation modalities, Top Clini Nurs 1(1), 1-29, 1979.

*References preceded by an asterisk are particularly well suited for students.

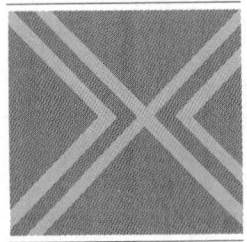

CHAPTER 10

Stress and Coping

PAMELA HOLSCLAW MITCHELL

CHAPTER OBJECTIVES

After studying this chapter, the student should be able to:
1. Analyze the concepts of stress, adaptation, and coping for their usefulness in nursing practice.
2. Analyze the adaptive functions of human behavior.
3. Analyze the consequences of alternative coping strategies.
4. Analyze nursing situations to identify potential stressors.

Stress, adaptation, and coping are words commonly used in both lay and professional writings to refer to problematic life situations and the ways of dealing with them. These terms are entrenched in nursing writings to the extent that it is now axiomatic that a major function of nursing is to help people cope with stress and adapt to stressful situations.

Yet, when attempting to define these terms in order to study and understand them better, we find that there is no scientific consensus as to their meanings. Since this is the case, how can these terms be used professionally to understand the nature of human problem-solving behavior? Why have they come to such prominence in the helping professions? Is there a set of related phenomena that these terms describe, or should they be abandoned as bad jargon?

The position is taken here that these terms are in the literature to stay and that they describe similar phenomena regarding the ways humans and nonhumans deal with life's changing events. The terms each provide a general reference point to approach common experiences of living systems interacting with their environments even though precise definitions acceptable to most investigators have been elusive. At best, one may recognize common themes that emerge from the multiple perspectives of those who have tried to define these terms precisely.

Stress is a general term describing patterns of psychologic and physiologic responses to a variety of emotional and physical stimuli. Stress responses occur when the ordinary capacity to adapt to life's demands is

taxed. Stress can thus be seen *as a subset of the concept adaptation*—or the processes of maintaining psychobiologic equilibrium during interaction with the environment. *Coping* comprises those strategies by which adaptation to ordinary or extraordinary environmental demands is accomplished. In this chapter the common themes that have emerged from the scientific study of stress, adaptation, and coping will be presented. These themes will then be applied in a framework useful for helping people in health, in acute illnesses, and in chronic illnesses throughout the life cycle.

ADAPTATION

Adaptation is a term that implies a variety of processes, depending on the differing perspectives of the discipline defining the term. In the colloquial or common meaning, adaptation connotes individual adjustment or compromises to meet the demands of a situation. To anthropologists, adaptation is defined in terms of the evolution of populations or groups to meet changing environmental demands—the survival of species.[36] Biologists tend to view adaptation as processes that restore homeostasis or balance to internal environmental systems when the system is perturbed. At the *biologic* level, adaptation is directed toward survival or stability of internal processes. At the *psychologic* level, the goal of adaptation is preservation of self-identity and self-esteem. At the *social* level, adaptation provides (1) definition of modes of adaptation for individuals, (2) support systems for coping endeavors, and (3) anticipation of common developmental tasks.[10]

Adaptation as a concept in nursing is tied most closely to Roy's[32] conceptualization. In Roy's view, adaptation is defined as processes, in interaction with environmental demands, that promote integrity of the individual with respect to survival, growth, reproduction, and self-mastery. Responses that do not contribute to these goals are termed *ineffective* (older formulations of the theory used the term *maladaptive*). Adaptation, or positive responses to environmental demands, is linked to health. Roy's adaptive modes consist of physiologic needs, self-concept, role function, and interdependence relations.

Although the literature regarding adaptation is extensive and the definitions and variations vary, common threads do emerge, however. These can guide health workers as they seek to help individuals, groups, and populations in interaction with their environments.

ADAPTATION AS INTERACTION WITH THE ENVIRONMENT

Adaptation was defined by Simpson[36] as both the processes and the outcome (end point) that create and maintain useful relationships between an organism or population of organisms and the environment. Nonliving systems are not regarded as adapting, because they do not change or grow to meet the demands of changing environments. Living systems, in contrast, are capable of seeking and using information, both biologically and cognitively, to effect change in response to changing environments. Living systems are not only acted on by external environments, but also can act on the envi-

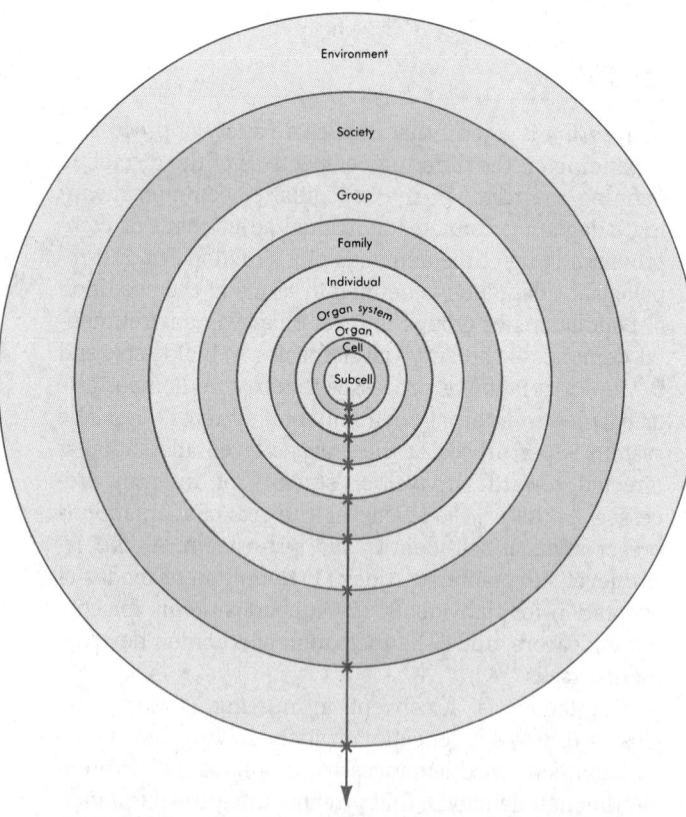

FIGURE 10-1 Person-environment interactions. There are many environments, both inside and outside an individual, with which the person interacts. Each environment could be considered part of a larger environment.

ronment to further adaptation. As a simple example, humans in northern climates create more comfortable winter environments by building shelters, making clothing, and using parts of the environment for fuel to warm the shelters. To the extent that these components of the environment are not renewable, people may be faced in the near future with the need to adapt life-styles to a markedly changing environment.

Human beings and other organisms adapt biologically and socially as well as technologically to changing environments. The Tierra del Fuegans, the inhabitants of the tip of South America, startled Darwin by their seeming imperviousness to severe cold and snow. More modern scientists have found that these people conserve heat far more efficiently than persons adapted to more temperate climates.[8] Various species of monkeys have adapted anatomically as well as biologically to their environments. For example, the gibbon has long, very strong arms that are well suited to swinging through the dense forests in which it lives. In contrast, the patas monkey has developed protective coloration to camouflage itself in the grasslands and social habits that allow quick dispersion should there be an attack in so open a place.[38]

If human beings are constantly interacting with their environments, it follows that adaptation must be a constant and dynamic factor of living. If adaptation is viewed as including growth as well as maintenance, it becomes a central concept in understanding living systems. All life processes then support the person-environment interaction. In the framework of adaptation, all person-environment interactions are intimately tied to interactions with successfully larger environments (Figure 10-1).

ENVIRONMENTS: INTERNAL AND EXTERNAL

Nurses frequently work with individuals, families, or small groups. Consequently, the interaction of these entities with their immediate environments becomes the most common unit of analysis for nursing. However, in living systems, including human beings, there are many environments, both internal and external to the whole organism.[25] The cell, which is often considered a fundamental unit of analysis, has an internal environment—the mitochondria, ribosomes, and other machinery of replication and metabolism. It also has many external environments—the immediate fluid environment, the organ and organ system of which it is a part, and the whole organism in which it resides. This organism in turn has the cell, its organ and organ systems, and integrating mechanisms as an internal environment and an external environment consisting of all the animate and inanimate entities outside its skin. These entities may constitute a physical environment of such elements as heat, light, sound, form, and motion and a sociocultural environment composed of the social groupings, institutions, and cultures through which many adaptive strategies are transmitted. Finally, one may consider cultures or nations as the systems of analysis, with terrestial and supranational environments as external to the system and nations, economic cartels, and racial subgroups as the internal environments.

For the most part, the medical-surgical nurse is concerned with an individual or a family attempting to maintain health or to adapt to an episode of acute or chronic illness. Consequently, evaluation of adaptive demands and strategies will most often occur in relation to an individual and his or her immediate physical and sociocultural environment. It is important, however, to be aware that these immediate environments are influenced by considerably larger environments.

ADAPTIVE STIMULI: DEVELOPMENTAL AND SITUATIONAL

Although by definition any changing environmental stimulus initiates adaptive processes, two classes of events create major adaptive demands for individuals or groups. These have been termed *developmental crises* and *situational crises*. Adams and Lindeman[1] define a crisis as any situation that requires an individual or a group to mobilize new resources or master new skills. Developmental demands are those which predictably occur in a given culture as the individual moves from one state of development to another; for example, the transition from childhood to adolescence or from early to middle adulthood. Many of these transitions are marked by biologic as well as psychologic changes accompanying maturation (see Chapter 11).

Situational crises, in contrast, do not occur predictably in relation to the maturational development of people (although most people face many situational crises at some times during their lives). Illness, accidents, loss, divorce, a new job, and fame are all examples of events that can produce situational adaptive demands. Note that not all the examples are negative or "bad" events; the common denominator is the demand for new resources or mastery of new skills.

For a given individual or family, situational crises interact with the state of development or maturation of the individual or family. The biologic and social capacity to cope with the demands of the situation depend in part on (1) the state of maturation and (2) the social and physical support systems available in the environment. For example, short-term malnutrition may permanently alter the intellectual capacity of the child whose brain is still developing but cause only temporary apathy in an adult. That same child, however, may become a contributing member of society, with appropriate social support systems such as sheltered workshops and special education.

STABILITY AND GROWTH

The notion that adaptation involves meeting developmental as well as situational demands stems from the concept that adaptation is concerned with more than just organismic stability. In sensory physiology, adaptation refers to the decrement in response to a prolonged stimulus, implying a return to stability after perturbation.[24] Many sources have criticized the concept of adaptation as being too limited because there is no room for growth if the end result is always stability.[6,11,31] However, all accounts of evolutionary and social adaptation, of necessity, include growth as organisms and species develop new ways of behaving both biologically and socially. Dubos[5] likens this process to a spiral as each adaptation creates demands for further adaptation on successively higher planes. Living creatures as open systems behave in ways that not only preserve or protect their existence (survival), but also that permit growth and striving.[41]

STRESS

HISTORICAL PERSPECTIVE

The term *stress* has been used colloquially for centuries to refer to mental and emotional strain or pressure. In physics stress has a precise mechanical meaning—the force put on an object. The resulting deformation or response is designated as *strain*. Selye[34] was the first to use the term stress in a biological context—the nonspecific response of the body to a variety of noxious stimuli. He termed the stimulus the *stressor*. Initially, Selye[35] avoided the term stress because of its common use in connoting emotional turmoil. However, as he came to see that many strong stimuli were capable of provoking the general adaptation syndrome (discussed below), he postulated that emotional stimuli were equivalent to physical stressors (for example, heat, cold, trauma) in evoking the response, and he began to use stress as synonymous with the general adaptation syndrome.[34]

The notion of a general integrated and mutually interacting biologic and psychologic response to a variety of environmental stimuli was not unique to Selye. In fact, his work was preceded by the philosophic writings of James[17] and Lange,[25] who proposed that the perception of visceral responses to emotional events *was* the emotion, by the experiments of Cannon,[3] who observed the similarity of physiologic responses of the sympathetic nervous system during a variety of emotional states, and by Jacobsen,[16] who documented responses of the sympathetic nervous system and skeletal muscles to emotional states. Jacobsen also demonstrated mutual influences of these subsystems by decreasing sympathetic arousal through therapy directed at relaxing skeletal muscle.

Selye's work led him to describe the *general adapta-*

tion syndrome, a classic triad of changes in internal organs seen following a wide variety of noxious stimuli such as heat, cold, skin trauma, and forced immobilization. Hypertrophy of the adrenal gland, ulceration of the stomach, and atrophy of the thymus constituted this triad. The pituitary-adrenocortical axis of the neuroendocrine system was found to be the mediator of these responses, thus setting the stage for development of the understanding of neuroendocrine response. Cannon's work forms the basis for understanding sympatheticadrenal medullary responses.

Selye's work had two major effects: addition of the neuroendocrine dimension to biologic manifestations of arousal and addition of the term stress to the list of words by which we categorize knowledge about integrated psychobiologic responses to our environments. Selye used the term stress to present the concept that there are a variety of internal and external environmental stimuli that can lead to similar protective biologic responses. Further, he proposed that continued intense stimulation would lead to depletion of the biologic ability to respond and to diminished ability to respond to additional challenges.

CONCEPTUALIZATIONS OF STRESS

These early ideas have led to a vast research and clinical literature regarding stress as a common denominator in causation of illness and as an impediment to recovery from illness. Despite the nearly 50 years that stress has been used as a research concept, investigators do not agree on its definition or measurement. Some have suggested discarding the term altogether.[14] Overlapping of concepts is evident in the multiple headings under which one may find studies and reviews relevant to the phenomenon: emotion, anxiety, stress, psychophysiology, arousal, activation, and adaptation. Three major approaches have been used: stress as the stimulus, stress as the psychologic response (or appraisal of threat), and stress as the psychobiologic response that exceeds normal adaptive capacities.

Early workers in the area of psychologic stress tended to view *events* or stimuli as stressful in themselves; however, it has become increasingly evident that the critical factor is the psychologic meaning attached to the stimulus.[9,20,25] Some theorists contend that the stimulus must symbolize threat to be stressful, thus emphasizing the stimulus and its appraisal.[2,7,15,22] Others note similar biologic responses to both threat and pleasure, thus defining stress from the standpoint of biologic *response.*[22] Lazarus and associates integrate these approaches by suggesting that the key is the psychobiologic appraisal of stimuli that are highly relevant to one's welfare, whether this relevance be positive or negative.[22]

A third approach is to define stress as existing when *adaptive capacities are exceeded,* thus suggesting an interactive state between stimulus and response.[7,19,24] The more complete theories in this perspective emphasize biologic as well as psychosocial responses and initiating stimuli. Examples of events that exceed adaptive capacity in most people are widespread infection, trauma, and surgery.

Distinguishing the different ways in which stress is conceptualized is important because the way we think about stress influences the way we use the concept in clinical work with both well and ill people. If we think of stress as a defined set of biologic events happening *to* people, we may not appreciate gradations of response or the influence of an individual's perceptions on the intensity or even presence of the response. Further, if we consider stress as external to the person, we may not consider using measures that help people manage their own perceptions and responses to the changing environment.

INTEGRATED PSYCHOBIOLOGIC RESPONSE

Some commonalities emerge, however, from the differing perspectives from which stress has been approached. First, Selye's observation that many different stimuli are capable of producing a common physiologic response has stood the test of time. There are, however, important qualifiers regarding when and to what degree diverse stimuli elicit this response.

Henry and Ely[13] and Mason[25] present convincing evidence that psychologic appraisal of any stimulus as challenging or threatening is the key mediator of the multiple neuroendocrine responses to stimuli. The multiple physiologic responses to acute stressors constitute a pattern called the *alarm response:* simultaneous activation of the sympathetic-adrenal medullary system and the pituitary-adrenocortical system. These physiologic responses promote energy use in a "fight-or-flight" reaction. Anxiety, hyperarousal, and sense of distress are psychologic responses that may accompany the physiologic components. If stimuli such as heat, cold, or even trauma can be introduced in such a way that the organism is unaware of the change,* only the response specific to the stimulus is elicited and not the multiple endocrine stress response. Physical immobility, surgery, fear, anger, and inescapable noxious stimuli have all been shown to be capable of eliciting this multisystem response. The intensity of response depends on a combination of (1) intensity of stimulus, (2) duration of stimulus, and (3) perception of control over the stimulus.

---

*Trauma can be introduced so that an experimental animal is unaware of it. For example, limb that has no nervous connections to the rest of the body (a denervated limb) may be injured.

INTENSITY OF STIMULUS

Intense physical and psychologic stimuli such as trauma, forceful immobilization, and strong fear lead to stress responses in most organisms—human and non-human. In experimental situations in which intense stimuli can be gradated, as in trauma or burns, the intensity of the multisystem response is also gradated in proportion to the stimulus.[33] A similar graded response is at least partially evident in human response to various traumas and surgical procedures. For example, the metabolic response to a burn over 40% of the body area is considerably greater than that to a hernia repair. The psychologic component (threat, fear, inescapability, lack of control) is also greater for the patient with a burn than for the person experiencing elective surgery.

DURATION OF STIMULUS

Some investigators have suggested that although most organisms may have similar emergency responses to acute and intense stimuli, ongoing stimuli may elicit different individual responses. The adaptive response of one organism to ongoing stimuli may either resemble or differ from the response of another organism. Henry's work with colonies of mice is the most extensive long-term investigation of the physiologic responses of animals to their ordinary social interactions.[13] As these animals established their social dominance hierarchy, those who became the dominant animals exhibited primarily sympathetic–adrenal medullary activation, characterized biochemically by elevated catecholamine levels, behaviorally by muscular activity, and symptomatically by hypertension. In contrast, the animals at the bottom of the social hierarchy showed primarily a pituitary-adrenocortical response: elevated corticosteroid

RESEARCH

Lanuza DM and Marotta SF: Endocrine and psychologic responses of patients to cardiac pacemaker implantation, Heart Lung 16:496-505, 1987.

Both physiologic and psychologic manifestations of the stress response were measured preoperatively and postoperatively in 28 patients undergoing cardiac pacemaker implantation. It was hypothesized that structured patient teaching about the procedure, device function, and expected sensory experiences would reduce both physiologic and psychologic stress responses. Although the experimental group had significantly greater knowledge about the pacemaker, indicators of sympathetic-adrenal medullary response (catecholamines) and pituitary-adrenocortical response (cortisol) increased similarly in both groups postoperatively. It is likely that the physical stimulus of surgery masked any differential physiologic response to patient teaching. ■

levels, withdrawn behavior, and ultimately enlarged adrenal glands and stomach ulcers. The animals who challenged the dominant animals had profiles midway between the two groups. While this study is not presented to suggest that socially dominant people will become hypertensive, it does support the notion that in ordinary daily living organisms, including humans, tend to respond in a characteristic mode. This mode is partially dependent on genetic factors, social position, and learned modes of coping with or responding to everyday events.

PERCEPTION OF CONTROL

Perception of control over a situation and relevant feedback regarding the effect of one's behavior on the stimulus appear to be potent factors regulating the multihormonal stress response. When a dominant animal from Henry's mouse colony was put into a colony in which dominance had already been established, the previously dominant mouse became submissive, and its behavior and physiologic response became that of the submissive mice. One could argue that the mouse perceived itself as no longer being in control. Parachutists in training in Norway exhibited all the characteristic neuroendocrine stress responses before their first jump but rapidly returned to baseline values in subsequent jumps. Their subjective fear decreased as their sense of mastery and control over the task increased.[24] Weiss[40] presents an excellent summary of animal research demonstrating that control over aversive stimuli (shock) and relevant feedback regarding one's efforts reduced and even prevented pathologic physiologic stress responses in a variety of situations.

The concepts of hardiness and resilience in human beings have been shown to be important factors in maintaining health in stressful situations.[18,29] Perception of control of life situations is a key component of these concepts. Stress has been linked both in the popular press and in scientific literature with disease, presumably caused by prolonged or excessive physiologic responses to a variety of situations. It should be evident from the foregoing, however, that it is not the situations by themselves that create the stress response, but rather the combination of psychologic appraisal and sense of control.[4,19] These concepts lead logically to the notion of coping with change: the perception and appraisal of some relevant but challenging situation, and the psychobiologic responses emanating from that perception.[22,29]

COPING

The definitions of *coping* are as many and varied as those for adaptation and stress. White[41] considers coping the *strategies* of adaptation—the means by which adaptation takes place. It is often defined as involving problem-solving efforts in situations that are perceived as being highly relevant to the individual and that tax adaptive resources.[22] While many persons explicitly or implicitly consider coping to be primarily a cognitive process, some authors recognize the interrelationship between physiologic and cognitive responses to adverse circumstances. Levine, Weinburg, and Ursin[24] define the ultimate goal of coping processes to be reduction of physiologic activation, whereas Murphy[28] divides coping processes into coping I, the capacity to deal with the changing environment (action and cognition), and coping II, the capacity to maintain the internal environment.

In general, then, coping refers to *processes or skills that individuals use to deal with events, circumstances, or situations that are out of the ordinary*. It is an integrated psychobiologic process in which "gut" feelings influence cognition of the need to cope and coping efforts influence the state of arousal of the internal environment. Stimuli to coping may arise in the external environment in the form of physical stimuli, interpersonal relationships, or community and international events. Similarly, stimuli may arise in the internal environment in terms of thoughts, feelings, and physical illness.

GENERAL THEMES IN COPING

Coping processes enable us to learn from new situations strategies that may be useful in the future, and they arise from what has been learned in the past. Coping processes may thus be considered the major means for growth in the continual process of adaptation. When various perspectives on coping are evaluated, recurrent themes are evident: (1) coping stems from appraisal of relevant situations, (2) there is motivation to change, (3) information must be sought and used, (4) either action is practiced and tried or attitudes are changed, (5) there must be relevant feedback regarding coping efforts, and (6) coping takes place in a social context that defines appropriate and inappropriate coping and that transmits coping strategies from one generation to the next. People tend, over time, to develop coping styles, using strategies that have served them well in the past to reduce physiologic arousal and to meet the developmental challenges of maturation.

Coping strategies have been categorized as those involving direct action on oneself or on the environment or involving intrapsychic processes.[22] With direct action one may change the environment or oneself or in some way directly confront, avoid, or sidestep the situation out of which the need to cope arises. Intrapsychic processes are largely cognitive ways of changing the meaning of the situation or of dealing with the emotions that arise from the situation. Many investigators have found that those who are judged as coping most successfully with a variety of situations are flexible in using strate-

gies from both categories rather than rigidly repeating the same strategies in each new situation.[39]

COPING IN ILLNESS AND DISABILITY

Illness often represents a crisis that challenges comfortable coping styles. Chronic illness and physical disability demand the development of new coping skills. As with all coping, the individual's appraisal of the meaning of the illness and disability determines the extent to which these situations represent a crisis. However, the characteristics of a given illness or disability together with societal expectations of related behaviors add a new dimension to previously learned coping skills.

Adams and Lindemann[1] define four mechanisms fundamental to successful coping with the environment: movement, sensing, energy production, and cerebral integration. Impairment of any of these leaves an individual with a diminished capacity to cope with the environment and thus with a disability. All acute and chronic illnesses affect one or more of these fundamental functions and thus by their nature diminish the available capacity for coping. When experiencing acute or chronic illness, people have two sets of adaptive tasks, as defined by Moos[27]: general tasks, as in any life crisis, and illness-related tasks. The *general tasks* defined by many authors include maintaining a sense of personal worth or self-esteem, maintaining a reasonable emotional balance, maintaining or restoring relationships with significant persons, and preparing for an uncertain future. *Illness-related tasks* include dealing with pain and incapacitation, enhancing the recovery of body functions, dealing with the hospital environment, and developing adequate relationships with hospital personnel. The latter two are integral to increasing the likelihood of the individual's return to a valued and socially accepted life-style after maximal physical recovery. These tasks are quite similar to the appropriate "sick role" behavior described by Parsons.

Chronic illness or *disability* imposes additional adaptive tasks.[37] These tasks include the prevention of medical crises, control of ongoing symptoms, carrying out treatment regimens, adjustment to changes in the disease course, obtaining funding for survival and ongoing treatment, adapting to or preventing social isolation, normalizing relationships with others, and confronting psychologic, marital, and familial problems (see Chapter 13).

A number of coping skills are as relevant to dealing with illness and disability as they are to general crisis situations. They relate to both action (problem-focused) or intrapsychic (emotion-focused) strategies.

Action-focused strategies include seeking relevant information about the illness or disability, learning procedures or tasks specifically related to it, setting concrete and realistic goals, and rehearsing alternative out-

RESEARCH

Roberts J et al: Coping revisited: the relation between appraised seriousness of an event, coping responses and adjustment to illness, Nurs Pap 19:45-54, 1987.

Adjustment to burn injury was studied in 256 adults in a regional burn center. Coping strategies of information seeking about their injuries, emotional discharge, and avoidance were used significantly more often by those who rated their burns as more serious than by those perceiving less seriousness to the event. Furthermore, those who perceived their injuries as more serious also perceived a significantly more negative impact on many areas of their daily living. ■

comes.[27] For example, a person faced with long-term hemodialysis for renal failure may cope with this major change in life-style and threat to life by learning everything possible about home dialysis and how others have managed and about the procedures that must be mastered to safely accomplish it. Information regarding expected energy levels, time required for dialysis, and duration between treatments may help the individual set realistic goals for employment or education. While the intended goal of home dialysis is to allow continued life and reasonable functioning, it is possible that the condition will worsen and less and less time off dialysis will be possible. Rehearsal of alternative outcomes is a strategy by which such possible outcomes are thought about, discussed, and possible options considered (for example, kidney transplant or death). Rehearsal is one strategy by which all of us "practice" behaviors for anticipated circumstances.

Coping strategies are not entirely rational, however. Emotional responses to crises are dominant and interact with action responses at all points. *Emotional strategies* that serve to protect us, consciously or unconsciously, from severe distress or anxiety have often been called defense mechanisms. Denying, minimizing, and dissociating oneself from situations are mechanisms that serve to reduce anxiety and often are helpful in buying time as one prepares to face the situation (see Chapter 2). However, when such strategies are prolonged, they may serve to prevent the gaining of needed information or learning necessary skills.

Other *intrapsychic strategies* include reframing the problem or finding some meaning or general purpose in it. If the event is explicable in the context of some larger purpose or understanding of life, distressing emotions may become more manageable and energy can be freed to focus on the problem itself. Simultaneously, one may be requesting reassurance and emotional support from others in the environment. Such support helps reaffirm

a sense of personal worth in the face of major change.

There is no one specific or best way to cope with any given situation. What is useful to one individual may be inappropriate for another. The nature of the particular illness, the state of development of the individual, the social and cultural environment, and the physical and interpersonal resources available all influence the style and effectiveness of coping strategies. In nursing, as in other helping relationships, it is most useful to assist a person to cope in ways that are congruent with previously established styles. Weisman[39] suggests seven simple questions that can garner a great deal of information about coping strategies:

1. What problems, if any, do you see this illness creating?
2. How do you plan to deal with them?
3. When faced with a problem you must do something about, what do you do?
4. How does it usually work out?
5. To whom do you turn when you need help?
6. What has happened in the past when you have asked for help?
7. What kinds of problems usually tend to get you upset or down?

These questions establish perception of the current problem (numbers 1 and 2), usual style of dealing with problems (numbers 2, 3, and 4), sources of help and response to help (numbers 5 and 6), and recurrent trouble areas (number 7).

STRESS, ADAPTATION, AND COPING: APPLICATION TO NURSING

Stress, adaptation, and coping are related concepts pervasive in everyday life. In *health,* people turn to the helping professions most often when they desire assistance in developing new coping strategies for developmental crises. For example, prospective parents are taught information and specific skills in childbirth education classes or parenting skills and tactics for coping with different ages in rearing children. Physical fitness classes and stress management classes are other examples of help provided to people who are not ill. Nursing roles with respect to coping and stress in the well person are primarily educative, facilitating the ability of individuals and groups to identify sources of and to manage stress by themselves, to identify common crises in ordinary living, and to facilitate coping.

In *acute illness,* the illness itself poses a major crisis for the person. Nursing roles are twofold: managing the environment to prevent the addition of further challenges to the person's equilibrium and supplementing, insofar as possible, the person's own adaptive responses. This supplementation may consist of care and comfort measures designed to reduce fear, pain, and anxiety as well as therapeutic activity within the patient's adaptive tolerance.

Chronic illness implies reduced adaptive capacity in one or more areas. Thus, although the individual may cope adequately with ordinary living demands, the compensatory reserve for adjusting to unusual circumstances may not be available. For example, persons with compensated congestive heart failure may have no difficulty doing their own laundry when the equipment is all on the same floor as the living areas. However, they might be unable to cope with this simple part of living if forced to use a laundromat located down one flight of stairs. Nursing roles in chronic illness are both supportive and educative: helping the person identify usual limits of adaptive capacity, helping the person learn ways to reach goals within adaptive limits, and locating resources to supplement the person's capacities.

CHAPTER SUMMARY

🗸 Adaptation is a process that characterizes living systems in interaction with their environments.

🗸 These environments may be internal or external to the living system.

🗸 Stimuli resulting in adaptation may be developmental (maturational) events or situational crises that occur in day-to-day living.

🗸 The processes of adaptation can lead to growth and autonomy, as well as to preservation and stability.

🗸 Stress and coping are concepts related to adaptation: stress connotes responses that tax adaptive capacities, and coping comprises the strategies of adaptation.

🗸 Stress is an integrated psychobiologic response that depends on the intensity and duration of the stimulus and the degree of perceived threat and control of the situation.

🗸 Coping comprises the processes or skills that individuals use to deal with events, circumstances, or situations that are out of the ordinary.

🗸 Coping strategies include those which are action focused (such as information seeking) and those which are emotion focused (such as avoidance or reassurance seeking).

QUESTIONS TO CONSIDER

▪ What determines if a given life event, for example, starting a new job, will be stressful?

▪ Name some illness events that are likely to produce stress responses in most people.

▪ If some degree of stress response is inherent in acute illness, how might the nurse minimize additional stress response during hospitalization?

▪ What common nursing interventions act to support action-focused coping strategies? Emotion-focused coping strategies?

REFERENCES AND SELECTED READINGS

1. *Adams J and Lindemann E: Coping with long-term disability. In Coehlo GV, Hamburg DA, and Adams JE: Coping and adaptation, New York, 1974, Basic Books, Inc, Publishers.
2. *Benner P and Wrubel J: The primacy of caring: stress and coping in health and illness, Menlo Park, Calif, 1989, Addison-Wesley Publishing Co, Inc.
3. Cannon WB: The wisdom of the body, New York, 1939, WW Norton & Co, Inc.
4. Dixon JP, Dixon JK, and Spinner J: Perceptions of life-pattern disintegrity as a link in the relationship between stress and illness, Adv Nurs Sci 11(2):1-11, 1989.
5. Dubos R: Man adapting, New Haven, Conn, 1965, Yale University Press.
6. *Duffy ME: The concept of adaptation: examining alternatives for the study of nursing phenomena. Scholar Inquir Nurs Pract 1(3):179-196, 1987.
7. *Eisdorfer C: The conceptualization of stress and a model for further study. In Zales MR, editor: Stress in health and disease, New York, 1985, Brunner/Mazel, Inc.
8. Follinsbee FJ: Environmental stress, New York, 1978, Academic Press, Inc.
9. Frankenhauser M: Psychoneuroendocrine approaches to the study of stressful person-environment interactions. In Selye H: Selye's guide to stress research, vol 1, New York, 1980, Van Nostrand Reinhold.
10. Grinker RR: Foreword. In Coehlo GV, Hamburg DA, and Adams JE, editors: Coping and adaptation, New York, 1974, Basic Books Inc, Publishers.
11. Hall BA: The change paradigm in nursing: growth versus persistence, Adv Nurs Sci 3:1-6, 1981.
12. Hassett J: A primer of psychophysiology, San Francisco, 1978, WH Freeman & Co, Publishers.
13. Henry JP and Ely DL: Physiology of emotional stress: specific responses, J SC Med Assoc 75:501-508, 1979.
14. Hinkle LE: The concept of stress in the biological and social sciences, Int J Psychiatry Med 5:335-337, 1974.
15. *Hyman RB and Woog P: Stressful life events and illness onset: a review of crucial variables, Res Nurs Health 5:155-163, 1982.
16. *Jacobsen E: Progressive relaxation, Chicago, 1938, University of Chicago Press.
17. James W: What is emotion? Mind 19:188-205, 1884.

*References that are preceded by an asterisk are particularly well suited for student reading.

18. Kadner KD: Resilience: responding to adversity, J Psychosoc Nurs 27(7):20-25, 1989.

19. Kemp VH and Hatmaker DD: Stress and social support in high-risk pregnancy, Res Nurs Health 12:331-336, 1989.

20. Lader M and Tyer P: Vegetative system and emotion. In Levi L, editor: Emotions: their parameters and measurement, New York, 1975, Raven Press.

21. Lanuza DM and Marotta SF: Endocrine and psychologic responses of patients to cardiac pacemaker implantation, Heart Lung 16:496-505, 1987.

22. *Lazarus RS and Folkman S: Stress, appraisal and coping, New York, 1984, Springer Publishing Co, Inc.

23. Levi L: Stress and distress in response to psychosocial stimuli, Int Ser Monographs Exp Psych, vol 17, 1972.

24. Levine S, Weinberg J, and Ursin H: Definition of the coping process and statement of the problem. In Ursin H, Baade E, and Levine S, editors: Psychobiology of stress: a study of coping men, New York, 1978, Academic Press, Inc.

25. Mason JW: A historical view of the stress field, J Human Stress 1(1):6-12; 1(2):22-36, 1975.

26. Miller J: Living systems, New York, 1979, McGraw-Hill Book Co.

27. Moos R: Coping with physical illness, ed 2, New York, 1985, Plenum Publishing Corp.

28. Murphy LP: Coping, vulnerability and resilience in childhood. In Coehlo GV, Hamburg DA, and Adams JE, editors: Coping and adaptation, New York, 1974, Basic Books Inc, Publishers.

29. *Pollock SE: The hardiness characteristic: a motivating factor in adaptation, Adv Nurs Sci 11(2):53-62, 1989.

30. *Roberts J et al: Coping revisited: the relation between appraised seriousness of an event, coping responses and adjustment to illness, Nurs Pap 19:45-54, 1987.

31. Rogers M: An introduction to the theoretical basis of nursing, Philadelphia, 1970, FA Davis Co.

32. Roy C and Roberts SL: Theory construction in nursing: an adaptation model, Englewood Cliffs, NJ, 1981, Prentice-Hall, Inc.

33. Salo M: Endocrine response to anaesthesia and surgery. In Watkins J and Salo M, editors: Trauma, stress and immunity in anaesthesia and surgery, London, 1982, Butterworth Publishers.

34. Selye H: The stress of life, New York, 1956, McGraw-Hill Book Co.

35. Selye H: A syndrome produced by diverse nocuous agents, Nature 138:32-35, 1936.

36. Simpson GG: Behavior and evolution. In Roe AR and Simpson GG, editors: Behavior and evolution, New Haven, Conn, 1958, Yale University Press.

37. Strauss A et al: Chronic illness and the quality of life, ed 2, St Louis, 1984, The CV Mosby Co.

38. Washburn SL, Hamburg DA, and Bishop NH: Social adaptation in nonhuman primates. In Coehlo GV, Hamburg DA, and Adams JE, editors: Coping and adaptation, New York, 1974, Basic Books Inc, Publishers.

39. Weisman A: Coping with cancer, New York, 1979, McGraw-Hill Book Co.

40. *Weiss JM: Psychological factors in stress and disease, Sci Am 226(6):104-113, 1972.

41. White RD: Strategies of adaptation: an attempt at systematic description. In Coehlo GV, Hamburg DA, and Adams JE, editors: Coping and adaptation, New York, 1974, Basic Books Inc, Publishers.

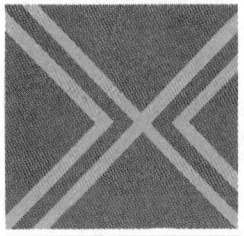

CHAPTER 11

Stress Management

PATRICIA A. BETRUS

CHAPTER OBJECTIVES

After studying this chapter, the student should be able to:
1   Analyze client situations as a basis for recommending stress management therapies.
2   Develop a personal stress management program.
3   Analyze deterrents to successful therapy for stress disorders.

THE NEED FOR STRESS MANAGEMENT

Stress is an integral part of daily life. Stress motivates, stimulates, and challenges individuals to engage in activities and interactions with others. Individuals must consistently develop new coping skills to respond to the challenges of stress. Economic demands, dual roles for women (career/homemaking), family interactions, pollution, and daily hassles all increase the stress experienced by individuals.

Every individual has a baseline of stress within which the homeostatic process operates normally. The boundaries of normal homeostasis are unique to the individual and are defined by the individual's genetic background, environment, and appraisal of events.[5] Figure 11-1 illustrates the relationship between stress and the homeostatic process.

It has been estimated that 50% to 85% of all illnesses are stress aided or stress induced.[6] Traditionally, stress and its effects have been treated within the framework of the medical model. Within this framework, amelioration of the effects of stress is achieved by the use of drugs. For example, insomnia, an affliction linked to stress, is often treated by the prescription of sleep medications. A survey of persons with insomnia in the San Francisco area indicated that 40% used sleep drugs nightly, and another 26% used sleep drugs occasionally. It was also found that in this sample 33% used alcohol to induce sleep, and another 14% used a combination of drugs and alcohol to get to sleep.[4]

Often when medications are used to diminish the stress response, the side effects of the medications become new stressors to the individual. The iatrogenic effects (side effects) of medical treatment for stress are often controlled by prescribing additional medications. The use of drugs to control the side effects of drugs used to diminish the effects of stress has been referred to as the domino theory approach to managing stress.[22]

The use of medications to diminish the effects of the stress response is not always inappropriate. Drugs can be of use, especially for short-term intervention. Drug usage for stress becomes problematic when it becomes chronic and physiologic or psychologic dependence results. Dependence on drugs, with all the accompanying medical problems, also prevents the individual from exploring new coping strategies and utilizing internal resources.[22]

STRESS MANAGEMENT THERAPEUTICS

In response to the problems inherent in the traditional approach to stress reduction, alternative strategies have been developed. These strategies utilize physiologic, cognitive, or behavioral techniques to diminish the effects of stress. Stress management as a therapeutic process has proliferated in the past 2 decades. Many of its techniques have been scrutinized carefully, and research documents the efficacy of these procedures in the management of stress.

The traditional mode of care in nursing has focused on providing direct care to patients. The direct care mode focuses on the nurse's knowledge and ability to identify and intervene to promote patient health. Patient health in this mode reflects the action and ability of the nurse to monitor, direct, and control the change process. Effective stress reduction is a function of everyday living. It is under the control of the individual patient. Intervention using direct care is inadequate for stress reduction, except for brief time-limited problems, such as control of anticipatory vomiting in cancer patients. For stress management to be effective in health maintainence and promotion, another mode of care must be implemented.

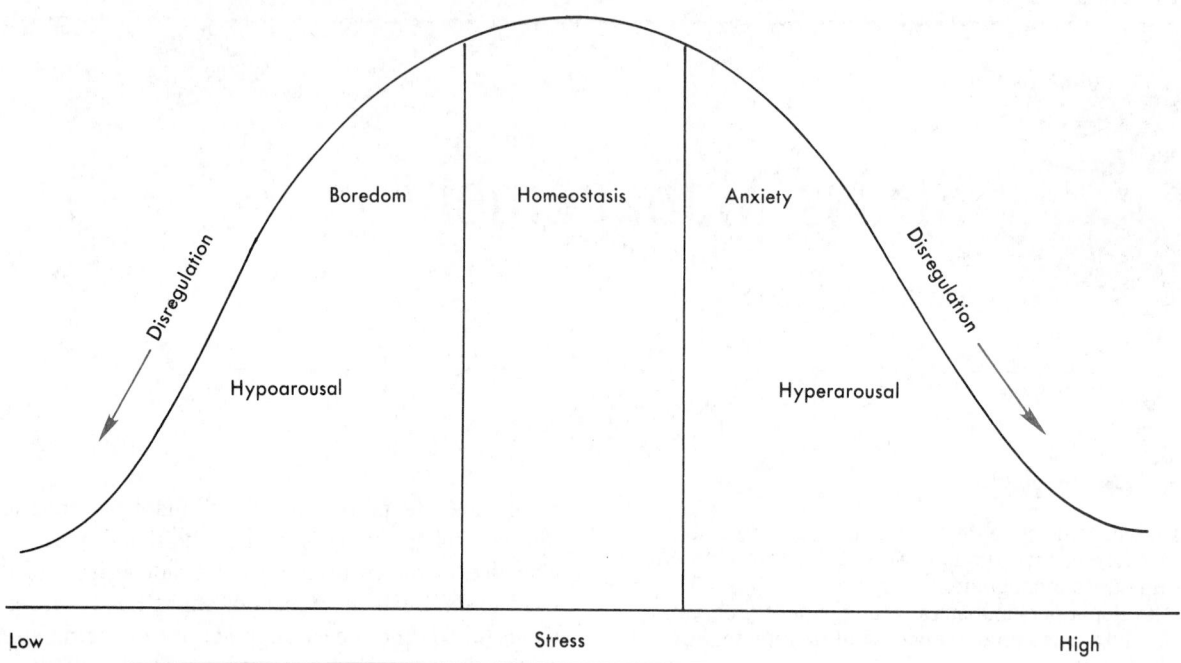

FIGURE 11-1 Stress and the homeostasis process.

Stress management embraces a self-management orientation, emphasizing individual responsibility and participation in treatment.[14] The goal of treatment for the nurse therapist is to provide the behavioral, cognitive, and psychophysiologic skills necessary for individuals to manage their own stress responses. In contrast to the traditional relationship between the individual and health care practitioner, which focuses on "compliance," individuals receiving stress management are active change agents. The stress management therapist, adhering to the self-management model, is cognizant of the limitations of his or her own therapeutic role. Ideally, the stress management therapist is a proficient therapist who acts as an instigator, facilitator, and model to assist the individual in the acquisition of relaxation and related stress management skills. The stress management therapist assumes the responsibility for designing a structured, realistic program of change, but it is the individual's responsibility to implement and maintain the program.[17] Table 11-1 contrasts the use of direct care and self-management.

The specific goals of a comprehensive stress manage-

TABLE 11-1 Contrast of direct care and self-management according to care characteristics

	Direct Care	Self-Management
Locus of control	Professional dominance	Predominantly patient, but nurse takes responsibility for imparting knowledge, skills, and feedback
Problem awareness and assessment	Usually depends on clinical observations and judgment of nurse	Self-awareness and self-assessment, with guidance from nurse
Goal setting	Most care based on end goal determined by nurse	Negotiation of goals of both patient and nurse
Change agent	Action by nurse is medium by which changes are generated	Predominantly patient action or skills to achieve changes
Knowledge	Predominantly nurse; knowledge is premise for care	Knowledge is transmitted to patient to use for developing skills to generate care
Feedback	Not central for effectiveness of care	Crucial for effectiveness of care and promoting change

From Kogan H and Betrus P: Self-management: a nursing mode of therapeutic influence, Adv Nurs Sci 6(4):55-73, 1984.

RESEARCH

Kogan H and Betrus P: Self-management: a nursing mode of therapeutic influence, Adv Nurs Science 6(4):55-73, 1984.

This study was undertaken to determine whether self-management training—which places responsibility on the patient for setting goals, monitoring health and illness signs, and evaluating the success of the change program—would be successful in altering physiological processes, cognitions, behavioral habits, and emotions. Application of self-management training to individuals (n = 322) with stress-related disorders produced significant changes in a number of outcomes, including symptoms of stress, EMG levels, and peripheral skin temperature when compared to individuals who were enrolled in a delayed treatment group. Moreover, the improvements persisted for 6 months beyond the initial self-management therapy period. ▪

ment program are to assist the individual in the following ways:

1. Developing an awareness of the stressors present in the environment
2. Recognizing his or her own specific response to stress
3. Developing and testing new coping behaviors
4. Gaining voluntary self-control over physiologic processes
5. Generalizing stress reduction skills and strategies to activities of daily living

Self-management training does not make any attempt to eliminate stress from the life of the individual. As stated earlier, stress is essential for life, and stress management training is designed to enhance the individual's ability to take charge of his or her own wellness-illness behaviors.

PSYCHOPHYSIOLOGIC STRESS MANAGEMENT STRATEGIES

PROGRESSIVE RELAXATION

Progressive relaxation was developed by Jacobson and described in *Progressive Relaxation,* his classic book of 1938. The major premise of the progressive relaxation strategy is that anxiety and muscular relaxation are mutually exclusive events. Thus anxiety does not and cannot exist when the muscles of the body are relaxed.[3]

The procedures involved in Jacobson's progressive relaxation are fundamentally simple. People typically have little or no awareness of the sensation of relaxation. In progressive relaxation the individual first tenses a specific set of muscles as hard as possible and acknowledges the feelings of tenderness, tension, and even pain in those muscles. Then the person relaxes the muscle group as much as possible and focuses on the

feelings of relaxation. Furthermore, the individual is taught to recognize the difference in sensations between the tension and the relaxation states. This pattern of tensing and relaxing muscle groups is repeated systematically throughout the musculoskeletal system of the body.

The systematic application of progressive relaxation has three major effects:

1. Muscle groups are relaxed more and more with each practice.
2. Each of the major muscle groups is relaxed one after the other. As a new muscle group is added, the individual simultaneously relaxes the other parts he or she has already learned to relax.
3. More and more total body relaxation is experienced as the person moves into the relaxation phase and progresses toward a relaxed state that is maintained beyond the relaxation period.[5]

The benefit derived from practicing progressive relaxation is that it sensitizes the individual to recognize mounting muscular tension. Increases in muscular tension are signals of increasing stress responses. When progressive relaxation is practiced and incorporated into the individual's life-style, it can help neutralize some of the effects of the stress response.

BIOFEEDBACK

Biofeedback arose from a debate between classical and operant conditioning theorists. Classical conditioning, introduced by Pavlov, refers to learning that takes place when a conditioning stimulus is paired with an unconditioned stimulus. Operant conditioning, introduced by Skinner, refers to learning that occurs without a known stimulus, usually through the receiving of rewards. The debate between the theorists focused on how many kinds of learning there were. Skinnerians claimed that only operant learning existed and that it involved voluntary processes. Other theorists stated that operant learning could also involve the involuntary processes of the autonomic nervous system. Miller,[19] in his classic experiments, taught curarized rats to raise and lower their heart rates, blood pressure, renal blood flow, and so on through operant rewards.[13] This initial research was rapidly expanded and applied to humans experiencing psychophysiologic disregulation caused by stress.

Simply stated, biofeedback is a process for learning voluntary control over autonomically regulated body functions. We have all received biofeedback in its simplest form during our lives. When we step on a bathroom scale, we get direct feedback regarding our weight. When we think we have a fever and place a thermometer in our mouths, the reading (feedback) tells us something of what is going on inside us.[6]

Biofeedback as a strategy for stress management is used to reduce tensions and anxiety that are manifested

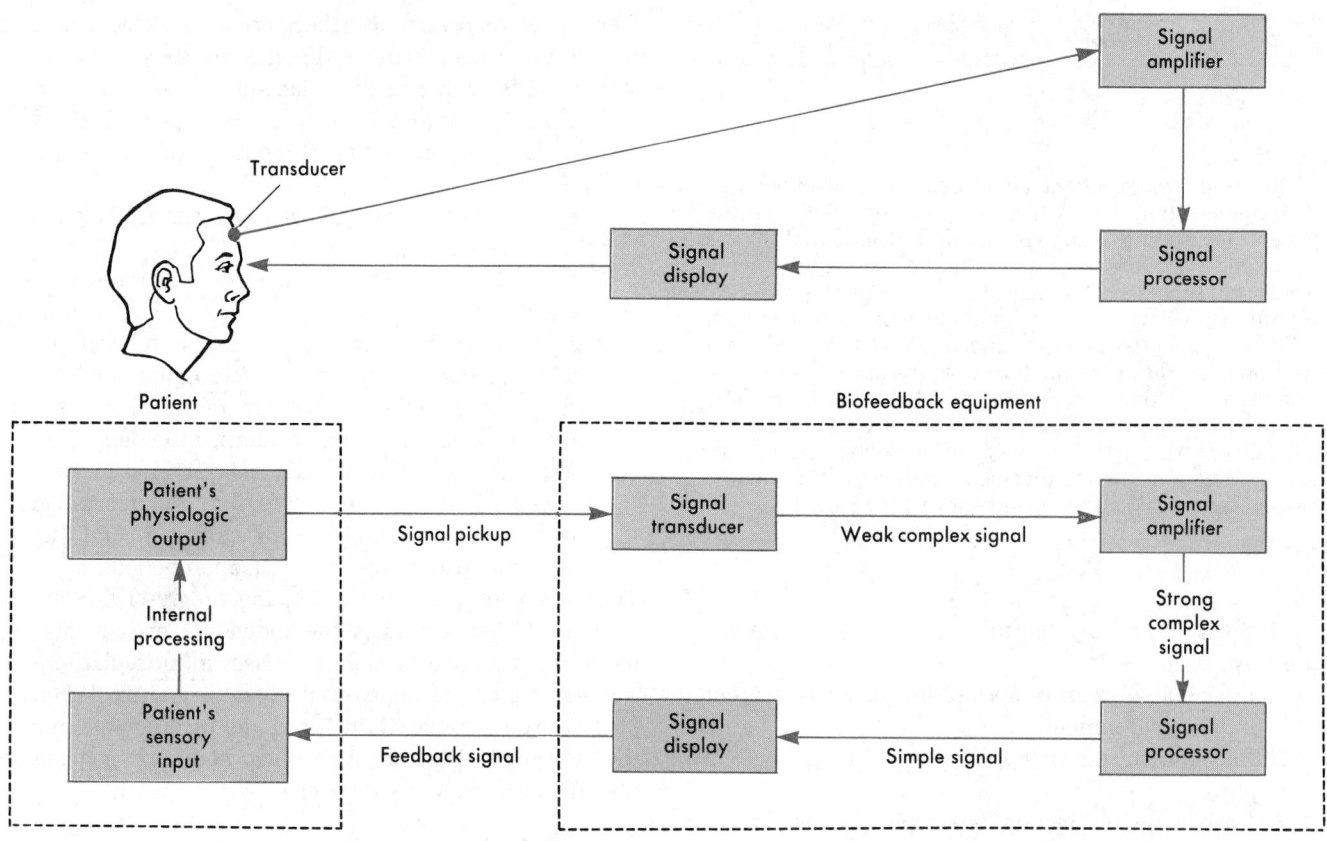

FIGURE 11-2 Elements of biofeedback system. (From Gaarder K and Montgomery P: Clinical biofeedback: a procedural manual, Baltimore, 1977, The Williams & Wilkins Co. © 1977, The Williams & Wilkins Co., Baltimore.)

in increased sympathetic arousal. Biofeedback therapy, then, is a technique in which a physiologic function of an individual, such as heart rate, muscle activity, or skin temperature, is monitored by an instrument. This information is then amplified within the instrument and presented to the individual in an auditory or visual display to reflect the changes in the individual's physiologic activity.[3] The basic elements of a biofeedback system are presented in Figure 11-2.

Biofeedback therapy is a learning process. The basic premise of biofeedback is that when individuals are presented information about their physiologic functioning, the knowledge acts as reinforcement to change those processes. With practice, the individual incorporates internally an awareness of his or her own physiologic responses and how to modulate them, thus making the biofeedback machinery unnecessary. This process of weaning the individual from reliance on the machinery is crucial. The goal of biofeedback therapy is to provide temporary assistance via instruments so that the individual will be able to monitor the physiologic response to stress and replace it with nonphysiologic arousal.[11]

METHODS OF BIOFEEDBACK

EMG Biofeedback

Muscle activity is monitored and measured by an electromyograph (EMG). Electrodes are placed on the skin over the selected muscle group. These electrodes monitor the electrical activity of the underlying muscle group and send this information to the biofeedback instrument. The instrument converts the raw signal into a display that is then fed back to the individual in the form of visual or auditory information. Muscle tension is an indication of stress. Utilizing the EMG biofeedback information, individuals are able to reduce muscle tension and replace it with muscular relaxation.

Peripheral Skin Temperature Biofeedback

Peripheral skin temperature reflects patterns of vascular constriction and dilation. A thermistor or sensor is placed on an area of skin (generally a finger or toe) to measure changes in temperature. Measurement of absolute temperature or a change in temperature is then fed back to the individual. Low skin temperatures are associated with stress; increasing skin temperature reflects relaxation.

Skin Conductance Biofeedback

Skin conductance is a measure of sweat level activity. Two electrodes are placed on hairless skin (typically the palm of the hand or fingers) and a tiny electrical current is passed between the two electrodes. When an individual becomes stressed, perspiration tends to increase. The increased moisture heightens the electrical conductance between the electrodes. When an individual relaxes, there is decreased conductance. These changes in conductance are fed back to the individual.

Other Forms of Biofeedback

Other physiologic forms of feedback that are used clinically and for research purposes are heart rate, blood pressure, pulse wave velocity, stomach acidity levels, and respiration feedback.[6]

BIOFEEDBACK PROGRAM

In stress management training the aim of biofeedback is to produce the physiology of relaxation. Merely presenting feedback in a selected system (i.e., muscle) or in a specific site does not guarantee generalization to other systems or sites. A comprehensive biofeedback training program includes monitoring and providing feedback of multiple systems and sites. Only through the use of multimodal sequencing of biofeedback can the acquisition of total body relaxation be accomplished.[17]

COGNITIVE-BEHAVIORAL STRESS MANAGEMENT STRATEGIES

MEDITATION

For centuries the art of meditation has been practiced in the East. Proponents of meditation techniques claim that meditators can control physiologic processes, some as dramatic as voluntarily stopping heart beats.[1] There are many different types of meditation with differing goals and foci, including Zen Buddhism, yoga, and transcendental meditation. Research has focused on transcendental meditation (TM) because it is one of the most practiced forms of meditation in the West.

TM is not a complicated process. The individual is given a word, a mantra, which is to be repeated silently. The individual sits in a comfortable position and focuses attention on breathing and repeating the mantra. The purpose of the mantra is to enhance a passive attitude and prevent distracting thoughts. Meditators are instructed to practice twice daily for at least 20 minutes. The physiologic relaxation that is produced during meditation generalizes to the individual's life as a protection against the effects of stress.

BENSON'S RELAXATION RESPONSE

The relaxation response was adapted by Benson[1] from transcendental meditation. The advantage of this method is that it is easy to learn and teach to others. There are four basic components necessary to elicit this response:

1. *Quiet environment.* Choose a quiet, calm environment with as few distractions as possible.
2. *Mental device.* To shift the mind from logical, externally oriented thought, there should be a constant stimulus: a sound, word, or phrase repeated silently or aloud, or fixed gazing at an object. Attention to the normal rhythm of breathing is also useful and enhances the repetition of the sound or word.
3. *Passive attitude.* Adopt a "let it happen" attitude. When distracting thoughts occur, they are to be disregarded and attention redirected to the repetition or gazing.
4. *Comfortable position.* A comfortable posture is important so that there is no undue muscular tension. Feeling comfortable and relaxed is essential.

The relaxation response produces physiologic responses similar to those in transcendental meditation. Daily use of the relaxation response is an effective mechanism to counteract the effects of stress.

ABDOMINAL BREATHING

A simple method for relaxation is a breathing technique. The focus of this technique is to take several slow, deep abdominal breaths. The individual is instructed to place one hand on the lower abdomen and slowly take in a breath to the count of four. This breath is held to the count of four, and then it is slowly expelled to the count of four. This process should be repeated several times. Often individuals are taught to use cognitive messages to accompany this technique. One such cognitive strategy is for the individual to repeat silently with each inspiration, "I will not let this problem bother me." With the expiration a simple message is, "Out goes all my stress and tension." This is an easy strategy to learn, and many people find it extremely successful when they use it frequently each day or in anticipation of a stressful situation or encounter.

BEHAVIORAL CHANGE PROGRAMS

Behavioral change programs typically focus on eliminating a specific stress-related activity such as smoking or overeating. The specific components of a behavioral program[14] are as follows:

1. *Self-monitoring of behaviors.* Monitoring of behaviors involves determining the frequency, duration, and intensity of the behavior. Furthermore, any antecedent behaviors or situations associated with the behaviors are recorded.
2. *Target behavior.* Identify in precise and measurable terms the final outcome behavior that is desired.

3. *Contracting.* Create a formal (usually written) contract between the individual and therapist. The contract should include:
   a. *Goals.* Time-limited goals (daily/weekly) related to the target behavior.
   b. *Contingency management.* The selected application of rewards and punishments used to increase or decrease behaviors. Also, the use of operant procedures, such as stimulus control and shaping.
   c. *Evaluation.* Established points of time used to evaluate progress of the change project. At these preset evaluations, the contract can be redesigned if it is found lacking.
   d. *Follow-up contingencies.* Future planning for reactivation of change program if undesirable behaviors recur.[14]

Behavior change programs are best directed to individuals who are highly motivated to make changes. The nurse assists in designing and evaluating the change program, but the responsibility for change lies with the individual.[14]

SYSTEMATIC DESENSITIZATION

Systematic desensitization is most effective for individuals with a single, circumscribed phobia (fear). Developed by Wolpe,[24] this technique is an attempt to counter-condition anxiety habits. The aim is to replace the anxiety reactions of individuals to a set of circumstances with relaxation.

Systematic desensitization involves a number of sequential stages:
   Stage 1: acquisition of adequate relaxation skills. Deeply relaxed musculature is an example.
   Stage 2: hierarchy construction. With the help of the individual, stimuli eliciting anxiety are arranged from least to most threatening; commonly a series of 8 to 12 graded images is generated.
   Stage 3: systematic desensitization proper. The person is instructed to relax while imagining progressively more threatening circumstances.[24]

The efficacy of this technique rests on the concept of a "competing response," a basic principle of behavior therapy. Here an individual is asked to engage in a behavior that is incompatible with a given problem behavior. For example, an individual cannot be anxious and relaxed at the same time; relaxation "competes" with the phobic anxiety.[17]

ATTITUDINAL RESTRUCTURING

The basic premise of rational-emotive therapy, developed by Ellis,[9] is that much if not all emotional suffering (stress) is due to the irrational ways people perceive the world. The assumptions that people make lead to self-defeating internal dialogues or negative self-talk.[26]

The goal of therapy is to replace negative self-statements with positive self-statements. Changing self-talk involves three steps: identifying self-talk, evaluating it, and replacing it with more appropriate self-talk.

Detection of self-talk may be difficult at first because it is "inaudible." Detection of self-talk usually involves keeping a daily log to identify specific thoughts and feelings.

Self-talk often distorts reality or arrives at false conclusions. The following five questions are useful in examining self-talk and the situations that are antecedent to it:
1. Have I disregarded an important aspect of the situation?
2. Have I exaggerated the meaning of an event?
3. Are my perceptions of the situation overly simplified or rigid?
4. Have I drawn conclusions where evidence is lacking or where evidence supports a contrary conclusion?
5. Have I overgeneralized or generated a false conclusion?

The answers to the five questions should reveal when self-talk is inappropriate and how to restructure it. Negative internal dialogues are probably a major source of stress to many individuals.[2]

AUTOGENIC TRAINING

Autogenic training, developed by Schultz and Luthe,[21] teaches cognitive behavior change simultaneously with physiologic behavior change. The autogenic state involves a significant reduction in sympathetic nervous system activity. The procedure applies the principles of self-management and training in passive concentration (not unlike transcendental meditation) through six standard physiologically oriented steps[2,6]:

Physiologic States	Repeated Statement
1. Heaviness in extremities	"My right arm is heavy."
2. Warmth in extremities	"My right arm is warm."
3. Regulation of cardiac activity	"My heart beat is calm and regular."
4. Regulation of respiration	"My breathing is calm and regular."
5. Abdominal warmth	"My solar plexus is warm."
6. Cooling of forehead	"My forehead is cool."

It generally takes 3 to 6 months to go through the six phases of autogenic training. An accomplished practitioner of autogenics should be able to induce a state of relaxation in any environment or situation.

STRESS INOCULATION

Individuals who undergo stress inoculation are provided with a prospective defense or a set of skills to deal with future stressful situations.[7] Stress inoculation training involves three phases:

I. Educational phase. This phase is designed to provide the individual with a conceptual framework for understanding stressful situations. The individual is provided with an explanatory scheme for understanding his or her specific responses to stress.

II. Rehearsal phase. During this phase individuals are provided with a variety of coping techniques. These coping techniques include both direct action and cognitive coping skills.

III. Application training. The individual tests out and practices the coping skills by actually employing them under stress situations.

Stress inoculation therapy has proved to be useful, especially in situations of extreme stress or anxiety.[7]

OBSTACLES TO AND BENEFITS OF SUCCESSFUL STRESS MANAGEMENT

Several factors may impede the progress of stress management training. Recognition of these factors assists the nurse therapist in selecting the appropriate stress management technique. The common obstacles to change are as follows:

1. *Secondary gain.* The individual may have been or may currently be rewarded for maintaining stress symptoms, for example, by significant others or by monetary reward.
2. *Social Support dynamics.* One or more members of the social support system (family, friends, coworkers) of the individual may have a vested interest in the maintenance of a particular illness behavior or symptom.
3. *Life-style habit patterns.* A client's occupation or leisure pursuits may have inherent stressors. These are relevant topics for stress counseling.
4. *Change represents the unknown.* Therefore it is frightening. There is often a cognitive and emotional reluctance to change because of this fear.
5. *Relevancy.* The therapy may not be seen as relevant to the problem at hand. An alcoholic, for example, may wonder what EMG training has to do with abstinence.[17]
6. *Physical or mental status of individual.* In some situations, individuals who are experiencing extreme levels of stress that require continual coping are "too stressed" to benefit from a program in stress management. For example, individuals undergoing chemotherapy intervention for cancer may be too physically fatigued with inadequate coping resources to engage in a stress management program for control of nausea/vomiting related to chemotherapy.

Stress management has rapidly been gaining popularity as a training modality in recent years. Research has demonstrated its effectiveness in alleviating discomfort

RESEARCH

Kogan-Nakagawa H, Garber A, Jarrett M, Egan K, and Hendershot S: Self-management of hypertension: predictors of success in diastolic blood pressure reduction, Res Nurs Health 11:105-115, 1988.

The purpose of this study was to determine if borderline hypertension subjects were successful in self-regulating blood pressure after receiving self-management therapy. A second purpose was to compare individuals who were successful in reducing blood pressure after treatment with individuals who were non-succeeders to distinguish if any psychologic or physiologic variables predicted success. Participants in the study were 34 white, male, unmedicated, borderline hypertensive individuals. The subjects participated in 14 sessions of biofeedback/cognitive-behavioral self-management treatment. The hour-long sessions were held twice weekly. The first four sessions consisted of EMG biofeedback, sessions five through seven were augmented with temperature or galavanic skin response; the final sessions included pulse wave velocity training and self-regulation of sympathetic arousal. A program of relaxation training was included as a counter-response to arousal states. Subjects were instructed to practice relaxation at home twice daily. Behavioral analysis was used to identify stressors and analyze emotional responses and appraisals of events. A variety of cognitive strategies was used to assist subjects in achieving their goals. Of the 34 participants, 22 subjects (65%) exited treatment with consistent diastolic pressure below 90 mm Hg; 12 subjects (35%) exited with diastolic pressure equal to or above 90 mm Hg. The successful group began and ended the treatment with lower psychologic distress than did the unsuccessful group; however, both groups demonstrated significantly reduced psychologic distress after treatment. A discriminant analysis revealed that the group with successfully reduced blood pressure had lower scores on psychologic indexes (anxiety, hostility, and interpersonal sensitivity), lower systolic blood pressure, and higher heart rates when challenged mentally (silent serial subtraction) before treatment than the group that did not reduce blood pressure ($p < .02$). The results of this study support self-management treatment as a clinical intervention for the treatment for borderline hypertension. Although diastolic blood pressure was not reduced for all individuals, this was only one facet of change during treatment. All subjects showed a reduction of psychologic distress after treatment. The reduction of diastolic blood pressure for 65% of the subjects and enhancment of effective coping for the entire sample is of prime clinical importance. ■

in a number of illnesses. The box on p. 204 lists several of the effective applications of stress management.

No one strategy or technique should be viewed as a panacea for stress reduction. Rather, a comprehensive stress management program recognizes the ubiquitous nature of stress, and a program should be individually tailored. Many individuals benefit from a combination of several stress management strategies. Furthermore,

STRESS-RELATED ILLNESSES FOR WHICH STRESS MANAGEMENT HAS BEEN EFFECTIVE

Muscle tension	Dysmenorrhea
Insomnia	Menopausal hot flashes
Hypertension	Tension headaches
Stuttering	Bruxism
Asthma	Chronic pain
Raynaud's disease	Arthritis
Migraine headaches	Cardiac arrhythmias
Colitis	Dermatitis
Ulcers	Incontinence
Neuromuscular tics	Hyperhydrosis
Gastrointestinal distress	Tinnitus
Anxiety	Nausea and vomiting
Phobias	

stress management strategies are often enhanced by adjunctive techniques such as imagery, directed fantasy, catharsis, thought stopping, and insight. The decision as to which strategies are likely to be effective is determined by the therapist after a complete assessment has been made of the individual and his or her response to stress.

STRESS MANAGEMENT: NURSING IMPLICATIONS

Stress management techniques have become firmly established therapeutic approaches in the past decade. The strategies have been employed by nurses in both hospital and outpatient clinical settings. The use of these strategies by nurses is growing rapidly. Most skilled nurse therapists obtain specialized training in stress reduction techniques. Several graduate training programs in nursing now include stress management training as a course of study.

Stress management techniques have been applied and researched by nurses in hospital settings for diverse patient populations, such as for patients receiving preoperative and postoperative care,[10] as stress inoculation for anticipatory vomiting of patients receiving chemotherapy,[8,20] to manage patient and family stress during recovery from coronary bypass surgery,[12] and to facilitate childbirth.[23] Continued development of nursing expertise in stress management therapies will extend the application of these strategies into other areas of nursing care.

Nursing is in the forefront in integrating stress management in outpatient settings. The focus of stress management by nurses in outpatient clinics has been health promotion/prevention and the treatment of psychophysiologic stress disorders. One example of this trend is the Management of Stress Disorders Clinic at the University of Washington. The clinic was established in the late 1970s as a center for graduate study and research.

In subsequent years the clinic has offerred treatment to individuals with stress-related disorders including hypertension, migraine headaches, chronic muscle tension pain, ulcers, gastrointestinal distress, and insomnia. The focus of treatment is self-management techniques with either biofeedback or systematic relaxation strategies as physiologic intervention. This program has treated over 900 patients with dramatic results and serves as one model of the effect that nursing care can have on the provision of health care.[16]

CHAPTER SUMMARY

- Stress is necessary for survival; only when stress exceeds the individual's coping abilities do problems arise.
- A successful stress management program uses strategies that diminish stress by focusing on cognitive, physiologic, and behavioral interventions.
- A variety of physiologic and cognitive techniques can be used by a trained nurse therapist to help individuals cope effectively with stress.
- The nurse must recognize that obstacles to successful treatment of stress disorders exist and must be considered when planning interventions.

QUESTIONS TO CONSIDER

- What is the nursing role in stress management therapy?
- Identify one obstacle to successful stress management and consider what strategies you would use to overcome this problem.
- Think of a recent stressful experience and your response to the situation. Consider which stress management techniques would have helped you cope more effectively.

REFERENCES AND SELECTED READINGS

1. *Benson H: The relaxation response, New York, 1975, William Morrow & Co Inc.
2. Betrus P and Kogan H: Stressors in nursing: causes, results and interventions. In Stressors in nursing: responses and resolutions, Seattle, 1981, University of Washington Press.
3. Brown B: Stress and the art of biofeedback, New York, 1977, Harper & Row, Publishers Inc.
4. *Coates T and Thoresen C: How to sleep better, Englewood Cliffs, NJ, 1977, Prentice Hall.
5. Curtis J and Detert R: How to relax, Palo Alto, Calif, 1981, Mayfield Publishing Co.

*References preceded by an asterisk are particularly well suited for student readings.

6. Danskin D and Crow M: Biofeedback: an introduction and guide, Palo Alto, Calif, 1981, Mayfield Publishing Co.

7. Davidson P: Behavioral management of anxiety, depression and pain, New York, 1976, Brunner/Mazel Inc.

8. *Donovan M: Relaxation with guided imagery: a useful technique, Cancer Nurs pp. 27-32, Feb 1980.

9. Ellis A: Reason and emotion in psychotherapy, New York, 1962, Lyle Stuart Inc.

10. *Flaherty G, and Fitzpatrick J: Relaxation technique to increase comfort level of postoperative patients: a preliminary study, Nurs Res 27(6):353-355.

11. Gaarder K and Montgomery P: Clinical biofeedback: a procedural manual, Baltimore, 1977, Williams & Wilkins.

12. *Gilliss C: Reducing family stress during and after coronary artery bypass surgery, Nurs Clin North Am 19(1):103-111, 1984.

13. Hassett J: A primer of psychophysiology, San Francisco, 1978, WH Freeman & Co Publishers.

14. *Kanfer F and Goldstein A: Helping people change, New York, 1975, Pergamon Press Inc.

15. Jacobsen E: Progressive relaxation, Chicago, 1938, University of Chicago Press.

16. Kogan H and Betrus P: Self-management: a nursing mode of therapeutic influence, Adv Nurs Sci pp. 55-73, July 1984.

17. Kogan H et al: Therapeutic manual for the management of stress response, Seattle, 1980, University of Washington.

18. *Meichenbaum D: Cognitive-behavior modification: an integrative approach, New York, 1977, Plenum Publishing Corp.

19. Miller N: Learning of visceral and glandular responses, Science 163:434-445, 1969.

20. Moore K and Altmaier E: Stress inoculation training with cancer patients, Cancer Nurs pp. 389-393, Oct 1981.

21. Schultz J and Luthe W: Autogenic training: a psychophysiologic approach in psychotherapy, New York, 1959, Grune & Stratton Inc.

22. *Sutterley D and Donnelly G: Stress management, Top Clin Nurs 1(1):1-104, 1979.

23. Sullivan M: Effect of psychophylatic method of prepared childbirth on specific muscle relaxation to command, Communicating Nursing Research, vol 12, Sept 1979, pp. 60-63.

24. Wolpe J: Psychotherapy by reciprocal inhibition, Stanford, Calif, 1958, Stanford University Press.

COMMON PSYCHOPHYSIOLOGIC STRESSORS

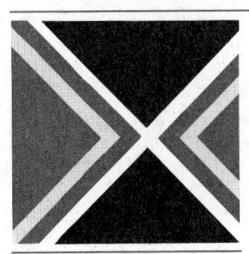

CHAPTER 12

Sensory Overload and Sensory Deprivation: Hazards of Caregiving Environments

SHARON FOUGHT
MARIANN DIMINNO
JUDITH OZUNA

CHAPTER OBJECTIVES

After studying this chapter, the student should be able to:
1 Relate sensory processes to sources of sensory deprivation and overload in caregiving environments.
2 Identify factors that predispose selected clients to sensory deprivation or sensory overload.
3 Distinguish conditions of chronic versus acute overload or deprivation.
4 Assess the consequences of sensory overload or deprivation for clients.
5 Design nursing interventions to provide meaningful stimuli, facilitate input of stimuli from a variety of sources, clarify meaning of the environmental stimuli to clients, and facilitate healthy adaptation.

Individuals continuously interact with their internal and external environments. Their boundaries, as unique systems, have been developmentally defined through their sensory apparatus. It is through their senses that individuals learn to differentiate themselves as separate entities.

Infants initially respond to the environment almost exclusively through their skin, since the first nerve endings to be myelinated are those of touch, temperature, and pain.[9] Eventually, as the sensory apparatus develops and refines, children perceive their boundaries as separate from the environment and learn to use their senses to expand their knowledge of the world. It is this very process of receiving and responding to environmental cues that an individual uses throughout the life cycle to form the basis for adaptive responses.

Since sensation is such an integral part of the ability to perceive and interact with the environment, it follows that any alteration of this process will result in the potential for system disequilibrium. As open systems, individuals constantly receive inputs or cues from the environment. If these inputs were suddenly altered, either diminished or increased radically in some way, the nor-

mal method of receiving environmental cues would be affected and the individual would have to adapt to this sudden change. If an individual is unable to adapt, sensory overload or deprivation may result in disequilibrium. An organism adapts to a significant decrease in or loss of sensation in one modality by obtaining data through another modality. For example, when children play games involving blindfolding, such as "Pin the Tail on the Donkey," the immediate response of the blindfolded individual is to place the arms in a frontal position to obtain tactile clues from the environment that are not available through vision.

Clients in health care settings may also experience system disequilibrium. The mechanized hospital environment may result in altered sensory input and may be compounded further by the physiologic alterations of illness, which add further stress to the client system.

Interest in the area of sensory alteration began in the 1950s. Early experiments manipulated the environment in an attempt to seek some answers to the phenomena of brainwashing and the effects of monotony on an individual's performance.[45] The findings indicated that by manipulating the amount of sensory-perceptual inputs, behavioral changes could be elicited from experimental subjects. When exposed to sensory and perceptual deprivation, subjects experienced hallucinations, difficulty in cognitive tasks, disorientation, anxiety, and somatic complaints.

Since these first studies, interest in sensory deprivation has grown considerably. Nursing therapies have been developed that might be effective in preventing or diminishing sensory deprivation or overload. Although the nursing profession requires additional rigorous clinical research to substantiate some of the nursing interventions or therapies proposed for clients with a sensory alteration, it is useful to consider a model of sensory overload and deprivation for clients whose behavior may seem confusing, perplexing, or not supportive of health adaptation. The nurse can use a systematic approach to assess potential inputs that could be possible system stressors and intervene to assist the client in making healthy, adaptive responses.

The purpose of this chapter is to explore sensory alteration and its resultant disequilibrium for both theoretical and clinical perspectives.

SENSORY PROCESS

SENSORY PERCEPTION

Humans orient themselves to their environment through their ability to receive and organize sensory stimuli. This *reception* and *organization of stimuli* is collectively known as *sensory perception*. The process of sensory perception depends on several factors: a stimulus, adequate sensory receptors, intact neural pathways, and adequate processing by the brain to interpret the stimulus input.

A stimulus is received by a sensory receptor, which then synapses with a cranial, peripheral, or autonomic nerve. The nerve then either synapses with sensory nerve tracts in the spinal cord or with areas of the brain. The exact mechanism by which the brain interprets sensory input is not known, but there is evidence that the *reticular formation* (RF) plays an integral role in processing sensory input. The RF is composed of a network of neurons that forms a central core extending from the medulla of the lower brain to the thalamus in the diencephalon.[37]

The RF can be stimulated by two major sources of stimuli, external and internal. External stimuli include cortical impulses and sensory stimulation from visual, auditory, and olfactory sources; and internal stimuli include somatic and visceral sources (muscles and joints).[6] The RF controls general central nervous system activity and selectivity of attention or arousal.

The RF serves a monitoring function for both inputs and outputs to the human system. The reticular activating system (RAS), a part of the RF extending from the midpons region to the thalamus and hypothalamus, is considered essential for maintaining consciousness.[37]

It is believed that the RF in conjunction with the thalamus and hypothalamus collects and combines sensory input. *Perception* takes place when the sensory input is received, decoded (synthesized), and interpreted by the cortex. When interpretation occurs, a conscious awareness of sensation begins. Perception provides the individual with an awareness of the environment, which then serves as a basis for determining if an adaptive response is required to maintain equilibrium. To clarify this further, consider the following example: if the cortex interprets an auditory stimulus to be loud, unpleas-

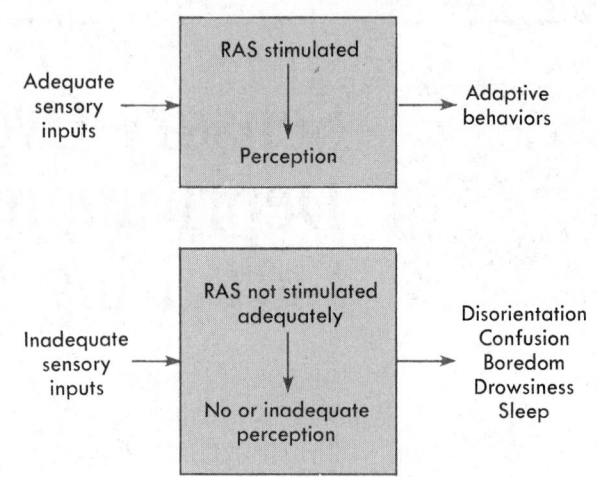

FIGURE 12-1 Relationship among sensory inputs, arousal, and outcome.

ant, and painful, the individual becomes consciously aware of the discomfort and may adapt by covering the ears or moving to a quieter environment. If the cortex interprets an auditory stimulus to be pleasant, the client becomes consciously aware of this sensation and may utilize a maintenance action of remaining stationary in the pleasant environment.

It is important to note that without the function of the ascending reticular activating system, perception does not occur. Lindsley[49] gives the example of an individual who is under barbiturate anesthesia: the sensory pathways can conduct their messages to the primary receiving areas, but discrimination and perception do not occur. Thus it is seen that the RAS not only plays an important role in providing a mechanism for general arousal and alerting of the individual, but it must also be stimulated for perception to take place.

If sensory inputs are adequate, the RAS is stimulated and an alert aroused state is created in the individual—a state that allows perception and adaptive responses to occur.

If the RAS is inadequately stimulated, disorientation, confusion, boredom, and drowsiness may occur (Figure 12-1). Sleep is a normal, rhythmic alteration in arousal.

From a systems perspective, the stimulus serves as an input; the sensory receptors, neural pathways, and cerebral decoding necessary for processing (the RAS) are throughput; and the resulting adaptive response or behavior of the individual is output (Figure 12-2).

SENSORY APPARATUS AND MODALITIES

The sensory apparatus provides stimulus inputs into the system; the eyes, ears, nose, skin, tongue, muscles, and visceral organs all provide information relevant to the functioning of the system. If one of the sense organs is

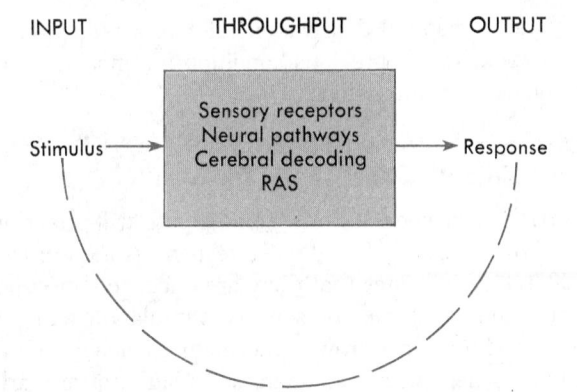

FIGURE 12-2 Sensory process from a systems perspective.

TABLE 12-1 Sources of sensory inputs, modalities, and their functions

Source and Function of Stimulus Inputs	Sense Organs	Modality
Internal		
Provide internal environmental cues	Viscera	Kinesthetic
	Joints	Visceral
	Muscle and specialized neural tissue	Visual
		Auditory
	Hollow organs	Olfactory
		Tactile
		Gustatory
External		
Provide external environmental cues	Eyes	
	Ears	
	Nose	
	Skin	
Internal and external		
Provide internal and external environmental cues		

no longer providing cues about the environment, functions and situations of everyday life are altered.

Sensory *modalities* can be broadly classified as either originating internally or externally (Table 12-1). The internal sources of stimuli are *kinesthetic,* such as those arising from muscles and specialized neural tissue, or *visceral,* originating from hollow organs. These internal sensations provide information about placement of the body and its position relative to space; that is, where parts of the body are in relation to one another. Kinesthetic stimuli are primarily involved with the sensations of pain and with the regulatory mechanisms of the internal environment of the body.

The external sources of stimulation arise from the eyes, ears, nose, and skin, whereas the tongue provides both internal and external inputs of stimulation.

It is important to emphasize that sensation has both internal and external components, since both sources contribute to the overall sensory information processed by the brain. An alteration in the amount of stimulation received from either an internal or external source will affect the amount of sensory input to the brain and may necessitate an adaptive response. The importance of this will be more evident in the discussion of the clinical applications of sensory alteration.

SENSORISTASIS

Schultz[42] has defined *sensoristasis* as a drive state of cortical arousal that propels the awake individual to seek an optimal level of sensory variation. In other words, each individual has a drive or need for a constant range of varied sensory input. This varied input is required for the organism to function optimally. Schultz compares sensoristasis as being similar to the homeostasis concept of Cannon[31]—a dynamic changing condition that adapts to subject and task variables but that also has a relatively constant pattern. The RAS appears to play a monitoring function by its mediation of system

inputs and outputs in maintaining the sensoristatic equilibrium. This equilibrium, however, can be disturbed under conditions of sensory restriction or overload, and the organism must then use adaptive behaviors to restore the balance. For example, if sensory stimulation is below the optimal level, the organism will adapt to seek alternative stimuli or become more sensitized to existing stimuli. If stimulation is greater than the optimal level, the organism will adapt by attempting to decrease system inputs.

Schultz[42] lists four major corollaries of his sensoristatic model:

1. The drive or need mechanism implemented in the sensoristatic concept is equivalent with arousal as mediated by the RAS.
2. An optimal range of external stimulation exists that influences cortical arousal. Only when this optimal level is maintained can the organism function adaptively with its environment. If there is alteration of stimulation, there is a disruption of learned responses and prevention of new learning.
3. An organism behaves in a way that will maintain this optimal arousal level.
4. The optimal range of sensory stimulation can alter depending on several factors: the task to be performed, the present status of the organism, and the preceding level of stimulation. Also, there may be individual differences in need for sensory inputs and differences over time within the same individual.

There seems to be general agreement that an optimal level of arousal is required to maintain perceptual and adaptive functions; however, it is still unclear what the exact limits of normal sensory stimulation are. What is considered optimal seems to vary widely among individual subjects.

DEPRIVATION AND OVERLOAD

DEFINITIONS

The term *sensory deprivation* has been used synonymously in the literature with many different terms, ranging from social deprivation to restricted stimulation and solitude. For the purposes of this discussion, *sensory deprivation* is defined as a state of being in which the amount or intensity of sensory inputs is below the individual's range of tolerance. Tolerance is the unique range each person has for coping with a type of sensation, enabling each person to function in a healthy manner. The state of being in which the sensory inputs exceed the optimal range of tolerance is termed *overload*.

Deprivation refers to the general concept of decreasing sensory inputs. In the specific case of a reduction in the pattern of meaningfulness of stimuli, the term *perceptual deprivation* is employed. This occurred in experimental studies when subjects wore translucent goggles or translucent halved Ping-Pong balls as eye shields to produce diffused, unpatterned light. The subject saw light, but the form and pattern did not alter. Another example is the consistent hum of a monitor in the intensive care unit (ICU). The state of being in which the patterning of sensory input is below the individual's optimal range of tolerance is defined as *monotony;* that which is above the optimal range is termed *mutability* (Figure 12-3). It should be emphasized that both sensory and perceptual deprivation refer to a reduction of stimulation from a previous condition and not the total absence of all stimulation.

EFFECT OF EARLY ALTERATION ON GROWTH AND DEVELOPMENT

Deprivation or overload of system inputs will affect an individual's capacity for adaptive responses. Experimental literature indicates that there are effects on adult behavior from alteration of sensory stimulation early in life.[39,49] The normal growth and maintenance of neural structures depend on adequate stimulation at an early level of development.[41,39] Experimental work with cats, monkeys, and chimpanzees demonstrated that organisms reared in restricted sensory environments show perceptual visual deficits, which may never be eliminated.[14,39] The primates also reacted violently to a marked increase in stimulation.

From these studies it appears that the adaptive capacity and neurologic structures of an organism can be severely affected when there is early sensory deprivation. Although deprivation can limit sensory development, it can also lead to physiologic adaptation. The findings of Freeman and Bradley[18] on monocularly deprived humans suggest that although the affected eye has an irreversible deficit (decreased ability to activate cortical neurons) the unaffected eye has increased visual sensitivity in alignment discrimination.

Studies of institutionalized children reveal that early childhood deprivation results in behavioral changes and developmental problems. When children who spent their first 3 years in an institution before being placed in a foster home were compared with children reared con-

---

Ballard KS: Identification of environmental stressors for patients in a surgical intensive care unit, Issues in mental health nursing 3:89-108, 1981.

The stressful factors associated with the environment of a surgical intensive care unit were reported by 22 adult subjects who had planned surgeries. All subjects were in multi-bed rooms and recorded onto Q sort cards the events they felt to be of high, medium, or low stress. The cards were then sorted into three piles. Highest ranking events that were reported included "being tied down by tubes," "being in pain," "being thirsty," missing their spouse, wearing oxygen masks, and having restricted mobility of hands or arms because of IV lines. The ranking of 40 items indicated which subjects may be at risk for or were experiencing isolation, immobilization, and sleep or sensory deprivation. Listing stressful situations and events indicates areas in which nurses can assess for cases of altered perception, sensory deprivation, or sensory overload and intervene to enhance healthy adaptation. ■

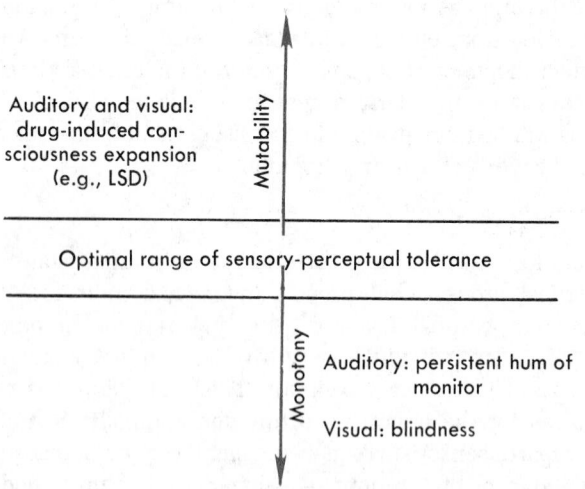

FIGURE 12-3 Sensory-perceptual deprivation. Change in patterning of sensory input may create mutability or monotony.

tinuously in a foster home, the children who were institutionalized experienced less intellectual and emotional capacity.[20] The institutionalized children demonstrated aimlessness, poor concentration, poor impulse control, and a decreased capacity for abstract thinking as compared with the control group. Thus it is evident that a decrease in critical inputs from a consistent source, such as a mother, adversely influenced the emotional and intellectual development of these children.

Another study compared the developmental patterns of institutionalized children with children reared in their own homes for the first year of life. Children were observed in two different institutions. The first was a foundling home where children had only minimal brief contacts with a nurse. The other institution was a nursery located in a penal institution for delinquent girls, where the children had consistent, frequent contacts with their own mothers.[46] The children reared in a foundling home began at a normal development level but did not maintain it and eventually fell behind the other children in social, perceptual, and motor development. Both of these studies indicate the critical nature of early sensory inputs from a consistent source and the importance of perceptual and social stimulation to normal human development.

Others investigated the effects of increased sensory

RESEARCH

Reimer M: Sleep pattern disturbance: nursing interventions perceived by patients and their nurses as facilitating nocturnal sleep in hospital. In McLane A, editor: Classification of nursing diagnoses, proceedings of the seventh conference, St Louis, 1987, The CV Mosby Co.

A study of patient and nurse perceptions of interventions that facilitate nighttime sleep included data from 143 patients and 157 nurses in 13 medical surgical units of a large hospital. Patients and nurses completed written questionnaires. Patients reported interesting differences in their own home and hospital sleeping patterns, including time awake at night, 60.2 minutes in the hospital versus 17.5 minutes at home (t (63) = 4.74, $p < .001$); more awakenings at night in the hospital than at home; and double the amount of daytime sleep in hospital versus that at home (t (89) = 3.66, $p < .001$). Finding a comfortable position and the presence of pain were the two most frequently reported stimuli that disrupt sleep. Interventions delineated as "very important" for facilitating sleep included pain medications, sleep medications, turning the lights down, the security or awareness that a nurse was available, and back rubs. Additionally, 16.9% of the patients stated that sleep would likely improve if they were fatigued or stayed up later. Frequently reported external and internal environmental stimuli that disturb sleep can be diminished or eliminated, and interventions can be implemented to facilitate the onset of sleep. ∎

inputs on infants. They found that infants who had experienced increased handling and exposure to objects within their visual field demonstrated "visually directed reaching" and "visual attentiveness" earlier than infants who had not been exposed to such stimuli.[52]

Early environmental inputs also affect the infant's ability for self-soothing, first as a child and later as an adult. For example, the sensory stimulation of a mother soothing a child through holding and rocking becomes an internalized structure, which the adult draws on later in times of distress. It has been hypothesized that the self-soothing psychic structure of the adult is linked to early repetition of infant satisfaction from the environment in meeting basic biologic needs and the supportive sensory inputs provided by a parent. Deficits in this early process adversely affect the adult's ability for psychic self-soothing.

It has been suggested that early levels of stimulation influence the optimal level of sensory variation in the adult. The child's level of stimulus variation will influence the arousal of the RAS for adaptive behavior as an adult. Thus adaptation levels may be determined by the amount of variety of early sensory input. This may explain individual differences in the optimal level of stimulation within which the organism can function effectively.[42]

The fact that early sensory input is critical to the normal growth and development of children has definite implications for nurses, who may be called on assess the amount of stimulation available to an infant in the home environment.

The same assessment process is called for when children are hospitalized. Nurses are entrusted with the care of hospitalized children whose needs include a stimulating sensory environment to enhance normal development. Contact with families, other children, play therapy and various sensory stimulators such as mobiles, toys, colors and patterns on walls, curtains, and furniture all contribute to adequate sensory inputs.

ADAPTIVE AND MALADAPTIVE RESPONSES

When system inputs either exceed or fall short of the optimal range for the organism, the overload or deprivation state is considered a system stressor. Any conditions that alter sensory inputs would also be considered stressors. These can be environmental, social, physical, psychologic, or developmental factors. For example, anxiety, immobilization, paralysis, flotation mattresses, body casts, isolation, and neurologic deficits alter sensory inputs and can be categorized as system stressors. The degree to which each individual tolerates system stressors differs, and this influences how a client will respond—whether in an adaptive or maladaptive manner. Roy[40] defines adaptation as a human's positive response to a changing environment. An adaptive response main-

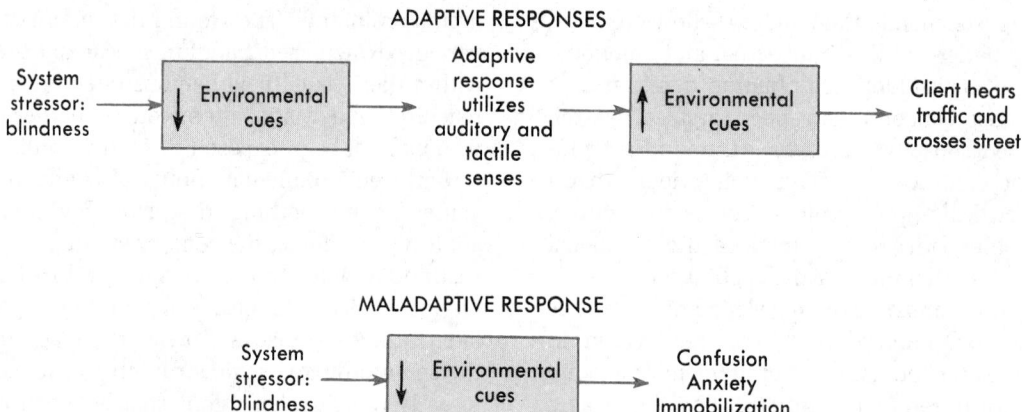

FIGURE 12-4 Adaptive versus maladaptive responses to blindness.

tains client integrity; a maladaptive response does not and is disruptive to the individual.

Mitchell[35] cites examples of adaptive behaviors by newly blinded individuals who can no longer see traffic lights. These individuals can adapt and obtain environmental cues through other sensory modalities, such as their auditory sense by listening to traffic patterns to determine if traffic has stopped, or through their sense of touch by becoming aware of the motion against their person as the crowd begins to move across the street. A maladaptive response to the same situation would occur if this individual became anxious, confused, and immobilized on the street corner and unable to utilize alternative environmental cues (Figure 12-4).

Stressors that exceed the optimal tolerance level of the client will result in maladaptive responses, which can be cognitive, perceptual, motor, or affective disturbances.

Cognitive changes experienced by subjects range from poor concentration, altered sequencing of thoughts, or unusual ideas to bizarre or primary process thinking— defined as the instinctual thought patterns experienced in dreams. There is also alteration in ability to perform unstructured cognitive tasks.[42]

Perceptual changes include visual and auditory distortions, perceived movement of stable objects, warping and curvature of surfaces and lines, changes in color and form, and changes in bodily sensations such as numbness. More elaborate distortions have also been reported where clients perceive their bodies to be floating or experience olfactory sensory distortions—exemplified by cooking or burning odors.[14,16,26] There is a difference of opinion among researchers as to whether these can be considered hallucinatory experiences, since they are not psychotic episodes but more accurately episodic occurrences where the subjects are aware that their experiences are not truly reflective of reality. It has been

contended that the term *perceptual distortions* is more accurate a description than hallucinations. Ellis[16] uses the term *indeterminate stimulus experience* (ISE) to describe such distortions where a perceptual disturbance occurs for which there is no known stimulus. This can occur without disorientation to time, place, or person.

The experimental literature supports the contention that sensory and perceptual alteration will produce changes in *motor* coordination. Dexterity, other measures of eye-hand coordination, balance, and body coordination have been found to be negatively affected by deprivation conditions.[51,58]

Affective disturbances noted by researchers include anxiety, fear, mood swings, irritability, depression, exaggerated emotional responses, and anger.[42] The intensity of the disturbances varies from mild discomfort to panic.

Additional responses include somatic complaints and noncompliant behavior. Noncompliant behavior would include actions clients display that are contrary to the instructions of health care providers and detrimental to the client. A study of postoperative eye surgery patients identified behaviors such as removing eye patches and getting out of bed as noncompliant.[55]

It should be emphasized that clients may not openly or easily share with staff some of these disturbances, such as perceptual distortions, because of the anxiety or embarrassment that may accompany such experiences. The nurse must be alert for maladaptive responses and investigate further, seeking additional data from the client if the situation warrants intervention.

It is also important for the nurse to be aware that clients in a hospital setting can display maladaptive behaviors in response to an altered sensory environment. It is not unlikely that the nurse may be in a situation where an apparently "normal" client is exhibiting psychotic-like behavior such as confusion, noncompliance, disorientation, anxiety, mood swings, or perceptual distortions. This does not mean the client has suddenly become psychotic, toxic, or senile but that he or she may be responding to an altered sensory environment. However, in applying research findings to the clinical situation, certain limitations must be noted. Although it is hypothesized that responses are correlated with alterations in sensory inputs, this hypothesis needs further testing. It is not a ready explanation but a framework to use in attempting to assess and understand client behavior.

Goals of nursing are to promote harmonious interaction between humans and their environment, to strengthen the integrity of the individual, and to direct and redirect patterning for maximal health potential.[40] With this aim in mind, the nurse must assess each individual client for unique responses to stressors and if maladaptive behaviors are exhibited, the nurse must intervene to assist the client in achieving an adaptive state.

CLIENTS PREDISPOSED TO SENSORY PERCEPTUAL ALTERATIONS

It appears that many clinical situations contain elements of sensory deprivation or overload. It also appears that certain clients are prone to developing cognitive and behavioral impairments. There is no research to support specific predictions of exactly who will experience the effects of sensory alteration, evidence suggests the categories of clients that might be considered as possible risks.

Clients experiencing *eye surgery* are most commonly discussed in clinical literature in which the majority of these persons have had cataract surgery.[25] These clients were relatively immobilized postoperatively and wore eye patches, a combination that greatly reduced sensory input. They experienced anxiety, perceptual and thought disturbances, and confusion. They also exhibited noncompliance behavior such as getting out of bed and removing their bandages.[25,27]

Immobilized clients also experienced sensory impairments. The hallucinatory behavior of clients with bulbar poliomyelitis confined to tank-type respirators has been described as exemplifying the possible effects of sensory alteration.[31] It has been suggested that immobility with the reduction of kinesthetic input produces perceptual and motor abnormalities. Downs[11] investigated the effects of bed rest on young, healthy adults. The subjects, who were relatively immobile for a fixed period of time, experienced difficulty in concentration, disorientation in time and place, olfactory distortions, and "indeterminate stimulus experiences" (ISEs). Similar effects may also be seen in orthopedic clients immobilized for long periods of time.

ENVIRONMENTAL FACTORS

Another category discussed in the literature are those clients placed in *intensive care units* (ICUs). The environment of the ICU has received attention as a possible stressor. Clients stated that they felt restricted by the monitoring equipment and experienced a feeling of being trapped. Researchers have also found that noise levels of the ICU and recovery room environment have potential for both sensory overload to the client and as a possible stressor for the staff's own work environment.[36,52] The psychotic-like symptoms exhibited by open heart surgery clients have prompted researchers to analyze the ICU for psychologic hazards.[28] It has been found that approximately 10% to 20% of persons experiencing open heart surgery develop ICU syndrome. This is manifested by decreased intellectual functioning, decreased orientation and memory, agitation, and confusion. It ranges from mild disorientation to psychotic episodes and can last from 2 to 14 days. Generally, the condition resolves with sufficient sleep and a return to a more normal routine.[15]

Eye surgery, immobilization, and exposure to the ICU or geographic, social, or protective isolation are the primary alterations considered in the clinical literature for client predisposition to sensory alteration. However, we can hypothesize that the research results are also applicable to other clients. This would encompass clients with a sudden alteration in one or more sensory modalities such as clients with acute blindness, neurologic impairments, spinal cord injuries, strokes, and cancer[11]; surgical clients who may be experiencing multiple stressors; clients in drug-induced states that alter their perception of the environment; and clients experiencing social isolation.

Two variables are considered when assessing the effect of environment on sensory input: (1) the amount and intensity of environmental inputs and (2) the increase or reduction of pattern or meaningfulness of sensory inputs from the environment. It is important to assess whether these two variables are sufficient to maintain an aroused state in the individual in which adaptive responses occur.

Much of the clinical literature focuses on two alterations that can occur in the environment of the client. The environment can be analyzed on the basis of being either a therapeutically or socially restricted environment.[15,35]

THERAPEUTICALLY RESTRICTED ENVIRONMENT

Clients who are kept isolated in sterile environments to protect themselves or others from pathogenic organisms constitute one major category of persons in a therapeutically restricted environment. Their surroundings are generally unchanging, and contacts with staff are minimal and are often directed through gowns and masks.

Clients with orthopedic or neurologic injuries are often immobilized or placed in traction, casts, or therapeutic beds. Although these devices are therapeutic, they limit mobility and prevent access to a variety of meaningful stimuli. For example, clients who have a spinal cord injury or are in a rehabilitation facility have been identified as being at risk for sensory perceptual alterations. Clients who have restricted movement can also have a limited visual perspective, since their position may not allow them to see a changing environment. They may be positioned, for example, on their backs with the major visual field being the ceiling.

Clients who are in a therapeutically restricted environment are often removed from familiar surroundings because of an acute crisis that did not allow time for client preparation or a transitional period. They are exposed to unfamiliar repetitive sounds, constant light and activity, immobilization, and strange equipment.

It has been suggested that critical care areas be designed to promote the client's sense of well-being and to promote appropriate adaptive response. Health care providers should influence decisions regarding architectural details, such as isolating utility areas from client areas, providing adequate privacy for individual clients, and utilizing carpeting and drapes to absorb sound. Interventions can also be initiated by staff to promote client adaptation. Appropriate interventions are preparing the client for the ICU environment when required (prescheduled surgery, for example), freeing the client from restrictive equipment as soon as possible, or placing equipment in such a way to diminish noise levels, limiting conversation to that which is essential, and speaking in a normal tone (see Chapter 80).

SOCIALLY RESTRICTED ENVIRONMENT

Several variations of a socially restricted environment have been cited:[16,18]

1. Infants reared in nonstimulating institutions who have minimal contact with care givers, or infants raised by families who do not provide an adequately stimulating environment
2. Institutionalized individuals of any age whose living situation is devoid of adequate social or perceptual inputs
3. The depressed or psychotic client, the elderly, and the chronically ill individual (these persons constitute another group who may live in their own homes but are physically, socially, or emotionally unable to venture out or whose home environment is restricted or monotonous).
4. Persons isolated by disfigurement. (These persons may also have restricted interaction with their environment. Persons with cancer of the head and neck, for example, contend not only with the physical impact of the disease but also with the psychologic trauma and social stigmatization.[16])

Also, clients who are cared for in the home setting and have oncologic or cancer-related diagnoses frequently have sensory perceptual alterations.[43] In summary, when all factors are considered, both individual and environmental variables should be assessed as possible contributory factors to sensory alteration.

■ ASSESSMENT

The nurse includes both individual and environmental variables as input when assessing sensory alterations in the client. Additionally, a variety of physiologic phenomena, such as hypoxia, profound anemia, central nervous system disorders, fluid and electrolyte imbalances, and toxic inhalations or ingestions, can affect the ability to process or "throughput" the sensory stimuli accurately. Subjective and objective data can be collected either by direct questioning or by assessment of the client and the client's behavior.

INDIVIDUAL FACTORS
SUBJECTIVE DATA

The nurse should investigate problems a client has with diminished concentration, problem solving, rest or sleep, or the frequency or intensity of environmental stimuli. Ask the client about his or her perceived ability to understand and follow directions for simple tasks. Determine what the client feels is an appropriate activity during daylight and awake hours. Is the person engaged in activity that is personally meaningful or interesting?

OBJECTIVE DATA

Following are individual factors to be considered:

1. *Sensory status of visual, auditory, olfactory, gustatory, and tactile modalities:* Does the client have normal visual and auditory functions? Are there any impairments,[19,24] defects, or corrective devices required such as glasses or a hearing aid? Can the client discriminate between odors and various taste sensations? Can the client perceive changes in temperature, feel pain, and discriminate between various forms of touch such as sharp and light? Does the client have the ability to define placement or position in space?
2. *Neurologic status:* What is the client's level of consciousness? (See Chapter 31.) Are the normal pathways and processing functions intact? Are there any neurologic conditions that would affect sensory inputs, such as peripheral neuropathies, spinal cord disease, or cerebral disease that would cause either excessive stimulation or suboptimal sensory input?
3. *Motor status:* Is the client capable of independent movement? Is there any alteration as a result of illness, such as paralysis, casts, or immobilization?

4. *Cognitive status:* Can the client perceive, process information, and respond appropriately to the environment? Is memory, insight, judgment, planning intact? Is the client oriented to time, place, person? Is the client able to solve problems at the usual level of functioning? Can the individual concentrate on the task at hand?

5. *Communication status:* Is the ability to communicate within normal range? Can the client understand and initiate speech and respond to verbal communications? Is there any impairment of speech organs or neural pathways necessary for verbal communications? Can the client read or write and follow simple commands?

6. *Age and developmental level:* Is the client's behavior normal in terms of age and developmental level?

7. *Psychologic status:* Is the client an independent, self-reliant person? What coping mechanisms are used? Does the client appear anxious, irritable, angry?

8. *Utilization of drugs:* Has the client been exposed to central nervous system depressants, such as alcohol or narcotics, which decrease awareness of the environment? Have stimulants, such as amphetamines, or consciousness-expanding drugs that would alter perception, such as LSD, been used?

9. *Presence of maladaptive behaviors:* Are there any cognitive, perceptual-motor, or affective disturbances noted?

10. *Presence of specific stressors:* Are there any additional specific stressors to which the client is exposed that would alter sensory input further? This could include pain, drug toxicity, immobilization, isolation, or specific system disorders such as alterations in gas exchange or regulatory mechanisms.

■ DATA ANALYSIS: NURSING DIAGNOSES

Nursing diagnoses are determined from assessment of patient data. Possible nursing diagnoses for the person with sensory deprivation or overload may include, but are not limited to, the following:

Diagnostic Title	Possible Etiologies
Injury, potential for, related to altered sensory function and protective ability	CVA with weakness, numbness, pr visual field changes; diminished visual, auditory, or sensory function occurring with aging; medications such as sedatives
Sensory/perceptual alteration, related to an excessive/insufficient amount of or change in pattern of meaningful stimuli	ICU admission; constant, unusual, or meaningless environmental stimuli; protective isolation (bone marrow transplant recipients, infants in isolettes); social isolation
Sensory/perceptual alteration, related to impaired functioning of sensory organs (auditory, gustatory, kinesthetic, olfactory, tactile, or visual sensory systems)	Cataract surgery, severe burns to hands, acoustic neuroma (cannot receive input)
	Language barrier, CNS lesion, altered level of consciousness (cannot process or throughput the stimuli)
Sleep pattern disturbance, related to environmental stimuli	Admission to hospital or ICU; pain; anxiety; immobility secondary to cast or therapeutic bed; medications such as sedatives, hypnotics, steroids

---

RESEARCH

Hilton A: Noise in acute patient care areas, Res Nurs Health 8:283-291, 1985.

A study of sound levels in acute patient care areas (four intensive care and two general care units within three hospitals) included measurement of sound levels in decibels [dB(A)] and equivalent continuous sound pressure levels (LEQ) for 24 hours and interviews with 25 patients to determine their perceptions of sound effects. In the larger hospital's open heart surgical recovery room and intensive care units, continuous high noise levels were found [48.5 to 68.5 dB(A), 15-minute LEQ] lower levels in the smaller hospital's intensive care units [32.5 to 57 dB(A)] and varying levels in the general ward areas [34.25 to 62.5 dB(A)]. Equipment generated decibel levels as high as 90 dB(A). Patients' perceptions ranged from content to highly perturbed. Many sources of noise were adaptable, preventable, or reducible. ■

RESEARCH

Mitchell PH et al: Critically ill children: the importance of touch in a high-technology environment, Nurs Admin Q 9:38-46, 1985.

A spects of touch by parents and nursing staff were summarized in a study of the influence of nursing activities on intracranial pressure in critically ill children. Staff other than nurses rarely touched the patients except to do physical examinations. Nurses touched children most often when performing procedures. Parents touched children more often than did nurses, particularly the more severely ill children. Touch alone (not related to procedures) never raised intracranial pressure beyond an individual's own physiologic variability. The data suggest that nurses are not touching these critically ill children very much, except as needed for procedures. However, the data also suggest that it is safe to increase nonprocedural touching of critically ill children and it is safe to allow and encourage parents to touch and stroke their children. ■

■ PLANNING: EXPECTED PATIENT OUTCOMES

Expected patient outcomes for the person with sensory deprivation or overload may include, but are not limited to, the following:

1. The client will experience no fall or injury.
2. The client will use sensory aids (glasses, hearing aid, walker) to ensure safety.
3. The client will demonstrate use of call bell or light to request assistance.
4. The client will be oriented to person, place, time, and patient/client role responsibilities.
5. The client will be able to participate in own care.
6. Client will identify sensory-perceptual function as decreased or absent.
7. Client will demonstrate alternate methods to access and throughput meaningful stimuli.
8. Client's behavior will indicate adjustment to sensory perceptual alteration.
9. The client will identify factors that enhance and inhibit sleep.
10. The client will report that the quality/quantity of sleep and rest is adequate.

■ IMPLEMENTATION

The following nursing interventions are appropriate for most persons with sensory deprivation or overload:

Intervention	Rationale
Provide client with glasses, hearing aid, walker as needed	Use sensory aids to enhance accurate inputs
Orient client to use of call bell or light	Use of safety features and assistance results in fewer injuries
Bed rails up	
Instruct family, client regarding measures to keep environment safe (remove obstacles, objects on floor)	
Assess at least q 8 hr for status and client interpretation of level of stimuli	Provide accurate, concrete feedback to the client facilitates orientation to reality and healthy adaptive responses to stimuli
Provide feedback to client regarding meaning of environmental stimuli	
Orient client to room, ongoing procedures	Use a variety of sensory stimuli to facilitate several "inputs"
Make frequent, meaningful contact with client	
Use radio, television, calendar, significant others to facilitate orientation	
Decrease/diminish the number of continuous and intermittent noises, lights, noxious odors	Diminish the number or intensity of stimuli to decrease the number of inputs
Identify self to client	
Orient client to setting by using touch, voice, visual cues; orient to time frequently	Speak clearly and frequently to the client so that a firm basis for adaptation to deficit is provided.

Intervention	Rationale
Position client for appropriate input—so he or she can see out window, have night light, face care provider; have personal items within reach	Facilitate adaptation to sensory perceptual alteration
Provide materials to facilitate communication verbally, in writing, or by pointing at symbols or pictures	Provide alternative to sensory input
Provide sensory assistance devices (glasses, hearing aid)	Provide ability to process foreign stimuli
Provide translator as needed	
Provide structure, daily routine, and regular socialization	
Identify and diminish or remove factors inhibiting sleep (decrease noise, light; use earplugs; provide privacy; provide relief from pain and anxiety)	Reduce intensity or frequency of stimuli to facilitate rest/sleep
Plan care to facilitate uninterrupted 90 min sleep intervals, avoid noncritical procedures; limit visitors as needed	Use of routine, usual bed time or sleep rituals facilitates adaptation to environment and return to usual sleep pattern
Use sleep rituals to facilitate initiation of sleep (PM hygiene, reading, snack, television, comfortable position, stay with client, use massage)	Planned, uninterrupted periods for nighttime rest will facilitate usual sleep pattern
Plan daytime activity to decrease opportunity for sleep, particularly in afternoons	

INTERVENTION

There are no clear-cut differences between clinical manifestations of sensory deprivation or overload. The nurse may be in a position where an individual client's unique situation must be assessed and the nurse must utilize professional judgment in making a decision to either increase or decrease sensory inputs as an intervention measure. It may be a trial-and-error approach until the client responds adaptively.

In managing manifestations of sensory alteration, the logical first step in the process is to perform an assessment including both individual and environmental variables, as discussed previously in this chapter. In addition, the nurse would consider the temporal variable. Is it an *acute* manifestation or is it indicative of a *chronic* condition, such as social restrictions that can occur with institutionalization?

SPECIFIC CLIENT PROBLEMS
PERCEPTUAL DISTURBANCES

Clients experiencing hallucinations or perceptual disturbances are often frightened and anxious, even when the client has an awareness that the experience is not based in reality. The nurse should not indulge or appease the client in an attempt to allay anxiety. A more useful intervention is to encourage the client to describe the experience and to allow opportunities to ventilate feelings. It may also be helpful to the client for the nurse to clarify possible environmental stimuli that were misinterpreted, such as an intercom message, and for the nurse to remain in the room with the client to provide reassurance.

DELUSIONAL THINKING

Clients may articulate beliefs that are contrary to reality, such as that the staff is persecuting or mistreating them. This generally is an episodic occurrence that passes when the client becomes reoriented. The client should not be ridiculed, dismissed, or strongly confronted when such beliefs are expressed. Instead, it would be more helpful to allow the client to verbalize thoughts and, when appropriate, be presented with the nurse's perception of the facts.

CONFUSED, COMBATIVE CLIENTS

When the patient's behavior indicates confusion or combativeness, attempts should be made to reorient the client repeatedly to time, place, and person. Explanations should also be provided regarding identification of staff, tasks to be performed, and environmental stimuli to which the patient is exposed. If the client is combative and requires restraints, the rationale for the restraints should be given and reassurance provided that the client is not being punished. Restraints that allow the most freedom in movement (body versus limb restraints) should be used, and safety measures should be taken regarding careful supervision and protection of the client. *Restraints should not be used indiscriminately, but only when the client's condition absolutely necessitates it.*

DECREASED SENSORY INPUTS

As stated throughout this chapter, nurses have many options at their disposal to increase sensory inputs when conditions necessitate such interventions. In summary, the nurse can intervene with both individual and environmental variables. Visual inputs can be increased through the utilization of mobiles, pictures, greeting cards, flowers, color, or something as simple as providing the patient with glasses to see the environment clearly. Auditory inputs can be increased through the use of radio, television, and increased verbal interaction with staff, family, or other clients. Tactile stimulation can be provided by administering back rubs or allowing the client to explore objects in the environment through the sense of touch. Social contacts can be initiated through group activities. Group sessions with the chronically ill have been described as one way to increase so-

cial interactions.[33] Also, using natural meeting places in the hospital environment, such as a solarium or day room, for staff and patients appears to increase social stimulation and client satisfaction. Clarifying and providing meaning to the environment through the use of calendars, clocks, and other measures to provide reality orientation are additional sources of increasing sensory inputs.

INCREASED SENSORY INPUTS

If inputs are above the client's range of tolerance, the nurse can intervene to reduce the amount and intensity of stimuli by reducing noise, light, or social contacts. The pattern of stimuli may also require a change. It appears that this is most problematic in critical care areas where the client's condition often necessitates constant monitoring.

CHAPTER SUMMARY

✔ Assess the client for predisposing factors that place the person at risk for sensory deprivation and overload.

✔ Determine if the sensory perceptual alteration you are observing is acute or chronic in nature.

✔ Assess the client's perspective of sensory-perceptual alteration, the extent to which the client believes it is influencing daily activity, and the plans the client has for adapting to the alteration.

✔ Focus nursing interventions on care that provides meaningful stimuli, facilitates input of stimuli from a variety of sources, and facilitates healthy adaptation.

QUESTIONS TO CONSIDER

■ How would your nursing care differ for your client who has burned both hands and who is also blind? Would you assign this client to a private or semi-private room? Why?

■ What approaches to nursing care would you consider for a client who states, "it is so noisy and disruptive around here all the time—I cannot sleep"?

■ How would you alter your plan of care for an elderly, 85-year-old client who has had surgery to replace a left hip, and you discover that the client's right side is numb because of a previous stroke?

■ What nursing care would you provide for a client who has both eyes patched after surgery to prevent injury? How might this plan be different if the client is 30 years old versus one who is 8 years old?

REFERENCES AND SELECTED READINGS

1. Bellak L: Overload, New York, 1975, Human Sciences Press.
2. *Berrien KF: General and social systems, New Brunswick, NJ, 1968, Rutgers University Press.
3. *Brownfield CA: Isolation: clinical and experimental approaches, New York, 1965, Random House, Inc.
4. *Cannon W: The wisdom of the body, New York, 1932, WW Norton & Co, Inc.
5. *Carlson S: Selected sensory input and life satisfaction of immobilized geriatric female patients. In ANA clinical sessions, New York, 1968, Appleton-Century-Crofts.
6. Carpenter MB and Sutin J: Human neuroanatomy, Baltimore, 1983, Williams & Wilkins.
7. *Chodil J and Williams B: The concept of sensory deprivation, Nurs Clin North Am 5:453-459, 1970.
8. *Cockburn K: Sensory stimulation in the nursing care of chronic schizophrenic patients. In ANA regional clinical conference, New York, 1967, Appleton-Century-Crofts.
9. *Cohen S: Contact deprivation in infants, Psychosomatics 7:85-88, 1966.
10. *Cullinan J: Quality of life is the challenge—not quantity, Nurs Times 76:1604-1605, Sept 11, 1980.
11. Daw NW and Ariel M: Properties of monocular and directional deprivation, J Neurophysiol 44:280-293, 1980.
12. DeKonninck J, Gagnon P, and Lallier S: Sleep positions in the young adult and their relationship with the subjective quality of sleep, Sleep 6:52-59, 1983.
13. *DeMeyer J: The environment of the intensive care unit, Nurs Forum 6:262-272, 1967.
14. Downs F: Bed rest and sensory deprivation, Am J Nurs 74:434-438, 1974.
15. Eisendrath SJ: ICU syndromes: their detection, prevention and treatment, Crit Care Update 7:5-8, 1980.
16. Ellis R: Sensory and thought disturbances after cardiac surgery, Am J Nurs 72:2021-2025, 1972.
17. Falk SA and Woods NF: Hospital noise: levels of potential health hazards, N Engl J Med 289:274-281, 1973.
18. Freeman RD and Bradley A: Monocularly deprived humans: nondeprived eye has supernormal Vernier acuity, J Neurophysiol 43:1645-1653, 1980.
19. Goldberg H: Hearing impairment: a family crisis, Soc Work Health Care 5:33-40, Fall 1979.
20. *Goldfarb W: Emotional and intellectual consequences of psychological deprivation in infancy: a reevaluation: psychopathology of childhood. In Proceedings of The American Psychopathological Association, New York, 1955, Grune & Stratton, Inc.
21. Gowan NJ: The perceptual world of the intensive care unit: An overview of some environmental considerations in the helping relationship, Heart Lung 8:2, 340-344, 1979.
22. Haslam P: Noise in hospitals: its effect on the patient, Nurs Clin North Am 5:715-724, 1970.
23. Hearth K: Beyond the curtain of silence, Am J Nurs 74:1060-1061, 1974.
24. Heppen CJ and Petersen SB: Visual impairment: facing possible blindness, Soc Work Health Care 5:41-49, 1979.
25. *Jackson CW: Clinical sensory deprivation: a review of hospitalized eye-surgery patients. In Zubek JP, editor: Sensory deprivation: 15 years of research, New York, 1969, Appleton-Century-Crofts.
26. Jackson CW and Ellis R: Sensory deprivation as a field of study, Nurs Res 20:49, 1971.
27. *Jackson CW and O'Neil M: Experiences associated with sensory deprivation reported for patients having eye surgery. In Jeffries JE, editor: Disturbances in sensory input in nursing practice and research, Columbus, Ohio, 1966, Ross Laboratories.
28. Kaplan BE and Hurley FL: Head and neck cancer: a threat to life and social functioning, Soc Work Health Care 5:51-58, Fall 1979.
29. *Kornfeld D, Maxwell T, and Momrow D: Psychological hazards of the intensive care unit, Nurs Clin North Am 3:41-51, 1968.
30. *Kornfeld D, Zimberg S, and Malm J: Psychiatric complications of open-heart surgery, N Engl J Med 273:287-292, 1965.
31. *Leiderman H, et al: Sensory deprivation: clinical aspects, Arch Med 101:389-396, 1958.
32. *Lindsley D: Common factors in sensory deprivation, sensory distortion and sensory overload. In Solomon, P, et al: Sensory deprivations, Cambridge, Mass, 1961, Harvard University Press.
33. Lierman LM: Phantom breast experiences after mastectomy, ONF 15, 1:41-44, 1988.
34. Lipowski ZJ: Sensory overloads, information overloads and behavior, Comp Psychiatry 16:199-220, 1975.
35. Mitchell PH: Concepts basic to nursing, ed 3, New York, 1981, McGraw-Hill Book Co.
36. Perron D: Deprived of sound, Am J Nurs 74:1057-1059, 1974.
37. Plum F and Posner JB: Diagnosis of stupor and coma, Philadelphia, 1980, FA Davis Co.
38. Rogers M: An introduction to the theoretical basis of nursing, Philadelphia, 1970, FA Davis Co.
39. *Riesen A: Excessive arousal effects of stimulation after early sensory deprivation. In Solomon P et al: Sensory deprivation, Cambridge, Mass, 1961, Harvard University Press.
40. Roy C: Introduction to nursing: an adaptation model, Englewood Cliffs, NJ, 1975, Prentice-Hall, Inc.
41. Sackett G: Innate mechanisms, rearing condition, and a theory of early experience effects in primates. In Jones M: Miami Symposium on the Prediction of Behavior, Coral Gables, Fla, 1970, University of Miami Press.
42. *Schultz D: Sensory restriction, New York, 1965, Academic Press, Inc.
43. Sheppard KC: Evaluation of the NANDA Taxonomy I as an assessment guideline in an oncology setting. In Johnson, editor: Classification of Nursing Diagnoses, Proceedings of the Eighth Conference, St Louis, 1988, The CV Mosby Co.
44. *Snyder-Halpern R: The effect of critical care unit noise on patient sleep cycles, Crit Care Quarterly 7:4, 41-51, 1985.
45. *Solomon P et al: Sensory deprivation, Cambridge, Mass, 1958, Harvard University Press.
46. *Spitz R: Hospitalism: an inquiry into the genesis of psychiatric conditions in early childhood, Psychoanal Study Child 1:53-74, 1945.
47. Suedfeld P: The benefits of boredom: sensory deprivation reconsidered, Am Sci 63:60-69, 1975.
48. Thompson LR: Sensory deprivation: a personal experience, Am J Nurs 73:266-268, 1973.
49. *Thompson WR and Schaefer T: Early environmental stimulation. In Fiske DW and Maddi SR, editors: Functions of varied experience, Stonewood, Ill, 1961, Dorsey Press.
50. Tolpin M: On the beginnings of a cohesive self, Psychoanal Study Child 26:316-352, 1971.
51. *Vernon J et al: The effect of human isolation upon some perceptual and motor skills. In Solomon, P et al: Sensory deprivations, Cambridge, Mass, 1961, Harvard University Press.
52. White BL: Human infants: experience and psychological development, Englewood Cliffs, NJ, 1971, Prentice-Hall, Inc.

*References preceded by an asterisk are particularly well suited for student reading.

53. *Winnicott DW: The maturational processes and the facilitating environment, New York, 1965, International Universities Press, Inc.

54. Woods NF and Falk SA: Noise stimuli in the acute care area, Nurs Res 23:144-150, 1974.

55. *Ziskind E: A second look at sensory deprivation, J Nerv Ment Dis 64:223-230, 1964.

56. *Ziskind E et al: Observations on mental symptoms in eye patched patients: hypnogogic symptoms in sensory deprivation, Am J Psychiatry 116:893-900, 1960.

57. *Zubek J, editor: Sensory deprivation: 15 years of research, New York, 1966, Appleton-Century-Crofts.

58. *Zubek JP, Sansom W, and Prysiaznuik A: Intellectual changes during prolonged perceptual isolation, Can J Psychol 14:233-243, 1960.

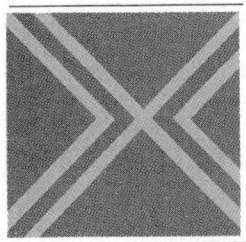

CHAPTER 13

Chronic Illness

WILMA J. PHIPPS

CHAPTER OBJECTIVES

After studying this chapter, the student should be able to:
1 Differentiate between acute and chronic illness.
2 Describe factors that influence chronic illness.
3 Identify areas of assessment for the chronically ill person.
4 Describe physical and psychosocial interventions for patients with chronic illness.
5 Define rehabilitation and the roles of team members, especially the nurse, and the patient.
6 Describe different patterns and facilities for continuing care.
7 Identify major health goals related to chronic health problems to be achieved in the United States by the year 2000.

Prevention and control of chronic disease constitute one of the major health problems in the United States today. In the past the impact of chronic diseases on individuals, families, and communities has been overlooked. Recently, there has been an increasing awareness in the United States of great pockets of unmet needs among people with long-term health problems. These individuals have needs that extend beyond strictly medical ones. Their problems demand the use of many sources of help and care. In many cases the coping capacities of chronically ill individuals are reduced because of advancing age, serious functional impairment and disability, and limited personal, social, and financial resources.

Chronic disease is not an entity in itself but an umbrella term that encompasses long-lasting diseases, which are often associated with some degree of disability. Each chronic illness is unique and has a different impact on the individual, family, and community. Nevertheless, common problems and complications that accompany the various chronic health problems can be studied in general to help the nurse understand and care for individuals with specific long-term illnesses.

The incidence and prevalence of chronic diseases have increased since the beginning of the twentieth century. This increase has arisen from various developments, including decreased mortality from infectious diseases, improved sanitation, and the introduction of effective vaccines and mass immunizations. In 1986 only 8.5% of U.S. deaths resulted from infectious diseases, including acquired immunodeficiency syndrome (AIDS). In the same year more than one million persons in the United States died from nine chronic diseases: (1) stroke, (2) coronary heart disease, (3) diabetes, (4) chronic obstructive pulmonary disease, (5) lung cancer, (6) female breast cancer, (7) cervical cancer, (8) colorectal cancer, and (9) cirrhosis.[11a] These diseases were responsible for 52% of all U.S. deaths. It is estimated that many of these diseases could have been prevented by effective control of smoking, blood pressure, diet, and alcohol consumption.[7]

Even though cardiovascular and cerebrovascular diseases are still the major cause of death, the mortality from these diseases has declined in recent decades. In fact, 1977 was the first year in which cardiovascular disease was responsible for less than 50% of all deaths in the United States.

At the same time the National Health Survey of 1981 identified major disparities in the health of black Americans and other minorities in the United States when compared with the white populations.[27] As a result of these findings, the Secretary of the U.S. Department of Health and Human Services (DHHS) established the Task Force on Black and Minority Health. The findings of the task force are discussed on p. 225. Recent figures from the U.S. Bureau of the Census show that limitation in activity caused by chronic diseases in all age groups decreases as family income increases.[34] As expected, most persons with limited activity are age 65 years and older. Also, the percentage of persons with limitation in activity is greater in blacks than in whites (Table 13-1).

DEFINITIONS OF ACUTE AND CHRONIC ILLNESS

An *acute illness* is caused by a disease that produces symptoms and signs soon after exposure to the cause, that runs a short course, and from which there is usually a full recovery or an abrupt termination in death.

TABLE 13-1 Percentage of persons limited in activity because of chronic conditions, according to family income and selected characteristics: United States, 1979-1980

Characteristic	All Income Levels (%)	Less Than $5000 (%)	$25,000 and Over (%)
AGE (YEARS)			
All ages	14.5	29.3	8.7
Under 17	3.9	5.1	3.5
17 to 44	8.7	15.0	6.4
45 to 64	24.0	54.9	14.2
65 and over	45.6	55.3	37.8
SEX			
Male	14.7	28.9	9.0
Female	14.3	29.6	8.4
RACE			
White	14.5	30.9	9.0
Black	15.4	25.5	6.3
Other	9.1	23.1	4.3

From US Department of Health and Human Services: Health characteristics according to family and personal income, United States, 1979-1980, data from National Health Interview Survey, 1982.

Acute illness may become chronic. For example, a common cold may develop into chronic sinusitis.

A *chronic illness* is caused by disease that produces symptoms and signs within a variable period, that runs a long course, and from which there is only partial recovery. The National Health Survey defined chronic conditions as follows: (1) those first noticed 3 months or more before the date of the interview or (2) those belonging to a group of conditions (including heart disease, diabetes, and others) considered chronic regardless of when they began.[23] This follows the pattern of the Commission on Chronic Illness, which in 1949 defined chronic illness as any impairment or deviation from normal that has one or more of the following characteristics: it is permanent, leaves residual disability; is caused by nonreversible pathologic alteration; requires special training of the patient for rehabilitation; or may be expected to require a long period of supervision, observation, or care. This definition is still in use.

The symptoms and general reactions caused by chronic disease may subside with proper treatment and care. The period during which the disease is controlled and symptoms are not obvious is known as a *remission*. However, later the disease may become active again with recurrence of pronounced symptoms. This is known as an *exacerbation* of the disease.

Exacerbations of chronic disease often cause the patient to seek medical attention and may lead to hospitalization. The needs of a patient who has an acute illness may be very different from those of the patient with an

PROBLEMS FACED BY PERSONS WITH CHRONIC ILLNESS

1. Preventing and managing medical crises
2. Controlling symptoms
3. Following prescribed regimen
4. Maintaining normal interactions with others
5. Adjusting to recurrent patterns in the course of the disease
6. Arranging payment for treatment

exacerbation of a chronic disease. For example, a young person may enter the hospital with complaints of fever, chest pain, shortness of breath, fatigue, and a productive cough. If the diagnosis is pneumonia, the patient usually can be assured of recovery after a period of rest and a course of antibiotic treatment. However, if the diagnosis is rheumatic heart disease and if the patient is being admitted to the hospital for the third, fourth, or fifth time, the reassurance needed will not be so definite, clear-cut, or easy to give. In such a case it is necessary to begin planning care that will extend beyond the period of hospitalization, taking into consideration many aspects of the patient's total life situation. The concerns of the patient who has repeated attacks of illness will be very different from the concerns of the one who has a short-term illness.

Further, the needs of patients who are admitted to the hospital with an acute illness but who also have an underlying chronic condition must not be overlooked. For example, elderly patients who enter the hospital with pneumonia may receive treatment for the pneumonia and recover from their illness. However, they may still be hampered by the arteriosclerotic heart disease and arthritis that they have had for years. Also, these two chronic conditions may have been aggravated by the acute infection, or the return to former activity may be hindered by joint stiffness resulting from bed rest and inactivity. Consideration of a patient's several diagnoses can help in preventing new problems associated with the chronic illness.

Strauss et al.[32] have described some problems experienced by persons with chronic illness, which are listed in the box above. Emotional, social, and economic implications of chronic illness are discussed later in this chapter.

CHRONIC ILLNESS AS A FORCE IN SOCIETY

EXTENT AND EFFECTS OF CHRONIC ILLNESS

According to the National Health Survey of 1981, 80 million people had one or more chronic conditions. The survey classified chronic conditions in the following categories: (1) selected skin and musculoskeletal conditions; (2) impairments (visual, hearing, speech, paralysis, deformity, or orthopedic impairment); (3) selected digestive conditions; (4) selected conditions of the genitourinary, nervous, endocrine, metabolic, and blood and blood-forming systems; (5) selected circulatory conditions; and (6) selected respiratory conditions.[27]

In 1986, the number of persons with one or more chronic illnesses who died was 110 million.[11a]

Many of these conditions cause a limitation of activity, which affects the life-style of the chronically ill. One documented trend is that the impact of acute illness has seemed to diminish, whereas the burden of chronic health problems and related disability has increased. Limitation of activity is a measure of long-term disability resulting from chronic health problems or impairment and is defined as the inability to carry on the major activity for one's age group, such as cooking, keeping house, going to school, or going to work.

Approximately 15% of the population experience some limitations in their activities, whereas almost half the persons over 65 years of age are limited in their activities by one or more chronic conditions. Some activity limitations are associated with mental disabilities, but most are the result of physical handicaps caused by heart conditions and arthritis. Because chronic disability increases in direct proportion to age, persons over age 65 are most prone to severe chronic disability. As the population of the United States ages, the number of persons with chronic illness will continue to increase.

The inability to work or to move about greatly influences the type of medical treatment and health supervision needed by persons who have a chronic illness. Some persons need only periodic medical examinations and perhaps continuing treatment with medications; others may require complete physical care. Some have a disease that progresses very slowly without remissions; others may have episodes of acute illness and then seem comparatively well for a time. Each person requires a thorough assessment to determine the stage of the illness, the course the illness is likely to take, the type of care needed, and the method by which that care will be delivered if the individual is to be helped appropriately.

FACTORS INFLUENCING CHRONIC ILLNESS
AGE

Different age groups have different experiences with acute and chronic diseases. The young are more likely to experience short, intense, acute conditions that are quickly over. The elderly are more likely to have long, drawn-out chronic diseases. Nevertheless, anyone can have either an acute or a chronic disease at any age. Chronic illness and disability may date from birth (for example, spina bifida with neurologic damage), or it may originate in childhood, adolescence, or early adult life (for example, multiple sclerosis, rheumatoid arthritis). The major chronic illnesses among those 65 years

and over identified in the National Health Survey were arthritis, diabetes, heart disease, and hypertension.

Because of strides made in pediatric medicine, children who would have died 30 years ago because of lack of knowledge and treatment of diseases such as cystic fibrosis are now living longer with those chronic diseases. The reduction in death rates among the younger age groups has allowed a higher percentage of the population to reach the age of greatest risk from chronic diseases. Cancer develops far more frequently in older people. Because the average age of the U.S. population continues to rise, about 30% of people now alive will eventually contract cancer.[3]

Much remains to be learned about interactions of the normal, pathologic, and physiologic changes of aging with various diseases. A common question asked is, "When does aging end and illness begin?" Differences found in age groups or changes found in individuals as they age represent normal aging, that is, a universal, intrinsic process of growth and development that is inevitable, irreversible, unpreventable, but ultimately detrimental. Although aging (a normal process) is distinct from chronic disease (a pathologic process), chronic illness is often concomitant with aging. The problems of aging and chronic disease are influenced in major ways by each other; for example, the social problems confronting the aged are strongly influenced by the presence and severity of chronic disabilities. Remissions and exacerbations are possibilities with chronic illness; they are not with aging.

RACE AND ETHNICITY

Race or ethnic group membership is a factor that influences chronic health problems. Race-specific rates measure the association between disease occurrence and race. Data on specific conditions indicate not only that some problems are more prevalent among nonwhites (blacks, American Indians, Asians), but also that nonwhites fail to receive necessary care. For example, nonwhites are more than three times more likely to die of hypertension than whites of the same age group.[18] The findings of the Task Force on Black and Minority Health, which were released late in 1985, found that 60,000 excess deaths occur each year in minority populations. Six causes of death were identified that together account for more than 80% of the excess mortality. The health problems according to excess deaths are listed here in alphabetical order[6]:

1. Cancer—16% of excess mortality among black males under age 70 and 10% for black females.
2. Cardiovascular disease and stroke—24% of excess mortality among black males and 41% among black females.
3. Chemical dependency, measured by deaths resulting from cirrhosis of the liver, associated with ex-

TABLE 13-2 Number of selected reported chronic conditions per 1000 persons by race and age: United States, 1982

Type of Chronic Condition	White 65 Years and Over		Black 65 Years and Over	
	65-74	75 Years and Over	65-74	75 Years and Over
Arthritis	499.8	482.9	595.3	395.0
Diabetes	86.3	75.3	203.1	96.5
Heart disease	235.7	323.4	142.3	198.2
Hypertension	369.7	394.9	533.7	468.1

From National Center for Health Statistics, Division of Interview Health Statistics, data from National Health Interview Survey, 1982.

cessive use of alcohol—13% of excess mortality among Native American males and 22% among Native American females under age 70.

4. Diabetes—38% of excess deaths among Mexican-born Hispanic females.

5. Homicides and accidents (unintentional injuries)—60% of excess mortality among Hispanics under 65. Unintentional injuries cause 44% of excess death among male and 30% among female Native Americans. Homicides and unintentional injuries account for 19% of excess mortality among black males under age 70 and 38% for those under age 45. The figures for black females are 6% and 14%, respectively. A substantial portion of excess deaths in this category may be associated with excessive use of alcohol and other drugs.

6. Infant mortality—of excess deaths among black females up to age 45 years, death in the first year of life accounts for 35% of that excess.

Table 13-2 compares the rates of four major chronic illnesses for white and black Americans.

CULTURAL VALUES

Western culture tends to be *cure oriented;* therefore, health care for persons with acute conditions is often more valued than is health care for those who are chronically ill. In contrast to the exciting aspects of sophisticated and mechanical technology, caring for chronically ill persons is often considered boring. The continual struggle to cope with day-to-day living soon becomes tedious for ill persons, their families, and health professionals. The rewards of treating chronic illness cannot be measured by a cure but by the prevention of complications and by helping individuals function at their optimal level.

The cultural context has many symbolic meanings, beliefs, and values that health professionals need to understand to meet individual's health needs. Some individuals may view their chronic disease as a form of punishment from God. Thus they may experience a sense of guilt. Individuals who view their chronic disease as a "leper phenomenon" may experience a sense of social rejection. Others may see their chronic illness as a destructive force without meaning or simply as a physical response of their body. Appreciation of the person's beliefs and behavior in the context of his or her cultural heritage rather than denial of the cultural influence increases understanding between the health professional and the chronically ill person. Differences need not imply deviance. It is possible to introduce health practices in a manner congruent with the individual's cultural values.

COST OF DISABILITY

For the individual and family the costs of disability are temporal, emotional, and financial. The goal of maintaining the patient in the best possible condition relative to the illness must be the primary concern, since a good program of maintenance is the best way to help the patient avoid financial drain caused by unnecessary or preventable complications. Meeting the goal, however, can require that extensive time be spent on treatments, maintenance regimens, and follow-up appointments. Further, each chronically ill person and family are subjected to great personal and emotional losses that must be dealt with, including loss of self-esteem, loss of status within the family, loss of independence, feelings of rejection, and feelings of helplessness. These can be more devastating than economic deprivation.

The economic cost to the patient and family is considerable. The cost of hospitalization rises yearly. Frequent or extended hospitalization and medical expenses can be ruinous if the patient is inadequately insured or if he or she is unable to qualify for insurance programs. Many are forced to seek public assistance merely to survive. Placement in quality nursing homes is frequently financially impossible for patients or their families to manage. The cost of medications to control or maintain a patient's health status may require a major portion of the family budget. Additional expenses may include special diets and equipment, home modifications (for example, ramps or widening of doors for wheelchairs), transportation, and support services provided by homemakers, day or live-in attendants, or nurses.

The ability of the individual family to pay its own way is determined in part by which family member becomes disabled. Studies show that if the wife is disabled, the family suffers less economic deprivation than if the husband is disabled. However, three fourths of chronically ill persons unable to carry on their major activity are men.[27]

Some financial assistance is provided by Medicare. This federally administered program provides hospital and medical insurance protection for individuals 65 years of age and over as well as for people under 65 who are disabled and eligible for Social Security benefits. Persons under age 65 who are medically indigent because of health problems may be eligible for assistance through the Medicaid program.

However, recent changes in federal funding have altered Medicare and Medicaid programs. Persons over age 65 receiving Social Security have a higher fee deducted from their monthly payments to pay for their Medicare premiums. In addition, most persons covered by Medicare purchase supplemental health insurance to cover expenses not covered by Medicare.

There have been severe cutbacks in Medicaid, which is administered at the state level, and eligibility requirements have been made more stringent.

Thus persons with chronic illnesses may have considerable difficulty in paying for prescribed therapy. For example, antiinflammatory agents used to treat arthritis are very expensive. Many of these medications cost between $0.75 and $1.00 each, and the usual dose is three times daily.

In considering the cost of disability to the community, it must be realized that most individuals who are unable to work must be supported by others, either from private or from public funds. Three million adults between the ages of 18 and 64 years are unable to work because of chronic disabilities. An additional 9.4 million are partially limited in their ability to work.[34]

CHRONICALLY ILL PERSONS AND THEIR FAMILIES

The effects of chronic illness on individuals and their families are numerous and varied. The first impact of the disability may nearly immobilize them. Time must be provided them to talk through their concerns and fears before they can be expected to begin coping with their new situation.

Marked changes often take place, and are often required to take place, in family living as a result of chronic illness. Some families may find themselves drawn closer together. Other families may drift apart, the individual members being incapable of helping one another. At times chronic illness may threaten an individual's basic emotional stability, and the whole situation may be unbearable to others. Sometimes the individual's emotional needs may not have been apparent to the family early in the illness, but when such needs grow obvious, relatives feel inadequate to cope with the situation. The length of illness, periodic hospitalizations, and increased financial, emotional, and social burdens are stressors that threaten the family's integrity.

Many persons struggle on their own to assume the full financial burden of the illness and consequently expose other members of the family to lower standards of nutrition, housing, and care. Many times relatives move in with one another, arguments develop, and family ties are strained or broken. Public assistance may be acceptable to some families, whereas others find it impossible to accept.

Chronic illness imposes additional problems of learning how to cope with restrictions on activities of daily living, how to prevent or identify medical crises that occur, and how to carry out treatment regimens as delineated by the health care provider. Family members also need to learn about the restrictions, not only to be of assistance to the chronically ill person, but also because their own activity patterns may be disrupted.

Because chronic illness may have periods of exacerbation when symptoms become more acute and medical crises may occur, patients and family members need to know which symptoms must be reported to the health care provider as well as the time interval for reporting these symptoms. They also must know how to contact the provider and what measures to take if a medical crisis occurs. For example, the person who has a history of myocardial infarction and the family members must know what to do if the person experiences severe chest pain. Should the person be taken immediately to a hospital emergency room, or should the physician be contacted first? Patient and family should plan in advance the sequence of actions to take during a medical crisis, depending on the nature and extent of the presenting symptoms. (See Chapter 6 for further discussion of families and illness.)

EPIDEMIOLOGY

Epidemiology examines the distribution of chronic disease as well as the measurement of health status in the general population. It is both a body of knowledge and a method for obtaining knowledge. As a methodology, epidemiology can be used to assist in explaining the multifactorial causal patterns of chronic diseases.

PROBLEMS IN DETERMINING CAUSALITY OF CHRONIC DISEASES

Some of the factors that contribute to the difficulty of studying the cause of chronic disease are the following:

1. *Multifactorial nature of etiologic factors.* The operation of multiple factors is particularly important in chronic diseases. The interaction of factors may be purely additive or may be synergistic; that is, the combined potential for harm of many risk factors is more than the sum of the individual potentials. They interact, reinforce, and even multiply each other. Asbestos workers, for example, have increased lung cancer risk. Asbestos workers who smoke have 30 times more risk than co-workers who do not smoke and 90 times more

risk than people who neither smoke nor work with as-bestos.

2. *Absence of a known agent.* Because no specific di-agnostic test exists for many chronic diseases, the dis-tinction between diseased and nondiseased persons may be more difficult to establish than in most infectious dis-eases.

3. *Long latent period.* Many chronic diseases have a long latent period, which is the equivalent of the incu-bation period in infectious disease except that it is gen-erally longer. Because of the extended latency, it is of-ten difficult to link antecedent events with outcomes. However, increasing evidence shows that onset of ill health is strongly linked to influences of physical, social, economic, and family environments. It is easy to iden-tify the common exposure to chickenpox in a school set-ting, but it is much more difficult to identify the impact of drastic alterations in family circumstances and result-ing mental disorders or slow-onset physical illnesses.

4. *Indefinite onset.* The problem of pinpointing the initial occurrence of the disease exists with many chronic conditions, such as degenerative diseases and mental illnesses. Because of the vague onset of chronic illnesses, it is difficult to collect statistics on the number of new cases in any given year.

5. *Differential effect of factors on incidence and course of disease.* Factors in the socioeconomic environ-ment that affect health include income level, housing, employment status, culture, and life-style. For example, Mormons who abstain from smoking and alcohol have lower cancer rates than the general population as a whole.

6. *Disease-specific mortality rates.* These rates are difficult to determine with chronic illness because the cause of death may result from factors other than the chronic disease itself.

One approach for studying chronic illness from an epidemiologic viewpoint is to emphasize that interre-lated factors determine illness; that is, disease is a pro-cess that results from the breakdown of a multiplicity of factors: biologic, cultural, economic, emotional, and so-cial. The multiple interactions involving the *host,* the *environment,* and the *agent* are sometimes described as the "web of causation." With this approach an attempt is made to identify the multiple related factors that lead to the disease process. Until a disease can be understood as a *web of causation,* it is difficult to make rational de-cisions regarding therapeutic interventions, and it is even more difficult to identify early preventive actions. To develop a chain of causation, one must identify first the natural history of disease by systemic studies of groups of people.

NATURAL HISTORY OF DISEASE

All diseases have a natural history. For example, chronic diseases extend over time and develop through a sequence of stages. When people speak of the epide-miology of a disease, they are referring to its natural his-tory. That is, the outcomes of a particular disease are observed over time, and the numbers of the affected persons developing each outcome are measured. This information is used to predict an individual's possible future health. Knowledge of the natural history of dis-ease allows us to intervene to prevent or limit the effects of diseases. The stages involved in the natural history include the following:

1. *Stage of susceptibility.* The disease has not yet de-veloped, but the groundwork has been laid by the pres-ence of factors that favor its occurrence. These may be referred to as *risk factors.* The need to identify such factors is becoming more apparent as awareness grows that chronic diseases present our major health chal-lenge. Some major risk factors are environmental and behavioral and therefore are amenable to change; for example, smokers can be persuaded to give up smoking.

2. *Stage of presymptomatic disease.* No manifesta-tion of disease is present, but pathologic changes have begun. An example of presymptomatic disease is athero-sclerotic changes in coronary vessels before any overt signs or symptoms of illness appear.

3. *Stage of clinical disease.* By this stage sufficient anatomic or functional changes have occurred so that recognizable signs of disease exist. At present the natu-ral history of many diseases is incompletely understood. For example, it is not known why some individuals with several risk factors do not progress to clinical disease, whereas others with fewer risk factors develop disease.

4. *Stage of disability.* Disability, which can result from an acute or chronic condition, reduces a person's activity. The extent of protracted disability resulting from chronic disease is very significant to the person and society because of the person's reduced income, the impact on psychosocial roles, and the burden on com-munity resources.

The subtlety of the natural history of chronic dis-eases often leaves the person unaware of a disease pro-cess for an extended period. Recently, predisposing characteristics or habits that help identify the person at risk to develop a particular chronic disease have been studied extensively. By altering habits of eating, rest, activity, or smoking, the course of certain chronic ill-nesses such as emphysema, hypertension, or heart dis-ease may be changed. Unfortunately, many chronic conditions begin without the individual's awareness of significant physiologic changes. An important step in prevention is early detection of these changes.

PREVENTION

Because chronic disease evolves over time and patho-logic changes may become irreversible, the goal is to de-tect risk factors as early as possible. Although the de-generative diseases differ from their infectious disease predecessors in having more complex causes, it is now clear that many are preventable.

Generally, prevention means inhibiting the development of a disease before it occurs. More specifically, the term includes several levels of prevention to interrupt or slow the progression of disease: (1) primary prevention, (2) secondary prevention, and (3) tertiary prevention.

Primary prevention, appropriate in the stage of susceptibility, is concerned with health promotion and specific protection against diseases. *Secondary prevention,* applied in presymptomatic and clinical disease, includes early detection and prompt intervention to halt the progression of the disease. *Tertiary prevention,* appropriate in the stage of disability, uses rehabilitation activities to prevent further complications and to restore optimal functioning as much as possible.

Another way of looking at prevention has been identified by Albee.[1] He has developed a "prevention equation" for preventing dysfunction:

$$\text{Incidence of dysfunction} = \frac{\text{Stress} + \text{Constitutional vulnerabilities}}{\text{Social supports} + \text{Coping skills} + \text{Competence}}$$

The two major strategies for preventing dysfunction are decreasing the values in the numerator (that is, decreasing stress or constitutional vulnerabilities) and increasing the values in the denominator (that is, increasing social supports, coping skills, and competence). It is more difficult to have an impact on the numerator of the prevention equation because stress in our lives cannot always be controlled; however, creative ways to decrease individual and societal stress must continually be sought. It is easier to affect the denominator by strengthening social supports, coping skills, and competence.[1]

One valuable tool that has been developed to assist persons to identify their own risk factors and change their life-styles is the health hazard appraisal (HHA).[5] The HHA is a screening process that includes a comprehensive questionnaire and the taking of certain physical measurements. Based on probability tables, a risk assessment is then calculated from each person's profile along with goals that would result in risk reduction. Counseling and follow-up are provided to reinforce the data.

■ ASSESSMENT

Before a plan of nursing care can be devised for the chronically ill person, a thorough assessment of needs and capabilities must be carried out. Included in such an assessment are the individual's *physical, psychologic, social,* and *financial status.*

PHYSICAL STATUS

Because medical diagnoses do not accurately reflect the physical status and functioning of the chronically ill person, the use of a profile system or assessment tool may be instituted as a guide for those working with the patient. One such tool[22] provides a guide for grading the patient in six different categories: (1) physical condition, including cardiovascular, pulmonary, gastrointestinal, genitourinary, endocrine, and cerebrovascular disorders; (2) upper extremities, structure and function, including the shoulder girdle and cervical and upper dorsal spine; (3) lower extremities, structure and function, including the pelvis and lower dorsal and lumbar sacral spine; (4) sensory components relating to speech, vision, and hearing; (5) excretory function, including the bowels and bladder; and (6) mental and emotional status. The ability of the person to carry out activities of daily living (for example, dressing, feeding, bathing, brushing teeth, combing hair, toileting, and moving from place to place) specifically need to be assessed. The completed assessment should indicate in what areas the patient has difficulty and the extent of that difficulty. Such a guide can be used in planning goals, both immediate and long term, and is useful in assisting the individual and the family to make realistic plans for care. Because a chronic condition is not static, reassessment should be carried out at regular intervals whether improvement or regression occurs.

PSYCHOLOGIC STATUS

Assessment of the individual's psychologic needs and capabilities includes determining attitudes and stage of adaptation to the illness, feelings concerning how illness affects the family or significant others, and the person's own goals in regard to living with an illness. For example, individuals who are almost totally helpless as a result of an accidental spinal cord injury may seem to have no interest in learning ways to help themselves. Their families may react in the same manner and be of little help to them. Both the individuals and their families need interest and support from professional persons as they learn to cope with the change in their life situations.

Feelings of anxiety, frustration, irritability, bitterness, and guilt may be expressed by some chronically ill persons who face unending pain and loss of economic and social security. Some persons become obsessed with their health problems and spend much of each day thinking about what will happen and what to do. Guilt may result from being unable to work and support oneself or from the belief, as a result of a search for some purpose or reason for the affliction, that one must deserve the suffering.

SOCIAL AND FINANCIAL STATUS

Social and financial status must be considered, as they relate specifically to the type of support and resources available to the individuals in meeting their goals. It would be unrealistic, for example, to plan for a hydraulic bathtub chair if the patient could not afford it, family members were unavailable to help operate it, or the patient's apartment manager would not permit it to be installed. Alternative methods of helping the patient to take a tub bath would have to be explored.

The social assessment includes living arrangements, family roles, support of significant others, cultural and social group memberships, education, and vocational and avocational activities. The data collected through the performance of this type of thorough assessment would make it possible to devise a plan of care directed toward the accomplishment of attainable goals that are mutually acceptable to the patient, the family, and the caregivers.

■ DATA ANALYSIS: NURSING DIAGNOSES

Nursing diagnoses are determined from the assessment of patient data. Possible nursing diagnoses for the person with a chronic illness may include, but are not limited to, the following:

Diagnostic Title	Possible Etiologies
Activity intolerance	Bed rest, immobility, generalized weakness, sedentary lifestyle
Adjustment, impaired	Disability requiring change in lifestyle; inadequate support systems; impaired cognition, sensory overload; altered locus of control; incomplete grieving
Anxiety	Threat to self-concept; threat of change in health status, socioeconomic status, and role functioning
Breathing pattern, ineffective	Neuromuscular impairment, pain, musculoskeletal impairment
Communication, impaired verbal	Aphasia, physical impairment
Constipation	Change in lifestyle, immobility, inadequate nutrition, inadequate fluid intake
Coping, ineffective family: compromised	Inadequate or incorrect information, temporary family disorganization and role changes, prolonged disability of significant person
Diversional activity deficit	Long-term hospitalization
Fear	Loss of body part, long-term illness, pain, lifestyle changes
Health maintenance, altered	Altered communication skills, decreased motor skills
Home maintenance management, impaired	Insufficient family resources, lack of knowledge/role modeling, inadequate support systems
Hopelessness	Prolonged activity restriction, failing physical condition, long-term stress

Diagnostic Title	Possible Etiologies
Incontinence, functional	Altered environment; sensory, cognitive, or mobility deficits
Incontinence, reflex	Neurologic impairment
Injury, potential for	Sensory/motor deficits, lack of awareness of environmental hazards
Knowledge deficit	Lack of exposure/recall, cognitive limitation
Mobility, impaired physical	Intolerance to activity; decreased strength/endurance; pain/discomfort; cognitive, neuromuscular, or musculoskeletal impairment; depression; severe anxiety
Nutrition, altered: less than body requirements	Chewing or swallowing difficulties, inability to obtain food
Pain	Immobility, improper positioning, pressure points
Powerlessness	Health care environment, illness-related regimen, lifestyle of helplessness
Self-care deficit, bathing/hygiene, dressing/grooming, feeding/toileting	Intolerance to activity/fatigue, pain/discomfort, perceptional/cognitive impairment, musculoskeletal impairment, depression
Self-esteem disturbance	Severe trauma, change in body appearance, change in social involvement
Sexual dysfunction	Altered body structure, physiologic limitations
Skin integrity, impaired	Mechanical forces (pressure, shearing), immobility
Social interaction, impaired	Poor communication skills, self-concept disturbance, absence of supportive others, altered thought processes

■ PLANNING: EXPECTED PATIENT OUTCOMES

Outcomes for specific chronic diseases are discussed in the chapters dealing with those diseases. However, in general it may be stated that on discharge from the hospital, patients with chronic disease or their family members should be able to do the following:

1. Demonstrate or explain those measures that must be taken to avoid further preventable disability.
2. Demonstrate or explain those self-care activities of which they are capable.
3. Identify those activities for which help is needed.
4. Explain who will be available to help with those activities and on what basis that help will be available.
5. Explain what community resources are available and how to obtain them.
6. Discuss in reasonable detail their plans for follow-up care and reevaluation.

Chronically ill persons and their families require long-term care. A major focus of the nursing profession has been concern with chronic health problems and the challenge involved in providing long-term nursing care to chronically ill individuals and their families.

The American Academy of Nursing made this statement regarding long-term care:

Long-term care is the provision of that range of services—physical, psychological, spiritual, and social, including socio-economic—needed to help people attain, maintain, or regain their optimal level of functioning. It includes health maintenance throughout the life span as well as care during acute and protracted illness and disability. Such care is the legitimate province of nurses who now are making social contributions through health teaching and promotion, prevention of illness, and rehabilitation.[2]

The Academy has also proposed that "nursing assume major responsibility for health promotion, maintenance, and teaching within the context of nursing."[2]

■ IMPLEMENTATION

PHYSICAL CONSIDERATIONS
REDUCING DISABILITY

The first focus in intervention for the chronically ill person is on preventing and reducing disability and enabling the person to remain a socially functioning individual in every respect. Some disabilities among chronically ill persons might have been prevented if prompt, aggressive, suitable medical and nursing care had been available at the onset of the illness. Many of the difficulties that limit these individuals may not have been caused by the disease itself but may have developed because of immobility during the acute phase of the illness.

Keeping the person's body in good alignment, maintaining joint range and strength, and preventing decubitus ulcers are physical measures that must constantly be borne in mind. (For further information, see Chapter 70). A careful plan of rest and activity helps preserve physical resources and makes the day purposeful. If assistance is needed, it should be given until the persons can manage the activity by themselves or until an alternative method of management can be taught.

PROMOTING SELF-CARE

Recognizing what is meaningful to the individual is a primary step toward helping develop self-care. Physical needs are of paramount importance for chronically ill persons. Meeting these physical needs provides a way to convey to such individuals an interest in their progress and welfare. For chronically ill persons who must be hospitalized, it is important that they be allowed to perform as much of their own care as possible. Persons who have been independent in self-care before hospitalization should not be allowed to regress in these abilities

if at all possible. Helping them to take their own baths, attend to toilet needs, and groom themselves can give some sense of accomplishment and help them maintain their self-respect. Helping them to be dressed appropriately promotes a sense of wellness. Success in performing portions of their own self-care may be stimulating enough to strengthen ill persons' motivation; they and their families then may make amazing strides in thinking through and working out future problems themselves. For their planning to be realistic and ultimately functional, all health care personnel must teach chronically ill persons the total physiologic ramifications of their disability as well as methods of coping with those ramifications.

Persons who are in their homes or in substitute homes should be encouraged to dress in regular, comfortable street clothing rather than pajamas or gowns. Visitors to the home and family members who constantly see such individuals dressed in bedclothes think of them as sick and are reminded of their illness. Seeing them dressed as usual helps to maintain normal attitudes, relationships, and expectations.

PSYCHOSOCIAL CONSIDERATIONS

The care of chronically ill persons requires alertness in feeling, seeing, and hearing. Continued warmth and interest are necessary to the well-being of any chronically ill person. Very often a relationship based on an understanding of these requirements helps the individual to become highly motivated. It may be taxing to listen to the same questions and say the same things day after day, but the nature of chronic illness may require this attention, and the manner in which responses are given will convey warmth and interest. The world of chronically ill persons, whether they are in the hospital or elsewhere, becomes narrowed and circumscribed. They treasure and are interested in those things and those people who are close to them. Their conversations may be largely about themselves, their immediate environment, a few close objects, and the persons who are close to them. Although they may be confined to bed and to their room, others can keep them up-to-date on outside news. Depending on their level of adaptation to their illness, they may welcome hearing about outside events, or they may not be able to think beyond themselves. When they reach the stage of being able to look beyond themselves, newspapers, magazines, radio, television, or creating something with their own hands may help to keep up their interest in others and in outside events.

SUPPORTING COPING SKILLS

Coping skills may be challenged by persistent, ongoing problems such as chronic pain, recurring medical expenses, or continuing difficulties in carrying out activities of daily living. Usual coping methods may become impossible; for example, a person who usually copes by expending energy in physical activity may become unable to do so. The person who usually copes by discussing problems with family members will need to find an alternative method if family communication patterns break down. The person can be helped to identify usual coping methods and to explore alternative approaches when necessary.

It is important to recognize that chronically ill persons or their families may suffer from unresolved sadness known as *chronic grief*. Chronic grief may be defined as accumulated or prolonged grief. It extends over long periods, with permanent characteristics developing in many persons, and carries with it a potential for decreased functioning The causes are varied, and new waves of grief are constantly triggered. One example is grief caused by the losses associated with aging: youth, dreams, jobs, hair, friends, family, health, visual acuity, social role, money, body parts, and mobility. Each loss is accompanied by grief, which builds on previous grief like bricks in creating a wall. In chronic grief the person may be faced with repeated acute episodes. These episodes may coincide with exacerbation of the condition, facing a new limitation, or meeting new indignities. Each new episode requires a renewed struggle back and forth through the various stages of grief.[32]

The nurse can assist by listening and helping the person explore feelings and the content related to these feelings. Because the grief is ongoing, family members can also be helped to identify their feelings and strengthen the communication patterns within the family structure for mutual support of its members.

CLARIFYING NURSE-PATIENT VALUES

Nurses who work with chronically ill persons need to be able to distinguish between their own values, standards, and goals and those of the patient. In day-to-day contact with individuals who are making little or no progress, it is tempting to make plans for their future because of a sincere interest in helping them. This is particularly true when the patient's age is similar to one's own. There may be a feeling that something must be done to speed progress. One may become frustrated by the feeling of wanting to do something or wanting to see some marked change. However, the nurse must recognize that management of chronically ill persons requires a slow-moving, persistent pace with possibly little or no change for a long time. The person's physical and mental condition must be maintained at its present level or improved, and efforts must be made to progress and encourage the family's adaptation to the patient's condition. Eagerness and readiness to progress will be determining factors for the future. The "doing" in the care of the chronically ill person is not always a physical action with the hands. Often the maintenance of a positive approach and attitude and a demonstration of real interest

are the greatest help to the patient. Teaching patients to perform activities related to their own care independently rather than performing those activities for them may also lead to progress.

SUPPORTING THE PERSON WITH PROGRESSIVE DISABILITY

Health care personnel must also be prepared to provide care for patients whose disease will follow a course of progressive disability, as in multiple sclerosis or rheumatoid arthritis. In these instances, goals of care must be modified to retard the downhill progression of disability rather than to achieve maintenance or improvement of physical status. Helping the patient and family cope with progressive deterioration and in some cases eventual death is a demanding task. Those who wish additional information relating to this aspect of care are referred to the literature treating this subject.[32,37]

Persons with a disability, whether obvious to others

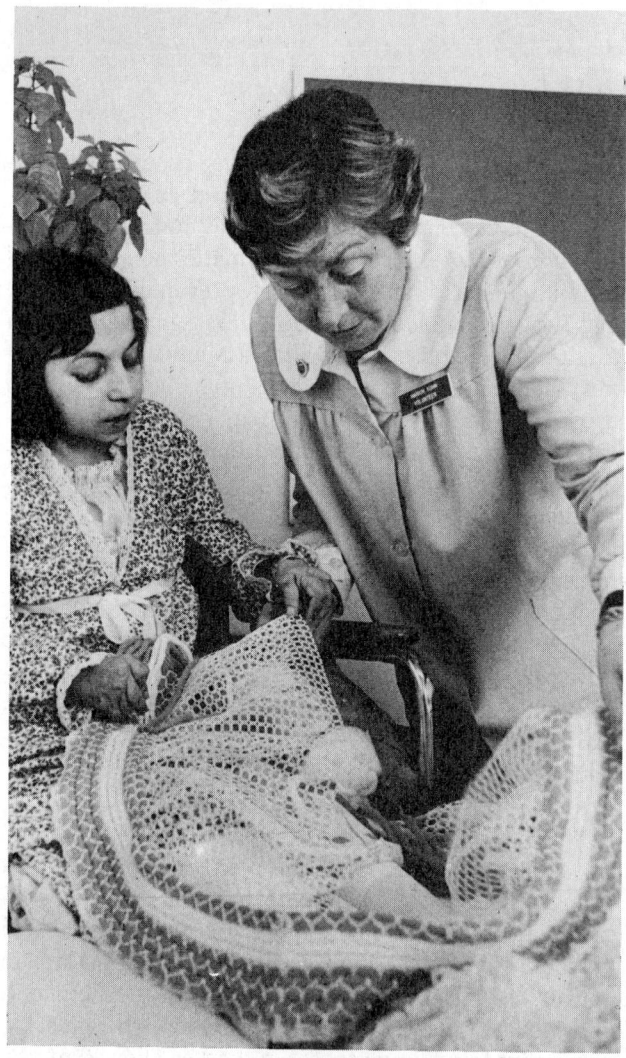

FIGURE 13-1 Volunteer helping patient who has a chronic illness with some handwork.

or unrecognizable, should not be viewed from the standpoint of their disability alone. Usually the greatest need is for comprehensive health services and continuing care. Comprehensive care is provided to patients according to their needs in an appropriate, continuous, and dynamic pattern. Accommodating the plan of care to the needs and goals of individual patients rather than to those of the providers is the essence of comprehensive care.

PROVIDING COMMUNITY RESOURCES

There has been an increasing interest in providing programs for chronically ill persons and in assisting them and disabled persons to assume a more active role in their communities. Volunteer workers may act as readers both in hospitals and in homes or may assist with other diversional activities (Figure 13-1). Institutions receiving federal funds are required to make aids such as ramps available to individuals who are unable to climb stairs or who are in wheelchairs. With the development of structural changes that facilitate mobility, some persons with physical limitations are more involved in local activities and associations. Nurses can assist by supporting the further development of these structural changes in all community buildings and by encouraging the participation of chronically ill persons in community activities of interest. Various information sources may be obtained from national organizations involved with chronic illness and disability. Many of these agencies have services available in the community (see the box on pp. 240 and 241). Programs, facilities, and legislation of this nature reflect the public's increasing awareness of the difficulties faced by chronically ill and disabled persons.

REHABILITATION

Rehabilitation is the process of assisting the individual with a handicap to realize his or her particular goals, physically, mentally, socially, and economically. As such, rehabilitation is an active concept and must be clearly differentiated from the concept of *maintenance* care. Following a thorough assessment of patients' disabilities and capabilities, assumptions can be made regarding the potential for improving their conditions. If improvement can be made, patients are candidates for rehabilitation. If improvement cannot be made, care is directed toward maintaining the current condition, that is, preventing further disability. The process of rehabilitation can be viewed more appropriately as patient *education* rather than patient "care." One must remember, however, that the rehabilitation of every patient will reach an end point, that is, a point at which no further progress is possible. At that time, the focus of care reverts to that of maintenance.

The purpose or extent of rehabilitation ranges from employment or reemployment for the handicapped person to the more limited achievement of developing self-care abilities. This latter accomplishment can be just as important to the individual as earning money and may represent that person's greatest life achievement. This might be true, for example, for a person who was born with a severe physical handicap such as cerebral palsy.

Success in learning to adjust to living with a disability depends on the person's premorbid personality, total life experience, and premorbid family relationships, as well as the person's current behavior and motivation. Certainly, some rehabilitation can occur in any health agency; nevertheless, the greater the number of rehabilitation disciplines made available as needed to individuals, the greater is their chance of achieving their highest potential. The rehabilitative process, as with any form of education, is involved as deeply in the motives and purposes of the teacher as in those of the learner.

Persons with disabilities, whether obvious to others or unrecognizable, should not be viewed from the standpoint of their disability alone. Usually the greatest need is for comprehensive health services and continuing care. Comprehensive care is that which is provided to patients according to their needs in an appropriate, continuous, and dynamic pattern. Accommodating the plan of care to the needs and goals of individual patients rather than to those of the providers of care is the essence of comprehensive care.

MULTIDISCIPLINARY APPROACH

The number of professional people required to assist the patient and family with rehabilitation will vary. Most often the patient, the family, the physician, and the nurse can work out a practical plan. If a patient's problems are complex, other members may be added to the team. Typically, such a team consists of a physician, nurse, medical social worker, vocational counselor, psychologist, speech pathologist, occupational and physical therapists, and a caseworker from the patient's social agency. Teamwork requires that members of the team be able to use their special knowledge and skill and understand the value of their contribution to the patient's care. In addition, team members need some understanding of each other's professional functions and contributions. One of the cooperative efforts of the involved team members is to meet regularly to evaluate patients and their abilities thoroughly. Based on this assessment, each patient and the team devise a plan to foster readjustment, compensation, and the learning of new ways to manage self-care and living.

REHABILITATION CENTERS

Persons with very complex problems of rehabilitation may need to receive care at specialized centers for rehabilitation, or they may receive care at home combined with visits to day rehabilitation centers. The variety of specialized centers includes teaching and research centers (centers located in and operated by hospitals and medical schools), community centers with facilities for inpatients, community outpatient centers, insurance centers, and vocational rehabilitation centers. In addition to centers that provide multiple services for the physically disabled, specialized centers provide rehabilitation for blind, deaf, mentally ill, and mentally retarded persons. Most centers offer a wide range of services that usually fall into the following three areas:

Physical area
Physical, nursing, and medical evaluation
Physical therapy
Occupational therapy
Speech therapy
Medical and nursing supervision of appropriate activities

Psychosocial area
Evaluation
Personal counseling
Social service
Psychometrics
Psychiatric service
Recreational therapy

Vocational area
Work evaluation
Vocational counseling
Prevocational experience
Industrial fitness of programs
Trial employment in sheltered workshops
Vocational training
Terminal employment in sheltered workshops
Placement

Several advantages exist for patients participating in organized programs for rehabilitation. They have an opportunity to see and be with others who have similar or more extensive disabilities. Often they progress more rapidly when they realize that others have similar difficulties and are overcoming them. Group therapy often arouses a competitive spirit, and a formerly reluctant person may become willing and diligent. On the other hand, all personnel need to be alert to those patients who have had the opposite reaction. Patients who see others advance in activity while they either do not improve or progress very slowly may become so discouraged that they give up trying.

On a rehabilitation unit activities are scaled so that individuals can see their own progress in comparison with their beginning abilities. Patients may take an active interest in keeping their own scores. After a program of therapy has been planned and is scheduled as to time of day, patients can help to keep themselves on the schedule by having a copy of it at the bedside. Individuals can then be assisted to gradually assume more

responsibility for readying themselves for scheduled activities. In addition, a master plan of activities for all patients on the unit can be a useful device for nurses, physicians, and therapists. The plan can be kept in a central place on the unit and should list name, activity, and time of activity for each patient. This type of plan is also helpful when a patient's progress is to be reevaluated.

A public program for vocational rehabilitation has been serving the United States since 1920. The program involves a partnership between the state and the federal governments. Services for disabled persons are provided by state divisions of vocational rehabilitation. The federal government, through the Social and Rehabilitation Service (SRS), administers grants-in-aid and provides technical assistance and national leadership for the program. Opportunities and services are available in all 50 states, the District of Columbia, and Puerto Rico. All persons of working age with a substantial job handicap resulting from either physical or mental impairment are eligible for help or assistance. The purpose of this service is to *preserve, develop,* or *restore* the ability of disabled persons to earn their own livings. The individual services offered are medical care, counseling and guidance, training, and job finding. All 50 states have separate rehabilitation programs for blind persons. Application for such services can be made to the SRS or to the agency in the state for serving the blind.

NURSE'S ROLE IN REHABILITATION

The concepts of comprehensive nursing care and rehabilitation can be considered synonymous. Helping the patient and family to help themselves is an integral part of nursing care. Nurses who work with patients who have disabilities have two major responsibilities: (1) to ensure that disability from disease is limited as much as possible and (2) to see that a rehabilitation program is planned and implemented. Details of the nurse's role and responsibilities are listed in the box on p. 235.

LIMITING DISABILITY

Limitation of disability requires attention to the prevention of complications, to the early recognition of symptoms of exacerbations or complications, and to the prevention of deformity. For patients with chronic illnesses, the onset of exacerbations or complications is frequently subtle, marked by minute changes in functional ability or general performance or attitude. Nurses, working closely with such patients and understanding the pathophysiology of their diseases, are frequently the first to recognize initial signs of difficulty and make provision for appropriate intervention. (See box on p. 235.)

PLANNING AND IMPLEMENTING REHABILITATION PROGRAM

The second responsibility, planning and implementing a program of rehabilitation in accordance with the patient's goals, is a process in which nurses are intimately

THE NURSE'S ROLE AND RESPONSIBILITIES IN REHABILITATION

I. Limit disability from disease as much as possible.
   A. Prevent complications.
      1. Ensure early recognition of symptoms of patient's condition worsening.
         a. Review signs and symptoms and pathology of the chronic illness to recognize changes.
         b. Review signs and symptoms of complications frequently associated with the chronic illness, such as infection.
      2. Prevent deformities.
         a. Maintain proper body alignment.
         b. Position limbs to prevent contractures.
         c. Turn frequently; keep skin clean and dry to prevent skin breakdown.
         d. Provide adequate nutrition.
         e. Provide adequate fluid intake to maintain bladder and bowel program.
         f. Take precautions to prevent infection.
II. Plan and implement rehabilitation program appropriate to patient.
   A. Determine patient's own goals for rehabilitation.
   B. Plan appropriate nursing interventions based on mutually agreed-on goals.
      Early in rehabilitation nurse may have to assume total responsibility for assisting with activities of daily living (ADL), bathing, intake of food and fluids, bowel and bladder programs, maintaining skin integrity, turning patient, and so on.
   C. Plan nursing interventions that encourage patient to assume responsibility for own ADL as soon as possible.
      1. Set short-term goals with patient.
      2. Goals should be realistic and attainable.
      3. Reinforce patient's progress (no matter how small) with positive feedback.
      4. Work with other members of the rehabilitation team in providing a consistent, coordinated rehabilitation plan.
      5. Keep patient's significant others informed of patient's progress so they can give positive feedback to patient.
      6. Reassess goals periodically and set new goals as appropriate.
      7. Teach patient, family, and, if necessary, the employer about patient's limitations and rehabilitative expectations.

involved. Nursing personnel are likely to be in contact with a patient and the family for a longer period of time each day than are members of any other discipline on the rehabilitation team. Both in the hospital and in the home, nurses are in an excellent position to plan a reasonable care program with the patient, as well as to teach the patient, the family, and, if necessary, the employer about the patient's limitations and rehabilitative expectations.

Much of the nursing activity in the rehabilitation process is no different from the nursing care given to all patients. Measures such as appropriate bowel and bladder programs, providing proper diet and fluid requirements, implementing new methods of bathing, and maintaining skin integrity fall within the domain of nursing concern and knowledge. Initially, nursing personnel may assume almost total responsibility for performing these activities for the patient. After assessing patient needs in these areas, nurses formulate, implement, and evaluate a teaching plan in much the same way as do therapists from other disciplines. The assistance nurses can give the patient and family depends on nurses' ability to understand themselves, personal feelings, and personal behavior as well as the behavior of the patient, family, and other professional team members.

One of the most important aspects of giving continuing care to a patient with a disability is the nurse's own attitude, perseverance, and expectations. Improvement may be slow, and patients may reach a plateau in their progress. Such a time can be critical for patients because they may become discouraged and not wish to continue with their program of care. Realistic encouragement can often sustain patients so that they will not regress before some improvement is noted.

Patients in a rehabilitation program must often learn and practice special physical techniques to strengthen muscles and to improve mobility. Such measures as physical exercise to improve walking, activities to improve self-care abilities, and the use of prostheses require the special knowledge and skills of physical and occupational therapists. To be effective in the rehabilitation process, nurses must have an understanding of the techniques used by the various therapists so that they can plan and work cooperatively with them in caring for the patient. This knowledge is also used to help the patient employ appropriate techniques in carrying out activities of daily living. (See box above.)

PATIENT'S ROLE IN REHABILITATION

The most important contributions to patients' rehabilitation are made by the patients themselves. The patient, the nurse, the physician, the social worker, the occupational therapist (Figure 13-2), and sometimes others planning together can arrive at the best plans for the future, but the patient's attitudes, acceptance, and direction of motivation are the most important considerations. If the patient cannot adjust to the disability,

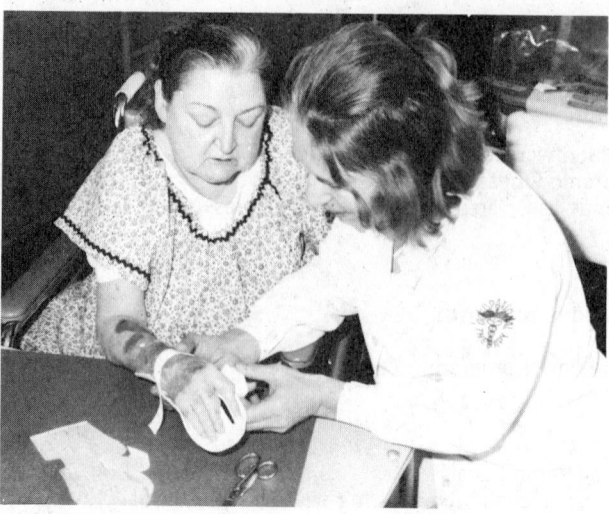

FIGURE 13-2 Occupational therapist makes resting splint for patient whose hands are severely deformed by rheumatoid arthritis. Splint will be worn by patient in effort to prevent further deformity.

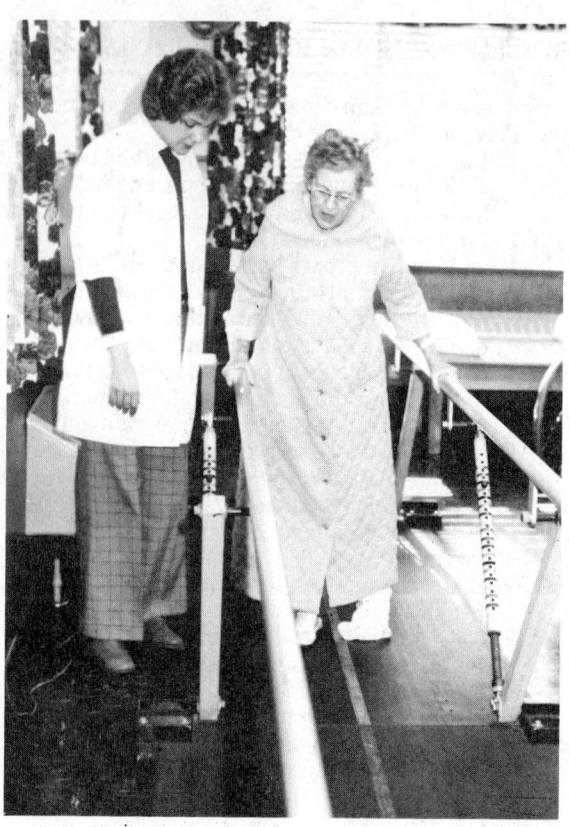

FIGURE 13-3 Physical therapist begins patient's ambulation training by teaching her to walk with support of parallel bars. Patient's left foot is wrapped in a towel to remind her not to bear weight on it.

whatever it is and however extensive, attempts at rehabilitation usually are hindered. Patients are the persons who really make the decisions, and they change at their own pace. If they are agreeable to suggestions but make little or no effort to try them, one should question if they really have accepted them.

Self-care is encouraged within existing limitations. The patient's behavior from day to day can be the first indication of the direction of positive motivation. For example, if the patient makes every effort to resume normal daily activities such as feeding, bathing, and dressing, one can be certain that the person has a sincere desire to be independent. As patients become ready for more advanced activities, such as ambulation and work in the occupational therapy shop, they need continuing genuine interest and support (Figure 13-3 and 13-4). As obstacles arise, patients may be able to accept and eventually overcome them. Patients who are truly motivated toward helping themselves never seem to give up, finding ways of accomplishing activities that professional personnel might believe impossible. Each person working with the chronically ill patient has seen that many times life has meaning for the individual even though it may not be readily apparent to others. Some patients, however, when faced with an added burden, cannot accept it and give up trying. Guidance and support for the families of such patients become tremendously important. Health care personnel who understand these attitudes and behaviors can help make life more satisfying for the chronically ill person and can positively influence the behaviors of the family, professional co-workers, and the public.

CONTINUING CARE

Traditionally, health care professionals have assumed responsibility for the patient's well-being within the hospital and little to no responsibility for the patient and family in the home setting. This dichotomy between health care in the home and hospital facility made little sense. With chronically ill individuals the dichotomy interferes with a smooth transition from hospital to home. The major portion of health care for persons with chronic illnesses occurs in the home; thus ongoing communications must exist between the patient and health professionals. Strauss et al.[32] advocate that sick people participate more in their care within health facilities and that health care professionals play a greater role in aiding chronically sick people *and* their families to cope with their problems at home. Social forces such as shorter hospital stays have made it necessary for nurses to be more aware of home health care needs.

HOME HEALTH CARE

Most persons with a chronic or long-term illness can care for themselves or be cared for at home, and most

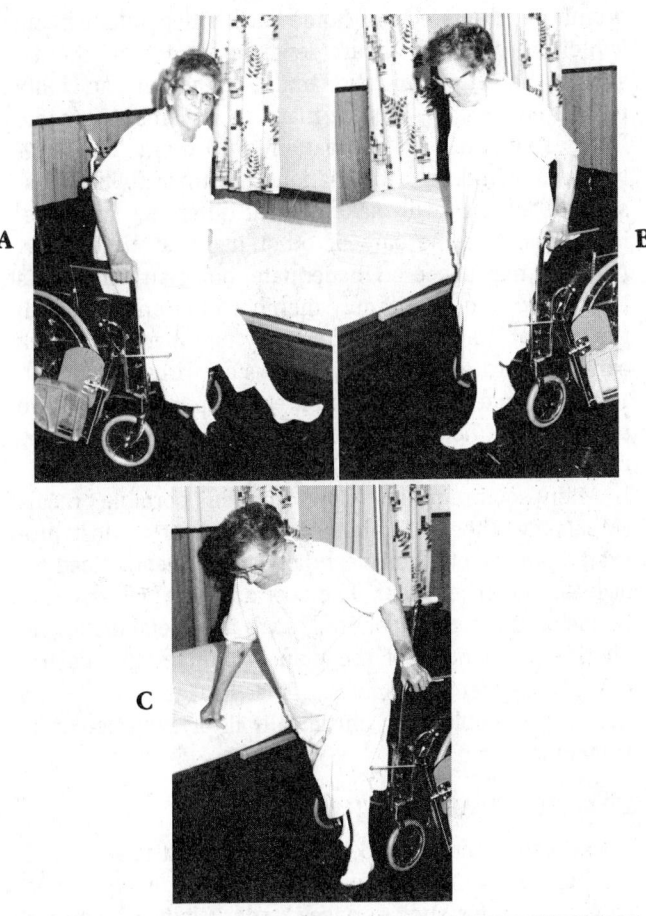

FIGURE 13-4 A, Patient executes transfer from bed to chair. She is not bearing weight on her left leg; thus she moves toward her right, or strong side. **B,** Patient moves back into bed from wheelchair, again leading with her right. She pushes up from chair, using arms of chair for support. **C,** Patient places her right hand on bed for support, pivots on her right foot, and sits down.

actually prefer to be at home, where family and friends are close by and where they can still participate in family life. Many chronically ill persons require health care supervision at home. The arrangements that can be made vary greatly and depend on the individual's needs and the facilities available. Many persons are ambulatory and during remissions are able to visit their local clinic. Others manage with visits from their personal physicians and with periodic workups in the physician's office. The assistance of a home health nurse or aide who goes into the home may also be necessary. Many chronically ill persons with disabilities also visit special rehabilitation units of hospitals or outpatient centers for daily or periodic instruction and practice in physical skills and job training.

Nurses from voluntary and official health agencies help chronically ill persons in their homes. Nurses who visit the home to assist the individual or family members to accomplish daily care need to understand the patient. Chronically ill persons are very often misjudged by even the closest family members because of blinding emotional ties or lack of knowledge and understanding. Families must be helped to understand the limitations and necessary restrictions on the patients. This process should begin while the patient is hospitalized, and it must continue in the home setting.

The benefits and the necessity of self-care as a valid part of the health care system are undergoing new recognition. Although the main impetus for this recognition has come from consumers, health care providers are increasingly incorporating self-care into the delivery of primary care. One definition of self-care is an action taken by the patient to reduce, to the degree possible, incremental debilitation resulting from chronic disease. The increasing prevalence and importance of chronic illness as a principal cause of disability and death place greater demands on the patient and family for involvement in self-care.

SELF-HELP GROUPS

Self-help groups are associated with self-care. These groups may or may not include the guidance of health care providers. They provide social support to their members through the creation of a caring community, and they increase members' coping skills through the sharing of information, experiences, and problem solving. Examples of self-help groups include those for women who have had mastectomies, for individuals who have colostomies or diabetes, and for obese persons.

FACILITIES FOR CONTINUING CARE

It is impossible to include here all the facilities that provide continuing care. Each of the programs mentioned has its own criteria for acceptance of patients for the services it renders. Before application for service is made, the individual patient's eligibility for that service must be determined.

AMBULATORY CARE

The term *ambulatory care* is used interchangeably with *outpatient care* and refers to first-contact health care services as well as to continuing contact services in settings that do not require overnight stays. The use of ambulatory care facilities has expanded because of the increase in chronic illness and the increase in cost of inpatient services. A good ambulatory care service constitutes one of the most important elements of the hospital's contribution to community health. There is a trend toward development of ambulatory care facilities in neighborhood health centers to assist disabled, aged, or disadvantaged persons to obtain needed health care.

An ambulatory care center usually provides long-term follow-up care needed by the person with a chronic illness, in addition to preventive health care, diagnostic workups, and treatment of acute illnesses for which hospitalization is unnecessary.

HOME CARE

Before World War II the home was the place where medical treatment was given. Well-to-do persons rarely went to a hospital; they received the services of a private physician in their own home, and the family was responsible for the day-to-day care. Poor families were among the first persons to use hospitals. The philosophy of home care can be traced as far back as 1796, when the Boston Dispensary provided medical care to the sick poor in their homes.

One of the most obvious reasons for the development of home care programs was to provide care to patients with long-term illnesses who did not need the around-the-clock services of an institution and yet who were too ill to go to an outpatient center. Caring for patients at home is often desired by the individual and family, and it also releases hospital beds for use by acutely ill patients.

Today home care is being provided for acutely ill patients discharged from the hospital more rapidly than in the past. The introduction of prospective reimbursement for hospitals under diagnosis-related groups (DRGs) has meant that many patients are being discharged while they still need skilled nursing care. As a result, many hospitals have set up home care programs to supply nursing care and other services to their patients after discharge. Hospitals that have not set up their own programs are contracting with the Visiting Nurse Association and other nursing agencies to supply nursing care for their patients after discharge.

Frequently the issue arises as to who should pay for home health services and who should be reimbursed for health care provided. The American Nurses Association's position is that reimbursement systems should foster care of individuals in their homes based on the following premises[4]:

1. Home care is humane and respectful of the individual's dignity and integrity.
2. Home care or care within the community can be less costly than institutional care.
3. Nursing care is the primary element in home care.
4. Payment systems for home care should recognize nurses as the major providers of home care, and as such their services should be reimbursed on their own authority.

Home care may not be possible for all patients. For those living in smaller dwellings, adequate space for the patient and other members of the family may be at a premium. The choice of home care, independent living center, or institutional care depends not only on the desires of the patient and the family, but also on the ability to finance the care. Despite many inconveniences, some families wish to have the patient with them. The family's understanding of the patient and their ability to assist one another will make a great difference in choosing between home care or other living arrangements. Not only may space be inadequate, but many times it is impossible to have a family member in attendance with the patient during the day. Family members who work cannot afford to sacrifice jobs to stay with the patient. However, many families find it easier financially to have the patient at home and are able to make satisfactory arrangements even though the facilities are limited.

Many communities now provide portable meals (Meals-on-Wheels) for homebound persons. Most programs provide one hot meal daily and unheated food for at least one other meal. The cost differs widely and depends on the services offered, such as special diets, and on the sponsorship of the plan. Volunteer groups frequently deliver the meals. This service alone often makes it possible for a chronically ill or aged person to remain at home.

HOME HEALTH AIDE SERVICES

Home health aide services were increased when Medicare came into existence. The greater number of persons eligible for such services under Medicare spurred their growth. The early discharge of patients from hospitals has increased the need for these services even more. Home health aides provide actual physical care to the patient after a registered nurse evaluates the home situation and the patient's need for physical personal care. The ongoing supervision of the home health aide is the responsibility of the nurse assigned by the agency providing the home care.

HOMEMAKER SERVICES

Homemaker services also have developed with the increased use of home care. These services are increasingly in demand in many communities and may be sponsored by a public or voluntary health or welfare agency or by a private agency that bills the family. Homemakers provide service to families with children and to the person who is convalescing, aged, or acutely or chronically ill. Homemakers are trained to assist in homes where the responsible family manager is temporarily unable to perform his or her usual responsibilities because of illness or absence.

DAY CARE CENTERS

In many communities some senior centers and nursing homes are expanding their facilities and services to include day care centers. Many chronically ill persons are able to live with their families but require 24-hour attendance. Often the caretaker in the family has to work. Homemaker or home health aide services are generally not available for the time the caretaker is at work. Day care centers provide a place where the chronically ill person can be looked after on a daily basis. Nursing services, physical and occupational therapy, recreational facilities, meals, and in some instances transportation to and from the center are provided. This form of service may allow a person to remain at home with the family rather than have to resort to institutional care.

RESPITE CARE CENTERS

Some nursing homes maintain a specified number of beds for respite care. As the name implies, these beds are available on a short-term basis to provide respite for families who have a chronically ill person at home. The day-to-day care of the patient, often 24 hours a day, is a very trying experience for any family. To provide the family or primary caretaker with a period free of this responsibility, respite care may be the answer. Usually the cost of respite care is not reimbursable; however, it may be the only alternative if the primary caregiver cannot continue to care for the family member without a break.

Community health agencies, such as the Visiting Nurse Association, are also providing respite services in some cities. They supply respite care in the patient's own home for part of a day, for 24 hours, or for extended periods depending on need. As mentioned, the cost of this service is usually not reimbursable.

INDEPENDENT LIVING CENTERS

Some persons with chronic illnesses may be unable to cope with the demands of maintaining a home but wish to live as independently as possible. Various options are available in some communities; these range from living units where persons cook their meals but have the unit maintained, to assisted units where persons can have their own physical living area but where one or more meals a day and other services are available. Living units are designed with such features as handrails for support in ambulation, wide doors to facilitate passage of wheelchairs, and emergency call systems.

FOSTER HOMES

Care in foster homes is a relatively new service that is now being widely used in many communities. Carefully selected families volunteer to take chronically ill persons into their own homes and provide the nonprofessional care needed. The family is paid either by the patient or the patient's family, from public funds, or by some social agency. The plan is primarily for those patients who have no family and cannot live alone, but who neither desire nor need institutional care.

INSTITUTIONAL CARE

Institutional care may be necessary when alternatives are not available, or the type of care needed by the patient requires close professional supervision. This include chronic disease hospitals, skilled care facilities, convalescent homes, rest homes, homes for the aged, and nursing homes. The patient's potential for rehabilitation, need for maintenance care, or the level of physical disability are factors that determine eligibility for placement in any of these facilities. A large or limited selection of outside facilities may be available, depending on the community.

NURSE'S ROLE IN CONTINUING HEALTH CARE

A nurse may be involved in continuing health care in several ways: (1) as an independent nurse practitioner assisting the person with chronic illness to cope with problems incurred by the illness; (2) as a public health nurse or visiting nurse involved in a primary rehabilitative program in the home; (3) as a supervisor of home health aides; or (4) as a nurse in a hospital concerned about the care patients will be receiving after they leave the hospital, particularly when the patient's rehabilitation program is not completed before discharge or when rehabilitation is not possible. Any of these nurses may also be involved in research pertaining to chronic illness. Some concepts that need further study in the area of chronic disease include social stigmatization, effects of isolation, and effects of chronic illness on the family, marriage, and domestic and occupational roles. Research will make a major contribution to clarification of these general concepts by identifying their relationship to chronic health problems.

Nurses must know the community resources available to patients to inform them and their families about what resources they might obtain, the types of service from which they may benefit, and what referrals they need for obtaining those services (see box on pp. 240 and 241 for a list of community resources). The hospital nurse should clearly communicate to the continuing care agency the data pertinent to the patient's care so that continuity is ensured. Teamwork and continuity are the keys to successful rehabilitation and management services for patients, and they must be practiced at all stages of care if patients are to realize their fullest potential.

FOCUS ON THE FUTURE

In 1979, the surgeon general's report established five goals concerned with major health problems in the United States. The time frame for the achievement of these goals was to be 1990.[35]

Although progress was made in meeting some of the 1990 goals, not all were met by 1990. Since the goals

COMMUNITY RESOURCES INVOLVED IN CHRONIC HEALTH PROBLEMS

Various types of information may be obtained by writing these national organizations. In addition, services of the various agencies are usually available at the local level.

GENERAL

Alzheimer's Disease and Related Disorders Association
360 N. Michigan Ave., Suite 601
Chicago, IL 60641

American Association of Diabetes Education
3553 W. Peterson Ave.
Chicago, IL 60659

American Association of Retired Persons
1909 K St. N.W.
Washington, DC 20006

American Cancer Society
159 9 Clifton Rd NE
Atlanta, GA 30329

American Diabetes Association
1 W. 48th St.
New York, NY 10020

American Heart Association
44 E. 23rd St.
New York, NY 10010

American Lung Association
1740 Broadway
New York, NY 10019

American Parkinson Disease Association
147 E. 50th St.
New York, NY 10022

Arthritis Foundation
221 Park Ave. S.
New York, NY 10003

Easter Seal Society for Crippled Children and Adults
2023 W. Ogden Ave.
Chicago, IL 60612

Juvenile Diabetes Foundation
23 E. 26th St.
New York, NY 10010

Leukemia Society of America, Inc.
211 E. 43rd St.
New York, NY 10017

Mental Health Materials Center
419 Park Ave. S.
New York, NY 10016

Muscular Dystrophy Association, Inc.
810 7th Ave.
New York, NY 10019

National Aid to Retarded Citizens
  (formerly N.A.R. Children)
2709 E. St.
Arlington, TX 76011

National Association for Down's Syndrome
628 Ashland Ave.
River Forest, IL 60305

National Association for Mental Health, Inc.
1800 N. Kent St.
Rosslyn Station
Arlington, VA 22209

National Association for Sickle Cell Disease, Inc.
945 S. Western Ave., Suite 206
Los Angeles, CA 90006

National Association for Visually Handicapped
305 E. 24th St.
New York, NY 10010

National Asthma Center
875 Avenue of the Americas
New York, NY 10001

National Council on the Aging
1828 L. St. N.W.
Washington, DC 20036

National Cystic Fibrosis Research Foundation
3379 Peachtree Rd. N.E.
Atlanta, GA 30326

National Epilepsy League
6 N. Michigan Ave.
Chicago, IL 60602

National Foundation–March of Dimes
1275 Mamaroneck Ave.
White Plains, NY 10605

National Genetics Foundation
250 W. 57th St.
New York, NY 10019

National Hemophilia Foundation
25 W. 39th St., Rm. 903
New York, NY 10018

National Kidney Foundation
116 E. 27th St.
New York, NY 10016

National Multiple Sclerosis Society
205 E. 42nd St.
New York, NY 10017

Nutrition Foundation, Inc.
489 5th Ave.
New York, NY 10017

Parents of Down's Syndrome Children
11507 Yates St.
Silver Spring, MD 20902

Shriners Hospital for Crippled Children
323 N. Michigan Ave.
Chicago, IL 60601

Stroke Clubs of America
805 12th St.
Galveston, TX 77550

United Cerebral Palsy Association, Inc.
66 E. 34th St.
New York, NY 10066

United Ostomy Association
1111 Wilshire Blvd.
Los Angeles, CA 90017

COMMUNITY RESOURCES INVOLVED IN CHRONIC HEALTH PROBLEMS—cont'd

REHABILITATION

American Coalition of Citizens with Disabilities
1346 Connecticut Ave. N.W., Rm. 817
Washington, DC 20036

Architectural and Transportation Barriers Compliance
  Board
330 C St. W.W., Rm. 1010
Washington, DC 20201

Closer Look, National Information Center for the Handi-
  capped
Box 1492
Washington, DC 20013

Mainstream, Inc.
1200 15th St. N.W., Rm. 403
Washington, DC 20005

National Center for a Barrier-free Environment
8401 Connecticut Ave.
Washington, DC 20015

National Center for Law and the Handicapped
1235 N. Eddy St.
South Bend, IN 46617

National Congress of Organizations of the Physically
  Handicapped
7611 Oakland Ave.
Minneapolis, MN 55432

National Paraplegia Foundation
333 N. Michigan Ave.
Chicago, IL 60601

Paralyzed Veterans of America
7315 Wisconsin Ave. N.W.
Washington, DC 20014

President's Committee on Employment of the Handicapped
111 20th St. N.W., Rm. 636
Washington, DC 20210

---

were formulated, new public health problems and challenges have arisen.[11] As this is being written, a draft of objectives for the year 2000 has been proposed. The goals to be achieved are:

1. To reduce infant mortality to no more than 7 deaths per 1000 live births (baseline: 10.4 per 1000 in 1986).
2. To increase life expectancy to at least 78 years (baseline: 74.9 in 1987).
3. To reduce disability caused by chronic conditions to a prevalence of no more than 6% of all persons (age-adjusted baseline: 8.9%).
4. To increase years of healthy life to at least 65 years (baseline: an estimated 60 years in 1987).
5. To decrease disparity in life expectancy between white and minority populations to no more than 4 years (baseline: 5.8 years in 1987).

The year 2000 draft contain 339 goals (compared to 226 objectives established for 1990). The year 2000 goals are characterized by (1) an increased emphasis on prevention of disability and morbidity, (2) greater improvements in health status of groups at highest risk for premature death, disease, and disability, and (3) inclusion of more screening interventions to detect asymptomatic disease and conditions early enough to prevent early death or disability.[11]

Even though we can identify health goals for a nation, it is far more difficult to carry them out so that the effect is noticeable to the individual seeking health care.

Problems that interfere with the achievement of these goals include (1) the increasing number of homeless people, who receive little or no health care; (2) medically indigent persons who work but cannot afford health insurance; (3) the greater number of infants born addicted to drugs, especially crack cocaine; and (4)

failure of certain segments of the population to reduce behavioral risk factors. The Centers for Disease Control includes the following as behavioral risk factors that affect morbidity and mortality in the United States: smoking, sedentary life-style, binge drinking, heavier drinking, drinking and driving, and seatbelt use. Nurses and other health care providers need to be active in assisting persons to examine their health practices and in teaching them ways to improve these practices.

The challenge of providing health care to all people includes the challenge to promote the full participation of individuals with physical and mental disabilities. The United Nations proclaimed 1981 as the International Year of Disabled Persons (IYDP). The U.S. Council for the IYDP has worked to strengthen public understanding of the needs and contributions of 35 million disabled people. The council has defined the following long-term national goals of and for disabled persons:

1. Expanded educational opportunities
2. Improved access to housing, buildings, and transportation
3. Greater opportunity for employment
4. Broader recreational, social, and cultural activities
5. Expanded and strengthened rehabilitation programs and facilities
6. Increased biomedical research aimed at conquering major disabling conditions
7. Reduced incidence of disability through accident and disease prevention
8. Increased application of technology on behalf of persons with disabilities
9. Expanded international exchange of information and experience to benefit disabled people everywhere

Almost 10 years later, not all these goals have been met. Thus all citizens have a responsibility to seek improvements that will assist chronically disabled persons to be more self-sufficient.

CHAPTER SUMMARY

✔ Chronic health problems are one of the major health problems in the United States.

✔ The incidence and prevalence of chronic diseases have increased in this century and can be expected to increase even more as the population ages.

✔ The Bureau of the Census estimates that approximately 110 million persons in the United States have one or more chronic illnesses.

✔ Major disparities exist in the health of black Americans and other minorities in the United States when compared with the white population.

✔ The characteristics of chronic illnesses include one or more of the following: (1) illness or impairment that is permanent, (2) residual disability, and (3) nonreversible pathologic alteration, which requires a long period of care.

✔ Chronic illnesses may be present from birth or develop during childhood, adolescence, early adult life, or old age.

✔ Today some children with chronic illnesses such as cystic fibrosis live into early adulthood because of more effective treatment (see Chapter 34).

✔ Major chronic illnesses of adults include arthritis, diabetes, heart disease, and hypertension. The rates for arthritis and hypertension are higher in blacks than in whites.

✔ Cultural values determine how both nurses and patients view chronic illness.

✔ The economic costs of chronic illness are considerable, and many persons require some type of financial assistance.

✔ It is important that nurses be involved in prevention of chronic illness.

✔ The three levels of prevention are primary, secondary, and tertiary; the nurse has an important role to play at each level.

✔ Primary prevention involves health promotion and specific protection against disease, such as immunization against poliomyelitis.

✔ Secondary prevention includes early detection of disease and prompt intervention to halt progression of disease.

✔ Tertiary prevention includes rehabilitation appropriate to the stage of disability, prevention of further complications, and restoring optimal functioning to the highest possible level.

✔ Depression is common among chronically ill persons, especially those who feel powerless about controlling or overcoming what has happened to them.

✔ Rehabilitation is best carried out in a setting where a multidisciplinary team of nurses, physicians, physical and occupational therapists, social workers and, when necessary, speech therapists are available to work together in planning the therapeutic regimen for the patient and in assisting and supporting the patient with the prescribed therapy.

✔ The two major roles of the nurse working with persons with disabilities are (1) to limit disability from disease as much as possible and (2) to see that the rehabilitation program is planned and implemented.

✔ The nurse should be familiar with the facilities for continuing care in his or her community and the eligibility requirements for each facility.

QUESTIONS TO CONSIDER

- What types of patients do you think are most in need of rehabilitation? Outline the rehabilitation needs of a patient you are now caring for or have cared for in the past.

- What proportion of the patients on the hospital unit to which you are assigned have a chronic illness as either their primary or secondary diagnosis? What proportion has more than one chronic health problem? What age group is affected most by more than one chronic health problem?

- What resources are available in your community for the care of chronically ill persons? Are the facilities adequate for the number of persons needing care? How are these facilities supported financially?

- From what you have learned in anatomy, outline in detail the physical movements necessary to rise from a sitting position in a chair to a standing position. Describe how you would assist a patient to stand while allowing him or her to be as independent as possible.

REFERENCES AND SELECTED READINGS

1. Albee G: In Curtis N, editor: Self help reporter 3(4), 1977.
2. American Academy of Nursing: Long-term care: some issues for nursing, Kansas City, Mo, 1976, American Nurses Association.

*References preceded by an asterisk are particularly well suited for student reading.

3. American Cancer Society: 1990 Cancer facts and figures, New York, 1990, The Society.

4. American Nurses Association: A national policy for health care: principles and positions, 1977, The Association.

5. *Anderson SV and Bauwens EE: Chronic health problems: concepts and application, St Louis, 1981, The CV Mosby Co.

6. Centers for Disease Control: MMWR 35(8), 1986, Massachusetts Medical Society.

7. *Centers for Disease Control: MMWR 38(S-1), 1989, Massachusetts Medical Society.

8. *Centers for Disease Control: Progress in chronic disease prevention, MMWR 38(8), Massachusetts Medical Society.

9. *Centers for Disease Control: MMWR 38(12), 1989, Massachusetts Medical Society.

10. *Centers for Disease Control: MMWR 38(57), 1989, Massachusetts Medical Society.

11. *Centers for Disease Control: Progress in chronic disease prevention, MMWR 38(37), 1989, Massachusetts Medical Society.

12. Crate M: Nursing functions in adaptation to chronic illness, Am J Nurs 65:72-76, 1965.

13. Dittmar S: Rehabilitation nursing, St Louis, 1989, The CV Mosby Co.

14. Expectation of life in the United States at a new high, Stat Bull 61(4):13-15, 1980.

15. *Johnson JH, editor: Rehabilitation nursing, Nurs Clin North Am 15:2, 1980.

16. Kottke F, Stillwell GK, and Lehman J: Krusen's handbook of physical medicine and rehabilitation, ed 3, Philadelphia, 1982, WB Saunders Co.

17. *Lambert VA and Lambert CE, editors: Adaptation to chronic illness, Nurs Clin North Am 22:527-644, 1987.

18. Lefkowitz B: Health differentials between white and nonwhite Americans, Washington, DC, 1977, US Government Printing Office.

19. Leslie PM: Nursing diagnosis: use in long-term care, Am J Nurs 81:1012-1014, 1981.

20. Lubkin IM: Chronic illness: impact and interventions, Boston, 1986, Jones & Bartlett Publishing, Inc.

21. Morris R, editor: Allocating health resources for the aged and disabled, Lexington, Mass, 1981, Lexington Books.

22. Moskowitz E and McCann CB: Classification of disability in the chronically ill and aging, J Chronic Dis 5:342-346, 1957.

23. National Center for Health Statistics: Vital statistics of the United States, 1980, vol 11, Mortality, Part B, DHHS, Pub No (PHS) 85-1102, Washington, DC, 1985, US Government Printing Office.

24. *Olson EV, editor: The hazards of immobility, Am J Nurs 67:780-797, 1967.

25. Pollock SE: Human responses to chronic illness: physiologic and psychosocial adaptation, Nurs Res 35:90-95, 1986.

26. Public Health Service: Vital and health statistics: health characteristics of persons with chronic activity limitations (1979), US Department of Health and Human Services, series 10, no 137, Rockville, Md, 1981.

27. Public Health Service: Vital and health statistics: current estimates from the National Health Interview Survey (1981), US Department of Health, Education and Welfare, series 10, no 141, Rockville, Md, 1982.

28. *Ryan S and Wassenberg C, editors: Community health and home care nursing, Nurs Clin North Am 15:2, 1980.

29. Shamansky SL, editor: Home health care, Nurs Clin North Am 23(2):305-445, 1988.

30. *Sorensen K and Armis DB: Understanding the world of the chronically ill, Am J Nurs 67:811-817, 1967.

31. *Stewart Al et al: Functional status and well-being of patients with chronic conditions, JAMA 262(7):907-913, 1989.

32. Strauss AL et al: Chronic illness and the quality of life, ed 2, St Louis, 1984, The CV Mosby Co.

33. Thom A: Home health care agencies in the 1980s, Home Health Care Serv Q 3:5-24, 1982.

34. US Bureau of the Census: Statistical abstract of the United States, 1986, annual ed 107, Washington, DC, 1987, US Government Printing Office.

35. US Department of Health, Education and Welfare: Healthy people: the surgeon general's report on health promotion and disease prevention, Washington, DC, 1979, US Government Printing Office.

36. *Van Horne WA and Tonnesen TV, editors: Ethnicity and health, Madison, 1988, The University of Wisconsin System Institute on Race and Ethnicity.

37. *Wright BA: Value-laden beliefs and principles for rehabilitation, Rehabil Lit 12:266-269, 1981.

CHAPTER 14

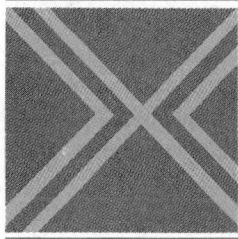

Loss, Dying, and Death

BENITA C. MARTOCCHIO
SR. KARIN DUFAULT

CHAPTER OBJECTIVES

After studying this chapter, the student should be able to:

1. Identify prevailing societal attitudes that influence how nurses, patients, and families respond to situations in which someone is dying or has died.
2. Compare and contrast the Kubler-Ross Stages of Dying and Martocchio's Patterns of Living-Dying as sensitizing schemes.
3. Describe the role of confidant to the dying person and how it differs from the role of friend.
4. Identify factors to consider in assessing whether a dying person might be cared for successfully in the home.
5. Describe the process of normal grieving and the behavioral manifestations of each phase.
6. Describe nursing strategies useful in assessing and intervening with individuals who are grieving.
7. Recognize the positive functions of after-death rituals for survivors.
8. Discuss how issues surrounding the care of the dying often present ethical dilemmas for caregivers.
9. Identify factors to consider in understanding what constitutes quality of life for a person in the last phases of life.

Throughout time people have been concerned with questions regarding life and death and mortality and immortality. Philosophers, poets, and scientists have attempted to understand and even to control death. Death, however, remains a part of life. The fact that humans are finite creates anxiety but also gives meaning to life.

The thoughts people have about death affect living in many ways. Some are beneficial and inspiring, whereas others are anxiety provoking and threatening. Koestenbaum[47] reiterates the many ways that death beneficially affects perceptions of life:

Death helps one savor life.
It provides an opposing standard against which to judge being alive.
It gives a sense of individual existence.
It helps give meaning to life.
It allows one to evaluate personal achievements.
It allows retrospective analysis of one's life.
It gives one strength to express convictions.
It reveals the importance of intimacy.

On the other hand, thoughts of death, especially one's own death or the deaths of close friends or relatives, can be anxiety provoking. Conceiving of a time with no future arouses anxiety. Death threatens all that we know and value.

Our personal thoughts about death and how we adapt to these thoughts significantly influence our lives, feelings, and behavior. Some people refuse to talk about death or acknowledge its existence. Consequently they avoid attending funerals or other death-related events, having annual physical examinations or participating in other health-promoting activities, and making a will.

People recognize mortality in different ways. Some perceive life on earth to be a transient state, a prelude to a better and more joyful life; and thus they downplay the importance of worldly goods and emphasize the tenets of a particular religious group that include a life after death.

Other people seek to control death. They may place themselves in dangerous situations occupationally or socially. They may ignore signs of illness or instructions to care for a serious illness.

Still others accept the finite nature of their lives but search for immortality in other ways. They may leave a legacy of artistic works or a long line of heirs, or they may search for a means to preserve their bodies after death to be revived at a future time.

One thing is certain: All persons react to the knowledge that life is finite, and how they react to this knowledge influences how they live *and* die. Nurses' and health professionals' reactions to dying, death, loss, and grief also affect the care of dying persons and their families.

Even though dying and grief are personal and vary from one individual to another, it is the purpose of this chapter to share understandings and to offer general guidelines that assist in caring for persons who are dying and in helping family members who are sharing the experience. Loss is the underlying theme. Perhaps the most beneficial way to learn to effectively care for dying persons and their families is to understand our own perspectives and those of others on loss, dying, and death.

DYING: A PART OF LIVING

Despite the amazing advances of science, technology, nursing, and medical knowledge, dying is and will continue to be a part of living. The fact is that at some future time we will cease "to be." In a sense we are dying even as we are living. To conceptualize living and dying as the opposite ends of a continuum creates a false dichotomy. Living and dying are not opposite ends of a continuum; they *are* the continuum. When we interact with persons who are known to have a life-threatening disease, we are more directly confronted with their dying and our own finiteness. This confrontation evokes anxiety, and thus we become more aware of the dying component of living. Although we may identify with the suffering and sorrow of persons as they live their dying, we interact with living persons. To appreciate our own and others' responses to loss, dying, and death, we need an understanding of the context in which they occur and of our own views and reactions within varying contexts.

SOCIETAL, CULTURAL, AND SOCIAL PERSPECTIVES

DYING AND DEATH ARE DIFFERENT

Dying is different from death. Dying, a part of living, is a process—the process of coming to an end. Death, the permanent cessation of all vital functions, the end of human life, is an event and a state. The event is the moment of death; the state is that of being dead.[55,56]

Both dying and death have unique aspects that evoke fears, anxieties, and uncertainties. Some aspects of dying such as physical and emotional pain, the loss of others, and the inability to function in familiar ways may also occur under other circumstances (for example, illness, retirement, or relocation) and therefore are not unique to dying. The unique aspect of dying is that it ends in death. People have no prior experiences to help them understand what it means to be dead. Questions surface: Can dead persons think? Can they have feelings? What is it like to be dead? Is there another life? Where will they go?

At the same time that death is a unique event, it is a universal. Because it is a universal, each society has had to develop its own beliefs, norms, mores, restrictions, and standards related to loss, dying, and after-death practices. Appropriate ways to respond in one societal or cultural group may be inappropriate in another. Each

society dictates the standards and practices that it will support. Thus members of societies have a prescribed set of behaviors from which to choose.

In general, the dominant view of dying, death, and loss of persons in any one society is a function of how death fits into the teleologic view of life. Individual responses reflect the dominant societal view. However, the repertoire of responses of dying persons or the survivors is also determined by personal beliefs and subcultural group (for example, social, cultural, religious) affiliations. For instance, Americans may view dying similarly, but their responses may be influenced by their religious beliefs, their views of life after death, their social class, and their occupations.

PREVAILING SOCIETAL ATTITUDES

Death denial, death defiance, death desire, and death acceptance are four prevailing societal attitudes toward death. As these general attitudes are discussed, it is important to remember that they may vary in different situations, depending on whose death is involved.

Recognition of the prevailing attitudes and their differences helps health care professionals to understand the process of dying, serves them as a guide when interacting with others, helps them to avoid conflicts among themselves, and, most important, enhances their communication abilities and thus patient care. Quality care for dying persons and family members must remain the constant goal of health professionals.

No attitude is good or bad; attitudes are merely different. Our behavior reflects our attitudes. If we recognize our own attitudes toward dying and death in a particular situation, as well as those of other individuals involved, we may better understand why all of us feel the way we do and why we are acting the way we are. This recognition and understanding may not always lead to agreement, but it can contribute to modifications of behavior and to decreased conflict in decision making. These attitudes are explored briefly in the following sections.

DEATH DENIAL

Western society has been described as a death-denying society.[10] Many people avoid the subject of dying and death. Health professionals, particularly physicians, have been described as being unwilling to talk to patients about their dying.[29] Both health professionals and family members often justify their stance by expressing the belief that they are "protecting" the dying person.

The question is, whom are they really protecting? In most situations they are protecting themselves; that is, consciously or unconsciously, they weigh the impact on themselves and decide—or choose—not to act because of fear of the reaction or response. The following questions often arise: What will happen to me? Will I lose emotional control? Will the other person shout, cry, or become angry? Will the family become angry? Will the physician become angry? Will I know what to do or say? What if they do not react at all?

In nursing, a death-denying attitude has taken on a negative connotation. But *no attitude in and of itself is good or bad—it just is*. The actions and consequences of an attitude can be evaluated as good or bad. For example, a death-denying attitude may contribute to a lack of open communication about dying, but it may also contribute to continuing care in bleak situations. On the other hand, a behavior or action such as continuation of care may reflect more than one attitude; for example, it may reflect both death denial and death defiance.

DEATH DEFIANCE

Death defiance is a part of the Judeo-Christian heritage. Throughout the ages people have fought for causes or ideologies, even though they knew that they might die in the attempt. This attitude is reflected in hospitals, especially in critical care units or during emergency situations. The cause is saving a life; the battle is with death.

Although it is not the staff who die in the battle, they are open to loss. If the patient dies, the staff lives with the sense of a battle lost. Moreover, they face once again the finiteness of their own lives and the inevitability of death, despite modern technology.

Death defiance is helpful as we fight for life. It is not helpful when we do not also attend to the realities of the situation.

DEATH ACCEPTANCE

Death acceptance is viewing death as a normal, natural, and integral part of living. Becker,[10] a prominent philosopher, defined the resignation to and acceptance of our limited existence as the central task for achieving maturity. With this acceptance, death becomes the conclusion of life's plan. It sounds so simple. Intellectually, it calms the fears and pains of dying and of facing our own mortality. But like the other attitudes toward death, this attitude is not a panacea. In fact, Schneidman[85,87] helps us to regain our perspective when he points out how romantic this attitude can be.

For some, death acceptance is the ultimate achievement of maturation, a form of self-actualization. The dying person must achieve this attitude himself or herself, it cannot be forced on him or her by others.

The value of the death-acceptance attitude can be judged by actions and behaviors of the dying person.

DESIRE FOR DEATH

The fourth attitude, the *desire for death,* is more common in our society than people generally know or like to admit. People may desire their own deaths or the death of others.

Many circumstances give rise to the desire to die or for someone else to die. One major reason is the search for relief from misery. Misery takes many forms; pain, loneliness, disability, fear, uncertainty, and economic and emotional crises are but a few.

Other reasons contributing to the desire to die may be associated with a relief from misery but are expressed in a different way. Some persons search for reunion with loved ones. Still others look forward to death as a last phase in the fulfillment of life.

Recognition of how people express their desire to die is important. In many instances the expression of the desire to die is the dying person's or family member's way of confirming his or her recognition that death is inevitable within a predictable period of time in the near future.

MY DEATH: YOUR DEATH

The knowledge that death is imminent or probable within a predicted period of time adds reality to feelings of fear, anxiety, and uncertainty.[45,55] As a result, persons facing imminent death experience these emotions differently than do healthy persons who are speculating about what it is like to be dying. Healthy persons speak of death in the abstract; they talk about the death of another or project it into the distant future. Casual comments such as, "We all have to die someday," "We are all dying from the time we are born," or "Everyone has to die of something," reflect what Freud[31] called "unconscious immortality." The fact that people can continue to think about others who have died causes them to unconsciously believe in their own immortality. But hearing of someone else's dying or death forces them to face their own finiteness.

Neither the casual comments nor the unconscious belief in our own immortality are good or bad in and of themselves. However, they offer little in the way of understanding or support when made to a dying person or to his or her family. The statements are usually in response to the discomfort we feel when someone tells us that death is imminent. A more understanding response might be "I'm sorry to hear that."

Views toward dying and death vary considerably, depending on whether the discussion is about "my death" or "your death" or whether the discussion is about a member of "my family" or "your family," or someone dear to me or to you. Even when we are discussing hypothetical situations, our closeness to dying or to a dying person can influence our views and our responses. The same data are seen differently from different perspectives. We can use age as a common factor and consider how our responses may change. For example, my father is 75 years old, and your father is 75 years old.

When death appears imminent, our thoughts may vary, depending on the referent of my father or your father. For example, my father is still young; your father has lived a long and a good life.

It is important to identify the referent under discussion whether we are talking in theoretic terms or about practical situations. In other words, from whose perspective are we evaluating the situation: my perspective, your perspective, the patient's perspective, or a family member's perspective? Lack of recognition of different perspectives leads to poor communication, faulty nursing judgments, and inappropriate nursing interventions.

RIGHTS OF DYING PERSONS

Some health care consumers are demanding that dying and death no longer be hidden behind closed doors. As a consequence, there is a movement to recognize that dying persons have rights.[19] One right of dying persons is the right to know that they are seriously ill and that they may die. The assumption is that such information will

---

EXAMPLE OF A LIVING WILL

To my family, my physician, my lawyer, my clergyman
To any medical facility in whose care I happen to be
To any individual who may become responsible for my health, welfare, or affairs

Death is as much a reality as birth, growth, maturity, and old age—it is the one certainty of life. If the time comes when I, (name), can no longer take part in decisions for my own future, let this statement stand as an expression of my wishes, while I am still of sound mind.

If the situation should arise in which there is no reasonable expectation of my recovery from physical or mental disability, I request that I be allowed to die and not be kept alive by artificial means or "heroic measures." I do not fear death itself as much as the indignities of deterioration, dependence, mental incapacity, and hopeless pain. I therefore ask that medication be mercifully administered to me to alleviate suffering even though this may hasten the moment of death.

This request is made after careful consideration. I hope you who care for me will feel morally bound to follow its mandate. I recognize that this appears to place a heavy responsibility on you, but it is with the intention of relieving you of such responsibility and of placing it on myself in accordance with my strong convictions that this statement is made.

Witnessed

_____

_____

Copies to:
(names of persons)

_____

_____

_____

---

ensure that they will have more control over what happens to them. As a result, they can participate more fully in decisions about their care and will have the opportunity to complete unfinished business.

Another right is the right to die in an atmosphere of hopefulness. Persons have a right to die in peace and dignity, surrounded by loved ones and unencumbered by tubes and machines. They have a right to privacy. Dying persons are entitled to be cared for by sensitive, caring, knowledgeable people who attempt to understand them and their loved ones. They are entitled to die as free from pain or other discomforts as is possible. Comfort contributes to dying with a sense of self-esteem and gives meaning to life.

ADVANCED DIRECTIVES

Concern that patients be allowed to die in a dignified manner has led to the development of the living will, or *advanced directive,* as it is referred to in many Natural Death Act state statutes. *Living wills* direct decisions for withholding or withdrawing life-sustaining treatment when the patient is in a terminal condition and death is imminent. Traditionally, life-sustaining treatment has included cardiopulmonary resuscitation and mechanical treatment such as a ventilator. However, with the growing number of court cases, questions have arisen about inclusion of nutrition and hydration.[40,43,61]

Living wills are written documents that address any individual who may become responsible for the person's health, welfare, or affairs, such as family members, lawyers, physicians, clergy, or representatives of any medical facility in which the person may be. These documents advise them on health care preferences. Living wills include directives to physicians and durable power of attorney.

Living wills generally request that under conditions when (1) an individual can no longer take part in decisions about his or her own future and (2) there is no reasonable expectation for recovery, the individual be allowed to die and not be kept alive through the use of artificial or extraordinary means. Most wills also request that the person be kept free of suffering and pain, even though the medications administered for pain relief may hasten the moment of death.

Several states have enacted legislation that permits designation of a *durable power of attorney for health care,* a form of advanced directive that enables one to choose an agent to act as decision maker if one becomes too incapacitated to responsibly participate in one's own health care decisions. Included are special directions for life-sustaining treatments and hydration/nutrition issues.[32]

At the present time, living wills are not legally enforceable in all states. In addition, there are many questions related to the conditions under which a living will can or should be honored. What is important for purposes of this chapter is that a living will can help caregivers and family members know what the dying person's wishes were, at least at the time of the writing.

Copies of living wills are usually given to family members, physicians, the person's attorney, and a member of the clergy. People are advised to sign and date them, at least yearly. The wills are likely to be honored if they are written or signed immediately before a person becomes unable to express his or her own wishes about dying care. The box on p. 248 is an example of a living will.

In those states where advanced directives are included in state law, mandated forms may be required. Consult the state statute when advising people and when acting on the directive. Ordinarily, other documents or statements of one's choosing can be added to the mandated form.

A sharing of philosophy of life desires related to the process of dying with loved ones and primary health care providers is perhaps the most effective way of ensuring a meaningful death—or what has been referred to as a "good" death.

GOOD DEATH/BAD DEATH

Many nurses, in fact people in general, express concern over dying with dignity or dying a "good" death. Is there such a thing as a good death? There is no one good death, rather there are many. There is no one right way to die, just as there is no one right way to live. Dying with dignity, or a good death, is really an ideal. The terms offer little in the way of guiding care.

There are many views about what constitutes a good death: to die as one lived, to die without pain, to die in the company of loved ones are all answers.

There are many ways to die well. A good death involves individual perceptions of the living-dying process as well as shared observations of the death event. A death is more likely to be labeled as good when dying is viewed as a part of living and not as a separate phenomenon. A good death is also associated with the way all persons involved interact with each other preceding and during the event; that is, if there is harmony rather than conflict.

Sometimes nurses refer to deaths as normal or abnormal. Deaths are perceived as normal or good when most or all persons involved perceive that all was done that could be done, and that the actions were appropriate and accepted by most persons involved. In these instances there is a sense of loss, but the loss is accompanied by a sense of fulfillment and closure. Nurses label deaths as bad or abnormal when there is conflict over the type or length of treatment, and when there are bad feelings about a lack of honesty, especially with family members.

Whether a death is seen as good or bad does not always have to do entirely with the way the person died. Sometimes it has to do with who is present and how they interpret what is happening in the situation. People's attitudes toward dying and when people should die, as well as the characteristics of the dying person, influence how they interpret the situation and how they act and interact with others.

AGE AND PREMATURE DEATH

There was a time when people did not make a connection between aging, loss of body function, or general progressive debilitation and dying. For example, primitive people believed that if there were no accidents or magically induced illnesses, no one would die.

The expectations of living have changed as life expectancies have changed. During the Roman period, life expectancy was 20 years and increased to about 35 during the Middle Ages. By the late 1800s Americans could anticipate living 50 years; few persons lived past the age of 60 or 70. In contemporary American life, people not only anticipate living more than 70 years, they expect to do so as active, functioning individuals.

Many people believe that any age is too young to die. In contemporary society death is perceived as premature and clinically unnecessary. The concept of clinical death is well entrenched.[39] Some perceive that people do not die of natural causes or of old age; people die from accidents, homicides, and suicides. They die while receiving treatment for a recognized, diagnosed clinical problem such as heart disease, stroke, disseminated intravascular coagulation (DIC), or total body failure. As a consequence, most deaths can be interpreted as avoidable, unnecessary, and premature. If death is always interpreted as avoidable, unnecessary, or premature, it follows that someone must be blamed. Who can be blamed—the physician, the hospital, society? Perhaps it is the fault of the person who died for not getting help sooner. It is this interpretation of death as always being avoidable that contributes to conflict and guilt. People die; death is a part of living. People can receive the best care possible and still die. In fact, sometimes the very treatments that save lives create dilemmas by prolonging life or perhaps even by prolonging dying.

PROLONGED DYING

Just as there is concern over premature death, there is concern over prolonged dying. Through modern technology and therapy we have become adept at maintaining life in the desperately ill person. Unfortunately, at times the same techniques used to maintain life during temporary crises create dilemmas related to what constitutes life. When are we prolonging dying rather than life? Our ability to prolong dying leads to many moral and ethical issues related to life and death. For example, what is quality of life? What is the definition of death?

Tension rises as involved individuals grapple with questions about what constitutes therapy and whether that therapy should be continued or not. For example, is administration of food a therapy? If feeding causes discomfort, should it be stopped? Should brain-dead persons be denied tube feedings? What constitutes euthanasia? What are dying persons' roles? How are they to be included in decision making? Do we sometimes stop treatment too soon? The ethical perspective is discussed in greater depth later in this chapter.

PERSPECTIVES OF DYING PERSONS

Thus far we have discussed dying and death in somewhat general terms. Now let us turn more directly to a discussion of dying persons and their characteristics, which will form a base for nursing assessment.

CHRONICITY OF DYING

The nature of dying has changed. Because of modern therapies and technology, patterns of illness have shifted from acute infectious diseases to chronic conditions; as a result, dying has become a chronic process. With the exception of some acute problems such as myocardial infarction, severe infections, fatal accidents, homicides, and suicides, most dying persons experience chronic problems with multiple pathophysiologic alterations. These alterations are usually permanent and result in disability with a need to adjust to loss and to accommodate change. Multiple series of losses can affect a person's behavioral responses and ability to cope.

Dying takes on many characteristics of chronic illness. Dying persons, just as do other chronically ill persons, express feelings of being socially displaced or isolated. They grieve over the loss of former activities and abilities. They express sorrow over the continued loss of friends, business associates, and acquaintances. They talk of being alive and yet not able to live. They are expected to be present- rather than future-oriented.

Whenever the anticipated life span is *perceived* as *shortened*, persons, even though they are healthy, may be viewed as chronically ill or dying and treated accordingly. For example, some elderly persons are perceived and perceive themselves as not having enough time left to make future-oriented plans or decisions. The same perception is associated with some persons with diagnoses of such illnesses as cancer, stroke, and multiple sclerosis. Some people with shortened life spans may perceive themselves or be perceived by others as not deserving of services or not being worthy of the efforts of others, since they will not live long; thus they may become displaced, isolated individuals, not allowed to live their living. Furthermore, the chronicity of their dying may force them into experiencing a social death while they are functionally and biologically very much alive.

KÜBLER-ROSS'S STAGES OF DYING

Shock and disbelief	Bargaining
Denial	Depression
Anger	Acceptance

Many factors contribute to promoting social dying long before the event of death; these factors are discussed.

STAGES AND PHASES OF DYING

One factor that may hasten social dying is indiscriminantly applying theoretical findings based on groups to individuals. Kübler-Ross[48] described a series of stages through which people pass in response to their dying (see the box above).

Physicians and nurse scientists, family members, and dying persons have challenged the accuracy and, more important, the usefulness of the stages of dying for guiding care.[35,55,69,88,99] Both Weisman[99] and Pattison[69] suggest, instead, phases of dying.

These challenges do not mean that Kübler-Ross had no contribution to make. Rather, they show that the stages should be used as *guidelines* of how some people may respond, *not* as rigid categories into which *all* people will or *should* be placed.

The theoretical stages and phases of dying are sensitizing schemes to help us remain open to assessing what is "going on" in a situation so that we may understand it better. Our ultimate goal is quality care for dying persons and their families. Understanding, observation, and assessment assist in determining appropriate intervention to better achieve that goal.

PATTERNS OF LIVING-DYING

Another tool to help understand the nature of dying is the patterns of living-dying.[22,55,57]

The four major patterns and their various combinations are based on the clinical courses of dying patients (Figure 14-1). They describe what has occurred, not what will occur. In other words, they are descriptive, not predictive. They are useful for understanding the variations of behavior among dying persons. They also demonstrate the futility of expecting persons to pass through a series of stages of behavior in any fixed sequence.

PEAKS AND VALLEYS PATTERN

The pattern of peaks and valleys is characterized by periods of greater health (peaks) and periods of crises (valleys). Dying persons refer to the peaks as "hopeful highs" and the valleys as "terrible or depressing lows." Although there are times of greater health, the overall course is downward to the event of death. Many hospitalizations and many moments of increased expectation

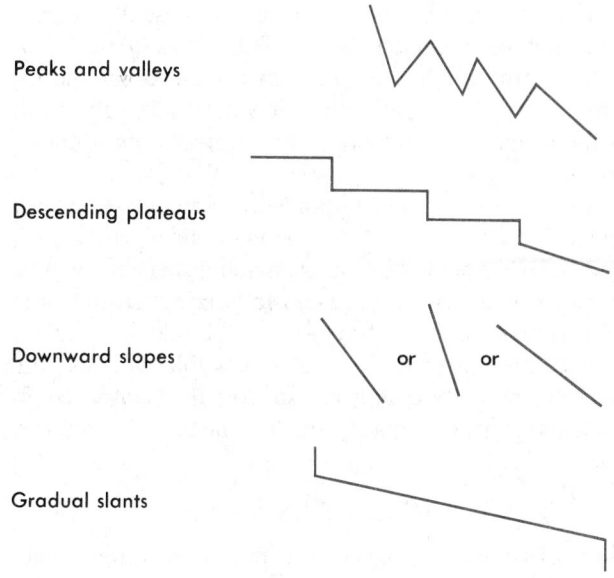

Peaks and valleys

Descending plateaus

Downward slopes   or   or

Gradual slants

FIGURE 14-1 Martocchio's patterns of living-dying.

and dashed hopes are associated with the experience of dying in this pattern. The uncertainties are great; fluctuations in behavior and difficulties in planning and adjustment are to be expected as goals and plans change.

DESCENDING PLATEAUS PATTERN

The pattern of descending plateaus is characterized by an unpredictable number of progressive degenerative steps with plateaus (periods of stable health) lasting an indeterminate period of time. Again, the overall general course is downward. People do not return to their former level of health or functioning after each crisis. Like the peaks and valleys pattern, the course is fraught with uncertainty and anxiety about whether another crisis will occur and cause more debilitation.

This pattern is associated with expressions of futility and anger. Dying persons and family grieve over the fact that functional ability is lost in spite of concerted rehabilitative efforts to maintain or regain it.

DOWNWARD SLOPES PATTERN

The downward slopes pattern is characterized by a consistent, persistent, easily discernible downward course. Unlike the other patterns, death is expected within a predictable period of time measured in hours or days. In most instances, the dying person loses consciousness, and there is little time to prepare family members for the death of their loved one. These deaths usually occur in critical care units.

GRADUAL SLANTS PATTERN

The fourth pattern of living-dying, gradual slants, is characterized by a low ebb of life, gradually and almost imperceptibly culminating in death. Generally these

persons experience a debilitating bodily insult from which there is little recovery. In many instances the person is no longer conscious, and life is maintained by life-support systems such as respirators. This pattern is associated with many of the following questions:

When should life-support system be discontinued?

Where should these persons be cared for?

Who should be responsible for their care?

In reality, many combinations of the four patterns may occur in one person's experience of living-dying. For example, a person's pattern may change from peaks and valleys to a downward slope, or from a downward slope to a gradual slant.

CHOICE: A RIGHT

All dying persons eventually learn of their fate. They should be free to choose what role, if any, they will play in the circumstances and manner in which they learn.

Dying persons describe a system of filtering out, or listening only to what they want to know or to realize. They tell us of how they listen to or look at the facts initially but do not hear or see them until later. People allow the facts to permeate their minds at their own pace. Dying people, or any person facing an extreme crisis, can describe reaching an emotional readiness when they suddenly hear or see the facts and wonder how long they have been there. Sometimes facts have to be introduced more than once by various people and in various ways. Sometimes patients look for confirmation of what they heard or what they saw; that is, of what they think they know.

The person who recognizes that death is imminent but is not allowed to talk about it is locked behind an impermeable wall of silence with no way to escape to the comfort of loving arms or to the closeness of a relationship with a loved one. No one should be condemned to such total isolation. No rationalization or self-protection exists to support such punishment of dying persons or their loved ones.

How does this happen? Fear is probably the greatest cause. Families and health care providers blunder into subterfuge and thus tragedy. No one anticipates all the additional lies that will be needed to support the first lie. No one anticipates the energy that will be spent futilely guarding the secret that all know.

There is tremendous hurt and anger when the truth is recognized. Would the person have chosen to live differently during the time that can never be returned? What happens to the confidence the person may have had in the nurses, physicians, and health system—the confidence that has been betrayed?

On the other hand, there are patients who sincerely choose not to see or to hear, who choose not to know. If that is their *informed* choice, then it is inappropriate to push them to know that which they do not want to see or hear. To force them to see or hear what they wish to deny is as cruel and inhumane as the conspiracy of silence. The refusal of the patient to know or to discuss the facts creates its own set of problems. The foremost problems, both with lying to patients and with refusal by patients to acknowledge or discuss the facts of dying, are the creation of barriers to comforting and supporting care and communication among interactors and the inability to share feelings and concerns on the basis of the reality of the situation.

ROLE OF CONFIDANT

Nurses can introduce the element of choice by fulfilling the patient's need for a confidant who will initiate and allow honest talk. The role of confidant is a necessary but difficult role. Talking of dying is not easy, and periods of awkwardness and expressions of fear are inevitable.

Dying persons look to the confidant for honesty and acceptance as they search for understanding of their state. They are not searching for pity, consolation, or sympathy. They are uncomfortable with the helplessness that they see in the eyes of others. The length of time that relationships exist with patients who have long-term chronic illnesses provides both the opportunity and the obligation for nurses to establish authentic relationships with dying patients, relationships in which nurses can be viewed as confidants.[52]

The confidant is one to whom patients can voice their deepest fears. They do not voice such fears to business associates; they cannot expect casual friends to understand. They do not reveal their most terrible anxieties to those they love; they protect loved ones from their panic. There are great risks in seeking information about that which they most dread, because what they most dread might be confirmed. There is also the superstition that lurks in their minds that what is said aloud might happen or come true; therefore, if they do not talk about it, it will not happen. The result may be fear and silence.

The role of the confidant is primarily to listen and to reassure as the dying person grapples with the experience of dying. The confidant can help to make the period of shifting from living to dying a time for a deepening feeling of closeness, a time for reinforcing family relationships, and a time to say what needs to be done and said.

Acting as a confidant does not mean that the relationship with the patient is a friendship. A true friendship is characterized by mutuality, with each party having equal rights and equal obligations to be sensitive and concerned for the needs and desires of the other. In contrast, in the nurse/patient relationship, the needs and desires of the patient are the primary concern and provide direction for interaction. Although not a friendship, an atmosphere of emotional closeness is a significant part of the relationship. Within this context, patients can develop and share their agendas for the future, for quality of life, and for what they truly want, without fear of protecting the nurse from difficult truths.[52]

Dying persons do not confide in every nurse, nor will the person they select as confidant necessarily be a nurse. Dying persons, just as any other persons, will be selective. Nurses are obligated to offer opportunities to be selected; to demand to serve in the role of confidant is not only inappropriate, but impossible. Nurses who may not be a confidant can support the chosen confidant and learn information that can be useful in guiding care.

DYING: AN ACHIEVEMENT OR A FAILURE

Although most dying people express resentment, fear, or sorrow over the major changes that are forced on their lives by their progressive debilitation, some view dying as an achievement.

Some persons, especially those with a prolonged course of living with dying, focus on living their dying so as to die well. They speak about their dying to selected people and at selected times. People who believe that dying well is an achievement are sometimes described by health professionals as denying or defying death. These people recognize their dying but choose therapy or choose to go home and participate in their customary activities. If you listen carefully to what they tell you, you will see that they intend to live their dying the way they wish, and thus from their own perspective they die well. These persons seem to do more than adjust or accommodate. They rise to an unseen challenge and in so doing expand their living rather than extend their dying.

A minority of persons may perceive dying as a personal failure or may attribute it to external forces. Some dwell on all they could have accomplished were it not for their illness. They usually exude a sense of powerlessness and futility and express overt anger. Others appear depressed, helpless, and resigned to their situation.

Remember that how people perceive their dying may change throughout the course of their dying. Attitudes, like physical capabilities, do not remain static. Dying encompasses the whole person; it is an emotional, behavioral, and physical process.

PERSPECTIVES OF FAMILY

Thus far we have focused on the dying person, but the impact of the knowledge that death is imminent extends beyond the dying person to their families, social groups, and the society in which they live.

COHESIVE OR DISRUPTIVE FORCE

The experience of dying may serve as a cohesive force in some families and a disruptive force in others. In general, families who have responded to stresses or crises as a unified force in the past will offer each other strength and support. For families who have strained relationships, the dying experience may promote further strain.

Family members generally express remorse over the fact that a family member had to come face-to-face with death before they realized how much they needed each other or cared for each other. But unless this recognition is coupled with assistance in learning how to make the relationship grow, it will not necessarily lead to greater social and emotional solidarity.[57]

FAMILY CONTROL

Dying persons, at times, use their dying to control the behaviors of family members. When dying persons use dying as a mean of control for self-gain or as a weapon, the result is anger, resentment, and perhaps retaliation by family members. Retaliation usually takes the form of not visiting, not phoning, or visiting for only short periods. It is an attempt to protect themselves from the tyranny of the dying person even while they wish to be close and loving.

The problem becomes more serious for the family members and dying person alike if the dying person is being cared for at home. The dying person usually recognizes the antagonism of family members but may interpret it as inappropriate, since, after all, he or she is dying. More frequently, the dying person may feel rejected and unloved and may not understand that the family loves the person but not the person's behavior.

Family members may recognize their own behavior as a response to the dying person's manipulation, but at the same time they feel guilty about their responses because the other person is dying and because they do care. The problem is best addressed openly and honestly, but it is usually difficult to resolve. It is difficult to deal with expressions of anger, resentment, and long-term depression under the best of circumstances. They are almost impossible to deal with when one person is dying. In either case, the focus must be on love for the dying person but displeasure with the offending behavior.

AN UNREASONABLE SITUATION

Although biomedical technologic advances continue to shift the locus of dying to the institution, the hospice movement is attempting to deinstitutionalize dying. The American Nurses' Association's *Standards and Scope of Hospice Nursing Practice*[4] provides an overview of hospice care in the United States and describes nursing as the cornerstone of hospice care. The standards provide a useful guide to those interested in understanding the special responsibilities of hospice nurses and the criteria for evaluating care.

With the increased emphasis on hospice care and the pressures by Medicare and other insurers to discharge patients as soon as aggressive treatment is discontinued, more and more persons are encouraged to die in the privacy of their own homes surrounded by family.

To have those we love die at home, cared for by family, may fulfill the romantic ideas we have surrounding dying; but it takes proper, careful, and advanced planning. Two major factors are usually considered: the economic situation and the dying person's wishes. Other important factors to be considered pertaining to environment and available caretakers are addressed in the box below. Unless all factors are discussed in advance, family members may be ill-prepared to deal with the most simple tasks. They may not know how to change an occupied bed. They may be concerned about how, what, or even whether to feed the dying person. Nurses choose to become nurses and have been educated to nurse. Family members are expected suddenly to assume nursing responsibilities that they may not desire or feel prepared to do, such as change dressings, irrigate wounds, and administer medications.

When families are asked to do more than they believe they can accomplish, especially when they do not have readily available assistance, they may feel trapped in an unreasonable situation. Feelings of entrapment lead to anger, frustration, depression, fear, and despair.

Family members who are prepared to care for dying persons in the home need planned times for their own social activities, as well as for grocery shopping and other necessities. Visitors and other family members, as well as the dying person, need help in actively supporting the caretaker.

Nurses can help caregivers by providing time off and giving them credit for what they are doing.

FACTORS TO CONSIDER IN HOME CARE OF THE DYING PERSON

Who will be the caretakers?

Who will relieve the caretakers?

How is the home arranged?

Are the doors large enough to accommodate wheelchairs?

Can rooms be arranged to accommodate commodes or other necessary equipment?

Would a hospital bed or other hospital equipment be helpful?

Are the people in the home prepared for the changes they must make in their own life-styles?

Was the decision made a family decision?

NURSING PERSPECTIVES

Although each person's experience of dying and grieving is unique and personal, there are similarities. Knowledge of the uniqueness of the perceived experience coupled with knowledge of some expected common responses assist nurses in assessing each situation, planning care, intervening, and evaluating both the plan of care and the interventions for dying people and their families and friends. Nurses who do not consider family members, as well as the dying person, as the focus of their care will not achieve the best possible quality of care for the dying person.

A REALISTIC PERSPECTIVE

To be of most assistance to dying persons and their families, nurses must be realistic about how much they can relieve suffering. Nurses cannot stop the dying or bring back the dead loved one. Nor can they take away the pain of loss. A realistic perspective helps make the experience better and facilitates appropriate grief. Nurses can *reach out* if they objectively accept the fact that pain and the often volatile responses to it are a natural part of the interaction.

ASSESSMENT: YOUR PERSPECTIVES

The role of the nurse is to help the dying person and family members to cope. Philosophic or religious tenets, (for example, "It's God's will," and "Everything happens for a reason") may assuage the nurse's feelings but are not helpful to others who need to ventilate their feelings and thoughts. A difficult situation is made less difficult by being honest and forthright, that is, by acknowledging that the situation is painful and does not make sense. It is not improved by rationalizing or trying to paint a rosy picture. It is good to plant seeds of hope regarding the meaning of life at a future time while acknowledging the despair of the present. Sometimes it helps to show emotion, to allow others to cry, or to ask the dying person or family members privately and as a group to talk about what is or will happen. By listening, the nurse can then help them separate fact from fiction. It may be a helpful way to begin assessment.

NURSING PRACTICE CONSIDERATION

■ ASSESSMENT

Nursing assessment is an ongoing process throughout the term of the dying person-family-nurse relationship. It will continue and become the family-nurse relationship at the death of the patient. A thorough initial assessment with direct input from the dying person and significant others provides the basis for relationships. Assessment parameters are listed in the box on p. 255.

■ DATA ANALYSIS: NURSING DIAGNOSES

As one reviews the various nursing assessment parameters in caring for dying people and their significant others, it becomes clear that analyses of the data may lead to identification of nearly all the NANDA[64] nursing diagnoses over the course of the dying process. The complex physiologic, psychological, social, and spiritual dynamics accompanying dying help explain the presence of the multiple primary and secondary nursing diagnoses. Perhaps the greatest challenge to nurses is prioritizing—which nursing diagnoses should be addressed and in which order?

Among the most important diagnoses to address are those related to symptom management and anticipatory grief. The physical symptoms accompanying the dying process are dependent on the particular pathophysiology of the disease responsible for the life-threatening state and the interface with other preexisting emotional and physical health problems. Assessing and understanding the cause of the symptoms is central to determining appropriate interventions. Following is a brief outline of some of the most common nursing diagnoses associated with care of dying persons as they relate to major symptoms/problems. A more complete discussion of the topic can be found in Amenta and Bohnet.[1]

Diagnostic Title	Possible Etiologies
Anorexia problems	
Nutrition, altered: less than body requirement	Nausea and vomiting secondary to chemotherapy, medication interactions, obstructions in the gastrointestinal tract, anxiety; altered taste secondary to dysphagia, weakness; depression
Body movement problems	
Activity intolerance	Depression, shortness of breath
Injury, potential for	Secondary to metastases to bone, confusion, seizures
Mobility, impaired physical	Weakness, contractures, pain, infection, semicomatose/comatose state, paralysis
Bowel elimination problems	
Constipation	Medication reaction, poor fluid-dietary intake, immobility
Diarrhea	Impaction, disease process
Incontinence, bowel	Secondary to weakened state; semicomatose/comatose state
Fluid balance problems	
Fluid volume deficit	Low fluid intake secondary to weakness, fever, reduced extracellular fluid volume, dysphagia, gastrointestinal fluid losses, oliguria, polyuria
Fluid volume excess	Altered cardiac output; effects of medication

NURSING ASSESSMENT

INPUT FROM DYING PERSON AND SIGNIFICANT OTHERS
General Perception of Each Individual

Awareness of clinical diagnosis and prognosis
Philosophy of living while dying and views regarding
  dying
Perceptions of self and effect on self of the dying process
Expected physiologic and behavioral changes
Past experiences with major illnesses or crises
Shared experiences with major illnesses or crises

Perceived Strengths, Desires, and Hopes

Personal abilities and coping techniques
Personal support systems
Availability of resources
Beliefs; religious convictions; cultural views of dying,
  death, and bereavement
Past experiences with death
Expectations about care and dying, use of life supports
  (present and future)

INPUT FROM NURSE

Beliefs, values, attitudes, responses
Support systems: personal and professional
Expertise, including incorporating others in care

Diagnostic Title	Possible Etiologies
Mouth symptoms	
Oral mucous membrane, altered	Disease secondary to impaired immune system, decreased protein intake; effects of treatment such as chemotherapy, radiation, and continuous oxygen
Pain	Stomatitis secondary to dehydration, continuous mouth breathing and local trauma
Respiratory/ventilation symptoms	
Airway clearance, ineffective	Inability to eliminate secretions
Breathing pattern, ineffective	Dysphagia, pain, rales/rhonchi, obstruction, semicomatose/comatose state
Gas exchange, impaired	Shortness of breath
Tissue perfusion, altered	Respiratory distress syndrome
Skin problems	
Skin integrity, impaired	Edema; immobility; urinary incontinence; sweating; cachexia; fungating tumors;
	Complications of treatment, reaction to medications
	Poor tissue perfusion secondary to infrequent turning/repositioning; circulatory impairment

Diagnostic Title	Possible Etiologies
Sleep & rest problems	
Sleep pattern disturbance	Fear of dying; uncertainty about the future; pain; shortness of breath; metabolic effects of disease; drug interactions/untoward drug reactions; night sweats; restlessness; depression
Temperature problems	
Body temperature, altered	Medication reaction, decreased fluid intake, altered metabolic rate, sedation
Urinary problems	
Urinary elimination, altered patterns	Reaction to medications, obstruction of the urinary tract, reduced fluid intake, nausea, urinary tract infection

In addition to the nursing diagnoses associated with physical symptoms, other nursing diagnoses associated with dying persons relate to psychosocial and spiritual dimensions. The following are examples that may be evident:

Diagnostic Title	Possible Etiologies
Coping, ineffective family: disabling	Conflicting perceptions among members; maladaptive coping styles
Coping, ineffective individual	Pain, effects of medication, lack of family or social support
Diversional activity deficit	Total focus on pain, effects of medication
Family process, altered	Patient's or other family member's inability to fulfill accustomed roles secondary to pain and disability
Grieving, anticipatory	Association of existence of pain and dysfunction with imminent death
Knowledge deficit	Patient and family lack of awareness of availability of modern methods of palliation
Powerlessness	Dependence on others for care secondary to pain and effects of medication
Social isolation	Inability of patient to focus away from symptoms, discomfort of others when confronted with patient's symptoms and dying
Spiritual distress	Association of symptoms with punishment, imminence of death, and sense of abandonment by God

---

TIMING PLANNED NURSING INTERVENTIONS

Times for physical care
Social interaction times
Times for privacy for family members and patient
Quiet times alone for reflection, grieving, or rest
Times for reassessment
Times for group planning and evaluation

■ **PLANNING**

As with assessment, planning is a joint venture. Successful planning incorporates the goals of the family and the dying person as well as goals of nurses and other health care providers.

The expertise of the nurse is of special importance in anticipating the dying person's various needs as his or her physical state declines. This expertise is needed to identify the neighbors, church groups, and family members who may serve as support persons and to help them to know when and how they may be of assistance to the dying person and to each other. These persons can participate with the nurses in planning the timing of nursing interventions (see the box above) and identifying alternative interventions.

Nurses need to plan for their own health maintenance (see the box below). This planning is done in relation to each individual situation involving a dying person or the significant others of dying persons.

The care of dying persons and their families is best accomplished by a team of caregivers. Planning care, therefore, must include obtaining input from and relying on and listening to others in the situation, if comprehensive care is to be achieved.

■ **IMPLEMENTATION**

The nursing needs of dying individuals are the nursing needs of living individuals. The range of activities are as broad as for any diverse population of patients, family, and significant others. Nursing intervention may occur in a variety of settings, either at home or in various institutional settings.

Direct physical care is a major part of caring for dying persons. Maintenance of comfort, both physical and emotional, is of the essence. Teaching others involved in direct care how to maintain the patient's comfort al-

---

PLANS FOR NURSE'S HEALTH MAINTENANCE

Time commitments
Support from other professionals or own significant others
Considerations of actual or potential value conflicts and
    means of dealing with conflicts

---

lows their participation and promotes their feelings of competence and well-being.

Health teaching may include teaching such measures as breathing exercises, relaxation techniques, and coping strategies to the dying person and to significant others for use throughout their grieving process. Teaching how dying persons may use medication for comfort and at the same time dispelling expressed fears of patient addiction may help the dying person and family alike. One should recognize and respect cultural differences and fears about addiction. Addiction in dying persons is improbable and in the last days of living, inconsequential.

Another nursing responsibility is to be well-informed about organized support systems, agencies, and independent resources within the community and to be prepared to assist patients and their families in contacting and using these resources. Inquiries related to the many alternative modes of care for dying persons such as hospice and other forms of home care, nursing home care, and other forms of institutional care, should be answered openly and honestly. If the nurse cannot answer the patient's or family's questions, they should be referred to those who can supply the answers.

Nursing intervention may include participation in resuscitative efforts and the maintenance of dying patients on life-support systems. Along with direct patient care in these circumstances, nurses are responsible for communicating with and supporting family members or for assuring that someone is providing this service.

In essence, nurses assist patients and families in maintaining control over their individual lives as much as is possible to ensure dignity and self-esteem. This control is accomplished through the actions discussed above.

If nurses are to care effectively for patients and families, they need to maintain their own well-being. Planned confidential sessions to discuss thoughts and feelings about a particular situation may be helpful. Recognition that others (other health professionals, volunteers, and family members) have much to contribute and are as committed and concerned about the patient's welfare is of importance. There is a tendency for each person to believe he or she is alone in the situation.

Withdrawal from a situation may be necessary in some rare situations, but it should occur only when other nursing personnel are available to maintain the care of the patient and significant others.

EVALUATION

Each nurse is responsible for evaluating his or her own practice as it relates to each situation. Comfort and satisfaction of the patient may be used as criteria. Nursing intervention may be evaluated through a preestablished evaluation system. Use of these systems contributes to the development and feelings of well-being of nurses by affording support in the decision process.

1. Evaluation methods in the care of dying persons
   a. Care of patient and significant others
   b. Observation of responses to interventions
   c. Discussion of goals and how they have been achieved
   d. Discussion of alternative methods to achieve goals more effectively
   e. Mutual evaluation of continued appropriateness of goals
   f. Mutual identification of new or revised goals and means to achieve these goals
2. Preestablished nursing evaluation systems
   a. Formal and informal peer review of goals and interventions
   b. Open discussion of problems
   c. Venting of feelings
   d. Sharing of positive responses
   e. Special criteria developed by groups of nurses involved in caring for dying persons

A nurse will experience loss when a nurse-patient relationship concludes with the death of the patient. Evaluation of his or her contribution to the relationship gains importance, especially for each nurse's well-being. Recognition of specific successful interventions and contributions leads to feelings of achievement and success. Lack of this recognition may lead to perceiving consecutive losses as a sign of failure.

Peer support is most beneficial to nurses caring for dying persons. Peer support may be accomplished through formal and informal groups. In addition to groups, one-to-one interactions with a trusted peer or personal significant other may alleviate some of the stress related to working with dying persons. More important, such relationships serve as an appropriate avenue for recognizing and reinforcing the inherent rewards of providing nursing care for people who are living their dying and for those who are sharing the experience.

FUNERALS AND AFTER-DEATH RITUALS

All societies have funeral practices associated with care and disposal of the body and with the expected behavior of the bereaved. Although there have been scathing attacks on the funeral industry,[58] funerals and after-death rituals serve many positive functions for the bereaved.[71] They include the following:

1. Focus on the bereaved by a gathering of friends and family offers sympathy, a recognition of the loss, communication of caring; in short, social support. Wakes, viewings, and visitations are forms of gatherings for family and friends. Nurses and other health professionals accomplish similar

tasks by reviewing together what occurred and sharing past experiences about the person who died or others who died.
2. Use of ritual, which is often religious in nature, offers some reason or lends some meaning to death.
3. Visual display of the dead body assists survivors with reaching closure or accepting the finality of death.
4. There is opportunity to display grief publically in a procession ending at the place of final disposition.
5. Burial, entombment, cremation, or some kind of sanitary disposition of the body reinforces the perservance of life on earth and for some provides a place to return for prayer or reminiscence.
6. Material expenditure for funerals is one way to communicate "the loss of the bereaved to society."

All major changes in life have rituals to help individuals and society adapt to the changed state and cope with the disequilibrium that occurs during the transition from one state to another (for example, birth, marriage, and death). Funerals serve as a rite of passage[95] from life to death. They function to validate the life of the deceased[78] and act as a testimony that a life has been lived.

During the funeral the bereaved begins the process of emancipation from the bondage of the deceased, readjustment to an environment in which the deceased is missing, and incorporation to a new state. The bereaved publically appears without the living loved one, to be reincorporated into their previous social group in a changed state. The deceased is removed from the social group and admitted to the land of the dead by internment, entombment, or cremation. The relationships are publicly declared changed.

During the funeral, society bestows rank on the deceased for the last time. The specifics of the ritual (for example, 21-gun salute), the number of mourners, and the impact of the death on society all reflect the value of the deceased individual.

Funerals meet the needs of mourners and society. They are for the living, not the dead. They offer spiritual, psychologic, and social benefits to the survivors and therefore are important.

PERSPECTIVES OF SURVIVORS

People experience many losses throughout their lifetimes; the longer a person lives, the more losses they will experience. Not all losses are attributable to deaths, but the most disruptive losses are associated with the deaths of loved ones, because of the many life changes imposed on the survivors. The most profound loss is the death of a spouse or of a child because of the closeness and intertwining nature of the relationship.

GRIEF, BEREAVEMENT, AND MOURNING

Grief and bereavement are frequent companions of adulthood. Loss occurs with increasing frequency as people age. Loss is so common among the elderly that Butler and Lewis[12] suggest that grief caused by loss is a predominant factor in aging. *Bereavement* is the response to loss caused by *death*. It is a subjective state that occurs as a result of having suffered the loss of a person with whom there had been a significant loving relationship. *Grief,* or perhaps more accurately stated, the *process of grieving* is the *total response* (thoughts, feelings, and behaviors) to the emotional suffering caused by loss.[54] Grieving has somatic as well as psychologic dimensions. *Mourning* is behavior that is shaped by cultural values, norms, and mores.

GRIEF: HISTORICAL PERSPECTIVE

As early as 1915, Freud described grief as a process of gradual withdrawal of the energy that ties the bereaved person to the lost object (person who died). Eliot[26,27] and Falconer[28] did empirical studies on grief in the 1930s and 1940s. More recent authors[41,54,79] who have described general patterns of the grieving process suggest an uncomplicated grief syndrome that has a more or less predictable course and distinctive symptoms. In general, the symptoms include a period of shock and somatic distress, feelings of hostility, guilt, and abandonment, interruption of life's usual activities, preoccupation with thoughts of the deceased, and finally a recovery period, or a working through to a state of healthy integration. Although Lindemann[49] suggested that people could recover from grief as quickly as within a few weeks, more recent research findings suggest that bereavement is more appropriately measured in years rather than weeks or months.

RESPONSES BY SURVIVORS

Although it is possible to describe clusters and phases of grief on the basis of how groups of people have responded to the loss of loved ones, manifestations of grieving are likely to vary greatly among and between individuals.[92] As in caring for the dying, understanding the process of grieving and recognizing the behavioral manifestations that usually occur can assist nurses to prepare survivors for what they can expect or to help them understand their feelings or somatic symptoms. Timing of the sharing of information, as well as the type and amount of information given at any one session, are important. Understanding the various processes and behaviors, both anticipated and unexpected, of bereaved persons may help to avert misunderstandings, strengthen the survivors, and help them to grow during the period of grieving. Grieving persons are helped by sharing their experiences. Recognizing the "normal" nature of their experiences, even those that seem somewhat bizarre, opens the way for sharing.

SHOCK AND DISBELIEF

The initial response begins at the time of death and usually lasts for several weeks beyond the funeral.[34] Regardless of whether the death was anticipated or not, the immediate response is shock, numbness, and disbelief. The survivors may feel a sense of unreality, and as a consequence, they may appear to be "taking the death well." After the funeral this feeling of unreality or numbness changes to feelings of pain and separation. Survivors may experience some somatic symptoms including muscular weakness, tremors, and tightness of the throat. They may become diaphoretic, sigh deeply, have cold or clammy sensations, become anorexic, or feel exhausted. Bereaved persons exhibit extremes of behavior. They may become sedentary; they do little or nothing except nap. On the other hand, they may be so hyperactive that they are unable to sit quietly or to sleep. They may experience extremes of mood such as profound sadness, anger, depression, or guilt or find themselves laughing without an explanation. They may have difficulty in concentrating. Coupled with these extremes in mood and behavior may be a continuance of disbelief, although the death is comprehended intellectually. "Searching behaviors" are common. These include dreams in which the deceased is alive and experiences of "seeing" the deceased or "feeling" the deceased's touch. During this phase offers of comfort are often rejected because the bereaved is focusing on the deceased.

YEARNING AND PROTEST

For several weeks the bereaved have feelings of yearning and protest. They may feel anger toward the deceased for leaving them, toward God for allowing the death to occur, toward the caregivers for not returning the deceased to health. They may be jealous of others who still have their loved ones. They may wish they had been the one to die. During this period they may find it difficult to share their feelings or thoughts with others because they question their own sanity. Knowing that others have had similar thoughts and feelings sometimes is beneficial.

ANGUISH, DISORGANIZATION, AND DESPAIR

As the bereaved begin to focus more on themselves and as the numbness and rage begin to fade, the reality and permanence of the loss begins to be recognized. New feelings and accompanying behaviors emerge. The bereaved may experience a sense of confusion, aimlessness, an inability to make decisions, a loss of motivation or interest, and a loss of confidence. During this period, they feel lonely and depressed and experience a general loss of meaning to their lives.

All those experiences that they formerly shared with the deceased now seem irrelevant. They experience extremes of mood. The intensity of their feelings often is frightening to them. Memory lapses and difficulty in concentrating, although common and temporary, increase their feelings of anguish. They fear they will lose emotional control and as a defense become centered on themselves. Family members and friends may interpret this behavior as selfish and either reprimand them or withdraw. Neither behavior is helpful to the bereaved.

The experience of anguish leads to a new awareness of the preciousness of life. Life appears fragile. The bereaved may display intense fears of their being hurt or worry over the welfare of family members. At the same time they may smoke or excessively use chemicals such as drugs or alcohol. Other health-risking behaviors, such as lack of rest, may be usual.

The wish and need to cry fulfills an important function in acknowledging the loss and in receiving support from others. Memories and mental images of the deceased are void of negative characteristics. Feelings of guilt, remorse, fear, and regret may surface. Opportunities to reminisce and to share feelings with others are helpful.

IDENTIFICATION

The bereaved may adopt the behavior, admired qualities, and mannerisms of their lost beloved ones. Some may take on the symptoms of the last illness of the lost loved one. Care must be taken to distinguish symptoms associated with physical illness from those associated with loss. Symptoms associated with loss will abate as the loss is resolved.

REORGANIZATION AND RESTITUTION

The feelings and symptoms of grieving gradually subside; they do not suddenly disappear. Bereaved persons tell us they have periods of depression, as well as periods of well-being, as life begins to make sense once again. Reorganization and restitution generally begin approximately 6 months after the loss and last for a few years. The process may be considerably longer or shorter and still be within normal range. Contrary to old popular beliefs, although life stabilizes, the pain of loss may remain for a lifetime. Reactions to loss recur around circumstances that are poignant reminders of the deceased—birthdays, anniversaries, and holidays.

FACTORS AFFECTING THE SURVIVOR'S RESPONSE

Many factors combine to affect the degree of stress and the particular response of survivors to a death. The major factors include (1) the type of relationship lost, (2) the nature of the death, (3) the characteristics of the survivor, (4) the social and cultural milieu, and (5) the nature of the support network.

TYPE OF RELATIONSHIP

The loss of someone—spouse, parent—upon whom one has been dependent leaves an expected void and feelings of helplessness. Not as expected is the intense void that accompanies the loss of the survivor's role as a caring wife, husband, or daughter when the loved one dies.

The greater the reliance on the lost person for validation of self, identity, role, meaningful activities, and links to social and friendships networks, the greater the impact on life-style and the more profound the feelings of loss. Generally, therefore, the loss of a spouse is the most emotionally devastating.[18]

THE BEREAVED AND DECEASED

Identities and roles are related. A survivor—widow, widower, daughter, son—is left with incomplete skills because the usual division of labor in everyday life is lost. Loss of children creates its own special problems. The normal course of life events is disrupted when the young die before the old. Feelings of guilt and self blame may be more pronounced.[91]

NATURE OF THE DEATH

The nature of the death and the circumstances following a death affect the grieving process. The closer the circumstances are to what the survivors would perceive as a "good" death, the more comforting it will be. Anticipatory grieving or grieving that began prior to a loss may ease the transition once a loss is complete. However, too much anticipation and repeated cycles of anticipatory grief may deplete a survivor's energy to complete the grieving process when the death finally occurs.

PERSONAL CHARACTERISTICS AND RISK FACTORS

Individual characteristics of survivors such as age, personality attributes, physical and mental health, and the number and nature of grief and crises experienced have impact on grief responses. Various factors associated with high risk in widowers and widows have been identified[54] from the literature:

1. Loss of socioeconomic status
2. Poor health before the loss
3. Sudden death or short illness
4. Perceived lack of social support
5. Perceived lack of supportive family
6. Family who discourage expression of grief
7. Extreme clinging to the deceased before death
8. Preoccupation with the image of the deceased
9. Strong reactions of anger, distress, or self-reproach
10. History of psychiatric illness or suicidal ideation

NURSING STRATEGIES FOR THE BEREAVED

Jackson[42] states that the role of the caregiver is to assist the griever in releasing emotional ties to the deceased despite the discomfort and sorrow it causes and in subsequently replacing the type of interaction lost. The griever must be persuaded to participate in grief work that entails *accepting the pain of looking realistically and actively at the loss.* There are a number of strategies that assist grievers. Rando[78] groups these in broad phases that roughly correspond to the process of grief from shock to reintegration. These activities are useful to health professionals *in helping others* to help the bereaved. Some are neither feasible nor appropriate for health professionals to perform themselves.

■ ASSESSMENT

Planning interventions for helping grieving persons help themselves must be preceded by accurate assessment of where persons are in their grief, as well as what factors are influencing their grief. The preceding sections, responses by survivors, and factors affecting the survivors' responses, provide a framework for gathering subjective and objective data associated with grief. Intervening without understanding the grieving situation and the factors influencing it can introduce more harm than good. Raphael[79] suggests the following assessments of the bereaved that yield information but also facilitate the expression of emotion and promote the grieving process:

1. Tell me a little about the death? What happened?
   These questions give the griever permission to talk about the death while providing information about the nature and circumstances of the death. At the same time the griever's feelings, ability to talk about the death, stresses related to it, and whether the griever had the opportunity to say good-byes can be evaluated.

2. Tell me about (name the deceased) and about your lives together or relationship together from the beginning.
   This opening allows the caregiver to evaluate the relationship, its quality, and the interactions associated with it. It also provides the opportunity to evaluate a griever's degree of denial of the loss and the degree to which he or she speaks of the loss in realistic terms. In addition, risk factors can be assessed.

3. What has been happening since the death? How have things been with your family and friends?
   This question provides the opportunity to explore patterns of family and social support that the bereaved perceive to be available. It also provides the opportunity to assess other crises that may affect the grieving process.

4. Have you been through any other bad times recently or when you were younger?
   This offers the opportunity to explore past experiences and concurrent crisis. It also opens the way to help the bereaved identify past successful ways of coping and new ways of coping.

Any assessment needs to be continually updated and revised. Fluctuations in the experiences of the bereaved are to be expected. Interventions that are appropriate for one person are not useful or may even be harmful to another person. Reassessment may address such major topics as:

1. Acceptance of the reality of the loss
2. Evaluation for need of medical attention and treatment
3. Identification of unresolved grief
4. Detection of illogical thoughts

People, especially under stress, attempt to impute cause. They may believe their actions in some way contributed to the death; for example, they didn't get to the hospital soon enough, or they didn't prepare a diet properly. Such beliefs can lead to unresolved feelings of guilt.

Instruments have been developed to identify individuals at risk for difficulty in the grieving process or to identify the problems of individuals who experienced prolonged bereavement-related distress with widowhood. The Grief Resolution Index, a screening instrument developed by Remondet and Hansson[81] includes four measures of short-term adjustment (survival expectation, fear, preparation, and desperation indexes) and four measures of long-term adjustment (depression inventory, anxiety, adjustment of widowhood, and health indexes).

■ DATA ANALYSIS: NURSING DIAGNOSES

Human responses to the loss of a loved one are varied. While other nursing diagnoses may be present, the most commonly recognized one among individuals who experience loss is *grieving*. To date, NANDA[64] has not approved the nursing diagnostic category of grieving. This may be because grieving is a normal healthy process, whereas nursing diagnostic categories usually focus on dysfunctional behaviors. For purposes of this chapter, grieving is an appropriate diagnostic category for those seeking to promote wellness and to facilitate healing associated with significant loss. At the same time, normal grieving may be associated with dysfunctional or distorted behaviors[1] that can be recognized in a variety of secondary diagnoses as illustrated in the following list:

Primary Diagnostic Title	Possible Etiologies
Grieving	Loss of loved one
Secondary Diagnostic Title	
Alteration in thought processes	Grief, anxiety, insomnia; guilt; loneliness; substance abuse; hallucinations
Anxiety	Loneliness, social isolation; self-reproach; fear of the unknown; financial insecurity; fear of own death

Secondary Diagnostic Title	Possible Etiologies
Coping, ineffective individual	Depression in response to loss
Hopelessness	Separation from significant other; inability to achieve goals in life associated with loss; loss of belief in God's care
Nutrition, altered	Anxiety; grief; loss of meal time companion; inertia due to fatigue; feeling of tightness in throat
Self-care deficit	Depression; anxiety; fatigue; social isolation
Self-esteem, disturbance	Hallucinations of the deceased; anger; anxiety; preoccupation with the deceased; social isolation; substance abuse; fear of loss of control
Sleep pattern disturbance	Anxiety; hyperactivity; agitation; fear of nightmares; substance abuse
Social isolation	Withdrawal; uncontrolled anger; knowledge deficit regarding support resources; housebound state (unemployed; young children); rejection by significant others
Spiritual distress	Inability to understand meaning of loss; anger at God; anxiety; depression

Grieving is the ultimate price of loving, of attachment, of a meaningful relationship.[54,86] In some instances the person is unable to mourn in a manner that allows for resolution of the grief and reinvestment in life, and this may result in dysfunctional grief.

NANDA has approved two independent nursing diagnostic categories in relationship to grieving: (1) anticipatory grieving and (2) dysfunctional grieving.[20] *Anticipatory grieving* is defined as "a condition in which the individual grieves before an actual loss,"[20] and *dysfunctional grieving* is defined as "a condition in which the individual experiences delayed or exaggerated response to a perceived, actual, or potential loss."[20]

Diagnostic Title	Possible Etiologies
Grieving, anticipatory	Perceived loss of: a significant other; physiopsychosocial well-being; personal possesions
Grieving, dysfunctional	Actual or perceived object loss; thwarted grieving response to loss; absence of anticipatory grieving; chronic fatal illness; loss of others; loss of physiopsychosocial well-being; prolonged denial; intense pining and yearning; ambivalent relationship with the deceased; severe self-reproach; multiple crises; lack of support from family

For some, the grieving process is extended or excessively intense, making reorganization and restitution improbable or impossible.[68] The bereaved in this situation has been described as "dying of a broken heart." The anger, guilt, depression, and self-blame are more intense and time offers no relief. Carpentino[14] defined the nursing diagnosis of unresolved grief as a "pathological response of prolonged denial of the loss or a profound psychotic response." Since the range of normality differs in each case of grief, it is difficult to describe dysfunctional grief. Much research remains to be done to clarify the expected duration of uncomplicated grief, the phenomenology of unresolved grief, and valid and reliable methods of assessing grief.

■ PLANNING: EXPECTED PATIENT OUTCOMES

The expected outcomes associated with grief and the work that is entailed in the grieving process has been described by Nichols and Nichols[62]: to remember the loved one without emotional pain and to reinvest emotional energy in life so that the capacity to love is not lost. Cantor[13] speaks of the same outcome as "enriched remembrance" that may not preclude sadness. To achieve these outcomes, six "tasks" of grief work must be satisfied.[41] The individual:

1. Faces the pain.
2. Permits the emotional expression of the full range of feeling.
3. Achieves emancipation from bondage.
4. Adjusts to an altered environment.
5. Renews or forms new relationships.
6. Is able to live with memories.

■ IMPLEMENTATION

Understanding the grieving process as a normal part of loving provides the basis for nursing assessments and interventions. Nursing actions in response to the bereaved call for a delicate blending of being present, listening, expressing honest feelings, and inviting the bereaved to share their experiences and emotions.

Some interventions are appropriately directed at supporting the caregivers and alleviating their stress while caring for the needs of dying relatives, which in turn enhances or promotes the caregiver's health following the death.[63] The National Hospice Study bereavement interview data revealed that health problems in the bereaved before the loved one's death was the key determinent of health care use and morbidity after the death.[59] In addition to assessing health of the caregiver before the death, nurses can learn about other existing resources available to the caregiver and reinforce them before and following the death. These resources include interpersonal support (provision of information, material goods and services, emotional support), religious-spiritual beliefs, and intrapersonal coping (cognitive and behavioral strategies).[82]

After the death, the following nursing interventions may be appropriate:

1. Make contact and assess.
   a. Establish a relationship; simply be present.
   b. Assess the bereaved in her or his grief to plan appropriate future interventions.
2. Reach out.
   a. Take the initiative; reach out in a concrete way. Don't say "call me if you need me." Do be specific in how you can assist or get others to assist. For example: "How about if I call your sister to accompany you to select the casket?" "Suppose I arrange for you to attend a widow-to-widow meeting?"
   b. Do not take refusals personally or give up.
   c. Repeat offers of assistance. Grievers initially may be unable to respond to and appreciate offers of help but will benefit over time.
3. Be physically and emotionally present to offer security and support.
   a. Do use physical contact, hugging, touching, hand-holding. These actions are important early in the process to convey that the griever is not alone. There may be exceptions. Some people do not like to be touched. You can sit nearby if that is more comforting.
   b. Social supports generally are decreased weeks or months after a death, when the bereaved is forced to resume life without the loved one. Encourage family members to be present after all the intensity of the funeral has subsided.
   c. Encourage regular expression of feelings to help minimize the tendency to become overwhelmed and unable to function.
   d. Encourage others to take charge of routine functions and responsibilities of the bereaved; for example, run errands, prepare meals.
   e. Provide for security through direction concerning meals, rest, priorities of activities for the day or week.
   f. Help family members focus on one problem at a time.
   g. Address problems to which practical solutions can be found before addressing more complicated problems.
4. Give people "permission" to grieve.
   a. Display nonjudgmental attitudes and behaviors. Be neutral.
   b. Communicate compassionate support through verbal and nonverbal behavior, for example, when the griever's voice cracks, facial muscles quiver, eyes water, and the bereaved turns to the caregiver, lean forward, relax, do not turn away, allow the griever to cry. Display your comfort and approval through your body language. Your actions will speak louder than your verbalizations.
5. Do not allow grievers to remain isolated.
   a. Be present and have others present.
   b. Suggest self-help groups and assist grievers to attend.
6. Maintain a family perspective.
   a. Remember that the family is changed.
   b. Help the bereaved reassess.

When unresolved grief is evident, psychiatric intervention may be required. Volkan[98] and Parkes[67] identified the following characteristics that require psychiatric care:

1. An extreme depressive reaction manifested by persistent sadness with no shifts to a normal state; an unresponsiveness to warmth; extreme expressions of guilt and of identification symptoms
2. Psychotic break with reality (neurotic anxiety; obsessions; phobic, hysteric, or schizophrenic reactions; acting and speaking as though the deceased was still present)
3. Suicidal tendencies (self-punitive acts, often to expiate guilt)
4. Excessive drinking, drug abuse, or promiscuity (as substitutes for the deceased)

Although the discussion in this section focused primarily on the survivors, all involved are experiencing loss. The dying person, perhaps, is facing the greatest loss of all. All people involved are grieving. The principles apply to all from different perspectives. Nursing care of dying persons includes multiple clients and multiple processes.

Dying persons and their families and friends may or may not experience the grieving process in the same way. Dying people may grieve over the loss of physical function, the loss of past abilities, the ultimate loss of life, and separation from all they know and love. At the same time, significant others may grieve over the potential loss of the loved one, the hurt they feel, and the emptiness they anticipate.

ETHICAL PERSPECTIVES

To help a person die well is to support that person's sense of self-respect, dignity, and choice until the last moment of life. Achivement of this goal entails skilled and compassionate nursing care to maximize comfort and minimize suffering. The goal is to provide calm, sensitive, individualized nursing care to each person so that dying, the final human experience, is as free from pain and anxiety as possible.[3]

Historically, the profession and activities of nursing have been concerned with life and based on two fundamental principles. These principles were that all people should (1) live as whole persons and (2) should live long and healthful lives. The expectation has been that nurses and physicians would help to fulfill these principles.[8]

In the past, nurses and physicians fulfilled their obligations by striving to save lives. There were no miracle drugs, life-sustaining machines, transplant surgeries, or radiation therapies. Intensive and continuous nursing care was the main hope of saving lives. Modalities such as heat, cold, food, fluid, rest, exercise, and maintenance of a sanitary environment were used. Physicians and nurses relied on the natural healing powers of the body. If a body failed to heal despite the efforts of nurses and physicians, the patient died. The power of medicine and nursing simply was no match for the diseases that people experienced. Death often was caused by infection and communicable disease. Many people died at young ages.

With the advent of miracle drugs and advances in anesthesia, surgical techniques, and life-sustaining technologies, persons who would have succumbed to life-threatening illnesses now seek treatment to restore health and function. The capacity to prolong life and to ease the pain and suffering of seriously ill persons has improved to a great extent. The improvement has been accompanied by some difficult consequences. Increasingly, deaths occur in institutions. In many instances, deaths occur in critical care units to the sound of monitors. More and more often death is caused by someone's decision rather than the failure of the heart to pump blood or the lungs to breathe.

Death becomes impersonal when the body and the tubes and machines become one and when there is only a deteriorating organ system present. The situation becomes so confusing that those involved have conferences to determine whether life or death is being prolonged.

When a dying person has been termed a nonperson and seems neither dead nor alive, all involved persons search for resolution of a situation where neither grief nor hope is appropriate. Family members long to return to normal living. They search for help in making life and death decisions for loved ones who are no longer able to contribute to decision making. Staff members search for relief from a situation fraught with dilemmas.

The dying person does not have to be completely incoherent or comatose for ethical issues to arise. Many ethical issues are inherent in the situation. For example, modern technology has made possible successful treatment of diseases that formerly resulted in fairly immediate death. Now cures from diseases such as cancer are possible. In many instances there are no cures, but there are temporary reprieves; for example, the mechanical ventilator can prolong life. In situations when there is great ambiguity regarding the result of therapy, when that therapy is associated with great discomfort to

the patient or the family, such as with bone marrow transplants, or when there is great expense and limited supply, such as in the case of the artificial heart, conflict arises over the course of care a person should receive and who should be involved in making decisions about that care.

Discussions of such issues as "quality of life," "right to die," "death with dignity," "living wills," and "informed consent" in lay as well as professional literature demonstrate the extent and awareness of the conflicts associated with modern therapies that extend life but at great cost. Concern over decisions regarding life and death issues has led to the development of organizations that represent differing views. The Hemlock Society,*[38] the Society for the Right to Die,[90] and the Americans United for Life are examples of a few of these organizations.

The question of who should decide under what circumstances is important. There are other important questions. What is death? What constitutes informed consent? When are therapies ordinary and when are they extraordinary? Should all life be preserved, regardless of quality? Should pain be treated, even though the medication may decrease the life span? What constitutes euthanasia? Is there a distinction between active and passive euthanasia? Is suicide a person's right? All these questions create ethical dilemmas.[21,23]

WHAT IS AN ETHICAL DILEMMA?

The questions posed above create ethical dilemmas because they generate emotions and because there are no clear-cut right answers to govern action. The reasons supporting each side of the argument for action are logical and appropriate. Each reason cited is a good reason in and of itself, but one reason may conflict with another when they are looked at as a whole. In addition, all reasons have equal merit. Further, the actions associated with any response are desirable in some respects and undesirable in others. In other words, *ethical dilemmas arise when on the basis of moral considerations an appeal can be made for taking each of two opposing courses of action.*[9]

The box on p. 264 represents the situation leading to an ethical dilemma. Of importance is the fact that *the actor must perceive the possibility of two responses;* otherwise there will be no dilemma, at least for that actor. For example, intentionally terminating a life-support system creates a dilemma for an individual who perceives the action as right in terms of death with dignity and wrong in terms of preservation of life. In most circumstances *taking no action is an action.* In this example, making no deliberate decision and therefore not terminating life support is an action. It is right in terms

---

*Hemlock Society, P.O. Box 66218, Los Angeles, CA, 90016.

SITUATION OF AN ETHICAL DILEMMA

1. Some evidence indicates that act x is morally right and some evidence indicates that act x is morally wrong.
2. Evidence on both sides is inconclusive.
3. The actor perceives that he or she ought and ought not perform the act.
4. Some action must be taken.
5. No action is an action.

LEVELS OF MORAL JUSTIFICATION[23]

Judgment = Decision
Rules = Fundamental Guides
Principles = More General Fundamental Guides
Theories = Foundation of Rules and Principles

of preservation of life but wrong in terms of death with dignity.

Intentionally terminating life-support systems does not create a dilemma for the individual who perceives the action only in terms of death with dignity. Terminating the life-support system may never enter the minds of some people who consider only preserving all life at all costs. For them, just as for those who consider only dignity of death, there is no dilemma.

ETHICS AS A GUIDE FOR JUDGMENTS AND ACTIONS
THEORIES, PRINCIPLES, AND RULES

Although no attempt will be made here to discuss ethical theories in great depth, it is important, at least, to understand the distinction among theories, principles, and rules; these provide the bases for making judgments and taking actions. Beauchamp and Childress[9] depict moral reasoning or justification in the form of hierarchical tiers, which they call levels of moral justification. According to these authors, judgments about what ought to be done in particular situations are justified by moral rules, which in turn are grounded in principles and ultimately in ethical theories (see the box above, right).

In brief, a *judgment* is a decision or verdict about a particular action. *Rules* tell what ought or ought not to be done in terms of right and wrong. For example, it is wrong to kill. *Principles* generally are more general and fundamental than rules. In addition, principles serve as the foundation of rules. Respect for other people is an example of a principle. It may be the grounds for the rule that it is wrong to kill. Theories are bodies of principles and rules that are more or less systematically related.[9] It is the principles and rules that serve as action guides.

MORALITY AND NORMATIVE ETHICS

Normative ethics is a field of inquiry that attempts to identify which action guides are worthy of moral acceptance and why. Morality is concerned with relations between people and how they behave toward one another to live in harmony and to protect important values cherished by society and its members. *Values* are the properties, qualities, skills, liberties, and other *goods* cherished by individuals. Quality of life, freedom to choose a style of life or a style of death, freedom to vote, freedom of choice, and health are all goods. Almost all people try to act morally in their personal and professional lives, but there are situations when it is difficult to know what actions are morally correct. Deliberation about some situations sometimes gives rise to more questions than it does to solutions. It is in these situations that an understanding of ethics can be helpful.

Ethics is that part of philosophy that deals with systematic consideration of situations where it is difficult to know what is morally correct. In this section, understandings from normative ethics will be used to identify guides for making judgments and decisions for action.

Normative ethics is concerned with more concrete questions than other forms of ethics and thus will be more useful to nurses and others who must take action. Normative ethics addresses such questions as what types of acts are morally right or wrong? What types of values are morally good or bad for the functioning of society and the welfare of individuals?[75]

MORAL JUDGMENT AND NURSING ASSESSMENT

In general, good clinical nursing is ethical nursing. Ethics are inextricably linked to a nurse's primary task, that of deciding upon and carrying out the best nursing care for a particular person in a particular environment under a particular set of circumstances. Just as systematic assessments are completed to decide on appropriate nursing diagnoses and related actions, organized systematic assessment can assist in making moral judgments or ethical decisions. The following scheme, similar to that of Jonsen, et al.[44] should help in gathering data, arranging questions, focusing on central points, excluding extraneous information, and weighing evidence. *It will not dictate conclusions or give definitive answers.* Conclusions can be drawn by the nurse after using the method to clarify and consolidate thinking.

The method consists of putting all considerations into one of three categories. Considerations include all direct and indirect observations, including facts, opinions, and circumstances that persons involved in a particular situation are likely to bring forth. The categories

CONSIDERATIONS FOR ETHICAL DECISIONS

Indications for medical/nursing intervention
  (Principle: beneficence/nonmaleficence)
Patient preference and quality of life
  (Principle: autonomy)
External factors
  (Principle: justice)

are (1) indications for medical and nursing intervention, (2) patient preferences and quality of life, and (3) external factors. Each category reflects certain major moral theories, rules and principles (see the box above) that are considered important in the ethics of health care. For example, the principle of "Beneficence/Nonmaleficence" underlies indications for medical and nursing intervention.

The principle of *beneficence/nonmaleficence* is expressed in the Hippocratic maxim: be of benefit and do no harm. It expresses the duties of assisting others in need and avoiding harm.

The principle of *autonomy* addresses the individual's right to control his or her own fate through decision making. Considerations of quality of life must be interpreted in light of the individual's preferences. The willingness to let the individual make decisions is a way of affirming that person's autonomy.

External factors include such elements as cost to the health care system, drain on family resources, and competing needs of other patients for care or resources. The application of the principle of *justice* provides a way to address fairness in distributing costs and resources.

In addition to evaluating each category of data by reference to these principles, an ethical theory may be used. For example, each category may be evaluated through application of utilitarian theory. *Utilitarianism* is a theory that states, in essence, that the best action is that which promotes the greatest good for the greatest number. The other major ethical theory relevant to clinical decision making is *deontology*. Deontologic systems recognize supreme principles, such as autonomy, that supercede any consideration of results of actions. In today's complex world, it is rarely possible to strictly adhere to one theory in its purest form.

Assessing the importance of the facts, opinions, and circumstances in light of the categories is a difficult task. When they are enmeshed in the categories, they are called ethical considerations. Generally, the priority that persons give the considerations reflects their own ethical system. However, it is not that simple. Some clinical situations exist in which the indications for treatment are questionable or the preferences of the patient undiscernible.[66]

ETHICAL ISSUES

Many ethical issues evolve around indications for medical and nursing interventions. These issues arise from such questions as the following: When should medical therapies be started or stopped? When should life supports be discontinued? What constitutes death? Who should decide?

WITHHOLDING OR WITHDRAWING TREATMENT

Appropriate consideration of withholding or withdrawing specific therapy occurs when (1) the therapy offers no reasonable expectation of the patient's attaining any human awareness, (2) the therapy is proving medically ineffective and useless after sufficient trial, or (3) therapy is perceived from the expressed point of view of the patient (or the decision-making representative) to be cummulatively a greater burden than a benefit.[51,60]

When decisions are made to withhold or withdraw life-sustaining treatment, the goal of medical and nursing care focuses on keeping the patient comfortable, avoiding suffering and pain, and providing support, comfort, and care on a physical, emotional, and spiritual level. It becomes more difficult once medical procedures designed to prolong life are withheld or withdrawn, to distinguish which procedures are not directed to supportive care and may be omitted. Perhaps the most controversial area is that of determining the proportionate benefit and burden of medical (artificial) nutrition and hydration.[33,36,40,43,61,89] The issue of withdrawing treatment, once started, is also present.

The American Nurses' Association Committee on Ethics has prepared guidelines to assist nurses in sorting through the concerns related to withdrawing or withholding food and fluids.[6] The document reflects principles of the Nursing Code of Ethics, as well as other ethical, medical, and legal considerations. Examining questions of if and when to discontinue treatment presents issues surrounding euthanasia.

EUTHANASIA

Euthanasia comes from the Greek words meaning good or pleasant death. It implies that under some circumstances death may be preferable to life for an individual. Euthanasia, or "mercy killing," is a topic surrounded by controversy. At the present time, there is no agreement on whether death is ever preferable to life for an individual or on what constitutes euthanasia. In fact, Curtin and Flaherty[16] provides 16 different definitions of the term.

The more common distinctions made when discussing euthanasia are those of *active and passive* and *voluntary and involuntary* (see the box on p. 266). Active euthanasia refers to an act that directly and intentionally shortens a person's life. It is an act of commission. Passive euthanasia, an act of omission, usually refers to

EUTHANASIA DISTINCTIONS

Active/Passive
Commission/Omission
Killing/Letting Die
Voluntary/Involuntary

EUTHANASIA CONTINUUM

Antieuthanasia: treating at all costs
Passive euthanasia: letting die
Active euthanasia: ending life

letting die by either withholding or withdrawing a treatment that might prolong a person's life.

Voluntary euthanasia refers to the involvement of the dying person in the manner and procedures leading to his or her death. The involvement may be through active participation during the dying period or by making his or her wishes known through a living will or other means prior to the period of imminent death. Sometimes it is necessary to presume the intent of voluntary euthanasia by considering what the patient would have wanted if he were able to participate in the decisions regarding the circumstances of his death. The latter is especially true in unexpected events such as accidents, strokes, and cardiac disease, in which the patient may have lost consciousness and may not have shared his or her wishes regarding the circumstances of dying. Under such circumstances, clearly written living wills that are carried out in good faith serve as a safeguard of a dying or incompetent person's rights. A poorly written living will can be used to hasten the death of an unwanted individual and thus detract from rather than strengthen the person's interests.

In looking at questions related to euthanasia, there is a continuum ranging from a strict belief in the sanctity of life (antieuthanasia, treating at all costs) to passive euthanasia (letting die) to active euthanasia (ending life, killing) (see the box above, right).

A persistent moral issue is the question of whether letting die is morally equivalent to killing, or omission equivalent to commission. Remember, no action is an action. Active and passive euthanasia are intentional choices. The distinction seems to be that of the intent of the action. The 1986 statement by the AMA Council on Ethical and Judicial Affairs holds that the patient and/or immediate family can decide to "discontinue all means of life-prolonging medical treatment," even "if death is not imminent but a patient's coma is beyond doubt irreversible."[2] The New Jersey Supreme Court implicitly invoked this distinction when it held that judgments about therapy should be made in terms of the degree of invasiveness of the treatment and its chance of success.[11] Ethicists have distinguished ordinary treatment from extraordinary treatment by stating ordinary treatments offer a reasonable prospect of benefit for the patient without excessive pain, expense, or inconvenience.[73]

In more direct terms, killing is wrong, but letting die in the sense of not instituting extraordinary efforts or by discontinuing extraordinary treatments is morally permissible. In fact, most physicians accept that killing a patient is morally wrong and thus not permissible, but in some circumstances it may become morally required to let a patient die.[11] Nurses generally accept the same view.

Rachels[76] argues that the distinction between active and passive euthanasia is not a morally justifiable one. Citing the example of a family's refusal to allow surgery for esophageal atresia on a child with Down's syndrome, Rachels argues that the refusal to perform this simple lifesaving surgery is no different from killing the child. Rachels' active/passive equivalency seems appropriate in this instance and may be under other circumstances where the distinction between killing and letting die is called upon as a pretext for not saving a life. Rachels does not take into consideration that the intent and the consequences of passive or active euthanasia are not always the same. There are situations in which there is a morally important difference between killing and letting die.[94]

In some circumstances, to let die instead of to kill implies that there is some possibility that the patient may recover, go into remission, or survive long enough for some new therapy to be discovered. It is an attempt to "buy time" for the patient. The difficult question is: Is the bought time quality time; that is, is it a meaningful enriching experience, or is it a hard time filled with meaningless suffering?

Active euthanasia may include such actions as giving a patient the means to kill himself.[17] If a patient takes his own life, it is a form of active voluntary euthanasia or suicide.

SUICIDE

Quality of living and quality of dying may be closely associated. A person with terminal illness may assess the situation and decide that living with pain, disability, or despair is not living. He may ask the question: Is it better to take measures to bring about a peaceful death than to continue in such a state?

Suicide or voluntary euthanasia carried out by the individual on his own behalf has been seen as an affirmation of life, a denial of life, and a questioning of life. The traditional religious teaching of the Western world since St. Augustine has condemned all forms of self-destruction. Suicide was and still is considered by some to be a sin and an interference with God's will.[17] According to Kant,[46] individuals do not have the power of disposal of their bodies. They can only treat their bodies as they choose in relation to self-preservation. These views are being challenged in society today as they have been in the past. Suicide is no longer considered a crime according to the Act of 1961.[100] Heifetz and Magel[37] suggest that under some circumstances, when death is imminent, individuals who are severely ill should be helped by their physicians to commit suicide. They distinguish this element of the population from the lonely, elderly, and physically handicapped, for whom they do not advocate assisted euthanasia. They point out that, although laws do not exist in the United States covering physician participation, they do exist in Uruguay, Switzerland, Peru, Japan, and Germany. Some cultures such as the Japanese and, regardless of culture, some individuals favor suicide over other negative values such as dishonor. Brutus preferred suicide to the disgrace of being marched through Rome as a vanquished hero.

Individual and societal views and practices regarding suicide run the gamut from opposition to suicide under all conditions and at all costs, to suicide as justifiable under some conditions, to suicide as a person's right. The question of an individual's right to autonomy or self-determination is a basic consideration in discussing suicide. Those who oppose suicide under all conditions usually use some form of the argument that "life is a gift, and no one has the right to take a life." Those at the opposite end of the continuum argue that a person has the right to determine his or her own fate, even if it means destroying his or her own life. Other considerations in arguments opposing suicide include viewing suicide as cowardly, a crime against society, an insult against humanity, and an act that brings great pain to the survivors.

Suicide is of particular concern to health professionals who may be in a position to offer other alternatives and thus prevent it. It is difficult to evaluate what constitutes suicide. Is refusal to eat or to continue with prescribed therapies a form of suicide, or must there be an overt act such as overdosing on medications? Is suicide always a voluntary act, or is a person driven to suicide by rejection of others or by pain that might have been controlled? When is suicide justifiable in the known dying person? What do you do when a patient who is dying all too slowly and painfully asks for your assistance in ending it all? Of interest is Rollin's[80] account of what she did when her mother, who was slowly dying of cancer and in unrelenting pain expressed her desire to commit suicide and asked her to assist. Rollin did assist, to her own peace of mind and satisfaction, as well as her mother's.

Nurses and physicians, however, are committed to another imperative—that is to *never abandon care*.[77] Never to abandon care includes ensuring that a dying person is not alone, that others are aware of his or her dying, and that he or she is free from pain and anxiety. It is not an obligation to assist in ending life. In fact, the ethical basis for suicide prevention is the psychologic thesis that a suicide attempt is often a cry for help rather than an unambivalent decision to end one's life. Thus nurses and physician have a legal and ethical obligation to assess and recognize suicidal risk and depression in patients and to make efforts to assist them in receiving counseling.[84] Often suicide is not an act of autonomy but rather is caused by impaired capacity that, in turn, is caused by an underlying emotional conflict or extreme physical discomfort. But what about instances of prolonged dying where it is medically impossible to control pain in spite of the positive impact of the hospice movement? Life for some dying people does become more of a burden than a gift. Ramsey[77] suggests the formulation of a moral rule that unrelenting and medically uncontrollable pain is the only circumstance under which positive action might be taken to hasten a person's death. Such a rule would not lessen the dilemma for nurses. It still leaves questions about the strength of the lifesaving ethic. In addition, impact of pain is really a quality of life question that can best be evaluated by the dying individual bearing the pain. If quality of life is determined by the person living the life, is suicide a purely personal decision? It seems that the quality of life of survivors also should be considered. When the survivors have had no prior warning or a part in the decision, and when the suicide is not perceived as an action to achieve comfort, the anguish to the survivors is great. For some the anguish never ends. Their grief is compounded by guilt, shame, and even anger. In some instances the survivors become victims of a society that condemns the act as a crime.

Even in such a limited discussion of suicide, and even when addressing persons known to be dying, it becomes evident that suicide is an issue about which health professionals and others disagree. It is an issue to be discussed with understanding and openness to better determine appropriate interventions.

Suicide may be a form of control in the dying situation or it may be a form of escape. Sometimes dying people seek an escape from loss of control over the event of dying; other times they seek an end to suffering. Nurses can be influential in providing dying persons and their families a sense of control by assisting with such problems as pain control, bowel and bladder control, and depression. They can decrease the uncertainty of the situation by explaining what the dying person and family can anticipate over the coming days. In other words, they can assist in promoting quality of life.

QUALITY OF LIFE

What constitutes quality of life? Who can predict what quality of life is or will be during the dying process? Can one person judge the quality of life of another, especially if the other is dying?

Much has been written on what constitutes quality of life from the research perspective, but there is little on what constitutes quality of life for the dying person. In fact, it has been suggested that, if the known instruments were used to measure quality of life, most dying persons would receive low scores, since most instruments focus on objective physical, behavioral, psychologic, and economic results of disease and treatment and less on measures of a general sense of well being, happiness, or satisfaction.[52] Dying persons may perceive quality of life differently than those who are living with an acute or chronic illness or who are well. What constitutes quality of life differs from person to person and for any one person during the various stages of life. What contributes to the *meaningfulness of life* may be a more cogent question than what constitutes quality of life when considering the dying person. For example, depression can be expected but how much and for how long? A person can live with pain, anxiety, and fear but how much and for how long? How much control does the person have over the situation? Can we increase the control they can have in the situation, although they have lost control over dying? Do the symptoms detract from the meaning of life from the perspective of the dying person? Sometimes trials and tribulations contribute to the growth of an individual.

Many ethical principles and rules are called into play when considering meaningfulness of life. Dying persons must have freedom to choose a style of dying and then be assisted in that choice. Patient preferences are important because they make explicit the values of personal autonomy and self-determination. Respect for the patient's *autonomy is the moral stance that deters a person from interfering with another person's beliefs and actions.* The legal counterpart of autonomy is *self-determination or the legal right of every human being of adult years and of sound mind to determine what shall be done with his or her body.*[44] Determining what shall be done implies making *informed* choices. Meaningful information presented in an understandable fashion is necessary to make informed choices or to give what is referred to as *informed consent.*

Informed consent, then, becomes an important factor in supporting meaningfulness of life. It includes giving dying people sufficient information about their diagnoses, prognoses, and possible therapies so that they make informed choices about how they will live or die and about who will help them and in what ways. Informed consent is a person's agreement to allow something to happen on the basis of a full disclosure of facts needed to make an intelligent decision. Informed consent reinforces the value of personal autonomy. It assumes that the person has the emotional and mental ability to understand, to process data, assessing benefits and burdens, and to make decisions. This ability is sometimes referred to as competence or mental capacity.

Competence and incompetence are used in many ways in everyday life to infer that a person is capable in some way, that is, clinically competent. Actually, the terms competence and incompetence are best reserved as legal terms. As such they infer reasoning ability and emotional stability sufficient to appreciate the nature and consequences of making decisions regarding such things as wills, contracts, or being a parent. A judge or other proper legal authority makes the judgment of whether or not a person is competent. If a person is judged incompetent, he or she is assigned a guardian. The guardian may be responsible for all decisions for another person, or his power may be restricted to *one area* of the dying person's affairs. For example, a person may be deemed incompetent in matters of business but may retain the mental capacity allowing autonomy in decisions about medical treatment.

In the health care setting, use of the terms mental capacity rather than competence or incompetence offers some clarity. *Mental capacity* refers to the ability to understand the situation and voluntarily make decisions about it. The mentally capable dying person has the right to refuse or to request treatment. When the request is based on an informed choice it should be respected, thus reinforcing the value of autonomy. As in other situations, it is not a simple matter. What makes a person mentally capable or incapable? The box below suggests some of the components of a systematic assessment of mental capacity or mental incapacity and factors that could influence judgments. Nurses can enhance the mental capacity of dying patients by educating them about their illnesses and treatments and assisting them to formulate questions for the health care team. They can also provide a safe environment as patients deal with uncertainty.

ASSESSMENT OF MENTAL CAPACITY AND FACTORS INFLUENCING JUDGMENT

Orientation to time, place, person, and situation
Ability to recall recent and past events, to logically sequence events, to understand abstract ideas, to make reasoned judgments
Psychological state, mood, and affect that may affect the ability to make choices; e.g., anxiety, fear, depression, suicidal ideation, hallucinations, delusions, illusions
Prior history of psychiatric disorders that could impact on present judgments

A significant ethical and legal problem associated with the principle of autonomy is the problem of *paternalism.* Paternalism is "a refusal to accept or acquiesce in another person's wishes, choices, or actions for that person's own benefit."[15] Laws passed with the intent of protecting people can be paternalistic. The Food and Drug Act prohibiting the prescription of laetrile for treating persons with cancer is an example. Traditionally medical practice and, by association, nursing practice has been paternalistic. Physicians have concealed diagnoses and prognoses from patients "for their own good." Nurses, although often not in agreement with concealing information, act in a paternalistic way by participating in the subterfuge to "protect the patient from conflict." The ethical questions are: Is paternalism ever justified? If so, under what circumstances? More specifically, should all dying persons be told they are dying? When, by whom, and in what manner should they be told? Does lack of total disclosure constitute paternalism?

DEFINITIONS OF DEATH

Much controversy surrounds the question, "What is death?" Is death the irreversible cessation of respiration and circulation, or is death the irreversible cessation of all functions of the entire brain, including the brain stem?

The term *brain dead,* introduced a decade ago, causes much confusion. Originally it referred to a person whose heart and lungs were activated by a respirator but whose centers in the brain stem were destroyed. Removal from the support system would end in death caused by the inability of the person to resume spontaneous breathing. In addition, brain dead means that the person is dead in the sense that a functioning brain is the seat of identity. What decision can be made about persons in a "persistent vegetative state"? They show no evidence of cortical functioning, but continue to have sustained capacity for spontaneous breathing and heartbeat.

Use of different definitions are appealed to as rationale for different actions. Each appeal or action has its own consequences. For example, the use of brain dead definitions provides more latitude for organ transplants and experimentation. The rationale for this latitude is that "harvesting organs" is done to aid the living. A worthy endeavor, but does retrieving organs lead to violation of the dead? What are the constraints? Are the bodies being used with the consent of the donor, or is consent necessary once a person is dead?

The 17th century philosopher Descartes (1596-1650) said that, for a human being, to exist is to think; and that, for a human being, not to think is not to exist. In this regard, Bandman and Bandman[8] raise the practical issue of "can one be a 'nonthinking person'?" They ar-

gue that if the answer is "no," the brain dead definition is morally acceptable, and one is free to treat the remains as any other objects. If the answer is "yes," the world will soon be overpopulated with brainless or mindless beings who may not be tampered with because they are not considered to be dead. In addition, they must be cared for by others and receive the benefits of scarce resources.

There are no clear rules that dictate decisions in these matters. Decisions depend upon discretion and reflection on basic values. They are accompanied by conflict, insecurity, and discomfort. The conflict and emotions that accompany decisions about the life or death of another are entirely appropriate, since they are irreversible.

The important things in any ethical dilemma, regardless of whether it is dealing with euthanasia, suicide, or treatment decisions, is to be aware of the values or forces that lead us to make the decisions we do. An understanding of our own values and perspectives, as well as of formal ethical systems, do not give explicit answers to dilemmas. They do, however, help us to be consistent and to communicate with others in a way that is understandable. This does not ensure agreement, but it does facilitate discussion and attention to multiple perspectives and to the consequences of actions.

ETHICS CONSULTATION

The ethical dilemmas experienced by nurses caring for dying patients and their families are shared by other members of the health care team. Mechanisms have been developed to facilitate discussion of the ethical and medical complexities surrounding these issues. They deal with the ethical/value tensions and conflicts in the decision-making process and strive to approach consensus.

Among the mechanisms are interdisciplinary ethics committees that have increased significantly in acute and long-term care facilities following the work of the President's Commission for the Study of Ethical Problems in Medicine and Biomedical Research, published in 1984.[73,74] Policies not only guide the committees' deliberations but foster the institution of sound ethical decision making in such areas as withholding resuscitation or withdrawing life-sustaining treatment. Education often centers around models for decision making, ethical analysis, group dynamics, and conflict resolution. Case consultation can be prospective, concurrent, or retrospective. Guidance for development of committees is present in medical, nursing, hospital, and ethics literature.[7,50,73,96]

Some nursing departments have developed Nursing Ethics Committees to provide opportunities for greater numbers of nurses to participate in ethics education and case discussion as a means of improving ethical decision making.[25] Such a forum can serve as preparation for nurses to serve as representatives to interdisciplinary committees.

In addition to the committee structure, ethical decision making has been aided in health care institutions by a growing number of ethics consultants or ethicists hired by the facility or health care system on a part-time or full-time basis. Services include regular ethics rounds conducted on nursing units, guidance for ethics committees, and individual case consultation. Nurses with advanced preparation in ethics are among the most respected consultants. The situations demanding the most frequent assistance of the ethicists are those surrounding care of the dying.

CHAPTER SUMMARY

✔ Dying is an integral part of living.

✔ Prevailing societal attitudes toward death include death denial, death defiance, death desire, and death acceptance.

✔ Living wills are one vehicle used to communicate one's desires related to the process of dying.

✔ With advances of modern therapies, dying has taken on many characteristics of chronic illness with its resultant challenges.

✔ Understanding the stages and phases of dying can aid in assessing the diversity of responses among dying people and their families.

✔ Discussions with family members and patients are critical in determining the likelihood of families being able to offer care in the home during the final phases of dying.

✔ The complex physiologic, psychological, social, and spiritual dynamics accompanying dying help explain the presence of the multiple primary and secondary nursing diagnoses and challenge nurses to prioritize among them for interventions.

✔ Bereavement is the subjective state that occurs as a result of having suffered the loss of a significant person whereas grieving is the total response (thoughts, feeling, and behaviors) to the emotional suffering caused by a loss.

✔ Normal grieving includes behavioral manifestations—of shock and disbelief, yearning and protest, anguish, disorganization and despair, identification, reorganization and restitution—that are often frightening and misunderstood by the grieving person.

✔ Some individual characteristics of survivors are associated with a high risk for problems with the grieving process.

✔ Many ethical issues and dilemmas surround care and treatment of dying persons and their families

and call for an exploration of the values, perspectives, and ethical systems leading to decisions.

QUESTIONS TO CONSIDER

- How can the concepts presented by Martocchio help you understand the experience of the dying person?

- What support services are available to dying persons and their families in your community?

- What are some of your own values regarding withholding or withdrawing treatment? What are some difficulties that may occur if your values differ with those of the patient, the family, or institutional policies? What support services are available to nurses in your institution for dealing with ethical decisions?

REFERENCES AND SELECTED READINGS

1. Amenta MO and Bohnet NL: Nursing care of the terminally ill, Boston, 1986, Little, Brown & Co.
2. American Medical Association Council on Ethical and Judicial Affairs: Current opinions: opinion 2.18, Chicago, 1986, The Association.
3. American Nurses Association: Code for nurses with interpretative statements, Kansas City, 1985, The Association.
4. American Nurses Association: Nursing practice in the care of the dying, Kansas City, 1982, The Association.
5. American Nurses Association: Standards and scope of hospice nursing practice, Kansas City, 1987, The Association.
6. American Nurses Association Committee on Ethics: Guidelines on withholding or withdrawing food and fluids, Kansas City, 1988, The Association.
7. Aroskar MA: Institutional ethics committees and nursing administration, Nurs Econ 2(2):130-136, 1984.
8. *Bandman B and Bandman E: Nursing ethics in the life span, Norwalk, Conn, 1985, Appleton-Century-Crofts.
9. Beauchamp, TL, and Childress JF: Principles of biomedical ethics, ed. 2, New York, 1983, Oxford University Press, Inc.
10. †Becker E: The denial of death, Riverside, NJ, 1973, The Free Press.
11. †Branson R and Casebeer K: The Quinlan decision: observing the role of the physician, Hastings Cent Rep 6(1):8-11, Feb 1976.
12. †Butler RN and Lewis MI: Aging and mental health, ed 2, St Louis, 1977, The CV Mosby Co.
13. †Cantor RC: And a time to live: toward emotional well being during the crisis of cancer, New York, 1978, Harper & Row.
14. Carpenito LJ: Nursing diagnosis: application to clinical practice, ed 3, Philadelphia, 1989, JB Lippincott Co.
15. Childress JF: Who should decide: paternalism in health care, Oxford, 1982, Oxford University Press, Inc.
16. Curtin L and Flaherty MJ: Nursing ethics: theories and pragmatics, Bowie, Md, 1982, Robert J Brady Co.

*References preceded by an asterisk are particularly well suited for student reading.
†References preceded by a dagger are classic readings.

17. *Davis AJ and Aroskar MA: Ethical dilemmas and nursing practice, ed 2, New York, 1983, Appleton-Century-Crofts.

18. Diamond M: Bereavement and the elderly: a critical review with implications for nursing practice and research, J Adv Nurs 6:461-470, 1981.

19. Donovan ML and Girton SE: Cancer care nursing, ed 2, New York, 1984, Appleton-Century-Crofts.

20. Duespohl TA: Nursing diagnosis manual for the well and ill client, Philadelphia, 1986, WB Saunders Co.

21. *Dufault K: Helping patients and families make life-sustaining treatment decisions, AORN J 39(7):1132-1133, 1984.

22. Dufault K: Hope and elderly persons with cancer, unpublished doctoral dissertation, Cleveland, 1981, Case Western Reserve University.

23. *Dufault K: What is nurse's role when adults forego treatment? Am Nurse 16(2):5, 23, 1984.

24. Editorial: Acts and omissions: killing and letting die, J Med Ethics 10(2):59-60, 1984.

25. *Edward BJ and Haddad AM: Establishing a nursing bioethics committee, J Nurs Adm 18:30-33, 1988.

26. †Eliot T: The adjustive behavior of bereaved families: a new field of research, Soc Forces 8:543-549, 1930.

27. †Eliot T: The bereaved family, Ann Am Acad Polit Soc Sci 160:184-190, 1932.

28. †Falconer D: The adjustive behavior of some recently bereaved spouses, unpublished doctoral dissertation, Evanston, Ill, 1942, Northwestern University.

29. †Feifel H: The functions and attitudes toward death and dying: attitudes of patient and doctor, New York, 1965, Group for Advancement of Psychiatry.

30. †Fletcher J: Ethics and euthanasia, Am J Nurs 73:670-672, 1973.

31. †Freud S: Instincts and their vicissitudes: collected papers, New York, 1915, Basic Books, Inc.

32. Fowler M: Appointing an agent to make medical treatment choices, Columbia Law Rev 84:985-1031, 1984.

33. *Fry ST: Ethical aspects of decision-making in the feeding of cancer patients, Semin Oncol Nurs 2(1):59-62, 1986.

34. †Glick I, Weiss RS, and Parkes CM: The first year of bereavement, New York, 1974, John Wiley & Sons Inc.

35. Graham J: In the company of others, New York, 1982, Harcourt Brace Jovanovich Inc.

36. Grant ER and Forsythe C: A plight of the last friend: legal issues for physicians and nurses in providing nutrition and hydration, Issues Law Med 2(4):279-299, 1987.

37. †Heifetz MS and Magel C: The right to die, New York, 1975, GC Putnam & Sons.

38. Hemlock Society: Supporting the option of active voluntary euthanasia for the terminally ill, Los Angeles, 1985, The Society.

39. †Illich I: Medical nemesis: the expropriation of health, New York, 1976, Pantheon Books.

40. Illinois Supreme Court: Brief in re: Estate of Longeway (Bonnie Keiner, appellant, v Community Convalescent Center, appellee), Nov 13, 1989.

41. †Jackson EN: Grief. In Grollman E: Concerning death: a practical guide for living, Boston, 1974, Beacon Press.

42. †Jackson EN: Understanding grief: its roots, dynamics and treatment, Nashville, Tenn, 1957, Abingdon Press.

43. Johnson SH: The Cruzan case: who has the right to decide, Health Prog 89(11):22-25, 1989.

44. Jonsen AR, Siegler M, and Winslade WJ: Clinical ethics, ed 2, New York, 1986, Macmillan Publishing Co.

45. †Kalish RA: Death and dying in a social context. In Binstock RH and Shanes E: Handbook of aging, New York, 1976, Van Nostrand Reinhold Co.

46. †Kant I: Duties towards the body in regard to life. In Gorovitz S, et al: Moral problems in medicine, Englewood Cliffs, NJ, 1976, Prentice-Hall Inc.

47. †Koestenbaum P: Is there any answer to death? Englewood Cliffs, NJ, 1976, Prentice-Hall Inc.

48. †Kubler-Ross E: On death and dying, New York, 1969, Macmillan Publishing Co.

49. †Lindemann E: Symptomatology and management of acute grief, Am J Psychiatry 101:141-148, 1944.

50. Lo B: Promises and pitfalls of ethics committees, N Engl J Med 317:46-50, 1987.

51. Lynn J and Childress J: Must patients always be given food and water? In Friedman E, editor: Making choices: ethics issues for health care professionals, Chicago, 1986, American Hospital Association.

52. Martocchio BC: Agendas for quality of life, Hospice J 2(1):11-21, 1986.

53. *Martocchio BC: Authenticity, belonging, emotional closeness, and self-representation, Oncol Nurs Forum 14(4):23-27, 1987.

54. *Martocchio BC: Grief and bereavement: healing through hurt, Nurs Clin North Am 20(2):327-341, 1985.

55. *Martocchio BC: Living while dying, Bowie, Md, 1982, Robert J Brady Co.

56. †Martocchio BC: The social processes surrounding the dying person, unpublished doctoral dissertation, Cleveland, 1975, Case Western Reserve University.

57. *Martocchio BC and Dufault K: Dying, a part of living. In Diamond M, editor: Advances in geriatrics, long-term care nursing, vol 1, New York, 1983, Pro Scientia, Inc.

58. †Mitford J: The American way of death, New York, 1963, Simon & Schuster Inc.

59. Mor V, McHorney C, and Sherwood S: Secondary morbidity among the recently bereaved, Am J Psychiatry 143(2):158-163, 1986.

60. *Mumma CM: Withholding nutrition: a nursing perspective, Nurs Adm Q 10(3):31-38, 1986.

61. National Hospice Organization: Amicus curiae: Cruzan v. Harmon v. McCanse, Washington, DC, 1989, The Organization.

62. †Nichols R and Nichols J: Funerals: a time for grief and growth. In Kubler-Ross E, editor: Death: the final stage of growth, Englewood Cliffs, 1975, Prentice-Hall Inc.

63. *Norris FH and Murrell SA: Older adult family stress and adaptation before and after bereavement, J Gerontol 42(6):606-612, 1987.

64. North American Nursing Diagnosis Association: Proceedings of the seventh conference, St Louis, The CV Mosby Co (in press).

65. *O'Mara RJ: Ethical dilemmas with advance directives: living wills and do not resuscitate orders, Crit Care Nurse 10(2):17-28, 1987.

66. *Otte DM and Allen KS: Ethical principles in the nursing care of the terminally ill adult, Oncol Nurs Forum 14(5):87-91, 1987.

67. †Parkes CM: The first year of bereavement: a longitudinal study of the reaction of London widows to the death of their husbands, Psychiatry 33:444-457, 1970.

68. Parkes CM and Weiss RS: Recovery from bereavement, New York, 1983, Basic Books, Inc.

69. †Pattison EM: The experience of dying, Englewood Cliffs, NJ, 1977, Prentice-Hall Inc.

70. Petrosino BM, editor: Nursing in hospice and terminal care: research and practice, New York, 1986, Haworth Press.

71. †Pine VR: Comparative funeral practices, Pract Anthropol 16:49-62, 1969.

72. †Pollack GH: Mourning and adaptation, Int J Psychoanal 42:341-361, 1961.
73. President's Commission for the Study of Ethical Problems in Medicine and Biomedical and Behavioral Research: Deciding to forego life-sustaining treatment, Washington, DC, 1983, Government Printing Office.
74. President's Commission for the Study of Ethical Problems in Medicine and Biomedical and Behavioral Research: Summing up: final report on studies of the ethical and legal problems in medicine and biomedical and behavioral research, Washington, DC, 1983, Government Printing Office.
75. Purtillo RB and Cassel CK: Introduction to ethical dimensions in the health professions, Philadelphia, 1981, WB Saunders Co.
76. Rachels J: Active and passive euthanasia. In Levine C, editor: Taking sides: clashing views on controversial bio-ethical issues, Guilford, CT, 1984, Dushkin Publishing Group Inc.
77. *Ramsey P: The patient as person: explorations in medical ethics, New Haven, 1970, Yale University Press.
78. Rando TA: Grief, dying and death, Champaign, Ill, 1983, Research Press Co.
79. Raphael B: The anatomy of bereavement, New York, 1983, Basic Books Inc.
80. Rollin B: Last wish, New York, 1985, Simon & Schuster Inc.
81. *Remondet JH and Hansson RO: Assessing a widow's grief—a short index, J Gerontol Nurs 13(4):30-34, 1987.
82. *Richter JM: Support: a resource during crisis of mate loss, J Gerontol Nurs 13(11):18-22, 1987.
83. Ross JW: Handbook for hospital ethics committees, Chicago, 1986, American Hospital Association.
84. *Saunders JM and Valente SM: Cancer and suicide, Oncol Nurs Forum 15:575-581, 1988.
85. †Schneidman ES: On the deromantization of death, Am J Psychoanal 25:4-17, 1971.
86. Schneidman ES: Reflections on contemporary death. In Corr CA, Stillion JMK, and Ribar MC, editors: Creativity in death education and counseling, Lakewood, Ohio, 1983, Forum for Death Education and Counseling.
87. Schneidman ES: Voices of death, New York, 1980, Harper & Row, Publishers Inc.
88. †Schultz R and Aderman D: Clinical research and stages of dying, Omega 7:137-143, 1974.
89. Siegler M and Weisbard AJ: Against the emerging stream: should fluids and nutritional support be discontinued? Arch Intern Med 145:125-128, 1985.
90. Society for the Right to Die: Support of dying with dignity, New York, 1985, The Society.
91. Stringham J, Riley JH, and Ross A: Silent birth: mourning a stillborn baby, Soc Work Health Care 27:322-327, 1982.
92. †Switzer DK: The dynamics of grief, New York, 1970, Abingdon Press.
93. Thomasma DC: Ethics and professional practice in oncology, Semin Oncol Nurs 5(2):89-94, 1989.
94. Thomasma DC: The range of euthanasia, Am Coll Surg Bull 73(8):3-13, 1988.
95. †Van Jennap A: The rites of passage, Chicago, 1960, University of Chicago Press.
96. Vaux KL and Savage TA: Initiating and maintaining an ethics committee, Semin Oncol Nurs 5(2):82-88, 1989.
97. Varricchio CG and Jassak P: Informed consent: an overview, Semin Oncol Nurs 5(2):95-98, 1989.
98. †Volkan VD: Typical findings in pathological grief, Psychiatr Q 44:231, 1970.
99. †Weisman AD: The realization of death: a guide for psychological autopsy, New York, 1974, Jason Aronson.
100. *Williams G: The right to commit suicide. In Gorovitz S, et al: Moral problems in medicine, Englewood Cliffs, NJ, 1976, Prentice-Hall Inc.

CHAPTER 15

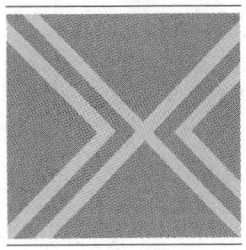

Infection

GRACE A. ROTTER

DORA RICE

CHAPTER OBJECTIVES

After studying this chapter, the student should be able to:
1 Describe the chain of infection.
2 Identify high-risk factors for infection.
3 Describe host response to infection.
4 Identify community approaches to infection control, and describe immunization programs.
5 Identify measures to prevent and control nosocomial infections (for example, bacteremia; urinary, wound, and respiratory infections).
6 Identify two systems of isolation precautions, and describe general approaches for each.

HISTORICAL PERSPECTIVE

Infection control has become a recognized discipline only in the last 20 years, although the principles governing it have been in existence for some time. In the middle of the nineteenth century Semmelweiss, an obstetrician in Vienna, demonstrated the significance of handwashing in combating the transmission of infection. He observed that the incidence of puerperal fever, a major cause of postpartum mortality, was much higher on the ward where the medical students trained than on the ward attended by the midwives. Although the role of microorganisms in causing infection was not yet realized, Semmelweiss believed that somehow the medical students could be transmitting disease from the autopsy suite to maternity patients. He showed that when the students and physicians were required to wash their hands and rinse them in a chlorinated lime solution before a delivery, the incidence of puerperal fever decreased greatly. The idea that handwashing alone could prevent the spread of disease met with much opposition by his colleagues. Better acceptance came after Pasteur, Lister, and Koch developed the germ theory of disease and related asepsis to the prevention of the spread of disease. At about the same time, Nightingale made significant contributions to sanitation and isolation practices. From this evolved an era in which medical asepsis was practiced more by ritual than with the true under-

standing of the scientific principles on which it was based.

A turning point came during World War II, when the sulfonamides and penicillin were first used successfully to treat infections. As new antibiotics were developed, a false sense of security developed about infection control. It soon became apparent, however, that antibiotics were not the sole answer to infection control. Organisms once well controlled by antibiotics, demonstrated the ability to develop resistant strains. In the late 1950s and the 1960s, outbreaks of penicillin-resistant *Staphylococcus aureus* infections were common, and gram-negative organisms such as *Pseudomonas*, which were previously considered nonpathogenic (incapable of producing disease), were suddenly implicated as the cause of infections acquired in the hospital. Along with drug resistance and the emergence of newly recognized pathogens, the number of persons at risk of secondary infections increased. A longer life expectancy, the use of immunosuppressive agents, and an increase in the use of invasive procedures to diagnose and treat disease all increased the risk of infection in certain persons.

The rise in hospital infections made it necessary to examine preventive and control measures, including a reemphasis on aseptic techniques. In 1970 an international conference to address the problem of hospital-acquired (nosocomial) infections was held in Atlanta. As a result, the Centers for Disease Control (CDC) in Atlanta set forth guidelines for prevention and control of infections in hospitals. The CDC is constantly updating and revising its recommendations based on epidemiologic studies and research findings. The American Hospital Association (AHA) and the Joint Commission on Accreditation of Hospitals (JCAH, since renamed the Joint Commission on Accreditation of Healthcare Organizations [JCAHO]), a major private accrediting agency, looked at the ethical and economic issues concerning nosocomial infections and established standards for programs in infection control. The purpose of these programs is to decrease morbidity and mortality from infections as well as reduce the cost of infections that could have been prevented. Consumer awareness of the problem also contributed to the attention given the issue of infection control. In the early 1970s only 10% of U.S. hospitals had infection surveillance and control programs, whereas by the end of that decade nearly all had them.

The field of infection control is challenging, with the identification of new pathogens and advances in research uncovering new information that may change current thinking and practices. Discovery of the human immunodeficiency virus (HIV) as the pathogen responsible for the current epidemic of acquired immunodeficiency syndrome (AIDS) has provided the incentive to develop safer practices to protect health caregivers from all blood-borne pathogens. Determining the modes of transmission of HIV has helped the CDC and infection control practitioners (ICPs) to develop new systems (universal precautions and body substance isolation) for staff to use when caring for all patients. Unfortunately the dissemination of misinformation about the spread of AIDS has caused some nurses and physicians to believe that complete isolation precautions are necessary when caring for these patients. It is well documented that HIV is not transmitted by casual contact and that it is easily killed by household disinfectants. Hospital staff are most at risk for infection with HIV from needle stick injuries. Programs to prevent needle stick injuries and to present factual information are essential. (See Chapter 77 for more information about AIDS.)

ICPs serve as a valuable resource as they interact with hospital departments, surveying for infections and teaching prevention and control. When a question or problem about infection control arises, the ICP should be contacted without hesitation. Questions may deal with clinical procedures, products for cleaning and disinfection, waste disposal, isolation systems, or personnel health issues.

This chapter presents an overview of the role of the nurse in the prevention and control of infection. For further information regarding a specific infectious disease, the reader should consult the chapter in which the site of the disease is discussed; for example, Chapter 39 for hepatitis, Chapter 33 for tuberculosis, and so on.

INFECTIOUS DISEASE PROCESS

DEFINITIONS

A *pathogen* is a microorganism or substance that is capable of producing disease. This discussion is concerned with microorganisms as pathogens. Factors that affect the microorganism's *pathogenicity*, or capacity to infect and produce disease, are shown in the box above.

Infection is the presence in the body of a pathogen

FACTORS AFFECTING PATHOGENICITY OF A MICROORGANISM

Ability to live and multiply outside its host
Its virulence
Its host specificity
Resistance of the host

---

that multiplies and produces effects that are injurious to the host. This injury may result from the presence and spread of the microorganism through the body tissues, known as the pathogen's *invasiveness,* or from the effects on the body of toxins produced by the microorganism, known as its *toxigenicity.* Some organisms, such as pneumococci, are highly invasive and virtually nontoxigenic, whereas others, such as *Clostridium tetani,* present the other extreme of high toxicity but low invasiveness. An infection may be *apparent,* thus causing clinical signs and symptoms, or *inapparent,* in which no perceivable signs or symptoms are present (asymptomatic).

Pathogenic organisms that are present in the body but do not produce injury or incite an injurious body response are said to be *colonizing* the body. Patients who have an endotracheal or tracheostomy tube often have colonization with microorganisms. Another example is the person whose nasal passages or skin surfaces are colonized with *Staphylococcus aureus.* The question of whether a person has an infection or colonization can be difficult to answer. What is important to realize is that persons who are colonized, as well as infected persons, can easily serve as a source of infection to themselves and others at risk.

CHAIN OF INFECTION

Essential to appropriate intervention in the prevention and control of infection is an understanding of the infectious disease process. With all infectious diseases, a common sequence of events occurs (Figure 15-1).

First, a *causative agent,* or pathogen, must exist. This can be a bacterium, virus, fungus, rickettsial organism, protozoa, or helminth (worm). Second, there must be a *reservoir* where the agent can be found. The reservoir can be animate (human, animal) or inanimate (soil, water, intravenous solutions, equipment, and so on). Human reservoirs can be persons with an acute clinical infection, with colonization, or who are asymptomatic carriers. Carriers can (1) be *incubating* the agent before the onset of signs and symptoms, (2) have an inapparent (*subclinical*) infection, (3) be in the *convalescent stage* of an infection, or (4) be *chronic carriers* of the agent. Viral hepatitis B is an example of an infectious disease that can be transmitted by human

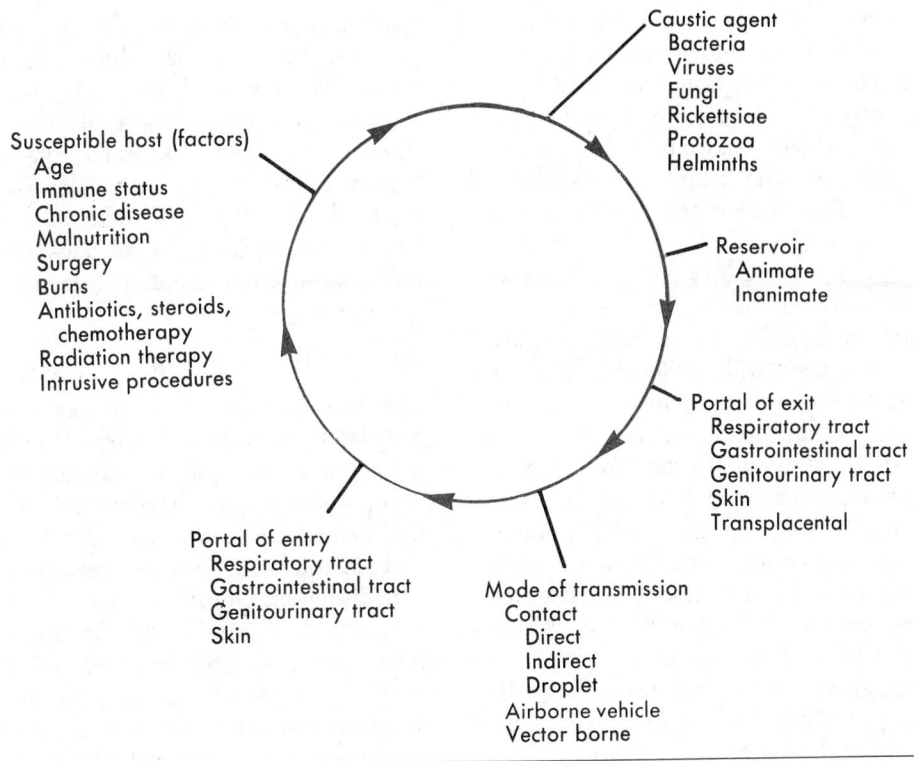

FIGURE 15-1 The infectious disease process.

carriers in all these stages. Often the reservoir of an agent responsible for an outbreak of an infection is not readily apparent and may never be identified. If the process of infection is well understood, however, appropriate and effective control measures can be instituted, even though the original source of the causative agent is not known.

The agent must have a *means of exit* from the reservoir. If the reservoir is human, the exit can be (1) the respiratory tract, (2) the gastrointestinal (GI) tract, (3) the genitourinary tract, (4) open lesions on the skin, or (5) across the placenta.

Once the agent has left the reservoir, it needs a *mode of transmission* to a host. Transmission can be by direct contact, by airborne vehicle, or by vectors. *Contact transmission* includes direct, indirect, or droplet contact. *Direct contact transmission* occurs when there is spread of infection from the source to the host without the presence of an intermediate object. This happens when there is physical contact with or skin shedding onto the host. Gonorrhea is an example of a disease transmitted by direct contact.

Indirect contact transmission has an intermediate object between the source and the host. This intermediary can be the contaminated hands of a person who has had contact with an infected source and then touches a susceptible host without washing the hands. An inanimate object that has been contaminated by an infec-

tious source is known as a *fomite*. Bed linen, respiratory therapy equipment, tissues, and silverware are examples of fomites that can be responsible for the indirect transmission of an infectious agent.

Droplet transmission occurs when the infectious agent is expelled from the reservoir in the form of droplets, as happens with a sneeze or cough toward a nearby recipient. These droplets do not become airborne but settle on surfaces about 3 to 4 feet from their source. Meningococcal meningitis and influenza are examples of diseases transmitted in this manner.

Airborne transmission occurs when the infectious agent expelled from the source remains suspended in the form of droplet nuclei or dust in the air. The agent is then inhaled by a host. These droplet nuclei are 1 to 5 μ in size and are smaller than the droplets discussed in droplet transmission, and they can thus be carried by air currents. Chickenpox (varicella zoster) and tuberculosis are diseases that can be spread by this route.

Common vehicle transmission occurs when a contaminated inanimate vehicle acts as the intermediary for the infectious agent from the source to multiple hosts. Contaminated water, food, and intravenous fluids are common vehicles. Salmonellosis and hepatitis B are examples of diseases that can be transmitted in this way.

Vector-borne transmission occurs when there is an animate intermediary from the source to the recipient. For example, mosquitos are the intermediary in the transmission of malaria, and ticks serve as the intermediary in the spread of Rocky Mountain spotted fever.

Once the infectious agent has been transmitted to a host, it must gain entry into the host. The *portals of entry* are similar to the modes of exit from the human reservoir mentioned previously and include the respiratory tract, the GI tract, the genitourinary tract, and breaks in the skin or mucous membranes.

The final step in the process after the inoculation of the host is the *maturation* and *multiplication* of the infectious agent. Entry of an infectious agent into a host does not mean that the agent will proliferate and cause infection. Infection depends on the agent's dose, the organism's virulence, and the host's susceptibility. The healthy human body is extremely resistant to infection; however, when the basic biologic defense mechanisms of the body are compromised, an organism has a much greater chance of causing an infection. Chapter 8 deals with many biologic defense factors exhibited by the host to prevent infection and injury. Some of the factors that affect host susceptibility to infection are (1) age (very young and very old persons being more susceptible); (2) immune status (certain disease states such as HIV infection, diabetes, cancer, or other chronic diseases can impair the immune status); (3) therapeutic treatments such as radiation and certain drugs, especially antibiotics, steroids, and chemotherapeutic agents; (4) surgery; (5) burns; (6) poor nutritional status; and (7) invasive procedures (intravenous catheters, chest tubes, urinary catheters) that break through the normal external defense barriers.

From this discussion of the infectious disease process, it becomes evident that no one factor is responsible for an infection. Rather, such variables as the *agent,* the *environment,* and the *host* determine the outcome. To intervene effectively in the infectious disease process, it is important that all these concepts be understood.

CLINICAL MANIFESTATIONS

Once a pathogen gains access to a susceptible host, a time known as the *incubation period* passes before the clinical symptoms of the disease appear. During this period the organism is establishing itself, spreading to target organs or tissues, and proliferating within various body sites. This incubation period varies depending on the condition of the host but is often predictable and diagnostically significant. The appearance of symptoms depends on the type of injury elicited by the virulent pathogen and the site of the organism within the body. The disease may be described as being *localized* (a focal point of symptoms or injury) or *generalized* (systemic involvement). The course of the disease may be *acute* or *chronic*. An acute disease often incites an immediate violent host response. The outcome of the infection

(pathogen over host or host over pathogen) is determined within a relatively short time, as seen in mumps, plague, or smallpox. Conversely, in a chronic infection the pathogen establishes itself more insidiously within the host, does not cause immediate damage, and tends to provoke less of a host response, as in tuberculosis and aspergillosis. Although chronic and acute are generally useful in describing the relationship between the host and a pathogen, many acute infections become chronic, and vice versa.

SIGNS AND SYMPTOMS

The establishment of an infection within the human body leads to several specific and generalized manifestations. The exact signs and symptoms elicited in the host depend on the agent responsible for the infection and the site of the infection. (For details on host response to specific infectious disease, see the particular chapter that discusses the disease site.) Some general subjective, objective, and diagnostic findings can alert the nurse to suspect an infection, even if the causative agent is not known. Recognition of the patient with a suspected infection is a crucial step in initiating early prevention and control measures.

Examples of data that would make the nurse suspect the patient may be developing an infection are listed in the box on p. 277.

For generalized infections the symptoms may be even more vague. The earliest clinical manifestations of an infection are generally sensed within the host as nondescript, nonspecific reactions such as weakness, headache, light-headedness, congestion, muscle aches, pain in the joints, decreased appetite, or malaise. These sensations are broadly referred to as *prodromal symptoms* (preceding the infection). As the infection progresses, other manifestations develop. These include fever, increased pulse rate, hypotension, altered mental status, or even jaundice, shock, confusion, and convulsions.

Of all the clinical symptoms mentioned, fever *(pyrexia)* is one of the most valuable diagnostic indicators of infection, although not all fevers are the result of an infectious process. Most persons with an infectious disease develop fever as a generalized response to the infectious agent.

Another systemic response to infection is the variation in leukocytes (white blood cells [WBCs] in peripheral circulation. The normal WBC count in blood is 5000 to 10,000 WBCs/mm^3. With the presence of a serious infection the number of WBCs rises above 10,000/mm^3 in response to the infectious inflammation. Leukocyte values between 10,000 and 20,000 are considered slightly elevated; 20,000 to 40,000 moderately elevated; and more than 40,000 greatly elevated. In a few infectious diseases the number of WBCs in circulation actu-

SUBJECTIVE AND OBJECTIVE DATA SUGGESTING INFECTION

LOCALIZED INFECTION

Subjective	Objective
Pain	Inflammation
Tenderness	Edema
Warmth	Redness
Swelling	Warmth
Itching	Exudate or drainage
	Amount
	Color
	Consistency

RESPIRATORY TRACT INFECTION

Subjective	Objective
Sore throat	Redness of throat
Congestion	Rales
Cough	Rhonchi
Sputum production	Cough
Chest pain	Type
Stuffy nose	Frequency
Runny nose	Sputum
	Amount
	Color
	Consistency

GI TRACT INFECTION

Subjective	Objective
Anorexia	Vomitus
Nausea	Frequency
Vomiting	Amount
Diarrhea	Color
	Consistency
	Diarrhea
	Frequency
	Amount
	Color
	Consistency

GENITOURINARY TRACT INFECTION

Subjective	Objective
Urgency	Frequency
Frequency	Amount
Burning or painful urination	Color
	Odor
Change in color or smell of urine	Purulent, foul discharge
Flank or pelvic pain	Presence of WBCs and bacteria
Discharge	Urinalysis
Itching	Culture

GENERALIZED INFECTION

Subjective	Objective
Malaise	Fever
Muscle aches	Elevated WBC count
Headache	Hypotension
Weakness	Altered mental status
Joint pain	Confusion
Anorexia	Convulsions
	Shock

ally drops, which is also significant diagnostic data.

Five types of mature WBCs are found in circulation: *neutrophils, eosinophils, basophils, lymphocytes,* and *monocytes.* Each type plays a more or less specific role in body defense (see Chapter 8); therefore different diseases produce different reactions among the WBC populations in the blood. These changes in patterns of distribution are detected not only by counting the total number of WBCs in a stained blood smear, but also by classifying them according to morphology and calculating the relative percentage of each cell type present. This type of count is known as a *differential count.* The differential count may provide information that can be correlated with other clinical data to help diagnose an infection. Table 15-1 provides some general correlations between leukocyte response and infectious diseases.

None of the signs and symptoms present in localized or generalized infections is diagnostic by itself. Many can be demonstrated by other disease processes. They can, however, serve as helpful clues in the diagnosis of a suspected infectious process.

DIAGNOSTIC TESTS

Diagnostic tests are an important adjunct in the diagnosis of an infection. Some of the diagnostic tests used to obtain data include skin tests, radiologic tests, gallium scans, ultrasound, computed tomography (CT scan), magnetic resonance imaging (MRI), microbiologic cultures, serologic antibody titers, and complete blood count (CBC). Examples of data obtainable from such tests include leukocytosis; anemia; increase in erythrocyte sedimentation rate (ESR); appearance of C-reactive protein; proteinemia; positive bacterial, viral, and fungal cultures; and positive radiologic findings, all of which may indicate the presence of an infection.

Proper collection and handling of laboratory specimens are essential to ensure accurate laboratory results. Inappropriate collection or handling of specimens may lead to unnecessary delays in test results or inaccurate results, thus affecting the patient's therapy. When an infection is suspected, cultures are taken of the suspected site. In the patient who has a fever and in whom the site of infection is unknown, cultures typically are taken of the blood, urine, sputum, and any other possible sites of infection. This may include spinal fluid cultures, aspirates of body fluid, or intravenous catheter tips. *It is imperative that these cultures be obtained before the initiation of antibiotic therapy because antibiotics can suppress any bacteria present and give inaccurate or false-negative culture results.* Cultures should be obtained in a manner that avoids contamination. Aseptic preparation of the site to be cultured, observance of aseptic technique, and placing specimens in an appropriate container are crucial factors to be observed

TABLE 15-1 White blood cell response to infections

Leukocyte Response	Associated Infectious Process
Increase in neutrophils (neutrophilia)	Typical in many acute local and systemic infections caused by bacteria (especially pyogenic bacteria), rickettsia, some viruses, and a few protozoa
Decrease in neutrophils (neutropenia)	Frequent in salmonellosis, brucellosis, whooping cough, overwhelming bacterial infections, influenza, infectious mononucleosis, hepatitis A infection, mumps, rubella, rubeola, and some rickettsial and protozoan diseases
Increase in eosinophils (eosinophilia)	Frequent in allergic reactions, chronic skin disease, helminthic infections, and scarlet fever
Increase in lymphocytes (lymphocytosis)	Frequent in chickenpox, mumps, measles, infectious mononucleosis, influenza, whooping cough, syphilis, tuberculosis, salmonellosis, viral hepatitis, and viral pneumonia; sometimes in convalescent phase of acute bacterial infection
Increase in monocytes (monocytosis)	Common in tuberculosis, chickenpox, brucellosis, mumps, syphilis, and certain rickettsial diseases; may occur in certain viral and protozoan diseases and in convalescent phase of acute bacterial infections
Decrease in lymphocytes (lymphocytopenia)	AIDS/AIDS-related complex (ARC)

in ensuring the best sample. Once obtained, the specimen must be properly stored and transported promptly to the laboratory. Each institution should have guidelines for the proper method for collecting and handling specimens for the laboratory. All specimens must be accompanied by the correct requisition and include the following information: (1) patient's name, (2) date and time of collection, (3) test requested, (4) type of specimen, (5) how specimen was obtained (clean void or catheter urine, expectorated sputum, tracheal aspirate), and (6) where the results are to be sent. A record of all tests is kept to avoid unnecessary duplication of tests.

Interpretation of laboratory results is sometimes difficult. Certain body sites have bacteria known as *normal flora,* which reside there in a commensalistic (intimate) relationship with the host. The skin, upper respiratory tract, vagina, urethra, and bowel are examples of body sites in which normal bacterial flora can be found. The bacteria found vary from site to site, and knowing the normal flora is helpful in discerning the significance of laboratory culture results. *A Clinician's Dictionary of Bacteria and Fungi*[20] is an excellent publication that lists in detail the normal flora of various sites. It must be emphasized that laboratory results alone cannot be used to make diagnostic and therapeutic decisions. Rather, they are used in conjunction with the patient's clinical status to make appropriate diagnostic and therapeutic decisions.

Knowledge about the infectious disease process and how to recognize or suspect an infectious process is vital to the prevention and control of infectious diseases in both community and hospital settings. Prevention and control of disease are addressed in the remainder of this chapter.

INFECTION CONTROL IN THE COMMUNITY

An infectious disease is termed a *communicable disease* when it is highly transmissible to other persons. Smallpox is an example of a communicable disease that, through cooperative efforts worldwide, has been successfully eradicated.[12] The methods used to eradicate smallpox throughout the world can serve as a model of how to eliminate other communicable diseases. The eradication of smallpox also demonstrates the importance of accurate reporting of communicable diseases to the proper authorities so that appropriate prevention and control measures can be instituted.

Efforts are now underway to eliminate rubella and measles (rubeola) in the United States. Rubella vaccine was licensed in 1969, and since then widespread epidemics of rubella and congenital rubella syndrome (CRS) have been successfully prevented. The continued occurrence of rubella in women of childbearing age has led to recommendations for immunization of both males and females in institutional settings such as hospitals and colleges to prevent outbreaks.

The original vaccine against rubeola licensed in 1963 was successful in reducing the incidence of measles by 99% until 1986. Since 1986 the outbreaks have increased, especially among unvaccinated preschool children and among vaccinated school-age children and college students. Outbreaks in students vaccinated before 1978 to 1980 are thought to result from instability of the vaccine manufactured before 1980. Current recommendations are for a two-step vaccination for infants in inner-city areas (at 9 and 15 months) and for revaccination of students in outbreaks (if vaccinated before 15 months of age or before 1980). Many schools and colleges now require proof of immunization before enrollment.

On the international level the World Health Organization (WHO), a special agency of the United Nations, has as its primary purpose the improvement and standardization of measures to prevent and control disease throughout the world. Its Epidemiological Intelligence Service in Geneva receives immediate notification of large-scale outbreaks of infectious diseases throughout the world and advises the world community of impending epidemics. *The Weekly Epidemiological Record* is an official publication of the agency.

On the national level the Centers for Disease Control (CDC) is responsible for programs for the prevention and control of communicable and other preventable disease in the United States. The CDC provides epidemiologic and laboratory services to state health facilities on request. It enforces quarantine regulations, conducts foreign quarantine activities; administers international activities for the control of malaria, smallpox, and measles; and provides consultation to other nations in the control of preventable diseases. It also collects, tabulates, and assesses data on reportable diseases from state health departments and publishes the findings in the *Morbidity and Mortality Weekly Report* (MMWR). Through its continuous surveillance, the CDC is able to detect new cases of diseases and intervene to control disease outbreaks. In addition, the CDC is instrumental in providing guidelines and recommendations for infection control.

In the United States the control of infectious diseases is the responsibility of each state. State health officers usually delegate this responsibility to a division of communicable diseases. A staff of physicians, nurses, veterinarians, and sanitary engineers works closely with a state epidemiologist in detection, assessment, and control of specific reportable diseases.

Local public health departments work in conjunction with their state health departments in this effort. The community health nurse plays a vital role in the collection of data, surveillance activities, immunization programs, education, and other control measures. Physicians and health care facilities have a responsibility to report communicable diseases promptly to the health department. Health agencies in the community can use the reported data to determine potential or real problems, identify the causative agent and hopefully its source, and identify the population at risk. A method to control the problem, care for those exposed, and protect the population at risk can then be devised and implemented.

PREVENTION AND CONTROL MEASURES

One method of prevention and control of disease in the community involves environmental control measures such as sanitation techniques that ensure a pure water supply and proper disposal of sewage and other potentially infectious materials. These measures have been legislated into building codes, state laws, and federal regulations. Similarly, regulations address health practices in institutions that handle, package, and prepare foods. Another environmental control measure is spraying a designated area to kill mosquitos, which are implicated in the spread of viral encephalitis. Spraying usually is done only after an outbreak has been identified.

Depending on the communicable disease, care of exposed persons and protection of the population at risk for contracting the disease may entail prophylaxis, immunization, or only careful monitoring of new cases. Often, simple adherence to basic principles of hygiene is sufficient. Determination of additional required measures should be made by the local or state health department. Attempts are made to reach those at risk and inform them of the preventive measures. Education of the public is a key component of these efforts.

In the United States a marked reduction has occurred in the incidence of infectious diseases that can be prevented by immunization. Concern is being expressed, however, about the decrease in the number of children presently being immunized, despite that these immunizations can often be obtained free. Additionally, many are concerned that federal monies used to support local immunization efforts will be reduced to such a level that free immunizations will no longer be equally available in all 50 states. Infections formerly seen only in children are now being seen more frequently in adults because of the failure of the population to develop acquired immunity during early childhood. This reduction in childhood infections is believed to be directly related to improved sanitary conditions.

Because of air travel, a more recent concern is the elimination of the barriers of time and distance. Thus a person with an infectious disease may be brought from a remote area of the world to a major population center where the disease can be readily spread to a susceptible public.

Several infectious diseases have been dramatically controlled by the development and use of various *inactivated vaccines* and *live attenuated antigens*. The potential for eradication of common infectious diseases brings with it major responsibilities for public health agencies, physicians, and nurses. Ways must be found not only to carry out planned programs of immunization, but also to educate the public to the hazards of apathy and failure to maintain proper levels of immunization. Continued progress in control and eradication requires continued commitment to increase knowledge about immunization patterns, to evaluate effectiveness and risks of antigens used, and to monitor the levels of protection in a population.

IMMUNIZATION PROGRAMS

Immunization programs have played and continue to play a primary role in the control of infectious disease throughout the world. The body can be stimulated to produce antibodies against some specific diseases without actually having the disease (*active artificial immunity*). Temporary protection sometimes can be provided by injecting antibodies produced by other persons or animals into the bloodstream of a human being (*passive artificial immunity*).

Recommendations concerning current immunization schedules are found in the *Red Book* published by the Committee on Infectious Diseases of The American Academy of Pediatrics and in *Morbidity and Mortality Weekly Reports,* which present recommendations of the U.S. Public Health Service's Advisory Committee on Immunization Practices (ACIP). The reader should refer to these resources when questions arise about proper immunization practices, prophylaxis, interruption in immunization schedules, or adverse reactions and side effects.

ACTIVE IMMUNIZATION

Active immunity can be acquired by artificially injecting small numbers of attenuated (weakened) or dead organisms of specific types or modified toxins from the organisms (toxoids) into the body. This procedure is known as *inoculation.* If 90% of the population is protected against organisms that require continued passage through humans to reproduce and live, the disease caused by the organism can be virtually eliminated because there are too few susceptible hosts for organism spread. Smallpox has been eliminated from the world in this way. This type of group protection is called *herd immunity.* It is ineffectual, however, against organisms such as tetanus bacilli that can exist indefinitely (in the soil), and in this instance each person must be immunized to be protected. If the disease is not prevalent in the environment, such as diphtheria in the United States, or is not spread from person to person by direct contact, such as tetanus, the inoculation must be repeated at regular intervals to maintain protection. This inoculation is called a *booster dose,* and usually one tenth of the original inoculating dose is sufficient.

An inoculation often causes a local tissue response. Symptoms of *inflammation* (redness, tenderness, swelling, sometimes ulcerations) appear at the site of the injection, and symptoms of *widespread tissue involvement* (slight febrile reactions, general malaise, muscle aching) for 1 or 2 days are common. The initial inoculation produces delayed symptoms because the immune response system must become sensitized to the antigen. Usually an accelerated, less severe systemic reaction to subsequent inoculations occurs because the immune response is stimulated at once. The local reaction also is less severe than that following the initial inoculation because the organisms have less opportunity to produce inflammation.

Active artificial immunization against many bacilli and viruses is now available. All persons should be encouraged to avail themselves of the protection advised by local health officials. They also should be advised to keep a permanent record of the date of each immunization.

In the United States the ACIP recommends that all children be immunized against diphtheria, pertussis (whooping cough), tetanus, mumps, rubella, poliomyelitis, and measles.

PRIMARY IMMUNIZATION SCHEDULES

The immunization schedule for diphtheria, pertussis, tetanus (DPT) begins with one dose of combined toxoid and vaccine when an infant is 6 weeks to 2 months old (Table 15-2). The next two doses are given at 4- to 8-week intervals thereafter. The fourth dose is administered about 1 year after the third dose. This schedule maintains adequate antibody levels until the child enters kindergarten, when a booster immunization is given. Thereafter, booster doses of tetanus and diphtheria are given only every 10 years (see Table 15-2).

Oral poliovirus vaccine (OPV), trivalent, is a live vaccine containing all three strains of poliomyelitis virus. OPV is the vaccine recommended for infants and children. Inactivated poliovirus vaccine (IPV) is preferred after age 18 years. IPV is also preferred for immunocompromised persons and their household contacts because it eliminates the theoretic risk to the *vaccinee* and prevents the spread of vaccine virus to immunocompromised persons. The primary series of OPV consists of three doses. The first is usually given at the same time the DPT series is begun (6 to 12 weeks of age). The next dose is administered 6 to 8 weeks later, and the third dose at least 6 weeks and preferably 8 to 12 months after that. A fourth dose is given just before entry into school.

A single dose of measles, mumps, rubella (MMR) virus vaccine, live, is given when the child is 15 months old. As mentioned previously, in urban outbreaks the first dose of monovalent measles vaccine, a live attenuated vaccine, may be given at age 9 months, followed by a dose of MMR at 15 months. Children who have not been vaccinated as infants can be vaccinated at any age.

Mumps vaccine, also live attenuated, should not be administered before 12 months of age because of the persistence of maternal antibodies, which may interfere with seroconversion. Mumps vaccine is usually given in a combined vaccine with measles and rubella (MMR) at 15 months of age. All susceptible children, adolescents, and adults should be vaccinated.

A single dose of rubella vaccine as part of MMR is

TABLE 15-2 Recommended schedule for active immunization of normal infants and children (See individual ACIP recommendations for details.)

Recommended Age	Vaccine(s)*	Comments
2 months	DTP #1, OPV #1	Can be given earlier in endemic areas
4 months	DTP #2, OPV #2	Six-week to 2-month interval desired between OPV doses
6 months	DTP #3	Additional dose of OPV at this time optional in areas with high risk of polio exposure
15 months	MMR, DTP #4, OPV #3	Completion of primary series
18 months	HbCV	Conjugate preferred over polysaccharide vaccine (HbPV)
4 to 6 years	DTP #5, OPV #4	At or before school entry
14 to 16 years	Td†	Repeat every 10 years throughout life

From Centers for Disease Control: Recommendations of the ACIP: general recommendations on immunization, MMWR 38(13):210, 1989.
*DTP, Diphtheria, tetanus, pertussis; OPV, oral poliovirus vaccine; MMR, measles, mumps, rubella; HbCV, vaccine composed of Haemophilus b polysaccharide antigen conjugated to protein carrier.
†Tetanus and diphtheria toxoids, adsorbed (for use in persons age 7 years and older); contains same amount of tetanus toxoid as DTP but reduced dose of diphtheria toxoid.

recommended for children after 12 months of age for maximal seroconversion. As previously discussed, most cases of measles are now seen in young adults, whereas before the vaccine became available in 1969, most cases occurred in school-age children. Females in childbearing years should be tested for rubella antibodies if they cannot document immunization, since rubella infection in the first trimester of pregnancy is associated with neonatal morbidity and mortality (congenital rubella syndrome). If antibodies are not present, vaccination is recommended. Because of the theoretic risk to the fetus, females of childbearing age are vaccinated only if they are not pregnant, and they are counseled not to become pregnant for 3 months following vaccination.

Haemophilus influenzae b vaccine with polysaccharide conjugated to protein (HbCV) is recommended at 18 months of age. Children less than 5 years of age previously vaccinated with polysaccharide vaccine (HbPV) should be revaccinated with a single dose of HbCV if at least 2 months have elapsed since they received HbPV.

Routine vaccination against *smallpox* is no longer recommended by the Public Health Service because the side effects and complications of the vaccine are greater than the danger of acquiring the disease. The vaccine is indicated only for laboratory workers who are directly involved with smallpox or closely related orthopox viruses.

At present, immunization against *typhoid fever* is recommended only when exposure to a typhoid carrier occurs in the household, when an outbreak of typhoid occurs in a community, or when a person travels to countries where typhoid is *endemic* (always present).

Immunization to protect against other diseases is given on a selective basis; that is, groups at a high risk are immunized.

Because of the prevalence of *influenza* and its poten-

tial for causing death, the ACIP recommends immunization against influenza for all individuals at increased risk of adverse consequences from infection of the lower respiratory tract. This includes persons over 60 years of age and those over 2 years of age who have chronic cardiac, respiratory, metabolic, or renal disease or diseases that impair the immune system. Initial protection is obtained by giving two injections of influenza vaccine 4 weeks apart beginning in October or November. Infants and children up to 6 years old who are at risk are given a subviron, split-virus vaccine in two doses 4 weeks apart. A yearly booster dose is needed to maintain and update immunity. Persons who are allergic to eggs or egg products should not be immunized because of the danger of hypersensitivity reactions.

The newest pneumococcal vaccine is a 23-valent polysaccharide vaccine licensed in 1983. It is recommended for adults and children over 2 years of age with chronic illness who are at increased risk for pneumococcal disease or its complications. It is also recommended for adults over 65 years of age who are otherwise healthy and for persons of any age with asymptomatic or symptomatic HIV infection. In general, revaccination of persons who received the previous 14-valent vaccine is not recommended because of the reported increase in adverse reactions.

Table 15-3 summarizes various vaccines.

PASSIVE IMMUNIZATION

Antibodies produced by other persons or by other animals such as the horse, cow, and rabbit can be introduced into a person's bloodstream for protection against attack by a pathogen. This protection is *temporary*, usually lasting only a few weeks, and stimulates no production of antibodies by the recipient. It is called *artificial passive acquired immunity*. Artificial passive immuni-

TABLE 15-3 Description of selected vaccines

Vaccine	Description	Comments
DPT		
Diphtheria	Toxoid Inactivated Diphtheria toxin	Booster dose every 10 years
Tetanus	Inactivated Tetanus toxoid	Booster dose every 10 years For contaminated wound management, additional booster given if more than 5 years since last booster dose
Pertussis	Killed whole *Bordetella pertussis*	Not recommended for individuals over 7 years of age because risk of pertussis low and reaction possibly severe
Measles	Live attenuated virus vaccine	Contraindications: pregnancy, immunocompromised state, history of anaphylactic reaction to eggs
Mumps	Live attenuated virus vaccine	Contraindications: pregnancy, immunocompromised state, history of anaphylactic reaction to eggs
Rubella	Live attenuated rubella virus grown in human diploid cells	Contraindications: pregnancy, immunocompromised state
Polio		
OPV	Live attenuated oral poliovirus vaccine	Contraindications: pregnancy, immunocompromised state
IPV	Inactivated poliovirus vaccine	Administered by subcutaneous injection, contraindicated in pregnancy
Influenza	Inactivated whole or disrupted (split) influenza viruses	Antigenic content annually changed to reflect influenza A and B virus strains in circulation; administered annually; contraindication: history of anaphylactic hypersensitivity to eggs
Pneumococcal	Purified preparation of 23 different types of pneumococcal capsular polysaccharide	Should be given only once to adults because of possible adverse reactions; data are not currently available regarding revaccination of children; should be given only to children 2 years and older who have chronic illnesses specifically associated with increased risk for pneumococcal disease
Hepatitis B		
Recombinant deoxyribonucleic acid (DNA)	Purified surface antigen of virus produced by recombinant yeast cells	Given in series of three injections; first followed by other two 1 and 6 months later; indicated for persons who have routine or frequent contact with blood and body fluids; contraindicated for persons allergic to yeast
Human serum	Purified, inactivated surface antigen of virus from plasma of human carriers	Administration schedule same as for recombinant DNA form; recommended for hemodialysis patients
Haemophilius influenzae b (HbCV)	Bacterial polysaccharide conjugated to protein	Administered at age 18 months to 5 years, up to sixth birthday

zation is given to a person who has been exposed to a disease and has no natural or artificial active immunity. It usually is administered before the disease develops but may be given to modify disease symptoms. However, for effectiveness after the disease has developed, it must be administered early, before extensive damage to body tissue.

Passive immunization usually is reserved for situa-tions in which the disease would be detrimental to the person. For example, it is rarely given to prevent a disease such as chickenpox or mumps in children because they are at an optimal age for the body to respond immunologically with minimal inflammatory response. On the other hand, an adult exposed to the same diseases often would be given antibodies because adults may have a severe pathologic response. Immunization is given to all age groups exposed to pathogens that cause serious diseases such as hepatitis, poliomyelitis, diphtheria, tetanus, or rabies. *Antivenins,* which are given to people bitten by poisonous snakes or black widow spiders, are other examples of passive immunologic products.

Products used for passive immunization may be specific to the disease. *Antitoxins* and *immune animal* and *human sera* are examples. These materials contain elevated levels of immune globulins, which can specifically detoxify the toxin, neutralize the virus, or inactivate the bacterium. The whole blood of a patient who has recently recovered from a disease against which antibodies are produced also may be used. Antitoxins are available for diphtheria, tetanus, botulism, gas gangrene, and the venom of snakes. Human immune serum is available for mumps, measles, pertussis, poliomyelitis, tetanus, and rabies.

Immune serum globulin (ISG), or gamma globulin (γ-globulin), is an antibody-rich fraction of pooled plasma from normal donors. The rationale for pooling plasma is that someone among the donors will have had the diseases and will have developed antibodies against them. The *globulin fraction* of the plasma carries the antibodies, and because it is known not to transmit the virus of hepatitis, it is considered safe to use. Because of occasional side effects, it is now recommended that the use of ISG be limited to those disorders in which its efficacy has been definitely established. These are measles prophylaxis or modification, viral hepatitis type A prophylaxis or modification, and immunodeficiency diseases. ISG is considered to be of questionable value in the following situations: (1) prevention of rubella in the first trimester of pregnancy, (2) prevention or modification of varicella in certain high-risk patients, (3) prevention or modification of viral hepatitis type B (serum hepatitis) after accidental inoculation, and (4) life-threatening bacterial infections.

Special human ISGs are derived from the sera of persons previously immunized or convalescing from specific diseases. Tetanus immune globulin (human) is of value in prophylaxis and treatment of tetanus in persons who have not received prior immunization. Pertussis immune globulin (human) and mumps immune globulin (human) are of uncertain or unproved value in the prevention and treatment of pertussis and mumps, respectively. Hepatitis B immune globulin (human) is available for prophylaxis after exposure to hepatitis B. Zoster immune globulin (human) is available for restricted use for prophylaxis against chickenpox.

NURSING RESPONSIBILITIES IN IMMUNIZATION

Probably the greatest responsibility of the nurse in immunization programs is to teach the public the advantages of immunization and encourage widespread participation in programs recommended by the local public health officer.

Teaching

In teaching it is advisable to provide the public with the following information: against what disease protection is being given, why immunization is desirable, and when booster doses should be obtained. The relative safety of the immunization and the advantages of immunization early in life should also be stressed.

The nurse is responsible for assessing persons before immunization because some contraindications exist to receiving certain immunizing substances. Those that are prepared in chicken or duck embryos may cause an allergic reaction in persons allergic to eggs. Many people are allergic to horse serum, and substances containing horse serum, such as tetanus antitoxin, should never be given unless a small amount of the substance has been injected intradermally (a *sensitivity test*) and no "hive" reaction about the injection site has been produced after 20 minutes. *Active immunologic products* should not be given while a person has a cold or other infection because the inflammatory reaction from the immunization will be greater than usual.

Children with histories of allergy often are *not* given routine immunization against diseases for which there is herd immunity because the danger of severe allergic response to the immunization is greater than the danger of contracting the disease. These children should be immunized against diseases such as tetanus, however, and immunization is achieved by giving the vaccine or toxoid in small doses over several weeks or months. The package inserts accompanying the immunologic product should always be read carefully to determine the indications, precautions, and side effects.

Live attenuated virus vaccines should not be given to persons with alterations in the immune status, since virus replication after administration may be unchecked in these individuals. As noted earlier, OPV viruses are excreted by the recipient of the vaccine and are communicable to other persons. Thus individuals who live with an immunocompromised person should receive IPV instead of OPV. If a person has a febrile illness, it is usually best to wait until recovery before vaccination is given. Pregnant women should not receive live attenuated virus vaccines because of the theoretic risk to the fetus. Live attenuated virus vaccines should not be given at the same time as passive immunization, since passively acquired antibodies can interfere with the response to live attenuated virus vaccines.

Before leaving the clinic, the person or family members should be instructed as to the expected effects of an inoculation and told to contact the physician or to report to a hospital emergency room if any other symptoms develop. The person is cautioned not to scratch any lesion produced by an inoculation. If a severe local reaction with redness, swelling, and tenderness occurs, the physician may order the application of hot, wet dressings. If the lesion is open, these dressings should be sterile.

When antitoxins, antisera, or antivenins are given, the patient is kept under observation for 20 to 30 minutes. Symptoms of severe allergic response usually will appear within that time. Epinephrine 1:1000 should be available for immediate administration if an allergic response occurs.

Persons employed in health care facilities should be evaluated for immunity against chickenpox, rubella, measles, polio, diphtheria, tetanus, and hepatitis B. Persons at risk for occupational hepatitis B infection should be offered vaccine at the time of employment. Persons with negative tuberculin skin tests should be retested every 6 to 12 months, depending on the prevalence of tuberculosis in the area. Yearly chest roentgenograms are no longer recommended for the routine management of persons with positive tuberculin skin tests. After the initial roentgenogram following a skin test conversion, annual ones have not been shown to be of significant clinical value and are not cost effective in monitoring persons for early disease.

Home Care

Persons with infections are frequently cared for at home. The community health nurse is often asked to teach family members how to care for the patient and how to protect family members, friends, and neighbors. Many of the same principles of infection control apply in the home as in the hospital. Some general principles for home care of persons with an infection are discussed here.

Handwashing is considered the most effective measure in preventing the spread of infection in the home. Hands should be washed before care and after contact with body substances (blood, urine, feces, sputum, vomitus, wound drainage, and so on). Caregivers should wear a smock or coverall to protect their clothes. Gloves should be worn when handling body substances. Soiled dressings, used disposable gloves, and other disposable items that contain body substances should be put in plastic bags before being discarded in the trash. All liquid waste can be flushed down the toilet. Used needles and syringes should be put in a glass jar or can, which is tightly closed before discarding in the trash. Disposable dishes are not required. Dishes and linen should be washed in hot soapy water. A cup of bleach should be added to the detergent to disinfect laundry soiled with blood. Blood and body substance spills should be cleaned up using an effective household disinfectant. If gloves are not available, plastic bags can be worn to protect the caregiver's hands. All persons should be taught

to cover the nose and mouth when coughing. In general, it is not considered necessary for the caregiver to wear a mask in the home. The special problems the nurse encounters in controlling hospital-acquired infections are the focus of the remainder of this chapter.

INFECTION CONTROL IN THE HOSPITAL
SCOPE OF THE PROBLEM

A *nosocomial* infection is not present or incubating when a person is admitted to the hospital but develops after admission. A *community-acquired infection* is present or incubating at the time of admission to the hospital. The nurse should be aware of the problem of nosocomial infections; their effects on patient morbidity, mortality, and increased hospital costs; and the related legal aspects. The nurse also should be knowledgeable about the types of infections seen most often, the common pathogens and how they are transmitted, factors that predispose a patient to a nosocomial infection, how to recognize persons at risk of infection, and the prevention and control measures necessary to decrease the incidence of nosocomial infections.

At least 2 million persons, or about 5% of all patients admitted to United States hospitals each year, develop nosocomial infections. In addition to the considerable morbidity and morality caused by these infections, their diagnoses and treatment, including additional days of hospitalization, cost more than 1 billion dollars per year.[22] The JCAHO develops and publishes standards for infection control in the *Accreditation Manual for Hospitals*. These standards are designed to help an institution improve its quality of patient care. The JCAHO requires that those institutions seeking accreditation have an effective, hospital-wide program for surveillance, prevention, and control of infection. The AHA and the CDC have developed guidelines for the prevention and control of infectious diseases for use in patient care centers. Because of these external forces, as well as to provide the best possible care for their patients, hospitals are recognizing the need to increase infection surveillance and upgrade programs to prevent nosocomial infections.

As seen in Figure 15-2, , the incidence of *nosocomial* infections varies with the type of hospital. This can be attributed to differences in the size of hospitals, the severity of illness in the patient population, susceptibility of the patient population, and the number of personnel who have hands-on contact with the patients. The patient with the greatest risk of developing a nosocomial infection has a chronic illness, a prolonged hospital stay, and the most direct contact with various hospital personnel (physicians, students, nurses, therapists, and so on.) These factors hold true for variations in infection rates not only from institution to institution but also within an institution. Certain patient care areas are considered to be *high-risk areas* for developing nosocomial infections. These areas are where patients who have decreased host defenses or who receive invasive procedures and devices are given care. Areas generally considered to be high risk are (1) intensive care units (including neonatal units), (2) burn units, (3) dialysis units, and (4) oncology units. The infection rate in these areas may be well over 20%.

PERSONS AT RISK

The nurse must recognize patients at the greatest risk of a nosocomial infection. Some of the factors that predispose a person to infection were mentioned previously. Briefly, these include (1) the age of the patient, the very young and the very old being the most susceptible; (2) impairment of normal immune defenses because of an underlying disease process, such as cancer, chronic renal disease, chronic lung disease, diabetes, or AIDS; (3) impairment of the normal immune defenses because of the therapy being given, such as radiation, steroids, or chemotherapy; (4) use of antibiotics, which can eliminate the patient's normal flora, providing opportunity for colonization with pathogenic and drug-resistant organisms that may then progress to cause infection; (5) use of invasive diagnostic and therapeutic procedures and devices, which bypass the patient's normal defense barriers and thus provide a portal of entry into the body (for example, indwelling urinary catheters, monitoring devices, intravenous catheters, respiratory

assistive devices); (6) surgery; (7) burns; and (8) length of hospitalization. Probably the most important factor predisposing a patient to acquiring a nosocomial infection is the severity of the patient's underlying disease.

A patient admitted to the hospital with an infection may develop a *superinfection* with another organism during the hospitalization. Often this superinfection is with a more virulent or drug-resistant organism. For example, a patient admitted with a leg ulcer infected with *Staphylococcus aureus* may develop further infection (not colonization) with *Pseudomonas aeruginosa*. Furthermore, if this infection progresses to involve the bloodstream, a *secondary bacteremia* has occurred. Infection can occur secondary to (1) an existing infection, (2) an underlying disease process, or (3) an anatomic defect that may be causing obstruction. An example of this is the man who has benign prostrate hypertrophy (BPH) and who develops a urinary tract infection secondary to the obstruction caused by the BPH. These concepts are the most helpful ones when seeking to determine the cause of a particular infection.

Hospitals participating in the National Nosocomial Infection Study (NNIS) provide the only source of recurring nationwide data on nosocomial infections. According to the 1984 NNIS data, the highest nosocomial infection rates occur in large teaching hospitals (Figure 15-2). This increased risk is attributed to differences in patients' severity of disease and in the use of invasive procedures in this category of hospitals.[10]

The most common site for a nosocomial infection is

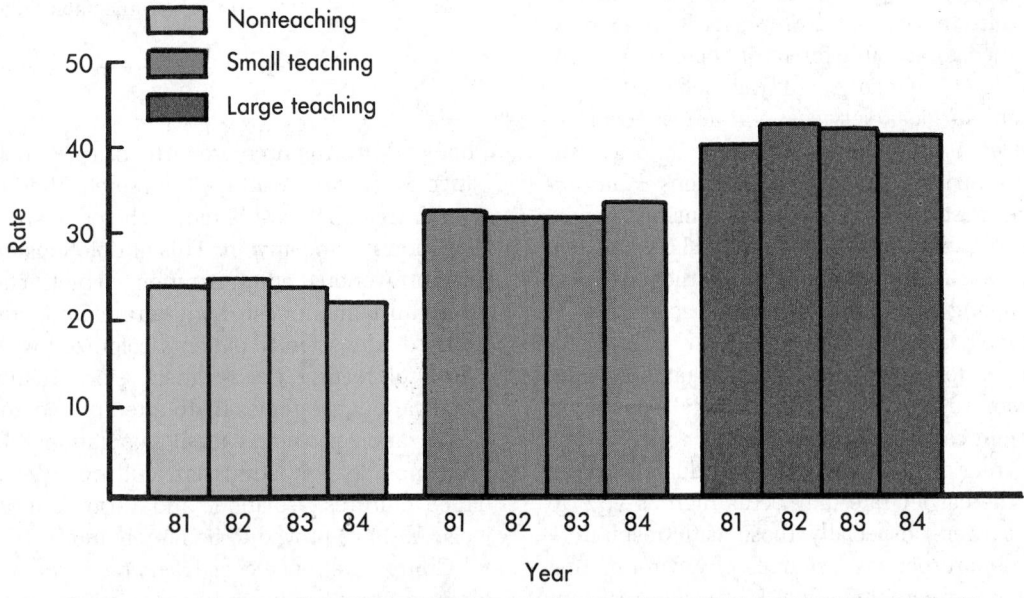

FIGURE 15-2 Infection rates per 1000 discharged patients from National Nosocomial Infection Study (NNIS) hospitals, by hospital category, 1980 to 1984. (From Centers for Disease Control: National Infection Surveillance, 1980-1982, MMWR CDC Surveill Summ 32:445, 1983; and National Infection Surveillance, 1984, MMWR CDC Surveill Summ 35:18, 1986.)

TABLE 15-4 Infection rates per 1000 discharged patients by site and hospital category, 1984

Hospital Category	Site (%)*					
	UTI	SWI	LRI	BACT	CUT	Other
Nonteaching	9.9	3.6	4.2	1.3	1.1	2.0
Small teaching	13.9	6.0	5.4	1.9	1.8	4.7
Large teaching	14.2	6.6	7.7	3.9	2.6	6.4
Total	12.9	5.6	6.0	2.5	1.9	4.6

From Centers for Disease Control: Nosocomial infection surveillance, MMWR 35(SS-1):19, 1986.
*UTI, Urinary tract infection; SWI, surgical wound infection; LRI, lower respiratory tract infection; BACT, primary bacteremia; CUT, cutaneous infection.

the urinary tract; 75% of these infections are related to instrumentation, including indwelling urinary catheters, catheterizations, and urologic procedures. Infected surgical wounds, followed by lower respiratory tract infections, cutaneous infections, and bloodstream infections (some associated with the use of intravascular lines), are the next most frequently encountered types of nosocomial infections. Together these sites account for about 35% of all nosocomial infections (Table 15-4).

PATHOGENS CAUSING NOSOCOMIAL INFECTIONS

The types of pathogens typically responsible for nosocomial infections and their usual reservoirs are listed in Table 15-5. In 1984, the most frequently reported nosocomial pathogens were *Escherichia coli, Pseudomonas aeruginosa, Enterococcus,* and *Staphylococcus aureus.* *E. coli* continued to account for most reported nosocomial urinary tract infections but was followed by *P. aeruginosa* on surgical services and enterococci on medical services. *S. aureus* was still the main organism causing nosocomial surgical wound infections. *P. aeruginosa* was the most common pathogen causing nosocomial pneumonia on all services. Coagulase-negative staphylococci and *S. aureus* were the pathogens most frequently causing nosocomial primary bacteremia on surgical and medical services.

The reservoir for *S. aureus* is the respiratory tract and skin. From 10% to 15% of the general population can be persistent carriers of this organism, which is harbored in the anterior nares. Among individuals working in hospitals, the carrier rate may be as high as 25% to 30%. Nasal carriers, especially those with respiratory tract infections, are potential sources of environmental and human contact contamination. Methicillin-resistant *S. aureus* (MRSA) especially causes concern among caregivers. Methicillin is one of the penicillins specifically developed to treat *S. aureus* infections. *S. aureus* is a common surgical wound and cutaneous pathogen. Al-

TABLE 15-5 Modes of transmission of some common pathogens

Pathogen	Common Reservoir
Gram-positive cocci	
Staphylococcus aureus	Contaminated objects, hands, and nasal tracts of health care workers, air, self
Group A *Streptococcus* organisms	Direct contact, air, hands, rarely objects
Enterococcus organisms	Self, hands of health care workers, environmental surfaces
Gram-negative rods	
Escherichia, Klebsiella, Enterobacter	Self, hands of health care workers, contaminated solutions
Proteus, Salmonella, Providencia, Serratia, Citrobacter	Contaminated food and water, hands of health care workers, self
Pseudomonas	Contaminated environment, hands, self
Anaerobic bacteria	
Clostridium, Bacteroides	Self, contaminated environment, hands
Fungal organisms	
Yeasts	Self, hands of health care workers
Fungi	Air, contaminated environment
Viruses	
Varicella	Air, direct contact
Herpes	Self, direct contact, air
Rubella	Direct contact, air
Hepatitis B	Contaminated instruments or injectables, direct contact

though MRSA is no more virulent than methicillin-sensitive *S. aureus* (MSSA), it is more difficult and expensive to treat. The antibiotic of choice for treating MRSA infection is vancomycin. This antibiotic is only available for intravenous administration, which contributes to overall treatment cost. Long-term care institutions have refused admission to patients colonized with MRSA because of fear of cross-transmission. Institutions have used various strategies in an attempt to eradicate MRSA colonization in their patient populations. These strategies include new admission cultures, periodic surveillance cultures, isolation, and various antibiotic protocols. All have proved to be largely ineffective.

Group A streptococci (*Streptococcus pyogenes*) are gram-positive organisms seen in nosocomial infections. Strains of these organisms cause streptococcal sore throat, scarlet fever, and streptococcal skin infections. Streptococci are found in animate reservoirs, particularly the pharynx and nares of personnel and patients.

Other organisms involved in nosocomial infections include gram-negative coliforms, *Escherichia, Klebsiella,* and *Enterobacter,* which live in the human intestinal tract. Although these organisms are usually susceptible to antibiotics, they have the capacity to develop antibiotic resistance. The large reservoir of coliform organisms within the general population can be a source for self-infection or for cross-infection from the hands of hospital personnel through the ingestion of foods or through the contamination of other materials. Some strains of these organisms are more likely to produce infection than others. The more pathogenic strains seem to gain the ascendency in patients who are receiving antibiotic therapy; immunodeficient patients are particularly susceptible to infection by the coliforms.

Although *Salmonella* organisms are usually acquired outside the hospital, the organism is readily transmissible and can be the cause of nosocomial infection. It is transmitted by direct or indirect contact with an infected person or through food (especially raw eggs), dairy products, or water contaminated with the organism. The CDC recommends that no one eat raw eggs. Patients with sickle cell disease or malignancies are more vulnerable to infection from these organisms.

P. aeruginosa, a gram-negative organism, is present throughout the hospital environment, especially where water is always present (in sinks, irrigating solutions, nebulizers). It is more frequently found in patients with *leukopenia* secondary to burns, leukemia, cystic fibrosis, and various immunodeficiency syndromes. It is also known to be a significant cause of infection in patients receiving prolonged courses of antibiotics, immunosuppressive drugs, and inhalation therapy. *P. aeruginosa* can be a threat to patients undergoing instrumentation (tracheostomy, urinary tract catheterization) and receiving renal transplants. Neonates, particularly premature infants, as well as elderly and debilitated persons, are the most vulnerable.

Serratia marcescens and *Serratia liquefaciens* are gram-negative organisms seen with increasing frequency in nosocomial infections. The reservoirs for these organisms are soil and water, and they are found in the hospital in similar reservoirs as *Pseudomonas.* Previously thought to be nonpathogenic, *S. marcescens* was used because of its red pigmentation to mark air flow and settling patterns of bacteria. It is now recognized as a pathogen that can cause severe infection in a susceptible host. One problem with *Serratia* has been its ability to develop resistance to antibiotics rapidly. This can have devastating consequences in an intensive care or burn unit when an outbreak occurs. Because its mode of transmission is through direct or indirect contact on the hands of personnel or on contaminated articles, good handwashing and aseptic techniques are the most effective measures to prevent outbreaks of infection.

Candida albicans is a yeastlike fungus that can cause infection, especially in immunocompromised patients or those receiving antibiotics. These patients have a decrease in the normal flora, which provides a niche for the *Candida* to settle in and proliferate. Antibiotics suppress bacterial growth but do not affect fungal growth; special antifungal agents are necessary to control these infections unless the normal flora return following discontinuance of the antibiotics.

PREVENTION AND CONTROL MEASURES

In the hospital many potential sources of infection exist, including patients, personnel, visitors, equipment, linen, and so on. Patients may become infected with organisms either from the external environment (*exogenous*) or, as is often seen in the severely immunocompromised host, from their own internal organisms (*endogenous*). Virtually any microorganism can be a potential pathogen to the immunocompromised patient. Most of the causative organisms are present in the patient's external environment and are introduced into the body through direct contact or contaminated materials. In many instances nosocomial infections could be prevented by strict aseptic technique when giving care and by greater restraint in the use of invasive procedures and antibiotics. Some specific infection control measures follow.

CONTROL OF EXTERNAL ENVIRONMENT

Health care providers should be in good health and keep their immunization status up to date. They should report to the employee health service when they feel ill. Visitors also should be in good health and should be limited to prevent overcrowding in the patient's room. Personnel should wear clean clothing and observe good personal hygiene practices, especially *thorough handwashing,* which decreases transient and resident flora on the hands and thus acts as a deterrent to cross-infection via the hands. Friction and rinsing are the two most important components of good handwashing. Ample handwashing facilities are necessary throughout the hospital and should be used by all personnel before and after patient contact; after contact with excretions, secretions, wound drainage, or any contaminated articles; and before any clean or sterile procedure or contact with clean or sterile equipment. *Handwashing is the most effective method for preventing nosocomial infection.*[23] Dermatologic conditions of the hands should be corrected, because dry, cracked skin can more readily become colonized with pathogens and broken skin is more difficult to rid of transient and resident flora. The person with a skin problem on the hands also tends to avoid proper handwashing, because it can further increase dryness and irritation. The person with active herpes simplex infection of the hand (*herpetic whitlow*) should not give direct patient care until the lesion has healed.

Housekeeping and sanitation practices should be strictly observed to reduce dust and environmental reservoirs of organisms, especially in high-risk areas such as nurseries, operating rooms, and intensive care units. Spills of blood or other body fluids should be cleaned up promptly with an approved hospital disinfectant or a 1:10 dilution of 5.25% sodium hypochlorite (household bleach and water). Linens should be changed with as little contact with the nurse's uniform as possible; linen should not be thrown on the floor or shaken in the air, because this not only will further contaminate the linen but also will stir up dust particles and create air currents that can transmit pathogens. Waste products should be disposed of in the appropriate receptacle. State and federal laws regulate the disposal of infectious waste from health care institutions. Items such as needles and syringes, laboratory cultures and tissue specimens, and other disposable items that are saturated with blood or body substances are considered infectious waste. *Infectious waste must be incinerated or treated (to render it noninfectious) before disposal.* Other waste materials from patient rooms may be disposed of as regular trash. Proper cleaning and sterilization of contaminated reusable articles and equipment are essential. A program should exist to monitor the effectiveness of these practices; however, routine culturing of the environment is not advocated.

Air is generally not considered an important factor in nosocomial cross-infection. However, in the case of *Aspergillus* spores and *Mycobacterium tuberculosis*, adequate air exchanges are necessary to reduce the number of organisms. Minimal standards for air exchanges in patient care areas are published by the Department of Health and Human Services. Minimal air changes of outdoor air per hour range from two in patient rooms to 15 in operating rooms.

CONTROL OF INTERNAL ENVIRONMENT

Reducing the *endogenous* sources of infection is more difficult than control of the external environment. Often the source is the patient's own normal flora, and these infections are not directly preventable by the nurse. Preventive measures are aimed at increasing the patient's defense mechanisms and thus decreasing the risk of the infection. Teaching the patient about good nutrition and personal hygiene is a practical measure that is part of nursing care. Maintaining the patient's normal flora and preventing colonization with pathogens that can serve as a source of infection are other effective measures. These, however, are not always possible when patients are receiving antibiotics or undergoing chemotherapy, because these measures may disrupt the normal flora and provide for colonization. Appropriate use of antibiotics for prophylaxis and treatment helps prevent colonization with pathogens and decreases the incidence of infection with drug-resistant organisms. Good handwashing by all who have contact with the patient decreases the possibility of the patient's inoculation with pathogenic organisms. Personnel should develop the habit of working from clean procedures to dirty procedures when delivering patient care. For example, the nurse should adjust the intravenous infusion rate and check the intravenous site *before* changing the bed of an incontinent patient.

PREVENTION OF URINARY TRACT INFECTIONS

As mentioned previously, urinary tract infections (UTIs) are the most common nosocomial infections seen in the hospital. Most of these infections are associated with catheterization and instrumentation of the urinary tract. Urinary catheters should be used only when absolutely necessary. If a catheter must be used, it should be discontinued as soon as medically feasible, because the longer the catheter is in place, the greater the risk of developing an infection. Strict aseptic technique is necessary when inserting the catheter to prevent transmission of bacteria into the bladder. Bacteria that are present around the catheter-meatal junction can also be transmitted on the tip of the catheter into the bladder along the thin layer of mucus that surrounds the catheter in the urethra. For this reason, the catheter should be securely anchored to prevent it from moving in and out of the urethra. Movement of the catheter can track bacteria into the urethra and up into the bladder along the mucous sheath. Furthermore, the catheter-meatal junction should be kept clean; the patient incontinent of stool can pose a problem in this regard. In some institutions, antiseptic agents are used to cleanse the meatus, and antimicrobial agents are applied around the catheter-meatal junction. *Both these practices are considered controversial.* Good handwashing techniques by personnel, cleansing of the patient's meatal area with soap and water, and proper anchoring of the catheter are considered effective ways to reduce the incidence of UTIs in patients with indwelling catheters.

Another portal of entry for bacteria is through the distal catheter–proximal drainage tube junction. Every time the system is disconnected, the risk of introducing bacteria into the system increases; thus a closed drainage system should be maintained. Bladder irrigations should not be a routine practice. If irrigation is necessary, a sterile disposable syringe and sterile solution should be used. If frequent irrigations are necessary, such as in patients who have had a transurethral prostatectomy (TURP), in which blood clots are common, a three-way catheter drainage system with continuous bladder irrigation is recommended. In this way a closed system is maintained. Urine specimens should be obtained from the rubber portal on the drainage tubing.

The portal should be cleansed with an antiseptic before insertion of the needle into the portal.

Another portal of entry of bacteria into the system is through the collection bag. The bag should be kept below the bladder level at all times to prevent reflux of urine into the bladder. It also should be kept off the floor, and the emptying spout should be cleansed with an antiseptic after the urine is emptied from the bag. The container used to collect the urine from the bag must be used for only one patient; it should not be shared between patients.

A final control measure in preventing nosocomial UTIs is to place patients with urinary catheters in separate rooms. This is helpful in preventing cross-infection between patients.

PREVENTION OF SURGICAL WOUND INFECTIONS

Surgical wound infection is primarily related to (1) the degree of contamination, endogenous or exogenous, during the surgical procedure and (2) specific host factors (underlying illnesses and the presence of a remote untreated infection at the time of surgery). The degree of contamination is related to the anatomic wound site, the wound classification, and the duration of surgery. Procedures involving the abdominal cavity, as well as wounds classified as contaminated or dirty, increase the patient's risk of surgical wound infection. Surgical procedures lasting longer than 2 hours have been shown to be the second best predictors of postoperative infection after controlling for the anatomic location of the surgery.[32] The duration of the procedure is often considered a function of the surgeon's skill and experience. The surgical wound infection rate is rarely affected by the postoperative nursing care because the closed wound serves as a barrier to further contamination from exogenous organisms. However, handwashing and aseptic technique during dressing changes are important for all personnel having contact with the surgical wound.

Studies have shown that the most effective approach to reducing surgical wound infection in both high- and low-risk patients involves two components. The first consists of (1) an ongoing surgical wound infection surveillance and control program and (2) the routine reporting of surgical wound infection rates back to the surgeons. The second component is the use of a hospital epidemiologist with specific training in hospital infection control who is an active member of the hospital infection control committee. Findings from the Project Study on the Efficacy of Nosocomial Infection Control demonstrated that hospitals with programs featuring both components had a 35% reduction in high-risk and 41% reduction in low-risk surgical wound infection rates.[31] Keeping the surgeons and operating room nurses informed about specific infection rates heightens awareness of the importance of aseptic technique and efficiency during surgery. Other measures that minimize the risk of infection include the appropriate use of prophylactic antibiotics, limiting the preoperative hospital stay, preoperative bathing with antiseptics, hair removal (preferably by depilatory or clipping) immediately before surgery, and traffic control in the operating room.

PREVENTION OF RESPIRATORY TRACT INFECTIONS

Nosocomial pneumonia occurs in approximately 0.6% of hospitalized patients (6 cases per 1000 hospital discharges) and is associated with the highest mortality rate of all nosocomial infections.[10] A major risk factor is respiratory intubation as endotracheal, nasotracheal, and tracheostomy tubes bypass the patient's defense mechanisms of the upper respiratory tract. The importance of proper maintenance and decontamination of respiratory therapy equipment in preventing nosocomial pneumonias is well established. Handwashing is essential before and after contact with patients and respiratory assist devices, which contain moisture and are ideal reservoirs for organisms, especially gram-negative species such as *Pseudomonas* and *Serratia*. Suctioning is a sterile procedure necessitating the use of sterile equipment and irrigants (see Chapter 34). Surgical procedures that lead to impaired coughing are also a risk factor. Preoperative patient teaching stressing the importance and proper technique of coughing and deep breathing is essential to the success of postoperative pulmonary toilet. Inappropriate use of antibiotics should be avoided to minimize oropharyngeal colonization with gram-negative bacteria; if aspirated, these may lead to a more serious pneumonia. Debilitated patients should be protected from the hazards of aspiration, especially while eating.

PREVENTION OF BACTEREMIAS

Many blood infections (bacteremias) occur secondary to infections at another site; thus prevention may depend greatly on control of the underlying infection. Some bacteremias are the result of the use of intravascular devices and systems. The sources of infection in these instances are the hands of personnel, the patient's skin, or infusions contaminated either from mishandling by hospital personnel or, less often, at the time of manufacture. Intravenous and intraarterial catheters should be inserted under aseptic conditions, and catheter insertion sites should be cared for aseptically. The insertion site is treated as an open wound and is inspected frequently for any sign of infection, such as redness, swelling, exudate, purulence, or warmth. The patient may also complain of pain at the site.

Central lines should have a sterile dressing to prevent contamination of the insertion site. A controversy exists over the use of transparent dressings rather than gauze dressings. Studies have shown an increase in site colonization and catheter-related infection with the use of transparent dressings.[21] Peripheral catheters should be changed every 48 to 72 hours or more often if a complication such as infiltration or phlebitis occurs. The catheter is secured to prevent in-and-out movement and tracking of bacteria into the cannula site. Aseptic technique should be followed when mixing and adding drugs, changing the infusion, or manipulating connections or stopcocks. It is recommended that the tubing also be changed every 48 to 72 hours.

Before hanging a solution, the nurse should check it for turbidity, particulate matter, and leaks in the system. Solutions should be discarded after 24 hours. Hyperalimentation solutions require special adherence to these practices because they are composed of nutrients that are an excellent culture media for organisms. *Candida* infections are frequently seen in patients receiving hyperalimentation, particularly those who are immunocompromised.

PROTECTION BY ISOLATION

The purpose of isolation is to protect both the caregiver from exposure to infectious agents and the patient from cross-infection. In 1983 The CDC published revised guidelines for isolation precautions in hospitals. Two systems were offered for use. One was based on categories of isolation, and the other listed disease-specific isolation precautions. Hospitals were advised to choose the system most appropriate for their needs. Hospitals were also given the option of devising their own system of isolation using the information and recommendations in these guidelines. The system listed seven major categories of isolation: *strict, contact, respiratory, tuberculosis (AFB), enteric, drainage/secretion,* and *blood/body fluids.* Protective isolation was eliminated as a category because it has not been shown to reduce the risk of infection in the immunocompromised patient.

The current AIDS epidemic has emphasized *the need for caregivers to consider the blood and body fluids of all patients as potentially infectious.* Although it has been shown that the risk of HIV transmission to caregivers is low, other pathogens (hepatitis A virus; hepatitis B virus; non-A, non-B hepatitis virus; cytomegalovirus; herpes simplex virus; Epstein-Barr virus; *S. aureus*) are more easily transmitted in health care settings. Infections with these agents are frequently undiagnosed at the initial contact with the patient. Therefore, taking precautions with the body fluids of all patients will protect the caregiver and reduce nosocomial transmission of pathogens. In August 1987 the CDC published new recommendations for the prevention of HIV transmission in health care settings. These guidelines recommended the elimination of a separate blood/body fluid category because these precautions are

to be taken with all patients. Some hospitals have eliminated all the isolation categories and implemented a system called *body substance isolation* (BSI). Following BSI principles will protect both the caregiver and the patient because it does not depend on diagnosis to initiate precautions. The following sections explain (1) category-specific isolation with universal blood/body fluid precautions and (2) BSI.

Table 15-6 lists information about isolation for patients with specific diseases.

CATEGORY-SPECIFIC ISOLATION WITH UNIVERSAL BLOOD/BODY FLUID PRECAUTIONS

Strict Isolation

Strict isolation is recommended only for highly transmissible diseases that are spread by direct contact and airborne routes of transmission. Some examples of disease requiring strict isolation are burn or skin wounds infected with *S. aureus* or group A *Streptococcus* organisms, when the wound drainage cannot be adequately contained by a dressing; diphtheria; disseminated herpes zoster; and staphylococcal pneumonia. Strict isolation requires that (1) the patient be in a private room with the door kept closed; (2) gowns, masks, and gloves are worn by all persons entering the room; (3) hands are washed on entering and leaving the room; and (4) all articles in the room must be placed in impervious plastic or paper bags and double bagged for disinfection or sterilization.

Respiratory Isolation

Respiratory isolation is recommended to prevent transmission of infectious diseases that primarily are carried for only short distances through the air (droplet transmission). Direct and indirect contact transmission occurs with some infections in this category but infrequently. The precautions to be practiced in respiratory isolation include placing a patient in a private room; however, patients infected with the same organism may generally share the same room. Masks are to be worn by personnel who come close to the patient, usually estimated to be within an arm's length. Gown and gloves are not indicated. Contaminated articles should be discarded or placed in a labeled plastic bag before being sent for decontamination. Personnel must wash their hands after touching the patient or potentially contaminated articles and before taking care of another patient.

Tuberculosis Isolation (AFB Isolation)

Tuberculosis isolation is indicated for patients with pulmonary tuberculosis who have a positive sputum smear for AFB or a chest roentgenogram that strongly suggests active tuberculosis. Laryngeal tuberculosis is also included in this isolation category. (See Chapter 33 for discussion and care of the patient with pulmonary tu-

TABLE 15-6 Disease/category-specific isolation with universal blood/body fluid precautions

Disease	Category	Infective Material	Duration of Precautions
Abscess, minor or limited	Drainage/secretion	Pus	Duration of illness (DOI)
AIDS	*	Blood/body fluids	DOI
Amebic dysentery	Enteric	Feces	DOI
Babesiosis	*	Blood	DOI
Burn infection, minor or limited	Drainage/secretion	Drainage	DOI
Cholera	Enteric	Feces	DOI
Colorado tick fever	*	Blood	Duration of hospitalization
Conjunctivitis			
Pink eye	Drainage/secretion	Purulent exudate	DOI
Gonococcal	Drainage/secretion	Purulent exudate	For 24 hours after effective therapy
Coxsackievirus disease	Enteric	Feces, respiratory secretions	For 7 days after onset
Creutzfeldt-Jakob disease	*	Blood, brain tissue, cerebrospinal fluid	DOI
Decubitus ulcer, infected, minor or limited	Drainage/secretion	Pus	DOI
Dengue	*	Blood	Duration of hospitalization
Diarrhea, acute, infectious cause suspected	Enteric	Feces	DOI
Diphtheria			
Cutaneous	Contact	Lesion secretion	Until 2 lesion cultures (taken 24 hours apart after antibiotics discontinued) are negative for *Corynebacterium diphtheriae*
Pharyngeal	Strict	Respiratory secretions	Same as cutaneous, except cultures obtained from nose and throat
Echovirus disease	Enteric	Feces, respiratory secretions	For 7 days after onset
Encephalitis, infectious cause suspected	Enteric	Feces	DOI or 7 days after onset
Endometritis, group A *Streptococcus*	Contact	Vaginal discharge	For 24 hours after start of effective therapy
Enterocolitis: *Clostridium difficile* or *Staphylococcus*	Enteric	Feces	DOI
Enteroviral infection	Enteric	Feces	For 7 days after onset
Epiglotitis caused by *Haemophilus influenzae*	Respiratory	Respiratory secretions	For 24 hours after start of effective therapy
Erythema infectiosum	Respiratory	Respiratory secretions	For 7 days after onset
Gastroenteritis	Enteric	Feces	
Campylobacter			DOI
Clostridium difficile			DOI
Cryptosporidium species			DOI
Dientamoeba fragilis			DOI
Escherichia coli (enteropathogenic, enterotoxic, or enteroinvasive)			DOI
Giardia lamblia			DOI
Rotavirus			DOI
Salmonella species			DOI
Shigella species			Until 3 consecutive stool cultures (taken after antimicrobials discontinued) are negative
Vibrio parahaemolyticus			DOI
Viral			DOI
Yersinia enterocolitica			DOI

From Garner JS and Simmons BT: Infect Control 4:261-283, 1983.
*Previously listed as blood/body fluid precaution category. Implementation of universal blood/body fluid precautions for all patients eliminates the need for this category.

Continued.

TABLE 15-6 Disease/category-specific isolation with universal blood/body fluid precautions—cont'd

Disease	Category	Infective Material	Duration of Precautions
Hand-foot-and-mouth disease	Enteric	Feces	DOI
Hepatitis, viral			
Type A (Infectious)	Enteric	Feces	For 7 days after onset of jaundice
Type B (serum, including hepatitis B surface antigen [HB$_s$Ag] carrier)	*	Blood/body fluids	Until HB$_s$Ag negative
Non-A, non-B	*	Blood/body fluids	DOI
Herpangina	Enteric	Feces	For 7 days after onset
Herpes simplex			
Disseminated, primary, or severe	Contact	Lesion secretion	DOI Until all lesions are crusted
Mucocutaneous, recurrent (skin, oral, genital)	Drainage/secretion	Lesion secretion	Until all lesions are crusted
Herpes zoster (varicella zoster): disseminated or localized in immunocompromised patient	Strict	Lesion secretion and possibly respiratory secretions	DOI Until all lesions are crusted
Impetigo	Contact	Lesions	For 24 hours after start of effective therapy
Lassa fever	Strict	Blood/body fluids, respiratory secretions	DOI
Leptospirosis	*	Blood, urine	Duration of hospitalization
Malaria	*	Blood	DOI
Measles (rubeola)	Respiratory	Respiratory secretions	For 4 days after start of rash; DOI in immunocompromised patients
Meningitis			
Aseptic	Enteric	Feces	For 7 days after onset
H. influenzae	Respiratory	Respiratory secretions	For 24 hours after start of effective therapy
Neisseria meningitidis (meningococcal)	Respiratory	Respiratory secretions	For 24 hours after start of effective therapy
Meningococcal pneumonia	Respiratory	Respiratory secretions	For 24 hours after start of effective therapy
Meningococcemia	Respiratory	Respiratory secretions	For 24 hours after start of effective therapy
Multiply-resistant bacteria, infection or colonization at any site with any of the following: 1. Gram-negative bacilli resistant to all aminoglycosides tested 2. Staphylococcus areus resistant to methicillin 3. Pneumococcus resistant to penicillin 4. H. influenzae resistant to ampicillin	Contact	Site of positive culture	Until antimicrobials discontinued and culture negative
Mumps	Respiratory	Respiratory secretions	For 9 days after onset of swelling
Pediculosis	Contact	Infested area	For 24 hours after start of effective therapy
Plague, pneumonic	Strict	Respiratory secretions	For 3 days after start of effective therapy
Pleurodynia	Enteric	Feces	For 7 days after onset

TABLE 15-6 Disease/category-specific isolation with universal blood/body fluid precautions—cont'd

Disease	Category	Infective Material	Duration of Precautions
Pneumonia			
S. aureus	Strict	Respiratory secretions	For 48 hours after start of effective therapy
Streptococcus, group A	Strict	Respiratory secretions	For 24 hours after start of effective therapy
Poliomyelitis	Enteric	Feces	For 7 days after onset
Rabies	Contact	Respiratory secretions	DOI
Rat-bite fever	*	Blood	For 24 hours after start of effective therapy
Relapsing fever	*	Blood	DOI
Ritter's disease (staphylococcal scalded skin syndrome)	Contact	Lesions	DOI
Rubella	Contact	Respiratory secretions	For 7 days after onset of rash
Scabies	Contact	Infested area	For 24 hours after starting effective therapy
Skin, wound, or burn infection			
Minor or limited	Drainage/secretion	Pus	DOI
Major	Contact	Pus	DOI
Smallpox	Strict	Lesions, respiratory secretions	DOI Room with special ventilation required
Syphilis, primary and secondary with skin and mucous membrane lesions	*	Lesions, blood	For 24 hours after start of effective therapy
Tuberculosis, pulmonary	Tuberculosis (AFB)	Airborne droplet nuclei	Usually within 2-3 weeks after chemotherapy begun and guided by clinical response and reduction of AFB on sputum smear; private room with special ventilation required
Typhoid fever (*Salmonella typhi*)	Enteric	Feces	DOI
Varicella (chickenpox)	Strict	Lesions, respiratory secretions	Until all lesions are crusted
Viral pericarditis	Enteric	Feces, possibly respiratory secretions	For 7 days after onset

berculosis.) In general, infants and young children with active pulmonary tuberculosis do not require isolation because they rarely cough and their broncheal secretions do not contain many AFB.[29]

The precautions to be practiced in tuberculosis isolation include placing the patient in a private room with the door closed. The room should be equiped with special ventilation so that the room air is exhausted to the outside and not recirculated through the hospital. Masks are indicated if the patient is coughing and does not reliably cover the mouth. Gowns and gloves are not routinely indicated. Proper handwashing is required before touching articles. Procedures such as bronchoscopy and dental examinations are generally postponed until the patient has received approximately 2 weeks of appropriate antituberculosis therapy and is no longer considered infectious.

Contact Isolation

Contact isolation is designed to prevent transmission of infectious diseases or multiply-resistant microorganisms that are spread by close or direct contact. Personnel are advised to wear a mask, gown, and gloves when in close or direct contact with a patient who has an infection or colonization that requires contact isolation. A private room is required; however, patients with identical infections may share the same room. Patients colonized with epidemiologically important multiply-resistant microorganisms (*Serratia marcescens*, methicillin-resistant *S. aureus*) generally require contact isolation for the duration of the hospital stay. The infection control practitioner can help in determining which patients have the same strains, as determined by an identically matching antibiotic-sensitivity pattern.

Enteric Precautions

Enteric precautions are designed to prevent transmission of disease through direct or indirect contact with infected feces or heavily contaminated articles. Pathogens are spread from contaminated hands to mouth, where they are ingested. Precautions to be practiced primarily consist of thorough handwashing after any patient contact. Gloves should be worn when handling infective excreta or objects contaminated with feces. Masks are not required. Gowns are indicated only if clothing may be soiled with feces. A private room is required when the patient does not practice good hygiene measures, such as handwashing after using the bathroom.

Drainage/Secretion Precautions

Drainage/secretion precautions are designed to prevent the transmission of microorganisms from the direct contact with a patient's wound drainage. The infectious diseases included in this category result in the production of purulent drainage from any body site that does not require more extensive precautions. Infected wounds are generally minor or limited, in which the drainage is contained within the dressing. Personnel are advised to wear gloves when in direct contact with the infective material. Contaminated articles should be discarded or placed in a plastic bag, which is labeled before sending for decontamination. Gowns are indicated if clothing is likely to become contaminated with the infective material. Masks are not required. The patient does not require a private room for this category of isolation.

Universal Blood/Body Fluid Precautions

Universal precautions are intended to protect health caregivers from exposure to blood-borne pathogens. The body fluids to which universal precautions apply are blood, semen, vaginal secretions, cerebrospinal fluid, synovial fluid, pleural fluid, peritoneal fluid, pericardial fluid, amniotic fluid, tissues, and other body fluids containing visible blood. These precautions are to be used in the care of all patients. This practice consists of wearing protective barriers and depends on the anticipated contact with blood and the body fluids mentioned. Gloves are worn for touching blood/body fluids and are changed after each patient contact. Masks and protective eyewear or face shields should be worn during procedures likely to generate droplets of blood/body fluids to prevent exposure of mucous membranes of the mouth, nose, and eyes. Gowns or aprons are worn during procedures likely to cause splashes of blood/body fluids. Hands and other body surfaces should be washed if contaminated with these fluids. Care should be taken to prevent injuries from needles or other contaminated sharp instruments. Contaminated needles should not be recapped, bent, or broken; removed from disposable syringes; or otherwise manipulated by hand. Used needles and other sharp items (scalpel blades, lancets) should be placed in puncture-resistant containers, which should be located as close to the point of use as possible.

BODY SUBSTANCE ISOLATION

In 1984 Jackson and Lynch[33] described a system of isolation that emphasizes precautions with the body substances (blood, sputum, urine, feces, pus, drainage, and so on) of *all* patients. They recognized that the colonized patient, not only the diagnosed patient, is a potential source of cross-infection. Therefore the practice of BSI provides better protection for patients and caregivers against the transmission of unrecognized communicable disease.

TABLE 15-7 Body substance isolation (BSI) techniques

Item	Precautions
Gloves	Worn for contact with mucous membranes, non-intact skin, and moist body substances; changed after each patient contact
Gown or plastic apron	Worn if soiling of clothing is likely
Mask and eye protection	Worn if mucous membranes may be splashed with body substances
Private room*	Indicated if personal hygiene is poor or if body substances contaminate the environment
Needles	Disposed of uncapped and unbent at point of use in puncture-resistant container
Soiled linen	Placed in leak-proof bags; gown and gloves worn by laundry workers sorting all soiled linen
Reusable equipment	Bagged for transport to decontamination area; gown, gloves, mask, and eye protection worn by decontamination workers
Trash	Bagged to prevent leakage; sharp items, laboratory waste, and disposable items saturated with body substances discarded in infectious waste containers

Modified from Lynch P and Jackson M: Isolation practices: how much is too much or not enough? Asepsis: Infect Control Forum 8(4):2-5, 1986.
*Airborne-transmitted diseases still necessitate private patient room with sign to alert persons entering. Special ventilation such as negative pressure indicated. Mask is required to enter room of patient with pulmonary tuberculosis or meningococcal disease. Only immune persons should enter room of patient with chickenpox.

Precautions should be determined by the anticipated interactions with a patient's body substances. Under this system, labeling patients with diagnosed infections would be a hindrance and support a double standard of practice. For example, a double standard exists when caregivers wear gloves when handling the urine of a patient with diagnosed *Serratia* UTI but not when handling the urine of other patients. Any patient may carry this or other resistant pathogens which are never diagnosed unless a urine culture is obtained. (See Table 15-7 for BSI techniques.)

GENERAL PRINCIPLES OF ISOLATION

Some general principles apply regardless of the type of isolation. Barriers such as gowns, gloves, and masks should be used only once and then discarded in an appropriate receptacle before leaving the patient's room. These barriers should be conveniently available for each patient room. *Hands must be washed before and after each patient contact even when gloves are worn.*

One can see the similarities between the CDC's universal blood/body fluid precautions and BSI. The difference is that BSI does not require the other categories except for airborne-transmitted diseases because BSI technique will prevent the transmission of diseases in the other categories. Redundancy exists in the CDC's category-specific and universal blood/body fluid precaution system. Nurses will need to determine which system is being used in their health care setting.

CHAPTER SUMMARY

- Infection control programs exist to decrease morbidity, mortality, and cost of nosocomial infections.
- The sequence of events in the chain of infection involve (a) a causative agent, (b) a reservoir, (c) a portal of exit, (d) a mode of transmission, (e) a portal of entry, and (f) a susceptible host.
- Modes of transmission are (a) contact (direct, indirect, droplet), (b) airborne, (c) vehicle, and (d) vector.
- Fever and a WBC count greater than 10,000/mm³ may indicate a generalized infection.
- When possible, appropriate cultures should be obtained before initiating antibiotic therapy.
- In the United States the ACIP recommends that children be immunized against diphtheria, tetanus, pertussis (DTP); measles, mumps, rubella (MMR); poliomyelitis (OPV); and *haemophilus influenzae* (HbCV).
- Health caregivers who have frequent contact with blood and body fluids should be immunized against hepatitis B virus.

- Passive immunity is temporary, lasting a few weeks without stimulating antibody production in the recipient.
- In general, live attenuated virus vaccines should not be given to persons with alterations in immune status.
- A nosocomial infection is not present or incubating when a person is admitted to the hospital but develops after admission.
- Handwashing is the most important measure in preventing cross-infection.
- Urinary catheterization is associated with increased risk for nosocomial urinary tract infection.
- Nosocomial pneumonia occurs in approximately 0.6% of hospitalized patients and is associated with the highest mortality rate of all nosocomial infections.
- Aseptic technique is an important factor in preventing nosocomial infection.
- Two systems of isolation are (1) category-specific isolation with universal blood/body fluid precautions and (2) body substance isolation (BSI).
- Adherence to universal blood/body fluid precautions or BSI is the best protection that caregivers have from occupationally acquired blood-borne infections.
- Caregivers should direct problems concerning any aspect of infection control to the infection control nurse, the hospital epidemiologist, or the infection control committee in their institution.

QUESTIONS TO CONSIDER

- Define the following terms: (1) active immunity, (2) active acquired immunity, (3) passive immunity, and (4) herd immunity.
- What is the danger in giving live virus vaccines to immunocompromised persons?
- List six factors that place a hospitalized patient at risk for developing a nosocomial infection.
- What is the most common nosocomial infection? What measures could nurses take to reduce the incidence of this nosocomial infection?
- What measures can nurses take to prevent occupationally acquired infectious diseases?

REFERENCES AND SELECTED READINGS

1. Albert RK and Condie F: Handwashing patterns in medical intensive care units, N Engl J Med 304:1465-1466, 1981.
2. American Academy of Pediatrics: Report of the Committee on the Control of Infectious Diseases, ed 19, Evanston, Ill, 1982, the Academy.
3. American Hospital Association: Infection control in the hospital, ed 4, Chicago, 1979, The Association.
4. American Public Health Association: Control of communicable disease in man, ed 14, New York, 1985, The Association.
5. Band JD and Maki DG: Safety of changing intravenous delivery systems at intervals longer than 24 hours, Ann Intern Med 91:173, 1979.
6. Bennett JV and Brachmann PS, editors: Hospital infections, Boston, 1986, Little, Brown & Co.
7. Berg R, editor: The APIC Curriculum for Infection Control Practice, vol III, Dubuque, Iowa, 1988, Kendall/Hunt Publishing Co.
8. Buxton J et al: Contamination of intravenous infusion fluids: effects of changing administration sets, Ann Intern Med 90:764, 1979.
9. Castle M: Hospital infection control, New York, 1980, John Wiley & Sons, Inc.
10. Centers for Disease Control: National infection surveillance, 1980-1982, MMWR CDC Surveill Summ 32:445, 1983, and National infection surveillance, 1984, MMWR CDC Surveill Summ 35:18, 1986.
11. Centers for Disease Control: Recommendations of the Advisory Committee on Immunization Practices (ACIP): update: pneumococcal polysaccharide vaccine usage, MMWR 33(20):273-281, 1984.
12. Centers for Disease Control: Recommendations of the ACIP: smallpox vaccine, MMWR 34(23):341-342, 1985.
13. Centers for Disease Control: Nosocomial infection surveillance, 1984, MMWR 35(SS-1):17-29, 1986.
14. *Centers for Disease Control: Recommendation of the ACIP: update on hepatitis B prevention, MMWR 36(23):353-366, 1987.
15. *Centers for Disease Control: Recommendations for prevention of HIV transmission in health-care settings, MMWR 36(S-2), 1987.
16. *Centers for Disease Control: Update: universal precautions for prevention of transmission of human immunodeficiency virus, hepatitis B virus, and other bloodborne pathogens in health-care settings, MMWR 37(24):377-388, 1988.
17. Centers for Disease Control: Recommendations of the ACIP: measles prevention: supplementary statement, MMWR 38(1):11-14, 1989.
18. Centers for Disease Control: Recommendations of the ACIP: general recommendations on immunization, MMWR 38(13):205-227, 1989.
19. Centers for Disease Control: Recommendations of the ACIP: prevention and control of influenza. Part 1. Vaccines, MMWR 38(17):297-311, 1989.
20. A clinician's dictionary of bacteria and fungi, Indianapolis, 1986, Eli Lilly Co.
21. *Conly JM, Grieves K, and Peters B: A prospective, randomized study comparing transparent and dry gauze dressings for central venous catheters, J Infect Dis 159(2):310-319, 1989.
22. Dixon RE, editor: Nosocomial infections, New York, 1981, Yorke Medical Books.
23. Dixon RE: Nosocomial respiratory infections, Infect Control 4:376-381, 1983.
24. Farke BF, Kaiser DL, and Wenzel RP: Relationship between surgical volume and incidence of postoperative wound infection, N Engl J Med 305:200-204, 1981.
25. Fernsebner B: Antimicrobial therapy for surgical patients, AORN J 36:479-486, 1982.
26. Fernsebner B: Patients at risk for nosocomial infections, AORN J 38:613-620, 1983.
27. Friedland, GH and Klein, RS: Transmission of human immunodeficiency virus, N Engl J Med 317(18):1125-1135, 1987.
28. Garbaldi RA et al: Meatal colonization and catheter-associated bacteremia, N Engl J Med 303:316-318, 1980.
29. Garner JS and Simmons BP: Guidelines for isolation precautions in hospitals, Infect Control 4(4):245-325, 1983.
30. *Gerberding JL et al: Risk of transmitting the human immunodeficiency virus, cytomegalovirus, and hepatitis B virus to health care workers exposed to patients with AIDS and AIDS-related conditions, J Infect Dis 156(1):1-8, 1987.
31. Haley RW et al: The efficacy of infection surveillance and control programs in preventing nosocomial infections in US hospitals, Am J Epidemiol 121(2):182-205, 1985.
32. Haley RW et al: Identifying patients at high risk of surgical wound infection, Am J Epidemiol 121(2):206-215, 1985.
33. *Jackson MM and Lynch P: Infection control: too much or too little? Am J Nurs 84:208-210, 1984.
34. *Jackson MM et al: Why not treat all body substances as infectious? Am J Nurs 87(9):1137-1139, 1987.
35. Kunin C: Detection, prevention, and management of urinary tract infections, ed 4, Philadelphia, 1987, Lea & Febiger.
36. Larson E: Clinical microbiology and infection control, St Louis, 1984, Blackwell Scientific Publications.
37. Mandell GL, Douglas RG, and Bennett JE: Principles and practice of infectious diseases, ed 3, New York, 1990, Churchill Livingstone, Inc.
38. Mooney BR and Armington LC: Infection control—how to prevent nosocomial infections, 50(9): 20-23, 1987.
39. Simmons BP et al: CDC guidelines for the prevention and control of nosocomial infections—guidelines for the prevention of intravascular infections, Am J Infect Control 11(5):1983-1999, 1983.
40. Smith PW, editor: Infection control in long-term care facilities, New York, 1984, John Wiley & Sons, Inc.
41. Soule BM, editor: The APIC Curriculum for Infection Control Practice, vols I and II, Dubuque, Iowa, 1983, Kendall/Hunt Publishing Co.
42. Williams WW: Guideline for infection control in hospital personnel, Infect Control 4(4):326-349, 1983.
43. Wong ES: CDC guidelines for the prevention and control of nosocomial infections: guidelines for prevention of catheter associated urinary tract infections, Am J Infect Control 11(1):26-36, 1983.

*References preceded by an asterisk are particularly well suited for student reading.

CHAPTER 16

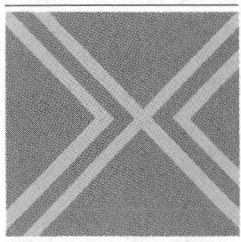

Pain

VIRGINIA BURKE KARB

CHAPTER OBJECTIVES

After studying this chapter, the student should be able to:
1 Provide a definition of pain.
2 Give examples of terms used to describe pain.
3 Identify factors that influence pain.
4 Define *pain threshold*.
5 Discuss perception of pain and reaction to pain.
6 Discuss the influence of fear on pain.
7 Elaborate on factors that influence a nurse's reaction to pain.
8 List three theories of pain transmission, and elaborate on the gate control theory as the most widely utilized.
9 Explain endorphins and enkephalins.
10 Differentiate between types of pain, including somatic, visceral, referred, psychogenic, and others.
11 Outline one taxonomy of pain.
12 Describe subjective and objective data appropriate to the nursing assessment of the patient in pain.
13 Give examples of pain rating scales.
14 Develop nursing diagnoses for the patient in pain.
15 Develop realistic patient outcomes for the patient in pain.
16 Outline examples of nursing interventions that may be used to assist the patient in pain. These interventions can be grouped under three headings: those that modify the pain stimulus; those that alter the mode of transmission; and those that modify the reaction to pain.
17 Describe treatment approaches used at pain clinics.

Pain is a two-edged sword. On the one hand, it warns us to move away from heat, cold, and sharp objects before injury occurs, and it makes us aware of the presence of disease and tissue damage; thus it usually influences us to seek medical attention. On the other hand, fear of pain may cause us to delay medical treatment, and if its cause cannot be located and relieved, its presence serves no useful purpose and it becomes harmful. Continuous, severe pain eventually causes physical and mental exhaustion and prevents the individual from functioning productively. Pain accompanies almost all illnesses, and perhaps no sensation is more dreaded by patients undergoing medical treatment or surgery.

Pain has never been satisfactorily defined or understood. It is an unpleasant feeling, entirely subjective, which only the person experiencing it can describe. It can be evoked by many stimuli (chemical, thermal, electrical, or mechanical), but the reaction to it cannot be measured objectively. Pain is a learned experience that is influenced by the entire life situation of each person. What is perceived as pain and the reaction to that pain differ among people and sometimes differ in the same person from one time to another.

Care of patients suffering pain demands skill in both the science and the art of nursing. The nurse's responsibility is to make the patient as comfortable as possible and to observe and report findings so that they may help the physician to make a correct diagnosis and prescribe appropriate treatment.[6,20]

CONCEPTS OF PAIN

DEFINITION OF PAIN

Sternbach[85,86] describes pain as an abstract concept that refers to sensation, stimulus, and response. There is also an emotion of pain in addition to the sensation of pain. It is probably not necessary to have an elaborate definition of pain in order to provide nursing care to a patient in pain. McCaffery states: "Pain is whatever the experiencing person says it is, existing whenever he says it does."[49,50] The nurse frequently sees patients in pain and must learn to use effective strategies to describe or eliminate pain and to help patients cope with pain.

SIGNIFICANCE AND FREQUENCY OF PAIN

Pain serves a major function by alerting us to possible harm or damage. It may or may not influence us to seek medical attention. Pain may have other meanings for an individual: the possible loss of mobility or activity, the recurrence of a particular disease, or the reminder that the individual is aging. Pain may precipitate feelings of fear, anger, uneasiness, challenge, or punishment. Other individuals may see pain as an opportunity for creative expression, for self-searching, for self-testing, or for fostering an appreciation of what less fortunate patients have gone through.

In general, however, most persons view pain as a negative experience. Below is a list of the top 20 words used to describe pain as listed by 148 patients.[13]

Treacherous	Hidden	Variety of words mean-
Mean	Obnoxious	ing satanic
Hateful	Faceless	Nasty
Detestable	Degrading	Sharp
Sneaky	Cruel	Cunning
Intense	Inconsiderate	Nervous
Dark	Invading	Persistent

Factors that influence the meaning of pain to an individual are many and varied. Some of these include age,[8] sex,[55] cultural background,[43,55,60,77] psychosocial factors,[55,60] environmental factors, expected response, setting,[55] and other assorted problems and diagnoses.

The setting in which pain occurs may be important. For example, a professional athlete injured in an athletic event may be in such pain that he has to withdraw from the event. A soldier injured in wartime activities may see injury and concomitant pain as relatively minor if the injury also means relief from the pressure of battle and a possible return home.[6]

Pain is experienced by most individuals at various times throughout life. It may be the result of or associated with such factors as trauma, exposure to excessive heat or cold, excessive strain or use of body parts (as in the person who exercises vigorously), normal body functions such as labor and delivery, and surgical intervention. Most individuals try to avoid pain but at the same time expect that it will occur with various activities.

PAIN THRESHOLD

Pain threshold refers to the intensity of the noxious stimulus necessary for the person to perceive pain. For many years, it was felt that the pain threshold was approximately the same for all individuals, but it is now recognized that the pain threshold is highly subjective.[49] It is important to note that the intensity of the pain is not related to the intensity of the noxious stimulus, and furthermore, most experts in the field agree that pain can exist without tissue damage or demonstrable noxious stimulation.[24,31] For example, the *severe pain of tic douloureaux* can be initiated by only a light touch on the face. The tolerance for pain, on the other hand, refers to "the duration time or the intensity of which a subject accepts a stimulus above the pain threshold before making a verbal or overt pain response."[85] McCaffery defines tolerance for pain as "the greatest stimulus intensity causing pain that a subject is prepared to tolerate."[49]

Tolerance of pain may be raised by alcohol, drugs, hypnosis, warmth, rubbing, or distracting activities.

Strong beliefs and faith seem to increase tolerance for pain, and it is sometimes difficult to judge how much pain a patient with a deep religious faith is actually experiencing. Fatigue, anger, boredom, and apprehension may decrease one's ability to tolerate pain. Pain tolerance also is lowered by persistent pain such as that sometimes experienced by patients with far-advanced carcinoma. A weak, debilitated patient usually tolerates pain less well than a healthy person, although increasing debility will eventually cause mental dulling with a resultant decrease in pain perception.

PERCEPTION OF PAIN

The perception of pain, or the actual feeling of pain, takes place in the cerebral cortex. It is known that a functioning frontal lobe of the brain is required to experience the full suffering and worry that result from pain. The reaction to the same stimuli differs widely among people and in the same person from one time to another because the final perception of pain depends more on the interpretation in the cerebral cortex than on the characteristics of the original stimuli. What the cerebral cortex interprets as pain depends on childhood training, previous experience, cultural values, religious beliefs, physical and mental health, knowledge and understanding, attention and distraction, fatigue, anxiety, tension, fear, state of consciousness, and the frequency and intensity of pain impulses.

Atrophy of nerve endings, degenerative changes in the pain-bearing pathways, and decreased alertness may reduce the perception of pain in the elderly, and more stimulation may be required to evoke a response. Elderly persons therefore may fail to perceive tissue damage that normally would cause pain and thus alert a younger person.

The perception of a pain stimulus may be altered at many points by both normal and abnormal conditions. A pleasant environment, an enjoyable book, stimulating conversation, or other distracting activities of a pleasing nature may serve to lessen the sensation of pain. Tissue damage or inflammatory conditions at the site where the stimuli originate may increase or decrease the impulse. For example, slapping a person who has a sunburn may set off a far greater impulse than if the person were not sunburned. On the other hand, if the local nerve endings have been damaged by a severe burn, the patient may not respond at all to what would ordinarily be painful stimuli. Abnormal conditions within the spinal cord such as inflammatory diseases, tumors, or injuries may prevent transmission of nerve impulses. This may occur at either the spinal or the thalamic relay stations. The impulse may also be altered at either of these two relay stations by other activity going on simultaneously within the spinal cord. This probably accounts for the fact that bruises and cuts sustained during absorbing activities sometimes go unnoticed until the activity is over. Perception of pain by the cortex may be influenced by abnormal conditions such as inflammatory processes, degenerative changes, and depression of brain function, which may alter the original signal pattern. Anesthesia and analgesia also cause depression of sensory perceptions.

REACTION TO PAIN

Meaning and perception of pain are accompanied by reaction to pain. Reaction to pain also is influenced by such factors as past experience, conditioning, cultural values, and physical and mental health. Consequently, people respond differently to the same stimuli. Some may be fearful, apprehensive, and anxious, whereas others are tolerant and optimistic. Some weep, moan, scream, beg for relief or help, threaten to destroy themselves, thrash about in bed, or move about aimlessly while they are in severe pain. Others lie quietly in bed and may only close their eyes, grit their teeth, bite their lips, clench their hands, or perspire profusely when experiencing pain.

Some people, by training and example, are taught to endure severe pain without reacting outwardly. American Indian men undergo rites in which they show their strength by the amount of pain they can endure. Such individuals probably tolerate pain from disease or injury better than those from a culture in which free expression of feelings is encouraged. Persons from cultures in which health teaching and disease prevention are emphasized tend to accept pain as a warning to seek help and expect that the cause will be found and cured.

Parents' attitudes toward pain may determine their children's lifelong reaction to pain. In the American culture, parents usually begin to teach their children what is expected of them in regard to courage and self-control at about 2 or 3 years of age. They try not to appear too concerned about minor injuries and usually encourage their children not to cry when they are hurt. Children try very hard to be brave, especially in the presence of other children.

The setting in which injury occurs may influence the external response to pain. A child may feel, for example, that the pain suffered from injury during a hockey game, although perhaps severe, should nevertheless be borne quietly, whereas pain resulting from an automobile accident can be expressed freely.

INFLUENCE OF FEAR

Morbid fear of a disease may intensify pain caused by it, or it may lead individuals to deny pain in their eagerness to believe that nothing is wrong.[84] Anticipation of pain based on past experience often intensifies pain. For example, a boy who enters the hospital for the last of several operations may react more vigorously to postop-

erative pain then he did on his first encounter with the sensation.

One's personality also influences reaction to pain. A person who reacts hysterically to trying situations may find even a small amount of pain intolerable. People may sometimes use moderate pain as an escape from unacceptable life situations, or they may try to use it to control situations around them. This latter reaction is often demonstrated both in the hospital and at home.

There is more reaction to pain during the night and early morning hours when the person's physiologic processes are at a low ebb and there is little distracting activity. Patients' thoughts may easily turn to concern for themselves and loved ones, and worrying may increase their reaction to pain.

Age affects the patient's reaction to pain. The young fear it because it may represent an unfamiliar experience, and they frequently respond to it by crying. Older persons may know what to expect and accept it, or they may be withdrawn and quiet while experiencing it because of emotional exhaustion.

THE NURSE'S REACTION TO PAIN

Just as the patients who experience pain are products of their age, culture, religion, environment, and other factors, the nurses working with them are also products of comparable factors.[20,33,75] Nurses must learn to recognize personal biases and expectations about patients to improve their objectivity and ultimately their nursing care. For example, a nurse who personally values an approach to pain described as "suffering in silence" may be unconsciously intolerant of the patient who expresses pain by crying and complaining.

Another problem the nurse must be alert to is the tendency to categorize patients on the basis of a certain criterion and then to assume that all patients meeting this criterion respond the same way. Examples of this include expectations that Oriental persons are always stoic, that American Indians do not express pain openly, that Puerto Ricans are always emotionally expressive, or that patients with low back pain complain a lot.[15,43,77,100] If a nurse meets a patient who does respond according to the stereotype, the stereotype is reinforced. The danger is that the nurse will administer care on the basis of category rather than on the basis of individualized assessment.

Some nurses also begin to develop expectations about the amount of pain the patient can be expected to have on the basis of the diagnosis and are intolerant of patients who exceed these expectations. Consider the following true example.

An elderly woman who fell and broke her hip was medicated liberally, when she requested it, for the first 2 days following surgery to repair the fracture. When, after 6 days, she continued to request frequent medication for pain, she found the nurses hostile, sarcastic, purposely slow in preparing and administering medication, and making statements such as, "You're 6 days post-op, you don't need all this medication." In addition, the nurses discussed the patient's apparent addiction to narcotics. The physician, too, was intolerant of the patient's requests for medication. It was then discovered that the surgically implanted hip prosthesis had slipped out of place. The patient had been forced to endure an improperly fitting prosthesis, which caused continued pain, as well as inappropriate remarks from the nurses.

Although this story illustrates several unfortunate problems, it points out that the nurses failed to remember that pain exists whenever the patient says it does, and also that *each* patient must be assessed on an individual basis *each* time the patient reports the existence of pain.

These examples are included as a reminder that the nurse must be vigilant about personal expectations, biases, and factors that may interfere with the nurse's ability to deliver individualized nursing care. A recent research report discusses the effect of a patient's culture on the nurse's inference of suffering (see the research box below).

THEORIES OF PAIN TRANSMISSION

People have been studying pain and attempting to develop theories of pain transmission for centuries. Three major theories are mentioned briefly; the specificity theory, the pattern theory, and the gate control theory. None of these provides all the answers to explain pain transmission, but many recent experiments in pain therapy have been based on the gate control theory.

The *specificity theory* holds that there are certain specific nerve receptors that respond to noxious stimuli and that these noxious stimuli are always interpreted as pain. In addition, this theory states that pain impulses are carried by pain fibers—fast, myelinated alpha-delta (A-δ) fibers and more slowly conducting unmyelinated C fibers—to the lateral spinothalamic tract in the spinal cord to a pain center in the thalamus. Impulses are then sent to the cerebral cortex by way of the corticothalamic tract, where the actual perception of pain takes place (Figure 16-1). Opponents of this theory point out that

---

RESEARCH

Davitz LL and Davitz JR: Culture and nurses' inferences of suffering. In Copp LA, editor: Recent advances in nursing, vol 11, New York, 1985, Churchill Livingstone.

In the first part of this study, practicing nurses were asked to read a vignette describing a patient and injury and to rate the degree of physical pain and psychologic distress that they felt the patient was experiencing. The vignettes described patients from six backgrounds (Oriental, Mediterranean, Black, Spanish, Anglo-Saxon/Germanic, and Jewish) and three levels of injury—mild, moderate, and severe. The study found that the background of the patient was a statistically significant factor that nurses used in determining the degree of suffering by these patients. In other words, when physical condition, age, and sex of the patient were controlled for, nurses judged patients of different backgrounds to have different degrees of suffering.

In the second part of the study, 1440 nurses from 13 countries rated 60 vignettes, with the research question asking: Do nurses from country X caring for a patient from country X with a certain medical problem assess the patient's degree of suffering the same as nurses from country Y might assess a patient from country Y with the same medical problem? The researchers found that nurses from different countries differ in their assessment of suffering.

These studies support the idea that nurses may generalize about the degree of suffering patients experience based on knowledge of the person's ethnic or cultural background and that nurses from different cultures may have different beliefs about the severity of pain experienced by patients. Nurses must examine their own beliefs about pain in order to be more objective in assessing the pain of others. ■

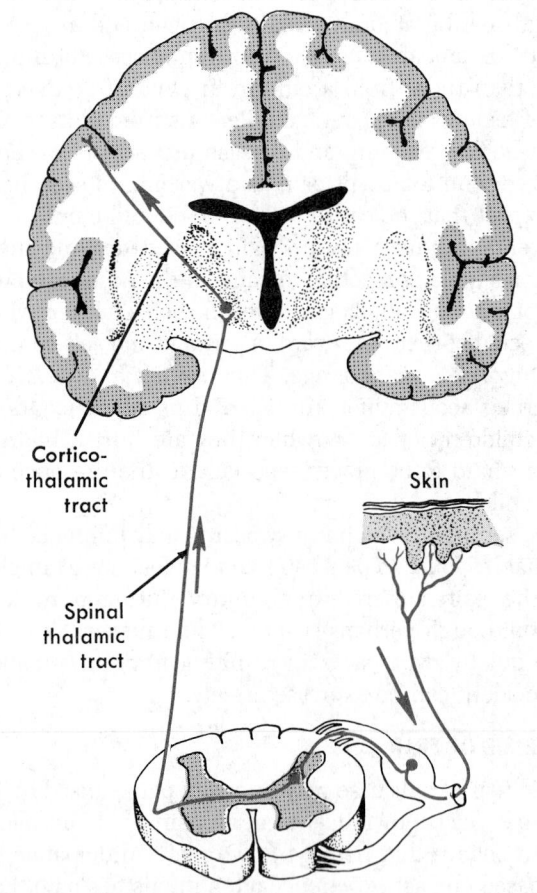

FIGURE 16-1 Pathways of pain transmission according to specificity theory.

specific pain receptors have not been identified and that the body does not always interpret certain stimuli as noxious.

In the *pattern theory,* it is thought that pain results from the combined effects of stimulus intensity and a critical summation of these impulses in the dorsal horns of the spinal cord. In other words, a pattern of impulses is transmitted to the cortex and is there perceived as pain.[9,36,62] This theory is considered to be vague.[9]

In 1965, Melzack and Wall[62] proposed the *gate control theory,* which has been revised or modified several times since then.[57,59,60,82] This theory proposes that pain and its perception depend on the *interaction of three systems*: the *substantia gelatinosa* in the dorsal horn of the spinal cord, which modulates impulses entering the spinal cord; a *central control system in the cortex and thalamus,* which influences the impulses reaching the brain; and the *neural system associated* with *perception of pain.* The theory proposes that pain impulses are conducted over small-diameter fibers to the spinal cord, travel across an "opened gate" in the substantia gelatinosa to the anterolateral spinothalamic tract, and then ascend the tract to the thalamus and cortex, where pain perception and interpretation occur. The "gate" in the substantia gelatinosa can be "closed" (Figure 16-2) so that no contact is made, thus interrupting the pain impulse. This gate can be closed by conflicting impulses from the skin conducted over large-diameter fibers, by impulses from the reticular formation in the brainstem, or by impulses from the entire cortex or thalamus (central control system). Thus impulses from the peripheral fibers, brainstem, thalamus, or cortex can effectively block the transmission of pain impulses or can intensify the impulse. In this manner, such variables as thoughts (cognition) and past experiences can modify or intensify the pain experience.

Although the gate control theory was revolutionary and has become a classic pain theory, it does not completely explain pain transmission. Newer research has focused on studying nerves and nerve transmission. The term *nociceptor* is used to describe the receptors that detect tissue injury.[67] In a cutaneous nerve, about 50% of the sensory fibers have nociceptive function.[11] Both A-δ and C fibers are involved in nociceptive input.[42]

Other factors now being studied include the neurotransmitters involved in nociceptive processing. Included in these transmitters are H^+ ions, serotonin, histamine, bradykinin, prostaglandins, and substance P, all of which have excitatory effects on nociceptors.[11] Some readers will recognize that many categories of medications have effects on one or more of these substances. For example, antihistamines block some actions of histamine, and salicylate, a product of the hydrolysis of aspirin, is a reversible inhibitor of prostaglandin synthesis. Further research into these neurotransmitters may provide help in understanding pharmacologic interventions for pain relief.[36]

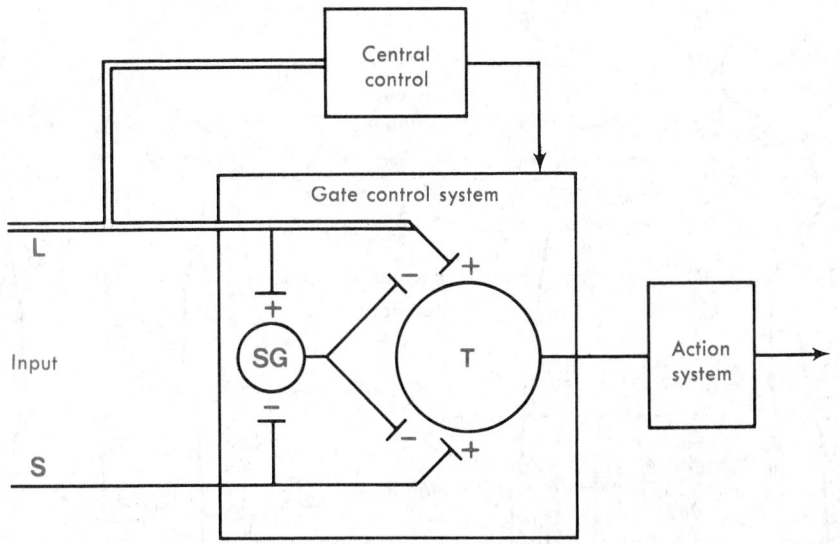

FIGURE 16-2 Schema of gate control theory of pain mechanisms. *L,* Large-diameter fibers; *S,* small-diameter fibers. Fibers project to substantia gelatinosa *(SG)* and first central transmission *(T)* cells. Inhibitory effect exerted by SG on afferent fiber terminals is increased by activity in L fibers and decreased by activity in S fibers. Central control processes project to gate control system. They include fibers from brainstem, which have predominantly inhibitory effect, as well as fibers from cortex. T cells project to entry cells of actions system. +, Excitation; −, Inhibition. (From Weisenberg M: Pain: clinical and experimental perspectives, St Louis, 1975, The CV Mosby Co; after Melzack and Wall.)

ENDORPHINS

The brain and spinal cord contain receptors to which morphine binds. Discovery of these receptors led researchers to seek endogenous substances resembling morphine that would also bind to these receptors. In 1975, researchers discovered small polypeptides called enkephalins that appeared to have morphinelike action. Further research led to the discovery of larger peptides labeled endorphins (a combination of the words *endogenous* and *morphine*).

It is now known that the opioid receptor system is more complex than first thought. There are two recognized opioid peptide systems in the brain. The enkephalins are found in the corpus striatum, periaqueductal gray matter of the brainstem, and dorsal horns of the spinal cord. The enkephalins have a short half-life and are concerned with pain modulation. The peptide β-endorphin is found in the anterior pituitary gland, medial thalamus, and central brainstem and has a much longer half-life than the enkephalins.

The complete significance of the endorphins is still unclear, but studies show that they may influence or be associated with pain relief from analgesics, electrical stimulators, acupuncture, and other methods. Patients with chronic pain may have lower levels of endorphins.[95]

TYPES OF PAIN
SOMATIC PAIN

Pain may originate in superficial structures, such as the skin and subcutaneous tissue, or in deeper structures, such as muscles or bone. Cutaneous pain may be either sharp and well localized if conducted by the fast A-δ fibers or diffuse and dull-aching if conducted by the slower C fibers. Deep somatic pain is poorly localized and may be accompanied by nausea, diaphoresis, and blood pressure changes.[67]

VISCERAL PAIN

Pain from the viscera is poorly localized, is associated with nausea and autonomic symptoms, and often radiates or is referred. Visceral pain is rarely caused by stimulation at a single point but responds to stimulation at many sites. For example, the intestines could be cut without the person experiencing pain, whereas pressure at many sites, such as occurs with distention of the viscera, causes pain. Other causes of visceral pain are ischemia, spasms, or chemical irritants. Visceral pain may initiate contractions of adjacent muscles, such as the abdominal wall; thus abdominal rigidity may be observed with inflammation of abdominal viscera.

REFERRED PAIN

Referred pain is pain that is felt in areas other than those stimulated. It may occur when stimulation is not perceived in the primary area. For example, the person experiencing a heart attack may complain only of pain radiating down the left arm when in fact the tissue damage is occurring in the myocardium.

Referred pain seems to occur most often with damage or injury to visceral organs, and the pain is referred

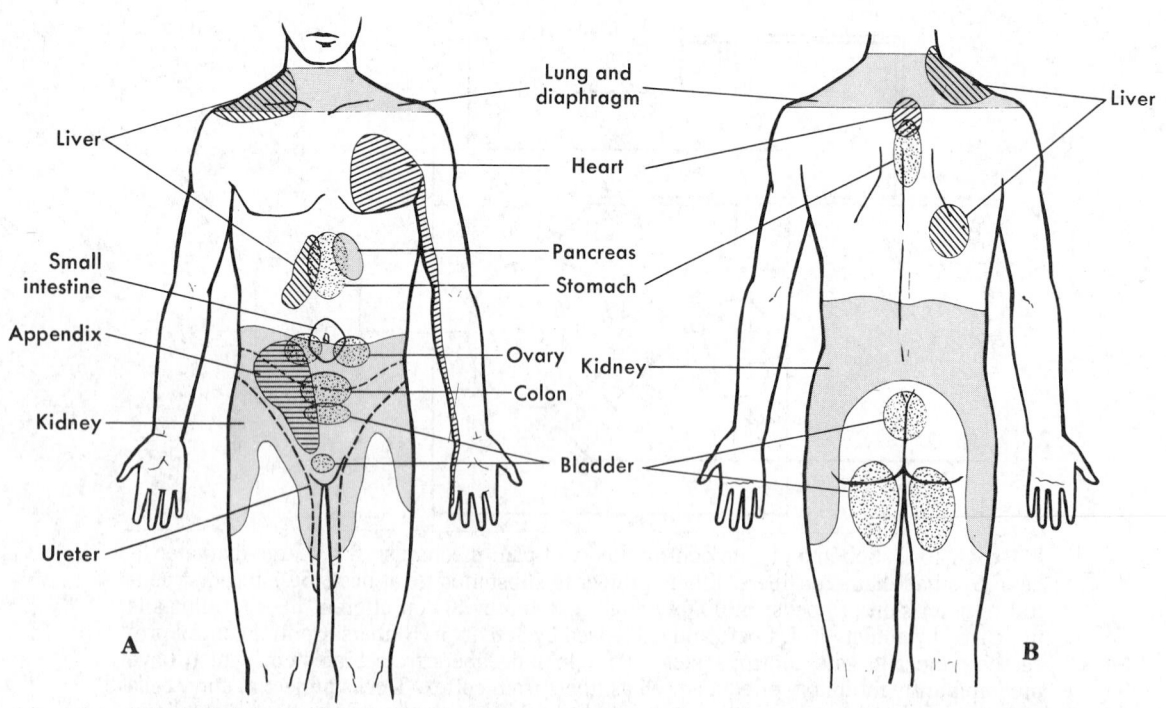

FIGURE 16-3 Referred pain, **A,** Front. **B,** Back.

to cutaneous surfaces (Figure 16-3). The exact physiologic mechanism that occurs during referred pain is not clearly understood but may relate in part to the lack of sensory nerve endings near visceral organs. The cutaneous pattern of various referred pains is fairly constant and frequently seen in practice. The nurse should be able to recognize the possibility of visceral organ disease in patients with appropriate complaints of cutaneous pain.

PSYCHOGENIC PAIN

The concept of psychogenic pain is difficult to understand and thus to treat. Psychogenic pain appears to have no physiological basis; rather, it seems to originate in the mind or the psychological state of the patient. Because all pain has a psychological component, it is difficult to distinguish somatic from psychogenic pain.[55] It is important to remember, however, that the patient feels the pain; that is, it is not imaginary to the patient.[31] Occasionally, psychogenic pain may be hysterical in origin or hypochondriacal; it may be associated with depression. Pure psychogenic pain, that is, pain with absolutely no physiologic basis, is rare. More often, the psychogenic pain seems to have a much larger psychological basis than apparent physical basis.[49]

In treating the patient with psychogenic pain, the nurse should remember what McCaffery points out: "Calling pain imaginary does not make it go away."[49] Although certain therapies traditionally used for pain relief may have limited value for these patients (for example, use of narcotics), careful planning and assessment of the patient by the health care team are necessary so that the patient will receive pain relief, if possible.

OTHER TYPES OF PAIN

Some types of pain are not completely explained by present theories of pain transmission and present specific management problems. *Phantom limb* pain refers to pain or discomfort perceived by the individual to be in an extremity that has been amputated. Phantom limb pain is not the same as phantom limb sensations, which include tingling, itching, and sweating in the missing limb. Phantom limb sensations occur in most patients after amputation. Phantom limb pain may occur briefly in up to 30% of patients, but persistent pain may occur in as few as 2% of patients.[55] It is known that phantom limb pain:

1. Has no single cause
2. Endures long after healing of the injured tissues
3. Is more likely to develop in patients who suffered pain in the limb before amputation
4. May be associated with trigger zones that, when stimulated, result in the perception of this pain (the trigger zones may spread to healthy areas on the same or opposite sides of the body)

5. Is influenced by emotional factors and sympathetic nervous system, but neither cause it[57]

Phantom limb pain may be very difficult to treat, probably because it is not clearly understood.

Another unusual type of pain is *causalgia,* which is a severe, burning pain sometimes associated with nerve injuries. This type of pain may gradually disappear, but a significant number of patients may still complain of pain a year after injury. An unusual feature of this type of pain is that it may sometimes be triggered by normally *nonnoxious stimuli,* such as the noise created when planes fly overhead.[57]

Neuralgia is pain that has a segmental or peripheral nerve distribution. Causalgia may be thought of as a type of neuralgia, but the converse is not true. *Trigeminal neuralgia* is intense pain over the distribution of one or more divisions of the trigeminal nerve. *Postherpetic neuralgia* may follow infection by the herpes zoster-varicella virus (shingles).

Headache is another type of pain that may vary significantly from one individual to another. The causes of certain headaches are fairly well understood, such as tension, increasing intracranial pressure as a result of a mass lesion, and infection. The migraine headache is less clearly understood, as is the cluster headache characterized by severe localized pain that is intense, of long duration, and difficult to treat (see Chapter 62).

A TAXONOMY OF PAIN

It has long been recognized that there are differences between acute and chronic pain (see Table 16-1). Crue, whose work has focused on chronic pain, has developed a taxonomy based on the length of time that pain has lasted.[18,19] *Acute* pain, which generally lasts for a few days, is caused by tissue injury and can be expected to end when the source of the injury is removed. An example of acute pain is pain caused by a kidney stone. *Subacute* pain is similar to acute pain but persists for days to weeks. The problem of *recurrent acute* pain is illustrated by rheumatoid arthritis, migraine headaches, and trigeminal neuralgia. In recurrent acute pain, flare-ups of chronic disorders are usually the cause, although the disorder may not be known, as with migraine headaches.

Ongoing cancer pain is the next category in Crue's taxonomy. In ongoing cancer pain, the pain is usually caused by a progressive disorder. (Cancer pain is discussed in Chapter 17). The final two categories are concerned with intractable pain. In *chronic intractable benign pain with adequate patient coping,* the pain is apparently continuous, but the person is able to live a productive life. The final category is *chronic intractable benign pain syndrome (CIBPS) with poor patient coping.* Patients in this category may be completely disabled by the pain or pain experience. These patients

TABLE 16-1 Comparison of acute and chronic pain

Characteristic	Acute Pain	Chronic Pain
Experience	An event	A situation, state of existence
Source	External agent or internal disease	Unknown; or if known, changes cannot occur or treatment is prolonged or ineffective
Onset	Usually sudden	May either be sudden or develop insidiously
Duration	Transient (up to 6 months)	Prolonged (months to years)
Pain identification	Pain versus nonpain areas generally well identified	Pain versus nonpain areas less easily differentiated; intensity becomes more difficult to evaluate (change in sensations)
Clinical signs	Typical response pattern with more visible signs	Response patterns vary; fewer overt signs (adaptation)
Meaning	Meaningful (informs person something is wrong)	Meaningless; person looks for meanings
Pattern	Self-limiting or readily corrected	Continuous or intermittent; intensity may vary or remain constant
Course	Suffering usually decreases over time	Suffering usually increases over time
Actions	Leads to actions to relieve pain	Leads to actions to modify pain experience
Prognosis	Likelihood of eventual complete relief	Complete relief usually not possible

may be the recipients of multiple, unsuccessful nerve blocks, surgical interventions, and multiple drug therapies. They may manifest preoccupation with pain, withdrawal, despair, depression, anxiety, and altered sleep patterns.[10,19,23,87,89] The use of this or other taxonomies may be helpful in understanding the many facets of pain, but the plan of care for a patient experiencing pain must be based on individualized patient assessment.

■ ASSESSMENT

SUBJECTIVE DATA

Assessment of the person undergoing pain begins with a careful history. Information to elicit includes characteristics and description of the pain. The person is asked to describe the pain, and the nurse should take care to validate with the person the exact meaning if it is unclear to the nurse. The characteristics may include the site, severity, duration, and location of pain. If the person is asked what may be causing the pain, some light may be shed on other possible topics for further elaboration.

The person also should be asked what does and what does not help relieve the pain. Careful questioning may also elicit the person's expectations of the health care team in relation to the relief of pain. Some persons hope for elimination of pain; others hope only for some relief from pain. Other helpful questions are: How has the pain interfered with your life-style? What activities would you like to be able to do if the pain is relieved? What do you expect might be done to relieve your pain? Would surgery be acceptable to you if it might relieve your pain?

Appropriate sociocultural data to include are the person's age, religion, usual reaction to pain, position in the family (for example, breadwinner or homemaker), and the responsibilities associated with that position. Some persons are able to describe their usual coping mechanisms and the expectations that they and their families or friends may have about how one should act when in pain.[14,22]

If medications are being taken for pain, what is the medication, in what dose and with what frequency is it taken, and does it provide relief?

The nurse should decide how and when data is obtained from the patient. Obviously, patients who are critically ill should be asked only a few key questions rather than subjected to a long list of questions at one time.

The nurse who has an opportunity to work with the patient on an ongoing basis can begin to assess the patient's pain and response to it over time and during various circumstances. The ongoing assessment should still include subjective data about the location, duration, and intensity of pain. The nurse and patient may also determine that there are factors associated with the pain experience, such as time of day, week, or month; certain body positions or actions; and certain environmental situations. In every case the nurse should convey trust and interest so that the patient feels free to discuss concerns with the nurse.

There has been interest recently in developing tools specifically for assessment of pain.* Nurses who are frequently faced with difficulties in assessing pain may wish to use one of the currently available tools or to develop one. One effective method of identifying pain intensity is the McGill Pain Scale.[58] The person is asked to rate the pain on a scale of 0 to 5 as described below:

_____

*References 32, 50, 56, 57, 58, 76, 94.

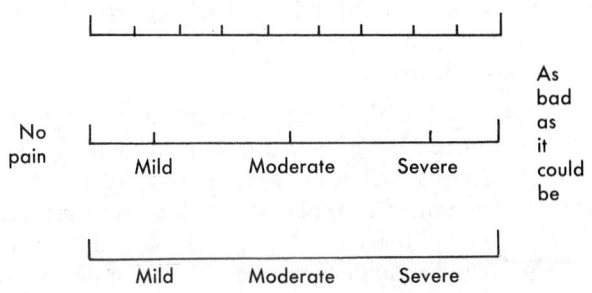

FIGURE 16-4 Visual analog pain scales. Patient marks line describing intensity of pain.

0 No pain
1 Mild pain
2 Discomforting
3 Distressing
4 Horrible
5 Excruciating

Visual analog scales can also be used (Figure 16-4) and may be helpful for comparison of a person's concept of the pain intensity over time.

OBJECTIVE DATA

The nurse should make careful objective observations of all patients. The objective data may help clarify the subjective response, or it may be the only way the nurse becomes aware of the patient's pain.

Physiologic signs of pain may include increased heart rate; increased frequency or depth of respiration, or both; diaphoresis; increased systolic and diastolic blood pressure; pallor; dilated pupils; increased muscle tension; and piloerection (goose bumps). The patient may complain of nausea or of feeling weak or sick.

If the pain is chronic or less severe, the physiologic manifestations may be less prominent and less severe. Instead, the nurse may notice changes in facial expression, such as frowning or gritting of teeth. Some persons clench their fists and withdraw inwardly when in pain. Others may complain bitterly, cry, moan, toss about in bed, assume a fetal position, or clutch at the affected body part. Still others pace up and down, if they have the energy to do so. Some patients in pain want someone in constant attendance, whereas others want to be left alone.

Nurses must be able to assess patients' pain and their emotional responses to it in a nonjudgmental manner. The way patients act when in pain is influenced by their life experiences and cannot be voluntarily modified with ease. Regardless of the cause of the pain or the person's behavior, the immediate goal is to relieve or modify the pain. Knowing how the person feels about pain helps the nurse initiate appropriate comfort measures.

There are times when the patient's subjective responses to questions about pain differ from the objective signs the nurse might expect to see. For example, the patient may request an analgesic, a back rub, or other measures to relieve pain. As the nurse arrives to carry out the request, the patient is found to be asleep. Some nurses feel that sleeping (or laughing or reading) or other behaviors indicate that the patient is not really in pain. It is important to reiterate that pain is what the patient says it is, and although objective data may assist in confirming the existence of pain, the nurse should not believe that there is a certain way the patient ought to behave when in pain. In the above example, the patient may have been exhausted by the pain and fallen asleep or the ability to sleep may be totally unrelated to the continuing presence of pain.

The need to assess the person with pain is ongoing, yet the nurse must also begin to plan an approach to the person and the pain. The nurse is able to function independently with many interventions, but careful planning with other members of the health care team should ensure that all have the same patient outcomes or goals in mind.

■ DATA ANALYSIS: NURSING DIAGNOSES

Nursing diagnoses are determined from the assessment of patient data. Possible nursing diagnoses may include, but are not limited to, the following:

Diagnostic Title	Possible Etiologies
Knowledge deficit	Lack of previous instruction; misunderstanding
Pain (indicate whether acute or chronic)	Disease process (specify if possible); surgery; trauma; diagnostic studies; immobility; other causes

Other nursing diagnoses may be appropriate after analysis of the subjective and objective data. Examples include, but are not limited to:

Activity intolerance related to pain
Mobility, impaired physical, related to pain
Sleep pattern disturbance related to unrelieved pain

■ PLANNING: EXPECTED PATIENT OUTCOMES

Possible outcomes for the patient with pain may include, but are not limited to, the following:
1. The person states that comfort has improved.
2. The person or significant others can:
   a. Describe general measures for relief of pain:
      (1) State rationale for therapy
      (2) Demonstrate exercises or other activities that have proved successful in pain control (for example, satisfactory biofeedback or self-hypnosis)

      (3) Describe method and frequency of specific measures

    b. Explain prescribed medications:

      (1) State actions, dosage, frequency, and side effects

      (2) Describe when to seek medical assistance if pain is not relieved as expected

    c. Demonstrate correct use of transcutaneous electrical stimulator, if prescribed:

      (1) State method and location for applying electrode

      (2) Describe how to adjust the frequency and amplitude controls

      (3) Demonstrate how to clean electrodes and how to change electrodes or batteries

      (4) Explain safety measures (for example, checking for loose wire connections; not bathing while apparatus is in use)

3. The person demonstrates increased tolerance for pain as manifested by return to full- or part-time employment, decreased analgesic consumption, and independence in activities of daily living.

■ IMPLEMENTATION

The first step in developing and implementing the plan of care is to obtain the patient's trust. Ideally, the nurse begins the initial assessment of the person with this need for trust in mind. As mentioned earlier, the nurse must remember that the pain is whatever the experiencing person says it is and that it exists whenever the person says it does.[49,50] Thus the nurse may not always anticipate when the patient will manifest pain. Being patient, conveying interest, being willing to help, and avoiding prejudging the patient are helpful. Prejudging implies tending to look for behavior associated with acute pain.

Careful patient assessment and planning should help the nurse to choose among many possible ways to relieve pain and to try them systematically. One aspect of the treatment plan that is often forgotten or omitted is the incorporation of measures the patient thinks may help relieve the pain, even if these measures are different from those usually employed or carried out in that institution. Without the nurse's encouragement, the patient may hesitate to mention these possible remedies. Examples include nonprescription liniments, special applications of heat or cold, unusual positioning, or favorite homemade foods or drinks. As long as there are no contraindications to the remedy the patient wishes to try, the health care team may consider using it before trying other measures to relieve pain.

Interventions for pain relief fall into three categories: (1) those that modify the pain stimulus, (2) those that alter the mode of transmission, or (3) those that modify the reaction to pain.

MODIFYING THE STIMULUS: CHANGING THE COGNITIVE OR SENSORY INPUT
PATIENT TEACHING

As the result of the nursing assessment, it may become clear that the patient's response to pain is really the manifestation of a lack of knowledge about the cause of the pain. Sometimes a simple explanation about what is causing the pain and how long it will last is all that is necessary. Understanding that pain or discomfort is to be expected may relieve anxiety or help the patient to alter expectations and be better prepared for what will happen. In all cases, an explanation that includes information about pain is given before each diagnostic test. An example might be the pain associated with a lumbar puncture or bone marrow biopsy.

PROMOTING AUTONOMY

Allowing the individual to retain some control over daily activities may allow for better control over pain. If possible and within limits, the patient should be allowed to make decisions about the frequency of certain tasks such as exercises and turning and the order of such daily events as the bath, getting out of bed, and so on. If the patient has delineated the least painful way of doing a certain activity, such as turning, this method is recorded on the plan of care and everyone working with the patient is expected to follow this method.

In some situations it may be appropriate for the patient to help plan the use of pain relief measures. An example would be the patient with cancer who wishes to receive parenteral analgesics at bedtime to improve sleep and to receive a less potent medication that causes less drowsiness before family members visit. Consult Chapter 17 about management of pain in the terminally ill patient with cancer.

PROMOTING CONSISTENCY

Planning for the same health care team members to care for the patient regularly should result in a more consistent approach and plan of care. Between the small group of health care team members and the patient, a plan of care can be developed in which the patient's decisions are honored, the day-to-day activities are put in order, and a daily routine can be devised that reduces anxiety and frustration about constant changes. This plan should include, if appropriate, such items as a specified time for analgesic administration before uncomfortable procedures, specified blocks of time for rest or napping, and coordination between various departments such as physical therapy and occupational therapy. For some patients, fatigue is a great problem, so regular visits to off-unit departments should be interspersed with rest periods throughout the day; for other patients the most beneficial plan includes ensuring that they go directly from one department to the next, so that time is not wasted getting in and out of bed or performing other painful maneuvers.

PROVIDING FOR DISTRACTION

Many individuals can be distracted from constant preoccupation with discomfort. Distraction interferes with the pain stimulus, thereby modifying the awareness of the pain. Mild or moderate pain can be modified by focusing on activity in the environment. A very quiet environment providing little or no sensory input can actually intensify the pain experience because the individual has nothing to focus on but the painful stimulus.

Severe pain requires more active participation by the individual in an effort to block out the painful stimulus. This can be enhanced by involving two or more sensory modalities such as vision, hearing, touch, or movement.[49,50] The distracters must be powerful enough to involve the individual's total interest without resulting in fatigue. Pain of long duration requires a variety of meaningful distracters.

Careful assessment may indicate ways in which the patient can be distracted, for example, playing games such as chess or checkers, watching television, or getting away from a particular setting. Music therapy provides several types of distraction. Individuals may be able to tolerate pain better if they become involved as a regular performer or listener of favorite music.[2] Simply talking with someone may be a sufficient distraction for some persons, and allowing time for this in a patient's daily routine may be very helpful. This same intervention can easily be used during some diagnostic procedures. With careful goal-directed questions and comments, the nurse may be able to take the patient's mind off the test. Discomfort will probably still occur, but preoccupation with the pain may be lessened.

Another form of distraction that may help involves the use of *rhythmic breathing*. There are many variations to this technique. McCaffery describes several forms, including "he-who" rhythmic breathing. In this approach, the patient takes a slow, deep breath at the beginning of the period. The patient is then instructed to whisper "he" during exhalation, inhale again, then whisper "who" during exhalation. The words are alternated with each exhalation. The nurse remains with the patient, repeating the instructions: "Inhale, he, inhale, who, inhale, he, inhale, who," and so on. The rate can be increased to a maximum of 60 breaths per minute as the intensity of the pain increases. For variations on this exercise and for other rhythmic breathing exercises, consult references 48 and 50.

In using distraction with patients, remember that not all persons can use it successfully and that it may become more effective with practice. On the other hand, the person need not perform the technique perfectly to achieve success. Finally, recall that although distraction can provide relief, other therapies may be necessary and useful for severe or ongoing pain.

PROMOTING EXERCISE

In selected situations, exercise is prescribed to assist in the alleviation of discomfort. The patient may need frequent encouragement to perform exercises that may actually be painful or that may not seem to be working as well or as quickly as anticipated.[3] The patient should be supervised occasionally while doing the exercises to ensure that they are being done correctly and are not causing unnecessary difficulty.

Working, dressing, and eating may be strenuous exercises for someone who has been unable to perform these and other activities of daily living. Reasonable expectations should be determined for the rate and frequency of exercising. Actually doing the exercises may serve as a form of distraction. Patients may volunteer to accept responsibility for remembering to do them, which will increase their independence and control.

PROMOTING REST, RELAXATION, AND SLEEP

If the patient has not been able to sleep because of pain or if daily activities are so strenuous or hectic as not to allow rest periods, the response to the pain may reflect exhaustion or fatigue. The nurse may be able to assist in several ways. Determine the patient's usual rest and sleep patterns, decide if they are adequate now, and analyze why the patient is not getting sufficient rest. Develop a plan in consultation with the patient to provide for more rest. This plan might include decreasing the number of interruptions during the night to check vital signs and for other activities, ensuring that the environment is quiet after a certain hour, providing a warm, noncaffeinated drink before sleep, providing rest periods during the day, and administering a sleeping medication or analgesic at a regular time each night.

The nurse may need to assist the patient to relax. The approach will be different with each individual but may include the following. Direct the person to assume a comfortable position (the nurse may have to assist). Make certain that this position is one that can be maintained for 2 to 3 hours. Also make certain the sheets are not constricting, the patient is warm enough, and so on. Instruct the patient to concentrate on each extremity, one at a time, to focus on how light and relaxed each extremity is, and to begin to breathe slowly but fully, allowing no other thoughts to enter the mind. With practice, the above approach can be used by the patient when going to sleep.

The Lamaze method of childbirth and other forms of relaxation combined with exercise are examples of ways the patient may be assisted to relax. Success with Lamaze depends partly on how well the woman has practiced the exercises and relaxation, and the same is true of the person in pain. The patient should not be led to expect success on the first couple of tries; the nurse and the patient may have to work together for a period of time before the best method for relaxation is achieved. A variety of specific relaxation techniques are now described in the literature.[16,25,41,48,49,50,63,71,90]

TEACHING WAKING-IMAGINED ANALGESIA

Waking-imagined analgesia[49] is defined as "imagining a pleasant situation when a noxious stimulus is applied." This intervention is similar to distraction, except that with this approach the person concentrates on trying to relive the sensations that occurred during a previous pleasant experience rather than only on enumerating the events that took place. McCaffery points out that only a small percentage of the population in pain can actually use this method of analgesia; more derive benefit from distraction alone.

REDUCING SOCIAL ISOLATION

The patient in pain may be socially isolated for a variety of reasons: the serious nature of a patient's disease may necessitate being in a private room for an extended period; isolation to prevent spread of infection may have confined the patient to a single room; hospitalization far away from home may mean few family members and friends can visit; extended periods of hospitalization may result in friends losing interest in visiting; or the patient may complain so much that no one cares to visit.

Each of the above causes of isolation may have a different solution. In any event, careful assessment by the nurse may indicate that social isolation is a problem for the patient. Before determining the plan for addressing this problem, the patient should be consulted about the desire and need to alter the present situation.

In the hospital, careful selection of roommates may provide natural support for any two or more patients. When actual isolation is required, more frequent visits by the health care team members may help. The nurse can assist a patient to write or telephone often to family and friends so they will keep in close touch. In many cases, the hospital staff almost becomes a family for the patient; each day a staff member fails to stop in to talk may contribute to feelings of loneliness for the patient.

Whether the person is hospitalized or at home, it may be possible to contact friends and arrange a time for them to visit regularly or even occasionally. It may be that certain friends are reluctant to come because they feel unsure of their role; the nurse may be able to reassure them or clarify expectations with them before their visits.

A careful but frank discussion with the patient about behavior around guests and family may be necessary. The nurse may be able to help the patient develop new methods for coping with constant pain; this assistance coupled with genuine interest and support from the nurse may help reduce the patient's social isolation.

PROVIDING CUTANEOUS STIMULATION

For some individuals, a change in the type of stimulation at the site of pain may result in pain relief. For example, lightly rubbing the affected area may cause significant pain reduction. The *gate control theory* would support changing the amount and type of sensory receptor stimulation, and the nurse with the help of the patient may be able to find a satisfactory and relatively simple stimulus modification to ease the patient's discomfort.

Associated with sensory input modification at the site of discomfort are other forms of cutaneous stimulation. Back rubs can aid in distraction and relaxation. Massage of various body parts (for example, feet, forehead, or arms) accomplishes the same thing (although massage of lower extremities in immobilized patients should be avoided because it may predispose patients to release of emboli).

The application of heat or cold is also a form of cutaneous stimulation. Most nurses recognize the value of heat or cold applied to the site of injury or inflammation, but heat or cold may also be helpful if applied elsewhere.[74,96] Ice packs (cold packs) can be placed at the site of pain, between the pain and the brain (for example, on the forearm between the brain and the hand, for hand pain), on the contralateral side of the body at the same site as the pain, or anywhere else that the patient might suggest. Ice massage (rubbing an ice cube directly on the skin for a 5- to 7-minute period) may also be helpful. Research has shown that ice massage of the web of the hand between the thumb and index finger helped relieve tooth or mouth pain on that side of the body.[61] Ice massage of areas on the lower back was found as effective as transcutaneous electrical nerve stimulation (TENS) for relief of low back pain.[59] Finally, gentle cool sponge baths or whirlpool massage may also be helpful. As with most treatments, patients vary in their responses to the application of heat or cold.

REDUCING PAINFUL STIMULI

With skill and adequate help the nurse usually can move the patient without causing excessive pain. Proper technique when handling the patient with generalized pain or a painful limb or other body part is important. Support to painful parts of the body is essential. Supporting the trunk and limbs in good body alignment prevents increasing the pain by unnatural pulling on muscles, joints, and ligaments. A "turning sheet" is often useful to prevent uneven lifting or pull on patients with severe neck, back, or general trunk pain. Painful joints may be moved with less discomfort if they are placed on a pillow or otherwise supported rather than being lifted directly. If there is tenderness or pain in the shaft of the bone, in muscles, or in large skin areas, the limb should be supported at the joints when the patient moves to prevent additional pain.

Binders, surgical belts, and girdles give support to the abdomen. Body casts, corsets, and braces are used to immobilize the vertebral column and thus decrease pain. A firm bed gives support and thereby lessens pain both when patients are at rest and when they move about in bed. Traction, splints, casts, and braces are used to immobilize a painful part of the body such as an ankle. Special beds (for example, Stryker frame, Foster bed, Circ-Olectric bed, and Bradford frame) allow movement with minimal handling of the body and thereby help lessen pain. If the nurse who is caring for a patient in pain feels that any of these devices would be of benefit, the suggestion should be discussed with the physician.

REDUCING AUDITORY AND VISUAL STIMULATION

The patient may be suffering from sensory overload. If nurses could stand still for 5 minutes in the patient's environment and watch and listen, they might understand that some patients are simply bombarded with noise and visual stimulation. If these are problems, it may be possible to change the environment. Changes include moving the individual away from a busy nurses' station or, in the home, away from a busy family room. Try to ensure that the lights are turned out or at least significantly dimmed at night. In the home or in the hospital, those around the patient's room may need to be reminded to talk and move more quietly at night.

Television and radio can serve as wonderful distracters, but most individuals tire of them after 14 to 18 consecutive hours. It may be possible to determine a schedule based on the likes and dislikes of family members or roommates that would include periods of silence during the day. Radio and television volume should be at a comfortable level.

Overtalkativeness and overoptimism are often annoying to the person in pain. This is particularly true when the patient knows or suspects that the prognosis is poor. Florence Nightingale gave the following advice on this subject:

But the long chronic case, who knows too well himself, and who has been told by his physician that he will never enter active life again, who feels that every month he has to give up something he could do the month before—oh! spare such sufferers your chattering hopes. You do not know how you worry and weary them. Such real sufferers cannot bear to talk of themselves, still less to hope for what they cannot at all expect.[66]

Plans should be made so that a minimal number of persons enter the room of the patient in severe pain.

The patient cannot possibly learn to know and trust all the individuals who enter the hospital room each day. Unless some effort is made to control traffic in and out of the room, the patient may be unable to relax and rest. The same principle applies to care of the individual at home, where the problem of too many visitors is frequently a real one. The nurse, of all members of the health care team, is in the best position to give attention to this crucial need of the patient. Some patients in pain welcome interruptions and distractions, whereas others prefer privacy and seclusion. The nurse should see that the patient's wishes are respected.

THERAPEUTIC TOUCH

A less traditional therapy, that of therapeutic touch, may be helpful to patients in pain. The rationale for the success of this therapy is not clearly understood. The nurse trained in therapeutic touch undergoes a brief period of meditation before coming in contact with the patient. During this period the nurse quiets inner energy, then touches the patient, channeling universal energies to effect a healing process in the patient. Few nurses are trained in the use of therapeutic touch as described here. It does seem to be helpful for some patients and some kinds of pain; it certainly seems to do no harm.[50]

ALTERING PAIN TRANSMISSION WITH MEDICATIONS

The nurse needs to know the precise effect on the body of medications used to treat pain (Table 16-2). The time curve of beginning effect, height of effectiveness, and declining effect must be understood. In addition, the effects of the medication may vary according to the time of day it is administered and the physiologic status of the individual. A brief summary of several categories of drugs is presented here; for a more definitive discussion and elaboration of appropriate nursing measures, refer to pharmacology texts.

MEDICATIONS TO RELIEVE THE CAUSE OF PAIN

Pain may be treated by drugs that help to relieve the cause of pain. For example, the belladonna group of drugs (atropine) or synthetic substitutes such as propantheline bromide (Pro-Banthine), which cause relaxation of smooth muscle, may diminish pain caused by spasm of the gut. If pain is caused by impaired circulation, drugs that dilate the blood vessels such as papaverine hydrochloride, nitroglycerin, and tolazoline hydrochloride may do more good than analgesic drugs. A final example includes antibiotics used to treat an infection that may be causing pain. Specific drugs are chosen based on the nature of the infection, the sensitivity of the organism to the antibiotic, and the general condition of the patient.

TABLE 16-2 Commonly used analgesics

Generic Name	Trade Name	Usual Dosage*	Route	Onset	Peak	Duration
NARCOTICS (OPIATE AGONISTS)						
Morphine sulfate	—	5-20 mg q 3-4 hr	SC, IM	5-10 min	60 min	4-6 hr
Codeine sulfate	—	15-60 mg q 3-4 hr	SC, PO	5-30 min	30-60 min	3-4 hr
Hydromorphone hydrochloride	Dilaudid	2-4 mg q 4-6 hr	IV, IM, SC, PO	5-15 min	1 hr	4-6 hr
Meperidine hydrochloride	Demerol	50-150 mg q 3-4 hr	IV, IM, SC, PO	10-15 min	30-60 min	2-4 hr
Methadone	Dolophine	2.5-10 mg q 3-4 hr	IM, SC, PO	10 min	1-2 hr	4-6 hr
MIXED AGONIST-ANTAGONISTS						
Buprenorphine	Buprenex	0.3-0.6 mg q 6-8 hr	IM	15 min	1 hr	6 hr
Butorphanol	Stadol	1-4 mg q 3-4 hr	IM	10-30 min	1 hr	4 hr
		0.5-2 mg q 3-4 hr	IV			
Nalbuphine	Nubain	10 mg q 3-6 hr	IV, IM, SC	2-15 min	1 hr	3-6 hr
Pentazocine	Talwin	15-30 mg q 3-4 hr	IV, IM	10-30 min	1 hr	2-3 hr
		50-100 mg q 3-4 hr	PO			
NONNARCOTICS						
Acetylsalicylic acid	Aspirin	300-1000 mg q 3-4 hr	PO	15-30 min	1 hr	3-4 hr
Acetaminophen	Tylenol, Datril	325-650 mg q 4-6 hr	PO	15-30 min	1-2 hr	4-6 hr
Ibuprofen	Motrin, Advil, Nuprin	200-600 mg q 4-6 hr	PO	15-30 min	1-2 hr	3-4 hr

*Must be individualized.

Salicylates and Acetaminophen

One of the most widely used analgesic drugs is acetyl-salicylic acid (aspirin). This is the safest of the coal-tar products; it usually relieves headache, muscle ache, and arthritic pain. The specific action of aspirin on pain is not known, but it does block *prostaglandin* production and thus may decrease the pain associated with inflammation. Aspirin does not cloud the sensorium, and this is an advantage over many other analgesics. Aspirin is highly effective when given with a narcotic, the combined effect being superior to the use of either drug alone. The nurse needs to be constantly aware that some persons are allergic to aspirin. Death can occur when aspirin is given to such individuals. Common side effects of acetylsalicylic acid are irritation of the gastric mucosa, ulceration of the gastric mucosa, and reactivation of peptic ulcers. For these reasons, aspirin should never be taken on an empty stomach; it should be taken after meals or with a snack such as a glass of milk. Sal-

icylism can occur in persons who take large doses of aspirin over long periods of time. Nausea, vomiting, ringing in the ears, deafness, and severe headache are common manifestations. An increased bleeding time, prolonged prothrombin time, and inhibition of platelet aggregation may also occur, depending on the dose, and may contribute to bleeding manifestations.

Aspirin products are available in a variety of combinations and forms such as timed-relief aspirin, enteric-coated aspirin, and aspirin buffered with antacids. Individuals vary widely in their response to these products, but there have been few conclusive data to indicate that any form or combination is best. Aspirin is also widely used to reduce fever and inflammation.

Acetaminophen (Tylenol, Datril), a paraaminophenol derivative with salicylate-like analgesic effects, has achieved wide popularity because it causes less alteration of the prothrombin level and fewer side effects. It can, however, cause severe liver damage and should not be used indiscriminately. This drug has antipyretic action but little antiinflammatory action. It is frequently prescribed for persons for whom aspirin is contraindicated.

Nonsteroidal Antiinflammatory Agents

Phenylbutazone (Butazolidin) is prescribed to relieve symptoms of an acute episode of gout. It has potent antiinflammatory properties but is poorly tolerated by many persons and has numerous side effects including hematologic changes, gastric irritation, and fluid and electrolyte disturbances.

Indomethacin (Indocin) is also an effective analgesic and antiinflammatory drug with antipyretic action. It has many side effects but may be helpful in decreasing pain in persons with rheumatoid arthritis, osteoarthrosis, and ankylosing spondylosis.

Fenoprofen calcium (Nalfon), *naproxyn* (Naprosyn), *sulindac* (Clinoril), *tolmetin sodium* (Tolectin), *piroxicam* (Feldene), and *ibuprofen* (Motrin, Advil) are just some of the nonsteroidal antiinflammatory drugs (NSAIDs). These chemically related drugs have analgesic, antipyretic, and antiinflammatory properties. They act by inhibiting an enzyme that is key to the formation of prostaglandins. They are used in rheumatoid arthritis, osteoarthritis, and in other orthopedic or arthritis-type conditions. As with other drugs in this category, gastric irritation is common, as are changes in hematologic values. These are just a few of the drugs available in this category. (For additional information, see Chapter 70.)

Counterirritants

Ointments, emollients, and liniments such as ethyl aminobenzoate and methyl salicylate (oil of wintergreen) are counterirritants that may be applied locally to alleviate pain. Oil of clove, used for toothaches, is another example.

MEDICATIONS TO CONTROL PAIN

Other types of pain medications are effective through modification of the response of the person experiencing the pain rather than altering the transmission of the pain stimuli. Many of these are thought to act at opiate receptor sites in the brain; these drugs are the exogenous morphines (see discussion of endorphins, p. 302). A discussion of these medications serves as a useful reference source for the reader.

Narcotics

The opiates are the drugs most widely recognized and used for the control of pain. Morphine and codeine are examples of opium alkaloids commonly used. Synthetic narcotic drugs such as meperidine hydrochloride (Demerol) and methadone hydrochloride (Dolophine) are also widely used. All of these drugs are termed *narcotic agonists;* that is, they have affinity for certain receptors and are efficacious in producing the effects desired of narcotics. When given in therapeutic doses, narcotics act by depressing brain cells involved in pain perception without seriously impairing other sensory perceptions. They also affect to some extent the patient's feeling about pain and thus affect both physical pain and the reaction to it. In addition, the synthetic narcotic drugs have some antispasmodic action and may encourage relaxation.

The effects of narcotics vary with the physiologic state of the patient. The very young and the very old are quite sensitive to the effects of narcotics and require smaller doses to obtain relief from pain.[78] A person of any age may be more depressed physically and emotionally by narcotics during the early morning hours (1 to 6 AM) than at any other time of the day and therefore should be watched carefully for untoward effects.

Narcotics can cause lowering of the blood pressure and general depression of vital functions, including respiratory depression, bradycardia, and drowsiness. Some of these reactions can be an advantage in treating a condition such as hemorrhage, in which some lowering of blood pressure may be desirable. Hypotension may be a disadvantage of treating the debilitated patient, who may go into shock from an excessive dosage of a drug. The narcotic drugs are less likely to cause shock if the patient is up and moving about and taking food and fluids, because these activities tend to maintain the blood pressure at a safe level. Other common side effects include nausea, vomiting, constipation, and occasionally allergic-type reactions. The appearance of side effects is influenced by such factors as dose, route of administration, relation to mealtimes, other medications, and drug idiosyncrasy.

Meperidine shares the general characteristics of the narcotic analgesics. With repeated administration, however, it may cause central nervous system excitation, probably because of the accumulation of normeperidine, a metabolite of meperidine.[91] This excitation may appear as shakiness, tremors, or even seizures.[51] Although the concomitant presence of renal failure may contribute to normeperidine accumulation, the excitatory effects have been seen in patients with normal renal function. If central nervous system excitation from meperidine is suspected, the drug should be discontinued and another analgesic used, Naloxone (Narcan), usually administered to treat narcotic overdose, should *not* be used, because it has no effect on normeperidine.[91]

Methadone, long used in treatment for narcotics addiction, is very useful in treatment of pain because of its long half-life, which is about 10 times that of morphine. Consequently, a dose of methadone needs to be taken only every 8 to 12 hours instead of every 3 to 4 hours as is true of morphine. A completely different situation would be the use of narcotic analgesics with the patient with advanced terminal cancer. In this patient fears of addiction are irrelevant. Some of these patients may require narcotics as often as every hour or even via continuous intravenous infusion.

Another group of drugs that shares many of the pain-relieving properties of the narcotic agonists is the mixed agonist-antagonist group, including pentazocine, buprenorphine, butorphanol, and nalbuphine. These drugs can produce analgesia, but are less likely to produce respiratory depression than the narcotic agonists. Tolerance to the analgesic effects of these drugs is supposed to develop more slowly with the mixed agonist-antagonists. Side effects of these drugs can include hallucinations, vivid daydreams, delusions, and other psychological effects. When mixed agonist-antagonists are administered to patients tolerant to the narcotic agonists, narcotic withdrawal symptoms may be produced. For this reason, narcotic agonists and mixed agonist-antagonists should never be administered concurrently to the same patient.[17] (For further discussion of narcotic antagonists, see a pharmacology text.) Pentazocine is often prescribed in place of morphine or meperidine for the relief of moderate to severe pain. It is given orally or parenterally. The most commonly occurring reactions are vertigo, nausea, and euphoria. Because sedation and dizziness have been noted in some instances, patients receiving pentazocine should be warned not to operate machinery, drive cars, or unnecessarily expose themselves to hazards. Pentazocine is contraindicated in persons with increased intracranial pressure, head injury, or pathologic brain conditions in which clouding of the sensorium is particularly undesirable.

Nalbuphine, buprenorphine, and butorphanol are available for parenteral administration only, so are used less often outside the hospital setting. These drugs are less likely than pentazocine to produce psychological side effects. The mixed agonists-antagonists are thought to have less abuse potential than the narcotic agonists. Pentazocine is a schedule IV drug; buprenorphine is a schedule V drug; butorphanol and nalpbuphine are not schedule drugs. In practice, however, pentazocine is frequently abused.

Propoxyphene hydrochloride (Darvon) and propoxyphene napsylate (Darvon-N) are related chemically to methadone and are widely used analgesics. They are said to be as potent as codeine, but some trials have indicated that they have little more than placebo effect. Propoxyphene is considered nonaddictive, but dependence may occur after repeated use of high doses. Side effects include dizziness, headache, gastrointestinal disturbances, and rashes. The effectiveness of either drug may be enhanced by use of combination preparations containing propoxyphene.

The danger of addiction. So much emphasis has been placed on the danger of addiction with use of the narcotics that nurses sometimes withhold narcotic drugs needlessly.[45,47] Studies have shown repeatedly that the danger of addiction resulting from the administration of narcotics to patients in the hospital is minimal. Porter and Jick[73] identified four cases of probable addiction resulting from narcotics administered in the hospital setting, but this was out of a total of 11,882 patients! McCaffery[50] reports that studies have shown that probably less than 1% of patients become addicted to narcotics from medications received in the hospital.

One reason for the concern about addiction may be related to a misunderstanding about the meaning of tolerance, physical dependence, and addiction.[17] *Tolerance* refers to the need for an increase in dose or frequency of dosing to achieve the same degree of pain relief. The rate of developing tolerance varies among patients, but if the severity of the pain remains unchanged, tolerance to the dose of analgesic always develops. *Physical dependence* refers to the body's physiologic adjustment to repeated doses of opiate drugs. After repeated, prolonged use of a narcotic drug, abruptly stopping the drug produces withdrawal symptoms, including lacrimation (tearing), runny nose, sweating, yawning, irritability, dilated pupils, gooseflesh, sneezing, diarrhea, nausea, vomiting, and bone and muscle pains. Physical dependence always develops with long-term use of opiates and should be expected. Anyone who receives narcotics for longer than 7 days should have the dose tapered to prevent withdrawal symptoms. For most patients this tapering occurs as the patient requires less frequent doses of narcotic as pain diminishes. *Addiction* is characterized by overwhelming involvement with the procurement and use of a drug.[17] (See Chapter 19 for more information on addiction.)

It is important for the nurse to evaluate the patient each time a medication for pain is requested. However, the nurse must remember that the majority of patients stop taking medications for pain when the pain is gone. Recall, too, that patients may request a dose of pain medication as soon as it may next be administered because they are not receiving an adequate dose of medication and have not had adequate pain relief. Finally, some patients have had the unfortunate experience of waiting an hour or longer after requesting a pain medication. It is not surprising then that they conclude that the best way to get any response to their requests is to ask for medication as soon as they can have it.[9]

It is also important that the nurse understand the goals of analgesic therapy for each patient, because there is wide variation in how analgesic drugs should appropriately be used. For example, in postoperative patients, the best pain relief is usually achieved by giving

TABLE 16-3 Approximate equivalent doses of oral analgesics for mild to moderate pain

Generic Name	Trade Name	Dose (mg)
Acetylsalicylic acid	Aspirin	650
Acetaminophen	Tylenol	650
Codeine	—	32
Meperidine	Demerol	50
Oxycodone	—	5
Propoxyphene napsylate	Darvon-N	100

TABLE 16-4 Approximate equianalgesic doses* of selected analgesics used for severe pain

Generic Name	IM Dose (mg)	PO Dose (mg)
Codeine	120	200
Hydromorphone	1.5	7.5
Meperidine	75	300
Methadone	10	20
Morphine sulfate	10	60
Oxycodone	15	30
Pentazocine	60	180

*References 5, 34, 52, and 78.

an ordered dose of narcotic every 3 to 4 hours (as often as permitted) around the clock for 24 to 48 hours before reducing the frequency to patient requests for the drug. This method takes advantage of the fact that it is easier to prevent pain than to treat it after it has become severe. In addition, the patient may be better able to cooperate with necessary postoperative routines if not in severe pain. This procedure does not increase the incidence of narcotic addiction.

A completely different situation would be the use of narcotic analgesics for patients with advanced terminal cancer. For nurses caring for these patients, fears of addiction are irrelevant. Some of these patients may require narcotics as often as every hour or even by means of continuous intravenous infusion.

Adequate doses of medication. Unfortunately, patients frequently suffer because the ordered dose of medication is inadequate.[5,35,47] This is probably caused by many factors, including inadequate knowledge on the part of physicians and nurses about pain and the drugs administered for pain, fear of addiction on the part of the patient and the health care providers, and switching dosage forms without readjusting the dose. Table 16-3 illustrates the approximate equivalent doses of oral analgesics used for mild to moderate pain. Table 16-4 delineates approximate equianalgesic doses of selected intramuscular and oral analgesics used for severe pain.

The American Pain Society recommends a step-wise approach to pain management.[78] The first step is to try a nonnarcotic analgesic, assessing its effectiveness. If pain relief is not adequate, add a weak narcotic agonist, such as oxycodone or codeine. If pain relief is still not adequate, switch to a stronger narcotic. Assess the patient's response, both subjectively and objectively, at each step. Generally, it is better to *slightly overmedicate* a patient, then taper back to a lower dose, especially if the patient has had continuous, unrelieved pain.

Treatment of overdose. Although sufficiently high doses of narcotics should be used, the nurse must be alert to

the possibility of administering an overdose. The first symptom of an overdose is respiratory depression. The respiratory status of all patients receiving narcotics must be monitored frequently. Other signs of overdose include central nervous system depression resulting in hypotension, lethargy, and drowsiness. In acute intoxication, pinpoint pupils and coma may be present. Narcotic overdose is treated with naloxone (Narcan) administered intravenously.

Newer routes of administration. Formerly, patients receiving analgesics were limited to the standard intramuscular, subcutaneous, or oral routes. Rarely were patients discharged from the hospital with medications to be taken other than by mouth.

Research has demonstrated that there are easier or more effective ways to provide analgesia. In the hospital, morphine is frequently administered by constant intravenous infusion to treat persons with intractable pain.[72] Morphine has also been administered by continuous intraspinal infusion, in which a small catheter is surgically placed to release the dose of morphine into the intraspinal (either intrathecal or epidural) space. Initially, the intraspinal approach was used only in hospitalized patients with acute pain, but now the catheter can be connected to a subcutaneously implanted infusion device.[26,29,30,64,68,80] This infusion device needs to be refilled only at intervals (such as every 2 weeks). It releases morphine continuously until the reservoir is empty.[1,69] Morphine can also be administered subcutaneously by infusion pumps.

Oral forms of therapy are also being updated. The original Brompton cocktail, which contained oral narcotics, has been revised numerous times. The concurrent use of oral narcotics with aspirin or nonsteroidal antiinflammatory drugs has improved pain relief. Sustained-release formulations of oral morphine (MS Contin; Roxanol SR) have been developed that allow for slow release of the drug over 8 to 12 hours. Newer uses of drugs are also being tested, such as intranasal cocaine for some kinds of myofascial pain.[46]

One of the challenges in pain control is switching the patient from intravenous medications to adequate oral doses. A frequently encountered error is prescribing the same dose of oral medication as was used intravenously. To provide equivalent analgesia, the oral dose must often be significantly higher than the intravenous dose.[51] This can be seen in Table 16-4.

Patient-controlled analgesia (PCA) *currently is more widely used.* In this approach, a syringe pump containing a drug such as morphine is connected to the patient's intravenous line. The patient activates the pump as needed to deliver a predetermined dose of analgesic. The pumps usually have devices that limit the total amount infused over several hours and that control the frequency of administration to prevent an overdose. For example, a patient's PCA pump may deliver 2 mg of morphine per dose, no more often than every 10 minutes, with a maximum dose of 20 mg every 4 hours. These doses and parameters are ordered by the physician. The doses are individualized based on patient needs and can be changed according to the patient's response.[4,38,69]

Research has indicated that patients using PCA report better pain relief, may have fewer postoperative complications, and require *less total analgesic* medication than patients receiving medication only as needed. In addition, patients have a much greater sense of control over their pain.[38]

Sedatives

Sometimes the patient needs a sedative drug instead of additional analgesics. This type of drug may permit enough drowsiness and relaxation for the analgesic to be effective. Phenobarbital, for example, often enables the patient to be comfortable with a lower narcotic dose than might otherwise be necessary. The patient with a severe emotional reaction to illness often receives relief when analgesic drugs are interspersed with sedative drugs. This arrangement has been found useful when the narcotic or other analgesic drug does not quite seem to "hold" the patient for the desired interval. The effect of sedative drugs, similar to narcotics, may be increased by the slowing down of physiologic response. In the presence of fever they sometimes produce excitement rather than relaxation. This effect is seen most often in older patients. Because barbiturates may make some patients less aware of their surroundings, side rails and constant nursing supervision may be necessary to protect them from injuries such as occur from falls.

Antianxiety Agents

Antianxiety agents, which affect the mood of the patient, have been found helpful in the treatment of pain,

particularly when given in combination with narcotics. This combination of drugs tends to separate the perception of pain from the reaction to pain. The sensation of pain appears less acute, and therefore the reaction to it becomes less severe. When fear and apprehension appear to be the most striking features of the patient's reaction, tranquilizers alone may be sufficient to achieve relaxation. Diazepam (Valium) and chlordiazepoxide hydrochloride (Librium) are examples of commonly used tranquilizers. If these drugs cause lethargy and failure of normal responses, this should be reported to the physician at once. The physiologic state of the person may cause a variance in response to these drugs similar to that seen with narcotics.

Antiemetics

Antiemetics, particularly of the phenothiazine group (haloperidol [Haldol] and prochlorperazine [Compazine]) and the antihistaminic group (hydroxyzine [Vistaril] and promethazine [Phenergan]) are often ordered to be administered concomitantly with parenteral analgesics, or they may be ordered to be given as necessary to the patient. The antiemetics are not potentiators of analgesic activity.[50] They do, however have *additive effects in producing sedation and central nervous system depression.* In addition, the antiemetics may help prevent or reduce nausea and vomiting, frequent side effects of narcotic analgesics.

McCaffery[49] points out that the sedated or sleeping patient should not be equated with the pain-free patient. On the contrary, severe pain may contribute to overwhelming fatigue, and sleep, when it occurs, may be most welcome by the patient and family. In some patients, nausea may be the only subjective complaint when the problem is actually one of pain. This reinforces the need for individualized patient assessment and care.

The side effects of individual antiemetic drugs vary, but they usually include sedation, hypotension, dry mouth, hematologic changes, and extrapyramidal side effects.

Antidepressants

Antidepressants may be prescribed for two reasons. Some patients, especially those with chronic pain, may have clinical depression severe enough to warrant treatment with antidepressant medications, in association with other psychiatric therapies. In addition, some antidepressants may have analgesic properties themselves.[54] The tricyclic antidepressants, including amitriptyline, desipramine, doxepin, imipramine, and nortriptyline have been used to treat a variety of painful conditions.

Side effects of tricyclic antidepressants include drowsiness or, occasionally, excitement and insomnia. Other side effects include anticholinergic effects: dry

FLOW SHEET—PAIN

Patient _____ Date _____

*Pain rating scale used _____

Purpose: To evaluate the safety and effectiveness of the analgesic(s).

Analgesic(s) ordered: _____

Time	Pain rating	Analgesic	R	P	BP	Level of arousal	** Other	Plan and comments

* Pain rating: A number of different scales may be used. Indicate which scale is used and use the same one each time. Two common examples:
- 0 to 10 with 0 being no pain and 10 being as bad as it can be.
- Melzack's scale:
0 = no pain; 1 = mild; 2 = discomforting; 3 = distressing; 4 = horrible; 5 = excruciating
** Possibilities for other columns: bowel function, activities, nausea and vomiting, other pain relief measures. Identify the side effects of greatest concern to patient, family, physician, nurses, etc.

FIGURE 16-5 Flow sheet for monitoring patient's response to pain. (Copyright M Mc-Caffery. From Meinhart NT and McCaffery M: Pain: a nursing approach to assessment and analysis, Norwalk, Conn, 1983, Appleton-Century Crofts. Used by permission.)

mouth, blurred vision, constipation, and urinary retention. Also, some patients experience skin changes, including rashes and photosensitivity.

Placebos

Placebos are sometimes used for their psychogenic effect in relieving pain, but they should never be given without a physician's order. Although the most usual response to a placebo is positive, some persons have negative reactions and may report intensified pain or other symptoms. Therefore when a placebo is being used, the nurse should observe the patient carefully and share with the physician any information that will help determine the best treatment for the patient. Favorable response to a placebo should not lead the nurse to ignore complaints of pain, because the individual who responds to placebos is as much in need of the nurse's interest and support as any other patient. Furthermore, the patient may have a new physical pain that needs to be evaluated.

Nurses and physicians often tend to underestimate how many patients will have a positive response to a placebo and instead reserve the use of placebos for patients who are disliked, are thought to be suffering from primarily psychogenic pain, exaggerate their pain, or are otherwise atypical in their response to pain. It is important for the nurse to remember that a positive response to a placebo is not related to the cause of the patient's pain or to the patient's subjective feelings about the pain.

Monitoring the Response to Drug Therapy

Developing a plan of care that incorporates the appropriate dosages and timing of analgesics or other medications can be difficult without sufficient data. One method for monitoring the patient's response to pain is illustrated in Figure 16-5. Although originally designed to monitor the response to analgesics, the tool can be modified by changing column titles to monitor the response to any pain relief measure.

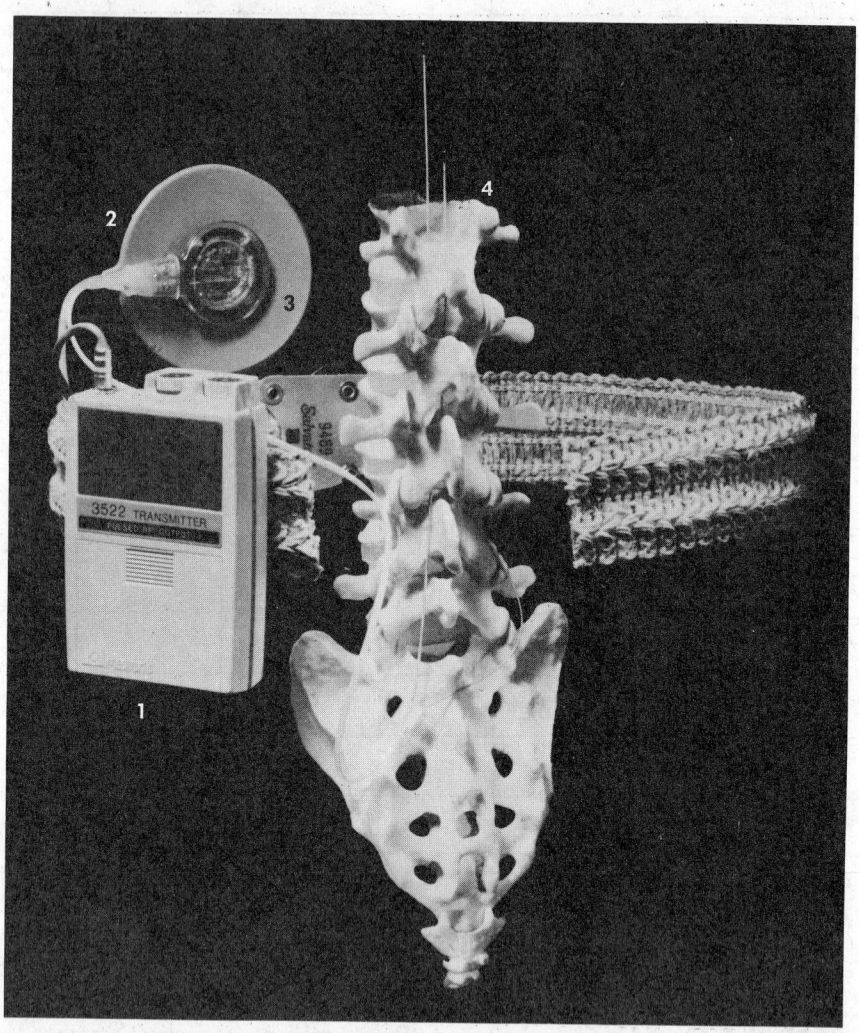

FIGURE 16-6 PISCES spinal cord stimulator. *1*, Simulation transmitter. *2*, Receiver-extension. *3*, Antenna. *4*, Leads. (Courtesy Medtronic, Inc, Minneapolis.)

TRANSCUTANEOUS ELECTRICAL NERVE STIMULATORS

A transcutaneous electrical nerve stimulator (TENS unit) is a battery-powered stimulator worn externally by the patient. Two or more electrodes attached to the battery box are applied on, around, or near the site of pain. The patient then manually regulates the power source to vary the amplitude and frequency of electrical stimulation passing between the electrodes. The goal of the device is to modify the sensory input by blocking or changing the painful stimulation with stimulation perceived as less painful or nonpainful. Success with this device may come only after repeated trials with various electrode placements or battery-box manipulations. The nurse may be very valuable in encouraging patients and assisting them to make these small manipulations.

Because the TENS is noninvasive in its application, it may be particularly useful for the person who cannot tolerate more extensive procedures.[27,53,92]

SPINAL CORD STIMULATORS

Spinal cord stimulators are similar to the TENS except that the electrodes are placed around or near the spinal cord. When spinal cord stimulation was first used, electrodes were surgically implanted over the dorsal column of the spinal cord through laminectomy, while the transmitter was worn externally. Later research indicated that, if the electrodes were placed over the ventral surface of the spinal cord or percutaneously through the back into the epidural space, the same degree of pain relief was obtained. Because percutaneous placement of electrodes can be performed under local anesthesia, it is preferred over surgical placement of the dorsal-column stimulator electrodes.[40] Figure 16-6 illustrates a percutaneous implanted spinal cord epidural stimulation (PISCES) system.

NEUROSURGICAL PROCEDURES

Constant, relentless pain that cannot be controlled by analgesics (intractable pain) may be reduced or abolished by one of several neurosurgical procedures.

Neurectomy

When pain is localized to one part of the body, it can sometimes be relieved by interruption of the peripheral or cranial nerves supplying the area. The nerve fibers to the affected area are severed from the cord (cell body) in an operation known as neurectomy. Not only pain fibers are interrupted by these procedures, but also fibers controlling movement and position sense. Therefore this type of treatment cannot be used to control pain in the extremities. A neurectomy probably is most often performed to relieve the pain of persons with trigeminal neuralgia, in which case it is referred to as a *fifth-nerve resection*. A neurectomy may also be performed to control incapacitating dysmenorrhea and is called a *presac-*

ral neurectomy. One of the difficulties with a neurectomy is that peripheral nerves regenerate, making this type of surgery questionable at times.

Rhizotomy

Resection of a posterior nerve root just before it enters the spinal cord is known as a rhizotomy (Figure 16-7). This procedure frequently is used in controlling severe pain in the upper trunk, such as that caused by carcinoma of the lung. It is also used to relieve severe spasticity in persons with paraplegia. However, it cannot be used to relieve pain in the extremities, because position sense is lost. The incision is made high in the thoracic or low in the cervical area and involves a laminectomy. Rhizotomy may be carried out lower in the cord, but when this is done bowel, bladder, and sexual function problems are frequent complications.[40]

The postoperative observations and care are similar to those necessary for any patient who has had a laminectomy, except that the patient who has had a rhizotomy is usually a poorer operative risk and may be suffering from a severe debilitating disease and therefore developing complications such as decubiti more easily. It is important for both the patient and the nurse to realize that this operation will not prevent pain at the level of the incision because the resected nerves affect only the area below the incision. Nursing intervention involves the usual postlaminectomy care. Teaching patients what to expect is important so that they can adjust expectations accordingly. Patients must understand that the loss of sensory transmission from the area of the rhizotomy interferes with the ability to perceive heat and cold. Care must be taken when the affected area is exposed to extremes in temperature (for example, heat used for cooking and baking).

Cordotomy

A cordotomy is an *operation performed to relieve intractable pain*. The advantages of cordotomy include a wide sense of analgesia below the surgical site while other sensory and motor functions are preserved. Cordotomy is most often performed on patients with extensive carcinoma of the pelvis. The incision is made high in the thoracic area, two laminae are removed, and the pain pathways in the spinothalamic tract (anterior and lateral aspect of the cord) on the side opposite the pain are severed (Figure 16-7). If the pain is in the midline, the interruption must be made bilaterally. However, the two operations must be performed separately to avoid extensive damage to the cord from edema.

Following surgery, nursing care is similar to that given a patient who has had a cervical laminectomy for removal of a protruded nucleus pulposus. Frequently, temporary paralysis, or at least leg weakness, and loss of bowel and bladder control follow a cordotomy; these re-

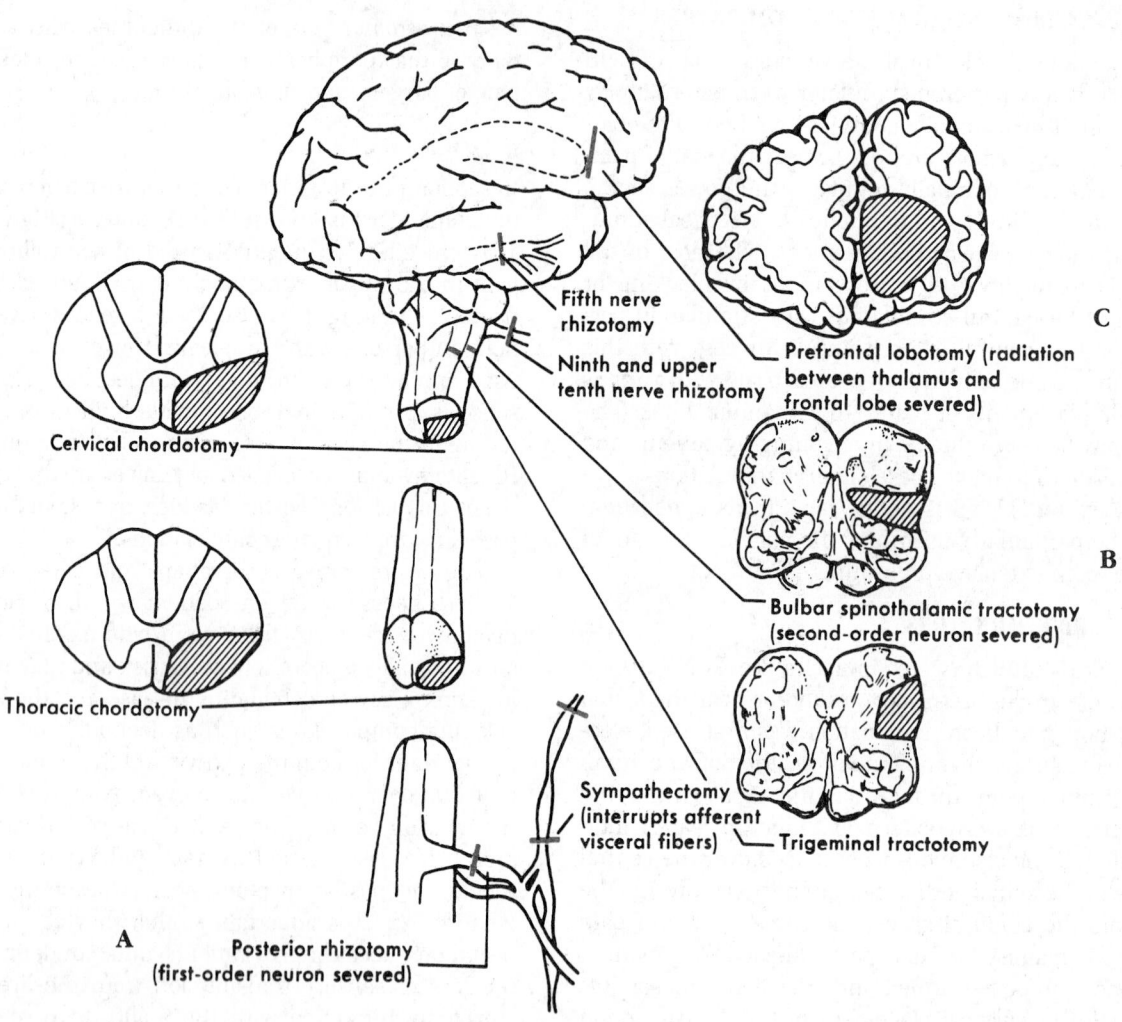

Fifth nerve rhizotomy

Ninth and upper tenth nerve rhizotomy

Cervical chordotomy

Thoracic chordotomy

Prefrontal lobotomy (radiation between thalamus and frontal lobe severed)

C

B

Bulbar spinothalamic tractotomy (second-order neuron severed)

Sympathectomy (interrupts afferent visceral fibers)

Trigeminal tractotomy

A

Posterior rhizotomy (first-order neuron severed)

FIGURE 16-7 Neurosurgical procedures for pain relief. **A,** Rhizotomy; sympathectomy, cordotomy. **B,** Tractotomy. **C,** Prefrontal lobotomy. (From Conway-Rutdowski BL: Carini and Owens' neurological and neurosurgical nursing, ed 8, St Louis, 1982, The CV Mosby Co.)

sult from edema of the cord and will gradually disappear in about 2 weeks. During the period of paralysis, the patient may be helped out of bed by using a hydraulic lift (Figure 16-8). Back care with special attention to pressure points should be given every 2 or 3 hours, because position sense is lessened and the patient is often debilitated. It is advisable to use an alternating air-pressure mattress, water mattress, or some other measure to reduce pressure until the patient is allowed out of bed. Sometimes a Foster bed or a Stryker frame enables the nurse to give the patient better care. Because of the decreased position sense, special attention should be given to placing the patient in proper body alignment. If quadriceps-setting exercises are begun in the early postoperative period, retraining in walking will be less difficult. It is usually easier for patients to use a walker when they begin ambulation and then progress to a cane.

Physical therapy activities that provide for hip and knee flexion, such as riding a stationary bicycle, may be used to strengthen leg muscles. Therapy can be started as soon as the patient can be out of bed comfortably for at least 2 hours at a time.

Because *temperature sensation is permanently lost,* the nurse must be careful to avoid burning or otherwise injuring the patient's trunk and legs and must teach the patient and family how to avoid injury to the patient. The lower portions of the body, especially the feet, are inspected routinely for any breaks in the skin or unnoticed infection.

Percutaneous cordotomy. *Percutaneous cordotomy,* which permits more precise control of the size and site of the surgical lesion, may be used instead of the direct thoracic approach. It is less traumatic surgically for the

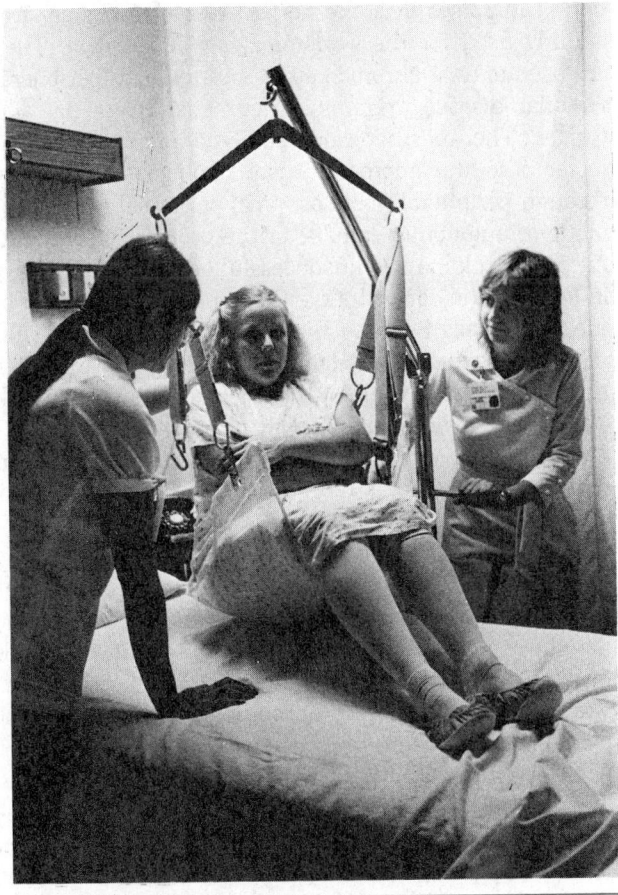

FIGURE 16-8 Hydraulic lift can be used to move paralyzed patient from bed to chair.

debilitated person who has often been on continuous analgesic therapy for long periods.[54,69]

The procedure consists of inserting a spinal lumbar puncture needle laterally between the cervical (C1 and C2) level. A wire electrode is then inserted into the anterior cord and a lesion is made at a designated site, under radiologic and stereotactic control, in order to destroy the ascending pain fibers. The procedure is performed with the patient under local anesthesia, and a sensation of tingling in the corresponding body area is noticed when the electrode is stimulated minimally. This assists the surgeon in locating the exact site for the surgical lesion.

Preoperatively, patients are evaluated carefully as to their candidacy for this type of surgery and to establish baseline data. It is important to identify and exclude persons whose pain is more functionally based. Cordotomy in this instance would not be successful in relief of the pain. Pulmonary function is also carefully evaluated to establish a baseline to be used for comparison postoperatively. The risk of respiratory complications, especially in patients who undergo *bilateral* percutaneous

cordotomy, is great. Regional anesthetic blocks (with an epidural catheter) are often evaluated before surgery for a 24-hour period or longer to test the benefits. Placebo blocks with normal saline solution are also done, and the results are compared with the anesthetic block. The patient is carefully monitored by the nurse during the regional blocks for hypalgesia and analgesia responses.

Postoperatively, patients are observed closely for postural hypotension when they initially ambulate. The sympathetic fibers in the cord controlling blood pressure may be affected for a period of time. Temperature sensation is also expected to be lost after this type of surgery. Bladder function and motor function may also be affected and should be observed carefully by the nurse following surgery. Usually such deficits do not increase following unilateral cordotomy but may after bilateral cordotomy. The value of accurate presurgical baseline data of all components is particularly necessary for good postsurgical care of the patient with a cordotomy.

Interruption of Nerve Pathways in the Brain

Numerous attempts have been made to alter the transmission of pain and the response to pain by surgical or stereotactic interruption of pathways in the brain. Lesions have been placed in the thalamus, the cingulum, the mesencephalon, the medulla, and the frontal lobe. The success rate has varied considerably depending on the skill of the surgeon, the type of pain, and the patient's general physical and emotional condition.[88]

These surgeries may have complications, particularly changes in the personality of the patient. Although the assistance of a psychiatrist is helpful in managing all patients with chronic pain, it is highly recommended for any surgery that may change the patient's personality.

A variety of other neurosurgical procedures may be helpful for specific problems. *Hypophysectomy* (destruction or removal of the pituitary gland) is sometimes helpful in patients with pain, particularly bone pain, caused by cancer of the breast or prostate gland. *Sympathectomy* (excision or destruction of one or more sympathetic ganglia or nerves) is useful in cases of true causalgia and pain that is secondary to vascular insufficiency of the extremities.

INTRATHECAL PHENOL OR ALCOHOL

Another medical intervention used at some institutions is the injection of hyperbaric phenol or hypobaric alcohol into the subarachnoid space by means of lumbar puncture. The patient is positioned carefully, the desired substance is injected, and the nerve roots involved in the pain transmission are destroyed. The effect is analogous to a chemical posterior rhizotomy, and effects may last from several weeks to months. Side effects are common and include bladder and bowel dysfunction and various degrees of lower extremity weakness. The value of this intervention is that no major surgery is required, but its use is limited to pain in the trunk, abdomen, and lower extremities. Nursing intervention includes that given a patient undergoing lumbar puncture.[44]

NEUROAUGMENTATION

The term *neuroaugmentation* is a broad one that includes the use of spinal cord stimulators. In neuroaugmentation procedures electrical stimulation is used to produce pain relief, but destruction of nerve function does not occur. In addition to spinal cord stimulation, electrodes have also been stereotactically placed in the thalamus. Although apparently similar to dorsal column stimulators in action, the use of electrodes in the thalamus may in fact work by *stimulating production of endorphins.*

NERVE BLOCK

A nerve block involves the injection of substances such as local anesthetics or neurolytic agents (for example, alcohol or phenol) close to nerves to block the conduc-

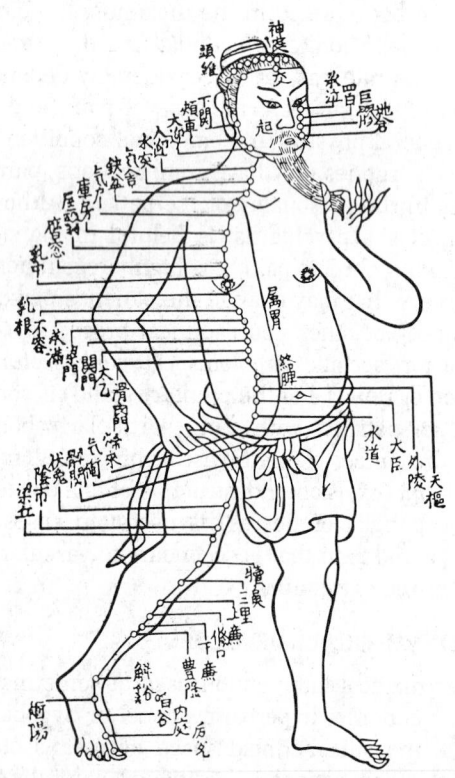

FIGURE 16-9 Acupuncture chart showing sites for insertion of needles along several body meridians. After two or more needles are inserted, electrical current is usually passed through needles for about 20 minutes. Resulting analgesia can permit major surgery. (From Weisenberg M: Pain: clinical and experimental perspectives, St Louis, 1975, The CV Mosby Co; courtesy *Abbottempo,* vol X, no. 1.)

tion of impulses over the nerves. Nerve blocks are frequently used for the symptomatic relief of pain. They are used to treat chronic pain associated with peripheral vascular disease, trigeminal neuralgia, causalgia, and cancer. The anesthetic or neurolytic agent can be injected into the appropriate site to block conductivity through peripheral fibers of spinal or cranial nerves, somatic or autonomic ganglia, or the posterior nerve root. A nerve block may be unsuccessful because of difficulty in locating the correct nerve fiber and the complexity of the pain itself. Because the nerve fibers, ganglia, and roots being injected contain other fibers than those for pain and because some of the injected agents may leak out of the injection site and affect other nerves, recipients of the nerve block usually experience other types of neurologic deficit.[44,81]

ACUPUNCTURE

Acupuncture is an ancient form of disease treatment that can be used for pain relief. Only recently, however, has the method been used in Western countries. Small needles are skillfully inserted and manipulated at specific body points, depending on the type and location of pain, producing often immediate and continued relief of pain (Figure 16-9). The gate control theory provides the best explanation for the success of acupuncture: the local stimulation of large-diameter fibers by the needles "closes the gate" to pain. It is not known to what extent the psyche and the power of suggestion contribute to effectiveness of this therapy. Nursing intervention includes careful patient assessment and teaching.[39,83]

MODIFYING THE RESPONSE TO PAIN
DECREASING PATIENT AND FAMILY ANXIETY

The patient in pain is often afraid. Fear may be allayed in part by the nurse's calm, quiet manner and particularly by a demonstration of competence. Confidence in the persons who care for them is a tremendous help to patients. It is a great comfort to the patient to know, for example, that the nurse will not hurry while giving nursing care, thus increasing pain, or be so busy that pain medication is not given at the prescribed intervals.

Sometimes preparation for pain helps to increase acceptance of it and in turn produces relaxation, which decreases pain. An example is the benefit derived from special preparation for childbirth. Fear and irritability can sometimes by allayed by explaining to patients why they have pain. This knowledge may let them relax somewhat and thereby lessen their discomfort. If patients can be told honestly that the pain will probably be of short duration, this should be done. Postoperative pain is often aggravated by movement. Therefore, when certain activities such as turning and coughing are necessary to prevent complications, the nurse explains this to the patient. Older patients may be comforted by having someone sit quietly with them, and some patients benefit from the personal contact of holding another's hand.

It is understandable that the family will be upset when the patient is in pain. Prompt attention to the patient's needs helps reduce the family's concern, and the patient's behavior should be interpreted to family and friends, as necessary, with simple, clear explanations. Regardless of explanations, persons who are emotionally close to the patient may need time to accept changes in the patient's behavior. Reassurance of family members is an essential part of nursing care because it may prevent them from communicating their concern to the patient. Expressions of concern by others may make the patient increasingly tense, which in turn lowers tolerance to pain. Helping family members understand the patient's behavior often reduces their demands for the patient to relate to them as usual and may help the patient feel less guilty about not being able to respond to them in the usual way.

TEACHING

Teaching as a nursing role has been mentioned frequently in relation to helping the person who has pain. Just as each plan of care should be individualized, so should the teaching within that plan of care. Careful assessment of the person's willingness and interest in learning and of mental and physical ability to tolerate teaching is made before teaching is initiated. Teaching varies with each patient but may include the cause of the pain, even at the physiologic level if the patient wishes to know; why or how various attempts at pain relief could or should work; and alternate ways to perform daily activities that might be less painful or consume less energy. Various nursing measures, even if not primarily for pain relief, are explained.

In preparation for surgery or diagnostic procedures, the patient should be told honestly what to expect in terms of the duration and intensity of pain *usually* experienced and what measures will be available to assist with this discomfort. If the patient must actually perform certain maneuvers or treatments, it is helpful for the patient to practice these before the procedure, for example, to cough and deep breathe preoperatively. If at all possible the family should be included in these teaching sessions, not only so they can support and assist the patient but also so they will understand what the patient will be expected to do.

SPIRITUAL ASSISTANCE

Even if no estimate can be made as to the duration of pain, patients should be given encouragement that the problem will not become too great for them to accept with the assistance that is available. Many patients who have prolonged pain with no hope of relief can and do derive benefit from their religious faith. This may help them to consider pain in a more positive way and thus make it more bearable for them. The nurse can arrange for the appropriate religious advisor to be available to the patient who indicates such a desire.

In addition, the nurse may become involved in doing such things as sharing in a prayer with the patient, reading from the Bible or another meaningful book, ensuring that meaningful religious medals or statues are within reach or sight, and so on.

PSYCHIATRIC ASSISTANCE

In some situations the medical team will ask a psychiatrist to evaluate the patient and perhaps begin ongoing psychiatric care. The *individual suffering from chronic or intractable pain may appear sad, hostile, or anxious.* These persons often have spent years undergoing various diagnostic and surgical procedures and have seen many different physicians without significant pain relief.[57]

For many individuals, psychiatric care is still not as acceptable as other kinds of medical care. The nurse should be supportive and help them understand why this type of therapy may be helpful. Careful recording and reporting of objective data about the patient's behavior, including interactions with family members and others, is important.

BEHAVIOR MODIFICATION

Whether used as part of the psychiatrist's plan of care or not, the nursing plan of care may outline a program designed to increase more acceptable or pleasing behavior or performance in the patient and reduce unpleasant or undesirable behavior. The basis for this therapy is the idea that "a behavior will tend to occur more frequently if it is consistently followed by a reward such as praise."[49] Forms of this behavior therapy are used unconsciously all the time: a young boy "throwing a tantrum" may be ignored, but as his behavior becomes more appropriate his mother may point this out and reward him with her time and attention.

Behavior modification can be used frequently with persons in pain. For example, the nurse may praise and congratulate a patient for performing postoperative exercises. If the patient is being encouraged to try a new pain relief measure such as relaxation, it is hoped the ultimate reward will come in the form of pain relief. During the practice and learning phase, however, *positive reinforcement and verbal praise and encouragement by the nurse* when the patient does try relaxation should stimulate the patient to practice the new method regularly.

In using behavioral methods in altering pain-associated behavior or in encouraging patient activities, success occurs only with a consistent approach on the part of the nurses and the health care team. Although patients should always be praised for their efforts to comply with or assist with treatment regimens, a *true behavior modification program requires careful analysis of patient behavior and the development of a specific and comprehensive treatment plan.*[23]

BIOFEEDBACK AND AUTOGENIC TRAINING

Some persons are able to alter body functions through mental concentration. Biofeedback is a general term that includes a group of techniques in which an individual learns to control bodily activities usually considered involuntary.[23,87] In learning these techniques, the patient may be connected to devices that monitor heart rate, respiratory rate, muscle tension (electromyograph), cerebral activity (electroencephalograph), and galvanic skin response. The patient then concentrates on lowering his or her heart rate, galvanic skin response, or other parameters to a level at which pain is less intense. The goal is to become adept at this and thus suppress pain. It may take months of regular practice to achieve the desired level of control. The nurse can be very helpful in encouraging and praising the patient's efforts.[12,79]

In autogenic training the same type of self-regulation is used to alter various autonomic nervous system functions such as pulse, blood pressure, and muscle tension. *Practiced use of transcendental meditation and other methods of concentration and self-control may achieve the same degree of autoregulation without the use of sophisticated physiologic monitoring equipment.* As can be seen from the discussion, many of the pain relief therapies combine distraction, relaxation, self-control, and forms of behavior modifications.

HYPNOSIS

Hypnosis has been used for decades in the treatment of various conditions, particularly when these conditions are aggravated by tension and stress. This therapy helps individuals to alter their perception of pain through the acceptance of positive suggestions made to the subconscious, and many patients are able to learn the technique of self-hypnosis. In addition to improved control of pain, some patients may be able to use hypnosis to help reduce nausea, improve appetite, or assist in controlling other problems. Persons vary in their suggestibility and readiness to try this approach. The skill of the hypnotist is also important. The nurse's most helpful role may be to support the patient's desire to make hypnotism work.[28,70,87]

PROMOTING NUTRITION

Appetite is affected by pain. When one is in continuous pain nothing, including meals, seems quite right. Care should be taken that foods the patient likes are prepared in a desired way. Appetite may be improved by small, attractive servings and by a sincere interest in the patient's reactions to food. Foods that patients do not like or that they believe disagree with them should not be offered. Very gratifying improvement in appetite has followed the control of intractable pain by surgical procedures that interrupt sensory pathways transmitting the painful sensation.

PROMOTING ELIMINATION

The patient with moderate to severe pain may be suffering from constipation, which adds to general discomfort and anxiety. Many factors may contribute to constipation, including the use of narcotic medications, inactivity, and inadequate nutritional intake. The nurse must monitor the frequency of bowel movements or instruct the patient and family to do so. The patient should increase the daily fluid intake to 2500 to 3000 ml if possible and should ambulate frequently. The inclusion in the diet of fruits or fruit juices, bran or fiber, or other foods known by the patient to stimulate defecation should also be tried. See Chapter 44 for further discussion of this problem.

PREVENTING SUICIDE

When caring for the patient who is experiencing severe, continuous, or intractable pain, the nurse must keep in mind the possibility of suicide. Pain is wearing and demoralizing, especially when it is difficult to control with medications and when the individual knows or suspects that no permanent relief will be forthcoming. Patients may dread the danger of growing dependence on drugs, they may fear that drugs will no longer help, and they may be depressed by thoughts of being a burden and an expense to their families. They may appear to tolerate pain quite well but at the same time may be planning their own destruction. Plans for protection should be individualized for each patient and depend on such factors as whether the patient is confined to bed. (For further discussion on patients who commit suicide, see specialized texts.)

PAIN CLINICS

In recent years the knowledge that pain has both a physical and an emotional component, combined with increased understanding of patients' needs and the treatments available, have resulted in the establishment of pain clinics. Most pain clinics or rehabilitation centers use a team approach. Physicians, including internists, dolorologists (specialists in pain), surgeons and psychiatrists, nurses, physical and occupational therapists, social workers, psychologists, vocational rehabilitation counselors, and others may be available to help the patient. Treatment may be on an inpatient or outpatient basis, with family members encouraged to participate in various aspects of the program.

Typical patient goals of therapy are withdrawal from drugs, increased physical activity, improved emotional well-being, and a reduction in pain by 50% to 100%. Each patient's needs and goals are assessed and a plan for care based on these is established. The plan involves most if not all of the following: progressive exercise, massage, application of heat and cold, acupuncture, external electrical stimulation, counseling, and autogenic biofeedback training.

Each pain clinic is organized slightly differently, placing greater emphasis on various aspects of pain relief and manifestation. Many of the clinics with inpatient services employ various forms of behavior modification.[21,93]

The responsibility of the nurse may vary according to the team members available but often includes assisting in assessment of the patient, documenting observations, creating and maintaining a therapeutic milieu, providing emotional support to the patient and family, and teaching the patient, family, and other nursing team members about the interventions planned for the patient. Nurses who work in pain clinics need to be skilled in interpersonal interactions, be knowledgeable about the mechanisms of pain and the effectiveness of various treatment modalities, and possess patience and understanding as they assist patients to reach their goals.

CHAPTER SUMMARY

- Pain is a subjective sensation that warns us that something is wrong, yet fear of pain may cause patients to delay seeking health care assistance.

- McCaffery's definition of pain is the most workable in guiding nursing care: "Pain is whatever the experiencing person says it is, existing whenever he says it does."[49,50]

- Pain has many meanings, including possible loss of mobility or occupation, deterioration of a health condition, or even relief of stress. The meaning of pain is influenced by age, sex, cultural background, psychosocial factors, setting, and other factors.

- Pain thresholds vary from person to person, and tolerance to pain may be altered by alcohol, drugs, hypnosis, warmth, rubbing, distraction, and other activities.

- Pain is perceived in the cerebral cortex.

- The patient's reaction to pain is influenced by many factors, including setting, parents' attitudes, associated fear, and cultural background.

- The nurse's reaction to pain is also influenced by many factors, including personal expectations, biases, and cultural background. Unless the nurse is careful, personal biases and expectations may interfere with individualized patient assessment and care.

- Two older theories of pain transmission are the *pattern theory* and the *specificity theory*. Currently, the *gate control theory* is widely accepted. This theory contends that pain perception depends on the interaction of three systems: the substantia gelatinosa, a central control system in the cortex and thalamus, and a neural system associated with perception. The theory explains the success of many forms of pain treatment.

- Endorphins and enkephalins both influence pain perception.

- A few examples of types of pain include somatic pain, visceral pain, referred pain, psychogenic pain, phantom limb pain, neuralgia, and headache.

- Crue has developed a taxonomy of pain that differentiates between acute, chronic, intractable, and other types of pain.

- The nursing assessment should begin with thoughtful questioning about the location, severity, and duration of pain, as well as relief measures that have been tried and their success. Specific pain rating scales may be used, and these may vary from elaborate questionaires to simply asking patients to rate pain from 1 to 10, with 10 being the most severe pain and 1 being no pain at all.

- Objective assessment includes observation of any abnormalities, vital signs, observation of behavior, and patient response to questions.

- Goals should be established after consultation with the patient and should be individualized for each person.

- Interventions that are focused on modifying the stimulus—changing the cognitive or sensory input—include patient teaching, promoting autonomy, promoting consistency, providing for distraction, promoting exercise, promoting rest, relaxation and sleep, teaching waking-imagined analgesia, reducing social isolation, reducing painful stimuli, reducing auditory and visual stimulation, and using therapeutic touch.

- Interventions that alter pain transmission include using medications (salicylates, nonsteroidal antiinflammatory agents, counterirritants, narcotics, sedatives, antianxiety agents, antiemetics, antidepressants); transcutaneous electrical nerve stimulators, spinal cord stimulators, neurosurgical procedures, intrathecal phenol or alcohol, neuroaugmentation, nerve block, and acupuncture.

- Placebos should be used with caution, if at all.

- Patient-controlled analgesia (PCA), which allows the patient to self-administer pain medication, is becoming widely used in hospitals.

✔ Interventions that modify the response to pain include decreasing patient and family anxiety, teaching, spiritual assistance, psychiatric assistance, behavior modification, biofeedback and autogenic training, hypnosis, promoting nutrition, promoting elimination, and preventing suicide.

✔ Pain clinics are specifically designed for a team approach to working with patients whose pain has been difficult to relieve or control.

QUESTIONS TO CONSIDER

- Think about your own ideas about pain and how openly you feel pain should be expressed. All nurses have ideas about pain. Can you identify some of your biases about pain?

- What factors should influence the nurse to administer "as necessary" (prn) medications for pain?

- In what ways could you involve the family in the care of the patient with pain?

REFERENCES AND SELECTED READINGS

1. Alberico JG: Breaking the chronic pain cycle, Am J Nurs 84:1222-1225, 1984.
2. *Bailey LM: Music therapy in pain management, J Pain Symp Manag 1(1):25-28, 1986.
3. Barbour LA, McGuire DB, and Kirchhoff KT: Nonanalgesic methods of pain control used by cancer outpatients, Oncol Nurs Forum 13(6):56-60, 1986.
4. Barkas G and Duafala ME: Advances in cancer pain management: a review of patient controlled analgesia, J Pain Symp Manag 3(3):150-160, 1988.
5. †Beaver WT: Managment of cancer pain with parenteral medication, JAMA 244:2653-2657, 1980.
6. †Beecher HK: Relationship of significance of wound to pain experienced, JAMA 161:1609-1613, 1956.
7. †Blaylock J: The psychological and cultural influences on the reaction to pain: a review of the literature, Nurs Forum 7:262-274, 1968.
8. Bond MR: Pain: its nature, analysis and treatment, ed 2, New York, 1984, Churchill Livingstone.
9. †Bonica JJ, editor: Pain. In Association for Research in Nervous and Mental Disease: Research publications, vol 58, New York, 1980, Raven Press.
10. Brena SF and Chapman SL, editors: Management of patients with chronic pain, New York, 1983, SP Medical and Scientific Books.
11. Bromm B, editor: Pain measurements in man, Amsterdam, 1984, Elsevier Science Publishers.
12. Cleeland CS: Nonpharmacological management of cancer pain, J Pain Symp Manag 2(suppl 2):23-28, 1987.
13. †Copp LA: The spectrum of suffering, Am J Nurs 74:491-495, 1974.
14. Copp LA: Pain coping model and typology, Image 17(3):69-71, 1985.
15. Copp LA, editor: Recent advances in nursing: perpectives on pain, New York, 1985, Churchill Livingstone.
16. *Cotanch PH and Strum S: Progressive muscle relaxation as antiemetic therapy for cancer patients, Oncol Nurs Forum 14(1):33-37, 1987.
17. Coyle N: Analgesics and pain, Nurs Clin North Am 22(3):727-741, 1987.
18. †Crue BL, editor: Chronic pain, New York, 1978, SP Medical and Scientific Books.
19. Crue BL: The neurophysiology and taxonomy of pain. In Brena SF and Chapman SL, editors: Management of patients with chronic pain, New York, 1983, SP Medical and Scientific Books.
20. †Davitz LL, Davitz JR, and Higuchi Y: Cross-cultural inferences of physical pain and psychological distress, Nursing Time 73:556-558, 1977.
21. Dickerson CC: Pain centers: a survey and analysis of past, present and future functioning. In Tollison, CD, editor: Handbook of chronic pain management, Baltimore, 1989, Williams & Wilkins.
22. Geach B: Pain and coping, Image 19(1):12-15, 1987.
23. Gildenberg PL and DeVaul RA: The chronic pain patient: pain and Headache, vol 7, Basel, Switzerland, 1985, S Karger AG.
24. †Goodwin JS, Goodwin JM, and Vogel AV: Knowledge and use of placebos by house officers and nurses, Ann Intern Med 91:106-110, 1979.
25. *Graffam S and Johnson A: A comparison of two relaxation strategies for the relief of pain and its distress, J Pain Symp Manag 2(4):229-231, 1987.
26. Haight K: What you should know about epidural analgesia, Nursing 17(9):58-59, 1987.
27. *Harrison M and Cotanch PH: Pain: advances and issues in critical care, Nurs Clin North Am 22(3):691-697, 1987.
28. Hilgard ER: Hypnosis and pain. In Sternbach RA, editor: The psychology of pain, ed 2, New York, 1986, Raven Press.
29. Inbar G: Pain management with intraspinal morphine sulfate injection, Perioper Nurs Q 2(4):64-67, 1986.
30. Inturrisi M, Camenga CF, and Rosen M: Epidural morphine for relief of postpartum, postsurgical pain, JOGNN 17(4):238-243, 1988.
31. †Jacox AK, editor: Pain: a sourcebook for nurses and other professionals, Boston, 1978, Little, Brown & Co.
32. *Jacox AK: Assessing pain, Am J Nurs 79:895-900, 1979.
33. *Kahn DL and Steeves RH: The experience of suffering: conceptual clarification and theoretical definition, J Adv Nurs 11:623-631, 1986.
34. Kaiko RF: Controversy in the management of chronic cancer pain: therapeutic equivalents of IM and po morphine, J Pain Symp Manag 1(1):42-45, 1986.
35. Kanner RM: Are the people who need analgesics getting them? Am J Nurs 86:589, 1986.
36. Kim S: Pain: Theory, research and nursing practice, Adv Nurs Sci 2:43-59, 1980.
37. *Kleiman RL, et al: PCA vs. regular IM injections for severe postop pain, Am J Nurs 87(11):1491-1492, 1987.
38. *Kleiman RL, et al: A comparison of morphine administered by patient-controlled analgesia and regularly scheduled intramuscular injection in severe postoperative pain, J Pain Symp Manag 3(1):15-22, 1988.
39. Laborde JM: Acupuncture treatment: a perspective, J Pain Symp Manag 1(4):232-234, 1986.

*References preceded by an asterisk are particularly well suited for student reading.
†References preceded by a dagger are classic readings.

40. Lamb S and Barbaro NM: Neurosurgical approaches to the management of chronic pain syndromes, Orthop Nurs 6(1):23-29, 1987.

41. *Levin RF, Malloy GB, and Hyman RB: Nursing management of postoperative pain: use of relaxation techniques with female cholecystectomy patients, J Adv Nurs 12(4):463-472, 1987.

42. Levine J: Pain and analgesia: the outlook for more rational treatment, Ann Intern Med 100:269-276, 1984.

43. Lipson JG and Meleis AI: Culturally appropriate care: the case of immigrants, Top Clin Nurs 7(3):48-56, 1985.

44. Lipton S: Neurodestructve procedures in the management of cancer pain, J Pain Symp Manag 2:219-229, 1987.

45. *Lisson EL: Ethical issues related to pain control, Nurs Clin North Am 22(3):649-659, 1987.

46. Marbach JJ and Wallenstein SL: Analgesic, mood, and hemodynamic effects of intranasal cocaine and lidocaine in chronic facial pain of deafferentation and myofascial origin, J Pain Symp Manag 3(2):73-79, 1988.

47. †Marks RM and Sachar EJ: Undertreatment of medical patients with narcotic analgesics, Ann Intern Med 78:173-181, 1973.

48. Mast D, Meyer J, and Urbanski A: Relaxation techniques: self-learning module for nurses, Cancer Nurs 10(3):141-147, 10(4):217-225, 10(5):279-285, 1987.

49. †McCaffery M: Nursing management of the patient with pain, Philadelphia, 1972, JB Lippincott Co.

50. †McCaffery M: Nursing management of the patient with pain, ed 2, Philadelphia, 1979, JB Lippincott Co. (The first and second editions cover different topics.)

51. *McCaffery M: Giving meperidine for pain: should it be so mechanical? Nursing 17(4):60-64, 1987.

52. *McCaffery M: A practical, "postable" chart of equianalgesic doses, Nursing 17(8):56-57, 1987.

53. *McCaffery M: When your patient is a drug abuser, Nursing 18(11):49, 1988.

54. *McGuire DB: Advances in control of cancer pain, Nurs Clin North Am 22(3):677-690, 1987.

54a. McGuire L: Administering analgesics—which drugs are right for your patient, Nurs '90 20(4):34-41, 1990.

54b. McGuire L: The power of non-narcotic pain relievers, RN 53(4):28-34, 1990.

55. Meinhart NT and McCaffery M: Pain: a nursing approach to assessment and analysis, Norwalk, CT, 1983, Appleton-Century-Crofts.

56. †Meissner JE: McGill-Melzack pain questionnaire, Nursing 10(1):50-51, 1980.

57. †Melzack R: The puzzle of pain, New York, 1973, Basic Books.

58. Melzack R, editor: Pain measurement and assessment, New York, 1983, Raven Press.

59. Melzack R: Neurophysiological foundations of pain. In Sternbach RA, editor: The psychology of pain, ed 2, New York, 1986, Raven Press.

60. Melzack R and Wall PD: The challenge of pain, New York, 1983, Basic Books.

61. †Melzack R, Guite S, and Gonshor A: Relief of dental pain by ice massage of the hand, Can Med Assoc J 122:189-191, 1980.

62. †Melzack R and Wall PD: Pain mechanisms: a new theory, Science 59:97-979, 1965.

63. *Miller TW and Jay LL: Cognitive-behavioral and pharmaceutical approaches to sensory pain management, Top Clin Nurs 6(4):34-43, 1985.

64. *Moulin DE and Coyle N: Spinal opioid analgesics and local anesthetics in the management of chronic cancer pain, J Pain Symp Manag 1(2):79-86, 1986.

65. †Neal H: The politics of pain, New York, 1978, McGraw-Hill Book Co.

66. †Nightingale F: Notes and nursing: what it is, and what it is not, Philadelphia, 1957, JB Lippincott Co.

67. Olsson G and Parker G: A model approach to pain assessment, Nursing 17(5):52-58, 1987.

68. Paice JA: Intrathecal morphine sulfate for intractable cancer pain, J Neurosurg Nurs 16(5):237-140, 1984.

69. *Paice JA: New delivery systems in pain management, Nurs Clin North Am 22(3):715-725, 1987.

70. Patterson DR, Questad KA, and Boltwood MD: Hypnotherapy as a treatment for pain in patients with burns: research and clinical considerations, J Burn Care Rehabil 8(4):263-268, 1987.

71. Pearson BD: Pain control: An experiment with imagery, Geriatr Nurs 8(1):28-30, 1987.

72. Portenoy RK: Continuous infusion of opioid drugs in the treatment of cancer pain: guidelines for use, J Pain Symp Manag 1(4):223-228, 1986.

73. *Porter J and Jick H: Addiction rare in patients treated with narcotics, N Engl J Med 302:123, 1980, (letter to the editor).

74. Ramler D and Roberts J: A comparison of cold and warm sitz baths for relief of postpartum perineal pain, JOGNN 15(6):471-474, 1986.

75. Rankin MS and Snider B: Nurses' perceptions of cancer patients' pain, Cancer Nurs 7:149-155, 1984.

76. Reading AE: A comparison of pain rating scales, J Psychosom Res 24:119-124, 1980.

77. Reizian A and Meleis AI: Arab-Americans' perceptions of and responses to pain, Crit Care Nurse 6(6):30-37, 1986.

78. *Relieving pain: an analgesic guide—principles of analgesic use in the treatment of acute and chronic cancer pain, Am J Nurs 88(6):815-826, 1988.

79. Roberts AH: Literature update: biofeedback and chronic pain, J Pain Symp Manag 2(3):169-171, 1987.

80. *St. Marie B and Henrickson K: Intraspinal narcotic infusions for terminal cancer pain, J Intraven Nurs 11(3):161-163, 1988.

81. Schroeder ME: Neurolytic nerve block for cancer pain, J Pain Symp Manag 1:91-94, 1986.

82. *Siegele DS: The gate control theory, Am J Nurs 74:498-502, 1974.

83. Smith G and Covino BG, editors: Acute pain, London, 1985, Butterworth & Co, Ltd.

84. Spross JA: Cancer pain and suffering: clinical lessons from life, literature and legend, Oncol Nurs Forum 12(4):23-31, 1985.

85. †Sternbach RA: Pain: a psychophysiological analysis, New York, 1968, Academic Press Inc.

86. †Sternbach RA: Pain patients: traits and treatment, New York, 1974, Academic Press Inc.

87. Sternbach RA: Clinical aspects of pain. In Sternbach RA, editor: The psychology of pain, ed 2, New York, 1986, Raven Press.

88. Stimmel B: Pain, analgesia, and addiction: the pharmacologic treatment of pain, New York, 1983, Raven Press.

89. Swerdlow M, editor: Relief of intractable pain. In Monographs in Anaesthesiology, vol 13, New York, 1983, Elsevier Publishing Co.

90. Swinford P: Relaxation and positive imagery for the surgical patient: a research study, Perioper Nurs Q 3(3):9-16, 1987.

91. †Szeto HH, et al: Accumulation of normeperidine, an active metabolite of meperidine, in patients with renal failure or cancer, Ann Intern Med 86:738:747, 1977.

92. Taylor AG: Pain, Annu Rev Nurs Res 5:24-43, 1987.

93. Tollison CD: Assessment and treatment at Pain Therapy

Centers programs. In Tollison CD, editor: Handbook of chronic pain management, Baltimore, 1989, Williams & Wilkins.

94. *Vandenbosch TM: How to use a pain flow sheet effectively, Nursing 18(8):50-51, 1988.

95. Wall PD and Melzack R, editors: Textbook of pain, New York, 1984, Churchill Livingstone.

96. †Waterson M: Hot and cold therapy, Nursing 8(10):46-49, 1978.

97. *Watt-Watson JH: What do we need to know about pain-?...assessing pain and giving narcotics, Am J Nurs 87(9):1217-1218, 1987.

98. Whipple B: Methods of pain control: review of research and literature, Image 19(3):142-146, 1987.

99. *Wright SM: The use of therapeutic touch in the management of pain, Nurs Clin North Am 22(3):705-713, 1987.

100. *Zborowski M: People in pain, San Francisco, 1969, Jossey-Bass Inc.

AUDIOVISUAL MATERIALS

Pain management: Margo McCaffery discusses new concepts, New York, 1984, American Journal of Nursing Co., Educational Services Division. (Four-part videotape series: (1) Nursing assessment and management of the patient with acute pain; (2) Special issues in using analgesics; (3) Special pain problems: the pediatric patient and the elderly patient; (4) New developments in nursing management of pain. Each program is 30 minutes.)

CHAPTER 17

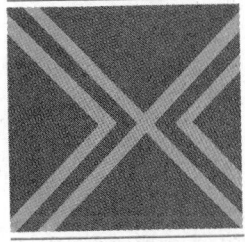

Cancer

ROSEMARIE HOGAN

CHAPTER OBJECTIVES

After studying this chapter, the student should be able to:
1 Describe epidemiologic factors related to cancer.
2 Identify the nurse's role in prevention of cancer and in health education.
3 Describe the pathophysiology of cancer including the characteristics of malignant cells, growth of neoplasms and nature of metastases.
4 Identify the factors related to carcinogenesis.
5 Relate the pathophysiologic changes that cause clinical manifestations of cancer.
6 Apply the nursing process to identify care of the patient in the diagnostic and treatment phases of cancer.
7 Explain the rationale for the four major types of cancer therapy and discuss nursing care of patients receiving these therapies.
8 Formulate a plan of care for patients with advanced cancer.

Cancer was recognized in ancient times by skilled observers who gave it the name "cancer" (L., *cancri,* crab) because it stretched out in many directions like the legs of a crab. The term is somewhat general and is used interchangeably with malignant tumor and malignant neoplasm. It denotes a tumor caused by cell growth. Forms of cancer are found in plants and in humans and other animals.

Few diseases cause greater feelings of anxiety and apprehension than cancer. Its physiologic and psychologic impact on patients and their families results in profound changes in their life-styles. Cancer may spell death to some and mutilation to others. The legends surrounding malignant disease, often focusing on incurability, help foster feelings of hopelessness and dread. Yet much progress has been made in prevention, early detection, and treatment of cancer, and research continues in these areas.

Nurses too may have the same negative attitudes that exist in society. For this reason it is extremely important that all nurses examine their own feelings about cancer and try to work them through, both by increasing their knowledge of the disease and its treatment and by discussing feelings openly with members of the health team. Nurses who have worked through their feelings are more able to help patients and their families than nurses who have not done so.

The nurse's role in helping cancer patients is broad in scope and areas of influence. The nurse must have correct knowledge of prevention, control, and treatment of cancer and be able to apply this information in a variety of settings. Teaching about cancer is not limited to the hospital or clinic setting but takes place in industry, at PTA meetings, and at other public forums. In addition to teaching about prevention, the nurse has an active role in treatment and control programs in all settings in which clients are found. Patients and their families look to the nurse for assistance and guidance in all phases of this illness, from detection to terminal care.

To be effective as a helping person the nurse must be aware of the emotional impact that the diagnosis of cancer has on the patient and family because this emotional response affects every aspect of nursing care. Cancer nursing is a challenge to the creativity, skill, and commitment of the nurse.

EPIDEMIOLOGY

The study of epidemiology is essential to identify patterns of cancer occurrence that help determine research, treatment, and financial priorities in cancer care. Cancer affects humans wherever they live and whatever their race, color, cultural background, or economic status.

Cancer ranks second to heart disease as the cause of death in the United States, but significant progress has been made in prevention and treatment. Five-year survival rates have risen to almost 50% for newly diagnosed cancer patients, and there is reason to believe that these rates will increase.[92] Success can be attributed to (1) the diagnosis of more cancers in the early localized stage, (2) the treatment of more patients within 4 months of diagnosis, and (3) the development of new diagnostic and treatment modalities, especially chemotherapy.

Despite these advances, in 1989 an estimated

TABLE 17-1 Reference chart: leading cancer sites, 1989*†

Site	Estimated New Cases 1989	Estimated Deaths 1989	Warning Signals (If You Have One See Your Doctor)	Safeguards	Comment
Breast	142,900	43,300	Lump or thickening in breast or unusual discharge from nipple	Regular checkup, monthly breast self-examination, mammograms	Leading cause of cancer death in women
Colon and rectum	151,000	61,300	Change in bowel habits, bleeding	Regular checkup including proctoscopy, especially for those over 40	Considered a highly curable disease when digital and proctoscopic examinations are included in routine checkups
Lung	155,000	142,000	Persistent cough or lingering respiratory ailment	80% of lung cancers would be prevented if no one smoked cigarettes	Leading cause of cancer death among men and rising mortality among women
Oral (including pharynx)	30,600	8650	Sore that does not heal, difficulty in swallowing	Regular checkup	Many more lives should be saved because the mouth is easily accessible to visual examination by physicians and dentists
Skin	27,000‡	8200	Sore that does not heal or change in wart or mole	Regular checkup, avoidance of overexposure to sun	Skin cancer readily detected by observation and diagnosed by simple biopsy
Uterus	47,000§	10,000	Unusual bleeding or discharge	Regular checkup including pelvic examination with Papanicolaou test	Uterine cancer mortality has declined 70% during the last 40 years with wider application of Papanicolaou test; postmenopausal women with abnormal bleeding should be checked
Kidney and bladder	70,200	20,200	Urinary difficulty, bleeding, in which case consult physician at once	Regular checkup with urinalysis	Protective measures for workers in high-risk industries are helping to eliminate one of the important causes of these cancers
Larynx	12,300	3700	Hoarseness, difficulty in swallowing	Regular checkup including laryngoscopy	Readily curable if caught early
Prostate gland	103,000	28,500	Urinary difficulty	Regular checkup including palpation	Occurs mainly in men over 60; disease can be detected by palpation at regular checkup
Stomach	20,000	13,900	Indigestion	Regular checkup	63% decline in mortality in 25 years for reasons yet unknown
Leukemia	27,300	18,100	Leukemia is a cancer of blood-forming tissues and is characterized by the abnormal production of immature white blood cells. Acute lymphocytic leukemia strikes mainly children and is treated by drugs that have extended life from a few months to as much as 10 years. Chronic leukemia usually strikes after age 25 and progresses less rapidly.		
Other blood and lymph tissue	51,800	27,400	These cancers arise in the lymph system and include Hodgkin's disease and lymphosarcoma. Some patients with lymphatic cancers can lead normal lives for many years. Five-year survival rate for Hodgkin's disease increased from 25% to 54% in 20 years.		

*From American Cancer Society: 1989 Cancer facts and figures, New York, 1989, The Society.
†All figures rounded to nearest 1000. Incidence estimates based on rates from NCI SEER Program (Surveillance, Epidemiology, and End Results), 1982-1984.
‡Melanoma only.
§Invasive cancer only.

502,000 persons died of cancer. Many might have been cured by early detection followed by prompt treatment.[4] In 1989 the probabilities of developing or dying of cancer seemed to increase, but these increases reflected the growing number of people who have survived other diseases and who are "available" or at risk for the development of cancer.

Although in general cancer does not show respect for distinctions based on economic or social status, there are some variables with regard to sex, site, age, race, and geographic location.

SEX AND SITE

The chance for developing cancer is greater for males than for females. White males now show the highest probability at birth of eventually developing cancer. By site, the largest probabilities are for the development of lung, skin, and prostate cancers in males. For women the largest probabilities are for breast, colorectal, and lung cancer. In both groups the largest increases are seen for lung cancer and cancer of the colon-rectum[92] (Table 17-1).

Overall survival rates for some cancers have increased, such as those for cervical cancer, whereas rates for most other cancers have leveled off in the past 25 years. Increases in survival have occurred for cancers of the prostate gland, uterine corpus, thyroid gland, kidney, bladder, and larynx, and for melanoma of the skin, Hodgkin's disease, and chronic leukemia. The survival rates for lung cancer have improved only slightly over a 10-year period; only 13% of these patients live 5 or more years after diagnosis.[4]

The average cancer mortality in developed countries is higher for men than for women. During the past 40 years there has been a decrease of 13% in mortality from cancer among American women because of a sharp reduction in mortality from uterine cancer. It is revealing to note that there has been an increase in the incidence of lung cancer in women; by 1989 this disease surpassed breast cancer as the number one killer of women. This appears to be related to increased cigarette smoking by American women.[4]

The death rate from cancer involving the female genital tract has dropped from between one third to one half the rate of 25 years ago. There is ample evidence that the increased use of the Papanicolaou test to detect lesions of the cervix before symptoms develop has resulted in early treatment and a higher rate of cure (Figure 17-1).

AGE

Fifty-two percent of all cancers occur in persons over 65 years of age. Cancer has been called a disease of aging, although it is the leading cause of death in women 35 to 74 years of age. Some researchers believe that if people live long enough, they will eventually develop cancer because of the decreased function of the immune system that accompanies aging (Table 17-2).

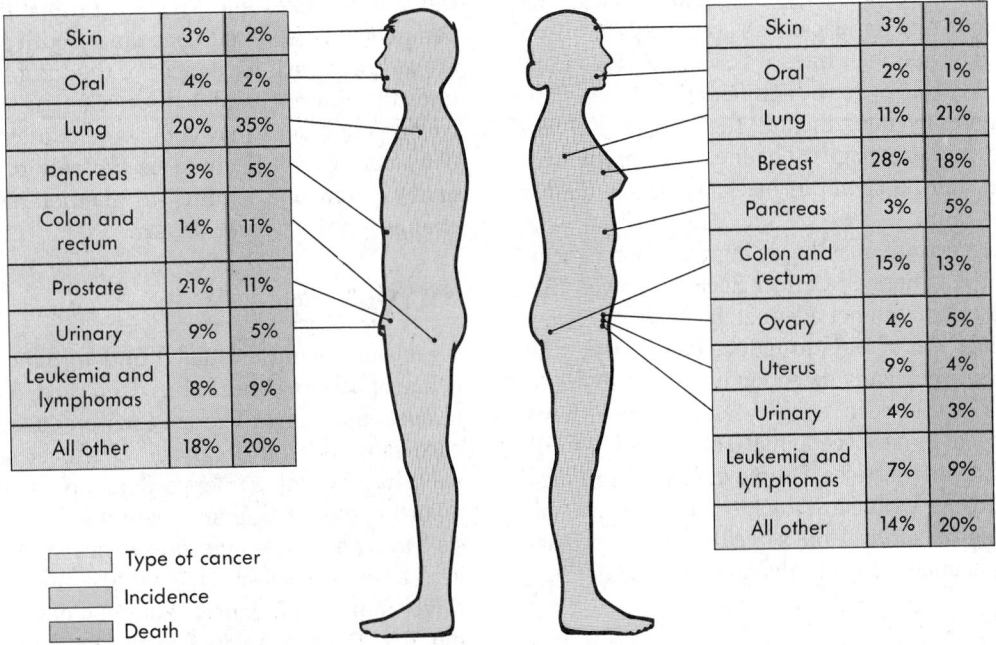

FIGURE 17-1 Comparison of cancer incidence and deaths by site and sex (1989 estimates). (From American Cancer Society, 1989, Cancer facts and figures, New York, 1989, The Society.)

TABLE 17-2 Mortality for the five leading cancer sites in major age groups by sex (United States, 1989)

Age	Males	Total	Females	Total
Under 15	Leukemia	418	Leukemia	296
	Brain and CNS	230	Brain and CNS	192
	Non-Hodgkin's lymphomas	66	Bone	41
	Connective tissue	50	Non-Hodgkin's lymphomas	36
	Bone	30	Bladder	36
15-34	Leukemia	679	Breast	649
	Skin (melanoma)	469	Leukemia	347
	Brain and CNS	444	Uterus	347
	Non-Hodgkin's lymphomas	438	Brain and CNS	321
	Hodgkin's disease	301	Non-Hodgkin's lymphomas	202
35-54	Lung	8926	Breast	8297
	Colorectal	2247	Lung	4960
	Brain and CNS	1272	Colorectal	1911
	Non-Hodgkin's lymphomas	1214	Uterus	1778
	Skin (melanoma)	1208	Ovary	1666
55-74	Lung	53,756	Lung	24,322
	Colorectal	14,749	Breast	20,301
	Prostate	10,488	Colorectal	12,200
	Pancreas	6652	Ovary	6380
	Stomach	4485	Pancreas	5542
75+	Lung	20,996	Colorectal	14,542
	Prostate	15,132	Breast	11,131
	Colorectal	10,422	Lung	9279
	Pancreas	3672	Pancreas	5211
	Bladder	3380	Ovary	3346

From Cancer statistics 1989, CA 39(1):7, 1989.

RACE

The cancer incidence rate and death rate are higher for blacks than for whites for both males and females. The overall incidence rate for blacks has gone up 27% over a 30-year period, while for whites it increased 12%. Cancer sites where blacks have significantly higher incidence and mortality rates include the lung, colon-rectum, prostate, and esophagus. The incidence of invasive cancer of the uterine cervix in black women is double that in whites.[4]

Hispanic-Americans may be at high risk for cancer. A survey for the American Cancer Society showed that Hispanic-Americans are not adequately aware of cancer warning signals and of ways to reduce cancer risk, and they tend not to seek early detection or treatment.[4]

Cancer survival and, in some cases incidence, however, are related to socioeconomic factors such as the availability of health services. Ethnic differences in cancer are secondary. Estimates suggest that at least half the differences in survival rates result from late diagnoses among economically disadvantaged persons.[4]

GEOGRAPHIC FACTORS

Differences in the geographic distribution of cancer occur. For example, primary cancer of the liver is common in Indonesia and parts of Africa and Asia but rare in other regions. Cancer of the breast is more frequent in the United States and Western Europe than it is in Japan. Ugandans, Nigerians, and South African blacks are at lowest risk for cancer of the lung, stomach, large intestine, uterus, and kidney. Genetic differences between populations may contribute to international variations but are not likely to be the only reason since migration from one country to another results in major changes in the cancer pattern.

FACTORS AFFECTING PROGNOSIS

Trends are being evaluated to determine why the incidence of certain cancers has decreased, increased, or remained the same. There is reason to believe that the cure rate and the prognosis of cancer would improve substantially with earlier recognition and more complete reporting of early signs. Patient delay in seeking diagnosis for symptoms suggesting cancer reduces chance of long-term survival by 10% to 20%. From one fourth to three fourths of cancer patients delay more than 3 months. Delay is related to the patient's *perception* of (1) the chance of cancer, (2) possibility of early detection and treatment, (3) inconvenience of examination,

(4) need for relief of symptoms, and (5) need for reassurance.

Reducing "hassle," providing accurate information in the event that a symptom does represent cancer, providing information on the benefits of early detection, and reducing fear and denial will all shorten delay and increase chance of cure.[32]

Success in treating many cancers awaits better and more sensitive diagnostic aids to detect lesions in their early stages. In some parts of the body such as the skin and cervix, early recognition and prompt treatment often result in cure.

The prognosis is also affected by the intrinsic characteristics of the tumor, such as histologic type and grade, size, and rate of growth. Another important factor is age and the general condition of the patient. The presence of debilitating conditions, such as infection, diabetes, or malnutrition, may adversely affect the outcome.

PREVENTION AND HEALTH EDUCATION

HEALTH TEACHING

Nurses have a major responsibility in the prevention of cancer. Because of their knowledge about the disease and their opportunity for contact with the public in the inpatient and outpatient setting, nurses have the opportunity to teach about cancer and to help motivate patients to seek treatment.

Risk factors must be identified and moderated. Three types of risk factors for cancer have been identified: *Life-style* factors are those over which the individual has some control, especially tobacco use, diet, alcohol, sunlight exposure, and sexual practices. *Environmental* factors include exposure to carcinogens and are at times beyond the individual's control. *Genetic* factors, conditions inherited at conception, are not usually controllable except through genetic counseling services.[5] High risk families, especially those at risk for breast, colorectal, and lung cancers, are being identified and have received intervention that includes assessment, screening, referral, education, and follow-up.[7]

Case finding is a responsibility of all nurses. The nurse must be able to (1) counsel and direct patients to the proper sources of help, (2) have information about those conditions that are known to predispose individuals to the development of the disease, and (3) educate the public about these factors. In addition, the nurse must be sensitive to the needs of patients who may be afraid and embarrassed when confronted with the possibility of cancer.

EARLY DETECTION AND TREATMENT

The approach to early detection of cancer is worldwide. General criteria for cancer screening and testing programs have been drawn up by the epidemiology section of the American Public Health Association, and these criteria have been adapted by the World Health Organization. Multiphasic screening and a periodic health examination are being accepted by the public. In some cases diagnosis can be made months before the development of symptoms causes the person to seek care.

Cancer detection is expensive. Education of the public often includes convincing them that a periodic health examination is a sound investment. Some cities have cancer detection centers where a complete physical examination including chest radiograph, Papanicolaou smear, breast examination, proctoscopy, urinalysis, and blood count are performed for a moderate fee. Nurses should be aware of clinics in their area where persons needing such resources may be referred. Knowledge is not in itself protection against adverse life-style habits. An appropriate attitude is essential. Many people believe that "everything causes cancer" and that there is not much a person can do to prevent it.[13] Nurses work with individuals to change these attitudes.

The American Cancer Society has revised its guidelines for cancer-related checkups to provide essentially the same benefits with greatly reduced cost, risk, and inconvenience. Protocols for the early detection of cancer in asymptomatic persons are listed in Table 17-3. In general, persons over 20 years of age should have a cancer-related health checkup every 3 years, and those over 40 years old should have one every year. These checkups should also involve health counseling including information about personal cancer risk factors.[104] Women should request that the Pap test (Papanicolaou stain) be done if it was inadvertently overlooked by the health care provider. If the test is done early, cancer may be diagnosed before metastasis occurs (see Chapter 53).

Early detection of cancer can decrease mortality. The nurse must know and be able to explain the significance of the seven warning signs of cancer (see the box below), stressing that any of these signs should be reported immediately to a physician. It should be emphasized that any of these signs should be investigated medically (see Table 17-1), but their occurrence does not necessarily mean that the person has cancer.

All persons should know the most common sites of

SEVEN WARNING SIGNS OF CANCER

1. Change in bowel and bladder habits
2. A sore that does not heal
3. Unusual bleeding or discharge
4. Thickening or a lump in the breast or elsewhere
5. Indigestion or difficulty in swallowing
6. Obvious change in a wart or mole
7. Nagging cough or hoarseness

TABLE 17-3 Guidelines for cancer related checkups*

Test or Examination	Sex	Age (Years)	Recommendation
Papanicolaou test	Female	Over 20; under 20 if sexually active	Every 3 years after two initial negative tests 1 year apart
Pelvic examination	Female	20-40	Every 3 years
		Over 40 or at menopause	Yearly
Endometrial tissue sample	Female	At menopause if high risk	High risk: history of infertility, obesity, failure of ovulation, abnormal uterine bleeding, estrogen therapy
Breast self-examination	Female	Over 20	Monthly
Breast physical examination	Female	20-40	Every 3 years
		Over 40	Yearly
Mammogram	Female	35-40	One baseline mammogram
		Over 50	Yearly
Stool guaiac slide test	Male and female	Over 50	Yearly
Digital rectal examination	Male and female	Over 40	Yearly
Sigmoidoscopic examination	Male and female	Over 50	Every 3-5 years after two initial negative examinations 1 year apart

*American Cancer Society recommendations.

cancer. In women these are the breast, uterus (cervix), lung, and gastrointestinal tract (Figure 17-1). Women should be taught to examine their breasts each month immediately after the menstrual period or, if postmenopausal, on a designated day each month. Such self-examination is a much better method of detecting early breast cancer than an annual physical examination.

Women of all ages should know the importance of reporting any abnormal vaginal bleeding or other discharge occurring between menstrual periods or after menopause (see Chapter 55 for details of early symptoms of cancer of the female reproductive system). (Further information about cancer of specific organs can be found in appropriate chapters of this book.)

Two common misconceptions that lead the person to ignore symptoms should be corrected. The first is a belief that a disease as serious as cancer must be accompanied by weight loss. Weight loss is usually a late symptom of cancer. Another reason for neglect of cancer is the belief that absence of pain means than an indisposition is minor. It must be repeatedly emphasized to the public that pain is not an early sign of cancer and that cancer often is far advanced before pain occurs.

Nurses also have a role in prevention and early detection of genetic cancer. They systematically obtain family cancer histories, teach about health maintenance, and do genetic counseling. They may be involved in centralized familial cancer registries analogous to the monitoring of communicable diseases by health departments. Familial cancer registries would be helpful in pooling data on suspected cancer-prone families, as well as in disseminating current methods of surveillance and management of the conditions.

FACTORS THAT INTERFERE WITH HEALTH-SEEKING BEHAVIORS

Even though knowledge of cancer is more widespread than before, a more positive attitude toward the disease is essential if individuals are to follow good health practices and seek help when warning signs of cancer are noted. Factors that may interfere with health-seeking behaviors include underestimation of the incidence of cancer and negative views about conventional therapies. Less-educated people and men in general are less likely to have physical examinations.[104] These are all factors that may interfere with health-seeking behaviors.

Unfortunately, anxiety and fear may immobilize the individual. Despite all the public announcements that have been made in the last few decades, there are still people who think cancer must be hidden from others. This attitude stems partly from the fact that cancer in its terminal stages may be a painful and demoralizing disease that is sometimes accompanied by body odor and other signs of physical debility that are deeply etched on the consciousness of friends and relatives. Actually, there is no characteristic odor of cancer, although diseased tissue that breaks down and becomes infected with odor-producing organisms will be as unpleasant as any other infected wound. The essential point—so often missed by the public—is that this tragic situation is by and large an unusual one.

Some people fear cancer and shun persons who have the disease because they believe it is contagious. Scientific speculation on the possibility that a virus may be the cause has added to this fear. At this time, there is no conclusive evidence that cancer can be spread among humans in a way similar to the spread of infectious diseases.

The positive aspects of cancer care should be emphasized. It is estimated that approximately one third of the persons for whom a diagnosis is made are cured by medical treatment. Another one third could perhaps be cured by medical treatment if the cancer is diagnosed early enough. Only a third have cancer occurring in locations in which the disease advanced beyond permanent medical aid before sufficient signs appeared to warn the patient of trouble. In spite of these facts, some persons think it is useless to report symptoms early, since they believe that if they do have cancer they cannot be cured. It can only be hoped that the recent publicity given to well-known persons who have been treated for cancer will help overcome some of these beliefs. If nothing else, the open discussion of the diagnosis and treatment in all types of media should result in a better informed public than ever before.

CANCER QUACKERY

Fatal delay in seeking medical care may occur because of the patient's reliance on a "quick, painless cure." Despite public education and efforts of the medical profession to control extravagant claims of a few unethical practitioners, cancer quackery still exists, feeding on the ignorance and fear of the cancer patient and family.

Quacks rely on testimonials of people they have "cured." Books and testimonials in magazines may be so appealingly written that the reader gets the impression that the content is factual and accurate. Electronic gadgets, dietary regimens, and various drugs and enzymes have all been purported to cure cancer.

Two drugs still available mostly outside the United States are krebiozen and laetrile, a substance derived from apricot kernels. Use of laetrile for cancer therapy has been outlawed by the FDA, whose regulations prohibit the transportation of laetrile across state lines. Neither drug has been scientifically demonstrated to result in objective benefit to the person or show evidence that metastatic growth has been controlled. Based on a study of 156 patients at 4 medical centers, investigators of the National Cancer Institute in 1981 reported that laetrile was a failure as a cancer treatment.

Other drugs that have no benefit for cancer cure include iscador, an extract of mistletoe, and dimethyl sulfoxide (DMSO) either by itself or combined with laetrile and procaine hydrochloride (KH3). The tragedy in the use of these drugs is the false sense of security the treatment creates in patients. This sense of security may cause patients to delay in seeking medical care until it is too late.

The most common treatment being used now is so-called metabolic therapy, a combination of special diet, detoxification by internal cleaning, spiritual and emotional healing, and high-dose vitamins and minerals.

Diet treatment may be a variety of therapies from the grape cure to raw foods to wheatgrass extract. The macrobiotic diet is the most commonly adopted dietary remedy touted in the United States. This unproven therapy has its own diagnostic technique, ideology that involves looking at the iris of the eye, each pie-shaped segment of which is supposed to represent a different organ and enable diagnoses of cancer of that area.

The megavitamin approach involves consumption of large qualities of high-dose vitamins believed to increase the body's ability to kill cancer cells.

Mental imagery requires the patient to visualize or imagine destruction of the cancer cells.[9] The acceptance by patients of these therapies is based on *unfounded* messages about the causes of cancer. People view positively any simple notions of causality.

CANCER RESEARCH

Just as research is the basis of nursing practice, so research is the basis of cancer control and cure. The National Cancer Institute has recognized the need for community participation in clinical trials. Cancer research is multifaceted and is ongoing in all facets of cancer control, education, intervention, screening, treatment, and patient care[33] (Figure 17-2).

Research on the cause of cancer has explored the effect of several factors acting together to stimulate aberrant cell growth, the role of chemicals and other environmental pollutants, genetic factors, and the role of viruses in the development of cancer.

Many investigators are focusing their interest on subcellular components. There is increasing interest in changes in the chromosome and in the nucleic acids, essential cell constituents, DNA, and RNA. In addition, investigations using animals yield much useful information. For example, a strain of mice has been developed in which all the mice develop breast cancer. Evidence obtained through animal experimentation, however, does not necessarily prove that human beings react in the same way, but it raises the possibility that they may do so.

Immunologists in cancer research have become increasingly aware of the role of the immune system in both the natural history and the therapy of malignant disease. They suggest that it is possible to strengthen the body's natural responses so that the body would be able to destroy malignant cells when they first appear. The discovery that human neoplasms contain tumor-specific antigens not found in normal cells has opened up new avenues of therapy in controlling the progression and in inducing the regression of human neoplasms.

Around the world many research centers are developing better treatment modalities. Use of a combination of surgery, radiation, and chemotherapy has shown that there may be significant prolongation of life and in some

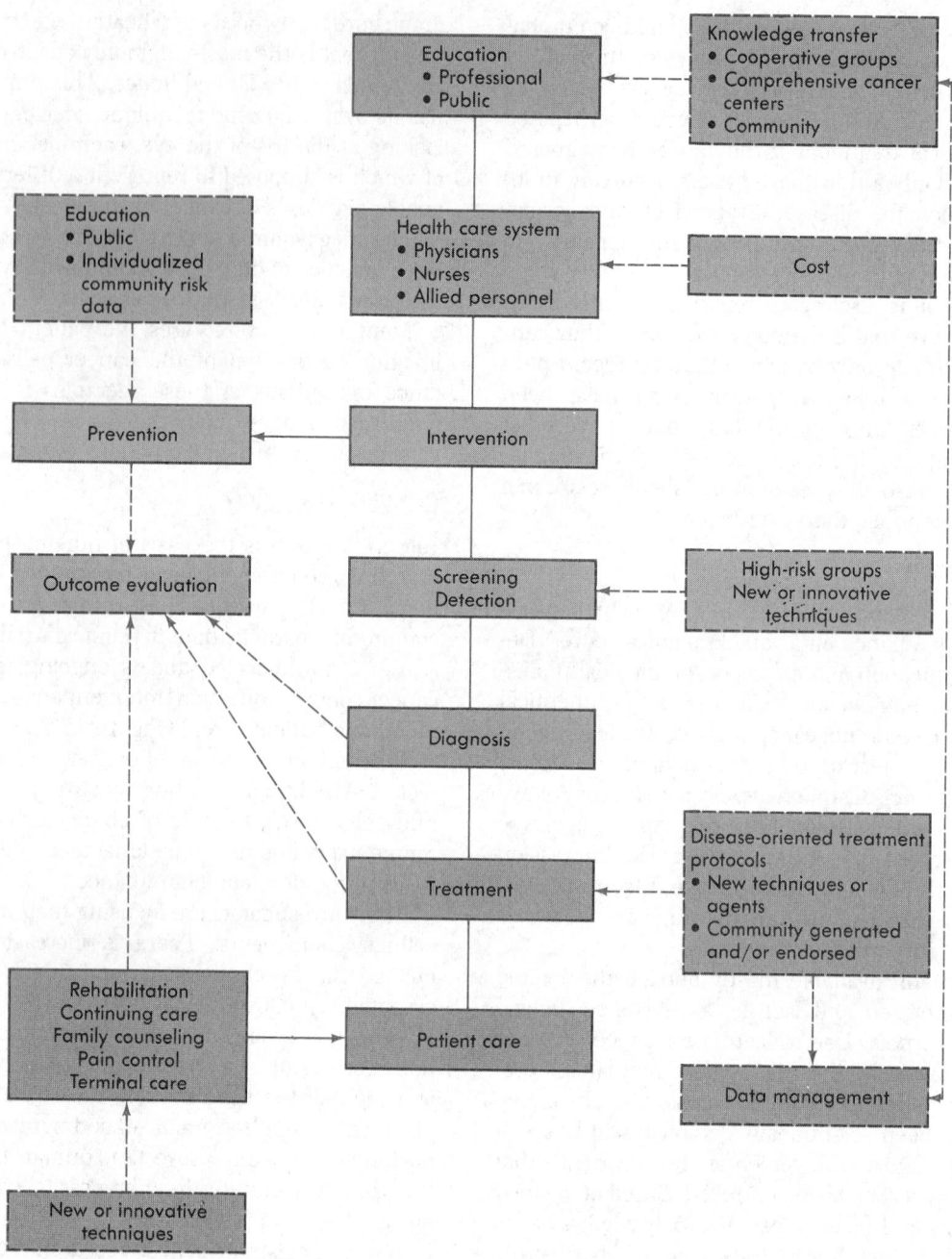

FIGURE 17-2 Model of the relationship between cancer control and clinical research in the community. Critical components of cancer control are outlined in the solid-line boxes, and clinical research elements are enclosed within dashed-lined boxes. (From Enck RE: Interrelationships of cancer control and clinical research in the community, CA 34:342, 1984.)

instances complete cure of children with Wilms' tumor, an extremely malignant embryonal tumor of the kidney. Continued study of the use of chemotherapeutic drugs has resulted in effective new combination therapies for many types of cancer.

Future research against cancer will probably be directed toward developing and screening new drugs that can act alone or with other drugs; applying new forms of radiation such as laser beams that spare normal tissue and are not carcinogenic themselves; developing forms of immunotherapy, both alone and in combination; developing new combinations of known effective drugs; and combining treatment modalities such as surgery, irradiation, chemotherapy, and immunotherapy.

The major focus of nursing research has been on clinical care of the patient. Continued work is directed toward developing the scientific foundation on which cancer nursing is based. At present, the largest number of studies relate to psychosocial responses of individuals and their families to cancer, to nursing interventions, and to terminal care. Nurses also investigate topics such as nausea and vomiting, nutrition, pain, stomatitis, alopecia, local tissue damage from drug extravasation, and patient teaching.[47] Studies concerned with education have focused on both patients and nurses.

Cancer nursing research has expanded because of educational opportunities in cancer care and active support from organizations such as the American Cancer Society. Nurses are continuing to look at priorities in cancer nursing research.

ORGANIZATIONS INVOLVED IN CANCER EDUCATION, DETECTION, AND REHABILITATION

FEDERAL ORGANIZATIONS

Federal recognition of the need to give intensive assistance to educational programs in cancer began in 1926 when Congress proclaimed April of each year as National Cancer Control Month. In 1937 the National Cancer Institute was created within the National Institutes of Health. This institute conducts an extensive program of research in the field of cancer.

Cancer patients may also obtain help from both Medicare and Medicaid. The Community Services Administration provides services through state agencies such as Welfare and Aging or by direct grants. The Rehabilitation Services Administration will arrange and pay for services that help the cancer patient return to productive living. With the passage of the National Cancer Act of 1971, impetus was given for the development of Cancer Clinical Research Centers. The goal was to translate research results into medical practice so that no one will be denied professional advice and care because of lack of facilities and knowledge. These centers combine research capability, demonstration of recent techniques and therapy, and community outreach programs.

Nurses can be articulate speakers for the cause of cancer care and cure, since they are intimately aware of the effects of cancer in threat to life and cost in dollars, disrupted lives, and human suffering. Nurses must assertively express to their representatives in government the importance of a combined effort to eradicate cancer.

AMERICAN CANCER SOCIETY

The American Cancer Society, Inc. (ACS), a large national voluntary organization, has branches in all states and in 11 major cities. This huge organization, which is supported by voluntary gifts, has three main objectives: research, education, and services to cancer patients.

Research is a major focus, and the Society finances studies that seek the cause of cancer and the development of better methods of treatment. As part of its education efforts, ACS publishes booklets and pamphlets for the use of health care providers, and it stimulates better preparation of professional persons in the care of patients with cancer by sponsoring institutes and other programs for these special groups. Information about available teaching materials may be obtained from the main office of the Society or from state or local offices.*

In addition, the American Cancer Society strives constantly to *educate* the public. It works intensively through magazines, radio, television, clubs, insurance companies, state departments of health, and medical and nursing organizations in an effort to reach all the population with the educational message of how cancer may be prevented and controlled. A large amount of literature for the laity is prepared and distributed annually. Also, many excellent films for use in public education may be borrowed from the Society.

The Society also performs *services* for patients and their families. Branches in most communities provide assistance for cancer patients who cannot afford to pay for adequate care and for those who, although they can presently afford to pay, will eventually leave their families with too great a financial burden. Depending on how much community support is given to the society, the services may include dressings, transportation to and from clinics and physicians' offices, special drugs such as expensive hormones, blood, prostheses, and the loan of equipment such as hospital beds. In some communities homemaking, visiting nurse, and rehabilitation services are also provided. Patients and their families should know about these services before their own resources are depleted, and local citizens should be urged to support the Society.

OTHER VOLUNTARY ORGANIZATIONS

Cancer Care, a large voluntary organization in New York City, confines its activities solely to the tremendous needs of patients with advanced cancer and to the needs of their families. The nurse who works in a small community or a rural area may learn of the resources available to cancer patients through local or state health departments.

Some insurance companies, such as the Metropolitan Life Insurance Company and the John Hancock Insurance Company, prepare very useful pamphlets on control of cancer and the care of persons who have the disease. These pamphlets are useful to nurses in conducting health education programs and in teaching relatives care of a patient with cancer.

---

*Headquarters: 90 Park Ave, New York, NY 10016.

RESEARCH

Rogers TF, Bauman LJ, and Metzger L: An assessment of the Reach to Recovery program, CA 35(2):116-124, 1985.

This study is based on data obtained from 652 mastectomy patients interviewed about their recovery from mastectomy (about 1 year previously) and their experience with the Reach to Recovery program. Almost all of the patients who saw a Reach to Recovery volunteer perceived the visit as helpful regardless of age, level of education, employment status, number of physical problems after surgery, or the availability of emotional support from family. Few women had criticisms of the program, and there was no evidence that the visit harmed any patient. The clinical implications are that patients benefit from contact with others who have had the same experience and that most will find the visit helpful. ■

CANCER PATIENTS' GROUPS

Patient groups have been organized to help others with the same disability. Lost Chord Clubs (laryngectomy patients), Encore and Reach to Recovery (both for mastectomy patients), and ostomy clubs have been formed in many cities. Individuals share what they have learned about coping with the problems resulting from therapy for their conditions. They visit patients either in the hospital or at home and hold regular group meetings (see the research box).

PUBLIC HEALTH AGENCIES

Many other agencies may be needed for the rehabilitation of the cancer patient. Community health nurses have a vital role in helping patients and families adjust after the cancer patient returns from the hospital. It is by the coordinated effort of hospital and community nurses that the patient and family can return to a satisfying and fulfilling life.

PATHOPHYSIOLOGY

Knowledge of pathophysiology is essential if nurses are to understand the rationale for the prevention and treatment of cancer. In addition, some patients and families want and need explanation of the disease process and how the various therapies will aid in cure.

CHARACTERISTICS OF NORMAL CELLS

Normal tissue contains large numbers of mature cells of uniform size and shape, each containing a nucleus of uniform size. Within each nucleus are the chromosomes, a specific number for the species, and within each chromosome is *deoxyribonucleic acid* (DNA). DNA is a giant molecule whose chemical composition

CELL REPLICATION: INTERPHASE AND MITOSIS

INTERPHASE	Two centrioles (small cell structures) begin to move apart. Microtubules grow radially away from centrioles, some penetrating cell nucleus, some connecting the centrioles forming a spindle. Within nucleus each chromosome splits to form two new chromosomes.
MITOSIS **Prophase**	Nuclear envelope dissolves and some of the microtubules become attached to the chromosomes.
Metaphase	The two centrioles are pushed further apart by the growing spindle, pulling the chromosomes to center of cell.
Anaphase	Each pair of chromosomes breaks apart; 46 daughter chromosomes are pulled toward one mitotic spindle and the other 46 chromosomes to the other spindle.
Telophase	The two sets of chromosomes are pulled completely apart and are enveloped by new nuclear membranes. The cell then separates into two cells with a nucleus in each cell.

controls the characteristics of *ribonucleic acid* (RNA), which is found both in the *nucleoli* of cells and in the cytoplasm of the cell itself and which regulates cell growth and function. When ovum and sperm unite, the DNA and RNA within the chromosomes of each will govern the differentiation and future course of the trillions of cells that finally develop to form the adult organism. In the development of various organs and parts of the body, cells undergo differentiation in size, appearance, and arrangement; thus the histologist or the pathologist can look at a piece of prepared tissue through a microscope and know the portion of the body from which it came.

MITOSIS

Mitosis refers to the splitting of one cell into two cells. In the normal cell, multiplication takes place by an orderly process. Reproduction begins in the nucleus by duplication (replication) of the 23 pairs (46) of chromosomes, as well as the genes within the chromosomes. This duplication is followed by the division of the two sets of chromosomes into two separate nuclei and finally splitting of the cell to form two daughter cells. Mitosis, which is preceded by a phase called *interphase,* consists of four phases: prophase, metaphase, anaphase, and telophase (see the box above and Figure 17-3).

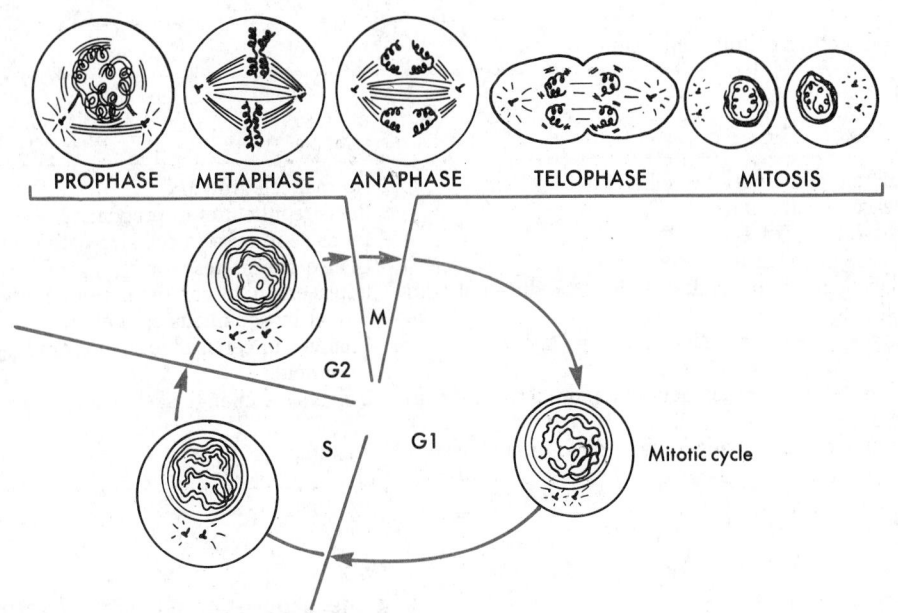

FIGURE 17-3 Cell cycle. *G1*, RNA/protein synthesis; *S*, DNA synthesis; *G2*, RNA/protein synthesis and interphase; and *M*, mitosis. (Adapted from Krakoff I: Cancer chemotherapeutic agents: American Cancer Society professional education publication, New York, 1977, American Cancer Society.)

CELL CYCLE TIME

The concept of cell cycle time is pertinent to understanding normal cell replication and has implications for drug use in cancer therapy (p. 361). Cell cycle time may be described as the interval from mitosis of a cell to its mitosis into daughter cells. Initially there is a stationary period (G_0) of apparent rest after mitosis takes place. The cells are not in the cycle but are viable and capable of undergoing mitosis if necessary. The cell cycle is divided into four phases (Figure 17-3): (1) a quiescent phase consisting of G_1 (G denotes a gap) in which RNA and protein synthesis begin; (2) S_1, a period of DNA synthesis; (3) G_2, further RNA and protein synthesis and the development of the mitotic spindle; and (4) mitosis (M). These processes of normal cell multiplication take place in response to a need and then stop.

DIFFERENTIATION

Another characteristic of normal cell growth and cell division is cell differentiation. Changes in physical and functional properties of cells occur in the embryo to form different organs and tissues. Differentiation of cells, consequently, refers to the extent to which the cells resemble their normal forebears and thus have fully mature, specialized function and morphology. For example, all kidney cells are similar but are different from muscle cells, and each type has its specialized function. In malignant cells, changes in differentiation take place.

The method by which differentiation takes place is unknown. One current thought is that all cells carry the same genetic material but that selective repression of different genetic characteristics occurs because of buildup of different repressor substances in the cytoplasm. Different cells repress different genetic characteristics.

NORMAL ALTERATIONS IN CELL GROWTH

Some abnormal changes in cell growth are malignant growths (neoplasias). Other types of cellular growths are benign. *Hyperplasia* is an increase in cell number, whereas *hypertrophy* is an increase in cell size but not in number. Although many neoplasms are characterized by hyperplasia, many normal tissues may also undergo increase in cell number. Wound healing, callus formation, and growth of embryonic tissue are all normal forms of hyperplasia.[28]

Metaplasia is a reversible process in which one adult cell type in an organ is replaced by another adult cell type. The new cell type usually is not one normally seen in the area in which metaplasia occurs. The most common type of epithelial metaplasia is the change of columnar or pseudostratified columnar epithelium of the respiratory tract to squamous epithelium or squamous metaplasia. *Dysplasia* is an alteration in adult cells characterized by changes in their size, shape, and organization (Table 17-4).

TABLE 17-4 Terms denoting cellular changes

Type of Cellular Change	Definition	Example
Mitosis	Formation of new cell by cell division	Normal cell growth
Hyperplasia	Increase in cell number	Breast epithelium in pregnancy
Hypertrophy	Increase in cell size	Increase in muscle cell size with exercise
Atrophy	Decrease in cell size	Disuse of muscles
Metaplasia	Replacement of one adult cell type by a different adult cell type	Replacement of columnar epithelium of respiratory tract by squamous epithelium
Dysplasia	Changes in cell size, shape, and organization	Changes in cervical epithelium in long-standing cervicitis
Anaplasia	Reverse cellular development to a more primitive cell type	Irreversible change accompanying cancer
Neoplasia	Abnormal cellular changes and growth of new tissues	Malignancies

BENIGN TUMORS

Benign (nonmalignant) tumors involve cellular proliferation of adult or mature cells growing slowly in an orderly manner in a capsule. These tumors do not invade surrounding tissue but may cause harm through pressure on vital structures within an enclosed structure such as the skull. Benign tumors remain localized, do not metastasize (spread), and do not recur once they are completely removed (see the box below).

CHARACTERISTICS OF MALIGNANT CELLS
CELLULAR CHANGES

A malignant cell is one in which the basic structure and activity have become deranged in a manner that is unknown and from a cause or causes that are still poorly understood. It is believed, however, that the basic process involves a disturbance in the regulatory functions of DNA. It is known that the DNA molecule is affected by radiation in certain instances, and it is speculated that it may be affected by other factors as well.

DIFFERENCES BETWEEN BENIGN AND MALIGNANT NEOPLASMS

BENIGN	MALIGNANT
Limited growth potential	May proliferate rapidly or grow slowly
Localized	Spreads (metastasizes) throughout the body
Fibrous capsule	No enclosing capsule
Rarely recurs after removal	May recur even after treatment
Usually regular in shape	Irregular shape with poorly defined border
Cells similar to cell of parent tissue (well differentiated)	Cells much different from parent cells (poorly differentiated)
Expansive growth	Infiltrative growth

In the neoplastic cell, normal restraints on growth are defective. It is believed that malignant neoplasms occur as the result of faulty mechanisms inside the cell nucleus.

DNA, the permanent genetic material in nuclear chromosomes, contains information necessary for cell replication: the chemical code for cell growth and development. To convey this information, RNA serves as a messenger. Any small change in DNA (mutation) causes a distortion of biologic information, which results in the affected cells running wild. Malignant neoplasm is the result. The malignant cells lose the normal specialized function of the normal cell or may take on new characteristics and functions.

A characteristic of malignant cells that can be observed through a microscope is a loss of differentiation, or a likeness to the original cell (parent tissue) from which the tumor growth originated. Cancer cells may vary in their likeness to the tissue of origin. They may be well differentiated (very similar to the tissue of origin), moderately well differentiated (somewhat similar to the tissue of origin), or poorly differentiated (little similarity to the tissue of origin). Generally the cancer with more poorly differentiated cells has a poor prognosis because of a higher degree of malignancy.

This loss of differentiation is called *anaplasia* and is characterized by alterations in intracellular macromolecular synthesis and intercellular relationships and associations. Two types of anaplasia have been identified. In positional or organizational anaplasia, the usual distinct histologic patterns in tissues are altered. In cytologic anaplasia there is increased or altered nucleic acid synthesis in growing tissues. Anaplasia is seen only in cancers and does not appear in benign neoplasms.

In many cancer cells the chromosomes that carry genes are abnormal. They may be broken apart, have pieces missing or flipped over, or be shuffled among

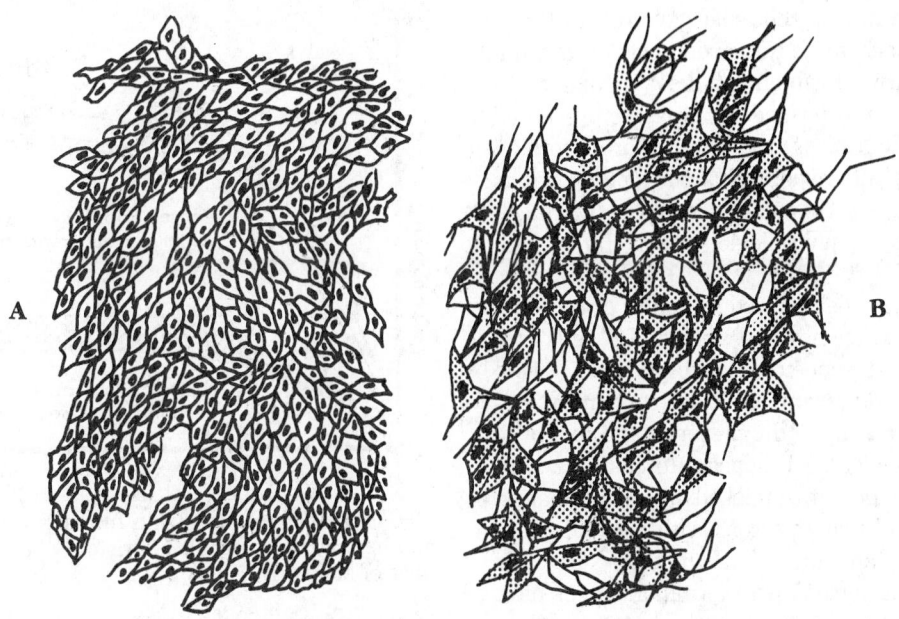

FIGURE 17-4 A, Normal cell appearance. **B,** Abnormal cell appearance.

chromosomes. The terms *translocation* or *deletion* are used to describe the alteration in position or the absence of parts of chromosomes.[86]

Other characteristics of malignant cells that can be seen through a microscope are the presence of nuclei of various sizes, many of which contain unusually large amounts of chromatin (hyperchromatic cells), and the presence of mitotic figures (cells in the process of division), which denotes rapid and disorderly division of cells (see the box for characteristics of malignant cells).

Tumor cells show less contact inhibition in vitro and therefore "pile up" in cultures, suggesting that surface properties of cancer cells are different from normal cells (Figure 17-4). In addition, the proportion of cancer cells actively proliferating in malignant tumors is generally greater than that of normal cells in benign tumors.[28]

Malignant tumors have no enclosing capsule; thus they invade adjacent or surrounding tissue, including lymph and blood vessels, through which they may spread to distant parts of the body to set up new tumors (*metastases*). Unless completely removed or destroyed, they tend to recur after treatment, and their continued presence causes death by replacing normal cells and by other means not fully understood.

GROWTH OF NEOPLASMS

The term *neoplasm* has been defined as a relatively autonomous growth of tissues—*autonomy* meaning that a malignant tumor is not subject to the "rules and regulations" that govern cells and cell interaction of the healthy individual. This autonomy is relative in that the

tumor is not completely independent of the tissue from which it arose.

There are considerable differences in the rate of growth of malignant tumors. Occasionally one grows so slowly that it can be removed completely after a long period of time. This characteristic probably accounts for the good results obtained in a few circumstances even when treatment has been delayed. However, no physician ever relies on this possibility to justify delay in treatment. Occasionally a malignant tumor grows slowly for a long time and then undergoes change, and the rate of growth increases enormously.

Factors Causing Tumor Growth

The first overt cellular change in the development of cancer is transformation. Transformed cells are morpho-

---

CHARACTERISTICS OF NEOPLASTIC CELLS[28]

1. Nuclei are larger and irregular in shape.
2. DNA is coarsely distributed and tends to appear near nuclear membrane.
3. Nucleoli are large, usually increased in number, and contain more chromatin than usual.
4. Mitosis is increased and atypical in appearance.
5. Abnormal multipolar mitoses and multinucleated cells may appear.
6. Cytoplasm is comparatively scanty and stains more deeply than normal cytoplasm, indicating greater RNA concentration.
7. Cells vary in size from normal cells.
8. Chromosome parts are deleted or translocated.

logically different from the cells that gave rise to them. Whether the cells become a tumor depends on a number of factors, many of which are host mediated (p. 344). Replication of transformed cells may be prevented if the immune system recognizes the tumor as foreign and destroys the cells, a hypothetical concept known as "immune surveillance." This ability decreases with age, since it depends on the physiologic state of the individual (p. 346).

Several factors may be involved in failure of immune surveillance: (1) a deficiency in T cells and B cells (see Chapter 8), (2) the presence of "blocking factor," which binds tumor cells and prevents their destruction by sensitized lymphocytes, and (3) the presence and extent of "recognition factor" (RF). RF appears to combine with tumor cells before they are attacked by macrophages. Healthy persons and many persons with nonmalignant diseases have large amounts of RF in their serum. It has been found that persons with terminal cancer have less RF than do those with less advanced disease. Failure of the recognition mechanism may play a role in growth of tumors.

Factors Inhibiting Tumor Growth

Some tumor growth may be checked by lack of vascularization. One researcher has shown that some tumors produce an angiogenesis factor that attracts capillaries to the tumor. Tumors will not grow over a diameter of 3 to 4 mm unless this vascularization occurs.[28]

Growth of tumors that arise in tissues regulated by sex hormones may be affected in positive or negative ways. For example, breast cancers that occur during pregnancy often grow rapidly but tend to grow less rapidly after delivery.

There are also a number of growth-inhibiting factors called *chalones*. For example, epithelial cells produce a glycoprotein chalone that interacts with adrenalin to inhibit proliferation. Some experimental tumors have been inhibited by a tissue-specific chalone from which the tumor arose.

Although it is rare, tumors have regressed spontaneously, in some cases as a result of maturation and differentiation of tumor cells. This happens most frequently in neuroblastoma, a tumor of embryonic neuroblasts. The cause and physiologic action of spontaneous maturation are not known.

Factors Affecting Rate of Tumor Growth

Most tumors continue to grow and evolve, and when a large number of rapidly growing cells are present, additional mutation and arrangement of chromosomes may occur. Stem cells, a subpopulation of tumor cells with an extreme ability to proliferate, develop and may eventually be the predominant tumor cells. Different stem lines have marker chromosomes, large chromosomes

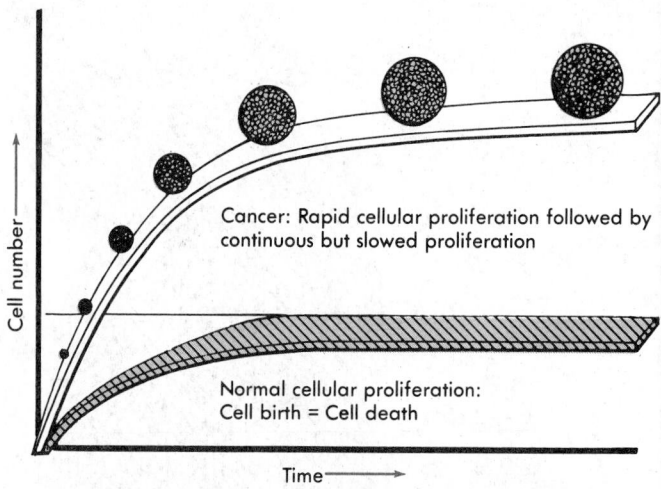

FIGURE 17-5 Gompertzian function. (From Cancer: chemotherapy and care, Pt I, Bristol Laboratories, Division of Bristol-Myers Co.)

with unusual morphologies. The ability to metastasize may be the result of the production of a stem cell line with greater invasive properties.[28]

The rate of growth of a tumor is expressed in terms of volume doubling time. Human tumors generally have a long doubling time, from 1 week to more than 1 year with a median time of about 60 days. Since tumors contain many different types of cells, the length of the cell cycle time (median generation time) varies and is 2 to 3 days among the various cells.

In normal adult tissue, cell birth is equal to cell death. In contrast, cancer cell division continues indefinitely. When the tumor is small and growing rapidly, a relatively high proportion of cells are undergoing division and tumor doubling time is rapid. As the tumor increases in size with a larger cell population, a larger doubling time is needed. This growth pattern is known as *Gompertzian function* (Figure 17-5).

Three factors affect *rate* of tumor growth: (1) the rate of replication of proliferating cells (cell cycle time, p. 337), (2) the proportion of total cell population that is actively proliferating (growth fraction), and (3) the rate of cell loss from the tumor, which depends on the type and age of the tumor. Cell cycle time is relatively constant in tumors of similar histology, but there is considerable difference between normal and tumor tissue. Tumor doubling time is influenced by the cell cycle time. Although early tumor growth is exponential, this soon stops and the required time for doubling increases with tumor age. For a given cycle time, a tumor with a high growth fraction will double faster than a tumor with a low growth fraction.

Cell loss may be caused by cell death as a result of senescence and differentiation, nutrient deficiency (including oxygen deprivation), and destruction of stem

CANCER SPREADS IN MANY WAYS:

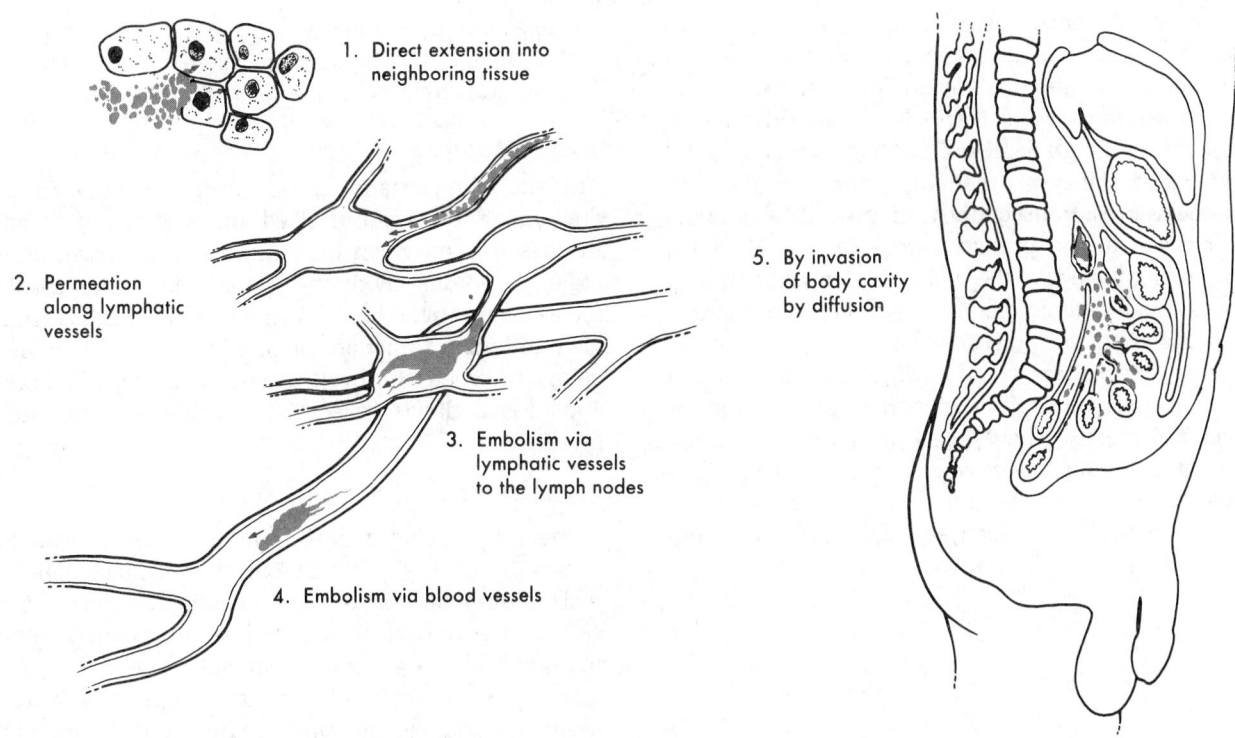

1. Direct extension into neighboring tissue

2. Permeation along lymphatic vessels

3. Embolism via lymphatic vessels to the lymph nodes

4. Embolism via blood vessels

5. By invasion of body cavity by diffusion

FIGURE 17-6 Modes of dissemination of cancer.

cells by host defense mechanisms. Cells also may be lost by their moving out of the tumor through exfoliation and metastasis. Knowledge of cell population kinetics is important, since the sensitivity of the cell to chemotherapy and radiotherapy depends heavily on the proliferative state of the cell at a specific time. In addition, study of cell cycle kinetics will help increase understanding of tumor growth and regulation, laying the foundation for better methods of controlling tumor cells.

Tumor size may also be increased by hemorrhage, by accumulation of a secretion such as mucin, or by some degenerative process. Escape of these secretions into the body may produce profound local or general symptoms such as endocrine disturbances and neurologic degeneration.

METASTASIS

Types of Metastases

The rate of growth of a tumor determines its capacity to metastasize (spread). Cancer spreads in several different ways (Figure 17-6).

Local spread involves infiltration into surrounding tissues and may involve hemorrhage, necrosis, ulceration, and fibrous replacement of the involved tissues. This produces the typical local effects of ulcerating, bulky, hemorrhagic masses or indurative, fibrosing lesions with tissue fixation, distortion of the structure,

and the pitting of the skin that may be seen in some cancer of the breast. Infection may accompany this local infiltration. The cancer cells tend to spread along the path of least resistance, in tissue clefts, along blood vessels or the perineural spaces. The fibrous capsule that covers some organs may limit growth. For example, primary tumors of the kidney, liver, or testes may increase the size of the organ without destroying the capsule. Local spread is not an orderly process, but stages of penetration can be identified, serving as a method of classifying extent of spread (pp. 342-343). Loss of cell cohesiveness, ameboid movements, alteration in cell membranes, and loss of contact inhibition may all play a role in local spread. Because of local spread, any cancer excision must include a margin of surrounding tissues to ensure removal of all malignant cells.

Cancer also spreads by *lymphatic permeation* and *embolization*. Once cells have invaded the lymph vessels, they then may detach and become emboli, which lodge in the lymph node, forming a metastatic lesion. Spread continues to the next group of nodes and into the other organs. The presence of cancer in the lymph nodes is certain evidence of spread, but even if there is no lymph node metastases, there still may be dissemination of malignant cells. The cell may pass through the lymph node without leaving a trace, to grow in other areas. *Vascular embolism* of malignant cells may occur through the veins to any part of the body but particularly to the lungs, the bone, and the liver.

Blood-borne cancer cells escape from the bloodstream by a process of attachment and invasion through endothelial cells lining the blood vessel (Figure 17-7).

In *disseminative metastasis* (distant spread) there is almost always a high degree of histologic, cytologic, and functional similarity between the primary cancer and these metastases. Consequently, the type of cell and the probable site of the primary tumor can be identified from the morphology of the metastasis. In addition, metastases usually mimic the primary tumor in the formation of cell products and secretions.

Finally, cancer can spread by *diffusion,* the spread of clumps of cancer cells from the surface of the tumor by mechanical means. This type of spread is particularly prevalent in serous cavities such as the abdominal or the pleural cavity. In the peritoneal cavity, cells tend to gravitate to the pelvis. Cancer cells can also be im-

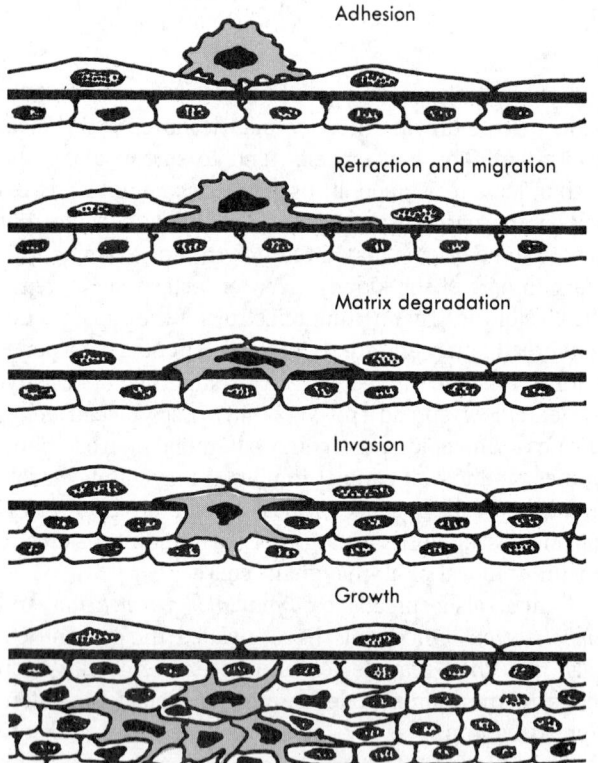

Adhesion

Retraction and migration

Matrix degradation

Invasion

Growth

FIGURE 17-7 Cancer cells exit from bloodstream. (Reprinted with permission from Rawls RL: In search of cancer control: understanding metastasis is crucial, Chem Eng News 63:11, 1985. Copyright © 1985 American Chemical Society.)

planted by the surgeon into the operative area, causing metastatic lesions.

Metastasis may regress or disappear without apparent cause and may be dormant for many years, only to resume growth years later.

Sites of Metastases

The site of metastatic spread depends on the venous drainage of the organ involved, the type of cancer, and the tissue from which the cancer arises. Cancer of an organ that ordinarily drains into systemic veins usually metastasizes to the lungs. Various body tissues seem to have different attraction for metastases, common sites being, in order, the liver, lungs, bone marrow, brain, and adrenal glands. Spleen, muscle, and skin are rarely involved.

CLASSIFYING AND NAMING NEOPLASMS

Tumors derive their names from the types of tissue involved (Table 17-5), but classification of malignant tumors is difficult, since many contain several types of cells and may have benign tissue incorporated within them as well. In general, the names of benign tumors carry the suffix *-oma* following the name of the parent tissue, for example, neuroma or fibroma; there are some exceptions.

Cancers may be classified according to cell type origin. Two main types are those of epithelial and of mesenchymal (connective tissue) origin. The term *carcinoma* denotes a malignant tumor of epithelial cells, and the term *sarcoma* denotes a malignant tumor of connective tissue cells. When a malignant tumor contains all three types of embryonal tissue, it is called a *teratoma.*

Tumors are also classified according to cellular maturity. When there is complete loss of identity with the tissue of origin, the tumor is called *undifferentiated* (anaplastic). Some tumors are known by the names of the scientists who first described them, for example, Hodgkin's disease and Wilms' tumor. Other tumors are named after the organ from which they arise, for example, hepatoma and thymoma.

METHODS OF CLASSIFYING DEGREE OF MALIGNANCY

The degree of malignancy (grade) may be estimated by histologic criteria. Tumors may be graded by arabic numerals into four grades; the higher the grade, the worse the prognosis. A grade 1 tumor is the most differentiated (most like the parent tissue) and therefore the least malignant, whereas grade 4 is the least differentiated (unlike parent tissues) and has a high degree of malignancy. These classifications are useful to the physician in knowing whether the tumor may be expected to respond to radiation treatment and in planning all other aspects of the patient's treatment. Usually, malignant

TABLE 17-5 Classification of neoplasms

Parent Tissue	Benign Tumor	Malignant Tumor
EPITHELIUM		
Skin and mucous membrane	Papilloma Polyp	Squamous cell carcinoma Basal cell carcinoma Transitional cell carcinoma
Glands	Adenoma Cystadenoma	Adenocarcinoma
ENDOTHELIUM		
Blood vessels	Hemangioma	Hemangioendothelioma Angiosarcoma
Lymph vessels	Lymphangioma	Lymphangiosarcoma
Bone marrow		Multiple myeloma Ewing's sarcoma Leukemia Lymphosarcoma Lymphangioendothelioma
Lymphoid tissue		Reticular cell sarcoma (difficult to classify because of cell embryology) Lymphatic leukemia
CONNECTIVE TISSUES		
Embryonic fibrous tissue	Myxoma	Myxosarcoma
Fibrous tissue	Fibroma	Fibrosarcoma
Adipose tissue	Lipoma	Liposarcoma
Cartilage	Chondroma	Chondrosarcoma
Bone	Osteoma	Osteogenic sarcoma
Synovial membrane	Synovioma	Synovial sarcoma
MUSCLE TISSUE		
Smooth muscle	Leiomyoma	Leiomyosarcoma
Striated muscle	Rhabdomyoma	Rhabdomyosarcoma
NERVE TISSUE		
Nerve fibers and sheaths	Neuroma Neurinoma (neurilemoma) Neurofibroma	Neurogenic sarcoma Neurofibrosarcoma
Ganglion cells	Ganglioneuroma	Neuroblastoma
Glial cells	Glioma	Glioblastoma Spongioblastoma
Meninges	Meningioma	
PIGMENTED NEOPLASMS		
Melanoblasts	Pigmented nevus	Malignant melanoma Melanocarcinoma
MISCELLANEOUS		
Placenta	Hydatidiform mole Dermoid cyst	Chorion-epithelioma (choriocarcinoma) Embryonal carcinoma Embryonal sarcoma Teratocarcinoma

tissue is slightly more sensitive to irradiation than normal tissue.

Staging is a form of classification describing the extent (spread) of disease rather than histologic criteria (appearance):

Stage 0	Cancer in situ
Stage I	Tumor limited to the tissue of origin; localized tumor growth
Stage II	Limited local spread
Stage III	Extensive local and regional spread
Stage IV	Metastasis

TNM STAGING CLASSIFICATION SYSTEM

TUMOR

T0	No evidence of primary tumor
TIS	Carcinoma in situ
T1, T2, T3, T4	Ascending degrees of tumor size and involvement

NODES

N0	No regional nodes demonstrably abnormal
N1a, N2a	Demonstrable regional lymph nodes, metastasis not suspected
N1b, N2b, N3	Demonstrable regional lymph nodes; metastasis suspected
Nx	Regional nodes cannot be assessed clinically

METASTASIS

M0	No evidence of distant metastasis
M1, M2, M3	Ascending degrees of metastatic involvement of the host including distant nodes

Determination of the extent of the spread of cancer (staging) and the site of the original tumor is vital for planning therapy. The International Union Against Cancer has devised the TNM system of classification: *T*, tumor; *N*, regional lymph nodes; *M*, distant metastases. Cancer has devised the TNM system of classification: *T*, tumor; *N*, regional lymph nodes; *M*, distant metastases.

Adding a number to the letters (e.g., T1, T2, N1, N2) indicates the extent of the malignancy (see the box). This system provides a type of "shorthand" notation to describe the particular tumor. The purpose of the TNM system is to define categories for all cases and also to allow subsequent and more detailed information to be added. A TNM classification has been identified for major cancer sites. It is important for treatment, planning, end-results reporting, communication, and for the conduct of clinical trials.

NURSE'S RESPONSIBILITY REGARDING PATHOPHYSIOLOGY

As individuals take more responsibility for their own health care and as their knowledge of disease processes grows, they want more explanations of and information about their illness. Physicians may give adequate explanation about cancer and its treatment, but the patient may not understand because of anxiety or misinterpretation of vocabulary. The nurse can clarify information for both patient and family, using appropriate but understandable terms and illustrations. If there is any question of the patient's or the family's understanding of the information given by the physician, the nurse clarifies with the physician what the patient and family have been told. The nurse may also interpret to the physician the patient's or family's readiness for more information.

ETIOLOGY: CARCINOGENESIS

The factors that contribute to the development of cancer are many and at the present time not fully understood; however, certain health practices are known to decrease the possibility that cancer may occur. Factors involved in carcinogenesis include oncogenes, host susceptibility, environmental carcinogens, habits and customs, and viruses.

ROLE OF ONCOGENES

In the early 1970s, *oncogenes* (specific genes that can trigger cancer cell growth) were discovered. Thirty of these cancer genes have now been identified. For 15% to 20% of cancers, the activity of one oncogene is enough to transform normal cells to cancer cells. These oncogenes are similar, if not identical, to genes normally present in the cell. It appears now that cells carry certain normal genes that, when activated by radiation, chemicals, or viruses, are transformed to a malignant state. It is unclear yet if oncogenes are involved in all or just some cancers, or how they fit into the overall pattern of carcinogenesis, which is a complex process involving many steps and often taking 20 years.[86]

The cancer-causing genes and normal genes appear to be virtually the same but their functions are drastically different. While the activation of an oncogene may be part of the process of carcinogenesis, it is not in itself enough to cause cancerous growth. It is possible that tumors grow from the concerted effort of a number of oncogenes, each representing one of the multiple steps of carcinogenesis. The activation of one oncogene may trigger the next oncogene, resulting in a cascade of reactions. It is too soon to predict how the knowledge of oncogenes can be used to treat, cure, or prevent cancer.

HOST SUSCEPTIBILITY
GENETIC FACTORS

Certain conditions and predispositions of the individual seem to contribute to the development of cancer. Studies of genetic factors have focused on specific cancer sites and the disease in general. Chromosomes have been studied to find evidence of the genetic origin of cancer. Human carriers seem to have an abnormal number of chromosomes, usually approximate multiples of the diploid state. The question is whether these changes are the cause or the effect of cancer. Abnormalities in chromosomes number 7 and 17 have been found in cells with malignant characteristics. These experiments, however, involved studying simian viruses, not human chromosomal changes.

A second indication of genetic origin is that cancer

cells are a population of cells descendant from a single cell of origin (clones). Future generations of cancer cells are always malignant; they inherit and pass on the trait.

Finally, there is the possibility that cancer arises from an innate genetic inability, possibly a defect in mitotic regulation. Theoretically, in normal cells mitosis is either inhibited or induced by diffusible substances. The repressor substances are called chalones. Cancer cells may fail to be regulated by the chalones either because the chalones may not be secreted, or if they are, they fail to respond.

Hereditary cancer has certain general characteristics: (1) an early age of onset, occurring 20 or more years earlier than in the general population, (2) a marked incidence of bilateral cancer in paired organs—for example, breasts, kidneys, thyroid glands, (3) multiple primary or multicentered cancers with greater frequency than expected, and (4) well-established autosomal recessive sex-linked and cytogenic cancer and precancerous disorders. In addition, in many cases there is evidence of vertical transmission in consecutive generations with autosomal dominant inheritance.

About 5% of cancers are purely hereditary. It is also possible to inherit a condition that increases the risk that an individual will get a certain type of cancer. Untreated ulcerative colitis results in cancer of the colon in almost 100% of all cases, as does familial polyposis (an inherited disease).

True "cancer families" are rare and are different from normal families who seem to develop many cancers. Cancer families tend to inherit the same cancer and get the disease at an early age (see the box). Studies have shown that the pattern of inheritance is not usually that of a single mendelian gene, and it is still not known whether the incidences of many specific cancers are a result of a combination of genetic or environmental factors.

HORMONAL FACTORS

Some evidence suggests that hormones may in some way be connected with the development of certain cancers. In addition, some metabolites of cancers may also act as antihormones or have new physiologic effects. Hormones do not appear to be primary carcinogens, but rather they seem to influence carcinogenesis in three ways: (1) by a preparative action on the target tissues making them susceptible to the carcinogenic agent, (2) by a "permissive" influence on carcinogenesis allowing the process to progress, and (3) by a conditioning effect on the tumor. Hormones are capable of restraining or enhancing growth of tumors that have developed. Hormone therapy (p. 377) and some surgical therapies (hypophysectomy and oophorectomy) are based on this fact.

CANCERS ASSOCIATED WITH GENETIC FACTORS

TYPE OF CANCER	CHARACTERISTICS
Wilms' tumor	Purely hereditary
Familial polyposis of colon	Precursor of cancer
Breast cancer	High incidence in vertical line of descent (mother to daughter)
Bronchogenic cancer	Seems to develop from synergistic effect of heredity and cigarette smoking
Cancer family syndrome (CFS): adenocarcinoma of colon and endometrium, sometimes of stomach, breast, and ovaries	Autosomal dominant inheritance, transmitted vertically
Familial atypical multiple mole—melanoma (FAMMM) syndrome	Familial disease; genetic factors predispose individuals
Multiple endocrine adenomatosis (MEA)	Familial; involves endocrine glands
Retinoblastoma, hemachromatosis, multiple exostosis	Autosomal dominant disorders
Gonadal dysgenesis	Autosomal recessive disorder
Xeroderma pigmentosum and disseminated superficial actinic porokeratosis	Autosomal recessive disorders, skin cancer precursors

There is evidence that tissues that are endocrine responsive (for example, breasts, endometrium, and prostate) do not develop cancer unless they are stimulated by their growth-promoting hormones. Estrogens have been associated with cancers such as adenocarcinoma of the vagina, hepatic tumors, breast tumors, and uterine cancer.

In addition to tissue stimulation by the hormone, carcinogenesis may be determined by the length of time of the hormonal effect. The longer the preparative influence of the hormone, the greater is the chance of cancer development.

PRECANCEROUS LESIONS

Certain benign lesions and tumors have a tendency toward malignant change. These cancers are preventable if minor precursor conditions are treated carefully. These precancerous conditions include polyps of the colon and rectum, certain pigmented moles, dysplasias of the cervical epithelium, Paget's disease of the bone, and radiodermatitis and senile keratosis.

Senile (solar) keratoses are thickened patches on the skin of the face and hands of those who are exposed to sunlight. Xeroderma pigmentosum, a rare congenital hypersensitivity to light, results in warty precancerous elevations of the skin in childhood. Epidermal carcinoma or malignant melanoma frequently develops. Leukoplakia, precancerous white thickened patches, may occur on the mucous membranes of the lips, mouth, tongue, vulva, and cervix.

Precancerous lesions are a large and heterogeneous group; in some, cancer is inevitable, whereas in others the risk is so low that medical management disregards the cancer risk. For example, the risk of cancer is high in xeroderma pigmentosum but low in leukoplakia of mucous membranes, especially of the oral cavity, larynx, and vulva.

CHRONIC IRRITATION

It is also known that cancer may follow chronic irritation of any part of the body. Effort is being made in industry to protect workers from coal-tar products known to contain carcinogens. Masks and gloves are recommended in some instances, and workers are urged to wash their hands and arms thoroughly to remove all irritating substances at the end of the day's work. Industrial nurses participate in intensive educational programs to help workers understand the need for carrying out company rules that may help prevent cancer.

Prolonged exposure to wind, dirt, and sun may also lead to skin cancer. Skin cancer of the face and hands is particularly frequent among farmers and cattle ranchers who have fair complexions and who do not protect themselves from exposure.

Any kind of chronic irritation to the skin should be avoided, and moles that are in locations where they may be irritated by clothing should be removed. Shoelaces, shoetops, girdles, brassieres, and shirt collars are examples of clothing that may be a source of chronic irritation. Glasses, earrings, dental plates, and pipes that are in repeated contact with skin and mucous membrane may contribute to cancer. Chewing food thoroughly is recommended to lessen irritation in the throat and stomach. Cancer of the mouth is sometimes associated with rough jagged teeth and the constant irritation of tobacco smoke. The habit of drinking scalding hot or freezing cold liquids is also thought to be irritating to the mouth and to the esophagus. Indiscriminate use of laxatives is believed to have possible carcinogenic effects on the large bowel.

IMMUNOLOGIC FACTORS

Immunologists have been increasingly aware of the role of the immune system in the natural history of malignant disease. It may be possible that failure of the normal immune mechanism may predispose to certain cancers. The change from normal to malignant cells is relatively common. These new cells are antigenically different and are recognized as such by the body's immune system. If the immune response is initiated, the malignant cell will be destroyed. That a kind of immune surveillance system may exist is suggested by the following evidence: (1) The two peaks of high incidence of tumors in humans are in early childhood and old age, periods when the immune system is weak. (2) Individuals with rare immunodeficiency diseases in which there is a defect in cellular immunity have increased evidence of tumor development. (3) Individuals who are receiving immunosuppressive drugs to prevent organ transplant rejection have an increased evidence of neoplasia.

The question arises, if a surveillance system exists, why do initial tumor cells progress to clinical cancer? There are no clear-cut answers but some are suggested. Some tumors arise in areas that are poorly served by the immune system, areas such as the central nervous system or the retrobulbar aspect of the eye. Some tumors do not stimulate antibody formation because they are so similar to normal cells. The normally occurring system, called suppressor lymphocytes, which checks the immune response, may become overly active and overwhelm the immune system. The problem may reside in individuals who do not have the same genetic ability for immune response as others have, just as not all have the same physical strength. A problem of time also exists, since the immune system can handle only about 10 million cells. A 1 cm tumor mass contains over 1 billion cells; therefore it is not controlled by normal immunologic response. Consequently a tumor that develops faster than the immune system can respond to it will escape destruction.

Cancer appears to suppress the immune response early in the disease as well as late in its progression. It has not been definitely established that cancer develops because of failure in immune surveillance and at the present time there is not enough data to make a strong case, but investigations continue.[118] (The role of the immune system and cancer therapy is discussed later in this chapter and in detail in Chapter 8.)

DRUG THERAPY

There is strong evidence that oral contraceptives decrease the risk of benign breast disease. However, several studies suggest that persons with prior benign breast disease or a family history of cancer are susceptible to malignant tumors after taking oral contraceptives.[92]

A rare form of vaginal cancer in women has been linked to the ingestion by their mothers of diethylstilbestrol (DES), which was prescribed to prevent spontaneous abortion.

Of 20,000 drugs available in the United States, some have been identified as human oncogens (causing cancer) (see the box on p. 347). Cancer therapy itself may increase the risk for other cancers. Intensive alkylating agent therapy is accompanied by significant subsequent risk of acute leukemia. Consequently its use is limited when no comparable alternative therapy exists. Further

---

DRUGS THAT MAY BE ONCOGENIC TO HUMANS[92]

1. Cytotoxic agents
2. Immunosuppressive agents
3. Estrogens
4. Oral contraceptives
5. Androgenic anabolic steroids
6. Methoxypsoralen
7. Phenacetin-containing analgesics

---

research of disease response to drugs and drug-radiation interactions is needed to prevent long-term risks of cancer treatment.[87]

ENVIRONMENTAL FACTORS

Many years ago it was observed that skin cancers developed more often in men who were employed as chimney sweeps in English homes in which coal was burned in fireplaces. It was then learned that when the suspected substance (methylcholanthrene) contained in the sweepings was repeatedly painted on the ears of experimental animals, cancer developed.

It has been estimated that 70% to 90% of human cancers result from environmental factors and that we have the knowledge to prevent 30% to 40% of cancers in the United States. One to five percent of human cancer is caused by occupational exposure, and the Environmental Protection Agency indicates that as many as 50,000 chemical substances, *excluding* pharmaceuticals and food additives in common use, are carcinogenic.

The Occupational Safety and Health Act of 1970 authorized the Occupational Safety and Health Administration to enforce maximal allowable concentrations of exposure to carcinogens (threshhold limit values [TLVs]). The National Institute for Occupational Health and Safety at present believes that it is not possible to show precise tolerance levels of chemical carcinogens and consequently stresses that exposure to any known or suggested carcinogens must be reduced to the least possible level by any means available.

There are several types of chemical and physical carcinogens (cancer-producing substances). Various carcinogens may have an additive or enhancing effect on one another, and even small amounts of these substances in the environment may constitute a hazard. Carcinogens act on different organs depending on the portal of entry and the distribution in the body.

IONIZING RADIATION

Radiographs and radium may cure cancer, but in other cases they cause it. Ionizing radiation consists of electromagnetic waves or material particles that have sufficient energy to ionize atoms or molecules (i.e., remove

electrons from them) and thereby alter their chemical behavior. In adequate amounts it destroys the cells.

Every living thing from the beginning of time has been exposed to small amounts of radiation from the sun and from certain natural elements in the earth, such as uranium, that emit gamma-rays (γ-rays) in the process of their decay. This is called natural background radiation. No problem regarding radiation existed until after 1895, when the roentgen-ray (x-ray) machine was developed and became widely used in diagnosis of disease. The development of this machine was followed by the discovery of radium and the use of both radium and radiographs for treatment of diseases such as cancer. With developments in the field of nuclear energy, it has been possible to produce radioactive isotopes of a number of the elements, although only a few of them, such as gold, iodine, cobalt, and phosphorus, have medical application at the present time.

The problem of overexposure and possible harm to patients and to personnel caring for them has increased greatly with the increased use of radiographs, and the more recent use of radioisotopes, in diagnosis and treatment. Also, radiation in the environment resulting from atomic testing has become a widely feared and much debated subject in many parts of the world.

No one really knows how much exposure to radiation is safe for persons working with patients and for patients having repeated radiographs taken for various purposes. Relatively small amounts of exposure have produced serious damage in experimental animals, but humans have not lived through enough generations of relatively high exposure for conclusive evidence of safe levels to be obtained. It is reasonable to assume that the less exposure one has the better.

The ionizing effect of radiation on the body cells remains, so that exposure is cumulative throughout life. Exposure of the entire body enormously increases the amount of radiation received. For this reason all of the body except the part being treated is protected from exposure when relatively high doses are given for therapeutic purposes.

The National Academy of Science's Advisory Committee on Radiation has recommended that the exposure limit for the population be set at 170 mrem per year per person. It has been calculated that an exposure of 500 mrem per year could be allowed for an occasional individual. At this level it was felt that there might be some increase in mutation rate but not sufficient to cause a significant increase in genetic disease. Scientists no longer assume nor can they prove that there is a threshold below which there is no radiation damage. There are certain effects of radiation that do show a threshold but scientists suspect that some irreparable residual damage exists at even the smallest dose. They postulate that a damaged cell might ultimately become cancerous. There is no assumption that any level of radiation is completely safe, but present arguments focus on how large a risk arises in the dose of natural background radiation.

The amount of exposure the patient receives from a series of radiographs taken for diagnostic purposes depends on the machine used and the technical skill involved. Usually, the fluoroscopic examination entails more exposure than radiography. The exposure of the average nurse working in a hospital and occasionally assisting a patient while a radiograph is taken is almost negligible.

Radiation Effects

Systemic reactions to excessive radiation exposure are leukopenia, leukemia, bone cancer, and sterility or damage to the reproductive cells. Leukemia and skin cancer are occupational diseases among radiologists. Because of the increased risk, badges are worn by persons whose daily work exposes them to radiation. The badge, which contains photographic film capable of absorbing radiation, is developed each month. A darkening or blackening of the film indicates excessive exposure. Personnel who are becoming overexposed are removed, at least temporarily, from direct contact with radiation.

Because of the possible danger to the fetus, particularly between the second and sixth weeks of life, radiographs are seldom taken of pregnant women. If they must be taken, the lower abdomen is carefully protected. Also, pregnant women usually are not employed in radiology departments or in caring for patients receiving radioactive materials internally.

Nurses who work where they are exposed to x-rays repeatedly or who care for patients receiving radioactive substances must take responsibility for learning how to protect themselves from too much exposure.

Effects of the Sun

Our society at times seems sun-addicted, and a tanned skin is eagerly sought by many, yet sunlight is the most universal carcinogen.[32] Skin cancer occurs mostly in people who work in the open air, such as sailors and farmers, and on areas of the body most exposed to sunlight. Light-complexioned individuals are the most cancer susceptible.

CHEMICAL POLLUTANTS

Air pollution and exposure to other chemicals has been blamed for the rising incidence of cancer in the twentieth century. The polycyclic hydrocarbons have been recognized as carcinogenic (see the box above).

Many nitrosamines cause a variety of cancers in different species. Nitrates are commonly used as food additives, whereas nicotine may be a source of amines. A liver carcinogen, aflatoxin 13, has been isolated from a

---

CHEMICAL CARCINOGENIC AGENTS

1. Polycyclic aromatic hydrocarbons (tar, pitch): skin cancer
2. Arsenic: skin cancer
3. Aromatic amines: bladder cancer
4. Chromium compounds: lung cancer
5. Asbestos: respiratory and lung cancer
6. Benzol inhalation: leukemia
7. Nitrosamines (food additives, nicotine)
8. Chloromethyl methyl ether and vinyl chloride (polyvinyl plastics)
9. Some hair dyes

---

common mold that grows on peanuts, soybeans, fruit, some meats, and mild and cheddar cheese.

Cyclamates previously used as a sugar substitute have been banned because they may be potentially carcinogenic. Saccharin has also been identified as being carcinogenic in a study of rats, and the Food and Drug Administration (FDA) has recommended that it not be used as an artificial sweetener. Some hair dyes have been implicated in certain cases of cancer.

NURSING IMPLICATIONS

Some people argue that some degree of carcinogen risk is acceptable; others say that no level is acceptable and that all risks must be eliminated from the environment no matter what the cost. Most agree that some level of regulation is necessary, but the mechanisms and standards for these regulations have not been delineated.

Nurses, as patient advocates, can give information about health hazards in the workplace and can assess past and present exposures and signs and symptoms of work-related diseases. Appropriate agencies such as the Environmental Protection Agency (EPA), Occupational Safety and Health Association (OSHA), or a trade union are contacted regarding health-related problems.

Nurses teach about health hazards, dispel myths and misconceptions, and give workers information about self-protection when working with hazardous materials.[36]

HEALTH PRACTICES
SMOKING, TOBACCO USE

Cigarette smoking is linked with the increased incidence of lung cancer. More reports are appearing that incriminate moderate and heavy cigarette smoking as a predisposing factor in the development of lung cancer, which now causes 14 times as many deaths each year as it did 30 years ago. In 1989 lung cancer killed approximately 142,000 persons in the United States.[4] Although the rate of lung cancer in men has been alarming, studies have noted a proportionately greater rise in the rate of lung cancer in women. The rise appears to parallel an increase in recent years of women smokers, particularly teenage girls.

It has also been demonstrated that there is a correlation between cancer mortality and the number of cigarettes smoked daily, the number of years an individual has smoked, and the age at which he or she began to smoke cigarettes. Smoking has also been connected with esophageal cancer and possibly bladder cancer.[4] If smoking is discontinued even after a habit of 30 years, there is a decrease in the evidence of lung cancer.

In 1964 the National Interagency Council on Smoking and Health was formed after the release of the Surgeon General's Report on Smoking and Health. This group has produced films and other educational materials that are available to schools, organizations, and individuals. Assistance in securing films and other materials can be obtained from the Library, National Interagency on Smoking and Health.* One of the main concerns of the Interagency Council is how to convince young people not to start smoking. A film, *Breathing Easy,* was produced by the American Lung Association† especially for the preteen group. The American Cancer Society is designing stop-smoking clinics for places of employment and for schools.[4] Antismoking education drives in schools are conducted through school courses, assemblies, and exhibits.

Since January 2, 1971, no cigarette advertising has been permitted on either television or radio. On the same date the warning on packages was changed from "Caution: cigarette smoking may be hazardous to your health" to either "Warning: the Surgeon General has determined that cigarette smoking is dangerous to your health" or a more definitive statement, asserting that smoking may cause cancer, heart disease, and emphysema. Although the campaign to convince people to stop smoking has been slow and arduous, changes have been noted in smoking patterns. There is a trend toward increased use of filter cigarettes and pipes among smokers. The two thirds of the population who are nonsmokers have been active and in some instances successful in getting smokers to refrain from smoking in public places such as specified sections of airplanes and public buildings. In 1972 the Surgeon General of the United States declared that smoking in the presence of a nonsmoker might be considered an act of aggression. Experiments have shown that cigarette smokers in a crowded, ill-ventilated room or an automobile can raise the level of carbon dioxide to the point that all within the area can experience trouble discriminating time intervals and visual and sound cues, as well as difficulty

*American Heart Association, 7320 Greenville Ave, Dallas, TX 75231.
†1740 Broadway, New York, NY 10019.

METHODS TO CONTROL SMOKING

1. Encourage young people not to start
2. Educate public on the hazards of smoking with the aim of getting the smoker to quit
3. Provide self-help materials
4. Work with the media
5. Recruit exsmoker volunteers to provide one-to-one help for smokers trying to quit
6. Encourage industries, hospitals, and organizations to conduct their own stop-smoking programs
7. Make available FRESH START, the American Cancer Society quit-smoking program
8. Support legislation to restrict smoking in public places

with eye-hand coordination. Action in the form of bills, ordinances, and restrictions on smoking and the sale of tobacco in places of public assembly are being instituted at all government levels on a nationwide basis.

Nurses have a responsibility, both as well-informed citizens and as professional persons, to be aware of the most recent antismoking programs, to be active in these programs, and to interpret them to the public (see the box above).

As a substitute for smoking, some individuals have turned to the use of snuff or chewing tobacco. The use of these products, however, has been associated with a high incidence of oral cancer, and the risk increases with length of use.[75,117]

NUTRITION

Nutritional habits are increasingly being investigated and implicated in the cause of cancer. A high incidence of cancer of the colon occurs in populations whose diet is high in refined food and low in nonabsorbable cellulose "roughage" or fiber. Evidence indicates that a low incidence of colonic carcinoma exists among persons who eat a largely vegetarian diet that has relatively few animal products and is especially low in fats. Breast cancer appears to be associated with a diet high in animal fat, but the precise relationship has not been identified.

Many nutritional substances are being investigated for their effects on carcinogenesis (see the box on p. 350). Nutritional excesses and deficiencies may also be carcinogenic. Breast and colon cancers have been correlated with nutritional deficits, especially with vitamins A, B (riboflavin), and C, although these may play an indirect role.[113] Ingestion of smoked foods, which contain benzopyrene, has been correlated with an increased incidence of stomach cancer. Some epidemiologic and experimental evidence suggests that high caloric intake may lead to cancer and calorie deprivation may prevent it. Obesity may increase the risk of endometrial cancer.

EFFECTS OF NUTRITIONAL SUBSTANCES BEING INVESTIGATED AS CARCINOGENIC

PRACTICE	EFFECTS
Food additives (chemicals to improve color and flavor)	Some believed carcinogenic, others protective
Vitamin E	No evidence it gives protection
Selenium	Too little evidence of protection to recommend dietary increase
Saccharin	Long-term effects cannot be predicted in humans
Other noncaloric sweeteners	Long-term effects not studied in humans
Coffee	Inconclusive evidence as a risk factor (no recommendation against moderate use)
Cholesterol	Little evidence as a risk factor for cancer
Meat and fish cooked at high temperature (frying, broiling)	Increases number of mutagens; has induced cancer in animals
Fats	Increase risk of colon, breast, rectum, and prostate cancer

NUTRITIONAL PRACTICES TO PREVENT CANCER[49,113]

1. Avoid obesity: associated with high risk of cancer of uterus, gallbladder, kidney, colon, and breast
2. Decrease total fat intake: fat increases chance of cancer of breast, prostate, colon
3. Eat more high-fiber foods (whole-grain cereals, fruits and vegetables)
4. Include foods rich in vitamins A and C (dark green and deep yellow vegetables): lowers risk of cancer of larynx, esophagus, and lung
5. Include cruciferous vegetables (cabbage, broccoli, Brussels sprouts, kohlrabi, cauliflower); reduces risk of gastrointestinal and respiratory cancer
6. Drink alcohol only in moderation
7. Eat salt-cured, smoked, and nitrite-cured foods (bacons, some sausages) only in moderation

Some foods may protect against cancer. The food additives BHA (butylated hydroxyanisole) and BHT (butylated hydroxytoluene) seem to inhibit cancer. Although reports are conflicting, some investigators believe vitamins A, B, and C actually have anticancer effects.[49] The *Lactobacillus bulgaris* and *Streptococcus thermophilus* microorganisms found in yogurt have been found to inhibit tumor cell proliferation.

Although their effects are still under study, micronutrients such as Vitamins C and E, folates, and carotenoids (chemicals related to Vitamin A), appear to have a protective action, and the National Research Council recommends an increase in their intake.

Nurses have an opportunity to teach about nutritional practices that help prevent cancer no matter where their practice setting (see the box above right).

The Delaney Amendment to the federal Food, Drug and Cosmetic Act requires that no substance producing tumors in experimental animals should be permitted in food for human beings. The problem is that effects from ingesting carcinogenic agents may not be seen for decades because of the long latency periods. Childhood exposure, particularly, may provide the time for cancer to appear.

ALCOHOL

There is a significant association between high alcohol intake and cancer of the mouth, pharynx, larynx, and esophagus. However, alcoholism is often associated with smoking and with vitamin and dietary deficiencies, whose roles as etiologic factors of cancer are not known. It is speculated that alcohol and nutritional deficiencies enhance carcinogenesis by increasing the metabolic activities of specific tobacco carcinogens. Tumors of the involved sites occur with greater frequency in men, blacks, lower socioeconomic groups, increasingly urbanized societies, and the elderly.

SEXUAL PRACTICES

Carcinoma of the uterine cervix is less common in virgins than in married women. It is higher in those who have first coitus at an early age, who have an early first marriage, and who have had multiple sex partners. Cervical cancer is more frequent in women who have had multiple pregnancies, but this factor decreases in importance when the groups of women compared started their sex life at the same age. The development of cancer seems to be connected with coitus rather than pregnancy.

Carcinoma of the penis is virtually unknown among circumcised men. The means by which circumcision provides protection is not clear, but it is probably related to better hygiene. There is also a lower incidence of cancer of the uterine cervix in women whose sexual partner has been circumcised and in cultures in which the men, even though not circumcised, have a high standard of genital hygiene.

The correlation with sexual experience and breast cancer is the reverse of that for the uterine cervix. Breast cancer patients usually have been married and become pregnant later in life. Lactation may provide some protection against breast cancer, since women who have breast-fed their infants show a lower incidence of breast malignancy. Cancer of the breast is reported to be unknown among Eskimo women and to be

TABLE 17-6 Prevention: Objectives of the National Cancer Institute for the year 2000[50]

Risk Factor	Reduction Activities
Smoking	Reduce smoking among all levels of smokers (heavy, moderate, light), the rate of decline 4% or more per year.
Diet	Change dietary habits to increase the per capita consumption of fiber from grains, fruits, and vegetables to 15 g or more per day.
	Decrease fat consumption to below 35% of total calories.
	Increase dietary micronutrients (vitamins C and E, folate) and the carotenoids (chemicals related to vitamin A).
Alcohol	Reduce excessive consumption.
Occupational exposure	Control or eliminate exposure to asbestos, benzene, arsenic and its compounds (soots, tars and oils, vinyl chloride, etc.)
	Require companies with more than 500 employees to have a hazard control plan for processes associated with carcinogens.
	Require that at least 25% of all workers be informed of their occupational health, risks, and consequences before employment.
	Teach employees about life-style and other factors that interact with work factors that increase risk.
	Require that at least 70% of primary health care providers question patients about hazardous exposure in the work environment and interpret information to patients in an understandable manner.

latively rare among Japanese women; both cultures actice breast-feeding.

The National Cancer Institute of the National Institutes of Health has developed objectives to decrease risks of cancer from life-style and environmental factors. Their goal in the prevention of cancer is to decrease the cancer incidence and its mortality by changing these factors.[50] (See Table 17-6)

VIRUSES

Studies in animals have established that there is a viral role in carcinogenesis, but proof that humans are affected has not been definitely established. Viruses have been isolated and identified as the cause of cancer in mice, rabbits, and frogs.

Cervical cancer may result from a virus introduced into the cervix during sexual intercourse. This virus may be a member of the herpes group, *herpesvirus hominis* (HV-2). Carriers of HV-2 in the population are generally uncircumcised males with poor personal hygiene.

Herpeslike viruses have been visualized by electron microscopy in Burkitt's tumor and Hodgkin's disease cells. Investigators, however, have been unable to dem-

onstrate human oncogenic viruses from human tumors. This may be a technical problem, since the ideal laboratory conditions for the isolation of tumor viruses have not been found. In addition, the long latency period in humans makes study of viruses difficult.

The viruses found in animal tumors indicate that viruses may act individually or as co-carcinogens in causing malignancy in humans. Viruses are involved in the cause of cancer but they do not appear to have a major role.[86]

PSYCHOSOCIAL FACTORS

Stressors such as life changes, loss of a significant other, and personality variables have been suggested as etiologic factors in the development of cancer. A "cancer-prone" personality has also been suggested but considerable research is needed to determine if there is such a personality. Some researchers believe that even if such a personality is identified, there is little possibility of practical application of the information, since it is extremely difficult to change behavior.

The role of "psychological" treatments in "curing" cancer is also poorly investigated. Information about the relationship of positive attitude to the outcome of cancer is sparse, one study finding no relationship between the two factors. Little is known, also, about the effect of states of mind on the immune or hormonal systems that may affect the disease,[114] although depression has been suggested as causing a change in immune mechanisms that protect against cancer.

Social support in the form of institutions, family, and friends also may be an important variable. The individual with low social support and high need may be at a higher risk for developing cancer. In addition, lack of social support may adversely affect coping responses to therapy and to the illness. At the present time, however, how one defines the nature of social support and the degree to which it is present or lacking is unclear.

CONCLUSIONS

Carcinogenesis is a dynamic process that is influenced by many independent and poorly defined variables. The initial molecular changes are irreversible, but they may not be expressed when cooperative conditions are absent. Changes in these conditions may alter the carcinogenic process, resulting in either acceleration, inhibition, or even reversal of the process. Etiologic agents may be co-carcinogens. A genetic predisposition for a "weak" immune system along with a viral infection may lead to cancer, or oncogenic viruses may act as suppressants of the immune system. Chemical carcinogens may activate latent viral genes or inhibit the immune system's effectiveness in destroying cancer cells. Figure 17-8 illustrates the relationship among various carcinogenic factors as causes of cancer.

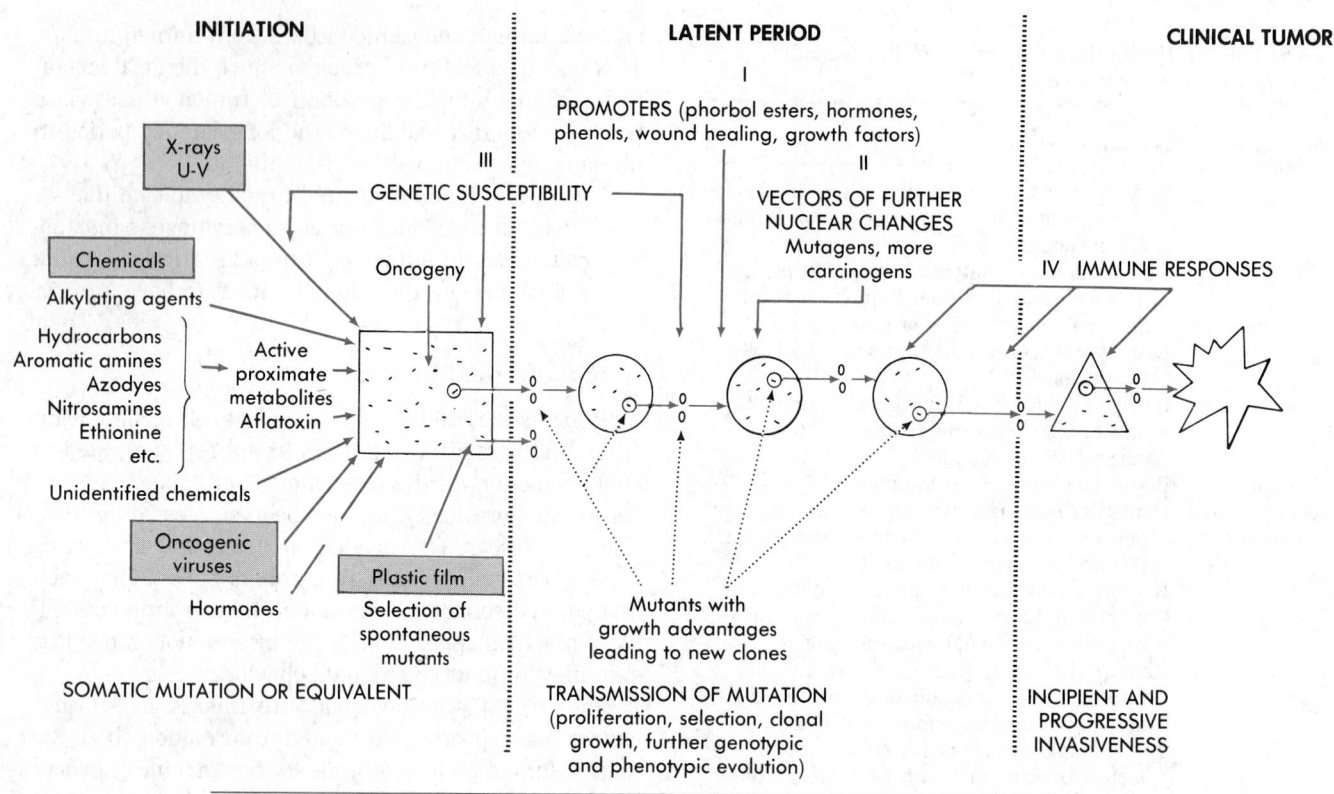

FIGURE 17-8 Physical, chemical, and viral carcinogens may cause damage in cells of target organs (*dots in square*). Changes are transmitted by cell division resulting in clones of modified cells (*small circles*). These cells undergo further genotypic and phenotypic changes as a result of exposure to same or different carcinogens. Promoters of proliferation, whether chemical, hormonal, or viral, enhance carcinogenic process. Successive selection of new clones (*large circles*) leads to premalignant state. From complex interplay of host and tumor, affected by genetic, endocrine, immunologic, and other environmental factors, populations of cells characteristic of clinical tumors arise. (From Ryser HJ: Special report: chemical carcinogenesis, CA 24:358-359, 1974).

TABLE 17-7 Systemic effects of cancer

Category	Problems	Cause
Hematologic	Anemia, leukopenia, thrombocytopenia	Replacement of bone marrow by cancer cell
Immunologic	Infection	Deficiency of T and B cells
Vascular	Hemorrhage	Blood vessel erosion by tumor, DIC
Hormonal and endocrinologic	Syndromes such as Cushing's hyperthyroidism	Tumors of endocrine glands cause increased secretions; malignant lung tumors secrete trophic hormones
	Cachexia	Hypermetabolism of tumors
		Increased gluconeogenesis
Neuromuscular	Weakness, cerebellar disease, peripheral neuritis	Degenerative changes in DNS and peripheral nervous system
	Poor pulmonary respiration, stasis of secretions and pneumonia	Destruction of muscle protein, impaired cellular respiration, and failure of abdominal and intercostal muscles
	Urinary tract infection and constipation	Failure of smooth muscle in bladder and GI tract
Skin and connective tissue	Dermatomyositis	—
Gastrointestinal	Weakness, fatigue, weight loss	Malabsorption, chronic blood loss, impaired digestion
General disorders	Ascites	Metastatic implant in abdomen
	Pleural effusion	Metastatic implant in pleural cavity

CLINICAL MANIFESTATIONS OF CANCER

The clinical manifestations of cancer may be diverse and affect multiple systems depending on the site and size of the tumor. Nurses need to be aware of these signs and symptoms to aid in early detection of cancer and to monitor the effects of therapy in relation to these manifestations.

The physician obtains a medical history to identify those persons with a familial tendency for cancer; a social history, marital and sex history, past medical history, as well as information about habits and occupation. These data may provide clues to identify the presence of cancer. Depending on the size and location of the tumor, many different signs and symptoms may be present.

LOCAL EFFECTS

Benign tumors cause serious problems if they obstruct the lumen of tubular structures such as the ureter, trachea, or intestinal tract. Intraspinal and intracranial tumors cause problems because of the pressure they exert in a closed space. Tumors may also degenerate or by the pressure they exert cause atrophy and ulceration of overlying epithelium.

Malignant tumors may produce the same problems as benign tumors. In addition, because of their size and ability to infiltrate and destroy surrounding tissue, symptoms of obstruction, hemorrhage, ulceration, and secondary infection may be present.

SYSTEMIC EFFECTS

The term *paraneoplastic syndrome* is used to describe the systemic effects of cancer. These can be divided into the following categories: (1) hematologic, immunologic, and vascular abnormalities; (2) hormonal and endocrinologic effects; (3) neuromyopathies; (4) skin and connective tissue disorders; (5) gastrointestinal disorders; and (6) general and metabolic disorders.[28] These effects do not occur in every patient but vary depending on the location and activity of the tumor (Table 17-7).

CACHEXIA

Cachexia is usually a sign of advanced cancer. It was once thought to be the result of a progressive starvation of the patient. Although decreased food intake is a factor, it appears to be a complex derangement of the patient's metabolism. Clinical signs of cachexia are anorexia, early satiety, gradual or rapid weight loss, anemia, and asthenia (see the box above).

Four etiologic factors are involved in cachexia:

1. It is possibly caused by inhibition of the hypothalamic appetite center. Appetite may fail to increase in the face of the increased nutrient needs of the tumor.

CLINICAL SIGNS OF CACHEXIA

SIGNS	CAUSE
Anorexia	Metabolites produced by cancer, food aversions caused by decreased taste and smell and by therapy
Early satiety and early filling	Cause unknown—patient is hungry but after a few bites feels full
Weight loss	Impaired digestion and absorption, hypermetabolism, negative nitrogen balance
Anemia	Decreased RBC production, increased RBC destruction or loss
Asthenia (marked feeling of muscle weakness, easily tired)	Biochemical alterations

2. There is altered gastrointestinal function, malabsorption of nutrients, especially in the small intestine, and exudation of protein and electrolytes.
3. There is increased utilization of nutrients by some tumors that require more amino acids and vitamins than do normal tissues. There may also be insufficient utilization of available nutrients.
4. There is increased excretion of nutrients such as urinary excretion of electrolytes and metabolic products.[28]

In addition, other factors that may be implicated include immobilization, drugs, and reactive depression that may accompany metastatic cancer. Along with this may be insomnia and a feeling of hopelessness, which also may contribute to anorexia and cachexia. There is an increased susceptibility to infection.

Therapy for the cachectic state is rarely successful unless the underlying cancer is treated. Glucose plus insulin, or androgens for males, may stimulate anabolism.

Pain does not always occur with cancer; when it does occur, it is usually a late sign. Cancer pain is described later in the chapter (p. 391).

DIAGNOSTIC STUDIES

The nurse needs to be able to give a simple description of various diagnostic procedures to patients and families. The tests may involve the use of complex equipment, as well as the injection or ingestion of various substances. The patient's anxiety may be high, and the nurse's ability to give factual information often will help decrease anxiety. Several of the most widely used tests are presented in the following discussion.

LABORATORY TESTS

Cancer tumors produce hormones or proteins that may be detected by blood tests. Measurement of an enzyme, acid phosphatase, which is produced almost entirely by the prostate gland, gives evidence of the extent of prostatic disease. Another enzyme, alkaline phosphatase, is elevated in individuals with bone metastases and sometimes in those with liver metastases. Blood in the stool, identified by the guaiac test, may be a sign of gastrointestinal cancer. Calcitonin increase has been shown to be a good indicator of thyroid and lung cancer.

Cytology

In 1942 Dr. George Papanicolaou demonstrated that the diagnosis of cancer can be made from the study of cells that have sloughed or exfoliated from a tumor. These cells are found in body secretions such as cervical discharges, sputum, gastric washings, pleural fluid, and urinary washings. The secretion is spread on a slide, stained, and examined by a pathologist. The main use of the Pap smear, as it is often called, is to diagnose cancer in an asymptomatic person and to identify precancerous lesions or noninvasive cancer. If suspect cells are found, a biopsy must be performed to diagnose cancer.[4] The Pap smear is most widely used in routine examination of cervical washings.

RADIOLOGIC TESTS

X-Ray and Scanning Procedures

X-ray studies are usually ordered. Chest radiography is absolutely necessary if the patient is a smoker. Gastrointestinal series, intravenous pyelogram, and mammography may be done depending on areas where lesions are expected to be present.

The scanning technique, which permits the mapping of organs, plays an important part in the evaluation of the patient with cancer.[20] Some of these procedures are described in Table 17-8.

Radioisotope Studies

Various scanning procedures that involve the introduction of a radioactive substance into the body are used to detect primary or metastatic cancer. The radioisotope either concentrates in the tumor and shows up as a "hot spot" in the scan of the organ, or the tumor does not concentrate the isotope and a "cold spot" surrounded by normal tissue that did concentrate the isotope is found. Radioisotopes used include the following:

1. Radioactive iodine: oral or by injection; used for diagnosis of thyroid disease
2. Radioactive iodine-tagged albumin: injected IV; used for locating brain tumors and to determine blood volume.

Ultrasound

Ultrasound probing, or *echography,* is done by an electronic instrument that detects and records echoes of sound when they are reflected at the junction of tissue with different densities. The procedure is helpful in differentiating between cystic and solid tumors.

SPECIAL TEST: BIOPSY

Biopsy is the only definitive way that cancer can be diagnosed. *Incisional biopsy* is the surgical removal of a section of the neoplasm. If the tumor is small, the entire growth may be removed, a procedure called an *excisional biopsy.* When possible, an *aspiration biopsy,* removing a small plug of tumor by use of a needle or syringe, is used to avoid the larger incisional or excisional biopsy.

The biopsy specimen is examined under a microscope to obtain a histologic diagnosis as to the type of

---

TABLE 17-8 X-ray and scanning procedures

Study	Procedure	Comment
Lymphangiography	Vital blue stain and Novocain injected in skin of web between first and second toes or index and second fingers to show lymphatic drainage of extremities	Use in diagnosing lymph and metastatic cancer. Lymphomatous nodes have "foamy" or "lacy" structure. Metastatic nodes have "moth-eaten" appearance. Skin discoloration from dye may last 1 week.
Xeroradiography	X-ray on plate of selenium-coated metal	Obtain picture of soft tissue
Tomography	X-ray with ability to penetrate dense shadows	Obtain picture of soft tissue
Thermography	Constructs photographic images of surface temperature	Identifies skin temperature elevations over inflammatory or malignant lesions
Computerized axial tomography (CAT scan)	X-ray beam and use of computer	Produces images of plane sections of body; identifies size and location of tumors
Magnetic resonance imaging (MRI)	Magnetic fields	Produces a cross-sectional image of the body; spares patient from x-rays
Positron-emission tomography (PET)	Scanners that rotate around patient; image formed by positrons emitted by isotope injected into or inhaled by patient	Allows viewing of brain and body processes in three dimensions; gives a picture of biochemical and metabolic processes

cancer. In some cases it may be possible to determine the degree of malignancy.

Contrary to a belief sometimes expressed by patients, a biopsy, properly taken, adds little or no risk of causing the spread of cancer. Nurses must be careful to dispel the idea that biopsy should be avoided.

ENDOSCOPY

Hollow metal tubes equipped with a light are used to illuminate various body cavities and to permit visual inspection of the interior of the cavity being examined. These instruments are commonly referred to as scopes and are named for the organs they are to visualize. Thus a bronchoscope is used to examine the bronchus, a gastroscope is used to visualize the stomach, and a proctoscope to visualize the anus and sigmoid colon. A biopsy of tissue or secretions is usually obtained during these endoscopic procedures. A local anesthetic that diminishes the gag reflex is used before bronchoscopy or gastroscopy. Usually, no anesthetic is necessary for sigmoidoscopy. Peritonoscopy, which is employed to examine the peritoneal cavity, is particularly helpful in visualizing peritoneal metastasis. A local anesthetic is used with this procedure.

NURSING INTERVENTION DURING DIAGNOSTIC PHASE

The emotional climate produced during the period of diagnostic examination and initial treatment is very important in determining whether patients will continue diagnostic examination, treatment, or repeated follow-up care after discharge. The care they receive in the hospital may shape their attitudes toward the disease and may determine whether they can return home and either care for themselves or be cared for by the family.

Many patients must undergo extensive diagnostic examinations and surgery in large medical centers a long distance from their homes. Some patients have reported that, although they were confident that they were in "good medical hands," such confidence did not make up for the feelings that they were not always known as individuals. They needed desperately to feel that at least one person knew and understood them. Some patients experience near panic at the thought of their loved ones coming to visit and being unable to locate them. The nurse who works with the patient in the community, in the small hospital, or in the physician's office can help patients by preparing them for what they may experience in the large medical center. In most instances it is best for the patient to be accompanied by a relative or a close friend. It should also be recognized that even a patient in familiar surroundings may feel very much alone when awaiting diagnostic tests or surgical treatment for known or suspected cancer.

Members of the family often need direction in their activity when they have just learned that a loved one has cancer. They may need to talk over immediate and long-term plans with someone not close to the family situation. The nurse can sometimes be this listening person. At other times the family can best be served by a social caseworker, who will help them talk through and think through a course of action.

GENERAL NURSING CARE DURING TREATMENT PHASE

■ ASSESSMENT

It is especially important that the nurse obtain baseline data in relation to the cancer patient's health and health habits, since the treatment of cancer often involves complex changes in the patient's ability to meet psychologic, physiologic, and sociologic health needs. By careful collection of data the nurse can plan and carry out the complex nursing that may be needed by the patient with cancer.[119] Data pertaining to physiologic needs are described in the box below.

INITIAL DATA

Some initial psychosocial data are also needed to plan care (see the box on p. 356). The first important question to be answered is whether the patient knows the diagnosis. This information should be recorded on the nursing care plan and discussed with other health team members. This will ensure that the person does not receive different answers to the same questions from the health care providers. Some hospitals have partially overcome this problem by having regular meetings of all the members of the professional staff at which the information given to each patient is reviewed. If meetings of this type are not being held, nurses should take the initiative in planning such a meeting.

The nurse should also elicit from both the patient and the physician what the patient has been told. Because of anxiety and the need for denial to protect the ego, the patient may have only heard part of the information given by the physician or may have misinterpreted the information. The nurse can identify any discrepancies to plan the care on the basis of the patient's perceptions of the illness.

Members of the medical profession differ in their

INITIAL DATA TO MEET PHYSIOLOGIC NEEDS

1. General health
2. Activity: exercise, mobility (including oxygenation, self-care ability)
3. Cognition, perception
4. Elimination
5. Health perception, health management
6. Nutrition, metabolism
7. Sexuality
8. Sleep, rest

INITIAL DATA TO MEET PSYCHOSOCIAL NEEDS

SELF-PERCEPTION, SELF-CONCEPT

Does the patient know the diagnosis?
What has the patient been told about cancer, its treatment, prognosis?
How long has the patient known the diagnosis?
Has the cancer metastasized and does the patient know it?
How aware is the patient of his/her feelings?

ROLES, RELATIONSHIPS

What kind of support can be expected from family, friends?

COPING, STRESS

What are the patient's coping skills and usual responses to stress?
What are the patient's talents, strengths, assets?
What are the patient's and family's interpersonal, physical, and financial resources?

VALUES, BELIEFS

What is the patient's lifestyle, motivation, and interests?
What are the patient's spiritual, philosophical beliefs and values?
How important are religious practices to the patient?

opinions regarding whether the patient with cancer should be told the diagnosis. The decision is usually made by the physician after consultation with the patient's family.

The guiding principle in identifying how much the cancer patient should know and decide is respect for persons, which means that competent persons have the right to know and decide. In addition, family wishes, in general, do not set the limit on what the competent patient should know and decide. Over the past 25 years physicians have changed their attitude toward disclosure to cancer patients.

In a 1979 study 98% of physicians surveyed had a policy of informing the cancer patient. In addition, clinicians' fears that information about risks of treatment will cause the patient to refuse treatment are not sufficient reason to withhold information. However, competent patients may waive rights to know and decide.[91]

Patients may not want to know the diagnosis and may ask and then answer their own questions negatively. Some do not ask for the diagnosis because they do not wish to have confirmed what they already suspect. Some insist on knowing the diagnosis and are preoccupied with every detail of their progress and treatment in a detached but completely abnormal fashion. Finally, there are some who wish to know the facts and who can accept them in a realistic way when given an opportunity to discuss their feelings with others. Some physicians prepare the patient over a period of time and

tell the complete truth when they feel the patient is ready to accept it.

When patients are not informed, the reasons seem to be related much more to the physician's own attitudes and emotional reactions than to concern about patients' reactions. The nurse may help by discussing with the physician the reactions of the patient and the feelings expressed. It is the nurse's responsibility and sometimes a challenge to work effectively for the ultimate benefit of the patient within the seeming limitation it may impose.

It is also important to determine how long the patient has known the diagnosis. The patient who has just been told may be going through the initial grief reactions. The person who has known for many years may have made a realistic adaptation and may see cancer as a chronic disease and not as a death sentence. The nurse should ascertain from the physician whether the cancer has already metastasized and, if so, whether the patient is aware of this fact. Responses of the patient with metastatic cancer will be different from those of the patient who can be more hopeful of a cure.

COPING SKILLS

Coping skills should be identified, for in no other disease are the person's inner resources and those of friends and families tested to a greater degree. Some persons cope by directly verbalizing fears and seeking support from others, whereas other persons are less direct. Some deal with problems with a problem-solving approach, whereas others try to avoid dealing with the problem.

The patient's and family's interpersonal, physical, and financial resources must be determined. What kind of support can be expected from the family? The financial burden the patient anticipates because of the therapy may affect the reaction to the disease.[66]

PSYCHOLOGIC RESPONSE TO CANCER

Patients and families may be overwhelmed and immobilized. Not all patients openly express feelings so it may be difficult to gather data and plan interventions. Collection of data to identify psychologic responses is an ongoing process, since these responses may change throughout the treatment period.

Some individuals are stoic, feeling it is a sign of weakness to display their psychologic devastation in public. The nurse must be alert for subtle cues that may indicate that intervention is needed.

Grief

The general psychologic responses to a diagnosis of cancer are those accompanying the grieving process (see Chapter 14). The patient and family may go through a period of denial, during which there may be a delay in beginning therapy. Anxiety, depression, regressive behavior, and anger may all be manifested.

To many the diagnosis of cancer signifies the end of life itself, the ultimate loss. Nurses must be careful that they do not communicate any negative reactions to cancer. Beginning practitioners must look at their own attitudes toward the disease.

Guilt

Guilt is also a frequent psychologic response. Cancer patients may feel that the disease is punishment for actions during their life. They may also feel guilty if they have delayed seeking treatment.

Sense of Isolation

Perhaps one of the most prevalent reactions described by patients with cancer is a sense of isolation, of being cut off from those persons and things that are important to them. Patients with cancer may report that there is a gradual break in relationships. In some cases the isolation is patient initiated; in others it may result from actions of significant others because of their negative attitude toward the disease. Perhaps the most profound isolation is psychologic isolation, an inability to relate to and derive comfort from others.

Sexual Dysfunction

Nurses must be comfortable with their own sexuality and sensitive to the patients' responses, which may indicate that sexual tension is present.

Cancer is particularly destructive to the sexual relationship. It may so occupy the patient's life that all energy is directed to the illness. Sexual roles change. There may be fear that sexual activity may either cause the cancer to spread or that the well partner may "catch" it. Treatment modalities that affect the genital organs may cause loss of sexual drive, sexual dysfunction, and the psychologic responses of anxiety, anger, depression, and body image disturbance may severely damage the sexual relationship[55] (see Chapter 52).

Fantasies of Death and Dying

Some patients report that they are overwhelmed with fantasies of death and dying. Most patients are more concerned about the process of dying, fearing pain, mutilation, and deterioration in both their physiologic and psychologic status, than with death itself. Patients may be open about their fantasizing, but they are more apt to communicate this in less obvious ways. Patients may focus their attention and discussion on the suffering and pain of others. They may express concern about the future of their families and may speculate what will happen to their loved ones. The nurse must be alert to these signs that patients need to talk about their view of their future (see Chapter 14).

■ DATA ANALYSIS: NURSING DIAGNOSES

Nursing diagnoses are determined from assessment of patient data. Possible nursing diagnoses may include but are not limited to the diagnoses listed in Table 17-9. Some cancer patients have few diagnoses; others have many.

■ PLANNING: EXPECTED PATIENT OUTCOMES

Patient outcomes for specific nursing diagnoses are listed in Table 17-9. Four principles should be considered by the nurse when planning nursing interventions that are patient- or client-centered:

1. Patients have a right to be part of the treatment team.
2. Patients have the right to choose the desired degree of privacy or communication.
3. The nurse must respect the coping mechanisms of patients who are trying to maintain themselves through a difficult illness.
4. The nurse must remember not to give the appearance of hurrying, thus blocking communications and "turning the patients off."

■ IMPLEMENTATION
CHARACTERISTICS OF THE NURSE CARING FOR CANCER PATIENTS

A sound personal philosophy and an objective, positive attitude toward cancer based on knowledge will help the nurse who is caring for the patient with cancer. Cancer

RESEARCH

Derdiarian AK: Informational needs of recently diagnosed cancer patients, Nurs Res 35:276-281, 1986.

Informational needs of 60 recently diagnosed cancer patients were identified in relation to the disease and to personal, family, and social concerns by using the Derdiarian Informational Needs Assessment. The need for information about treatment was significantly greater than for any other factor related to cancer, followed by prognosis. In addition, significantly more importance was attached to these two needs than to diagnosis (i.e., nature and extent of cancer) and to tests.

In the personal category the need for information on physical well-being was significantly greater than for information on job/career and on plans/goals. Psychologic well-being ranked second. In social relationships more information was needed about job/career relationships than about leisure and special interest relationships. Finally more information was needed about spouses than about children or parents.

The implication is that information needed by patients appears to be associated with harms, threats, and resources associated with the diagnosis. Nurses should assess these needs and intervene even when it appears that the physician has informed the patient about them. ■

TABLE 17-9 Nursing diagnoses and expected outcomes for patients with cancer

Problem Area and Nursing Diagnosis	Possible Etiologies	Expected Outcomes: Patient/Family
INFORMATION		
Knowledge deficit (disease process, treatment methods, self-care activities)	Lack of exposure, recall, cognitive limitation	Describes their role in self-care during various therapies Participates in self-care
COPING		
Coping, ineffective (individual/family)	Maladaptive coping styles, temporary family disorganization, prolonged disability of significant person	Participates in care and decision making Uses support resources or identified alternative support systems
Grieving, dysfunctional	Loss of loved one, of health, of independence	Describes loss and feelings about loss Work together to overcome losses
COMFORT, REST		
Pain	Pathophysiologic changes, improper administration of pain medication, psychologic stress	States that pain is gone or is tolerable Identifies measures to reduce pain
Sleep pattern disturbance	Pain, anxiety, environmental changes	Uses pain medication, relaxation techniques appropriately to induce sleep and relieve pain
NUTRITION		
Nutrition, altered: less than body requirements	Anorexia, nausea and vomiting, swallowing difficulties, anxiety, depression	Identifies foods that are tolerated Selects foods that provide sufficient nutrients Returns to near normal weight or exhibits no further weight loss
Fluid volume deficit	Nausea and vomiting, abnormal fluid loss (diarrhea etc.) decreased intake	Maintains or regains fluid volume, (normal serum electrolytes, serum osmolality, tissue turgor) Maintains balanced intake and output Maintains moist membranes
PROTECTIVE MECHANISMS		
Injury, potential for: physical	Sensory, motor deficits, decrease in platelets, lack of awareness of environmental hazards	Shows no evidence of physical injury, bleeding, trauma
Infection, potential for	Lack of knowledge, decreased nutrition, decreased immune response	Lists measures to prevent infection Identifies signs and symptoms of infection States measures to control infection Develops no evidence of infection
Skin integrity, impaired, potential	Immobility, inadequate nutrition, mechanical forces (pressure, shearing), radiation	Describes measures to prevent skin breakdown Maintains intact skin and mucous membranes States measures to care for skin breakdown (includes mucosa of mouth and vagina)
Oral mucous membrane, altered	Oral cavity radiation chemotherapy, dehydration, ineffective oral hygiene, decreased salivation	Develops moist, intact mucous membranes
MOBILITY		
Mobility, impaired physical	Activity intolerance; perceptual/cognitive, neuromuscular impairment; pain, depression, severe anxiety	Maintains optimal level of mobility for physical condition Uses methods to increase mobility Uses activities to prevent complications of immobility
Self-care deficit	Activity intolerance, fatigue, pain; perceptual/cognitive, neuromuscular, musculoskeletal impairment; depression, severe anxiety	Participates in self-care (eating, bathing, dressing, grooming, toileting) consistent with health status

TABLE 17-9 Nursing diagnoses and expected outcomes for patients with cancer—cont'd

Problem Area and Nursing Diagnosis	Possible Etiologies	Expected Outcomes: Patient/Family
ELIMINATION		
Bowel elimination, alteration: Constipation Diarrhea	Change in life-style, immobility, drugs, inadequate nutrition (roughage, fluids)	States actions to decrease constipation/diarrhea Develops normal bowel elimination pattern
Urinary elimination, pattern altered: incontinence	Altered environment, sensory cognitive or mobility deficits	Develops control of urination or describes methods to cope with incontinence
VENTILATION		
Airway clearance, ineffective	Decreased energy, fatigue, tracheobronchial infection, perceptual/cognitive impairment	States methods to maintain clear airway Describes methods to cope with altered airway
Breathing pattern, ineffective	Neuromuscular, musculoskeletal, perceptual/cognitive impairments; pain, anxiety, decreased energy	Exhibits effective breathing pattern (clear chest; normal TPR; respirations clear, unlabored)
Gas exchange, impaired	Ventilation-perfusion imbalance, impaired alveolar membranes, pulmonary circulation	Exhibits no signs of hypoxia (confusion, restlessness, increased Pco_2, decreased Po_2)
SEXUALITY		
Sexual dysfunction	Altered body structure and/or function due to chemotherapy, radiation therapy, lack of knowledge, privacy, anxiety, fear	Identifies and uses alternate methods of expressing sexuality Expresses satisfaction with sexuality
SELF-PERCEPTION, SELF-CONCEPT		
Anxiety (mild, moderate, severe)	Threat to self-concept, life, health, economic status, role functioning, crises of cancer, unmet needs	States not feeling anxious or worried Exhibits no signs of anxiety (restlessness, increased psychomotor activity)
Fear	Loss of function, long-term illness, treatments, pain, life-style changes, lack of knowledge	States not feeling afraid States source of fear and how to manage feelings
Body image disturbance	Loss of body parts/functions, change in body appearance (alopecia, ostomies, facial trauma, etc.)	States feeling comfortable with altered body structure or function
Depression	Cancer diagnosis, change in role, discomfort related to cancer therapy; loss of status, control	Interacts with family and health team Participates in activities of daily living States feeling in control
Self-esteem disturbance	Trauma, change in body appearance/function, inability to carry out roles	Expresses feeling of self-worth Expresses no feelings of guilt or self-blame
ROLE-RELATIONSHIP PATTERN		
Social isolation	Self-concept disturbance, therapeutic isolation, immobility	Interacts with family, friends, health team members
Independence-dependence conflict, unresolved	Cancer pathophysiology, therapy	Verbalizes comfort with need for dependence in situation that requires dependence
VALUES, BELIEFS		
Spiritual distress	Loss of hope, faith; depression	Verbalizes satisfaction with beliefs, values, spiritual practices Expresses belief in the meaning of life and death

nursing demands not only caring *for* the patient but also caring *about* the patient, who may be angry, depressed, and perhaps physically unattractive because of the effects of the disease or its treatment.

Situations found most stressful to cancer patients may include care by an inexperienced nurse, emergency situations on the hospital division that cause delay in answering call lights, and lack of knowledge about tests and procedures they may be facing (see research box on p. 357). Consequently, nurses caring for cancer patients must be knowledgeable and skillful, recognizing the wide range of emotions experienced by cancer patients. Most important, nurses must be able to listen to and empathize with the patient and family.

Persons working with these patients must have confidence in themselves and the ability to suspend their own concerns, needs, and desires to concentrate on patients' problems. To do this one must be able to tolerate a high level of anxiety and to look at problems on both a feeling (affective) and a thinking (cognitive) level.

HELPING THE PATIENT AND FAMILY COPE

Since the threat to life and the potential for other losses are great for patients with cancer, they need especially to have their existing coping mechanisms supported or to receive support if coping mechanisms are inadequate to meet their needs.

Each patient's reaction to cancer is unique, so there can be no easy formula for care. The nurse must be able to work with and accept the patient's behavior and coping style. At times patients may deny their illness; at other times they may want to talk about it. When patients complain, perhaps the best response is "Tell me how you feel. Perhaps we can do something about it." Guidelines for helping patients meet psychosocial needs are listed in the box below).

The nurse also tries to know the family and their reactions. Families may need to be reminded not to cut the patient off from family activities and concerns. In their desire to help their loved ones, families may unintentionally contribute to the patient's sense of isolation by shielding him or her from family concerns (see research box below).

NURSING INTERVENTIONS TO MEET PHYSIOLOGIC NEEDS

Nursing care to meet the physiologic needs in the treatment phase are discussed in relation to the medical therapies: radiation, chemotherapy, and immunotherapy.

INTERDISCIPLINARY APPROACH TO CARE

The skills of many members of the health team may be required to meet the needs of the cancer patient. Clear, concise communication of ideas about care and planned interventions is essential for coordination, continuity, and integration of care. Team conferences are helpful to promote the sharing of expertise. The social worker, occupational therapist, minister, and psychologist may all be needed to contribute to the patient's well-being. The nurse, who spends the most time with the patient, may be the first to recognize that the patient and family may need the services of other team members.

CARE AFTER HOSPITAL DISCHARGE

Ambulatory health care services are now the major source of care for individuals with cancer. With the shortening of hospital stays, most treatment, follow-up, and symptom management are provided in ambulatory settings.

After discharge, nurse-led programs such as "I Can Cope" have proven very effective in teaching patients and significant others about the disease and in helping

---

GUIDELINES FOR CARE OF PERSONS IN THE TREATMENT PHASE OF CANCER: MEETING PSYCHOSOCIAL NEEDS

1. Identify existing coping mechanisms (spiritual, cognitive, psychomotor, interpersonal).
2. Support existing mechanisms.
3. Provide psychologic support by working with the patient's behavior.
4. Avoid false reassurance.
5. Allow patients and families to express feelings.
6. Be open, honest, creative in approach to problems.
7. Support hope (p. 397) but avoid giving false hope.
8. Trust the patient's resilience and will to try.
9. Foster the patient's independence.
10. Allow patients to participate in decision making.
11. Listen carefully and attentively.
12. Answer questions and give information about tests, treatments.
13. Consult with other health professionals as necessary, including oncology nurse specialists.
14. Do not push patients and families into responsibilities they cannot handle.
15. Validate assumptions and assist patients to describe, clarify, and identify reasons for feelings; get feedback.
16. Make explanations clear and uncomplicated.
17. Let patients and families know that their feelings are normal.

RESEARCH

Tringali CA: The needs of family members of cancer patients, Oncol Nurs Forum 13(4):65-69, 1986.

This study explored perceptions of family members of cancer patients to determine their most important needs. Twenty-five family members rated the importance of 53 need statements using a Likert-type scale. For data analysis, subjects were grouped according to phase of illness (initial, recurrent, and follow-up), and need statements were divided into cognitive, emotional, and physical categories. Analysis of findings indicated that cognitive needs were perceived as most important (for example, to have questions answered honestly, to be informed of changes in the patient's condition). The highest marked emotional need varied across phase of illness. The category of physical needs contained none of the needs ranked most important for family members. Since information-seeking is one of the general coping strategies used by individuals, nurses must meet the challenge of family-oriented practice and deal with these needs. ■

them cope. It is recommended that they participate in the therapeutic sessions.

CANCER REHABILITATION

Rehabilitation is an essential component of cancer care and begins when patients are first diagnosed so they can maintain their highest level of physical, psychological, spiritual, and social well-being.[31] With the advent of new and effective therapies for cancer, patients are recovering or living longer and in better health. Society's negative attitudes that must be overcome include the view of cancer as terminal rather than a curable or chronic disease. Emphasis should be on quality of life regardless of anticipated length of life.

Specific goals are established early in the disease process and are best based on interdisciplinary team assessment, of which the patient and family are essential members. Comprehensive rehabilitation services, however, are often lacking for cancer patients. There is lack of identification of patient problems and the absence of referrals.[31]

Nurses are involved in prevention and health promotion as part of the rehabilitation process. The nurse's role in prevention consists of promoting new behaviors in the cancer survivor for risk-factor reduction for second malignancies and for other preventable diseases. Health-promoting behaviors are those that sustain or increase the levels of well-being, self-actualization, and fulfillment of the individual, an approach to living that leads individuals to their highest potential of well-being no matter what their diagnoses.[35] Activities that are health promoting include exercise, interpersonal support, adequate nutrition, stress management, health responsibility to identify activities to promote health, and finally achieving self-actualization through respect for accomplishments and worth along with a positive attitude.[31]

Nurses must convince other nurses, the public, and other health care professionals that cancer is a chronic disease and that patients have rehabilitation needs. Some rehabilitation objectives and interventions are listed in Table 17-10.

TABLE 17-10 Interventions to enhance cancer rehabilitation

Objectives	Methods to Achieve Goals
1. Promote a positive attitude toward cancer rehabilitation.	1. Emphasize that cancer is a chronic disease, not a terminal one. 2. Disseminate the improvements in cancer care and increased survival statistics in the lay literature.
2. Promote the positive aspects in cancer care.	1. Incorporate potential long-term and short-term rehabilitation needs as part of initial patient assessments in acute care settings and outpatient clinics. 2. Provide inservice programs for nurses and non-professional staff on prolonged survival and improved quality of life for cancer patients. 3. Increase the number and focus of publications reflecting the positive results in cancer care.
3. Promote positive attitudes in nursing students toward cancer care.	1. Arrange for student experiences with patients who have survived cancer. 2. Provide opportunities for students to have positive experiences helping patients manage side effects of cancer treatment. 3. Provide a balance of experiences with survivors of cancer and those in terminal stages.
4. Promote positive self-care and independence of patients with cancer.	1. Encourage participation in programs designed to help cope with cancer (e.g., I Can Cope, Living with Cancer). 2. Use referrals to other disciplines, (O.T., P.T., social work) as indicated for individual patients. 3. Inform patients regarding programs of American Cancer Society, such as Reach to Recovery, CanSurmount, Ostomy Rehabilitation Program.
5. Promote successful integration in the workplace.	1. Provide opportunities for patients to role play how they will handle information about their diagnosis with coworkers. 2. Discuss patient's employment setting and routines to determine potential problems and solutions related to cancer-related disabilities.

From Dudas S and Carlson S: Cancer rehabilitation, Oncol Nurs Forum 15:187, 1988.

MEDICAL MANAGEMENT

Medical management of the patient with cancer is complex and often involves multiple therapies. The nurse is often the health care professional who augments the physician's explanation of the treatments and their benefits. In addition, in many cases it is the nurse who carries out or assists in the therapeutic interventions. The nursing diagnoses and expected patient/family outcomes listed in Table 17-9 (p. 358) are pertinent for care of the patient receiving cancer therapy.

THERAPEUTIC REGIMENS

Often several physicians are involved in determining the appropriate treatment for cancer. The medical team chooses treatment on the basis of the biologic characteristics of the tumor, its clinical stage (p. 343), and the condition of the patient. The histologic type of tumor is particularly important in determining the treatment to be used.

Therapy may be curative (removal of all traces of the disease from the body) or palliative (directed only toward relieving symptoms). At the present time there are four major forms of treatment: surgery, radiotherapy, chemotherapy, and immunotherapy. The latter is the newest form of treatment for cancer. Combinations of the four treatment modalities are often employed to achieve the best results for each patient.

Data from the National Cancer Institute indicates a 49%, 5-year relative survival rate among all patients diagnosed between 1976 and 1981, compared with 48% for patients diagnosed between 1973 and 1975. This trend reflects better diagnostic actions and more effective treatment. Most recently, the results from surgery, chemotherapy, and radiation therapy support the idea that multidisciplinary therapy should result in even greater patient survival and decreased morbidity.[50]

SURGICAL INTERVENTION

Surgery, the oldest method of treating cancer, may be either curative or palliative. The best treatment for cancer at the present time is complete surgical removal of all malignant tissue before metastasis occurs. Surgery must often be extensive and may require adjustments beyond that needed in many other conditions. There may not be time to accustom oneself gradually to the idea of surgery and the effect it can have on one's body and on one's life-style. The individual often faces the prospect of mutilating surgery with only the hope that it will cure the cancer and be lifesaving. Concern about what will happen to the family may be utmost in the patient's mind. Obviously, the individual and family need empathy and understanding as they attempt to accept the recommendations for immediate surgery.

The interaction of surgical treatment with radiation and chemotherapy is now more carefully planned both for primary and metastatic cancer. Greater attention is paid on restorative procedures for many types of cancer. The nutritional, immune, and metabolic status of the patient are also being given more attention before surgery is used.[118] The operative procedures used to treat various types of cancer are discussed in later chapters under the particular systems.

RADIOTHERAPY

Radiotherapy, or the use of radiation in the treatment of disease, has been used in the treatment of cancer for about 80 years. The principal radiation agents are: (1) x-ray, which consists of electromagnetic radiation produced by waves of electrical energy traveling at a very high speed; (2) radium, which is a radioactive isotope occurring freely in nature; and (3) the artificially induced radioactive isotopes produced by bombarding the isotopes of elements with highly energized particles in a cyclotron. The most common sources of radiation for external beam therapy are the linear accelerator, the cobalt-60 teletherapy machines, and the betatron. These machines produce radiation of varying types of energy, which control the depth of penetration of the x-rays into tissues.[120]

Radiotherapy is effective in curing cancer in some instances; in other instances it controls the growth of cancer cells for a time. Because it may deter the growth of cancer cells, it may relieve pain even when extension of the disease is such that cure is impossible.

Radiation therapy is increasingly being used in lieu of surgery, particularly in patients with cancer of the larynx, prostate, and breast and in malignant melanoma of the eye. Research is directed toward modifying radiosensitivity and toward improving radiation therapy's effects on hypoxic tumor cells.

TUMOR RESISTANCE

Tumor resistance to radiation is a major problem. Tissue hypoxia is one of the major factors contributing to radio-resistance. Efforts to overcome the problem include use of hyperbaric oxygen (HBO) or hypoxic cell sensitizers and use of high linear energy transfer (LET) particle beams, such as neutrons, pi mesons and heavy charged particles.[120] *Neutrons* are uncharged nuclear particles that, like x-rays, deposit their energy as they pass through tissue. They have no advantage over standard x-rays but do, however, produce more dense ionizations than do x-rays, gamma and beta rays. Consequently they are less oxygen-dependent, and the effect of low oxygen is reduced 50% when compared with x-rays.

Low LET rays are cell-cycle dependent with cells in S and G2 less responsive to these beams. *High LET beams* are effective independent of the cell cycle phases

TERMS RELATED TO RADIATION

Roentgen	Amount of radiation exposure in the air
Rad	Amount of radiation absorbed per dose
Gray (GY)	(International measure) 1 gray = 100 rads
Rem	Unit of measure used to express the biologic effect of one rad of x-rays
Sievert (SV)	(International measure) 1 SV = 100 rems

and are theoretically more effective against slowly proliferating, relatively hypoxic bulky tumors. High LET irradiation's potential benefit lies in improving control of cancers resistant to conventional radiation either alone or with other forms of treatment.

PRINCIPLE UNDERLYING RADIOTHERAPY

Radiotherapy is based on the fact that rapidly reproducing malignant cells are more sensitive to radiation than are normal cells. Therapeutic doses of radiotherapy are calculated to destroy or delay the growth of malignant cells without destroying normal tissue. Rotation of either the target site in the patient or the radiation beam makes it possible to deliver a high total dose to the tumor while at the same time only part of the dose reaches the noncancerous tissue surrounding it.

Radiation dose is measured by the amount of radiant energy absorbed by tissues and is expressed in the unit "rad" (see box). One rad is the absorption of 100 ergs/g of irradiated tissue. Common radiotherapy regimens deliver 200 rads/day. The amount of radiation given to an individual, however, depends on the dosage required to kill cancer cells and the length of time between treatments.[122] Most cells are killed as they go through the S or M phases of cell division (see Figure 17-3).

The treatment can range in time from 1 minute to a few minutes. The exact time is dependent on the dose to be delivered, the energy, the type of radiation beam, and the depth of the tumor. Frequency of treatment varies, with some patients being treated daily, five times per week.

In some cases patients may receive a "split course" of therapy by receiving part of the total dose followed by a rest of 1 to 2 weeks until the final high dose is achieved. The total radiation dose delivered is about 40 to 70 GY (4000 to 7000 rad).[69]

The radiation used medically consists of alpha- (α-), beta- (β-), and gamma- (γ-) rays (Figure 17-9). α- and β-rays cannot pass through the skin. γ-Rays, however, have been found to penetrate several inches of lead, although lead shielding offers a considerable degree of protection. X-rays, which are similar to γ-rays, require lead protection.

Radiation can be delivered to the patient *externally* by exposure to rays, such as from an x-ray machine or from cobalt-60, or *internally*, either by placing radioac-

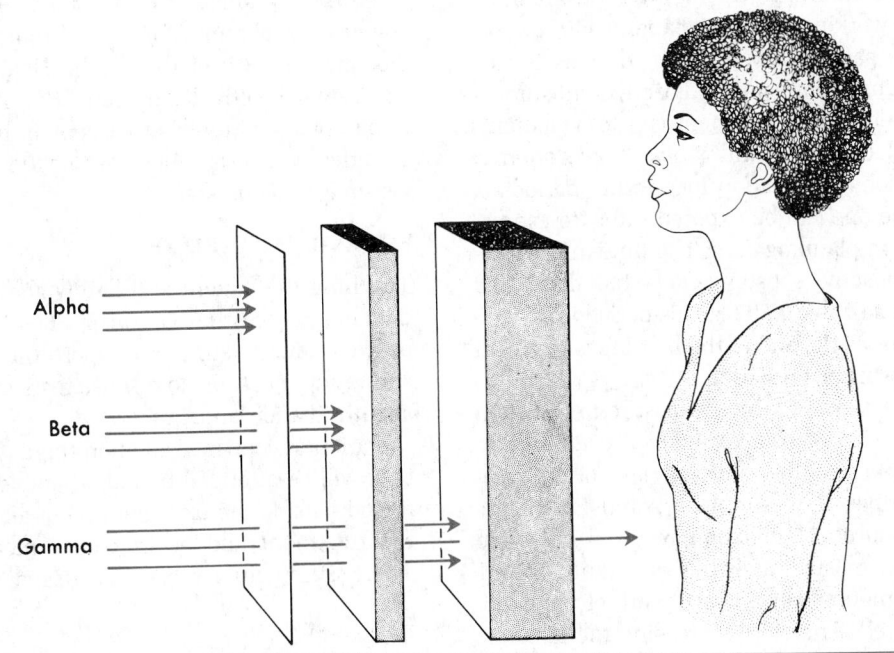

FIGURE 17-9 Relative penetrating power of three types of radiation. (From Bouchard-Kurtz R and Speese-Owens N: Nursing care of the cancer patient, ed 4, St Louis, 1981, The CV Mosby Co.)

TABLE 17-11 Characteristics and uses of some commonly used radioactive agents

Radiation Source	Half-Life (Where Applicable)	Rays Emitted	Appearance or Form	Method of Administration
X-ray	—	γ	Invisible rays	X-ray machine
Radium	1600 yr	α β γ	In needles, plaques, molds	Interstitial (needles) Intracavitary (plaques, mold)
Radon	4 days	α β γ (low intensity)	In seeds, needles	Interstitial (seeds, needles)
Cesium (137-Cs)	33 yr	β γ	In needles, capsules	Interstitial (needles) Intracavitary (capsules)
Cobalt (60-Co)	5 yr	β γ	External (cobalt unit) Internal (needles, seeds, molds)	Machine (teletherapy) Interstitial (needles, seeds)
Iodine (131-I)	8 days	β γ (low intensity)	Clear liquid	By mouth
Phosphorus (32-P)	14 days	β	Clear liquid	By mouth, intracavitary, intravenous
Gold (198-Au)	3 days	β γ	Purple liquid	Intracavitary
Iridium (192-Ir)	74 days	β γ (low intensity)	In needles, wires, seeds	Interstitial
Yttrium (90-Y)	3 days	β	Beads, needles	Interstitial

tive material such as radium within the tissues or body cavity (sealed internal radiation) or by administering the materials intravenously or orally so that they are distributed throughout the body (unsealed internal radiation).

PROTECTION OF HEALTH PROFESSIONALS FROM RADIATION HAZARDS

Radiation delivered externally (including x-rays) can do harm to persons working with the patient *only during* the time that the patient is being treated. This is true also of the radiation from some radioactive substances used for other methods of treatment (p. 367). Patients with internal radiation who emit γ-rays, however, may expose other persons to radiation for varying periods of time, and the time one can be exposed safely to the patient is important in planning care. The time interval required for the radioactive substance to be half dissipated is called its *half-life* (Table 17-11). This period varies extremely widely, but as the end of the half-life is reached, danger from exposure decreases.

There are three ways by which exposure to radiation can be controlled: *time, distance,* and *shielding.* All emanations are subject to the physical law of inverse-square. For example, a person who stands 2 meters away from the source of radiation receives only one fourth as much exposure as when standing only 1 meter away. At 4 meters only one sixteenth of the exposure will be received. Therefore increasing the distance from the emanations decreases the exposure (Figure 17-10). *Lead-lined gloves and a lead apron, which act as a shield to reduce exposure, should be worn by anyone who attends patients during x-ray treatment or during examination by fluoroscopy.*

When the nurse knows the kind of substance used, the kind and amount of rays it emits, its half-life, and its exact location in the patient and considers these facts in relation to control of exposure, safe and adequate care for the patient can be planned.

Nurses wishing to know about radioactive substances can obtain information from the Division of Radiological Health of the Public Health Service or from their state health department. Several drug companies also publish pamphlets that contain helpful information. In cities with large medical facilities a radiation physicist may be consulted.

EXTERNAL RADIOTHERAPY

Teaching the patient and family about all aspects of radiotherapy (see the box on p. 366) is an important aspect of care. There is an opportunity during individual and group meetings to discuss fears and misconceptions about radiation and cancer.[102]

Patients receiving radiation therapy should know that they will be attended by radiotherapists who will be stationed outside the treatment room and who will observe the treatment and be in communication at all times. There is no pain associated with radiation therapy.

Procedure

In giving treatment, rays can be directed at the tumor from several different angles so that normal tissue receives a minimum of exposure. The areas through

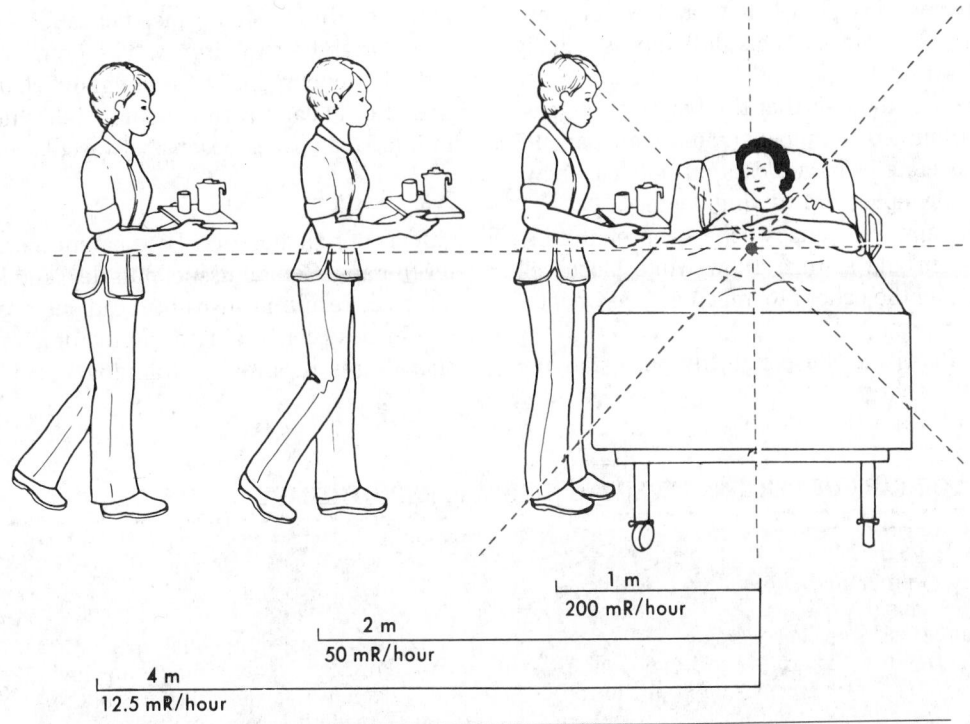

1 m
200 mR/hour

2 m
50 mR/hour

4 m
12.5 mR/hour

FIGURE 17-10 Nurse nearest source of radioactivity (patient) is exposed to more radio-activity. (Adapted from Bouchard-Kurtz R and Speese-Owens N: Nursing care of the cancer patient, ed 4, St Louis, 1981, The CV Mosby Co.)

which rays pass are known as *ports*. Different ports may be used on different days, or the position may be changed at intervals during a daily treatment so that only a certain amount is given through each of several ports. The patient may be placed on a rotating device such as a rotating chair so that although the tumor mass receives the full dose of radiation, skin areas receive less exposure.

In medical centers where hyperbaric oxygen chambers are available, patients may receive radiation therapy while receiving hyperbaric oxygen. The rationale for this combined therapy is that malignant cells, in which the oxygen tension is increased, are more susceptible to the effects of radiation. At the same time the sensitivity of normal cells to the radiation effects is not increased.[120]

Early Reaction

Radiation affects DNA of normal cells differently from DNA of cancer cells. Normal tissue can recover more effectively from radiation than can cancer cells. Effects are seen more rapidly in cells that have a high mitotic index (those that are rapidly dividing, such as skin, mucous membranes, and hair follicles), and seen later in cells that divide more slowly (muscles and vascular system). Early side effects are usually reversible, whereas late effects are more permanent.

When radiation therapy is used, some degree of radi-

ation reaction may occur. Early reactions include blanching or erythema of the skin and mucous membranes, possibly progressing to dry or moist desquamation. Recovery after most desquamation usually takes 2 to 4 weeks and is usually complete. After 2 to 3 months, the new pink skin has gradually returned to normal.[69] If the mucosa of the mouth, pharynx, bladder, or rectum is affected, there may be pain, inhibition of the normal secretions, and impairment of functions.

When treatment is directed toward abdominal organs or any deep tissues there is almost always some skin reaction. There may be itching, tingling, burning, oozing, or sloughing of the skin. The term *burn* should never be used in referring to this reaction, since it implies incorrect dosage. Reddening may occur on or about the tenth day, and the skin may turn a dark plum color after about 3 weeks. The skin may also become dry and inelastic and may crack easily.

Sloughing of tissue and subsequent hemorrhages are complications that must be considered when radiation is used in any form. Hemorrhage is not mentioned to the patient, but ambulatory patients are told that they should call the physician at once should any sloughing of tissue occur.

Gastrointestinal reactions to radiation therapy are more common when treatment includes some part of the gastrointestinal tract or when the ports lie over this system. The patient may have nausea, vomiting, anorexia, malaise, and diarrhea. This difficulty is usually not discussed with the patient before treatment is started because it is thought that the power of suggestion may contribute to symptoms. Almost all patients who receive moderate or large doses of radiation, however, have these symptoms in varying degrees.

Radiation therapy also causes depression of the hematopoietic system and in turn a low white blood cell count, predisposing the patient to infection (see Chapter 30).

Pulmonary effects include cough, dyspnea, fatigue, and sore throat. Acute radiation effects are a result of vascular and airway injury. The primary acute effect is radiation pneumonitis. Swelling and sloughing of endothelial cells causes an exudate while fluid accumulates in interstial spaces because of vascular damage.[102]

Late Reaction

Effects of radiation may be apparent months or years after therapy. Genital tissue, muscles, and kidneys may be affected, resulting in painful radionecrosis.[69] Radiation causes destruction of fine vasculature, and the skin may show signs of atrophy (thinning and blanching), pig-

---

GUIDELINES FOR CARE OF PERSONS RECEIVING EXTERNAL RADIOTHERAPY

1. Teach the patient:
   a. Orientation programs, information booklets, group sessions
   b. Scheduling, when to seek assistance
   c. How the treatment is given, need to lie still, possible use of sandbags, pillows, or straps for positioning
   d. Early and late signs and symptoms of reactions
   e. Type of clothing to wear (no girdle, tight pantyhose, tight trousers or belt during treatment to trunk) and for several weeks thereafter
   f. Avoidance of excess cold or heat to skin during treatment period (*no* hot water bottle or ice caps)
   g. Caution regarding use of cosmetics if x-ray is to face (may contain irritating oils)
   h. Wig, if alopecia occurs
   i. Cooler baths or showers; avoid sunbathing or extremes of temperature if blanching or discoloration of the skin has occurred
2. Prepare the skin:
   a. Remove ointments and dressings and thoroughly cleanse skin; apply alcohol (follow institution guidelines)
   b. Do not wash off skin marks placed by radiologist
   c. Use sponge baths instead of shower or tub after skin marks are placed
3. Prevent skin breakdown:
   a. Apply ointments (if ordered)
   b. Do not use solutions or ointments containing heavy metals (zinc)
   c. Use cornstarch instead of powder
4. Promote healing of irritated skin after therapy is completed:
   a. Cleanse area gently with a solution of 30 ml hydrogen peroxide in 100 ml water (or follow institution guidelines)
   b. Do *not* remove crusts
   c. Pat area dry
   d. Leave area uncovered as much as possible
   e. Use saline soaks, antibiotic ointments, or steroid creams for moist desquamation[57]
   f. Apply ointments by spreading on sterile gauze and fastening to patient's clothing or bandaging loosely and anchoring to healthy skin
   g. Use a nonirritating tape
   h. Apply dressing loosely to avoid pressure and allow air circulation
5. Decrease gastrointestinal upset:
   a. Provide rest before mealtime and after eating to decrease nausea and vomiting
   b. Provide frequent small meals
   c. Avoid food 2 to 3 hours before and 2 hours after treatment
   d. Give sour beverages and effervescent liquids for nausea
   e. Breakfast may be the best meal; make it substantial
   f. Try high protein, high-carbohydrate, low-residue diet[1]
   g. Give low roughage diet, increased calories and fluids for diarrhea
   h. Give IV glucose in normal saline solutions as ordered
   i. Administer antiemetics as prescribed (dimenhydrinate [Dramamine], chlorpromazine [Thorazine], trimethobenzamide hydrochloride [Tigan])
   j. Administer antidiarrhetics as prescribed (camphorated tincture of opium [paregoric], kaolin and pectin [Kaopectate], diphenoxylate hydrochloride [Lomotil])
6. Prevent infections:
   a. Avoid persons with respiratory tract or other infections
   b. Do not place in hospital room with a patient with infection
   c. Provide private room or protective isolation if white blood count is low
   d. Administer prophylactic antibiotics as prescribed during or after treatment
7. Decrease pulmonary effects[102]
   a. Give cough suppressants, especially at night
   b. Use oxygen judiciously
   c. Use humidifier to liquefy secretions
   d. Position patient in high Fowlers
   e. Teach pursed lip breathing

mentation, and telangiectasis. If there is severe vascular damage or if there are other complications that require further surgery, the irradiated tissues may fail to heal.

Nursing Interventions for Patients Receiving External Radiation

Nursing diagnoses are determined from assessment of patient data. Refer back to Table 17-9 (p. 358) for possible nursing diagnoses and expected patient outcomes. Some of the more common nursing diagnoses for the person receiving external radiotherapy include the following:

Knowledge deficit
Infection, potential for
Nutrition, altered: less than body requirement
Skin integrity, impaired
Diarrhea

Specific nursing interventions are listed in the box on p. 366. The nurse may prepare the skin for treatment as described in the same box.

After this preparation nothing should be used on the skin. The area to be treated is usually outlined by the radiologist at the time of the first treatment. Occasionally, a small tattoo mark is used instead of the conspicuous skin markings when treatment is given to exposed parts of the body. Marks must not be washed off until the treatment is completed because they are important guides to the radiologist (Figure 17-11).

The radiologist is consulted about skin care when a local radiation reaction occurs. Healing usually starts in the fifth week of treatment and should be complete about a month later. When treatment is given to any part of the head, there may be loss of hair or loss of beard, depending on the amount of radiation.

Depending on the area treated, other side effects include gastrointestinal tract upset and infection if the hematopoietic system is depressed. Problems related to specific radiation therapy are discussed in appropriate sections of the text.

INTERNAL RADIOTHERAPY

Internal radiation may be delivered by sealed or unsealed methods. In either type special precautions may be necessary, depending on the amount of radioactive material used, its location, and the kind of rays being emitted (Table 17-11). Special precautions may be taken if more than a tracer diagnostic dose has been given. Hospitals in which therapeutic doses of radioactive isotopes are administered are required to have a radiation safety officer. Quite often this person is a physicist. The radiation safety officer determines the precautions to be observed in each situation. Most hospitals have printed instruction sheets stating the precautions to be followed for each substance used. Personnel should be fully acquainted with all precautions and should be supervised in carrying them out. Generally, the patient will be placed in a single room or in a double room with another patient who is also receiving radiation therapy. A radiation precaution sign should be placed on the door to the patient's room, and visitors should be restricted.

Sealed Internal Radiotherapy (Brachytherapy)

Brachytherapy is used to deliver a concentrated dose of radiation directly to the malignant lesion or tumor area. Usually this involves insertion of radioactive substances within hollow cavities or within tissues. The radioactive isotopes commonly used are cobalt-60, iridium-192, iodine-125, phosphorus-32, cesium-137, gold-198, and radium-226. These radioactive substances may be used in the form of molds, plaques, needles, wires, special applicators, or ribbons that are carefully placed and left in position for a specified length of time (Figure 17-12). Emanations from the radioactive substances may also be sealed in tiny gold tubes (seeds) and left indefinitely within the tissues into which they are inserted (Figure 17-13). The half-life of the seeds is much less than that of substances from which their emanations come.

A fairly common site for the implantation of seeds is the mouth. Plaques and molds also are used for lesions in the mouth. Sealed internal radiation also is used widely in treatment of cancer of the cervix.

Prevention of radiation hazards: sealed radiotherapy. Safe practice for the nurse caring for a patient receiving sealed internal radiotherapy depends on the principles of time, distance, and shielding (p. 364). Radioactive

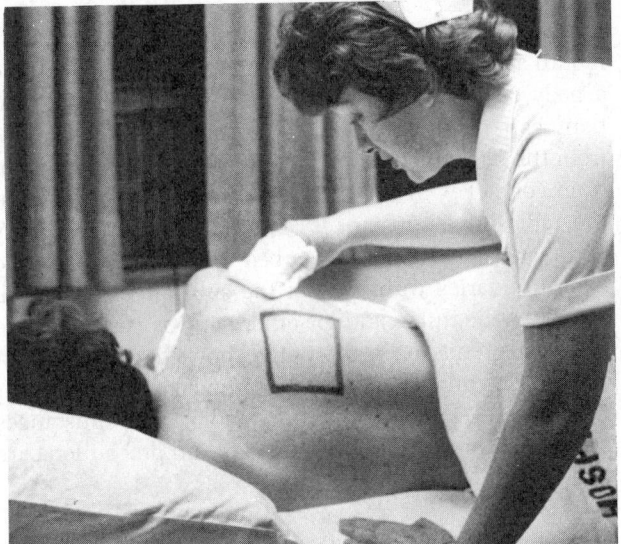

FIGURE 17-11 When a bath is given, care must be taken not to remove skin markings used to guide the radiologist in giving x-ray treatments.

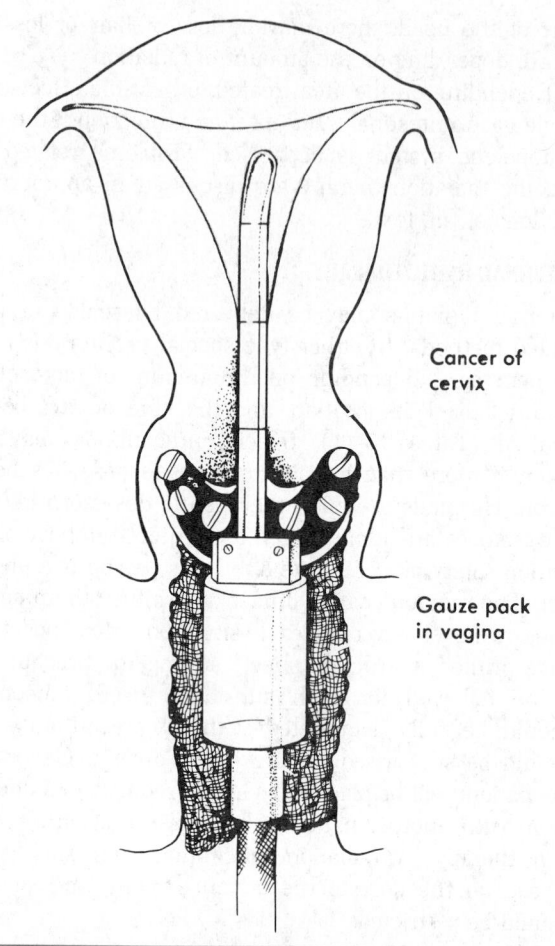

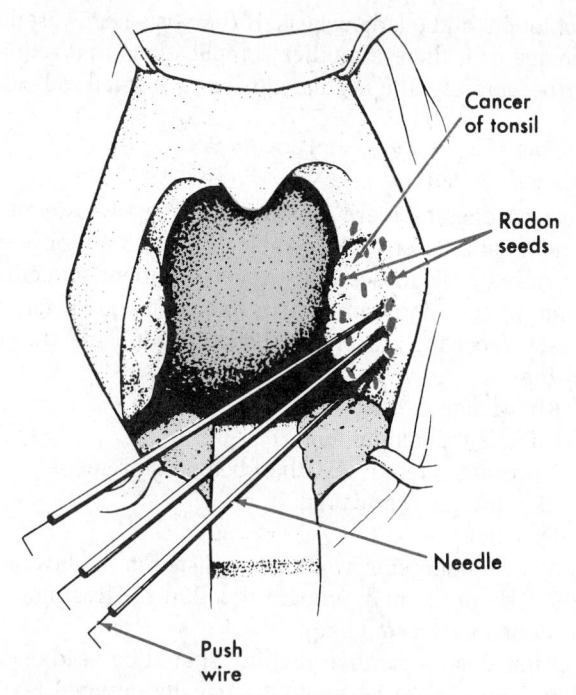

FIGURE 17-13 Radium emanations may be sealed in tiny gold tubes (radon seeds) and left indefinitely within tissue into which they are inserted. Schema shows insertion into tonsil.

FIGURE 17-12 Ernst applicator in place for treatment of cancer of the cervix. Note gauze packing in the vagina to help maintain applicator in position.

materials for sealed internal therapy usually are kept in a lead-lined container in the radiology department and are inserted into the patient in the operating room. They should never be touched with bare hands.

Various types of applications are used to insert radioactive substances to ensure they remain in site and to reduce radiation exposure to the staff. These applications allow direct positioning of the radioactive substance (the Fletcher-Suit application) or allow remote control positioning of the material (the cathetron, the Curieton, and the Selectron) so that staff do not have to come in contact with the radioactive substance.[69]

Sealed radioactive material is often reused. Even if it is not to be reused, it is returned in a lead-lined container (see the box p. 369, left).

Exposure is sometimes termed *external* in that it can occur only by direct exposure to the encased radioactive substance. It cannot result from contact with linen, vomitus, or urine or from touching the patient. Knowing where the radioactive material is implanted helps the

nurse to plan activities of care. If, for example, the substance is in the patient's mouth, there is less exposure if one stands toward the foot of the bed. If it is in the uterus or bladder, standing at the head of the bed is safer.

Unsealed Internal Radiotherapy

Unsealed internal radiation is delivered to the patient by mouth as an "atomic cocktail" or as a liquid instilled into a body cavity. Exposure for persons caring for the patient can result from direct contact with emanations from the substance of the patient (external exposure) or from contact with the patient's discharges that contain the radioactive substances (internal exposure). It may be inhaled, ingested, or absorbed through the skin. The exposure varies with each of the substances used, and safety for the nurse and for other persons caring for the patient depends on a thorough knowledge of the substance used and its action within the body. If only tracer doses (very small amounts) of radioactive substances are used, as for diagnostic purposes, no precautions are necessary.

Prevention of radiation hazards: unsealed radiotherapy. *Radioactive iodine* (iodine-131) is a clear liquid with a half-life of 8.1 days. It is often used, however, in conjunction with surgical removal of the thyroid gland.

PREVENTION OF RADIATION HAZARDS: SEALED INTERNAL RADIOTHERAPY

1. Use forceps to handle material: *do not* touch with hands
2. Cleanse radioactive material after removal using institution protocols
   a. Use basin of water, *not sink*, to prevent loss
   b. If brush is used for cleansing, grasp brush with forceps
3. Return radioactive materials to radiology department in lead-lined container immediately after removal from body
4. Check all bed linen and patient clothing for possible dislodged material before discarding linens in hamper
5. Use principles of time, distance, and shielding (p. 364) when giving care

Most of the radioactive iodine is eliminated through the kidneys, but small amounts will be present in sputum, vomitus, perspiration, and feces. An indwelling catheter may be inserted before the radioactive iodine is given, and urine may be released at intervals directly into the lead-lined container. It is important that all urine be collected carefully, because it is the quantitative determination of the amount of radioactive substance excreted that determines when the patient may be removed from isolation (see the box at right).

Radioactive phosphorus (phosphorus-32) is a clear liquid with a half-life of 14 days. It is used in the treatment of polycythemia vera and leukemia. It may be given intravenously, orally, or directly into a body cavity. Sources of contamination are vomitus and seepage from wounds. There is no danger from external exposure because the β-rays emitted by this substance are absorbed by the patient's body.

Radioactive gold (gold-198) is a purple liquid with a half-life of 2.7 days. It is used largely for treatment of cancer of the lung that has caused effusion into the pleural cavity and for peritoneal ascites from generalized carcinoma. It is injected into the body cavity, and the patient is turned every 15 minutes for 2 hours so that the radioactive gold will spread evenly within the cavity. In addition to β-rays, the substance emits x-rays, so that special isolation precautions may be necessary to prevent external exposure.

If a purple stain appears, it indicates that some of the radioactive gold is escaping from the wound or the site of injection.

The patient who receives radioactive gold is usually terminally ill. If he dies soon after receiving gold-198, a notation that the patient was receiving radioactive gold immediately before death is made on a tag, and the tag should be conspicuously placed on the body for the protection of the coroner and the mortician. If the nurse

PREVENTION OF RADIATION HAZARDS: UNSEALED INTERNAL RADIOTHERAPY

1. Radioactive iodine
   a. Use special precautions for urine
      (1) Collect in lead-lined container, label
      (2) Take to radioisotope laboratory for disposal
      (3) Follow approved institution protocols for spilled urine
   b. Monitor linen and equipment for contamination, using a Geiger-Muller counter, before removal from room
   c. Label and store radioactive linen in lead containers or burn
   d. Use paper dishes and burn after use
   e. Wash skin and equipment with soap and water, if contaminated, then monitor
   f. Wear gloves when handling linen
   g. Air room for at least 24 hours or until monitoring shows radioactivity is negligible
2. Radioactive phosphorus
   a. Follow skin and equipment contamination procedures as for radioactive iodine
   b. Place vomitus and dressings in lead-lined container, label, and take to radioisotope laboratory for disposal
3. Radioactive gold
   a. Place contaminated linen in container, label, send to radioisotope laboratory
   b. Burn dressings and tissues or send to laboratory for disposal

has any questions about precautions that should be taken, the radiation safety officer is consulted.

Nursing Interventions for Persons Receiving Internal Radiotherapy

Refer to Table 17-9 (p. 358) for possible nursing diagnoses and expected patient outcomes.

Nursing interventions are primarily directed toward teaching the patient about the radiation treatment and the protocols involved, decreasing patient isolation, and promoting comfort of the patient (see the box on p. 370).

CHEMOTHERAPY
BENEFITS

Advances in knowledge of cancer growth and chemotherapeutic agents have led to concomitant advances in cancer treatment. Improvement in overall survival and longer disease-free intervals can be directly ascribed to the use of chemotherapeutic agents, particularly in combination chemotherapy regimens and as adjuvant therapy.

Chemotherapy may be curative, palliative, or have negligible or uncertain effects depending on the type of cancer (see Table 17-12). Patients and families may be told that "incurable" does not mean untreatable or uncontrollable.

NURSING INTERVENTIONS FOR THE PERSON RECEIVING INTERNAL RADIOTHERAPY

1. Teaching the patient
   a. The routine and reason for precautions
   b. Isolation is temporary; restrictions will be removed on a specified date
   c. Nursing staff is available but will work quickly, remain in room only for essential activities
   d. Visitors will be restricted
   e. Methods by which the substance is eliminated, to decrease fear of danger to other people after discharge
2. Decreasing patient isolation
   a. Provide a radio, television, telephone
   b. Interact with patient from doorway at frequent intervals if possible
   c. Plan so one trip allows longer interactions with patient rather than several brief trips
3. Promoting comfort
   a. Provide for a complete bath before therapy (bathing usually not permitted during therapy)
   b. Make up bed with clean linen before therapy
   c. Place turning sheet if patient is very ill or weak
   d. Provide pillows for support of trunk or extremities if indicated

In the care of an individual patient with cancer, the expected benefit of chemotherapy (cure, control, or palliation) should be known by the physician, nurse, and patient. This allows for realistic goal setting by the care givers, patients, and family. Such background also provides a perspective from which to view side effects. The potential for cure, prolonged disease-free survival, or reduction of symptoms is a benefit that most often outweighs the risk and discomfort of short-term toxicity and side effects. *Conditions in which risk may outweigh benefits* include overt or occult infections, bleeding dyscrasias, bone marrow depression, severe metabolic disturbances, renal or liver dysfunction, and pregnancy.

In addition, analogs of existing drugs have decreased the toxicity of some drugs. Carboplatin and iproplatin are "second generation" platinum compounds. Epirubicin and idarubicin are analogs of doxorubicin and daunorubicin and are thought to be less cardiotoxic. Many of these second generation drugs are still in clinical trials.

Adjuvant chemotherapy refers to chemotherapy administered after surgical removal of all known cancer present in the body. It is aimed at the destruction of micrometastases thought likely to be present but too small to be detected by current diagnostic techniques. Left untreated, the micrometastases have a high potential for tumor growth and cancer recurrence. With the use of chemotherapy at a time when the malignant cell popu-

TABLE 17-12 Neoplastic disease response to chemotherapy[65]

Response	Neoplastic Disease
Cures in advanced cancer	Gestational trophoblastic tumors Acute lymphoblastic leukemia Acute myeloblastic leukemia Hodgkin's disease Non-Hodgkin's lymphoma (children) Diffuse histiocytic lymphoma Burkitt's lymphoma Testicular tumors
Cures with adjuvant chemotherapy	Wilms' tumor Osteogenic sarcoma Rhabdomyosarcoma
Minor responses with chemotherapy/adjuvant chemotherapy; no demonstrable prolongation of life	Head and neck cancer Large bowel cancer Liver cancer Pancreatic cancer Cervical cancer Melanoma Cancer of the adrenal cortex Soft tissue sarcoma
Complete and partial remissions with uncertain prolongation of survival with chemotherapy/adjuvant chemotherapy	Chronic granulocytic leukemia Multiple myeloma Ovarian cancer Endometrial cancer Neuroblastoma
Complete remissions and increased survival with chemotherapy/adjuvant chemotherapy	Breast cancer Small cell lung carcinoma Acute myeloblastic leukemia Non-Hodgkin's lymphoma, indolent Prostate cancer

lation is small and likely to be susceptible, complete tumor cell eradication is possible. The goal is cure.

A feeling of well-being and knowledge that all diagnostic tests are negative for cancer understandably may cause the patient to question the need for adjuvant therapy. This is emphasized when side effects are experienced. A sensitivity to these feelings, coupled with the knowledge of the expected benefit of therapy, is the basis for both patient teaching and the supportive encouragement often needed for continued therapy.

Despite an intellectual understanding of the benefits of chemotherapy, it is sometimes difficult for a nurse to maintain an appropriately optimistic and realistic outlook if all one sees are those patients who did not respond to or are no longer responsive to therapy, manifest severe toxicity, or are dying. The practitioner must take into account the setting in which patients are seen. Hospital-based nurses tend to see patients at the time of diagnosis, when they are critically ill, or during the final days of life. The community nurse may see the patient

TABLE 17-13 Phases of clinical trials for chemotherapeutic drugs

Phase	Action
I	Identify toxic reactions; determine optimal dose within safe limits and set schedule
II	Determine extent of antineoplastic activity
III	Compare action of new drug with standard antineoplastic drugs
IV	Determine effect on advanced cancer, effect of combined therapy with other antineoplastic drugs, and effect with adjuvant therapy

at comparable points of illness while providing nursing care in the home. Discussion between the nurse and primary physician, contact with the outpatient clinic, and readmission to the same nursing unit are useful ways of acquiring a more complete picture of an individual's response to treatment. Such positive experiences are a means of nurturing one's own beliefs in therapy so that a realistic and at times very optimistic approach to caring for, supporting, and teaching the chemotherapy patient exists.

CLINICAL TRIALS

The general public and, at times, health professionals outside of oncology view chemotherapy as a mystique and have some feelings of it being experimental. The patient may ask, "Am I a guinea pig?" For this reason it is helpful for the nurse to be able to explain that chemotherapeutic drugs are carefully tested before being identified as an acceptable mode of treatment. Chemotherapeutic drugs reach a phase of clinical trial in humans according to a drug-screening process established by the National Cancer Institute. This screening process identifies compounds with antitumor activity, demonstrates the activity in animals, studies and determines all of the pharmacologic aspects of the drug (kinetics, absorption, dose, metabolism, and excretion), and defines toxicity. The drugs next go through the four phases of clinical trial outlined in Table 17-13. The effectiveness of the new agent is then compared with standard therapy to determine if the new drug is equal to or better than drugs currently used.

PATHOPHYSIOLOGIC PRINCIPLES OF CHEMOTHERAPY

Normal and malignant cells progress through various phases in the cell cycle as they replicate (Figure 17-3) (p. 337). Cancer chemotherapy is based on the actions of certain drugs, creating changes in the cell cycle phases. Figure 17-14 summarizes how some of the commonly used chemotherapeutic agents interrupt cell growth and replication. Drugs such as antimetabolites

and vinca alkaloids that are effective during a particular point of the cell cycle are said to be *phase-specific drugs* (Figure 17-15). Drugs that are active throughout the cell cycle (*phase-nonspecific drugs*) include the alkylating agents, antibiotics, nitrosoureas, procarbazine, and dacarbazine (DTIC-Dome). Combinations of cycle-specific and cycle-nonspecific drugs have proved useful in constructing treatment regimens. One major factor that influences the response of a cancer to chemotherapy is the fraction of tumor cells in replication at a given time, a percentage that varies among different tumors, among individual patients, and at different times in the same patient.

Cell Population Growth

Chemotherapy is more effective when the tumor is small and growing rapidly, a time when a relatively high proportion of cells are undergoing division. At this time, tumor cells are more sensitive to chemotherapeutic agents that are toxic to dividing cells (phase-specific drugs). Larger, slower-growing tumors respond better to drugs that are effective regardless of whether a cell is dividing (phase-nonspecific drugs). Consequently the physician chooses the appropriate drug or combination of drugs, depending on tumor size and rate of growth.

Combination Chemotherapy

Increased knowledge of how specific cytotoxic drugs exert their effect and of the potential for the emergence of tumor cells resistant to a specific therapy, similar to antibiotic resistance, has led to the use of combination chemotherapy. Combination chemotherapy demonstrates a therapeutic effect superior to single agent therapy for many cancers. Drugs considered for combination chemotherapy are those that:

1. Are active when used alone
2. Have different mechanisms of action
3. Have a biochemical basis for possible synergism
4. Do not produce toxicity in the same organs
5. Produce toxicity at different times after administration

Repeated brief courses of drug therapy are given to reduce immunosuppressive effects. Principles of chemotherapy administration are listed in the box on p. 373.

Cell-Kill Hypothesis

The cell-kill hypothesis explains why patients must often have several or more courses of chemotherapy. Chemotherapy is thought to kill a fixed percentage of the total number of cancer cells. Theoretically, if a drug had a 90% cell rate and one million cells were present, the first therapeutic regimen would kill 900,000 cancer cells, leaving 100,000. The second treatment would again destroy 90% of the cells, leaving 10,000. Again, theoretically, after a number of chemotherapy treat-

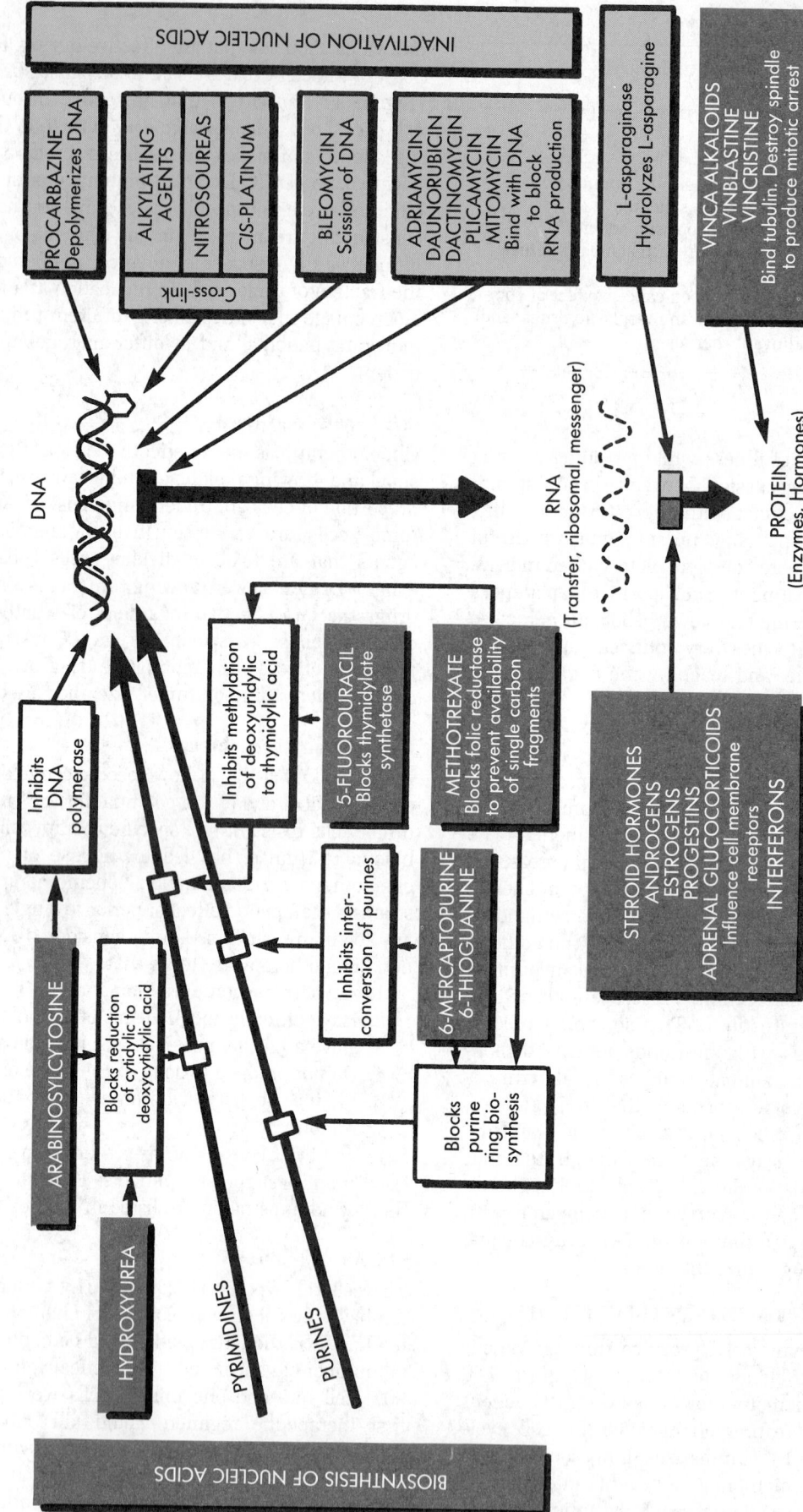

FIGURE 17-14 Mechanism of action of anticancer drugs. (From Krakoff I: Cancer chemotherapeutic agents, CA 37:93-105, 1987.)

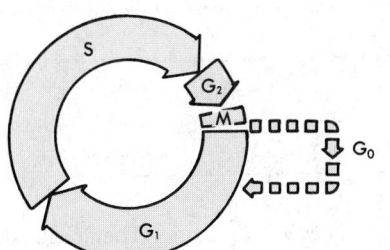

S-phase dependent
Antimetabolites
 Cytarabine
 Diglycoaldehyde
 Fluorouracil
 Mercaptopurine
 Methotrexate
 Thioguanine
Hydroxyurea
Prednisone
Procarbazine

M-phase dependent
Vinca alkaloids
 Vincristine
 Vinblastine

Colchicine derivatives
 Trimethylcolchicinic acid

Podophyllotoxins
 Etoposide (VP-16)
 Teniposide (VM-26)

Have greatest effects in S phase
and possibly late G_2; cell blockade
or death, however, occurs during
early mitosis.

G_1-phase dependent
Asparaginase
Corticosteroids
Diglycoaldehyde (also in early
 S-phase)

G_2-phase dependent
Bleomycin

FIGURE 17-15 Cell cycle phase-specific chemotherapeutic drugs. (Reprinted by permission of the publisher from RT Dorr and WI Fritz, Cancer Chemotherapy Handbook, p 7. Copyright 1980, by Elsevier Science Publishing Co, Inc.)

PRINCIPLES OF CHEMOTHERAPY ADMINISTRATION[65]

1. Combination chemotherapy is far superior to single agent chemotherapy.
2. Complete remission is the minimum requisite for cure and even increased survival.
3. First attempt at chemotherapy offers the best chance for significant benefit; therefore the initial therapy should be the type with maximum effectiveness.
4. Maximum doses of drugs are used to attain maximum tumor cell kill. Dose reduction to minimize toxicity has been called "killing patients with kindness."

ments only one cell would remain and that would be killed by the body's immune system (Figure 17-16).

PROTECTION OF HEALTH PROFESSIONALS FROM CHEMOTHERAPY HAZARDS

Some chemotherapeutic drugs are fetotoxic and carcinogenic. Nurses who handle antineoplastic drugs can be exposed to low doses of the drug by direct contact, inhalation, and injection. The National Institutes of Health (NIH) Division of Safety, along with the NIH clinical pharmacy and the nursing staff of the National Cancer Institute, have identified protective measures on the preparation, administration, and disposal of these drugs for personal and environmental safety.[109] In addition, in 1986 the Occupational Safety and Health Administration (OSHA) of the U.S. Department of Labor gave recommendations generally consistent with these earlier guidelines (see box on guidelines for safety in handling chemotherapeutic agents, p. 376). It is essential that nurses in all settings follow these guidelines to prevent injury to themselves or others.

CHEMOTHERAPEUTIC AGENTS

Drugs may be classified as alkylating agents, antimetabolites, plant (vinca) alkaloids, antibiotics, and steroids (Table 17-14). Abbreviations of common chemotherapeutic drugs are listed in the box on p. 377.

Alkylating Agents

The alkylating agents are cell cycle nonspecific and act against already formed nucleic acids by cross-linking DNA strands, thereby preventing DNA replication and the transcription of RNA.

Antimetabolites

The antimetabolites act by interfering with the synthesis of chromosomal nucleic acid. Antimetabolites are analogs of normal metabolites and block the enzyme necessary for synthesis of essential factors or are incorpo-

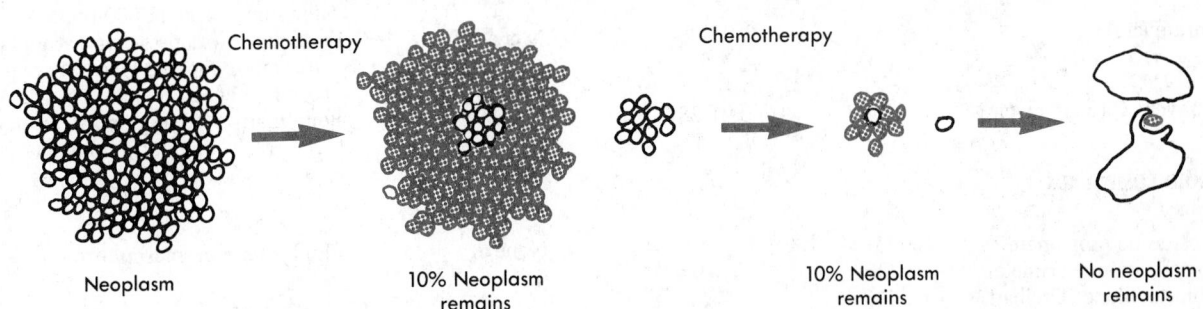

Chemotherapy

Chemotherapy

Neoplasm

10% Neoplasm
remains

10% Neoplasm
remains

No neoplasm
remains

FIGURE 17-16 Cell-kill theory. Chemotherapy destroys 90% of neoplasm; repeated chemotherapy repeats process until last neoplastic cell is killed by body's immune response. (From Cancer: chemotherapy and care, Pt I, Bristol Laboratories, Division of Bristol-Myers Co.)

TABLE 17-14 Specific agents used in cancer chemotherapy

Agents	Principle Route of Administration	NADIR* (Days)	Acute Toxic Signs	Major Toxic Manifestations
ALKYLATING AGENTS				
Mechlorethamine (HN$_2$, Mustargen)	IV	7-10 and 24-30	N & V†	Therapeutic doses moderately depress peripheral blood cell count; excessive doses cause severe bone marrow depression with leukopenia, thrombocytopenia, and bleeding. Maximum toxicity may occur 2 or 3 weeks after last dose. Dosage, therefore, must be carefully controlled. Alopecia and hemorrhagic cystitis occur occasionally with cyclophosphamide
Chlorambucil (Leukeran)	Oral	7-14	None	
Melphalan (Alkeran)	Oral	7-14	None	
Cyclophosphamide (Endoxan, Cytoxan)	IV Oral	7-14	N & V	
Triethylthiophosphoramide (TSPA, Thio-TEPA)	IV	14-28	None	
Busulfan (Myleran)	Oral	10-30	None	
ANTIMETABOLITES				
Methotrexate	Oral IV	7-14	None	Oral and digestive tract ulceration; bone marrow depression with leukopenia, thrombocytopenia and bleeding. Toxicity enhanced by impaired kidney function
6-Mercaptopurine (6-MP, Purinethol)	Oral	5-10	None	Therapeutic doses usually well tolerated; excessive doses cause bone marrow depression
6-Thioguanine (6-TG, Thioguan)	Oral	8-14	None	
5-Fluorouracil (5-FU, Fluorouracil)	IV	7-14	None	Stomatitis, nausea, GI injury, bone marrow depression
Cytarabine (Ara-C, Cytosar-U)	IV	7-14	N & V	Bone marrow depression, megaloblastosis, leukopenia, thrombocytopenia
Floxuridine (FUDR)	IA	—	N & V	Stomatitis, GI injury, bone marrow depression, alopecia
ANTIBIOTICS				
Adriamycin	IV	10-14	N & V	Stomatitis, GI disturbances, alopecia, bone marrow depression. Cardiac toxicity at cumulative doses over 500 mg/M^2
Bleomycin (Blenoxane)	IV SC	—	N & V, chills, fever	Mucocutaneous ulcerations, alopecia, pneumonitis and pulmonary fibrosis in cumulative doses over 400 μ
Dactinomycin (Cosmegen)	IV	10-15	N & V	Stomatitis, GI disturbances, alopecia, bone marrow depression
Daunorubicin	IV	10-14	N & V, fever	Bone marrow depression with leukopenia and thrombocytopenia, alopecia, stomatitis, cardiac toxicity at total lifetime dosage of 600 mg/M^2
Mithramycin	IV	21-30	N & V	Bone marrow depression, particularly thrombocytopenic bleeding, hypocalcemia, hepatic toxicity at large doses
Mitomycin C (Mutamycin)	IV	21-28	N & V	Bone marrow depression, GI injury, hypercalcemia, lung problems
STEROID COMPOUNDS **Androgen**				
Testosterone propionate	IM	—	None	Fluid retention, masculinization
Fluoxymesterone (Halotestin)	Oral			
Dromostanolone (Drolban)	IM			
Testolactone (Teslac)	Oral			
Methyltestosterone	Oral			

Modified from Krakoff IH: Cancer chemotherapeutic agents, CA 37:93, 1987.
*Lowest point of leukocyte and thrombocyte count and greatest risk of infection and bleeding.
†Nausea and vomiting.

TABLE 17-14 Specific agents used in cancer chemotherapy—cont'd

Agents	Principle Route of Administration	NADIR* (Days)	Acute Toxic Signs	Major Toxic Manifestations
Estrogen				
Diethylstilbestrol	Oral	—	Occasional N & V	Fluid retention, feminization Uterine bleeding
Ethinyl estradiol (Estinyl)	Oral			
Antiestrogen				
Tamoxifen citrate (Nolvadex)	Oral	—	N & V	Hot flashes, skin rash, hypercalcemia, increased vaginal secretions
Leuprolide acetate (Lupron)	SC			
Progestin				
Hydroxyprogesterone caproate (Prodrox)	IM	—	None	
Megestrol acetate (Megace)	Oral		None	
Medroxyprogesterone acetate (Provera)	IM		None	
Adrenal Cortical Compounds				
Cortisone acetate	Oral	—	None	Fluid retention, hypertension, diabetes, increased susceptibility to infection
Prednisone (Meticorten)	Oral			
Dexamethasone (Decadron)	Oral			
Methylprednisolone sodium succinate (Solu-Medrol)	IM IV			
Hydrocortisone sodium succinate (Solu-Cortef)	IV			
Antiadrenal				
Aminoglutethimide (Cytadren)	Oral	—	None	Adrenal insufficiency
VINCA ALKALOIDS				
Vinblastine (Velban)	IV	5-10	N & V	Alopecia, areflexia, bone marrow depression
Vincristine (Oncovin)	IV	3-5	None	Areflexia, muscular weakness, peripheral neuritis, paralytic ileus, mild bone marrow depression, SIADH
MISCELLANEOUS DRUGS				
L-Asparaginase	IV	—	N & V, fever, hypersensitivity reactions	Anorexia, weight loss; somnolence, lethargy, confusion; hypoproteinemia, hypolipidemia, abnormal liver function tests; azotemia; granulocytopenia, lymphopenia, thrombocytopenia
Carmustine (BCNU)	IV	12-14 and 26-32	Fever chills	Bone marrow depression
Lomustine (CCNU)	Oral	12-20 and 35-45	N & V	Bone marrow depression with leukopenia and thrombocytopenia; gonadal suppression
Streptozocin (Zanosar)	IV	—	N & V	Hypoglycemia
Mitotane (Lysodren)	Oral	—	N & V	Skin eruptions, diarrhea, mental depression, muscle tremors
Dacarbazine (DTIC-Dome)	IV	14-25	N & V	Bone marrow depression
Hydroxyurea (Hydrea)	Oral	2-10	None	Bone marrow depression, stomatitis, dysuria
Etoposide (VP-16)	IV	—	N & V	Alopecia
Cisplatin (Platinol)	IV	7-14	N & V	Bone marrow depression, renal tubular damage, deafness
Procarbazine (Matulane)	Oral	20-35	N & V	Bone marrow depression with leukopenia and thrombocytopenia, mental depression
Quinacrine (Atabrine)	Intrapleural	—	Local pain, fever	

GUIDELINES FOR SAFETY IN HANDLING CHEMOTHERAPEUTIC AGENTS[51]

A. Prevention of inhalation of aerosols
1. Mix all drugs in an approved Class II biologic safety cabinet (these contain a vertical laminar air-flow hood) with the gloves on at all times.
2. Prime all IV bags containing drugs under the hood, if possible; use a maintenance bag of normal saline or D5W to prime the tubing and all the chemotherapy bags afterwards.
3. Use a needle with a hydrophobic filter to remove drugs from vials when in settings without a safety cabinet. Mix in a well-ventilated area with a pattern of air-flow away from the drug preparer's face.
4. Break ampules by wrapping a sterile gauze pad or alcohol wipe around the neck (decreases chance of droplet contamination).
5. Vent vials with a hydrophobic filter needle (equalizes internal pressure).
6. Do not clip needles, break syringes, or remove needles from syringes when disposing of them.
7. Use a gauze pad when removing syringes and needles from IV injection parts or spikes from IV bags.

B. Prevention of drug absorption through the skin
1. Wear surgical latex gloves and a gown made of low permeability fabric with a closed front and cuffed long sleeves.
2. Change gloves every 30 minutes if working consistently with drugs.
3. Remove gloves immediately after spilling drug solution on them or puncturing or tearing them.
4. Wash hands before putting on gloves and after removing them.
5. Cover the work surface with a plastic-backed absorbent pad; change pad when cabinet is cleaned or after a spill.
6. Clean all surfaces of the biologic safety cabinet before and after drug preparation: use 70% alcohol and a disposable towel. Discard towel in a leak-proof chemical-waste container.
7. Use syringes and IV sets with Luer-Lock fittings.
8. Place an absorbent pad under injection sites to catch accidental spillage.
9. Label all antineoplastic drugs with a chemotherapy hazard label.
10. Wash skin areas thoroughly with soap and water as soon as possible in the event of skin contact with drugs.
11. Flush eyes with eye solution or clean water in the event of eye contact; seek medical attention.

C. Prevention of ingestion
1. Do not eat, drink, chew gum, apply cosmetics, or smoke in drug preparation areas.
2. Keep all food and eating items from the preparation area.
3. Do not place food or drink in the same refrigerator with drugs.
4. Wash hands before and after preparing or giving drugs.
5. Avoid hand-to-mouth or hand-to-eye contact when handling the drugs.

D. Ensuring safe disposal
1. Discard gowns and gloves after contamination in a waterproof container marked as contaminated waste.
2. Discard and identify waste products in leak-proof, sealable plastic bags that are marked with a color and label to indicate contents.
3. Use puncture-proof containers for noncapped, nonclipped needles, and sharp, breakable items.
4. Keep waste containers in labeled, covered waste containers for disposal.
5. Housekeeping personnel should be instructed in safe procedures and wear surgical latex gloves and gowns.
6. Place all drugs used in home chemotherapy in a leak-proof container, remove from home to a designated disposal area.

E. Prevention of contamination by body fluids
1. Provide tight-fitting lid for urinals.
2. Wear latex surgical gloves when handling body fluids.
3. Place waterproof pad over toilet bowl before flushing to avoid splashing.
4. Empty waste products into the toilet by pouring close to the water to avoid splashing. Close the lid and flush two to three times (in the home).[77]
5. Wear gloves and gown when handling linen soiled with body fluids; place in isolation linen bag for separate laundry.
6. Place soiled linens in separate, washable pillow cases and wash twice, separately from other household linens (in the home).

rated into the DNA or RNA and thus prevent replication. Most antimetabolites are pyrimidine analogs, purine analogs, or folic acid antagonists and are, in general, cycle specific.

Vinca Alkaloids

Vincristine sulfate and vinblastine sulfate are plant alkaloids that act as mitotic inhibitors. These agents exert their cytotoxic effect by binding to proteins within the cells causing metaphase arrest. The vinca alkaloids are cell cycle specific. Although these two agents are similar in composition, mechanism of action, and metabolism, their antitumor spectrum, dose, and clinical toxicity differ.

Antibiotics

Those antibiotics that demonstrate antitumor activity appear to affect either the function or synthesis of the

ABBREVIATIONS OF COMMON CHEMOTHERAPEUTIC DRUGS

Adria	Adriamycin
Alk agents	Alkylating agents
L-Asp	L-Asparaginase
BCNU	1,3-*bis* (B-chloroethyl)-1-nitrosourea (carmustine)
Bleo	Bleomycin
CF	Citrovorum factor (Leucovorin calcium)
CLB	Chlorambucil
CPDD	*cis*-Platinum II diamine dichloride
CTX	Cyclophosphamide
Dact	Dactinomycin
Daun	Daunorubicin
o,p-DDD	o,p-Dichlorodiphenyldichloroethane
DTIC	5-(3,3-Dimethyl-1-triazene)-imidazole-4-carboxamide
5FU	5-Fluorouracil
HN2	Nitrogen mustard (Mustargen)
5HP	5-Hydroxypyrinaldehyde-thiosemicarbazone
HU	Hydroxyurea
MeCCNU	1-(B-chloroethyl)-3-(4-methocyclohexyl)-1-nitrosourea
Mith	Mithramycin
Mito	Mitomycin C
6 MP	6-Mercaptopurine
MTX	Methotrexate
NFX	Nafoxidine
PDN	Prednisone
Procarb	Procarbazine
STZ	Streptozotocin
TMX	Tamoxifen
6TG	·6-Thioguanine
VCR	Vincristine
VLB	Vinblastine
VP-16	Etoposide

nucleic acids. In addition, antimitotic and cell surface effects may be caused by these agents. The cytotoxic antibiotics are cell cycle nonspecific agents.

Steroids

The corticosteroids are produced by the adrenal cortex and include mineralocorticoids and glucocorticoids. It is the glucocorticoids that, in addition to their use in numerous nonmalignant diseases, are effective in the treatment of many neoplastic disorders. In some malignancies (e.g., lymphomas, breast cancer, multiple myeloma, acute lymphocytic leukemia, and chronic lymphocytic leukemia) steroids exert a direct antitumor effect. Steroids are also able to reduce edema and inflammation around a tumor and therefore are useful for symptom relief. There are many side effects associated with long-term steroid use, most notably a compromised immunologic response to infection, osteoporosis, and a cushingoid syndrome. Steroids in cancer treatment reg-

imens are often given intermittently and for short periods of time and are not often associated with the debilitating side effects associated with chronic, long-term use. Patients often describe an improved sense of well-being and an increased appetite while on prednisone. With completion of a prescribed course of therapy, a brief period of fatigue, malaise, and emotional lability may be experienced.

Hormonal alteration may be a desired therapeutic goal when tumor growth is directly influenced by certain hormones. The mechanism whereby the steroid hormones stimulate or inhibit cellular growth is not clear; an important mechanism may be interference or alteration at the cell membrane.

Estrogen receptor assays are now routinely done at the time of mastectomy for breast cancer. This technique has made it possible to evaluate the ability of a breast tumor to bind estrogen and thus project the probable sensitivity of the tumor to hormonal therapy.

DOSE CALCULATIONS

The dosage range for a particular drug is determined at the time of clinical trial and regimen development. Given these guidelines, the dosage for a specific individual must be calculated before starting therapy. Although some regimens may still prescribe milligrams per kilogram, drug doses are usually stated in terms of body surface area, and therefore the doses are given in milligrams per square meter (mg/M^2). An individual's height and weight are used to determine body surface; therefore it is very important that height and weight are measured *accurately*.

CRITERIA TO MEASURE TUMOR RESPONSE

Criteria have been established to measure chemotherapy effectiveness and include: (1) improvement in survival rates, (2) degree of response or remission, (3) duration of response, and (4) degree of toxicity. Complete remission (CR) refers to disappearance of all clinical signs of a tumor for a given time period. A partial response (PR) indicates a reduction in tumor mass of greater than 50% of the original size for more than a month. Progressive disease refers to evidence of advancing disease in the presence of therapy; the chemotherapy is ineffective.

METHODS OF ADMINISTERING CHEMOTHERAPEUTIC AGENTS

The route of administration is based on the metabolism and absorption of a given drug. The route of choice is that which will deliver the optimal amount of drug to the tumor. Chemotherapeutic agents are given orally, intravenously, intramuscularly, intraarterially, and by local instillation (i.e., intrapleurally and intrathecally). If tumor cells are in an area that drugs cannot reach, cancer cells will survive with a consequent increase in disease recurrence.

Before administering a cytotoxic drug, the nurse consults a reference for usual dosage, acceptable routes of administration, and any precautions that should be taken for that particular drug. Since protocols may deviate from drug manufacturers' guidelines, discussion with the prescribing physician may also be indicated.

Oral Administration

Many cytotoxic drugs are given in pill form. Since these may be prescribed on a daily basis to be taken at home, careful instructions need to be given to patients.

Subcutaneous Administration

The patient may be taught to administer chemotherapy at home by subcutaneous infusions through an automatic syringe subcutaneous infusion pump (see p. 380).

Intravenous, Intraarterial Administration

The nurse must know specific properties for each drug to be administered. Parenteral chemotherapeutic agents can be classified as nonvesicants, irritants, and vesicants depending on their potential to cause tissue damage when extravasated (infiltrated from vessel to subcutaneous tissue). Nonvesicants do little damage to soft tissues. Irritants produce burning or minor inflammation without necrosis. Vesicants cause soft tissue necrosis (see the box below).

The intravenous site is evaluated before the administration of vesicant drugs. If any suspicion of an infiltration or leak exists, the site is changed. Most often, vesicant drugs are given via the side arm of a running IV. If extravasation occurs, immediate action is taken to minimize damage. Guidelines vary but may include the administration of methylprednisolone (Solu-Medrol) or sodium bicarbonate to the area of infiltration and the intermittent application of ice for a 24-hour period.

Double-lumen Hickman/Broviac catheters. Double-lumen Hickman or Hickman/Broviac catheters are frequently used (Figure 17-17). These allow administration of total

parenteral nutrition (TPN) and of medications through the larger diameter Hickman catheter.[5]

Problems that can occur with the catheter include malfunctioning, breakage, and infections. The most common malfunction is catheter blockage caused by drug precipitate, blood clot, or development of a fibrin sheath. Occasionally, a catheter is broken or accidentally cut, but these can be repaired.

Infections may vary in severity and may occur at the catheter site. More serious infections are those in which organisms have colonized the catheter and are in the bloodstream. The patient may complain of tenderness along the tract and in the shoulder. Meticulous aseptic technique following established protocols are observed in changing the dressing and irrigating the catheter[39] (see the box on p. 379).

For other patients with poor venous access, a single-lumen indwelling Hickman catheter may be used for chemotherapy administration.

Groshong catheter. The Groshong catheter is a soft, flexible, elastic catheter whose distal end and lateral surface are radiopaque to aid in verification of placement. The closed distal end has a pressure-sensitive two-way valve that eliminates the need for heparin flushing and a two-way clamp. A removable tab at the proximal end allows easy repair. The catheter is available in single, double, or triple lumen. Care of the catheter is similar to that of

---

CHEMOTHERAPEUTIC DRUGS CLASSIFIED ACCORDING TO POTENTIAL LOCAL TISSUE DAMAGE

NONVESICANTS	IRRITANTS	VESICANTS
Bleomycin	Carmustine	Dactinomycin
Cisplatin	Dacarbazine	Daunorubicin
Cyclophosphamide		Doxorubicin
Cytarabine		Mechlorethamine (nitrogen mustard)
5-Azactidine		Mithramycin
5-Fluorouracil		Mitomycin
Floxuridine		Vinblastine
Methotrexate		Vincristine

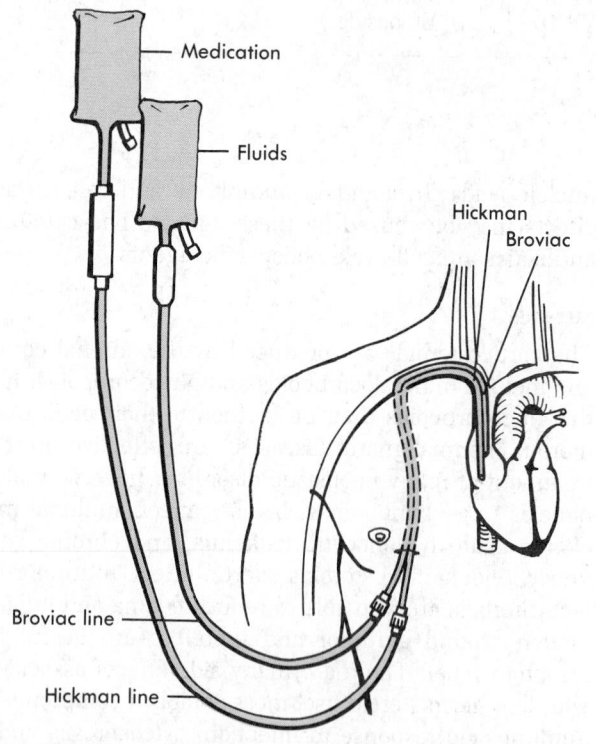

FIGURE 17-17 Double-lumen Hickman/Broviac catheters.

other central venous catheters in terms of dressing changes and aseptic techniques. Avoid using acetone during site care since it can weaken the catheter. There are other differences, however, in the care of the catheter[17]:

1. Flushing: irrigate *briskly* with 5 ml normal saline every seven days. After administration of viscous liquids (lipids for example) flush briskly with 20 ml normal saline.

2. Blood withdrawal: withdraw and discard 5 ml of blood, draw the sample, flush briskly with 20 ml normal saline (brisk flushing causes a swirling effect at distal end of the catheter).

3. Injection caps: place in the distal end of the catheter when the catheter is not in use; caps changed as needed (the valve will not open nor will fluid escape).

4. Never use sharp instruments near the catheter. If a tear occurs, sterile technique is used to repair the catheter with a bit from the manufacturer.*

Implantable vascular access systems. Vascular access systems (Figure 17-18) can be implanted in a subcutaneous pocket with the catheter inserted in the subclavian vein or the brachial artery. There is less danger of blood vessel or catheter occlusion, catheter displacement, or infection as compared to an externally inserted catheter. The system can be used for bolus injections and short-term continuous infusions. Special needles (Huber needles) must be used to prevent perforation of the infusion port (Figure 17-19). Instructions for maintenance of infusion ports are listed in the box below, right).

_____

*Catheter Technology Corporation, Salt Lake City, UT.

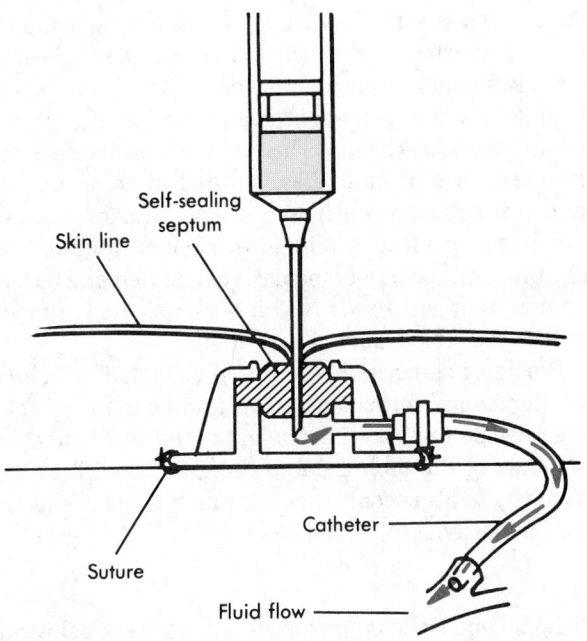

FIGURE 17-18 Drugs are administered through self-sealing infusion port.

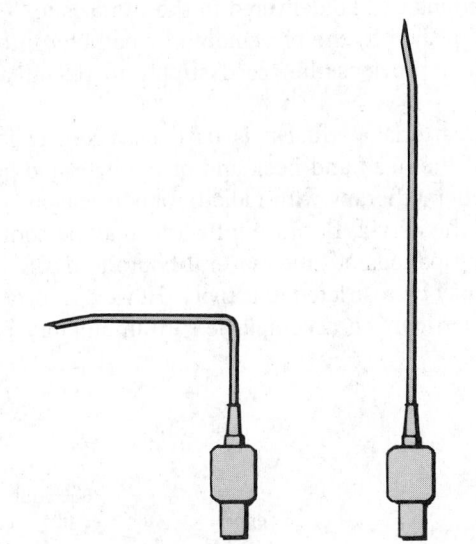

FIGURE 17-19 Special Huber needles used to inject medication through infusion port to prevent perforation of port.

CARE OF HICKMAN OR OTHER ATRIAL CATHETERS

1. Inspect skin around catheter for redness, swelling, or drainage
2. Change dressing as ordered using meticulous aseptic technique
3. Monitor patient for signs of systemic infection
4. Irrigate catheter daily with 3 ml heparin/saline solution (10 U heparin/ml) to prevent clotting
5. Notify physician if resistance is met in irrigation; lumen may be occluded
6. Irrigate briskly—may help prevent outflow obstruction[45]
7. Clamping is *not* recommended; clamp over protective covering if necessary[32]
8. Change dressing every other day for 2 to 3 weeks after insertion, then apply Band-aid to exit site
9. Prevent undue tension on catheter; tape to patient at all times
10. Change cap(s) every 7 days
11. Obtain repair kit for catheter from manufacturer

MAINTENANCE OF IMPLANTED INFUSION PORTS[45]

1. Puncture with Huber point needle only
2. Irrigate every 4 weeks with 3 to 5 ml heparin/saline solution (100 U heparin/ml)
3. Use 20 ml normal saline flush after blood drawing
4. Irrigate arterial ports once a week with 3 to 5 ml heparin/saline solution (100 U heparin/ml)
5. Flush catheter after each use
6. No restrictions on patient because port is implanted

Vascular access graft. To solve the problem of starting IVs on patients who have repeated chemotherapy infusions, a totally subcutaneous arteriovenous (AV) shunt or vascular access graft is used, especially for patients without readily accessible veins. The AV graft is inserted into the upper arm or groin area, sutured to an artery, and then run subcutaneously to a 4-inch straight line or a 7-inch loop to a nearby vein, to which it is sutured. Usually bronchial artery-bronchial vein or femoral artery-femoral vein are used. Needles are inserted into the graft to draw blood and give IV fluids.

Problems associated with the graft include thrombosis, hematoma formation, extravasation from use of a large needle that has torn the graft, and graft infection. Ischemia of the limb distal to the graft, the "steal syndrome," can also occur when too much blood is shunted from the arterial to the venous side.[94]

Perfusion

Regional and isolation perfusion is a means of delivering a high dosage of a drug directly to a tumor. The rationale for regional chemotherapy is that many solid tumors are unresponsive to drug levels that can be safely obtained by systemic administration. Higher drug concentrations can be delivered to the tumor site.[10] This is accomplished by the placement of a catheter into an artery that provides the blood supply to the area being treated.

Intraarterial perfusion is used occasionally for cancers of the head and neck and of the liver and as adjuvant chemotherapy with radiotherapy for advanced cancer of the cervix. Because infusions may be continuous for long periods of time (several hours to days), the patient may be restricted in activity. However, intraarterial perfusion can be accomplished in ambulatory patients by means of a portable infusion pump. Aspects of nursing care include assessment of the catheter insertion site, care of the line to maintain placement and prevent infection, and observation for bleeding. Outpatients need careful and detailed instruction so that these same criteria can be maintained in the home. Hospital nurses involved in the discharge planning of such patients need to ensure that the community-based nurse is also informed of these details.

Implantable drug delivery systems are now available for delivering cytotoxic drugs to target sites (Figure 17-20). The infusion pump is a totally implantable system that decreases risk of infection or perforation without the physical limitations and discomfort of extracorporeal pumps. Drugs are added percutaneously through a central inlet septum with a special needle. The intrinsic source of energy is an inexhaustible charging fluid permanently sealed in the pump. Drug refills are usually needed every 2 weeks on an ambulatory basis.

The most common complication is development of a seroma over the pump pocket. This is an accumulation of sterile fluid that may be either aspirated by the physician or allowed to be absorbed by the body. Pump pocket infection is rare but may require the pump to be removed. Patients are taught to resume activities as soon as the incision heals. Written instructions are given to the patient including telephone numbers of health care professionals who can be consulted. The importance of keeping appointments for pump refilling is emphasized (see box p 381, at left).

Intrathecal Administration (Ommaya Reservoir)

Direct access to the cerebrospinal fluid (CSF) for administration of drugs was devised by a neurosurgeon, A.K. Ommaya. The Ommaya reservoir is now used to

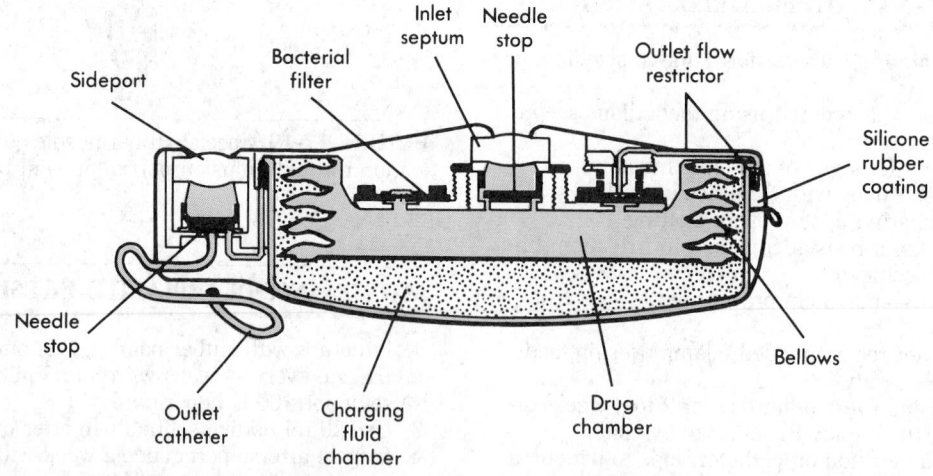

FIGURE 17-20 Implantable drug-delivery system for ambulatory persons. (Courtesy Infusaid Corp, Norwood, Mass 02062.)

administer antibiotics, analgesics, and cancer drugs to treat CSF malignancies and to prevent leukemic spread into CSF. The reservoir also permits measuring of CSF pressure, draining of excess CSF to reduce intracranial pressure, or sampling of CSF.[82]

The Ommaya reservoir is a mushroom-shaped, self-sealing silicone dome with a catheter attached. The catheter is surgically guided into the lateral ventricle. The reservoir is inserted beneath the scalp flap and over the burr hole. The reservoir should function for months or years, barring any complications. Care of the reservoir is as follows:

1. Dilute the drugs with nonbacteriostatic sterile water, normal saline without preservative, or Elliot B's solution.
2. Check patient's TPR, BP, and neurologic status before giving drug.
3. Assess for drug side-effects (headache, fever, nausea, change of mental status).
4. Assess for inflammation, swelling, tenderness, warmth, or drainage at the injection site. Teach patient to report headache, fever, neck stiffness, signs of CNS infection.
5. Check catheter function by pumping the reservoir (a finger is placed on top and gentle pushing down and releasing is done—usually done by the physician. One can feel the CSF fill the reservoir, indicating proper placement and function. (Slowed or absent filling indicates the reservoir is blocked.)

TEACHING THE PATIENT WHO HAS AN IMPLANTABLE INFUSION PUMP[99,109]

1. Avoid contact sports or activities that may cause blunt trauma to the pump.
2. Avoid activities that cause an increase in body temperature (long, hot baths, saunas) or atmospheric pressure (stay in high altitude areas): flow rate of pump may increase.
3. Keep appointments for pump refilling: catheter occlusion may occur due to complete emptying of pump reservoir (newer implantables have low-reservoir alarms).
4. Watch for infection, which is rare but may occur: the pump is a foreign body and chemotherapy-induced myelosuppression or sepsis predisposes to infection and inflammation.
5. Be alert for malfunction of pump: usually caused by motor failure, indicated by absence of backflow into a syringe or release of manual pressure after injection of 5 to 10 ml of fluid. In externally programmable pumps, failure is caused by computer operating system or microcomputer circuits.
6. Be alert for catheter occlusion: usually caused by drug incompatibility, resulting in precipitation in the drug chamber.

CARE OF PATIENTS ON CHEMOTHERAPY

■ Assessment

There is always some degree of injury to normal cells with treatment by cytotoxic drugs, normal cells with a high rate of growth being particularly susceptible.[45] Bone marrow, gastrointestinal epithelium, and hair follicles are most sensitive to chemotherapy. Side effects and toxicity may include pulmonary toxicity, cardiac toxicity (congestive heart failure), genitourinary toxicity (cystitis, renal damage, sterility), neurotoxicity (numbness and tingling of the hands and feet and motor weakness), and hepatic toxicity. (See Table 17-14 on p. 374 for toxicities associated with specific drugs.)

Assessment should be made for signs of *bone marrow suppression:* neutropenia, thrombocytopenia, and anemia. Blood counts are done before administration and at regular intervals to identify nadir effect, the times that the blood count is lowest and the patient is

ASSESSMENT OF THE PATIENT RECEIVING CHEMOTHERAPY

IDENTIFICATION OF MARROW SUPPRESSION

1. WBC, platelet count, hemoglobin, hematocrit
2. Signs of bleeding (petechiae, ecchymosis, etc.)

IDENTIFICATION OF INFECTION

1. Inspect skin and mucous membranes daily (especially mouth, axillae, and perineum)
2. Auscultate respiratory tract
3. Monitor temperature, pulse, respiration
4. (Most important) Monitor neutrophil count:
   a. A count of $500/mm^3$ to $1000/mm^3$ indicates moderate risk of infection
   b. A count of less than $500/mm^3$ indicates severe risk of infection

IDENTIFICATION OF OTHER ORGAN TOXICITIES

1. Gastrointestinal toxicity
   a. Inspect mouth for white patches or ulcers
   b. Monitor weight, fluid, and electrolytes
   c. Assess for constipation, decreased bowel sounds
2. Liver toxicity: monitor liver enzymes
3. Cardiac toxicity
   a. Obtain baseline echocardiogram
   b. Check apical pulse for arrhythmias
   c. Monitor for signs of congestive heart failure
4. Pulmonary toxicity
   a. Auscultate lungs
   b. Monitor for shortness of breath and cough (especially with bleomycin)
5. Urinary toxicity
   a. Monitor urine for blood
   b. Monitor for signs of cystitis (frequency with dysuria)
   c. Evaluate renal function by either serum creatinine or 24-hour urine for creatinine clearance
   d. Keep accurate intake and output
6. Neurotoxicity: assess for paresthesia and motor weakness

1. Teaching the patient and significant others:
   a. Signs and symptoms of infection, thrombocytopenia
   b. How to read a thermometer (if appropriate) and when to notify the physician
   c. Good hygiene practices:
      (1) Cleanse the perineum from front to back
      (2) Change underwear daily
      (3) Hand washing
   d. Information about prescribed drugs: name, dose, side effects, importance of taking as prescribed
   e. Use of antiemetics
   f. Importance of medical follow-up and blood studies
   g. Available support groups for chemotherapy patients
2. Preventing infection:
   a. Good hygiene, *especially hand washing* (patient, family, health professionals)
   b. Prevent exposure to people with known infection (other patients, staff, family, friends)
   c. Meticulous aseptic technique during intravenous infusions and dressing changes
      (1) Use povidone iodine for skin preparation (Center for Disease Control also considers alcohol, tincture of iodine, and chlorhexidine effective)
      (2) Use one tourniquet for patient's exclusive use
      (3) Use gloves for procedures
   d. No aspirin or acetaminophen (prevent masking fever)
   e. Maintain intact skin and mucous membranes:
      (1) Avoid bumping and breaking the skin
      (2) No injections
      (3) Keep fingernails short to prevent small skin breaks (nurse, patient, other caregivers)
      (4) Avoid anal intercourse
      (5) Avoid enemas, rectal medications, rectal thermometers
      (6) Avoid excessive friction and provide vaginal lubrication during sexual intercourse (use water-soluble jelly, if necessary)
   f. Maintain fastidious oral hygiene:
      (1) Maintain teeth and gums in good condition, see dentist
      (2) Use mouth wash or oral irrigations (normal saline), mild peroxide solution (1 tablespoon in 240 ml water), sodium bicarbonate (1 teaspoon baking soda in 240 ml water)
      (3) Use mycostatin tablets or suspension, as necessary
      (4) Relieve dryness: drink water and other fluids
      (5) Use artificial saliva, as needed, in form of spray (Moi-Stir, Salivart, Ora-lub)
      (6) Stimulate saliva with gum, candies, buttermilk, yogurt
      (7) Brush teeth with soft toothbrush (small soft bristles) or use foam stick or swab
      (8) Brush teeth in short horizontal strokes at least 3 to 4 minutes, at least 3 times a day
      (9) Use fluoridated toothpaste or rinse, to prevent caries
      (10) Use Water Pik under low pressure or irrigation, if platelet count is low

   g. Use life islands or laminar airflow rooms as indicated
   h. Maintain optimal respiratory function: turn, cough, and deep breathe patients confined to bed
3. Maintaining optimal gastrointestinal function:
   a. Give antidiarrheal medication as needed
   b. Plan daily bowel regimen for constipation, give stool softeners as prescribed
   c. Treat stomatitis:
      (1) Oral nystatin (Mycostatin) or other antibiotics as prescribed
      (2) Milk of magnesia or Kaopectate to coat lesions
      (3) Dyclone (dyclonine hydrochloride), Orabase, Xylocaine viscous 2% (lidocaine), as local anesthetic before meals and as necessary
      (4) KY jelly, mineral oil, to coat lips and oral mucosa
      (5) Vaseline (petrolatum) to coat lips (not if neutropenic)
      (6) Benadryl (diphenhydramine hydrochloride) alone or in combination with Maalox and Kaopectate, as a rinse
      (7) Oral irrigations (see under infection) every 2 hours
      (8) Soft, bland foods, cold liquids tolerated by some persons
   d. Treat nausea and vomiting:
      (1) Give antiemetics 30 to 45 minutes before chemotherapy; use large doses
      (2) Use auditory or diversional stimulation (music, slides, photographs)
      (3) Give antiemetics around the clock for severe nausea and vomiting
      (4) Use relaxation techniques, self-hypnosis, therapeutic touch
      (5) Eat foods that minimize nausea
4. Minimizing or preventing alopecia:
   a. Apply ice pack to cover entire head 10 minutes before drug administration and 30 minutes after (for doxorubicin [Adriamycin])
   b. Use scalp tourniquet for vincristine if patient desires while drug is being administered
   c. Urge use of wigs, scarves, eyebrow pencil, false eyelashes
   d. Avoid frequent shampooing, combing, or brushing
   e. Use soft bristle hair brush
   f. Advise against permanents and hair coloring (increase rate of hair loss)
5. Minimizing or preventing urinary effects: hemorrhagic cyctitis, renal toxicity:
   a. Force fluids when taking cyclophosphamide
   b. Take cyclophosphamide early in the day
   c. Check serum creatinine or 24-hr urine for creatinine clearance before giving *cis*-platinum and streptozotocin.
6. Minimizing effects of sterility:
   a. Provide birth control information and reproductive counseling
   b. Provide information about sperm banking before initiation of therapy for male patients

most susceptible to infection and hemorrhage. Assessment is also made for signs and symptoms of other organ toxicity (see the box on p. 381). Nursing care of patients with neutropenia, thrombocytopenia, and anemia is discussed in Chapter 30.

■ Data Analysis: Nursing Diagnoses

Multiple nursing diagnoses may be identified for the patient receiving extensive chemotherapy. Nursing diagnoses for the patient with cancer are listed in Table 17-9, p. 358. Some of the more common nursing diagnoses for the patient receiving chemotherapy may include but are not limited to the following:

Activity intolerance
Body image, disturbance in
Comfort, alteration in
Constipation
Diarrhea
Fluid volume deficit
Infection, potential for
Knowledge deficit
Mobility, impaired physical
Nutrition, altered: less than body requirements
Self-care deficit
Sensory perceptual alteration
Sexual dysfunction
Skin integrity, impaired
Tissue perfusion, altered
Urinary elimination, altered patterns

■ Planning: Expected Patient Outcomes

Expected patient outcomes for specific nursing diagnoses are listed in Table 17-9. Those outcomes of specific importance for the diagnosis of *knowledge deficit* for the person receiving chemotherapy include the following:

The patient or significant others can:
1. State the name of chemotherapeutic drugs and any special instructions related to each
2. State the importance of close medical follow-up, especially for blood studies
3. Describe interventions for anticipated side effects of prescribed drugs
4. State person to call if side effects persist or new symptoms occur
5. Describe how to contact support groups for chemotherapy patients

■ Implementation

Interventions for the patient receiving chemotherapy are given in the box on p. 382.

Prevention of infection. The prevention of infection is of utmost importance in the care and teaching of cancer patients. A cold or flu in a person with neutropenia may result in septicemic shock in a few hours. Intact skin and mucous membranes are first-line defenses against infection, so care is directed to prevent breaks in skin integrity (see the box on p. 382). Persons receiving chemotherapy are susceptible to middle-ear infections, sinusitis, and pharyngitis. Pneumonia is especially prevalent in patients with leukemia and in elderly persons.

In addition, signs of early infection may be absent. Alkylating agents and antimetabolites cause depression or complete absence of delayed hypersensitivity (T cell defect). There may also be inhibition of the primary antibody response (B cell defect) and bone marrow hypoplasia (reduction in polymorphonuclear [PMN] cells).[52]

Localized inflammatory response may not occur in patients with severe leukopenia (<1000 cells/mm^3). The absence of PMNs prevents the formation of pus. Localized tenderness or pain may be the only sign of a skin or wound infection, followed by later signs of tachypnea, tachycardia, confusion, or restlessness.[52]

Reverse isolation may be ordered but it is not usually effective unless life islands or laminar airflow units are used. The *life island* consists of a special large plastic canopy placed around and over the patient's bed. All equipment is sterilized and the air is filtered to remove airborne bacteria. Objects are passed in and out through locks irradiated by ultraviolet light. Patient contact is through arm-length gloves built into the side of the canopy.

Laminar airflow units are rooms that have a constant flow of purified air flowing across the width and breadth of the room (Figure 17-21). Anyone in the room remains "downstream" from the patient. If the patient must be touched, a mask, cap, and gown are worn. The advantage of the laminar airflow room is that it is large and allows more freedom of movement than the life island.

One problem with any type of isolation is that the patient may experience psychotic episodes because of sensory deprivation. In addition, patients may react adversely when allowed out of the unit. They may feel unsafe, vulnerable, and angry because they are removed from the protected environment.

Decreasing gastrointestinal effects. Changes in bowel habits commonly occur but usually do not require intervention. Alertness to the possibility of bleeding or ulceration must be part of the assessment of diarrhea or cramping. Vincristine may cause paralytic ileus, therefore persons receiving this drug are specifically instructed to report constipation. Persons receiving narcotic-based pain medications may have constipation as a result and a daily bowel regimen program may be indicated.

A side effect of some chemotherapeutic drugs (see the box on p. 384) is *stomatitis*, an inflammation of the oral mucous membranes that may range from an erythema to mild or severe ulcerations. Thorough cleansing of the

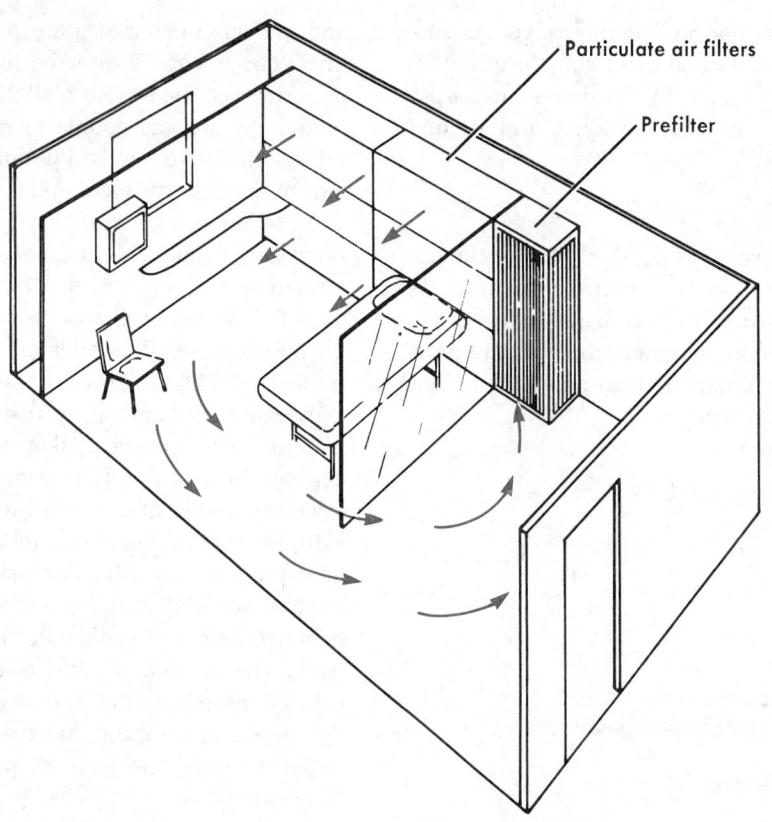

FIGURE 17-21 In laminar airflow units a constant flow of purified air flows across width and breadth of room. (From American Cancer Society: Proceedings of the National Conference on Cancer Nursing, New York, 1973, The Society.)

mouth and dental prophylaxis to prevent dental caries or gum disease provides the first line of defense against stomatitis. Various mouthwashes may be used (see the box on p. 382). Patients may also develop a superimposed *Candida* infection of the mouth and esophagus.

Nausea and vomiting. Oncology nurses and patients often identify nausea and vomiting as one of the most uncomfortable and distressing side effects of chemotherapy.[63] Four emetic syndromes have been identified in patients with cancer: (1) chemotherapy-induced emesis, (2) delayed emesis that occurs 1 to 4 days after treatment, (3) anticipatory emesis that occurs before the next scheduled therapy, and (4) emesis caused by fac-

tors other than chemotherapy, such as intestinal obstruction or other drug therapy (e.g., opiates). Depending on the type of emesis, different therapies are indicated. Relaxation techniques can be effective.

For the ambulatory patient, nausea may interfere with the ability to continue daily work. Persistent vomiting may result in fluid and electrolyte imbalance, general weakness, and weight loss. Decline of nutritional status renders the person more susceptible to infection and perhaps less able to tolerate therapy. Such physiologic symptoms can accompany or precipitate psychologic responses that might include depression, withdrawal, and humiliation. The onset and duration of both nausea and vomiting vary greatly from patient to patient and with the drugs given (see research box).

The success of antiemetics varies. The dose and schedule of antiemetic administration is important to its effectiveness. Many drugs give relief at high doses but are of only limited effect at lower doses that are considered standard. Tetrahydrocannabinol (THC) taken in pill form produces an antiemetic effect in some patients who have not benefited from prochlorperazine (Compazine). Common antiemetic protocols contain high dosages of Reglan, Decadron, Benadryl, and Ativan.

DRUGS CAUSING STOMATITIS[8]

Bleomycin (Blenozane)
Doxorubicin (Adriamycin)
Ara-C (Citarabine)
Cyclophosphamide (Cytoxan)
Daunorubicin (Cerubidine)
Methotrexate
5-Fluorouracil

RESEARCH

Rhodes VA, et al: Patterns of nausea, vomiting and distress in patients receiving antineoplastic drug protocols, Oncol Nurs Forum 14(4):35-44, 1987.

Nausea and vomiting (N & V) are some of the most distressing side effects of chemotherapy, yet patterns of occurrence have not been described. Research also indicates that antiemetics alone are sometimes unable to control the symptoms. The purpose of this study was to describe patterns of nausea and vomiting and distress after six consecutive cycles of selected chemotherapeutic drug regimens to identify patterns of symptoms, the relationship of the pattern to duration, frequency, and distress from N & V to specific chemotherapy drug combinations, and to determine if the experience of N & V is altered with repeated cycles of drug administration. Findings revealed that for 84% of the 309 subjects, vomiting was well controlled 48 hours after therapy, while 71% had little or no nausea. In the remaining sample three antiemetic drug resistent nausea patterns emerged: intense nausea, latent nausea (dramatic increase in nausea after 24 hours) and 24-hour nausea that peaked in 24 hours but then dropped dramatically. Vomiting experiences indicated three patterns: latent vomiting, i.e., low vomiting for 36 hours but climaxing at 48 hours; declining vomiting from high incidence 12 hours after therapy; and minimal vomiting, little or no vomiting in the 48 hours after treatment. Statistically significant relationships between nausea and vomiting and antineoplastic drug protocols were found. However, there was no increase of symptoms across drug cycles. Since the predominant pattern was minimal occurrence of nausea and vomiting in 75% of the subjects, this information should be shared with other patients who may be told to expect nausea and vomiting. ■

Reducing alopecia. Alopecia may occur by two mechanisms. If the hair roots are atrophied, alopecia occurs readily and hair either falls out spontaneously or from combing, often in large clumps. If the hair shaft is constricted because of atrophy or necrosis, the hair will break off very near the scalp. The root remains in the scalp and a patchy thinning pattern of hair loss occurs.

In addition to scalp hair, body hair, pubic hair, and chest hair may also be affected. Loss of leg, arm, and facial hair is seen less often although loss of eyebrows and eyelashes may occur. The pattern and extent of hair loss cannot be accurately predicted for a given patient. However, when treatment is given with a drug known to cause alopecia (see the box above), the patient needs to be told that severe hair loss can begin within a few days or weeks of treatment and that partial or complete baldness can quickly ensue. *Drug-induced alopecia is never permanent.* Occasionally, hair growth may return while chemotherapy treatment continues.

Besides the initial diagnosis of cancer, alopecia may be the most traumatic psychologic side effect cancer pa-

DRUGS COMMONLY CAUSING ALOPECIA

Bleomycin	ICRF-159
Cyclophosphamide	Hydroxyurea
Dactinomycin	Methotrexate
Daunomycin hydrochloride	Mitomycin
Doxorubicin hydrochloride	VP-16-213
5-Fluorouracil	Vincristine

From Knopf, M., et al.: Cancer chemotherapy treatment and care, New Haven, Conn., 1979, Yale Comprehensive Cancer Center.

tients may experience. It is a constant reminder of their disease, makes the illness visible to others, and may result in a significant change in body image. Efforts have been made to minimize hair loss by use of scalp tourniquets and scalp hypothermia with varying success.[41] The negative effects of hair loss can be minimized by covering the head in various ways, such as with wigs and scarfs.

Preventing skin breakdown. Vesicant drugs may cause severe tissue necrosis if infiltration should occur (p. 378). Other skin reactions that might occur are hyperpigmentation, nail changes, and an increased sensitivity to the sun (photosensitivity).

Organ toxicities. *Liver toxicity* is uncommon but may occur. Alteration in liver function has been associated with Ara-C, methotrexate, and 6-mercaptopurine. Two forms of *cardiac* damage may occur: arrhythmias, most commonly associated with a preexisting cardiac disease, and a delayed moderate to severe congestive heart failure. Drugs associated with potential cardiac toxicity include doxorubicin, daunorubicin, and high-dose cyclophosphamide (Cytoxan). *Pulmonary* toxicity occurs most commonly with bleomycin; it may also occur with methotrexate and some of the alkylating agents. Pulmonary fibrosis can occur and may be irreversible. *Urinary* effects include hemorrhagic cystitis, occurring occasionally with cyclophosphamide, and renal toxicity, associated primarily with *cis*-platin and streptozotocin. (See the box on p. 382 for ways to minimize these effects.)

Sterility. Cancer chemotherapy reaches the reproductive organs at dose levels similar to those achieved at the site of the target tumor. The potential exists for a disruptive effect on genetic and fetal development. It is recognized that chemotherapy, particularly some of the alkylating agents, may cause transient or permanent sterility. Persons receiving chemotherapy need to be informed of the known and possible effects on fertility. Following completion of chemotherapy, conception and the birth of normal, healthy children are possibilities for couples. It is customary to recommend that procreation be avoided until at least 18 months after completion of treatment.

BONE MARROW TRANSPLANTATION

Bone marrow transplantation (BMT) following treatment with high-dose chemotherapy or radiotherapy is being used in patients with a variety of hematologic malignancies and solid tumors. This is a "rescue" technique that allows administration of what would be toxic doses of drugs and/or radiation when best effect is achieved with high doses.[93]

There are three types of tissue or bone marrow donors: allogeneic, usually from a sibling who has a close human leukocyte antigen (HLA) match (Chapter 76); syngeneic, from an identical twin; or the most recent type used, autologous bone marrow transplantation (ABMT) in which patients serve as their own donors. ABMT has been useful because it is frequently difficult to get a donor that has a close HLA match.[93]

In ABMT the patient's marrow is usually disease free or has been purged of tumor cells before reinfusion. The rationale for ABMT is based on the knowledge that higher doses of chemotherapy or radiation will increase the number of tumor cells killed in a logarithmic fashion; that is, doubling the dose may result in 10 times or more the number of tumor cells killed. Large doses of drugs can be given because ABMT provides a rescue for bone marrow depression.

Autologous bone marrow "harvest" (the term used for donating the bone marrow) is done when the patient is in remission or when the tumor burden is small and bone marrow involvement cannot be microscopically identified. The purpose of the harvest is to collect enough stem cells (pluripotent cells) to reconstitute the hematopoietic system after therapy. (See Chapter 30 for discussion of the hematopoietic system.)

The marrow is obtained by multiple needle aspirations from the posterior iliac crest under general or spinal anesthesia, although the anterior iliac crest and sternum may also be used. The amount of marrow extracted is usually 600 to 1000 to 2500 ml for the average adult.

After processing, the marrow is given to the patient intravenously through a transfusion bag or it can be frozen at $-140°$ C although $-196°$ C is preferred (cryopreservation). Marrow can be kept for a period of 3 years or more.

If there is a possibility that malignant cells may be present, bone marrow purging, to remove the residual cells, may be done. This may be done by one of three methods: separation of malignant cells from the marrow based on density differences between malignant and normal cells (physical); use of immunotoxic or monoclonal antibodies (immunologic); use of drugs such as mercocyanine 540, mafosfamide or 4-hydroperoxcyclophosphamide (pharmacologic).

Complications of BMT, whether autologous or allogeneic, are often caused by the high-dose chemoradiotherapy and the toxicity to the gastrointestinal tract, lungs, liver, kidneys, and other organs. The effects are caused by nonfunctioning bone marrow. Another complication of BMTs is venoocclusive disease (VOD) of the liver. This results from the narrowing or fibrous obliteration of the terminal hepatic venules and sublobular veins from reticulin-collagen deposits in the veins. Symptoms of VOD usually occur 1 to 4 weeks after reinfusion and include ascites, hepatomegaly, elevated SGOT, alkaline phosphatase and bilirubin levels, jaundice, and coagulation difficulties.

Other complications include hemorrhagic cystitis and graft-versus-host-disease (GVHD) if allogenic BMT is used. In addition, if allogenic BMT is used, a conditioning regimen must be initiated to permit acceptance of the foreign tissue by the patient's body. Early regimens included total body irradiation in combination with drugs such as cyclophosphamide. New regimens include fractimated or hypofractimated irradiation, total lymphoid irradiation, busulfan, and arabinosylcytosine.[105]

Marrow grafting is costly because inpatient hospital stay may run from $50,000 to $100,000, but BMT has been established as a treatment for a wide range of diseases.[105]

The procedure often involves psychologic stress in patient, family, and nursing staff who may try to be positive about the outcome. It cannot be overemphasized that hope has a major role with BMT. The involvement of staff and patient is intense in a BMT unit and nurses may be placed in the paradoxic situation of providing hope to dying patients.[12] (See Chapter 14 for discussion of hope.)

TEACHING THE BONE MARROW HARVEST PROCEDURE TO THE PATIENT

1. Explain that bone marrow forms special stem cells that produce all blood cells.
2. Discuss special preparation, for example, shower with antiseptic soap the evening before harvest.
3. Describe the harvest procedure:
   a. General or spinal anesthesia is used
   b. Needle placed through skin in back side of hip bone
   c. If transplant is autologous, filtered bone marrow is frozen until needed
   d. If transplant is allogeneic or syngeneic, marrow is transferred to blood transfusion bag and given immediately through an intravenous line
4. Explain what happens after recovery.
   a. Pain in harvest sites can be relieved by medication
   b. Patient is out of bed the night of the harvest
   c. Pressure dressing is removed the day after harvest
   d. Surgical sites are kept clean and covered for 3 days; on each day clean the sites, apply Betadine ointment, and cover with adhesive bandage

Teaching donors and patients about the bone marrow harvest procedure minimizes anxiety and helps increase participation in their recovery. (See box on p. 386).

IMMUNOTHERAPY
PATHOPHYSIOLOGY

The role of immunotherapy in the prevention and treatment of cancer is being studied. Many scientists believe cancer occurs in the body more frequently than once in a lifetime; however, in most cases clinical evidence of the disease is not apparent. It is postulated that there is a natural immunity against the development of the disease and that cancer cells are destroyed almost as fast as they develop. Clinical malignancy may occur as a result of failure in the immunologic surveillance system of the body (see p. 346).

Studies of cancer in lower animals and in humans show that when the normal cell becomes malignant it often undergoes biochemical changes resulting in formation of new cellular antigens that cause an immune response.

This response has two major components. The first, or *cellular immune response* (see Chapter 8), produces lymphocytes capable of destroying tumor cells on contact. These lymphocytes (T cells) undergo division and are released into the bloodstream when stimulated by an antigen. In addition to destroying cancer cells on contact, T cells may release cytotoxins, which cause holes in the cell membrane, eventually resulting in lysis or death of the malignant cell.

Another important cell, which collaborates with the T cell, is the macrophage. The macrophage, which is attracted to the immune lymphocyte, is immobilized in its vicinity and then activated by the lymphocyte. It is a relatively nonspecific cell that seems to have the ability to kill selectively malignant cells with which it comes in contact.

The second component of the immune response is *antibody production* resulting from activation of lymphocytes (B cells). When stimulated by antigen, B cells proliferate and differentiate into plasma cells, which are the major source of antibody production.

In addition to B cells and T cells, a third immunologic component, natural killer (NK) cells, has been discovered in animals having natural resistance to tumors.

The cells involved in the immune response interact and seem to exchange signals at both cellular and humoral levels. At the present time the immune response can handle only a limited number of tumor cells, up to 10 million. After a growth to 100 million cells the immune response is not capable of preventing further growth. Once the cancer is large, it cannot be totally controlled by the immune system, so immunotherapy cannot be the primary mode of cancer therapy at the present time. It is used after surgery, radiotherapy, and chemotherapy have removed the bulk of the tumor.

APPROACHES USED IN IMMUNOTHERAPY

Immunologic treatment of cancer may involve active immunotherapy, either specific or nonspecific. Passive or adoptive immunotherapy may also be specific or nonspecific (Table 17-15).

Nonspecific immunotherapy using the Bacillus Calmette-Guérin (BCG), *Corynebacterium parvum,* or specific allogeneic or autologous vaccines were the first attempts at immunotherapy in the 1960s. BCG has had some success against melanoma and bladder cancer, but its ability to prolong survival has not been proven.[70]

Other substances have been used to stimulate the immune system. The first group was derived from microorganisms, the second includes synthetic compounds such as azimexon and isoprinosine, and the third includes conventional chemotherapeutic agents (cyclophosphamide, doxorubicin, and the vinca alkaloids).[70]

The newest approach to immunotherapy is use of biologic response modifiers.

BIOLOGIC RESPONSE MODIFIERS

Biologic response modifiers (BRM) can be classified into three types: agents that restore, strengthen, or modify the immune system (such as interferon); cells that have direct antitumor activity (such as monoclonal antibodies); agents that have other biologic effects, such as interfering with cells' ability to metastasize or survive, or interfering with transformation of normal cells to cancer cells.

The BMRs include three species of interferon (alpha, beta, and gamma), interleukin-2, and tumor necrosis factor (TNF). In addition, lymphokine-activated killer cells (LAKC) are being used for adoptive immunotherapy.[70]

TABLE 17-15 Immunotherapy for cancer[70]

Specificity	Active	Passive
Specific	Inactivated tumor vaccines (autologous, allogeneic)	Monoclonal antibodies
		Human heterologous antiserum
	Human tumor hybrids	T lymphocytes
		Monoclonal lymphocytes
		Bone marrow transplants
Nonspecific	Chemical immunostimulants	Lymphokine-activated killer cells (LAKC)
	Biologic immunostimulants (such as BCG, *C. parvum*)	Activated macrophages
	Cytokines (interferon, IL-2, TNF)	
	Chemotherapy	

Interferons

Interferons (IFNs) are a family of secretory glycoproteins produced by leukocytes in response to viral infections or other stimuli. All nucleated cells are capable of interferon production, which can be induced by natural or synthetic agents. INFs are now produced by recombinant DNA technology by insertion of genes for an INF of each class in *Escherichia coli.*

Interferons have four major actions; first, an *antiviral* action by inhibiting the replication of DNA in a virus that has invaded a cell. The second action is *immunomodulatory* by directly interacting with T lymphocytes to stimulate the formation of cellular products that signal monocytes, natural killer cells, and other T lymphocytes to recognize and destroy the tumor cells. A third action is *antiproliferative* in that it directly inhibits the growth and division of tumor cells. Finally, it *stimulates* the expression of HLA and tumor-associated antigens in tumor cells, making them more recognizable.[57]

Tumors most responsive to interferon are hematologic malignancies, especially hairy cell leukemia, but IFN has also been effective against nodular lymphomas, cutaneous T cell lymphoma, and chronic myeloid leukemia.[44] Interferon has demonstrated only moderate effectiveness against Kaposi's sarcoma, melanoma, and renal cancer. The most common cancers, such as breast cancer, show little response.

A number of clinical questions must be answered before wide use of interferons begins: (1) optimal dose and schedule, (2) specific application of each interferon, (3) mechanism of antitumor action, and (4) effective combinations with other modalities of therapy.[64]

Interferon works best in conjunction with other therapy and has been particularly effective in use with an agent called *tumor necrosis factor* (TNF). INFs may also work synergistically with certain cancer drugs and with radiation therapy. INFs hold the most promise for patients whose immune systems have not been weakened by chemotherapy and radiation.

Nursing assessment of the patient receiving interferon therapy includes knowledge about the patient's emotional status, family and community support systems, previous therapy, and general condition.

Side effects include chills and fever beginning 3 to 6 hours after administration and myalgias that last 5 to 10 days. Higher doses may produce the following effects:

1. Severe muscle contractions and chronic fatigue
2. GI effects: nausea, altered taste, early satiety, anorexia, weight loss[57]
3. Cardiovascular changes: pallor, tachycardia, cyanosis, rapid breathing, orthostatic hypotension
4. Neurologic toxicity: depression, low motivation, paranoia, cognitive impairment
5. Renal function: compromised (IFN is cleared primarily by kidneys)

TEACHING INTERFERON THERAPY TO THE PATIENT

1. Explain treatment regimen
2. Explain and describe side effects, and reassure person that these effects lessen as treatment continues
3. Teach method of giving subcutaneous injections (if pertinent)
4. Assist in planning for management of side effects of therapy

---

At some centers nurses teach the patients to give their own intravenous injections (see box). It is important not to raise false hopes in persons who may view interferon as a last-resort therapy.

Interleuken-2

Interleuken-2 (IL-2) is a lymphokine that helper T cells produce in response to antigenic stimulation. It has four functions in relation to the immune response: (1) enhances production of T lymphocytes, (2) augments activity of natural killer (NK) cells and cytotoxic T cells, (3) stimulates responses of B and T cells, and (4) induces production of lymphokine-activated killer (LAK) cells.[59,70] It has been effective for melanoma and renal cell carcinoma.

IL-2 may be given by IV bolus, subcutaneous injection, continuous IV infusion, or by intrahepatic or peritoneal infusion. It may be given tid, by 24-hour infusion twice weekly, by weekly IV bolus, or by continuous IV infusion for a period of 5 to 6 days.[59] IL-2 may be toxic to every body system and many toxicities relate to dosage levels; most symptoms disappear within 96 hours after IL-2 is stopped. Complications of IL-2 therapy with related nursing care is described in Table 17-16.

IL-2 and Lymphokine-Activated Killer Cells

Although IL-2 transforms peripheral lymphocytes into lymphokine-activated killer (LAK) cells that attack cancer cells, administration of LAK cells alone does not produce the same effect; therefore clinical trials combining LAK cells with IL-2 are underway. Patients are given IL-2 intravenously for 3 days, followed by a 24- to 36-hour-rest period to allow the LAK-cell precursors and lymphocytes to rebound. The leukocytes are collected by leukopheresis (Chapter 76) and are incubated with IL-2 to increase the production of LAK cells. The LAK cells are then given to the patient through a central venous catheter or large peripheral vein.

The advantage of this therapy is that lower doses of IL-2 can be used to avoid the severe toxicities that may accompany use of high-dose IL-2. Clinical trials indicate positive responses in patients with melanoma, colorectal carcinoma, and non-Hodgkin's lymphomas.[70]

TABLE 17-16 Toxic effects of Interleukin-2 and nursing interventions

System	Toxic Effects	Pathophysiology	Interventions
Neurological	Confusion Disorientation Combativeness Psychosis Anxiety	Unknown, perhaps multiple causes; may result from sleep deprivation or stress of intensive care.	Assess neuro status before starting IL-2 therapy. Reassure patient/family that symptoms are reversible. Explain that symptoms may be dose related and that IL-2 treatments may be interrupted or stopped. Observe for subtle changes in patient's personality and notify MD if they occur. Provide for patient safety.
Renal	Oliguria Creatinine rise BUN rise Proteinuria	Direct action by IL-2 on kidneys; related to cumulative levels of IL-2.	Monitor intake and output q4h during infusion and for 24 hours thereafter. Test urine for protein after every voiding. Monitor BUN and creatinine weekly; notify MD of abnormalities.
Hematologic	Anemia Thrombocytopenia	Related to cumulative IL-2 levels.	Monitor CBC daily. Check for petechiae, bruising, bleeding gums, or other bleeding. Test all stool, urine, and emesis for blood. If platelets <65,000, prohibit rectal suppositories, rectal temperatures, and IM injections.
Hepatic	Elevated bilirubin, SGOT, SGPT, LDH	Unknown.	Note pretreatment values. Monitor bilirubin, SGOT, SGPT, and LDH weekly.
Skin	Erythematous rash Pruritus Skin desquamation	Unknown.	Give prophylactic diphenhydramine (Benadryl) 25-50 mg PO q6h during infusion. Assess skin daily. Apply water-based lotion or cream to body twice daily. Tell patient to avoid scrubbing and to pat skin dry after bathing.
Gastrointestinal	Nausea Vomiting Diarrhea Mucositis Reduced appetite	Unknown.	Monitor intake and output q4h during infusion and for 24 hours thereafter. Give prophylactic antiemetic as prescribed. Give antidiarrheal agents as needed. Assist patient with oral hygiene q2h while awake. (Rinse mouth with 1 teaspoon baking soda dissolved in 1 cup water.) Assess oral mucosa daily. Encourage patient to eat six small meals rather than three full meals.
Cardiovascular/ Pulmonary	Hypotension	Reduced systemic vascular resistance.	Monitor vital signs every 1 to 4 hours during treatment; notify MD if BP <100/70. Give 5% albumin, dopamine, or phenylephrine to maintain systolic BP>100 or as prescribed.
	Weight gain Peripheral edema Ascites Arrhythmia Pulmonary edema Dyspnea	Capillary-permeability syndrome with extravasation of fluid into extravascular space or fluid shifts due to eosinophilia.	Monitor fluid intake and output q4h. Weigh daily. Measure abdominal girth q8h if ascites is present. If peripheral edema is present, elevate extremities. Monitor O_2 saturation; if <90%, notify MD. Note shortness of breath or altered breathing.

From Jassek PF and Spiewak PL: Interleukin-2, Am J Nurs 87:466-477, 1987.

Continued.

TABLE 17-16 Toxic effects of Interleukin-2 and nursing interventions—cont'd

System	Toxic Effects	Pathophysiology	Interventions
Other	Fever	It is speculated that IL-2 may affect the hypothalamic regulatory centers or that IL-2 stimulates other lymphokines and monokines that act on the hypothalamus	Give acetaminophen PO or rectally q4h prophylactically. Monitor temperature every hour during infusion and for 24 hours thereafter. If temp ≥38.5°C (101.3°F), culture blood and urine specimens. Provide cooling mattress if needed. Give meperidine (Demerol) 25-50 mg IV push at onset of chills or rigors. If symptoms persist after discharge, tell patient to rest at home and to continue to take acetaminophen PO q4h as needed.
	Chills		
	Headache	Unknown.	
	Malaise		
	Flulike syndrome		
	Nasal congestion		
	Glossitis		
	Xerostomia		

Monoclonal Antibodies

Monoclonal antibodies (MoAbs) are produced by hybridoma techniques that involve immunizing animals (usually mice) with antigen, then fusing B cells from the mouse's spleen with tumor cells to make hybrid cells. MoAbs can be produced to bind with almost any antigen. They are effective in the serologic detection of tumors since cells that have undergone malignant transformation often express antigens that are not found frequently on the surfaces of normal cells. A tumor marker for colon, breast, and lung cancer carcinoembryonic antigen (CEA) is a tumor specific MoAb. These markers may be sensitive to detection of early cancer and to monitor the cause of disease in patients undergoing therapy.[70,85]

Cancer therapy with MoAbs is in its early trials. Some tumor responses have occurred, but MoAbs alone are not toxic enough to kill tumor cells. Immunoconjugate therapy, however, shows much promise. Anticancer drugs, radioisotopes, other biologic response modifiers may be attached to MoAbs and targeted directly to tumor cells bypassing normal cells.

MoAbs are usually given intravenously by slow infusion using a pump or intraarterially through the hepatic artery to treat liver metastasis. Side effects, usually caused by an allergic reaction to the mouse protein used in manufacture, include fever, chills, headache, flushing, urticaria, rash, bronchospasm, dyspnea, hypotension, tachycardia, and anaphylactic reactions.[85]

Care of patients receiving monoclonal antibodies includes the following:

1. Remain near the patient's bedside; assess the skin for erythema, rash or hives.
2. Take vital signs every 15 minutes during the first hour, every 30 minutes during the second.
3. Keep emergency drugs (epinephrine), hydrocortisone (solu-cortef and diphenhydramine), normal saline, and resuscitation equipment at the bedside in case of anaphylaxis.
4. Answer patient's questions to allay apprehension.

FUTURE OF IMMUNOTHERAPY

In the future it appears that biologic agents such as IL-2 will be most effect as the fourth type of cancer therapy in combination with other agents. Much research is needed to identify significant unanswered questions about their use (See reference 70).

NEW APPROACHES IN CANCER THERAPY
HYPERTHERMIA

Clinical data suggest that there is a synergistic effect between temperatures of 41° C to 42° C and radiation therapy, as well as some chemotherapy. The field of systemic hyperthermia is young. Future investigation will study optimal sequencing of heat alone, of heat plus chemotherapy, and of heat plus radiation therapy as a means of augmenting treatment of deep tumors.[16,100]

Four methods are used for local or regional hyperthermia: (1) ultrasonic (US) devices, (2) devices using ultramagnetic waves (EMW), (3) devices that use alternating EM fields to heat by induction of electrical currents, and (4) devices using direct coupling of EM currents between needles or plates encompassing the tissue to be heated.

These methods may be noninvasive; that is, they do not use materials to enter the body, or invasive, such as by needle implants, interstitial seeds, and interstitial and intracavity application of small antennae emitting electromagnetic waves. Whole body hyperthermia has been achieved by immersing the patient in liquid wax, circulating hot water in a special suit, or a heated cabinet.[100]

PHOTODYNAMIC THERAPY

Researchers are experimenting with the use of dye and light, a process called photodynamic therapy. The dye is injected into a vein and spreads throughout the body. After a few days it remains only in the cancer cells. A red light produced by a laser is then used. The dye in the cell absorbs the light, causing a photochemical reaction that destroys the cells.

ONCOLOGIC EMERGENCIES

Oncologic emergencies may occur as a result of the disease process or of its treatment. These emergencies include obstructions (increased intracranial pressure, spinal cord compression, superior vena cavae syndrome, tracheal or bowel obstruction), metabolic syndromes (hypercalcemia, tumor lysis syndrome, syndrome of inappropriate antidiuretic hormone secretion, hyperviscosity, anaphylaxis, septic shock, disseminated intravascular coagulation), and cardiac toxicities (pericardial tamponade, cardiomyopathy with congestive heart failure) as described in Table 17-17. The oncology nurse is the health care professional frequently in a position to recognize these emergencies. A careful history and ongoing monitoring for signs and symptoms alerts nurses to life-threatening conditions. Nursing care of these problems is described in chapters related to the organ system involved.

CANCER PAIN

Pain is one of the most feared effects of cancer, although contrary to popular belief, it is frequently the last symptom to appear. Pain is not a problem for the majority of persons in the early stages of cancer. About 5% to 10% of patients with solid tumors have pain that interferes with activity or mood. When metastatic disease occurs, about 1 in 3 persons has significant pain. In a comprehensive survey of 1103 advanced cancer patients, the most common symptom encountered and the one that counted for the greatest amount of fear was pain. With *advanced* disease 60% to 90% report a problem with pain. In this group 73% had pain, and in a little more than half of this group, the pain was severe.[48] The cause of cancer pain is complex, since it has physical, psychologic, social, and spiritual aspects.[21,81]

STAGES OF CANCER PAIN

Three stages of cancer pain have been described: early, intermediate, and late. Early pain usually occurs after initial surgery for diagnosis or treatment and usually subsides after the third day; thus this pain is an acute episode, that is, short-term and temporary.

Intermediate-stage pain results from postoperative contraction of scars and nerve entrapment or from cancer recurrence or metastasis. This pain may subside or may be controlled by palliative therapy such as radiation, chemotherapy, neurosurgery, and analgesics. Therapy itself may initiate the pain.

Late-stage pain occurs in terminal cancer when therapy no longer controls the disease. This pain is chronic, may slowly increase in intensity, and at times may be intractable.

PATHOPHYSIOLOGY

Malignant neoplasms cause pain by five physiologic changes: bone destruction (the most frequent cause), obstruction of lumens (viscera or vessels), peripheral nerve involvement, pressure of growing tumors causing ischemia or distention and inflammation, infection or necrosis of tissue (see the box below).

PSYCHOSOCIAL ASPECTS

The psychologic component of cancer pain is associated with the patient's perception of the threat and stress of cancer and varies from individual to individual. Three categories of stressors have been identified: injury or threat of injury as a result of the cancer, loss or threat of loss (body part or death), and frustration of drives as a result of disabilities from the cancer per se or from the effect of therapies. Patients may respond with depression, decreased self-esteem, hostility, and irritability.

The sociologic effects include decreased interaction and participation in activities of daily living. There is de-

---

PATHOPHYSIOLOGY OF CANCER PAIN

CAUSE	TYPE OF PAIN
Bone destruction with infraction (fracture without displacement)	Increased sensitivity over area or sharp continuous pain
Obstruction of a viscus (gastrointestinal or genitourinary tract)	Severe, colicky, crampy-type pain, may be dull, diffuse, poorly localized
Obstruction of an artery, vein, or lymphatic	Dull, diffuse, aching (caused by arterial ischemia, venous engorgement, edema)
Infiltration, compression of peripheral nerves or nerve plexus	Continuous, sharp, or stabbing pain; sometimes hyperesthesia or paresthesia
Infiltration or distention of integument, fascia, or tissue (e.g., ascites)	Localized, dull aching pain
Inflammation, infection, and necrosis of tissue	Varied pain caused by pressure or ischemia

TABLE 17-17 Oncologic emergencies

Type	Pathophysiology	Clinical Manifestations
OBSTRUCTIVE		
Increased intracranial pressure	Increased brain mass from tumor, hemorrhage, or edema. Alteration in internal jugular vein flow caused by head/neck tumor or by surgical resection, cause alteration in function	Change in mental status, vomiting, headache, dizziness, seizures (see Chapter 62)
Spinal cord compression	Primary or metastatic lesions causing disruptions of reflexes and motor function because of neuron impairment and interruption of motor or sensory nerve fibers. Symptoms depend on location	Flaccid paralysis, paresthesias, locomotion difficulties, respiratory impairment at C-5 level (see Chapter 63)
Superior vena cava syndrome (SVC)	Obstruction of the SVC caused by primary (usually lung CA) or metastatic tumors in the mediastinal or paratracheal nodes	Dyspnea, facial and neck swelling, chest pain, cough, dysphagia, ruddy edematous face
Tracheal obstruction	Reduction in lumen from tracheal stenosis, extrinsic compression, or mass in lumen	Signs and symptoms of inadequate gas exchange and respiratory function (see Chapter 33)
METABOLIC EMERGENCIES		
Hypercalcemia[23]	Bone disease or metastasis increase bone resorption with bone destruction and release of calcium in the ECF. Release of prostaglandin from the tumor causes an increase in serum calcium. Osteoclast activity factors lead to secretion of parathyroid-type hormone	N & V, constipation, muscle weakness, coma, arrhythmias, polyuria, nephrolithiasis (see Chapter 23)
Tumor lysis syndrome (TLS)	Rapid tumor cell destruction after cytotoxic chemotherapy may result in release of intracellular electrolytes. May occur in malignancies characterized by rapid cell growth (leukemia and lymphomas)	Hyperphosphatemia, (oliguria, azotemia), hyperkalemia, hyperuricemia (N & V, lethargy, anuria, azotemia), hypocalcemia (see Chapter 23)
Syndrome of inappropriate antidiuretic hormone secretion (SIADH)	Increase in ADH seen in malignancies such as lung carcinoma (especially oat cell), duodenal and pancreatic carcinoma, thymoma, lymphomas, uterine carcinoma, and CNS tumors. May also occur with some chemotherapeutic agents (cyclophosphamide, vincristine)	Fluid and electrolyte changes and neurologic changes (see Chapter 36)
Hyperviscosity	Increased blood viscosity from increase in cell number, loss of flexibility of cells, or overproduction of serum proteins. This causes increased resistance to blood flow	Bleeding from GI or urinary tracts or puncture sites; visual disturbance, headache, dizziness, weakness, dyspnea, distended neck veins
Anaphylaxis	Hypersensitivity responses (I, II, III, IV) caused by chemotherapeutic agents (asparaginase, cisplatin, neocarzinostatin, VM-26, doxorubicin, daunorubicin, bleomycin, cyclophosphamide, methotrexate, melphalan)	Signs of anaphylactic reactions (see Chapter 76)
Septic shock	Increased susceptibility to infection from impaired immune system or effect of immunosuppressive agents, leading to bacterial septicemia	Signs and symptoms of septic shock (see Chapter 25)
Disseminated intravascular coagulation (DIC)	Chronic bleeding consumes all clotting factors; may also result from sepsis	Thrombocytopenia, bleeding of mucous membranes and tissues (see Chapter 30)
CARDIAC TOXICITIES		
Cardiac tamponade	Intrapericardial pressure increases from accumulation of fluid from direct tumor invasion, metastatic lesion, infection, or from pericardial thickening after radiation. Results in decreased diastolic ventricular filling and decreased stroke volume and cardiac output	Dyspnea, cough, chest pain, muffled heart sounds, cyanosis, edema, decreased systolic pressure, decreased CVP (see Chapter 28)
Cardiomyopathy with congestive heart failure	Chemotherapeutic drugs (such as anthracyclines, mithramycin, mitomycin, and cyclophosphamide) appear to damage cardiac myofibrils, causing sarcoplasmic reticular swelling that leads to destruction of the myofibril; hypertrophy of the heart muscle ensues with decreased function	Acute: tachycardia, arrhythmias Chronic: signs of CHF (see Chapter 28)

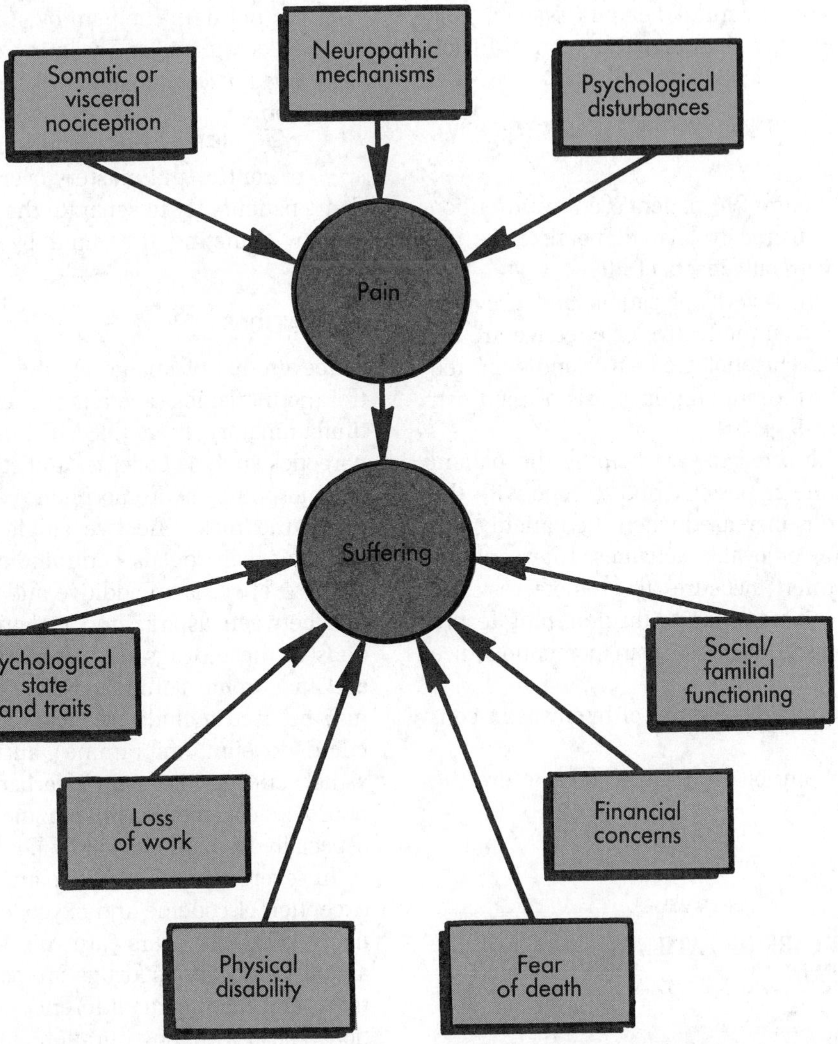

FIGURE 17-22 Model of factors associated with pain. (From Portenoy RK: Practical aspects of pain control in the patient with cancer, CA 138:332, 1988, and the American Cancer Society.)

creased productivity characterized by absence from work, economic problems, and deterioration in family relationships. The spiritual effects of pain are evidenced by loss of hope and trust and an overwhelming feeling of despair, rejection, and sense of isolation (Figure 17-22).

Side effects of cancer pain include fatigue, sleeplessness, anorexia, and decreased movement followed by the complications of immobility, namely muscle weakness, decubiti, contractures, and respiratory dysfunction.

MEDICAL THERAPY

Medical therapy in early-stage pain focuses on therapy directed at the cancer per se. Late-stage pain is treated symptomatically by analgesia, neurosurgery, and nerve blocks. Surgical procedures to relieve the pain include simple intercostal nerve block where feasible, surgical section of posterior sensory roots adjacent to the spinal cord, and spinothalamic tractotomy (interruption of pain- and temperature-conducting tracts). Dorsal column stimulators and transcutaneous electrical nerve stimulators (TENS) (Chapter 16) may be helpful in selected cases.[81]

Another method for the control of chronic pain is to flood the related nerve fibers with a drug by means of a continuous extravascular infusion (CEI) that delivers an anesthetic such as bupivacaine (Marcaine) or an analgesic such as meperidine for a period of 5 to 7 days. The local anesthetic blocks the sympathetic nervous system locally and also reduces conduction of the nerve fiber peripherally. Narcotics act by stimulating the opiate receptor sites in the central nervous system. The continuous drug flow is maintained by an infusion pump.[1]

NURSING CARE OF THE PATIENT WITH CHRONIC CANCER PAIN

Cancer pain may occupy the patient's entire attention and, unless treated vigorously, may demoralize the patient and interfere with all aspects of life.

The type, duration, severity, location, and previous measures that have been ineffective or effective are assessed. (Chapter 16). The etiologic factors and expected patient outcomes for the nursing diagnosis of pain can be found in Table 17-9, p. 358.

Nursing care is directed toward helping the patient to live as normal a life as possible and to cope with the pain. Pain tolerance is increased when the patient's energy is preserved for enjoyable activities. Interventions include general comfort measures to promote rest and sleep, good body positioning, and nutrition, plus teaching various methods to decrease pain perception (see the box below).

Three principles underlie the use of hypnosis in controlling pain[96]:

1. Filter the hurt out of the pain, to restructure the experience of it.

GUIDELINES FOR CARE OF PATIENTS WITH CANCER PAIN

1. Promote comfort:
   a. Meticulous hygiene
   b. Clean, dry, bed linen
   c. Control of odors
   d. Good body positioning such as with pillows, bed cradle, foot boards for the bedfast person
2. Maintain nutrition (pp. 398-399)
3. Provide diversionary activities for distraction to decrease pain perception:
   a. Physical activities (for example, working, walking, gardening, swimming)
   b. Mental relaxation activities (for example, watching TV, reading, crafts, listening to music, comedy cassettes)
   c. Social (for example, visits from family, friends)
4. Suggest and teach forms of noninvasive pain relief[115]:
   a. Guided imagery (waking-imagined analgesia)
   b. Hypnosis
   c. Progressive muscle relaxation
   d. Transcendental meditation
5. Teach patients and families physiologic and pharmacologic effects of analgesic drugs
6. Give pain medication in high enough doses continuously over the 24-hour period
7. Provide psychologic support to help patients cope

---

2. Do not fight the pain by struggling with it, having talks with it, or becoming angry since the resulting muscle tension will increase the pain sensation.
3. Use self-hypnosis because it gives a greater sense of control and mastery over the pain.

Some patients try to separate the pain from their bodies, thereby "quieting the mind by letting the body drop away."

MEDICATIONS

Three groups of analgesics may be used for pain control: nonnarcotics (acetaminophen and nonsteroidal antiinflammatory drugs [NSAID], including aspirin), weak narcotics such as codeine, and strong narcotics (including morphine, hydromorphone, and methadone). Aspirin is the most effective single analgesic for mild to moderate pain but is contraindicated if platelet counts are low. There is an additive and perhaps synergistic effect between aspirin and codeine; therefore combinations of these drugs are useful in moderate acute pain and in chronic aching pain. Adjuvant analgesics that may be used include tricyclic antidepressants (amitriptyline, doxepin, imipramine), anticonvulsants for paroxysmal cutting-like pain (carbamazepine, phenytoin), neuroleptics (methotrimeprazine), and corticosteroids, especially for pain caused by bony metastasis.

In severe chronic cancer pain, the narcotics, with the exception of codeine and oxycodone, are the most effective. Although there are no significant differences among the various drugs in potency or side effects, there are significant differences in the duration of action. Those with long duration of action are preferred for the relief of chronic cancer pain. Tolerance and dependence in these drugs are less common with cancer pain than when the narcotics are used for acute pain.

There are three important principles in administration of narcotics that relate to dose level and frequency of administration (see the box below). Prevention of pain recurrence usually requires less analgesia than treatment of pain after it has recurred.

Oral administration is preferred. Parenteral therapy produces higher initial serum and tissue levels of the

---

PRINCIPLES OF ADMINISTRATION OF NARCOTICS FOR CANCER PAIN

1. Determine optimal dose and give larger doses of narcotics for initial control.
2. Start with a dose that is too high, since the patient may become anxious if there is no pain relief despite medication (anxiety increases pain).
3. Administer the narcotic regularly, *not* PRN, so each dose is given before previous dose loses its effect.

narcotic, but the oral doses are as effective as parenteral doses in maintaining drug levels in the body. Intramuscular and subcutaneous injections are more difficult to administer and are painful to patients with marked muscle wasting. In addition, parenteral administration may make the patient dependent on others for drug administration.[111]

There are, however, numerous other routes of administration of opiates if the patient cannot tolerate oral medication (See Table 17-18). Continuous infusion with a portable infusion pump attached to a needle placed in the subcutaneous tissue has been found to be safe and effective for home and the hospital. This method avoids repeated IM or subcutaneous injections and the need for intravenous access, and provides continuous levels of pain control.[24]

Analgesic drug "cocktails," such as Brompton's cocktail mixture, have become less widely used. This liquid commonly contains morphine, cocaine, alcohol, syrup, and chloroform water. Oral morphine gives just as effective analgesia, controlling intense pain for about 4 hours. Only persons with gastrointestinal upsets or who are unable to take oral medications need parenteral administration, which has the disadvantage of producing higher untoward effects. An exception to these side effects is the continuous intravenous or subcutaneous administration of morphine. For persons who do not get pain relief from oral morphine, hydromorphone (Dilaudid) IM may be preferred because a smaller volume of solution is needed.

Some hospitals prepare the morphine in chloroform water, which improves the taste and prevents bacterial growth. The effective dose of morphine in aqueous solution is 5 to 180 mg every 4 hours. It has been found that 70% of those with advanced cancer never need more than 20 mg every 4 hours.[111]

PRN administration is not effective for chronic severe pain and contributes to tolerance and dependence. The patient loses confidence in the staff and a vicious cycle of relief-pain-relief is set up.

There has been controversy about the use of diamorphine (heroin). Heroin may be more potent in smaller doses but when equipotent doses are administered, there is no difference in the drugs in level of analgesia or in side effects.

It is not always necessary to administer an antiemetic unless an additional sedative or antianxiety effect is desired. Tolerance is not a problem with consistent oral administration. It occurs with PRN parenteral intramuscular injection, which also increases drug dependency. Respiratory depression is not a problem with oral administration because of tolerance to the respiratory depressant effect of morphine during long-term use.

Morphine sulfate sustained-release tablets are now available. These tablets maintain blood levels of morphine for 8 hours and are particularly helpful for night pain relief.

One of the newest programs for pain relief is *patient-controlled analgesia* (PCA), an intravenous drug delivery system that allows patients to control their own narcotic analgesics (see Chapter 16). Patients using PCA report better pain relief than from intramuscular injections, feel less sedated, and have fewer periods of intense pain.[61]

Pain management programs have been developed that include several types of therapy: physical therapy, occupational therapy, relaxation therapy, nutrition, education, individual and marital counseling, and family education. The goal of these programs is to help patients cope with the pain and problems the pain has caused in their lives.

Pain is often not effectively managed at home, resulting in decreased functional ability of the patient. Common reasons for not taking medications included fear of addiction or tolerance, misunderstanding dosages, and feeling that pain could not be treated.[34] Nurses give information to family or patient to prevent these misconceptions that result in inadequate pain control.

TABLE 17-18 Routes of administration of opioid drugs

Route	Comment
Oral	Preferred, if feasible
Buccal	Potentially effective if drug exposed to oral mucosa for prolonged period; not clinically available
Sublingual	Buprenorphine effective, but not yet available in U.S.; clinical efficacy of other drugs controversial
Rectal	Morphine, oxymorphone, and hydromorphone available; very few studies, but generally believed to be equianalgesic to oral route
Subcutaneous: repetitive, continuous	Outpatient continuous infusion now possible with ambulatory pumps
Intramuscular	Limited role in chronic administration of opioids
Intravenous: repetitive, continuous, patient-controlled	Cost and need for manual dexterity and intact cognition may limit utility of patient-controlled pumps for many with cancer pain
Spinal: epidural (repetitive, continuous), intrathecal	Well-accepted, but many facets controversial including indications, best site of administration, appropriate timing of therapy, best technique for implantation, and best drug
Intraventricular	Effective, but should be considered experimental

From Portenoy, RK: Practical aspects of pain control in the patient with cancer, CA 38:343, 1988.

HOME AND AMBULATORY CARE

The settings for care of patients with cancer have changed; now more patients receive care at home or as a cancer outpatient rather than in the acute care setting.

Ambulatory services have been described as the mainstay of cancer nursing care.[14,79] Three factors have made ambulatory care a major method of providing services: advances in cancer therapy, technology, and quality of life. New technology has eliminated some of the early problems in teaching patients in ambulatory settings or at home. Procedures adopted for the home include glucose monitors, pump-driven tube feedings, peritoneal dialysis systems, ventilators, suctioning machines, intravenous therapy, chemotherapy, and total parenteral nutrition.[53] Ambulatory oncology centers are often associated with hospitals so that patients can continue therapy begun as an inpatient while living at home.

There are stressors associated with home care. Patients may feel stress because of uncertainty about the treatment, physical restrictions, anger or depression, and isolation. They may feel lack of support from family members who also express stress.

Caregivers describe treatment uncertainty, role conflict, and worry about the added responsibilities of their loved one's care. They may feel guilty, and be afraid of being alone without support. They may also complain of lack of information and, with the patient, worry about transportation to clinics and the financial burden of therapy.[9]

Nurses must do family assessments to identify the patient's and the caregiver's ability to cope with the stress that may accompany home and ambulatory care. For further information on home care, see Chapter 78.

SUPPORTIVE CARE OF THE PATIENT WITH ADVANCED CANCER

When all possible surgery and maximal chemotherapy and radiation therapy have failed to control the spread of cancer, the patient and family have many special problems. They need encouragement and help in living as normally as possible, in planning for the late stages of the patient's illness, and in adjusting to death and its implications for the family.

Before nurses can help the patient and family, they must have developed a mature philosophy that allows acceptance of death as an eventual reality for everyone. This philosophy is not acquired overnight. The nurse needs the opportunity to discuss feelings about caring for the patient whose death is imminent, since the nurse's attitude toward death and suffering will affect the ability to plan and give care to the person with ad-

vanced cancer. (See Chapter 14 for discussion of death and dying.)

No one can say with certainty when death will come. The patient may ask about the length of time remaining, but no absolute answer can be given. Physicians may have made a statement to the patient about life expectancy.

■ ASSESSMENT

Even if done earlier, a complete assessment of the patient and family is needed before planning care after a diagnosis of advanced cancer is made. (See guidelines on pp. 355-356). Other factors to consider include the patient's and significant others' feelings about death and chronic illness, since these feelings will color other responses. In addition, the patient's and others' willingness to participate in care may be influenced by their perception of life expectancy.

■ DATA ANALYSIS: NURSING DIAGNOSES

Any or all of the nursing diagnoses in Table 17-9 may be identified on the basis of a complete physiologic, psychologic, sociocultural, and spiritual assessment. Those nursing diagnoses most often seen in advanced cancer are listed in the box.

■ PLANNING: EXPECTED PATIENT OUTCOMES
PLANNING FOR HOME CARE

At least half of all deaths from cancer occur in the patients' homes. Planning for home care of the patient without completely disrupting the rest of the family takes the concerted efforts of many people. Patients must always be consulted, and their wishes should be respected in the early stages of the disease. In the final stages they may be too ill to be bothered or concerned with making decisions. The physician, the social

---

COMMON NURSING DIAGNOSES FOR THE PATIENT WITH ADVANCED CANCER

Airway clearance, ineffective
Constipation
Coping, ineffective family and individual
Family process, altered
Fear (specify type)
Gas exchange, impaired
Grieving, anticipatory, dysfunctional
Nutrition, altered: less than body requirements
Oral mucous membrane, altered
Pain
Powerlessness
Self-care deficit, total
Skin integrity, impaired
Social isolation
Spiritual distress

worker, and the nurse must work together with the local community agencies, such as the American Cancer Society, to ensure continuity of care from the hospital to the home.

The principles governing suitability for home care are similar to those for any patient receiving home care, although the patient with cancer may not live as long as many others with chronic long-term illnesses. Medical and nursing supervision must be available; it must be possible for required care to be given; both patient and family must want the patient home; and home facilities must be suitable. Rehabilitation teams may also be sent into the home to help the patient and family.

Outcome criteria for patients with advanced cancer include:

1. The person makes his or her own decisions and participates in care as long as desired
2. Skin does not break down
3. The patient states that:
   a. Pain is absent or bearable
   b. She or he can cope with the illness and dying

HOSPICE

Hospice is a program of care designed to meet the needs of those who are dying and of those close to them. The emphasis is on home care, and efforts are directed toward keeping patients at home as long as possible and allowing them to die at home if that is their wish. The goals of hospice are short-term and directed toward relief of symptoms and palliation. Hospice requires a high degree of skilled professional care in which nurses play the pivotal role on the interdisciplinary team. Nurses are the patient/family advocates and managers of the team.

Patients and their families are the participants in hospice care. Facilitation of the autonomy of the dying person is a primary goal so that nurses share relevant information to help the patients make decisions about their care. (See the box for components of hospice.) The

---

COMPONENTS OF HOSPICE CARE[15]

1. Coordinated home care with inpatient beds available under an autonomous hospice administration
2. Control of symptoms (physical, psychologic, sociologic, spiritual)
3. Physician services
4. Care by interdisciplinary team
5. Services available 24 hours a day, 7 days a week with emphasis on nursing and medical skills
6. Patient and family regarded as unit of care
7. Bereavement follow-up
8. Use of volunteers as part of the team
9. Structured personal support and communication systems
10. Patients accepted into the program on the basis of health care need rather than ability to pay

---

major purpose is to maintain the quality of life by assisting patients and their families to live life to its fullest.[90]

Hospice care also emphasizes the health of family members and caregivers who, in addition to care, may have responsibilities for household activities and holding a job. Health status of family members is assessed, recommendations are made for their health care, and their coping strategies are supported by nurses.

High technology is also being associated with hospice. Although hospice principles preclude therapies directed toward cure, symptom control is a major emphasis of hospice care so that technology such as infusion pumps for pain control or fluid provision may be used to maintain patient comfort.[53]

Programs may be acute care hospital-based, long-term care facility-based, community-based home health care agencies, and community-based independent hospices. Planning that includes provision for care and support of the hospice team helps meet the goals of nursing care to relieve physical, mental, and spiritual distress.

■ IMPLEMENTATION
MEETING PSYCHOLOGIC NEEDS
Maintaining Hope

One of the most difficult nursing tasks is helping the patient and family maintain hope and avoid despair. There are many manifestations of hope. Generalized hope is a sense of some future beneficial developments. Particularized hope is concerned with a particularly valued outcome, goal, or state of being. Both are important for the cancer patient.[30] Hope can be structured and

---

STRATEGIES TO INSPIRE HOPE[73]

1. Emphasize sustaining relationships, the will to live by relating to someone to live for.
2. Tell patients that loss of control is temporary (if true).
3. Radiate hope—view the health problem as an opportunity for growth and adaptation, not as an impossible situation.
4. Expand the patient's coping mechanisms, the cognitive, affective, and motor activities individuals use to deal with difficulties.
5. Teach reality surveillance by analyzing past events and assigning logic and reasoning to them (compare oneself with others with the same problem, plan for realistic resumption of self-care).
6. Help the patient identify and revise goals that reflect progress and that are achievable.
7. Help the patient renew the spiritual self by creating an environment in which spiritual beliefs may be expressed and practiced.
8. Maximize esthetic experiences (savoring the taste of food, feeling the warmth of the sun, studying a painting).
9. Guard against despair by renewing appreciation and pleasure from the beauty of the moment.

supported by nursing interventions (see the box on p. 397). The nurse must, however, avoid encouraging false hopes. Patients may come to accept their prognosis with hope that a cure for cancer may be found. Nurses also must be careful that they do not have false hope. The inability to fulfill the hope that the patient will live may make it more difficult for nurses to accept the patient's death and they may see themselves as having failed.

Meeting Spiritual Needs

Patients and families are faced with an intense personal crisis at many times during the cancer experience. Some may be crushed by the burdens they face, but others learn the real purpose of being and how best to live a rewarding life. They confront their mortality, submit to the future, transcend early priorities, and cherish their life each day. Nurses should not be surprised when patients return to religious traditions and describe personal "religious experiences." These are not psychologic phenomena. Nurses should be comfortable with patients' overt religious practices, support them, and not be content to refer religious concerns only to a hospital chaplain. Nurses, through listening skills, genuine openness, and tolerance, can encourage the spiritual experiences of patients.[15,108]

Encouraging Social and Vocational Activities

Patients with advanced cancer should resume their regular work if they can possibly do so, for work makes them feel as though they are still an active part of their group and worthy of the approval of others. It was said many centuries ago that employment is a person's best physician, and this concept applies particularly to persons whose existence is seriously threatened by cancer.

Social activities and all experiences associated with normal family life should continue whenever possible. There is probably no greater service the nurse can give patients with uncontrollable cancer than to help them continue everyday life in any way possible. Family members often need guidance in seeing the patient's need to live as normally as possible. Sometimes the patient appears almost unduly concerned with the details of some aspect of the immediate treatment and almost oblivious to the entire problem. Such a patient senses that success with the immediate treatment is the only way to remain up and about or to carry on at that time.

Decreasing Fear of Helplessness and Dependency

Patients may be haunted by fear of brain involvement, loss of mental faculties, and becoming completely helpless and dependent on others. Through these fears they express a basic human wish: to leave the world with as much dignity as possible. The nurse can urge the patient and family to discuss such fears with the physician. The patient may feel that the physician is too busy and that questions are too trivial to justify the use of the

physician's time, but satisfactory answers to questions add greatly to the patient's peace of mind.

Metastasis to the brain in persons who have other metastases is somewhat rare, and some patients suffer more from fear of damage to the brain than is justified. The patient should know that good hygiene, good nutrition, being up and about for part of each day, and doing deep-breathing exercises with attention to posture all help to prevent helplessness. A positive approach to all problems certainly shortens the time of helplessness and makes the patient more content.

MEETING PHYSIOLOGIC NEEDS

Every effort is expended to meet the patient's physiologic needs so that higher psychologic needs may be expressed. The patient who is in pain or feels "dirty" will have difficulty expressing concerns and fears. Research has shown that families believe that availability of nursing service, the ability to answer questions, allowing patient self-care when possible, and teaching family to give physical care rank highest as most helpful nursing behaviors (see the research box).

Increasing Comfort

Good nursing care of the patient with advanced cancer is challenging. Promoting the patient's comfort should be high on the list of goals. Nursing measures that increase rest and sleep and reduce pain will help maintain the patient's physical and psychologic well-being.

Maintaining Nutrition

Cachexia is a frequent problem. Anorexia may accompany therapy, and the increased protein needs of the

---

RESEARCH

Skorupka, P., and Bohnet, N.: Primary caregivers' perceptions of nursing behaviors that best meet the needs in a home care hospice setting, Cancer Nurs. 5:371-374, 1982.

This exploratory study provided baseline data to determine what nursing behaviors are perceived to be most helpful to primary caregivers in a home hospice program. The most helpful behaviors in rank order were: (1) provide the patient with emergency measures if needed; (2) assure the patient that nursing services will be available 24 hours a day, 7 days a week; (3) answer questions honestly, openly, and willingly; (4) allow the patient to do as much for self as possible; and (5) teach me how to make the patient physically comfortable. The findings suggest that primary caregivers found nursing behaviors related to the patients' physical and emotional needs more helpful than those related to the primary caregivers' emotional needs. The care plan should provide technical skills and teach those skills to the patient and family. The primary caregivers need information and skill to enhance their sense of security and sense of control. ■

REFERENCES AND SELECTED READINGS

1. *Alberico JG: Breaking the chronic pain cycle, Am J Nurs 84:1222-1225, 1984.
2. *Amenta MO: Hospice in the United States: multiple and varied programs, Nurs Clin North Am 20:269-280, 1985.
3. American Cancer Society: Nutrition and cancer: cause and prevention, CA 34:121-128, 1984.
4. American Cancer Society: 1989 Cancer facts and figures, New York, 1989, The Society.
5. *Anderson MA, Aker SN, and Hickman RO: The double-lumen Hickman catheter, Am J Nurs 82:272-273, 1982.
6. *Baird SB: Economic realities in the treatment and care of the cancer patient, Top Clin Nurs 2:67-80, 1981.
7. *Beck S et al: The family high-risk programs: targeted cancer prevention, Oncol Nurs Forum 15:301-306, 1988.
8. *Bersani G and Carl W: Oral care for cancer patients, Am J Nurs 83:533-536, 1983.
9. Blank JJ, Clark L, Longman AJ, and Atwood JR: Perceived home care needs of cancer patients and their caregivers, Cancer Nurs 12:78-84, 1989.
10. Boddie AW: Regional chemotherapy using surgical drug delivery systems, Nursing Intervention in Oncology, MD Anderson Case Reports and Review 7-10, 1989.
11. *Boxley KO et al: Alopecia: effect on cancer patients' body image, Cancer Nurs 7:499-503, 1984.
12. *Brack G, LaClave L, and Blix S: The psychological aspects of bone marrow transplant, Cancer Nurs 11:221-229, 1988.
13. Brown HG: Attitudes of the public and health professional influencing cancer prevention and detection. In Proceedings of the Fourth National Conference on Human Values and Cancer, New York, 1984, American Cancer Society.
14. Brown JK: Ambulatory services: the mainstay of cancer nursing care, Oncol Nurs Forum 12:1, 57-59, 1985.
15. Burns N, Carney K, and Brobst B: Hospice: a design for home care of the terminally ill, Holistic Nurs Pract 3(2):65-76, 1989.
16. Bull JMC: Whole body hyperthermia as an anticancer agent, CA 32:123-127, 1982.
17. Camp LD: Care of the Groshong catheter, Oncol Nurs Forum 15:745-748, 1988.
18. *Carlson AC: Infection prophylaxis in the patient with cancer, Oncol Nurs Forum 12:53-64, 1985.
19. Cassileth BR and Brown H: Unorthodox cancer medicine, CA 38:176-186, 1988.
20. Chasen MH: Imaging primary lung cancer, pleural cancers, and metastatic disease, CA 37:194-210, 1987.
21. *Cleeland CS: The impact of pain on the patient with cancer, Cancer 54:2635-2641, 1984.
22. *Cobb SC: Teaching relaxation techniques to cancer patients, Cancer Nurs 7:157-161, 1984.
23. Coward DD: Hypercalcemia knowledge assessment in patients at risk of developing cancer-related hypocalcemia, Oncol Nurs Forum 15:471-476, 1988.
24. Coyle N et al: Continuous subcutaneous infusions of opiates in cancer patients with pain, Oncol Nurs Forum 13(4):53-57, 1986.
25. Cozzi E et al: Nursing management of patients receiving hepatic arterial chemotherapy through an implanted infusion pump, Cancer Nurs 7:229-234, 1984.
26. *D'Agostino NS: Managing nutrition problems in advanced cancer, Am J Nurs 89:50-56, 1989.
27. Derdiarian AK: Informational needs of newly diagnosed cancer patients, Nurs Res 35:276-281, 1986.
28. DeVita VT, Hellman S, and Rosenberg S: Cancer: principles and practices of oncology, Philadelphia, 1985, JB Lippincott Co.
29. Donovan ML: Cancer care: a guide for patient education, New York, 1984, Appleton-Century-Crofts.
30. *Dufault K and Martocchio BC: Hope: its spheres and dimensions, Nurs Clin North Am 20:379-391, 1985.
31. Dudas S and Carlson CE: Cancer rehabilitation, Oncol Nurs Forum 15:183-188, 1988.
32. Eddy DM and Eddy JF: Delay factors in the detection of cancer. In Proceedings of the Fourth National Conference on Human Values and Cancer, New York, 1985, American Cancer Society.
33. Enck RE: Interrelationship of cancer control and clinical research in the community, CA 34:340-342, 1984.
34. *Ferrell BR and Schneider C: Experience and management of cancer pain at home, Cancer Nurs 11:84-90, 1988.
35. *Frank-Stromberg M: Health promotion behaviors in ambulatory cancer patients: fact or fiction? Oncol Nurs Forum 13:37-43, 1986.
36. Frank-Stromberg M et al: Carcinogens: are some risks acceptable? Am J Nurs 83:814-817, 1986.
37. *Fredette SL and Gloriant FS: Nursing diagnosis in cancer chemotherapy, Am J Nurs 81:2013-2023, 1981.
38. Gahart BL: Intravenous medications: a handbook for nurses and other allied health personnel, ed 5, St Louis, 1989, The CV Mosby Co.
39. Garvey E and Kramer R: Improving cancer patients' adjustment to infusion chemotherapy: evaluation of a patient education program, Cancer Nurs 6:373-378, 1983.
40. *Geltman RL and Paige RL: Symptom management in hospice care, Am J Nurs 83:78-84, 1983.
41. Giaconne G et al: Scalp hypothermia in the prevention of doxorubicin-induced hair loss, Cancer Nurs 11:170-173, 1988.
42. *Glasgow M, Halfin V, and Althouser AF: Sexual response and cancer, CA 37:322-333, 1987.
43. Glover DJ and Glick JH: Metabolic oncologic emergencies, CA 37:302-320, 1987.
44. Goldstein D and Laszlo J: The role of interferon in cancer therapy: a current perspective, CA 38:258-277, 1988.
45. Goodman MS and Wickborn R: Venous access devices: an overview, Oncol Nurs Forum 11:15-22, 1984.
46. Gordon M: Manual of nursing diagnosis, New York, 1987, McGraw-Hill Book Co.
47. Grant MM and Padilla GV: An overview of cancer nursing research, Oncol Nurs Forum 12:28-39, 1985.
48. Gray G et al: A clinical data base for advanced cancer patients, Cancer Nurs 11:77-83, 1988.
49. Greenwald P: Manipulation of nutrients to prevent cancer, Hosp Prog 19:119-134, 1984.
50. Greenwald P and Sondik EJ, editors: Cancer control objectives for the nation 1985-2000, Division of Cancer Prevention Control, National Cancer Institute, Bethesda, Md, 1986, US National Institutes of Health.
51. Gullo SM: Safe handling of antineoplastic drugs: translating the recommendations into practice, Oncol Nurs Forum 15:596-602, 1988.
52. Gurevich I and Tafuro P: The compromised host: deficit-specific infection and the spectrum of prevention, Cancer Nurs 9:263-275, 1986.
53. *Hays JC: High technology and hospice home care: strange bedfellow, Nurs Clin North Am 23:329-340, 1988.
54. Henk JM: Does hyperbaric oxygen have a future in radiation therapy? Int J Radiat Oncol Biol Phys 7:1125-1128, 1981.

*References preceded by an asterisk are particularly well suited for student reading.
†References preceded by a dagger are classic readings.

55. Hogan R: Human sexuality: a nursing perspective, ed 2, New York, 1985, Appleton-Century-Crofts.

56. Holcombe A: Bone marrow harvest, Oncol Nurs Forum 14(2):63-65, 1987.

57. *Hood LE: Interferon, Am J Nurs 87:459-464, 1987.

58. *Jarvis W: Helping your patients deal with questionable cancer treatments, CA 36:293-301, 1986.

59. *Jassok PF and Spiewak PL: Interleuken-2, Am J Nurs 87:464-467, 1987.

60. Johnstone JD: Infrequent infections associated with Hickman catheters, Cancer Nurs 5:125-129, 1982.

61. Kane NE et al: Use of patient-controlled analgesia in surgical oncology patients, Oncol Nurs Forum 15:29-37, 1988.

62. Kaszyk LR: Cardiac toxicity associated with cancer therapy, Oncol Nurs Forum 13(4):81-88, 1986.

63. *Kennedy M et al: Chemotherapy related nausea and vomiting: a survey to identify problems and interventions, Oncol Nurs Forum 8:19-22, 1981.

64. Kirkwood VM and Ernstoff MS: A clinical update: the role of interferon in the biotherapy of solid tumors, Oncol Nurs Forum (suppl) 15(6):3-6, 1988.

65. Krakoff IH: Cancer chemotherapeutic agents, CA 37:93-105, 1987.

66. *Krumm S: Psychosocial adaptation of the adult with cancer, Nurs Clin North Am 17:729-737, 1982.

67. Larson PJ: Cancer nurses' perceptions of caring, Cancer Nurs 9:86-91, 1986.

68. *Lewandowski W and Jones SL: The family with cancer: nursing interventions throughout the course of living with cancer, Cancer Nurs 11:313-321, 1988.

69. Lewis F and Levita M: Understanding radiotherapy, Cancer Nurs 11:174-185, 1988.

70. Lotze MT and Rosenberg SA: The immunologic treatment of cancer, CA 38:68-94, 1988.

71. *Martocchio B: Grief and bereavement: healing the hurt, Nurs Clin North Am 20:327-342, 1985.

72. McKinstry DW: Implanted drug delivery system for regional cancer chemotherapy, Res Resources Reporter, 5:1-5, 1981, Washington, DC, US Dept Health and Human Services.

73. *Miller J: Inspiring hope, Am J Nurs 85:22-28, 1985.

74. Miller SA et al: Cancer chemotherapy: guidelines and recommendations for nursing, education, and practice, Pittsburgh, 1984, Oncology Nursing Society.

75. National Institutes of Health Consensus Development Conference statement: Health implications of smokeless tobacco use, CA 36:310-316.

76. Nunnally C, Donoghue M, and Yosko JM: Nutritional needs of cancer patients, Nurs Clin North Am 17:557-578, 1982.

77. Ohio State University Hospitals Department of Nursing: Helpful hints: chemotherapy safe handling in the hospital and chemotherapy safe handling in the home, Columbus, Ohio, 1987, Ohio State Hospital.

78. Oncology Nursing Society and ANA Division on Medical-Surgical Nursing Practice: Outcome standards for cancer nursing practice, Kansas City, Mo, 1987, The American Nurses Association.

79. Pluth N: A home care transfusion program, Oncol Nurs Forum 14(5):43-46, 1987.

80. Poe CM and Taylor LM: Syndrome of inappropriate antidiuretic hormone: assessment and nursing implications, Oncol Nurs Forum 16:373-386, 1989.

81. *Portenroy RK: Practical aspects of pain control in the patient with cancer, CA 38:327-352, 1988.

82. Rahr V: Giving intrathecal drugs, Am J Nurs 86:829-831, 1986.

83. Rawl RL: In search of cancer control: understanding metastasis is crucial, Chem Eng News 63:10-17, 1985.

84. Richter MP et al: Current status of high linear energy transfer irradiation, Cancer 54:2814-2822, 1984.

85. *Rieger PT: Monoclonal antibodies, Am J Nurs 87:469-473, 1987.

86. Roberts L: Cancer today: origins, prevention, and treatment, Washington, DC, 1984, National Academy Press.

87. Rodman MJ et al: Pharmacology and drug therapy in nursing, Philadelphia, 1985, JB Lippincott Co.

88. Rose MA: Health promotion and risk prevention: applications for cancer survivors, Oncol Nurs Forum 16:335-340, 1989.

89. †Rumerfield PS and Rumerfield MJ: What you should know about radiation hazards, Am J Nurs 70:780-786, 1970.

90. *Saunders JM and McCorkle R: Models of care for persons with progressive cancer, Nurs Clin North Am 20:365-377, 1985.

91. *Schoene-Seifert B and Childress JF: How much should the cancer patient know and abide? CA 36:85-94, 1986.

92. Schottenfeld D: Cancer risks of medical treatment, CA 32:258-275, 1982.

93. Schryber S, Lacasse CR, and Barton-Burke C: Autologous bone marrow transplantation, Oncol Nurs Forum 14(4):74-80, 1987.

94. Schulmeister L: Vascular access grafts in cancer chemotherapy, Am J Nurs 82:1388-1389, 1982.

95. Souba WW and Copland EM: Hyperalimentation in cancer, CA 39:105-113, 1989.

96. *Spiegel D: The use of hypnosis and controlling cancer pain, CA 35:221-231, 1985.

97. Squier CA: Smokeless tobacco and oral cancer: a cause of concern, CA 34:242-247, 1984.

98. Stam HJ and Challis G: Rating the toxicities of cancer drugs, Am J Nurs 88:1362-1363, 1988.

99. Stewart CD: Nursing interventions in regional chemotherapy using surgical drug delivery systems. In Nursing Interventions in Oncology, MD Anderson Case Reports and Review, Newton, Pa, 1989, Associations in Medical Marketing Co, Inc.

100. Stewart VR and Gibbs FA: Hyperthermia in the treatment of cancer, CA 54:2823-2830, 1984.

101. *Sticklin LA: Interleuken-2 and killer T-cells, Am J Nurs 87:468-469, 1987.

102. Strohl RA: The nursing role in radiation oncology: symptom management of acute and chronic reactions, Oncol Nurs Forum 15:429-434, 1988.

103. Suppers VJ and McClamrock EA: Biologicals in cancer treatment: future effects on nursing practice, Oncol Nurs Forum 12:27-32, 1985.

104. Survey of physicians' attitudes and practices in early cancer detection, CA 35:197-213, 1985.

105. Thomas ED: Bone marrow transplantation, CA 37:291-301, 1987.

106. *Thorne SE: Helpful and unhelpful communications in cancer care: the patient's perspective, Oncol Nurs Forum 15:167-169, 1988.

107. *Valanis B and Shortridge L: Self-protective practices of nurses handling antineoplastic drugs, Oncol Nurs Forum 14(3):23-27, 1987.

108. *Vastyan EA: Spiritual aspects of the care of cancer patients, CA 36:110-114, 1986.

109. vonRoemeling E et al: Chemotherapy via implanted infusion pump: new perspectives for delivery of long-term continuous treatment, Oncol Nurs Forum 13(2):17-24, 1986.

110. †Warren W: Ionizing radiation and medicine, Sci Am 201:154-176, 1959. (Entire issue devoted to radiation, including how it affects the cell, evolution, and the whole animal.)

111. Walsh TD: Common misunderstanding about the use of

CHAPTER 18

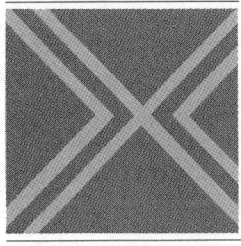

Altered Body Image

DOROTHY J. BRUNDAGE
DEBRA C. BROADWELL

CHAPTER OBJECTIVES

After studying this chapter, the student should be able to:
1 Analyze the concept of altered body image.
2 Compare different human responses to altered body image.
3 Analyze the basis for the individual's and others' responses to altered body image.

Body image is the mental idea a person has of his or her body at any moment based on past as well as present perceptions. This mental picture of one's body develops over time and is derived from internal sensations, postural changes, contact with outside objects and people, emotional experiences, and fantasies.[48] Body image is formed by the interaction between the perceptual pool and the experiential pool.[18,41] The perceptual pool consists of all present and past sensory experiences, whereas the experiential pool consists of all experiences, affects, and memories.

Body image is influenced by cognitive growth as well as by changes in the body that give rise to physical stimuli.[35] These stimuli may be internal or external to the body and include stimuli from the social and physical environment.

Three levels of body experiences play a role in the development of body image: somatic, behavioral, and topologic.[41] Somatic stimuli include neurologic, metabolic, endocrine, and hormonal sensations. This sensory level of experience is observed in infants as they respond to internal stimuli. As a toddler becomes aware of separateness from the environment, behavioral aspects of the development of body image that involve perceptual, cognitive, motor, and personality variables become evident. During adolescence, topologic stimuli such as superficial sensations and physical characteristics of the body surface become influential. Modification of one's body image occurs with new percepts and new experiences.[40] Throughout all stages of growth and development and with changes in health stage, body image is continually being altered.

Body image makes up one aspect of the individual's self-concept. The importance of body image within the self-concept will vary mainly according to the nature and intensity of values and emotions invested in it.[47] Self is what a person is, whereas self-image is what a person thinks of self. An essential factor in the development of self-image is body image. Body image is an intrapersonal experience of the body, including one's attitudes and feelings. One's body image becomes a standard that influences performance and self-concept.

Many societal and cultural standards influence the development of body image.[41] The attitudes of society, parents, and peers will be reflected in the way persons view their bodies. There has been much discussion of the emphasis on youth, wholeness, and beauty in the American culture. Body image includes both reality and ideality[14]; thus body image does not always coincide with objective body.[3] Components of a person's ideal body image may be youth, slenderness, or beauty. Individuals may incorporate so much ideal into their body image that when confronted by the reality of a videotape or a mirror they are genuinely shocked. They do not feel older, and the face in the mirror does not seem to belong.[14]

Since body image is a dynamic, constantly changing perception, change in the structure, function, or appearance of the body requires modification of the image an individual has. The idea of body image disturbances arises from observations that persons with altered structure, function, or appearance may fail to perceive the changes and to adapt to the body as it exists. Attempts have been made to measure body image and to assess the impact of alterations in structure, function, and appearance.[1,7,31,38,57] Current clinical literature related to persons with altered structure, function, or appearance includes studies of patients with alopecia,[2,50,57] amputation,[19,34] breast and gynecologic cancer,[6,31,50] depression,[39] facial disfiguration,[13,22] heart attack,[53] obesity,[27,38] and pregnancy.[16] Such studies frequently have direct application to patient assessment and intervention by a variety of the health professions involved in rehabilitation of the physically disabled. Body image alterations are a concern in critical as well as chronic illness.[4,42,43,45] A major assumption underlying this chapter is that physical disability or a change in body structure that results in altered function or appearance or both is accompanied by an alteration in the person's body image. Interventions by the health team to help the patient manage the results of the physical change must include help in the psychosocial areas of life also affected. Much of the effort made in this latter area is focused on helping the patient recognize, accept, and live with the change in self-concept, which includes both body image and self-esteem. These conditions occur not only in the young but also in the older person.

Alteration in body function or appearance usually is not an isolated problem. People are often faced with high hospital costs and long-term use of medications and prosthetic devices. The chronicity of the problem may affect the entire family. Change in body image often creates anxiety, distortion of self, self-depreciation, and mourning for a loss.[29]

This chapter will focus on (1) physical causes of alterations in body image; (2) reactions to such alterations; (3) responses to physical disability by the patient, family, health team, and community; and (4) nursing interventions and desired patient outcomes when changed body image occurs. The content of this chapter will be limited to acquired physical alterations. Please refer to pediatric texts for information about congenital problems.

PHYSICAL DISABILITY AND CHANGE IN BODY IMAGE

The nature of the change causing altered body image may include (1) altered appearance; (2) altered patterns of eating, breathing, communicating, and eliminating; (3) action and motion limitation; (4) deformity; (5) discomfort; (6) stigma; (7) social isolation; and (8) vocational threat.

ALTERED STRUCTURE: CHANGE IN FUNCTION AND APPEARANCE

Physical disability is often associated with a change in body image. Physical changes in body structure may be temporary or permanent. An example of a temporary change is a temporary colostomy, which may be done for a variety of reasons such as diverticulitis or gunshot injuries. Many patients tolerate the change because it is temporary. Problems in management of the physical care can develop, however, when a patient refuses to participate in self-care because the change is temporary. Additional problems may develop if the temporary

RESEARCH

Baxley K et al: Alopecia: effect on cancer patients' body image, Cancer Nurs 7(6):499-503, 1984.

Alopecia is felt by many cancer patients to be the most traumatic side effect of chemotherapy. Because hair contributes substantially to an individual's body image, it is likely that alopecia should alter the person's body image. A body image scale administered to 40 cancer patients receiving chemotherapy differentiated the body image of patients with and without alopecia, confirming the predicted response. ▪

change becomes permanent.[20] The major problems requiring body image alteration are the result of permanent changes in structure. These alterations may be readily visible, as in an amputation of an extremity, in alopecia, or in facial disfigurement, or they may be invisible, as in impaired cardiac function after myocardial infarction.

Physical disability can cause loss of function or change in appearance or both. Loss of function occurs in paraplegia, hemiplegia, and chronic renal failure. Partial loss of function occurs in chronic respiratory insufficiency and chronic cardiac disease. Renal, respiratory, and cardiac problems show relatively few visible signs of their presence until the problems are far advanced. Appearance is modified in paraplegia as the muscles of the legs atrophy and contractures occur. Facial muscles may droop, and the hands may appear flaccid or spastic on the affected side of a patient with hemiplegia. Change in appearance without loss of function occurs with a traumatic injury to the external ear that leaves hearing unimpaired and with facial scarring after multiple lacerations received in an automobile accident. Enucleation of the eye and amputation of an extremity cause marked changes in both function and appearance.

While some physical changes are immediately visible, some must be disclosed during the activities required to replace the functional loss or to improve appearance. A patient with chronic renal failure who requires hemodialysis two or three times a week cannot hide this fact except from strangers. The person with an artificial eye, ear, or nose may under some circumstances, such as hospitalization, be forced to share this information.

Although health care professionals often discuss and initiate intervention for body image alteration following traumatic injuries, cancer surgeries (mastectomies, laryngectomies, colostomies), and paralysis, it is important to remember that obesity, pregnancy, and aging also result in body image alteration. Nathan[38] found

SELECTED CAUSES OF BODY IMAGE ALTERATIONS

Injuries from accidents and war
    Amputation
    Burns: scars and contractures
    Lacerations: scars

Sensorimotor system disease
    Paralysis: paraplegia, hemiplegia
    Blindness, deafness
    Parkinsonism, muscular dystrophy, multiple sclerosis

Change in body structure
    Cardiac, renal, respiratory disease
    Cushing's syndrome
    Rheumatoid arthritis
    Cancer: colostomy, ileostomy, laryngectomy
    Excessive overweight or underweight

that obese subjects failed to develop an organized, differentiated, and inner sense of self and of integrity. Wagner and Bye[56] found that patients with chemotherapy-induced alopecia refocused on spiritual values and inner worth as opposed to physical appearance.

CAUSES OF BODY IMAGE ALTERATION

Major causes of conditions that result in physical disability and altered body image are (1) injuries from accidents and war, (2) diseases of the sensorimotor systems, and (3) changes in body structure from toxic or metabolic disorders (see the box above). Body image changes related to these conditions may also include the need to incorporate prosthetic devices or a donated body part.

THE INDIVIDUAL'S RESPONSE TO BODY IMAGE CHANGES AND LOSSES

Individuals are disturbed when serious threats to or actual deficits in the structure, function, or appearance of the body occur. They must revise long-accepted assumptions about their bodies. Life patterns may need to be changed. The patient faces problems regarding work, social activities, and family. Sexual activities may require modification. Patients may believe that goodness is lost, the ability to accomplish is lost, and that valued skills and talents are impaired. They may feel they are receiving "deserved punishment." One reaction that may interfere with recovery is expectation of rejection and separation. The individual also may feel vulnerable, resigned, rebellious, defiant, rejected, dependent, avoided, resentful, timid, self-conscious, unhappy, humiliated, stigmatized, inferior, and hypersensitive. Indecision, decreased self-respect, bitterness, and cynicism also occur. The hostility of a disabled person toward the healthy may interfere with communication. The atti-

RESEARCH

Glockner MR: Perceptions of sexual attractiveness following ostomy surgery, Res Nurs Health 7:87-92, 1984.

Home interviews conducted with 40 persons who had ostomy surgery an average of 4.6 years earlier revealed that perceptions of attractiveness decreased in the first year after surgery but continued to improve with time. Most responses related to body image during the first year were negative. Women more often than men saw themselves as most sexually attractive at the time of the interview, whereas men had seen themselves as most sexually attractive before surgery. No matter when they occurred, management problems with the ostomy decreased feelings of sexual attractiveness significantly. People with ileostomies who had been ill for 10 years or more before their surgery had enhanced feelings of sexual attractiveness at the time of the interview when compared to those persons with other types of surgeries and lengths of illness. ∎

tudes of disabled persons toward themselves are more important than the nature of their disabilities.

IMPORTANT DETERMINANTS OF RESPONSES

Regardless of the body image alteration, the response of the person will depend on (1) the personal meaning and the significance of the change, (2) the responses of significant others, (3) the availability of help for the person and the family, (4) previous coping behaviors, and (5) the availability of positive role models. The outcome of the alteration in body image is also influenced by the physiologic status of the person, that is, the amount of pain present, the extent of the change or disability, and the realistic expectations of therapy. The physiologic status is relatively fixed for the specific disability; therefore this section will explore the broader psychosocial factors that are amenable to intervention by health care professionals.

MEANING OF THE CHANGE

The value the individual assigns to what was lost, the meaning the part or the function has, and the intensity of the person's feelings about the loss all influence how the individual will respond. A person may attribute successes in life to specific body features. When there is an overvaluation and reliance on security through physical beauty or activity, alteration in the body image is likely to cause severe emotional disturbances. Women appear to be less disturbed by threats to the body than men.[17] Women are often concerned about cosmetic effects.[49]

The self-concept is closely linked to sexuality and perception of body image. The response to mastectomy is in part a response to the culture's preoccupation with the breast as a symbol of femininity. This represents the integration of the ideal into the body image. Thus the loss of a breast is often followed by lowered self-esteem, postoperative depression, and concerns of psychosexual role and sexual functioning. The ability of a woman to accept the trauma of loss of her breast depends on her reactions (real, perceived, or anticipated), and the acceptance of her partner.[31,50] Her response reflects the value she assigns to the loss, rehabilitation and reinforcement from health professionals, and positive role models.

Men are often concerned about their ability to work and their earning capacity. The loss of earning power and the resultant loss of self-esteem are important determinants of family relationships. Dyk and Sutherland[8] reported that after ostomy surgery, the reduction in housework seemed to be more acceptable to wives than the reduction in gainful employment was to husbands. Most men expressed fears of dependence on spouse or children. The thought of getting old and being ill can be disabling; however, when fears of ostomy spillage and other problems are added, the older person with a stoma may view the burden as insurmountable. Work is important to a sense of achievement, and many persons express who they are in terms of their work.

Social interactions are also affected. Dropkin[13] reported that social interactions decreased after head and neck surgery as the deformity became more pronounced. To varying degrees everyone has a need to feel that the presentation of one's body is acceptable to others. The person who has sustained facial alterations may feel isolated, excluded, stigmatized, helpless, or ashamed. Physical unattractiveness is often associated with social devaluation, denied opportunities, inaccurate judgments of worth, and low self-esteem. The individual with a low need for social approval does not rely as heavily on others to maintain body image, but a low need for social approval does not preclude fear of social rejection. This individual, however, may show earlier signs of integration through early efforts toward self-care.[13]

RESEARCH

Sutherland S: Burned adolescents' descriptions of their coping strategies. Heart Lung 17(2):150-157, 1988.

Lazarus' model of problem-focused and emotion-focused coping is used to describe the strategies employed by eight adolescents in response to the physical changes caused by burns. A semistructured interview was used, and the investigator identified themes in the responses that were classified as problem- or emotion-focused. The identification of such responses supports anticipatory guidance and planning for nursing interventions. ■

The meaning of the disability is also influenced by the expected duration of the change and its permanency. A body image alteration resulting from a diagnosis of cancer involves the fear of recurrence or death. The alteration in the body function or structure may be of lesser significance if the person equates the change with an extension or saving of life.

The rapidity of onset is another variable, and a sudden unexpected change may be devastating. A traumatic injury that results in sudden loss of mobility may completely alter a person's life goals; for example, a football player with a spinal cord injury must find a new career in addition to coping with everything else. A slow, progressive change, as in rheumatoid arthritis or chronic ulcerative colitis, may allow time for anticipatory mourning.

The source of the change, its type, and the opinions of others are important. Hirschfield and Behan[25] describe acceptable and unacceptable disability following accidents. Changes resulting from heroic sacrifice are viewed differently from changes resulting from socially unacceptable activities. The loss of a leg saving a comrade in battle is viewed quite differently from loss of a leg in a motorcycle accident during a high-speed chase from the scene of a crime. Sterility following venereal disease may be viewed as deserved punishment, whereas sterility caused by exposure to prescribed radiation therapy carries no stigma. The cause of the disability (active combat injury versus the sequelae of venereal disease), the type of disability (paralysis versus weakness or anxiety), and the opinion of others (sympathy versus scorn) make a difference in the meaning of disability.

RESPONSES OF SIGNIFICANT OTHERS

Satisfactory social adaptation to a body change depends to a great extent on family relationships and cultural attitudes toward the body structure involved. The sociocultural milieu plays an important role in the acceptance of the change.

What are the attitudes of others, including parents, siblings, and peers, toward physical disability? The sociocultural milieu is important. What are the specific body values of the subculture of the patient? What prejudices are there that are related to wholeness, independence, and attractiveness?

Does stigma accompany the change? A stigma is an attribute that is deeply discrediting. Goffman[21] discusses the idea of being discredited (having a disability fairly readily noted) and being discreditable (having a disability that may be discovered).

Myths and misconceptions abound regarding one whose body is scarred or misshapen by disease or is distorted during movement. There is an overabundance of largely unfounded opinion and folklore regarding physical disability. A strange belief exists that suffering and misfortune somehow make one "a better person." It is also believed that the disabled person mysteriously develops untapped assets and achieves a new depth of understanding and sensitivity.

HELP AVAILABLE TO PATIENT AND FAMILY

How a client deals with the loss may well depend on the kind of help available. The help available from the health team and specifically the nurse's role in helping clients with altered body image is discussed later in this chapter. Much of the outcome will depend on whether the client can and does make use of the help offered.

The rehabilitation program generally has as its goal the recovery of physical function. Psychosocial diagnoses and psychosocial therapy are often secondary. Consider the person needing rehabilitation as a complete person with a partial disability. Make attempts to strengthen the individual's inner resources and the relationship between the individual and the immediate family. A family assessment should be made and family therapy instituted, if necessary.

The family needs help from health care providers to be supportive during this time of change. The reactions of patients discussed earlier also apply to the family. Their reaction will depend on the meaning of the threat, their coping patterns, available resources, and positive role models. They also are frightened by the altered appearance of the patient or the loss of function. They wonder and speculate about the significance of the change on their lives. Since their response plays a significant role for the patient in the integration of the body image alteration and rehabilitation, the family cannot be ignored.

Patient care conferences that involve physicians, nurses, social workers, and the family are extremely beneficial in delineating the reality of the situation and the available resources. Rehabilitation centers often use these conferences appropriately when the patient is admitted. More acute care centers are holding patient care conferences throughout the patient's hospitalization. Involvement of the patient and family is encouraged.

COPING BEHAVIORS

Health problems have different meanings at different stages in the life cycle; however, the same problem may be perceived quite differently by persons of the same age. By 4 years of age body image is becoming stabilized and can be affected by body changes. Special care must be taken to assess a child's perception of body image, because it influences personality organization and ego strength. The level of psychosocial development, the quality of the child's relationship with the parents, and previous adjustment are important. In adolescence the body image undergoes a massive upheaval. Physical

changes in the body as a result of accident or illness place an enormous strain on the coping abilities of the young person. Surgical intervention for congenital craniofacial lesions *before* school age is more likely to allow for normal development of body image.[35]

The young adult needs independence. The nurse who "does for" the young adult rather than permitting self-care may precipitate conflicts. Young war veterans with disabling injuries experienced at a time of high physical abilities find adjustment very difficult, and aggressive behavior is common. Concern for sexual identity is prominent. Older persons face the changes of aging: physical deterioration, social losses, and death. Esberger[14] describes a phenomenon known as "body monitoring" found most often in older persons, because the body at this time requires more care to maintain adequate performance. Because older persons have more health problems, they often require daily medications, more frequent contacts with health care agencies, special diets, and prosthetic aids. It often becomes more difficult for the older person to maintain activities and hobbies that contribute to a positive self-concept.

As a result of their life history, all persons have a well-developed and predictable pattern of coping with threats, real or perceived. Some people immediately begin to problem solve, looking for alternatives; others are immobilized and require help to return to a balance.[54]

POSITIVE ROLE MODELS

The use of positive role models in the rehabilitation plan following body image alteration has increased significantly. Trained visitation programs sponsored by the American Cancer Society have resulted in Reach to Recovery, Ostomy Visitors, and Laryngectomy Visitors. The value of visitors and self-help groups is readily apparent in the growth of these services around the country.

Patients gain from talking with someone who has been through a similar situation and has coped and adapted well. One important aspect is the timing of the visit. The nurse needs to assess each person carefully and offer the choice of a preoperative or postoperative visit. The visitor should be close to the patient's age and have had a similar diagnosis and surgery. Most important, the visitor should have reached a successful level of rehabilitation, know how to talk with others, and be prepared for a mixed reaction from the patient.

ADAPTIVE RESPONSES

Those responses in which the patient works through and accepts the loss are considered adaptive. Any situation perceived by a person as resulting in a major body change and profoundly affecting body image may precipitate a crisis. Most commonly the period of crisis is followed by unrealistic defenses, gradual acceptance, and then reduction of the problem to manageable proportions. Responses depend on the number and intensity of the stresses in comparison to the degree of emotional support and the strength of personal attributes. Patients are helped to meet the challenge of disability if they are mature and secure from the start. An acute sense of proportion helps them recognize reality. A sense of humor helps them live with reality. The urge to fight back and pick up the pieces of an interrupted life may motivate the patient. Hunt[26] has edited a series of essays written by persons with disabilities that provide profound insights into their perceptions of living with disability.

Several authors note that the loss of a valued body part or function is followed by a period of reaction and adjustment that can be compared to the grief and mourning process that follows the death of a loved one (see also Chapter 13). Grief is the subjective state of one who has sustained the loss of a valued object, in this instance, physical function or body appearance or both. Mourning is the psychologic process by which one works through to acceptance (ideally) of the loss. The subjective reactions to grief include helplessness, loneliness, hopelessness, sadness, guilt, and anger. Mourning usually leads to relinquishing that which was lost. Eventually the person looks at the past realistically and comfortably.

Rubin[46] describes the losses associated with body image change as the loss of the *capacity for functioning* and the loss of the capacity for *control of functioning* in time and place. A sense of shame accompanies such losses. This reaction reflects a private judgment of failure. The intensity of the emotional response seems to be related to the intensity of the struggle to maintain control.

An individual facing a real or threatened change or loss may experience several stages of grieving, including (1) shock and panic, (2) defensive retreat, (3) acknowledgment, and (4) adaptation. During the first stage the person may be unable to understand or comprehend the event, its meanings, and its implications. During defensive retreat the person acknowledges the event but is unable to cope with the meaning and implications. The retreat provides time and distance and may appear as denial. Acknowledgment is the recognition of the reality of the situation, its meaning, and its significance. Adaptation is the integration of the change or loss in a way that is supportive of functional living. The person is realistic about the event, its meaning, and its significance.

The reactions of individuals are different throughout the grief process. Some people may lack initiative during shock, have high energy levels during panic, and demonstrate goal-directed behavior later. Other people may feel helpless, angry, guilty, or lost.

MALADAPTIVE RESPONSES

When a person is unable to accept the reality of the situation, the response is maladaptive. Patients may deny the change in appearance or the loss of function. They may completely deny the change, may appear withdrawn and aloof, may joke and laugh, or may present a pseudo-self-confidence. They may use a variety of defense mechanisms such as denial, projection, repression, or regression.

The loss may be acknowledged, but its significance denied and the situation intellectualized. The person may project concern onto others: "My wife is very upset about my having to change jobs." Tasks may be avoided. Overcompensation for the loss may occur. Patients may project hostile feelings that interfere with acceptance. The resumption of a social, sexual, and emotional life may be impossible. Some may reject others out of a fear of being rejected themselves.[27]

Some persons may try to hide the disability to forget it, and they often pay a high price for such a futile endeavor. Exaggerated independence, overdependence, and pseudocooperation are responses that interfere with the necessary acceptance of help from the family and health care team.

Occasionally, the disability may be used as a crutch, and if the defect is corrected, problems may occur. For example, a person may attribute failures in life to an external facial feature; when this feature is changed by plastic surgery, the person may be forced to examine the realities. A similar situation may exist after changes resulting from illness and injury, and in both cases extreme emotional upsets are possible.

Another strategy is to focus attention on a healthy part to deny or shut out the damaged part. Idealizing normal standards commits the disabled person to repeated feelings of inferiority. On the other hand, overidentification with the disabled may limit efforts toward achievable levels of rehabilitation. The patient may use the disability as the excuse for early retirement. A return to work can thus be avoided. Another defensive response is the illusion of restoration of the part (phantom). A complete rejection of reality is a psychotic response and may require intense therapy.

The effects of the disability may spread beyond the specific structure, function, or change in appearance to other areas of life and activity and increase the patient's limitations. Perceptions of being incompetent, unlovable, insecure, and unworthy reflect low self-esteem. The person's perception of the situation, the responses received from others, and previous experience with losses determine the level of self-esteem and affect coping mechanisms.

The initial response of the family to the loss depends on many factors already discussed, The *rapidity of onset,* the *specific loss,* and *its meaning* are especially important. The patient is the center of attention, and the family is unified by dread, numbness, a sense of unreality, and the shared threat of loss. During the time the patient is denying the situation, the family may also be denying it. Fear and anger may be directed at the staff. The family may lose interest and patience. They may urge the patient to make a more rapid recovery.

The *degree and quality of support* are important. Sometimes families deal well with the immediate threat but have difficulty with the kinds of long-term help needed. The family must acknowledge the change in the patient, their way of life, and the patient's reactions. Family conflicts over the prescribed regimen occur. Families may use the patient's changed state to keep the patient dependent. Rejection by the family complicates the life of a disabled person. The family may attempt to conceal the defect by avoiding and isolating the patient. They may be angry, blaming, and rejecting or indifferent. Ambivalence is not uncommon.

The family must acknowledge the change in the patient and deal with changes in the interpersonal reactions within the family. Constructive, supportive attitudes in the family increase the possibilities for successful adaptation and for compensatory development without personality disorder. As patients move to reorganize their lives, their families should reexamine interactions, modify living arrangements, encourage social activities, and try to improve family relationships.

OTHERS' RESPONSES TO BODY IMAGE ALTERATIONS

COMMUNITY RESPONSES

Society values youth and beauty, attractive facial features, physical wholeness, and activeness. Social discrimination against those who are different is common. Physical disability provokes stereotyped responses in the public. The type of deformity rather than its severity evokes the stereotypic response. Subtle and overt negative reactions occur. Repulsion, revulsion, rejection, contempt, ridicule, taunts, discrimination, patronizing aversion, tactless curiosity, staring, questioning, and devaluing pity are frequent.

Goffman[21] describes two sets of sympathetic others: those who share the stigma and the "wise" who are normal but are acquainted intimately with the secret life of the stigmatized. The latter includes family members and professional persons involved in the patient's care.

Reactions to one who is physically disabled may range from overly sympathetic to unsympathetic. Because one takes on the attitude of others toward one's body, negative feelings already present about one's body may be reinforced by society.

Visible handicaps alter social and psychologic functioning in important ways. Confronting a damaged face disrupts one's sense of inner security. The thought of disfigurement or scarring causes fear of public reaction in most people, and not without cause. Social ostracism is a real possibility. Physical disability is accompanied by a fear of being unable to perform one's regular routines and the fear of loss of control. If the disability is not visible, it may not be considered important by others.

The part of the body that is lost or nonfunctioning will also influence the reactions of others. People are usually very uncomfortable discussing ostomies or the wearing of a pouch. Loss of sexual function is not usually easily accepted. Others will often respond with comments such as "he should be thankful he's alive," showing a lack of concern for the values of the individual.

Some disabilities are more acceptable than others. Breast cancer and mastectomies have received recent national television coverage. Several movies have been made about recoveries following spinal cord injuries. Recovery from drug abuse has made headlines as television stars seek help for drug and alcohol problems. Yet there are many other disabilities that are poorly understood by the public.

Attitudes toward body structures affect responses to those with physical disabilities. The attitudes of well people affect the social adaptation of those with body defects. Disapproval may be present when those persons with disability do not appear to be helping themselves. Generalized indifference rejects the reality of the person facing real threats. Studies show that women are more accepting of persons with disabilities than men are, whereas adolescents are less accepting than those of college age. No significant difference in attitude was found according to socioeconomic status.

HEALTH TEAM RESPONSES

Members of the health care team are not immune to negative attitudes toward the disabled. They may subscribe to certain stereotypes, especially with regard to sexual functioning in persons with disabilities. Condescension, resentment, insensitivity, and aloofness can be found in those "dedicated to help." The health team may expect a passive, compliant, dependent patient. They may feel protective, or they may react with superiority. Examples of negative attitudes are reflected in the use of such labels as "unmotivated" as justification for closing a case. The use of stereotype labels—"CPs," "CVAs," "quads"—reflects obvious disregard for the individuality of the patient. The reactions of health professionals may include embarrassment, undefined anxiety, relief if the patient is cheerful, abandonment by disregarding stress signals, and maintenance of a superficial atmosphere to being thoughtful, understanding, and helpful. Anger at being unable to help is a recurring phenomenon.

Health professionals can contribute to a patient's

lowered self-esteem when they express openly or covertly negative reactions to the change in structure, function, or appearance. A patient's loss of control threatens the health professional's control. Sarcasm covered with saccharine sweetness and teasing may be signs of displaced anger. People reject what they cannot cope with, and they may withdraw from the situation. Health professionals should honestly explore their feelings toward the patient with body changes.

Little investigation of health care team attitudes has been done. This is unfortunate, because the health care team probably is more important in shaping the patient's response than any other group.[33] Persons who work with the disabled should try to be as sensitive and perceptive as possible about their own responses to disability and the disabled and about the patient's emotional reactions to problems. Recently, group experiences have been made possible so that health care providers can explore their feelings and be better able to facilitate rehabilitation. Specialization in certain areas has occurred within nursing as people identify those patients with whom they are best capable of working. Values clarification is one method of helping nurses identify their values and the effect of personal values on the care provided.

NURSING PROCESS FOR PERSONS WITH ALTERED BODY IMAGE

Persons with changes in structure, function, and appearance face problems related to (1) physical limitations and failures; (2) discomfort from appliances, abnormal sensations, and fatigue; (3) visual or auditory perception changes; (4) vocational and economic limitations; and (5) social interaction limitations.

■ ASSESSMENT

Bernstein and Cope[3] have delineated six axes for adjustment to disability: (1) active coping—passive surrender; (2) leading and comanaging treatment—resisting treatment; (3) loving exchange—rage; (4) denial—overawareness; (5) adaptive defenses—maladaptive defenses; and (6) mental (activity) mode—physical (activity) mode. Along each axis are important variables. Complex interwoven patterns form within a matrix of factors including money, education, family support, religious help, and rehabilitation services. Bernstein and Cope have found this framework helpful in looking at the catastrophe of burn disfigurement.

The patient's perception of the situation and usual pattern of adapting must be considered in planning nursing intervention. How does the patient deal with stress? What threats are seen as dangerous? What are the patient's goals? Consider the patient's personality, values, needs, and readiness for learning.

Does the patient cry? If not, consider the following possibilities. The patient cannot cry or does not want to cry, or perhaps feels no need to cry. Usually, however, there is ambivalence with feelings of guilt and shame.

Recognize the energy used to handle the enforced awareness of the disability. Be aware of how far the patient has come and the distance yet to go.

Appraise the response of family members and significant others. Identify the patient's support systems—those people and resources that may assist during the period of adaptation. Consider the importance of the patient's peers.

Transitional points of entry and termination are critical points of emotional adjustment—they reflect periods of change. The move from rehabilitation center to home for a patient with paraplegia or the first hemodialysis treatment at home for a patient with chronic renal failure are examples of such points.

The nurse's ability to assess accurately the patient's response and adaptation to loss requires an understanding of (1) the visibility of the loss, (2) the loss of function, and (3) the patient's emotional investment in the part affected.[12] This information is useful in predicting (1) the patient's and the family's coping abilities, (2) the nature of assistance needed for adaptation, and (3) the identification of those persons who can provide the assistance.

■ DATA ANALYSIS: NURSING DIAGNOSES

Diagnostic Title	Possible Etiology
Body image disturbance	Changes or losses in body structure, function, or appearance, for example, injuries from accidents or war; sensorimotor system diseases; other major organ system diseases

■ PLANNING: EXPECTED PATIENT OUTCOMES

1. The patient effectively integrates the change in body image into his or her self-concept.
2. The patient exhibits positive attitudes toward rehabilitation, the staff, and the program of help.
3. The family supports patient efforts to deal with altered structure, function, and appearance.

■ IMPLEMENTATION

Nursing care is important during the *acute, convalescent,* and *rehabilitative* phases following disability. During the acute phase the nursing focus is on activities such as life-saving techniques, assisting with diagnosis, and preoperative and postoperative care. Most frequently the patient is hospitalized. The goal is to save life, halt illness, and to prevent helplessness and deformity.

During the convalescent phase nursing activities in-

ADAPTATION PROCESS

I. Shock and panic (message: "Oh!")
A. Shock
  1. Critical issue: the mind is communicating an inability to integrate the critical event, its meaning, and its implications.
  2. Thought process: immobilized, devoid of problem-solving ability, decision making difficult.
  3. Physical behavior: immobilized, responsive primarily to external suggestions. May have difficulty caring for self. (At times, the individual may appear to be functional in problem solving and self-care because "automatic" survival response occurs.)
  4. Affect: blunted or devoid of affect.
  5. Intervention: dependent on an accurate assessment of the individual's mental, physical, and affectual status. Individuals in shock respond to directive interventions and supports that provide for very basic physical and psychosocial needs.
B. Panic
  1. Critical issue: the mind is communicating an inability to integrate the event, its meaning, and its implications.
  2. Thought process: scattered thoughts, often tangential in nature. They may also be in the form of "racing thoughts," numerous, constant, repetitive questioning with limited or no ability to integrate answers or data in response to questioning.
  3. Physical behavior: extensive energy release through nondirected or non–goal-oriented behavior; high-level motor activity.
  4. Affect: obviously anxious.
  5. Intervention: Allow opportunity for physical release and expression of energy and anxiety. Provide very calm, accepting environment. Provide appropriate intervention for client safety.

II. Defensive retreat (message: "No")
A. Critical issue: the mind is communicating an acknowledgment of the critical event or situation and an inability to integrate or cope with the affectual meaning and implications of the event. The retreat acts as a time and distance maneuver, allowing the individual the space and opportunity to integrate the psychosocial impact of the critical event.
B. Thought process: denial is an unconscious process that protects the individual from further intrusion of fearful or threatening implications related to the critical event. Specific information related to the critical situation or the event itself may be negated as nonexistent. In rationalization/intellectualization the critical event and related information are treated with seeming objectivity and distance. Request for information is seemingly appropriate to resolution of the "problem."
C. Physical behavior: appears goal-directed, reasonable and logical excepting those areas of information that may be negated as nonexistent with denial.
D. Affect: may appear to be minimal or at least cautiously covered. Affectual responses of fear or anxiety minimally acknowledged.
E. Intervention: acknowledge to yourself as therapist that significant affect is being defended against, not that information has not been received. Do not challenge the areas of information being denied or negated. This will only precipitate the strengthening of this defense. Acknowledge to the individual the normalcy of his difficulty in integrating this "confusing and upsetting" information and your willingness to be available to discuss feelings. Provide open-ended opportunities for feeling expression without being intrusive. Use feeling words that are nonspecific and nondiagnostic in encouraging feeling expression, for example, "You seem a bit confused or upset by all this information" rather than "You seem to be denying very important aspects of your diagnosis and treatment." It is imperative that the therapist keep in mind that effective feeling expression will diminish the need for defensive retreat mechanisms. Often time and distance (if realistic to the critical nature of the situation) will themselves give the individual the opportunity to integrate the meaning and implications of the critical situation.

III. Acknowledgment (message: "Yes, but I don't want it!")
A. Critical issue: the mind has integrated the critical event, its meaning, and its implications in a way that is supportive of functional living.
B. Thought process: equilibrium has returned, effective problem solving is in process, learning of new information related to the integration of the situation is more possible.
C. Physical behavior: returned to previous function with the integration of necessary alterations related to critical change or loss.
D. Affect: hopeful and realistic. Life is now worth living. Feelings of sadness and anger may be experienced from time to time, but the individual is not immobilized or ruled by his feelings.
E. Intervention: effective teaching and learning may now occur. Anticipate with the individual the possibility of emotional upset in the future, which is normal rather than regressive. Be available over time (4 to 6 months at least) for further follow-up and exploration of the adjustment process.

From Sultenfuss S: Psychosocial issues and therapeutic intervention, In Broadwell DC and Jackson BS: Principles of ostomy case, St Louis, 1982, The CV Mosby Co.

clude assisting the patient to adjust to change; maintaining physical abilities through occupational therapy and physical therapy; and home planning with the family, community health nurse, and social worker. During this phase patients may still be hospitalized, but some individuals may be at home. The goal is to prepare for the rehabilitative phase. Patient education plays an important role in the rehabilitation of persons with altered body image. Patients need the information necessary for self-care to recognize signs and symptoms of potential problems and to identify which person to see for additional supportive services.

Rehabilitation includes the coordination of a number of specialized services. Rehabilitation should focus on physical, social, emotional, and sexual aspects of the person's life. The patient's response and needs will vary in each stage of adaptation (see box on p. 413). Assist the patient in identifying reasonable goals and objectives; then carefully plan ways of implementing a sequence of events that will enable the person to complete the goals successfully.

The person with a disability needs understanding. Assume that such patients are coping with an overwhelming experience, support the self-esteem necessary for them to reorganize the body image, and permit crying in such a manner that patients still have a sense of self-respect and worthiness. Give patients time, and help them confront the problem in manageable steps. Acknowledge appropriate feelings, recognize assets and strengths, and provide support to the extent needed, that is, the degree mutually agreed upon.

Let the patient ventilate, helping clarify misconceptions. Promote a sense of trust, respect, security, and comfort. It is essential for the patient to come to terms with the change. Reassurance that "you'll be as good as new" delays adjustment and raises false hopes. Do not encourage the patient to blame others; rather, assist the patient to accept help with everyday tasks. Counteract the effects of deprivation and immobilization by helping the patient understand what is occurring and by maintaining the remaining body integrity. The focus of care is on what is left—not what is lost.

Be accepting within appropriate limits. Assure the patient that grief is normal. The patient must also accept the fact that permanently unattainable goals exist. Privacy and a safe environment are necessary for the patient to achieve control of a lost or altered body function. Avoid overprotection and unnecessary restrictions. Work on exploring realistic alternatives rather than being overly optimistic or pessimistic. Help the patient find the facts, since speculating can be worse than the truth. Help the patient develop compensatory personality traits.

Predict the occurrence of body image problems, prevent them where possible, and be ready to intervene to help solve them when necessary. Anticipatory guidance and preventive intervention help to promote the capacity of individuals to cope with life crises. Prepare patients before surgery or before receiving drugs that alter body image. Consider various influencing factors. Recognize the need for grief and mourning. Help the patient strengthen both coping mechanisms and problem-solving skills.

HEALTH CARE TEAM

All the health team members must work through their feelings regarding loss, disability, and disfigurement, and examine their behaviors used in coping with such threats. If this conscious self-examination is omitted, feelings and behaviors may interfere with the patient's rehabilitation and may result in the professional's leaving this field of service. Staff responses to persons with disability should be honest, patient, consistent, realistic, and firm, but not hostile. Often they must accept the patient despite his hostility and rejection toward them. Every effort must be made to avoid reinforcing the person's low self-esteem. Special preparation is needed for open, honest discussion of the patient's problems with sexuality. Consistent support promotes the trust vital to learning to cope with altered structure, function, and appearance.

EVALUATION

Positive attitudes of the patient toward rehabilitation, the staff, and program of help are desirable. Acceptance and use of prosthetic devices are expected. Desired patient outcomes include self-assurance, confident behavior, self-reliance, stable motivation, self-acceptance, and adequate social interactions. It is generally accepted that a person is happier if involved in productive activities.

Siller[52] suggests that one outcome measure of the acceptance of the loss is the degree that the reconstituted self is oriented toward self-approval and is responsive to reality.

Some dependency may be legitimate, and some physical help may be needed. Retirement from gainful employment may be required, or reduced household responsibilities and a sharp curtailment of social activities may be unavoidable.

Litman's study[30] of family disruption because of disability shows no significant relationship between the degree of family solidarity and rehabilitation response. However, family support during rehabilitation has a significant effect on the patient's response to the program. The family consequently reexamines and probably reorients interpersonal relationships and readjusts living arrangements.

Employment, school attendance, or home responsibilities are insufficient measures of outcomes for many patients. Areas to be considered include cognition, activities of daily living, home activities, activities outside the home, and social interaction. Evaluation is best accomplished after the patient is discharged. Many tools have been designed to assist in measuring body image, but there is no one tool that adequately measures the whole of body image.[15] Most tools measure body perception or body attitude. Body perception is the mental experience of the body's physical appearance. Body attitude reflects feelings, attitudes, and emotional reaction toward the body. Champion, Austin, and Tzeng[10] examined self-concept and body image for their interrelationships to provide a base for developing nursing interventions. Since patients are not regularly tested, behavioral responses are usually used to evaluate the effectiveness of the integration of a change in body image. A therapeutic relationship established early in the rehabilitative phase is often beneficial in evaluating change.

The change in body image does not occur quickly. Adaptation to a change may take a year or longer, but that does not signify maladaptation. The integration of a new mental image takes time and a reorganization of thoughts and images.

CHAPTER SUMMARY

- Body image is a dynamic, changing perception.
- Changes in structure, function, and appearance require modification in body image.
- The patient's perception of the situation and pattern of coping affect his or her responses.
- The family's response and ability to support the patient are important to outcomes.
- The patient and family responses determine the nature of assistance needed.
- Adaptation to changes in body image takes time.

QUESTIONS TO CONSIDER

- How might a patient's response differ if a below-the-knee amputation was caused by a motor vehicle accident as compared with a similar amputation for diabetic gangrene in one foot?
- How might the family response differ if the cause of a patient's altered function was related to alcoholism versus long-term employment in a textile mill?
- What interventions might be particularly useful for a patient scheduled for an ileostomy?

REFERENCES AND SELECTED READINGS

1. Baird SE: Development of a nursing diagnosis assessment tool to diagnose altered body image in immobilized patients, Orthop Nurs 4(1):47-54, 1985.
2. Baxley KO et al: Alopecia: effect on patients' body image, Cancer Nurs 7(6):499-503, 1984.
3. Bernstein NR and Cope O: Emotional care of the facially burned and disfigured, Boston, 1976, Little, Brown & Co.
4. Brundage DJ: Self-concept alterations: theory and assessment. In Thelan LT, Urden LD, and Davies JK, editors: Nursing diagnosis in critical care, St Louis, 1990, The CV Mosby Co.
5. *Darlington-Fisher CS: Impairment of body image. In Jacobs M and Geels W: Signs and symptoms: interpretations and management, Philadelphia, 1985, JB Lippincott Co.
6. Derogatis LR: The unique impact of breast and gynecologic cancers on body image and sexual identity in women: a reassessment. In Vaeth JM, editor, Body image, self-esteem, and sexuality in cancer patients, ed 2, Basel, 1986, Karger.
7. Diekmann JM: Measuring body image. In Frank-Stromberg M: Instruments for clinical nursing research, Norwalk, Conn, 1988, Appleton & Lange.
8. Dyk RB and Sutherland A: Adaptation of the spouse and other family members to the colostomy patient, CA 9:123-125, 1956.
9. Canaday ME: Anorexia nervosa: distorted body image, Issues in Health Care of Women 3:281-286, 1981.
10. Champion VS, Austin JK, and Tzeng, O: Assessment of relationship between self-concept and body image using multivariate techniques, Issues in Mental Health Nursing 4:(4):299-315, 1982.
11. Compton CY: War injury: identity crisis for young men, Nurs Clin North Am 8:53-66, 1973.
12. *Donovan MI and Pierce SG: Cancer care nursing, Norwalk, Conn, 1984, Appleton & Lange.
13. Dropkin MJ: Rehabilitation after disfigurative facial surgery. Plast Surg Nurs 5(4):130-134, 1985.
14. Esberger K: Body image, J Gerontol Nurs 4(4):35-38, 1978.
15. Fawcett J and Frye S: An exploratory study of body image dimensionally, Nurs Res 29:324-327, 1980.
16. Fawcett J et al: Spouses' body image changes during and after pregnancy: a replication and extension. Nurs Res 35(4):220-223, 1986.
17. Fisher S: Body experience in fantasy and behavior, New York, 1970, Appleton-Century-Crofts.
18. Fujita MT: The impact of illness or surgery on the body image of the child, Nurs Clin North Am 7:641-649, 1972.
19. Garrett JF and Levine ES: Rehabilitation practices with the physically disabled, New York, 1973, Columbia University Press.
20. Glockner MR: Perceptions of sexual attractiveness following ostomy surgery, Res Nurs Health 7(2):87-92, 1984.
21. Goffman E: Stigma: notes on the management of spoiled identity, Englewood Cliffs, NJ, 1963, Prentice-Hall.
22. Goin JM and Goin MK: Changing the body: psychological effects of plastic surgery, Baltimore, 1981, Williams & Wilkins.
23. Gruendemann BJ: Problems of physical self: loss. In Roy SC: Introduction to nursing: an adaptation model, Englewood Cliffs, NJ, 1976, Prentice-Hall.
24. Harris R: Cultural differences in body perception during pregnancy, Br J Med Psychol 52:347-352, 1970.
25. Hirschfield AH and Behan RC: The accident process: disability, acceptable and unacceptable, JAMA 197:85-89, 1966.
26. Hunt P, editor: Stigma: the experience of disability, London, 1966, Geoffrey Chapman Publishers.

*References preceded by an asterisk are particularly well suited for student reading.

27. Kaplan SP: Some psychological and social factors present in the condition of obesity, J Rehabil 45(3):52-54, 1979.

28. *Lacey JH and Birtchnell SA: Review article: body image and its disturbances. J Psychoso Res 30(6):623-631, 1986.

29. Liss JL: Psychiatric issues in ostomy management. In Broadwell DC and Jackson BS: Principles of ostomy care, St Louis, 1982, The CV Mosby Co.

30. Litman TJ: The family and physical rehabilitation, J Chronic Dis 19:211-217, 1966.

31. May HJ: Psychosexual sequelae to mastectomy: implications for therapeutic and rehabilitative intervention, J Rehabil 46(1):29-31, 1970.

32. McCrea CW, Summerfield AB, and Rosen B: Body image: a selective review of existing measurement techniques, J Med Psychol 55:225-233, 1982.

33. McDaniel JW: Physical disability and human behavior, New York, 1969, Pergamon Press Inc.

34. Mital MA, and Peirce DS: Amputees and their prostheses, Boston, 1971, Little, Brown & Co.

35. Murray J et al: Twenty year experience in maxillocraniofacial surgery, Ann Surg 190:320-331, 1979.

36. *Murray RLE: Body image development in adulthood, Nurs Clin North Am 7:617-630, 1972.

37. *Murray RLE: Principles of nursing intervention for the adult patient with body image changes, Nurs Clin North Am 7:697-707, 1972.

38. Nathan S: Body image in chronically obese children as reflected in figure drawings, J Pers Assess 37:456-463, 1973.

39. Noles SW, Cash TF, and Winstead BA: Body image, physical attractiveness and depression, J Consult Clinical Psychol 53(1):88-94, 1985.

40. Norris CM: The professional nurse and body image. In Carlson CE: Behavioral concepts and nursing intervention, ed 2, Philadelphia, 1979, JB Lippincott Co.

41. *O'Brien J: Mirror, mirror, why me? Nurs Mirror 150(17):36-37, 1980.

42. *Platzner H: Body image—a problem for intensive care patients (Part 1), Intensive Care Nurs 3:61-66, 1987.

43. *Platzner H: Body image (Part 2): Helping patients to cope with changes—a problem for nurses, Intensive Care Nurs 3:125-132, 1987.

44. *Price B: Body image: keeping up appearances. Nurs Times Oct 1:58-61, 1986.

45. Roberts SL: Behavioral concepts and the critically ill patient, ed 2 Norwalk, Conn, 1986, Appleton & Lange.

46. Rubin R: Body image and self esteem, Nurs Outlook 16:20-23, 1968.

47. Safilios-Rothschild C: The sociology and social psychology of disability and rehabilitation, New York, 1981, University Press of America Inc.

48. Salkin J: Body ego technique, Springfield, Ill, 1973, Charles C Thomas, Publisher.

49. Schoenburg B et al., editors: Loss and grief: psychological management in medical practice, New York, 1970, Columbia University Press.

50. Scott DW: Quality of life following the diagnosis of breast cancer, Top Clin Nurs 4(4):20-37.

51. Sekelman J: The development of body image in the child: a learned response, Top Clin Nurs 5(1):12-21.

52. Siller J: Psychosocial aspects of physical disability. In Mesilin J: Rehabilitation medicine and psychiatry, Springfield, Ill, 1976, Charles C Thomas, Publisher.

53. Smith C: Body image changes after myocardial infarction, Nurs Clin North Am 7:663-688, 1972.

54. Sultenfuss S: Psychosocial issues and therapeutic intervention. In Broadwell DC, and Jackson BS: Principles of ostomy care, St. Louis, 1982, The CV Mosby Co.

55. Sutherland S: Burned adolescents' descriptions of their coping strategies. Heart Lung 17(2):150-157, 1988.

56. Wagner L and Bye MG: Body image and patients experiencing alopecia as a result of cancer chemotherapy, Cancer Nurs 2:365-369, 1979.

57. Williamson ML: The nursing diagnosis of body image disturbance in adolescents dissatisfied with their physical characteristics. Holistic Nurs Pract 1(4):52-59, 1987.

58. Woods NF: Human sexuality in health and illness, ed 3, St Louis, 1984, The CV Mosby Co.

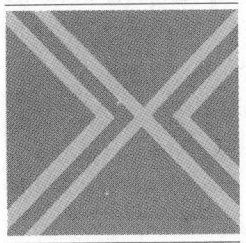

CHAPTER 19

Addictive Behaviors

ELIZABETH SCHENK

CHAPTER OBJECTIVES

After studying this chapter, the student should be able to:
1 Name four negative compulsions that are considered addictions.
2 Define the difference between tolerance (behavioral, pharmacologic, and cross tolerance) and dependence (physical, psychological, and cross-dependence).
3 Name one legal effort and one educational effort to prevent alcoholism and chemical dependency.
4 Define the terms *enabling* and *intervention*.
5 State two theories of the development of alcoholism.
6 Name five disorders directly associated with alcoholism.
7 Discuss alcohol withdrawal, including delirium tremens, and actions taken to prevent or reduce withdrawal symptoms.
8 Define drug addiction and drug habituation.
9 Name the six basic types of drugs, citing examples, how they are used, and their street names, effects and side effects, pathophysiologic factors, and symptoms of overdose.
10 Discuss why nurses are at increased risk for chemical dependency.
11 Differentiate between anorexia nervosa and bulimia nervosa.

The subject of substance abuse is gaining increased attention. Treatment centers have emerged in many localities, and growing numbers of nurses are becoming involved in this specialty. There is a recognition that substance abuse entails a complex set of behaviors that are covered under the term *addiction*. Persons may experience one or more of these addictions concurrently. An example is the alcoholic who also is a drug addict and a compulsive overeater.

Alcoholism and drug addiction are now commonly brought together under the term *chemical dependency*. This is in recognition that alcohol is a drug, and that the person addicted to alcohol also is at great risk for drug addiction.

Most modern definitions of dependence consist of two components—physical and psychological dependence. Physical dependence refers to a physiologic state where continuous and prolonged consumption of a drug or alcohol leads to the user adapting to its presence. Tolerance then develops. If use of the drug is interrupted, withdrawal symptoms occur. Psychological dependence refers to craving for the drug. See the box below for a description of terms used to describe responses to drugs and alcohol.

This chapter deals with four addictions or examples of substance abuse: drug addiction, alcoholism, eating disorders, and codependency.

ALCOHOLISM

Alcoholism is very common and may compound the problems of persons with other health disorders. Excessive alcohol intake may lead to coma or near death from acute alcohol poisoning, or if it occurs over a period of

TERMS USED TO DESCRIBE RESPONSES TO DRUGS/ALCOHOL

Tolerance	Decreased susceptibility to effects because of long-term ingestion of drugs/alcohol
Behavioral tolerance	Few changes in social behavior or activities despite ingestion of large amounts of drugs/alcohol
Pharmacologic tolerance	Adaptive metabolic changes despite ingestion of large amounts of drugs/alcohol
Cross-tolerance	Decreased sensitivity to other drugs as a result of tolerance to drugs/alcohol
Dependence	Need to continue use of drugs/alcohol to prevent symptoms
Physical dependence	Withdrawal symptoms occur when the drug/alcohol is withheld
Psychologic dependence	Need to take the drug/alcohol to prevent occurrence of symptoms
Cross-dependence	Suppression of abstinence symptoms by withdrawal of another drug

time, it may lead to numerous other health disorders. Alcoholism is recognized today as a treatable disease. Significant changes in the identification and treatment of alcoholism point toward advances that are having an important impact on this major health problem.

EPIDEMIOLOGY

Alcoholism is said to be the third major health problem in the United States. Conservative estimates are that about 90 million people use alcohol and at least 9 to 10 million persons are alcoholics or "problem drinkers." In addition, alcoholism adversely affects the mental health or functioning of another 30 million friends and relatives of alcohol abusers.[26]

It has been estimated that 70% of alcoholics are male. The number of female alcoholics, however, is increasing. Research has demonstrated that women are more likely to hide their problem drinking. In addition, women are not as likely as men to be involved in the three major systems that give external motivation for treatment (industrial programs, public intoxication and drunk driving laws, and the criminal justice intervention system).[26,32]

Industries lose at least $43 billion annually because of alcoholism. This figure includes medical expenses, lost wages, decreased industrial productivity, motor vehicle accidents, violent crime, fire loss, and social responses.[26]

The use of alcohol predates recorded history. Cultures the world over have developed their own alcoholic beverages. These beverages have been used in rites of passage, to celebrate significant events, and to mourn the dead. They have also been used as magic, medicine, and as part of worship services.

There have been many changing attitudes and laws about the use of alcoholic beverages in American history. In 1642, Maryland made drunkenness punishable by a fine. In 1790, the U.S. Government passed a law that gave every soldier a daily portion of hard liquor. In 1919, a law that prohibited the production and sale of alcoholic beverages in the United States was passed. This was repealed in 1933.[40]

Current laws concerning drunk driving focus both on the need of the person to be educated about the disease and on the need to suffer the consequences of the actions caused by the alcoholism.

ETIOLOGY

Alcohol abuse can become a problem over a long or short period of time after the beginning of excessive drinking. The alcoholic begins to develop an increasing physical dependence on and tolerance for alcohol. Drinking behavior becomes uncontrollable and secretive. Blackouts (loss of memory from episodes of drinking) may start to occur. Guilt, shame, and remorse are feelings that occur frequently; the alcoholic then drinks more to relieve such feelings. As the drinking becomes more frequent, symptoms increase and relationships with others degenerate.

THEORIES OF THE CAUSE OF ALCOHOLISM

Numerous theories have been advanced to explain the cause of alcoholism. Research is being done to advance the known knowledge about alcoholism. Thus far, no one theory can completely explain the syndrome.

Current theories can be divided into the following three main categories[40]:
1. Physiologic theories of the cause
2. Psychological theories of the cause
3. Sociocultural-etiologic theories (also known as cultural-etiologic theories)

Physiologic Theories of Etiology

These theories operate on the belief that persons are predisposed to develop alcoholism because of some organic defect.

Genetotropic-etiologic theories. These theories suggest that alcoholism is related to a genetically determined biochemical defect. The desire to drink is believed to be an inner urge mediated by the nervous system, perhaps in the hypothalamus of the brain. These nerve structures are influenced by alcohol and malnutrition.

Much research has been carried out in the past 10 years on endorphins, the body's natural opiate. There is some evidence to suggest that the alcoholic may manufacture endorphins in different amounts, as well as use them to react to drugs and alcohol differently, than other persons.[17]

Endocrine-etiologic theories. These theories hypothesize that dysfunction of the endocrine system leads to the development of alcoholism. A pituitary-adrenocortical deficiency results in hypoglycemia that is believed to cause symptoms that stimulate drinking.

Genetic theories. There is evidence that alcoholism is in part genetically determined. The incidence of alcoholism is high in families, and the risk of sons of impaired alcoholic men developing alcoholism over their lifetime is 30% to 50%.[32] Studies of twins who have been adopted also have shown that the identical twins of an alcoholic will be alcoholic in 60% of the cases, whereas only 30% of the fraternal twins of an alcoholic will be alcoholic. Studies of children of alcoholic parents who were adopted shortly after birth and reared separately from the natural parents indicate that those who were adopted had a higher rate of alcoholism than normal control subjects.[26,40]

Psychological Theories of Etiology

These theories are based on the assumption that some element in the personality structure and development leads to the development of alcoholism. Although there has been a search for the "alcoholic personality," most studies have failed to find any specific personality traits that clearly differentiate alcoholics from normal drinkers. Certain common personality traits have been identified as occurring in alcoholics. These include low stress tolerance, dependency, negative self-image, and feelings of insecurity and depression. It is not clear whether these traits precede alcoholism or are a result of it.

Oral fixation. The oral fixation theory is a psychoanalytic theory first advanced by Freud. According to this theory, trauma affects the infant in the earliest stage of psychosexual development, at a time when stimulation of the oral cavity is a method of release of tension and gaining of security. Because of an absent or uncaring mother, the infant is deprived of a warm, loving relationship with a mother figure and therefore seeks to gratify primary emotional hunger. The person becomes fixated at the oral stage of development and develops a desire for warmth and nuturing that is not satisfied in normal interpersonal relationships. The alcoholic seeks to fill this void with alcohol, which generates a sensation of warmth and satisfaction. The alcoholic's feelings of rage and anger at the parents who failed him or her are redirected at self, and, as a result of this rage, alcohol is consumed.[40]

Behavioral learning theory. This psychological model of alcoholism focuses on observable behavior and on the environmental conditions that serve to cause or maintain excessive drinking. This can also be called the reinforcement theory. According to this theory, the association of alcohol ingestion with a positive experience is a cause of alcoholism. This theory also suggests that alcoholics drink because alcohol consumption is followed by a reduction in anxiety, stress, and tension. Prolonged heavy alcohol ingestion produces alterations in the metabolic system that creates physiologic addiction. When this state is reached, withdrawal symptoms that occur when alcohol consumption is reduced automatically reinforce the drinking.

Sociocultural- or Cultural-etiologic Theories

These theories postulate a relationship between various groups in society and the incidence of alcohol use. For instance, Jews, Mormons, and Moslems have a very low rate of alcoholism,[40] whereas the French have the highest rate. Individual attitudes toward alcohol and alcoholism to a large extent reflect the attitude of one's culture toward drinking. Another part of these theories is that stress factors in cultures may contribute to alcoholism.

One theory that is no longer recognized as valid is the moral etiologic theory. This theory held that alcoholism was either a moral fault or a sin of the alcoholic. Much of the early treatment of alcoholics was based on this theory. This theory is still held by some groups, often by fundamentalist religious organizations.

PREVENTION

Prevention of alcoholism is a complex issue. Legally, efforts have been made to restrict the sale of alcohol to minors, as well as to institute fairly stringent legal consequences of use by minors. Unfortunately, many of these efforts have not been very effective.

The key to prevention seems to be grounded in education. This education includes the teaching of fairly young children about the dangers of alcohol use and abuse. Many elementary schools now start these programs as early as the first or second grades. In addition, work may be done with children to increase their self-esteem, so that they may be better able to avoid peer pressure to drink as they become older.

Another attempt to educate persons involves families and employers of alcoholics. They are taught that alcoholism is a disease that needs treatment, but at the same time the person who is an alcoholic may need to suffer the consequences of the use so that help may be sought at an earlier time. This has sometimes been called "raising the bottom." The alcoholic usually is surrounded by persons who *enable* his use and abuse; for example, the wife who calls in to work for her drunk husband and tells the employer that he is sick with the flu. Without this *enabling behavior,* the alcoholic might be forced to seek help earlier.

The importance of secondary prevention cannot be denied. Prompt diagnosis and treatment can be important in assisting alcoholics to once again become productive members of society and thus save themselves and others from much heartache and expense.

PATHOPHYSIOLOGY

Alcohol is a central nervous system (CNS) depressant. It affects the brain by suppressing the activity of the neurotransmitter gamma aminobutyric acid (GABA). GABA is an inhibitory neurotransmitter. Thus alcohol inhibits the inhibitor. The so-called stimulating effects of alcohol occur because the first areas affected by the suppression of GABA are the higher centers of the brain governing self-control and judgment, which are inhibitory functions. Slowing the release of GABA to those areas results in a seemingly "stimulating" effect. As alcohol continues to accumulate in the brain, areas of the limbic system and brainstem become inhibited. Unconsciousness may set in. In fact, the brain may become so overwhelmed by alcohol that it can stop functioning permanently. Other organ systems are also affected. See

TABLE 19-1 Normal function, primary pathophysiology, and clinical picture in alcoholism

Normal Function	Primary Pathophysiology	Clinical Picture
Gamma aminobutyric acid (GABA)— (neurotransmitter)	Activity of GABA is inhibited	Lessening of inhibitory functions; self-control and judgment lessened
Pancreas—synthesizes protein	Activation of proteolytic enzymes with autodigestion of pancreatic tissue	Epigastric pain; vomiting and rigidity of abdominal muscles
Liver—provides glucose during fasting; during carbohydrate ingestion removes glucose and stores it as glycogen	Infiltration of liver parenchymal cells with fat	Jaundice, enlarged liver, increased bleeding time, ascites, possible hepatic coma
	Glucose broken down to acetaldehyde to acetic acid	
Stomach and esophagus—normal food ingestion	Increased acid production; irritation of mucosa	Bleeding ulcers, gastritis; cancer of esophagus and mouth
Intestine—absorption of vitamins and minerals	Decreased absorption of thiamine, folic acid, and vitamin B_{12}	Malabsorption syndrome, skin conditions, Wernicke-Korsakoff syndrome
Immunologic system—protection against infection	Decreased susceptibility to infection	Infections and illness
Neuromuscular system—transmission of impulses	Abnormal transmission of impulses	Neuropathies and myopathies

Table 19-1 for a comparison of normal function, pathophysiology, and clinical picture of alcoholism.

The active ingredient in alcoholic beverages is ethyl alcohol or ethanol. Most American beers contain 3% to 6% alcohol, wine 2% to 21% alcohol, and hard liquors contain 40% to 50% alcohol. A 12-ounce bottle of beer, a 4-ounce glass of wine and 1½ ounces of hard liquor contain similar amounts of alcohol.

Alcohol does not require digestion and is absorbed in both the stomach and intestine. Absorption is accelerated by increased alcohol concentrations and an empty stomach. After absorption, alcohol is distributed equally throughout body fluids, passing across all membranes. About 2% to 10% is lost through the lungs through breathing and by urination. About 90% of alcohol is disposed of by metabolic processes that occur mainly in the liver (Figure 19-1).

Alcohol has a diuretic effect, partly caused by the increased amounts of fluids ingested. Increased amounts of electrolytes, particularly potassium, magnesium, and zinc, may be excreted in the urine of heavy drinkers. Prolonged use of alcohol has a toxic effect on the intestinal mucosa that results in decreased absorption of thiamine, folic acid, and vitamin B_{12}.

Because alcohol is not converted to glycogen, it cannot be stored, and it provides calories but no minerals or vitamins. One ounce of alcohol provides 200 kcal. Most of the ingested alcohol is metabolized in the liver at a rate of 10 g/hr. The excess remains in the bloodstream where it acts as a depressant and an anesthetic, which in turn slows down cellular metabolism. The anesthetic action of alcohol can have serious consequences. The margin of safety for the person anesthetized by alcohol is very small.

Blood alcohol levels depend on the amount ingested and the size of the individual. Most laws designate blood alcohol serum levels of 100 mg/100 ml (0.1%) as the legal limit for driving a motor vehicle. Increasing blood alcohol levels have increasingly more serious side effects (Table 19-2).

CLINICAL MANIFESTATIONS

Habitual drunkenness is the main symptom of alcoholism. Usually alcoholism develops slowly, over a period of 10 to 20 years, until the person reaches a point where he "drinks to live and lives to drink."

Several clinical features have been found to occur with alcoholics[26]:

1. Chronicity as a disease or disorder of behavior
2. Undue preoccupation with the intake of ethyl alcohol
3. Loss of control over the drinking pattern itself
4. Use of alcohol in a way that is dangerous to the drinker's physical health, interpersonal relationships, and/or economic functioning
5. Use of alcohol as a universal solution to problems

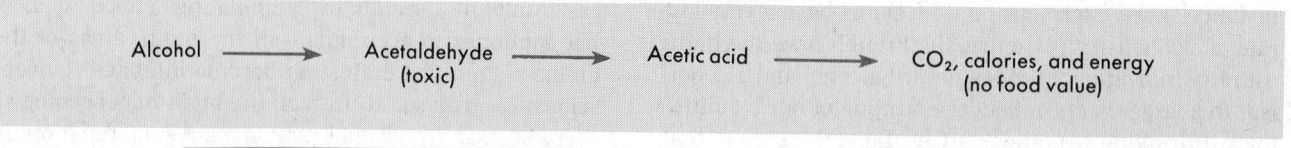

Alcohol → Acetaldehyde (toxic) → Acetic acid → CO_2, calories, and energy (no food value)

FIGURE 19-1 Metabolism of alcohol.

TABLE 19-2 Effects of blood alcohol levels on average-sized nontolerant adult

Blood Alcohol Levels (per 100 ml of Blood)	Effects
50-75 mg	Pleasant relaxed state, mild sedation, loosening of inhibitions
100-200 mg	Overt signs of intoxication: loosening of tongue, clumsiness, beginning emotional changes
200-400 mg	Severe intoxication: difficulty speaking, stumbling, emotional lability
400-500 mg	Stupor, coma
Over 500 mg	Usually fatal

DISORDERS ASSOCIATED WITH ALCOHOLISM

Hepatic	Alcoholic hepatitis, Laënnec's cirrhosis, fatty liver
Gastrointestinal	Gastritis, pancreatitis, duodenal ulcers, malabsorption syndromes, cancer of mouth and esophagus
Neurologic	Peripheral neuropathy, Wernicke-Korsakoff's syndrome, organic brain disease
Cardiovascular, hematologic	Cardiomyopathy, hypertension, familial type-IV hyperlipidemia, hypoglycemia, anemia, hyperuricemia, coronary artery disease, congestive heart failure
Musculoskeletal	Skeletal myopathies
Immunologic	Increased susceptibility to infections

6. Incorporation of denial and other defense mechanisms as a necessary component of the disease
7. Loss of ability to express feelings

In addition, frequent intoxication affects multiple body systems. (See box above, right for details of these effects.)

FETAL ALCOHOL SYNDROME

Women who drink during pregnancy have a higher incidence of children with birth defects. The children of women who drink several times a day throughout pregnancy may be born with fetal alcohol syndrome. The syndrome can include the following:

1. Mental retardation
2. Microcephaly
3. Growth deficiencies
4. Facial abnormalities
5. Malformations of skeletal, urogenital, and cardiac systems

An increase in spontaneous abortions, stillbirths, and infant deaths is also associated with heavy drinking during pregnancy. Even moderate drinking can result in the birth of children with significant lags in mental and motor development.[26]

ALCOHOL WITHDRAWAL

With continued drinking, a physiologic dependency on alcohol and tolerance for increasing amounts of it occur. Symptoms range from mild tremors to severe agitation and hallucinations when alcohol is withheld. The type and severity of symptoms depend on several factors. Alcoholics at higher risk of experiencing severe withdrawal symptoms are those who are older, who have had previous convulsive seizures or delirium tremens (DTs), and who have coexisting acute illnesses or nutritional deficiencies.

The alcohol withdrawal syndrome includes the following[26]:

1. Diaphoresis, tachycardia, and elevated blood pressure
2. Tremors
3. Nausea or vomiting
4. Anorexia
5. Restlessness
6. Hallucinations
7. Convulsions
8. Delirium tremens

Tremors

Tremors may be observed 6 to 48 hours after withdrawal of alcohol and may persist for 3 to 5 days. The hands are involved first, but the tremors may become generalized with involvement of the extremities, tongue, and trunk.

Seizure Disorders

Seizures may occur 12 to 24 hours after abstinence. Usually auras do not precede the grand mal seizures, but postictal stupor usually follows them.

Delirium Tremens

Delirium tremens, or DTs, is an acute complication of alcohol withdrawal that is a true emergency. It is a pathologic state of consciousness resulting from interference with brain metabolism. DTs that are treated carry a 5% mortality rate, whereas untreated DTs have a 15% mortality rate. The nurse is often in a position to assess the signs of impending alcohol withdrawal. These signs frequently include restlessness and irritability, headache, nausea, insomnia, and nightmares. Before the onset of full-blown DTs, withdrawal signs may include visual and tactile hallucinations that are followed by seizures.

The onset of DTs is often sudden and dramatic. It usually occurs 3 to 4 days after abstinence. The condi-

SYMPTOMS OF DELIRIUM TREMENS (DTs)

Increased psychomotor activity and tremulousness
Confusion and disorientation
Fearfulness
Signs of vasomotor lability
Tachycardia
Temperatures 37° C to 40.5° C (100° to 105° F)
Illusions and hallucinations (visual and tactile, including
    terrifying animal images and crawling skin sensations)

tion usually lasts from 2 to 3 days to a week, but at times it can last as long as 4 to 5 weeks. The cause of DTs is thought to be sudden withdrawal from alcohol, although physical trauma, infection, and various metabolic disorders have been found to have an influence. See the box above for the symptoms of DTs.[26]

Wernicke-Korsakoff's Syndrome

Symptoms of Wernicke-Korsakoff's syndrome include ocular disturbances such as nystagmus and paralysis of the lateral rectus muscle of the eye. Ataxia is usually present along with symptoms of disturbed mental functioning. The latter can include symptoms of delirium tremens, as well as apathy, listlessness, psychosis, and severe confusion. Memory problems and confusion are commonly seen. At one time this syndrome was felt to be the result of neurologic damage from long-term alcohol use. It is now known, however, that *nutritional deficiency* is the causative factor. The specific nutritional deficiency is thiamine.

With Wernicke-Korsakoff's syndrome, the patient may recover from the initial illness, but amnesia and psychosis may continue. If the residual mental illness is severe, the person may require close supervision and intensive care.

DIAGNOSTIC TESTS

Routine blood tests often reveal abnormalities that are directly related to alcoholism. These include elevated liver enzymes; that is, serum glutamic-oxaloacetic transaminase (SGOT), serum glutamic pyruvic transaminase (SGPT), alkaline phosphatase, and bilirubin. Hypoglycemia may also be present if glycogen stores have been depleted. In addition, hypoalbuminemia and hyperglobulinemia are also present in patients with cirrhosis of the liver. Magnesium is often decreased in persons who are alcoholic, usually because of poor dietary intake. It is not uncommon to find anemias and other indicators of poor nutrition in alcoholic patients. Patients who are alcoholics often have an increased mean corpuscle volume (MCV) when the complete blood

count (CBC) is done. This and an elevated gamma glutamyl transferase (GGT) are strong indicators of a possible diagnosis of alcoholism.

Other diagnostic tests demonstrate the concomitant diseases that usually accompany alcoholism.

DIAGNOSTIC CRITERIA

The diagnosis of psychoactive substance dependence, including alcoholism, has been established to include the following:

1. At least three of the following:
    a. Substance often taken in larger amounts or over a longer period than intended.
    b. Persistent desire for the substance or one or more unsuccessful efforts to cut down or control substance use.
    c. A great deal of time spent in activities necessary to get the substance, taking the substance, or recovering from its effects.
    d. Frequent intoxication or withdrawal symptoms when expected to fulfill major role obligation at work, school, or home.
    e. Important social, occupational, or recreational activities given up or reduced because of substance use.
    f. Continued substance use despite knowledge of having a persistent or recurrent social, psychological, or physical problem caused or exacerbated by the use of the substance.
    g. Marked tolerance: Need for markedly increased amounts of the substance to achieve intoxication or the desired effect.
    h. Characteristic withdrawal symptoms.
    i. Substance often taken to relieve or avoid withdrawal symptoms.
2. Some symptoms of the disturbance have persisted for at least 1 month or have occurred repeatedly over a longer period of time.[3]

MEDICAL MANAGEMENT

Medical management of the alcoholic patient in acute withdrawal focuses on restoration of nutritional and metabolic equilibrium, prevention of seizures, and safe withdrawal from alcohol. Medication is used as needed, often in large doses because of the tolerance of the alcoholic for other mood-altering chemicals. These medications are discussed later in this chapter.

Successful treatment of the alcoholic usually demands a multidisciplinary approach to care. The physician plays an extremely important part as a key member of this team, which often includes social service, counseling, pastoral care, recreational therapy, and nutritionists, in addition to nurses.

Many patients may benefit from psychotherapy with

a physician or psychologist who is knowledgeable about the disease of alcoholism. This is most helpful when used in conjunction with self-help groups.

■ ASSESSMENT

Both subjective and objective data are important to assess in the patient with alcoholism. The nurse is reminded that two cardinal symptoms of the untreated alcoholic are *denial* and *delusion*. Therefore the information gathered from the patient may not always be accurate.

SUBJECTIVE DATA

Subjective data include the following:
1. Normal using or drinking patterns
2. Date of last use or drink
3. Substance used
4. Quantity used
5. Past history of blackouts, tremors, hallucinations, or DTs
6. Past periods of abstinence
7. Normal dietary pattern
8. Legal problems
9. Family problems
10. Occupational problems
11. Family history of alcoholism
12. Other medications used

The nurse may wish to validate information gathered with a family member or significant other. The first five questions are important in all settings; the others may be asked at the discretion of the nurse.

OBJECTIVE DATA

Objective data are as follows:
1. Abnormal response to preoperative medication, anesthesia, or sedatives
2. Presence of tremor (usually worse in the morning)
3. Morning nausea
4. Abnormal laboratory studies
5. Symptoms of vitamin deficiency (pellagra or polyneuropathy)
6. Body weight in relation to height
7. Mental functioning
8. Memory loss
9. General behavior
10. Vital signs
11. Presence of ascites
12. Positive blood alcohol or urine alcohol level
13. Petechiae

■ DATA ANALYSIS: NURSING DIAGNOSES

Nursing diagnoses are determined from assessment of patient data. Possible nursing diagnoses for the person with alcoholism may include, but are not limited to, the following:

Diagnostic Title	Possible Etiologies
Activity intolerance	Generalized weakness
Adjustment, impaired	Required change in life-style
Cardiac output, alteration in: decreased	Stress of alcohol withdrawal
Coping, ineffective individual	Situational crises
Denial, ineffective	Threat to life
Disuse syndrome, potential for	Weakness
Fluid volume deficit, actual or potential	Decreased fluid intake and abnormal fluid loss
Hopelessness	Lost beliefs
Infection, potential for	Decreased nutrition and immune response
Injury, potential for	Sensory/motor deficits
Knowledge deficit	Lack of exposure, cognitive limitation
Mobility, impaired physical	Decreased strength and endurance
Nutrition, altered: less than body requirements	Anorexia
Powerlessness	Illness-related regimen
Self-care deficit	Cognitive impairment, depression
Social isolation	Alteration in mental status, unaccepted social behaviors
Spiritual distress	Separation from religious ties
Thought processes, altered	Neurologic disorders, depression, isolation
Violence, potential for: self-directed or directed at others	Inability to control behavior

■ PLANNING: EXPECTED PATIENT OUTCOMES

Expected patient outcomes for the person with alcoholism may include, but are not limited to, the following:
1. Activity tolerance is increased.
2. Adjustment to sobriety is improved.
3. Cardiac output is maintained.
4. Denial as a defense mechanism is minimized or eliminated.
5. Disuse syndrome is prevented.
6. Fluid volume is maintained.
7. Hopelessness is minimized.
8. Patient can verbalize the need to attend aftercare, including Alcoholics Anonymous (AA) meetings.
9. Patient can verbalize importance of family members receiving help.
10. Patient can verbalize powerlessness over alcohol and the importance of abstaining completely from alcohol or mood-altering chemicals.

11. Patient can verbalize recognition of over-the-counter products to avoid.
12. Patient's mobility is improved.
13. Nutritional status is improved.
14. Patient is able to care for self.
15. Patient verbalizes sense of less social isolation.
16. Patient verbalizes less spiritual distress.
17. Thought processes are maintained.
18. Patient's safety is maintained.
19. Abstinence from alcohol or mood-altering substances occurs.
20. Patient has made contact with AA.
21. Patient can verbalize importance of being honest with physician or dentist.

■ **IMPLEMENTATION**
MANAGEMENT OF ACUTE WITHDRAWAL

Detoxification entails withdrawing alcohol in a controlled environment.

Medication

Medication usage in the initial detoxification from alcohol includes the following.
1. Chlordiazepoxide (Librium) or similar drug
   a. Chlordiazepoxide is used in decreasing doses for its sedating and anticonvulsant effect during detoxification.
   b. See the box below for an example of a protocol to be used for alcohol withdrawal.
2. Anticonvulsant therapy such as magnesium sulfate (2 ml of a 50% solution every 8 to 12 hours for several doses)
   a. Phenytoin (Dilantin) may be used for a longer period of time if the patient has a prior history of seizures or DTs.
3. Multivitamin supplement
   a. Multivitamin supplements usually are given, at least for the first 3 to 5 days.
   b. Thiamine, 1 g every day is usually given, along with other B-complex vitamins.
   c. Patients may not have been eating a balanced diet for a long period of time and may have nervous system involvement.

The specific medication used may differ from setting to setting. However, one concept that is important for the nurse to remember is that many alcoholics need to receive medication for safe and effective detoxification.

PROTOCOL FOR WITHDRAWAL FROM ALCOHOL USING LIBRIUM

50 mg every 3 hr p.r.n. for the first 24 hr
50 mg every 6 hr p.r.n. for the next 24 hr
50 mg every 8 hr p.r.n. for the next 24 hr

There is no reason for the alcoholic to suffer needlessly because health professionals may feel that the alcoholic deserves to suffer. In actuality, detoxification can be dangerous and requires diligent observation by the nurse. Medication should be used freely in the first several days of treatment.[44]

Management of Delirium Tremens

Treatment of DTs consists of the use of tranquilizing drugs such as chlordiazepoxide or diazepam and sedatives such as paraldehyde given rectally, intramuscularly, or orally. High-caloric and high-vitamin diets may have to be given by nasogastric tube. The patient must be protected from physical injury and observed carefully for signs of cardiac failure. If at all possible, restraints should be avoided, because they increase agitation.

Promoting Nutrition

Many alcoholics enter treatment with a history of poor nutritional habits. Often, they have consumed many calories from alcohol but have received no nutritional protein or other nutrients. In the initial detoxification period, diet is as tolerated, including liberal fluids. Intravenous fluids are usually not necessary. As the condition of the alcoholic improves, the appetite also usually improves. The emphasis is on three well-balanced meals a day, with free access to snacks. Many patients find that they crave sugar during this initial period. Usually this is not discouraged, because withdrawal from alcohol is the first priority.

Patients usually benefit from an assessment by a nutritionist or dietician. Education about the importance of improved nutrition is essential.

If the alcoholic patient has developed liver involvement with cirrhosis, dietary modifications may become necessary. The reader is referred to Chapter 39 for further information on cirrhosis.

Management of Wernicke-Korsakoff's Syndrome

Treatment of Wernicke-Korsakoff's syndrome includes strict abstinence from alcohol and the administration of large dosages of B-complex and C vitamins. When severe brain damage has occurred, long-term custodial care may be required. Family members who assume the care of this type of patient require much support and education.

Promoting Safety

It is important for the nurse to be aware of safety concerns of the alcoholic patient. Because of the effects of alcohol or other drugs, the person may become violent and attempt to hurt themselves or others. The behavior of the person may be erratic and unpredictable. If necessary, restraints may be used until the person passes through the detoxification process. Side rails are also important to prevent the patient from falling from bed. If the patient has a history of seizures, the side rails should be padded.

Because alcohol withdrawal may cause hallucinations or other mental problems, it is important to remove items from the area of the patient that could be harmful or destructive, including matches and sharp objects. The room of the patient should be adjacent to the nursing station for ease of observation.

LONG-TERM CARE

The object of all treatment is to assist patients to stop drinking alcohol. When alcoholics do stop drinking, they can never take one single drink without serious danger of relapsing. Studies have tried to demonstrate that alcoholics may be taught to control their drinking or to become so-called social drinkers, but this has not been substantiated.[40] Alcoholics who are not currently drinking are never considered cured, only recovering. Various methods of long-term treatment are used. These include the methods described below.

Behavior Modification

In the treatment of alcoholism, behavior modification methods may be attempted to discourage drinking behaviors. The best-known aversive agent used is disulfiram (Antabuse), which blocks the enzymatic action necessary to metabolize alcohol. Taken on a regular basis, the drug causes symptoms of nausea, vomiting, palpitations, and general prostration in the person who takes even a small sip of alcohol. The person is then conditioned to avoid alcohol. Disulfiram is usually used as an adjunct to other therapy. Sometimes it is also useful to provide a somewhat forced period of sobriety for an alcoholic who is unable to abstain in any other way.

Group Therapy

Much of the goal of group therapy with the alcoholic is to enable the person to see the relationship between the use of alcohol and the negative consequences that have been suffered. This in one sense is also a form of behavior modification. When the alcoholic becomes sober, he or she can see that many negative consequences and problems decrease.

Many alcoholics are socially isolated. Group therapy may also assist the person to begin to relate to others in a caring and supportive environment. The group members can help the person look at issues that are still a concern in recovery.

Associating with people who drink or use drugs should be discouraged for the newly recovering person. They may need assistance in planning ways of meeting new people with whom they can form healthier relationships.

An important part of the treatment of the acoholic is positive reinforcement. This usually occurs in the context of interpersonal relationships with the counselors and nurses, as well as with the other patients. Caring, emotional support, and encouragement are very important.

Rehabilitation Groups

Alcoholics Anonymous (AA) is a group of self-acknowledged alcoholics whose aim is to stay sober and to help other alcoholics gain sobriety. There are AA groups who meet regularly in most communities. Meetings are of various types. Open meetings may be attended by anyone, not just the alcoholic. Closed meetings are limited to persons who are alcoholic. There are "lead" meetings, in which a recovering alcoholic tells his or her personal story of alcoholism, or meetings in which the members present discuss a topic. There are meetings in most communities for women only, men only, gay persons, young people, and, in larger communities, the deaf. There is no charge for attendance at the meetings—a free will offering is usually taken.

Local groups are sometimes listed in the telephone directory, and larger communities publish directories of meetings for distribution. A phone call to AA (often the central office) will bring help in the form of telephone conversation, or an AA member will visit the alcoholic desiring help.

In some communities there is a reluctance on the part of AA members to have persons with other addictions attend meetings. This is partly because of lack of information about the disease of chemical dependence; it is also based partly on fear. With improved methods of diagnosing drug abuse and alcoholism, especially among younger persons, many AA groups are faced with the addition of many younger people who have not suffered the same number or kind of consequences that the older members may have.

The AA philosophy focuses on the opportunity for the alcoholic to share personal experiences of alcohol abuse and control. Participation in AA may or may not be accompanied by the participation of the patient in other treatment modalities. AA has the highest success rate of any treatment program. The success of AA has led to the formation of other groups that share the same 12-step spiritual approach (see the box on p. 426). These groups include Al-Anon, Families Anonymous, Narcotics Anonymous, Overeaters Anonymous, Emotions Anonymous, Cocaine Anonymous, and Gamblers Anonymous.

Many communities have alcoholic clinics where medical and psychiatric help is available. In addition, many industries have employee assistance programs to aid impaired employees. Treatment centers that offer a variety of inpatient and outpatient programs are also more readily available now than ever before. Informa-

TWELVE STEPS OF ALCOHOLICS ANONYMOUS

1. We admitted we were powerless over alcohol—that our lives had become unmanageable.
2. Came to believe that a power greater than ourselves could restore us to sanity.
3. Made a decision to turn our will and our lives over to the care of God as we understood Him.
4. Made a searching and fearless moral inventory of ourselves.
5. Admitted to God, to ourselves, and to another human being the exact nature of our wrongs.
6. Were entirely ready to have God remove all these defects of character.
7. Humbly asked him to remove our shortcomings.
8. Made a list of all persons we had harmed, and became willing to make amends to them all.
9. Made direct amends to such people whenever possible, except when to do so would injure them or others.
10. Continued to take personal inventory and when we were wrong promptly admitted it.
11. Sought through prayer and meditation to improve our conscious contact with God as we understood Him, praying only for knowledge of His will for us and the power to carry that out.
12. Having had a spiritual awakening as a result of these steps, we tried to carry this message to alcoholics, and to practice these principles in all our affairs.

From Alcoholics Anonymous: New York, 1976, Alcoholics Anonymous World Sources, Inc.

tion on alcoholism and programs for alcoholics and others are available for interested individuals and groups.

Promoting Health

The alcoholic often enters the treatment process in a state of poor health. As a result, they may need assistance in planning a program that will help them regain mobility and self-care skills. A program of regular exercise that is adapted to the person's level of endurance and health status can be helpful.

The patient may also need assistance in planning healthy alternatives to their former patterns of drinking and/or using drugs. If they have used intravenous drugs, they should be tested for acquired immune deficiency syndrome (AIDS), as this disorder commonly occurs in this group. The patient should choose a physician and dentist who are aware of the diagnosis of alcoholism and who have a knowledge of treating alcoholics and drug addicts.

Reestablishment of regular patterns of sleep and adequate rest are important for regaining health.

Facilitating Coping

The patient will need assistance in learning to deal with life without the crutch of alcohol or drugs. This includes helping them to find a sense of spirituality and perhaps become reconnected with a religious organization or leader. Decision making may be difficult at first and the person may require support to look at options. Just because the person becomes sober does not mean that all problems will be gone.

Allowing the person to vent emotions and responding with empathy (not sympathy), may assist them in letting go of anger or resentment. If needed, the nurse may suggest professional counseling for the alcoholic.

It is not uncommon for the alcoholic to have problems with intimacy and sexuality. They need to learn to trust others and to risk becoming vulnerable with another person. Marriage counseling may be necessary to help a couple regain a healthy marriage, especially if there has been a long history of problems as a result of alcoholism or drug addiction.

PROMOTING TREATMENT

Some still believe that it is only when alcoholic patients truly desire and seek help with their alcoholic problem that treatment is useful. This is true in some cases, but, often by the time an alcoholic person seeks help, he or she has lost almost everything. Recently, there has been emphasis on the use of a process called *intervention* to assist the alcoholic to receive help. Part of the reason for intervention is that the disease of alcoholism causes delusions or impairs judgment that keeps harmfully dependent persons locked into self-destructive patterns.

Interventions are *planned confrontations* by individuals who care about the persons. Rules for conducting interventions have been summarized as follows[31,53]:

1. Meaningful persons must present the facts or data. The most meaningful may be the person's employer.
2. The data presented should be specific and descriptive of events that have happened or conditions that exist.
3. The tone of the confrontation should not be judgmental.
4. The chief evidence should be tied directly to drinking, whenever possible.
5. The evidence of behavior should be presented in some detail and very explicitly.
6. The goal of the intervention is to have the alcoholic see and accept reality so that the need for help can be accepted.
7. The choices available for treatment should be offered. If possible, immediate help should be available.

The nurse can also do much to encourage treatment of alcoholism by first recognizing that many patients in the hospital may be alcohol- or drug-addicted, even when this is not listed as a diagnosis.

NURSING CARE PLAN

PERSON WITH ALCOHOLISM

DATA: Mrs. Brown is a 67-year-old retired school teacher who has lived alone since the death of her husband 5 years ago. She retired from teaching 2 years ago. She has three children, but they all live out of town, and she sees them about two or three times a year. Her health has been good except for some aches and pains that she has treated with "a stiff drink." Before her husband died, she had been a social drinker, having one or two drinks a week. Her alcohol consumption has now increased to at least a pint each day. She admits to using alcohol to ease her loneliness and help her sleep, but does not see her drinking as a problem. She was seen in the clinic because of a fall that caused a severely sprained ankle. Her laboratory tests indicate elevated liver function studies and anemia.

The nursing history identified the following:
- She has suffered from at least three falls in the past 6 months.
- She has lost about 10 lbs in the past year and she gives a sporadic history of eating.
- She has stopped seeing many of her friends because, she says, "They are too busy for me."

Further investigation indicates that alcoholism is a problem. The nurse assists in setting up an intervention, which is successful in getting Mrs. Brown into a hospital for detoxification. Collaborative nursing activities include those to assess (1) Mrs. Brown's potential for alcohol withdrawal and (2) the presence of any complications associated with her alcoholism. She expresses a great deal of remorse about her "problem." Nursing actions include:
- Monitoring vital signs
- Assessing for signs and symptoms of alcohol withdrawal
- Assuring safety during detoxification
- Administering libirium to treat the withdrawal
- Allowing Mrs. Brown time to vent her feelings about her drinking
- Administering vitamins and thiamine

NURSING DIAGNOSIS

Adjustment, impaired related to use of alcohol to ease feelings of loneliness

Expected Patient Outcomes	Nursing Interventions	Rationale
Patient begins to learn alternative ways to cope with stress	Explore with patient times when she feels need to drink	Needs to learn substitutes for handling stress to stay sober

NURSING DIAGNOSIS

Injury, potential for, related to alcohol withdrawal

Expected Patient Outcomes	Nursing Interventions	Rationale
Patient will not experience seizures	Keep siderails up while in bed	To prevent falling from bed if seizure occurs
Patient will pass through detoxification without injury	Medicate as ordered and PRN as needed	Alcoholics may require large amounts of medication to prevent dangerous withdrawal
	Observe for signs of increasing tremors or confusion	Tremors and confusion that increase may lead to DTs.

NURSING DIAGNOSIS

Nutrition, altered: less than body requirements related to drinking instead of eating

Expected Patient Outcomes	Nursing Interventions	Rationale
Patient will begin to eat a normal diet	Provide small, frequent meals with adequate liquids	Nausea may be a problem and patient may be dehydrated from diuretic effect of alcohol
	Give vitamins as prescribed	Alcoholism interferes with absorption of vitamins through intestine

NURSING DIAGNOSIS

Knowledge deficit (alcoholism as a disease) related to lack of exposure to information and denial

Expected Patient Outcome	Nursing Interventions	Rationale
Patient can verbalize disease nature of alcoholism	Teach patient about disease	Education will help diminish shame and guilt
Patient can verbalize need to stay sober	Have patient attend AA meeting in hospital	Can help patient learn from others
Patient can verbalize physical problems related to drinking	Teach about physical problems such as falls, liver disease	Will help patient break through denial

Continued.

NURSING CARE PLAN

PERSON WITH ALCOHOLISM—cont'd

NURSING DIAGNOSIS

Social isolation related to shame and guilt and negative behavior that occurred with drinking

Expected Patient Outcomes	Nursing Interventions	Rationale
Patient attends AA and relates to at least one other person	Encourage patient to attend AA	Will help ease feeling of isolation
Patient tells family of alcoholism	Assist patient in telling family	Support of family will ease shame and guilt

---

PATIENT TEACHING

Education about the disease of alcoholism is extremely important for the alcoholic. The necessary elements of this education include the following:

1. Disease concept of alcoholism
2. Medical aspects of the disease
3. The need for continued abstinence
4. The importance of expressing feelings to stay sober
5. Drugs to avoid
6. Products such as mouthwash to avoid
7. Importance of being honest with physician and dentist
8. Signs and symptoms of impending relapse
9. Importance of aftercare (including AA)

Any education of the alcoholic should also include the family or significant others. The alcoholic became "sicker" in the midst of persons who cared about him or her. These persons also become "sick" and need understanding and education to help themselves and the alcoholic to recover.

Many over-the-counter drugs contain alcohol, for instance, mouthwash. The alcoholic also needs to know that the use of any mood-altering chemical may lead to relapse.

DRUG ABUSE

Since alcohol is in itself a drug, alcoholism and drug abuse are not mutually exclusive. There is an increasing tendency for persons who abuse substances to mix a variety of drugs and alcohol. Much of the information already covered in the section on alcoholism also pertains to drugs.

The history of nonmedical drug use is thousands of years old. As early as 5000 BC, the Sumerians referred to a "joy plant." This is believed to be a reference to the opium poppy plant.[41] Since then drugs have played a significant role in almost every culture. Even the results of historic events may have been altered, because the persons involved were under the influence of drugs. Different drugs have assumed importance in different periods of history. For instance, currently cocaine is more problematic than ever before. The newest problem drugs are the so-called designer drugs many of which were unheard of several years ago.

EPIDEMIOLOGY

In recent years drug abuse has risen sharply. There are no reliable statistics on drug abusers, and experts disagree as to what actually constitutes drug abuse. Some include repeated use of any drug, whereas others limit it to those drugs that; used repeatedly, lead to habituation or addiction.

Use of drugs has increased among adolescents and young adults. Drugs are readily available in most elementary and secondary schools and on most college campuses.

The terms habituation and addiction have been used to define the nature and extent of drug use. Drug *habituation* includes repeated use of a drug to a point where there is psychological dependence. Drug *addiction* involves craving, psychological dependence, and physical dependence. The latter includes development of *tolerance* for increasing dosages of the drug and the appearance of withdrawal symptoms on cessation of the drug. Drug dependence is another term that is used. This refers to a psychological or physical dependence on a drug that is taken regularly.[26]

According to the Controlled Substance Act of 1971 there are five basic kinds of drugs:

1. Stimulants
2. Depressants
3. Hallucinogens
4. Narcotics
5. Cannabis

To this list could be added deliriants such as glue and paint thinner. Each of these classifications is discussed in Table 19-3.

TABLE 19-3 Effects of mood-altering drugs

Drug	Tolerance	Physical Dependence	Psychological Dependence
Narcotics	High	High	High
Barbiturates	Moderate	High	High
Methaqualone	Moderate	High	High
Tranquilizers	Moderate	Moderate	High
Amphetamine	High	Low to moderate	High
Cocaine	Low	Low to moderate	High
Lysergic acid diethylamide (LSD)	Moderate	None	Moderate
Mescaline	Low	None	Moderate
Phencyclidine (PCP)	Low	None	Low
Marijuana	Low	None	Moderate

SPECIFIC DRUGS
STIMULANTS

Stimulants are both natural and synthetic drugs that have a strong stimulating effect on the central nervous system. They are accompanied by a feeling of alertness and self-confidence. Drugs included in this category are:

1. Amphetamines
2. Cocaine
3. Caffeine
4. Nicotine

Amphetamines

Epidemiology/etiology. Amphetamines and amphetamine-like drugs are synthetic psychoactive drugs that are available legally by prescription. They are available in both capsule and tablet forms. A powdered or crystalline line form of amphetamine is methamphetamine, which must be injected. It is no longer legally produced in injectable form.

Medical uses of amphetamines include the treatment of narcolepsy, obesity, fatigue, and depression. Ritalin, an amphetamine-like drug, is used to treat children who are hyperactive. Common brand names of amphetamines include dextroamphetamine (Dexedrine), methamphetamine (Methedrine), and amphetamine (Benzedrine).

Street names for amphetamines vary, but include the following:

Street Names for Stimulants

Pep pills	Ups	Meth
Dexies	Speed	Whites
Bennies	Crystal	

Pathophysiology/clinical manifestations. Amphetamines are CNS stimulants. When swallowed or injected, they speed up the activity of the heart and brain. They dilate the pupil of the eye and increase the pulse rate and blood pressure. The use of amphetamines also reduces fatigue, increases concentration, and reduces appetite. However, the feeling of alertness, often coupled with a sense of confidence and well being, wears off, and the person experiences fatigue and depression.

Amphetamines have the potential to produce tolerance. The abrupt discontinuation of amphetamines usually does not produce physical withdrawal, although many persons have psychological dependence on these drugs.

Side effects of amphetamine usage include restlessness, dizziness, insomnia, headaches, diarrhea, constipation, and lack of appetite. Persons who ingest a large amount of amphetamines over a period of time may experience extreme agitation and anxiety. They may become paranoid and suffer from a temporary paranoid psychosis that is a psychiatric emergency. Death by overdose does not usually occur. However, cerebral hemorrhage or heart attacks have been precipitated by the use of amphetamines. Also, because use hides a sense of fatigue, persons can collapse from exhaustion after use.

Withdrawal from the drug often leads to profound depression and may lead to suicide.[41]

Cocaine

Epidemiology/etiology. Cocaine is a psychoactive drug that comes from the leaves of the South American coca bush. It was first used by the members of early South American tribes. When the Spanish conquistadores discovered the Inca empire, they also found cocaine. They encouraged its use when they found that the natives worked longer and harder and needed less food when it was used. The active ingredient of cocaine was isolated in its pure form in the nineteenth century. During that time the drug was also used as an ingredient of many products, including syrups, nasal sprays, cigarettes, and liquors. At one time it was an ingredient of Coca-Cola and was also recommended as a treatment for alcoholism. In 1914 the nonmedical use of cocaine was prohibited by the Harrison Narcotic Act. During the last 15 years, cocaine has become increasingly popular as a recreational drug.[28]

Medical uses for cocaine include use as an anesthetic of choice for certain procedures and surgery involving the nose, throat, larynx, and lower respiratory passages. It may also be used as an ingredient in Brompton's mixture, which is used for terminal cancer patients.

Cocaine is used by sniffing, smoking, or injecting. When it is sniffed or snorted, the effect of the drug is realized when the cocaine is absorbed into the nose. Cocaine may also be free-based. This is a process of heating the drug to separate it from whatever adulterants it may contain. When free-base cocaine is injected, it produces a high that is more intense and more short-lived than when cocaine is smoked.

Crack is a mixture of cocaine and common baking soda and water. It gets its name from the sound it makes as it cooks. Crack is smoked, much like free-basing, and creates an intoxication more intense than cocaine alone. It is quicker, causes more euphoria, and is instantly addictive.

Street Names for Cocaine

Blow	Flake	Superblow
Coke	Nose candy	Toot
Crack	Rock	White
Dust	Snow	White girl

Pathophysiology/clinical manifestations. Cocaine acts as a CNS stimulant. It stimulates respiration and heart rate. It raises blood pressure and blood sugar levels and suppresses the appetite. Other physical symptoms include dilation of the eyes, constriction of certain blood vessels, increased physical activity, insomnia, and trembling. Sensations of extreme euphoria and feelings of energy, power, confidence, and talkativeness have been found with the use of cocaine. There is a letdown effect of "cocaine crash" that occurs when the effect of the drug wears off.[28]

Chronic sniffing of cocaine can destroy the nasal tissues. Smoking it can cause lesions in the lungs. Tolerance and psychological dependence can develop, and an overdose can cause convulsions, respiratory paralysis, and death. A cocaine psychosis has been reported that is characterized by a loss of pleasure, loss of orientation, hallucinations, insomnia, concern with minor details, stereotyped behavior, and an increased potential for violence. Treatment with an antipsychotic medication may be necessary.

Abrupt withdrawal from cocaine does not lead to physical symptoms of withdrawal.

Caffeine

Epidemiology/etiology. Caffeine is the most accepted and used psychoactive substance in the United States. Many beverages and other products contain caffeine. Because of its availability and widespread use, most persons do not view caffeine as a drug.

The use of tea leaves in China dates back at least 4000 years. In the 1200s the Arabians used coffee. Caffeine was first isolated from coffee in 1820. In its pure state, caffeine is a white powder or white needle-shaped crystals. It has been used as an additive in carbonated beverages since the early 1900s.

Medically, caffeine is present in many headache remedies, cold medications, diuretics, diet aids, and other prescriptions. (See the following box for the amount of caffeine in commonly used beverages.)

CAFFEINE CONTENT OF PRODUCTS

Coffee	
Brewed per cup	75 to 155 mg
Instant	60 to 90 mg
Decaffeinated	2 to 4 mg
Carbonated sodas	30 to 70 mg
(all colas, Dr. Pepper, Mountain Dew, Sunkist Orange)	
Chocolate	
Hot cocoa	30 to 70 mg
Candy (1 oz)	6 mg
Over-the-counter drugs	16 to 65 mg
Anacin, Excedrin, Vanquish, Doan's Pills	
No-Doz, Vivarin	100 to 200 mg
APC tablets	30 to 100 mg
Diet Aids	
AYDS, Dexatrim, Prolamine	140 to 200 mg
Tea, per cup	25-75 mg

Pathophysiology/clinical manifestations. Caffeine stimulates the CNS, as well as the digestive system and the kidneys. Body metabolism is increased, and the blood pressure is raised. Urination is also increased, and the secretion of gastric acid is stimulated. Large doses of caffeine cause tachycardia, headaches and nervousness, insomnia, and stomach distress. Physical dependence occurs with regular intake of 350 mg for an adult. The withdrawal symptoms include severe headaches, irritability, and tiredness.[6]

Caffeine makes most people feel energetic and alert. Too much caffeine can precipitate an anxiety attack. Long-term involvement can lead to depression, persistent anxiety, low-grade fever, nausea, ringing in the ears, and chronic insomnia. A fatal dose of caffeine is considered to be about 10 g, or 10,000 mg.

Early research seems to indicate that excessive use of caffeine may contribute to the development of heart disease as well as to bladder cancer.[6]

Nicotine

Epidemiology/etiology. Over 50 million Americans smoke more than 600 billion cigarettes yearly. It is one of the most physically damaging and addictive habits that a large number of people engage in. Smoking has been linked to heart and blood vessel disease, chronic bronchitis and emphysema, and cancer of the lungs, larynx, mouth, esophagus, bladder, pancreas, and kidneys. It is far easier to become addicted to cigarettes than to alcohol or other drugs.[5]

Tobacco is used by smoking, chewing, or inhaling. Snuff is usually placed between the gums and the cheek.

The tobacco plant belongs to the genus *Nicotiana*, a

member of the nightshade family. Evidence has been found that cigarette smoking occurred as far back as 200 AD. When Columbus reached the New World, the sailors saw the natives smoking and soon picked up the habit. The cigarette-rolling machine was invented in the 1880s. This added greatly to the number of people who abused tobacco. In 1964, the Surgeon General of the United States issued the now-famous report that linked smoking with several diseases. Cigarette packages are now so labeled. Some experts believe that cigarette smoking is the chief preventable cause of death in our society.[5]

Pathophysiology/clinical manifestations. The nicotine in tobacco acts as a stimulant to the CNS. Nicotine is present in the brain within a few seconds of the beginning of smoking. Smokers claim that smoking produces relaxation; however, smoking releases epinephrine, which may create physiologic stress. Nicotine acts as an appetite suppressant. In large doses it produces tremors, decreased urine, and a rapid respiratory rate.

Withdrawal symptoms occur with the stoppage of cigarette smoking. These include the following:
1. Decrease in heart rate
2. Weight gain
3. Impairment of psychomotor performance
4. Nervousness and anxiety
5. Headaches
6. Fatigue
7. Insomnia
8. Constipation or diarrhea

The craving for a cigarette often continues for an extended period of time.[5]

DEPRESSANTS

Depressants are synthetic drugs that have a depressant action on the CNS. Drugs included in this category are:
1. Sedatives or methaqualone
2. Barbiturates
3. Tranquilizers

Sedatives or Methaqualone

Epidemiology/etiology. Methaqualone is a nonbarbiturate sedative-hypnotic. It is the active ingredient in the drugs Quaalude and Mequin. It is available as a prescription drug but has also become a common and popular street drug. It is taken orally. Because of its nonsoluble nature, it cannot be injected.

Common Street Names for Methaqualone

Ludes	Love drug
Soaps, soapers, or sopes	Wallbangers
714s	Lemons

Methaqualone was first made in the early 1950s as a treatment for malaria in India. In the 1960s it was used

as a sedative in Europe; 1965 saw it manufactured in the United States. It was at first thought not to be addicting. Its use as a street drug began in the 1960s and 1970s. This drug is no longer available through legitimate channels, but it is available on the street.

Pathophysiology/clinical manifestations. Methaqualone is a CNS depressant that is unrelated to other sedatives or barbiturates. It slows the CNS and impairs coordination, walking, and talking. It also possesses anticonvulsant, anesthetic, and cough-suppressant effects. Its primary effect is drowsiness. If the user resists the sleep-inducing effects of the drug, he or she experiences a relaxed, mellow sense of well-being.

The repeated use of methaqualone produces tolerance, as well as physical and psychological dependency. Withdrawal from the drug produces headache, fatigue, dizziness, nausea, anxiety, skin problems, abdominal cramps, seizures, and vomiting if the withdrawal is not medically supervised.

Overdoses occur when the CNS-depressing effects of the drug slow down the person's rate of breathing to the extent that consciousness is not possible. Most overdoses occur when the drug is combined with other drugs such as alcohol that potentiate its action. Symptoms of overdose include delirium, coma, restlessness, convulsions, and vomiting.[45]

Withdrawal from methaqualone requires the use of medication, which may include diazepam or phenobarbital.

Barbiturates

Epidemiology/etiology. Barbiturates are synthetic drugs that are classified as "sedative hypnotics." They arise from barbituric acid. They are used medically to treat high blood pressure, epilepsy, insomnia, and to sedate patients before and during surgery. Barbiturates are also commonly used street drugs.

Barbiturates are swallowed (capsule or elixir), used as a suppository, or injected. The drug was first synthesized in the early 1900s by two German scientists. Currently about 10 derivatives of barbituric acid are in use.

There are many common names for barbiturates. The names usually refer to the drug type, the drug effect, the drug name, or the color of the particular capsule.

Pathophysiology/clinical manifestations. Barbiturates cause depression of the CNS, including slowing of physical and mental reflexes. The continued use of these drugs can cause physical and psychological dependence as well as tolerance. Barbiturates produce a feeling of well-being, euphoria, and relief from anxiety. Some side effects of barbiturates include difficulty in breathing, lethargy, allergic reactions, nausea, and dizziness.

Common Street Names for Barbiturates

Yellow jacket (pentobarbital)	Barbs
Red devil (secobarbital)	Downs or downers
Phennie (phenobarbital)	Rainbows
Blue heaven or blue devil (amobarbital)	Blues
	Goof balls

Alcohol and other CNS depressants tend to potentiate the effects of barbiturates. Accidental overdoses are common. A person who is physically dependent on barbiturates will experience various withdrawal symptoms. Mild withdrawal includes irritability, restlessness, anxiety, and sleep disturbances. An extreme form of barbiturate withdrawal can be life threatening and includes symptoms of convulsions, delirium, and hyperpraxia. Detoxification includes appropriate medication, which may be a long-acting barbiturate given in diminishing dosages.[41]

Tranquilizers

Epidemiology/etiology. Minor tranquilizers are psychoactive drugs that are taken to reduce anxiety. They may also be used as a muscle relaxant. *They are the most commonly prescribed drugs in the world today.* Tranquilizers are available in prescription form in capsule, tablet, and liquid forms. Illicitly, they are sometimes injected. Common types of tranquilizers are those found in the benzodiazepine family and include the following:

1. Chlordiazepoxide
2. Diazepam (Valium)
3. Prazepam (Antrax or Vestran)
4. Oxazepam (Serax)
5. Lorazepam (Ativan)
6. Clorazepate (Tranxene)

These drugs are relatively new; the first tranquilizer was developed in 1950. Diazepam was first marketed in 1963.

Pathophysiology/clinical manifestations. Minor tranquilizers slow the activities of the CNS. They also have anticonvulsant and muscle-relaxant properties and produce a sense of relaxed well-being. When the effects of the drug wear off, however, users frequently experience an increased level of anxiety. Tranquilizers cause physical and psychologic dependence, and tolerance to them can develop.

Side effects reported for these drugs include skin rash, headache, nausea, impairment of sexual function, dizziness, and light-headedness. Other CNS-depressing drugs potentiate the action of the tranquilizers. Signs of an overdose include sleepiness, confusion, loss of consciousness, and diminished reflexes.

Withdrawal symptoms of minor tranquilizer use may not appear for a week after cessation of the drug. These symptoms include anxiety, sweating, insomnia, vomiting, tremors, delirium, and seizures. The patient must be detoxified with medication in a controlled environment.

HALLUCINOGENS

Hallucinogens are natural and synthetic drugs that affect the mind and produce changes in perception and thinking. Drugs included in this category are phencyclidine (PCP), which is discussed separately from the hallucinogens.

Epidemiology/Etiology

Hallucinogens include lysergic acid diethylamide (LSD), mescaline, psilocybin, and 3,4-methylenedioxyamphetamine (MDA). They are found on the streets in a wide range of forms, including powder, peyote buttons, mushrooms, capsules, and tablets. LSD may be found as tablets, pellets, blotter paper, chips, and sheets of paper containing tattoos or stamplike pictures of cartoon figures. Hallucinogens are taken orally, although MDA can be sniffed and injected. They may be put on sugar cubes or mixed in other food.

Common street names for these drugs are found below.

Psilocybin and mescaline have been used in religious rites by cultures in the Western hemisphere for centuries. MDA was first synthesized in the 1930s and used as an appetite suppressant. LSD was first synthesized in 1938, and the first "trip" that was documented occurred in 1943 when the drug was accidently ingested.

The use of LSD was prohibited in 1965. Before that time, it had been used as a therapeutic treatment for neurotic and psychotic patients. Some experiments have also been conducted in the use of this drug with alcoholics and terminal cancer patients.[46]

Pathophysiology/Clinical Manifestations

Most of the effects of hallucinogens are psychological, although nausea and vomiting are not uncommon possible reactions. These drugs act as stimulants at first, and produce anxiety, depressed appetite, dilated pupils, and increases in body temperature, heart rate, and respirations. With psilocybin, dizziness, numbness of the face, and shivering may also occur. Tolerance to these drugs occurs rather quickly (usually after 3 days of use), and there is cross-tolerance among the four drugs.[46]

Common Street Names of Hallucinogens

LSD	Acid, barrels, blotter, domes, microdots, purple haze, windowpane
Mescaline	Buttons, cactus, mesc, mescal buttons
MDA	Love drug, mellow drug of America
Psilocybin	Magic mushroom, shroom

Hallucinogens also have a profound psychological effect on most people. The effect has been described as a process of amplifications, with the drug being a catalyst. Hallucinogens amplify the users' experience of the environment and put them in touch with thoughts and feelings. In low doses, MDA produces a peaceful euphoria. With higher doses, it mimics LSD experiences minus the hallucinations.

All four drugs produce altered sensory awareness. The senses become more acute, and it is thought that colors can be heard and sounds seen. Fantasies and illusions occur, along with hallucination-like happenings, although the user is aware that they are not real. With LSD the mood changes can be rapid. Past and present experiences meld together, and some have described a feeling of oneness, compassion, and love for all things.

The feelings brought on by MDA, mescaline, and psilocybin lasts from 6 to 8 hours, whereas those of LSD usually last 8 to 12 hours. Toward the end of the "trip," the person will gradually reenter reality. A person's attempts to resist the effects of the drug seem to increase the chances of a negative experience, or a "bad trip."[41]

Flashbacks may occur with use of the hallucinogens. In these, the user reexperiences the effects of the drug without having taken it. Bad trips are described as being characterized by tremendous confusion, unpleasant sensory images, and extreme panic. Care during these situations includes getting the person into a nonstimulating environment and staying with the person until the effects of the trip wear off. Reassurance of the fact that the person is experiencing a drug trip is helpful. Some sources cite the giving of niacin (500 mg) as a way to bring the person down from a bad trip.[41]

Although there have been no reports of deaths from LSD, there have been documented instances in which the person died as a result of trying to do something impossible while on a trip. An example is trying to fly; that is, the person actually believes he or she will be able to fly.

PHENCYCLIDINE

Phencyclidine (PCP) is a synthetic drug that is generally described as an anesthetic-hallucinogen. However, it is chemically unrelated to hallucinogens such as LSD and mescaline.

Epidemiology/Etiology

PCP was first synthesized in 1957 and tested as a general anesthetic for humans. Testing stopped in the mid-1960s because of side effects of agitation and delirium. It presently is available as an anesthetic agent used by veterinarians. In the late 1960s and 1970s the drug became available as a street drug. It was banned from legal manufacture in 1978, but is still produced illegally.

PCP, produced as a white or yellowish-white powder, has a variety of forms, including tablets and capsules. As angel dust, it is sprinkled on tobacco or marijuana and smoked. It may also be snorted or injected.[46]

Common Street Names for PCP

Angel dust	Embalming fluid
Animal tranquilizer	KJ killer
Crystal	Peace pill
Dust	Synthetic marijuana
Hog	

Pathophysiology/Clinical Manifestations

Different doses of PCP provide different physical effects. These can be found in the box below.

Psychological effects of PCP ingestion last from 1 to 6 hours, with 24 hours needed to return to baseline. Research seems to indicate that the bad trip rate of PCP is five times that of other drugs. Chronic users may experience flashbacks. The dose of PCP may indicate the nature of the effects. These are found in the box on p. 434.

Although there is disagreement about whether PCP is physically addicting, there is wide agreement that it is psychologically habit-forming.

PCP overdoses are dangerous, because the person may die as a result of respiratory or cardiac arrest. Symptoms of PCP intoxication include a variable response. These include the following:

1. Violent or combative to nearly unconscious
2. Little or no pain response
3. Inability to speak
4. Elevated blood pressure and pulse rate with slight fever[47]

DOSE-RELATED PHYSICAL EFFECTS OF PCP

DOSE	EFFECTS
5 mg	Physical sedation
	Numbness of extremities
	Loss of muscle coordination
	Dizziness
	Constricted pupils, blurred or double vision, and involuntary eye movement
	Flushing and profuse sweating
	Nausea and vomiting
	Increase in blood pressure, heart rate, and respiratory rate (breathing is shallow)
5 to 10 mg	Marked drop in blood pressure, breathing, and heart rates
	Shivering, increased salivation, and watering of the eyes
	Loss of balance, dizziness, and rigidity of muscles
	In some cases, repetitive movements, such as rocking
	Analgesic and anesthetic properties apparent
Over 10 mg	Extreme agitation followed by seizures or coma
	Symptoms similar to mental confusion and delusion of schizophrenia

---

From Scott L: PCP (pamphlet), Charlotte, NC, 1981, Charlotte Drug Educational Center, Inc.

DOSE-RELATED PSYCHOLOGICAL EFFECTS OF PCP

DOSE	EFFECTS
Low	Euphoria and sense of alcohol-like intoxication
	Changes in body image
	Mood swings from ecstasy to panic
	Hallucinations and confusion about time and space
	In final stage in some cases, a sense of despair and emotional isolation, possibly leading to a feeling of paranoia and a sense of impending death
Moderate	Increase in effects felt at low dose
	Loss of sense of contact with environment
High	Symptoms of mental and emotional confusion similar to schizophrenia

From Scott L: PCP (pamphlet), Charlotte, NC, 1981, Charlotte Drug Educational Center, Inc.

The person intoxicated by PCP becomes more agitated by noise, bright lights, and talking.

PCP may result in psychosis that lasts from several days to 2 weeks. It is often mistaken for acute schizophrenia. Individuals may be actively suicidal and become depressed when the acute psychosis has passed.

NARCOTICS

Narcotics are drugs that are derived from the opium poppy or produced synthetically. The use of these has been recorded far back in history. Synthetic production of narcotics has occurred in the past 30 to 50 years. In general, narcotics lower the perception of pain.

Epidemiology/Etiology

Heroin is one narcotic that is abused to a large extent. There has been a shift toward younger addicts and an increase in the percentage of whites using heroin. On the streets, heroin is known as "H," horse, junk, hard stuff, smack, or scag.

There are several different forms of narcotics. See Table 19-4 for a listing of these drugs, their medical use, and route of administration.

Pathophysiology/Clinical Manifestations

Effects of the use of narcotics include shallow breathing; reduced hunger, thirst, and sexual drive; and drowsiness. The person may also experience euphoria, lethargy, heaviness of limbs, and apathy. There is a loss of ability to concentrate and a loss of judgment and self-control. Overdoses of narcotics can cause coma, convulsions, respiratory arrest, and death. As in the case of heroin, when the drug is injected, there are associated risks of hepatitis, acquired immune deficiency syndrome (AIDS), and other infections such as septicemia. Narcotic addicts develop both tolerance and physical

TABLE 19-4 Narcotics

Name	Medical Use	Route of Administration
Heroin	None in the United States	By injection or sniffing
Morphine	Ease pain	By mouth smoking, or injection
Opium	Ease pain, treat diarrhea, and suppress cough	By mouth or smoking
Codeine	Suppress cough and reduce pain	By mouth or injection
Meperidine	Relieve pain	By mouth or injection
Methadone	Ease pain and to help those dependent on heroin	By mouth or injection

From O'Brien R and Cohen S: The encyclopedia of drug abuse, New York, 1984, Facts on File, Inc.

and psychological addiction. Withdrawal may be painful and should be done under medical supervision. Clonidone (Catepres) is often used for purposes of detoxification from narcotics. The heavier the usage, the longer detoxification may take. Symptoms of withdrawal may include nausea, cramps, chills, sweating, watery eyes, running nose, and restlessness.[41]

Heroin is an expensive habit; addicts may resort to crime to support it.

Methadone Maintenance

One approach to the treatment of narcotic addiction is the methadone maintenance program. The drug is given legally as a part of a rehabilitation program. The drug reduces the severity of the heroin withdrawal but must itself be tapered off. There are many controversies surrounding methadone programs, and many professionals discourage its use, recommending instead detoxification leading to abstinence.

CANNABIS

Epidemiology/Etiology

Cannabis, or marijuana, comes from the Indian hemp plant. It can grow wild or is fairly easily cultivated. Marijuana is usually smoked as a cigarette (joint, reefer) or in a pipe. Other paraphernalia may be used, including "bongs." There are many slang terms for marijuana, including the following: dope, grass, herb, joint, pot, reefer, roach, smoke, stuff, and weed.

Marijuana has been used as both a medical and nonmedical drug for more than 3000 years. It has been used since the 1850s in the United States. Its popularity as a street drug began to occur in the twentieth century. It is still one of the most popular and commonly abused drugs, especially among young people.

Hashish, or hash, is a resinous extract of the leaves and flowering part of the marijuana plant. It is more concentrated than marijuana and has more intense effects.

Marijuana is being evaluated in research studies to reduce eye pressure in glaucoma patients and to control side effects of cancer chemotherapy.

Pathophysiology/Clinical Manifestations

Physical effects of marijuana include drying of the eyes and mouth, increase in appetite, reddening of the eyes, and impairment of short-term memory. It also influences the way stress affects the heart and circulation, and it raises the heart rate and blood pressure. Lowered body temperature, loss of coordination, and possible confusion and distortion of reality may occur. In addition, research indicates that marijuana may affect chromosome segregation during cell division. Since marijuana is a fat-soluble molecule, parts of it may be stored in the body for up to 30 days or more.[41]

Psychological effects of marijuana include an altering of perception (that is, an altering of sight, sound, touch, sense of time, and taste). The user usually experiences a feeling of well-being and intoxication, although depression and panic may occur. Psychological addiction develops in users. Crisis situations may occur in the form of an anxiety reaction to the marijuana high. A calming and reassuring approach has been found to be helpful.

DELIRIANTS

Epidemiology/Etiology

Deliriants are any chemicals that give off fumes or vapors that, when inhaled, produce symptoms similar to intoxication. They may also be called inhalants. Vasodilators such as amyl nitrate and butyl nitrite are also considered inhalants.

The fumes or vapors from inhalants are sniffed through the nose, or the vapors are put into a bag or captured in a balloon to increase the concentration of the inhaled fumes.

The history of the use of inhalants is traced back to ancient Greece. Sniffing commercial products and solvents was first documented in the 1950s. No medical use exists for commercially prepared inhalants. Of course, the vasodilators and anesthetic agents have a legitimate medical purpose.

The deliriants or inhalants have a psychoactive or mood-altering effect when the vapors are inhaled or sniffed. Most fall into one of three categories:

1. Solvents
2. Aerosol sprays
3. Anesthetics

Solvents include commercial products that are not commonly thought of as drugs. These include glue, gaso-line, kerosene, lighter fluid, paint products, lacquer thinner, spot-remover, and nail polish remover. Products such as hair spray, deodorant, insecticides, and cookware coating sprays are examples of aerosols. Anesthetics that are used recreationally include ether, chloroform, and nitrous oxide.

Typically, solvent and aerosol users are among the youngest drug users.

Pathophysiology/Clinical Manifestations

Almost all inhalants are CNS depressants that slow the user's heart rate, brain activity, and breathing. Other effects include slurred speech, blurred vision, inflamed mucous membrane, light-headedness, ringing in the ears, watering eyes, loss of coordination, and excessive nasal secretions. With high doses, the user may lose consciousness or experience seizures. The effects are immediate and usually last 20 to 45 minutes.

Symptoms of inhalant use include bloodshot eyes, nosebleed, and bad breath. The prolonged use of inhalants may lead to liver, kidney, blood, and bone marrow damage. The sniffing of toluene, found in gasoline and commercial cleaners, has been demonstrated to cause irreversible brain damage. This may be demonstrated as forgetfulness, inability to think clearly, depression, irritability, hostility, and paranoia.[41]

Some inhalants cause tolerance. Physical dependency is a possibility. Symptoms of withdrawal have included chills, hallucinations, headaches, stomach pains, cramps, and delirium tremors.

The psychological effects of deliriants include a feeling of stimulation and energy. At higher doses, the user may feel intoxicated. The development of psychological dependency is a real possibility.

Use of large amounts of aerosols or solvents can cause death as a result of cardiac arrest following arrhythmias. Death from inhalants is usually caused by suffocation because of the displacement of oxygen in the lungs. Sniffing inhalants from a bag or balloon increases the risk of suffocation. Misuse of commercial aerosol products used to chill food have been reported to cause death by freezing the lungs of the user.

The CNS effects of inhalants are potentiated by other CNS depressants. This increases the chances of overdose.

■ ASSESSMENT

Most early indications of drug use have been covered in the preceding description of individual classes of drugs. The reader is also referred to the assessment section under the section on alcoholism. Breaks in the skin are an objective sign that must be noted when assessing for drug addiction. If the person has been "mainlining" (that is, injecting the drug directly into the vein), needle marks, scars, or small scabs can be seen on the hands

TABLE 19-5 Acute intoxication and withdrawal of mind-altering drugs

| Drug Group | Acute Intoxication | | Withdrawal Symptoms |
	Symptoms	Treatment	
Narcotics	Respiratory depression, bradycardia, hypotension, cold clammy skin, decreased body temperature; deep sleep, stupor, or coma; pin-point pupils	Maintain ventilation, provide oxygen Give narcotic antagonist: naloxone (Narcan) 0.4 mg IV Monitor vital signs every 15-30 min until patient is conscious Treat for shock	(Not life-threatening) Early: restlessness, irritability, drug craving, yawning, lacrimation, diaphoresis, rhinorrhea; followed by "yen" sleep (intense desire to sleep; sleeps restlessly) Later: awakens with more severe symptoms, nausea, vomiting, anorexia, abdominal cramps, bone and muscle pain, tremors, piloerection (gooseflesh)
Other CNS depressants	Same as narcotics (above)	Lavage if recent oral ingestion Maintain ventilation, provide oxygen Monitor vital signs every 15-30 min until patient is conscious Position patient side-lying or prone, not supine Treat for shock Hemodialysis for renal shutdown	(May be life-threatening) Insomnia, restlessness, tremors, anorexia, followed by convulsion, and symptoms similar to DTs (confusion, visual and auditory hallucinations), fever, dehydration
CNS stimulants	Labile cardiovascular symptoms (flushing or pallor, pulse and blood pressure changes, arrhythmias), hyperpyrexia, mental disturbances (agitation, paranoia, hallucinations), convulsions, circulatory collapse	Give chlorpromazine, 25-50 mg IM Provide a quiet environment Orient patient to reality Monitor vital signs until stable	(Withdrawal is not severe) Somnolence, apathy, irritability, depression, fatigue
Hallucinogens	Physiologic toxicity low at doses that produce strong psychological effects Acute panic reaction (bad trip) may lead to suicide "Flashback" episodes Prolonged psychotic disorders (paranoia, depression) Phencyclidine: CNS depression or stimulation may lead to death	Provide quiet, supportive environment and constant attention Give diazepam (Valium), 2-10 mg IM for severe anxiety	No evidence of withdrawal symptoms
Cannabis	Adverse reactions infrequent Simple depression, paranoid ideation, confusion, disorientation, hallucinations	Provide support and reassurance Give tranquilizer for agitation	(Withdrawal symptoms rare) Insomnia, anorexia
Deliriants	Slowing of heart rate, brain activity, and breathing Slurred speech, blurred vision, inflamed mucous membranes, excessive tearing, and nasal secretions With high doses, loss of consciousness and seizures may occur Brain damage may occur (memory loss, depression, paranoia, hostility) Feeling of stimulation and energy Death may occur from suffocation or cardiac arrest	Maintenance of airway Maintain respirations Provide quiet environment and provide support Monitor vital signs Orient patient to reality	Chills, hallucinations, headaches, stomach pains, cramps, and delirium tremors

and forearms or instep. However, many other veins are used as points of entry to conceal addiction, including the dorsal vein of the penis or the conjunctival artery of the eyelid.

The reader is referred to the section on assessment of the alcoholic for other relevant subjective and objective data, nursing diagnoses, and specific outcomes.

Because of the expense involved, users often sell their belongings, steal, or become prostitutes to get money to supply their drug habit. Each day abuse of drugs costs the American economy millions of dollars.

■ IMPLEMENTATION

The treatment of withdrawal from drug abuse has been discussed in each section under the specific drugs. (See Table 19-5 for more detail on acute intoxication and withdrawal.) General rehabilitation follows the guidelines for treatment of the alcoholic. This can be found in the section on alcoholism. Today, most treatment centers treat alcoholics and drug addicts side-by-side. In fact the majority of persons receiving treatment for chemical dependency today have a history of abuse of both alcohol and drugs.

One difference between drugs and alcohol is that in most cases the possession and use of drugs is illegal. In the United States the addiction to narcotics has been considered a crime ever since the passage of the Harrison Narcotic Act of 1914. Education is making the public more aware of the primary nature of the disease of drug addiction.

EATING DISORDERS

Eating disorders such as anorexia nervosa and bulimia nervosa has been known since ancient times, when they were described as "nervous consumption" and "anorexia hysteria."[21] Compulsive overeating is also considered an eating disorder, but is not be discussed in this chapter.

EPIDEMIOLOGY/ETIOLOGY

The incidence of eating disorders, especially anorexia and bulimia, is high in certain subpopulations where maintenance of excessively low weights is required. These include models, ballet dancers, and flight attendants. Adolescent girls often have a preoccupation with losing weight. It is estimated that from 5% to 15% of this group meet the criteria for bulimia. Although the incidence of eating disorders is much higher in females, some males also experience anorexia and/or bulimia.

PREVENTION

Prevention of eating disorders is difficult. It is generally recognized that this activity is a way of coping with stress and relieving tension; aiding the young person to develop a healthy self-concept and positive ways to express tension and stress may help. The reader is referred to the discussion on prevention in the section of this chapter referring to alcoholism (p. 419).

Currently, eating disorders are more promptly recognized by both health professionals and the general public. Teachers in high schools and colleges may also play a significant role in diagnosis of this condition.

PATHOPHYSIOLOGY

The pathophysiology occurring with bulimia is related to the constant purging of the gastrointestinal system. If laxatives are used in large amounts, the individual may experience a loss of rectal tone and the loss of great amounts of minerals with diarrhea. If the person purges by vomiting, loss of enamel on the teeth is common, leading to decay and to infection of the mouth and gums. Gastrointestinal bleeding may also occur, along with gastritis or esophagitis, from the contact of the mucosa with stomach acids. Malnutrition is common.

With anorexia, the patient suffers from frank malnutrition. This leads to depletion of muscle mass, skin lesions, loss of hair, neuromuscular abnormalities, and cessation of menses in females.

Bulimia or anorexia becomes a way to "anesthetize" intense feelings and to cope with stress and relieve tension. The person, who does not have adequate coping skills, attempts to deny difficult events, minimize distress, and rationalize stress. When tension builds to high levels, food (or lack of food) serves as a coping mechanism.

Control is a recurring theme for persons suffering from eating disorders. They fear losing control and being spontaneous. These fears cause them to set up rules and regulations (ritualistic behaviors) for everything they do. Restrictive eating and purging are attempts made by the bulimic to control the body, especially after an eating binge. Restrictive eating often functions as evidence of willpower and control over the body. Purging is seen as a way to bring the body back under control. There is a vicious cycle of binging and purging in many of these persons.

CLINICAL MANIFESTATIONS

The signs and symptoms of eating disorders may mask themselves with similar symptoms of other disorders. Suspicion should be aroused if the person develops amenorrhea, exhibits hyperactivity with no apparent fatigue, shows agitated behavior or disorganized thinking, or experiences excessive weight loss, sleep disturbances, or physical complaints, especially epigastric pain.

ANOREXIA NERVOSA

With anorexia nervosa, weight loss leads to a body weight at least 15% less than the expected norm based on age and height. The person is intensely fearful of becoming obese, and the menstrual cycle usually is absent. The person experiences a distortion of body image and feels fat even when emaciated.

BULIMIA NERVOSA

Bulimic patients present with episodes of binge eating during which they feel a lack of control. This has been defined as at least two binging episodes a week for at least 3 months. The patient attempts to prevent weight gain through regular self-induced vomiting or the use of laxatives, restrictive dieting, fasting, and increasingly vigorous exercise. The patient shows an excessive concern with body shape and weight.[21]

MEDICAL MANAGEMENT

The medical management of the patient with anorexia or bulimia often centers around nutritional management. Intravenous therapy, hyperalimentation, or tube feedings may be necessary to sustain life. Supplemental vitamins are usually administered and infections are treated if present. It is not helpful to use psychoactive drugs with these patients. They need to regain coping abilities without the use of medications. Psychotherapy is often imperative to enable the person to face the truth of his or her behavior and to curb the need to be in control at all times.

■ ASSESSMENT

Both subjective and objective data are important to assess in the patient with bulimia or anorexia. These patients are similar to the alcoholic patient in that they may manifest a strong sense of denial of their problem. Information should be validated with a family member if possible.

SUBJECTIVE DATA

1. Typical eating patterns
2. History of binging or purging
3. Laxatives used—type and quantity
4. Patient's perception of weight and body image
5. Family history of eating disorders
6. Family problems
7. Past problems with eating disorders
8. Average weight
9. Use of drugs or alcohol
10. Complaints of problems, especially gastrointestinal problems
11. Exercise pattern
12. Sleep disturbances

OBJECTIVE DATA

1. Presence of low weight in relation to height
2. Evidence of loss of tooth enamel
3. Amenorrhea
4. Hyperactivity or agitated behavior

■ DATA ANALYSIS: NURSING DIAGNOSES

The reader is referred to the section of this chapter concerning alcoholism (p. 423).

■ PLANNING: EXPECTED PATIENT OUTCOMES

The reader is referred to the section of this chapter concerning alcoholism (p. 423).

■ IMPLEMENTATION
MAINTAINING NUTRITION

Efforts must be made to support the nutritional status of the patient until a more normal eating pattern is restored. If needed, tube feedings, intravenous feedings, or hyperalimentation may be prescribed. The nurse must be aware that the patient may try to sabotage efforts to restore nutrition. Weights are obtained at frequent intervals as a measure of the success of the plan of care. A written contract may be used with the patient to aid in behavioral change.

The goal of nutritional therapy is to assist the patient in learning to eat a well-balanced diet with an adequate caloric count. A consultation with the dietitian is usual. The patient is given extra support before, during, and after meals.

PROMOTING HEALTH

In addition to nutritional counseling, the patient must learn to cope with stress in healthier ways. If exercise has been excessive, the nurse assists the patient in planning a more healthy and realistic exercise schedule. The patient is assisted in facing fears and in confronting the need to be in control at all times. Often group therapy is very effective, especially when combined with individual counseling.

The nurse can do a great deal in terms of role modeling with the patient. This may include eating with the patient and demonstrating that a meal can be enjoyed without the constant struggle and fear of gaining weight.

Often the patient with anorexia or bulimia is socially isolated. Encouragement is needed to encourage the patient to socialize with and begin to trust others. The patient should be referred to Overeaters Anonymous (OA).

PATIENT TEACHING

Educating the patient about the eating disorder is important. Elements of the teaching include the following:

1. Disease concept of eating disorders
2. Medical aspects of the disease
3. The need for an adequate and prudent diet
4. The importance of finding healthy ways to cope with life
5. The awareness of an increased tendency to transfer obsessions
6. Signs and symptoms of relapse
7. Importance of aftercare

CODEPENDENCY

Codependency often has been used to describe a person who is emotionally involved with a chemically dependent person. The codependent is someone who develops an unhealthy pattern of coping as a reaction to someone else's drug or alcohol use. Recently, however, the definition of codependency has been expanded. It is now seen as a disease entity with a definable onset, a set of physical and psychological symptoms, and a predictable medical course.

Definitions of codependency vary, but there is agreement that the person manifests dysfunctional responses to life and that they derive their self-esteem from their ability to control themselves and others.

Characteristics of codependency include the following[27]:

1. Perfectionism
2. Denial
3. Poor communication
4. Caretaking
5. Inability to identify, express, and manage feelings
6. Difficulty forming and maintaining close relationships
7. Feeling responsible for others' behavior or feelings
8. Constantly seeking approval of others
9. Feelings of powerlessness
10. Feeling morally superior
11. Difficulty in setting limits
12. Feeling "super responsible" or "super irresponsible"
13. Martyrdom
14. Need to control
15. Any addictive behavior
16. Stress-related illness

Many nurses suffer from the disease of codependency. It is thought to be a chief cause of "burn-out." Nurses who give too much become depleted.

Recovery from codependency starts with the person learning to care for themselves. The use of a journal to record feelings may be helpful. Breaking through the denial of the codependent is often difficult. The person also requires help to learn to set appropriate boundaries, grieve past losses, and acquire the skill of reparenting. Daily affirmations may be used to reinforce the self-worth of the person.[8,27]

IMPAIRED NURSES

Over the last several years many states have developed programs to assist the nurse who is impaired by either alcoholism or drug addiction. One of the main reasons for the establishment of these programs is that the rate of chemical dependency in the nurse or other health professional is greater than in the general public, principally because these persons have greater access to mood-altering substances. For instance, nurses may handle narcotics every day and may succumb to the temptation to use them. Before the inception of peer assistance programs (through either the state boards of nursing or state nursing associations), the nurse often was fired and then was free to migrate to another facility, where the cycle might start over again.

In March 1978 nurses from several states attended a meeting held in Manhattan to discuss the problem of the alcoholic nurse. By 1980 two organizations of nurses interested in alcoholism were active in encouraging help. These were the Drug and Alcohol Nursing Association (DANA) and the National Nurses Society on Addiction (NNSA). In 1981 the American Nurses Association (ANA) created a Task Force on Addiction and Psychological Disturbance to formulate guidelines for state nursing associations to develop programs to help the impaired nurse. At their 1982 convention, the American Nurses Association adopted a resolution that recognized its responsibility to assist the nurse who is impaired.

In 1980 two states, Maryland and Ohio, had peer assistance programs in place. This effort has grown so that almost every state now has a program.[2,9]

The peer assistance programs have several goals: (1) to assist the nurse who is impaired to receive treatment; (2) to protect the public from the untreated nurse; (3) to help the recovering nurse reenter nursing in a systematic, planned, and safe way; and (4) to assist in monitoring the continued recovery of the nurse for a period of time. The reentry of the nurse may include a restriction from handling of controlled drugs for a period of time.

The basis of these programs is one nurse helping another. Many volunteers in these programs are nurses who are themselves recovering or who are working in the field of chemical dependency.

CHAPTER SUMMARY

- Examples of addictions include alcoholism, drug addiction, eating disorders (anorexia nervosa and bulimia nervosa), and compulsive gambling.

- Alcoholism and drug addiction are considered diseases and are commonly referred to as chemical dependencies.

- Dependency includes physical and psychological dependency and is defined as the need to continue use of the substance to prevent withdrawal symptoms.

- Tolerance, a decreased susceptibility to the effects of a substance, develops with increased use of alcohol and drugs.

- Enabling behavior by family, friends, or co-workers

enables the alcoholic or drug addict to continue the use of the substance.

✔ Alcoholism is the third major health problem in the United States and affects more than 10 million persons.

✔ An estimated 7% of the adult population suffer from the disease of chemical dependency.

✔ Theories concerning the cause of alcoholism include physiologic, psychological, and sociocultural theories.

✔ Alcohol is a central nervous system depressant that affects the brain by suppressing the activity of the neurotransmitter gamma aminobutyric acid (GABA).

✔ The so-called stimulating effects of alcohol occur because the first areas of the brain affected are the higher centers that affect judgment and self-control.

✔ Ninety percent of alcohol is metabolized in the liver.

✔ The amount of alcohol in the blood at any one time is called the blood alcohol level.

✔ Alcohol withdrawal includes symptoms ranging from mild tremors to severe agitation and hallucinations.

✔ Delirium tremens (DTs) is an acute complication of alcohol withdrawal that requires aggressive therapy to prevent mortality and morbidity.

✔ Medication used in the initial period of detoxification includes chlordiazepoxide (Librium), phenytoin (Dilantin), magnesium sulfate, and multivitamins.

✔ Wernicke-Korsakoff's syndrome is a complication of alcoholism that includes symptoms of psychosis, amnesia, and apathy.

✔ Alcoholics Anonymous (AA) is a group of self-acknowledged alcoholics whose aim is to stay sober and to help other alcoholics gain sobriety.

✔ Drug habituation is the repeated use of a drug to the point of psychological dependence.

✔ Drug addiction includes craving, psychological dependence, and physical dependence.

✔ The basic categories of drugs of abuse include stimulants, depressants, hallucinogens, cannabis, and deliriants.

✔ Caffeine is the most accepted and widely used psychoactive substance in the United States and is found in many beverages and health products.

✔ Drug addicts who use drugs intravenously are at increased risk for the development of AIDs and hepatitis.

✔ It is not unusual for persons with chemical dependency to also experience symptoms of a psychiatric disorder.

✔ A codependent is a person who has let someone else's behavior affect him or her and is obsessed with controlling other people's behavior.

✔ The diagnosis of eating disorders includes anorexia nervosa, bulimia nervosa, and compulsive overeating.

✔ Nurses and other health professionals are at increased risk for the development of chemical dependency.

QUESTIONS TO CONSIDER

■ What factors make the diagnosis of chemical dependency difficult to establish?

■ In what situation would an "intervention" be useful and how would you prepare for it?

■ Why do alcoholics fail to stay sober?

■ Why is Alcoholics Anonymous helpful in treating the alcoholic patient?

■ What common factors do all addictive behaviors share and what treatment modalities do they have in common?

REFERENCES AND SELECTED READINGS

1. Alcoholics Anonymous: New York, 1976, Alcoholics Anonymous World Services, Inc.
2. *American Nurses Association: States start assistance programs for impaired nurses, Am Nurse 15:6, 1983.
3. American Psychiatric Association: Diagnostic and statistical manual of mental disorders, ed 3, Washington, DC, 1987, American Psychiatric Association.
4. Arundell R: Barbiturates, Charlotte, NC, 1981, Charlotte Drug Educational Center, Inc.
5. Arundell R: Tobacco, Charlotte, NC, 1982, Charlotte Drug Educational Center, Inc.
6. Arundell R: Caffeine, Charlotte, NC, 1981, Charlotte Drug Educational Center, Inc.
7. Bean M: Alcohol and adolescents, Minneapolis, 1982, Johnson Institute.
8. *Beattie M: Co-dependent no more: how to stop controlling others and start caring for yourself, Center City, Minn, 1987, Hazelton Foundation.
9. Bissell L and Haberman P: Alcoholism in the professions, New York, 1984, Oxford University Press, Inc.
10. *Bluhm J: When you face the chemically dependent patient: a practical guide for nurses, St Louis, 1987, Ishiyaku Euroamerica, Inc.
11. Blume S: Alcoholism and depression, Minneapolis, 1984, Johnson Institute.
12. Brisbane F and Womble M, editors: Treatment of black Americans, New York, 1985, The Haworth Press.
13. *Brodsley L: The hospitalized alcoholic: avoiding a crisis Am J Nurs 82:1865-1873, 1982.
14. Captain C: Family recovery from alcoholism: mediating family factors, Nurs Clin North Am 24(1):55-68, 1989.

*References preceded by an asterisk are particularly well suited for student reading.

15. Caroselli-Karinja M: Drug abuse and the elderly, J Psychosoc Nurs Ment Health Serv 23:25-30, 1985.
16. *Cohn L: The hospitalized alcoholic: the hidden diagnosis, Am J Nurs 82:1861-1864, 1982.
17. Davis J: Endorphins: new waves in brain chemistry, Garden City, NY, 1984, The Dial Press.
18. Deutsch C: Broken bottles and broken dreams: understanding and helping the children of alcoholics, New York, 1982, Teachers College Press.
18a. Dubiel D: Action stat! Cocaine overdose, Nurs '90 20(3):33, 1990.
19. Effinger J: Women and alcoholism, Top Clin Nurs 4:10-19, 1983.
20. *Fitzgerald L: Alcoholism: the genetic inheritance, New York, 1988, Doubleday.
21. *Flood M: Addictive eating disorders, Nurs Clin North Am 24(1):45-54, 1989.
22. Geller A: Alcohol and sexual performance, Minneapolis, 1984, Johnson Institute.
23. Geller A: Alcohol and anxiety, Minneapolis, 1983, Johnson Institute.
24. Goby M, editor: Alcoholism, treatment, and recovery, St. Louis, 1984, The Catholic Health Association.
25. *Green P: The chemically dependent nurse, Nurs Clin North Am 24(1):81-94, 1989.
26. Haber J, et al: Comprehensive psychiatric nursing, ed 2, New York, 1983, McGraw-Hill Book Co.
27. *Hall S and Wray L: Codependency: nurses who give too much, Am J Nurs 89(11):1456-1461, 1989.
28. Hankes L: Cocaine: today's drug, J Fla Med Assoc 71:235-239, 1984.
28a. House M: Cocaine, Am J Nurs 90:40-45, 1990.
29. Hughes T: Models and perspectives of addiction: implications for treatment, Nurs Clin North Am 24:(4):1-12, 1989.
30. Jack L: Use of milieu as a problem solving strategy in addiction treatment, Nurs Clin North Am 24(1):69-80, 1989.
31. *Johnson V: I'll quit tomorrow, San Francisco, 1980, Harper & Row, Publishers.
32. Joyce C: The Woman Alcoholic, Am J Nurs 89(10):1314-1318, 1989.
33. Kimball B: The alcoholic woman's mad, mad world of denial and mind games, Center City, Minn, 1987, Johnson Institute.
34. *Kirk E and Bradford L: Effects of alcoholism on the CNS: implications for the neuroscience nurse, J Neurosci Nurs 19:6:326-335, 1987.
35. Mann M: Marty Mann's new primer on alcoholism, New York, 1981, Holt, Rinehart, & Winston.
36. Milkman H and Shaffer H, editors: The addictions: multidisciplinary perspectives and treatments, Lexington, 1985, DC Heath & Co.
37. Newman S: Amphetamines, Charlotte, NC, 1981, Charlotte Drug Educational Center, Inc.
38. Newman S: Cocaine, Charlotte, NC, 1981, Charlotte Drug Educational Center, Inc.
39. *Nuckols C and Greeson J: Cocaine addiction: assessment & intervention, Nurs Clin North Am 24(1):33-44, 1989.
40. O'Brien R and Chafetz M: The encyclopedia of alcoholism, New York, 1982, Facts on File Publications, Inc.
41. O'Brien R and Cohen S: The encyclopedia of drug abuse, New York, 1984, Facts on File Publications, Inc.
42. *Pires M: Substance abuse: the silent saboteur in rehabilitation, Nurs Clin North Am 24(1):291-296.
43. Reed M: The dependent nurse: drugs or alcohol, Nurs Times 79:19-25, 1983.
44. Rich J: Action stat: acute alcohol intoxication, Nurs '89 19(9):33, 1989.
45. Scott L: Quaaludes, (pamphlet), Charlotte, NC, 1982, Charlotte Drug Educational Center, Inc.
46. Scott L: PCP, Charlotte, NC, 1981, Charlotte Drug Educational Center, Inc.
47. *Sullivan E, et al: Chemical dependency in nursing, Menlo Park, California, 1988, Addison Wesley Publishing Co.
48. Sullivan E: A descriptive study of nurses recovering from chemical dependency, Arch Psychiatr Nurs 1(3):194-200, 1987.
49. Talbot GD: Substance abuse and the professional provider: the need for new attitudes about addiction, Ala J Med Sci 21:150-155, 1984.
50. Talbot GD: The disease of alcoholism and drug addiction in physicians, nurses, pharmacists, dentists and other health professionals, Smyrna, Ga, 1985, Caduceua Foundation, Inc.
51. *Tweed S: Identifying the alcoholic client, Nurs Clin North Am 24(1):13-32, 1989.
52. Twerski A: It happens to doctors too, Center City, Minn, 1982, Hazelton Publications.
53. *Williams E: Strategies for intervention, Nurs Clin North Am 24(1):95-108, 1989.
54. *Zerwekh J and Michaels B: Co-dependency: assessment and recovery, Nurs Clin North Am 24(1):109-120, 1989.
55. Zimberg S: The clinical management of alcoholism, New York, 1982, Brunner Mazel, Inc.

SURGERY: PERIOPERATIVE NURSING

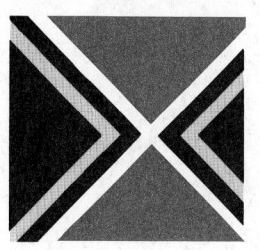

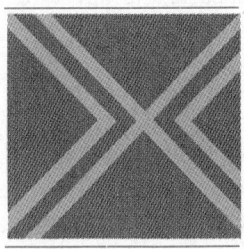

CHAPTER 20

Preoperative Nursing

BARBARA C. LONG

CHAPTER OBJECTIVES

After studying this chapter, the student should be able to:
1 Identify different types of surgeries.
2 Describe the neuroendocrine and metabolic responses to surgery.
3 Identify factors affecting patient responses to surgery.
4 Explain the concept of "informed consent."
5 Describe psychologic and physiologic preparation of the patient for surgery.

Surgery is a unique experience for each patient, depending on the underlying psychosocial and physiologic factors present. Thus no two persons respond alike to similar operations, nor does one person respond in like manner to different surgeries.

The preoperative period is from the time the decision is made for surgery through transportation to the operative suite. This chapter discusses the following:
1. Types of surgery
2. Effects of surgery as a stressor
3. Factors that affect patient responses to surgery
4. The meaning of "informed consent" for surgery
5. Psychologic preparation for surgery
6. Physiologic preparation for surgery
7. Patient care on the operative day

TYPES OF SURGERY

Most surgical procedures are given names that describe the site of the surgery and the type of surgery performed. For example, appendectomy refers to removal (-ectomy) of the appendix. Common surgical suffixes are listed in the box on p. 446. Some surgeries carry the name of the surgeon who developed the technique, such as the Billroth procedures (partial gastrectomies). Surgeries may be classified according to the extent, purpose, or body site of the surgery, or the timing or physical setting.

EXTENT

Surgeries may be divided into minor and major surgeries. *Minor surgery* is simple surgery that presents little risk to life. It may be performed in a surgeon's office, clinic, or outpatient or inpatient surgical suite. Many minor surgeries are performed using local anesthesia although general anesthesia may be used (Chapter 21). Although the operation is termed "minor," it is rarely viewed as a minor episode by the patient and may evoke some fears and concerns.

Major surgery is performed in a surgical suite, usually in a hospital setting, although in selected instances (such as for hernia repair) it may take place in ambulatory surgical centers. Major surgery is usually performed using general or regional anesthesia. It is more serious than minor surgery and may involve risk of life.

PURPOSE

Surgery may also be classified according to the various reasons it is performed.
1. Diagnostic: determine cause of symptoms (e.g., biopsy, exploratory laparotomy)
2. Curative: remove diseased part (e.g., appendectomy)
3. Restorative: strengthen weakened area (e.g., herniorrhaphy), rejoin disconnected or injured area (e.g., bone pinning), or correct deformities (e.g., mitral valve replacement)
4. Palliative: relieve symptoms without curing disease (e.g., sympathectomy)
5. Cosmetic: improve appearance (e.g., face lift)

BODY SITE

Surgery may performed externally or internally. In *external surgery* the skin or underlying tissues are readily accessible to the surgeon. Plastic surgery (Chapter 73) is an example of external surgery. *Internal surgery* involves deep penetration of the body, such as surgery of organs, major blood vessels or bone structure.

Surgery may also be classified by location of body parts or systems, such as cardiovascular surgery, chest

COMMON SURGICAL SUFFIXES

-ectomy:	Removal of an organ or gland
-rrhaphy:	Suturing or stitching
-ostomy:	Providing an opening (stoma)
-otomy:	Cutting into
-plasty:	Formation or plastic repair
-scopy:	Looking into

surgery, intestinal surgery, or neurologic surgery. Information specific to these types of surgery can be found in appropriate chapters elsewhere in the text.

TIMING OR PHYSICAL SETTING

Surgery may be planned or unplanned. An example of unplanned surgery is *emergency surgery,* such as that which follows major trauma or hemorrhage of internal organs. Although the same principles related to preoperative care apply in both planned and unplanned surgery, modifications must be made for emergency surgery because of the limited preoperative time period.

Ambulatory surgery is that which does not require overnight hospital admission. The patient is admitted to the surgical center (either in a hospital or ambulatory surgical center) on the day of surgery, remains there for postoperative care, and is discharged before the end of the day (Chapter 22).

In the past, all patients were admitted to the hospital for preparation 1 or more days before major surgery. The newest trend, mainly because of economics, is *same day surgery*. The patient is admitted on the same day of the planned surgery to a regular inpatient unit or to a special same day surgery unit. Nurses on the special unit may be involved in patient assessment and preoperative teaching that is carried out on an outpatient basis before the hospital admission. Patients are responsible for their own preparation for surgery; therefore these patients must receive the necessary preoperative teaching and counseling well before admission. Upon admission to the inpatient unit, interventions pertinent to the operative day (p. 461) are carried out. Following surgery, the patient is sent to the appropriate patient care unit.

SURGERY AS A STRESSOR

Although some operations are considered minor procedures by hospital personnel, surgery is always a major experience for the patient and family. Surgery is a stressor that produces both psychologic stress reactions (anxiety, fear) and physiologic stress reactions (neuroendocrine responses). Surgery is a potential or actual threat to a person's bodily integrity and can interfere with need gratification during any phase of surgery.

ANXIETY

Anxiety is a normal adaptive response to the stress of surgery. Anxiety occurs in the preoperative phase as the patient anticipates the surgery or postoperative problems such as pain and discomfort, changes in body image or function, increased dependency, loss of control, family concerns, or potential changes in life-style. Anxiety may be decreased if the patient perceives the surgery as having positive results, such as curing disease, relieving discomfort, or creating a more attractive physical appearance. On the other hand, anxiety is usually increased when the underlying pathologic condition is or is believed to be a malignancy or life-threatening (e.g., open heart surgery). Assessment of and interventions for preoperative anxiety are discussed on p. 452.

NEUROENDOCRINE RESPONSES TO SURGERY

Neuroendocrine responses play a major role in the reaction of a patient to the stress of surgery. The responses include stimulation of the autonomic nervous system (primarily the sympathetic nervous system) and stimulation of selected hormones (primarily aldosterone and glucocorticoid hormones from the adrenal cortex, and antidiuretic hormone from the posterior pituitary) (Table 20-1).

SYMPATHETIC NERVOUS SYSTEM

Stimulation of the sympathetic nervous system serves to protect the body from further damage. Vasoconstriction of peripheral blood vessels enables the body to compensate for blood loss and redirect blood flow to critical areas such as the heart and brain. Increased cardiac output also helps to maintain blood flow. Severe trauma or excessive blood loss, however, will overwhelm the compensatory mechanisms and blood pressure will fall. Certain types of anesthetics or high spinal anesthesia may also interfere with the compensatory vasoconstriction, producing hypotension. The patient's blood pressure is therefore monitored closely during the intraoperative and early postoperative phases.

One aspect of the sympathetic response that may produce undesirable effects is the decrease in gastrointestinal activity. Psychologic stress in the preoperative period may lead to anorexia and constipation. Following the trauma of surgery the patient may experience anorexia, gas pains, and constipation from diminished peristalsis in the gastrointestinal tract. Peristalsis may cease completely after abdominal surgery following manipulation of abdominal organs.

HORMONAL RESPONSE

Adrenocortical activity is increased, producing greater amounts of aldosterone and glucocorticoids. Aldosterone enhances sodium reabsorption by the kidney. This serves to retain fluid to compensate for fluid lost

TABLE 20-1 Effects of endocrine changes associated with surgery

Physiologic Changes	Results	Effect on Surgical Patient
↑ Norepinephrine secretion	Peripheral vasoconstriction	Helps maintain blood pressure when circulating volume is decreased
	↓ Gastrointestinal activity	May lead to anorexia or constipation
↑ Aldosterone secretion	Sodium retention	Maintains blood circulating volume
		Increases susceptibility to fluid overload
		Decreases urinary output
↑ Glucocorticoid secretion	Gluconeogenesis	Provides energy to meet stress of surgery
	↑ Protein catabolism	Provides an additional energy source
		Provides amino acids for cell synthesis following tissue destruction
	Ketogenic effect	Provides fat as an energy source
	Antiinflammatory effect	Increases susceptibility to infection
	↑ Platelet production	Promotes clotting to prevent bleeding
		Contributes to development of thrombophlebitis
↑ ADH secretion	Water reabsorption in the kidney tubules	Maintains blood circulating volume
		Increases susceptibility to fluid overload
		Decreases urinary output

through blood loss, diaphoresis, and respirations. When sodium is reabsorbed by the kidneys, potassium is excreted; thus after surgery there is a loss of potassium. The potassium is excreted regardless of the body's need for it.

The increase in the amount of glucocorticoid from the adrenal cortex is thought to mobilize cellular stores of fats and amino acids for energy and protein synthesis.[13] Healing tissues require protein. Glucose is released for energy with resultant hyperglycemia and glycosuria. Patients who have diabetes must be carefully monitored during the early postoperative phase for signs of ketosis.

In addition to the increase in adrenocortical hormones, there is an increase in antidiuretic hormone (ADH) by the neurohypophysis (posterior pituitary gland) during the first 24 to 48 hours after surgery. Water is reabsorbed by the kidney, and renal output is decreased. Following surgery the increased production of aldosterone and ADH is evidenced by a *decreased urinary output as compared with fluid intake*. Spontaneous diuresis occurs as the amount of ADH is decreased, usually in about 24 to 48 hours.

METABOLIC RESPONSES TO SURGERY

It can be said that after surgery the patient is in a relative state of starvation; metabolism is increased, while nutrient intake is decreased.

CARBOHYDRATE METABOLISM

As a result of the increased production of glucocorticoid hormones, there is an increase in the carbohydrate metabolism following the stress of surgery. With major surgery there are periods when the patient is not permitted to eat and is given dextrose by intravenous fluids. This is not adequate to meet the body's energy needs (Chapter 42). Anorexia may also occur as part of the stress response, thus adding to the problem of inadequate carbohydrate intake even if food is permitted by mouth. The body must supply its glucose needs by the breakdown of stored liver glycogen or by the synthesis of glucose from noncarbohydrate sources (gluconeogenesis) (Figure 20-1).

FAT METABOLISM

Glucocorticoids also have a ketogenic effect; that is, they increase the rate of mobilization of fat from the cells to make fat available as an energy source. With the decreased intake of carbohydrates and fats after surgery, body fats are metabolized for energy and the patient loses weight.

PROTEIN METABOLISM

Body proteins consist of combinations of amino acids, of which nitrogen is an essential component. When tissues break down during catabolism following surgery, some of the nitrogen is lost. As new tissue is formed, essential amino acids are needed. If none of these amino acids are taken in, as by ingestion, the body will continue to break down existing tissue proteins to obtain the amino acids that it needs for healing. The "leftover" amino acids not used at that time are broken down to the nitrogen end products such as urea and are excreted. A *negative nitrogen balance* results; nitrogen loss exceeds nitrogen intake. If there is little or no protein intake following surgery, nitrogen balance will be further compromised; the patient will continue to lose

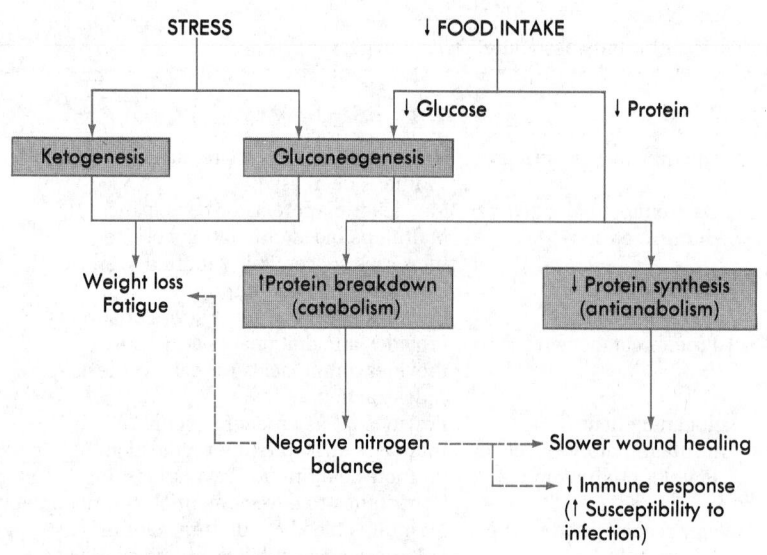

FIGURE 20-1 Metabolic responses to surgery.

weight and healing will be delayed. Nitrogen is also needed for production of white blood cells and fibroblasts needed to resist infection and to repair tissue.

FACTORS AFFECTING PATIENT RESPONSES TO SURGERY

No two persons respond to surgery in exactly the same way. A number of variables influence physiologic and psychologic responses throughout the entire surgical experience. These include age, nutritional status, effectiveness of neuroendocrine responses, presence of disease or limiting conditions, surgical procedure performed, complications, and previous experience with surgery.

AGE: ELDERLY

Surgery can be performed on persons of any age, from the newborn to the very elderly. Persons at the extremes of age are less able to tolerate stress such as tissue trauma (surgery) or infection. (Consult a pediatrics textbook for the effects of surgery on an infant or child.)

The ability of the elderly patient to tolerate surgery depends on the extent of physiologic changes that have occurred with the aging process, the duration of the surgical procedure, and the presence of one or more chronic diseases.

Elderly persons vary greatly in the extent to which physiologic changes occur. The very elderly (over age 80) generally have a greater number of changes than those in their 60s or 70s. The changes that affect responses to surgery involve all of the body systems (Table 20-2). The greater the number of changes, the greater the potential for the patient to develop a postoperative complication. Note in Table 20-2 that the more

common postoperative complications in the elderly are atelectasis, pneumonia, shock, thrombosis with pulmonary emboli, hypervolemia, delayed wound healing, and infections. Careful monitoring of the elderly person receiving fluids parenterally is important to prevent overhydration (either water intoxication or pulmonary edema).

Cardiovascular changes affect mechanisms that help the body compensate for the sympathetic nervous system response to stress. Because heart rate changes in the elderly occur more slowly than in younger persons, pulse rates may not be a good index in assessment of shock, and a longer period of time may be necessary for pulse stabilization after activity.

Elderly persons tolerate stress less effectively; therefore the duration of the surgery can affect the response. Surgery of short duration is more easily tolerated. Presence of chronic diseases, such as pulmonary, cardiac, or central nervous system disease, limits the elderly person by prolonging recovery or increasing the risk of mortality. The safest type of surgery for elderly persons is surgery that does not involve enforced immobility, infections, areas close to the diaphragm, or the need for considerable narcotics.

NUTRITION

Malnourished persons with nutrition deficits or excesses are poorer surgical risks than the well-nourished and are more likely to develop postoperative complications.

NUTRITIONAL DEFICIENCY

Persons most likely to have nutritional deficiencies are the aged and the chronically ill, particularly those with gastrointestinal tract conditions or malignancies. The

TABLE 20-2 Physiologic changes related to the aging process that can affect surgery

Physiologic Changes	Effects	Potential Postoperative Complications
CARDIOVASCULAR		
↓ Elasticity of blood vessels	↓ Circulation to vital organs	Shock (hypotension), thrombosis with pulmonary
↓ Cardiac output	Slower blood flow	emboli, delayed wound healing, postoperative con-
↓ Peripheral circulation		fusion, hypervolemia, decreased response to stress
RESPIRATORY		
↓ Elasticity of lungs and chest wall	↓ Vital capacity	Atlectasis, pneumonia, postoperative confusion
↑ Residual lung volume	↓ Alveolar volume	
↓ Forced expiratory volume	↓ Gas exchange	
↓ Ciliary action	↓ Cough reflex	
Fewer alveolar capillaries		
URINARY		
↓ Glomerular filtration rate	↓ Kidney function	Prolonged response to anesthesia and drugs, overhy-
↓ Bladder muscle tone	Stasis of urine in bladder	dration with IV fluids, hyperkalemia, urinary tract
Weakened perineal muscles	Loss of urinary control	infection, urinary incontinence
MUSCULOSKELETAL		
↓ Muscle strength	↓ Activity	Atelectasis, pneumonia, thrombophlebitis, constipa-
Limitation of motion		tion or fecal impaction
GASTROINTESTINAL		
↓ Intestinal motility	Retention of feces	Constipation or fecal impaction
METABOLIC		
↓ Gamma globulin level	↓ Inflammatory response	Delayed wound healing, wound dehiscence or evis-
↓ Plasma proteins		ceration
IMMUNE SYSTEM		
Fewer killer T-cells	↓ Ability to protect against invasion	Wound infection, wound dehiscence, pneumonia,
↓ Response to foreign antigens	by pathogenic microorganisms	urinary tract infection

person who is emaciated or cachectic or who has lost considerable weight below an acceptable level usually has a prolonged postoperative recovery (see box on p. 450).

The *undernourished* person already has diminished reserves of carbohydrates and fats. Body proteins will be utilized to provide the necessary energy requirement to maintain metabolic functioning of cells. Nitrogen imbalances (p. 447) will be greater than normal, and less protein will be available for healing. Collagen, the connective tissue that is the substance of scar tissue, is a protein. Wound healing therefore becomes considerably delayed, and wound separation and infection may occur.

If the surgery is not an emergency and can be delayed for several weeks, the undernourished patient is preoperatively placed on a high-protein, high-carbohydrate diet. In the preoperative or postoperative period total parenteral nutrition (TPN) may be given until the patient is able to tolerate a high-protein, high-carbohydrate diet by mouth. High protein intake will not result in increased body protein unless there is sufficient carbohydrate to provide the necessary energy. Activity or exercise also is required for protein synthesis (see Chapter 40).

Nutrition-depleted patients usually have a deficiency of vitamins. Vitamins B_1, C, and K are necessary for wound healing and clot formation, and supplemental vitamins will be prescribed.

NUTRITIONAL EXCESS

The *obese* patient presents several risk factors for surgery, including enlarged organs such as heart, kidneys, and liver. During surgery fluctuations of vital signs are more common in the obese person, resulting from the excessive demands on the cardiovascular system. The surgeon incising through layers of fatty tissue has to exert more traction on the tissues to expose the surgical site; this increases trauma to the tissues. Incisional hernias may occur at a later date.

During the immediate postoperative period these patients often require more assistance with turning, coughing, and deep breathing. Excess fat deposits often limit movement of the diaphragm, thereby decreasing ventilation. It is also more difficult for obese persons to move about, and they may require additional assistance. Both decreased activity and decreased diaphragm expansion are contributing factors to development of postoperative pulmonary complications. Decreased activity also predisposes to thrombophlebitis.

PERSONS AT HIGH RISK FOR DELAYED POSTOPERATIVE RECOVERY RESULTING FROM MALNUTRITION[1]

PREOPERATIVE MALNUTRITION	POSTOPERATIVE MALNUTRITION
Chronic infection	Abdominal trauma
Inflammatory bowel disorders	Severe multiple trauma (especially pelvic, hip, and leg fracture)
Chronic pancreatitis	Major burns
Carcinoma of stomach or colon	Wound sepsis
Liver disease	Acute pancreatitis
Renal disease	Small bowel fistulas
Congestive heart failure	Severe peritonitis
Weight loss (10% of body weight in 3 months before surgery)	

The obese person is more likely to develop wound separation and infection. Good circulation is important to bring to the wound the white blood cells, fibrocytes, and nutrients necessary for healing. Since fatty tissue has a decreased number of blood vessels, wound healing may be impaired.

NEUROENDOCRINE RESPONSE INEFFECTIVENESS

The neuroendocrine response assists the body in coping with the stress of surgery. If this response is ineffective, postoperative complications such as shock and delayed wound healing may occur. In addition, anesthesia may be tolerated poorly, and fluid and electrolyte imbalances are more likely to occur. Persons with diseases of the adrenal gland or the sympathetic nervous system or those who are under a great deal of stress before surgery may do less well postoperatively. Infants and the elderly also have diminished neuroendocrine response.

CHRONIC DISEASES OR DISABILITIES

The existence of one or more chronic diseases does not necessarily increase surgical risk. The nature and extent of the disease or diseases and the degree to which they are under control are the important variables.

Pulmonary disease, such as chronic obstructive pulmonary disease (COPD), may affect the person's response to the anesthetic and ability to cope with respiratory problems after surgery (see Chapter 33). In preparation for surgery the pulmonary status of persons with COPD will be carefully evaluated and measures will be instituted to improve ventilation. In persons with a history of recent respiratory infection surgery will be delayed until they are in optimal condition. Most surgeons prefer that persons who are heavy smokers decrease

their smoking for a few days before surgery since smoke irritates the tracheobronchial tree, resulting in increased secretions that impinge on the airway and decrease ventilation.

Persons with chronic pulmonary problems must be monitored very carefully during surgery and in the early postoperative period to prevent atelectasis, respiratory insufficiency, and respiratory acidosis.

Cardiovascular disease can affect the individual's response to surgery. A heart that pumps effectively and blood vessels that constrict effectively are necessary for the prevention of shock and fluid imbalances. Body responses to hemorrhage and inflammation depend on an adequate supply of red and white blood cells. Surgery is usually postponed if possible when the cardiovascular functioning of the patient is not at the optimal level. Measures are instituted to improve the cardiovascular status and reduce the risk of surgery. Careful monitoring for potential problems is carried out by both physician and nurse during the intraoperative and postoperative phases.

Renal insufficiency can increase the risk of surgery because of difficulty in removing increased amounts of electrolytes, especially potassium, and waste products from catabolism. Persons with renal disease are prone to develop fluid overload from parenteral fluids if urine production is not adequate.

Endocrine diseases that are influenced by hormonal changes occurring with the stress response can affect the patient's response to surgery. The patient with diabetes mellitus should be well controlled before surgery and monitored closely during and after surgery. Glucocorticoid activity and potassium changes following surgery can influence insulin utilization (see Chapter 37). If the wound is in an area where the patient may have impaired circulation, such as legs and feet, healing may be delayed. In persons who have increased levels of adrenocortical hormones such as occurs in pituitary or adrenocortical disease or for those receiving exogenous hormones, healing may be delayed because of an antiinflammatory response. In contrast, patients with Addison's disease (hypofunction of the adrenal cortex) or patients receiving hormonal replacement will require additional replacement therapy because of the stress of surgery.

Disabilities that can influence response to surgery include those that affect or limit activity. Inability to ambulate, to exercise, or to move about freely in bed increases the risk of postoperative atelectasis, pneumonia, or thrombophlebitis.

SURGICAL PROCEDURE
SITE

Surgery that is performed on body areas that are visible to others may leave scars that are perceived by the patient or significant others as disfiguring. Surgery of vital organs such as the heart, lungs, and kidneys may be threatening to the patient in terms of survival. Surgery of the mouth or throat may create temporary breathing problems that can be perceived as threatening. Surgery of the extremities may create permanent changes in life-style, especially in activities of daily living (eating, bathing, dressing, walking). Surgery on body areas that have special meaning to the person such as the breast, genitalia, or reproductive organs will have differing effects and responses.

TYPE AND EXTENT OF SURGERY

Removal of organs can be perceived as a threat (especially if there is considerable meaning attached to the organ by the patient) or can create changes in life-style. Surgery that creates an artificial opening, such as a colostomy, is highly stressful to the patient and produces differing responses. The more extensive the surgery, the greater the physiologic responses that will occur. Psychologic responses are not directly related to the extent of the surgery, since they are influenced by the patient's past experiences, perceptions of what the surgery means to self-image, and possible changes in life-style.

POSTOPERATIVE COMPLICATIONS

Occurrence of postoperative complications will delay recovery. Wounds that separate or become infected may take considerable time to heal, especially if other complicating factors such as inadequate nutrition are also present. Shock, cardiac aberrations, fluid and electrolyte imbalances, atelectasis or pneumonia, or thrombophlebitis can all prolong the postoperative course. These complications are discussed in more detail later in this chapter and in later chapters of this book.

PREVIOUS EXPERIENCES WITH SURGERY

The patient who has had previous experience with surgery may respond either positively or negatively to the present surgery. A previous negative experience can be transferred to the present experience and increase anxiety. On the other hand, a previous negative experience is sometimes viewed by the patient as an entirely separate event that happened under different circumstances and thus may not influence the present experience.

INFORMED CONSENT

Before surgery, the patient is asked to sign a statement indicating consent to have the operative procedure performed. The consent implies that the patient has been provided with the knowledge necessary to understand the nature of the procedure as well as the known and possible consequences of the procedure.

The physician has the duty to provide the patient with sufficient information to weigh the risks and benefits of the proposed surgery (disclosure duty). The data usually include the nature of the surgery with its benefits and risks, alternatives to the surgery with their benefits and risks, and prognoses if treatment is withheld.[7] Risks include bodily harm or death but not the common possible postoperative complications such as infection. *Legal responsibility for obtaining informed consent from the patient, therefore, resides with the physician.* Oral consent is as binding as written consent.[7] Physicians will document that the necessary information has been provided the patient.

Signing of the official consent form is primarily evidence that the *consent process* has occurred and that the patient is aware of the concept of informed consent. The signatures of the health care personnel (as required by specific states or hospitals) merely provide witness to the signature of the patient or family member. Thus the nurse's signature does not reflect the substance of the informed consent process.

What then is the role of the nurse in the decision-making process? In the role of patient advocate, the nurse verifies that the patient has discussed with the physician the risks and benefits of the procedure and the alternatives. If this has not been done, the nurse consults with the physician. The professional nurse then uses skills of teaching and counseling to clarify any patient misconceptions and to facilitate the decision-making process. This process should occur before the patient receives any sedation. Patients may decide to refuse surgery and it is their right to do so. Nurses have the responsibility to see that the decision is an *informed* decision.

If an adult is incapable of giving informed consent, consent must be obtained from the next of kin. The order of kin relationship for an adult, as determined from legal intestate succession, is usually spouse, adult child, parent, sibling.[39] A parent or legal guardian usually provides consent for a minor child. "Emancipated minors," that is, persons who are married or earning their own livelihood and retaining the earnings, can sign their own permit. The signature of the husband or wife of a married minor is also acceptable.

In an emergency situation, the surgeon may operate without written permission of the patient or family, although every effort is made to contact a family member or guardian if time permits. Consent in the form of a telephone call is permissible in this situation.

PSYCHOLOGIC PREPARATION FOR SURGERY

For clarity of understanding, psychologic preparation for surgery is discussed separately from physiologic preparation for surgery. A nursing process format is used for each of these topics. It must be remembered, however, that people respond to stressors (such as surgery) as a cohesive whole; therefore actions are taken concurrently.

COMMON FEARS RELATED TO SURGERY

The patient facing surgery has numerous anxiety-provoking decisions to make. The first decision may be whether to seek medical advice (fear of the unknown). Decisions may have to be made concerning having specific tests made (fear of discomfort, fear of the unknown). The decision to have surgery may be the most difficult. Having major surgery involves putting one's life under the control of others and subjecting oneself to intrusion into the body and possible pain. It may also involve permanent changes in life-style.

Some of the fears underlying preoperative anxiety are elusive, and the patient may not be able to identify their causes. Others are more specific (see box below). Fear of the unknown is the most common. If the diagnosis is uncertain, fear of malignancy is frequent regardless of its probability. Fears concerning anesthesia are usually related to dying; a frequent example is "going to sleep and never waking up." Fears concerning pain, disfigurement, or permanent disability may be realistic or may be influenced by myths, lack of information, or lurid stories recited by friends. The patient may also have other concerns related to hospitalization, such as job security, income, and care of family.

Most surgeons will cancel surgery for a patient who is extremely anxious. Patients with anxiety levels so high that they cannot discuss and begin to cope with their anxiety before surgery frequently experience difficulty in the postoperative period. They are more apt to be angry, resentful, confused, or depressed. They are also more vulnerable to psychotic reactions than are patients with lower levels of anxiety.

Lack of any emotional response to surgery may indicate denial; this precludes dealing with and coping with the anxiety before surgery. A moderate amount of anxiety enables the individual to identify and begin to cope with feelings. These patients usually experience a smoother postoperative course.

FEARS RELATED TO SURGERY

GENERAL	SPECIFIC
Fear of unknown	Diagnosis of malignancy
Loss of control	Anesthesia
Loss of love from significant others	Dying
	Pain
Threat to sexuality	Disfigurement
	Permanent limitations

■ ASSESSMENT

If the patient facing possible surgery has contact during the prehospitalization period with a professional nurse, data should be collected at that time to identify potential or actual sources of preoperative anxiety, and interventions to assist the patient in coping with the threat of surgery should begin. Communication of the data to the nurse in the hospital can provide for continuity of care. If preadmission data are not available, the hospital admission or primary care nurse assesses the patient's psychologic readiness for surgery.

SUBJECTIVE DATA

Much of the data concerning knowledge and perceptions of the coming event will be obtained directly from the patient (see box below). It is necessary to know the level of the patient's understanding of the surgical event before any teaching can take place. Since persons respond on the basis of their perceptions, it is important to find out exactly how the surgery is perceived. Patients may not be able to identify specific concerns, and further exploration may be indicated. If the nurse has identified cues on which conclusions are drawn, these conclusions should be validated with the patient.

Knowledge of the meaning of religion for the patient

ASSESSMENT OF PREOPERATIVE ANXIETY

SUBJECTIVE DATA

1. Understanding of proposed surgery
   a. Site
   b. Type of surgery to be done
   c. Information from surgeon regarding extent of hospitalization, postoperative limitations
   d. Preoperative routines
   e. Postoperative routines
   f. Tests
2. Previous surgical experiences
   a. Type, nature
   b. Time interval
3. Any specific concerns or feelings about present surgery
4. Religion, meaning for patient
5. Significant others
   a. Geographic distance
   b. Perception as source of support
6. Changes in sleep patterns

OBJECTIVE DATA

1. Speech patterns
   a. Repetition of themes
   b. Change of topic
   c. Avoidance of topics related to feelings
2. Degree of interaction with others
3. Physical
   a. Increased pulse and respiratory rates
   b. Increased hand movements and perspiration
   c. Increased activity level
   d. Increased voiding frequency

can help the nurse identify a possible source of support. The effect of family members or significant others on the patient's level of anxiety needs to be determined. Some significant others increase the patient's anxiety by transmission of their own anxiety by hovering over the patient, displaying anxious behaviors, or by offering false reassurances. Others are calm, and it is observed that the patient's anxiety is reduced when they are present.

Changes in sleep patterns also provide clues about increased anxiety. Major causes of insomnia are worry, fear, and concerns about the future.

OBJECTIVE DATA

Signs of anxiety in the presurgical patient are no different than in other persons. Signs vary from person to person and can be observed in a number of ways. Highly anxious persons may talk rapidly, ask many questions without waiting for answers, repeat the same questions, or change topics frequently during the interaction. They may deny that they have any worries or fears, but their actions belie this. Some patients will not talk about the forthcoming surgery, responding only in monosyllables, while others cry and display anger; both behaviors are overt signs of anxiety. Physical signs include increased pulse and respiratory rate, moist palms, constant hand movements, and restlessness.

■ DATA ANALYSIS: NURSING DIAGNOSES

Nursing diagnoses are determined from assessment of patient data. Possible nursing diagnoses related to psychologic readiness for surgery may include but are not limited to the following:

Diagnostic Title	Possible Etiologies
Anxiety	Threat of death, threat to role functioning, threat of unmet needs, fear of unknown
Fear	Anesthesia, surgery (type), loss of body part, anticipated pain, possible life-style changes
Knowledge deficit (procedural, sensory)	Lack of exposure to surgery
Powerlessness	Loss of control from anesthesia or forced dependency

■ PLANNING: EXPECTED PATIENT OUTCOMES

Expected patient outcomes related to psychologic readiness for surgery may include, but are not limited to, the following:

1. Signs of anxiety/fear are decreased.
2. The patient or significant others can identify concerns related to surgery and explain events that will occur.
3. The patient and significant others are relaxed.
4. The patient participates in decision making when feasible.

■ IMPLEMENTATION

PROVIDING FOR EXPRESSION OF CONCERNS

Having opportunities to talk with a supportive, knowledgeable person will help patients begin to identify the reasons for their anxiety and to marshal coping responses. It is helpful for the nurse to plan for a quiet unhurried time to sit down with the patient and give an opportunity to ask questions and talk about concerns.

Touch is often a helpful form of communication, sending the message, "I care," and some patients will talk more readily while receiving a back rub. Knowing that a nurse is interested and cares helps to reduce anxiety. If the patient knows also that anxiety is a normal reaction to the threat of surgery, it may help to remove the often self-imposed expectation, "I shouldn't be nervous." Emphasis should be on accentuating the positive and helping patients identify their own strengths and coping responses.

Preoperative visits by the operating room nurse are helpful in many instances, especially in those situations when a great deal of anxiety may be expected, such as in heart surgery. The visit promotes the feeling that "someone in surgery knows me as an individual and will look after me." If it is known that the patient will be in intensive care for a period of time after surgery, a visit by a nurse from the intensive care unit may also help to allay anxiety.

SUPPORTING FAMILY/FRIENDS

Persons who have close ties with the patient are also frequently anxious. This anxiety can be transmitted to patients, increasing their anxiety level. The same principles described in exploring concerns and giving information to the patient hold true for significant others. If the patient needs assistance in meeting physical needs, receptive family members or friends can be shown how they can effectively participate if they so desire. This can reduce some of their own anxiety.

PROVIDING A MEANS OF CONTROL

Loss of control is one of the fears associated with surgery. Allowing patients to participate in decision making concerning care when feasible helps them partially meet the needs for control. Identifying and carrying out measures to help the person meet physical needs in the preoperative phase may help to provide a feeling of security about having postoperative needs met and thus allay some anxiety. Protection of the patient's privacy and modesty may also help.

Teaching relaxation methods (see Chapter 11) as a

method of decreasing the perception of pain in the postoperative period is another way of giving the patient a means of control. Relaxation exercises appear to reduce primarily the psychologic component of pain.

PATIENT TEACHING
PREOPERATIVE TEACHING GOALS

The purpose of preoperative teaching is to help decrease patient anxiety and to prepare the patient for surgery. The patient needs to learn (1) what to expect of surgical procedures or routines, and of sensations that may be experienced (such as pain); (2) measures to decrease anxiety; and (3) activities to enhance postoperative recovery (as described on p. 459).

Considerable nursing research has focused on preoperative patient teaching.[37] In general, research has demonstrated that preoperative teaching is effective in (1) decreasing patient anxiety, (2) altering unfavorable attitudes, (3) influencing postoperative recovery, and (4) promoting satisfaction with care.[37]

TYPES OF PREOPERATIVE TEACHING

Anxiety and fear experienced before surgery may be decreased by different approaches: explanations about what will occur during the expected surgery (*procedural*), what the patient may experience during the perioperative period (*sensory*), and what actions may help to decrease the anxiety (*psychologic*).[37] Fear of the unknown may be partly relieved by knowing what to expect. Procedural information generally has a positive effect by changing the unknown to the known. If the patient is highly anxious, however, too much information may serve only to increase the anxiety.

The amount of information to give preoperatively depends on the background, interest, and stress level of the patient. A good way to decide is to ask patients what they would like to know about the forthcoming surgery and to base responses on the types of questions asked. Persons under considerable stress, such as those in moderate to severe pain, cannot cope with much added stimuli, and simple explanations are indicated. A highly anxious person has a narrow perceptual field and may not perceive concurrent events and information. It is also important to remember that giving someone information does not necessarily mean that the information has been perceived or understood.

The preoperative information helpful to most patients relates to preoperative tests and activities, events related to the surgery, and expectations about what will happen postoperatively (see box above, right). Most patients are less anxious and participate more effectively if they know the reasons for tests and preoperative activities.

Patients experiencing high anxiety may benefit from learning about *sensations* that may be experienced during the perioperative period, such as drowsiness after

___

PREOPERATIVE TEACHING TO DECREASE ANXIETY

1. Preoperative tests—reasons, explanations of the tests
2. Preoperative routines
3. Schedules—time of surgery, probable length, time in recovery room
4. Recovery
   a. Place where patient will awaken
   b. Close nursing supervision
   c. Frequent monitoring of vital signs
   d. Return to room when vital signs are stable
5. Family directions
   a. Time patient will leave for surgery (visiting time)
   b. Where family may wait during surgery
   c. Procedure for notification of results of surgery (by physician)
   d. Procedure of notification of patient's return to unit
6. Probable postoperative therapies
   a. Anticipated treatments (such as IV, nasogastric tube)
   b. Need for increased mobility as soon as possible
   c. Need for breathing and coughing routines, even though these may be uncomfortable
   d. Pain medication routines (timing, sequence, "as needed" [prn] status)

___

premedication, coldness in the surgical suite (blankets will be applied), no discomfort before general anesthesia (except for needle prick from the IV through which the initial anesthesia will probably be given), and discomfort in the early postoperative period (medication will be given). It may be helpful to explain the expected pain relief routines, so the patient knows to ask for medication *before* pain becomes very severe (see Chapter 22).

The patient may also be taught *activities* that help decrease anxiety. The most common approaches are deep breathing, other relaxation exercises, and patient imagery (Chapter 11). A more recent approach is the use of music therapy (see research box).

TIMING AND METHODS OF PREOPERATIVE TEACHING

Preoperative teaching is done as early in the preoperative period as possible to permit time for the patient to learn. *Preadmission* teaching has been found to be effective for patient learning, and it requires less admission teaching time.[35] Booklets and pamphlets have proved effective. Preadmission teaching has been a major approach in recent years since the advent of ambulatory surgery or same day admission. Teaching during the 24 hours before surgery is less effective. Review or reinforcement of previously learned materials during this time, however, is effective.

Some patients may be admitted several days before surgery, and in these situations an *individual* teaching plan can be devised or the patient may be asked to attend a class (such as before heart surgery). *Group*

RESEARCH

Moss VA: Music and the surgical patient, AORN J 48:64-68, 1988.

Sedative music has been shown to decrease sympathetic nervous system activity. It was hypothesized in this study that introduction of sedative music as a nursing intervention would decrease anxiety in the patient undergoing surgery. The sample consisted of 17 patients ages 20-24 admitted for elective arthroscopic surgery to be performed using general anesthesia. The experimental group listened to sedative music of choice through a headset. The music was played from the time of the preoperative injection until the patient entered the postanesthesia care center. Data was collected pre- and postoperatively by a written State-Trait Anxiety Inventory (STAI), and by a postoperative interview in which the patients were asked their feelings about the musical experience. Postoperative anxiety was significantly decreased in the experimental group but not in the control group. Subjective comments from the experimental group were favorable to the experience. Further study is suggested for the use of music as a means of decreasing preoperative anxiety, but this research shows that music may be an additional method that nurses could use to help decrease preoperative anxiety. ■

teaching is effective but does not always present what the patient wants to know; therefore group discussions can be planned following lectures or AV presentations to give patients an opportunity to ask questions.

PHYSIOLOGIC PREPARATION FOR SURGERY

Preoperative intervention by both physician and nurse is directed toward making the surgical experience safe and comfortable for the patient (Table 20-3).

MEDICAL MANAGEMENT
MEDICAL ASSESSMENT

After the decision has been made for surgery, the physician collects additional data to identify the patient's physical readiness for surgery. Assessment usually includes emphasis on the patient's respiratory, cardiovascular, renal, and metabolic status (Table 20-4). Some operative and postoperative complications can be prevented or ameliorated if patients who are at high risk of developing these complications are identified early and measures are taken to try to prevent the complications.

Respiratory Status

A chest x-ray examination may be ordered to identify the presence of lung disease. If interference with pulmonary function is suspected, additional tests will be ordered, such as vital capacity tests, pulmonary function tests, and blood gas studies. If signs of upper respiratory

TABLE 20-3 Preoperative management

Physician	Nurse
COLLECT DATA	
Aid in medical diagnosis	Identify psychologic readiness for surgery
Determine need, type, and extent of surgery	Assess knowledge of events that will occur
Identify potential complications requiring medical intervention	Identify potential complications requiring nursing intervention
Obtain baseline data for future comparison	Obtain baseline data for future comparison
PSYCHOLOGIC PREPARATION	
Explain need, type, and extent of surgery to patient and significant others	Verify patient's understanding and clarify as indicated
	Give explanations about tests
	Give opportunities to express feelings and concerns
	Support significant others
PHYSICAL PREPARATION	
Prescribe and/or carry out tests	Assist patient and physician in carrying out tests
Prescribe diet, drugs	Assist patient to meet basic needs in preparation for surgery
Prescribe actions to ensure safety and comfort during surgery	Assist patient in carrying out physician's orders

infection are present (rhinitis, pharyngitis, sore throat, fever, cough), surgery will be postponed, if possible, until the symptoms abate.

Cardiovascular Status

Medical assessment of the cardiovascular status identifies signs of heart disease that need correction before surgery is carried out. An electrocardiogram (ECG) is often ordered for persons over age 40 to detect signs of cardiac arrhythmia or heart damage. Blood studies (Table 20-4) may indicate presence of blood dyscrasias, liver disease, or electrolyte imbalances as well as serving as baseline data. Blood volume studies or central venous pressure measurements may be ordered when there is known or suspected heart disease or if the patient is elderly and fluid overload is a potential problem.

If surgery is to be performed on major blood vessels or on the extremities, presence and strength of peripheral pulses are recorded. Comparison of preoperative and postoperative findings helps determine adequacy of circulation. If the patient has a low hematocrit or blood hemoglobin level or if major surgery that may involve considerable blood loss is planned, blood is drawn for typing and cross-matching so that blood will be available for transfusion as necessary.

TABLE 20-4 Preoperative tests to establish baselines and detect presence of diseases that can affect patient responses in intraoperative or postoperative phases

System	Test	Disease or Condition
Respiratory	Chest x-ray	Tuberculosis or other pulmonary disease
	Vital capacity	
	Pulmonary function	Tuberculosis, chronic obstructive lung disease, bronchitis, asthma
	Blood gas studies	
Circulatory	Electrocardiogram	Cardiac arrhythmias, myocardial damage
	Blood studies	
	WBC and differential	Chronic infection
	RBC, hemoglobin, hematocrit	Anemia
	Electrolytes	Electrolyte imbalances
	Platelet count, bleeding and clotting times, prothrombin	Liver disease, blood dyscrasias
	Typing and cross-matching	Compatibility for transfusion
	Blood volume	Heart disease
Renal	Urine studies	
	Bacteria	Urinary tract infection
	Albumin, specific gravity	Kidney disease
	Blood studies	
	Creatinine, BUN, NPN, electrolytes	Kidney disease
Metabolic	Blood sugar, urine sugar, acetone	Diabetes mellitus Starvation

Renal Status

Good renal function is necessary to maintain fluid and electrolyte balance postoperatively. Urinalysis will be ordered routinely on all patients. Presence of albumin or a low specific gravity may indicate the possibility of kidney disease, and further evaluation will be necessary. If urine sugar is noted, a blood sugar level will be obtained to ascertain the possibility of diabetes mellitus. Acetone in the urine may indicate diabetes mellitus or starvation. Signs of urinary tract infection include bacteriuria, fever, urgency, frequency, and burning on voiding. Urinary tract infection is treated with antibiotics before surgery if possible. Men with a history of prostatic enlargement may have difficulty voiding postoperatively.

MEDICAL INTERVENTIONS

Prevention of Postoperative Difficulties

Postoperative complications can be minimized if existing medical conditions are treated or well-controlled before surgery. Treatment of wound infections is carried out before secondary closure or skin grafting. Dehydra-

tion from vomiting and diarrhea is treated with parenteral fluids to reestablish fluids and electrolyte balance.

Patients with chronic diseases should be at their optimal level of health before surgery. The undernourished patient is placed on a high-protein, high-carbohydrate diet rich in vitamins B_1, C, and K. Supplementary vitamins may be prescribed. Total parenteral nutrition may be instituted for a severely undernourished person. The obese patient is placed on a weight-reducing diet. Both undernourished and obese patients should understand the rationale for the diets, and they may need considerable support and encouragement to maintain the diets.

Patients with chronic obstructive pulmonary disease (COPD) are frequently placed on vigorous respiratory therapy to ensure maximal ventilation and to decrease postoperative respiratory complications. This therapy usually includes postural drainage, aerosol inhalations, and antibiotics. Smoking is discouraged for all patients preoperatively, especially for patients with chronic obstructive pulmonary disease (COPD). Diabetes mellitus should be under good control.

Diet

On the day before surgery there is usually no change in the patient's dietary intake. One exception is bowel surgery, in which case patients may be placed preoperatively on a low-residue diet.

If general anesthesia is planned, food and fluids are usually not permitted for 4 to 8 hours before surgery. Presence of food or fluids in the stomach increases the possibility of aspiration of gastric contents should the patient vomit while under anesthesia. This can lead to aspiration pneumonia. If it should be discovered that the patient has consumed food or fluids when ordered "nothing by mouth" (NPO), the surgeon is notified, since this may require rescheduling the surgical procedure. If a local or spinal anesthetic is planned, a light meal may be permitted.

Patients who are dehydrated will have parenteral fluids initiated before surgery. If it is anticipated that the patient may have decreased peristalsis after surgery (such as after gastrointestinal surgery), a nasogastric tube may be inserted before surgery.

Bowel Preparation

Cleansing the bowel preoperatively by means of enemas is not a routine procedure. The surgeon makes the decision based on the surgical site and type of surgery to be performed. Preoperative enemas may be ordered before gastrointestinal tract surgery or surgery on the pelvic, perineal, or perianal areas. The purpose of the preoperative enema is to prevent injury to the colon and to provide better visualization of the surgical area. Enemas should be given if a patient has had x-ray studies involving barium immediately before surgery, because barium remaining in the intestinal tract may predispose to postoperative fecal impactions. Enemas given preoperatively should be effective.

If enemas are to be given until the returns are clear, it is important to remember that fluid excess and potassium deficits can occur with repeated enemas. It is common practice to check with the physician if returns are not clear after the third enema. One method is to give up to three enemas the evening before surgery, and then, if the returns are still not clear, to repeat the enemas the following morning. Repeated enemas are very tiring to the patient and may irritate rectal and bowel mucosa.

Controversy exists regarding the benefits of antibiotic enemas, because of the disturbance of the ecology of the bowel flora.[1] If antibiotic enemas are ordered, synthesis of vitamin K by intestinal bacteria may be inhibited; supplementary vitamin K may therefore be given to prevent increased bleeding after surgery.

Skin Preparation

The skin is the body's first defense against invading microorganisms. Any break in the continuity of the skin presents the potential for infection. The purpose of preoperative skin preparation is to decrease the risk of postoperative wound infection by (1) removing soil and transient microbes from the skin, (2) decreasing the resident microorganisms to subpathogenic amounts in a short time with the least amount of tissue irritation, and (3) inhibiting rapid regrowth of microorganisms.[34] The normal flora of even very clean skin contains several types of microorganisms, including staphylococcus and streptococcus.

The skin can never be completely rid of microorganisms, but the numbers can be considerably reduced by thorough cleansing or showering, especially with use of medicated bar soap or 4% chlorhexidine gluconate.

It is recommended that hair be removed only when it is so thick that it interferes with the surgical procedure.[34] Hair can be removed by one of three methods: depilatory, electric clipper, or razor. The first two methods are preferred. All hair removal articles should be either *disposable* or *terminally sterilized* between patients to avoid cross-contamination. The *depilatory* can be used safely before the patient goes to the operating room; the *clipper* and *razor* are best used in the operating holding room to minimize the time between hair removal and surgery (Chapter 21).

Shaving hair from the operative site has been shown to increase the incidence of postoperative wound infection (see research box), and regrowth of pubic hair is uncomfortable for many patients. Before shaving, the hair is well wetted to make it softer and easier to remove and to reduce the likelihood of skin abrasion. Hair on

RESEARCH

Cruse PS and Foord R: The epidemiology of wound infection, Surg Clin North Am 60(1):27-40, 1980.

The purposes of this study were to determine the extent of postoperative wound infection and to determine factors that influenced infection rate. Over a 10-year period, 63,000 wounds were inspected by nurses during the patient's hospital stay. There was a follow-up call to the surgeon's office after 28 days. The overall infection rate was 4.7%, but the percentage of infections was directly related to the character of the wound: clean wounds 1.5%, clean-contaminated wounds (minimal spillage of organs) 7.7%, contaminated wounds (gross spillage of organ or inflammation without pus at time of surgery) 15.2%, and dirty wounds (pus at operation or perforated viscus) 40%. A wound that became infected was found to increase a hospital stay by a mean of 10.1 days.

The major factors found to influence the occurrence of wound infection were preoperative skin preparation and the length of preoperative hospitalization. The wound infection rate for the person who had showered with hexachlorophene was 1.3%, compared to showering with soap 2.1%, and no shower 2.3%. The wound infection rate after shaving with a razor was 2.5%. The rate dropped to 1.7% when pubic hair was clipped, 1.4% after shaving with an electric razor, and 0.9% when the hair was neither shaved nor clipped.

In reference to the length of preoperative hospitalization, the longer the patient's preoperative stay, the greater was the infection rate. ◾

certain areas of the body, such as face, head, and pubic areas, may have a special meaning for some persons. If the entire head is to be shaved, the procedure is usually performed after the patient has been anesthetized.

◾ ASSESSMENT

The nurse collects physiologic data in the preoperative phase for two reasons: to obtain baseline data for comparison during the intraoperative and postoperative phases and to identify potential problems that may require preventive nursing interventions before surgery. If the patient has been hospitalized, the admission nursing history and physical assessment should contain much of the pertinent data that can serve as baseline data for surgery. Data of pertinence for the surgical patient are listed below. Recording of the data is important for comparison when changes occur during the perioperative period and for planning nursing care.

SUBJECTIVE DATA

Subjective physiologic data for the preoperative patient include the following:

   1. Medications that may interfere with anesthesia or

TABLE 20-5 Medications that can adversely affect anesthesia or surgery

Medication	Effect
Antibiotics	Potentiate muscle relaxants
Anticoagulants	Increase bleeding and hemorrhage
Antihypertensives	Affect anesthesia and compensatory ability (hypotension may occur)
Aspirin	↓ Platelet aggregation
	Potentiates effect of anticoagulants
Diuretics (thiazides)	Possible potassium imbalance
Steroids	↓ Neuroendocrine response
	Antiinflammatory effect, may delay wound healing
Tranquilizers	Potentiate effect of narcotics and barbiturates
	Hypotension

TABLE 20-6 Risk factors in development of postoperative pulmonary complications

Risk Factors	Effect
INCREASED RESPIRATORY SECRETIONS	
Smoking	Irritation of lining of tracheobronchial passages
Intubation	
Inhalant anesthetics	Decreased ciliary action to remove secretions
Chronic lung disease	
Upper respiratory infection	Secretions will block bronchial passages or alveoli
DRY STICKY SECRETIONS	
Chronic lung disease	Difficult to cough up secretions
Dehydration	
	Secretions will block bronchial passages
DECREASED THORAX EXPANSION	
Pain (chest, upper abdomen)	Lung does not expand fully, resulting in hypoventilation of alveoli
Obesity	
Age (elderly)	
Tight binders or casts	
Skeletal abnormalities (for example, scoliosis)	
DECREASED DIAPHRAGM MOBILITY	
Abdominal distention	Decreased lung expansion, leading to hypoventilation
Surgery of chest or upper abdomen	
Muscle relaxants	
Neurologic deficit	
DEPRESSION OF RESPIRATORY CENTER	
Sedatives	Depressed respirations result in hypoventilation
Narcotics	
Acid-base imbalance	
ASPIRATION OF GASTRIC CONTENTS	
Vomiting	Causes aspiration pneumonia

contribute to postoperative complications (Table 20-5)

2. Allergies: medications, soaps, adhesive tape
3. Sensory: difficulties with vision or hearing
4. Prosthetic devices: dentures, artificial eye or limb
5. Motor: difficulties with ambulation, movement of arms and legs, arthritis, previous orthopedic surgery (joint replacement, spinal fusion)
6. Nutrition: adequacy of dietary intake (food, fluids), nausea
7. Elimination: problems with constipation
8. Comfort: ability to sleep, presence of pain or discomfort, expectations regarding relief of postoperative pain
9. Knowledge of postoperative exercises

OBJECTIVE DATA

Objective physiologic data for the preoperative patient include the following:

1. Vital signs
2. Height and weight
3. Skin: turgor, bruising, presence of lesions, rashes
4. Sensory: ability to see and hear
5. Mouth: dentures, condition of teeth and mucous membranes
6. Chest: breath sounds (presence, character), chest expansion, ability to do diaphragmatic breathing
7. Extremities: muscle strength (especially legs), character of peripheral pulses prior to vascular or limb surgery, coordination with ambulation

Ventilation

Decreased ventilation resulting in atelectasis or pneumonia is the most common postoperative complication. A preoperative baseline assessment of the person's ventilatory status is important for early identification of de-

creased postoperative ventilation. Patients who are at high risk for developing postoperative pulmonary complications must be identified (Table 20-6). Patients at high risk include: (1) those scheduled for upper abdominal or thoracic surgery, (2) those to be administered inhalant anesthesia, (3) the obese, (4) smokers, (5) patients suffering from chronic lung disease, and (6) the elderly.

Nutrition

Because undernourished or obese patients have a greater potential for developing postoperative complications, it is important to identify them before surgery by comparing weight with height and bone structure (see Chapter 40). Diet histories should be taken for high-risk patients to determine dietary preferences and usual food habits. Excessive preoperative nausea and vomiting will dehydrate the patient and cause electrolyte imbalance.

Signs of dehydration (decreased skin turgor, dry mucous membranes, high hematocrit level) should be noted.

Elimination

A history of chronic constipation is noted for vigorous follow-up in the postoperative period when decreased activity may further complicate the problem. Methods that the patient has found effective in the past to control constipation are noted. Diarrhea is reported to the physician because this may lead to dehydration and electrolyte imbalances.

Mobility

Baseline data on the patient's muscle strength and ability to move the extremities and to ambulate are important data for the care of the patient in the operating room and postoperatively. Any limitations are carefully recorded.

■ DATA ANALYSIS: NURSING DIAGNOSES

Nursing diagnoses are determined from assessment of patient data. Possible nursing diagnoses related to physiologic preparedness for surgery may include but are not limited to the following:

Diagnostic Title	Possible Etiologies
Knowledge deficit (prevention of postoperative complications)	Lack of exposure/recall, information misinterpretation
Injury, potential for	Hazards of surgery
Fatigue	Lack of sleep or rest

■ PLANNING: EXPECTED PATIENT OUTCOMES

Expected patient outcomes for physiologic preparation for surgery may include, but are not limited to the following:

1. The patient can demonstrate and explain the rationale for exercises to prevent postoperative complications:
   a. Deep breathing and coughing exercises
   b. Leg exercises
   c. Turning and moving in bed
2. Injury or nosocomial infection does not occur.
3. The patient sleeps well the night before surgery and is relaxed during transportation to surgery.

■ IMPLEMENTATION
PATIENT TEACHING

Much preoperative teaching focuses on information or activities that may help to decrease patient anxiety (p. 454). Additional teaching includes activities that enhance physiologic healing by preventing postoperative complications. Because of short postoperative hospital stays, discharge teaching must be initiated during the preoperative period.

It is important to find out first what the patient already knows. Previous experiences, level of understanding, level of anxiety, and presence of distractors such as pain are assessed. Explanations are kept simple, but the rationale for what is being taught and how it will later affect the patient is given. Planning ahead may be necessary so that a quiet area conducive to teaching is available. Patients are asked to repeat in their own words what they have learned or to demonstrate how to do an activity such as coughing or leg exercises.

DEEP BREATHING AND COUGHING EXERCISES

Deep breathing facilitates oxygenation and removal of residual inhalant anesthetics. It also prevents alveolar collapse that leads to atelectasis. Coughing removes secretions that may block the airways. All patients potentially at risk of developing postoperative pulmonary complications (see Table 20-6) are taught deep breathing and coughing exercises before surgery. Waiting to do so until the patient is awakening from anesthesia decreases the possibility that these exercises will be carried out effectively; anesthesia and postoperative pain decrease the ability to retain information.

The patient needs to know how to perform correct diaphragmatic breathing, since this increases lung expansion by permitting the diaphragm to descend fully. Many males normally breathe diaphragmatically, whereas few females do. With diaphragmatic breathing, the *abdomen rises with inspiration and falls with expiration*. The nurse assesses the patient's normal breathing pattern by placing a hand lightly on the patient's abdomen and asking the patient to take a deep breath. If diaphragmatic breathing does not occur naturally, the patient can be taught to inspire deeply while pushing the abdomen up against the hand.

DEEP BREATHING AND COUGHING EXERCISES

DEEP BREATHING

1. Lie in semi-Fowler's or high Fowler's position with knees flexed to relax abdomen and allow full chest expansion.
2. Place a hand lightly on the abdomen.
3. Breathe in slowly through nose, letting chest expand and feeling abdomen rise against hand.
4. Hold breath for 3 seconds.
5. Exhale slowly through pursed lips (abdomen contracts).
6. Repeat deep breathing three times, then cough (see below).

COUGHING

1. Breathe in as described above.
2. Count to 3.
3. On "3," cough *deeply* three times.
4. If unable to cough deeply, do repeated "huff" coughs (forced expiration with glottis open).

Deep breathing and coughing exercises are described in the box on p. 459. It is important for the patient to hold the breath for 3 seconds for most effective alveolar expansion. If there is difficulty with a deep cough, encourage the patient to do a "huff" cough (see box); repeated huff coughs often stimulate a deep cough. The patient is also shown how to splint an incision with a pillow, towel, or hands to help decrease pain while coughing.

LEG EXERCISES

Venous stasis in the postoperative period may lead to thrombophlebitis (blood clot). Patients at high risk include those who (1) will have decreased mobility after surgery, (2) have a history of decreased peripheral circulation, or (3) experience cardiovascular or pelvic surgery. These patients will need to carry out exercises postoperatively to prevent venous stasis in the legs. Leg exercises (Figure 20-2) help to prevent venous congestion by "pumping" the blood along the veins. Valves in the veins prevent backflow of blood.

MOBILITY

Moving and turning in bed help to prevent pulmonary and circulatory complications, prevent decubiti, stimulate peristalsis, and decrease pain. During the preoperative period, patients can be taught how to use the side rails effectively for turning and how to sit up on the side of the bed with the least amount of pull on the incision.

To turn to right side:
1. Slide hips to left side of bed
2. Support incision with right hand
3. Flex left knee
4. Grasp right side rail with left hand
5. Pull with left hand while pushing with left leg to turn

To sit up on side of bed before ambulation:
1. Move to edge of bed
2. Raise head of bed to high Fowler's position
3. Drop feet over side of bed
4. Push up to sitting position with hand closest to edge of bed (other hand can support the incision)

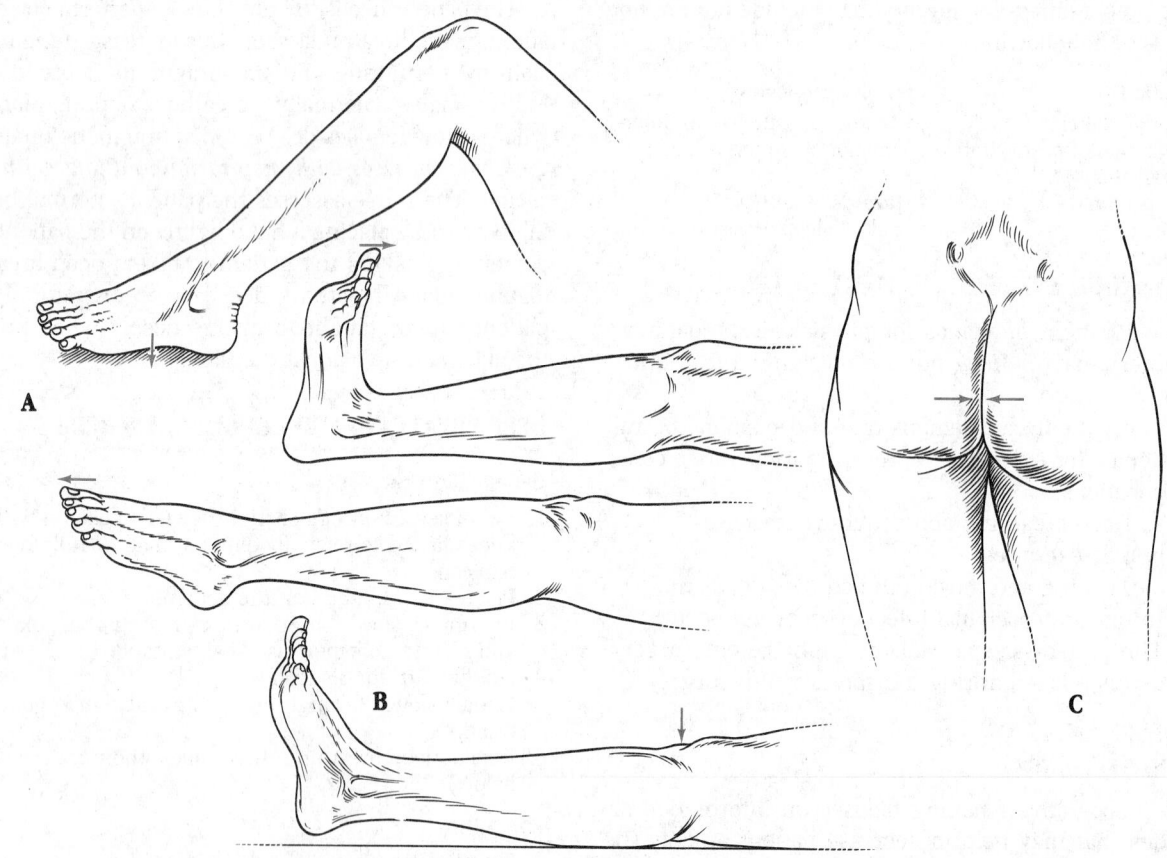

FIGURE 20-2 Exercises to strengthen muscles for ambulation and to prevent thrombus formation. **A,** Knees and ankles are flexed and extended. **B,** Knee is pressed against bed and heel is lifted off bed (quadriceps setting). **C,** Buttocks are pinched together and relaxed (gluteal setting).

PATIENT CARE ON OPERATIVE DAY

Promoting Rest and Sleep

Because surgery is trauma and therefore stressful, energy is required for coping. Sleep and rest conserve energy and thus are important before surgery. A sedative is usually ordered on the night before surgery to ensure a good night's rest. If additional sedation or medication for pain is given during the night, it must be given at least four hours before the preoperative medication.

The preadmitted patient should be permitted to sleep on the morning of surgery for as long as possible and to rest undisturbed until shortly before administration of the preanesthetic medication. Many patients therefore prefer to take their bath or shower the evening before surgery rather than in the morning. The patient who has bathed the night before is given an opportunity to wash hands and face and to perform mouth care. The patient is reminded not to swallow any water if fluids by mouth are not permitted. A hospital gown is worn to surgery.

Comfort implies readiness for surgery and ability to marshal effective coping mechanisms. The patient should have an opportunity to have last-minute questions answered. Explanations for last-minute routines are given if this was not done previously. If the surgery is to be delayed even for a short time, both the patient and family should be informed.

It is advisable that the patient not be unduly stimulated by visitors before surgery. The patient's choice of who he or she wants to see should be taken into consideration, whether it be family members or a close friend. The patient's family or close friends who plan to be present the day of surgery are made aware of the time for surgery and when the patient will be transported, to permit time for a visit. They are also informed where they may wait while the patient is in surgery and when to expect to receive information about the patient's condition. The patient may also desire a visit from a chaplain on the morning of surgery.

Preventing Injury or Loss

Final assessment. Vital signs are taken for identification of significant changes. It is normal for the pulse rate and systolic blood pressure to be increased from baseline levels as a result of the immediacy of the stressful situation; however, significant changes are reported to the surgeon. Other data to be reported are temperature elevation (possible infection) or expressions of a new or different type of pain.

The patient's identification band is checked for accuracy, legibility, and firmness of attachment. The band will be checked additionally by the nurse in the operating room suite. This action protects the patient from receiving surgery designated for another person.

Removal of accessories. *Hairpins* are removed because they may become dislodged and injure the scalp. *Wigs* are removed because they may become lost. A disposable cap is worn by the patient during surgery to protect the hair should the patient vomit and to facilitate easy access to the patient's face by the anesthesiologist.

Nail polish is removed to facilitate assessment of capillary filling for circulatory status. *Dentures* are removed because they may fall away from the gums and drop back into the pharynx, causing respiratory obstruction when the muscles of the jaw relax under anesthesia.

Any *hearing aid is left in place*. It is important that the operating room staff be able to communicate with the patient in the crucial minutes before surgery. The operating room nurse is informed that the hearing aid is in place. If the patient does not speak English, an attempt should be made to locate an interpreter who can accompany the patient to the operating room and remain until anesthesia is induced. Many larger hospitals have foreign language registries of employees who can be called on for such assistance.

Application of antiembolic stockings. Antiembolic stockings or elastic bandages are applied to legs of high-risk persons (see box below). The stockings or bandages compress superficial veins and increase blood flow through deep veins by counterpressure, thus preventing venous stasis. This in turn helps to prevent thromboembolism and shock.

Bladder emptying. The patient is asked to void immediately before leaving for the operating room. An empty bladder permits better visualization of abdominal organs and decreases the chances of inadvertent injury to the bladder. A patient who has voided shortly before being asked to do so may not be able to void again because of fluid restrictions. If the bladder must be kept in a collapsed state throughout the surgery or if the patient has a condition that will interfere with postoperative urination, an indwelling catheter is inserted and attached by tubing to a closed drainage system. This is frequently carried out in the operating room to ensure asepsis.

HIGH RISK FACTORS FOR POSTOPERATIVE THROMBOEMBOLISM

Age: elderly

Marked varicosities

Pelvic surgery

Time-consuming surgery

Prolonged postoperative bed rest

TABLE 20-7 Commonly used preanesthetic medications

Generic Name	Trade Name	Desired Effects	Undesired Effects
NARCOTICS			
Meperidine hydrochloride	Demerol	Reduce anxiety, promote relaxation, decrease preoperative pain	Depress respiration, circulation and gastric motility; may cause nausea and vomiting
Morphine sulfate	—		
BARBITURATES			
Butabarbital sodium	Butisol	Reduce anxiety, promote relaxation and sleep	May cause excitement or confusion in elderly persons or those with severe pain
Pentobarbital sodium	Nembutal		
Secobarbital sodium	Seconal		
BENZODIAZEPINES			
Chlordiazepoxide hydrochloride	Librium, Libritabs	Reduce anxiety, promote relaxation	Dizziness and headache, especially in the elderly person
Diazepam	Valium		
Lorazepam	Ativar		
NEUROLEPTANALGESIC AGENT			
Fentanyl and droperidol	Innovar	General quiescence; state of indifference; decreased motor activity; analgesia; antiemetic	Respiratory depression; muscle rigidity; hypotension

Safeguarding of personal belongings. Objects or prostheses taken to the operating room with the patient may become lost or damaged. Prostheses such as dentures or false limbs or eye are removed, labeled, and placed in safekeeping. Patients who want to take religious medals to the operating room can be advised that in many instances paper emblems may be obtained from their priest. All jewelry and money should be sent home with the family, if possible, or removed from the bedside and locked up. Because a ring can catch on objects and cause injury, it should be removed. If the patient is permitted to wear a wedding ring, it should be taped or tied securely to the hand.

Preanesthetic Medication

The term *premedication* is used to signify medication that is given 1 to 2 hours before induction of anesthesia, which is usually given immediately before the patient is transferred to surgery. The purposes of premedication are (1) to decrease anxiety and provide sedation, (2) to induce amnesia, (3) to decrease secretion of saliva and gastric juices, and (4) to prevent allergic reaction to anesthetic drugs.[39] Commonly used preanesthetic medications include barbiturates, narcotics, and benzodiazepines (Table 20-7).

The combination and dosages of the premedication vary based on factors identified by the anesthesiologist. Adults frequently receive a combination of drugs depending on body size. Dosages are often decreased for the elderly. Narcotics have a number of disadvantages that cause some disagreement as to their use as preanesthetic medications. Anticholinergic drugs, such as atropine and scopolamine, are used rarely because of the more effective techniques of anesthetic administration and more rapid inductions that lessen secretion formation.

Preanesthetic medications are usually administered intramuscularly 60 to 90 minutes before the induction of anesthesia so that the maximal effect takes place. Any delay in giving the medication should be reported to the anesthesiologist. All preoperative routines should be completed before the preanesthetic medication is given. Noise and confusion are avoided to achieve maximal effect. It must be reemphasized that psychologic preparation of the patient for surgery is the most effective approach to help allay anxiety. Studies have shown that the administration of preanesthetic medication without any attempt at psychologic preparation may render the patient drowsy but does not reduce anxiety.

Recording of Final Data

Data relevant to the care of the patient in the intraoperative and postoperative phases are recorded. Having a form with the important data highly visible and accessible facilitates continuity of care and easy retrieval of data for later use.

Two types of forms are commonly used. One provides pertinent nursing assessment and problem identification (see box on p. 463); the second form is a checklist identifying completion of preoperative routines (see check list box on p. 463).

SAMPLE PREOPERATIVE NURSING ASSESSMENT FORM

Directions: Complete form day before surgery. Fill in or check off appropriate data.

Name _____
Age _____ Height _____ Weight _____
Vital sign range: T _____ P _____ R _____ BP _____
Consciousness: Alert _____ Confused _____ Disoriented _____
　　　　　　　Semicomatose _____ Comatose _____
Anxiety level: Mild _____ Moderate _____ Severe _____
Language: English speaking _____ If not, other: _____
Speech: Distinct _____ Other _____
Hearing: Can understand direction without aids _____ Deaf _____
　　　　　Decreased: Left _____ Right _____ Hearing aid _____
Vision: Can distinguish people/objects without aids _____
　　　　Glasses _____ Contacts _____ Blind: Left _____ Right _____
Skin: Intact _____ Other _____
Respiration: Character: Normal _____ Dyspeneic _____ Orthopneic _____
　　　　　　Breath sounds: Clear all lobes _____
　　　　　　Other findings: _____
　　　　　　Chest expansion: Full _____ Restricted _____
Pulse strength: Full _____ Weak _____ Absent in: _____
Drainage systems present: _____
Allergies: _____
Knows postoperative exercises: DB&C _____ Leg exercise _____
Comments:

Date _____ Signature _____

Transportation to Operating Room

The surgical patient is usually transported to the operating room on a mobile stretcher unit or in some instances in bed. To protect the patient from falling, each stretcher has body restraint straps and side rails.

Personnel transporting the surgical patient identify themselves to the clinical unit nursing staff and request assistance. The unit nurse assigned to prepare the patient for surgery checks the patient record, accompanies the transportation attendant to the patient's bedside, and signs the patient identification form. Before the patient is transported from the room the patient identification form is attached to the stretcher or bed. The patient is made comfortable with a pillow under the head and a blanket as a cover. Woolen or synthetic blankets should never be sent to the operating room because they are a source of static electricity. All patients should be protected from drafts, and if the patient holding area in the operating room is kept cool, additional blankets may be needed.

SAMPLE PREOPERATIVE CHECK LIST FORM

NAME _____

PREOPERATIVE LAB RESULTS	SAFETY	PREOPERATIVE ROUTINES
CBC _____	Identification bracelet _____	Operative permit _____
Urinalysis _____	Voided _____	Skin prep _____
Chest x-ray _____	Nail polish removed _____	Preanesthetic medication given _____
EKG _____	Valuables secured _____	Time _____
Type and cross-match _____	Place _____	Drug(s) _____
	Objects _____	
	Dentures removed _____	
Date _____ Time _____	Signature _____	

CHAPTER SUMMARY

- Surgery may be diagnostic, curative, restorative, palliative, or cosmetic.

- Neuroendocrine responses to surgery include vasoconstriction, increased cardiac output, decreased GI activity, increased glucocorticoid secretions, and increased ADH secretion.

- Increased aldosterone and ADH secretions lead to decreased urinary output compared to fluid intake for 24-48 hours after surgery.

- Metabolic responses to surgery include ketogenesis, gluconeogenesis, and protein breakdown, as well as reduced protein synthesis. These responses explain the weight loss, fatigue, negative nitrogen balance, slower wound healing, and increased susceptibility to infection that may occur after surgery.

- The ability of the elderly to tolerate surgery varies; however, physiologic changes in most body systems make the elderly more susceptible to atelectasis, pneumonia, shock, thrombosis, hypervolemia with IV fluids, infection, confusion, and constipation.

- Patients must know about the nature and risks of the proposed surgery and available options for care before signing a consent form (informed consent). The physician is responsible for obtaining informed consent; the nurse facilitates the process and ensures that the consent form has been signed before surgery.

- Anxiety and fear are common responses to anticipated surgery. Persons with severe anxiety are poor candidates for surgery.

- The patient's preoperative anxiety can be decreased by providing for expression of concerns, allowing access to supporting family members, providing means to achieve control, and providing patient teaching.

- Most preoperative patients have decreased anxiety if they understand the procedures and routines that will occur in the perioperative period. Highly anxious persons, however, may respond better to learning about the sensations that they will be experiencing and how these can be modified.

- Preoperative medical care includes assessment and treatment of existing medical conditions to minimize postoperative complications.

- Dietary restrictions for adults having major surgery usually include no food for 8 hours and no fluids for 4 hours before surgery.

- The skin is prepared for surgery by careful cleansing to remove soil and to lessen transient microorganisms to subpathogenic levels. Hair is not generally removed unless there is sufficient hair to interfere with surgery. Depilatories and electric hair clippers are preferred to shaving. Shaving can cause breaks in the skin and serve as a potential source of infection.

- Risk factors for postoperative complications include increased respiratory secretions, dry sticky secretions, decreased thorax expansion, decreased diaphragm motility, depression of the respiratory center, and aspiration of gastric contents.

- Exercises that can help to prevent postoperative complications should be taught preoperatively, as appropriate, and should include deep breathing and coughing exercises, leg exercises, and methods of turning in bed.

- Final preparations before the patient is transported to surgery include removing nonattached objects, ensuring proper patient identification, providing a hair cap, asking the patient to void, and giving the prescribed preanesthetic medications.

- Preanesthetic medications are given to decrease anxiety, provide sedation, induce amnesia, decrease secretions, and prevent allergic reactions to anesthetics. Commonly used preanesthetic medications include barbiturates, narcotics, and benzodiazepines.

QUESTIONS TO CONSIDER

- If you were scheduled for major surgery tomorrow, what concerns would you have?

- How do you think preoperative concerns might be similar or different among a 30-year-old mother of two young children, a 45-year-old factory maintenance foreman, and a 75-year-old widow?

- How would you explain Figure 20-1 to a lay person?

- Examine Table 20-2. How do the effects result from the physiologic changes?

REFERENCES AND SELECTED READINGS

1. American College of Surgeons Committee on Pre- and Postoperative Care: Manual on preoperative and postoperative care, ed 3, Philadelphia, 1983, WB Saunders Co.
2. *Blackwood S: Back to basics: the preop exam, Am J Nurs 86:39-44, 1986.
3. Clark JB, Queener SF, and Karb VB: Pharmacological basis of nursing practice, ed 3, St Louis, 1987, The CV Mosby Co.
4. Connaway CA and Blackledge D: Preoperative testing center: central location to evaluate and educate patients, AORN J 43:666-670, 1986.

*References preceded by an asterisk are particularly well suited for student reading.

5. Cramer C: Preoperative care unit: an alternative to the holding unit, AORN J 45:464-472, 1987.

6. *Crawford FJ: Ambulatory surgery: the elderly patient, AORN J 41:356-369, 1985.

7. *Cushing M: Informed consent: an MD responsibility? Am J Nurs 84:437-440, 1984.

8. *Fraulini DE: Coping mechanisms and recovery from surgery, AORN J 37:1198-1208, 1983.

9. *Fuchs P: Before and after surgery, stay right on respiratory care, Nursing '83 13(5):47-50, 1983.

10. Garibaldi RA et al: The impact of preoperative skin disinfection on preventing wound contamination, Infect Control Hosp Epidemiol 9(3):109-115, 1988.

11. *Greenwood BS: Check out your patient's presurgery fears, Nursing '82 12(7):34-35, 1982.

12. Gruendemann BJ and Meeker, MH: Alexander's care of the patient in surgery, ed 8, St Louis, 1987, The CV Mosby Co.

13. Guyton A: Textbook of medical physiology, ed 7, Philadelphia, 1986, WB Saunders Co.

14. Hathaway B: Effect of preoperative instruction on postoperative outcomes: a meta-analysis, Nurs Res 35:269-275, 1986.

15. Hinshaw AS et al: The use of predictive modeling to test nursing practice outcomes, Nurs Res 32:35-42, 1983.

16. *Hogue E: What you should know about informed consent, Nursing '86 16(6):47-48, 1986.

17. *Jackson MF: High risk surgical patients, J Gerontol Nurs 14(1):8-15, 1988.

18. Johnston M: Preoperative emotional states and postoperative recovery, Adv Psychosom Med, 15:1-22, 1986.

19. Kaplan EB et al: The usefulness of preoperative laboratory screening, JAMA 253:3576-3581, 1985.

20. *Kathol DK: Anxiety in surgical patients' families, AORN J 40:131-137, 1984.

21. *Kennedy-Caldwell C: The morbidly obese surgical patient, Crit Care Nurs 7(5):87-89, 1987.

22. Kneedler J and Dodge G: Perioperative patient care, ed 2, Boston, 1987, Blackwell Scientific Publications Inc.

23. Knight CG and Donnelly MK: Assessing the preoperative adult, Nurs Pract 13(1):6-17, 1988.

24. Kupferer RN, Uebele JA, and Levin DF: Geriatric ambulatory surgery patients: assessing cognitive functions, AORN J 47:752-764, 1988.

25. *Latz PA and Wyble SJ: Elderly patients: perioperative nursing implications, AORN J 46:238-252, 1987.

26. Lindeman CA: Patient education (review), Annu Rev Nurs Res 6:29-60, 1988.

27. Luce JM: Clinical risk factors for postoperative pulmonary complications, Resp Care 29:484-495, 1984.

28. *Mackie RM and Peddie RP: Perioperative careplan guides, AORN J 40:192-201, 1984.

29. *McHugh NG, Christman JN, and Johnson JE: Preparatory information, what helps and why, Am J Nurs 82:780-782, 1982.

30. *Miller KM: Deep breathing relaxation: a pain management technique, AORN J 45:484-488, 1987.

31. *Moss VA: Music and the surgical patient: the effect of music on anxiety, AORN J 48:64-68, 1988.

32. *Murphy EK: Informed consent, Pt I, AORN J 47:1009-1016, 1988, Pt II, AORN J 47:1295-1298, 1988.

33. Nyamathi A, and Kashiwabara A: Preoperative anxiety: its affect on cognitive thinking, AORN J 47:164-170, 1988.

34. Proposed recommended practices: preoperative skin preparation, AORN J 46:719-723, 1988.

35. Rice VH and Johnson JE: Preadmission self-instruction booklets, postadmission exercise performance, and teaching time, Nurs Res 33(3):147-151, 1984.

36. Rogers M and Reich P: Psychological intervention with surgical patients: evaluation outcomes, Adv Psychosom Med 15:23-50, 1986.

37. *Rothrock JC: Perioperative nursing research: preoperative psychoeducational interventions, AORN J 49:597-616, 1989.

38. Torrington KG et al: Perioperative respiratory therapy (PORT): a program of preoperative risk assessment and individualized postoperative care, Chest 93:946-951, 1988.

39. Way LW: Current surgical diagnosis and treatment, ed 8, Norwalk Conn, 1988, Appleton & Lange.

40. *Weaver TE: New life for lungs . . . through incentive spirometers, Nursing '81 11(2):54-58, 1981.

41. White HE et al: Body temperature in elderly surgical patients, Res Nurs Health 10:317-321, 1987.

42. Wong J et al: A randomized trial of a new approach to preoperative teaching and patient compliance, Int J Nurs Stud 22(2):105-115, 1985.

43. Worley B: Preadmission testing and teaching: more satisfaction at less cost . . . surgical admissions, Nurs Manage 17(12):32-33, 1986.

CHAPTER 21

Intraoperative Nursing

JUDITH C. GREIG

CHAPTER OBJECTIVES

After studying this chapter, the student should be able to:
1 Identify roles of operating room team members.
2 Identify basic rules of surgical asepsis.
3 Explain the rationale for proper operating room attire and personnel health habits.
4 Identify factors promoting patient safety and protection.
5 Describe different methods of anesthesia and stages of general anesthesia.
6 Describe monitoring methods used during anesthesia.

Patients bring with them to the operating suite a unique set of feelings and values that must be considered in planning nursing care during the intraoperative period. The operating room nurse functions as the patient's advocate during surgery. This role has been viewed in the past as being entirely technical in nature. One cannot deny that an operating room nurse must possess knowledge of skills, procedures, instruments, and supplies to function as an effective team member. All of operating room nursing, however, is not technical, and the integration of nursing process into this arena of care has become the accepted standard for operating room nurses. These nurses are responsible for providing a safe, caring, and efficient environment in which the surgical team can function to provide the best outcome for each patient.

CONCEPTS BASIC TO OPERATING ROOM NURSING

PERIOPERATIVE NURSING

The perioperative role of the operating room (OR) nurse consists of nursing activities performed by the professional operating room nurse during the operative phases of the patient's surgical experience (Figure 21-1). The extent of activities depends on the nurse's knowledge and skill, varying from a level of basic competency to a level of excellence.

Each phase of this role begins and ends at an appointed time in the chain of events involved in surgical intervention, and each includes a variety of nursing activities that can be performed utilizing nursing process. The *preoperative phase* begins when the decision for surgical intervention is made and ends when the patient is transferred to the operating room table. The scope of nursing activities involved can be as broad as beginning assessment of the patient in the clinic or at home through a preoperative interview, or as limited as doing a preoperative assessment in the holding area of the surgical suite.

The *intraoperative phase* begins when the patient is transferred to the operating table and ends with transfer to the recovery area. Again, the activities performed by the nurse can be as broad as recognizing the patient's potential for skin breakdown in certain areas and taking special precautions, or as limited as simply positioning the patient on the table according to the basic principles of good body alignment.

The *postoperative phase* begins with admission of the patient to the recovery area and ends with a follow-up evaluation. The scope of care can be as broad as seeing the patient at home or in a clinic setting, or as limited as communicating pertinent information about the patient's surgery to personnel in the recovery area. Table 21-1 is a sample list of nursing activities in the three phases of perioperative nursing.

The practice of perioperative nursing is envisioned as a goal for care given by operating room nurses. The role has been developed by the Association of Operating Room Nurses (AORN), a voluntary organization of registered nurses concerned with the care of patients before, during, and after surgery. By practicing the perioperative role, the OR nurse combines traditional and extended nursing activities during the intraoperative period with the more recently developed preoperative and postoperative assessment, teaching, and evaluation functions, thus integrating both technical and professional functions.

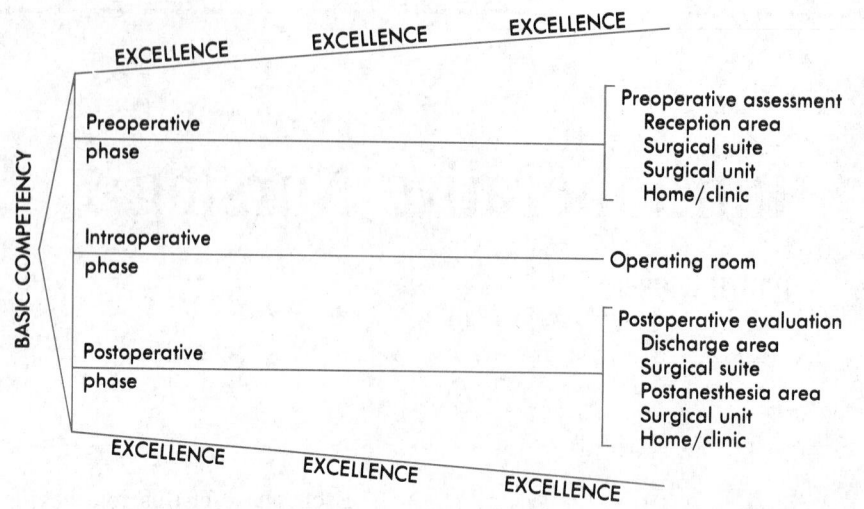

STANDARDS OF PERIOPERATIVE NURSING PRACTICE

Standards have been developed to guide the practice of operating room nursing.[5] These standards are based on nursing process and serve as a model to measure the quality of patient care delivered. The standards include all aspects of nursing process (assessment, planning, implementation, and evaluation) pertinent to the planned surgical intervention.

Standards of care and the use of nursing process during the intraoperative period pave the way for nurses in the operating room to expand knowledge, to increase sensitivity to individuals' needs, and to be accountable to patients as consumers. Standards of care are also a means to provide continuity of care in an integrated manner using preoperative assessment, intraoperative intervention, and postoperative evaluation.

INTRAOPERATIVE PATIENT CARE TEAM MEMBERS
OPERATING TEAM

The intraoperative patient care team members are commonly subdivided into two basic categories—scrubbed sterile members and nonsterile members.

The *scrubbed sterile* team members usually include:
1. Primary surgeon
2. Assistants to the surgeon (May vary in number and qualifications; however, most medical staff bylaws state, "A qualified physician shall assist during all major operations."[6]) A recent addition has been the RN First Assistant (p. 469).
3. Scrub nurse or technician

The *nonsterile* team members may include:
1. Anesthesiologist or anesthetist
2. Circulating nurse

3. Others (technicians to operate complicated monitoring devices or equipment, such as the heart-lung machine, biomedical engineers, or pathologist if a frozen section is necessary)

SCRUB NURSE

Nursing responsibilities in the operating room are commonly divided into the roles of scrub nurse and circulating nurse. The scrub nurse may or may not be a nurse, because this role can be carried out by a registered nurse, practical or vocational nurse, or a trained technician. Scrub nurse activities may include:
1. Preparing sterile supplies and equipment needed for the operation
2. Assisting the surgeon and surgical assistants during the procedure
3. Teaching new personnel, if qualified to do so
4. Assisting in accounting for needles, sharps, sponges, and instruments used during the procedure, using the established "count" procedure

To carry out these activities effectively, the scrub nurse must possess thorough knowledge of aseptic technique, manual skill and dexterity, physical stamina, the ability to work under pressure, and a sincere concern for accuracy and accountability in achieving optimal patient care.

CIRCULATING NURSE

The circulating nurse plays a role in the overall management of the operating room. This person is vital to the effective flow of patient care before, during, and after the surgical procedure. Although the surgeon is in charge of the operative site, the circulating nurse is relied on to coordinate all activities of the room and to

TABLE 21-1 Examples of nursing activities in perioperative nursing practice

Preoperative Phase	Intraoperative Phase	Postoperative Phase

Preoperative assessment
Home/clinic
1. Initiates initial preoperative assessment
2. Plans teaching methods appropriate to patient's needs
3. Involves family in interview
Surgical unit
1. Completes preoperative assessment
2. Coordinates patient teaching with other nursing staff
3. Explains phases in perioperative period and expectations
4. Develops a plan of care
Surgical suite
1. Assesses patient's level of consciousness
2. Reviews chart
3. Identifies patient
4. Verifies surgical site
Planning
1. Determines a plan of care
Psychologic support
1. Tells patient what is happening
2. Determines psychologic status
3. Gives prior warning of noxious stimuli
4. Communicates patient's emotional status to other appropriate members of the health care team
	Maintenance of safety
	1. Ensures that the sponge, needle, and instrument counts are correct
	2. Positions the patient
	  a. Functional alignment
	  b. Exposure of surgical site
	  c. Maintenance of position throughout procedure
	3. Applies grounding device to patient
	4. Provides physical support
	Physiologic monitoring
	1. Calculates effects on patient of excessive fluid loss
	2. Distinguishes normal from abnormal cardiopulmonary data
	3. Reports changes in patient's pulse, respirations, temperature, and blood pressure
	Psychologic monitoring (before induction and if patient is conscious)
	1. Provides emotional support to patient
	2. Stands near/touches patient during procedures/induction
	3. Continues to assess patient's emotional status
	4. Communicates patient's emotional status to other appropriate members of the health care team
	Nursing management
	1. Provides physical safety for the patient
	2. Maintains aseptic, controlled environment
	3. Effectively manages human resources
		Communication of intraoperative information
		1. Gives patient's name
		2. States type of surgery performed
		3. Provides contributing intraoperative factors (drain, catheters)
		4. States physical limitations
		5. States impairments resulting from surgery
		6. Reports patient's preoperative level of consciousness
		7. Communicates necessary equipment needs
		Postoperative evaluation
		Recovery area
		1. Determines patient's immediate response to surgical intervention
		Surgical unit
		1. Evaluates effectiveness of nursing care in the OR
		2. Determines patient's level of satisfaction with care given during perioperative period
		3. Evaluates products used on patient in the OR
		4. Determines patient's psychologic status
		5. Assists with discharge planning
		Home/clinic
		1. Seeks patient's perception of surgery in terms of the effects of anesthetic agents, impact on body image, distortion, immobilization
		2. Determines family's perceptions of surgery

From A model for perioperative nursing practice, AORN J 41:92-193, 1985.
Reprinted with permission from AORN, Inc, 10170 E Mississippi Ave, Denver, CO, 80231. All rights reserved.

manage the nursing care required for the patient. The circulating nurse is often the one team member who is in a position to have an overall picture of patient care needs and to be the patient's advocate. Consistent with such responsibility, it is considered vital to the perioperative role that this individual be minimally prepared as a registered professional nurse.

Circulating nurse activities may include the following:

1. Assessing, planning, implementing, and evaluating nursing activities to meet individualized patient needs
2. Creating and maintaining a safe and comfortable environment for the patient. This often involves diligent observation for breaks in aseptic technique and initiation of appropriate measures to correct the situation.

3. Providing assistance to any team member as necessary (directing and anticipating the performance and needs of the scrub nurse and providing extra supplies and equipment as needed to any team member)
4. Maintaining communication among team members in the operating room and any necessary contact with other health care professionals and patient's family
5. Identifying any potential environmental dangers or traumatic situations involving the patient or team members and taking appropriate action to correct or assist with the problem

RN FIRST ASSISTANT (RNFA)

The RN First Assistant is a newly recognized addition to the personnel of the operating room. This role has been approved by the Association of Operating Room Nurses and endorsed by the American College of Surgeons. Specific qualifications and training must be achieved to perform in this role. This person practices under the direct supervision of the surgeon and may carry out such functions as using instruments, suturing, providing exposure, and hemostasis.[34,40,41]

ALLIED PERSONNEL

There are a number of other persons who are not involved in the operation per se but who contribute to the needs of each surgical patient. These persons may include clerical personnel, blood bank employees, laboratory technicians, nursing assistants, pharmacists, central service employees, pathologists, radiologists, and laundry personnel.

OPERATING ROOM SUITE DESIGN

The design of an operating room suite offers a challenge to the planning team to optimize efficiency by creating realistic traffic and workflow patterns for patients, personnel, and supplies. Designs must allow for flexibility for future needs. Because no one plan meets all hospitals' requirements, each OR suite is designed on an individual basis to meet projected and specific community needs.

Specific *traffic patterns* are determined dependent on the entrances and exits for both personnel and materials. Traffic control can be aided by designating a 4-zone concept that includes a protective area, clean area, sterile area, and dirty area (see the box below).

Infection control practices that are related to design may include but are not limited to the following:

1. Smooth, easily washable walls
2. Cabinets recessed to facilitate cleaning
3. No windows
4. Sliding doors (as opposed to swinging doors) to decrease air turbulence
5. Adequate air filtration system
6. Ceiling-mounted lighting units on a single post as opposed to lights on tracks (ceiling light tracks are not readily accessible for cleaning, and handles are likely to become contaminated)
7. Uniform disposal systems for contaminated equipment

OPERATING ROOM ZONES

Protective	Locker rooms, lounges, offices, patient receiving areas
Clean	Clean storage areas, scrub areas, recovery room
Sterile	Operating rooms, storage of sterile supplies
Dirty	Disposal area for all used materials

Temperature and *humidity* are also important design factors. High relative humidity should be maintained; moisture provides a relatively conductive medium, allowing static to leak to earth as fast as it is generated. Temperature is purposely kept cool to deter bacterial growth. The combination of increased humidity and decreased temperature is also desirable to prevent drying of the patient's exposed tissue.

A *communication system* is a vital link to summon routine or emergency assistance or to relay appropriate information to and from the operating room team. An intercom system is commonly used, but team members must be aware of the type of information that is shared over an intercom if the patient is awake. Call light systems outside the operating room door may be used to summon selected persons such as attendants or housekeeping personnel.

ASEPTIC TECHNIQUE AND INFECTION CONTROL

Modern surgery is based on aseptic technique. Asepsis means the absence of any infectious agents, and therefore aseptic technique is aimed at eliminating microorganisms present in the surgical environment. This also includes those microorganisms living harmlessly on the body surface or within, which must be prevented from reaching the open wound to allow healing by first intention (Chapter 22).

Principles of bacteriology and microbiology are applied in developing infection control programs to be followed by all operating room personnel. Such programs involve specific guidelines for OR attire, sterilizing and packaging supplies, scrubbing, gowning and gloving, and methods of housekeeping.

When one is following infection control principles, self-discipline and a surgical conscience are imperative. A surgical conscience may be described as a Surgical Golden Rule: that is, "Do unto the patient as you would have others do unto you."[6] This implies that the nurse takes appropriate action to rectify any break in technique, whether the person is alone or observed by others. Thus the nurse must be as conscientious about monitoring his or her own technique as when observing other team members.

BASIC RULES OF SURGICAL ASEPSIS

Definite rules must be followed during surgery to create and maintain a sterile field with a well-defined margin of safety for the patient. Strict adherence to these rules eliminates or minimizes possible contamination.

1. Only sterile materials may be used within a sterile field. If there is any doubt about the sterility of an item, it is considered unsterile.
2. Gowns of scrubbed team members are considered sterile in the *front from shoulder to waist level and sleeves to 2 inches above the elbow.* Unsterile areas of

gowns are shoulders, neckline, axillary region, and back. Scrubbed persons should not allow their hands or any sterile item to fall below waist or table top level.

3. Draped tables are considered to be sterile on the top surface only. Any item that extends over the table edge is considered contaminated and cannot be brought back up to table top level.

4. Sterile surfaces should contact only other sterile areas. Unsterile team members must avoid reaching over a sterile field. Scrubbed persons should stay close to the sterile field and if they change positions, they should turn back to back or face to face.

5. Edges of any sterile package or container are considered unsterile. Sterile boundaries are not always well defined; therefore the following rules are accepted guidelines:

   a. Cap edges of a bottle of sterile solution are considered contaminated once the cap is removed. Because the cap cannot be replaced without contaminating the pouring edges, the sterility of the bottle contents is no longer certain and the remainder is discarded.

   b. Package wrappers are usually considered to have a 1-inch safety margin around the edge. The flap ends are secured in the hand of the person opening them to avoid dangling the flap ends loosely (Figure 21-2).

   c. Peel-back packages should not be torn open but rather pulled back to expose sterile contents. The inner edge of the heat seal is considered to be the boundary between sterile and unsterile.

6. The sterile field should be created as close to the time it is going to be used as possible. The degree of contamination is proportional to the length of time items are left uncovered. Sterile areas are kept continuously in view and once supplies are opened, someone must remain in the room to ensure sterility.

7. Sterile barriers that have been permeated are considered contaminated. Filtration of airborne microorganisms through materials (as when an item is dropped on the floor), passage of liquids through materials, and undetected holes are modes of contamination.

OPERATING ROOM ATTIRE AND PERSONNEL HEALTH HABITS

Adherence to proper practices regarding the attire worn by health care workers within the operating room greatly lessens the risk of their serving as potential sources of infection for the patient. It is known that large quantities of bacteria are present in the nose and mouth, on the skin, and on the wearing apparel of persons who enter the operating room. For this reason, areas must be provided for staff members to remove personal attire, to put on appropriate OR attire, and to enter the operating room suite directly without passing through a contaminated area.

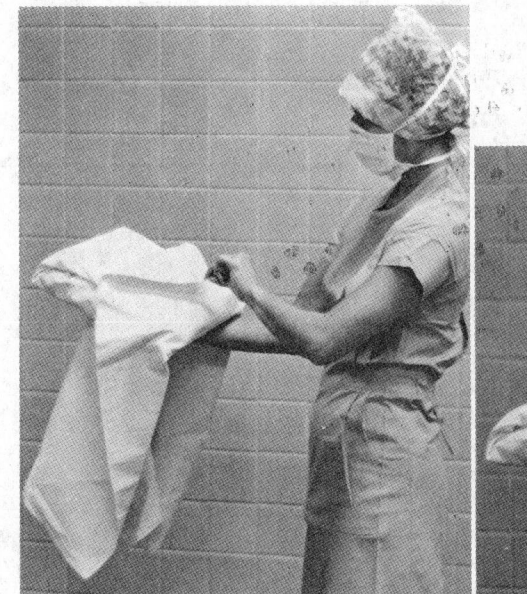
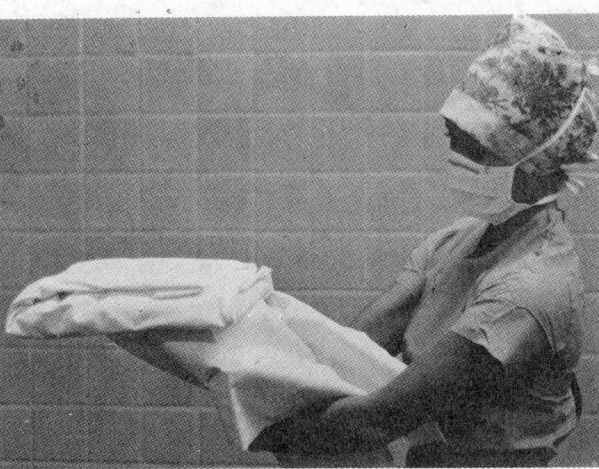

FIGURE 21-2 A, When opening sterile package, circulating nurse opens corner nearest body last to avoid potential contamination of inner pack. **B,** To prevent unsterile corners of outer wrapper from touching scrub nurse or sterile field, circulating nurse draws back corners of opened wrapper when presenting inner package. (From Gruendemann BJ and Meeker MH: Alexander's care of the patient in surgery, ed 8, St Louis, 1987, The CV Mosby Co.)

Daily body hygiene practices and clean hair also help prevent wound infections. Hair is a fertile source of bacteria, and other body areas may shed bacteria and dead cells into an open wound. Policy should restrict personnel with active infections of any kind or known carriers from entering the operating room suite.

UNIFORM

Street clothes should not be worn in restricted areas of the surgical suite. There should be a visible line beyond which no one may go without proper attire (Figure 21-3). Clean operating room apparel made of fabric that meets the National Fire Protection Association standards should be available to anyone requiring entrance into restricted areas. Scrub pants with close-fitting cuffs are superior to scrub dresses; such cuffs prevent the liberation of bacteria from the perineal and thigh area. Shirts are tucked inside pants to prevent accidental contact with sterile areas and to contain skin shedding. It is also recommended that nonsterile team members wear long-sleeved warm-up jackets to prevent shedding from bare arms. If scrub dresses are worn, they are secured at the waist and panty hose are worn to reduce bacterial shedding. Operating room attire that becomes visibly soiled or wet is changed, and all OR apparel is laundered by the hospital laundering facilities.

Head Coverings

All possible head and facial hair, including sideburns and neckline, is completely covered before donning other OR attire. This prevents the possibility of hair or dandruff being shed onto the scrub suit. Caps should be flame resistant and comfortable and should fit snugly. Cleanliness of homemade caps is debatable, and if they are used, it is recommended that they be laundered by hospital facilities. Disposable head coverings are discarded in designated containers before leaving the operating room suite.

Masks

All personnel should wear disposable high-filtration masks in specified restricted areas of the surgical suite. The mask must completely cover the mouth and nose and be secured as to allow no venting to occur at the sides. This prevents droplets from the oropharynx or nasopharynx from being expelled into the surgical environment. Masks must also be handled properly during and after use. Masks should be either on or off and not

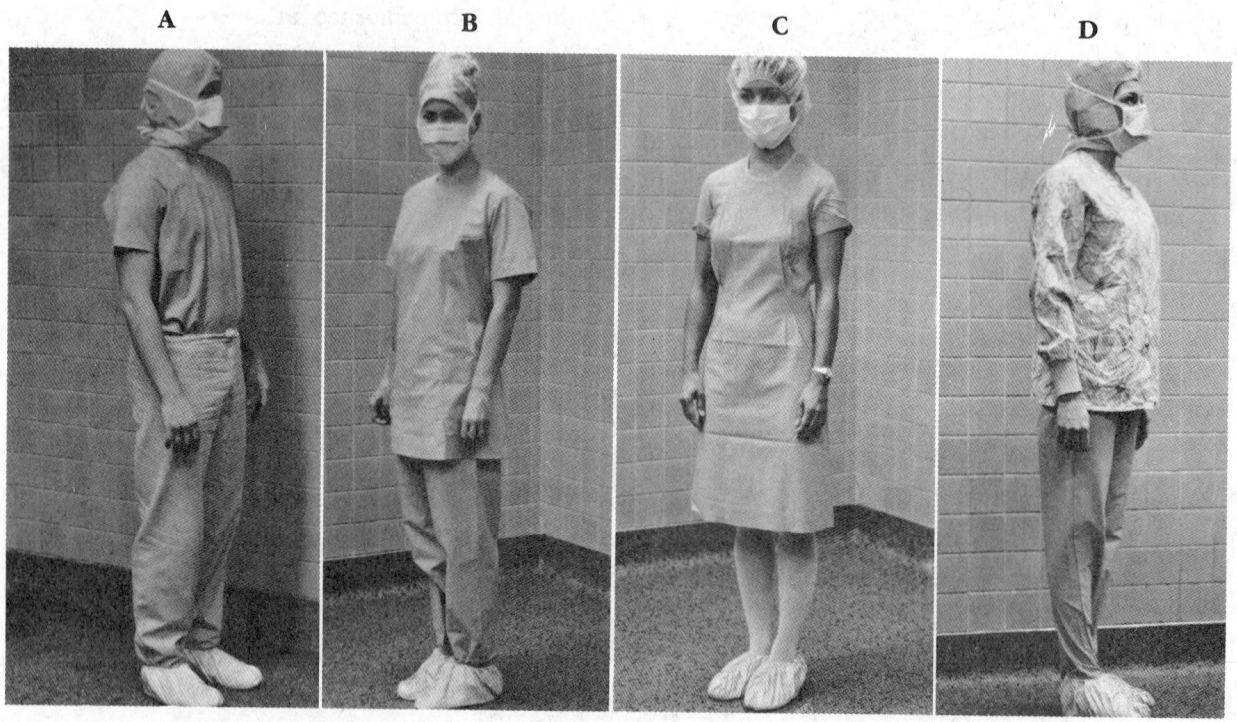

FIGURE 21-3 Proper operating room attire. **A,** Scrub top should be tucked into pants or, **B,** should conform to waist to reduce dispersal of bacteria. Ankle closures on scrub pants ensure containment of potential contaminants. **C,** Scrub dress should be secured at waist. Advocates of scrub dresses believe that bacteria can be contained as effectively with panty hose as with pantsuits. **D,** Warm-up jacket worn over scrub suit provides maximum coverage of skin. (From Gruendemann BJ and Meeker MH: Alexander's care of the patient in surgery, ed 8, St Louis, 1987, The CV Mosby Co.)

dropped loosely around the neck; if this is done, bacteria that have been filtered onto the mask will become dry and airborne. When masks are removed, only the strings are touched to reduce contamination of the hands from the nasopharyngeal area. Masks are changed between cases and more often if they become moist during a long case.

Shoe Coverings

All persons entering the restricted areas of the surgical suite should wear shoe covers. When the same shoes are worn in the OR for successive operations, they will have a very high bacterial count with the potential for cross-infection.

Shoe covers must be conductive in areas where static spark is a hazard, and conductivity is checked when entering the restricted area and at intervals throughout the tour of duty. Care must be taken to make sure that the black carbon strip is placed inside the shoe between the sock or hose in good contact with the inner sole to provide conductivity or an electrical ground for the wearer.

Shoe covers are removed when leaving restricted areas, and clean ones are reapplied upon returning. This prevents cross-contamination with other areas of the hospital. In the interest of safety, clogs, sandals, and tennis shoes should not be worn in the operating room. Clogs can be a hazard when a person tries to move quickly, and if sharp objects are accidentally dropped, sandals and tennis shoes provide little protection.

Other Considerations

Additional considerations in relation to OR attire include the amount and type of jewelry that may be worn. Dangling necklaces and earrings may fall into the sterile field. Excessive numbers of rings or rings with sharp stones interfere with good handwashing technique as well as possibly injuring patient skin during transfers.

No operating attire, including surgical uniforms, caps, and shoe covers, should be worn outside the surgical suite, because this creates a two-way hazard. Any contaminants coming in contact with the operating room team members can become airborne and find susceptible hosts outside the surgical suite. Conversely, bacteria present outside the suite may be carried back on the OR attire. If this practice is not feasible, head and shoe coverings are removed and the scrub clothes are covered by a clean, buttoned lab coat when a person leaves the suite. On return, the scrub clothes are changed.

SCRUBBING, GOWNING, AND GLOVING

Only personnel who are free of upper respiratory infections and skin problems should scrub. Abrasions and cuts tend to ooze serum that may serve as a medium for bacterial growth.

The major objective of the surgical scrub is to reduce the microbial skin count as much as possible and to leave an antimicrobial residue on the skin to prevent regrowth. This is achieved by mechanically cleansing the hands and lower arms to remove skin oil, dirt, and microbes.

The exact procedure to be followed and the selection of materials used may differ among hospitals. The most frequently used antimicrobial agents include povidone iodine, hexachlorophene, and chlorhexidene gluconate. When scrubbing, it is recommended that light friction be applied as opposed to hard scrubbing. This will produce dilation of blood vessels with better circulation, which helps recondition the skin, whereas scrubbing with harsh bristles can cause desquamation of the dermis. Synthetic disposable sponges, rather than brushes, have become popular. However, reusable or disposable nylon brushes have been shown to be equally effective.

The actual scrub procedure may be based on the "time method" or the "anatomical brush-stroke method." Both methods are effective if properly carried out. The time method involves scrubbing the fingers, hands, and arms for an allotted period of time for each area. The brush-stroke method prescribes a number of brush strokes to be applied lengthwise with the brush or sponge for each surface of the fingers, hands, and arms. There is no difference in microbial reduction whether the scrub is of 5 or 10 minutes in duration. The same scrub procedure should be used consistently, whether it is the first or last scrub of the day.

Before beginning the scrub, the hands are inspected for cuts or skin problems. Nails should be short to avoid glove puncture, and no polish is preferred to prevent a harbor for microbes. The head covering is adjusted to ensure that all hair is contained, and a fresh mask should be properly applied. (Surgical scrub guidelines are described in the box on p. 474).

After the scrub, the team member is ready to put on sterile gown and gloves. The procedure for gowning and gloving may vary, depending on the type of materials used (linen or disposable) and gown design, and whether the gloving will be done by self or by another team member. Sterile gloves may be applied using an open or closed method. The closed method is usually preferred, since bare skin on the hands and wrists is not exposed during the process. (For a detailed discussion on the procedures, see references 6 and 24.)

NURSING PRACTICE IN THE OPERATING ROOM

■ ASSESSMENT

When patients are admitted to the operating room suite, the first area they usually enter is the holding area. The circulating nurse is generally responsible for assessing the patient's emotional and physical status and confirming the information on the preoperative checklist. Ide-

SURGICAL SCRUB GUIDELINES

SUGGESTED ACTION	RATIONALE
1. Remove all hand jewelry. Make last minute adjustments of head covering, mask, and eyeglasses.	1. Jewelry harbors microorganisms and is also a potential source of foreign bodies in the operative wound.
2. Adjust water to a comfortable warm temperature. (Most scrub sinks have automatic or knee controls for water flow.)	2. Warm water has a lower surface tension than cold, which is believed to enhance cleansing action.
3. Wet hands and forearms and apply antimicrobial soap or detergent into palms via foot control. Rub palmar surfaces together and add water as needed to make a lather.	3. Detergents and soaps lower surface tension of water and emulsify oil.
4. Using friction, wash the hands and arms thoroughly to a level at least 2 inches above the elbow. The amount of time required may vary with the cleansing agent used and the amount of soil present.	4. Microbes are removed by physical, mechanical separation as well as chemical antisepsis. By washing one hand-breadth above contaminated areas, recontamination of hands and forearms during rinsing and drying is more readily avoided.
5. Hands and arms should be rinsed thoroughly, being careful to keep the hands higher than elbows. Avoid splashing water onto clothing.	5. This allows water to run off at the elbow and prevents contaminated water from above the elbow from running down onto scrubbed hands. If the scrub attire becomes wet, the moisture may cause contamination of the sterile gown by wicking action.
6. A sterile brush or sponge (either prepackaged or from a dispenser) should be obtained. A metal or plastic nail cleaner should be included and used to clean under the fingernails while hands are held under running water.	6. Special attention should be given to the subungual space where microbes can accumulate. Orangewood sticks should not be used because they cannot be sterilized properly afterwards.
7. An antimicrobial agent should be applied to the brush or sponge if not already impregnated. Starting at the fingertips, the nails and subungual area should be scrubbed vigorously with the brush held perpendicular to them. All sides of each finger are scrubbed, followed by the back and palm of the hand.	7. and 8. Hospital policy should be established, and the procedure posted in the scrub area. The individual's conscientious attention to detail is of utmost importance.
8. The arms are scrubbed on each side with a circular motion to 2 inches above the elbow. (The time spent in steps 7 and 8 may be established by setting a time limit for the scrubbing of one part after another or by counting a particular number of strokes for each side of each part.)	
9. The hands and arms are rinsed thoroughly with the brush being discarded into the proper container. Hands and arms are held up in front of the body with elbows slightly flexed as the person enters the operating room.	9. Rinse procedure should be followed as in step 5. Same rationale applies.

ally the nurse will have information recorded by an OR nurse from a preoperative visit, but this is not always possible. During the time in the holding area, the nurse must quickly assess the patient's status, paying particular attention to any factors that would increase surgical risk. The nurse continues to assess the patient's status during the patient's transfer into the operating room, positioning on the operating room table, induction of anesthesia, and draping. Assessment of the patient's status is ongoing during the surgical procedure. The nurse also monitors the equipment needed to maintain patient safety.

■ DATA ANALYSIS: NURSING DIAGNOSES

During the intraoperative period, nursing diagnoses may be identified for a number of actual or potential problems. Possible nursing diagnoses for the intraoperative patient may include, but are not limited to the following:

Diagnostic Title	Possible Etiologies
Anxiety or fear	Anesthesia, local/regional procedures
Aspiration, potential for	Decreased level of consciousness
Breathing patterns, ineffective	Anesthesia
Cardiac output, decreased	Anesthetics, decreased mobility, venous pooling
Fluid volume deficit	Loss of blood
Fluid volume excess	Excess fluid intake (IV)
Hypothermia	Environmental changes, preoperative medications, anesthetics

Diagnostic Title	Possible Etiologies
Infection, potential for	Body intrusion
Injury, potential for (foreign body, burn, hemorrhage, neuromuscular trauma)	Positioning, fall, emboli/thrombi formation, surgical procedure, electrical equipment
Oral mucous membrane, altered	Dehydration, anesthetics
Pain	Surgical manipulation, decreased mobility, local/regional procedures
Powerlessness	Decreased consciousness, decreased mobility
Skin integrity, impaired potential	Positioning, decreased mobility
Tissue perfusion, altered (cerebral, cardiopulmonary, renal, peripheral)	Decreased blood flow, hypothermia, immobility, anesthetics

■ PLANNING: EXPECTED PATIENT OUTCOMES

Although desired outcomes will vary depending on the individual needs that are assessed for each patient, the following outcomes may be desirable for any surgical patient:

1. Signs of anxiety/fear are decreased; the patient rests quietly in the holding area.
2. Aspiration does not occur.
3. Adequate respiratory function is maintained throughout the procedure.
4. Adequate cardiac output is maintained.
5. The patient is hydrated without excess fluid.
6. A body temperature within normal range is maintained.
7. No injury results from a foreign body left in a wound, improper positioning, restraints, electrical equipment, solutions used to prepare the skin, or improper application of the surgical dressing.
8. The patient experiences minimal pain and exposure during transfer to and from the OR table and during the procedure as a result of positioning.
9. Tissue perfusion is maintained.

■ IMPLEMENTATION

To promote patient safety and comfort and to achieve the other desired patient outcomes, operating room nurses have a variety of responsibilities in planning care. The following areas of discussion focus on those responsibilities.

ADMITTING PATIENT TO THE OPERATING ROOM AREA

Most hospitals have an established procedure for admission into the holding area of the OR suite. The holding area is ideally a quiet, restful area where patients can gain optimal benefit from any premedication they have received. However, this is also an area where patients may feel terribly alone. They now come face to face with their impending surgery. Separation from family members has become a reality, and any fears the patient might have are likely to resurface.

The professional nurse's first goal is to establish a positive relationship with the patient. The nurse greeting the patient can decrease the patient's apprehension by introducing herself or himself and talking to the patient in a positive manner. The patient is told that the circulating nurse will be in constant attendance once the patient is admitted to the surgical room, and what is being done in preparation for the surgery is explained. If the nurse treats the patient with respect and warmth, answering any questions and seeing to the patient's comfort at this time, much will be accomplished toward instilling in the patient security and confidence in the entire OR team. Any necessary delays are explained and also relayed to the waiting family.

The circulating nurse also has a number of important observations to make when admitting the patient to the operating room.

1. Ask the patient to state his or her name, the operative procedure to be done, and the side of the operation, if pertinent.
2. Check the patient's name and hospital number on the chart and compare it with the name and number on the patient's identification band.
3. Check for the signature on the operative permit and determine whether it has been properly signed, dated, and witnessed. The procedure on the permit must agree with the scheduled procedure.
4. Review the chart, checking for:
   a. The history and physical, which must be completed before surgery begins
   b. Laboratory reports and x-ray film (abnormalities are reported to the surgeon and anesthesiologist)
   c. Availability of blood if the patient was typed and cross-matched
   d. Allergies and any previous reactions to anesthesia or transfusions
5. Check for jewelry, wigs, contact lenses, prostheses, dentures, and objects in the mouth.
6. Observe the patient for any signs of adverse reactions to preoperative medication and ask patient if anything has been taken by mouth if an NPO order was written.

TRANSFERRING AND POSITIONING PATIENT FOR SURGERY

Based on the scheduled procedure and the surgeon's preferences, the circulating nurse should be able to anticipate the basic patient position required. The final responsibility for the position of the patient on the OR table is one shared by the nurse, surgeon, and anesthesiologist. During the preoperative assessment, the patient's height, weight, and individual health problems that may relate to safe transfer and positioning have been determined and recorded.

No matter what position is to be assumed, good positioning is important to:

1. Adequately expose the operative area
2. Make the patient accessible for induction of anesthesia and administration of intravenous solutions or drugs
3. Minimize interference with circulation as a result of pressure on a body part
4. Provide protection from injury to nerves as a result of improper positioning of arms, hands, legs, or feet
5. Provide for maintenance of respiratory function by avoiding pressure on the chest to allow for adequate lung ventilation and by holding the jaw forward to keep it from dropping on the chest
6. Provide for patient's privacy by proper draping and avoiding unnecessary exposure

Specific nursing care planning may involve deciding the appropriate method of transfer, determining needed equipment and positioning aids, and whether additional personnel will be needed to carry out the plan safely. Implementation of the plan includes certain safety measures, which may include:

1. The OR table and transfer cart are securely locked.
2. A physician assumes responsibility for movement of an unsplinted fracture.
3. All muscles, nerves, and bony prominences are positioned or padded to avoid injury.
4. Heavily sedated patients and the elderly are moved slowly and gently to prevent shearing forces on the skin and to allow the circulatory system to adjust.
5. Care is taken to see that no tubings (for example, intravenous lines, urinary catheters) are dislodged or obstructed.
6. The restraint is placed snugly over a blanket covering the patient, avoiding contact with the skin. The strap should not interfere with circulation or exert pressure on nerves or bony prominences.
7. Sterile tables are positioned high enough to prevent any pressure on the patient's body.
8. Sterile team members are reminded not to lean on any part of the patient.

The patient may be positioned on the operating room table in a number of different positions (see Table 21-2 and Figures 21-4 and 21-5). Whatever the position, special attention is given to prevent injury to arms and legs and to prevent pressure on any one given area.

One major problem that may occur is the pooling of blood in dependent areas. Sudden shifting of blood when the supine position is reassumed following surgery may place a strain on the cardiovascular system with a precipitous drop in blood pressure. For this reason, the patient is always returned *slowly* from the operative position to the supine position. Elderly persons and persons with preexisting cardiovascular problems are at high risk and are monitored carefully.

SKIN CLEANSING AND PREPARATION

The purpose of preoperative skin preparation is to establish an operative site as free as possible from dirt, skin oils, and transient microbes, as well as reducing the resident microbial count to as low as possible. This should

TABLE 21-2 Commonly used operative patient positions

Position	Description	Comments
Supine	Flat on back with arms at side, palms down, legs straight with feet slightly separated (Figure 21-4, A)	Most commonly used position; used for hernia repair, exploratory laparotomy, cholecystectomy, gastric and bowel resection, and mastoidectomy
Prone	Patient lies on abdomen with face turned to one side, arms at side with palms pronated, elbows slightly flexed; feet elevated on pillow to prevent plantar flexion (Figure 21-4, B)	Patient is anesthetized in supine position, then placed prone; used for surgery on back, spine, and rectal area
Trendelenburg	Head and body are lowered into a head-down position and held in place with padded shoulder braces; knees are flexed by "breaking" table (Figure 21-4, C)	Respiratory excursion is decreased from upward movement of viscera; used for surgery on lower abdomen and pelvis
Reverse Trendelenburg	Head is elevated and feet lowered	Used for biliary surgery
Lithotomy	Patient lies on back with buttocks to edge of table; thighs and legs are placed in stirrups simultaneously to prevent muscle injury; head and arms are secured to prevent injury (Figure 21-5, A)	Used for perineal, rectal, and vaginal surgery; elastic wraps may be used on legs to prevent thrombus formation
Lateral	Patient lies on side; table may be "bent" in middle (Figure 21-5, B)	Used for renal surgery

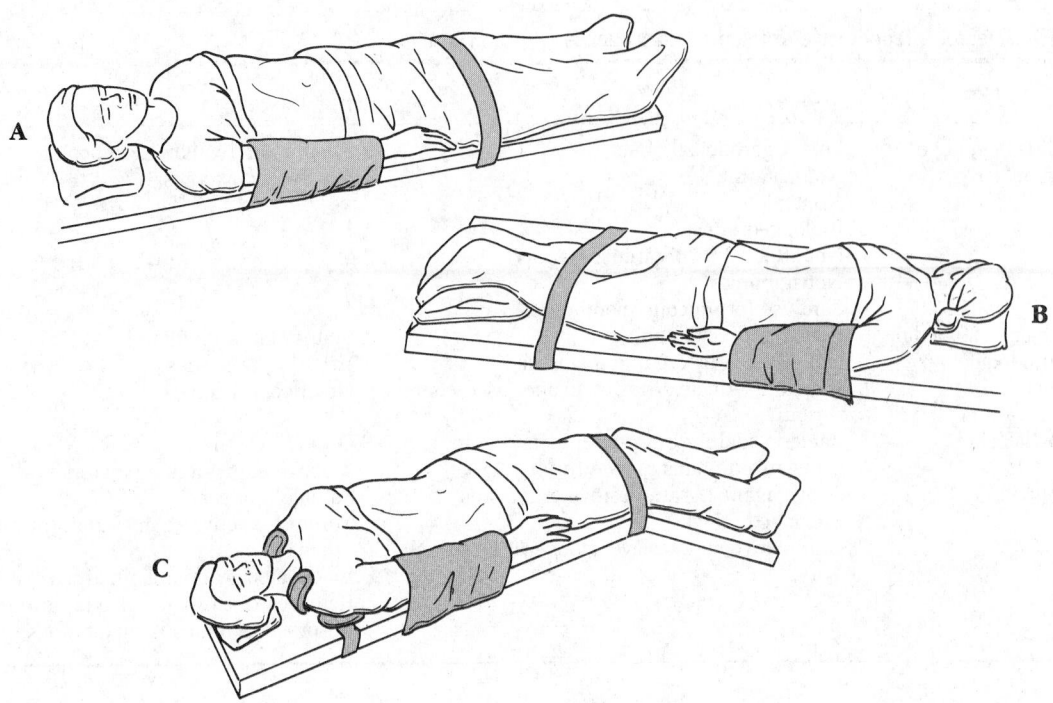

FIGURE 21-4 Three commonly used operative positions. **A**, Supine. **B**, Prone. **C**, Trendelenburg.

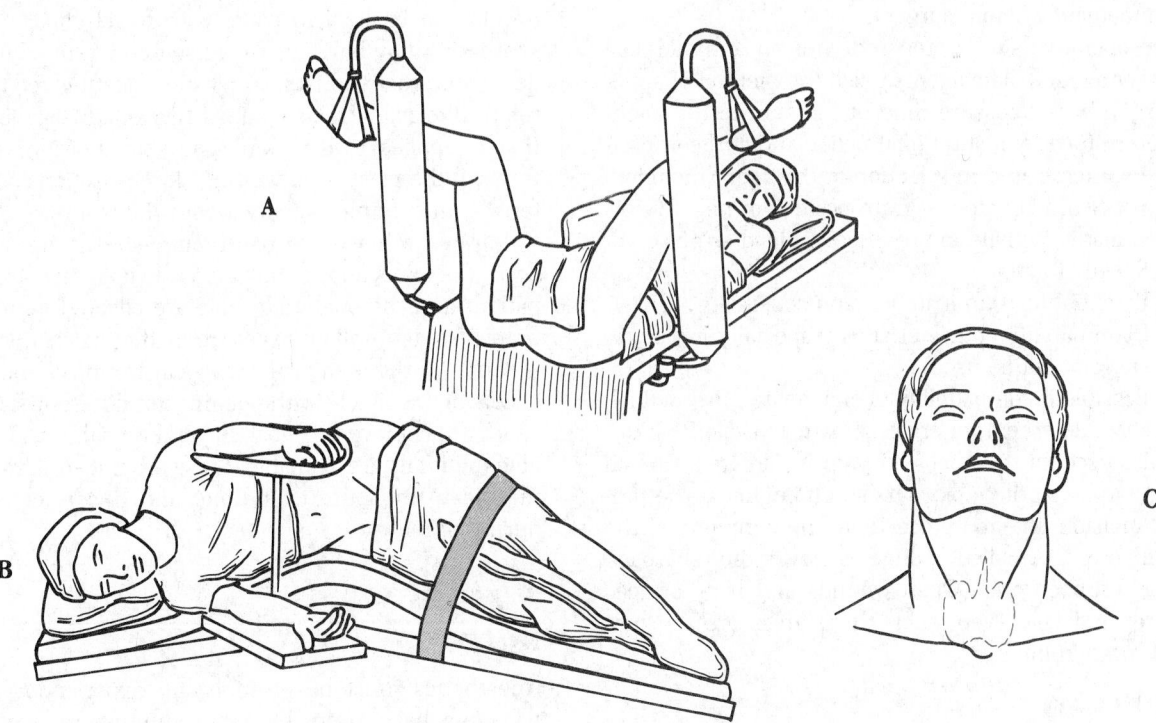

FIGURE 21-5 Three operative positions for specialized surgery. **A**, Lithotomy. **B**, Lateral. **C**, Thyroid exposure.

TABLE 21-3 Selected preoperative antiseptic skin agents

Antiseptic Agent	Advantages	Disadvantages
Povidone-iodine (Betadine, PVP, Isodine)	Potent germicidal effect Nonirritating Nontoxic Prolonged effect Not affected by organic materials Nonstaining Safe use for mucous membranes	Should not be allowed to pool No effect on spores
Tincture of iodine (2% iodine), 2.4% sodium iodide, 46% ethyl alcohol	Potent germicidal effect Not affected by organic materials Increases effectiveness of alcohol used concurrently	Stains skin and linens Irritating to tissues No effect on spores
70% Isopropyl alcohol	Bacteriocidal for gram-positive and gram-negative organisms and fungi	Drying to skin Inactivated by organic material
Hexachlorophene	Active against gram-positive organisms Prolonged effect Cumulative suppressive action with frequent use	Soluble in alcohol Minimally active against gram-negative organisms Inactivated by organic material Requires rinsing after use to prevent absorption Absorbed by mucous membranes

be accomplished in the shortest period of time with the least amount of tissue irritation. If the skin "prep" is to be done while the patient is awake, the nurse explains the procedure to the patient, providing for comfort and minimizing exposure. Hair removal may be done before the patient arrives at the OR (see Chapter 20) or in the OR immediately before surgery.

The operative site is prepared with an antimicrobial agent (or agents). The agents used, the method of application, and the exposure time of the skin to the agent are determined by institutional policy and surgeon preference. Criteria used in selection of the agent include:

1. Spectrum of activity (gram positive or negative organisms, activity in presence of blood or pus)
2. Speed of action
3. Potential for skin irritation and sensitivity
4. Flammability characteristics (especially if electrosurgery will be used)
5. Possible incompatibility or inactivation by alcohol, soap, detergent, or organic matter (Table 21-3)

Supplies used for the final skin preparation are arranged on a separate sterile table. The scrub begins at the proposed incision line and proceeds to the periphery of the area involved. A soiled sponge is never brought back over a scrubbed area. Open wounds and body orifices are prepared last, even when these areas are the proposed incision line.

STERILE DRAPING

The purpose of draping is to create a sterile field around the operative site. An effective barrier will eliminate the passage of microorganisms between sterile and nonsterile areas and will leave a minimal area of skin exposed.

Towels or self-adhering plastic sheeting are commonly used to drape the area immediately surrounding the operative site. Towels may be made of cotton muslin or synthetic disposable materials. If muslin is used, the towels will be held in place with towel clips, whereas synthetics may have their own self-adherent edge. Sterile, waterproof, antistatic, plastic sheeting, commonly referred to as an "incise drape," has an adhesive backing that is applied to dry skin. The skin incision is made through the plastic, preventing skin excretions and bacteria from coming in contact with the wound.

Various other sizes of draping sheets are used to cover the areas above and below the operative area. The patient and the operating table are covered with sterile drapes so as to allow exposure of the surgical site and isolation of the area of the surgical wound. Fenestrated sheets are available with openings of different sizes and shapes to achieve this goal. Several reusable and disposable materials are available; these are not equally impermeable to moisture over time, and this is considered during draping.

ANESTHESIA

USAGE

Anesthetics must be given by an experienced person who has been trained in the administration of anesthetic agents. This may be an *anesthesiologist* who is a physician certified by the American Board of Anesthesi-

EFFECTS OF ANESTHESIA

Amnesia	Loss of memory
Analgesia	Insensibility to pain
Hypnosis	Artificially produced sleep
Muscle relaxation	Rendering a part of the body less firm or rigid

ology, or a certified registered nurse anesthetist (CRNA). A CRNA renders nursing and anesthesia services to patients requiring a combination of those services that are medically delegated under the direction of a licensed physician.

Although surgical nurses do not administer anesthetic agents, they may be called on to assist the physician on the clinical unit or in a specialized area of the hospital. It is essential for the nurse to have an understanding of drug interactions, the preanesthetic preparation of the patient, and the effects of anesthetic agents given during the operative phase to provide effective nursing care in the postoperative period.[3,16,17]

The effects of anesthesia are listed in the box at left. Anesthetic agents may be given to produce unconsciousness (general anesthesia) or to produce loss of sensation in specific body areas (regional anesthesia). "Local" anesthesia can be considered a form of regional anesthesia (Table 21-4). Hypnoanesthesia (usually hypnosis) is rarely used without supplemental drugs in the United States. In China, acupuncture is commonly used in combination with narcotics. It may be used in modern operating rooms by using needles or surface electrodes that are connected to a machine that creates current flow between the electrodes. Acupuncture is also believed to cause the release of endorphins, which are naturally occurring morphinelike substances in the human body.

CHOICE

The choice of an anesthetic is based on many factors: the physical condition and age of the patient; the presence of coexisting diseases; the type, site, and duration of the operation; and the personal preferences of the anesthetist. When feasible, the patient's preference is also considered. The anesthesiologist evaluates each pa-

TABLE 21-4 Types of anesthesia

Type	Action and Effect	Method of Administration	Definition
General	Blocks awareness centers in brain; produces unconsciousness, body relaxation, loss of sensation	Inhalation	Vapors from liquids and gases under pressure, administered through a tube and/or mask
		Intravenous	Drug given directly into vein, usually used for induction
Regional	Inhibition of excitatory process in nerve endings or fibers; analgesia over a specific body area with consciousness retained	Nerve block	Injection of drug to anesthetize an isolated nerve
		Intravenous regional block with tourniquet (Bier block)	Injection of drug intravenously into an extremity
		Field block	Series of injections of drug into tissues surrounding the operative site
		Spinal (intrathecal)	Injection of drug into subarachnoid space of spinal cord (Figure 21-6)
		Epidural	Injection into space surrounding dura mater without breaking dural membrane
Local	Blocks transmission of nerve impulses at site of action; analgesia over limited tissue area with consciousness retained	Topical	Drug applied directly to surface, mucous membrane, or open wound
		Infiltration	Injection of drug into tissue at site of incision
Hypnoanesthesia	Artificially induced passive state of consciousness in which there is increased amenability to suggestions and commands, reduced awareness, and restricted attentiveness	Hypnosis	Induction of the anesthetic state of hypnosis; may be combined with use of small dose of IV anesthetic or muscle relaxant
Acupuncture	Blocks painful stimuli by "gate control theory" and by stimulating release of endorphins with consciousness retained	Use of needles or surface electrodes	Needles or electrodes are connected to an electronic machine that creates current flow between these electrodes

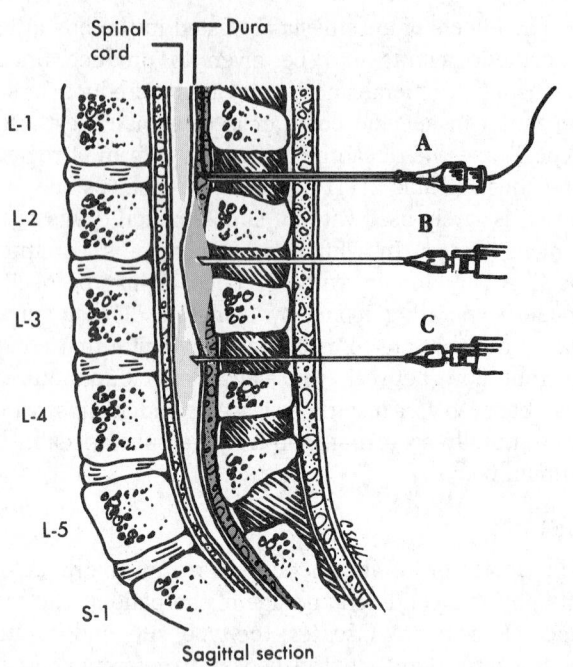

Spinal cord — Dura

L-1
L-2
L-3
L-4
L-5
S-1

A
B
C

Sagittal section

FIGURE 21-6 Position of needles and injection sites. **A,** Epidural catheters. **B,** Epidural anesthesia. **C,** Spinal anesthesia. (From Gruendemann BJ and Meeker MH: Alexander's care of the patient in surgery, ed 8, St Louis, 1987, The CV Mosby Co.)

ient carefully and selects the drugs best suited for that individual considering the physical and mental state.

PREPARATION OF THE PATIENT FOR ANESTHESIA

Patients have many anxieties related to anesthesia (see the box above, right). Most anxieties can be dispelled if the patient and family are well informed about the anesthetic selected for use and the care taken by the physician and nurse in assessing the patient's physical condition. The patient is encouraged to discuss any questions or concerns about the anesthetic with either the anesthesiologist or the surgeon.

The patient can be assured that there will be close surveillance during anesthesia and in the immediate postoperative period. Very few patients talk while under anesthesia, and what is said is usually unintelligible so that talking need not be of great concern to the patient. Persistent anxiety on the part of the patient regarding the anesthetic should be discussed with the surgeon and the anesthesiologist.

A premedication is commonly ordered to assist in sedating the patient, and if necessary, in drying secretions that may interfere with safe deliverance of a general anesthetic. This is usually administered before arrival at the operating room suite (see Chapter 20), but may be given there in an emergency situation.

After the patient is transferred to the operating room

FEARS RELATED TO ANESTHESIA

Going to sleep
Not waking up
Fear of the unknown
Effectiveness of the anesthetic
Pain during the surgical procedure
Postoperative nausea and vomiting
Talking, revealing personal information while anesthetized
Mask over face

---

table, an intravenous infusion is started and any necessary noninvasive monitoring equipment is connected (for example, electrocardiogram leads, blood pressure cuff, stethoscope). The desired anesthetic will then be administered.

It is very important that the circulating nurse remain near the patient during induction of the anesthetic. The nurse may be called on to protect the patient physically if an untoward reaction occurs. It is possible for the patient to become excited and move excessively, requiring additional restraint to prevent self-injury. Stimulation of the patient in the form of noise or moving body parts is avoided as this may cause vomiting, retching, or laryngospasm, which in turn may lead to hypoxia. If this occurs, the anesthesiologist may require the nurse's assistance with suctioning equipment and with observing the monitors. Emotional support can be very important, and simply holding the patient's hand has been reported by many to be a great comfort.[58]

GENERAL ANESTHESIA

General anesthesia is produced by inhalation or by injection of anesthetic drugs into the bloodstream. The muscle relaxation that occurs during general anesthesia results from depression of neuromuscular transmission and loss of skeletal muscle tone. This ultimately leads to sufficient relaxation for endotracheal intubation and intraabdominal or thoracic surgery.

Anesthesia induction is the procedure of taking the patient from a conscious state to one in which surgery can be initiated. Ultra–short-acting barbiturates such as thiopental (Pentothal) and methohexital (Brevital) are the most commonly used induction agents for adults. However, these drugs may cause severe cardiovascular depression, which may require the use of an alternative agent. The benzodiazepines, diazepam (Valium) and midazolam (Versed), may be used and are less likely to cause cardiovascular depression.

Short-acting anesthetic narcotics may be used for induction and their analgesic effect, or as an adjunct to general anesthesia. Use of short-acting narcotics such as fentanyl (Sublimaze), sufentanil (Sufenta), and alfentanyl (Alfenta) requires a reduction in dose of other

TABLE 21-5 Comparison of selected anesthetic agents

Name	Method of Administration	Advantages	Disadvantages	Special Postoperative Care
Enflurane (Ethrane)	Inhalation	Rapid induction and recovery; some muscle relaxation on its own; nonflammable	Circulatory/respiratory depression (dose dependent); expensive; shivering with emergence	Monitor vital signs frequently
Halothane (Fluothane)	Inhalation	Rapid induction; low incidence of postoperative nausea/vomiting; nonirritating; nonflammable	Shivering with emergence; circulatory/respiratory depression; reduces urinary output; hepatic toxicity; associated with hyperpyrexia	Monitor vital signs closely; report any alteration in liver function
Isoflurane (Forane)	Inhalation	Smooth and rapid induction; good muscle relaxation; nonirritating; cardiovascular stability	Expensive	Hypotension may occur
Nitrous oxide	Inhalation	Rapid induction and recovery; nonirritating; nonflammable but supports combustion	Possible hypoxia with excessive amounts	Monitor for signs of hypoxia and administer supplemental oxygen for about 10 minutes following surgery
Alfentanil (Alfenta)	Intravenous	Very brief duration of action	Elimination is slow, and repeated doses exert more prolonged effect	Be alert for signs of respiratory depression and be prepared to treat it
Droperidol and fentanyl (Innovar)	Intravenous	Rapid, smooth induction and recovery; nontoxic to liver, kidneys, or heart; less analgesia required postoperatively	Hypoventilation; hypotension and skeletal muscle rigidity may occur	Monitor for decreased respiratory depth and rate; decrease postoperative narcotics to ⅓ to ¼ usual dose
Etomidate (Amidate)	Intravenous	Fewer adverse cardiopulmonary effects	Venous pain on injections; myoclonic muscle movements	Same as for thiopental sodium (see below)
Fentanyl (Sublimaze)	Intravenous or intramuscular	Abolition of stress response; very potent analgesic	Respiratory depression; muscle rigidity and bradycardia may occur	Monitor for decreased respiratory rate and depth and decreased blood pressure
Ketamine (Ketalar)	Intravenous or intramuscular	Profound analgesia with no loss of consciousness; amnesia for surgical event	Unpleasant dreams in early postoperative period and sometimes later; does not block visceral pain	Maintain quiet environment postoperatively
Midazolam (Versed)	Intravenous	Induction achieved within narrow dose range and short period; high incidence of partial or complete impairment of recall for several hours	Depresses respiration and causes fluctuation of vital signs	Monitor for respiratory depression and hypotension
Sufentanil citrate (Sufenta)	Intravenous	Rapid onset producing hypnosis and anesthesia without use of additional agents; inhibits sympathetic response to surgical stress	Respiratory depression and skeletal muscle rigidity	Monitor for muscle rigidity of chest wall and respiratory depression; have naloxone available to reverse respiratory depression
Thiopental sodium (Pentothal sodium)	Intravenous or rectal (children)	Rapid, smooth induction and recovery	Laryngospasm with stimulation of larynx; respiratory depression with high doses; blood pressure may drop suddenly	Monitor for signs of stridor, neck tissue retraction, cyanosis; monitor vital signs for decreased respiratory depth or decreased blood pressure
Procaine Cocaine Tetracaine Dibucaine Lidocaine Carbocaine Bupivacaine Chloroprocaine	Tissue injection (local) spray	No loss of consciousness	CNS stimulation or seizures; cardiac depression; absorbed into bloodstream	Monitor for excitability, twitching, pulse or blood pressure changes, pallor, respiratory difficulty

TABLE 21-6 Stages and planes of ether anesthesia and selected central nervous system effects

| Central Nervous System Effects | Stage 1 | Stage 2 | Stage 3 Planes | | | | Stage 4 |
			1	2	3	4	
Consciousness	Maintained Analgesia Euphoria Some distortion of perceptions Variable amnesia	Lost	Absent	Absent	Absent	Absent	Absent
Respiration	No alteration or increased rate with some irregularity	Rapid, irregular	Regular	Regular, but expirations longer than inspirations	Diaphragmatic	Thoracic ceased Diaphragmatic depressed	No respiratory movement Respiratory paralysis
Skeletal muscles	Normal tone	Tone increased	Small muscles relaxed	Large muscles relaxed	Complete relaxation	Complete relaxation	Diaphragm paralyzed
Eyes							
Pupils	Reaction to light	Dilated	Constriction	Mid-dilation		Dilated	Dilated
Movements	Unchanged	Increased	Increased	None	None	None	None
Tear secretion				Decreased	Decreased	Absent	
Reflexes							
Lid	Present	Present	Absent	Absent	Absent	Absent	Absent
Corneal	Present	Present	Present	Absent	Absent	Absent	Absent
Pharyngeal or "gag"			Absent				
Laryngeal				Absent			
Cough					Absent in large bronchi	Absent in small bronchi	
Heart rate		Increased	Decreased				
Blood pressure	Unchanged	Increased	Normal	Normal	Decreased	Decreased	Decreased
Venous pressure	Unchanged	Increased	Unchanged				Increased

From Hahn AB, Barkin RL, and Oestreich SJK: Pharmacology in nursing, ed 15, St. Louis, 1982, The CV Mosby Co.

induction agents. These drugs are particularly useful for patients in whom it is critical to maintain a stable cardiac output. Muscle relaxants may also be administered during induction of such procedures as a tracheal intubation.

After induction, general anesthesia is usually maintained with combinations of agents listed in Table 21-5. The choice of agents depends on the anesthesiologist's judgment and the individual patient's and surgeon's needs. Use of a combination of inhalation anesthetic agents, along with muscle relaxants, narcotic analgesics, barbiturates, and other neuroleptic and antiemetic drugs is referred to as *balanced anesthesia*. It is important to note that rapid intravenous induction, along with extensive use of intravenous adjuncts, has led to the need for increased technology in monitoring anesthetic depth. This monitoring is primarily aimed at assessing pulmonary and cardiovascular function.[50]

STAGES OF GENERAL ANESTHESIA

The stages of anesthesia may vary, depending on the drug used, the rapidity of induction, and the skill of the anesthesiologist. Because current practice is to induce anesthesia with a rapid-acting intravenously administered drug before inhalation anesthesia, a rapid transition through the early stages may occur. The classic, distinct stages are best seen when diethyl ether is used. All stages will not be observable with all anesthetics (Table 21-6). Characteristics of each stage are listed in the box on p. 483).

STAGES OF ANESTHESIA

Stage I	Extends from beginning of administration of anesthetic to beginning of loss of consciousness
Stage II	Extends from loss of consciousness to loss of eyelid reflexes; often called the stage of *excitement or delirium*
Stage III	Extends from loss of eyelid reflex to cessation of respiratory effort; called stage of *surgical anesthesia*. Patient is unconscious; muscles are relaxed; reflexes are abolished
Stage IV	Stage of *overdose or danger;* death will follow if anesthetic is not immediately discontinued

INHALATION ANESTHESIA

Inhalation anesthesia is produced by having the patient inhale the vapors of certain volatile liquids or gases. Oxygen is always given with these anesthetic agents. The gas mixture may be administered by mask or into the lungs through an endotracheal tube inserted into the trachea through either the nose or mouth. The use of endotracheal intubation ensures that an airway can be maintained when the chest wall is open. The endotracheal tube may have a balloon that is inflated after insertion; the balloon fills the tracheal space, lessening the chance of aspiration of gastric contents. Regardless of the skill of the anesthesiologist, an endotracheal tube may cause some irritation to the trachea and subsequent edema. If it is difficult to intubate the patient, which may occur as a result of anatomic differences, it is not uncommon for the patient to complain of a sore, irritated throat postoperatively.

Some of the more common inhalant anesthetics are described in Table 21-5. The use of *nitrous oxide* alone is limited because it cannot be administered in adequate concentrations to produce deep muscle relaxation. Nitrous oxide is additive with other anesthetics, and it is used extensively as an adjunct to halothane, enflurane, and isoflurane. Its greatest use is as an agent for induction and as a component of balanced anesthesia for prolonged or complicated surgery. In low concentrations, nitrous oxide may provide adequate anesthesia for intraabdominal procedures in patients who are in profound shock, debilitated, or who are critically ill and cannot tolerate other anesthetic agents. It is also used for dental surgery.

Increasing concern exists regarding long-term health problems from occupational exposure to nitrous oxide. It has been noted that long-term exposure can produce neurologic syndromes consistent with vitamin B_{12} deficiency. Some studies suggest increased rates of spontaneous abortion in female operating room and dental personnel. More recent studies, however, indicate that occupational exposure to trace amounts of nitrous oxide does not carry a significant health risk.[57] Further research is needed in this area, but for the time being, personnel working around inhalation anesthetics should be aware of careful evaluation and use of scavenging systems to minimize levels of gas in their environment.

Halothane (Fluothane) is easily inhaled and very widely used. Advantages include rapid onset of action and fairly rapid elimination of effect. This allows the anesthesia depth to be easily controlled with reasonably rapid arousing when the drug is stopped. Hepatic toxicity of halothane has resulted in a decline in its use in favor of newer agents; however, it remains widely used in pediatrics because toxicity is rare in children. The vapors do not irritate the respiratory mucosa, and because it tends to dilate the bronchi, halothane is a preferred anesthetic for asthmatic patients. Separate muscle relaxants may need to be used, because halothane does not produce adequate relaxation of abdominal and other skeletal muscles.

Enflurane (Ethrane) is a newer anesthetic that is approximately half as potent as halothane. Induction and recovery is more rapid than with halothane, and enflurane does not sensitize the myocardium to catecholamines as halothane does. Enflurane also provides skeletal muscle relaxation. Deep anesthesia with enflurane is associated with circulatory and respiratory depression. It may also cause increased intracranial pressure (ICP), and seizure activity has occurred with high concentrations of the drug. Metabolites of enflurane include the fluoride ion, which can be nephrotoxic.

Isoflurane (Forane) has become the most widely used anesthetic agent because of several properties. In comparison to halothane and enflurane, isoflurane is minimally metabolized and most of the drug eliminated quickly via the lungs. A significant reduction in hepatic and renal damage is also noted. Of the three drugs, isoflurane causes the least amount of myocardial depression and reduces cardiac workload by dilating the coronary arteries. Effects on skeletal muscle are similar to those caused by enflurane, and neuromuscular blockers may be needed for intraabdominal surgery; however, required doses are lower. Rapid elimination means that the patient awakens faster, thus experiencing surgical discomfort early in the recovery period. This usually requires the administration of IV narcotics in the recovery room.

Cyclopropane, methoxyflurane (Penthrane), and ether are seldom used in the United States today. *Cyclopropane* is highly flammable and requires extreme care to prevent any electrical charge during administration. Because of its potential for nephrotoxicity, *methoxyflurane* is rarely used except for obstetric anesthesia.

Ether is also highly flammable and has disagreeable side effects, but because of its wide margin of safety, it may be used in areas of the world where sophisticated monitoring equipment is unavailable.

MALIGNANT HYPERTHERMIA (HYPERPYREXIA)

No discussion of general anesthesia would be complete without the mention of malignant hyperthermia, which is a life-threatening complication of anesthesia. The physical signs of malignant hyperthermia commonly include unexplained tachycardia, unstable blood pressure, tachypnea, muscle rigidity, cyanotic skin mottling, rapidly rising body temperature (sometimes higher than 46° C). The condition may occur at induction or at any time postoperatively, although usually in the immediate recovery period.

Malignant hyperthermia is usually triggered by anesthetic agents in patients who have an inherited defect in the membrane of the skeletal muscle. The defect is believed to be present in the sarcoplasmic reticulum, where the triggering agent sets off the release of calcium. The high intracellular calcium level of the muscle cells accelerates their metabolic rate dramatically. A number of resultant chemical changes take place that, if not controlled, may lead to renal failure, neurologic damage, heart failure, and disseminated intravascular coagulation (DIC).

Although malignant hyperthermia is a rare occurrence, every facility that administers anesthetic agents should have a protocol for dealing with this crisis. The primary treatment modalities include packing the patient in ice, chilled intravenous fluids, administering diuretics, steroids, and dantrolene (Dantrium).[24]

INTRAVENOUS ANESTHESIA

Thiopental sodium (Pentothal sodium) is the drug used most frequently for induction of anesthesia. It produces unconsciousness quickly and may be used in combination with other drugs for many kinds of surgery. Intermittent intravenous injection of thiopental along with nitrous oxide and oxygen may be used for brief surgical procedures such as closed reduction of a fracture or incision and drainage of an abscess. The rapid onset of action also carries with it potential dangers; medullary paralysis may develop rapidly with an overdose. Special care is required to prevent leakage of concentrated intravenous solutions into surrounding tissues, because the high alkalinity of thiopental can cause severe pain and damage.

Thiopental is detoxified chiefly in the liver with metabolized products excreted by the kidney, resulting in a prolonged emergency phase. Thiopental is also used to treat acute convulsive states caused by overdoses of CNS-stimulating drugs such as local anesthetics. Rectal administration is sometimes used to produce basal narcosis in children.

Innovar injection is a combination of droperidol, a neuroleptic (antipsychotic) drug, and fentanyl, a powerful narcotic analgesic. This combination is used primarily for procedures that require the patient's cooperation. The condition produced is referred to as *neuroleptanesthesia,* a state in which patients are neither asleep nor awake but experience profound analgesia and psychomotor sedation. Innovar has lost some of its original popularity, because of the depression of alveolar ventilation and respiratory rate that persists longer than the analgesic effect.

Ketamine (Ketalar) is a rapid-acting nonbarbiturate that produces an anesthetic state termed *dissociative anesthesia.* It produces a cataleptic state in which the patient appears to be awake and yet is unaware of surrounding events and unresponsive to pain. Ketamine is chemically related to hallucinogens, and some patients become confused and excited during emergence from the drug. It is not a desirable agent for routine use but is very useful for selected situations, such as for burn patients; ketamine's combination of an amnesic and an analgesic is beneficial for debridement, painful dressing changes, and skin grafting procedures. It is also of value with asthmatic patients, because of its bronchodilating properties, and with high-risk patients who are hypovolemic or hypotensive, because it activates the sympathetic nervous system. Ketamine increases ICP and should be avoided for neurosurgical procedures. Avoidance of excessive stimulation is important in the immediate postoperative period to lessen such side effects as delusions and disorientation.

Fentanyl citrate (Sublimaze) is a short-acting narcotic that is 50 to 80 times the potency of morphine. Fentanyl is used as an analgesic supplement for regional and general anesthesia; it can be used as a primary anesthetic for selected procedures. Fentanyl is widely used for induction and maintenance of anesthesia of patients with severe peripheral vascular, cardiovascular, carotid, or coronary-occlusive diseases. Side effects may include nausea and vomiting, mood changes, pruritus, hypotension, and severe respiratory depression. Fentanyl also depresses the coughing center, which may reduce the patient's ability to clear secretions postoperatively.

Sufentanil citrate (Sufenta) is 5 to 10 times more potent than fentanyl and provides profound analgesia with significantly more sedation. It may be used as an analgesic adjunct, in the maintenance of balanced general anesthesia, or as a primary agent with 100% oxygen for the induction and maintenance of anesthesia in patients undergoing cardiovascular or neurosurgical procedures. It is cleared from the bloodstream more quickly than fentanyl, which allows for a more rapid recovery. The most common adverse reactions are respiratory depression and skeletal muscle rigidity.

Alfentanil (Alfenta) has only one fourth the potency

of fentanyl and is considered to be an ultra–short-acting narcotic. It is frequently administered via continuous IV infusion to maintain continuous action. Although alfentanil has a brief duration of action, the elimination of its clinical effect takes much longer than that of fentanyl and prolonged respiratory depression may occur.

Etomidate (Amidate) is classified as an ultra–short-acting induction anesthetic that differs chemically from barbiturates and benzodiazepines. Etomidate lacks analgesic or muscle-relaxing properties frequently requiring the concomitant use of neuromuscular blockers if endotracheal intubation is required. Only slight cardiovascular and respiratory depression occur, which makes etomidate useful in high-risk patients. Myoclonus and pain on injection are the most common side effects; however, the drug's ability to cause adrenal suppression can also limit its clinical use.

Midazolam (Versed) is a benzodiazepine that is particularly useful in producing anesthesia. Its primary effects include sedation and amnesia; however, it also reduces neuronal activity, cerebral blood flow, and ICP. It lacks analgesic properties, is only a mild cardiovascular depressant, and has only minor effects on the lungs, liver, kidneys, and skeletal and smooth muscles. It is used primarily as a preanesthetic but can also be used as an intraoperative sedative and amnesic. Side effects include respiratory depression, apnea, and disorientation. Effects are greatly intensified in the elderly or in any person receiving other sedative and analgesic drugs.

MUSCLE RELAXANTS

Skeletal muscle relaxants (neuromuscular blocking agents) are frequently employed in combination with anesthetics. These drugs have the following uses:
1. Facilitating endotracheal intubation
2. Preventing laryngospasm
3. Producing adequate muscle relaxation during anesthesia
4. Reducing the amount of general anesthetic needed

Nondepolarizing agents, such as metocurine, pancuronium bromide, gallamine triethiodide, atracurium besylate, vercuronium bromide, and tubocurarine chloride, may be referred to as stabilizing agents and are preferred in longer procedures. Depolarizing blocking agents, such as succinylcholine and decamethonium bromide, are used in shorter procedures.

Muscle relaxants cause respiratory depression or paralysis; thus the patient must be observed closely for signs of *respiratory distress* during and after administration of the drug. Patients developing respiratory problems will require intubation and mechanical ventilatory assistance.

Delayed recovery can result in patients who have received nondepolarizing relaxants along with certain other drugs. Drug interactions may occur with the use of antibiotics, causing a synergistic effect in which paralysis will be prolonged. This is more likely to occur if the antibiotics are given intravenously or if the peritoneal cavity is irrigated with antibiotic solution. Synergism also occurs with inhalation anesthetics and the nondepolarizing agents. (For more complete discussion, refer to a current pharmacology text.)

REGIONAL ANESTHESIA

Regional anesthesia is produced by the injection or application of a local anesthetic agent along the course of a nerve or at the site of the stimulus, thus abolishing the conduction of all impulses to and from the area supplied by that nerve. The patient experiences no pain in the operative area and remains awake during the entire procedure because the anesthetic affects a particular region only; it does not affect cortical functions. Regional anesthesia is used for treatments, diagnostic measures, examinations, and surgery.

The drugs used to produce regional anesthesia are usually called local anesthetics (Table 21-5). Care is taken that the drugs are given in a localized area in the smallest dose necessary to produce anesthesia, because absorption in the bloodstream may cause CNS stimulation and depression of the heart. Epinephrine may be added to the solution of local anesthetic drugs to produce vasoconstriction in the area of injection. Vasoconstriction tends to reduce the rate of absorption, to extend the length of anesthesia, and to reduce hemorrhage.

At the first sign of toxic reactions (see the box below), an intravenous injection of a short-acting barbiturate such as thiopental sodium is administered. Oxygen may also be necessary, and it is important that a patent airway is maintained. If the reaction is caused by an idiosyncrasy to the drug, circulatory failure may occur, and emergency measures such as CPR must be started. Patients should be questioned preoperatively regarding any previous sensitivity to these drugs.

Regional anesthesia may be given by infiltration, by nerve block, by epidural block, by spinal injection, or topically (see Table 21-4).

Spinal anesthesia is not used for surgery of the upper

SIGNS OF TOXIC REACTION TO LOCAL ANESTHETICS

Excitability (laughing, crying, excessive talking)
Twitching
Pulse or blood pressure changes
Pallor of the skin
Respiratory difficulties

part of the body because it causes paralysis of the diaphragm and the intercostal muscles used in respiration. With spinal anesthesia the patient may be conscious of pulling sensations throughout the operation but experiences no pain. Occasionally a feeling of faintness and nausea may result from these sensations. Because of the sympathetic blockade, hypotension may occur with both spinal and epidural anesthesia.

One of the limitations of spinal anesthesia is that the patient may be awake during the operation, although the preoperative medication may decrease awareness of the surroundings. A screen restricts the patient's vision from the surgical area and a towel may be placed over the eyes. The conversation and activities of the members of the operating room staff should be carried on with the patient's consciousness in mind.

Following spinal anesthesia the patient should be quiet in bed in a supine position. Turning from side to side is permitted. Safety needs must be considered, since sensation may not return to the anesthetized area for 1 or 2 hours. The patient is monitored for signs of respiratory or circulatory depression.

Headache may occur following spinal anesthesia and is thought to result from leakage of spinal fluid at the puncture site. The headache usually occurs 24 hours after the puncture and may last several days or a week, occasionally longer. It may be prevented by keeping the patient flat and quiet after surgery and promoting hydration to replace the lost spinal fluid.

SPECIAL CONSIDERATIONS RELATED TO GERONTOLOGIC PATIENTS

With the upward trend in the length of life, increasing numbers of older patients are coming to the operating room. Because of the normal aging process, these patients may face higher risks, many of which are related to medications they will receive in the OR. Elderly patients generally require less anesthesic agents, and it takes longer for these agents to be distributed and eliminated. A change in body composition is one reason why this occurs. A decrease in lean body mass, along with increased body fat, increases the uptake of lipid-soluble drugs by fatty tissue. Anesthetic agents tend to be lipid soluble and will concentrate in body fat, thus prolonging the drug action. Reduced blood flow and impaired renal function from aging also cause inefficient and slowed drug excretion. The presence of acute and chronic illness may further alter pharmacokinetics in elderly persons.

Older patients undergoing surgery are also at high risk for developing hypothermia. This can occur because of cold operating rooms, cold solutions being used, lack of covering, and impaired heat regulation from preoperative medications. Ideally, operating rooms should be maintained at higher temperatures for the el-

derly, and skin prep solutions should be warmed. A study by Biddle & Biddle[8] indicates that heat loss can be prevented by simply using a disposable plastic bag as a cap to cover the patient's head during the surgical procedure.

OTHER TYPES OF ANESTHESIA

Induced Hypothermia

Hypothermia refers to the reduction of body temperature below normal to reduce oxygen and metabolic requirements. Extracorporeal cooling, a method of bloodstream cooling, consists of removing the blood from a major vessel, circulating it through coils immersed in a refrigerant, and returning it to the body through another vessel. Bloodstream cooling is the fastest method for producing hypothermia and is used primarily for patients undergoing surgery, particularly open-heart surgery. The patient is given heparin to prevent the blood from clotting during surgery.

The most widely accepted method of nonintrusive hypothermia today is the use of cooling blankets (Figure 21-7). The patient is placed on and may be covered by body-sized vinyl pads containing many coils. The pads

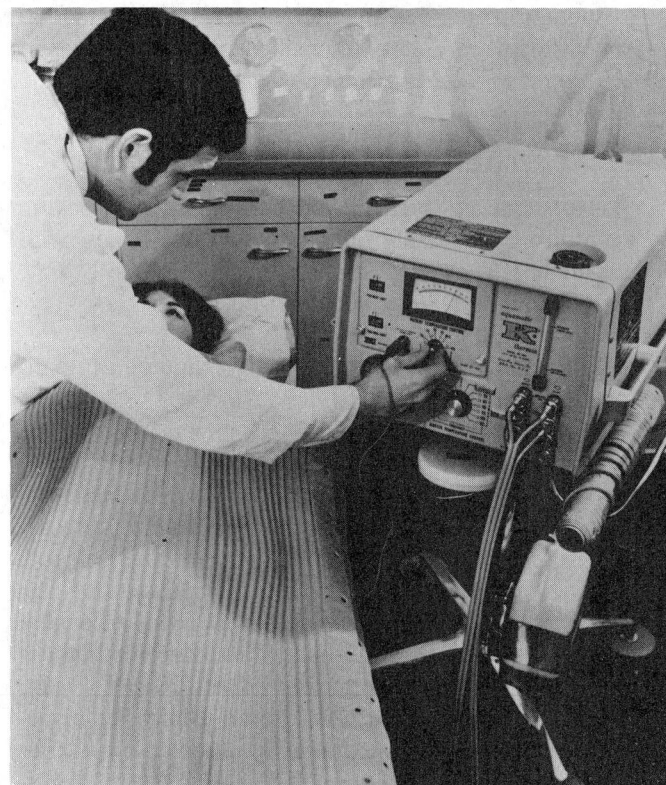

FIGURE 21-7 Hypothermia can be produced by means of a cooling blanket. Cold alcohol and water are circulated through the coils by a pressure pump. (Courtesy Hamilton Industries, Two-Rivers, Wisconsin.)

are connected to a reservoir filled with alcohol and water. A pump fills the coils and circulates the solution through the coils. A recording thermometer monitors the patient's temperature, and an electric unit heats or cools the solution to a preset temperature. Hypothermia may be used for a variety of illnesses when extremely high temperatures occur.

The care of the person who is experiencing prolonged hypothermia is described in the box below.

Induced Hypotension

Hypotension may be induced for the purpose of decreasing bleeding at the operative site in selected instances such as radical head and neck or pelvic surgery. Hypotension can be induced by deep anesthesia with an inhalant anesthetic such as halothane or by an intravenous anesthetic that affects the autonomic nervous system. Vital signs are monitored closely in the early postoperative period.

MONITORING PATIENT DURING ANESTHESIA

Monitoring Methods

During surgery requiring anesthesia, the patient's body is subjected to a variety of stressors. Potent drugs, required body positions, aggravation of preexisting disease processes, and bleeding may all contribute to situations that interfere with respiration and circulation and contribute to altered physiology.

Many devices are now available to augment the measurement of patients' responses to these stressors (see

---

CARE OF PATIENT DURING PROLONGED HYPOTHERMIA

1. Prepare patient for procedure
2. Give complete bath before procedure; protect skin with a thin coating of emollient
3. Insert indwelling catheter (if ordered) for monitoring urinary output
4. Monitor patient
   a. Monitor vital signs for sudden increases or decreases or rapid fluctuations
   b. Note shivering and give prescribed medication (usually chlorpromazine hydrochloride)
   c. Observe skin for signs of pressure, edema, discoloration
5. Turn patient every 2 hours and maintain good body alignment
6. Provide fluids and nutrients as ordered (usually by intravenous or tube feedings)
7. Provide good oral hygiene
8. Cleanse and protect eyes if corneal reflexes and eye secretions are decreased
9. When hypothermia is terminated:
   a. Apply blankets to rewarm patient
   b. Monitor return of normal body temperature and remove blankets as necessary

---

Table 21-7). Most of this equipment is expensive, takes up extra space in the operating room, and may constitute an electrical safety hazard. Involved personnel must still use skills of looking, listening, and palpating even when sophisticated monitoring equipment is in use.

A variety of other monitoring devices may be used depending on the complexity of the procedure being performed and the physical condition of the patient. Computers are being used more extensively today in monitoring and processing patient data, and greater use of the computer is envisioned in the future.

Electrical Safety Hazards

Monitoring of patient safety during anesthesia must also take into consideration electrical safety hazards. The operating room is an area containing many potential life-threatening and mechanically injurious situations related to electrical shock, burns, fire, and explosions. It is imperative that team members have current knowledge of the equipment and supplies most often involved in such incidents.

Federal regulations govern the marketing and safety standards of electronic devices used in operating rooms, and the Joint Commission on Accreditation of Hospitals has standards that must be met. The most significant hazards, however, are inadequately trained personnel, malfunctioning equipment due to improper maintenance, inappropriate design of operating room suites, and inappropriate surveillance by team members.

TERMINATION OF SURGERY

One of the most crucial periods for the surgical patient is the immediate postoperative phase during the time after surgery has been completed and the patient is transferred to the appropriate recovery area. During this period, the operating room nurse may be involved in a variety of activities related to providing effective patient care.

DRESSINGS AND DRAINS

The circulating nurse will assist in the application of the outer layer of any necessary dressings. Dressings are used to protect the wound from trauma and contamination, to absorb drainage, and to support or immobilize the incisional area. Pressure dressings may be applied to aid in minimizing edema and to assist with hemostasis.

A wide variety of gauzes, pads, and tapes are available for use. The type used will depend on the area of the body involved, the amount of drainage anticipated, and the pressure that is necessary. Montgomery straps may be used if frequent dressing changes or wound inspections are anticipated. In some instances the application of a splint or cast will be required.

TABLE 21-7 Monitoring during anesthesia

Parameter	Method	Comments
Arterial blood pressure	Sphygmomanometer (indirect)	Used in all situations
		Automatic equipment available
		Arm is protected from injury
	Arterial catheter (direct)	Catheter usually inserted percutaneously in radial artery
		Used for continuous monitoring in complex procedures and for induced hypotension
Cardiac	Stethoscopy	Stethoscope taped to chest
		Pressure sensitive units may be placed in esophagus
		Units attached to anesthesiologist's ear by indwelling ear piece
	ECG	Usually consists of a screen and print-out system
		Chest and extremity electrodes used
		Other electrosurgical equipment may affect ECG recordings
Central venous pressure	Water manometer	Used for evaluation of overall circulatory status
		Serves as a guide during blood and fluid administration
		Aids in preventing too rapid fluid replacement that could lead to pulmonary edema
Arterial blood gases	Blood samples	Used for evaluation of acid-base status and pulmonary gas exchange
Body temperature	Thermistor	Thermistor inserted in esophagus or rectum
		Used for events that are preceded by hypopyrexia or hyperpyrexia
Urinary output	Indwelling urinary catheter	Hourly measurements made
		Used for evaluation of blood volume and fluid administration
Blood loss	Weighing of blood-soaked sponges	Used to estimate blood loss from surgical procedure
		Dry weight of sponges is subtracted from wet weight
	Measurement of blood in suction systems	Estimate is also made of blood on drapes and team members' gowns

Some surgeons prefer that the wound be covered with a transparent spray dressing. This commonly stays on for 3 to 6 days and may either peel off or be removed with solvent. This type of dressing is particularly suitable for areas where gauze dressings could become contaminated with urine or feces.

Other surgeons prefer that the wound be left uncovered and open to the air to allow the incisional area to heal with the aid of air and light. This also allows for easy observation, prevents possible tape reactions, and increases comfort and maneuverability for certain patients.

A variety of drains may also be inserted at the time of surgery (see Chapter 22). Drains are used to expedite the removal of air and fluids such as blood, serum, bile, and pus from the involved site. The type and exact location of the drains are recorded and reported to the recovery room nurses.

DOCUMENTATION

Written documentation is important for communicating to other health team members the nursing actions that were performed in the intraoperative period and the patient outcomes. If the perioperative role is to be effectively implemented, operating room nurses must be accountable by documenting what they do.

Some facilities have the operating room nurse document information on the same form used for all nursing notes. Others have found it more expedient to develop a separate form that combines a checklist format along with areas for narrative comments.

TRANSFER OF PATIENT TO RECOVERY ROOM

After appropriate dressings have been applied, the circulating nurse checks to see that the patient is clean. A clean gown and blanket are applied.

Special care must be taken in moving the patient from the operating room table to the recovery stretcher or bed. At least four people are usually required to transfer the unconscious patient safely while keeping the body in proper alignment. Care must be taken not to allow the patient to slip between the table and the stretcher and that no body tissues have shearing forces applied to them. Arms and legs must be carefully supported and intravenous sites splinted to prevent dislodging the needle. The anesthesiologist protects the head and neck from injury during the transfer. A patient-lifting frame or roller device is very helpful when moving heavy patients.

The patient is lifted or rolled slowly to avoid circulatory depression, and the actions of all involved persons are carefully synchronized. The patient is placed in a comfortable position appropriate for maintaining an unobstructed airway and adequate circulation. It is important that the patient be constantly observed during this time, because changes in position can stimulate vomiting or cause respiratory obstruction, hypotension, or cardiac arrest.

Before the stretcher or bed is moved, side rails are pulled up and restraint straps fastened. Drainage systems are connected as indicated, and drainage bags are kept below the level of tubing to prevent retrograde flow.

The patient chart and nursing care plan are sent with the patient, together with any other supplies that will be needed. In some hospitals the circulating nurse accompanies the patient and anesthesiologist to the recovery room so that a nursing report can be given to the nurse admitting the patient. Various other personnel may go along during the actual transfer depending on the condition of the patient.

CHAPTER SUMMARY

✔ Members of the scrubbed sterile team include the primary surgeon, assistant surgeons or RN first assistant, and scrub nurse or technician.

✔ Members of the nonsterile surgical team include an anesthesiologist or anesthetist, circulating nurse, and such other persons as technicians, biomedical engineer, or pathologist.

✔ The scrub nurse or technician prepares supplies and equipment for surgery, assists the surgeon and surgical assistants during the procedure, and assists with counting procedures.

✔ The circulating nurse prepares the patient for surgery, maintains patient safety and comfort, and provides assistance and communication for scrubbed team members.

✔ Basic rules of surgical asepsis must be maintained in the OR to prevent infection.

✔ Rules for wearing correct OR attire and following good health habits are essential for lessening the risk of personnel serving as loci of infection.

✔ The use of the nursing process is as important in nursing care of patients in the operating room as it is elsewhere.

✔ Procedures for scrubbing before surgery differ among health care agencies; however, persons should always be free of upper respiratory infections and skin problems that could serve as a medium for bacterial growth.

✔ Factors that promote patient safety in the OR include reducing patient anxiety, following correct procedures for patient identification, reviewing the chart for completeness of necessary information and for identification of allergies, checking for possible hazards, and observing the patient for adverse effects of preoperative medication.

✔ Some commonly used operative positions include supine, prone, Trendelenburg, reverse Tredenlenburg, and lateral. Care must be taken in placing persons in each position to prevent patient injury.

✔ Anesthesia may be general, regional, or local; it may be administered by inhalation or intravenously or localized by regional block, field block, spinal, epidural, topical, or infiltrative means. Hypnosis or acupuncture may also be used.

✔ Anesthetic agents may produce amnesia, analgesia, hypnosis, or muscle relaxation, thus decreasing either the awareness of or the sensation to pain or both.

✔ Four stages can be noted with some types of anesthetics (especially diethyl ether); the extent to which the states manifest depends on the drug used, the rapidity of induction, and the skill of the anesthesiologist or anesthetist.

✔ Older patients generally require less anesthetic, and it takes longer for it to be distributed and eliminated. Older patients are also at high risk for developing hypothermia.

✔ Parameters monitored during anesthesia include arterial blood pressure, cardiac arrhythmias, arterial blood gases, central venous pressure, body temperature, urinary output, blood loss, and patient safety.

✔ After the surgical procedure, nursing activities include applying external dressings (as necessary), connecting drainage tubes, moving the patient to the recovery stretcher, monitoring the patient, documenting actions and the nursing care plan, transferring the patient to the recovery room, and reporting on the patient's condition and special needs.

QUESTIONS TO CONSIDER

■ Examine the charts of several patients who have undergone surgery and document the type of anesthetic used. What special care needs would that patient have had as a result of the chosen anesthetic?

■ What special precautions and activities are necessary to attend a patient going to surgery and to observe the surgical procedure? What is the purpose of each of these activities?

REFERENCES AND SELECTED READINGS

1. Altemeier WA, American College of Surgeons Committee on Control of Surgical Infections of the Committee on Preoperative and Postoperative Care: Manual on control of infection in surgical patients, ed 2, Philadelphia, 1984, JB Lippincott Co.
2. Association of Operating Room Nurses Proposed recommended practices: Surgical attire, AORN J 50:409-415, 1989.
3. Association of Operating Room Nurses Recommended Practices: Monitoring the patient receiving local anesthesia, AORN J 50:624-626, 1989.
4. Association of Operating Room Nurses Recommended Practices: Sponge, sharp, and instrument counts, AORN J 49:1638-1643, 1989.
5. Association of Operating Room Nurses, Inc: AORN Standards and recommended practices for perioperative nursing, Denver, 1989, The Association.
6. Atkinson LJ and Kohn ML: Berry and Kohn's introduction to operating room technique, ed 6, New York, 1986, McGraw-Hill Book Co.
7. Bargagliotti LA: Perioperative nursing research. VIII. Issues in perioperative nursing, AORN J 50:613-622, 1989.
8. *Biddle CA and Biddle WL: A plastic headcover to reduce surgical heat loss, Geriatr Nurse 6:39-41, 1985.
9. *Breslow MJ, Miller CF, and Rogers MC: Perioperative management, St Louis, 1990, The CV Mosby Co.
10. *Brown, DG, Wetterstroem N, and Finch J: Anesthetic gas exposure: protecting the OR environment, AORN J 41:590, 1985.
11. Centers for Disease Control: Update: universal precautions for prevention of transmission of immunodeficiency virus, hepatitis B virus, and other bloodborne pathogens in health-care settings, MMWR 37:377-388, 1988.
12. Centers for Disease Control: Update: human immunodeficiency virus infections in health-care workers exposed to blood infected patients, MMWR 36:1S-16S, 1987.
13. Christ MA and Hohloch F: Gerontologic Nursing: a study and learning tool, Springhouse, Penn, 1988, Springhouse Publishing Co.
14. Copp G et al: Covergowns and the control of operating room contamination, Nurs Res 35:263-268, 1986.
15. Copp G et al: Footwear practices and operating room contamination, Nurs Res 36:366-369, 1987.
16. Crow S: False nails increase risk of faulty handwash, Hosp Infect Contr 12:99, 1985.
17. Dripps RD, Eckenhoff JE, and VanDam LD: Introduction to anesthesia, ed 7, Philadelphia, 1988, WB Saunders Co.
18. *Felver J and Pendarvis JH: Electrolyte imbalances: intraoperative risk factors, AORN J 49:992-1008, 1989.
19. Fernsebner B: Infection control education, AORN J 43:898-899, 1986.
20. Garner JS: Guidelines for prevention of surgical wound infections. In Hospital Infection Program Center for Infectious Diseases, Atlanta, 1985, Centers for Disease Control.
21. Gaskey NJ et al: Use of fentanyl markedly increases nausea and vomiting in gynecologic short-stay patients, AANA J 54:309-311, 1986.
22. *Gillette MK and Caruso C: Intraoperative tissue injury: major causes and preventive measures, AORN J 50:66-78, 1989.
23. Greany D and Brown MM: Malignant hyperthermia: a concern for critical care nurses, Focus Crit Care 13:52-57, 1986.
24. Gruendemann BJ and Meeker MH: Alexander's care of the patient in surgery, ed 8, St Louis, 1987, The CV Mosby Co.
25. Guidelines for prevention of surgical wound infections, Atlanta, 1985, US Department of Health and Human Services.
26. Henschel EO, ed: Malignant hyperthermia: current concepts, New York City, 1987, Appleton-Century-Crofts.
27. Jacobson G et al: Handwashing: ring-wearing and number of microorganisms, Nurs Res 34:186-188, 1985.
28. Julien RM: Understanding anesthesia, Redwood city, Calif, 1984, Addison-Wesley Publishing Co.
29. Keith KS and Pieper B: Perioperative blood glucose levels: a study to determine the effect of surgery, AORN J 50:103-110, 1989.
30. King PL: Quality assurance guidelines: developing standards for a freestanding ambulatory surgery unit, AORN J 50:98-102, 1989.
31. *Kleinbeck SV: Developing nursing diagnoses for a perioperative care plan, AORN J 49:1613-1625, 1989.
32. Kneedler J and Dodge GH: Perioperative patient care: the nursing perspective, ed 2, Boston, 1987, Blackwell Scientific Publications.
33. Kneedler JA and Purcell SK: Perioperative nursing research. III. Potential intraoperative biological hazards to personnel, AORN J 49:1066-1082, 1989.
34. *Leske JS and McKnight EA: First assisting for RN's, AORN J 42:185-192, 1985.
35. *Malen AL: Perioperative nursing diagnoses: what, why, and how, AORN J 44:829-839, 1986.
36. Marchette L and Faulconer DR: Perioperative nursing research: a study of priorities, AORN J 44:387-394, 1986.
37. Mathias JM: Ambulatory surgery meeting stresses quality of care, AORN J 45:1191-1200, 1987.
38. McKenry L and Salerno E: Mosby's pharmacology in nursing, ed 17, 1989, St. Louis, The CV Mosby Co.
39. Nelson AH and Hanson RL: Perioperative functions: classification of knowledge and required skills, AORN J 41:1078-1088, 1985.
40. Palmer P: Nonphysician first assistants topic of collaborative meeting, AORN J 49:1645-1646, 1989.
41. Patterson RE and Daake JW: First assisting, Today's OR Nurse 7:10-16, 1985.
42. Pearce J: Current electrosurgical practice: hazards, J Med Eng Tech 9:107-111, 1985.
43. Pestana C: Fluids and electrolytes in the surgical patient, ed 4, San Antonio, Tex, 1989, Williams & Wilkins.
44. RN first assistant survey, AORN J 41:169-179, 1988.
45. *Rothrock JC: Perioperative nursing research. I. Preoperative psychoeducational interventions, AORN J 49:597-619, 1989.
46. Sack RA and Kroener WF: Hypokalemia of various etiologies complicating elective surgical procedures, Am J Obstet Gynecol 149:74-78, 1984.
47. Schaffner W: The evolution of hospital infection control policies concerning AIDS: the current United States debate, J Hosp Infect Supplement A:11, 1988.
48. Schwartz SE et al: Principles of surgery, ed 4, New York, 1984, McGraw-Hill Book Co.
49. Shlafer M and Marieb EN: The nurse, pharmacology, and drug therapy, Redwood City, Calif, 1989, Addison-Wesley Publishing Co.
50. Shoup A: The nurse as circulator, AORN J 47:1231-1240, 1988.
51. Silo HM: Perioperative nursing research. V. Intraoperative recommended practices, AORN J 49:1627-1636, 1989.
52. Spry C: Essentials of perioperative nursing: a self-learning guide, Rockville, Md, 1988, Aspen Publishers, Inc.
53. Stanfield V: Perioperative documentation: integrating nursing diagnosis on the patient record, AORN J 46:699-704, 1987.

*References preceded by an asterisk are particularly well suited for student reading.

54. *Stewart TP and Magnano SJ: Burns or pressure ulcers in the surgical patient, Decubitus 1:36, 1988.

55. Stoelting R: Basics of anesthesia, ed 2, Indianapolis, 1989, Churchill Livingstone, Inc.

56. *Sullivan D: Complications from intraoperative positioning, Orthop Nurs 4:56-59, 1985.

57. Tannenbaum TN and Goldberg RJ: Exposure to anesthetic gases and reproductive outcome, J Occup Med 27:659-668, 1985.

58. *Tovar MK and Cassmeyer VL: Touch: the beneficial effects for the surgical patient, AORN J 49:1356-1361, 1989.

59. Unexplained skin injuries may be pressure sores, OR Manager 2:1, 6-8, 1986.

60. Wehmer MA and Baldwin BJ: Inadvertent hypothermia: clinical nursing research, AORN J 44:788-796, 1986.

61. Wetchler BV, editor: Anesthesia for ambulatory surgery, Philadelphia, 1985, JB Lippincott Co.

62. *Wheeler BR: Crisis intervention: recognizing and helping patients overcome anxiety, AORN J 47:1242-1248, 1988.

63. Wlody GS: Malignant hyperthermia—potential crisis in patient care, AORN J 50:286-298, 1989.

CHAPTER 22

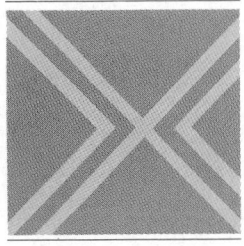

Postoperative Nursing

BARBARA C. LONG

CHAPTER OBJECTIVES

After studying this chapter, the student should be able to:

1 Describe wound healing in terms of pathophysiology, influencing factors, and complications.
2 Describe care of the surgical wound.
3 Identify nursing interventions to meet patient needs in the postanesthetic period.
4 Identify important factors of postoperative nursing assessment.
5 Identify common concerns of postoperative patients.
6 Describe pathophysiology, assessment, and nursing interventions of common postoperative alterations in aeration, circulation, fluid and electrolyte balance, nutrition, elimination, mobility, and comfort.
7 Describe the special needs of ambulatory surgery patients.

The goal of the postoperative phase is the patient's return, as quickly as possible, to an optimal level of functioning. Wound healing should be promoted and postoperative complications should be prevented. Nursing has a vital role during the postoperative period in promoting a rapid, smooth, and comfortable patient recovery from the traumatic effects of surgery.

This chapter begins with a discussion of wound healing, including the care of the surgical wound and problems of delayed healing. Postanesthesia care is described in a separate section because this care is generally performed in a postanesthesia (recovery) room. A nursing process approach is used to describe care of the postoperative patient on the surgical unit.

WOUND HEALING

Understanding of the pathophysiology of wound healing and the factors that influence wound healing provides the basis for postoperative nursing care, particularly wound care, dietary requirements, and need for patient activity.

PATHOPHYSIOLOGY
METHODS OF WOUND HEALING

When cells are injured and die, tissue repair may result in either *regeneration* of the tissue with little if any evidence that injury occurred, or in *scar formation*. The type of cells that constitute the tissue determines the end result (Figure 22-1).

There are three types of cells: labile cells, stable cells, and permanent cells. *Labile* cells multiply throughout life, constantly replacing similar cells that are being destroyed. Regrowth is through regeneration of marginal cells. Examples of labile cells are those of the skin and mucous membranes and the blood cells. *Stable* cells, occurring in bone or functional cells of glandular organs, do not usually multiply vigorously but will do so if injured. Both labile and stable cells require an underlying structure; they will not grow across an empty space. Thus if the framework is intact, there will be regeneration of normal structure. If the framework is destroyed, scarring will occur.

Permanent cells are the main constituents of muscle and nerve tissues. These cells rarely undergo mitotic division and are unable to regenerate. Muscle cells in striated, smooth, and cardiac muscles therefore do not regenerate. Satisfactory performance may result by hypertrophy of the preserved marginal cells. Nerve cells of the *central nervous system* do not regenerate. In the *peripheral nervous system* there is no regeneration if the cell body is destroyed. If the axon is injured, there is degeneration of the injured part to the closest node of Ranvier; then regeneration will occur. The discovery of nerve growth factors has led to research on new methods that could improve nerve regeneration.[59] Destruction of permanent cells results in scarring. A typical surgical incision cuts into muscle tissue. Although the epithelial cells regenerate over the scar tissue, the epithelial layer is so thin that the scar tissue is visible.

TYPES OF WOUND HEALING

Tissues may heal by one of three ways: primary, secondary, or tertiary intention. Most surgical wounds heal by *primary* intention. The incision is a clean straight line and all layers of the wound (muscle, subcutaneous tissue, and epithelial tissue) are well approximated by suturing (Figure 22-2). These wounds, if they remain free of infection and do not separate, heal quickly with a minimum of scarring.

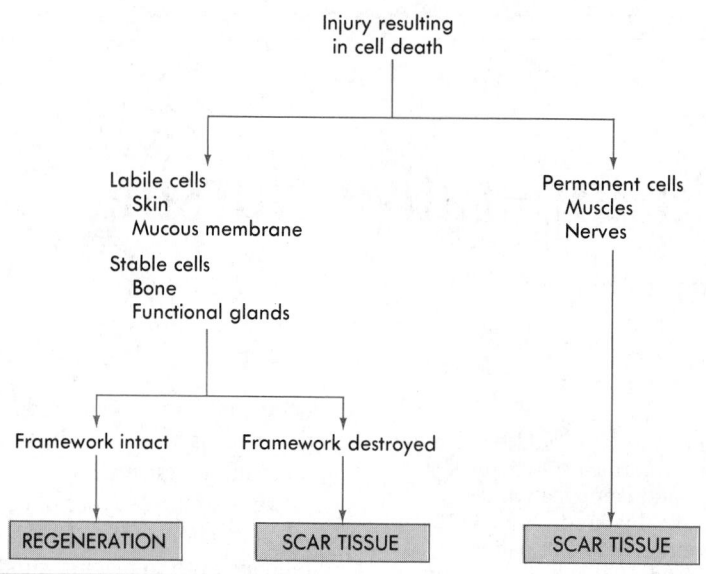

FIGURE 22-1 End results of wound healing.

Healing by *secondary* intention is seen in wounds such as ulcers with edges that cannot be approximated. Healing occurs by a filling in of the wound by granulation tissue over a larger area. Because these wounds are more open, they have a greater possibility for infection. More granulation tissue is formed than in healing by primary intention; therefore more scarring occurs.

Healing by *tertiary* intention occurs when there is a delay between injury and suturing. The time period permits more microorganisms to penetrate the wound; therefore there will be a greater inflammatory reaction. More granulation tissue will be formed than with healing by primary intention but less than by secondary intention (Figure 22-2).

PROCESS OF WOUND HEALING

When there is injury to tissue, two major responses occur: the stress response and the inflammatory response (Figure 22-3). If microorganisms enter the wound, a third response, the immune response, occurs. The inflammatory response is the first phase of wound healing.

Wound healing progresses through three overlapping phases: inflammation, proliferation, and maturation. Regardless of the type of wound healing, the process is the same. The difference is in the length of time for each phase of healing and in the extent of granulation tissue formed.

Inflammation

In surgical wounds the first phase occurs from the time of incision through the fourth day. The focus of this phase is on hemostasis and phagocytosis. *Hemostasis* results from aggregation of platelets that plug bleeding vessels and form a clot to seal the wound.

The inflammatory response (see Chapter 8) is immediate and prepares the tissue so that healing can ensue. Plasma fills the wound, bringing required substances for healing. During the cellular exudation, leukocytes or white blood cells invade the injured area to ingest the bacteria and debris (phagocytosis). Neutrophils, the most common leukocytes, appear within 6 hours after wounding.

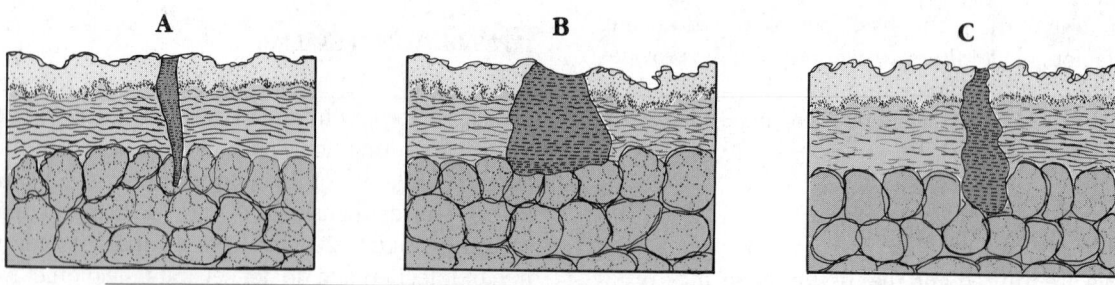

FIGURE 22-2 Types of wound healing. **A,** Primary. **B,** Secondary. **C,** Tertiary.

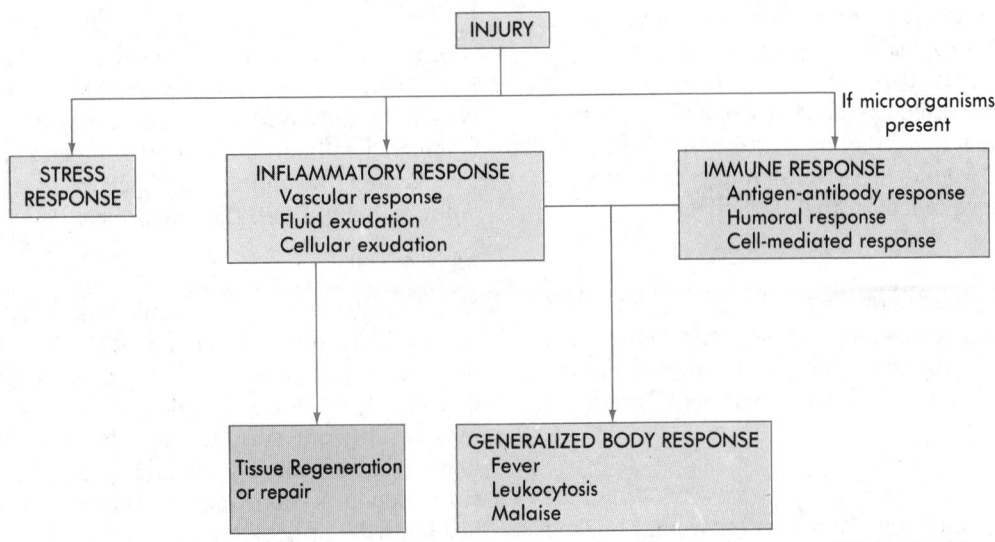

FIGURE 22-3 Response of the body to injury.

Proliferation

Proliferation begins on the second day, during the inflammatory phase, and continues to about the twenty-fourth day.[63] The major actions of the proliferative phase are epithelization, neovascularization, and collagen synthesis.[47]

Epithelization is the process of wound covering by epithelial (skin) cells; this begins on day two. The cells are formed at the margins of the wound and slide leapfrog fashion over each other across the top of the clot or wound plug. The epithelial cells secrete a fibrinolytic enzyme that permits advancement of the cells over the wound. Within 48 hours there is a thin layer of epithelial cells closing the wound to the external environment.

Neovascularization is the formation of new capillaries across the wound. It begins on day two and is completed by day seven. Fibroblasts migrate from blood vessels and deposit fibrin, a threadlike substance that stretches across the wound. Capillaries adjacent to the wound begin to develop buds similar to those of plants. The buds grow across the wound, using the fibrin threads for support. When the capillary branches reach other capillary branches, they cannulize, opening up blood flow across the wound. The new capillaries bring oxygen and nutrients that are necessary for tissue healing; capillaries give the pink color to the wound margins.

Collagen synthesis is the production by fibroblasts of collagen, a white protein fiber. Collagen is first laid down as precollagen material starting on day two, and the tensile strength of the new tissue increases as the collagen continues to be deposited. Collagen synthesis peaks during days five to seven, although it is deposited for up to 1 year.[63] The collagen fibers are initially laid down in a crisscross fashion, but as the fibers aggregate and become thicker and stronger, more orderly layers are produced to form scar tissue.

The various layers of epithelial tissue are regenerated in about 1 week. Since the grayish epithelial layer is thin, it does not alter the color of the underlying new tissue. This new tissue, called *granulation* tissue, is a highly vascular connective tissue that is reddish in color from the numerous blood vessels. If scraped, this tissue will bleed readily. During this period the patient begins to look and feel better.

Maturation

The final phase of wound healing starts with the fourth week and may last for up to 2 years. During this period new collagen fibers are modeled along lines of mechanical tension while other fibers are broken down and removed.[63] The new collagen compresses the newly formed blood vessels, and blood flow across the wound decreases and finally ceases.

During the early part of this period the wound looks like a broad, pinkish, raised scar; heavy use of the affected muscles should be avoided before the sixth week. Although collagen continues to be deposited after the sixth week, there is shrinkage and *contraction* of the wound. If the wound is near a joint, contractures may occur. Because of the shrinkage, the wound becomes a concave thin white line. The scar tissue is acellular, avascular collagen tissue. It will not tan with exposure to sunlight, nor will it sweat or produce hair.

FACTORS INFLUENCING WOUND HEALING

Some of the factors that affect patient responses to surgery (see Chapter 20) are directly related to wound healing. Research in wound healing is centered primarily on growth factors that may increase wound tensile strength more rapidly, thereby *enhancing* wound healing.[63] Major factors that can *delay* wound healing are age, nutrition, circulation, endocrine function, presence of foreign bodies, infection, dead space, and irradiation. Enzymatic activity in wounds is highest during the early stages of wound healing; therefore new wounds are more sensitive to factors that delay healing.

AGE

Wounds in children normally heal more rapidly than those in adults because of increased metabolism and good circulation. Wounds in the elderly often heal more slowly because of decreased fibroblastic activity and impaired circulation.

NUTRITION

One of the most important nutrients for wound healing is *vitamin C,* which is necessary to form collagen and to maintain the integrity of the capillary walls. Vitamin C may be depleted in the surgical patient because of inadequate dietary intake in the early postoperative period and because large amounts of vitamin C in the adrenal cortex are rapidly depleted under stress.[59]

Protein insufficiency will also delay wound healing since collagen is a protein. Other nutrients necessary for healing include vitamin A, vitamin B complex, zinc, magnesium, and copper. Vitamin A is important for epithelial growth.

CIRCULATION

Adequate circulation to the injured tissue is important to provide the white blood cells, fibroblasts, and nutrients needed for healing and to remove the debris after phagocytosis. Subcutaneous tissue is poorly supplied with blood vessels; therefore wounds of obese patients may heal more slowly. Persons with peripheral vascular disease have impaired circulation to the legs causing delayed healing of leg ulcers.

ENDOCRINE FUNCTION

Corticosteroids delay wound healing because of their antiinflammatory effect. They limit capillary budding, inhibit fibroblast proliferation, decrease the rate of epithelization, decrease the rate of collagen synthesis, and impair wound contraction. Persons with *diabetes mellitus* often have delayed healing because of decreased movement of leukocytes to the site and because of impaired circulation.

FOREIGN BODIES

Most foreign bodies are not sterile and create an excessive inflammatory reaction and infection when present in a wound. Foreign bodies are usually removed unless removing them will cause more damage than leaving them in the tissue.

INFECTION

A contaminated wound usually becomes infected. There is a greater inflammatory response as the white blood cells fight the invading microorganisms. A wound that is infected will not heal until the infection is eliminated. The greater the number of bacteria or amount of necrotic tissue present, the longer healing will be delayed.

DEAD SPACE

If fluid collects in a closed area where tissue has been removed, a space will occur where tissue healing does not take place. Cells above this dead space may break down in the absence of underlying support. Dead space may result from surgical procedures such as mastectomy, radical neck dissection, or arthroplasty. Low-pressure suction is often used to remove the fluid so that healing will not be delayed.

RADIATION

Large doses of radiation affect the fibroblasts' ability to divide, migrate, and produce collagen.[1] Direct irradiation of the wound after surgery may slow the development of blood vessels through the wound. Heavy irradiation may cause necrosis of the wound. If required after surgery, irradiation is usually postponed for at least 1 week to provide time for the fibroblastic activity to be established.[1]

CARE OF A SURGICAL WOUND
WOUND CLOSURE

Closure of the wound following surgery is achieved by sutures, wires, staples (Figure 22-4), metal clips, or tape. Closure of choice for the skin is tape (steri-strips) because of decreased probability of infection; sutures, staples, metal clips, and wires penetrate the skin, thus creating possible foci of infection. Tapes are ineffective if the wound is actively bleeding or if the surface is uneven. The time of removal for staples or silk sutures depends on the development of sufficient tensile strength to hold the wound edges together. Although this time varies among patients, depending on factors such as age and nutritional status, most skin sutures or staples are removed by 1 week to prevent suture marks. Sutures on the face and neck are often removed earlier because there is increased vascularization and less stress on the wound in these areas. Underlying tissues are closed with various types of absorbable or nonabsorbable sutures that are not removed.

TUBES AND DRAINS

Excess fluid accumulation interferes with oxygen delivery to cells, alters collagen organization, disrupts lymph flow, and creates a dead space, thus leading to delayed healing. If it is anticipated that fluid may collect in a body area near the wound postoperatively, the surgeon

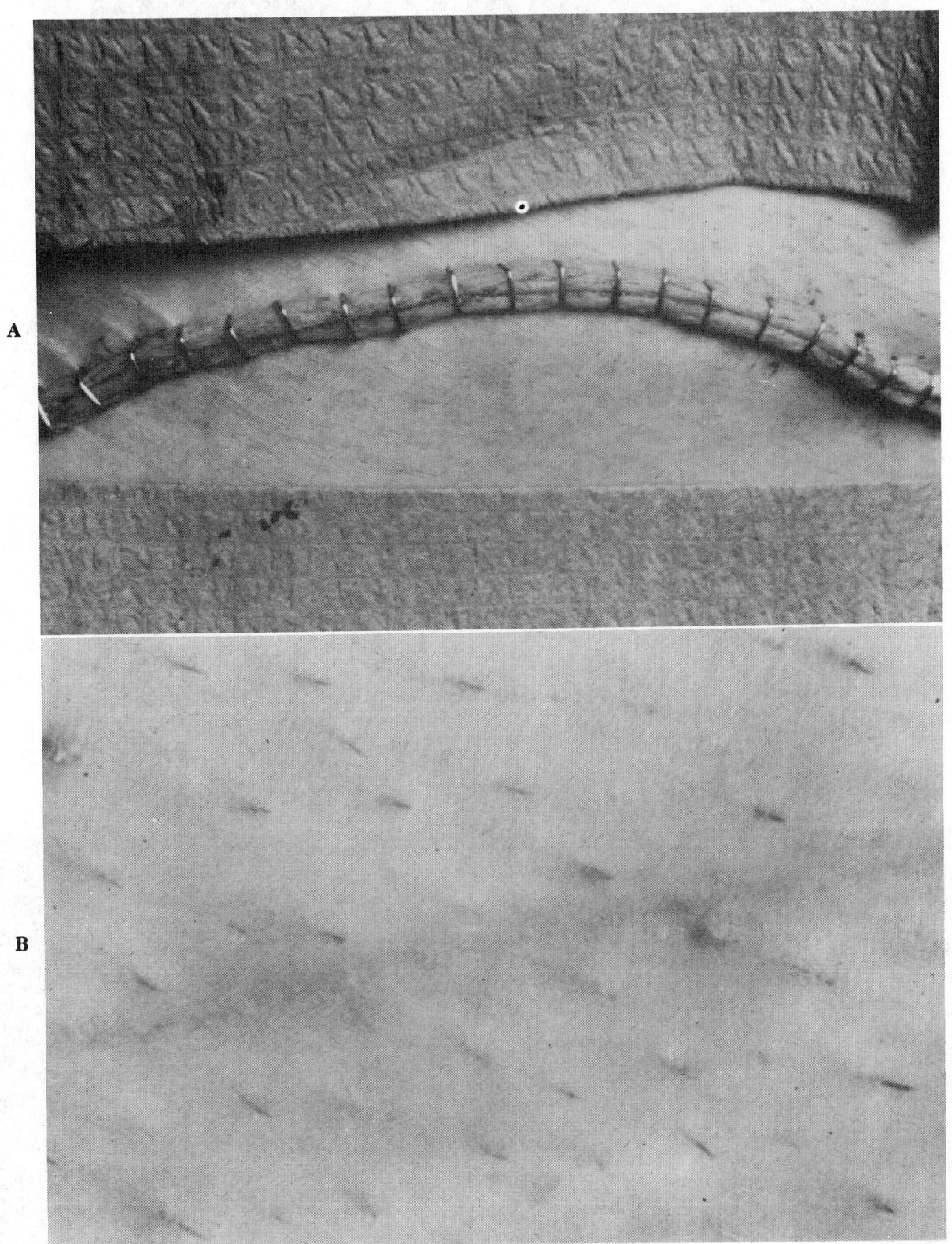

FIGURE 22-4 Skin staples used for wound closure. **A,** Immediately after surgery. Note staples grasping only superficial layer of skin. **B,** Same site 6 months later. (Courtesy Ethicon Inc, Somerville, NJ)

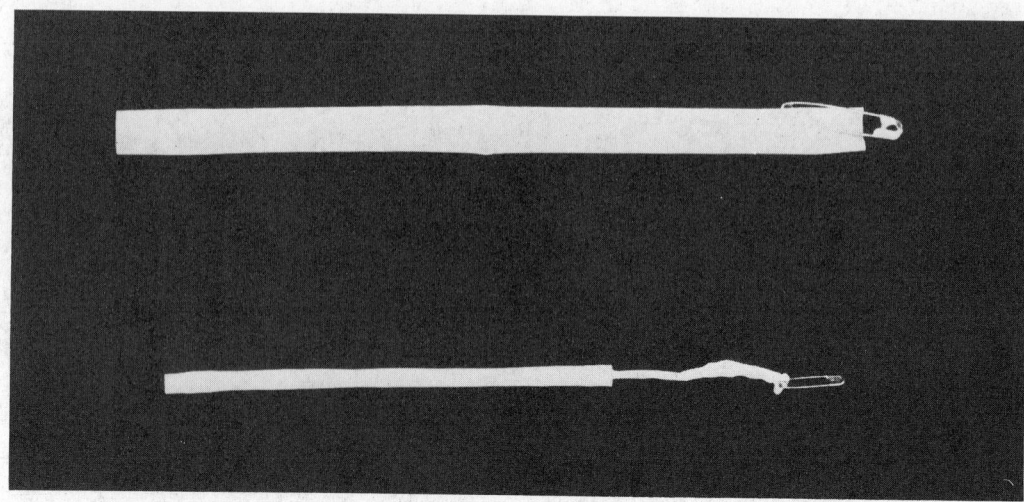

FIGURE 22-5 Wound drains. *Top,* Penrose drain. *Bottom,* Cigarette drain.

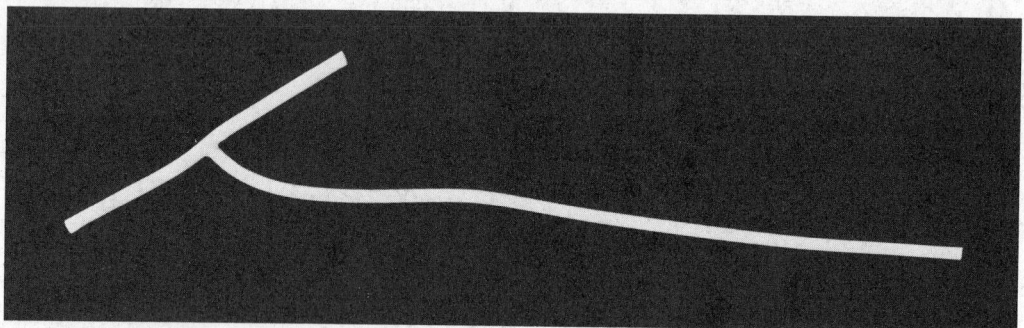

FIGURE 22-6 T tube for draining common bile duct.

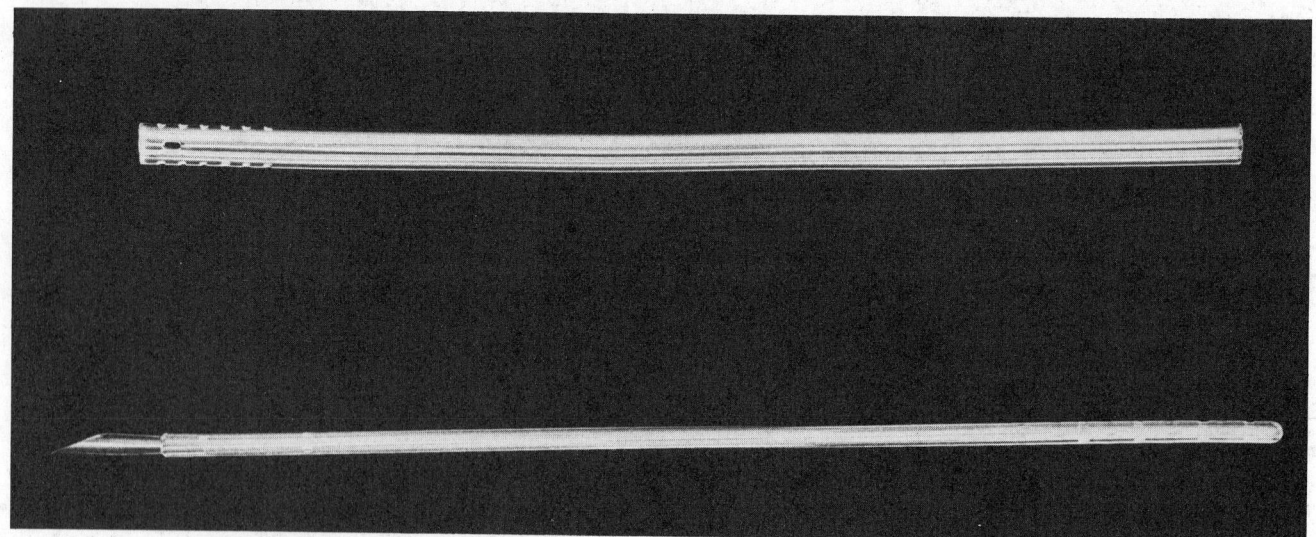

FIGURE 22-7 Surgical drain tubes. *Top,* Abramson all-purpose drain has three lumens: for aspiration, irrigation, and instillation. *Bottom,* Saratoga sump drain has a tube within a tube for low-pressure suction.

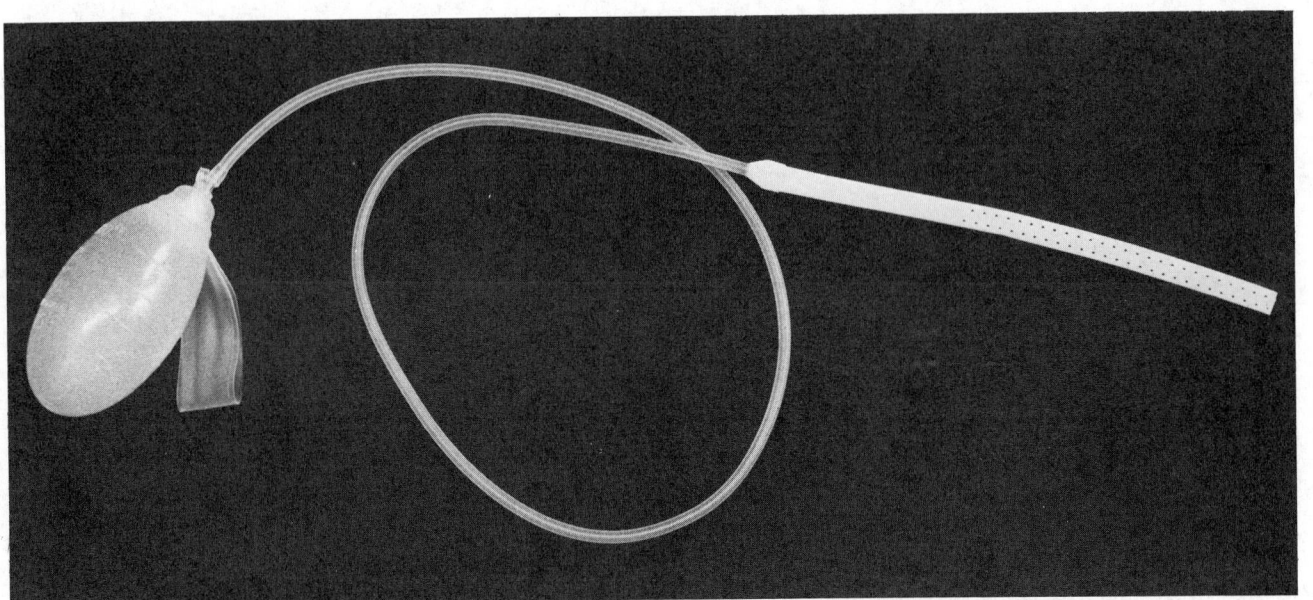

FIGURE 22-8 Jackson-Pratt wound suction apparatus. After emptying through spout, reservoir bulb is kept compressed until spout is closed. Slow expansion of bulb creates low-pressure suction.

usually inserts a tube or drain to permit the fluid to escape. One end of the tube or drain is placed in or near the organ or cavity to be drained and the other end is passed through the body wall, usually through a separate "stab wound."

Drains are made of soft rubber material, and the ends are left bound within the dressing. The two most commonly used drains are the *Penrose drain* and the *cigarette drain* (a gauze wick covered by a Penrose drain) (Figure 22-5). A safety pin is attached to the external end of the soft rubber drain to prevent the drain from sliding back into the cavity. The skin under the external end of the drain is protected by a double fold dressing. A drainage bag is placed over the wound to protect the skin if there is a large amount of drainage.

Tubes are usually inserted to prevent blockage of a passageway, such as the common bile duct (Figure 22-6), or when suction is desired (Figure 22-7). To help prevent infection, tubes with closed drainage systems are preferred to open drains when profuse drainage is expected. Tubes draining wound cavities are usually attached to a constant suction device to provide *negative* pressure. Suction creates a vacuum in the tissue and helps to hold the tissue layers together for healing. Suction draining devices include *manual* devices such as the Jackson Pratt (Figure 22-8), *spring* devices such as the hemodrain (Figure 22-9), and *portable* and *wall* vacuum control systems. Manual and spring devices provide between 60 mm Hg and 125 mm Hg of negative pressure,[17] but when the collection device fills, the suction decreases. The portable and wall vacuum sys-

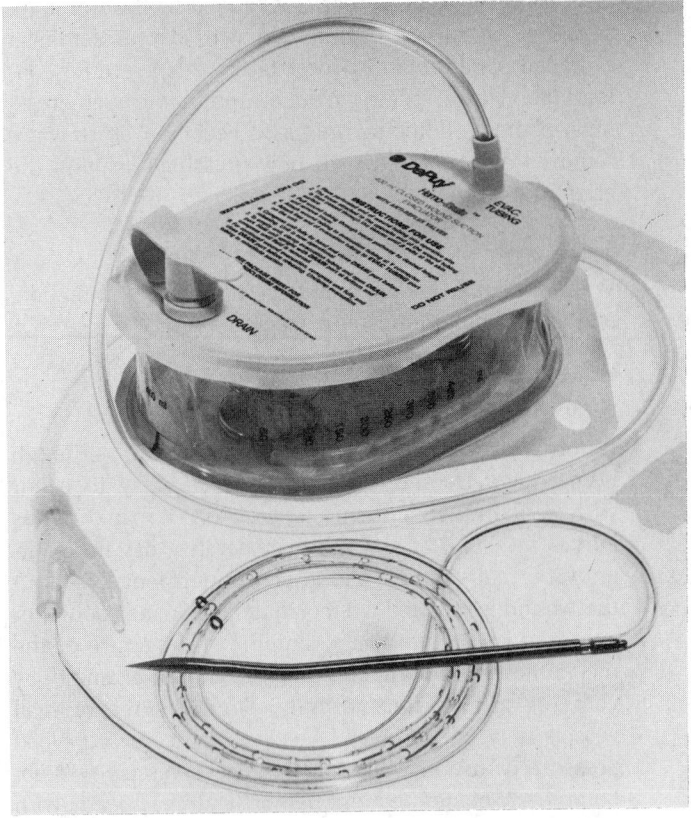

FIGURE 22-9 Hemodrain for low-suction wound drainage. Unit is compressed, then drain cap closed. Inner spring expands slowly creating suction through tube. (Courtesy De Puy Co, Warsaw, Inc)

tems provide 10 mm Hg to 360 mm Hg and are more precisely regulated.[17] The higher pressures are used when large amounts of fluid must be removed or when active adhesion formation between healing surfaces is desired.[17]

DRESSINGS

For psychologic reasons and to prevent trauma, the wound is usually covered in the operating room with a dry sterile dressing. After 72 hours, dressings provide little protection because of the epithelial covering of the incision. Staples closing an incision are usually covered to prevent the staples from catching on linens. Medicated sprays forming a transparent film on the skin may be used as a dressing over clean incisions. The film lasts 3 to 4 days; it may be removed with acetone or will flake and peel off eventually. Polyurethane dressings may also be used. Occasionally surgeons leave an operative wound uncovered, believing that healing progresses best when the wound is exposed to the air.

After most types of surgery, the surgeon usually changes the dressing for the first time. Many incisions do not need further dressings. If drainage is present, the dressing is changed as often as necessary to prevent injury to the underlying skin and to promote patient comfort. Dressings that cannot be changed by the nurse for specified reasons are reinforced with dry dressings if drainage penetrates the outer layer; this prevents contamination by capillary action through the wet dressings. If these additional dressings become wet, they are removed and replaced with new dressings, leaving the original dressing intact.

COMPLICATIONS OF WOUND HEALING

Wound complications include hemorrhage, infection, and wound dehiscence or evisceration.

HEMORRHAGE

Pathophysiology

External or internal hemorrhage may occur. Although hemorrhage from the wound is most likely to occur within the first 48 hours postoperatively, it may occur as late as the sixth or seventh postoperative day in apparently normal wounds and after a much longer time if the wound is infected. Hemorrhage occurring soon after surgery may be due to the slipping of a ligature or the mechanical dislodging of a clot, caused, for example, by vomiting after a tonsillectomy. During surgery small vessels may go unnoticed because of decreased blood pressure or use of a tourniquet. These vessels will not be properly obliterated and hemorrhage may occur with the reestablishment of blood flow. Hemorrhage after a few days may be caused by sloughing of a clot or of tissue, to infection, or to erosion of a blood vessel by a drainage tube.

Assessment

Dressings are checked at frequent intervals during the first 48 hours and at least once every 8 hours thereafter. Subjectively, the patient may complain of a wet sensation on the skin or dressing or of feeling restless or weak. Any postoperative patient who complains of an uneasy, restless feeling, such as "Something is wrong, but I don't know what," should be checked for signs of hemorrhage.

Objective data include signs of shock (tachycardia, weak thready pulse, cold clammy skin, fall in blood pressure or central venous pressure or decreased urinary output). Bright red blood may be present on the dressing or coming from a drainage tube.

Intervention

The physician is notified of any signs of increased bleeding or shock. A small amount of bleeding on the dressing is outlined with a pen and rechecked at 10- to 15-minute intervals for signs of change. If there is bleeding from a tube into a container, the drainage is marked with the time and the amount so that the rapidity of bleeding can be determined at frequent intervals. If the bleeding is profuse, measures to control bleeding are instituted if possible; for example, a pressure dressing is applied over the existing dressing and measures to treat shock are started immediately (see Chapter 25). Constant monitoring of vital signs is important. A calm environment is necessary so that increased anxiety does not add further stress to the patient's system.

The patient who is bleeding internally or in profuse amounts externally is usually returned immediately to surgery where the incision is opened and the bleeding vessel is ligated. If a preanesthetic medication is ordered, the time when the last narcotic was given should be checked. Under pressure of the emergency there is danger of the patient receiving an overdose of narcotics. It should also be remembered that during shock peripheral circulation is decreased, resulting in poor absorption of medication from the tissue. Respiratory depression can occur when the shock is corrected and narcotics in the tissue from previous injections are rapidly absorbed.

INFECTION

Pathophysiology

Wound infection is a major cause of nosocomial infections. The incidence ranges from 1.5% in clean wounds to as high as 17% in contaminated wounds; the average is about 7%.[1] *Staphylococcus* and *Streptococcus* (Table 22-1) have been the more frequent causes of infection but Gram-negative organisms, such as *Pseudomonas* and *E. coli,* have become more frequent. Anaerobic rods, such as *Clostridia* or *Bacteroides* may also be the cause of wound infections.

TABLE 22-1 Characteristic signs of postoperative wound infections[1]

Organisms	Cardinal Signs of Inflammation	Other Signs	Discharge
Staphylococcus aureus	Usually present, but may be absent	May occur at a later date Seen after "clean" surgery or with trauma	Pus formation Odorless
Streptococcus	Yes	Blisters may be present	Thin, watery discharge Odorless
Clostridia	Usually not red or painful	Wound is boggy Seen mostly with colon or biliary tract surgery or with trauma	Brownish discharge Odor: sweet
Anaerobic	Minimal	Tissue may look necrotic Seen with GI surgery	Pus formation Odor: foul

Whether a wound becomes infected depends on factors intrinsic to the patient, factors that can delay healing, and the aseptic technique utilized by health personnel (physician, nurse). Whenever there is an open or draining wound, aseptic technique must be scrupulously followed. Infection control teams in hospitals are responsible for monitoring the incidence of wound infections (see Chapter 15).

Assessment

The patient may complain of persistent pain in the incisional area and a feeling of general malaise. Pain is caused by stimulation of the nerve endings from the increased inflammation and by pressure from edema. The malaise is a systemic reaction to infection.

Objective signs include fever after the third postoperative day, increased white blood cell count (leukocytosis), incisional swelling, and erythema. There may be purulent drainage on the dressing. Wound culture and sensitivity studies should be obtained from the infected wound to determine the causative organism.

Intervention

Some surgeries, such as total hip replacement or vascular grafts, may be severely compromised if an infection does occur. In these situations antimicrobial prophylaxis may be instituted *preoperatively* to achieve adequate antibiotic levels before contamination occurs. The antimicrobial therapy is terminated either during surgery or within the first 24 hours after surgery to lessen the possibility of resistant bacterial strains. Commonly used antimicrobials are the cephalosporins, the semisynthetic penicillins, erythromycin, and clindamycin.

Prevention of wound infection is an important nursing measure. Carry out all open wound dressing changes under sterile conditions. Use sterile gloves or instruments when cleaning an open wound and applying the sterile dressings. Change soiled wet dressings immediately to prevent tissue breakdown from maceration and infection. Cover sterile moist dressings with a dry sterile cover.

If a wound infection does occur, the physician may open the wound to facilitate drainage if spontaneous drainage has not already taken place. Wound discomfort usually disappears after the wound has drained. A small drain may be placed in the wound to facilitate drainage, and irrigations may be ordered to wash away debris of infection. Purulent drainage is cleansed from the skin since pus contains proteolytic enzymes that can cause skin breakdown. The pus is sent to the laboratory for culture and sensitivity studies before antibiotics are given to control the infection. To maintain adequate blood levels the antibiotics must be given at the scheduled times.

WOUND DEHISCENCE AND EVISCERATION

Pathophysiology

Wound disruption (dehiscence) is a partial to complete separation of the wound edges. Wound evisceration is protrusion of abdominal viscera through the incision and onto the abdominal wall (Figure 22-10).

Wound separation that occurs during the first 3 days is usually related to technical factors such as the suturing. From the third to the fourteenth day, dehiscence is usually associated with postoperative complications such as distention, vomiting, excessive coughing, dehydration, or infection. Many of these complications can be prevented by careful assessment and continued monitoring and by the institution of vigorous preventive measures (ventilatory exercises, ambulation, adequate fluid intake, aseptic technique) on the part of the nurse. Wound separation after 2 weeks is usually associated with metabolic factors such as cachexia, hypoproteinemia or avitaminosis, increased age, decreased resistance

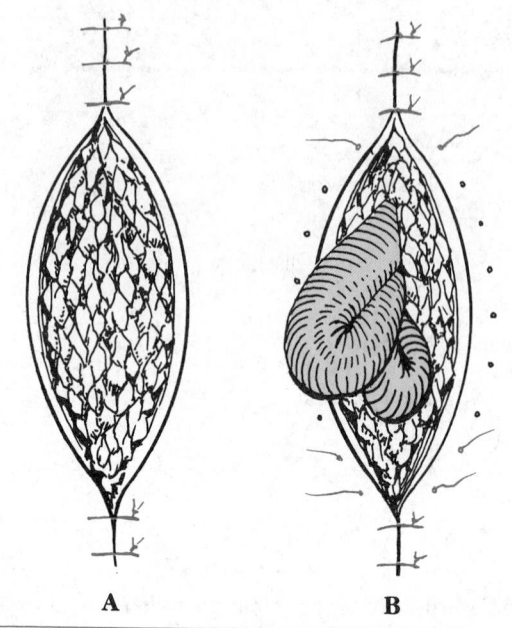

FIGURE 22-10 A, Wound dehiscence. **B,** Wound evisceration.

to infection, malignancy, multiple trauma, or hypothermia. These factors can also cause wound separation at an earlier time.

Assessment

Subjectively, the patient may complain of a "giving" sensation at the incision or a feeling of wetness. If evisceration has occurred and if a loop of bowel has obstructed, the patient will complain of severe localized pain at the incision. The dressing will be saturated with clear pink drainage. The wound edges may be partially or entirely separated, and loops of intestine may be lying on the abdominal wall. Signs of shock may be present.

Intervention

A patient who experiences either a wound dehiscence or wound evisceration is put to bed in low Fowler's position and told to remain quiet, not to cough, and not to eat or drink anything until the surgeon arrives. Protruding viscera are covered, preferably with a warm, sterile saline dressing. Interventions for shock are initiated if signs of shock are present. The surgeon will cover the wound after inspection.

The treatment for wound dehiscence and wound evisceration is immediate closure of the wound under local or general anesthesia. If the patient is in shock, the preanesthetic medication may be omitted. Convalescence is generally prolonged, although the wound usually heals surprisingly well after secondary closure.

POSTANESTHETIC PHASE

It is the practice in most hospitals that any patient who has received general, dissociative, or regional anesthesia is taken to a postanesthesia recovery room after surgery where continuous attention can be given for a period of time. In some instances the patient who has had local anesthesia but who requires close observation in the immediate postoperative period may also be cared for in the recovery room. In such an area, specially prepared nursing personnel and all the equipment that may be necessary for the care of the patient in the postanesthetic phase are readily available. Ideally, the recovery room is located in the immediate vicinity of the operating rooms.

▪ ASSESSMENT

The patient is accompanied to the recovery room or to the clinical unit by the anesthesiologist and another member of the operating room professional staff. While the anesthesiologist remains at the bedside, the nurse begins assessment of the patient by obtaining *vital signs*. *Level of consciousness*, ability to follow commands, and adequacy of *ventilatory* and *circulatory* functions are also rapidly assessed. The patient is usually asleep or responding to oral commands. Within an hour, most patients are oriented but fall asleep readily, although they will respond to oral or tactile stimulation.

The nurse receives a report on the patient's condition from members of the operating room team before assuming responsibility for patient care (see box on p. 503). A quick review is made of the pertinent preoperative summary, obtained preoperatively by unit nurses or nurses from the operating room or recovery room staffs (see Chapter 20).

Following the report, the nurse completes the overall patient assessment:

1. Temperature
2. Inspection of surgical site dressings for drainage or frank bleeding
3. Patency of tubes and catheters (including IV fluids)
4. Connection of drainage tubes to containers; character of drainage
5. Ability to move extremities and recognize touch of areas anesthetized by regional anesthesia
6. Assessments specific to surgical procedures performed

The physician's order sheet is then checked for other instructions and orders for treatments and medications.

RECORDING

A complete and accurate recording during the immediate postanesthetic course is essential so that those who continue management of the patient have a reference

DATA TO BE OBTAINED WHEN PATIENT IS ADMITTED TO THE RECOVERY ROOM

1. Current medical diagnosis
2. Surgical procedure performed
   a. What; why
3. Agents administered
   a. Anesthetic
   b. Narcotic
   c. Muscle relaxant
   d. Muscle relaxant reversal agent
   e. Antibiotic
   f. Other (e.g., digitalis preparation, diuretic)
4. Complications during surgery
   a. Type
   b. Treatment instituted
5. Fluids
   a. Estimated blood loss (EBL)
   b. Blood and fluid administered
6. Pertinent preoperative problems
   a. Physical
   b. Psychologic

for comparison of patient data. The recording starts with a summary of the patient's status when admitted from the operating room; this provides a baseline assessment. Thereafter, notations are made concerning changes in the patient's status as determined by frequent reassessments. All medications, fluids, and treatments received by the patient are also recorded.

■ DATA ANALYSIS: NURSING DIAGNOSES

Nursing diagnoses are determined from assessment of patient data. Possible diagnoses for the postanesthesia patient may include, but are not limited to, the following:

Diagnostic Title	Possible Etiologies
Anxiety	Pain, strange environment, possible results/effects of surgery
Airway clearance, ineffective	Secretions from anesthesia, tongue blocking airway, improper positioning
Aspiration, potential for	Decreased consciousness
Cardiac output, decreased	Hypotension
Fluid volume excess	Excess intravenous fluids
Gas exchange, impaired	Drugs, incisional pain, constrictive dressings
Injury, potential for	Sensorimotor deficits
Pain	Surgical incision

■ PLANNING: EXPECTED PATIENT OUTCOMES

Expected patient outcomes for the postanesthesia patient may include, but are not limited to, the following:
   1. The patient is sleepy and is not restless or showing signs of anxiety.
   2. Breathing is quiet and regular at preoperative rate.

3. Pulse is at preoperative rate and regularity; blood pressure returns to preoperative level.
4. The patient shows no signs of fluid overload (rapid moist breathing, mental confusion).
5. No injury results from improper positioning or other environmental factors.
6. No signs of severe pain are present (facial grimacing, crying and holding the painful area, diaphoresis).

■ IMPLEMENTATION
MAINTAINING AERATION

The goal of respiratory care for the postanesthetic patient is to maintain pulmonary ventilation that is adequate to prevent hypoxemia (a deficiency of oxygen in the blood) and hypercapnia (an excess of carbon dioxide in the blood). In the immediate postanesthetic period, two of the most common causes of inadequate pulmonary exchange are airway obstruction (ineffective airway clearance) and hypoventilation (impaired gas exchange).

Airway Patency

Airway obstruction most frequently occurs as a result of the tongue, which is relaxed from anesthesia, falling back against the pharynx (Figure 22-11) or as a result of secretions or other fluids collecting in the pharynx, trachea, or bronchial tree. All noisy breathing (for example, snoring, gurgling, wheezing, crowing) is indicative of some type of airway obstruction. Obstruction can occur, however, without being accompanied by noise.

Artificial airway. The patient usually arrives in the recovery room with an airway in place, either pharyngeal (mouth or nose to pharynx) or endotracheal (mouth or nose to just above the bifurcation of the trachea). The *pharyngeal* airway (Figure 22-12) is most commonly used. It keeps the air passage open and the tongue forward until pharyngeal reflexes have returned. Pharyngeal airways may be made of rubber, plastic, or metal. They are removed as soon as the patient begins to awake and has regained cough and swallowing reflexes. After this time their presence can be irritating and can stimulate vomiting or laryngospasm.

The *endotracheal* airway not only prevents the tongue from falling back but also prevents airway obstruction resulting from laryngospasm. The endotracheal tube is removed when the patient is awake and able to maintain the airway, as evidenced by the patient's ability to raise the head and grip a hand and by normal blood gas levels.[39]

If the artificial airway is ineffective (or if one is not in place), the majority of obstructions due to the tongue falling back can be alleviated by holding the patient's jaw up and forward or by the side-lying position. When

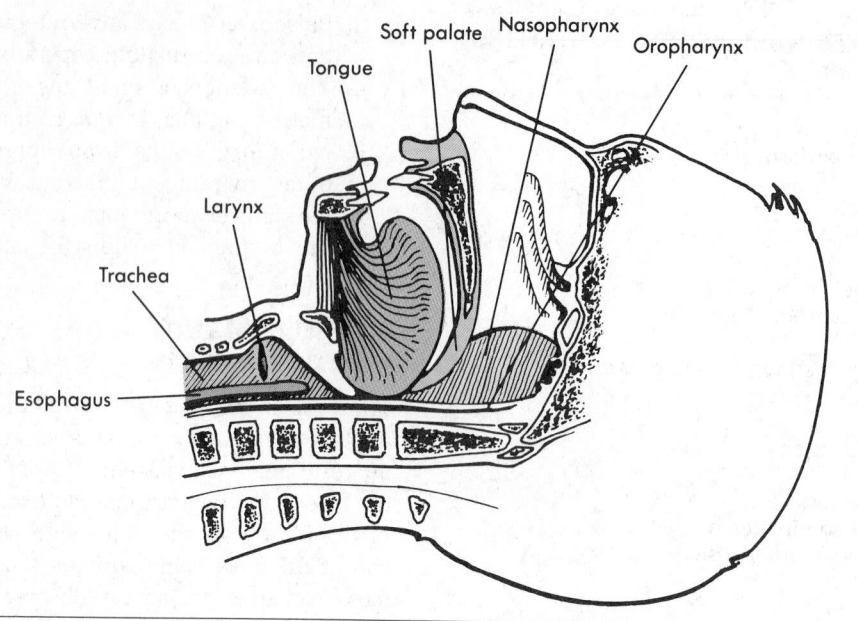

FIGURE 22-11 Obstruction of airway by tongue blocking oropharynx in unconscious person lying in supine position.

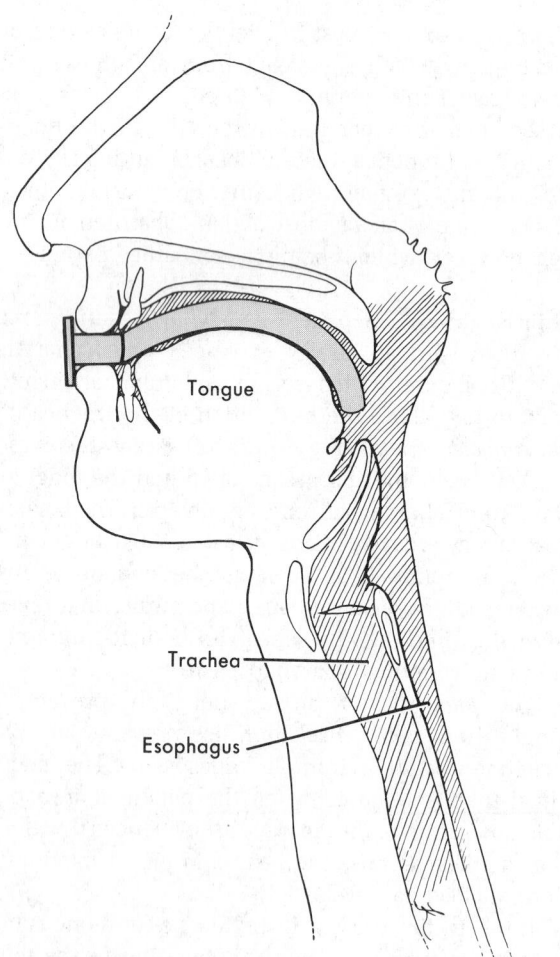

FIGURE 22-12 Pharyngeal airway in place to prevent tongue from blocking oropharynx.

absolutely necessary to clear the airway, the nurse can open the patient's mouth by pushing at the angle of the jaw with the thumbs and have someone insert a padded tongue depressor between the back teeth. The tongue can then be brought forward by grasping it with a piece of gauze.

Positioning. The most desirable position to ensure maintenance of a patent airway depends on the size and condition of the patient, the anesthesia used, the surgery performed, and the amount of experienced nursing care available. Ideally, the patient should be in a position to breathe normally with full use of all portions of the lungs and so that vomitus, blood, and mucus can drain out and will not be aspirated.

Until protective reflexes have returned, the best position for the majority of patients is a *side-lying* or *semi-prone* position with the head tilted back and the jaw supported forward. Aspiration can occur unless the *whole body* is turned. Turning the patient's head when the chest and shoulders remain in the back-lying position is useless. The disadvantage related to diminished chest expansion in the side-lying position can be minimized by turning the patient frequently and by raising the flexed upper arm and placing it on a pillow.

The supine position with head hyperextended permits fullest expansion of the lungs, but it is dangerous because of its potential for aspiration or obstruction from secretions. If the supine position must be used before pharyngeal reflexes have returned and the patient can manage secretions, suctioning equipment must be

CAUSES OF POSTANESTHETIC HYPOVENTILATION

1. Drugs given preoperatively, intraoperatively, or postoperatively
   a. Anesthetic agents (inhalation, IV)
   b. Muscle relaxants
   c. High spinal or epidural anesthesia
   d. Narcotics
   e. Tranquilizers
   f. Sedatives
2. Incisional pain
3. Obesity
4. Chronic lung disease
5. Gastric dilation
6. Constrictive thoracic or abdominal dressings

available at the bedside and the patient should be monitored frequently.

Removal of secretions. Excessive secretions from the nasopharynx or tracheobronchial mucosa can also lead to partial or complete airway obstruction. Unless the patient can manage these secretions by coughing them up and expectorating them, they must be removed by suctioning. Pharyngeal suctioning is often all that must be done. If intratracheal suctioning is necessary, the patient should be hyperventilated with 100% oxygen before and after each introduction of the catheter into the trachea. When thick secretions are a problem, the humidity of the air breathed is increased to keep secretions as thin as possible and to prevent dry air from further irritating the respiratory passages.

Promoting Gas Exchange

Postoperative hypoventilation results from respiratory depression or from interferences with chest expansion (see box above). Ventilation is promoted in the postanesthetic phase by oxygen therapy, breathing exercises, and other therapies.

Oxygen therapy. Oxygen is usually given postoperatively because after anesthesia almost all patients have decreased pulmonary expansion and areas of atelectasis (p. 513), both of which result in hypoxemia. Oxygen is administered by nasal prongs, disposable face mask, or endotracheal or tracheostomy tube if one is in place.

How long postoperative oxygen therapy should be continued depends on the individual patient. As a general rule, all patients should receive oxygen at least until they are conscious and able to take deep breaths on command. Prolonged oxygen therapy should be guided by arterial blood gas determinations. Patients with thoracic or upper abdominal incisions or with preexisting pulmonary disease may be given oxygen for several hours, perhaps until the next day. Special care must be

taken when administering oxygen to patients with chronic obstructive pulmonary disease so that hypoxemia, which is their stimulus to breathe, is not entirely removed (see Chapter 33). Any patient experiencing shivering, which increases oxygen consumption, should receive oxygen therapy until the shivering ceases.

Breathing exercises. To help maintain normal levels of arterial blood gases and to counteract hypoventilation, all patients need to be encouraged to breathe deeply at frequent intervals (see Chapter 20). Ideally, during the postanesthetic phase, the patient will take 3 or 4 deep inhalations every 10 to 15 minutes. If the patient is unconscious or will not breathe deeply when stimulated, the lungs can be hyperventilated passively with a breathing bag and mask.

Other therapies. Additional therapies to promote ventilation may include the following:
1. Respiratory assistance if hypercapnia is present
2. Drug therapy
   a. Narcotic antagonists (nalorphine, naloxone, levallorphan) to counteract respiratory depression from opiates
   b. Reversal agents (such as neostigmine, edrophonium) to counteract effects of nondepolarizing muscle relaxants
   c. Narcotics if pain is causing patient to splint respirations
3. Elevation of head of bed with obese patient, to relieve pressure on diaphragm
4. Nasogastric tubes to relieve gastric distention
5. Loosening of constricting dressings
6. Intubation and mechanical ventilator assistance if treatment is ineffective to relieve hypoventilation

MAINTAINING CIRCULATION

Hypotension and cardiac arrhythmias are the most commonly encountered cardiovascular complications of the immediate postanesthetic period. Early recognition and management of these complications before they become serious enough to diminish cardiac output depends on frequent assessment of the patient's vital signs.

The routine for taking blood pressure, pulse, and respirations varies. One of two approaches is commonly used:
Method 1:
1. Every 15 minutes while patient is in recovery room
2. Every 15 minutes for 1 hour after return to clinical unit, then
3. Every 4 hours until otherwise indicated
Method 2:
1. Every 15 minutes until signs are stable, then
2. Every 30 minutes for 2 hours, then
3. Every 4 hours until otherwise indicated

POSSIBLE CAUSES OF POSTOPERATIVE HYPOTENSION

1. Moving patient from operating room table to bed
2. Jarring of patient's bed during transport
3. Drugs, anesthesia
4. Loss of blood and other body fluids
5. Cardiac arrhythmias
6. Cardiac failure
7. Inadequate ventilation
8. Pain
9. Residual sympathectomy from conductive anesthesia

The rate, volume, and rhythm of the pulse are carefully observed.

Hypotension

A number of factors in the early postoperative period cause circulatory changes that may result in lowering the blood pressure (see box above). A mild decrease in blood pressure from the normal preoperative range is not uncommon during the early postoperative period. It is usually well tolerated in healthy patients and does not require treatment.

Shock, however, must be prevented because the brain, heart, kidneys, and other vital organs do not tolerate long periods of hypoxemia. A weak, thready pulse with a significant drop in blood pressure may indicate hemorrhage or circulatory failure. The surgeon, anesthesiologist, or both are notified at once if any of these signs occur, especially if the skin becomes cold, moist, pale, or cyanotic, or if the patient suddenly becomes restless or apprehensive. Oxygen therapy is started to increase the oxygen saturation of the circulating blood. Other therapies to treat shock (see Chapter 25) are also initiated.

Cardiac Arrhythmias

When a cardiac arrhythmia is detected, it is important to ascertain if the patient has a history of such a disturbance. Arrhythmias unchanged from those that existed preoperatively usually do not require treatment. When there is no history of a cardiac irregularity but one has developed postoperatively, the patient is assessed to determine if ventilation is adequate. Oxygen is started while the physician is being notified. A patient who is exchanging gases poorly should receive ventilatory assistance with a bag and mask.

Hypoxemia and hypercapnia are common causes of postoperative cardiac arrhythmias, especially premature beats and sinus tachycardia. These arrhythmias often can be suppressed by adequate ventilation. Frequent premature beats of ventricular origin that are not decreased by oxygen therapy are usually treated with drugs such as intravenous lidocaine (Xylocaine) or procainamide (Pronestyl). The sinus bradycardia that may follow the administration of neostigmine (Prostigmine) or edrophonium (Tensilon) is countered by the administration of atropine. Other common causes of postoperative cardiac arrhythmias include pain, hypovolemia, gastric distention, and acidosis. In the event of a life-threatening arrhythmia, such as ventricular fibrillation or cardiac asystole, resuscitation efforts are started immediately.

MAINTAINING FLUID AND ELECTROLYTE BALANCE

Most patients admitted to the recovery room will receive intravenous fluids to maintain fluid and electrolyte balance. The exact amount and type of fluid administered depends on the surgical procedure as well as the patient's preoperative status, intraoperative course, and individual response to stress. Careful monitoring of the patient's intravenous fluid administration is essential to ensure adequacy of replacement and prevention of fluid overload (p. 518).

PREVENTING INJURY

Stupor and muscle weakness are major nervous system complications that may occur in the postanesthesia period. Failure to awaken promptly or completely is usually the result of a residual effect of the anesthetic. Maintenance of pulmonary and circulatory function helps to eliminate most residual agents. Other causes of stupor include severe hypoxia, hypothermia, metabolic imbalances, hyponatremia, hyperglycemia, and severe hypercapnia.

Muscle weakness usually results from prolonged effects of muscle relaxants. Renal failure and electrolyte imbalances may delay recovery from muscle relaxants.

Following anesthesia, side rails on the stretcher or bed are generally raised until the patient is fully awake. The patient is turned frequently and placed in good body alignment to prevent nerve damage from pressure and to prevent muscle and joint strain caused by lying in one position for a long time. Unconscious patients and those recovering from spinal or epidural anesthesia have loss of sensation and are unable to indicate discomfort. Heating pads, heat lamps, or cast driers must be used with great care to prevent burns in these cases.

PROMOTING COMFORT

Incisional pain is probably the most significant postoperative problem from the patient's point of view. In the immediate postanesthetic period, narcotic analgesics are given for pain when warranted, with the realization that pronounced depression of the respiratory, circulatory, or central nervous systems may follow. Because the patient generally has not completely recovered from the effects of anesthesia, the first postoperative dose of a narcotic is usually reduced to about one half the dose to be received after full recovery from anesthesia. Pain medication for restlessness is given only after it has been determined that the restlessness is not a result of hypoxia.

Analgesics may be given intramuscularly or intravenously. The intramuscular route may be used for patients with stable circulatory functions. If circulation is decreased, as with shock, medication given intramuscularly may remain in the tissue and then be absorbed suddenly when circulation is restored, leading to overdosage. The intravenous route is safer and faster and is often preferred. Morphine sulfate and meperidine are the more commonly used narcotics. If electrodes for a transcutaneous electrical nerve stimulator (TENS) for relief of pain (p. 520) have been placed after surgery, the TENS may be initiated in the recovery room in conjunction with analgesics.

RELIEF OF ANXIETY

The immediate postanesthetic period is often a frightening time for the patient. Psychologic support is imperative for physical and emotional well-being. While awakening from anesthesia, the patient needs frequent orientation to place and reassurance of not being alone. The patient also needs to know that the operation is over and that recovery from anesthesia is satisfactory. Careful explanations of procedures being carried out are given even when it appears that the patient is not alert. The need for privacy should be considered at all times. Patients who receive this type of support frequently recover from anesthesia faster, with fewer complications, and with less incisional pain. The patient who has had regional anesthesia needs the same information and needs to be reassured that the sensation and movement in the extremities will return.

It is also important that the patient's routine hygiene needs are not overlooked. The skin is inspected; excess tape, electrode paste, and skin preparations are removed; and soiled areas are washed. Mouth care should be provided. Meeting these hygiene needs enhances the patient's comfort and assists in maintenance of dignity as a human being.

DISCHARGE FROM RECOVERY ROOM

Multiple criteria are used to determine when a patient has sufficiently recovered from anesthesia to be transferred from the recovery room. Some recovery rooms use discharge criteria scoring systems. In general, the following outcomes are expected:

1. Vital signs are stable and indicate adequate respiratory and circulatory function.
2. The person is awake or easily aroused and can call for assistance if needed.
3. Postsurgical complications have been thoroughly evaluated and are under control.
4. The person who has had regional anesthesia has motor as well as partial sensory return to all anesthetized areas.

Complications that must be under control include excessive wound drainage, vomiting, fever, pain, or inadequate urinary output as well as complications specific to the type of surgery performed. Acutely ill patients who cannot adequately fulfill these criteria are usually transferred to an intensive care unit. All pertinent information concerning the patient's status must be communicated to the nurse who will be continuing to provide postoperative nursing care.

RETURN OF PATIENT TO CLINICAL UNIT
EQUIPMENT

Before the patient returns to the clinical unit from the postanesthesia recovery room, the patient's room is prepared to facilitate meeting the patient's needs in the immediate postoperative period. The bed is made so that the patient can be moved easily from stretcher to bed. The bed should have added protection in areas where drainage may be expected to occur and sufficient covers to ensure patient warmth.

The patient's room is cleared of any unnecessary equipment and a clear passageway is provided for approach to the bed by the stretcher. Equipment that will be needed is placed in readiness. This equipment will depend on the type of surgery and might include such items as an intravenous pole, emesis basin, tissues, and sphygmomanometer. The recovery room nurse alerts the unit staff of any specialized equipment such as for suction or oxygen that may be needed.

FAMILY

The family is kept informed of the patient's progress in the recovery room, particularly when the patient's return to the unit has been delayed. Information that can be shared with the patient's family helps to lessen their anxiety.

Most surgeons discuss the results of the operation with the family immediately after the surgery and also visit the patient, briefly telling what was found and providing reassurance. The family is frequently highly anxious concerning the patient's condition and may not perceive or understand all that the surgeon tells them. Patients frequently experience periods of amnesia during the hours when they first regain consciousness and may not remember what they have been told. The nurse needs to know what information was given the patient and family to be able to answer their questions. The family also needs to know what to expect when the patient returns to the unit.

DATA FROM PATIENT'S CHART

Selected data from the patient's chart will be particularly important to the nurse on the clinical division. The data are collected from the surgeon's orders, the surgeon's surgical notes, and the recovery room nurse's summary of care given.

Surgeon's Orders

Data from the surgeon's orders that are of importance for planning immediate postoperative care include the following:

1. *Activity:* The range of activity can be from strict bed rest to up as desired. The order should state clearly the extent of activity allowed.
2. *Fluids, food:* Orders for fluids to be given intravenously should include type, amount and rate. Orders for fluid or food to be taken orally should include type and time these can be started.
3. *Medications:* An order for pain medication should be included if pain is a possibility. Other medications that need to be reinstituted or started immediately are noted.
4. *Other orders:* These orders depend on the type of surgery and anesthesia. The nurse should understand the rationale for each order.

Surgical Notes

The surgeon writes a note on the progress sheet providing information about the surgery. Data of specific relevance for postoperative care include the following:

1. *Postoperative diagnosis:* Patient or family may need interpretation regarding what the surgeon has told them
2. *Type of surgery:* Patient or family may need interpretation; type of surgery may give direction to nursing care
3. *Anesthetic:* May give direction to nursing care
   a. Inhalants: need for active deep-breathing measures
   b. Muscle relaxants: assess for respiratory distress
   c. Spinal: supine position postoperatively; headaches may occur
4. *Estimated blood loss and fluid replacement:* Potential for fluid and electrolyte imbalance or delayed transfusion reactions
5. *Drains:* Drainage on the dressing can be expected with drains; tubes need to be connected to drainage receptacles

Recovery Room Summary

The summary notes written by the recovery room nurse provide baseline data for comparison of new data obtained by the division nurse. Data of specific importance include the following:

1. *Vital signs before discharge:* Changes in vital signs and baseline at discharge from recovery room
2. *Patient progress:* Problems that may persist during postoperative period
3. *Medications given:* Type, dosage, time given and response of patient

4. *Urinary output:* Amount and character of last voiding to be used for comparison during the first 24 hours

■ POSTOPERATIVE NURSING ASSESSMENT

The areas of nursing assessment and observations to be made during the early postoperative period are described in Table 22-2. Many of these assessments are initiated during the postanesthetic period. A complete assessment is done when the hospitalized patient returns to the clinical unit or during the patient's stay in an ambulatory surgical center.

PATIENT ASSESSMENT
SUBJECTIVE DATA

The patient's level of alertness can be quickly ascertained by asking the patient about symptoms of discomfort. An indirect question such as, "How do you feel?" will elicit data concerning nausea or pain without focusing on a specific area where there may be no discomfort. Frequently there is an increase in pain perception when the patient is transferred from the transportation cart to the bed. If pain is experienced, further data are collected concerning the nature and location. The assumption should not be made that the origin of the pain is incisional. General discomforts may be experienced from poor body positioning.

Postoperative nausea occurs less frequently with the use of newer anesthetics. There is greater possibility of nausea when the stomach has been manipulated extensively during the surgical procedure or if considerable amounts of narcotics have been administered.

OBJECTIVE DATA
Neurologic Status

Level of consciousness is determined by the patient's response to oral or tactile stimulation (see Chapter 60). Variations in consciousness level from alertness to drowsiness will be observed. If the patient is not easily aroused, the data is compared to the earlier status as documented in the records. A decrease in status may indicate shock and should be reported to the surgeon.

Following regional anesthesia, such as spinal or epidural, the legs are assessed for movement and sensation. Nerve injury is rare but may occur.

Respiratory Status

Respiratory assessment is particularly important in the early postoperative period because of the high incidence of postoperative atelectasis resulting from decreased ventilation of the alveoli (p. 513). Hypoventilation (Table 22-3) is characterized by rapid shallow respirations and absent or diminished breath sounds in the lower lobes. Depth of respiration is an important criterion be-

TABLE 22-2 Early postoperative patient assessment

Area of Assessment	Observations
Neurologic status	Level of consciousness
	Ability to follow commands
	Sensation and ability to move extremity following regional anesthesia
Respiratory status	Patency of airway
	Respirations: depth, rate, character
	Breath sounds: presence, character
	Chest expansion
	Patient position to facilitate ventilation
	Ability to deep breathe and cough
Circulatory status	Blood pressure, temperature
	Pulse: rate, strength (presence distal to limb surgery)
	Skin: color, temperature
	Capillary filling
Urinary status	Urine output >30 ml/hr
Comfort	Pain: presence, character, severity
	Nausea/vomiting
	Warmth
	Patient position of comfort
Safety	Necessity for side rails
	Call cord within reach
Mobility	Ability to turn self
	Ability to do leg exercises
Monitoring systems	Connected and functioning
Intravenous fluids	Rate, amount in bag, patency of tubing
Dressings	Drainage; frank bleeding
Drainage systems (e.g., nasogastric, chest, urinary)	Type, patency of tubes; connection to collection containers
	Character and amount of drainage

TABLE 22-3 Some causes of vital sign changes in early postoperative phase

Vital Sign	Increase	Decrease
Temperature	Stress reaction (low-grade fever)	Cold operating room and recovery room
Pulse rate	Jarring during transfer	Digitalis overdose
	Shock, hemorrhage	Cardiac arrhythmias
	Hypoventilation, hypoxemia	
	Acute gastric dilation	
	Fluid imbalances, acidosis	
	Pain	
	Anxiety	
	Cardiac arrhythmias	
Respiratory rate	Hypoventilation: poor positioning, tight chest or upper abdominal dressing, obesity, gastric dilation	Drugs: anesthetics, narcotics, sedatives
Blood pressure	Anxiety ($\uparrow$ systolic) Pain	Jarring during transfer
		Severe pain
		Cardiac arrhythmias
		Shock: fluid loss, hemorrhage, acute gastric dilation

cause the alveoli are poorly ventilated when respirations are shallow.

Pain, constrictive chest or abdominal dressings, obesity, or gastric dilation may result in decreased chest expansion leading to a decrease in vital capacity and thus inadequate ventilation. Chest expansion is observed during inspiration; if the chest is held fairly rigid, there will be decreased ventilation.

The lungs are auscultated to establish a baseline for future comparison and to identify adventitious sounds. Findings may include the following:

1. Absent breath sounds: hypoventilation of that lobe
2. Coarse rales: secretions in air passages.

The lungs should be free of rales but diminished breath sounds may be present during the first 24 hours after surgery.[59]

Respiratory distress is characterized by noisy respirations heard without the aid of a stethoscope, decreased depth of respirations, decreased breath sounds, use of accessory muscles for breathing, pallor or cyanosis, and restlessness. It is caused by the tongue (Figure 22-11) or secretions blocking the airway. Signs of respiratory distress are reported immediately and actions are taken to improve airway patency by side-lying position and hyperextension of the neck (p. 504) unless contraindicated.

Presence of a productive cough during the first few postoperative days is a positive sign that the patient is able to clear the bronchial secretions that might otherwise block the bronchioles. The productiveness of the cough usually decreases as secretions diminish.

Circulatory Status

Adequate circulation is important in the postoperative period to provide adequate oxygenation to all tissues, especially to the traumatized tissue for commencement of wound healing.

Pulse. The pulse is assessed for rate and quality. The pulse rate may be increased or decreased (Table 22-3). A rapid, weak, thready pulse may indicate bleeding. If this is a change from the baseline data, other signs of shock and bleeding are assessed and reported to the physician.

The presence and strength of peripheral pulses distal to an operative site or cast on an extremity are used to measure adequacy of circulation. If the pulse is weaker and the dressing is too tight, the dressing should be loosened, if this is permissible, or the condition should be reported at once to the physician.

Blood pressure. Blood pressure is monitored carefully in the early postoperative period (p. 505). Changes in blood pressure readings are more significant than consistent high or low readings. An increase in systolic pressure may be related to anxiety or pain. Hypotensive changes may be caused by shock, although other signs of shock usually appear before changes in blood pressure occur.

Temperature. A subnormal temperature in the early postoperative period may be related to the cool, air-conditioned operative or recovery room suites. A slight rise in body temperature to about 38° C (100° F) is commonly observed during the first 24 hours after surgery as a result of the stress reaction to the trauma of surgery. Fever is suggestive of atelectasis after the second postoperative day and of wound infection after the fifth day.[59]

Skin color and temperature. Pallor in light-skinned patients and a dullness or decrease in red tones in dark-skinned patients indicates decreased circulation to the skin. Pallor in dark-skinned patients may be more easily assessed by examining the mucous membranes of the mouth. Vasoconstriction may result from cold temperatures or a decrease in the amount of circulating blood as a result of blood loss or from the neuroendocrine response to stress. The nail beds are checked for capillary return. If circulation is adequate, pinkness should return to the nail after it is "flicked" by the examiner's finger.

Warm moist skin may be secondary to vasodilation from excessive warmth applied after surgery or to overhydration from excess fluid replacement. In this situation, the intravenous fluid intake is assessed.

Body Position

Body position should be one that facilitates ventilation and does not place strain on the area surrounding the incision. Pillows should not exert pressure on the popliteal area (behind the knee) since this leads to venous obstruction. Most patients prefer the bed with the head slightly elevated. The bed is usually kept flat for a period of time following certain types of eye surgery or neurosurgery or following spinal anesthesia.

Dressings

The entire dressing is inspected with the covers pulled back or the patient turned as necessary. A dressing applied to the side, such as for kidney surgery, may appear dry on the top visible area if the patient is supine but may have excess drainage on the lower portion as a result of gravity. An excess of drainage is reported immediately. If small amounts of unexpected drainage occur, especially bright red drainage, the area can be outlined with a pen on the dressing so that the rate or increase can be easily determined.

Elimination

Urinary output is closely monitored after surgery until normal urinary function is reestablished. A urinary output of at least 30 ml/hour is required to maintain kidney function to excrete wastes, but 50 ml/hr is desirable. Urinary output will be less than fluid intake during the first 24 hours and the specific gravity will be high. The bladder is palpated for distention when output is low to identify possible urinary retention. The distended bladder rises out of the pelvis just above the symphysis pubis; it may be difficult to palpate when the patient is obese. Occasionally, the overdistended bladder expels just enough urine to relieve the pressure within it temporarily and the patient voids frequently in small amounts but without discomfort (retention with overflow).

Bowel movements may be small and infrequent or even absent for 2 or 3 days following major surgery, but normal bowel patterns are usually reestablished as the person becomes more active and eats better. Peristalsis may be absent for a period of time following gastrointestinal surgery (see Chapter 44). Return of peristalsis of the lower gastrointestinal tract is indicated by presence of bowel sounds, gas pains, and passing of flatus. Absence of bowel sounds does not indicate absence of peristalsis because the sounds may be occurring only occasionally and may be missed. The presence of bowel sounds usually indicates gas moving in segments of the bowel.

Mobility

Leg exercises need to be performed by the patient who will have decreased activity following surgery. These exercises help to prevent thrombophlebitis and to strengthen muscles for walking. Knowledge and ability to carry out these exercises (see Chapter 20) is assessed.

If the patient has been inactive for a period of time, sitting ability and muscle strength of the legs need to be assessed. The quadriceps muscles are tested by the patient flexing and extending the leg against resistance provided by the nurse's hand. Weak quadriceps muscles indicate decreased ability to stand and walk. Sitting ability is assessed by asking the patient to maintain an upright position while being gently pushed sideways.

ASSESSMENT OF ENVIRONMENTAL FACTORS
EQUIPMENT

Equipment connected to the patient by means of tubes or lines is checked for proper connection, patency, and functioning. Visual patterns on monitors should be in working order.

Fluids may be ordered to be given to the patient intravenously or instilled in body cavities for irrigation, as in the bladder. The contents of the fluid containers, the patency of the tubing, and the rate of fluid administration are checked. Intravenous fluids are usually given at rates ranging from minimal (to keep the line open, K/O) to 3 ml/min. If the fluid is running in at a rate greater than 3 ml/min, the rate is slowed, the order is checked immediately, and the rate is adjusted appropriately. Rate of administration varies with the amount of fluid lost, size and age of the patient, and the underlying illness (see Chapter 23). Amount and character of drainage in fluid receptacles from fluids draining from the patient are also monitored.

SAFETY FACTORS

Following major surgery, the patient is often weak and has increased potential for falling. If the patient is only partially conscious or confused, side rails may be necessary. The call cord should be within the reach of the bedfast patient. The room is examined for possible physical causes for falls, such as equipment or footstools in the path of ambulation to the patient's chair, door, or bathroom, or water spilled on the floor.

■ DATA ANALYSIS: NURSING DIAGNOSES

Nursing diagnoses are determined from assessment of patient data. Possible nursing diagnoses for the postoperative patient may include, but are not limited to, the following:

Diagnostic Title	Possible Etiologies
Airway clearance, ineffective	Secretions
Anxiety	Threat to self-concept, health status, socioeconomic status, role functions
Breathing pattern, ineffective	Incisional pain, sedation
Constipation	Stress of surgery, anesthetic, narcotics, decreased mobility, inadequate nutrition
Fluid volume excess	Compromised regulatory mechanisms
Knowledge deficit (postoperative routines, preventive measures, specific care requirements)	Lack of exposure/recall, misinterpretation of information

Diagnostic Title	Possible Etiologies
Mobility, impaired physical	Decreased strength and endurance, pain/discomfort
Nutrition, altered: less than body requirements	Decreased peristalsis, anorexia, nausea, pain
Pain	Incision, tight bandages/casts, abdominal distention, vomiting, hiccoughs
Sexual dysfunction	Altered body structure, lack of knowledge, psychologic stress
Tissue perfusion, altered: peripheral	Immobility, pressure
Urinary retention	Recumbent position, anesthetic, drugs, pain

■ PLANNING: EXPECTED PATIENT OUTCOMES

Planning includes not only the immediate postoperative period but also the discharge period. Plans for the patient's discharge are considered during the preoperative period, but most of the teaching, arrangements, and preparations are done after surgery. Because hospitalization stays have been shortened for most surgical patients, early planning for discharge is imperative.

Expected patient outcomes for the postoperative patient may include, but are not limited to, the following:
1. Avoidable complications (atelectasis, pneumonia, thrombophlebitis, overhydration) do not occur.
2. The incision heals normally without infection or dehiscence.
3. Weight loss is minimal or stabilized.
4. Elimination patterns are reestablished.
5. The patient ambulates (if permitted) and carries out activities of daily living at an optimal level, although fatigue may still be present.
6. Signs of pain are decreased.
7. The patient has an opportunity to explore individual concerns, including sexual concerns.
8. At discharge, the patient and significant others can explain:
   a. Treatment to be continued at home
   b. Community resources for supplies
   c. Activity limits and prescriptions
   d. When and where to go for follow-up care

■ IMPLEMENTATION

General nursing care of the postoperative patient is summarized in the box on p. 512. Care is focused on relieving anxiety, maintaining aeration, circulation, nutrition, fluid and electrolyte balance, urinary and bowel elimination; and promoting activity and comfort.

RELIEVING ANXIETY

Some of the concerns that were present in the preoperative period may continue into the postoperative period.

GUIDELINES FOR POSTOPERATIVE NURSING CARE

1. Maintain aeration
   a. Encourage deep breathing and coughing exercises and yawn maneuvers for all persons following inhalant anesthesia
   b. Use additional ventilatory maneuvers, such as incentive spirometer for persons at high risk for pulmonary complications
   c. Encourage body position changes at least every 2 to 3 hours for bed patients
   d. Encourage maximum activity within prescribed limits
   e. Monitor breath sounds until patient is ambulatory
2. Maintain circulation
   a. Provide elastic stockings for persons at high risk for thrombophlebitis
   b. Encourage bed exercises and ambulation within prescribed limits
   c. Instruct patient to elevate legs when sitting, unless contraindicated
   d. Avoid postoperative leg massage
3. Maintain fluid and electrolyte balance
   a. Monitor intake and output until patient is taking oral fluids equal to at least 1200 ml output
   b. Monitor intravenous fluid flow to provide required fluids evenly spaced
   c. Assess patients for fluid overload, especially small elderly patients; monitor body weight
   d. Encourage oral fluids as soon as permitted
   e. When oral intake is permitted encourage high protein foods and fresh fruits to supply needed potassium
4. Maintain nutrition
   a. Teach patients to select foods high in protein and vitamin C to enhance wound healing
   b. Encourage carbohydrate intake for energy supply
   c. Suggest more frequent, smaller meals for the anorexic person
5. Maintain elimination
   a. Encourage micturition in the early postoperative period
   b. Encourage fluids and maximal activity within prescribed limits to prevent constipation
   c. Use measures to encourage defecation if patient has not had a bowel movement 2 to 3 days after peristalsis returns
6. Promote activity
   a. Encourage leg exercises for the bed patient and during the early postoperative period
   b. Encourage patient to carry out ADL and to turn self in bed within the limitations of pain and fatigue
   c. Encourage progressive ambulation as soon as permitted
7. Promote comfort
   a. Teach pain-relieving measures such as relaxation exercises and position changes
   b. Remove causes of pain other than incisional, such as loosening tight bandages
   c. Encourage use of TENS if electrodes have been applied after surgery
   d. For 48 hours following major surgery, offer prescribed analgesics at regular intervals before pain becomes severe
   e. Carry out usual comfort measures if vomiting occurs
   f. Encourage ambulation and exercises, and consider use of rectal tube if gas pains are present
   g. Give patient opportunities to talk about concerns related to surgery
8. Teach patient
   a. Care of self according to specific surgery performed
   b. Community resources available for assistance as needed
   c. Dietary and activity restrictions according to surgery performed
   d. Gradual resumption of normal activities
   e. Avoidance of heavy lifting, pushing, or pulling for at least 6 weeks after major surgery
   f. Importance of medical follow-up visits

These concerns generally focus on the performed surgery, loss of body part, or effect of the surgery.

PSYCHOLOGIC FACTORS

Concerns Specific to the Surgery Performed

Sometimes patients doubt the information that they have been given. They may wonder if surgery was really needed. They may still worry that they have cancer but that nobody is telling them the truth. If they do have cancer, they may think that it is more extensive than they are being told.

Concerns Over Loss of a Body Part

Surgery frequently means removal of tissue. If an organ such as the uterus or part of the colon is removed or if part of a limb, breast, or face is removed, patients are faced with a change in self-image (Chapter 18). They may experience grief over the lost part (Chapter 14). For complete recovery the patient needs to identify feelings and cope with the perceived changes.

Concerns About the Future

The patient may have concerns about changes in sexuality, economic status, prognosis, or permanent effects. Sexuality may be threatened by the enforced absence from home or a specific surgery such as a colostomy. These concerns may center around the effect of the surgery on the spouse or parent relationship or on the effect of surgery on sexual performance itself. Economic worries center mainly on loss of income during hospitalization and cost of the surgery. Fears also exist relating to prognosis. Is the surgery really going to correct the original problem? Am I going to die? Will the problem recur? Will there be more pain? What permanent effects will occur? How will my life change?

ASSESSMENT

Anxieties will be expressed in many different ways. It must be remembered that expressions such as anger, resentfulness, crying, excessive joking, inappropriate laughter, or withdrawal may all be signs of anxiety and are often seen in the postoperative period. Some of these feelings may be projected against the surgeon, nurse, housekeeping aide, food, and so forth.

SUPPORTING EXPLORATION OF CONCERNS

Sitting down and talking with surgical patients about their concerns is as important a nursing action in many instances as any of the physical activities. Time must be planned for this. If a specific concern is expected, such as sexual functioning after a perineal prostatectomy, the topic may have to be introduced by the nurse who has established rapport with the patient to let the patient know that it is permissible to talk about this topic.

Some patients will talk freely about the cancer or the heart operation but never really face their feelings about the surgery. The patient is not forced to do so, but the alert nurse will watch for cues that the patient is beginning to move from a cognitive thinking level to a feeling level and may need some support while identifying and learning to cope with these feelings.

MAINTAINING AERATION

Pulmonary complications, primarily atelectasis and pneumonia, are the most common postoperative complications. Nursing management plays an important role in the prevention of these complications.

PATHOPHYSIOLOGY

Atelectasis is a Greek term meaning "incomplete expansion" and refers to collapse of alveoli in the lungs. The atelectasis may be regional (involvement of a specific small or large area) or it may involve widespread small alveoli (microatelectasis). Microatelectasis occurs frequently, often producing no overt symptoms despite the hypoventilation. Atelectasis may result from either obstruction of air passages or from progressive regional hypoventilation.

Obstructive Atelectasis

Obstruction of alveoli is caused by blockage of the air passages by mucous plugs. When alveolar ducts are blocked, the alveolus distal to the block may remain aerated with *deep inspiration* by means of interalveolar ducts (Figure 22-13). If respirations are shallow, the

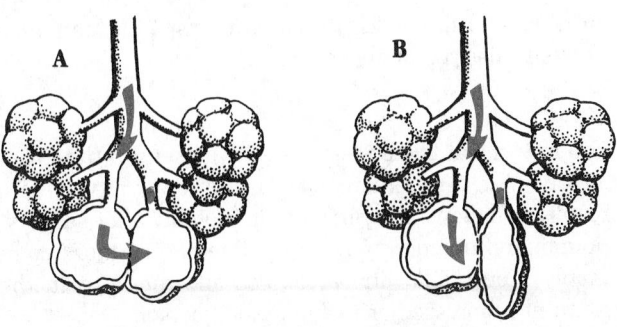

FIGURE 22-13 Mucous plug blocking alveolar duct in obstructive atelectasis. **A,** Aeration of blocked alveolus through interalveolar duct with deep inspiration. **B,** Collapse of blocked alveolus with shallow inspiration.

connecting alveolar ducts remain closed and the alveolus distal to the mucous plug will collapse as all of the air is absorbed. Collapse of many alveoli results in hypoventilation. A bronchus or bronchiole may also become blocked; the lung tissue distal to the blockage then becomes atelectatic.

Various factors can cause secretions to block the air passages (see the box below). Blockage can be prevented by keeping secretions moist, taking deep breaths, and coughing up the secretions.

Hypoventilatory Atelectasis

Microatelectasis may also occur from a decrease of *surfactant,* a phospholipid produced by alveolar cells. Surfactant acts by reducing the surface tension of pulmonary liquids. Normally, when the volume of an alveolus decreases with expiration, the proportion of surfactant increases and prevents the alveolus from collapsing. Surfactant also decreases the force necessary for reexpansion. Surfactant formation is stimulated by deep breaths.[26] Normally, people take periodic "sighs" or deep breaths. Sighing occurs less frequently after surgery as a result of sedation or incisional pain. Shallow breathing without sighs may result in progressive alveolar collapse within 1 hour.[26] Smoking also decreases

---

FACTORS CONTRIBUTING TO DEVELOPMENT OF ATELECTASIS

---

1. Anesthetic: decreased ciliary action
2. Narcotics, sedatives: decreased cough and respirations
3. Smoking: decreased ciliary action, decreased surfactant
4. Immobility: pooling of secretions
5. Dehydration: secretions become thickened
6. Pain: shallow respirations, weak cough
7. Abdominal distention: shallow respirations

---

surfactant. Taking deep breaths or yawning can help prevent this type of atelectasis.

Pneumonia

Oropharyngeal bacteria are usually present in the lower airway. When secretions pool in the lower airway as a result of shallow breathing and immobility after surgery, pulmonary infection may occur. Pneumonia more commonly occurs following prolonged anesthesia or in the immunosuppressed or malnourished person.

ASSESSMENT

Early in the postoperative period the patient is assessed to determine the risk for developing a pulmonary complication. Data are collected to identify high-risk factors that are present. The greater the number of risk factors, the greater the risk for developing a pulmonary complication if preventive measures are not taken. Risk factors include the following:

1. Inhalant anesthesia
2. High abdominal or thoracic surgery
3. Age: elderly
4. Presence of chronic obstructive lung disease
5. Smoking
6. Medications that decrease respirations or cough: narcotics, sedatives
7. Breath sounds: decreased in upper lobes; decreased in lower lobes after 24 hours; presence of rales
8. Shallow respirations; decreased chest expansion
9. Presence of pain that limits chest expansion or mobility
10. Decreased patient mobility; recumbent body position
11. Dehydration; decreased skin turgor.

An unexplained rise in temperature is often the first sign of atelectasis. Pulse and respiratory rates increase. If a large bronchus is blocked, the patient may exhibit dyspnea and cyanosis and signs of shock. Diagnosis is confirmed by chest radiography. Pneumonia also produces fever, dyspnea, chest pain, and a cough productive of mucopurulent sputum.

VENTILATORY MEASURES

The use of postoperative "routines" without identifying specific patient needs is *not* quality nursing care. It is common to find postoperative routines that read "Turn, cough, and deep breathe every 2 hours"; the order is never changed. In reality, some patients need ventilatory exercises more often than every 2 hours, others less often. After general anesthesia, most patients will need to ventilate their lungs well at least every 1 to 2 hours the first postoperative day, and then every 3 to 4 hours while awake for several days if not active. The decision for the type and frequency of preventive respiratory measures should be based on each patient's risk factors and hour-by-hour and day-by-day response. Measures that work effectively in increasing ventilation in one patient may be less effective in another.

A plan that best meets oxygen needs should be developed for each patient. For example, an elderly patient with a history of lung disease, who smokes and has just had high abdominal surgery with an inhalant anesthetic, may need to carry out ventilatory maneuvers as often as every 30 to 60 minutes during the first few postoperative hours. A young patient with no history of smoking or lung disease, who had preoperative medication and an inhalant anesthetic and who is up ambulating frequently after surgery, may need breathing exercises only every 2 to 3 hours the first day and none thereafter. Reassessment of patient status is important, and the plan of care should be updated as the risk factors change.

Persons at low risk for developing postoperative pulmonary complications should carry out deep breathing and coughing exercises and yawn maneuvers. Persons at greater risk (several risk factors present) usually need additional measures, such as the incentive spirometer. The nurse may initiate any of the ventilatory measures. Many patients are drowsy or have periods of amnesia during the early postoperative period, so that frequently the instructions must be repeated. Persons who have had good instruction in the preoperative phase are usually better able to carry out the measures postoperatively.

The most effective position for ventilatory exercises is high Fowler's, since this decreases the pressure of the abdominal contents on the diaphragm and permits better thorax expansion. If the patient must remain flat in bed, restraining bedclothes and pillows are removed from around the chest.

Deep Breathing

If carried out correctly and at appropriate intervals depending on the degree or risk, deep breathing is a very effective method of preventing atelectasis and pneumonia. Patients should learn deep-breathing exercises during the preoperative period to facilitate initiation of deep breathing shortly after awakening from anesthesia. The deep-breathing exercises are described in detail in Chapter 20.

Yawn Maneuver

The yawn maneuver leads to full alveolar inflation, thus stimulating surfactant production. Once the alveoli are fully inflated, they will remain open for at least 1 hour.[5]

The initiation of the yawn maneuver by the patient is easy, especially if demonstrated by the nurse because the yawn is often initiated by seeing another person do it. The patient is asked to take a deep breath with the

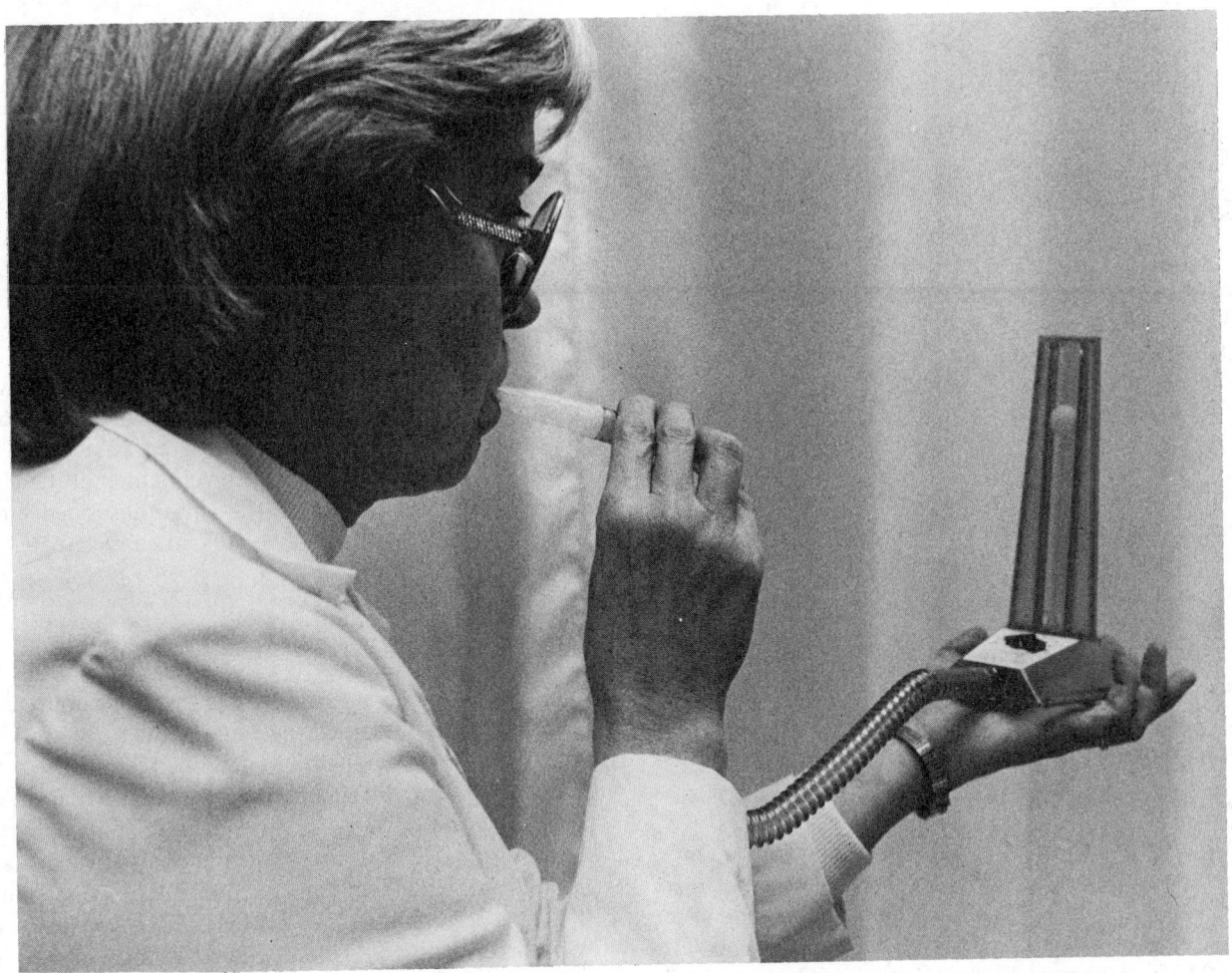

FIGURE 22-14 Incentive spirometer. Ball rising with inspiration is a visual cue for patient. Ball remains up as patient holds breath for 3 seconds.

mouth open and to hold the breath for more than 3 seconds. The yawn is spontaneous; once it starts, it is difficult to stop from taking a deep inspiration.

Incentive Spirometer

The incentive spirometer is a mechanical device that promotes *sustained maximal inspiration*. Several incentive spirometers are on the market, and each has some way of demonstrating to the patient how much volume has been inspired, to encourage the patient to expend still greater inspiratory effort (Figure 22-14).

Maximal effect occurs when the full inspiration is held for at least 3 seconds. Only minimal patient instruction is required. The patient breathes in through the mouthpiece as deeply as possible and holds the breath for at least 3 seconds if possible. Expiration is passive. The patient should take three to five normal breaths between each deep breath to prevent dizziness and light-headedness. Use of the incentive spirometer at mealtimes may cause nausea.

Coughing

All of the ventilatory measures used by the surgical patient are followed by *deep coughing* to remove any secretions that have been loosened. Deep breathing in itself often stimulates coughing. Coughing may be contraindicated in a few instances, such as following brain, spinal, or eye surgery, because of the increased intracranial or intraocular pressure that can result.

A shallow cough is ineffective in mobilizing secretions and produces fatigue; therefore the patient is encouraged to cough deeply and productively. Patients with incisions can be told that it may be painful to cough but that assistance will be given. Narcotics given before ventilation exercises may facilitate cooperation of the patient; on the other hand, narcotics decrease the cough reflex and depress respirations. A patient who will not cough deeply because of pain is encouraged to "huff" cough (see Chapter 20).

Some patients feel that the incision may split open with deep coughing; they may be encouraged to cough

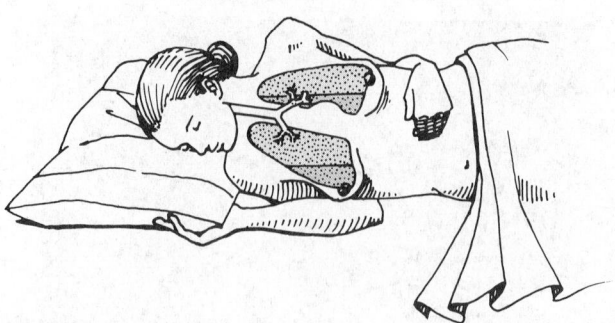

FIGURE 22-15 Schematic of lungs illustrating pooling of secretions in dependent alveoli.

deeply by splinting the incision with a drawsheet, towel, small pillow, or placement of the hands firmly on either side of the incision with exertion of slight pressure. Such splinting prevents excessive muscular strain around the incision.

The lungs are auscultated before and after ventilatory measures to determine effectiveness. If the patient has noisy breathing but is unable to cough up secretions, respiratory tract suctioning may be required.

POSITIONING AND TURNING

If the patient lies in one position with continuous pressure from body weight against the chest wall, proper ventilation and drainage of secretions on that side of the chest are not possible and atelectasis can develop (Figure 22-15). Turning and changing of position frequently (at least every 2 to 3 hours) provides for better ventilation of the lungs. The patient should be encouraged to help in turning. Most patients assume a supine position

and are not eager to change position because of the increased pain during movement. They may find side rails useful for turning during the early postoperative period. Assistance can be given by supporting a limb or helping the patient to turn in one smooth movement. Alternating the height of the bed is useful: high Fowler's position facilitates diaphragm movement; low Fowler's or a flat position facilitates drainage and expectoration of respiratory secretions.

ACTIVITY

Stimulation of the respiratory center occurs with activity because of the increased need for oxygen at the cellular level. The more active the patient, the greater will be the depth of respirations and the ventilation of the alveoli. Activity is encouraged within the prescribed limits and depending on the patient's tolerance of activity.

MAINTAINING CIRCULATION
PATHOPHYSIOLOGY

Oxygen is needed by tissue cells for metabolism. It cannot reach the cells if blood flow to the part is curtailed. The formation of clots in the veins of the pelvis and the lower extremities, impairing circulation, is a fairly common and potentially serious postoperative complication.

Blood clots develop because of a roughness in the vessel wall such as occurs with trauma from venous stasis (slowing of blood flow), and with hypercoagulability. Platelets adhere to the vessel wall, and the resulting inflammatory response stimulates blood coagulation and fibrin development, resulting in a blood clot on the vessel wall (thrombophlebitis) (Figure 22-16). Postoperatively, the clot often forms in a vein of the foot, calf, thigh, or pelvis. The clot grows, usually in the direction

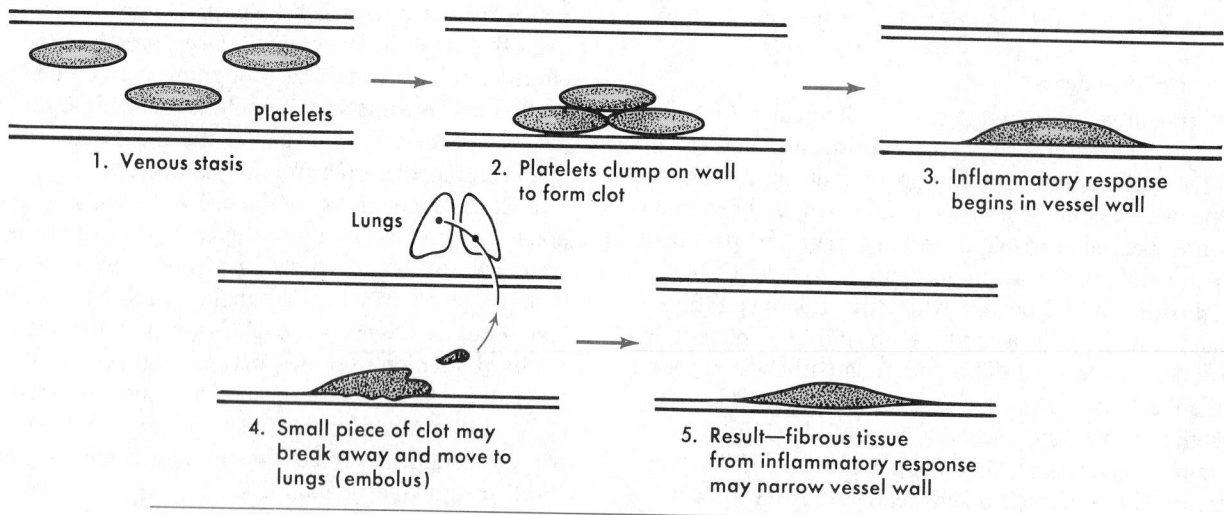

Platelets

1. Venous stasis

2. Platelets clump on wall to form clot

3. Inflammatory response begins in vessel wall

Lungs

4. Small piece of clot may break away and move to lungs (embolus)

5. Result—fibrous tissue from inflammatory response may narrow vessel wall

FIGURE 22-16 Diagram illustrating formation of thrombus on wall of vein following venous stasis resulting in narrowing of blood vessel.

RISK FACTORS FOR DEVELOPMENT OF POSTOPERATIVE VENOUS THROMBOSIS

INTRINSIC FACTORS

Older age
Obesity
Malnutrition
Contraceptive use

PATHOLOGIC CONDITIONS

Malignancy
Congestive heart failure
History of previous deep vein thrombosis
Polycythemia

TYPE OF SURGERY

Pelvic surgery
Abdominal or thoracic surgery
Fracture of hip or lower extremities

EFFECTS OF SURGERY

Anesthesia
Shock
Decreased mobility
Prolonged sitting with legs dependent
Pressure on popliteal area (pillows, chair)
Intestinal distention
Tight dressings or cast on lower extremities

of the slow-moving blood. It can occur in either a deep or superficial vein. In about 1 of every 10 instances[23] the clot or a portion of it breaks away and flows through the heart into the pulmonary circulation until it occludes a pulmonary vessel (pulmonary embolism) (see Chapter 33).

Venous stasis occurs postoperatively for a number of reasons (see the box above). A major contribution to venous stasis is inactivity of the legs. Every time the leg is moved, the muscle compresses the vein, pushing the blood toward the heart (venous pump); valves prevent the blood from moving backward. Exercise therefore promotes return of venous blood to the heart and prevention of venous stasis.

ASSESSMENT

A venous blood clot may develop without any local symptoms (*phlebothrombosis*), and the first indication of difficulty may be a pulmonary embolism. Homan's sign (pain on dorsiflexion of the foot) indicates a phlebothrombosis, but this may not always be present. Pain and local tenderness in the leg are signs of thrombophlebitis.

If a superficial vein is inflamed, *thrombophlebitis* can be noted as a reddened line along the vessel route, which feels firm on gentle palpation. If it forms in the femoral or iliac veins, the entire limb becomes swollen,

pale, and cold. There is usually extreme tenderness along the course of the vein. The swelling and coldness are caused by lymphatic obstruction and arterial spasm. The body temperature often rises. If the thrombophlebitis is confined to the saphenous vein, the accompanying edema is not so marked, but pain and tenderness are just as severe, and heat and redness can be noted along the inflamed vein.

Signs of a *pulmonary embolism* depend on the size of the blood vessel that has been occluded. Any complaints of sudden sharp thoracic or upper abdominal pain or dyspnea or any signs of shock should be reported immediately to the physician.

PREVENTION

Postoperative thrombophlebitis often may be prevented by nursing management. Patient education in the causes of thrombophlebitis will help ensure greater participation in preventive measures. Elastic stockings or bandages should be worn both in and out of bed by high-risk patients. These stockings compress superficial veins, increase blood flow through deep veins by pressure, and prevent venous pooling. The stockings are removed at least once daily to permit washing and inspection of the legs.

Patients should not sit in one position for a long time and should elevate their feet on a stool to facilitate venous return by gravity. No pressure should be permitted on the popliteal area. When supporting legs on pillows, pressure should be equally distributed along the entire leg. Because of the danger of dislodging a clot, *the muscle portion of a patient's leg should not be massaged postoperatively.* A patient who is rubbing a leg should be questioned about discomfort.

Bed exercises (Figure 20-2) and early ambulation are known to minimize the effects of venous stasis caused by bed rest, and they usually are contraindicated only in the presence of thromboembolic diseases or after vascular surgery such as anastomosis of a blood vessel. Specific exercises for the upper extremities are not usually necessary because the patient uses the arms in eating, bathing, combing hair, and reaching for articles on the bedside stand or overbed table.

Medical preventive measures in high-risk patients include (1) heparin prophylaxis given 2 hours preoperatively and 8 to 12 hours postoperatively, (2) aspirin in instances when heparin is contraindicated such as for hip surgery, (3) dextran, or (4) warfarin. *Intermittent external pneumatic compression* to the legs may also be prescribed. This consists of a pneumatic cuff that extends from the feet to below the knee. The cuff is inflated rapidly to 40 to 50 mm Hg pressure, held for 10 to 12 seconds, and then deflated for 45 seconds. This procedure is not uncomfortable and has demonstrated marked effectiveness in high-risk patients.[59]

INTERVENTION FOR POSTOPERATIVE THROMBOPHLEBITIS

At the first sign of a possible thrombophlebitis the patient should return to bed and remain there until seen by a physician. Rest, leg elevation, and elastic bandages are usually prescribed. The patient may also be given anticoagulant therapy (see Chapter 29).

MAINTAINING FLUID AND ELECTROLYTE BALANCE
PATHOPHYSIOLOGY

Fluids are lost during surgery through blood loss and increased insensible fluid loss (by hyperventilation and exposed skin surfaces). Fluids may also be "lost" to the circulation following major surgery in which tissue dissection was extensive, because of fluid retention at the surgical site or in the intestines by ileus (third spacing).

Following surgery for at least 24 to 48 hours, fluids are retained by the body because of the stimulation of antidiuretic hormone (ADH) as part of the stress response to trauma and the effect of anesthesia. During surgery there is also renal vasoconstriction and increased aldosterone activity leading to increased sodium retention with subsequent water retention. *Overhydration* can occur with vigorous fluid replacement, especially in the small elderly patient. Both water intoxication and pulmonary edema can occur depending on the type and amount of fluids given. (For further information on fluid overload see Chapter 23.)

The major *electrolyte* disturbances are sodium and potassium deficits and acidosis (see the box above). Note that loss of large amounts of gastrointestinal fluids is a major cause of sodium and potassium imbalances. Hyponatremia is more frequently seen in elderly persons because of the higher incidence of renal dysfunction in this population.[1]

Increased amounts of potassium enter the circulation following surgery or trauma because of catabolism (tissue breakdown) but this potassium is then excreted in the urine regardless of the body's need for potassium. Potassium serum levels are generally adequate during the first 24 hours after surgery; potassium excess may occur if supplementary potassium is given then.

Acid-base imbalances may also occur postoperatively. *Alkalosis* occurs more frequently than acidosis but is usually well tolerated by the patient and requires no specific therapy.[1] Hypoventilation is a major cause of postoperative *acidosis* and can be prevented by ventilatory measures (p. 514).

ASSESSMENT

All patients who have had major surgery and those receiving fluids intravenously after surgery need careful monitoring of fluid balance. Fluid intake will exceed fluid output during the first 24 to 48 hours. After this initial period, fluid intake should essentially equal fluid output for the patient taking solid foods.

PATHOGENESIS OF POSTOPERATIVE ELECTROLYTE IMBALANCES

SODIUM DEFICIT (HYPONATREMIA)

Vomiting, diarrhea, prolonged nasogastric intubation: loss of GI secretions high in sodium
Preexisting renal disease: inability to concentrate urine with loss of sodium
Head injury: inappropriate ADH secretion leading to water retention

POTASSIUM DEFICIT (HYPOKALEMIA)

Vomiting, diarrhea, prolonged nasogastric intubation: loss of GI secretions high in potassium
Stress: retention of sodium with excretion of potassium
Prolonged administration of potassium-free IV solutions

ACIDOSIS

Incisional pain, abdominal distention: hypoventilation
Shock: lactic acidosis from decreased circulation
Diabetes mellitus: ketosis during catabolism
Preexisting renal disease: inadequate excretion of inorganic acids

ALKALOSIS

Pain, anxiety, ventilatory therapy: hyperventilation
Nasogastric intubation: loss of hydrogen ions
Large numbers of blood transfusions: oxidation of citrate to bicarbonate
Stress: decreased renal excretion of bicarbonate

The patient receiving fluids intravenously is monitored for signs of pulmonary edema (dyspnea, cough) or water intoxication (change in behavior, confusion, warm moist skin). Weight gain is the earliest sign of excessive infusion; therefore accurate daily weights are taken for those patients receiving intravenous fluids for several days. Small elderly patients may need central venous pressure monitoring of fluid volume. The patient is also monitored for signs of sodium and potassium deficit and for acidosis (see Chapter 23). Extra potassium may be necessary to replace losses by gastric secretion.

FLUID AND ELECTROLYTE REPLACEMENT

Fluid volume deficits require fluid replacement given intravenously following major surgery. The amount of fluid prescribed depends on the patient's age, sex, weight, and body surface in addition to needs from additional losses. Daily maintenance requirements are about 1500 to 2500 ml. A rough measure consists of 30 ml times body weight in kilograms (for example, a person weighing 60 kg needs 1800 ml/day [30 ml × 60 kg ≥ 1800 ml]. A solution of 5% dextrose in 0.45% sodium chloride is commonly given. Lactated Ringer's solution may be given for prolonged periods to supply the necessary electrolytes (see Chapter 23). Potassium may be added after the first 24 hours.

Intravenous fluids are monitored carefully to provide

an even distribution of fluid over the entire 24-hour period. Fluids are started orally as soon as the patient can tolerate them and if active peristalsis is present. Sips of water are offered first. Some persons cannot tolerate iced fluids but can tolerate sucking on ice chips, which must be recorded as intake (2 parts ice equal 1 part water). High protein foods and fresh fruits, which are high in potassium, are encouraged when foods are permitted by mouth.

MAINTAINING NUTRITION
PATHOPHYSIOLOGY

Most persons can begin to eat within 24 hours after surgery unless the abdomen has been opened. Peristalsis is decreased when the abdominal contents are handled. Postoperative ileus (cessation of peristalsis) is usually of short duration following uncomplicated abdominal surgery[1] but may last for several days following surgery of the stomach or colon.

The best way to supply essential foods is orally. Solid food can promote the flow of saliva during mastication, aiding digestion and encouraging the stomach to empty. This process in turn stimulates peristalsis of the lower gastrointestinal tract. Ingestion of solid food also helps to prevent the occurrence of nonepidemic parotitis, an inflammation of the salivary glands that occurs occasionally in debilitated patients who have poor oral hygiene and who also may be dehydrated.

Two food substances of special importance in wound healing are protein and vitamin C (p. 496). During catabolism in the early postoperative period a negative nitrogen balance occurs; more nitrogen is lost than is taken in (see Chapter 20). Protein intake is necessary to restore nitrogen balance and to provide the necessary amino acids for anabolism.

Patients lose weight following surgery because body resources are used to provide the necessary energy. This weight loss is rarely a problem in well-nourished persons because weight will be restored within a few weeks with an adequate dietary intake. Persons who are malnourished preoperatively do not have the necessary resources and thus have a greater incidence of infection and wound dehiscence and a prolonged recovery.

ASSESSMENT

The presence of bowel sounds, passing of flatus, or belching indicates the return of peristalsis. Daily weight measurement for patients not eating a full meal at least three times a day will give an indication of the degree of tissue loss. Rapid weight gain indicates fluid retention; rapid loss indicates dehydration. A gradual loss of about 0.15 to 0.25 kg (⅓ to ½ lb) per day indicates tissue loss. There is usually an increase in blood urea nitrogen (BUN) levels during catabolism, but unless the patient has renal insufficiency the excess urea is excreted in the urine. Meal trays of surgical patients should be inspected to identify those patients who are not eating foods high in protein and vitamin C.

DIET

Patients receiving standard intravenous fluids containing dextrose do not have sufficient caloric intake. This is essentially a "starvation diet." As soon as fluids can be tolerated, foods are started. Most patients quickly resume their usual diet. Elderly patients or patients who have had stomach surgery may tolerate a soft diet and six small feedings more easily than a standard diet. Urging solid food when the patient has no appetite may induce vomiting and may lessen the desire to eat. The anorexic patient is encouraged to select preferred foods that are high in protein and vitamin C. Carbohydrate is also needed to provide energy expended in early ambulation. After even a few days of enforced starvation the patient may be somewhat indifferent to food, and it may take 2 to 3 days on a well-balanced diet to overcome this. The patient who was malnourished before surgery and who has extensive gastrointestinal surgery is a candidate for total parenteral nutrition.

The usual home diet of elderly persons living alone is often low in protein and vitamins. Patient education concerning the increased need for these food substances in the weeks after surgery may be indicated.

MAINTAINING URINARY ELIMINATION
PATHOPHYSIOLOGY

A patient who is well hydrated usually voids within 6 to 8 hours after surgery. Although 2000 to 3000 ml of intravenous fluid usually is given on the operative day, the first voiding may not be more than 200 ml and the total urinary output for the operative day may be less than 1500 ml. The decreased amount of urinary output results from the loss of body fluid during surgery, increased insensible fluid loss, vomiting, and increased secretion of ADH. As body functions stabilize, fluid and electrolyte balance returns to normal within 48 hours.

Urinary retention, the inability to void, may occur in the early postoperative period. The difficulty may be due to the following:

1. Recumbent position
2. Nervous tension
3. Effects of anesthetics that interfere with bladder sensation and the ability to void
4. Pain caused by movement
5. Pain at the surgical site following bladder or urethral surgery

Inability to void is a common occurrence following spinal anesthesia or surgery of the rectum, colon, or gynecologic structures, as a result of temporary disturbance of the innervation of the bladder musculature or from local edema.

Urinary tract infections may occur in patients who have indwelling catheters inserted following surgery, particularly after pelvic surgery. Prolonged bed rest leading to urinary stasis may also be a contributing factor.

ASSESSMENT

Urinary output is closely monitored after surgery until normal urinary function is reestablished. Urinary *retention* is characterized by the voiding of little or no urine over a 6 to 8 hour period. Light palpation of the bladder over the lower abdomen just above the symphysis pubis usually elicits discomfort, and distention may be observed. Signs of urinary tract *infection* include frequency with dysuria; fever may also be present. Patients who exhibit signs of urinary tract infection should have a urine specimen sent to the laboratory for culture and sensitivity.

PROMOTING URINARY ELIMINATION

Voiding may be facilitated by measures such as offering fluids, getting the patient up to the bathroom or commode as permitted, running water in the bathroom, pouring water over the perineum, and assuring the patient of time and privacy. Men can void more easily if they are allowed to stand to void.

If the above measures are not effective, the physician may order catheterization. Because of the possibility of reproductive tract infections in men and the danger of urinary tract infection in all patients, catheterization may be delayed longer than the usual 8 hours postoperatively in the hope that the patient will void normally. Bethanechol chloride (Urecholine) may be ordered by the physician for acute postoperative retention. It may be given orally or subcutaneously but not by intramuscular injection because this may induce circulatory collapse.

An indwelling catheter may be necessary if the inability to void persists. Indwelling catheters are inserted at the time of surgery following those procedures, such as pelvic surgery, that frequently lead to urinary retention. Good catheter care is imperative. Fluids are encouraged up to 3000 ml unless contraindicated, to prevent urinary stasis.

MAINTAINING BOWEL ELIMINATION
PATHOPHYSIOLOGY

Decreased peristalsis from the neuroendocrine response to the stress of surgery, from the effect of anesthesia or narcotics, or from hypokalemia may lead to constipation in the early postoperative period. Inactivity and decreased intake of foods that provide roughage are contributing factors. Peristalsis will be decreased for at least 24 hours in all patients with abdominal or pelvic surgery, and for 3 to 4 days following surgery of the stomach or colon. Following surgery of the rectum, bowel movements may be painful and the patient may be reluctant to defecate.

Patients receiving intravenous fluids may have bowel movements if peristalsis is present. Because of the lack of ingested roughage, the stools will occur less frequently and be small and hard.

ASSESSMENT

Bowel elimination is monitored after surgery until normal bowel patterns have been reestablished. After major surgery, bowel sounds are auscultated and the patient questioned about passing flatus. Signs indicating the return of intestinal peristalsis are recorded after abdominal surgery. Assessment is made of the frequency with which narcotics are given, extent of activity, amount of fluid intake, and previous bowel problems to determine the patient's potential for developing constipation.

Stool is examined for amount and consistency; small, dry, hard stool indicates constipation. A small amount of diarrhea may be indicative of fecal impaction. Digital examination of the rectum is contraindicated following rectal surgery.

PROMOTING BOWEL ELIMINATION

No attempt is made to hasten bowel evacuation for the first 2 or 3 days after peristalsis fully returns, but preventive measures are instituted. Fluids are encouraged to 2000 to 3000 ml per day unless contraindicated. Maximal activity is encouraged within the prescribed limits. Bathroom privileges are provided as early as possible.

If there are no results after 3 or 4 days, a mild laxative may help reestablish function. Fruit juices, especially prune juice, may be effective. If these are not effective, a hypertonic (Fleet) enema will usually stimulate defecation. Patient teaching is carried out, particularly for those patients who are discharged early following surgery.

PROMOTING ACTIVITY
PATHOPHYSIOLOGY

Early ambulation is a significant factor in hastening postoperative recovery and preventing postoperative complications. Numerous benefits accrue from the exercise of getting in and out of bed and walking during the early postoperative period (Figure 22-17). Increases in rate and depth of breathing improve ventilation, helping to prevent atelectasis and hypostatic pneumonia. Oxygen intake increases and with the increased circulation more oxygen reaches the brain, increasing mental alertness. Cardiac output increases; more blood flows through the capillaries, providing the wound with substances needed for healing, and venous return is enhanced, decreasing venous stasis. Kidney function is enhanced because of the increased circulation. Activity also promotes micturition.

Metabolism increases as muscles are stimulated, pre-

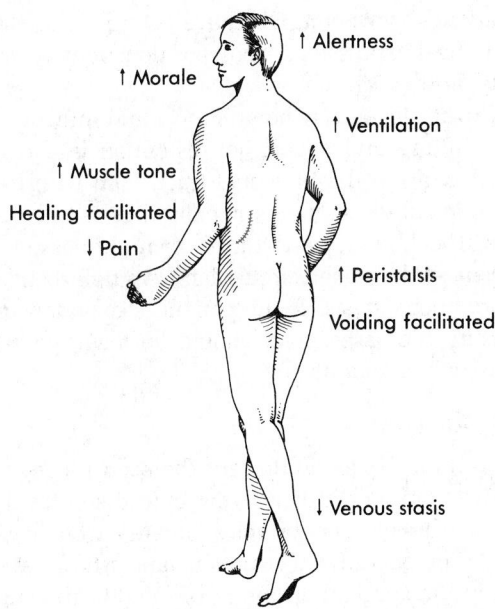

↑ Alertness

↑ Morale

↑ Ventilation

↑ Muscle tone

Healing facilitated

↓ Pain

↑ Peristalsis

Voiding facilitated

↓ Venous stasis

FIGURE 22-17 Benefits from early postoperative ambulation.

POSTOPERATIVE LEG EXERCISES

MUSCLE PUMP EXERCISES
1. Contract calf and thigh muscles
2. Relax leg muscles
3. Rest
4. Repeat at least 10 times

QUADRICEPS DRILL
1. Bend knee with foot flat on bed
2. Straighten leg on bed
3. Lift heel, pressing back of knee against bed
4. Repeat at least 5 times

GLUTEAL TIGHTENING EXERCISES
1. Pinch buttocks together
2. Attempt to move leg to side of bed
3. Relax
4. Repeat at least 5 times

venting loss of muscle tone. Nitrogen loss is decreased, thus helping to restore nitrogen balance. Activity stimulates peristalsis in the gastrointestinal tract, promoting passage of fluids and gas and thus helping to prevent abdominal distention, gas pains, and constipation. Pain is decreased over time as the chemical stimuli are removed through increased circulation, and strained muscles around the incision, neck, back, and legs relax. Morale is also affected as the patient sees function returning. Ambulation is usually contraindicated when there is a severe infection or thrombophlebitis.

Exercises in bed facilitate strengthening of muscle tone. Moving around in bed, if carried out actively by the patient with minimal help, will offer some of the same benefits but to a lesser extent. Moving to different positions also helps prevent tissue ischemia from pressure and pooling of secretions in the lungs.

ASSESSMENT

A postoperative patient who is to get out of bed needs to be alert enough to follow directions. Asking the patient to answer simple questions or to follow simple commands will help to determine the level of alertness.

Assessment of the patient's cardiovascular status includes obtaining baseline pulse and respiratory rate and rhythm. A change in position from supine to sitting or standing may produce orthostatic hypotension. Pulse and respiratory rates will increase as the result of sympathetic stimulation. Pallor and dizziness may be present. Ambulation should not be attempted until the pulse and respirations stabilize at close to their baseline

level. Elderly patients may require additional time to become stabilized.

Muscle strength and sitting ability are assessed (p. 510) before the patient sits or walks for the first time. Sitting ability gives an indication of the patient's ability to maintain balance while ambulating. Preoperative mobility limitations may affect the patient's ability to ambulate postoperatively. The patient with arthritis or arteriosclerosis may take longer to move and to adjust to standing and walking. The patient who used a walker preoperatively will need assistance for a longer time before progressing to using the walker again.

ENCOURAGING ACTIVITY

Muscle-strengthening exercises are encouraged for patients who are not permitted to or who cannot ambulate for a period of time (see the box above). Exercises of the lower extremities will also prevent venous stasis. Bed exercises should be carried out several times a day. If the patient is unable to do active exercises, passive range-of-motion exercises are carried out.

Patients are encouraged to ambulate as soon as permitted. The word *ambulate* means to move from place to place, to walk; sitting in a chair is not considered ambulation. Treatments need not interfere with ambulation. Intravenous fluid bags are hung on movable IV poles. Nasogastric tubes can usually be clamped and disconnected for a short period of time while the patient is walking. Urethral catheters remain connected to closed drainage bags that may be carried or fastened to the inner side of the patient's robe during ambulation.

When patients are permitted out of bed, they are first assisted to sit up on the side of the bed and to dangle the legs over the side to become accustomed to an upright position. Orthostatic hypotension may occur at this time. After the pulse has stabilized and the patient is ready to move, assistance is given to help the patient stand and walk a few steps. Ample space should be available for walking. A weak patient may need two helpers, one to assist the patient and the other to manage the intravenous pole or other equipment. The patient is assisted and supervised in getting out of bed and walking until able to do this without difficulty or danger of injury. Goals can be set to increase the amount walked each day to give the patient something to work for and a sense of achievement.

After ambulating, the patient may sit in a chair if permitted but should be advised to stand and walk at intervals and to elevate the legs while sitting to prevent venous pooling in the extremities. Sitting in a chair for long periods is to be avoided.

PROMOTING COMFORT
POSTOPERATIVE PAIN
Pathophysiology

Pain is a common occurrence after nearly all types of surgical procedures in which there has been cutting, pulling, or manipulating of tissues and organs. Postoperative pain is most severe following intrathoracic, intraabdominal, and major orthopedic surgeries. It may result from stimulation of nerve endings by chemical substances released at the time of surgery or from tissue ischemia caused by interference of blood supply to the part, such as by pressure, muscle spasm, or edema. Trauma to the nerve fibers in the skin produces sharp localized pain. Extensive dissection and prolonged retraction of muscle and fascia produce deep long-lasting pain. Pain originating in the visceral organ may be referred to a distant portion of the body surface or deeply in a different area. It is usually characterized as a deep, aching pain. A hollow visceral organ such as the ureter or bile duct can develop muscle spasms characterized as cramping pain.

Following surgery other factors can add to the pain sensation: pressure from tissue edema, infections, distention, muscle spasms surrounding the incisional area, and tight dressings or casts. Postoperative pain usually lasts 24 to 48 hours but may continue longer depending on the extent of the surgery, the pain threshold of the patient, and response to pain. (See Chapter 16 for a discussion of the pain syndrome.) The presence of pain can prolong convalescence, because it may interfere with return to activity.

Assessment

When the patient complains of pain in the postoperative period, one must not assume that the pain is incisional in nature. It is important to try to ascertain the possible cause of the pain. Subjective data include origin, area involved, nature of the pain, and possible cause from the patient's viewpoint. Objective data include observation of facial expressions, body position, activity, muscle rigidity, and pulse rate.

Pain with fever may be due to wound infection. Pain with vomiting and abdominal distention is a result of gas collecting in the intestinal tract. Pain with fullness about the symphysis pubis is caused by a full bladder. Pain with coldness, paraesthesia, or numbness of a part is a result of decreased circulation from tight bandage or cast or venous stasis. If the patient is experiencing severe pain, the assessment should be made gently and quickly but thoroughly.

Pain Alleviation

It is often impossible to prevent the occurrence of postoperative pain, but it can be minimized so that the patient is relatively comfortable. Patients who have had adequate preoperative instructions and who have confidence in the surgeon, in the nurse, and in the outcome of the surgery usually have less postoperative pain than the apprehensive patient because they have less tension. Measures to reduce anxiety and apprehension will also help reduce and pain that is present.

General measures. If the cause of pain is determined to be other than incisional, measures are taken to relieve the cause. Emptying a full bladder can relieve what was thought to be pain from a lower abdominal incision. Elevation of a part may relieve venous stasis. Loosening of a tight bandage if permissible will relieve ischemic pain.

Incisional pain can be relieved by nursing measures and by analgesics. Spasms and pain from surrounding muscles being continually contracted contributes to incisional pain. Many patients find a position that is tolerable and then hesitate to move for fear of increased pain. Muscles used to hold this position and guard the incision become strained. If the patient understands what is occurring and is helped and encouraged to move frequently, pain will be decreased. Patients with surgery of the trunk should avoid twisting the body; they may be more comfortable if the trunk is moved as one unit. Side rails are helpful for the patient to hold onto when turning over. A limb that has been operated on should be supported. If hands are used for supporting a limb, the broad palms rather than fingers, which dig into painful tissue, are more comfortable for the patient. Pillows serve as useful "splints" during movement of a limb. Autogenic techniques for control of pain, such as the relaxation response technique or deep breathing may be helpful for some patients (see Chapter 16).

Transcutaneous electrical nerve stimulation (TENS). The TENS is a useful adjunct for control of postoperative pain. It is a simple noninvasive method of pain control (see Chapter 16). There are a number of TENS devices on the market, consisting of a battery-powered portable pulse generator about the size of a pocket paging device. This is connected by a pair of cables to electrically conductive tape electrodes placed on either side of the incision after surgery. The TENS delivers a balanced biphasic potential in a wave form.

For relief of postoperative pain, a *high frequency, low intensity* impulse (Table 22-4) appears to be the most effective.[57] The intensity is determined preoperatively on a trial and error basis by the patient who locates a point just below the threshold of discomfort. A tingling sensation may be experienced. The patient can vary the intensity according to the pain level. The best results are obtained when the TENS is used at periodic intervals, such as for a 60-minute period, rather than continuously. It may be helpful to provide stimulation for about 30 minutes prior to painful activities, such as coughing exercises or ambulation.

TENS is not for all patients. Effectiveness appears greater for relief of muscle or bone pain and lesser for poorly localized visceral pain.[57] Patients using TENS require decreased amounts of analgesic medications postoperatively (see research box below, right). TENS has been shown to decrease postoperative complications such as atelectasis[57] by alleviating incisional pain. It permits earlier ambulation and decreases the side effects of narcotics. TENS should not be used with demand cardiac pacemakers or during the first trimester of pregnancy.

Medications. It is usually necessary to administer a narcotic during the first 48 hours after major surgery. The goal is to keep the patient fairly comfortable without overmedication. Analgesics have greater effect if they are administered before pain becomes severe. If severe pain is expected, medication should be offered to the patient at regular intervals within the prescribed limits before it is requested.

One method being used by some hospitals is the administration of narcotics by *patient controlled analgesia* (PCA). The patient receives a predetermined bolus of narcotic intravenously by activating a hand control when pain relief is desired (see Chapter 16). The mech-anism is set to prevent repeated dosages at too frequent intervals. (Usually 10 minutes is required before another dose can be given.) Persons using PCA usually take lower dosages when they can have control over their pain relief.[58]

Another method of administering postoperative narcotics is delivery directly into the epidural or subarachnoid space. This is often performed by an anesthesiologist. Epidural narcotics produce analgesia for 15 to 16 hours without respiratory depression or sympathetic, motor, or sensory disturbances.[59] Epidural analgesia is very effective for major orthopedic surgery of the lower extremities.

Addiction is not a probability when narcotics are given for severe pain during the first few postoperative days. Thus narcotics should not be withheld or delayed by the nurse for fear of patient addiction. Pain is a powerful respiratory stimulant; therefore postoperative narcotics rarely produce respiratory depression.[59] Relief of pain may encourage the patient to move and breathe more deeply, thus preventing postoperative complications. During early ambulation patients receiving meperidine hydrochloride (Demerol) may develop orthostatic hypotension.

The amount of analgesic medication required by patients varies according to age (see research box on p. 524) and type of surgery in addition to the variables related to pain perception and reaction. In general, after the first 48 to 72 hours following most surgeries, pain usually decreases in severity and may be controlled by a less potent analgesic. It is the custom in some hospitals for physicians to write "prn" orders for different analge-

TABLE 22-4 Use of the TENS for postoperative pain relief

Term	Description	Measurement
Pulse width	Duration of the impulse	60-150 μsec
Frequency	Number of impulses delivered	80-100 Hz
Intensity or amplitude	Amount of current delivered	12-20 mamp at 1000 ohm

RESEARCH

Taylor AG et al: How effective is TENS for acute pain? Am J Nurs 83:1171-1174, 1983.

The purpose of this study was to determine the effectiveness of transcutaneous electrical nerve stimulation (TENS) for relief of postoperative pain. A total of 77 post-abdominal surgery patients were placed in 3 study groups: functional TENS unit (FT), sham TENS unit (ST), and usual narcotic analgesic regimen. Patients in both the FT and ST groups were offered medication if the TENS did not provide relief. Patients in both TENS groups showed significantly more pain relief and required significantly less narcotic analgesic than patients treated with narcotics alone. There were no significant differences between the two TENS groups. The authors suggest that this may have been because of placebo effect of the sham TENS that may have stimulated release of endogenous opiates for pain relief in addition to giving patients an increased feeling of control over the pain. Significantly greater physiologic depression as evidenced by decreased patient ambulation and slower return of normal bowel sounds was demonstrated by the group receiving narcotics alone. ∎

RESEARCH

Faherty BS and Grier MR: Analgesic medication for elderly people post-surgery, Nurs Res 33(6):369-372, 1984.

The purpose of this study was to determine if elderly patients receive less analgesic medication postoperatively than do younger patients. A random sample of hospital records of patients experiencing abdominal or pelvic surgery was reviewed. There were seven 10-year age groups (age range 25-107) and a total of 142 subjects (75F, 67M). Data included analgesic medication prescribed and administered for 48 hours postoperatively, and the patient's weight. Older patients were prescribed and were administered less analgesic medication than younger patients. The decreases in mean amounts of analgesic medication were significant after age 55 for prescription and after age 45 for administration. For all subjects, more analgesic medication was prescribed during the first 24 hours than the second, but more analgesic medication was administered during the second 24 hours. Age more than weight was the variable influencing the amount of analgesic medication administered. ■

sics, thus permitting the nurse to select the one that best meets the patient's immediate needs. Some communities do not permit this practice, considering it to be prescription of drugs and therefore not under the legal jurisdiction of nursing.

POSTOPERATIVE VOMITING

Pathophysiology

Nausea and vomiting in the postoperative patient may be related to a number of factors: effect of certain anesthetics on the stomach, decreased peristalsis producing a collection of fluid and gas in the stomach, drinking fluids before peristalsis returns, psychologic factors in patients who anticipate postoperative vomiting, drug idiosyncrasies, pain, or disturbances in electrolyte balance.

Persistent postoperative vomiting is usually a symptom of pyloric obstruction, intestinal obstruction, or peritonitis. Vomiting tires the patient, puts a strain on the incision, and causes excessive loss of fluids and electrolytes. Choking while vomiting may lead to aspiration pneumonia.

Promoting Comfort and Safety

Postoperative vomiting is one of the most distressing problems that a patient encounters. To prevent possible aspiration, the patient who is vomiting should lie on the side. Food and fluid are omitted for several hours, and the patient is advised to lie quietly in bed. The emesis basin and soiled linen are cleaned and changed. Frequent oral care is provided. When vomiting has subsided, and unless contraindicated, sucking on ice chips,

taking sips of ginger ale or hot tea, or eating small amounts of dry solid food may relieve nausea. Antiemetics such as trimethobenzamide hydrochloride (Tigan), prochlorperazine dimaleate (Compazine), or Benzquinamide (Emete-Con) may be administered by injection. Because vomiting can be a sign of drug idiosyncrasy, presence of other side effects should be observed and the pattern of vomiting in relation to administration of drugs noted. Accurate recording of intake and output of fluids and electrolyte balance is important.

HICCOUGHS

Pathophysiology

Hiccoughs interfere with eating and sleeping and are among the most exhausting postoperative complications. The exact cause of postoperative hiccoughs is not known, but it is known that dilation of the stomach, irritation of the diaphragm, peritonitis, and uremia cause either reflex or central nervous system stimulation of the phrenic nerve. Fortunately, hiccoughs are not a common postoperative complaint. They usually disappear within a few hours.

Relief of Hiccoughs

Hiccoughs may be relieved by such a simple measure as having the patient rebreathe carbon dioxide at 5-minute intervals by inhaling and exhaling into a paper bag held tightly over the nose and mouth. Carbon dioxide inhalations, using 5% carbon dioxide and 95% oxygen, may also be ordered for 5 minutes every hour. If dizziness occurs, they should be discontinued because an overdose of carbon dioxide may cause convulsions and coma. Aspiration of the stomach will stop hiccoughs caused by gastric dilation. Chlorpromazine hydrochloride is used to treat mild cases of hiccoughs. If the hiccoughs are persistent and do not respond to these treatments, local infiltration of the phrenic nerve with 1% procaine may be necessary, or in extreme cases surgical crushing of the phrenic nerve may be done.

ABDOMINAL DISTENTION AND GAS PAINS

Pathophysiology

Postoperative distention is a result of an accumulation of nonabsorbable gas in the intestines caused by a reaction to the handling of the bowel during surgery, by swallowing of air during recovery from anesthesia and as the patient attempts to overcome nausea, and by passing of gases from the bloodstream to the atonic portion of the bowel. Distention will persist until the tone of the bowel returns to normal and peristalsis resumes. It is experienced to some degree by most patients after abdominal and renal surgery.

Gas pains are caused by contractions of the unaffected portions of the bowel in an attempt to move the accumulated gas through the intestinal tract.

Assessment

Patients with abdominal distention complain of diffuse abdominal pain. High distention may cause dyspnea by pressure on the diaphragm and may lead to atelectasis. Abdominal girth is increased because of the collection of gas; this can be measured with a tape measure to determine progress. Percussion produces a drumlike (tympanic) sound as compared with a dull sound occurring with ascites or obesity. Acute gastric dilation may produce signs of shock (restlessness; rapid, weak, thready pulse; hypotension) and overflow vomiting. Gas pains in the intestinal tract usually occur as peristalsis is beginning to return, and these can be extremely painful. Bowel sounds are usually audible on auscultation.

Relief of Discomfort

Ambulation is one of the most effective means for stimulation of peristalsis and expulsion of flatus. Dilation of the stomach can be relieved by aspiration of fluid or gas with a nasogastric tube. Hot or cold liquids tend to cause gas buildup and thus should be avoided when peristalsis is sluggish; ice chips do not have the same effect because the water warms before it reaches the stomach.

Exercises can be performed by the patient to help move the gas through the colon to be expelled (see box below). If the exercises are not effective, a rectal tube may be used to stimulate lower colonic peristalsis and permit easy passage of the gas beyond the anal sphincter. A lubricated rectal tube is inserted just past the rectum and left there for 10 to 20 minutes. Heat to the abdomen may be used in conjunction with the rectal tube; heat expands the gas, thus stimulating peristalsis. If these measures fail, a prescribed enema may be given to stimulate peristalsis.

PATIENT TEACHING

During the postoperative period, the patient and family are prepared for care that must be continued at home. Patients are helped to become as self-sufficient as possible before being discharged so that they do not have to depend any more than necessary on the assistance of others.

All treatments to be done at home are taught early enough for the patient or family members to practice the skills while nursing help is available. Previous teaching is reinforced. Written instructions are provided as a resource to be used at home. If dressings are needed, the patient may be given a 48-hour supply for home use unless a family member has already obtained the supplies. Referrals are made to community nurses as needed. Patients who have been under the care of a clinical nurse specialist may be instructed on how to consult the nurse should the need arise.

An appointment is made for a follow-up examination in the surgeon's office or clinic, usually within 1 to 2 weeks after discharge. Following major surgery, most patients are able to return to their usual activities and occupations within 2 to 4 weeks. Normal activities should be resumed gradually; driving is usually permitted after 2 weeks, but the patient should avoid any heavy lifting, pushing, or pulling for at least 6 weeks.

AMBULATORY SURGERY

Many surgeries are performed as outpatient (ambulatory) surgery. Ambulatory surgical centers may be freestanding or may be located at a hospital. Ambulatory surgery is effective for healthy persons requiring uncomplicated surgery. The surgery itself must not require expert postoperative care. The patient receives preoperative testing and instructions before the day of surgery. On the day of surgery the patient reports to the ambulatory surgical center at the assigned time, is prepared for surgery, and is taken to the ambulatory center operating room for surgery. Following surgery, the patient recovers in a postanesthesia room until discharge on the same day. Principles of preoperative and postoperative care are followed as appropriate. Success in ambulatory surgery depends on several factors, including the patient's physical status, preoperative testing and teaching, and the home care support persons.

EXERCISES TO STIMULATE PERISTALSIS FOR PASSAGE OF FLATUS

1. Exercise to Stimulate Movement of Gas from Right to Left Colon[46]
    a. Lie on back with legs extended and pillow under knees
    b. Bend right knee, moving it toward abdomen
    c. Put hands on knee and pull down toward abdomen
    d. Hold position to count of 10
    e. Lower leg slowly
    f. Take two to three slow deep breaths
    g. Repeat action with left leg
    h. Repeat steps *b* through *g* three to four times
2. Pelvic Rock to Stimulate Peristalsis[27]
    a. Lie on back
    b. Exhale slowly while contracting abdominal muscles, simultaneously pressing small of back to bed
    c. Relax and then repeat action several times
3. Abdominal Massage to Help Push Gas Along Colon[46]
    a. Make fists with both hands
    b. Place one fist on lower right abdomen, rolling knuckles upward
    c. Keeping first fist in place, place second fist above it and roll upward
    d. Work hand over hand up to lower edge or ribs, across abdomen, then down left side (following course of colon)

PHYSICAL STATUS

Most ambulatory surgical patients either are healthy or have a mild systemic disease, such as diet-controlled diabetes mellitus, moderate obesity, chronic bronchitis, past myocardial infarction, or mild hypertension. In selected instances persons with a severe systemic disease who are in stable condition may be considered.[61] Persons who are poor risks for ambulatory surgery include those with brittle diabetes mellitus, those with morbid obesity, or those with a systemic disease that places them in constant threat, such as cardiac, pulmonary, renal, hepatic, or endocrine insufficiency.

Old age is not a limiting factor; in fact, many elderly persons have increased benefits from ambulatory surgery versus inpatient surgery. Benefits for the elderly include decreased risk of complications such as pneumonia or infection, increased mental and physical functioning because the environment is less foreign, decreased cost, and maintenance of contacts with family and friends.[9] Additional care requirements may exist for elderly persons, including providing time and attention needed for adjustment.

PREOPERATIVE TESTING

Preoperative screening is performed several days before the date of surgery. The extent of the preoperative testing depends on the nature of the surgery and the patient's physical status. The present trend is based on cost versus benefits; it is moving away from extensive preoperative testing in the absence of data from the medical history and physical examination. The type of anesthesia to be given is discussed with the patient by the physician and anesthesiologist; general, regional, or local anesthesia may be used.

PREOPERATIVE PATIENT TEACHING

Patient teaching is especially important before ambulatory surgery, because the patient must follow any necessary preoperative routines at home and must rely on home support persons for any necessary postoperative care. Most ambulatory surgical centers give booklets to the patient in advance of surgery, providing the necessary instructions and attempting to answer probable questions that patients may have. A telephone number is usually provided in case the patient has additional questions. Some centers follow this up with a preoperative telephone call after the patient has had time to review the instructions.

The minimum preoperative information includes the following:

1. Arrival date and time
2. Clothes to wear
3. Restrictions (food, fluids)
4. Necessity for a responsible person to accompany the patient to and from the surgical center
5. Expected activity in the surgical center
6. Postoperative routines (in center and at home)
7. Type of home support needed

DAY OF SURGERY

Presurgical preparations are usually similar to those of inpatient surgeries, such as removal of loose prostheses, wearing of identification band, presurgical voiding, and preanesthetic medication. The physician and anesthesiologist do a final physical checkup before surgery.

In the postoperative period, patients often are not routinely given medication for postoperative pain, because pain is frequently not severe and because the person must not be sedated or dizzy before leaving for home. Some surgeons administer long-acting local anesthetics to reduce postoperative pain.

Most ambulatory surgical centers have specific criteria that must be met before the patient is discharged. Vital signs must be stable, and the patient must be fully awake. Nausea, vomiting, and dizziness should be absent or at least minimal, and there should be no respiratory distress. The person must be able to swallow and cough, and to ambulate at the preoperative level. Home care instructions are provided in writing and are repeated, preferably with the home caregiver. The patient and caregiver must know what specific signs and symptoms to watch for, what to do if these occur, and the specific person or agency to notify.

CHAPTER SUMMARY

✔ Wounds may heal by regeneration or scarring, depending on the types of cells involved and the presence of underlying structures.

✔ Healing by primary or tertiary intention involves suturing of the incision, immediate or delayed; healing by secondary intention consists of the area being filled in from the bottom.

✔ Wound healing progresses through three overlapping phases: inflammation, proliferation (epithelization, neovascularization, collagen synthesis), and maturation.

✔ Wound healing is delayed in aged persons and those with malnutrition, impaired circulation, increased corticosteroids, diabetes mellitus, foreign bodies, wound infection, and dead space, and in persons receiving radiation therapy.

✔ Excess fluid accumulating in the wound area interferes with oxygen delivery to cells, alters collagen organization, disrupts lymph flow, and creates a dead space, thus delaying healing.

✔ Drains and tubes are used to remove excess fluid from wound areas. Drains remove fluid by gravity or capillary action; suction is used with tubes.

- Complications of wound healing include hemorrhage, infection, and wound separation. Wound dehiscence or evisceration may be prevented by early institution of ventilatory exercises, ambulation, adequate fluid intake, and aseptic technique during dressing changes.

- Nursing interventions in the postanesthetic period include activities to relieve anxiety, maintain airway patency, promote gas exchange, prevent hypotension, identify cardiac arrhythmias, promote fluid balance, prevent injury, and promote comfort.

- Early postoperative patient assessment includes determination of the patient's neurologic, respiratory, circulatory, and urinary status; appraisal of mobility, comfort, and safety; and evaluation of monitoring systems, intravenous fluid flow, dressings and drainage systems.

- The most common postoperative pulmonary complications include atelectasis and pneumonia. Atelectasis refers to collapse of alveoli in the lungs from either obstruction of air passages or progressive regional hypoventilation.

- Persons at high risk for postoperative pulmonary complications are those with increased or dry respiratory secretions, decreased thorax expansion, decreased diaphragm mobility, depressed respiratory center because of drugs, or aspirated gastric contents.

- Measures to prevent postoperative pulmonary complications include instituting ventilatory therapy, positioning and turning the patient, and encouraging activity.

- Measures to prevent postoperative thrombophlebitis include providing elastic stocking for persons at high risk, avoiding pressure on popliteal area or leg massage, and encouraging leg exercises and early ambulation.

- Most fluid lost during surgery is replaced by intravenous infusion until the patient can drink sufficient fluids. Overhydration can occur with vigorous fluid replacement, especially in the small elderly patient.

- Postoperative patients should consume foods high in protein, carbohydrates, and vitamin C for promotion of healing and prevention of weight loss.

- The patient is monitored in the early postoperative period for urinary retention; measures are taken to encourage voiding.

- Constipation is a common postoperative problem resulting from the effects of anesthesia and narcotics, decreased dietary intake, and inactivity. It may be prevented postoperatively by encouraging maximal fluids and ambulation, as permitted, and by providing bathroom privileges as early as possible.

- Early ambulation is a significant factor in hastening postoperative recovery and preventing postoperative complications. Ambulation increases alertness, morale, ventilation, muscle tone, and peristalsis; decreases pain; facilitates voiding and wound healing; and prevents venous stasis.

- Incisional pain may be relieved or modified by medication or TENS, by encouraging position changes and deep breathing or relaxation exercises, and by supporting injured body parts.

- For relief of postoperative pain by TENS, a high frequency, low intensity impulse appears to be the most effective.

- Addiction is not a probability when narcotics are given for severe postoperative pain. In addition, respiratory depression is less likely to occur because pain is a powerful respiratory stimulant.

- Gas pains may be relieved by ambulation, avoidance of very hot or cold liquids, specific exercises or massage to help move the gas, rectal tubes, heat to the abdomen, or enemas.

- Ambulatory surgery is usually performed either on persons who are healthy or on those who may have a mild systemic disease that is under control. Elderly persons may benefit more from ambulatory surgery than inpatient surgery.

- Patient teaching is especially important for ambulatory surgery patients because preoperative preparation and ongoing postoperative care will be done in the home.

QUESTIONS TO CONSIDER

- As you examine a postoperative incision, describe the wound and explain the pathophysiologic process that is occurring at that time.

- Compare the charts of several patients who have had the same type of surgery. In what ways were postoperative needs and nursing care similar or different? What were the reasons for the differences? What conclusions can you draw?

- Role play a patient with an upper abdominal incision on the first postoperative day. Carry out the different types of ventilatory measures. Which methods do you think would most effectively provide the best ventilation of deep alveoli? Imagine that you have had a narcotic for pain and are sleepy; what nursing interventions would help you achieve maximal ventilation?

- Role play the same patient as in question 3. Tape an IV line to your arm. Pretend that you are fatigued and uncomfortable. Walk from a bed to a chair. What type of nursing assistance do you think would be most helpful? What would you say to a patient who did not want to get out of bed and walk? Would your statement encourage you to ambulate in the same situation?

REFERENCES AND SELECTED READINGS

1. American College of Surgeons: Manual of pre- and postoperative care, ed 3, Philadelphia, 1983, WB Saunders Co.
2. *Bray CA: Postoperative pain: altering the patient's experience through education, AORN J 43:672-683, 1986.
3. *Brozenec S: Caring for the postoperative patient with an abdominal drain, Nursing '85 15(4):55-57, 1985.
4. *Burge S et al: How painful are postop incisions? Am J Nurs 86:1263-1265, 1986.
5. *Cahill CA: Yawn maneuver to prevent atelectasis, AORN J 27:1000-1004, 1978.
6. *Carroll PF: Artificial airways: real risks, Nursing '86 16(8):56-59, 1986.
7. *Cerrato PL: What diet does for wound healing, RN 51(6):73-77, 1988.
8. Coleman DL: Control of postoperative pain: nonnarcotic and narcotic alternatives and their effect on pulmonary functioning, Chest 92:520-528, 1987.
9. Crawford FJ: Ambulatory surgery: the elderly patient, AORN J 41:356-369, 1985.
10. *Crocker CG: Acute postoperative pain: cause and control, Orthop Nurs 5(2):11-15, 1986.
11. David JA: Wound Management, Springhouse Pa, 1988, Springhouse Corp.
12. *Deters GE: Managing complications after abdominal surgery, RN 50(3):27-32, 1987.
13. Drain CB: Comparison of two inspiratory maneuvers on increasing lung volumes in postoperative upper abdominal surgical patients, AANA J 52:379-388, 1984.
14. Drain CB and Christoph SS: The recovery room: a critical care approach to postanesthesia nursing, ed 2, Philadelphia, 1987, WB Saunders Co.
15. Equipment: wound care, taking a drain check, Am J Nurs 84:1039-1040, 1984.
16. *Faherty BS and Grier MR: Analgesic medication for elderly people post-surgery, Nurs Res 33:369-372, 1984.
17. *Fay MF: Drainage systems: their role in wound healing, AORN J 46:442-455, 1987.
18. *Flynn ME: Influencing repair and recovery, Am J Nurs 82:1550-1558, 1982.
19. *Fraulini KE and Borchardt AC: Guide to solving postanesthesia problems, Nursing '88(5):66-86, 1988.
20. *Fuchs P: Before and after surgery, stay right on respiratory, Nursing '83 13(5):47-50, 1983.
21. *Greenwood BS: The before and after of good postoperative pulmonary care, Nursing '82 12(12)68-69, 1982.
22. Gruendemann BJ and Meeker MH: Alexander's care of the patient in surgery, ed 8, St Louis, 1987, The CV Mosby Co.
23. Guyton A: Textbook of medical physiology, ed 7, Philadelphia, 1986, WB Saunders Co.
24. Hargreaves A and Lander J: Use of transcutaneous electrical nerve stimulation for postoperative pain, Nurs Res 38(3):159-161, 1989.
25. *Howie JN: How and when should I respond to postop fever? Am J Nurs 89:984-986, 1989.
26. *Hughes JM: Postoperative pulmonary care: past, present, future, Crit Care Q 6(2):67-71, 1983.
27. *Kearns PC: Exercises to ease pain after abdominal surgery, RN 49(7):45-48, 1986.
28. *Keithley JK: A unified approach to assessment of the surgical patient, Am J Nurs 82:612-614, 1982.
29. Kennedy-Caldwell C: The morbidly obese surgical patient, Crit Care Nurse 7(5):87-89, 1987.
30. *Kleinbeck SVM: Simplifying postoperative assessment, AORN J 38:344-348, 1983.
31. Kneedler J and Dodge D: Perioperative patient care, ed 2, Boston, 1987, Blackwell Scientific Publications, Inc.
32. *Kresl JS: Patient-controlled analgesia, AORN J 48:481-487, 1988.
33. *Latz PA and Wyble SJ: Elderly patients: perioperative nursing implications, AORN J 46:238-253, 1987.
34. Lemmink JA: Infection control: when a surgical wound becomes infected, RN 50(9):24-27, 1987.
35. Luce JM: Clinical risk factors for postoperative pulmonary complications, Resp Care 29:484-495, 1984.
36. Marini JJ: Postoperative atelectasis: pathophysiology, clinical importance, and principles of management, Resp Care 29:516-528, 1984.
37. *Matheney NM: Fluid and electrolyte balance: nursing considerations, Philadelphia, 1986, JB Lippincott Co.
38. *McCaffery M: Narcotic analgesia for the elderly, Am J Nurs 85:296-298, 1985.
39. *McConnell EA: After surgery: how can you avoid the obvious and not so obvious hazards, Nursing '83 13(2):74-84, 1983.
40. *Miller KM: Deep breathing relaxation: a pain management technique, AORN J 45:484-488, 1987.
41. *Montanari J: Wound dehiscence, Nursing '86 16(2):33, 1986.
42. Mortenson M and McMullin C: Discharge score for surgical outpatients, Am J Nurs 86:1347-1348, 1986.
43. *Neary JM: Transcutaneous electrical nerve stimulation for the relief of post-incisional surgical pain, AANA J 49:151-155, 1981.

*References preceded by an asterisk are particularly well suited for student reading.

44. *Neuberger GB: Wound care: what's clear, what's not, Nursing '87 17(2):34-37, 1987.

45. *Neuberger GB and Richling JB: A new look at wound care, Nursing '85 15(2):34-41, 1985.

46. *Nichols RR: Simple remedies for postoperative gas pain, RN 49(2):42-44, 1986.

47. Peacock E: Wound repair, ed 3, Philadelphia, 1984, WB Saunders Co.

48. *Robusto N: Advising patients on sex after surgery, AORN J 32:55-61, 1980.

49. Roth RA and Verbridge N: Surgical wound surveillance, AORN J 47:722-729, 1988.

50. Schomburg FL and Carter-Baker SA: Transcutaneous electrical nerve stimulation for post laparotomy pain, Phys Ther 63:188-193, 1983.

51. *Shea M and McCreary M: Early postoperative feeding, Am J Nurs 83:1171-1174, 1983.

52. *Smith CE: Detecting acute abdominal distention: what to look for, what to do. In The Nursing Institute's CE test handbook, vol 3, Hicksville, NY, 1988, Springhouse Corp.

53. Stone HH: Infection in postoperative patients, Am J Med 81(1A):39-44, 1986.

54. *Taylor AG et al: How effective is TENS for acute pain? Am J Nurs 83:1171-1174, 1983.

55. Torrington KG et al: Perioperative respiratory therapy (PORT): a program of preoperative risk assessment and individualized postoperative care, Chest 93:946-951, 1988.

56. Tyler ML: The respiratory effects of body positioning and immobilization, Resp Care 29:477-480, 1984.

57. Warfield CA and Stein JA: Pain relief by electrical stimulation, Hosp Prac 18:207-218, 1983.

58. Warfield CA and Warfield GR: Postoperative analgesia, Hosp Prac 19:85-92, 1984.

59. Way LW: Current surgical diagnosis and treatment, ed 8, Norwalk, Conn, 1988, Appleton & Lange.

60. *Weaver TE: New life for lungs through incentive spirometers, Nursing '81 11(2):54-58, 1981.

61. Wetchler BV: Patient selection criteria for 1987: Ambulatory surgery, AORN J 44:30-36, 1987.

62. *Wound management: update 88, Nursing '88 18(6):33-37, 1988.

63. *Wysocki AB: Surgical wound healing, AORN J 49:502-518, 1989.

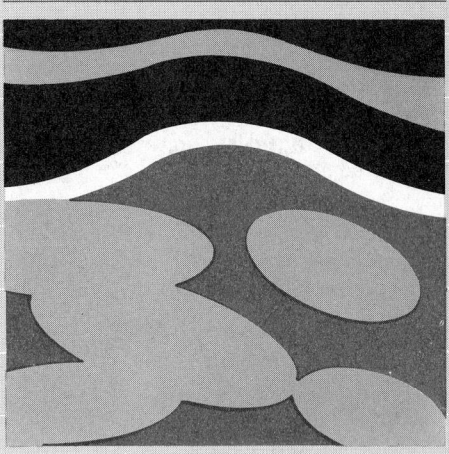

UNIT VI

ALTERATIONS OF FLUID/GAS TRANSPORT

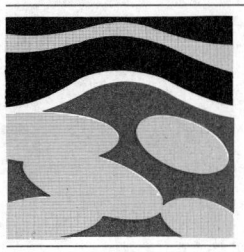

CHAPTER 23

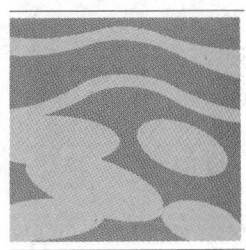

Fluid and Electrolyte Imbalance

MARY KAY LEHMAN
BARBARA SOLTIS
VIRGINIA L. CASSMEYER

CHAPTER OBJECTIVES

After studying this chapter, the student should be able to:
1 Describe the mechanisms for maintaining fluid and electrolyte balance.
2 Describe the mechanisms and effects of fluid deficit and excess.
3 Describe the mechanisms and effects of deficits and excesses of sodium, potassium, calcium, and magnesium.
4 Identify data indicating fluid and electrolyte imbalances.
5 Develop a nursing care plan for a patient with a fluid and electrolyte imbalance.

The body fluids of humans have been described as "a sea within." Like sea water, these fluids are composed of water containing dissolved electrolytes and other substances. The amount and location of the water and its constituents are constantly changing, that is, they are being taken in, used, shifted among compartments, and excreted, but ever maintained in the delicate balance dictated by nature, a dynamic equilibrium. When diseases and their medical or surgical treatments interrupt this healthful state, fluid and electrolyte imbalances occur. These imbalances are manifest as excesses, deficits, or abnormal shifts among body compartments.

This chapter reviews normal fluid and electrolyte balance and describes the causes, prevention, assessment, and management of imbalances of body fluids, sodium, potassium, calcium, magnesium, and hydrogen ions. Each imbalance is discussed separately, although in most instances a disturbance in the balance of one is accompanied by a disturbance in the balance of one or more of the others.

Although a physician prescribes medical therapy to prevent and treat imbalances, nurses must carry out the following vital functions:
1. Recognizing situations likely to cause imbalances
2. Intervening to prevent imbalances

3. Carrying out preventive and therapeutic measures prescribed by the physician and monitoring patients' responses to these measures
4. Recognizing signs and symptoms of fluid and electrolyte disturbances
5. Monitoring patients to prevent and recognize imbalances related to their specific conditions or treatments
6. Alleviating the effects of disturbances on the comfort and safety of patients

MAINTENANCE OF FLUID AND ELECTROLYTE BALANCE

BODY FLUID AND ELECTROLYTE COMPARTMENTS, DISTRIBUTION, AND FUNCTIONS

BODY FLUIDS

Fluid and electrolytes are found in the body either within the cell (*intracellular*) or outside the cell (*extracellular*). The extracellular fluid (ECF) is contained in two compartments: the *interstitial* fluid (fluid between the cells) and *intravascular* fluid (fluid in the blood vessels). A third type of fluid, *transcellular*, denotes fluid separated by a layer of epithelial cells from other ECF.[26] Transcellular fluid includes digestive juices, water, and solutes in the renal tubules and bladder; intraocular fluid; and cerebrospinal fluid. Some authorities consider this to be a part of the extracellular compartment, and others consider it to be a separate compartment. Transcellular fluid makes up 1% to 3% of body weight.

Body water is the largest single constituent of the body, representing 45% to 75% of body weight. The volume and distribution of body water vary with age and sex (Figure 23-1). In the newborn infant, almost three fourths of the body weight is water, with the greatest percentage found in the extracellular compartment. The volume and distribution change over time, and by adulthood in the young male only 60% of body weight is wa-

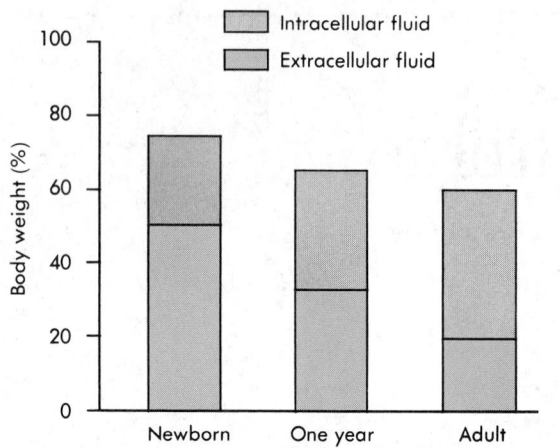

FIGURE 23-1 In newborn, more than half of total body fluid is extracellular. As child grows, proportions gradually approximate adult levels.

TABLE 23-1 Normal electrolyte content of body fluids*

Electrolytes (Anions and Cations)	Extracellular		Intracellular (mEq/L)
	Intravascular (mEq/L)	Interstitial (mEq/L)	
Sodium (Na^+)	142	146	15
Potassium (K^+)	5	5	150
Calcium (Ca^{++})	5	3	2
Magnesium (Mg^{++})	2	1	27
Chloride (Cl^-)	102	114	1
Bicarbonate (HCO_3^-)	27	30	10
Protein ($Prot^-$)	16	1	63
Phosphate ($HPO_4^=$)	2	2	100
Sulfate ($SO_4^=$)	1	1	20
Organic acids	5	8	0

*Note that the electrolyte level of the intravascular and interstitial fluids (ECFs) is approximately the same and that sodium and chloride contents are markedly higher in these fluids, whereas potassium, phosphate, and protein contents are markedly higher in ICF.

ter, and two thirds of this is in the intracellular compartment. In the average young female only approximately 50% of body weight is water. This difference between men and women is caused by an increased amount of fat in women. Fat is essentially water free.

Body water has multiple functions. The extracellular water maintains blood volume and serves as the body's transport system to and from cells. Intracellular fluid (ICF) provides the internal aqueous medium for cellular chemical function. Adequate body water balance is also necessary for the maintenance of normal body temperature and for the elimination of waste products.

ELECTROLYTES

All body fluids contain electrolytes, which are chemical compounds in solution that have the ability to conduct an electrical current. In solution, electrolytes break into charged particles called *ions*. Positively charged ions are called *cations*, and negatively charged ions are called *anions*. Electrolytes are distributed in different concentrations in the intracellular, intravascular, and interstitial compartments (Table 23-1).

The electrolyte quantities given in Table 23-1 are in milliequivalents per liter. A *milliequivalent* is a unit of measurement of chemical activity. It is important to remember that 1 mEq of any specific ion is chemically equal to 1 mEq of any other ion. When electrolytes are measured in milliequivalents, the number of cations equal the number of anions. Electrolytes can also be measured in terms of weight such as in milligrams per 100 ml. When the electrolytes are measured in this way, the number of cations does not equal the number of anions, because the weights are not the same. For example, 1 mEq of hydrogen equals 1 mg of hydrogen, whereas 1 mEq of chloride equals 35.5 mg of chloride;

1 mEq of hydrogen has the same chemical activity as 1 mEq of chloride, but the weights (in milligrams) are different. At times nurses need to be able to make conversions between the two systems of measurement. The box on p. 537 gives the formulas for these conversions.

Transcellular fluids have very distinct patterns of electrolyte concentration. For example, gastric secretions have a high hydrogen ion concentration, pancreatic secretions have a high bicarbonate concentration, and renal tubular and bladder fluids vary on a daily basis. Gastric, pancreatic, and intestinal juices and bile all contain high concentrations of sodium. Although the concentration of electrolytes vary, electrical neutrality is maintained in all fluid compartments; that is, the solution contains equal quantities in terms of chemical activity (milliequivalents per liter) of anions and cations.

Each electrolyte has specific functions. The general functions of all electrolytes are to (1) promote neuromuscular irritability, (2) maintain body fluid volume and osmolality, (3) distribute body water between fluid compartments, and (4) regulate acid-base balance.

OSMOLALITY/OSMOLARITY

Before normal fluid and electrolyte balance are discussed, the terms osmolality and osmolarity need to be defined, even though they are frequently used interchangeably in a discussion of body fluids. *Osmolality* is an expression of the concentration of solution in terms of 1000 g of *water*. Neither the temperature (which can affect volume) nor the amount of solute has an effect on the osmolality of a solution. A 1 osmol solution is made by adding 1 g mole of solute to exactly 1000 g of water. The volume of the solution is then greater than 1 L.

FORMULAS FOR CALCULATING MILLIEQUIVALENT QUANTITY OF AN ION AND OF A SALT FROM WEIGHT (IN MILLIGRAMS) AND CONVERSION BETWEEN MILLIEQUIVALENTS PER LITER AND MILLIGRAMS PER 100 MILLILITERS

CALCULATION OF MILLIEQUIVALENT QUANTITY OF AN ION

$$mEq = \frac{\text{Atomic weight of ion}}{\text{Valence}}$$

CALCULATION OF MILLIEQUIVALENT QUANTITY OF A SALT FROM WEIGHT IN MILLIGRAMS

$$mEq = \frac{\text{Weight in milligrams}}{\text{Atomic weight}} \times \text{Valence}$$

Example: 0.5 g of NaCl = 500 mg; molecular weight of NaCl = 23 (atomic weight of Na^+) + 35.5 (atomic weight of Cl^-) = 58.5; Valence = 1

$$\text{Thus } \frac{500}{58.5} \times 1 = 8.5, \text{ or 500 mg of NaCl}$$

$$= 8.5 \text{ mEq of NaCl}$$

CONVERSION OF MILLIEQUIVALENTS PER LITER TO MILLIGRAMS PER 100 ML

$$mg/100 \text{ ml} = \frac{mEq/L \times \text{Atomic weight}}{10 \times \text{Valence}}$$

CONVERSION OF MILLIGRAMS PER 100 ML TO MILLIEQUIVALENTS PER LITER

$$mEq/L = \frac{mg/100 \text{ ml} \times 10 \times \text{Valence}}{\text{Atomic weight}}$$

Osmolarity is an expression of concentration in terms of 1000 ml of *solution*. Temperature and the amount of solute affect the amount of water in 1000 ml of solution. A 1 osmolar solution is made by placing 1 g mole of solute in a container and then adding water sufficient to make exactly 1 L of solution.

From the above, it can be seen that 1 osmolar solution and 1 osmol solution are not exactly the same. However, if the concentration of solute is small and the temperature is within normal body temperature range, the difference is negligible. This is why the difference between osmolarity and osmolality is negligible in normal body fluids.

NORMAL EXCHANGE OF FLUID AND ELECTROLYTES

In the healthy human, body fluids (water and electrolytes) are constantly being lost and must be replaced to maintain normal processes. The fluid that is lost is not pure water but always contains some electrolytes; thus both water and electrolytes must be replaced daily. By knowing the concentration of fluid and electrolytes in the various compartments, the nurse can anticipate which fluid and electrolyte imbalance will most proba-

TABLE 23-2 Normal fluid intake and loss in an adult consuming 2500 calories per day (approximate figures)

	Intake		Output	
Route	Amount of Gain (ml)	Route		Amount of Loss (ml)
Water in food	1000	Skin		500
Water from oxidation	300	Lungs		350
Water as liquid	1200	Feces		150
		Kidney		1500
TOTAL	2500	TOTAL		2500

bly occur if abnormal losses occur from any particular site.

In a state of health, body fluids are lost daily from the kidneys, lungs, gastrointestinal tract, and skin, with negligible amounts being lost in saliva and tears. Two processes demand continual expenditure of water: control of body heat and excretion of metabolic waste products. The volume of fluid used in these processes depends on such things as external temperature, humidity, metabolic rate, and physical activities. In normal fluid balance the output of fluid equals the intake of fluid. In addition, a balanced diet provides excess amounts of electrolytes; the excess is excreted, and electrolyte balance is maintained.

Table 23-2 summarizes the normal routes of gains and losses of fluid in an adult consuming approximately 2500 calories per day. It should be noted that approximately two fifths of the normal fluid intake is obtained from water in food, or "preformed water." Solid foods such as meat and vegetables are 60% to 90% water. The fact that a large quantity of water is obtained from food has important implications if a person's food intake decreases substantially.

Approximately two fifths of the fluid lost daily is lost through the insensible route (skin, lungs, and gastrointestinal tract). Insensible loss through the skin refers to invisible perspiration. When visible perspiration occurs, such as that following heavy physical activities or with shock, the loss of water through the skin is greater than the normal 500 ml. Fecal loss increases in the presence of diarrhea or watery stools. Persons with certain pulmonary problems lose more than the normal amount of fluid (350 ml) from the lungs. Increased loss of fluids through these insensible routes also results in the loss of electrolytes.

INTERNAL REGULATION OF BODY WATER AND ELECTROLYTES

Fluid and electrolyte balance depends on an adequate intake and output. This means that the intake must equal the output. The control of intake and output is regulated by various internal mechanisms. In this section the regulation of body water and major electrolytes is discussed. The reader is referred to physiology texts for a more in-depth review.

SODIUM AND WATER

Thirst

The major control of actual fluid intake is thirst. The thirst center is located in the ventromedial nucleus of the hypothalamus. Impulses from this center can stimulate the cerebral cortex, which interprets this stimulation as the perception of thirst. The thirst center is stimulated by hypertonic body fluid, isoosmotic contraction, decreased blood pressure, decreased cardiac output, dryness of the mouth, and angiotensin (p. 539). How these factors cause the thirst center to be stimulated is not fully understood. It is thought that the dehydration (shrinkage) of cells in the thirst center causes stimulation of the neurons, which transmit the impulse to the cerebral cortex, which translates the sensation to that of thirst. Most of the time thirst is not thought of as a control of water intake, because social and cultural habits greatly influence the quantity of liquid humans drink. Persons who depend on others to supply their intake of fluid or persons who have a sudden increase in fluid loss (bleeding, increased sweating) will complain of being thirsty. Some evidence suggests that humans also have a salt appetite, which may be important in times of extreme sodium depletion such as with prolonged heat exposure and perspiration.

Kidney

The major organ controlling output is the kidney, which is under the influence of several control mechanisms. The kidney is responsible for regulating the volume and osmolality of body fluids. The osmolality of body fluids depends predominantly on sodium and its associate anions. The maintenance of water and sodium balance depends on glomerular filtration rate (GFR), antidiuretic hormone (ADH), and the aldosterone-renin-angiotensin system.

Glomerular filtration in the kidney is an involved topic (see Chapter 47). Three factors determine glomerular filtration: glomerular capillary blood pressure, Bowman's capsule hydrostatic pressure, and plasma protein concentration. Many factors and pathophysiologic states can affect these three factors and thus change glomerular filtration. Conditions such as shock and hypertension change glomerular capillary blood pressure. Changes in Bowman's capsule pressure can be caused by urinary obstruction. A decrease in plasma protein concentration can occur with increased loss, decreased intake, or decreased production of proteins.

Antidiuretic Hormone

Antidiuretic hormone (ADH) is a hormone produced by the supraoptic and paraventricular nuclei of the hypothalamus and released from the posterior pituitary gland. The neurons in the hypothalamus receive input from volume receptors in the left atrium and great veins and from osmoreceptors in the hypothalamus. Volume receptors are stimulated by changes in atrial blood volume or blood pressure. Impulses from the volume receptors are transmitted by afferent nerve fibers to the hypothalamus. Increased blood volume or increased blood pressure increases the firing of the volume receptors, stimulates the hypothalamus, and inhibits ADH production. Conversely, decreased blood volume or blood pressure decreases the firing of the volume receptors and increases ADH production.

Osmoreceptors are stimulated by changes in cell size. The addition of pure water to the body fluids increases the size of the cells in the osmoreceptors and

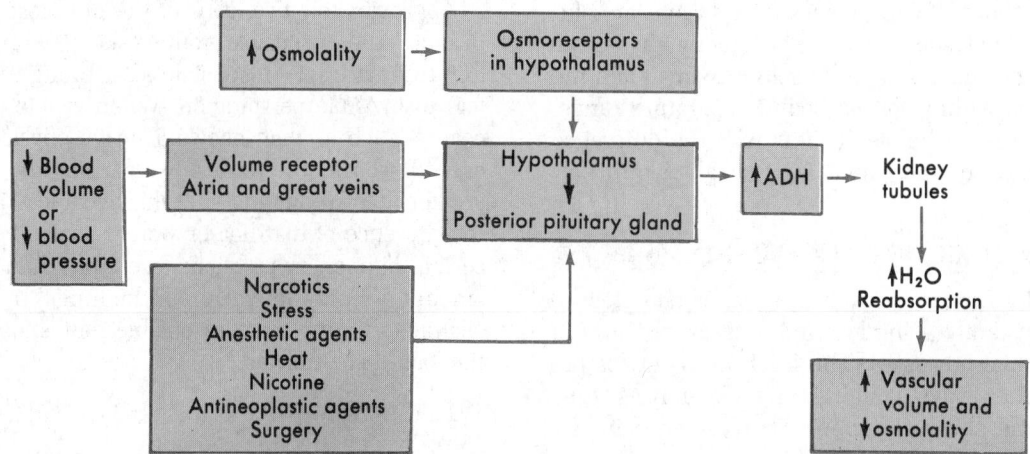

FIGURE 23-2 Factors and mechanisms involved in ADH production, and effect of ADH.

leads to the inhibition of ADH production. A loss of pure water causes the cells to shrink and stimulates the secretion of ADH. ADH secretion is also stimulated by angiotensin, narcotics, stress, heat, nicotine, antineoplastic agents, and anesthetic agents. Figure 23-2 depicts the factors and mechanisms involved in ADH production and the results of ADH production.

ADH acts on the kidney cells by stimulating 3'5'-cyclic adenosine monophosphate (AMP) release, and the cyclic AMP causes appropriate cellular metabolism. In the kidney, ADH causes increased water reabsorption in the distal convoluted tubules and collecting ducts. It also may stimulate the pumping of sodium in the loop of Henle and regulate the rate of blood perfusion, both of which would lead to increased water reabsorption. In the presence of ADH, the kidney can concentrate urine to 1200 mOsm/kg H_2O.

The conservation of water increases blood volume and blood pressure and decreases osmolality. Because ADH can be secreted in response to factors other than a deficit of water (narcotics, anesthetic agents, stressors), fluid overload can occur. Patients who are at high risk of inappropriate ADH secretion need to be monitored closely by the nurse. This includes postoperative patients (see Chapter 22).

Aldosterone-Renin-Angiotensin System

Aldosterone is a hormone produced by the zona glomerulosa of the adrenal cortex. It increases the kidney's reabsorption of sodium and thus water in the proximal tubules and the distal convoluted tubules. In the complete absence of aldosterone a person may excrete 25 g of sodium per day, whereas if large quantities of aldosterone are present no sodium will be excreted.

The major stimulus for aldosterone production is a reflex initiated by the kidney. Cells in the kidney monitor sodium levels and blood volume. When the serum sodium level or the blood volume decreases, the juxtaglomerular cells in the kidney secrete a protein, *renin*. Renin acts on *angiotensinogen*, a plasma protein formed in the liver, to form *angiotensin I*. Angiotensin I is converted to *angiotensin II* by another enzyme. Angiotensin II stimulates the adrenal cortex to secrete aldosterone. Aldosterone causes the retention of sodium by the kidneys, intestines, and sweat and salivary glands. In addition, angiotensin II causes vasoconstriction of arterial smooth muscles, thus decreasing the GFR.

Some aldosterone may be secreted in response to adrenocorticotropic hormone (ACTH). Another important fact is that aldosterone is catabolized by the liver, and with liver failure, because of ineffective catabolism, inappropriate amounts of aldosterone may lead to sodium and water retention. Figure 23-3 depicts the factors and mechanisms involved in aldosterone production and the effects of aldosterone production.

Third Factor

Glomerular filtration, ADH, and the aldosterone-renin-angiotensin system do not explain the kidney's complete control of sodium and water reabsorption and excretion. It is hypothesized that a third factor is involved in the control of sodium and water balance.[28] The term *third factor* is used because little is known about this mechanism. Three other factors seem to assist in the control of sodium and water: (1) a natriuretic hormone, (2) intrarenal physical factors, and (3) redistribution of blood flow. Research is ongoing in these areas.

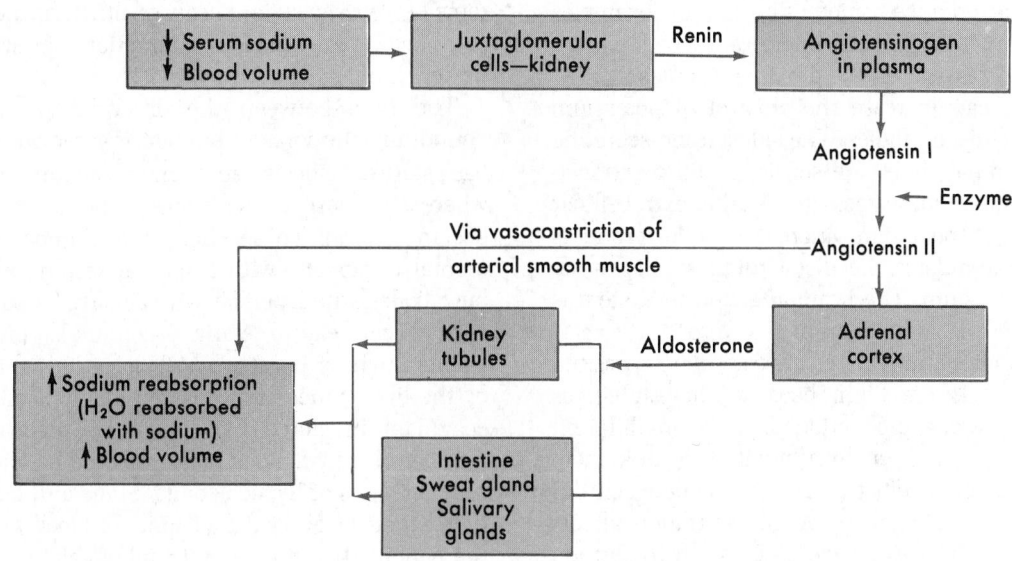

FIGURE 23-3 Factors and mechanisms involved in aldosterone production, and effects of aldosterone production.

POTASSIUM

Potassium (K^+) is the major intracellular cation and regulates *intracellular* osmolality. Potassium is very important in the conduction of nerve impulses and promotion of proper skeletal and cardiac muscle activity. Because of potassium's role in the excitability of nerves and muscles, it is important that the extracellular concentration of potassium be maintained within the normal range.

The major excretion site of excess potassium is the kidney. The majority of excess potassium (80% to 90%) is excreted in the urine, and the remainder is excreted by the gastrointestinal tract. Potassium is completely filtered by the kidney, but most of the filtered potassium is reabsorbed in the proximal tubules and the loop of Henle. Glomerular filtration of potassium plays only a minimal role in normal potassium excretion. The control of renal excretion of potassium resides in the ability of the distal tubular cells to secrete potassium into tubular fluid. As extracellular potassium levels rise, more potassium moves into all cells, including the distal tubular cells. This higher concentration in the cells facilitates potassium secretion into tubular fluid because of the gradient difference between the distal tubular cells and the fluid in the tubular lumen. Conversely, if potassium intake is low or if there is increased loss of potassium through the gastrointestinal tract, the potassium level in the distal tubular cells is decreased. This causes a decrease in the gradient, and less potassium is secreted.

Even though glomerular filtration plays only a minimal role in the amount of potassium excreted in the urine, it is an important point to remember. Certain situations interfere with the reabsorption of the filtered potassium in the proximal tubules, and this can lead to an increased loss of potassium. Osmotic diuretics and disease states that produce osmotic diuresis are examples of situations in which there is interference with the reabsorption of potassium in the proximal tubules.

Aldosterone can increase the amount of potassium secreted by the distal tubules. The aldosterone-secreting cells of the adrenal cortex are sensitive to the extracellular concentration of potassium. If the extracellular concentration of potassium increases, aldosterone is secreted and stimulates the distal tubular cells to secrete more potassium. The renin-angiotensin system is not involved in this stimulation of aldosterone.

It is apparent that a conflict arises when potassium and sodium levels are high, because these changes stimulate aldosterone production to move in different ways. What happens in such a situation is unknown. This is not the only conflict that can arise between different electrolytes. Hydrogen ion concentration affects potassium levels. The existence of a low hydrogen ion concentration increases potassium excretion and leads to potassium depletion (hypokalemia). The presence of a high hydrogen ion concentration decreases potassium excretion and can cause potassium excess (hyperkalemia).

Factors Influencing Distribution

Calcium (Ca^{++}) plays a major role in the promotion of neuromuscular irritability and muscular contractions. Calcium and phosphorus are found primarily in the bones and teeth (99%) and dissolved in the blood (1%). The amounts of dissolved calcium and phosphorus are in an inverse relationship. As one increases, the other decreases. The inverse relationship must be maintained because if both are elevated at the same time, they form an insoluble precipitate. The dissolved portion of calcium is carried in the blood in two forms: bound to protein, particularly albumin, and ionized. The serum levels that are usually reported are measures of total dissolved calcium (both bound and ionized). The ionized fraction can be measured separately, but this is a more expensive test and is not routinely done. Only the ionized fraction is involved in the promotion of neuromuscular activity.

The ionized portion must be maintained within fine limits because a decrease in ionized calcium has profound effects on the body such as *tetany* (p. 556). In a person with normal serum protein and albumin levels and a normal calcium level, the ionized fraction is usually a little greater than 50% of the total dissolved level. Because part of the dissolved calcium is bound to protein, the concentration of serum calcium varies as the protein level varies. If the total protein and albumin levels fall, the total serum calcium level will fall. Persons with serum calcium levels below normal resulting from a decrease in protein or albumin may exhibit no symptoms of *hypocalcemia*, because, although their total calcium level is low, the ionized fraction may still be within normal limits.

The ratio between the dissolved calcium that is bound and the ionized fraction is affected by the acid-base status. Acidosis causes more calcium to be ionized, whereas alkalosis causes more of the ionized fraction to become bound. These changes are probably not detrimental to persons with a normal serum calcium level, but alkalosis in a person who already has a low serum calcium can lead to tetany. Calcium also binds to other agents such as citrate, which is normally metabolized by the liver. Since citrate is commonly used as an anticoagulant in stored blood, persons receiving a large number of transfusions rapidly should be watched carefully for signs of hypocalcemia. Some authorities recommend that for every 3 to 4 units of blood given rapidly, the patient should receive 10 ml of calcium gluconate.[8]

Control of Calcium Levels

The level of calcium depends on three hormones: parathormone, vitamin D, and calcitonin. *Parathormone* is a hormone produced by the parathyroid gland, and decreased calcium levels stimulate its production. Parathormone causes increased movement of calcium from the bone, increased absorption of calcium from the gastrointestinal tract, and increased reabsorption of calcium in the renal tubules, all of which lead to an increase in serum calcium levels. Parathormone also increases the excretion of phosphorus by the kidneys.

Vitamin D is a hormone that is formed by the action of sunlight on a provitamin that is present in the skin or is obtained from dietary sources. Vitamin D is hydroxylated by reactions in the liver and kidney to its active form. Vitamin D is essential for the absorption of calcium from the gastrointestinal tract. Parathormone cannot increase the absorption of calcium from the gastrointestinal tract unless activated vitamin D is present. Vitamin D significantly increases the effectiveness of parathormone in bone resorption. In addition, vitamin D and parathormone are interlinked in another way. The major control point for the blood concentration of active vitamin D is the hydroxylation step in the kidney, which is stimulated by parathormone. Therefore a low calcium level stimulates the secretion of parathormone, which then activates vitamin D; both then increase the absorption of calcium from the gastrointestinal tract and the resorption of calcium from the bone.

Calcitonin, a hormone produced by the thyroid gland, decreases calcium levels by preventing bone resorption of calcium. It opposes the effects of parathormone and vitamin D on bones. High calcium levels stimulate the thyroid gland to release calcitonin, which inhibits the release of calcium from the bone and thus lowers serum calcium levels.

MOVEMENT OF FLUIDS BETWEEN COMPARTMENTS

The preceding discussion has referred to the fact that water and solutes are in various compartments. The water and solutes in these compartments are not static but are constantly moving between compartments. Movement of water and solutes is how needed materials are carried to and waste products removed from the cells.

FLUID AND SOLUTE TRANSPORT BETWEEN EXTRACELLULAR AND INTRACELLULAR COMPARTMENTS

Fluids and electrolytes flow between the extracellular and intracellular compartments by passive or facilitated diffusion, osmosis, and active transport. Some electrolytes and other solutes flow between the two compartments with a concentration gradient by the process of passive or facilitated *diffusion.* For other solutes to move into the cell, they must flow against a concentration gradient by *active transport.* Active transport is not

well understood, but it implies that solutes are moving against a concentration gradient or an electrical potential gradient. The mechanism involves the expenditure of energy. It has been shown that with the expenditure of one high-energy phosphate bond from adenosine triphosphate (ATP), three sodium ions move out of the cell, and two potassium ions move into the cell. Active transport uses a large percentage of the energy formed each day, because sodium is constantly diffusing into the cell and potassium is constantly diffusing out of the cell. Active transport is required to keep the concentration of the two electrolytes in the appropriate amounts within the cell.

Water, like solutes, moves between the extracellular compartment and the intracellular compartment. The movement of water is controlled by the osmolality of the two compartments. Sodium is the main regulator of extracellular osmolality, and potassium is the main regulator of intracellular osmolality.

Water moves from an area of high concentration of water (low concentration of solutes) to an area of low concentration of water (high concentration of solutes). This process is called *osmosis.* The movement of water will continue until the osmolality between the two compartments is approximately equal. Therefore if the water content increases in the extracellular compartment or the solute concentration decreases in the extracellular compartment, water moves into the cells to equalize the osmolality. Likewise, if the water content decreases in the extracellular compartment or the solute concentration increases in the extracellular compartment, water moves from the cells to equalize osmolality. Solutes move back and forth between the two compartments, but the cell membrane is more permeable to water than it is to solutes.

The mechanisms that control water and sodium levels control osmolality and thus the movement of fluid between the extracellular compartment and the intracellular compartment. Various disease states can change the osmolality and cause cellular edema or cellular dehydration.

FLUID TRANSPORT BETWEEN VASCULAR AND INTERSTITIAL SPACES

The control of fluid movement between the vascular and interstitial spaces is governed by Starling's law of the capillaries. Two different types of pressure influence the flow of fluid between the vascular space and the interstitial space. These are hydrostatic pressure and colloid osmotic pressure (oncotic pressure). *Hydrostatic pressure* is that pressure caused by the blood pressing against the walls of the blood vessels. Hydrostatic pressure also exists in the tissue but is minimal (5 torr or less), and some authorities believe that the hydrostatic pressure in the tissue is actually a negative pressure.[10]

Hydrostatic pressure effectively pushes fluid out of the vascular bed into the interstitial space.

Colloid osmotic pressure is the pressure needed to overcome the pull of the proteins, especially albumin, in the blood. The proteins do not pass freely through the walls of the capillaries because of their size. A few proteins are present in the interstitial space, but a much larger concentration is in the vascular space. The colloid osmotic pressure within the vascular space serves as a force to *pull* or *absorb* fluid from the interstitial space.

The difference between the vascular hydrostatic pressure and the vascular colloid osmotic pressure determines the movement of fluid between the vascular and interstitial spaces. For example, in Figure 23-4, the tissue hydrostatic pressure and tissue colloid osmotic pressure would be zero. The hydrostatic pressure at the arteriole end of the capillary (approximately 40 torr) is greater than the hydrostatic pressure at the venule end of the capillary (approximately 10 torr). The colloid osmotic pressure stays approximately the same throughout the vascular bed and equals about 25 torr.

The difference between the hydrostatic pressure and colloid osmotic pressure at the arteriole end of the capillary is +15 torr (40 torr − 25 torr = 15 torr) and favors the movements of fluid out of the vascular compartment. The difference between the hydrostatic pressure and colloid osmotic pressure at the venule end of the capillary is −15 torr (10 torr − 25 torr = −15 torr) and favors the movement of fluid into the vascular compartment (Figure 23-4).

Overall, this system allows fluids high in nutrients and oxygen to diffuse out of the vascular bed at the arteriole end of the capillary and fluids containing waste products to move back into the vascular bed at the venule end of the capillaries. The system is not perfect, however, and some excess fluid is left in the interstitial

space. In addition, some proteins may escape from the vascular bed and, if allowed to accumulate, act as a force to pull even more fluids from the vascular bed. The lymphatic system picks up the excess fluid and the escaped proteins and returns them to the vascular space.

Multiple factors affect the hydrostatic pressure. At the arteriole end of the capillary, the hydrostatic pressure depends on the volume of blood, viscosity of the blood, force of the heart, and resistance of the blood vessels. Hydrostatic pressure at the venous end depends on the venous pressure. The venous pressure in turn depends on the condition of the veins, respiration, and skeletal muscle contractions. The colloid osmotic pressure depends on the protein level, which depends on the dietary intake, the liver's ability to produce proteins, and the fact that excess proteins are not lost from the body. Various disease states can interfere with any of these multiple factors and result in edema. Damage to the lymphatic system can also cause edema.

FLUID IMBALANCE

As previously noted, the osmolality of the ECF varies proportionally with its sodium concentration. Sodium and its anions (chloride and bicarbonate) make up 90% to 95% of the total solute in the ECF. When a change occurs in the sodium-to-water ratio, a disturbance in osmolality results; that is, the ECF becomes more dilute (*hyposmolar*) or more concentrated (*hyperosmolar*) than normal. A considerable change in the concentration of solutes other than sodium in the ECF can also cause osmolar disturbances.

Hyposmolality of the ECF causes water to move into body cells by osmosis to equalize the concentration of fluid on both sides of the cell membrane. Hyperosmola-

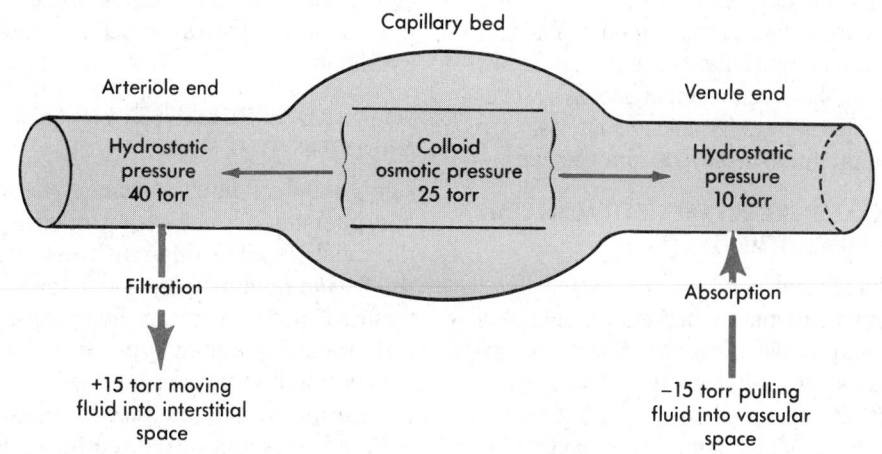

FIGURE 23-4 Pressure difference across capillary provides for movement of fluid, nutrients, and waste between interstitial and vascular space.

TABLE 23-3 Water and sodium imbalances

Osmolar Imbalances				Isotonic Volume Imbalances	
Hyperosmolar		Hyposmolar		Volume Excess	Volume Deficit
Water deficit: water ↓ in relation to sodium and other solutes	Sodium or solute excess: sodium or other solutes ↑ in relation to water	Water excess: water ↑ in relation to sodium and other solutes	Sodium deficit: sodium ↓ in relation to water	ECF volume excess (edema): water and sodium ↑ proportionally	ECF volume deficit: water and sodium ↓ proportionally

lity of the ECF causes water to move out of the cells to dilute the ECF and to equalize the concentration of solutes in both compartments.

When there are changes in the volume of ECF but no change in osmolality, an *isotonic* volume disturbance results. There is no significant change in the sodium-to-water ratio; sodium deficits or excesses are accompanied by proportional water deficits or excesses. There is no appreciable movement of water between the ICF and ECF compartments, and the imbalance is essentially restricted to the ECF compartment. Table 23-3 shows the types of fluid imbalances that are likely to occur.

HYPEROSMOLAR IMBALANCE: EXTRACELLULAR WATER DEFICIT AND SOLUTE EXCESS

An extracellular water deficit occurs when the amount of water in the extracellular compartment is diminished in proportion to the solutes contained therein. An increase in solutes in proportion to water produces the same imbalance, known as hyperosmolar or hypertonic imbalance, in which the serum osmolality is above the normal 275 to 290 mOsm/kg. Dehydration is often used to describe any type of volume depletion; however, the precise definition of dehydration is water loss without electrolyte loss.

ETIOLOGY

Imbalances may originate in either the fluid or the solute portion of the ECF. There may be (1) decreased intake of water, (2) excess loss of water without proportional loss of solutes, (3) increased solute intake without sufficient water, and (4) excess accumulation of solutes secondary to a particular disease condition.

Any person who does not have fluids available to drink, who cannot take fluids independently, or who does not respond to thirst is likely to develop a water deficit.

In a disaster such as a flood or an earthquake, a supply of drinkable water or fluids may not be available and would lead to a water deficit. Patients who are unable to ask for fluids, to identify their need for fluid, or to swallow easily may develop a fluid deficit. Thus a patient

with a cerebral vascular accident and aphasia may not be able to communicate a desire for fluids or may have difficulty swallowing fluids that are offered. A confused or disoriented patient may not be aware of thirst. Patients who are comatose, weak, or catatonic may also develop fluid deficits because of the inability to ask for fluids, swallow, or respond to thirst.

Although loss of body water is usually accompanied by loss of electrolytes, there are a number of conditions in which water is lost in excess of electrolytes. These include increased loss through the lungs in hyperventilation or in secretions from a tracheostomy, through the skin with a high fever, through the gastrointestinal tract when there is watery diarrhea, or in urine when the kidneys fail to concentrate solutes.

PREVENTION

Prevention is crucial in the nursing care of patients who are at risk of developing a water deficit. The nurse is alert to those patients who may not be receiving adequate fluid intake, monitors their intake and output, and plans a schedule for offering fluids to them. Patients who are hyperventilating for long periods of time, regardless of the reason, should have their fluid intake increased somewhat, because they are losing more fluid than usual through the lungs. Those receiving high-protein tube feedings need sufficient water to prevent osmotic diuresis and water deficit.

PATHOPHYSIOLOGY

When solutes are taken in without sufficient water, (such as occurs with intake of tube-feeding solutions that are high in protein, dextrose, and electrolytes), hyperosmolality results. The excess of solutes causes an *osmotic diuresis*, that is, the body's attempt to excrete a solute load through the kidneys by excreting a large volume of urine. Formation of the urine in this process requires the use of a great deal of water, interferes with the normal water conservation mechanisms, and results in a water deficit.

Several conditions lead to endogenous (internal) addition of excess solutes—large amounts of glucose can accumulate in the blood in diabetes mellitus, and glucose and ketone bodies can accumulate in the blood in diabetic ketoacidosis (see Chapter 37). A large volume of nitrogenous waste products results from metabolism of a high-protein diet. All of these solute excesses cause large water losses from osmotic diuresis.

When an extracellular water deficit occurs, water moves out of the cells to replace water lost from the extracellular compartment, thus maintaining an adequate circulating blood volume. If the water deficit is not corrected, the cells eventually become unable to compensate for extracellular losses; cellular dehydration ensues, and circulation begins to fail. As both ICFs and ECFs decrease, cell function is impaired, because food, oxygen, and waste products are diffused inadequately. Brain cells are particularly sensitive to these changes, and a disruption of brain cell function develops, manifested as mental changes in the patient.

CLINICAL MANIFESTATIONS

Thirst and weight loss are early symptoms of water deficit and become more pronounced as the deficit increases. Body temperature begins to rise as less water is available for temperature regulation. When cells are unable to continue providing water to replace ECF losses, signs of collapse of the circulatory system appear. A dry mouth and throat cause difficulty with speech. Signs and symptoms of water deficit are shown in Table 23-4.

INTERVENTIONS

Goals of therapy are to treat the underlying causes to prevent further water loss and to replace lost fluid.

TABLE 23-4 Signs and symptoms of water deficit

	Moderate Deficit	Severe Deficit
Skin	Flushed, dry	Cold, clammy
Mouth	Dry mucous membranes	Dry, cracked tongue
Eyes	Decrease in tears	Soft, sunken eyeballs
Cardiovascular system	—	Tachycardia, low blood pressure, rapid respirations
CNS	Apprehension, restlessness	Lethargy, coma
Blood	—	Hemoconcentration, increase in hematocrit, BUN, electrolytes
Urine	High specific gravity, scant amount (except with osmotic diuresis)	Oliguria, highly colored urine
Other	Thirst, weight loss	Thirst, weight loss, fever

The physician can use several methods, such as those based on serum sodium concentration or change in the patient's weight, to calculate the volume of water loss.[9] For instance, if a patient has lost 4 kg of body weight, the fluid deficit equals 4 L (1 kg weighs 1 L). Therapy will require replacement of the volume lost plus about 1.5 L of fluid to supply current daily need. Often the replacement is administered over a period of several days, because too rapid infusion of fluid may cause sudden intercompartmental shifts of water and pulmonary edema.

When the water deficit is not severe, fluids can be replaced orally if the patient is able to drink fluids. Otherwise, intravenous fluids are given.

Intravenous glucose and water are usually given first to replace the water loss and increase urinary flow. Urinary output must be adequate so that electrolytes in excess of body needs can be excreted. Solutions containing electrolytes are therefore not given until renal function is established. Normal saline or half-strength saline (0.45%) can be given with other ions—potassium, calcium, and lactate—as needed.

In addition to providing fluids and participating in the treatment of conditions underlying water loss, nurses use measures to decrease discomfort and ensure patient safety. *Mouth care* is especially important to relieve dryness of mucous membranes and remove debris on lips and teeth. Safety measures such as side rails on beds are necessary for patients who have developed restlessness, confusion, lethargy, or other mental changes as a result of water deficit. Monitoring intake and output and changes in the patient's weight and vital signs will indicate whether the patient's condition is improving or deteriorating.

A state of adequate hydration is evidenced by mental alertness, moist mucous membranes, and urinary output that is approximately equal to fluid intake.

HYPOSMOLAR IMBALANCE: WATER EXCESS OR WATER INTOXICATION

When there is an excess of water in relation to solutes in the ECF, a hyposmolar (hypotonic) imbalance known as *water excess* or *water intoxication* (cellular edema) exists. Although this imbalance is not common, it can develop when water intake exceeds the ability of the kidneys to excrete it. Usually there is a concomitant increase in secretion of ADH, which promotes water retention and aggravates the water excess.

Under normal conditions, a decrease in osmotic pressure suppresses ADH production and permits free water to be excreted by the kidneys.

ETIOLOGY

One or more of the following conditions exists when water intoxication develops: (1) excess intake of electrolyte-free fluid, (2) increased secretion of ADH, or (3) decreased or inadequate output of urine.

Water excess can be caused by ingestion of large amounts of tap water, a behavior called *psychogenic polydipsia*. The ingestion of frequent sips of tap water by one who is not able to tolerate food or other fluids because of illness can also lead to water excess. Some treatments that lead to excessive water intake are multiple tap water enemas and absorption of water from irrigating solutions during transurethral resection of the prostate gland.

Excess or inappropriate secretion of ADH occurs in response to stressors, drugs, and anesthetics. It can also accompany inflammatory conditions of the lung (tuberculosis, pneumonia) and brain (encephalitis, meningitis), endocrine disturbances, and tumors in the lungs (especially oat cell carcinoma), pancreas, duodenum, and other body organs.[8] Inadequate kidney function or renal failure potentiates the development of water excess.

A low serum sodium or sodium deficit can also produce a hyposmolar imbalance. This condition is discussed under "Sodium deficit" (p. 550).

PREVENTION

Water intoxication can be anticipated by identifying patients who present one or more risk factors. Daily weights and careful monitoring of intake and output will help to detect the problem before it becomes severe.

PATHOPHYSIOLOGY

When water intoxication occurs, hyposmolar water excess in the extracellular compartment quickly becomes an *intracellular water excess*. A lesser concentration of solutes is present in the ECF as compared to that in the ICF; therefore water moves into the cells to equalize concentration on both sides of the cell membranes, causing the cells to swell.

CLINICAL MANIFESTATIONS

Since brain cells are particularly sensitive to the increase in intracellular water, the most common signs are manifestations of changes in the patient's *mental status*.

In acute water intoxication, there is swelling of the cells, which may develop rapidly and dramatically. Signs of water intoxication are listed in the box above.

When the condition develops more slowly, there may be apathy, sleepiness, anorexia, nausea, and vomiting. A low serum sodium concentration is a usual finding.

INTERVENTIONS

The primary intervention for water intoxication is water restriction. In severe cases of hyposmolarity, when the serum sodium is critically depressed(<116 mEq/L), ad-

---

SIGNS OF ACUTE WATER INTOXICATION

Changes in behavior: confusion, incoordination, convulsions
Hyperventilation
Sudden weight gain
Warm, moist skin
Increased intracranial pressure: slow bounding pulse with an increase in systolic and decrease in diastolic blood pressures
Peripheral edema, usually not marked

---

ministration of furosemide (Lasix) and infusion of 3% to 5% hypertonic saline may be used. The saline raises the sodium level, while the diuretic causes water loss. Administration of saline without diuretics does not maintain the sodium level because sodium will continue to be excreted by the kidneys. Furosemide inhibits some of this urinary sodium excretion and assists in preventing hypervolemia.

During treatment, hourly intake and output measurements are necessary. Infusions should be given by use of a controlled infusion device to prevent too rapid administration. Daily body weight, serum sodium levels, and neurologic status should also be assessed.

Providing for the safety of patients with this imbalance is a priority nursing function, because of the confusion and other mental changes that occur. Any patient who is receiving a large amount of water orally, rectally, or intravenously should be monitored carefully for signs of water intoxication, especially if a condition of excess ADH prevails.

ISOTONIC VOLUME DEFICIT: EXTRACELLULAR FLUID DEFICIT

Conditions causing a loss of water together with a loss of electrolytes lead to *isotonic volume deficit*, also known as *ECF depletion*.

ETIOLOGY

Water and electrolytes are lost in hemorrhage and profuse sweating. About 8 L of fluid circulate through the gastrointestinal tract per day (Table 23-5). These fluids are derived from the ECF; therefore vomiting, diarrhea, draining intestinal fistulas, and surgical openings such as ileostomy and cecostomy result in ECF loss. Severe losses can deplete the extracellular compartment rapidly.

PREVENTION

Nurses are responsible for identifying and monitoring patients at risk of developing isotonic fluid deficit. Taking postural vital signs is one method used to detect this deficit before cardiovascular symptoms develop. *Pos-

TABLE 23-5 Fluid composition of total internal secretions*

	Approximate ml of Fluid (Daily)
Saliva	1500
Gastric juice	2500
Intestinal juice	2000
Pancreatic juice	1500
Bile	500
TOTAL	8000 ml/24 hr

*Note that approximately 8 L of fluid are used daily for digestive purposes. Normally, most of this fluid is reabsorbed. Some of each of the ions found in blood plasma is present in each of the fluids listed, but the individual concentration varies with each fluid.

tural vital signs are the comparison of a person's blood pressure and pulse measured from a lying position to a sitting or standing position. A drop in blood pressure of 10 torr or more with an increase in pulse rate indicates postural hypotension and signals a state of isotonic fluid depletion.

The healthy person who is perspiring profusely needs extra dietary salt and should drink extra fluids. Patients on low-sodium diets and those with draining gastrointestinal fistulas are prone to develop sodium depletion. They should always be taught to increase their salt intake slightly whenever they perspire profusely. Patients who have hot packs applied to large areas of the body also lose sodium and water, although the loss may not be readily noticeable as perspiration. Attention to ingesting more salt and water than usual in situations of excessive heat may prevent heat exhaustion.

PATHOPHYSIOLOGY

In isotonic volume deficit, the extracellular osmolality does not change, because sodium, the chief contributor to extracellular osmolality, is lost along with water. Consequently, water content of the cells is not affected, and the deficit remains restricted to the extracellular compartment. Fluid movement is from the extracellular compartment to outside the body, depleting vascular and interstitial volumes.

CLINICAL MANIFESTATIONS

The most prominent signs of volume depletion manifest in the cardiovascular system. Following is a list of the symptoms of ECF depletion:

1. Skin: poor turgor
2. Mouth: dry mucous membranes
3. Cardiovascular: postural hypotension (early), low blood pressure, tachycardia, increased respiration, decreased vein filling
4. Weight: loss
5. Urine: low output, increased specific gravity

INTERVENTIONS

Treatment consists of identifying and correcting the underlying cause to prevent further fluid and electrolyte loss and of replacing those fluids and electrolytes that have been lost. Hemorrhage must be controlled. Vomiting may be treated with antiemetics such as trimethobenzamide hydrochloride (Tigan) and prochlorperazine (Compazine), and diarrhea with antidiarrheal drugs, that is, diphenoxylate (Lomotil), paregoric, and kaolin and pectin (Kaopectate).

Any patient who is losing body fluids through perspiration, fever, or loss of gastrointestinal fluid should be given salty fluids to drink. Meticulous mouth care relieves the discomfort of dry mucous membranes.

As blood volume decreases, postural hypotension develops, and the patient's safety may be threatened by the resultant weakness, dizziness, or fainting on standing upright. Loss of fluid through a tracheostomy can be minimized with humidity therapy.

ISOTONIC VOLUME EXCESS: EXTRACELLULAR FLUID EXCESS AND EDEMA

If there is an excess of body water with a concomitant increase in sodium, the excess fluid will be retained in the *extracellular* compartments and lead to the formation of edema. *Edema* is the accumulation of fluid in the interstitial spaces.

ETIOLOGY

Edema can be produced by any of the following: increase in capillary fluid pressure, decrease in capillary oncotic pressure, increase in interstitial oncotic pressure, and any condition that increases the amount of aldosterone circulating in the blood. Causes of edema with clinical examples are shown in Table 23-6.

PREVENTION

The possibility of overhydration is considered whenever intravenous fluids are being given and during planning of "forced fluid" regimens. Persons with renal or circulatory impairment can easily be overhydrated. Usually such persons must restrict fluid and sodium intake.

Patients on a low-sodium diet need to know which foods to avoid. They should read labels on all prepared foods, because many contain large amounts of sodium, and they may need assistance in planning ways to adhere to fluid restriction. When medications are prescribed to be taken at home, patients are taught the purpose of each drug and its usual side effects. They should also record the fluid taken with medications, monitor their weight daily, and notify the physician if there is a significant change.

TABLE 23-6 Causes of edema according to underlying physiologic mechanism

Fluid Pressure	Oncotic Pressure
INCREASED CAPILLARY FLUID PRESSURE **Increased Venous Pressure**	**DECREASED CAPILLARY ONCOTIC PRESSURE** **Loss of Serum Protein**

Vein obstruction
  Varicose veins
  Thrombophlebitis
  Pressure on veins from casts, tight bandages, or garters
Increased total volume with decreased cardiac output
  Congestive heart failure
Fluid overloading
	Burns, draining wounds, fistulas
	Hemorrhage
	Nephrotic syndrome
	Chronic diarrhea

	Decreased Intake of Protein
	Malnutrition Kwashiorkor
Sodium and Water Retention, Increased Aldosterone	**Decreased Production of Albumin**

Decreased renal blood flow
  Congestive heart failure
  Renal failure
Increased production of aldosterone
  Cushing's syndrome
Aldosterone added to system
  Corticosteroid therapy
Inability to destroy aldosterone
  Cirrhosis of liver
	Liver disease

	INCREASED INTERSTITIAL ONCOTIC PRESSURE **Increased Capillary Permeability to Protein**

	Burns
	Inflammatory reactions
	  Trauma
	  Infections
	Allergic reactions (hives)

	Blocked Lymphatics: Decreased Removal of Tissue Fluid and Protein
	Malignant diseases Surgical removal of lymph nodes Elephantiasis

PATHOPHYSIOLOGY

According to Starling's law of the capillaries (p. 551), an equilibrium exists between the forces filtering fluid out of the capillary and the forces absorbing fluid back into the capillary (see Figure 23-4). Three changes that can alter this equilibrium and lead to increased interstitial fluid (edema) are (1) an increase in capillary fluid pressure, (2) a decrease in capillary colloid osmotic (oncotic) pressure, or (3) an increase in interstitial oncotic pressure.

Increased Capillary Fluid Pressure

Increase in capillary fluid pressure results from the overloading of the vascular compartment. The high pressure pushes fluid out of the vessels into the surrounding interstitial tissues. More important, if the increase in hydrostatic pressure is great enough, large amounts of fluid will be pushed across the alveolar-capillary membrane into the alveoli of the lungs. *Pulmonary edema* can occur unless this process is reversed.

Overloading of the vascular system may be caused by giving too much fluid within a short period of time to a person who, because of circulatory or renal disease, cannot dispose of the surplus. Elderly people tolerate increases in blood volume very poorly, because with in-

elastic vessels only relatively small increases in volume are needed to markedly increase the hydrostatic pressure. Monitoring the central venous pressure (see Chapter 26) is one method used to determine if overloading is occurring. Retention of sodium and water, which occurs in cardiac and renal dysfunction, is one of the most common causes of increased vascular volume and results in high capillary fluid pressure and edema.

Overloading of the vascular system may also be caused by giving solutions high in proteins so rapidly that the body cannot dispose of protein that is in excess of its need. This overloading causes fluids to be pulled into the intravascular compartment from other body fluid compartments. The blood volume increases rapidly, neutralizing the oncotic pressure but increasing the hydrostatic pressure of the vascular system. Fluid is then pushed back into the tissues. Overloading the vascular system is a risk when fluids such as plasma, plasma expanders, albumin, or blood are given to any person regardless of age or state of health.

Decreased Capillary Oncotic Pressure

Proteins in the blood (particularly albumin) are necessary to create the oncotic pressure that holds fluids in the vessels. When the capillary oncotic pressure is decreased, fluid moves out of the vascular compartment into the interstitial spaces. When serum proteins are low because of inadequate intake (severe malnutrition), excess loss from burns or renal disease, or decreased production in the liver, edema results.

Increased Interstitial Oncotic Pressure

An increase in interstitial oncotic pressure increases the pull of fluid from the vascular compartment into the interstitial spaces. Proteins may leak out of blood vessels because of increased capillary permeability such as occurs in inflammatory or allergic reactions. In the healthy person, edema does not develop immediately after the initial movement of fluid into the interstitial spaces because of the body's compensatory mechanisms, which include the existing low interstitial fluid pressure and the lymph system, which removes excess fluids and proteins.

Fluid Collection in Potential Fluid Spaces

The same mechanisms that create edema in the interstitial spaces can create fluid collection in potential fluid spaces—that is, in spaces between two membranes that normally contain only traces of fluid (Table 23-7). The symptoms of fluid collection in these spaces are caused by the pressure of the collected fluid on adjoining organs or walls. Large amounts of fluid can collect in an operative site and in tissues surrounding an injury. An accumulation of fluid in all body tissues is called generalized edema, or *anasarca*.

CLINICAL MANIFESTATIONS

In general, *weight gain* is the best indicator of an extracellular volume excess, because several liters of fluid can be retained without visible evidence of edema. Because hydrostatic pressure in the capillaries is greatest in the lower parts of the body, edema collects in these areas. This is called *dependent* edema. When one is standing or sitting with feet on the floor, edema develops in the ankles and feet; when in a supine position, edema fluid collects in the sacral area of the back.

If a finger is pressed over an edematous area, the in-

dentation made by the finger will remain briefly as the fluid is pushed to another area; this is called *pitting edema*. Fluid refills the interstitial place in the "pit" area gradually. A subjective measure is sometimes used to describe pitting edema on a scale from "one plus" (+) to "four plus" (++++), with the latter indicating severe pitting edema, because it takes longer for displaced fluid to move back into the pit area. Skin over parts of the body with marked edema is usually tight, smooth, and shiny. It is cool and pale because of poor circulation. If edema is very severe, fluid will leak out of pores when the skin is pressed. This is called *weeping* edema.

Overhydration causes neck vein engorgement, so that these veins appear distended even when the patient is in an upright position (see Figure 26-12). Clothing and shoes may begin to feel tight and uncomfortable.

INTERVENTIONS

The treatment of edema depends on the condition that has caused it. Congestive heart failure is usually treated with digitalis, diuretics, and sodium and fluid restriction. Cirrhosis of the liver is also treated with sodium and fluid restriction and possibly mild diuretics. Renal failure requires severe restrictions of water and electrolytes or their removal by dialysis.

Reducing sodium intake alone may reduce edema, because the supply of body sodium is reduced and that which remains appears to be needed to maintain isotonicity of the blood.

Malnutritional edema responds to adequate dietary intake, especially to the addition of protein to the diet, unless the condition is far advanced, as occurs in starving children and adults in famine areas where kwashiorkor is a common cause of death. Edema associated with infections and burns resolves over time as the underlying cause responds to treatment.

Excess fluid in the tissues results in poor cellular nutrition as cells are pushed further apart and away from capillaries. Normal exchange of nutrients and wastes is interrupted. Edematous tissues therefore are poorly nourished, are susceptible to trauma and infection, and heal poorly. Caution must be taken to protect edematous parts of the body from prolonged pressure, injury, and extremes of heat and cold. Skin over these parts should be kept well lubricated to prevent dryness. If edematous areas are exposed to extensive moisture from incontinence or perspiration, they should be dried frequently to prevent maceration.

When edema is caused by venous stasis, elevating dependent body parts and applying supportive stockings to the legs help promote venous return. Extremities that become edematous as a result of surgery or trauma should also be elevated and supported.

Great care must be taken if intravenous fluids are being administered to an edematous person. The use of an

TABLE 23-7 Fluid collection in potential fluid spaces

Potential Fluid Space	Location	Fluid
Intrapleural	Between lung and chest wall	Pleural effusion
Pericardial	Between heart and pericardial sac	Pericardial effusion
Peritoneal	Between intestines and abdominal wall	Ascites

intravenous administration pump will add a margin of safety to the control of solution flow rate.

Diuretics

Edema is often treated with diuretics that act on the kidneys. Thiazide diuretics, the most commonly used, inhibit reabsorption of sodium and chloride in the proximal renal tubules and thus promote excretion of sodium and water, or *diuresis*. Potassium is usually lost along with sodium and water unless a potassium-sparing diuretic is used. Fluid and electrolyte imbalances are undesirable but rather common side effects of diuretic therapy. When diuretics are given, a large amount of fluid is lost from the vascular compartment, decreasing its hydrostatic pressure and causing fluid to be pulled back into it from the interstitial compartment.

Before excess fluid in the interstitial spaces can be excreted, it must be moved back into the vascular compartment; otherwise, diuresis causes serious vascular depletion. Table 23-8 shows some diuretics and their effects.

ELECTROLYTE IMBALANCE

As noted earlier, sodium, potassium, calcium, and magnesium are the principal cations in the body. Chloride, bicarbonate, and phosphate are the principal anions. Although these electrolytes make up less than 5% of the total body weight, life cannot be sustained unless body fluids contain exactly the right amount of each in the right concentration within each of the fluid compartments.[26] In addition, no single electrolyte can be out of balance without causing other electrolytes to be out of balance also.

Sodium, potassium, and calcium are all essential for the passage of nerve impulses. Whenever the concentration of any of these cations is increased or decreased in body fluids, the increase or decrease is reflected in the stimulation of muscles by nerves. The muscles may become weak and atonic because of inadequate stimulation, or they may become somewhat spastic because of excess stimulation.

TABLE 23-8 Common diuretics and their effect on fluid and electrolyte balance

Generic Name	Trade Name	Method of Administration	Peak Effect	Probable Effects on Fluid and Electrolyte Balance
Thiazides				
Chlorothiazide	Diuril	Oral	4 hr	Hyponatremia Hypokalemia ↓ ECF volume Hyperglycemia Hyperuricemia
Hydrochlorothiazide	Esidrix HydroDiuril	Oral	3-4 hr	Hypomagnesemia
Loop diuretics (act mainly on ascending loop of Henle)				
Furosemide	Lasix	IM or IV Oral	½ hr 2-4 hr	Hypokalemia Hyperuricemia ↓ ECF volume
Ethacrynic acid	Edecrin	Oral IV	2-4 hr ½ hr	Hyponatremia
Bumetanide	Bumex	Oral	½-1 hr	Hypokalemia Hypouricemia
		IM	40 min	Hyponatremia Hypocalcemia
		IV	5 min	Hypochloremia
Aldosterone antagonist (opposes potassium-losing action of aldosterone)				
Spironolactone	Aldactone	Oral	72 hr	Hyperkalemia Hyponatremia
Potassium-conserving action				
Triamterene	Dyrenium	Oral	4-8 hr	Hyperkalemia
Osmotic agent				
Mannitol	Osmitrol	IV infused over 24-hr period	—	Hyponatremia Hypochloremia ↑ ECF volume

SODIUM

The normal concentration of sodium in the blood is 138 to 145 mEq/L. Sodium is the most prevalent cation in the ECF and controls the osmotic pressure of this compartment. It is essential for neuromuscular functioning, for many intracellular chemical reactions, and for helping to maintain acid-base balance in the body. The sodium gradient theory states that sodium must be present for glucose to be transported into cells.

As previously mentioned, aldosterone causes reabsorption of sodium in the kidney tubules (p. 539). When the sodium supply becomes low, renal loss of sodium drops to zero. Aldosterone does not greatly influence sodium *concentration,* however, because as sodium is reabsorbed, water is also reabsorbed in equal proportions.

SODIUM DEFICIT

A low sodium level in the blood, *hyponatremia,* can result from either a sodium loss or a water excess (p. 544).

Etiology

The treatment of cardiac conditions and hypertension with diuretics and restricted sodium intake is a frequent cause of hyponatremia. The minimum daily requirement for sodium is 2 g/day. Sodium depletion also results from loss of gastrointestinal or biliary drainage and draining fistulas. Diseases interfering with aldosterone secretion, such as Addison's disease, result in excessive losses of sodium and water.

Sodium depletion can also occur in the shifting of body fluids so that the sodium and water are "trapped" in certain body areas and are not accessible for use. This can occur in massive edema, ascites, burns, or small bowel obstruction.

Anyone who is perspiring profusely because of climate, exercise, or fever is losing large amounts of both sodium and water. A form of chronic renal disease, "salt-wasting nephritis," also causes large daily losses of sodium ions. Sodium depletion caused by any of the above conditions is aggravated by a low-sodium diet.

Prevention

Athletes and persons who work in very hot environments are advised to ingest fluids containing sodium and to add some salty foods to their diets. If salt is not replaced along with water, that is, if thirst is quenched by drinking large amounts of tap water alone, water intoxication (p. 544) can occur. Salt tablets may be taken during the period of adaptation to an exceptionally hot environment. Diuretics such as the thiazides eventually may cause sodium depletion; therefore the patient who is receiving extensive diuretic treatment should be observed for symptoms of sodium depletion. Because many patients receiving diuretics are at home, they should be taught to report symptoms of sodium depletion to the physician. These patients should not be on severely restricted sodium diets.

When a nasogastric tube needs to be irrigated, normal saline should be used in preference to water. Plain water irrigation washes sodium out of the stomach and leads to hyponatremia.

Pathophysiology

Sodium loss from the intravascular compartment causes fluid from the blood to diffuse into the interstitial spaces. As a result, the sodium in the interstitial fluid is diluted. In response to this reduction in sodium concentration in the ECF, potassium moves out of the ICF. Therefore the patient with a sodium imbalance is also likely to have a potassium imbalance.

The decreased osmolality of ECF that exists with sodium loss creates a condition similar to water excess, that is, water moves into the cells by osmosis and leaves the extracellular compartment depleted. It differs from water intoxication because there is not an excess of total body water but an intercompartmental movement of water and depletion of the extracellular compartment.

The laboratory test for plasma sodium does not always give an accurate indication of total body sodium. Some clinical conditions in which the level of serum sodium is not an accurate indicator of total body sodium can be seen in Table 23-9. Sodium readily combines with bicarbonate or chloride to help maintain acid-base balance.

TABLE 23-9 Comparison of serum sodium levels with total body sodium*

Condition	Serum Sodium	Total Body Sodium
Prolonged sweating	Low (hyponatremia)	Low
Diuretics and low-sodium diets	Low	Low
Addison's disease	Low	Low
Edema (cardiac, renal hepatic disease)	Low or normal	High
Excretion of dilute urine, early stages of gastrointestinal sodium loss	Normal	Low
Excess oral or IV sodium intake	High (hypernatremia)	High
Water and sodium loss with water loss > sodium loss	High	Low

*Note that a low or high serum level does not necessarily correspond with total body sodium.

SIGNS AND SYMPTOMS OF HYPONATREMIA

Headache
Muscle weakness
Fatigue and apathy
Postural hypotension
Anorexia, nausea, and vomiting
Abdominal cramps
Weight loss

Clinical Manifestations

The signs and symptoms of hyponatremia are listed in the box above. As the sodium loss becomes more severe, the increase in ICF and decrease in circulating blood volume produce symptoms of mental confusion, delirium, coma, and shock. If the onset of sodium depletion is rapid, shock can ensue quickly from the sudden decrease in blood volume.

Interventions

Treatment of shock, if present, is the first concern. Saline solution, usually 0.9% sodium chloride, is given intravenously at a rapid rate. Plasma expanders may also be infused.

If other electrolytes (potassium, calcium, bicarbonate) have been depleted, these also need to be replaced. Treatment that alleviates the underlying cause will prevent further sodium loss. Salt or salty foods are added to the diet for sodium depletion, which develops slowly or follows profuse perspiration (diaphoresis) or vomiting. (See Chapter 25 for a more detailed description of the treatment.)

Safety measures, such as the use of side rails on the bed, supervision of ambulation, and frequent observation, are necessary if the patient becomes weak or confused or experiences marked hypotension.

SODIUM EXCESS

A serum sodium level greater than 145 mEq/L is known as *hypernatremia*. There are actually two kinds of sodium excess, edema or hypernatremia. When there is a sodium and water excess, edema exists; when there is an excess of sodium in relation to water in the extracellular compartment, hypernatremia exists. As seen in Table 23-9 hypernatremia does not necessarily indicate an excess of total body sodium.

Etiology

Hypernatremia occurs when more water than sodium is lost from the body and sodium concentration in the blood rises. It can also result from an abnormally large oral intake of sodium such as when a child accidentally eats many salt tablets or when intravenous saline is infused so rapidly that the body cannot excrete the amount not needed.

Prevention

Sodium excess can be prevented in persons whose ability to excrete it is impaired. Persons with kidney failure, congestive heart failure, or increased aldosterone production need to have sodium intake restricted. Whenever intravenous electrolyte solutions are being given, the urinary output must be adequate so that portions of the electrolytes not needed by the body can be excreted. This usually means that fluid intake should not exceed urinary output.

Pathophysiology

If sodium becomes concentrated in ECF, osmolality rises, water leaves the cells by osmosis and enters the extracellular compartment to dilute fluids there, and the cells are water-depleted. The presence of hypernatremia suppresses aldosterone secretion, and sodium is excreted in the urine.

Clinical Manifestations

Hypernatremia causes dry, sticky mucous membranes, low urinary output, and firm, "rubbery" tissue turgor. If adequate fluid is not given to dilute the sodium and if excretion of sodium is not increased, severe fluid and electrolyte imbalances will occur, and manic excitement, tachycardia, and eventual death will ensue.

Interventions

Water alone is given to treat sodium excess. If cardiac and renal function are normal, a liberal amount of water is administered orally, or 5% dextrose in water is given intravenously. In the absence of normal cardiac and renal function, hydration must be carried out with caution to prevent fluid overloading in the patient.

Diuretics are of value in removing sodium. If sodium excess is severe, with or without excess water retention, and does not respond to other treatment, renal dialysis may be necessary.

POTASSIUM

The normal concentration of potassium in the blood is 3.5 to 5.0 mEq/L. Because most of the potassium in the body is intracellular, the serum potassium level does not necessarily indicate the total body potassium content. Maintenance of serum potassium within normal range, however, is vital to normal body functions.

Potassium has a direct effect on the excitability of nerves and muscles, contributes most to the intracellular osmotic pressure, and helps maintain acid-base balance and normal kidney function. A potassium deficit is associated with excess alkalinity (alkalosis) of the body fluids, and a potassium excess accompanies an excess of acid (acidosis). These conditions are discussed in Chapter 24.

Potassium is the major cation of the cells. During the formation of new tissues (anabolism) or when glucose is converted to glycogen, potassium enters the cell. With tissue breakdown (catabolism) such as occurs with trauma, dehydration, or starvation, potassium leaves the cell. The body conserves potassium less effectively than it conserves sodium, and the kidneys excrete potassium even when the body needs it. Normally about 5% of the total body potassium is excreted each day.

POTASSIUM DEFICIT

A low level of serum potassium, below 3.5 mEq/L, is known as *hypokalemia*.

Etiology

The patient who has food withheld for several days, is dehydrated, or is given large amounts of parenteral fluids with no replacement of potassium develops potassium depletion. The parenteral administration of 5% dextrose in water without the addition of potassium tends to dilute the potassium in the extracellular tissues. This dilution, in addition to the lack of a balanced diet and to potassium loss caused by catabolism of body proteins, accounts for many instances of electrolyte imbalance in the postoperative patient. Persons who eat an inadequate diet, who take no food for an extended period of time, or who are losing large amounts of fluid from the gastrointestinal tract through vomiting, diarrhea, or a draining fistula usually are given intravenous solutions containing potassium.

The practice of giving multiple enemas is becoming much less common, because it is now known that some of the enema fluid is absorbed through the bowel wall and dilutes the potassium in the interstitial compartment. Hypertonic enema solutions may damage cells in the bowel mucosa, causing potassium loss. Figure 23-5 summarizes the causes and effects of hypokalemia.

Prevention

Hypokalemia can be prevented by being alert to the conditions that cause potassium depletion (vomiting, diarrhea, and diuretics) and by monitoring the patient for early warning signs. If there is an order for enemas until results are clear, the nurse should not give more than three enemas to a patient without consulting the physician, because this treatment may result in water intoxication and potassium loss.

Pathophysiology

Movement of sodium (inward) and potassium (outward) across the cell membrane causes depolarization of the membrane and initiates an action potential—this creates nerve and muscle activity. When extracellular po-

tassium is low, the resting membrane potential increases (hyperpolarization), and the cell becomes less excitable. For this reason the major symptoms of hypokalemia are muscle weakness and atony.

Potassium is involved in acid-base balance, because it moves out of the cells when hydrogen ions move into the intracellular compartment in acidosis; therefore hyperkalemia accompanies acidosis. As the acidosis is treated, potassium moves back into the cells, and hypokalemia may develop. In alkalosis, hypokalemia usually develops because of movement of potassium into cells and also because potassium is excreted by the kidneys while hydrogen ions are being retained.

Whenever sodium is retained in the body through reabsorption by the kidney tubules, potassium is excreted. Thus whenever aldosterone secretion is increased, such as during the stress response, potassium is excreted. Potassium may also be lost in the urine when there is considerable urinary output and as a result of certain diuretics (the thiazides, furosemide) and the corticosteroids.

Clinical Manifestations

The patient with potassium deficit shows characteristic electrocardiographic changes, flattened or inverted T waves with prolonged QT segments and prominence of a U wave. (See Chapter 26 for discussion of a normal ECG.) The most striking symptom of hypokalemia is muscle weakness. Other symptoms are apathy, abdominal distention, anorexia, vomiting, and paralytic ileus.

Digitalis toxicity can occur in persons taking digitalis if they develop hypokalemia. Persistent potassium deficit may cause kidney and heart damage.

Interventions

With severe hypokalemia the patient may die unless potassium is administered promptly. The safest way to administer potassium is orally. When potassium is given intravenously, the rate of flow must be monitored closely to prevent hyperkalemia and atrial arrest. The usual rate of infusion should not exceed 20 mEq/L of potassium per hour. Since potassium is irritating to the veins, it is given very diluted, usually 20 to 40 mEq/L of intravenous solution. In some instances potassium is given at a greater concentration (40 mEq/100 ml) over a 4-hour period. When potassium is administered in this concentration, it should be delivered by a controlled infusion pump such as an IVAC or IMED. Because of the potential cardiovascular complications that can occur with this concentration of potassium, the patient can be put on a cardiac monitor so that changes in cardiac status will be identified immediately.

Persons who are receiving potassium-losing diuretics should be instructed to include foods high in potassium in their diet (Table 23-10). If low serum potassium levels are shown to result from diuretic therapy, a potas-

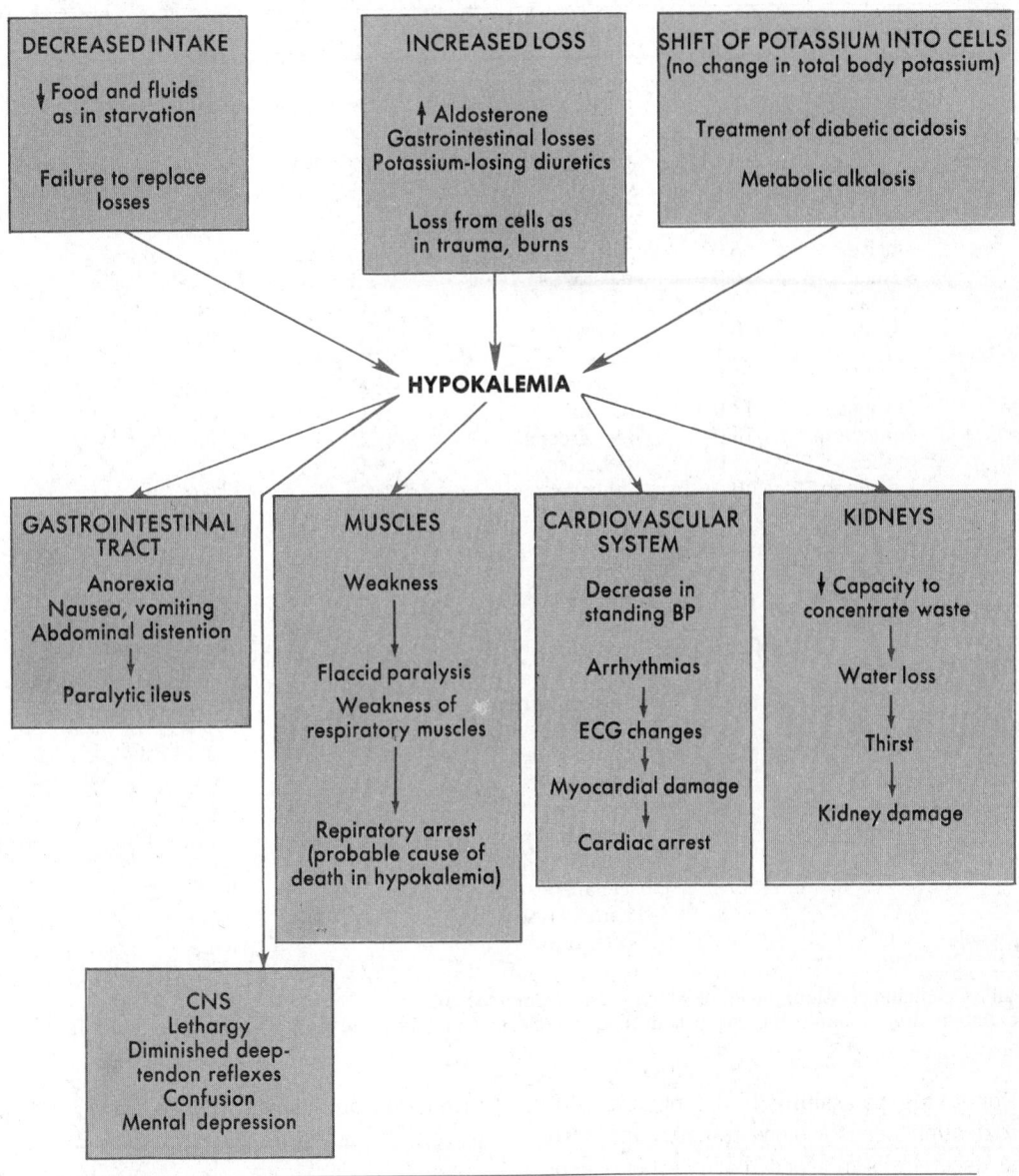

FIGURE 23-5 Causes and effects of hypokalemia.

sium supplement may be prescribed, usually in the form of potassium chloride (elixir of potassium chloride), or a potassium-sparing diuretic such as triamterene (Dyrenium) may be used. Persons taking diuretics at home should be taught to recognize symptoms of potassium depletion, such as muscle weakness, anorexia, nausea, and vomiting, and to report these symptoms to the physician. Because potassium supplements are irritating to the gastrointestinal tract, they should be given with at least one-half glass of water.

POTASSIUM EXCESS

A serum potassium level greater than 5 mEq/L is termed *hyperkalemia*. This condition does not occur as

frequently as hypokalemia, especially if renal function is normal.

Etiology

As previously stated, whenever severe tissue damage is present, potassium is released from the cells into ECF. If it is not excreted quickly, hyperkalemia results.

Shock, which often accompanies tissue damage, reduces renal function, thus promoting hyperkalemia. Great danger exists in giving extra potassium to any patient with poor renal function. If the patient is dehydrated or has lost vascular fluid, glucose and water or plasma expanders usually are given until renal function returns. Untreated adrenal insufficiency also is a con-

TABLE 23-10 Foods high in potassium

Fruits			Buttermilk	1 C	8.5
Apricots			Skim	1 C	8.8
Canned	½ C	6.0	Powdered, skim	¼ C	13.5
Dried	4 halves	5.0	Vegetables*		
Fresh	3 small	8.0	Asparagus		
Banana	1 small	9.6	Fresh	½ C	4.7
Strawberries	1 C	6.3	Frozen	½ C	5.5
Grapefruit sections	¾ C	5.1	Beans		
Melon			Dried, cooked	½ C	10.0
Cantaloupe	½ small	13.0	Lima	½ C	9.5
Honeydew	¼ medium	13.0	Beet greens	½ C	8.5
Watermelon	½ slice	5.0	Broccoli	½ C	7.0
Nectarine	1 medium	6.0	Cabbage, raw	1 C	6.0
Orange	1 medium	5.1	Carrots, raw	1 large	8.8
Orange juice	½ C	5.7	Celery, raw	1 C	9.0
Peach			Collards	½ C	6.0
Dried	2 halves	5.0	Mushrooms, raw	4 large	10.6
Fresh	1 medium	6.2	Mustard greens	½ C	5.5
Protein foods			Peas, dried	½ C	6.8
Beef	3 oz	8.4	Potato		
Chicken	3 oz	9.0	Baked, white	½ C	13.0
Frankfurters	1	3.0	Boiled, white	½ C	7.3
Liver	3 oz	9.6	Baked, sweet	½ C	8.0
Pork	3 oz	9.0	Spinach	½ C	8.5
Veal	3 oz	11.4	Tomatoes	½ C	6.5
Scallops	1 large	6.0	Brussels sprouts	⅔ C	7.6
Turkey	3 oz	8.4	Squash, winter, baked	½ C	12.0
Milk			Miscellaneous†		
Whole	1 C	8.8	Peanut butter	2 tbsp	5.0
Powdered, whole	¼ C		Nuts, unsalted	25	4.5

*Most raw vegetables contain potassium, much of which is lost during cooking.
†Beverages that contain large amounts of cocoa, cola drinks, and dry, instant coffee and tea.

traindication for giving potassium. If the patient with potassium intoxication needs a blood transfusion, fresh blood must be used. Cells in blood that has been kept for several days tend to release potassium during storage. Administration of stored blood may increase the person's blood potassium level still further. Figure 23-6 shows the causes and effects of hyperkalemia.

Time is an important factor in the development of hyperkalemia. A rise of serum potassium of only 1 to 3 mEq/L that occurs rapidly can be lethal. On the other hand, some persons with renal failure develop severe hyperkalemia slowly and seem to be able to adjust to the potassium excess with few symptoms. Because there are huge stores of potassium inside the cells, the kidney's efficient excretion of potassium is a safety factor that reduces hyperkalemia when there is a rapid shift of potassium into the extracellular compartment where the excess becomes dangerous.

Prevention

Hyperkalemia can be anticipated and prevented in persons who for any reason have a significant decrease in urinary output, especially if they are receiving oral or intravenous potassium preparations.

Pathophysiology

Hyperkalemia in ECF has the opposite effect from hypokalemia on the resting cell membrane. The membrane potential is decreased (partially depolarized), and the cell becomes more excitable. Potassium excess therefore causes nerve and muscle irritability. Severe hyperkalemia, however, soon leads to muscle weakness and flaccid paralysis.

Clinical Manifestations

The person with potassium intoxication develops spasticity of muscles because of their overstimulation by nerve impulses. Nausea, colic, diarrhea, and skeletal muscle spasms are common. The muscles later become weak, because overstimulation produces an accumulation of lactic acid and because potassium is lost from the muscle cells.

If the condition is not controlled, overstimulation of the cardiac muscle will cause the heartbeat to become

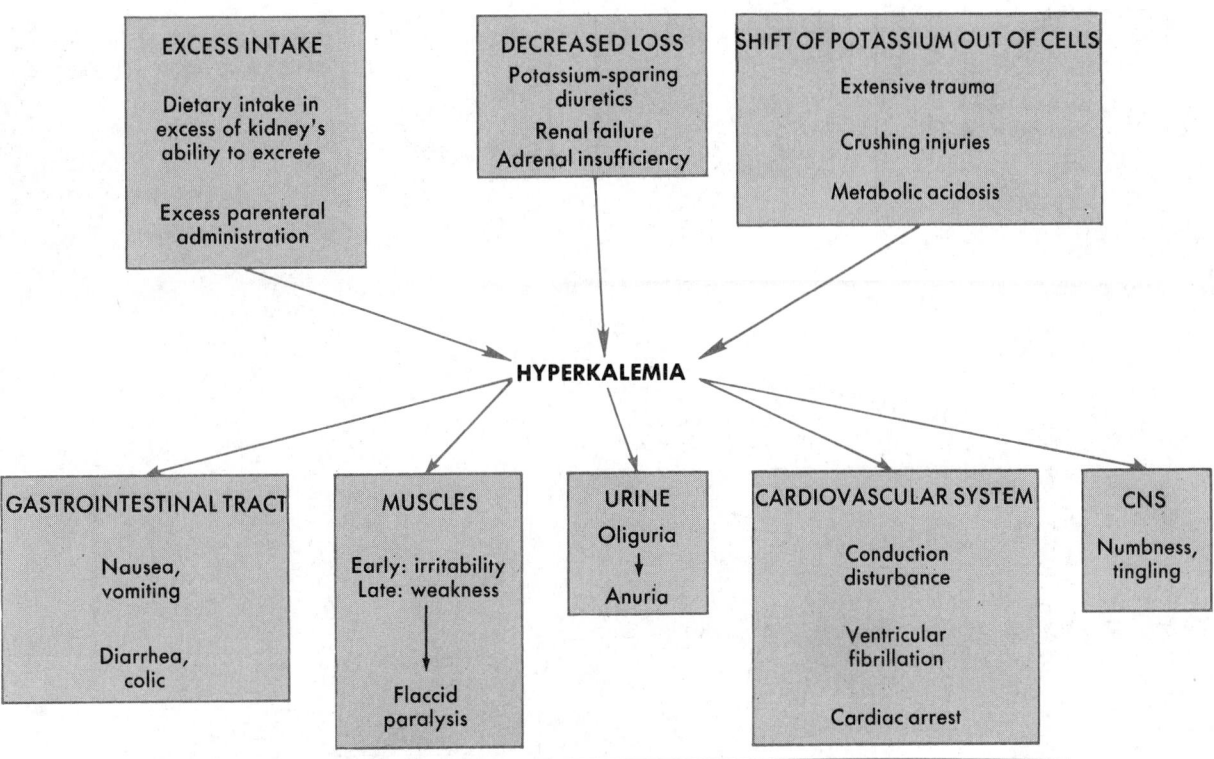

FIGURE 23-6 Causes and effects of hyperkalemia.

irregular and eventually stop. Electrocardiographic evidence of potassium elevation includes tall, peaked, symmetric, or tented T waves with a short QT segment. As the blood potassium level increases further, the QRS complex spreads, and atrial arrest occurs.[33]

Interventions

When potassium intoxication occurs, the person is allowed nothing orally, and an infusion of 10% glucose with regular insulin may be given to induce transfer of potassium from the serum to ICF. If the patient is in acidosis, correction of the acidosis will result in movement of potassium back into the cell (p. 541). A cation exchange resin such as polystyrene sulfonate (Kayexalate) may also be given. It works by exchanging other cations in the resin for potassium in the intestine. The potassium is then excreted in the stool. Good bowel function must be maintained if this therapy is to be effective. If the patient is in acute renal failure, dialysis is necessary. Calcium given intravenously antagonizes the effect of potassium on the heart.

Persons with potassium intoxication are placed on bed rest and receive complete nursing care until the potassium blood level returns to normal. Those persons who retain potassium secondary to renal failure or to a decrease in aldosterone will need instruction in restricting foods high in potassium (see Table 23-10). If salt substitutes are being used, patients need to be aware that these usually contain potassium as a substitute for sodium.

CALCIUM

The normal calcium level in the blood is 4.5 to 5.8 mEq/L. Calcium in the blood is in two forms: ionized and bound to plasma proteins. Free, ionized calcium is needed for (1) blood coagulation; (2) smooth, skeletal, and cardiac muscle function; (3) nerve functions; and (4) bone and teeth formation. Only the ionized calcium is physiologically active.

Both vitamin D and parathyroid hormone must be present for calcium to be absorbed from the gastrointestinal tract. Parathyroid hormone maintains the serum calcium level within normal limits by mobilizing calcium from bone. Calcium is excreted principally through the gastrointestinal tract, with normally only very small amounts being lost in the urine.

CALCIUM DEFICIT

Hypocalcemia is a decrease of the serum calcium level to below 4.5 mEq/L.

Etiology

Calcium deficit results from inadequate intake, vitamin D deficiency, hypoparathyroidism, interruption of normal calcium absorption from the gastrointestinal tract, and excess loss of calcium through the kidneys.

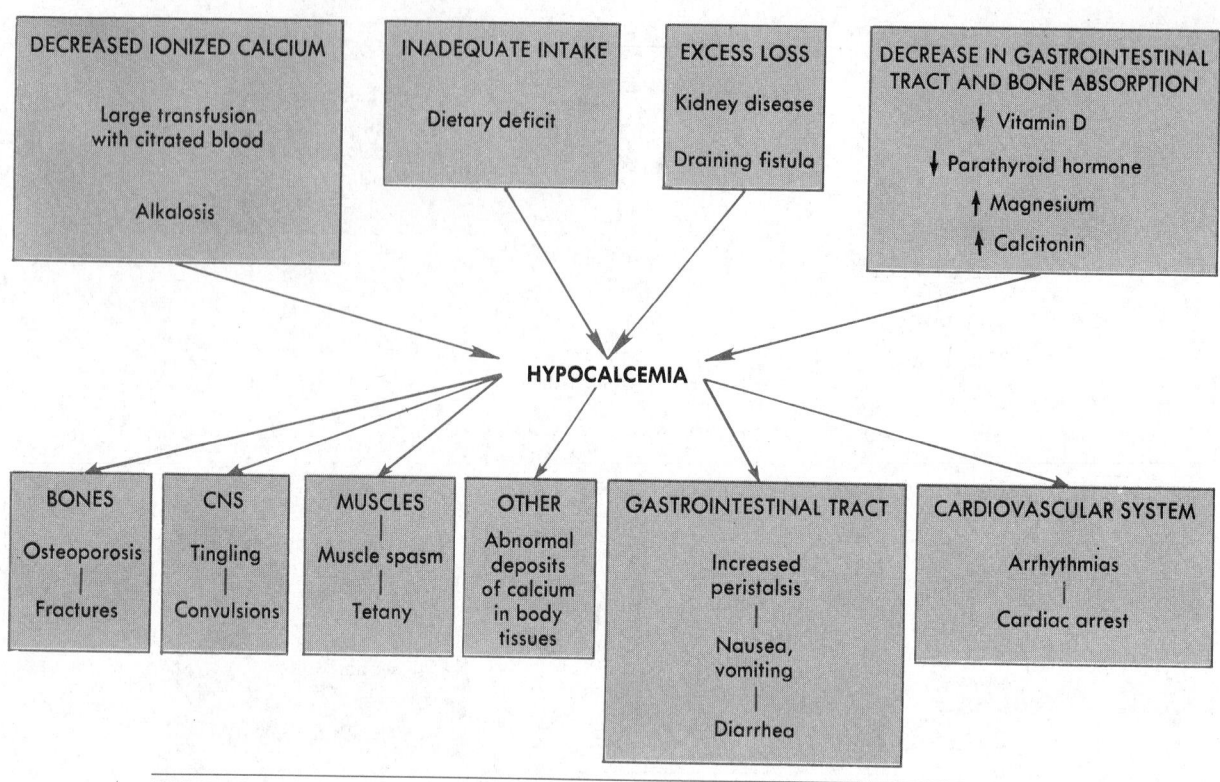

FIGURE 23-7 Causes and effects of hypocalcemia.

Patients with pancreatic disease or disease of the small intestine may fail to absorb calcium normally from the gastrointestinal tract, and they may excrete large amounts of calcium in the feces. Persons with chronic pancreatitis have persistent hypocalcemia. Draining intestinal fistulas also cause excess calcium loss. These causes and effects are shown in Figure 23-7.

Prevention

Calcium deficiency can be prevented by alertness to conditions of inadequate intake, excess calcium loss, or vitamin D deficiency. Patients who are on extremely poor diets or who have calcium-depleting conditions should be monitored for signs of hypocalcemia. Teaching persons with a low intake of calcium and vitamin D to include more of these nutrients in the diet is an important nursing action.

Pathophysiology

It is thought that calcium ions line the pores of cell membranes. Since both calcium and sodium ions carry a positive charge, they tend to repel each other. The presence of calcium in the pores of cells (especially neurons) through which sodium must pass for depolarization to take place has a blocking effect on this permeability to sodium. When calcium levels in the blood are low, this blocking effect is minimized, sodium moves more easily into the cell, and depolarization with result-

ing action potential takes place more readily.[10] The result is increased excitability of the nervous system leading to muscle spasm, tingling sensations, and, if severe, to convulsions and tetany. Skeletal, smooth, and cardiac muscle function are all affected by overstimulation.

Clinical Manifestations

Tetany is the most characteristic sign of severe hypocalcemia. The patient who has calcium deficiency usually complains first of numbness and tingling of the nose, ears, fingertips, or toes. If calcium is not given at this time, painful muscular spasms (tetany), especially of the feet and hands, muscle twitching, and convulsions may follow.

There are two tests used to elicit signs of calcium deficiency. *Trousseau's sign* is elicited by grasping the patient's wrist or inflating a blood pressure cuff on the upper arm to constrict the circulation for a few minutes. If the hand goes into a position of palmar flexion (carpopedal spasm), the person probably has a serious calcium deficit. *Chvostek's sign* is elicited by tapping the patient's face lightly over the facial nerve (just below the temple). A calcium deficit is probably present if the facial muscles twitch.

Interventions

The drug of choice in treating calcium deficiency is a 10% intravenous solution of calcium gluconate given slowly.[11] In milder cases, a high calcium diet or oral calcium salts may be sufficient. When decreased parathyroid hormone or vitamin D is the causative factor, these substances must be supplied. When the serum phosphorus level rises, the calcium level falls; aluminum hydroxide gel can be given to lower a high serum phosphorus concentration.

Any patient who has had thyroid surgery must be watched very closely for symptoms of calcium deficiency (tetany), because of the possibility that parathyroid glands may have been inadvertently removed with the thyroid tissue or may be temporarily suppressed by local edema.

Because chronic hypocalcemia can result in loss of calcium from bone to replenish low serum calcium, persons with this condition must be carefully moved, turned, or ambulated to prevent fractures of the demineralized bone. Calcium preparations must be given with caution to cardiac patients, because calcium has an effect on the heart similar to digitalis.

Osteoporosis

In recent years a great deal of interest and information has been generated regarding osteoporosis, a condition prevalent in postmenopausal women (see Chapter 53).

Normally in young persons, the constant processes of bone formation and resorption are in equilibrium, but after age 40 resorption becomes greater, causing structural weakness of bones and increased risk of fracture. The problem is compounded because calcium intake and absorption in the intestine decrease with age, creating a negative calcium balance over time. To correct the deficit, calcium is released from bone to make it available for vital nerve and muscle function. If there is a long-term deficiency, the calcium-depleted bones become porous and brittle.

To prevent osteoporosis, young women are advised to have an adequate daily intake of calcium and vitamin D, to exercise regularly, to avoid smoking, and to decrease phosphorus and caffeine intake. After menopause, the usual recommended daily allowance of 1000 mg of calcium should be increased to 1500 mg.[26] Vitamin D, which increases calcium absorption, may also need to be added to the daily regimen of postmenopausal women.

Long-term therapy with corticosteroids is another cause of osteoporosis, because the corticosteroids promote calcium mobilization from bones and inhibit calcium absorption.

CALCIUM EXCESS

A serum calcium level above 5.8 mEq/L is called *hypercalcemia.*

Etiology

Hypercalcemia can result from excessive intake of calcium, especially in milk and absorbable calcium-containing antacids (milk-alkali syndrome), from excessive vitamin D intake, and from conditions that promote release of calcium from the bones into ECF. These causes and their effects are shown in Figure 23-8.

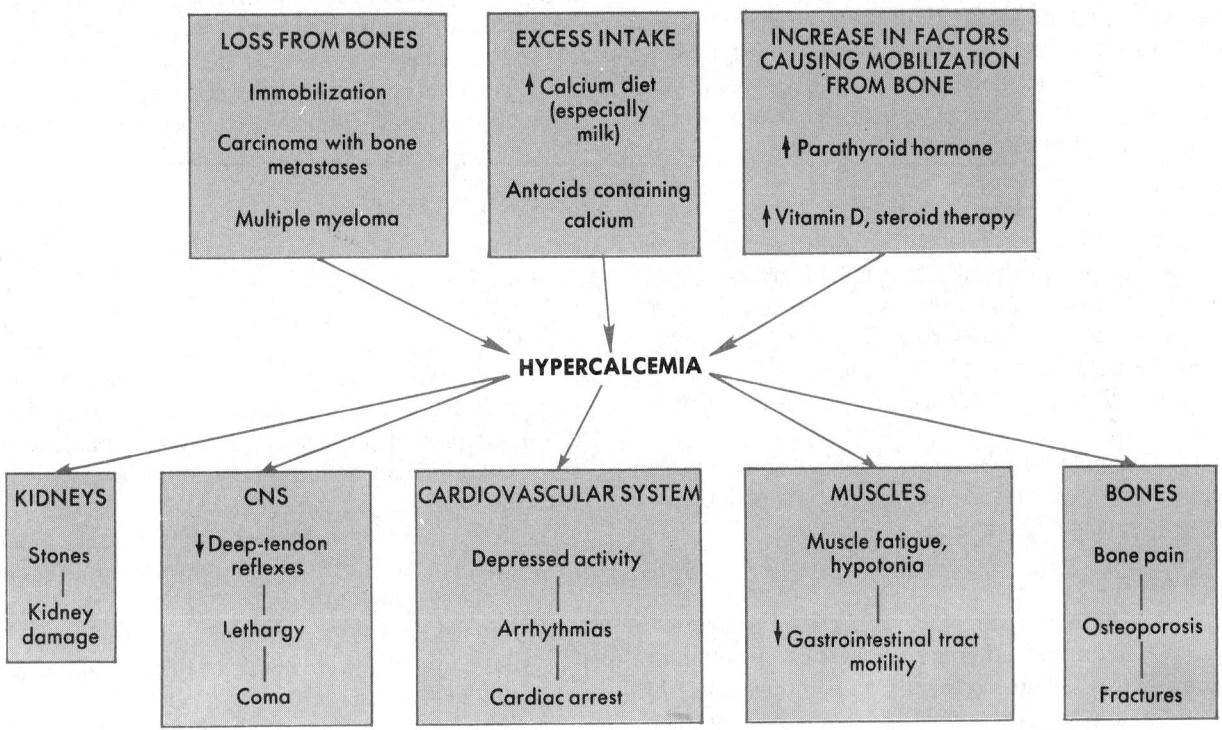

FIGURE 23-8 Causes and effects of hypercalcemia.

Prevention

Hypercalcemia can be alleviated in persons who are immobilized by helping them to exercise muscles in uninvolved parts of the body. A tilt table may be used to put a patient who is unable to stand unassisted in an upright, weight-bearing position so as to provide pressure on the bones. Patients who are immobilized in a back-lying position should be encouraged to use a trapeze bar, and all patients who are able should move about as much as possible and, with the use of side rails and other means, engage in activities that require muscle action.

Pathophysiology

The blocking effect of calcium on cell membrane permeability is accentuated in the presence of high serum calcium levels. Nerve and muscle activity is depressed. The activity of cardiac muscle is depressed, gastrointestinal motility decreases, and skeletal and smooth muscles become fatigued. Deep tendon reflexes are decreased or absent.[26]

When a person is immobilized for any reason, calcium leaves the bone and concentrates in ECF. Normal retention of calcium in the bones is believed to be caused by the pressure exerted on bones by active movement or exercise. When a large amount of calcium accumulates in ECF and passes through the kidneys, calcium can precipitate and form stones (calculi), a not infrequent complication of immobilization.

Calcium precipitates more readily in alkaline solution. This can be a problem in a urinary tract infection, which increases the alkalinity of the urine, because renal calculi are more likely to be formed. Metastatic carcinoma, multiple myeloma, hyperparathyroidism, and other diseases with extensive bone involvement also produce marked hypercalcemia.

Clinical Manifestations

The person with hypercalcemia commonly complains of polyuria and severe thirst. Gastrointestinal symptoms, including anorexia, nausea, vomiting, and constipation, may also develop. Without treatment the patient may become lethargic, confused, and comatose. Deep bone pain and radiographic evidence of bone cavitation may be present.

Hypercalcemic crisis is an emergency condition that is signaled by intractable nausea and vomiting, dehydration, stupor, coma, and azotemia.[18]

Interventions

The only definitive treatment is removal of the cause. Because calcium excretion is promoted by excretion of sodium, hypercalcemia is treated with intravenous saline and a diuretic (furosemide). If this treatment fails, inorganic phosphate preparations given orally or intra-venously may be effective. Mithramycin (Mithracin), a potent antitumor drug, has been used successfully to reduce serum calcium. If the hypercalcemia is caused by multiple myeloma or other cancers, glucocorticoids may be effective in reducing hypercalcemia, either because they decrease the size of the tumor or because the effect of the tumor on bone is reduced.

Because persons with marked hypercalcemia often are losing calcium from their bones or have malignant involvement of bone, special care should be taken to prevent pathologic fractures. Even the pressure used in giving a back rub must sometimes be avoided.

Careful attention must be directed to the prevention of calcium stone formation in the kidneys. Acid-ash fruit juices, cranberry and prune juice, or ascorbic acid can be given to promote urinary acidification and discourage stone formation. Urinary tract infections must be avoided. Good perineal care and meticulous technique in caring for Foley catheters are mandatory.

Unless they are contraindicated, persons with hypercalcemia are encouraged to drink 3000 to 4000 ml of fluids per day to reduce the possibility of renal calculi and to overcome the thirst that accompanies hypercalcemia.

MAGNESIUM

The normal serum magnesium level is within the range of 1.5 to 2.5 mEq/L. About 50% of magnesium is located in bones, 5% in ECF, and the remaining 45% in the intracellular compartment. It functions in the activation of enzymatic reactions, especially in carbohydrate metabolism. Magnesium has a sedative effect on the central nervous system similar to that of calcium. It has been used successfully to prevent convulsions in toxemia of pregnancy. High serum levels result in vasodilation with lowering of blood pressure.

MAGNESIUM DEFICIT

Hypomagnesemia is a serum magnesium level below 1.5 mEq/L.

Etiology

Hypomagnesemia is most frequently caused by disturbances in the gastrointestinal and renal systems (Figure 23-9). Chronic alcoholism is usually accompanied by a severe magnesium deficit. Magnesium levels decrease with the following conditions:

1. Loss of intestinal fluids through draining fistulas, diarrhea, steatorrhea, and gastrointestinal suction
2. Prolonged malnutrition
3. Renal disorders
4. Drug therapy with aminoglycosides and loop diuretics
5. Endocrine disorders such as increased secretion of ADH, aldosterone, and thyroid hormone[21]

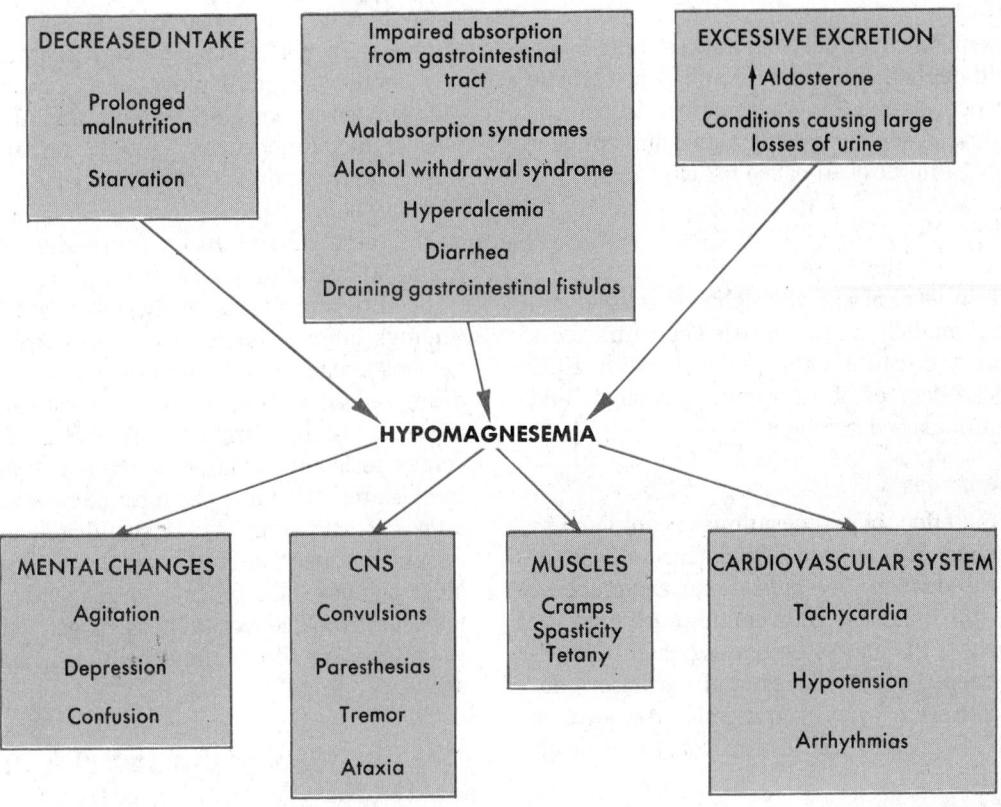

FIGURE 23-9 Causes and effects of hypomagnesemia.

Prevention

Dietary teaching and management can help prevent magnesium deficit, especially in persons with magnesium-depleting conditions. Fruits, green vegetables, whole grain cereals, milk, meats, and nuts are good dietary sources of magnesium.

Pathophysiology

A low serum magnesium level leads to increased neuromuscular irritability by increasing acetylcholine release, increasing the sensitivity of the myoneural junction to acetylcholine, diminishing the threshold of excitation of the motor nerve, and enhancing the force of contraction of the myofibril.[14]

In the presence of a large amount of calcium in the gastrointestinal tract, calcium is absorbed in preference to magnesium, and the magnesium is excreted. Conversely, low calcium levels increase magnesium absorption. The kidneys effectively conserve magnesium when intake is low. Hypocalcemia and hypokalemia that are unresponsive to therapy may indicate hypomagnesemia.

Metabolically, magnesium is closely interrelated with both calcium and potassium. Magnesium inhibits transport of parathyroid hormone from the glands, causing a decrease in the amount of calcium being released from bone, resulting in a calcium deficit. Hypomagnesemia potentiates the action of digitalis, leading to toxicity.[21]

Clinical Manifestations

Hypomagnesemia is usually manifested by behavioral and neurologic symptoms such as confusion, hallucinations, convulsions, increased reflexes, tremors, muscle spasms, and parathesias.

Interventions

The treatment of magnesium deficit consists of the correction of the underlying cause and of the administration of magnesium salts orally or parenterally. Oral magnesium sometimes causes diarrhea; therefore it is often replaced by intravenous or deep intramuscular injection.

Providing for the safety of the patient until the magnesium deficit is corrected is the prime nursing responsibility. Carefully observing and supervising the person who is confused or hallucinating and taking protective measures for persons who develop convulsions will prevent injury.

MAGNESIUM EXCESS

Hypermagnesemia represents a serum magnesium level greater than 2.5 mEq/L.

Etiology

Hypermagnesemia seldom develops unless there is renal failure, although it has been identified in diabetic ketoacidosis where there is severe water loss. In persons with renal failure, frequent use of magnesium-containing antacids or cathartics can cause toxicity.

Pathophysiology

Magnesium acts on the myoneural junction where a high magnesium level blocks acetylcholine release and decreases the excitability of the muscle cells. An excess of magnesium can cause cardiac effects with ECG changes, various degrees of atrioventricular block, and premature ventricular contractions.[8]

Clinical Manifestations

The vasodilating effect of magnesium is accentuated in hypermagnesemia and can lead to hypotension because of peripheral vasodilation. The person may experience a sense of heat, thirst, nausea, and vomiting with mild hypermagnesemia. If the excess becomes greater, drowsiness, loss of deep tendon reflexes, and respiratory depression occur. Severe hypermagnesemia, at a level as high as 15 to 20 mEq/L, will lead to coma and death from cardiac arrest.[8]

Interventions

Correction of the underlying cause corrects the magnesium excess. If renal failure is present, dialysis is necessary. Intravenous calcium gluconate may be a useful temporary treatment, because calcium has an antagonistic effect on magnesium.

FLUID AND ELECTROLYTE PROBLEMS OF THE ELDERLY

Elderly persons are particularly vulnerable to fluid and electrolyte disorders because of the following changes:

1. Less total body water
2. Decline in function of vital regulatory organs
3. High incidence of chronic illnesses
4. Diminished ability to reestablish homeostasis when an imbalance has occurred

The kidneys and lungs, which are the organs most involved with maintenance of fluid, electrolyte, and acid-base balance, steadily lose functional ability with aging. Kidney function in a 90-year-old person is normally about half of what it was at age 30. Similarly, there is a gradual decline in lung function with aging.

Elderly persons readily become *dehydrated* when they experience physiologic stressors from imposed water restrictions (for tests or x-ray films) or from fever, diarrhea, infections, and diuretic therapy. There is less body water to compensate for decreased intake and excess losses. Water depletion often goes unrecognized for many reasons: the sense of thirst is blunted, the need for water is not recognized and interpreted correctly, and swallowing difficulties may exist.[3] In addition, many older persons deliberately limit fluid intake for fear of incontinence or frequent urination. Hypernatremic dehydration is a frequent cause for admission of nursing home patients to a general hospital. In one study, these patients had serum sodium levels ranging from 150 to 202 mEq/L.[13]

Sodium and potassium depletion are both common findings among the elderly. *Hyponatremia* in elderly persons usually results from the use of potent diuretics, decreased dietary intake, excess intestinal loss from laxatives or diarrhea, and congestive heart failure that becomes resistant to diuretics. *Hypokalemia* may result from diuretic therapy, but most often it is caused by an intake of potassium that is insufficient to replace daily losses. Frequent enemas, which are common among older persons, also produce hypokalemia. Some symptoms of hypokalemia such as apathy, confusion, and weakness, are all too often mistakenly attributed to old age.

ASSESSMENT OF FLUID AND ELECTROLYTE IMBALANCE

The nurse needs to recognize the symptoms of fluid and electrolyte imbalance and make ongoing physical assessments of those patients who have a potential for fluid and electrolyte imbalances (Table 23-11). For subjective data such as headache, thirst, nausea, or dyspnea, time of onset and extent of symptoms are ascertained. Objective data can be compared to baseline assessments made at the time of the patient's entry into the health care system.

Data of particular importance in assessing fluid and electrolyte imbalance are comparison of fluid intake to output and changes in the patient's weight. Acutely ill medical patients and patients undergoing major surgery should have their fluid intake and output and daily weight closely monitored. If patients and families are given explanations, they can participate, when appropriate, in measuring and recording the intake and output. Totaling the fluid intake and output every hour, every 8 hours, or every 24 hours gives the nurse and physician additional data to determine if the patient may have a fluid imbalance.

Since symptoms of fluid and electrolyte imbalance are sometimes not very specific, a good rule is to be alert for any changes in behavior, level of consciousness, vital signs, skin turgor, muscle strength, and condition of mucous membranes. Baseline observations made during the first encounter with a patient are essential for comparison with subsequent observations to be able to detect changes.

TABLE 23-11 Assessment of fluid and electrolyte imbalance

	Fluid Excess	Fluid Loss/Electrolyte Imbalance
Behavior	Change in behavior, confusion, apathy	Change in behavior, confusion, apathy
Head, neck	Facial edema, distended neck veins	Headache, thirst, dry mucous membranes
Upper gastrointestinal tract	Anorexia, nausea, vomiting	Anorexia, nausea, vomiting
Skin	Warm, moist, taut, cool feeling where edematous	Dry, decreased turgor
Respiration	Dyspnea, orthopnea, productive cough, moist breath sounds	Changes in rate and depth of breathing
Circulation	Tires easily, loss of sensation in edematous areas, pallor*	Pulse rate changes, arrhythmias, postural hypotension
Abdomen	Increased girth, fluid wave	Distention, abdominal cramps
Elimination	Oliguria, constipation	Oliguria, diarrhea, constipation
Extremities	Dependent edema, "pitting," discomfort from weight of bedclothes	Muscle weakness, tingling, tetany

*Pallor-edema decreases the intensity of skin color by decreasing the distance between the skin surface and the pigmented or vascular areas. In the dark-skinned individual, pallor is observed by absence of underlying red tones that give brown and black skin "glow." The brown skin appears more yellow-brown, and the black skin appears more ashen gray.[22]

INTAKE AND OUTPUT MONITORING
INTAKE RECORD

The intake record should show the type and amount of all fluids the patient has received and the route by which these were administered. This includes fluids given orally, parenterally, rectally, or by tubes. A record of solid food intake is sometimes necessary, especially with very young children. Foods that are eaten in a semisolid state but which are basically liquid such as gelatin or ice cream are recorded as fluids. Ice chips are recorded by dividing the amount of chips by one half (60 ml of chips would equal 30 ml of water). Patients may receive a considerable amount of fluid intake through the frequent sucking of ice chips.

URINARY OUTPUT

Urinary output is recorded by recording time and amount of each voiding. If renal function is a major concern, as in a severely burned patient, an indwelling catheter is used so that the amount of urinary drainage can be recorded every hour and fluid intake regulated accordingly. It has been said that nothing is more difficult to obtain in a modern hospital than an accurate record of urinary output, and unfortunately this statement is often true. Conspicuous signs posted on the patient's chart and in the utility room and bathrooms help to prevent the discarding of urine before it is measured. Flow sheets kept close to the patient's room facilitate recording of intake and output and other patient data.

Specific gravity of urine, normally 1.010 to 1.030, is an indicator of fluid balance. A high specific gravity is indicative of fluid depletion, and a low specific gravity accompanies fluid excess. Oliguria, a urine output of less than 20 ml/hr, also signals a fluid-depleted state.

WOUND DRAINAGE

All drainage from body orifices or artificial openings should be measured. This would include such drainage as that from an ileostomy, from a T tube following exploration of the common bile duct, or from any catheter draining a surgical area. If there is excessive drainage from a wound, it may be necessary to weigh the dressings. Fluid loss is the difference between the wet weight and the dry weight of the dressing.

GASTROINTESTINAL OUTPUT

Vomitus, gastrointestinal drainage, and liquid stools are measured as accurately as possible and are described by color, content, and odor. Gastric secretions are watery and pale yellowish green; they usually have a sour odor. However, if the acid-base balance has been upset, gastric secretions may have a fruity odor because of the presence of ketone bodies (acetone). Bile is somewhat thicker than gastric juice and may vary from bright yellow to dark green in color. It has a bitter taste and acrid odor. Intestinal contents vary from dark green to brown in color, are likely to be quite thick, and have a fecal odor. The amount of fluid retained during irrigation of nasogastric tubes is added to "intake" and needs to be subtracted from total drainage before it is recorded.

It is difficult to determine accurately the amount of water lost in the stools, but a description of their consistency and a record of the number of stools passed gives a good estimate. The color of stools is also recorded.

OTHER OUTPUT

Fluid aspirated from any body cavity such as the abdomen (paracentesis) or pleural spaces (thoracentesis) must be measured. The fluid contains not only electrolytes and water but also proteins. Blood loss from any part of the body is measured carefully.

Diaphoresis is difficult to measure without special laboratory equipment; however, it may be important to estimate the loss of fluid by this route in some patients. Careful note of excessive perspiration and its duration is made. If the clothing and linen become saturated, dry and wet weights may be taken. Accurate recording of body temperature helps the physician determine how much fluid should be replaced, since fluid loss through the skin and lungs increases as temperature rises. A patient who has a high fever and is breathing rapidly can lose as much as 2500 ml/day through the lungs.[8]

DAILY WEIGHT

The daily weight record is often the best way to determine the onset of dehydration or the accumulation of fluid either as generalized edema or as "hidden" fluid in body cavities. An increase of 1 kg in weight is equal to the retention of 1 L (1000 ml) of fluid in the edematous patient. If the weight record is to be accurate, the patient must be weighed on the same scale and at the same hour each day and must be wearing the same amount of clothing. Circumstances that may affect the weight should be kept as nearly identical as possible from day to day. Usually weights are taken in the early morning before the patient has eaten or defecated, but after voiding. When extremely accurate measurements are needed, all clothing and even wound dressings are removed before the patient is weighed. A person maintained on intravenous fluids alone can be expected to lose approximately 0.2 to 0.5 kg/day.

LABORATORY VALUES

Laboratory determinations of serum levels of the specific electrolytes help in making decisions concerning electrolyte excesses or deficits. When there is water excess, hemodilution occurs and the hematocrit, hemoglobin, blood-urea nitrogen (BUN), and electrolyte levels are decreased. With excessive fluid loss there is hemoconcentration; and the hematocrit, hemoglobin, BUN, and electrolyte levels are increased.

LUNG AUSCULTATION

Regular auscultation of the lungs helps identify states of fluid excess. Moist breath sounds (crackles) that do not clear when the person coughs, indicate a collection of fluid in the alveoli.

REPLACEMENT AND MAINTENANCE OF WATER AND ELECTROLYTES

GENERAL PRINCIPLES

Replacement of the water and electrolyte losses from the body and the necessary daily intake of these sub-

stances and other nutrients are usually accomplished by one of the following methods: (1) oral intake, (2) tube feeding (gavage), (3) intravenous infusion, and (4) total parenteral nutrition.

The best way to administer water, electrolytes, and nutrients is to give them orally. When fluids can be tolerated by the stomach but cannot be swallowed, a nasogastric tube may be passed, and fluids containing all the essentials of a balanced diet may be given through it. Normal saline solution or plain water also may be given by slow drip through the tube to replace fluid loss and provide for daily fluid needs.

If it is not possible for a patient to take food or fluid through the alimentary tract, the most common method of replacement is by intravenous infusion. A vein in the leg or arm is commonly used. An intravenous infusion may be given by introducing a needle or intracatheter into a vein and taping them in place or by making an incision (cutdown) and threading a polyethylene catheter (intracatheter) into the vein. The intracatheter is the method of choice for total parenteral nutrition (TPN) in which a concentrated nutrient solution is infused into the superior vena cava. (For further information on TPN, see Chapter 42.)

Fluids given by any route should be spaced throughout the 24-hour period. Not only does this practice help to maintain normal body fluid levels, but it also provides for better regulation of the electrolyte balance by the kidneys and prevents the end products of metabolism and toxic materials from being excreted in concentrated form. In this way the danger of renal damage, formation of calculi, and irritation of the lower urinary tract is reduced. In addition, fluid spacing prevents overloading of the circulation, which may result in dilution of body fluids, with resultant fluid and electrolyte shifts, the most serious of which causes pulmonary edema (Chapter 28).

Concentrated solutions of sugar or protein should always be given slowly and in small amounts at a time, because they require body fluids for dilution. Hypertonic saline solution may cause fluid to diffuse from the tissues to equalize the concentration of salt in the vascular compartment; therefore it too should be given slowly and in small amounts. Because of the rapid dilution by the larger amounts of blood at the superior vena cava, it is the preferred site for infusions of hypertonic solutions given by parenteral hyperalimentation.

Giving concentrated solutions rapidly and in large amounts into the alimentary tract causes a rapid shift of fluid from the vascular compartment into the intestinal lumen and a resultant decrease in blood volume, which can lead to shock. The "dumping syndrome," which sometimes occurs after a gastric resection, is caused by this abnormal shift of fluid. Concentrated solutions sometimes are given intentionally to reduce cerebral edema. Giving large amounts of fluid either orally or parenterally is potentially dangerous even in a healthy person, and therefore fluids of any kind should never be replaced faster than they are lost.

The size of the patient should be considered when administering fluids. The small adult normally has less fluid in each body compartment, especially in the intravascular system. This person therefore becomes seriously dehydrated more quickly than a larger adult and needs to have fluid losses replaced more promptly. People with small or inelastic vascular systems also become overhydrated easily. It is important to remember that the vascular system of a person who has had a large portion of the body such as a limb removed either by surgery or trauma is not the same size as previously.

ORAL INTAKE

Adults who have no circulatory or renal malfunction usually are given between 2500 and 3000 ml/day. Precautions should be taken so that the overzealous patient does not drink too much fluid in a day or does not take too much (3 to 4 glasses) at one time. Excessive water intake may cause water intoxication.

When they are ill, many persons find it difficult to eat or drink even though they are allowed to do so. There are many ways that the nurse can help the patient take adequate food and fluids orally and thus avoid the need for parenteral fluids. Fruit drinks, tea, coffee, ginger ale, or other soft drinks may be substituted for part of the water. Soup, bouillon, milk, eggnog, and cocoa provide both fluid and nutrients. Juicy fruits and other semisolid foods with a high fluid and nutrient content such as custard, ice cream, or gelatin may be more palatable than regular meals and tap water. Care must be taken, of course, that any substitutions are allowed on the diet prescribed for the patient. If a fluid record is needed, the amount of fluid given in semisolid form is estimated and recorded.

The methods used in presenting food and fluids to patients may influence their consumption; often a small amount of either food or fluid offered at frequent intervals is more acceptable than is a large amount presented less often. Serving foods that the patient likes may improve appetite. For example, carbonated beverages may be better tolerated by patients who are nauseated. Consideration should always be given to the cultural and esthetic aspects of eating.

Vomiting and diarrhea are common symptoms of many illnesses, and most people suffer from them from time to time. Sodium and some potassium are lost in vomiting and diarrhea, whereas chloride is lost only in vomitus. As soon as fluids are tolerated, the patient who has vomiting or diarrhea should be served salty broth and tea or another fluid high in potassium (see Table 23-10) to replace the losses. This measure often helps the patient feel less weak and exhausted. Dry soda crackers often are tolerated when fluids are not and can be used to replace sodium.

A patient with a draining fistula from any portion of the gastrointestinal tract loses sodium, calcium, and potassium, and dietary supplements are necessary. Extra milk will replace all the losses, and the patient is instructed to increase milk intake somewhat above normal levels. For the body to use the calcium, vitamin D also must be available, but most milk is now fortified with vitamin D. Persons with a permanent fistulous opening, such as an ileostomy, need to be especially careful to supplement sodium and potassium when vomiting, diarrhea, or fever add to their already unusually large loss of electrolytes.

The nurse needs to know which foods contain large and small amounts of various essential nutrients, minerals, and vitamins (see Chapter 40). When losses must be restored, the patient needs more than is required in the usual adequate diet. It is especially important to know which foods and fluids are high or low in potassium and sodium and which foods are complete proteins. Bananas, citrus fruits, all fruit juices, many fresh vegetables, coffee, and tea are relatively high in potassium and low in sodium content. Salty broths and tomato juice provide extra sodium but have a high potassium content. Meat, milk, and eggs are all complete protein foods and contain relatively large quantities of both sodium and potassium. Current nutrition literature and the dietitian or nutritionist should be consulted as necessary.

The nurse frequently has an order to "force fluids." Because the amount required depends on the size of the patient, the amount of fluid loss, and the patient's circulatory and renal status, no standard amount can be given. The nurse must therefore make a judgment as to the desirable amount and inform members of the nursing team or family members who will care for the patient. If there is any question, the physician is consulted.

If an elderly person living at home complains of pronounced weakness without apparent cause, the nurse should ask whether cathartics or enemas have been taken. If so, stopping this procedure, eating foods with high sodium and potassium content, and increasing the fluid intake may relieve the symptoms. Methods to combat constipation without purging should be taught.

Any patient with renal or circulatory impairment, as may occur in shock, cardiac decompensation, or constriction of blood vessels because of disease, may develop electrolyte imbalance. Sodium and water may be held in the tissues, the potassium level of the blood may rise, acidosis may develop from inadequate tissue oxygenation, or the kidneys may be unable to excrete waste products properly. Patients with cardiac and renal impairment are instructed to avoid taking too much food containing sodium, potassium, or bicarbonate.

GAVAGE (TUBE FEEDING)

Water, a physiologic solution of sodium chloride, high-protein liquids, or a regular diet that has been passed through a blender and diluted is often given by gavage to older children and adults (see Chapter 42). As previously mentioned, high-protein tube feeding can cause water deficit through osmotic diuresis. A need to increase water intake along with the tube feeding should be considered when (1) the patient complains of thirst, (2) protein content of the tube feeding is high, (3) the patient has a fever, (4) urinary output is decreased or very concentrated, and (5) signs of water deficit develop.[15]

PARENTERAL FLUIDS
TYPES OF SOLUTIONS

The nurse needs to know the common solutions used parenterally (Table 23-12). A solution of 5% dextrose in distilled water is often used to maintain fluid intake or to reestablish water volume. Ascorbic acid and vitamin B (Solu-B) are frequently added. Dextrose, 5%, in saline solution may be given depending on the serum levels of sodium and the vascular volume, and potassium chloride may be added to meet normal intake needs of potassium and to replace losses. A physiologic solution of sodium chloride is given primarily when sodium chloride has been lost in large amounts such as in loss of gastrointestinal fluids or in burns and when patients have vascular volume deficits. A one-sixth molar lactate solution may be ordered when sodium, but not chloride, needs replacement; ammonium chloride solution may be used to replace chlorides when added sodium is undesirable. Balanced solutions containing several electro-

lytes may be used to replace fluid loss in surgical patients. Ringer's solution and lactated Ringer's solution are examples.

Body needs for carbohydrates may be partially met by giving fructose or 10% or 20% glucose in distilled water, but these solutions are hypertonic and require additional water for excretion.

Amino acid preparations (Aminosol) are seldom given by standard intravenous methods. Whole blood is the fluid of choice to replace blood loss, but plasma, 25% salt-poor albumin, or plasma volume expanders can be given to substitute for blood protein loss and are used to reestablish normal blood volume and prevent shock. Dextran is the most generally accepted plasma volume expander. It increases the oncotic pressure of the blood, thus increasing the reabsorption of fluid from interstitial spaces and increasing plasma volume. Low-molecular-weight dextran decreases the viscosity of the blood, allowing greater flow of blood through the capillaries; thus it is useful in treating cardiogenic, hemorrhagic, or septic shock (see Chapter 25). It may cause a prolonged bleeding time and should not be used if renal disease with severe oliguria or anuria is present or during pregnancy.[8]

INTERVENTIONS

Intravenous fluids containing electrolytes should be run slowly to allow the body to regulate their use. The patient is watched carefully for untoward signs (excess of fluids or electrolytes). Increased serum potassium (hyperkalemia) can be particularly dangerous, because it may cause cardiac arrest. When solutions containing electrolytes are given, the nurse monitors the urinary output carefully and reports any marked decrease in the amount to the physician. Because the kidneys select the ions needed and excrete surplus ones, a normal output

TABLE 23-12 Solutions for intravenous use

	Contents of Solutions								
	Cations (mEq/L)					Anions (mEq/L)			
Type of Solution	Na⁺	K⁺	Ca⁺⁺	Mg⁺⁺	NH₄⁻	Cl⁻	HCO₃⁻ Lactate	PO₄⁻	Glucose (g/L)
5% Dextrose in water									50
10% Dextrose in water									100
Normal saline (0.9%)	154					154			
3% Saline	513					513			
Ringer's solution	147	4	4			155			
5% Dextrose in Ringer's lactate	130	4	3			109	28		50
Ringer's lactate	130	4	3			109	28		
Ammonium chloride (0.9%)					170	170			
Sodium lactate ⅙ molar	167						167		
5% Dextrose in 0.2% saline	34					34			50
5% Dextrose in 0.45% saline	77					77			50

is essential. If the nurse is planning the sequence of intravenous fluids, hydrating fluids such as one-half strength physiologic solution of sodium chloride or glucose in water solution should be given first if the patient primarily has a water deficit. Renal failure and untreated adrenal insufficiency are contraindications for the use of potassium. If these conditions are known or suspected to exist, the nurse should verify orders for its administration. Many physicians do not start intravenous therapy for the day until blood chemistry results have been reported.

Usually the rate of administration of fluids is ordered by the physician and depends on the patient's illness, the kind of fluid given, and the patient's age. An infusion is rarely run at a rate faster than 4 ml/min. If it is given continuously or if it is given when there is impaired renal function or impaired cardiac function, it is rarely run faster than 2 ml/min. The usual rate for replacement of fluid loss is 3 ml/min. This rate allows time for the fluid to diffuse into ECF compartments and avoids overloading the circulation or raising the blood volume high enough to produce a diuretic effect. The equipment used for fluid administration may have varying numbers of drops per milliliter, and the nurse needs to check the equipment used to determine the rate of delivery, because it is not the drops per minute but the milliliters per minute that are important.

Nurses should question the advisability of the rather common practice of speeding up the rate of flow of solutions given intravenously primarily to complete the treatment at a specified time. Every nurse should recognize the initial signs of pulmonary edema (bounding pulse, engorged peripheral veins, hoarseness, dyspnea, cough, or pulmonary rales) and should watch closely for them in those patients who are receiving concentrated solutions, those who must be given any intravenous solution rapidly, and those whose age or physical condition makes them special risks. At the first signs of increased blood volume, the rate of flow of the infusion should be reduced to a "keep open" rate or barely running at 5 to 6 drops/min, and the physician notified. Special care needs to be taken in giving fluids to infants, elderly patients with circulatory impairment, patients whose hearts are decompensated, those with renal impairment, those who have had plasma shifts such as burned patients, and those with extensive tissue trauma from other causes. Patients whose plasma has shifted need to be watched especially carefully because after a few days the plasma tends to shift back suddenly from the interstitial tissue to the blood, potentially producing an increase in blood volume with resulting pulmonary edema.

It is imperative that the nurse check the labels of fluid bottles carefully for correctness of content and record accurately the fluids given. (For details of equipment and nursing techniques needed in parenteral fluid administration, refer to a textbook on fundamentals of nursing.)

Patients who are receiving fluids intravenously are observed frequently so that symptoms indicating the need to slow down, speed up, or stop the infusion may be noted (Table 23-13). The tissue at the site of the inserted needle or catheter is checked at intervals for signs of infiltration or inflammatory reaction. If infiltration occurs, the infusion should be stopped at once and plans made to restart it. Solutions containing potassium are very irritating, and extravasation may cause tissue necrosis. When dextran or other protein solutions are being given, the patient is observed for signs of anaphylactic reaction (apprehension, dyspnea, wheezing respirations, tightness of chest, itching, hypotension) (Chapter 76).

RELIEF OF SYMPTOMS

Persons with fluid and electrolyte imbalance often have extreme thirst, nausea, and vomiting. These symptoms are distressing, and the nurse should know measures that can be used to give the patient relief.

THIRST

Thirst, the first and most insistent sign of dehydration, sometimes causes the patient more misery than surgery or the symptoms of a disease. It may develop even when fluids have been withheld only for a number of hours. If fluids are being withheld intentionally, thirst often is made more bearable by explaining to the patient why the fluids are being withheld and when they will be reinstituted.

Usually, thirst is relieved readily by taking fluids. When fluids cannot be taken orally, the administration of fluids parenterally usually gives relief. It is often helpful to explain this to the patient. Mouth care will allay some of the discomfort from thirst. This care includes cleansing the tongue, teeth, and mucous membranes lining the oral cavity. It may be necessary to repeat the procedure every hour. Solutions containing glycerine or alcohol should be avoided because of their drying effect. A mixture of hydrogen peroxide and saline is effective in removing dried secretions.

When fluids are not permitted, the water pitcher at the bedside is removed, and if the patient cannot be relied on not to get up and drink at a water tap, special provisions such as insistence on bed rest may be necessary. Thirst sometimes compels the patient to obtain water in any way possible.

Pronounced and continued thirst despite the administration of fluids is not normal and should be reported. In the immediate postoperative period, this kind of thirst suggests internal hemorrhage, elevation of temperature, or some other untoward development. In the chronically ill patient it may indicate the onset of disease such as

TABLE 23-13 Complications of intravenous fluid therapy

Complication	Observations	Nursing Actions
Circulatory overload	Bounding pulse, venous distention, hoarseness, dyspnea, cough, pulmonary rales, restlessness	Notify physician Reduce flow to "keep open" rate Raise head of bed to facilitate breathing
Local infiltration	Decreased rate or cessation of fluid flow Tissue around needle or catheter site cold, pale, swollen, hard Complaint of local pain	Stop infusion Arrange to restart infusion at another site Apply moist heat Elevate lower arm
Thrombophlebitis	Pain, redness, warmth, edema along vein	Same as for local infiltration Cold compresses may be applied initially
Pyrogenic reaction	Fever, chills, general malaise, nausea, and vomiting 30 min after infusion started Hypotension (if severe)	Switch to another infusion solution and run at "keep open" rate Notify physician Monitor vital signs Save infusion fluid for culture
Anaphylactic reaction (with proteins)	Apprehension, dyspnea, wheezing, tightness of chest, itching, hypotension	Switch infusion to nonprotein solution and run at "keep open" rate Notify physician Monitor vital signs

diabetes mellitus in which extra water is used by the kidneys to eliminate glucose in the urine. It is also a symptom of hypercalcemia.

NAUSEA AND VOMITING

Fluid and electrolyte imbalances may cause nausea and vomiting. Vomiting in turn frequently leads to further fluid and electrolyte imbalances as a result of the loss of gastric secretions. A vicious cycle may be set up:

Vomiting → Losses → Vomiting → (and so on)

Treatment of severe nausea and vomiting is by replacing the fluids and electrolytes by parenteral methods and by the use of antiemetic medications. The care of the person experiencing nausea and vomiting is described in Chapter 42.

CHAPTER SUMMARY

- Internal regulation of sodium and water is controlled by thirst, the kidney, ADH, the aldosterone-renin-angiotensin system, and third factor.

- When a change in the sodium-to-water ratio occurs, a disturbance in osmolality results; that is, the ECF becomes dilute (hyposmolar) or more concentrated (hyperosmolar) than normal.

- When the concentration of sodium, potassium, or calcium is increased or decreased in body fluids, the increase or decrease is reflected in the stimulation of muscles by nerves.

- Losses of fluid and electrolytes occur through the skin by diaphoresis and oozing from severe wounds or burns; from gastrointestinal drainage and ene-

mas; from the kidneys because of diuretic use and polyuria; from hemorrhage; and through the trapping of fluids by wound swelling, edema, ascites, and intestinal obstruction.

- Elderly persons are particularly vulnerable to fluid and electrolyte disorders because of the following changes: (1) less total body water; (2) declines in the function of vital regulatory organs; (3) the high incidence of chronic illnesses; and (4) a diminished ability to reestablish homeostasis when an imbalance has occurred.

- Assessment of fluid and electrolyte balance includes the monitoring of laboratory values, fluid intake, fluid output (urinary output, wound drainage, gastrointestinal drainage, fluid from any body cavity, diaphoresis), daily weight, and urine specific gravity.

QUESTIONS TO CONSIDER

- What measures would you recommend to young women to prevent osteoporosis?

- How would you explain a low potassium diet to an elderly patient with a hearing deficit?

- Explain the relationship between vitamin D, parathyroid hormone, and calcium absorption.

- Why are the elderly at particular risk of dehydration?

- What is the best method to administer water, electrolytes, and nutrients? Why?

REFERENCES AND SELECTED READINGS

1. Ashby D: Balancing fluids and electrolytes in the PACU, J Post Anesth Nurs 2(2):114-116, 1987.
2. *Barta M: Correcting electrolyte imbalances, RN 50(2):30-34, 1987.
3. Brocklehurst JC and Allen S: Geriatric medicine for students, ed 3, New York, 1987, Churchill Livingstone.
4. *Calloway C: When the problem involves magnesium, calcium, or phosphate, RN 50(5):30-36, 1987.
5. *Felver L and Pendarvis J: Electrolyte imbalances: intraoperative risk factors, AORN J 49(4):992-1008, 1989.
6. Fishback F: A manual of laboratory diagnostic tests, Philadelphia, 1984, JB Lippincott Co.
7. Folk-Lighty M: Solving the puzzles of patients' fluid imbalance, Nursing 14(2):34-41, 1984.
8. Goldberger E: A primer of water, electrolyte and acid-base syndromes, ed 7, Philadelphia, 1986, Lea & Febiger.
9. Groer M and Shekelton ME: Basic pathophysiology: a holistic approach, St. Louis, 1989, The CV Mosby Co.
10. Guyton A: Textbook of medical physiology, ed 7, Philadelphia, 1986, WB Saunders Co.
11. Hahn AB, Barkin RL, and Oestreich SJK: Pharmacology in nursing, ed 16, St Louis, 1985, The CV Mosby Co.
12. *Hennessy L: HHNK dehydration, Am J Nurs 83:1425-1426, 1983.
13. Himmelstein DV, et al: Hypernatremic dehydration in nursing home patients, J Am Geriatr Soc 31:466-471, 1983.
14. Krupp M and Chatton M: Current medical diagnosis and treatment, ed 26, Los Altos, Calif, 1986, Appleton & Lange.
15. Kubo W, et al: Fluid and electrolyte problems of tube-fed patients, Am J Nurs 76:912-916, 1976.
16. Lucas CF and Ledgerwood AM: The fluid problem in the critically ill, Surg Clin North Am 63:439-454, 1983.
17. *Mathewson M: Intravenous therapy, Crit Care Nurs 9(2):21-23, 26-28, 30-36, 1989.
18. Methany NM: Fluid and electrolyte balance: nursing considerations, ed 3, Philadelphia, 1987, JB Lippincott Co.
19. Methany NM: Preoperative fluid balance assessment, AORN J 33:51-56, 1981.
20. Miller G: Osteoporosis: is it inevitable? J Gerontol Nurs 11(3):10-15, 1985.
21. Quinlan M: Would you recognize this dangerous electrolyte imbalance? RN 46(3):51-55, 1983.
22. Roach FB: Color changes in dark skin, Nursing 2:20-22, 1972.
23. Robinson SB and Demuth P: Diagnostic studies for the aged: what are the dangers? J Gerontol Nurs 11(6):6-12, 1985.
24. Sabiston DC, editor: Textbook of surgery, ed 13, Philadelphia, 1986, WB Saunders Co.
25. Stroot V, Lee C, and Schaper C: Fluids and electrolytes: a practical approach, ed 3, Philadelphia, 1984, FA Davis Co.
26. *Symposium on fluid, electrolytes, and acid-base balance, Nurs Clin North Am 22(4):749-872, 1987.
27. *Valle G and Lemberg L: Electrolyte imbalances in cardiovascular disease: the forgotten factor, Heart & Lung 17(3):324-329, 1988.
28. Vander AJ, Sherman JH, and Luciano DS: Human physiology: mechanisms of body functioning, ed 3, New York, 1980, McGraw-Hill Book Co.
29. Wade JF: Comprehensive respiratory care, ed 3, St Louis, 1982, The CV Mosby Co.
30. Williams S: Essentials of nutrition and diet therapy, ed 4, St Louis, 1986, The CV Mosby Co.
31. Winters B: Nursing implications of hyperosmolar coma, Heart Lung 12:439-446, 1983.
32. *Woodward W and Woodward T: Management of dehydrating diarrhea, Hosp Pract 21(3):60, 63, 67-68, 1986.
33. Wyngaarden JB and Smith LH, editors: Textbook of medicine, vol 1 and 2, ed 18, Philadelphia, 1988, WB Saunders Co.
34. *Young M and Flynn K: Third-spacing: when the body conceals fluid loss, RN 51(8):46-48, 1988.

*References preceded by an asterisk are particularly well suited for student reading.

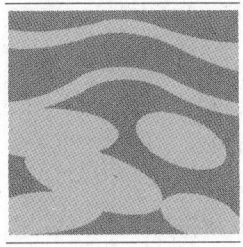

CHAPTER 24

Acid-Base Imbalance

MARY KAY LEHMAN

CHAPTER OBJECTIVES

After studying this chapter, the student should be able to:
1. Describe the mechanisms that maintain acid-base balance.
2. Differentiate between metabolic and respiratory acidosis and alkalosis, and describe the causes and effects of each type.
3. Identify data indicating acid-base imbalances.
4. Describe the management of patients with acid-base imbalances.

This chapter reviews the regulation of normal acid-base balance. Mechanisms that regulate acid-base balance, including chemical buffer systems, the respiratory system, and the kidneys, are explored. Causes, prevention, clinical manifestations, and interventions for acid-base imbalances are discussed.

Although the prescription of medical therapy to prevent and treat imbalances is the responsibility of the physician, nurses must carry out the following vital functions:

1. Recognizing situations likely to cause imbalances
2. Intervening to prevent imbalances
3. Carrying out preventive and therapeutic measures prescribed by the physician and monitoring patients' responses to these measures
4. Recognizing signs and symptoms of acid-base disturbances
5. Monitoring patients to prevent and recognize imbalances related to their specific conditions or treatments
6. Alleviating the effects of disturbances on the comfort and safety of patients

ACID-BASE BALANCE AND IMBALANCES

REGULATION OF ACID-BASE BALANCE

Hydrogen ions are vital to life and health. The concentration of hydrogen in the body is less than that of other ions (0.00004 mEq/L). Hydrogen ion concentration is expressed as pH. Normal arterial body pH is 7.35 to 7.45. A reading of less than 7.35 is present in acidosis,

and a reading greater than 7.45 is present in alkalosis. Limits of pH compatible with life are 7 to 7.8.

Hydrogen circulates throughout the body fluids in two forms: the volatile hydrogen of carbonic acid and the nonvolatile form of hydrogen in organic acids such as sulfuric, pyruvic, phosphoric, and lactic acids. In a day's time many acids are produced as the end products of metabolism. In the normal person, the lungs excrete 13,000 to 30,000 mEq/day of the volatile hydrogen in carbonic acid (H_2CO_3) as CO_2, and the kidneys excrete approximately 50 mEq/day of nonvolatile acids.

Mechanisms that regulate acid-base balance include chemical buffer systems, the respiratory system, and the kidneys (Table 24-1).

CHEMICAL BUFFER SYSTEMS

The body cells are very sensitive to changes in pH, and the pH is kept relatively constant by the buffer systems in the body. A buffer is a substance that can act as a chemical sponge, by either soaking up or releasing hydrogen ions so that the pH remains stable. The main buffer systems of the body are the carbonic acid–bicarbonate system, the phosphate system, and protein. The carbonic acid–bicarbonate buffer system is the system that is monitored clinically. If this buffer system is stable, the other buffer systems are stable.

Carbonic Acid–Bicarbonate Buffer System

The carbonic acid–bicarbonate system is present in extracellular fluid (ECF). Carbonic acid is formed by the combination of carbon dioxide and water: $CO_2 + H_2O \rightleftarrows H_2CO_3$. When a strong base is added to the body fluids, it is buffered by carbonic acid to a bicarbonate salt and water: $H_2CO_3 + NaOH \rightarrow NaHCO_3 + H_2O$. When a strong acid is added to the system, the bicarbonate buffer changes it to a salt and carbonic acid: $HCl + NaHCO_3 \rightarrow NaCl + H_2CO_3$. This carbonic acid then dissociates into carbon dioxide and water and can be excreted by the lungs and kidneys.

The ability to maintain a stable pH relies essentially on maintenance of the normal ratio of 20 parts bicar-

TABLE 24-1 Mechanisms regulating acid-base balance

	Action Time	Effect
Chemical buffers in cells and ECF	Instantaneous	Combine with acids or bases added to the system to prevent marked changes in pH
Respiratory system	Minutes to hours	Controls CO_2 concentration in ECF by changes in rate and depth of respiration
Kidneys	Hours to days	Increases or decreases quantity of $NaHCO_3$ in ECF Combines HCO_3^- or H^+ with other substances and excretes them in urine

bonate to 1 part carbonic acid. The normal serum bicarbonate is 24 to 28 mEq/L. The carbonic acid level is determined by taking the P_{CO_2} (normally 40 torr) and multiplying it by the constant 0.03. This constant is the dissolvability factor of CO_2. This computation gives an approximate figure of 1.2. From these figures it can be seen that the normal bicarbonate–carbonic acid ratio is 20:1 (Figure 24-1).

This ratio of 20:1 is maintained by the lungs and the kidneys. The carbonic acid concentration is controlled by excretion by the lungs of the gas carbon dioxide. The depth and rate of respiration change in response to changes in carbon dioxide. The bicarbonate concentration is controlled by the kidneys, which selectively retain or excrete bicarbonate in response to the body's needs.

Phosphate Buffer System

The phosphate buffer system is present in cells and ECF; it is especially active in the kidneys. Like bicarbonate, phosphate can "mop up" spare hydrogen ions. Conversely, 1 molecule of phosphoric acid can donate up to 3 hydrogen ions to make up for any hydrogen ion deficits. Phosphate groups may occur free in plasma or bound to certain organic compounds. Even when bound, phosphate can exert some buffering influence.[6]

The phosphate system is composed of sodium and other cations in combination with $H_2PO_4^-$ and $HPO_4^=$. When a strong acid is present, the following action takes place: $Na_2HPO_4 + HCl \rightarrow NaCl + NaH_2PO_4$. A hydrogen ion is excreted via the urine in the NaH_2PO_4. A strong base is buffered in the following reaction: $NaOH + NaH_2PO_4 \rightarrow Na_2HPO_4 + H_2O$. Na_2HPO_4 is a weak base and minimizes the pH change.[5]

Protein Buffer System

The protein buffer system is located in the plasma and inside cells; the protein hemoglobin in red blood cells is one of the proteins involved. Although most protein buffers are intracellular, they assist in buffering ECF. Some of the amino acids in proteins contain free acid radicals, $-COOH$, which can dissociate into $CO_2 + H$,

thus adding a hydrogen ion. Other proteins have basic radicals, $-NH_3OH$, which can dissociate into NH_3^+ and OH^-; the OH^- combines with a hydrogen ion to form water, thus removing one hydrogen ion from body fluid. The protein buffer system is the most plentiful buffer system in the body.[5]

RESPIRATORY CONTROL OF pH

The respiratory control center in the brain responds to increases of carbon dioxide and hydrogen ions in body fluids. Rate and depth of respiration are in turn controlled by the respiratory control of pH as follows: (1) when pH decreases (more acid), respiratory rate and depth are increased, and there is greater excretion of carbon dioxide through the lungs; thus less carbon dioxide is present to produce carbonic acid by the reaction: $CO_2 + H_2O \rightleftarrows H_2CO_3$, and the pH increases toward alkalinity; and (2) when pH rises above the normal range (more alkaline), the respiratory center is depressed, rate and depth of respiration decrease, carbon dioxide is retained, and more carbonic acid is formed, moving the pH toward acidity.

Because carbon dioxide is constantly being formed as a product of metabolism, the concentration of carbon dioxide in ECFs must be continuously balanced between the rate of metabolism and the rate of pulmonary excretion. The buffering capacity of the respiratory system is more than double that of all the chemical buffers combined.

RENAL REGULATION OF pH

Both chemical buffers and respiratory regulation have limited ability to make complete adjustments in pH, and it remains for the kidneys to make permanent adjustments in the pH of body fluids. The renal regulation of pH is affected by control of the retention or excretion of bicarbonate and hydrogen ions. The kidneys usually excrete an acid urine because of the excess of acid metabolic products (nonvolatile acids), which must be eliminated by the renal route. Normally, almost all of the bicarbonate formed by the kidneys is retained.

Hydrogen ions secreted by kidney tubule cells and

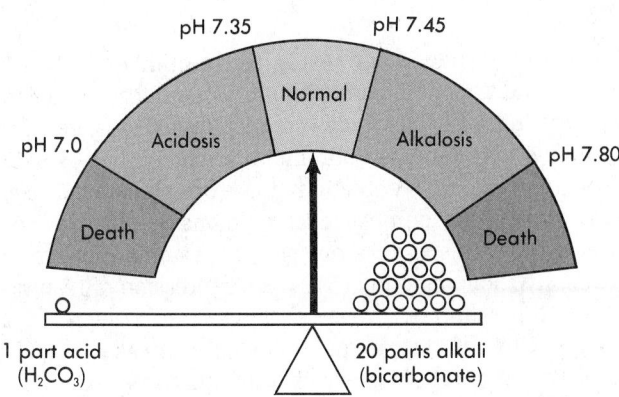

Carbonic acid-base bicarbonate balance

FIGURE 24-1 Note that relationship of 1 part carbonic acid to 20 parts bicarbonate maintains hydrogen ion concentration (pH) within normal limits. Increase in H_2CO_3 or decrease in HCO_3^- causes acidosis; similarly, decrease in H_2CO_3 or increase in HCO_3^- causes alkalosis. (Redrawn from Abbott Laboratories: Fluid and electrolytes, North Chicago, 1970, Abbott Laboratories.)

bicarbonate filtered into the glomerular filtrate combine in the kidney tubules to form carbon dioxide and water, which is excreted through exhalation (CO_2) and in urine (H_2O). In acidosis, excess hydrogen ions are secreted into the kidney tubules, where they combine with buffers and are excreted in the urine. In alkalosis, bicarbonate ions enter the tubules, where there exists a lack of the hydrogen ions with which they normally combine to form carbonic acid; the bicarbonate ions combine instead with sodium or other cations and are excreted in the urine. Hydrogen ions can be exchanged for sodium and potassium ions in the kidney tubules; therefore excretion or conservation of hydrogen ions can result in imbalances of sodium and potassium.

COMPENSATION

The kidneys and lungs serve a compensatory function in relation to maintaining acid-base balance. In a disease state that leads to an acid-base imbalance, the normal bicarbonate–carbonic acid ratio of 20:1 is lost. In compensation, the kidneys attempt to compensate for changes in blood CO_2 by making a corresponding change in blood *bicarbonate*, and the lungs attempt to compensate for abnormal changes in blood bicarbonate by making corresponding changes in blood CO_2. Compensation is an effort to maintain the normal 20:1 ratio. Figure 24-2 illustrates what happens in metabolic acidosis and how compensation of acid-base imbalance can occur.

The extent of change in either bicarbonate or P_{CO_2} that will be needed for compensation to take place can

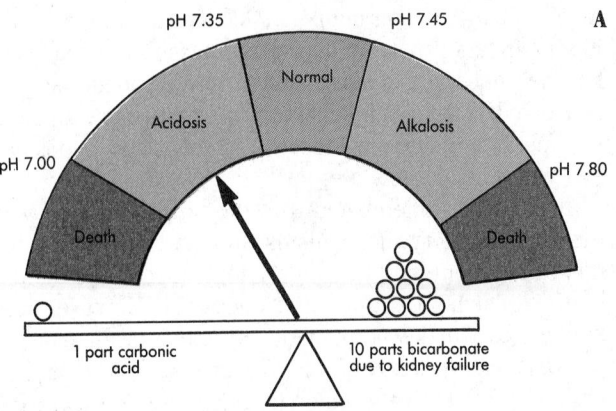

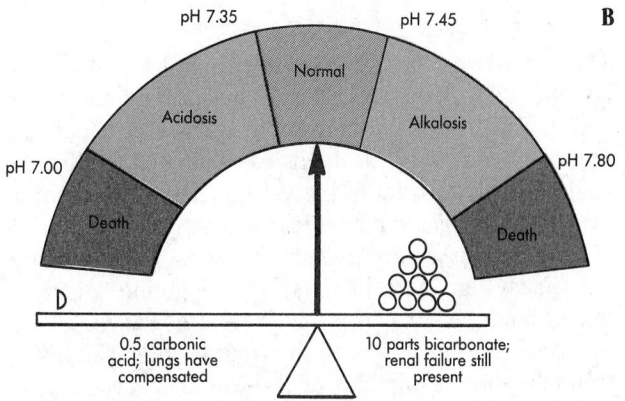

FIGURE 24-2 A, Example of metabolic acidosis. Bicarbonate decreased because of renal failure. Carbonic acid to bicarbonate ratio is 10:1; acidosis is present. **B,** Example of compensation. Note that bicarbonate is still decreased, but now carbonic acid is also decreased. Ratio returned to 20:1; pH is normal.

be calculated.[3] For example, a patient who has a P_{CO_2} of 30 would need a bicarbonate of 18 to bring the pH into normal range:

$$(P_{CO_2})\ 40:30 = (HCO_3)\ 24:x$$
$$40x = 30(24)$$
$$40x = 720$$
$$x = 18$$

Another compensatory mechanism that can be used by the body in the presence of acid-base problems is *shifting of hydrogen ions from the extracellular to the intracellular compartment or vice versa.* When there is an increased level of hydrogen ions (metabolic acidosis), these ions can be shifted into the intracellular compartment in exchange for *potassium.* This shift alone increases the pH of the blood. In addition, because the hydrogen ion concentration is now higher in the renal tubule cells, hydrogen is excreted in exchange for the reabsorbed sodium. In *metabolic alkalosis*, hydrogen ions are pulled from the intracellular compartment, and potassium ions are shifted into the intracellular compartment. Again, this shift alone helps to lower the pH.

Also, because potassium ion concentration is now higher in the renal tubule cells, potassium is excreted for the conserved sodium, and hydrogen ions also are conserved. These compensatory mechanisms can lead to hyperkalemia when acidosis is present and hypokalemia when alkalosis is present.

It must be remembered that the buffer systems and the compensatory mechanisms provide for only temporary adjustment, and the underlying cause of the disturbance must be identified and corrected. However, the kidneys can make permanent adjustments as seen in persons who have respiratory acidosis as a result of chronic obstructive pulmonary disease (see Chapter 33).

TYPES OF ACID-BASE DISTURBANCES

There are two types of acidosis (respiratory and metabolic) and two types of alkalosis (respiratory and metabolic). Table 24-2 shows the four types that occur and their compensatory mechanisms. The major effect of acidosis is depression of the central nervous system as evidenced by disorientation followed by coma (Table 24-3). Alkalosis is characterized by overexcitability of the nervous system, and the muscles may go into a state of tetany and convulsions. Acid-base imbalance always produces an imbalance of the body's other cations as well; therefore symptoms of these imbalances also occur.

LABORATORY TESTS

The following laboratory values are used in diagnosing and monitoring acid-base disturbance:

pH (normal): 7.35 to 7.45

P_{CO_2} (normal): 38 to 42 torr

Plasma bicarbonate (normal): 23 to 25 mEq/L

Both pH and P_{CO_2} are determined from a sample of arterial blood, a blood gas analysis.

Table 24-4 shows whether laboratory values characteristic of the four types of acid-base disturbances are increased or decreased and the results of the body's compensatory efforts when partial compensation occurs.

RESPIRATORY ACIDOSIS: CARBONIC ACID EXCESS

Any factor that decreases the rate of pulmonary ventilation increases the concentration of dissolved carbon dioxide, carbonic acid, and hydrogen ions and results in *respiratory acidosis*. An excess of carbon dioxide (hypercapnia) can cause carbon dioxide narcosis. In this condition carbon dioxide levels are so high that they no longer stimulate respirations but depress them. Associated with the decreased respiratory rate are lack of oxygen and hypoxia. During respiratory acidosis, potassium moves out of the cells, producing hyperkalemia. Ventricular fibrillation may occur if the blood potassium level is greatly increased.

ETIOLOGY

Respiratory acidosis can result from a number of pathologic conditions: (1) damage to the respiratory center in the medulla; (2) obstruction of respiratory passages, for example, pneumonia, chronic bronchitis; (3) loss of lung surface for ventilation, for example, atelectasis, pneumothorax, emphysema, pulmonary fibrosis; (4) weakness of respiratory muscles, for example, poliomyelitis, hypokalemia; and (5) severe depression of respirations, for example, overdose of respiratory depressant drugs. Chronic obstructive pulmonary disease (COPD) is the most common cause of respiratory acidosis.

PREVENTION

Persons with diseases such as emphysema that limit lung excursion and therefore limit gaseous exchange should not take carbonated beverages or bicarbonate of soda. These substances tend to make the blood more alkaline than normal, and respirations are depressed in an effort to correct this imbalance. Depression of respirations is highly undesirable for these patients.

Any person with symptoms of inadequate oxygenation or carbon dioxide retention requires medical treatment. Early recognition and treatment of the primary condition often prevent its becoming complicated by acid-base imbalance. Therefore any person with symptoms suggestive of anemia, cardiac insufficiency, or chronic bronchitis, emphysema, asthma, or other obstructive diseases of the bronchioles should receive medical attention. These conditions are discussed in detail in later chapters of the book.

CLINICAL MANIFESTATIONS

Signs and symptoms of respiratory acidosis include hyperpnea, visual disturbances, and headache. Later, confusion, drowsiness, and coma can ensue. Ventricular fibrillation may be the first sign noted in some cases.

INTERVENTIONS

Treatment is aimed at increasing the alveolar ventilation rate to improve the exchange of carbon dioxide and oxygen. This objective is accomplished by using respiratory treatments with bronchodilators, postural drainage, and chest clapping in persons with obstruction of respiratory passages. Because the respiratory center is narcotized by the increased amounts of carbon dioxide, the lowered oxygen tension of the blood is the stimulus for respiration. If a patient whose respiratory drive is dependent on a low P_{O_2} is given large amounts of oxygen, the stimulus for breathing is removed, and respirations will cease. For this reason, uncontrolled oxygen delivery is never used with patients with carbon dioxide narcosis. Low-flow oxygen (1 to 3 L/min) is given to a patient with chronic pulmonary disease who maintains a chronically high P_{CO_2}. Respiratory treatments are usually

TABLE 24-2 Types of acid-base disturbances and compensatory mechanisms

Disturbance	Physiologic Causes	Method of Compensation
Respiratory acidosis	Carbonic acid excess: lungs not removing sufficient CO_2 (hypoventilation)	Bicarbonate production by kidneys increased; bicarbonate retained and chloride excreted instead by kidneys; secretion and excretion of hydrogen ions in urine increased
Respiratory alkalosis	Carbonic acid deficit: lungs removing too much CO_2 (hyperventilation)	Kidneys increase excretion of bicarbonate ions
Metabolic acidosis	Bicarbonate deficit: retention of acid metabolites, diabetic ketoacidosis, excess acid intake (salicylate poisoning), hyperkalemia, or loss of bicarbonate	Increased rate and depth of respiration cause increased excretion of CO_2 by lungs; formation of bicarbonate ions in the kidneys increased

Metabolic alkalosis	Bicarbonate excess:
	    excess intake (sodium bicarbonate, carbonated drinks) or retention of bicarbonate
	    Potassium depletion
	    Loss of acid
		Rate and depth of respiration decreased; lungs retain more CO_2; kidneys excrete bicarbonate

TABLE 24-3 Major signs and symptoms and therapy for acid-base imbalances

Imbalance	Signs and Symptoms	Therapy
Respiratory acidosis	Hyperpnea Visual disturbances Headache Ventricular fibrillation Late: confusion, drowsiness, coma Potassium excess	Bronchodilators Postural drainage Chest clapping Sodium bicarbonate for ventricular fibrillation or potassium excess
Respiratory alkalosis	Lightheadedness Numbness or tingling of fingers or toes Late: tetany, convulsions Potassium deficit	Treatment of underlying condition
Metabolic acidosis	Headache and mental dullness Kussmaul's respirations Late: disorientation, coma Potassium excess	Treatment of underlying condition Sodium bicarbonate(IV) Fluid and electrolyte replacement
Metabolic alkalosis	Confusion, dizziness Numbness or tingling of fingers or toes Late: tetany, convulsions Potassium deficit	Treatment of underlying condition Diuretic:acetazolamide (Diamox) Fluid and electrolyte replacement

TABLE 24-4 Laboratory values in uncompensated and partially compensated acid-base disturbances

	pH	P_{CO_2}	HCO
Respiratory acidosis			
Uncompensated	Below 7.35	↑	Normal
Partially compensated	Move toward normal, but still ↓	↑	↑
Respiratory alkalosis			
Uncompensated	Above 7.45	↓	Normal
Partially compensated	Move toward normal, but still ↑	↓	↓
Metabolic acidosis			
Uncompensated	Below 7.35	Normal	↓
Partially compensated	Move toward normal, but still ↓	↓	↓
Metabolic alkalosis			
Uncompensated	Above 7.45	Normal	↑
Partially compensated	Move toward normal, but still ↑	↑	↑

given using compressed air or room air instead of oxygen in these situations.

If ventricular fibrillation or severe potassium excess exists, it may be necessary to administer sodium bicarbonate intravenously.

The major nursing responsibility is to recognize patients who have the potential for developing respiratory acidosis because of conditions that interfere with normal respiratory gas exchange. A patient whose airway is compromised by the presence of secretions must be encouraged to cough frequently or may need to undergo nasopharyngeal or tracheal suctioning.

RESPIRATORY ALKALOSIS: CARBONIC ACID DEFICIT
ETIOLOGY

Excessive pulmonary ventilation decreases hydrogen ion concentration and thus causes *respiratory alkalosis*. A common cause of respiratory alkalosis is *hyperventilation*. A person who hyperventilates blows off large amounts of carbon dioxide. Hyperventilation may be caused by anxiety, pain, hypoxia, or lesions affecting the respiratory center in the medulla (brain tumor, encephalitis). Other causes of respiratory alkalosis are conditions that greatly increase metabolism (hyperthyroidism) and the overventilation of patients with mechanical respirators.

PREVENTION

Respiratory alkalosis can be prevented in a person who is hyperventilating from anxiety or pain by administering a few whiffs of carbon dioxide or by having the person breathe into a paper bag and then rebreathe the exhaled carbon dioxide. Care should be taken in adjusting mechanical respirators so that the patient is not being forced to take breaths too deeply or rapidly. Correction of hypoxia prevents respiratory alkalosis in these situations.

CLINICAL MANIFESTATIONS

The patient may complain of lightheadedness and numbness or tingling of the fingers and toes. If the alkalosis becomes more severe, tetany and convulsions may be present. These manifestations are due to an increase binding of serum calcium and a decrease in ionized calcium. Serum potassium levels will be decreased because the kidneys retain hydrogen ions and excrete potassium instead.

INTERVENTIONS

Treating the underlying condition usually effectively resolves the respiratory alkalosis. Respiratory alkalosis becomes especially dangerous when it leads to cardiac arrhythmias caused partly by a decreased serum potassium level. If a patient who is receiving assisted ventilation complains of dizziness or shows any signs of muscle irritability, it is likely that the depth of respira-

tion is too great, and the respiratory rate of the machine should be decreased. If tetany is present, calcium gluconate is given intravenously (p. 556). Renal function must be maintained to promote renal compensation of the disturbance.

METABOLIC ACIDOSIS: BICARBONATE DEFICIT

When excess organic acids are added to the body fluids or when bicarbonate is lost, a *metabolic acidosis* or nonrespiratory acidosis results.

ETIOLOGY

In some conditions such as uncontrolled diabetes mellitus or starvation, glucose either cannot be used or is not available for oxidation. The body compensates for this by the use of body fat for energy, producing abnormal amounts of ketone bodies in the process. In an effort to neutralize the ketones and maintain the acid-base balance of the body, plasma bicarbonate is exhausted. The resultant acid-base imbalance is called metabolic acidosis or *ketoacidosis*. This condition can develop in anyone who does not eat an adequate diet and whose body fat must be burned for energy. It is the reason why extremely low-carbohydrate or high-protein–no carbohydrate reduction diets are criticized by nutrition experts.

Metabolic acidosis can also develop whenever excessive amounts of lactic acid are produced, such as in prolonged strenuous muscle exercise or when oxidation takes place in cells without adequate oxygen such as occurs in heart failure and shock. Loss of large amounts of alkaline intestinal secretions such as in severe diarrhea or through fistulas can also create a bicarbonate deficit.

The normal functioning kidney excretes an excess of hydrogen ions in conditions of acidosis and, in so doing, retains potassium so that hyperkalemia, as well as acidosis, is present. In kidney failure, metabolic acids accumulate in the bloodstream. Causes of metabolic acidosis are listed in the box below.

CAUSES OF METABOLIC ACIDOSIS

Diarrhea or draining intestinal fistulas (loss of bicarbonate)
Renal failure
Ureteroenterostomy (retention of Cl^- ions)
Diabetic ketoacidosis
Lactic acidosis
Salicylate intoxication
Starvation (increased breakdown of body fat or protein)
Surgical anesthesia
Conditions that greatly increase the body's metabolic needs (high fever, infectious disease, thyrotoxicosis)
Shock
Convulsions

PREVENTION

Metabolic acidosis can be prevented by careful medical management or, when possible, by prevention of the conditions that lead to acidosis.

CLINICAL MANIFESTATIONS

Headache and mental dullness are early signs of acidosis. The patient in acidosis is hyperpneic and has deep respirations (Kussmaul's respirations). This breathing pattern represents an attempt to blow off carbon dioxide, thus compensating for the acidosis. If the condition is untreated, disorientation, stupor, coma, and death occur.

Hyperkalemia results from the movement of potassium out of the cells as hydrogen ions move in and from the retention of potassium by the kidneys. Aside from laboratory evidence, there may be few indications of the acidosis until the pH falls to 7.1 or lower.

INTERVENTIONS

Treatment of acidosis is directed toward the underlying cause and restoration of electrolyte balance. If the acidosis is severe, intravenous sodium bicarbonate is sometimes given. Bicarbonate preparations must be administered with caution because they can induce a metabolic alkalosis and lead to tetany and convulsions. When acidosis is caused by renal failure, renal dialysis is necessary.

As the acidosis is corrected, potassium moves back into cells, and hypokalemia develops. If a patient being treated for acidosis needs to receive potassium, it is given after the acidosis has been partially corrected and as pH is returning to normal. It is important to bear in mind that even though acidosis is accompanied by hyperkalemia, the patient may be potassium-depleted. The potassium leaves the cells in exchange for the hydrogen ions, and much of it is excreted.

Maintenance of good respiratory function in a patient with metabolic acidosis facilitates the excretion of carbon dioxide. If the kidneys are functioning well, they can help correct the acidosis by producing more bicarbonate. Since some conditions that lead to metabolic acidosis cause a hyperosmolar state as well, osmotic diuresis will take place, and the patient will need fluid replacement along with careful monitoring of intake and output. If changes in the sensorium have resulted, safety precautions are instituted.

METABOLIC ALKALOSIS: BICARBONATE EXCESS

When excessive amounts of acid substance and hydrogen ions are lost from the body or when large amounts of bicarbonate or lactate are added orally or intravenously, the result is an imbalance in which there is an excess of base elements, called *metabolic alkalosis*. This type of imbalance does not occur as often as metabolic acidosis. In alkalosis, potassium enters the cells and hypokalemia results. A potassium loss causes a metabolic alkalosis, whereas an alkalosis causes hypokalemia.[4] An excess of bicarbonate in distal tubular fluid causes obligatory potassium loss.

ETIOLOGY

Metabolic alkalosis can occur in the following conditions: (1) loss of hydrochloric acid from the stomach caused by vomiting or gastric drainage from a nasogastric tube (loss of chloride leaves more sodium to combine with and retain bicarbonate in the kidneys); (2) loss of potassium ions through intestinal fistulas or diarrhea or in the urine; (3) ingestion of large amounts of sodium bicarbonate or other systemic antacids to treat indigestion or ulcers; (4) infusion of excessive amounts of bicarbonate or lactate intravenously; (5) diuretic therapy; and (6) excessive mineralocorticoids.

PREVENTION

Persons must be cautioned against the excessive use of sodium bicarbonate to alleviate indigestion. Controlling the conditions that can cause metabolic alkalosis can prevent this imbalance from developing. If drug therapy is causing the alkalosis, these drugs should be discontinued and others substituted where possible.

CLINICAL MANIFESTATIONS

In metabolic alkalosis, breathing becomes depressed in an effort to conserve carbon dioxide for combination with water in the blood to raise the blood level of carbonic acid. Symptoms that can occur are mental confusion, dizziness, numbness and tingling in extremities, muscle twitching, and later, tetany and convulsions. Electrocardiographic changes consistent with hypokalemia may be present.

INTERVENTIONS

Treatment is aimed at correcting the cause of the metabolic alkalosis. Sodium chloride or ammonium chloride may be given orally or intravenously. If the condition is associated with loss of sodium chloride, potassium must be restored because it is lost with the sodium. It is given in the form of potassium chloride. A diuretic that acts as a carbonic anhydrase inhibitor (Diamox) may help relieve the alkalosis by increasing excretion of bicarbonate by the kidneys.

The nurse assists in maintenance of good respiratory function so that compensation can take place through this mechanism. Careful monitoring of the patient for adequate renal function and safety precautions are important in the nursing care of patients with metabolic alkalosis. Because convulsions may occur, precautions are taken for the patient's protection.

CHAPTER SUMMARY

- ✔ Mechanisms that regulate acid-base balance include chemical buffer systems, the respiratory system, and the kidneys.

- ✔ The respiratory control center in the brain responds to increases of carbon dioxide and hydrogen ions in body fluids by changing the rate and depth of respiration.

- ✔ The renal regulation of pH is affected by control of the retention or excretion of bicarbonate and hydrogen ions.

- ✔ The major effect of acidosis is depression of the central nervous system as evidenced by disorientation followed by coma.

- ✔ Alkalosis is characterized by overexcitability of the nervous system, and the muscles may go into a state of tetany and convulsions.

- ✔ Any factor that decreases the rate of pulmonary ventilation increases the concentration of dissolved carbon dioxide, carbonic acid, and hydrogen ions and results in respiratory acidosis.

- ✔ Excess pulmonary ventilation decreases hydrogen ion concentration and thus causes respiratory alkalosis.

- ✔ When excess organic acids are added to the body fluids or when bicarbonate is lost, metabolic acidosis results.

- ✔ When excessive amounts of organic acid substance and hydrogen ions are lost from the body or when large amounts of bicarbonate or lactate are added, the result is an imbalance in which there is an excess of base elements, or metabolic alkalosis.

QUESTIONS TO CONSIDER

- ■ Why is low-flow oxygen (1 to 3 L/min) given to patients with obstructive pulmonary disease?

- ■ Explain one common method of preventing respiratory alkalosis.

- ■ Which acid-base imbalance occurs frequently in persons with diabetes mellitus? Why?

- ■ What is the role of potassium in acid-base balance?

- ■ Kussmaul's respirations are an indication of which acid-base imbalance? What does this breathing pattern indicate?

REFERENCES AND SELECTED READINGS

1. Buddle N: Arterial blood gases: a simple method for interpretation, J Post Aneseth Nurs 2(4):227-229, 1987.
2. Cogan MG, et al: Metabolic alkalosis, Med Clin North Am 67:903-914, 1983.
3. Glass L and Jenkins C: The ups and downs of serum pH, Nursing 13(9):34-41, 1983.
4. Goldberger E: A primer of water, electrolyte, and acid-base syndromes, ed 7, Philadelphia, 1986, Lea & Febiger.
5. Guyton A: Textbook of medical physiology, ed 7, Philadelphia, 1986, WB Saunders Co.
6. Knepil J: Biochemistry: the buffering and excretion of acids, Nurs Mirror 156(17):41-43, 1983.
7. Mathewson M and Mathewson R: Establishing acid-base balance, Crit Care Nurs 7(5):77-86, 1987.
8. *Metabolic acid-base disorders. I. Chemistry and physiology (programmed instruction), Am J Nurs 77:1619-1950, 1977.
9. *Metabolic acid-base disorders. II. Physiology abnormalities and nursing actions (programmed instruction), Am J Nurs 78:87-108, 1978.
10. *Metabolic acid-base disorders. III. Clinical and laboratory findings (programed instruction), Am J Nurs 78:443-460, 1978.
11. Middaugh R, Middaugh D, and Menk E: Current considerations in respiratory and acid-base management during cardiopulmonary resuscitation, Crit Care Nurs 10(4):25-33, 1988.
12. *Symposium on fluid, electrolytes, and acid-base balance, Nurs Clin North Am 22:749-872, 1987.
13. Tannen R: Ammonia and acid-base homeostasis, Med Clin North Am 67:781-798, 1983.

*References preceded by an asterisk are particularly well suited for student reading.

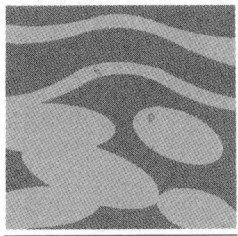

CHAPTER 25

Shock

GAIL OSTERFIELD

CHAPTER OBJECTIVES

After studying this chapter, the student should be able to:
1. Contrast three major types of shock.
2. Describe early and late pathophysiologic changes that occur with shock.
3. Describe organ damage that may occur with shock.
4. Describe different methods of monitoring for shock.
5. Describe methods of fluid replacement during shock.
6. Identify effects of pharmacologic agents used to treat shock and nursing measures for patients receiving drug therapy.
7. Describe therapeutic measures for shock other than fluids and drug therapy.

Shock is a syndrome characterized by hypoperfusion of body tissues. Any condition that prevents cells from receiving an adequate blood supply can interfere with their metabolism and produce shock.

Blood flow depends on pressure changes within the vascular compartment. Blood flows from areas of greater pressure to areas of lesser pressure. In the systemic circulation, the mean pressure is highest in the aorta, where the blood leaves the left ventricle, and lowest in the right atrium. For the necessary pressure gradients to exist so that blood can flow, the following three factors are necessary:
1. An adequate amount of blood for the heart to pump around the body
2. Ability of the heart to pump blood
3. Blood vessels with good tone, able to constrict and dilate to maintain normal pressure

Shock results from the disruption of one or more of these factors.

ETIOLOGY

Shock may be classified as hypovolemic, cardiogenic, or vasogenic (see box at right).

HYPOVOLEMIC SHOCK

Hypovolemic shock is the most common type of shock. Any condition that reduces the *volume* within the vas-

cular compartment by 15% to 25% can result in hypovolemic shock. Common causes include the following:
1. Excessive blood loss: trauma (most common cause), gastrointestinal (GI) bleeding, coagulation disorders, surgery
2. Loss of body fluids other than blood: excessive diuresis (diabetic ketoacidosis or other hyperosmolar states), plasma loss from excessive vomiting or diarrhea
3. Movement of fluid from the vascular compartment to a body compartment that does not usually contain a large amount of fluid, such as the peritoneal cavity or the interstitial space. With a bowel obstruction, 5 to 10 L of fluid may collect in the bowel. Peritonitis may result in the accumulation of 4 to 6 L of fluid in the peritoneal cavity within 24 hours. The collection of a large amount of fluid in a body compartment other than the vessels or the cells is referred to as *third spacing of fluid.*

CARDIOGENIC SHOCK

Cardiogenic shock results from the inability of the heart to pump sufficient blood to perfuse the cells of the body. Because cardiac output is the product of stroke volume and heart rate, a decrease in stroke volume will be accompanied by an increase in heart rate. Initially this will maintain cardiac output. Tachycardia, however, can have a deleterious effect on the heart. Oxygen consumption is increased, and because the coronary arter-

TYPES OF SHOCK

Hypovolemic	Shock from loss of fluid from vascular system (through blood loss or fluid loss)
Cardiogenic	Shock from inability of heart to pump blood to tissues (decreased cardiac output)
Vasogenic	Shock from massive vasodilation (from interference with sympathetic nervous system or effects of histamine or toxins)

ies fill during diastole, the filling time is decreased. The heart thus needs more oxygen and receives less.

Although cardiogenic shock may be caused by various cardiac conditions, including cardiac tamponade, restrictive pericarditis, pulmonary embolism, severe valvular disease, or dysrhythmia (arrhythmia), the most common cause is myocardial infarction. Studies have shown that in most patients who die from cardiogenic shock, at least 40% of the left ventricle was damaged by a recent infarction or by a recent infarction plus a previous scar. Despite improvements in managing cardiogenic shock, the mortality still remains greater than 80%.

VASOGENIC SHOCK

Vasogenic shock is caused by massive dilation of the blood vessels, resulting in disproportion between the size of the vascular space and the amount of blood contained in it. As vessels dilate, blood pressure falls and blood pools in dilated vessels, resulting in a decrease in venous return to the heart and a fall in cardiac output.

In the early stage of vasogenic shock, the extremities are warm and pink because of vasodilation. As the cardiac output decreases and tissue perfusion is reduced, compensatory vasoconstriction causes the limbs to become cool and blanched.

Loss of vascular tone, which causes vasodilation, may result from several conditions. *Neurogenic shock* results from interference with the sympathetic nervous system, which helps maintain vasomotor tone. Spinal cord injury, spinal anesthesia, and, rarely, brain damage are among the causes. *Anaphylactic shock,* which is a type of allergic reaction, may occur when a sensitized person has contact with an antigen. Vasoactive substances, including histamine, kinins, and prostaglandins, are released and cause massive vasodilation in the body. The endothelial cells that line the capillaries separate and expose the basement membrane, which is permeable to fluid and plasma proteins. Large quantities of fluid may leak out of the capillaries, causing severe hypovolemia.[9]

SEPTIC SHOCK

Septic shock is another form of vasogenic shock that may result from various infections, including those caused by both gram-positive and gram-negative bacteria, viruses, and fungi. Gram-negative bacteria, including *Escherichia coli, Klebsiella-Enterobacter-Serratia* (KES), *Pseudomonas,* and *Proteus,* are the most frequent causative organisms in septic shock. Infections anywhere in the body can result in septic shock. The most common sites are the urinary tract, respiratory tract, and blood. Some gram-negative organisms that may cause sepsis and septic shock are normal flora of the intestinal tract. As long as they remain in the intestinal tract, they do no harm and are even beneficial.

However, if these organisms enter the bloodstream, they are lysed by leukocytes and release an endotoxin. Septic shock may result.

Conditions that predispose to septic shock include the following:

1. Extremes of age; that is, the very young and the very old
2. Immunosuppressive and steroid therapy
3. Chronic illness
4. Urologic and GI surgery
5. Poor nutritional status
6. Use of invasive devices
7. Pregnancy

Elderly men with benign prostatic hypertrophy are particularly susceptible to septic shock, because they have a high incidence of urinary tract infections and are often subjected to invasive urologic procedures.

The release of the endotoxin from the gram-negative organism into the bloodstream causes the release of numerous vasoactive substances within the body, including histamine, prostaglandins, serotonin, bradykinin, and endorphins. Some cause massive vasodilation, others cause selective vasoconstriction, and some cause an increase in capillary permeability. The result is major fluid shifts and maldistribution of blood within the body. The massive vasodilation results in hypotension despite the cardiac output usually being very high in the early stages. The high cardiac output (hyperdynamic state) is thought to cause the warm, flushed skin in early septic shock. As septic shock progresses, cardiac output falls and the clinical picture resembles other types of shock.

Septic shock is of particular importance because it has a high mortality rate and is likely to have resulted from a hospital-acquired infection. It has been estimated that 1 in every 100 persons admitted to hospitals in the United States acquires gram-negative sepsis (not all develop septic shock) and that more than 100,000 deaths occur annually in the United States from septic shock.[33]

PATHOPHYSIOLOGY

EARLY STAGE

In the early stage of shock the body responds to hypoperfusion as it would to any other stressor. Many changes that occur are mediated through the sympathetic nervous system. Stimulation of the sympathetic nervous system results in secretion of norepinephrine from the sympathetic fibers and epinephrine and norepinephrine by the adrenal medulla. Both α- and β- adrenergic receptors are stimulated throughout the body. α-Receptors respond by causing vasoconstriction; β-receptors respond by causing vasodilation (β_1) and increased rate and strength of contraction of the heart (β_2). Other organs with β_2-receptors are also stimulated (**respiratory sys-**

tem). The skin and the abdominal organs, which are rich in α-receptors, receive a decreased blood supply because of vasoconstriction. The heart and skeletal muscles, which are rich in β-receptors, receive an increased blood supply because of vasodilation. The heart beats faster and harder, and the respiratory rate increases in response to β-stimulation, thereby increasing oxygen delivery to the tissues. All the compensatory responses mediated through the sympathetic nervous system occur rapidly.

The overall effect of the sympathetic nervous system response in hypovolemic and cardiogenic shock is an increase in systemic vascular resistance (SVR). The widespread vasodilation characteristic of septic shock negates the effect of norepinephrine, resulting in a decreased SVR.

Another compensatory response, mediated through the renin-angiotensin system, occurs more slowly. As cardiac output falls, the blood flow to the kidneys decreases. The juxtaglomerular cells respond by secreting renin, which acts on a plasma protein, converting it to angiotensin I. This is converted to angiotensin II, which has two major effects: it causes vasoconstriction and causes the adrenal cortex to secrete aldosterone. Aldosterone causes the kidneys to retain sodium and water and secrete potassium, resulting in an increased blood volume. The secretion of potassium may result in *hypokalemia* during this stage of shock. In addition, de-

creased cardiac output results in decreased hydrostatic pressure in the capillaries, causing fluid to shift from the interstitial space into the capillaries. This also improves blood volume.

For a short period the compensatory mechanisms have a beneficial effect. The most vital organs, the heart and the brain, receive an adequate blood supply at the expense of the less vital organs, such as the kidneys, and other abdominal organs. This allows time for the underlying cause of shock to be corrected. However, if the underlying problem is not or cannot be corrected, the compensatory mechanisms will not be able to continue to perfuse vital organs sufficiently, and the mechanisms themselves will have a deleterious effect on the body. Shock will then progress to a later stage. Table 25-1 summarizes the pathophysiologic changes in early and late shock.

LATE STAGE

As shock progresses, blood flow to all body tissues becomes impaired. Cells in vasoconstricted organs receive insufficient oxygen, and aerobic metabolism is replaced by anaerobic metabolism. Energy in the form of adenosine triphosphate (ATP) is produced very inefficiently. Only 2 mol of ATP are produced for each mole of glucose metabolized, in contrast to 38 mol in aerobic metabolism. In addition, lactic acid is formed and cannot be further metabolized in the absence of oxygen. Acido-

TABLE 25-1 Major pathophysiologic changes in shock

Change	Effect
EARLY STAGE (COMPENSATORY STAGE)	
Increased epinephrine and norepinephrine	Increased cardiac output to send more blood to tissues
α- and β-Receptors stimulated	
Alpha effects: skin and most viscera	Vasoconstriction and decreased blood supply
Beta effects: heart and skeletal muscles	Vasodilation and increased blood supply and heart rate
Renin-angiotensin response	Vasoconstriction and secretion of aldosterone; sodium and water retention and potassium loss
Increased glucocorticoids and mineralocorticoids	Sodium and fluid retention to increase intravascular volume Potassium loss
Hypoxemia	Hyperventilation; provides more oxygen to tissues; may cause respiratory alkalosis
Decreased hydrostatic fluid pressure	Fluid shifts from interstitial space to capillaries to increase vascular volume
LATE STAGE (NONCOMPENSATORY STAGE)	
Decreased blood flow to heart	Impaired cardiac pumping ability (decreased cardiac output); blood pressure decreases
Anaerobic metabolism	Acidosis; decreased adenosine triphosphate; failure of cellular sodium-potassium pump (potassium leaves cell; sodium and water enter cell); cellular damage
Arteriolar dilation and venule constriction	Fluid shift from intravascular to interstitial space
Decreased blood flow to kidney	Decreased kidney function (oliguria or anuria, retention of nitrogenous waste products and potassium)
Decreased blood flow to pancreas	Production of myocardial depressant factor (MDF)

sis and energy deficiency result. Without enough energy, the sodium-potassium pump fails. Potassium leaves the cells, and sodium and water enter, damaging various organelles. Lysosomes, which have an important role in phagocytosis, contain digestive enzymes that are ordinarily contained within a wall. When the lysosome is damaged, the digestive enzymes spill into the rest of the cell and destroy it. As these enzymes come in contact with adjacent cells, they also are destroyed and release their digestive enzymes. Cellular death results in organ death.

Acid metabolites cause dilation at the arteriole end of the capillaries (precapillary sphincter) and constriction at the venule end (postcapillary sphincter). Increased hydrostatic pressure within the capillary results and causes fluid to shift from the capillary into the interstitial space; the blood volume is decreased even further. In addition to the increase of presure within the capillaries, increased capillary permeability may occur. This

is most likely to occur in *septic shock* because of the release of large amounts of histamine and serotonin in response to the presence of gram-negative toxins. Proteins are able to leak through the capillary walls, increasing the osmotic pressure in the interstitium. This causes a further shift of fluid out of the capillaries. Longstanding hypoxemia of the capillaries can also result in capillary permeability, so that in the late stages of *cardiogenic* and hypovolemic shock, this type of fluid shift may also occur. Decreased blood supply to the kidneys results in oliguria or anuria. The serum creatinine and the blood urea nitrogen (BUN) levels increase. The kidneys are not able to excrete the increasing amounts of potassium that are accumulating in the blood as a result of cellular damage, and hyperkalemia results, which is worsened by the acidosis. *Hyperkalemia* depresses the conduction and contractility of the heart.

Vasoconstriction of the splanchnic vessels in response to sympathetic stimulation causes ischemia of

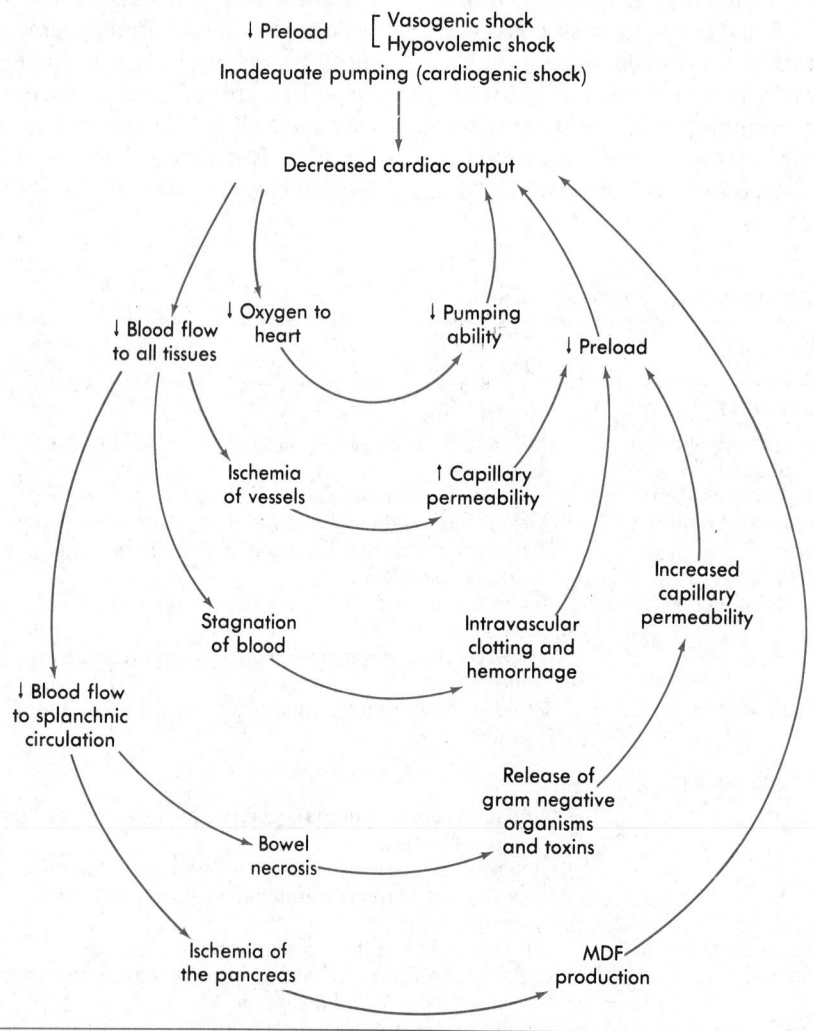

FIGURE 25-1 Shock causes shock.

the abdominal organs. Of particular importance is the pancreas. In response to hypoxemia, the pancreas forms and secretes a substance called *myocardial depressant factor* (MDF), which depresses the contractility of the heart. As cardiac output continues to fall, the heart itself, despite the compensatory mechanisms, receives an inadequate blood supply. This further impairs its electrical and mechanical activity.

Shock is a dynamic process, with shock itself causing shock[13] (Figure 25-1). At some point a cycle begins that cannot be interrupted, and an irreversible stage of shock develops. Even if the primary problem is corrected and good supportive care is given, the patient will die. However, the exact point at which shock becomes irreversible is not known. Regardless of the symptoms, all efforts should be made to reverse the progression of shock.

ORGAN DAMAGE
KIDNEYS

The kidneys contain about 2.4 million nephrons, each of which is capable of forming urine. Each nephron is composed of a glomerulus that is made up of capillaries and collecting tubules (see Chapter 47). Under normal conditions the pressure within the glomerulus is sufficiently high to force fluid out of the capillaries into the collecting chamber. When the systolic pressure falls below 70 torr, glomerular filtration ceases, and the body is unable to rid itself of fluid and nitrogenous wastes. Urinary output is decreased in both the early and the late stages of shock. In the early stage, low output is the caused by sympathetic stimulation of the α-receptors in the kidneys, resulting in vasoconstriction and a fall of pressure within the glomeruli. Decreased pressure causes a drop in the glomerular filtration rate.

As shock progresses, the tubules, which are perfused by the peritubular capillaries, begin to suffer from a lack of oxygen and nutrients, and acute *tubular necrosis* develops. The tubular epithelial cells slough and block the tubules, causing loss of nephron function.

BRAIN

Blood flow to the brain is under the control of local influences rather than the autonomic nervous system. In response to decreased blood flow, the vessels dilate so that the brain, as with the heart, is preferentially perfused. As shock progresses, however, inadequate perfusion of the brain occurs. Cerebral *hypoxia* results in *lethargy* and eventually *coma*. The accumulation of toxic substances and acidosis may compound the symptoms of hypoxia.

HEART

Although deterioration of cardiac function is a primary problem only in cardiogenic shock, the heart eventually is affected in all types of shock. As cited earlier, in the early stage of shock the heart is spared. As shock increases, the pumping ability of the heart is affected and cardiac output decreases. As the heart muscle becomes increasingly hypoxic, it begins to show disturbances of electrical activity. Dysrhythmias have a detrimental affect on cardiac output, and some may be fatal. In the later stages of shock, deterioration of myocardial function is probably the most important factor in the further progression of shock.[13]

LUNGS

The effect of shock on the lungs has been determined only more recently. During the Vietnam War, many victims of traumatic shock survived the early complications because of the use of massive blood transfusions and renal dialysis. The effect of shock on the lungs surfaced as a later complication. The pulmonary condition that results from hypoperfusion of the lungs has been known by various names, including shock lung, white lung, and Da Nang lung. It is now generally known as *adult respiratory distress syndrome* (ARDS) (see Chapter 33).

ARDS can result from any condition that causes hypoperfusion of the lungs but is seen most often with hemorrhagic, anaphylactic, traumatic, or septic shock.[30] It is characterized by increased permeability of the pulmonary capillaries to proteins and water, resulting in noncardiac pulmonary edema. Type 2 pneumocytes are destroyed, impairing the production of surfactant that normally prevents collapse of the alveoli. Alveoli either become filled with fluid or collapse, and lungs become stiff.

In the early stages, hypoxemia results from impaired gas exchange, and hyperventilation occurs, resulting in hypocapnia and respiratory alkalosis. Platelet aggregation in the pulmonary capillaries further damages the lungs. Hypoxemia persists despite administration of increasing amounts of oxygen. As shock progresses, ventilation is impaired, and carbon dioxide is retained. Respiratory acidosis results. As hypoxemia increases, platelet aggregation increases, and a destructive cycle is initiated.

GASTROINTESTINAL TRACT

Sympathetic stimulation, which occurs early in shock, causes vasoconstriction and therefore decreased blood supply to the organs of the GI tract. Bowel function decreases, and paralytic ileus may result. If the blood supply is severely impaired for a time, necrosis of the intestinal mucosa may occur. Microorganisms that are normally found in the bowel lyse and release endotoxins when they are attacked by the leukocytes in the blood. Shock, from whatever cause, will now also have a septic component. The gastric mucosa commonly ulcerates when it becomes ischemic, which may result in occult bleeding or massive hemorrhage.

LIVER

Sympathetic stimulation causes vasoconstriction in the liver. In the early stages of shock this can be beneficial. Normally the liver is capable of storing large amounts of blood in its veins. With vasoconstriction it can release up to 350 ml of blood into the general circulation, resulting in improved cardiac output. With continued sympathetic stimulation and decreased blood flow, liver tissue is affected. In septic shock there is an increase in oxygen uptake and a decrease in energy production in the liver. All types of shock affect the metabolic functions of the liver, including the excretion of bile and cholesterol, gluconeogenesis, detoxification, and protein synthesis.[20]

The sinusoids of the liver are lined with Kupffer cells, which are part of the reticuloendothelial system (RES). These cells are very powerful phagocytes and destroy the many bacteria from the colon that reach the liver by way of the portal system. Normally, only a very few bacteria get past the RES. With the destruction of the RES, bacteria enter the general circulation and produce toxins, which under normal circumstances would be detoxified by the liver. The liver can no longer perform this function, and overwhelming infection and toxicity result.

BLOOD

Disseminated intravascular coagulation (DIC) (see Chapter 30) can cause or result from shock. It is characterized by intravascular clotting, resulting in the formation of microthrombi in the capillaries. Clotting factors in the blood may be activated by acidosis, stagnation, and procoagulation substances. Acidosis and stagnation are common in all forms of shock. Therefore DIC may occur with all types of shock. In septic shock, however, the bacterial toxins and the prostaglandins that are released enhance coagulation and make DIC even more likely. Clotting in the capillaries causes a depletion of clotting factors in the rest of the body. Hemorrhage may then occur from surgical incisions, injection sites, intravenous insertion sites, or the GI tract. Intravascular clotting results in a further decrease in tissue perfusion and acidosis, and a vicious cycle ensues. The hemorrhage caused by DIC decreases the cardiac output even further and worsens tissue perfusion. The mortality in patients with DIC in association with infection and shock is very high.

CLINICAL MANIFESTATIONS

The signs and symptoms of shock are summarized in Table 25-2. There are few observable signs in the early stage; the patient may be restless, and the pulse and respiratory rates may be increased. Cool, clammy skin;

TABLE 25-2 Comparison of signs and symptoms in early and late shock by body system

	Early Shock	Late Shock
Respiratory system	Hyperventilation; ↑ minute volume; ↓ Pco_2; normal Po_2*	Respirations shallow; breath sounds may suggest congestion; ↑ Pco_2; ↓ Po_2*
Cardiovascular system	Blood pressure normal to slightly lowered; ↑ diastolic pressure; ↓ pulse pressure; tachycardia; cardiac output normal in hypovolemic shock, slightly decreased in cardiogenic shock, and increased in septic shock; mild vasoconstriction in hypovolemic and cardiogenic shock; vasodilation in septic shock	↓ Blood pressure; ↓ cardiac output; tachycardia continues; vasoconstriction worsens in hypovolemic, cardiogenic, and septic shock
Renal system	Decreased urine output; ↑ urine osmolality; ↓ urine sodium concentration; hypokalemia	Oliguria or complete renal shutdown; hyperkalemia; buildup of waste products
Acid-base balance	Respiratory alkalosis	Metabolic acidosis; respiratory acidosis
Vascular compartment	Fluid shift from interstitial space to vascular compartment; thirst	Fluid shift from vascular space to interstitial and intracellular spaces, causing edema
Skin	Minimal to no changes in hypovolemic and cardiogenic shock; warm, flushed skin in septic shock	Cool, clammy skin in hypovolemic, cardiogenic, and septic shock; cool, mottled skin in neurogenic and vasogenic shock
Hematologic system	Release of red blood cells (RBCs) from bone marrow to increase vascular volume; platelet aggregation	Disseminated intravascular coagulation (DIC)
Mental-neurologic system	Restless; alert; confused	Lethargy; unconsciousness
GI-hepatic system	No obvious changes	Perfusion decreases; bowel sounds possibly diminished

*Pco_2, Carbon dioxide pressure; Po_2, oxygen pressure.

PARAMETERS FOR ASSESSING STATUS OF PATIENT IN SHOCK

HEMODYNAMIC MONITORING	FLUID AND ELECTROLYTE MONITORING	NEUROLOGIC MONITORING
Blood pressure (cuff and/or intraarterial)	Serum electrolytes	Alertness
Pulse	Blood lactate and pyruvate levels	Orientation
Central venous pressure	Intake	Confusion
Pulmonary artery pressure	By mouth	
Pulmonary wedge pressure	Intravenous	**HEMATOLOGIC MONITORING**
Cardiac output	Nasogastric	
Electrocardiogram	Irrigation solutions	Erythrocytes
	Solution in medications	Hematocrit and hemoglobin levels
RESPIRATORY MONITORING	Output	Leukocytes
	Urinary	Platelets
Respiratory rate, depth	GI tract	Prothrombin and partial thromboplastin
Breath sounds	Sweating	times
Blood gases	Dressings	Clotting time
pH	Weight	Fibrin degradation factor
Po_2	Serum creatinine level	
Pco_2	BUN level	**OTHER MONITORING**
Percent O_2 saturation	Serum and urinary osmolality	
	Urinary specific gravity	Bowel sounds
		Skin temperature

decreased blood pressure; and lethargy or unconsciousness are signs in the later stage. The physiologic status of patients in shock is monitored by various methods.

MEDICAL MANAGEMENT

Medical management is determined by the stage of shock and the patient's signs and symptoms. The details of treatment are included under the implementation section later in this chapter.

■ ASSESSMENT

The parameters for assessing patients in shock are summarized in the box above and then discussed in more detail.

HEMODYNAMIC ASSESSMENT

Hemodynamic alterations are often the first sign of the onset of shock. The patient's hemodynamic status can be assessed at various levels (Figure 25-2).

VITAL SIGNS

Vital signs are assessed frequently. In the early stages of shock the pulse is usually increased. As shock progresses, the pulse becomes quite rapid and difficult to palpate. Irregularities in the pulse may develop as cardiac dysrhythmias occur.

Early in shock the blood pressure may be normal, slightly decreased, or even elevated because of compensatory vasoconstriction. Blood pressure can be heard without difficulty at this stage. As shock progresses, the blood pressure may be difficult to auscultate, and it may

be possible to obtain the systolic pressure only by palpation. If intraarterial pressure monitoring is not instituted, Doppler ultrasound may be helpful in obtaining the blood pressure.

Venous pulsation in the neck is noted. Both the external and the internal jugular veins should be examined. Generally the external jugular vein is easier to see, but the internal jugular is more reliable as a sign of elevated right atrial pressure. Normally, venous pulsations are visible when the patient is lying flat but not when the heart is elevated to 45 degrees (Figure 25-3). Neck veins that are not visible when the patient is in the horizontal position may indicate an abnormally low intravas-

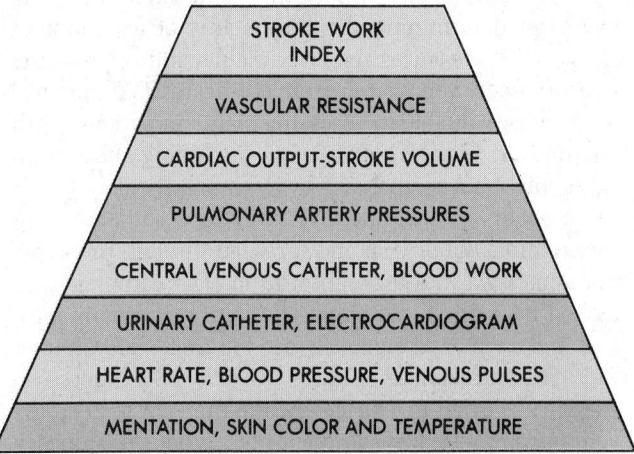

FIGURE 25-2 Levels of hemodynamic monitoring. (From Ellerbe S: Fluid and blood component therapy in the critically ill and injured, New York, 1981, Churchill Livingstone, Inc.)

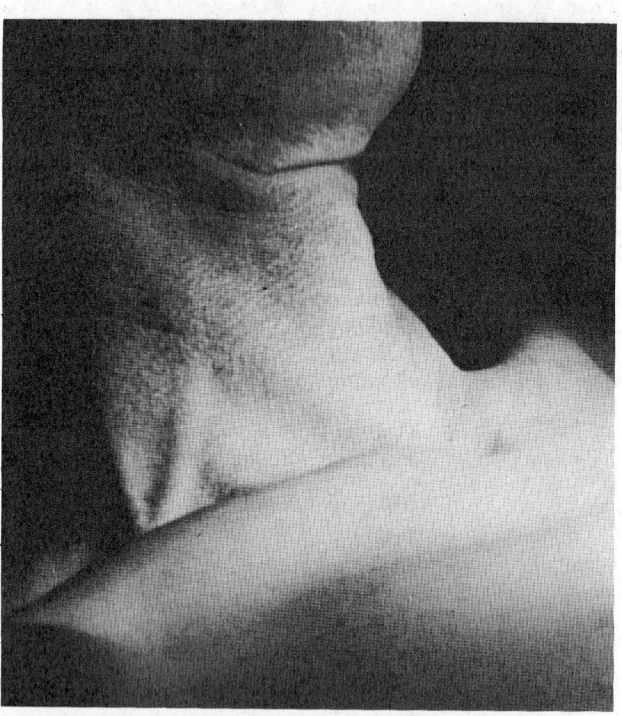

FIGURE 25-3 Distended external jugular neck vein of a patient with right-sided heart failure. (From Daily EK and Schroeder J: Techniques in bedside hemodynamic monitoring, ed 2, St Louis, 1981, The CV Mosby Co.)

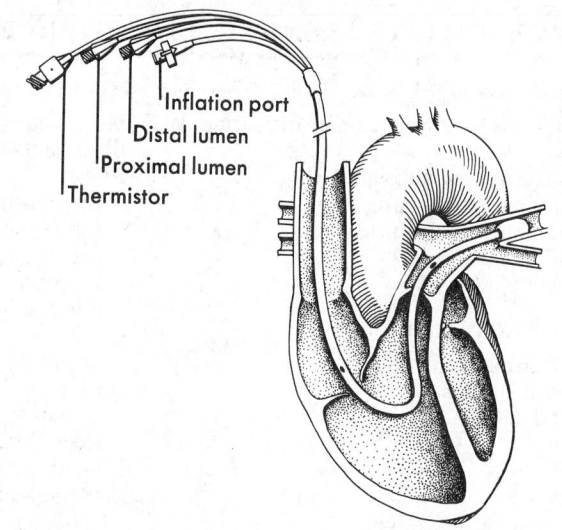

FIGURE 25-4 Placement of Swan-Ganz catheter.

cular volume. This may be seen in both hypovolemic and vasogenic (distributive) shock. In cardiogenic shock the neck veins are often distended, even when the head of the patient's bed is elevated more than 45 degrees. This indicates excessive fluid volume.

CENTRAL VENOUS PRESSURE

Central venous pressure (CVP) is a more accurate means of determining the fluid status of a patient in shock. CVP measures right ventricular filling pressure, which reflects venous return to the heart. CVP monitoring is most valuable in assessing status in patients with absolute or relative hypovolemia, including those with vasogenic, neurogenic, and hypovolemic shock.

To obtain an accurate CVP reading, a catheter is inserted into a major vein and threaded through the superior vena cava into the right atrium. The catheter is attached by a three-way stopcock to an intravenous infusion and a water manometer (see Figure 26-15, Chapter 26). The intravenous solution (usually 5% glucose in water) is allowed to drip slowly into the vein to keep the vein open. When a reading is to be taken, the stopcock is opened to the manometer, and the manometer is filled with the intravenous solution. The stopcock is then turned to the venous opening of the patient. The fluid level in the manometer should fluctuate with each

respiration. The fluid is allowed to stabilize before a reading is taken, and the highest level of the fluid fluctuating in the column is used for the CVP reading. As soon as the reading is taken, the stopcock is returned to the solution position, and the infusion is continued.

For the CVP reading to be accurate, the patient must be relaxed, and the zero point of the manometer must always be at the level of the right atrium, which in most people is level with the midaxillary line. If the patient cannot lie flat in bed, the zero point on the manometer is adjusted to the level of the right atrium in a sitting position. Any change in the patient's position requires that the zero point be reset. The initial CVP reading and the position that the patient was in when it was taken should be recorded, because these will serve as a baseline for comparison with subsequent readings. The patient should be placed in the same position for each reading because even a slight change in position alters the CVP.

A range of 5 to 15 cm of water is usually considered normal. In hypovolemic shock the CVP is usually very low because the blood volume is decreased. In vasogenic shock the CVP would also be low, because the blood has pooled in the expanded vascular space and fluid has been lost into the interstitium as a result of increased capillary permeability. In cardiogenic shock the CVP is likely to be high because of the excess intravascular fluid. It is important to note that a change in the trend of the CVP is more important than a numeric reading.

Central venous catheters can also be used to obtain blood samples, to assess venous oxygen saturation determinations, and to administer fluids. The catheter insertion site should be kept scrupulously clean to minimize the possibility of phlebitis. Patient movement is not restricted as long as the catheter and tubing are secured adequately and intravenous flow is maintained.

PULMONARY ARTERY PRESSURES

The status of the left side of the heart can best be evaluated by the measurement of *pulmonary artery pressure* (PAP) and *pulmonary capillary wedge pressure* (PCWP). A mean PAP of less than 10 mm Hg may indicate decreased blood volume, resulting in decrease preload in the left ventricle. A mean PAP of more than 20 mm Hg may indicate poor myocardial contractility and left ventricular overload.

These pressures are measured with a special balloon-tipped (Swan-Ganz) catheter (Figure 25-4). The catheter is inserted into a vein, usually the subclavian, and advanced to the atrium. The balloon is inflated and carried by the blood flow into the right ventricle and then to the pulmonary artery. The balloon is then deflated, and the tip of the catheter is left in the pulmonary artery. The other end of the catheter is connected to low-compliance tubing, which in turn is connected to a transducer. The transducer converts the pressure that it senses through the catheter to an electrical signal, which is displayed on a monitor. Thus the pressure in the pulmonary artery can be monitored continuously. A continuous flush system usually is used to maintain patency of the catheter.

In individuals without lung or pulmonary vascular disease, PAP is a good indicator of how well the left side of the heart is functioning. Pressure changes in the left ventricle are reflected in the left atrium and back to the pulmonary artery. However, if any disease exists in the lungs, as frequently occurs in shock, the PAP does not accurately reflect left ventricular pressure. In this case the PCWP should be obtained. By inflating the balloon, which is near the tip of the catheter, the pulmonary artery can be occluded. This blocks communication between the pulmonary artery and the lumen of the catheter, allowing for pressure that is ahead of the occluded artery to be transmitted through the catheter. The PCWP is *identical* to the *left atrial pressure*.

The nurse caring for the patient with PAP monitoring must be aware of the common complications that can occur with this type of invasive monitoring (Table 25-3). The appearance of either a *right ventricular* or *PCWP waveform* on the monitor can have serious consequences for the patient. Dislodgement of the tip of the catheter from the pulmonary artery into the right ventri-

TABLE 25-3 Complications of pulmonary artery pressure (PAP) monitoring

Complication	Indications	Interventions
Infection	Chills Headache Malaise Generalized aching Flushed face Warm skin Elevated temperature	1. Notify physician immediately. 2. Prepare for removal of catheter. 3. Administer antibiotics as ordered. 4. Provide symptomatic relief.
Ventricular dyshythmias: premature ventricular beats (PVBs), or short runs of ventricular tachycardia	"Skipped heartbeats" Irregular pulse PVBs noted on cardiac monitor	1. Notify physician immediately. 2. Prepare for repositioning of catheter. 3. Administer antidysrhythmic drugs if problem persists after repositioning.
Sustained ventricular tachycardia or ventricular fibrillation	Lightheadedness, progressing to loss of consciousness Loss of consciousness Pulselessness Dysrhythmia noted on cardiac monitor Respiratory arrest	1. Notify physician immediately. 2. Prepare for repositioning of catheter. 3. Defibrillate.
Pulmonary infarction	Chest pain Hemoptysis Fever Friction rub Elevated lactate dehydrogenase (LDH) Area of opacity on chest roentgenogram Decreased Pao_2	1. Notify physician immediately. 2. Administer oxygen. 3. Prepare for repositioning or removal of catheter. 4. Provide symptomatic relief.
Valvular damage	Depends on extent of damage Patient may be asymptomatic or may develop symptoms of congestive heart failure or new murmur	1. Notify physician of development of new murmur or new symptoms.

Modified from Asheervath J and Belvins D: Handbook of clinical nursing practice, Norwalk, Conn, 1986, Appleton-Century-Crofts.

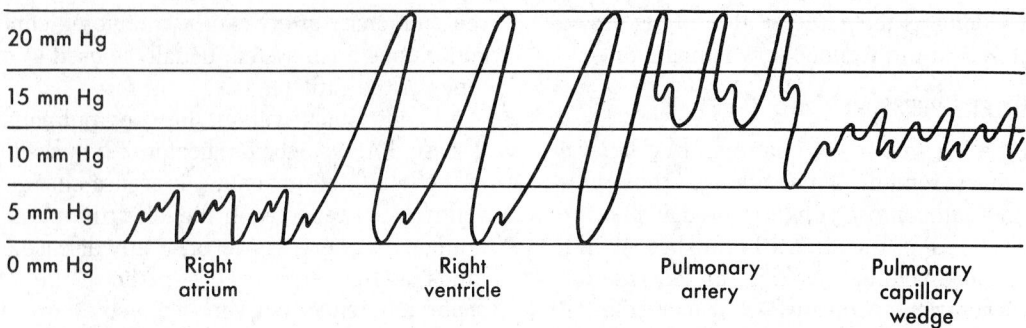

20 mm Hg				
15 mm Hg				
10 mm Hg				
5 mm Hg				
0 mm Hg	Right atrium	Right ventricle	Pulmonary artery	Pulmonary capillary wedge

FIGURE 25-5 Characteristic waveforms of pulmonary artery pressure (PAP) monitoring. (From Asheervath J and Blevins D: Handbook of clinical nursing practice, 1986, Norwalk, Conn, Appleton-Century-Crofts.)

cle can result in the occurrence of *premature ventricular beats* (PVBs) or even *ventricular tachycardia.* Progression of the catheter into a small vessel in the pulmonary vasculature can occlude the vessel and result in *pulmonary infarction.* Prolonged inflation of the balloon can have the same effect. The nurse must be able to distinguish the normal PAP waveform from both right ventricular and PCWP waveforms (Figure 25-5). It is essential that sterile technique be maintained during insertion of the PAP catheter and during dressing changes.

INTRAARTERIAL MONITORING

Intraarterial monitoring is usually instituted along with PAP monitoring. A catheter is inserted into a radial, brachial, or femoral artery and attached to a transducer in much the same way as the pulmonary artery catheter (Figure 25-6). Because hemorrhage is a possible complication, the insertion and connections in the system must be monitored frequently. The extremity distal to the insertion site must be monitored for signs of arterial occlusion (color, temperature, movement, presence or absence of pulses, pain). It is essential that sterile technique be maintained during insertion of the catheter and during dressing changes. A patient who is ill enough to require hemodynamic monitoring has little reserve to fight infection.

CARDIAC OUTPUT AND CARDIAC INDEX MONITORING

Some pulmonary artery catheters allow for cardiac output and cardiac index to be monitored at the bedside. Such catheters have a port through which fluid can be injected into the right atrium. A thermistor is located at the tip of the catheter and attached to a wire that runs through the catheter and is attached to a cardiac output computer. Iced or room-temperature saline solution is injected into the right atrium. The solution travels with the blood into the pulmonary artery. The thermistor senses the extent of temperature change, and from this data the computer is able to calculate cardiac output. Complications of PAP monitoring are listed in Table 25-3.

OXYGEN UTILIZATION MONITORING

In all types of shock a discrepency exists between the amount of oxygen delivered to the cells and the amount

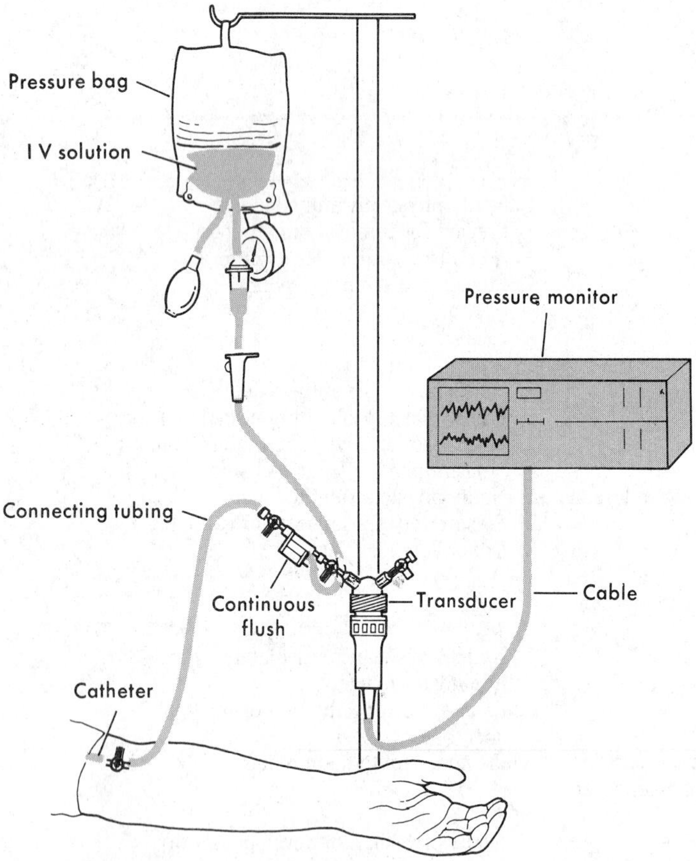

FIGURE 25-6 Connections between intraarterial catheter, transducer, monitor, and fluid. (From Daily EK and Schroeder J: Techniques in bedside hemodynamic monitoring, ed 3, St Louis, 1985, The CV Mosby Co.)

they need. Oxygen delivery is affected by cardiac output, serum hemoglobin concentration, and the amount of oxygen in the blood (measured by arterial oxygen pressure, or Pao_2). If any of these decreases, the cells normally compensate by extracting more oxygen than normal from the blood as it passes by them. Blood in the veins then has a lower-than-normal oxygen content. By sampling blood that is a mixture of venous blood from the entire body, oxygen utilization by the body can be determined. Blood in the pulmonary artery is used for this purpose. The difference between the oxygen saturation of arterial blood (Sao_2) and the oxygen saturation of the mixed venous blood (Svo_2) reflects cellular utilization of oxygen. In both hypovolemic shock and cardiogenic shock the fall in cardiac output causes the cells to extract more oxygen, with a resultant decrease in Svo_2. In septic shock, however, especially in the early stages, this is not the case. The Svo_2 may be abnormally high despite the cells not apparently receiving enough oxygen. This may be a result of the high cardiac output seen in early shock. Other possible reasons include inability of the cells to extract oxygen because of the effects of endotoxins on them and the passage of blood through some organs, with little gas exchange occurring because of clogged capillaries.

The Svo_2 can be measured by withdrawing blood from a pulmonary artery catheter. However, the preferred way is to monitor the Svo_2 by use of a fiberoptic pulmonary artery catheter, which will display a continuous value on a monitor.

Table 25-4 lists the hemodynamic parameters found in various types of shock.

RESPIRATORY ASSESSMENT

As cited earlier, hypoperfusion of the lungs, which frequently occurs in shock, may result in ARDS. This may be suspected very early in the course of the disease from changes in the patient's mentation, as caused by hypoxemia. The patient is observed for *cough* and *dyspnea*, which develop as ARDS progresses. Changes in respiratory rate and in the color of the mucous membranes and skin are important indicators of pulmonary status. Breath sounds are auscultated. Early in the course of the disease the lungs may be clear, but, as ARDS progresses, rales and rhonchi may be heard.

If the patient is receiving mechanical ventilation, the amount of pressure required to deliver a specific tidal volume is noted. As the lungs become increasingly stiff, the pressure required to deliver the volume increases. With ARDS, the PAP may rise, although the PCWP remains normal.[30]

Arterial blood gases may provide valuable information and are monitored as indicated depending on the patient's condition. Characteristically with ARDS, the Pao_2 falls, in spite of ventilation with increasing amounts of oxygen, because of physiologic shunting of blood through the lungs to the left side of the heart. Physiologic *shunting* occurs because many alveoli are either collapsed or filled with fluid, and diffusion cannot occur as the blood passes through them. In the earlier stages of ARDS, when a sufficient number of alveoli are functioning, the arterial carbon dioxide pressure ($Paco_2$) is usually normal or more likely low because of the rapid diffusion of carbon dioxide and the hyperventilation that results from hypoxia.

However, as ARDS progresses and the lungs become increasingly stiff, an acute restrictive condition occurs and ventilation and diffusion are impaired. In this stage the $Paco_2$ as well as the Pao_2 are affected. The $Paco_2$, which was decreasing as a result of hyperventilation, begins to increase as a result of hypoventilation.

Arterial blood gas determinations are also used to assess the acid-base balance of the patient. In the early stages of shock, mild respiratory alkalosis typically occurs from the hyperventilation that is part of the stress response.

FLUID AND ELECTROLYTE ASSESSMENT

The urinary output and the CVP most accurately reflect fluid status. An indwelling urinary catheter is usually inserted, and the urine output is measured hourly. Other output, such as GI drainage, wound exudate, or perspiration, is measured or estimated as accurately as possible. Body weight often gives a more accurate assessment of fluid changes than the measurement of intake and output; however, this can be an inaccurate determinant of intravascular volume when third spacing of fluid occurs. Noting the presence of edema, auscultating the chest for the presence of fluid, and measuring the abdominal girth for the development of ascites are means of assessing fluid collection in the third space.

In the early stages of shock the serum potassium concentration may be abnormally low as a result of in-

TABLE 25-4 Hemodynamic parameters in various types of shock

	Hypovolemic	Cardiogenic	Septic*
Cardiac output	Low	Low	High
Pulmonary capillary wedge pressure (PCWP)	Low	High	Low
Mixed venous oxygen saturation (Svo_2)	Low	Low	High
Systemic vascular resistance (SVR)	High	High	Low

*In the late stage of septic shock, severely depressed cardiac function results in a clinical picture similar to that of cardiogenic shock.

creased levels of aldosterone in response to stress. However, as shock progresses, the serum potassium level may become abnormally high as damaged cells release potassium. As urinary output falls, the body is unable to eliminate the excess amounts of potassium accumulating in the serum. If potassium is administered in the early stage of shock, it is extremely important that the urinary output and serum electrolytes be monitored frequently.

The concentration of other serum electrolytes may be abnormal as a result of acid-base abnormalities, altered renal function, or fluid therapy. Serum enzymes may be elevated because of ischemia and damage to the heart, liver, and pancreas.

NEUROLOGIC ASSESSMENT

In shock the brain may be adversely affected by hypoxia, acid-base imbalance, or toxins. Often, subtle changes in mentation are the earliest signs of cerebral hypoxia. The patient is observed for increasing restlessness. Sedation should not be given until the patient's status has been assessed further and it has been determined that the restlessness does not have an organic cause. In the late stages, when perfusion of the brain is severely impaired, loss of consciousness occurs. Vital signs and arterial blood gas determinations can aid in assessing the cause of subtle neurologic changes.

HEMATOLOGIC ASSESSMENT

The hemoglobin and hematocrit levels are valuable tools for assessing blood loss in hypovolemic shock secondary to hemorrhage. It must be remembered, however, that the hemoglobin and hematocrit levels do not drop immediately with loss of an excessive amount of blood, because plasma is lost along with the blood cells. The blood that remains in the intravascular compartment initially will have a normal concentration of RBCs. Within a few hours after a blood loss, the hemoglobin and hematocrit levels begin to decrease as the kidneys retain water and electrolytes in response to low perfusion. An increase in hemoglobin and hematocrit levels may be seen in some types of shock. Increased capillary permeability, which occurs primarily in septic and anaphylactic shock, permits water and electrolyes to move out of the capillaries, leaving behind blood with a high concentration of cells.

Patients in shock are assessed for the development of DIC. The nurse may be the first to observe that the patient is bleeding for an excessively long time after a venipuncture or that blood is oozing from an incision. If DIC is suspected, laboratory studies are initiated; clotting factors (including fibrinogen and platelet counts) are decreased, prothrombin time (PT) and partial thromboplastin time (PTT) are prolonged, and fibrin degradation products are increased.

ABDOMINAL ASSESSMENT

Abdominal assessment is important for the patient in shock. Decreased blood flow to the intestines may result in decreased peristalsis or paralytic ileus (see Chapter 44). Decreased or absent bowel sounds are noted. Gastric drainage and stools are assessed for occult blood because of the high incidence of GI tract bleeding with shock.

■ DATA ANALYSIS: NURSING DIAGNOSES

Nursing diagnoses are determined from assessment of patient data. Possible nursing diagnoses for the person with shock include, but are not limited to, the following:

Diagnostic Title	Possible Etiologies
Activity intolerance	Imbalance between oxygen supply and demand
Airway clearance, ineffective	Decreased energy, endotracheal intubation
Anxiety	Threat of death
Breathing pattern, ineffective	Inadequate perfusion of respiratory muscles
Cardiac output, decreased	Myocardial hypoxia, myocardial depressant factor
Fluid volume deficit (2)	Blood loss, increased capillary permeability, vasodilation
Gas exchange, impaired	Decreased lung compliance, interstitial edema
Infection, potential for	Invasive monitoring, Foley catheterization, decreased immune response
Oral mucous membrane, altered	Endotracheal intubation
Sleep pattern disturbance	Intensity of nursing care
Tissue perfusion, altered cardiopulmonary	Hypovolemia, decreased cardiac output, redistribution of blood

■ PLANNING: EXPECTED PATIENT OUTCOMES

Expected patient outcomes for the person with shock may include, but are not limited to, the following:

1. Patient will be able to tolerate activity involved in care without an increase in pulse rate of more than 20 per minute.
2. Patient's airway will remain free from secretions.
3. Patient and significant others will remain free of avoidable anxiety.
4. Patient will have a respiratory rate and tidal volume within normal limits.
5. Patient will make his or her needs understood by verbal or alternate means of communication.
6. Intravascular volume will return to normal.
7. Blood gases will be within normal limits.
8. Patient will be free from infection.
9. Oral mucous membrane will remain moist and intact.

10. Patient will have undisturbed periods of sleep.
11. Patient will be alert and oriented.
12. Urinary output will be within normal limits.
13. Patient will remain free from avoidable injury.

■ IMPLEMENTATION

Treatment of shock will vary to some extent, depending on the cause. The cause of the shock must be treated first. Blood must be given if the patient has hemorrhage, antibiotics are given if an infection is present, and epinephrine is given if anaphylaxis has occurred. However, all types of shock have enough in common that certain forms of treatment are typically administered. In most types of shock, fluid replacement is the first therapeutic measure to be instituted, followed by administration of vasoactive drugs.

PROMOTING FLUID BALANCE AND CARDIAC OUTPUT
FLUID REPLACEMENT

The need to administer fluids to the patient with hypovolemic shock is obvious. At times, fluid replacement is the only therapy needed in this type of shock. Vasogenic and septic shock are accompanied by hypovolemia because fluid is leaking out of the capillaries. Fluids are always part of the treatment. However, patients with cardiogenic shock *may* also require fluid therapy, although many may require fluid *restriction* or removal of fluid. Before fluid therapy is instituted for cardiogenic shock, a pulmonary artery catheter is inserted, and the pulmonary end-diastolic pressure measured. If the pressure is less than 20 torr, fluid therapy may be beneficial.[24]

Various fluids may be given to the patient in shock. It is generally agreed that the patient who has sustained a large blood loss will require whole blood replacement. Much disagreement surrounds what other types of fluids should be used to treat shock. Both advantages and disadvantages exist to all types of resuscitative fluids, including blood.

Table 25-5 lists fluids used for replacement therapy in shock.

Whole Blood

The administration of whole blood has the obvious advantage of increasing the oxygen-carrying capacity of the blood. It also has many disadvantages (transmission of diseases, transfusion reactions, cost). If massive transfusions are given, additional problems may result. Because blood for transfusion contains an anticoagulant to prevent it from clotting while it is being stored, the patient who receives large amounts of blood may develop clotting defects. Stored blood is also deficient in platelets and other clotting factors. Massive transfusions of cold blood can result in hypothermia, which can cause cardiac dysrhythmias.

Stored blood also contains some debris resulting from the aggregation of platelets, leukocytes, and fibrin. It is believed that some of this debris is able to pass through standard blood filters and is eventually filtered out of the blood by the pulmonary capillaries. This probably causes little difficulty in the patient who receives only a few units of blood, but it is likely to cause a problem for the patient who receives massive transfusions. It is recommended by some that microfilters be used when large quantities of blood are transfused.[27]

The pH in stored blood is lower than that in normal blood. The added anticoagulant makes the blood more acid. Also, because blood is stored in an airtight bag, the metabolism that continues is anaerobic, and the end products are lactic and pyruvic acid. Despite all the disadvantages, until a blood substitute is available for general use, blood must be given to maintain relatively normal hemoglobin and hematocrit levels.[17]

Some patients who are losing large amounts of blood may be given transfusions with their own blood, which has been collected from the bleeding site with special equipment. *Autotransfusion* has been used in patients bleeding massively from an uncontaminated wound as well as in patients who bleed excessively during surgery. Although it does eliminate transfusion reactions and hepatitis associated with blood transfusions, it is not without risks. Some of the complications of autotransfusion are sepsis and emboli.[27] Its main use is in patients who are bleeding so rapidly that the supply of stored blood is becoming depleted.

Other Types of Fluid Therapy

Fluids are generally classified as either cystalloid or colloid solutions (see Table 25-5). Controversy over which of these is better for the treatment of shock has existed since the 1960s. In theory, colloids would seem to be superior because they should have the ability to hold fluid within the vascular compartment. However, when shock results in increased capillary permeability, the colloidal particle may leak into the interstitium and be followed by water. Another important consideration is cost. Colloids are generally much more expensive than crystalloids and therefore should be used only if their effect can be shown to be clearly superior to that of crystalloids.[16,39]

Regardless of the type of fluid that the patient receives, the nurse must carefully monitor the rate at which it is administered. The patient is assessed frequently for signs of hypovolemia or fluid overload (see Chapter 28). Neck veins are observed for distention, and lungs are auscultated for signs of fluid (rales, rhonchi).

FLUID REDISTRIBUTION

Another way in which fluid resuscitation may be accomplished is by the use of the military antishock trousers

Text continued on p. 594.

TABLE 25-5 Fluids used for replacement therapy in shock

Type	Uses/Indications	Advantages	Disadvantages	Special Considerations
BLOOD AND BLOOD PRODUCTS				
Whole blood	Replace blood volume and maintain hemoglobin (Hb) at 12-14 g/100 ml	Provides intravascular volume Increases oxygen-carrying capacity of blood	Potential associated risks of hepatitis and allergic reactions Delayed administration because of necessary typing and cross-matching Possibility of type and crossmatch errors	Whole blood should be stored at 0°-10° C (32°-50° F), but warmed at least 20-30 min before administration (*never* infuse cold blood). Use *fresh* whole blood whenever possible to avoid adverse metabolic changes related to stored blood.
RBCs (packed, concentrate) Fresh, frozen (also called leukocyte-poor)	Increase hematocrit to minimum level of 30% Correct RBC deficiency and improve oxygen-carrying capacity of blood	Concentrated form helps prevent excess fluid administration in patients with cardiogenic shock (increases oxygen-carrying capacity with less volume loading) Associated with fewer risks of metabolic complications when compared to stored whole blood (decreased amount of transfused antibodies, electrolytes, and so on) Provides economic use of blood as a resource; frees other blood components such as platelets and clotting factors to be concentrated and stored	Slow infusion rate because of increased viscosity Decreased content of plasma proteins and coagulation factors when compared to whole blood Inadequate (alone) for volume replacement and correction of hypovolemia Altered blood clotting with administration of more than 20 units; for every 4 units of RBCs over 20, 1 unit of fresh frozen plasma should be administered to replenish clotting factors High cost of frozen (thawed) RBCs	Administer via Y-connector tubing with normal saline to increase infusion flow rate. Washed RBCs (resuspended in saline) can be given in shock to decrease red cell adhesiveness (washing decreases cell's fibrinogen coating).
Human plasma (fresh, frozen, or dried)	Restore plasma volume in hypovolemic shock without increasing the hematocrit Restore clotting factors (except platelets)	Effective for rapid volume replacement Contains clotting factors	Expensive Deficient of RBCs	Human plasma carries risk of viral hepatitis and allergic reactions. Administer fresh frozen plasma promptly after thawing to prevent deterioration of clotting factors V and VIII.

From Rice V: Shock: shock, a clinical syndrome, the clinical continuum of septic shock, shock management, Secaucus, NJ, 1985, Critical Care Nurse/Hospitals Publications, Inc.

TABLE 25-5 Fluids used for replacement therapy in shock—cont'd

Type	Uses/Indications	Advantages	Disadvantages	Special Considerations
COLLOID SOLUTIONS				
Plasma protein fraction (Plasmanate, Plasma-Plex)	Expand plasma volume in hypovolemic shock (while cross-matching being completed) Increase serum colloid osmotic pressure	Can be used interchangeably with 5% human serum albumin Osmotically equivalent to plasma Associated with low risk of hepatitis	Expensive Deficient of clotting factors Associated with more side effects such as hypotension and hypersensitivity, than those reported with 5% albumin (because of presence of globulins) Hypotension induced by rapid intravenous administration (greater than 10 ml/min)	Plasma protein fraction is prepared from pooled plasma heated to 60° C (140° F) for 10 hr. This procedure reduces risk of transmission of hepatitis viruses. Rapid administration of large dosages can alter blood coagulation. This solution should be used cautiously in patients with congestive heart failure (caused by added fluid and rapid plasma volume expansion) and in patients with renal failure (caused by added proteins).
Albumin 5% 25% (salt poor)	Increase plasma colloid osmotic pressure Rapidly expand plasma volume	Rare allergic reactions (less than 0.01% in all albumin solutions combined) Rare transmission of hepatitis virus	Potential leakage from capillaries in shock states associated with increased capillary permeability Possible precipitation of congestive heart failure following rapid infusion in patients with circulatory overload and compromised cardiovascular function	Albumin does not contain preservatives; therefore each opened bottle should be used at once. Rate of administration of 5% albumin should not exceed 2-4 ml/min. Rate of administration of 25% albumin should not exceed 1 ml/min. 25% albumin is reserved for use in patients with pulmonary or peripheral edema and hypoproteinemia. Administer with a diuretic to ensure diuresis.

Continued.

TABLE 25-5 Fluids used for replacement therapy in shock—cont'd

Type	Uses/Indications	Advantages	Disadvantages	Special Considerations
PLASMA EXPANDERS				
Dextran Low-molecular-weight dextran (LMWD; dextran 40, Rheomacrodex, Gentran 40) High-molecular-weight dextran (HMWD; dextran 70, Gentran 70 and 75, Macrodex)	Rapidly expand plasma volume	All dextrans: associated with low incidence of anaphylactic reactions; less expensive than protein solutions LMWD: associated with fewer allergic reactions than HMWD; facilitates blood flow by decreasing RBC adhesiveness HMWD: leaks from the capillaries less readily than LMWD; can effectively increase plasma volume for up to 24 hr	LMWD: 70% excreted unchanged in urine, so urine osmolality and specific gravity are altered; potential osmotic nephrosis and renal tubular shutdown; possible bleeding from raw surfaces caused by decreased platelet adhesiveness; side effects include decreased hemoglobin, hematocrit, fibrinogen, and clotting factors V, VIII, and IX HMWD: 50% excreted unchanged in the urine, so urine osmolality and specific gravity altered; higher incidence of allergic reactions when compared to LMWD; increases blood viscosity and platelet adhesiveness	Avoid use of dextran in patients with active hemorrhage, hemorrhagic shock, coagulation disorders, and thrombocytopenia. Bleeding times can be prolonged when the correct dose of dextran 70 (1.2 g/kg/day) or dextran 40 (2 g/kg/day) are exceeded. Administer dextran in dextrose solutions to patients with sodium restriction.
Hetastarch (Hespan, Volex)	Expand plasma volume	Same volume expansion characteristics of albumin but with a longer duration of action (up to 36 hr) Associated with low risk of allergic and anaphylactic reactions (0.085%) Cost of hetastarch is about one-half that of plasma protein fraction and albumin Nonantigenic No danger of transmission of hepatitis virus	Potential dilution of plasma proteins and decreased plasma colloid osmotic pressure Potential dilution of clotting factors with resultant coagulation changes Potential circulatory overload in patients with severe congestive heart failure and compromised renal function Increased serum amylase level (>200 mg/100 ml), peaking within 1 hr of intravenous administration of hetastarch and persisting for 3-4 days (caused by action of amylase in hetastarch degradation)	Do not use if solution is cloudy or deep brown or if it contains crystals. Monitor clotting studies and platelet counts, observing for prolonged PT and PTT and thrombocytopenia. Safety and compatibility of additives with hetastarch have not been established; manufacturer recommends infusing hetastarch through separate line, when possible, or piggybacking second drug. Maximum infusion rate in acute hemorrhagic shock is 20 ml/kg/hr. Monitor serum albumin; if it falls below 2 g/100 ml, consider substituting albumin for hetastarch.

TABLE 25-5 Fluids used for replacement therapy in shock—cont'd

Type	Uses/Indications	Advantages	Disadvantages	Special Considerations
Mannitol (Osmitrol)	Raise intravascular volume Reduce interstitial and intracellular edema Promote osmotic diuresis	Reduce intracellular swelling Increases urinary output	Potential circulatory overload in patients with congestive heart failure, pulmonary congestion, and renal dysfunction	
CRYSTALLOID SOLUTIONS (ISOTONIC)				
Normal saline	Raise plasma volume when RBC mass is adequate Replace body fluid	Considered by some to be most important salt for maintaining and replacing extracellular fluid Increases plasma volume without altering normal sodium concentration or serum osmolality	Potential fluid retention and circulatory overload caused by sodium content	
Lactated Ringer's solution (Hartmann's solution)	Replace body fluid Buffer acidosis	Lactate converted to bicarbonate in liver, which buffers acidosis Lactate replaces bicarbonate, preventing precipitation of calcium bicarbonate and calcium carbonate Lactate more stable than bicarbonate and more compatible with ions present in solution	Increased lactic acidosis in shock caused by lactate Fluid retention and circulatory overload caused by sodium content	Lactate conversion requires aerobic metabolism; therefore it should be used cautiously in shock and other hypoperfusion states.
Ringer's solution	Replace body fluid Provide additional potassium and calcium	Does not contain lactate, so can be given to patients with hypoperfusion	Potential hyperchloremic metabolic acidosis caused by high chloride concentration Potential fluid retention and circulatory overload caused by sodium content	
CRYSTALLOID SOLUTIONS (HYPOTONIC)				
One-half normal saline	Raise total fluid volume		Potential interstitial and intracellular edema caused by rapid movement of this fluid from vascular space Dilution of plasma proteins and electrolytes	
5% dextrose in water (D5W)	Raise total fluid volume Provide calories for energy (200/1000 ml)	Distributed evenly in every body compartment (acts as free water) Reverses dehydration Prevents hyperosmolar state Maintains adequate renal tubular flow (facilitates water excretion)	Dilution of plasma proteins and electrolytes caused by rapid metabolism of glucose and resultant free water	

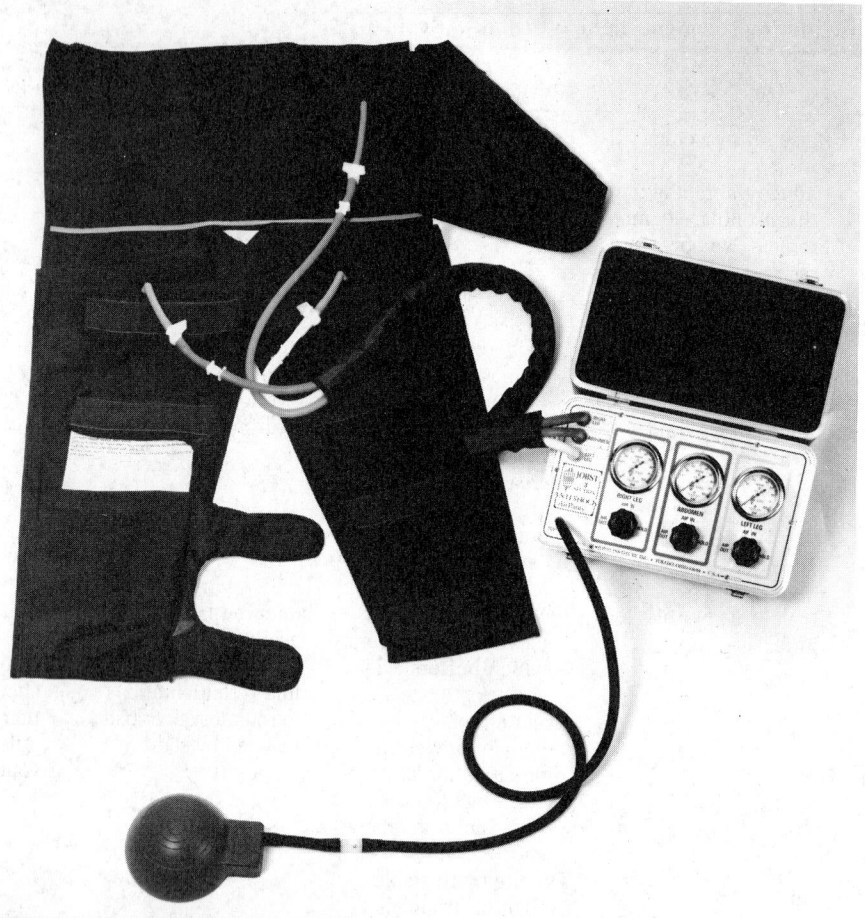

FIGURE 25-7 Military antishock trousers (MAST) with inflation device and manometers. (Courtesy The Jobst Institute, Inc, Toledo, Ohio; from Burrell LO and Burrell AL: Critical care, St Louis, 1982, The CV Mosby Co.)

(MAST). The suit consists of three inflatable parts, one for each leg and one for the abdomen (Figure 25-7). When they are inflated, the trousers autotransfuse the upper circulation with up to 2 L of blood from the lower extremities, redirecting blood to the heart, lungs, and brain.[26] The trousers also increase peripheral resistance, which helps compensate for decreased blood volume. If bleeding in the lower extremities is present, the MAST helps to control bleeding by tamponade (counterpressure). The suit is used as a temporary measure until adequate fluid can be administered. When the suit is to be removed, it must be deflated gradually to prevent a sudden fall in peripheral resistance and a return of shock.

MEDICATIONS

If fluid therapy alone is not sufficient to reverse the shock state, vasoactive drugs may be given. Most vasoactive drugs are catecholamines, which stimulate α-or β-receptors in the body. Generally, stimulation of α-receptors causes vasoconstriction, and stimulation of β-re-

ceptors also causes the heart to increase its rate (*chronotropic effect*) and strength of contraction (*inotropic effect*). The abdominal viscera, skin, and muscles respond primarily to the alpha effects of the catecholamines.

Mixed α- and β-adrenergic drugs are used most often (Table 25-6). In the very early stage of shock, particularly shock characterized by vasodilation, the patient may benefit from drug therapy that results in vasoconstriction. This would enhance the body's normal compensatory mechanisms and increase the blood supply to the brain and the heart, allowing time for the primary problem to be corrected. However, if the primary problem is not or cannot be corrected, compensatory vasoconstriction itself can harm the body. *Vasoconstrictive drugs*, if used after the early stages of shock, *may harm the kidneys* and result in *renal failure*. They may also cause *ischemia* of *the bowel, resulting in bowel necrosis and sepsis*, and *ischemia of the pancreas, resulting in the release of MDF*.

Vasodilatory drugs may be effective in counteracting

TABLE 25-6 Vasoactive drugs frequently used to treat shock

	Effect	Advantages	Disadvantages
MIXED α- AND β-ADRENERGIC DRUGS			
Norepinephrine (levarterenol)	β_1: pronounced effect in low doses Positive inotropic and chronotropic effects	May improve cardiac output by increasing rate and stroke volume.	Increase O_2 need of heart
	β_2: weak effect Dilation of coronary arteries	May improve blood flow to heart	
	α: pronounced effect, especially in higher doses Vasoconstriction	May improve oxygenation of heart by increasing coronary artery perfusion pressure, especially in presence of hypotension	May decrease cardiac output by increasing afterload Increases O_2 need of heart
Metaraminol (Aramine)	Same as norepinephrine Acts by releasing catacholamine stores in body	Same as norepinephrine	Same as norepinephrine
Epinephrine	β_1: pronounced effect Positive inotropic and chronotropic effect	May improve cardiac output by increasing stroke volume and rate	Increases O_2 need of heart
	β_2: pronounced effect, especially in lower doses Dilates coronary arteries and vessels in skeletal muscles	May increase blood supply to heart	May shunt blood away from vital organs because of dilation of vessels in skeletal muscles
	α: pronounced effect in higher doses	May improve oxygenation of heart by increasing coronary perfusion pressure	May decrease cardiac output by increasing afterload Increases O_2 need of heart
Dopamine	Dopaminergic receptors: pronounced effect in low (2-5 μg/kg/min) and moderate doses (5-10 μg/kg/min); α effect in high doses (>10 μg/kg/min)	Improves perfusion of kidneys and abdominal viscera	
	β_1: pronounced effect in moderate dose range Positive inotropic and chronotropic effect	Improves cardiac output	Increases O_2 need of heart
	β_2: moderate effect Dilates coronary arteries	Increased blood supply to heart	
	α: pronounced in high doses Offsets dopaminergic and beta effects Vasoconstriction	May improve oxygenation of heart by increasing coronary perfusion pressure	May decrease cardiac output by increasing afterload Increases O_2 need of heart
Dobutamine	β_1: pronounced effect Positive inotropic effect Minimal chronotropic effect	Improves cardiac output by increasing stroke volume Lack of rate increase allows more coronary filling time than other inotropic drugs	Increases O_2 need of heart
	β_2: weak effect Some dilation of coronary arteries α: minimal effect	May improve coronary artery blood flow	
β-ADRENERGIC DRUGS			
Isoproterenol	β_1: very pronounced effect Strong positive inotropic and chronotropic effects	Increases cardiac output by increasing stroke volume and rate	Pronounced increase in O_2 need of heart Cardiac dysrhythmias
	β_2: very pronounced effect Dilates coronary arteries and vessels in skeletal muscles Lowers peripheral resistance	May increase blood supply to heart May improve cardiac output by decreasing afterload	Decreased blood pressure may decrease coronary artery perfusion pressure
VASODILATORS			
Nitroprusside	Acts directly on smooth muscle, dilating both veins and arterioles	Decreases O_2 need of heart by decreasing both preload and afterload Decreases pulmonary congestion by decreasing preload Increases cardiac output by decreasing afterload	Decreases in peripheral resistance can decrease coronary artery perfusion pressure
Nitroglycerine	Acts directly on smooth muscle Effect on veins—pronounced Effect on arterioles—weak	Decreases O_2 need of heart by decreasing both preload and, to a lesser extent, afterload	Decrease in preload can decrease cardiac output and coronary artery perfusion pressure

the adverse effects of the body's compensatory mechanisms. They also decrease the pressure against which the failing heart has to pump, thereby decreasing the oxygen needs of the heart. However, they are not without danger. They may cause a fall in an already low arterial pressure, reducing coronary artery filling and making the heart even more hypoxic. Fluid therapy must be given with vasodilator drugs to maintain cardiac output. *Dopamine*, the most frequently used drug in the treatment of shock, has a variable effect depending on the dose administered. In certain dosage ranges it *increases cardiac output* by an *inotropic effect* on the heart and at the same time *selectively dilates the renal and mesenteric vessels, increasing perfusion of the kidneys and the abdominal viscera.* Selecting the proper drug depends to some extent on the cause of shock and how far it has progressed.

A combination of drugs may be given. Dopamine and nitroprusside may be given together to increase cardiac output by combining the inotropic effect of dopamine with the decreased peripheral resistance effected by nitroprusside. Low-dose dopamine may be given for its effect on renal and mesenteric perfusion along with dobutamine for its inotropic effect.

Patients receiving vasoactive drugs require very careful monitoring. Ideally, intraarterial and pulmonary pressure monitoring should be instituted. If the blood pressure is being measured by both cuff and intraarterial line, the two readings may vary. It is imperative that everyone working with the patient use the same measurements in adjusting the rate of drug infusion.

Steroids are often administered to patients in shock; however, *their use is controversial.* Many benefits from their use have been suggested, the most important being stabilization of lysosomal membranes, thereby preventing the leak of destructive enzymes.[20]

CARE OF PATIENTS RECEIVING VASOACTIVE DRUGS

1. Monitor blood pressure every 5 to 15 minutes at the beginning of the infusion and every 15 minutes thereafter to maintain a *mean* blood pressure at prescribed level, usually 80 mm Hg.
2. Drug must be diluted in a compatible solution and administered slowly by intravenous pump (for control).
3. Observe peripheral site of infusion (if used) frequently for signs of infiltration; necrosis and sloughing of tissues may occur with infiltration.
4. If infiltration occurs, infiltrate area around site with norepinephrine blockers (phentolamine [Regitine]) as prescribed.
5. Monitor urinary output.
6. When discontinuing drug infusion, taper infusion slowly while continuing to monitor blood pressure every 15 minutes.

Many drugs are being used experimentally in the treatment of shock, particularly in septic shock. These include naloxone, calcium channel blockers, prostaglandin inhibitors, nonsteroidal antiinflammatory drugs, and endotoxin antibodies.[6,17,36]

Care of patients receiving vasoactive drugs is summarized in the box below.

ASSISTING WITH CARDIAC SUPPORT

When the left ventricle becomes severely impaired, as in cardiogenic shock or in the late stages of any type of shock, its function may be augmented by the use of the intraaortic balloon pump (see Chapter 28). A balloon-tipped catheter is inserted into the aorta by way of the femoral artery. The catheter is attached to a machine that inflates and deflates the balloon in synchrony with the patient's cardiac cycle. During systole the balloon is deflated as the heart pumps blood into the aorta. During diastole the balloon inflates, enhancing blood flow to the heart, which is perfused during diastole, and to the rest of the body. During the next period of systole the balloon deflates again, leaving a space in the aorta that must be filled. This causes a reduction in resistance, which allows the heart to eject a larger quantity of blood with less effort than would normally be required.

Complications may occur with use of the balloon pump, the most common being vascular insufficiency of the extremity distal to the insertion site. Frequent assessments are made of the pulses, color, temperature, movement, and sensation of the extremity, and any abnormality is reported immediately. Infection may occur with this procedure, as with any invasive procedure; therefore the patient's temperature is also monitored.

The use of the intraaortic balloon is a temporary measure used to enhance cardiac output only until the heart is able to function adequately on its own.

ASSISTING WITH RESPIRATORY SUPPORT

Most patients in shock have some degree of hypoxemia. Oxygen is usually administered because tissues are already suffering from oxygen deprivation caused by decreased blood flow. Because the energy system of the body is impaired, the muscles used in ventilation may not function adequately, and breathing may have to be assisted. If symptoms of ARDS develop, positive end-expiratory pressure (PEEP) may have to be used. Positive pressure at the end of expiration prevents surfactant-deficient alveoli from collapsing, resulting in atelectasis. Coughing and deep breathing are important. If the patient is too weak to cough or if an endotracheal tube is in place, suctioning is necessary to keep the airway free of excessive secretions. Meticulous mouth care is necessary while the endotracheal tube is in place, because the mouth remains open and swallowing may be difficult. The patient with an endotracheal tube in place be unable to talk, therefore, a nonverbal method such as a magic slate must be used.

PROMOTING SAFETY

In the early stages of shock the patient may exhibit restlessness, which may then progress to confusion. During this time, injury is likely to occur if preventive measures are not taken. If the patient attempts to remove or disconnect life-saving equipment, soft restraints may have to be applied.

Infections occur often in patients with shock because of the many invasive procedures that are performed. Some potential sources of infection are indwelling catheters, arterial lines, pulmonary artery catheters, intravenous lines, endotracheal tubes, surgical incisions, and traumatic wounds. Meticulous sterile technique must be used with endotracheal suctioning, dressing changes, tubing changes, and urinary catheter care. Patients who are receiving steroids or who have experienced excessive blood loss are at increased risk for developing infection.

Complications of immobility must be prevented. The patient in shock may remain in one position for an extended period because of the constant activity occurring at the bedside. This immobility can predispose the patient to thrombi, pneumonia, and decubitis ulcers.

PROMOTING COMFORT AND REST

The patient should be kept as comfortable as possible. In the past, patients in shock were kept in Trendelenberg's position (head down), but this is no longer recommended. It is usually suggested that the patient remain flat, with the legs elevated if necessary. If a patient in shock has difficulty breathing, a small pillow may be used to elevate the head slightly.

Rest is important. All nonessential activities should be eliminated because activity increases the body's need for oxygen and nutrients, substances already deficient in the cells of the patient in shock.

Ambient temperature should be kept at a comfortable level. Excessive warmth increases the metabolic rate of the tissues, thereby increasing their oxygen need. Excessive coolness may cause the blood to flow even more sluggishly through the microcirculation, enhancing the formation of microthrombi. Patients with an endotracheal tube in place or who are very lethargic may not be able to express how they feel. Covers should be used according to the room temperature.

Both the conscious patient and the family will probably experience considerable anxiety. The nurse should remain calm and explain all interventions whenever possible. It may be necessary to repeat explanations frequently to both patient and family, because anxiety can interfere with their ability to comprehend and to remember.

CHAPTER SUMMARY

- ✔ Shock is a syndrome characterized by hypoperfusion of body tissues.
- ✔ The major classifications of shock are hypovolemic, cardiogenic, and vasogenic shock.
- ✔ Shock results in a derangement of cellular metabolism; if not treated in the early stages, it can affect all body systems.
- ✔ The early stage of shock is characterized by a stress response.
- ✔ At some point in the progress of untreated shock, the process becomes irreversible and no treatment can save the patient.
- ✔ The management of shock includes the following:
  a. Fluid therapy—colloids, crystalloids
  b. Drug therapy—vasodilators, vasoconstrictors, inotropes
  c. Supportive care—cardiac support, respiratory support, prevention of injuries

QUESTIONS TO CONSIDER

- How would you expect your assessment findings of a patient in cardiogenic shock to differ from those of a patient in hypovolemic shock?
- What would you include in your assessment to determine whether or not a patient was receiving adequate fluid replacement?
- How would you assess the comfort of a patient with an endotracheal tube?
- How would you assess the effect of vasoactive drugs on your patient?

REFERENCES AND SELECTED READINGS

1. Asheervath J and Blevins D: Handbook of clinical nursing practice, Norwalk, Conn, 1986, Appleton-Century-Crofts.
2. Bihari DJ and Tinker J: The therapeutic value of vasodilator prostaglandins in multiple organ failure associated with sepsis, Intensive Care Med 15(1):2-7, 1988.
3. Bonato J: Blood transfusions: are they safe? Crit Care Nurs 9(7):40-46, 1989.
4. Brandstetter RD: The adult respiratory distress syndrome—1986, Heart Lung 15(2):155-164, 1986.
5. Bulle TM and Rogers WJ: Cardiogenic shock. In Hardaway RM: Shock: the reversible stage of dying, Littleton, Mass, 1986, PSG Publishing Co, Inc.
6. Calandra T et al: Treatment of gram-negative septic shock with human IgG antibody to *Escherichia coli* J5: a prospective, double-blind, randomized trial, J Infect Dis 58(2):312-319, 1988.

*References preceded by an asterisk are particularly well suited for student reading.

7. Clowes GHA, Jr: Trauma, sepsis and shock: the physiological basis of therapy, New York, 1988, Marcel Dekker, Inc.

8. Danner RL and Parrillo JE: The role of endotoxin in human septic shock: therapeutic potential of lipid A analogs, Prog Clin Biol Res 286:183-200, 1989, Alan R Liss, Inc.

9. *Dickerson M: Anaphylaxis and anaphylactic shock, Crit Care Nurs Q 11(1):678-674, 1988.

10. *Dislet L et al: Cardiogenic shock in evolving myocardial infarction, Heart Lung 16:649-651, 1987.

11. *Dunham CM and Cowley RA: Shock trauma/critical care handbook, Rockville, Md, 1986, Aspen Systems Corp.

12. Fowler NO: Examination of the heart: inspection and palpation of venous and arterial pulses, New York, 1978, American Heart Association.

13. Guyton AC: Textbook of medical physiology, ed 7, Philadelphia, 1986, WB Saunders Co.

14. *Halfman-Franey M: Current trends in hemodynamic monitoring of patients in shock, Crit Care Nurs Q 11(1):9-18, 1988.

15. Hammerschmidt DE and Vercellotti GM: Granulocytes of mediators of tissue injury in shock: therapeutic implications, Prog Clin Biol Res 236A:19-32, 1987, Alan R Liss, Inc.

16. *Hancock BG and Eberhard NK: The pharmacological management of shock, Crit Care Nurs Q 11(1):19-29, 1988.

17. Hardaway RM: Shock: the reversible stage of dying, Littleton, Mass, 1986, PSG Publishing Co, Inc.

18. Hesselvik JF and Brodin B: Low dose norepinephrine in patients with septic shock and oliguria: effects on afterload, urine flow, and oxygen transport, Crit Care Med 17(2):179-180, 1989.

18a. *Houston MC: Pathophysiology of shock, Crit Care Nurs Clin N Am 2(2):143-149, 1990.

19. *Jeffries PR and Whelan SK: Cardiogenic shock: current management, Crit Care Nurs Q 11(1):48-56, 1988.

20. Jurkovich GJ, Moore EE, and Eiseman B: The liver in shock. In Hardaway RM: Shock: the reversible stage of dying, Littleton, Mass, 1986, PSG Publishing Co, Inc.

20a. *Lancaster LE and Rice V: Nursing care planning overview and application to the patient in shock, Crit Care Nurs Clin N Am 2(2):279-286, 1990.

21. Lefer AM and Hock CE: Vascular mediators in circulatory shock. In Hardaway RM: Shock: the reversible stage of dying, Littleton, Mass, 1986, PSG Publishing Co, Inc.

22. *Littleton MT: Pathophysiology and assessment of sepsis and septic shock, Crit Care Nurs Q 11(1):30-47, 1988.

23. *Littleton MT: Prostaglandins and leukotrienes as mediators of shock and trauma, Crit Care Nurs Q 11(2):11-20, 1988.

24. MacLean LD: Shock, Br Med Bull 44(2):437-452, 1988.

25. *Martin E et al: Autotransfusion systems, Crit Care Nurse 9(7):65-73, 1989.

26. McSwain NE: Pneumatic anti-shock garment: state of the art, 1988, Ann Emerg Med 17(5):506-526, 1988.

27. Millar S: AACN procedure manual for critical care, Philadelphia, 1985, WB Saunders Co.

28. Nagy S: Cardiodepressant and cardiostimulant factors in shock, Prog Clin Biol Res 236A:599-610, 1987, Alan R Liss, Inc.

29. Parrillo JE: The cardiovascular pathophysiology of sepsis, Ann Rev Med 49:469-485, 1989.

30. *Perry AG: Shock complications: recognition and management, Crit Care Nurs Q 11(1):1-8, 1988.

31. Perry AG and Potter PA: Shock: comprehensive nursing management, St Louis, 1983, The CV Mosby Co.

32. Rackow EC, Astiz ME, and Weil MH: Cellular oxygen metabolism during sepsis and shock, JAMA 259(13):1989-1993, 1988.

33. Rice V: Shock: shock, a clinical syndrome, the clinical continuum of septic shock, shock management, Secaucus, NJ, 1985, Critical Care Nurse/Hospitals Publications, Inc.

34. *Schedel I: New aspects in the treatment of gram-negative bacteremia and septic shock, Infection 16(1):4-7, 1988.

35. Schumer W: Coticosteroids in the treatment of shock, Prog Clin Biol Res 236B:249-259, 1987, Alan R Liss, Inc.

36. Soulioti AM: Naloxone for septic shock, Lancet 2(8620):1133-1134, 1988.

37. *Strange JM, editor: Shock trauma care plans, Springhouse, Pa, 1987, Springhouse.

37a. Stroud M, Swindell B, and Bernard GR: Cellular and humoral mediator of sepsis syndrome, Crit Care Nurs Clin N Am 2(2):150-161, 1990.

37b. *Summer G: The clinical and hemodynamic presentation of the shock patient, Crit Care Nurs Clin N Am 2(2):161-166, 1990.

38. Tilkian SM, Conover MB, and Tilkian AG: Clinical implications of laboratory tests, ed 4, St Louis, 1987, The CV Mosby Co.

39. Weil MH and Rackow EC: Colloid osmotic pressure and its implication for the fluid management of patients in shock. In Hardaway RM: Shock: the reversible stage of dying, Littleton, Mass, 1986, PSG Publishing Co, Inc.

CHAPTER 26

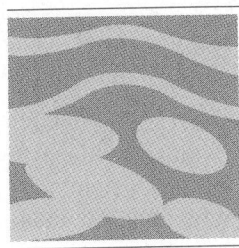

Assessment of the Cardiovascular System

TERRI ABRAHAM
JOAN M. KAVANAGH

CHAPTER OBJECTIVES

After studying this chapter, the student should be able to:

1. Describe the basic structure and function of the heart.
2. Describe the conduction system of the heart in relation to the cardiac cycle.
3. Identify factors that affect cardiac output.
4. Describe physiologic changes that occur in the cardiovascular system with aging.
5. Identify common manifestations of altered cardiac functioning.
6. Identify diagnostic tests used to assess cardiac functioning and the significance of each.
7. Describe nursing care of a patient experiencing cardiac catheterization and electrophysiologic study.

Since the 1970s in the United States, deaths from myocardial ischemia and its complications have decreased significantly. Contributing factors for this decline are (1) an overall increase in health awareness, including increased interest in exercise or fitness and improved nutritional habits; (2) reduction in cigarette use; (3) improved screening and treatment of hypertension; and (4) advances in medical and surgical treatment of heart disease.

In 1987 it was estimated that approximately 1.5 million people in the United States sustained a myocardial infarction and that 540,000 (36%) of them died. Of those deaths, 350,000 people died before reaching the hospital.[1] In essence, more than half of cardiac deaths occur within 2 hours of the onset of symptoms and take place outside the hospital. These statistics strongly support the need for educating the public to recognize cardiac emergencies and to employ basic cardiac life-support measures as soon as possible.

Mortality from coronary disease has also greatly declined for patients with acute myocardial infarction who reach the hospital. Expedient resuscitative measures in emergency departments and coronary care units, as well as improved antiarrhythmic drug therapy for the prevention of fatal ventricular dysrhythmias, play a crucial role in mortality reduction. Other therapies further reduce mortality from acute ischemic heart disease when initiated within the first 6 hours of the onset of chest pain or infarct-related symptoms.

This chapter is the first of three chapters that focus primarily on the heart. A review of anatomy and physiology of the heart, physiologic changes with aging, and cardiac assessment, including diagnostic tests, are included in this chapter. Cardiac dysrhythmias and cardiac disorders are discussed in Chapters 27 and 28.

ANATOMY AND PHYSIOLOGY

BASIC STRUCTURE

The heart is a relatively small organ that weighs 300 g and is approximately the size of a fist. It is located in the middle of the mediastinum, where the lungs partially overlap it. This pulsatile four-chambered pump beats approximately 72 times/minute, pumping more than 5 L of blood each minute, or about 2000 gallons per day. It continually propels oxygenated blood into the arterial system and receives poorly oxygenated blood from the venous system. The heart muscle rests on the diaphragm and is tilted forward and to the left so that the apex of the heart is rotated anteriorly.

The heart is enclosed by the *pericardium*, which consists of two layers: the inner layer (visceral pericardium) and the outer layer (parietal pericardium). The two pericardial surfaces are separated by a pericardial space that normally contains approximately 10 to 20 ml of thin, clear pericardial fluid. This lubricating fluid moistens the contacting surfaces of the pericardial layers and serves to reduce the friction produced by the pumping action of the heart. The visceral pericardium actually encases the heart and extends several centimeters onto each of the great vessels. The parietal pericardium is attached anteriorly to the manubrium and xiphoid process of the sternum, posteriorly to the vertebral column, and inferiorly to the diaphragm.

There are three layers of cardiac tissue: *epicardium*—the outer layer of the heart, which is the same structure as the visceral pericardium; *myocardium*—the middle layer of the heart, which is composed of striated muscle fibers and is responsible for the heart's contractile force; and *endocardium*—the innermost layer of the heart, which consists of endothelial tissue. The endocardium lines the inside of the heart's chambers and covers the heart valves.

CHAMBERS

The heart is divided into two halves by a muscular wall (*septum*) (Figure 26-1). Each half has an upper collecting chamber (*atrium*) and a lower pumping chamber (*ventricle*). Oxygen-poor venous blood enters the right atrium, flows from the right atrium to the right ventricle (mainly by gravity) when the tricuspid valve is opened, and is pumped into the pulmonary artery to the lungs. Oxygen-rich blood returns from the lungs to the left atrium, enters the left ventricle when the mitral valve is opened, and is ejected into the aorta for distribution to the peripheral tissues.

The *right atrium* is a thin-walled structure that serves as a reservoir for venous blood returning to the heart. Venous blood returns to the heart via the superior and inferior vena cava and the coronary sinus, which drains venous blood from the heart muscle. Blood is temporarily stored in the right atrium during right ventricular systole (contraction). During ventricular diastole (filling), approximately 80% of the venous return to the right atrium flows by gravity into the ventricle through the tricuspid valve. The remaining 20% of the venous return is delivered to the ventricles during atrial systole. This additional 15% to 20% of the venous return, which is actively propelled into the ventricles, is called the "atrial kick."

The *right ventricle* is normally the most anterior structure of the heart and is situated immediately beneath the sternum. The right ventricle receives venous blood from the right atrium during ventricular diastole and then propels this blood through the pulmonic valve into the pulmonary artery and then to the lungs. Be-

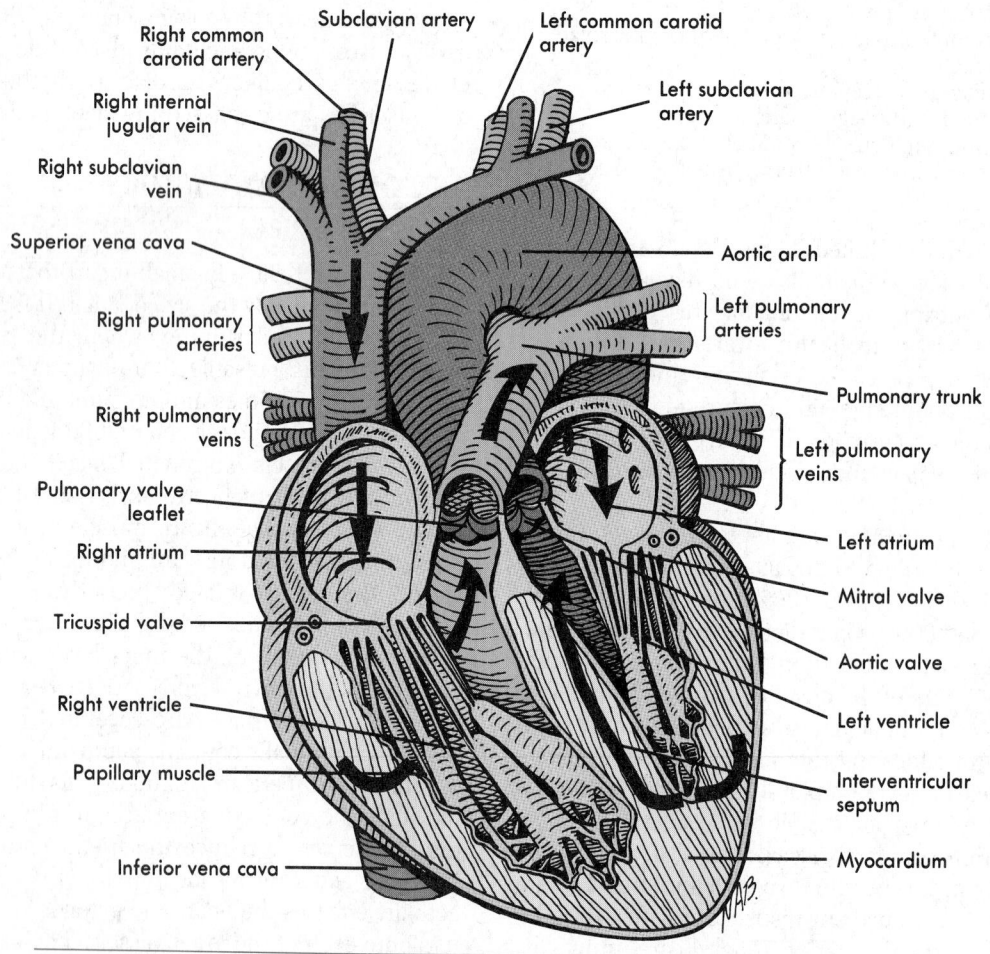

FIGURE 26-1 Heart in frontal section; course of blood through the chambers.

cause the pulmonary system is a low-pressure system, the overall workload of the right ventricle is much lighter than that of the left ventricle. The right ventricle has a crescent-shaped chamber and a thin outer wall that is 4 to 5 mm thick. This thin structure is suitable for right ventricular systole, because the right ventricle contracts against low resistance.

The thin-walled *left atrium* receives oxygenated blood from the four pulmonary veins and serves as a reservoir during left ventricular systole. Blood flows by gravity from the left atrium into the left ventricle through the opened mitral valve during ventricular diastole. Left atrial contraction then propels the remaining 20% of the venous return and provides a significant increment of blood volume to the left ventricle. This atrial kick serves to stretch the ventricle and prime it for ventricular ejection.

The *left ventricle* receives blood from the left atrium through the opened mitral valve during ventricular diastole. Blood is then ejected through the aortic valve into the systemic arterial circulation during ventricular systole. The left ventricle must contract against a high-pressure systemic circulation to deliver blood flow to the peripheral tissues. Therefore the left ventricular chamber is surrounded by 8 to 15 mm of thick musculature, which is approximately 2 to 3 times the thickness of the right ventricle. The thick musculature and ellipsoidal

sphere shape contribute to the powerful expulsive ability of the left ventricular chamber during systole.

VALVES

The four cardiac valves are flaplike structures that function to maintain unidirectional (forward) blood flow through the heart chambers. These valves open and close in response to pressure and volume changes within the cardiac chambers. The cardiac valves can be classified into two types: the atrioventricular (AV) valves, which separate the atria from the ventricles; and the semilunar valves, which separate the pulmonary artery and the aorta from their respective ventricles.

ATRIOVENTRICULAR VALVES

The AV valves are the *tricuspid* valve, located between the right atrium and the right ventricle, and the *bicuspid* (or *mitral*) valve, located between the left atrium and left ventricle. The tricuspid valve contains three leaflets held in place by fibrous cords called the *chordae tendineae,* which in turn are anchored to the ventricular wall by the papillary muscles. The mitral valve on the left side of the heart is a bicuspid valve with two valve cusps or leaflets. It also is attached to strands of fibrous tissue called chordae tendineae, which extend to the papillary muscles (Figure 26-2). The chordae tendineae are extremely important because they support the AV

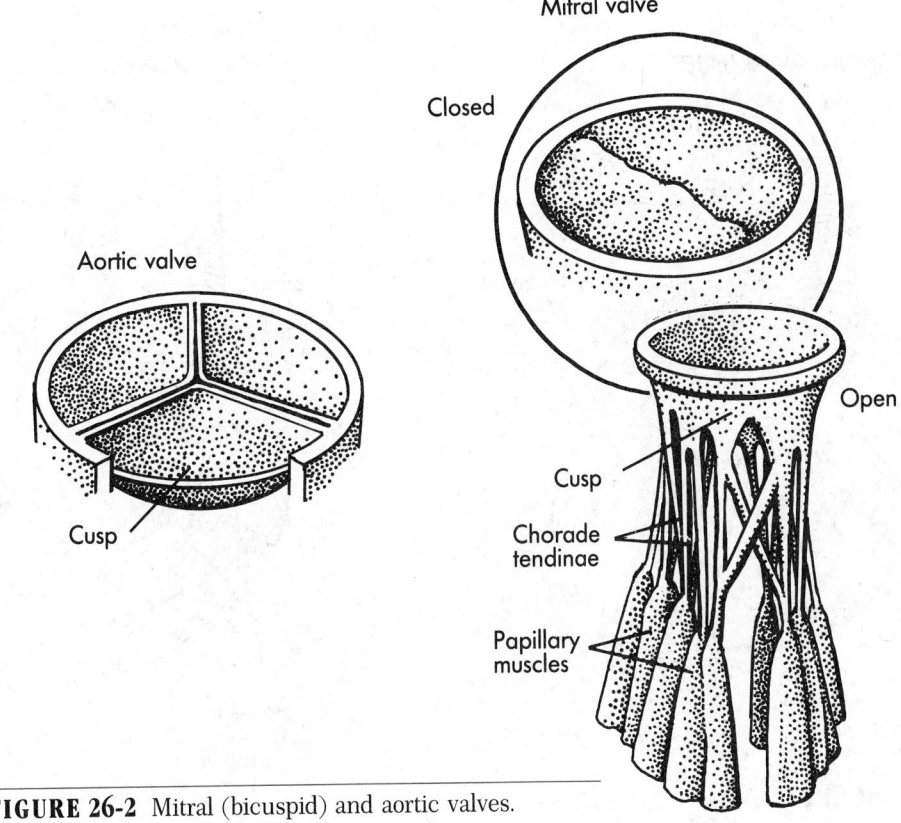

FIGURE 26-2 Mitral (bicuspid) and aortic valves.

valves during ventricular systole to prevent valvular prolapse into the atrium. Some leaflet overlapping occurs during closure of the AV valves, which helps to prevent the backward flow of blood. Damage to the chordae tendineae or to the papillary muscles would permit valvular regurgitation of blood back into the atrium during ventricular systole. During diastole the AV valves serve as a type of funnel as they allow blood to flow from the atria to the ventricles. The diameter of the AV cusps is almost double that of the orifice that they occlude. In general, the AV valves are structurally much more complex than the semilunar valves.

SEMILUNAR VALVES

The semilunar valves include the *aortic* and *pulmonic* valves. The structural design of the semilunar valves is quite different from the AV valves; each consists of three cuplike cusps (Figure 26-2). The pulmonic valve lies between the right ventricle and pulmonary artery. The aortic valve lies between the left ventricle and aorta. These valves are open during ventricular systole (contraction) to permit blood flow into the aorta and pulmonary artery. They are closed during diastole (relaxation) to prevent retrograde flow from the aorta and pulmonary artery back into the ventricle when it is relaxed.

CORONARY ARTERIES

The coronary arteries arise from the aorta (just behind the cusps of the aortic valve) in an area known as the

Valsalva's sinuses. The function of the coronary artery system is to provide an adequate blood supply to the myocardium. Despite scientific advances in the field of cardiology, coronary artery disease and its complications remain the leading cause of death in the United States (see Chapter 28).

There are two main coronary arteries, the *left* and the *right* (Figure 26-3). The left main coronary artery (LCA) divides into two branches: the left anterior descending (LAD) artery and the circumflex coronary artery (CCA). The LAD branch supplies the left ventricular myocardium, the septum, anterior papillary muscle, and portions of the right ventricle. In addition, the LAD artery usually supplies the anterior apex as well as some portion of the posterior apex. The CCA typically emerges at a sharp 90-degree angle from the LCA and is then directed toward the lateral left ventricle and apex. The CCA and its branches supply most of the left atrium, the lateral wall of the left ventricle, and part of the posterior wall of the left ventricle. Diagonal branches arise between the LAD artery and the CCA and are distributed along the free wall of the left ventricle.

One should look for two important external landmarks when tracing coronary circulation. These anatomic landmarks are sulci or grooves and include the following: the *atrioventricular groove,* which encircles the heart between the atria and the ventricles; and the *interventricular groove,* which divides the right and left

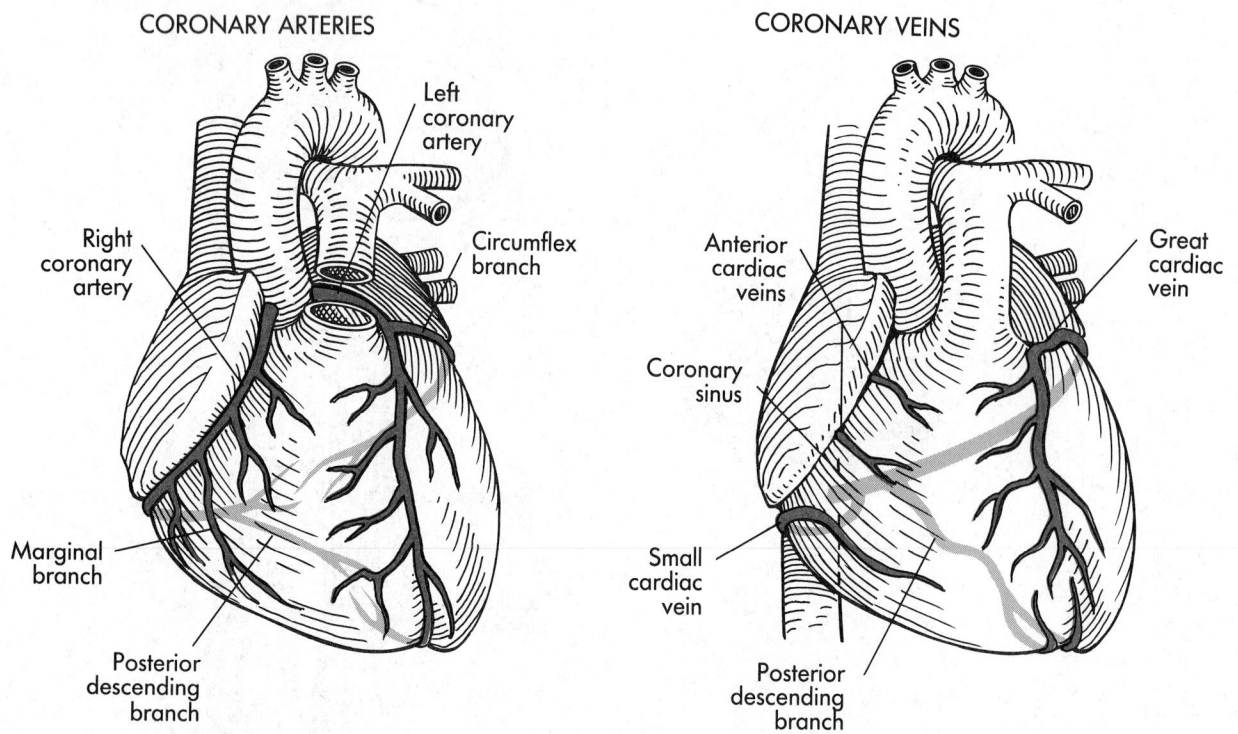

FIGURE 26-3 Coronary blood vessels.

ventricles. The meeting of the two anatomic grooves on the posterior side of the heart is known as the *crux* of the heart. The location of the crux is significant because this is where the AV node is located. The phrases "dominant left" circulation and "dominant right" circulation refer to whether the right or the left coronary artery turns at the crux of the heart and supplies the posterior interventricular groove. Therefore, if the CCA extends as far as the posterior interventricular groove, the circulation is considered to be dominant left. This condition occurs in only 10% to 15% of all individuals.

The right main coronary artery (RCA) arises from the right Valsalva's sinus off the aorta and courses around the right AV groove. Its branches supply the right ventricle, a portion of the septum, and in more than 50% of all individuals, the sinoatrial (SA) node. In approximately 67% of all individuals, the RCA turns at the crux of the heart and descends in the posterior interventricular groove. These individuals are classified as "right dominant." The posterior descending branch of the RCA then supplies the posterior aspect of the septum and the posterior left papillary muscle before terminating in several branches to the left ventricular wall.

Great variation exists in the branching pattern of the coronary arteries. In approximately 18% of the population, the CCA also reaches the crux of the heart with the RCA; this is the so-called balanced coronary artery pattern. In the remaining individuals, no true posterior interventricular branch exists; rather, many branches from either main coronary artery supply the posterior septum.

Coronary artery blood flow to the myocardium occurs almost exclusively during diastole, when coronary vascular resistance is diminished. During systole, coronary vascular resistance is increased because of the increased ventricular wall tension produced by ventricular contraction. During diastole, blood enters the coronary arteries at the pressure that exists at the moment in the aortic arch. This particular pressure is termed the *aortic diastolic pressure*.

Coronary venous drainage is accomplished via three subdivisions of the heart's venous system: (1) the thebesian veins drain a portion of the right atrial and right ventricular myocardium; (2) the anterior cardiac veins drain a large portion of the right ventricle; and (3) the coronary sinus and its branches drain the left ventricle and most myocardial venous return.

CONDUCTION SYSTEM
PROPERTIES OF CARDIAC MUSCLE

The mechanical contraction of the heart is the product of a stimulus-response process. The following properties are integral components of the electromechanical events in the heart.

Automaticity

The ability of the heart to initiate impulses regularly and spontaneously is known as automaticity, or rhythmicity. Although most cardiac cells have this ability, it is the prominent property of the SA node, making it the dominant pacemaker in the normal heart. Pacemaker cells are known to have lower resting membrane potentials than other myocardial cells and exhibit *spontaneous* depolarization.

Excitability

The ability of cardiac cells to respond to a stimulus by initiating a cardiac impulse is known as excitability. It should be noted that excitatory cells differ from pacemaker cells in that pacemaker cells do not require a stimulus to initiate an impulse.

Conductivity

The ability of cardiac cells to respond to a cardiac impulse by transmitting the impulse along cell membranes is referred to as conductivity. Cells specialized in this function are found in the conduction system. The arrangement of cells outside the conduction system ensures rapid conduction through intercalated disks joining adjacent cells.

Contractility

The ability of cardiac cells to respond to an impulse by contracting is known as contractility. Contractile cells compose the largest mass of the myocardium.

ANATOMY OF CONDUCTION SYSTEM

The pacemaking center of the normal heart is the SA, or "sinus," node (Figure 26-4). It is composed of a group of highly specialized tissues located in the right atrium adjacent to the superior vena cava. Automatically and at regular intervals, an electrical impulse is emitted from the SA node at a rate of 60 to 100 beats per minute. The atria are then depolarized, and the impulse travels to the AV node via three tracts designated as anterior, middle, and posterior *internodal tracts*. A fourth tract, called Bachmann's bundle, branches off the anterior nodal tract and transmits the impulse to the left atrium.

The three internodal tracts meet at the atrionodal junction. The junctional area refers to the region where atrial and ventricular tissues merge. This junction contains the AV node. The junctional cells above and below the AV node are capable of pacemaking activity under many circumstances (for example, failure of the SA node to fire).

The AV node itself is located on the right side of the interatrial septum. These cells lack the ability to initiate electrical impulses (that is, automaticity), but they are uniquely responsible for a brief physiologic delay in the conduction of the impulse to the ventricles.

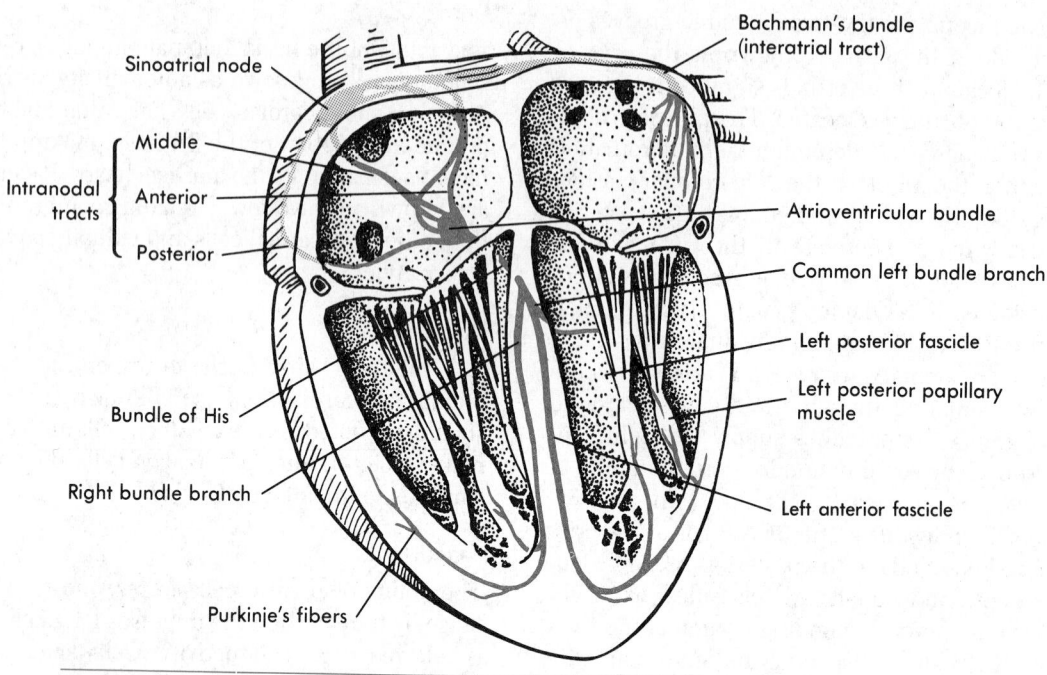

FIGURE 26-4 Schematic diagram of heart illustrating the conduction system.

The *bundle of His* begins anatomically as the "tail" of the AV node. It is a short, thick cable of fibers separated by collagen septa that bifurcates into the right and left bundle branches (RBB and LBB).

The RBB extends down the right side of the interventricular septum and is covered by a connective tissue sheath. It extends to reach the anterior papillary muscle of the right ventricle, where it merges with the Purkinje system. It lies close to the septal surface for much of its length, and therefore its functional ability is vulnerable to right ventricular pressure changes.

The LBB bifurcates into anterior and posterior fascicles. The anterior fascicle extends anteriorly down the left side of the interventricular septum to reach the anterior papillary muscle. The posterior fascicle is shorter and thicker and extends to the posterior papillary muscle of the left ventricle. Both fascicles connect with the Purkinje system and equally share in the spread of the impulse to the left ventricle.

Purkinje's fibers lie as a network on the endocardial surface and penetrate the myocardium of both ventricles. They are responsible for the transmission of the impulse to both ventricular free walls. Purkinje's cells are elongated and contain intercalated disks, which contributes to the superiority of conductivity in myocardial tissue.

Cells outside the conduction system also play a role in the conduction of an impulse. A surface membrane, the sarcolemma, surrounds each cell and acts as a selectively permeable barrier to sodium and potassium ions. Adjacent myocardial cells are connected end to end by a thickened portion of the sarcolemma known as an intercalated disk. These disks act as low-resistance pathways to the transmission of an impulse between cells.

SEQUENCE OF CARDIAC ACTIVATION

Depolarization is initiated by an impulse from the SA node. The impulse first spreads through the right atrium and then activates the left atrium. Atrial activation is normally accomplished in 0.11 second or less.

Shortly after the impulse reaches the left atrium, it also activates the junctional region and subsequently the AV node. The AV node delays the impulse about 0.1 second before the impulse enters the bundle of His.

On reaching the bundle of His, the impulse is transmitted along to the bundle branches. Within the ventricles, the first structure to be activated is the ventricular septum. The septum is activated by the impulse traveling from the left side to the right side (Figure 26-5).

The impulse then continues down the remaining length of the bundle branches and into the Purkinje network, thus activating the free ventricular walls almost simultaneously. Activation of the ventricular muscle proceeds from the apex toward the base of the heart to complete the process.

Depolarization of cardiac musculature proceeds from endocardium to epicardium. Repolarization in the atria follows this same pathway. In contrast, repolarization of ventricular musculature proceeds from epicardium to

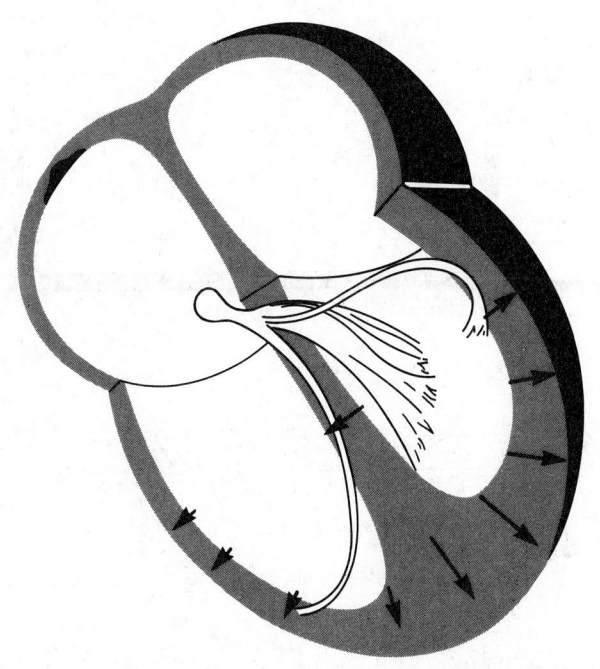

FIGURE 26-5 Sequence of electrical activation in the heart. (From Conover MB: Understanding electrocardiography: arrhythmias and the 12-lead ECG, ed 5, St Louis, 1988, The CV Mosby Co.)

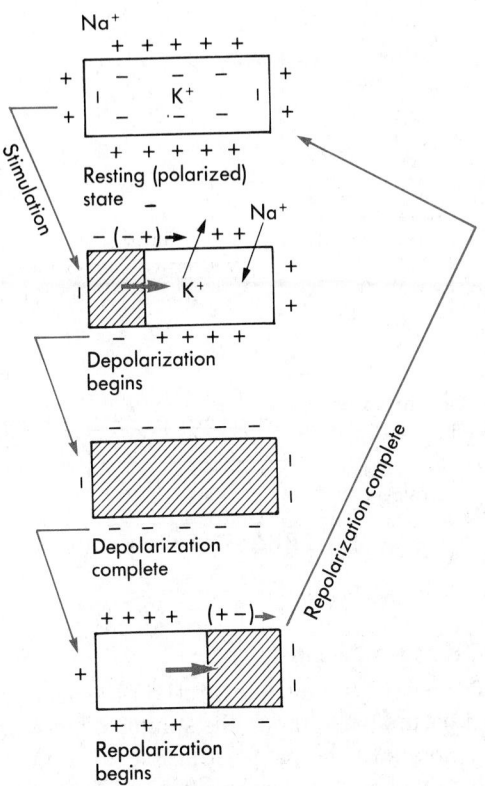

FIGURE 26-6 Schematic diagram illustrating process of depolarization and repolarization.

endocardium. Knowledge of the sequence of activation is fundamental to analysis of the electrocardiogram (ECG).

Action Potential

The resting myocardial cell has a membrane potential (that is, an electrical charge) as a result of the relative distribution of sodium and potassium ions extracellularly. Whenever the cell is stimulated, the membrane potential undergoes a change. A graphic record of this change forms the basis for an ECG. The change in electrical potential in response to a stimulus is known as the action potential. The two components of the action potential are *depolarization* and *repolarization*.

Resting Membrane Potential

In the resting state the inside of the cell is negative with respect to the outside (Figure 26-6). Initiation and conduction of cardiac impulses depend on the cell's ability to maintain an electrical potential gradient when the cell is at rest. The main factor that contributes to the −90 mV resting membrane potential is the cell's permeability to potassium and not to sodium. The sodium-potassium exchange pump is responsible for actively transporting sodium out of the cell and potassium into the cell. The hydrolysis of the high-energy phosphate adenosine triphosphate (ATP) provides the energy for the functioning of this pump. Because more sodium is

pumped out of the cell than potassium is moved in, a net outward current of positive ions further enhances the cell's negativity during the resting phase.

Depolarization

The initiation of a cardiac impulse begins with the process of depolarization. Depolarization indicates the rapid reversal of the resting membrane potential, which results from the following sequence of events: (1) the cell membrane permeability to sodium increases spontaneously (as in pacemaking cells) or in response to a stimulus; (2) a rapid influx of sodium occurs; and (3) potassium moves out of the cell. This movement of ions across the membrane creates an electrical current. When the amount of sodium entering the cell reaches a critical level, an electrical impulse is generated. The impulse may spread as a wave of depolarization to adjacent cells.

Repolarization

Repolarization is the process by which the cell is returned to the resting state. The following sequence occurs: (1) the cell membrane permeability to sodium decreases; and (2) sodium leaves the cell, whereas potassium returns through an active ion transport system.

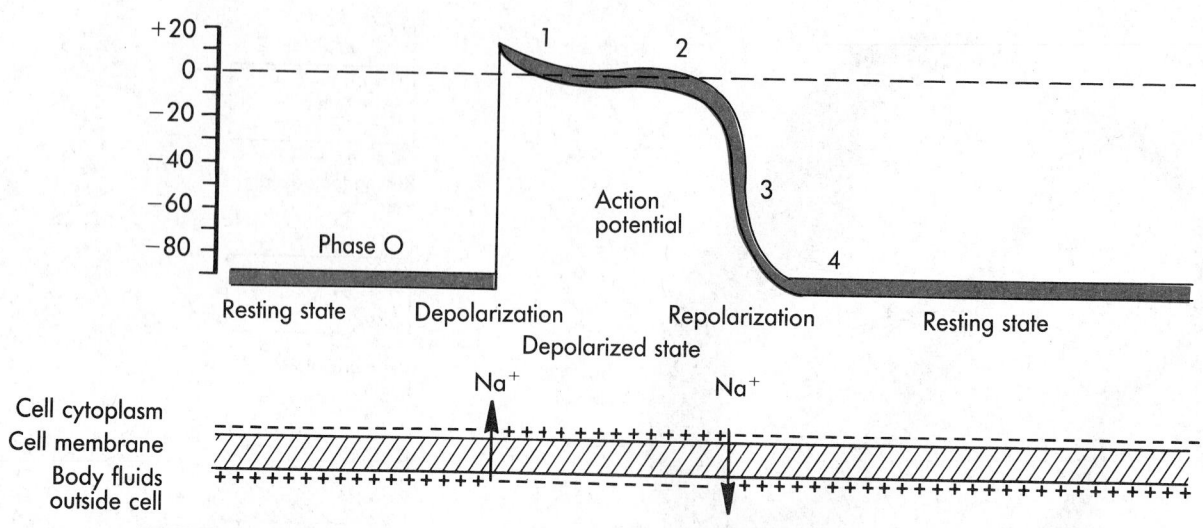

FIGURE 26-7 Phases of the action potential of cardiac muscle.

Phases of Action Potential

Phase 0. Phase 0 is the tall upstroke of the action potential that occurs when the cell is stimulated, causing the cell membrane to become permeable to sodium ions. Fast sodium channels open to allow sodium to rush into the cell, creating a positive intracellular membrane potential of 0 to +20 mV (Figure 26-7).

Phase 1. Phase 1 represents a brief period of rapid repolarization secondary to an outward positive current carried mainly by potassium ions. Further, sodium influx is abruptly terminated as soon as the cell depolarizes. These two factors cause a slight decline in intracellular positivity.

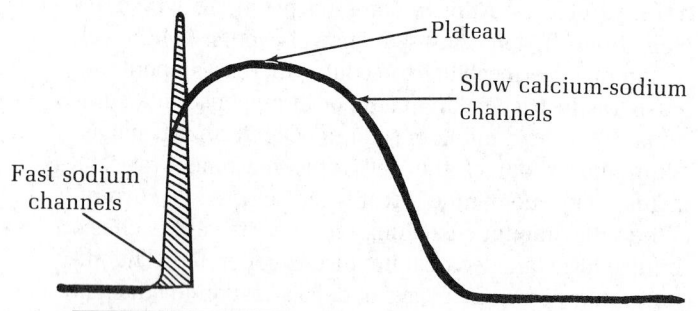

FIGURE 26-8 The differing effects of the fast sodium channels and the slow calcium-sodium channels on the action potential. The flow of sodium through the fast sodium channels initiates the action potential, and then these channels close (*shaded area*). The flow of current through the slow calcium channels is responsible for the plateau and duration of the action potential. (From Conover MB: Understanding electrocardiography: arrhythmias and the 12-lead ECG, ed 5, St Louis, 1988, The CV Mosby Co.)

Phase 2. Phase 2 of the action potential is often referred to as the *plateau phase*. It is sustained by an influx of positive ions, primarily calcium, through the slow calcium channels into the cell (Figure 26-8). This inward current results in prolonged refractory by maintaining the cell in a depolarized state, allowing time for completion of muscular contraction. This channel supplies the cell with calcium necessary for contraction. The effects of calcium channel blocker drugs on myocardial contractility and conduction are discussed in Chapters 27 and 28.

Phase 3. During phase 3 the sodium pump, along with the increased loss of intracellular potassium, causes a rapid restoration of negativity to the cell.

Phase 4. Phase 4 is the return of the cell to the resting membrane potential.

Refractoriness

The inability of cardiac cells to respond to successive stimuli is known as refractoriness. During the *absolute refractory period,* no stimulus will produce a response. This period begins with depolarization and extends through a portion of the repolarization period until the sodium ion carrier sites are again free to transport the sodium ions necessary for depolarization (Figure 26-9).

Refractoriness progressively diminishes in the *relative refractory period,* which occurs in the final stage of repolarization. During this interval, a stimulus of sufficient strength will produce a response. When the resting state is attained, the cell is no longer refractory. During the latter period, a mild stimulus will initiate a cardiac impulse. This is known as the *supernormal period.*

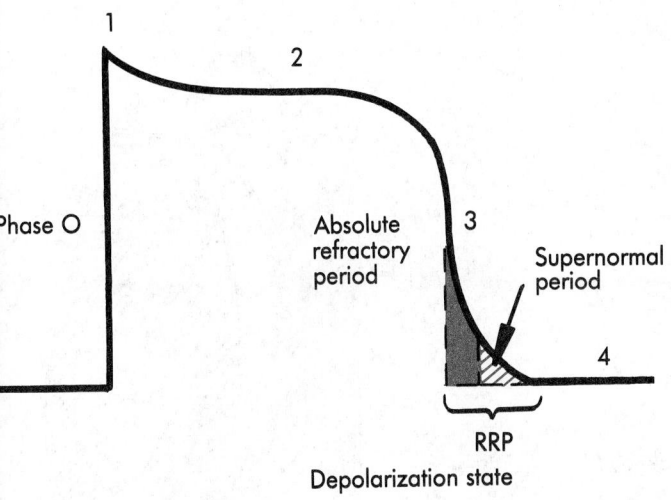

FIGURE 26-9 Schematic of the action potential showing the absolute and relative refractory period (RRP). A strong stimulus will produce a response in the first part of the RRP and a mild stimulus in the latter part (supernormal period).

CARDIAC CYCLE

The action potential itself does not cause the myofibrils to contract. The electrical stimulation initiates muscular contraction by stimulating the release of calcium ions in the sarcoplasmic reticulum of the muscle. Calcium ions then catalyze the chemical reaction that promotes the interdigitating and sliding of the actin and myosin filaments along each other, producing muscle contraction (see Chapter 68).

The cardiac cycle has two phases, diastole and systole. Relaxation and filling of both atria and then both ventricles take place during diastole. Contraction and emptying of both atria and then both ventricles occur during systole.

DIASTOLE

The diastolic phase of the cardiac cycle is subdivided into the following phases: (1) isovolumetric ventricular relaxation, (2) rapid ventricular filling, (3) slow ventricular filling, and (4) atrial systole (Table 26-1 and Figure 26-10, *A*).

The initial phase of *isovolumetric ventricular relaxation* begins as soon as the aortic valve and pulmonic valve close. During this time the myocardial muscle relaxes, and ventricular pressure falls. However, the falling ventricular pressure is still higher than atrial pressure; therefore the AV valves remain closed. Because

TABLE 26-1 Events during the cardiac cycle

Phase	Valves		Actions	Pressure (P) Changes
	Pulmonary and Aortic	Mitral and Tricuspid		
DIASTOLE				
Isovolumetric relaxation	Closed	Closed	Blood collects in atria.	Atrial P increases until greater than ventricular P.
Rapid ventricular filling	Closed	Open	Blood flows rapidly into ventricles from pressure differential.	Atrial P decreases; ventricular P increases.
Slow ventricular filling	Closed	Open	Blood flows passively into ventricles.	Same as for rapid filling.
Atrial systole	Closed	Close	Atrial contraction pushes additional blood into ventricles.	Ventricular P becomes greater than atrial P.
SYSTOLE				
Isovolumetric contraction	Closed	Closed	Myocardial tension increases.	Ventricular P increases; aortic P decreases until ventricular P greater than aortic P.
Maximal ventricular ejection	Open	Closed	Blood is pumped from ventricles into pulmonary artery and aorta.	Ventricular P decreases.
Reduced ventricular ejection	Open, then close	Closed	Some blood ejected.	Ventricular pressure decreases rapidly when ventricles relax.

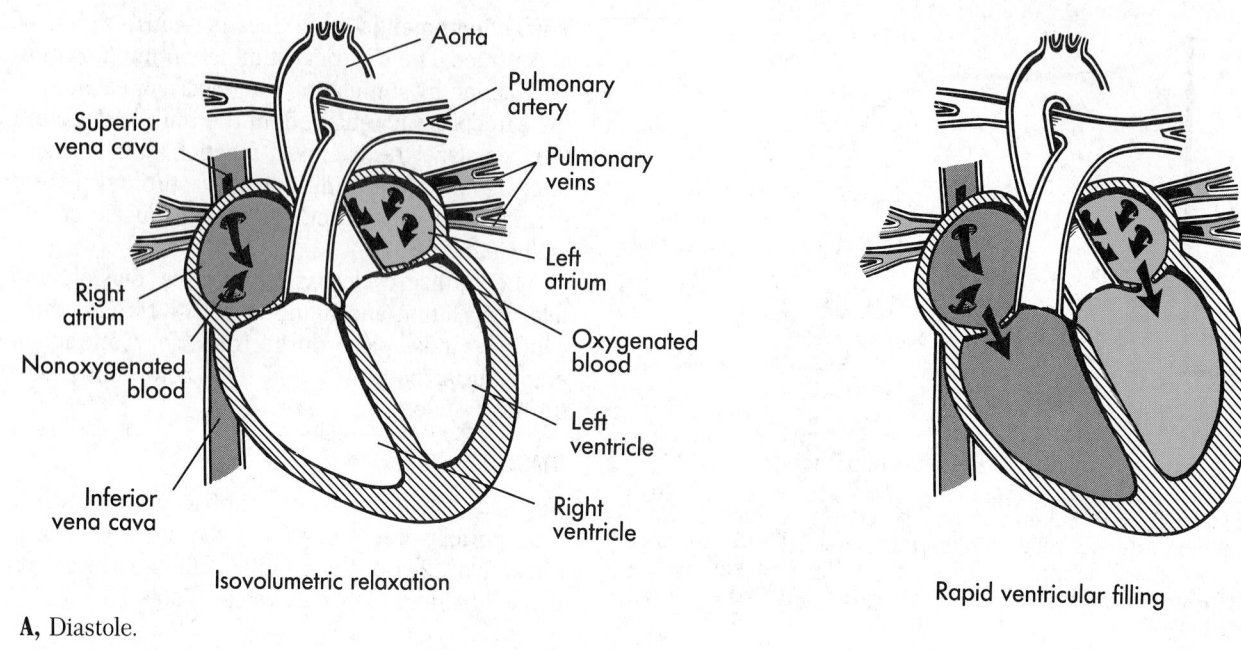

A, Diastole.

FIGURE 26-10 Events during the cardiac cycle.

these valves remain closed, a large amount of blood collects in the atria. As ventricular pressure begins to drop more rapidly to its low diastolic level, the higher pressure in the atria pushes the AV valves open and allows blood to flow rapidly into the ventricular cavity. This second phase of diastole, *rapid ventricular filling*, lasts for approximately the first third of diastole and causes intraventricular pressures to rise. As ventricular pressure increases, it impedes further rapid filling, and the resultant slowing of ventricular filling marks the third phase of diastole. This phase of *slow ventricular filling* is referred to as *diastasis*. Both the atrial and the ventricular chambers are relaxed, and blood entering the atria flows passively into the ventricles. During the phase of *atrial systole*, electrical depolarization spreads through the atria and pauses at the AV node for 0.10 second. The atrial musculature then contracts, propelling an additional 20% to 30% of blood into the ventricle before ventricular contraction.

SYSTOLE

The ventricular systolic phase of the cardiac cycle is subdivided into phases of isovolumetric ventricular contraction, maximal ventricular ejection, and reduced ventricular ejection (Table 26-1 and Figure 26-10, *B*).

During the *isovolumetric ventricular contraction* phase, myocardial tension and intraventricular pressure increase, whereas no change occurs in blood volume or muscle fiber length. At this time the aortic valve is closed because pressure in the aortic root exceeds left ventricular pressure. The higher pressure in the aortic root is the result of a previous systole that has just ejected blood into the aorta. As this aortic blood is distributed to the periphery, aortic pressure falls slowly. At the same time, intraventricular pressure and tension are increasing. When intraventricular pressure exceeds aortic root pressure, the aortic valve opens and *maximal ventricular ejection* begins. Blood from the ventricles is pumped into the pulmonic and systemic circulations. As the ejection rate starts to slow, the phase of *reduced ventricular ejection*, or *protodiastole*, begins. The ventricles remain contracted, but little blood is being ejected from the ventricle into the aorta. Ventricular pressure actually falls slightly below aortic root pressure, but some blood is still being ejected simply because of the momentum built up by the contraction. At the end of systole, ventricular relaxation begins suddenly, and a rapid decrease in intraventricular pressure occurs. The higher pressure in the large arteries and in the aortic root immediately pushes blood back toward the ventricles, thus snapping shut the semilunar valves.

CARDIAC OUTPUT

The *amount of blood ejected from the left ventricle into the aorta per minute* is called the cardiac output. Although the right ventricle ejects an equivalent amount of blood into the pulmonary artery, it is not included in the measurement of total cardiac output. Rather, car-

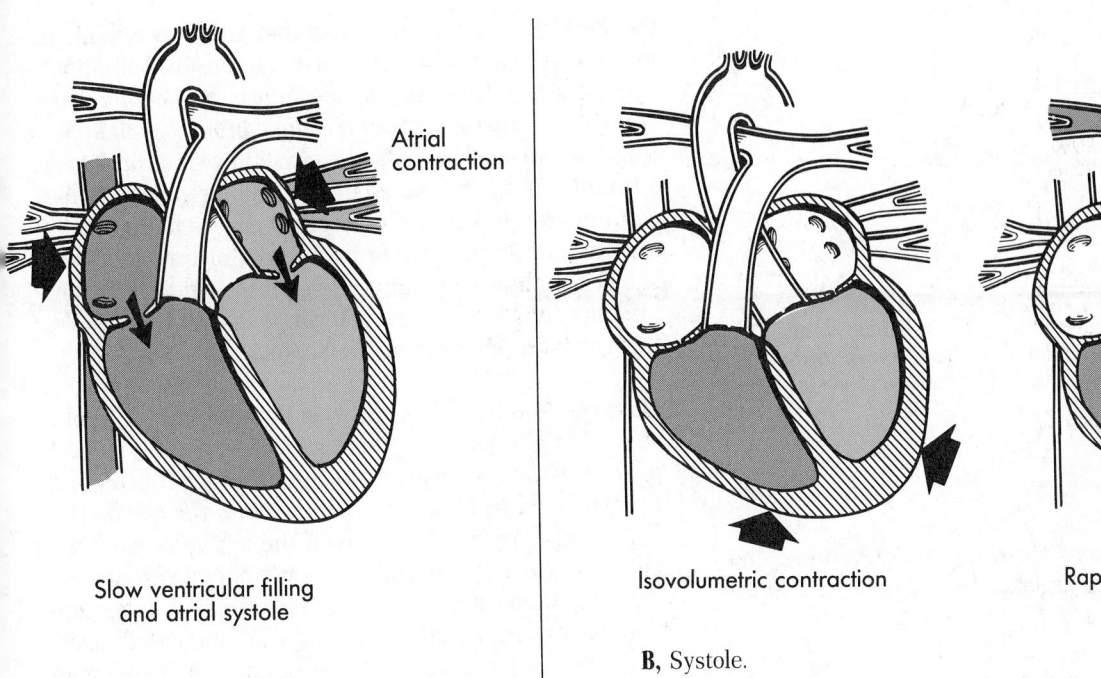

Atrial
contraction

Slow ventricular filling
and atrial systole

Isovolumetric contraction

Rapid ventricular ejection

B, Systole.

diac output (CO) is equivalent to stroke volume (SV) (volume of blood ejected from the left ventricle with each contraction) times heart rate (HR) (number of heartbeats per minute):

$$CO = SV \times HR$$

The average cardiac output is 5.6 L/minute in the average man. However, during periods of strenuous exercise, the cardiac output may reach 20 to 25 L/minute. Since cardiac requirements will vary according to individual body sizes, a more accurate means of assessing tissue perfusion is to compute the cardiac index. The *cardiac index* is obtained by dividing the cardiac output by the patient's total body surface area:

$$\text{Cardiac index} = \frac{\text{CO (L/min)}}{\text{Body surface area (m}^2)}$$

Therefore the cardiac index represents the cardiac output in terms of liters per minute per square meter of body surface. This corrects an individual's cardiac output to match body size. The normal range for cardiac index is 2.4 to 4.0 L/minute. The cardiac output is based solely on the amount of blood ejected by the left ventricle into the systemic circulation. The average 70 kg man will have an approximate cardiac index of 3 L/minute.

STROKE VOLUME

Stroke volume is the *amount of blood ejected by the left ventricle into the aorta per beat.* At the completion of each filling phase, or diastole, the ventricle contains approximately 120 ml of blood (end-diastolic volume [EDV]) (Figure 26-11). Under normal circumstances, the heart ejects approximately two thirds of the end-diastolic volume. The portion of blood that is ejected is termed the ejection fraction. The volume of residual blood in the ventricle at the end of systole is known as the end-systolic volume (ESV). Therefore stroke volume can be defined as the difference between the volume of blood contained in the ventricle at the end of diastole and the volume of blood remaining at the end of systole:

$$SV = EDV - ESV$$

CONTROL OF CARDIAC OUTPUT

Cardiac output depends on the relationship between two important variables—stroke volume and heart rate. Despite fluctuations in one of these two variables, cardiac output can be maintained at relatively constant levels by compensatory adjustments made in the other variable. For example, if the heart rate slows, the time for ventricular filling (diastole) is lengthened. This lengthened period allows for an increase in preload and a subsequent increase in stroke volume. Conversely, if the stroke volume falls, the heart rate can increase to compensate temporarily and maintain cardiac output. Therefore the actual determinants of cardiac output are the mechanisms regulating stroke volume and heart rate.

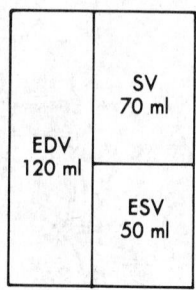

FIGURE 26-11 Representation of normal ventricular function, illustrating relationship between end-diastolic volume (*EDV*), stroke volume (*SV*), and end-systolic volume (*ESV*).

Control of Stroke Volume

Three significant factors affecting stroke volume and thus cardiac output are preload, contractility, and afterload.

Preload. Starling's law of the heart states that myocardial fiber responds with a more forceful contraction when it is stretched. An example of this phenomenon is that of increasing the stretch of a rubber band to obtain a more forceful recoil when the rubber band is released. Myocardial fibers can be stretched by increasing the volume of blood delivered to the ventricles during diastole. The degree of myocardial stretch before contraction is expressed in terms of preload. Preload is related to the *volume of blood distending the ventricles at the end of diastole.* Preload is determined by the amount of venous return and the ejection fraction, which determines the amount of blood left in the ventricle at the end of systole.

According to Starling's law, increasing venous return and thereby increasing left ventricular end-diastolic volume (preload) facilitates ventricular contraction and promotes increased ventricular function by stretching the myocardial fibers. Stretching of the sarcomeres increases the number of interaction sites for actin-myosin linkages and therefore increases ventricular contraction. Under normal conditions the sarcomere is stretched to 2 mm during ventricular diastole. Maximal ventricular force is developed at a sarcomere length of 2.2 mm. At this length, actin and myosin are able to use the most interaction sites. When myocardial stretching exceeds 2.4 mm, the myofilaments become partially disengaged, and fewer contractile sites are activated. Since Starling's length-tension relationship is only functional within physiologic limits, it is important to note that prolonged, excessive stretching of the myocardial fibers will eventually lead to a decrease in cardiac output by reducing the stroke volume (as in ventricular hypertrophy).

Contractility. Contractility is another major mechanism involved in the control of stroke volume. By definition, contractility refers only to *a change in the inotropic state of the muscle without a change in myocardial fiber length or preload.* Increased contractility (inotropism) is a function of the increased intensity of interaction at the actin-myosin linkages. Contractility can be increased by sympathetic stimulation or by the administration of substances such as calcium or epinephrine. Increased contractility improves ventricular emptying during systole, thereby increasing the stroke volume.

Afterload. Another factor involved in the control of stroke volume is afterload. Afterload is defined as the *amount of tension the ventricle must develop during contraction to eject blood from the left ventricle into the aorta.* The major impedance against which the left ventricle must pump is primarily determined by peripheral vascular resistance. Increase in pressure resulting from hypertension or vasoconstriction produces an increased resistance to pumping and will necessitate an increase in ventricular tension to eject blood. The afterload on the heart is affected not only by the amount of aortic pressure, but also by the size of the heart. This relationship between ventricular tension, arterial pressure, and ventricular size is known as Laplace's law:

Ventricular tension = Arterial pressure × Ventricular radius

As this simplified version of Laplace's law indicates, both hypertension and dilation of the ventricular chamber increase ventricular tension (increase afterload). Therefore, if arterial pressure increases, the ventricle must pump against higher resistance to empty adequately. Also, if ventricular radius increases, ventricular volume will increase. Thus at the same level of aortic pressure, the afterload against which an enlarged or dilated left ventricle must work is higher than that encountered by a normal-sized ventricle.

Excessive elevation of the afterload may impair ventricular emptying, thereby reducing stroke volume and cardiac output.

Control of Heart Rate

The autonomic nervous system (ANS) regulates the heart through two distinctly opposing sets of nerves, the sympathetic and the parasympathetic nervous systems. Afferent fibers accompany the efferent fibers of both these systems.

The sympathetic fibers arise from the thoracic spinal cord and reach the entire atria and ventricles as well as the SA and the AV nodes. The control of the ANS on the heart is mediated by neurotransmitters. The sympathetic nervous system neurotransmitter is norepinephrine. The *sympathetic fibers* have both *positive chrono-*

tropic (increase rate) and *inotropic* (increase force) effects. Therefore with an increase in sympathetic stimulation, the neurotransmitter norepinephrine is released from the nerve endings and produces the following effects: increase in heart rate, increase in atrial and ventricular contractility, and increase in the speed of electrical conduction through the AV node.

The parasympathetic fibers originate in the medulla and have their innervation primarily in the atrial musculature and in the SA and AV nodes; however, parasympathetic stimulation has been shown to reach the ventricles. The *parasympathetic fibers* have a *negative chronotropic* effect and may exert a slightly negative inotropic effect; however, in the healthy circulatory system, this negative inotropic effect is compensated for by the increased filling that occurs as a result of a lengthened diastole. Stimulation of the parasympathetic system causes the release of the neurotransmitter acetylcholine at the vagal nerve endings and has basically the opposite effect of norepinephrine. Parasympathetic stimulation causes a decrease in the rate of discharge of the SA node, a decrease in the rate of conduction from the atria to the ventricles, and a decrease in the force of atrial contraction and probably also of ventricular contraction. The final effect of ANS control on the heart is the balance between these two opposing nervous systems at any one time. It is thought that the heart is normally under the control of vagal inhibition and maintains a resting heart rate of 65 to 75 beats/minute.

The effects of the ANS can be greatly influenced by several additional factors, such as the central nervous system (CNS) and pressoreceptor reflexes. Impulses from the cerebral cortex can have a significant effect on the heart rate. Pain, fear, anger, and excitement can all cause substantial increases in the heart rate. Also, reflex changes caused by stimulation of the pressoreceptors can influence heart rate. The *baroreceptor reflex,* with afferent branches in the aortic arch, carotid sinus, and other pressoreceptor zones, functions as a negative feedback mechanism to regulate pressure in the arteries and regulate the resistance of vessels in the vasculature. Consequently, an episode of hypotension would cause a sudden drop of blood pressure in the aorta or carotid sinus and would stimulate the pressoreceptors less intensely. The cardiac inhibitory center would then be stimulated less, and the result would be a reflex increase in the heart rate.

Many other important factors are involved in the control of heart rate, including body temperature, medication, catecholamines, arterial blood gas tensions, hormones other than epinephrine, and plasma electrolyte concentrations.

In summary, ventricular function and thus cardiac output are influenced by heart rate and stroke volume.

Heart rate is primarily controlled by the ANS, and stroke volume depends on the three distinct variables of preload, contractility, and afterload.

PHYSIOLOGIC CHANGES WITH AGING

The number one cause of death in individuals who are 65 years or older is cardiovascular disease. Age-related changes take place in the chemical composition, cells, and tissues of the heart and blood vessels and influence many aspects of cardiovascular functioning. However, despite the physiologic changes of aging, the heart is able to meet the day-to-day demands and function adequately. It is only under unusual circumstances or increased stress that the deteriorating function of the heart is most apparent. For instance, asymptomatic ischemia may cause significant functional impairment. Not only is coronary atherosclerosis more prevalent in the elderly, but it frequently manifests as an occult (hidden) disease. It is crucial to detect the occult form of this disease to determine necessary interventions such as pharmacotherapy and alterations in life-style.

With advancing age, life-styles often change with regard to eating, drinking, smoking, and physical activity. A sedentary life-style versus habitual exercise can produce a significant difference in cardiac output.

HEART

Progressive left ventricular hypertrophy with age occurs concomitantly with a rise in arterial systolic blood pressure. Interestingly, heart weight increases in women but not in men. Ventricular septal thickness and the circumference of all four cardiac valves increase. By age 40 years the circumference of the aortic valve generally surpasses that of the pulmonic valve. In both sexes the leaflet thickness of the mitral and aortic valves increase progressively and significantly with advancing age. These rigid valves can lead to audible systolic murmurs, usually of an ejection nature.

An increase in average myocyte size primarily explains the increase in heart mass; however, the simultaneous change in the amount and functional properties of myocardial collagen plays a key role in causing physiologic cardiovascular abnormalities of aging. The increased connective tissue contributes to myocardial stiffness and decreased cardiac compliance. The amount of subendocardial fat also increases, and the endocardium undergoes fibrosis, thickening, and sclerosis (Table 26-2).

A decreased peak-systolic left ventricular wall stress occurs with aging. Increasing left ventricular wall thickness and increasing body surface area with age are presumed to be a contributing factors. The isovolumetric relaxation period is also prolonged, resulting in incomplete relaxation during early diastolic filling. However,

TABLE 26-2 Physiologic changes of cardiovascular system with aging

Source	Changes	Possible Outcome
Heart	Increased subendocardial fat Increased deposition of lipofuscin pigment in cardiac cells Increased amounts of connective tissue and changes in properties of connective tissue	Decreased cardiac output Decreased compliance Less efficient pump
Valves	Thickening, calcification and fibrosis, particularly in aortic and mitral valves	Systolic murmurs (usually ejection) Possible disturbance in blood flow to coronary arteries
Rate and rhythm	Increased amounts of connective tissue in SA nodes, internodal tracts, AV nodes, and bundle branches Atrial atrophy	High rate response to exercise/stress is less effective and takes longer to return to normal Sinus dysrhythmias, atrial flutter, extrasystoles
Arteries	Thickening of intima Thinning and fragmentation of elastin, leading to arterial stiffening Increase in absolute number of collagen fibers	Reduced compliance of blood vessels and peripheral vascular resistance (PVR) Increased pulse wave velocity Less effective baroreceptor response Slight increase in blood pressure; increase in systolic and slower rate of increase in diastolic

enhanced ventricular filling occurs later in diastole as a result of a compensatory, augmented atrial contribution to ventricular filling.

ARTERIES

Both the aorta and its branches and the major pulmonary arteries and their branches undergo progressive dilation and elongation with age. Because the enlargement is both transverse and longitudinal, the aorta tends to become tortuous. The major pulmonary arteries, however, appear to be too short with too low a pressure to dilate longitudinally. These alterations are caused by fragmentation, degeneration, and reduction in the amount of elastic tissue, as well as by increased collagen amount and structural changes. Because of decreased vascular distensibility, arterial pulse pressure increases secondarily to increased systolic pressure (with less change in diastolic pressure). A larger portion of forward blood flow is imposed on the left ventricle because of decreased aortic size during diastole, resulting in increased impedance to blood flow and decreased cardiac output. The generalized loss of elasticity in the arterial system can lead to a sluggish baroreceptor response. The baroreceptors are then less able to modulate blood pressure, particularly during rapid postural change.

EXERCISE AND CARDIOVASCULAR RESPONSE

As stated earlier, age-related changes in the cardiovascular system are significantly more pronounced in response to exercise. The overall increase in heart rate during vigorous exercise is less in elderly persons. Older people without significant coronary artery disease may demonstrate increases in stroke volume greater than in younger individuals to compensate for the lesser increases in heart rate. Persons of all ages exhibit comparable increases in left ventricular end-diastolic volume during upright exercise at low workloads. At higher workloads, in older persons whose heart rate increase is less, increases in left ventricular volume and stroke volume may continue throughout physical exercise. In contrast, younger individuals at higher workloads tend to exhibit accelerated heart rates, decreased end-diastolic and end-systolic volumes, and plateaued stroke volumes.

Left ventricular ejection fraction has been shown to decrease, or fail to increase, with more exercise in persons with coronary artery disease. Similarly, reductions in left ventricular ejection fraction from rest to exercise could also be attributed to aging.

PURPOSE OF CARDIAC ASSESSMENT

Systematic cardiac assessment provides the nurse with baseline data useful for identifying the physiologic and psychosocial needs of the patient and for planning appropriate nursing interventions to meet these needs. The nurse is in a unique position of ongoing patient monitoring and thus is able to take immediate action when signs occur that indicate alterations of cardiac function.

SUBJECTIVE DATA

Subjective data obtained by means of a detailed patient history are as diagnostically significant as laboratory data and ECG recordings in the assessment of the patient with suspected cardiac disease. Accurate assessment data are necessary to develop a profile of the cardiac risk factors operating in any individual situation, as well as to determine the psychodynamic family relationships that must be addressed throughout the diagnostic, treatment, and follow-up phases.

The cardinal symptoms of heart disease include *dyspnea, chest pain* or discomfort, *edema, syncope, palpitations,* and excessive *fatigue.* Cyanosis is usually a sign rather than a symptom, but it also may be an important feature of the patient's history, particularly in patients with congenital heart disease. An important principle of cardiovascular evaluation is that cardiovascular function, which may be adequate at rest, may be insufficient during exercise or exertion. Therefore careful attention should be directed to the effects of activity on the patient's symptoms.

DYSPNEA

Dyspnea is one of the most common and distressing symptoms of cardiopulmonary disease. It is described as an abnormally uncomfortable awareness of breathing. The patient complains of shortness of breath. Since dyspnea is associated with a variety of diseases as well as with anxiety, the history is a necessary tool in evaluating the etiologic factors.

Several different types of dyspnea exist; therefore the history must include factors that precipitate and relieve dyspnea and data regarding the patient's body position when dyspnea occurs.

Dyspnea on exertion is a common symptom of cardiac dysfunction. In the early stages of heart failure, dyspnea is usually provoked only by effort and is relieved promptly by rest. It is important to identify the amount of exertion necessary to produce dyspnea, because the less the cardiac reserve (heart's ability to adjust and adapt to increased demands), the less effort is required to precipitate dyspnea.

Orthopnea refers to dyspnea in the recumbent position. It is usually a symptom of more advanced heart failure than is exertional dyspnea. Patients relate that they may use two or more pillows to sleep restfully in a semiupright position. When an individual assumes the recumbent position, gravitational forces redistribute blood from the lower extremities and splanchnic bed, increasing venous return. The augmentation of intrathoracic blood volume elevates pulmonary venous and capillary pressures, resulting in a transient pulmonary congestion. Orthopnea is usually relieved in less than 5 minutes after the patient sits upright.

Paroxysmal nocturnal dyspnea, also known as cardiac asthma, is characterized by severe attacks of shortness of breath that generally occur 2 to 5 hours after the onset of sleep. This condition is frequently associated with sweating and wheezing and wakens the patient from sleep. These frightening attacks are precipitated by an increased blood volume caused by the reabsorption of edema that was pooled in dependent portions of the body during the day. When the patient lies in a recumbent position, there is a redistribution of the increased intravascular volume with a specific rise in intrathoracic blood volume. The diseased heart is unable to compensate for this increase in blood volume and unable to pump extra fluid into the circulatory system; therefore pulmonary congestion results. Paroxysmal nocturnal dyspnea is relieved by having the patient sit on the side of the bed or even get out of bed. However, unlike simple orthopnea, 20 minutes or more may be required for the patient with paroxysmal nocturnal dyspnea to obtain relief.

CHEST PAIN

Although pain or discomfort in the chest is one of the cardinal symptoms of cardiac disorders, it is essential to recognize that chest pain can be precipitated by various conditions. For example, chest pain may be caused by ischemic heart disease, acute dissection of the aorta, or acute pericarditis, or it may occur in pulmonary disorders (for example, pleurisy and pulmonary embolism). The most common cause of chest pain, however, is not associated with cardiovascular disease, but rather with anxiety. Therefore, to evaluate chest pain correctly, the following list of characteristic symptoms should be addressed during a thorough history.

1. Onset	When was chest pain first noticed?
2. Manner of onset	Did the pain or discomfort start suddenly or gradually?
3. Duration	How long did the pain last?
4. Precipitating factors	Ask patient to describe possible precipitating factors (for example, exertion, food, anxiety, emotions).
5. Location	Where did the pain originate? Did it radiate? To what area?
6. Quality	Ask patient to describe how symptoms feel (for example, sharp, dull).
7. Intensity	Ask patient to describe severity of the pain (for example, if pain interfered with any activities).
8. Chronology and frequency	Has this pain occurred in the past? If so, how often?
9. Associated symptoms	Do any other signs or symptoms occur at the same time?
10. Aggravating factors	What makes the pain worse?
11. Relaxing factors	What makes symptoms less intense?

WEIGHT GAIN

Edema is defined as an accumulation of excess fluid in the interstitial spaces. The retention of considerable amounts of extracellular fluid may occur without associated edema. In fact, weight gains of up to 7 kg of water can occur before the abnormality is detected. Because early manifestations of edema may be subtle, careful comparison of daily weights is required to determine weight gains resulting from fluid retention. Normally, basal body weight varies little from day to day; therefore subtle weight gains resulting from fluid retention are readily detectable.

The numerous causes of edema include congestive heart failure, fluid overload, and obstruction of venous drainage. Therefore, depending on the specific cause of the edema, it may be localized to one particular body part, organ, or tissue; or it may have a generalized distribution. (For a more in-depth discussion of edema, see Chapter 23.)

SYNCOPE

Syncope is defined as a generalized muscle weakness with an inability to stand upright, accompanied by loss of consciousness. The most common cause of syncope is decreased perfusion to the brain. Any condition that results in a sudden reduction of cardiac output and therefore reduced cerebral blood flow could potentially cause a syncopal episode. In patients with cardiovascular disorders, conditions such as orthostatic hypotension, hypovolemia, or a variety of dysrhythmias (for example, heart block and severe ventricular dysrhythmias) may precipitate syncope.

PALPITATIONS

Palpitation is a common subjective phenomenon defined as an unpleasant awareness of the heartbeat. It may be precipitated by a change in cardiac rate or rhythm or by an increase in myocardial contractility. Patients may describe their heartbeat as "pounding," "racing," or "skipping." Palpitations that occur either during or after strenuous activity are considered physiologic and represent an awareness of the overactivity of the heart. Palpitations that occur during mild exertion may suggest the presence of heart failure, anemia, or thyrotoxicosis. Other noncardiac factors that may precipitate palpitations include the following: nervousness, heavy meals, lack of sleep, and a large intake of coffee, tea, alcohol, or tobacco.

FATIGUE

Fatigue and lassitude have many causes, and therefore these symptoms are not diagnostic of cardiovascular disorders. However, fatigue as a symptom associated with heart failure may result from such states as nocturia, insomnia, and nocturnal dyspnea. In addition, fatigue may be a direct consequence of the heart failure itself. The exact physiologic mechanism responsible for fatigue related to heart failure is not known, but it is probably a consequence of an inadequate cardiac output. Such fatigue can occur during effort or at rest and generally worsens as the day progresses. Fatigue that occurs after mild exertion may indicate a low cardiac reserve if the heart is unable to meet even small increases in metabolic demands.

OBJECTIVE DATA

PHYSICAL ASSESSMENT OF CARDIAC FUNCTION

Physical examination of the cardiovascular system includes the use of inspection, palpation, percussion, and auscultation. The following is a description of the essential components in cardiovascular assessment. For a detailed description of the techniques involved, the reader is referred to a physical assessment textbook.

INSPECTION

Skin Color

The color of the patient's skin and mucous membranes should be noted (see the box below). A person's "normal" color depends on race, ethnic background, and life-style and is an indication of adequate cardiac output and circulation. Pallor may indicate anemia, hypoxia, or peripheral vasoconstriction. *Cyanosis*, a bluish discoloration of the skin, is most easily observed by examining the earlobes, oral mucosa at the base of the tongue, the lips, and the nail beds.

There are two types of cyanosis, central and peripheral. In central cyanosis the tongue is characteristically cyanotic. This form of cyanosis is caused by low arterial oxygen saturation and is generally seen in some patients who have congenital heart defects with left-to-right shunts or in those with pulmonary diseases that interfere with ventilation or diffusion.

Peripheral cyanosis results from low cardiac output and is generally accompanied by decreased skin temperature and mottling. In contrast to central cyanosis, no cyanosis of the tongue is present. (For further information on skin color, see Chapter 71.)

PHYSICAL INSPECTION FOR ASSESSMENT OF CARDIAC FUNCTION

Skin color
Neck vein distention
Respiratory rate and character
Location of point of maximal impulse (PMI)
Presence of edema
Nail clubbing
Capillary filling

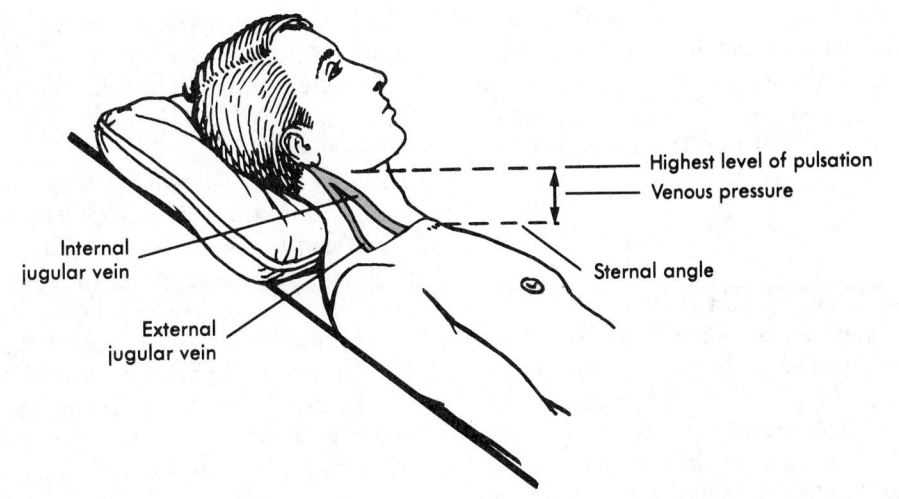

FIGURE 26-12 Position of internal and external jugular veins, used in measuring venous pressure.

Neck Vein Distention

A general estimate of venous pressure can be obtained by observation of the neck veins (Figure 26-12). Normally, when an individual is in a supine position, the neck veins are distended. However, when the head of the bed is elevated at a 45-degree angle, the neck veins are collapsed. The jugular veins reflect venous tone, blood volume, and right atrial pressure. Therefore distended neck veins suggest increased venous pressure, which may be caused by right-sided heart failure, circulatory volume overload, superior vena caval obstruction, or tricuspid valve regurgitation.

Respirations

Next, the rate and character of the patient's respirations are assessed. Normally, an adult breathes comfortably at a rate of 12 to 20 times/minute. Particular attention is paid to the ease or difficulty in breathing and noting the patient's general demeanor.

Point of Maximal Impulse

Inspection of the anterior chest is best accomplished with the patient lying in a supine position, either flat or with the head slightly elevated. Observe the precordium for the point of maximal impulse (PMI), which is a faint heaving of the chest wall caused by the forward thrusting of the ventricles during systole. The location of the PMI helps to locate the apex of the heart, which lies approximately 0.5 cm to the left of the PMI. The PMI is normally located in the left fifth intercostal space in the midclavicular line or 8 to 10 cm to the left of the midsternal line. Any pulsation noted below the third intercostal space on the left precordium is known as the PMI; any pulsation above the third intercostal space is generally not related to the heart but rather to the great vessels. The PMI is not always visible, but it is usually palpable.

Peripheral Edema

An important indicator of cardiovascular function is the presence or absence of peripheral edema, especially in the feet, ankles, legs, and sacrum. Edema that disappears on elevation of the body part may be caused by gravity flow or by interruption of the venous return to the heart as a result of constricting clothing or pressure on the veins of the lower extremities.

In contrast, *pitting edema* does not disappear with elevation of the extremity or body part, and it may indicate fluid overload or a pathologic condition (for example, congestive heart failure) when cardiac pumping efficiency is impaired. Edema is identified by inspection and palpation. Pitting edema is present if an indentation is left in the skin after a thumb or finger has been used to apply gentle pressure (see Chapter 23).

The nutritional state of the hair, skin, and extremities is also assessed. Nutritional deficiencies caused by decreased circulation can produce dry skin, thickened nails, brittle hair, and occasional hair loss in an extremity (characteristic of peripheral vascular disease).

The nails must also be assessed for clubbing and capillary refill. The exact cause of *clubbing* is not known at present; however, clubbing of the fingers is typical of congenital heart defects and pulmonary arterio-venous (A-V) fistulas with right-to-left shunting. *Capillary filling,* usually called blanching, is an indicator of peripheral circulation to the fingers and toes and can be tested in all nail beds. This maneuver is done by pressing the examiner's thumbnail against the edge of a patient's fingernail or toenail and then quickly releasing it. The normal response is whitening (blanching) of the area when pressure is applied and brisk return of color when pressure is released. Lack of the blanching response may indicate lack of circulation to the finger or toe because of arterial insufficiency secondary to atherosclerosis or spasm. It may also be a reflection of severe vasoconstriction.

PALPATION

Peripheral Pulses

One method for evaluating the arterial flow of the vascular system is to palpate the extremities and the peripheral pulses. The peripheral pulses are evaluated bilaterally on the basis of their absence or presence, rate, rhythm, amplitude, quality, and equality. It is recommended that each pulse, except the carotids, be palpated on the left and right sides simultaneously to evaluate contralateral symmetry.

Pulses are rated on a scale of 0 to +4 as follows:

$$0 = \text{Absent}$$
$$+ = \text{Palpable, but diminished}$$
$$+ + = \text{Normal, or average}$$
$$+ + + = \text{Full and brisk}$$
$$+ + + + = \text{Full and bounding, often visible}$$

Apical Impulse

Normally, the apical impulse is felt as a single, light tap. The presence of anything other than a single, light tap may suggest a myocardial pathologic condition and should be reported to the physician. A thrill, or palpable murmur, indicates the presence of significant turbulent blood flow across an intracardiac shunt or a severely stenotic valve. A thrill has been described as a vibration similar to that of a cat's purr. A thrill is more readily palpated after the patient exhales forcefully. Frequently, having the patient in a left lateral position or leaning forward will accentuate the vibration.

PERCUSSION

The use of percussion for detecting cardiac enlargement has generally been replaced by the more accurate use of palpation. Therefore the use of percussion in the cardiovascular examination is considered to be somewhat limited. Usually, only the left border of cardiac dullness can be determined, since this is located near the PMI, or within the midclavicular line. Cardiac dullness noted below the fifth intercostal space, beyond the left midclavicular line, or to the right of the sternum is characteristic of cardiac hypertrophy. Unfortunately, mild to moderate degrees of cardiac hypertrophy or dilation are not usually detectable by percussion.

AUSCULTATION

Auscultation of heart sounds enables a nurse to establish baseline data for identifying current and future cardiac problems that require nursing intervention. Cardiac auscultation also assists the nurse in evaluating a patient's progress (for example, effect of activity on heart rate) or in monitoring responses to medications (for example, quinidine or digitalis preparations).

Heart Sounds

The *first heart sound* (S_1) is generally thought to be produced by the almost simultaneous closures of the mitral and tricuspid valves. Closure of the mitral valve slightly precedes closure of the tricuspid valve, but the combined closure is usually heard as one sound. S_1 lasts approximately 0.10 second and signals the onset of ventricular systole. S_1 is generally loudest at the apex but can be heard over the entire precordium. S_1 is longer and lower pitched than the *second heart sound* (S_2), and S_1 corresponds with the beat of the carotid pulse. S_2 is mainly caused by the closure of the semilunar valves (aortic and pulmonic). Because the mechanical events in the right side of the heart are slightly slower than those in the left side, the aortic valve closes just before the pulmonic valve. S_2 is usually loudest at the base of the heart and is described as shorter, higher pitched, and "snappier" than S_1. The sounds of the cardiac cycle are depicted in Figure 26-13.

The diaphragm chest piece is most useful in listening to high-pitched sounds and murmurs. These include such sounds as S_1, S_2, and ejection sounds and clicks. The diaphragm should be placed firmly on the chest wall so that when it is removed, an indentation is present on the patient's skin. The bell chest piece is most useful in detecting low-pitched sounds and murmurs. These include the third heart sound (S_3), the fourth heart sound (S_4), and mitral and tricuspid diastolic rumbles. The bell should be placed lightly on the chest wall, barely creating an airtight seal. If the bell is placed firmly on the skin, it will act as a diaphragm.

Splitting of S_1 and S_2. The two main components of S_1 (closure of the mitral and tricuspid valves) are asynchronous, because left ventricular contraction usually occurs slightly ahead of right ventricular systole. The S_1 may be split in individuals who have RBB block, left-sided mechanical defects (for example, mitral stenosis),

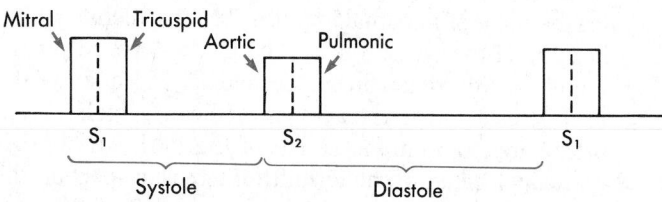

FIGURE 26-13 Heart sound S_1 is the closure of mitral and tricuspid valves; S_2 is the closure of aortic and pulmonic valves. Systole is the interval between S_1 and the start of S_2; diastole is S_2 to the start of S_1. Diastole is longer than systole.

or tricuspid valve dysfunction associated with pulmonary hypertension.

Since left ventricular contraction slightly precedes right ventricular contraction, the aortic valve normally closes slightly before the pulmonic valve. On inspiration, intrathoracic pressure decreases and facilitates an increase in venous blood return to the right side of the heart. This increased blood return delays the closure of the pulmonic valve and results in a normal physiologic, split S_2. On expiration, closure of the aortic and pulmonic valves occurs almost simultaneously and is therefore heard only as a single sound. In conditions of increased blood flow or increased right ventricular pressure (atrial septal defect or pulmonary artery stenosis), there may be a "fixed" splitting of S_2; that is, both components of S_2 are heard in both inspiration and expiration. A fixed split is considered abnormal and may occur in RBB block, pulmonary hypertension, and right ventricular failure related to atrial or ventricular septal defects.

Extra heart sounds. Extra heart sounds include ejection sounds (systolic clicks), opening snaps, and S_3 and S_4. Of these sounds, the two that occur most frequently and discussed here are S_3 and S_4 (see Figure 26-14).

Ventricular diastolic gallop, or S_3, is a faint, low-pitched sound produced by rapid ventricular filling in early diastole. This occurs when the volume of early filling is increased or a decrease occurs in ventricular compliance. Ventricular "gallop" describes the canter of a horse, which is frequently mimicked at heart rates greater than 100. When this sound is present in healthy children and young adults, it is almost always a normal condition and is referred to as a *physiologic* S_3. A physiologic S_3 results from the transition from rapid to slow filling in a healthy compliant ventricle. An S_3 heard in an older person is usually a pathologic sign and is frequently one of the first signs of serious heart disease or cardiac decompensation, as seen in congestive heart failure. An audible S_3 is associated with elevated middiastolic left ventricular filling pressures. S_3 is typically present in such states as left-to-right shunts, mitral regurgitation, congestive heart failure, and constrictive pericarditis.

Atrial diastolic gallop, or S_4, is a low-frequency sound that occurs under circumstances of altered ventricular compliance, either left or right. S_4 occurs late in diastole when atrial systole ejects blood into a noncompliant ventricle. Because the presence of an audible S_4 is related to a decrease in left ventricular compliance and an increase in left ventricular end-diastolic pressure, it is often heard in hypertensive cardiovascular disease and idiopathic hypertrophic subaortic stenosis. An S_4 is frequently identified in patients with acute myocardial infarctions and in patients with coronary artery disease, especially during an attack of angina pectoris. In addition, an S_4 may be present when cardiac output and stroke volume are increased, such as in severe anemia, thyrotoxicosis, and large A-V fistulas. Although the S_4 sound occurs close to S_1, it can be easily differentiated because S_4 is lower pitched than S_1.

Murmurs

Murmurs are audible vibrations of the heart and great vessels that occur because of turbulent blood flow. Turbulent blood flow may be produced by hemodynamic events or by structural alterations occurring in the heart or in the walls of the great vessels. In general, murmurs are heard most distinctly over the area of the valve or altered cardiac structure responsible for the vibrations. The major factors involved in the production of cardiac murmurs include the following: (1) increased velocity of blood flow through normal or abnormal valves; (2) forward flow through a stenotic or irregular valve orifice; (3) backward (regurgitant) blood flow through an incompetent valve, septal defect, or patent ductus arteriosus; and (4) turbulent blood flow produced in a dilated chamber, such as in a ventricular or aortic aneurysm.

Murmurs are generally characterized according to timing (position in the cardiac cycle), intensity, quality, pitch, location, and direction of radiation. These characteristics provide data concerning the location and nature of the cardiac abnormality.

Pericardial Friction Rub

A pericardial friction rub is an extra heart sound originating from the pericardial sac. This rub may be a sign of inflammation, infection, or infiltration. It occurs as the heart moves. Pericardial friction rubs may have specific subcomponents (different sounds), each associated with a particular cardiac movement. The heart moves with atrial and ventricular systole and with ventricular diastole. Each of the sound components of a pericardial friction rub corresponds to a movement of the cardiac cycle and is described as a short, high-pitched, scratchy sound.

ABNORMAL PULSES

A *hypokinetic* (weak) pulse signifies a narrowed pulse pressure, that is, decreased difference between systolic

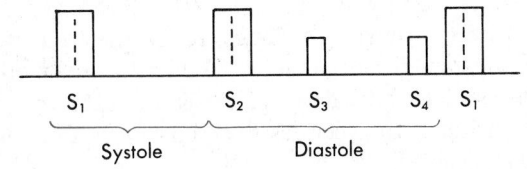

FIGURE 26-14 Location of extra heart sounds during cardiac cycle.

and diastolic pressures. It is usually produced by a low cardiac output and is associated with increased peripheral vascular resistance. This type of pulse may be palpable in such conditions as severe left ventricular failure, hypovolemia, or mitral and aortic valve stenosis.

A *hyperkinetic* (bounding) pulse represents a widened pulse pressure. It is usually associated with an increased left ventricular stroke volume and a decrease in peripheral vascular resistance. This type of pulse is frequently found in hyperkinetic circulatory states caused by exercise, fever, anemia, and hyperthyroidism.

Pulsus alternans is a condition in which the heart beats regularly, but the pulses alternate in amplitude. It is caused by an alternating left ventricular contractile force and usually indicates severe depression of myocardial function. Pulsus alternans may be detected by palpation but is more accurately assessed by auscultation of the blood pressure.

Pulsus paradoxus signifies a reduction in the amplitude of the arterial pulse during inspiration. Variations in pulse strength can be palpated, but a paradoxical pulse is most readily detected by sphygmomanometry. The difference between the peak systolic pressures at which sounds are audible *only* during expiration and later when sounds are audible during both inspiration and expiration is a measure of the magnitude of the paradoxical pulse. Normally the difference between these two pressures should not exceed 8 mm Hg.

Pulsus paradoxus is an accentuation of the normal decrease in systolic arterial pressure with inspiration. This is a result of decreased left ventricular stroke volume and the transmission of negative intrathoracic pressure to the aorta. Pulsus paradoxus may occur in conditions such as cardiac tamponade and constrictive pericarditis, but it may also be found in patients with chronic obstructive airway disease who have wide swings of intrapleural pressure during respiration.

DIAGNOSTIC TESTS

Cardiovascular diseases are usually diagnosed by correlating laboratory test results with findings from the patient interview and the physical examination. The laboratory tests ordered most frequently in patients with heart disease or suspected heart disease include the following: blood tests, urinalysis, electrocardiography (see Chapter 27), invasive hemodynamic monitoring, sonic studies, dynamic studies, radiography, scintigraphic studies, and angiography.

The nurse may be directly or indirectly involved in these tests and procedures and should understand why a particular test or examination is being performed and what it will contribute to the patient's diagnosis. This information enables the nurse to prepare the patient adequately before any diagnostic procedure and to observe

and record signs and symptoms while caring for the patient.

LABORATORY TESTS

A complete blood count (CBC) is ordered on all patients with documented or suspected heart disease for evaluation of the overall health status. Data concerning red and white blood cells (*RBCs* and *WBCs*) are helpful in diagnosing infectious heart diseases and myocardial infarctions (Table 26-3). RBCs may be elevated as a physiologic response to inadequate tissue oxygenation. The *erythrocyte sedimentation rate* (ESR) is a measurement of the rate at which RBCs "settle out" of anticoagulated blood in an hour. The rate of RBC settling is increased if the proportion of globulin to albumin increases or if fibrinogen levels are excessively increased. Nonspecific increases in globulin and fibrinogen levels occur when the body responds to injury or inflammation, as seen with infectious heart disorders or myocardial infarction.

Blood coagulation tests, including prothrombin time (PT) and activated partial thromboplastin time (APPT), indicate the rapidity of blood clotting. These tests are useful during anticoagulation therapy (Table 26-3). *Blood urea nitrogen* (BUN) is primarily useful as an indicator of renal function. Prerenal factors, such as decreased cardiac output leading to a low renal blood supply and concomitant reduction in glomerular filtration rate, will elevate the BUN.

BLOOD LIPIDS

The blood (plasma) lipids are composed mainly of cholesterol, triglyceride, phospholipid, and free fatty acids, all of which are insoluble in water and require a "carrier" to transport them. The carriers for plasma lipids are the proteins to which they are bound, thus the name *lipoproteins.* There are four major classes of lipoproteins: chylomicrons, very low-density lipoproteins, low-density lipoproteins, and high-density lipoproteins, all of which contain varying levels of cholesterol, triglycerides, and phospholipids.

Chylomicrons are composed mainly of triglycerides and originate in the intestine following the absorption of dietary fat. Chylomicrons should not be found in the plasma after 12 to 14 hours of fasting. Studies to date have not shown elevated chylomicron levels to be associated with premature coronary artery disease.

Very low-density lipoproteins (VLDLs) are composed primarily of triglycerides and are synthesized in the liver. Sustained elevations of VLDLs have sometimes been associated with atherosclerosis; however, the exact relationship of triglycerides to coronary heart disease is not yet clear.

Low-density lipoproteins (LDLs) are composed of approximately 50% cholesterol and are thought to have

TABLE 26-3 Selected laboratory tests for cardiovascular disorders

Test	Normal Values	Significance in Heart Disorders
Serum RBC	Men: 4.7-6.1 million/mm^3 Women: 4.2-5.4 million/mm^3	Decreased in subacute endocarditis Increased with inadequate tissue oxygenation Decreased in some congenital heart disease with right-to-left shunt
Serum WBC	5000-10,000/mm^3	Increased in acute and chronic heart inflammations and in acute myocardial infarction
Erythrocyte sedimenatation rate (ESR)	Men: up to 15 mm/hr Women: up to 20 mm/hr	Increased in acute myocardial infarction and infectious heart disease
Prothrombin time (PT)	11-12.5 sec 100% compared to control	Indicates rapidity of blood clotting; used to monitor anticoagulant therapy with coumarin and warfarin sodium
Activated partial thromboplastin time (APPT)	30-40 sec	More sensitive than PT; used to monitor heparin therapy
Blood urea nitrogen (BUN)	5-20 mg/100 ml	Increased with decreased cardiac output
Serum proteins	6-8 g/100 ml	Levels below 5 g/100 ml seen with edema

the greatest correlation with coronary artery disease. According to the insudation theory of atherogenesis, LDLs can enter the arterial intima and produce arterial endothelial injury, which can lead to progressive atherosclerotic plaque formation and eventually produce clinical manifestations, including ischemic heart disease.

High-density lipoproteins (HDLs) are composed of mostly protein with a modest amount of cholesterol and a considerable amount of phospholipids. This lipoprotein appears to have the lowest atherogenic potential. In fact, recent studies have demonstrated that HDLs are inversely associated with coronary heart disease. In vivo tests indicate that HDLs may carry cholesterol away from tissues, including atheromatous plaques. It appears that HDLs may even protect individuals against coronary heart disease.

Before blood tests are performed for the detection of elevated lipids, the patient must fast for 12 hours. No alcoholic beverages or lipid-influencing drugs (for example, estrogens, oral contraceptives, steroids, salicylates) may be taken, with the exception of insulin for the diabetic patient. If the patient is under stress or has any acute illness, the tests should be postponed. Since lipid levels may fluctuate greatly from day to day, repeated blood samples are obtained before a definitive diagnosis of hyperlipidemia is assigned. Disorders of lipid metabolism are classified according to their lipoprotein pattern and are discussed in Chapter 28.

BLOOD CULTURES

Blood culture tests are crucial in the diagnosis of infective diseases of the heart such as endocarditis. Blood cultures are obtained by venipuncture, and special care should be taken not to contaminate the cultures. Re-

sults of these blood cultures will identify the organism responsible for the infective process and the organism's sensitivity to various antibiotics. This information will aid the physician in planning an effective course of antibiotic therapy.

ENZYME STUDIES

Enzymes, which are located in all tissues, catalyze the biochemical reactions of the body. When cell membranes are damaged, such as in myocardial infarction, enzymes leak out of the damaged myocardial cell and escape into the serum. The serum enzyme measurements that are used to detect myocardial necrosis are serum aspartate aminotransferase (AST) (formerly serum glutamic oxaloacetic transaminase [SGOT]), creatinine phosphokinase (CPK), lactic dehydrogenase (LDH), and hydroxybutyrate dehydrogenase (HBD). Since these enzymes are located in various body tissues, numerous conditions other than myocardial damage may produce enzyme elevations; for example, the brain, pancreas, and liver are all rich sources of AST. If an individual were to develop chest pain concurrently with pancreatic or liver disease, an elevated AST may be mistaken for myocardial necrosis. Fortunately, two of the enzymes, CPK and LDH, have isoenzymes that are thought to be present almost exclusively in myocardial muscle.

The CPK molecule has two subunits, which have been identified as follows: M, associated with muscle; and B, associated with brain. The brain and gastrointestinal tract contain modest amounts of the BB dimer, and skeletal muscle contains large amounts of the MM form. Heart muscle contains huge quantities of MM, but it also contains the MB hybrid form of CPK. Because CPK_{MB} is not found in any other tissue, its presence in the serum is a sensitive indicator of myocardial damage.

Of the five LDH isoenzymes, LDH_1 has been found to be the most sensitive indicator of myocardial damage. Specifically, the LDH_1/LDH_2 ratio is very helpful in distinguishing myocardial infarction from other causes of chest pain or vascular instability. Normally the LDH_1 value is less than LDH_2; however, in the presence of acute myocardial infarction, LDH_1 is not only elevated, but also exceeds LDH_2. (For further discussion of cardiac enzymes, see Chapter 28.)

URINALYSIS

A routine urinalysis is done to determine the effects of cardiovascular disease on renal function and to determine the existence of concurrent renal or systemic diseases, such as glomerulonephritis, hypertension, or diabetes. Mild to moderate proteinuria (usually albuminuria) can be seen in patients with malignant hypertension and venous congestion of the kidneys secondary to congestive heart failure or constrictive pericarditis. The presence of RBCs in the urine may indicate infective endocarditis or an embolic kidney disease.

Recently the detection of myoglobin in the urine (myoglobinuria) has been useful in the diagnosis of myocardial infarction. At present, clinical experience with this test remains limited; however, it may prove to be a sensitive indicator of myocardial damage. Destruction of infarction of striated muscle liberates myoglobin; and because of its small size, the molecule filters through the glomerulus and is excreted in the urine.

SEROLOGIC TESTS

Syphilis can play an important role in the development of aortic disorders. The patient may have aortic insufficiency, aortic aneurysms, or disease of the ostia of the coronary arteries. Because of the relationship between syphilis and heart disease, a routine VDRL (Veneral Disease Research Laboratories) test is performed on all cardiac patients.

INVASIVE HEMODYNAMIC MONITORING

Invasive monitoring techniques used to evaluate the hemodynamic status of the critically ill patient have greatly increased the data base on which health professionals can plan and evaluate therapeutic modalities. Numerous devices are used in hemodynamic monitoring. (For a detailed description of this particular aspect of care, see reference 8.)

CENTRAL VENOUS PRESSURE

Central venous pressure (CVP) measurements reflect the pressures in the right atrium and provide information regarding changes in right ventricular pressure.

For many years it was thought that CVP accurately reflected changes in left ventricular function. However, it has now been documented that although the CVP may provide information about left-sided heart pressures, the CVP is not as accurate as other methods in reflecting rapid changes in cardiovascular status.

The primary factors affecting CVP are the circulating blood volume, right-sided pump function, and the degree of peripheral vasoconstriction. Therefore the CVP is best utilized in *monitoring blood volume and adequacy of the venous return to the heart*. Since the CVP reflects the pressure in the great veins as blood returns to the right side of the heart, a low (or falling) reading may indicate an inadequate blood volume (hypovolemia), and fluid replacement may be necessary. A high (or rising) CVP is usually secondary to left-sided pump failure. This decrease in cardiac contractility may lead to congestive heart failure and pulmonary edema. Unfortunately, the patient's hemodynamic status may be severely altered before representative changes in the CVP are evident.

The normal values for CVP will vary with the use of different equipment; however, a range of 5 to 15 cm of water is acceptable. It is important to note that a change or a trend in the CVP is more important than the actual numeric value. For example, if the CVP of a patient who has had a myocardial infarction should change from 5 to 10 cm in a 30-minute period, the physician should be notified. Even though both 5 cm and 10 cm are "normal" values, it is crucial to monitor the trend of a rising CVP. (For additional information in CVP, see Chapter 25.)

INTRAARTERIAL BLOOD PRESSURE MEASUREMENT

In the critically ill patient, the stroke volume and thus the cardiac output may be decreased to such an extent that cuff blood pressure readings may be inaccurate. As the stroke volume falls, Korotkoff sounds become increasingly more difficult to auscultate, and a wide range in the blood pressure readings have been found to be in error by as much as 25 mm Hg. In this particular patient population, invasive arterial blood pressure monitoring will more accurately reflect actual blood pressure.

Arterial catheters may be placed in a variety of arteries; however, the radial, brachial, and axillary arteries are used most often. Normally the arterial catheter is attached to a transducer, which converts the mechanical pressure of the pulses to electrical impulses, which can be viewed as waveforms on an oscilloscope. Generally the arterial line is also used to obtain blood samples for arterial blood gas determinations. Catheter patency is maintained with the use of an arterial flush system.

The patient with an arterial line requires frequent observation. It is essential that the extremity with the arterial line be kept uncovered so that the site can be monitored for bleeding caused by loose connections in the system. Also, the pulse, color, and temperature of the extremity distal to the catheter should be assessed every 2 hours so that early signs of circulatory compromise or thrombosis may be detected.

PULMONARY ARTERY AND PULMONARY CAPILLARY WEDGE PRESSURES

To obtain essential information regarding left ventricular function, a balloon-topped catheter (Swan-Ganz catheter) may be introduced into the pulmonary artery. The pulmonary artery catheter permits the measurement of the pulmonary artery end-diastolic pressure (PAEDP) and the pulmonary capillary wedge pressure (PCWP) (Table 26-4).

The best indicator of left ventricular function is the left ventricular end-diastolic pressure (LVEDP). Since a direct relationship exists between the PAEDP, the PCWP, and the LVEDP, an elevated PAEDP or PCWP reflects an elevated LVEDP. Elevations in LVEDP result from impaired left ventricular contractility, which does not permit adequate emptying of the ventricles.

In the healthy individual the PAEDP and the PCWP will be similar. However, in the presence of increased peripheral vascular resistance such as that found in pulmonary embolism, the PAEDP will rise while the PCWP remains normal. Therefore, to evaluate the true LVEDP accurately, the PCWP must be monitored. The PCWP is a critical factor affecting the transudation of fluid from the vascular space to the interstitial and alveolar in the lungs. Normally the PCWP ranges from 4 to 12 mm Hg. PCWP exceeding 25 mm Hg suggests imminent pulmonary edema.

TABLE 26-4 Pulmonary artery and capillary wedge pressures

Type	Common Abbreviation	Normal Values
Left ventricular end-diastolic pressure	LVEDP	12-15 mm Hg
Pulmonary artery end-diastolic pressure	PAEDP	4-12 mm Hg
Pulmonary capillary wedge pressure	PCWP	4-12 mm Hg

Insertion of the pulmonary artery catheter is often accomplished through a small incision (cutdown) made in an antecubital vein. The catheter is threaded into the vein, through the superior vena cava, through the tricuspid valve, and into the pulmonary artery. One of the lumens of the pulmonary artery catheter is attached to a monitor that usually presents a numeric reading as well as a display of waveforms indicating the location (capillary bed, pulmonary artery, or right ventricle) of the catheter. The balloon is then inflated so that it wedges the catheter in a distal branch of the pulmonary artery (Figure 26-15). Once the balloon is inflated, it occludes the pressure produced by the right side of the heart. The reading (or measurement) obtained when the balloon is inflated is the PCWP and reflects pressures in the pulmonary capillary bed and left-sided heart function. The balloon must be deflated quickly and should never be left inflated for more than a few seconds so that damage to the pulmonary circulation does not occur. The nurse usually obtains measurements of the

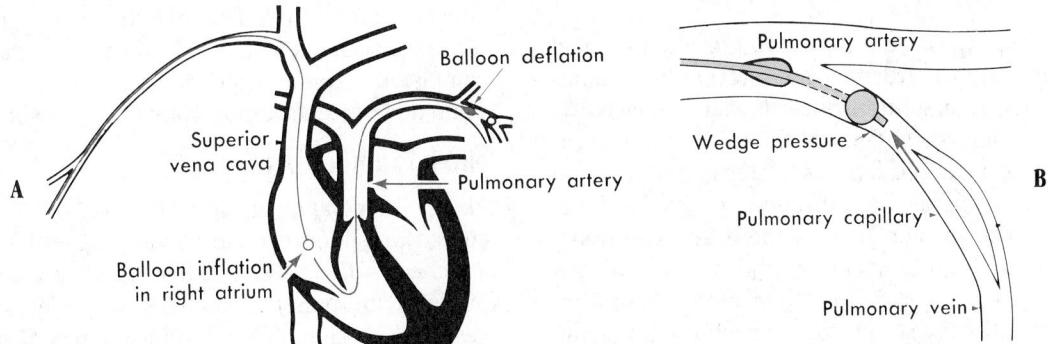

FIGURE 26-15 A, Flow-directed, balloon-tipped catheter showing inflation of balloon in right atrium and consequent "floating" of catheter through right ventricle and out to distal pulmonary artery branch. Balloon is deflated, advanced slightly, and reinflated slightly to obtain pulmonary capillary wedge pressure (PCWP). **B,** During initial positioning of balloon-tipped catheter in pulmonary artery, balloon is deflated. Catheter is then advanced and balloon is reinflated just enough to obtain PCWP. (From Schroeder J and Daily L: Techniques in bedside hemodynamic monitoring, St Louis, 1976, The CV Mosby Co.)

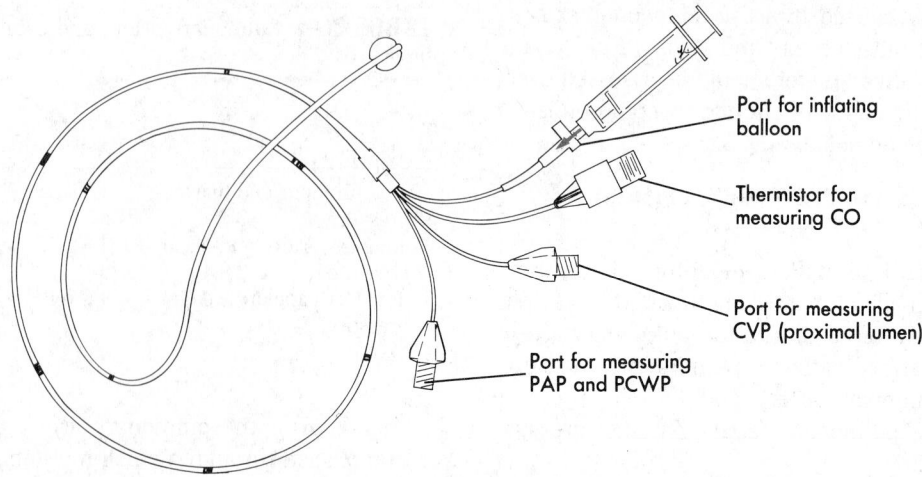

FIGURE 26-16 Four-lumen thermodilution pulmonary artery catheter for measuring cardiac output *(CO)*, central venous pressure *(CVP)*, pulmonary artery pressure *(PAP)*, and pulmonary capillary wedge pressure *(PCWP)*.

PCWP every few hours or more frequently if the patient's condition is unstable or if pharmacologic modifications of preload and afterload are being used.

The type of pulmonary artery catheter used will determine what hemodynamic measurements other than PAEDP and PCWP can be obtained. Some catheters have a third lumen that contains a thermistor. This is used to determine cardiac output by the thermodilution technique. A fourth (proximal) lumen ends at the level of the right atrium and is used to monitor CVP and to obtain blood samples. A four-lumen thermodilution catheter is illustrated in Figure 26-16.

SONIC STUDIES
ECHOCARDIOGRAPHY

Echocardiography uses ultrasound to provide a method for assessing cardiac structure and mobility in a noninvasive manner. A small transducer is usually placed on the patient's chest at the level of the third or fourth intercostal space near the left lower sternal border. The technician then angles the transducer in varying directions to visualize specific areas of the heart. The transducer transmits high-frequency sound waves and then receives these waves back from the patient as they are reflected off different structures. The ultrasonic beam, which is reflected back from the patient's heart, produces "echoes" that are viewed as lines and spaces on an oscilloscope. These lines and spaces represent bone, cardiac chambers and valves, the septum, and muscle. A copy of the echocardiogram is recorded on paper and becomes a permanent graphic record of the findings.

Since echocardiography is a noninvasive procedure, it is safer than cardiac catheterization; thus whenever possible, echocardiography is carried out first and then followed with cardiac catheterization as necessary. There are virtually no contraindications to performing an echocardiogram. In fact, for the critically ill patient, portable echocardiography can be performed at the bedside. No special preparation is necessary for the test; the patient can eat and take medications as usual. Patient teaching regarding the echocardiogram should include not only the purpose of the test but also that it is painless and takes approximately 30 to 60 minutes to complete. During the procedure the patient will have to lie quietly. The position assumed for the test is lying supine, turned slightly onto the left side with the head elevated 15 to 20 degrees. Since no adverse or untoward effects occur from echocardiography, the patient may resume normal activities as soon as the examination is completed. Numerous conditions can be detected or evaluated by echocardiography (see box above, right).

PHONOCARDIOGRAPHY

Phonocardiography involves the use of electrically recorded amplified cardiac sounds. Special microphones attached to the patient's chest pick up cardiac sounds produced by pressure changes in the heart and great vessels. The sounds are graphically recorded on special phonograph paper so that a permanent record is available. Phonocardiography can be helpful in determining the exact timing and characteristics of murmurs and extra heart sounds. Frequently, phonocardiograms are used in conjunction with echocardiograms so that a comparison can be made between sound (phono) and motion (echo). Patient preparation is similar to that described for the echocardiogram.

CONDITIONS DETECTED OR EVALUATED BY ECHOCARDIOGRAPHY

Abnormal pericardial fluid
Valvular disorders, including prosthetic valves
Ventricular aneurysms
Cardiac tumors, such as atrial myxomas
Some forms of congenital heart disease, such as atrial septal defects
Cardiac chamber size
Stroke volume and cardiac output
Some myocardial abnormalities, such as idiopathic hypertrophic subaortic stenosis (IHSS)

INDICATIONS FOR PERFORMING A STRESS TEST

Evaluation of the patient with symptoms suggestive of coronary artery disease
Determination of the patient's physical work capacity and aerobic capacity
Determination of the patient's functional capacity following a myocardial infarction and as an aid in planning an exercise rehabilitation program
Evaluation of exercise-induced dysrhythmias
Evaluation of the asymptomatic individual over 40 years of age at risk for coronary artery disease
Evaluation of pharmacologic interventions for dysrhythmias, angina, or ischemia

DYNAMIC STUDIES
HOLTER MONITOR

Resting ECGs supply much valuable information about an individual's cardiovascular status. However, for some people who may experience cardiovascular symptoms (chest pain, palpitations) only during exertion or while performing daily activities, a more dynamic method for studying the ECG is necessary.

At present the Holter monitor is being used to obtain a continuous graphic tracing of a patient's pulse while performing daily activities. The Holter monitor is a small, portable ECG monitor about the size of a large transistor radio. The patient is attached to the monitor by a precordial lead system and the monitor itself can be carried with the use of a shoulder strap. Generally the patient is attached to the Holter monitor for approximately 24 hours. During this time the patient is required to keep a log or diary of daily activities. The log should include the time, present activity, any medication taken, and any unusual sensations experienced while attached to the monitor. When the monitoring period is completed, the physician compares the ECG with the patient's log to determine if any correlations exist between the ECG and the patient's activities. The Holter monitor is helpful in documenting transient or episodic dysrhythmias and is sometimes used to evaluate patients for pacemaker therapy.

STRESS TESTING

Stress testing (ECG during exercise) or exercise testing is a noninvasive test to evaluate cardiovascular response to a progressively graded workload. Stress testing may be done for a variety of reasons (see the box above, right).

The exercise test can be performed with a bicycle ergometer (stationary bicycle with adjustable resistance to pedaling) or a treadmill (moving belt that can be adjusted so that the individual either walks or runs on a gradient). The patient's blood pressure and ECG are monitored closely during and after the stress test. Since the stress test is designed to progressively increase myocardial oxygen demand, some patients may experience untoward effects, and the test may need to be terminated. Conditions necessitating termination include the following: (1) ventricular tachycardia, (2) fall in peak systolic blood pressure and/or fall in heart rate despite increased workload, (3) vertigo, (4) frequent premature ventricular beats, (5) chest pain (angina), (6) severe dyspnea, (7) severe anxiety, and (8) diagnostic ST segment depression.

The manifestations of an abnormal stress test reflect an imbalance between supply and demand for myocardial oxygen caused by myocardial ischemia. Many criteria exist for evaluating a stress test as positive and may vary with individual patients. The most common criteria are listed in Table 26-5.

Adequate preparation for stress testing is extremely important. Although the procedure is not considered painful, it can be extremely fatiguing; patients may become anxious because they will be exercising at a level that might produce such cardiovascular symptoms as dyspnea, palpitations, and chest pain. After reviewing the purpose and method of stress testing, the patient should be advised to do the following:

1. Get adequate rest the night before the test.
2. Avoid coffee, tea, and alcohol the day of the test.
3. Avoid smoking and taking nitroglycerin during the 2 hours immediately before the test.
4. Eat a light breakfast or lunch at least 2 hours before the test.
5. Wear comfortable, loose-fitting clothes. (Women should be advised to wear a bra for support.)
6. Wear sturdy, comfortable walking shoes.
7. Consult with the physician about taking medications before the test. (Digoxin, propranolol, and vasodilators may affect the results of the stress test.)

TABLE 26-5 Criteria for evaluating a stress test

Assessment Parameters	Possible Indicators of Positive Stress Test
ECG	ST segment depressions 1 mm or more are generally regarded as indicative of ischemia. Dysrhythmias: exercise-induced premature ventricular beats in the healthy individual are of little prognostic significance unless they occur in conjunction with ST segment depression; individuals with both exercise-induced ventricular dysrhythmias and significant ST depression are likely to have severe coronary artery disease.
Hemodynamics	An exercise-induced, sustained reduction of peak systolic blood pressure of 10 mm Hg or more may be an inappropriate blood pressure response to stress testing and is a highly specific sign of multivessel coronary artery disease. An inappropriate heart rate response to exercise may correlate with impaired left ventricular function.
Symptoms	Typical anginal pain induced by exertion is a reliable symptom of coronary artery disease
Cardiac auscultation	Development of S_3 suggests advanced coronary artery disease and myocardial dysfunction Development of transient S_4 following stress testing may result from increased turbulence and volume of blood flow. Development of systolic murmurs is often caused by papillary muscle dysfunction, which suggests coronary artery disease.

8. Inform the physician if any unusual sensations develop during the test (for example, chest pain, dizziness).
9. Rest after the test. (Do *not* take a hot shower; a bath in warm water 1 to 2 hours after the test is permitted.)

RADIOLOGIC TESTS
CHEST ROENTGENOGRAMS

A roentgenogram (x-ray film) of the chest may be taken to determine overall size and configuration of the heart as well as individual cardiac chamber size. Most abnormalities of heart size can be detected with a standard posteroanterior and lateral view of the chest. Calcifica-

tions in the pericardium, heart muscle, valves, or large blood vessels can also be visualized in such a cardiovascular film.

CARDIAC FLUOROSCOPY

Cardiac fluoroscopy facilitates observation of the heart from varying views while the heart is in motion. Fluoroscopy can be used to detect ventricular aneurysms, which appear as a paradoxical bulging during systole. In addition, fluoroscopy is used to monitor prosthetic valve movement and to assess the position of cardiac calcifications during the cardiac cycle. Because of the increased risk of exposure to radiation during fluoroscopy, many institutions no longer use this diagnostic technique; rather, procedures such as echocardiograms and phonocardiograms are used more frequently.

SCINTIGRAPHIC STUDIES
MYOCARDIAL IMAGING

Presently, myocardial imaging is used to identify myocardial infarctions, evaluate myocardial perfusion, and assess left ventricular function. This technique can provide invaluable information in the presence of conflicting data. For example, if a patient has recently undergone coronary artery bypass surgery, the cardiac enzymes may already be elevated and may complicate the diagnosis of a new infarction. Also, certain ECG abnormalities (for example, LBB block, pacer-induced beats) may complicate the usual ECG indicators of a new infarction. Unfortunately, at times a patient is either unable to supply a history or presents conflicting data about a cardiovascular episode. In all these examples, myocardial imaging can provide a relatively safe and noninvasive technique for evaluating myocardial function.

Static Myocardial Imaging

Two basic techniques are used to produce a static picture of a myocardial image: stannous pyrophosphate scan and thallium imaging.

Pyrophosphate scan. The pyrophosphate scan, referred to as "hot spot" imaging, typically uses the agent technetium-99m stannous pyrophosphate. A minute dose of the radioisotope is injected into an antecubital vein. The patient then waits approximately 2 hours while the renal system clears the unbound technetium so that the heart can be visualized. In the healthy myocardium, there will be a homogeneous tracer distribution of the radiopharmaceutical. In the damaged heart however, the uptake to the radioactive material will increase. A gamma (γ-) scintillator camera is used to identify the area of increased uptake (hot spot). This type of scanning plays a less significant role in imaging acute myocardial infarction because of technical difficulties. For example, false-positive results can occur if the scan is performed too early because the isotope failed to clear the intravascular volume. This problem is magnified if the patient also has renal failure. The test is best performed 1 to 3 days after the infarction. Because such a minute isotope amount is administered during the examination, no toxic or allergic reactions have been noted, and it is considered radioactively safe for both patient and staff.

Thallium imaging. Thallium imaging can be referred to as "cold spot" imaging because the isotope is taken up by healthy myocardial tissue and not by the infarction area; thus this area remains a "cold spot." A γ-scintillator is used to detect the distribution of the radioisotope. Thallium imaging is most often used with exercise testing, but it can provide valuable information regarding myocardial infarction. Because the radioisotope is a potassium analog, it behaves as an intracellular monovalent cation. The isotope is actively transported across healthy myocardial cells, where extraction by these cells is significantly high. With ischemia, blood supply is diminished and thus a lesser amount of the isotope is delivered to such areas. Therefore an area of diminished thallium uptake (cold spot) surrounded by an area of normal myocardial uptake results. Cellular release of the isotope exceeds its accumulation after the initial uptake, resulting in washout of the tracer from the perfused areas with redistribution of the isotope to the ischemic areas. Ischemic and infarcted tissue can then be differentiated because the infarcted myocardium is unable to take up the redistributed tracer.

Thallium scanning can be helpful in quantifying the amount of myocardium at risk during acute infarction by using two resting scans to localize the affected area. The resting scan is obtained in the very early phase, whereas a redistribution scan is obtained 3 to 4 hours later. The total area of ischemia and infarction is visible on the initial scan. During the period before the redistribution scan, a border zone area has an opportunity to extract the isotope. Thus a smaller cold spot is visible when redistribution occurs. This technique is useful in assessing the efficacy of therapeutic interventions, such as thrombolytic therapy, as well as providing direction for further treatment based on the degree of myocardium still in jeopardy.

Because the amount of thallium used is small, the risk is considered to be minimal.

MUGA Scanning (Dynamic Scan)

A second way of imaging myocardial function is the use of a dynamic scan to assess cardiac wall motion and global left and right ventricular function. The easiest method for performing this type of imaging is to use *multiple-gated acquisition cardiac blood pool imaging*

(MUGA scanning). This technique lends itself well to the portable imaging techniques required to scan acutely ill patients with myocardial infarction. Furthermore, neither type of static scan, pyrophosphate or thallium, gives any information about the systolic or diastolic performance of the infarcted heart. MUGA scanning has the capability of demonstrating cardiac wall motion to enable assessment of injury as well as capacity of cardiac function.

Gated blood pool imaging is a noninvasive radionuclide method. ECG leads are attached to the patient, and the ECG is then synchronized to a computer and a γ-camera. A small amount of technetium-99m (attached to either human serum albumin or to autologous RBCs) is injected intravenously. After the radioactivity reaches a state of equilibrium (approximately 3 to 5 minutes), the patient is placed in a supine position with the γ-camera positioned over the precordium. The computer then constructs an average cardiac cycle that represents the summation of several hundred heartbeats. Enough data are generated so that an outline of the left side of the heart in all phases of the cardiac cycle can be seen.

Gated blood pool imaging offers several advantages in assessment of patients with myocardial infarction in addition to assessment of ventricular and segmental wall function. Because all RBCs are tagged, their counts reflect blood volume. Thus, if the heart can be positioned on the scan so that the left ventricle is isolated from the other chambers, left ventricular ejection function can be determined from left ventricular counts. The ejection fraction, calculated from the computer-reconstructed image of end diastole and end systole, may provide an early indicator of deteriorating cardiovascular functioning in patients with congestive heart failure, with low cardiac output, or who are at risk of developing cardiotoxicity caused by high doses of adriamycin (Doxorubicin). Right ventricular ejection fraction can also be determined, but it is less accurate because of difficulty in separating right atrial counts.

Mild injury of the cardiac wall is reflected in MUGA scanning as hypokinesia or mild depression of myocardial contraction versus a more severe disturbance producing akinesia or dyskinesia. Clinical interventions are determined according to improvement or deterioration of global function and wall motion segments. Other important information, such as recognition of right ventricular infarction and aneurysm formation, can be easily recognized. In addition, the effects of pharmacotherapeutics (for example, nitroglycerin, vasodilators) on ventricular function can be evaluated.

Stress-testing ventriculography can also be performed to evaluate the ejection fraction during exercise. Some patients with coronary artery disease demonstrate a normal resting ejection value. However, under maximal stress, the ejection fraction may decrease, or an abnormality in a specific region of the heart may become apparent.

POSITRON-EMISSION TOMOGRAPHY

Positron-emission tomography represents a radionuclide-based imaging technique that uses short-lived radionuclides as tracers to report both perfusion and metabolic events. These tracers are generally given by intravenous injection or inhalation and only occasionally by intraarterial injection. Myocardial uptake is proportional to the quantity of tracer delivered by the amount of blood flow, by the fractional extraction, and by the loss of tracer through decay, metabolism, and flow. The tracer elements readily pass through the tissues and are simultaneously detected by counters placed on opposite sides of the body, a process known as *annihilation coincidence detection*.

Under normal circumstances the well-perfused, aerobically metabolizing myocardium prefers free fatty acids for energy production from oxidative metabolism. When ischemia is present, more glucose and less fatty acid tend to be utilized. Positron-emission tomography is particularly useful in demonstrating this process by incorporating radioisotopes into biochemically relevant components (such as C palmitate or F-2-fluoro-2-deoxyglucose) used in the study and by demonstrating myocardial flow deficits in patients with coronary disease.

CARDIAC CATHETERIZATION

Cardiac catheterization is an extremely valuable diagnostic tool for obtaining detailed information about the structure and function of the cardiac chambers, valves, and great vessels. Cardiac catheterization may include studies of the right side of the heart, the left side of the heart, and coronary arteries. Studies of the coronary arteries are done to detect the presence and extent of coronary artery disease and to evaluate the effects of medical and surgical treatment of the disease. There are many indications for performing a cardiac catheteriza-

---

REASONS FOR PERFORMING A CATHETERIZATION

Confirmation of the presence of suspected heart disease, including congenital heart disease, valvular disease, and myocardial disease.

Determination of the location and severity of the disease process

Preoperative assessment to determine if cardiac surgery is indicated

Evaluation of ventricular function following surgical revascularization

Evaluation of the effect of medical treatment modalities on cardiovascular function

Performing specialized cardiac techniques such as the placement of an internal pacemaker

---

tion (see the box below). Often, individuals will have undergone several other diagnostic procedures before being evaluated for catheterization.

RIGHT-SIDED HEART CATHETERIZATION

Right-sided heart catheterization is performed when congenital heart disease is suspected or to evaluate certain acquired conditions, such as tricuspid stenosis or valvular incompetence. Blood samples and blood pressure readings are taken, ECG studies are done, and cineradiographs of the right chambers of the heart and the pulmonary arterial circulation are made.

To perform a catheterization of the right side of the heart, a catheter is inserted via cutdown into a large vein (for example, the medial cubital or brachial vein). The catheter is then threaded with the use of fluoroscopy into the superior vena cava, the right atrium, the right ventricle, the pulmonary artery, and pulmonary capillaries. As the catheter is passed through the various chambers and vessels, blood samples are obtained to determine the oxygen content and saturation. In the presence of a left-to-right atrial shunt, blood samples would indicate a higher oxygen content in the right atrium than in the superior or inferior vena cava. Blood pressure measurements are also recorded (Figure 26-17). Normal blood pressures in the heart vary among the chambers. The pressure is highest in the left ventricle because of the stronger ventricular contractions. Normally the pulmonary artery pressure (PAP) is approximately 25/10 mm Hg or approximately one fifth of the systemic blood pressure. Elevations in chamber pressures such as an elevated left atrial pressure can indicate mitral stenosis or insufficiency and possibly left ventricular failure.

LEFT-SIDED HEART CATHETERIZATION

Left-sided heart catheterization is performed to evaluate pressures of the left side of the heart, valvular competency, and left ventricular function. A catheter is passed into the aorta from either the brachial or the femoral artery with the use of fluoroscopic visualization. After the catheter reaches the aorta, it is manipulated around the aortic arch, down the ascending aorta, and through the aortic valve into the left ventricle. Pressure-gradient measurements are obtained to detect pressure changes across the valves. In the presence of a stenotic valve, the chamber pressure proximal to the stenosis will be significantly higher than the pressure in the distal chamber. Pressure gradients are recorded by taking continuous pressure measurements while simultaneously pulling the catheter back through a valve. Normally a pressure gradient exists across the mitral and tricuspid valves (Figure 26-17). Therefore a decrease in the gradient is indicative of stenosis. Conversely, no pressure gradient exists across the aortic and pulmonic

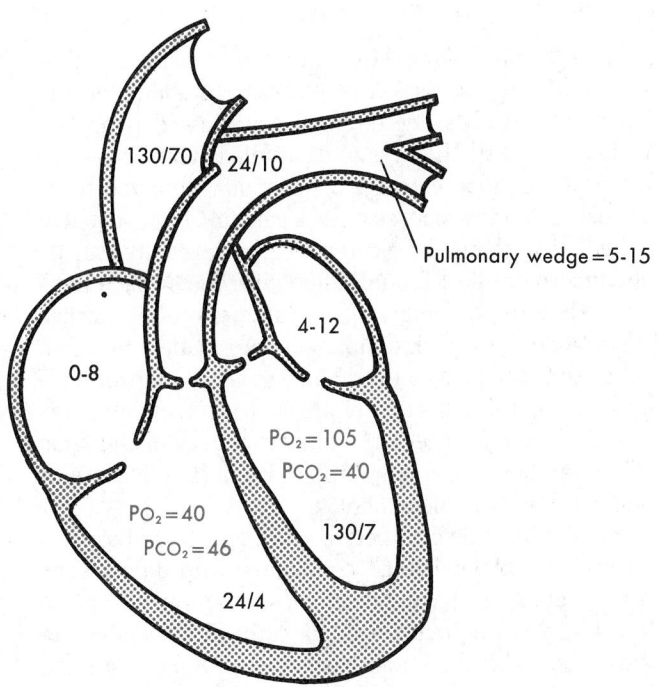

FIGURE 26-17 Pressure readings and blood gases in millimeters of mercury (mm Hg) in chambers of heart and major blood vessels.

valves; therefore, if a gradient is present, it is of diagnostic importance.

VENTRICULAR ANGIOGRAPHY

Ventricular angiography may be performed during the left-sided heart catheterization. This procedure involves the injection of contrast material into the ventricle while concomitant roentgenograms are taken. Information about contractility, aneurysm formation, valvular disorders (for example, mitral regurgitation), and the ejection fraction can be obtained.

CORONARY ARTERIOGRAPHY

Selective coronary arteriography may also be completed during the left-sided heart catheterization. A catheter is introduced into the arterial system through either a femoral or a brachial arteriotomy. The catheter is threaded (using fluroscopy) to the aortic root; the tip of the catheter is then advanced into the right and left coronary ostia. Approximately 2 to 5 ml of contrast medium is injected into each coronary artery, and cineangiographic films are taken to monitor the progression of the dye. The contrast medium outlines the entire coronary circulation and enables the examiner to evaluate the anatomy of the coronary arteries as well as stenotic segments and collateral vessels.

The introduction of contrast material into the coronary arteries may produce transient chest pain or discomfort. The presence of the dye may temporarily displace coronary artery blood flow, producing transient ischemia. Sublingual nitroglycerin is frequently administered to relieve the anginal discomfort. In addition, medications such as isosorbide (Isordil) may be given to dilate vessels so that greater visualization of the coronary arteries may be achieved. Occasionally the injection of contrast material into the right coronary artery may suppress the SA node, producing bradydysrhythmias, and intravenous atropine may be required.

PATIENT PREPARATION

Preparation for cardiac catheterization is extremely important. Even after careful explanations, most patients are somewhat apprehensive. It is important to include the family in the instructions to alleviate their anxiety; this will facilitate their support of the patient. The patient may be concerned about both the procedure and the results. Preparation should include information about the procedure and the more common sensations that may be experienced during the catheterization. The material is presented as reassuring information so the patient understands the various sensations experienced are expected. The patient is questioned concerning any history of drug allergy, especially to contrast media.

Usually the meal before the procedure is withheld. If the procedure is scheduled for later in the day, the patient may be permitted a clear liquid breakfast. A mild sedative may be given before the procedure, and an antibiotic may be ordered as a prophylactic measure.

For adults, a local anesthetic is injected over the vein to be used, and a small cutdown is performed. Relatively little discomfort is involved in a right-sided heart catheterization, although the patient may feel pressure in the femoral or antecubital area. During a left-sided heart catheterization with ventricular angiography, the patient may experience a warm, flushing sensation as the contrast medium is injected. This flushing sensation lasts for approximately 30 seconds. The patient may also experience nausea and "fluttering" sensations produced by ectopic beats from catheter manipulation or from catheter advancement as it is threaded through the heart. The small amount of contrast material injected into the coronary arteries during coronary arteriography does not produce the warm, flushing sensation noted in ventriculography, although the patient may experience some pain or tightness in the chest.

If chest discomfort or alterations in blood pressure occur, the patient is instructed to cough as fast and as hard as possible. This coughing maneuver facilitates the clearing of the contrast material from the coronary arteries and also acts as a mechanical stimulus to the heart if ectopic beats occur. In addition, coughing appears to help alleviate the feelings of lightheadedness and nausea that might result after injection of the dye.

The body's physiologic responses to cardiac catheterization are numerous and vary with each individual. It is therefore essential that the patient understand the importance of alerting the physician to any unexpected or unusual sensations that might arise during the catheterization.

NURSING CARE AFTER CATHETERIZATION

Regardless of the type of cardiac angiographic study performed, the postoperative nursing care will be the same. These procedures generally last from 1 to 3 hours and can be tiring for the patient. Following the examination, many patients like to rest or sleep, but they may resume usual activities as soon as their vital signs are stable.

The patient's *pulse* (on the operative side) and *blood pressure* (on the opposite side) are monitored every 15 minutes for 1 hour and then every 30 minutes for 3 hours. It is essential to check the pulses distal to the catheter insertion site to determine the patency of the cannulated artery. Occasionally the amplitude of the pulse may be slightly diminished for approximately 24 hours because of arterial spasm or edema at the site. At times thrombus formation may totally obliterate the distal pulse, and surgical correction may be necessary to detect any sign of impaired circulation. The cutdown site should be closely monitored for signs of bleeding, inflammation, tenderness, or swelling.

If a *femoral* approach was used, the patient is kept on bed rest for 12 to 24 hours. Frequently the patient will return from the catheterization with either a weight, sandbag, or ice applied to the femoral site. The patient should not have the head of the bed elevated more than 30 degrees and should avoid flexing the femoral area. If the *brachial* site is used, the arm is kept straight for several hours (with the use of an armboard), but the patient can be up in the room as soon as vital signs are stable. If any bleeding occurs from the cutdown site, firm pressure is applied directly over the site, and the physician is notified. For the first 24 hours after catheterization, intake and output are monitored.

Hypotension may develop as a result of the sometimes profound diuretic effect of the contrast material used during angiography. Complications during cardiac catheterization are infrequent; however, cardiac dysrhythmias, including ventricular fibrillation, can occur. Following the procedure, the development of tachycardia or any other dysrhythmia is reported to the physician immediately.

To reduce stress for the patient, many cardiac catheterization laboratories now permit patients to wear their glasses, dentures, and watches during the procedures. They may also have piped-in music or allow patients to bring a radio or favorite records with them.

ELECTROPHYSIOLOGIC STUDY

The electrophysiologic (EP) study is a technique that systematically assesses the electrical stability of the heart. The study's degree of invasiveness depends on which area of the heart is to be studied. This procedure requires electrode catheter placement within the heart to record intracardiac electrical activity. More detailed information about the heart's electrical activity can be obtained with the EP study than with the surface ECG because of the proximity of the catheters to the cardiac conduction system. Examples of information that can be gained include exact sequence of atrial and ventricular activation, localization of areas of conduction disturbances (such as accessory pathways, areas of ischemia and infarction, dysrhythmia foci), and effectiveness of antiarrhythmic management.

Similar to cardiac catheterization, an EP study is performed under laboratory conditions with fluoroscopy used to guide the pacing electrodes into position. Vascular sites most frequently used for catheter placement are the femoral, brachial, and basilic veins. Subclavian and jugular veins are rarely used, whereas arterial cannulation is performed only when left ventricular stimulation is necessary.

For the initial EP study especially, antiarrhythmic drugs are usually discontinued for approximately five half-lives to prevent pharmacologic interference with the study. Drugs typically tested include amiodarone, encainide, flecainide, tocainide, mexiletine, quinidine, bretylium, lidocaine, procainamide, disopyramide, propranolol, and phenytoin. Three to six intracardiac pacing catheters connected to a multichanneled electrogram may be used depending on the information to be obtained. A surface ECG is usually recorded simultaneously for comparison and evaluation. Atrial and bundle of His electrograms are typically recorded, as well as various measures of the conduction system. When indicated, dysrhythmias may be initiated by applying a series of programmed extra stimuli to areas of the heart. Pacing may also be done to terminate a tachycardia by inhibiting impulse transmission in conduction pathways.

The EP study usually lasts 2 to 4 hours. At the completion of testing, catheters are removed and pressure is applied at the insertion site for at least 10 minutes, followed by application of antiseptic ointment and a dry, sterile pressure dressing. Depending on the severity of dysrhythmia, patients must be continuously monitored in a telemetry or intensive care unit, where they can be closely observed and have rapidly accessible emergency equipment.

An EP study may also be performed intraoperatively, requiring placement of electrodes directly on the endocardium. This technique is sometimes used for the patient with a ventricular aneurysm to facilitate localization of the dysrhythmia substrate, which can be removed along with the aneurysm. Another use is localization of an accessory pathway before surgical removal.

Complications of EP studies are similar to those of cardiac catheterization and include hemorrhage, perforation, hematoma, pulmonary emboli, deep vein thrombus, pneumothorax, phlebitis, infection, cerebrovascular accident (stroke), angina with resultant ischemia or infarction, dysrhythmia, and death. The few published reports of death associated with EP studies are estimated at less than 0.01%.[22]

The many nursing responsibilities for these patients are challenging. Patients referred for EP studies may experience fear, anxiety, frustration, and depression. For some the EP study may be perceived as experimental, especially if various antiarrhythmic medication regimens were unsuccessful. Others have survived sudden cardiac death, perhaps more than once. In essence, each patient's psychoemotional needs will be unique and frequently complex. A thorough nursing history and physical assessment is important in establishing a data base so a comprehensive plan of care can be formulated.

Nurses play a key role in preparing patients for the EP study. Reinforcing physician information about the indications for the test, the procedure itself, rationale, and risks may allay anxiety for the patient as well as the family. A description of the equipment used and the room's appearance may also be helpful. It is important to inform patients that they will be awake throughout the procedure, thus providing the opportunity to ask questions and follow the instructions of the EP team.

Postprocedural observations for complications include assessment and documentation of vital signs; peripheral pulses; insertion site; and color, warmth, and sensation of extremities. Initially these observations are done every 15 minutes and gradually increased to every 4 hours. The extremity used for the study is immobilized, and the patient is placed on bed rest for 4 to 6 hours if venous access was used or 6 to 12 hours for arterial access. Observations for signs and symptoms of drug toxicity and allergy are critically important, especially if new antiarrhythmic drugs are prescribed. The nurse must be aware of the drug protocol as well as potential drug interactions and incompatibilities. Documentation of stability or changes in rhythm and frequency of ectopy is essential.

Discharge planning includes a review of medications, indications for use, directions for administration, and side effects, as well as signs and symptoms associated with the medical condition and dysrhythmia. The family and patient are instructed to contact the physician if the patient experiences new or increased chest pain, syncope, dyspnea, diaphoresis, or palpitations.

CHAPTER SUMMARY

✓ Electrophysiologic properties of the heart include automaticity, excitability, conductivity, and contractility.

✓ The action potential has two components, depolarization and repolarization. The main ions involved in this process include sodium, potassium, and calcium.

✓ Phases of the cardiac cycle include diastole (isovolumetric relaxation, rapid and slow ventricular filling, atrial systole) and systole (isovolumetric contraction, maximal and reduced ventricular ejection).

✓ Determinants of stroke volume include preload, afterload, contractility, and heart rate.

✓ Physiologic changes of the cardiovascular system with aging include increased amounts of fat and connective tissue as well as calcification and fibrosis of valves, leading to possible decreased cardiac output and reduced vascular compliance.

✓ Cardiovascular disease is the number one cause of death in individuals 65 years or older.

✓ The cardinal symptoms of heart disease include dyspnea, chest pain or discomfort, edema, syncope, palpitations, and excess fatigue.

✓ Methods to assess cardiovascular functioning include laboratory tests, invasive hemodynamic monitoring, sonic studies, dynamic studies, radiologic tests, scintigraphic studies, cardiac catheterization, and electrophysiologic studies.

QUESTIONS TO CONSIDER

- How does the ionic environment affect contractility and, subsequently, cardiac output?

- What factors contribute to an increase or decrease in preload, afterload, contractility, and heart rate?

- How would you care differently for an elderly person with heart disease?

- How does anxiety affect myocardial oxygen supply?

REFERENCES AND SELECTED READINGS

1. American Heart Association: Textbook of advanced cardiac life support, Dallas, 1987, The Association.
2. American Heart Association: Heart facts, Dallas, 1989, The Association.

*References preceded by an asterisk are particularly well suited for student reading.

3. Andreoli KG et al: Comprehensive cardiac care: a text for nurses, physicians, and other health practitioners, ed 6, St Louis, 1987, The CV Mosby Co.

4. Bates B: A guide to physical examination, ed 4, Philadelphia, 1987, JB Lippincott Co.

5. Berne RM and Levy MS: Cardiovascular physiology, ed 5, St Louis, 1986, The CV Mosby Co.

6. Braunwald E: Heart disease: a textbook of cardiovascular medicine, ed 3, Philadelphia, 1988, WB Saunders Co.

7. Conover MB: Understanding electrocardiography: arrhythmias and the 12-lead ECG, ed 5, St Louis, 1988, The CV Mosby Co.

8. Darovic GO: Hemodynamic monitoring: invasive and noninvasive clinical application, Philadelphia, 1987, WB Saunders Co.

9. *Finesilver C: Reducing stress in patients having cardiac catheterization, Am J Nurs 80:1085-1087, 1980.

10. *Fletcher GF: Exercise and exercise testing: current state of the art, Heart Lung 13:5-6, 1984.

11. Gardin JM et al: Effects of aging on peak systolic left ventricular wall stress in normal subjects, Am J Cardiol 63:998-999, 1989.

12. Gore JM et al: Handbook of hemodynamic monitoring, Boston, 1985, Little, Brown & Co.

13. Guyton AC: Textbook of medical physiology, ed 7, Philadelphia, 1986, WB Saunders Co.

14. Haughey BP: Holter monitoring: a method for nursing research, Nurs Res 32(1):59-60, 1983.

15. *Humbrecht A and Parys E: How to use heart and breath sounds as part of your nursing care plan, Nursing '82 12(4):34-41, 1982.

16. *Hurst JW et al: The heart, ed 6, New York 1986, McGraw-Hill Book Co.

17. Kohn RR: Heart and cardiovascular system. In Finch C and Hayflick L: Handbook of biology of aging, New York, 1987, Van Nostrand Reinhold.

18. Kutcher KL: Cardiac electrophysiologic mapping techniques, Focus Crit Care 12(4):26-30, 1984.

19. Lakatta EG et al: Human aging: changes in structure and function, J Am Coll Cardiol 10(2):42A-47A, 1987.

20. Lipid Research Clinics Program: The Lipid Research Clinics coronary prevention trial results: reduction in incidence of coronary heart disease, JAMA 251:351-364, 1984.

21. *Marinelli-Miller D: What your patient wants to know about angiography, but may not ask, RN 46:52-54, 1983.

22. *Mercer ME: The electrophysiology study: a nursing concern, Crit Care Nurse 7(2):58-65, 1987.

23. Roberts WC: The aging heart, Mayo Clin Proc 63:205-206, 1988.

24. *Saul L: Heart sounds and common murmurs, Am J Nurs 83:1679-1689, 1983.

25. Schelbert HR et al: Regional myocardial metabolism by positron tomography. In Heiss HW, editor: Advances in clinical cardiology, vol III, Mahwah, NJ, 1987, Foundation for Advances in Clinical Medicine, Inc.

26. *Selwyn AP and Smith TW: Current and future directions for clinical investigation of the heart with positron-emission tomography, Circulation 72(11)(suppl IV):31-38, 1985.

27. Sokolow M and McIlroy MB: Clinical cardiology, ed 5, Norwalk, Conn, 1989, Appleton & Lange.

28. Tilkien A and Conover M: Understanding heart sounds and murmurs, ed 2, Philadelphia, 1984, WB Saunders Co.

29. *Winters WL and Cahien WR: Imaging techniques in patients with acute myocardial infarction, Heart Lung 14:259-264, 1985.

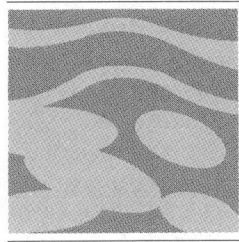

CHAPTER 27

Management of Persons with Cardiac Dysrhythmias

TERRI ABRAHAM

JOAN M. KAVANAGH

CHAPTER OBJECTIVES

After studying this chapter, the student should be able to:

1 Recognize common dysrhythmias associated with the cardiac conduction system, as obtained from a 12-lead ECG or electrocardiographic signal averaging.
2 Explain the arrhythmogenic mechanisms responsible for the manifestations of dysrhythmias.
3 Describe treatment modalities for patients with cardiac dysrhythmias.
4 Identify teaching needs of patients receiving antiarrhythmic therapy.
5 Identify nursing needs for patients requiring temporary or permanent pacemakers.
6 Explain nursing implications during cardioversion or defibrillation.
7 Describe the technique of basic life support.

Persons with heart disease or with conditions that can affect heart function may experience cardiac dysrhythmias, which in certain situations may lead to cardiac arrest. Although the term *dysrhythmia* is preferred to denote a disturbance or variation from normal heart rhythm, the term *arrhythmia* can be used interchangeably with dysrhythmia. This chapter describes the electrocardiogram (ECG), electrocardiographic signal averaging, and some common cardiac dysrhythmias and their management and reviews the techniques of cardiopulmonary resuscitation (CPR).

At present, various pharmacologic agents, cardiac pacemakers, and electrical stimulation techniques are useful in the control of dysrhythmias. These methods and salient features of the common dysrhythmias are presented here. Since the care of persons with cardiac dysrhythmias is complex, the review that follows is not sufficient for the nurse with primary responsibility for monitoring patients in an intensive care setting. For further study, the reader is referred to more specialized texts.

DETECTION OF CARDIAC RHYTHM

ELECTROCARDIOGRAM

The ECG is a graphic representation of the electrical forces produced within the heart. It is a necessary component in the assessment of cardiovascular status, but it is important to remember that this tool has limitations. For example, a resting ECG may be normal, even in the presence of heart disease. Conversely, abnormal variances may be seen in the ECG of a normal heart. It is therefore essential that the ECG be used in conjunction with data obtained from the patient history, physical assessment, and laboratory tests.

There are numerous indications for recording an ECG (see the box below). Continuous electrocardiographic monitoring for dysrhythmia detection is possible in the inpatient setting.

It is important to prepare the patient before any type of electrocardiographic procedure. Those patients who are unfamiliar with the procedure may fear receiving a shock or being electrocuted. The patient should be informed of the step-by-step procedure and assured of its safe, painless nature. Once the ECG is taken, the correct interpretation is based on knowledge of the electro-

MOST COMMON EXAMPLES OF ECG USE

Evaluation of tachycardia, bradycardia, or dysrhythmias
Sudden onset of dyspnea
Evaluation of pain occurring in the upper trunk and extremities
Evaluation of syncopal episodes
Evaluation of shock state or coma
Preoperative evaluation
Evaluation of postoperative hypotension
Evaluation of hypertension, murmurs, or cardiomegaly
Evaluation of artificial pacemaker function

mechanical system of the heart as well as the significance of each portion of the ECG tracing.

STANDARD 12-LEAD ECG

The electrocardiographic tracing represents the net electrical activity or electrical potential variations of the atria and ventricles as each depolarizes and repolarizes. The electrical currents passing through the heart are subsequently conducted to the body surface. These currents can be detected by electrodes and then measured when they reach the surface.

Basically the ECG machine is a galvanometer designed to measure the electrical potential difference between two locations on the body surface. The conventional 12-lead system uses several electrode sites to record potential differences at the body surface. A pair

of electrodes, consisting of a positive and a negative terminal, constitutes an ECG lead.

The patient is first attached to the ECG machine as the examiner places electrode plates or suction cup electrodes on the upper and lower extremities. These are designated as right arm (RA), left arm (LA), right leg (RL), and left leg (LL). The chest (or precordial) electrode is placed and moved across the chest wall six times during the latter portion of the ECG. These 10 sites are combined in pairs through a switching network connected to the lead selector switch. The operator of the ECG machine need only select the desired lead with the selector switch.

Effective contact between the skin and the electrode is facilitated by the use of electrode jelly, which contains electrolytes and an abrasive to interrupt the water-

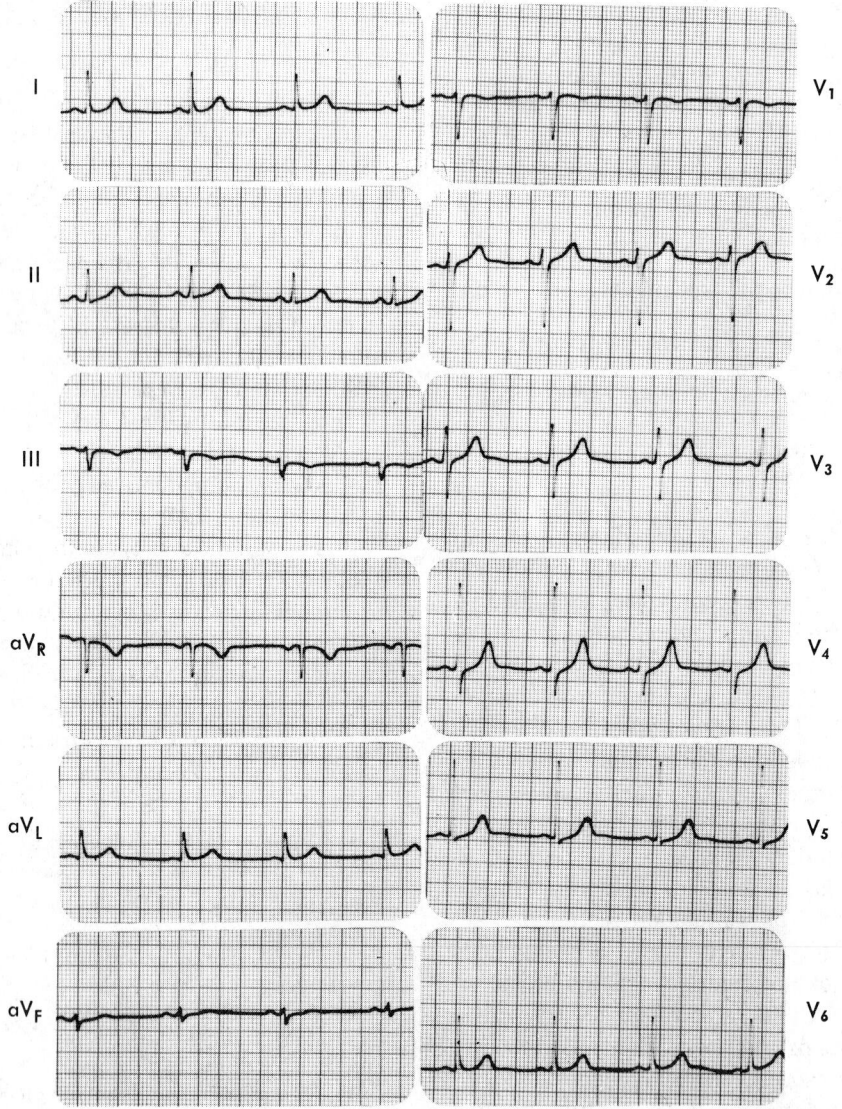

FIGURE 27-1 Twelve-lead ECG showing normal sinus rhythm. (From Andreoli KG et al: Comprehensive cardiac care, ed 6, St Louis, 1987, The CV Mosby Co.)

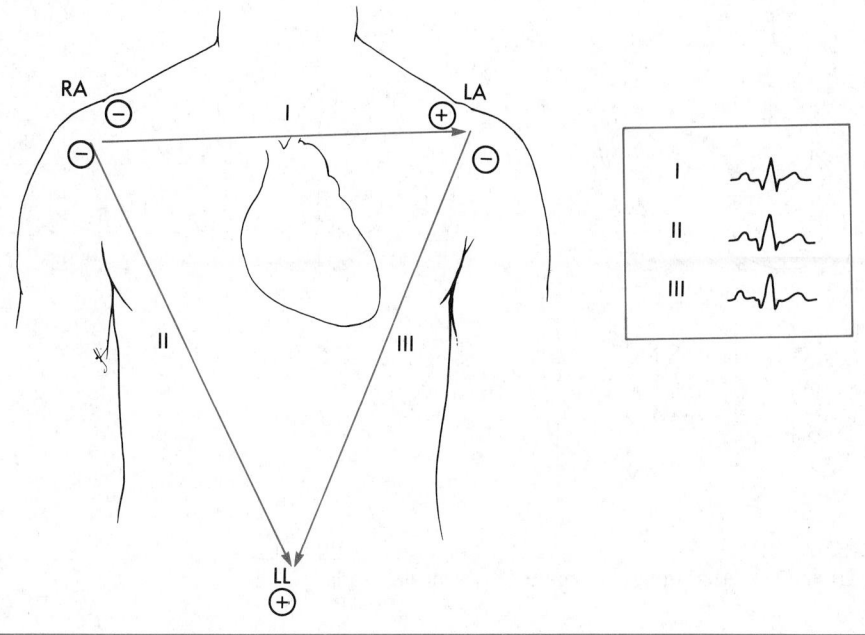

FIGURE 27-2 Schematic representation of standard limb lead system.

proof layer of the skin. In addition, the position of the patient should be uniformly flat if possible. Assuming a sitting or side-lying position severely alters the position of the heart relative to the electrodes. The discussions that follow clarify the individual leads and their respective electrode sites (Figure 27-1).

Standard Limb Leads

The standard limb leads, designated by Roman numerals I, II, and III, are obtained by using electrodes applied to the right arm (RA), left arm (LA), and left leg (LL) (Figure 27-2). The right leg (RL) electrode acts only as a grounding electrode. The limb leads are

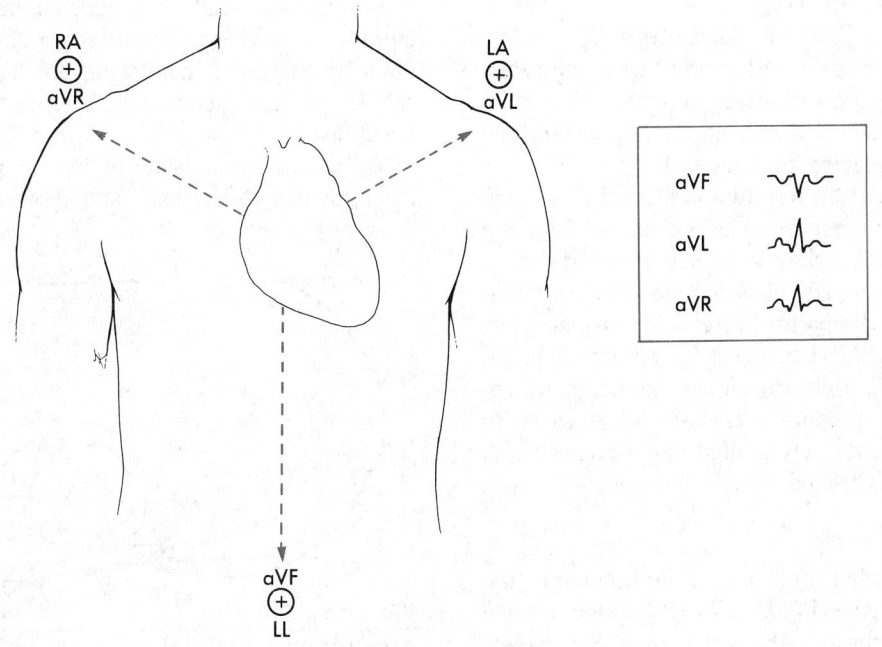

FIGURE 27-3 Schematic representation of augmented unipolar limb lead system.

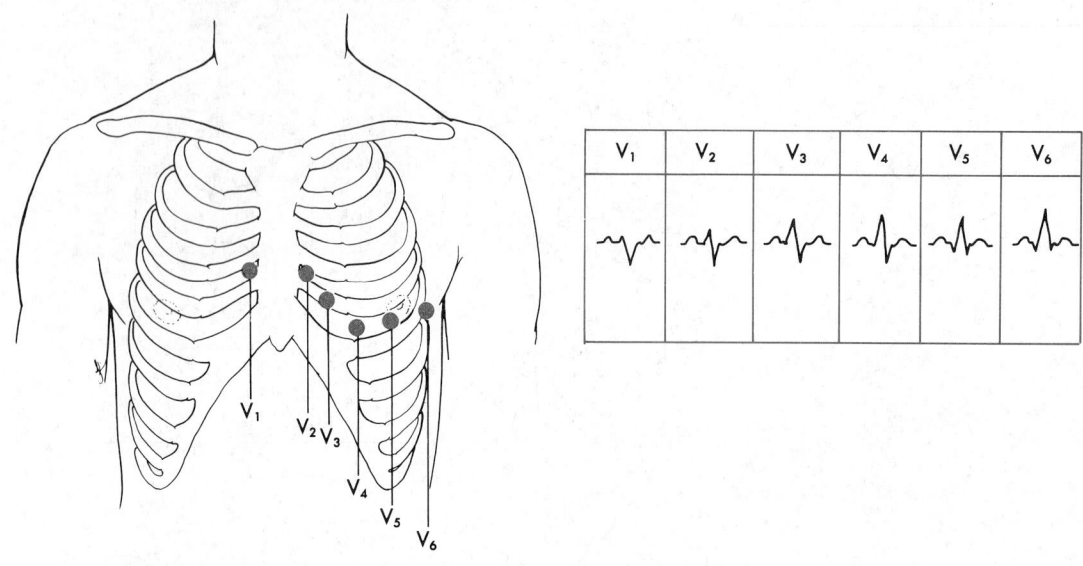

FIGURE 27-4 Anatomic placement of precordial leads.

termed *bipolar leads* because each registers the electrical potential difference between two anatomic sites.

 Lead I records the difference between the RA and LA potentials. The LA electrode is positive. (The importance of the positive electrode is more apparent in later discussions.)

 Lead II records the difference between the RA and LL potentials. The LL electrode is positive.

 Lead III records the difference between the LA and LL potentials. The LL electrode is positive.

Augmented Unipolar Limb Leads

The augmented unipolar limb leads are designated by the abbreviated forms aVR, aVL, and aVF (a represents augmented; V represents unipolar). For these leads the right arm (R), left arm (L), and left leg (F) become the respective positive electrodes (Figure 27-3).

 The negative (central) terminal is formed by electrically joining the remaining two limb electrodes. Such a connection essentially nullifies any potential variation at the negative terminal. The electrical potential variation is only recorded by the positive electrode, thus the term *unipolar lead.* For clinical purposes the amplitude of the recordings from these electrodes is augmented by approximately 50% to produce a tracing that is easier to interpret. Together, the augmented and standard limb leads provide the six frontal plane leads.

Precordial Unipolar Leads

There are six precordial or chest leads designated by the symbols V_1 through V_6 (Figure 27-4). V designates the unipolar design of these leads, which register the electrical variations of the heart in the horizontal plane (Figure 27-5). The negative (central) terminal of each V lead is formed by the joining of the three limb lead electrodes. The positive or "exploring" electrode is a suction cup electrode that is moved to six different sites across the chest. As in the case of the limb leads, these connections are made automatically when the lead selector is turned to "V".

MONITORING

To perform continuous cardiac monitoring and to provide for patient mobility during hospitalization, the conventional ECG leads have been modified to eliminate cumbersome wiring. The most popular leads for continuous dysrhythmia monitoring are lead II and lead V_1 (MCL_1: M for modified; CL for bipolar hookup [not chest lead]).

 During the monitoring period the patient wears two, three, or five electrodes; each consists of a conducting

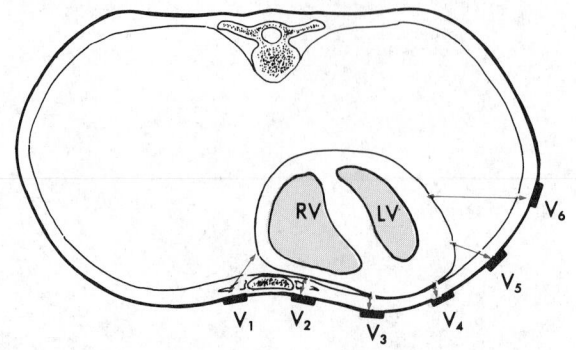

FIGURE 27-5 Cross section of heart showing precordial leads V_1 through V_6 in a horizontal plane.

gel pad surrounded by an adhesive. These electrodes are attached by small lead wires to a cable connected to a wall-mounted monitor. The monitor consists chiefly of an oscilloscope screen (for the ECG tracing display), a lead selector switch, and a heart rate indicator. This is sometimes known as a "hardwire" monitor.

An alternative type of continuous monitoring is known as *telemetry*. The telemetry system requires no cables that would restrict patient mobility; instead, electrical impulses are transmitted by antennae to an oscilloscope at the nurses' station.

Lead II is produced by placing the negative electrode on the right arm (modified and placed near the right shoulder below the clavicle) and the positive electrode on the lower left rib cage (eighth intercostal space).

Lead V_1 is produced by placing the negative electrode on the left arm (modified and placed near the left shoulder below the clavicle) and the positive electrode at the fourth intercostal space to the right of the sternum. With these modifications, V_1 is known as MCL_1. MCL_1 is the most helpful lead for (1) determining the origin of premature beats, (2) determining the presence of bundle branch blocks, and (3) visualizing atrial activity. (For further discussion, see Chapter 28.)

ECG PAPER

The electrocardiographic tracing is recorded on graph paper that passes by a heated pen at a speed of 25 mm/second. The graph paper is divided into millimeter squares. The millimeter squares are grouped and divided into larger squares by thick lines occurring every fifth square (Figure 27-6).

Horizontally, each millimeter square represents 0.04 second of time elapsed. Each thick line denotes the passage of 0.20 second. Fifteen hundred (1500) small, or 300 large, squares represent 1 minute. With this information, one can measure the duration of any complex or interval by determining the number of small squares and multiplying by 0.04 second.

Heart rate may be measured or estimated quickly by any of the following three methods:

1. Measure the interval between consecutive complexes, determine the number of small squares, and divide 1500 by that number.
2. Measure the interval between consecutive complexes, determine the number of large squares, and divide 300 by that number.
3. Determine the number of complexes occurring between two slash marks found along the top of the ECG paper, and multiply by 20. (The interval between two slash marks represents 3 seconds elapsed.) This is a most helpful method when the heart rate is very irregular.

Vertically, each small square is 1 mm in height and represents 0.1 mV of voltage. Thus each large square represents 5 mm or 0.5 mV. The ECG machine is standardized so that 1 mV produces a 10 mm deflection before its use.

The voltage or amplitude of a wave or complex in a given lead indirectly indicates the electrical activity of

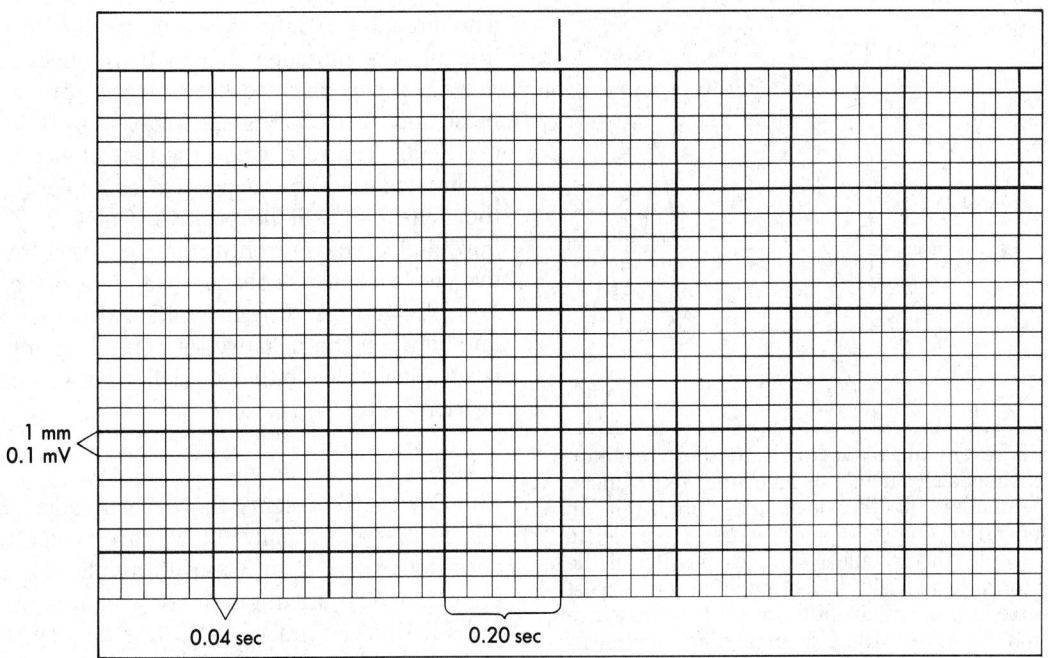

1 mm
0.1 mV

0.04 sec   0.20 sec

FIGURE 27-6 Components of ECG paper.

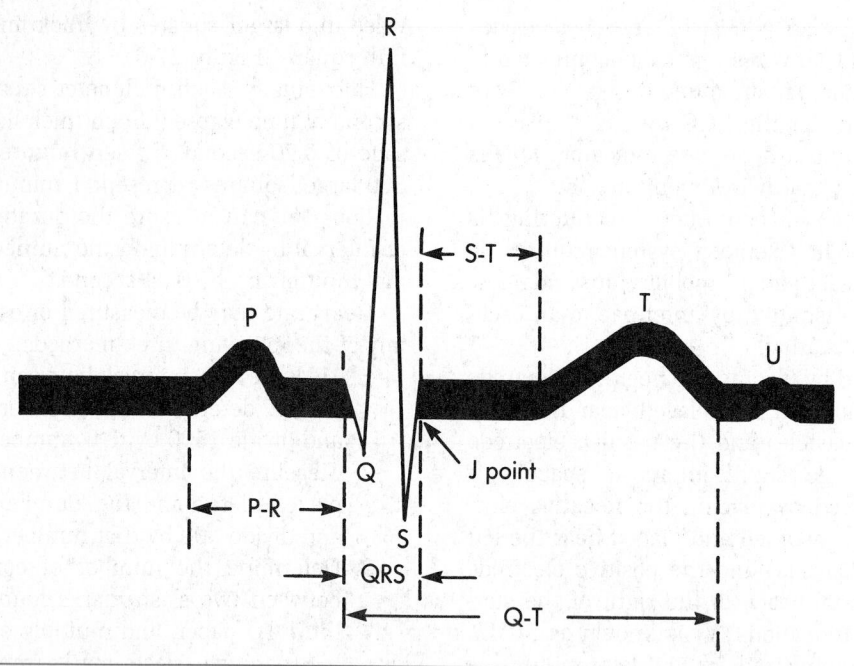

FIGURE 27-7 Schematic drawing of ECG waves produced by the cardiac cycle.

the muscle below the exploring or positive electrode. For example, hypertrophied myocardium will produce abnormally high voltage in some leads, whereas infarcted myocardium could produce no voltage or low-voltage waves. The reader is referred to a coronary care text for a more detailed discussion of the significance of voltage.

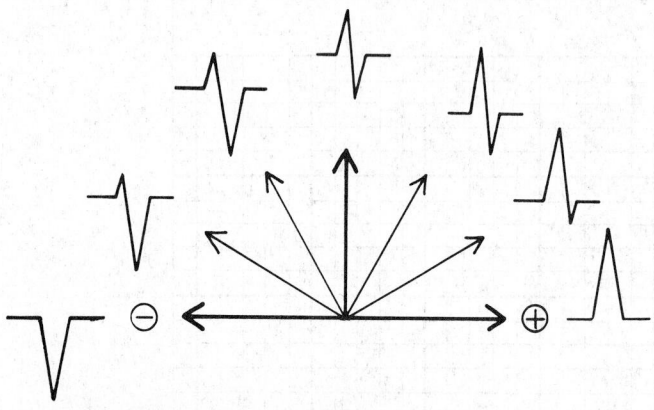

FIGURE 27-8 Several mean vectors and their resultant ECG complex. Especially note the following: (1) a mean current perpendicular to the lead axis produces an equiphasic deflection, and (2) a mean current parallel to the lead axis results in the tallest complex possible if the current flows toward the positive electrode and the deepest complex possible if the current flows toward the negative electrode. (From Conover MB: Understanding electrocardiography: arrhythmias and the 12-lead ECG, ed 5, St Louis, 1988, The CV Mosby Co.)

WAVES, COMPLEXES, AND INTERVALS

The waves recorded electrocardiographically have been arbitrarily designated by the letters *P, Q, R, S, T,* and *U* (Figure 27-7). A discussion of each wave will be presented after the basic concept of wave generation.

The baseline of the ECG tracing is known as the *isoelectric line* (Figure 27-8). Waves are deflections, either above (positive) or below (negative) the isoelectric line. The direction of deflection is determined by the following: (1) the direction in which the electrical impulse flows, (2) the distance between the source of the impulse and the exploring electrode, and (3) the site of the electrode. As a rule, when the flow of electrical current is directed toward the positive or exploring electrode, the deflection will be positive. Conversely, when the flow of electrical current is directed away from the positive electrode, the deflection will be negative. When the flow of electrical current is directed perpendicular to a line between the negative (or central) terminal and the positive electrode, either no deflection or a biphasic deflection occurs.

P Wave

The P wave represents the depolarization of the atria (Table 27-1). Normally the P wave is gently rounded, does not exceed 2 to 3 mm in amplitude, and is 0.11 second or less in duration. It is normally positive in leads I, II, aVF, and V_4 to V_6. It is negative in aVR and variable in all other leads. A P wave that does not comply with these criteria may be diagnostic of atrial en-

TABLE 27-1 Electrical activity of the heart and resultant ECG findings

Electrical Activity of Heart	ECG Events
SA node fires	Not recorded
Wave of depolarization spreads through atria	P wave
Slight pause at AV node	Isoelectric baseline between P wave and QRS complex
Atrial repolarization	Not recorded; overpowered by electrical activity of ventricles
Ventricular depolarization	QRS complex
Ventricular repolarization	T wave

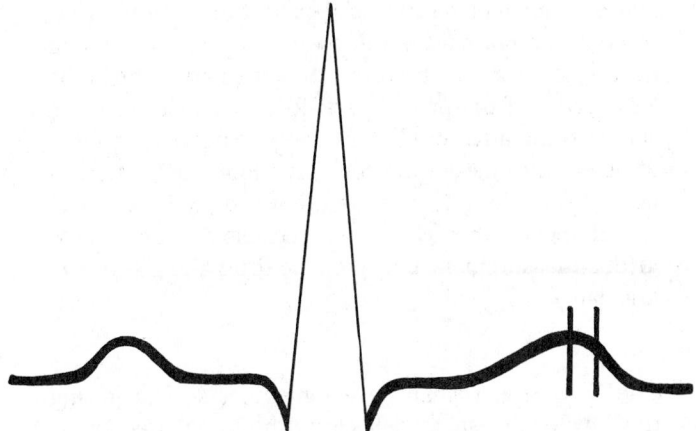

FIGURE 27-9 Approximate location of the vulnerable period. (From Conover MB: Understanding electrocardiography: arrhythmias and the 12-lead ECG, ed 5, St Louis, 1988, The CV Mosby Co.)

largement or hypertrophy or denote the presence of a pacemaker other than the sinoatrial (SA) node. Repolarization of the atria also produces a wave, but it is generally hidden within the QRS complex.

PR Interval

The PR interval is a measurement of the amount of time taken for the impulse to travel from the SA node to the ventricular musculature. It includes the normal physiologic delay of impulse conduction by the atrioventricular (AV) node. The interval is measured from the beginning of the P wave to the beginning of the QRS complex. Normally the PR interval measures from 0.12 to 0.20 second.

QRS Complex

The QRS complex represents depolarization of the ventricles and thus is often the most significant portion of the ECG. It is important to note that the Q, R, and S waves are separate waves and must be named correctly. If the first deflection from the isoelectric line is negative, it is a Q wave (Q waves are not always present). The first positive deflection from the isoelectric line is an R wave. The negative deflection following an R wave is an S wave. A small Q wave of less than 0.04-second duration is a normal finding in leads I, II, III, aVL, aVF, and V_4 to V_6. The full duration of the QRS complex is measured from the first deflection from the isoelectric line (whether it is a Q or an R wave) to the junction point (J-point). The *J-point* is where the QRS complex ends and the ST segment begins. The normal QRS complex is 0.05 to 0.10 second.

ST Segment

The ST segment represents the plateau (phase 2) of the action potential. It is normally isoelectric because no difference exists in electrical potential among the action potentials of the heart. No current flow occurs because

all cells are at zero potential. Normally there may be slight elevation not greater than 1 mm or subtle depression not greater than 0.5 mm. Abnormal elevations or depressions of the ST segment can occur as a result of derangement in the action potential. Some causes include myocardial muscle injury, conduction disturbances, preexcitation, hypertrophy, tachycardia, and digitalis effect.

T Wave

The T wave represents phase 3 of the action potential, when the ventricles are being rapidly repolarized. It is normally rounded, slightly asymmetric, and of the same polarity as the QRS complex. The height of the T wave should not exceed 5 mm in a limb lead or 10 mm in a precordial lead. It is normally a positive wave in leads I, II, and V_3 to V_6. The T wave is a negative deflection in lead aVR and variable in all other leads.

The effective refractory period is present during the beginning of the T wave. At the peak of the T wave, more of the fast sodium channels have recovered and therefore a stronger-than-normal stimulus can produce a successful action potential. However, some fibers are still unresponsive, and conduction velocity is very slow. Electrical chaos and subsequent ventricular fibrillation may occur. The approximate location of this vulnerable period is illustrated in Figure 27-9. Some causes of T wave abnormality include ischemia, ventricular hypertrophy, quinidine therapy, digitalis therapy, acid-base imbalance, hyperkalemia, and ventricular extrasystoles.

QT Interval

The QT interval is measured from the beginning of the QRS complex to the end of the T wave. It represents the entire duration of ventricular depolarization and repolarization. The normal QT value varies with age, sex, and heart rate. As a rule, however, the QT interval should be less than half the preceding R-R interval. Because the actual termination of the T wave is sometimes difficult to determine, measuring the QT interval accurately is not always easy. It is important, however, to be aware of any change in the QT interval because an abnormality in this measurement may indicate drug and electrolyte imbalances.

U Wave

The U wave is a small wave sometimes seen following the T wave. It usually deflects in the same direction as the T wave and is best seen in lead V_3. It has been suggested that the U wave represents late repolarization of papillary muscle. The U wave is affected by many drugs and conditions but is best known for its prominence in hypokalemia.

ELECTROCARDIOGRAPHIC SIGNAL AVERAGING

Signal averaging of the surface QRS complex is now being used to detect low-amplitude, high-frequency signals in the terminal portion of the QRS complex or in the early ST segment. It is a new, noninvasive, computerized method of analyzing standard ECGs that identifies patients at risk for ventricular tachycardia. Although late potentials have been reported in patients with ventricular tachycardia, the independent role of quantitative, signal-averaged variables alone or in combination with other diagnostic predictors of arrhythmogenesis has yet to be established.

Electrocardiographic signal averaging involves amplification of electrical signals from the heart that have a voltage too small to be recorded by a standard ECG. Ischemia and infarction can cause the extreme slowing of conduction that results in this delayed activity, which can be recognized in the terminal portion of the QRS complex or early portion of the ST segment. Typically, approximately 200 identical QRS complexes are grouped and averaged, resulting in a waveform that appears smooth and continuous. Signal averaging minimizes the level of noise that contaminates the ECG signal and thereby exposes signals of a microvolt level normally hidden within noise, such as skeletal muscle noise, especially from respiratory muscles, and noise from electrical equipment, amplifiers, and electrodes.

Equipment necessary to perform signal averaging includes ECG leads, an amplifier, an analog-digital converter, and a personal computer with software to average the QRS waveforms and store data. Patient interface with the electrodes is of primary importance for acquisition and analysis of data. Cleansing and mildly abrading the skin are necessary before attachment of the electrodes.

Probably the most significant contribution of the signal-averaged ECG will be in the management of patients after acute myocardial infarction (see Chapter 28). The rate of postinfarction sudden death precipitated by ventricular tachycardia that degenerates into ventricular fibrillation is approximately 10% to 15%; these deaths usually occur within 2 years after the myocardial infarction. Because of a 15% probability of developing prodysrhythmia, antiarrhythmic therapy for all patients after infarction is unwarranted and obviously may be harmful. Thus identification of these patients who will need treatment is critical for overall management.

TYPES OF CARDIAC DYSRHYTHMIAS

The term *dysrhythmia* (also called arrhythmia) refers to the presence of a heart rate and rhythm other than normal sinus rhythm. There are many types of dysrhythmias (Table 27-2), which are grouped in the following discussion according to anatomic origins. Abbreviations typically used to name specific dysrhythmias are listed in the box below. The mechanisms that underlie the dysrhythmias are discussed before the specific dysrhythmias.

ARRHYTHMOGENIC MECHANISMS

Most dysrhythmias are believed to be caused by (1) abnormalities in *impulse formation* because of (a) altered automaticity (enhanced or abnormal automaticity) or (b) triggered activity (early or delayed afterdepolarizations), (2) abnormalities of *conduction* caused by a block or reentry, or (3) a combination of these. The following is a brief discussion of these mechanisms.

ALTERED AUTOMATICITY

Cardiac cells are able to maintain an electrical potential across their cell membranes. When an impulse of sufficient magnitude that exceeds their threshold potential arrives, these cells depolarize. Some cardiac cells have

---

ABBREVIATIONS DENOTING CARDIAC DYSRHYTHMIAS

SSS	Sick sinus syndrome
PAB	Premature atrial beat
PAT	Paroxysmal atrial tachycardia
PJB	Premature junctional beat
SVT	Supraventricular tachycardia
PVB	Premature ventricular beat
VT	Ventricular tachycardia
RBBB	Right bundle branch block
LBBB	Left bundle branch block
LAH	Left anterior hemiblock
LPH	Left posterior hemiblock

TABLE 27-2 Comparison of selected cardiac dysrhythmias

Dysrhythmia	Description	Etiology	Symptoms/Consequences	Treatment
DYSRHYTHMIAS OF SINUS NODE				
Sinus dysrhythmia	Phasic shortening then lengthening of P-P and R-R interval	Respiratory variation in impulse initiation by SA node	Usually none	Usually none
Sinus tachycardia	P waves present followed by QRS Rhythm regular Heart rate 100-150 beats/min	Increased metabolic demands Decreased oxygen delivery, congestive heart failure, shock, hemorrhage, anemia	May produce palpitations Prolonged episodes may lead to decreased cardiac output	Treat underlying cause Occasionally sedatives
Sinus bradycardia	P waves present Rhythm regular Heart rate <60	Physical fitness Parasympathetic stimulation (sleep) Brain lesions Sinus dysfunction Digitalis excess	Very low rates may cause decreased cardiac output: light-headedness, faintness, chest pain	Atropine if cardiac output is decreased Pacemaker Treat underlying cause if necessary
ATRIAL DYSRHYTHMIAS				
Premature atrial beats	Early P wave QRS may or may not be normal Rhythm irregular	Stress, ischemia, atrial enlargement, caffeine, nicotine	May produce palpitations Frequent episodes may decrease cardiac output Is sign of chamber irritability	Sedation Quinidine May require no treatment
Atrial tachycardia	P wave present (may merge into previous T wave), QRS usually normal, rapid heart rate usually >150/min	Sympathetic stimulation, chemical stimuli (caffeine, nicotine), drug toxicity	Palpitations Possible anxiety	Usually none Prolonged episodes may require carotid sinus pressure, vagal stimulation, verapamil, digitalis, or beta blockers
Atrial fibrillation	Rapid, irregular waves (> 350/min) Ventricular rhythm irregularly irregular Ventricular rate varies, may increase to 120-150/min if untreated	Rheumatic heart disease Mitral stenosis Atrial infarction Coronary atherosclerotic heart disease Hypertensive heart disease Thyrotoxicosis	Pulse deficit Decreased cardiac output if rate is rapid Promotes thrombus formation in atria	Digitalis Quinidine Cardioversion
VENTRICULAR DYSRHYTHMIAS				
Premature ventricular beats (PVBs)	Early wide bizarre QRS, not associated with a P wave Rhythm irregular	Stress, acidosis, ventricular enlargement Electrolyte imbalance Myocardial infarction Digitalis toxicity Hypoxemia, hypercapnia	Same as for premature atrial beats	Procainamide Quinidine Disopyramide (Norpace) Lidocaine Oxygen Sodium bicarbonate Potassium Treat congestive heart failure
Ventricular tachycardia	No P wave before QRS; QRS wide and bizarre; ventricular rate >100, usually 140-240	PVB striking during vulnerable period; hypoxemia; drug toxicity; electrolyte imbalance; bradycardia	Decreased cardiac output, hypotension, loss of consciousness, respiratory arrest	Lidocaine Procainamide Bretylium Cardioversion

Continued.

TABLE 27-2 Comparison of selected cardiac dysrhythmias—cont'd

Dysrhythmia	Description	Etiology	Symptoms/Consequences	Treatment
VENTRICULAR DYSRHYTHMIAS—cont'd				
Ventricular fibrillation	Chaotic electrical activity No recognizable QRS complex	Myocardial infarction Electrocution Freshwater drowning Drug toxicity	No cardiac output Absent pulse or respiration Cardiac arrest	Defibrillation Epinephrine Sodium bicarbonate Bretylium CPR
Ventricular standstill	Can be distinguished from ventricular fibrillation only by ECG P waves *may* be present No QRS "Straight line"	Myocardial infarction Chronic diseases of conducting system	Same as for ventricular fibrillation	CPR Pacemaker Intracardiac epinephrine Isoproterenol
IMPULSE CONDUCTION DEFICITS				
First-degree atrioventricular (AV) block	PR interval prolonged, >0.20 sec	Rheumatic fever Digitalis toxicity Degenerative changes of coronary atherosclerotic heart disease Infections Decreased oxygen in AV node	Warns of impaired conduction	Usually none as long as it occurs as an isolated deficit
Bundle branch block	Same as normal sinus rhythm (NSR) except QRS duration >0.10	Hypoxia, acute myocardial infarction, congestive heart failure, coronary atherosclerotic heart disease, pulmonary embolus, hypertension	Same as first-degree AV block	Usually none unless severe blockage of left posterior division (see text)
Second-degree AV blocks	P waves usually occur regularly at rates consistent with SA node initiation. (Not all P waves followed by QRS; PR interval may lengthen before nonconducted P wave or may be consistent; QRS may be widened.)	Acute myocardial infarction	Serious dysrhythmia which may lead to decreased heart rate and cardiac output	May require temporary pacemaker
Complete third-degree AV block	Atria and ventricles beat independently P waves have no relation to QRS Ventricular rate may be as low as 20-40/min	Digitalis toxicity Infectious disease Coronary artery disease Myocardial infarction	Very low rates may cause decreased cardiac output: light-headedness, faintness, chest pain	Pacemaker Isoproterenol to increase heart rate Epinephrine if isoproterenol ineffective

the additional property of *automaticity* (ability to depolarize spontaneously without external stimulation). Control of the cardiac conduction system belongs to the cells with the most rapid, spontaneous depolarization, normally those of the *sinus node*. The rate of discharge of the sinus node may be altered by any condition that enhances automaticity or causes automaticity to be abnormal.

Automaticity is enhanced if phase 4 accelerates in latent pacemaker cells, that is, those below the SA node. Premature beats or tachycardia of atrial, junctional, or ventricular origin may occur. Some causes for this ac-

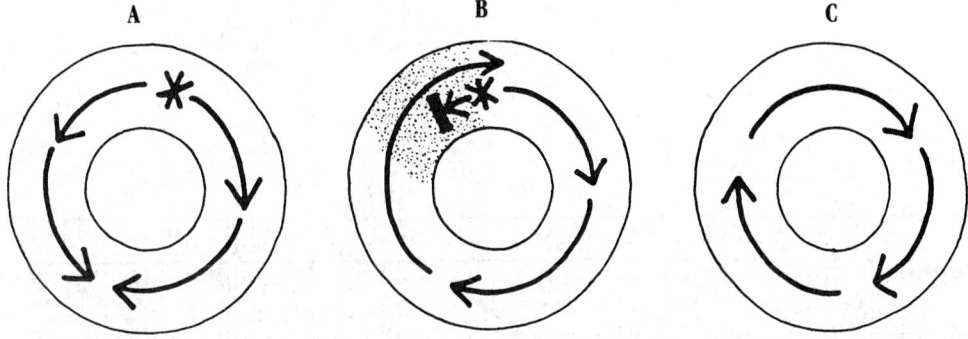

FIGURE 27- 10 Mechanism of reentry. In **(A)** the impulses travel from the stimulus in opposite directions around the ring to meet and cancel each other out. In **(B)** pressure has been applied at the shaded area in the ring, at which point the impulse is blocked and travels only in the opposite direction. Pressure is then removed, and the impulse continues around and around **(C)** on its one-way journey as long as refractory tissue is not encountered. (From Marriott HJL and Conover MB: Advanced concepts in arrhythmias, ed 2, St Louis, 1989, The CV Mosby Co.)

celeration include hypoxia, catecholamines, hypokalemia, hypocalcemia, atropine, heat, trauma, and digitalis toxicity.

Abnormal automaticity may occur in both pacemaker and nonpacemaker cells. Usually a significantly reduced membrane exists (−60 mV) so that resulting dysrhythmias are not easily suppressed. Causes of reduced membrane potential include ischemia, infarction, hypokalemia, hypocalcemia, and cardiomyopathy.

TRIGGERED ACTIVITY (LATE POTENTIALS)

Triggered activity refers to repetitive ectopic firing, which is the result of afterdepolarizations. These afterdepolarizations occur either during or after repolarization; thus they are not the same as altered automaticity and are not sustained by a reentry circuit. It is only when the afterdepolarization achieves threshold potential that triggered activity results. The afterdepolarization may reach threshold because of a shortening of the cycle length or increased levels of catecholamines. Researchers have demonstrated not only that a relationship exists between this delayed activation and ventricular dysrhythmias, but also that this delayed activation represents the substrate for reentry ventricular tachycardia.[7,22]

REENTRY

Reentry occurs when an impulse is delayed long enough within a pathway of slow conduction that it is still viable when the remaining myocardium repolarizes. The impulse then reenters surrounding tissue and produces another impulse. The initiating impulse may either be normal sinus or ectopic (Figure 27-10). One-way conduction is necessary because without it the impulse would cancel itself out within the area of slow conduction. Any condition that decreases the amplitude of the action potential, such as ischemia, hypercalcemia, or calcification of the conducting fibers, can cause cardiac conduction disturbance, resulting in either heart block or a reentry rhythm.

DYSRHYTHMIAS ORIGINATING IN SINOATRIAL NODE

SINUS DYSRHYTHMIA

Sinus dysrhythmia is the most frequently noted dysrhythmia. It is typically found in young adults and the elderly. The P waves are of sinus origin and have a constant morphology. The PR intervals are within normal limits and constant. The P-P or R-R intervals vary by at least 0.16 second (Figure 27-11).

There are two forms of sinus dysrhythmia, respiratory and nonphasic. In the respiratory form the cyclic pattern of changing P-P or R-R intervals correlates with the patterns of inspiration and expiration. During inspiration the intervals shorten as the heart rate increases. Conversely, the intervals lengthen during expiration. This phenomenon results from a reflex inhibition of vagal tone, an enhancement of sympathetic tone, or both. Its occurrence is favored by slower heart rates and ingestion of drugs, such as digitalis, that enhance vagal tone. The nonphasic form has no correlation to respiration. It may be caused by vagal stimulation from other vagally innervated organs.

Sinus dysrhythmia is a benign rhythm that usually requires no treatment. With slower heart rates, some patients may experience palpitations or dizziness if the P-P intervals are unusually long. In such cases, exercise or medications that increase the heart rate will abolish the dysrhythmia.

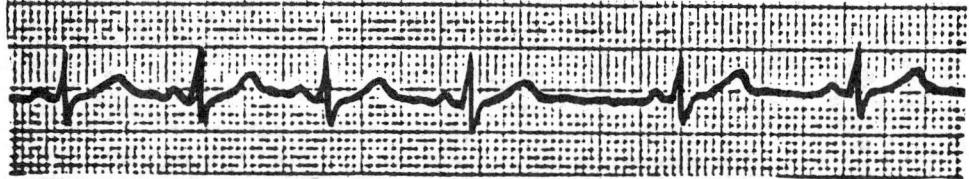

FIGURE 27-11 Sinus dysrhythmia. Lead II showing atrial and ventricular rate, 78 to 58 beats/minute, irregular rhythm; PR interval, 0.16 second; and QRS complex, 0.08 second.

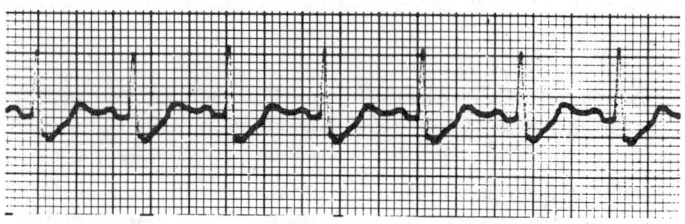

FIGURE 27-12 Sinus tachycardia. Lead II showing heart rate of 115 beats/minute, regular rhythm, normal PR interval, and normal QRS duration.

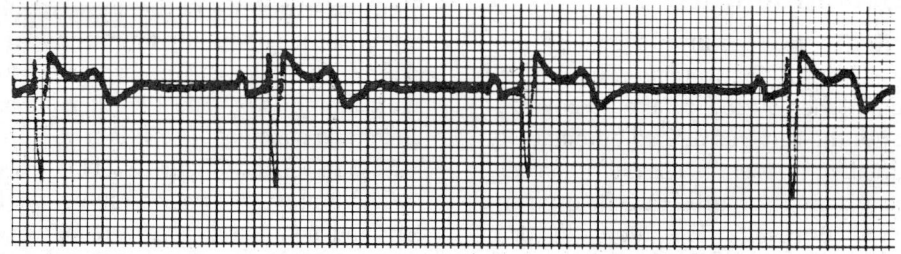

FIGURE 27-13 Sinus bradycardia. Lead V_1 showing heart rate of approximately 44 beats/minute, regular rhythm, normal PR interval, and normal QRS duration.

V_1

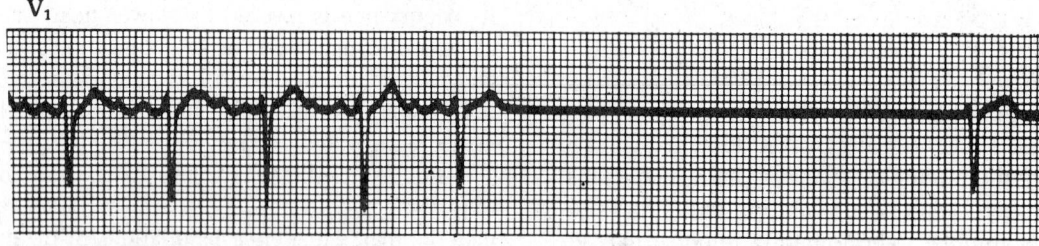

FIGURE 27-14 Sick sinus syndrome (SSS) caused by bradycardia/tachycardia. (From Marriott HJL and Conover MB: Advanced concepts in arrhythmias, ed 2, St Louis, 1989, The CV Mosby Co.)

SINUS TACHYCARDIA

Sinus tachycardia (Figure 27-12) is characterized by an atrial and ventricular rate of 100 beats/minutes or more. Generally the upper limit with sinus tachycardia is 160/minute, but the rate may increase to 200 under extreme exertion. The P waves are sinus in origin, but they may appear more peaked than usual with very high rates. Intervals and complexes are within normal limits. A QRS complex follows each P wave. The onset of sinus tachycardia is gradual.

Sinus tachycardia is associated with the ingestion of alcohol, tea, coffee, or tobacco. It is a normal physiologic response to exertion, fever, fear, excitement, or any condition that requires a higher basal metabolism. Clinically, it is a short-term compensatory mechanism associated with heart failure, hypovolemia, and hypotension. It is also often seen with hyperthyroidism and may be produced by drugs such as atropine, epinephrine, and isoproterenol.

Generally, sinus tachycardia is a benign rhythm. The patient may complain of palpitations or be asymptomatic. In the patient with a compromised myocardium, the tachycardia may cause a decrease in cardiac output with resultant lightheadedness and heart failure. Treatment is directed toward correction of the underlying cause.

SINUS BRADYCARDIA

Sinus bradycardia (Figure 27-13) is characterized by atrial and ventricular rates of less than 60 beats/minute. It should be noted that some researchers use a rate of 50 or below as an indication of bradycardia. In all other respects, sinus bradycardia has the normal parameters for sinus rhythm. It may develop gradually or occur suddenly for a brief period.

Bradycardia generally results from increased vagal tone or decreased sympathetic tone. It is frequently seen in the elderly and in athletes. It is associated with sleep, vomiting, eye surgery, intracranial tumors, and myocardial infarction. Carotid sinus stimulation and parasympathomimetic drugs induce sinus bradycardia in many patients.

Generally, sinus bradycardia is a benign rhythm. Often in association with myocardial infarction, it is a beneficial rhythm because it reduces myocardial oxygen demand. If the heart rate is too slow to maintain adequate cardiac output, the patient may be predisposed to syncope and congestive heart failure. Administration of atropine or isoproterenol is usually effective in increasing the heart rate. The patient with refractory bradycardia who is symptomatic may require a permanent implantable pacemaker (see p. 657).

SICK SINUS SYNDROME

Sick sinus syndrome (SSS) is a term describing several clinical disorders of SA node function. The SA node dysfunction is often accompanied by depressed automaticity of lower pacemakers (for example, AV junction) as well as conduction disturbances in the atria, AV node, bundle branches, or ventricles.

The *tachycardia-bradycardia syndrome* is the most common type of SSS (Figure 27-14). Typically, it is characterized by the presence of a sinus bradycardia with intermittent episodes of atrial tachydysrhythmias. The episode of tachydysrhythmia is often followed by a long pause before returning to sinus bradycardia. Complications of this inefficient rhythm include congestive heart failure and cerebrovascular accidents resulting from thromboembolisms. In addition, cerebral blood flow may be decreased, producing symptoms similar to senility in the elderly person.

Some patients may remain asymptomatic or complain only of palpitations. For the severely symptomatic patient, the heart rhythm should be stabilized by the use of a permanent implantable pacemaker.

DYSRHYTHMIAS ORIGINATING IN ATRIA
PREMATURE ATRIAL BEAT

The premature atrial beat (PAB) is initiated by an ectopic focus in the atria (Figure 27-15). It is characterized by a premature P wave with a contour different from that of a sinus P wave. The QRS complex may or may not be normal, and the PAB is followed by a pause approximately equal to the sinus cycle (measured R to R). The atrial impulse may be nonconducted (blocked) because of refractoriness of the ventricles at the time the impulse arrives. The nonconducted atrial beat (blocked PAB) is the most common cause of irregularities in the heart rhythm.

The PAB may be associated with stress or the use of caffeine or tobacco products. It is also seen in the clinical setting with infection, inflammation, and myocardial ischemia. Frequent PABs may warn of impending atrial fibrillation or tachycardia.

In the absence of organic disease, no treatment is required. Often the omission of caffeine and tobacco will suppress the atrial focus. If symptoms are present or organic disease is known, PABs may be suppressed by digitalis, quinidine, or procainamide.

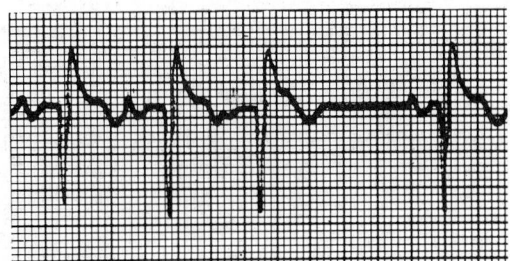

FIGURE 27-15 Premature atrial beat (PAB). Lead V_1 showing third beat is PAB with abnormal early P wave followed by normal QRS complex.

V₁

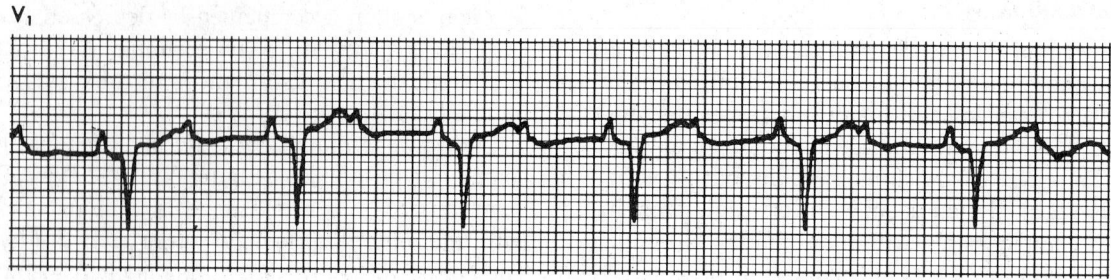

FIGURE 27-16 Atrial tachycardia (130 beats/minute) with 2:1 AV conduction. (From Conover MB: Cardiac arrhythmias, ed 2, St Louis, 1978, The CV Mosby Co.)

ATRIAL TACHYCARDIA

In atrial tachycardia the atrial rate is approximately 150 to 250 beats/minute. In contrast to atrial flutter or fibrillation, P waves are present but may be hidden in the T waves of the preceding beats when the ventricular rate is high. The QRS complex is generally normal, and the ventricular rate is regular.

When atrial tachycardia occurs suddenly, it is called *paroxysmal atrial tachycardia* (PAT). Transient episodes of PAT may occur in children and young adults in the absence of heart disease. When underlying disease is present, it is usually rheumatic heart disease.

The patient may complain of palpitations and experience anxiety during a tachycardic episode. Short, infrequent episodes require no treatment. Generally, hemodynamic changes are not severe unless the episode is persistent, the rate is greater than 200/minute, or underlying disease exists. Lengthy paroxysms may require carotid sinus pressure, vagal stimulation, or intravenous administration of verapamil, digitalis, or beta blockers to slow the rate or restore sinus rhythm. Some patients may benefit from receiving instruction in the performance of Valsalva's maneuver to cause slowing of the rate. Digitalis and propranolol are the drugs of choice if vagal stimulation is unsuccessful. Should hypotension or congestive heart failure (CHF) complicate the dysrhythmia, cardioversion is indicated.

Atrial tachycardia *with block* (see p. 649) is characterized by the same rapid atrial rate. The AV nodal conduction ratio is usually 2:1, producing a ventricular rate of 75 to 125/minute (Figure 27-16). This dysrhythmia is associated with organic heart disease. Digitalis toxicity and potassium depletion in the patient receiving digitalis are two conditions that also favor its development. The treatment depends on the clinical picture and is often aimed at correcting the underlying cause.

ATRIAL FLUTTER

The hallmark of atrial flutter is the presence of a saw-tooth pattern of rapid atrial activity (Figure 27-17). The atria depolarize at a rate of 250 to 350 beats/minute. The atrial depolarizations produce flutter (F) waves that give the baseline a sawtooth appearance. The QRS configurations are normal. There is no true PR interval because it is often difficult to determine electrocardiographically which atrial impulse is actually conducted to the ventricles. Physiologically the AV node generally prevents conduction of each atrial impulse to the ventricles although increased conduction may occur in hyperthyroidism. Despite this protective mechanism, the ventricular rate is often greater than 150/minute if untreated (2:1 conduction).

Atrial flutter is seen less often than atrial fibrillation but usually indicates underlying disease. It is associated most frequently with coronary atherosclerotic heart disease (CAHD), pulmonary embolism, mitral valve disease, and thoracic surgical procedures.

The potentially rapid ventricular rate of atrial flutter

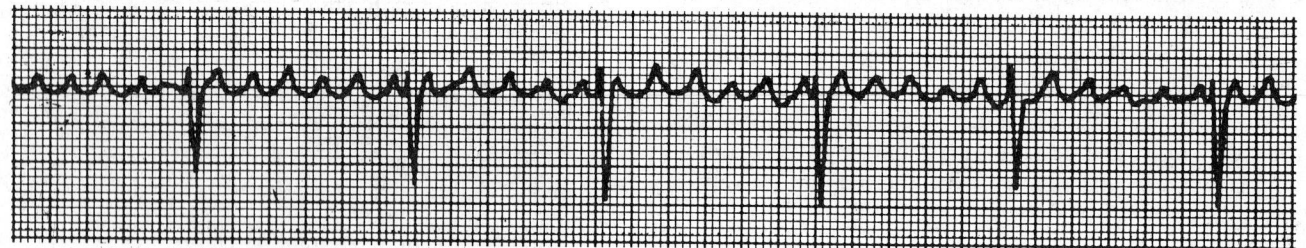

FIGURE 27-17 Atrial flutter (lead V₁). Rate of atrial flutter waves is 300 beats/minute. Ventricular rate is 50 to 75/minute.

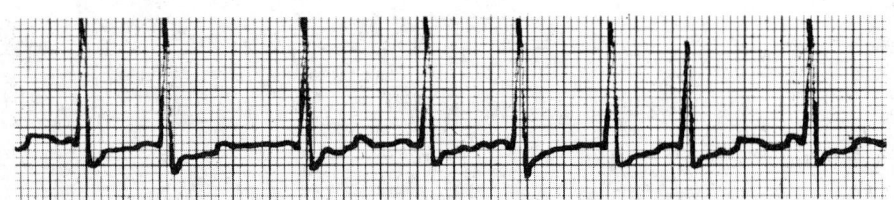

FIGURE 27-18 Atrial fibrillation (lead II). Atrial rate is rapid with varying conduction to ventricles, irregular rhythm, normal QRS complex, no definite P waves visible, and PR interval not measurable.

may result in a decrease in cardiac output. The major goal of treatment is conversion to sinus rhythm or control of the ventricular rate. Direct current cardioversion (see p. 659) is the treatment of choice in the patient with an acute myocardial infarction to protect an already compensated myocardium from the metabolic demands of rapid contractions.

Cardioversion is highly successful in converting atrial flutter to sinus rhythm, often with 50 watt-seconds (joules) or less. If cardioversion is unsuccessful or if atrial flutter is recurrent, digitalis usually succeeds in slowing the ventricular rate by lengthening AV nodal conduction time. In some cases the addition of quinidine, procainamide, or propranolol to digitalis therapy may result in conversion to sinus rhythm. Atrial pacing may be used in patients for whom pharmacologic and external cardioversion methods have been unsuccessful.

ATRIAL FIBRILLATION

Atrial fibrillation (Figure 27-18) is the most rapid of atrial dysrhythmias. The atria beat chaotically at rates of 350 to 600 beats/minute. The baseline is characteristically composed of irregular undulations without definable P waves. The QRS complex is usually normal, but the ventricular rhythm is irregularly irregular. If untreated, the ventricular rate will generally be 100 to 180/ minute.

Atrial fibrillation may be paroxysmal and transient, or it may be chronic. The latter generally indicates underlying heart disease. It is typically associated with pericarditis, thyrotoxicosis, cardiomyopathy, CAHD, hypertensive heart disease, and rheumatic mitral valve disease. Its development is also related to atrial infarction.

Because of ventricular rhythm irregularity and the loss of synchronous atrial contractions *(atrial kick),* cardiac output is decreased and a pulse deficit often exists. In the presence of mitral stenosis, thrombi may form in the atria and cause embolisms affecting the lungs or periphery. The goal of therapy is to prevent these complications through the control of the ventricular rate and the use of anticoagulants in certain patients.

The treatment for atrial fibrillation depends on the circumstances. Often, correction of the underlying con-

dition will convert the rhythm to sinus rhythm. If the patient's condition deteriorates hemodynamically with symptoms of CHF and hypotension, immediate intervention with cardioversion is highly successful. Cardioversion is contraindicated in several conditions, including digitalis toxicity, AV block, and SSS. If the patient is hemodynamically stable, digitalis is the drug of choice. Propranolol may be added to the regimen. The goal is to attain a resting heart rate of 60 to 80 beats/minute or restoration of sinus rhythm. The patient must be monitored for heart rate and blood pressure until stable.

DYSRHYTHMIAS ORIGINATING IN ATRIOVENTRICULAR JUNCTION
PREMATURE JUNCTIONAL BEATS

The premature junctional beat (PJB) arises from an ectopic focus either (1) at the junction of atrial and AV nodal tissue or (2) at the junction of AV nodal tissue and the bundle of His. If the PJB arises from the first junction, the P wave will be inverted, premature, and precede the QRS complex. In the second case, the P wave is either hidden in the QRS or is inverted and follows the QRS (Figure 27-19). The abnormal timing and the inversion of the P wave are caused by depolarization of the atria in a retrograde fashion. The QRS is normal, but the PR or RP (when P waves follow the QRS) interval is less than 0.12 second.

PJBs may occur in the normal heart. They are also associated with CHF and digitalis toxicity. Treatment, when needed, is directed toward correcting the underlying cause. Quinidine, propranolol, and procainamide may suppress PJBs. Phenytoin (Dilantin) is particularly useful in the suppression of PJBs secondary to digitalis toxicity.

JUNCTIONAL RHYTHMS

When the SA node fires at a rate less than 40 to 60 beats/minute, the automatic cells in the AV junction may initiate impulses (escape beats) to stabilize the rhythm. If a single junctional escape beat occurs, the cycle length is longer than the longest sinus cycle. A succession of beats from the junction is a *junctional escape rhythm.*

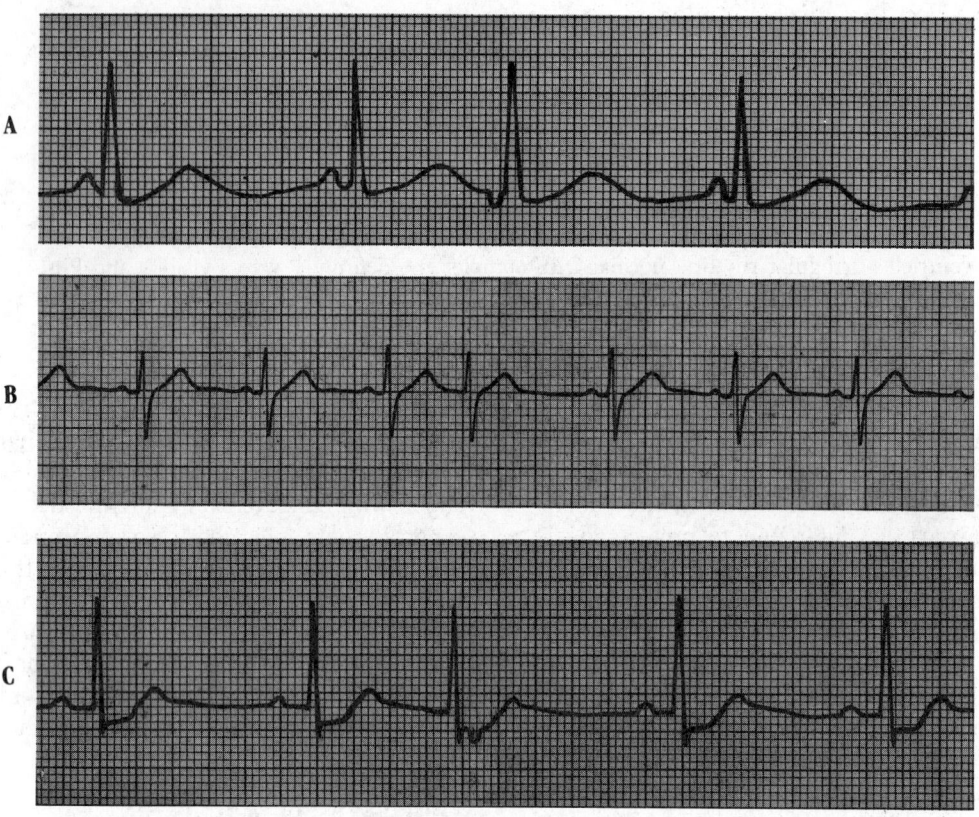

FIGURE 27- 19 Premature junctional beats (PJBs). **A,** Inverted P wave (third QRS complex). **B,** P wave hidden in fourth QRS complex. **C,** P wave follows third QRS complex. (From Conover, MB: Understanding electrocardiography: arrhythmias and the 12-lead ECG, ed 5, St Louis, 1988, The CV Mosby Co.)

The P waves may occur before, during, or after the QRS. The QRS is normal, and the ventricular rhythm is regular. Junctional escape rhythm is occasionally found in the well-trained athlete with sinus bradycardia. It is also found when sinus bradycardia complicates an acute inferior wall myocardial infarction. Junctional escape rhythm is generally not treated unless the loss of atrial kick produces symptoms of low cardiac output. In such a case, the patient may require artificial pacing.

When the automaticity of a junctional pacemaker increases to a rate greater than 60/minute, it may usurp the SA node as the pacemaker of the heart. At a rate of 60 to 100/minute, the rhythm is called *accelerated* junctional rhythm.

A *junctional tachycardia* exists when the rate exceeds 100/minute. Junctional tachycardia is associated with digitalis toxicity, acute inferior myocardial infarction, acute rheumatic fever, and open heart surgical procedures. Digitalis is the drug of choice to slow the ventricular rate. If digitalis toxicity is present, phenytoin or propranolol is effective.

Junctional tachycardia may occur paroxysmally. Be-

cause of the rate, it is often difficult to distinguish it from PAT. Both premature junctional tachycardia and PAT are often referred to as supraventricular tachycardia (SVT), indicating that the rhythm originates above the ventricles (Figure 27-20).

DYSRHYTHMIAS ORIGINATING IN VENTRICLES
PREMATURE VENTRICULAR BEATS

The premature ventricular beat (PVB) arises from an ectopic focus in the ventricles. The characteristic wide, bizarre QRS (usually greater than 0.12 second) makes the PVB readily identifiable on the ECG tracing (Figure 27-21). There is no associated P wave preceding the QRS complex, and the T wave is in the opposite direction from the main QRS deflection. Most PVBs are followed by a compensatory pause such that the interval from the beat preceding to the beat following the PVB is equal to two sinus cycles.

If several PVBs of different configuration are noted in an ECG tracing, they are said to be *multiform*. This indicates the presence of more than one ectopic focus in the ventricles or one ectopic focus but multiple reentry

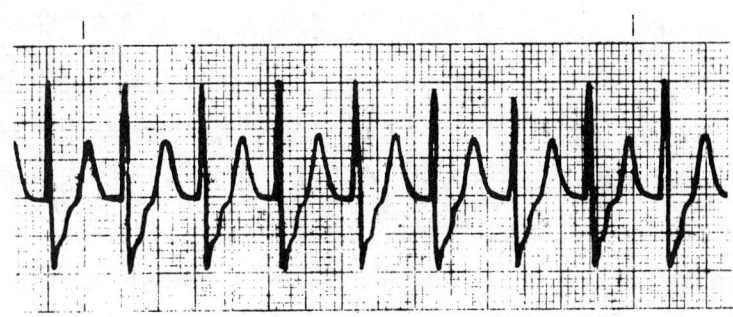

FIGURE 27-20 Supraventricular tachycardia (SVT). Origin is atrial or junctional. If P waves are present, they are not visualized; they may be present in preceding T wave.

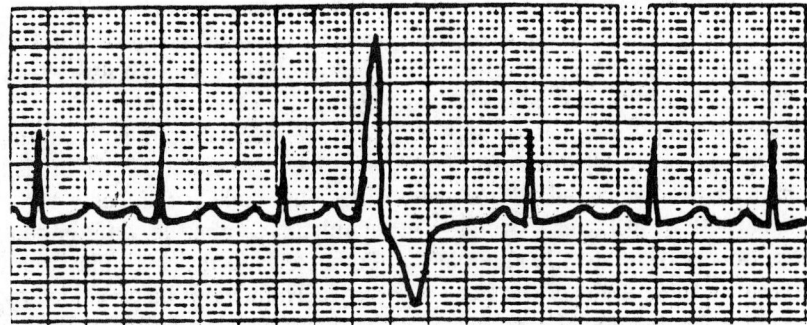

FIGURE 27-21 Premature ventricular beat (PVB). Lead II showing fourth beat is a PVB with wide early QRS complex; no P wave associated with beat.

pathways within the ventricle, thus producing complexes of differing forms. PVBs may also have various degrees of prematurity. It is important to note the relationship of the PVB to the Q, R, S, and T waves of the preceding beat. Remember that an electrical impulse of any kind that stimulates the heart near the peak of the T wave (vulnerable period; see Figure 27-9) may precipitate a more dangerous or lethal dysrhythmia.

Even in the absence of heart disease, PVBs occur often and increase in number with a person's age. The incidence and frequency of occurrence are higher, however, for the population with heart disease. The patient with an acute myocardial infarction must be monitored closely for the presence of PVBs. Clinically, PVBs are also associated with CHF, digitalis toxicity, and electrolyte imbalances. In the latter cases treatment of the underlying cause may abolish the dysrhythmia. Pharmacologic suppression of PVBs is most often accomplished with lidocaine, procainamide, quinidine, or disopyramide.

PVBs occurring in conjunction with an acute myocardial infarction may lead to more serious dysrhythmias and must be suppressed. Lidocaine is an intravenous preparation that is a first-line choice for immediate

suppression of ventricular irritability. After initial suppression, PVBs may be controlled on a long-term basis with the oral antiarrhythmics. Most authors agree that in the face of an acute myocardial infarction, PVBs should be treated if they (1) are greater than 5/minute, (2) fall in the vulnerable period (known as the R-on-T phenomenon), (3) are multiform, (4) occur in pairs or multiples, or (5) are accompanied by a history of ventricular tachycardia or fibrillation.[4]

VENTRICULAR RHYTHMS AND TACHYCARDIA

If the SA node and AV junction fail to initiate impulses, a ventricular pacemaking cell will automatically begin to initiate impulses at an inherent rate of 20 to 40 beats/minute. This is known as *idioventricular* rhythm.

If the rate of the ventricular-initiated rhythm increases to 40 to 100/minute, it is known as an *accelerated* idioventricular rhythm (commonly misnomered slow ventricular tachycardia). It may be seen in digitalis toxicity or as a complication of an acute myocardial infarction. Generally, neither of these rhythms is treated except to correct underlying abnormalities. Suppression of the heart's dominant and perhaps only rhythm could be hazardous. If the cardiac output is low and symp-

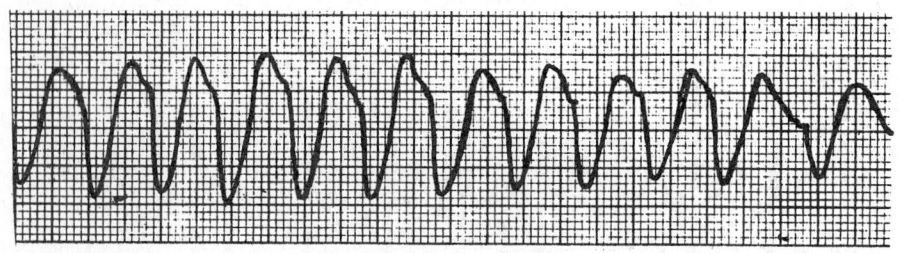

FIGURE 27-22 Ventricular tachycardia at a rate of approximately 150 beats/minute; rhythm is slightly irregular.

toms of CHF, syncope, or hypotension develop, the patient may require temporary or permanent artificial pacing. Atropine may also be helpful in stimulating the return of SA node activity.

By definition, three or more successive PVBs constitute *ventricular tachycardia* (Figure 27-22). The ventricular rate is greater than 100/minute and is usually 140 to 240. The rhythm is regular or slightly irregular. P waves may be present but are not associated with the QRS complexes. Ventricular tachycardia may complicate any form of heart disease and be a direct result of a PVB striking during the heart's vulnerable period. Conditions that favor its occurrence include hypoxemia, drug toxicity, electrolyte imbalance, and bradycardia. Some patients may tolerate ventricular tachycardia without loss of consciousness, particularly if the heart rate is closer to 100/minute. If the patient remains stable, treatment may include intravenous lidocaine, procainamide, or bretylium to break the tachycardia. If pharmacologic measures are unsuccessful, the alternative is cardioversion.

Because of the high ventricular rates and the loss of atrial kick, other patients may experience severe hypotension, loss of consciousness, and respiratory arrest. CPR should be administered immediately until emergency defibrillation can be performed. Once conversion to sinus rhythm is accomplished, intravenous lidocaine is generally administered to prevent recurrence. Maintenance suppression is obtained with oral antiarrhythmics.

VENTRICULAR FIBRILLATION AND STANDSTILL

In ventricular fibrillation the ventricles twitch chaotically, much as the atria do in atrial fibrillation. The ECG tracing consists of a bumpy line of unidentifiable waves (Figure 27-23). The fibrillatory waves may be coarse (as pictured) or fine (smooth).

In ventricular standstill (asystole) the ECG tracing is a flat line. No electrical activity is noted; all pacemaking cells have failed. Clinically, ventricular fibrillation and standstill cannot be differentiated without the ECG. Both are fatal dysrhythmias requiring immediate measures. The patient has no blood pressure, pulse, or audible heartbeat; respirations quickly cease. CPR must be instituted immediately and defibrillation performed within 1 minute to prevent biochemical derangements that further compromise the patient.

Coarse ventricular fibrillation is most likely to respond to defibrillation. Intracardiac administration of epinephrine or intravenous isoproterenol (Isuprel) and calcium is useful in producing a positive response to defibrillation of fine fibrillation or standstill. Unfortunately, the patient most vulnerable to these dysrhythmias has suffered an acute myocardial infarction complicated by CHF. Because of these factors, resuscitation efforts are less likely to be successful.

CONDUCTION ABNORMALITIES
ATRIOVENTRICULAR BLOCK

A block to conduction of an impulse may occur at any point along the conduction pathways. One common

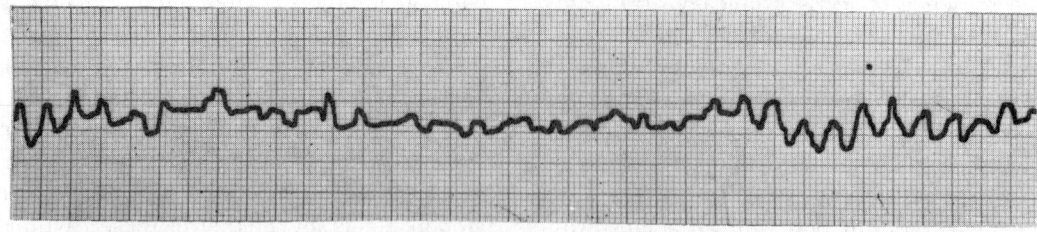

FIGURE 27-23 Ventricular fibrillation (lead II). Rate is rapid, rhythm irregular, no QRS complexes, and no definite P waves visible. Tracing shows electrical chaos in myocardium.

area of block is the atrioventricular (AV) junction. The severity of the block is identified by degrees; first-, second-, or third-degree AV block.

First-degree AV block is present when the PR interval is prolonged to greater than 0.20 second, indicating a conduction delay in the AV node (Figure 27-24). It is usually found in association with rheumatic fever, digitalis toxicity, and the degenerative changes of CAHD in the conducting tissue. When a first-degree AV block occurs as an isolated defect, no treatment is necessary.

Second-degree AV block may be divided into two categories. Type I (Wenckebach or Mobitz I) is character-

ized by a PR interval that progressively lengthens until a P wave is not followed by a QRS complex (Figure 27-25). The nonconducted beat is the result of the arrival of the impulse during the refractory period of the AV node. The ratio of P waves to QRS complexes may be 5:4, 4:3, 3:2, or 2:1. Any drug that slows AV conduction may cause a type I block, but such blocks are most often seen in the patient with an acute inferior wall myocardial infarction. Type I blocks are often transient and reversible. Generally, no treatment is required unless the patient becomes symptomatic because of the slow ventricular rate induced by 2:1 conduction.

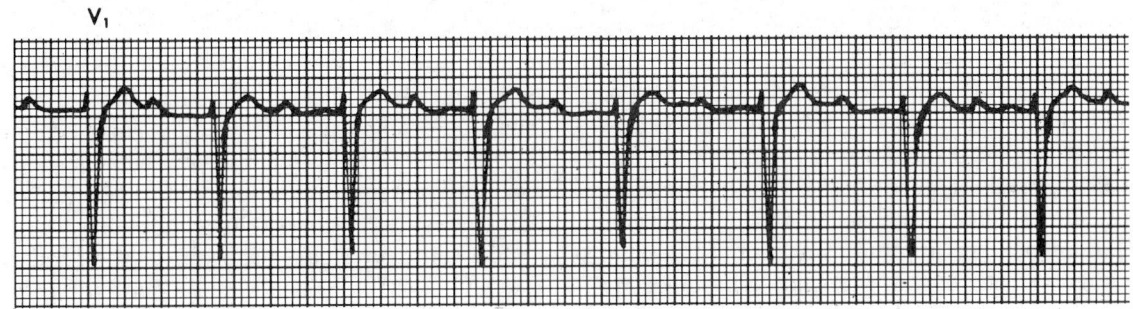

FIGURE 27-24 First-degree AV block. PR interval is an overlong 0.33 second. (From Conover MB: Cardiac arrhythmias, ed 2, St Louis, 1978, The CV Mosby Co.)

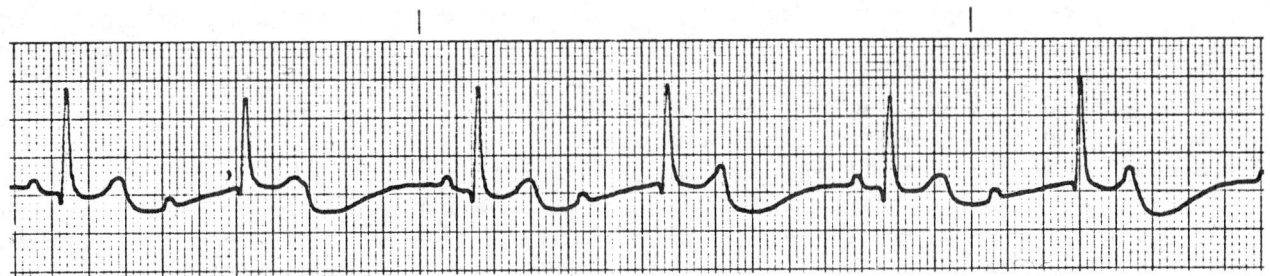

FIGURE 27-25 Second-degree AV block, type I (Wenckebach). Every third P wave is hidden in preceding T wave; conduction is 3:2. Note progressive lengthening of PR interval before dropped QRS complex.

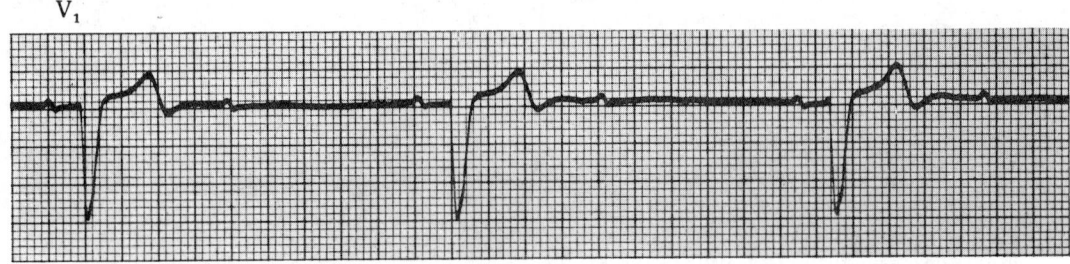

FIGURE 27-26 Second-degree AV block, type II with 2:1 conduction. (From Conover MB: Understanding electrocardiography: arrhythmias and the 12-lead ECG, ed 5, St Louis, 1988, The CV Mosby Co.)

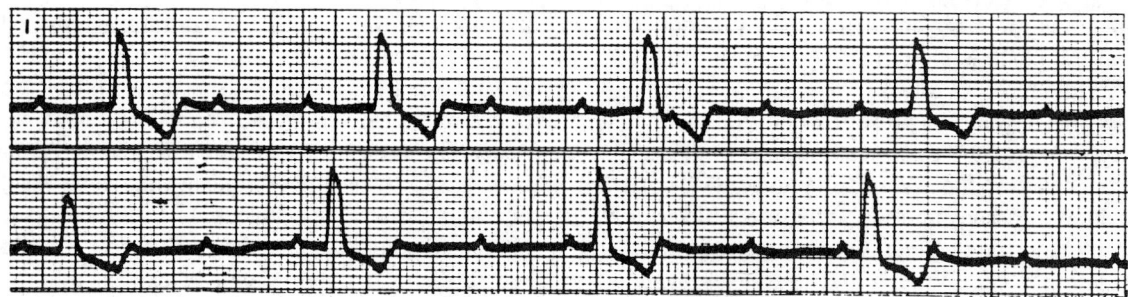

FIGURE 27-27 Complete (third-degree) AV block. The strips are continuous. In the presence of sinus tachycardia (rate, 108/minute), an independent idioventricular rhythm occurs (rate, 36/minute). Note that the ventricular rhythm is absolutely regular, whereas the P-to-R relationship is constantly changing. (From Marriott HJL and Conover MB: Advanced concepts in arrhythmias, ed 2, St Louis, 1989, The CV Mosby Co.)

Type II (Mobitz II) second-degree AV block is less common but more serious than type I. A type II block is characterized by nonconducted sinus impulses despite constant PR intervals (Figure 27-26). Usually the QRS complexes are widened because of a bundle branch block. The dropped beat represents a form of intermittent blockage of both bundle branches. The defect is found in either the bundle branches or the bundle of His. Type II blocks are most often seen in the patient with an acute anterior wall myocardial infarction and are a warning of an impending third-degree block. A temporary pacemaker is usually inserted prophylactically until the conduction stabilizes. If the block is persistent, the patient will benefit from a permanent implantable pacemaker.

In *third-degree AV block* (complete heart block) all the sinus or atrial impulses are blocked, and the atria and ventricles are forced to beat independently. The ventricles are driven by either a junctional or a ventricular pacemaker cell. The usual lesion is in the bundle of His or the bundle branches but may also be AV nodal. The rate and dependability of the ventricular rhythm are related to the level of the lesion. If a junctional pacemaker drives the ventricles, the ventricular rate will be at least 40 to 60 beats/minute, indicating that the block

is located above the bifurcation of the bundle of His. The QRS complexes are typically narrow (Figure 27-27). This block may be a transient complication of inferior posterior myocardial infarction or digitalis toxicity. Atropine is useful in restoring conduction.

If a ventricular pacemaker drives the ventricles, the rate will be 20 to 40 beats/minute, and the patient may experience syncope, CHF, altered mentation, or angina. The QRS complex is abnormally wide, indicating that the block lies below the AV node (Figure 27-28). The prognosis is more serious if complete heart block accompanies anterior myocardial infarction. Generally the patient will require a permanent artificial pacemaker. Epinephrine or isoproterenol administered intravenously may increase the ventricular rate temporarily until artificial pacing can be instituted.

BUNDLE BRANCH BLOCK

A bundle branch block (BBB) occurs as a permanent defect or as a transient block secondary to tachycardia, CHF, acute myocardial infarction, pulmonary embolus, hypoxia, or metabolic derangements. In all these cases, the electrical impulse spreads from one ventricle to the other by abnormal pathways, thus producing distinct ECG tracings.

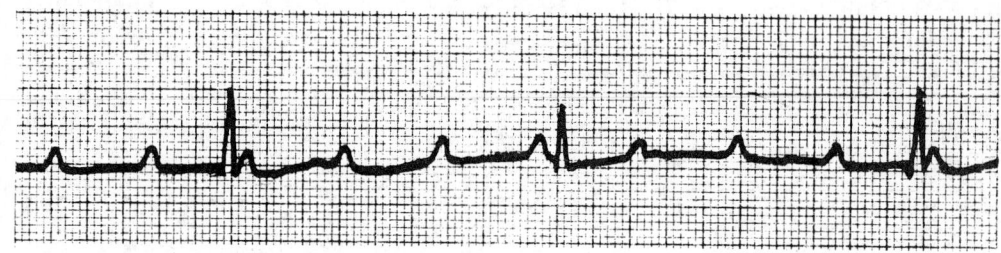

FIGURE 27-28 Third-degree (complete) AV block. Atrial rate is 105 beats/minute and ventricular rate, 33/minute; an idioventricular rhythm.

The *right bundle branch* is the more delicate structure of the two bundles and has a longer refractory period in some individuals. In the younger patient right bundle branch block (RBBB) often results from right ventricular hypertrophy, whereas CAHD is usually the cause in the older patient. The QRS complex is widened to 0.10 second or greater. Among the most classic ECG changes is the M-shaped QRS in V_1 and V_2. In the absence of other conduction defects, no intervention is necessary.

The *left bundle branch* has a main trunk that bifurcates into the left anterior and left posterior divisions. A block may occur in the main trunk or in either of the divisions. A block in the main trunk produces a complete left bundle branch block (LBBB) resulting in a QRS greater than 0.12-second duration, large R waves in V_5 and V_6, and deep wide S waves in V_1 through V_3. LBBB is associated with severe CAHD, valvular disease, hypertensive disease, cardiomegaly, and acute anterior wall myocardial infarction. It may also occur secondary to the degenerative changes in the conduction system.

Blocks of the anterior or posterior division are known as *left anterior hemiblock* or *left posterior hemiblock,* respectively. Because the left posterior division is the sturdier, its blockage carries a poorer prognosis. It is important to determine *all* blocks to conduction that may coexist. Whenever sufficient blockage is present to leave the heart dependent on one fascicle for conduction to the ventricles, the patient is a candidate for a permanent artificial pacemaker.

■ ASSESSMENT

Depending on the person's physical condition and the severity of the dysrhythmia, varying clinical effects may be experienced. Careful data collection is essential to assess the overall impact produced by a disorder of the heartbeat. A heart rhythm that is benign to one person may be life threatening to another. The key lies in recognizing the many factors that may be pertinent to the occurrence of an dysrhythmia. Although dysrhythmias most frequently occur in persons with underlying heart disease, some are noted in the absence of disease.

A careful history, physical assessment, and dysrhythmia interpretation provide the optimal evaluation of potentially dangerous cardiac events.

SUBJECTIVE DATA

Subjective data obtained by means of a detailed patient history (see Chapter 26) are as diagnostically important as laboratory data and ECG recordings in the assessment of the person with a cardiac dysrhythmia. A history should include the following:

1. Subjective complaints or symptoms
2. Activities or situations that may have precipitated or preceded the symptoms

ONE APPROACH FOR SYSTEMATIC INTERPRETATION OF ECG TRACING

1. Rate (atrial and ventricular)
2. Rhythm (atrial and ventricular)
3. Presence or absence of P waves
4. PR interval
5. QRS complex
6. Relationship of QRS to P wave
7. QT interval
8. Interpretation

NOTE: A normal sinus rhythm has an atrial (P) and ventricular (QRS) rate of 60 to 100 beats/minute, a regular rhythm (constant P-P and R-R intervals), and a P wave before every QRS.

3. Onset of the dysrhythmia (gradual versus sudden)
4. Current medications
5. Presence of the six cardinal symptoms of altered cardiovascular status: dyspnea, chest pain or discomfort, palpitations, edema, syncope, and excessive fatigue
6. Concerns or anxious feelings

OBJECTIVE DATA

Objective data consist of monitoring the patient in addition to monitoring ECG tracings and include the following:

1. Circulatory changes
   a. Changes in cardiac rhythm; irregular heartbeat
   b. Abnormal pulses
   c. Murmurs or extra heart sounds
   d. Blood pressure changes
   e. Delayed capillary refill
   f. Cyanosis
   g. Edema
2. Respiratory changes
   a. Respiratory rate
   b. Respiratory effort with activity
   c. Breath sounds: presence of rales or rhonchi
3. Neurologic: change in level of consciousness
4. Body temperature; diaphoresis
5. Electrolyte imbalances
6. State of hydration
7. Behavior, appearance
8. ECG tracing: changes in conduction (see the box above for one suggested approach to reading the ECG tracing).

■ DATA ANALYSIS: NURSING DIAGNOSES

Nursing diagnoses are determined from assessment of patient data. Possible nursing diagnoses for the person with cardiac dysrhythmias may include, but are not limited to, the following:

Diagnostic Title	Possible Etiologies
Activity intolerance	Generalized weakness, imbalance between myocardial oxygen supply and demand, immobility, bed rest
Anxiety	Threat of death, threat/change in health status/socioeconomic status/role, threat to self-concept
Cardiac output, decreased	Bradycardia, tachycardia, heart block, CHF, shock, reduced stroke volume
Knowledge deficit (cardiovascular disease process and treatment)	Lack of exposure/recall, information misinterpretation, cognitive limitation, unfamiliarity with information sources
Pain	Coronary artery occlusion or vasospasm, hypoxia, overactivity, diagnostic tests, immobility/improper positioning
Tissue perfusion, altered cardiovascular	Decreased cardiac output, coronary artery disease, myocardial infarction, angina, CHF, pulmonary edema

■ PLANNING: EXPECTED PATIENT OUTCOMES

Expected patient outcomes for the person with cardiac dysrhythmias may include, but are not limited to, the following:

1. Patient identifies factors that increase cardiac workload.
2. Patient demonstrates cardiac tolerance to increased activity (stable pulse and blood pressure)
3. Patient identifies factors that reduce activity intolerance and progresses to highest level of mobility possible.
4. Patient demonstrates improved peripheral circulation (decreased chest pain, dyspnea, and lightheadedness).
5. Patient uses effective coping mechanisms in managing anxiety.
6. The patient can:
   a. Describe underlying disease process.
   b. Describe purpose, rationale, and preparation for diagnostic testing.
   c. Assess pulse rate and rhythm accurately.
   d. Describe events that may precipitate dysrhythmias.
   e. Describe the medication regimen for managing the dysrhythmia.
   f. Indicate plans for medical follow-up.

■ IMPLEMENTATION

Certain nursing interventions are appropriate for most persons with a cardiac dysrhythmia. Some persons, however, may require artificial pacemakers to control the dysrhythmia. When the dysrhythmia leads to an unstable condition, cardioversion or defibrillation may be required for conversion to a hemodynamically stable rhythm. These measures are discussed here.

GENERAL NURSING INTERVENTIONS
PROMOTING ADEQUATE CARDIAC OUTPUT

The following interventions are directed toward ongoing monitoring of the status of the dysrhythmia, its effect on the patient's cardiac output, and how this facilitates therapy:

1. Monitor for dysrhythmias on ECG tracings.
2. Assess vital signs for changes; document rate and rhythm of pulse.
3. Monitor effects of daily activities on cardiac status, occurrence of dysrhythmias, and need for oxygen.
4. Monitor for signs of fluid overload and electrolyte imbalance.
5. Administer prescribed pharmacotherapy (see Tables 27-3 and 27-4).
6. Encourage appropriate increases in activity and ambulation to prevent overwhelming increases in cardiac workload.

PROMOTING ACTIVITY AND REST

Enhance the patient's activity tolerance by encouraging slower activity or shorter periods of activity with more rest periods. The pulse increases by 50 beats/minute with strenuous activity. This rate is safe provided it returns to the resting pulse within 3 minutes. Plan nursing strategies to promote rest and minimize unnecessary disturbances.

PROMOTING TISSUE PERFUSION

Instruct patient to avoid becoming overly fatigued and to stop activity immediately in the presence of chest pain, dyspnea, lightheadedness, or faintness, indicating insufficient oxygen reaching the tissues because of decreased cardiac function. Decreased tissue perfusion causes cellular hypoxia with subsequent ischemia, cellular swelling, and cellular death.

PROMOTING COMFORT

Chest pain results from inadequate circulation to the heart muscle. The degree of pain perception and tolerance can be influenced by psychologic as well as physi-

TABLE 27-3 Antiarrhythmic agents

Drug	Action	Indications	Dosage	Side Effects
Procainamide (Pronestyl)	Slows conduction; prolongs the refractory period; depresses spontaneous depolarization and automaticity	Ventricular tachydysrhythmias, especially after lidocaine or cardioversion breaks tachycardia; SVT, particularly atrial fibrillation	IV: 100 mg every 2-4 min, not to exceed 1 g; or 2-6 mg/min by drip PO: 250-500 mg q4-6h	Nausea, vomiting, fever, leukopenia, lupus erythematosus, AV block
Quinidine	Anticholinergic effect; prolongation of refractory period of atria; same but less effect on ventricular refractory period	Conversion of atrial fibrillation or flutter to sinus rhythm; PAB, PVB; more effective in suppressing SVT than ventricular tachycardia	PO: 275-825 mg q3-4h until normal rhythm restored; maintenance; 275 mg bid or tid 1	Thrombocytopenia purpura, nausea, vomiting, diarrhea, skin rashes, fever
Propranolol (Inderal)	Inhibition of β-adrenergic stimulation; reduction of automaticity; prolongation of atrial and AV conduction times	Tachydysrhythmias, especially digitalis induced; catecholamine-induced dysrhythmias (exercise, emotion, sympathetic stimulation)	IV: 1-3 mg, not to exceed 10 mg PO: 10-30 mg tid or qid	Hypotension, CHF, bradycardia, nausea, vomiting, mental depression
Phenytoin (Dilantin)	Depressed automaticity of pacemaker cells; shortens refractory period and action potential duration; may improve depressed conduction	Digitalis-induced dysrhythmias (atrial and ventricular)	IV: 125-250 mg slowly until dysrhythmia terminates PO: 200 mg, then 100 mg q4-rh	Nausea, vomiting, drowsiness, ataxia, vertigo, gum hyperplasia, blurred or double vision, hallucinations, convulsions
Disopyramide (Norpace)	Similar to procainamide and quinidine	Ventricular and supraventricular tachydysrhythmias; PVB; helpful in patients who are not helped by all the above drugs; contraindicated in severe CHF, glaucoma, second-or third-degree AV block	PO: 200-300 mg loading dose, then 100-150 mg q6h	Dry mouth, urinary hesitancy or retention, N & V, diarrhea, abdominal pain
Verapamil	Calcium channel blocker; slows SA node discharge rate and prolongs AV conduction time, depresses myocardial contractility	Termination of paroxysmal SVT; slows ventricular rate of atrial fibrillation or flutter; coronary vasodilator	IV: 5-10 mg over 2 min PO: 80-100 mg q6-8h	Headache, dizziness, nausea, constipation, bradycardia, hypotension, second- or third-degree AV block
Lidocaine	Similar to procainamide and quinidine; depresses spontaneous depolarization and automaticity in ventricles	PVB; ventricular tachycardia; contraindicated in severe liver or renal disease	IV: 75-100 mg bolus (1-1.5 mg/kg), then 2-4 mg/min	Hypotension, dizziness, drowsiness, confusion, convulsions, respiratory depression, coma
Bretylium tosylate (Bretylol)	Raises ventricular fibrillation threshold; lengthens action potential and effective refractory period of ventricles; interferes with release of norepinephrine and uptake of catecholamines by nerve endings	Ventricular tachydysrhythmias and fibrillation; refractory to other drug therapy or cardioversion	IV: 5-10 mg/kg IV bolus over 10 min, then 1-2 mg/min IM: 5-10 mg/kg q1-2h, then q6-8h	Severe hypotension, dizziness, lightheadedness, nausea, vomiting, fainting
Esmolol (Brevibloc)	Ultra-short-acting β-adrenergic blocking agent; cardioselective; significant prolongation of sinus cycle length; significant decrease in AV conduction	Supraventricular tachydysrhythmias; perioperative tachycardia and hypertension	Consult pharmacology source	Hypotension: self-limiting; resolves within 30 min after discontinuation of infusion

TABLE 27-4 New and investigational antiarrhythmic drugs

Drug	Action	Indications	Dosage	Side Effects
Amiodarone (Cordarone)	Prolongs action potential duration and refractiveness of both atrial and ventricular myocardium and Purkinje's fibers	SVT; VF; recurrent atrial flutter; atrial fibrillation; serious atrial and ventricular tachydysrhythmias refractory to other drug therapy	IV: loading, 5-10 mg/kg; maintenance: 0.005 mg/kg/min PO: loading, 200-1200 mg qd; maintenance, 200-600 mg qd	Corneal microdeposits, transient increase in hepatic enzymes, visual disturbances, pulmonary fibrosis, bradycardia, PVCs, sinus arrest
Encainide (Enkaid)	Decreases action potential duration; slows conduction; inhibits automaticity; prolongs refractory periods	Limited to treatment of life-threatening dysrhythmias such as sustained ventricular tachycardia and ventricular fibrillation	IV: loading, 0.6-0.9 mg/kg PO: maintenance, 25-75 mg q6-8h	Worsening of ventricular tachycardia, metallic taste, dizziness, chest pain, palpitations, blurred vision
Flecainide acetate (Tambocor)	Depresses conduction throughout heart, with greatest effect on bundle of His—Purkinje system	Suppression of complex ventricular dysrhythmias resistant to conventional drug therapy	PO: 100-200 mg bid	Worsening of ventricular dysrhythmias, dizziness, blurred vision, hypotension, bradycardia
Mexiletine (Mexitil)	Similar to lidocaine; depresses conduction throughout heart	Ventricular dysrhythmias	IV: loading, 0.5-1.5 mg/min PO: maintenance, 200-400 mg q8h	Neurologic, GI, and cardiovascular symptoms
Propafenone (Rythmol)	Decreases maximal rate of depolarization, slows bundle of His—Purkinje conduction, causing a widening of QRS complex	Chronic, recurrent supraventricular and ventricular tachydysrhythmias	IV: should be adjusted to each patient's needs; 1-2.5 mg/kg PO: 300-900 mg qd, divided doses	Worsening of ventricular dysrhythmias, conduction abnormalities, dizziness, visual disturbances, metallic taste, nausea, constipation
Tocainide (Tonocard)	Similar to lidocaine; is effective orally, therefore suitable for long-term therapy	Drug-resistant PVBs; ventricular tachycardia; ventricular dysrhythmias	IV: 0.5-0.75 mg/kg/min for 15 min PO: 400 mg q8h	GI, neurologic, and cardiovascular symptoms

cal factors (see Chapter 16). Assess for causes of decreased pain tolerance, such as lack of knowledge, fear, or fatigue. Reduce or eradicate factors contributing to increased discomfort. All pain is authentic regardless of etiology. Provide a calm environment to decrease stress and anxiety, and provide rest periods if fatigue is present during physical activities. Evaluate effects of pain intervention measures (including prescribed pharmacologic agents.

PROMOTING RELIEF OF ANXIETY AND FEELING OF WELL-BEING

Facilitate a reduction in the patient's present level of anxiety. Anxiety varies in intensity depending on the severity of the threat as perceived by the individual as well as the individual's success in coping. Measures to reduce anxiety and stress are discussed in Chapter 11.

PROMOTING PATIENT/FAMILY LEARNING

Delay teaching until the individual is ready. The patient needs to be relatively free of pain and excessive anxiety

to learn. Teaching includes the following:
1. Nature of the dysrhythmia in terms of the patient's level of understanding
2. How to assess pulse rate and rhythm
3. Nature and treatment regimen of underlying disease process
4. Lifestyle modifications, coping strategies, and support networks
5. Symptoms requiring medical intervention and precipitating factors
6. Medication regimen
7. Need for medical follow-up

PACEMAKERS
INDICATIONS FOR USE

The artificial pacemaker has become a leading modality in the control of potentially dangerous dysrhythmias. Pacemakers may be temporary (Figure 27-29) or permanent (Figure 27-30). Indications for artificial pacemakers are summarized in the box on p. 656. Some of these conditions require only temporary pacing. Permanent

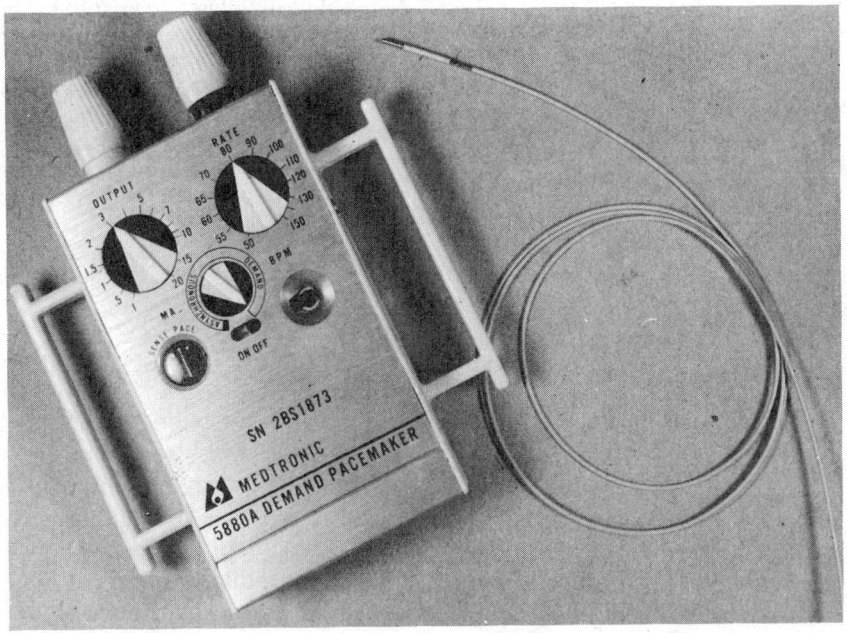

FIGURE 27-29 Temporary (external) pacemaker. Pulse generator is battery powered. Electrode is passed into heart before being attached to pulse generator.

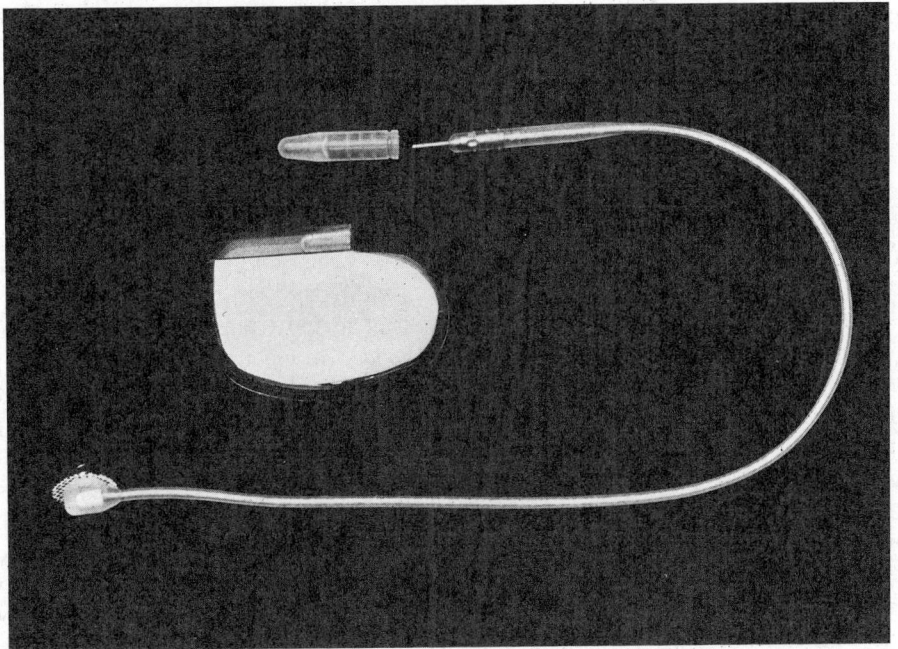

FIGURE 27-30 One type of implantable permanent pacemaker (pulse generator), usually implanted subcutaneously in right anterior chest below clavicle.

INDICATIONS FOR ARTIFICIAL PACEMAKERS

1. Adams-Stokes attack (syncope secondary to third-degree AV block)
2. Third-degree AV block with slow ventricular rate
3. Acute myocardial infarction (MI) with Mobitz II AV block
4. Right bundle branch block plus left anterior hemiblock or left posterior hemiblock (particularly with acute MI)
5. New left bundle branch block associated with acute MI
6. Symptomatic sinus bradycardia unresponsive to medical therapy
7. Atrial fibrillation with slow ventricular rate in the patient who requires digitalis therapy
8. Carotid sinus syncope
9. Suppression of dysrhythmias (atrial or ventricular tachydysrhythmias)
10. Dysrhythmias occurring during or after cardiac surgery
11. Sick sinus syndrome
12. Prophylaxis before anesthesia and surgery in patients with history of cardiac arrest or AV blocks

TYPES OF PACEMAKERS

1. Stimulation of ventricles only
   a. QRS-inhibited (demand) pacing
   b. P wave–triggered ventricular pacing (SA node still determines heart rate and atrial kick is maintained)
2. Stimulation of atria only (requires the presence of a normal conduction system below the atria)
3. Stimulation of both atria and ventricles (simulates the normal impulse formation and conduction; has artificial PR interval to maintain synchronous contraction of the cardiac chambers)

pacing is an option when the condition is recurrent or persistent.

The artificial pacing system consists of a battery-powered generator and a pacing wire that delivers the stimulus to the heart to control heart rate. The pacing unit initiates and maintains the heart rate when the natural pacemakers of the heart are unable to do so.

PULSE GENERATOR

The pulse generator is powered by battery cells. Technologic advances have occurred in both power sources and electronic circuitry, and currently lithium batteries lasting 6 years or more are used in most pacemakers. Research is directed toward power sources that may function for extended periods. For example, nuclear-powered pacemakers (plutonium-238 source) can last 20 years or more. Other pacemakers can have their batteries recharged externally.[18] For most pacemakers in which lithium or the older mercury-zinc battery is used, battery exhaustion is inevitable. When the generator battery fails, the implantable unit that contains the batteries must be replaced surgically.

The pulse generator has several controls, including energy output, heart rate, and mode of pacing. In a temporary pacemaker system, these controls can be easily regulated, and because of technologic advances in permanent pacers, selected persons are supplied with "programmable" pacers that can be controlled outside the body.

Energy Output

Energy output refers to the intensity of the electrical impulse delivered by the pulse generator to the myocardium. The amount of output is measured in milliamperes (mA). The mA setting is regulated by the physician at the time of pacemaker insertion and is set at the lowest level that will produce depolarization. A setting of 1.5 mA is usually sufficient to cause depolarization. However, depending on the condition of the individual and the placement of the pacer wire, a higher mA setting may be necessary.

Heart Rate

Heart rate is set according to the desired therapeutic aim and the clinical condition of the patient. With few exceptions the heart rate is usually set between 70 and 80 beats/minute. If the purpose of inserting a pacemaker is to suppress dysrhythmias, the rate is usually set higher, often 100 to 120 beats/minute.

Mode of Pacing

There are two basic modes of artificial pacing: fixed rate (asynchronous) or demand mode. In the *fixed-rate mode* the pacemaker fires electrical stimuli at a preset rate regardless of the person's inherent rhythm. Because of the hazards of a pacing stimulus falling within the vulnerable period, asynchronous pacing is rarely used today.

The most popular mode is the *demand* or *standby mode*. An electrode at the tip of the pacing wire is able to sense the person's own heartbeats. The pacemaker produces a stimulus only when the person's own heart rate drops below the rate per minute preset on the generator by the physician. Some types of pacemakers currently available are described in the box above.

It should be noted that the temporary pacemaker is limited to atrial or ventricular stimulation. The potential for maximizing the person's hemodynamic status is much greater with the various types of permanent pacemakers.

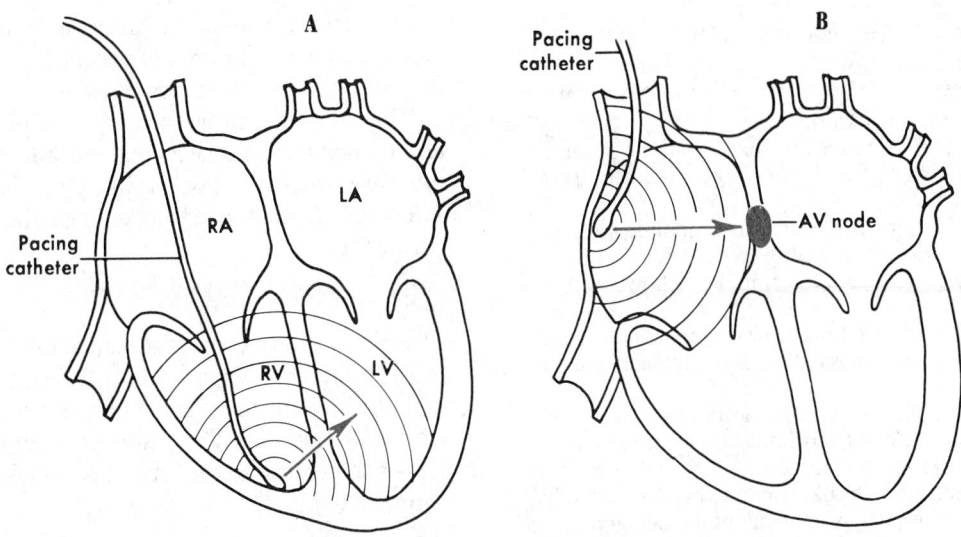

FIGURE 27-31 A, Ventricular pacing. Impulses are initiated in ventricle. **B,** Atrial pacing. Impulses are initiated in atrium and travel to ventricles by normal conduction system.

If an individual has a functioning conduction system below the atrium but has difficulty in impulse formation from the SA node, a pacing catheter may be placed in the atrium. Atrial pacing has been somewhat difficult to achieve; however, it more closely approximates the normal electrical activity of the heart (Figure 27-31). Ventricular pacing results in a retrograde depolarization, which does not mimic the normal conduction system. Despite this retrograde stimulation and depolarization, most individuals achieve a cardiac output sufficient for their physiologic needs.

COMPLICATIONS OF PACEMAKER THERAPY

The use of artificial pacemakers is not without potential complications. Complications usually arise because of improper pacer functioning and the presence of the pacemaker wires as a foreign object in the body.

Infection

For the person with a temporary pacemaker, local infection or hematoma formation may occur at the venous cutdown site. With a permanent pacemaker, local infection at the suture line or sepsis may occur. The person is monitored daily for any signs of inflammation or infection.

Dysrhythmias

The pacemaker wire and electrode can irritate the ventricular wall, producing ectopic activity. Less frequently the pacer electrode may dislodge and move about, producing electrical stimulation and potential dysrhythmias. The most common causes of pacemaker failure

are displacement of the pacing wire electrode and battery failure. Both these situations require minor surgery to make repairs.

Electrical Interference

Interference from electrical sources is a particular area of concern for the person with an external (temporary) pacemaker. The person must be careful to avoid contact with any electrical machinery that is not properly grounded. A small electrical charge passing via the pacer wire directly into the heart could initiate lethal dysrhythmias.

TEMPORARY PACEMAKERS

For temporary pacing the pacer wire is usually passed transvenously to the right atrium or ventricle (Figure 27-31). This procedure can be performed at the bedside or using fluoroscopy in a special procedure room. The wire connects externally to a generator, as seen in Figure 27-29. If the antecubital fossa is used as the insertion site for the pacer wires, the pacemaker may be secured to the person's arm. If a subclavian site is used, the pulse generator may be secured to the person's chest or placed in a specific "pacemaker pocket" available or cut in hospital gowns. Nursing care for persons with temporary external pacemakers is summarized in the box on p. 658.

PERMANENT PACEMAKERS

The same pacemaker system exists for permanent pacing, except that the generator itself is more compact and may be implanted subcutaneously (see Figure 27-

NURSING CARE OF THE PERSON WITH A TEMPORARY PACEMAKER

1. Monitor pacemaker performance:
   a. Assess heart rate to ensure that it has not fallen below preset level. *If heart rate is below preset level, notify physician.*
   b. Using an ECG tracing or cardiac monitor, note the presence of pacing stimulus "pace spikes" and whether a P wave or QRS complex follows each stimulus.
   c. Assess the person for signs of pacemaker malfunction, such as weakness, dizziness, hypotension, or fainting.
2. Maintain pacemaker system integrity:
   a. Ensure that catheter terminals are securely connected to the pulse generator.
   b. Ensure that the external pacemaker is adequately secured to the person so accidental dislodgement of the system is avoided.
3. Assess patient safety and comfort:
   a. Monitor for signs of inflammation or infection at the catheter insertion site.
   b. If clinically permitted, assist the person with range of motion exercises for the involved extremity.
   c. Ensure that the person avoids contact with any improperly grounded electrical equipment.
   d. Explain the purpose of the pacing unit to decrease anxiety.
   e. Explain any prescribed restrictions in physical activity.

30). The permanent pacing generator may be implanted in the right or left subclavicular areas, and the pacing wire is passed through the major veins to the right side of the heart (transvenous or endocardiac). Alternatively, the generator may be implanted subcutaneously in the abdomen, with the pacing wire passed upward and sutured to the left ventricle (epicardial).

Permanent pacemakers are inserted in the operating room or in a special procedure room. The transvenous approach to insertion does not require general anesthesia, which greatly decreases the risk of this procedure. In epicardial pacing, however, the electrode is passed transthoracically to the myocardium, where it is sutured in place. This procedure requires general anesthesia, because a thoracotomy is required to provide access to the heart.

Immediate Nursing Care

Immediate nursing care for the person with a permanent pacemaker includes connecting the person to a cardiac monitor or ECG machine to assess pacemaker function. An intravenous line is maintained should the person require fluids or medications, including antiarrhythmic drugs. Data about the person's pacemaker should be clearly identified in the patient's chart and include the type and model of pacemaker, its location, the mA setting, rate, and mode of pacing.

The incision site is covered by a pressure dressing and is monitored for bleeding and infection. Safe nursing care also includes ensuring that only electrically safe equipment is used on or near the person with a pacemaker.

ECG Tracing

The ECG appearance of pacemaker-stimulated heartbeats is shown in Figure 27-32. Paced beats are readily identified by the sharp spike that precedes a paced ECG complex. The skilled practitioner is able to analyze an ECG and determine the type of pacemaker and where it is implanted.

Assessment of Pacemaker Function

All persons with permanent pacemakers need to have the function of their pacemakers assessed at varying intervals. Pacemaker clinics are available to assess pulse generators and to warn persons of low or failing batteries. For persons who may not have access to pacemaker clinics, telephone transmission of pacer functioning is one way of ensuring follow-up assessment. By means of special equipment, the sound tone of a pacemaker can be transmitted over the telephone to special recording equipment. The pacemaker tone is electronically converted into a signal that is recorded on an ECG strip. With a brief telephone call, the pacemaker rate and other data concerning pacemaker function can be assessed.

Patient Teaching

The following instructions concerning pacemaker function and care should be given to the patient:

1. Check pulse daily for 1 full minute at relatively the same time.
2. Report any sudden slowing or increase in pulse rate.
3. Notify physician of any pain or redness over incision site.
4. Wear loose-fitting clothing around the pacemaker area for increased comfort.
5. Have pacemaker function checked at special centers (in person or by telephone) at instructed intervals.
6. Carry an identification card or an emergency alert identification tag specifying the type of pacemaker, name of manufacturer, settings, name of hospital where implanted, and name of physician; keep duplicate card at home.
7. Show the identification card to airport employees at the safety detection station so a hand scanner can be used rather than conventional detectors.

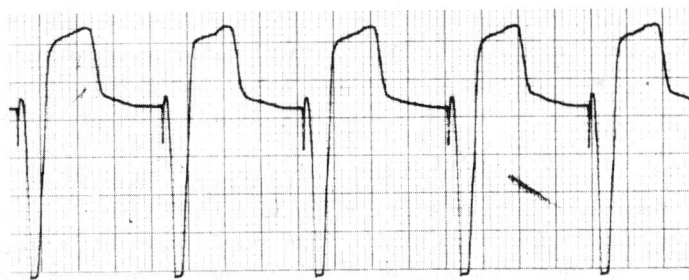

FIGURE 27-32 Pacemaker ECG (lead V_1). Rate is 78, rhythm regular, QRS complex wide, and no P waves visible. Pacing stimulus (spike) precedes each QRS.

EXTERNAL TRANSCUTANEOUS PACEMAKERS

External pacemakers were first introduced in the 1950s. The device was refined since its invention and was generally successful in restoring cardiac rhythm, but the external stimulation was often painful. Thus it was largely replaced by the internal pacemaker in 1959. In the 1980s, external pacemakers and pads were improved to ensure cardiac stimulation at lower current levels. They are now being used again, particularly in emergency situations.

External pacing, as a temporary treatment modality, can correct the same dysrhythmias as endocardial pacemakers. Examples of indications for use include (1) overdrive suppression of ventricular tachydysrhythmias; (2) restoration or acceleration of rhythm when asystole or bradycardia occur because of drug effect, myocardial infarction, or heart block; (3) in the presence of thrombocytopenia or leukopenia when endocardial pacing is contraindicated; (4) during emergencies when there is a time constraint against inserting a pacemaker wire; and (5) as a prophylaxis during invasive procedures, such as pulmonary artery line insertion, cardioversion, or electrophysiologic studies.

Pacing is usually achieved by application of two electrodes to the chest wall, one over the cardiac apex and the other on the back beneath the left scapula. An electrical current is delivered between the electrodes via an output pulse delivered in milliamperes controlled by the operator. Most devices function in the demand mode and are equipped with a built-in oscilloscope to allow monitoring of pacer activity.

CARDIOVERSION AND DEFIBRILLATION

Cardioversion is the use of electrical energy to convert a cardiac dysrhythmia (other than ventricular fibrillation) to one that is more hemodynamically stable, preferably a sinus rhythm. *Defibrillation* generally applies to unsynchronized electrical countershock during a ventricular fibrillation emergency. Cardioversion differs from defibrillation in that the electrical discharge is synchronized with the R wave to avoid triggering ventricular fi-

brillation by accidental discharge during the ventricular vulnerable period.

Electrophysiologically, the electrical countershock produces a simultaneous depolarization of a critical mass of cardiac fibers, thus halting the asynchronous chaos of a fibrillation or the rapid firing of a tachycardia. In some cases, especially in elective cardioversion, the shock will be delivered more than once until the correct level of voltage is reached. Once the heart is fully depolarized, the SA node is better able to resume control of the heart.

For emergency defibrillation, the paddles from the defibrillator are placed at the third intercostal space to the right of the sternum and the fifth intercostal space on the left midaxillary line. Either conducting gel or saline pads must be applied between the paddles and the skin to ensure conductance and minimize skin burning. The button on each paddle is depressed simultaneously to release 200 to 360 watt-seconds (joules) to the patient. Defibrillation must be performed rapidly for ventricular fibrillation and most cases of ventricular tachycardia.

When the cardioversion is elective (for example, conversion of atrial flutter, atrial fibrillation, or PAT), the procedure differs slightly. The patient should have nothing by mouth for 8 hours in advance. In many cases the daily digitalis dose may be withheld that day or for several days in advance. Selected patients who are receiving anticoagulants should continue to receive this therapy. Oral antiarrhythmics (see tables 27-3 and 27-4) are also frequently given in advance.

Patients should be prepared psychologically for what to expect and be reassured that they will remember none of it. The atmosphere should be quiet. The patient is generally given intravenous diazepam (until sleepy) for its amnesic effect. The defibrillator is synchronized such that when the buttons are pressed, the impulse is not initiated until the next R wave. Because of this precaution, the danger of entering the vulnerable period is eliminated. For most elective procedures, the amount of watt-seconds or joules required for conversion is lower than that required for defibrillation. The patient is monitored after cardioversion until vital signs are stable and the gag reflex has returned.

RECENT ADVANCES IN DEFIBRILLATION

Current-Based Defibrillation

Recent studies have shown that current is a better descriptor of defibrillation than energy, favoring the use of a current-based approach.[13,14] The higher the energy level or frequency of shocks, the greater is the amount of myocardial damage that can occur. If transthoracic impedance could be accurately determined before defibrillation or cardioversion, inappropriately high or low energies could be avoided in patients with high transthoracic impedance. Recently, Hewlett Packard defibrillators have been modified to allow advanced prediction of transthoracic impedance. Once impedance is determined, the defibrillator automatically selects the energy necessary to provide the specified current. Although still under investigation, this approach to defibrillation and cardioversion may develop as the safest and most effective method to restore rhythm and hemodynamic stability with reduced risk of profound myocardial damage and deterioration.

Automatic Implantable Cardioverter Defibrillator

More than half the deaths from coronary artery disease in the United States each year are sudden deaths occurring within 24 hours of the onset of symptoms and frequently before the patient reaches the hospital. The pathophysiology of sudden cardiac death remains obscure. Numerous studies have shown that pathologic evidence of acute myocardial infarction or fresh thrombi is often absent. Furthermore, the severity of the coronary artery disease present in patients who die suddenly is sometimes less than that in patients who survive longer or equal to that found in patients dying of other causes. Many researchers conclude that the cause of sudden cardiac death is not occlusive thrombosis or myocardial damage, but a derangement in the heart's electrical stability, most often deteriorating into ventricular fibrillation.

After several years of research and development, Mirowski and others[16] performed the first permanent implantation of an automatic defibrillator in 1980. This device automatically senses ventricular fibrillation and, within approximately 15 to 20 seconds, delivers an electrical countershock. It is also capable of identifying and correcting ventricular tachycardia via cardioversion. One advantage is that defibrillatory energy requirements are considerably less because the shock is being applied directly within the heart. With conventional transthoracic defibrillation, a large amount of energy is necessary because dissipation occurs before the charge reaches the heart.

The automatic implantable cardioverter defibrillator (AICD) system consists of a pulse generator and two lead or sensing systems that continuously monitor heart activity and automatically deliver a countershock to correct a dysrhythmia as necessary. The device is implanted surgically, usually through a median sternotomy or lateral thoracotomy approach. The AICD has been approved by the Food and Drug Administration (FDA) for two categories of patients: (1) those who have survived one or more episodes of sudden cardiac death resulting from ventricular tachycardia or ventricular fibrillation, with episodes not associated with acute myocardial infarction; and (2) those who have experienced recurrent, refractory, life-threatening ventricular dysrhythmias and can be induced into sustained hypotensive ventricular tachycardia, ventricular fibrillation, or both, despite conventional antiarrhythmic drug therapy. In the future, it is conceivable that selection criteria may be broadened.

CARDIOPULMONARY RESUSCITATION

Myocardial infarction (heart attack) is the leading cause of death in America. The American Heart Association estimates an incidence of 1.5 million victims per year, of whom approximately 540,000 (36%) will die. Of these deaths, 350,000 take place outside the hospital and usually occur within 2 hours after the onset of symptoms.[4] Thus sudden death from ischemic heart disease is the most serious and most important medical emergency today. It seems reasonable to assume that many of these deaths might be prevented by prompt and appropriate interventions that provide either rapid entry into the emergency medical system (see Chapter 79) or cardiopulmonary support using CPR.

Cardiopulmonary arrest is recognized by the cessation of breathing and circulation and signifies a state of clinical death. Immediate and definitive action must be instituted within 4 to 6 minutes following the arrest or biologic death will occur.

CLINICAL MANIFESTATIONS

The person who has suffered a cardiac arrest appears clinically dead. Unresponsiveness, cessation of respirations, development of pallor and cyanosis, absence of heart sounds and blood pressure, loss of palpable pulse, and dilation of the pupils are present. (Pupillary response can be misleading in patients who are receiving drugs such as atropine or opium derivatives or in the presence of corneal pathologic conditions.) If a hospitalized patient is being monitored by means of an ECG machine or cardiac monitor, the ECG pattern of *ventricular fibrillation* or, less often, *ventricular asystole* will appear.

TABLE 27-5 Sequence of cardiopulmonary resuscitation (CPR)

Findings	Action	ABCs of Action
No response		
Absence of respira- tions; cyanosis, dilated pupils	Open airway	A—Open Airway
Respirations still absent	Initiate artificial ventilation	B—Restore Breathing
Carotid pulse not palpable	Initiate external cardiac compres- sions	C—Restore Circu- lation
ECG; ventricular fibrillation	Drug therapy; de- fibrillation	D—Provide Definitive treat- ment

TECHNIQUES OF BASIC LIFE SUPPORT

Basic life support is an emergency procedure that consists of recognizing an arrest and initiating proper CPR techniques to maintain life until the victim either recovers or is transported to a medical facility where advanced life-support measures are available (Table 27-5).

STEP I—ASSESS LEVEL OF CONSCIOUSNESS

Persons may appear to be unconscious when in fact they are either asleep, deaf, or possibly intoxicated. Unconsciousness is confirmed by shaking the victim's shoulders and shouting, "Are you OK?" If the person does not respond, help is summoned and the victim is placed in the supine position on a *firm* surface.

STEP II—OPEN THE AIRWAY

The tongue is the most common cause of respiratory obstruction in the unconscious person. The head tilt–chin lift (Figure 27-33) and the jaw thrust (Figure 27-34) are the two recommended methods for opening and maintaining the airway. Jaw thrust (without head tilt) is the safest first approach to opening the airway of a victim with a suspected neck injury. The head must be carefully supported to avoid turning from side to side or tilting it backward. While maintaining an open airway, the rescuer should take 3 to 5 seconds to *look, listen,* and *feel* for spontaneous breathing. The rescuer places an ear over the victim's nose and mouth while looking at the victim's chest. The rescuer looks to see if the chest moves with respiration, listens for air escaping during exhalation, and feels for air movement against the face.

STEP III—INITIATE ARTIFICIAL VENTILATION
Mouth-to-Mouth Ventilation

If the victim is not breathing, two mouth-to-mouth breaths are given. To perform mouth-to-mouth resuscitation, the head tilt–chin lift position is maintained while the victim's nostrils are gently pinched off so that no air escapes. The rescuer places the mouth around the outside of the victim's mouth, forming a tight seal, and gives two full breaths. One to one and one-half seconds are allowed for each breath. The rescuer takes a breath after each ventilation.[21] If the lungs are being adequately ventilated using mouth-to-mouth resuscitation, the rescuer should be able to (1) observe the rise and fall of the chest during respiration, (2) hear and feel air escape as the victim passively exhales, and (3) feel in the rescuer's own airway the resistance of the victim's lungs as they expand.

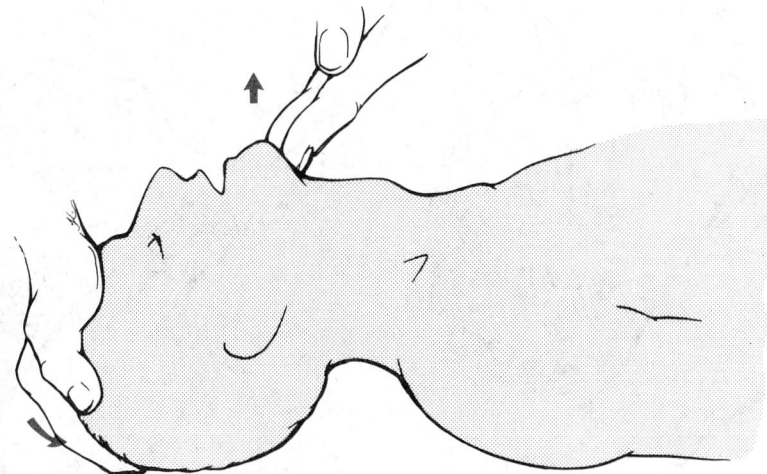

FIGURE 27-33 Head tilt–chin lift maneuver for opening airway. Place one hand on forehead and place tips of fingers of other hand under lower jaw near chin. Bring chin forward while pressing forehead down.

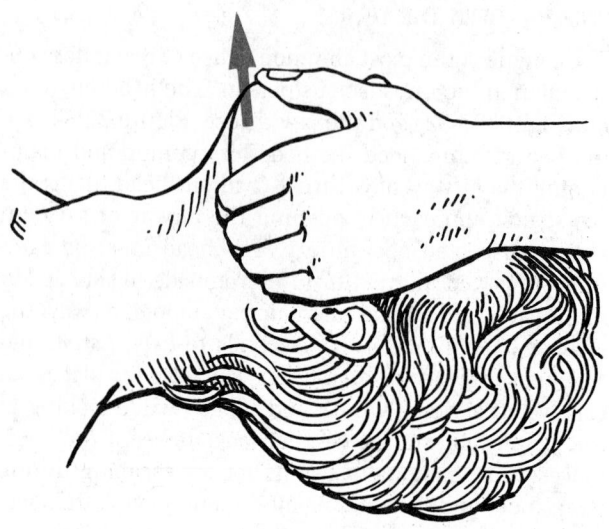

FIGURE 27-34 Jaw thrust maneuver for opening airway.

Mouth-to-Nose-Ventilation

Mouth-to-nose ventilation is indicated when it is impossible to open the victim's airway, if the mouth is seriously injured, or if a tight seal cannot be established around the mouth. The rescuer places one hand on the forehead to tilt the head back and uses the other hand to lift the lower jaw and close the mouth. After taking a deep breath, the rescuer seals the mouth around the victim's nose and begins blowing until the lungs expand. Occasionally, when mouth-to-nose ventilation is used, it may become necessary to open the victim's mouth or lips to allow air to escape on exhalation because the soft palate may produce nasopharyngeal obstruction.

Mouth-to-Stoma Ventilation

Direct mouth-to-stoma artificial ventilation should be performed for the laryngectomy patient. For the patient with a temporary tracheostomy tube, mouth-to-tube ventilation should be initiated after the cuff is inflated.

STEP IV—ASSESS CIRCULATION

The carotid pulse is palpated rapidly to determine if cardiac compression is needed. The carotid pulse is located by finding the larynx and then sliding the fingers laterally into the groove between the trachea and the sternocleidomastoid muscle (Figure 27-35). If the carotid pulse is not palpable in 5 to 10 seconds, help is again summoned and cardiac compressions are initiated. The carotid pulse is palpated because the rescuer will already be at the victim's head and generally no clothing has to be removed to assess the pulse. In addition, the carotid arteries are central, and sometimes these pulses will persist when more peripheral pulses have diminished and are no longer palpable. If a pulse is palpable but breathing is absent, rescue breathing should be initiated at a rate of 12 times per minute after the initial two breaths of 1 to 1½ seconds each. If the pulse is absent, cardiac arrest is confirmed and external chest compression must be initiated after the initial two breaths.

STEP V—INITIATE EXTERNAL CARDIAC COMPRESSION

External cardiac massage is the rhythmic compression of the heart between the lower half of the sternum and the thoracic vertebral column. This intermittent pressure compresses the heart, raises intrathoracic pressure, and produces an artificial pulsatile circulation. Correctly performed cardiac compressions can produce a peak systolic blood pressure of more than 100 mm Hg, but

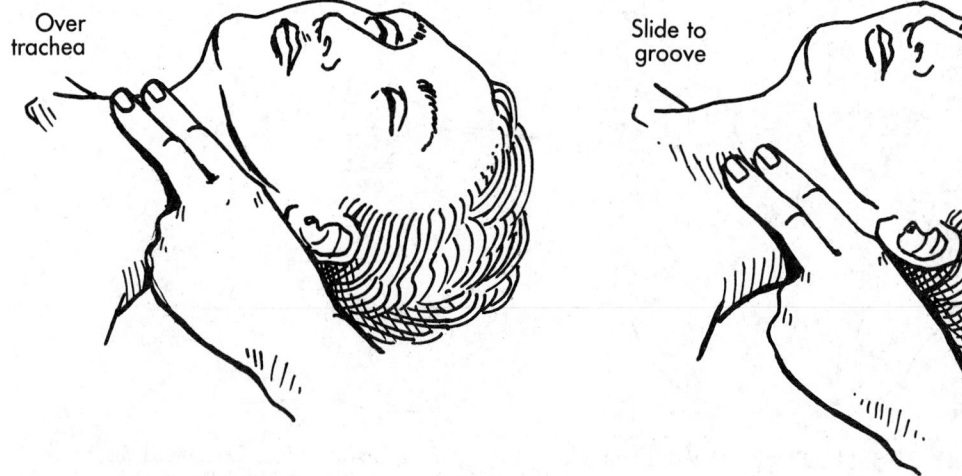

Over trachea

Slide to groove

FIGURE 27-35 Locating carotid artery.

the diastolic pressure is close to zero and the mean blood pressure in the carotid arteries is approximately 40 mm Hg, or one-fourth to one-third normal. The technique for performing external cardiac compression is outlined in the following four stages:

1. The rescuer is positioned close to the victim's side. Using the middle finger of the hand closest to the victim's feet, the rescuer locates the xiphoid process (Figure 27-36, *A*). The index finger of the same hand is then placed on the victim's sternum directly next to the middle finger. Using the index finger as a landmark, the heel of the opposite hand is placed next to the index finger on the sternum (Figure 27-36, *B*). The first hand is then removed from the landmark position and placed on top of the hand on the sternum, so that the heels of both hands are parallel and the fingers are pointing

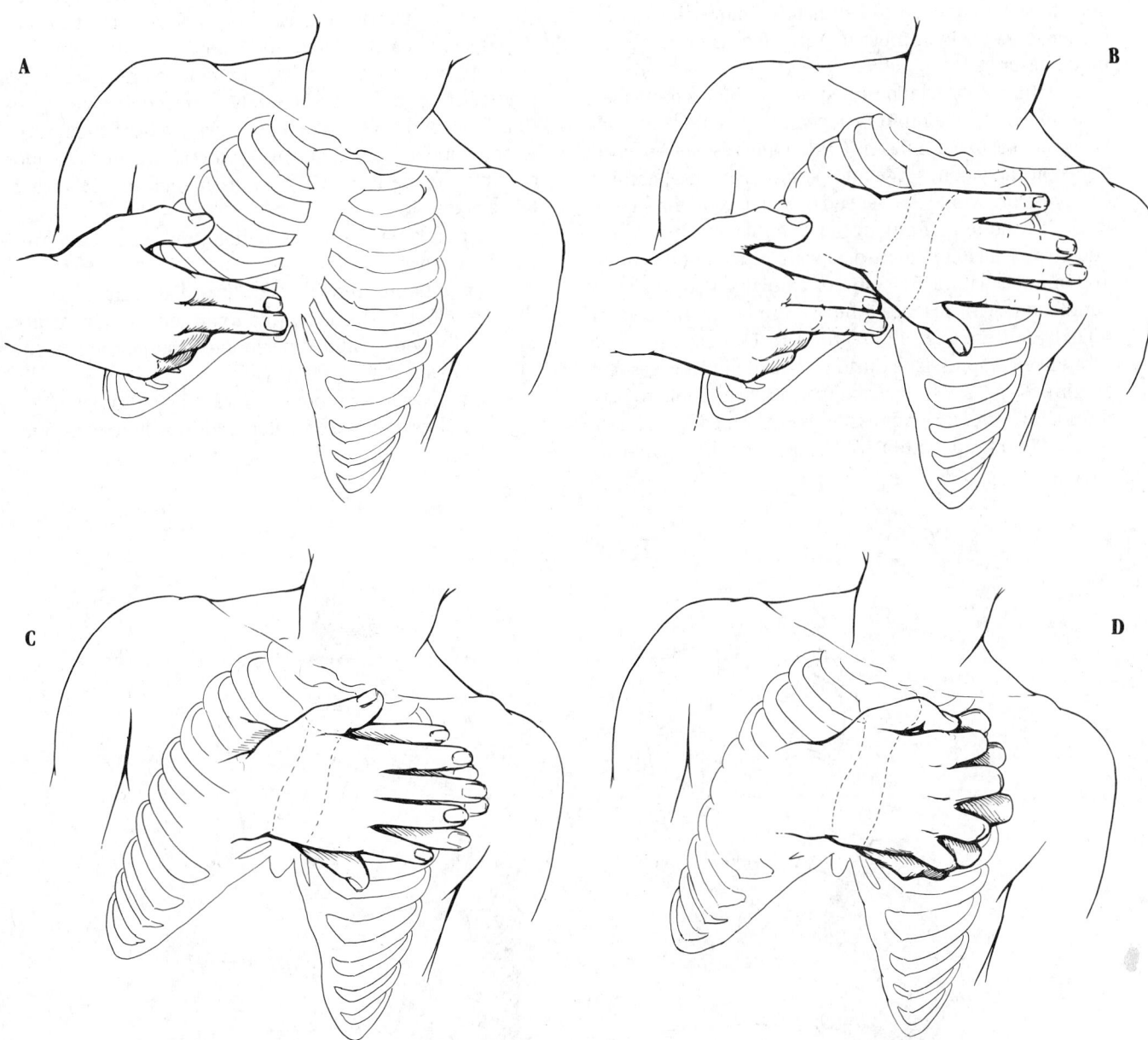

FIGURE 27-36 Positioning of hands on sternum in external cardiac compression. **A,** Middle finger locates xiphoid process; index finger is positioned next to middle finger. **B,** Heel of opposite hand is placed on sternum next to index finger. **C,** First hand is removed from landmark position and placed on top of other hand so heels of both hands are parallel and fingers point away. **D,** Fingers may be interlocked to avoid pressure on ribs.

away from the rescuer (Figure 27-36, C). Fingers may be interlocked to avoid putting pressure on the patient's ribs (Figure 27-36, D).

2. To perform effective external cardiac compression, the rescuer must position the shoulders directly over the victim's sternum and, while keeping elbows locked in a straight position, depress the lower sternum 1½ to 2 inches. The compressions should be regular, smooth, and uninterrupted. Following each compression, the rescuer must release the pressure completely to allow the heart to refill. The rescuer's hands should not ordinarily leave the chest or change position. If hand position must be changed to ventilate or move the victim, proper hand position must be relocated using the technique described.

3. Artificial circulation must always be accompanied by artificial ventilation. It is hoped that two rescuers will be available to administer CPR. One rescuer is positioned at the victim's side and performs external cardiac compression while the second rescuer remains at the victim's head to perform artificial ventilation. If two rescuers are available, the cardiac compression rate is 80 to 100/minute, with a 5:1 ratio of cardiac compression to ventilation. The rescuer who is ventilating the victim quickly delivers one full breath (1 to 1½ seconds) after every five compressions during a pause in compressions (Figure 27-37, B). If only one rescuer is available to perform CPR, cardiac compression is performed at a rate of 80 to 100/minute, with a 15:2 ratio of cardiac compres-

sion to ventilation. The rescuer delivers two full breaths after every 15 compressions (Figure 27-37, A). The victim is reassessed after four cycles of compression and ventilation. If the pulse is still absent, CPR is resumed, beginning with ventilation.

4. After the first minute of CPR, the carotid pulse is palpated to assess the effectiveness of CPR and to check for the return of spontaneous circulation. If two rescuers are performing CPR, the person ventilating the victim can also assess pulses, monitor for the return of spontaneous breathing, and assess pupillary response to light. If the victim's brain is being adequately oxygenated, the pupils will constrict in response to light. If the pupils are grossly dilated and nonreactive to light, severe brain damage may be imminent or may have already occurred. CPR should be stopped for no more than 7 seconds every 4 to 5 minutes to assess the return of spontaneous pulse and respiration. Rescuers should continue to perform CPR until one of the following takes place:

   a. Spontaneous circulation and ventilation return.
   b. Another rescuer takes over basic life support.
   c. Victim is transported to an emergency facility where qualified personnel assume the responsibility for CPR.
   d. Victim is pronounced dead by a physician.
   e. Rescuer is exhausted and unable to continue.

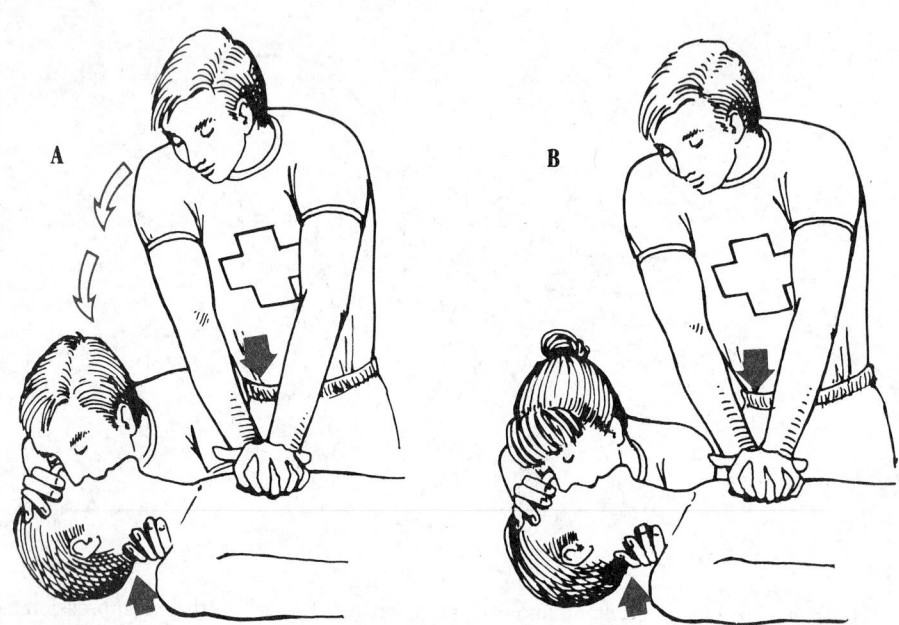

FIGURE 27-37 A, One-person rescuer CPR. The person delivers two rapid inflations after every 15 compressions. **B,** Two-person rescuer CPR. One rescuer delivers one breath after every five compressions given during a pause by other rescuer.

TABLE 27-6 Drugs commonly used in cardiac resuscitation

Drug	Route and Dosage	Actions and Indications
Atropine sulfate	0.5 mg by IV bolus; may be repeated at 5-min intervals	Reduces vagal tone; enhances AV conduction; accelerates heart rate in cases of pronounced sinus bradycardia
Bretylium tosylate (Bretylol)	5 mg/kg by IV bolus followed by defibrillation; may be increased to 10 mg/kg and repeated at 15- to 30-min intervals until maximal dose of 30 mg/kg has been given	For ventricular fibrillation and tachycardias that have not responded to other forms of therapy
Calcium chloride, 10% solution	2-4 mg/kg by IV bolus; may repeat at 10-min intervals	To increase myocardial contractile function; no significant beneficial effect during CPR; use during resuscitation limited to treat calcium channel blocker toxicity and acute hyperkalemia or hypocalcemia
Dobutamine hydrochloride (Dobutrex)	2.5-20 μg*/kg/min by IV	Used to treat refractory pump failure; direct receptor stimulating agent; increases myocardial contractility
Dopamine hydrochloride (Intropin)	5 μg/kg/min by IV drip; may be increased up to 20-50 μg/kg/min; a range of 5-30 μg/kg/min is usually required in arrest situations	Actions depend on dosage; 2-10 μg/kg/min generally has β-receptor stimulating action on heart with resultant increase in cardiac output; greater than 10 μg/kg/min has α-receptor stimulating action with resultant peripheral vasoconstriction
Epinephrine hydrochloride (Adrenalin), 1:10,000 solution	0.5-1.0 mg IV push; repeat every 5 min as needed; If used endotracheally, use full 1 mg	Positive inotropic and chronotropic action; peripheral vasoconstrictor; converts fine ventricular fibrillation to coarse, making it more amenable to defibrillation; increases perfusion pressure of cardiac compressions
Isoproterenol hydrochloride (Isuprel)	2-10 μg/min by IV bolus or intracardiac; dosage should be titrated to heart rate and blood pressure response	Potent inotropic and chronotropic agent; may induce or exacerbate myocardial ischemia caused by greatly increased myocardial oxygen requirements; no appreciable effect in cardiac arrest from asystole or electromechanical dissociation; recommended only in hemodynamically significant and atropine-refractory bradycardia on temporary basis until pacemaker can be implanted
Levarterenol bitartrate (Levophed)	2 μm/min as initial dose; average adult dose, 2-12 μm/min; should be titrated to blood pressure response	Potent vasopressor and positive inotropic effects; increases peripheral resistance; used in severe hypotension with low total peripheral resistance
Sodium bicarbonate (50 mEq)	1 mEq/kg by IV bolus; may repeat maximum of one-half this dose; further doses governed by arterial blood gas and pH determinations	To counteract metabolic acidosis
Lidocaine hydrochloride (Xylocaine)	Initial bolus 1 mg/kg; additional boluses of 0.5 mg/kg may be given at 8 min intervals up to total of 3 mg/kg if needed	Antiarrhythmic; shortens refractory period and suppresses automaticity of ectopic foci; useful in treatment of both ventricular tachycardia and fibrillation

*μg (micrograms) is sometimes written *mcg.*

IN-HOSPITAL CARDIAC ARRESTS

Many hospitals have prepared teams of personnel, including physicians, nurses, anesthesiologists, and technicians, who can be called to give immediate and complete care in the event of a cardiac arrest. Most hospitals are equipped with a cardiac arrest tray or have access to a specially equipped cart on which all necessary emergency items are available. Equipment needed includes an ECG machine, a suction device, oxygen, defibrillator, airway and Ambu or other breathing bag, laryngoscope, a variety of endotracheal tubes, cutdown set, intravenous fluids, and tracheostomy set.

Medications usually administered during a cardiac arrest are generally available on the emergency cart. Some of these medications are described in Table 27-6.

For a more detailed discussion of basic life support and for information on advanced life support, see reference 21.

COMPLICATIONS OF CARDIOPULMONARY RESUSCITATION

The most common complication of external cardiac massage is fracture of the ribs. This may occur in some individuals even though the technique of external cardiac compression was performed correctly. Other possible complications despite correct CPR technique include fractured sternum, costochondral separation, and lung contusions. If medications were injected into the heart during the resuscitative effort, the patient is monitored carefully for signs of hemothorax, pneumothorax, or pericardial tamponade. Any indication of labored respiration, paradoxical pulse, muffled heart sounds, tachycardia, decreased breath sounds, or drop in blood pressure is reported to the physician immediately. Laceration of the liver may also occur as a result of compressions performed over the xiphoid process.

INTERNAL CARDIAC COMPRESSION

In this seldom-used method of cardiac massage, a thoracotomy is performed and the heart is massaged with the hands or stimulated with an electric current. In most cases, open heart compression will not succeed when proper external compressions coupled with appropriate drug therapy and ventilation have failed. Internal compression is necessary in some instances or conditions, such as in cardiac tamponade, in crushing or penetrating chest injuries, and in the presence of an anatomic chest deformity that precludes adequate and effective compression by external cardiac massage.

CHAPTER SUMMARY

✔ An ECG is a graphic record of the electrical activity of the heart muscle; it is recorded on a grid that allows measurement of time and voltage. A 12-lead ECG provides 12 different views of cardiac electrical activity.

✔ A normal cardiac complex consists of a P wave, a QRS complex, and a T wave. The exact configuration varies according to the lead being recorded.

✔ Electrocardiographic signal averaging is a noninvasive, computerized method of analyzing standard ECGs.

✔ The mechanisms responsible for the genesis of dysrhythmias include altered automaticity, triggered activity, and reentry.

✔ Dysrhythmias originating in the sinoatrial node include sinus dysrhythmia, sinus tachycardia, sinus bradycardia, and sick sinus syndrome.

✔ Dysrhythmias originating in the atria include premature atrial beat, atrial tachycardia, atrial flutter, and atrial fibrillation.

✔ Dysrhythmias originating in the atrioventricular (AV) junction include premature junctional beat and junctional rhythms.

✔ Dysrhythmias originating in the ventricles include premature ventricular beat, ventricular rhythms and tachycardia, and ventricular fibrillation and standstill.

✔ Conduction abnormalities include AV block and bundle branch block.

✔ Two life-threatening dysrhythmias are ventricular fibrillation and ventricular standstill; CPR must be initiated and maintained until definitive treatment is effective.

✔ Treatment for cardiac dysrhythmias involves identification and elimination of the cause (if possible), drugs or electrical suppression of ectopic impulse initiation, and modalities to regulate heart rate (drugs, regulation of oxygen demand, artificial pacemakers).

✔ General nursing interventions for persons with dysrhythmias include promoting adequate cardiac output, activity and rest, tissue perfusion, comfort, relief of anxiety and a feeling of well-being, and patient/family learning.

✔ Artificial pacing may be by temporary or permanent pacemakers; the basic modes of pacing include fixed-rate mode and demand or standby mode. Complications include infection, dysrhythmias, and electrical interferences.

✔ Cardioversion and defibrillation are two methods for using electrical energy to convert a cardiac dysrhythmia to one that is more hemodynamically stable. Defibrillation is unsynchronized electrical countershock, whereas cardioversion synchronizes with the R wave to prevent accidental discharge during the ventricular vulnerable period.

✔ The automatic implantable cardioverter defibrillator (AICD) is an implanted device that automatically delivers a countershock when sensing ventricular fibrillation.

✔ Steps of basic life support include assessment of level of consciousness, opening of airway, initiation of artificial ventilation, assessment of circulation, and initiation of external cardiac compressions.

QUESTIONS TO CONSIDER

- How would electrolyte imbalance contribute to arrhythmogenesis?
- How do the principles of automaticity and excitability relate to cardioversion/defibrillation?
- What symptoms can a person experience as a result of decreased cardiac output?

REFERENCES AND SELECTED READINGS

1. Alpert JS and Rippe JM: Manual of cardiovascular diagnosis and therapy, ed 3, Boston, 1988, Little, Brown & Co.
2. American Heart Association: Instructor's manual for BLS, Dallas, 1987, The Association.
3. American Heart Association: Textbook of advanced cardiac life support, Dallas, 1987, The Association.
4. American Heart Association: Heart facts, Dallas, 1989, The Association.
5. *Andreoli KG et al: Comprehensive cardiac care: a textbook for nurses, physicians, and other health practitioners, ed 7, St Louis, 1987, The CV Mosby Co.
6. Berne RM and Levy MN: Cardiovascular physiology, ed 5, St Louis, 1986, The CV Mosby Co.
7. Breithardt G and Borggrefe M: Recent advances in the identification of patients at risk of ventricular tachyarrhythmias: role of ventricular late potentials, Circulation 75:1091-1096, 1987.
8. Carpenito LJ: Nursing diagnosis: application to clinical practice, ed 3, Philadelphia, 1989, JB Lippincott Co.
9. *Conover MB: Understanding electrocardiography: arrhythmias and the 12-lead ECG, ed 5, St Louis, 1988, The CV Mosby Co.
10. Dunn DL and Gregory JJ: Noninvasive temporary pacing: experience in a community hospital, Heart Lung 18:23-28, 1989.

11. Echt DS and Winkle RA: Management of patients with the automatic implantable cardioverter/defibrillator, Clin Prog 3(1):4-16, 1985.
12. Hanon DWG and Brogden RN: Propafenone: a review of its pharmacodynamic and pharmacokinetic properties and therapeutic use in the treatment of arrhythmias, Drugs 34:617-647, 1987.
13. Hopson JR, Hopson RC, and Kerber RE: The role of energy and current in successful defibrillation and cardioversion: C16 arrhythmias and conduction disturbances, Cardiol Board Rev 6(5):31-45, 1989.
14. Kerber RE et al: Energy, current, and success in defibrillation and cardioversion: clinical studies using an automatic impedance-based method of energy adjustment, Circulation 77:1038-1046, 1988.
15. *Marriott HJL: Practical electrocardiography, ed 8, Baltimore, 1988, Williams & Wilkins.
16. Mirowski M et al: Termination of malignant ventricular arrhythmias with an implanted automatic defibrillator in human beings, New Engl J Med 303:322-324, 1980.
17. Moser SA, Crawford D, and Thomas, A: Caring for patients with implantable cardioverter defibrillators, Crit Care Nurse 8(2):52-65, 1988.
18. *Purcell JA and Burrows SG: A pacemaker primer, Am J Nurs 85:553-568, 1985.
19. Purdy RE and Boucek RJ: Handbook of cardiac drugs, Boston, 1988, Little, Brown & Co.
20. Restrictions on use of flecainide and encainide, FDA Drug Bull 19(2):16, 1989.
21. Standards and guidelines for cardiopulmonary resuscitation (CPR) and emergency cardiac care (ECC), JAMA 255:2905-2973, 1986.
22. Vatterott PJ et al: Signal-averaged electrocardiography: a new noninvasive test to identify patients at risk for ventricular arrhythmias, Mayo Clin Proc 63:931-942, 1988.
23. *Weller S and Noone J: Mechanisms of arrhythmias: enhanced automaticity and reentry, Crit Care Nurse 9(5):42-66, 1989.
24. Winkle RA: The implantable defibrillator in ventricular arrhythmias, Hosp Pract 18:149-165, 1983.
25. Winkle RA et al: Practical aspects of automatic cardioverter/defibrillator implantation, Am Heart J 108:1333-1346, 1984.
26. Zipes DP: Genesis of cardiac arrhythmias; electrophysiological considerations: management of cardiac arrhythmias, diagnosis and treatment. In Braunwald E: Heart disease: a textbook of cardiovascular medicine, ed 3, Philadelphia, 1988, WB Saunders Co.
27. Zipes DP: Cardiac electrophysiology: promises and contributions, J Am Coll Cardiol 13:1329-1352, 1989.

*References preceded by an asterisk are particularly well suited for student reading.

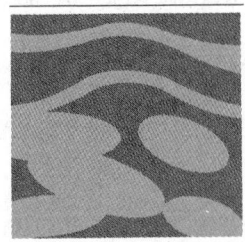

Management of Persons with Cardiovascular Problems

TERRI ABRAHAM
AUDREY BAKANAUSKAS
JOAN M. KAVANAGH

CHAPTER OBJECTIVES

After studying this chapter, the student should be able to:
1. Differentiate between the different inflammatory heart diseases and valvular heart diseases.
2. Identify behavioral and psychosocial influences on the genesis of coronary artery disease.
3. Explain the pathophysiology, clinical manifestations, and medical and nursing interventions for inflammatory heart diseases, valvular heart diseases, aneurysms, angina pectoris, myocardial infarction, and congestive heart failure.
4. Describe the method and purpose for cardiopulmonary bypass used during some cardiac surgeries.
5. Describe method and purpose of different cardiovascular surgeries and modalities, including valvular surgery, resection of aneurysm, coronary artery bypass surgery, percutaneous transluminal coronary angioplasty (PTCA), intravascular stenting, laser therapy, and thrombolytic therapy.
6. Describe preoperative and postoperative nursing care for cardiovascular surgery.

Heart disease is a major cause of death in industrialized nations. Unfortunately, noninvasive diagnostic techniques have not yet been perfected for mass screening for all types of cardiovascular disorders. Therefore many persons are not even aware that they have heart disease until severe symptoms develop. This chapter discusses the following major cardiovascular disorders:
1. Inflammatory heart diseases
2. Valvular heart diseases
3. Aortic aneurysms
4. Coronary artery diseases (angina pectoris and myocardial infarction)
5. Congestive heart failure
6. Acute pulmonary edema (resulting from left ventricular failure)

Heart surgery, including types and nursing care, is also included.

EPIDEMIOLOGY OF HEART DISEASE

In the United States cardiovascular disorders cause more deaths than all other diseases combined. Nearly 66 million Americans (more than one in four persons) have some form of cardiovascular disease. In 1986, almost 1 million Americans died of heart and blood vessel disease. This figure represents almost as many deaths from cancer, influenza, accidents, pneumonia, and all other causes combined.[2]

The type of cardiovascular disorder that causes death varies with age. In the United States, congenital heart disease and closely related vascular disorders are responsible for disabling 25,000 newborns each year. The most common cause of death from heart disease after the age of 25 years is coronary atherosclerotic heart disease (CAHD). CAHD strikes a significant number of persons without any warning and causes prolonged suffering and disability in even larger numbers. In 1987 it was estimated that approximately 15 million people in the United States would sustain a myocardial infarction, and an estimated 540,000 of them would die.[3]

Other cardiovascular disorders with substantial morbidity and mortality include hypertensive heart disease, rheumatic heart disease, and cerebrovascular disease. Fortunately, despite the discouraging statistics related to the incidence of cardiovascular disorders, there has been a steady reduction in mortality from cardiovascular disease. In the United States the past decade has witnessed a tremendous expansion in cardiovascular research and much progress has been made in preventing and treating cardiovascular disease. This reduction in mortality suggests an effective application of increased knowledge regarding the causes, diagnosis, treatment, and, most significantly, the prevention of heart disease.[11]

Although the exact pathogeneses of many types of heart diseases are not yet known, extensive epidemiologic studies are in progress in an attempt to delineate further preventive measures. Observational epidemiologic studies have identified numerous risk factors for cardiovascular disease. The implication is that with pharmacologic interventions and behavior modification, especially in regard to changes in life-style, the manifestations of cardiovascular disease may be decreased, delayed, or even eliminated.[32] Further definitive research protocols are now being developed to study the validity of these implications. Presently it is felt that screening and public education can effect a significant reduction in the morbidity and mortality from cardiovascular disorders.

CLASSIFICATION OF HEART DISEASE

Heart diseases may be divided into two general groups: those that are *congenital* and those that are *acquired* after birth. Congenital heart disease follows an abnormality of structure caused by error in embryologic development of the heart. Acquired disease may affect the heart either suddenly or gradually. There may be damage to the heart from bacteria, chemical agents, or diminished blood supply. For example, inflammation may cause scarring of heart valves, muscle, or outer coverings that may impair the heart's function. Any changes in the coronary vessels supplying the heart muscle may decrease its efficiency.

Heart disease may also be classified according to a specific cause such as rheumatic fever, infective endocarditis, or hypertension. It is also classified according to anatomic change such as valvular scarring. Progression of any of these diseases may lead to cardiac failure. Varying degrees of cardiac arrhythmia and cardiac failure are the cause of many of the symptoms commonly associated with the various cardiac diseases, but with early diagnosis and treatment these complications may be prevented or controlled.

INFLAMMATORY HEART DISEASES

PERICARDITIS
ETIOLOGY

Pericarditis may occur as a result of bacterial, viral, or fungal infection; it may occur as a complication of a systemic disease such as rheumatoid arthritis, systemic lupus erythematosus, scleroderma, uremia, or myocardial infarction, or as a result of trauma.

PATHOPHYSIOLOGY

Pericarditis is an inflammatory process of the visceral and or parietal pericardium. It can often result in compression of the heart (*cardiac tamponade*) causing a decrease in venous return to the heart and a decrease in ventricular emptying, which may lead to cardiac failure.

Pericarditis may be acute or chronic in nature and may spread from or to the myocardium. *Acute pericardi-*

tis is further classified as fibrinous or exudative. The exudate accompanying acute pericarditis may be serous, purulent, or hemorrhagic. When fluid accumulates in the pericardial sac, cardiac tamponade may occur with impairment of ventricular filling and emptying. If not diagnosed and treated promptly, the severe reduction in cardiac output can result in shock and death. Chronic pericarditis is referred to as chronic constrictive or adhesive pericarditis. If the pericardium becomes a constrictive band surrounding the heart, it will prevent adequate filling and emptying of the ventricles, ultimately producing cardiac failure.

ACUTE PERICARDITIS
Clinical Manifestations

A predominant clinical manifestation of acute pericarditis is a *pericardial friction rub* along with severe precordial chest pain, which may closely resemble that of acute myocardial infarction. The patient may complain of pain over the left shoulder (left trapezial ridge), which may radiate to the neck and down the left arm; it is intensified when lying supine and is relieved by sitting. The pain may also intensify when the patient coughs, swallows, or breathes deeply. Dysphagia is commonly experienced.

Typically, the temperature is elevated and a leukocytosis of 10,000 to 20,000 is present. In the exudative form of acute pericarditis, the electrocardiogram (ECG) may show a bradycardia with low-voltage QRS complexes caused by attenuation of the pericardial fluid or an atrial fibrillation or flutter. Occasionally, electrical alternans secondary to the heart changing position as it beats in the pericardium may be evident on the ECG.

Symptoms of cardiac tamponade may include diminished or absent point of maximal impulse (PMI) and peripheral pulses. Distended neck veins secondary to increased central venous pressure and decreased blood pressure secondary to ineffective pumping action may be noted. A narrowing pulse pressure is a sign of cardiac tamponade. Heart sounds may be diminished, and the pulse is paradoxic.

Radiographs may show a pericardial effusion, although an echocardiogram is more diagnostic. If the accumulation of pericardial fluid is gradual, little pain may be noticed by the patient. As much as 1 L of clear or serosanguineous fluid may accumulate.

Interventions

A known etiologic disease process or agent is treated specifically, such as with antibiotic therapy if indicated. Otherwise, the clinical symptoms of fever, malaise, and pain are treated.

If the pericardial effusion is small or absent, therapy for pericarditis is supportive with salicylates or indomethacin (Indocin) to decrease inflammation. If the effusion is large, the physician may perform a pericardiocentesis (pericardial tap). Caution is exercised to avoid puncture of the heart wall. Occasionally, after removal of the fluid the physician will instill antibiotics directly into the pericardial sac. A pericardial fenestration (pericardial window) may be performed to provide continuous drainage of pericardial fluid. Complications may include atelectasis and introduction of infectious agents. Corticosteroids may be administered to reduce inflammation.

CHRONIC PERICARDITIS

Chronic constrictive pericarditis may result from fibrosing of the pericardial sac secondary to trauma or neoplastic disease. The thick fibrous pericardium tightens around the heart and decreases its efficiency as a pump.

Clinical Manifestations

Chronic constrictive pericarditis is three times more prevalent in males than in females. Patients may complain of dyspnea and fatigue and exhibit symptoms of congestive heart failure secondary to the diminished ability of the heart to function as a pump.

Interventions

Removal of the pericardium (pericardiectomy) may be necessary to restore cardiac function. Postoperative care is similar to that of other heart surgery (p. 697). Other measures to restore more efficient pumping include digitalization, diuretic therapy, and a low-sodium diet.

MYOCARDITIS
EPIDEMIOLOGY/ETIOLOGY

Myocarditis is an inflammatory disease of the myocardium that causes an infiltrate in the myocardial interstitium and injury to adjacent myocardial cells atypical of infarction. Myocarditis may be primary with an unknown etiology or secondary from an identifiable cause such as drug hypersensitivity or toxicity and infection. Very often this inflammatory process develops secondary to acute endocarditis or pericarditis. Myocarditis may be classified as acute (benign or fulminant) or chronic.

Infection may result in one of three ways: invasion of the myocardial tissue by organisms, production of toxins (diphtheria), or an autoimmune reaction (rheumatic fever, systemic lupus erythematosus). Worldwide, the most frequent infectious agents are rickettsiae, bacteria, protozoans, and metazoans. In North America infection is most often caused by a virus, including coxsackievirus, echovirus, viral encephalitis, rabies, and herpes simplex.

PATHOPHYSIOLOGY

Although a wide variety of organisms are linked to the development of myocarditis in human beings, the correlation between viruses and myocarditis is primarily circumstantial, because viruses have been isolated from the human myocardium in only a few cases. Myocarditis is difficult to study in human beings, because it frequently remains undiagnosed until chronic cardiac dysfunction and congestive heart failure become clinically obvious. Animal studies, especially the mouse (murine) model, have been particularly helpful in aiding understanding resulting from similarities between murine and human myocarditis.

Research has shown that mice infected with coxsackievirus B_3 manifest an acute and chronic phase of the illness.[72] During the acute phase (7 to 10 days after infection), the virus can be directly cultured from the myocardium. Chronically, antibodies directed against the virus remain for several months; inflammation may persist for up to 6 months. Fifteen months after the initial infection cardiac damage is characterized by mural thrombi, cardiac chamber dilation, scarring (fibrosis), and hypertrophy and disintegration of heart muscle cells. This second chronic phase is possibly mediated by the immune system and results in cardiac dilation and failure similar to that seen in human dilated cardiomyopathy. Furthermore, the significant incidence of dilated cardiomyopathy after recovery from acute viral myocarditis provides evidence linking these disease processes.

Clinical Manifestations

Symptom manifestation may be divided into two distinct phases: an acute viral phase and a chronic phase with symptoms unrelated to the viral infection. During the acute phase symptoms are flulike and include fever, lymphadenopathy, pharyngitis, myalgias, and GI complaints. Hepatitis, encephalitis, nephritis, and orchitis can also occur.

The most common cardiac symptom during the acute phase is pericardial pain, which may be associated with a friction rub because the pericardium is so inflamed. Other cardiac manifestations include signs of congestive heart failure, syncope, pericardial effusion, and ischemia. ECG changes include ST-segment elevation, T-wave flattening or inversion, appearance of Q waves, and QT-interval prolongation. Ventricular ectopy may include multiple morphologies of premature ventricular beats and ventricular tachycardia. ECG abnormalities may disappear after recovery or persist for several years.

Preliminary laboratory findings are nonspecific, including elevation of the erythrocyte sedimentation rate, viral titers, and levels of various enzymes (such as lactic dehydrogenase, creatinine phosphokinase, and the transaminases). Mild to moderate leukocytosis with atypical lymphocytes may be seen. Chest radiographs may show the heart size normal or enlarged. In the fulminant form of acute myocarditis, pulmonary rales may be auscultated.

INTERVENTIONS

Patients with myocarditis are often treated with bed rest and digitalis to prevent heart failure and cardiogenic shock. Immunosuppression may be beneficial in reducing myocardial inflammation and in preventing irreversible myocardial damage. Medical therapy also involves treatment of the underlying disease with antibiotics, conventional therapy for congestive heart failure, and management of dysrhythmias.

ALCOHOLIC CARDIOMYOPATHY

ETIOLOGY

When any form of ethanol (the chief substance in alcoholic beverages) is consumed in large quantities over a period greater than 5 years, it has a direct toxic effect on cardiac tissue. Additives in alcoholic beverages may also create their own toxic effects. Persons with alcoholic cardiomyopathy are usually well-nourished individuals; only 15% of these patients have thiamine deficiency as is seen in many alcoholics.

CLINICAL MANIFESTATIONS

The onset of alcoholic cardiomyopathy is usually gradual with nonspecific fatigue and dyspnea on exertion. Physical examination may reveal pulmonary rales, cardiac murmur, edema, and increasing blood pressure and central venous pressure (CVP). ECG changes may show low-voltage QRS complexes and ST-segment abnormalities. Conduction defects and arrhythmias may also occur. Symptoms progress to congestive heart failure and thromboemboli, but liver enlargement is not usually present.

Electron microscopic studies of heart tissue may show fatty degeneration of myocardial cells and the heart itself may become flabby.[11] Chest radiographs show an enlarged heart with hypertrophic left ventricle and general pulmonary congestion.

INTERVENTIONS

Medical treatment is primarily symptomatic. Vasodilator therapy may be helpful, and prolonged bed rest is thought by some to reduce the size of the enlarged heart.

More than 10% of the adult population is involved in "heavy" alcohol consumption. It is therefore not surprising that alcoholic cardiomyopathy is such a major health problem. Nurses have an important role in stressing the need for moderation in ethanol intake and in teaching patients that complete abstention from alcohol may halt the progression or even reverse alcoholic cardiomyopathy.

INFECTIVE ENDOCARDITIS

Infective endocarditis is an infection of the endocardium and most often of the heart valves. The disease has commonly been classified in the past on the degree of acuteness. *Acute endocarditis* occurs rapidly, often on normal heart valves, and if untreated may cause death within days to weeks. Even with treatment the mortality is high.[11] *Subacute bacterial endocarditis* (SBE) develops more gradually, usually on previously damaged heart valves, and responds well to treatment.

ETIOLOGY

The more recent method of classification of infective endocarditis is on the basis of the causative organism. The viridans streptococci are the major causative organisms, especially in the subacute form. Other major infective agents include staphylococci, such as *S. aureus* or *S. epidermidis,* and enterococci. Major causes of underlying cardiac pathologic conditions include rheumatic valvular disease, congenital heart disease, and degenerative heart disease. In some cases, endocarditis is preceded by intrusive procedures such as dental procedures, minor surgery, gynecologic examinations, and insertion of indwelling urinary catheters or renal shunts. Other persons at high risk include those who "mainline" street drugs (inject drugs directly into the veins), because of the possibility of bacteremia from contaminated needles and syringes.

PATHOPHYSIOLOGY

A previously damaged cardiac valve or a ventricular septal defect produces turbulent blood flow, allowing bacteria to settle on the low-pressure side of a stenotic valve or a ventricular septal defect. The hallmark of endocarditis is the platelet-fibrin-bacteria mass on the valve constituting a vegetation. A Venturi effect is set up around the anomalies, and the organisms bombard the heart valves, become embedded in the valve matrix, and result in vegetative growths that may scar and perforate the leaflets. One to four percent of persons who have artificial heart valve implants will develop endocarditis.

Further risk results if the vegetative growths break free of the valves, enter the bloodstream, and cause emboli. If the vegetative emboli enter such organs as the spleen and kidney, abscesses may form.

PREVENTION

Prevention of infective endocarditis should include correction of any underlying cardiac defect, if possible, as well as utilization of measures to prevent bacteremia. For persons with underlying cardiac disease, early and vigorous treatment of infections, maintenance of oral hygiene, avoidance of intraarterial or intravenous catheters, and prophylactic use of antibiotics when undergoing dental treatment or a surgical procedure are important.

CLINICAL MANIFESTATIONS

The onset of SBE is gradual, and the patient reports malaise and general achiness. Low-grade fever is usually present, although a high fever usually occurs if *S. aureus* is the causative organism. Other frequently reported symptoms include arthralgias, arthritis, low back pain, myalgias, disk-space infection, tenosynovitis, anorexia, weight loss, chest pain, and occasional hemoptysis. Physical examination may reveal splenomegaly, clubbing of the fingers, the presence of Osler's nodes on fingers or toe pads, and small capillary hemorrhages (petechiae) in the conjunctiva, mouth, and extremities. On auscultation, murmurs may be audible over the cardiac valves. A normocytic normochromic anemia is usually present.

INTERVENTIONS

In infective endocarditis the affected areas have impaired cellular or humoral host defenses; therefore the major aim of therapy is to eliminate all microorganisms from the vegetative growths and to prevent the development of complications. If symptoms go untreated for weeks or months, the incidence of embolic complications and progressive involvement of the heart valves are greatly increased. Therefore, after several blood cultures have been drawn and the infecting organism identified, intravenous antibiotic therapy is initiated. It is important that antibiotic therapy be continued *for a prolonged time,* even after symptoms abate, to eradicate all organisms. Abscesses may require surgical drainage. When necessary, deteriorated heart valves are surgically replaced with prostheses.

Measures are also taken to prevent further infection. Good oral hygiene is imperative, and all intrusive approaches, such as catheterization, are avoided if possible. The patients need to learn the importance of obtaining prophylactic antibiotic therapy before any dental procedures, genitourinary or gastrointestinal procedures, or surgeries are performed.

RHEUMATIC HEART DISEASE

Rheumatic heart disease is an acute inflammatory reaction. It may involve (1) the lining of the heart, or endocardium (endocarditis), including the valves, resulting in scarring, distortion, and stenosis of the valves, (2) the heart muscle (myocarditis), or (3) the outer covering of the heart (pericarditis) where it may cause adhesions to surrounding tissues. The development of symptoms of chronic rheumatic heart disease in later life depends on the location and severity of the damage and other factors. Somewhat less than 10% of persons with rheumatic fever develop rheumatic heart disease, and about one half of those with rheumatic heart disease have *mitral stenosis* (p. 674). It is possible for rheumatic fever and rheumatic heart disease with mild

symptoms to go undiagnosed, or the disease may be subclinical with no noticeable symptoms. Thus the discovery of rheumatic heart disease is made years later. Careful recall of illness in childhood may include a recollection of "growing pains," confirming the likelihood that the patient had rheumatic fever during childhood.

Prophylactic penicillin is prescribed during acute episodes of rheumatic fever and for several years thereafter. Continuous antibiotic prophylaxis for life may be necessary for those persons with significant rheumatic heart disease. In persons with significant carditis during acute rheumatic fever, corticosteroids may be prescribed to decrease the cardiac inflammation. If congestive heart failure occurs during this period, bed rest, sodium and fluid restrictions, diuretics, and digoxin are usually prescribed.

SYPHILITIC CARDIOVASCULAR DISEASE

Syphilitic cardiovascular disease usually occurs from 10 to 20 years after the primary syphilitic infection. Since the highest incidence of primary syphilis is among persons in their early 20s, persons with symptoms of syphilitic heart disease are usually over 30 to 50 years of age.

PREVENTION

It is the aim of health organizations and medical personnel to treat all persons with syphilis before they develop cardiovascular disease or any of the other complications of late syphilis. Primary syphilis can be arrested; however, once syphilis has affected the aorta and the valves of the heart, little can be done except to treat the patient symptomatically.

PATHOPHYSIOLOGY AND CLINICAL MANIFESTATIONS

In cardiovascular syphilis the spirochetes attack the aorta, the aortic valve, and the heart muscle. The portion of the aorta nearest the heart is usually affected, and the elastic wall of the aorta becomes weakened and bulges. This bulge is known as an *aneurysm.* As the aneurysm grows it may press on neighboring structures such as the intercostal nerves and cause pain. Aneurysms may also be present without symptoms. Evidence may be discovered on radiographic examination. There is a possibility that the aneurysm may rupture as it increases in size, and the person is encouraged to avoid strenuous activities that might cause a sudden increase in the pressure exerted against the bulging vessel. Surgical resection of the aneurysm sometimes is possible (p. 686).

Syphilis may also attack the aorta more diffusely, causing *aortitis.* The aorta becomes dilated, and small plaques containing calcium are laid down. There may be complaints of substernal pain associated with exertion caused by constriction at the orifices of the coronary arteries. Thrombi may develop along the aorta, and emboli may occur, resulting in severe complications such as myocardial infarction or cerebral emboli.

Spirochetes may also attack the aortic valve, causing it to become scarred. This causes *aortic insufficiency*, and the person may have a bounding pulse and a high systolic blood pressure because of the extra effort demanded of the ventricles to pump blood into the systemic circulation. Heart failure eventually occurs.

INTERVENTIONS

The use of penicillin in the treatment of the patient with cardiovascular syphilis is thought to possibly prolong life, since penicillin destroys any active organisms and permits healing to occur. Treatment at this stage, however, will not restore damaged aortic tissue or damaged aortic valves, and extensive scarring may occur. The person with syphilitic heart disease should be given guidance in planning activities of daily living and in selecting work that places the least possible burden on the damaged heart and aorta. In certain cases of aortic insufficiency, surgery is possible.

CARDIOVASCULAR EFFECTS OF COCAINE ABUSE

Despite the widespread use of cocaine, medical investigation of its systemic effects in humans is sparse and frequently controversial. Cocaine is classified as a local anesthetic (Chapter 21) and a sympathomimetic drug. It is a tropane alkaloid of the evergreen shrub, *Erythroxylon coca*, which is cultivated extensively in Bolivia and Peru. Crack cocaine is a heat-stable, freebase form of cocaine that is suitable for smoking and which causes an almost immediate, often intense, response.

Cocaine is metabolized rapidly in the liver by hepatic enzymes and in the bloodstream by plasma cholinesterase. Individuals with impaired liver function are subject to the prolonged effects. Depending on the urine acidity (enhanced excretion occurs with a decreased urine pH), 10% to 20% of the drug is excreted unchanged. Cocaine toxicity is characterized by generalized stimulation including hyperthermia, acute agitation, tachycardia, hypertension, diaphoresis, and acidosis. Fatal pulmonary edema has been associated with cocaine intoxication, as well as seizure activity, cardiac dysrhythmias, and respiratory arrest with doses approaching 1 g.

Cardiovascular collapse is secondary to a combination of hyperthermia, hypoxia, acidosis, and CNS stimulation. Myocardial ischemia and infarction have been associated with cocaine use. The pathogenesis remains uncertain; hypotheses include coronary artery thrombosis, embolus, or spasms; increased thrombogenicity; and increased myocardial oxygen demand. Treatment options include beta blockers for ventricular dysrhythmias, nitrates and calcium channel blockers if coronary artery pathogenesis is suspected, and aspirin or other thrombolytic agents for acute ischemic events. (For fur-

ther discussion on substance abuse and nursing implications, see Chapter 19).

VALVULAR HEART DISEASE
PATHOPHYSIOLOGY

Healthy and competent heart valves facilitate unidirectional blood flow through the heart. The atrioventricular valves (AV) (mitral and tricuspid) prevent blood from flowing back into the atria from the ventricles during systole. During diastole, blood flows through the AV openings and passively opens the AV valves. During systole, the intense ventricular contractions force the valve flaps back into a closed position. Simultaneous contraction of the papillary muscles and the resultant tension on the chordae tendineae prevent the valve flaps from being forced back into the atria (see Figure 26-1). The semilunar valves (SV) (aortic and pulmonic) prevent blood from flowing back into the ventricles from the aorta and pulmonary artery during diastole.

When the atrioventricular or semilunar valves become diseased, they may become stenosed and obstruct the normal flow of blood through the heart, or they may become insufficient and cause regurgitation or backflow of blood into the cardiac chamber from which the blood was previously propelled (Figure 28-1). Initially, the heart can compensate for the stenosed or insufficient valves through gradual hypertrophy of the myocardium. Medical treatment can facilitate a more effective compensation for the dysfunctional valve for years. However, if the stenosis or insufficiency worsens, congestive heart failure will eventually ensue, and valve replacement or repair is indicated.

MITRAL VALVULAR DISEASE
MITRAL STENOSIS
Etiology

Two thirds of all persons with mitral stenosis are females. Mitral stenosis, the most common disease of the mitral valve, is predominantly an acquired disease. Rheumatic fever, which is the primary cause of mitral stenosis, causes adhesions or fibrosis of the chordae tendineae or commissures. Nonrheumatic causes include atrial myxomas, bacterial vegetation, thrombus formation, or calcification of the mitral annulus.

Pathophysiology

Rheumatic fever can cause valve thickening by calcification and fibrous tissue formation. The valve leaflets or commissures are fused together and become stiffened, resulting in a progressively narrowed and immobile valve. The chordae tendineae will also shorten and thicken, and the mitral orifice may decrease in size from its normal 4 sq cm to 6 sq cm to less than 1 sq cm. Progressive stenosis of the mitral aperture causes increas-

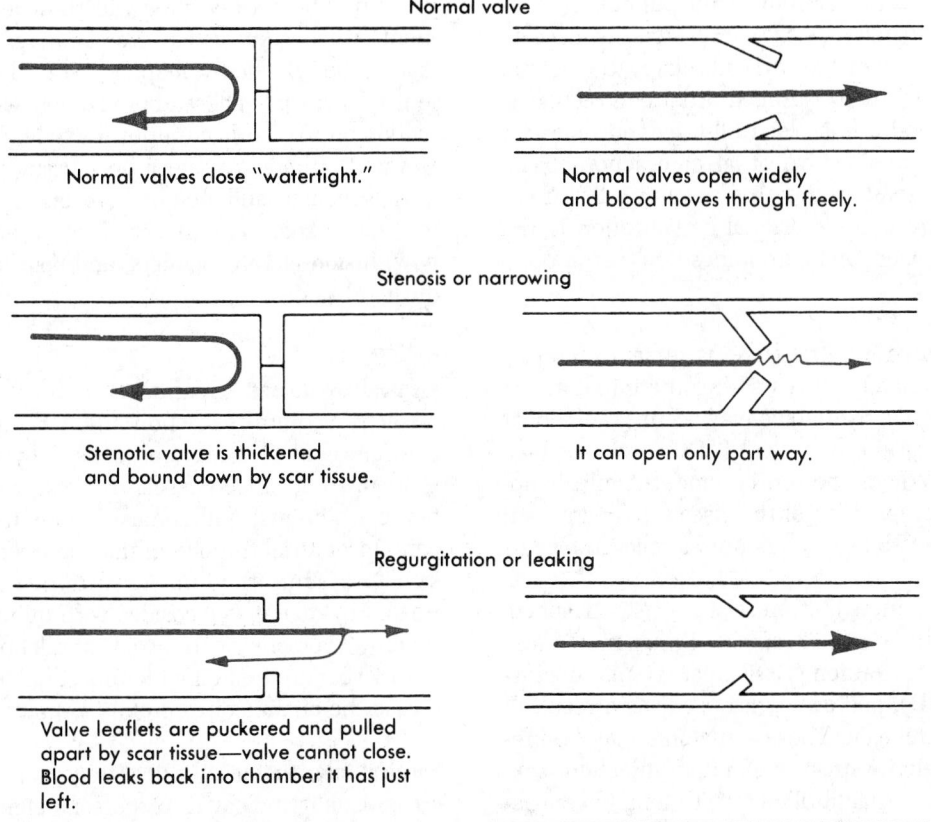

FIGURE 28-1 Diseases of heart valves. (From Phibbs B: The human heart: a guide to heart disease, ed 4, St Louis, 1979, The CV Mosby Co.)

ingly elevated left atrial pressures as a result of the additional trapped blood in the left atrium (Figure 28-2).

Hypertrophy of the left atrium develops as the heart compensates for the increased contractile strength needed to propel the blood through the stenosed valve. The elevated left atrial pressure causes pulmonary hypertension and congestion. As the stenosis becomes

more severe, higher pulmonary artery pressures will impede right ventricular function and will precipitate right-sided heart failure. The left ventricle receives insufficient end-diastolic blood volumes, leading to a decrease in the cardiac output and eventual left ventricular atrophy.

To complicate further the hemodynamic status from

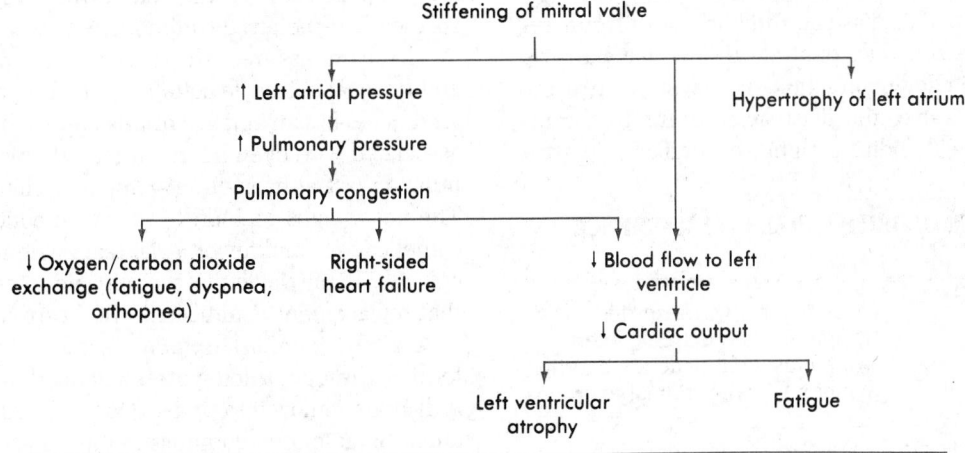

FIGURE 28-2 Pathophysiology of mitral stenosis.

inadequate left ventricular filling and pulmonary congestion, 50% of persons with mitral stenosis develop atrial fibrillation. When the atria fibrillate, the normal end-diastolic "kick" from a unified atrial contraction is eliminated and again, less blood fills the ventricles for systole. Without an effective atrial contraction, blood may pool and stagnate in the atria, resulting in thrombus formation and possible arterial embolization to the brain, kidneys, spleen, and extremities.

Clinical Manifestations

Many individuals with mitral stenosis remain asymptomatic for approximately 20 years after the initial attack of rheumatic carditis. Symptoms may occur gradually or abruptly depending on the severity of the stenosis (see the box below). When a person becomes acutely symptomatic, a rapid progression of the disease to death usually occurs between 5 to 10 years unless relieved by surgical intervention.

The principal symptom of mitral stenosis is dyspnea, which is largely the result of reduced compliance of the lungs. Dyspnea on exertion (DOE), paroxysmal nocturnal dyspnea (PND), and orthopnea occur as a result of pulmonary hypertension. These symptoms may be precipitated by emotional stress, respiratory infection, sexual intercourse, or atrial fibrillation with a rapid ventricular response. Some people may experience a dry cough, dysphagia, or bronchitis because of bronchial irritation as a result of an enlarged left atrium. Pressure exerted on the laryngeal nerve by an enlarged pulmonary artery will cause hoarseness. Excessive fatigue and weakness occur secondary to a decreased cardiac output. Other symptoms include peripheral and facial cyanosis. Hemoptysis, usually a late sign, is due to the rupture of a bronchial vein. Eventual right-sided heart failure will lead to jugular vein distention, pitting edema, and hepatomegaly.

Diagnosis of mitral stenosis is established by clinical symptoms, such as an opening snap (OS), created by the forceful opening of the mitral valve, followed by a diastolic rumbling. This diastolic rumbling or murmur results from increased velocity of blood flow that narrows after left ventricular contraction. However, with a severely calcified valve, the diastolic murmur is absent. ECG changes will indicate right ventricular hypertro-

phy, and chest x-ray films will show left atrial enlargement. Mitral stenosis can also be diagnosed with a cardiac catheterization (Chapter 26) to determine the extent of stenosis. The catheterization will provide information on the cardiac output, valve leaflet function, and elevated pulmonary artery pressures (Table 28-1). The most sensitive and noninvasive diagnostic indicator is the echocardiogram that will show an impedance of flow, fusion of valve leaflets, and poor leaflet separation during diastole.

Interventions

Medical treatment. Treatment of the disease is initially medical. Sodium restriction and oral diuretics can help alleviate clinical symptoms caused by pulmonary congestion. In advanced cases, bed rest or the sitting position can diminish pulmonary venous hypertension. Recent onset atrial fibrillation may be treated by cardioversion to a sinus rhythm. Atrial fibrillation may also be treated by digitalis glycosides with quinidine as adjunct therapy. Persons with atrial fibrillation lasting more than 1 year are treated with anticoagulant therapy to decrease the chance of thrombus formation.

Surgical intervention. Surgical treatment for mitral stenosis is usually indicated for persons significantly limited in activity despite appropriate medical treatment. Surgical options include commissurotomy (repair) or valve replacement.

Mitral commissurotomy is the separation or incision of the stenosed valve leaflets at their borders or commissures. There are two techniques used for a commissurotomy—open or closed. Controversy exists over the two methods, with an open commissurotomy being the procedure of choice.

An *open commissurotomy* is usually done through a median sternotomy or a right anterolateral thoracotomy incision. This allows for proper visualization of the mitral valve. A cardiopulmonary bypass pump is used, and after the incision of the left atrium, the valve is inspected and the atrial thrombus removed.

The commissures are then incised with a scalpel, and new mobilized leaflets are attached to the chordae tendineae. Disadvantages of this approach include those associated with open heart surgery, that is, difficult cannulation of the heart-lung pump and clotting problems. The advantages include fewer thrombotic and embolic complications and fewer atrial tears with resultant hemorrhage. If the valve disease appears to be so advanced that replacement is indicated, the heart is already open.

A *closed* commissurotomy (without bypass) is performed through a left posterolateral thoracotomy. The fifth rib is removed to prepare for a closed or open operation. Some closed commissurotomies are performed in the fourth and fifth interspace with a transection of a

---

EFFECT OF MITRAL ORIFICE SIZE ON EMERGENCE OF SYMPTOMS

> 2.6 sq cm	No symptoms with exertion
2.1-2.5 sq cm	Symptoms with extreme exertion
1.6-2.0 sq cm	Symptoms with moderate exertion
< 1.5 sq cm	Symptoms with minimal exertion

From Hurst JW (editor): The heart, ed. 6, New York, 1986, McGraw-Hill Book Co.

TABLE 28-1 Findings in valvular heart disorders

Disorder	Chest Radiograph	ECG	Echocardiogram	Cardiac Catheterization
Mitral stenosis	Left atrial enlargement Mitral valve calcification Right ventricular enlargement Prominence of pulmonary artery	Left atrial hypertrophy Right ventricular hypertrophy Atrial fibrillation	Thickened mitral valve Left atrial enlargement	Increased pressure gradient across valve Increased left atrial pressure Increased PCWP Increased right heart pressure Decreased CO
Mitral regurgitation	Left atrial enlargement Left ventricular enlargement	Left atrial hypertrophy Left ventricular hypertrophy Atrial fibrillation Sinus tachycardia	Abnormal mitral valve movement Left atrial enlargement	Mitral regurgitation Increased atrial pressure Increased LVEDP Increased PCWP Decreased cardiac output
Aortic stenosis	Left ventricular enlargement Aortic valve calcification May have enlargement of left atrium, pulmonary artery, right ventricle, right atrium	Left ventricular hypertrophy	Thickened aortic valve Thickened ventricular wall Abnormal movement of aortic leaflets	Increased pressure gradient across valve Increased LVEDP
Aortic regurgitation	Left ventricular enlargement	Left ventricular hypertrophy Tall R waves Sinus tachycardia	Left ventricular enlargement Abnormal mitral valve movement Increased movement of ventricular wall	Aortic regurgitation Increased LVEDP Decreased arterial diastolic pressure
Tricuspid stenosis	Right atrial enlargement Prominence of superior vena cava	Right atrial hypertrophy Tall peaked P waves Atrial fibrillation	Abnormal valvular leaflets Right atrial enlargement	Increased pressure gradient across valve Increased right atrial pressure Decreased CO
Tricuspid regurgitation	Right atrial enlargement Right ventricular enlargement	Right ventricular hypertrophy Atrial fibrillation	Prolapse of tricuspid valve Right atrial enlargement	Increased atrial pressure Tricuspid regurgitation Decreased CO

PCWP = pulmonary capillary wedge pressure; CO = cardiac output; LVEDP = left ventricular end-diastolic pressure.

rib, if necessary. After the incision is made, the atrium is palpated to detect any thrombi. If a thrombus is present, the procedure is converted to an open procedure to remove the clot. Otherwise, the surgeon inserts a finger through a small incision, dividing the papillary muscle longitudinally from the apex toward the base. The atrium is digitally examined for thrombi, and the valve is examined for calcium particles. Some surgeons may digitally open the fused commissures and use a dilator to open the valve and relieve the stenosis. The advantages of the closed approach include a shorter operating time, greater simplicity, and less blood replacement. Systemic emboli, atrial wall tears, inadequate alleviation of the stenosis, and mitral regurgitation are all risks of this method of commissurotomy.

One major advantage of mitral valve repair over a mitral replacement is the mortality rate. The operative mortality for a commissurotomy is 1% to 2%, compared with 10% for a mitral valve replacement.[19]

Mitral valve replacement is considered when the valve is so stenosed and calcified that repair would not achieve long-term relief of obstruction. The site of incision can be any of those discussed; however, most frequently the heart is approached via a median sternotomy. The extracorporeal bypass pump is used in an open procedure. The diseased valve leaflets are excised at the annulus, and the remaining annuli are sized with an obturator. The loose chordae are excised to avoid their becoming tangled in the new valve. The prosthetic valve is sutured into the new annulus. The mortality rate with a mitral valve replacement is roughly 5% to 10%, and the overall survival rate is approximately 70%.

MITRAL REGURGITATION

Etiology

Mitral regurgitation is more commonly found in males than in females. Similar to mitral stenosis, rheumatic heart disease is the predominant cause of mitral regurgitation, but there are many other factors, both acquired and congenital, that contribute to its cause. *Mitral valve prolapse* is a form of mitral insufficiency seen most often in thin, young females; it is often asymptomatic. Weakness, rupture, or fibrosis of a papillary muscle secondary to ischemic coronary artery disease, ventricular aneurysm, or myocardial infarction can cause mitral regurgitation. Papillary muscle dysfunction allows the valve leaflets to flop in the direction of the left atrium during systole, and the blood flows backward. Other acquired factors include trauma and dysfunction of a prosthetic mitral valve. A person with idiopathic hypertrophic subaortic stenosis (IHSS) can develop mitral regurgitation as a result of displacement of the anterior leaflet of the mitral valve during systole. Bacterial endocarditis may cause erosion of the cusps or chordae tendineae, resulting in mitral regurgitation.

Pathophysiology

In chronic mitral insufficiency or regurgitation a variable amount of blood from the left ventricle is shunted back through the mitral orifice to the left atrium. This backflow of blood will cause both the left atrium and left ventricle to dilate and hypertrophy. In response to increasing preload and left atrial pressure, the pulmonary venous and arteriolar pressures also rise and eventually will cause right-sided heart failure (Figure 28-3). As the ventricle hypertrophies, it becomes dysfunctional and the cardiac output decreases. Concurrently, the left atrium is often fibrillating, diminishing the cardiac output even further.

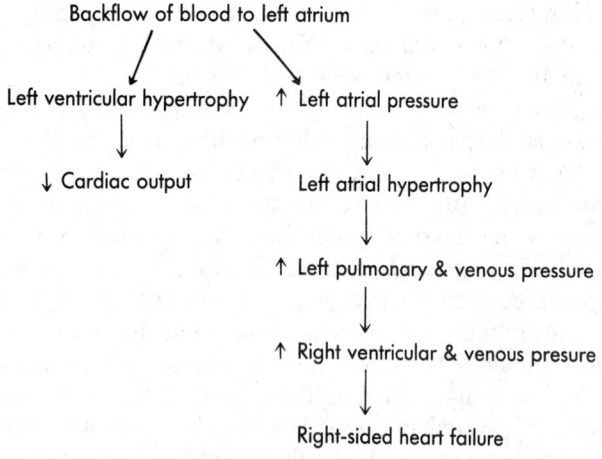

FIGURE 28-3 Pathophysiology of mitral regurgitation.

Clinical Manifestations

In persons with mitral regurgitation, fatigue and weakness related to a decreased cardiac output are the predominant complaints. Right-sided heart failure with its sequelae of hepatic congestion, edema, ascites, and distended neck veins occurs in severe mitral regurgitation. Some persons experience palpitations (from atrial fibrillation) or paroxysmal nocturnal dyspnea.

In acute mitral regurgitation, progressive dyspnea on exertion and frequent pulmonary edema from an elevated left atrial pressure are the primary symptoms. The atrial pressure is transmitted immediately to the pulmonary veins, causing the congestive symptoms. Because the ventricle has not yet hypertrophied, the cardiac output remains sufficient and the fatigue is not a problem. Although persons with mitral regurgitation commonly have atrial fibrillation, thrombus formation in the atria is less common than with mitral stenosis because of backflow and resultant turbulence of blood.

The diagnosis of mitral regurgitation is made by the presence of clinical symptoms and auscultation of a blowing, high-pitched systolic murmur and third heart sound. The first heart sound (S_1) may not be heard, depending on the severity of regurgitation. A chest x-ray film will reveal left atrial enlargement and occasional left ventricular dilation. ECG tracings will show left ventricular hypertrophy and, less commonly, right ventricular hypertrophy (Table 28-1). The echocardiogram may identify mitral valve cusp prolapse, ruptured chordae tendineae, and enlargement of the left atrium and left ventricle. A vectorcardiogram will indicate left ventricular hypertrophy. Definitive diagnosis is made by a cardiac catheterization or left ventricular angiography, which will assess left ventricular function and the degree of regurgitation.

Interventions

Medical treatment. Initial treatment of mitral regurgitation is medical and is similar to that of mitral stenosis. Restricting physical activities that produce fatigue, weakness, and dyspnea; decreasing sodium intake; and using diuretics and afterload reducers are common. Anticoagulant therapy is not usually necessary until end stages of the disease, because of the turbulence of the blood in the left atrium. Because the left ventricle is more burdened in mitral insufficiency than in mitral stenosis, digitalis glycosides are important in augmenting the output of the left ventricle. Vasodilators may also be instituted to decrease left-sided heart failure.

Surgical intervention. As with mitral stenosis, when physical limitations become significant despite appropriate medical intervention, surgical intervention is inevitable. The surgical treatments for mitral regurgitation are all open heart procedures using either a median sternotomy or left thoracotomy approach. Valve replacements are the most common choice of treatment. The patient is placed on cardiopulmonary bypass, the native valve is excised, and the remaining annuli are sized. A prosthetic valve is then inserted and sutured into place. The operative mortality for this procedure ranges from 5% to 10%.

Valvuloplasty (repair or reconstruction) is also indicated for mitral regurgitation, especially for solitary cusp perforation seen with bacterial endocarditis and for simple valve clefts. In this procedure, direct suture repair of torn leaflets or clefts is done. In patients for whom such simple repair is needed, valvuloplasty may be recommended as the treatment of choice over replacement. Life expectancy with valvuloplasty is the same as that with replacement, although the reoperation rate is higher. The big advantage of valvuloplasty, however, is its 0.4% thromboembolic rate per year without anticoagulation versus a 3% to 6% rate with anticoagulation of mechanical valves.

Annuloplasty (repair of the annulus) is a procedure to reduce the enlarged annulus. This surgical procedure involves using a prosthetic ring and suturing the ring into the circumference of the mitral annulus. The stitches are pulled together toward the prosthesis, reducing the size of the valve orifice.

AORTIC VALVULAR DISEASE
AORTIC STENOSIS
Etiology

Aortic valvular disease is less common than mitral disease and occurs in about 25% of all persons with chronic valvular heart disease. Eighty percent of adults with aortic stenosis are men.

Aortic stenosis can be rheumatic in origin, since myocarditis invades the valve, causing edema, inflammation, formation of granulation tissue, scarring, and, finally, fusion of the leaflets. Rheumatic aortic stenosis is almost always concomitant with rheumatic disease of the mitral valve. Atherosclerosis in elderly persons also

causes aortic stenosis and is also called idiopathic calcific aortic stenosis.

Congenital valvular disease or malformation is the predominant etiologic factor in aortic stenosis. A congenitally deformed valve may remain asymptomatic for several years; however, it is more susceptible to bacterial endocarditis, rheumatic fever, and calcification.

Pathophysiology

When the aortic valve becomes stenosed, thus obstructing left ventricular outflow during systole, left ventricular hypertrophy develops as a compensatory mechanism to continue pumping the same blood volume through the narrowed opening. As the stenosis progresses, cardiac output decreases. The left atrium cannot empty adequately, and thus the pulmonary system becomes congested. The hypertrophied left ventricle elevates myocardial oxygen needs and at the same time compresses the coronary arteries at a pressure exceeding coronary perfusion pressure. Thus myocardial oxygen needs increase and the supply decreases. This phenomenon gives rise to the myocardial ischemia and angina that are characteristic of more severe aortic stenosis. Eventually, right-sided heart failure will ensue (Figure 28-4).

Aortic stenosis rarely becomes significantly debilitating until the aortic orifice is about one third its normal size. Symptoms occur late in the disease even with severe stenosis, because the hypertrophied left ventricle is able to generate pressures strong enough to maintain an adequate cardiac output and because the mitral valve prevents the high intraventricular pressures from affecting the atrium and pulmonary vasculature. When the mitral valve is also diseased, the onset of symptoms may be more rapid and may be compounded.

Clinical Manifestations

Gradually increasing obstruction without clinical symptoms usually occurs until 40 to 50 years of age in most persons. There are three characteristic symptoms of aortic stenosis: exertional dyspnea, angina pectoris, and ex-

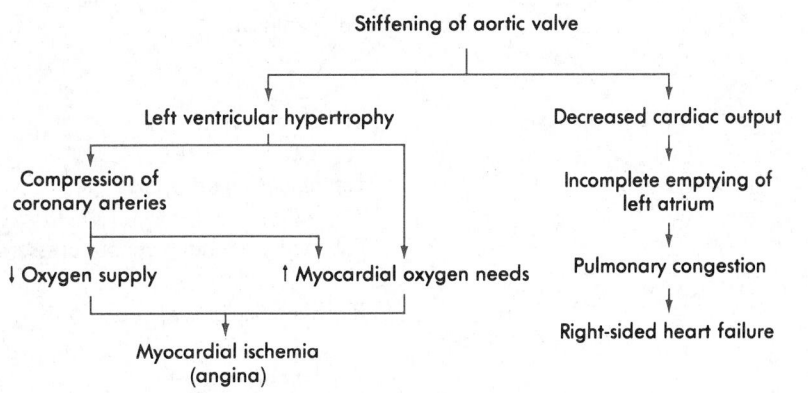

FIGURE 28-4 Pathophysiology of aortic stenosis.

ertional syncope. Exertional dyspnea is secondary to diminished cardiac reserve and elevation of the pulmonary capillary pressures. Angina pectoris (p. 706) is secondary to diminished coronary perfusion and increased myocardial oxygen needs. Exertional syncope is caused by a decline in arterial pressure secondary to vasodilatation in exercising muscles and a fixed cardiac output.

Other symptoms that also only occur in the late stages of the disease include fatigue, weakness, orthopnea, paroxysmal nocturnal dyspnea, and pulmonary edema. Symptoms of right-sided heart failure (that is, hepatomegaly, atrial fibrillation, systemic venous hypertension) are usually end-stage symptoms. If aortic stenosis goes untreated, the survival rate is 1.5 to 3 years.

Aortic stenosis is diagnosed by a harsh, rough, midsystolic murmur and a systolic thrill over the aortic area, by clinical symptoms, and by cardiac catheterization and angiography (Table 28-1).

Interventions

Treatment of aortic stenosis is initially medical. Avoidance of strenuous activity is advocated as is the use of digitalis glycosides, a sodium restriction, and diuretics for the treatment of congestive heart failure. Nitroglycerin is used to treat angina.

As symptoms increase in severity, surgical treatment consisting of valve replacement is the treatment of choice, and symptomatic improvement occurs. The 8-year survival rate following surgery is roughly 65%. Valve replacement of the aortic valve is similar in technique to mitral valve replacement.

AORTIC REGURGITATION
Etiology

Aortic regurgitation occurs less frequently than stenosis, and about 75% of those persons with aortic regurgitation are male. Etiologic factors may be congenital or acquired. The disease is rheumatic in origin in 80% of the cases. Rheumatic disease thickens, deforms, and contracts the valve leaflets. Dilation of the annulus may also occur to produce insufficiency. In persons with isolated aortic regurgitation (that is, without associated mitral disease) rheumatic heart disease does not play such a prominent causal role.

Syphilis is a rarely seen cause of dilation of the annulus and widening of the commissures. Less than 5% of the cases of aortic insufficiency in the United States are related to syphilis. Bacterial endocarditis can cause bacterial vegetation on valve leaflets, which initiates the inflammatory response and can cause erosion of the valve.

Marfan's syndrome is another etiologic factor related to aortic regurgitation. As a generalized, systemic disease of connective tissue, it can cause necrosis of the aorta, dilation of the aortic ring, and aneurysm formation, thus causing insufficiency. Another cause is congenital malformation, which, as with aortic stenosis, renders the aortic valve more susceptible to endocarditis and rheumatic fever and can thus cause aortic insufficiency.

Pathophysiology

When the aortic valve is deformed congenitally or by infectious processes, the leaflets may not close properly and the annulus may be dilated, loose, or deformed. This allows a regurgitation of blood from the aorta back into the left ventricle during diastole. The ventricle dilates and hypertrophies with this greater volume of blood and thus compensates with a more forceful and rapid ejection (Figure 28-5).

Studies have indicated that greater than 50% of the left ventricular ejection volume must reflux into the left ventricle before a person becomes symptomatic. Because of this cardiac compensation, symptoms in un-

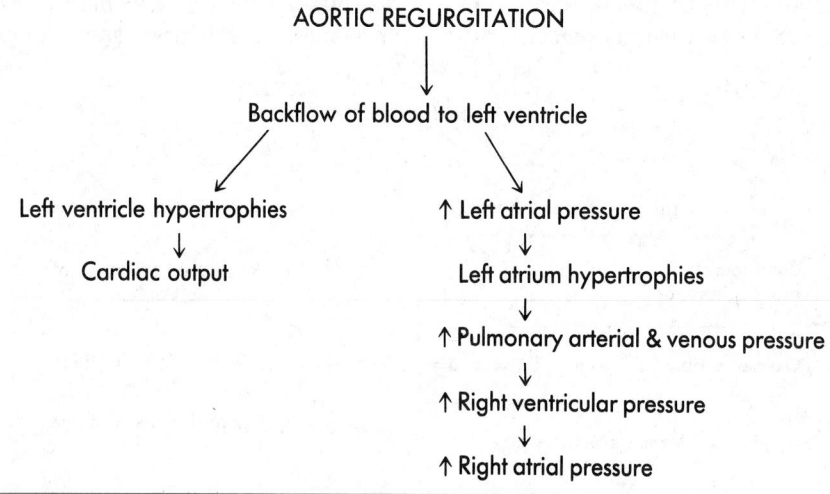

FIGURE 28-5 Pathophysiology of aortic regurgitation.

complicated aortic insufficiency are rare until left ventricular failure is imminent.

Clinical Manifestations

People with aortic regurgitation remain asymptomatic for years because of the myocardium's ability to hypertrophy. Symptoms usually begin with an awareness of the heart beat, which is uncomfortable and more prominent on the left side-lying position. Sinus tachycardia may occur with exertion or stimulation, and premature ventricular beats occur. Exertional dyspnea secondary to cardiac decompensation, orthopnea, paroxysmal nocturnal dyspnea, and diaphoresis always indicate impending left-sided heart failure. Angina may develop at rest or with exertion secondary to myocardial ischemia or pounding on the chest wall by the heart. End-stage disease is indicated by hepatomegaly, ankle edema, and ascites.

Diagnosis is made from clinical findings of a soft, blowing aortic diastolic murmur and a widened pulse pressure. The ECG will indicate left ventricular hypertrophy with ST-segment depression and T-wave inversion. Cardiac catheterization will determine the severity of the valve disease (Table 28-1). Echocardiogram indicates the amount of ventricular volume overload, the stroke volume, and ejection fraction. Angiography may be used to determine the severity of coronary artery disease.

Interventions

As with other valvular disease, medical therapy is used initially to reduce congestion secondary to increasing left ventricular workload. Digitalis, a sodium-restricted diet, diuretics, and vasodilators are often used. Although it is not as effective as with aortic stenosis, nitroglycerin is used for decreasing anginal pain.

Valve replacement is usually necessary; however, surgical treatment does not always restore normal ventricular function. Valvuloplasty is rarely a viable alternative when just one valve leaflet is torn or perforated.

TRICUSPID VALVULAR DISEASE
TRICUSPID STENOSIS
Etiology

Tricuspid stenosis is a more uncommon valvular disease that occurs four to five times more frequently in women than in men. This lesion is rarely isolated and usually occurs with mitral stenosis or aortic stenosis but usually not with mitral regurgitation. Rheumatic heart disease is the usual cause of tricuspid stenosis.

Pathophysiology

The fusion of the commissures and shortened and fused chordae tendineae cause the tricuspid orifice to narrow. Blood is blocked returning to the heart. The systemic pressure is increased as a result of the obstruction, and there is a reduced right ventricular output.

Clinical Manifestations

Symptoms of right heart failure in the patient with tricuspid stenosis include hepatomegaly and jugular vein distention, as well as cardiac cirrhosis and resulting jaundice. The decrease in blood volume returned to the heart decreases cardiac output and causes fatigue, weight loss, and hypotension.

Interventions

Medical treatment includes digitalis, a low-sodium diet, and diuretics. Surgical treatment may include commissurotomy (p. 676) or replacement of the valve. This is usually performed simultaneously with repair or replacement of the mitral or aortic valve when valvular diseases occur concomitantly.

TRICUSPID REGURGITATION

Tricuspid regurgitation is uncommon, because normal valve leaflets are very small and valve closure is primarily reliant on the contraction of the valvular ring. Consequently, tricuspid insufficiency caused by rheumatic, carcinoid, or bacterial destruction of the leaflets is rare. Right ventricular dilation from any cause may dilate the tricuspid ring or displace the papillary muscles and cause regurgitation. An insufficient tricuspid valve allows blood to flow back into the right atrium, causing venous engorgement and diminishing right ventricular output (Table 28-1).

PULMONIC VALVULAR DISEASE
PULMONARY STENOSIS

Pulmonary stenosis is a rare valvular disease that is usually congenital in origin, although it may be caused by cancer or rheumatic fever. In pulmonary stenosis, the pulmonic valve narrows, causing less blood to flow forward. As a result, blood flows back into the right ventricle and right atrium. Both the right ventricle and atrium hypertrophy to compensate for the volume of blood received. Symptoms of pulmonary stenosis include a harsh systolic murmur, fatigue, and dyspnea on exertion. As the condition worsens, the patient will present symptoms of hepatomegaly, ascites, and edema.

PULMONARY REGURGITATION

Pulmonary regurgitation is also a rare condition caused by infective endocarditis, tumors, or rheumatic fever. The pulmonic valve leaflets become incompetent and fail to close. Blood flows back into the right ventricle during systole. The right ventricle and right atrium hypertrophy. The patient will exhibit symptoms of right-sided heart failure similar to those of pulmonary stenosis. The treatment of pulmonary valvular disease includes digitalis, diuretics, a low-sodium diet, and vasodilators to reduce failure.

■ ASSESSMENT

Many of the symptoms of valvular heart disease are related to decreased cardiac output. Therefore the assessment data that the nurse obtains are essentially the same for any person with valvular heart disease.

SUBJECTIVE DATA

Persons with different types of valvular disease will exhibit different symptoms.
1. Fatigue and weakness: In severe valvular disease the fatigue may be overwhelming
2. Dysnea: occurrence, type
   Many persons experience DOE, orthopnea, or PND, depending on the extent of ventricular involvement and failure
3. Angina: occurrence, location, quality, and measures to relieve pain
4. Palpitations: occurrence, precipitating condition or events, such as lack of sleep, dietary intake of caffeine
5. Syncope: occurrence
6. Peripheral edema: site, extent, time of day, alleviating factors

OBJECTIVE DATA

Objective data are collected by inspection, auscultation, and palpation.
1. Observation/inspection
   a. Body posture/position and comfort level
   b. Character and rate of respirations, flaring of nostrils
   c. Use of supplemental oxygen
   d. Skin color and temperature, including presence of cyanosis, mottling, petechiae, and other skin discolorations
   e. Nail bed color and capillary refill
   f. Neck vein engorgement
   g. Myocardial heaves (can be observed in severe left ventricular hypertrophy)
   h. Diaphoresis
2. Auscultation
   a. Cardiac rate and rhythm
   b. Heart sounds (murmurs, S_3, S_4) (Table 28-2)
   c. Breath sounds, comparing contralaterally
   d. Presence of adventitious sounds (rales, rhonchi)
3. Palpation
   a. Temperature of extremities
   b. Pulse rate and rhythm: irregular, fast pulse is often palpable in persons with mitral stenosis who experience atrial fibrillation
   c. Equality and symmetry of pulses; pulse deficit or pulse alterans, widened pulse pressure
   d. Presence of edema, pitting or nonpitting
   e. Signs of phlebitis (increased calf diameter, positive Homan's sign)

■ DATA ANALYSIS: NURSING DIAGNOSES

Nursing diagnoses are determined from assessment of patient data. Possible nursing diagnoses for the patient with valvular heart disease may include, but are not limited to:

Diagnostic Title	Possible Etiologies
Activity intolerance	Weakness, imbalance between oxygen supply/demand
Anxiety	Threat to health status
Breathing pattern, ineffective	Decreased cardiac output, fatigue
Fluid volume, excess	Decreased cardiac output
Knowledge deficit	Lack of exposure/recall
Sleep pattern disturbance	Dypsnea, anxiety

■ PLANNING: EXPECTED PATIENT OUTCOMES

Expected patient outcomes for the person with valvular heart disease during the medical phase of treatment may include, but are not limited to, the following:
1. The patient states feeling comfortable; signs of anxiety decrease.
2. The patient rests between activities.
3. The patient states that breathing is easier and fatigue occurs less frequently with activity.
4. The patient can:
   a. Explain the nature of the valvular disease.
   b. State the name, purpose, dosage, frequency, and side effects of any medication therapy.

TABLE 28-2 Auscultatory difference in valvular heart disease

Valvular Disorder	General Findings	Murmurs
Mitral stenosis	S_1 snapping, louder Palpable thrill at apex	Soft, low-pitched, rumbling Diastolic
Mitral regurgitation	S_1 soft or absent S_3 present Palpable thrill at apex	High-pitched, blowing Pansystolic
Aortic stenosis	S_2 soft Left-sided S_4 Systolic thrill at heart base	Low-pitched, harsh, rasping Midsystolic
Aortic regurgitation	S_3 present Systolic thrill over aortic area	High-pitched, blowing Diastolic
Tricuspid regurgitation	Systolic thrill at lower left sternal border	High-pitched, blowing Pansystolic

c. Explain any prescribed dietary sodium modifications.

d. Describe a work, rest, and activity program to conserve energy and decrease exertional dyspnea.

e. Describe the rationale for and the type of surgery to be performed, if surgery is indicated.

f. State plans for continued medical therapy.

▪ IMPLEMENTATION

Because heart failure may be present, the care of the person with valvular heart disease who is receiving medical therapy may be similar to that for heart failure (p. 723). Nursing activities center primarily on continued monitoring and on patient teaching. Fluid balance is monitored by daily weights, intake and output, and inspection of neck veins. Auscultation of heart and breath sounds is continued from the initial assessment. The skin is observed for changes in appearance, capillary perfusion, and the presence and extent of edema. The person's tolerance is monitored during any activity as evidenced by dyspnea on exertion, fatigue, or chest pain. Rest periods are planned between activities.

Patient teaching includes the following:

1. General anatomy of the heart and the function and purpose of the cardiac valves
2. Effect of medications: diuretics, cardiac glycosides, anticoagulants, and antibiotics
3. Prophylactic use of antibiotics before and after dental work and surgical procedures, if there is a prior history of rheumatic fever
4. Effect of a sodium- or fluid-restricted diet on cardiac function, if prescribed
5. Assessment of fluid formation in the extremities
6. Need to plan for a work, rest, and activity program to conserve energy and to identify intolerance to activity

TYPES OF VALVE REPAIR

Annuloplasty	Repair of ring or annulus of incompetent or diseased valve
Valvuloplasty	Repair of valve, suturing of torn leaflets
Commissurotomy	Dilation of valve; repair of a leaflet or commissure, fibrous bond or ring

(DOE, fatigue, pulse that does not return to baseline within 10 minutes following activity)

7. Purpose and procedures for diagnostic tests in preparation for surgery, if appropriate
8. Purpose and nature of surgical intervention, if appropriate.

SURGICAL TREATMENT OF VALVULAR DISEASE

Cardiac valves may be repaired or replaced, depending on the severity of the diseased valve. Three types of valvular repair are annuloplasty (p. 679), commissurotomy (p. 676), and valvuloplasty (p. 679) (see the box above). Variables affecting the results of the valve replacement include the patient's general clinical condition and level of myocardial functioning before surgery and the type of valve used. Care of the patient undergoing cardiac surgery is described on p. 687.

TYPES OF VALVES

The ideal valve used for replacement should include the following characteristics: durable, hemodynamic accuracy, nonhemolytic, nonthrombogenic, easily inserted, anatomically suitable, and a low incidence of endocarditis.[71] There are a wide variety of prosthetic valves avail-

TABLE 28-3 Types of prosthetic cardiac valves

Type	Examples	Advantages	Disadvantages
Caged ball	Starr-Edwards Smeloff Braunwald-Cutter McGovern-Cromie	Durable, low incidence of endocarditis	Large size that may create obstruction to blood flow
Caged disk	Beall Hufnagel Cross-Jones Kay-Shiley	Low incidence of thromboemboli	Disk may stick, causing severe obstruction of blood flow
Tilting disk	Bjork-Shiley Wada-Cutter St. Jude Lillehei-Kaste	Central blood flow, low incidence of hemolysis	Higher incidence of thrombus
Stenting allograft	—	Central blood flow, low incidence of hemolysis, no thromboemboli	High incidence of regurgitation
Xenograft	Porcine	Silent valves, low incidence of thromboembolism or hemolysis	High incidence of calcification over time

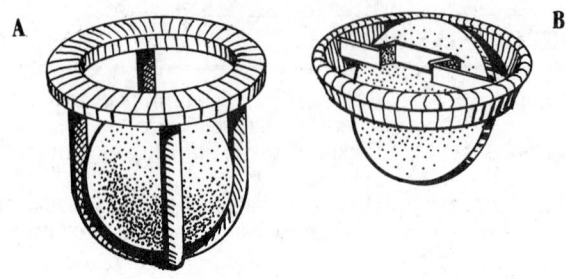

FIGURE 28-6 Heart valve prosthesis. **A,** Caged ball valve. **B,** Tilting-disk valve.

able. The advantages and disadvantages of each valve type are listed in Table 28-3.

Caged-ball prosthetic valves consist of a metal cage with a synthetic, freely moving ball inside; the cage is attached to a sewing ring (Figure 28-6, *A*). The ring and struts of the cage are covered by a synthetic cloth. The cloth-covered ring is sutured carefully into the existing valve annulus. Within 2 to 3 months, tissue covers the cloth and the incidence of thromboembolism decreases. Caged-ball valves come in various sizes and slightly varying designs and materials.

Caged-disk prosthetic valves occupy less space in the ventricles than other valves and require less force to move the occluding disk. This type of valve creates the most obstruction to blood flow than other types of valves. If the disk "sticks" in the cage, causing total obstruction of blood flow, hemodynamics are seriously compromised.

Tilting-disk valves have occluders that tilt or pivot within a ring rather than balls or disks that pop back and forth in a cage (Figure 28-6, *B*). This type of valve produces nearly central blood flow through its orifice, providing more normal blood flow. However, the valve may develop areas under the pivoting points where thrombi can form as a result of the blood stasis.

Stented allografts are human heart valves that are supported or "stented" by an underlying frame. Allografts provide relatively normal hymodynamic characteristics with central flow, no thromboemboli, and little hemolysis. Allografts are difficult to procure in quantity, however.

Xenograft bioprosthetic valves are composed of valves from species other than human, are more easily available than other valves, and can be obtained in all sizes. *Porcine* xenograft valves (Figure 28-7) are most frequently used. The hemodynamic performance has been similar to that of human heart valves. Many patients with this type of valve may not require anticoagulants. Approximately 70% to 80% of patients over 35 years of age are free of primary tissue failure at 10 years. After 10 to 12 years, the process will accelerate calcification on the valve.[46] Porcine valves are now used less often in young persons or in patients with renal failure requiring dialysis, because of a higher incidence of calcification over a long period.

ANTICOAGULATION

Patients with mechanical or bioprosthetic valves are at a high risk for systemic emboli. Antithrombotic agents are used to decrease the incidence of thrombi developing. A major risk to patients receiving antithrombotic agents is bleeding. Warfarin (Coumadin) is the most common antithrombotic medication used with both kinds of valves. Maintenance of warfarin is based on the prothrombin time (PT); a therapeutic PT is 1.5 to 2.5 of the control time. If bleeding occurs while the patient is taking warfarin, the dosage may be lowered or other medications

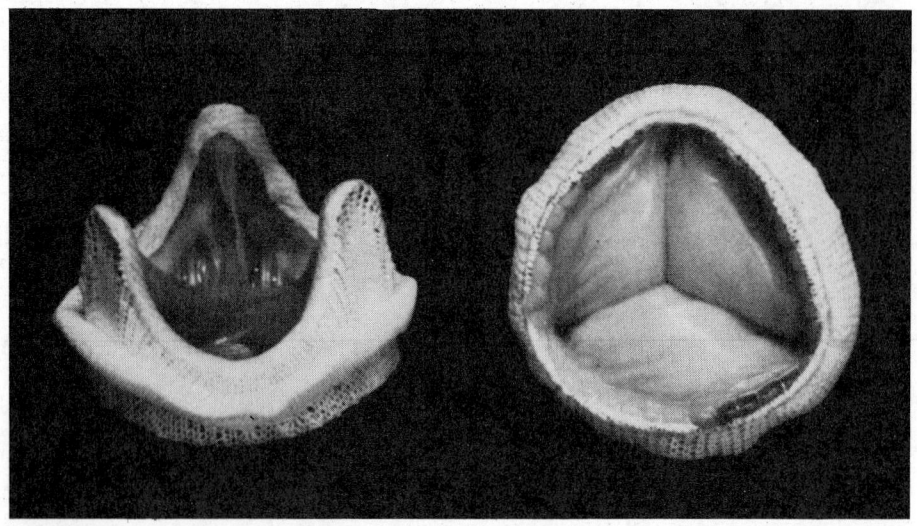

FIGURE 28-7 Porcine valve prosthesis (two views).

added. Dipyridamole (Persantine) is another type of antithrombotic agent. It inhibits platelet aggregation while not affecting the PT. Dipyridamole may be used in conjunction with warfarin to prevent embolization. The normal dose to reduce platelet aggregation is 225 mg to 400 mg/day; orthostatic hypotension may occur.

ANEURYSMS

ETIOLOGY

An aneurysm is a localized or diffuse enlargement of an artery at some point along its course. Aneurysms occur when the vessel becomes weakened from trauma, congenital vascular disease, infection, or atherosclerosis. Syphilitic aneurysms of the arch of the aorta are rare with the vast majority of aneurysms.

PATHOPHYSIOLOGY

Although the pathologic processes involved in the formation of an aneurysm are varied, certain factors are common to all. Once an aneurysm develops and the arterial tunica media (the middle coat composed of layers of smooth muscle and elastic tissue) is damaged, there is a tendency toward progressive dilation, degeneration, and a risk of rupture. Aneurysms may develop in any blood vessel, but the most common site is the aorta.

A *saccular* aneurysm involves only part of the circumference of the artery. It takes the form of a sac or pouchlike dilation attached to the side of the artery. A *fusiform* aneurysm is spindle shaped and involves the entire circumference of the arterial wall (Figure 28-8). A *dissecting* aneurysm involves hemorrhage into a vessel wall, which splits and dissects the wall causing a widening of the vessel. Dissecting aneurysms are caused by a degenerative defect in the tunica media and tunica intima (innermost layer) as a result of the great hemodynamic stresses to which it is subjected. Dissecting aneurysms of the aorta are classified into three categories (see the box at right).

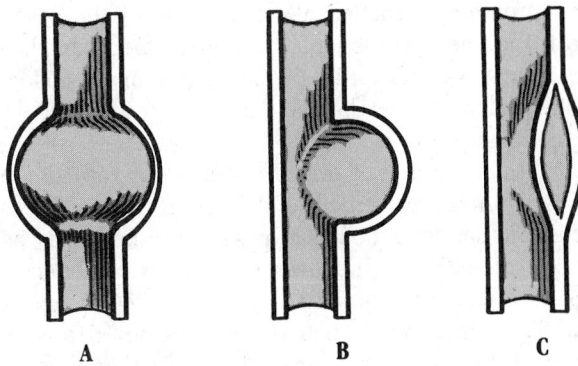

FIGURE 28-8 Types of aneurysms. **A,** Fusiform. **B,** Saccular. **C,** Dissecting.

DIAGNOSTIC TESTS
RADIOGRAPHY

Routine chest and abdominal radiographs have proved to be very helpful in case finding and preliminary diagnosis of aortic aneurysms. Such studies frequently reveal a ring of calcification outlining the aneurysm and displacement of surrounding structures.

ANGIOGRAPHY

Angiographic studies are usually conducted to provide the surgeon with a definite diagnosis, accurate location, and delineation of the lesion. An *aortogram* reveals whether an aneurysm is leaking, expanding, or dissecting. This procedure is performed by inserting a catheter into the femoral, brachial, or axillary artery. A contrast dye is injected to outline the aorta, and then subsequent radiograms are taken to determine an accurate flow study. This procedure involves minimal discomfort, but persons may experience a slight burning sensation as the contrast dye is injected.

Following the procedure, bed rest is suggested for 6 to 12 hours, with minimal flexion of the cannulated joint. Vital signs are monitored every 15 minutes for the first 2 hours. Ongoing assessment of the patient's skin color, temperature, pulses, discomfort, and any numbness distal to the cannulation site is continued for 12 hours. The cannulation site is inspected for the presence of bleeding, swelling, or hematoma whenever vital signs are monitored.

SONOGRAPHY

Ultrasound is useful in determining the size, shape, and location of the aneurysm. After conducting gel is applied to the skin, a Dopler probe is placed over the gel to intensify pulse sound vibrations. Blood flow and the presence of a bruit are detected. Since this is a noninvasive procedure, no special precautions or posttest care is required.

THORACIC AORTIC ANEURYSMS

Aneurysms in the thoracic area occur most frequently in hypertensive men between the ages of 40 and 70.

CLASSIFICATION OF DISSECTING ANEURYSMS OF THE AORTA

Type I	Dissection of ascending aorta and aortic pouch extending to iliac bifurcation
Type II	Limited to ascending aorta
Type III	Originates at or distal to left subclavian artery and extends distally for varying distances, but does not involve aorta proximal to left subclavian artery

From DeBakey M et al: Surgical management of dissecting aneurysms of the aorta, J Cardiovasc Surg 49:130-149, 1965.

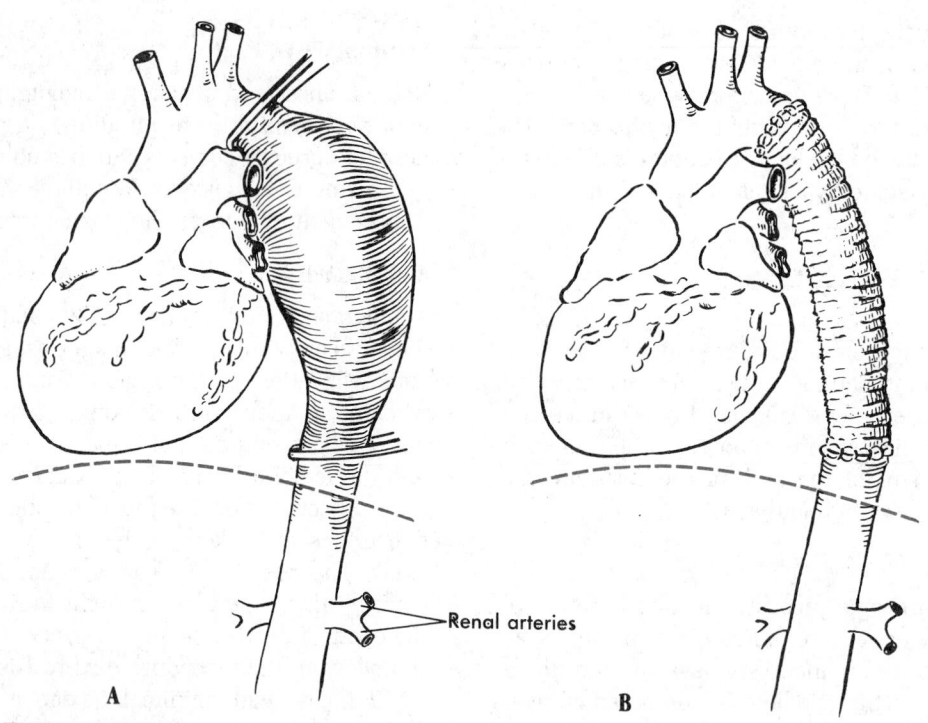

—Renal arteries

A

B

FIGURE 28-9 Aneurysm of descending thoracic artery. **A,** Resection of thoracic aorta with cardiovascular clamps in place. **B,** Permanent replacement graft after resection of aneurysm. (Redrawn from Bloodwell RD et al: Surg Clin North Am 46:901-911, 1966.)

These aneurysms can develop in the ascending, transverse, or descending aorta and are the most likely aneurysms to dissect. Most persons are asymptomatic, but symptoms may occur depending on how rapidly the aneurysm dilates and whether the mass is impinging on surrounding intrathoracic structures. Chest pain is usually the most frequent symptom, but it may only be perceived when the person is in a supine position. Other symptoms may include cough, dyspnea, hoarseness, or dysphagia, all related to pressure from the sac of the aneurysm pressing against internal structures.

Operative mortality is highest in those persons who have an acute onset of symptoms and in whom a dissecting aneurysm begins in the ascending aortic arch and causes insufficiency of the aortic valve. Cardiopulmonary bypass (p. 693) is needed to maintain tissue oxygenation when the aorta is clamped. Hypothermia may be used to decrease the need of tissues for oxygen and thus decrease metabolic waste production (Chapter 21). After the chest is opened, the aneurysm exposed, and an extracorporeal bypass instituted to produce a satisfactory flow of oxygenated blood, cross-clamps are applied proximal and distal to the lesion (Figure 28-9). The aneurysm is then resected and replaced with a Teflon or Dacron prosthesis. Nursing care after surgery is the same as for cardiac surgery (p. 697).

ABDOMINAL AORTIC ANEURYSMS

The most common site for the formation of an aortic aneurysm is the abdominal aorta below the renal arteries. The person may be asymptomatic and the condition evident only as a pulsatile abdominal mass, which may be found on a routine physical examination. At other times the person may have pain or tenderness in the mid- or upper abdomen.

The prognosis for a person with an abdominal aortic aneurysm depends not only on the size and location of the defect, but also on the extent of arteriosclerotic disease. The aneurysm may extend to impinge on the renal, iliac, or mesenteric arteries. The stasis of blood favors thrombus formation along the wall of the vessel, and if the aneurysm is large the most feared complication is aneurysmal rupture. An aneurysm of the abdominal aorta is a serious disease entity and the mortality is high with rupture.

Treatment of an abdominal aneurysm is resection of the lesion and replacement with a graft. Extracorporeal perfusion (cardiopulmonary bypass) is *not* necessary because arterial flow to the lower extremities can be interrupted safely for the time needed to complete the operation. The aneurysm is opened, the clots and debris are removed, the graft replacement is inserted, and the remaining arterial wall is closed over the graft (Figure 28-10).

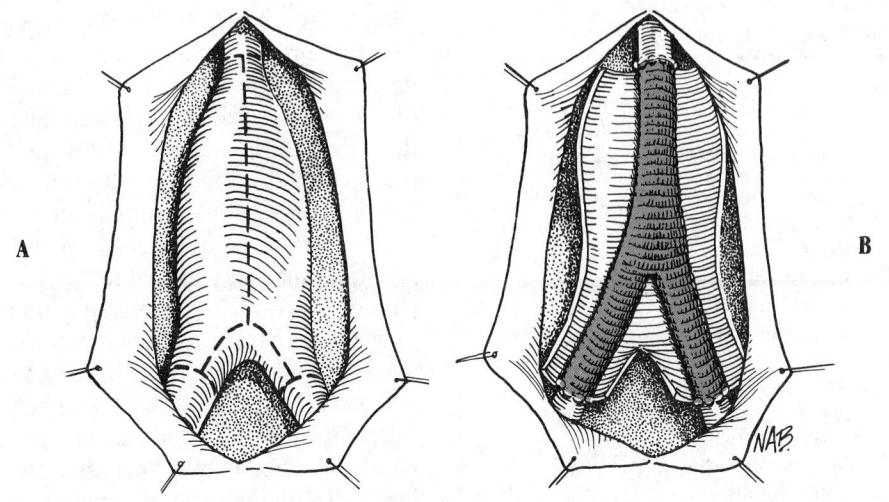

FIGURE 28-10 A, Abdominal aneurysm of aorta and iliac arteries. **B,** Bifurcation graft used to replace excised aneurysm.

Postoperative care following resections of an abdominal aneurysm is summarized in the box at right. Monitoring is an essential component for the immediate postoperative period. Pulmonary hygiene is important, because the abdominal incision restricts full lung expansion.

INTERVENTIONS FOR THE PERSON REQUIRING HEART SURGERY

In the third decade of this century, the first heart surgery procedure was performed on a human patient in England. It consisted of a closed repair of a stenosed mitral valve, or mitral commissurotomy. Since that time great progress has been made in a variety of heart surgery procedures, including valve repairs and replacements, structural defect and congenital anomaly repairs, coronary artery bypass grafting, and total heart transplants (Table 28-4). Currently, research is being done to implant and test prosthetic heart chambers and total prosthetic hearts. Today's surgeon has the advantage of a highly sophisticated technology to aid in performing these extremely delicate yet vital procedures, a technology advanced enough to allow many Americans to undergo heart surgery each year.

One term frequently used to describe heart surgery is also commonly misused; the term *open heart surgery* is often used in referring to any surgical procedure performed on the heart. Strictly speaking, however, open heart procedures are those in which the heart muscle itself is incised and the internal heart structures are directly visualized. A coronary artery bypass procedure is not, therefore, a true open heart procedure. True open heart procedures always involve the use of extracorporeal circulation. It is perhaps best to avoid the term open heart surgery entirely and instead to refer specifically to

NURSING CARE OF THE PATIENT AFTER SURGERY FOR ABDOMINAL ANEURYSM

1. Monitor during immediate postoperative period:
   a. Vital signs, including apical pulses, every 15 minutes until stabilized
   b. CVP, LAP, PAP, PCWP—observe for decrease indicating hypovolemia
   c. Dysrhythmias
   d. Peripheral pulses (posterior tibial and dorsalis pedis) every 1-2 hours
   e. Neurologic: level of consciousness and ability to move lower extremities, every 1-2 hours
   f. Signs of arterial occlusion:
      1. Poor perfusion: decreased blood pressure; weak, thready pulse
      2. Advanced occlusion: legs pale or mottled, bluish and cool to touch; numbness of one or both legs
   g. Intake and output: accurate hourly measurements; report output <30-50 ml/hr from indwelling urinary catheter; monitor BUN and creatinine
   h. Blood loss: monitor chest tube output every hour; report drainage of >100ml/hr × 3 hrs
   i. Electrolytes: hypokalemia, hypocalcemia; supplement when necessary
   j. Back pain: may occur from retroperitoneal hemorrhage or thrombus at graft site
   k. Postoperative ileus or distention: monitor NG output, bowel sounds, abdominal pain or discomfort
2. Encourage respiratory exercises to prevent pulmonary complications
3. Bed rest in flat position
   a. Avoid flexion of hip or knee (pressure on femoral or popliteal arteries)
   b. Turn patient gently side to side
   c. Encourage patient to dorsiflex and extend feet at regular intervals to prevent venous congestion
4. Give prescribed analgesics liberally during first few days for postoperative pain
5. Encourage ambulation, when permitted

TABLE 28-4 Types of cardiac surgery

Action	Surgical Procedures	Use of Extracorporeal Circulation
Repair or replacement	Correction of congenital defects; valve replacements; valvuloplasty; thoracic aortic aneurysm repair	Yes
Vascular bypass	Coronary artery bypass	Yes
Release of constriction	Pericardial fenestration; pericardiectomy; closed mitral commissurotomy	No
Replacement of diseased heart with healthy heart	Transplantation	Yes

the actual procedure being performed, particularly when speaking with the patient and family. It is not uncommon to find patients scheduled for coronary artery bypass grafting who believe that their heart will be opened during the procedure.

PREOPERATIVE CARE

All of the preparations necessary for a person about to undergo a surgical procedure (see Chapter 20) apply to the patient being prepared for heart surgery. In addition, there are a number of specific considerations that are pertinent to the cardiac surgical patient.

HISTORY

Persons being admitted for cardiac surgery may have exhibited cardiac and pulmonary symptoms for months or years before this admission. They will have undergone extensive testing to establish the underlying pathologic condition and to delineate the severity of the condition. Testing may have included chest x-ray films, cardiac catheterization, coronary angiography, echocardiography, phonocardiography, nuclear cardiac studies, electrocardiogram, stress testing, and blood serum analyses.

It is necessary for the nurse caring for the heart surgery patient to understand each patient's pertinent medical history in order to individualize care appropriately. It is necessary to know the underlying nature of the heart condition, how long it has been diagnosed, and the particular surgical procedure chosen to correct it. The relative degree of cardiac impairment will be demonstrated in the patient's limitations in life-style. The current manifestations of the illness may range from no

symptoms to intermittent pain to debilitating heart failure. It is important to be aware of past cardiopulmonary or circulatory conditions or disorders, such as myocardial infarction, bacterial endocarditis, pulmonary embolus, blood clotting abnormalities, and a history of smoking, that might place the individual at higher risk for developing postoperative complications.

The patient's current medical regimen is very important, and medications or therapeutic measures that the patient was utilizing before admission must be noted. It may be necessary to modify some of these measures once the patient is hospitalized, and all such changes in medication, diet, activity, and other areas must be carefully explained. Without an adequate explanation, the patient or family may feel that such changes during hospitalization are an indictment of the care provided at home, rather than seeing them as necessary preoperative preparations.

PHYSIOLOGIC PREPARATION

Despite the fact that the person scheduled for heart surgery may have suffered from the cardiac condition for years, it is desirable to have the person in the best physical condition possible at the time of surgery. This is one goal of patient care during the preoperative period, however short or long that may be. Efforts will have been made to help the overweight patient reach a safe body weight, to assist the patient who smokes to stop or nearly stop, to eliminate or reduce edema and establish body fluids and electrolytes in normal balance, to correct or control cardiac arrhythmias, to eliminate any signs of infection, in short, to achieve the healthiest state possible in light of the severity of the illness and the urgency of the surgery.

Therefore, along with a thorough knowledge of the patient's history, as mentioned above, it is necessary to obtain a complete data baseline to document the patient's condition just before surgery. While many of the preoperative tests and preparations may have been performed in the days or weeks before the scheduled surgery, the person is usually admitted to the hospital at least 1 or 2 days before the planned procedure. At this time, a chest x-ray film, an ECG, and full laboratory screening will be performed. For selected individuals, arterial blood gas analyses and even pulmonary function studies may be obtained to help establish a baseline of respiratory status and to plan appropriate and aggressive preoperative, intraoperative, and postoperative pulmonary care. Baseline vital signs (including apical and radial heart rates and bilateral arm blood pressures), integrity of all pulses (both proximal and distal), neurologic status, height, weight, nutritional status, elimination patterns, and psychologic status are all carefully assessed and recorded in the immediate preoperative period.

PREOPERATIVE TEACHING FOR THE PERSON UNDERGOING CARDIAC SURGERY

1. General information
   a. Places of care during hospitalization
      (1) CCU or ICU after surgery
      (2) Return to general patient care division in 2 to 3 days
   b. Visiting hours and location of waiting rooms
2. Description of surgery
   a. Simple explanation of anatomy of heart and effect of the patient's cardiovascular disorder (e.g., incompetent valve, obstructed coronary artery)
   b. Explanation of surgical procedure
   c. Definition of an unfamiliar terms: bypass, extracorporeal
   d. Length of time in surgery: 2 to 4 hours
   e. Length of time until able to see family (usually 1½ to 2 hours after surgery)
3. Preparation for surgery
   a. Shower or bath night before surgery with special antimicrobial soap
   b. Surgical shave: shaving of entire chest and abdomen neck to groin and left midaxillary line to right
   c. Legs shaved if saphenous vein grafts will be used
   d. Preoperative medication
4. Explanation of monitors
   a. Round patches on chest connected to a cardiac monitor which records patient's heart beats
   b. Monitor makes beeping sound all the time
5. Explanation of lines
   a. Intravenous routes for fluid and medications
   b. Central venous line in neck or chest to monitor fluid status
   c. Swan-Ganz line in chest or neck to measure pulmonary pressures and monitor fluid status
   d. Plastic connector line to obtain blood samples without a needle stick
6. Explanation of drainage tubes
   a. Indwelling urinary catheter
   b. Chest tube: bloody drainage is expected
7. Explanation of breathing tube
   a. Tube in windpipe connected to machine called ventilator
   b. Unable to speak with tube in place, but can mouth words and communicate in writing
   c. Tube is removed when patient is fully awake and stable
   d. Secretions in lungs or tube removed by nurse using a suction catheter
   e. Food and oral fluids not permitted until breathing tube is removed
8. Explanation and demonstration of activities and exercises
   a. Purpose of activity is to promote circulation, keep lungs clear, and prevent infection
   b. Activity includes:
      (1) Turning from side to side in bed
      (2) Sitting on edge of bed
      (3) Sitting in chair the night of or the morning after surgery
   c. Range-of-motion exercises
   d. Deep breathing using sustained maximal inspiration
   e. Tubes and lines will restrict movement somewhat, but nurse will assist patient
9. Relief of pain
   a. Some pain will be experienced, but it will not be excruciating (different pain than original angina if this was present)
   b. Frequent pain medication will be given to help relieve the pain, but patient should always tell nurse when pain is present

PATIENT TEACHING

In the past several years preoperative teaching programs for heart surgery patients have become well established. These fairly structured approaches still allow the nurse to individualize a teaching plan for any particular patient and yet ensure that all necessary topics are covered in a consistent manner for all patients (see the box above).

General Information

While most persons admitted for heart surgery have undergone previous hospitalizations, there will be significant differences in this particular stay, and an initial overview of general information is helpful to most patients and families. Frequently, the family will be requested to identify one spokesperson who will be told where to meet the surgeon after the operation and who will be allowed to call the intensive care unit (ICU) nurses at any time for information. This serves to enhance the consistency and thoroughness of information given to the family while reducing the interruptions from multiple sources.

Information Concerning the Intensive Care Unit

Many patients and family members benefit from a tour of the ICU, both to familiarize them with the equipment and to locate important areas such as waiting rooms and restrooms. Such a tour should always be conducted by ICU personnel who can accurately yet reassuringly describe the myriad of sights and sounds that assail the untrained observer. Timing of the tour must be convenient for the ICU personnel, who should greet the patient and family when they arrive, without appearing so rushed that the patient and family feel that they are imposing.

At times a tour may be omitted depending on the acuity of the ICU patients and the level of critical activity in the unit. If there is any possibility that a tour might prove distressing or unusually anxiety provoking to the patient or family, it should be replaced with a general description of the sights, sounds, and activities that the patient is likely to encounter. It is important that all discussions of the stay in the ICU center about the unique attention and in-depth care that the patient will receive from specially qualified nurses.

Description of Surgery

Specific instruction must be given concerning the particular type of heart surgery that the patient will undergo. Simple diagrams or plastic heart models can be used to illustrate what type of cardiac problem the patient has and how the surgery will correct it. The type of chest incision to be made should be described: most commonly, a median sternotomy is performed for all bypasses and some valve procedures, whereas a left anterior axillary chest approach is used for certain selected repair procedures. In addition, the internal thigh incision for obtaining vein grafts is described for selected coronary artery bypass patients.

Explanation of Preoperative and Postoperative Procedures

It is important to describe the types of interventions and equipment that are made necessary by the intricacy of heart surgery. Specific aspects of the equipment and techniques that will be of special significance to the patient are described (Table 28-5).

Explain that the patient will receive continuous observation in the ICU and may at times be awakened to receive necessary nursing care, such as taking vital signs, obtaining blood specimens, taking x-ray films, turning, coughing, and deep breathing. Demonstrate the types of exercises in which the patient will be expected to participate actively. Document the patient's preoperative ability to cough and use assistive breathing

TABLE 28-5 Techniques and equipment commonly used after cardiac surgery

Technique/Equipment	Purpose
Intubation; ventilator for 12-24 hours	Maintain open airway and ventilation
Cardiac monitoring	Identify arrhythmias
Chest tubes (one to four)	Drain blood and air from chest
Intravenous lines	Replace fluids; monitor CVP
Intraarterial lines	Monitor blood pressure; obtain arterial blood samples
Pulmonary artery line (Swan-Ganz)	Monitor pulmonary artery and capillary wedge pressure; monitor cardiac output
Indwelling urinary catheter (Foley)	Monitor urinary output for signs of impaired renal function

devices for later comparison and encouragement postoperatively.

Teaching Approaches

Initial assessment of the patient's knowledge and ability to learn is essential to planning a thorough, individualized teaching plan. Continued reassessment of the patient's readiness to learn and retention ability is important throughout the preparative education period. Teaching sessions should be conducted at planned times and in a quiet area. The pace must be adapted to the patient's interest and ability to master the information presented. Opportunities should be allowed for the patient to demonstrate understanding of concepts and techniques. Adjunctive printed information should be given to all patients to reinforce what has been taught verbally (see the nursing care plan on p. 692).

PSYCHOLOGIC PREPARATION

Patients scheduled to undergo heart surgery are usually aware that they are facing a potentially life-threatening situation; however, no two patients will manifest this awareness in the same way. A complete psychosocial evaluation is becoming a routine part of the preparative care of heart surgery patients in medical centers throughout the country. This evaluation is one part of the multidisciplinary team approach, which usually consists of the medical referral physician, cardiac surgeon, psychologist, clinical nurse specialist or practitioner, social worker, and dietitian.

The psychosocial evaluation looks at patients and significant others in relation to the presence of support mechanisms, the use of defense mechanisms (long-standing versus situational), and established methods of adaptation. Combined with an assessment of the patients' basic levels of understanding of the experience they are about to undergo, a sound plan can be developed to enhance patients' preoperative and postoperative psychologic well-being.

It has been established that a small amount of anxiety enhances learning, whereas too much anxiety blocks learning. The highly anxious individual may benefit from limited and carefully worded preoperative teaching, with an emphasis on a simple understanding of the surgical procedure. Highly fearful or anxious patients are most prone to serious misconceptions about their illness, the surgical procedure itself, and the anticipated outcome. It is very important to include significant others in the preoperative teaching plan when the patient is unusually worried or appears to have significant misconceptions. It is also very important to address patients' fears very seriously, no matter how unusual they might sound. Patients must be given frequent opportunity to vent their concerns to supportive, understanding staff members.

Patients who consistently reject the offer of information about their illness and impending surgery also need a supportive environment in which they feel safe. Information should not be pressed on those who truly do not wish to hear it; for them, such defense mechanisms may be tremendously important. Rather, a complete psychosocial evaluation may point out ways in which staff and significant others can assist in maintaining the psychologic well-being both before and after surgery. Conversely, it may also reveal that for some patients, highly restricted visiting and family contact may be desirable for a few days postoperatively.

Finally, as more and more patients have relatives and friends who have undergone heart surgery, they may be concerned about postoperative psychologic problems that they have observed. The health professional will exercise judgment in introducing this topic in preoperative teaching, but when it appears indicated or if the topic arises, an explanation should be given of the factors that may precipitate a postoperative or ICU psychosis: sleep deprivation, stress, and sensory overload from continuous environmental stimuli. Patients who develop the psychosis may complain of depression, inability to sleep, or of having "bad dreams" when they do sleep. These symptoms usually disappear after the patient's condition will allow a few lengthy intervals of undisturbed sleep. For some patients, preoperative awareness of the effects of such stressors may prevent the patients

from fearing that they are "losing their minds" if such symptoms arise. A sedative may be given the night before surgery to aid the patient in maintaining a calm state and obtaining a restful night's sleep despite a normal amount of apprehension.

INTRAOPERATIVE PERIOD

The preoperative medications frequently include a narcotic analgesic, a sedative, an anticholinergic agent, and sometimes an antibiotic. The patient's skin is often prepared in a specially designated area, adjacent to the operating room. A light analgesic is given first, followed by insertion of various intravenous and intraarterial lines. The patient is monitored during the insertion of the lines. When the patient is fully anesthetized, the patient is intubated and placed on mechanical ventilation.

If the cardiac surgery to be performed is a coronary artery bypass, either autologous superficial saphenous vein segments or an internal mammary artery is used for grafts, which are "harvested." With saphenous veins, portions of the veins are removed from one leg using longitudinal, interrupted incisions. The internal mammary artery (IMA) is retrieved by retracting the sternum and entering the pleural space. The tissue is dissected to obtain the IMA (Figure 28-11). Studies have shown that 40% to 50% of saphenous vein grafts close within 10 years, whereas 90% of IMA grafts remain patent 10 years after the operation (see the research box below).

The heart is exposed through either a midline sterno-

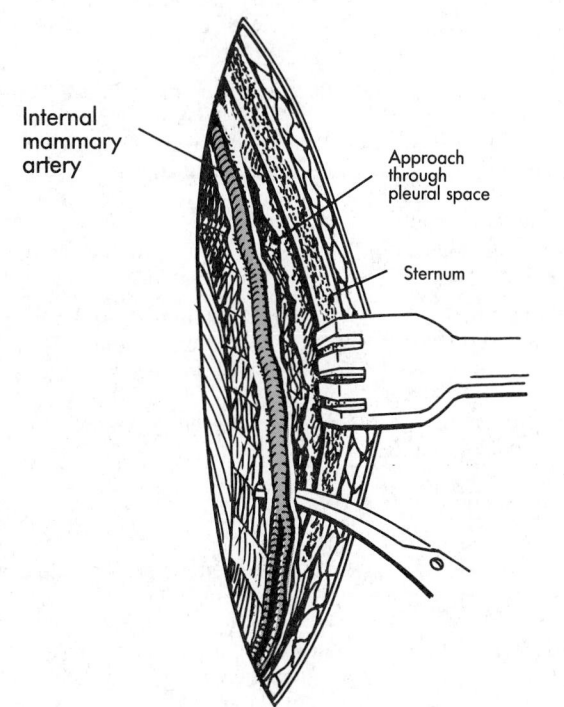

FIGURE 28-11 The internal mammary artery (IMA) is resected from the inner chest wall.

Internal mammary artery

Approach through pleural space

Sternum

RESEARCH

Loop F et al: Coronary bypass surgery: the total experience at the Cleveland Clinic Foundation, Clinical Essays of the Heart 2:131-138 1984.

This study examined the patency rate of saphenous vein and internal mammary artery grafts during the years of 1972 to 1982. The severity of lesions, number of operable vessels, change in activity, unstable angina, and left main coronary artery disease were the most common reasons for surgical referral. Patients with saphenous vein grafts or internal mammary artery grafts were studied in relation to their patency rates over a course of several months to years. The number of subjects with saphenous vein grafts were 6968 (11,655 grafts), whereas those with internal mammary artery grafts were 2110 (2127). Patency of the grafts was evaluated based on cardiac catheterizations over a period of months. Approximately 4 years after surgery, 80% of saphenous vein grafts were patent. However, 96% of those patients with internal mammary artery grafts remained patent. When comparing the saphenous vein graft and internal mammary artery graft for the repair at the anterior descending artery, 83% of the saphenous vein grafts versus 96% of the internal mammary artery grafts remained patent. ■

NURSING CARE PLAN

PERSON PREOPERATIVE FOR CARDIAC SURGERY

DATA: Ms. Philips is a 40-year-old stockbroker who was admitted to the hospital for a mitral valve repair. She has a history of rheumatic fever as a child and mitral stenosis. Six months ago, Ms. Philips was admitted to the hospital for chest pain, dyspnea, and tachyarrhythmia (atrial fibrillation). A cardiac catheterization revealed a narrowed orifice of the mitral valve (2.2 cm sq). A loading dose of digoxin was given, with a maintenance dose of 0.125 mg daily. Ms. Philips was an avid runner, averaging 3 miles/day before this hospitalization.

Over the course of the past 6 months, Ms. Philips has been unable to maintain any activity level and has complained of severe dyspnea and fatigue. During this hospital admission, tests revealed the mitral orifice now to be 2.0 cm sq. It was decided that surgery was warranted.

The nursing history identified the following:
- Ms. Philips has a limited understanding of the surgical procedure and of invasive lines.
- She states she is willing to undergo the procedure but is concerned because she has a low pain threshold.

Nursing activities include monitoring the following:
- Heart rhythm and rate: opening snap, S_3
- Breath sounds
- Intake and output
- Serum electrolytes: potassium, calcium
- Activity tolerance

NURSING DIAGNOSIS

Knowledge deficit related to the surgical procedure and invasive lines

Expected Patient Outcomes	Nursing Interventions	Rationale
Ms. Philips describes the anatomy of the heart and valve repair.	Describe the anatomy of the heart and valve repair in simple terms using a model.	Use of models can facilitate learning.
Ms. Philips describes events pertaining to the surgery.	Discuss events related to the surgery: ■ Shower night before surgery ■ Preoperative medication ■ Length of surgery (2-4 hours) ■ Family visitation (2 hours after surgery) ■ Length of ICU stay (1-2 days) ■ Patches placed on chest	Knowing what to expect helps to decrease preoperative anxiety. Preoperative medication is given before line insertion. Early family visitation decreases patient's anxiety. Patches will monitor heart rate and rhythm.
Ms. Philips describes purpose of lines.	Explain purpose of lines: 1. IV for fluids and medications 2. Line in neck or chest to monitor fluid status (CVP) and pulmonary pressures (PAP) 3. Arterial line to measure blood pressure and obtain blood samples without a needle stick 4. Epicardial pacing wires placed before closure of chest (may require pacing postbypass)	Because of the many lines in place postoperatively, advance knowledge will help decrease postoperative anxiety. Wires are used to improve conduction and cardiac output.
Ms. Philips describes events related to breathing tube.	Explain events related to breathing tube: 1. Tube in windpipe connected to a ventilator 2. Patient unable to talk 3. No food or drink given before tube removal 4. Tube removed when patient is fully awake (about 14-16 hours after surgery) 5. Secretions are removed using a suction catheter	Awakening to find a ventilator tube in place can be frightening unless advance knowledge is given. This will prevent aspiration.
Ms. Philips describes drainage tubes.	Describe drainage tubes: 1. NG tube placed in nose to remove gastric contents 2. Indwelling urinary catheter 3. Chest tubes	NG tube prevents gastric reflux during ventilation. Indwelling urinary catheter will accurately measure fluid output. Chest tubes remove bloody drainage.

NURSING CARE PLAN
PERSON PREOPERATIVE FOR CARDIAC SURGERY—CONT'D

NURSING DIAGNOSIS
Anxiety related to ability to tolerate postoperative pain

Expected Patient Outcomes	Nursing Interventions	Rationale
Ms. Philips expresses less concern about postoperative pain.	Describe postoperative pain: will become apparent after the anesthetic wears off and will be different than original pain	Knowledge of what to expect can decrease anxiety.
	Describe measures to reduce pain: 1. Tell nurse about the pain before it becomes severe 2. Medication will be given frequently during the first 2 days, then when necessary 3. Relaxation will help to decrease pain and help breathing	Knowing what to expect about the pain and measures that can be taken for pain relief can decrease anxiety and perception of pain postoperatively. Pain will cause patient to splint chest, affecting breathing and pulse (tachycardia).

tomy or anterolateral thoracotomy incision, and retractors are used to hold the chest open.

CARDIOPULMONARY BYPASS

Some heart surgery procedures can be performed without artificial ventilation and circulation, but most procedures require either partial or total cardiopulmonary bypass. In *partial*, or left heart, bypass, blood is drained from the left atrium and ventricle and is passed through a pulsatile pump or roller pump, which returns the blood to the common femoral artery or the descending aorta. In this type of bypass, the pulmonary circulation is not interrupted.

In *total* cardiopulmonary bypass both oxygenation and circulation of the blood are performed by the bypass machine. Venous blood is removed from the body via cannulas placed in either the right atrium or the inferior and superior venae cavae (Figure 28-12). The blood passes through the oxygenating mechanism of the bypass machine, is oxygenated, and is then pumped back into the arterial circulation of the body through cannulas placed either in the ascending aorta (most common) or in the femoral artery. A venting tube is usually introduced through the apex of the left ventricle or left atrium and is connected to the pump to aspirate intracardiac blood and maintain decompression.

The bypass pump circuits must be primed before use with a fluid volume of approximately 2500 ml. In the past a large portion of that volume was composed of cross-matched type-specific whole blood. Currently, more centers are using an entirely blood-free hemodilution primer consisting mainly of lactated Ringer's solution. The advantages of the nonblood primer include decreased viscosity, limited hemolysis, and no risk of transfusion reaction and hepatitis from the primer solution. The main concern in using a nonblood primer is maintenance of an adequate hematocrit. This can be achieved by intermittent additions of blood to the system during the cardiopulmonary bypass process.

In addition to performing blood oxygenating and circulating functions for the body, the bypass machine has two other distinct functions. It can act as a source for the direct administration of medications into the systemic circulation. It is also able to provide systemic hypothermia by cooling the perfusate to temperatures that range from mildly (30° to 34° C) to profoundly (15° C) below body temperatures. Hypothermia decreases the tissue's metabolic needs, thereby lowering the body's overall oxygen consumption. A reduced need for oxygen enhances myocardial tissue preservation during times such as when the aorta is cross-clamped.

Cold Cardioplegia

Myocardial tissue preservation is of primary concern in all cardiac surgery procedures and especially in surgery for ischemic heart disease. In recent years a clearer understanding of the principles involved in myocardial tissue preservation has resulted in the widespread use of cold cardioplegia solutions.

Cold cardioplegia consists of infusing an alkaline hyperosmotic solution containing potassium, calcium chloride, mannitol, and other substances into the aortic root. It is usually infused for a few minutes immediately after aortic cross-clamping and again after about 30 to 45 minutes or when myocardial temperatures rise above 19° C. External cardiac cooling is achieved by a continuous infusion of lactated Ringer's solution at about 4° C into the pericardium. Several variations of the cold car-

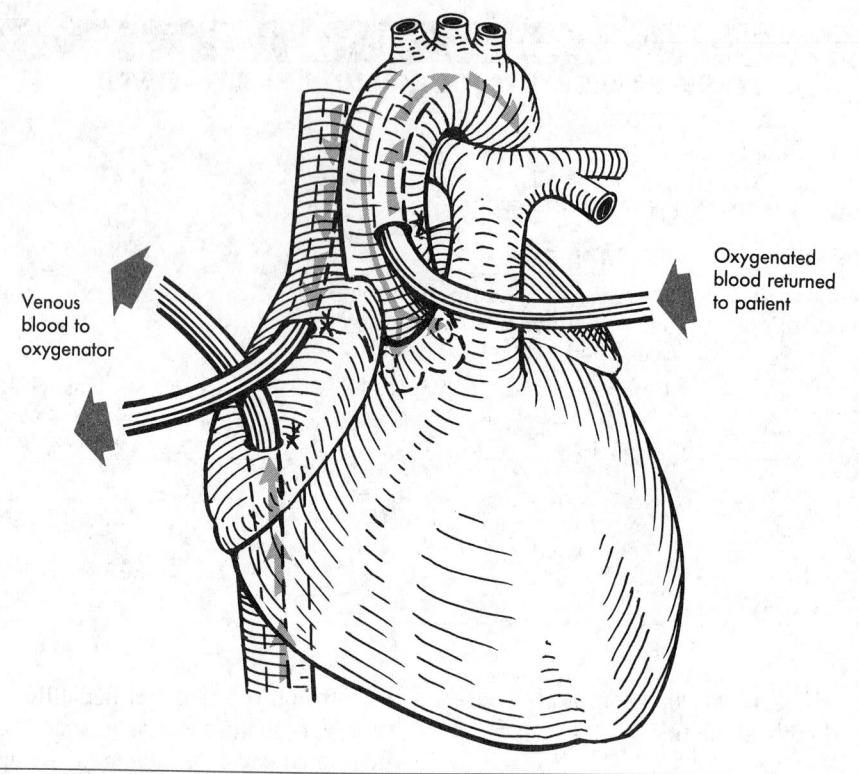

Venous
blood to
oxygenator

Oxygenated
blood returned
to patient

FIGURE 28-12 Cardiopulmonary bypass.

dioplegia technique are in use, and it appears that this development has significantly improved myocardial tissue preservation in the intraoperative phase by supercooling the myocardium and drastically reducing its oxygen requirements.

Termination of Procedure

Once the surgical repair has been executed, the cardioplegia infusion is terminated. The blood in the bypass pump is slowly rewarmed, and the patient's body temperature is brought back to near normal. If the aorta was cross-clamped, it is unclamped at this time and the heart, which had been stopped while on hypothermia, is restarted. The lungs are reexpanded, and when the cardiac rhythm is good, weaning from the bypass machine is begun. Blood volume is given back to the patient from the bypass machine, and the patient remains on decreasing amounts of partial bypass until weaning is complete. Systemic heparinization, which was done to promote blood flow while on bypass and to prevent blood from clotting quickly in the operative field, is reversed with protamine.

Epicardial pacing wires may be attached directly to the right ventricular wall, the right atrial wall, or the internal chest wall and are then brought through the incision to the chest surface. There they may be used for temporary cardiac pacing if needed during the postoperative period. Chest tubes are inserted as indicated for blood drainage and air evacuation, if necessary. The incisions are closed and dressed, and the patient is taken to the recovery room.

Side Effects of Cardiopulmonary Bypass

Although cardiopulmonary bypass has been the most significant advance in the rapidly growing area of safe and effective cardiac procedures, it has a number of specific, potentially deleterious side effects. It creates a shocklike state, in which there is a functionally low hematocrit (produced by hemodilution), decreased platelets (shearing forces during bypass), decreased systemic arterial pressures, and decreased perfusion to major organs (Figure 28-13). A prolonged decrease in blood pressure may result in neurologic changes, such as encephalopathy or cerebral anoxia. Decreased perfusion to the vital organs may also contribute to neurologic changes or renal ischemia, leading to acute renal failure.

Some patients may experience difficulties in being weaned from extracorporeal circulation. These persons may require circulatory assistance, such as the intraaortic balloon pump (IABP) to temporarily augment their circulatory system.

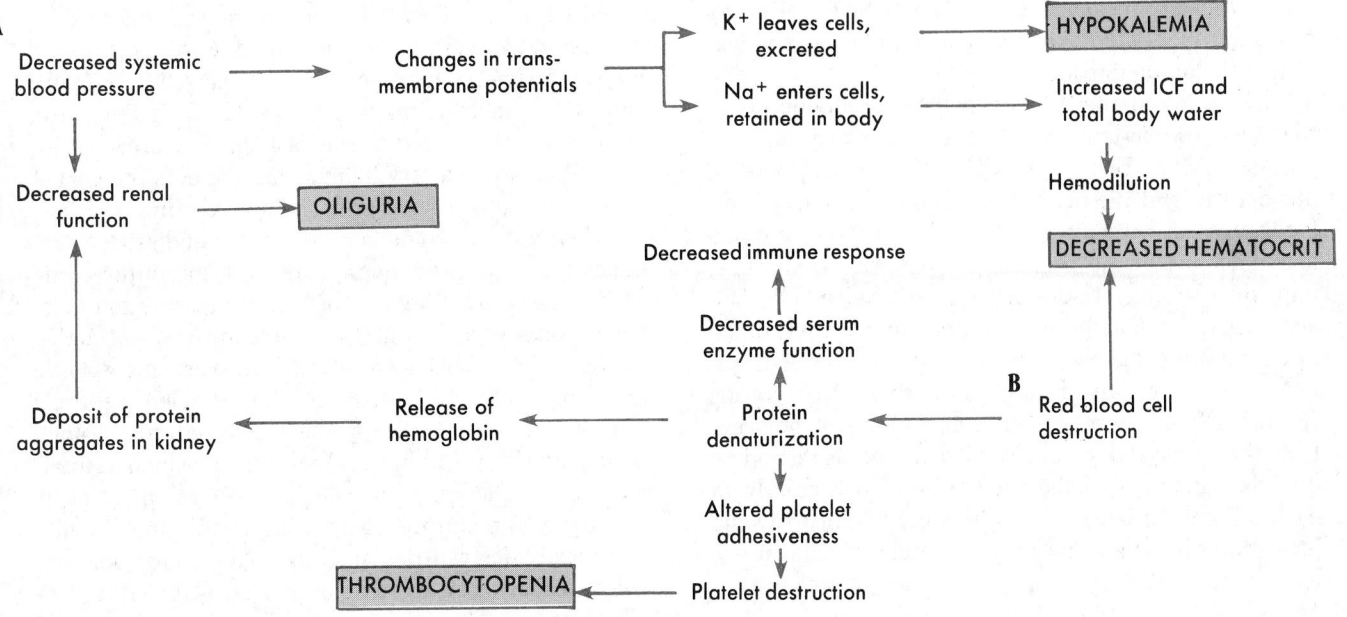

FIGURE 28-13 Some effects of the shocklike state, **A,** and red blood cell destruction, **B,** that may occur with cardiopulmonary bypass. Clinical signs are indicated in boxes.

INTERVENTION FOR THE PERSON WITH INTRAAORTIC BALLOON COUNTERPULSATION

A counterpulsation device is one that assists the circulation of blood through the body by pumping when the heart is in ventricular diastole. The hemodynamic result of this action is to augment intraaortic blood pressure during diastole. The physiologic effects of counterpulsation are therefore an increase in coronary artery perfusion, a decrease in preload (the degree to which the myocardium is stretched before contracting), and a decrease in afterload (the resistance against which blood is expelled).

The two primary goals in the use of circulatory assist devices are to provide temporary assistance to the patient's circulation until the pathophysiologic condition is corrected and to afford optimal conditions for repair or resting of the heart until it can provide adequate circulation unaided. The IABP is a counterpulsation device capable of achieving these goals in selected patients.

Indications for Use

The various situations in which counterpulsation has been found useful are listed in the box at right. In all cases, the timeliness of its application is essential to reduce the workload of the heart and halt the progressive deterioration of the myocardium. Individuals have been maintained on IABP assistance for periods of several hours to several months; however, the usual time is from 2 to 3 days. The IABP is not indicated for persons whose underlying pathologic condition is so severe that eventual weaning from the IABP is considered impossible, unless the individual is being seriously evaluated for a heart transplant. Absolute contraindications are few; the two primary ones are aortic valve incompetence and aortic aneurysm.

Technique

The intraaortic balloon is inserted percutaneously or by cutdown into the right or left femoral artery. It is advanced into the thoracic aorta and is sutured into place at the insertion site after the balloon tip has been correctly positioned just distal to the left subclavian artery.

INTRAAORTIC BALLOON COUNTERPULSATION: INDICATIONS FOR USE

Cardiogenic shock secondary to acute myocardial infarction
Other low cardiac output states
During emergency diagnostic procedures on unstable cardiac patients
In unstable cardiac patients before and during open heart surgery
Assistance in removing patients from cardiopulmonary bypass postoperatively
Drug-resistant, life-threatening arrhythmias
Unstable angina pectoris
Severe acute myocardial infarction

The end of the balloon catheter is attached to a pump console, which alternately inflates and deflates the balloon with carbon dioxide gas.

The timing of the inflation-deflation sequence is of the utmost importance in obtaining maximal counterpulsation effect. Using the ECG to trigger the pumping mechanism and the arterial waveform to determine effectiveness of the counterpulsation, the balloon is timed to inflate just at the beginning of ventricular diastole, immediately after closure of the aortic valve. The balloon remains inflated during diastole and is then timed to deflate immediately before the next ventricular systolic ejection or just before the aortic valve reopens (Figure 28-14). Improper balloon timing not only defeats the purpose of counterpulsation, but also could be directly damaging to the myocardium, particularly in early inflation or late deflation in which the heart would be ejecting blood against a partially inflated balloon.

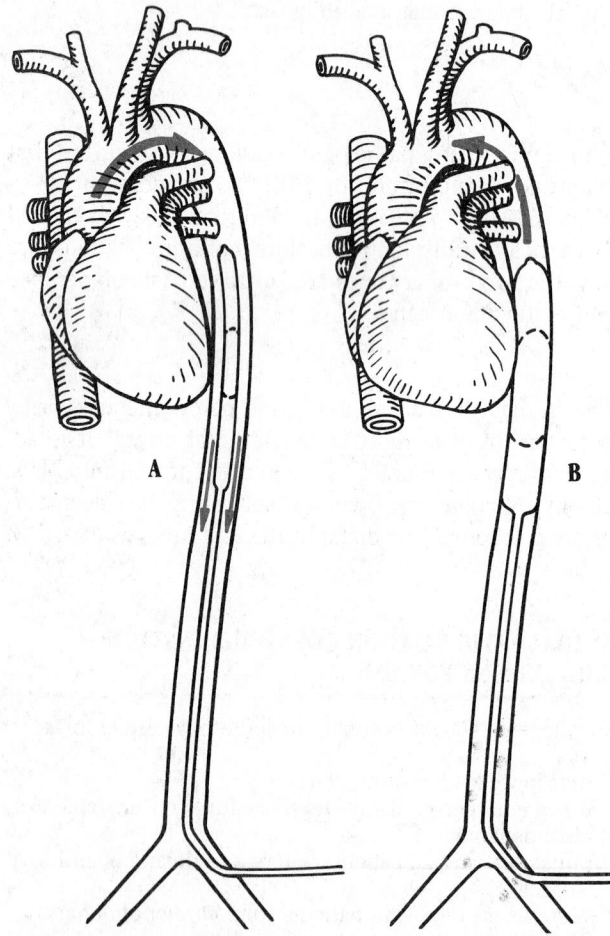

FIGURE 28-14 Representation of intraaortic balloon positioned just distal to left subclavian artery. **A,** Balloon is deflated, allowing forward blood flow during systole. **B,** Balloon is inflated to increase coronary perfusion during diastole.

When the balloon is inflated during diastole, it causes an intraaortic pressure rise known as *diastolic augmentation*. This heightened diastolic pressure caused by balloon inflation forces blood in the aortic arch to flow in a retrograde fashion and provides increased coronary artery filling. This achieves the goal of improving oxygen delivery to the myocardium.

When the balloon deflates at the end of diastole, it reduces pressure in the aorta, causing blood in the aortic arch to move from an area of higher pressure to one of lower pressure and to fill the space previously occupied by the balloon. This decreases the pressure in the aortic arch, reducing the resistance that the left ventricle must overcome in order to eject blood during systole; hence afterload is reduced. A sustained reduction in afterload will allow the left ventricle to eject more of its stroke volume during each contraction, thus leaving more space for ventricular filling. This will usually result in a secondary decrease in preload as the left ventricle becomes and remains more efficient.

Nursing Interventions

The patient undergoing IABP counterpulsation requires intensive nursing observation and care. All vital signs and indices of cardiac function must be observed continually and recorded; frequently the patient will be receiving vasopressor and antiarrhythmic drugs, and it is the nurse's responsibility to titrate these for the desired effects. The patient may be intubated and be dependent on ventilatory support. All such factors require meticulous nursing intervention.

In addition, the patient with an IABP in place requires specific observation and care to prevent possible complications, such as circulatory insufficiency in the catheterized leg, aortic damage, and infection. Circulation checks of all pulses in both lower extremities are performed before insertion and hourly thereafter until the balloon is removed. No hip flexion is allowed on the catheterized side; well-padded leg restraints must be used if the patient is unable to cooperate. The head of the bed is not elevated more than 30 degrees to prevent balloon migration upward in the aorta. The patient should be tilted and carefully positioned on alternate sides every 2 hours to prevent skin breakdown and other consequences of limited mobility. The dressing on the balloon insertion site must be kept clean and dry and should be changed every 24 to 72 hours using sterile technique.

Considerable psychologic support is necessary for the patient and family during such critical therapy. Not only is the physical size and noise of the pump console very intimidating, but its presence only reinforces everyone's awareness of the frailty of the patient's heart and uncertainty about the future. Careful but simple explanations of the pump's action are necessary for those patients who are alert enough to understand; it is important that they not get the mistaken idea that the pump is working instead of their heart. Some patients with this type of misunderstanding fear that they will die if the pump stops even momentarily. Such terrific fear makes them anxious and restless and further increases the body's demand for oxygen. Continuous reassurance and repeated simple explanations are essential; some patients may benefit from mild sedation.

VENTRICULAR ASSIST DEVICES

An alternative approach for patients in ventricular failure is left- or right-ventricular assist devices (L-VAD or R-VAD). These devices provide rest for the ventricles while artificially replacing systemic pumping.[11] They are generally indicated for profound intraoperative myocardial depression with failure to wean from the cardiopulmonary bypass. Patients requiring this type of assistance are critically ill and require care in an intensive care unit. For further information see Chapter 80.

POSTOPERATIVE CARE

After the conclusion of the heart surgery, patients are transferred to the postanesthesia recovery area or directly to a cardiovascular or surgical ICU where they will typically remain for 1 to 2 days. During this time the patient will need continuous observation and professional nursing care to promote optimal recovery and prevent complications, which are most serious in the first 48 hours after surgery (see the box below).

NURSING CARE OF THE PATIENT AFTER CARDIAC SURGERY

1. Monitoring
   a. Cardiovascular
      1. Blood pressure and pulse (rate, pulse deficit)
      2. Pulmonary artery pressure (PAP), pulmonary capillary wedge pressure (PCWP), cardiac output (CO), central venous pressure (CVP), left atrial pressure (LAP)
      3. ECG for signs of dysrhythmias
      4. Body temperature
      5. Skin color, temperature, capillary filling
      6. Signs of hypovolemic shock (decreased CVP, decreased LAP, decreased PCWP, decreased cardiac output)
      7. Signs of cardiac tamponade (cessation of chest drainage, restlessness, decreased blood pressure, increased CVP, increased PAP, increased LAP)
   b. Respiratory
      1. Respirations: rate, depth, quality
      2. Breath sounds
      3. Chest tubes for patency and drainage
      4. Autotransfuse chest tube drainage
   c. Neurologic
      1. Level of consciousness
      2. Pupillary size and reaction
      3. Orientation
      4. Movement and sensation of extremities
   d. Urinary
      1. Output (amount)
      2. Color
      3. pH and specific gravity
   e. Fluid & electrolyte balance
      1. Intake/output balance
      2. Daily weights
      3. Serum potassium and calcium levels
   f. Presence of discomfort: pain, fatigue
   g. Ability to sleep
   h. Behavior: depression, fear, disorientation, hallucinations
2. Promoting oxygen/carbon dioxide exchange
   a. Preoxygenation and suction during intubation; suction as necessary after extubation
   b. Position with head only slightly elevated; turn side to side
   c. Encourage breathing exercises
   d. Medicate before breathing and coughing exercises
   e. Encourage range-of-motion exercises and progressive activity
3. Promoting fluid and electrolyte balance
   a. Record accurate intake and output
   b. Maintain prescribed flow rates of parenteral fluids
   c. Give prescribed supplemental IV potassium chloride
4. Promoting comfort
   a. Give narcotic analgesics every 3 hours during the first 24 hours, then as needed
   b. Give frequent mouth care
   c. Control environment for comfort
   d. Change bed linens when diaphoresis is present (assure person that this is common)
   e. Plan activities to permit periods of sleep
   f. Provide back rubs for backache
   g. Splint incision during coughing
   h. Encourage patient to share feelings and experiences
5. Promoting activity
   a. Provide for passive then active range-of-motion exercises
   b. Encourage ambulation when permitted
6. Teaching
   a. Progressive return to physical activity as recommended by the physician
   b. Rehabilitation exercise program
   c. Sexual activity usually permitted in 3 to 4 weeks
   d. Signs of overexertion include fatigue, dyspnea, pain
   e. Eat a balanced diet with any prescribed modifications (such as no added salt or low cholesterol)
   f. Medications
      1. Name, dosage, schedule, action, and side effects of prescribed medications
      2. Use of prescribed medications as needed
   g. Signs that may persist: dyspnea, pain, night sweats
   h. Signs requiring medical attention (fever, increasing dyspnea, or chest pain with minimal exertion)
   i. Need for ongoing medical care

Complete observation, thorough assessment, careful planning, and knowledgeable intervention may be organized through a systems approach to care.

CARDIOVASCULAR SYSTEM

One of the major goals of patient care in the immediate postoperative period is to promote cardiovascular function, adequate tissue perfusion, and stabilization of vital signs. To evaluate cardiovascular function thoroughly, the patient will have an intraarterial line and a pulmonary artery catheter (Swan-Ganz), each connected to a pressure transducer and continuous monitor; a CVP line connected to a water manometer or a pressure transducer and monitor; and a continuous electrocardiograph monitor.

Promoting Cardiac Function

Blood pressure and heart rate are monitored continuously and are recorded every 15 minutes until stable, then every hour thereafter. *CVP, pulmonary artery pressure, pulmonary capillary wedge pressure,* and *cardiac output* measurements are obtained every 2 to 4 hours as indicated by changes in the patient's condition. The radial pulse is checked for rate, rhythm, and volume, with bilateral comparisons made. The apical and radial pulses are checked simultaneously for any differences (pulse deficit), which could be indicative of such complications as atrial fibrillation. Distal peripheral pulses, either posterior tibial or dorsalis pedis, are checked for strength and bilateral equality.

The *cardiac pattern* is monitored continuously for the first several days postoperatively, and the ECG pattern is compared with the preoperative baseline to detect any changes. Cardiac dysrhythmias are very common in the immediate postoperative period; they may be the result of operative trauma from incision of the left ventricle, prolonged use of anesthesia, extracorporeal circulation, and alterations in potassium levels, hypotension, hypovolemia, or hypoxia.

The treatment for dysrhythmias depends on the cause and the type of dysrhythmia produced. Treatment modalities include antiarrhythmic drugs such as lidocaine and procainamide (Pronestyl), cardiotonics such as digoxin, potassium replacement, and temporary pacing. With the increasing use of computerized monitoring systems, the nurse has a highly sophisticated adjunct to help obtain, store, and analyze ECG information when it is most vital. If the ECG status remains somewhat uncertain as recovery progresses, the patient may be transferred from the ICU to a cardiac step-down unit or telemetry unit for several days so that the ECG pattern may continue to be monitored closely.

Body temperature can be an important indication of cardiovascular function. The skin should be warm and dry, although immediately after surgery the skin may still be quite cool as a result of intraoperative hypothermia. Once the body temperature has warmed, cool or diaphoretic skin may be an indication of shock. It is not uncommon for the body temperature to rise above normal and remain elevated for the first day or two postoperatively. This is usually attributed to the time spent on cardiopulmonary bypass.

As with skin temperature, *skin color* is indicative of the patient's perfusion state. The nailbeds should be pale pink, blanch easily, and return to pink color quickly, indicating good capillary refill. Cyanosis, either central or peripheral, can indicate poor perfusion, poor oxygenation, or both. The causative agent must be quickly differentiated and eliminated. Although cyanosis is not usually an early or reliable indicator of blood oxygen concentration, it can develop rapidly in the acutely ill patient and must be immediately reversed.

Maintaining Chest Drainage

Blood loss will directly affect the systemic perfusion status, and both the chest incision and the chest tubes must be observed frequently for signs of unusually profuse drainage. Chest tubes are connected to a collection apparatus and a low level of suction (Chapter 34). Autotransfusion is a relatively new method of collecting blood from chest tubes via a reservoir, then transfusing the drainage back into the patient. It has little risk for transfusion reactions and provides patients with inexpensive volume replacement (Chapter 76). Mediastinal chest tubes are placed for the sole purpose of evacuating excess blood from the pericardial and mediastinal areas. The tubes are "stripped" by hand every 15 to 30 minutes for the first few hours after surgery to promote drainage. Drainage should be slow and fairly consistent and does not usually exceed 100 ml/hour after the first 2 hours postoperatively. The patient is routinely turned from side to side every 2 hours to assist in proper chest drainage. The total blood drainage over the first 24 hours will usually average 500 ml.

A change in chest drainage color to a very bright red from a dark red, a sustained hemorrhage that lasts for over 1 minute, or a sudden cessation of chest drainage are all abnormal findings that must be reported immediately. Cessation of chest drainage within the first few hours postoperatively usually indicates clotting of the chest tube within the mediastinum. This could predispose the patient to *cardiac tamponade*, a life-threatening emergency. Tamponade indicates a compression of the heart caused by excessive amounts of blood or blood clots collecting between the heart and the anterior chest wall. The return of venous blood to the right atrium and the cardiac output can be significantly impaired. Other signs of cardiac tamponade, in addition to minimal or no chest tube drainage, include sudden increase in bleeding from the midline incision, restlessness, decreased blood pressure, increased CVP and PAP, and decreased urinary output. The physician must be notified at once, and cardiac decompression by needle aspiration or other methods will be undertaken.

Maintaining Blood Pressure

Maintenance of a stable systemic blood pressure in the postoperative period may be difficult in some patients. *High* blood pressure must be controlled so that the weakened heart muscle does not have to work excessively hard to maintain an adequate cardiac output. Excessive myocardial workload increases myocardial oxygen demands, which may not be met. Pharmacologic intervention may be necessary in the form of vasodilators, such as sodium nitroprusside, which reduce vascular resistance and decrease afterload, thereby decreasing myocardial workload and oxygen demands.

More difficult to control and potentially more life threatening is the *unstable low* blood pressure, which could be indicative of hypovolemia or shock. Hypovolemia is not uncommon after cardiac surgery and is usually corrected with blood or plasma transfusions or plasma volume expanders (for example, low-molecular weight Albumisol and Hespan) rather than with large volume noncolloidal solutions. "Fluid pushes" are rarely used to increase systemic blood pressure, because of the sudden extra workload created for the heart.

A postoperative shock state not caused by hypovolemia may be cardiogenic in nature. *Cardiogenic shock* (p. 715) is caused by an impairment of the pumping action of the heart muscle and results in inadequate cardiac output and tissue perfusion. Specific impairments may include myocardial depression as a result of anesthetics and hypothermia, trauma of surgery, mechanical impedance to contraction caused by an implanted prosthetic valve, decreased compliance of the ventricle because of scar tissue or hyperthrophy, preexisting heart disease not corrected by surgery, or arrhythmias associated with an inadequate stroke volume.

Therapy for cardiogenic shock is directed toward improvement in myocardial contractility. Correction of any specific underlying cause will be attempted, as in eliminating cardiac arrhythmias. Pharmacologic support may include vasoconstrictors such as dopamine hydrochloride to raise arterial pressure, although care must be taken not to increase undue blood return to the heart and peripheral resistance unless cardiac output is increased. Sympathetic agents such as epinephrine may be used for their cardiotonic effects. Isoproterenol is a preferred catecholamine, because it combines inotropic with chronotropic effects and decreases peripheral and pulmonary vascular resistance. Frequently, a combination of medications will be used to achieve the desired result of improving cardiac output with a minimum of side effects. Drug dosage administration is individually

titrated to obtain desired effects. Whenever cardiac and vasopressor medications are given by continuous intravenous infusion, the patient must remain under close observation and the medications should always be administered via intravenous infusion pumps.

If pharmacologic support is inadequate in reversing or minimizing cardiogenic shock, a temporary mechanical assistive device may be employed to reduce the cardiac workload. *Intraaortic balloon counterpulsation* (p. 695) may be used for several hours or several days and may be inserted at any time that its use is indicated in the preoperative, intraoperative, or postoperative period. Circulatory assistance may also be obtained through the use of *left ventricular assist devices* (p. 697).

Prophylaxis

Finally, some patients may receive prophylactic medications in the postoperative period. Antibiotics may be initiated just before surgery and continued for 3 to 5 days postoperatively to help prevent infection from numerous potential sources in the perioperative period. Anticoagulants will be given, starting about the third postoperative day, to patients receiving prosthetic mechanical valve implantations. The anticoagulation is necessary to prevent embolus formation on the surface of the valves and will be continued after the patient's discharge.

RESPIRATORY SYSTEM

All patients receiving general anesthetics, especially those having undergone cardiopulmonary bypass, require meticulous attention to maintaining a clear and patent airway. Removal of excess pulmonary secretions, proper aeration of lungs and oxygenation of blood, and maintenance of chest tube patency are essential.

The rate, depth, and quality of respirations are monitored and recorded, and also the patient's breath sounds are obtained through chest auscultation. While intubated, the patient should be preoxygenated and suctioned as frequently as necessary to clear secretions. The patient is turned from side to side every 2 hours; positioning and chest percussion are used to help loosen and mobilize secretions. Arterial blood samples are obtained for blood gas analysis to document the status of the patient's systemic oxygenation. Drainage and patency of chest tubes are noted, particularly when there is a known pleural leak. Daily chest x-ray films are obtained as ordered or more frequently if a sudden change is noted. Lungs are auscultated frequently while the patient is intubated to detect any shift in endotracheal tube placement.

After extubation it is important to observe the patient for any signs of respiratory distress. The patient is helped to splint the incision, and cough and deep breathe at least every 2 hours while awake. Medicating the patient before coughing may help increase the effort to cough, but some patients may require nasotracheal suctioning even after extubation. Preoperative instructions that were given regarding incentive spirometry or nebulization devices should be reinforced as the patient is assisted in utilizing them. Aggressive pulmonary hygiene must be maintained for the first week postoperatively.

NEUROLOGIC SYSTEM

Following surgery the patient's neurologic status must be carefully assessed, including level of consciousness, pupil size and reaction, orientation, and movement and sensation of extremities.

Patients usually begin to awaken within 1 to 2 hours after surgery. Failure to awaken may be the result of unusually deep anesthesia or of embolization of air, calcium, fat, or thrombotic particles to the brain. A return of consciousness that seems sluggish and in which the patient does not seem to regain full alertness after a day or two may have been caused by poor cerebral perfusion or microembolization during cardiopulmonary bypass.

Pupil size, equality, and reaction to light are checked frequently in the immediate postoperative period. Pupil dilation may be caused by excessive carbon dioxide in the blood or by such cardiac medications as atropine. Constricted pupils may be caused by dopamine. Disorientation and restlessness may be signs of hypoxia or embolization to the brain in addition to being symptoms of fatigue, fear, or sensory overload. Impaired sensation or muscular control of any portion of the body postoperatively indicates a neurologic deficit that will require careful observation and complete evaluation by specialists.

RENAL SYSTEM

Careful observation of hourly urinary output as well as urine color, pH, and specific gravity will give essential information about renal function. Adequate urinary output is at least 20 to 30 ml/hour. It is common for the urine to demonstrate increased sugar and acetone for the first several hours after cardiopulmonary bypass. This elevation is not usually treated unless it coincides with sustained elevated serum glucose levels. Specific gravity may be elevated, because of oliguria or the presence of red blood cells as a result of extracorporeal circulation.

Renal insufficiency in the patient after heart surgery is always caused by complications of extracorporeal circulation. The destruction of red blood cells can cause sludging in the kidneys. If low-perfusion states occurred during the surgical procedure, the kidneys themselves may have been damaged, resulting in acute tubular necrosis. This is marked by oliguria with increased blood urea nitrogen and serum creatinine levels. If the acute tubular necrosis is severe and prolonged, temporary re-

nal replacement therapy or membrane hemodialysis will be initiated to sustain the patient through the acute phase. Return of kidney function after acute tubular necrosis is usually gradual but complete. Up to 25% of postbypass patients may encounter some form of renal failure.

FLUID AND ELECTROLYTE BALANCE

The patient will receive necessary blood products after heart surgery to maintain a stable hematocrit. Plasma and plasma expanders such as Albumisol and Hespan will be given to avoid hypovolemia while maintaining a normal osmotic gradient. Crystalloid intravenous solutions are given to maintain adequate circulating volume.

Extremely *accurate recording of intake and output* is essential for the first few days postoperatively. Fluids will be limited to reduce the chance of fluid overload and increased work for the heart. Daily weights are obtained, and diuretics are administered if fluid retention occurs. Intravenous fluids must be titrated very carefully, and this is usually accomplished with the aid of intravenous infusion pumps.

Serum electrolytes are obtained several times during the first 24 hours and at least daily thereafter. Initially, the serum glucose level may be grossly elevated; this is transient. Particular attention is paid to the *serum potassium level*, and supplemental intravenous potassium chloride is usually given in the immediate postoperative period, particularly in conjuction with diuretic use. Hematocrit, hemoglobin, and prothrombin time are obtained daily to assess the extent of blood loss and the effect of replacement therapy.

The patient is usually allowed sips of water 1 hour after endotracheal extubation and progresses to a clear liquid, full liquid, and then solid diet as tolerated. Solid food is usually restricted to a specific daily sodium intake while hospitalized, and the restrictions may be continued after discharge. Although few patients have much appetite initially, there is rarely any difficulty maintaining adequate nutrition within a few days.

COMFORT, REST, AND SLEEP

Alleviation of pain is very important in the postoperative period, and patients should be kept as comfortable as possible. Narcotic analgesics are administered every 3 hours for the first day and then offered to the patient as needed after that. Keeping the patient comfortable not only adds to a sense of security, but reduces the stress on the heart, decreases the need for oxygen, and promotes healing. Other comfort measures are routinely employed, such as positioning in bed, controlling environmental temperature, and giving frequent oral hygiene.

The postoperative heart patient will be quite weak and will tire from activity very quickly. Activity periods should be organized so that rest periods may be frequent (even if brief) and uninterrupted. While patients are in the ICU, it is very difficult for them to obtain sufficient restful sleep. Sleep deprivation, particularly of REM sleep, is a serious problem, and significant efforts should be made to allow occasional intervals of uninterrupted sleep at least 90 minutes long.

PSYCHOLOGIC RESPONSE

The psychologic ramifications of heart surgery, sleep deprivation, and sensory overload can be overwhelming. Some persons experience a period of depression or disorientation after surgery, whereas others may become unreasonably fearful or experience hallucinations. The disorientation may even progress to panic. The nurse should be alert to subtle behavioral changes and reassure the person and family that these reactions are common and do not mean that the patient is "losing his mind." At the same time, physiologic causes of the behavior must be ruled out.

It is very helpful to the patient and family if the nursing staff attempt to personalize the patient's experience as much as possible. It is rather easy to lose sight of the person behind the monitoring equipment in an ICU. Calling the patient by name, using frequent physical contact when orienting the patient to time and place, and including the patient in any discussions that are held at the bedside will all help to decrease the sense of isolation.

ACTIVITY

Passive arm exercises are started shortly after surgery, followed by active exercises as the person gains strength. Mobilization of the person depends on the operation and the status of the heart.

In general, persons who have had surgery of the aorta are kept flat in bed for several days to prevent unnecessary strain on the vessel (the blood pressure is lower when the patient is flat). Before getting out of bed, the person must gradually become accustomed to having the head of the bed elevated. When this procedure is first attempted, dizziness and faintness may be experienced; if this happens, the person is returned to a flat position, and elevation is attempted again later.

Persons who have had surgery for patent ductus arteriosus and mitral stenosis may be kept in Fowler's position postoperatively and are encouraged to move their arms and legs. Backache from lying flat on the back, even for short periods, is common.

The time of ambulation for each patient depends on the patient's progress and condition, but (other than the above exceptions) it usually proceeds as follows: The first day the feet are dangled over the side of the bed for 15 minutes in the morning and afternoon, and the person is allowed to sit in a chair at the side of the bed for 15 minutes in the afternoon and evening. Walking around the room is permitted by the third day. The fourth day the patient is allowed to walk around the room and to sit in the chair for gradually increasing periods of time. By the fifth day walking longer distances is encouraged. During ambulation, close supervision is necessary and activity that causes excessive fatigue, dyspnea, or an increased pulse or respiratory rate is discontinued. If any of these symptoms appear, the patient is returned to bed, and the physician is consulted before further activity is attempted.

PATIENT TEACHING

Definite instructions must be provided regarding when the person may attempt to climb stairs. The activity should be done slowly. Only two or three steps should be attempted the first time, after which the number of steps is gradually increased. The patient should rest two or three times while climbing one flight of stairs.

The person and family need to be told that no marked improvement will be noticed after the operation—that it will be at least 3 to 6 months before the full result of the surgery can be ascertained. It is essential that all persons be given this information so that they will not be depressed by dyspnea or pain that may still be present postoperatively.

In preparation for discharge from the hospital, the person is asked to make a list of normal daily activities. This list is discussed with the physician to determine

---

RESEARCH

Clancy CA, Way JM, and Guinn GA: The effect of patients' perceptions on return to work after coronary bypass surgery, Heart Lung 13:173-176, 1984.

The purpose of this study was to examine the relationship between return to work after coronary artery bypass surgery (CABS) and patients' perceptions on their return to work. Subjects consisted of 69 post-CABS male patients who had not retired before surgery. Questionnaires were distributed or mailed 1 year after CABS. Significant relationships were found between return to work and five of the six variables (patients' perceptions) studied: (1) perceived physicians' instructions regarding return to work, (2) perceived physical ability to return to work, (3) perceived ability to tolerate physical activity, (4) perceived improvement in overall physical ability, and (5) perceived current health status. No significant relationship was found between return to work and the perceived contribution of the job to the occurrence of heart disease.

The authors suggest that since perceptions are a variable over which the patient has some control and which could be changed, misperceptions could be altered through a patient education program, direct discussion by the physician on the patient's return to work, and referral of patients to structured rehabilitation programs. ▪

the activities that are appropriate. Sexual intercourse is usually permitted within 3 to 4 weeks postoperatively. Patients are usually advised to start activities slowly and progress gradually to more energy-consuming tasks. The physician will want the patient to return for frequent medical follow-up examinations, at which time advice will be given regarding additional activities. The person is allowed to do anything that does not cause fatigue or pain but must be kept from attempting too much too soon.

The family should be aware of how much the person may be encouraged to do. Since the patient may have been an invalid preoperatively, the family may be as fearful as is the person about an increase in activity. Persons are encouraged to return to work as soon as permitted. To prevent misunderstandings, physicians need to give the person specific directions regarding return to work (see research box on p. 701).

HEART TRANSPLANTATION

Heart transplantation may be considered for persons under age 55 who have end-stage cardiac ischemia or cardiomyopathy. The one-year survival rate is presently 80%, and the five-year rate 50%.[50] The donor heart is from a person under age 35 with a comparable body weight and ABO compatibility (see Chapter 76) with the recipient. The heart must be transplanted less than 8 hours (preferably 3 to 4 hours) from procurement.

Surgery consists of removal of the diseased heart (leaving the posterior walls of the person's atria to spare the SA node) followed by anastomosis of the atria, aorta, and pulmonary arteries (Figure 28-15). Steroids and cyclosporine are used for immunosuppression (see Chapter 76). Cyclosporine, which maintains the natural defense mechanisms, is started before transplantation and is continued by daily oral doses for the remainder of the person's life.[50] Complications of cyclosporine therapy may include hypertension, myocardial fibrosis, and transient kidney or liver dysfunction. Infections occur less frequently with the use of cyclosporine than with other immunosuppressants, such as azathioprine.[49]

Rejection of the new heart during the first 3 months is a possibility as with any other graft. During the early stages, rejection may be reversible with appropriate therapy. With irreversible rejection, the patient will die unless mechanical intervention is used to sustain the person temporarily until a new heart is obtained. Permanent mechanical hearts are still experimental.

Postoperative care of the person with a transplanted heart is the same as that for other heart surgery. Isolation precautions are not necessary with the use of cyclosporine. Inotropic drugs may be given during the

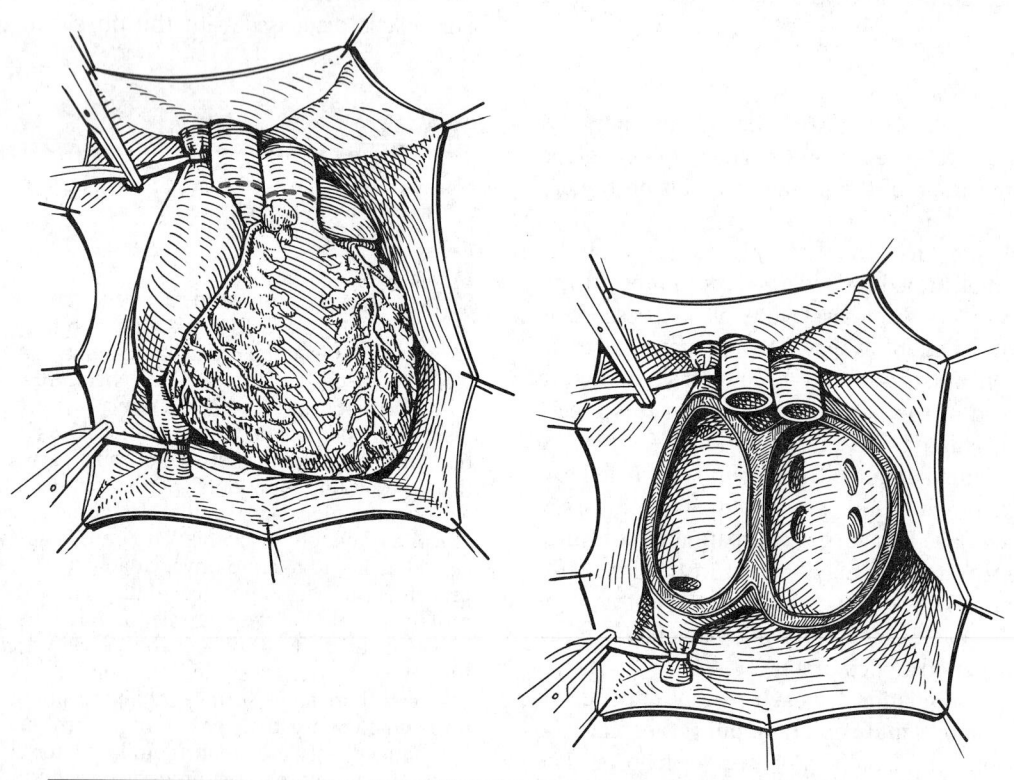

FIGURE 28-15 Heart transplantation. The diseased heart is removed, leaving the posterior walls of the atria. The new heart is then anastomosed to the atrial walls and great vessels.

first 48 hours to improve cardiac function. Radionuclear imaging and right cardiac catheterization may be performed weekly for the first 4 weeks to assess graft viability.[50] Long-term therapy, in addition to steroids and cyclosporine, includes antiplatelet agents and a low-cholesterol, low-sodium diet.

CORONARY ARTERY DISEASE: CORONARY ATHEROSCLEROTIC HEART DISEASE

DEFINITIONS

The term *coronary artery disease* (CAD) is a generic designation for many different conditions that involve obstructed blood flow through the coronary arteries. Some texts refer to coronary artery disease as coronary heart disease (CHD) and/or ischemic heart disease (IHD); however, these terms are not specific and are gradually being abandoned. Coronary atherosclerotic heart disease (CAHD) is the most common type of coronary artery disease and will be presented in this text. For a discussion of the more unusual nonatherosclerotic forms of coronary artery disease, the reader is referred to specialized texts.

EPIDEMIOLOGY

Coronary atherosclerosis is recognized as the leading cause of death in the industrialized Western world. In the United States, CAHD (angina, sudden death, myocardial infarction) has reached epidemic proportions. Each year approximately 1 million Americans die from the disease and another 2.5 million are disabled by it. The annual economic cost is overwhelming, averaging tens of billions of dollars.

The increased incidence of CAHD over the last 60 years has been causally linked to affluence and prosperity. There are many factors involved in this increase,

however, such as increased longevity and improved recognition of the disease.

Epidemiologic studies have shown that the incidence of coronary atherosclerosis is much higher in men than in women of childbearing age, in older individuals, and in the affluent. Nutrition has become a key factor in epidemiologic studies, forming the link between affluence and an increased rate of coronary atherosclerosis. In such countries as the United States and Finland, where diets are high in calories, total fat, cholesterol, and refined carbohydrates, the incidence of coronary atherosclerosis is extremely high, whereas in a country such as Japan, where the diet is low in calories, total fat, and cholesterol, coronary atherosclerosis is infrequent or rare.

RISK FACTORS: GENERAL CONSIDERATIONS

Although a tremendous amount of research (both epidemiologic and experimental) is being conducted in order to learn the cause of CAHD, the exact cause remains unknown. Certain characteristics, however, have been singled out as being common in persons who have or are at risk of developing coronary atherosclerosis (see box below and Figure 28-16). These common characteristics or risk factors have evolved from many different types of research studies and therefore require special interpretation.

Although risk factors help to screen individuals who are at high risk for developing CAHD, the presence of a risk factor does not definitively indicate the presence or severity of coronary atherosclerosis. Conversely, the absence of risk factors for CAHD does not mean that an

---

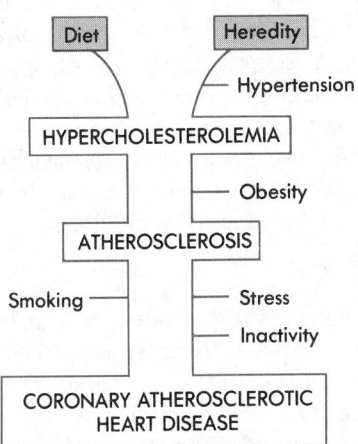

FIGURE 28-16 Predisposing factors in the development of coronary atherosclerotic heart disease (CAHD).

RISK FACTORS FOR DEVELOPING CORONARY ATHEROSCLEROTIC HEART DISEASE

NONMODIFIABLE RISK FACTORS

1. Age
2. Sex
3. Race
4. Family history

MODIFIABLE RISK FACTORS

5. Major risk factors
   a. Elevated serum lipid levels (hyperlipoproteinemia)
   b. Habitual diet high in calories, total fats, cholesterol, refined carbohydrates, sodium
   c. Hypertension
   d. Obesity
   e. Glucose intolerance
   f. Cigarette smoking
6. Minor risk factors
   a. Personality type
   b. Sedentary living
   c. Psychologic stress
   d. Oral contraceptive use

individual will necessarily be free from coronary atherosclerosis. At the present time there is strong evidence supporting a prudent approach to the prevention of coronary atherosclerosis. It is felt that the three major risk factors in CAHD are high blood pressure, hypercholesterolemia, and cigarette smoking.[26] Cessation of smoking, a lowering of blood lipids by diet, and a reduction in blood pressure can reduce the risk of CAHD. Prevention efforts require identification of risk factors and efforts to correct or alter those risk factors that can be modified.

NONMODIFIABLE RISK FACTORS

Age and Sex

Clinical evidence of coronary atherosclerosis may occur in the second and third decades of life. Although women seem somewhat immune until after menopause, the disease is already a major cause of death for men aged 35 to 44 years. The mortality in CAHD rapidly increases with age, so that by age 55 to 64, 40% of all deaths among men are caused by this single disease. Although there seems to be a strong and constant relationship between age and the onset of CAHD, this may simply reflect prolonged exposure to other atherogenic factors.

Race

Before 1968, nonwhites tended to have lower mortality rates from CAHD than whites. Since that time there has been a higher mortality rate in nonwhites who are less than 65 years of age. The fact the black Americans have a 45% greater chance of developing hypertension may play a significant risk in these statistics.[2]

Family History

A family history of CAHD occurring in parents or siblings (before the age of 50) increases the risk of developing premature atherosclerosis. This familial disposition is thought to be related to both genetic and environmental factors. It is not clear to what extent genetic elements act in combination with environmental factors such as nutrition, socioeconomic status, and other risk factors. In addition, other mechanisms of genetic transmission are not yet known.

MAJOR MODIFIABLE RISK FACTORS

Hyperlipoproteinemia

Strong evidence indicates that an elevated cholesterol, triglyceride, or phospholipid level is a major risk factor in the development of atherosclerosis. These plasma lipids are bound to specific proteins, hence the term *lipoproteinemia*. If only one component is elevated, it is referred to as *hyperlipidemia*.

The five basic groups of lipoproteins include the chylomicrons, very low-density lipoproteins (VLDL), low-density lipoproteins (LDL), intermediate-density lipoproteins (IDL), and high-density lipoproteins (HDL) (see Chapter 26). These lipoprotein complexes transport the plasma lipids including triglycerides and cholesterol.

Cholesterol and LDL, or β-lipoproteins, have been found to have a higher associative and predictive value for CAHD than triglycerides. Cholesterol in the body comes from two sources: it can be taken into the body directly in food, or it can be manufactured by the liver and intestine. Approximately 0.8 g of cholesterol is manufactured by the liver each day. Cholesterol is involved in lipid transport and is excreted with bile salts into the intestine to participate in the digestion and absorption of fats. The complex process by which cholesterol is manufactured, distributed, and eliminated is not very well understood, although it is widely believed that the inherited endocrine system plays a definite part because of its effect on the metabolic processes. Studies have shown that when a large amount of saturated fat is eaten, the cholesterol level in the blood tends to rise. When the saturated fats are replaced by polyunsaturated fats, the blood cholesterol level tends to fall.

Individuals with serum cholesterol levels greater than 300 mg/dl have been found to have four times more risk of CAHD than those individuals with levels less than 200 mg/dl. It would therefore appear prudent to take measures to decrease or maintain serum cholesterol levels below 200 mg/dl. The upper limit of normal for serum cholesterol is 220 to 240 mg/dl.

LDL, or β-lipoprotein, is most directly associated with CAHD. As a molecule LDL is approximately 50% cholesterol by weight. Other lipoproteins contain cholesterol, but it is in lesser amounts.

Recently, investigations have indicated a tremendous difference between HDL and LDL as predisposing factors to heart disease. Unlike LDL, HDL is inversely related to CAHD risk. In fact, HDL may serve to remove cholesterol from tissues.

The hyperlipoproteinemias have been classified on the basis of clinical and laboratory data into five types with recommendations for therapy (Table 28-6). The conditions may be primary (familial) or secondary to some other condition or process. The goal of therapy for the majority of patients is reduction of the rate of development of atherosclerosis. Many physicians are urging that blood lipid testing be done periodically and that preventive therapy begin early in childhood.

Dietary Patterns

The contemporary American diet, rich in total calories, total and saturated fats, cholesterols, refined sugars, and salt, is a significant coronary risk factor. The national dietary average for fat consumption is still very high in the United States, with approximately 50% of our dietary calories being derived from fats. Studies indicate that populations that consume low-fat diets generally

TABLE 28-6 Types of hyperlipoproteinemias

Type	Abnormality	Clinical Features of Elevated Levels
I	↑ Chylomicrons	Eruptive xanthoma, pancreatitis, organomegaly
IIa	↑ LDL	Premature atherosclerosis, corneal arcus, tendinous and tuberous xanthomas
IIb	↑ LDL and VLDL	
III	↑ IDL	Glucose intolerance, hyperuricemia, premature atherosclerosis
IV	↑ VLDL	Glucose intolerance, hyperuricemia
V	↑ VLDL and chylomicrons	Hepatosplenomegaly, eruptive xanthoma, glucose intolerance

have been found to have lower serum cholesterol levels than those consuming high-fat diets. In addition, populations consuming diets reduced in calories, total fats, saturated fats, and cholesterol not only have a lower cholesterol level but also have a lower incidence of and mortality from preventive CAHD.

The American Heart Association[2] has endorsed a policy recommending some modification in diet for everyone: reducing the fat content of the diet, substituting polyunsaturated fat for saturated fat, and maintaining body weight at normal levels. Some sources of polyunsaturated fat are corn, cottonseed, soy and safflower oils, and margarines incorporating these oils in liquid form. Oils that have been hydrogenated contain more saturated fat, as do coconut oil, butterfat, and animal fats.

Hypertension

Elevated blood pressure, either systolic or diastolic, is a significant risk factor in association with coronary atherosclerosis. However, many studies suggest that hypertension seems to accelerate atherosclerosis only in the presence of hyperlipidemia.

Obesity

Although obesity has been frequently cited as a significant coronary risk factor, its independent effect in predisposing an individual to CAHD is controversial. Obese individuals are more prone to diabetes, hypertension, glucose intolerance, and hyperlipidemias. These associated factors may in fact be the link between obesity and CAHD.

Carbohydrate Intolerance

Individuals with diabetes mellitus have been found to have a greater prevalence and severity of coronary atherosclerosis. However, it is difficult to isolate diabetes mellitus as a single factor since it is well established that hypertension, obesity, and hyperlipidemia are also frequent in individuals with impaired carbohydrate tolerance.[33]

Cigarette Smoking

In general, the risk of death from CAHD is two to six times higher in smokers than in nonsmokers, and the risk is proportional to the number of cigarettes smoked per day. Fortunately, individuals who stop smoking have a lesser risk of developing CAHD than those who continue to smoke. Pipe and cigar smokers have been found to have only a slightly increased risk of cardiovascular death and morbidity.

The relationship between cigarette smoking and CAHD is not totally clear, but it has been suggested that the adverse effects of cigarette smoking on the heart and blood vessels involve the effects of nicotine and carbon monoxide. Specific changes include increased myocardial oxygen demand induced by nicotine, interference with oxygen supply by carboxyhemoglobin, and adhesion of platelets. In addition, cigarette smoking has itself been associated with decreased levels of HDL compared with levels for nonsmokers and ex-smokers.[11]

PSYCHOSOCIAL INFLUENCES

There is significant evidence of behavioral and other psychosocial influences on the course of atherosclerosis and CAHD. Furthermore, smoking behavior and diet patterns notably change depending on the degree of stress an individual perceives is being experienced.

Low socioeconomic status was assigned highest priority by Tyroler and associates.[66] There is an inverse relationship between morbidity and mortality associated with CAD and socioeconomic status. This process is not completely understood, but one possibility is that it could be linked to other risk factors. For example, it is known that persons in lower socioeconomic positions are more obese, smoke more heavily, and have higher blood pressures and serum cholesterols when compared with individuals in higher socioeconomic positions. Social support systems and level of education may also affect this variable. Minimal social resources, as well as occupations with low autonomy and high demand, are associated with increased risk of CAHD. The stress response appears to play a focal role between physical and behavioral components.

Increased plasma levels of circulating cortisol and catecholamines have been associated with the development of hypertension and atherosclerosis. Catecholamines have known effects on platelet aggregation and lipid metabolism, both of which are involved in the genesis of CAHD. Cortisol enhances the sensitivity of arterioles to catecholamines, influences cholesterol and triglyceride levels, and affects sodium retention.

The association between behavioral patterns and the incidence of CAHD has been made. In early studies, people with type A personality characteristics were found to have twice the risk of developing CAHD compared with the type B personality, which has totally opposite characteristics. However, several recent prospective studies fail to confirm these earlier findings. In fact, it now appears that not only is the global type A behavior pattern not a reliable indicator of subsequent development of CAHD, but it actually may even represent a positive and healthy coping pattern.[29,65]

PATHOPHYSIOLOGY

The exact cause of atherosclerosis is still unknown. Coronary atherosclerosis involves the localized accumulation of lipid and fibrous tissue within the coronary arteries, resulting in arterial narrowing and possible occlusion. As the atherosclerosis progresses, the narrowing of the lumen is accompanied by vascular changes that affect the functional ability of the coronary arteries to dilate. The result of this atherosclerotic process is a variable reduction of blood flow to the myocardium.

Manifestations of coronary atherosclerosis are the result of an imbalance between myocardial oxygen supply

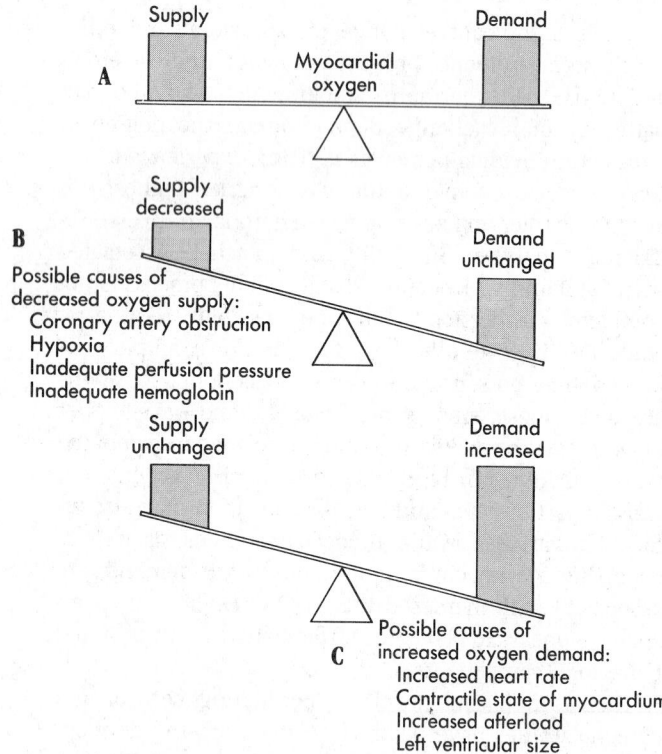

FIGURE 28-17 Balance between myocardial oxygen supply and myocardial oxygen demand (mVO$_2$). **A,** Normal balance. **B,** Imbalance: supply is decreased, while demand remains unchanged. **C,** Imbalance: supply unchanged, but demand is increased. Atherosclerotic coronary vessels are limited in ability to increase oxygen supply.

and myocardial oxygen demand. These manifestations, such as angina or coronary insufficiency, generally do not appear until the atherosclerotic process is well advanced. Despite alterations in vessel architecture and function, often greater than 75% of the coronary vessel is occluded before myocardial ischemia or dysfunction is produced. Coronary ischemia implies a relative deficit in myocardial oxygen to supply the normal aerobic metabolism of a functioning myocardium. The balance between myocardial oxygen supply and demand may be altered by a number of factors, as illustrated in Figure 28-17.

Atherosclerotic lesions usually occur near the origin and bifurcation of the main coronary vessels in the epicardial segment of the coronary artery. These lesions tend to be localized and focal; however, in advanced coronary atherosclerosis, diffuse involvement of the coronary arteries can be seen.

Therefore the primary significance of coronary atherosclerosis is that the lesion, either alone or in conjunction with coronary occlusion, causes *myocardial ischemia.* Myocardial ischemia is then responsible for producing the clinical manifestations of CAHD: (1) *angina pectoris,* (2) *acute myocardial infarction,* and (3) *sudden cardiac death.* (See Chapter 27.)

ANGINA PECTORIS
ETIOLOGY

Angina pectoris occurs when myocardial oxygen demand exceeds myocardial oxygen supply. Although it is usually caused by atherosclerosis of the coronary vessels, the incidence of angina pectoris is high in persons with hypertension, diabetes mellitus, thromboangiitis obliterans, polycythemia vera, periarteritis nodosa, and aortic regurgitation caused by syphilis or rheumatic heart disease. Typically, angina is triggered by exercise, cold, or anything that increases the work of the heart and myocardial consumption.

CLINICAL MANIFESTATIONS

Angina pectoris is characterized by paroxysmal retrosternal or substernal pain, often radiating down the inner aspect of the left arm. The left submammary region is seldom involved. The patient frequently describes the pain as a heaviness or tightness of the chest, and at times it may be interpreted by the patient as indigestion. The pain is usually diffuse and can rarely be pinpointed at a specific site. The patient may be observed gripping the sternum with one or both hands. The pain is often associated with exertion and is relieved by rest or vasodilation by means of medication. It is believed to be caused by a *temporary* inadequacy of the blood supply in meeting the needs of the heart muscle. The location and severity of the pain vary greatly, but the same pattern recurs repeatedly in a given individual. The frequency and severity of the attacks usually increase over a period of years, and less and less exertion may cause pain. No matter how mild the attacks, they may be complicated at any time by acute myocardial infarction, cardiac standstill, or death.

MEDICAL MANAGEMENT

Medical therapy is aimed at reducing myocardial oxygen demand. The precipitating factors that bring on an attack of angina are identified and avoided if possible. Risk factors that may aggravate the person's condition (for example, hypertension, obesity) should also be corrected, if possible.

Drug therapy consists of vasodilators (nitrates, especially nitroglycerin), β-adrenergic blocking agents, and calcium channel blockers (Table 28-7). The calcium channel blockers inhibit the movement of calcium ions across cell membranes via the calcium channel. Under normal circumstances, ions cannot penetrate the lipid membrane of either heart or smooth muscle cells. However, with appropriate electrical or chemical stimulation, molecular channels are formed that permit ion passage into the cell through a gating mechanism. Unlike the rapid sodium ion channel that permits inward depolarization, the calcium ion channel is much slower and ionic current is much smaller, hence the term *slow* channel. The exact mechanism by which these new drugs block the calcium channel pathway is not yet clear, but inotropic and chronotropic activity are depressed. By reducing the cardiac activity, a balance can be achieved between myocardial oxygen supply and demand. Decreasing the heart rate also allows for prolonged diastole, which augments perfusion of the coronary arteries. Another benefit of calcium blockers is their potent vasodilatory effects. Exaggerated release of substances such as catecholamines and prostaglandins is known to produce vasoconstriction. Calcium channel blockers interfere with vasoconstriction and have been shown to be effective in reducing coronary vasospasm.

SURGICAL MANAGEMENT

Coronary Artery Bypass Surgery

Because surgical intervention does not alter the atherosclerotic process, the choice between medical or surgical management for CAHD is sometimes controversial. Generally, medical therapy is effective in the earlier phases of CAHD. It can decrease anginal pain and decrease the workload of the heart while at the same time increasing the oxygen and blood supply to the myocardium.

Surgical intervention in the form of coronary artery bypass graft (CABG) may not prolong life or reduce the occurrence of myocardial infarction, but it does reduce angina and improve activity tolerance. Therefore, as CAHD progresses, many patients and physicians will choose bypass surgery to improve the quality of life. Coronary artery bypass surgery is a dramatically effective treatment for severe coronary disease. If severe narrowing of one or more branches of the coronary arteries exists, as indicated by coronary arteriography, a CABG may be recommended as a prophylactic measure.

The purpose of coronary artery bypass (jump graft) surgery is to increase blood flow to the myocardium (myocardial revascularization). Many persons show marked improvement after this surgery and usually do not require nitrates to maintain relief of symptoms.

The surgical technique varies somewhat among surgeons, and some surgeons routinely use extracorporeal circulation during the operation, whereas others do not. When the saphenous vein is used for the graft, one end is sutured to the aorta and the other end is sutured to the coronary artery distal to the occlusion (Figure 28-18). When an internal mammary artery is used, the distal end of this vessel is freed from the anterior chest wall and sutured in place distal to the occlusion in the coronary artery. Coronary bypass surgery is performed on the right coronary artery (RCA), the left anterior descending (LAD) artery, and the circumflex coronary artery (CCA) and their major branches. The care of the

---

TABLE 28-7 Drugs commonly used to treat angina pectoris

Type	Agents	Effect
Vasodilator	Nitroglycerin Amyl nitrate Isosorbide (Sorbitrate)	Peripheral vasodilation to decrease peripheral resistance, decrease systolic blood pressure, produce venous pooling, and decrease preload
β-adrenergic blocking agents	Propanolol (Inderal) Metoprolol (Lopressor) Nadolol (Corgard) Atenolol (Tenormin) Esmolol (Brevibloc)	Decrease myocardial oxygen demands to decrease heart rate, blood pressure, myocardial contractility, and calcium output
Calcium channel blockers	Verapamil (Calan, Isoptin) Nifedipine (Procardia) Diltiazem (Cardizem)	Inhibit calcium ion transportation into myocardial cells to depress inotropic and chronotropic activity, decreasing cardiac workload; also have vasodilatory effects

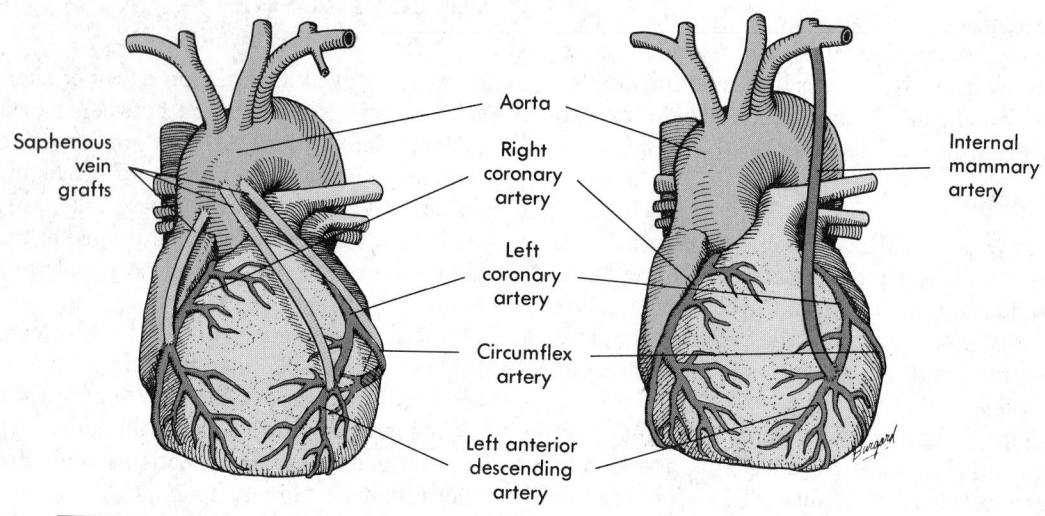

FIGURE 28-18 Coronary artery bypass grafts.

person undergoing coronary artery surgery is similar to that of those having other cardiac surgery (p. 687).

Percutaneous Transluminal Coronary Angioplasty

An alternative approach to coronary bypass surgery for selected persons with single-vessel coronary artery disease is percutaneous transluminal coronary angioplasty (PTCA). The procedure consists of mechanically dilating the coronary vessel wall by compressing the atheromatous plaque. During PTCA, a specially designed balloon-tipped catheter is inserted under fluoroscopy (similar to cardiac catheterization) and advanced to the site of the coronary obstruction. Once in position, the balloon on the catheter is inflated to provide compression and rupture the atheromatous plaque.

The complications associated with PTCA include sudden occlusion of the coronary artery through spasm, clot, or collapse. Arterial dissection or rupture may occur, and there is always the possibility of myocardial infarction. About 5% to 10% of persons undergoing PTCA require emergency coronary bypass surgery because of coronary occlusion; therefore preparation is similar to preparation for coronary bypass surgery.

Following a successful PTCA most patients are hospitalized for 2 to 4 days in either a cardiology unit or an intensive care unit. Anticoagulants are administered prophylactically to prevent thrombosis, and ECG monitoring is maintained for the first 24 hours to monitor any signs of myocardial ischemia or arrhythmias.

Intravascular Stenting

Restenosis persists as the single greatest limitation of percutaneous transluminal coronary angioplasty. Despite acceptable short-term rates of successful vein graft dilation, stenosis recurs in 30% to 60% of patients depending on the location of dilation within the graft. A recent approach to solving the dilemma of restenosis has been to seek ways of "stenting" or maintaining the cylindrical lumen produced by the balloon. Two techniques are currently being investigated. The first is to produce a "biologic stent" during balloon dilatation through coagulation of collagen, elastin, and other tissues in the vessel wall by *laser photocoagulation* or *radio-frequency–induced heat*. Preliminary results with the laser technique appear most encouraging.

The second technique has been to develop *prosthetic intravascular cylindrical stents* capable of maintaining good luminal geometry after balloon deflation and withdrawal. To date, this approach has had the widest clinical application, both in preventing acute closure and limiting late restenosis.

Laser Therapy for Cardiovascular Disease

Light is a form of electromagnetic energy that lasers use under controlled conditions. Over the past few years a number of percutaneous devices for use in peripheral and coronary arteries have undergone clinical trials. As laser light interacts with tissue, it is transmitted, scattered, reflected, or absorbed. A thermal reaction occurs when target tissue absorbs the laser light. This thermal reaction produces necrosis, hemostasis, coagulation, evaporation of tissue, cutting, or vaporization, depending on the time of application, power density, and focusing of spot size.

Each medium produces a specific wave length and affects a different tissue response to laser radiation. The *carbon dioxide* laser is absorbed by water, causing intracellular water temperature elevation to the boiling point. This thermal reaction causes cell vaporization and coagulation. The *argon* laser is large and bulky, requiring higher voltage than ordinary electrical outlets provide. Areas of current research in the treatment of cardiovascular disease include transluminal and percutaneous laser angioplasty, myocardial revascularization, and percutaneous resection of an aberrant conduction pathway, valvular calcium, or hypertrophic myocardium.

Nursing care after laser angioplasty is similar to postcatheterization care. Cardiac rehabilitation after laser therapy is important to heighten patients' awareness of the value of risk-factor reduction to prevent the advance of coronary artery disease.

■ ASSESSMENT

Subjective Data

Data collected for the person with angina pectoris include the person's knowledge of the disorder, presence of risk factors, and perception of the anginal pain. Specific data related to pain include the following:

1. Location and radiation to other sites
2. Quality of pain
   a. Tightness or heaviness in chest
   b. Pressure or squeezing pain
3. Onset and duration of pain
4. Precipitating factors: exertion, exposure to cold, exposure to heat or humidity, stress, heavy meal
5. Relieving factors: rest, nitroglycerin

Objective Data

When anginal pain is present, data are collected regarding the person's behavior, increases in vital signs, and changes in cardiac rhythm. During an anginal attack, the person may become apprehensive and press the hands against the chest.

■ DATA ANALYSIS: NURSING DIAGNOSES

Nursing diagnoses are determined from assessment of patient data. Possible nursing diagnoses for the person with angina pectoris may include, but are not limited to, the following:

Diagnostic Title	Possible Etiologies
Activity intolerance	Sedentary life-style, generalized weakness, imbalance between oxygen supply and demand, bedrest, immobility, pain, fatigue
Anxiety	Threat of or actual change in health status, role functioning, socioeconomic status; threat to self-concept; threat of death
Knowledge deficit: disease process, prognosis, treatment	Lack of exposure/recall, information misinterpretation, language differences, unfamiliarity with information sources, lack of interest, cognitive limitation
Pain/discomfort	Coronary artery occlusion, vasospasm, decreased coronary blood flow, hypoxia, diagnostic tests, overactivity
Tissue perfusion, altered: cardiovascular	Hypertension, angina, coronary artery occlusion

■ PLANNING: EXPECTED PATIENT OUTCOMES

Expected patient outcomes for the person with angina pectoris may include, but are not limited to, the following:

1. Patient states feeling more comfortable.
2. Patient demonstrates cardiac tolerance to increased activity, that is, stable pulse and blood pressure.
3. Patient identifies factors that reduce activity tolerance and progesses to highest level of mobility possible.
4. Patient identifies factors that increase cardiac workload.
5. Patient describes:
   a. Disease process, causes, variables contributing to symptoms, and interventions for disease or symptom control.
   b. Events that may precipitate attacks.
   c. Medical regimen.
   d. Plans to participate in a regular exercise program.
   e. Rationale for and type of surgery to be performed, if surgery is indicated.
   f. Plans for medical follow-up.
6. Patient uses effective coping mechanisms in managing anxiety.

■ IMPLEMENTATION

Promoting Comfort

Reduce or eradicate any known factors (physiologic or psychologic) that are contributing to increase in pain. Assess for causes of decreased pain tolerance, such as fatigue, lack of knowledge, or anxiety. Fatigue from increased oxygen demands with a decreased oxygen supply increases pain perception; therefore take measures to reduce fatigue, such as providing rest periods if fatigue is present during physical activities. Provide a calm environment to decrease stress and anxiety that can increase the pain experience.

Nitroglycerin remains the drug of choice for treatment of pain from acute ischemic attacks. A nitroglycerin tablet placed sublingually and allowed to dissolve in the saliva will often relieve the pain of angina within 1 to 2 minutes. The person should experience a burning sensation on the tongue and may experience a throbbing sensation in the head. Some persons frequently experience flushing and headache from the vasodilation properties of nitroglycerin. Fortunately, these side effects diminish as the person develops a tolerance for the drug. If the pain does not subside after the nitroglycerin is given three times, the person is instructed to call the physician or go to the nearest medical center.

Long-acting forms of nitrates are being used more commonly to diminish attacks and increase exercise capacity. Nitroglycerin ointment can be applied to any surface of the body that is not hairy. This cream is prescribed in doses of one half to several inches and is spread on cellophane-like paper and placed on the person's chest or another part of the body. The cream is absorbed slowly through the skin over many hours. The site of application is changed daily. An easier method of transdermal application is by means of a commercially prepared transdermal system. The date and time of application is noted on the transdermal unit, and the unit is changed every 24 hours. Nitroglycerin oral spray has also been shown to be effective in relieving anginal attacks.

A variety of medium- and long-acting β-adrenergic blocking agents are currently in use in the management of angina pectoris (see Table 28-7). Beta blockers prevent angina by reducing myocardial oxygen requirements during stress or exertion. Intravenous beta blockers such as esmolol hydrochloride (Brevibloc) are ultra–short-acting and also cardioselective. Brevibloc is administered as a continuous infusion. Beta blockade is abolished within minutes of terminating the infusion, as a result of rapid degradation of the drug by tissue and serum enzymes. Several clinical situations offer appropriate indications for such an agent, such as for patients with angina pectoris and a history of bronchial asthma, COPD, or previous heart failure. If heart failure or wheezing develops in these patients, the drug is discontinued and reversal of the untoward reaction is initiated immediately.

Promoting Tissue Perfusion

Instruct patient to avoid becoming overly fatigued and to stop activity immediately in the presence of chest pain, dyspnea, light-headedness, or faintness, indicating low tissue perfusion. Decreased tissue perfusion causes cellular hypoxia with subsequent ischemia, cellular swelling, and cellular death.

Promoting Activity and Rest

Enhance the patient's activity tolerance by encouraging slower activity or shorter periods of activity with more rest periods. Pulse increases of 50/min occur with strenuous activity; this rate is safe provided it returns to the resting pulse within 3 minutes. Most persons with angina pectoris can tolerate mild exercise such as walking and playing golf, but exertion such as running, climbing hills or stairs rapidly, and lifting heavy objects causes pain. Anginal pain is likely to be evoked more easily in cold weather, since the vessels normally constrict to conserve body heat. When persons with angina pectoris must be exposed to the cold, they should err on the side of being too warmly clothed. It is unwise to sleep in a cold room, and walking against the wind and uphill should be avoided because these activities increase the workload of the heart and cause pain.

If possible, the person should participate in a regularly scheduled exercise program, spacing exercise periods with rest periods. A "trained" individual experiences less of a rise in blood pressure and pulse rate on exertion. The result is a decrease in myocardial oxygen demand and an increase in the amount of exercise or work the individual can do before an imbalance occurs between myocardial oxygen supply and demand. Some persons may have to take nitroglycerin prophylactically before they engage in exercise, but the key to healthful activity is to avoid overexertion.

Promoting Patient/Family Learning

Delay teaching until the individual is ready. The patient needs to be relatively free of pain and excessive anxiety in order to learn. Promote a positive attitude and active participation of the patient and family to encourage compliance. Points to be included in the teaching are listed in the box below.

Promoting Relief of Anxiety and Feeling of Well-Being

Facilitate a reduction in the patient's present level of anxiety. Because excessive emotional strain also causes vasoconstriction by releasing epinephrine into the circu-

---

TEACHING THE PERSON WITH ANGINA

1. Rationale for symptoms and prevention of anginal pain
   a. Avoid excessive activity in cold weather, especially activity against resistance
   b. Avoid overeating
   c. Sleep in a warm room
   d. Minimize exposure to stressful situations when possible
   e. Use stress-reducing activities such as relaxation exercises when stress is present
2. Medications
   a. Nitroglycerin tablets
      (1) Carry tablets for immediate use if necessary
      (2) Keep tablets in original container tightly closed
      (3) Store tablets in a cool, dry place
      (4) Inspect expiration date and have replacement available
   b. β-adrenergic agents and calcium channel blockers
      (1) Monitor pulse and report to physician a pulse rate less than 50/min
      (2) Take β-adrenergics with food
      (3) Take calcium channel blockers 1 hour before or 2 hours after meals
      (4) Check with physician before omitting medication
      (5) Avoid driving if dizziness is present
3. Activity
   a. Plan for a regular activity program
   b. Increase extent of exercises gradually
   c. Avoid overexertion
   d. If necessary, take nitroglycerin before exercise if pain is anticipated
   e. Space exercise with rest periods
4. Medical follow-up
   a. Continue medical follow-up as instructed
   b. Report to physician if anginal pain increases

lation, emotional outbursts, worry, and tension should be minimized. Persons with angina may need continuing help in accepting situations as they find them. The family, the spiritual adviser, business associates, and friends can sometimes help. An optimistic outlook helps to relieve the work of the heart. Many persons who learn to live within their limitations live out their expected life span despite the disease.

UNSTABLE ANGINA

Unstable angina is frequently referred to as preinfarction angina, crescendo angina, or intermittent coronary syndrome. Unstable angina is characterized by an increase in the frequency, severity, or duration of symptoms or prolonged ischemic pain without infarction. Most patients with unstable angina have severe diffuse disease and need to be closely monitored in the coronary care unit. Therapy includes bed rest, sedation, supplemental oxygen, nitrates, and beta blockers. Intraaortic balloon pumping (p. 695) may be indicated for the severely compromised and symptomatic patient. Coronary arteriography is indicated, and depending on the results of the procedure or the patient's response to medical treatment, coronary bypass surgery is considered.

Theoretically, severe coronary artery stenosis will produce turbulent flow and stasis, which may increase platelet aggregation. Aspirin and heparin are two agents frequently used to prevent reductions in coronary blood flow and distal coronary perfusion pressure due to platelet accumulation at the site of stenosis. Cigarette smoking is a known risk factor for coronary disease. Platelet aggregation may be enhanced by nicotine stimulation of catecholamine secretion.

As with unstable angina before infarction, recurrent angina shortly after infarction is due to either a transient decrease of myocardial oxygen supply or to a transient increase of myocardial oxygen demand under the condition of a fixed coronary reserve. Decreased myocardial oxygen supply can be due to transient thromboses or platelet aggregation in severely diseased vessels, as well as excessive constriction of arteries proximal to the site of atherosclerotic narrowing. Factors that may increase myocardial demand include tachydysrhythmias, hypermetabolic states, hyper- or hypotension, anemia, drugs, hyper- or hypovolemia, mitral regurgitation, ventricular aneurysm, ventricular septal defect, and severe left ventricular failure.

MYOCARDIAL INFARCTION
ETIOLOGY

Acute myocardial infarction (MI) is caused by sudden blockage of one of the branches of a coronary artery. It may be extensive enough to interfere with cardiac function and cause immediate death, or it may cause necrosis of a portion of the myocardium with subsequent healing by scar formation or fibrosis. *Coronary occlusion* is a general term for blockage of a coronary artery. The blockage may be caused by formation of a thrombus in the coronary artery *(coronary thrombosis),* sudden progression of atherosclerotic changes, or prolonged constriction of the arteries.

PATHOPHYSIOLOGY

Infarction is not immediately total and complete; rather, ischemic injury evolves over several hours toward complete necrosis and infarction. During an acute ischemic process, the subendocardial layer of the myocardium is most susceptible to hypoxia, and cellular ischemia usually manifests itself in this area before it involves the full thickness of the ventricular myocardium. Ischemia almost immediately alters the integrity and the permeability of the cell membrane to vital electrolytes, thereby producing depressed myocardial contractility. The autonomic nervous system attempts to compensate for the depressed cardiac performance, resulting in a further imbalance between myocardial oxygen supply and demand (Figure 28-19).

Prolonged ischemia lasting more than 35 to 45 minutes produces irreversible cellular damage and necrosis of cardiac muscle. Contractile function in the necrotic area ceases permanently. The infarcted or necrotic area is surrounded by a zone of ischemia, made up of potentially viable tissues. The final size of the infarct depends on whether the marginal area in the ischemic zone succumbs to prolonged ischemia or is able to develop and maintain collateral circulation. The prognosis after an acute myocardial infarction reflects the degree of functional impairment of the heart.

The clinical features of acute myocardial infarction are determined by both the anatomic location and the extent of occlusive coronary disease. Knowledge of the anatomic location of the MI enables one to anticipate whether arrhythmias, conduction disturbances, and congestive heart failure are likely to occur. The location of the infarct is, of course, directly related to the disease in a particular region of the coronary circulation. An *anterior wall myocardial infarction* results from lesions in the left anterior descending (LAD) branch of the left main coronary artery (Chapter 26). Because the LAD branch supplies most of the left ventricle, an anterior infarct is often associated with a substantial loss of left ventricular muscle mass and can result in severe hemodynamic disturbances. An *inferior wall myocardial infarction* is most often caused by occlusion of the right coronary artery (RCA). Since the RCA is often proximal to the origin of both the AV node and the SA node arteries, it is frequently accompanied by ischemia of the AV node, the proximal bundle of His, and the SA node as well. Abnormalities of impulse conduction and formation caused by ischemia or infarction are primary factors

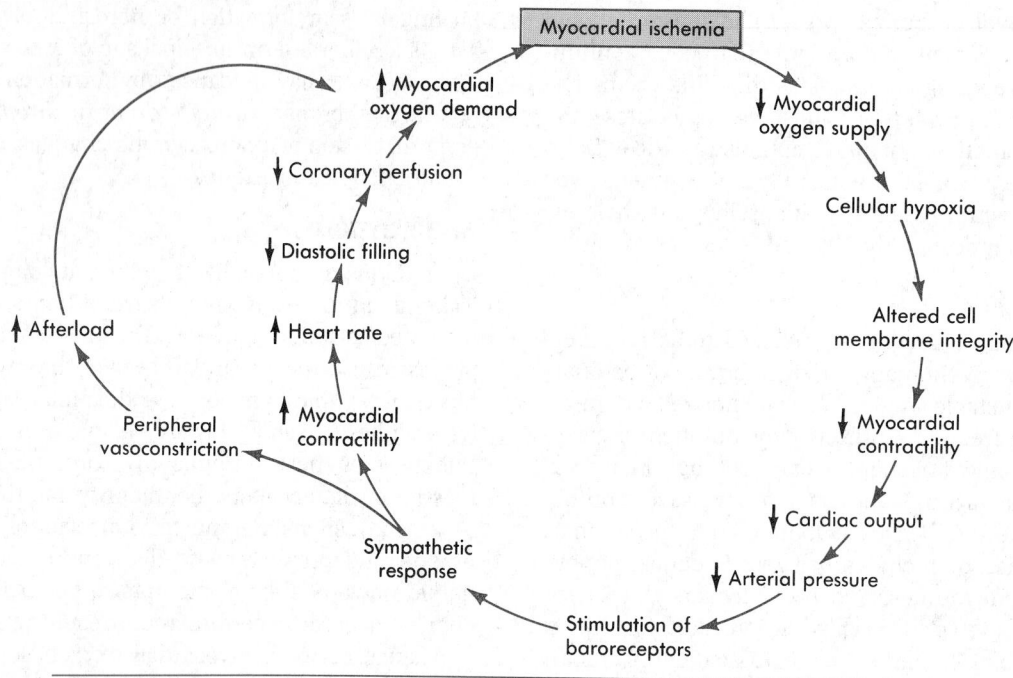

FIGURE 28-19 Effects of prolonged myocardial ischemia.

contributing to the development of serious arrhythmias early in the course of inferior infarction.[11] *Lateral wall* infarcts are usually caused by occlusion of the left circumflex coronary artery and may be complicated by the hemodynamic changes similar to an anterior infarction when a large mass of myocardium is disrupted.

PROGNOSIS

The mortality for persons with acute MI is high, ranging from 30% to 40%; however, a substantial number of these deaths take place before the patient reaches the hospital. Among those patients who reach the hospital, approximately 80% survive. Most in-hospital deaths from myocardial infarction take place during the first 3 to 4 days.

The person who has had a myocardial infarction is at high risk for recurrent heart attacks. In the past, antithrombotic therapy has been given in attempts to prevent recurrences. β-adrenergic blocking drugs, such as timolol, have been found to decrease the incidence of death in the months after myocardial infarction.[11]

CLINICAL MANIFESTATIONS

Pain is the most frequent complaint of the patient with an MI. The individual typically complains of sudden, severe, crushing, or viselike pain in the substernal region. This pain may radiate into the left and sometimes the right arm and up the sides of the neck (Figure 28-20). At other times it may simulate indigestion or a gallbladder attack with abdominal pain and vomiting. Persons

often become restless and fear that they are dying. They may become short of breath and cyanotic and show signs of severe shock. On auscultation, rales or rhonchi may be audible. The pulse is usually rapid, and it may be barely perceptible. The blood pressure usually falls, and the patient may collapse. S_1 and S_2 heart sounds are often faint; S_4 can often be heard; and at times an S_3 (gallop rhythm), which indicates left ventricular failure, may be evident. A soft systolic murmur may be heard at the apex. The symptoms of cardiogenic shock (p. 715) occur as a result of inadequate cardiac output from decreased myocardial contractility and ineffective pumping.

Although pain is the most common initial complaint, it is not necessarily present. Approximately 15% to 20% of myocardial infarcts may be painless. The incidence of painless infarcts increases with age, and in the elderly, the chief complaint may be sudden shortness of breath. Other less common presenting symptoms include confusion, sudden dysrhythmia, unexplained drop in blood pressure, or sudden loss of consciousness.

DIAGNOSTIC TESTS

Laboratory tests used in diagnosing the presence of a myocardial infarction can be divided into three categories: nonspecific indicators of tissue necrosis and inflammation, ECG, and serum enzymes. Other diagnostic procedures include myocardial scintigraphy, myocardial perfusion imaging, and gated pool imaging (see Chapter 26).

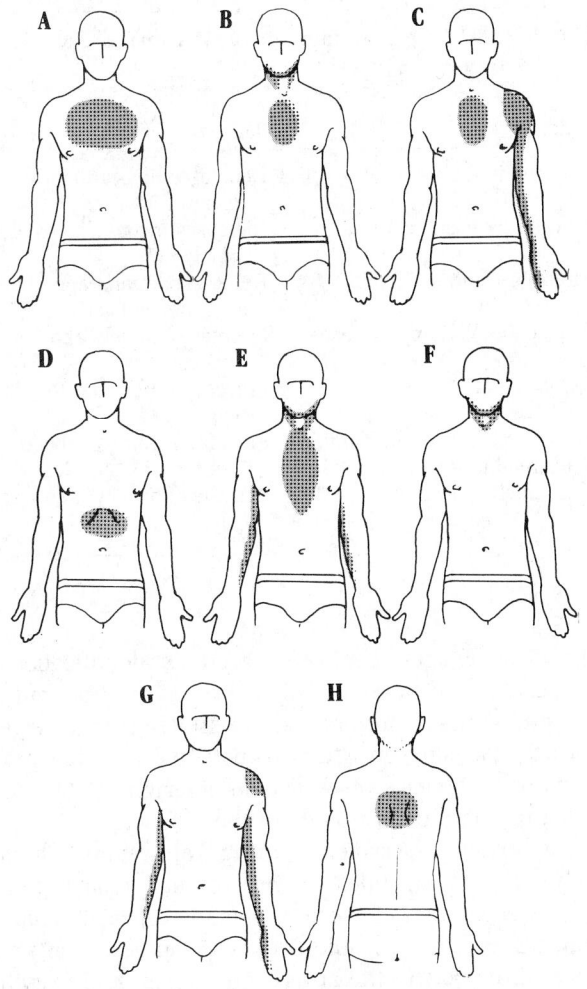

FIGURE 28-20 Sites where ischemic myocardial pain may be referred. **A,** Upper chest. **B,** Beneath sternum radiating to neck and jaw. **C,** Beneath sternum radiating down left arm. **D,** Epigastric. **E,** Epigastric radiating to neck, jaw, and arms. **F,** Neck and jaw. **G,** Left shoulder, inner aspect of both arms. **H,** Intrascapular.

Nonspecific Indicators

The nonspecific reaction to myocardial injury is a *leukocytosis* that begins within a few hours after the onset of pain. This leukocytosis often reaches 12,000 to 15,000/cu mm and lasts for approximately 3 to 7 days. In general, high white blood cell (WBC) counts are associated with larger infarcts. The *erythrocyte sedimentation rate* (ESR), another nonspecific indicator, rises during the first week after infarction and remains elevated for several weeks.

Electrocardiogram

The term *transmural myocardial infarction* denotes that the full thickness of the wall of the myocardium has been involved. If an infarct does not involve the entire thickness of the myocardium, it is termed *nontrans-*

mural or *subendocardial.* In this situation there are no Q waves present and the characteristic ECG changes are limited to the ST segment and the T wave. It must be emphasized the ECG does not always provide definitive evidence of the ischemic process. However, pronounced Q waves, ST-segment elevation, and T-wave abnormalities are often evident during acute infarction. These ECG changes are apparent in the leads overlying the area of myocardial necrosis.

Serum Enzymes

When cardiac muscle cells die, certain enzymes are released into the blood stream via the coronary lymphatic drainage. These enzymes include creatine phosphokinase (CPK), serum glutamic-oxaloacetic transaminase (SGOT) (also termed serum aspartate amino-transferase [AST]), and lactic dehydrogenase (LDH).

A pattern of enzyme elevations following an acute MI is a valuable diagnostic indicator. However, enzyme interpretation is somewhat limited in that enzyme elevations are not solely specific to myocardial damage. For example, SGOT is found mainly in heart muscle, but it is also present in the liver and to some extent in the skeletal muscle. LDH is found in the heart, liver, kidney, brain, skeletal muscle, and erythrocytes. CPK occurs in heart, skeletal muscle, and brain cells. Because of the lack of specificity of these enzymes, coexisting processes such as cirrhosis of the liver may produce misleading enzyme elevations.

To increase the specificity of these enzymes, measurements of the enzyme fractions or isoenzymes are taken. Fractionating the CPK enzyme into isoenzymes is the most specific enzymatic indication of myocardial infarction. CPK_1 (BB) is found in brain, lungs, bladder, and bowel; CPK_2 (MB) is found almost exclusively in the myocardium; and CPK_3 (MM) is found in the serum of all patients for 48 hours after a transmural infarction, but it may also be elevated in the individual with crescendo, or unstable angina, even in the absence of true infarction. The total CPK value is elevated within 3 to 6 hours after an acute myocardial infarction, peaks in 12 to 18 hours, and returns to normal in 3 to 4 days (Figure 28-21).

Because of the extensive tissue distribution of LDH, it can be elevated in a variety of disorders. Fractionating LDH into its five isoenzymes allows for greater specificity. Normally, LDH_2 is most prominent in the serum. The myocardium is especially rich in LDH_1, so that when an infarction occurs the serum level of LDH_1 becomes higher than that of LDH_2 and the LDH pattern is said to be "flipped."

MEDICAL MANAGEMENT

Medical interventions include promoting oxygenation of the tissues, relieving pain, preventing further tissue

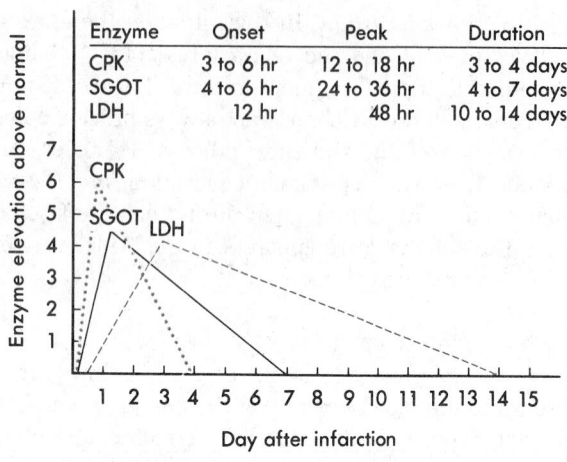

Enzyme	Onset	Peak	Duration
CPK	3 to 6 hr	12 to 18 hr	3 to 4 days
SGOT	4 to 6 hr	24 to 36 hr	4 to 7 days
LDH	12 hr	48 hr	10 to 14 days

FIGURE 28-21 Patterns of serum enzyme levels after myocardial infarction.

TABLE 28-8 Medical interventions for myocardial infarction in acute phase

Actions	Rationale
Bed rest initially	Decreases myocardial oxygen demand
Oxygen by nasal cannula	Increases myocardial oxygen supply
Morphine sulfate (IV, IM)	Relieves pain and apprehension; prevents shock
Diazepam (Valium) as needed	Decreases anxiety and restlessness
Lidocaine (IV)	Prevents ventricular fibrillation
Heparin (IV) (may be omitted for mild cases)	Prevents thromboembolic events
Thrombolytic therapy	Activates fibrinolysis to lyse clot

damage, promoting improved coronary circulation, and preventing complications (Table 28-8).

Analgesic drugs such as morphine sulfate or meperidine hydrochloride can be administered for the relief of pain. Myocardial tissue oxygenation can be improved with supplemental oxygen. When relaxation occurs with pain relief and with improved tissue oxygenation, cardiac workload is thereby reduced. Cardiac monitoring is used to detect the occurrence of dysrhythmias.

The size of the infarct is an important prognostic indicator; that is, the larger the infarct, the poorer the prognosis. The course of recovery may also be complicated by extension of the original infarct or early reinfarction. Goals for treatment include prevention of further tissue injury and limitation of infarct size. Interventions are aimed at maximizing myocardial tissue perfusion and reducing myocardial energy demands. β-adrenergic blocking agents are used to reestablish the balance between myocardial oxygen supply and demand. As previously discussed (p. 707), reperfusion of the myocardium can be achieved by coronary artery bypass surgery with grafts. The reopening of an occluded artery can also be done with thrombolytic agents that are injected into the vascular system or with percutaneous transluminal coronary angioplasty (PTCA) (p. 708).

Thrombolytic Therapy

Thrombolytic agents such as streptokinase, urokinase, and tissue plasminogen activator (TPA), activate fibrinolytic processes to lyse the clot. The value of thrombolytic therapy is its ability to be administered within the crucial period between coronary artery occlusion and actual myocardial tissue necrosis. This period can range between 3 to 6 hours after the initial infarction has occurred. Nursing implications for the use of any

thrombolytic agent begin with accurate identification of candidates and prompt implementation of treatment. A thorough nursing history and assessment should be performed, focusing on actual or potential bleeding problems or tendencies. Assessments for signs of bleeding must be continued throughout the infusion.

Additional assessment during intravenous thrombolytic therapy includes noninvasive markers of reperfusion. Recognition of these markers is especially important for documenting the patient's response to intravenous thrombolytic therapy. For instance, rapid resolution of ST-segment elevation signals recanalization of the infarcted artery; thus the choice of a monitoring lead that demonstrates ST-segment elevation is recommended.

Observation for occult bleeding is crucial during and after thrombolysis. The patient must be continuously assessed for changes in neurologic status, evidence of gastrointestinal bleeding, or signs and symptoms of cardiac tamponade. If these occur, the physician must be notified because a decision to discontinue thrombolytic therapy, reverse anticoagulation, or administer blood products must be accomplished quickly to avoid life-threatening complications.

The primary goal during the immediate postthrombolytic period is to maintain arterial patency. Anticoagulants, antiplatelet medications, and mechanical interventions have been used to achieve this end.

COMPLICATIONS OF MYOCARDIAL INFARCTION

The more common complications of MI are arrhythmias (Chapter 27), cardiogenic shock, and congestive heart failure (p. 720). Other complications include ventricular aneurysm, postmyocardial infarction syndrome, pericarditis (p. 670), and embolism (Chapter 29).

Cardiogenic Shock

Cardiogenic shock is a shock state of primary cardiac origin. It is most frequently caused by myocardial infarction, but it may also be the result of critical aortic stenosis, intractable dysrhythmias, ruptured aortic aneurysm, obstruction to flow between cardiac chambers (atrial myxoma), severe congestive heart failure, massive pulmonary embolism, or cardiac tamponade.

Pathophysiology. Shock occurs in approximately 15% of all patients hospitalized with the diagnosis of acute myocardial infarction. When cardiogenic shock follows a myocardial infarction, it is the result of severe left ventricular failure. So much myocardium has been damaged (usually more than 40% of the left ventricle) that inadequate systemic perfusion occurs secondary to low cardiac output. As the shock state progresses, there is decreased coronary artery perfusion, leading to the development of extended areas of cardiac muscle ischemia and necrosis throughout both ventricles. This progressive ischemia and infarction lead to further deterioration of left ventricular function, and, if unchecked, to death. The mortality for cardiogenic shock is very high; 80% to 90% do not survive.

Clinical manifestations. The severe organ hypoperfusion is characterized by metabolic acidosis (caused by anaerobic metabolism and lactate production), hypotension with a systolic blood pressure less than 90 mm Hg, tachycardia, urinary output less than 20 ml/hour, cold clammy skin, and mental confusion or lethargy.

Interventions. Cardiogenic shock is a medical emergency that requires immediate intervention and constant attention to prevent irreversible cell damage and death. Therapy is aimed at correcting factors that contribute to decreased tissue perfusion, such as cardiac dysrhythmias, hypoxemia, and pain. Lactic acidosis may be partially compensated for through use of hyperventilation and buffering agents such as sodium bicarbonate. Invasive monitoring lines that are usually placed include catheters in the pulmonary artery, systemic artery, and urinary bladder. The left ventricular end-diastolic pressure is reflected in the pulmonary capillary wedge pressure, which is used as a guide to fluid therapy. Hypovolemia must be carefully corrected without inducing a fluid overload, which could result in acute pulmonary edema.

Vasopressors and cardiotonic agents are chosen to raise the systemic arterial pressure without increasing the workload (and therefore the oxygen requirements) of the myocardium. Dopamine and norepinephrine are frequently used to raise the systemic arterial pressure and cardiac output. Nitroprusside may be added in small amounts to decrease afterload and to reduce systemic vascular resistance. Every effort is made to maintain systemic arterial pressure at an absolute minimum of 60 mm Hg, preferably 90 mm Hg; total coronary artery collapse occurs at approximately 40 mm Hg.

Unless the shock state can be reversed with reinstatement of adequate cardiac output and tissue oxygenation, the patient will continue to deteriorate and death will ensue. Patients who require extensive pharmacologic support and in whom it is felt sufficient myocardium remains undamaged to allow for eventual recovery may benefit from initiation of intraaortic balloon counterpulsation (p. 695).

Ventricular Aneurysm

Aneurysms of the ventricular myocardium are predominantly a result of transmural myocardial infarctions. Traumatically induced or congenitally formed aneurysms are very rare. In 12% to 15% of people sustaining myocardial infarctions, the resultant myocardial necrosis and scar formation develop a weakened ventricular wall. During systole the high pressures within the ventricle cause the weakened myocardium to bulge outward. Blood collects in the aneurysm or outpouched area and is a potential source of emboli. Cardiac output may be compromised. If symptomatic, the patient usually has congestive heart failure and recurring dysrhythmias. Symptoms usually occur when 20% or more of the ventricle has been involved. The majority of ventricular aneurysms occur in the apex and anterior part of the heart.

Diagnosis is usually made in the presence of a ventricular gallop, persistent ST elevations following a myocardial infarction, a chest x-ray film showing an enlarged left ventricle, a paradoxic expansion of the aneurysmal sac during systole on fluoroscopy, and cardiac catheterization.

Treatment consists of a ventricular aneurysmectomy in which the aneurysm sac is excised and the ventricle sutured together. If the area excised includes part of a coronary artery, bypass surgery is done simultaneously. Operative mortality is less than 5%.

Postmyocardial Infarction Syndrome (Dressler's Syndrome)

A few patients develop a syndrome approximately 1 to 6 weeks after an acute myocardial infarction, characterized by pleural pain, joint pains, and fever. It is thought to be due to an autoimmune reaction to the myocardial necrosis. Aspirin is usually effective for the discomfort, and more severe symptoms usually respond quickly to a short intensive course of corticosteroids.

■ ASSESSMENT
Subjective Data

During the acute phase of myocardial infarction, pertinent subjective data include the patient's perception of the cardiac pain and both the patient's and family's feelings about the patient's condition.

1. Patient's perception of pain
   a. Location and radiation to other sites
   b. Quality of the pain
   c. Onset and duration
   d. Associated factors: exertion, stress, at rest
   e. Relieving factors
2. Presence of associated symptoms: dyspnea, nausea, dizziness, weakness, sleep disturbances
3. Feelings of patient and family
   a. Uneasiness or feelings of impending doom
   b. Fear of death
   c. Possible denial or depression

Objective Data

Monitoring objective data of the patient's response to the MI both physically and psychologically and for signs of complications is an important part of the nursing care of the person with MI. The patient is monitored constantly for *dysrhythmias*. One of the most serious threats to the person during the acute phase is ventricular fibrillation (Chapter 27), often heralded by premature ventricular beats (PVBs). Other objective data include the following:

1. Behavior: signs of anxiety
2. Changes in vital signs: increased pulse rate, decreased blood pressure
3. Associated signs: diaphoresis, vomiting, sudden dysrhythmias
4. Breath sounds: presence or rales or rhonchi
5. Serum enzyme levels (p. 713).

■ DATA ANALYSIS: NURSING DIAGNOSES

Nursing diagnoses are determined from assessment of pertinent data. Possible nursing diagnoses for the person with myocardial infarction may include, but are not limited to, the following:

Diagnostic Title	Possible Etiologies
Activity intolerance	Dysrhythmias, CHF, angina, electrolyte imbalance, sedentary life-style, decreased mobility
Anxiety	Threat of death; threat/change in health status, socioeconomic status/role; threat to self-concept
Cardiac output, altered: decreased	Reduced stroke volume, CHF, cardiogenic shock, valvular stenosis/insufficiency, bradycardia, tachycardia, heart block
Knowledge deficit (disease process, prognosis, treatment)	Lack of exposure/recall, information misinterpretation, ineffective coping patterns

Diagnostic Title	Possible Etiologies
Pain/discomfort	Coronary artery vasospasm or occlusion, hypoxia, immobility, overactivity, diagnostic tests, improper positioning
Tissue perfusion, altered: cardiovascular	Decreased cardiac output, pulmonary edema, CHF, angina, coronary artery disease, vasospasm or vasoconstriction

■ PLANNING: EXPECTED PATIENT OUTCOMES

Expected patient outcomes for the person with myocardial infarction may include, but are not limited to, the following:

1. Patient demonstrates cardiac tolerance to increased activity (stable pulse and blood pressure).
2. Patient identifies factors that increase cardiac workload.
3. Patient states breathing is easier and fatigue is decreased.
4. Patient identifies factors that reduce activity tolerance and progresses to highest level of mobility possible.
5. Patient participates in a program of progressive activity.
6. Patient states feeling more comfortable.
7. Patient can describe:
   a. Nature of myocardial infarction and how the healing process relates to the treatment regimen.
   b. Variables contributing to symptoms and interventions for disease or symptom control.
   c. Risk factors that can be modified and plans to alter life-style (if appropriate).
   d. Plans to participate in a regular exercise program.
   e. Rationale for and type of surgery, if surgery is indicated.
   f. Any dietary restrictions.
   g. Plans for ongoing medical care.

■ IMPLEMENTATION DURING ACUTE PHASE

The patient is admitted to a coronary care unit (CCU), which is equipped with special systems for monitoring cardiac rhythms and vital signs (Chapter 80). The unit is staffed by nurses with expertise in cardiovascular nursing. Guidelines for care of the person with a myocardial infarction are listed in the box on p. 717.

Promoting Oxygenation/Tissue Perfusion

Instruct the patient to avoid becoming overly fatigued and to stop activity immediately in the presence of chest pain, dyspnea, light-headedness, or faintness. Decreased tissue perfusion causes cellular hypoxia with subsequent ischemia, cellular swelling, and cellular death. Oxygen is administered by nasal cannula for the

GUIDELINES FOR CARE OF PERSONS DURING THE ACUTE PHASE OF MYOCARDIAL INFARCTION

1. Monitor for cardiac dysrhythmias; notify physician if increased ventricular irritability (coupling of premature ventricular beats [PVBs]) are present
2. Monitor vital signs for signs of cardiogenic shock (hypotension, weak thready pulse, cold clammy skin, mental confusion)
3. Monitor breath sounds for signs of respiratory congestion (rales, rhonchi)
4. Administer prescribed medications: intravenous morphine, intravenous lidocaine, anticoagulants, thrombolytics, tranquilizers, or sedatives
5. Administer supplemental oxygen as needed; maintain oxygen therapy in the presence of persistent pain, hypotension, dyspnea, or dysrhythmias
6. Position patient in semi-Fowler's position to enhance oxygenation
7. Maintain patient on prescribed bed rest for 24 to 48 hours; encourage progressive ambulation when permitted
8. Maintain patient on prescribed low-cholesterol, low-salt diet; avoid extremes of hot or cold foods
9. Administer stool softener to prevent constipation from effects of opiates and decreased mobility and to prevent Valsalva maneuver
10. Start patient teaching as described on p. 718

TABLE 28-9 Interpretation of changes in vital signs during an acute myocardial infarction

Vital Sign	Change	Interpretation
Blood pressure	High	Increased myocardial oxygen demand
	Low (>80 mm Hg)	Decreased coronary perfusion with further myocardial ischemia
Heart rate	Increased	Possible shock
Heart rhythm	Irregular	Potential life-threatening dysrhythmia
Respirations	Slow	Possible morphine toxicity
	Gurgling (rales)	Pulmonary edema

first 24 to 48 hours and longer if persistent pain, hypotension, dyspnea, or dysrhythmias occur. Monitor vital signs carefully for changes indicating possible complications (Table 28-9). Position the patient in semi-Fowler's position to permit greater diaphragm expansion, thus improving lung expansion and better CO_2/O_2 exchange.

Promoting Adequate Cardiac Output

1. Monitor the patient for the following parameters:
   a. Dysrhythmias on ECG tracings
   b. Vital signs
   c. Effects of daily activities on cardiac status, as evidenced by occurrence of dysrhythmias and need for oxygen
   d. Signs of fluid overload and electrolyte imbalance
2. Document rate and rhythm of pulse.
3. Administer pharmacotherapy as prescribed.
4. Plan nursing strategies to promote rest and minimize unnecessary disturbances.

Promoting Comfort

The amount of pain and discomfort an individual will experience is highly variable. Some persons experience severe pain, and others have minimal discomfort. After an intravenous route is established, the patient is given

morphine sulfate to relieve pain and apprehension and also to produce vasodilation. Continued episodes of chest pain may be related to the size of the infarction, the relative lack of collateral circulation, and an increased myocardial oxygen demand. Control of this pain is essential to provide comfort and rest and also to decrease sympathetic stimulation, which increases myocardial oxygen demands.

Providing Rest

To limit the size of the infarction and to prevent any complications, the patient is usually placed on bed rest with commode privileges for 24 to 48 hours. Assistance with activities of daily living (ADL) is given during this period. Sedation with diazepam (Valium) or an equivalent may be prescribed to relieve anxiety and restlessness in the crisis situation and to promote sleep. Rest and reassurance are essential. Patients are assured that the most dangerous stage of the MI has passed and that the purpose of the CCU is for continued monitoring and safety during the early recovery period. The nurse plays an integral role in providing support not only to the patient, but also to the family. Displaying calmness and competence can be extremely reassuring.

Promoting Activity

After the first 24 to 48 hours, patients are usually encouraged to increase their activity gradually depending on the extent of the infarction. The patient usually first sits on a chair for increasing periods of time and then begins ambulation by the fourth or fifth day. During this period the person is continually monitored for signs of dysrhythmias, presence of cardiac pain, and changes in vital signs.

Promoting Nutrition and Elimination

Fluids are provided initially followed by resumption of a regular diet according to the patient's needs. Extremely hot or cold foods are avoided initially, and small frequent feedings may be better tolerated. Salt restrictions may be prescribed, particularly for those persons with signs of heart failure, and low-caloric, low-cholesterol diets are often prescribed.

A stool softener is prescribed from the beginning, since constipation is common from the effects of narcotics and decreased activity. Use of bedpans and straining should be avoided because Valsalva's maneuver causes changes in blood pressure and heart rate, which may trigger ischemia, dysrhythmias, pulmonary embolus, or cardiac arrest.

Promoting Relief of Anxiety and Feeling of Well-Being

Anxiety varies in intensity contingent on the severity of the threat as perceived by the individual, as well as the person's success in coping. Provide the patient and family with opportunities to explore their concerns and to explore alternative methods of coping, if appropriate.

Promoting Patient/Family Learning

Teaching is delayed until the individual is ready. The patient needs to be relatively free of pain and excessive anxiety to learn. Promote a positive attitude and active participation of the patient and family. Both patient and significant others need to know the nature of myocardial infarction, risk factors, variables contributing to symptoms, and the interventions for disease or symptom control. Teaching is similar to that for angina (see the box p. 710).

CARDIAC REHABILITATION

Cardiac rehabilitation is a process by which a person is restored to and maintains optimal physiologic, psychosocial, vocational, and recreational status. This process of rehabilitation involves progressive activity and exercise and education of the patient and family. Rehabilitation of the person who has suffered a myocardial infarction begins the moment the person is admitted to the hospital for emergency care and may continue for months and even years after discharge from the hospital.

Progressive Activity

During the 1960s, 2 to 3 weeks of bed rest were recommended for the person who had myocardial infarction. Today the hazards of prolonged bed rest are well documented, and patients with uncomplicated myocardial infarctions (no evidence of severe dysrhythmias, congestive heart failure, or shock) progress rapidly through a supervised program of increased activity. Activity progression is based on METs, a term used to describe the energy expenditure for various activities. An MET is a metabolic equivalent that can be assigned to activities regardless of a person's weight. One MET represents the energy expenditure of a person at rest; it equals approximately 3.5 ml/O_2/kg of weight per minute.

A hospitalized myocardial infarction patient is usually limited to activities with low MET levels (that is, 1 to 3 METs). For example, using a bedside commode requires 3 METs and using a bedpan requires 4 METs. Champion athletes can perform at equal to or greater than 20 METs, whereas the average middle-aged man following an uncomplicated MI is capable of performing at a level of 8 to 9 METs.

Over 50% of all myocardial infarctions are uncomplicated, and these patients will be discharged from the hospital in 7 to 14 days. Since most patients will need to do 3 to 4 MET level activities when they return home, in-hospital activities should be geared toward reaching this level. In some institutions it is the physical therapist who supervises the exercise program, working closely with both the medical and nursing personnel to coordinate activities. During the first few days after an uncomplicated myocardial infarction, the patient is instructed and encouraged to perform lying or sitting exercises (arms, legs, and trunk) at low MET levels. Then exercises progress to standing and slow walking in the hall. Patients are supervised constantly during these activities, and their vital signs and heart rhythms are constantly monitored.

Patients are taught early in the exercise program how to check their own pulses. This enables them to become familiar with the normal rate, rhythm, and response to exercise. Normally, patients can expect to have an increase in heart rate and systolic blood pressure with exercise. An exercise session is terminated if any of the following abnormal responses occur during exercise:

1. Cyanosis, cold sweat, faintness, extreme fatigue, severe dyspnea, marked pallor, ataxia, chest pain
2. Resting heart rate greater than 100 or an increase in heart rate greater than 20 over resting pulse; decrease or no change in heart rate despite exercise
3. Dysrhythmias, frequent PVBs, supraventricular tachycardia, various AV blocks, tachycardia greater than 120
4. Resting blood pressure greater than 160/95 mm Hg or an increase in systolic blood pressure of more than 40 mm Hg; decrease or no change in systolic pressure despite exercise

Progressive exercise is continued throughout the hospitalization. The nurse may be an integral member of the interdisciplinary team involved in instructing and supervising the program. Patients should exercise twice a day for approximately 20 minutes. Patients who will need to climb stairs at home gradually progress so that they can climb stairs in the supervised hospital environment. There are many psychologic as well as physiologic benefits to early and progressive activity. Most patients feel that activity is a positive sign and that they are making progress and are recovering from their infarction. Exercise also gives the patients a sense of control over their bodies and tends to decrease anxiety and depression during the convalescent period.

Home Exercise Program

During the posthospitalization convalescent period, many patients are encouraged to begin a 2- to 12-week walking program. This is a structured program designed to have the patient walk 2 miles in less than 60 minutes by the end of the 12 weeks. Individuals are encouraged to work through this program at their own rate until they have achieved a pace just below a slow jog and their heart rate is below the prescribed rate set by the cardiologist.

After completion of the walking program, some individuals will progress to a supervised outpatient exercise training program. Physical conditioning improves the maximal oxygen uptake (Vo_2 max), which is a measure of the maximal rate at which oxygen can be delivered to the tissues. Unfortunately, not all postinfarction patients are physiologically capable of participating in a rigorous exercise program. Eventually, most patients are encouraged to participate in a maintenance (lifetime), unsupervised, home-based exercise program designed specifically for them.

Teaching and Counseling

Education of the patient and family enables them to assume a more active role in their own health care (see the research box). A great deal of anxiety and apprehension can be allayed by providing information about the cardiac condition and its management. Although teaching methods and the amount of information presented may vary, several key concepts need to be presented (see the box on p. 720).

The patients and their partners may need teaching and reassurance regarding resumption of *sexual activity*. Many feel that after MI their sex life is over, fearing a second MI during intercourse. Approximately 80% of all postcoronary patients will be able to resume sexual activity without serious risk. The other 20% need not totally abstain, but their sexual activity should be limited according to their cardiac capacity. Once patients with an uncomplicated MI are capable of walking two flights of stairs without difficulty, they are generally able to perform sexual intercourse safely. In many hospitals, exercise stress tests are done to help the physician determine the patient's cardiac capacity and when sexual activity can be resumed. Coital positions that require less effort on the part of the post-MI person can be suggested. Persons can be encouraged to participate in sexual closeness (such as cuddling) until intercourse is permitted. The person should report adverse signs occurring during intercourse to the physician.

During the hospitalization period many patients ex-

RESEARCH

McCance KL et al: Preventing coronary heart disease in high-risk families, Res Nurs Health 8:413-420, 1985.

This experimental study examined the effects of preventive nursing intervention to reduce risk of coronary heart disease (CHD). The sample consisted of 58 relatives (spouses, siblings, parents, and children) of 19 victims (aged 30 to 55) of sudden death from coronary occlusion. The experimental groups were visited in their homes 3 to 5 months later. Interventions consisted of education/information about cardiovascular risk factors and methods of decreasing risk (blood pressure control, smoking effects, and dietary control of cholesterol, alcohol, and sodium) provided on an individualized supportive approach. The control group received questionnaires on the same time frame; information for blood pressure and cholesterol screening was attached to the first questionnaire. Reduction of CHD risk was measured at 7 months by reported changes in high-risk CHD behaviors, changes in health beliefs, and reported participation in blood pressure and serum cholesterol screenings.

No overall main effects of nursing interventions were demonstrated for health beliefs between the experimental or control groups except for sibling groups. There were greater decreases of alcohol and high-fat meat intake and higher rates for blood pressure and serum cholesterol screening by the experimental group receiving nursing intervention. ■

perience denial, depression, and anxiety. Generally, patients tend to become more anxious on the second day of hospitalization, after the immediate threat of death from the infarction has passed. Depression may begin several days later and may continue after the person is discharged. About 50% of persons continue to experience irritability and tension up to 1 year following an MI.[55] If the spouse is either overprotective or overcritical of the patient's behavior or of changes in the marriage roles and functions during the recovery period, the marriage may deteriorate.[55] The spouse is therefore included in teaching and counseling sessions, and both patients and families are encouraged to talk about their feelings and concerns. Often in group sessions, a feeling of camaraderie develops as several individuals face similar problems.

Physical symptoms may persist during the year following an MI and include excessive fatigue, chest pain, or dyspnea. Persons experiencing these symptoms often learn how to manage their symptoms and resume normal activities. Over 85% of all patients with uncomplicated MI are able to return to work, and this, along with resuming normal sexual functioning and usual activities, aids tremendously in the adjustment period.

TEACHING THE PERSON WITH A MYOCARDIAL INFARCTION

1. Effect of myocardial infarction and healing process
2. Prevention of further risks
   a. Discontinue smoking
   b. Correct existing hypertension with continued medical follow-up
   c. Eat a diet low in calories, saturated fats, and cholesterol; decreased salt, if hypertensive
   d. Participate in a weight reduction program, if appropriate
   e. Take prescribed prophylactic medications (β-blockers)
3. Effect of activity on heart and participation in planned program of increased activity under medical supervision
4. Resumption of sexual activity (if appropriate)
   a. Abstention from sexual intercourse as directed, usually for 4 to 6 weeks
   b. Reporting to physician the following symptoms occurring during or following intercourse
      (1) Dyspnea or increased heart rate continuing for more than 15 minutes after intercourse
      (2) Extreme fatigue
      (3) Chest pain during intercourse
      (4) Palpitations for more than 15 minutes after intercourse
      (5) Insomnia after intercourse
5. Effect of stressors on the heart and benefits of stress management techniques (for example, relaxation exercises)
6. Benefits of participation in group counseling sessions for both patient and spouse
7. Benefits of return to usual home activities and relationships as soon as possible
8. Benefits of return to work at earliest opportunity as prescribed specifically by physician

HYPERTENSIVE HEART DISEASE

Hypertensive heart disease refers to changes in the heart from prolonged sustained hypertension, which increases afterload. The heart enlarges (as seen on radiographic examination) in an attempt to compensate for the increased cardiac workload. If the underlying hypertension is untreated, cardiac failure results. Hypertension is discussed in Chapter 29.

CONGESTIVE HEART FAILURE

Heart failure (also known as congestive heart failure, cardiac decompensation, cardiac insufficiency, and cardiac incompetence) has been described clinically, physiologically, and biochemically, yet no definition has been accepted universally. One widely accepted definition of heart failure is a state in which the heart no longer is able to pump an adequate supply of blood to meet the demands of the body.

Heart failure can be classified as acute or chronic.

Acute heart failure develops quickly and often without warning. The clinical picture may include syncope, shock, cardiac arrest, or sudden death. These outcomes are clearly the results of the myocardium failing to function adequately. Acute heart failure may result from decreased effectiveness of the heart after myocardial infarction. *Chronic* heart failure, on the other hand, develops gradually and the patient is seen initially with milder symptoms. The heart has the capability to compensate for the decreased performance, thus lessening the severity of symptoms.

ETIOLOGY

The causes of heart failure can be divided into three groups. The first group is made up of conditions that result in direct damage to the heart and includes myocardial infarction, myocarditis, myocardial fibrosis, and ventricular aneurysm.

The second is made up of conditions that result in ventricular overload (Chapter 26). Overload can be described in two subgroups:

1. *Preload.* Preload is the ventricular blood volume at end-diastole, the maximal ventricular blood volume for that beat of the heart. According to Starling's law, once the preload has reached a given limit, the effectiveness of the contraction diminishes resulting in heart failure. Increased preload can result from mitral or aortic regurgitation, atrial or ventricular septal defects, or rapid infusion of intravenous solutions.

2. *Afterload.* Afterload is the force that the ventricle must develop to eject blood into the circulatory system. This is the pressure against which the heart must work. Increased afterload may develop from aortic or pulmonary valve stenosis, systemic hypertension, or pulmonary hypertension.

The last major group of conditions that can lead to heart failure are those resulting in constriction of the ventricle, which limits ventricular filling and thus decreases stroke volume. Constriction can result from cardiac tamponade, constrictive cardiomyopathies, and pericarditis.

PATHOPHYSIOLOGY

CARDIAC COMPENSATORY MECHANISMS

Three mechanisms of compensation that enable the weakened heart to continue to meet the metabolic demands of the body are tachycardia, ventricular dilation, and hypertrophy of the myocardium.

Tachycardia

By increasing the heart rate, cardiac output is also increased (see Chapter 26 for discussion of cardiac output). As the heart rate continues to increase, however, diastole is shortened to the point where an inadequate filling of the ventricles occurs and cardiac output actually decreases.

Ventricular Dilation

The myocardium has been demonstrated to function according to Starling's law of the heart, which states that within certain limits, cardiac muscle fibers contract more forcibly the more they are stretched before contraction. By increasing venous return to the heart, the fibers are stretched, which allows for a more forceful contraction, thus increasing stroke volume. This mechanism then results in increased cardiac output.

Hypertrophy of the Myocardium

Hypertrophy, which is an increase in the diameter of muscle fibers, is seen as a thickening in the walls of the heart. This increase in muscle mass results in more effective contraction of the heart, further increasing cardiac output. The greatest limitation to hypertrophy as a compensatory mechanism is that the muscle mass outgrows the coronary artery supply, resulting in hypoxia and decreased effectiveness.

HOMEOSTATIC COMPENSATORY MECHANISMS

When cardiac compensatory mechanisms become inadequate to continue to meet the metabolic needs of the body, homeostatic compensatory mechanisms are activated. Knowledge of these physiologic responses is essential in understanding the treatment modalities for congestive heart failure.

Vascular System

As the circulating blood volume is decreased, sympathetic stimulation and release of norepinephrine result in generalized vasoconstriction. Both arterial circulation and venous circulation are affected.

Kidneys

Vasoconstriction and low cardiac output have a profound effect on renal perfusion. When cardiac output falls to one half to two thirds of normal, complete anuria can occur. As arterial pressure in the kidneys is diminished, glomerular filtration is reduced, resulting in retention of sodium and water. Aldosterone secretion by the adrenal cortex is stimulated, resulting in further reabsorption of sodium by the renal tubules. Osmotic pressure is increased by the rising sodium concentration, leading to release of antidiuretic hormone by the hypothalamus. The end result is increased tubular reabsorption of water, leading to fluid overload and edema (Figure 28-22).

Liver

The venous volume increases to such an extent that hepatic congestion develops, resulting in decreased effectiveness of all hepatic functions. The liver normally metabolizes aldosterone and antidiuretic hormone. Since the congested liver has a reduced ability to metabolize these substances, hepatic congestion serves to further compound heart failure.

CLASSIFICATIONS OF HEART FAILURE

Heart failure has been classified into three main categories. These include backward versus forward, left versus right, and low versus high output heart failure.

Backward Versus Forward Heart Failure

Backward versus forward heart failure is perhaps the oldest method of classifying heart failure. Backward failure is said to be the result of damming up of blood in

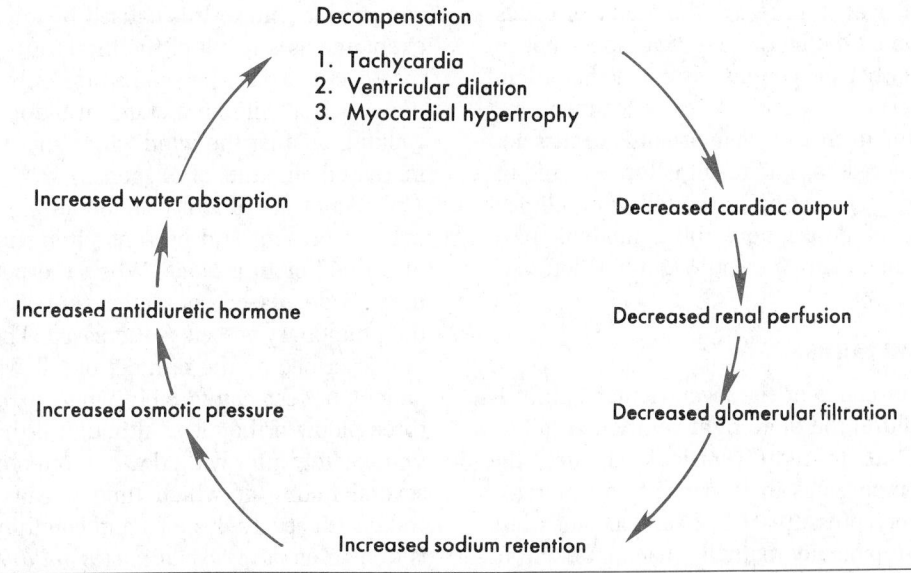

FIGURE 28-22 Sequelae compounding decompensation in chronic heart failure.

the vessels proximal to the heart. Forward heart failure, conversely, is the result of the inability of the heart to maintain cardiac output. It should be emphasized that since the heart is part of a closed system, forward failure and backward failure will always be associated with each other.

Left Versus Right Heart Failure

The most common event would be for one ventricle to fail before the other. Since the left ventricle is most often affected by coronary atherosclerosis and hypertension, heart failure usually begins there. Left ventricular failure is usually signaled by pulmonary congestion and edema. Right ventricular failure is most often triggered by left ventricular failure. Right ventricular failure usually leads to systemic venous congestion and peripheral edema. However, when the patient usually seeks health care, signs and symptoms of both right and left heart failure are present.

Low- Versus High-Output Heart Failure

With the development of diagnostic tools that allow for the measurement of cardiac output (cardiac catheterization), heart failure can be classified by the effectiveness of the heart as a pump. When cardiac output remains normal or above normal but the metabolic needs of the body are not met, the heart failure is termed *high output*. Causes of high output failure include hyperthyroidism, anemia, Paget's disease, and arteriovenous fistula. When cardiac output falls below normal, the results are termed *low-output heart failure* and can result from arteriosclerosis, hypertension, myocardial infarction, and valvular disorder.

CLINICAL MANIFESTATIONS

The symptoms of heart failure are the result of excessive fluid retention by the body. The congestion that results can involve either the venous system or the pulmonary system and eventually both. As the effectiveness of the heart as a pump decreases, venous stasis occurs and venous pressure increases. The result is further fluid retention by the kidneys, leading to the following clinical picture. For ease of description, the symptoms have been described individually for both right and left ventricular failure.

RIGHT VENTRICULAR FAILURE

The most common cause of right ventricular failure is left ventricular failure; therefore right ventricular failure is rarely seen alone. In right ventricular failure, the right ventricle compensates in response to an increase in pulmonary artery pressure. The heart becomes less effective and is unable to maintain adequate output against the increased resistance. This results in blood damming back into the systemic circulation, leading to

peripheral edema. This *edema* is of the *pitting* type and is nontender. It is also known as dependent edema, because it occurs in dependent parts of the body such as the legs or sacrum. As the edema becomes more pronounced, it progresses up the legs into the thighs, external genitalia, and lower trunk. As the tissue becomes extremely engorged, the skin cracks and fluid may "weep" from the tissues.

The *liver* may also become engorged with intravascular fluid, resulting in *enlargement* and tenderness in the right upper quadrant of the abdomen. As the venous stasis increases, pressure within the portal system becomes so great that fluid is forced through the blood vessels into the abdominal cavity. The collection of fluid *within the abdomen*, known as *ascites*, can reach volumes of more than 10 L. This great volume of fluid can displace the diaphragm, resulting in severe respiratory distress. A paracentesis (Chapter 39) may be required to relieve the pressure on the diaphragm. *Distended neck veins* as a result of the increased systemic venous pressure are usually observed when the patient is in a sitting position (see Figure 26-12).

LEFT VENTRICULAR FAILURE

In left ventricular failure, the left ventricle cannot pump oxygenated blood coming from the lungs at a volume necessary to meet the demands of the body. Symptoms are the result of congestion of the lungs with fluid that is forced from the pulmonary circulation into the pulmonary tissues, causing pulmonary edema (p. 731) and pleural effusion. Fluid may be present in the interstitial tissues, alveoli, bronchioles, or pleural space.

Respiratory Signs and Symptoms

Dyspnea, labored breathing, is an early symptom of left ventricular failure. It is caused by interference with gas exchange as a result of the fluid in the alveoli. Dyspnea may occur or may become worse only on physical exertion, such as climbing stairs, walking up an incline, or walking against the wind, since these activities require increased amounts of oxygen.

Orthopnea, difficulty in breathing when lying flat, may be present and persons often must sleep propped up in bed or in a chair. When the person is lying flat, there is decreased ventilation and the blood volume in the pulmonary vessels is increased. The orthopnea is often described by the number of pillows required for the patient to rest comfortably when in bed, for example, three-pillow orthopnea. Although orthopnea may occur immediately after lying down, it often does not occur for several hours, at which time it causes the person to wake with severe dyspnea and coughing. This condition is known as *paroxysmal nocturnal dyspnea* and results from the accumulation of fluid in the lungs as the person is lying in bed. The patient usually experiences a feeling of suffocation and often awakens in panic.

In heart failure the patient may experience alternating periods of *apnea* and *hyperpnea* (Cheyne-Stokes respirations). Often because of respiratory insufficiency, an inadequate amount of oxygen is delivered to the brain. The decrease in oxygen makes the respiratory center in the brain insensitive to the amounts of carbon dioxide in the arterial blood, and respirations cease either until the carbon dioxide content in the arterial blood increases enough to stimulate the respiratory center or until the oxygen level in the blood drops to a level that is low enough to stimulate the respiratory center. This results in hyperpnea. These periods of overbreathing result in greater than normal decreases in carbon dioxide content of arterial blood, producing another period of apnea. Periodic overbreathing often begins as the patient goes to sleep and decreases as sleep deepens and ventilation decreases. Cheyne-Stokes respiration can often be improved by administration of morphine sulfate, which suppresses respirations. The use of morphine sulfate has the added advantage of reducing patient anxiety. High concentrations of oxygen generally are contraindicated, since this would prevent the reflex stimulus to respiration caused by low oxygen content in the blood.

A persistent hacking *cough* is often a symptom of left-sided heart failure. The cough is usually productive of large quantities of frothy sputum, which is occasionally blood tinged. Coughing results from congestion of trapped fluid, which is irritating to the mucosal lining of the lungs and bronchi. On auscultation, *rales* can be heard. Rales are the moist popping and crackling sounds heard most often at the end of inspiration.

Fatigue

Persons with heart failure commonly note fatigue following activities that ordinarily are not tiring. The fatigue results from impaired blood circulation to tissues as a result of the decreased cardiac output. The reduction in tissue oxygen decreases the aerobic production of adenosine triphosphate (ATP), the immediate energy source for muscle contractions. Also the impaired circulation decreases removal of metabolic waste products, resulting in further decreased muscle function.

Pain

Cardiac pain is *not* a typical symptom of heart failure; however, angina pectoris can occur from the decrease in cardiac output. Cardiac pain associated with congestive heart failure is most likely to occur in patients with coronary artery disease. Coronary artery disease increases the patient's sensitivity to a deficiency in the oxygen content of the circulating blood. As heart failure develops, the blood is less effectively oxygenated and angina occurs. As the fluid overload state is corrected, the chest pain resolves.

Anxiety

Most persons are aware of the importance of an effective functioning heart to maintain life, and persons are acquainted with symptoms that indicate a failing heart. Therefore anxiety usually occurs when symptoms of heart failure are present. Anxiety can cause increased breathlessness, which is then interpreted by the patient as an increase in the severity of the heart failure, and this in turn increases the anxiety.

DIAGNOSTIC TESTS

The most common diagnostic tests for the person experiencing congestive heart failure include a chest roentgenogram, ECG, echocardiogram, and cardiac catheterization (see Chapter 26).

MEDICAL THERAPY

Medical therapy for congestive heart failure consists of reducing oxygen requirements of the body through oxygen therapy and rest and of optimizing cardiac output with digitalis, diuretics, vasodilators, and a sodium-restricted diet.

DIGITALIS THERAPY

Digitalis is the major therapeutic approach in the treatment of congestive heart failure. Digitalis and its derivatives usually are effective in improving myocardial function in persons with congestive heart failure. The positive inotropic action of digitalis preparations enhances mechanical performance by strengthening the force of myocardial contraction. This leads to increased cardiac output and increased blood flow to the kidneys. Digitalis preparations also decrease heart rate (automaticity) and cardiac conduction velocity, which permits the ventricles to relax more to allow time for better filling of the ventricles with blood.

When acute congestive heart failure occurs, the physician usually orders an *optimal therapeutic dose* of a digitalis preparation to slow the ventricular rate and decrease symptoms. This larger dose given over a short period of time, usually 24 to 48 hours, is called a *load-*

SIGNS AND SYMPTOMS OF DIGITALIS TOXICITY

Cardiovascular effects	Neurologic effects
Bradycardia	Headache
Tachycardia	Double vision
Bigeminy	Blurred or colored vision
Ectopic beats	Drowsiness, confusion
Pulse deficit	Restlessness, irritability
Gastrointestinal effects	Muscle weakness
Anorexia	
Nausea and vomiting	
Abdominal pain	
Diarrhea	

ing, or *digitalizing,* dose. In some instances the dose may approach the toxic level, and the person is observed carefully for signs and symptoms of toxicity (see the box on p. 723). The full effect of the digitalizing drug is realized when the heart and circulation return to normal under treatment, and the symptoms of toxicity are more evident at this time. Since digitalis preparations have a *cumulative effect* and are slowly eliminated, early recognition of toxic symptoms and discontinuance of the drug will decrease their severity. After the optimal therapeutic dose has been determined, the person is given a daily maintenance dose of digitalis.

Several factors predispose the person to digitalis toxicity. One of the most common is hypokalemia, which potentiates the effects of digitalis. When potassium is depleted in the body or myocardium, the heart becomes more excitable and dysrhythmias may occur. Decrease in potassium levels below the normal range of 4.0 to 5.4 mEq/L can occur whenever excess potassium is lost from the body such as occurs in vomiting and diarrhea or induced diuresis. Most of the diuretics used to treat congestive heart failure result in the loss of potassium along with sodium and water. To replace the potassium lost through diuresis, persons are often placed on a supplemental form of potassium such as potassium chloride. Some diuretics have potassium added to them, but many physicians prefer to order the diuretics and potassium separately. In addition, foods such as orange juice or bananas, which are high in potassium and low in sodium content, are encouraged.

Other predisposing factors to digitalis toxicity include severe liver and kidney disease, since the liver inactivates the drug and the kidney excretes it, and primary myocardial disease, which makes the myocardium more sensitive to the drug. Increased toxicity also occurs with alkalosis, hypercalcemia, hypomagnesemia, and hypothyroidism. If digitalis toxicity occurs, the medication is stopped at once and other therapy instituted as necessary. This often includes administration of procainamide and potassium chloride.

Numerous types of digitalis preparations may be used (Table 28-10). For rapid digitalization in emergency situations, deslanoside (Cedilanid-D) or G-strophanthin (Ouabain) is usually selected. Digoxin or digitoxin is most commonly used for maintenance drug therapy. Digoxin has a more rapid effect than digitoxin yet has sufficient duration for adequate maintenance therapy. If given intramuscularly, digoxin should be injected deeply and the area massaged after injection because the drug is a tissue irritant. Powdered digitalis is highly toxic and is therefore rarely used.

Before a digitalis preparation is given, the apical pulse rate is taken. If this rate is below 60 the medication should be withheld until the physician has been consulted. The pulse is also evaluated for changes in rhythm. The pulse rate of persons with irregular rhythm should always be taken for a full minute for accuracy. Response to digitalis is evaluated on the basis of relief of symptoms, that is, decreased edema, loss of weight, fluid output greater than fluid intake, and no dyspnea or cyanosis.

DIURETIC THERAPY

Diuretic therapy is not a substitute for digitalis therapy, which has a direct action on the myocardium. Diuretics are potentially dangerous medications and their use is

TABLE 28-10 Digitalis preparations

Generic Name	Trade Name	Digitalizing Dose (time)	Route	Maintenance Dose (mg)	Onset	Peak	Duration (days)
Purple foxglove							
Powdered digitalis	Digifortis Digiglusin	1.0-2.0 g (24-48 hr)	Oral	100-200	2-4 hr	12-14 hr	14
Digitoxin	Crystodigin Purogidin	1.2-1.6 mg 0.5-0.6 mg (24-48 hr)	Oral IV	0.1-0.2	1-4 hr 1-2 hr	8-14 hr 4-12 hr	14
Gitalin	Gitaligin	2.5-6.0 mg (3-4 days)	Oral	0.5	2-4 hr	8-12 hr	12
White foxglove							
Digoxin	Lanoxin	1.0-1.5 mg 0.25-0.5 mg (12-24 hr)	Oral IV	0.125-0.50	1-2 hr 15-30 min	6-8 hr 1-5 hr	6
Deslanoside	Cedilanid-D	0.8-1.6 mg (12 hr)	IV, IM	0.25-0.5	10-30 min	1-3 hr	2-5
Lanatoside-C	Cedilanid	10 mg (4 days)	Oral	0.5	1-2 hr	4-6 hr	3-6
Strophanthus gratus							
G-Strophanthin	Ouabain	0.25-0.5 mg (12-24 hr)	IV	—	3-10 min	½-2 hr	1-3

instituted only after symptoms of heart failure persist following digitalization and sodium restriction. The purpose of diuretic therapy is to decrease cardiac workload by reducing circulating volume and thus reduce preload.

Essential to proper initiation of diuretic therapy is determining how much fluid should be removed from the patient by establishing a "dry weight," or edema-free weight. This can be accomplished by gradually removing fluid by use of diuretics and assessing the patient's blood pressure. When the patient becomes hypotensive, particularly orthostatic, this signals the physician that too much fluid has been removed. The patient is then permitted to reaccumulate a small amount of fluid until hypotension no longer occurs. The weight at which this occurs is then considered the patient's dry weight. This can all be accomplished by adjusting the dose of diuretics. Adjustments in diuretic therapy can best be accomplished while the patient is hospitalized; however, changes in the patient's dry weight when discharged will affect the equilibrium obtained while the patient is hospitalized.

Diuretics function by increasing the urinary output, which decreases blood volume, thereby reducing cardiac workload. This is accomplished primarily by inhibiting the reabsorption of sodium by the kidneys. Mercurial diuretics affect the proximal tubules; furosemide and ethacrynic acid affect the ascending loop of Henle, thiazides and triamterene affect the distal tubule, whereas spironolactone exerts its effect on the collecting duct. Dosages and side effects of these diuretics are listed in Table 28-11).

Currently, the *thiazides* are the diuretics of choice in the treatment of heart failure. The thiazides are inexpensive, easy to take, and effective when taken over a long period. Because these patent drugs can lead to electrolyte imbalance, serum chemistry levels should be observed closely, particularly at the onset of therapy. The major complication is hypokalemia, which can be prevented by the intake of foods high in potassium or by potassium supplements.

If thiazides are ineffective, an oral aldosterone antagonist, such as spironolactone (Aldactone) or triamterene (Dyrenium), may be given with the thiazide. These drugs work by competitive inhibition of aldosterone, resulting in retention of potassium and excretion of sodium and water.

The most potent diuretics currently available are furosemide (Lasix) and bumetanide (Bumex). These medications are reserved for severe congestive heart failure or when other forms of treatment are ineffective in relieving symptoms. These agents also increase renal blood flow and therefore may prove effective in treating heart failure when renal function is also impaired. Therapy is best initiated in the hospital setting so that electrolyte and acid-base balance may be monitored.

OTHER DRUGS

Vasodilators may be used to decrease afterload by decreasing resistance to ventricular emptying. The more commonly used agents are nitroprusside, hydralazine (Apresoline), and prozosin (Minipress). Nifedipine, a calcium channel blocker, also has vasodilator effects. Captopril (Capoten), a newer drug with antihyperten-

TABLE 28-11 Diuretics used in the treatment of heart failure

Type	Example	Onset/Peak/Duration	Dose	Side Effects
Thiazide	Chlorothiazide (Diuril)	2 hr/4 hr/6-12 hr	0.5-1.0 g once or twice a day	Gastrointestinal upsets (can be minimized by taking medication with meals); hypokalemia; hyperglycemia
	Hydrochlorothiazide (Esidrix, Hydrodiuril)	2 hr/4 hr/6-12 hr	25-100 mg/day	
Loop	Furosemide (Lasix)	1 hr/1-2 hr/6-8 hr	20-80 mg/day orally (may be given intravenously in doses up to 600 mg in 24 hr to treat pulmonary edema)	Similar to thiazide diuretics; also ototoxicity and blood dyscrasias
	Bumetanide (Bumex)	Oral: 30-60 min/1-2 hr/4-6 hr IV: within minutes/15-30 min	Oral 0.5-2 mg qd IV/IM 0.5-1 mg (may be repeated at 2-3 hr intervals ×2; maximum 10 mg qd)	
Potassium sparing	Spironolactone (Aldactone)	Gradual/3 days/2-3 days after therapy discontinued	25-50 mg four times a day	Gastrointestinal irritation; hyperkalemia
	Triamterene (Dyrenium)	Rapid/7-9 hr/12-16 hr	150-200 mg once a day	

sive properties, is also a vasodilator and blocks sodium retention by suppressing aldosterone. Vasodilators are more effective in the treatment of acute rather than chronic heart failure.

■ ASSESSMENT
SUBJECTIVE DATA

Data are collected concerning the person's perception of breathing ability, fluid retention, and response to activity, and to the person's knowledge and response to the cardiac failure.

1. Shortness of breath and presence of cough
2. Presence of orthopnea (number of pillows needed for sleep)
3. Recent weight gain
4. Edema, especially pedal
5. Dizziness or confusion
6. Fatigue
7. Exercise or heat intolerance
8. Discomfort: anginal or abdominal pain
9. Concerns, anxieties
10. Knowledge of condition
11. Usual coping skills

OBJECTIVE DATA

Objective data focus primarily on signs of fluid retention and include the following:

1. Respiratory distress, increased effort, and respiratory rate
2. Neck vein distention: presence, degree
3. Adventitious breath sounds
4. Heart sounds: presence of S_3 or gallop rhythm
5. Edema: site and degree of pitting
6. Coolness of extremities
7. Pulse changes
8. Abdominal distention
9. Daily weights
10. Level of consciousness

■ DATA ANALYSIS: NURSING DIAGNOSES

Nursing diagnoses are determined from assessment of patient data. Possible nursing diagnoses for the person with congestive heart failure may include, but are not limited to, the following:

Diagnostic Title	Possible Etiologies
Anxiety	Threat of death; threat/change in health status, socioeconomic status, role; threat to self-concept
Cardiac output, altered: decreased	Reduced stroke volume, cardiogenic shock, tachycardia, valvular insufficiency, hypertension
Fatigue	Decreased oxygenation, muscle weakness, inadequate rest, inadequate nutrition

Diagnostic Title	Possible Etiologies
Gas exchange, impaired	Ventilation/perfusion imbalance
Knowledge deficit	Lack of exposure/recall, information misinterpretation, cognitive limitation
Tissue perfusion, altered: decreased	Decreased blood flow, hypervolemia, immobility, pulmonary edema
Thought process, altered	Hypoxia, depression, anxiety, psychologic stress, neurologic disorders

■ PLANNING: EXPECTED PATIENT OUTCOMES

Expected patient outcomes for the person with congestive heart failure may include, but are not limited to, the following:

1. Patient uses effective coping mechanisms in managing anxiety.
2. Patient identifies factors that increase cardiac workload.
3. Patient performs ADL without undue fatigue.
4. Normal respiratory rate is achieved without use of supplemental oxygen, patient states breathing is easier, confusion is decreased.
5. Patient demonstrates cardiac tolerance to increased activity (pulse and blood pressure are stable).
6. Patient differentiates between reality and fantasy, describes any problems in relating with others, and identifies situations that evoke anxiety.
7. The patient can:
   a. Describe a modified plan for activity that avoids fatigue or dyspnea.
   b. Plan a diet in accordance with prescribed sodium or fluid restrictions.
   c. Describe the medication therapy, including adverse side effects.
   d. State plans for follow-up medical care.
8. If the patient is discharged with supplemental oxygen therapy, the person can describe usage and precautions.

■ IMPLEMENTATION

At many acute care hospitals, patients with acute congestive heart failure are admitted to medical or cardiac intensive care units if the institution has such a facility. Occasionally, the physician may elect to place the patient in the usual room accomodations where the environment is less stressful and where family members can visit more routinely. The decision about room placement is made on the basis of degree of failure and specific responses of the individual patient to the acute situation.

Care of the person with congestive heart failure is summarized in the box on p. 727.

GUIDELINES FOR CARE OF THE PERSON WITH CONGESTIVE HEART FAILURE

1. Provide oxygenation
   a. Administer oxygen by nasal cannula at 2-6 L/min as prescribed
   b. Give oxygen as needed for dyspnea
   c. Patient should be well supported in semi-Fowler's or high Fowler's position
2. Provide rest and activity
   a. Reinforce importance of conservation of energy and planning for activities that avoid fatigue
   b. Encourage activity within prescribed restrictions; monitor for intolerance to activity (dyspnea, fatigue, increased pulse rate that does not stabilize)
   c. Assist with ADL as necessary; encourage independence within patient's limitations
   d. Provide diversional activity that will assist in conservation of energy
3. Monitor for signs of fluid and potassium imbalance; record daily weights
4. Provide skin care, particularly over edematous areas; use prophylactic measures to prevent skin breakdown
5. Assist in maintaining an adequate nutritional intake while observing prescribed dietary modifications (sodium restrictions)
6. Monitor for constipation; give prescribed stool softeners
7. Give prescribed medications
   a. Digitalis (take apical pulse before administration)
   b. Diuretics (assess for hypokalemia)
   c. Vasodilators
   d. Drugs to reduce anxiety and promote sleep
8. Provide patient/family opportunities to discuss their concerns
9. Teach patient about the disorder and self-care (see the box on p. 729).

PROVIDING OXYGENATION

In heart failure the oxygen content of the bloodstream may be markedly reduced because of the less effective oxygenation of the blood as it passes through the congested lungs. The patient may be more comfortable and better able to rest when receiving oxygen, since it helps in reducing dyspnea and fatigue. Oxygen is usually administered by nasal cannula at 2 to 6 L/min. Baseline arterial blood gas levels are obtained at initiation of oxygen therapy and intermittently during therapy to assess effectiveness of the treatment. Breathing is often made easier by maintaining the patient in semi-Fowler's or high Fowler's position. These positions maximize oxygenation by permitting greater lung expansion.

PROMOTING REST AND ACTIVITY

Reducing the requirements of the body for oxygen can best be effected by providing the patient with the degree of activity that does not compromise myocardial function, as demonstrated by the presence of symptoms. If the degree of heart failure is mild, with only edema of the legs or minimal pulmonary congestion, the patient may be treated on an ambulatory basis with only a regimen of less strenuous activity and more rest than usual.

If the degree of heart failure is severe, a program of bed rest or limited activity may be necessary until symptoms abate. The amount of activity permitted each person is a function of the extent of symptoms such as dyspnea and fatigue. A careful assessment must be made each day to determine to what extent the person can perform ADL such as eating and bathing. Most patients prefer to maximize their independence, and this is encouraged within the limitations of their symptoms.

Sedation is used judiciously for patients with heart failure, since oversedation may mask symptoms of increasing failure. In addition, immobility increases the risk of venous thrombosis and embolus. Patients with heart failure are often apprehensive and may have difficulty relaxing; thus diazepam (Valium), 2 to 10 mg three to four times a day, may be prescribed. Chloral hydrate or flurazepam hydrochloride (Dalmane) may be used if the person is unable to sleep despite nursing measures to promote rest.

The patient is often orthopneic and tends to be more comfortable sitting than lying in bed. If the patient is placed in a chair, the feet are elevated to reduce pooling of fluid in the dependent limbs. When the patient is placed on bed rest, the high Fowler's position is often most comfortable. A pillow may be placed lengthwise behind the shoulders and back in such a manner that full expansion of the rib cage is possible. A foot block can be used to keep the patient from slipping toward the foot of the bed. The arms may also be supported on pillows to reduce the pull on the shoulder muscles (Figure 28-23). An over-the-bed table may be placed close to the patient to allow resting the head and arm.

Ambulation

Ambulation is started slowly to avoid overloading the heart and to determine how much activity the heart can tolerate without again showing signs of failure. The regimen varies depending on individual patient response. When a patient has been on restricted bed rest, activities progress slowly through stages of dangling, sitting up in a chair, and then walking increased distances under close supervision. The patient is assessed for signs indicating that activity cannot be tolerated, including dyspnea, fatigue, and increased pulse rate that does not stabilize readily. If these signs or symptoms occur, the person is returned to bed. If dyspnea is present, the

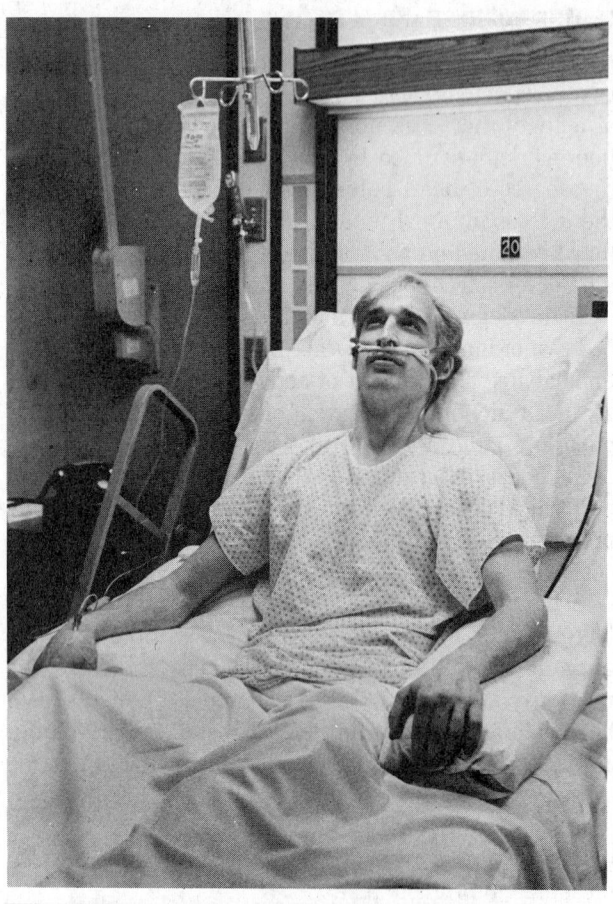

FIGURE 28-23 Patient sitting upright with pillows under head and each arm to promote chest expansion and comfort.

head of the bed is elevated and oxygen is administered at a low flow of 1 to 3 L/min. The physician is consulted before further ambulation is attempted.

The plan for increased activity is explained to the patient and family. They should understand that if activity tires the person excessively, it may be curtailed. Overactivity can produce physical and mental setbacks that delay ultimate recovery. In the early stages of ambulation, it is important to begin stressing the importance of the rate of activity; that is, the demand on the heart is decreased when a normal activity is performed more slowly than before.

PROVIDING EMOTIONAL SUPPORT

The goal of intervention is to help break the anxiety—increased symptoms—anxiety circle by helping the patient (1) identify feelings and the content related to those feelings, (2) identify strengths that can be used for coping, and (3) learn what can be done to decrease the anxiety. Learning about measures to control heart failure and measures to reduce stress may be helpful. Working with family members in the same manner is

also helpful to decrease their anxiety so that they can be of greater support to the patient.

MONITORING DAILY WEIGHTS

Although careful records of intake and output are kept on most patients with cardiac failure, the best method to estimate progress and response to prescribed diet, medications, and other forms of treatment is daily monitoring of the patient's weight. Weight gain indicates fluid retention; 1 kg of weight gain represents 1 L of fluid retention. The weight is carefully recorded on admission and then daily while the patient is hospitalized.

The patient with severe heart failure is weighed on a litter scale, which contains a stretcher to minimize exertion. The patient should be weighed at the same time of day with the same amount of clothing. A good practice is to weigh the patient each morning after the bladder has been emptied and before breakfast is eaten. The patient is also encouraged to continue to take his or her weight daily after being discharged to provide weight gain information for the health care provider.

PROVIDING SKIN CARE

Edematous skin is poorly nourished and very susceptible to breakdown. Edema of the sacrum is prevalent in patients with heart failure restricted to bed rest, and decubiti can develop quickly. The patient is carefully positioned and turned frequently to minimize breakdown. Measures to prevent skin breakdown are instituted early, since prevention is more cost effective for both patient and care provider in addition to promoting patient comfort, both physical and mental. Flotation mattresses and water beds are of assistance in preventing decubiti; however, neither eliminates the need for turning the patient.

PROMOTING NUTRITION

During the acute stage of congestive heart failure the diet should be bland, low-calorie, low-residue with vitamin supplement. Anorexia is often present because of edema in the gastrointestinal tract, dyspnea, fatigue, and the effect of medications. Frequent small feedings minimize exertion and reduce gastrointestinal blood requirements, which can tax the failing heart. Care must be taken in providing a diet that meets the metabolic demands of the body so that body wasting does not occur.

Sodium Intake

Edema is often effectively controlled in patients with heart failure by restriction of sodium intake. The degree of restriction depends on the severity of the failure and the extent of diuretic therapy. The severely restricted sodium diet is rarely prescribed, since the diet is unpalatable and expensive, resulting in poor patient compliance.

The amount of sodium in the normal diet is 3 to 10 g/day. Sodium restriction in persons receiving diuretics may not be dropped below 3 to 5 g/day, because of the dangers of hyponatremia from removal of sodium as well as water by the action of the diuretic on the kidneys. In mild cardiac failure, sodium may be restricted to 1 to 2 g/day. This is known as a "no added salt" (NAS) diet and is essentially a normal diet except that no extra salt is added to prepared foods, and obviously salted foods such as potato chips are omitted. For moderate or severe heart failure, the amount of sodium permitted is specifically prescribed. Vitamin supplements are usually required when severely restricted sodium diets are prescribed.

Low-sodium diets can be made more appealing by adding salt substitutes to food in place of table salt. Since many salt substitutes contain potassium, the patient's need for potassium must be assessed. Often the increased intake of potassium is beneficial when the patient is on diuretic therapy. The use of herbs, such as basil, dill, bay leaves, garlic (powder not salt), and taragon, often makes the food more appetizing.

Fluids

Fluid restriction is less commonly instituted than in the past as long as the person is on a sodium-controlled diet and is receiving diuretics or digitalis or both. When sodium intake is controlled, patients usually do not experience thirst and will control their own fluid intake. The kidneys will also remove water from the body to maintain proper sodium concentration. If fluids are restricted, the amount of fluid permitted is prescribed by the physician and a plan is made, in conjunction with the patient if possible, to space the fluids over the day depending on patient preferences. Usually one half of the fluids are planned for meals and the other half for between meals. If thirst does present a problem, frequent mouth care may add to patient comfort.

Nutrition Education of Persons and Family

The rationale for dietary and fluid restrictions must be explained to both the patient and the family. The family must understand the necessity for these restrictions so they do not present the patient with food or fluids that are unacceptable. The patient needs to learn early about the food and fluid restrictions to be followed after discharge. This allows time for answering questions and planning menus. The ambulatory patient may need frequent interactions with the dietitian or nurse before being able to follow the diet adequately.

PROMOTING ELIMINATION

It is advisable for the person with cardiac disease to avoid straining at defecation, since it places an extra burden on the heart. During straining against a closed glottis (Valsalva's maneuver), venous return to the heart is decreased as a result of increased intrathoracic pressure. When this pressure is released after straining, a large amount of venous return creates an increased workload on the heart.

The feces can be kept soft by giving a mild cathartic such as milk of magnesia, a mild bulk cathartic such as psyllium (Metamucil), or a stool-softening agent such as sodium docusate (Colace). If an enema becomes necessary, it should be of low volume and given with a small rectal tube inserted only 3 to 4 inches.

The use of a bedpan is often uncomfortable and does not facilitate bowel evacuation. The necessity for use of a bedpan often will create anxiety in the patient. For these reasons the patient is usually permitted to use a bedside commode. The patient should be assisted to and from the commode.

TEACHING THE PERSON WITH CONGESTIVE HEART FAILURE

1. Monitor for signs and symptoms of recurring congestive heart failure and report these signs and symptoms to the physician or clinic:
   a. Weight gain of 1-1.5 kg (2-3 lb) over a short period of time (about 2 days)
   b. Loss of appetite
   c. Shortness of breath
   d. Orthopnea
   e. Swelling of ankles, feet, or abdomen
   f. Persistent cough
   g. Frequent nighttime urination
2. Avoid fatigue and plan activity to allow for rest periods
3. Plan and eat meals within prescribed sodium restrictions
   a. Avoid salty foods
   b. Avoid drugs with high sodium content (for example, some laxatives and antacids, Alka-Seltzer)—read the labels
   c. Eat several small meals rather than three large meals per day
4. Take prescribed medications
   a. If several medications are prescribed, develop a method to facilitate accurate administration
   b. Digitalis: check own pulse rate daily; report a rate of less than 60/min to physician and signs and symptoms of toxicity
   c. Diuretics
      (1) Weigh self daily at same time of day
      (2) Report weight gain to physician
      (3) Eat foods high in potassium and low in sodium (such as oranges, bananas)
   d. Vasodilators
      (1) Report signs of hypotension (light-headedness, rapid pulse, syncope) to physician
      (2) Avoid alcohol when taking vasodilators
5. Report to physician for follow-up as directed

NURSING CARE PLAN

PERSON WITH CONGESTIVE HEART FAILURE

DATA: Mr. A. is a 65-year-old white man with congestive heart failure who was admitted to the hospital with increased fluid retention. He has a history of hypertension and atherosclerotic heart disease. He has felt tired for several weeks and has experienced increased dyspnea on exertion, vertigo, and syncope. He has had two myocardial infarctions, the most recent being 6 months before admission. A cardiac catheterization performed several months previously revealed triple vessel disease, decreased left ventricular function with an ejection fraction of 25%, and poorly developed collaterals. He has been on a regimen of antianginal medications that have kept him painfree, although he has been cognizant of progressive intolerance to exertion and increasing peripheral edema. On admission, his medication included bumetanide 20 mg bid, captopril 25 mg tid, digoxin 0.25 mg qd, diltiazem 90 mg q6h, and nitroglycerine ointment 2% in a 2-inch patch q6h.

The nursing history identified the following:
- Mr. A. has very little understanding of his medications and his low-sodium, low-cholesterol diet.
- The episodes of dyspnea have been increasingly anxiety provoking.
- Mr. A. does not understand the need to take his medication, especially when he does not feel sick.
- Mr. A. has had increasing weight gain, approximately 10 pounds before admission.

Collaborative nursing activities include those to assess Mr. A.'s response to current therapeutic regimen and those to assess the presence of any complications associated with the regimen. Nursing actions include monitoring the following:
- Daily weights and intake/output
- Vital signs
- Breath sounds
- Response to exertion
- Heart rate and rhythm
- Serum electrolytes

NURSING DIAGNOSIS

Altered cardiac output, decreased, related to reduced stroke volume, resulting in a compromised state

Expected Patient Outcomes	Nursing Interventions	Rationale
Mr. A.'s pulse and respirations are within normal limits.	Organize care to provide scheduled periods for rest and to minimize unnecessary disturbances.	Exercise and physical activity increase cardiac output, heart rate, and blood pressure.
Mr. A. identifies factors that increase cardiac workload.	Explain and encourage increases in activity and ambulation to prevent a sudden increase in cardiac workload.	Regular exercise makes the heart more efficient, so stroke volume increases and heart rate is not appreciably altered.
	Monitor respirations q4h for increased effort, pulse for tachycardia.	
	Monitor heart sounds q4h for presence of gallop rhythm.	
	Teach Mr. A. to avoid Valsalva's maneuver.	Surge of blood to heart after intrathoracic pressure decreases causes increase in cardiac workload

NURSING DIAGNOSIS

Tissue perfusion, altered, related to decreased blood flow to tissues and edema

Expected Patient Outcomes	Nursing Interventions	Rationale
Mr. A. has fewer episodes of syncope and vertigo.	Encourage movement and activity as tolerated.	Movement promotes circulation to tissues.
	Assess neck vein distention, edema of extremities and coolnes of skin q4h; weigh daily.	Assessment will provide information on fluid overload.
Skin breakdown does not occur.	Eliminate or reduce pressure points by changing position frequently, use of pressure mattress, etc.	Excess interstitial fluid interferes with diffusion of oxygen to cells. Cellular nutrition and respiration are dependent on adequate blood flow. Hypoxia causes cellular swelling and injury.
	Give diuretics and sodium-restricted diet as prescribed.	

NURSING CARE PLAN

PERSON WITH CONGESTIVE HEART FAILURE—cont'd

NURSING DIAGNOSIS

Activity intolerance related to imbalance between oxygen supply and demand

Expected Patient Outcomes	Nursing Interventions	Rationale
Mr. A. progresses to highest level of mobility possible with less fatigue and dyspnea.	Encourage rest periods according to daily schedule and during the first hour after meals.	Any factor that compromises cardiovascular function reduces tolerance to activity.
Mr. A. identifies factors that reduce his activity intolerance.	Assess Mr. A.'s response to activity (pulse, blood pressure, respirations).	
	Increase Mr. A.'s tolerance for activity by having him perform activity more slowly or for a shorter period of time with more rest periods.	Pacing of activity decreases myocardial oxygen demand.
	Explain the effects of increased oxygen demand with decreased oxygen supply.	

NURSING DIAGNOSIS

Knowledge deficit (pathophysiology of heart failure, rationale for therapy) related to lack of recall, poor understanding

Expected Patient Outcomes	Nursing Interventions	Rationale
Mr. A. describes the pathophysiology, symptoms, and rationale for therapy of CHF.	Discuss with Mr. A.: 1. Basis of the symptoms and rationale for therapy. 2. Self-monitoring for recurring signs of CHF. 3. How to be active yet avoid fatigue. 4. Management of prescribed sodium-restriction diet. 5. Need for follow-up care.	If Mr. A. understands reasons for the symptoms and how therapy will modify the symptoms, he will be more ready to learn about his care and to follow through with prescribed care.
	Examine Mr. A.'s health beliefs and past experiences related to illness and assess the impact on his desire/ability to learn.	Learning is influenced by values, beliefs, and previous experiences.

PATIENT TEACHING

Teaching is initiated early in the person's hospitalization to permit time for learning and asking questions. Many episodes of recurring congestive heart failure might be prevented if patients were able to follow the prescribed drug therapy, avoid dietary indiscretions, avoid excessive physical activity, and recognize and report recurring symptoms to their physician. Repeated episodes of congestive heart failure can lead to serious consequences such as liver cirrhosis, pulmonary fibrosis, and enlargement of the spleen and kidneys. Guidelines for patient teaching are listed in the box on p. 729. (See the nursing care plan on pp. 730-731).

ACUTE PULMONARY EDEMA
ETIOLOGY

Acute pulmonary edema is a medical emergency arising from severe left ventricular failure. It usually results from prolonged strain on a diseased heart. It may also result from inhalation of irritating gases or from too rapid administration of plasma, serum albumin, whole

blood, or intravenous fluids; or it may be associated with barbiturate or opiate poisoning.

PATHOPHYSIOLOGY

In pulmonary edema caused by heart failure, cardiac output is decreased, resulting in an increase in left atrial pressure. This results in an increase in pulmonary vein and capillary pressure. As the pulmonary capillary pressure exceeds the intravascular osmotic pressure, serous fluid is rapidly forced into the alveoli. Fluid rapidly reaches the bronchioles and bronchi, and patients literally begin to drown in their own secretions.

CLINICAL MANIFESTATIONS

Signs and symptoms of pulmonary edema include restlessness and vague uneasiness at the onset. As pulmonary edema progresses, the patient develops profound dyspnea, pallor, cough productive of large quantities of blood-tinged frothy sputum, audible wheezing, and cyanosis. Tachycardia is often present.

INTERVENTIONS

The goals in the treatment of acute pulmonary edema include physical and mental relaxation, relief of hypoxemia, retardation of venous return, and improvement of cardiovascular function.

The patient with acute pulmonary edema is placed in bed in *high Fowler's position,* and the physician is summoned immediately. Treatment is usually begun by administering *morphine sulfate,* 10 to 15 mg intravenously. The intravenous route is preferred, since vascular collapse may hinder its absorption from subcutaneous tissues. Anxiety is relieved by morphine, which increases venous capacitance and lowers left atrial pressure and which may decrease ventilation.

To relieve hypoxemia, the physician often orders *oxygen* at 40% to 70% to be delivered by face mask. Humidification is desirable to keep secretions moist and facilitate mobilization of these secretions. Occasionally, the patient with severe pulmonary embarrassment will require intubation to deliver adequate tidal volumes and oxygen concentration. Intubation also aids in removing secretions by suctioning. The patient is often extubated within hours of the initiation of therapy. *Aminophylline* may also be administered intravenously in the treatment of pulmonary edema to dilate the bronchi, increase urinary output, and increase cardiac output.

The treatments described earlier for congestive heart failure are also implemented for pulmonary edema, including rapid *digitalization,* institution of diuretic therapy using *furosemide* or *bumetanide,* and *vasodilators.* Serum potassium levels are obtained immediately, since these patients have large diuresis and lose large amounts of potassium.

Two more radical and controversial treatments that may be used when the preceding regimens fail include phlebotomy and rotating tourniquets. The purpose of phlebotomy is to decrease the amount of circulating blood to decrease pulmonary engorgement; however, this removes hemoglobin that may further contribute to hypoxemia.

The purpose of rotating tourniquets is to pool blood in the extremities, thus reducing cardiac overload. As much as 1 L of blood may be trapped in the extremities when tourniquets are used. The tourniquets are placed on three extremities at one time. Every 15 minutes in clockwise or counterclockwise order, one tourniquet is placed on the extremity that has no tourniquet and one tourniquet is removed. Thus each extremity is occluded for 45 minutes. A rotating tourniquet machine uses blood pressure cuffs as tourniquets and automatically pumps and deflates the cuffs to obtain the desired effect. Since the purpose of this therapy is to occlude venous blood, the tourniquets should not obliterate arterial pulses in the extremity. If an extremity does not return readily to normal color on release of a tourniquet, the physician is informed. When the procedure is terminated, the tourniquets are released, one every 15 minutes to prevent a sudden increase in venous return and recurrence of pulmonary edema.

CHAPTER SUMMARY

✔ All layers of the heart (pericardium, myocardium, and endocardium) may become inflamed. Patients with these conditions have the usual signs of inflammation and may also develop heart failure. Measures to prevent further episodes are important aspects of the treatment regimen.

✔ Mitral and aortic valvular disease occur more frequently than do pulmonic and tricuspid valvular disease. Rheumatic fever is a common precursor. The two basic problems that compromise normal functioning of the valves are stenosis and regurgitation (insufficiency). Stenosis causes a narrowing of the valvular orifice and impedes the forward flow of blood. Regurgitation causes incomplete closure of the valve and allows blood to flow backward.

✔ Cardiac murmurs are a common physical finding in patients with valvular heart disease. Depending on the severity of the disease, the patient may develop such clinical symptoms as those associated with heart failure.

✔ Treatment of valvular disease involves management of clinical symptoms. Surgical repair of the valve or replacement of the valve with an artificial valve may be necessary.

✔ An aneurysm is a localized or diffuse enlargement of an artery, most commonly seen in the thoracic or abdominal aorta. Depending on the location and size of the aneurysm, surgical resection may be necessary.

✔ Types of heart surgery include repair or replacement of valves, repair of ventricular aneurysms, coronary artery bypass, release of constriction, or heart transplantation.

✔ Teaching is a major preoperative nursing intervention for cardiovascular surgery and includes information about the ICU, surgery, and pre- and postoperative procedures.

✔ In total cardiopulmonary bypass, both the oxygenation and circulation of the blood are bypassed and performed by the bypass machine, thus permitting the heart to be incised and opened for surgery. The machine also permits administration of medications and can provide systemic hypothermia. Side effects of the procedure include hemodilution, decreased platelets, shock, and decreased perfusion to major organs.

✔ Intraaortic balloon counterpulsation is a method by which a balloon is inserted into the thoracic aorta as temporary assistance for circulation. When inflated, the balloon forces blood retrograde to increase coronary filling; when deflated, it decreases pressure in the aortic arch, thus facilitating afterload.

✔ Postoperative nursing care after cardiovascular surgery includes monitoring cardiovascular, respiratory, neurologic, and urinary systems; monitoring and promoting fluid and electrolyte balance and oxygen/carbon dioxide exchange; promoting patient comfort and activity; and patient teaching.

✔ Nonmodifiable risk factors for CAHD include advancing age, sex (males), race, and a positive family history of CAHD.

✔ Major modifiable risk factors for CAHD include hyperlipidemia, hypertension, diabetes mellitus, and cigarette smoking; a diet high in cholesterol and saturated fats contributes to the risk.

✔ Behavioral and psychosocial influences are strongly correlated with the occurrence of CAHD.

✔ Angina pectoris is chest pain caused by reversible myocardial ischemia. Treatment involves increasing myocardial blood and oxygen supply (with medications or surgery) and reducing myocardial oxygen demands. The most commonly used drugs for treating angina pectoris are vasodilators, β-adrenergic blocking agents, and calcium channel blockers.

✔ Coronary artery bypass graft (CABG) consists of circumventing a coronary occlusion using a saphenous vein or internal mammary artery graft.

✔ Intravascular stenting consists of maintaining the cylindrical lumen of the coronary artery (following CABG) by laser photocoagulation or radio-frequency–induced heat.

✔ Myocardial infarction is the result of prolonged myocardial ischemia, which causes irreversible cellular damage. The clinical consequences depend on the location of the coronary artery occlusion and the extent of necrosis.

✔ Diagnosis of MI is based primarily on the clinical picture, ECG findings, and elevation of serum enzymes. Medical interventions include promotion of improved coronary circulation and tissue oxygenation, relief of pain, and prevention of further tissue damage and complications.

✔ Thrombolytic agents to activate fibrinolytic processes to lyse the clot must be given within 3 to 6 hours after an initial infarction.

✔ Complications of MI include dysrhythmias, cardiogenic shock, CHF, ventricular aneurysm, postmyocardial syndrome, pericarditis, and embolism.

✔ Nursing interventions for MI include promoting oxygenation, tissue perfusion, adequate cardiac output, comfort, activity, nutrition, and elimination; providing rest; promoting relief of anxiety; and patient teaching. During cardiac rehabilitation, patients are encouraged to participate in a planned activity program.

✔ Congestive heart failure (CHF) refers to a state of circulatory congestion resulting from heart failure and its compensatory mechanisms. Symptoms may involve the pulmonary circulation, the systemic venous circulation, or both.

✔ Medical therapy for CHF consists of reducing oxygen requirements through oxygen therapy and rest, optimizing cardiac output with medications (digitalis, diuretics, vasodilators), and providing a sodium-restricted diet plan.

✔ Nursing interventions for CHF consist of providing oxygenation; promoting rest and activity, nutrition, and elimination; providing skin care and emotional support; and patient teaching.

✔ Pulmonary edema represents the most severe form of congestion resulting from left ventricular failure; it requires immediate medical and nursing intervention.

QUESTIONS TO CONSIDER

- How do pathophysiology and therapy differ among mitral and aortic stenosis and regurgitation?

- How would you explain to a patient the difference between congestive heart failure and myocardial infarction?

- What electrocardiographic criteria must be considered to differentiate myocarditis from an acute myocardial infarction?

- What nursing measures are crucial to limiting the size of the myocardial damage with an acute myocardial infarction?

- What important preventive nursing measures should be implemented for the patient receiving thrombolytic therapy?

REFERENCES AND SELECTED READINGS

1. *Alpert JS: The pharmacologic management of coronary artery disease in 1986, Heart Lung 15:558-561, 1986.
2. American Heart Association: Heart facts, Dallas, 1989, The Association.
3. American Heart Association: Heart valve surgery, Dallas, 1987, The Association.

*References preceded by an asterisk are particularly well suited for student reading.

4. American Heart Association: Textbook of advanced cardiac life support, Dallas, 1987, The Association.

5. *Bakanauskas A: Abdominal aortic aneurysms. In Von Ruedden, K: Case studies in critical care, Rockville, Md, 1989, Aspen Publishers.

6. Bergan J and Yao J: Aneurysms: diagnosis and treatment, New York, 1982, Grune & Stratton, Inc.

7. Berne RM and Levy MN: Cardiovascular physiology, ed 5, St Louis, 1986, The CV Mosby Co.

8. *Bitran E et al: Intraortic balloon counterpulsation in acute myocardial infarction, Heart Lung 10:1020-1027, 1981.

9. *Borders CR: When the bypass patient returns home: problems your bypass patients fare after discharge, Patient Care 19(13):65-76, 1985.

10. *Brannon P and Tower S: Ventricular failure: new therapy using the mechanical assist device, Crit Care Nurse 6(2):70-85, 1986.

11. Braunwald E: Heart disease: a textbook of cardiovascular medicine, ed 3, Philadelphia, 1988, WB Saunders Co.

12. *Cantwell JD: Exercise and coronary heart disease: role in primary prevention, Heart Lung 13:6-13, 1984.

13. Carpenito LJ: Nursing diagnoses: application to clinical practice, ed 2, Philadelphia, 1989, JB Lippincott Co.

14. Cavello G: Person with valvular disease. In Guzetta K and Dossey B: Bodymind tapestry, St Louis, 1984, The CV Mosby Co.

15. Chatterjee K: Ischemia, silent or manifest: does it matter? JACC 13:1503-1505, 1989.

16. *Cohen S: New concepts in understanding congestive heart failure. I. How the clinical features arise, Am J Nurs 81:119-142, 1981.

17. *Cohen S: New concepts in understanding congestive heart failure. II. How the therapeutic approaches work, Am J Nurs 81:357-380, 1981.

18. *Conti CR: Advances and controversies: laser therapy for cardiovascular disease, Heart Lung 16:465-473, 1987.

19. Cosgrove D et al: Results of mitral valve reconstruction, Circulation 74(suppl I):182-187, 1986.

20. *Deans K and Hartshorn J: Use of antithrombotic agents in valvular heart disease, J Cardiovasc Nurs 1(3):65-69, 1987.

21. DeBakey M et al: Surgical management of dissecting aneurysms of the aorta, J Cardiovasc Surg 49:130-149, 1965.

22. Diehl J et al: Complications of abdominal aortic reconstruction, Ann Surg 197:49-56, 1983.

23. Duncan C et al: Effect of chest tube management on drainage after cardiac surgery, Heart Lung 16:1-9, 1987.

24. Flameng W et al: Intermittent aortic cross-clamping versus St Thomas' Hospital cardioplegia in extensive aorta-coronary bypass grafting, J Cardiovasc Surg 88:164-173, 1984.

25. Fletcher GF: Exercise and exercise testing: current state of the art, Heart Lung 13:5-6, 1984.

26. Fletcher GF: Long-term exercise in coronary artery disease and other chronic disease states, Heart Lung 13:28-46, 1984.

27. Gottlieb SV: Ischemia as an indicator of future adverse events in patients with coronary artery disease, J Myocard Ischemia 1:20-28, 1989.

28. *Grady KL and Costanzo-Norden MR: Myocarditis: review of a clinical enigma, Heart Lung 18:347-354, 1989.

29. Groer MW and Shekleton ME: Basic pathophysiology: a holistic approach, ed 3, St. Louis, 1989, The CV Mosby Co.

30. Grunkmeier G and Starr A: Late ball variance with model 1000 Starr-Edwards aortic valve prosthesis, J Cardiovasc Surg 91:918-923, 1986.

31. Henderson E: Assessment of successful reperfusion after thrombolysis, Heart Lung 17:761-771, 1988.

32. Hurst AH: Mitral valve prolapse: physical assessment, complications, and management, Nurs Pract 10(4):15-17, 1985.

33. Hurst JW: The heart, ed 6, New York, 1986, McGraw-Hill Book Co.

34. Ismal M, Hannachi N, and Abid F: Prosthetic valve endocarditis, Brit Heart J 58:72-77, 1987.

35. Izor-Povenmire K and House MA: Acute crack cocaine intoxication: a case study, Focus Crit Care 16:112-119, 1989.

36. Jeffrey D et al: Results of coronary bypass surgery in elderly women, Ann Thoracic Surg 42:550-553, 1986.

37. *Johnston BL: Exercise testing for patients after myocardial and coronary surgery: emphasis on predischarge phase, Heart Lung 13:18-27, 1984.

38. *Kern K: Advances in the surgical treatment of coronary artery disease, J Cardiovasc Nurs 1(1):1-14, 1986.

39. Kinney M: Priorities in the nursing management of patients after open heart surgery, Curr Rev Recovery Room 5(5):35-40, 1983.

40. Kleven MR: Comparison of thrombolytic agents and mechanisms of action, efficacy and safety, Heart Lung 17:750-755, 1988.

41. *Kretten C and Bass L: Valvular heart disease, surgery, and postop care, RN 50(12):38-43, 1987.

42. Krone R: Valvular heart disease. In Ahumadr G: Cardiovascular pathophysiology, New York, 1988, Oxford University Press.

43. Loop F et al: Coronary bypass surgery: the total experience at the Cleveland Clinic Foundation, Clinical Essays Heart 2:131-138, 1984.

44. Loveys BJ: Physiologic effects of cocaine with particular reference to the cardiovascular system, Heart Lung 16:175-182, 1987.

45. *Lovvorn J: Coronary artery bypass surgery: helping patients cope with postop problems, Am J Nurs 82:1973-1075, 1982.

46. Magilliland D et al: The porcine bioprosthetic valve, J Thoracic Cardiovasc Surg 89:499, 1985.

47. *Marrie TJ: Infective endocarditis: a serious and changing disease, Crit Care Nurs 7(2):31-46, 1987.

48. McElliott M: Person undergoing cardiovascular surgery. In Guzetta K and Dossey B: Bodymind tapestry, St Louis, 1984, The CV Mosby Co.

49. *Misenski M: Pathophysiology of acute myocardial infarction: a rationale for thrombolytic therapy, Heart Lung 17:743-750, 1988.

50. *Painvin G et al: Cardiac transplantation: indications, procurement, operation, and management, Heart Lung 14:484-489, 1985.

51. *Parent D et al: Developing a cardiac teaching program, Can Crit Care Nurse 1(1):22-23, 1984.

52. *Penckofer S and Holm K: Hopes and fears after coronary artery bypass surgery, Prog Cardiovasc Nurs 2(4):139-146, 1987.

53. Reuvelta J et al: The Ionescu-Shiley valve: a solution for the small aortic root, J Thorac Cardiovasc Surg 88:234-237, 1984.

54. Roubin GS: Intracoronary stenting, percutaneous placement of intracoronary prostheses: new solutions and new problems, J Invasive Cardiol 1(1):1-6, 1988.

55. *Runions J: A program for psychological and social enhancement during rehabilitation after myocardial infarction, Heart Lung 14:117-125, 1985.

56. *Russell A and Blake S: Aortic valvuloplasty: potential nursing diagnoses, DCCN 8(2):72-82, 1989.

57. *Ruzevich SA, Swartz MT, and Pennington DG: Nursing care of the patient with a pneumatic ventricular assist device, Heart Lung 17:399-405, 1988.

58. Sakallares BR: Advances and controversies: laser therapy for cardiovascular disease, Heart Lung 16:464-473, 1987.

59. Sanborn TA: New interventional techniques for atherosclerotic disease, Prim Cardiol 15(8):21-28, 1989.

60. Schakenbach L: Physiological dynamics of acquired valvular heart disease, J Cardiovasc Nurs 1(3):1-17, 1987.

61. *Seifert P: Surgery for acquired valvular heart disease, J Cardiovasc Nurs 1(3):26-40, 1987.

62. Sheldon W and Loop F: Coronary artery bypass surgery: Cleveland Clinic experience 1967-1982, Postgrad Med 75(6):108-121, 1984.

63. Singh R and Taylor P: Use of the right mammary artery for coronary bypass, Vasc Surg 21(5):1-2, 1987.

64. *Spodick DH: Acute pericardial disease, Heart Lung 14:599-604, 1985.

65. Teoh K et al: Accelerated myocardial metabolic recovery with terminal warm blood cardioplegia, J Thorac Cardiovasc Surg 91:888-895, 1986.

66. Tyroler HA et al: Task force: environmental risk factors in coronary heart disease, Circulation 76(suppl I):I139-I144, 1987.

67. Urban P et al: Intravascular stenting for stenosis of aortocoronary venous bypass grafts, JACC 13:1085-1091, 1989.

68. *VanMeter M: Balloon flotation catheters today: what they tell you, why they're vital, RN 46:36-41, 1983.

69. *Weiland A: A review of cardiac valve prostheses and their selection, Heart Lung 12:498-504, 1983.

70. *Wenger N: Early ambulation, physical activity: myocardial infarction and coronary artery bypass surgery, Heart Lung 13:14-18, 1984.

71. *Whitman G: Prosthetic cardiac valves, Prog Cardiovasc Nurs 2:116-123, 1987.

72. Woodruff JF: Viral myocarditis, Am J Pathol 101:427-479, 1980.

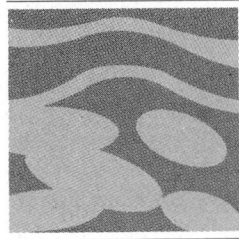

CHAPTER 29

Management of Persons with Peripheral Vascular Problems

M. EILEEN WALSH

CHAPTER OBJECTIVES

After studying this chapter, the student should be able to:
1. Identify risk factors associated with the development of peripheral vascular disorders.
2. Differentiate the pathophysiologic effects of arterial and venous disorders.
3. Describe the pathophysiology of and medical and nursing interventions for persons with arterial, venous, and arteriovenous disorders, and for those with leg ulcers and lymphedema.
4. Describe nursing interventions for persons having surgery for arterial or venous disorders.
5. Identify risk factors associated with hypertension, and describe the pathophysiology and management.

Problems of the peripheral vascular system include a variety of conditions that disrupt blood flow through the arteries and veins of the upper and lower extremities. This chapter excludes those disorders that affect blood flow in the coronary arteries and aorta (Chapter 28) and cerebral vessels (Chapter 62). The following disorders are discussed in this chapter:
1. Arterial disorders: arteriosclerosis obliterans, Raynaud's phenomenon, thromboangiitis obliterans, arterial embolism
2. Venous disorders: thrombophlebitis, varicose veins
3. Arterial and venous problems: arteriovenous fistulas, leg ulcers
4. Lymphedema
5. Hypertension

This chapter discusses lymphedema because the lymphatic system complements the function of the vascular system. Hypertension is also discussed because it is one of the major causes of peripheral vascular disorders.

INTRODUCTION TO PERIPHERAL VASCULAR PROBLEMS

To fully understand the causes and pathophysiologic changes of peripheral vascular disorders, it is important to know the normal structures and functions of the peripheral vascular system; a brief review follows.

STRUCTURE AND FUNCTION

Body cells depend on an intact and functioning vascular system. This vascular system is a closed circuit consisting of the systemic and pulmonary circulations. Blood circulates from the left side of the heart to the tissues and back to the right side of the heart. It then flows through the lungs and back to the left side of the heart. The main components of the vascular system are the arteries, capillaries, and veins.

ARTERIES

Arteries are thick-walled vessels that transport oxygen and blood via the aorta away from the heart and to the tissues. As the arteries approach the tissues, they branch into smaller vessels called arterioles (Figure 29-1). Arteries are composed of three tissue layers.
1. Inner layer of endothelium (intima)
2. Middle layer of connective tissue, smooth muscle, or elastic fibers (media)
3. Outer layer of connective tissue (adventitia)

The media forms the major part of the vessel wall. In the large arteries the media is primarily composed of elastic and connective tissue that enables the artery to respond to alteration of blood volume while maintaining a constant flow. There is much less elastic fiber in the smaller arteries and arterioles; these vessels have smooth muscle that contracts and relaxes via nervous, chemical, and hormonal factors.

CAPILLARIES

Capillaries, composed of a single layer of cells, are minute, thin-walled vessels located in the tissues. The capillaries connect the arterioles to the smallest veins and venules, allowing for the exchange of essential cellular products. Nutrients, oxygen, and regulatory substances move into the cells, whereas waste products, carbon dioxide, and cellular secretions move from the cells into the blood.

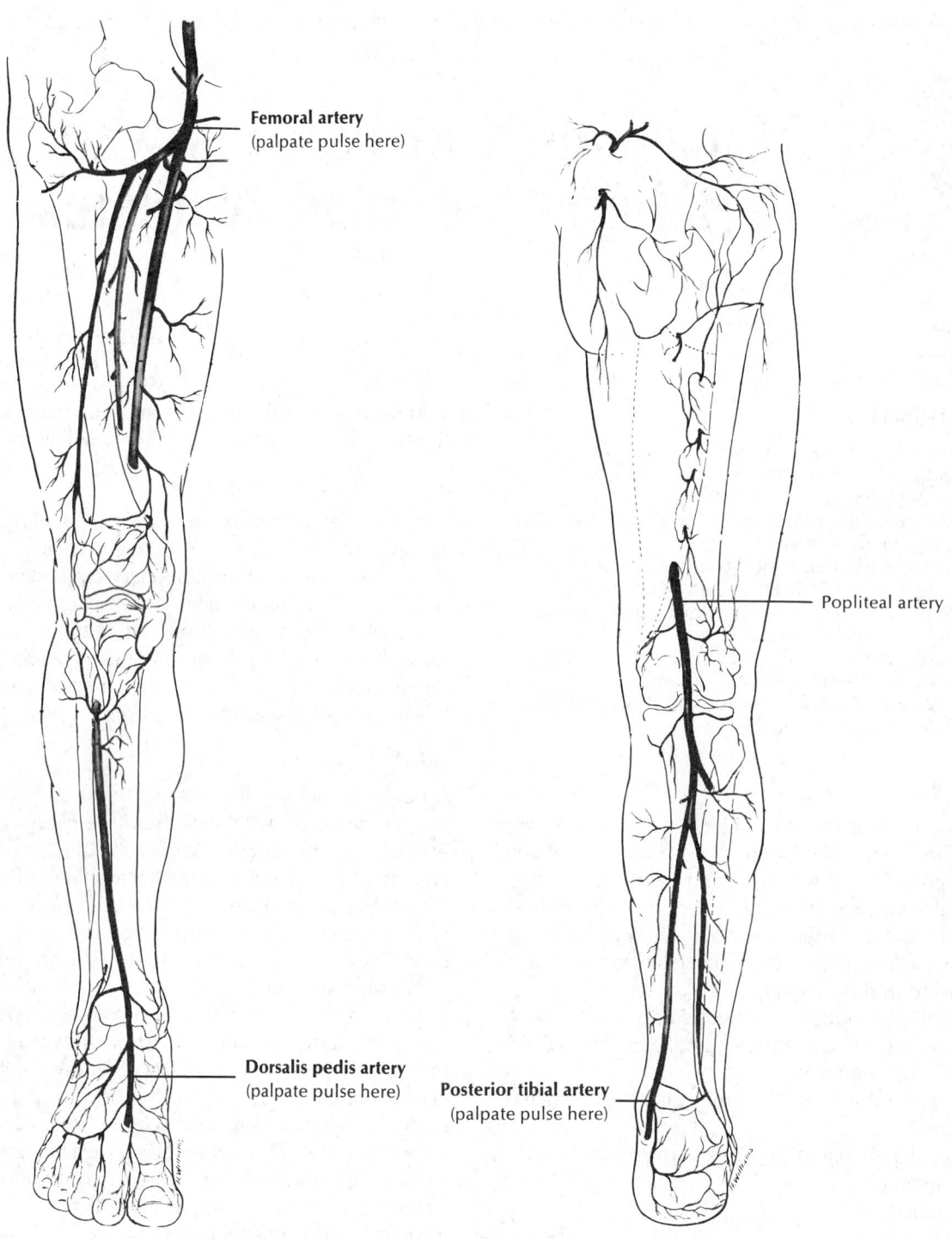

FIGURE 29-1 Arteries of the lower extremity. (Modified from Francis CC and Martin AH: Introduction to human anatomy, ed 7, St Louis, 1975, The CV Mosby Co.)

VEINS

Veins are thin-walled vessels that transport deoxygenated blood from the capillaries back to the right side of the heart. They are composed of three layers: intima, media, and adventitia. These layers differ from arterial walls in that there is little smooth muscle and connective tissue. This makes the veins distensible so that they can accumulate large volumes of blood. The sympathetic nervous system innervates the veins and causes venoconstriction, decreased venous volume, and increased circulating blood volume. Major veins, particularly those in the lower extremities, have one-way valves that allow blood flow against gravity.

EPIDEMIOLOGY/ETIOLOGY

All peripheral vascular disorders are characterized by a reduction in blood flow and hence oxygen through the peripheral vessels. As the need of the tissues for oxygen exceeds the supply, areas of ischemia and ultimately necrosis will develop. It is the extent to which the tissues are deprived of oxygen that gives rise to the manifestation of symptoms. Furthermore, the inherent ability of the vascular system to develop collateral circulation, or alternate circulatory pathways, affects this process.

Several factors can contribute to the development of peripheral vascular disorders. Pathologic changes within the blood vessels, including atherosclerotic changes, thrombus formation, and embolization, are the most common causes. Other factors such as increased coagulability of blood, blood pressure changes, and inflammatory processes affect peripheral circulation in some of these disorders. Heart failure can also impede peripheral blood flow from a reduction in cardiac output with resultant systemic venous congestion. Finally, mechanical or chemical trauma can be implicated in peripheral vascular disorders.

PATHOPHYSIOLOGY
PHYSIOLOGIC CHANGES WITH AGING

Degenerative changes occur in the vascular system as part of the normal aging process. These changes affect the walls of the blood vessels and can cause problems in the transport of blood and nutrients to the tissues. There is increased thickness in the intimal wall resulting from fibrosis. Further wall stiffness is caused by an accumulation of collagen and calcium in the intima and media. The elastic fibers of the media become thin and calcified. These changes greatly decrease the elasticity and flexibility of the vessels and hence increase peripheral vascular resistance. The result is a rise in blood pressure. There is less blood flow through the vessels, leading to a decreased supply of oxygen and nutrients to the tissues coupled with an accumulation in the tissues of cellular secretions, waste products, and carbon dioxide.

Atherosclerosis, a type of arteriosclerosis, occurs normally with aging and is characterized by the accumulation of fatty materials (lipids), fibrous tissues, and cell debris within the arterial wall, specifically the intimal wall.

Although the exact pathogenesis of atherosclerosis is unclear, the following specific changes occur:

1. Injury to the intimal cell wall causing increased cell permeability
2. Accumulation of smooth muscle cells and lipids that produce a fatty streak

3. Formation of fibrous plaque from smooth muscle cells, lipids, collagen fibers, and plasma components
4. Development of a complicated lesion from calcified fibrous plaque

The complicated lesion that is usually associated with complete arterial occlusion may rupture and greatly increase the risk of spasm, thrombus formation, and embolization. Fatty streaks primarily composed of cholesterol have been found in persons of all ages, although they do not necessarily progress to produce disease. The formation of the fibrous plaque is thought to be an irreversible process, and hence plaque is most characteristic of atherosclerosis. These atherosclerotic lesions primarily affect the larger arteries, particularly those in the descending aorta. Smaller arteries are usually impaired at their bifurcation. The coronary arteries are frequently affected (see Chapter 28). Atherosclerosis is more commonly seen in males.

EFFECTS OF ARTERIAL AND VENOUS INSUFFICIENCY

Disorders of the peripheral vascular system generally interfere with circulation to the tissues, leading to characteristic clinical manifestations. With *arterial* insufficiency, there is decreased blood flow to the tissues, producing *ischemia*. Pulses are usually diminished or absent, and sharp, stabbing pain occurs because of the ischemia, particularly with activity. There is interference with nutrients arriving to the tissues, leading to ischemic ulcers and changes in the skin (Table 29-1). In *venous* insufficiency, blood reaches the tissue but blood return to the heart is diminished, leading to venous *congestion* and *stasis*. Pulses are present. The venous congestion leads to edema, skin changes, and stasis ulcers.

PREVENTION
PRIMARY PREVENTION

Primary prevention is the most important means for reducing the incidence of peripheral vascular disorders. Nurses in all clinical settings can provide health education about the risk factors that affect development of peripheral vascular disorders. Because these disorders normally develop with advancing age, all individuals, and particularly older adults, can benefit from this information. The risk factors are similar to those associated with other forms of cardiovascular diseases (see the box on p. 740).

Cigarette smoking is one of the major contributory factors in the development of peripheral vascular problems. Nicotine causes vasoconstriction and spasms of the arteries, thus reducing circulation to the extremities. The carbon dioxide inhaled in cigarette smoke reduces oxygen transport to the tissues.

Hypertension causes the elastic tissue in the arteries

TABLE 29-1 Differentiating characteristics of arterial and venous disorders

Parameter	Arterial Disease	Venous Disease
Skin	Cool or cold; hairless, dry, shiny; pallor on elevation and rubor on dangling	Warm; tough, thickened; mottled, pigmented areas
Pain	Sharp, stabbing; worsens with activity and walking; lowering feet may relieve pain	Aching, cramping; activity and walking sometimes help; elevating feet relieves pain
Ulcers	Severely painful; pale, gray base; found on heel, lateral malleolus, toes, and dorsum of foot	Moderately painful; pink base, with irregular, pigmented skin edge; found on medial aspect of ankle
Pulses	Often absent or diminished	Usually present
Edema	Infrequent	Frequent, especially at end of day and in areas of ulceration

to be replaced by fibrous collagen tissue. This makes the arterial wall less distensible and increases the resistance to blood flow (p. 766).

Hyperlipidemia refers to the elevation of lipid levels, such as cholesterol and triglycerides, within the blood. Cholesterol and triglycerides contribute to the development of atherosclerotic plaque in the vessels (see Chapter 28).

Obesity, or excess body weight in relation to height (Chapter 42), places an added burden on the heart and blood vessels. Excess fat compromises blood vessels and contributes to increased venous congestion. Obese individuals are also more prone to physical inactivity, diabetes, hypertension, and hyperlipidemia.

Physical activity promotes muscle contraction and relaxation. It improves the return of venous blood to the heart by the pumping of muscle on the veins and aids in the development of collateral circulation, which is useful for venous return when veins are blocked. *Physical inactivity,* therefore, may compromise circulation.

Emotional stress stimulates the sympathetic nervous system and causes peripheral vasoconstriction. Stress can also cause increased cholesterol and platelet levels, decreased clotting time, and sustained high blood pressure.

The exact mechanisms by which *diabetes mellitus* contributes to the development of peripheral vascular disorders are unknown. The changes in glucose and fat metabolism are thought to affect the atherosclerotic processes.

RISK FACTORS FOR PERIPHERAL VASCULAR DISORDERS

Age (elderly)	Obesity
Sex (male)	Lack of exercise
Cigarette smoking	Emotional stress
Hypertension	Diabetes mellitus
Hyperlipidemia	Family history of atherosclerosis

SECONDARY PREVENTION

Secondary prevention is also important because peripheral vascular disorders can become chronic and potentially disabling diseases. Persons with peripheral vascular disorders are subject to periods of exacerbation and complications such as infection, injury, thrombosis, and amputation. Persons with early symptoms are encouraged to seek medical care. Increasing the person's knowledge of the specific disorder and preventing future occurrences is essential.

ARTERIAL DISORDERS

Any disturbance in the structure of the arteries interferes with transport of blood from the heart to the tissues. The symptoms of arterial disease are not caused by the degree of obstruction or narrowing but by the degree to which the involved body part is deprived of circulation. This in turn is affected by such factors as blood pressure and presence or absence of collateral circulation. The following arterial disorders are discussed: arteriosclerosis obliterans, thromboangiitis obliterans, Raynaud's phenomenon and disease, and arterial embolism.

ARTERIOSCLEROSIS OBLITERANS
EPIDEMIOLOGY/ETIOLOGY

Arteriosclerosis obliterans is a disorder in which there is segmented arteriosclerotic narrowing or obstruction of the tunica intima and tunica media. It is the most common cause of arterial obstructive disease in the extremities of individuals over 30 years of age. This disorder affects men more often than women, with clinical symptomatology evident in individuals between 50 to 70 years of age. The lower extremities are involved more frequently than the upper extremities. Common sites of this disease process include the femoral artery, iliac arteries, and popliteal arteries. The presence of diabetes mellitus has been found to further this disease process. In the diabetic, the disease becomes more progressive, affects the smaller arteries, and more often involves vessels below the knee.

PREVENTION

Health teaching for prevention of peripheral vascular disease is important. Persons at high risk are older persons, males, and persons with diabetes.

PATHOPHYSIOLOGY

The primary lesion of arteriosclerosis obliterans is plaque formation on the intimal wall that causes partial or complete occlusion. In addition, there is calcification of the media and a gradual loss of elasticity that further weakens the arterial walls and predisposes to aneurysmal dilation or thrombus formation.

As a result of these physiologic changes, the artery is unable to transport an adequate blood volume to the tissues during exercise or rest. Symptoms of arteriosclerosis obliterans gradually appear when the blood vessels can no longer provide enough blood to supply oxygen and nutrients and remove metabolic waste products.

CLINICAL MANIFESTATIONS

The most common symptom occurs with exercise and is termed *intermittent claudication*. This is pain that develops in a muscle that has an inadequate blood supply and is stressed during exercise. It is described as a cramp that disappears within 1 or 2 minutes after cessation of the exercise. This pain is usually bilateral but may be unilateral. The muscles of the calf are more frequently affected, since the femoral artery is often involved.

Pain at rest is indicative of severe disease. This pain is usually described as gnawing or burning, occurring more frequently at night. Accompanying symptoms such as feelings of coldness, numbness, and tingling may also be present. In advanced arteriosclerosis obliterans the ischemia may lead to necrosis, ulceration, and gangrene, particularly of the toes and distal foot.

Diagnostic Tests

Several tests may be indicated in the diagnosis of arteriosclerosis obliterans. Most of these tests are useful in the diagnosis of other disorders that affect the arterial system (Table 29-2). Noninvasive techniques include Doppler ultrasonography (Figure 29-2), segmental limb pressure, pulse volume recordings, and exercise testing.

MEDICAL MANAGEMENT

Medical management for arteriosclerosis obliterans is directed toward prevention of vessel occlusion. Drug therapy with vasodilators, although controversial, may be of benefit to some individuals. Surgical intervention is indicated for patients who have advanced peripheral vascular disease in which ischemic changes are present or for those whose pain severely impairs activities. These surgical procedures include embolectomy or endarterectomy, arterial bypass, percutaneous transluminal angioplasty, or amputation.

Embolectomy and Endarterectomy

An embolectomy is the removal of a blood clot and is most often used when large arteries are obstructed. An endarterectomy is the removal of a blood clot and stripping of atherosclerotic plaque along with the inner arterial wall (Figure 29-3).

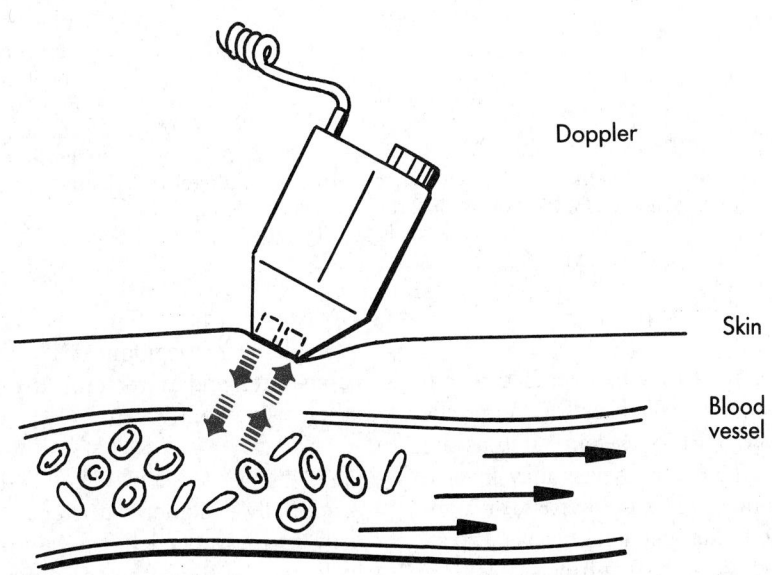

Doppler

Skin

Blood vessel

FIGURE 29-2 Doppler effect showing RBCs reflecting sound.

TABLE 29-2 Diagnostic tests for arterial disorders

Test	Purpose	Procedure	Comments
Doppler ultrasonography	Evaluate vascular network (arteries, veins) Measure blood flow through vessels Monitor status of bypass grafts	High-frequency sound waves directed to artery or veins through hand-held transducer moved evenly across skin surface; audible tone produced proportional to blood velocity	No discomfort experienced Noninvasive
Segmental limb pressure	Evaluate arterial occlusion	Systolic pressure readings from each limb segment obtained by pneumatic pressure cuffs and Doppler probe; readings compared	Noninvasive
Pulse volume recordings	Substantiate diagnosis of arterial stenosis and occlusion	Pneumatic pressure cuffs attached to extremities; pressure changes recorded by pressure transducer as wave forms during cuff inflation and deflation	Useful to assess areas such as foot and toes, not easily evaluated by segmental limb pressure
Exercise testing	Determine amount of exercise that precipitates ischemia and claudication	Ankle pressure, pulse volume, and blood pressure measured while person walks on treadmill at specific speed for about 5 min or until onset of leg pain	Exercise should be stopped at onset of pain
Radionuclide scan	Visualize vascular system and detect changes in blood vessels Assess arterial blood flow; determine perfusion pressure Identify arterial obstruction or vascular abnormality Determine patency of bypass graft	Injection of radionuclide followed by scanning of area at predetermined intervals to determine accumulation of radionuclide	Explain to patient that radiation dose is usually less than that received from diagnostic x-rays
Arteriography (angiography)	Visualize arterial system and detect vascular changes Assess arterial blood flow Identify arterial obstruction, vascular abnormality, or aneurysm	Dye inserted through catheter inserted into femoral or brachial artery, followed by x-ray films	Transient flushing and burning sensation felt when dye is inserted Post-test assessment includes the following: 1. Injection site for bleeding and hematoma 2. Peripheral pulses distal to site qh for 4-8h 3. Allergic reaction to dye (dyspnea, flushing, hives, nausea, vomiting) 4. Sensation distal to site Encourage patient to drink fluids to facilitate excretion of dye
Digital subtraction angiography	Visualize vascular system Determine presence and extent of occlusion	Dye injected through catheter inserted into blood vessel; x-ray signals are digitized	Same as for arteriography

Arterial Bypass Surgery

An obstructed arterial segment may be bypassed by using prosthetic material such as Teflon or Dacron or autogenous (the patient's own) artery or vein, such as the saphenous vein (Figure 29-3). The bypass may involve the aorta itself, as with an aortofemoral bypass, or more distal vessels such as the femoropopliteal bypass. Procedures that are performed either in conjunction with a bypass or by themselves include *patchgrafting* (replacing a damaged segment of the arterial wall with a vein patch) and endarterectomy using balloon catheters or other instruments.

Percutaneous Transluminal Angioplasty

A specially designed catheter is inserted under fluoroscopy and advanced to the site of the obstruction. The balloon tip of the catheter is inflated to provide compression and to rupture the atherosclerotic plaque. Throm-

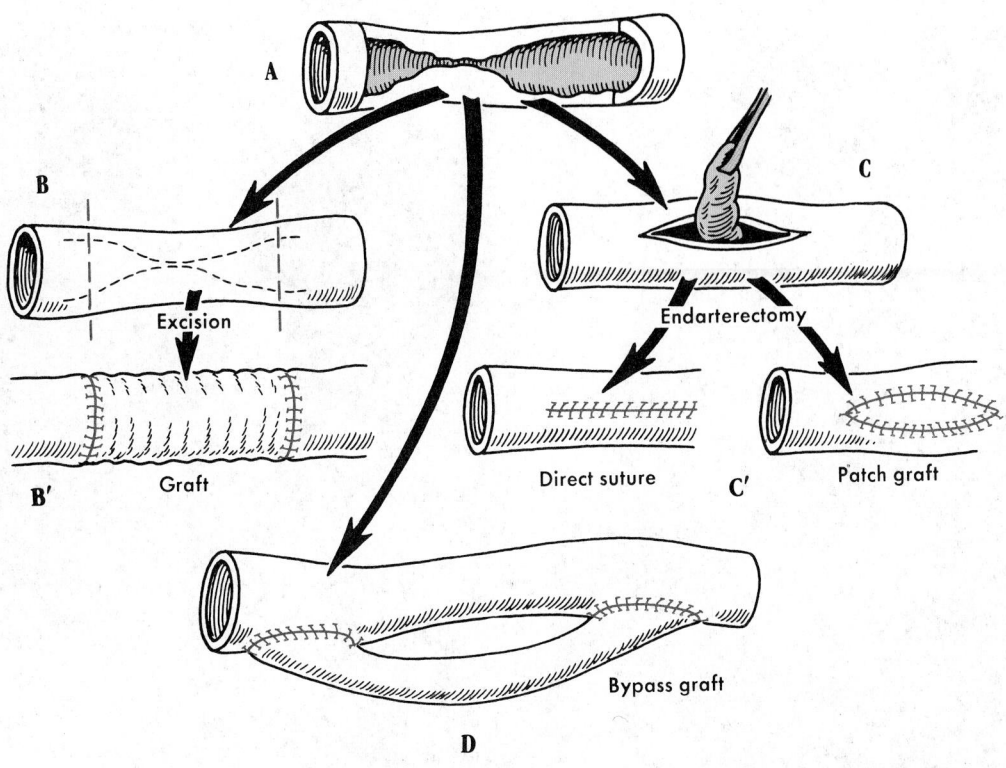

FIGURE 29-3 A, Obstructed artery. Methods of restoring arterial blood flow include: **B,** excision; **B′** graft; **C,** endarterectomy; **C′,** direct suture and patch graft reconstruction; and **D,** bypass graft. (Redrawn from Fairbairn JF et al: Peripheral vascular disease, Philadelphia, 1972, WB Saunders Co.)

bosis may occur after treatment; therefore anticoagulants are usually prescribed.

Amputation

Although a partial or complete amputation of an extremity may be necessary as a result of sarcoma or trauma, most amputations are indicated for patients with advanced atherosclerosis and gangrene of the extremities. The majority of amputations are of the lower extremity; the toes are the most often amputated part of the body. An amputation may also be offered as an option to improve functional ability with a prosthesis.

The surgical goal is to remove the least amount of tissue possible and to create a stump adequate for the fitting of a prosthesis. The specific level of the amputation is determined by the extent of the disease process. Below-knee (BK) amputations maintain knee function and allow for greater stability with a prosthesis. This type of amputation is usually performed in the lower third of the leg, leaving a 12 to 18 cm stump. An above-knee (AK) amputation may be made at any level, although it is frequently below the middle of the thigh to preserve an adequate stump for satisfactory use of a prosthesis (Figure 29-4). AK amputations are often indicated after unsuccessful BK amputations.

■ ASSESSMENT

Subjective data are collected about the perception of pain, associated factors, and relieving factors.

1. Gradual or sudden onset of pain in extremity, primarily in calf muscles (gradual or sudden occlusion)
2. Presence of pain while at rest or during exercise (extent of occlusion)
3. Type of pain: cramping, burning, gnawing
4. Changes noted in temperature of extremities: coldness (indicating obstruction)
5. Presence of additional symptoms indicating advanced stages of ischemia: numbness, tingling, pallor
6. Effect of relieving factors: rest, drug therapy

Objective data include observation of the skin, assessment of circulatory status, and presence of risk factors.

1. Condition of skin: shiny, taut, absence of hair growth (indicates poor circulation)
2. Ulcerations or necrotic tissue (advanced stages of ischemia)
3. Extremity cold to touch
4. Quality of peripheral pulses: diminished, weak, absent, bilateral inequality (Figure 29-5)
5. Prolonged (>3 sec) or absent capillary refill of nailbeds

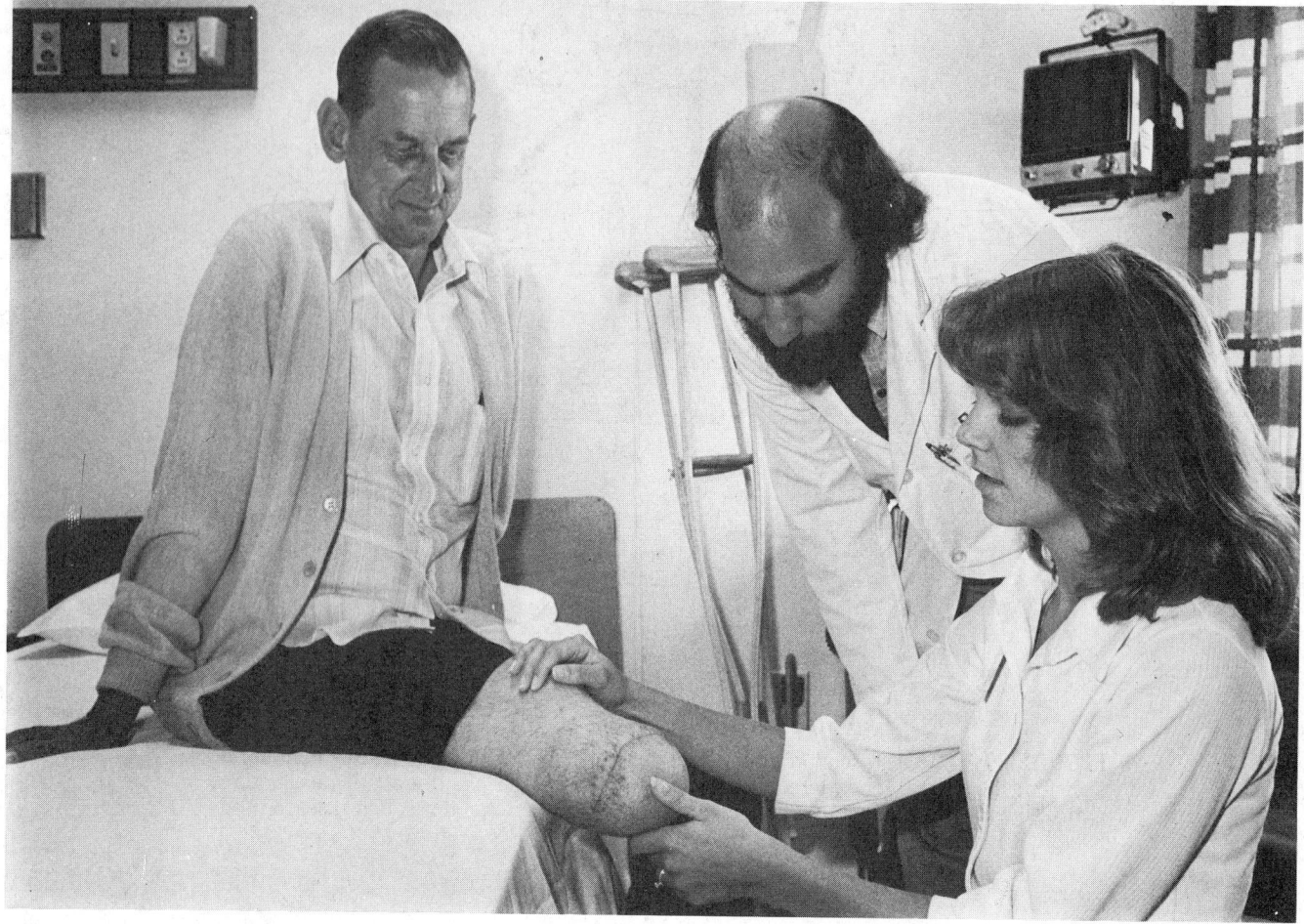

FIGURE 29-4 Nurse and physician examine the well-healed stump of a patient with AK amputation.

6. Loss of muscle tone or weakness
7. Presence of risk factors (see the box on p. 740)

■ DATA ANALYSIS: NURSING DIAGNOSES

Nursing diagnoses are determined from assessment of patient data. Possible nursing diagnoses for the person with arteriosclerosis obliterans may include, but are not limited to, the following:

Diagnostic Title	Possible Etiologies
Activity intolerance	Immobility, imbalance between oxygen supply/demand
Infection, potential for	Lack of knowledge
Injury, potential for	Sensorimotor deficit, lack of awareness of environmental hazards
Knowledge deficit: risk factors, medications, diagnostic test, surgery	Lack of exposure/recall, unfamiliarity with information sources
Pain: extremities	Ischemia of tissue
Skin integrity, impaired, potential	Ischemia, immobility
Tissue perfusion, altered, peripheral	Decreased arterial blood flow

■ PLANNING: EXPECTED PATIENT OUTCOMES

Expected patient outcomes for the person with arteriosclerosis obliterans may include, but are not limited to, the following:

1. Describes plans to participate in a regular exercise program or activity with adequate provision for rest
2. States measures to decrease potential risk for infection
3. Describes risk factors of arteriosclerosis obliterans and plan to modify these
4. Describes pharmacotherapy and postoperative surgical care, as appropriate
5. States that he or she experiences reduced pain
6. Describes measures to promote skin integrity and increase peripheral tissue perfusion

■ IMPLEMENTATION

Preventive Care

Actions to prevent further progression of existing disease are an important part of the care of the person with

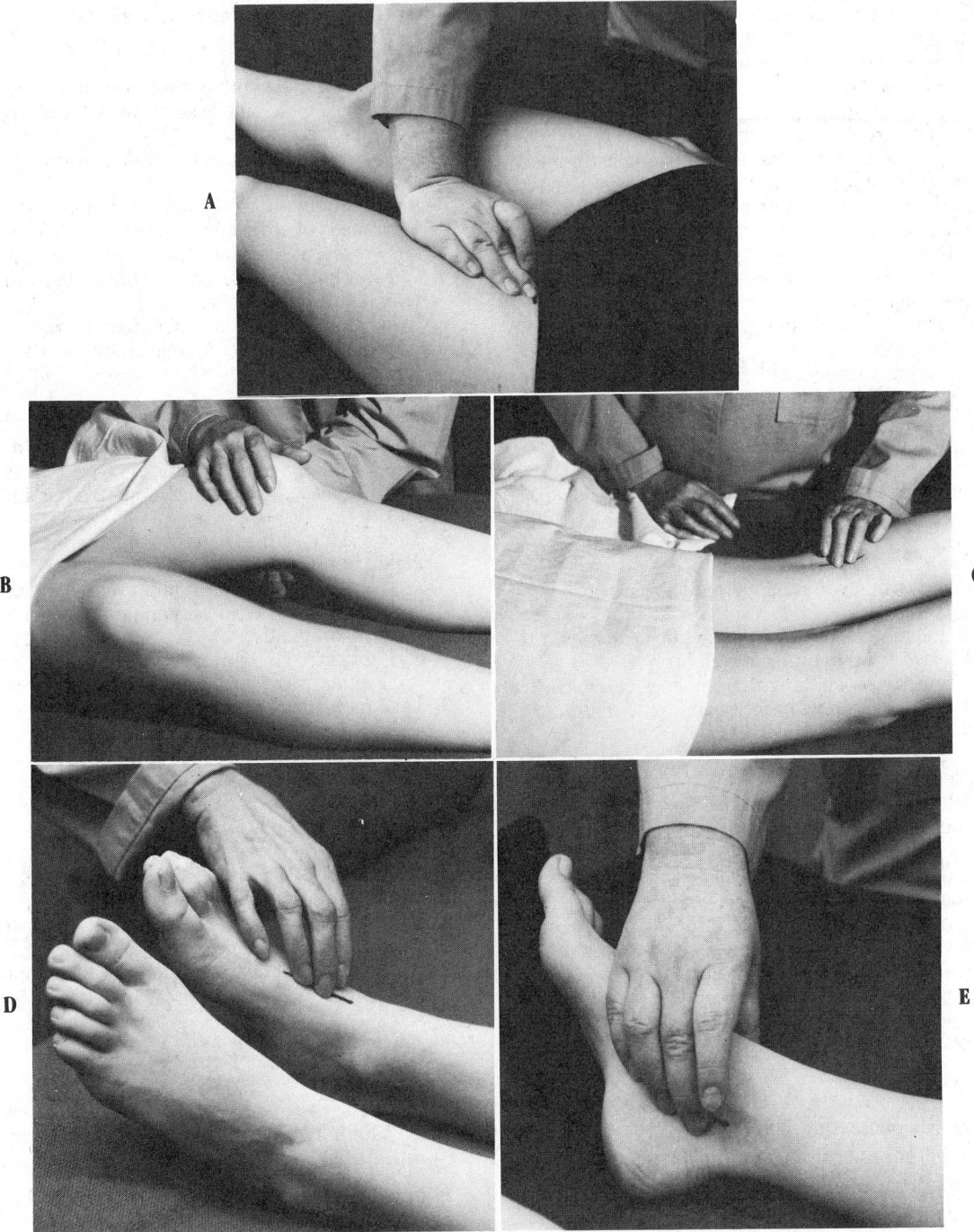

FIGURE 29-5 A, Palpation of femoral pulse. **B,** Palpation of popliteal pulse with patient in the dorsal recumbent position. **C,** Palpation of popliteal pulse with patient in the prone position. **D,** Palpation of dorsal pedal pulse. **E,** Palpation of posterior tibial pulse. (From Malasanos L et al: Health assessment, ed 4, St Louis, 1990, The CV Mosby Co.)

PREVENTIVE CARE FOR ARTERIAL DISORDERS

PROMOTING ACTIVITY AND REST

1. Engage in a regular aerobic exercise program (exercise stimulates collateral circulation and improves circulation through muscle contraction and relaxation).
   a. Include activities such as walking, swimming, jogging, or bicycling.
   b. Do 30-45 minutes of activity with warm-up and cool-down procedures on three alternate days.
2. Allow adequate time for rest between aerobic exercise program; walk at a slow pace on a daily basis.
3. Perform Buerger-Allen exercises on a daily basis:
   a. Lie flat with legs elevated above heart level for 2 to 3 minutes.
   b. Next sit for 2 to 3 minutes with legs relaxed and slightly dependent.
   c. Flex, extend, invert, and evert feet for 30 seconds in each position.
   d. Last, lie flat with legs at heart level and cover with warm blanket for approximately 5 minutes.
4. Avoid sitting positions that require full dependency of legs (contributes to venous congestion).
5. Perform other specific exercises such as ankle rotations, ankle pumps, and knee extension on a daily basis.

PROMOTING TISSUE PERFUSION

1. Maintain warm environmental temperature of 21° C (70° F).
2. Avoid chilling (causes vasoconstriction) and exposure to cold; layer clothing in cold weather.
3. Avoid constrictive clothing that impedes circulation: rolled garters, socks with tight banding, girdles, tight waistbands, and tight shoelaces.
4. Avoid crossing legs at knees (places pressure on arteries of legs).
5. Avoid sitting or standing for prolonged periods of time (impedes circulation through venous congestion).
6. Place legs in *slight dependency* (uses gravity to enhance tissue perfusion) and avoid elevation of legs (impedes arterial flow).
7. Quit smoking (nicotine causes vasoconstriction and vasospasms; inhaled carbon monoxide reduces oxygen-carrying capacity of blood).
8. Avoid pressure on affected extremity; use padding for severe ischemia.

9. Avoid vigorous massage of extremities (may promote embolus formation).
10. Engage in activities as specified above.

PREVENTING INJURY

1. Wear comfortable protective shoes at all times; alternate shoes on a daily basis to allow for airing.
2. Trim nails carefully.
   a. Cut at regular intervals; soak in warm water to soften nails.
   b. Use straight nail clippers; avoid using scissors.
3. Seek medical advice for thickened or deformed nails, blisters, corns, calluses, and ulcerations.
4. Check water temperature carefully; ability to sense temperature may be decreased.
5. Avoid scratching and rubbing feet to prevent abrasion.
6. Keep pathways in home free of clutter to avoid possible injury.

MAINTAINING SKIN INTEGRITY AND PREVENTING INFECTION

1. Assess skin on a daily basis for intactness, dryness, redness, and lesions; use mirror to inspect areas that are difficult to see, such as heels and plantar surface of toes.
2. Take a daily bath in tepid water (three times per week if skin is very dry).
   a. Use a neutral pH soap to prevent skin irritation.
   b. Wash gently; avoid scratching and vigorous rubbing.
   c. Dry skin gently.
   d. Lubricate skin with moisturizing agent; avoid using alcohol (dries skin).
3. Take meticulous care of feet.
   a. Bathe each toe and dry well.
   b. Use only prescribed foot powders.
   c. Wear clean cotton socks and change daily (synthetic fibers can cause irritation and do not absorb moisture).
4. Avoid wearing shoes that do not "breathe," such as those made of synthetic materials (prevents evaporation and contributes to fungal infections).
5. Avoid application of direct heat such as hot water.
6. Contact health care professional at onset of skin breakdown such as abrasions, lesions, or ulcerations.

---

arteriosclerosis obliterans. The focus of prevention is on activity and other measures to promote tissue perfusion, to get adequate rest between activities, to prevent injury and infection, and to maintain skin integrity (see the box above). Note that in the sitting position the legs should be kept *slightly dependent* (not fully elevated) to encourage optimal tissue perfusion with the aid of gravity yet avoid venous congestion.

Acute Care

Monitor the limb distal to the affected site for changes in color or temperature. When arterial flow is reduced,

skin is initially pale and cool; as blood flow reduction continues, the skin becomes bluish in light-skinned persons and darker or duller in dark-skinned persons. If blood flow ceases, tissue becomes necrotic and black.

Preventive measures should continue during acute episodes; activities that cause pain should be avoided. Give vasodilators, if prescribed, to provide relaxation of vascular smooth muscle. Explain to the patient that medications are to reduce the pain. Comfort measures include (1) an overbed cradle to protect the leg and foot from pressure of bed linens, (2) proper body positioning to decrease pressure on affected areas, and (3) a soft cotton bath blanket or acrylic pad directly under affected areas.

Postoperative Care for Arterial Surgery

After surgery such as embolectomy, endarterectomy, or arterial bypass surgery, the patient is monitored for signs of decreased circulation in the affected limb, and interventions are instituted to promote circulation and comfort. These activities include the following:

1. Assess and report changes in skin color and temperature distal to the surgical site (every hour for 12 hours, then q 2-4 h following arterial bypass surgery).
2. Assess peripheral pulses.
   a. Sudden absence of pulse may indicate thrombosis.
   b. Mark location of peripheral pulse with a pen to facilitate frequent assessment.
   c. Use a Doppler probe (Figure 29-2) if pulses are difficult to palpate.
3. Assess surgical wound for redness, swelling, and drainage.
4. Promote circulation.
   a. Reposition patient every 2 hours.
   b. Tell patient not to cross legs.
   c. Use a footboard and overbed cradle to keep linens off extremity.
   d. Encourage progressive activity when permitted.
5. Medicate with analgesics to reduce pain.

Additional interventions after *arterial bypass surgery* include the following:

1. Assess sensation and movement in the distal limb.
2. Monitor extremity for edema.
3. Monitor and report immediately signs of complica-

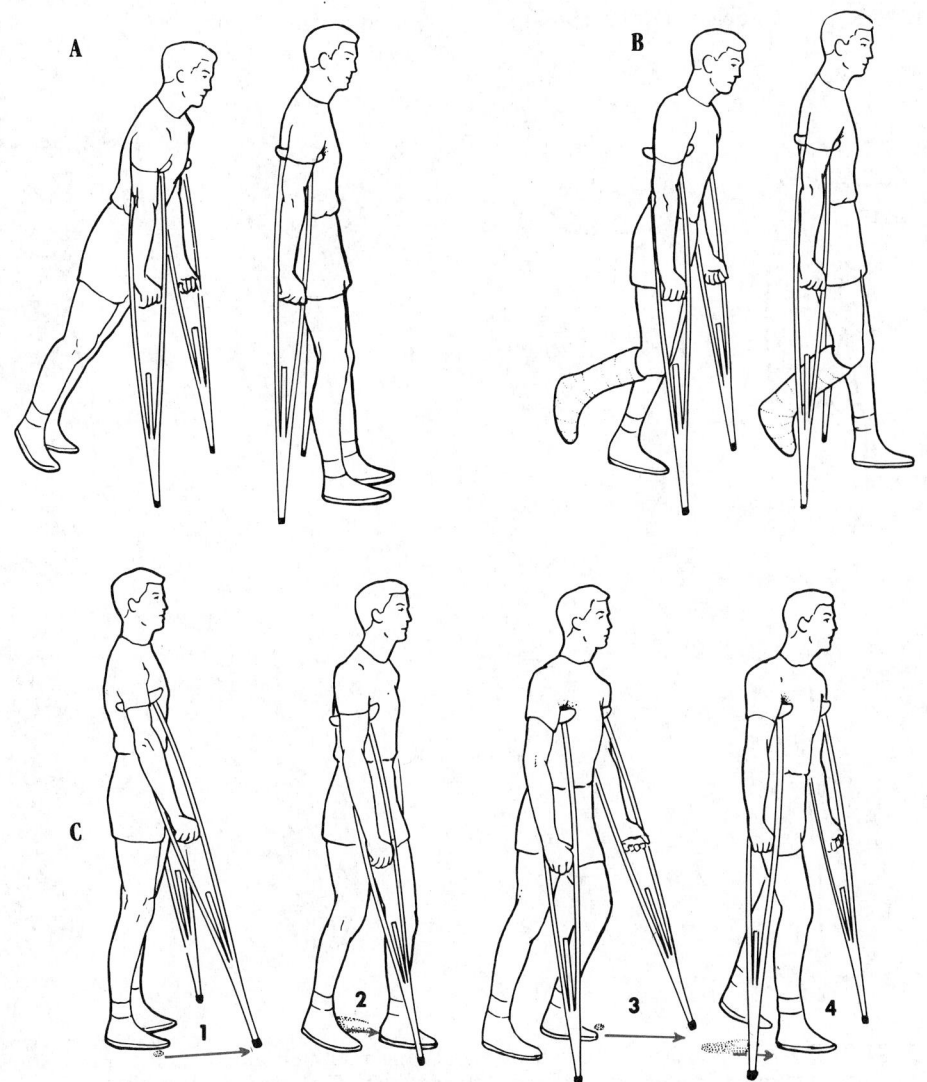

FIGURE 29-6 A, Swing-through gait. **B,** Swing-to gait. **C,** Four-point gait.

tions such as increasing pain, fever, and limitation of movement or paresthesia.

4. Avoid sharp flexion in the area of the graft to prevent decreased circulation to the graft.

Nursing Care of the Patient Undergoing Amputation

Preoperative care. Because of the seriousness of amputation and its impact on the patient, preoperative nursing care is of major importance. The two areas of greatest significance are the patient's emotional readiness for amputation and physical readiness for rehabilitation (postoperative exercises to strengthen arm and leg muscles).

The initial response on learning of the need for amputation is usually distress, anger, or grief. Loss of a leg means loss of ease of locomotion. Loss of an arm means difficulties in performing activities of daily living and other activities. Whether the amputation is sudden or planned, it will have an impact on the individual's *body image* (see Chapter 18.) The feedback or information re-

ceived from others concerning the impact of this body change is a major determinant of the success of the patient's efforts and resultant attitude. The nurse therefore must not only be sensitive to the patient's needs and questions but must also help the family or significant others work through their own feelings so that they can support the patient.

Phantom limb pain is the sensation that the painful limb is still present after amputation. The patient may have a sensation of tingling, burning, pressure, or pain in the absent limb postoperatively; the sensation is often similar to that experienced before the limb was removed. *Theories* regarding this sensation include interpretation in the cerebral cortex of stimuli from the nerve endings as similar to stimuli received before amputation or as patient feelings of guilt, anger, or denial expressed as pain. Patients should be told that most persons do experience some sensations postoperatively and that these will decrease, particularly if active postoperative rehabilitation is carried out.

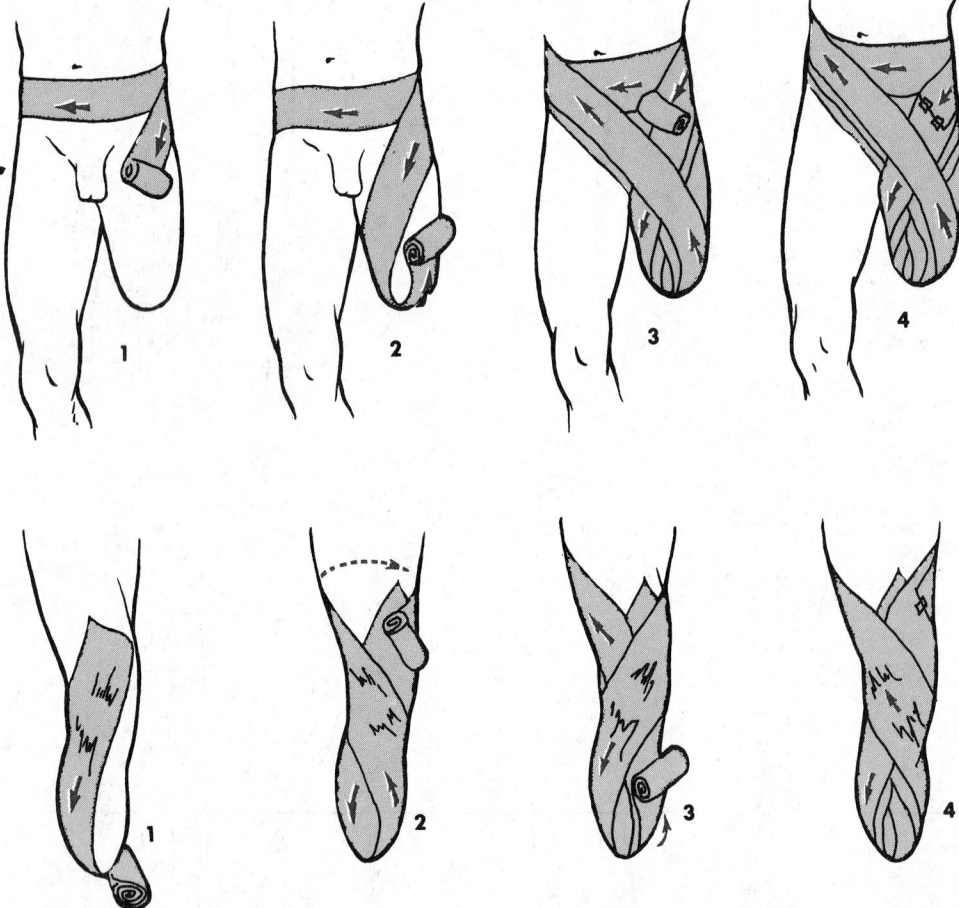

FIGURE 29-7 *Top,* Correct method for bandaging midthigh amputation stump. Note that bandage must be anchored around patient's waist. *Bottom,* Correct method for bandaging midcalf amputation stump. Note that bandage need not be anchored around the waist.

Preoperative interventions for amputation include the following:

1. Assess patient's and family's knowledge of the expected surgical procedure; answer questions and validate information.
2. Assist patient and family to express feelings, concerns, and fears; accept patient reaction of anger, discouragement, and grief.
3. Discuss possibility of phantom limb sensation.
4. Discuss and demonstrate postoperative regimen:
   a. Frequent repositioning to promote circulation
   b. Exercises to strengthen arm muscles for use of crutches: pushups and weight lifting
   c. Exercises to strengthen leg muscles to prevent knee and hip contractures and to promote ambulation: ankle rotations, ankle pumps, and quadriceps sets (Chapter 20)
5. Teach crutch walking (Figure 29-6), if appropriate (usually done by physical therapist).

Postoperative care. Chances for success with a BK amputation can be greatly improved by applying a rigid dressing that can be used with a temporary prosthesis to facilitate early ambulation. A rigid dressing may also be used with an AK amputation but is less effective. The rigid dressing also helps to prevent edema and trauma. Early ambulation is a psychologic boost for patient morale and facilitates early rehabilitation with fewer complications. Complications include nonhealing or infection of the stump, thromboembolism, and flexion contractures. Nursing interventions include the following:

1. Assess stump and monitor catheter drainage for color and amount; report signs of increased drainage.
2. Position patient with no flexion at hip or knee to avoid contractures; encourage prone position
3. Maintain patient in low-Fowler's or flat position following AK amputation.
4. Support stump with pillow for first 24 hours (according to physician preference and avoiding flexion); place rolled bath blanket along outer aspect to prevent outward rotation.
5. Encourage exercises to prevent thromboembolism.
   a. Active ROM of unaffected leg, ankle rotations and pumps
   b. Use of overhead trapeze when moving in bed
   c. Push-ups from sitting position and bed
   d. Quadriceps sets (Chapter 20)
   e. Lifting stump and buttocks off bed while lying flat on back to strengthen abdominal muscles
6. Teach care of stump.
   a. Inspect for redness, blister and abrasions.
   b. Wash stump with mild soap, rinse with water, and pat dry.

c. Avoid use of alcohol, oils, and creams.
d. Remove stump bandage or stump sock and reapply as needed; use firm smooth figure-eight ace wrapping (Figure 29-7) to reduce swelling and shape stump (if rigid dressing not used).

7. Encourage patient to ambulate using correct crutch-walking technique.
   a. Keep elbows extended; limit elbow flexion to 30° or less.
   b. Avoid pressure on axilla.
   c. Bear weight on palms of hands, not on axilla.
   d. Maintain upright posture (head up, chest up, abdomen in, pelvis in, foot straight (Figure 29-8).
8. Monitor patient's ability to use a prosthesis (Figure 29-9).

THROMBOANGIITIS OBLITERANS
EPIDEMIOLOGY/ETIOLOGY

Thromboangiitis obliterans (Buerger's disease) is an obstructive arterial disorder caused by segmented inflam-

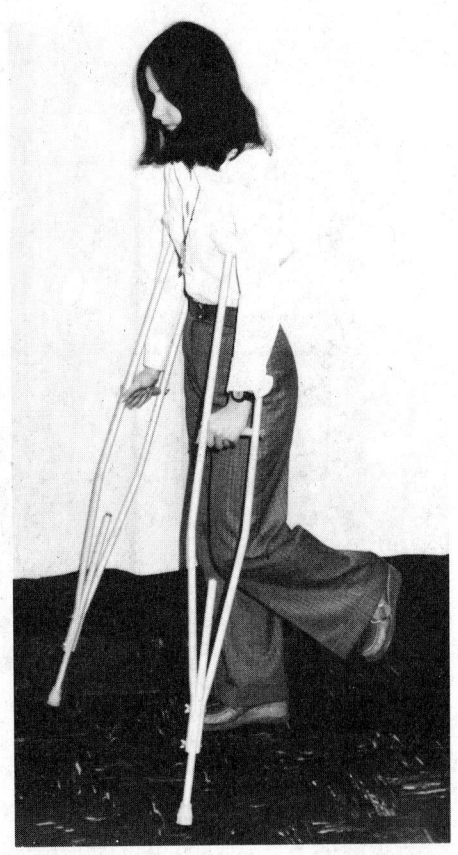

FIGURE 29-8 Axillary crutches are ambulatory aids best used by young persons or persons with good motor ability, particularly if the patient is nonweightbearing on one leg. This patient has good balance and erect posture.

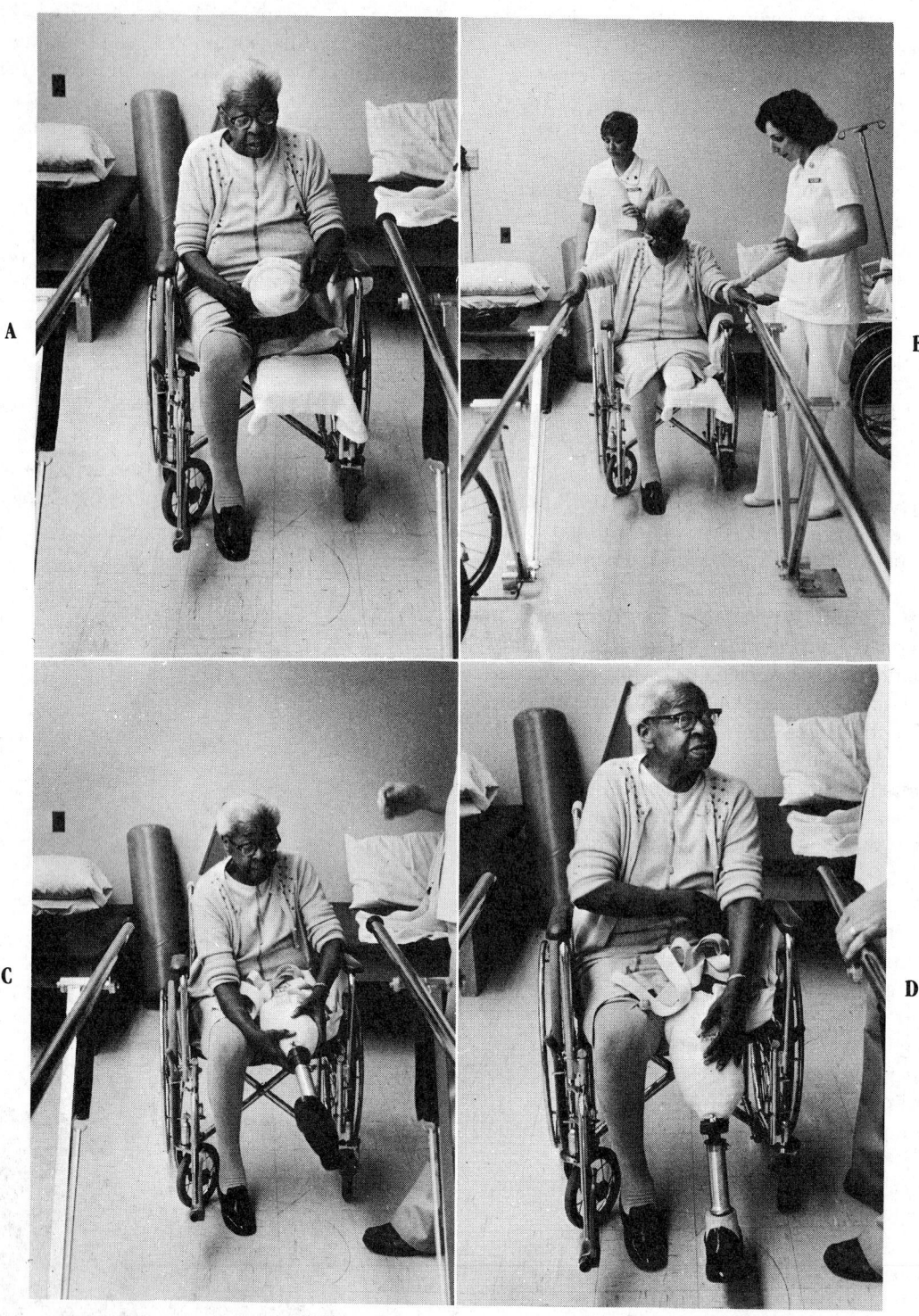

FIGURE 29-9 A, Patient uses care in putting on stump sock. **B,** Patient makes sure that she is close enough to bars to have secure grip. Note smooth fit of socks. **C,** Prosthesis is slipped over sock. **D,** Patient seeks more information about buckle on prosthesis.

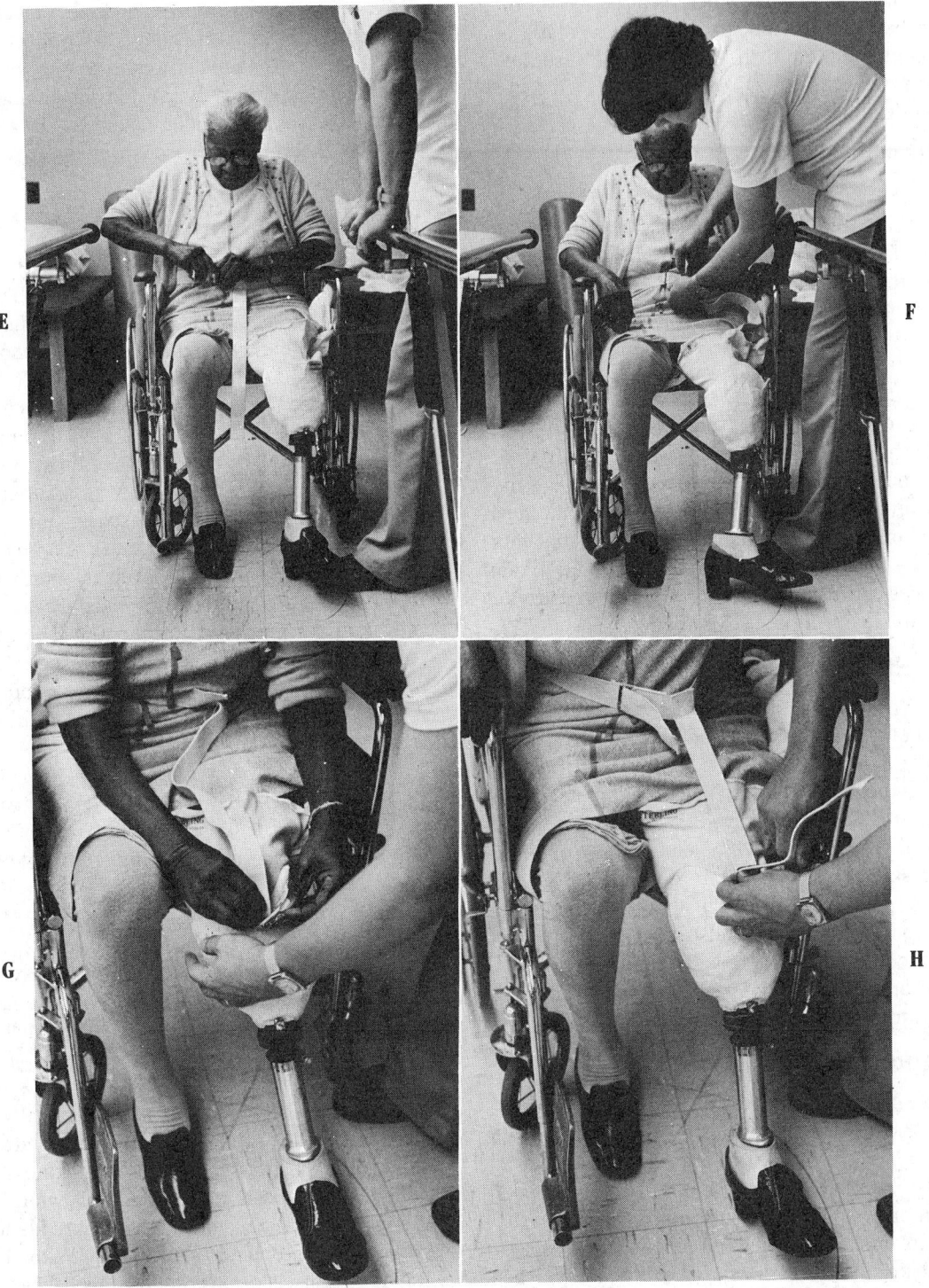

FIGURE 29-9, cont'd E, Belt is secured around waist. **F,** Fit of belt is checked. It must be secure enough to support weight of prosthesis but loose enough for comfort. **G,** Strap is buckled to prosthesis. **H,** Length of strap is adjusted.

mation in the arteries and veins. This disorder typically occurs in men between the ages of 20 and 40 and has been reported in all races, with a higher prevalence in Israel, the Orient, and India. There is also a very strong association between thromboangiitis obliterans and cigarette smoking. Although the cause of the disorder is unknown, a hypersensitivity reaction to tobacco and an alteration in cellular and humoral immunity have been suggested.

PREVENTION

Health teaching about risk factors associated with development of peripheral vascular problems (p. 740) is essential in the prevention of thromboangiitis obliterans. High risk factors include race (see above), sex (male), and cigarette smoking.

PATHOPHYSIOLOGY

In contrast to arteriosclerosis obliterans, this disorder develops in the small arteries and veins, primarily in the feet and hands although the wrists and lower leg may also be involved. The main characteristic is inflammatory infiltration of vessel walls. Different segments of arteries may be involved, becoming occluded. The inflammatory process is intermittent, and the occluded arteries may recannulize during quiescent periods.

CLINICAL MANIFESTATIONS

The most common symptom is pain that results from ischemic changes. Pain with exercise in the arch of the foot or instep claudication may be present. Calf claudication is an atypical finding, since the femoral and popliteal arteries are not involved. With involvement of the hands the pain is usually bilaterally symmetric. Changes in skin color or temperature, sensitivity to cold, and ulcers or gangrene of the digits may be present. Superficial thrombophlebitis may also exist.

Diagnostic tests may include arteriography, digital subtraction angiography, Doppler ultrasonography, and exercise testing (see Table 29-2).

MEDICAL MANAGEMENT

The goal of medical management is to halt further progression of the disease. A major effort is directed toward modification of risk factors; the primary focus is on reducing cigarette smoking because it is directly related to progression of symptoms. Drug therapy using vasodilators is controversial. Vasodilators affect healthy vessels and thus cause blood to flow to healthy rather than compromised tissues. *Surgery* may be indicated in some cases. A sympathectomy, removal of sympathetic ganglia and nervous tissues to eliminate vasospasms, may be performed. In advanced stages amputation of ulcerated fingers or toes may be necessary.

NURSING MANAGEMENT

Nursing care of persons with thromboangiitis obliterans is similar to that for persons with other types of arterial disorders. These activities include preventing injury, promoting tissue perfusion and comfort, and patient teaching. The patient is monitored for signs of thrombophlebitis (redness, heat) and for changes indicating arterial obstruction (pallor, coldness). In addition, interventions to prevent vasoconstriction (p. 753) are instituted.

RAYNAUD'S PHENOMENON AND DISEASE
EPIDEMIOLOGY/ETIOLOGY

Raynaud's phenomenon is a condition characterized by episodic arterial spasms of the extremities, predominantly of the hands. Raynaud's phenomenon is the term used to connote that it is a disorder secondary to another disease process, for example, occlusive arterial diseases, connective tissue disease, trauma from occupational hazards, or neurogenic lesions. When this phenomenon occurs in the absence of another vascular insult, it is termed Raynaud's disease.

Raynaud's disease, the most common cause of Raynaud's phenomenon, develops more frequently in women between 20 and 40 years of age and is more prevalent during the winter months. The exact cause of this is unknown, although immunologic factors, alterations in sympathetic innervation, emotional stress, and a hypersensitivity to cold have been postulated.

PREVENTION

As with other arterial disorders, health teaching about prevention, particularly to young females living in cold climates, is important to modify the effects of this disorder.

PATHOPHYSIOLOGY

Few pathologic changes occur in the early stages. With advancing stages of the disease, the intimal wall thickens, and there is hypertrophy of the medial wall.

CLINICAL MANIFESTATIONS

Individuals with Raynaud's disease typically complain of chronically cold hands and feet. During arterial spasms sluggish blood flow causes pallor, coldness, numbness, cutaneous cyanosis, and pain. Following the spasms, the involved area becomes intensely reddened, with tingling and throbbing sensations. With longstanding Raynaud's disease, ulcerations can develop on the fingertips and toes.

A cold stimulation test is used to diagnose Raynaud's phenomenon. Skin temperature changes are recorded by a thermistor attached to each finger. The patient's hand is submerged in an ice-water bath for 20 seconds, and ongoing temperature recordings are obtained. A comparison is then made with baseline values.

MEDICAL MANAGEMENT

Medical management is primarily aimed at prevention. The person is advised to protect against exposure to cold and to quit smoking. Drug therapy with calcium antagonists, vascular smooth muscle relaxants, and vasodilators may be prescribed to promote circulation and reduce pain. Biofeedback techniques to increase skin temperature and thereby prevent spasms have been beneficial in some cases. A sympathectomy may be indicated to relieve symptoms in the early stage of advanced ischemia. If ulcerations and gangrene occur, the involved area may need to be amputated.

NURSING MANAGEMENT

Nursing care of persons with Raynaud's phenomenon or disease is similar to that for patients with other arterial disorders. Data collection includes the effect of associated factors (emotional stress, exposure to cold, cigarette smoking) and the effect of relieving factors such as warmth. In addition to interventions to prevent injury and promote tissue perfusion and comfort, the following interventions are emphasized:

1. Teach patient the effects of smoking on arterial flow (nicotine causes vasoconstriction); recommend techniques such as behavior modification, stimulus control, biofeedback, nicotine gum, and hypnosis to quit smoking.
2. Discuss ways of avoiding exposure to cold.
   a. Wear adequate clothing to promote warmth.
   b. Layer clothes as needed.
   c. Wear gloves and socks during winter months.
   d. Use caution when cleaning refrigerator and freezer.
   e. Wear gloves when handling frozen foods.
   f. Avoid occupations that require constant exposure to cold.
3. Caution patient to avoid drugs that will cause vasoconstriction, such as birth control pills, β-adrenergic blockers, and ergotamines.
4. Suggest antiinflammatory analgesics to promote comfort.

ARTERIAL EMBOLISM
EPIDEMIOLOGY/ETIOLOGY

Arterial emboli are blood clots floating in the circulating arterial blood. These clots most commonly originate in the heart as a result of atrial fibrillation, myocardial infarction, congestive heart failure, or vascular disease, and have been associated with anemia and dehydration. Arterial emboli also tend to develop in individuals who are immobile for long periods.

PATHOPHYSIOLOGY

A blood clot, or thrombus, may become detached from the site of origin and travel through the arterial circulation. The embolus is frequently a fragment of arteriosclerotic plaque loosened from the aorta. Emboli tend to lodge in the bifurcation of arteries, especially in the femoral or popliteal arteries. Blood flow to sites distal to the lodged embolus is impaired and ischemia ensues.

CLINICAL MANIFESTATIONS

The signs and symptoms of arterial embolism depend on the size of the embolus, the presence of collateral circulation, and the proximity to a major organ. There is an abrupt onset of severe pain from the sudden cessation of circulation. Muscular weakness and burning, aching pain occur distal to the occlusion. Distal pulses are absent, and the extremity becomes cold, numb, and pale. Signs and symptoms of shock may develop if a saddle embolus blocks a large artery.

MEDICAL MANAGEMENT

Medical therapy for acute arterial embolism includes bed rest, drug therapy, treatment for shock (Chapter 25), and surgery. *Anticoagulants* (heparin and warfarin sodium) (Table 29-3) prolong the clotting time of the blood and are used to prevent clot extension and new clot formation. *Fibrinolytics*, or thrombolytics, (Table 29-4) are useful for dissolving existing thrombi when rapid dissolution of the clot is required to preserve organ and limb function. Streptokinase and urokinase impair hemostasis by increasing fibrinolytic activity. After the infusion of fibrinolytics, the patient is started on heparin or oral anticoagulants to prevent extension of existing clots or formation of new clots. Blood or blood products may be used to counteract effects of a fibrinolytic if hemorrhage occurs. Aminocaproic acid, a fibrinolysis inhibitor, may be given.

An *embolectomy*, the removal of a blood clot, is most often used when large arteries are obstructed. The success of the surgery depends on the length of time the extremity was ischemic. Surgery must be performed within 6 to 10 hours to prevent muscle necrosis and loss of the extremity. An endarterectomy may also be performed (p. 741).

NURSING MANAGEMENT

Monitor the patient during the acute phase for changes in skin color and temperature of the extremity distal to the embolus. Increasing pallor, cyanosis, or coldness of the skin indicates vessel occlusion. Keep the extremity warm but do not apply heat; avoid chilling. Also monitor the peripheral pulses for presence, quality, and bilateral symmetry.

Keep the patient on complete bed rest to prevent fur-

TABLE 29-3 Anticoagulants used in treatment of vascular disorders

Drug	Action	Dosage	Side Effects
Heparin	Forms complex with antithrombin III which inhibits thrombin action Intravenous route produces immediate action; duration is 2 h Subcutaneous route used for maintenance and prophylaxis	Intravenous: Loading dose 5000 U Continuous drip: 20,000-30,000 U/day at 0.5 U/kg/min in 5% dextrose or NS Intermittent: initial loading dose, then 5000-10,000 U q4h Subcutaneous: 5000 U 2 h before surgery and every 8-12 h thereafter Other: 10,000-12,000 U q8h 14,000-20,000 U q12h NOTE: dosage adjusted to maintain APTT at 2-2.5 times laboratory control Normal APTT = 33-45 sec Prolonged APTT = 60-100 sec	Hemorrhage, spontaneous bleeding, epistaxis, bleeding gums, hematoma, GI bleeding with black tarry stools
Warfarin sodium (Coumadin, Panwarfin)	Inhibits vitamin K dependent clotting factor synthesis (factors II, VII, IX and X) Depresses prothrombin activity Peaks in 36-72 h Duration is 2-5 days	Oral 10 to 15 mg/day until prothrombin time within therapeutic range Then 2 to 10 mg/day NOTE: dosage adjusted to maintain prothrombin time (PT) at 1.2 to 1.5 times laboratory control Normal PT = 11-12 sec Prolonged PT = 17-19 sec	Same as for heparin

ther progression of the embolism. Keep the affected extremity flat or in a slight dependent position to promote circulation, as indicated by the physician. Use an overbed cradle to protect the affected extremity from pressure of bed linens. Monitor anticoagulant and fibrinolytic therapy and assess for bleeding (see the box at the top of p. 755).

Patient teaching following the acute phase of arterial embolism includes information regarding measures to prevent further arterial problems (see the box on p. 746). Additional teaching is related to oral anticoagulant therapy (see the box at the bottom of p. 755).

VENOUS DISORDERS

Venous problems arise when there is alteration in the transport of blood from the capillary beds back to the heart. Changes in smooth muscle and connective tissue make the veins less distensible with limited recoil capacity. Valves in the veins may malfunction, causing

TABLE 29-4 Fibrinolytics used in treatment of vascular disorders

Drug	Action	Dosage	Side Effects
Streptokinase (Streptase, Kabikinase)	Synthetic protein derived from streptococcal bacteria Activates plasminogen by forming streptokinase-plasminogen complex	IV: Loading dose 250,000 IU over 30 min Then 100,000 IU/h for 24-72 h (arterial thrombosis) or 72 h (deep vein thrombosis)	Bleeding, bronchospasm, rash, urticaria
Urokinase (Abbokinase, Breokinase, Win-Kinase)	Human proteolytic enzyme derived from cultured kidney cells Directly converts circulating plasminogen to plasmin	IV: Loading dose 4100 IU/kg over 10 min Then 4400 IU/kg/h for 12-24 h	Same as for streptokinase

GUIDELINES FOR CARE OF THE PERSON RECEIVING ANTICOAGULANT OR FIBRINOLYTIC THERAPY

1. Monitor the infusion accurately; maintain desired therapeutic rate of units per minute or hour.
2. Assess skin for signs of bleeding: bleeding gums, nosebleeds, petechiae (pinpoint red areas on skin), ecchymosis (bruising), hematoma formation, and venipuncture sites.
3. Monitor urine, stool, emesis, and gastric secretions for blood.
4. Avoid administration of medications by intramuscular route to prevent bleeding.
5. Avoid unnecessary bleeding.
   a. Use a soft toothbrush and brush teeth gently.
   b. Use an electric razor rather than razor blade for shaving.
   c. Avoid use of rectal thermometers (may cause mucosal bleeding).
6. Special care with *anticoagulant therapy*
   a. Give heparin by deep subcutaneous injection; use a fine gauge needle at a 90 degree angle; do not aspirate nor massage site after injection (can result in bleeding); rotate sites on a regular basis.
   b. Administer protamine sulfate, if necessary, as a heparin antagonist to reverse anticogulant effects.
   c. Hold pressure for 3 to 5 minutes on venipuncture sites.
   d. Monitor results of blood work: a partial thromboplastin time should be 2 to 3 times normal level (normal APTT is 33 to 45 seconds); a prothrombin time (PT) should be 1.2 to 1.5 times normal level (normal PT is 11 to 12 seconds).
   e. Avoid use of aspirin; aspirin inhibits platelet adhesion, thus having an anticoagulant effect.
7. Special care with *fibrinolytic therapy*
   a. Assess patient for signs of intracranial bleeding: headache, vomiting, disorientation, mental confusion.
   b. Assess patient for signs of retroperitoneal bleeding: low back pain, muscle weakness, or numbness in lower extremity.
   c. Assess patient for allergic reaction: chill, bronchospasm, rash, malaise; an IV steroid may be given to counteract potential allergic reaction.
   d. Avoid insertion of unnecessary venous and arterial lines; insert before initiation of therapy if necessary.
   e. Hold pressure on all venipuncture or other bleeding sites for 20 to 30 minutes to promote blood clotting.
   f. Give antiulcer medication, if prescribed, as a prophylactic measure.

---

backflow of blood. The major venous disorders are thrombophlebitis and varicose veins.

THROMBOPHLEBITIS
EPIDEMIOLOGY/ETIOLOGY

Thrombophlebitis is a common disorder more frequently occurring in women. It affects people of all races, and the incidence increases with advancing age. The primary factors associated with the development of thrombophlebitis include venous stasis, damage to the vessel wall, and hypercoagulability of the blood. This disorder is common in hospitalized patients, particularly those who have undergone major surgery (especially pelvic surgery and total hip replacement) or who have sustained a myocardial infarction. Hypercoagulability may also occur with the use of oral contraceptive drugs (especially in women over age 30) and with adenocarcinoma.

TEACHING THE PATIENT ON ORAL ANTICOAGULANT THERAPY

1. Know general action and side effects of oral anticoagulants and drug interactions (such as with aspirin).
2. Take oral anticoagulant at the same time every day; do not stop taking it unless advised by physician.
3. Inspect for signs of bleeding (bleeding gums, nosebleeds, bruising, red areas on skin, cuts that do not stop bleeding, blood in urine or stool); report these signs promptly to health care professional.
4. Wear a Medic Alert bracelet or carry an identification card containing the drug name, dosage, and physician name and phone number in case of emergency.
5. Have the prescribed blood tests (APTT, PT) that are used to adjust drug dosage on a regular basis.
6. Reduce intake of dark green and yellow vegetables, which are sources of vitamin K (counteracts the anticoagulant effects of coumadin).
7. Refrain from alcohol intake (increases anticoagulant effects).

PATHOPHYSIOLOGY

Thrombophlebitis develops in both the deep and superficial veins of the lower extremity. The most common deep veins affected are the femoral, popliteal, and small calf veins. The saphenous vein (Figure 29-10) is a frequent site of superficial thrombophlebitis.

Thrombi form in the veins from the accumulation of platelets, fibrin, WBCs and RBCs. Deep vein thrombophlebitis (DVT) tends to occur at bifurcations of the deep veins, which are sites of turbulent blood flow. A major risk during the acute phase of thrombophlebitis is dislodgement of the thrombus, forming an embolus. A pulmonary embolus (Chapter 33) is a frequent and serious complication arising from DVT of the lower extremities (Figure 29-11).

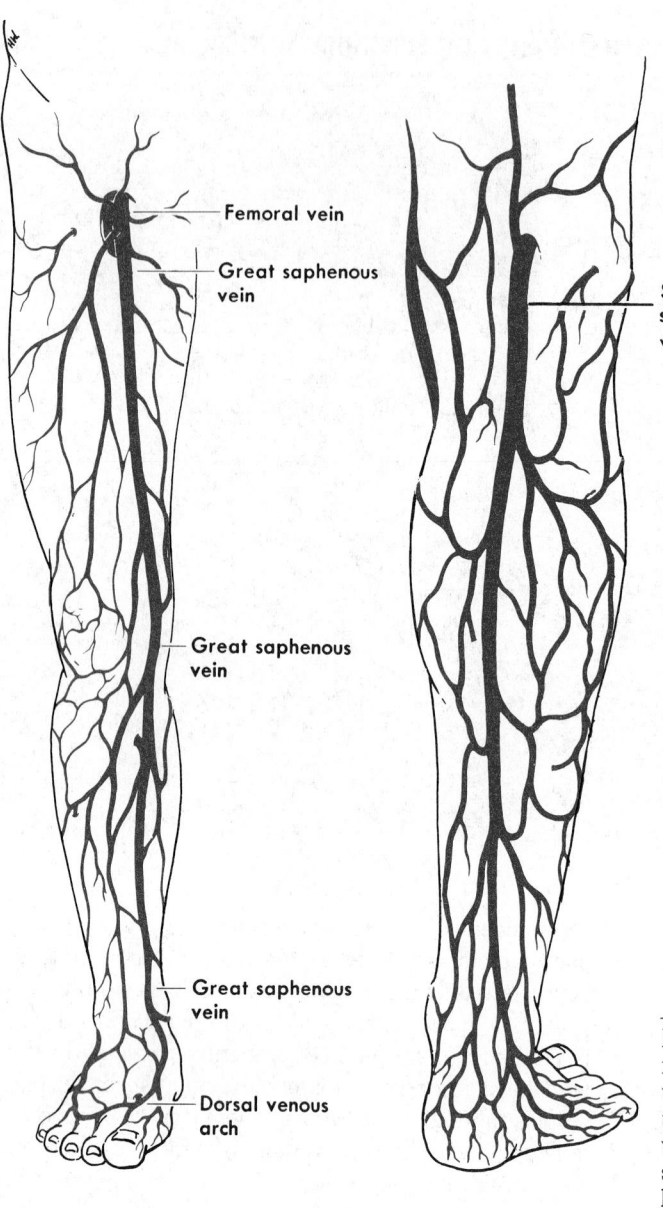

Femoral vein

Great saphenous vein

Great saphenous vein

Great saphenous vein

Dorsal venous arch

Small saphenous vein

FIGURE 29-10 Superficial veins of the leg and foot. (From Anthony CJ and Thibodeau GA: Textbook of anatomy and physiology, ed 13, St Louis, 1990, The CV Mosby Co.)

FIGURE 29-11 Development of thromboemboli with arrows indicating direction of blood flow. **A,** Thrombus in a valve pocket of a deep vein with blood flowing beside thrombus. **B,** Thrombi tend to form at bifurcations of deep veins with some slowing of blood flow. **C,** Complete occlusion of the vein by a thrombus forcing backflow of blood. **D,** An embolus that has broken off from a thrombus and is floating in the bloodstream could migrate to the lungs and cause pulmonary embolus.

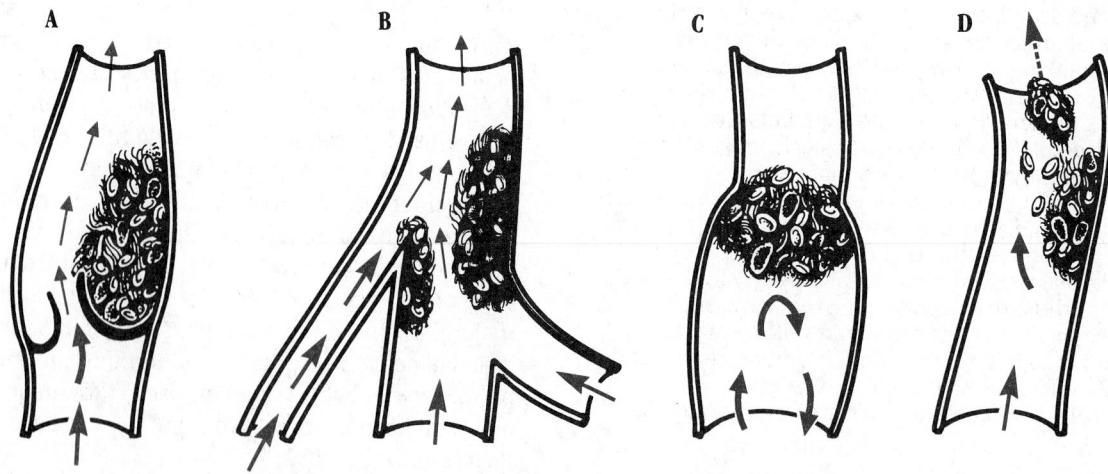

A   B   C   D

TABLE 29-5 Diagnostic tests for venous disorders

Test	Purpose	Procedure	Comments
Venography	Identify thrombi or obstruction in veins of lower extremities	Radiopaque dye inserted through superficial vein in foot, followed by x-ray films	Transient flushing and burning sensations when dye injected Assess for allergic reaction to dye (dyspnea, rash, urticaria)
Radionuclide scan	Visualize vascular system and detect changes in veins Assess venous blood flow	Injection of radionuclide followed by scanning over area 24 h after injection; accumulation of isotope indicates degree of obstruction	Explain to patient that radiation dose is usually less than that received from diagnostic x-rays
Impedance plethysmography	Measure variations in electrical resistance due to changes in blood volume in deep vein thrombophlebitis	Pressure cuff applied to thigh and electrodes applied to calf; measurements taken during inflation and deflation	Noninvasive
Doppler ultrasonography	(See Table 29-2)		

CLINICAL MANIFESTATIONS

Venous flow is usually obstructed with DVT, leading to pain and edema of the extremity. An increase in circumference of the calf or thigh (depending on location of the thrombus) may be noted. Ongoing calf or thigh measurements should be taken at the same sites; these sites should be marked with pen. Active dorsiflexion of the foot often produces calf pain (Homan's sign). Do not check for Homan's sign if DVT is known to be present, because this increases risk of embolization. Some individuals with DVT have no symptoms until a pulmonary embolism occurs.

Because superficial veins are closer to the surface, inflammation may be noted on inspection if superficial thrombophlebitis is present. Signs include redness, warmth, and tenderness along the course of the vein. The affected superficial veins feel hard and thready, and are sensitive to pressure.

Several diagnostic tests may be used to determine the diagnosis and extent of thrombophlebitis. These tests include venography, radionuclide scan, and impedance plethysmography (Table 29-5). Doppler ultrasonography (see Table 29-2) may also be used.

MEDICAL MANAGEMENT

Superficial thrombophlebitis is generally treated with bed rest with legs elevated and moist heat applied. Hospitalization is generally not required. Resolution of the inflammation may be enhanced by nonsteroidal antiinflammatory drugs (NSAIDS). Ligation and division of the saphenous vein may be indicated if the saphenofemoral junction is involved.

Deep vein thrombophlebitis usually requires hospital-ization, and therapy includes the following:

1. Bed rest with legs elevated 15 to 20 degrees above heart (knees slightly flexed), trunk horizontal (head may be raised) to promote venous return (help prevent further emboli) and prevent edema
2. Application of warm moist heat to reduce pain
3. Elastic stocking or bandage
4. Anticoagulants, initially with intravenous heparin, then coumadin
5. Fibrinolytic to resolve the thrombus
6. Vasodilator if needed to control vessel spasms and improve circulation

Surgery

If the thrombus is recurrent and extensive or if the patient is at high risk for pulmonary embolism, surgery may be necessary. A thrombectomy or a vena caval interruption may be performed. *Thrombectomy* consists of incising the common femoral vein in the groin and extracting the clots. *Vena caval interruption* consists of the transvenous placement of a grid or umbrella filter in the vena cava to block the passage of emboli (Figure 29-12). This is used when a patient has DVT or pulmonary emboli. The filter is passed through a small incision in the internal jugular vein. This procedure usually takes place in a cardiac catheterization laboratory equipped with fluoroscopy. If the femoral vein is used as the insertion site, the procedure is done in the operating room to faciliate surgical repair of the vein.

■ ASSESSMENT

Data to be collected include signs and symptoms of thrombophlebitis, extent of circulatory involvement, and signs of a developing embolism. *Subjective data* include the following:

1. Characteristics of pain in extremity
2. Onset and duration of symptoms
3. History of thrombophlebitis or other venous disorders; effects of previous therapies; use of preventive measures

Objective data include the following:

1. Color and temperature of the extremity (pale and cold if vein is occluded; red and warm if superficial vein is inflamed)
2. Edema of calf or thigh (use tape measure and mark site for future measurements, if indicated); measurement of both legs for comparison

■ DATA ANALYSIS: NURSING DIAGNOSES

Nursing diagnoses are determined from assessment of patient data. Possible nursing diagnoses for the person with thrombophlebitis may include, but are not limited to, the following:

Diagnostic Title	Possible Etiology
Knowledge deficit: prevention, pharmacotherapy, surgery	Lack of exposure/recall, unfamiliarity with information sources
Pain: leg	Inflammation, edema, venous stasis
Tissue perfusion, altered peripheral	Decreased venous blood flow, immobility

■ PLANNING: EXPECTED PATIENT OUTCOMES

Expected patient outcomes for the person with thrombophlebitis may include, but are not limited to, the following:

1. Patient can describe:
   a. Preventive measures
   b. Major action and side effects of anticoagulants, fibrinolytics and vasodilators
   c. Surgical intervention, if indicated
   d. Signs and symptoms of pulmonary embolism
2. Patient states that leg pain is reduced.
3. Patient can describe measures to increase perfusion of lower extremities, including rationale for activity limitation.

■ IMPLEMENTATION

Preventive Care

The major emphasis of nursing interventions for the patient with a chronic venous disorder is patient teaching. Important topics include measures to prevent recurrence of thrombophlebitis and measures to increase tissue perfusion.

1. Maintain desired weight for height to prevent excess pressure on legs and excess workload on heart.
2. Modify life-style to prevent long periods of standing or sitting that impair venous return.
3. Elevate legs when sitting; dorsiflex both feet at regular intervals when sitting or lying down to prevent

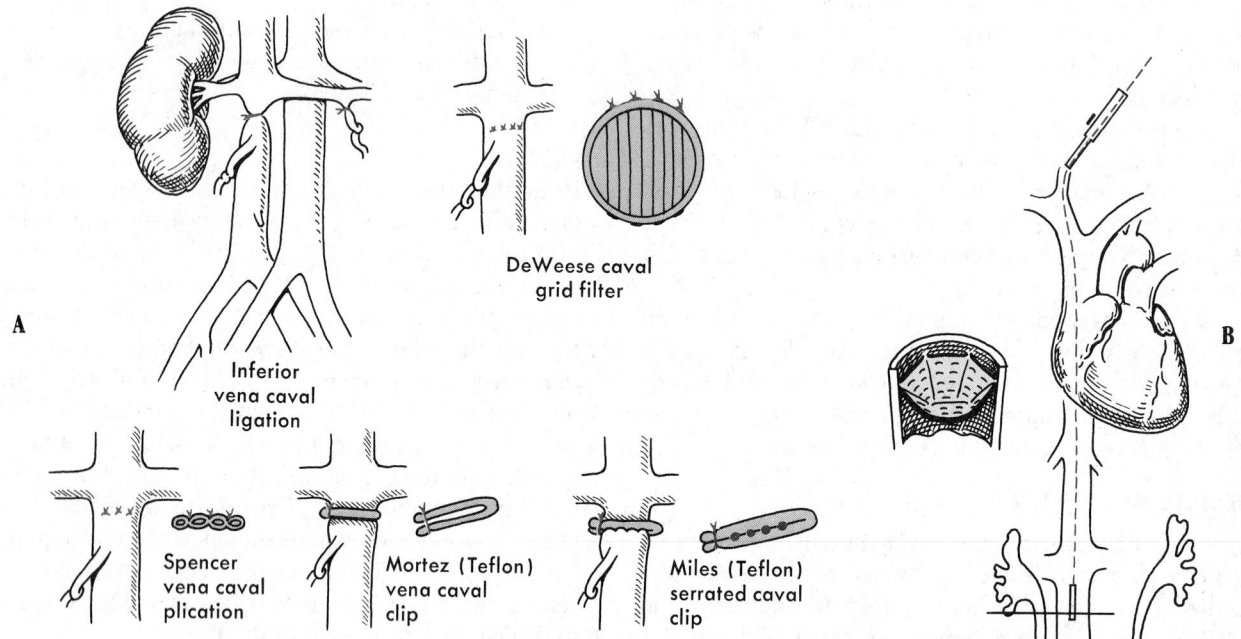

FIGURE 29-12 A, Various surgical techniques for preventing embolism of pelvic and lower extremity veins. **B,** Transvenous method of vena caval interruption with caval prosthesis of umbrella design. Insert illustrates open umbrella. (Redrawn from Fairbairn JF et al: Peripheral vascular disease, Philadelphia, 1972, WB Saunders Co.)

venous pooling; if edema occurs, elevate above heart level when possible.

4. Engage in a regular aerobic exercise program (such as swimming, jogging, fast walking, or bicycling) to promote circulation.
5. Avoid crossing legs at the knee; this impairs circulation.
6. Avoid wearing constrictive clothing such as tight bands around socks or garters.
7. Wear elastic stocking on affected leg, especially when sitting or standing for prolonged periods (see the box below).
8. Do leg exercises and wear elastic stockings during periods of enforced immobility, such as following surgery or during long airplane or automobile trips.
9. Report signs of vein inflammation to physician.

Acute Care

When the patient is hospitalized for DVT, explain the purpose of bed rest to prevent embolization, and of leg elevation to prevent further thrombus formation. Elastic stockings are preferred to Ace bandages because they maintain a more even pressure. Carry out nursing interventions for the person receiving anticoagulation and fibrinolytic therapy (p. 755). Monitor for signs of pulmonary embolus: sudden onset of chest pain, dyspnea, rapid breathing, and tachycardia. Nursing interventions for the person requiring surgery for vena caval interruption are listed below:

1. Assess insertion site; if there are signs of bleeding or hematoma, apply pressure over site and notify surgeon.
2. Keep patient on bed rest for first 24 hours; encourage ROM exercises to promote venous return.
3. Assist patient in ambulation when permitted; elevate legs when sitting or lying to promote circulation.
4. Keep elastic bandage snug and without wrinkles to maintain even pressure on leg veins.
5. Medicate with prescribed analgesics and antiinflammatory agents to promote comfort.

TEACHING THE USE OF ELASTIC STOCKINGS

1. Use correct size (see instructions on box or consult medical supply person) and length (to knee or groin) as prescribed.
2. Apply stocking before getting out of bed.
3. For ease of application, turn all but foot of stocking inside out, slide foot into stocking, and pull stocking over leg.
4. Remove stocking at bedtime if desired; if leg aches at night, stocking may be of benefit if worn in bed.
5. Keep a second stocking on hand for use when the other is being laundered.

VARICOSE VEINS
EPIDEMIOLOGY/ETIOLOGY

Varicose veins are abnormally dilated veins with incompetent valves, occurring most often in the lower extremities and lower trunk. At least 20% of the total U.S. population is affected. The highest incidence is in the third to fifth decades of life and in women. Varicose veins can develop from the congenital absence of a valve or acquired incompetence of the valve. They often occur as a result of external pressure on the veins from pregnancy, ascites, or abdominal tumors. They may also arise from sustained elevations in venous pressure related to chronic diseases such as heart disease and cirrhosis.

PREVENTION

Persons with early varicosities, especially if there is a family history of varicosities, should wear elastic stockings during activities requiring long periods of standing or when pregnant. Moderate exercise and elevation of the legs when sitting help to prevent venous congestion. No continual pressure should be applied to the veins.

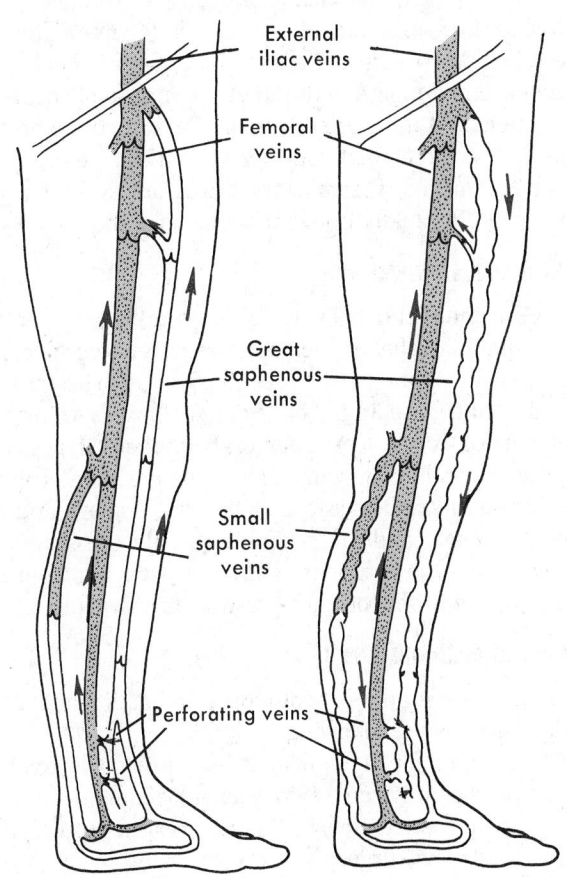

FIGURE 29-13 *Left,* Venous flow in normal veins. *Right,* Venous flow in varicose veins. (Redrawn from Fairbairn, JF et al: Peripheral vascular disease, Philadelphia, 1972, WB Saunders Co.)

PATHOPHYSIOLOGY

The great and small saphenous veins are most often involved (Figure 29-13). The precipitating factor in varicose vein development is simply a weakening of the vein wall. Because the vessel is weak, it does not withstand normal pressure and dilates with pooling of blood. As the vessel dilates, the valves become stretched and incompetent. This results in an inability to support a column of blood, and more venous pooling occurs.

CLINICAL MANIFESTATIONS

Varicose veins may be primary or secondary. *Primary* varicosities have a gradual onset and affect the superficial veins. Often there are no accompanying symptoms except the appearance of darkened tortuous veins. Symptoms include dull aches, muscle cramps, pressure, heaviness, or fatigue arising from reduced blood flow to the tissues. *Secondary* varicosities affect the deep veins and occur as a result of chronic venous insufficiency or venous thrombosis. Symptoms of edema, pain, changes in skin color, and ulceration may occur from venous stasis.

Trendelenburg's test is a simple noninvasive diagnostic tool to assess the competency of the venous valves through measurement of venous filling time. The patient lies down with the affected leg raised to allow for venous emptying. A tourniquet is then applied above the knee, and the patient stands. The direction and filling time are recorded both before and after the tourniquet is removed. Incompetent valves are evident when the veins fill rapidly from backward blood flow.

MEDICAL MANAGEMENT

Surgical intervention for varicose veins is indicated for prevention or relief of edema, for recurrent leg ulcers or pain, or for cosmetic purposes. Surgery consists of vein ligation and stripping. The great saphenous vein is ligated (tied) close to the femoral junction, if possible. The great and small saphenous veins are then stripped out through small incisions at the groin, above and below the knee, and at the ankle. Sterile dressings are placed over the incisions, and an elastic bandage extending from the foot to the groin is firmly applied.

NURSING MANAGEMENT

Nursing care for the patient after vein ligation and stripping includes the following:
1. Monitor for signs of bleeding, especially on first postoperative day. If incisional bleeding occurs, elevate the leg, apply pressure over the wound, and notify the surgeon.
2. Keep patient flat in bed for first 4 hours after surgery; elevate leg to promote venous return when lying or sitting.
3. Medicate 30 minutes before ambulation and assist patient as necessary.

4. Keep elastic bandage snug and wrinkle-free to maintain even pressure on veins; do not remove bandage for daily care.

Because venous disorders are usually chronic conditions, the person must know how to prevent venous stasis and encourage return of venous flow. Preventive measures are listed on p. 758.

ARTERIOVENOUS DISORDERS

ARTERIOVENOUS FISTULAS
EPIDEMIOLOGY/ETIOLOGY

An arteriovenous fistula is an abnormal direct communication between an artery and vein caused by a congenital anomaly or an acquired disorder. Most acquired arteriovenous fistulas develop secondary to penetrating injuries from trauma. A single arteriovenous fistula is rare. More often, multiple fistulas affect circulation to an entire region or area such as the arm or leg.

PATHOPHYSIOLOGY

In an arteriovenous fistula the high arterial blood flow bypasses the capillary network and goes into the veins. This causes an increase in venous pressure that predisposes to venous engorgement, dilatation, and aneurysm development. The veins become thickened as the artery thins and loses its elastic and muscular properties.

CLINICAL MANIFESTATIONS

Signs and symptoms of arteriovenous fistulas may include pain at the site of a fistula; edema, varicosities, and asymmetry of an extremity; tortuous, dilated superficial veins; venous pulsations; and venous bruit and thrill. Testing includes arteriography and Doppler ultrasonography.

MEDICAL MANAGEMENT

Small peripheral arteriovenous fistulas may not require intervention. Surgical intervention may be indicated when ulceration, bleeding, or severe arterial or venous insufficiency occur. The most common procedure is embolization consisting of closing the fistula with embolic material such as Gelfoam, glass beads, or muscle. Large fistulas may be repaired or resected, or the involved artery may be ligated.

NURSING MANAGEMENT

Nursing management is primarily related to teaching and support. Teaching includes information about the underlying disease and measures to prevent symptoms of venous insufficiency and promote venous return (p. 758). Elastic stockings can help prevent discomfort and edema. Postoperative care includes assessing skin color and temperature and peripheral pulses in the limb distal to the surgery, and ensuring a wrinkle-free elastic wrap.

LEG ULCERS

ETIOLOGY

Most leg ulcers occur from chronic deep vein insufficiency or severe varicose veins. Less frequently, they develop from arterial insufficiency resulting from arterial obstruction. Other causes include burns, leg trauma, and neurogenic disorders. Persons with diabetes mellitus are at high risk for development of leg ulcers because of vascular insufficiency.

PATHOPHYSIOLOGY

A leg ulcer is an open necrotic lesion that results from inadequate exchange of oxygen and other nutrients to the tissues because of decreased circulation. The same underlying pathophysiologic changes that contribute to the development of chronic venous or arterial insufficiency are involved. Secondary bacterial infection occurs because the circulatory factors necessary for preventing infection are diminished. Infection delays healing and contributes to frequent leg ulcer recurrences.

CLINICAL MANIFESTATIONS

Clinical signs vary, depending on the underlying problem. A *venous ulcer* (stasis ulcer) is usually moderately painful and located on the medial aspect of the ankle. Edema and pigmentation are common around the area of ulceration. Most venous ulcers heal with therapy. An *arterial ulcer* (ischemic ulcer) causes more pain and has a more necrotic, pale gray base; it frequently develops on the heel, lateral malleolus, toes, and dorsum of the foot. Pale or mottled skin is common around the base of the ulcer. Edema is infrequent, and peripheral pulses are diminished or absent.

MEDICAL MANAGEMENT

Medical management of the patient with a leg ulcer is directed at wound healing and prevention of infection. Necrotic tissue is debrided by mechanical, chemical, or surgical means. A wet-to-dry dressing may be applied to debride the wound *mechanically*. The dressing is applied damp then removed when dry, pulling off the debris that has adhered to the dressing. *Chemical* beads such as Debrisan, and enzyme ointments such as fibrinolysins (Elase), may be placed over the ulcer (avoiding healthy tissue) to break down the debris. Necrotic tissue can also be cut away with the aid of *surgical* instruments, usually a scalpel.

Topical and systemic antibiotics may be prescribed to prevent infection; systemic antibiotic therapy is the most effective route. Periodic culture of wound drainage may be ordered to monitor effectiveness of the antibiotics.

A *boot* may be applied to cover small, newly formed ulcers in ambulatory persons (Figure 29-14). This boot protects the ulcer and provides constant, even support to the area. The boot is made from a special type of impregnated gauze (using Unna paste) that hardens after it is wrapped around the patient's leg. The Unna boot is generally left on for 1 to 2 weeks, although it may be changed more often if copious drainage occurs. Elastic bandages are applied to the leg after the ulcer has healed.

■ ASSESSMENT

Subjective data for the person with a leg ulcer include the following:
1. Leg discomfort or pain: aching, heaviness
2. Onset and duration of symptoms (usually chronic)
3. History of venous insufficiency: thrombophlebitis, arterial insufficiency, diabetes

Objective data include the following:
1. Skin color: pale, gray, mottled
2. Location and extent of ulceration and necrosis
3. Presence of edema and drainage
4. Quality of peripheral pulses

■ DATA ANALYSIS: NURSING DIAGNOSES

Nursing diagnoses are determined from assessment of patient data. Possible nursing diagnoses for the person with a leg ulcer may include, but are not limited to, the following:

Diagnostic Title	Possible Etiologies
Infection, potential for	Lack of knowledge, decreased cellular nutrition
Knowledge deficit: ulcer care, prevention	Lack of exposure/recall, misinterpretation of information
Pain: ulcer	Inflammation, necrosis
Tissue perfusion, altered peripheral	Decreased blood flow (arterial or venous)

■ PLANNING: EXPECTED PATIENT OUTCOMES

Expected patient outcomes for the person with a leg ulcer may include, but are not limited to, the following:
1. Ulcer shows signs of healing and absence of further breakdown.
2. Patient states that discomfort is lessened.
3. Patient can describe the following:
   a. Measures to prevent infection
   b. Care of the ulcer
   c. Measures to increase tissue perfusion

■ IMPLEMENTATION

Preventive Care

Nursing interventions for patients with leg ulcers are similar to those for patients with other venous or arterial problems. Teaching includes proper foot care to decrease the incidence of infection and measures to promote tissue perfusion:
1. Assess skin condition on a daily basis.
2. Keep skin clean and dry.
3. Avoid wearing rubber-soled shoes because they

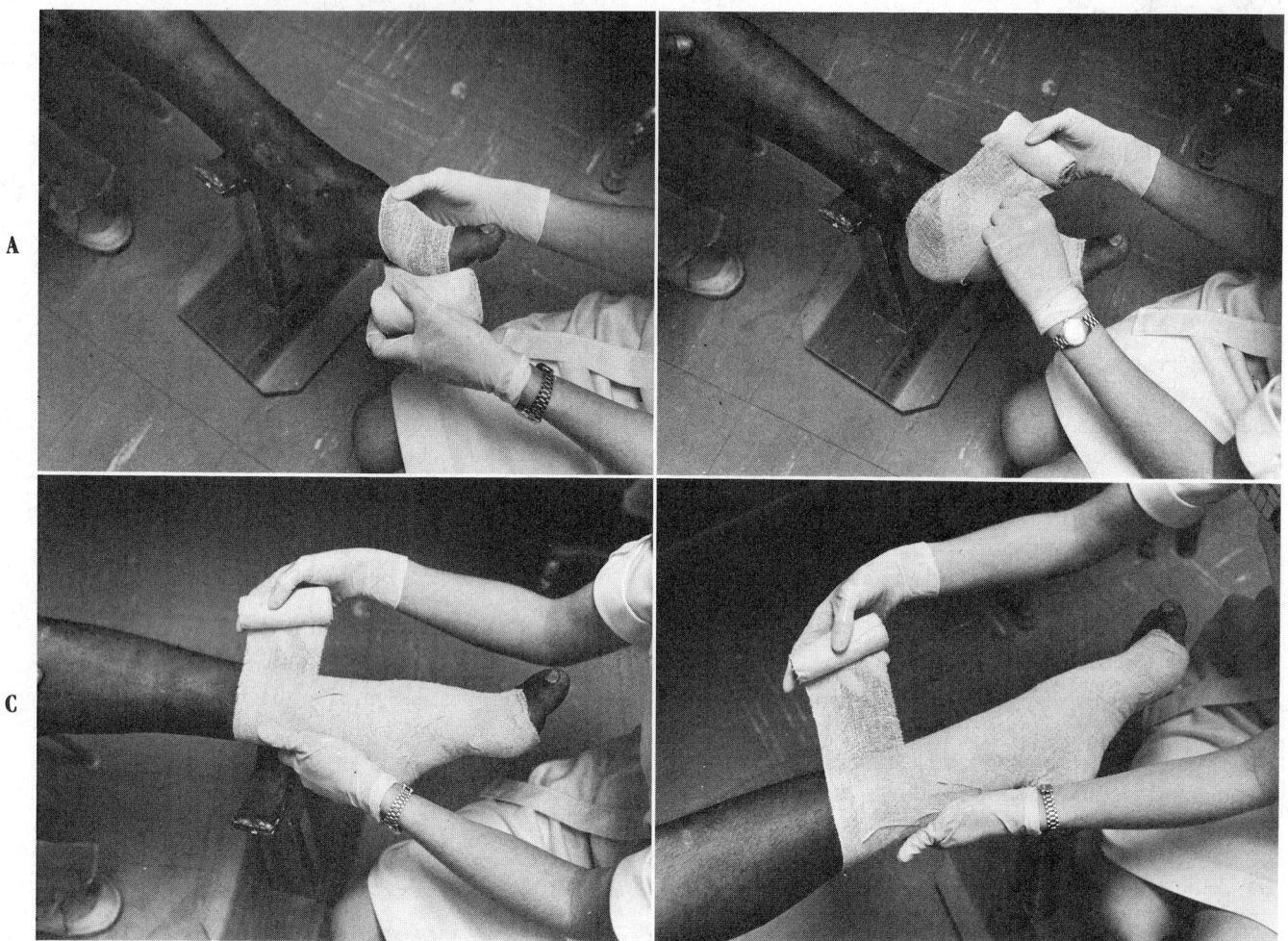

FIGURE 29-14 Nurse applying Unna paste boot using specially impregnated gauze. Note ulcers on inferior aspect of patient's foot.

prevent evaporation and thus contribute to foot infection.

4. Wear cotton socks and change daily.
5. Use only prescribed ointments and antibiotic creams on legs and feet.
6. Keep pathways in home free of clutter to avoid possible injury to legs and subsequent infection.
7. Contact health care professional at onset of skin breakdown.
8. Engage in regular aerobic exercise to promote circulation to the legs and feet.

Acute Care

Care for the hospitalized patient with a leg ulcer includes care of the ulcer, promotion of comfort, and positioning to facilitate circulation. If the dressing change is painful, medicate patient about 20 to 30 minutes before the dressing change. Avoid application of debriding agents on healthy tissue. Use cotton between toes to prevent pressure on other toe ulcers. Maintain proper body positioning to decrease pressure on affected areas and to promote comfort. An overbed cradle may help protect the leg from bed linens. For an arterial ulcer, elevate head of bed on 3 to 6 inch blocks to promote circulation. For a venous ulcer, elevate lower extremities on pillows to decrease edema and promote venous return.

LYMPHEDEMA

EPIDEMIOLOGY/ETIOLOGY

Lymphedema is the swelling of soft tissue as a result of the collection of interstitial fluid secondary to obstruction of lymph vessels. Primary lymphedema results from an abnormal development of the lymph vessels at birth or during puberty. Secondary lymphedema is caused by

TYPES OF LYMPHEDEMA

PRIMARY LYMPHEDEMA

(*abnormal development of lymph vessels*)
Hypoplastic development of lymph vessels
Congenital
Lymphedema precox (puberty)

SECONDARY LYMPHEDEMA

(*inflammatory or mechanical obstruction of lymphatics as a result of*)
Mastectomy with excision of lymph nodes
Trauma
Malignant tumors
Tissue inflammation
Filariasis (transmitted by mosquitos)

obstruction, inflammation, or infection (see the box above). The disorder is more commonly seen in young females.

PATHOPHYSIOLOGY

The lymphatic vessels carry lymph from the tissues back into the venous circulation. This system is made up of small thin vessels that are found throughout the body in close proximity to the veins. The lymphatics begin as capillaries that drain the tissues of lymph (a fluid similar to plasma) and tissue fluid that contains cells, cellular debris, and proteins. The lymph flows through oval bodies called *lymph nodes*, which remove noxious agents such as bacteria and toxins. The flow then drains into the thoracic duct and the right lymphatic duct, which empty into the junction of the internal jugular vein and subclavian vein (Figure 29-15).

Pathophysiologic changes may include (1) roughening of the surface of the lymphatic vessel, (2) dilation of some lymph channels with thickening and edema of the lymphatic tissue, and (3) fibrosis and separation of elastic fibers that may be present in inflammatory states. Recurrent episodes of lymphedema may cause fibrosis and hyperplasia of lymph vessels, leading to a severe enlargement of the extremity, called elephantiasis.

CLINICAL MANIFESTATIONS

Lymphedema of the lower extremities begins with mild swelling on the dorsum of the foot, usually at the end of the day, which gradually extends to the entire limb. Initially, the edema is soft and pitting but then progresses to firm, rubbery, nonpitting edema. The condition is aggravated by the following:

1. Prolonged standing
2. Pregnancy
3. Obesity
4. Warm weather
5. Menstrual period

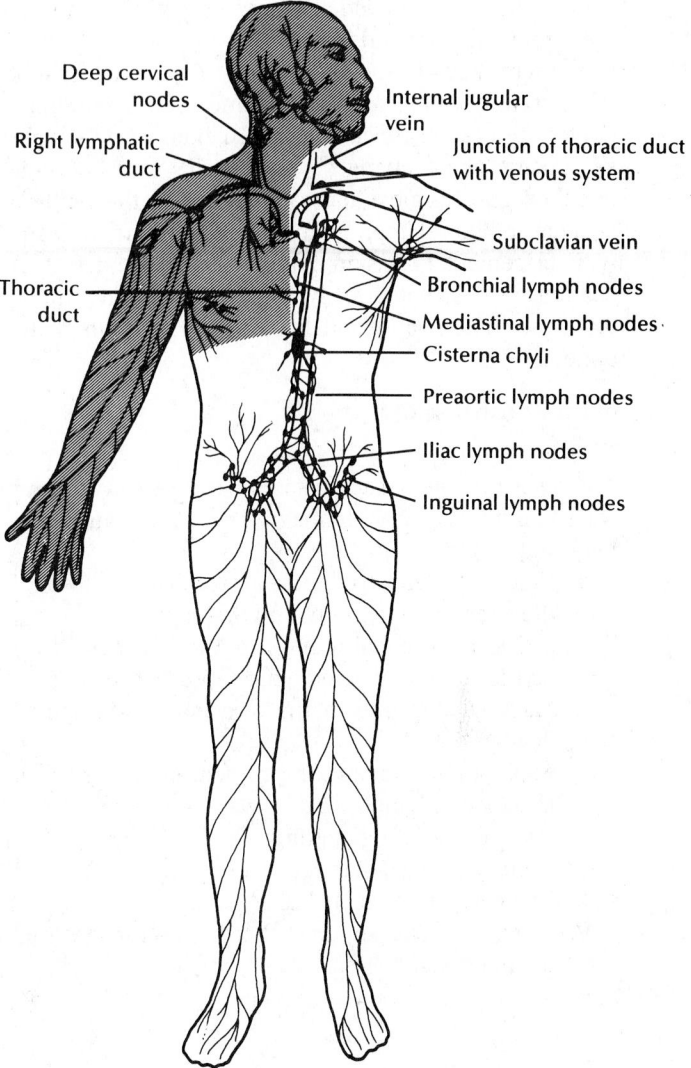

FIGURE 29-15 Lymph pathways of the lower limb drain into the subclavian vein. (From Hamilton WJ: Textbook of human anatomy, ed 2, St Louis, 1976, The CV Mosby Co.)

Diagnostic tests include lymphangiography, the injection of a contrast medium directly into the lymphatic vessels to detect lymph node defects and lymph node involvement in metastatic cancer.

MEDICAL MANAGEMENT

Medical management includes measures to encourage lymph flow and drug therapy to reduce edema and prevent infection.

1. Physical therapy
   a. Massage in direction of lymph flow
   b. Active and passive exercises to assist the movement of lymph fluid into the bloodstream
   c. Mechanical pulsatile pressure devices
2. Drugs
   a. Diuretics to temporarily decrease size of limb

b. Long-term antibiotic therapy for control of recurrent cellulitis and infection

Surgery may also be necessary to (1) reduce size of the extremity, (2) improve appearance of the extremity, (3) reduce the incidence of inflammations, and (4) limit secondary skin changes associated with chronic lymphedema. Surgical approaches include the removal of hypertrophied lymph channels and disfigured tissue with placement of a skin graft to cover the defect. A conduit is constructed for lymphatic drainage by transfer of the superficial lymphatics into the deep lymphatic system.

NURSING MANAGEMENT

Patient Teaching

The goal of patient teaching is for the person to learn ways to improve lymph drainage. Teaching includes the following:

1. Elevate the involved extremity above the level of the heart to increase lymph drainage.
   a. Elevate the foot of the bed 4 to 8 inches.
   b. Elevate the affected extremity when sitting.
2. Massage the limb in the direction of the lymph flow.
3. Apply an elastic stocking to help prevent reaccumulation of lymph fluid.
4. Avoid constricting clothing.
5. Avoid prolonged standing.
6. Exercise on a regular basis.
7. Avoid salty or spicy food that predisposes to fluid retention and edema.

TABLE 29-6 Classification of blood pressure* (age 18 and older)[38]

Range (mm Hg)	Classification
DIASTOLIC	
<85	Normal blood pressure
85-89	High normal blood pressure†
90-104	Mild hypertension
105-114	Moderate hypertension
>115	Severe hypertension
SYSTOLIC	
<140	Normal blood pressure
140-159	Borderline isolated systolic HTN‡
>160	Isolated systolic HTN‡

*Based on average of two or more readings on two or more occasions.
†High normal blood pressure takes precedence over normal [systolic] blood pressure when both occur in same person.
‡Borderline isolated systolic HTN or isolated systolic HTN take precedence over high normal blood pressure when both occur in same person.

HYPERTENSION

Hypertension can be considered with peripheral vascular disorders because they both involve problems of peripheral circulation and are affected by similar factors. Hypertension itself is a risk factor in atherosclerosis, the major cause of peripheral vascular disease.

EPIDEMIOLOGY/ETIOLOGY

Hypertension is defined as a consistent systolic blood pressure >140 mm Hg and/or a consistent diastolic blood pressure >90 mm Hg. A more complete classification of blood pressures is listed in Table 29-6. This classification was developed by a national task force to assist in a more universal diagnosis of hypertension. It must be emphasized that the categorical classification is based on the average of two or more blood pressure readings, not a single elevated reading.

The incidence of hypertension (HTN) increases with age (see the research box) and varies considerably among different groups. Hypertension occurs more often in men than in women. It is nearly twice as prevalent among blacks as whites. Hypertension in blacks is usually more severe than it is in similar hypertensive whites. There is increased incidence and severity of HTN in blacks living in the southeastern United States compared with blacks residing in other areas.

More than 58 million Americans have been diagnosed with elevated blood pressure or are taking antihypertensive medications. Additionally, it is estimated that another 50% of adults in the United States are undiagnosed hypertensives.[8] The exact number is unknown because most individuals are symptom-free and some persons avoid pursuing treatment.

Hypertension may be primary (essential, idiopathic), or secondary, occurring as a consequence of another condition (Table 29-7). Essential hypertension accounts

RESEARCH

Dannenberg AL, Garrison RJ, and Kannel, WB: Incidence of hypertension in the Framingham study, Am J Pub Health 78:676-679, 1988.

The incidence of identified hypertension by age and sex was pooled for 15 2-year periods within the 30 year follow-up of 5209 subjects in the Framingham Heart Study. Hypertension incidence per biennium increased with age in men and women at ages 30 through 39 and 70 through 79. The proportion of hypertensive subjects on antihypertensive medications increased consistently from 1954 to 1958 and 1979 to 1981. Because hypertension incidence and antihypertensive medications increased, this data may be helpful in determining the impact of future primary prevention strategies. ∎

for 90% to 95% of all types of HTN. Although there is no generally accepted cause of essential hypertension, several theories have been postulated, including arteriolar changes, alterations in sympathetic tone, hormonal influences, and genetic factors.

Malignant hypertension is a severe, rapidly progressive elevation in blood pressure that causes damage to the small arterioles in major organ systems (heart, kidneys, brain, and eyes). A primary distinguishing finding is inflammation of the arterioles (arteriolitis) in the eyes. Retinitis and papilledema occur in later stages. This type of HTN is most common in black males under age 40. Unless medical treatment is successful, the course is rapidly fatal. The most common causes of death are myocardial infarction, congestive heart failure, stroke, or renal failure.

PREVENTION

Hypertension is a major risk factor in the development of cardiovascular, renal, and cerebral diseases. Thus it is important to control HTN through primary and secondary prevention strategies.

Primary prevention is aimed at the reduction of risk factors associated with hypertension (see the box at right). Health education programs include teaching about moderate sodium intake, a decreased saturated fat diet, maintenance of optimum body weight for height, cessation of cigarette smoking, moderate consumption of alcohol, and the use of effective coping strategies.

Secondary prevention is focused on identification and control of HTN in high risk groups, such as blacks (especially males), obese individuals, and blood relatives of known hypertensives. A major effort should be made to contact people who have a limited access to health care because of geographic or economic constraints. Mass blood pressure screenings are currently not recommended. Most often these screenings occur at large-scale gatherings where environmental conditions may cause inaccurate blood pressure readings. In addition, these sites tend to be frequented by the same people. Adults should have their blood pressure checked at regular intervals, depending on the findings (see Table 29-8).

PATHOPHYSIOLOGY

Blood pressure is the pressure exerted by the blood on the vessels through which it flows. The pressure during ventricular contraction is the systolic pressure and that during ventricular relaxation is the diastolic pressure. Blood pressure is regulated by two factors: blood flow and peripheral vascular resistance. Factors that determine blood flow are the volume of blood ejected from the left ventricle with each contraction (stroke volume) and the heart rate (Chapter 26). Peripheral vascular resistance is affected primarily by the diameter of the

TABLE 29-7 Causes of secondary hypertension

Disorder/Condition	Mechanism
Kidney	
Renal parenchymal disease (glomerulonephritis, renal failure)	Most often cause a renin or sodium dependent HTN; physiologic changes relate to type of disease and severity of renal insufficiency
Renovascular disease	Decrease in renal perfusion from atherosclerotic or fibrotic narrowing of renal arteries; causes marked increase in peripheral vascular resistance and cardiac output
Adrenal cortex	
Cushing's syndrome	Increase in blood volume
Primary aldosteronism	Increase in aldosterone, causing sodium and water retention that increase blood volume
Pheochromocytoma	Excess secretion of catecholamines (norepinephrine increases peripheral vascular resistance)
Coarctation of aorta	Causes marked elevated blood pressure in upper extremities with decreased perfusion in lower extremities
Head trauma or cranial tumor	Increased intracranial pressure reduces cerebral blood flow; resultant ischemia stimulates medullary vasomotor center to raise blood pressure
Pregnancy-induced HTN	Cause unknown; generalized vasospasm may be a contributing factor

RISK FACTORS IN ESSENTIAL HYPERTENSION

Age: advancing
Sex: male
Race: black
Family history: hypertension
Obesity: associated with increased intravascular volume
Atherosclerosis: narrowing of arteries increases blood pressure
Smoking: nicotine constricts blood vessels
High salt diet: sodium causes water retention, increasing blood volume
Alcohol: increases plasma catecholamines
Emotional stress: stimulates sympathetic nervous system

TABLE 29-8 Recommendations for follow-up of initial blood pressure measurements in adults (over age 18)[38]

Range (mm Hg)	Recommended Follow-up*
DIASTOLIC	
<85	Recheck within 2 yr
85-89	Recheck within 1 yr
90-104	Confirm within 2 mon
105-114	Evaluate or refer to source of care within 2 wk
>115	Evaluate or refer immediately to source of care
SYSTOLIC	
<140	Recheck within 2 yr
140-199	Confirm within 2 mon
>200	Evaluate or refer to source of care within 2 wk

*If recommendations for follow-up of diastolic and systolic blood pressure are different, the shorter recommended time for recheck should take precedence.

blood vessel and to a lesser degree by the viscosity of the blood. Increased peripheral vascular resistance as a result of narrowing of the arterioles is the most common characteristic in hypertension.

Dilation and constriction of the peripheral arterioles are controlled by several mechanisms, in particular, the sympathetic nervous system and the renin-angiotensin system. The vasomotor center in the medulla can be stimulated by the baroreceptors (Figure 29-16) or by psychogenic stress. Impulses are then carried through the sympathetic nervous system, causing the release of catecholamines. Norepinephrine is released from the postganglionic nerve fibers, causing blood vessel constriction and increased peripheral resistance. Epinephrine is secreted by the adrenal medulla and causes vasoconstriction. Epinephrine also causes an increased ventricular contraction force and increased cardiac output.

Renal regulation is an essential component of blood pressure control (Figure 29-17). Activation of the renin-angiotensin system occurs when there is reduced blood flow to the kidneys. Renin leads to the formation of angiotensin, a potent vasoconstrictor. Angiotensin also stimulates the secretion of aldosterone to promote retention of sodium and water.

COMPLICATIONS

With prolonged hypertension, the elastic tissue in the arterioles is replaced by fibrous collagen tissue. The thickened arteriole wall then becomes less distensible, offering even greater resistance to the flow of blood. This process leads to decreased tissue perfusion, especially in the target organs of high blood pressure, that is, in the heart, kidneys, and brain. Atherosclerosis is also accelerated in persons with high blood pressure.

In the cardiovascular system, decreases in coronary perfusion may lead to angina pectoris or myocardial infarction. Congestive heart failure can result from left ventricular hypertrophy, which occurs as the heart is forced to work against any elevated aortic pressure for long periods of time.

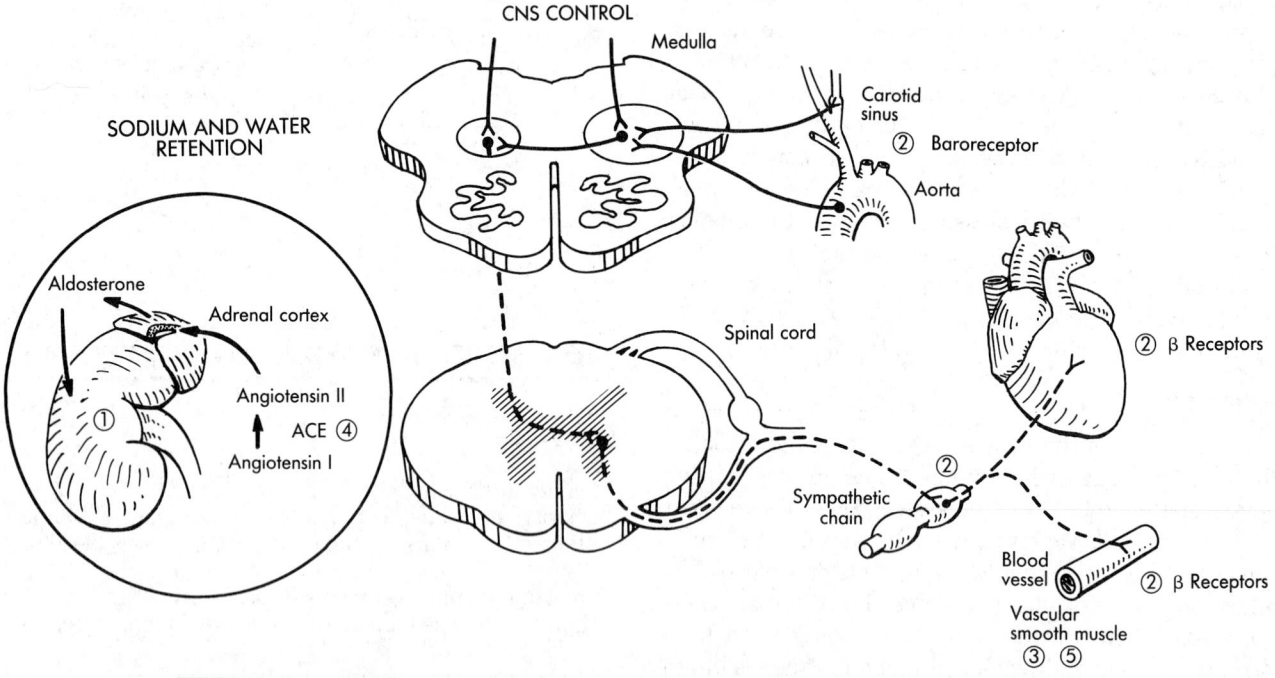

FIGURE 29-16 Sites of blood pressure regulation and action of antihypertensive drugs. ①, Diuretics. ②, Adrenergic inhibitors. ③, Vasodilators. ④, ACE inhibitors. ⑤, Calcium antagonist.

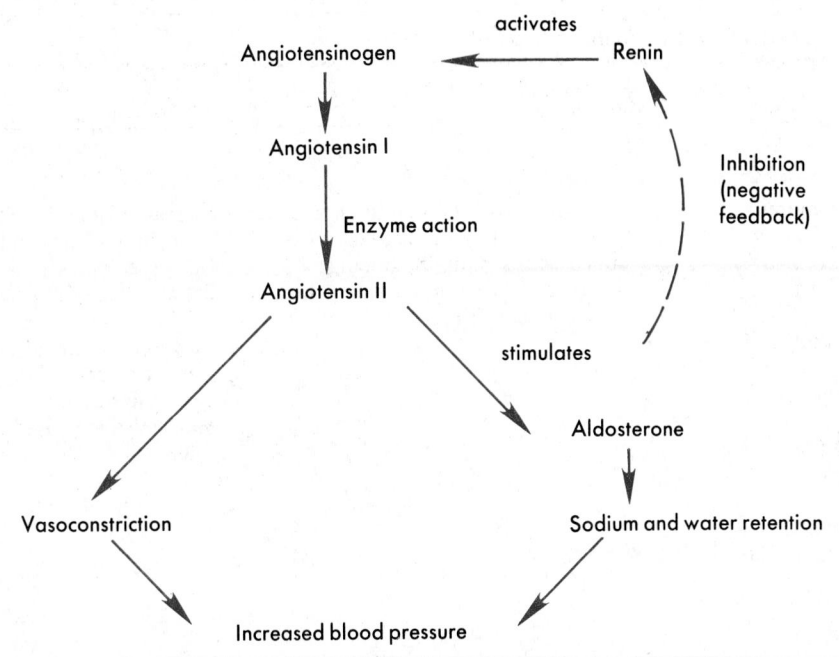

FIGURE 29-17 Diagram of the effect of the renin-angiotensin system on blood pressure.

When renal vessels thicken and perfusion diminishes, the glomerulus is deprived of its blood supply. Permanent kidney damage and possible renal failure result.

Cerebral ischemia and arteriosclerosis can occur as a result of the progressive effects of hypertension. Strokes can occur as the result of arteriosclerosis or hemorrhage from a leaking cerebral vessel.

CLINICAL MANIFESTATIONS

Hypertension is essentially a disease without symptoms. When symptoms do occur, they are usually indicative of advanced hypertension. Signs and symptoms may include early morning headache, unsteadiness, blurred vision, depression, and spontaneous epistaxis. Evidence of the effects of advanced HTN on cerebral blood vessels and the cardiovascular system may include nausea and vomiting, confusion, chest pain, and peripheral edema.

Diagnostic tests used to determine the possible cause of HTN and the extent of the disease on other organ systems, or to provide baseline information, may include the following:

1. Serum levels of sodium, potassium, calcium, and creatinine, as well as hemoglobin and hematocrit (severity and possible causes)
2. Urinalysis, BUN, and uric acid levels (effect on kidneys and as baseline for drug therapy)
3. Total cholesterol, triglycerides, high-density and low-density lipoproteins, fasting blood glucose, and ECG (presence of cardiovascular risk factors and baseline values for drug therapy)

4. Intravenous pyelogram (IVP) (extent of renal damage)

MEDICAL MANAGEMENT

Medical management is directed at control of HTN and the prevention of associated diseases. The primary goal is to maintain a systolic blood pressure of less than 140 mm Hg and a diastolic pressure of less than 90 mm Hg. The decision to treat HTN is based on degree of the blood pressure elevation, presence of risk factors, and extent of damage to associated organ systems. In most instances both nonpharmacologic and pharmacologic measures are needed.

NONPHARMACOLOGIC MEASURES

Measures to aid in lowering blood pressure without use of drugs include the following:

1. Weight control
2. Restriction of dietary sodium and saturated fats
3. Cessation of cigarette smoking
4. Restriction of alcoholic beverages
5. Maintenance of a regular aerobic exercise program
6. Use of biofeedback techniques

DRUG THERAPY

Drug treatment has been shown to successfully lower a consistent diastolic blood pressure of 94 mm Hg and greater. Antihypertensive medications have a protective effect against the progressive development of strokes, congestive heart failure, and renal failure in patients with mild hypertension. An individual decision is made

TABLE 29-9 Oral medications for treatment of hypertension

Drug	Action*	Side-effects*
DIURETICS		
Thiazide/Thiazide-like Diuretics		
Bendroflumethiazide (Naturetin)	Block sodium reabsorption in cortical portion of ascending tubule; water excreted with sodium, producing decreased blood volume. NOTE: thiazides ineffective in renal failure	Increased BUN, uric acid, blood glucose, calcium, cholesterol, and triglycerides
Benzthiazide (Aquatag, Exna)		Decreased potassium
Chlorothiazide (Diuril)		Possible postural hypotension in summer from sodium loss.
Chlorthalidone (Hygroton)		GI upset, dry mouth, thirst weakness, muscle aches, fatigue, tachycardia
Cyclothiazide (Fluidil)		Sexual dysfunction
Hydrochlorothiazide (Esidrix, Hydrodiuril)		May cause increased blood levels of lithium
Hydroflumethiazide (Saluron)		
Indapamide (Lozol)		
Methyclothiazide (Enduron)		
Metolazone (Zaroxolyn)		
Polythiazide (Renese)		
Quinethazone (Hydromox)		
Trichlormethiazide (Diurese, Metahydrin)		
Loop Diuretics		
Bumetanide (Bumex)	Block sodium and water reabsorption in medullary portion of ascending tubule; causes rapid volume depletion	Decreased potassium
Ethacrynic acid (Edecrin)		Thirst, skin rash, postural hypotension, nausea, vomiting
Furosemide (Lasix)		
Potassium-sparing Diuretics		
Amiloride (Midamor)	Inhibit aldosterone; sodium excreted in exchange for potassium	Drowsiness, confusion
Spironolactone (Aldactone)		Increased potassium levels
Triamterene (Dyrenium)		Diarrhea
		Gynecomastia with Aldactone
ADRENERGIC INHIBITORS		
Beta-adrenergic Blockers		
Acebutolol (Sectral)	Block beta-adrenergic receptors of sympathetic nervous system, decreasing heart rate and blood pressure.	Bronchospasms
Atenolol (Tenormin)		Bradycardia, fatigue, insomnia
Metoprolol (Lopressor)		Sexual dysfunction
Nadolol (Corgard)	NOTE: beta blockers should not be used in patients with asthma, COPD, CHF, and heart block; use with caution in diabetes and peripheral vascular disease	Peripheral vascular insufficiency
Pindolol (Visken)		Increased triglycerides
Propranolol (Inderal)		
Timolol (Blocadren)		
Centrally Acting Alpha Blockers		
Clonidine (Catapres)	Activate central receptors that suppress vasomotor and cardiac centers, causing a decrease in peripheral resistance.	Drowsiness, sedation
Guanabenz (Wytensin)		Dry mouth
Guanfacine (Tenex)		Fatigue
Methyldopa (Aldomet)	NOTE: rebound hypertension may occur with abrupt discontinuation of drug (except with Aldomet)	Sexual dysfunction
		Orthostatic hypotension
		Positive Coomb's test with Aldomet
Peripheral-acting Adrenergic Antagonists		
Guanadrel (Hylorel)	Deplete catecholamines in peripheral sympathetic postganglionic fibers	Orthostatic hypotension
Guanethidine (Ismelin)		Lethargy, depression
Rauwolfia serpentina (Raudixin)	Block norepinephrine release from adrenergic nerve endings	Sexual dysfunction
Reserpine (Serpasil)		Nasal congestion (with Raudixin and Serpasil)

*Primary actions and most common side effects are included and are related to entire drug category; consult a drug reference or drug package insert for more specific information.

TABLE 29-9 Oral medications for treatment of hypertension—cont'd

Drug	Action*	Side-effects*
Alpha-1-adrenergic Blockers		
Prazosin (Minipress) Terazosin (Vasocard, Hytrin)	Block synaptic receptors that regulate vasomotor tone; reduce peripheral resistance by dilating arterioles and venules	"First dose" syncope, orthostatic hypotension, weakness, palpitations, decreased low density lipoproteins
Combined Alpha- and Beta-Adrenergic Blockers		
Labetalol (Normodyne, Trandate)	Same as for beta blockers	Bronchospasm, orthostatic hypotension, peripheral vascular insufficiency
VASODILATORS		
Hydralazine (Apresoline) Minoxidil (Loniten)	Dilate peripheral blood vessels by directly relaxing vascular smooth muscle NOTE: usually used in combination with other antihypertensives as they increase sodium and fluid retention and can cause reflex cardiac stimulation	Headache, dizziness Tachycardia, palpitations, fatigue, edema
ACE INHIBITORS		
Captopril (Capoten) Enalapril maleate (Vasotec) Lisinopril (Prinivil)	Inhibit conversion of angiotensin to angiotensin II thus blocking the release of aldosterone, thereby reducing sodium and water retention	"First dose" hypotension, headache, dizziness, fatigue Increased potassium Cough, skin reactions
CALCIUM ANTAGONISTS		
Diltiazem (Cardizem) Nifedipine (Procardia) Nitrendipine Verapamil (Calan, Isoptin) Verapamil SR	Inhibit influx of calcium into muscle cells; act on vascular smooth muscles (primary arteries) to reduce spasms and promote vasodilation	Dizziness, fatigue, nausea, headache, edema

to treat patients with diastolic blood pressure readings between 90 and 94 mm Hg.

Several medications are available to treat HTN (Table 29-9). Drug selection is determined by use of a step-care approach. Initial therapy is started with a small dose of a less potent drug. Additions of drugs, substitutions, and dosage adjustments are based on the person's response. The step-care approach is as follows:

1. Use a diuretic, beta blocker, calcium antagonist, or angiotensin converting enzyme (ACE) inhibitor.
2. If ineffective after 1 to 3 months, increase dosage of drug, add a second drug of a different class, or substitute another drug.
3. Add a third drug of a different class or substitute a second drug.
4. Add a fourth drug of a different class or substitute a third drug; evaluate further and refer to a specialist if ineffective.

After 1 year of satisfactory blood pressure control, a stepdown approach may be effective in patients also adhering to nonpharmacologic measures.

HYPERTENSIVE CRISIS

Hypertensive emergency or crisis refers to a situation that requires immediate blood pressure lowering. Although such cases are relatively uncommon, prompt recognition and management are essential to prevent organ dysfunction. Clinical conditions that may precipitate a hypertensive crisis include hypertensive encephalopathy, intracranial hemorrhage, left ventricular heart failure, dissecting aortic aneurysm, severe hypertension of pregnancy, head trauma, extensive burns, unstable angina, or acute myocardial infarction. It may also occur in patients with poor hypertensive control and in those who abruptly discontinue their medications. Parenteral drug administration through IV and IM routes is used to quickly lower markedly elevated blood pressure. Intravenous medications are administered by drip and titrated according to the patient's response. Common drugs used in the treatment of hypertensive emergencies are listed in Table 29-10.

TABLE 29-10 Medication for treatment of hypertensive emergencies

Drug	Action*	Side Effects*
VASODILATORS		
Sodium nitroprusside (Nipride, Nitropress) Nitroglycerine Diazoxide (Hyperstat) Hydralazine (Apresoline)	Dilate peripheral blood vessels by relaxing vascular smooth muscle	Headache, dizziness Tachycardia, palpitations, fatigue, nausea, edema NOTE: thiocyanate toxicity may occur with sodium nitroprusside
ADRENERGIC INHIBITORS		
Phentolamine (Regitine) Trimethaphan camsylate (Arfonad) Labetalol (Normodyne, Trandate) Methyldopa (Aldomet)	Block adrenergic receptors of sympathetic nervous system, thereby dilating peripheral blood vessels and reducing peripheral vascular resistance	Tachycardia, orthostatic hypotension

*Primary action and common side effects are included and are related to entire drug category; consult drug reference or drug package insert for more specific information.

■ ASSESSMENT

SUBJECTIVE DATA

Subjective data are collected about the presence of any symptoms, history of HTN, and patient knowledge of HTN. These data may include the following:

1. Presence of symptoms indicative of advanced HTN (p. 767)
2. Presence of risk factors: intake of sodium and saturated fats, weight for height, smoking history, exercise level, and alcohol consumption
3. Presence of stress in occupation and personal life
4. Family history of HTN and cardiovascular diseases
5. Course and compliance with therapy for previously diagnosed HTN
6. Current knowledge of HTN: definition of high blood pressure; meaning of systolic and diastolic readings; and effects of high blood pressure on heart, kidney, and brain

OBJECTIVE DATA

Two or more blood pressure measurements are taken in both arms with the patient in both supine and sitting positions. Height and weight are also recorded. Additional objective data may be collected by a nurse clinician or a physician:

1. Examination of neck for carotid bruits and abdomen for abdominal bruits
2. Auscultation of heart for abnormal heart sounds (S_3, S_4, murmurs)
3. Palpation of peripheral pulses: rate, amplitude, bilateral symmetry
4. Presence of peripheral edema
5. Funduscopic examination for presence of arteriolar narrowing or hemorrhage

■ DATA ANALYSIS: NURSING DIAGNOSES

Nursing diagnoses are determined from assessment of patient data. Possible nursing diagnoses for the person with hypertension may include, but are not limited to, the following:

Diagnostic Title	Possible Etiologies
Knowledge deficit: hypertension, drug therapy	Lack of exposure/recall, misinterpretation of information, unfamiliarity with information sources
Noncompliance: drug regimen, ongoing care	Patient value system, treatment side effects
Sexual dysfunction	Lack of knowledge of effects of medication

■ PLANNING: EXPECTED PATIENT OUTCOMES

Expected patient outcomes for the person with hypertension may include, but are not limited to, the following:

1. Defines HTN; explains meaning of systolic and diastolic blood pressure readings and effects of HTN on heart, kidney, and brain
2. Demonstrates correct procedure for self-measurement of blood pressure
3. States name, general action, dosage, and major side effects of each prescribed medication
4. Explains actions to prevent and control side effects of medications
5. Describes plans to reduce dietary salt, saturated fats, calories, and alcohol
6. Describes plans for a regular aerobic exercise program
7. Identifies sources of occupational and personal stress and methods to reduce the stress
8. Explains the effects of specific antihypertensives on sexual function (as appropriate)

■ IMPLEMENTATION

Nursing interventions for the person with HTN are primarily focused on patient teaching and counseling. Teaching is directed toward increasing knowledge about hypertension, risk factors, associated diseases, and the treatment regimen. Other efforts are intended to assist the person in making behavioral changes to further reduce, control, or maintain blood pressure at acceptable levels.

KNOWLEDGE OF HYPERTENSION

The individual needs to know the concepts of blood pressure and hypertension. Use simple terms to define systolic and diastolic blood pressure. Explain the effects of HTN on the heart, kidneys, and brain. Many persons can be taught self-monitoring of their blood pressure. Advise the person to purchase a reliable instrument and discourage use of coin-operated machines because these are often inaccurate. Have the patient keep a written record of blood pressures, including date and any pertinent information if elevated or lowered.

TEACHING ABOUT RISK FACTORS

Discuss *dietary modifications*. Explain that excess salt intake will contribute to fluid retention. Teaching should include the following:

1. Do not add salt to foods at the table.
2. Avoid highly salted foods, such as potato chips, pretzels, nuts, canned soups, and packaged luncheon meats.
3. Minimize eating "fast foods."
4. Reduce intake of saturated fats to maintain body weight and control atherosclerotic changes; avoid foods with visible fat, fried foods, certain dairy products, and saturated oils (palm, kernel, coconut).
5. Use moderation in alcohol consumption; alcohol may potentiate certain antihypertensive medications in addition to raising blood pressure.
6. Reduce body weight to a healthy level.

Other factors to discuss include smoking, exercise, and stress. Explain the effects of *nicotine* on blood vessels; suggest use of behavior modification, group therapy, or hypnosis as means of stopping smoking. Discuss need to participate in a regular *aerobic exercise program* three times a week, consisting of 20 to 45 minutes of activity with warm-up and cool-down procedures. Help patient identify sources of *stress;* demonstrate relaxation techniques such as deep breathing, progressive muscle relaxation, and imagery that can help lower blood pressure (see the research box).

MEDICATIONS

Patients who are prescribed medications to control their blood pressure should know the name and type of drug,

RESEARCH

Pender NJ: Physiologic responses of clients with essential hypertension to progressive muscle relaxation training, Res Nurs Health 7:197-203, 1984.

This study examines the effects of progressive muscle relaxation on blood pressure of hypertensive clients. After baseline data were collected, 22 clients received group relaxation training followed by individual monitoring sessions over a 6-week span of time. The control group consisting of 22 persons did not receive relaxation training. At the 4-month follow-up, the group instructed in relaxation had a lower mean systolic pressure than the nontrained group. The difference between trained and nontrained groups at follow-up was not significant, but the group trained in relaxation showed a significant decrease in diastolic pressure from baseline to follow-up. Relaxation, taught initially in group sessions with individual follow-up, resulted in continued practice of relaxation and subsequent lowering of blood pressure in subjects with essential, uncomplicated hypertension. ■

general action, dosage, and administration schedule. Provide the patient with written information, if possible. Common side effects include orthostatic hypotension, potassium depletion, and sexual dysfunction (see below). *Potassium depletion,* seen mostly with use of diuretics, can be avoided by eating foods high in potassium, or by taking a multivitamin that contains potassium or a potassium supplement. *Orthostatic hypotension* is a common side effect of antihypertensive therapy. It is often worse in the mornings (when blood pressure is normally lower), after alcohol ingestion (vasodilator), and during immobility that follows exercise. Orthostatic hypotension may be avoided by the following:

1. Rise slowly from a lying or sitting position to standing.
2. Sit down immediately if feeling faint.
3. Avoid long periods of standing (blood pools in legs, thereby temporarily causing hypovolemia).
4. Avoid very hot showers or baths (cause vasodilation, temporarily decreasing blood pressure).
5. Take medication at bedtime if drug can cause "first dose" hypotension or syncope.

SEXUAL DYSFUNCTION

Sexual dysfunction is a potential side effect of sympatholytic drugs which include the adrenergic inhibitors. In general, beta-adrenergic blockers and alpha blockers decrease ejaculation ability. Beta blockers also depress libido. Specific drugs such as clonidine interfere with erection. The nurse must discuss these adverse effects that may contribute to noncompliance. Define terms of sexual dysfunction in simple language: libido, erection, ejaculation. Identify the importance of sexual function to the patient, considering age and frequency of sexual activity. Encourage patient to report promptly any problems to a health care professional, and include the patient's sexual partner in the teaching process if possible. If necessary, consult with physician to determine an alternate medication regimen to counteract effects on sexual functioning.

NONCOMPLIANCE

Noncompliance is a major reason for inadequate HTN control. One reason is the absence of symptoms until advanced stages; hence the individual may not perceive a need to adhere to therapy. A second factor is the experience of unpleasant side effects of medications and unwillingness to seek professional follow-up. If several medications are prescribed, it is sometimes difficult to remember to take the medications correctly. Well-controlled hypertensives have been found to have fewer HTN-related problems and lower blood pressures (see the research box).

Measures to help increase compliance with therapy include the following:

1. Be sure patient understands that absence of symptoms does not indicate control of blood pressure; remind patient that symptoms do not occur until advanced stages of the disease.
2. Advise patient against abrupt withdrawal of medication; rebound hypertension can occur.
3. Encourage patient to discuss unpleasant side effects of medication and other nonpharmacologic therapies with a health care professional.
4. If remembering to take the medications is a problem, discuss alternate ways to remember, such as taking them with certain meals or placing medica-

tions in separate containers for certain times of the day.
5. Advise patient of need for regular health care follow-up.
6. Include family and significant others in the teaching process to provide support and promote adherence.
7. Contact patients who consistently cancel follow-up appointments.

CHAPTER SUMMARY

- Risk factors associated with the development of peripheral vascular disorders include cigarette smoking, hypertension, hyperlipidemia, obesity, physical inactivity, emotional stress, diabetes mellitus, and a family history of atherosclerosis.
- Primary prevention through health education about risk factors is the most important means to reduce the incidence of peripheral vascular disorders.
- Arterial disorders occur when any disturbance in the structure of the arteries causes diminished blood flow and decreased oxygen and nutrients to the tissues.
- The symptoms of arterial disorders are not caused by the degree of obstruction but by the extent to which the involved body part is deprived of circulation.
- Medical therapy for patients with atherosclerosis obliterans includes smoking cessation, low-fat–low cholesterol diet, weight reduction, regular exercise, control of associated diseases, and control of emotional stress.
- Intermittent claudication is a symptom of arterial disorders. This term is used to describe a cramplike muscle pain that develops during exercise and ceases 1 to 2 minutes after stopping the exercise. It is usually unilateral and affects primarily the calf muscles.
- Peripheral pulses may be absent or diminished in patients with arterial disorders.
- Anticoagulants such as heparin and warfarin sodium (Coumadin) prolong clotting time, prevent extension of an existing clot, and inhibit further clot formation.
- A teaching plan for a patient receiving Coumadin must include the prevention of bleeding.
- Protamin sulfate is a heparin antagonist, and vitamin K counteracts the effects of Coumadin.
- Fibrinolytics such as streptokinase and urokinase dissolve existing thrombi.
- Nursing interventions for the patient undergoing arterial bypass surgery include frequent assessment of peripheral pulses and the graft site, avoidance of flexion in the area of the graft, and position changes to promote circulation.

RESEARCH

Powers MJ and Jalowiec A: Profile of the well-controlled, well-adjusted hypertensive patient, Nurs Res 36:106-110, 1987.

The purpose of this study was to identify factors to predict blood pressure control and adjustment to chronic illness in hypertensive patients. A random selection of 450 hypertensive patients underwent structured interviews with the investigators, had their medical charts reviewed, and completed a 45-item Psychosocial Adjustment to Illness Scale (PAIS). Investigators found the well-controlled hypertensive patients to have more satisfaction with health care. They were knowledgeable about their medication side effects and had lower blood pressure readings. In addition, they reported fewer hypertension-related problems, and blood pressure was under control despite fewer medications. They were also less likely to worry and rated stress lower. ∎

✔ Positioning a patient with an arterial disorder may include placement of the extremity flat in bed or in a slightly dependent (15 degree) position to promote circulation. Elevation is contraindicated in arterial disorders.

✔ An important nursing intervention for the patient undergoing amputation surgery is to avoid flexion of the hip or knee to prevent contractures.

✔ A teaching plan for a patient with arterial problems includes measures to prevent infection and injury, interventions to maintain skin integrity and increase peripheral tissue perfusion, and methods to alter risk factors.

✔ Thrombophlebitis can affect the superficial or deep veins. Thrombophlebitis in a deep vein can lead to a pulmonary embolus.

✔ Deep vein thrombosis is treated by bed rest with periodic elevation of the affected extremity above heart level to prevent venous stasis and reduce edema.

✔ Patients with chronic venous disorders such as varicose veins should be taught measures to increase peripheral perfusion. These include avoiding constrictive clothing, never crossing legs at the knee, avoiding long periods of sitting or standing, elevating legs when sitting, and wearing elastic stockings.

✔ An arteriovenous fistula is an abnormal direct connection between an artery and a vein; it can lead to arterial and venous insufficiency.

✔ Leg ulcers can develop secondary to arterial or venous disorders. Primary treatment goals are to promote wound healing and prevent infection.

✔ Wet-to-dry dressings and debriding chemicals remove necrotic tissue from leg ulcers. A special protective boot (Unna paste boot) may be applied over ulcers for ambulatory patients. Arterial bypass surgery or amputation may be necessary for nonhealing chronic ulcers.

✔ Lymphedema results from interference with the drain of interstitial fluid from the tissues through the lymph system; the affected part becomes greatly edematous.

✔ A teaching plan for the patient with lymphedema includes elevating the affected extremity, wearing elastic stockings, taking diuretics as ordered, and avoiding an excess intake of foods high in sodium.

✔ Hypertension is generally considered to be present when blood pressure levels persistently exceed 140/90. Most hypertension is idiopathic. It is a major cause of coronary artery disease, cardiac failure, strokes, and renal failure.

✔ Drugs to control hypertension include diuretics (especially thiazides), peripheral and central acting adrenergics, beta-blockers, vasodilators, ACE inhibitors, and calcium antagonists. Medications are added in steps, as necessary, to control the blood pressure within normal limits.

✔ Persons with hypertension should monitor their own blood pressure, continue prescribed medications, exercise, avoid salty foods, stop smoking, and continue with follow-up care.

QUESTIONS TO CONSIDER

■ What are the similarities and differences in patient teaching for persons with arterial and venous disorders?

■ How would you position the leg of a person with an arterial problem? Does this positioning differ from that for a venous problem? What is the physiologic basis for the positioning?

■ How would your nursing care be altered for the patient undergoing a below knee amputation if the patient were 40 years old versus age 75?

■ What approaches might you use to assist an elderly hypertensive patient who is noncompliant in taking prescribed medications?

REFERENCES AND SELECTED READINGS

1. *Adelman EM: When the patient's blood pressure falls: what does it mean? what should you do? Nursing '87 17(10):66-73, 1987.
2. *Bartucci MR et al: Factors associated with adherence in hypertensive patients, ANNA J 14:245-248, 1987.
3. *Baum PL: Heed the early warning signs of peripheral vascular disease, Nursing '85 15:50-57, 1985.
4. *Beaver BM: Health education and the patient with peripheral vascular disease, Nurs Clin North Am 21:265-272, 1986.
5. Brengman SL and Burns MK: Hypertensive crisis in L & D, Am J Nurs 88:325-328, 1988.
6. Cahill M et al: Cardiovascular systems. In Diagnostics: the nurses' reference library, Springhouse, Penn, 1987, Intermed Communications, Inc.
7. Cline WT et al: Considerations in diagnosing deep vein thrombosis, Infect Surg 2:596-607, 1983.
8. Cotran RS et al: Robbin's pathologic basis of disease, Philadelphia, 1989, WB Saunders Co.
9. Craeger MA: Preventing and treating deep vein thrombophlebitis, Drug Ther 15:16-25, 1985.
10. Crockett, F: Varicose veins as a cause of venous ulceration, Pract Cardiol 11:191-199, 1985.
11. Cunningham SG: Nonpharmacologic management of blood pressure, J Cardiovasc Nurs 23(4):18-22, 1987.
12. Daeschner SA: Action stat! pulmonary embolism, Nursing '88 18(9):33, 1988.
13. *David JA: Wound management update 88, Nursing '88 18(6):33-37, 1988.

*References preceded by an asterisk are particularly well suited for student reading.

14. *Dixon MB et al: Arterial reconstruction for atherosclerotic occlusive disease, J Cardiovasc Nurs 1(2):36-49, 1987.

15. *Doyle JE: Treatment modalities in peripheral vascular disease, Nurs Clin North Am 21:241-253, 1986.

16. *Ekers MA: Psychosocial considerations in peripheral vascular disease: cause or effect? Nurs Clin North Am 21:255-263, 1986.

17. *Foreman MD: Arterial prosthetic graft infections: the pathophysiologic basis of nursing care, Focus Crit Care 12:23-28, 1985.

18. Ganong WF: Review of medical physiology, ed 14, Norwalk, Conn, 1987, Appleton & Lange.

19. *Gerdes L: Recognizing the multisystemic effects of embolism, Nursing '87 17(12):34-41, 1987.

20. Goldberg K, editor: Vascular problems, Springhouse, Penn, 1986, Springhouse Corp.

21. *Henneman EA and Henneman PL: Intricacies of blood pressure measurement: reexamining the rituals, Heart Lung 18(3):263-271, 1989.

22. *Herman JA: Nursing assessment and nursing diagnosis in patients with peripheral vascular disease, Nurs Clin North Am 21:219-231, 1986.

23. *Hill MN and Cunningham SL: The latest words for high BP, Am J Nurs 89:504-509, 1989.

24. Hurst JW et al: The heart, ed 7, New York, 1990, McGraw-Hill Inc.

25. Kerr JA: Adherence and self-care, Heart Lung 14:24-41, 1985.

26. *Kleven MR: Comparison of thrombolytic agents: mechanisms of action, efficacy, and safety, Heart Lung 17(6):750-755, 1988.

27. *Kline E: Management of bleeding in the patient receiving thrombolytic therapy for acute myocardial infarction: a nursing perspective, Heart Lung 17(6):771-777, 1988.

28. *Krakosky JN and Vanscoy GJ: Running an anticoagulation clinic, Am J Nurs 89:304-306, 1989.

29. *Massey JA: Diagnostic testing for peripheral vascular disease, Nurs Clin North Am 21:207-218, 1986.

30. McCarthy WJ and Williams LR: Femoral artery reconstruction, Crit Care Q 8:39-48, 1986.

31. *McMahan BE: Why deep vein thrombosis is so dangerous, RN 51:20-23, 1987.

32. *Miller RA and Evans WE: Immediate postop prosthesis, Am J Nurs 87:310-311, 1987.

33. Moake JF and Levine JD: Clinical symposia: thrombotic disorders, Summit, NJ, 1985, Ciba-Geigy Corp.

34. *Moore LD and Pulliam CB: An on-the-spot guide to antihypertensive drugs, Nursing '86 16(1):54-57, 1986.

35. Moore WE, editor: Vascular surgery: a comprehensive review, Orlando, Fla, 1986, Grune & Stratton Inc.

36. Pender NJ: Health promotion in nursing practice, ed 3, Norwalk, Conn, 1987, Appleton & Lange.

37. *Ramsey R: Adjusting drug dosages for critically ill elderly patients, Nursing '88:47-49, 1988.

38. Report of the Joint National Committee on Detection, Evaluation and Treatment of High Blood Pressure, US Department of Health and Human Services, Public Health Services, Bethesda, MD, 1988, National Institutes of Health.

39. *Sands D and Holman E: Does knowledge enhance patient compliance? J Gerontol Nurs 11:23-29, 1985.

40. Schwartz SI et al: Principles of surgery, ed 5, New York, 1989, McGraw-Hill Inc.

41. Sobel BE: Fibrinolysis and activators of plasminogen, Heart Lung 17(6):775-779, 1987.

42. Spittell JA: Medical treatment of arteriosclerosis obliterans, Drug Ther 15:12-18, 1985.

43. Swearingen PL, editor: Manual of nursing therapeutics: applying nursing diagnoses to medical disorders, Menlo Park, Calif, 1986, Addison-Wesley Publishing Co Inc.

44. *Swithers CM: Tools for teaching about anticoagulants, RN 51(1):57-58, 1988.

45. Swonger AK and Matajski MP: Nursing pharmacology, Glenview, Ill, 1988, Scott, Foresman & Co.

46. *Turner JA: Nursing interventions in patients with peripheral vascular disease, Nurs Clin North Am 21:233-240, 1986.

47. *Vitello-Ciccio J: Thrombolytic therapy: urokinase, J Cardiovasc Nurs 1(2):59-62, 1987.

48. *Wagner MM: Pathophysiology related to peripheral vascular disease, Nurs Clin North Am 21:195-205, 1986.

49. Wyngaarden JB and Smith LH: Cecil textbook of medicine, ed 18, Philadelphia, 1988, WB Saunders Co.

CHAPTER 30

Management of Persons with Hematologic Problems

KATHRYN SABO THOMPSON
ROSEMARIE M. HOGAN

CHAPTER OBJECTIVES

After studying this chapter, the student should be able to:
1. Assess persons with suspected hematologic disorders.
2. Compare and contrast different types of anemias in terms of pathophysiology, assessment, and interventions.
3. Explain the genetic factors of sickle cell disease and describe the nature of and nursing care for patients with sickle cell crisis.
4. Compare and contrast disorders of hemostasis, platelets, and coagulation (thrombocytopenia, thrombocytosis, hemophilia, vitamin K deficiency, disseminated intravascular coagulation) and describe nursing interventions.
5. Identify four types of leukemia, therapeutic modalities, and nursing interventions.
6. Differentiate between Hodgkin's disease and non-Hodgkin's lymphoma and describe related interventions.

Diseases associated with the reticuloendothelial system (RES) are diverse in their underlying pathologic manifestations, disease course, and response to treatment. Most often the symptoms manifested are the result of interference with the normal development and function of the blood components: erythrocytes (red blood cells, RBCs), platelets, leukocytes (white blood cells, WBCs), and altered hematopoiesis (blood cell production). Normally, homeostasis is maintained through a balance between the rate of production of normal blood cells and the rate of destruction. Disorders of the blood are manifested when this balance is lost. Disturbances in the coagulation mechanism also result in blood disorders.

COMPONENTS OF THE HEMATOPOIETIC SYSTEM

The hematopoietic system includes blood and its components, as well as the RES, which is located through-out the body. Its function is phagocytizing foreign materials and lysing (breaking down) RBCs.

BLOOD

Blood is an aqueous solution (plasma) that contains proteins, electrolytes, and inorganic and organic constituents. Solids make up 7% to 9% of the blood.

The cell components of blood include erythrocytes, leukocytes, and thrombocytes or platelets (Table 30-1). All normal cells are derived from a single stem cell that can divide into lymphoid and blood stem cells, which in turn become progenitor cells that divide along a specific single pathway (Figure 30-1). This process is known as *hematopoiesis* and takes place in the *bone marrow* of the skull, vertebrae, pelvis, sternum, ribs, and proximal epiphysis of long bones. Production may occur in all the long bones during periods of increased demand, such as with hemorrhage or during cell destruction (hemolysis).

RED BLOOD CELLS (ERYTHROCYTES)

An RBC is a nonnucleated biconcave disk that is soft and pliable, which enables it to change its shape during passage through the microcirculation. The RBC's major component is hemoglobin (Hb), a protein that transports oxygen and carbon dioxide and maintains normal pH through a series of intracellular buffers (see Chapter 24). The Hb molecule contains globin (two pairs of polypeptide chains) and four heme groups, each one containing an atom of ferrous iron. Thus each Hb molecule can unite with four oxygen molecules to form oxyhemoglobin (a reversible reaction). Carbon dioxide is carried by the globin portion of the Hb molecule.

Maturation of RBCs in the bone marrow requires adequate amounts and use of vitamin B_{12}, folic acid, proteins, enzymes, and minerals (iron, copper). *Erythropoiesis* (RBC formation) can be greatly stimulated by the secretion of a hormone *erythropoietin* from the kidneys when RBCs decrease in number below normal (such as with severe blood loss) or when demand for ox-

TABLE 30-1 Laboratory tests for hematologic assessment

Blood Cell	Function	Diagnostic Test
Erythrocytes (RBCs)	Mediate the exchange of oxygen and carbon dioxide between lungs and tissue	RBC, hemoglobin (Hb), hematocrit (Hct), reticulocyte count Blood indices: Hb, mean corpuscular hemoglobin concentration (MCHC), mean corpuscular volume (MCV), mean corpuscular hemoglobin (MCH) Red cell fragility Morphologic description in stained smear
Platelets	Platelet plug; promotion of thrombin production	Platelet aggregation Platelet count Bleeding time
Leukocytes (WBCs)		WBC
Granulocytes		WBC with differential
Neutrophils	Phagocytosis	
Eosinophils	Allergic responses, parasitic infestation	
Basophils	Immunologic responses	
Lymphocytes	Formation of immunoglobulins	
Monocytes	Phagocytosis	

ygen increases (tissue hypoxia). RBCs circulate for 120 days and are then destroyed by the macrophages of the RES. Most of the iron is removed from the heme and can be used to form new heme groups. Small amounts of iron lost daily in urine and feces and through menstrual flow must be replaced by iron ingestion (see p. 792). The remainder of the heme is broken down to form bilirubin and is secreted into the bile. Energy in the form of adenosine triphosphate (ATP) is required to maintain cell membrane integrity and the relatively low sodium and high potassium content of the RBC and as a defense against oxidation and other environmental stressors.

WHITE BLOOD CELLS (LEUKOCYTES)

WBCs may be classified into two groups as follows: *granular leukocytes* (also called *polymorphonuclear* [PMN] *leukocytes*), consisting of neutrophils, eosino-

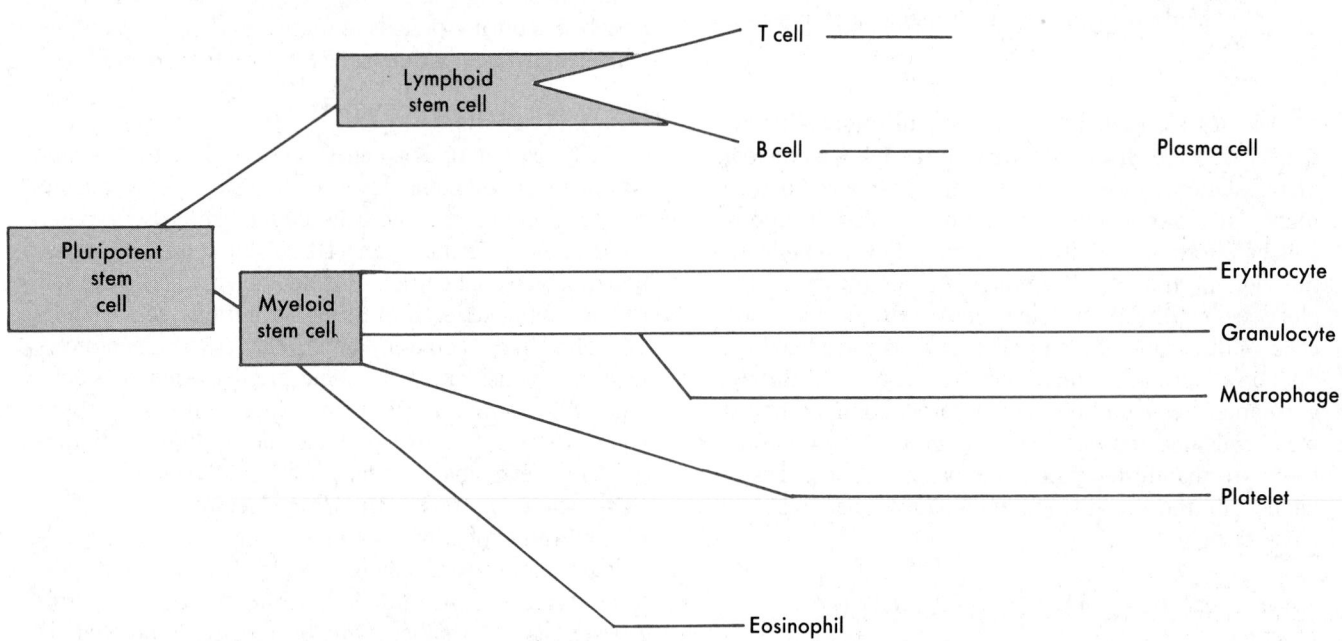

FIGURE 30-1 Scheme of stem cell differentiation showing typical progenitor cell for erythrocytes, granulocytes, and platelets. (Adapted from Clinc M and Golde D: Blood 53:157, 1979).

phils, and basophils; and *nongranular leukocytes,* consisting of monocytes and lymphocytes. The granulocytes contain enzymes that kill and digest bacteria with degranulation of the cells.

Neutrophils are present in the circulation or along the capillary walls (the margination pool). They move into the tissues and mucous membranes and serve as the body's primary defense against bacterial infection through the process of phagocytosis (see Chapter 8). *Eosinophils* are involved in allergic responses and destruction of parasitic worms. *Basophils* respond similar to mast cells in immunologic reactions.

Monocytes are larger than neutrophils and have one large, folded or kidney-shaped nucleus. They leave the circulation and become tissue *macrophages,* which also have phagocytic action, removing dead and injured cells, cell fragments, and microorganisms.

Lymphocytes are mononuclear with a round or oval nucleus. They originate primarily in lymphoid tissue (lymph nodes) but also in the bone marrow. There are two types of lymphocytes, the long-lived circulating T lymphocytes (from the thymus) and short-lived noncirculating B lymphocytes. T lymphocytes initiate the cellular immune response, whereas B lymphocytes (immunoglobulins) initiate the humoral immune response (see Chapter 8).

PLATELETS

Platelets (thrombocytes) are not cells but granular, disk-shaped, nonnucleated cell fragments. One third of all platelets are in the spleen as a reserve pool, and the remainder are in circulation. Platelets are also derived from the stem cells and are essential to hemostasis and coagulation. Hemostasis results from the adhesion and aggregation capabilities of platelets to plug small breaks in blood vessels. Platelets also release thromboplastin (factor III), which, in the presence of calcium ions, converts prothrombin into thrombin in the first step of the coagulation mechanism (Figure 30-2). In the second

COAGULATION FACTORS

Factor I	Fibrinogen
Factor II	Prothrombin
Factor III	Thromboplastin, tissue thromboplastin
Factor IV	Calcium
Factor V	Proaccelerin, labile factor
Factor VII	Serum prothrombin conversion accelerator (SPCA)
Factor VIII	Antihemophilic globulin (AHG) Antihemophilic factor (AHF)
Factor IX	Plasma thromboplastin component (PTC), Christmas factor
Factor X	Stuart-Prower factor
Factor XI	Plasma thromboplastin antecedent (PTA)
Factor XII	Hageman factor, contact factor
Factor XIII	Fibrin-stabilizing factor, fibrinase

step of the coagulation mechanism, thrombin promotes the conversion of fibrinogen (a soluble plasma protein) into fibrin (an insoluble strand). Step one requires coagulation factors IV, V, VIII, IX, X, XI, and XII; whereas step two requires factors IV and XIII (see box). (For further discussion on hemostasis, see p. 794).

RETICULOENDOTHELIAL SYSTEM

The RES, also called the mononuclear phagocyte system or macrophage system, includes circulating monocytes and their precursor cells in the bone marrow. It also includes more or less fixed mononuclear phagocytic cells found in blood channels in the spleen and liver (Kupffer cells), in the lymphatic system, in serosal cavities of the body, in the lungs, in general connective tissue, and in the bone marrow (see Chapter 8).

In addition to phagocytosis, the RES processes the Hb of RBCs that have reached the end of their life span, splitting Hb into an iron-containing substance and bilirubin.

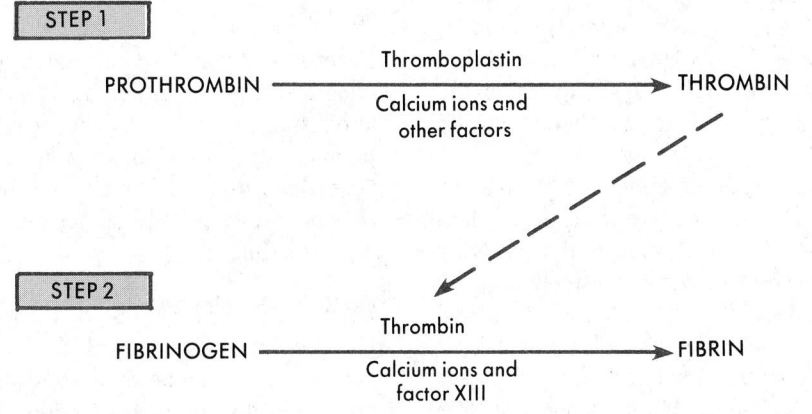

FIGURE 30-2 Basic steps in coagulation process.

PHYSIOLOGIC CHANGES WITH AGING

The effect of aging on hematopoiesis is still being studied, with findings that are sometimes ambiguous or of questionable clinical significance. Evidence from studies of mouse marrow show that stem cells have a limited capacity to proliferate. Findings from animal studies suggest that changes related to aging do not have clinical significance.[45] The cellularity of human marrow decreases with age, but this may be the result of an increase in fat from osteoporosis rather than a decrease in hematopoietic cells.

In humans the total number of leukocytes and differential counts shows no variation through middle age and no gross changes in old age. In general the leukocyte count does not rise as high in response to infection, and studies suggest that the elderly have a diminished marrow granulocyte reserve.

The Hb level decreases after middle age, although the decrease in women seems to be relatively less than that in men. Unexplained anemia in the elderly has been noted, but iron absorption is not impaired; however, use of orally administered iron is reduced. This anemia does not appear to be related solely to age.[45] Serum iron and iron-binding capacity decrease in the elderly, and low serum vitamin B_{12} and folic acid levels occur in a significant proportion of elderly people but without anemia.

No age-related changes in platelets have been reported. RBC sedimentation rate increases significantly, but this rate is of limited value in detecting disease in the elderly. Some of the plasma coagulation factors have been reported to increase with age (factors I, V, VII, and IX). Partial thromboplastin time (PTT) may be shortened.[45]

ASSESSMENT OF PERSONS WITH SUSPECTED HEMATOLOGIC DISORDERS

A variety of disorders affect the hematopoietic system. In addition to primary hematologic disorders, secondary effects from disease of another body system may manifest themselves in abnormal hematologic findings. For example, the anemia associated with azotemia is the consequence of disease outside of the hematopoietic system.

The cause of any hematologic abnormality must be assiduously pursued. The importance of accurate diagnosis combined with the very diverse and frequently nonspecific signs and symptoms makes it likely that the person will become involved in an arduous diagnostic process. At the time of initial contact the patient is already experiencing the stress of sudden onset of illness or the gnawing fear or suspicion that all is not well. The explanations offered and the time allowed for verbaliza-tion and questions are means of providing a positive foundation for the long-term care that may follow.

SUBJECTIVE DATA

A thorough history includes detailed information about the person's symptoms and a thorough review of systems. In the history taking of a person with suspected hematologic disease, other key points to include are family history, drug history, exposure to chemicals, and general nonspecific complaints offered by the patient.

FAMILY HISTORY

The existence of inherited hematologic disorders, such as sickle cell disease and malignancies, necessitates a detailed family history. Questions regarding disease or presence of symptoms among relatives should include reference to parents, siblings, grandfathers, uncles, and nephews. Questions should explore instances of severe or prolonged bleeding after minor trauma, dental extractions, or surgery. The occurrence of jaundice or anemia in relatives should also be ascertained.

DRUGS AND CHEMICALS

Drugs may induce or potentiate hematologic disease (see box on p. 779). Most notable are the hematologic effects of the cytotoxic drugs used in cancer chemotherapy and the neutropenia associated with chloramphenicol. A thorough history of drugs ingested by a person is a crucial part of assessment. Many persons regularly ingest "something to help me sleep," "something to calm me down," or "just aspirin." Analgesics, tranquilizers, laxatives, and sedatives are often overlooked by persons when asked about drugs. Specific, often rephrased questioning is necessary to obtain a complete drug history.

Certain chemicals may exert a potentially harmful effect on the hematopoietic system. To obtain a history of exposure to chemicals, an occupational history is useful. In addition, such common practices as the use of hair dye should also be explored.

FEVER

Fever is a common manifestation of many of the hematologic disorders and is an important question to be asked during the history. Fever typically occurs in lymphoma, primarily Hodgkin's disease and leukemia. Severe chills may accompany hemolytic disorders. Night sweats are frequently associated with both lymphoma and leukemia.

FATIGUE AND MALAISE

Fatigue and malaise are difficult symptoms to evaluate because they frequently accompany many physical and emotional disorders. Information regarding the occurrence of these symptoms should be included in the his-

SOME DRUGS IMPLICATED IN HEMOPOIETIC SUPPRESSION*

Acetophenetidin (1, 3)	Cycloheximide (3)	Para-aminosalicylic acid (3, 4)
Acetylsalicylic acid (aspirin) (1, 2, 3)	Dextromethorphan HBr (2)	Penicillin (1, 2, 3, 4)
Acetyl sulfisoxazole (3)	Diethylstilbestrol (2)	Phenobarbital (1, 2, 3, 4)
Aminosalicylic acid (3, 4)	Diphenylhydantoin (Dilantin) (4)	Phenylbutazone (Butazolidin) (1, 2, 3)
Ammonium thioglycolate (3)	Dipyrrone (3)	Pipamazine (1)
Amodiaquin HCI (3)	Ethinamate (2)	Primidone (1)
Arsenicals (1, 2, 3, 4)	Fumagillin (3)	Prochlorperazine (Compazine) (2, 3)
Arsphenamine (1, 2)	γ-Benzene hexachloride (1, 3)	Pyrimethamine (Daraprim) (1, 2, 3)
Atabrine (1, 2)	Hair lacquer (3)	Quinidine (2)
β-Naphthoxyacetic acid (2)	Imipramine HCI (3)	Quinine (2, 3)
Benzene (1, 2, 3, 4)	Iproniazid (1)	Reserpine (2)
Bishydroxycoumarin (3, 4)	Isoniazid (1, 3, 4)	Stibophen (2)
Carbamide (2)	Lead (1)	Streptomycin (1, 2, 3)
Carbon tetrachloride (1)	Lithium carbonate (1)	Sulfamethoxypyridazine (Kynex) (2, 3, 4)
Carbutamide (Orabetic) (2)	Mephenytoin (Mesantoin) (1, 2)	Tetracycline (3)
Chloramphenicol (1, 2, 3, 4)	Meprobamate (1, 2, 3)	Thenalidine tartrate (3)
Chlordane (1)	Methaminodiazepoxide (Librium) (3)	Thioridazine HCI (3)
Chlorophenothane (DDT) (1, 2)	Methapyrilene HCI (4)	Tolazoline HCI (1, 2)
Chlorothiazide (3)	Methylpromazine (3)	Tolbutamide (1, 2, 3)
Chlorpheniramine maleate (3)	Mezapine (2)	Tolbutamide (Orinase) (2)
Chlorpromazine (Thorazine) (3)	Nitrofurantion (4)	Trifluoperazine (1, 3)
Chlorpropamide (2)	Novobiocin (4)	Trifluoperazine (Stelazine) (3)
Chlortetracyline (1, 3)	Nystatin (2)	Trimethadione (Tridione) (1, 2)
Cinophen (3)	Oxyphenabutazone (2)	
Coldricine (2, 3)		

From Miale J: Laboratory medicine: hematology, ed 6, St Louis, 1982, The CV Mosby Co.)
*More than 500 are listed in the latest report of the American Medical Association Subcommittee on Blood Dyscrasias. The drugs listed in this table are those that have produced dyscrasias when given alone. 1 = pancytopenia; 2 = thrombocytopenia; 3 = leukopenia; 4 = anemia.

tory. When combined with physical and laboratory findings, they are of some diagnostic value. In addition, the person's subjective description of such symptoms lends some insight into perception of the illness, the extent to which the illness is affecting daily living, and the ability to adapt.

OBJECTIVE DATA

A thorough physical examination is performed in the assessment of a person with a hematologic disorder. It is useful to recognize target organs and alterations that may reflect hematologic disease.

SKIN

Skin manifestations of hematologic disease are often readily visible. *Petechiae, ecchymoses,* and *purpura* are associated with decreased platelets (thrombocytopenia) and other bleeding disorders. *Jaundice,* when observed, may be associated with pernicious anemia or hemolytic disease. *Pallor* is typically associated by the layperson with disorders of the blood. Pallor as a criteria for assessment may be deceptive, since many healthy persons have pale complexions, whereas some severely anemic patients may have ruddy complexions.

Changes in skin texture may also be observed. Except in severe cases, the patient will most likely observe such changes. With iron deficiency anemia the patient may notice dry skin, dry hair, and brittle nails. Severe itching is often associated with Hodgkin's disease and may also occur with polycythemia vera, especially after bathing. In persons with leukemia and lymphoma, infiltrative lesions of the skin may be observed on any portion of the body.

HEAD AND NECK

The sclerae of the eyes are examined for jaundice and the conjunctivae for pallor. Retinal hemorrhages may occur in persons with severe anemia and thrombocytopenia. Questions may also elicit a history of visual disturbances.

The oral mucosa is observed for pallor, bleeding tendency, and ulceration. The tongue may be very smooth in association with both pernicious anemia and nutritional deficiencies.

The neck is observed primarily for evaluation of lymph nodes. Nodes may be so large as to be visible. A "lump" on the neck is often the reason for seeking medical attention.

CHEST

Firm pressure with the fingertips is exerted along the sternum and ribs to elicit any tenderness that may be present. Such tenderness may reflect a leukemic process or multiple myeloma.

ABDOMEN

The abdomen is percussed and palpated with special attention to the liver and spleen. Both organs are prone to enlargement in association with hematologic disease.

BACK AND EXTREMITIES

The skeletal system is evaluated primarily for pain, joint deformity, and arthritis. Bone pain may be associated with hematologic malignancies. In persons with hemolytic processes and some hematologic malignancies, there is increased uric acid production and a corresponding increase in the incidence of gout. Joint deformities are associated with bleeding disorders.

LYMPH NODES

Lymph nodes are widely distributed in the body and are routinely examined by palpation of the body part being examined. In the healthy adult the only palpable nodes are in the inguinal region and less often in the axilla. With disease the cervical and supraclavicular nodes may become palpable. Further evaluation of lymph nodes requires x-ray examination and lymphangiography. It is important to recognize that any enlarged lymph node may reflect a disease process and should be evaluated thoroughly.

NERVOUS SYSTEM

Many neurologic abnormalities may be manifested in persons with hematologic disorders. These catastrophic complications are caused by bleeding or infection within the central nervous system. Infiltration of malignant leukemic or lymphomatous cells may produce signs and symptoms of cerebral tumor. In addition, some of the lymphomas, especially Hodgkin's disease, may produce a dementia as a remote effect. Initial physical examination should therefore include assessment of mental status, cranial nerve function, sensory function (pain, touch, position, vibratory sensation), and motor function (strength, reflexes, plantar response).

DIAGNOSTIC STUDIES

Extensive blood examinations are performed as part of the diagnostic workup of a person suspected of having a hematologic disorder. The most frequent laboratory tests include Hb and hematocrit (Hct) levels, red blood cell indices, and peripheral smear. The information obtained from such studies provides important clues as to the pathology of the disorder. In addition to their diagnostic value, blood studies are used to monitor an individual's progress and response to treatment. The final diagnosis of a hematologic disease often depends on an examination of a peripheral blood smear and the bone marrow.

TABLE 30-2 Normal values of cellular blood components

Type	Normal Values
RBCs	Male: 4.6-6.1 million/mm^3
	Female: 4.0-5.4 million/mm^3
WBCs	5000-10,000/mm^3
Neutrophils	55%-70%
Eosinophils	1%-4%
Basophils	0%-1%
Monocytes	2%-6%
Lymphocytes	25%-40%
Platelets	150,000/mm^3
Hematocrit (Hct)	Male: 45%-52%
	Female: 37%-48%
Hemoglobin (Hb)	Male: 13-18 g/100 ml
	Female: 12-16 g/100 ml
Mean corpuscular volume (MCV)	80-95 μm^3
Mean corpuscular Hb concentration (MCHC)	32%-36%

Differential blood count—totals 100% (Neutrophils, Eosinophils, Basophils, Monocytes, Lymphocytes)

HEMOGLOBIN AND HEMATOCRIT

An Hb test measures the amount of Hb in circulation. The packed red blood cell volume, or Hct, is the ratio of RBC volume to the whole blood volume (Table 30-2).

RED BLOOD CELL INDICES

The RBC indices consist of the mean corpuscular volume (MCV), mean corpuscular hemoglobin (MCH), and the mean corpuscular hemoglobin concentration (MCHC). The MCV estimates the average size of the RBC. Both the MCH and the MCHC measure the content of the Hb in RBCs. The MCHC is considered more accurate than the MCH because it measures the entire blood volume of Hb rather than just from a single cell. The RBC indices provide a differential diagnosis of the type of anemia. Normal values are indicated in Table 30-2.

PERIPHERAL BLOOD SMEAR

Each blood cell possesses microscopic features that identify and set the cell apart from other cell types. Examination of the peripheral blood smear provides information concerning the etiology of an anemia. The size and shape of the RBC is observed (see box on p. 781). Alteration in the size of the RBC is classified as *anisocytosis;* alteration in shape of the RBC is noted as *poikilocytosis.* The WBC may be examined to provide information about adequate bone marrow production. Often this information, when combined with data from the history, physical examination, and other laboratory tests, determines the medical diagnosis.

DESCRIPTIVE CELL CHARACTERISTICS IN ANEMIA

Size	Macrocytic (large)
	Normocytic
	Microcytic (small)
Hb	Normochromic
	Hypochromic (decreased)

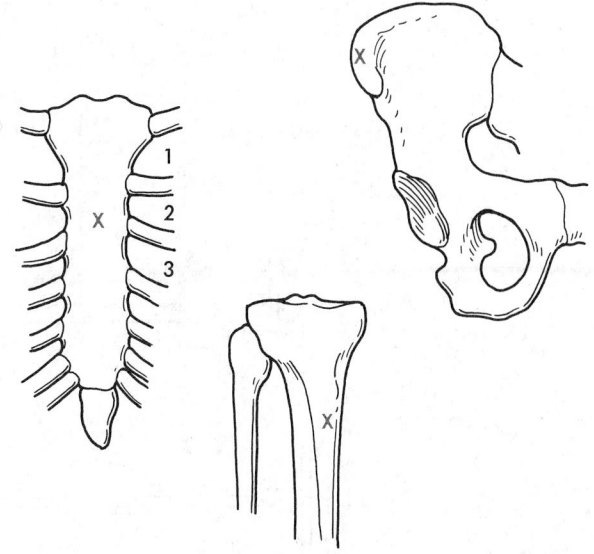

FIGURE 30-3 Sites for bone marrow aspiration: sternum, iliac crest (most common), and tibia.

BONE MARROW EXAMINATION

An adjunct to the peripheral blood smear is the bone marrow examination. Generally the bone marrow is examined when the diagnosis is not clearly established from the peripheral blood smear or when further information is needed. A bone marrow specimen is obtained by bone marrow aspiration or bone marrow biopsy.

Bone Marrow Aspiration

Aspiration is the most common procedure for obtaining a bone marrow sample. The procedure is possible because normal bone marrow is soft and semifluid and can therefore be removed by aspiration through a needle. Bone marrow aspiration is most likely to be performed in persons with severe anemia, neutropenia (decreased number of WBCs), acute leukemia, and thrombocytopenia (decreased number of platelets).

Procedure. The skin surrounding the puncture site (Figure 30-3) is shaved, if necessary, and cleansed with an antiseptic such as povidone-iodine complex (Betadine). Sterile towels are placed around the site. The skin and periosteum are anesthetized to avoid pain. First, the most superficial layer of the skin is infiltrated with procaine. After a few seconds the needle is further advanced until bone is touched. Procaine is then injected to anesthetize the periosteum.

The marrow aspiration needle is inserted; when the marrow cavity is entered, the marrow stylet is removed from the needle, and a sterile syringe is attached. The syringe plunger is drawn back until marrow appears in the syringe. As the plunger is drawn back, the person will experience a brief, sharp pain, sometimes described as a burning sensation. The pain is caused by the suction exerted as the plunger is pulled back. At this point the nurse's hands placed gently on the person's shoulder and a calm warning coupled with a reminder to lie still serve well to prevent a sudden jerk or movement by the person.

After the needle is removed, pressure is applied briefly over the aspiration site to arrest the minimal bleeding that occurs. If the patient is thrombocytopenic, pressure is applied for 3 to 5 minutes.

Some persons may complain of tenderness at the aspiration site for a few days. Most often, no pain or discomfort is experienced following the procedure.

Bone Marrow Biopsy

A bone marrow biopsy is indicated when a large sample of bone marrow is needed. Persons most likely to undergo a bone marrow biopsy are those with pancytopenia (more than one altered cell type), myelofibrosis, metastatic tumor, lymphoma, and multiple myeloma. The most common site for bone marrow biopsy is the posterosuperior iliac spine. (The sternum is also used.) The initial steps in the biopsy procedure are similar to those outlined for bone marrow aspiration. The use of a Jamshidi needle allows for a core of marrow to be collected (Figure 30-4).

After a bone marrow aspirate or biopsy, patients are assessed for bleeding from the site. Other comfort measures, such as assisting the person to freshen up, are often needed to help the person relax and rest comfortably.

From microscopic examination of the bone marrow, iron stores can be determined, as can the morphology of the progenitor cell. Megaloblastic changes may be observed; infiltration with leukemic cells and absence of cells, as in aplastic anemia, can be determined.

Other diagnostic tests are discussed throughout the text along with the specific disorder to which they pertain.

PREVENTION AND HEALTH EDUCATION

Exposure to certain chemicals and drugs places individuals at high risk for hematologic disorders, especially

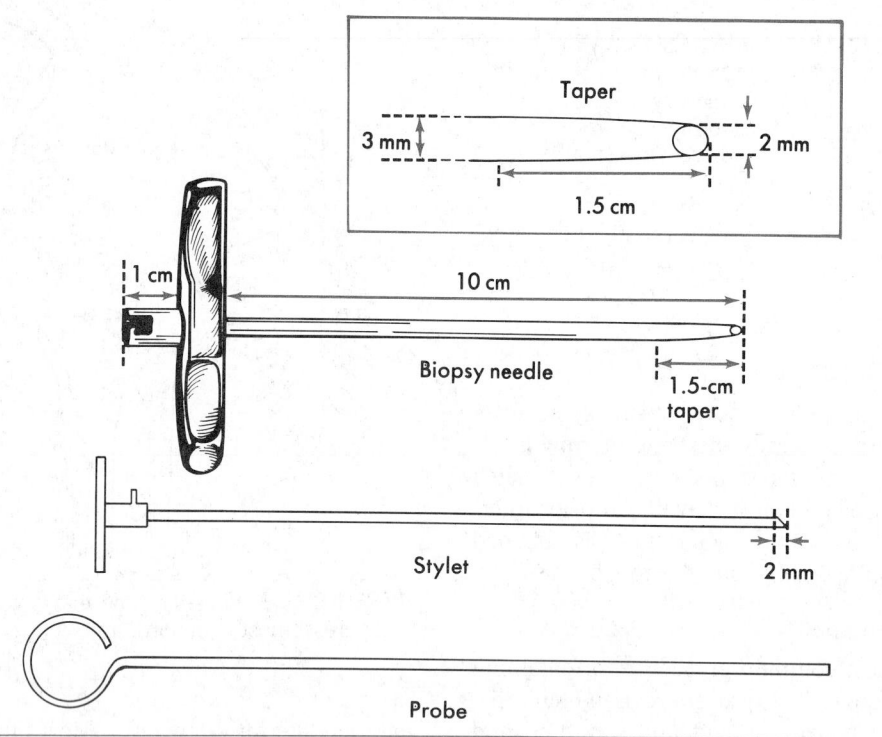

FIGURE 30-4 Bone marrow biopsy needle showing shape and size.

aplastic anemia and the leukemias. Individuals with inadequate dietary intake of iron and vitamins (for example, folic acid and B_{12}), alcoholics, and others with poor dietary habits because of inadequate knowledge or low income are particularly susceptible to anemia. Women who have long-term blood loss because of heavy menstrual bleeding (menorrhagia) are also at risk for anemia, as are other persons with long-term, slow blood loss.

Other diseases such as sickle cell anemia, the thalassemias, and hemophilia are hereditary; therefore marriage between carriers of defective genes may result in children with the disease.

Health teaching involves identifying persons at high risk and ways in which the risk factors can be mitigated. Occupational health nurses are involved in identifying industrial chemicals or processes that place workers in danger and in working with companies to minimize those risks. Nurses in all settings teach about dietary needs for iron and other vitamins. An important facet of this teaching is helping those persons with low incomes to identify inexpensive sources of the vitamins and minerals necessary for hematologic health. Nurses also may become politically active in order to ensure that there is adequate government funding for food stamps and other low-cost nutritional programs for those persons who have marginal incomes.

One of the most difficult and sensitive roles for nurses is that of genetic counselor, communicating to individuals with hereditary problems the risk factors involved and possibility of having children with severe hematopoietic disease. The persons are allowed to make their own decisions after information has been shared with them, a decision that can be devastating to the individual, no matter what it is.

DISORDERS ASSOCIATED WITH ERYTHROCYTES

The major health problems associated with erythrocytes are the anemias (including hemoglobinopathies) and erythrocytosis (polycythemia).

ANEMIA

Anemia refers to a deficiency of RBCs, as reflected in a decreased Hb level, packed cell volume (Hct), and RBC count. Anemias may be divided into those that are the result of blood loss, impaired production of RBCs, increased destruction of RBCs, or nutritional deficiency. The anemias are summarized in Table 30-3.

Anemia may also be differentiated by examining the size of a red cell and the amount of Hb contained. The suffix *-cytic* refers to RBC size and *-chromic* refers to amount of Hb (see box on p. 781).

ANEMIA SECONDARY TO BLOOD LOSS
Etiology and Clinical Manifestations

Acute blood loss. The anemia associated with acute blood loss is the direct result of the decrease in circulat-

TABLE 30-3 Types of anemia

Type	Causes	Clinical Manifestations
SECONDARY TO BLOOD LOSS		
Acute	Hemorrhage	Early: weakness, cool moist skin, tachycardia, hypotension; late: decreased Hb and Hct
Chronic	Gastrointestinal or other malignancy, bleeding ulcers, bleeding hemorrhoids, menorrhagia	Decreased RBC, Hb, Hct, MCV, and MCHC; fatigue
SECONDARY TO IMPAIRED PRODUCTION OF RBCS		
Aplastic anemia	Drugs, chemicals, radiation, chemotherapy, virus, congenital, autoimmune mechanism	Pallor of skin and mucous membranes, fatigue, palpitations, exertional dyspnea, pancytopenia, bleeding tendency, infections
Chronic anemia	Chronic illness, renal disease	Decreased serum iron concentration, fatigue
HEMOLYTIC ANEMIAS		
Hereditary spherocytosis	Genetic: inherited as autosomal dominant trait	Spherocytes and increased reticulocytes on peripheral blood smear; fatigue, exertional dyspnea
Thalassemia	Genetic: decreased synthesis of one of globin chains of Hb	Microcytosis, hypochromic RBC, decreased growth at pubescence, eventual cardiac failure
Sickle cell disease	Genetic hemoglobinopathy	Painful episodes; vaso-occlusive crises; chronic leg ulcers, chronic renal and ocular problems; sickled cells on peripheral blood smears
Enzyme deficiency anemia	Genetic: deficiency of glucose-6-phosphate dehydrogenase (G6PD)	Episodic hemolytic episodes, decreased levels of G6PD
Acquired hemolytic anemia	Drug-induced or autoimmune response	Presence of RBC antibody on antiglobin or Coombs' test
NUTRITIONAL ANEMIAS		
Iron deficiency anemia	Chronic blood loss, inadequate intake	Fatigue, exertional dyspnea; microcytosis; low serum iron concentration
Megaloblastic anemia	Deficiency in vitamin B_{12} or folic acid	Macrocytosis; glossitis and neurologic abnormalities with vitamin B_{12} deficiency

ing RBCs. The adult of average build has a total blood volume of approximately 6000 ml. Usually an adult can lose 500 ml of blood without serious or lasting effects. If the loss reaches 1000 ml or more, serious acute consequences may result.

Signs and symptoms include those associated with hypovolemia and hypoxemia. Weakness, stupor, irritability, and cool moist skin may be observed. Vital signs demonstrate hypotension and tachycardia. Decreased hemoglobin and hematocrit may not be evident until several hours after the blood loss has occurred. The severity of the patient's symptoms correlates with the severity of the blood loss.

Chronic blood loss. The body has remarkable adaptive powers and may adjust fairly well to a severe reduction in RBCs and Hb, provided the condition develops gradually. A person may remain asymptomatic even though the total RBC count may drop to almost half its normal amount. With chronic anemia, RBC counts, Hb and Hct levels, MCV, and MCHC are important diagnostic tests.

All indices are usually below normal (see Table 30-2 for normal values).

Chronic blood loss is the most common cause of iron deficiency anemia. When blood loss is continuous and moderate in amount, the bone marrow may be able to keep up with the losses by increasing the production of RBCs. Eventually, if the cause of chronic blood loss is not found and corrected, the bone marrow will not be able to keep pace with the loss, and symptoms of anemia appear.

Interventions

Medical management. Sucessful treatment for anemia secondary to blood loss requires immediate identification of the source of the loss and the institution of appropriate treatment. In addition, transfusion therapy or iron supplements may be needed.

Transfusion therapy is usually not indicated in asymptomatic persons with chronic anemia because it unnecessarily exposes the person to risks associated with transfusion (see Chapter 76). Transfusion of erythrocytes is reserved for those patients whose cardiovascular system is compromised by the anemia and in whom rapid correction by other means is not possible.

Transfusion of whole blood may be used in the treatment of anemia secondary to acute blood loss. For virtually all other anemias, packed red cells rather than whole blood are used in transfusions because the total blood volume is generally normal and administration of whole blood may produce circulatory overload and pulmonary edema.

Iron supplements may be needed by the person with anemia from chronic blood loss because of depletion of iron stores. The iron is usually given in the form of ferrous sulfate (see p. 792).

Nursing management. Nursing interventions for acute blood loss are the same as those for hypovolemic shock (see Chapter 25). The person receiving blood transfusions is monitored for signs of transfusion reactions.

If the Hb count is very low, weakness and fatigue may be present. Nursing interventions include scheduling of activities to promote rest and to prevent falls.

APLASTIC ANEMIA

Etiology

Aplastic anemia affects all age groups and both genders. The incidence is 1:100,000 of the population. In approximately one half of patients with aplastic anemia in the United States, no etiologic agent is identifiable. Predictable bone marrow depression occurs with antineoplastic drugs. Aplastic anemia may follow exposure to certain drugs, including chloramphenicol, sulfonamides, phenylbutazone (Butazolidin), and anticonvulsant agents such as mephenytoin (Mesantoin). Insecticides such as DDT and chemicals, particularly benzene, are also thought to cause aplastic anemia. Infections associated with the pathogenesis of aplastic anemia include hepatitis (types B and non-A, non-B), Epstein-Barr virus, cytomegalovirus, and miliary tuberculosis. The defect leading to aplastic anemia is most likely injury or destruction of a common stem cell (see Figure 30-1) affecting all subsequent cell populations. Aplastic anemia may also be congenital.

Pathophysiology

Aplastic anemia (anemia secondary to impaired erythrocyte production) is usually characterized by depression or cessation of activity of all blood-producing elements. There is a decrease in WBCs (leukopenia), a decrease in platelets (thrombocytopenia), and a decrease in the formation of RBCs leading to an anemia (Table 30-4).

Clinical Manifestations

Symptoms of aplastic anemia usually develop gradually over weeks or months but may appear suddenly. Pallor of the skin and mucous membranes is characteristic, in

TABLE 30-4 Normal function, primary pathophysiology, and clinical picture in aplastic anemia

Normal Function	Pathophysiology	Clinical Picture
RED BLOOD CELLS		
Major component is Hb, which provides transportation of oxygen and carbon dioxide to cells	Reduction or depletion of hematopoietic stem cells with decreased production of erythrocytes, platelets, and leukocytes Decreased tissue oxygenation	Pallor of skin and mucous membrane; fatigue and exertional dyspnea Low Hb and Hct levels
PLATELETS		
Adhesion and aggregation capabilities to plug small breaks in small blood vessels Release of thromboplastin, which, in presence of calcium ions, converts prothrombin into thrombin in initial step of coagulation process	Fewer platelets available for blood coagulation	Bleeding tendency, as evidenced by ecchymosis purpura, and petechiae Bleeding from nose, mouth, vagina, and rectum Low platelet count
WHITE BLOOD CELLS		
Neutrophils serve as primary defense against bacterial infection through phagocytosis *Monocytes* remove dead and injured cells, cell fragments, and microorganisms *Lymphocytes* participate in cellular immune response (T cell) and humoral immune response (B cell)	Fewer WBCs make a person more susceptible to infection (decreased phagocytosis, decreased immune response)	Complaints of many infections, frequent sick days Low WBC count

addition to fatigue, palpitations, and exertional dyspnea. Infections of the skin and mucous membranes occur with severe granulocytopenia; and hemorrhagic symptoms (bleeding into the skin and mucous membranes and spontaneous bleeding from the nose, gums, vagina, and rectum) occur with severe thrombocytopenia. Physical examination is often normal. The hemogram characteristically reveals a pancytopenia (a marked decrease in the numbers of all cell types). The reticulocyte count is low. Definitive diagnosis is made by bone marrow examination. Attempts at bone marrow aspiration may yield a "dry tap" because of hypocellularity and a decrease in active marrow. Bone marrow biopsy is often necessary for diagnosis of aplastic anemia.

Medical Management

The immediate treatment for aplastic anemia is the removal of the causative agent, if known. In the past, treatment for aplastic anemia was mainly aimed at stimulating hematopoiesis through the administration of steroids and androgen therapy. These agents have been shown to be of limited value and can produce toxic side effects. In recent years, bone marrow transplantation from a donor with identical human lymphocyte antigen (HLA) has emerged as the treatment of choice for persons under age 40 years with severe aplastic anemia. The remainder of persons are treated with immunosuppressive therapy. Transplant centers are reporting survival rates of 60% to 80%.[32]

The prognosis for aplastic anemia primarily depends on the severity of the anemia, method of treatment, and general supportive care. In addition, a higher treatment success rate occurs in patients who are transplanted early and have not received blood products, especially from the potential bone marrow donor. Transfused patients have a higher mortality rate from development of graft-versus-host disease. If transfusions are essential, then leukocyte-poor RBCs and platelets should be used (see Chapter 76). Patients who are not successfully treated often die from complications associated with repeated hemorrhage and infection.

■ Assessment

Subjective data include a history of exposure to chemicals (insecticides, benzene) and drugs, in addition to a family history of aplastic anemia. The person is questioned about the ability to carry out activities of daily living (ADLs) without dyspnea and fatigue. Physical examination includes monitoring for signs of infection (from the leukopenia) and bleeding (from the thrombocytopenia).

■ Data Analysis: Nursing Diagnoses

Nursing diagnoses are determined from assessment of patient data. Possible nursing diagnoses for the person with aplastic anemia include, but are not limited to, the following:

Diagnostic Title	Possible Etiologies
Activity intolerance	Imbalance between oxygen supply and demand
Infection, potential for	Decreased immune response
Injury, potential for (falls, bleeding)	Lack of awareness of environmental hazards, tissue hypoxia, syncope
Knowledge deficit	Unfamiliarity with information

■ Planning: Expected Patient Outcomes

Expected patient outcomes for the person with aplastic anemia may include, but are not limited to, the following:

1. Patient states that he or she is feeling rested.
2. Patient does not fall.
3. No nosocomial infections occur.
4. Bleeding is controlled.
5. Patient can explain measures to prevent hemorrhage and infection.

■ Implementation

Nursing care depends on the severity of symptoms. The patient may be critically ill. Prevention of infection and bleeding is the focus of nursing care.

Preventing infection. The following activities may be carried out for the hospitalized patient:

1. Place patient in private room; avoid contact with visitors or staff who have infection.
2. Place patient in protective isolation or laminar air flow room (see Chapter 17) if necessary.
3. Provide meticulous hygiene, including daily bath, careful oral hygiene, and perineal care; use antiseptic creams.
4. Avoid catheterization.
5. Use povidone-iodine skin cleansing 1 minute before parenteral injections (or other prescribed preparations).
6. Maintain a clean environment.
7. Provide emotional support for anxiety when infection occurs.

Preventing hemorrhage. Excessive bleeding may be prevented by the following actions:

1. Assess all sites for bleeding.
2. Test urine (Hemastix) and stool (guaiac) for blood.
3. Keep venipuncture and intramuscular injections to a minimum.
4. Apply pressure to venipuncture for 5 minutes, arterial puncture for 10 minutes.
5. Use soft toothbrush or swab for mouth care.
6. Keep mouth clean and free of debris with normal saline rinse if bleeding occurs.

PATIENT TEACHING FOR APLASTIC ANEMIA

1. Prevent infection
   a. Use good handwashing technique.
   b. Avoid contact with those who have infections.
   c. Avoid sharing eating utensils and bath linens.
   d. Take a bath every day (or every other day if skin is dry); keep perineal area clean.
   e. Use good oral hygiene.
   f. Eliminate intake of raw meats, fruits, or vegetables.
   g. Report signs of infection immediately to physician.
2. Prevent hemorrhage
   a. Observe for signs such as bloody urine, stool, and petechiae, and report these to physician.
   b. Use a soft toothbrush or swab for mouth care.
   c. Keep mouth clean and free of debris.
   d. Avoid enemas or other rectal insertions.
   e. Avoid picking or blowing the nose forcefully.
   f. Avoid trauma, falls, bumps, and cuts; avoid contact sports.
   g. Avoid use of aspirin or aspirin preparations (anticoagulant effect).
   h. Use an electric razor.
   i. Use adequate lubrication and gentleness during sexual intercourse.

7. Avoid taking rectal temperatures, administering rectal medications, or giving enemas.
8. Avoid invasive procedures.

Teaching the patient. All persons with aplastic anemia need to know how to protect themselves from infection and excessive bleeding. Points to emphasize are listed in the box.

HEMOLYTIC ANEMIA

Hemolytic anemia (anemia secondary to increased erythrocyte destruction) results when the RBCs are destroyed at such a rapid rate that the bone marrow is unable to compensate for the loss. The severity of the anemia is determined by the degree of lag between the rate of erythrocyte destruction (hemolysis) and the rate of bone marrow production of RBCs (erythropoiesis).

Hemolytic anemias are divided into congenital and acquired. *Congenital hemolytic anemias* include hereditary spherocytosis, the hemoglobinopathies, thalassemia, and enzyme deficiency anemia. *Hereditary spherocytosis,* inherited as an autosomal dominant trait, is characterized by a membrane abnormality that leads to osmotic swelling of the RBC and susceptibility to destruction by the spleen. It is usually detected in childhood but may appear initially in adulthood.

Diagnosis depends on observation of spherocytes on the peripheral blood smear and by demonstration of increased osmotic fragility of the RBCs in the laboratory. The reticulocyte count is usually elevated, as is the se-
rum bilirubin level. Bilirubin is derived from the breakdown of the hemoglobin released by the destroyed RBCs. Occasionally, red cell survival time will need to be determined. This is done by labeling the cells with radioactive chromium and measuring the rate of decrease of radioactivity for 1 to 2 weeks (chromium survival). Symptoms include those typically associated with anemia (pallor, fatigue, exertional dyspnea), jaundice from the increased serum bilirubin level, and an enlarged spleen from the increased RBC destruction.

Hereditary spherocytosis is almost invariably corrected by splenectomy.

THALASSEMIA

Etiology and Pathophysiology

Thalassemia is an inherited disorder affecting primarily Italians, Greeks, Chinese, Southeast Asians and blacks. It is characterized by a decreased synthesis of one of the globin chains of hemoglobin. The beta ($\beta-$) chain is most often affected (β-thalassemia). As a result, there is decreased synthesis of hemoglobin and an accumulation in the erythrocyte of the unaffected globin chain. These alterations result in decreased RBC production and a chronic hemolytic anemia.

Clinical Manifestations

The heterozygous state, *thalassemia minor,* is associated with a mild anemia that is usually asymptomatic; no therapy is required. The homozygous condition, *thalassemia major,* is characterized by a severe anemia. The RBCs are characteristically hypochromic (low MCH) and microcytic (low MCV). Hemoglobin electrophoresis is diagnostic. Growth failure begins about ages 10 to 12 years. Eventually, cardiac failure develops and death usually occurs between ages 17 and 30.[46]

Interventions

Currently, the only treatment available for thalassemia is transfusion therapy. The life span is usually significantly shortened. Transfusions may be administered either when severe symptoms occur or to maintain the Hb at a near-normal level continuously to allow for a more normal life-style. The latter approach incurs the risk of producing iron overload from frequent transfusions, a problem that can be ameliorated by the use of an iron-chelating agent such as deferoxamine.

ENZYME DEFICIENCY

Etiology and Pathophysiology

Deficiency of enzymes in the pathways that metabolize glucose and generate ATP (Embden-Meyerhof and pentose phosphate shunt pathways) frequently leads to premature RBC destruction. The most common clinically significant enzyme abnormality is that of *glucose-6-phosphate dehydrogenase* (G6PD). This disorder often

TABLE 30-5 Phenotypes for sickle cell

Genetic Relationship	Hemoglobin Alleles	Sickle Cell Disease
Homozygous dominant	Hb A, Hb A	No disease
Heterozygous	Hb A, Hb S	Sickle cell trait
Homozygous recessive	Hb S, Hb S	Sickle cell anemia

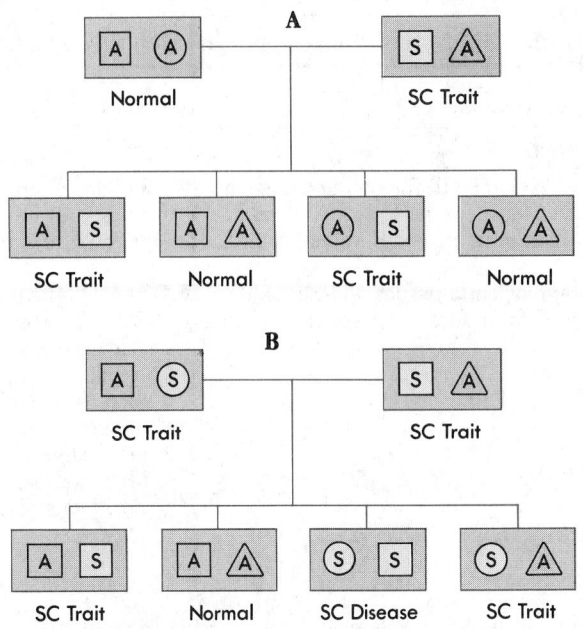

FIGURE 30-5 A, When one parent has sickle cell trait (Hb SA) and the other does not (Hb AA), a 50% probability (2/4) exists that a child will have sickle cell trait. **B,** When both parents have sickle cell trait, there is a 25% probability (1/4) that a child will have sickle cell disease and a 50% probability of sickle cell trait.

occurs in a mild form among the black population in the United States.

Clinical Manifestations

Anemia generally occurs in G6PD deficiency only when the patient is exposed to an oxidant drug (aspirin, sulfonamides, antimalarial drugs) following infection or during the newborn period, which places the cells under unusual stress with which they are unable to cope. Acute hemolysis of varying severity, which is generally self-limiting, results. The patient may experience back pain, jaundice, and hemoglobinuria as evidence of the hemolytic process. Diagnosis is established by assay for the enzyme.

Interventions

Treatment is recognition of the disorder and cessation of the offending drug. This disorder occurs in a more severe form in certain population groups in the Mediterranean area and may cause a chronic hemolytic anemia.

SICKLE CELL DISEASE: A HEMOGLOBINOPATHY

Normal Hb is composed of heme (red) and globin (protein component). The globin portion is comprised of two pairs of polypeptide chains, α and β. There is a specific amino acid sequence and number for each of the polypeptide chains. Any deviation in the normal number or sequence of essential amino acids results in abnormal Hb synthesis.

Disorders of abnormal hemoglobins are categorized as hemoglobinopathies. They result from abnormalities in one or both of the polypeptide chains (α or β) or in any one of the more than 500 amino acids. One of the most common hemoglobinopathies is Hb S disease (sickle cell anemia). Abnormalities in Hb are diagnosed through serum electrophoresis (see Chapter 76).

Etiology

Sickle cell anemia is the most common genetic disorder in the United States. Sickle cell disease is homozygous recessive (Table 30-5 and Figure 30-5) and is characterized by a chronic hemolytic anemia.

Sickle cell anemia occurs predominantly in the black population. It is estimated that there are 50,000 black

Americans with the disease. To a lesser extent, sickle cell disease also occurs in people from Asia Minor, India, the Mediterranean area, and the Caribbean area.

Pathophysiology

The basic abnormality lies within the globin fraction of the Hb, where a single amino acid (valine) is substituted for another (glutamic acid) in the sixth position of the β chain. This single amino acid substitution profoundly alters the properties of the Hb molecule (Table 30-6). Because of the intermolecular rearrangement, Hb S is formed instead of normal Hb A. Hb S has normal oxygen-carrying capacity.

However, when the oxygen tension decreases, Hb S polymerizes, causing the Hb to distort and realign the RBC into a sickle shape (Figure 30-6). The sickle cell in circulation leads to increased blood viscosity, which decreases circulation time. This decrease in circulation time causes an increase in the hypoxic time of the cell, promoting further sickling. The development of sickle cells leads to plugging of the small circulation, further decreasing cellular pH and oxygen tension (Figure 30-7).[32] This vicious cycle leads to further hypoxia, infarction of organs, and painful crisis. The affected cells have a shortened life span of 7 to 20 days, as compared to the normal 105 to 120 days.

Different terminologies are used with discussions of

TABLE 30-6 Normal function, primary pathophysiology, and clinical picture in sickle cell disease

Normal Function	Pathophysiology	Clinical Picture
HEMOGLOBIN		
Hb A is major Hb fraction in adults and consists of two α- and two β-chains, which form a smooth, round shape	Inheritance of homozygous Hb S interferes with function and structural integrity of Hb molecule	Chronic hemolytic anemia classified as normochromic and normocytic; peripheral blood smears demonstrate sickled RBC
Carry oxygen to tissues and carbon dioxide from tissues to be expelled by lungs	When cellular oxygen tension decreases, RBC distorts itself into sickle shape Sickle cell increases viscosity of the blood, slowing circulation and causing increased cellular hypoxia and plugging of circulation to the organs; infarcts can occur in central nervous system, eyes, lungs, liver, spleen, kidney, joints, and bone	Vaso-occlusive or "painful" crisis, cerebrovascular accident (CVA), retinal hemorrhage, pulmonary infarct, hepatomegaly, autosplenectomy, renal failure, enlarged heart, bone and joint abnormalities, leg ulcers

sickle cell anemia (Table 30-7). Only the homozygous condition of Hb SS describes the classic form of the disease called *sickle cell anemia*. The heterozygous state, Hb SA, refers to the often asymptomatic condition called *sickle cell trait*. In addition, a category of sickling disorders is associated with the presence of Hb S, called *sickling syndromes*.

Healthy Person With Sickle Cell Disease
The persons with severe complications increasingly represent a relatively small number of all patients with sickle cell disease.[44] Many sickle cell patients are quite healthy, seldom experience severe pain, and live nearly normal life spans. For the adult with sickle cell disease, it is hoped that issues of employment, insurability, and positive self-image will be improved through increased recognition of the healthy person with sickle cell disease.

Clinical Manifestations
Sickle cell disease (HB SS) is often diagnosed in early childhood. This form of the disease is often fatal by mid-

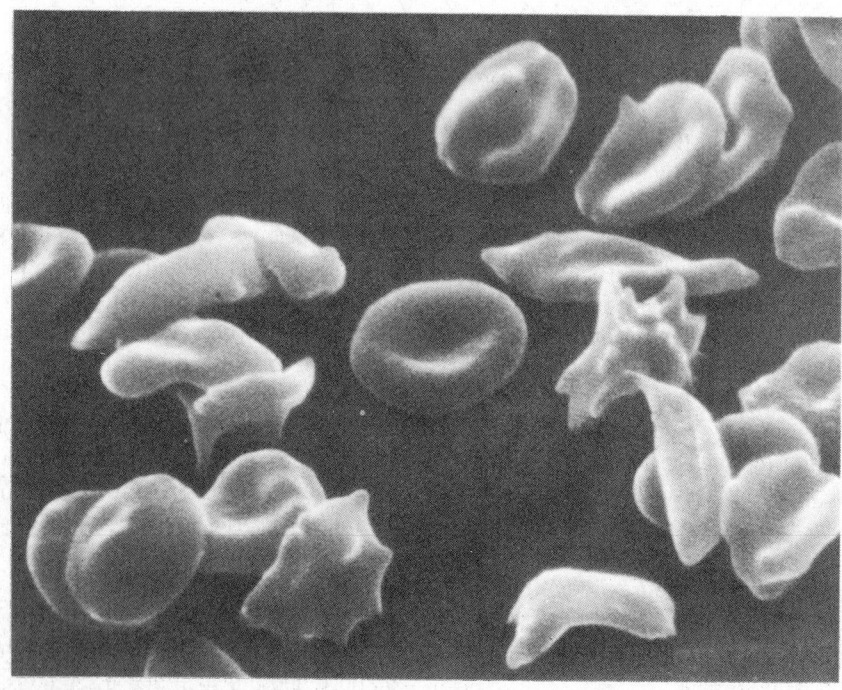

FIGURE 30-6 Sickled red cells.

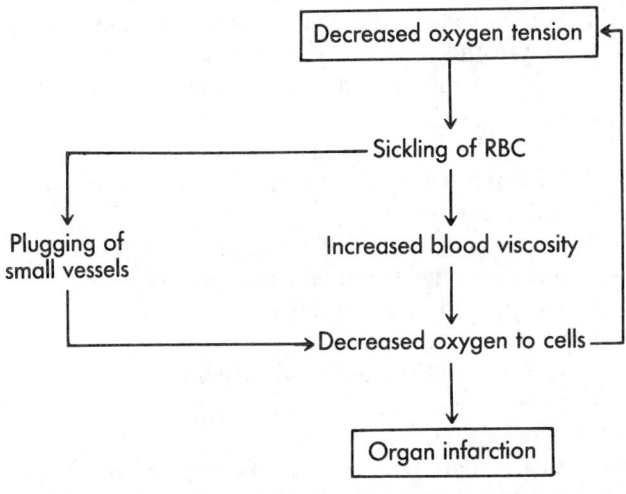

FIGURE 30-7 Physiologic effects of RBC sickling.

CLINICAL MANIFESTATIONS OF SICKLE CELL DISEASE

ACUTE EPISODES

Pain: usually in back, chest, or extremities; may be localized, migratory, or generalized
Fever: low grade, 1 to 2 days after onset of pain
Vaso-occlusive crises: occlusion of blood vessels by the sickled cells; may occur in areas such as the brain (CVA), chest, liver, or penis (priapism)

CHRONIC PROBLEMS

Leg ulcers: usually of the medial malleolus
Renal problems: renal insufficiency from repeated infarctions
Ocular problems: microinfarctions of the peripheral retina leading to retinal detachment and blindness

dle age. The gradations of sickling and symptoms vary both in occurrence and intensity. The complexity of this disorder and the problems that can arise from it make sickle cell disease a major health problem.

Anemia is usually severe, chronic, and hemolytic. When encountered in the health care setting, the person has one of many complications inherent in sickle cell disease (see box above, right).

The painful vaso-occlusive episode is the most common event in sickle cell disease. The pain is a manifestation of localized bone marrow necrosis affecting the juxtaarticular areas of the long bones, spine, pelvis, ribs, and sternum. Usually it is the event on which sickle cell patients and medical personnel focus their attention and concern.[37] The frequency of painful episodes varies greatly. Some patients experience one or two episodes per month, whereas others only have one or two a year. The duration of the episode also varies and may last from 1 to 10 days. Physical and probably emotional factors (stress) precipitate a painful episode. Physical factors include events that cause dehydration or change the oxygen tension in the body, such as infection, overexertion, weather changes (cold), high Hb levels, ingestion of alchohol, and smoking.[37]

Bacterial infection is a major cause of morbidity and mortality in patients with sickle cell disease. Persons with other hemoglobinopathies, such as Hb SC and Hb S, seem to be at lower risk for infection. Individuals with sickle cell disease are particularly susceptible, primarily because the majority experience functional asplenia (no spleen function). Meningitis, sepsis, pneumonia, and urinary tract infections are all potential risks for the person with sickle cell disease.

Sickle cell crisis. The sudden exacerbation of sickling can bring about a condition known as crisis. Sickle cell crisis may be thrombotic, aplastic, or megaloblastic. Vaso-occlusive, or *thrombotic*, crisis is the most common type and is caused by occlusion of blood vessels by the sickled cells. Pain is the primary symptom in thrombotic crisis. *Aplastic crisis* is most often secondary to infection and a temporary decrease in erythropoiesis resulting from the continuous stimulus for production of new RBCs. Because of the shortened RBC survival, the anemia rapidly worsens. Diagnosis may be made by bone marrow examination. *Megaloblastic crisis* appears in some cases to be caused by the depletion of bone marrow stores of folic acid. In such cases the crisis may

TABLE 30-7 Types of sickle cell disorders

Term	Characteristic	Hb Molecule
Sickle cell trait	Carrier of Hb S Persons are asymptomatic	Hb SA
Sickle cell disease	Presence of sickling with associated symptoms	Hb SS
Sickle cell syndromes	Diseases associated with presence of Hb S	Hb SC (sickle cell Hb C) Hb SD (sickle cell Hb D) Hb Sβ (sickle cell thalassemia)

be treated or prevented by administration of folic acid.

Splenic sequestration crisis occurs when the spleen suddenly increases in size, leading to pooling of blood and subsequent hypovolemia. Signs of shock are present.

Medical Management

No specific therapy is available to treat sickle cell disease. Transfusion therapy may be given; the blood products generally used are packed RBCs. The goal of transfusion therapy depends on the specific condition: replacing RBCs for anemia, lowering the percentage of Hb S in an infarction, and increasing the amount of circulating Hb and thus oxygen in overwhelming infections, leg ulcers, pregnancy, and preoperatively.

Analgesics, oxygen, and adequate hydration are given for vaso-occlusive episodes. Pneumococcal vaccine may be given to prevent pneumococcal infections. Therapeutic apheresis may also be initiated.

■ Assessment

Data are collected concerning the person's knowledge and feelings about the disease and factors that appear to precipitate crisis or exacerbate symptoms. Fatigue may be reported when anemia is severe. Data pertaining to pain characteristics are appropriate when pain is present.

■ Data Analysis: Nursing Diagnoses

Nursing diagnoses are determined from assessment of patient data. Possible nursing diagnoses for the person with sickle cell disease may include, but are not limited to, the following:

Diagnostic Title	Possible Etiologies
Activity intolerance	Imbalance between oxygen supply and demand
Anxiety	Threat of death; threat/change in health status, socioeconomic status, role functioning
Coping, ineffective family: compromised; ineffective individual	Crisis, prolonged disability
Gas exchange, impaired	Ventilation/perfusion imbalance
Infection, potential for	Decreased immune response
Knowledge deficit	Unfamiliarity with information
Pain	Imbalance between oxygen supply and demand
Sexual dysfunction (priapism)	Altered body structure
Tissue perfusion, altered	Decreased blood flow

■ Planning: Expected Patient Outcomes

Expected patient outcomes for the person with sickle cell disease may include, but are not limited to, the following:

1. Patient states that he or she is feeling comfortable and restful.
2. Patient/family say they are coping with the disease.
3. Patient states satisfaction with life and self.
4. Patient/partner state that the sexual relationship is satisfying.
5. Complications do not occur (infection, impaired gas exchange, impaired tissue perfusion).
6. Patient and family describe the following:
   a. Basis of the anemia
   b. Availability of genetic counseling

■ Implementation

Promoting comfort. The person who experiences weakness and fatigue from the anemia is assisted in planning daily activities to include rest periods. Oxygen is given for dyspnea or excessive fatigue with exertion.

Nursing care for painful episodes involves all the principles of pain management (see Chapter 16). The goal is to relieve the pain but not overmedicate. This usually involves the use of both narcotic and nonnarcotic analgesics. Astute evaluation of the effectiveness of pain medication is most important. Future trends in managing pain in sickle cell crisis may include the use of patient-controlled analgesia using an infusion device.

Promoting hydration. The vaso-occlusive nature of painful episodes requires adequate hydration to decrease blood viscosity. Patients who are supposedly in a steady state of their disease are advised to drink 4 to 6 quarts daily; this requirement increases to 6 to 8 quarts daily during a painful episode. If intravenous hydration is necessary, careful attention must be given to venous access, with avoidance of multiple punctures and infiltration. Use of a small-bore (no. 23) needle is recommended.[37]

General counseling. Sickle cell patients may sometimes be labeled as malingerers, because some of them demonstrate difficult behavior patterns that are influenced by anxiety over their chronic illness. Counseling and the use of support groups are encouraged to minimize behavioral dependency. In caring for this patient population, it is also helpful to maintain a sense of respect and consideration for persons who experience frequent crises and yet continue to try to live as normal a life as possible.

Family planning and genetic counseling. Many people are now deciding when or if they want to have children. This is increasingly true for persons with genetic disorders such as sickle cell disease. Some forms of birth control, such as the intrauterine device (IUD), are not as highly recommended as other forms, such as the dia-

NURSING CARE PLAN

PERSON WITH SICKLE CELL DISEASE

DATA: Mr. Lane, a 29-year-old bank teller with known sickle cell disease, was admitted to the hospital in acute distress with fever and abdominal pain. He is prescribed a folic acid supplement daily, which he takes sporadically. He is not taking any other medications. Mr. Lane has had a congested cough for 1 week. He has noticed a decrease in appetite and has had a 5-pound weight loss since his last clinic visit 1 month ago. He goes to the hospital to "get something to take away the pain." On physical examination, splenomegaly is evident, rhonchi are auscultated in his lungs, and he appears dehydrated. The patient has guarding with light abdominal palpation. His vital signs are temperature, 39.5° C; blood pressure, 140/90; pulse, 120; and respirations, 28. Laboratory examination revealed the following:

  Hb: 6.0 g/100 ml

  Hct: 17%

  RBC count: 1.6 million/mm^3

  WBC count: 23,000/mm^3

  Platelet count: 395,000

Following a 5 mg morphine sulfate (MSO_4) intravenous bolus and 2 mg MSO_4 every 4 hours, his pain is controlled. He is also started on intravenous antibiotic and hydration therapy.

The nursing history identified the following:
- Mr. Lane has little understanding of why he was prescribed the folic acid supplement.
- The episode of pain has been very frightening to Mr. Lane, and he fears that he is "going to die."
- He has little understanding of sickle cell disease and what is causing the pain.

Collaborative nursing activities include those to assess (1) Mr. Lane's response to the therapeutic regimen and (2) the presence of any complications associated with the regimen. Nursing actions include monitoring the following:
- Vital signs, especially respirations and blood pressure
- Lung sounds and sputum production
- Response to exertion: note postural vital signs and increased perception of pain
- Daily weights and intake and output measurements: assess hydration status
- Abdominal assessment: auscultate bowel sounds, response to palpation; assess for nausea/vomiting; measure girth
- CBC and differential
- Electrolytes, especially sodium and potassium

NURSING DIAGNOSIS

Pain related to imbalance between oxygen supply and demand (vaso-occlusive crisis)

Expected Patient Outcomes	Nursing Interventions	Rationale
Patient states he is free of pain.	Assess pain location, quality, duration, and contributing and alleviating factors. Monitor effectiveness of MSO_4 in relieving pain. Provide quiet, restful environment.	Patient's perception of pain provides avenues for intervention by nurse.

NURSING DIAGNOSIS

Knowledge deficit related to lack of recall of purpose for folic acid suplement and pathophysiology of sickle cell disease.

Expected Patient Outcomes	Nursing Interventions	Rationale
Patient can describe sickle cell disease and explain basis for symptoms experienced.	Explain purpose of normal Hb, abnormality of Hb in sickle cell disease, and effects of sickling: anemia, painful crisis, and splenic sequestration resulting in increased risk of infection. Teach about factors that can precipitate painful crisis: infection, dehydration, overexertion, cold weather, alcohol, and smoking.	Providing rationale for basis of symptoms allows persons to gain some control and feel less frightened.
Patient can explain rationale for folic acid supplement.	Teach relationship between folic acid and synthesis of new bone marrow elements.	Understanding of rationale for medication may improve compliance.

phragm or spermicides, for persons with sickle cell disorders. To make a wise decision about contraception, a couple must be provided with accurate information about side effects, risks, and options (see Chapter 54). Such family counseling must be performed by persons who are well versed and knowledgeable about the options.

Family planning for persons with sickle cell disease can be a most difficult issue. The fact that an individual carries a gene for the disorder makes it possible that this gene will be carried into the next generation. Although moral and ethical arguments can be made, it is ultimately the personal decision of the involved couple. Information about local services can be obtained from the National Association of Sickle Cell Disease.*

Teaching the patient. Teaching for the person with sickle cell disease includes the following:
1. Knowledge of the disease
2. Avoidance of situations that cause crisis (infection, overexertion, emotional stress, alcohol, cigarette smoking)
3. Importance of adequate fluid intake
4. Availability of psychologic support services and social resources
5. Need for medical follow-up

A nursing care plan for the patient with sickle cell disease can be found on p. 791.

ACQUIRED HEMOLYTIC ANEMIA

Etiology and Pathophysiology

Acquired hemolytic anemia is most often drug induced or is caused by an autoimmune disorder. In the latter case an antibody develops that is directed against an antigen on the individual's own erythrocytes. The antibody-coated RBCs are destroyed prematurely by reticuloendothelial cells, particularly in the spleen. This autoimmune disorder may occur secondary to lymphocytic lymphomas or chronic lymphocytic leukemia in the course of certain connective tissue disorders, or it may occur idiopathically. Diagnosis is confirmed by demonstrating the presence of the antibody on the RBCs (antiglobin or Coombs' test) (see Chapter 75).

Drugs produce hemolysis in various ways. Methyldopa (Aldomet) is associated with production of an autoantibody and a positive Coombs' test in approximately 20% of patients and a hemolytic anemia indistinguishable from an idiopathic autoimmune hemolytic anemia in 1%. More rarely, high-dose penicillin produces hemolysis through production of an antibody that requires the presence of penicillin on the RBC membrane for its effects to occur.

_____
*4221 Wilshire Blvd, Los Angeles, CA 90010.

Interventions

Therapy for autoimmune hemolytic anemia is with corticosteroids, which are beneficial in approximately 50% of patients, and with splenectomy in those patients not sufficiently responsive to steroids and more recently to the use of danazol, a gonadotropin inhibitor. In many cases, this disorder is fatal, in part because transfusion is often made difficult and dangerous by the autoantibody reacting not only with the patient's RBCs, but also with all donor cells.

IRON DEFICIENCY ANEMIA

Etiology and Pathophysiology

Iron is a fundamental part of the Hb molecule, and its deficiency leads to production of RBCs with a decreased amount of Hb and ultimately to fewer RBCs. The average adult body contains approximately 4 g of iron, 3 g of which are in Hb, 500 mg to 1 g in iron stores in the liver and bone marrow, and the rest in certain tissues and enzyme systems. Average daily loss of iron by the body is approximately 1.5 mg, which is compensated for by absorption from the diet of approximately that amount of iron daily. This tenuous balance may be compromised by chronic blood loss, which may be physiologic, such as in menstruation, or pathologic, as in gastrointestinal (GI) or other bleeding.

Clinical Manifestations

Gradual development of iron deficiency anemia may permit adaptation with few clinical signs of anemia. Some persons may develop fatigue and exertional dyspnea. With severe iron deficiency anemia, the nails become brittle and spoon shaped (concave) and develop longitudinal ridges. The papillae of the tongue atrophy, and the tongue has a smooth, shiny, bright-red appearance. The corners of the mouth may crack and become red and painful (cheilosis). The anemia, which is characteristically hypochromic and microcytic, may be detected by observation of the peripheral blood smear and/or by blood cell indices. Diagnosis may be confirmed by a low serum iron and elevated serum iron-binding capacity or by low serum ferritin or absent iron stores in the bone marrow.

Interventions

The treatment of iron deficiency anemia is to determine and correct the cause. Repletion of iron stores in the body may then be accomplished by the administration of iron. Oral iron supplement is usually given in the form of ferrous sulfate. If the person is to take the medication at home, patient instruction is necessary. Because it may be irritating to the GI tract, ferrous sulfate should be taken after meals. The person should also be told that stools will be black and that he or she should report to the physician any symptoms of diarrhea or nausea. When the person cannot tolerate oral preparations of iron, parenteral iron therapy is used. Parenteral therapy is also indicated when the person is unable to absorb iron properly from the GI tract.

Poor diet is rarely the sole cause of iron deficiency anemia, but it may be a contributing factor. All persons with iron deficiency anemia should be assessed for their knowledge of a well-balanced diet and their ability and willingness to provide themselves with such a diet. When indicated, follow-up through a clinic, home visits by a dietitian, and such community resources as Meals on Wheels can be effective ways of ensuring a well-balanced diet.

Megaloblastic anemia refers to anemias with characteristic morphologic changes caused by defective deoxyribonucleic acid (DNA) synthesis and abnormal RBC maturation. On the peripheral blood smear, macrocytic RBCs and hypersegmented neutrophils (increased number of nuclei) are present. In the bone marrow, erythroid precursors can be found that are two to three times larger than normal, with nuclei that are immature relative to their cytoplasmic development.

Etiology and Pathophysiology

Most megaloblastic anemias are caused by deficiency of either *vitamin B_{12}* or *folic acid* (see the following discussion). Both are essential in the synthesis of DNA, and their deficiency leads to impaired nuclear development in cells throughout the body. Deficiency of either leads to anemia and often leukopenia and thrombocytopenia. Administration of medication that interferes with DNA metabolism, such as chemotherapeutic agents and anticonvulsants, can also cause megaloblastic anemias.

Vitamin B_{12} Deficiency

Vitamin B_{12}, obtained from dietary sources, combines with intrinsic factor in the stomach and is carried to the ileum, where it is absorbed and transported by a carrier protein to the tissues of the body.

Clinical manifestations. Diagnosis of B_{12} deficiency is made by demonstration of a low serum vitamin B_{12} level in a patient with macrocytic anemia and megaloblastic bone marrow. In addition to the general symptoms associated with anemia, patients with B_{12} deficiency may manifest neurologic abnormalities; in particular, they may develop a peripheral neuropathy and a loss of balance resulting from an abnormality of the posterior and lateral columns of the spinal cord (subacute combined degeneration).

A deficiency of vitamin B_{12} may be the result of dietary deficiency, surgical removal of the stomach, malabsorption syndromes, or pernicious anemia. *Pernicious anemia* (PA) is caused by the absence of intrinsic factor. Dietary vitamin B_{12} therefore cannot be absorbed. Diagnosis of PA is confirmed by an abnormal Schilling test, which demonstrates the inability to absorb vitamin B_{12} unless intrinsic factor is also administered.

Interventions. Treatment of vitamin B_{12} deficiency consists of parenteral administration of vitamin B_{12}, usually once a month. The most common cause of relapse in persons with PA is their reluctance to continue therapy for life. Patient teaching is a focus of nursing care and discharge planning. The individual must be assisted to understand the nature of the illness and the absolute necessity for continued treatment.

Folic Acid Deficiency

Folic acid deficiency anemia may be caused by dietary deficiency, often in association with chronic alcoholism, overcooking of vegetables, malabsorption syndromes, and medications that inhibit the enzyme involved in normal folate absorption through the intestinal wall.[19]

Clinical manifestations. Signs and symptoms are associated with the underlying disease and anemia in general. Laboratory findings include macrocytic anemia, megaloblastic changes in the bone marrow, and a low serum folate level.

Interventions. Most people respond promptly to oral folic acid and a well-balanced diet. Return visits to nurse clinics and community health nurse home visits (will assist the person in incorporating dietary modifications into daily life. Patients who drink alcohol excessively may be referred to Alcoholics Anonymous.)

ERYTHROCYTOSIS

Erythrocytosis refers to an abnormal increase in erythrocytes. It may be caused secondarily by hypoxia (from high altitudes or from pulmonary and cardiac disease), by certain erythropoietin-producing tumors, or as a primary disorder (polycythemia vera). With hypoxia, RBCs increase as a compensatory mechanism to carry additional oxygen. Principal laboratory tests to determine the nature of erythrocytosis include determination of the arterial oxygen concentration, RBC volume, and plasma volume.

STRESS ERYTHROPOIESIS

Elevation of the Hb and Hct levels may occur when the total RBC mass volume is normal but the plasma volume is decreased, leading to a contraction of the plasma volume. This stress erythropoiesis occurs predominantly in middle-aged males who are obese, hypertensive, and smokers. It is self-limiting and requires no therapy.

POLYCYTHEMIA VERA

Pathophysiology

Polycythemia vera (primary polycythemia) is a bone marrow disorder characterized by erythrocytosis with usually a simultaneous leukocytosis and thrombocytosis. Hypervolemia, increased blood viscosity from the increased RBC mass, and platelet dysfunction occur. The etiology is unknown.

Clinical Manifestations

Symptoms are frequently absent in the early stages. As hypervolemia develops, symptoms include headaches, vertigo, tinnitus, and blurred vision. Thromboses with embolization may result from the increased blood viscosity, and the skin may develop a more reddened appearance. Platelet dysfunction may lead to nosebleeds, ecchymoses, and GI bleeding. Thromboembolic events occur frequently and generally account for the early mortality rate.

Splenomegaly is typically found in polycythemia vera on physical examination, but it is not common in other types of erythrocytosis. Laboratory tests demonstrate an increased total RBC volume and a plasma volume that is either increased or normal. The Hct at sea level is greater than 53%. Arterial oxygen concentration is usually normal.

Interventions

Usual treatment is periodic phlebotomy aimed at maintaining the Hct and Hb at a normal level. In some patients who need phlebotomy too frequently, other modes of therapy may be required, such as the use of radioactive phosphorus (32-P) or an alkylating agent such as busulfan. There is an increased incidence of other hematologic disorders arising in the course of polycythemia vera, especially acute leukemia, and this has been accentuated with the use of alkylating agents in the treatment regimen.

Teaching for the person with polycythemia vera includes the following:

1. Nature of the disorder
2. Importance of continued medical care, blood tests, and phlebotomy
3. Name, dosage, frequency, desired action, and side effects of prescribed medications
4. Signs of extremity thromboses (swelling, redness, pain) requiring immediate medical attention

DISORDERS OF HEMOSTASIS, PLATELETS, AND COAGULATION

PATHOPHYSIOLOGY

Normal hemostatic functioning is an intricate system that requires vascular integrity, normal numbers and functioning of platelets, and normal clotting factors. Although each of the essential components arises sepa-

---

DISORDERS ASSOCIATED WITH PLATELETS AND COAGULATION

PLATELETS

Thrombocytopenia	Decreased number of platelets
Thrombocytosis	Increased number of platelets
Bleeding syndromes	Disorders of platelet function

COAGULATION
Congenital

Hemophilia A	Decrease of factor VIII
Hemophilia B	Decrease of factor IX
von Willebrand's disease	Decrease of factor VIII and defective platelet aggregation

Acquired

Vitamin K deficiency	Decrease of factors II, VII, IX, and X
Disseminated intravascular coagulation	Stimulates first the clotting process, then the fibrinolytic process

---

rately and is independently regulated, the balanced interplay among these components is necessary to protect the body from excessive bleeding or excessive thrombi formation.

Primary hemostasis involves the formation of a platelet plug over a damaged area of endothelial cells lining a blood vessel. Primary hemostasis is completed with the formation of the platelet plug. Secondary hemostasis is the formation of a fibrin clot overlying the platelet plug. This process requires the sequential activation in the cascade of clotting factors (Figure 30-8). The major steps are the formation of thrombin from prothrombin leading to the formation of fibrin from fibrinogen.

A *fibrinolytic* mechanism exists to balance clot formation and leads to *clot lysis*. Two enzymes are involved in clot lysis, plasminogen and plasmin. Plasminogen is the inactive form that circulates in the blood. It is converted to plasmin by the action of active Hageman factor in addition to other factors. Plasmin then degrades and dissolves the clot. Streptokinase is an enzyme that is fibrinolytic.

Another balance to clot formation are substances called *anticoagulants*. A naturally occuring anticoagulant is heparin, which acts by interfering with activation of several coagulation factors, including activation of thrombin. Coumarin derivatives interfere with synthesis of coagulation factors II, VII, IX, and X in the liver by interfering with vitamin K.

Disorders of platelets and coagulation are listed in the box above.

THROMBOCYTOPENIA
ETIOLOGY AND PATHOPHYSIOLOGY

Thrombocytopenia is defined as a lower-than-normal number of circulating platelets. Laboratory values for a

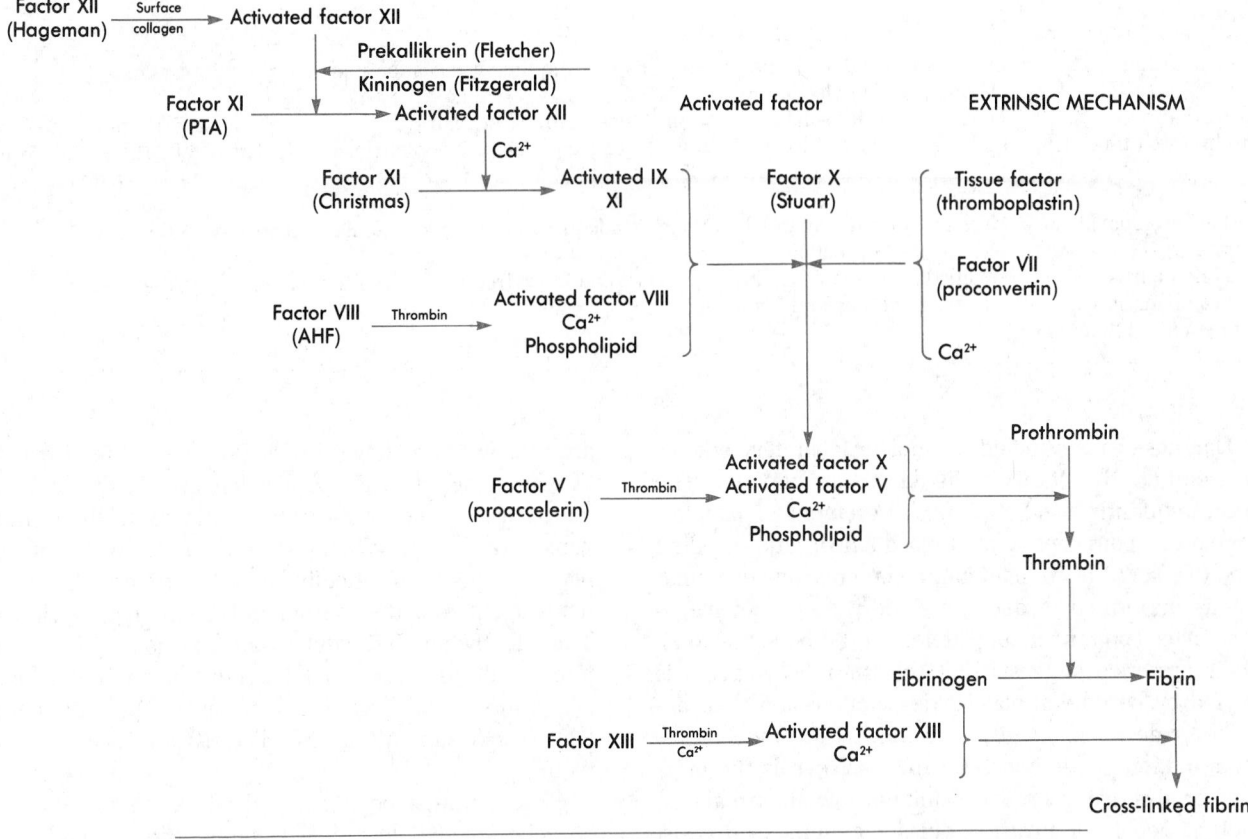

INTRINSIC MECHANISM

FIGURE 30-8 Mechanisms of blood coagulation. (Redrawn from Mountcastle VB: Medical physiology, ed 14, St Louis, 1980, The CV Mosby Co.)

normal adult platelet count range from 150,000 to 400,000/mm^3. The many types of thrombocytopenia may result from (1) decreased platelet production, (2) decreased platelet survival, (3) increased platelet destruction (most common form), or (4) sequestration of blood in the spleen.

The most common cause of increased destruction of platelets is *idiopathic thrombocytopenia purpura* (ITP), which also may be drug induced. Approximately 70 drugs (some of which are listed in the box below) have

been shown to induce thrombocytopenia.[46] Platelet counts generally return to normal within 1 to 2 weeks after the drug is withdrawn; some drugs such as gold salts may require several months.

ITP occurs most often in the second and third decades of life and is caused by production of an autoantibody (IgG) directed against a platelet antigen. It has thus been suggested that this disorder be named *autoimmune* thrombocytopenia purpura (ATP).[46]

Secondary thrombocytopenia may result from aplastic anemia, acute leukemia, and conditions causing splenomegaly (such as cirrhosis or lymphomas) that lead to sequestration of blood in the spleen.

CLINICAL MANIFESTATIONS

The major signs of thrombocytopenia observable by physical examination are petechiae, ecchymoses, and purpura on the skin. Petechiae occur only in platelet disorders. The person may give a history of menorrhagia, epistaxis, and gingival bleeding. The patient is questioned about recent viral infections, which may produce a transient thrombocytopenia; drugs in current use; and extent of alcohol ingestion.

SELECTED DRUGS TYPICALLY PRODUCING THROMBOCYTOPENIA

Alcohol	Oral hypoglycemic agents
Aspirin	Penicillin
Chemotherapeutic agents	Phenobarbital
Chloroquine	Quinidine
Digitoxin	Quinine
Gold salts	Rifampin
Methyldopa	Sulfonamides
Nonsteroidal antiinflammatory agents	Thiazides

TABLE 30-8 Common bleeding/coagulation blood tests

Test	Description	Normal Value
Bleeding time	Evaluation of vascular and platelet factors—the time it takes for a small stab wound to stop bleeding	2-9 min
Clotting time	Time required for solid clot to form (less sensitive test than PTT)	5-10 min
Prothrombin time (PT)	Indicates rapidity of blood clotting (indicative of adequacy of extrinsic coagulation pathway; factors I, II, V, VII, X)	11-16 sec; 100% as compared to control levels
Partial thromboplastin time (PTT)	More sensitive test than PT to evaluate adequacy of intrinsic coagulation pathway (fibrin clot formation)	60-90 sec
Activated partial thromboplastin time (APTT)	Modified PTT; more sensitive; quicker to perform; frequently used to monitor heparin therapy and hemophilia	26-42 sec

Diagnostic tests include complete laboratory studies to ascertain the status of all blood components. The most frequently used tests for assessment of platelets are platelet count, peripheral blood smear, and bleeding time (Table 30-8). In addition, a bone marrow examination is performed to determine the presence of megakaryocytes (precursors of platelets in the bone marrow). Their presence suggests that the thrombocytopenia is caused by peripheral platelet destruction, and their absence or decrease suggests a failure of thrombopoiesis. Examination of the bone marrow also reveals the presence or absence of primary bone marrow abnormalities, such as neoplastic invasion, aplastic anemia, or fibrosis.

INTERVENTIONS

Medical Management

The primary treatment modalities for ITP are corticosteroid therapy and splenectomy. Steroids appear to decrease both antibody production and phagocytosis of the antibody-coated platelets. Splenectomy removes the principal organ involved in destruction of the antibody-coated platelets. Other therapeutic modalities include danazol, γ-globulin, or immunosuppressive drugs. Plasma exchange, a form of experimental therapy, may have some efficacy in acute ITP.

Platelet transfusion. Transfusion with platelet concentrates may be used in persons with thrombocytopenic bleeding. It is not usually helpful for ITP because the transfused platelets are rapidly destroyed by the same mechanism as the person's own platelets and they have an extremely short survival. In conditions of impaired platelet production, the platelet concentrates increase the platelet count for 1 to 3 days.

Platelets may be obtained from random or HLA-compatible donors. Random donors are logistically easier to obtain and often provide effective platelets for considerable periods, but they may eventually lead to decreased efficacy because of antibody production. Since platelets are not always matched for ABO antigens (see Chapter 76), and since the infused platelets are usually contaminated with some erythrocytes, antibody to these antigens may develop. When production of antibody impairs platelet transfusion effectiveness, an attempt should be made to obtain platelets from an HLA-compatible donor. The effectiveness of platelet transfusions may be monitored by performing a platelet count before and 1 hour after transfusion. If no rise occurs in the platelet count, it may be assumed that the platelet transfusion is ineffective.

Platelets must be transfused within several days of collection or they lose their viability. Their survival in a recipient ranges from 48 to 72 hours. This compares with a normal platelet life span of 10 days. Transfusions often must be administered twice weekly.

Nursing Management

A primary concern in the nursing care of persons with decreased numbers of platelets is the concomitant bleeding tendency. Bleeding associated with trauma is likely with a platelet count less than 60,000/mm³. Spontaneous hemorrhage may be a life-threatening possibility when the platelet count is less than 20,000/mm³.

Ongoing nursing assessment of the patient is essential and includes alertness for increased ecchymoses, petechiae, bleeding from other sites, and any change in mental status. The need for avoidance of trauma is obvious. Bleeding precautions to institute for persons with counts below 20,000/mm³ include the following:

1. Test all urine and stools for blood (guaiac).
2. Avoid rectal temperatures.
3. Avoid intramuscular injections.
4. Apply pressure to all venipuncture sites for 5 minutes and to all arterial puncture sites for 10 minutes.

Patient teaching is an important component of patient care. Points to be included in the teaching are listed in the box on p. 797.

TEACHING THE PERSON WITH THROMBOCYTOPENIA

1. Nature of the disorder
2. Signs of decreased platelets (petechiae, ecchymoses, gingival bleeding, hematuria, menorrhagia)
3. Name, dosage, frequency, and side effects of prescribed medications (corticosteroids) and importance of not stopping corticosteroid medications suddenly
4. Measures to prevent injury
   a. Use a soft toothbrush or swab for mouth care.
   b. Keep mouth clean and free of debris.
   c. Avoid intrusions into rectum (for example, rectal medications, enemas).
   d. Use electric shaver.
   e. Apply direct pressure for 5 to 10 minutes if any bleeding occurs.
   f. Avoid contact sports, elective surgery, and tooth extraction.
5. Need for follow-up medical care

THROMBOCYTOSIS

Thrombocytosis is defined as the presence of an abnormally high number of platelets in the circulating blood. It may be seen in association with polycythemia vera, myelofibrosis, splenectomy, iron deficiency anemia, or chronic inflammatory diseases; or it may occur as a separate neoplastic disorder, hemorrhagic thrombocythemia.

The major problems incurred by persons with thrombocytosis are thrombosis or abnormal bleeding. Medical and nursing management is similar to that described for persons receiving anticoagulation therapy (see Chapter 29).

DISORDERS OF PLATELET FUNCTION

Mild bleeding syndromes may be caused by quantitatively normal but functionally defective platelets. The most common cause of such platelet abnormalities is drugs, particularly aspirin. Aspirin inhibits the release of intrinsic platelet adenosine diphosphate (ADP) and produces a defect in platelet aggregation. The defect remains for the life span of the platelet. A variety of familial and nonfamilial platelet disorders have also been described, and defective platelet function typically occurs in persons with uremia. The abnormality may be detected by a test of bleeding time or, more sensitively, by platelet aggregation tests. Disorders of platelet function have clinical manifestations and patient care needs similar to those of thrombocytopenia, although the bleeding abnormality is usually mild.

HEMOPHILIA

Hemophilia is a hereditary coagulation disorder. Both hemophilia A (factor VIII deficiency) and hemophilia B (factor IX deficiency) are inherited as sex-linked recessive disorders and are therefore almost exclusively limited to males. An example of the inheritance pattern of hemophilia is shown in Figure 30-9. The incidence of hemophilia A is 1:10,000, and for hemophilia B, 1:100,000 of the male population.

CLINICAL MANIFESTATIONS

The diagnosis of hemophilia is usually made in infancy or early childhood. The clinical history is one of lifelong bleeding tendency. A history of excessive bleeding following circumcision or dental extractions is frequently obtained. Individuals with hemophilia may give a history of bleeding into any part of the body, spontaneously or following trauma.

A diagnosis of hemophilia is made by specific assays for factors VIII and IX. The partial thromboplastin time (PTT), which reflects the intrinsic pathway of coagulation, is prolonged in both hemophilia A and hemophilia B. The platelet count and prothrombin time (PT) are normal.

Complications associated with hemophilia are the direct result of the bleeding tendency. Frequently the individual experiences repeated episodes of spontaneous bleeding into the joints, resulting in several joint deformities. Bleeding that is life-threatening involves retroperitoneal, intracranial, and paratracheal soft tissue hemorrhages.

INTERVENTIONS

Medical Management

Treatment consists of replacement of the deficient coagulation factor when bleeding episodes do not respond to local treatment (ice bags, manual pressure or dressings, immobilization, elevation, topical coagulants such as fibrin foam and thrombin). Because the deficient factors are contained in plasma, the treatment used for many years was fresh plasma and blood or fresh frozen plasma. In major hemorrhages, adequate blood levels were difficult to maintain without overloading the person's circulation with large volumes of blood and plasma. The discovery of cryoprecipitate in 1964 led the way to the development of commercially prepared concentrated preparations such as fibrinogen, factor VIII, and a concentrate containing the four vitamin K–dependent factors (prothrombin and factors VII, IX, and X). Concentrates avoid the problem of circulatory overload and produce fewer adverse effects (for example, urticarial or febrile reactions) in some patients. High cost and contamination with the virus of serum hepatitis or acquired immunodeficiency syndrome (AIDS) are drawbacks, however, to the use of some of the concentrates from pooled blood.

A number of persons with hemophilia A have developed AIDS from transfusions of factor VIII concentrate.

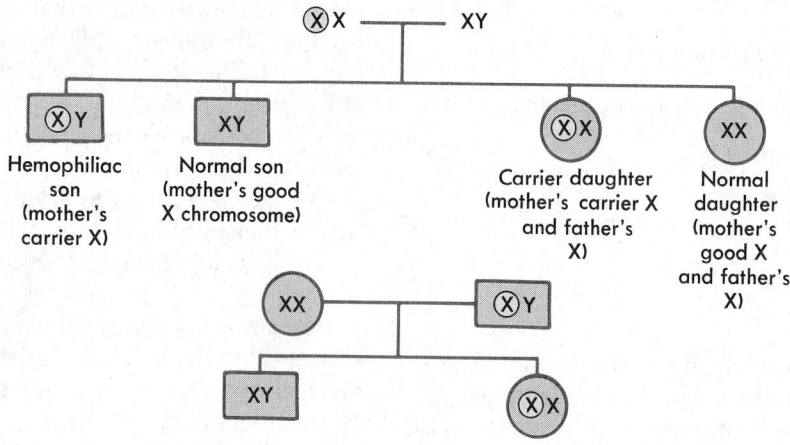

Defective gene is found on X chromosome.
When faulty X chromosome is present in a male,
the male will be a hemophiliac.

When faulty X chromosome is present in a female,
she will be a carrier of hemophilia.

In conception between a normal male and a carrier
female, four possibilities arise:

Hemophiliac
son
(mother's
carrier X)

Normal son
(mother's good
X chromosome)

Carrier daughter
(mother's carrier X
and father's
X)

Normal
daughter
(mother's
good X
and father's
X)

In conception between a hemophiliac male and a normal female,
son will be normal but daughter will be carrier.

FIGURE 30-9 Pattern of inheritance of hemophilia.

This problem should be obviated in the future with the testing of blood donors for evidence of the human immunodeficiency virus (HIV) virus and, more recently still, heat treatment of the factor VIII concentrates that kills the AIDS virus.

In classic hemophilia the treatment of choice for an acute bleeding episode is infusion of concentrates of the antihemophilic factor (factor VIII). One such concentrate is cryoprecipitate. This concentrate is made by slowly thawing previously frozen plasma at refrigerator temperature. Most of the factor VIII remains as a gel and can be separated from the rest of the plasma by centrifugation. The gel is reconstituted by the addition of saline solution. After the antihemophilic factor is extracted, the remaining plasma may be used for other purposes. This process results in a concentration of factor VIII as high as 15 to 40 times that of normal plasma. It can be produced and stored in any well-equipped blood bank at a cost well below that of other concentrates. Treatment with cryoprecipitate is being given in ambulatory care centers. Home infusion programs are a method of controlling bleeding episodes more quickly, thereby decreasing the need for hospitalization and long absence from school or work.

Recently, DDAVP (D-amino-8-D-arginine vasopressin) has been demonstrated to increase the factor VIII level in persons with von Willebrand's disease and mild hemophilia A. It is given intravenously and has been associated with few side effects. It does not carry the risk of transmitting hepatitis, AIDS, or other disorders and should play an increasingly significant role in the treatment of these disorders.

The outlook for the person with hemophilia has been greatly improved by the availability of transfusion therapy. In the past, many persons with factor VIII deficiency died in infancy or in the first 5 years of life. Surgical procedures can now be performed and joint deformity prevented, thus increasing quality of life. Today persons with moderate or mild hemophilia may live normal, productive lives.

Nursing Management

Adults with hemophilia are generally very knowledgeable about their disease. They must be aware of the possibility of hemorrhage after dental extraction, injury, or surgery. Persons who have hemophilia should carry a card or wear a Medic-Alert tag that includes their name, blood type, physician's name, and their disorder so that medical treatment will not be delayed if they should accidentally sustain injury and lose consciousness.

Pain control and the threat of spontaneous bleeding episodes are ongoing stressors the individual must confront. Those individuals who are able to meet the demands of their illness and adapt their life-styles accordingly are able to live productive lives as individuals, spouses, parents, and employees. Genetic counseling, aimed at explaining the pattern of inheritance of hemophilia, may be of great value to adults contemplating parenthood. Such counseling can serve to assist potential parents to evaluate realistically their ability to raise a child afflicted with hemophilia and to anticipate ways to meet the demands placed on both them and the child.

The National Hemophilia Foundation* is an organization established for persons with hemophilia and their families. There are 51 chapters across the United States. The basic function of the national organization is hemophilia research. In addition, it establishes standards for chapters, publishes literature, produces films, and promotes health care legislation in Washington, DC. Local chapter services include special camps for children with hemophilia; parent, child, and adult counseling; group therapy sessions for parents; and a newsletter that reports on advances in hemophilic care. A chapter may function as a liaison agent between hospitals and families with insurmountable bills for blood.

VITAMIN K DEFICIENCY
ETIOLOGY AND PATHOPHYSIOLOGY

Vitamin K, a fat-soluble vitamin, is a cofactor in the synthesis of clotting factors II, VII, IX, and X. Approximately 50% of required vitamin K is obtained from a normal diet, and 50% is produced by intestinal bacteria. Deficiencies in vitamin K can be anticipated in persons who have a decreased intake and who are given broad-spectrum antibiotics that decrease the growth of intestinal bacteria. Interference with vitamin K absorption occurs with primary intestinal disease (for example, ulcerative colitis, Crohn's disease, cystic fibrosis), biliary disease, and malabsorption syndromes. Drugs such as coumarin derivatives and large doses of salicylates, quinine, and barbiturates interfere with vitamin K function.

CLINICAL MANIFESTATIONS

Symptoms are those of hypoprothrombinemia superimposed on the underlying disease. Bleeding is similar to other coagulation disorders; that is, bleeding of the mucous membranes and into the tissues. Postoperative hemorrhage may be observed. In severe cases GI bleeding may be massive. PT is prolonged.

*110 Green St, Rm 406, New York, NY 10012.

INTERVENTIONS

Treatment consists of therapy for the underlying disorder and cessation of causative drugs. For mild disorders a water-soluble vitamin K preparation (menadione) is given orally or parenterally. In severe disorders a fat-soluble vitamin K preparation (phytonadione) may be given. Fresh frozen plasma will partially correct the disorder immediately, whereas vitamin K therapy takes 6 to 24 hours to be effective, but does not have the complications of fresh frozen plasma.

DISSEMINATED INTRAVASCULAR COAGULATION

Disseminated intravascular coagulation (DIC) is a response of the body's hemostatic mechanisms to a variety of diseases or injury. DIC is a complicated and potentially fatal process that is characterized initially by clotting and secondarily by hemorrhage. It almost always occurs in response to a primary disease.

ETIOLOGY

DIC is essentially an imbalance between the processes of coagulation and anticoagulation. Many disease states may alter the normal balance of clotting and fibrinolytic factors, which under normal conditions prevent bleeding while maintaining the fluidity of the blood. DIC may be directly or indirectly initiated by conditions that trigger at least one of three mechanisms: factor XII formation, tissue thromboplastin release, and activation of factors II and X (see box below).[32] Stimuli such as sepsis, anoxia, or burns most likely cause activation of the intrinsic clotting system by the release of factor XII following endothelial cell wall damage and platelet aggregation. DIC may be caused by factor VII activation from massive trauma or the release of tissue thromboplastin

---

PRECIPITATING CONDITIONS ASSOCIATED WITH DIC[32]

ENDOTHELIAL CELL WALL DAMAGE: FACTOR XII FORMATION

Anaphylaxis	Vasculitis
Systemic lupus erythematosus	Anoxia
Transfusion reaction	Acidosis
Sepsis	Liver disease
Burns	

TISSUE THROMBOPLASTIN RELEASE: FACTOR VII ACTIVATION

Carcinoma	Extracorporeal circulation
Leukemia	Abruptio placentae
Blunt trauma	Amniotic fluid embolus
Hemolytic anemia	Retained dead fetus
Sepsis	

ACTIVATION OF FACTORS II AND X

Snake venom	Pancreatitis
Liver disease	

from an amniotic fluid embolus entering the maternal circulation. Proteolytic enzymes in snake venom can cause direct activation of factors II and X.

PATHOPHYSIOLOGY

The primary disease causes the initiation of the clotting process. This response is generalized and occurs throughout the vascular system, creating a state of *hypercoagulability*. The fibrinolytic processes, which normally operate to limit clot extension and dissolve clots, are then stimulated. As clotting factors are depleted and fibrinolysis continues, a state of *hypocoagulability* develops.

The most common sequela of DIC is hemorrhage. This paradox is caused by decreased platelets and the depletion of clotting factors II, V, VIII, and fibrinogen in the clotting process and the production of fibrin degradation products (FDPs) through fibrinolysis. The FDPs act as anticoagulants, which increase the hemorrhagic tendency.

CLINICAL MANIFESTATIONS

Laboratory findings may be the only indications of DIC in the early stages and usually include thrombocytopenia, low levels of fibrinogen, and prolonged PT and PTT. In addition, low levels of factors V and VIII are present, and abnormal RBCs may be found on peripheral smear. Characteristically, there is evidence of fibrinolysis, which is reflected in increased fibrin split products, D-dimers, and prolonged thrombin time. As the disorder progresses, clinical manifestations may include bleeding of the mucous membranes and tissues (petechiae, ecchymoses). Oral, vaginal, and rectal bleeding and bleeding following injections and venipunctures may occur.

INTERVENTIONS

Medical Management

The management of DIC must always begin with treatment of the primary disease. Once this has been initiated, the goal is to control the bleeding and restore normal levels of clotting factors. Blood products such as platelet packs, cryoprecipitate, and fresh whole blood may be administered to replace the depleted factors. Heparin has been used to inhibit the underlying thrombotic process; however, it too often promotes rather than decreases bleeding, and its use is controversial.

Nursing Management

Nursing intervention in the care of the patient with DIC is extremely challenging. The person who develops DIC is critically ill and frequently has numerous sites of bleeding. The amount and nature of drainage from chest and nasogastric tubes, oozing from surgical incisions, or progressive discoloration of the skin should be noted and recorded.

Continual observation for new bleeding sites and for an increase or decrease in bleeding is an integral part of the nursing plan, especially if heparin therapy is being used. The susceptibility of these persons to bleeding presents special problems; medications should be given orally or intravenously if at all possible, and small-gauge needles used when other injections are necessary. The precautions previously described for thrombocytopenia are applicable to the patient with DIC (see box on p. 797).

Maintaining fluid balance assumes great importance. Persons with DIC usually lose large quantities of blood and receive frequent transfusions and other fluid replacement. In addition to monitoring blood infusion rates carefully, the nurse must be alert to signs of fluid overload such as increasing pulse rate and central venous pressure. Hourly urine output is recorded not only as another indication of cardiac function but also because of the possibility of renal thrombi formation and subsequent renal failure.

Frequently the patient is comatose, and the presence of purpura, numerous intravenous lines, and drainage tubes makes the patient's appearance especially upsetting to the family. Most of the primary conditions associated with DIC are of a sudden nature, and the family requires preparation and help in understanding this catastrophic occurrence and support during the long period of treatment.

DISORDERS ASSOCIATED WITH WHITE BLOOD CELLS

The WBC (leukocyte) system is comprised of neutrophils, lymphocytes, monocytes, basophils, and eosinophils. All but the lymphocytes are derived from a common stem cell. The primary function of WBCs is to provide for humoral and cellular response to infection. Neutrophils are primarily responsible for phagocytosis and the destruction of bacteria and other infectious organisms. Lymphocytes are the principal cells involved in immunity, which is responsible for the development of delayed hypersensitivity and the production of antibodies (see Chapter 8). Any compromise in the integrity of the WBC system renders the individual susceptible to infection.

NEUTROPENIA
ETIOLOGY AND PATHOPHYSIOLOGY

Neutropenia is defined as a neutrophil count of less than 2000/mm³. Neutropenia may occur as a primary hematologic disorder, but more often it is seen in association with other disorders, including malignant diseases of the bone marrow, aplastic anemia, megaloblastic anemia, use of chemotherapeutic agents, and hypersplenism. The degree of susceptibility to infection is in direct proportion to the degree of neutropenia. Individuals with severe neutropenia are at risk of contracting a life-threatening infection.

Severe neutropenia, sometimes referred to as *agranulocytosis,* occurs as a reaction to a variety of drugs and chemicals, including sulfonamides, propylthiouracil, and chloramphenicol. Specific treatment consists of removing the offending agent.

INTERVENTIONS

An individual with a compromised WBC system is highly susceptible to life-threatening infections. Nursing care is directed toward protecting the patient from potential sources of infection and assiduous monitoring to detect the earliest signs of infection so that prompt therapy may be instituted. Likewise, patients and families must be taught to recognize early signs of infection. Meticulous washing of the hands by medical and nursing personnel and strict asepsis are mandatory. The environment should be kept scrupulously clean and dustless, and no person with any type of infection should be allowed in contact with the patient. Family members and hospital personnel need frequent reminders of this. Mild colds and respiratory tract infections, taken for granted in daily life, are serious threats to patients with decreased numbers of WBCs.

Patients should be in private rooms. When this is not possible, cautious screening of roommates for a potential source of infection is mandatory.

Granulocyte transfusion may be used for the severely neutropenic patient.[46] This is usually reserved for life-threatening situations, such as when a extremely neutropenic patient acquires an infection. (Further discussion of the nursing care of patients with neutropenia is given in Chapter 17).

NEUTROPHILIA

Neutrophilia is defined as a neutrophil count greater than 10,000/mm^3. Such an increase is a normal response to infections, primarily bacterial infections. Prolonged elevation of the neutrophil count, especially in the absence of an apparent cause, demands a diligent search for the underlying cause. Persistent elevated neutrophil counts are associated with leukemia, polycythemia vera, myeloid metaplasia, and various systemic and inflammatory disorders.

LEUKEMIA
ETIOLOGY AND PATHOPHYSIOLOGY

Leukemias are malignant disorders of the hematopoietic system involving the bone marrow and lymph nodes; they are characterized by uncontrolled proliferation of leukocytes and their precursors. With rare exceptions, the bone marrow is involved at the onset, with infrequent manifestations in other hematopoietic organs leading to organ enlargement (splenomegaly, hepato-

megaly). The proliferation of one type of cell often interferes with the normal production of other hematopoietic cells, leading to the development of immature cells, thrombocytopenia, and anemia. The immaturity of the WBCs leads to decreased immunocompetence and inceased susceptibility to infections. The cause of leukemia is unknown.

Although the etiology leading to the development of acute leukemia in most patients has not been identified, some predisposing relationships have been discovered. Individuals with specific chromosomal aberrations, such as occurs with Down's syndrome, von Recklinghausen's neurofibromatosis, and Fanconi's anemia, have an increased incidence of acute leukemia. Chronic exposure to chemicals, such as benzene; drugs that cause aplastic anemia; and radiation exposure have been associated with an increased incidence of the disease. An increased risk for development of acute leukemia has been noted following cytotoxic therapy for Hodgkin's disease; non-Hodgkin's lymphoma; multiple myeloma; polycythemia vera; and breast, lung, and testicular cancers.

The leukemias are classified as acute or chronic and are further subdivided according to cell type or maturity. *Acute* leukemias involve immature cells and are categorized according to the predominant cell in the bone marrow. They are subclassified as acute lymphocytic leukemia (ALL) or acute nonlymphocytic leukemia (ANLL) according to the specific morphology of the leukemic cell. ANLL is further classified as acute myelogenous (AML), promyelocytic, monocytic, and other varieties according to cell type. Distinguishing between the various subclassifications of ANLL is difficult, but it is important to do so because newer chemotherapeutic agents appear to have more success against some types and almost none against others. *Chronic* leukemias may be lymphocytic, as in chronic lymphocytic leukemia (CLL); or granulocytic, as in chronic granulocytic or myelogenous leukemia (CML) (Table 30-9).

CLINICAL MANIFESTATIONS

Acute leukemias have a rapid onset and a short course ending in death if untreated. The paucity of normal WBCs leads to numerous infections such as pneumonia and septicemia. Early symptoms include fever, lymphadenopathy, pallor and fatigue from anemia, and ecchymoses. WBC count may be normal, decreased, or increased.

Chronic leukemias have a more insidious onset. Median survival of patients with CML is 3 to 4 years and with CLL, 2 to 10 years, depending on the stage at diagnosis. Early signs include fatigue, weakness, anorexia, and weight loss characteristic of a hypermetabolic state. An enlarged spleen and liver can usually be palpated. The WBC count is usually elevated.

TABLE 30-9 Characteristic signs and common chemotherapeutic agents used in different leukemias

Leukemia	Peak Age (Yr)	Characteristic Symptoms	WBC Level	Bone Marrow Cell Predominance	Common Chemotherapeutic Agents
Acute lymphocytic leukemia (ALL)	2-4	Fever, infections of respiratory tract, anemia, bleeding of mucous membranes, ecchymoses, lymphadenopathy	Decreased, normal, or increased	Lymphoblasts	Regimens with vincristine and prednisone, 6-mercaptopurine, methotrexate
Acute myelogenous leukemia (AML)	12-20, after 55	Same as ALL except less lymphadenopathy	Normal, decreased, or increased	Myeloblasts	Cytosine arabinoside, 6-thioguanine, doxorubicin (Adriamycin), daunomycin
Chronic lymphocytic leukemia (CLL)	50-70	Weakness, fatigue, lymphadenopathy, pruritic vesicular skin lesions, thrombocytopenia, anemia, splenomegaly	Increased (20,000-100,000)	Lymphocytes	Alkylating agents (for example, chlorambucil), glucocorticoids
Chronic myelogenous leukemia (CML)	30-50	Weakness, fatigue, anorexia, weight loss, splenomegaly	Increased (15,000-500,000)	Granulocytes	Busulfan

ACUTE LYMPHOCYTIC LEUKEMIA

Epidemiology

Of persons with ALL, 80% are children, with a peak incidence between 2 and 4 years and an extreme decrease after age 10.

Pathophysiology

ALL is a malignant disorder arising from a single lymphoid stem cell (see Figure 30-1), with impaired maturation and accumulation of the malignant cells in the bone marrow. Different stages of lymphoid development typically are found in the bone marrow, from very immature to almost normal cells. The degree of immaturity is a guide to the prognosis: the greater the number of immature cells, the poorer the prognosis.

Clinical Manifestations

Signs and symptoms of ALL include anemia, bleeding, lymphadenopathy, and a predisposition to infection. A blood smear may show immature lymphoblasts. The platelet count and Hct level are reduced in most patients. Diagnosis is confirmed by bone marrow aspiration or biopsy.

Interventions

Perhaps more dramatically than in any other malignant disorder, chemotherapy has improved the prognosis of children with ALL. Untreated patients have a median

survival time (MST) of 4 to 6 months. With current chemotherapy, the MST is close to 5 years, and approximately 50% of children with ALL can now be cured.

Complete remissions are obtained in more than 90% of patients treated with chemotherapeutic regimens, most of which include vincristine and prednisone. Maintenance of remission is accomplished with a combination of drugs, usually including the antimetabolites 6-mercaptopurine and methotrexate. In most regimens, vincristine and prednisone are administered intermittently during the maintenance program. Appropriate duration of therapy in patients who continue free of disease remains unsettled, but in most centers it is approximately 3 years. The use of "prophylactic" treatment of the central nervous system (that is, intrathecal administration of methotrexate with or without craniospinal radiation) has greatly diminished recurrences.

ACUTE MYELOGENOUS LEUKEMIA

Epidemiology and Clinical Manifestations

Acute myelogenous leukemia (AML) can occur at any age but occurs more often at adolescence and after age 55. It arises from a single myeloid stem cell and is characterized by the development of immature myeloblasts in the bone marrow.

Clinical manifestations are the same as for ALL. The WBC count may be low, normal, or high. Bone marrow aspiration reveals a marked increase in myeloblasts.

Interventions

In the untreated patient or in one who is nonresponsive to therapy, the MST is approximately 2 to 3 months. Current therapy includes the use of cytosine arabinoside, 6-thioguanine, and doxorubicin or daunomycin. Complete remission occurs in 50% to 75% of treated patients, and the MST is approximately 2 to 3 years. Approximately 20% of patients are in complete remission at 5 years and are capable of prolonged disease-free periods (remission). Although patients in remission clearly have an improved quality of life, induction of therapy is arduous, often requiring weeks in the hospital with the need for intensive supportive care (blood component replacement and antibiotic therapy). Bone marrow transplantation (see p. 804) with the use of HLA-identical allogenic bone marrow is being used with increasing frequency. Transplanting the patient's own (autologous) bone marrow obtained after a remission with chemotherapy or radiation therapy is another option.

CHRONIC LYMPHOCYTIC LEUKEMIA

Epidemiology

CLL occurs at any age but is found mainly between ages 50 and 70. It is three times more common in men.

Pathophysiology

CLL is characterized by a proliferation of small, abnormal mature B lymphocytes, often leading to decreased synthesis of immunoglobulins and depressed antibody response. The accumulation of abnormal lymphocytes begins in the lymph nodes, then spreads to other lymphatic tissues and the spleen. The number of mature lymphocytes in the peripheral blood smear and bone marrow is greatly increased.

Clinical Manifestations

The onset is insidious with weakness, fatigue, and lymphadenopathy. Symptoms include pruritic vesicular skin lesions, anemia, thrombocytopenia, and an enlarged spleen. The WBC count is elevated to a level between 20,000 and 100,000. Bone marrow biopsy shows infiltration of lymphocytes.

Interventions

The MST of persons with CLL is 4½ to 5½ years. As a general rule, persons are treated only when symptoms, particularly anemia, thrombocytopenia, or enlarged lymph nodes and spleen, appear. Chemotherapeutic agents used in the treatment of CLL are most often one of the alkylating agents, such as chlorambucil, and the glucocorticoids (see Chapter 17).

CHRONIC MYELOGENOUS LEUKEMIA

Epidemiology

CML occurs at any age but primarily from ages 30 to 50. The incidence is slightly higher in males.

Pathophysiology

The primary defect in CML is an abnormal stem cell leading to an uncontrolled proliferation of the granulocytic cells. As a result of this proliferation, there is a marked increase in the number of circulating granulocytes. In most cases a characteristic chromosomal abnormality, the *Philadelphia chromosome,* is present, involving deletion of a portion of one of the arms of chromosome 21 and its addition to another chromosome.

Clinical Manifestations

Characteristic symptoms of chronic leukemia occur: fatigue, weakness, anorexia, weight loss, and splenomegaly. Diagnosis of CML is made on the basis of an elevated WBC count (15,000 to 500,000), granulocytes on the peripheral blood smear that range in maturity from blast cells to mature neutrophils, and granulocytic hyperplasia in the bone marrow. The Philadelphia chromosome is present in 80% of patients.

CML frequently changes from a chronic indolent phase into an accelerated phase that progresses rapidly into a fulminant neoplastic process sometimes indistinguishable from an acute leukemia. The accelerated phase of the disease (blastic phase) is characterized by increasing numbers of granulocytes in the peripheral blood. Often there is a corresponding anemia and thrombocytopenia. The patient may also develop fever and adenopathy. Of patients with CMl, 50% to 60% progress to the blastic phase.

Interventions

Busulfan (Myleran), an alkylating agent, and hydroxyurea, both oral agents, are the most common drugs used. They are often effective in decreasing symptoms but have minimal impact on survival. Additional approaches include allogenic bone marrow transplantation in the chronic phase and autologous transplantation (see p. 804) in the acute blastic phase.

NURSING MANAGEMENT OF PERSONS WITH LEUKEMIA

Leukemia, by its nature, is a diverse illness. The varied courses and response or lack of response to treatment also add to the diversity. Nursing diagnoses, expected patient outcomes, and nursing interventions for persons with malignancies can be found in Chapter 17.

In acute phases of the disease and during aggressive chemotherapy, nursing care is aimed toward the prevention of complications and supportive therapy. Decreased WBC and platelet counts render the individual vulnerable to *severe infections* and *bleeding* episodes. Frequent transfusions of both whole blood and component therapy (platelets, WBC) are often necessary.[3,45] Many patients require the insertion of an indwelling central venous catheter for the administration of chemotherapy, total parenteral nutrition, and diagnostic blood work.

TEACHING THE PERSON WITH LEUKEMIA

1. Nature of the disease process and its effects
2. Prevention of infection
3. Drug regimen: name, side effects (see Chapter 17)
4. Method of arranging for chemotherapy administration and periodic blood counts
5. Symptoms requiring immediate medical attention (fever, bleeding)
6. Available community resources (American Cancer Society, Leukemia Society*)
7. Need for continual medical follow-up

*211 East 43rd St, New York, NY 10017.

Many foci of nursing care are beyond those found in the life-threatening situations. Each individual with leukemia responds in a different way. It cannot be predicted for certain if an individual will respond to a prescribed treatment or how long a remission will last. Likewise, how the individual incorporates the illness into life is also unique to each person. Nursing has a key role in patient education. Before discharge from the hospital, the person should possess basic knowledge of the disease process and the importance of continued medical follow-up. Knowledge of specific drug therapy and anticipated side effects is also a component of the teaching plan. Of utmost importance in learning is the ability of the person to identify the body's signals that blood abnormalities exist. Petechiae, ecchymoses, and gingival bleeding are again the hallmarks to seek prompt medical attention. Bone pain, often severe, may signal blastic crisis (acute proliferation of immature cells).

Individuals whose illness runs the course of several months to years often become very knowledgeable about their disease, blood components, related symptoms, and specific chemotherapeutic drugs. These persons sometimes discuss their progress in terms of changes in their blood counts. Over time many individuals become attuned to how such changes affect them. For example, they often can predict their count by how they feel. Many such persons respond well to being included in their plan of care during hospitalization and in preparation for discharge.

Time set aside for patient teaching (see box) also allows for a sharing time with the individual. This time may provide the foundation for an honest nurse-patient relationship from which emotional support may be given the person as attempts are made to adapt to the many stressors associated with leukemia.

BONE MARROW TRANSPLANTATION
USAGE

Bone marrow may be removed from one person and given intravenously to another person or withdrawn at one time and given to the same person at another time. It has been used increasingly in several hematologic malignancies following large doses of chemotherapy or radiation therapy. The amount of chemotherapy or radiation therapy that can ordinarily be administered is limited by toxicity to the bone marrow. By transplanting bone marrow following these therapeutic modes, much larger therapeutic doses can be administered.

Bone marrow transplantation is generally used (1) in children with ALL who have relapsed and have been reinduced into a second complete remission with chemotherapy, (2) in younger patients with ANLL in either a first or second remission, and (3) in persons with CML in the chronic phase who have either a syngeneic or allogeneic donor.

Among nonmalignant diseases, bone marrow transplantation has had its greatest impact with aplastic anemia.

TYPES OF BONE MARROW TRANSPLANTATION

Bone marrow transplantation is labeled *autologous* if the marrow has been obtained from the recipient, *syngeneic* if from an identical twin, and *allogeneic* if from a genetically different individual. Autologous and syngeneic transplants avoid the problems of transplant rejection and graft-versus-host disease (see Chapter 76). These problems become increasingly prevalent and severe as the HLA type of donor and recipient differ. The HLA system refers to genetic loci on chromosome 6 that govern tissue histocompatibility. One haplotype is acquired from each parent. Four possible combinations exist in the offspring of two parents; thus there is one in four chances that a sibling will have an identical HLA match.

Autologous transplantation is under extensive investigation. Marrow is withdrawn from the patient when the disease is in a complete remission and stored until needed. In leukemia, however, relapse and mortality increase with autologous transplantation, possibly because of the absence of mild graft-versus-host disease effects on residual leukemic cells.

PROCEDURE

The technique of obtaining bone marrow is by multiple bone marrow aspirations under general or spinal anesthesia, usually yielding 500 to 800 ml of marrow. There has been essentially no morbidity to the donor. The marrow is cryopreserved until used and then, after large particles are filtered out, administered intravenously through a central line to the recipient. The infused marrow repopulates the marrow of the patient after several weeks. Possible complications to the recipient include infections (particularly interstitial pneumonitis from cytomegalovirus, *Pneumocystis carinii*, or other organisms), marrow rejection, graft-versus-host disease, volume overload, and veno-occlusive disease of the liver.

DISORDERS ASSOCIATED WITH THE LYMPH SYSTEM

ASSESSMENT OF LYMPH NODES

The normal lymph node consists of connective tissue encapsulating a fine mesh of reticular cells. The reticuloendothelial cells function chiefly in the phagocytosis of cellular debris. The chief function of lymphocytes, which are the main cells comprising the lymph nodes, is to provide an immune response to antigens presented to the node from the structure being drained by the node.

Lymph node enlargement results from an increase in the number and size of lymphoid follicles with proliferation of lymphocytes and reticuloendothelial cells. Lymphadenopathy may also occur when the node is invaded by cells normally not present (leukemic cells, cancer cells). In the lymphomas the actual nodal structure is destroyed by the malignant cells.

Normally lymph nodes are not palpable. With disease and the consequent increase in size, the nodes become palpable. In a routine physical examination the lymph nodes are examined by palpation.

Lymphangiography is a radiologic technique used for evaluation of lymph nodes to detect the presence of disease. This procedure is especially valuable in the assessment of those nodes that are anatomically too deep in the abdomen to allow for evaluation by palpation (paraaortic). For this procedure a small incision is made on the dorsal surface of each foot so that the small lymph channels are made accessible. Dye is slowly instilled over a few hours. All lymph chains and nodes fill with dye and are then visible on roentgenograms. X-ray films are usually done immediately after the dye is absorbed and again at intervals of 24 and 48 hours after the procedure. In addition, because the dye remains in the lymph nodes for as long as 6 months after the initial study, disease status and response to therapy can be periodically evaluated with routine abdominal roentgenograms.

Computed tomography (CT scan) is also used to evaluate abdominal lymph nodes.

HODGKIN'S DISEASE
ETIOLOGY AND PATHOPHYSIOLOGY

Hodgkin's disease is a malignant disorder of lymph nodes. The etiology is unknown. Diagnosis requires biopsy and pathologic examination of the suspicious node. The presence of the Reed-Sternberg cell remains the pathologic hallmark of the disorder, but four pathologic variants of Hodgkin's disease have been recognized: *lymphocyte predominant, nodular sclerosis, mixed cellularity,* and *lymphocyte depletion.* The lymphocyte predominant and nodular sclerosis types have the best prognosis, and lymphocyte depletion has the worst. The most important prognostic indicator is the stage of the

disease at the time of diagnosis. Accurate staging is crucial to the subsequent treatment regimen. The diagnostic workup is often arduous and difficult, and explanation of the many facets of the complex diagnostic procedures helps provide the emotional support so often needed during this time.

CLINICAL MANIFESTATIONS

Systemic symptoms that may be associated with Hodgkin's disease include fatigue, weakness, anorexia, unexplained fever, night sweats, and generalized pruritus. Physical examination may show enlargement of lymph nodes, liver, and spleen. A chest roentgenogram may identify the presence of a mediastinal mass. A bone marrow biopsy is done to determine if there is marrow involvement. The liver and spleen are evaluated by radionuclide scanning or by CT scan. Lymphangiography is done to evaluate the intraabdominal nodes. A *staging laparotomy* is performed in some circumstances to obtain a biopsy specimen of retroperitoneal lymph nodes and both lobes of the liver and to remove the spleen. The rationale for this procedure is the limitations of nonsurgical diagnosis of liver, spleen, and intraabdominal node involvement.

The classification into stages allows for comparison of persons with similar disease involvement and their response to a given treatment regimen. Over time such comparisons have identified the treatment course most appropriate for a described disease. The revised Ann Arbor staging classification for Hodgkin's disease is shown in the box.

ANN ARBOR CLINICAL STAGING CLASSIFICATION OF HODGKIN'S DISEASE

STAGE DEFINITION

I   Involvement of a single lymph node region (I) or of a single extralymphatic organ or site (I_E)

II   Involvement of two or more lymph node regions on the same side of the diaphragm (II) or localized involvement of an extralymphatic organ or site and of one or more lymph node regions on the same side of the diaphragm (II_E)

III   Involvement of lymph node regions on both sides of the diaphragm (III), which may also be accompanied by involvement of the spleen (III_S) or by localized involvement of an extralymphatic organ or site (III_E) or both (III_{SE})

IV   Diffuse or disseminated involvement of one or more extralymphatic organs or tissues, with or without associated lymph node involvement

The presence or absence of fever, night sweats, or unexplained loss of 10% or more of body weight in the 6 months preceding admission are denoted by the suffix letters B and A, respectively. Biopsy-documented involvement of stage IV sites is also denoted by letter suffixes: M, marrow; L, lung; H, liver; P, pleura; O, bone; D, skin and subcutaneous tissue.

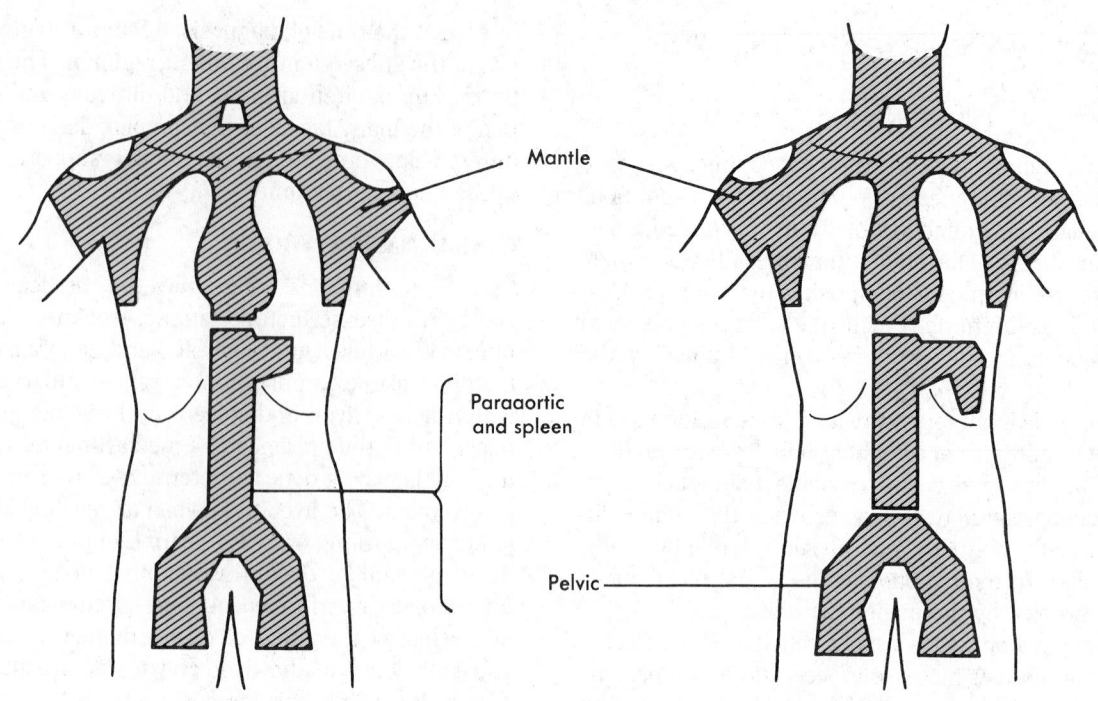

FIGURE 30-10 Diagram of mantle and inverted Y fields used in total lymphoid radiotherapy of Hodgkin's disease. (From Rosenberg SA and Kaplan HS: Calif Med 113:23, 1970.)

MEDICAL MANAGEMENT

Radiation therapy (Figure 30-10) is used for stages IA, IB, IIA, and IIB. This treatment yields a cure rate of approximately 90% for stage I and 80% for stage II. Combination chemotherapy is the treatment of choice for stages IIIB and IV. Therapy of stage IIIA is controversial and involves chemotherapy, radiation, or a combination of these therapies. The most frequently used combination is the MOPP regimen, which consists of nitrogen mustard, vincristine, procarbazine, and prednisone (Table 30-10). This regimen is administered in a 2-week course each month with prednisone added during the first and fourth course. The drugs are administered for at least 6 months or for two or three courses following the attainment of complete remission. Complete remis-

sions are achieved in approximately 80% of these patients; long-term, disease-free remissions and probable cures occur in half of this group. Continuing chemotherapy beyond the attainment of complete remission has not been shown to improve survival. Combinations such as ABVD (Table 30-10) are likely to be added to the treatment regimen if relapse occurs, and complete remission can again be attained. Initial use of alternating courses of MOPP and ABVD has increased response rates.

NON-HODGKIN'S LYMPHOMAS
ETIOLOGY AND PATHOPHYSIOLOGY

The non-Hodgkin's lymphomas include a broad spectrum of lymphoid malignancies with different histo-

TABLE 30-10 Chemotherapeutic regimens for treatment of Hodgkin's disease

Name	Drugs	Dosage	Method	Schedule	Cycle
MOPP	Mechlorethamine (nitrogen mustard)	6 mg/m^2	IV	Days 1 and 8	2 wk with 2-wk rest period
	Vincristine (Oncovin)	1.4/m^2	IV	Days 1 and 8	
	Prednisone	20 mg/m^2	Oral	Days 1-14	
	Procarbazine	100 mg/m^2	Oral	Days 1-14	
ABVD	Adriamycin	25 mg/m^2	IV	Days 1 and 15	2 wk with 2-wk rest period
	Bleomycin	10 mg/m^2	IV	Days 1 and 15	
	Vinblastine (Velban)	6 mg/m^2	IV	Days 1 and 15	
	Dacarbazine (DTIC)	150 mg/m^2	IV	Days 1-5	

NON-HODGKIN'S LYMPHOMAS

"FAVORABLE" HISTOLOGY

Nodular poorly differentiated lymphocytic lymphoma
(NLPD)
Nodular mixed lymphocytic and histiocytic lymphoma
(NML)
Well-differentiated lymphocytic lymphomas of the nodular
(NLWD) or diffuse (DLWD) type

"UNFAVORABLE" HISTOLOGY

Nodular histiocytic (NHL)
Diffuse poorly differentiated lymphocytic (DPDL)
Diffuse histiocytic lymphoma (DHL)
Diffuse mixed lymphoma (DML)
Diffuse undifferentiated lymphoma (DUL)

pathologies, disease courses, and responses to therapy. The cause is unknown, although viruses have been implicated. Accurate identification of the histopathology is crucial to the determination of the treatment plan. The classifications are reviewed here only briefly so that familiarity with terminology will allow the reader to review charts and treatment plans. Also, recognition of the diversity of the disease course, prognosis, and the importance of an extensive diagnostic workup is useful to the nurse for patient and family teaching.

One classification separates the non-Hodgkin's lymphomas into *lymphocytic, histiocytic,* or *mixed cell types,* each of which may appear as nodular or diffuse on microscopic examination. These have been subdivided into "favorable" and "unfavorable" histology (see box above). In general a nodular pattern of cell structures conveys a more favorable prognosis than a diffuse pattern. A lymphocytic cytology is more favorable than a histiocytic one, and a mixed cellularity–histiocytic is intermediate in its prognosis.

CLINICAL MANIFESTATIONS

Characteristically, patient's with non-Hodgkin's lymphoma have a median age of 50 to 60 years. Patients most often have nontender peripheral lymphadenopathy that may appear bulky. The liver and spleen may be moderately enlarged. Other symptoms that may occur include unexplained fever, night sweats, and weight loss.

The diagnosis of non-Hodgkin's lymphoma is made by examination of pathologic lymph node tissue. Accurate histologic classification is of importance, and often slides are sent to major cancer centers for consultation regarding the classification. Once the diagnosis is made, the extent of the disease (staging) must be determined. As with Hodgkin's disease, accurate staging is a crucial factor required to determine the treatment regimen. The staging workup is similar to that for Hodgkin's dis-

ease, except that staging laparotomies are less often needed. Explanations of the extensive workup and its importance in determining the treatment plan are an important focus of patient teaching during the diagnostic period.

MEDICAL MANAGEMENT

The complexity of the disease and the array of treatment regimens used encourages nurse-physician discussion of the treatment plan. It is especially important that the goals of therapy be shared, whether curative or only local or systemic palliation.

In general, radiotherapy is the initial treatment when the disease has a localized presentation. Local field radiation is used. Total nodal radiation is reserved for patients whose disease is more widespread. Chemotherapy is the mainstay of treatment of non-Hodgkin's lymphomas that are not localized (Table 30-11).

Nodular poorly differentiated lymphocytic lymphoma is the most frequently occurring non-Hodgkin's lymphoma. In some patients, observation is reasonable until the disease shows signs of progression. Treatment with a single alkylating agent, most often chlorambucil, is effective in that it produces a response rate that extends survival. Combination chemotherapy, however, produces higher response rates, including complete remissions, but are not yet shown to be curative. MST is 7 to 10 years.

In *diffuse histiocytic lymphoma,* which includes most of the cases previously designated as reticulum cell sarcoma, combination chemotherapy has been superior to single-agent therapy. Survival is significantly prolonged in those who demonstrate a complete response, and a significant minority of this group are cured. COP, COPP (COP and procarbazine), MOPP, and CHOP (M-BACOD and Pro-MACE MOPP) (Table 30-11), among other combinations, produce complete responses in 40% to 60% or more of patients, whose MST is well over 3 years.

Data are more limited in other types of lymphomas. In *nodular histiocytic* and *nodular mixed histiolymphocytic* types, complete responses have been achieved with single agents, and 50% to 70% of those treated with COP, COPP, MOPP, and other combinations have shown a MST of 55 months for those who attained a complete response and 13 months for those in whom only a partial response was attained.

■ ASSESSMENT

Subjective data include (1) knowledge of the disorder, (2) effect of fatigue on the ability to carry out ADLs, (3) appetite and present nutritional status, and (4) discomfort from night sweats or pruritus. *Objective* data specifically include condition of the skin (such as excoriations from scratching) and weight.

TABLE 30-11 Chemotherapeutic regimens for treatment of non-Hodgkin's lymphomas

Name	Drugs	Dosage	Method	Schedule	Cycle
COP	Cyclophosphamide (Cytoxan)	800 mg/m^2	IV	Day 1	2 wk
	Vincristine (Oncovin)	2 mg	IV	Day 1	
	Prednisone	60 mg/m^2	Oral	Days 1-5	
CHOP	Cytoxan	750 mg/m^2	IV	Day 1	3 wk
	Adriamycin	50 mg/m^2	IV	Day 1	
	Vincristine	1.4 mg/m^2	IV	Day 1	
	Prednisone	100 mg/m^2	Oral	Days 1-5	
CHOP-Bleo	Cytoxan	750 mg/m^2	IV	Day 1	3 or 4 wk
	Adriamycin	50 mg/m^2	IV	Day 1	
	Vincristine	2 mg	IV	Days 1 and 5	
	Prednisone	100 mg	Oral	Days 1-5	
	Bleomycin	15 U	IV	Days 1 and 5	
COPP	Cytoxan	650 or 600 mg/m^2	IV	Days 1 and 8	2 wk with 2-wk rest period
	Vincristine	1.4 mg/m^2 (max, 2 mg)	IV	Days 1 and 8	
	Procarbazine	100 mg/m^2	Oral	Days 1-10	
	Prednisone	40 mg/m^2	Oral	Days 1-14	
BACOP	Bleomycin	5 U/m^2	IV	Days 15 and 22	4 wk
	Doxorubicin (Adriamycin)	25 mg/m^2	IV	Days 1 and 8	
	Cytoxan	650 mg/m^2	IV	Days 1 and 8	
	Vincristine	1.4 mg/m^2 (max, 2 mg)	IV	Days 1 and 8	
	Prednisone	60 mg/m^2	Oral	Days 15-28	
Pro-MACE	VP 16	120 mg/m^2	IV	Days 1 and 8	2 wk with 2-wk rest period
	Cyclophosphamide	650 mg/m^2	IV	Days 1 and 8	
	Adriamycin	25 mg/m^2	IV	Days 1 and 8	Follow with MOPP regimen (see Table 30-10) then restart Pro-MACE
	Methotrexate	1.5 g/m^2	IV		
	Leucovorin	50 mg/m^2	IV	q6h for 5 days	
	Prednisone	60 mg/m^2	Oral	Days 1 to 14	
M-BACOD	Methotrexate	3 g/m^2	IV	Days 1 and 14	Repeat cycles every 3 wk × 10
	Bleomycin	4 mg/m^2	IV	Days 1 and 21	
	Adriamycin	45 mg/m^2	IV	Days 1 and 21	
	Cyclophosphamide	600 mg/m^2	IV	Days 1 and 21	
	Oncovin	1 mg/m^2	IV	Days 1 and 21	
	Dexamethasone	6 mg/m^2	Oral	Days 1 to 5 and 21 to 25	
MACOP-B	Methotrexate	400 mg/m^2	IV	Wk 2, 6, 10	Treatment completed in 12 wk
	Doxorubicin	50 mg/m^2	IV	Wk 1, 3, 5, 7, 9, 11	
	Cyclophosphamide	350 mg/m^2	IV	Wk 1, 3, 5, 7, 9, 11	
	Vincristine	1.4 mg/m^2	IV	Wk 3, 4, 6, 8, 10, 12	
	Bleomycin	10 U/m^2	IV	Wk 4, 8, 12	
	Prednisone	75 mg	Oral	Daily doses tapered over last 15 days	
	Co-trimoxazole (Bactrim)	2 tablets	Oral	Twice daily to prevent infection	

■ **DATA ANALYSIS: NURSING DIAGNOSES**

Nursing diagnoses are determined from assessment of patient data. Possible nursing diagnoses for the person with a lymphoma may include, but are not limited to, the following:

Diagnostic Title	Possible Etiologies
Activity intolerance	Generalized weakness, imbalance between oxygen supply and demand
Comfort, alteration in	Pruritus, night sweats
Knowledge deficit	Unfamiliarity with information

Other nursing diagnoses may be identified on the basis of effects of chemotherapy or radiation therapy (see Chapter 17).

■ **PLANNING: EXPECTED PATIENT OUTCOMES**

Expected patient outcomes for the patient with a lymphoma may include, but are not limited to, the following:

1. The patient will state that he or she is feeling comfortable.
2. Skin breakdown from scratching will be minimal.
3. The patient will be able to describe the following:
   a. Nature of the disorder
   b. Therapeutic regimen
   c. Need for continued medical follow-up
   d. Resources in community

■ **IMPLEMENTATION**

PROMOTING COMFORT AND SAFETY

Fever, pruritus, and profuse night sweats may lead to general discomfort. Measures to ease pruritus and prevent excoriations of the skin from scratching are instituted (see Chapter 73). Frequent changes of night clothing or bed linens may be necessary, and a high fluid intake is encouraged.

COUNSELING AND TEACHING

Hodgkin's disease most often affects young adults; therefore special attention needs to be given to minimizing the impact of the illness and its treatment on their lives, not only during the treatment period but later as well. Before the initiation of treatment, therapy-induced sterility should be discussed. For young women receiving radiation therapy alone, surgical relocation of the ovaries outside the field of radiation may be performed. Sterility frequently occurs in association with chemotherapy (see Chapter 17). For women, this is often temporary, and the ability to conceive and bear normal children often returns after therapy is completed. For men, sterility is more frequently permanent. For this reason the option of sperm banking should be discussed before beginning either radiation therapy or chemotherapy.

To allow for work and career development, every effort should be made to schedule treatment at those times and days of the week that least interfere with work and other important events in the person's life. The nurse has a crucial role in assisting individuals to develop a realistic approach to the illness and in successfully meeting the demands and limitations imposed by the illness and its treatment.

Persons with lymphomas have periods of remission and recurrence. Such peaks and valleys are stressful and disruptive. Many patients describe subsequent courses of treatment following a recurrence as more stressful than the initial treatment. Comments include "Is it worth it? I don't have the same faith." Other patients, realistically encouraged by the initial response to treatment, are able to express an optimistic outlook, "It worked the first time. It will work again." Recognition of the stress involved in therapy requires that support systems be available to the individual. The health care team can provide some of the needed support and guidance as the individual learns to incorporate the illness into daily life.

Patient teaching includes the following:

1. Knowledge of the disorder, its treatment, and prognosis
2. Name, dosage, frequency, and side effects of medications
3. Arrangements for chemotherapy or radiation treatments and for periodic blood counts
4. Symptoms requiring immediate medical attention (fever, bleeding)
5. Need for continued medical follow-up
6. Resources available in the community: financial assistance and local support groups (American Cancer Society)

INFECTIOUS MONONUCLEOSIS

EPIDEMIOLOGY AND ETIOLOGY

Infectious mononucleosis is an acute disease caused by a herpeslike virus, the Epstein-Barr virus. It occurs more often in young persons, the highest incidence occurring between 15 and 30 years of age.

CLINICAL MANIFESTATIONS

Signs and symptoms of infectious monoucleosis are varied. It is a benign disease with a good prognosis. Malaise is a frequent early complaint, and it is often accompanied by fever, enlargement of lymph nodes, sore throat, headache, generalized aches and pains resembling those of influenza, and moderate enlargement of the liver and spleen. Rupture of the spleen and encephalitis are rare complications. Diagnosis is established by the heterophil agglutination or Monospot blood test. This test is based on a certain substance being present in the blood of a person with infectious mononucleosis that causes clumping, or agglutination, of the washed erythrocytes (antigen) of another animal. The test is almost always positive after 10 to 14 days of the illness. Another laboratory finding is a great increase in the number of mononuclear leukocytes, which lends the name to the disease. At the height of the disease the WBCs may range between 10,000 and 20,000 cells/mm³.

INTERVENTIONS

Infectious mononucleosis is self-limiting, and with rest affected individuals will usually recover spontaneously within a few weeks. Nursing care is aimed at relief of symptoms and promotion of rest and comfort. The person is advised to avoid heavy lifting or contact sports when splenomegaly is present. Most persons can return to activities that do not require heavy exertion in 1 to 2 weeks and to normal activities in 4 to 6 weeks. Some persons have persistent fatigue for several months.

CHAPTER SUMMARY

- Diagnostic tests for hematologic disorders include tests for serum hemoglobin (Hb) and hematocrit (Hct), RBC indices (MCV, MCHC), peripheral blood smears, and bone marrow examinations.

- Major health problems of the hematopoietic system include RBC disorders (anemias, erythrocytosis); disorders of hemostasis, platelets, and coagulation; WBC disorders (neutropenia, neutrophilia, leukemia); disorders of the lymph system (lymphomas); and infectious mononucleosis.

- Anemias may be caused by blood loss, impaired RBC production, increased RBC destruction, or nutritional deficiencies.

- Weakness and fatigue are major signs of anemia as a result of decreased oxygenation from lack of Hb and increased energy needs required by increased RBC production.

- Aplastic anemia is anemia secondary to impaired RBC production and is characterized by pancytopenia. Treatment is by bone marrow transplantation or immunosuppressive therapy. Nursing interventions include preventing infection and hemorrhage.

- Sickle cell anemia is a hemolytic anemia with a genetic basis. A sickle cell crisis occurs when the RBCs become deoxygenated and sickle shaped, causing plugging of small vessels, leading to organ infarction and necrosis.

- Nursing interventions for sickle cell disease include promoting comfort and hydration, counseling, and teaching.

- Ingestion of iron compounds is part of the therapy for iron deficiency anemia only; it will not help the other types of anemias.

- Megaloblastic anemia is a macrocytic anemia from defective DNA synthesis and abnormal RBC maturation; causes include vitamin B_{12} and folic acid defi-

ciencies and administration of chemotherapeutic and anticonvulsant drugs.

- Erythrocytosis is an abnormal increase in RBCs, as seen with polycythemia vera.

- Thrombocytopenia is a decrease in the number of circulating platelets and leads to bleeding; persons with thrombocytopenia need to learn how to prevent injury and hemorrhage.

- Hemophilia is a hereditary coagulation disorder; hemophilia A is a lack of coagulation factor VIII, and hemophilia B is a lack of factor IX; maintenance therapy consists of blood factor replacement therapy and prevention of injury.

- Disseminated intravascular coagulation (DIC) is a coagulation disorder characterized initially by clotting and secondarily by hemorrhage, resulting from an alteration in the balance between clotting factors and fibrinolytic factors; the person is usually critically ill.

- Persons with alteration of WBCs are at a high risk of infection because leukocytes are a major factor in the body's defense against invading microorganisms.

- The leukemias are malignant disorders characterized by uncontrolled proliferation of WBCs and their precursors; the cause is unknown.

- Leukemias may be acute or chronic, lymphocytic or nonlymphocytic (primarily myelogenous). Acute leukemias have a rapid onset and a short course if untreated; chronic leukemias have a more insidious onset and longer course. The major therapies for leukemias are chemotherapy and bone marrow transplantation.

- Lymphomas (Hodgkin's disease and non-Hodgkin's lymphomas) are malignant disorders of the lymph system; radiotherapy and chemotherapy are the major medical treatments.

QUESTIONS TO CONSIDER

- How would your care differ if the patient with aplastic anemia said, "I feel so lonely and frightened when everyone has to wear masks and gloves when they come in to see me"?

- What approaches might you consider for teaching a person with hemophilia how to administer clotting factors at home?

- How would your care differ if the patient with Hodgkin's disease said, "When I go home, I'm not going to take this chemotherapy"?

- What approaches might you consider for teaching a person at risk measures to prevent infection and bleeding?

REFERENCES AND SELECTED READINGS

1. Alcorn R et al: Fluid therapy and exercise in the management of sickle cell anemia: a clinical report, Phys Ther 64:1520-1522, 1984.
2. Anionwu EN: Sickle cell disease: screening and counseling in the antenatal and neonatal period, Midwife Health Vist Comm Nurse 19:440-443, 1983.
3. *Barker SM: Blood cell products in the supportive care of patients with acute leukemia, Nurs Times 76(4):152-154, 1980.
4. Baum K et al: The painful crisis of homozygous sickle cell disease, Arch Intern Med 147:1231-1234, 1987.
5. *Beaudoin K: Going the distance with the patient who's a real fighter: this man who fought so valiantly against leukemia, Nursing '83 13(4):70-75, 1983.
6. *Beutler E: Iron. In Goodhart R and Shiels M: Modern nutrition in health and disease, ed 6, Philadelphia, 1980, Lea & Febiger.
7. *Borley D: Oncology nursing: leukemia and bone marrow transplant unit. Part 3, Nurs Mirror 160(6):30-34, 1985.
8. Brannan D and Guthrie T: Idiopathic thombocytopenic purpura in adults, South Med J 81(1):75-80, 1988.
9. *Brown M: Standards of care for the patient with graft vs host disease post bone marrow transplant, Cancer Nurs 4:191-198, 1981.
10. Brozovic M, Davies S, and Brownwell A: Acute admissions of patients with sickle cell disease who live in Britain, Br Med J 294:1206-1208, 1987.
11. DeVita V, Hellman S, and Rosenberg S: Cancer principles and practice of oncology, ed 2, Philadelphia, 1985, JB Lippincott Co.
12. Farfel MR and Holtzman NA: Education, consent and counseling in sickle cell screening programs: report of a survey, Am J Public Health 74:373-375, 1984.
13. *Fraser M and Tucker M: Second malignancies following cancer therapy, Semin Oncol Nurs 5(1):43-45, 1989.
14. *Freedman SL: An overview of bone marrow transplantation, Semin Oncol Nurs 4(1):3-8, 1988.
15. *Froberg J: The anemias: causes and courses of action, RN 52(1):24-29, 1989.
16. *Gibbons P: Transfusion therapy in sickle cell anemia, Nurs Clin North Am 18(1):201-215, 1983.
17. *Goodman M: Managing the side effects of chemotherapy, Semin Oncol Nurs 5(2):29-52, 1989.
18. *Hays K and Rafferty DC: Care of the patient with malignant lymphoma, Nurs Clin North Am 17(4):677-695, 1982.
19. Herbert C: Folic acid and vitamin B_{12}. In Goodhart R and Shiels M: Modern nutrition in health and disease, ed 6, Philadelphia, 1980, Lea & Lebiger.
20. *Huckstadt A: Hemophilia: the person, family and nurse, Rehabil Nurs 11(3):225-228, 1986.
21. *Hutchison MM and Itho K: Nursing care of the patient undergoing bone marrow transplantation for acute leukemia, Nurs Clin North Am 17(4):697-711, 1982.

22. *Hutchison MM and King AH: A nursing perspective on bone marrow transplantation, Nurs Clin North Am 18(3):511-522, 1983.
23. Johnson BL and Grass J: Handbook of oncology nursing, New York, 1985, John Wiley & Sons, Inc.
24. *Lakhani AK: Current management of acute leukemias, Nursing '88 (Lond) 3:755-758, 1988.
25. Lamb C: Managing sickle cell emergencies, Patient Care 19(1):92-95, 1985.
26. *Lewandowski W and Jones S: The family with cancer, Cancer Nurs 11(6):313-321, 1988.
27. Mauer AM: Acute lymphoblastic leukemia in a young adult, Hosp Pract 22(9):145-156, 1987.
28. *Myrie J: Family planning and genetic counseling, Nurs Clin North Am 18(1):174-183, 1983.
29. Naley RL, Fabry ME, and Kaul DK: New insights on sickle cell anemia, Diagn Med 7(5):26-33, 1984.
30. *Nauscher R et al: Bone marrow transplantation, Am J Nurs 84:764-772, 1984.
31. Panek D and Brown NC: Conflicts in practice: bone marrow transplantation, J Assoc Pediatr Oncol Nurs 2(1):37-40, 1985.
32. Pittiglio D and Sacher R: Clinical hematology and fundamentals of hemostasis, Philadelphia, 1987, FA Davis Co.
33. *Richardson EAW and Milne LS: Sickle cell disease and the childbearing family: an update, MCN 8(6):417-422, 1983.
34. *Rooks Y and Pack B: A profile of sickle cell disease, Nurs Clin North Am 18(1):131-138, 1983.
35. *Rooney A and Haviley C: Nursing management of disseminated intravascular coagulation, Oncol Nurs Forum 12(1):15-22, 1985.
36. *Ross MS et al: Biotherapy with interferon in hematologic malignancies, Oncol Nurs Forum (Suppl) 14(6):16-22, 1987.
37. *Rozzell MS, Hijazi M, and Pack B: The painful episode in sickle cell disease, Nurs Clin North Am 18(1):185-199, 1983.
38. *Simonson GM: Caring for patients with acute myelocytic leukemia, Am J Nurs 88:304-309, 1988.
39. *Smith D: Sexual rehabilitation of the cancer patient, Cancer Nurs 12(1):10-15, 1989.
40. *Terry BA: Hodgkin's disease and non-Hodgkin's lymphomas, Nurs Clin North Am 20(1):207-217, 1985.
41. Thomas ED: Bone marrow transplantation: present states and future expectations. In Isselbacker KJ et al, editors: Harrison's principles of internal medicine, ed 11, New York, 1987, McGraw-Hill Book Co.
42. *Trotta P: Nursing assessment of symptoms associated with hyperviscosity syndrome, Oncol Nurs Forum 14(1):21-27, 1987.
43. *Walters I, Baysinger M, and Buchanan I: Complications of sickle cell disease, Nurs Clin North Am 18(1):139-184, 1983.
44. *Williams I, Earles AN, and Pack B: Psychological considerations in sickle cell disease, Nurs Clin North Am 18(1):215-229, 1983.
45. Wintrobe MM et al: Clinical hematology, ed 7, Philadelphia, 1981, Lea & Febiger.
46. Wyngaarden JB and Smith LH: Cecil textbook of medicine, ed 18, Philadelphia, 1988, WB Saunders Co.

*References preceded by an asterisk are particularly well suited for student reading.

CHAPTER 31

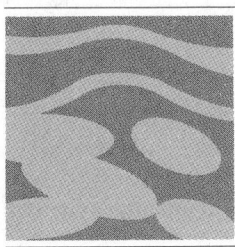

Assessment of the Respiratory System

JOSEPHINE BRUCIA

CHAPTER OBJECTIVES

After studying this chapter, the student should be able to:
1. Define selected terms.
2. Identify structural components of the upper and lower airways and their primary functions.
3. Describe the mechanisms of pulmonary ventilation, gas exchange, pulmonary circulation, and control of respiration.
4. Identify physiologic changes that occur in the respiratory system with aging.
5. Identify data to collect in a nursing history for the patient experiencing a pulmonary dysfunction.
6. Recognize major symptoms associated with respiratory disease and the significance of each.
7. Describe the technique of physical examination of the respiratory system.
8. Describe diagnostic tests used to diagnose problems of the respiratory system and nursing responsibility associated with each test.
9. Differentiate between respiratory acidosis and akalosis.

Breathing is an activity that most of us rarely think about throughout our daily lives. However, the ease or discomfort with which we breathe has a major impact on the quality of our daily activities.

The act of breathing involves the two interrelated processes of ventilation and respiration. *Ventilation* is the mass movement of air from outside the body through the conducting system to the alveoli. The conducting system includes both the upper and lower airways. *Respiration* consists of the dual processes of oxygen uptake and carbon dioxide elimination between the body and its environment. The only place respiration can occur is at the alveolar-capillary membrane where oxygen (from air) and carbon dioxide (from cellular waste) can move in and out of the body.

To effectively intervene with patients' pulmonary problems, nurses must be knowledgeable about the structure and function of the upper and lower airways, the major pulmonary signs and symptoms, and the implications of data gathered in the assessment process.

ANATOMY AND PHYSIOLOGY

UPPER AIRWAY

The upper airway consists of the nose and sinuses, the pharynx and tonsils, and the larynx and hypopharynx.

NOSE AND SINUSES

The nose is supported by the nasal bones, the nasal processes of the maxillary bones, the cartilaginous and bony parts of the septum, and the upper and lower nasal cartilages. Air enters the nose through the two nostrils (nares), which are separated by the septum. The septum, which is usually straight and thin in the child, is rarely straight in adults because in many cases, it has been injured.

The nasal cavities are located between the roof of the mouth and the frontal, ethmoid, and sphenoid bones. Three projections, lined with mucous membrane and called the turbinate bones, are located on the lateral walls of each nasal cavity (Figure 31-1). The turbinates provide a large surface area with a rich blood supply that warms and humidifies ambient air as it passes through this area. Large particles are filtered out of inhaled air by precipitation or by stimulation of mechanical receptors located in the nasopharynx, which results in the sneeze reflex.[9]

The vestibule of the nose is the anterior part of the nose. The vestibule extends posteriorly a short distance to a point at which its lining changes from skin to mucous membrane. This mucous membrane posterior to the vestibule contains cilia that beat in a constant wavelike motion to carry mucus into the nasopharynx. Trapped in the mucus are bacteria, dust, and other foreign matter entering the nose. The olfactory epithelium is located in a small area superiorly and provides the end-organ of smell. The lateral walls of the nose contain the opening for the paranasal sinuses and the nasolacrimal ducts. These openings provide a means of aeration of and mucus drainage from the sinuses. The blood sup-

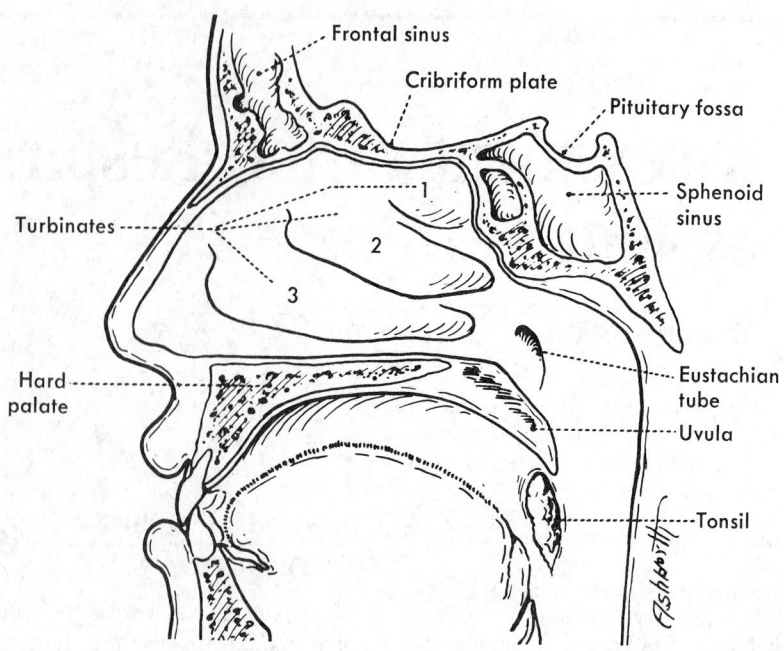

FIGURE 31-1 Turbinates of nose: 1, superior; 2, middle; 3, inferior. (From DeWeese DD and Saunders WH: Textbook of otolaryngology, ed 6, St Louis, 1982, The CV Mosby Co.)

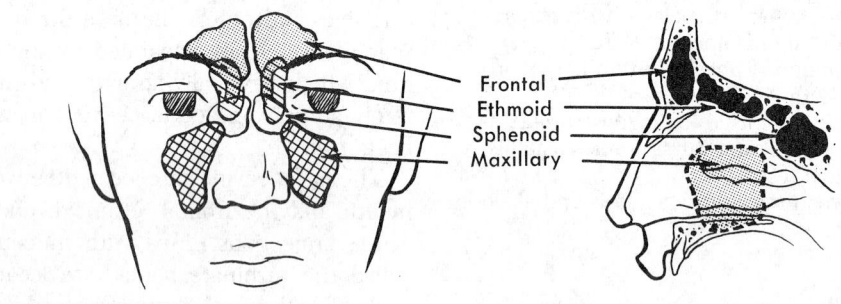

FIGURE 31-2 Location of sinuses.

ply to the nose comes from both the external and internal carotid systems.

Four sets of paranasal sinuses are located on either side of the head (Figure 31-2). These sinuses are air-filled spaces in the skull that serve to lighten the head. They drain into the nasal cavities through the openings behind the turbinates. The maxillary sinuses are the largest and most accessible. The sinuses are lined with mucous membrane that is continuous with that of the nose. The functions of the nose and nasal sinus are to warm, moisten, and filter air in preparation for the lungs; to house receptors for olfaction; and to promote vocal resonance.

UPPER THROAT: PHARYNX AND TONSILS

The pharynx is the space behind the oral cavity that extends from the base of the skull to the larynx. The phar-

ynx can be considered in three parts: the nasopharynx, the oropharynx, and the hypopharynx (Figure 31-3). It is lined with mucous membrane.

The adenoids are located in the nasopharynx, the palatine tonsils anterior to the oropharynx, and the lingual tonsils in the hypopharynx. The adenoids and tonsils are made up of lymphoid tissue that helps to filter the circulating lymph of bacteria or other foreign matter that penetrate the body, especially by way of the nose and mouth.

LOWER THROAT: LARYNX AND HYPOPHARYNX

The larynx forms the upper extremity of the trachea. The framework of the larynx is made up of several cartilages held together by muscle and ligaments (Figure 31-4). The cartilaginous framework of the larynx protects the vocal cords and affords a stiffness that permits

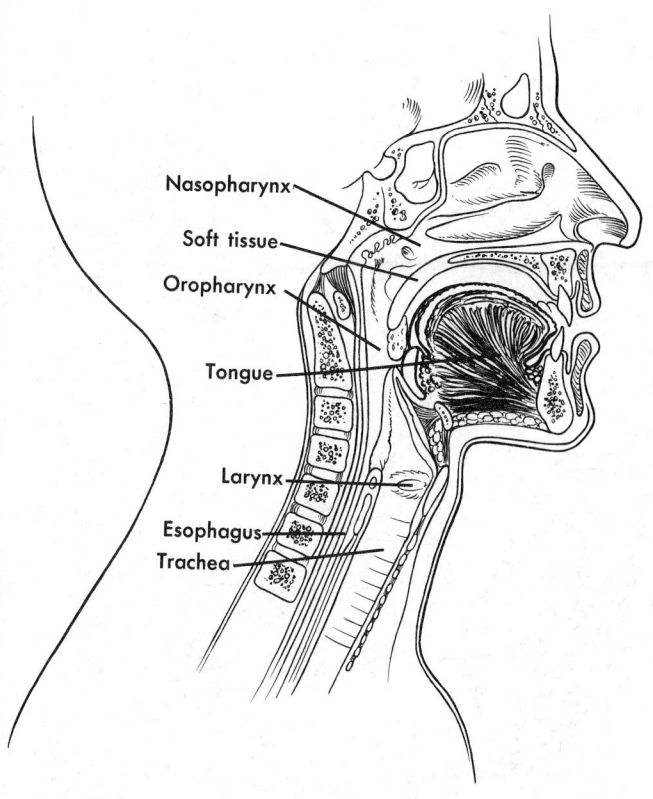

FIGURE 31-3 Sagittal section of head showing pharynx and larynx.

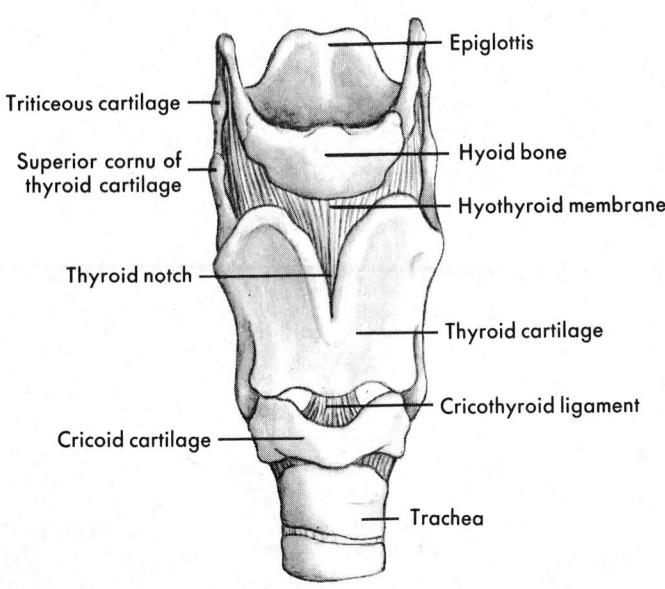

FIGURE 31-4 Anterior aspect of larynx. (From Francis CC: Introduction to human anatomy, ed 6, St Louis, 1975, The CV Mosby Co.)

an airway. The thyroid cartilage, commonly termed the "Adam's apple," is the largest cartilaginous element in the larynx and serves to protect the inner structures. The hyoid bone lies just above the thyroid cartilage and forms an attachment for the larynx and tongue. The cricoid cartilage lies just below the thyroid cartilage and articulates with the arytenoid cartilages, which swing in and out to open and close the vocal cords by opening and closing the glottis (the opening formed between the vocal cords). The larynx is lined with mucosa continuous with that of the hypopharynx and trachea. The vagus nerve innervates the larynx by means of the recurrent laryngeal nerve.

The chief function of the larynx is to serve as an airway between the pharynx and trachea. A leaf-shaped lid of fibrocartilage (epiglottis) protects the glottis by covering the entrance to the larynx during swallowing to prevent aspiration of food or fluids. The closing of the glottis also allows for an increase of intrathoracic pressure, which is needed, for example, in coughing or lifting. The cough reflex, like the sneeze reflex, helps remove inhaled particles from the respiratory tract.

This increased pressure gives added advantage to the use of the muscles of the shoulder and thorax. In addition to these, a most important function of the larynx is

phonation. The larynx creates sounds as a result of vocal cord vibrations that are formed into speech patterns by the movement of the pharynx, palate, tongue, teeth, and lips.

LOWER AIRWAY
STRUCTURE AND FUNCTION OF RESPIRATORY TRACT

The *conducting airways* (trachea, right and left mainstem bronchi, and bronchioles), which terminate into *respiratory units* (respiratory bronchioles, alveolar ducts, and alveoli), make up the lower airways (Figures 31-5 and 31-6).

In addition to providing a passageway for air, the conducting airways serve three functions: filtering, warming, and humidifying air. Air inspired through an intact respiratory tree is cleansed of all particles larger than 2 μm in diameter before reaching the alveolus. The removal of particulate matter such as dust and bacteria preserves the sterility of the alveolus. The removal of particulate matter, such as dust and bacteria, is accomplished by the *mucociliary system*, one of the lung's primary defense mechanisms. The mucociliary system consists of *cilia*, which line the respiratory tract from the hypopharynx through the terminal bronchioles, and a dual layered *fluid lining* secreted by *goblet cells* and *subendothelial glands*. The fluid lining that lies on top of the cilia, consists of a lower serous, and upper muco-polysaccharide (mucous) layer. Inhaled particles are trapped in the mucous layer and are propelled upward toward the pharynx by the continuous rapid beating of the cilia. After reaching the pharynx, mucus and parti-

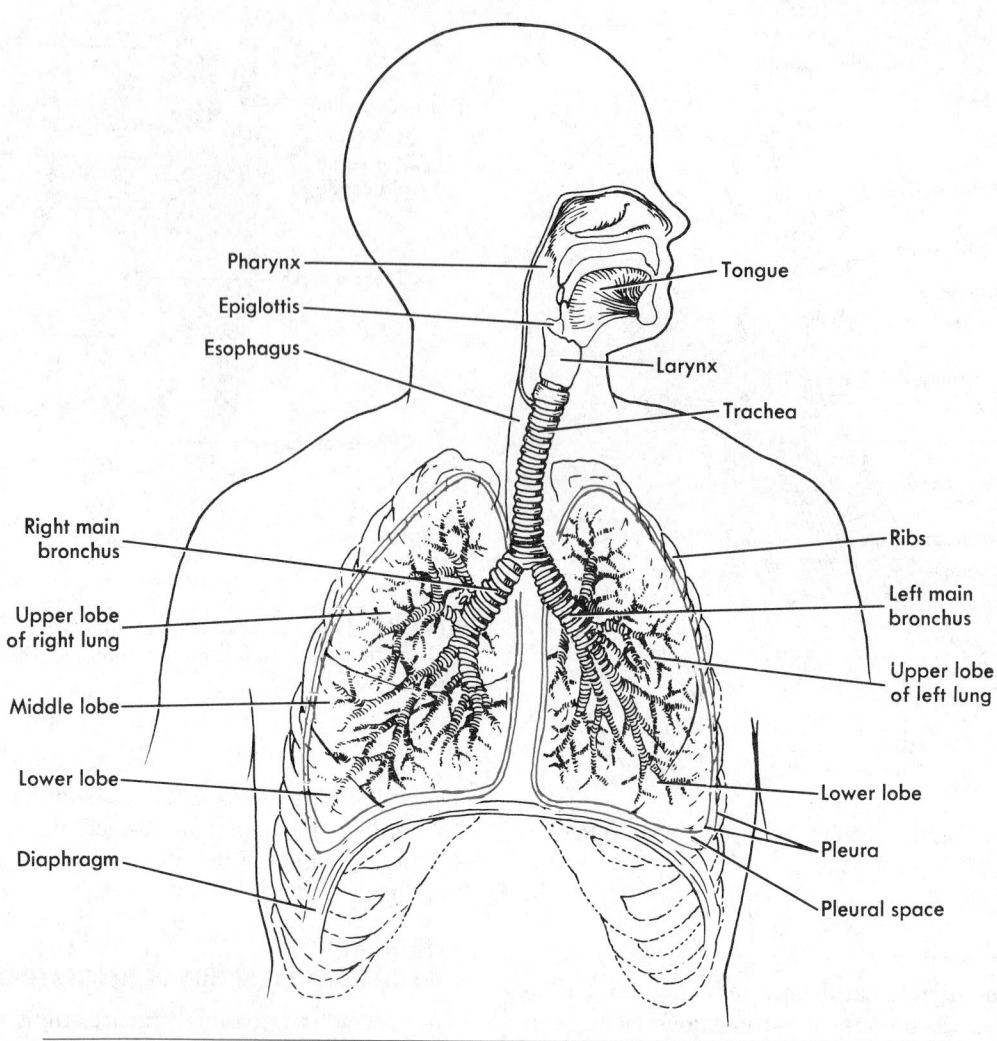

FIGURE 31-5 Anatomy of the thorax and lungs.

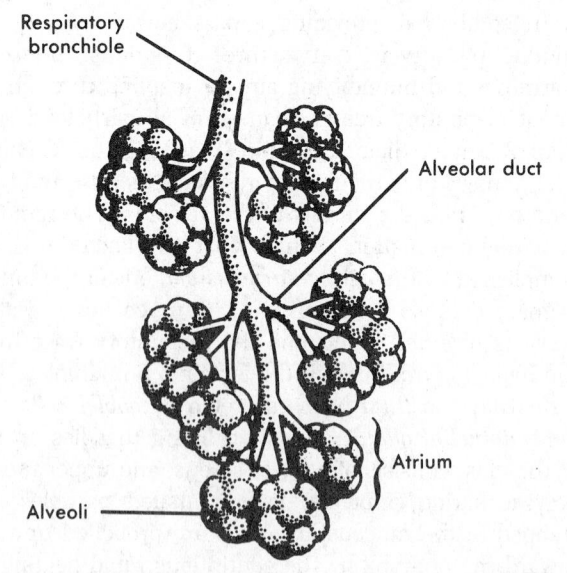

FIGURE 31-6 Respiratory unit.

cles are removed from the airways by swallowing, coughing, or sneezing. The process of particle removal by the mucociliary system is often referred to as the *mucociliary escalator*.

The warming and humidifying functions are made possible by the rich capillary blood supply in the submucosal layer of the airways. During inspiration, air is heated to body temperature, and up to 1000 ml/day of water is used to raise the humidity of the inspired air to at least 80%. On expiration, some of this water is reabsorbed, thus conserving fluid; an average of 300 ml/day is lost in normal respiration.

Within the respiratory unit, respiration occurs only in the alveoli. *Alveoli*, which number 300 million in adults, are minute sacs that arise from the walls of the respiratory bronchioles and alveolar ducts. The alveolus itself is composed of a single layer of squamous epithelium and an elastic basement membrane. These two layers, together with the interstitum and the endothelial and

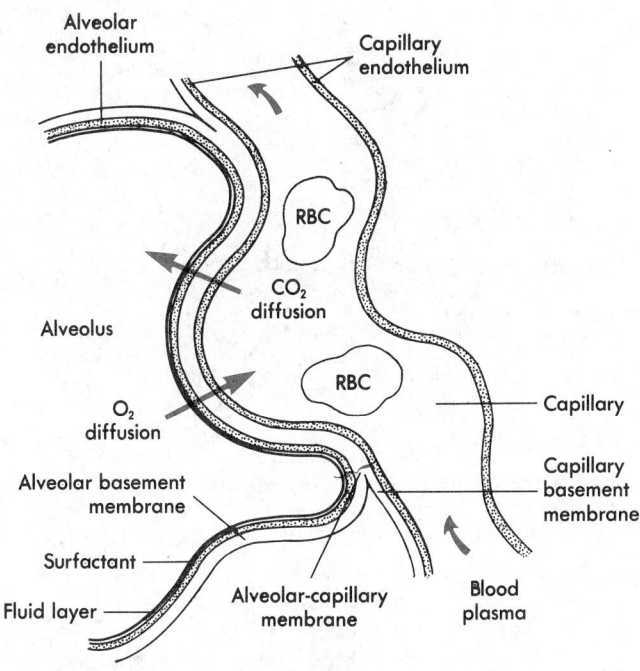

FIGURE 31-7 Alveolar-capillary membrane.

basement layers of the adjacent capillary, form the alveolar-capillary membrane or interface. It is across this membrane, a distance less than 1 μm, that *diffusion of carbon dioxide and oxygen occurs* (Figure 31-7). The spherical interconnected structure of the millions of alveoli provides a large (50 to 100 m) surface area for gaseous diffusion to occur.

In addition to their respiratory function, the alveoli prevent lung collapse by producing *surfactant,* a phospholipid that decreases surface tension and prevents interstitial fluid from traversing into the lung space. Any foreign matter that deposits in healthy alveoli is engulfed by macrophages and disposed of through the circulatory system.

LUNGS AND THORACIC CAVITY

The lungs themselves are subdivided into lobes. The right lung has three lobes: upper, middle, and lower. The left lung has only two lobes: upper and lower. Air is conducted to each lobe through lobar bronchi that branch off the main-stem bronchus. An important difference between the right and left lungs is the size of the airways leading to them. The right bronchus is significantly wider and shorter and extends at a straighter angle from the trachea, making it the more likely lodging point of aspirated material. The left bronchus is narrower and extends at more of a right angle off the trachea, making it more difficult to suction secretions from the left lung.

The thoracic cavity is lined with pleura. The pleura is a continuous *serous* membrane; one surface of it lines the inside of the rib cage (parietal pleura), and the other surface (visceral pleura) covers the lungs. The space between the two surfaces is known as a *potential space.* It normally contains a few milliliters of serous fluid that prevents friction rub when the two surfaces come together.

The lungs lie in and are protected by the thoracic cavity. This bony cage is composed of the sternum and ribs anteriorly and the ribs, scapulae, and vertebral column posteriorly. On the anterior surface, the apices of the lungs lie just above the clavicles and posteriorly extend to the eleventh or twelfth rib. Figures 31-8 to 31-10 illustrate the borders of each lobe.

RESPIRATORY MUSCLES

The major function of the respiratory muscles is to pump air in and out of the lungs, thereby maintaining arterial blood gases within acceptable limits.[22]

The primary muscles of *inspiration* include the *diaphragm, the external intercostals, the internal parasternal intercostals, and the scalene muscles.* The major inspiratory muscle is the diaphragm, which is innervated by the phrenic nerve.

Although normal quiet expiration does not require active muscle contraction, relaxation of the abdominal muscles at the far end of inspiration allows passive descent of the diaphragm during expiration. When expiration is active, for example as a result of exercise, the *internal intercostal and abdominal muscles* contract to assist expiration of air out of the lungs.

Accessory muscles that are used when breathing is labored include the *sternocleidomastoids, pectoralis major and minor, trapezii, and laryngeal muscles.* The scalene muscles were formerly thought to be accessory muscles, but recent research has demonstrated that the contraction of these muscles during inspiration is necessary for diaphragmatic descent to occur.[22]

MECHANISMS OF PULMONARY VENTILATION

Air moves in and out of the lungs as a result of the principle of gas flow; that is, movement is from an area of greater pressure to an area of lesser pressure. At the start of inspiration, the atmospheric air pressure is greater than alveolar pressure; therefore, air moves through the respiratory passageway into the alveoli. When the alveolar pressure exceeds atmospheric pressure, expiration occurs, and air moves out of the lungs into the atmosphere.

The pressure gradient between the alveoli and the atmosphere is established by changes in the size of the thoracic cavity. As the size of the thorax increases, pressure decreases, and air flows into the lung. Thoracic size is increased by contraction of the diaphragm and the external intercostal muscles. The diaphragm de-

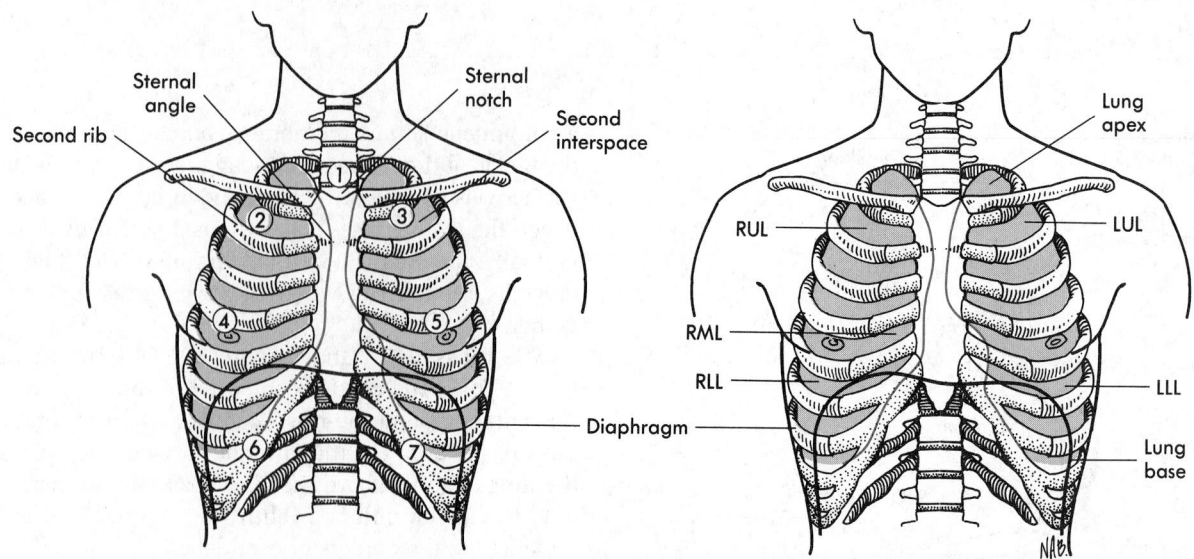

FIGURE 31-8 Anterior thorax showing position of lobes of lung. Numbers indicate stethoscope placement when listening to breath sounds.

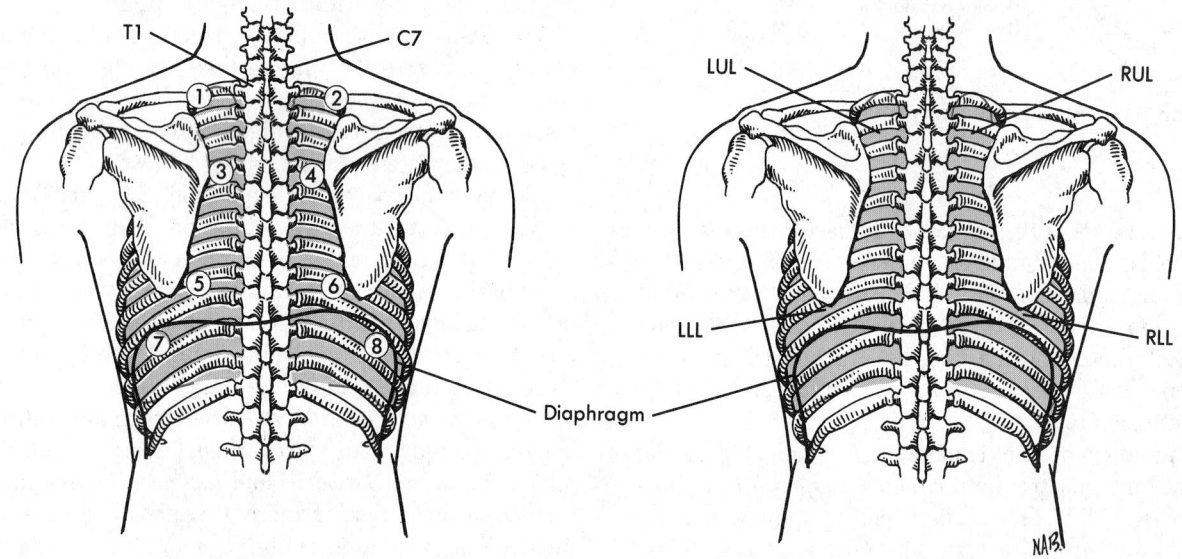

FIGURE 31-9 Posterior thorax showing position of lobes of the lungs. Numbers indicate stethoscope placement when listening to breath sounds.

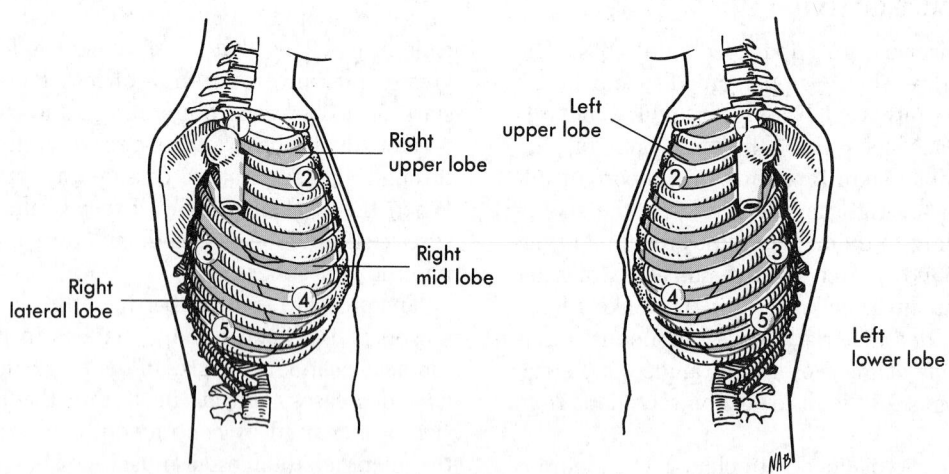

FIGURE 31-10 Lateral thorax showing position of lobes of the lungs. Numbers indicate placement of stethoscope when listening to breath sounds.

scends as it contracts and flattens, increasing the longitudinal diameter of the thorax. The external intercostals, parasternal internal intercostal, and the scalene muscles pull the ribs up and out, elevating the sternum and increasing both anteroposterior and lateral diameter of the chest.

As the thorax expands, it pulls the lungs with it because of cohesion between the moist surfaces of the lungs and chest wall. Expiration is normally a passive process that results from the elastic recoil of the lungs and thoracic muscles. It is this ability of the lungs to stretch and recoil that is evaluated by *pulmonary function testing* (see Table 31-7, *A* and *B*). The ability of the lungs to stretch is measured in terms of compliance. *Compliance* is the volume increase in lungs for every unit increase in intra-alveolar pressure. This relationship is defined by the formula:

$$\text{Compliance} = \text{Change in volume/Change in pressure}$$

Thus lungs with increased (high) compliance have a larger increase in volume for each unit of pressure. Lungs with increased compliance characterize a group of pulmonary disorders known as obstructive diseases. Lungs with decreased (low) compliance have a diminished volume for each unit of pressure. Decreased lung compliance characterizes lung disorders called restrictive diseases (see Chapter 33).

The other property that impacts on the ability of the lungs to ventilate is pulmonary resistance. This property is evaluated by measuring lung volume and airflow over time (see Table 31-7, *C*). *Pulmonary resistance is made up of tissue resistance and airway resistance.* Tissue resistance results from the friction created as tissues move against each other during lung expansion. Airway resistance results from friction encountered by air passing through the airways. The major factor affecting pulmonary resistance is the radius of the airways. The following factors alter airway radius: (1) bronchial innervation (for example: bronchospasm); (2) external compression (for example: thoracic tumor); and (3) internal obstruction (for example: mucus).

GAS EXCHANGE

In the alveoli, oxygen diffuses across the alveolar-capillary membrane from the alveoli into the blood because the partial pressure of oxygen (oxygen tension, PO_2) of *alveolar air* (100 torr*) is greater than the PO_2 of venous blood (40 torr). Carbon dioxide diffuses in the opposite direction, because the PCO_2 of *venous blood* (46 torr) is greater than the PCO_2 of alveolar air (40

torr). The pulmonary diffusion capacity for carbon dioxide is much greater than the capacity for oxygen, and thus carbon dioxide diffuses more readily.

Diffusion of oxygen is *decreased* by the following factors: (1) decreased atmospheric oxygen, (2) decreased alveolar ventilation, (3) decreased alveolar-capillary surface area, and (4) increased alveolar-capillary membrane thickness.

LUNG CIRCULATION

The lungs receive blood from the pulmonary circulation and the bronchial circulation. *Bronchial circulation* provides blood flow to the tissues of the tracheobronchial tree. *Pulmonary circulation* is made up of the entire blood volume received from the right ventricle of the heart. The deoxygenated blood from the right ventricle is carried through the main pulmonary artery to successively branching vessels that follow the bronchi to the respiratory units. Within the alveolar walls, the branching capillaries form a dense network that has been described as a sheet of blood. Thus the circulatory system matches the vast surface created by the alveoli to provide for the rapid efficient exchange of oxygen and carbon dioxide. Newly oxygenated blood then travels via the *four pulmonary veins* back to the left atrium where it is circulated throughout the body via the aorta.

In addition to its role in respiration, the pulmonary circulation serves four other functions:

1. Is a blood reservoir for the systemic circulation
2. Regulates certain metabolic substances
3. Matches blood flow to ventilation
4. Provides nutrition for blood tissue

VENTILATION PERFUSION RELATIONSHIPS

Exchange of oxygen and carbon dioxide between alveolar air and pulmonary capillary blood occurs by gaseous *diffusion*. It is imperative that lung *ventilation (airflow) and perfusion (bloodflow)* are relatively evenly matched so that adequate oxygen and carbon dioxide exchange can occur. Both airflow to the alveoli and blood flow to the pulmonary capillaries have volumes of 4 to 6 L/min. A normal ratio between ventilation and perfusion ranges from 0.8 to 1.2. A low ventilation-to-perfusion ratio exists when alveoli cannot receive ambient air. Blood flowing through the capillaries in contact with the occluded alveoli would have low oxygen and high carbon dioxide levels. A clinical situation that can cause low ventilation-to-perfusion ratios is when secretions block bronchioles leading to alveoli. A high ventilation-to-perfusion ratio exists when a pulmonary capillary is blocked. In this situation, oxygen and carbon dioxide levels in the alveoli remain the same as ambient air. A clinical situation that can cause high ventilation-to-perfusion ratios is pulmonary emboli.

---

*Although *mm Hg* is still widely used in practice, *torr* is becoming the accepted unit of pressure measurement in the scientific literature; 1 torr = 1 mm Hg.

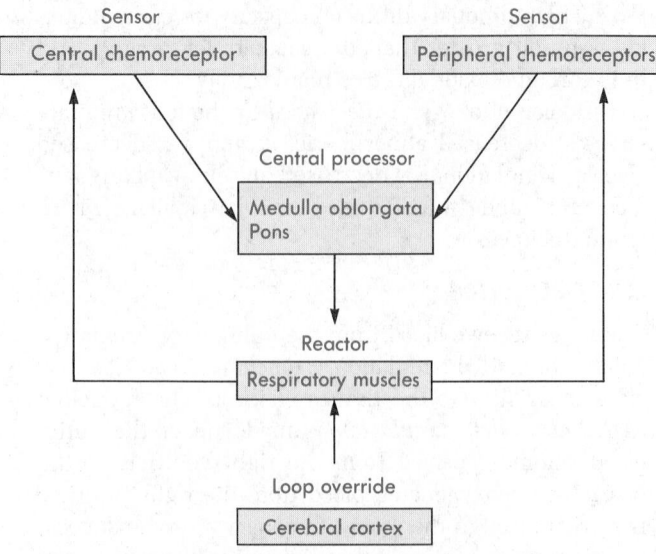

FIGURE 31-11 Respiratory control loop.

CONTROL OF RESPIRATION

Breathing is an automatic loop process by which multiple sensors (chemoreceptors) continually feed data to a central processor (medulla oblongata and pons), which then directs respiratory muscles that adjust ventilation to maintain homeostasis (Fig. 31-11). In addition, humans are equipped with an override feature (cerebral cortex) so that ventilatory patterns can be consciously altered.

The major sensors are the central and peripheral chemoreceptors. *Central chemoreceptors,* located near the medulla, are *sensitive to pH* and *carbon dioxide level changes* in the cerebral spinal fluid. The response can be summarized as:

Increased carbon dioxide = Decreased pH
= Increased respiration

Decreased carbon dioxide = Increased pH
= Decreased respiration

In healthy individuals, ventilation is regulated by the central chemoreceptor response to levels of CO_2. It is important to remember that after a few days of exposure to elevated carbon dioxide levels, the central chemoreceptor becomes ineffective (CO_2 narcosis).

Peripheral chemoreceptors, located in the carotid body and aortic arch, respond to low arterial blood oxygen levels. The peripheral sensor mechanism is believed to be a built-in backup mechanism, and it does not function under normal physiologic conditions (Fig. 31-11).

When the central chemoreceptor is not functioning because of elevated carbon dioxide levels of more than a few days' duration, the person's peripheral chemoreceptor response to a decreased oxygen level maintains respiration. Elevating the oxygen level without simulta-neous lowering of the carbon dioxide level will result in apnea and death.

PHYSIOLOGIC CHANGES WITH AGING

The nurse assessing the older adult's respiratory system will observe normal variations in clinical findings that are the result of anatomic and physiologic changes associated with aging.

The thorax becomes more rigid with diminished rib movement from cartilage calcification and partial muscle contraction.[57] Kyphosis (hunchback) results in an increased anteroposterior diameter. Muscle atrophy of the pharynx and larynx decreases the ability to cough and clear airways effectively. Lung elasticity is diminished, resulting in decreased pulmonary compliance. Airway resistance increases and blood flow to the pulmonary-capillary membranes decreases resulting in increased mismatch of air ventilation ($\dot{V}$) and blood perfusion ($\dot{Q}$).

An individual with these changes will present a clinical picture of *decreased vital capacity, decreased residual volume,* and *decreased forced expiratory volume.*[25] (See Table 31-2). The patient can be observed to have a slight increase in resting respiratory rate with a simultaneous decrease in tidal volume. Although arterial carbon dioxide tension does not change, arterial oxygen tension will be lower. The other classic variant resulting from pulmonary structural changes is that a larger interval will be required for return to resting respiratory rate after exertion.

SUBJECTIVE DATA
UPPER AIRWAY

Before the physical examination, the nurse elicits information specific to the upper airways. A detailed symptom analysis is required whenever the patient indicates a positive history for upper airway dysfunction (for specific symptom analysis refer to a basic nursing text).

NOSE AND SINUSES

Data relevant to assessment of the nose and sinuses can be obtained by asking questions about the following:
1. Obstruction of nares
   a. History of mouth-breathing (time of day or night, duration, and frequency)
   b. History of nasal surgery or injury to nose
   c. Use of nasal drops or spray (type, amount, frequency, and duration of use)
2. Nasal discharge
   a. Color, amount, and consistency of discharge
   b. Nasal bleeding (epistaxis)—one or both nares
   c. Presence of nasal crusting or pain
3. History of sinusitis
   a. Headaches (location and severity)

b. Relationship of sinusitis to certain seasons or types of weather

UPPER THROAT: PHARYNX AND TONSILS

Data relevant to dysfunction of the pharynx and tonsils can be obtained by asking questions about the following if the patient has a dry or sore throat:

1. Work or home environment (for example, exposure to recent illness, inhalation of fumes or dust, or humidity level)
2. Pain on swallowing (dysphagia)
3. History of alcohol use

LOWER THROAT: LARYNX AND HYPOPHARYNX

Questions related to dysfunction of the larynx and hypopharynx in a patient experiencing a change in voice (hoarseness) include the following:

1. Acute or chronic
2. Frequency
3. Smoking and alcohol use history
4. Excessive use of voice (that is, excessive speaking or shouting)

LOWER AIRWAY

Before the physical examination is performed, a nursing history is obtained. Elements critical to assessment of respiratory status are:

1. Exposure to known risk factors, such as cigarette smoke
2. Presence of common pulmonary symptoms
3. Impact of respiratory illness on functional capacity
4. Current medications and treatments, including prescription, nonprescription, and "folk" remedies
5. Acceptable level of health the patient hopes to attain

The major symptoms associated with respiratory disease are *cough, dyspnea, chest pain, sputum production, hemoptysis,* and *wheezing.* Whenever the patient indicates the presence of pulmonary symptoms, a full analysis of the symptoms is completed. Analysis of these symptoms is discussed next.

COUGH

Coughing, the explosive expulsion of air from the lungs, has two main functions: *It protects the lungs from aspiration, and it helps propel foreign matter and excess mucus up through the airways.* Coughing is also the most common symptom of respiratory disease. The box above lists terminology used to describe the types of cough.

One aspect of chronic cough that is difficult to assess is the actual time of onset. The individual is often not aware of its onset or attributes its presence to identifiable causes, such as smoking or sinusitis. A family member or close associate might be able to more accurately identify actual time of onset. It is important to

COUGH DESCRIPTORS

TIMING

1. Chronic
2. Acute
3. Paroxysmal (periodic forceful episodes which are difficult to control)

QUALITY

1. Productive-nonproductive
2. Dry-moist
3. Barking
4. Hoarse
5. Hacking

---

identify those factors the patient (and spouse or friend) believes contribute to the cough. Areas to explore include these factors commonly associated with *cough: activity, body position, environmental irritants, vocalization (normal speech, shouting, singing, whispering), weather, anxiety,* and *infection.*

DYSPNEA

Dyspnea is the highly individualized perception of *breathlessness* inappropriate to the level of exertion. Dyspnea involves both a physiologic and cognitive component. First, awareness of breathing must occur; then it must be interpreted as inadequate for the degree of activity. A retrospective descriptive study of peoples' sensations of dyspnea is presented in the research box below.

The physiologic component is not fully understood, but is appears that dyspnea is related more to the ventilatory component of breathing than to respiration.[26] Dyspnea associated with respiratory disease results from pathologic changes that increase airway resistance, decrease pulmonary compliance, alter the pulmonary vascular system, or weaken the respiratory muscles. Al-

RESEARCH

Janson-Bjerklie S, Carrieri VK, and Hudes M: The sensations of pulmonary dyspnea, Nursing Research 35(3), 154-159, 1986.

The study of a convenience sample of 68 subjects with a variety of pulmonary diseases compared recalled physical and emotional sensations during episodes of acute dyspnea. Although frequency of sensations were found to be similar across disease categories, some differences in magnitude and character of the dyspnea experience were found among disease groups. Physical sensations experienced during episodes of dyspnea clustered into categories of suffocation, tightness, and congestion. ■

DYSPNEA DESCRIPTORS

TIMING

1. Chronic or acute
2. Episodic or paroxysmal
3. Onset
4. Duration
5. Frequency

CHARACTERISTICS

1. Perceived severity
2. Phase of respiratory cycle when occurs
   a. Inspiratory
   b. Expiratory
   c. Throughout entire cycle
3. Other symptoms related to dyspnea
4. Associated factors
   a. Time of day
   b. Seasonal or weather changes
   c. Environmental irritants
   d. Anxiety
   e. Body position
      (1) Paroxysmal nocturnal dyspnea (PND): sudden onset while sleeping in recumbant position
   f. Orthopnea: breathlessness upon assuming recumbent position

TABLE 31-1 American Thoracic Society/Five-level scale of breathlessness, graded 1 to 5

Grade	Description
1	Are you troubled by shortness of breath during walking on the level or walking up a slight hill? Yes ____ No ____
2	Do you have to walk slower than people of your age on the level because of breathlessness? Yes ____ No ____
3	Do you ever have to stop for breath when walking at your own pace on the level? Yes ____ No ____
4	Do you ever have to stop for breath after walking about 100 yards or after a few minutes walking on the level? Yes ____ No ____
5	Are you too breathless to leave the house or breathless on dressing or undressing? Yes ____ No ____

though dyspnea is associated with many underlying cardiopulmonary diseases, two common mediating processes that are present, regardless of underlying pathology, are *increased respiratory muscle activity* and *respiratory muscle weakness.*

The box above presents those aspects of the patient's dyspnea that are important to assess.

Because of its insidious nature, the actual onset of chronic dyspnea is difficult to identify. Relatives or close associates of the person might be able to help in identifying the time of onset. Often it is helpful to offer suggestions such as having the person associate past birthdays or holidays with the presence of dyspnea. When assessing the severity of dyspnea, subjective terms such as mild, moderate, or severe should be avoided. A number of tools in the literature provide a means for the clinician to quantify the person's experience of dyspnea.[5,11,12,47] Many of these instruments provide a systematic magnitude estimate using the dyspneic person's verbal report; thus they are amenable to clinical assessment without requiring special equipment. The instruments often focus on the person's perception of dyspnea related to activities of daily living (ADL). An example of one of the magnitude scales is a scale developed by the American Thoracic Society (Table 31-1).

CHEST PAIN

Chest pain of pulmonary origin can derive from the chest wall, parietal pleura, visceral pleura, or the lung parenchyma itself. Table 31-2 summarizes the types of chest pain related to pulmonary conditions.

Whenever the patient indicates the presence of chest pain, the symptom requires detailed investigation. (Chapter 16 includes specific guidelines for pain assessment.)

TABLE 31-2 Thoracic-pulmonary chest pain

Origin	Characteristics	Possible Cause
Chest wall	Well-localized constant ache increasing with movement	Trauma, cough, herpes zoster
Pleura	Sharp, abrupt onset increasing with inspiration or with sudden ventilatory effect (cough, sneeze), unilateral	Pleural inflammation (pleurisy), pulmonary infarction, pneumothorax, tumors
Lung parenchyma	Dull, constant ache, poorly localized	Benign pulmonary tumors Carcinoma Pneumothorax

SPUTUM DESCRIPTORS

AMOUNT

1. Scant (few teaspoons)
2. Copious

CONSISTENCY

1. Thick
2. Viscous (gelatinous)
3. Tenacious (sticky)
4. Frothy
5. Mucoid (clear, thin to moderately thick)
6. Watery
7. Mucopurulent (thick, viscous; color: cream, yellow, or green)
8. Casts (from bronchioles, rubbery)

SPUTUM PRODUCTION

The lung *goblet cells* and *mucous glands* secrete mucus that coats the interior lung surface. Mucus is constantly propelled upward toward the pharynx by the lung cilia. Sputum, composed of mucus, cellular debris, microorganisms, blood, pus, and foreign particles, is the substance ejected from the lungs by coughing or clearing the throat.

It is important to clarify whether the patient is describing saliva or sputum. To accurately assess the type and amount of sputum production, specimen collection might be required (see p. 832). The patient's sputum production should be analyzed for onset, pattern or occurrence, exposure to risk factors, associated illnesses, consistency, odor, color, and amount. Common descriptors for sputum are presented in the box above, left.

HEMOPTYSIS

Hemoptysis is the coughing up of blood or bloody or blood-tinged sputum. The source of bleeding might be from anywhere in the upper or lower airways or from the lung parenchyma. The patient usually perceives hemoptysis as an indicator of serious illness and will often appear anxious or afraid. If hemoptysis is present, a description of onset, duration, amount, and color (for example, bright red or frothy) is obtained. As with any symptom, a full analysis is appropriate. *It is important to differentiate between hemoptysis and hematemesis.* This can be difficult if the patient has swallowed bloody sputum or conversely, aspirated bloody vomitus. If a specimen has been saved, it might be possible to assess its origin by criteria noted in the box above, right.

WHEEZING

Wheezing is a continuous sound produced when air passes through the smaller bronchi or bronchioles where there is increased airway resistance. Airway re-

BEDSIDE ASSESSMENT OF HEMOPTYSIS AND HEMATEMESIS

HEMOPTYSIS	HEMATEMESIS
Usually frothy	Never frothy
pH alkaline	pH acidic

sistance is increased by bronchoconstriction or an increase of mucus in the bronchi. Audible wheezing can be heard throughout the respiratory cycle or only during inspiration or expiration. When bronchoconstriction is present, wheezing will be greater on expiration. If wheezing is present, a full analysis of it is completed.

PULMONARY RISK FACTORS

Major risk factors associated with pulmonary disease are *smoking, history of previous pulmonary disorders, environmental irritants, and genetic predisposition.*

Smoking has been implicated as a major cause of lung disease. There is a strong relationship between smoking and the development or exacerbation of chronic bronchitis, emphysema, asthma, lung carcinoma, and respiratory infections.*

Passive smoking has been implicated as increasing the *nonsmoker's risk of developing carcinoma.* Maternal smoking is known to increase the incidence of respiratory illness in children and may be related to increased lung cancer risk in later life.[71] The known acute effects of cigarette smoking include increased airway resistance, increased mucus in small airways and later increased secretions in large airways, reduced lung recoil, vascular changes, and respiratory bronchiolitis.[8]

The nursing assessment should include the patient's current or previous type and mode of smoking. The patient's current or past history of smoking behaviors must be determined. The type of smoking material (e.g., tobacco, marijuana), the mode of smoking (pipe, cigarette, or cigar) should be identified. *It is also important to explore the use of smokeless tobacco, particularly in the younger male population because of its relationship to upper airway disorders.* Variable effects of smoking that should be assessed include an estimate of depth of inhalation, number of puffs per cigarette, use of a filter, brand of cigarette smoked, and presence of other risk factors.[41]

Questions relevant to smoking history are:

1. How long?
2. How much in pack-years? (see the following formula)

---

*The reader is referred to the Jan. 6, 1989 issue of the Journal of the American Medical Association, which is devoted entirely to the subject of the effects of smoking.

3. Is smoke inhaled?
4. How much of the cigarette (cigar, pipe) is smoked?
5. Have attempts been made to quit?
6. Is there a desire to quit?

The nurse can determine how much tobacco is smoked by the following equation (cigarettes are determined by "pack-years"; cigars, pipes, marijuana, and smokeless tobacco are determined as amount used per day):

"Pack-year" = Number of years smoked ×Number of packs smoked per day (for example, 20 years of 2 packs/day=40 pack years)

ENVIRONMENTAL IRRITANTS

This category includes atmospheric pollutants (dust, fungal spores, vapor, fumes, and gases), occupational contaminants (chemical fumes, coal dust, and molds), and environmental factors.

The following areas should be addressed during the nursing history:

1. Residence or work in heavy industry areas
2. Residence or work in area of heavy automobile traffic
3. Known high-risk occupations (for example, mining, foundry work, welding, textile, quarry work, wood and paper mills, farming, and chemical manufacturing)
4. Exposure to bird droppings in an enclosed space (for example, chicken house, old buildings being remodeled)
5. Travel and residential history, where person has lived or visited (certain pulmonary disorders such as histoplasmosis or "farmer's lung" related to geographic areas) (see Chapter 33)
6. History of previous pulmonary disorders; that is, a history of the following predisposing illnesses:

a. Childhood allergies and frequent pulmonary infections
b. History of influenza (especially *Haemophilus influenzae*), chronic sinusitis, frequent colds, pneumonia, and pleurisy
c. Chest surgery
d. Tuberculosis
e. Adult-onset allergies

GENETIC DISORDERS

A genetically predetermined deficiency in the proteinase inhibitors, α_1-antitrypsin, and α_2-macroglobulin is associated with a high risk of developing emphysema. To identify the possible presence of this risk, inquiry into the following areas is helpful:

1. Does the patient or any family member have a documented history of enzyme deficiency?
2. Is there a strong family history of chronic obstructive pulmonary disease (COPD)?
3. Has either the patient or any family member developed respiratory symptoms at an early age?
4. Does either the patient or any family member have a history of liver disease? NOTE:There is also a correlation between liver disease and α_1-antitrypsin deficiency.

ASSESSMENT OF FUNCTIONAL CAPACITY

Individuals experiencing pulmonary dysfunction tend to perceive their illness in terms of its impact on their ability to carry out activities of daily living (ADL). One study of persons with COPD found that participants would describe dyspnea as "weakness," "tiredness," or "loss of libido"; but in retrospect it is believed that these were the onset of COPD-related dyspnea. An example of a nursing assessment that identifies the functional area of locomotion, biofunctional activities, and vocalization is presented in the box below.

NURSING ASSESSMENT OF ACTIVITIES OF DAILY LIVING

Do any of the following make you short of breath?	YES	NO
a. Walking fast on flat ground (l)	_____	_____
b. Walking uphill (l)	_____	_____
c. Climbing stairs (l)	_____	_____
d. Bending over to do something such as tying shoes or picking up an object (l)	_____	_____
e. Any work requiring arms raised above chest such as combing your hair (l)	_____	_____
f. Talking (v)	_____	_____
g. Yelling (v)	_____	_____
h. Laughing (v)	_____	_____
i. Sleeping (b)	_____	_____
j. Eating (b)	_____	_____
k. Bowel movements (b)	_____	_____
l. Sexual activity (b)	_____	_____
m. Any other activity	_____	_____

From Brucia J: Unpublished master's thesis, 1982, p. 104.
b = Biofunctional; l = Locomotion; v = Vocalization.

MEDICATIONS AND TREATMENTS

In addition to obtaining information about all prescription and nonprescription medications and treatments, it is also important to ask about any additional methods used by the patient to treat illness. Patients are often unwilling to share folk remedies at their initial interview for fear of disapproval by caregivers. Patients must be approached in a nonjudgmental manner. A neutral inquiry such as, "Is there anything you have found that seems to help you feel better?" conveys receptiveness on the part of the interviewer.

ESTABLISHING THE PATIENT'S HEALTH GOAL

Since pulmonary disorders run the spectrum from total cure without residual damage to chronic terminal illness, the patient's goals for health will be highly individualized. A functional approach to defining the patient's health goals will provide visible meaningful goals for both caregivers and the patient. An example of a functional goal would be, "I want to be able to cook my meals."

OBJECTIVE DATA

UPPER AIRWAY

In addition to the interview, physical examination provides objective data necessary to identify specific upper airway disorders.

NOSE AND SINUSES

Inspection of the nose includes looking for deformities, asymmetry, and inflammation. Nasal mucosa is normally redder in appearance than oral mucosa. The inferior and middle turbinates are observed for color, edema, exudate, or polyps. The nasal septum is observed for deviation, bleeding, or perforation. Some septal deviation (Figure 31-12) is common in most adults and is usually asymptomatic, although it can produce nasal obstruction. Abnormal findings in assessing the nose include any excessive redness, edema, exudate, or bleeding, as well as the presence of any furuncles. Red, swollen nasal mucous membranes accompanied by watery to mucopurulent nasal discharge indicate *acute rhinitis*. Nasal mucosa that is swollen, pale, boggy, and usually gray to dull red is seen in persons with *allergic rhinitis*. Soft, pale gray mobile structures found in the middle meatus are polyps that can develop in persons with allergic rhinitis.

The sinuses are palpated for signs of tenderness of the frontal and maxillary areas when inspecting the nose. The normal frontal and maxillary sinuses can be visualized by illuminating them in a dark room with a specially shaped, lighted bulb or a lighted *transillumination* tip. This examination is referred to as transillumination. If disease is present, the light will not penetrate the sinuses, or it will reveal fluid levels indicative of obstruction to drainage of the sinuses. Roetgenologic examination of the sinuses can help establish the diagnosis of sinusitis. No physical preparation is necessary, and usually no contrast medium is used, because the normal sinus is filled with air, which in itself casts a shadow in contrast to surrounding structures.

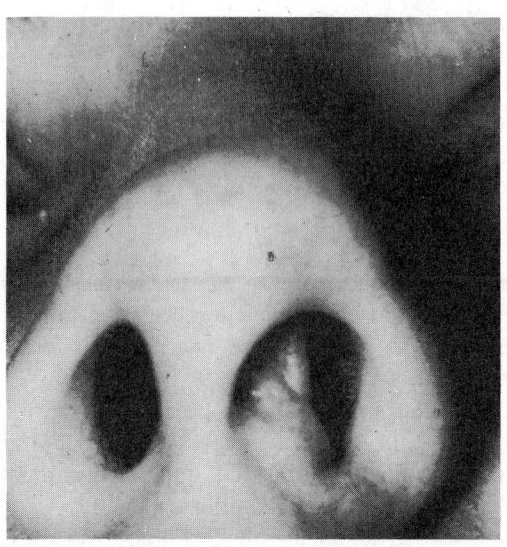

FIGURE 31-12 Septal deviation. Anterior end of septal cartilage is dislocated and projects into nasal vestibule. (From Saunders WH et al: Nursing care in eye, ear, nose, and throat disorders, ed 4, St Louis, 1979, The CV Mosby Co.)

PHARYNX AND TONSILS

The oropharynx, that portion of the pharynx directly posterior to the oral cavity bounded by the nasopharynx above and laryngopharynx below, is examined with a tongue blade and a mirror. The anterior and posterior tonsillar pillars, the uvula, the tonsils, and the posterior pharynx are inspected for color, symmetry, evidence of exudate, edema, ulceration, and tonsillar enlargement. Redness and swelling of the tonsils, pillars, and uvula with white or yellow exudate on the tonsils might indicate streptococcal infection. Tonsils can be enlarged without being infected.

LARYNX AND HYPOPHARYNX

The larynx can be examined by an *indirect laryngoscopy*; the person being examined sits in a chair with the head tilted back and is asked to stick out the tongue. The examiner then grasps it with a gauze sponge and pulls it forward and down. A warmed laryngeal mirror is introduced into the back of the throat until the larynx is visualized. It is examined at rest and during attempts to speak (phonation). If the gag reflex is very sensitive, the pharyngeal wall can be sprayed with a topical anesthetic such as 2% cocaine or 2% tetracaine (Pontocaine). Tetracaine is preferred by some physicians because it is less toxic than cocaine. A *direct laryngoscopy* is performed on children, on adults who are unable to cooperate for an indirect examination, and on all persons with suspicious lesions of the larynx.[24]

LOWER AIRWAY

Physical examination of the chest provides objective data that, along with information obtained during the interview, forms the database necessary to formulate nursing diagnoses appropriate to the individual. The pulmonary examination should be conducted with the person sitting upright on the edge of the bed, if possible. Adequate lighting and a relaxed, quiet environment are essential to obtain maximum information.

Detailed instruction on the techniques for performing the chest examination are beyond the scope of this book. The reader is referred to a textbook of physical assessment for in-depth information on the techniques of pulmonary physical assessment.

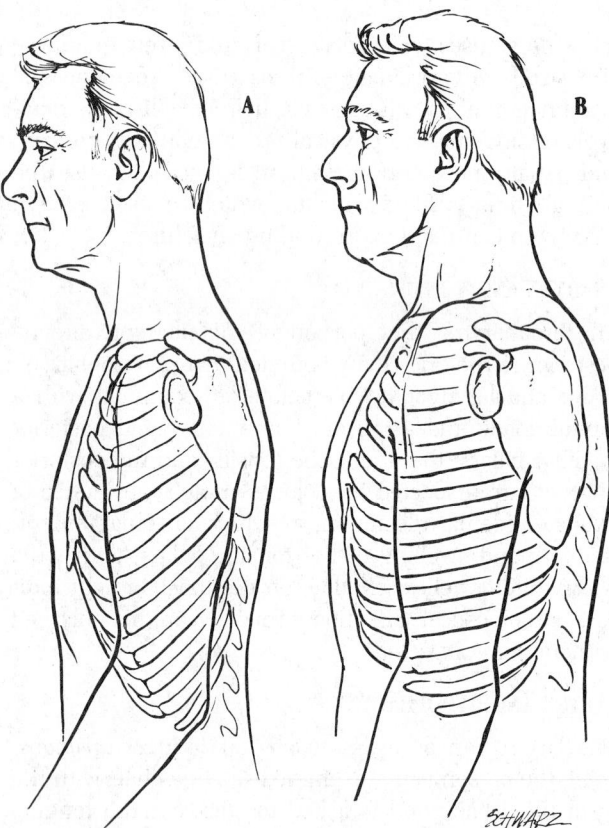

FIGURE 31-13 A, Normal thorax configuration. **B,** Increased anteroposterior diameter. Note contrasts in the angle of the slope of the ribs and the development of the accessory muscle of respiration in the neck. (From Malasanos L et al: Health assessment, ed 3, St Louis, 1986, The CV Mosby Co.)

INSPECTION

The patient is observed for general appearance, respiratory rate and pattern, and thoracic configuration (Figure 31-13, *A* and *B*). It is important to take adequate time to thoroughly observe the patient before moving to the "hands on" component of the examination. By observing general appearance, respiratory rate and pattern, the presence and character of the person's cough, and sputum production, the nurse can determine which components of the pulmonary examination are appropriate for assessing the patient's current respiratory status. Table 31-3 indicates the normal and abnormal findings for each component of inspection.

PALPATION

The chest is palpated to evaluate skin and chest wall status. Palpation of the chest and spinal column is a general screening technique to identify the presence of underlying abnormalities such as inflammation. The chest is also palpated for *fremitus,* which are vibrations felt on the chest surface when sound passes through underlying tissue and air- or fluid-filled space. Fremitus can be caused by secretions in the large airways, a pleural friction rub, or lung consolidation. Vocal (tactile) fremitus is normally present; thus it is necessary to determine whether fremitus is increased or decreased. The chest is also palpated for symmetry and degree of lateral chest expansion from maximal exhalation to maximal inhalation. Possible normal and abnormal findings are presented in Table 31-4.

PERCUSSION

Percussion is used to assess the lung fields and the position and movement of the diaphragm (excursion). Percussion notes are produced from vibration created by tapping the chest wall. The quality of the percussion note depends on the density of underlying tissue and the amount of air through which the vibration passes. Table 31-5 identifies common normal and abnormal percussion findings.

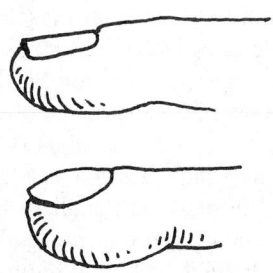

FIGURE 31-14 Comparison of normal nail (top) and digital clubbing (bottom).

TABLE 31-3 Possible findings by inspection in a pulmonary examination

Observe	Normal	Abnormal
General appearance	Quiet respiration Sitting or reclining without difficulty Skin translucent, appears dry Nailbeds pink Mucous membranes pink and moist* Cyanosis or pallor assessed by establishing an early individual baseline	Lips puckered when exhaling Restless and apprehensive Leans forward with hands or elbows on knees Skin: diaphoretic, dull pale, or ruddy Cyanosis: Skin or mucous membrane has bluish cast Central cyanosis: results from decreased oxygenation of blood† Peripheral cyanosis: result of local vasoconstriction or decreased output Nail clubbing: painless enlargement of terminal phalanges related to chronic tissue hypoxia (Figure 31-14)
Trachea	Midline in neck	Tracheal deviation; displacement either lateral, anterior, or posterior Jugular venous distension (see Chapter 26) Cough: strong or weak, dry or wet, productive or nonproductive Sputum production: amount, color, odor, consistency (p. 832)
Rate	Eupnea: 12 to 20	Tachypnea: rate >20 breaths/min Bradypnea: rate <10 breaths/min
Breathing pattern	Minimal effort with inspiration: passive, quiet expiration Inspiration/expiration ratio: 1:2 Male: diaphragmatic breathing Female: thoracic breathing	Hyperpnea: increased breathing rate Accessory muscle breathing Apnea: total absence of breathing Biots: irregular rhythm with periods of apnea Cheyne-Stokes: cyclical deeper and shallower breaths followed by periods of apnea Kussmaul's: deep, rapid and regular breathing Paradoxical: portion of chest wall moves in during inhalation and out during exhalation Stridorous: audible, loud, low-pitched sound with inhalation and exhalation
Thoracic configuration	Symmetric appearance Anteroposterior diameter (AP) less than transverse diameter Spine straight Scapulae on same horizontal plane Trachea midline (centered on suprasternal notch)	Chest expands unevenly Muscular development asymmetric Barrel chest: AP diameter increased in relation to transverse diameter (Figure 31-13) Kyphosis: increased thoracic curvature Scoliosis: increased lateral curvature Scapular placement *asymmetric* Trachea right or left of midline

*Dark-skinned people might have normal bluish pigmented mucous membranes.
†Central cyanosis is relevant to respiratory status. Observe nailbeds, mucous membrane, and lips.

TABLE 31-4 Possible findings by palpation in a pulmonary examination

Palpate	Normal	Abnormal
Skin and chest wall	Skin nontender, smooth, warm, and dry Spine and ribs nontender	Skin moist or exceedingly dry Crepitation—"crackling" when skin palpated—due to air leak from lung into subcutaneous tissue Localized tenderness
Fremitus*	Symmetric, mild vibrations felt on chest wall during vocalization	Increased fremitus—a result of vibration through more solid medium such as lung tumors Decreased fremitus—a result of vibration through increased space in the chest such as pneumothorax or obesity. Asymmetric fremitus is always abnormal
Lateral chest expansion	Symmetric 3 to 8 cm expansion†	Expansion less than 3 cm, painful or assymetric†

*Normal fremitus varies from person to person. An individual's baseline must be established.
†Reduced expansion can result from either an overexpanded chest (barrel chest) or from a restricted chest.

TABLE 31-5 Possible findings by percussion in a pulmonary examination

Percussion	Normal	Abnormal
Lung fields	Resonant-low-pitched, hollow, easily heard sounds; equal quality bilaterally	Hyperresonant: heard with air trapping or pneumothorax Dull or flat: results from decreased air in lungs (tumor, fluid)
Diaphragm position and movement	Resting diaphragm at 10th thoracic vertebrae Each hemidiaphragm moves 3-6 cm (Figure 31-15)	High position—stomach distension or phrenic nerve damage Decreased or no movement in either hemidiaphragm*

*Decreased excursion can result from hyperinflated lungs pushing down on diaphragm, diaphragmatic disorders, or loss of diaphragmatic innervation.

AUSCULTATION

Airway and lung status can be assessed by auscultating breath and voice sounds transmitted through the chest wall. The origin of breath sounds is unclear.[9]

In order to hear breath sounds throughout all lung spaces, the patient is instructed to take slow, moderate to deep breaths through the mouth. Breath sounds are assessed during both inspiration and expiration. The duration of inspiratory time to expiratory time, intensity, and pitch of breath sounds are assessed. Except for normally diminished breath sounds in the left upper lobe, breath sounds should be approximately symmetric in intensity and character when comparing the two lungs.

Changes in *breath sounds that may indicate underlying pathology include decreased or absent breath sounds, increased breath sounds, and superimposed breath sounds, also known as adventitious* sounds. Increased breath sounds are heard when conditions such as atelectasis or pneumonia increases lung tissue den-

sity. Decreased or absent breath sounds occur whenever transmission of sound waves through the lung tissue or chest wall are reduced. Conditions that decrease sound transmission include lung hyperinflation, air or fluid in the pleural space, shallow breathing, or increased chest wall thickness. Adventitious breath sounds can be caused by a variety of underlying pathologies that cause excess mucus or fluid, tissue inflammation, bronchospasm, or airway obstruction. Table 31-6 presents normal and abnormal sounds that may be heard during auscultation.

CLINICAL APPLICATION OF PULMONARY NURSING ASSESSMENT

The process of nursing assessment must be highly individualized (see box on p. 830). In view of the patient's current respiratory status, the nurse tailors the interview and physical examination to maximize data gathering without increasing respiratory distress. The follow-

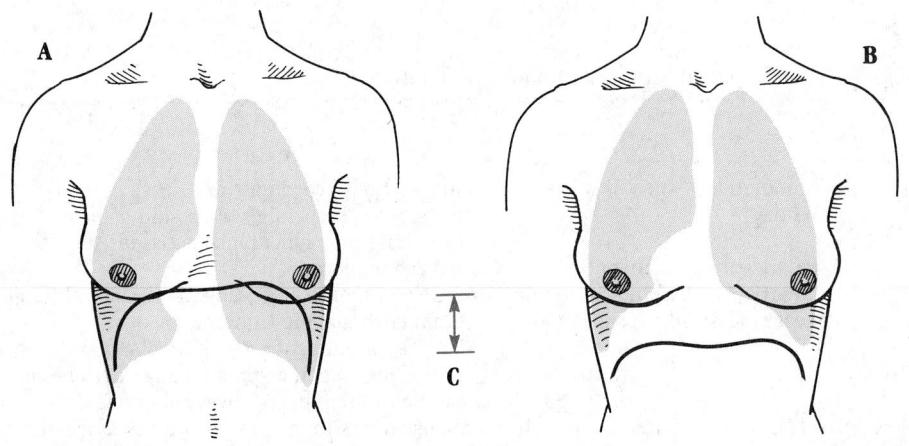

FIGURE 31-15 Diaphragmatic excursion. **A,** Full-end expiration. **B,** Full-end inspiration. **C,** Range of diaphragmatic movement—distance from A to B.

TABLE 31-6 Possible findings by auscultation in a pulmonary examination

Auscultation	Normal	Abnormal
Breath sounds (Figure 31-16)	*Vesicular:* soft, breezy low-pitched sound on inspiration; heard over peripheral lung area (away from bronchi) *Bronchovesicular:* medium in pitch and loudness, heard equally on inspiration and expiration, heard over major airways (that is, over the sternum and between the scapula) Bronchial: high-pitched and loud; heard only over trachea	Adventitious-sounds superimposed on breath sounds* Crackles: discontinuous, intermittent crackling or bubbling sound of short duration; caused by movement of excess secretions during inspiration and expiration or opening of closed airways during inhalation (can be in larger proximal bronchioles or peripheral bronchioles and alveoli); can be identified as inspiratory and expiratory, early inspiratory and late inspiratory; common underlying disorder—atelectasis Wheezes: continuous, high-pitched sound caused by turbulent air passing through compressed airway; common underlying disorder—asthma Rhonchi: continuous low-pitched sounds; common underlying disorder—bronchitis Bronchial: abnormal if heard anywhere other than over trachea; common underlying disorder—pneumonia Friction rub: crackling, grating sound often heard throughout respiratory cycle; originates in inflamed pleura; common underlying disorder—pleuritis

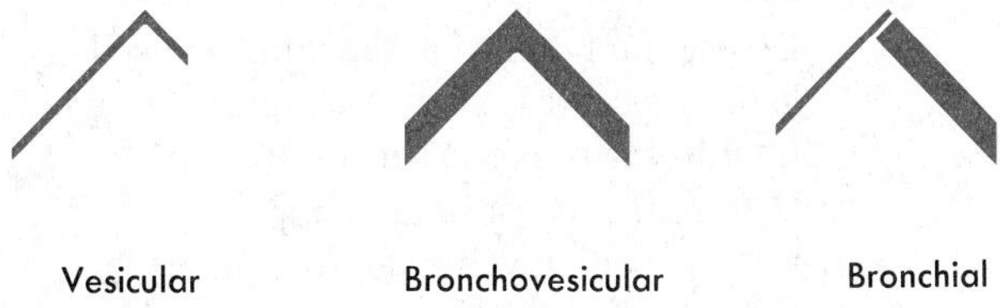

FIGURE 31-16 Schematic representation of three types of breath sounds.

Auscultation	Normal	Abnormal
Voice sounds	Patient instructed to vocalize specific sounds while examiner auscultates for characteristic changes when vocal sounds are transmitted through chest wall Egophony: instructed to say prolonged "e" Sound auscultated is muffled "e" Whispered pectoriloquy: instructed to whisper "1,2,3" Sound auscultated is muffled "1,2,3" Bronchophony: instructed to say "1,2,3" Sound auscultated is muffled "1,2,3"	Sound auscultated: "a" (indicates consolidation) Sound auscultated: loud, clear "1,2,3," (indicates consolidation Sound auscultated: loud, clear "1,2,3," (indicates consolidation)

*The terminology used to describe lung sounds is based on the 1981 report of the ATS-ACCP Ad Hoc Subcommittee on Pulmonary Nomenclature. Other terminology can be used, see Table 31-7.

ing information demonstrates how the nurse might select specific components of the pulmonary assessment on the basis of patient's respiratory status.

After initial assessment of the current respiratory status, the nurse selects components of the pulmonary examination appropriate to the patient's level of respiratory distress. Components of the pulmonary examination that should be included for each of the three respiratory distress categories previously identified are presented in the box below.

TABLE 31-7 Recommended terminology for lung sounds versus terminology in other publications

Recommended Term	Classification	Terms Used in Other Publications
Crackles	Discontinuous	Rales Crepitations
Wheezes	High-pitched, continuous	Sibilant rales Musical rales Sibilant rhonchi
Rhonchi	Low-pitched, continuous	Low-pitched wheeze Sonorous rales

From Willkins RL, Sheldon RL, Krider SJ: Clinical assessment in respiratory care, St Louis, 1985, The CV Mosby Co.

COMPONENTS OF PULMONARY EXAMINATION FOR RESPIRATORY DISTRESS

Acute respiratory distress	Inspection: all components Auscultation: breath sounds, abnormal sounds
Moderate respiratory distress	Interview: as tolerated; divide into several brief sessions Inspection: all components Palpation: thoracic expansion Percussion: to assess resonance Auscultation: breath sounds, abnormal sounds
Mild respiratory distress	All components of pulmonary examination

GUIDELINES FOR CLINICAL ASSESSMENT

Initial nursing assessment
Goal: to quickly determine the patient's respiratory status
Initial assessment components used include:
1. Determine chief complaint
2. Rapid inspection for:
   a. General appearance
   b. Respiratory rate/pattern
   c. Thoracic configuration
On the basis of clinical signs observed during the initial assessment, the patient's respiratory status might be categorized as one of the following:
1. *Acute respiratory distress*
   a. General appearance
      (1) Extremely apprehensive, restless or lethargic
      (2) Might verbalize, "Help, I can't get my air," or may be unable to speak
      (3) Skin diaphoretic, grayish, bluish, or a deep ruddy color
   b. Respiratory rate/pattern
      (1) Rate increased >20 or decreased <12
      (2) Shallow gasping
      (3) Might be any of abnormal pattern listed in Table 31-7
      (4) Inspiratory/expiratory (I:E) ratio prolonged
   c. Thoracic configuration
      (1) Accessory muscle breathing with noticeable clavicular lift, retracting intercostal muscles
      (2) Chest might appear asymmetric at rest or on expansion
2. *Moderate respiratory distress*
   a. General appearance
      (1) Somewhat apprehensive, restless, or might try to minimize respiratory distress
      (2) Skin might be diaphoretic, ruddy, or grayish in appearance
   b. Respiratory rate/pattern
      (1) Respiratory rate mildly elevated
      (2) Inspiratory/expiratory ratio might be slightly prolonged
   c. Thoracic configuration
      (1) Slight clavicular lift
3. *Mild respiratory distress*
   a. General appearance
      (1) Relaxed
      (2) Can verbalize detailed chief complaint
      (3) Skin translucent, color within normal limits
   b. Respiratory rate/pattern
      (1) Normal or slightly increased
   c. Thoracic configuration
      (1) Thoracic or diaphragmatic breathing
      (2) Chest expansion is symmetric

DIAGNOSTIC TESTS

ROENTGENOLOGIC EXAMINATION OF THE THORAX AND LUNGS

Patients are usually familiar with the roetgenologic examination. In recent years, there has been an increase in consumer awareness of the danger of excessive exposure to radiation. The patient should have a full explanation of the type of test to be performed and the benefits (knowledge gained) in relation to risk from radiation exposure.

Chest film studies are indicated for the following reasons:

1. Detect alterations of the lung caused by pathologic processes such as tumors, inflammation, fractures, fluid or air accumulation
2. Determine appropriate therapy
3. Evaluate effectiveness of treatment
4. Determine position of tubes and catheters
5. Provide a way of following the progression of lung disease[75]

CHEST FILMS

Chest film studies are best performed in the radiology department. However, if the patient is acutely ill, the test can be completed at the bedside with a portable x-ray camera. The x-ray camera moves from the front to the back of the body; that is, anteroposterior (AP). Standard chest x-ray films are preferably taken in the standing position, although the sitting or supine position can be used. The standard views are as follows:

1. Posteroanterior (PA)—x-rays pass through the back to the front of the body
2. Lateral—x-rays pass through the side of the body (usually left side)

Special views might be required to visualize specific parts of the chest. The special views include the following:

1. Oblique—x-ray films slanted at specific angles
2. Lordotic—x-ray films slanted at 45-degree angle from below to visualize lung apices
3. Decubitus—x-ray films taken with patient lying on either side to visualize free fluid in chest

See left box on p. 831 for details of preparation procedure.

TOMOGRAPHY

Tomography is a special technique that permits better visualization of a single layer or plane of the lungs. It is used to study cavities, neoplasms, and lung densities. The patient is required to lie still while an x-ray tube is rapidly moved over the lung at approximately 1 cm intervals. The procedure takes approximately 15 minutes.

COMPUTED TOMOGRAPHY

Computed tomography (CT) is rapidly replacing standard tomographic examination. Conventional tomogra-

PREPARATION OF PATIENT FOR RADIOGRAPHIC EXAMINATION

1. Explain specific procedure.
2. Instruct patient to remove all clothing above the waist and wear a gown open in the back. The patient must remove metal objects above the waist because metal restricts x-ray films from passing through the body.
3. The procedure is noninvasive and should cause no discomfort.
4. Patient will probably be alone in the room, but someone is nearby and always has voice contact.
5. Patient will probably be asked to take a deep breath and hold it.
6. If it is necessary for persons to be in the room while x-ray is being taken, they will wear lead apron to protect them from radiation exposure.

PREPARATION OF PATIENT FOR A BRONCHOGRAM

PREBRONCHOGRAM

1. Patient is instructed to do complete mouth care night and morning before procedure.
2. Patient does not eat or drink for 8 hours before procedure.
3. Dentures are removed. Document any loose teeth on preoperative sheet.
4. Shortly before the examination, patient receives a short-acting sedative and an antispasmodic.

POSTBRONCHOGRAM

1. Postural drainage is initiated unless contraindicated to assist removal of radiopaque substance.
2. Food and fluid are withheld until gag reflex returns.
3. Deep breathing, coughing, and movement are encouraged to maintain a clear airway.

phy resulted in a blurred film, except for the one plane being observed. CT scanning uses computer programming to enhance and process the x-ray film "slices" to produce a clear picture of the chest cavity structures.

FLUOROSCOPIC EXAMINATION

When dynamic information about the chest such as diaphragmatic movement is required, lung expansion and contraction, or cardiac action, fluoroscopy is the preferred examination.

ULTRASOUND (ECHOGRAM)

In an ultrasound examination, a harmless, high-frequency sound wave is emitted and penetrates the thorax. These sound waves bounce back and are converted by a transducer to a pictorial image of the area being studied. Ultrasound of the thorax can provide information about pleural effusion or opacities in the lung.

BRONCHOGRAPHY

A bronchogram enables the physician to visualize the bronchial tree by x-ray film after the introduction of an iodized radiopaque liquid, which coats the bronchial mucosa. The pharynx, larynx, and major bronchi are anesthetized with a topical anesthetic before introduction of a metal cannula into the trachea. The radiopaque substance is then introduced, and the patient is tilted in various positions to distribute the dye to the bronchi and bronchioles. A series of x-ray films are then taken. See box above, right for details.

ROENTGENOLOGIC EXAMINATION OF VENTILATION AND PERFUSION
LUNG SCAN (PULMONARY SCINTIPHOTOGRAPHY)

Lung scan procedures involve the use of a scanning device that records the pattern of pulmonary radioactivity after the inhalation or intravenous injection of gamma ray–emitting radionucleotides, thus providing a visual image of the distribution of ventilation or blood flow in the lungs. These studies provide valuable information about ventilation-perfusion patterns and aid in the diagnosis of parenchymal lung disease and vascular disorders such as pulmonary embolism. See the box below for preparation procedures.

In a *perfusion scan, radiopaque iodine is injected intravenously.* The lungs are then scanned, and the pattern of particle distribution in the lung vasculature is recorded. Areas of poor radionucleotide uptake are suggestive of pulmonary vascular disorders. In a *ventilation scan, the radioactive gas is inhaled, and the lungs are scanned to detect abnormal diffusion of the gas throughout the lungs.*

PULMONARY ANGIOGRAPHY

Pulmonary angiography is used to detect pulmonary emboli and a variety of congenital and acquired lesions of the pulmonary vessels. A radiopaque material is injected via a catheter into a systemic vein, the right chambers of the heart, or the pulmonary artery; and the distribution of this material is recorded on film.

PREPARATION FOR LUNG SCAN OR PULMONARY ANGIOGRAPHY

Radiopaque iodine is the radionucleotide usually used for both pulmonary angiography and lung scan. Always carry out the following activities.

1. Check patient for iodine allergy.
2. Obtain an order (often a standing order) to administer 10 drops of Lugol's solution several hours before the test to block thyroid uptake of radioactive iodine.

POSITRON EMISSION TOMOGRAPHY (PET)

PET uses the capability of computerization to study regional pulmonary perfusion and ventilation-perfusion relationships. A radioisotope that releases positrons (positively charged particles with the same mass as an electron) is inhaled by or injected into the individual. As the short-lived radioisotope decays, it releases gamma rays that are recorded by the computerized scanner.

EXAMINATION OF THE SPUTUM
SPUTUM ANALYSIS

Examinations of sputum are usually required when chest disease is suspected. The mucous membrane of the respiratory tract responds to inflammation by an increased flow of secretions that often contain causative organisms. The volume, consistency, color, and odor of the sputum are observed and recorded (see the box below).

Sputum examination includes the following tests:

1. *Gram stain* usually gives enough information about organisms and cells present to give a presumptive diagnosis.
2. *Culture* identifies specific organisms to enable making a definitive diagnosis. It should be collected before initiation of antibiotic therapy and thereafter to monitor effectiveness of antibiotic therapy.
3. *Sensitivity* serves as a guide to antimicrobial therapy by identifying antibiotics that prevent growth of the organism present in the sputum. It is collected before initiation of antibiotic therapy. Culture and sensitivity (C & S) are usually ordered together.
4. *Acid-fast bacilli* (AFB) determines the presence of mycobacterium tuberculosis which, after taking up a dye, is not decolorized by acid alcohol.
5. *Cytology* assists in identification of lung carcinoma. Sputum contains sloughed cells from tracheobronchial tree; thus malignant cells might be present. Although the presence of malignant cells indicates carcinoma, the absence of cells might indicate that either there is no tumor or that the tumor is not shedding cells.
6. *Quantitative test* is the collection of sputum over a period of 24 to 72 hours.

SPUTUM COLOR ANALYSIS

---

1. Colorless or clear mucoid: noninfectious process
2. Creamy yellow: staphylococcal pneumonia
3. Green: *Pseudomonas* pneumonia
4. "Currant jelly": *Klebsiella* pneumonia
5. Rusty: pneumococcal pneumonia
6. Pink frothy: pulmonary edema

SPUTUM COLLECTION

Tests to be performed on sputum are explained to the patient so that a suitable specimen will be obtained. The patient is instructed to collect only sputum that has come from deep in the lungs. When not instructed adequately, patients often expectorate saliva rather than sputum. They are likely to exhaust themselves unnecessarily by shallow, frequent coughing that yields no sputum suitable for study and that affords them little relief from discomfort. *The first sputum raised in the morning is usually the most productive of organisms.* During the night, secretions accumulate in the bronchi, and just a few deep coughs will bring them to the back of the throat. If patients do not know this fact, on awakening they may almost unconsciously cough, clear their throats, and swallow or expectorate before attempting to produce the specimen.

The patient should be supplied with a wide-mouthed container and instructed to expectorate directly into it. Because the sight of sputum is often objectionable to the patient and to others, the outside of a glass container is covered with paper or other suitable covering. Usually 4 ml of sputum is sufficient for laboratory tests and examinations. Nursing implications for sputum collection include the following:

1. Patients who have difficulty producing sputum or who have very tenacious sputum might be dehydrated. Encourage fluid intake.
2. Collect specimen before meals to avoid possible emesis from coughing.
3. Instruct patient to rinse mouth with water before collecting specimen to decrease sputum contamination.
4. Instruct patient to notify staff as soon as specimen is collected so that it can be sent to the laboratory as soon as possible.

Occasionally patients have difficulty producing sputum for examination. Inhalation of a hypertonic solution such as 10% saline in distilled water is used to temporarily stimulate sputum collection. Other methods to collect sputum include the following: (1) endotracheal aspiration with a suction catheter and special sputum collection container, (2) transtracheal aspiration (insertion of a needle with a catheter through the cricothyroid cartilage), and (3) fiberoptic bronchoscopy (p. 837).

GASTRIC WASHINGS

Gastric aspiration is occasionally used to collect gastric contents, which may contain swallowed sputum. It is usually performed when the diagnosis or suspected diagnosis is tuberculosis. Because most patients swallow sputum when coughing in the morning and during sleep, an examination of gastric contents can reveal causative organisms.

The procedure requires the following steps:

1. Breakfast is withheld before aspiration.
2. A nasogastric tube is passed into the stomach.
3. A large syringe is connected to the nasogastric tube, and a specimen of stomach contents is gently withdrawn.
4. The specimen is placed in a covered container.
5. The nasogastric tube is withdrawn.

SKIN TESTING

For various pulmonary disorders, the skin is tested for an antigen-antibody reaction to the proteins of the infectious agent. This cell-mediated or delayed hypersensitivity reaction is manifested by induration caused by cellular infiltration at the site of the injection in persons who have been sensitized to the proteins of the infectious agent. Skin testing for *Mycobacterium tuberculosis* with either tuberculin purified protein derivative (PPD) or old tuberculin (OT) is the most common type of test. However, skin testing also can be conducted for *atypical tubercule bacilli* and for *fungal infections* resulting from *coccidioidin*, *histoplasmin*, and *blastomycin*. The primary purpose of skin testing is to detect individuals who are infected with the suspect organism but who are not necessarily diseased. In this capacity, skin testing is primarily a screening device. Skin antigens can also be used for presumptive diagnosis; however, a positive skin test reaction must be substantiated with other diagnostic evidence before active disease can be confirmed. Skin testing can produce false-positive and false-negative results (usually in immunosuppressed, older, or newly infected people).

ADMINISTRATION TECHNIQUE FOR THE MANTOUX TEST

1. Draw up 0.1 ml of PPD, OT, atypical (tuberculin), or fungal antigen, using a tuberculin syringe and ½ inch 24- to 26-gauge needle.
2. Cleanse the site (dorsal surface of forearm).
3. Keeping skin slightly taut, insert the needle bevel upward just beneath the skin surface.
4. Inject the solution, creating a 6 to 10 mm wheal.
5. Read the test site with a millimeter ruler 48 to 72 hours after injection. The site should be lightly palpated to determine the presence or absence of induration. The largest diameter of induration should be measured and recorded in millimeters. Any erythema at the site should also be noted.
6. Interpretation of induration:
   a. 10 mm or more = highly significant for past or present infection.
   b. 5 mm through 9 mm = doubtful reaction.
   c. 0 through 4 mm = little or no sensitivity, however if patient's history indicates exposure, the test should be repeated.

SKIN TEST ADMINISTRATION

Skin tests can be administered by intracutaneous injection (Mantoux method), jet gun or multiple puncture tests (tine, mono-vacc, and heaf-type). The *Mantoux test is the only method used for diagnosis*. The jet gun or multiple puncture methods are used *only* for screening tests. (See box below for details of administration.)

PULMONARY FUNCTION TESTS

Pulmonary function testing is a noninvasive method of assessing the functional capacity of the lungs. These tests cannot be used by themselves to diagnose specific diseases, but they are an integral part of the diagnostic process. Pulmonary function tests (PFTs) are used for the following purposes:

1. Screening for the presence of pulmonary disease
2. Preoperative evaluation
3. Evaluating the patient's condition for weaning from a ventilator
4. Researching pulmonary physiology
5. Documenting the progression of pulmonary disease or effects of therapy
6. Studying the effects of exercise on respiratory physiology[75]

ASSESSMENT OF LUNG PROPERTIES

The functional ability of the lungs is assessed by measuring properties that affect ventilation and respiration.

1. Ventilation
   a. Static properties focus on lung distensibility; that is, on the bellows action of the thorax and lungs. Static properties are assessed through measurement of lung volumes and functional capacities (Table 31-8, *A* and *B*).
   b. Dynamic properties are those aspects of lung mechanics that affect the resistance within the airways. These properties are assessed by pulmonary function tests that measure volume/time relationships (Table 31-8, *C*).
2. Respiration
   a. Diffusion properties are those aspects of lung function that affect the ability of gas to move across the alveolar-capillary membrane (Table 31-8, *D*).
   b. Perfusion properties affect the supply of blood to the lungs (Table 31-8, *D*).

Normal values for pulmonary function tests are calculated by taking into consideration the following variables for each individual being evaluated: (1) age, (2) sex, (3) height and weight, and (4) individual effort in performing each test.

MEASUREMENT OF VENTILATION

Ventilatory studies are performed by having the patient breathe through a mouthpiece connected to a spirome-

TABLE 31-8 Definitions and implications of pulmonary function tests

Definitions		Clinical Implications	
		Obstructive Diseases	Restrictive Diseases
A. LUNG VOLUME (NONOVERLAPPING MEASURES)			
Tidal volume (TV)	Volume of gas inspired and expired with a normal breath	General measure of ventilatory ability	
Inspiratory reserve volume (IRV)	Maximal volume that can be inspired from the end of a normal inspiration	↓	↓
Expiratory reserve volume (ERV)	Maximal volume than can be exhaled by forced expiration after a normal expiration	Clinically useful when combined with RV-FRC	
Residual volume (RV)	Volume of gas left in lung after maximal expiration	↑	↓
B. LUNG CAPACITIES (COMBINATIONS OF VARIOUS VOLUMES)			
Inspiratory capacity (IC)	Maximal amount of air than can be inspired after a normal expiration (TV + IRV)	↓	↓
Functional residual capacity (FRC)	Amount of air left in lungs after a normal expiration (ERV + RV)	↑	↓
Vital capacity (VC)	Maximal amount of air that can be expired after a maximal inspiration (TV + IRV + ERV)	↓	↓
Forced vital capacity (FVC)	Maximal amount of air that can be expelled with a maximal effort after a maximal inspiration	↓	↓
Total lung capacity (TLC)	Total amount of air in lungs after maximal inspiration (TV + IRV + ERV + RV)	↑	↓
C. VOLUME/TIME RELATIONSHIPS			
Minute volume (MV)	Volume inspired and expired in 1 min of normal breathing	↑	↓
Forced expiratory volume in 1 sec (FEV_1)	Amount of air expelled in the first second of the forced vital capacity maneuver	↓	—
FEV_1/VC ratio	Amount of air forcefully expelled in 1 sec compared to total amount forcefully expelled	↓	—
Maximal voluntary ventilation (MVV), also termed maximal breathing capacity (MBC)	Amount of air exchanged per minute with maximal rate and depth of respiration	↓	—
D. DIFFUSION/PERFUSION MEASUREMENTS			
Diffusing capacity (D_x)	Assesses ability of gas molecules to cross alveolar-capillary membrane	↓	↓
Nitrogen washout (N_2)	Measurement of amount of nitrogen in lungs at end expiration; indicates uniformity of gaseous distribution in lungs	↓	↓

ter that measures the air moving through the apparatus. The spirometer is connected to a recording device that documents air volume, usually in liter measurements. Some measurements such as the residual volume cannot be measured directly and are calculated mathematically. The interrelationship of lung volumes and capacities that measure *static properties* is shown in Figure 31-17. The volumes and capacities are defined, and clinical implications of each measurement are given in Table 31-8.

Spirometric measurement of lung *dynamic properties* are of particular clinical significance because they relate the volume of air expired to the time required for expiration. One of the most meaningful clinical measurements is the forced expiratory volume (FEV). The FEV measures the amount of air in liters forcefully expired over 1, 2, or 3 seconds after a full inspiration. The FEV is an accurate indicator for obstructive diseases, since airway obstruction becomes worse on expiration and particularly when expiration is forceful and rapid. The FEV at 1 second is the most clinically accurate of the three measurements and is particularly useful when expressed as a percentage of the forced vital capacity (FVC). An FEV_1/FVC of 80% or greater is considered normal.

MEASUREMENT OF RESPIRATION

It is best to measure efficiency of respiration by both PFTs and other parameters such as arterial blood gas measurements. Two variables affecting respiration that

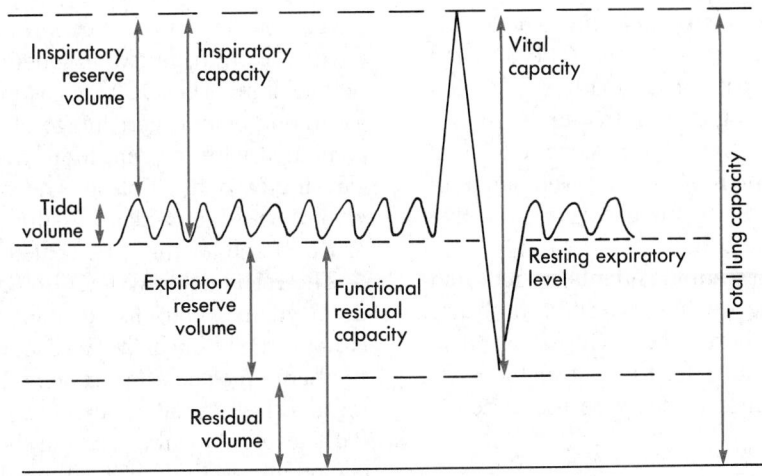

FIGURE 31-17 Lung volumes and capacities illustrated by spirography tracing. (Adapted from Wade JF: Respiratory nursing care, ed 2, St. Louis, 1977, The CV Mosby Co.)

PFTs can measure are the ability of gas to diffuse across the alveolar-capillary membrane and the ratio of ventilated alveoli to perfused capillaries.

ALVEOLAR-CAPILLARY DIFFUSION

The ability of gas to diffuse across the alveolar-capillary membrane is measured by a test called diffusing capacity (D_x). The patient breathes a measured amount of carbon monoxide from a closed system. The rate of carbon monoxide removal from the closed system indicates the status of the alveolar-capillary membrane.

VENTILATION-PERFUSION RELATIONSHIP

In order for the lung to perform gas exchange efficiently, the ventilation-perfusion ratio (V/Q ratio) must be balanced. That is, areas that receive ventilation should be well perfused with blood, and areas that receive blood flow should be capable of ventilation (Figure 31-18). Although in the normal lung with its many millions of gas exchange units some imbalance in ventilation and perfusion exists, this has little effect on overall gas exchange function. In fact, adaptive mechanisms appear to exist that divert blood flow to the best ventilated regions of the lungs or redirect ventilation away from nonperfused areas in order to maintain a normal ratio in the range of 0.8 to 1.2. Alteration in ventilation-perfusion relationships (either overall or in circumscribed areas of lung tissue) is largely responsible for the *hypoxemia* or *hypercapnia* seen in clinical practice. The nitrogen washout test measures ventilation/perfu-

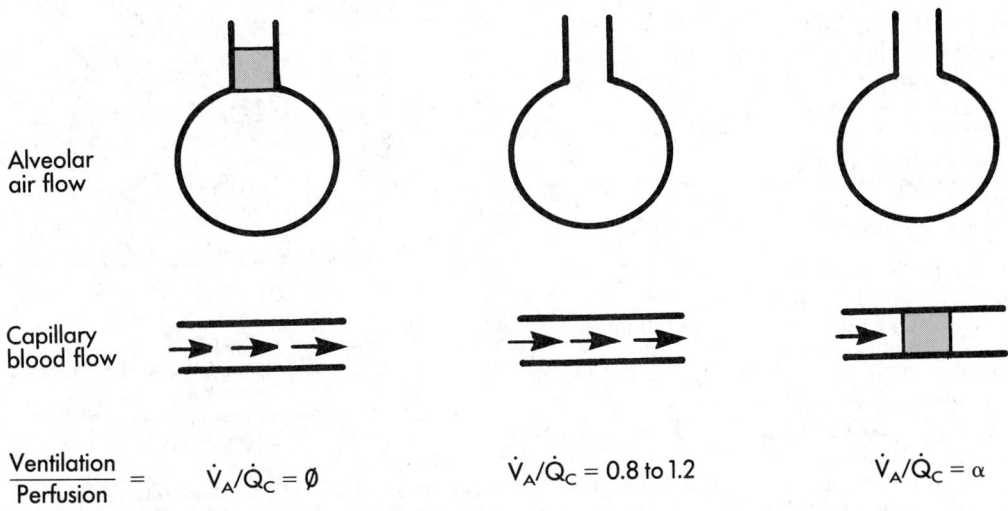

Alveolar air flow

Capillary blood flow

$\dfrac{\text{Ventilation}}{\text{Perfusion}} = \qquad \dot{V}_A/\dot{Q}_C = \emptyset \qquad\qquad \dot{V}_A/\dot{Q}_C = 0.8 \text{ to } 1.2 \qquad\qquad \dot{V}_A/\dot{Q}_C = \alpha$

FIGURE 31-18 Range of ventilation to perfusion ratios from zero to infinity. (Adapted from West JB: Ventilation, blood flow and gas exchange, ed 3, Oxford, 1977, Blackwell.)

sion relationships. Ambient air, and thus air in the lungs, is known to contain 80% nitrogen. The nitrogen washout test requires the patient to breathe 100% oxygen to wash out all the nitrogen from the lungs. After a measured period of time, the patient's expired air is measured for nitrogen content. Unevenly ventilated alveoli that receive less of the inspired oxygen will take longer to wash out lung nitrogen.

For pulmonary function testing, patients are required to breathe into a mouthpiece while wearing a noseclip; thus they often fear smothering or having a dyspneic episode. Thorough preparation for the test includes an explanation of the procedure to decrease the patient's apprehension.

ARTERIAL BLOOD GASES

Arterial blood gas analysis provides objective determination of the following: (1) arterial blood oxygenation, (2) gas exchange, (3) alveolar ventilation, and (4) acid-base balance. The arterial blood gas parameters that assess function of the respiratory system are shown in Table 31-9. A blood sample is obtained from a radial, brachial, or femoral artery with a preheparinized syringe to prevent clotting. The syringe is capped after obtaining the blood sample to prevent contact with air and is placed in an ice-water container until analyzed. Pressure is maintained over the puncture site for at least 5 minutes after needle withdrawal to prevent bleeding.

Patients with blood-clotting abnormalities may require that pressure be applied to the sample site for longer than 5 minutes. Nursing implications include assessing the site periodically and applying pressure for as long as necessary to prevent hematoma formation or bruising.

MEASUREMENT OF OXYGENATION

Both PaO_2 and SaO_2 are used to determine the adequacy of arterial blood oxygenation. The PaO_2 measures oxygen dissolved in the blood; however, the amount of oxygen carried in the blood in this form is small. Most oxygen is transported in chemical combination with hemoglobin. The SaO_2 measures the oxyhemoglobin saturation or that percentage of the hemoglobin that is combined with oxygen. More than 90% of the oxygen-carrying capacity of blood is accounted for by oxyhemoglobin, with the partial pressure of oxygen acting as the driving force for this chemical combination.

The relationship of PaO_2 to SaO_2 is demonstrated in the oxyhemoglobin dissociation curve. This relationship is not directly linear; many factors affect the affinity of the heme molecule for oxygen. The sigmoid curve represents the saturation percentages that occur at various PaO_2 levels. As can be seen in the oxyhemoglobin dissociation curve (Figure 31-19), in the upper portion of the curve, hemoglobin has an increased affinity for oxygen, so that large changes in PO_2 levels can be tolerated without significantly changing the saturation. For example, at a PO_2 of 100 torr, hemoglobin saturation is almost total, 97%; even if the PO_2 should fall to 70 torr, the saturation would only decrease to 94%. This serves as a protective mechanism that ensures adequate tissue oxygenation even when there is mild hypoxemia. It should be noted, however, that once the PO_2 level falls below 60 torr, saturation begins to decrease sharply, thus reducing the ability of the hemoglobin to transport oxygen.

The oxygen affinity of hemoglobin is influenced by various factors. Those factors that cause the curve to shift to the left (that is, hypothermia, alkalosis, and hypocapnia) increase the affinity of oxygen but diminish the release of oxygen to the tissues. Factors that cause a shift to the right are fever, acidosis, and hypercapnia.

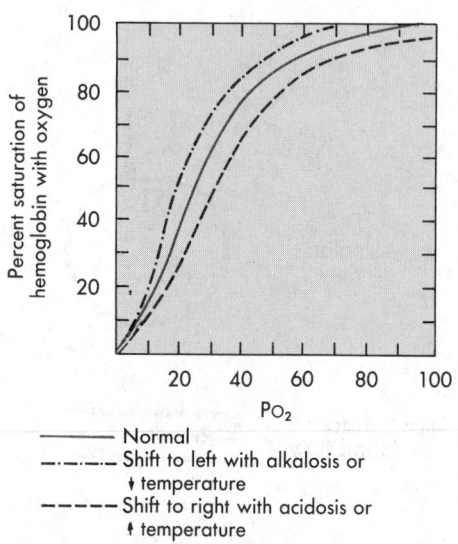

FIGURE 31-19 Oxyhemoglobin dissociation curve. (Reproduced with permission from Comroe JH Jr: Physiology of respiration, ed 2, 1974, Year Book Medical Publishers, Inc.)

TABLE 31-9 Arterial blood gases

Respiratory Function	Measurements	Normal Value
Acid-base balance	pH-hydrogen ion concentration	7.35-7.45
Oxygenation	PaO_2:partial pressure of dissolved O_2 in blood	80-100 mm Hg
	SaO_2:percentage of O_2 bound to hemoglobin	95%-98%
Ventilation	$PaCO_2$:partial pressure of CO_2 dissolved in blood	38-45 mm Hg

The primary impact of a shift to the right is reduced affinity of hemoglobin for oxygen.

The PaO_2 and SaO_2 must be evaluated in relation to the amount of hemoglobin. Since SaO_2 measures saturation of hemoglobin, an anemic person can have a normal saturation but still be inadequately oxygenated.

ASSESSMENT OF VENTILATION

The $PaCO_2$ is used as a measurement to determine the adequacy of ventilation and depends on the amount of carbon dioxide produced by the body and the ability of the lungs to eliminate it. *Hypoventilation* is shown by an elevated $PaCO_2$ and *hyperventilation* is indicated by a decrease in $PaCO_2$ below normal levels.

MEASUREMENT OF ACID-BASE BALANCE

Arterial blood pH is a measurement of hydrogen ion concentration. Because pH is expressed as a negative logarithm, as the hydrogen ion concentration increases and blood becomes more acid, the pH value falls. When the hydrogen ion concentration decreases, the blood becomes more alkaline, and the pH value rises.

The lungs play an important part in maintaining normal body pH (7.35 to 7.45) by regulating $PaCO_2$ through ventilation. The $PaCO_2$ is related to the pH be-the chemical reaction of carbon dioxide and water in the blood, which results in the formation of carbonic acid. Carbonic acid, in turn, dissociates to form hydrogen and bicarbonate ions, as illustrated in the following equation:

$$CO_2 + H_2O \rightleftarrows H_2CO_3 \rightleftarrows HCO_3^- + H^+$$

The maintenance of a normal pH depends on a ratio of 20 bicarbonate ions to 1 hydrogen ion. It can be seen from the equation that the presence of an elevated $PaCO_2$ shifts the equilibrium equation to the right and will result in an excess of H^+ ions. When this occurs, the pH falls, and the patient is said to be in *respiratory acidosis*. Conversely, when $PaCO_2$ is decreased, the equation shifts to the left, resulting in an increased pH and *respiratory alkalosis*.

ENDOSCOPIC EXAMINATION
BRONCHOSCOPY

A bronchoscopic examination is performed by passing a bronchoscope into the trachea and bronchi (Figure 31-20). By use of either a rigid bronchoscope or a flexible fiberoptic bronchoscope, the larynx, trachea, and bronchi can be visualized. Diagnostic bronchoscopic examination includes observation of the tracheobronchial tree for abnormalities, tissue biopsy, and aspiration of sputum for testing. Therapeutic bronchoscopic examination can be performed to remove a foreign body, to facilitate free air passage by removal of mucus plugs with suction, or to control bleeding.

Preparation for a bronchoscopy is similar to that for bronchography, except that postural drainage is less often ordered. If the patient is very apprehensive or if a sponge biopsy (abrasion of a lesion with a sponge) is to be performed or a tissue biopsy specimen is obtained, intravenous anesthetic can be used.

Nursing care for patients after bronchoscopy is as follows:

1. Patient is NPO until gag reflex returns.
2. Patient is positioned in semi-Fowler's position on either side to facilitate removal of secretions, unless physician specifies position.
3. All sputum is saved for culture and cytologic studies. Note: If bronchograms were performed, sputum cannot be used for cytologic examination, since the dye impedes cell fixation.
4. Patient is monitored for signs of laryngeal edema or laryngospasms such as stridor or increasing shortness of breath.
5. If lung tissue biopsy is taken, sputum is monitored for signs of hemorrhage. Note: Blood-streaked sputum can be expected for a few days after biopsy.

MEDIASTINOSCOPY

In mediastinoscopy a *mediastinoscope*, which is an instrument much like a bronchoscope, is inserted through

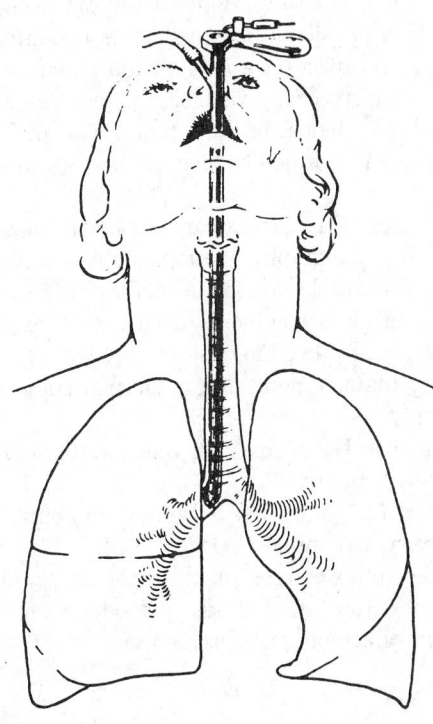

FIGURE 31-20 Bronchoscope inserted through trachea into bronchus. (From DeWeese DD and Saunders WH: Textbook of otolaryngology, ed 7, St Louis, 1988, The CV Mosby Co.)

a small incision in the suprasternal notch and advanced into the mediastinum where inspection and biopsy of the lymph nodes can then be carried out. Because these lymph nodes receive lymphatic drainage from the lungs, they are of diagnostic value for carcinoma, granulomatous infections, and sarcoidosis. This procedure is performed in the operating room, and the patient usually receives a general anesthetic.

LARYNGOSCOPY

Direct laryngoscopy is usually performed under local anesthesia with 10% cocaine or under general anesthesia. A sedative (for example, secobarbital, meperidine, or another narcotic) and atrophine sulfate are given 1 hour before the examination. Atropine is essential before administering both local and general anesthesia because it reduces the volume of secretions. For direct laryngoscopy, the person is placed in a reclining position, with the head in a head holder. If no head holder is available, the head is extended over the edge of the table and manually supported by a physician or nurse. In some cases, a suspension device can be applied to the laryngoscope so that the physician's hands are free for instrumentation or manipulation of the focus of the microscope. *Microlaryngoscopy* using an operating microscope is becoming more widely used. This method provides magnification and binocular vision.

The laryngoscope, a hollow, metal tube with a handle at the proximal end and a light at the distal end, is introduced by a physician through the mouth into the hypopharynx, elevating the epiglottis and making the interior of the larynx easily visible. Minor surgical procedures, such as a biopsy or the removal of a small benign tumor, can be performed by looking through this instrument.

The interior of the larynx can also be visualized by x-ray films and tomography. Radiopaque contrast material is instilled into the larynx (as in a bronchogram). These x-ray films are less commonly used than laryngoscopy. Xerography is also used to evaluate the larynx.

Nursing management after a laryngoscopy includes the following:

1. Patient is NPO until gag reflex returns (approximately 2 hours).
2. Check for gag reflex by gently touching back of throat with tongue blade.
3. If gag reflex is present, have patient try drinking water before other fluids or food is given in the event of accidental aspiration.

THORACENTESIS

Thoracentesis involves the insertion of a needle into the pleural space. Indications for a thoracentesis include the following:

1. Removal of pleural fluid for diagnostic purposes

NURSING CARE FOR PATIENT UNDERGOING THORACENTESIS

1. Explain procedure. Emphasize the importance of not moving, breathing quietly, and not coughing during the procedure to avoid damage to the pleura. Although a local anesthetic is used, discomfort might be felt when the needle enters the pleura.
2. Patient's respiratory status and vital signs are assessed before the procedure to collect baseline data.
3. If possible, the patient sits on the edge of the bed with feet supported on a chair. With the use of an elevated overbed table, the patient is helped to maintain a position with the head resting upon folded arms. Patients who are unable to sit up should be turned to the unaffected side with the head of the bed elevated 30 degrees.
4. Reassure and provide physical support, such as holding patient's hand, as needed.
5. Monitor vital signs, general appearance, and respiratory status throughout the procedure. No more than 1500 ml of pleural fluid should be removed within a 30-minute period because of the risk of intravascular fluid shift with resultant pulmonary edema.
6. After the needle is withdrawn, a sterile occlusive dressing and pressure is applied to the site.
7. After thoracentesis, the patient is positioned on the unaffected side with the insertion site up.
8. Monitor respiratory status, vital signs, and puncture site. Observe for signs of the following complications:
   a. Intravascular shift: hypotension, a rapid thready pulse, and increasing shortness of breath.
   b. Lung trauma: coughing paroxysms, bloody sputum, or tracheal deviation.

---

   a. The pleural fluid can be examined for specific gravity, white blood cell count, differential cell count, red blood cell count, protein, glucose, and amylase concentrations.
   b. The fluid can be cultured and checked for the presence of abnormal or malignant cells.
   c. The gross appearance of the fluid, the quantity obtained, and the location of the site of the thoracentesis should be recorded.
2. Biopsy of the pleura
3. Removal of pleural fluid when it is a threat to patient safety or comfort
4. Installation of medications into the pleural space

The box above contains the nursing care for a patient having a thoracentesis.

CHAPTER SUMMARY

↙ Breathing includes the movement of air in and out of the lungs (ventilation) and exchange of oxygen and carbon dioxide between capillary blood and alveolar air at the alveolar-capillary membrane (diffusion).

↙ Although normal changes associated with aging decrease lung function, the lungs have a large reserve capacity.

✔ A nursing history of the person with pulmonary problems includes information about risk factors, pulmonary symptoms, functional capacity, current treatment, and the person's desired level of health.

✔ The major pulmonary symptoms are cough, dyspnea, chest pain, sputum production, hemoptysis, and wheezing.

✔ Pulmonary physical assessment includes inspection of the chest and breathing patterns, palpation of the chest wall for fremitus, percussion of lung fields and diaphragm movement, and auscultation of breath and voice sounds.

✔ Pulmonary assessment must be tailored to accommodate the person's level of respiratory distress.

✔ Diagnostic testing is performed to assess the origin of pulmonary symptoms and to assess the ventilatory and respiratory capacity of the lungs.

QUESTIONS TO CONSIDER

- A new patient has arrived on your unit. When you approach her to carry out an admission assessment, you observe that she is sitting on the edge of the bed gasping for breath, is diaphoretic, and has audible wheezing. How would you organize and implement your pulmonary assessment?

- How would you collect a sputum specimen from a patient who continues to expectorate on the floor and in bed linens even though you have reminded her to use the sputum cup that you have placed at bedside.

- How would you prepare a patient for pulmonary function testing? What information about the procedure would you give the patient?

- What is the quality of air in the community in which you reside? If air pollution is a problem, what are the major contributing factors (industries, automobile exhaust, and so on)? Are there community groups working to improve air quality? If so, what activities are they involved in, and how might a nurse be helpful to their efforts?

REFERENCES AND SELECTED READINGS

1. Ahrens R, and Rutherford K: The new pulmonary math applying the a/A ratio, Am J Nurs 3:337-387, 1987.
2. Altose MD: Assessment and management of breathlessness, Chest 88:77S-82S, 1985.
3. American Thoracic Society: Cigarette smoking and health, 132:1133-1138, 1985.
4. American Thoracic Society: Chest x-ray screening statements, American Thoracic Society News, 10(2):14, 1984.
5. American Thoracic Society: Recommended respiratory disease questionaire for use with adults and children in epidemiological research, Am Rev Respir Dis 118(1):7-53, 1978.
6. American Lung Association: Diagnostic standards and classification of tuberculosis, New York, 1981, The Association.
7. Anderson S and Bouwens E: Chronic health problems: concepts and application, St Louis, 1981, The CV Mosby Co.
8. Bates B: A guide to physical examination, ed 3, Philadelphia, 1987, JB Lippincott Co.
9. Bates D: Respiratory function in disease, ed 3, Philadelphia, 1989, WB Saunders Co.
10. Bordow R and Moser K: Manual of clincial problems in pulmonary medicine, ed 2, Boston, 1988, Little, Brown and Co.
11. Borg G: Psychophysical bases of perceived exertion, Med Sci Sports Exerc, 14:377-381, 1982.
12. *Borg G: Physical performance and perceived exertion, Studia Psychol Paedagog, 11:1-64, 1962.
13. Boyce B: Nursing practice: respiratory care terminology, part 1, New York, 1976, American Lung Association.
14. *Brown M: Selecting an instrument to measure dyspnea, Oncology Nursing Forum, 12(3):98-100, 1985.
15. Brucia J: Self perception of premonitory cues signaling COPD onset, unpublished master's thesis, Cleveland, 1982, Case-Western Reserve University.
16. Canobbio M: Chest x-ray film interpretation, Focus on Critical Care 11(2):18-24, 1984.
17. Celli B: Respiratory muscle function, Clin Chest Med 7(4):567-580, 1986.
18. Cherniack R: Current therapy of respiratory disease −2, Toronto, 1986, BC Decker Inc.
19. *Cohen S: Pulmonary function tests in patient care: programmed instruction, Am J Nurs 80:1135-1161, 1980.
20. *Cosenza J, and Nortonk L: Secretion clearance: state of the art from a nursing perspective, Crit Care Nurse 6(4):23-36, 1986.
21. Cugell D: Lung sounds: classification and controversies. Semin Resp Med 6(3):180-182, 1985.
22. De Troyer A and Estenne M: Functional anatomy of the respiratory muscles, Clin Chest Med 9(2):175-193, 1988.
23. De Troyer A and Estenne M: Coordination of between rib cage muscles and diaphragm during quiet breathing in humans. J Appl Physiol 57:899, 1984.
24. DeWeese D, and Saunders W: Textbook of otolaryngology, ed 5, St Louis, 1977, The CV Mosby Co.
25. Ebersole P, and Hess P: Toward healthy aging, ed. 3, St Louis, 1990, The CV Mosby Co.
26. Edlund B and Wheeler E: Adaptation to breathlessness, Topics Clin Nurs 2(3):11-25, 1980.
27. Environmental tobacco smoke, Washington DC, 1986, National Academy Press.
28. Farer L: All about TB—what practicing physicians must know and can do about tuberculosis, Clinical Notes on Respiratory Diseases 16(4):3-15, 1978.

*References preceded by an asterisk are particularly well suited for student reading.

29. *Fuchs-Carroll P: Cyanosis: the sign you can't count on, Nursing 188(3): 50, 1988.

30. Gress T and Bahr R: The aging person. a holistic perspective. St Louis, 1984, The CV Mosby Co.

31. Guyton A: Textbook of medical physiology, ed 6, Philadelphia, 1981, WB Saunders Co.

32. Harper R: A guide to respiratory care physiology and clinical applications, Philadelphia, 1981, JB Lippincott Co.

33. Hodgkin J: Chronic obstructive pulmonary disease, Park Ridge, Ill, 1979, American College of Chest Physicians.

34. Howder C: Respiratory care: know the facts, Philadelphia, 1989, JB Lippincott Co.

35. Hunter P: Bedside monitoring of respiratory function, Nurs Clin North Am 16(2):211-224, 1981.

36. Janson-Bjerklie S, Carrieri GK, and Hudes M: The sensations of pulmonary dyspnea, Nursing Research 35(3):154-159, 1986.

37. Janson-Bjerklie S: Defense mechanisms: protecting the healthy lung, Heart Lung 12(6):643-649, 1983.

38. Johnson JT, Newman RK, and Olson JE: Persistent hoarseness: an aggressive approach for early detection of laryngeal cancer, Postgrad Med 67:122-126, 1980.

39. Kersten LD: Comprehensive respiratory nursing: a decision making approach, Philadelphia, 1989, WB Saunders Co.

40. Killian KJ, and Jones NJ: Respiratory muscles and dyspnea, Clin Chest Med 9(2):237-248, 1988.

41. Killian KJ: The objective measurement of breathlessness, Chest 88(2):84S-90S, 1985.

42. Levitzsky MG: Pulmonary physiology, ed 2, New York, 1986, McGraw-Hill Inc.

43. Lauden R: Cough: a symptom and a sign, Basics of RD 9,4:1-5, 1981.

44. Lyons H: Differential diagnosis of hemoptysis and its treatment, Basics of RD 5,(2):1-5, 1976.

45. Mahler DA, et al: The measurement of dyspnea, contents interobserver agreement, and physiologic correlates of two new clinical indexes, Chest 85(6):751-757, 1984.

46. Malasanos L, et al: Health assessment, ed 3, St Louis, 1986, The CV Mosby Co.

47. McCaffrey TV and Kern EB: Clinical evaluation for nasal obstruction: a study of 1000 patients, Arch Otolaryngol 105:542-545, 1979.

48. *McCauley K and Weaver T: Cardiac and pulmonary diseases: nutritional implications, Nurs Clin North Am 16(2):195-209, 1981.

49. Moser K: Fiberoptic bronchoscopy and other diagnostic procedures. In Isselbacher K, et al, editors: Harrison's principles of internal medicine, ed 9, New York, 1980, McGraw-Hill Inc.

50. Murray J: The normal lung: the basis for diagnosis and treatment of pulmonary disease, ed 2, Philadelphia, 1986, WB Saunders Co.

51. Pagana K, and Pagana T: Diagnostic testing and nursing implications a case study approach, St Louis, 1982, The CV Mosby Co.

52. Panicucci C: Functional assessment of the older adult in the acute care setting, Nurs Clin North Am 18(2):355-363, 1983.

53. Reischman R: Review of ventilation and perfusion physiology, Crit Care Nurse 8(7):24-28, 1988.

54. Reischman R: Impaired gas exchange related to intrapulmonary shunting, Crit Care Nurse 8(8):35-49, 1988.

55. Report of ATS-A CCP Ad Hoc Subcommittee on Pulmonary Nomenclature, ATS News 2(8), 1981.

56. *Rifas E: How you and your patient . . . can manage dyspnea, Nursing 80, 10(6):34-41, 1980.

57. *Roach L: Skin changes: the subtle and the obvious. In Assessing Vital Functions Accurately, Horsham, Pa., 1978, Intermed Communications Inc.

58. Rodarte J and Hyatt R: Respiratory mechanics, Basics of RD, 4(4):1-6, 1976.

59. Saunders W et al: Nursing care in eye, ear, nose and throat disorders, ed 4, St Louis, 1979, The CV Mosby Co.

60. Sbarbaro J: Are you up to snuff on TB skin tests, Patient Care 1:30-51, 1979.

61. Schweiger J: Oral assessment, Am J Nurs 80:654-657, 1980.

62. Slonem NB, and Hamilton LH: Respiratory physiology, ed 4, St Louis, 1981, The CV Mosby Co.

63. Stevens S and Becker K: How to perform picture-perfect respiratory assessment, Nursing '88, 18(1):57-63, 1988.

64. *Taylor D: Assessing breath sounds, Nursing '85 15(3):60-62, 1985.

65. The health consequences of involuntary smoking, Washington DC, 1986, US Dept of Health and Human Services.

66. Thompson J, and Bowers A: Clinical manual of health assessment, St Louis, 1980, The CV Mosby Co.

67. Tomashefski J: Chronic obstructive pulmonary disease; a perplexing and challenging spectrum, Post Grad Med 62(1):87-97, 1977.

68. *Traver G: Respiratory nursing: the science and the art, New York, 1982, John Wiley & Sons Inc.

69. Weiss ST: Passive smoking and lung cancer, Rev Respir Dis 133:1-3, 1986.

70. West J: Respiratory physiology—the essentials, ed 3, Baltimore, 1985, Williams & Wilkins Co.

71. *Westia B: Assessment under pressure: when your patient says "I can't breathe," Nursing '84, 14(5), 34-40, 1984.

72. Wilkens R, Sheldon R, and Krider S: Clinical assessment in respiratory care, St Louis, 1985, The CV Mosby Co.

73. Witkowski A: Pulmonary assessment a clincal guide, Philadelphia, 1985, JB Lippincott.

74. Zagelbaum G and Pare J: Manual of acute respiratory care, Boston, 1983, Little, Brown & Co Inc.

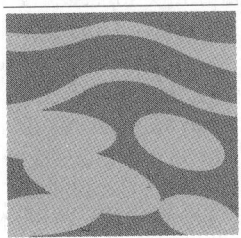

CHAPTER 32

Management of Persons with Problems of the Upper Airway

WILMA J. PHIPPS
LINDA ANNE BROSEMAN

CHAPTER OBJECTIVES

After studying this chapter, the student should be able to:
1. Describe the etiology, pathophysiology, clinical manifestations, and management of the patient with rhinitis and sinusitis.
2. Compare acute pharyngitis with acute follicular tonsillitis and peritonsillar abscess in relation to etiology, clinical manifestations, and management.
3. Describe the nursing care of the patient after nasal surgery.
4. Identify conditions that cause obstructions of the upper airway and their management.
5. Describe clinical manifestations and management of the patient experiencing epistaxis and malignancies of the upper airway.
6. Describe the nursing care of the patient after a partial laryngectomy and after a total laryngectomy with radical neck dissection.
7. Describe speech methods used for patients after a total laryngectomy.

The upper airway includes the nose and sinuses, upper throat (naso- and oropharynx and tonsils), and lower throat (hypopharynx and larynx). Disorders of the upper airway are very common, and patients often ask nurses to give them advice about these kinds of problems.

ANOSMIA

Disorders that affect the nose or olfactory nerve may lead to *anosmia,* or loss of the sense of smell. Anosmia may result from (1) nasal obstruction, which prevents air currents from reaching the olfactory epithelium; (2) skull fracture across the cribriform plate at the roof of the nose where part of the olfactory nerve enters the nose; (3) viral infections, which affect the olfactory nerve; or (4) some meningiomas, which may form in the olfactory area. A perverted sense of smell, called *parosmia,* may also be present during sinusitis or an upper respiratory tract infection.

INFECTIONS OF THE NOSE AND SINUSES

INFECTIONS OF EXTERNAL TISSUES ABOUT THE NOSE

The skin around the external nose is easily irritated during acute attacks of rhinitis or sinusitis. Furunculosis (boils) and cellulitis (see Chapter 72) occasionally develop. Infections around the nose are extremely dangerous because the venous blood supply from this area drains directly into the cerebral venous sinuses. Septicemia therefore can occur easily. No pimple or lesion in the area should ever be squeezed or "picked"; hot packs may be used. If any infection in or around the nose persists or shows even a slight tendency to spread or increase in severity, a physician should be consulted.

RHINITIS
ETIOLOGY AND PATHOPHYSIOLOGY

Rhinitis refers to inflammation of the mucous membrane of the nose. It may be acute or chronic.

Acute rhinitis (coryza, common cold) is an inflammatory condition of the mucous membranes of the nose and accessory sinuses caused by a filtrable virus. It affects almost everyone at some time and occurs most often in the winter, with additional high incidence in early fall and spring. Some of the known causes of the common cold are 100 serotypes of rhinoviruses, coronoviruses, adenoviruses, echoviruses, influenza and parainfluenza viruses, and coxsackievirus. The common cold is spread by droplet nuclei from sneezing and the condition is contagious for the first 2 to 3 days. Secondary invasion by bacteria may complicate the cold, causing pneumonia, bronchitis, sinusitis, and otitis media.

Allergic rhinitis (hay fever) can be acute and seasonal when caused by the pollens of grasses and flowers, or it may be chronic and perennial when associated with numerous allergens, such as house dust, animal dander, wool, and certain foods.

Chronic rhinitis is a chronic inflammation of the mucous membrane caused by repeated acute infections, by an allergy, or by *vasomotor rhinitis.* The cause of vasomotor rhinitis is unclear, but this condition may result from an instability of the autonomic nervous system caused by stress, tension, or some endocrine disorder. Often it is mistaken for nasal allergy, but an allergen cannot be identified. There is an increased formation of nasal mucus. Rhinitis can also be caused by the overuse of nose drops *(rhinitis medicamentosa);* a rebound phenomenon occurs after the immediate effect of the nose drops with the return to congestion. Discontinuing use of the nose drops usually clears up this condition within a week or two.

CLINICAL MANIFESTATIONS

All forms of rhinitis cause sneezing, nasal discharge with nasal obstruction, and headache, but the form of these symptoms varies with the different types of rhinitis (Table 32-1). Acute rhinitis also includes signs of acute inflammation (early chilliness followed by "feverishness" and malaise). A painful throat is not always associated with a cold. However, the pharynx may feel sore because of early dryness followed by irritation from postnasal drainage. If uncomplicated, the cold is usually self-limiting and lasts for about 1 week.

In chronic rhinitis, acute symptoms are absent. The chief complaint is nasal obstruction accompanied by a feeling of stuffiness and pressure in the nose. Polyp formation (p. 854) may occur and vertigo may be present.

INTERVENTIONS

Medical Management

No specific treatment is available for the common cold. Over-the-counter cold remedies usually contain one or more drugs, including antihistamines, sympathomimetics, and analgesics. Differences of opinion exist concerning the effectiveness of antihistamines in relieving cold symptoms. If taken during the onset of the cold, the allergic manifestations (sneezing, tearing, watery discharge) may be relieved; use during the latter stages may only cause drowsiness. Sympathomimetic drugs (such as phenylephrine [Neosynephrine] and phenylpropanolamine) are nasal decongestants and help to relieve the nasal stuffiness. Vitamin C has no significant protective or inhibitory effect on colds.[69] Antibiotics are used only for complicating secondary infections.

Nose drops are sometimes recommended for infrequent use (every 4 hours for a few days) if there is some nasal obstruction. Many otolaryngologists now believe that the frequent use of nose drops results in rhinitis medicamentosa, an "addiction" of the nasal mucosa to their use.[12] Some physicians believe that the obstruction of the nose may be a protective device that prevents the spread of infection to other parts of the body.

For allergic rhinitis, the treatment consists of maintaining an allergen-free environment (see Chapter 76). Hyposensitization or desensitization (administering the allergen in gradually increasing doses to establish an "immunity") may be helpful. Antihistamines give relief to most persons, but the effectiveness often decreases as the "hay fever season" continues.[40]

For chronic rhinitis, antihistamines may give relief. When nasal obstruction persists, surgery may be necessary to remove polyps (polypectomy) or to remove tissue obstruction (submucous resection or septoplasty, p. 852).

Nasal irrigations are now seldom used in the treatment of chronic rhinitis. Details of the procedure are described in texts on fundamentals of nursing or otolaryngology. Care should be taken to ensure that both nostrils are open and that the pressure in the nostrils is not excessive (the irrigating container should not be higher than 12 to 15 in above the level of the nose). Excess pressure may force infected material into the sinuses or the middle ear.

Nursing Management

Nursing management is directed toward patient teaching and includes the following:
1. Get additional rest
2. Drink at least 2 to 3 L fluid per day
3. Medications
   a. Antihistamines
      (1) Effective only during initial period of a cold
      (2) Be cautious about their sedative effects when driving or working with heavy machinery
   b. Nose drops: use correct procedure (see the box on p. 843)

TABLE 32-1 Symptoms of rhinitis

	Acute Rhinitis	**Allergic Rhinitis**	**Chronic Rhinitis**
Nasal discharge	Initially watery, then mucoid	Thin, watery	Serous, mucopurulent, or purulent
Eyes	Tearing during early phase	Tearing, itching	No tearing
Turbinates	Edematous	Pale, edematous, mucoid	Enlarged
Nasal polyps	No	Yes	Yes
Headache	Generalized	Frontal	Frontal

CORRECT ADMINISTRATION OF NOSE DROPS

1. Wash hands
2. Assume a position that will facilitate flow of medication
   a. Sit in chair and tip head well backward, or
   b. Lie down with head extended over edge of bed, or
   c. Lie down with pillow under shoulders and head tipped backward
3. Turn head to side that will receive the drops
4. Place no more than 3 drops of solution into each nostril at one time (unless otherwise prescribed)
5. Remain in position with head tilted backwards for 5 minutes to permit solution to reach posterior nares
6. If marked congestion is still present 10 minutes after nose drop insertion, another drop or two of solution may be administered (nasal constriction from first insertion may facilitate additional drops reaching posterior nares)

4. Prevention of further infection
   a. Blow nose with both nostrils open to prevent infected matter from being forced into eustachian tube
   b. Cover mouth with disposable tissues when coughing and sneezing to prevent droplet nuclei from entering the air.
   c. Dispose of used tissues carefully
   d. Avoid exposure when possible (that is, avoid crowds, people with colds, specific allergens). Elderly persons and those with chronic lung disease are particularly vulnerable
5. *Wash hands frequently and especially after coughing, sneezing, and so on. Recent evidence suggests that colds are transmitted from person to person by hand contact.* Seek medical attention when necessary for:
   a. High fever, severe chest pain, earache
   b. Symptoms lasting longer than 2 weeks
   c. Recurrent colds

SINUSITIS
ETIOLOGY AND PATHOPHYSIOLOGY

The sinuses are air-filled cavities lined with mucous membrane. Any inflammation of the mucous membranes of the sinuses is called *sinusitis*. This is still a frequent disorder, although it is less common since the advent of antibiotics. Often patients who complain of sinusitis do not have sinus infection but some other disorder. When an otolaryngologist refers to sinusitis, a bacterial invasion of the mucous membrane is implied. Only about 10% of the patients who consult an otolaryngologist because of "sinus trouble" are diagnosed as having sinusitis.

Sinusitis is classified as follows:
- acute suppurative

LOCATION OF PAIN WITH SINUSITIS

SINUS	PAIN LOCATION
Maxillary	Over cheek and upper teeth (Figure 32-1)
Frontal	Above the eyebrow (Figure 32-1)
Ethmoid	Medial and deep in the eye. (Figure 32-2)
Sphenoid	Deep behind the eye, over the occiput, or top of head

- subacute supportive
- chronic suppurative
- allergic
- hyperplastic

The most common cause of *acute suppurative sinusitis* is the obstruction of the paranasal sinuses that blocks the egress of secretions from the sinuses. These secretions become infected, giving rise to acute suppurative sinusitis. The organisms most often responsible are *Streptoccous pneumoniae*, beta-hemolytic *Streptococcus*, *Haemophilus influenzae*, coagulase-positive *Staphylococcus aureus*, and *Klebsiella pneumoniae*. More than 50% of maxillary sinus infections are caused by *S. pneumoniae* and *H. influenzae*. Another 30% are caused by anerobic bacteria, which are often dental in origin. *Cultures are not helpful* because multiple organisms are usually demonstrated.

CLINICAL MANIFESTATIONS
Acute Suppurative Sinusitis

The first symptom of acute sinusitis is usually a stuffy nose followed by slowly developing pressure over the involved sinus. Other symptoms include general malaise and toxicity, headache, slightly elevated or normal temperature, and mild leukopenia. Symptoms worsen over 48 to 72 hours until there is severe localized pain and tenderness over the involved sinus (see box above). The patient often believes that the pain is due to an infected tooth.

In acute frontal and maxillary sinusitis, pain usually does not appear until 1 to 2 hours after awakening. It increases for 3 to 4 hours and then becomes less severe in the afternoon and evening.

There may be bloody or blood-tinged discharge from the nose in the first 24 to 48 hours. The discharge rapidly becomes purulent and copious, blocking the nose. The throat may become inflamed and sore on one side because of the purulent discharge.

On examination, the involved nasal mucosa is hyperemic and edematous, and the turbinates are enlarged. X-ray films show that the involved sinus is clouded, and a fluid level is visible (Figure 32-3). Usually the diagnosis is established without x-rays. If there are recurrent episodes of acute sinusitis, x-rays or CT scan are indicated to rule out underlying pathology.

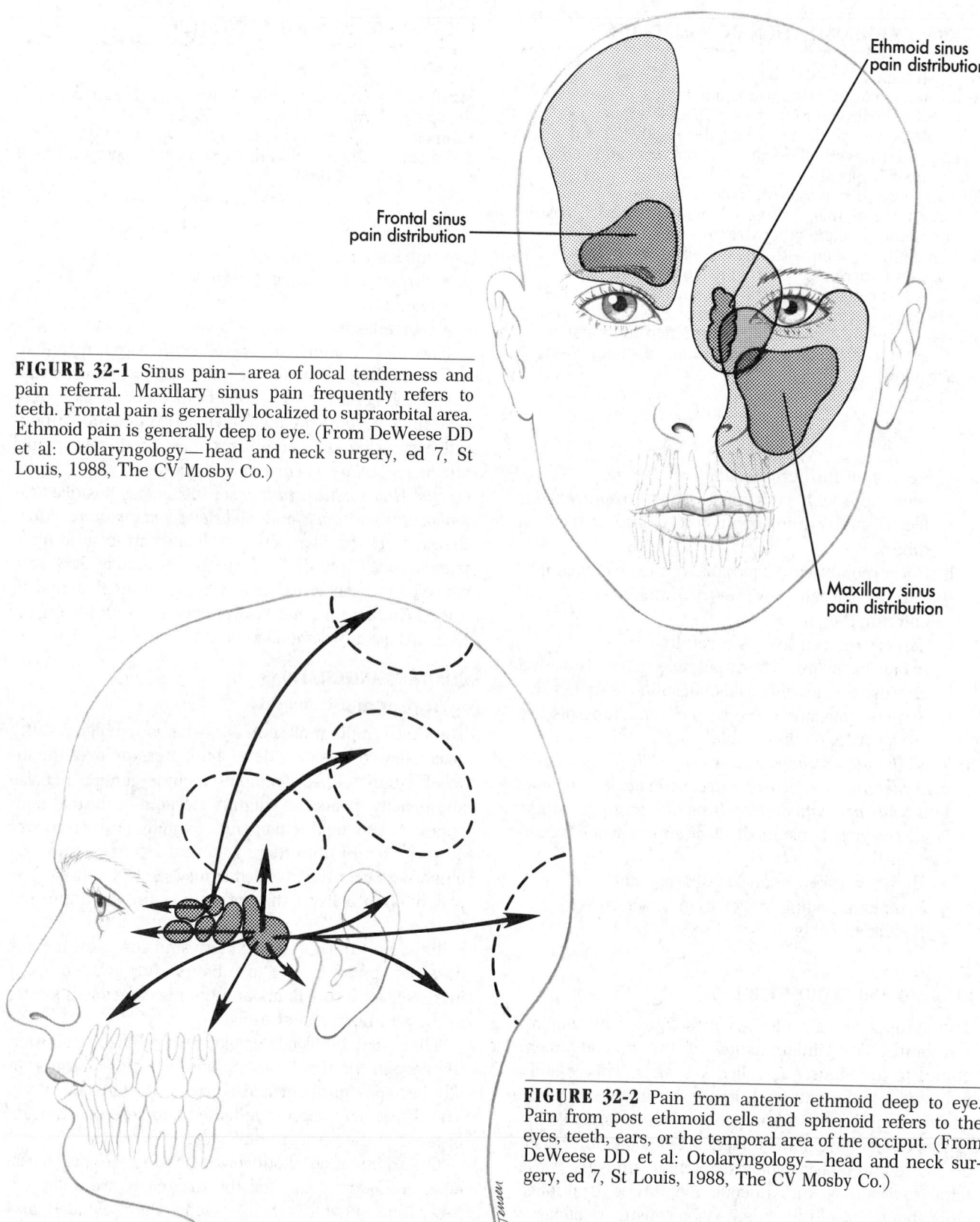

FIGURE 32-1 Sinus pain—area of local tenderness and pain referral. Maxillary sinus pain frequently refers to teeth. Frontal pain is generally localized to supraorbital area. Ethmoid pain is generally deep to eye. (From DeWeese DD et al: Otolaryngology—head and neck surgery, ed 7, St Louis, 1988, The CV Mosby Co.)

Ethmoid sinus
pain distribution

Frontal sinus
pain distribution

Maxillary sinus
pain distribution

FIGURE 32-2 Pain from anterior ethmoid deep to eye. Pain from post ethmoid cells and sphenoid refers to the eyes, teeth, ears, or the temporal area of the occiput. (From DeWeese DD et al: Otolaryngology—head and neck surgery, ed 7, St Louis, 1988, The CV Mosby Co.)

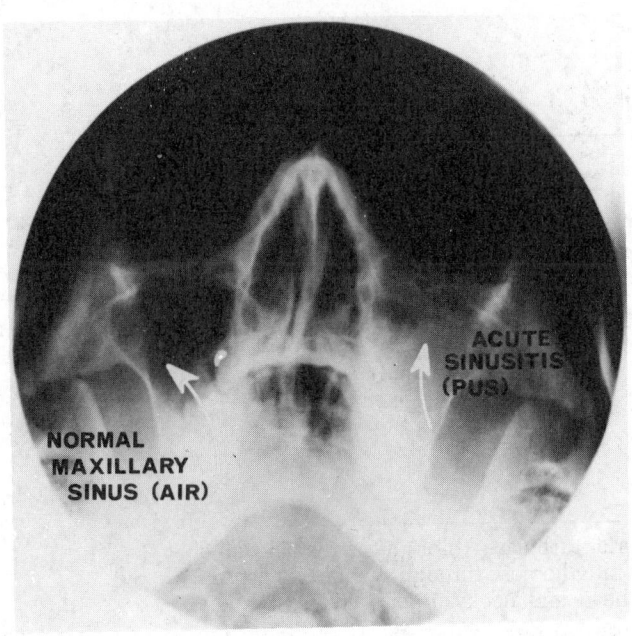

FIGURE 32-3 Roentgenogram of maxillary sinus showing normal sinus on left and acute sinusitis on right. (From Saunders WH, et al: Nursing care in eye, ear, nose, and throat disorders, ed 4, St Louis, 1979, The CV Mosby Co.)

MEDICAL MANAGEMENT

Management of *acute suppurative sinusitis* centers on relief of pain, shrinkage of the nasal mucosa, and control of infection. Codeine, meperidine (Demerol), or other narcotic analgesics may be required to control pain. They may need to be taken for several days. Symptomatic relief may be obtained from hot wet packs applied to the face or over the involved sinus either continuously or for 1 to 2 hours at a time, four times a day. Vasoconstrictive nose drops or nasal spray is used to keep the nose open. The most commonly used vasoconstrictors are ephedrine and phenylephrine (Neo-Synephrine). Symptomatic relief may be obtained from drugs containing antihistamine and a decongestant (Actifed, Co-Tylenol).[12]

Antibiotics are the treatment of choice in acute sinusitis. The most effective antibiotics are penicillin, ampicillin, amoxicillin, trimethoprim-sulfamethoxazole, and cefaclor. The cephalosporins and sulfas are used to treat persons who are sensitive to penicillin.[12]

Subacute Suppurative Sinusitis

The measures described above cure more than 90% of patients with acute suppurative sinusitis. A subacute infection persists in the remaining 10%. Persistent purulent discharge is the only constant symptom. An x-ray or CT scan is indicated to determine whether one or more sinuses are involved. Because it is uncommon for acute sinusitis to persist, the causative organism may be unusual.[12] Special culture techniques may be necessary and antibiotics sensitivity studies are essential. The most commonly isolated organisms are *H. influenzae*, *S. pneumoniae*, and *Branhamella catarrhalis*. *B. catarrhalis* is not sensitive to penicillin or amoxicillin, and treatment requires systemic sulfonamide therapy or erythromycin with a sulfonamide. Pain is not severe and requires no medication. Treatment consists of vasoconstriction of nasal mucosa, heat, and irrigation of the involved sinus. *Antral irrigation,* in which the anterior wall of the maxillary sinus is punctured, is the preferred treatment for subacute sinusitis. Anesthesia is obtained with an injection of 2 to 3 ml of 1% lidocaine (Xylocaine) with 1:100,000 epinephrine under the upper lip. A 16-gauge needle (with stylet in place) is rotated through the soft tissue and bone. (Figures 32-4 and 32-5). When proper placement of the needle is assured, saline solution is instilled to wash out the sinus. Antibiotic solutions may be used, but mechanical cleansing is more important than the solution used.[12]

It is not possible to irrigate the ethmoid sinuses directly and *ethmoiditis* is treated with systemic antibiotics. The antibiotics should be continued for 10 to 14 days.[12] Proper treatment of subacute sinusitis is the best means of preventing *chronic suppurative sinusitis*.

Chronic Suppurative Sinusitis

When suppurative sinusitis is not treated or is inadequately treated during the acute or subacute phase, or when the mucosa is damaged from recurrent attacks, permanent change may occur. Bacteria can invade the tissue of the sinuses, become walled off, and produce chronic inflammation. With prolonged infection of soft tissue, pathologic change may become irreversible and the patient has *chronic suppurative sinusitis*.[12]

The most common and sometimes only symptom is purulent nasal discharge. In a small percentage of patients, repeated irrigation, antihistamines, and antibiotics may cure the disease. However, most patients must be treated surgically.

The major nursing strategy for the patient with sinusitis who is not having surgery is teaching. Important points in teaching include the following:

1. Avoid factors that contribute to the sinusitis.
   a. Avoid chilling and cold, damp atmospheres.
   b. Avoid air conditioning when outside air is warm and moist, if this precipitates sinus irritation.
   c. Avoid smoking and being around smokers (further irritates damaged mucous membranes).
   d. Avoid fatigue.

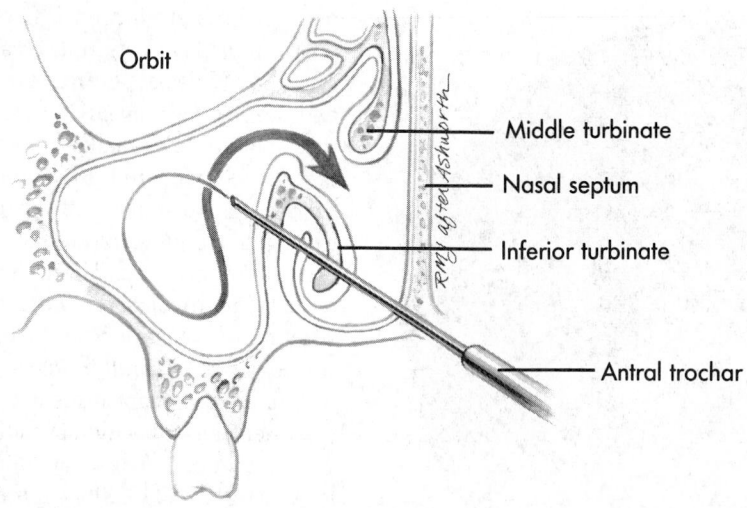

FIGURE 32-4 Trochar inserted under the inferior turbinate (through the medial wall of the antrum). Contents of the sinus are washed into the nose through the natural ostium. (From DeWeese DD et al: Otolaryngology—head and neck surgery, ed 7, St Louis, 1988, The CV Mosby Co.)

e. Try to avoid upper respiratory infections.

f. Protect nose during swimming; avoid diving.

g. Inform dentist of chronic sinus condition before tooth extraction.

2. Use acetaminophen rather than aspirin for pain relief; apply moist heat over sinus.

3. During an acute sinus infection, get additional rest and drink 2 to 3 L fluids per day.

4. Take antibiotic for prescribed time period, even if symptoms abate.

5. Keep room temperature constant (changes in room temperature aggravate sinusitis).

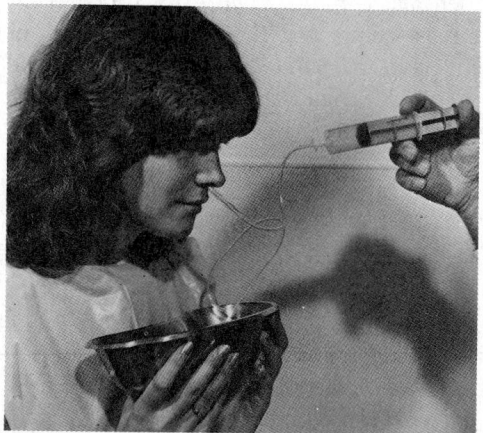

FIGURE 32-5 Irrigation of the maxillary sinus. With the head tipped forward, solution returns via the natural ostium and out the anterior nose for examination and/or culture. (From DeWeese DD et al: Otolaryngology—head and neck surgery, ed 7, St Louis, 1988, The CV Mosby Co.)

6. If allergens are a contributing factor, prepare an environmentally controlled bedroom (see Chapter 76).

Complications of Sinusitis

Complications of sinusitis usually are the result of inadequate therapy during the acute stage or by a delay in treatment.

According to DeWeese et al.[12] complications include:

1. Generalized persistent headache
2. Vomiting
3. Convulsions
4. Chills or high fever
5. Edema or increasing swelling of the forehead or eyelids
6. Blurring of vision, diplopia, or persistent retroocular pain
7. Signs of increased intracranial pressure
8. Personality changes or dulling of the sensorium
9. Increase in white cell count above 20,000

Orbital complications. Most orbital infections (75%) are caused by extension from paranasal sinusitis. Most frequently the ethmoid sinuses are involved. *Orbital complications* include *inflammatory edema, orbital cellulitis, subperiosteal abscess, orbital abscess,* and *cavernous sinus thrombosis.* Complications are treated vigorously with appropriate antibiotics and, in the case of abscess, incision and drainage.

Cavernous sinus thrombosis occurs when there is extension of infection through the venous pathways (usually the angular vein) to the cavernous sinus. The patient is very ill, with chills and a temperature as high

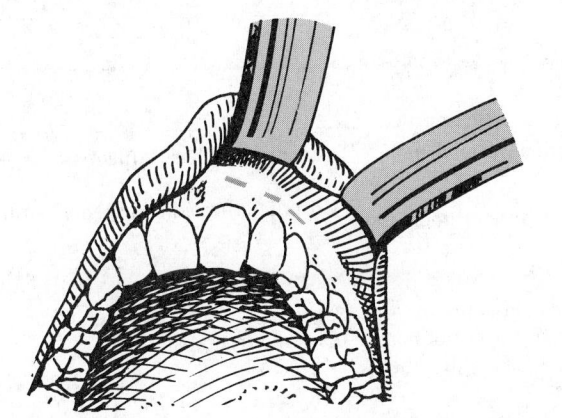

FIGURE 32-6 The incision into the maxillary sinus (Caldwell-Luc surgery) is made under the upper lip.

as 41°C(106° F). There is pain deep behind the eye and the patient becomes toxic and may become semicomatose.

Cavernous sinus thrombosis. This very serious complication of sinusitis can cause death in 48 to 72 hours if untreated. More than 25% of patients who develop this complication will die even when adequately treated. The primary treatment is with intravenous antibiotics.

SURGERY OF THE SINUSES

Treatment of *chronic suppurative sinusitis* involves surgery to remove all diseased soft tissue and bone, adequate postoperative drainage, and obliteration of the si-

nus cavity where possible. The goal of surgery is to eradicate infection and leave contiguous structures normal.

Caldwell-Luc Surgery

The Caldwell-Luc procedure is the generally accepted operative procedure for chronic maxillary sinusitis. It is also called a *radical antrum* operation. Local or general anesthesia may be used.

The procedure is performed through an incision under the upper lip (Figure 32-6). Part of the anterior bony wall of the antrum is removed, producing a permanent window (Figure 32-7). All of the diseased mucosa and periosteum is removed through the window. The bone of the lateral wall of the nose in the inferior meatus, which divides the nose from the antrum, is removed.[12] The mucous membrane and periosteum of the lateral wall of the nose are preserved, and fashioned into a hinged flap.

The antrum may be packed to prevent bleeding. Packing is removed through the nose 24 to 48 hours postoperatively. As the maxillary sinus heals, the exposed bone is covered by mucosa. Numbness of the upper lip and upper teeth may be present for several months after a Caldwell-Luc operation because some nerves to these structures pass through the site of the incision. Interference with eating will occur initially. Only liquids will be given for at least 24 hours, followed by a soft diet for several days.

In addition to general care of the patient following sinus surgery, patient teaching specific to Caldwell-Luc

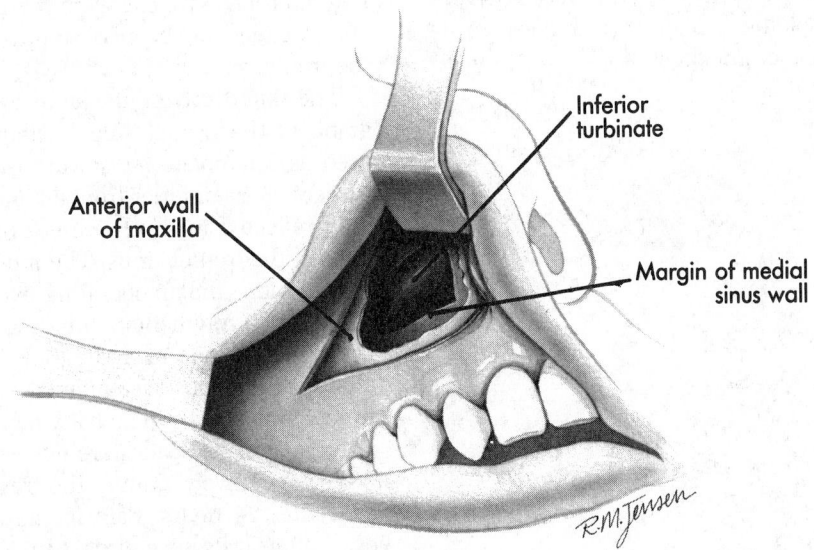

FIGURE 32-7 After removal of the sinus mucosa or polypoid tissue, a window is made into the nose along its floor, allowing dependent drainage from the maxillary sinus. Incision is closed with absorbable sutures. (From DeWeese DD et al: Otolaryngology—head and neck surgery, ed 7, St Louis, 1988, The CV Mosby Co.)

TABLE 32-2 Sinus surgery

Surgery	Procedure	Use
Caldwell-Luc (radical antrum operation)	Clearing out of maxillary sinus through incision under upper lip	Chronic maxillary sinusitis
Intranasal ethmoidectomy External ethmoidectomy Frontal ethmoidectomy	Various approaches used to excise ethmoid tissue or for ethmoidotomy	Chronic ethmoid or sphenoid sinusitis
Ethmoidotomy Osteoplastic flat	Drainage of ethmoid or sphenoid sinus Complete removal of diseased mucosa of both frontal sinuses; space is packed with subcutaneous fat from abdomen	Chronic ethmoid or sphenoid sinusitis Chronic frontal sinusitis

surgery includes the following:
1. Do not chew on affected side until incision heals.
2. Use caution with oral hygiene to avoid injury to the incision.
3. Avoid wearing dentures for about 10 days.
4. Avoid blowing nose for about 2 weeks after packing has been removed.

Ethmoidotomy and Ethmoidectomy

The external approach is preferred for ethmoid surgery because it allows better visualization and reduces the risks of complications such as damage to the optic nerve and central spinal fluid leak. Ethmoidotomy is an opening made for drainage, whereas an ethmoidectomy entails removal of ethmoid air cells (Table 32-2). The incision is made in the inner half of the eyebrow downward along the side of the nose (Figure 32-8).[31,52] Ethmoidectomy is performed for correction of nasal polyps, as well as for ethmoiditis because nasal polyps frequently originate in the ethmoid cells.

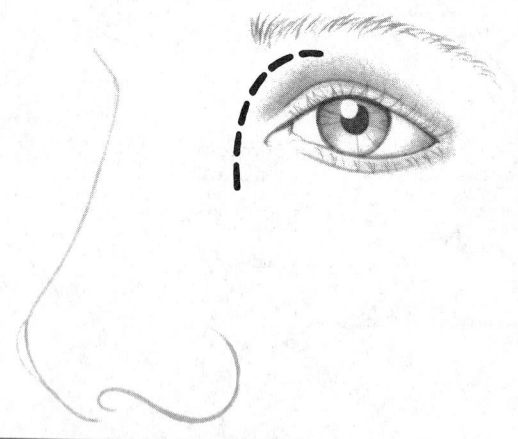

FIGURE 32-8 Medial canthal incision for external ethmoidectomy. (From DeWeese DD et al: Otolaryngology—head and neck surgery, ed 7, St Louis, 1988, The CV Mosby Co.)

Osteoplastic Flap Surgery

The advent of the osteoplastic flap operation makes frontal sinus surgery different from that performed on the other sinuses. Surgery of the other sinuses basically provides for an open, well-drained cavity, which in the past proved inadequate for the frontal sinuses because recurrence of disease was common. The osteoplastic flap operation allows for complete removal of diseased mucosa of the frontal sinus and for obliteration of the sinus so that it is no longer functional or continuous with the inner nose.

The osteoplastic flap procedure is performed through a "gull-wing" or "cross-bow" incision.[24] In men, the incision extends along the eyebrows and connects along the bridge of the nose. In women, where baldness is not a problem in later life, the incision connects both temporal areas a few centimeters posterior to the hairline. Both incisions give excellent postoperative cosmesis and are extended to the periosteum of the bone overlying the frontal sinus.

The skin overlying the sinus is reflected, and a radiograph of the frontal sinus (obtained preoperatively) is used as a template for sawing the lateral and superior borders of the anterior frontal bone. The anterior bone is then reflected inferiorly, thus exposing the entire contents of the frontal sinus. The mucosa is removed under direct vision, and an operating microscope is used to ensure that all fragments of mucosa are removed. An incision is then made in the left-lower-abdominal quadrant and subcutaneous fat obtained for placement into the frontal sinus cavity. The bony flap and skin are then repositioned. Nasal packs are not required.

Postoperatively, pain in the frontal area is not significant after 24 hours. Pain in the abdominal area, however, often lasts several days and serous drainage from this area is common after the drain is removed. Sutures are removed about the fifth postoperative day. Because nasal packs are not used, special oral hygiene care is not needed.

■ ASSESSMENT

Subjective Data

1. Obstruction of nares
   a. history of mouth breathing—time of day or night, duration, and frequency
   b. history of nasal surgery or injury to nose
   c. use of nasal drops or spray—type, amount, frequency, and duration of use
2. Nasal discharge
   a. color, amount, and consistency of discharge
   b. blood/drainage—one or both nares
   c. presence of nasal crusting or pain
3. History of sinusitis
   a. pain—location and severity
   b. relationship of sinusitis to certain seasons or types of weather
4. Other general symptoms such as malaise

Objective Data

1. Fever and drainage (serous, mucopurulent, purulent)
2. Polyps (pale, soft, edematous outpouching of nasal or sinal mucosa) may be present and are usually bilateral in inflammation of the nose and sinuses
3. Redness and edema of mucous membrane
4. Lack of energy

■ DATA ANALYSIS: NURSING DIAGNOSES

Nursing diagnoses are determined from assessment of patient data. Possible nursing diagnoses for the person with sinusitis may include but are not limited to:

Diagnostic Title	Possible Etiologies
Pain (headache, throat, sinus)	Inflammation in nose or sinuses
Knowledge deficit: condition and treatment	Lack of exposure to information

■ PLANNING: EXPECTED PATIENT OUTCOMES

Expected patient outcomes for the person with sinusitis may include but are not limited to the following:

1. Symptoms (headache and nasal drainage) are improved.
2. The patient can state ways to prevent further attacks by:
   a. avoiding crowds during periods of high incidence of infection
   b. getting adequate rest
   c. eating a well-balanced diet.
3. The patient demonstrates the correct use of nose drops.
4. The patient knows how to use prescribed medications and knows what over-the-counter medications to avoid.
5. The patient states plans for follow-up care.

PREOPERATIVE TEACHING FOR SINUS SURGERY

Determine what patient understands about the surgical procedure. Clarify misconceptions and answer patient's questions. Explain that he or she:
- Will have nothing to eat or drink 6 to 8 hours preoperatively.
- Will receive sedative medication before surgery.
- Will feel pressure, not pain, during surgery.
- Will have a nasal pack for 24 to 48 hours postoperatively.
- Will have a mustache dressing postoperatively.
- Will have some ecchymosis and swelling around the nose and eyes for 1 to 2 weeks postoperatively.

POSTOPERATIVE CARE FOR SURGERY OF SINUSES

1. After general anesthesia, position patient well onto the side to prevent swelling or aspiration of bloody drainage.
2. When the patient is awake, remind him or her to expectorate secretions and not swallow them.
3. Encourage mid-Fowler's position when fully awake to promote drainage and decrease edema.
4. Apply ice compresses over nose (or ice bag over maxillary or frontal sinuses) in the early postoperative period.
5. Monitor the patient for:
   a. Excessive bleeding from nose (may be evidenced by repeated swallowing).
   b. Decreased visual acuity, especially *diplopia,* indicating damage to optic nerve or muscles of globe of eye.
   c. Complaints of pain over the involved sinus, which may indicate infection or inadequate drainage.
   d. Fever—take temperature rectally.
6. Give frequent mouth care using a soft toothbrush. If there is an oral incision, mouth care is given before meals to improve appetite and after meals to decrease danger of infection.
7. Change nasal pad when it is soiled.
8. Apply ice compresses to ecchymotic areas to constrict blood vessels, decrease oozing and edema, and to help relieve pain.
9. Encourage liberal fluid intake. Patient may be very thirsty because of dry mouth from mouth breathing.
10. Teach patient to:
    a. Avoid blowing nose for at least 48 hours after packing is removed to prevent bleeding.
    b. Report signs of infection (fever, purulent discharge) to surgeon.
    c. Expect tarry stools from swallowed blood for a few days.
    d. Avoid constipation (Valsalva maneuver can cause bleeding).
    e. Expect that ecchymosis of nose and eyes will begin to change color over next 1 to 2 weeks.
    f. Take prophylactic antibiotics as prescribed. Do not stop until all medication is taken.

■ IMPLEMENTATION

Preoperative teaching and postoperative teaching for the patient having sinus surgery is outlined in the box on p. 849.

INFECTIONS OF THE PHARYNX AND LARYNX
ACUTE PHARYNGITIS
ETIOLOGY/EPIDEMIOLOGY

Acute pharyngitis is the most common throat inflammation. It may be caused by hemolytic streptococci, staphylococci, or other bacteria or filtrable viruses. There is increased evidence of gonococcal pharyngitis caused by the gram-negative diplococcus *Neisseria gonorrhoeae*. The disease is increasingly found in both men and women. When gonorrhea is suspected, a throat culture is indicated. A severe form of acute pharyngitis often is referred to as *strep throat* because of the frequency of streptococci as the causative organisms.

CLINICAL MANIFESTATIONS

Dryness of the throat is a common complaint. The throat appears red, and soreness may range from slight scratchiness to severe pain with difficulty in swallowing. A hacking cough may be present. Children often develop a very high fever, whereas adults may have only a mild elevation of temperature. Symptoms usually precede or occur simultaneously with the onset of acute rhinitis or acute sinusitis. Pharyngitis can occur after the tonsils have been removed because the remaining mucous membrane can become infected.[17] Pharyngitis is also a common manifestation of infectious mononucleosis.

INTERVENTIONS
Medical and Nursing Management

Acute pharyngitis usually is relieved by hot saline throat gargles. An ice collar may make the person feel more comfortable. The physician may prescribe acetylsalicylic acid administered orally as a gargle or in Aspergum. Lozenges containing a mild anesthetic may help relieve the local soreness. Moist inhalations may help relieve the dryness of the throat. A liquid diet usually is more easily tolerated, and fluids to at least 2.5 L per day are encouraged. Oral hygiene may prevent drying and cracking of the lips and usually refreshes the mouth. If the temperature is elevated, the patient should remain in bed and, even if ambulatory and afebrile, should have extra rest.

A throat culture is taken to identify the offending organism. If beta-hemolytic streptococci is identified, the drug of choice is penicillin. For the person allergic to penicillin, erythromycin or another antibiotic will be prescribed. As with other infections treated with antibiotics, the patient will need to understand the need to take the prescribed antibiotic until the course is completed. This will vary from 7 to 12 days, depending on the organism and the severity of infection. Patients must understand that they should continue therapy for the prescribed number of days, even if they are symptom-free.

Persons with a history of bacterial endocarditis or rheumatic fever are usually given penicillin prophylactically.

ACUTE FOLLICULAR TONSILLITIS
ETIOLOGY/EPIDEMIOLOGY

Acute follicular tonsillitis is an acute inflammation of the tonsils and their crypts. It is usually caused by the *Streptococcus* organism. It is more likely to occur when the person's resistance is low and is very common in children.

CLINICAL MANIFESTATIONS

The onset is almost always sudden, and symptoms include sore throat, pain on swallowing, fever, chills, general muscle aching, and malaise. These symptoms often last for 2 or 3 days. The pharynx and tonsils appear red, and the peritonsillar tissues are swollen. Sometimes a yellowish exudate drains from crypts in the tonsils. A throat culture usually is taken to identify the offending organism.

INTERVENTIONS
Medical and Nursing Management

The patient with acute tonsillitis is encouraged to rest and take generous amounts of fluids orally. Warm saline throat irrigation may be ordered, and antibiotics are given for streptococcal pharyngitis. Acetylsalicylic acid and sometimes codeine sulfate may be ordered for pain and discomfort. An ice collar may be applied to the neck.

Complications of untreated tonsillitis include heart and kidney damage, chorea, and pneumonia. Incidence of these complications is decreasing with the wide-

---

PATIENT TEACHING FOR PERSONS WITH PHARYNGITIS OR TONSILLITIS

1. Comfort measures: use warm saline gargles, ice collars, moist inhalations, mouth care
2. Need for fluid intake of at least 2 to 3 L/day
3. Symptoms of recurrence requiring medical attention: fever, excessive pain, pus, dysphagia
4. Rationale for prophylactic antibiotic therapy for pharyngitis in patients with a history of rheumatic fever or infective endocarditis to prevent reinfection

---

spread use of penicillin and early diagnosis. Most physicians believe that persons who have recurrent attacks of tonsillitis should have a tonsillectomy. This procedure is usually performed from 4 to 6 weeks after an acute attack has subsided.

Because the person with acute tonsillitis is usually cared for at home, the nurse should help in teaching the general public the care that is needed (see box on p. 850). The office nurse, the clinic nurse, the nurse in industry, the school nurse, and the community health nurse have many opportunities to do this teaching.

PERITONSILLAR ABSCESS

A peritonsillar abscess is an uncommon, local complication of acute follicular tonsillitis in which infection extends from the tonsil to form an abscess in the surrounding tissues. The presence of pus behind the tonsil causes difficulty in swallowing, talking, and opening the mouth; and the person may be unable to swallow. Pain is severe and may extend to the ear on the affected side.

INTERVENTIONS

Medical and Nursing Management

If antibiotics to which the offending organism is sensitive are administered early, infection subsides. If the peritonsillar abscess is caused by anaerobic organisms, hydrogen peroxide (an oxidizing agent) in the form of a mouth wash may help relieve symptoms. Acute streptococcal or staphylococcal tonsillitis may also cause a peritonsillar abscess to form. If an abscess forms, incision and drainage are necessary. During the operation, the patient's head usually is lowered, and suction is applied as soon as the incision is made to prevent the patient from aspirating the drainage. Warm saline irrigations, an ice collar, or narcotics may relieve discomfort. If acute follicular tonsillitis is treated adequately, peritonsillar abscess is unlikely to occur.

LARYNGITIS
SIMPLE ACUTE LARYNGITIS

Simple acute laryngitis is an inflammation of the mucous membrane lining the larynx accompanied by edema of the vocal cords. It may be caused by a cold, by sudden changes in temperature, or by irritating fumes. Symptoms vary from a slight huskiness to complete loss of voice. The throat may be painful and feel scratchy, and a cough may be present.

Laryngitis in adults usually requires only symptomatic treatment. The person is advised to remain indoors in an even temperature and to avoid talking for several days or weeks, depending on the severity of the inflammation. Steam inhalations may be soothing and cough syrups or home remedies for coughs provide relief to some patients. Smoking or being near others who are smoking should be avoided.

CHRONIC LARYNGITIS

Some people who use their voices excessively, who smoke a great deal, or who work continuously where there are irritating fumes develop a chronic laryngitis. Hoarseness usually is worse in the early morning and in the evening. There may be a dry, harsh cough and a persistent need to clear the throat.

Treatment may consist of removal of irritants, voice rest, correction of faulty voice habits, steam inhalations, and cough medications. The physician may order spraying of the throat with an astringent antiseptic solution such as hexylresorcinol (S.T. 37). To carry out this procedure properly, the patient must use a spray tip that turns down at the end so that the medication reaches vocal cords and is not dissipated in the posterior pharynx. The spray tip is placed in the back of the throat with the bent portion behind the tongue. The patient should then take one or two deep breaths and spray the medication on inhalation. This procedure may cause temporary coughing and gagging. Many medications used as throat sprays are sold in plastic squeeze bottles with tube and spray tip attached.

OBSTRUCTIONS OF THE UPPER AIRWAY
PATHOPHYSIOLOGY

The upper airway may become partly obstructed, leading to interference with breathing. Obstructions may occur in the nose (deviated septum, hypertrophied turbinates, or nasal polyps), pharynx (enlarged tonsils and adenoids), or larynx (laryngeal paralysis or edema).

CLINICAL MANIFESTATIONS

The signs and symptoms of upper airway obstruction include difficulty in breathing through the nose, dry mucosa, postnasal drip, nasal discharge, bleeding from the nose, and loss of sense of smell.

MEDICAL MANAGEMENT

Management is mainly surgical. The types of surgery are discussed under each of the obstructions.

■ ASSESSMENT
SUBJECTIVE DATA

Symptoms of nasal obstructions include presence or absence of and duration of the following:
- Noisy, difficult breathing
- Dry mucosa
- Postnasal drip
- Nasal discharge
- Anosmia (loss of sense of smell)
- Bleeding from nose

If nasal trauma is present, additional symptoms include displacement of the bones, cosmetic deformity, pain, and ecchymosis around the eyes or jaw.

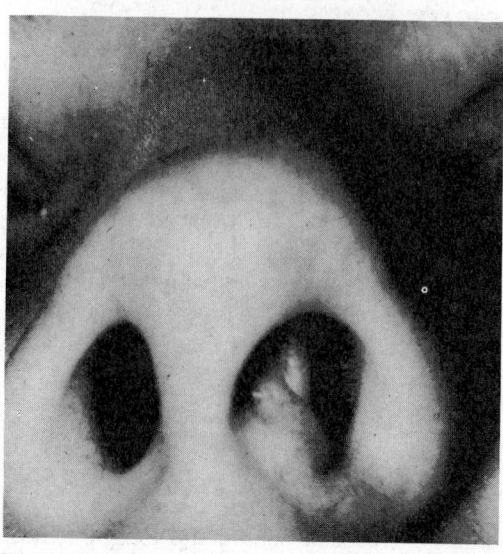

FIGURE 32-9 Septal deviation. Anterior end of septal cartilage is dislocated and projects into nasal vestibule. (From Saunders WH et al: Nursing care in eye, ear, nose, and throat disorders, ed 4, St Louis, 1979, The CV Mosby Co.)

OBJECTIVE DATA

- Inspection for deformity or asymmetry
- Some septal deviation is common in adults (Figure 32-9) and is asymptomatic
- Check for abnormal findings in nose
  a. Excessive redness
  b. Edema
  c. Exudate
  d. Bleeding

■ DATA ANALYSIS: NURSING DIAGNOSES

Nursing diagnoses are determined from an assessment of patient data. Possible nursing diagnoses for the person with obstruction of the nose and throat may include, but are not limited to, the following:

Diagnostic Title	Possible Etiologies
Body image disturbance	Severe trauma/disfiguring surgery
Knowledge deficit; condition and its treatment	Lack of exposure to information
Pain	Trauma/obstruction
Sensory/perceptual alterations: olfactory	Trauma/surgery

■ PLANNING: EXPECTED PATIENT OUTCOMES

Expected patient outcomes for the person with an obstruction of the nose or throat may include, but are not limited to, the following:

1. Patient feels comfortable.
2. Patient can state care required after surgery and discharge from hospital.

SURGERIES TO RELIEVE NASAL OBSTRUCTION OR TRAUMA

SURGERY	DESCRIPTION
Submucous resection	Removal of obstructive parts of cartilage and bone from nasal septum
Nasoseptoplasty	Reconstruction of nasal septum
Rhinoplasty	Reconstruction of external nose after trauma or for cosmetic reasons
Nasal polypectomy	Removal of polyps from nose

3. Patient knows how to prevent nosebleeds or to treat them if they occur.

DEVIATED SEPTUM

Deviated septum is a common cause of nasal obstruction in older children and adults. It may be congenital but usually is the result of an injury. The nasal septum, which is normally thin and straight, may be deviated from the midline and protrude more to one side of the nasal passage than to the other (Figure 32-9). The deviation may cause a *nasal obstruction that increases when infection or allergic reaction occurs* and that is evidenced by marked, noisy, and difficult breathing. There may be a postnasal drip or the mucosa may become so dry that crusts form. A broken nose can lead to chronic sinusitis if not treated, even though it may cause no immediate problem. Some persons may have a deviated septum that does not cause obstruction and, thus, surgery is not necessary.

Surgery is performed when obstruction occurs and consists of either a submucous resection or nasoseptoplasty (see the box above). *Submucous resection* usually is performed under local anesthesia. An internal incision is made on one side of the nasal septum from top to bottom. The mucous membrane is elevated away from the bone, the obstructive parts of the cartilage and bone removed, and the mucous membrane sutured back into place. Packing is placed in both nostrils to prevent bleeding and to splint the operative area. Commonly used gauze packs are ½-inch petrolatum-impregnated gauze, Adaptic gauze, iodoform gauze with bacitracin, and Cortisporin-impregnated gauze. The latter is particularly effective in reducing nasal pack odor. Nasal packing can be left in place from 24 to 48 hours, depending on the extent of surgery and the surgeon's preference.

Nasoseptoplasty involves reconstruction of the septum and is becoming more widely used to treat deviated nasal septum. Reconstruction of the external nose (*rhinoplasty*), often done for cosmetic reasons (see Chapter

POSTOPERATIVE CARE FOR NASAL SURGERY

1. Assessment
   a. Monitor for hemorrhage
      (1) Excessive blood on nasal dressing
      (2) Bright red vomitus
      (3) Repeated swallowing (check back of throat with penlight for blood running down throat)
      (4) Rapid pulse
   b. Monitor for infection: fever, elevated WBC
2. Discomfort
   a. Mid-Fowler's position to decrease local edema
   b. Ice compresses over nose for 24 hours prn
   c. Support and sedation for patient apprehension because of difficulty in breathing caused by blockage of nasal passages
   d. Frequent oral care
   e. Change dressing under nose prn
3. Nutrition
   a. Food as tolerated
   b. Encourage increased fluid intake
4. Patient teaching
   a. Avoid blowing nose for 48 hours after packing removed
   b. Avoid constipation (Valsalva maneuver) and vigorous coughing until healing occurs (can initiate bleeding)
   c. Expect stools to be tarry for several days
   d. Expect face to be discolored around eyes and nose for several days
   e. Cosmetic effect from nasal surgery cannot be judged for 6 to 12 months (time for tissue to return to normal and for scar resolution)

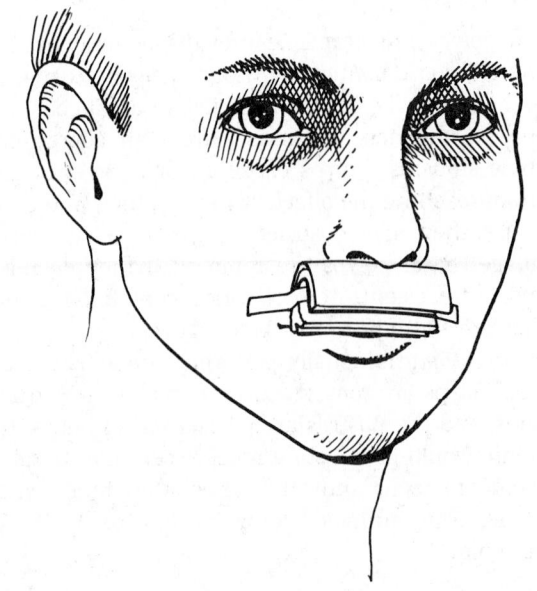

FIGURE 32-10 Dressing placed under nose for nasal drainage.

73), is often combined with septoplasty. It is usually performed under local anesthesia. With rhinoplasty, the nasal bones or cartilaginous framework of the nose are altered. The nose is usually protected with a plaster-of-Paris splint, adhesive tape dressing, or plastic mold following a plastic procedure on the nasal bones. Firm healing develops on about the tenth day. Usually only the surgeon changes a septoplasty or rhinoplasty dressing.

POSTOPERATIVE CARE FOR NASAL SURGERY

After nasal surgery, the patient is placed in mid-Fowler's position to decrease local edema, and ice compresses are usually applied to the nose to lessen the discoloration, bleeding, and discomfort. Patients can usually apply their own ice compresses.

The patient is monitored for signs of hemorrhage (see the box above on postoperative care). Some oozing on the dressing below the nose (Figure 32-10) is expected and this dressing may be changed as necessary. If bleeding becomes pronounced, the surgeon is notified and material for repacking the nose is prepared. This material consists of a hemostatic tray containing gauze packing, umbilical tape for posterior packing, a few small gauze sponges, small catheter (used for inserting

a postnasal plug), packing forceps, tongue blades, and scissors. The surgeon may require a head mirror, good light, epinephrine 1:1000 or other vasoconstrictor, 4% topical lidocaine (Xylocaine) or 4% cocaine solution, applicators, nasal speculum, and suction.

Because packing blocks the passage of air through the nose, a partial vacuum is created during swallowing, and the person may complain of a sucking action when attempting to drink. Postnasal drainage, the presence of old blood in the mouth, dryness of the mouth from mouth breathing, and loss of the ability to smell often lead to anorexia. Antihistamines may be prescribed to reduce nasal secretions and frequent mouth care is important. Patient teaching is described in the box on postoperative care above.

HYPERTROPHY OF THE TURBINATES

Enlarged inferior turbinates sometimes cause considerable nasal obstruction. Hypertrophied turbinates may be medically treated by the use of aerosols containing corticosteroids such as dexamethosone (Decadron, Turbinaire). These aerosols are used for their anti-inflammatory response and have proven to be effective for allergic and inflammatory nasal conditions as well as for treatment of nasal polyps.

Although not used as often since the advent of the corticosteroid aerosols, local surgery on the turbinates, such as cryosurgery or electric fulguration, may still be used to restore the airway. Debulking (resection) of the hypertrophied mucosa may be necessary.

NASAL POLYPS

Nasal polyps are grapelike growths of mucous membrane and loose connective tissue. They are usually bilateral and may be caused by irritation to mucous membranes of the nose or sinuses from an allergy or by chronic sinusitis. Polyps cause *anosmia* by preventing air from reaching the olfactory mucosa high in the nose. Because they may obstruct breathing or block sinus drainage, nasal polyps are removed if they do not respond to treatment. Aerosol sprays containing corticosteroids have also proven to be effective.

Polypectomy is usually performed under local anesthesia. Polyps are removed with a small snare or biting forceps, and the nostrils are packed for 24 hours. Polypectomy would give lasting relief except that nasal polyps tend to recur and often affect the sinus mucosa, thus requiring ethmoidectomy (p. 848) for more complete removal.

CHRONIC ENLARGEMENT OF TONSILS AND ADENOIDS

Tonsils and adenoids are lymphoid structures located in the oropharynx and nasopharynx. They reach full size in childhood and then begin to atrophy during puberty. When adenoids enlarge, usually as a result of chronic infections but sometimes for no known reason, they cause nasal obstruction. The person breathes through the mouth, may have a dull facial expression, and may have reduced appetite, because the blocked nasopharynx can interfere with swallowing. Hypertrophy of the tonsils does not usually block the oropharynx but may affect speech and swallowing and cause mouth breathing.

The tonsils and adenoids are removed when they become enlarged and cause symptoms of obstruction, when they are chronically infected, when the person has repeated attacks of tonsillitis, or after repeated peritonsillar abscesses. Chronic infections of these structures usually do not respond to antibiotics and may become foci of infection by spreading organisms to other parts of the body such as the heart.

TONSILLECTOMY

Tonsillectomy in adults may be performed under either general or local anesthesia. After the tonsils are removed, pressure is applied to stop superficial bleeding. Bleeding vessels are tied off with sutures or by electrocoagulation. The person is monitored carefully for hemorrhage (see the box above), especially when sleeping, because a very large amount of blood may be lost without any external evidence of bleeding. The physician may be able to control minor postoperative bleeding by applying a sponge soaked in a solution of epinephrine to the site. The person who is bleeding excessively often is returned to the operating room for surgical treatment to stop the hemorrhage.

POSTOPERATIVE CARE FOR TONSILLECTOMY

1. Position patient on side until fully awake after general anesthesia or in mid-Fowler's position when awake
2. Monitor for hemorrhage
   a. Frequent swallowing (inspect throat)
   b. Bright red vomitus
   c. Rapid pulse
3. Comfort
   a. Apply ice collar to neck (will also reduce bleeding by vasoconstriction)
   b. Use acetaminophen in place of aspirin
4. Food and fluids
   a. Give ice-cold fluids and bland foods during initial period (such as ginger ale, cold milk, custard, ice cream)
   b. Advance to normal diet as soon as possible
5. Patient teaching
   a. Avoid attempting to clear throat immediately after surgery (may initiate bleeding)
   b. Avoid coughing, sneezing, or vigorous nose blowing for 1 to 2 weeks
   c. Drink fluids (2 to 3 L/day) until mouth odor disappears
   d. Avoid hard scratchy foods, such as pretzels or popcorn, until throat is healed
   e. Report signs of bleeding to physician immediately
   f. Expect more throat discomfort between fourth and eighth postoperative day because of membrane separation
   g. Expect stool to be black or dark for a few days because of swallowed blood
   h. Resume normal activity immediately, as long as it is not stressful or requires straining

---

If sutures are used, the person will have more pain and discomfort than that occurring after a simple tonsillectomy and may be unable to take solid foods for several days. Some otolaryngologists prescribe acetaminophen instead of aspirin for pain after tonsillectomy because aspirin increases the tendency for bleeding.

The tough, yellow, fibrous membrane that forms over the operative site begins to break away between the fourth and eighth postoperative days, and hemorrhage may occur. The separation of the membrane accounts for the throat being more painful at this time. Pink granulation tissues soon become apparent, and by the end of the third postoperative week the area is covered with mucous membrane of normal appearance. Postoperative care is outlined in the box above.

LARYNGEAL PARALYSIS

Laryngeal paralysis may result from disease or injury of either the laryngeal nerves or the vagus nerve. Some causes include aortic aneurysm, mitral stenosis, bronchial carcinoma, neck injuries, and severing or stretching of the recurrent laryngeal nerve during thyroidectomy. The major diagnostic method is laryngoscopy.

Either one or both vocal cords may be paralyzed. If only one cord is affected, the airway is adequate and only the voice may be affected.[12] Efforts to improve the voice in persons with unilateral cord paralysis have been accomplished by injecting a small quantity of Teflon into the paralyzed cord. This swells the cord and pushes it toward the midline where the other cord can approximate it better during phonation.

Bilateral paralysis causes a poor airway that results in incapacitating dyspnea, stridor on exertion, and a weak voice. A sudden bilateral vocal cord paralysis is uncommon and is usually a result of a massive cerebrovascular accident or blunt trauma, both of which are usually incompatible with life. Treatment of bilateral cord paralysis is aimed at restoration of the airway, not at improvement of the voice. An arytenoidectomy may be performed, which consists of resection of one of the arytenoid cartilages, thus increasing the diameter of the posterior portion of the glottis sufficiently to improve breathing. Other procedures include external surgical approaches to lateralize (that is, hold vocal cords open by lateral fixation) the paralyzed vocal cord. A new technique of reinnervation of the paralyzed vocal cord restores cord function in some cases. If both cords are paralyzed and the airway is inadequate, a tracheostomy will be necessary to restore the airway (see Chapter 34).

LARYNGEAL EDEMA

Acute laryngeal edema is a medical emergency. It may be caused by anaphylaxis, urticaria, acute laryngitis, serious inflammatory disease of the throat, or edema after intubation. Acute laryngeal edema causes the airway to narrow or close and requires restoration of the airway. Treatment of acute laryngeal edema consists of administration of an adrenal corticosteroid or epinephrine. A tracheostomy or intubation may be necessary (see Chapter 34). Edema of the larynx may be chronic because of irradiation treatment of the larynx or tumors of the neck, thus requiring a tracheostomy.

TRAUMA OF THE UPPER AIRWAY

FRACTURES OF NASAL BONES AND SEPTUM

Fractures of the nasal bones and septum commonly occur from relatively minor injuries, such as falls, or from more severe injuries, such as automobile accidents or fights. If there is no displacement of the bone, no obstruction to the airway, and no cosmetic deformity, treatment is not needed. When airway obstruction or bone displacement occurs (Figure 32-11), simple reduction is performed. Most simple nasal fractures can be reduced by applying firm pressure on the convex side of the nose. Nasal fractures should be reduced within the first 24 hours if at all possible. Local anesthesia is used. After 24 hours the reduction becomes more difficult and may require general anesthesia.

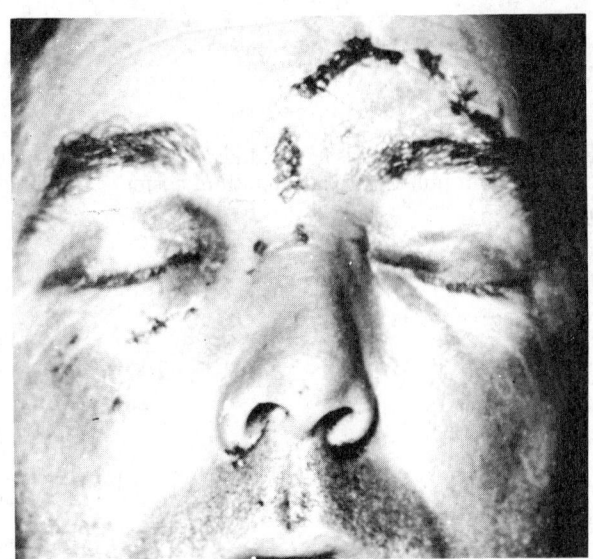

FIGURE 32-11 Laterally displaced fracture of nose secondary to trauma. Pressure on convex side will restore alignment. (From Saunders WH et al: Nursing care in eye, ear, nose, and throat disorders, ed 4, St Louis, 1979, The CV Mosby Co.)

FRACTURES OF THE MAXILLARY AND ZYGOMATIC BONES

Fractures of the maxillary and zygomatic bones are seen after automobile accidents and fights.[28] These fractures are generally reduced under anesthesia. Patients may also require wiring of the teeth with all the attendant problems of that procedure.

EPISTAXIS
ETIOLOGY/PATHOPHYSIOLOGY

Epistaxis (nosebleed) usually originates from the tiny blood vessels in the anterior part of the septum. Bleeding from the posterior part is more common in elderly persons and is more likely to be severe. In adults, nosebleeds are more common in men than in women.

The most common cause of epistaxis is trauma to the nasal mucosa from damage by a foreign object.[27] Other causes include picking the nose, local irritation of the mucous membrane from lack of humidity in the air, chronic infection, violent sneezing, or blowing of the nose. Systemic causes include coagulation defects such as hemophilia, leukemia, and purpura.

Although persons with hypertension do not have more nosebleeds than normotensive persons, they tend to bleed more profusely when they do have a nosebleed. Nosebleed is usually unilateral and some persons are more prone to nosebleed than are others. Persons with frequent nosebleeds should have a complete physical examination to see if a cause can be determined.

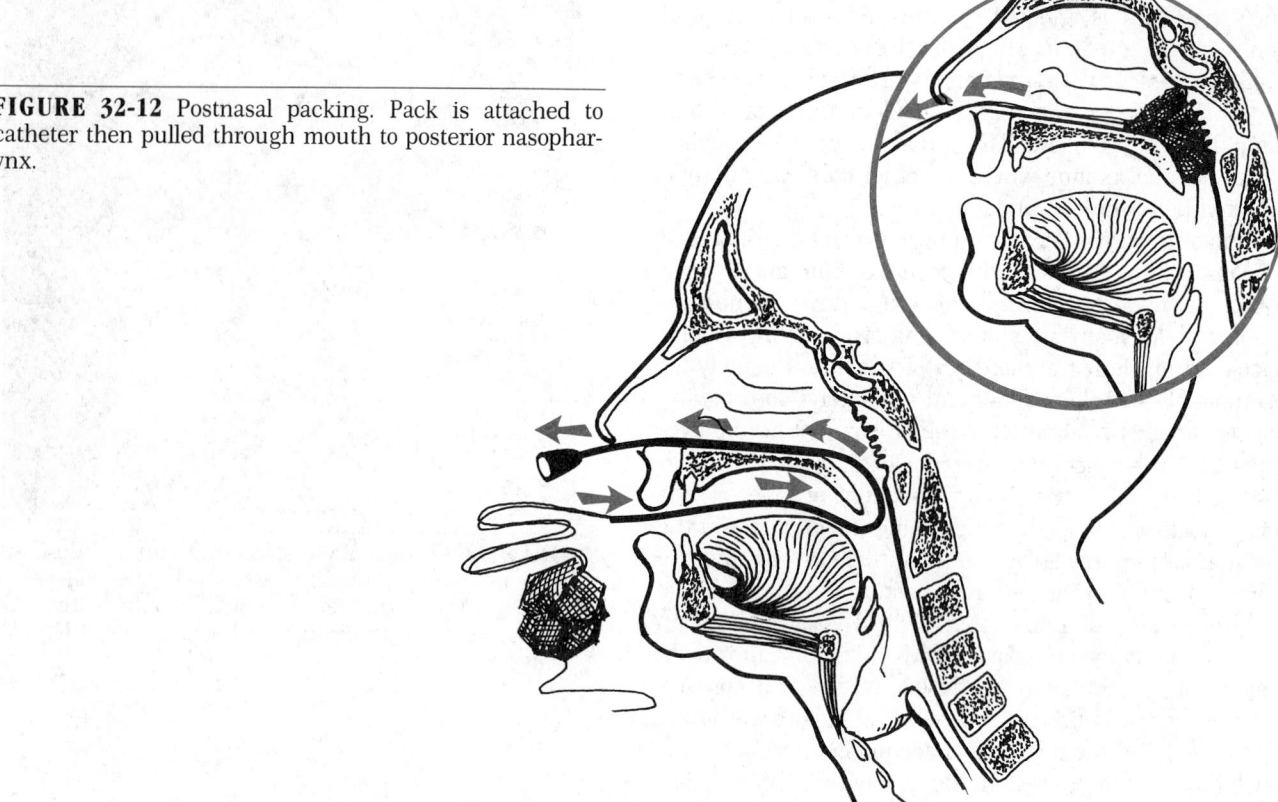

FIGURE 32-12 Postnasal packing. Pack is attached to catheter then pulled through mouth to posterior nasopharynx.

INTERVENTIONS
Medical Management

Most nosebleeds can be controlled with simple measures (see the box below). If these measures are ineffective, medical intervention should be obtained. After identifying the site of the bleeding, the physician cauterizes the bleeding point with a silver nitrate stick or electrocautery. If the bleeding point cannot be seen, a *postnasal pack* may be inserted (Figure 32-12). Because this procedure is extremely painful and some-

INITIAL INTERVENTIONS FOR EPISTAXIS

1. Have person sit up leaning forward with head tipped downward (prevents swallowing or aspiration of blood).
2. Compress soft tissues of nose against septum with finger and maintain pressure for at least 5 minutes.
3. Apply ice or cold compress to nose to constrict blood vessels.
4. If bleeding does not stop with direct pressure, place a cotton ball soaked in a topical vasoconstrictor (such as phenylephrine [Neo-Synephrine]) into nose and apply pressure.
5. Instruct person not to blow nose for several hours after a nosebleed.
6. Notify physician.

times causes complications, patients should be admitted to the hospital. Complications include confusion, hypoxia, hypotension, and possible death. The pack is left in place 3 to 5 days and then removed very gently. Medical management includes adequate oxygenation, humidification, analgesia, bed rest, blood transfusions, intravenous fluids, systemic antibiotics, and sedation. If the posterior pack fails to control the bleeding, another pack may be placed and the patient may be taken to surgery for ligation of the internal maxillary artery or to the x-ray department for embolization of the bleeding vessels.

Nursing Management

Severe epistaxis can cause apprehension because of the profuse bleeding not only from the nose but also flowing into the throat. The person is kept in mid-Fowler's position and is urged not to swallow blood because it may cause nausea and vomiting. The position of the postnasal pack must be checked frequently by viewing the posterior oropharynx for bleeding or slippage. Nasal packs may slip out of place and cause airway obstruction. The patient is monitored for signs of complications (confusion, agitation, increased lethargy, and changes in vital signs). Nasal packs also make eating and swallowing difficult; a liquid diet is usually more tolerable.

TABLE 32-3 Malignant disorders of nose and throat

Disorder	Description	Signs and Symptoms	Therapy
Nasopharyngeal carcinomas	Carcinomas that obstruct nose first on one side then the other	Nasal obstruction, early metastasis to neck, bleeding	Surgery; radiation therapy
Carcinoma of maxillary and ethmoid sinuses	Relatively uncommon	Loosening of upper teeth; nasal obstruction, nosebleeds, displacement of eye, anosmia, tearing and diplopia	Chemotherapy; radiation; surgery that removes entire upper jaw (maxillectomy) and one eye (orbital exenteration)
Cancer of tonsil	May be carcinoma, lymphoepithelioma, or lymphosarcoma	Local ulceration, enlarged tonsil, pain	Surgery; radiation
Carcinoma of larynx	Squamous cell carcinoma of vocal cords and surrounding tissue	Progressive hoarseness that lasts longer than 2 weeks	Partial or total laryngectomy; radiation therapy if limited to vocal cord

MALIGNANCIES OF THE UPPER AIRWAY

Malignancies may develop in the nasopharynx, sinuses, tonsils, and larynx (Table 32-3).

MALIGNANCY OF THE NASOPHARYNX

Tumors of the nasopharynx may be benign or malignant; both can produce nasal obstruction. Nasopharyngeal carcinomas obstruct the nose, at first on one side and then on both sides. These tumors metastasize early to the neck. Medical therapy consists of surgery and radiation therapy.

MALIGNANCY OF THE MAXILLARY AND ETHMOID SINUSES

CLINICAL MANIFESTATIONS

Malignant tumors of the maxillary and ethmoid sinuses are relatively uncommon. Carcinoma of the maxillary sinus presents no early symptoms. The first complaints are usually dental in origin; either the person complains of loosening of the upper teeth or of the upper plate no longer fitting if dentures are worn.[37] Other symptoms may include nasal obstruction caused by the tumor eroding into the nose, nosebleeds, and displacement of the eye.

Carcinoma of the ethmoid sinus presents no oral or dental symptoms. The tumor causes outward displacement of the eye, anosmia, and nosebleeds. Often tearing of the eye or diplopia occurs. The prognosis is grave.

INTERVENTIONS

Medical Management

Chemotherapy has become very useful in the management of carcinoma of the sinus, and is used in conjunction with *radiation* and *surgery*.

Surgery often consists of removal of the entire upper jaw (*maxillectomy*) removal of the entire palate (hard and soft), and one eye (*orbital exenteration*). Split-thickness skin grafts are usually applied to the operative area. Postoperatively, the deformity of the jaw is managed with a dental prosthesis that closes off the defect in the mouth (Figure 32-13). Radical surgery is required because of the danger of recurrence. Meningitis is a potential postoperative complication and prophylactic antibiotics are usually prescribed.

Maintenance of an airway postoperatively is critical for these patients and a tracheostomy is often performed. A nasogastric tube is inserted to ensure adequate liquid and caloric intake because eating is difficult until the prosthesis is fitted. Several different prostheses may be needed before a final one fits because of shrinking of the cavity as healing progresses.

NURSING MANAGEMENT

General postoperative care includes tracheostomy care (see Chapter 34) and routine care of the person with a nasogastric tube (see Chapter 43). The person is monitored for signs of meningitis (fever, headache, neck rigidity).

Mouth care for patients with this type of surgery is important. Sometimes a gentle spray or oral irrigation using saline with hydrogen peroxide, weak sodium bicarbonate, or antibiotic solution may be used. Because the person may have difficulty in swallowing, it may be necessary to aspirate the irrigating solution from the mouth; care must be taken to prevent trauma to the sutures by the suction. Management of saliva may also be a problem because of the swallowing difficulty.

Persons who undergo radical surgery of this type have a number of emotional adjustments to make. Alteration in their physical appearance is readily visible; the person feels conspicuous and different. In addition to disfigurement, these patients have all the normal fears of surgery and of cancer. Fear, anger, and grief are nor-

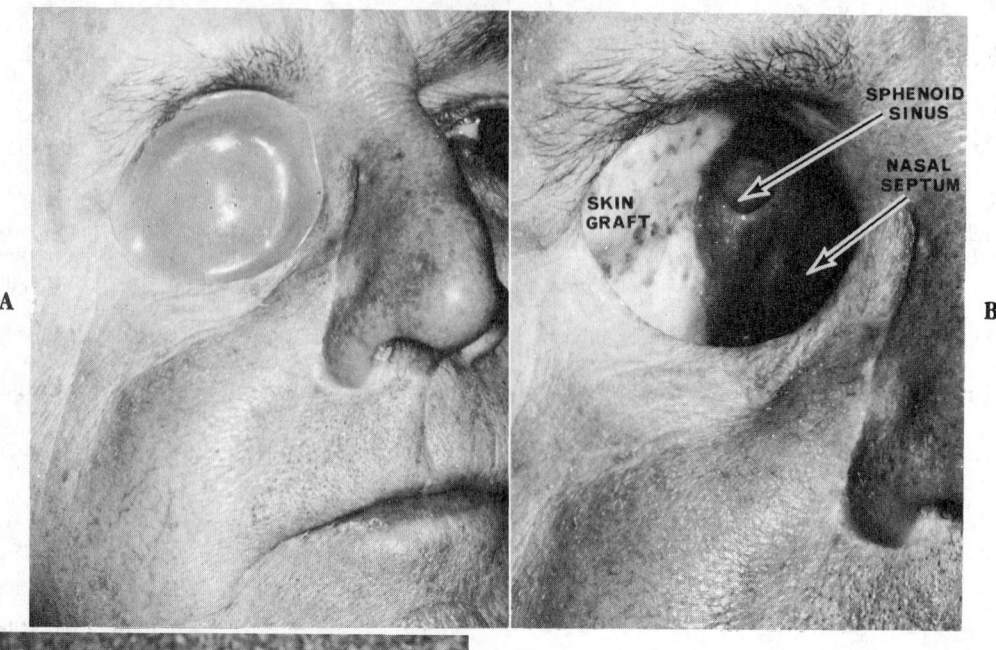

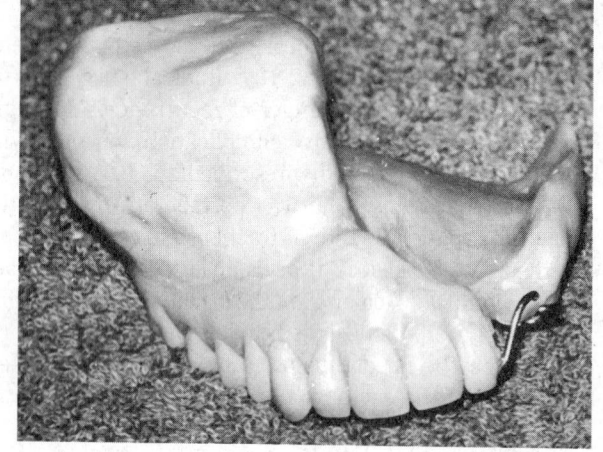

FIGURE 32-13 Patient after maxillectomy and orbital exenteration. **A,** Orbital prosthesis in place. Eyeglasses worn over this further improves appearance. **B,** Defect in orbit with skin graft lining upper and lateral wall of orbital-maxillary cavity. **C,** Upper denture worn with large obturator to fill in defect created by maxilectomy. (From Saunders WH et al: Nursing care in eye, ear, nose, and throat disorders, ed 4, St Louis, 1979, The CV Mosby Co.)

mal reactions to the situation. Fear is focused on concerns about the future, the ability to live normally, and of being rejected. Anger and grief are common responses to the loss and the helplessness to control the loss. Oral communication also may be a problem immediately after surgery, and every effort is made to allow the person to express needs and feelings by writing if necessary. Conveying compassion and concern to the person is important.

MALIGNANCY OF THE TONSILS

PATHOPHYSIOLOGY AND CLINICAL MANIFESTATIONS

Malignancy of the tonsils is second only to malignancy of the larynx in malignancies of the upper respiratory tract. The malignancy can be one of three types: *carcinoma, lymphoepithelioma,* or *lymphosarcoma.* Carcino-

mas are more common in men, possibly related to heavy smoking. The carcinomas spread upward into the soft palate and usually metastasize early to the neck. Local ulceration and otalgia (earache) are early symptoms. Lymphoepitheliomas often remain small and do not ulcerate, but neck metastasis occurs early. Lymphosarcomas produce large tonsils, usually without ulceration or pain, and metastasize early to the neck.

INTERVENTIONS
MEDICAL MANAGEMENT

Medical interventions for all tonsillar malignancies always include radiation in conjunction with an extensive surgical procedure to remove all the malignant tissue. Chemotherapy may be used. The cure rate is improved using this combined technique.[12] Recurrence often occurs locally or with distant metastasis.

MALIGNANCY OF THE LARYNX
ETIOLOGY AND PATHOPHYSIOLOGY

Squamous cell carcinoma of the larynx is increasing in frequency. It is estimated that in the United States over 12,300 new cases and over 3700 deaths occur every year.[1] Cancer of the larynx limited to the true vocal cords grows slowly because of the limited lymphatic supply. Elsewhere in the larynx (epiglottis, false vocal cords, and pyriform sinuses) lymphatic vessels are abundant, and cancer of these tissues often spreads rapidly and metastasizes early to the deep lymph nodes of the neck.

Cancer of the larynx is five times more common in men than in women, and it occurs most often in persons over 60 years of age. There appears to be some relationship between cancer of the larynx and heavy smoking, heavy alcohol intake, chronic laryngitis, vocal abuse, and family predisposition to cancer. Because of in the number of women who are heavy smokers, the incidence of carcinoma of the larynx among this group is increasing. Carcinoma of the larynx may invade deeper structures and cause vocal cord paralysis or metastasis to the neck.

CLINICAL MANIFESTATIONS

Any smoker who becomes progressively hoarse or is hoarse for longer than 2 weeks should be urged to seek medical attention at once. *Hoarseness is an early symptom of cancer of the vocal cords.* If treatment is given when hoarseness first appears (caused by the tumor's preventing the complete approximation of the vocal cord), a cure usually is possible. Signs of metastases of cancer to other parts of the larynx include a sensation of a lump in the throat, pain in the Adam's apple that radiates to the ear, dyspnea, dysphagia, enlarged cervical nodes, and cough. The diagnosis of cancer of the larynx is made from the history, from visual examination of the larynx with indirect laryngoscopy, and from a biopsy and microscopic study of the lesion.

INTERVENTIONS
MEDICAL MANAGEMENT

Treatment of carcinoma of the true vocal cord depends on the extent of the tumor involvement. If the tumor is limited to the true cord without limitation of cord movement, then radiation therapy is the best course of treatment, with cure rates of 80% to 90%. Surgical intervention is considered when extension of the tumor fixes

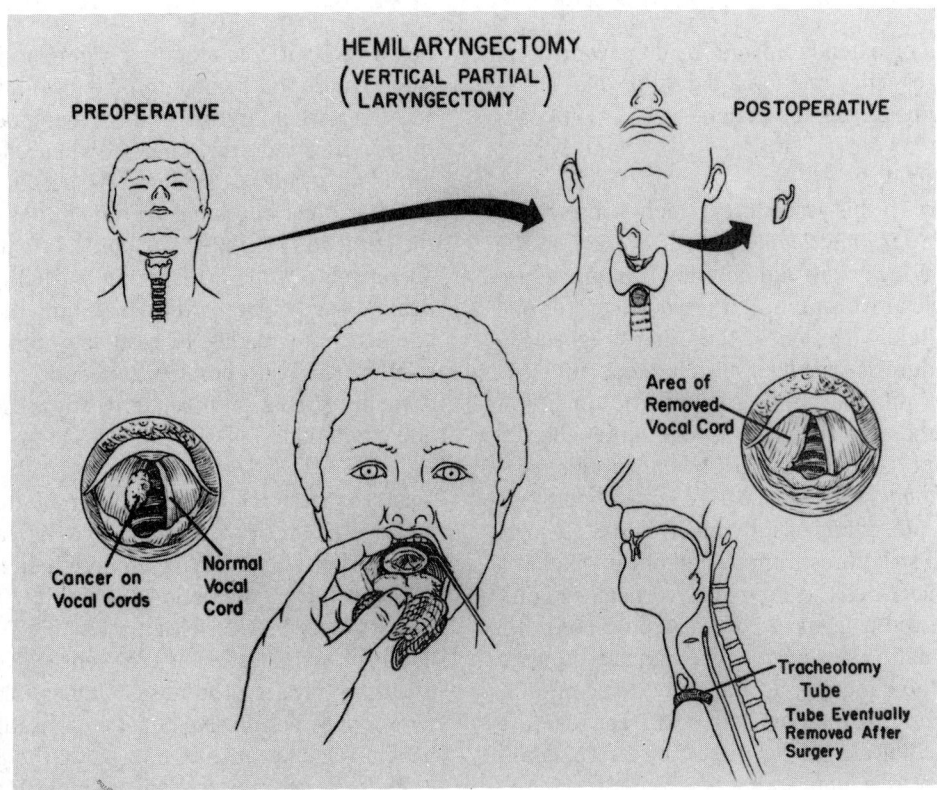

FIGURE 32-14 The technique of hemilaryngectomy. (From DeWeese DD et al: Otolaryngology—head and neck surgery, ed 7, St Louis, 1988, The CV Mosby Co.)

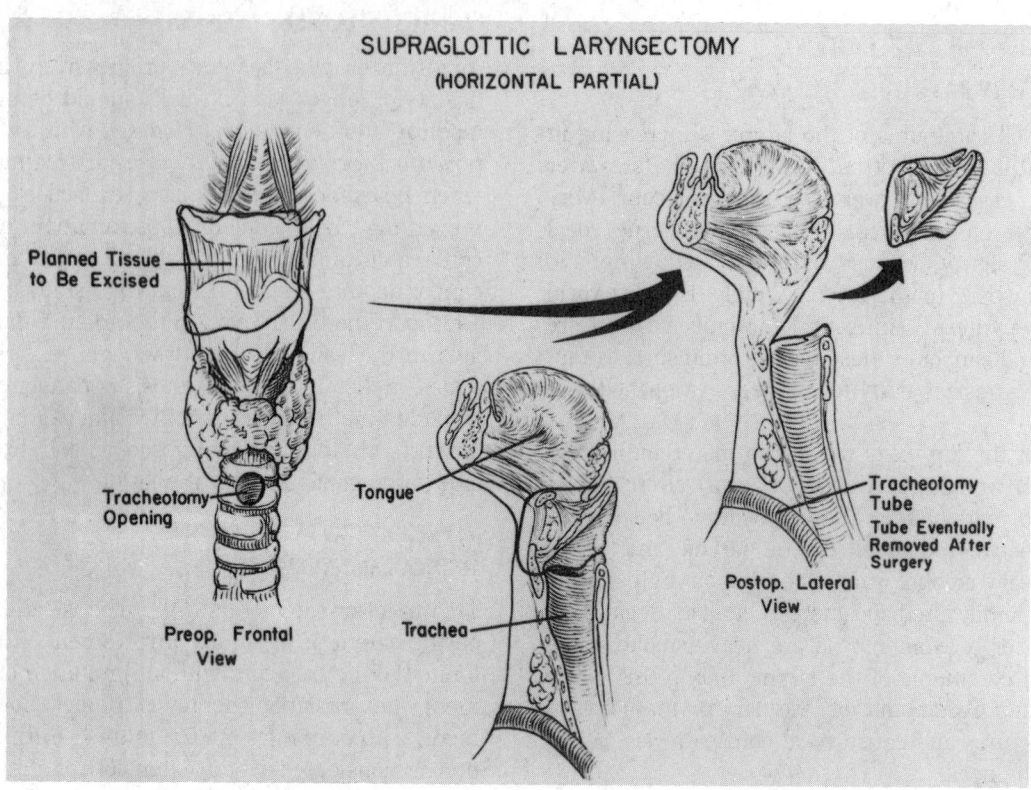

FIGURE 32-15 The technique of supraglottic laryngectomy. (From DeWeese DD et al: Otolaryngology—head and neck surgery, ed 7, St Louis, 1988, The CV Mosby Co.)

one of the cords or extends upward or downward from the larynx. Surgery may include a partial or total laryngectomy, or a radical neck dissection.

Parital Laryngectomy

Hemilaryngectomy. In this procedure, which is also called a *vertical partial laryngectomy,* one half or more of the larynx is removed. Persons suitable for this procedure have malignancies involving one true vocal cord or one true vocal cord and a portion of the other (Figure 32-14). This procedure is usually well tolerated; difficulty in swallowing is minimal; and although the quality of the voice is altered, it is adequate for communication.[12]

When the supraglottis is invaded by cancer, a *supraglottic laryngectomy* (horizontal partial laryngectomy) is performed. The procedure usually involves the removal of endolaryngeal structures from the tip of the epiglottis down to and including the laryngeal vertical. (Figure 32-15). Because the true vocal cords are preserved, the patient's voice quality is excellent. The major postoperative problem is the danger of aspiration because of difficulty in swallowing. Aspiration may occur because the major reflex arc that causes closure of the larynx is initiated by sensory receptors in the supraglottic larynx, which has been removed. These patients will need special swallowing training postoperatively. Although pa-

tients take variable amounts of time to learn to swallow safely, most will be able to take feedings by mouth.

After partial laryngectomy, a temporary tracheostomy tube is inserted and removed when edema in the surrounding tissues subsides. The person is not on absolute voice rest but is not permitted to use the voice until the surgeon gives specific approval (usually 3 days postoperatively). Only whispering is then permitted until healing is complete, after which time the person usually adjusts quite readily to relatively minor limitations of speech. The main problems encountered by persons undergoing partial laryngectomy are those of swallowing and aspiration.

Total laryngectomy. When cancer of the larynx is advanced, a total laryngectomy may be performed (Table 32-4). After a total laryngectomy, there is no connection between the trachea and the mouth; *a permanent tracheostomy is in place* (Figure 32-16). The presence of a tracheal stoma affects the sense of smell because breathing through the nose is impossible; therefore, the person does not receive olfactory sensations. The person has no voice because of removal of the larynx.

Radical neck dissection. A radical neck dissection may be performed along with a laryngectomy in patients whose risk of metastases to the neck from carcinoma of

TABLE 32-4 Laryngectomy surgery for cancer

Type	Description	Voice Result
CONSERVATION PROCEDURES WITH PRESERVATION OF PART OF LARYNX		
Hemilaryngectomy (vertical partial laryngectomy)	Removal of one-half or more of larynx	Adequate
Supralottic laryngectomy (horizontal partial laryngectomy)	Removal of supraglottal portion of larynx	Normal because true vocal cords preserved
CONSERVATION PROCEDURE *NOT* POSSIBLE BECAUSE OF INVASIVENESS OF TUMOR		
Total laryngectomy	Removal of all of larynx	No voice

the larynx is high. This includes primary tumors whose size and location are known to result in metastasis and palpable cervical lymph nodes at time of surgery. In a radical neck dissection the submandibular salivary gland, sternocleidomastoid muscle, internal jugular vein, and spinal accessory nerve are removed to assure complete removal of nodal-bearing tissue.[12] In some patients, a modification of a radical neck dissection will be performed. These are referred to as *modified, conservative,* or *functional* neck dissections and are used when the nodal metastatic disease is not far advanced. These

procedures cause atrophy of the trapezius muscle and the shoulder drops on the side of the surgery.

Patients can be taught to do exercises to gradually replace the function of the lost muscles with that of other muscles. A patient may have some difficulty lifting the head and can achieve this by placing the hands behind the head. The patient is more comfortable and can breathe better when placed in mid-Fowler's position. Pressure dressings are best avoided in radical neck dissection because they compromise the blood supply to the skin flaps protecting the vital neck structures. The

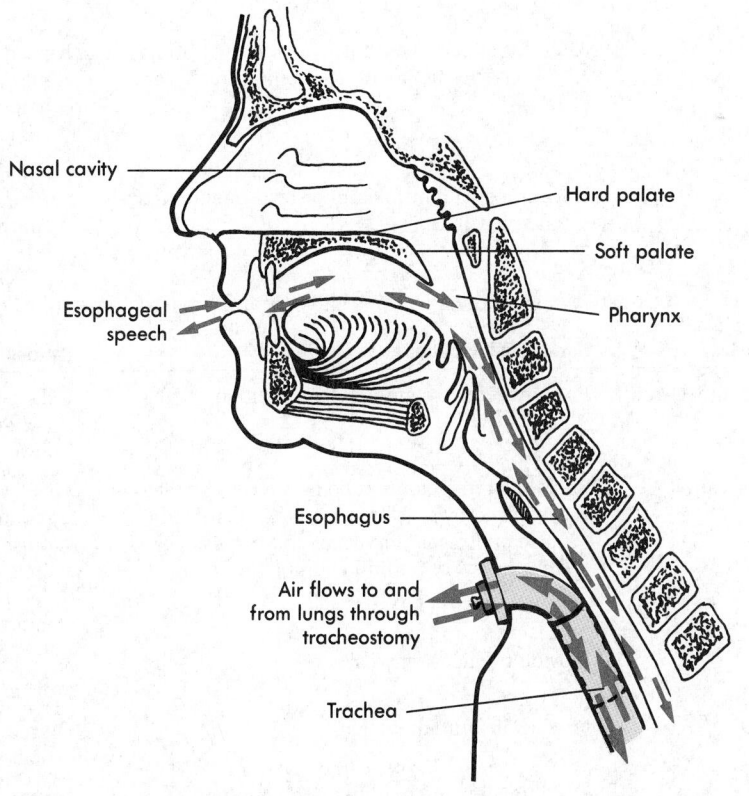

FIGURE 32-16 Permanent tracheostomy: no connection exists between trachea and esophagus.

PERSON WITH LARYNGECTOMY

DATA: Mr. Knox, a 68-year-old man, had noted progressive hoarseness for several months. Indirect laryngoscopy and biopsy confirmed cancer of the larynx and he was admitted for a total laryngectomy. His wife accompanied him to the hospital and planned to be with him as much as possible during his hospitalization. She was attentive and supportive.

The following pertinent data were identified on admission:
- He was visibly apprehensive (pacing the floor, restless, asking repeated questions).
- His major concerns centered on the extent of the cancer and on communication problems postoperatively.
- Height 175 cm (5 ft 10 in), weight 68 kg (150 lbs).
- He wears glasses; near vision is poor without glasses.

Before surgery, Mr. Knox's primary nurse spent time with him, encouraging him to explore his concerns and providing information about what to expect in the postoperative period and care that would be provided. After the interaction, Mr. Knox's restlessness decreased and he was observed talking quietly with his wife and watching TV.

During surgery, the larynx was removed; a permanent tracheostomy was performed with insertion of a temporary laryngectomy tube. A nasogastric tube was inserted, to be removed after Mr. Knox was swallowing well. During the first postoperative day, Mr. Knox again appeared apprehensive (restlessness, pointing frequently to his tracheostomy, pulling on wife's hand and pointing to call cord to call the nurse). Breath sounds in the upper lobes were clear but were absent in the lower lobes. Codeine and acetaminophen were prescribed for pain.

NURSING DIAGNOSIS

Anxiety related to breathing difficulties and inability to communicate

Expected Patient Outcomes	Nursing Interventions	Rationale
Patient rests quietly, does not call frequently for suctioning	Explain to patient and carry out regular, suctioning of tracheostomy	If patient knows tube will be suctioned frequently, fear of possible asphyxiation should decrease.
	Develop a means of communication (such as cards with needs printed clearly or paper for writing). Be sure patient wears glasses.	If patient can communicate needs, anxiety should decrease. His glasses are needed for visual communication.
	After initial period, and if wife is willing and able, teach her to help with suctioning tracheostomy.	Participating in husband's care may assist wife to feel she is helping, thus decreasing her anxiety (anxiety can be transmitted to patient).
	Encourage patient to care for own tracheostomy when feasible.	Self-care enhances feelings of control of situation.

NURSING DIAGNOSIS

Airway clearance, ineffective, related to secretions in upper airway and laryngectomy tube

Expected Patient Outcomes	Nursing Interventions	Rationale
Respirations effortless, quiet, and at baseline rate	Place patient in semi-Fowler's position	Uses gravity to help expand thorax and decrease pressure on lower lobes.
Breath sounds are clear at all lobes	Suction laryngectomy tube as often as needed as evidenced by noisy respirations, increased pulse and respiratory rate, and restlessness (may be every 5 minutes initially)	Air blowing through secretions produce noisy respirations; pulse and respirations are increased when oxygen intake is decreased; restlessness may indicate decreased oxygenation.
	Provide tracheostomy care	Keeping tube patent will facilitate air interchange.
	Provide air humidification	Humidity will help keep secretions liquid for easier removal.
	Encourage deep breathing and coughing	Deep breathing will help aerate lower lobes; coughing will help expel the secretions.

NURSING DIAGNOSIS

Pain related to surgery

Expected Patient Outcomes	Nursing Interventions	Rationale
Patient is relaxed and signals feeling comfortable	Give prescribed analgesic to prevent pain from becoming severe	Analgesics will decrease transmission and interpretation of pain stimuli.
	Encourage other pain-relieving measures such as relaxation exercises or distraction	Help to minimize pain perception.
	Provide nose and mouth care while nasogastric tube is in place	Tube may irritate nose; mouth becomes dry and uncomfortable from open mouth breathing and decreased lubrication (unable to swallow fluids).

NURSING DIAGNOSIS

Nutrition, alteration in: less than body requirements, related to difficulty swallowing

Expected Patient Outcomes	Nursing Interventions	Rationale
Weight is not less than 5 lbs from baseline	Give prescribed tube feedings via nasogastric tube until patient can swallow well	Tube feedings provide more adequate nutrients than IV fluids; swallowing is impaired initially from postoperative edema of lower pharynx.
	When nasogastric tube is removed, give fluids until patient is swallowing well	Fluids are easier to swallow initially past the edematous area.
	Explain anatomic changes to patient (no connection between esophagus and tracheostomy)	May help to decrease patient's concern of choking
	Stay with patient during initial eating of semi-solid and solid foods	He may fear choking and not be willing to swallow initially; encouragement by nurse with assurance of suctioning if necessary may give patient more confidence.
	Use measures to encourage eating as necessary (tray for wife so they can eat together, selection of desired foods, etc.)	Return to usual eating patterns may encourage patient to eat.
	Encourage him to monitor weight two to three times a week until baseline weight is regained	Participating in own weight monitoring may motivate him to eat.

NURSING DIAGNOSIS

Communication impaired, verbal, related to laryngectomy

Expected Patient Outcomes	Nursing Interventions	Rationale
Patient communicates with others	Encourage him to communicate via an established system (such as hand signals, writing) during initial period	With larynx removal, sounds cannot be made by previous method of vibrating vocal cords.
Patient begins speech rehabilitation using esophageal speech	Support activities of speech therapist: 1. Encourage him to practice burping as instructed	Burping provides air movement; esophageal tissue folds act as vibrating surface.
	2. Monitor for gastric flatus or gastric discomfort; explain that this may be due muscle strain or nervous tension	Excessive air may be swallowed when practicing burping and may discourage him from further practice; discomfort will decrease with practice.
	3. Discuss availability of mechanical devices for speech or telephone use	Until esophageal speech is perfected, mechanical devices can help him communicate verbally

Continued.

NURSING CARE PLAN

PERSON WITH LARYNGECTOMY—cont'd

NURSING DIAGNOSIS

Knowledge deficit related to lack of exposure/recall

Expected Patient Outcomes	Nursing Interventions	Rationale
Patient describes self-care	Teach patient: 1. Description of anatomic changes 2. Care of stoma, including self-suctioning 3. Methods to protect stoma 4. Availability of community resources	Providing own care will give him self-confidence; care is needed to keep the tracheostomy open for air exchange. He may be interested in the Lost Chord Club for sharing of experiences

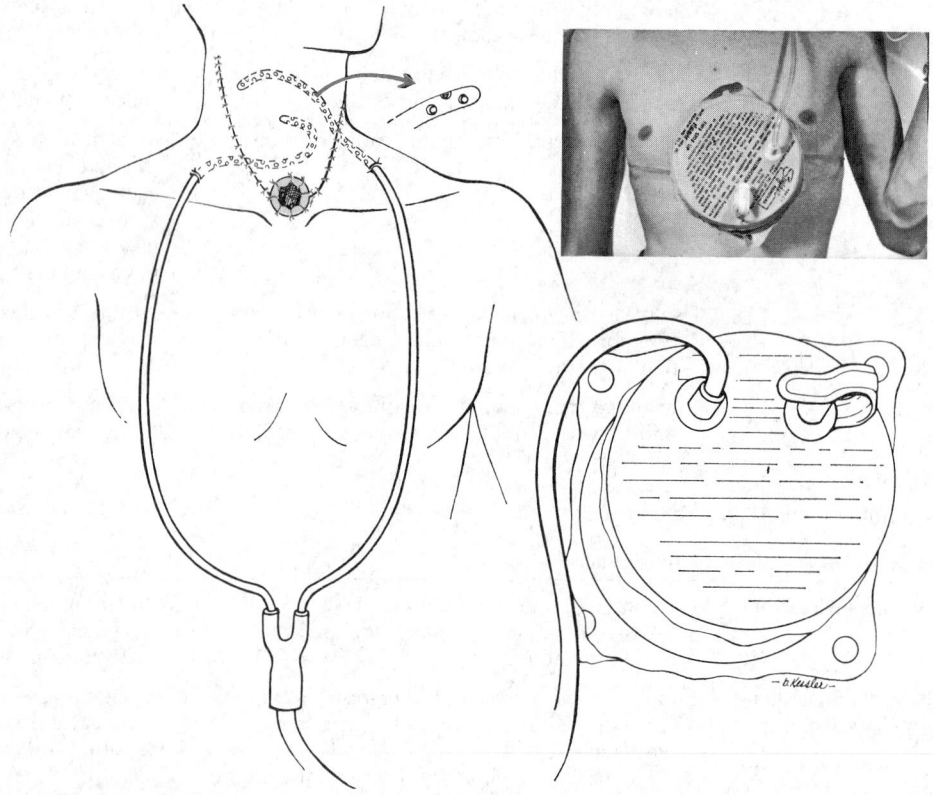

FIGURE 32-17 Hemovac apparatus for constant closed suction. In this system of wound drainage, suction is maintained by plastic container with spring inside that tries to force apart lids and thereby produces suction that is transmitted through plastic tubing. Neck skin is pulled down tight, and no external dressing is required. Container serves as both suction source and receptacle for blood. It is emptied as required, and drainage tubes are left in neck for 3 days. (From DeWeese DD and Saunders WH: Textbook of otolaryngology, ed 6, St Louis, 1982, The CV Mosby Co.)

Hemovac (Figure 32-17) is one device available to keep constant drainage from the neck wound without pressure on the flaps. The Hemovac must be checked to see that it is working properly and that there is no edema, which might indicate hematoma.

There is some readily visible alteration of appearance that may cause the person to feel somewhat conspicuous. Anger, grief, or denial may be part of the normal response to the change in body image. (For further information on body image, refer to Chapter 18.)

Radical neck dissection can be performed without laryngectomy for persons whose primary malignant lesion is in the tongue, tonsil, lip, nasopharynx, or thyroid. Often the procedure accompanies other procedures and is termed a *composite* resection. Composite resections may include radical neck dissection in addition to either the removal of the mandible; removal of the mandible and resection of the floor of the mouth; or removal of the mandible, floor of the mouth, and the tongue. The nursing care for these patients is similar to the care given for maxillectomy and orbital exenteration (p. 857).

Emotional reactions to this type of radical surgery may be profound. Disfigurement is readily visible, and reactions to the change in body image are marked. In addition to the usual fears of surgery and cancer, the patient having a composite resection may have fears of rejection and fears concerning the future.

An alternative to neck dissection is *radiation therapy*. According to some experts, occult nodal disease (nonpalpable nodes) can be treated just as effectively with radiation therapy as it can with surgery. However, as the size of the metastatic nodes increases, the effectiveness of radiation therapy decreases and surgery will be necessary.[12]

NURSING MANAGEMENT AFTER TOTAL LARYNGECTOMY

COPING WITH CHANGES FROM SURGERY

The patient who is to have a total laryngectomy is told by the physician that breathing will occur through a special opening made in the neck and that normal speech will not be possible. This is often depressing to the patient because it threatens economic status as well as life. The patient requires much empathic support during this period, as well as during the postoperative period.

In some instances, it is helpful to receive a visit from another person who has made a good recovery from laryngectomy and who has undergone rehabilitation successfully. In other instances, this visit may depress the patient further. Careful assessment must be made to determine if the patient will benefit from such a visit and whether the visit should be made preoperatively, immediately after surgery, or later in the recovery period. Often no one else can reassure a patient that speech can

be regained as well as a fellow patient. Many large cities have a "Lost Chord Club" or a "New Voice Club," and the members are willing to visit hospitalized patients. Information regarding these clubs may be obtained by writing to the International Association of Laryngectomees.* Local speech rehabilitation centers may supply instructive films and other resources. The local chapter of the American Cancer Society and the local health department also have information available.

INITIAL POSTOPERATIVE CARE

Postoperative care of the patient is essentially the same as that described for tracheostomy (see Chapter 34), except that these patients will have a laryngectomy tube in place—a tube that is shorter and wider in diameter than a tracheostomy tube. Some patients may not have a tube in the stoma after the operation because the stoma is a permanent one kept open initially by the sutures and because their surgeon believes that there is less tissue reaction and a better stoma if no tube is used. Most otolaryngologists believe that a laryngectomy tube is better than a tracheostomy tube because it is shorter.

*American Cancer Society, Inc, 1599 Clifton Road NE, Atlanta, GA 30329.

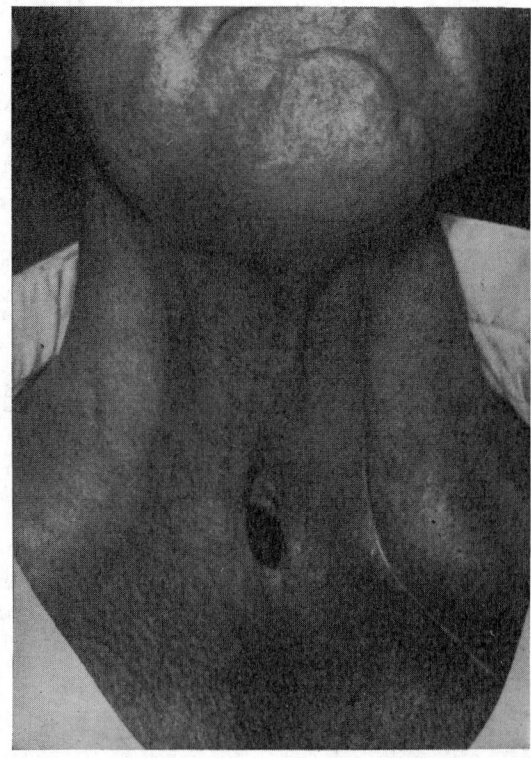

FIGURE 32-18 After laryngectomy. Note scars of bilateral radical neck dissections. (From DeWeese DD and Saunders WH: Textbook of otolaryngology, ed 6, St Louis, 1982, The CV Mosby Co.)

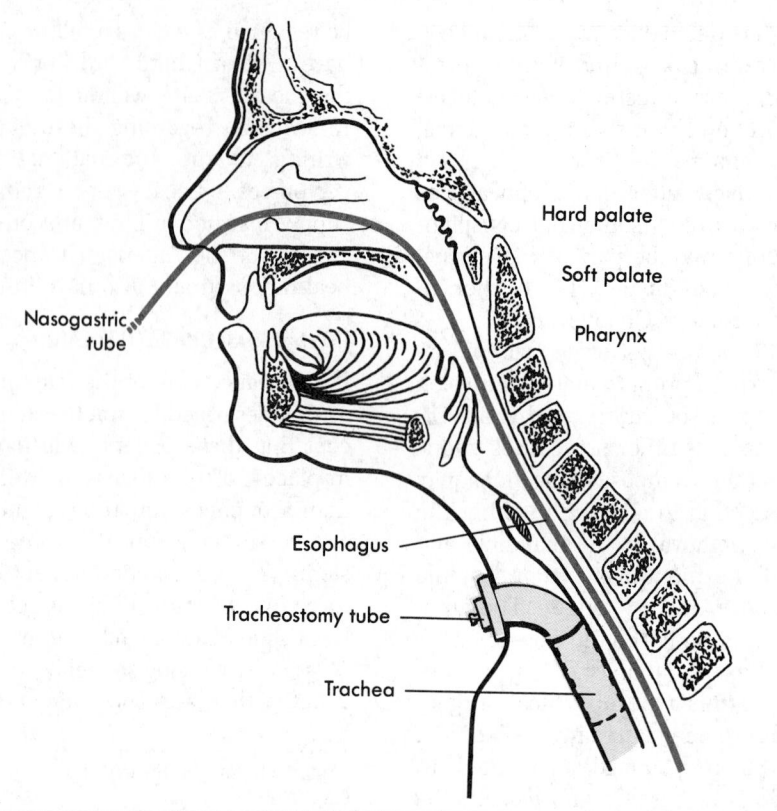

FIGURE 32-19 Position of tracheostomy tube and nasogastric tube after total laryngectomy.

The tube will remain until the wound is healed and a permanent fistula has formed, usually in 2 or 3 weeks (Figure 32-18). Frequent suctioning is necessary in the early postoperative period to keep the trachea free of secretions.

A nasogastric tube is usually inserted during the surgical procedure for the instillation of food and fluids at regular intervals postoperatively for about 10 days (Figure 32-19). The use of the tube to give food is thought to minimize contamination of the pharyngeal and esophageal suture lines and to prevent fluid from leaking through the wound into the trachea before healing occurs. The nasogastric tube is removed as soon as the patient can safely swallow. The patient then needs careful attention in the first attempts to swallow. There may be a sensation of choking as well as severe coughing that is frightening and painful. Aspiration cannot occur because the trachea no longer communicates with the esophagus.

SPEECH REHABILITATION

Until recently, *esophageal speech* was the primary speech method after laryngectomy. Although this method of speech was successful for many laryngectomees, others could never learn to use it. In addition, the increased use of radiation therapy after laryngectomy causes fibrous tissue to form, making *esophageal speech* less possible.

For a number of years, surgeons had been working to develop other forms of speech after laryngectomy. In 1980, the first successful procedure using surgical-prosthetic voice restoration was introduced. In this procedure, a *tracheoesophageal puncture* to create a tracheoesophageal fistula large enough to permit the insertion of a valve prosthesis is made. The prosthesis is a hollow tube open at the tracheal end and closed with a horizontal slit at the hypopharyngeal end. (Figure 32-20). When the patient talks, air pressure opens the closed end, permitting air to enter the hypopharynx. When the patient stops talking, the hypopharyngeal end closes preventing saliva from draining into the trachea. Because air is diverted from the trachea into the esophagus, this form of speech is referred to as *tracheoesophageal speech*.

The stoma must be occluded during speech, either by a finger placed over the opening or by a special tracheostomal valve inserted after the patient has learned to use the prosthesis. The patient or family must be taught to remove, clean, and reinsert the voice prosthesis rapidly so that stenosis of the fistula does not occur.

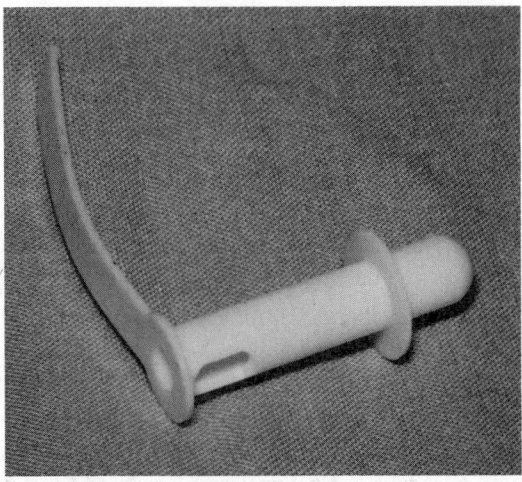

FIGURE 32-20 This vocal prosthesis allows for the passage of air from the trachea into the hypopharynx but prevents the opposite flow of saliva. (From DeWeese DD et al: Otolaryngology—head and neck surgery, ed 7, St Louis, 1988, The CV Mosby Co.)

Not all patients and families are comfortable with removing and cleaning the prosthesis, and considerable support by the speech pathologist may be necessary. Ideally, the patient should be able to use the prosthesis for speaking and be able to clean and reinsert it before discharge from the hospital.

Early evidence indicates that there are several advantages of tracheoesophageal speech. These include more rapid restoration of voice, speech that is closer to normal

SPEECH METHODS AFTER TOTAL LARYNGECTOMY

Tracheoesophageal speech	Formation of a tracheoesophageal fistula and insertion of a silicone prosthesis that allows speech when air is diverted from the trachea into the esophagus.
Esophageal speech	Speech produced by expelling swallowed air (burping) across constricted tissue in the pharyngoesophageal segment.
Electrolarynx	Battery powered electronic devices that assist the laryngectomee to speak (Figure 32-3).

in rate and phrasing, and speech that is more pleasing than speech with an electrolarynx. (Figure 32-21). Disadvantages include reliance on a prosthesis and the rapidity with which the tracheoesophageal fistula may undergo stenosis.[12] For this reason, all three methods of speaking are still in use, and none are mutually exclusive. In fact, some patients find it useful to use more than one of the methods (see box above).

Information about devices used to produce electronic speech can be obtained from the American Cancer Society or from the local telephone company. Information about esophageal speech can be obtained from the American Speech and Hearing Association,* the Inter-

*10801 Rockville Pike, Rockville, MD 20852.

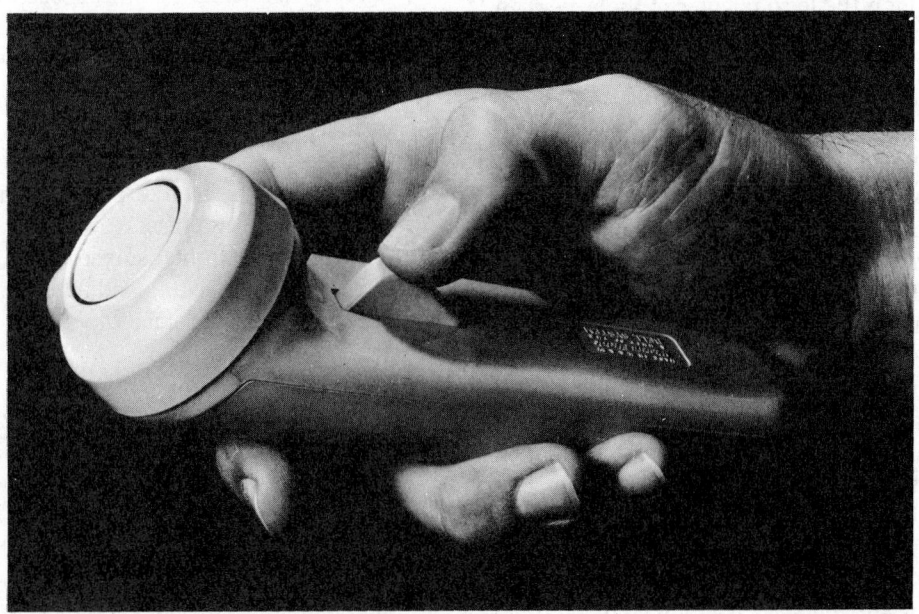

FIGURE 32-21 Battery-powered electronic artificial larynx for patient who has total laryngectomy and cannot learn esophageal speech. (Courtesy Illinois Bell Telephone Co.)

PATIENT TEACHING FOLLOWING TOTAL LARYNGECTOMY

1. Wear a scarf or shirt with closed collar of porous material (to warm and screen air over stoma).
2. Use caution while taking a bath or shower (to prevent aspiration of water into stoma).
3. Check with surgeon concerning swimming or boating; if swimming is permitted, use a special snorkle device designed for tracheostomies.
4. Use available community resources for support and speech rehabilitation as necessary (for example, laryngectomee clubs, American Cancer Society).
5. Seek immediate medical attention for respiratory tract infection or signs of stomal bleeding.
6. Continue medical follow-up per physician instructions.

national Association of Laryngectomies, and the American Cancer Society. No matter what form of speech rehabilitation is used, the patient will require careful teaching and follow-up by a speech pathologist.

PATIENT TEACHING

Persons with laryngectomies must take special precautions because of the permanent tracheostomy (see the box above). Usually by the time of discharge, patients with laryngectomies do not need suctioning of the tracheostomy, but can cough up secretions. If suctioning is deemed necessary, patients or their families need to be told where to secure the necessary suction equipment and how to care for themselves. Suction equipment can be rented for home use or obtained in many communities through the local chapter of the American Cancer Society.

RECONSTRUCTIVE SURGERY

Because of the extensive surgery required to treat malignancies of the head and neck, reconstructive surgery may be necessary. In the past, skin grafts and pedicle or rotation skin flaps were used for reconstruction. Today the *myocutaneous flap* is the major reconstructive flap used after radical neck dissection and traumatic defects of the head and neck.

Myocutaneous flaps use the axial blood supply that supplies muscle mass, as well as cutaneous and subcutaneous tissue. The inclusion of muscle with its blood supply when transferring the skin allows for a much greater range of rotation of the flap. The pectoralis major, the latissimus dorsi, the trapezius, and the sternocleidomastoid muscles can be used for myocutaneous flaps.

The care of these patients is complex and there are many nursing requirements both preoperatively and postoperatively. The reader is referred to two excellent articles on the nursing care of these patients for further information.[47,59]

CHAPTER SUMMARY

✔ The major infections of the nose and sinuses are rhinitis (common cold), allergic rhinitis (hay fever), chronic rhinitis secondary to repeated infections, or allergy; sinusitis caused by a bacteria or virus.

✔ Persons with allergic rhinitis (hay fever) are usually sensitive to pollen of grasses such as ragweed (see Chapter 76).

✔ It is important for persons who are allergic to know which allergens they are allergic to and to avoid these allergens if at all possible. For this reason, they need to know how to prepare an environmentally controlled bedroom (see Chapter 76).

✔ Persons with acute sinusitis usually have a severe headache and pain over the infected area. Fever is common and is related to the amount of sinus obstruction. If the sinus is abscessed, fever may be as high as 40°C (104° F).

✔ Subjective assessment of the person with a nose or sinus problem includes a careful history of previous infections, how they were treated, and self-treatment by the person including the use of over-the-counter medications.

✔ Acetaminophen is recommended instead of aspirin in persons with nasal problems because aspirin may be associated with nasal polyposis.

✔ Five surgical procedures may be used to treat chronic sinusitis: Caldwell-Luc procedure, ethmoidotomy, sphenoidectomy, ethmoidectomy, and osteopathic flap.

✔ Postoperative care for persons having sinus surgery includes the following:
   a. Place patient in side-lying position until reacted from anesthesia and then mid-Fowler's position.
   b. Apply ice compresses over nose or ice bag over maxillary or frontal sinuses.
   c. Monitor for bleeding and for decreased visual acuity, such as diplopia, which indicates damage to the optic nerve.
   d. Provide frequent mouth care.
   e. Change nasal pad when soiled.
   f. Teach patient not to blow nose for at least 48 hours *after* packing is removed.
   g. Instruct patient to avoid constipation because Valsalva maneuver can cause bleeding.

✔ The most common throat inflammation is acute pharyngitis. Hemolytic streptococci, staphylococci, and other bacteria and viruses may be the source of infection. Pharyngitis caused by *Neisseria gonor-*

rhoeae is being seen more commonly in both men and women.

✔ A throat culture is taken to obtain material for culture and sensitivity so that appropriate antibiotic therapy can be determined.

✔ To prevent superinfection, prophylactic antibiotics are often prescribed for persons with pharyngitis who have a history of rheumatic fever or bacterial endocarditis.

✔ Obstructions of the nose, such as a deviated septum, are often treated surgically by submucous resection or septoplasty.

✔ Postoperative care after nasal surgery includes the following:

a. Monitor for hemorrhage.

b. Place patient in mid-Fowler's position to decrease local edema.

c. Apply ice compresses over the nose for 24 hours, as needed.

d. Give food and fluids as tolerated.

e. Provide frequent oral care.

f. Change dressing under nose, as needed.

g. Teach patient to avoid blowing nose for 48 hours after packing is removed to prevent bleeding.

h. Teach patient to avoid constipation and vigorous coughing until healing occurs because they may initiate bleeding.

i. Explain that stools may be tarry for several days.

✔ Smokers with progressive or persistent hoarseness that lasts longer than 2 weeks require medical evaluation for cancer of the larynx.

✔ Carcinoma of the larynx is treated with a partial or total laryngectomy.

✔ Partial laryngectomy may be achieved by hemilaryngectomy, or supraglottic partial laryngectomy, after which the person will be able to speak.

✔ Total laryngectomy is necessary when cancer of the larynx is far advanced. Persons with total laryngectomy are unable to speak.

✔ Radical neck dissection is commonly performed along with total laryngectomy because of the possible metastasis to the neck.

✔ Postoperatively, the person will have a laryngectomy tube and a nasogastric tube in place.

✔ Communication is impaired because of the loss of ability to speak and the person will require speech rehabilitation.

✔ Tracheoesophageal speech is becoming more common. In this type of speech, a tube is inserted into a tracheoesophageal fistula, diverting air from the trachea into the esophagus.

✔ Persons with a total laryngectomy will have a perma-

nent tracheostomy and need to be taught certain precautions including:

a. wearing a scarf or shirt with a closed collar of porous material.

b. using caution when showering or bathing to prevent aspiration of water into stoma.

c. checking with surgeon about swimming or boating. A special snorkel device for use with a tracheostomy is available.

d. making them aware of support groups such as laryngectomy clubs.

✔ The myocutaneous flap is the major reconstructive flap used after radical neck dissection.

QUESTIONS TO CONSIDER

- What actions can you take to prevent spreading a cold to your patients?

- Discuss the postoperative care of a person having sinus surgery or nasal surgery.

- After a laryngectomy, how would you monitor the patient? Why?

- What resources are available in your community to assist the person who is unable to speak after a total laryngectomy?

REFERENCES AND SELECTED READINGS

1. American Cancer Society: 1990 Cancer facts and figures, Atlanta, 1990, The Society.

2. Anderson S and Bouwens E: Chronic health problems: concepts and application, St Louis, 1981, The CV Mosby Co.

3. Annvas AA et al: Groningen prosthesis for voice rehabilitation after laryngectomy, Clin Otolaryngol 9:51-54, 1984.

4. Argawal MK et al: Fibrosarcoma of nose and paranasal sinuses, J Surg Oncol 15:53-57, 1987.

5. Baker KH, and Feldman JE: Cancers of the head and neck, Cancer Nursing, 10(6): 293-299, 1987.

6. Brown PF and Coleman JJ: The role of radiotherapy and musculocutaneous flaps in oropharyngocutaneous fistulas, Am J Surg 156:256-260, 1988.

7. Burke RH: A simplified nasal packing. J Oral Maxillofac Surg 43:555, 1985.

8. Carroll PF: Laryngospasm. Nurs '86 16(5):33, 1986.

9. Causes of stuffy nose: external nasal deformity, Hosp Med 21(5):194-198, 1985.

10. *Chislolm S et al: Duck-bill prosthesis: words of hope for the laryngectomy patient, Nurs '86 16(3):29-31, 1986.

11. Clark KM: Hoarseness and laryngitis. In Rakel, RE editor: Conn's current therapy 1990, Philadelphia, 1990, WB Saunders Co.

12. *DeWeese DD, Saunders WH, Schuller DE, and Schleuning AJ: Otolaryngology—head and neck surgery, ed 7, St Louis, 1988, The CV Mosby Co.

*References preceded by an asterisk are particularly well suited for student reading.

13. Ebersole P, and Hess P: Toward healthy aging, ed 3, St Louis, 1990, The CV Mosby Co.

14. Eichel B: Ethmoiditis: pathophysiology and medical management, Otolaryngol Clin North Am 18(1):43-53, 1985.

15. Estelle R, Simons R, and Simons KJ: Pharmacologic treatment of rhinitis, Clin Rev Allergy 2:237-253, 1984.

16. *Feinstein D: What to teach the patient who's had a total laryngectomy, RN 50(4):53-57, 1987.

17. Fiumara NJ: Pharyngeal infection with *Neisseria* gonorrhea, Sex Transm Dis: 6:264-266, 1979.

18. Fosso BA: Sore throat, antibiotics and rheumatic fever, Fam Pract 2:101-107, 1985.

19. *Gannon EP: Giving your patient meticulous mouth care, Nurs '80 10(3):70-75, 1980.

20. Gantz NM: Streptococcal pharyngitis. In Rakel RE editor: Conn's current therapy 1990, Philadelphia, 1990. WB Saunders Co.

21. *Griffin CW et al: Learning to swallow again. Am J Nurs 87:314-315, 1987.

22. *Harris LL and Kraege J: After T-E puncture: relearning to speak, Am J Nurs 86(1):55-58, 1986.

23. Harold ML: Rehabilitation of the dysphagic client following ablative surgery for laryngeal cancer, J Soc Otorhinolaryngol Head Neck Nurses 5(2):16-18, 1987.

24. Hassard AD and Holness RO: The "crossbow" incision and nasal flap: its blood supply and clinical application, Head Neck Surg 7:135-138, 1984.

25. Hendrickson FR: Radiation therapy treatment of larynx cancers, Cancer 55:2058-2061, 1985.

26. Hillel AD, Kross H, Dorman J, and Medieros J: Radical neck dissection: a subjective and objective evaluation of postoperative disability, J Otolaryngol 18(1):53-61, 1989.

27. *Hirsch JE: Ear, nose and throat. In Thompson JM et al: Mosbys' manual of clinical nursing, ed 2, St Louis, 1989, The CV Mosby Co.

28. Holt JE: Orbital blowout fractures, Ear Nose Throat J 62:346-351, 1983.

29. *Hutton B and Hutton J: Living with facial prosthesis: a guide to patient care, Am J Nurs 84(1):50-52, 1984.

30. Innes AJ and Gates N: ENT surgery and disorders, with notes on nursing care and clinical management, London, 1985, Faber and Faber.

31. Jafek BW: Intranasal ethmoidectomy, Otolaryngol Clin North Am 18(1):61-67, 1985.

32. Johnson JT, Neman RK, and Olson JE: Persistent hoarseness: an aggressive approach for early detection of laryngeal cancer, Postgrad Med 67:122-126, 1980.

33. *Kane KK: Carotid artery rupture in advanced head and neck cancer patients, Oncol Nurs Forum 10(1):14-18, 1983.

34. *Kennedy DW et al: Endoscopic sinus surgery: ambulatory surgery, AORN J 42:932-936, 1985.

35. Kennedy DW and Shikhani AH: Sinusitis. In Rakel, RE editor: Conn's current therapy 1990, Philadelphia 1990, WB Saunders Co.

36. *Key G: Stopping nosebleeds in the elderly: pressure, cautery, or packing? Geriatrics 36:74-80, 1981.

37. Knegt PP et al: Carcinoma of the paranasal sinuses: results of a prospective pilot study, Cancer 56:57-62, 1985.

38. Konda M et al: Prognostic factors influencing relapse of squamous cell carcinoma of the maxillary sinus, Cancer 55:190-196, 1985.

39. Konrad HR: Carcinoma of the larynx, Hosp Med 20(8):165-179, 1984.

40. Krupp MA, Chatton MJ, and Werdegar D: Current medical diagnoses and treatment, 1985, Los Altos, Calif, 1985, Lange Medical Publications.

41. Larsen GL: Rehabilitation for the patient with head and neck cancer, Am J Nurs 82:119-120, 1982.

42. Lucente FE: Psychological problems in otolaryngology, Laryngoscope 83:1684-1689, 1973.

43. *Lyons RJ: Surgical implants: voice prosthesis, AORN J 37:1369-1373, 1983.

44. *Lyons RJ: The head and neck patient, AORN J 40:751-760, 1984.

45. Mack RM: Lessons from living with cancer, N Engl J Med 311:1640-1644, 1984.

46. Mandel JH: Pharyngeal infections: causes, findings, and management, Postgrad Med 77:187-193, 1985.

47. *Mahon SM: Nursing interventions for the patient with a myocutaneous flap, Cancer Nurs 10(1):21-31, 1987.

48. McCormick GP et al: Artificial speech devices, Am J Nurs 82:121-122, 1982.

49. Medina JE: Editorial: a rational classification of neck dissections, Otolaryngol Head Neck Surg 100(3):169-176, 1989.

50. Minx SM et al: Carcinoma of the parasinus: perioperative nursing responsibilities, AORN J 42:671-681, 1985.

51. Moore JC: Establishment of an outpatient ENT clinic, AORN J 31:620-626, 1980.

52. Neal GD: External ethmoidectomy, Otolaryngol Clin North Am 18:55-60, 1985.

53. Norante JD: Surgical management of sinusitis, Ear Nose Throat J 63:155-162, 1984.

54. Norris JL: Fiberoptic endoscopy: where to go from here, laryngoscopy, AANA J 52:611-613, 1984.

55. *Oser J: Oral cancer; coping with the changes, Am J Nurs 79:1418-1419, 1979.

56. Parsons JT et al: Neck dissection after twice-a-day radiotherapy: morbidity and recurrence rates, Head Neck, 11(5):400-404, 1989.

57. *Patry-Lahey R: Doing it better: helping a laryngectomy patient go home, Nursing '85, 15(3):63-64, 1985.

58. Richardson JL: Vocational adjustment after total laryngectomy, Arch Phys Med Rehabil 64:172-175, 1983.

59. *Rodzwic D and Donnard J: The use of myocutaneous flaps in reconstructive surgery for head and neck cancer, Oncol Nurs Forum 13(3):29-34, 1986.

60. Romm S: Cancer of the larynx: current concepts of diagnosis and treatment, Surg Clin North Am 66:109-118, 1986.

61. Schweiger J: Oral assessment, Am J Nurs 80:654-657, 1980.

62. Segal C, et al: Adenotonsillectomies on a surgical day-clinic basis, Laryngoscope 93:1205-1208, 1983.

63. Singer MI, Blom ED, and Hamaker RC: Voice rehabilitation after total laryngectomy, J Otolaryngol 12:329-334, 1983.

64. *Stephens DJ: An information guide for patients receiving head and neck irradiation, Oncol Nurs Forum 11(5):75-80, 1984.

65. *Ulbricht GF: Laryngectomy rehabilitation: a woman's viewpoint, Women Health 11:131-136, 1986.

66. Weingrad DN and Spiro RH: Complications after laryngectomy, Am J Surg 146:517-520, 1983.

67. Wetmore SJ et al: Long-term results of the Blom-Singer speech rehabilitation procedure, Arch Otolaryngol 111:106-109, 1985.

68. Wyngaarden JB and Smith LH: Cecil textbook of medicine, ed 18, Philadelphia, 1988, WB Saunders Co.

69. Yarington CT: The Calwell-Luc operation revisited, Ann Otol Rhinol Laryngol 93:380-384, 1984.

CHAPTER 33

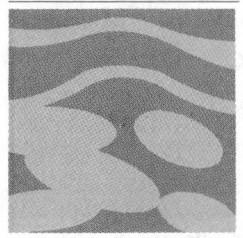

Management of Persons with Problems of the Lower Airway

JOSEPHINE BRUCIA
WILMA J. PHIPPS
DENISE KRESEVIC
MARY NACCAROTO

CHAPTER OBJECTIVES

After studying this chapter, the student should be able to:
1 Differentiate between restrictive and obstructive pulmonary disorders.
2 Describe the nature of viral respiratory infections and methods of assisting effective coughing.
3 Compare classic, atypical, aspiration, and hematogenous pneumonias.
4 Describe incidence, preventive measures, and therapeutic approaches to tuberculosis.
5 Compare fungal infections of the respiratory tract.
6 Explain the pathophysiology of adult respiratory distress syndrome (ARDS).
7 Describe incidence, prevention, and therapy for lung cancer.
8 Explain the pathophysiology of and interventions for chronic obstructive pulmonary disease.
9 Discuss the clinical manifestations of cystic fibrosis (CF) in adults.
10 Explain current therapy used to treat adults with CF.
11 Describe the nature of respiratory failure and the care of the patient with an artificial airway and mechanical ventilation.

Many diseases affect the respiratory system, including both acute (short-term) and chronic (long-term) diseases. Substantial changes in the relative incidence of diseases affecting the respiratory system have occurred in the past few decades. Although chronic infectious disorders, such as tuberculosis, lung abscess, and bronchiectasis, have decreased, persons with chronic bronchitis and emphysema now survive longer and constitute an increasing number of persons with chronic respiratory disease, along with those with environmental lung disease. In addition, modern intercontinental travel has increased the incidence of parasitic lung infestations in the western world. Also, the reduction of immunologic competence that occurs with cancer chemotherapy, immunosuppressant medications administered af-

ter organ transplantation, or with acquired immune deficiency syndrome (AIDS) has resulted in an increased incidence of opportunistic infections of the lungs with a variety of microorganisms that were rarely pathogenic in the past.

The most significant pulmonary diseases are those that are chronic and have increased dramatically in recent years. Current statistics indicate that 17 million Americans suffer from emphysema, asthma, and chronic bronchitis. This number can be expected to increase yearly as the number of elderly persons in our society increases. Since most diseases of the respiratory tract are not reportable, the full extent of both acute and chronic illness is difficult to estimate. However, known facts about disability from chronic pulmonary diseases indicate that they are a major health problem and that they cause tremendous losses in the nation's productivity. The Social Security Administration reports that disability payments to persons with chronic pulmonary problems are second only to payments to persons with heart problems. Whereas mortality from tuberculosis has declined, mortality from bronchitis, emphysema, and cancer of the lung has continued to rise yearly.

The objectives of health education in relation to pulmonary diseases are the same as for other diseases. Prevention, early diagnosis, prompt and often continued treatment, limitation of disability, and rehabilitation should be emphasized for all persons. Early symptoms of respiratory diseases are probably those most often ignored by the general population. With the exception of acute pulmonary disorders, the major factor preventing early diagnosis and treatment of pulmonary diseases is the insidious nature of their signs and symptoms. Nurses should encourage individuals and families to seek proper medical attention if they have symptoms such as *cough, difficulty in breathing, production of sputum, shortness of breath,* and *nose and throat irri-*

tation that do not subside within 2 weeks. These symptoms are suggestive of respiratory diseases and should be investigated.

In recent years, many organizations, most notably the American Lung Association (ALA), the American Cancer Society (ACS), and the federal government, have launched campaigns to reduce cigarette smoking in the United States. The stated objective of the federal government was to reduce the proportion of smokers in the national population to 25% by 1990. A major emphasis has been on preventing children and teenagers from beginning to smoke. These campaigns have been somewhat successful. Based on data from National Health Interview Surveys (1974 to 1985) it is estimated that by 1990 only 22% of the United States adult population will be smokers. The data indicate that differences in smoking prevalence has decreased between males and females, with females continuing to smoke. Additionally, although smoking has declined in general, it has declined less among the less well educated.[45,94]

National surveys have found that the percentage of adult male smokers has declined from 51% in 1965 to 34% in 1985. However, the percentage of women smokers has only decreased from 33% in 1965 to 28% in 1985. The small decrease in female smokers is a result of the large percentage (40%) of young women smokers. An unfortunate consequence of this relative shift in the proportion of smokers who are female has been an increase in morbidity and mortality from lung disease, especially cancer of the lung and COPD.

Along with the campaign to decrease smoking, there has been increased emphasis on reducing pollution in the environment, which has resulted in legislation such as the Clean Air Act. With the resurgent use of wood stoves, particularly in urban areas, wood smoke has become the nations's major source of pollutants suspected to be potent carcinogens (polycyclic organic matter). Under the auspices of the Clean Air Act, the U.S. Environmental Protection Agency has taken action to implement a nationwide emissions control program for wood stoves. Some of the measures taken to reduce pollution are presently under threat, since they are believed by some to be too costly for the benefits achieved. This issue will be at the forefront during the 1990s, and nurses as health professionals and concerned citizens will need to keep themselves informed about proposed changes and their effects on health.

Nurses seeking current information about respiratory diseases and their treatment are referred to the ALA and its local branches for information. The American Thoracic Society, the medical section of the ALA, publishes a journal* that is an excellent source of current information on all acute and chronic respiratory diseases. The ALA also publishes the *Bulletin,* many booklets and pamphlets, and newsletters that aid nurses in educating the public and in teaching patients.

CLASSIFICATION OF PULMONARY DISORDERS

One way to classify lung diseases is to differentiate the various pulmonary disorders on the basis of how they affect ventilation. This system divides pulmonary disorders into either restrictive or obstructive ventilatory defects. A third category of pulmonary disorders consists of those that affect the pulmonary vascular system and thus alter the ability of the lung to carry out respiration.

Although it is convenient to classify pulmonary disorders according to these categories, pulmonary diseases rarely fall exclusively into one of the three groupings. Of the three categories, *obstructive airway disease* (OAD), has been most criticized as being inaccurate and misleading because it implies that the primary pathology of diseases falling within this category is obstruction of the airways. For example, emphysema, a major obstructive airway disease, causes limitation to expiratory airflow by enlargement of alveolar airspace through tissue destruction, rather than by primary airway obstruction. Pulmonary experts have recommended that diseases resulting in diminished expiratory airflow be identified as syndromes of *chronic airflow limitation.* In the clinical setting, however, OAD or *chronic obstructive pulmonary disease* (COPD) continues to be the most common terminologies used to describe this group of pulmonary disorders.

Communication among health professionals is hampered by both the many terms used to label chronic airflow limitation and by inconsistent definition. Thus, pulmonary diseases fall under the classification umbrella of chronic airflow limitation, OAD, or COPD.

In *restrictive lung disease* there is a limitation to full expansion of the lungs. Static lung volumes are diminished as a result of decreased lung or thoracic compliance (Table 33-1).

TABLE 33-1 Comparison of pulmonary function test results in restrictive and obstructive disease

Test	Restrictive	Obstructive
FVC	Decreased	Decreased or normal
RV	Decreased	Increased
TLC	Decreased	Normal or increased
RV/TLC	Normal or increased	Significantly increased
$FEV_{1.0}$/FVC	Normal or increased	Decreased
$FEV_{3.0}$/FVC	Normal or increased	Decreased

From Morrissey W: Respiratory diseases. In Kaye D, and Rose LF (editors): Fundamentals of internal medicine, St Louis, 1983, The CV Mosby Co.

*American Review of Respiratory Diseases, published by the American Lung Association, 1740 Broadway, New York, NY.

Patients with a restrictive disorder may demonstrate respiratory alkalosis caused by a compensatory increase in respiratory frequency (rate) to offset diminished lung volumes. When the increased respiratory rate no longer adequately compensates for the diminished lung volumes, *hypoxemia* (low arterial blood oxygen) occurs. Clinically, persons with restrictive disorders exhibit some degree of dyspnea. Often they will become dyspneic only on exertion. However, as the restrictive disease progresses they will become dyspneic at rest. Additionally, persons with restrictive disorders often have a dry hacking cough. Major disorders that result in primarily restrictive ventilatory defects are indicated in the box below.

Obstructive airway disease includes any process that limits airflow on expiration. Both lung compliance (lung expansibility) and airway resistance are increased. These pathophysiologic changes alter the ability to move air out of the lungs, which results in characteristic changes in both static and dynamic lung volume measurement (see Table 33-1). Clinically, persons with obstructive airway disease may exhibit a prolonged expiration time, increased anterior-posterior thorax diameter, and hyperresonance upon percussion. Persons with pulmonary disorders characterized by the preceding description have been identified as having COPD, which has classically included any mixture of *emphysema,* *chronic bronchitis,* and *asthma,* although some experts believe that asthma should not be included. The ongoing controversy over what should or should not be included under COPD lends support to those who argue that the classic subdivisions of COPD be abandoned and that all be classified as chronic airflow limitation.[14,107] However, because COPD is the most commonly used terminology in the clinical setting, discussion of COPD in this chapter will include these three conditions.

The third category of pulmonary disorders that will be considered in this chapter is those identified as resulting in *pulmonary vascular disease.* Pulmonary vascular diseases include any process that results in the narrowing or occlusion of pulmonary blood vessels. In pulmonary vascular disease efficiency of pulmonary respiration is compromised, usually resulting in hypoxemia. Clinically patients present with *dyspnea, increased respiratory frequency, digital clubbing, atelectasis, and chest pain.* Pulmonary vascular disease may result from primary pulmonary hypertension or as a sequelae of either circulatory or lung disease. Only pulmonary vascular disease related to pulmonary emboli and pulmonary infarction will be discussed. In this chapter restrictive diseases are presented first, beginning with the infectious diseases. Obstructive lung diseases and pulmonary vascular diseases are discussed later in the chapter.

RESTRICTIVE LUNG DISEASE

INFECTIOUS DISEASES OF THE PULMONARY TRACT

The respiratory tract is in contact with the environment via inhalation of ambient air. Fortunately the lung has a variety of defense mechanisms to prevent contamination of the respiratory tract with infectious agents. These mechanisms are outlined in the box on pp. 874-875.

VIRAL INFECTIONS

Many acute respiratory disorders are caused by viral pathogens. Presently, over 30 have been found to be directly related to viral infections, and there are probably many more. Some diseases may be caused by one virus, or different viruses may cause the same symptoms. Although viral respiratory infections such as the common cold tend to be self-limiting, certain viral strains can induce life-threatening illness by themselves or as a result of secondary bacterial infections.

Common Cold, Influenza

Epidemiology and etiology. Few persons escape upper respiratory tract infections (URI). The average among the general population is three colds per person each year. Indeed, Americans spend more than 380 million days in bed each year because of colds and influenza.

Respiratory diseases, primarily virus infections, are responsible for 30% to 50% of time lost from work by adults and from 60% to 80% of time lost by children from school. The frequency of their occurrence, the number of people affected, the resulting economic loss, and the possibility that URI may lead to more serious diseases are reasons why colds and influenza merit serious attention.

The specific virus causing the common cold is unknown. Influenza is usually caused by one of three myxoviruses that are categorized as influenza types A, B, or C. Type A influenza virus has a greater tendency to mutate than the other viral types; thus it is more often the strain that causes worldwide epidemics.

RESTRICTIVE PULMONARY DISEASES

ALTERATION	DISEASE EXAMPLE
Parenchymal inflammation	Pneumonia, adult respiratory distress syndrome
Space occupying lesions	Tumors, malignancies
Diffuse pulmonary disease	Silicosis, fibrosis
Pleural disease	Pleural effusion
Lung collapse	Pneumothorax, atelectasis
Resectional surgery	Pneumonectomy
Neuromuscular disorders	Poliomyelitis, Guillain-Barré syndrome
CNS depression	Narcotics, cerebral edema

LUNG DEFENSE MECHANISMS*

1. Upper airway defenses against pulmonary infection
   a. Removing particulate matter from inspired air
      (1) Particles greater than 20 μm settle back on surfaces
      (2) Particles 5-10 μm deposited in nose
      (3) Particles 0.1-10 μm remain suspended in air for long periods and are then inhaled
      (4) Particles 1-5 μm deposited in tracheobronchial tree
         (a) Droplet nuclei 2-4 μm (dried particles from sneezing, coughing, talking)
         (b) May contain viruses or bacteria
         (c) Spread organisms from person to person
   b. Minimizing the microbial population on membranes of upper respiratory tract
      (1) Mucociliary transport
         (a) Posterior two thirds of nasal cavity, sinuses, and nasopharynx lined by *ciliated epithelium* covered with thin layer of mucus
         (b) Dense concentration of small blood vessels present beneath ciliated epithelium and mucous layers
         (c) Mucus and fluid produced = 1000 ml/24 hr in normal persons
         (d) Mucus and fluid carried at rate of 5-10 mm/minute back into hypopharynx by beating action of cilia
         (e) Substances in secretions inhibit microbial growth and prevent organisms from sticking to mucous membranes
            i. Immunoglobulins (secretory IgA)
            ii. Lysozyme
            iii. Complement
   c. Minimizing possibility of aspiration
      (1) Motor function of upper airway
         (a) Laryngeal mechanism—closes glottis when swallowing to protect larynx
            i. Gag reflex also closes glottis
            ii. Clearing throat, spitting, clears upper airway
      (2) Contamination of lower respiratory tract
         (a) Impaired clearance of particles in upper airway = spread of bacteria
         (b) Accumulation of debris and microbes → penetration of tissues = sinusitis, otitis media
         (c) Accumulation of debris and microbes → aspiration into trachea; lung abscess caused by anaerobic bacteria secondary to severe gingival disease
         (d) Intoxication or distraction → aspiration
         (e) Normal sleep → minor aspiration
         (f) Aspiration of pharyngeal contents → lung → bacterial pneumonia
2. Lower respiratory tract clearance mechanisms
   a. Pulmonary reflex
      (1) Cough—an involuntary reflex elicited by stimulation of irritant receptors in subepithelium of hypopharynx, larynx, and tracheobronchial tree: mediated by vagus nerve
         (a) Facilitator of mucociliary clearance
         (b) Aids in dealing with gross contamination from above larynx
      (2) Bronchoconstriction—reflex response to airway irritants
         (a) Decreased size of bronchus and forced expiration and cough propel debris toward mouth
         (b) Excessive bronchoconstriction (asthma) = decreased expiratory airflow, air trapped in lung, effective cough difficult
   b. Mucociliary clearance
      (1) Mucus secreted by epithelial goblet cells from submucosal glands 0.10-100 ml passes up trachea into hypopharynx and is swallowed; amount and nature of mucus secreted are controlled, in part, by parasympathetic nervous system affected by neurohumoral stimulation (adrenergic or cholinergic), and by direct mucosal irritation
      (2) Cilia (200 cilia/each cell surface) beat rhythmically 1200 beats/min mouthward beginning at terminal bronchioles → larynx; beating of cilia → overlying mucous layer → mouthward at rate of 0.5 mm/min in small airways to about 10 mm/min in major bronchi

*Adapted from Light B: Respiratory infections. In Kryger MH, editor: Pathophysiology of respiration, New York, 1981, John Wiley & Sons Inc.

LUNG DEFENSE MECHANISMS—cont'd

(3) Clearance increased by:
  (a) Bronchodilator drugs
    i. β-Adrenergic agents (ephedrine) stimulate transport of water and salt into mucus = ↓ viscosity of mucus
    ii. Methylxanthines (aminophylline)— ↑ mucus production and ciliary activity
(4) Ciliary function depressed by:
  (a) Chronic exposure to airway irritants—cigarette smoke and other irritants
  (b) Pharmacologic agents—100% O_2, anticholinergic agents, alcohol
  (c) Infection such as viral bronchitis
(5) Mucus production increased by:
  (a) Chronic irritation of respiratory tract → increase in number of mucus-secreting goblet cells = ↑ mucus
  (b) Inflammatory response to irritatin→ ↑ numbers of phagocytic cells and amount of cellular debris in mucus (especially DNA = ↑ viscosity of mucus, which is less readily moved along by ciliary action
(6) Immotile cilia—congenital impairment
  (a) *Kartagener's syndrome*—sinusitis, recurrent lung infection, and sinusitis
  (b) *Cystic fibrosis*—infection, chronic inflammatory increases in respiratory mucus volume and viscosity = impaired lung clearance and progressive lung damage
3. Intrapulmonary detoxification mechanisms
  a. Phagocytes
    (1) Alveolar macrophage
      (a) Phagocytosis of particles—inhaled particulate debris, bacteria, or cell constituents
      (b) Kills most microbes
    (2) Polymorphonuclear neutrophil present in blood (normally only small number in lung)
      (a) Avid phagocyte—kills microbes
      (b) Defends against established infectious processes
      (c) Infection—products of inflammation attract neutrophils to site of infection (chemotoaxis)
    (3) Factors interfering with phagocytosis
      (a) Inhibition of alveolar macrophage function
        i. Cigarette smoke
        ii. Other inhaled pollutants—ozone, nitrogen dioxide, oxygen
        iii. Drugs—corticosteroids, antineoplastic and antiinflammatory cytoxic agents, and ethanol (alcohol)
        iv. Metabolic derangements—uremia, hyperglycemia of diabetes mellitus
        v. Acquired granulocytopenia—bone marrow depression from cytotoxic drugs and other drugs
  b. Immunoglobulins
    (1) IgG and IgA—most important for lung defense; present in secretion of respiratory tract as well as in blood
      (a) IgA antibodies—specific for viral antigens; neutralize viruses and prevent infection
      (b) IgA predominates in terminal lung units; antigen-specific IgG contributes to local defense against bacterial infections (important in neutralizing highly pathogenic encapsulated bacteria (especially *Streptococcus pneumoniae* and *Haemophilus influenzae*), which are resistant to phagocytosis)
  c. Cell-mediated immunity (CMI)
    (1) One half of lymphocytes in and around airways are thymus-derived lymphocytes, or *T cells*
      (a) Found in lymphoid aggregates adjacent to bronchi (bronchus-associated lymphoid tissues, or BALT)
      (b) T cells important in:
        i. Resistance to some viral infections
        ii. Resistance to most fungal infections
        iii. Infections by organisms that survive and multiply inside host cells: *Mycobacterium* tuberculosis, *Brucella, Listeria monocytogenes,* and *Pneumocystis carinii*
    (2) Impaired CMI = ↑ susceptibility to infection
      (a) Deficient T cell function (anergy) associated with:
        i. Neoplasms—lymphoma
        ii. Cytotoxic or corticosteroid therapy
        iii. Systemic diseases—sarcoidosis, malnutrition
      (b) Some lung infections occur almost exclusively in severely impaired CMI—pneumonia caused by cytomegalovirus, herpes zoster, *Aspergillus* species, or *P. carinii*

SIGNS AND SYMPTOMS UPPER RESPIRATORY INFECTION

SIGNS	SYMPTOMS
Cough	General malaise
Nasal discharge	Rhinitis
Erythematous pharynx	Sore throat
Conjunctivitis	Watery eyes
Laryngitis	
Low-grade temperature	

MANAGEMENT OF UPPER RESPIRATORY INFECTION

1. Increased fluid intake (3 to 4 L/day)
2. Frequent rest periods
3. Medications:
   a. Antipyretics/analgesics: acetylsalicylic acid, acetaminophen
   b. Oral decongestants: pseudephedrine
   c. Nasal decongestants: ephedrine, 0.5% to 2% NOTE: use of nasal decongestants should be time limited to avoid increasing severity of nasal symptoms
   d. Cough suppressants: glycerol guaiacolate

Prevention. Colds and influenza are communicable diseases spread by droplet nuclei. The only known way to totally prevent spread of URIs from one individual to another is to isolate the infected person, which is extremely difficult in our society. However, there are several ways to minimize the spread of infection. Persons with colds should avoid crowded places such as theaters. The individual should particularly avoid contact with and, therefore, exposure of infants and young children, persons who have chronic lung diseases such as bronchitis and emphysema, those who have recently had an anesthetic, and elderly people. Covering the nose and mouth when sneezing and coughing prevents the contamination of the air breathed by others. Frequent *washing of hands, covering of coughs and sneezes,* and *careful disposal of waste tissues* are *protective health measures* that are advisable for everyone; but they become increasingly important when known respiratory tract infection exists. Because colds and influenza are communicable diseases, the principles for protection of oneself and others should be practiced.

Clinical manifestations. Symptoms of either a cold or influenca usually appear suddenly, and the infection may be full-blown within 48 hours. The signs and symptoms commonly associated with a URI are presented in the box above left.

The infected individual is contagious for 2 to 3 days after onset of symptoms. The course of a URI is variable but ordinarily lasts from 7 to 14 days. It is difficult to determine when a cold or influenza ends and when complications appear. Tracheobronchitis is a complication usually caused by a secondary bacterial infection. Acute sinusitis and otitis media may also follow a URI.

Medical and nursing management. Treatment of colds and influenza is directed toward relief of symptoms and control of complications. Persons considered to be at higher risk, such as those with chronic lung disease or those who are immunologically compromised, should be encouraged to seek medical assistance. Additionally, persons who display a continued temperature elevation,

headache, or muscular aches should seek the advice of a physician. General treatment of URI symptoms is indicated in the box above.

Additionally, influenza vaccine should be given yearly to all persons at high risk for developing complications of influenza. The vaccine is recommended for all persons with chronic heart or lung disease unless they are allergic to eggs or egg products or have had a previous reaction to the vaccine. It is also recommended for all persons age 65 or older since they are at high risk of developing complications from influenza.

Acute Bronchitis

Epidemiology and etiology. Bronchitis can be acute or chronic (chronic bronchitis will be discussed later in this chapter). Acute bronchitis is an inflammation of the bronchi and sometimes the trachea (tracheobronchitis). Although it occurs most often in persons with chronic lung disease, it also occurs as an extension of an upper respiratory infection in persons without underlying lung disease and is therefore communicable. It also may be caused by physical or chemical agents such as dust, smoke, or volatile fumes. As air pollution increases, the incidence of acute bronchitis increases. Acute bronchitis is typically viral in origin, but bacterial pathogens such as *Streptococcus pneumoniae* and *Haemophilus influenzae* may also cause bronchitis either as a primary or secondary infection.

Clinical manifestations. The signs and symptoms usually seen in a person with acute bronchitis are presented in the box on p. 877.

In addition to the signs and symptoms noted above, any of the signs and symptoms associated with the common cold or influenza may be present.

■ Assessment

Subjective data. Subjective data include the following:

1. Onset and duration of symptoms; pay particular attention to history of sputum; amount, consistency, and color changes; in persons with COPD,

SIGNS AND SYMPTOMS OF ACUTE BRONCHITIS

SYMPTOMS	SIGNS
Cough	Sputum production: Viral-clear to mucopurulent; bacterial-purulent
Chest pain	Tachypnea Diffuse rhonchi/wheezes Chest x-ray—clear, differentiates bronchitis from pneumonia

the only change in pulmonary status may be a change of sputum from thin and clear to purulent and tenacious

2. History of previous pulmonary illness
3. Self-care modalities used to treat the symptoms
4. History of exposure to lung irritants (smoking habits, occupational history)

Objective data. Objective data include the following:

1. Vital signs—possible temperature elevation; tachypnea frequent with severe bronchitis
2. Sputum color and consistency
3. Pulmonary examination (see Chapter 31)
   a. Inspection—observe for use of accessory muscle breathing
   b. Palpation—should be within normal limits
   c. Percussion—should be within normal limits
   d. Auscultation—vesicular and bronchovesicular breath sounds, normal voice sounds, adventitious sounds—diffuse rhonchi/wheezing

■ **Data analysis: nursing diagnoses.** Nursing diagnoses are determined from an assessment of patient data. Possible nursing diagnoses for the person with acute bronchitis may include but are not limited to:

Diagnostic Title	Possible Etiologies
Airway clearance, ineffective	Tracheobronchial infection
Breathing pattern, ineffective	Decreased energy/fatigue
Knowledge deficit: condition and its treatment	Lack of information
Pain	Inflammation of tracheobronchial tree

■ **Planning: expected patient outcomes.** Expected patient outcomes for the patient with acute bronchitis may include, but are not limited to the following:

1. Patient can describe the cause and factors contributing to the occurrence of acute bronchitis and name common symptoms of it
2. Patient can demonstrate effective cough with adequate sputum production
   a. Both cough and sputum production will decrease within 72 hours of treatment initiation.
   b. For persons with chronic lung disease, sputum

will become clear and thin (return to prebronchitis status).
3. Patient can demonstrate effective breathing patterns
4. Patient can demonstrate prebronchitis vital signs
5. Patient reports that chest pain is absent

■ **Implementation**

Viral acute bronchitis. Implementations for viral acute bronchitis are as follows:

1. Management is the same as for URI (see the box on p. 876).
2. Humidification of immediate ambient air
3. Promote effective coughing, breathing, and sputum production (see details in discussion on chronic obstructive pulmonary disease, p. 923)

Bacterial primary or secondary infection. Interventions for bacterial primary or secondary infections are as follows:

1. Same as for viral bronchitis
2. Antibiotic therapy
   a. Ampicillin, 250 mg, four times a day to 500 mg every 6 hours, or
   b. Tetracycline, 250 mg, four times a day or every 6 hours
3. Bronchodilator
   a. Aminophylline, 200 mg, four times a day

BACTERIAL INFECTIONS

Pneumonia

Epidemiology/etiology. Pneumonia is an acute inflammation of lung tissue resulting from inhalation or transport via the bloodstream of infectious agents or noxious fumes or from radiation treatment. Of all the infectious diseases, pneumonia is the leading cause of death in the United States. Over 3 million cases of pneumonia occur in the United States yearly.[17] Risk factors commonly associated with the incidence of various types of pneumonia are included in Table 33-2.

Most pneumonias are communicable diseases; the mode of transmission depends on the infecting organism. Pneumonia is classified according to the offending organism rather than the anatomic location (lobar or bronchial) as was the practice in the past. A recent classification of infectious pneumonia in adults is presented in the box on p. 880.

Prevention. Preventive measures differ, depending on the type of pneumonia that the person is at risk of developing within a given environment. Table 33-3 identifies the various preventive activities associated with certain pneumonia types.

Pathophysiology. Pneumonia results in inflammation of lung tissue. Depending on the particular pathogen and

TABLE 33-2 Etiology, signs and symptoms, and pharmacotherapy of pneumonia

Pneumonia	Etiology	Risk Factors	Signs and Symptoms	Pharmacotherapy
Typical syndrome	S. pneumoniae; uncomplicated	Sickle-cell disease; hypogammaglobulinemia; multiple myeloma	Sudden onset with shaking chill; fever (39° to 40° C; 102.2° to 104°), pleuritic chest pain, productive cough; Sputum—green and purulent and may be blood tinged, "rusty"; respirations—rapid and shallow with "grunting" at end of each breath; nasal flaring, intercostal rib retraction, use of accessory muscles, cyanosis may be present	Drugs of choice: penicillin G procaine, IM; aqueous crystalline penicillin G, IV; penicillin V Other effective drugs: erythromycin, clindamycin, cephalosporins, other penicillins, trimethoprim with sulfamethoxazole
	Streptococcus complicated (empyema, metastatic infection) H. influenzae S. aureus	Advanced age COPD Alcoholism Recent influenza		Drugs of choice: penicillin G; ampicillin Other effective drugs: chloramphenicol, cefamandole, trimethoprim with sulfamethoxazole nafcillin Other effective drugs: methicillin; oxacillin; cefazolin; cephalothin; vancomycin; clindamycin; vancomycin, IV; Cefazolin, IV; plus gentamicin or tobramycin
Atypical syndrome	Common causes: mycoplasma pneumonia, viral pathogens	Childhood Young adults	Onset gradual over 3-5 days Malaise, headache, sore throat, dry cough May have chest wall soreness from coughing	Drug of choice: erythromycin Other effective drugs; tetracycline
	Uncommon cause: Legionella pneumophila	Recent URI influenza	Above plus abdominal pain and diarrhea Temperature 40° C (104° F) or greater Shaking chills Respiratory distress Renal failure, hyponatremia hypophysphatemia, elevated creatine phosphokinase	None Drug of choice: erythromycin Other effective drugs: rifampin, gentamicin
	P. carinii	Renal transplantation Autoimmune disease Immunologic deficiency Debilitation	Rapid or gradual onset with increasing dyspnea, dry cough, tachypnea hypoxemia X-ray—diffuse interstitial involvement	Trimethoprim Pentamidine
Aspiration	Aspiration of: gram-negative bacilli; Klebsiella, Pseudomonas, Serratia, Enterobacter, Escherichia, Proteus; gram-positive bacilli;	Alcoholism Debilitation Hospitalization nosocomial infection	Mixed anerobic: At first gradual onset Low-grade fever, cough Sputum-increased production, musty smelling Chest x-ray—interstitial involvement in dependent portion of lung	Antibiotic therapy dependent on pathogen-causing infection

TABLE 33-2 Etiology, signs and symptoms, and pharmacotherapy of pneumonia

Pneumonia	Etiology	Risk Factors	Signs and Symptoms	Pharmacotherapy
	Staphylococcus Gastric acid aspiration	Altered consciousness	*Gram-negative or gram-positive infection:* May also present same clinical picture as classic pneumonia; sudden onset of respiratory distress, severe dyspnea, cyanosis, coughing, hypoxemia, followed by signs and symptoms of secondary infection	
	Aspiration of inert substances, water, barium, nutritional supplements			
Hematogenous	Occurs when pathogens are spread to lungs via bloodstream, *Staphylococcus*, *E. coli*, enteric anerobes	Infected intravascular catheter Endocarditis IV drug abuse Intra-abdominal abscess Pyonephrosis Empyema of gallbladder	Pulmonary symptoms minimal compared with the symptoms of septicemia; most common complaints— nonproductive cough and pleuritic pain similar to that seen in *pulmonary embolism*	Drugs of choice: Nafcillin, IV; ampicillin, IV; plus gentamicin or tobramycin; clindamycin, IV; plus gentamicin or tobramycin

TABLE 33-3 Preventive modalities

Specific Pneumonia	Modality	Specific Pneumonia	Modality
Streptococcal	Pneumonia polysaccharide vaccine for those at high-risk, effective 3 to 5 years against multiple strains of pneumococcal polysaccharides	Aspiration	Positioning patients with decreased consciousness to facilitate drainage of secretions Inflating endotracheal or tracheostomy cuff before feeding
Gram-negative and gram-positive	Frequent handwashing Adequate ventilation Every 24 hours: Change open container solutions Change respiratory equipment Tracheostomy and endotracheal airways treated with sterile technique Sterile technique when suctioning Turning and repositioning every 2 hours Necessity of not draining condensation in respiratory equipment back into liquid reservoir	Viral, mycoplasma, or *P. carinii*	Ensuring proper placement of nasogastric tube before giving tube feeding Always checking for gag reflex before feeding patient with decreased consciousness Prompt treatment of unresolved URI or acute bronchitis Limiting contact with people who have viral infections Maintaining optimal nutrition

ORGANISMS CAUSING INFECTIOUS PNEUMONIA IN ADULTS*

1. Typical or classic pneumonia syndrome
   a. Bacterial pneumonia
      (1) Common
         (a) *S. pneumoniae* (also known as pneumococcal)
      (2) Uncommon
         (a) *H. influenzae*
         (b) *Staphylococcus aureus*
2. Atypical pneumonia syndrome
   a. Common
      (1) Mycoplasma pneumoniae
      (2) Viral
   b. Uncommon
      (1) *Legionella pneumophila*
      (2) *P. carinii*
3. Aspiration pneumonia syndrome
   a. Hospitalized, debilitated, or antibiotic-treated person
      (1) Mixed anaerobic/aerobic pharyngeal flora
      (2) *S. aureus*
      (3) *Klebsiella pneumoniae*
      (4) *Pseudomonas aeruginosa*
      (5) *Serratia marcescens*
      (6) *Acinetobacter* species
      (7) Enteric gram-negative aerobes *Escherichia coli, Enterobacter, Proteus*)
   b. Outpatients with normal pharyngeal flora
      (1) Mixed anaerobic/aerobic pharyngeal flora
4. Hematogenous pneumonia syndromes
   a. *S. aureus*
   b. *E. coli*
   c. Enteric/pelvic anaerobes

*Adapted from Frame PT: Acute infectious pneumonia in adults, Basics RD 10:1-8, 1982.

the physical status of the host, the inflammatory process may involve different anatomic areas of the lung parenchyma and the pleurae. The normal function, primary pathophysiology, and clinical picture of pneumonia are listed in Table 33-4.

Clinical manifestations. Clinical signs and symptoms associated with the various types of pneumonia also can be found in Table 33-4.

Medical management. Pharmacotherapy appropriate to the different types of pneumonia is presented in Table 33-2. The process of medical diagnosis of pneumonia may include any of the following investigative modalities:

1. Patient history
2. Physical examination
3. Diagnostic studies
   a. Chest x-ray to confirm lung consolidation and distribution, pleural effusion
   b. Sputum studies for culture and sensitivity; if

unable to obtain specimen by usual means, may use:
      (1) Transtracheal aspiration
      (2) Bronchoscopy with aspiration, biopsy, or bronchial brushing
   c. Arterial blood gas studies
   d. Hematology
      (1) White blood cell (WBC) count for bacterial pneumonia
      (2) Cold agglutinins and complement fixation for viral studies
   e. Thoracentesis to obtain pleural fluid specimen if pleural effusion present

■ **Assessment**

Subjective data. Subjective data include the following:

1. History of character of onset and duration of:
   a. Cough
   b. Fever
   c. Shaking chills
   d. Chest pain
   e. Sputum production (amount, color, and consistency)
2. Self-care modalities used to treat symptoms
3. History of exposure to:
   a. Persons with infection
   b. Pulmonary irritants

Objective data. Objective data include the following:
1. Observe for signs of other chronic disease and general debilitation
2. Monitor vital signs
   a. Elevated temperature (39° C to 40° C; 102.2° to 104° F) or low-grade temperature elevation
      Tachycardia
      Tachypnea
3. Pulmonary examination
   a. Inspection
      (1) Accessory muscle retraction
      (2) Central cyanosis
      (3) Respiratory grunting on expiration
      (4) Restricted chest movement
   b. Palpation
      (1) Decreased expansion on affected side of chest
      (2) Increased tactile femitus
   c. Percussion
      (1) Dullness on percussion
   d. Auscultation
      (1) Bronchial breath sounds
      (2) Inspiratory crackles (rales)
      (3) Decreased vocal fremitus (pleural effusion)
      (4) Egophony (consolidation)
4. Assess laboratory findings
   a. Chest x-ray

TABLE 33-4 Normal function, primary pathophysiology, and the clinical picture of pneumonia

Normal Function	Pathophysiology	Clinical Picture
MUCOCILIARY SYSTEM		
Cleanses inhaled air by trapping particles	Hypertrophy of mucous membrane lung lining resulting in hypersecretion	Increased sputum production and cough Anaerobic-foul-smelling sputum *Klebsiella*-current jelly color *Staphlococcus*-creamy yellow *Pseudomonas*-green Viral-mucopurulent
	Bronchospasm from increased secretions	Localized or diffuse wheezing, dyspnea
ALVEOLAR-CAPILLARY MEMBRANE		
Oxygen/carbon dioxide exchange	Increased capillary permeability resulting in excess fluid in interstitial spaces	Chest x-rays: consolidation: localized-bacterial; diffuse-viral
	Decreased surface area for gas exchange	Hypoxemia
PLEURA		
Maintains close approximation of lungs and chest wall. Minimizes friction during lung expansion and contraction	Inflammation of pleurae	Chest pain Pleural effusion Dullness on percussion Decreased breath sounds Decreased vocal fremitus
RESPIRATORY MUSCLE		
Expands and contracts chest wall, and thus pleura and lungs	Hypoventilation Respiratory acidosis (in presence of underlying disease)	Decreased chest expansion Hypercapnia and low arterial blood pH
LUNG DEFENSE SYSTEM		
Protects the normally sterile lung from invasion by pathogens	Bacteremia	Elevated white blood count: leukocytes (15,000 to 25,000/mm^3), Neutrophilia Tachypnea, fever

Diffuse involvement—atypical pneumonia (Table 33-4)

Lobar involvement—typical pneumonia (Table 33-4)

   b. Hematology

     (1) WBC—elevated 15,000 to 25,000/mm^3

     (2) Cold agglutins—complement fixation/viral or *Mycoplasma pneumoniae*

   c. Arterial blood gas studies

     (1) Hypoxemia/respiratory alkalosis

     (2) If underlying chronic disease, respiratory acidosis

■ **Data analysis: nursing diagnoses.** Nursing diagnoses are determined from assessment of patient data. Possible nursing diagnoses for the person with pneumonia may include but are not limited to:

Diagnostic Title	Possible Etiologies
Airway clearance, ineffective	Decreased energy, fatigue, tracheobronchial inflammation

Diagnostic Title	Possible Etiologies
Gas exchange, impaired	Alveolar-capillary membrane changes, altered oxygen delivery
Infection, potential for	Compromised lung defense system
Knowledge deficit: conditions and its treatment	Lack of exposure to or unfamiliarity with information
Nutrition, altered less than body requirements	Increased metabolic needs Anorexia due to infectious process, sputum production
Pain	Pleural inflammation, coughing paroxysms

■ **Planning: expected patient outcomes.** Expected patient outcomes for the person with pneumonia may include, but are not limited to:

   1. The patient can describe the cause and factors contributing to the occurrence of pneumonia and name common symptoms indicating pneumonia

   2. The patient can demonstrate absence of infection

     a. White cell count or cold agglutins return to normal

b. Body temperature returns to normal for a minimum of 24 hours

c. Sputum production returns to prepneumonia level

d. Sputum specimen is negative for pathogens

3. Patient can demonstrate effective cough with adequate sputum production. (Both cough and sputum production will decrease within 72 hours of treatment initiation. Patient with chronic lung disease will return to prepneumonia status.)

4. Patient can demonstrate improved ventilation and adequate oxygenation of tissues

a. pH returns to within normal limits

b. PaO_2 during active disease—60 to 80 torr; after resolution of disease, process PaO_2 within normal limits

5. Patient reports absence of chest pain

6. Patient can maintain prepneumonia body weight

■ **Implementation.** Nursing interventions for patients with pneumonia are similar, regardless of the type of pathogen or source of infection, and are described below.

Monitoring the infection. The infection is monitored as follows:

1. Collect sputum for culture and sensitivity before initiation of antibiotic therapy in order to identify causative agent.

2. Collect blood for culture and sensitivity.

3. Monitor vital signs and respiratory status (see objective data).

4. Initiate antibiotic therapy as ordered by physician. Monitor for hypersensitivity to antibiotic.

5. Initiate respiratory isolation using the approved procedure of institution.

6. Wash hands before and after working with patient.

Maintaining effective airway clearance. Airway clearance is maintained as follows:

1. Monitor for increased respiratory distress.

2. Assist patient to cough effectively.

3. If unable to clear own airway, suction airway using sterile technique (see Chapter 34).

4. Assist with nebulizer therapy.

5. Administer bronchodilators as ordered. Monitor for side effects and response to therapy.

6. Change position frequently to assist in mobilizing secretions.

7. Ensure fluid intake adequate to thin secretions.

8. Assist with activities of daily living (ADL), pacing activities to prevent fatigue and respiratory distress.

Maintaining adequate gas exchange. Adequate gas exchange is maintained as follows:

1. Monitor arterial blood gas results, and assess respiratory status for signs of hypoxemia and hypoventilation.

2. Encourage patient to be as active as possible without increasing respiratory distress. If comatose, turn and reposition every 2 hours, with passive range of motion (ROM) every 4 hours.

3. Encourage deep breathing every 1 to 2 hours.

a. Incentive spirometer

b. Slow inhalation, hold for few seconds, slow exhalation

Promoting comfort. Comfort is promoted as follows:

1. Assess for character and location of chest pain.

2. Administer analgesics for chest pain.

a. Acetylsalicylic acid

b. Acetaminophen

c. Codeine

3. Splint chest when patient coughs (see Chapter 34).

4. Administer frequent mouth care. Protect lips and nares with lubricant.

5. Keep patient warm and dry and avoid chilling.

Promoting adequate hydration and nutrition. Adequate hydration and nutrition are promoted as follows:

1. Encourage oral fluids. If on IV fluids, monitor rate. Observe for signs of fluid volume deficit or excess.

2. Offer small frequent feedings. Encourage high-carbohydrate and high-protein foods.

Patient teaching. Patient teaching is carried out as follows:

1. Assess understanding of pneumonia with questions concerning such factors as how transmitted and risk factors.

2. Teach proper handling of secretions. Cover nose and mouth with tissue when coughing or sneezing. Expectorate into container provided.

3. Stress importance of hand washing after coughing, sneezing, and expectorating.

4. Reinforce importance of follow-up care.

The guidelines in the box below summarize the nursing care of the person with pneumonia.

GUIDELINES FOR CARE OF THE PERSON WITH PNEUMONIA

1. Limit the impact of infection
2. Maintain effective airway clearance
3. Maintain adequate gas exchange
4. Promote comfort
5. Promote adequate hydration and nutrition
6. Teach patient how to lower the risk of recurrence

Tuberculosis

Epidemiology/etiology. In 1900 tuberculosis was the leading cause of death in the United States. It remained a major cause of death until the introduction of antituberculosis drug therapy in the late 1940s and early 1950s. The most effective of these agents is isoniazid, which first became available clinically in 1952. The use of isoniazid in combination with two agents introduced earlier, streptomycin and para-aminosalicylic acid, resulted in a striking decrease in tuberculosis death rates. It also made it possible for patients with tuberculosis to be treated on an outpatient basis. However, some patients still have to be hospitalized during their illness, and most nurses will care for a patient with tuberculosis at some time during their careers.

Although tuberculosis is now considered a preventable and curable disease, it still is a disease requiring public health attention. In 1988, there were 22,436 cases of tuberculosis reported to the Centers for Disease Control (CDC).[1] These new cases were not evenly distributed throughout the population, however, and some differences bear mentioning. The highest number of cases were in the 25 to 44 year age group, which increased by 961 cases when compared with 1985. In all other age groups, the number of cases declined. In all age groups, cases *increased* among non-Hispanic blacks and Hispanics but *decreased* among non-Hispanic whites, Asian/Pacific Islanders, and American Indians/Alaskan natives (Figure 33-1). Increases in cases occurred among both males and females. In 1988, the tu-

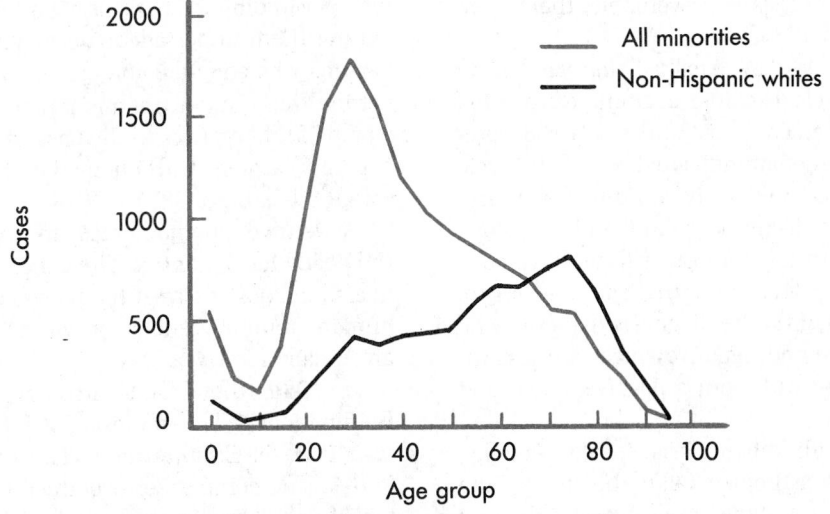

FIGURE 33-1 Frequency distribution of cases of tuberculosis by age, race, and ethnicity in the United States, 1988 (From Centers for Disease Control MMWR: update: tuberculosis elimination, United States MMWR 39(10):153-156, 1990).

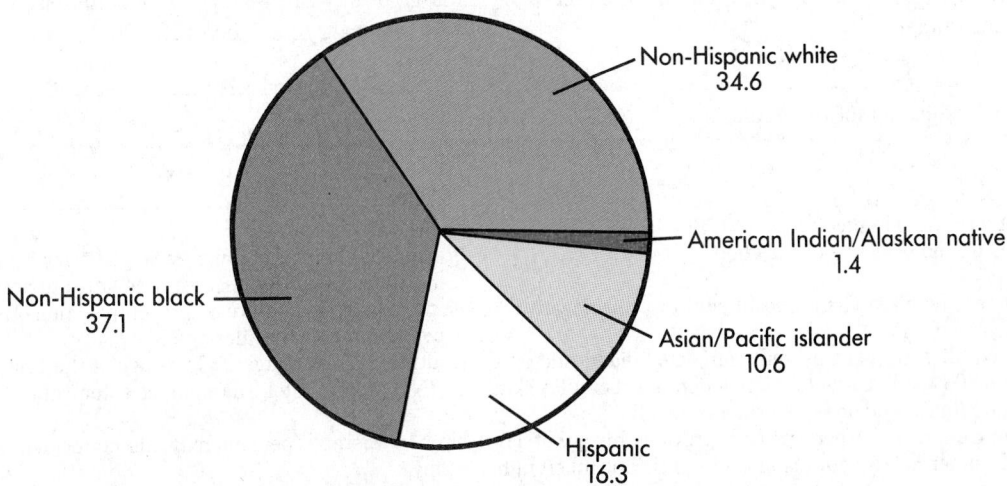

FIGURE 33-2 Percentage of cases of tuberculosis by race and ethnicity in the United States, 1988 (From Centers for Disease Control MMWR: update: tuberculosis elimination, United States MMWR 39(10):153-156, 1990).

berculosis case rate for racial/ethnic minorities was between four and nine times greater than for non-Hispanic whites (Figure 33-2). The increases in these racial/ethnic groups primarily reflects the increase in tuberculosis in persons infected with the human immunodeficiency virus (HIV).[27]

Because HIV infection is an important risk factor for developing clinically apparent tuberculosis among persons already infected with the tubercule bacillus, the CDC recommends that all HIV-infected persons be screened for tuberculosis and latent tuberculous infection and, if infected, placed on appropriate therapy. Also, persons with tuberculosis and known tuberculin-positive persons should be evaluated for HIV infection so that appropriate counseling and treatment can be given.

Even though tuberculosis is preventable, there were 1755 deaths from it in 1988.[27]

Tuberculosis is caused by bacillus, *mycobacterium tuberculosis,* or tubercle bacillus, a gram-positive and acid-fast organism. If microscopic study of a slide prepared from the sputum of an individual reveals tubercle bacilli, the individual is said to have positive sputum; and this confirms the diagnosis of tuberculosis. However, most persons with tuberculosis will not have positive sputum on smear, and a *positive sputum culture* will be necessary to confirm the diagnosis. Patients who have a positive culture and negative smear are less infectious than are those with both a positive smear and culture.

When a person with tuberculosis speaks, coughs, sneezes, or sings, minute droplets fall to the ground; the smaller ones evaporate, leaving *droplet nuclei* that remain suspended indefinitely in the air and are carried on air currents. Droplet nuclei are 1 to 10 μm in size and are small enough to be inhaled into the alveoli. Thus tuberculosis is transmitted by inhalation of tubercle-laden droplet nuclei.

Classification. The classification used by states and territories of the United States when reporting morbidity statistics to the CDC of the Public Health Service is outlined in Table 33-5. The six basic classifications cover the total child and adult population, those unexposed to tuberculosis, those uninfected even though exposed, those with evidence of tuberculosis infection without disease, those with current disease, those with evidence of tuberculosis without current disease, and those in whom tuberculosis is suspected (diagnosis pending).

Prevention. To eliminate tuberculosis, the organism must be prevented from being transmitted from one person to another. Preventive measures are directed toward the recommendations described under classification. Preventive therapy emphasis consists of the following: (1) finding all persons who have tuberculosis and getting them under adequate treatment, (2) identifying persons who should be on preventive chemotherapy and getting them under treatment, and (3) locating persons who had tuberculosis in the past who did not receive adequate treatment with chemotherapy and treating them (see the box on p. 885).

Preventive chemotherapy in the United States is INH daily for 6 months. The usual adult dose is 300 mg in a single dose daily. If the person has antibodies to the human immunodeficiency virus (HIV), isoniazid is given daily for 1 year.

In 1989, the CDC's Advisory Committee for the Elimination of Tuberculosis (ACET) published *A Strategic Plan for Elimination of Tuberculosis in the United States.* The committee recommended that a goal be established to eliminate tuberculosis by the year 2010. To achieve the goal, a case rate of 0.1 per 100,000 persons was set for the year 2010, with an interim goal of a case rate of 3.5 per 100,000 population by the year 2000. This goal may not be easy to accomplish, in view of the 1988 case rate of 9.1 per 100,000.[28]

TABLE 33-5 Classification of tuberculosis

Class	Description	Therapy
0	No TB exposure, not infected	None
1	TB exposure, no evidence of infection	Preventive chemotherapy may be given for persons converting their tuberculin test from negative to positive
2	TB infection, no disease, significant skin test but negative bacterial and x-ray	Isoniazid (INH) for 1 year (preventive chemotherapy) for *positive reactors* under age 35
3	TB: current disease (persons with completed diagnostic evidence of TB: both a significant reaction to tuberculin skin test and clinical and/or x-ray evidence of TB).	Antituberculosis drugs: at least two of the first-line drugs (INH, ethambutol, rifampin, streptomycin)
4	TB: no current disease (persons with previous history of TB or with abnormal x-ray films but no significant tuberculin skin test reaction or clinical evidence)	No new therapy (persons may still be receiving chemotherapy)
5	TB: suspect (diagnosis pending) (used during diagnostic testing of suspect persons, for no longer than 3 months)	Preventive chemotherapy may be instituted

PERSONS WHO SHOULD BE CONSIDERED FOR PREVENTIVE CHEMOTHERAPY

1. Persons known to be exposed to tuberculosis who may be in the process of converting their tuberculin test (recent converters under 35 years of age)
2. Household contacts of persons diagnosed as having tuberculosis, especially children under age 5
3. Positive reactors to the tuberculin test under age 35
4. Tuberculin reactors over age 35 who are at special risk:
   a. Those receiving corticosteroid therapy
   b. Those receiving immunosuppressive therapy
   c. Those having a disease that impairs the immune response
5. Persons with
   a. Leukemia or lymphoma
   b. Silicosis
   c. Diabetes mellitus
   d. Gastrectomy
   e. End-stage renal disease
   f. Antibodies to human immunodeficiency virus

Persons over 35 years of age without the risk factors listed in the box above are not given preventive chemotherapy because of the risk of isoniazid-associated hepatitis. Although the risk is small, it is age related and increases from less than 0.2% in those under age 20 to up to 2% to 3% in those 50 to 64 years of age.

If isoniazid-associated hepatitis occurs, the symptoms are quite mild and nonspecific and resemble those of any viral illness. (See Chapter 39 for a discussion of viral hepatitis.)

Contraindications to the use of isoniazid preventive therapy are (1) previous isoniazid-associated liver disease; (2) severe adverse reactions to isoniazid, including fever, chills, rash, and arthritis; and (3) *acute* liver disease of any cause.

Persons receiving isoniazid preventive chemotherapy should be seen monthly by a health care provider for the purpose of reinforcing the necessity of taking the chemotherapy regularly and to monitor the patient for any serious side effects.

Vaccination. Efforts continue in search of a more satisfactory tuberculosis vaccine. Presently, bacillus Calmette-Guérin (BCG) vaccine is in use in many countries throughout the world. The vaccine contains attenuated tubercle bacilli that have lost their ability to produce disease. It is administered only to persons who have a negative reaction to the tuberculin test. It is not widely used in the United States because of disagreements among physicians as to its safety and effectiveness. Also, vaccination with BCG induces hypersensitivity to tuberculin in vaccinated persons.

Most persons who have received BCG will have a skin test reaction of less than 10 mm. If a larger reaction occurs to puritive protein derivative (PPD), it can be assumed that the person has a TB infection.

Pathophysiology. When an individual with no previous exposure to tuberculosis (negative tuberculin reactor) inhales a sufficient number of tubercle bacilli into the alveoli, tuberculosis *infection* occurs. The body's reaction to the tubercle bacilli depends on the *susceptibility of the individual, the size of the dose, and the virulence of the organisms.* Inflammation occurs within the alveoli (parenchyma) of the lungs, and natural body defenses attempt to counteract the infection. Lymph nodes in the hilar region of the lung may be involved as they filter drainage from the infected site. The inflammatory process and cellular reaction produce a small, firm, white nodule called the *primary tubercle*. The center of the nodule contains tubercle bacilli. Cells gather around the center, and usually the outer portion becomes fibrosed. Thus blood vessels are compressed, nutrition of the tubercle is interfered with, and *necrosis* occurs at the center. The area becomes walled off by fibrotic tissue around the outside, and the center gradually becomes soft and cheesy in consistency. This latter process is known as *caseation*. This material may become calcified (calcium deposits), or it may liquefy and is known as *liquefaction necrosis*. The liquefied material may be coughed up, leaving a *cavity* or hole in the parenchyma of the lung. The cavity or cavities are visible on chest x-ray films and result in the diagnosis of *cavitary* disease. Most individuals who are exposed to tuberculosis and develop a tuberculosis infection (confirmed by a positive tuberculin test) do not develop an active case of tuberculosis. The only x-ray evidence of their tuberculosis infection is a calcified nodule known as the *Ghon tubercle*. The evidence on x-ray film of enlarged hilar lymph nodes and a Ghon tubercle is referred to as the *primary complex*.

Persons who have been exposed to the tubercle bacillus become sensitized to it, and this is confirmed by a positive tuberculin test. Sensitization, once developed, usually remains throughout life unless something interferes with the immune response. Evidence suggests that most tuberculin reactors who take isoniazid for 6 months convert back to negative test results. This protection is believed to last for life. A positive tuberculin test does not mean that one has tuberculosis, however, and nurses should explain this fact to persons undergoing the test.

Tuberculosis infection is unlike other infections. Usually, other infections disappear completely when overcome by the body's defenses and leave no living organisms and generally no signs of infection. However, a person who has been infected with tubercle bacilli harbors the organism for the remainder of his or her life. Tubercle bacilli remain in the lungs in a dormant,

TABLE 33-6 Drugs used to treat tuberculosis

Drug	Classification	Common Side Effects	Tests for Side Effects
Isoniazid (INH)	Bactericidal	Peripheral neuritis, hepatitis, rash, fever	SGOT/SGPT (not as routine)
Rifampin	Bactericidal	Hepatitis, febrile reactions, thrombocytopenia (rare), nausea, vomiting	SGOT/SGPT, platelet count (not as routine)
Ethambutol (EMB)	Bacteriostatic	Optic neuritis (reversible with discontinuation of EMB; very rare at 15 mg/kg, skin rash)	Visual acuity; red-green color discrimination
Pyrazinamide (PZA)	Bactericidal	Hyperuricemia, arthralgias hepatoxicity, GI distress	Uric acid, SGOT/SGPT
Streptomycin (SM)	Bactericidal	Eighth cranial nerve damage (vestibular); nephrotoxicity	Vestibular function audiograms; creatinine level determined before therapy started

walled-off, or so-called, resting state. When a person is under physical or emotional stress, these bacilli may become active and begin to multiply. If body defenses are low, active tuberculosis may develop. Most persons who have active tuberculosis developed it in this manner. However, it is generally accepted that only 1 out of 20 persons with a positive tuberculin test will ever develop active tuberculosis, and the incidence is expected to be much lower among those who receive preventive therapy with isoniazid.

Clinical manifestations. *Early* in the course of *tuberculosis,* the person may be *asymptomatic.* Later symptoms include cough with sputum production, afternoon temperature elevation, and night sweats. Blood-streaked sputum in the absence of pronounced coughing may be the first indication to the person that anything is wrong.

Diagnostic tests include:
1. Tuberculin skin testing
2. Sputum smear and culture
3. Chest x-ray films

These tests are discussed in detail in Chapter 31.

Medical management. Medical treatment is with antituberculosis drug therapy. The drugs used to treat tuberculosis, their classification, side effects, and tests for side effects can be found in Table 33-6. At least two drugs are given together to prevent the development of resistant strains of *M. tuberculosis.* A commonly used treatment schedule uses three drugs in combination: INH, 300 mg/day; rifampin, 600 mg/day for 6 months; and PZA, 15 to 30 mg/kg/day, up to 3 g maximum during the first 2 months of treatment.

When drug resistance develops, other drugs to which the patient's organisms are sensitive are prescribed. Some persons are infected with resistant strains of the tubercle bacillus. Resistance is most common to isoniazid and streptomycin. There are race/ethnic differences in rates for *primary drug resistance.* Asians and Hispanics have the highest rates, followed by blacks,

whites, and American Indians.[28] Primary drug resistance rates vary widely in the United States and Canada, and nurses need to know the local resistance rates for areas where they are working. It can be assumed that resistance rates will be highest in those areas where large numbers of Hispanics and Asian immigrants are living.

■ **Assessment**

Subjective data. It is important to determine whether the patient was exposed to a person with tuberculosis. Often the *source* of the infection is unknown and may never be determined. At the same time, close contacts of the patient need to be identified so that they may undergo follow-up to determine if they are infected and have active disease or a positive tuberculin test.

The patient complains of productive cough and night sweats.

Objective data. Objective data include the following:
1. Productive cough
2. Afternoon temperature elevation
3. Tuberculin skin test reaction of 10 mm induration or more (see Chapter 31)
4. X-ray film showing a pulmonary infiltrate (see Chapter 31)

■ **Data analysis: nursing diagnoses.** Nursing diagnoses are determined from assessment of patient data. Possible nursing diagnoses for the person with tuberculosis may include, but are not limited to:

Diagnostic Title	Possible Etiologies
Airway clearance, ineffective	Increased sputum, decreased energy/fatigue
Fear	Long-term illness requiring long-term chemotherapy, lifestyle changes until no longer infectious
Knowledge deficit about tuberculosis—spread and treatment	Lack of exposure to information

■ **Planning: expected patient outcomes.** Expected patient outcomes for the person with tuberculosis may include, but are not limited to, the following:

1. Patient can explain how tuberculosis is spread and those measures necessary to prevent spread of tuberculosis (remain on chemotherapy, cover mouth and nose when coughing or sneezing)
2. Patient can explain basic food groups and how a nutritionally adequate diet will be achieved
3. Patient can state name, dose, actions, and side effects of prescribed medications
4. Patient can state why two or three chemotherapy agents must be taken together
   a. Can explain drug-resistant organisms and relate this to the need to take chemotherapy as directed
   b. Can explain why the health care provider should be notified immediately if for any reason (for example, side effects) chemotherapy cannot be taken
5. Patient can state where to receive new supply of chemotherapy and date it is to be obtained
6. Patient can state plans for follow-up care
   a. Can list signs and symptoms that indicate need for immediate medical care (increased cough, hemoptysis, unexplained weight loss, fever, night sweats)
   b. Can state when next sputum test or x-ray film is to be taken and where
   c. Can state plans for ongoing follow-up care

■ **Implementation.** The major nursing responsibility is to teach the patient about tuberculosis and how it is transmitted. Preventing contamination of air with tubercle bacilli is accomplished by the following: (1) treating the patient with antituberculosis drugs and (2) preventing contamination of air with the tubercle bacilli. The most effective way to achieve both of the above is by patient teaching (see the box above, right).

Lung Abscess

Etiology and pathophysiology. A lung abscess is an area of localized suppuration within the lung. It usually is caused by bacteria that reach the lung through *aspiration*. Some experts suggest that it might better be called *aspiration lung abscess* because *aspiration* is the common factor. The infected material lodges in the small bronchi and produces inflammation. Partial obstruction of the bronchus results in retention of secretions beyond the obstruction and the eventual *necrosis of tissue*. The *necrotic lung tissue is coughed up,* and *an air-filled cavity is left in the lung.*

Food particles and perigingival debris, which contain both aerobic and anaerobic organisms, are the most commonly aspirated substances. Laboratory cultures of

---

PATIENT TEACHING TO PREVENT TRANSMISSION OF TUBERCULOSIS

1. Patient must take antituberculosis drugs as prescribed.
   a. Drugs are always taken in combination of two or three drugs.
   b. Drugs must be taken as prescribed.
   c. Both of the above are necessary to prevent development of resistant strains of *M. tuberculosis.*
2. Preventing contamination of air with *M. tuberculosis.*
   a. Cover nose and mouth with disposable tissues when coughing, sneezing, or laughing.
   b. Place used tissues in paper bag that will be burned.

---

sputum or transtracheal aspirates are necessary to identify the causative organism. When only normal oropharyngeal flora is found, aerobic cultures may demonstrate the presence of fusospirochetal organisms, peptostreptococci, and *Bacteroides* species. All of these organisms are commonly found in gingival infections. The most common aerobic bacteria causing lung abscess are S. *aureus* and K. *pneumoniae.* Aerobic gram-negative organisms are found most frequently in persons with nosocomial infections (see Chapter 15) or in persons who are immunosuppressed. Sputum should also be examined for tumor cells and for tuberculosis and fungal organisms. Before the advent of antibiotics and specific chemotherapy, lung abscess was a fairly frequent complication after pneumonia.

Lung abscess may follow bronchial obstruction caused by a tumor, foreign body, or stenosis of the bronchus. Children particularly may *aspirate foreign materials* such as a peanut, and a lung abscess results. *Metastatic spread of cancer cells to the lung parenchyma may also cause an abscess,* and occasionally the infection appears to have been *borne by the bloodstream.* In recent years, the incidence of lung abscess caused by infection has decreased, and secondary lung abscess after bronchogenic carcinoma has increased. Bronchoscopy may be used to identify the infected segment and to obtain specimens for culture.

Clinical manifestations. Symptoms of lung abscess include cough, elevation of temperature, loss of appetite, and malaise. Unless the abscess is walled off so that there is no access to the bronchi, the patient usually raises sputum. There may be hemoptysis, and often the patient raises dark brown ("chocolate colored"), foul-smelling sputum that contains both blood and pus.

Interventions

Medical management. The course of lung abscess is influenced by the cause of the abscess and by the kind of drainage that can be established. If the purulent material drains easily, *the patient may respond well to segmental postural drainage, antibiotic therapy, and good general supportive care.* When obstruction interferes with drainage into the bronchi, bronchoscopic procedures should be used not only to improve drainage but also to rule out obstructing foreign bodies or neoplasms. Today, surgical treatment to establish drainage has become increasingly less necessary; but, if after several weeks of medical treatment a cavity persists, a segmentectomy or lobectomy may be performed (Chapter 34).

Penicillin G is the drug of choice, and 2 g is given intravenously every 6 hours until the fever is relieved and the patient's condition shows marked improvement. Penicillin G (Penicillin V, ampicillin, or amoxicillin) in doses of 500 to 750 mg four times daily is then given orally. When the patient has a sensitivity to penicillin, clindamycin, 600 mg every 8 hours, is prescribed. For staphylococcal infections, oxacillin or nafcillin, 6 to 8 g intravenously in divided doses, is often prescribed. Lung abscesses caused by gram-negative organisms are treated with appropriate antibiotics as determined by in vitro sensitivity tests.

Antibiotic therapy is continued until all signs of the illness have subsided and the chest x-rays show that the cavity has completely disappeared or has reduced significantly in size. Most cavities close within 6 weeks, but occasionally a cavity may persist for months. Foul-smelling sputum usually disappears within a few days, whereas cough and nonfoul sputum may continue for a longer period. Usually the patient begins to feel better during the first week of therapy, but it may take up to 2 months for the temperature to return to normal.[62]

If the patient does not improve with the therapy discussed above, *bronchoscopy is performed to search for a possible obstruction* to drainage, such as carcinoma or a foreign body.

Medical treatment cannot cause a walled-off abscess to disappear, and surgery may be necessary. If surgery is necessary, the portion of lung containing the abscess is removed. If the abscess is caused by carcinoma, the surgery may be much more extensive.

Nursing management. The person with a lung abscess is very ill and will be admitted to the hospital. Other persons already in the hospital are at risk of aspiration and lung abscess. These include persons with suppressed levels of consciousness such as found in head injury, post anesthesia, cerebrovascular accident, alcoholism, seizure disorders, drug overdoses, persons with compromised immunologic defenses, and the elderly, especially if immobile.

Nursing responsibilities include the following:
1. Prevention of aspiration in hospitalized patients
   a. Monitoring patients who are at risk of aspiration
   b. Frequent mouth care to persons with diminished levels of consciousness

NURSING CARE OF PATIENTS WITH LUNG ABSCESS

ACTIVITY	RATIONALE
Monitor vital signs at least every 4 hours	Temperature may spike in afternoon and may persist for as long as 2 weeks.
Place patient in comfortable position	If patient is conscious, usually more comfortable with head rest at 45 to 90 degrees
Assist patient to cough up sputum	Helps to drain abscess
Collect sputum for culture and sensitivity tests	Culture and sensitivity to determine organism and antibiotic therapy. Also monitors effectiveness of therapy and whether resistant organisms are developing

   c. Close monitoring of persons receiving tube feedings to ensure that tube is in stomach
   d. If patient is vomiting place on side in post-anesthesia position to reduce aspiration
   e. If patient is unable to expectorate secretions from mouth and oropharynx, oral suctioning may be necessary
2. Care of patient with a lung abscess is outlined in the box above.

Bronchiectasis

Etiology and pathophysiology. Bronchiectasis is irreversible dilation of the bronchial tree. When infection attacks the bronchial lining, inflammation occurs, and an exudate forms. The progressive accumulation of secretions obstructs the bronchioles. The obstructed bronchioles then break down and ciliated columnar epithelium is replaced by nonciliated cuboidal epithelium and sometimes fibrotic tissue resulting in localized areas of dilation or saccules. The expulsive force of the bronchioles is diminished, and they may remain filled with exudate. Only forceful coughing and postural drainage will empty them. Bronchiectasis may involve any part of the lung parenchyma, but it usually occurs in the dependent portions or lobes. Before the widespread use of antibiotics in treating persons with respiratory tract infections, this disease began to develop in young people, with many showing symptoms in childhood or by age 20. Although the incidence of childhood bronchiectasis is decreasing, it is increasing in individuals with *cystic fibrosis, immunodeficiency diseases, or atopic asthma* in which repeated respiratory infections have been successfully treated with antibiotics. These persons now survive the acute episodes of bacterial infection that complicate their underlying disease but not infrequently develop bronchiectasis as a sequela.

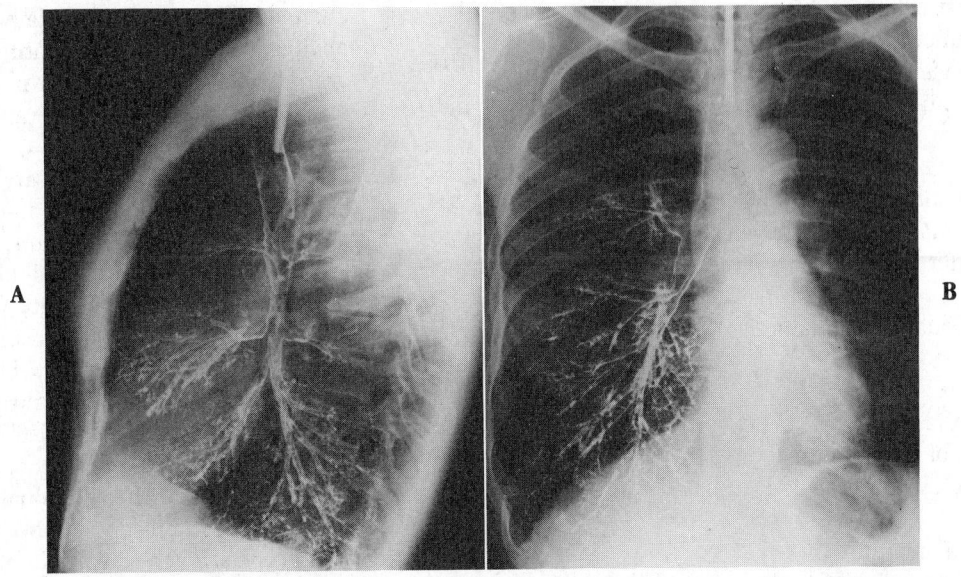

FIGURE 33-3 Normal bronchogram of right lung. **A,** Lateral view. **B,** Anteroposterior view (From DeWeese DD and Saunders WH: Textbook of otolaryngology, ed 6, St Louis, 1982, The CV Mosby Co.).

A contributing factor in bronchiectasis may be a congenital weakness in the structure of the bronchi that results in impairment of elasticity. Bronchiectasis may occur without previous pulmonary disease, but it usually follows such diseases as bronchopneumonia, lung abscesses, tuberculosis, cystic fibrosis, or asthma. A bronchogram in which radiopaque dye is instilled into the bronchial tree through a catheter shows trapping (puddling) of dye in the dilated bronchi (Figure 33-3).

Clinical manifestations. Signs and symptoms of bronchiectasis vary with the severity of the condition and may include the following:

1. Signs
   a. Cyanosis
   b. Clubbing of fingers
   c. Fine rales and coarse rhonchi
   d. Dull or flat sounds over areas of mucous plugs
   e. Increased vocal and tactile fremitus over middle and lower lobes
   f. Decreased diaphragmatic excursion
   g. Paroxsysms of coughing upon arising in morning and when lying down
2. Symptoms
   a. Severe coughing productive of copious amounts of purulent sputum
   b. Hemoptysis
   c. Dyspnea
   d. Fatigue and weakness
   e. Loss of appetite and weight loss

The condition may develop so gradually that the person is frequently unable to tell when the symptoms first began.

Interventions

Medical management. Treatment of bronchiectasis is not very satisfactory. Surgical removal of a portion of the lung is the only cure. Therefore, patients who have bronchiectasis that involves both lungs are not candidates for surgery and do not have a good prognosis. The life expectancy is considered to be no more than 20 years. Many patients develop cardiac complications (*cor pulmonale*) resulting from the extra strain on the heart caused by inability of the lungs to oxygenate the blood adequately.

Other therapy may include the following:

1. Antibiotics to prevent further infection or in preparation for surgery
2. Oxygen if there is widespread involvement in the lung
3. Postural drainage to assist in removing secretions and prevent coughing
4. Bronchoscopy to remove a mucous plug or to break up adhesions that may be blocking passage of secretions to the main bronchi

Nursing management. Nursing care should stress good general hygiene, which may contribute to relief of symptoms. Adequate diet, rest, exercise, and diversional activity are important; and avoiding superimposed infections such as colds should be emphasized. Frequent mouth care is essential, and cleansing the mouth with an aromatic solution before meals often makes food more acceptable.

Empyema

Epidemiology/etiology. Empyema is pus within a body cavity, usually the pleural cavity. Empyema occurs as a result of or in association with other respiratory diseases such as pneumonia, lung abscess, tuberculosis, and fungal infections of the lung and also after thoracic surgery or chest trauma. It now occurs fairly commonly as a complication of staphylococcal pneumonia.

Clinical manifestations. The patient with a lung infection or chest injury may develop empyema and should be observed closely for the following signs and symptoms of empyema:

1. Cough (usually nonproductive)
2. Dyspnea
3. Tachypnea
4. Tachycardia
5. Elevation of temperature
6. Unilateral chest expansion
7. Malaise
8. Decreased appetite

The diagnosis can usually be made from the signs and symptoms and the medical history, but it is confirmed by a chest x-ray that demonstrates the presence of a pleural exudate. A thoracentesis is performed to obtain a sample of the pus for culture and sensitivity studies and to relieve the patient's respiratory symptoms.

Interventions

Medical management. The aim of treatment of empyema is to drain the empyema cavity completely and thus obliterate the pleural space. The cavity can be drained in the following ways:

1. Initial treatment is often daily aspiration of the cavity and instillation of antibiotics into the pleural space. Oral or IV antibiotics may also be given. If the cavity cannot be evacuated within a few days or if the lung fails to reexpand to obliterate the space, surgery is necessary.
2. The type of surgery depends on the situation and may include the following:
   a. In *closed chest drainage*, a trochar is inserted between the ribs at the base of the cavity. A chest catheter is inserted through the trochar, the trochar is removed, and the tube is connected to water-seal drainage (see Chapter 34). Pus then drains from the cavity into the water-seal bottle. For closed drainage to be successful, the pus must be thin enough to drain out of the pleural space, and the lung must be able to reexpand to fill the pleural space.
   b. *Open chest drainage* will be necessary when empyema is chronic and the lung is incapable of reexpanding to obliterate the pleural space. A portion of one or two ribs is removed, and a large drainage tube is inserted into the empyema cavity. This allows pus to drain into a heavy chest dressing, which will need to be

changed once or twice daily. The tube is changed weekly. If the treatment is effective, granulation tissue will form in the space from the inside out, thus obliterating the pleural space.
   c. *Decortication* will be necessary in instances of chronic empyema where a fibrinous peel has formed on the visceral pleura, preventing the lung from reexpanding and filling the space left after the empyema cavity was drained. In decortication, the fibrinous peel is removed from the visceral pleura by blunt dissection, freeing the lung so that it can reexpand and fill the pleural space. Two chest tubes are inserted into the pleural space and connected to water-seal drainage with additional suction. See Chapter 34 for a discussion of chest drainage.
   d. *Thoracoplasty* (the removal of one or more ribs) may be necessary if none of the preceding procedures are successful in obliterating the pleural space. The removal of ribs alters the shape of the thorax, and the chest wall is brought inward to obliterate the pleural space (see Chapter 34).

Nursing management. Nursing care depends on the type and effectiveness of the procedure. In some cases, the patient will go through several treatments before the empyema space is closed. This can be frustrating, and the patient can become very discouraged. A major nursing role is to support the patient and family during the various procedures.

FUNGAL INFECTIONS

There are three major fungal infections of the lungs: *histoplasmosis, coccidioidomycosis,* and *blastomycosis.* They are classified as deep mycoses because there is involvement by the parasite of deeper tissues and internal organs. The etiology, epidemiology and prevention of these fungal infections are discussed in Table 33-7.

HISTOPLASMOSIS
PATHOPHYSIOLOGY

The spores are inhaled and phagocytized by alveolar macrophages within which they germinate. They form yeast cells and multiply by budding. In persons previously uninfected there is a primary or initial infection that resembles the infection in primary tuberculosis with involvement of regional lymphatics and early dissemination via lymphatics and blood to other organs. Yeast cells spread hematogenously and are phagocytized by reticuloendothelial cells in the liver, spleen, and bone marrow. *The process in the lung is similar to that seen in tuberculosis with necrosis and healing by fibrotic encapsulation.* Eventually, the original parenchy-

TABLE 33-7 Etiology, epidemiology, and prevention of fungal lung infections

Disease	Etiology	Epidemiology	Prevention
Histoplasmosis	Inhalation of spores of *Histoplasma capsulatum* Soil contaminated with fowl excreta; possibly bats infected and areas they inhabit [caves, attics, hollow trees] can be extremely infectious	Most common systemic mycotic disease in United States; endemic areas in Missouri, Kentucky, Tennessee, Southern Illinois, Indiana, and Ohio	Locate areas where soil is infected with fowl excreta. Teach public to avoid inhalation of dust from infected soil. Infants and elderly are especially susceptible.
Coccidioidomycosis (Valley fever, San Joaquin Valley fever)	Inhalation of spores of *Coccidioides immitis* Soil contaminated with spores; growth of fungus enhanced by heavy rainfall in desert; inhibited by sunlight; anthrospores which are inhaled, dispersed by liberation of dust in spring	Endemic to well-defined areas in southwestern United States, Mexico, and South America. In United States, endemic in San Joaquin Valley, Southern Arizona, New Mexico, and Southwestern Texas	Encourage wearing of masks by persons working in desert dust; archeologists, construction workers.
Blastomycosis	Believed to be inhalation of *Blastomyces dermatitidis* Soil contaminated with spores that are carried on air currents and inhaled by humans and animals; dogs can acquire the disease; not believed to be spread from animals to man; believed that both humans and animals infected by inhaling spores	Most prevalent in the United States and Canadian valley areas surrounding the Mississippi, Missouri, Ohio, and St. Lawrence rivers; also present in Africa, South America, and Mexico	Avoid inhalation of spores in areas where cases have been identified.

mal foci in the lung and in the hilar lymph nodes show calcification. Usually the initial infection is self-limiting, and does not require antifungal chemotherapy. However, some persons such as infants and adults with immunologic incompetence (lymphoma) may develop a rapidly progressive primary infection that will be fatal without antifungal therapy.

Reinfection histoplasmosis and *progressive histoplasmosis* can also occur. Reinfection with *Histoplasma* causes an illness resembling the initial infection. Since some degree of immunity to histoplasmosis is conferred by the initial infection, the extent of disease will be modified by the degree of fungal immunity.[2] Heavy inoculation may cause *pneumonitis*, which is usually self-limiting over days to weeks. The onset is acute with nonproductive cough, fever, malaise, and dyspnea. Some persons who are fully immune may develop a hypersensitivity-like pneumonitis with small, discrete granulomatous foci that may give a *miliary* appearance on x-ray examination. This means that the infection is spread throughout the lung, giving the appearance of the presence of small millet seeds throughout the lung.

Progressive histoplasmosis is usually chronic; chronic pulmonary histoplasmosis is the most frequently encountered symptomatic form of the disease. It develops almost exclusively in middle-aged white men who have chronic obstructive pulmonary disease. There are recurrent episodes of necrotizing segmental or lobar granulomatous pneumonitis, which have a tendency to cavity formation, contraction, fibrosis, and compensatory emphysema.

Progressive disseminated histoplasmosis usually occurs as a consequence of the initial infection in persons with very low resistance to the infection (infants, persons with immunologic incompetence). Rarely, it can occur in adults of both sexes and all ages with no known immune disorder. These persons have fever, weakness, weight loss, hepatosplenomegaly, leukopenia, and mucous membrane ulceration involving the oropharynx, tongue, or larynx. Adrenal insufficiency occurs in about 50% of these persons.[2]

COCCIDIOIDOMYCOSIS
PATHOPHYSIOLOGY

The process following inhalation of spores is believed to be very similar to that described under histoplasmosis.

The arthrospores reach the alveoli, where they are phagocytized. If the disease becomes disseminated there is marked hilar adenopathy, and fungi can be isolated from lymph nodes. A pneumonic disease with necrosis and cavitation may occur after development of delayed hypersensitivity.[121] The disease process is controlled and resolved in most persons as the result of cell immunity to infection. Thus progressive disseminated coccidioidomycosis or progressive pulmonary disease is found only in those persons whose ability to resist infection or develop immunity has been compromised in some way. Susceptibility to infection is in part genetically determined. Coccidioidomycosis is 50 times more common in Filipino men and 10 times more common in black men that it is in white men. This increased susceptibility to progressive disease in these groups of men parallels their susceptibility to tuberculosis. The increased susceptibility of some races to diseases such as coccidiodiomycosis and tuberculosis is believed to be the result of a genetically determined impairment of their capacity to develop cellular immunity to infection.[121]

Skin testing with coccidioidin 1:10 or 1:100, is available to test for the disease. The test is read in 48 hours. It takes 3 to 6 weeks after exposure for the test to become positive. In severe disseminated disease the test may be negative, indicating that the patient's immune system is no longer able to respond.

X-ray films of the chest may show pneumonic infiltrate, hilar adenopathy, pleural effusion, or a cavitary lesion.[69] About 5% of persons with primary pulmonary involvement will have residual lung lesions such as cavities or nodules. Only about 0.5% of infected individuals go on to develop a severe, progressive mycosis.

Extrapulmonary dissemination of coccidioidomycosis can occur. One of the most frequent sites of dissemination is the meningeal surfaces of the brain. If there is any indication of involvement of the central nervous system, a lumbar puncture is performed. A positive complement fixation titer in the spinal fluid is diagnostic of meningitis.[69]

Dissemination can also occur to skin, soft tissue, and bones; and the patient is monitored by physical examination of the skin, gallium scanning of soft tissues, and bone scans. A bone scan should be performed before starting amphotericin B therapy.

Surgical intervention for lesions that are localized may involve either excision or drainage to facilitate healing.

BLASTOMYCOSIS
PATHOPHYSIOLOGY

Although skin lesions are the first evidence of blastomycosis, it is believed that the initial site of infection is in the lung. It is assumed that spores are inhaled and phagocytzed in the alveoli as part of the primary infection.

Thus the pathogenesis of blastomycosis is similar to that of tuberculosis, histoplasmosis, and coccidioidomycosis. The infection is spread by the lymphatics and spread throughout the body. The skin lesions represent metastatic infection from the primary pulmonary disease.[121]

Acute pulmonary blastomycosis in the form of a self-limiting pneumonia can occur. Otherwise, blastomycosis is a chronic progressive disease with a mortality of about 90% when untreated. For this reason, treatment is recommended for every person in whom the diagnosis is established.[92]

CLINICAL MANIFESTATIONS OF FUNGAL DISEASES

The signs and symptoms and the medical therapy for the three fungal diseases are presented in Table 33-8.

Diagnostic tests include the following:

1. Direct demonstration of intracellular yeasts in smears of bone marrow and biopsy of lymph nodes, liver, and spleen; cultures of bone marrow, blood or sputum.
2. Serologic tests. (Aggulutination, precipitation and complement-fixation tests are used to help establish diagnosis of histoplasmosis and coccidioidomycosis. Serology tests become positive about 1 month after the primary infection. Titers of serial tests are used to determine activity of the infection.)
3. Skin testing. (Skin test for histoplasmosis is only used for screening purposes. In endemic areas between 90% and 95% of young adults have positive test results. The person should be tested with histoplasmin, tuberculin, blastomycin, and coccidiodin because of the likelihood of cross-reaction. The strongest reaction indicates the likely cause of the infection.)
4. In histoplasmosis and coccidioidomycosis, chest films demonstrate a nodular infiltrate similar in appearance to tuberculosis. In blastomycosis, chest films may be nonspecific.
5. WBC count is usually normal. In acute cases it may increase to 13,000/mm^2.
6. Leukopenia and anemia may be present in persons with disseminated disease.

■ ASSESSMENT
Subjective Data

Subjective data include the following:
1. History of exposure to soil contaminated with spores
2. Onset and duration of signs and symptoms

Objective Data

Objective data include the following:
1. Palpation of chest to check for limited expansion
2. Percussion of chest to check for dull or flat sounds

TABLE 33-8 Signs and symptoms and medical therapy for fungal lung infections

Type of Infection	Signs and Symptoms	Medical Therapy
Histoplasmosis	Severe infections; acute onset with fever, chest pain, dyspnea, prostration, weight loss, widespread pulmonary infiltrates, hepatomegaly, and splenomegaly. No symptoms in some persons, benign acute pneumonitis in others	Drug(s) of choice: amphotericin B (Fungizone intravenous); 75% of patients are cured Ketoconazole (Nizoral), 400 mg orally daily at bedtime or with meals; without treatment patient with disseminated disease will die.
Coccidioidomycosis (Valley fever, San Joaquin Valley fever)	Asymptomatic upper respiratory tract infection in about 60% of those who inhaled spores; 40% have symptoms ranging from flulike illness to frank pneumonia	Amphotericin B IV Therapy required for only 10% of those with symptoms; remainder have spontaneous remission Ketoconazole orally
Blastomycosis	Skin lesions that appear as small papular or pustular lesions on exposed parts of the body such as hands and face Peripheral development of lesions, may become raised and do not itch	Amphotericin B IV; mandatory in immunocomprised patients Ketoconazole orally Miconazole (only for patients who cannot tolerate amphotericin or ketoconazole)

3. Auscultation to check for type of breath sounds or adventitious sounds

■ DATA ANALYSIS: NURSING DIAGNOSES

Nursing diagnoses are determined from assessment of pertinent data. Possible nursing diagnoses for the person with severe mycotic infection may include but are not limited to:

Diagnostic Title	Possible Etiologies
Airway clearance, ineffective	Tracheobronchial infection/secretions
Anxiety	Change in health status/socioeconomic status
Breathing pattern, ineffective	Musculoskeletal impairment
Gas exchange, impaired	Ventilation/perfusion imbalance
Knowledge deficit: condition, how spread, and treatment	Lack of exposure to information

■ PLANNING: EXPECTED PATIENT OUTCOMES

Expected patient outcomes for the person with severe mycotic infection may include, but are not limited to, the following:

1. Patient can demonstrate cough with adequate sputum production
2. Patient can demonstrate improved ventilation and adequate oxygenation of tissues
3. Patient's temperature returns to normal
4. Patient knows source of infection and can teach others to avoid infection areas (Table 33-7)
5. Patient states plans for follow-up care

■ IMPLEMENTATION

Promoting Comfort

Promoting comfort includes the following:
1. Place patient in position to facilitate breathing.

2. Take measures to reduce fever (if present), such as use of cool sponge baths.
3. Maintain room temperature desired by patient.

Administering and Monitoring Medications

The role of the nurse is as follows:
1. Administer medications as prescribed and monitor patient for side effects.
   a. Amphotericin B (Fungizone IV) is the standard therapy for mycotic infection. The dose and length of therapy are determined by the difficulty in eradicating the infection and the likelihood of relapse.[2] The therapy may last 2 to 3 weeks or 2 to 3 months.
   b. Amphotericin B must be given intravenously and has many toxic properties, including local phlebitis, systemic reactions, renal toxicity, hypokalemia, and anemia. In rare instances anaphylaxis, bone marrow suppression, and cardiovascular and hepatic toxicity develop.
   c. Systemic toxicity (chills, fever, aching, nausea, and vomiting) can be lessened by premedication with 600 mg of aspirin along with 25 to 50 mg of diphenhydramine (Benadryl) or promethazine (Phenergan) or 10 mg of prochlorperazine (Compazine) orally.[2] Heparin and hydrocortisone succinate (Solu-Cortef) are sometimes added to the infusions to minimize phlebitis.
   d. A reversible azotemia occurs regularly when amphotericin B is administered. The level of azotemia is monitored by biweekly BUN or serum creatinine determinations. A BUN of greater than 40 or a creatinine nearing 3 indicates a need to temporarily reduce or stop the

drug. Therapy is not continued until the ax-otemia is improved. Serum potassium levels are checked biweekly, and hypokalemia is treated with oral potassium. Anemia is common, and the hematocrit usually stabilizes at 25% to 35%.[2]

e. Ketoconazole (Nizoral) is administered orally and is effective in the treatment of systemic mycotic infections. It is given daily for a minimum of 6 months. Toxicity appears to be minimal; pruritus, minor gastrointestinal intolerance, and liver function abnormalities have been reported.

2. Teach patient about medications and follow-up therapy.

Providing Emotional Support

Patients with mycotic infections can be quite ill and may require long-term therapy (as long as 2 to 3 months) with intravenous antibiotics. Because these diseases are not well understood by the public, the patient needs to feel free to discuss concerns with the nurse. The nurse needs to provide factual information, clarify misconceptions, and help the patient understand the disease and therapy.

OCCUPATIONAL LUNG DISEASES
EPIDEMIOLOGY AND ETIOLOGY

Many pulmonary diseases are believed to be caused by substances inhaled in the workplace. They are more common (1) in blue-collar workers than in white-collar workers, (2) in industrialized areas than in rural areas, and (3) in small and medium-sized businesses than in larger industrial plants.

In some instances it is debatable whether a person's lung disease is clearly occupation specific. This is especially true in cases of bronchitis, asthma, emphysema, or cancer, since all of these conditions can be caused or aggravated by several factors found in many different occupations and by nonoccupational factors such as smoking and pollution of the atmosphere.[3]

Millions of Americans are believed to be suffering from job-related diseases. Since these diseases are not reportable, exact statistics do not exist. The Department of Health and Human Services (HHS) has estimated that 400,000 persons develop job-related diseases each year. They also estimate that there are 100,000 deaths each year from occupational diseases. The National Heart, Lung, and Blood Institute reports that lung diseases cause more than half of these deaths. Over $5 billion a year is paid out in workers' compensation for job-related illnesses and injuries.[3]

PREVENTION

Occupational lung diseases are preventable. However, there must be a concerted effort by the public, governmental agencies, and industry if these diseases are to be prevented.

Governmental action has been slow and has only occurred, in some instances, in response to public interest groups that have lobbied for stricter regulation of harmful substances. However, countervailing political pressures have sometimes prevented laws from being passed or have resulted in less strict laws being passed because of the costs involved in meeting the strict standards required to control certain hazards.

The ALA recommends several measures to reduce the incidence of occupational-related lung diseases: (1) public education about the relationship between polluted air in the work place and lung diseases; (2) general commitment to reducing, eliminate, or avoid air pollution in the workplace; and (3) elimination of the most prevalent and notorious lung hazard: cigarette smoke.[3]

Education of the public includes not only employers and employees but also engineers and planners who design operations; buyers and purchasers who select ingredients, cleaning agents, and equipment; and physicians who see persons with occupation-related diseases. Many times workers who are instructed about the hazards involved in certain occupations and workplaces are helpful in deciding what preventive measures need to be taken to combat or minimize the effects of hazards. The commitment to reduce, eliminate, or avoid pollution of workplace air requires full consideration of possible health effects whenever operations are planned and improvement of conditions whenever possible.

It is well documented that smokers develop occupational lung diseases more often than nonsmokers and that smokers' lungs are more vulnerable to the effects of these diseases than are nonsmokers' lungs. The combined effects of cigarette smoke and industrial pollutants are very great. The risk of developing chronic bronchitis, emphysema, lung cancer, and heart disease is much increased when the worker smokes.[3] Some of these risks such as lung cancer in asbestos workers who also smoke are becoming more commonly known.

Occupational lung diseases can be divided into several categories. The major ones are (1) the pneumoconioses, including silicosis and coal miner's pneumoconiosis (black lung disease); (2) asbestos-related lung disease; (3) other pneumoconioses such as chronic berylliosis; (4) mixed-dust pneumoconioses; and (5) hypersensitivity diseases, including occupational asthma, allergic alveolitis (farmer's lung), and byssinosis (brown lung disease). The etiology, epidemiology, pathophysiology, clinical manifestations, and prevention of the major occupational lung diseases are presented in Table 33-9. *Text continued on p. 898.*

TABLE 33-9 Major occupational lung diseases*

Type	Etiology and Epidemiology	Pathophysiology	Clinical Manifestations and Prevention
PNEUMOCONIOSES†	1 million people in United States run risk of developing silicosis		
Chronic silicosis	Inhaled silica dust; commonest form seen in miners, foundry workers, and others who inhaled relatively low concentrations of dust for 10-20 yr	Dust accumulated in tissue → tissue reaction with whorl-shaped nodules throughout lungs	Breathlessness with exercise
Complicated silicosis	20%-30% of persons with chronic silicosis develop this	Progressive massive fibrosis (PMF) throughout lungs → ↓ lung function and cor pulmonale	Breathlessness, weakness, chest pain, productive cough with sputum, respiratory cripple, dies of heart failure
Acute silicosis	Rapidly progressive disease, leading to severe disability and death within 5 yr of diagnosis	Inflammatory reaction within alveoli, diffuse fibrosis	Early symptoms, difficulty in breathing, weight loss, fever, cough Prevention: dust control, wetting down of mines, and improved ventilation can reduce dust levels; sandblasters in enclosed spaces can use special suits and breathing apparatuses; some experts believe such protective measures are still inadequate
Coal worker's pneumoconiosis (CWP; "black lung disease")	150,000 coal miners in the United States at risk; amount, size, and nature of dust in air vary according to type of coal, machinery, and technique used, efficiency of ventilation, and other dust control measures; 10%-30% of all coal miners develop simple form of the disease, more prevalent in miners of anthracite or hard coal; other minerals found in miner's lung (silica, kaolin, mica, beryllium, copper, cobalt, and others); unknown whether these minerals contribute to development or progression of CWP	Simple CWP; dust accumulation in lungs visible on x-ray film; over years dust piles up, and respiratory bronchioles are dilated (called focal emphysema)	Simple CWP, no symptoms, no respiratory difficulty
Complicated CWP or progressive massive fibrosis (PMF)	3% of persons with simple CWP develop complicated form; more often occurs in miners with heavy deposits of coal dust in lungs; may appear suddenly years after miner has left the mines; can stop suddenly for no discernible reason; smoking seems to have no effect on development of CWP, but smoking has adverse effect on miners' health; miners who smoke have 5 to 6 times more lung obstruction than nonsmoking miners; cigarette smoking causes chronic bronchitis and emphysema as in nonminers	Fibrosis develops in some of dust-laden areas; fibrosis spreads and fibrotic areas coalesce; eventually most of lung is stiffened and useless; silica plays some role in fibrosis but despite international research, role of silica in CWP is not understood	PMF shortens life span; may die from respiratory failure, cor pulmonale, or superimposed infection Prevention: dust control; reduced levels of coal dust can lower simple CWP and reduce number of miners who develop complicated CWP

*From American Lung Association: Occupational lung diseases: an introduction, New York, 1979, The Association.
†Also known as "dust in the lungs."

TABLE 33-9 Major occupational lung diseases—cont'd

Type	Etiology and Epidemiology	Pathophysiology	Clinical Manifestations and Prevention
ASBESTOS-RELATED LUNG DISEASE‡	One of the most dangerous occupational hazards; can cause both fibrosis and cancer in asbestos workers; also a general environmental hazard because of its extensive use before health hazards were recognized; most dangerous to those who mine the ores and process the crude material into pure form; no asbestos mines in United States, but processed and used in United States; federal agencies and state governments have tightened controls on use of asbestos; lung cancer associated with all types of asbestos; 20%-25% of deaths of workers with heavy exposure are from lung cancer; cancer related to degree of asbestos and to *cigarette smoking, which enhances carcinogenic properties of asbestos,* asbestos worker who smokes is 90 times as likely to get lung cancer as smoker who never worked with asbestos	Asbestos occurs in several different forms or ores; commercially important ores are chrysolite, crocidolite, and amosite; most hazardous medically are crocidolite and amosite, fibrosis caused by asbestos is called *asbestosis;* asbestos fibers accumulate around terminal bronchioles; body surrounds fibers with iron-rich tissue = asbestos body with characteristic picture on x-ray film; more asbestos bodies as more fibers are inhaled; after 20-30 years of exposure, fibrosis begins in lungs, if heavy exposure, fibrosis appears in 4-5 years	After fibrosis begins, cough, sputum, weight loss, increasing breathlessness; most die within 15 years of first symptoms
	Mesothelioma (cancer of the pleura) accounts for 7%-10% of deaths of asbestos workers; inoperable and always fatal; can occur after very little exposure to crocidolite; has been reported in wives of asbestos workers and in persons living near asbestos plants; cigarette smoking not a contributing factor; only a few fine, straight crocidolite fibers are necessary; asbestos workers have higher incidence of other cancers (esophagus, stomach, and intestines); swallowing of asbestos-contaminated sputum responsible for these cancers.	Occurs in persons exposed to crocidolite fibers of a certain size; a few cases involve amosite fibers; needlelike shape of crocidolite fibers enables them to pass through lung tissue to pleura	Prevention: number of asbestos-related diseases has been increasing despite recognition of hazards and dust-control measures; much tighter controls are needed; some countries have taken such steps; there is need for massive efforts to educate general public of dangers of asbestos
SOME OTHER PNEUMOCONIOSES			
Aluminum	Inhaled particles of a certain size induce disease		
Beryllium	Greatest risk of exposure in plants that extract beryllium from crude ore; beryllium is metal used in metallurgy, certain machine tools, making of ceramics, and nuclear power industry	Affects most body systems; in lung produces a severe chemical pneumonia after acute exposure; chronic form is called *berylliosis*	

‡Asbestos is a fire-proofing and insulating agent.

TABLE 33-9 Major occupational lung diseases—cont'd

Type	Etiology and Epidemiology	Pathophysiology	Clinical Manifestations and Prevention
Chronic berylliosis	Disease of hypersensitivity; unrelated to level of exposure; beryllium exposure also associated with ↑ rates of cancer of lung, liver, and gallbladder	Diffuse fibrosis over 15-20 yr → cor pulmonale	Difficulty in breathing
Talc	Inhaled by miners and millers of crude ore and soapstone and by workers in cosmetic, paint, pottery, asphalt, and rubber industries; high incidence of lung cancer; not known whether high incidence is caused by asbestos in talc or whether increased incidence in those who smoke	*Pure* talc produces a characteristic pneumoconiosis; less fibrosis than with silica inhalation; evaluation of fibrosis is difficult because most talc contains traces of asbestos and silica	
MIXED-DUST PNEUMOCONIOSES	Many workers exposed to a mixture of dusts; foundry, steel, and iron workers inhale dust from a variety of ores and may also inhale fumes; miners exposed to mixed dusts; some workers are exposed to one dust, then change jobs and are exposed to another dust	Individual dusts usually deposit in patterns that can be recognized on x-ray film; mixed dusts result in different patterns; patient's work history important in diagnosing occupational lung diseases	
	Not known whether mixed dusts in lungs are additive $(1 + 1 = 2)$ or potentiating $(1 + 1 = 5)$	Amount of fibrosis present depends on amount of silica inhaled	
HYPERSENSITIVITY DISEASES	Hypersensitivity diseases fall into occupational category when antigen is found primarily in work place; lung hypersensitivity can occur in bronchi, bronchioles, or alveoli; coarse dust causes bronchial reactions; fine dust provokes small airway and alveolar reactions		
Occupational asthma	More common in the 10% of the population who are atopic (genetic tendency to develop an allergy); nonatopic persons can also become sensitized; substances with antigenic properties include detergent enzymes, platinum salts, cereals and grains, certain wood dusts, isocyanate chemicals used in polyurethane paints and other products, agents used in printing, and some pesticides	Hypersensitivity reaction mediated by histamine → bronchoconstriction and ↑ mucus production; repeated attacks if cause unrecognized and asthma is untreated; may lead to permanent obstructive lung disease; asthmatic response that is well established can be provoked by other factors (house dust, cigarette smoke) and by fatigue, breathing cold air, and coughing	Wheezing is major symptom Prevention: total elimination of antigen; desensitization not successful

Continued.

TABLE 33-9 Major occupational lung diseases—cont'd

Type	Etiology and Epidemiology	Pathophysiology	Clinical Manifestations and Prevention
Allergic alveolitis (farmer's lung)	Hypersensitivity disease caused by fine organic dust inhaled into smallest airways; cause of farmer's lung is moldy hay; other dusts can cause allergic alveolitis: these include moldy sugar cane and barley, maple bark, cork, animal hair, bird feathers and droppings, mushroom compost, coffee beans, and paprika; often disease is named for cause (mushroom worker's lung, etc.); fungus spores growing in the apparent antigen are thought in many cases to be real cause of the disease	Alveoli are inflamed, inundated by WBCs, sometimes filled with fluid; if exposure infrequent or level of dust low, symptoms are mild, and treatment not sought, chronic form develops over time; eventually, fibrosis occurs, and fibrosis may be so well established that it cannot be arrested	Symptoms begin some hours after exposure to offending dust and include fatigue, shortness of breath, dry cough, fever, and chills; symptoms may be severe enough to require emergency treatment and hospitalization; acute attacks treated with steroids; recovery may take 6 weeks, and patient may suffer residual lung damage; real cure is permanent separation of patient and antigen Prevention: properly dried and stored farm products (hay, straw, sugar cane) do not cause allergic alveolitis; presumably fungi only grow in moist conditions
Byssinosis (brown lung)	Occupational disease occurs in textile workers; mainly in cotton workers but also afflicts workers in flax and hemp industries; cause is found in bales of raw cotton that contain not only cotton fibers but fragments of cotton plant; something in plant matter, rather than pure cotton, is cause	Chronic bronchitis and emphysema develop in time; constriction of bronchioles in response to something in crude cotton; symptoms of asthma and allergy persist as long as there is exposure to cotton antigen	Tightness in chest on returning to work after a weekend away (Monday fever); strong relationship between amount of dust inhaled and symptoms; persistent productive tight chest with chronic bronchitis and emphysema; person leaves industry as respiratory cripple Prevention: dust control measures; pretreating bales of cotton by washing with steam and other agents may inactivate causative agent; try to detect persons who are likely to become sensitized to cotton dust and keep them out of high-risk areas

INTERVENTIONS

MEDICAL AND NURSING MANAGEMENT

Medical therapy and nursing care of these patients depends on the patient's signs, symptoms, and complications. The reader is referred to other sections of this chapter for discussion of these topics. The major role of nurses is to be knowledgeable about the cause and prevention of occupational lung diseases so that appropriate information and teaching can be presented to the public.

SARCOIDOSIS

EPIDEMIOLOGY AND ETIOLOGY

Although sarcoidosis is worldwide in distribution, it is most likely to be diagnosed where the medical community is alert to the disease and diagnostic facilities are available. It is most common in adults between 20 and 40 years of age. The incidence is almost equal in men and women, but it is twice as common in women in childbearing years. In the United States, it is 10 times more common in blacks than in whites. There is some evidence that the incidence is higher in blacks than whites in other parts of the world, especially if the disease is sought out.

PATHOPHYSIOLOGY

Sarcoidosis is a systemic granulomatous disease. Although the cause is unknown, there is evidence of an antigen-antibody reaction manifested by reticuloendothelial response in which both thymus-derived (T) cells and plasma (B) cells participate (see Chapter 76 for more information). It is believed that the antigen is airborne, because bilateral hilar lymphadenopathy is frequently present at the onset and bronchopulmonary macrophages are increased.

CLINICAL MANIFESTATIONS

The central pathologic event involves the growth of granulomas and proliferation of lymph tissue. Preliminary sarcoidosis commonly is seen on chest x-ray films as enlarged lymph nodes in the hilar area. The patient with sarcoidosis may initially complain only of *vague symptoms of malaise, fever, aching in the joints, or weakness*. In addition to mediastinal lymph node enlargement, ocular manifestations, such as uveitis and conjunctivitis, and dermatologic changes, such as erythema nodosum, are commonly found.

Diagnosis of sarcoidosis is based on x-ray film findings, organ biopsy, and positive skin test. The Kveim-Siltzback test involves the injection of sarcoid tissue; if the reaction is positive, a visible, palpable nodule develops at the site 3 to 6 weeks after the antigen is injected. A biopsy of the nodule is then performed to confirm the presence of granulomatous tissue. The Kveim-Siltzback test is not always used as part of the diagnostic process, however, because it is difficult to obtain the active antigen and because the test is associated with frequent false-negative results. Organ biopsy yields the most conclusive evidence of sarcoidosis and is most helpful in differentiating it from Hodgkin's disease and tuberculosis.

Newer diagnostic methods in pulmonary sarcoidosis include gallium scan and bronchoalveolar lavage (BAL) with flexible fiberoptic bronchoscopy. The fluid obtained from BAL is examined to determine the degree of active inflammation in the lung and need for therapy. The patient's symptoms and pulmonary function tests (especially lung volume) are still widely used, however, in deciding whether treatment is required.

INTERVENTIONS
MEDICAL AND NURSING MANAGEMENT

In many patients, sarcoidosis is a benign, self-limiting process that resolves with no residual damage within 2 years of diagnosis. Other patients will have an acute or chronic form of the disease.

Treatment of acute disease is with systemic steroids. Patients are treated with prednisone, 40 mg daily for 2 months, followed by 20 mg of prednisone daily for another 4 months. The steroids are then slowly tapered off. Most patients are treated for between 18 and 24 months. The patient is then followed medically for several years for signs of relapse. Relapse usually occurs within 3 to 6 months after the steroids are discontinued.

In chronic forms of sarcoidosis, patients are treated with small doses of steroids (5 to 10 mg every other day) for years.[97] About 10% of patients develop the chronic form of sarcoidosis in this form; the disease proceeds to nodular granulomatous depositions in lung tissue and eventual pulmonary fibrosis. In severe cases, pulmonary hypertension and cor pulmonale develop.

Nursing care depends on severity of patients signs and symptoms and medical therapy. Teaching the patient about the precautions and side effects of steroid therapy is a major nursing function.

FIBROSING ALVEOLITIS
EPIDEMIOLOGY AND ETIOLOGY

Fibrosing alveolitis (interstitial pneumonitis) is a disease of unknown cause with a poor prognosis. It occurs mainly in persons over 40 years of age, and men and women are equally affected.

PATHOPHYSIOLOGY

Fibrosing alveolitis is characterized by inflammation of the alveoli resulting in cellular thickening of alveolar walls with a tendency toward fibrosis. The cellular infiltrate contains lymphocytes, plasma cells, and granulocytes.[70] Serum rheumatoid factor, antinuclear factor, and circulating immune complexes are sometimes present. Fibrosing alveolitis can be associated with the collagen diseases. It is also known as interstitial fibrosis or *pulmonary fibrosis*.

CLINICAL MANIFESTATIONS

The patient becomes progressively short of breath because of the reduction in the size of the lungs and reduction in the amount of alveolar-capillary membrane available for gas exchange. Blood gas findings demonstrate hypoxemia and often hypercapnia. Clubbing of the fingers is common, and cardiac complications may develop.

INTERVENTIONS
MEDICAL AND NURSING MANAGEMENT

There is no cure and no specific treatment for fibrosing alveolitis because the cause is unknown. Persons who have circulating immune complexes or have abnormal cells on lung biopsy may show improvement if given adrenocorticosteroids. Patients usually must curb activities because of dyspnea, and they should be advised to guard against exposure to respiratory tract infections, because an infection could be fatal.

CANCER OF THE LUNG
EPIDEMIOLOGY AND ETIOLOGY

During the past 50 years there has been a startling increase in the incidence of cancer of the lung.

The ACS estimates 155,000 new cases in 1989 and 142,000 deaths. In 1986, cancer of the lung surpassed breast cancer to become the number one cancer killer of women. Thus lung cancer is now the leading cause of death from cancer in both men and women.

The increase in death rates for both men and women is directly related to cigarette smoking. A history of smoking, especially for 20 years or more, is considered to be a prime risk factor. Other risk factors include exposure to certain industrial substances such as asbestos, particularly in those who smoke.

The mortality of persons with lung cancer depends primarily on the specific type of cancer and the size of the tumor when detected. Squamous cell carcinoma is the most common, followed by adenocarcinoma; undifferentiated small cell (oat cell) carcinoma is the least common. Most people who develop the disease are over 50 years of age. Some of the factors believed to be involved in the increased incidence of cancer of the lung include an increase in smoking among women, more accurate diagnosis, and a tendency to name the lung as the primary site.

Only 13% of lung cancer patients live 5 years or more after diagnosis. The survival rate is 33% for cases detected in a localized stage; only 24% of lung cancers are discovered that early. Survival rates have improved only slightly over the past 10 years.[1]

Cancer of the lung may be either metastatic or primary. Metastatic tumors may follow malignancy anywhere in the body. Metastasis from the colon and kidney is common. Metastasis to the lung may be discovered before the primary lesion is known, and sometimes the location of the primary lesions is not determined during the person's life.

PREVENTION

The cause of cancer of the lung is closely related to cigarette smoking. Table 33-10 shows the extreme increase in mortality from lung cancer in those persons who smoke. Prevention is the best protection against cancer of the lung because early detection of the disease is difficult. The American Cancer Society estimates that cigarette smoking is responsible for 85% of lung cancer cases among men and 75% among women—about 83% overall. The cancer death rates for male cigarette smokers is more than double that for nonsmokers, and the rate for female smokers is 67% higher than that for nonsmokers.[1]

From available research data it seems evident that curtailing smoking is a primary preventive measure. The nurse should be active in teaching the dangers of smoking and should set a positive health example in this regard. It is especially important that teenagers be given specific facts about the dangers of cigarette smoking because they are not likely to be habitual smokers at that age. *Recent studies indicate that the incidence of smoking among teenagers is increasing.* People who are already habitual smokers should also be urged to stop

TABLE 33-10 Deaths caused by lung cancer, according to smoking habits*

	Deaths per 100,000 Population
Nonsmokers	3.4
10-20 cigarettes per day	54.3
20-40 (1-2 packs) per day	143.9
More than 40 (2 packs) per day	217.3

*From American Cancer Society: Cancer facts and figures, New York, 1976, The Society.

smoking, although it may be difficult for them to do so. Various types of programs to assist persons to stop smoking are available. Since air pollution affects the lungs and may predispose to the development of cancer, the nurse should encourage and actively support community programs to decrease the amount of air pollution.

PATHOPHYSIOLOGY AND CLINICAL MANIFESTATIONS

Because most new growths in the lungs arise from the bronchi, the term *bronchogenic carcinoma* is widely used. The signs and symptoms that a patient has depend on several factors including the location of the lesion.

Signs and symptoms of lesion in the bronchus and lung include the following:

1. Ten percent of patients are asymptomatic and are picked up on routine chest x-ray.
2. Seventy-five percent will have a cough.
3. Fifty percent will have hemoptysis.
4. Shortness of breath and a unilateal wheeze are common.

If peripheral pulmonary lesions perforate into the pleural space, there will be extrapulmonary intrathoracic signs and symptoms. These include:

1. Pain on inspiration
2. Friction rub
3. Pleural effusion
4. If the superior vena cava is involved, edema of face and neck
5. Fatigue
6. Clubbing of fingers

Diagnostic tests include:

1. Chest x-ray
2. Sputum cytology test
3. Fiberoptic brochoscopy (sometimes biopsy taken)

In the later stage of the disease, weight loss and debility usually indicate metastases, especially to the liver. Cancer of the lung may metastasize to nearby structures such as the prescalene lymph nodes, the walls of the

HISTOLOGIC SUBTYPES OF CANCER OF THE LUNG AND THE THERAPY OF EACH TYPE

TYPE	CLASSIFICATION AND PERCENTAGE OF CASES	THERAPY
Small cell carcinoma	Small cell lung cancer cancer (SCLC); 25% of cases	Combination chemotherapy such as (1) cyclophosphamide, doxorubicin, and vincristine, or (2) cyclophosphamide, doxorubicin, and etoposide, or (3) cisplatin plus etoposide
Squamous cell carcinoma Adenocarcinoma Large cell carcinoma	All three classified as non-small cell lung cancer (NSCLC); 75% of cases	Pulmonary resection—only one third are operable; one third unoperable because of advanced lung cancer; one third unoperable because of distant metastases

esophagus, and the pericardium of the heart or to distant areas such as the brain, liver, or skeleton.

MEDICAL MANAGEMENT

The treatment of lung cancer depends on the type and stage of the disease. Histologically, lung cancer is divided into four major subgroups: small cell carcinoma, squamous cell carcinoma, adenocarcinoma, and large cell carcinoma. The box above shows the types, percentage of cases in the subtypes, and recommended therapy. As with other types of cancer, lung cancer is staged

(see Chapter 17 for more details about staging). The international Tumor, Node, Metastasis (TNM) Staging for Lung Cancer is presented in the box below.

Because patients with early lung cancer have no symptoms, they are often inoperable by the time they are seen. Some patients with cancers of the lung are first diagnosed after a chest x-ray as part of a routine physical examination. Other patients are not diagnosed until they seek medical treatment for symptoms related to metastases.

INTERNATIONAL TNM STAGING FOR LUNG CANCER*

TUMOR SIZE (T)

TX = Occult carcinoma (cytologically positive; bronchoscopically and radiographically nondetectable)
T1 = Tumor 3 cm or less surrounded by lung or visceral pleura
T2 = Tumor more than 3 cm
T3 = Tumor of any size with direct extension into chest wall, or with 2 cm of the carina, or associated with atelectasis or obstructive pneumonia of the entire lung
T4 = Tumor of any size invading the mediastinal structures or vertebral body, or presence of malignant pleural effusion

NODAL STATUS (N)

N0 = No hilar or mediastinal nodal involvement
N1 = Ipsilateral hilar nodal involvement
N2 = Ipsilateral mediastinal nodal or subcarinal nodal involvement
N3 = Contralateral hilar or mediastinal nodal involvement, supraclavicular nodal involvement (ipsilateral or contralateral)

METASTASES (M)

M0 = No distant metastases
M1 = Distant visceral metastases present

STAGE

Occult carcinoma	TX, N0, M0
Stage I	T1-2, N0, M0
Stage II	T1-2, N1, M0
Stage IIIA	T3, N0-1, M0
	T1-3, N2, M0
Stage IIIB	T4, N1-3, M0
	T1-3, N3, M0
Stage IV	Any T, any N, M1

*Adapted from Mountain CF: A new international staging system for lung cancer; Chest 89(Suppl):2255, 1986.

FIVE-YEAR DISEASE-FREE SURVIVAL RATES FOR SURGICAL RESECTION IN PATIENTS WITH NON-SMALL CELL LUNG CANCER

	STAGE	5 YR DISEASE-FREE (%)
I	T1, N0, M0	70-85
	T2, N0, M0	55-65
II	T1, N1, M0	30-50
	T1, N2, M0	25-30
IIIA	T3, N0, M0	25-35
	T3, N1, M0	15-20
	T1-2N2, M0	9-24
	T3, N2	0-5

From Bonomi P: Primary lung cancer. In Rakel RE, editor: Conn's current therapy, 1990, Philadelphia, 1990, WB Saunders Co.

Survival rates of patients with non-small cell lung cancer (NSCLC) obviously depend on the size of the tumor, nodal status, and degree of metastases. The box above gives the 5-year survival rates for patients with non-small cell cancers.

Some patients who undergo surgical resection (pneumonectomy or lobectomy) may also receive radiation therapy or chemotherapy. These adjuvants are given mainly to treat metastases and in an attempt to relieve some of the patient's symptoms.

■ ASSESSMENT
SUBJECTIVE DATA

Subjective data include the following:
1. Onset and duration of signs and symptoms
2. What the patient understands about why he or she is hospitalized
   a. For diagnostic tests
   b. For chest surgery or radiation or chemotherapy
3. Whether the patient states that carcinoma of the lung is present or suspected
4. Smoking history
5. Occupational history of exposure to asbestos or other carcinogenic agents

OBJECTIVE DATA

Objective data include the following:
1. Presence of cough and whether or not productive of sputum
2. If sputum is present, whether blood-tinged
3. Hemoptysis
4. Shortness of breath when talking or on exertion
5. Unilateral wheezing on auscultation

■ DATA ANALYSIS: NURSING DIAGNOSES

Nursing diagnoses are determined from assessment of patient data. Possible nursing diagnoses of the person with bronchogenic carcinoma may include, but are not limited to, the following:

Diagnostic Title	Possible Etiologies
Airway clearance, ineffective	Decreased energy/fatigue
Anxiety	Threat of death, Threat/change in health status/scocioeconomic status/role functioning environment
Gas exchange, impaired	Ventilation/perfusion impairment
Knowledge deficit: about the disease and its treatment	Lack of exposure/ unfamiliarity with information sources
Pain	Pleuritic chest pain (if pleura involved)

■ PLANNING: EXPECTED PATIENT OUTCOMES

Expected patient outcomes for the person undergoing thoracic surgery may include, but are not limited to, the following: The patient or significant others can:
1. Explain recommended changes in ADL
   a. Which usual activities to limit and for how long
   b. Exercise program
2. Explain any changes required in lifestyle (reason and plans for changes in occupation and habits such as smoking, activity level, and so on).
3. State name, dose, action, and side effects of medications ordered
   a. How and when to use prn medications
   b. Schedule for other medications and how to take them
4. Describe professional and community resources necessary for structuring an environment compatible with convalescence
   a. Plans for obtaining assistance of agencies such as Visiting Nurses Association
   b. Plans for necessary modifications of home
5. Describe plans for follow-up care.
   a. Signs or symptoms requiring immediate medical assistance
   b. State plans for ongoing medical care

■ IMPLEMENTATION

Nursing care depends on whether the patient has been diagnosed and is undergoing treatment or whether the patient is admitted for treatment of metastases or for supportive care during the terminal stage of illness. Care of the patient undergoing chest surgery is discussed in Chapter 34.

All patients can be expected to be fearful and anxious and require considerable emotional support. The nurse and physician should discuss the treatment plan for the patient, so that all information given to the patient and family is carefully coordinated.

Because of the very poor survival rate in persons with lung cancer, a major role of the nurse is to teach the

PREVENTION AND EARLY DETECTION OF LUNG CANCER

1. Smoking control programs
   a. Encourage young persons not to start smoking.
   b. Educate public about hazards of smoking.
   c. Provide self-help materials to assist persons to quit smoking.
   d. Refer to stop-smoking programs sponsored by organizations such as the ACS, ALA, and American Heart Association.
   e. Stress that there is no such thing as a "safe cigarette," but that persons who smoke cigarettes lower in tar and nicotine find it easier to quit smoking.[1]
   f. Support nonsmoking areas in public places such as restaurants and meeting places.
   g. Support legislation to establish nonsmoking areas in public meeting places.
2. Urge all individuals over 40 years of age to have a chest x-ray periodically in addition to a yearly physical examination.
3. Know the cancer detection centers in your community or other resources to which persons can be referred for evaluation.

---

public how lung cancer can be prevented or at least diagnosed as early as possible. Points to be emphasized in teaching are listed in the box above, left.

ADULT RESPIRATORY DISTRESS SYNDROME

EPIDEMIOLOGY AND ETIOLOGY

Adult respiratory distress syndrome (ARDS) is the name given to a syndrome of acute hypoxemic respiratory failure without hypercapnia. The syndrome was first described by T.J. Petty in 1967. ARDS is often fatal and is characterized by severe dyspnea, hypoxemia, and diffuse bilateral pulmonary infiltrations after lung injury in previously healthy persons. Recently, the term hyperpermeability pulmonary edema (HPPE) has been used to describe the condition that affects between 150,000 and 200,000 critical care patients yearly.[100a] Causes of ARDS are presented in the box above right.

PREVENTION

Prompt treatment of the underlying cause of ARDS is the major focus of preventive care. Additionally, judicious use of the mechanical ventilator and oxygen therapy is required to avoid inducing ARDS as an untoward complication of these treatment modalities.

PATHOPHYSIOLOGY

The pathophysiologic alterations that result in ARDS are typically initiated by a major trauma to the body, often a physical insult to a body system other than the pulmonary system (see Fig. 33-4). The following physiologic alterations result in the clinical syndrome identified as ARDS:

CLINICAL CONDITIONS ASSOCIATED WITH ARDS/HPPE

1. Shock
   a. Septic
   b. Hemorrhagic
   c. Cardiogenic
   d. Anaphylactic
2. Trauma
   a. Pulmonary contusion
   b. Nonpulmonary, multisystem
3. Infection
   a. Pneumonia
      (1) Viral
      (2) Bacterial (staphylococcal or streptococcal)
      (3) Legionellosis
   b. Miliary tuberculosis
4. Disseminated intravascular coagulation (DIC)
5. Fat emboli
6. Near-drowning
7. Aspiration: highly acid gastric contents (pH <2.5)
8. Inhaled toxic agents
   a. Smoke
   b. Phosgene
   c. Oxides of nitrogen
9. Pancreatitis
10. Oxygen toxicity
11. Narcotic drug abuse
    a. Heroin
    b. Methadone
    c. Propoxyphene (Darvon)
12. Radiation pneumonitis
13. Drugs
    a. Ethchlorvynol
    b. Salicylates

Adapted from Petty TL: Adult respiratory distress syndrome. In Kryger M: Pathophysiology of respiration, New York, 1981, John Wiley & Sons, Inc.

1. As a consequence of the precipitating insult, the complement cascade is activated, which in turn increases capillary wall permeability.
2. Fluid, granular leukocytes, red blood cells, macrophages, cell debris, and protein leak into the interstitial spaces between the capillaries and alveoli, and ultimately into the alveolar spaces.
3. Because of the fluid and debris in the interstitium and alveoli, surface area for oxygen and carbon dioxide exchange is decreased resulting in low ventilation/perfusion ratios and hypoxemia.
4. Compensatory hyperventilation of functional alveoli occurs, resulting in hypocapnia and respiratory alkalosis.
5. Cells that normally line the alveoli are destroyed and replaced by cells that do not produce surfactant, thus increasing alveolar surface tension and resulting in atelectasis and increased alveolar opening pressures.

The normal function, pathophysiology, and clinical picture of a person with ARDS/HPPE is presented in Table 33-11.

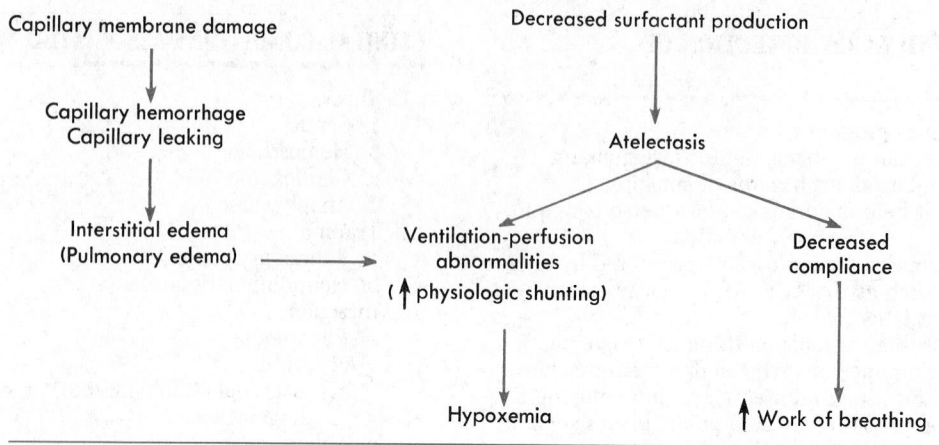

FIGURE 33-4 Pathophysiologic events in adult respiratory distress syndrome.

CLINICAL MANIFESTATIONS

ARDS usually occurs in a person who has had a recent physical trauma, although it can appear in persons who appeared to be healthy immediately before onset (for example, someone with sudden onset of an acute infection). There is usually a latent period of 18 to 24 hours from the time of lung injury to the development of symptoms. The syndrome runs a variable course from a few days to several weeks' duration. Patients who appear to be recovering from ARDS may suddenly relapse into acute pulmonary disease from secondary insult such as pneumothorax or overwhelming infection. Signs and symptoms of ARDS include the following:

1. Acute respiratory distress: tachypnea, dyspnea, accessory muscle breathing, and central cyanosis
2. Dry cough and fever that develop over a few hours or days
3. Fine crackles throughout both lung fields
4. Altered sensorium ranging from confusion and agitation to coma

Radiologic and laboratory findings include the following:

1. Chest x-rays—reveal diffuse, bilateral, and usually symmetric interstitial and alveolar infiltrations
2. Arterial blood gases
   Hypoxemia less than 50 torr
   Hypocapnia
   Respiratory alkalosis
   End-stage: hypercapnia and respiratory acidosis

MEDICAL MANAGEMENT

Patients with ARDS are critically ill and are best managed in an intensive care unit. Medical management focuses on the following aspects of care:

1. Oxygenation
   a. Initially may need to administer highest concentration of oxygen available (100%—using nonrebreathing facemask). However, oxygen delivered at levels greater than 50% are associated with oxygen toxicity that worsens already

TABLE 33-11 Normal function, pathophysiology, and clinical picture of a person with ARDS/HPPE

Normal Function	Pathophysiology	Clinical Picture
ALVEOLAR/CAPILLARY MEMBRANE Oxygen and carbon dioxide exchange between alveolar air and pulmonary capillaries	Increased capillary wall permeability blood plasma contents infiltrate interstitial and alveolar spaces, resulting in hypoxemia, alveolar hyperventilation and respiratory acidosis	$PaO_2 \downarrow$ $PaCO_2 \downarrow$ pH ↑ Fine crackles auscultated throughout lungs
LUNG PARENCHYMA Lung tissue that makes up the alveoli	Destruction of normal lung tissue, in particular, alveolar septal walls, normal cells replaced by nonsurfactant producing cells, and presence of edema and debris result in decreased lung compliance (stiff lung). Fibrosis may also develop.	Functional residual capacity and need to use high pressures to ventilate patient Dyspnea at rest

existing ARDS pathology. Oxygen concentrations can usually be lowered below 50%, by using positive end expiratory pressure (PEEP) to open closed alveoli for increased ventilation.

  b. Goal is PaO_2 = 50 to 60 torr.
  c. Gradually reduce FiO_2 while maintaining adequate arterial oxygen levels.

2. Ventilatory support

  a. If oxygen therapy alone is unsuccessful in providing adequate arterial oxygenation, the patient is intubated and placed on a mechanical ventilator.

   (1) A volume-limited ventilator is preferred.
   (2) Ventilator is set to provide tidal volume equal to 10-12 ml/kg body weight, respiratory rate equal to 10 to 14/min FiO_2 = 50%, PEEP used.
   (3) If individual's spontaneous respiration is adequate, intermittent mandatory ventilation (IMV) mode is used. When spontaneous ventilatory pattern interferes with providing adequate ventilation, the patient is sedated or paralyzed with Pavulon. The control mode is then used. See Chapter 34 for more information on care of the patient on a ventilator.

3. Fluid volume

  a. Insert balloon-tipped pulmonary artery catheter to measure pulmonary capillary pressure.
  b. Diuretics, fluid volume expanders, and hypotensive medications are administered as indicated to maintain optimal fluid volume.

4. Treat underlying cause of ARDS.

■ ASSESSMENT

Nursing assessment of the patient with ARDS must be tailored to maximize information obtained without increasing respiratory distress.

SUBJECTIVE DATA

Background information and history of present illness can be obtained from family members, since the patient is usually too ill to give details.

OBJECTIVE DATA

The process of gathering objective data is the same as that described for respiratory failure (see p. 944).

■ DATA ANALYSIS: NURSING DIAGNOSES

Nursing diagnoses are determined from assessment of patient data. Possible nursing diagnoses for the person with ARDS may include, but are not limited to, the following:

Diagnostic Title	Possible Etiologies
Gas exchange, impaired	Ventilation/perfusion inequality
Nutrition, altered: less than body requirements	Unable to take in adequate nutrition to meet increased metabolic workload from increased work of breathing
Anxiety	Threat of death
	Physiologic factors (arterial blood gas derangements
Tissue perfusion, altered (cardiopulmonary)	Fluid mobilization to (and from) third space (interstitium and alveolar space)

■ PLANNING: EXPECTED PATIENT OUTCOMES

Expected patient outcomes for the person with ARDS/HPPE may include, but are not limited to:

1. Improved ventilation and oxygenation

  a. PaO_2 is maintained at 50 to 60 torr during acute phase of illness.
  b. Upon resolution of ARDS PaO_2, pH, and PCO_2 return to acceptable baseline limits.
  c. Sensorium returns to preillness level.
  d. During acute phase of illness, patient is able to tolerate mechanical ventilatory assistance.
  e. Inspiratory to expiratory ratio is 5:10 seconds.
  f. Respiratory rate and tidal volume are within normal limits.
  g. Patient does not complain of dyspnea.

2. Adequate tissue perfusion

  a. Pulmonary capillary wedge pressure (measure of pulmonary capillary pressure) below 18 torr
  b. Urinary output of at least 30 ml/hr
  c. Peripheral pulses present and extremities warm to touch

3. Increased physiologic and psychological comfort

  a. Tolerates ventilator and artificial airway
  b. Acknowledges and expresses fears
  c. Communicates personal needs effectively with staff and family
  d. Cooperates and assists with care

4. Stable body weight within normal range

■ IMPLEMENTATION

Patients with ARDS are critically ill and are best cared for in an intensive care unit. Their care centers around the following measures.

MAINTAINING ADEQUATE GAS EXCHANGE

Oxygenation

1. Maintain oxygen therapy as ordered.
2. Monitor for signs of hypoxemia (p. 943).

Ventilatory Support

Provide ventilatory support as follows:

1. Maintain a patent airway.

NURSING CARE PLAN

PERSON ON MECHANICAL VENTILATION WITH PEEP

DATA: Mr. R. is a 28-year-old married male admitted to the Surgical Intensive Care Unit after a motor vehicle accident. Injuries sustained include a ruptured spleen and liver laceration resulting in hypovolemic shock. Mr. R. was taken to the operating room where his injuries were repaired and blood losses replaced. His early postoperative course was unremarkable. On Mr. R.'s third postoperative day, he began to experience some respiratory difficulties with a deterioration in his arterial blood gases. Due to severe hypoxemia, Mr. R. was intubated. His chest x-ray revealed diffuse interstitial and alveolar infiltrates. He had developed ARDS and eventually required 16 cm H_2) of PEEP.

Mr. R.'s wife visited her husband daily and often attempted to communicate with him. She would reassure and calm him when he got anxious and resisted the ventilator. Mrs. R. would ask the nurse many questions about her husband's status.

The nursing history identified the following:
- Mr. and Mrs. R. have been married 5 years; they have no children.
- Mr. R. has full hospitalization and medical coverage through insurance at work.
- Mr. and Mrs. R. come from large families that appear supportive.
- Mr. R. is a nonsmoker.

Collaborative nursing actions include those to assist in improving oxygenation through evaluating FiO_2 and levels of PEEP as well as techniques used to wean AR from the ventilator.

Nursing actions include:
- Supporting oxygenation and ventilation to maintain PaO_2 over 60 torr and to maximize functional residual capacity
- Weaning from FiO_2 and levels of PEEP gradually while monitoring arterial blood gases.
- Monitoring patient for signs of hypoxia.

NURSING DIAGNOSIS

Gas exchange, impaired, related to ARDS

Expected Patient Outcomes	Nursing Intervention	Rationale
Mr. R. will remain adequately oxygenated as evidence by: 1. PaO_2 on arterial blood gas >75 mm Hg 2. Adequate color 3. Adequate peripheral circulation	Monitor arterial blood gases to determine PaO_2 Suction AR only when necessary to prevent loss of PEEP secondary to disconnection from ventilator Monitor required levels of PEEP and FiO_2 Assess peripheral circulation for pulses, color of extremities and warmth Monitor mixed venous blood oxygen levels	ARDS is an acute lung injury that results in increased capillary permeability, which permits proteins and fluids to leak out into alveoli and interstitial spaces, thus preventing normal gas exchange to occur.

NURSING DIAGNOSIS

Cardiac ouput decreased, related to decreased venous return

Expected Patient Outcomes	Nursing Interventions	Rationale
Mr. R. will not experience hemodynamic compromise related to PEEP	Monitor vital signs every hour and as needed Monitor hemodynamic parameters for signs of decreased cardiac output, hypotension, elevated CVP, and oliguria Monitor intake and output Check peripheral circulation every 2 to 4 hr and as needed Elevate foot of bed 10 to 20 degrees to encourage venous return Perform passive range of motion exercises every 4 to 6 hr to encourage venous return Administer adrenergic agents as ordered to improve cardiac output Notify physician of hemodynamic complications	PEEP may cause decreased cardiac output by increasing intra-alveolar pressures, thereby decreasing venous return to the heart Ineffective breathing pattern related to altered lung/thoracic pressure relationship

NURSING DIAGNOSIS

Ineffective breathing pattern related to altered lung/thoracic pressure relationship

Expected Patient Outcomes	Nursing Interventions	Rationale
Mr. R. will not experience pulmonary complications secondary to PEEP 1. Atelectasis 2. Pneumothorax 3. Pneumomediastinum 4. Subcutaneous emphysema	Monitor respirations every hour and as needed Assess breath sounds for adventitious findings Administer pulmonary toilet every 2 hours and as needed 1. Frequent turning 2. Chest physiotherapy Monitor for signs of pulmonary complications and respiratory distress 1. Asymmetric chest excursion 2. Sudden sharp pain 3. Cyanosis 4. Anxiety Assess for subcutaneous emphysema Keep chest tube set up at bedside Monitor arterial blood gases as needed Notify physician of respiratory complications	When walls of alveoli cannot withstand the positive pressure from PEEP, perforation may occur. As a result, air leaks into the pleural space, mediastinum and/or its subcutaneous space. The result is a pneumothorax, pneumomediastinum or subcutaneous emphysema, respectively

NURSING DIAGNOSIS

Nutrition, altered: less than body requirements, related to intubation

Expected Patient Outcomes	Nursing Interventions	Rationale
Mr. R. will receive adequate nutritional intake while intubated	Administer hyperalimentation or arterial feedings as prescribed Intake and output Daily weights Administer albumin or volume expanders as prescribed Monitor serum albumin level	Nutritional status must be maintained to assist in weaning process; proteins and volume expanders will increase serum colloidal osmotic pressure thus maintaining fluid in the intravascular compartment

NURSING DIAGNOSIS

Anxiety, related to ARDS, intubation, and discomfort from PEEP

Expected Patient Outcomes	Nursing Interventions	Rationale
Mr. and Mrs. R. will exhibit behavioral signs of decreased stress and anxiety	Assess for signs of anxiety Explain ARDS to family, including rationale for mechanical ventilation and PEEP Allow Mr. and Mrs. R. to express concern and fears Explain procedures before performing them Provide comfort measures Provide for a means of communication between AR and his wife Attempt to anticipate their needs Administer light sedation/antianxiety medications if necessary, as ordered Attempt to calm and reassure Mr. R. if he begins to "buck" or resist the ventilator Provide AR and his wife distraction from the ICU environment ■ soft music, TV ■ breaks from the ICU for Mrs. R.	The Intensive Care Unit, mechanical ventilation, the inability to communicate, and fear of the unknown all contribute to feelings of stress and anxiety for the patient in the ICU as well as significant others Positive pressure exhalation is often uncomfortable for the patient who often responds by resisting ventilator

2. If artificial airway present (endotracheal tube or tracheostomy) provide necessary care.
   a. Secure tube to avoid movement either in or out of established position.
   b. Position patient for optimal oxygenation (see Chapter 34).
   c. Auscultate lungs hourly to assess placement of endotracheal tube (may slip into right mainstem bronchus).
3. Suction endotracheal tube as needed.
4. Administer bronchodilators as ordered.
5. Check ventilator settings frequently.

DECREASING PATIENT ANXIETY

1. Ensure proper ventilator function to deliver adequate tidal volume and oxygen concentration: If patient appears in respiratory distress although ventilator is functioning properly, assess arterial blood gas levels
2. Identify a way for patient to be able to communicate concerns and express feelings (if unable to verbalize due to intubation, try alternative ways of communication)
3. Provide simple explanations about procedures; orient patient to surroundings, and repeat explanations regularly.
4. Offer explanations of care routines and environment to family. Encourage family to approach, talk, and touch patient, as they desire.

MAINTAINING ADEQUATE TISSUE PERFUSION

The maintenance of adequate tissue perfusion is a nursing responsibility.
1. Monitor pulmonary capillary wedge pressure.
   a. Notify physician if pressure is above or below established range.
   b. If pressure is below established range administer plasma volume expanders or hypotensive medications as ordered.
   c. If pressure is high, administer diuretics or vasodilators as ordered.
2. Assess urine output, vital signs, and extremities hourly.

PREDISPOSING FACTORS IN THE OCCURRENCE OF PULMONARY EMBOLI

1. Thrombophlebitis
2. Immobility
3. Recent surgery
4. Obesity
5. Congestive heart failure/myocardial infarction
6. Recent fracture
7. Estrogen therapy

MAINTAINING ADEQUATE NUTRITION

Nutritional interventions for patients are the same as those for the patient with COPD (see nursing care plan for person on mechanical ventilation with PEEP on p. 906).

PULMONARY VASCULAR DISEASE

PULMONARY EMBOLI AND PULMONARY INFARCTION

EPIDEMIOLOGY AND ETIOLOGY

Pulmonary embolism is the lodging of a clot or other foreign matter in a pulmonary arterial vessel. Pulmonary infarction is the extravasation of blood and, rarely, the necrosis of lung parenchyma resulting from the occlusion of a medium-sized pulmonary artery.

Emboli formation rarely occurs without the presence of certain risk factors (see the box below).

Pulmonary emboli result from damage to blood vessel walls (surgery), blood stasis (varicosities), or blood hypercoagulability (estrogen therapy).

PREVENTION

The best treatment for pulmonary emboli is prevention. Preventive measures for hospitalized patients are presented under nursing interventions. The person at high risk of emboli should be counseled to:
1. Avoid prolonged sitting or standing
2. Avoid restrictive clothing
3. Consider smoking cessation

PATHOPHYSIOLOGY

Emboli travel from their site of origin through the right side of the heart and lodge in the pulmonary vasculature. The size of the pulmonary artery and the number of emboli determine the severity of symptoms.

Blood flow is obstructed, causing localized tissue hypoxia and ultimately a decrease in the pulmonary vascular bed. Pulmonary vessels vasoconstrict in response to the hypoxia. The resultant ventilation-perfusion inequality (ventilation greater than perfusion) causes arterial hypoxemia. The normal function, primary pathophysiology, and the clinical picture of a patient with pulmonary emboli is presented in Table 33-12.

CLINICAL MANIFESTATIONS

If the embolus blocks a larger vessel, the person may complain of sudden, sharp upper abdominal or thoracic pain, become dyspneic, cough violently, and have hemoptysis; shock may develop rapidly. If the area of infarction is small, the symptoms are much milder. The patient may have cough, tachypnea, pleuritic chest pain, slight hemoptysis, elevation of temperature and an increased leukocyte count. An area of dullness or crackles may be detected when checking breath sounds.

TABLE 33-12 Normal function, primary pathophysiology, and clinical picture of pulmonary embolism

Normal Function	Pathophysiology	Clinical Picture
PULMONARY VASCULATURE		
To carry venous blood received from right heart to alveolar-capillary membrane for oxygen/carbon dioxide exchange	Occlusion of pulmonary vessels in: increased vascular resistance, decreased cardiac output (usually occurs only in massive emboli), decreased lung perfusion	Elevated pulmonary artery pressure Dyspnea Hypotension Tachycardia High ventilation/perfusion ratio as shown on lung scan Hypocapnia and elevated arterial blood pH
AIRWAYS		
Carry oxygenated air to alveolar/capillary membrane and deoxygenated air out of lung	Airway constriction from lowered alveolar carbon dioxide levels	Underventilated lung areas as shown on lung scan Hypoxemia Tachypnea Cough
ALVEOLI		
Lung site where gas exchange takes place	Infarction of alveolar tissues due to complete obstruction, resulting in extravasation of blood cells into alveoli (note: occurs only in more severe cases)	Hemoptysis Radiologic opacity
PLEURA		
Maintain close approximation of lungs and chest wall Minimize friction during lung expansion and contraction	Transudate from damaged vascular structures	Pleural friction rub Chest pain during inhalation/exhalation

The diagnosis of pulmonary embolism is made by the clinical history, by changes in blood chemistries, and by chest films. Lung scans and pulmonary angiography are also performed; pulmonary angiography is a definitive diagnostic tool if a sharp cutoff is seen. Since recannulization often takes place rapidly, the procedure must be completed in the acute phase, or the results may be negative. The diagnosis of pulmonary embolism is often, of necessity, made on the basis of clinical criteria alone.

MEDICAL MANAGEMENT

The major component of medical treatment for pulmonary emboli is anticoagulant therapy. Anticoagulant therapy may be either prophylactic for high-risk persons or curative for the actual pathologic event (see the box at right).

When the patient is not responsive to heparin therapy or when anticoagulant therapy is contraindicated, surgical intervention may be required. Two procedures are used to treat pulmonary emboli:

1. Vena caval interruption: a filter device is placed inside the vena cava. This procedure may be carried out under local anesthesia.
2. Pulmonary embolectomy: pulmonary emboli are

extracted from the pulmonary vasculature. This procedure is usually performed under general anesthesia with the use of extracorporeal circulation, although it may be performed with a special intravenous suction catheter under local anesthesia.

■ **ASSESSMENT**

Subjective Data

Subjective data include the following:

1. Determine the presence of risk factors (see Prevention, p. 908).

ANTICOAGULANT THERAPY FOR PULMONARY EMBOLI

1. Prophylactic: often used for high-risk persons[87]
   a. Low-dose heparin—5000 U SQ every 12 hours
   b. Oral anticoagulants-warfarin 5-10 mg daily for 3 days then maintenance on the basis of prothrombin time
2. Curative treatment
   a. Heparin approximately 5000 to 15,000 U IV bolus, then continuous infusion approximately 1000 U every hour or 2500-5000 U IV every 4 hours
   b. Long-term treatment with warfarin 5-10 mg daily

2. Assess for the recent onset of any of the following symptoms.
   a. Dyspnea
   b. Substernal chest pain
   c. Hemoptysis
   d. Chest palpitations
   e. Pleuritic pain
   f. Cough
   g. Apprehension
   h. Diaphoresis

Objective Data

Objective data include the following:
1. Assess general appearance
   a. Patient will often appear apprehensive
2. Assess vital signs for the following:
   a. Tachypnea
   b. Tachycardia
   c. Elevated temperature
3. Pulmonary examination
   a. Inspection, palpation, and percussion usually normal unless there is an underlying pulmonary disease
   b. Auscultation, listen for
      (1) Pleural friction rub
      (2) Localized, decreased breath sounds and crackles
4. Assess laboratory findings for the following:
   a. Arterial blood gases
      (1) Hypoxemia
      (2) Respiratory alkalosis
   b. Chest x-ray
      (1) Often normal
   c. Lung scan
      (1) Perfusion scan positive
      (2) Ventilation scan may indicate underventilated areas
   d. Pulmonary angiography
      (1) If positive, is definitive for pulmonary emboli
      (2) Positive findings = vessel filling defect and cut-off (abrupt ending of vessel)

■ DATA ANALYSIS: NURSING DIAGNOSES

Nursing diagnoses are determined from assessment of patient data. Possible nursing diagnoses for the person with pulmonary emboli may include, but are not limited to, the following:

Diagnostic Title	Possible Etiologies
Gas exchange, impaired	High ventilation-to-perfusion ratio
Knowledge deficit: condition and its treatment	Lack of exposure or unfamiliarity with information sources
Pain	Pleural effusion
Tissue perfusion, altered in pulmonary vascular and lung	Vascular obstruction from emboli resulting in decreased or absent blood flow to region

■ PLANNING: EXPECTED PATIENT OUTCOMES

Expected patient outcomes for the person with pulmonary emboli may include, but are not limited to, the following:
The patient will:
1. Demonstrate adequate tissue perfusion
   a. Extremities warm and dry to touch, pulses present
   b. Coagulation studies: prothrombin (PT) time and partial prothrombin time (PPT) are within normal limits.
   c. Intravenous sites intact and nonreddened
2. Demonstrate adequate ventilation
   a. Pa_{O_2} = 80 to 100 torr
   b. Pa_{CO_2} = 40 torr
   c. pH = 7.35 to 7.45
3. State pain is relieved

The patient or significant others will be able to:
1. List behaviors that would increase the risk of pulmonary emboli
2. Identify the signs and symptoms of pulmonary emboli
3. State the reason for anticoagulant therapy, the prescribed dose and time of administration of medications, any adverse side effects, and need to take medications as prescribed
4. State plans for follow-up care, including periodic blood coagulation tests

■ IMPLEMENTATION

Nursing interventions for the person with a pulmonary embolism include the following.

Promoting Comfort

1. Elevate the head of the bed 30 to 40 degrees.
2. Maintain a quiet calm environment.
3. Administer pain medications as ordered.

Promoting Tissue Perfusion

1. Antiembolism stockings
2. Hourly active foot dorsiflexion
3. Elevating lower extremities (do not use Gatch bed)
4. Range of motion exercises
5. Assessing legs for adequate pulses and leg size (do not massage legs)
6. Inspecting IV sites regularly
7. Administering anticoagulants as ordered
8. Monitoring PT and PPT; withholding anticoagu-

lant and notifying physician if PT or PPT falls below accepted levels.

Promoting Gas Exchange

1. Assist patient to deep breathe hourly and to cough unless coughing is contraindicated.
2. Administer oxygen therapy as ordered.
3. Maintain prescribed activity while avoiding overexertion.

Patient Teaching

Teach patient about risk factors associated with emboli and how to avoid them.

1. Do not wear constrictive clothing such as rolled garters.
2. Avoid standing or sitting for prolonged periods. Be sure to move about at least every 2 hours. Do active dorsiflexion of feet while sitting.
3. Stop smoking. Refer to resource that assists patients to stop smoking.

The patient also needs to understand the common signs and symptoms of pulmonary emboli so immediate assistance can be sought if they occur. These include:

1. Dyspnea
2. Substernal chest pain
3. Hemoptysis
4. Chest palpitations
5. Cough
6. Diaphoresis
7. Apprehension

CHRONIC AIRFLOW LIMITATION— OBSTRUCTIVE LUNG DISEASE

CHRONIC OBSTRUCTIVE LUNG DISEASE
EPIDEMIOLOGY AND ETIOLOGY

As indicated at the beginning of this chapter, although chronic airflow limitation has been recommended as the most appropriate terminology, COPD and OAD continue to be used interchangeably with chronic airflow limitation. Chronic airflow limitation uses pathophysiologic

criteria to specify which disease entities should be included within this category (see box below, left). Based on criteria for chronic airflow limitation, more disease entities are included within this category than has traditionally been the case under the classifications of COPD or OAD. Table 33-13 compares the diseases that fall under chronic airflow limitation to those that are traditionally identified with COPD or OAD.

The disease entities identified as the components of COPD are the major airflow limitation diseases. Because COPD is the term most commonly used by clinicians, it will be used in this book to refer to a pathophysiologic state characterized by limitation to airflow on expiration. The major disease entities identified under the rubric of COPD include a variable combination of asthma, chronic bronchitis, and pulmonary emphysema (Table 33-14).

The processes that result in the pathophysiologic changes associated with COPD are neither static nor necessarily progressive. Thus all stages are possible, from reversible abnormalities to relentlessly progressive cardiopulmonary insufficiency.

COPD remains one of the United State's most critical health problems. Both morbidity and mortality are increasing at alarming rates. An estimated 10 million Americans suffer from COPD, and the number of deaths caused by COPD are increasing at an estimated 9% a year. In 1985 direct and indirect costs related to COPD was more than 8.1 billion dollars.[7] This increase in death rate from COPD is believed to be related to (1) the growing tendency of physicians to list it as a primary cause of death, (2) the greater use of pulmonary function testing, and (3) more emphasis in medical literature on the importance of this syndrome. Despite these facts, it is believed that the mortality rate is even higher than reported because many persons who were reported to have died from pneumonia, asthma, or con-

---

MAJOR PHYSIOLOGIC COMPONENTS OF CHRONIC AIRFLOW LIMITATION*

Chronic mucus hypersection (a clinical diagnosis based on history)

Pulmonary emphysema (destruction of parenchyma)

Airway hyperreactivity (asthma, reversible airflow limitation)

Changes in small airways (including respiratory bronchiolitis)

---

*Bates DV: Respiratory function in disease, ed 3, Philadelphia, 1989, WB Saunders.

TABLE 33-13 Comparison of disease entities included under the classification of chronic airflow limitation and COPD

Chronic Airflow Limitation*	COPD
Chronic bronchitis	Chronic bronchitis
Asthma	Asthma
Emphysema	Emphysema
Bronchiolitis	
Cystic fibrosis	
Parenchymal fibrosis or granulomatosis	
Pulmonary lymphangiomyomatosis	
Tracheal stenosis	

*Disease entities included under chronic airflow limitation are from Bates DV: Respiratory function in disease, ed 3, Philadelphia, 1989, WB Saunders.

NURSING CARE PLAN

PERSON WITH COPD

DATA: Mrs. Davis is a 54-year-old housewife with a past medical history of severe chronic obstructive pulmonary disease with cor pulmonale. She has a 75 pack year history of cigarette smoking and stopped smoking 2 years ago (husband still smokes). Patient states: "I am unable to walk back from the bathroom to the living room without a 30 to 60 minute rest." Lung sounds are diminished throughout. Chest x-ray indicates overinflation of the lungs. Pulmonary function tests show severe obstructive ventilatory dysfunction with hyperinflation. Arterial blood gases are: pH = 7.34, $PaCO_2$ = 48, PO_2 = 69, oxygen saturation = 94%. Current medications include metaproterenol inhaler, Theo-Dur, terbutaline, hydrochlorothiazide, K-Lyte, and nitroglycerin sublingual tablets as needed for chest pain. She is seeking outpatient rehabilitation, including muscle reconditioning and education.

The nursing history identified the following:

■ Mrs. Davis continues to be exposed to cigarette smoke because of her husband's continued cigarette smoking. Patient stated, "He's never without a cigarette in the house."

■ Mrs. Davis indicated that her husband's smoking makes it hard for her not to smoke. Patient indicated that she occasionally had a cigarette.

■ Mrs. Davis is fearful of becoming a "bedridden invalid like my mother." Patient's mother had COPD and in her last years had a cerebrovascular accident, which left her totally dependent on her daughter for care until her death 5 years ago.

Collaborative nursing activities include those to assess (1) Mrs. Davis's current pulmonary function status, (2) establish individualized rehabilitation, and (3) evaluate current theophylline levels. Nursing actions include the following:

■ Prepare patient for pulmonary function testing. Explain her role in the testing procedure and describe what she might expect to feel during testing.

■ Participate in rehabilitation team meetings for planning Mrs. Davis's program. Encourage Mrs. Davis to actively participate in the planning process to establish realistic individualized program goals. Elicit feedback to assess Mrs. Davis's understanding of the program activities and goals.

■ Assess theophylline blood levels and presence of any medication side effects.

NURSING DIAGNOSIS

Activity intolerance, related to tissue hypoxia associated with impaired gas exchange/fatigue

Expected Patient Outcomes	Nursing Interventions	Rationale
Mrs. Davis demonstrates increased tolerance for activity.	Provide frequent rest periods. Instruct patient in energy saving techniques. Reinforce use of pursed lip breathing. Gradually increase activity.	Improve activity tolerance.

NURSING DIAGNOSIS

Gas exchange, impaired related to decrease in effective lung surface

Expected Patient Outcomes	Nursing Interventions	Rationale
Mrs. Davis' dyspnea is decreased	Assess respiratory status	Obtain baseline information
	Provide prescribed low-flow oxygen	Many persons with COPD depend on hypoxemia as stimulus to breathe
	Provide breathing retraining	Decrease work of breathing
	Provide rest periods	Improve tolerance

NURSING DIAGNOSIS

Infection, potential for, related to increased secretions, decreased motility in lungs

Expected Patient Outcomes	Nursing Interventions	Rationale
Mrs. Davis' infections are minimized	Restrict persons with upper respiratory infections Teach patient measures to prevent infections Encourage patient to get annual influenza immunizations	Decrease exposure

NURSING CARE PLAN

PERSON WITH COPD—cont'd

NURSING DIAGNOSIS

Self-esteem disturbance, related to changes in lifestyle, dependence on others

Expected Patient Outcomes	Nursing Interventions	Rationale
Mrs. Davis participates in necessary activities	Give patient opportunities to express concerns about limitations.	Allow for communication
	Provide rationale for necessary activities.	Maintain sense of control.
	Discuss with family and friends the need for patient to maintain role relationships	Increase self-esteem
	Assist patient to identify personal strengths	
	Provide information about community resources.	

NURSING DIAGNOSIS

Knowledge deficit, related to lack of exposure/lack of recall.

Expected Patient Outcomes	Nursing Interventions	Rationale
Mrs. Davis describes therapeutic regimen and health maintenance	Teach Mrs. Davis: 1. Nature of COPD and need to follow prescribed therapy and activities 2. Home medication and treatment plans 3. Home exercise plan 4. Avoidance of respiratory irritants and infections 5. Signs requiring medical attention 6. Professional and community resources	Increase self-care abilities and self-esteem

gestive heart failure probably had COPD. In addition to improved reporting and the increased aging of the population, the major factor in this increase in mortality, is an increase in cigarette smoking. These diseases are more prevalent among men than women, but death rates are now showing a higher percentage rate of increase in women than in men. This is believed to be directly related to the increase in smoking among women.

Various causes are related to the onset of COPD. Table 33-15 identifies these causative factors on the basis of predominant obstructive disease with which they are associated.

Although asthma, chronic bronchitis, and emphysema are classified under the common category, it is clinically important to identify the predominant type of pulmonary disease that is the basis for the individual's COPD. Therefore, in the following presentation, COPD is divided into three major obstructive diseases: chronic bronchitis, emphysema, and asthma. Because the clinical management of chronic bronchitis and emphysema is similar, the care for patients with either of these diseases is presented together. (See nursing care plan for person with COPD on p. 912.)

TABLE 33-14 Possible variants of COPD*

Predominant Disease Entity	Associated Obstructive Disease		
	Asthma	Chronic Bronchitis	Emphysema
Asthma	Pure asthma	Asthma with bronchitis	Asthma with emphysema
Chronic bronchitis	Chronic bronchitis with asthma	Pure chronic bronchitis	Chronic bronchitis with emphysema
Emphysema	Emphysema with asthma	Emphysema with chronic bronchitis	Pure emphysema

*In addition to the nine variants above, the individual can have a combination of asthma, bronchitis, and emphysema.

TABLE 33-15 Factors in development of COPD*

Asthma	Chronic Bronchitis	Emphysema
Allergy	Cigarette smoking	Cigarette smoking
Hypersensitivity	Atmospheric contaminants	Atmospheric contaminants
Infection	Infection	Antienzyme and enzyme deficiencies (α, α_1, and α_2)
Environment	Chronic irritation	Advanced pulmonary fibrosis
Drugs	Gastroesophageal dysfunction	Destruction of lung parenchyma (necrosis, ischemia)
Emotions		
Social conditions		
Exercise		

*Tomashefski JF, editor: Chronic obstructive pulmonary disease: a perplexing and challenging spectrum: core curriculum symposium (pulmonary disease), Postgrad Med 62:87-151, 1977.

CHRONIC BRONCHITIS

Chronic bronchitis is defined *clinically* by hypersecretion of mucus and recurrent or chronic productive cough for a minimum of 3 months per year for at least 2 consecutive years in patients in whom other causes have been excluded. It is characterized *physiologically* by hypertrophy and hypersecretion of the bronchial mucus glands and structural alterations of the bronchi and bronchioles.

EPIDEMIOLOGY AND ETIOLOGY

As indicated in Table 33-15, chronic bronchitis is caused by the inhalation of physical or chemical irritants or by viral or bacterial infections. The most common inhaled irritant is cigarette smoke, and heavy cigarette smoking is believed to be the major cause of the disease. Occupations in which dust or other irritants are inhaled may cause bronchitis, but the evidence for this is not conclusive. However, in Great Britain it has been recognized for years that the highest incidence of bronchitis occurs in large industrial cities with high levels of air pollution.

PREVENTION

The overall focus for prevention of chronic bronchitis is to alleviate whatever irritant appears to be causing the associated symptoms in the individual. Of all the known risk factors, the most clearly implicated is smoking. The continued inhalation of tobacco smoke leads to worsening of bronchial inflammation and hypersecretion. Thus smoking cessation is an essential step for the prevention of chronic bronchitis. Additionally, such preventive measures as avoidance of repeated infections and prompt treatment of upper and lower respiratory infections are important steps to avoid disease progression. National standards for air quality and governmental actions related to improving the quality of the air we breathe should be of concern to everyone.

Progress in the prevention of chronic bronchitis has been impeded by the slow and insidious onset of the disease. Recent advances in pulmonary function testing have allowed identification of abnormalities in the small airways of the lungs.[58] It is believed that peripheral airway changes occur early in the development of obstructive lung disease. Research has indicated that some of the abnormalities associated with small airway changes may be reversible.[77] Thus if high risk populations could be identified and a feasible screening test developed, preventive measures could be instituted before permanent lung damage and chronic disease occur.

PATHOPHYSIOLOGY

The two pathologic changes that typify chronic bronchitis are hypertrophy of mucus-secreting glands and chronic inflammatory changes in the small airways. First, there is glandular hypertrophy. *Mucus gland hypertrophy* and *hyperplasia* from chronic irritation cause excessive mucus production. The excessive mucus and impaired ciliary movement associated with chronic bronchitis increase susceptibility to infection. Bacteria proliferate in the mucous secretions in the lumen of the bronchi. The most common infectious agents are *S. pneumoniae* and *H. influenzae*. As bacteria multiply, they exert a neutrophilic chemotaxis, and pus cells migrate from between bronchial epithelial cells to produce a mucopurulent exudate in the lumen, or the disease may progress to ulceration and destruction of the bronchial wall. The presence of granulation tissue and peribronchial fibrosis result in stenosis and airway obstruction. Small airways may be completely obliterated, and others may become dilated. This chain of events further traps secretions and promotes multiplication of bacteria. There is some evidence that the pathologic changes occur initially in small airways and move to larger bronchi.[116]

Second, persons with chronic bronchitis develop increased airway resistance as a result of bronchial wall tissue changes, mucosal edema, and excessive mucus production. Excess mucus in the airways not only obstructs airflow but also often causes bronchospasm, which further increases airway resistance.

Third, there is altered oxygen-carbon dioxide exchange. Airway obstruction resulting from all the pathophysiologic changes that increase airway resistance may impair the ability of the lungs to exchange oxygen and carbon dioxide. Obstructed airways cause ventilation-perfusion mismatching at the alveolar-capillary membrane by decreasing the amount of oxygenated air that reaches the alveoli. Additionally, the obstructed airways may lead to atelectasis, which further diminishes the surface area available for respiration. The result of these pathophysiologic alterations is hypercapnea, hypoxemia,

and respiratory acidosis (see discussion of arterial blood gases; see Chapter 34).

Fourth, right ventricular decompensation (cor pulmonale) may result. The hypercapnia and hypoxemia commonly associated with chronic bronchitis cause pulmonary vascular vasoconstriction. The increased pulmonary vascular resistance results in pulmonary vessel hypertension that in turn increases vascular pressure in the right ventricle of the heart.

CLINICAL MANIFESTATIONS

Signs and symptoms of chronic bronchitis are manifestations of the underlying physiologic abnormalities that have occurred. Table 33-16 relates normal function, pri-

TABLE 33-16 Normal function, primary pathophysiology, and the clinical picture in chronic bronchitis, emphysema, and asthma

Normal Function/ Pathophysiology	Clinical Picture		
	Chronic Bronchitis	**Emphysema**	**Asthma**
Bronchial mucus-*secreting glands* produce mucus to trap foreign particles and transport them out of lungs	Productive chronic cough, grayish-white sputum; when infected sputum is yellow, inspiratory; crackles (rales)		Inflammation, hypersecretion; eosinophilis in sputum
BRONCHI AND BRONCHIOLES			
Carry oxygenated air to alveoli and carry deoxygenated air out of lungs	Inspiratory, expiratory rhonchi; dyspnea: episodic or continual; ↓FEV, ↓VC with small response to bronchodilators*	Early onset dyspnea on exertion, which progresses to continuous dyspnea. Rhonchi, crackles, accessory muscle breathing ↓FEV, ↓VC with no response to bronchodilators	Episodic dyspnea, accessory muscle breathing; inspiratory/expiratory wheezing. ↓FEV ↓VC with good response to bronchodilators. ↑Work of breathing, pulsus paradoxus
ALVEOLAR-CAPILLARY MEMBRANE			
Semipermeable membrane where oxygen diffuses from alveoli to blood and carbon dioxide diffuses from blood to alevoli	Respiratory acidosis, hypoxemia, polycythemia, tachycardia, cyanosis	Early stage: normal or mild hypoxemia, respiratory alkalosis; late stage: hypoxemia respiratory acidosis, ↓diffusing capacity	Respiratory alkalosis with mild hypoxemia Status asthmaticus: respiratory acidosis with hypoxemia
RIGHT SIDE OF HEART			
Carries deoxygenated blood to pulmonary vasculature for oxygen/carbon dioxide exchange	Jugular vein distention hepatomegaly, peripheral edema	Right ventricular decompensation	
LUNG AND CHEST WALL COMPLIANCE			
The relationship between lung and chest wall ability to expand and contract curing inhalation and exhalation		↑A-P diameter, ↓lateral expansion, ↓diaphragmatic excursion, ↓breath, heart, and voice sounds, ↑RV, ↑FRC, ↑TLC hyperresonance, complaint of epigastric fullness	↓Fremitus, ↓lateral expansion, hyperresonance, ↓breath sounds, ↓diaphragmatic excursion

FEV, forced expiratory volume; VC, vital capacity.

mary pathophysiology, and the clinical picture observed in chronic bronchitis.

The earliest symptom of chronic bronchitis is a productive cough, especially on awakening. This symptom is often ignored by cigarette smokers who become so accustomed to an early morning cough that they take it for granted; and some of them even refer to it as their "cigarette cough."

Persons with chronic bronchitis often unconsciously adapt their activity level to accommodate their respiratory symptoms in their daily lives. Thus they do not seek medical help until they experience a severe exacerbation of their symptoms, usually precipitated by a respiratory infection.

Pulmonary function testing reveals a limitation to airflow on expiration as evidenced by a diminished FEV_1. Vital capacity is also reduced, indicating diminished air movement both in and out of the lungs. Lung volumes are usually within normal limits until later in the course of the disease, when the lung volumes may be increased. There usually is no loss of diffusing capacity.

Early in the course of chronic bronchitis, the symptoms tend to be episodic in nature. As the disease progresses in severity, the patient's symptoms are constantly present to some degree. The patient appears increasingly dyspneic, using accessory muscles to breathe. Chronic hypoxemia resulting in polycythemia causes the patient to appear to be cyanotic. Increased pulmonary vascular resistance caused by respiratory acidosis and hypoxemia increases pressure on the right side of the heart, ultimately resulting in right heart failure (cor pulmonale). The person with late-stage chronic bronchitis and cor pulmonale appears stout or overweight from edema. Because of the edema and dusky skin color these people are often referred to clinically as a "blue bloater." The person with preceding characteristic appearance is identified as a person with type B COPD.

Patients with chronic bronchitis complicated by cor pulmonale often have chronic respiratory failure (gradual onset of $PaO_2 < 50$ and a $PaCO_2 > 50$). They are also prone to develop acute respiratory failure (sudden onset of a $PaO_2 < 50$ and a $PaCO_2 > 50$) as a complication of a respiratory infection superimposed on their already diseased lung.

MEDICAL MANAGEMENT

The process of medical diagnosis of chronic bronchitis may include any of the following investigative modalities.

1. Patient history
2. Physical examination
3. Diagnostic studies
   a. Chest x-ray: typical findings with chronic bronchitis increased bronchovascular markings
   b. Sputum studies for culture and sensitivity: neutrophils and bronchial epithelial cells usually present in chronic bronchitis
   c. Arterial blood gas studies: see discussion under clinical manifestations
   d. Hematology studies: CBC
   e. Pulmonary function testing: see discussion under clinical manifestations

Effective health care management programs for persons who have chronic bronchitis or any of the variant combinations of pulmonary diseases that make up COPD requires a multidisciplinary approach. The multidisciplinary approach to the management of COPD is included in the discussion of implementation of care for patients with COPD later in this chapter.

Medical management of a person with chronic bronchitis is included in Table 33-17, which summarizes a typical multidisciplinary program for a person with COPD.

■ ASSESSMENT

Subjective Data

Subjective data include the following:
1. History of character of onset and duration of:
   a. Cough
   b. Sputum production (amount, color, and consistency)
   c. Dyspnea
   d. Pain in right upper quadrant (hepatomegaly)
2. Smoking history
3. Disease history
   a. Influenza
   b. Pneumonia
   c. Repeated respiratory tract infections
   d. Chronic sinusitis
4. Past or present exposure to environmental irritants at home or at work
5. Self-care used to treat symptoms
6. Medications taken and their effectiveness in relieving symptoms

Objective Data

Objective data include the following:
1. Assess general appearance
   a. Patient may appear overweight or bloated.
   b. Check for dependent edema and jugular vein distention
   c. Abdominal assessment may indicate heptomegaly
2. Assess vital signs
   a. Elevated temperature
   b. Tachycardia
   c. Tachypnea
3. Pulmonary examination
   a. Inspection

TABLE 33-17 Etiology, signs and symptoms, and medical therapy for chronic bronchitis and pulmonary emphysema

Bronchitis	Pulmonary Emphysema
ETIOLOGY	
Inhalation of physical or chemical irritants or viral or bacterial infections	Not known; believed that some change in the enzyme-inhibitor balance occurs, allowing proteolytic enzymes to attack lung tissue
Most common inhaled irritant—cigarette smoke	Not known why some smokers develop bronchitis and others develop emphysema. α-antitrypsin deficiency in some persons who develop severe, disabling emphysema early in life; familial tendency for this type of emphysema
SIGNS AND SYMPTOMS	
Early Symptoms	
Productive cough on awakening; often ignored by cigarette smokers who refer to it as their "cigarette cough"	Dyspnea on exertion, may be in acute respiratory distress
	Using accessory muscles to breathe; ruddy color
Later Symptoms	Thin with a "barrel chest"
Significant physical incapacity; breathlessness even when walking on a flat surface, noticeable shortness of breath (SOB) and use of accessory muscles to breathe; cyanosis common; ankle edema, bloated appearance, distended neck veins; sometimes referred to as "blue bloater"	Usually able to maintain resting PO_2
	Cyanosis uncommon
	Sometimes referred to as "pink puffer"
	Late in Disease
	$PCO_2 \uparrow$
	Cor pulmonale and respiratory failure possible complications
Late in Disease	
Frequent complications—cor pulmonale (right ventricular hypertrophy), right-sided heart failure, and respiratory failure	
PULMONARY FUNCTION TEST FINDINGS	
$\downarrow$ Expiratory flow rates	$\downarrow$ Expiratory flows rates, especially forced expiratory volume, and maximal mid-expiratory flow
$\downarrow$ Vital capacity	$\uparrow$ Total lung capacity
$\uparrow$ Residual volume	$\uparrow$ Residual volume
Total lung capacity usually within normal limits	Vital capacity normal or slightly reduced until late stages of disease, FEV_1/VC ratio changed.
ARTERIAL BLOOD GAS FINDINGS	
Low resting PO_2	PO_2 normal or slightly reduced at *rest* but falls during exercise
Elevated PCO_2 (if obstruction severe)	
During exercise $PCO_2 \uparrow$ and PO_2 may also $\uparrow$	Normal PCO_2
	Late in disease PCO_2 elevated

MEDICAL THERAPY

Medical therapy for chronic bronchitis and pulmonary emphysema is similar and depends on symptoms, pulmonary function test results and blood gas findings. Therapy may include all or some of the modalities outlined here.

SUPPORTIVE MEASURES

Education of patient and family about the following:
    Avoidance of cigarette smoke
    Avoidance of other inhaled irritants
    Avoidance of persons with upper respiratory infections
    Control of environmental temperature and humidity
    Proper nutrition
    Adequate hydration

SPECIFIC THERAPY

Medications
Bronchodilators (Table 33-18)
Antimicrobials
    Tetracycline or ampicillin usually prescribed to treat respiratory tract infections
Corticosteroids
    May be prescribed to alleviate acute symptoms; prednisone most often used
Digitalis
    May be prescribed to treat left ventricular failure

Continued.

TABLE 33-17 Etiology, signs and symptoms, and medical therapy for chronic bronchitis and pulmonary emphysema—cont'd

Bronchitis	Pulmonary Emphysema
RESPIRATORY THERAPY	
Aerosol Therapy	
Used to deliver bronchodilators through metered cartridge devices or hand-bulb nebulizers	
Oxygen Therapy	
Required for patients who are unable to maintain a PO_2 of 50 torr or more at rest or who cannot carry out ADL without becoming short of breath; 1 to 2 L of O_2 given by nasal prongs	
PHYSICAL CONDITIONING	
Relaxation Exercises	
Progressive relaxation exercises encouraged; best practiced before meals or 2 hours or more after eating, since digestion seems to interfere with ability to relax	
Meditation	
Meditation becoming more widely used to assist patients to relax	
Breathing Retraining	
Pursed-lip breathing Leaning forward position for exhalation Abdominal breathing Inhalation-exhalation exercises Exhalation with exertion	
Rehabilitation	
Muscle reconditioning programs specific for the patient	

     (1) Accessory muscle breathing
     (2) Forward leaning posture
     (3) Central cyanosis
     (4) Clubbing of fingers
     (5) Altered sensorium (restlessness or lethargy)
  b. Palpation
     (1) Increased tactile fremitus
  c. Percussion—normal
  d. Auscultation
     (1) Inspiratory crackles (rales)
     (2) Inspiratory and expiratory rhonchi
4. Assess laboratory findings
  a. Arterial blood gases
     (1) Respiratory acidosis
     (2) Hypoxemia
  b. Hematology
     (1) Elevated hemoglobin and hematocrit
     (2) Elevated WBC
  c. Pulmonary function tests
     (1) Decreased FEV_1
     (2) Normal diffusing capacity
     (3) Normal lung volumes (in end-stage chronic bronchitis lung volumes may appear similar to those found with emphysema)

■ **DATA ANALYSIS: NURSING DIAGNOSES**

Nursing diagnoses are determined from assessment of patient data. Possible nursing diagnoses for the person with chronic bronchitis include, but are not limited to, the following:

Diagnostic Title	Possible Etiologies
Activity intolerance	Imbalance between oxygen demand and requirement
Altered nutrition, less than body requirements	Dyspnea, anorexia, sputum production, medication side effects, fatigue
Fear	Long-term illness and disability, change in role functioning
Fluid volume excess	Pulmonary hypertension with resultant increased cardiac workload
Impaired gas exchange	Low ventilation/perfusion ratio
Ineffective airway clearance	Hypersecretion, tracheobronchial infection, decreased energy/fatigue
Ineffective breathing pattern	Decreased energy/fatigue, airway changes
Infection, potential for	Decreased lung defenses
Knowledge deficit: condition and its treatment	Lack of exposure/recall, cognitive limitation, unfamiliarity with information source

■ PLANNING: EXPECTED PATIENT OUTCOMES

Expected outcomes for patients with COPD are similar, regardless of the underlying obstructive airway disease. Thus outcomes for patients with chronic bronchitis are included later in this chapter under the outcomes for patients with COPD.

EMPHYSEMA

Emphysema is defined *pathologically* by destructive changes in alveolar walls and enlargement of air spaces distal to the terminal nonrespiratory bronchioles. It is characterized *physiologically* by increased lung compliance, decreased diffusing capacity, and increased airway resistance.

EPIDEMIOLOGY AND ETIOLOGY

Although it is not known when emphysema actually begins, there appear to be many years between the initial pathophysiologic changes and the onset of overt symptoms. Symptoms associated with emphysema usually appear in the fourth decade, and disability from disease usually occurs in the fifth or sixth decade of life. The typical individual with emphysema is a male of about 55 years of age with a history of tobacco smoking.

The cause of emphysema is not known; however, recent evidence suggests that proteases released by polymorphonuclear leukocytes or alveolar macrophages are involved in the destruction of the connective tissue of the lungs. Connective tissue in the lungs is primarily composed of elastin, collagen, and proteoglycan, which can be damaged and destroyed by enzymes such as proteases and elastase. It has been demonstrated that elastase (produced by alveolar macrophages) can destroy or damage the elastin in the connective tissue of the parenchyma of the lung.[9] Normally, inhibitors found in human serum, lung tissue, peripheral airways, and bronchial mucus protect the lung from the proteolytic enzymes. It is believed that some change in the enzyme-inhibitor balance occurs, which allows the proteolytic enzymes to attack lung tissue.

It has been known since 1965 that some persons have a deficiency of α_1-antitrypsin and that these persons develop severe, disabling emphysema early in life, usually of the bullous type. Recent studies indicate that cigarette smoke increases the amount of elastase secreted by the alveolar macrophages and neutrophils and that it impairs the inhibitor functions of α_1-antitrypsin.[37]

It is not known, however, why some smokers develop bronchitis and others develop emphysema. Differences in susceptibility and the predominant type of disease are believed to be influenced by hereditary or environmental factors or those related to the patient's history.[37] It is established, however, that there is familial tendency to α_1-antitrypsin deficiency and that relatives of persons with this type of emphysema should be screened and provided with counseling as discussed below.

PREVENTION

The cornerstone of prevention of emphysema is education. Public education must focus on the pulmonary health risks associated with inhaled irritants, regardless of their source. Increased public awareness of the vital role clean air plays in pulmonary health is essential for the success of any legislative actions promoting air quality standards. Individuals must also be educated to understand the importance of personal responsibility to decrease their own health risk through smoking cessation.

Persons with a family history of emphysema should be screened for α_1-antitrypsin deficiency. It is imperative that persons with this enzyme deficiency take active measures to prevent additive lung damage from smoking, air pollution, and infection. Persons identified as being at high risk for emphysema may require vocational counseling if their current work environment is known to have inhaled irritants. These individuals also should be counseled to receive the influenza and pneumonia vaccines.

PATHOPHYSIOLOGY

The type of emphysema can be determined only by descriptive morphology. There are two principal types of emphysema morphologically—*centrilobular* emphysema (CLE) and *panlobular* emphysema (PLE). In CLE, there is distention and damage of the respiratory bronchioles selectively. Openings develop in the walls of the bronchioles; they become enlarged and confluent and tend to form a single space as the walls enlarge. The disease tends to be unevenly distributed throughout the lung but usually is more severe in the upper portions.

In PLE, there is a more uniform enlargement and destruction of the alveoli in the pulmonary acinus. PLE is usually more diffuse and is more severe in the lower lung. It is found in elderly persons who have no evidence of chronic bronchitis or impairment of lung function.[4] It occurs just as commonly in women as in men, but PLE is less common than CLE. PLE is a characteristic finding in persons with homozygous α_1-antitrypsin deficiency.[4]

The clinical diagnosis of emphysema is inferred from the presence of signs and symptoms that are manifestations of known pathophysiologic changes associated with the disease. Physiologic abnormalities characteristic of emphysema include the following alterations:

1. Increased lung compliance. Loss of elastic recoil resulting from destruction of elastin in lung parenchyma causes the lungs to become permanently overdistended. Thus, compared to normal lungs, emphysematous lungs have a larger in-

crease in volume relative to the pressure change that occurs during inhalation.

2. Increased airway resistance. Destruction of elastic lung tissue causes the small airway to either collapse or narrow, particularly during expiration. Thus air becomes trapped in the distal airspaces, contributing to the lungs' overdistended state. The overdistended lungs press against the diaphragm, diminishing its ventilatory effectiveness. Accessory muscle breathing, which is a compensatory attempt to force the trapped air out of the lungs, causes an increase in intrapleural pressure, which further accentuates airway collapse.

3. Altered oxygen-carbon dioxide exchange. Destruction of alveolar and respiratory bronchiole walls decrease alveolar-capillary membrane surface area, which in turn may diminish gaseous diffusion. Persons with emphysema are able to compensate for these destructive changes by increasing their respiratory rate. Thus arterial blood gases remain relatively normal, although mild hypoxemia may be present. Late in the course of the disease, extensive surface area loss coupled with ventilation-perfusion inequalities usually cause respiratory acidosis and hypoxemia.

Normal function, pathophysiology, and clinical picture of emphysema is presented in Table 33-16.

CLINICAL MANIFESTATIONS

Typically, the first symptoms heralding the onset of emphysema is dyspnea on exertion (DOE), which progresses to continual dyspnea. Sputum production tends to be scant or absent. Persons with emphysema usually appear thin and manifest a "barrel chest" with an increased anteroposterior (AP) diameter from hyperinflation. The characteristic breathing pattern of the emphysematous individual includes accessory muscle

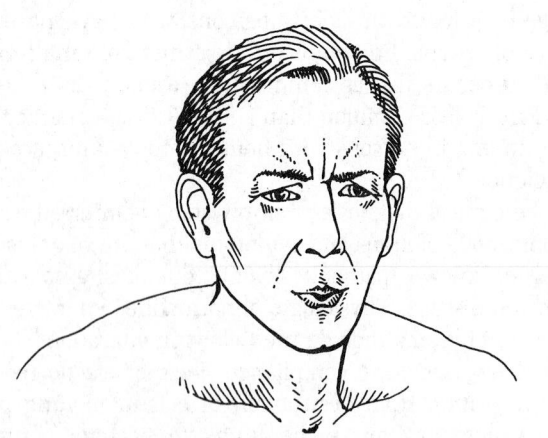

FIGURE 33-5 Pursed-lip breathing.

breathing, an increased respiratory rate, and a prolonged expiratory phase resulting from airway narrowing or collapse on expiration. These individuals will spontaneously exhibit pursed-lip breathing (Figure 33-5), which facilitates effective air exhalation. (Pursed-lip breathing elevates end-expiratory pressures, which inhibits airway collapse during expiration.)

Pulmonary function studies demonstrate an increased residual volume, functional residual capacity, and total lung volume. Diffusing capacity is significantly reduced because of lung tissue destruction. Diminished respiratory air flow is demonstrated by a decreased forced expiratory volume (FEV) and maximal midexpiratory flow rate (MMFR). The vital capacity (VC) may be normal or only slightly reduced until late in the disease progression; thus the FEV_1/VC ratio is decreased. The degree of respiratory impairment may be estimated on the basis of the ratio of FEV to FVC (see the box below). A significant finding that differentiates emphysema from the other obstructive airway pathologies is the failure to demonstrate improvement in pulmonary function test results in response to the administration of bronchodilators.

Arterial blood gases are often near normal because of the individual's ability to compensate through increased respiratory rate and tidal volume. Indeed, many people with emphysema overcompensate and develop a mild respiratory alkalosis from hyperventilation. Because resting hypoxemia is absent and ventilation is high, these individuals maintain a normal P_{CO_2} despite abnormal gas exchange and are described as "pink puffers." A person exhibiting these symptoms of pure emphysema is classified as having type A COPD. Late in the course of the disease the P_{CO_2} is elevated, which promotes the development of cor pulmonale and respiratory failure.

The terms "blue bloater" and "pink puffer" represent the two extremes seen in persons with chronic airway obstruction. Recently, it has been suggested that the underlying disease alone does not determine whether the person is "blue" or "pink," but rather the interaction between the lung disease and the person's drive to breathe. For example, the pink puffer may just fight harder to maintain a normal P_{CO_2}, whereas the blue bloater settles for less work and allows the P_{CO_2} to rise.

ESTIMATE OF PULMONARY DYSFUNCTION BASED ON FEV/VC RATIO

Normal lung function—greater than 80% predicted values

Mild impairment—65% to 85% of predicted values

Moderate impairment—50% to 64% of predicted values

Severe impairment—49% or less of predicted values

MEDICAL MANAGEMENT

The process of medical diagnosis of emphysema may include any of the following investigative modalities.

1. Patient history
2. Diagnostic studies
   a. Chest x-ray: positive finding = increased radiolucency of lungs with diaphragm in a low flat position
   b. Arterial blood gas studies
   c. Pulmonary function testing
   d. Hematology
      (1) α,-antitrypsin assay
      (2) CBC; usually normal
   e. Sputum for culture and sensitivity

Medical management of emphysema includes the same modalities as those used in the treatment of chronic bronchitis. Table 33-17 presents the components of medical therapy used in the treatment of both chronic bronchitis and emphysema.

■ ASSESSMENT

Subjective Data

Subjective data include the following:

1. History of character and onset of the following:
   a. Dyspnea—(important to investigate if patient correlates the occurrence of dyspnea with any specific illness or other life event; establish how the patient's dyspnea affects ADL)
   b. Cough—usually mild or may be absent
   c. Sputum production—usually scant white sputum
2. Smoking history
3. Family history of emphysema
4. Past or present exposure to environmental irritants at home or at work
5. Self-care modalities
6. Medications or other prescribed therapies and their effectiveness in relieving symptoms

Objective Data

Objective data include the following:

1. Assess general appearance
   a. Patient usually appears thin with a large chest. (Note: this is a normal variant in the elderly; thus it does not always signify pulmonary disease.)
2. Assess vital signs for:
   a. Tachycardia
   b. Tachypnea
3. Pulmonary examination
   a. Inspection
      (1) Accessory muscle breathing
      (2) Forward-leaning posture
      (3) Pursed-lip breathing
      (4) Prolonged expiration
      (5) Barrel chest, increased A-P diameter
   b. Palpation
      (1) Decreased lateral expansion
      (2) Decreased fremitus
   c. Percussion
      (1) Hyperresonance
      (2) Low diaphragm
      (3) Decreased diaphragmatic excursion
   d. Auscultation
      (1) Decreased breath and heart sounds
      (2) Late inspiratory crackles
      (3) Rhonchi (Note: adventitous sounds are often not present with emphysema.)
4. Assess laboratory findings
   a. Arterial blood gases
      (1) Early stage emphysema-respiratory alkalosis with mild hypoxemia
      (2) Late stage emphysema-respiratory acidosis with hypoxemia
   b. Hematology
      (1) Positive α_1 antitrypsin assay
   c. Pulmonary function
      (1) Decreased FEV_1, VC, and diffusing capacity (D_L)
      (2) Increased total lung capacity, functional residual capacity (FRC), residual volume (RV)

■ DATA ANALYSIS: NURSING DIAGNOSES

Nursing diagnoses are determined from assessment of patient data. Possible nursing diagnoses for the person with emphysema include, but are not limited to, the following:

Diagnostic Title	Possible Etiologies
Activity intolerance	Imbalance between oxygen supply and demand, dyspnea
Altered nutrition, less than body requirements	Anorexia, sputum production, medication side effects, fatigue, long-term illness and disability
Impaired gas exchange	Airway changes, low ventilation/perfusion ratio
Ineffective breathing pattern	Decreased energy/fatigue
Knowledge deficit: disease and its treatment	Lack of exposure/recall, cognitive limitation, unfamiliarity with information source

■ PLANNING: EXPECTED PATIENT OUTCOMES

The following expected patient outcomes and implementation sections apply to patients with chronic bronchitis, emphysema, or any combination of these two obstructive airway diseases.

The patient will:
1. Demonstrate an effective breathing pattern
   a. Inspiratory to expiratory ratio = 5:10 seconds
   b. Pursed-lip breathing (Fig. 35-5)
   c. Appropriate use of leaning forward postures
   d. Diaphragmatic breathing (abdominal muscle breathing)
   e. Exhales with activity
   f. Respiratory rate within near normal limits, moderate tidal volume
2. Demonstrate improved ventilation and oxygenation
   a. Arterial blood pH and Pco2 that returns or stays within acceptable baseline limits
   b. Pao2 at optimal level for individual
   c. Explains how and when to use oxygen therapy
3. Demonstrate adequate airway clearance
   a. Effective methods of coughing
   b. Appropriate use of nebulizers, humidifiers, mistometers, intermittent positive pressure breathing (IPPB) machine, and medications
4. List common signs and symptoms that require reporting to the health care provider
   a. Change in sputum color, amount, and consistency
   b. Increased coughing
   c. Change in behavior
   d. Increased fatigue
   e. Increased dyspnea
   f. Weight gain
   g. Peripheral edema
   h. Elevated temperature
5. Demonstrate how to carry out the specific exercise program to be followed at home including:
   a. Specific exercises to be completed
   b. Frequency of each exercise
   c. Criteria for monitoring physical response to exercises such as heart rate increase or perceived fatigue
6. Maintain or work toward an optimal activity level
   a. Pacing activities
   b. Planning for simplification of activities
   c. Participating in planned muscle conditioning program
7. Demonstrate comprehension of self-care activities
   a. Explain health maintenance or therapeutic follow-up program
   b. Describe any home medication or treatment program
   c. Explain exercise program to be followed at home
   d. Describe how to obtain professional and community resources necessary to structure a satisfactory environment at home
   e. State plans for ongoing follow-up care
8. Explain dietary changes required after discharge
   a. Explain food and fluid requirements and daily plan for achieving them
   b. List specific foods to be avoided
   c. Explain plan for frequent, small feedings that are soft and that do not require much chewing, and the need for increased time required for eating if indicated
   d. Maintain optimal weight for height, age, and gender
9. Demonstrate activities to control stress response to symptoms
   a. Muscle relaxation
   b. Meditation
   c. Participation in support group
10. Explain the following aspects of home medication or treatment regimens:
    a. State name, dose, action, and side effects of each medication to be used at home
    b. How and when to use medications ordered on an as needed basis (for example, bronchodilators, antibiotics, steroids, antacids)
    c. Techniques necessary for follow-up care (for example, segmental postural drainage, clapping and vibrating, inhalation therapy treatments
    d. How to obtain and maintain any needed equipment or supplies such as oxygen, nebulizers, humidifiers, mistometers, IPPB machine, syringes, and medications
11. List names and telephone numbers of appropriate community support services such as the Visiting Nurse Association and a home medical equipment supplier

■ **IMPLEMENTATION**

COPD and all of its actual or potential impact on the individual's life are most effectively managed by a multidisciplinary team. Pulmonary health care teams consisting of physicians, nurses, respiratory therapists, oc-

---

MULTIDISCIPLINARY PROGRAMS FOR PATIENTS WITH COPD[59]

Patient and family education
  Pharmacotherapy
  Conditioning exercises
    Cardiopulmonary conditioning
    General muscle conditioning
  Pulmonary hygiene modalities
  Relaxation training
  Counseling
    Psychosocial counseling
    Vocational counseling

---

cupational therapists, physical therapists, dieticians, social workers, and psychologists or psychiatrists, provide a comprehensive approach to assist patients to attain or maintain their optimal level of function within the constraints of their pulmonary disability.

A typical multidisciplinary program incorporates the areas listed in the box on p. 922.

Although it is difficult to measure the physiologic effects of these programs, hospitalization of patients who have participated in them is less frequent, and most people state that they feel better.

Although the complex multidisciplinary rehabilitation team is the ideal, the nurse functioning in a small community hospital or community team setting can provide effective rehabilitation activities for the person with COPD. The research box at right presents the results of a research study about the effectiveness of teaching patients with COPD.

Nursing interventions for chronic bronchitis and pulmonary emphysema are the same and center around the following.

Improving Efficiency of Breathing Patterns

Although patients with COPD often spontaneously use pursed lip breathing, it is important that patients' use of this effective intervention be reinforced and promoted (Figure 33-5). PEEP is slightly increased by exhaling against the pursed lips, thus increasing airway stability. Additionally, length of expiration is increased and respiratory rate is slowed, which results in a more effective ventilatory pattern.[72]

RESEARCH

Perry JA: Effectiveness of teaching in the rehabilitation of patients with chronic bronchitis and emphysema, Nurs Res 30(4):219-222, 1981.

The effectiveness of the educational component of a pulmonary rehabilitation program that used principles of adult learning was evaluated. Twenty participants ranging in age from 51 to 70 who were diagnosed with COPD were followed for 11 months. The participants were required to keep a symptom diary for the first 4 weeks of the program and for 8 weeks after completion of the program. The data from the two diaries were analyzed. The investigator found that after participating in the rehabilitation program, the participants reported a significant decrease in the number of symptoms and a significant increase in the number of self-care modalities used to treat symptoms. The study indicated that a rehabilitation program that used adult learning concepts promoted the participants' abilities to cope independently with their pulmonary symptoms. ■

A promising area of nursing research that may help patients with ineffective breathing patterns is the use of inspiratory muscle training. The goal of inspiratory muscle exercises is to strengthen and increase the endurance of respiratory muscles in order to help prevent muscle fatigue.

See the research presented in the box on p. 924 for details. Patients are taught to improve their breathing pattern by assuming a forward-leaning posture (Figure

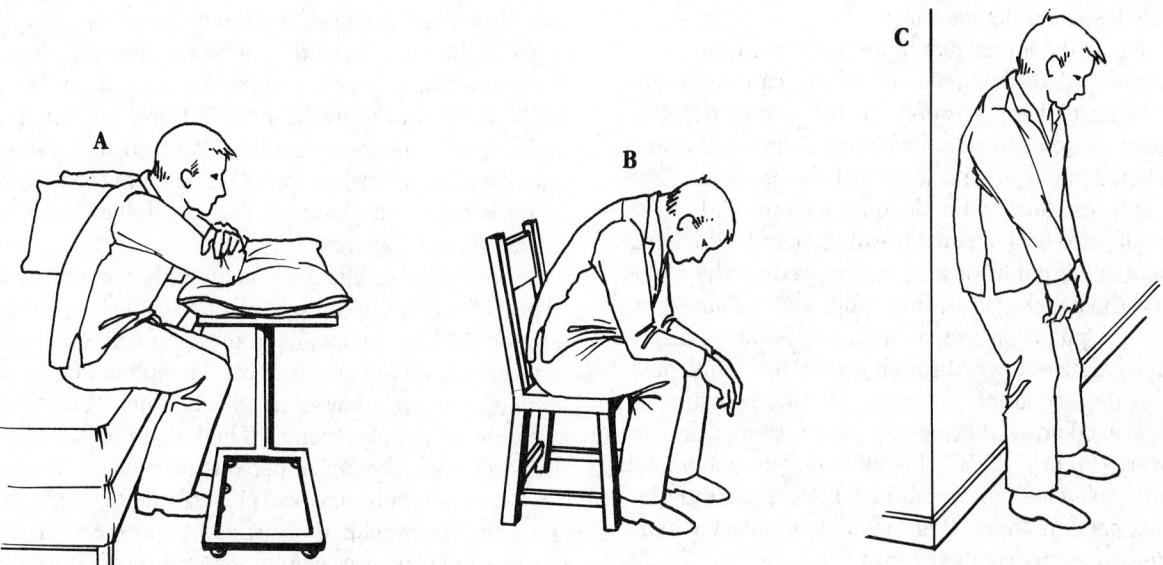

FIGURE 33-6 Forward-leaning position. **A,** Patient sits on edge of bed with arms folded on pillow placed on elevated bedside table. **B,** Patient in three-point position. Patient sits in chair with feet approximately 1 foot apart and leans forward with elbows on knees. **C,** Patient leans against wall with feet spread apart, allowing shoulders to sag forward with arms relaxed.

RESEARCH

Larson M, and Kim MJ: Respiratory muscle training with the incentive spirometer resistive breathing device, Heart Lung 13(4):341-345, 1984.

The effect of using an incentive spirometer for 15 minutes twice daily for 1 month was studied in nine people between 40 and 70 years of age with COPD. Inspiratory muscle strength, exercise performance, clinical condition, and ADL were compared in each individual before and after participating in the respiratory muscle training program. The results indicated that inspiratory muscle strength increased significantly, and that participants reported a marked improvement in sputum expectoration ability. No significant change was found in exercise performance, clinical condition, or ADL. ∎

TABLE 33-18 Bronchodilators commonly used to treat COPD

Name	Mode of Action
METHYLXANTHINES	
Aminophylline Theophylline Dyphylline	Block action of phosphodiesterase and interfere with degradation of cyclic AMP, resulting in bronchodilation
SYMPATHOMIMETICS*	
β_1-receptor sites Epinephrine (adrenaline HCL) Isoproterenol (Isuprel) β_2-receptor sites Terbutaline (Brethine) Metaproterenol (Alupent) Isoetharine (Bronkosol)	Activate adenylcylase leading to increased production of cyclic AMP, resulting in relaxation of smooth muscle of airway; increase in cyclic AMP also inhibits release of chemical mediators that cause bronchospasm (histamine and SRS-A)

*β-adrenergic drugs.

33-6). Leaning forward causes the patient to automatically shift from breathing with accessory muscles to breathing with the diaphragm. Along with the forward-leaning position they are taught to:

1. Inhale through the nose and exhale through pursed lips, with the lips assuming an elliptical "O" shape
2. Consciously slow respiratory rate and avoid inhaling large amounts of air; goal—inhalation to the count of 5 seconds and gently exhaling to the count of 10 seconds
3. Exhale with activity; for example, to tie shoes, the patient inhales normal breath through nose and exhales when bending over
4. Practice abdominal/diaphragmatic breathing

Abdominal (diaphragmatic) breathing can be taught in the sitting or lying position. In the sitting position, the patient sits on the side of the bed or in a chair and holds a small pillow or a book against the abdomen. The patient exhales slowly while leaning forward and pressing the pillow or book against the abdomen. In the lying position, a small pillow or a book is placed on the abdomen, and the patient is asked to "puff out" the abdomen and raise the pillow or book as high as possible. The patient then exhales slowly through pursed lips while pulling in on the abdominal muscles. Manual pressure on the upper abdomen during expiration facilitates this maneuver (Figure 33-7). In addition to abdominal breathing, exercises to strengthen abdominal muscles will assist patients to use their abdominal muscles more effectively in emptying their lungs.

Teaching patients to use conscious diaphragmatic breathing to counteract dyspnea has been criticized by some because people automatically assume accessory muscle breathing when they are dyspneic. By comparison, leaning-forward postures are believed to promote more effective breathing because they initiate automatic diaphragmatic breathing.

Medications. Two basic categories of bronchodilators—sympathomimetic (adrenergic) agents and xanthine compounds—are used to improve efficiency of breathing patterns. These bronchodilators act at different sites and appear to work synergistically when used together.[59] Table 33-18 lists the commonly used bronchodilators and their mode of action. Adrenergic agents that work at B_2 sites located in smooth muscles of the airways have fewer cardiac side effects than do B_1 agents with receptor sites in the myocardium. For this reason, isoetharine, metaproterenol sulfate, and terbutaline sulfate may be prescribed for COPD patients who have hypertension or who have excessive palpitations or tachycardia from B_1 agents.

The methylxathines are commonly prescribed for all types of COPD, although recent studies have demonstrated little or no benefit from theophylline in relieving irreversible airway obstruction. Theophylline-type medications are an effective medication for controlling reversible airway obstruction. The box on p. 925 discusses nursing management of persons on methyl xanthines.

Corticosteroids may be prescribed for patients with intermittent bronchial obstruction and blood or sputum eosinophilia whose conditions are not controlled by bronchodilators.[59] Corticosteroids are known to increase airway diameter through bronchodilation and by decreasing mucosal edema.[98] Usually a short course of corticosteroids is prescribed to alleviate acute symptoms. Prednisone is often given for a total of 7 to 10

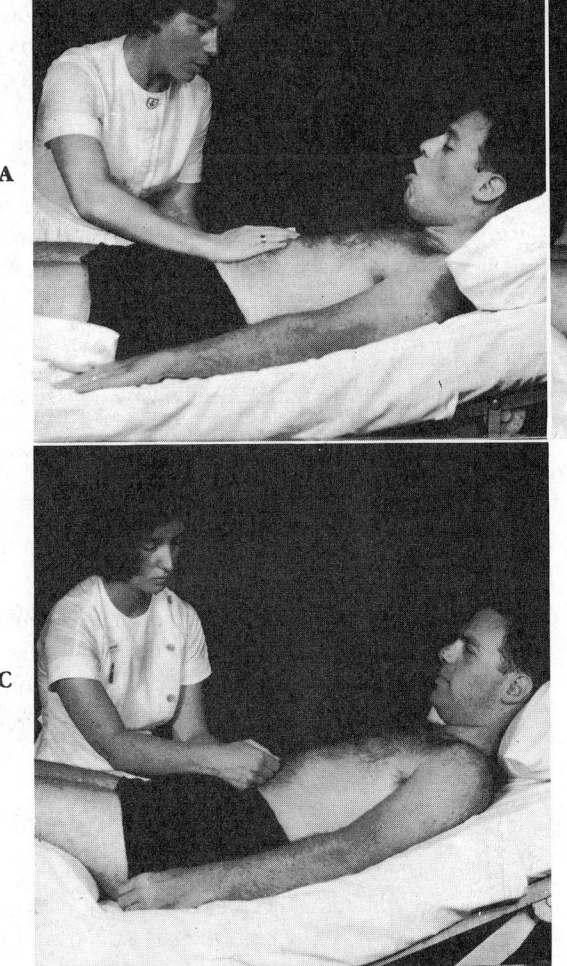

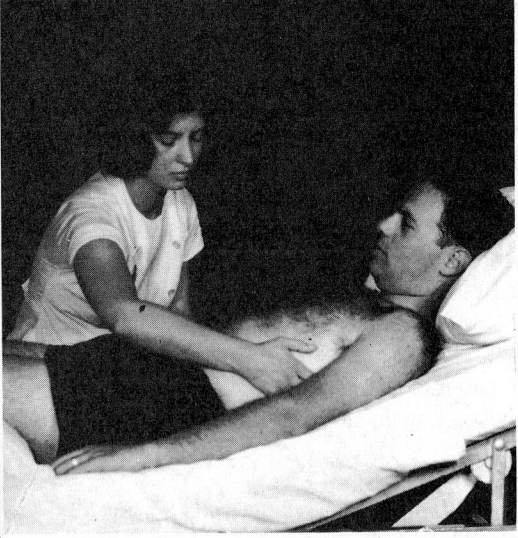

FIGURE 33-7 A, When made to breathe against the resistance offered by the therapist's hands, the patient is made aware of every phase of his respiration and use of muscle groups. **B,** The patient learns how to fully expand his lower lobes by breathing against counter-pressure applied to the side of the chest during inspiration. **C,** The patient is taught diaphragmatic control by breathing against a resistance applied in the costophrenic angle (From Bendixen HH et al: Respiratory care, St Louis, 1965, The CV Mosby Co.).

days. In some patients with asthma, a longer course of prednisone may be indicated and some patients will be on low maintenance dose (5 to 10 mg/day) for several months or even years. Long-term corticosteroid therapy is usually not recommended for patients with COPD unless their disease is rapidly progressing or other treatments have been ineffective.[59]

Persons should have a tuberculin test before initiation of long-term steroid therapy. Those with a tuberculin reaction of 10 mm or more are candidates for isoniazid therapy (see the box on p. 885).

Aerosol therapy. Aerosol therapy, one method to administer bronchodilators, can be delivered in several ways: a Freon-propelled, metered-dosage cartridge inhalator; hand-bulb nebulizer; compressor pump; or IPPB machine (see Chapter 34). In general, metered-dosage cartridge inhalators and hand-bulb nebulizers are used more commonly than IPPB. However, IPPB is still used

NURSING MANAGEMENT FOR PATIENTS RECEIVING METHYLXANTHINE MEDICATIONS

1. Monitor theophylline plasma level results.
   Therapeutic levels = 10 to 20 µg/ml, although individual response to theophylline levels varies. Notify physician if these levels are exceeded before administering the next dose of medication.
2. Certain types of theophylline formulations must be specifically taken with or without food. Food present in the stomach can either slow or speed up absorption of certain types of theophylline.
3. Cigarette or marijuana smoking significantly increases plasma clearance of theophylline. Patients who quit smoking may experience onset of side effects of higher levels of these medications. Counsel patients to notify their physician if they quit smoking.
4. Various medications interact with theophylline, altering plasma absorption rates. Counsel patients to inform their physician when they begin any new medication.
5. Liver cirrhosis, hepatitis, cardiac decompensation, cor pulmonale, and viral respiratory infections decrease plasma clearance of theophylline.

to deliver aerosols to persons who cannot inhale repetitively to near total lung capacity (TLC) or in those persons unable to use a hand-bulb nebulizer because of lack of coordination or fatigue. When administering bronchodilators, the solution should be diluted with either water or saline. Some experts recommend that the diluent be water. All bronchodilator solutions are high molecular weight, concentrated solutions and have a high solute content. When they are diluted with water, there is a maximal in solute concentration; thus smaller particle size and deeper deposition of the aerosol result.[59] Aerosol devices are excellent sites for bacterial growth, and patients using such equipment at home should be advised how to clean them appropriately.

Improving Gas Exchange

Arterial blood gases are monitored for indications of hypoxemia, respiratory acidosis, and respiratory alkalosis.

Hypoxemia and hypercapnea often occur simultaneously, and the signs and symptoms of each are similar. These include headache, irritability, confusion, increasing somnolence, asterixis (flapping tremors of extremities), cardiac arrhythmias, and tachycardia.

If hypocapnia is developing, tachypnea, vertigo, tingling of the extremities, muscular weakness, and spasm are commonly present. It is important to remember that the presence of signs and symptoms associated with altered levels of O_2 and CO_2 depend more on the *rate of change* than on the *degree of change* in the levels. Rapidly changing signs usually indicate a rapid worsening of the patient's condition. At the same time, patients with long-standing hypoxemia and hypercapnia may be relatively asymptomatic because they have physiologically accommodated to increased levels of CO_2 and decreased levels of O_2.

Oxygen therapy. Oxygen therapy is required for patients with COPD who are unable to maintain a Po_2 of greater than 55 mm Hg or an Sao_2 of greater than 85% or more at rest and for those who cannot carry out ADL (breathing, eating, dressing, toileting) without becoming very short of breath. In these instances, 1 to 2 L oxygen is usually given via nasal prongs to relieve hypoxemia, and decrease pulmonary hypertension which in turn, decreases the load on the right side of the heart. It has been demonstrated that patients receive the best benefits from oxygen therapy if the oxygen is used continuously.[88] A common misunderstanding expressed by patients requiring ongoing oxygen therapy is that they should only use their oxygen when they are symptomatic (i.e., short of breath) in order to avoid becoming habituated to the oxygen and thus requiring higher levels of oxygen. It is imperative that the nurse clarify the importance of continual oxygen use in order to receive maximal benefits of oxygen therapy.

Because many patients with COPD have chronic carbon dioxide retention, their stimulus to breathe is their low arterial oxygen level. It is of critical importance that patients understand that high flow rates of oxygen (greater than 6 L/min) and high concentrations (greater than 40%) may elevate their arterial blood oxygen to a level that removes the stimulus by which they breathe, resulting in respiratory failure (see section on respiratory failure later in this chapter).

Pursed-lip breathing is also helpful in improving gas exchange in people with COPD. It has been shown to decrease arterial carbon dioxide levels and improve arterial oxygen tension.[72]

Improving Airway Clearance

Patients can be taught the following measures to improve airway clearance:

1. Teaching effective coughing maneuvers: Have patient sit upright. Instruct patient to
   a. Inhale slowly through the nose.
   b. Lean forward and exhale slowly through pursed lips to promote open airways.
   c. Repeat these steps several times to mobilize secretions and move them upward in the airway.
   d. Take a slow maximal inhalation through the nose when secretions reach the oropharynx. During exhalation use short repeated coughs to minimize bronchospasm.
   e. Inhale maximally after coughing, to reinflate alveoli.
2. In order to thin secretions a fluid intake of 3 to 4 L has traditionally been encouraged unless contraindicated. However, evidence suggests that this quantity of fluids may not be needed to keep secretions mobile.[33]
3. Teach postural drainage, clapping, and vibration as discussed in Chapter 34.
4. Research indicates that airway clearance maneuvers may be enhanced by strengthening respiratory muscles. See the research box on p. 924 for details.

Although expectorants are sometimes prescribed, some experts believe they do more harm than good. Water is still considered to be the best expectorant, and adequate hydration without fluid overload should be encouraged.

Improving Activity Tolerance

Persons with COPD have increased dyspnea on exertion. The typical response to this symptom is to curtail activities to avoid dyspnea. The unfortunate result of this lowered activity level is muscle and cardiopulmonary deconditioning. To avoid this downward spiral of events, the patient must be encouraged to maintain or increase activity levels. The patient can be assisted to achieve this goal either through an organized rehabilitation program or through individual instruction.

Muscle reconditioning. Muscle reconditioning refers to a variety of exercises that will tone muscles. For patients who are able to be up and about, walking, using a treadmill, riding a bicycle, or general flexing and stretching exercises are helpful. The exercise period is started slowly and gradually increased, depending on the patient's physiologic response to the exercise. Criteria should be preestablished to assess the patient's response to the exercise regimen. Examples of criteria that might be used are a 70% to 85% increase in heart rate or signs of muscle fatigue, ashen gray color, clammy skin, or diaphoresis. The bedridden patient can be assisted to maintain muscle condition through active or passive range of motion exercises and muscle-resistive exercises. Encourage exercise before meals. Regular rest periods should be taken as needed. Patient should be taught to incorporate pursed-lip breathing while exercising (recall that the individual should exhale with activity).

Pacing and simplification of activities. Patients can often continue with their usual ADL if they pace their physical effort and take periodic rest pauses. Additionally, by planning ahead they can simplify the steps involved in a complex activity to maximize efficiency in completing a given task.[13]

Reducing Fear

Patients with COPD often experience a feeling of loss of control over their bodies and their lives related to their symptoms and disease progression. Even a basic requirement such as sleep often evades the individual with COPD. The following interventions increase the patient's perception of physical and emotional comfort.

Relaxation exercises. Various techniques may be used to induce a state of relaxation. Relaxation exercises are based on the holistic model of illness and health that presumes that the individual is an integrated psychobiologic entity. Thus physical status can be altered by the psychological state of the individual. By using relaxation techniques, persons with COPD can gain conscious control of certain aspects of their bodily response that can exacerbate their pulmonary symptoms (for example, the sympathetic nervous system response to stress that results in narrowing of the airways). An example of one approach that can be used to induce relaxation is presented in the box above.

Meditation. Meditation, like relaxation techniques, is based on the holistic perspective of human response to health and illness. The two techniques are often used

---

PROGRESSIVE RELAXATION EXERCISES[99]

1. Contract each muscle to a count of 10 and then relax it.
2. Do exercises in quiet room while sitting or lying in a comfortable position.
3. Do exercises to relaxing music, if desired.
4. Have another person serve as a "coach" by giving command to contract muscle, count to 10, and relax muscle.
5. The following are examples of exercises helpful to some persons with COPD:
   a. Raise shoulders, shrug them, and relax for 5 seconds; then relax them completely.
   b. Make a fist of both hands, squeeze them tightly for 5 seconds, and then relax them completely.

---

together, with meditation preceded by relaxation exercises. Meditation induces a state of relaxation that can be an end in itself. In the meditative state the mind is more receptive to suggestion (the individual remains totally in control, however); thus meditation is often combined with positive suggestion. Typical steps to induce meditation are presented in the box below.

Symptom diary. Events that may aggravate patient's symptoms can often be indentified by keeping a symptom diary. Steps can then be taken to modify the aggra-

---

MEDITATION EXERCISES

1. Sit or lie quietly with eyes closed and attempt to relax all muscles, beginning with feet and moving upward (see relaxation techniques at left).
2. Breathe in through the nose slowly (may help to count slowly to four on inhalation), exhale slowly through pursed lips (mentally count to six) with a natural rhythm, relaxed and peaceful (this can be coached or done privately).
3. Survey the body for points of tension. Consciously relax the tense areas. The body is peaceful and relaxed.
4. Continue breathing as above, aware of the feeling of well-being throughout your body. This can be continued for 10 to 20 minutes, or after 5 minutes go to step 5.
5. Listen for (or visualize) a special relaxing sound (or image) such as relaxing sound or picture. Listen to it closely (or visualize) all the while breathing as above.
6. At this point positive suggestion can be used; for example, "I am in control of my body. When I find myself getting tense I can take a moment to stop and breathe in all the air that I need and let the tension flow away."
7. After mental suggestion continue breathing easily and slowly come back to normal alert mental state.
8. Meditation can be used at any time to induce a relaxed state of mind (for example, to promote sleep).

vating event, thus giving the patient more control over the symptoms.

Support groups. Psychosocial motivation involves reinforcing the worth of the individual. Group meetings that provide mutual support are often helpful, and in some cities there are emphysema clubs sponsored by the local Christmas seal agencies, which are affiliates of the ALA. These clubs are open to persons with emphysema and their significant others.

Medications. Psychopharmacologic agents may need to be prescribed for some patients with severe emotional disturbances. The type of agent and size of dose are individually determined; but in general, the older the patient, the smaller the dose. When these agents are prescribed, a pharmacology book should be referred to for information about the side effects and precautions to be used in administering these medications.

Improving Nutritional Intake

Persons with COPD often demonstrate excessive weight loss. Some of the factors that may contribute to weight loss are:

1. A feeling of satiety with small amounts of food because of compression of abdominal contents by the flattened diaphragm
2. Dyspnea interfering with eating
3. Increased dyspnea when eating caused by stomach pushing against the diaphragm
4. Decreased appetite secondary to chronic sputum production
5. Gastric irritation associated with bronchodilators and steroids
6. Increased work of breathing requiring increased caloric intake to maintain weight[36]; imperative that the patient with COPD maintain adequate nutritional levels because:
   a. A diminished total weight is correlated with a dramatic decrease in respiratory muscle (especially the diaphragm) size and strength[101]
   b. Inadequate nutritional status and in particular deficiencies in vitamins A and C decrease resistance to infection
   c. Protein insufficiency decreases colloid osmotic pressure, which increases the risk of pulmonary edema

Nursing actions focused on assisting the patient with COPD to maintain adequate nutrition include the following:

1. Explore usual dietary habits (collect a 24-hour diet history).
2. Counsel patient to select foods that provide a high-protein, high-calorie diet (see the box above).
3. Encourage vitamin supplementation. It is impor-

FOODS TO INCREASE PROTEIN AND CALORIC INTAKE*

Offer frequent small feedings of foods high in protein and calories such as the following:
a. Milk shakes
b. Flavored gelatin or pudding with whipped cream
c. Cream soups made with half-and-half
d. Peanut butter spread on crackers, bananas, pears, or apples
e. Crackers and cheese, nuts, dried fruits, and ice creams readily available for snacks

*Excellent sources for suggestions to increase protein and calorie intake are McCauley K and Weaver R: Cardiac and pulmonary diseases-nutritional implications, Nurs Clin North Am 18:81-95, 1983; and Spector N: Nutritional support of the ventilator-dependent patient, Nurs Clin North Am 24:407-414, 1989; and Cerrato PL: The special nutritional needs of a COPD patient, RN 11:75-76, 1987.

---

tant to counsel the patient to select foods that provide higher calorie levels through higher fat content rather than by high carbohydrate levels. Persons with advanced COPD are unable to breathe off the excess carbon dioxide that is a natural end product of carbohydrate metabolism. Therefore, calories obtained from high carbohydrate foods may elevate arterial carbon dioxide levels in persons with COPD.
4. Prepackaged food supplements taken between meals provide an excellent source of protein and calories.
5. Smaller more frequent meals are often tolerated better than three large meals.
6. Consider financial and ethnic background when planning for meals.

Preventing Infection

The *most common complication of COPD*, and cause of hospital readmissions, is *respiratory infection*. Pulmonary system response to the infectious process includes increased respiratory rate, mucosal irritation, and increased mucus production. Because of these localized responses, patients may present with bronchospasm and a change in their pattern of sputum production (see list of signs and symptoms on p. 917). If the infection remains untreated, the end result is an overall increased work of breathing with eventual respiratory failure. Thus for the person with COPD, it is imperative that respiratory infections be avoided. The patient should be counseled to take the following steps to *decrease* the chance of contacting a pulmonary infection.

1. Avoid large crowds, especially during known influenza seasons.
   a. Avoid contact with people who have an upper respiratory infection.
   b. Get influenza and pneumonia immunizations

2. Contact health care provider if the following common signs and symptoms occur:
   a. Change in sputum color, amount and consistency
   b. Increased cough
   c. Change in behavior (e.g., more argumentive than usual)
   d. Increased fatigue
   e. Increased dyspnea
   f. Weight gain
   g. Peripheral edema
   h. Elevated temperature

Antimicrobial agents are prescribed to treat respiratory tract infections in persons with COPD. The most commonly used antimicrobials are tetracycline or ampicillin, 1 to 2 g/day for 7 to 10 days. Some patients have a prescription on hand and self-administer the antimicrobial agent after telephone consultation with their physician. Antimicrobials should be started within 24 hours of the first signs of a respiratory infection. Patients who are febrile or who have other signs and symptoms of infection that do not respond to the prescribed therapy should have a Gram stain and culture and sensitivity studies. When antibiotics are used inappropriately, especially in patients who are not adequately clearing their lungs of secretions, superinfection with bacteria or fungi may occur. Although these regimens of prophylactic treatment do not appear to decrease the incidence of infection, they do decrease the severity and duration of the infection.[87]

Preventing Fluid Volume Excess

Low arterial blood oxygen is a potent pulmonary vasoconstrictor. Pulmonary vasoconstriction increases pulmonary arterial pressure. If pulmonary hypertension exists for a prolonged period of time, the increased workload on the heart's right ventricle will ultimately result in *right ventricular failure* and what is known as pulmonary heart disease or *cor pulmonale*. Depending on its severity and duration, cor pulmonale may be characterized by neck vein distention, hepatomegaly, dependent peripheral edema, and, as oncotic pressure is exceeded, ascites and pleural effusions.[13,87] Nursing interventions for fluid volume excess resulting from cor pulmonale are based on the understanding that the disease is treated by intervening with the underlying cause of the pulmonary hypertension. Therefore, nursing interventions focus on promoting adequate ventilation for optimal oxygen/carbon dioxide exchange and relieving symptoms that result from the fluid volume excess. Thus a nursing plan of care for the person with COPD that promotes optimal ventilation also intervenes with fluid volume excess resulting from cor pulmonale. Additionally, interventions focused on the symptoms of fluid volume excess include:

1. Monitor intake and output accurately. (Note: Although it is unknown if fluid restriction is effective in the actual treatment of cor pulmonale, excess fluid intake may overwhelm an already compromised cardiac system.)
2. Encourage moderate exercise or change patient's position frequently to promote adequate perfusion in lung.
3. Measure abdominal girth at regular intervals to assess the possible presence or progression of ascites.
4. Administer diuretics as ordered. When diuretics are given, the patient should be carefully monitored for side effects. Those on thiazide diuretics will need to be taught about eating foods high in potassium such as bananas, oranges, prunes, and raisins.
5. Administer digitalis as ordered. (Note: Digitalis is of questionable usefulness in pure right-sided heart failure.) Persons receiving digitalis should be carefully monitored for side effects.

Patient Teaching

Persons with COPD play a major role in monitoring their own condition and in maintaining their physical and psychological functioning at the maximum possible level.

For these reasons, it is imperative that the nurse thoroughly assess the patient's knowledge about COPD, including its cause and treatment. Individualized teaching plans on the basis of the patient's knowledge level can then be developed. Areas that may be included in the teaching program are listed in the box on p. 930.

ASTHMA

Asthma is discussed separately from bronchitis and emphysema because it results in intermittent rather than continuous, irreversible airway obstruction. Its onset is sudden as opposed to the slow insidious progression of symptoms seen in bronchitis and emphysema. Asthma is characterized by increased responsiveness of the trachea and bronchi to various stimuli that cause narrowing of the airways and difficulty in breathing.

EPIDEMIOLOGY AND ETIOLOGY

Asthma is known to affect 9.6 million people in the United States, two thirds of whom are adults. Table 33-19 lists the traditional classification and general causative factors associated with asthma. In any type of asthma, the airway is in a state of easy provocation, and attacks may be precipitated by a variety of factors. Although the classification listed in Table 33-19 is still the most commonly used way of differentiating types of asthma, there is a move away from using this classification system. Clinically, most people with asthma fall

TEACHING THE PATIENT WITH COPD

The following areas should be addressed in a typical teaching program for persons with COPD:

1. Patients should be able to explain, in lay terms, the basic function and pathology of their lungs. The ALA offers several excellent booklets for the lay population. (Your local branch of the ALA can provide you with a complete listing of their various publications.)

2. The avoidance of respiratory irritants and maintenance of a proper environment should be emphasized to people with COPD. As discussed earlier, inhaled irritants (especially cigarette smoke) pose a serious threat to these persons. Steps the patient can take to reduce or avoid exposure to these irritants are listed below.

   a. Stop smoking. There are many community agencies, including the ALA, American Heart Association, and American Cancer Society that offer programs for persons who want to stop smoking. The nurse should be familiar with community programs and give a list of them to the patient.

   b. Ask other persons not to smoke in the immediate environment. Inhalation of secondary smoke can exacerbate symptoms.

   c. Pay heed to announcements on radio and television warning of pollution alerts. Do not go outside during an alert.

   d. Use an air conditioner or high-efficiency particulate air filter or electrostatic filter to remove particulate matter from air.
      1. Keep filters clean.
      2. Follow manufacturer's directions for use.

   e. Use an activated charcoal filter if offending odors or gas pollutants are a problem.

   f. Avoid abrupt environmental temperature or humidity changes because they can increase sputum production and cause bronchospasm.

1. Use an air conditioner in hot weather.
2. Use a face mask when going out in cold weather.
3. Use a dehumidifier or humidifier as appropriate to maintain a humidity of 30% to 50%.

   g. If air travel is required, check with physician about the need for supplemental oxygen.

   h. Avoid large crowds, especially during known influenza seasons.
      1. Avoid contact with people who have an upper respiratory infection.
      2. Get influenza and pneumonia immunizations.

3. The patient should be able to explain the following aspects of the home medication or treatment regimen.

   a. State name, dose, action, and side effects of each home medication.

   b. Explain how and when to use medications ordered on an as needed basis (for example, bronchodilators, antibiotics, steroids, antacids).

   c. Demonstrate techniques necessary for follow-up care (for example, postural drainage, clapping and vibrating, aerosol therapy).

   d. Describe how to obtain and maintain any needed equipment or supplies such as oxygen, nebulizers, humidifiers, aerosols, IPPB machines, syringes, and medications.

4. The patient should demonstrate how to carry out the specific home exercise program.

   a. Specific exercises to be completed

   b. Frequency of each exercise

   c. Criteria for monitoring physical response to exercises such as heart rate increase or perceived fatigue

5. The patient should be able to list the names and telephone numbers of appropriate community support services such as the visiting nurse association and a home medical equipment supplier.

---

into the mixed classification of asthma types; thus the traditional asthma classification is of limited usefulness in establishing individual treatment programs. Experts in asthma treatment are recommending that asthma be grouped as *syndromes* and *classified according to precipitating factors* and *individual response patterns to precipitating factors*.[98] Table 33-20 presents some of the common syndromes of asthma using the currently recommended classification.

PREVENTION

Prevention of immunologic (atopic) asthma is focused on identification of the allergens to which the person is sensitive. In nonimmunologic or mixed asthma, factors

---

TABLE 33-19 Asthma classification

Type	Immunologic (Allergic, Extrinsic)	Nonimmunologic (Nonallergic, Intrinsic)	Mixed (Combined Immunologic, Nonimmunologic)
Onset	Usually in childhood	Usually after age 35	Any age
Causative agent/precipitating	Any extrinsic protein (antigen)	Nonspecific stimulus	Allergen or nonspecific stimulus
Associated factors	Other allergic-based disorders (that is, eczema)	Respiratory infections, influenza	Nonspecific
	Elevated IgE (see Chapter 76)		

TABLE 33-20 Asthma syndromes classified by precipitating factor and response pattern

Asthma Syndromes	Characteristics
Atopic asthma	Childhood onset, allergic rhinitis, allergic dermopathy, identifiable environmental precipitating events
Exercise-induced asthma	Airway constriction after exercise
Aspirin-hypersensitivity triad	Presence of nasal polyps, urticaria, and asthma after aspirin ingestion
Bronchospasm associated with nonbacterial upper respiratory tract infections	As described
Industrial asthma	Bronchoconstriction associated with certain industrial precipitating factors

IDENTIFICATION OF FACTORS PRECIPITATING ASTHMA

1. Be alert for casual comments about daily activities the patient might consider insignificant.
2. Encourage patient to keep a symptom diary. Ask patient to perform the following tasks.
   a. Use a small notebook that can be carried at all times.
   b. Record everything that occurred and was present before (24 hours) and during the onset of the attack. When the attack began: What were you doing? Where were you? Who or what else was present? What was the weather like?
   c. Note the time and date that the attack occurred.
3. Write down what you think caused the symptoms to occur, even if it is a guess.
4. Observe patient's interaction with others and reaction to stressors that might aggravate and/or precipitate an attack.

precipitating the exacerbation of symptoms may be obscure. However, identification of causative or aggravating factors is still imperative in order to avoid or decrease the incidence of asthma attacks.

There is perhaps no disease in which knowing the patient well is more important than in asthma. Since sensitivity tests can be performed with only a very small fraction of the substances with which the patient is in contact, the physician usually makes the diagnosis on the basis of a careful history. Knowing about the person's lifestyle such as the type of work, leisure-time activities, and even food preferences may give useful clues as to what precipitates the asthmatic attack. Nursing strategies for identifying causes are included in the box above, right.

It is imperative to understand that even though psychological factors may precipitate an attack, the response to it is physiologic and requires the same treatment as that prescribed for an attack precipitated by an allergen or any other factor.

PATHOPHYSIOLOGY

An asthmatic attack results from several physiologic alterations, including altered immunologic response, increased airway resistance, increased lung compliance, impaired mucociliary function, and altered oxygen-carbon dioxide exchange. Each of these alterations is discussed below.

Altered Immunologic Response

Nor matter what the precipitating factors are, the basis of asthma appears to be genetic or immunologic factors. The basis of nonimmunologic asthma is less well understood than immunologic asthma.

Immunologic asthma is the result of an antigen-anti-

body reaction in which chemical mediators are released. The chemical mediators, which include histamine, slow-releasing substance of anaphylaxis (SRS-A), eosinophilic chemotactic factor of anaphylaxis (ECF-A), and perhaps others, cause three main reactions: (1) constriction of smooth muscles of both the large and small airways, resulting in bronchospasm; (2) increased capillary permeability that results in mucosal edema and further narrows the airways; and (3) increased mucous gland secretion and increased mucus production. As a result, the person with an asthmatic attack struggles to breathe through a narrowed airway that is in spasm. Because breathing is labored, the person breathes through the mouth, which dries the mucus and further occludes the airway.

Common precipitating factors are presented in the box below. Although allergic mechanisms are important in the pathogenesis of asthma, the many nonimmunologic precipitating factors indicate that other pathophysiologic processes, such as parasympathetic and sympa-

COMMON PRECIPITATING FACTORS OF ASTHMA

Environmental Factors
    Change in air temperature
    Change in humidity
    Irritating fumes
    Smoke
    Strong odors
    Pollutants (sulfur dioxide, sulfates, ozone, and particulates)[14]
Aspirin ingestion (prostaglandin inhibitor)
Exercise
Emotional stress
Infection (usually viral)

thetic nervous system reactivity, are active in the onset of asthma. Hypoxemia, hypercapnia, and overuse of bronchodilators may lead to an acute asthma attack.

Increased Airway Resistance

Increased airway resistance results from bronchial smooth muscle spasm, mucosal inflammation, and hypersecretion of mucus. These airway changes cause obstruction to airflow both in and out of the lungs.

Increased Lung Compliance

The lungs become hyperinflated during an acute asthmatic attack as a result of air that becomes trapped in the distal airspaces. During the acute attack the person with asthma demonstrates the same symptoms of increased lung compliance that are observed in the emphysematous patient (see Table 33-11).

Impaired Mucociliary Function

Hypertrophy of mucus-secreting glands, thickened mucus, and slowed ciliary movement are common findings in person's with asthma. During an asthma attack, increased mucus production combined with slowed clearance of mucus due to decreased ciliary movement results in increased water loss from mucus. Thus, the mucus becomes increasingly viscous and can ultimately result in the development of mucous plugs, which may block airways.

Altered Oxygen-Carbon Dioxide Exchange

Increased airway resistance and hyperinflation cause the respiratory muscles to work harder, resulting in muscle fatigue and ultimately exhaustion. In mild or short-term asthmatic attacks, the individual compensates with an increased respiratory rate, which results in respiratory alkalosis. Mild hypoxemia from altered ventilation-perfusion ratios usually accompanies the alkalosis.

In a severe or prolonged attack, if the increased work of breathing cannot be relieved, respiratory muscle exhaustion will result in hypoventilation, which in turn causes respiratory acidosis and severe hypoxemia.

CLINICAL MANIFESTATIONS

The signs and symptoms associated with asthma are correlated with normal lung functions, and underlying pathophysiologic origins (see Table 33-16). The character of asthmatic attacks can vary on a continuum from chronic or acute mild intermittent attacks to life-threatening *status asthmaticus.*

With chronic mild asthma, symptoms are not noticeable when the person is at rest. However, after exertion such as laughing, singing, vigorous exercise, or emotional excitement, dyspnea and wheezing develop rapidly. These attacks are controlled with medications, and·

patients usually can continue their mode of living with a few modifications and no serious lung changes. They are not hospitalized, but they sometimes come to outpatient clinics for medical supervision.

Acute asthmatic attacks often occur at night. The person awakens with a sensation of choking caused by the mucosal inflammation and hypersecretion. Bronchospasm, with resultant increased airway resistance, causes audible *expiratory* and *inspiratory wheezing.* During the acute attack patients appear to be in acute respiratory distress and typically demonstrate tachypnea, accessory muscle breathing, and nasal flaring. They appear to be apprehensive and diaphoretic, and their attention is totally focused on their breathing. The attack usually ends with the coughing up of large quantities of thick, tenacious sputum. Most attacks subside in 30 minutes to 1 hour, although repeated asthmatic attacks associated with infection may continue for days or weeks. The person is usually exhausted and should rest quietly after the attack.

Persons who are severely affected by asthma and who have attacks that are difficult to control with the usual medications may develop *status asthmaticus.* In this case, the symptoms of an acute attack continue despite measures to relieve them. Air trapping in the distal airspaces ultimately leads to respiratory muscle exhaustion and severe ventilation-perfusion abnormalities with resultant respiratory failure and hypoxemia.

Patients with status asthmaticus often demonstrate respiratory distress so severe that they are unable to talk. They may be moving minimal air in and out of the lungs; thus audible wheezing and adventitious lung sounds may *not* be present. During this phase of the attack the patient will appear cyanotic and may demonstrate both *pulsus paradoxis* and *sensorium changes.*

Repeated attacks of status asthmaticus may cause irreversible emphysema, resulting in a permanent decrease in total breathing capacity.

Pulmonary function studies characteristic of asthma show reduction in FEV_1. The FEV is usually markedly reduced in proportion to the FVC, although the FVC may also be decreased. Improved flow rates after administration of bronchodilators indicating reversible bronchospasm is a characteristic finding with asthma.

The results of arterial blood gas studies can vary from respiratory alkalosis with mild hypoxemia to severe respiratory acidosis with profound hypoxemia, depending on the severity and duration of the asthmatic attack.

MEDICAL MANAGEMENT

The objectives of medical management of asthma are to promote normal functioning of the individual, to prevent recurrent symptoms, prevent severe attacks, and prevent side effects from medication. The chief aim of various medications is to afford the patient immediate, progressive, and ongoing bronchial relaxation. Following are some approaches to therapy.*

1. Acute asthma
   a. Mild severity: treated safely on an outpatient basis.
      (1) Bronchodilators used alone, such as long-acting theophylline given orally
      (2) Or, occasional use of a sympathomimetic agent such as metraproterenol to control intermittent symptoms or prevent reaction to anticipated exposure to known precipitating factor
      (3) Or, cromolyn sodium used on a regular basis to reduce incidence of episodic attacks.
   b. Moderate severity: treated safely on an outpatient basis when *no danger signs* are present
      (1) Nasal oxygen
      (2) IV aminophylline in a loading dose
      (3) Sympathomimetic, such as isoproterenol or albuterol, given as an aerosol
      (4) If not responsive to bronchodilators, inhaled adrenocorticosteroid may be given to restore airway responsiveness to preceding medications (2 and 3 above).
      (5) Monitor FEV and symptoms; when they improve, begin oral therapy
      (6) Observe carefully for 48 hours and monitor for signs of relapse
   c. Severe attack with *one or more danger signs:* vital capacity <1.0 L, FEV_1 <0.5 L, Po_2 under 50 mm, increase in Pco_2, exhaustion, disturbed consciousness.
      (1) Hospitalize; give supplemental oxygen; intubate if necessary
      (2) Administer IV steroids (100 mg Solu-Cortef or equivalent every 6 hours for four doses); begin prednisone, 60 to 80 mg every 24 hours until FEV_1 nears best previous value, then reduce dose over next 2 to 3 weeks; begin use of beclomethasone inhaler
      (3) IV aminophylline in a loading dose and then in maintenance dose for 48 to 72 hours; monitor aminophylline blood levels
      (4) Administer β_2-adrenergic agents subcutaneously (terbutaline or epinephrine initially); inhalation therapy after 24 hours
      (5) IPPB may be used to deliver adrenergic agents and to facilitate bronchodilation
2. Chronic asthma
   a. Mild to moderate, or recurring: sympathomimetic in aerosol form, given alone or in combination with either or both cromolyn sodium and long-acting theophylline
   b. Moderately severe: add inhaled corticosteroid such as beclomethasone to medications given for mild chronic asthma
   c. Severe asthma causing interferences with work: give oral corticosteroids every other day in addition to medications indicated for mild to moderate asthma; try to switch patient to inhaled corticosteroid if possible

■ **ASSESSMENT**

Subjective Data

Subjective data include the following:
1. History of asthma onset and duration
2. Precipitating factors
3. Current medications
4. Medications used to relieve asthma symptoms
5. Any recent changes in medication regimen
6. Self-care methods used to relieve symptoms

Objective Data

Objective data include the following:
1. Assess general appearance.
   a. Does patient appear apprehensive?
   b. Is there any evidence of altered sensorium?
2. Assess vital signs.
   a. Tachycardia
   b. Pulsus paradoxus (diminished pulse with inspiration, confirmed by a 6 to 8 torr drop in systolic blood pressure during inspiration)
   c. Tachypnea
3. Pulmonary examination
   a. Inspection
      (1) Accessory muscle breathing
      (2) Forward leaning posture
      (3) Dyspnea
      (4) Prolonged expiration
      (5) Cyanosis
   b. Palpation
      (1) Decreased lateral expansion
      (2) Decreased fremitus
   c. Percussion
      (1) Hyperresonance
      (2) Decreased diaphragmatic excursion
   d. Auscultation (Note: as patient approaches exhaustion from increased work of breathing, breath sounds and adventitious sounds may be absent or faint)
      (1) Inspiratory and expiratory wheezing
      (2) Rhonchi
4. Assess laboratory findings
   a. Arterial blood gases
      (1) Short-term or moderate attack—respiratory alkalosis with mild hypoxemia

---

*Adapted from Cherniak RM: Current therapy of respiratory disease-2, Toronto, 1986, BC Decker Inc; and Dolovich J, and Hargreave FE: Strategies in the control of asthma, Med Clin North Am 65:1033-1043, 1981.

(2) Prolonged or severe attack—respiratory acidosis with severe hypoxemia
  b. Sputum—for eosinophilia
  c. Pulmonary function testing—decreased FEV, VC.

■ DATA ANALYSIS: NURSING DIAGNOSES

Nursing diagnoses are determined from assessment of patient data. Possible nursing diagnoses for the person with asthma may include, but are not limited to, the following:

Diagnostic Title	Possible Etiologies
Airway clearance, ineffective	Ineffective technique, decreased energy/fatigue, impaired mucociliary clearance mechanism, inadequate fluid intake
Anxiety	Threat of unknown or death
Breathing pattern, ineffective	Bronchoconstriction, underuse of bronchodilator medications
Gas exchange, impaired	Mucous plugs, ventilation/perfusion imbalance
Knowledge deficit of predisposing factors and prevention/treatment	Lack of exposure to information, unreceptiveness to information, unfamiliarity with information sources

■ PLANNING: EXPECTED PATIENT OUTCOMES

Expected outcomes for the person with asthma may include, but are not limited to, the following:
The patient will:
1. Demonstrate effective airway clearance
  a. Effective methods of coughing
  b. Appropriate use of medication and equipment
2. Demonstrate activities to control anxiety response to symptoms
  a. Muscle relaxation
  b. Medication
  c. Appropriate use of medications
3. Demonstrate effective breathing patterns
  a. Inspiratory to expiratory ratio = 5 seconds:10 seconds
  b. Respiratory rate within near-normal limits
4. Demonstrate improved ventilation and oxygenation
  a. Arterial blood pH and Pa_{CO_2} that returns or stays within acceptable limits
  b. Pa_{O_2} at optimal level for individual

■ IMPLEMENTATION

Nursing interventions for the person during an acute asthmatic attack include the following.

Improving Airway Clearance

During an asthmatic attack secretions tend to become viscous and can plug airways, causing increased airway obstruction. By mobilizing secretions, the need for intubation and artificial ventilation can often be prevented.
1. Ensure adequate systemic fluid intake (Note: Research findings suggest that overhydration may not increase secretion clearance above levels obtained by normal hydration levels)*
2. Provide adequate nutritional levels
3. Provide extra humidity
4. Medicate with bronchodilators
5. Teach effective cough maneuver (see p. 926)
6. If cough ineffective to produce sputum, administer chest physiotherapy (see Chapter 34).

Providing Emotional Support and Preventing Anxiety

1. Do not leave patient alone during an asthmatic attack
2. Encourage relaxation techniques
3. Guide/assist patient with respiratory maneuvers
4. Assess for possible medication overuse

Improving Breathing Patterns

The nursing role in improving breathing patterns and gas exchange is as follows:
1. Place in high Fowler's position
2. Encourage slow rhythmic breathing
3. Encourage patient to breathe through nose and exhale through pursed lips
4. Administer bronchodilator and anti-inflammatory medication as ordered. Monitor patient for both therapeutic response and side effects to medications. Table 33-21 lists medications, dosage, action, and side effects of medications commonly used to treat asthma.†

Improving Gas Exchange

Blood gas results should be monitored as follows:
1. If respiratory alkalosis is present, encourage slower breathing
2. If respiratory acidosis and hypoxemia are present
  a. Administer O_2 as prescribed
  b. If O_2 does not relieve the attack, intubation and ventilatory assistance may be required

Patient Teaching

After the patient has recovered from an acute attack, the patient's knowledge about asthma is assessed, and the following points are stressed.
1. Keep a symptom diary (p. 927) to help identify:
  a. Possible precipitating factors

---

*An excellent resource for nursing interventions to promote secretion clearance is Cosenza JJ, and Norton LC: Secretion clearance: state of the art from a nursing perspective, Crit Care Nurs 6:23-37, 1986.

†A comprehensive presentation of medications used to treat pulmonary problems including asthma can be found in reference 68.

TABLE 33-21 Medications used in treatment of asthma

Medications	Dosage	Action	Side Effects
Epinephrine 1:1000	0.3 to 0.5 ml subcutaneously, may need to repeat 2-3 times at 20-30 min intervals	Short-acting bronchodilator	Tachycardia Palpitations Elevated blood pressure
Ephedrine	25-50 mg PO q 4-6 hr	Long-acting bronchodilator	Cerebral agitation (often given with phenobarbital)
Terbutaline	2.5 mg PO	Bronchodilator	Tachycardia Tremors Headache Spasms in extremities
Isoproterenol .25% (Isuprel)	1-2 inhalations, q 3 hr (max. 8/day)	Bronchodilator	Headache Tremors
Metaproterenol (Alupent, Metaprel)	20 mg PO tid or 1-2 inhalations	Bronchodilator	Tachycardia Tremors Nausea
Cromolyn sodium (Intal)	20 mg qid inhaled	Antiasthmatic mast cell stabilizer used as prophylactic against asthma attacks	Nasal congestion Nausea Bronchospasm
Corticosteroids Hydrocortisone	200-400 mg IV (up to 1 gm first 24 hr) PO or IV	Anti-inflammatory	Corticosteroid withdrawal syndrome, sodium retention, GI disturbance
Dexamethasone	Varies with individual response and disease severity		
Beclomethasone Theophylline	Inhaled: 100 μg 3-4 times/day Dosage to maintain serum concentrations between 10-20 μg/ml	Bronchodilator	Nausea and vomiting CNS irritability Tachycardia Hypotension

b. Symptom patterns
c. Efficacy of self-treatment modalities (include time and dose of any medications self-administered)
2. Signs and symptoms
   a. Tightness in chest
   b. Restlessness or vague feeling of uneasiness
   c. Dyspnea
   d. Increased wheezing
   e. Productive cough
3. Self-treatment of signs and symptom
   a. Take bronchodilator as ordered.
   b. Take epinephrine if prescribed by physician.
   c. State conditions under which medication might be increased (infection-start or increase antibiotics; increased stress or worsening of symptoms)
   d. If another person is not present, call someone so patient will not be alone.
   e. Try to remain calm and breathe slowly; use relaxation techniques at first sign of attack
   f. If symptoms are not relieved, call physician or go to nearest emergency facility.
4. Know how to use special equipment (nebulizer,

aerosols, IPPB metered dose inhaler (see the box below) and peak flow meter (see research box on p. 936).
5. If asthma is immunologic, know how to prepare an environmentally controlled bedroom (see Chapter 76).
6. Understand postural drainage techniques (see Chapter 34).

CORRECT WAY TO USE A METERED-DOSE INHALER

1. Inhale through nose, then slowly breathe out completely.
2. Place mouthpiece in mouth.
3. Press down on inhaler, while simultaneously inhaling deeply. Breathe in air from around the mouthpiece while inhaling.
4. Hold breath for a few seconds, then exhale.
5. Repeat as ordered.

Caution: Some asthmatic individuals may experience bronchoconstriction after using a metered-dose inhaler. Patients who complain of chest tightness after using a metered-dose inhaler may be reacting to the propellant gases used to deliver metaproterenol.

RESEARCH

Janson-Bjerklie S and Shnell S: Effect of peak flow information on patterns of self-care in adult asthma, Heart Lung 17:543-549, 1988.

The purpose of this study was to identify self-care strategies used to control asthma symptoms and to determine the effect of peak flowmeter information on selection of self-care strategies. Twenty-eight adults with physician diagnosed asthma were randomly assigned to a control group (N=15). They were interviewed and instructed to keep an asthma care log. An experimental group (N=13) was interviewed, instructed to keep an asthma care log, and instructed to use and record peak flowmeter rate three times at the beginning and end of each asthma attack). Results indicated that subjects with access to peak flowmeter information used self-treatment strategies less frequently and believed their strategies were less effective than those subjects who depended solely on bodily or emotional sensations to assess their asthma status. The researcher speculated that the physiologic feedback about degree of airway obstruction provided by the peak flowmeter might have promoted more appropriate use of self-treatment modalities or may have limited subjects' use of additional information about their respiratory status that bodily sensations may have provided. The findings suggest that patients can use objective airway obstruction information to guide self-treatment. Patient teaching for people who use peak flowmeters to monitor asthma status needs to include instruction to pay close attention to body sensations and to correlate them with individual peak flow measurements. ▪

7. If on oral corticosteroid therapy, show card to be carried at all times giving data about drug, dose, and name of physician; alternatively, wear Medic-Alert bracelet.
8. State plans for ongoing follow-up care, including plans for desensitization if appropriate.

CYSTIC FIBROSIS
EPIDEMIOLOGY/ETIOLOGY

Cystic fibrosis (CF) continues to be the most common lethal genetic disease among whites. It is an autosomal recessive disease, and one of every 22 individuals carries the CF gene. When both parents are carriers (heterozygotes), there is a one in four chance with each pregnancy that their child will have CF (Figure 33-8).

Approximately 25,000 individuals with CF live in the United States. Of that population, 6500 individuals are adults according to the Cystic Fibrosis Foundation Patient Care Registry. More important, the number of adults with CF continues to increase steadily due to increased life expectancy and diagnostic advances. (Figure 33-9).

Two groups make up this adult CF population: Infants and children and adolescents and adults. Recent statistics indicate that approximately 20% of the adult CF population is diagnosed after age 15.[34]

Reaching adulthood is now a realistic expectation for infants and children with CF. The average life expectancy is 24 years with a maximum survival of 30 to 40

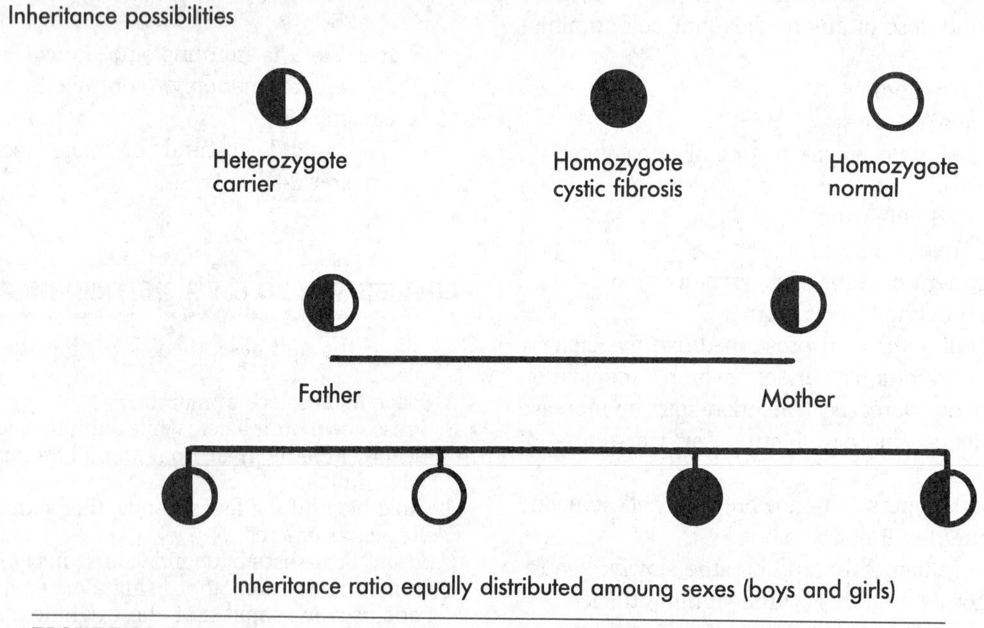

Inheritance possibilities

Heterozygote carrier

Homozygote cystic fibrosis

Homozygote normal

Father

Mother

Inheritance ratio equally distributed among sexes (boys and girls)

FIGURE 33-8 Inheritance of cystic fibrosis when both mother and father are carriers of cystic fibrosis gene (Adapted from CF Foundation Fact Sheet, 1980, Bethesda, Maryland).

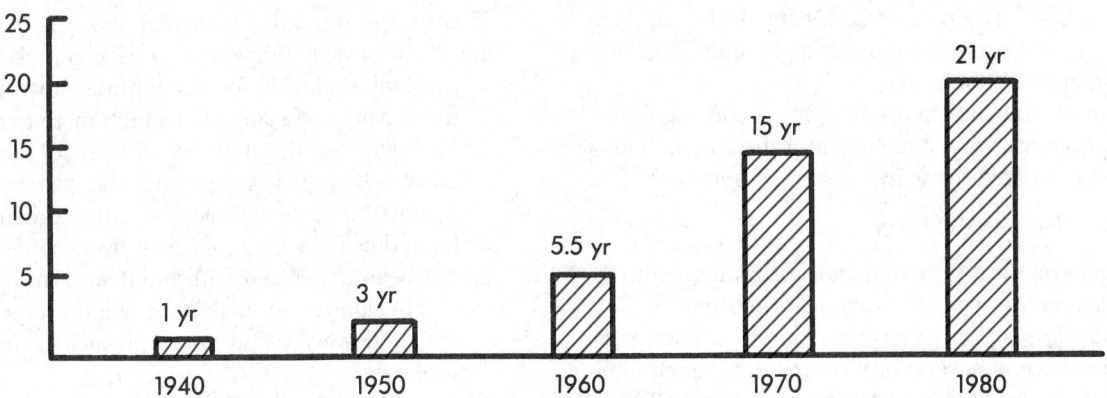

FIGURE 33-9 Life expectancy of children born with cystic fibrosis. The number of children surviving to adulthood continues to increase. (Adapted from CF Foundation Fact Sheet, 1988, Bethesda, Maryland).

years. The major contributing factors to this increased life expectancy include diagnostic advances and therapeutic interventions.

PREVENTION

Because CF is a genetically inherited disease, identification of carriers who may pass on the defect and disease to offspring remains the most important preventive strategy. Early identification of carriers combined with genetic counseling minimizes the chance of offspring inheriting this lethal genetic disease. Family histories of possible incidences of CF should be followed up by genetic testing.

PATHOPHYSIOLOGY

Cystic fibrosis is an exocrine gland disease involving various systems (pulmonary, pancreatic/hepatic, gastrointestinal, and reproductive). Obstruction of the exocrine gland ducts or passageways occurs in nearly all adult patients with CF.[120] Exocrine gland secretions are known to have a decreased water content, altered electrolyte concentration, and abnormal organic constituents (especially mucous glycoproteins); yet the specific biochemical or physiologic defect that leads to obstruction is not known.

The following physiologic alterations are found in adults with CF.

1. Pulmonary damage. Mucus obstruction, inflammation, edema, and smooth muscle restriction of airways are found in this chronic obstructive pulmonary disease. Changes in the airways predisposes the person to respiratory infection, which can be life-threatening. Frequent, recurrent pulmonary infections erode blood vessels. Brachial arteries branching from the aorta and the lung at high pressures are most at risk for bleeding (hemoptysis).

   Other complications of damage to the airways include *pneumothorax, respiratory insufficiency,* and *cor pulmonale.* These complications account for 95% of the deaths in adults with CF. The normal function primary pathophysiology and the clinical picture in CF is outlined in Table 33-22.

2. Gastrointestinal and pancreatic involvement. Intestinal obstruction occurs in 20% of adult patients with CF. Generally, pancreatic insufficiency predisposes to intestinal obstruction. Cramps and abdominal pain in adults with CF should arouse suspicion of intestinal obstruction. Pancreatic insufficiency is reported in 80% to 90% of adults

TABLE 33-22 Normal function, primary pathophysiology, and the clinical picture in cystic fibrosis

Normal Function	Pathophysiology	Clinical Picture
Mucus production by goblet cells lubricates airways and entraps foreign particles	1. Excessive amounts of mucus production 2. Inflammation of small airways, causing hyperinflation of alveoli 3. Chronic bacterial infections 4. Eroding of a major blood vessel secondary to infection	1. Increased cough and mucus production 2. Fatigue and shortness of breath 3. Fever, fatigue, shortness of breath 4. Hemoptysis

with CF.[34] The pathologic lesions in the pancreas decrease pancreatic enzyme production and lead to malabsorption of fat.

3 Glucose intolerance. About 40% of adults with CF have glucose intolerance caused by obstruction of islets of Langerhans by pancreatic fibrosis.[35,120]

CLINICAL MANIFESTATIONS

Three major clinical symptoms are associated with CF: *recurrent respiratory infections, malnutrition,* and *excessive salt losses*. Early identification of CF often rests on the presence of several otherwise unexplained clinical symptoms. In infants, clinical symptoms of CF may include meconium ileus and failure to thrive. Excessive salt losses in infants may first be detected by the infant's mother who reports that the child tastes salty when kissed. Older children should be suspected of having CF when *recurrent respiratory infections* and *failure to thrive* despite large appetites cannot otherwise be explained. *Excessive salt losses* in older children and young adults with CF may be manifested by *heat exhaustion* after exercise or exposure to hot weather, or *dehydration* after fevers. In young adults, the *only* clinical manifestation of CF may be *infertility*.

Specific clinical manifestation by system are listed below. Pulmonary signs and symptoms of CF include:

1. Chronic productive cough and/or recurrent bronchitis or pneumonia
2. Rales and rhonchi, decreased pulmonary compliance, digital clubbing
3. Shortness of breath and dyspnea on exertion, wheezing, and weight loss occur with respiratory complications and usually indicate need for vigorous therapy

Gastrointestinal signs and symptoms include:

1. Frequent, bulky, greasy stools
2. Weight loss
3. Cramps and abdominal pain—should arouse suspicion of obstructional obstruction

Glucose intolerance signs and symptoms include:

1. Polyuria, polydipsia, and polyphagia
2. Absence of ketoacidosis even with above signs

DIAGNOSIS

The diagnosis of CF is confirmed by the presence of *at least two* of the *following:*

1. A positive sweat test with a chloride level greater than 60 mEq/L
2. COPD
3. Exocrine pancreatic insufficiency
4. A positive family history of CF

MEDICAL MANAGEMENT

The goals of medical management of CF are to *minimize bronchial plugging and to inhibit bacterial colonization.*[32]

Measures to minimize bronchial plugging include:

1. Chest physiotherapy with chest percussion and postural drainage for 20 minutes two to three times daily and sometimes much more frequently.
2. Mucolytic agents may be ordered to thin secretions, although assuring that the patient is well hydrated may be sufficient to thin secretions.
3. Humidification of air is controversial because it has been associated with bronchospasm and bacterial colonization. It may be helpful for some patients, however, and some physicians may prescribe it.

To minimize bacterial colonization during acute phases of the disease, sputum should be cultured and tested for sensitivity. Antibiotics are prescribed based on the results of these tests. Combination therapy with two or three antibiotics is recommended to prevent bacterial resistance and is usually prescribed for 14 days. Shorter courses of antibiotic therapy are associated with reexacerbation of symptoms. Oral antibiotics may be prescribed for long-term therapy to inhibit bacterial colonization, although there is little scientific basis for this practice. Inhaled antibiotics are given in very high doses because only about 10% of the inhaled drug is absorbed.

COMPLICATIONS AND THEIR MANAGEMENT
PULMONARY INFECTIONS

Pulmonary infections compromise respiratory status and usually result in the patient being hospitalized for routine pulmonary physiotherapy or "clean out." This includes:

1. Vigorous postural drainage and clapping. Some patients will spend up to 8 hours a day consumed by clapping, vibrating, and postural drainage (see Chapter 34). Mechanical vibrators may be purchased by the patient with CF when physical therapists, nurses, respiratory therapists, or family members are not able to provide the necessary therapy. The majority of patients must have postural drainage with clapping every 4 hours. Respiratory personnel and nurses share the treatments.
2. Room humidification if ordered.
3. Aerosols with a bronchodilator such as Brokosol R or antibiotics may be administered before postural drainage and clapping.

HEMOPTYSIS

Hemoptysis occurs when a blood vessel is eroded as a result of pulmonary disease. The patient may expectorate as much as 300 to 500 ml of blood in 24 hours. When a patient with a pulmonary disease such as CF has an uncontrollable urge to cough, this usually indicates blood in the airways from hemoptysis. The patient will be very anxious and should not be left alone.

Nursing and medical care during hemoptysis includes the following:

1. Elevate head of bed 45 to 90 degrees.
2. Turn patient's head to left side.
3. Have emisis basin and tissues ready for expectoration of blood.
4. Provide clean basin frequently so that patient is not made more anxious by amount of blood.
5. Measure amount of hemoptysis and record time and amount.
6. Postural drainage and clapping are withheld during acute episodes of bleeding, usually for at least 24 hours.
7. Vitamin K_1, (Mephyton) is sometimes ordered by mouth or subcutaneously to control bleeding.
8. Stay with patient until bleeding has subsided and patient is made comfortable and is feeling less fearful.
9. Hemoptysis usually subsides without surgical intervention. If hemoptysis become life-threatening, surgical intervention, such as removal of the bronchiectatic lobe, may be necessary. Unfortunately, in most patients, the pulmonary disease is too extensive to permit surgery.[32]
10. Bronchoscopy with endobronchial tamponade may be successful in stopping bleeding in patients with minimal bleeding.

PNEUMOTHORAX

Pneumothorax occurs when apical cysts rupture, allowing air from the lung to enter the pleural space. Sudden sharp chest pain in adults with CF should suggest spontaneous pneumothorax. Pneumothorax occurs in 20% of adult CF patients and has a recurrence rate of 50%. Symptomatic pneumothoraces (increasing shortness of breath, mediastinal shift) are treated with intercostal drainage as follows:

1. Stab wound is made between ribs and chest tube is inserted.
2. Chest tube is connected to water-sealed drainage (see Chapter 34).
3. After lung is reexpanded, pleural sclerosis with tetracycline or guinacrine may be used. This procedure causes the visceral pleura to adhere to parietal pleura, obliterating the pleural space.
4. If there is a persistent air leak or pleural sclerosis fails, a partial pleurectomy should be performed.[32] In a partial pleurectomy, the portion of pleura overlying the cysts that ruptured is removed.

COR PULMONALE

As the airways become progressively plugged, *atelectasis* and *air trapping* occur. The result is a progressive ventilation/perfusion mismatch, resulting in progressive *hypoxemia*. Cor pulmonale can be expected to develop in patients with cystic fibrosis and advanced lung disease. A resting PaO_2 less than 50 mm Hg, and a $PaCO_2$ greater than 45 mm Hg usually indicate cor pulmonale.

Treatment of cor pulmonale includes the following:
1. Supplemental O_2 to help reverse pulmonary vasoconstriction caused by the hypoxemia and to improve myocardial performance. Oxygen therapy via cannula during sleep is commonly prescribed for patients with a daytime resting PaO_2 less than 60 mm Hg. Continuous O_2 is prescribed for patients with daytime resting PaO_2 less than 50 mm Hg.
2. Long-term diuretic therapy and fluid restriction may be effective therapy. The patient is monitored closely for electrolyte imbalances.
3. Digoxin is of questionable value in patients with right ventricular failure. However, many patients with CF have biventricular failure and digoxin may be of therapeutic value. Patients are monitored closely for hypoxemia and hypokalemia, which would increase the risk of digitalis toxicity.

GASTROINTESTINAL COMPLICATIONS

Gastrointestinal complications are common and are treated as follows:
1. Supplemental fat soluble vitamins are used to aid digestion and improve weight.
2. Most patients take multivitamins and Vitamin E.
3. Pancreatic enzyme supplement doses are individualized and titrated by patients to control fatty stools to less than three per day.
4. When a patient is NPO, minimal doses of pancreatic supplements are necessary
5. If adequate intake cannot be maintained orally, intravenous feedings or gastrostomy may be necessary.

■ ASSESSMENT

Assessment data need to be collected in three areas—pulmonary, nutritional/gastrointestinal, and psychosocial. Data to be collected in each of these areas are listed below.

PULMONARY

Subjective Data
1. Onset and description of symptoms such as shortness of breath, dyspnea on exertion, fatigue, and wheezing
2. Patient's understanding of CF pathophysiology and treatment regimens, including postural drainage and clapping, antibiotics, aerosol therapy, and nutritional supplements such as pancreatic enzymes and vitamins

Objective Data
1. Auscultation for adventitious breath sounds
2. Chest pain on inspiration
3. Cyanotic mucous membrane
4. Digital clubbing

5. Productive cough and color of sputum
6. Presence of fever, tachypnea
7. Review arterial blood gases (ABG) for indications of falling PaO_2 or rising $PaCO_2$; review results of pulmonary function tests (decrease in tidal volume, FEV_1 (forced expiratory volume in 1 minute)
8. Signs and symptoms of antibiotic toxicity that may cause renal toxicity
9. Side effects of aerosols (bronchodilators) that may cause tachycardia

NUTRITIONAL/GASTROINTESTINAL

Subjective Data

1. Patient's description of color, consistency, and frequency of stools
2. Patient's description of color, smell, and frequency of urination
3. Patient's description of appetite and ability to swallow food
4. Patient's description of daily eating pattern
5. Medications taken at home and their effectiveness in decreasing stool frequency
6. Onset and duration of abdominal discomfort
7. Signs or symptoms of gastric reflux
8. Weight loss; when began

Objective Data

1. Color, consistency, and frequency of stools
2. Weight loss
3. Presence of polyuria, polydipsia, or polyphagia
4. Dietary intake
5. Intensity, frequency, and location of abdominal pain
6. Absence of bowel sounds

PSYCHOSOCIAL

Subjective Data

1. Description of daily routines as it relates to work or school, pulmonary regimen, medications, and leisure activities
2. Description of current coping strategies and support network
3. Concerns about sexuality or fertility.
4. Method of financial support (job, family, other forms of assistance)
5. Patient and family's understanding of CF

Objective Data

1. Identify stage of grieving; symptoms that would infer that patient is grieving: anxiety, sleeplessness, hallucinations
2. Identify patient and family strengths
3. Identify patient support structure
4. Identify normal adult developmental needs (see Chapter 5).

5. Identify need for genetic counseling, career counseling, social services

■ DATA ANALYSIS: NURSING DIAGNOSES

Nursing diagnoses are determined from assessment of patient data. Possible nursing diagnoses for the adult with CF may include, but are not limited to:

Diagnostic Title	Possible Etiologies
Airway clearance, ineffective	Obstruction/thick secretions, tracheobronchial infection, hemoptysis
Fatigue	Decreased oxygenation, inadequate nutrition, inadequate rest
Gas exchange, impaired	Ventilation/perfusion imbalance
Grieving, dysfunctional	Loss of fertility/loss of independence/loss of job or role/loss of control of one's life; unhealthy grief work/withdrawal, preoccupation, sleeplessness.
Infection, potential for	Increased mucus in airway, decreased nutrition
Nutrition, altered: less than body requirements	Pancreatic insufficiency resulting in malabsorption, glucose intolerance/weight loss; shortness of breath makes eating difficult

■ PLANNING: EXPECTED PATIENT OUTCOMES

Expected patient outcomes for the person with CF may include, but are not limited to, the following:

1. Patient will have improved airway clearance
   a. Decreased mucus production
   b. Clear breath sounds
   c. Decreased fatigue and shortness of breath
   d. Absence of fever
   e. Absence of hemoptysis
2. Patient's fatigue will be improved
   a. Oxygenation will be improved and patient will have less shortness of breath
   b. Will be able to sleep better
3. Patient's gas exchange will be improved
   a. PaO_2 will be above 50 mmHg
   b. $PaCO_2$ will be less than 45 mmHg
4. Patient's grieving skills will be improved
   a. Verbalizes actual and potential losses
   b. Identifies own strengths and personal goals
   c. Identifies support person to assist with coping and achievement of goals
5. Patient's potential for infection is decreased
   a. Decreased mucus in airway
   b. Environment free of pathogenic bacteria
   c. Nutrition is improved
6. Patient demonstrates improved nutrition
   a. Maintains weight within 20% of ideal weight.
   b. Maintains normal blood glucose

c. Is able to eat small frequent feedings that permits eating when less fatigued and short of
breath

■ IMPLEMENTATION

Because the adult with CF is most commonly admitted
to the hospital when the airway is compromised, considerable nursing care will be necessary. The care of the
adult with CF centers around the following measures.

IMPROVING AIRWAY CLEARANCE

1. Provide with postural drainage with clapping every 2 to 4 hours, depending on the severity of the
   infection
2. Assist to cough effectively
3. Assess breath sounds before and after each treatment
4. Encourage patient to increase fluid intake to 3 to
   4 L every 24 hours unless contraindicated
5. Monitor food intake; provide frequent snacks
   when energy level is improved
6. Provide quiet environment with frequent monitoring and reassurance
7. Maintain cool room with temperature below 70° F.

MONITORING FATIGUE

The nurse is responsible for monitoring the patient's fatigue and instituting methods to improve it.
1. Assess fatigue frequently
2. Provide rest periods between activities.
3. Provide frequent small feedings, which will increase energy stores

IMPROVING GAS EXCHANGE

The nursing role is as follows:
1. Place in high Fowler's position.
2. Encourage slow rhythmic breathing.
3. Encourage patient to breathe through nose and
   exhale through pursed lips.
4. Monitor ABG findings.

HELPING THE PATIENT COPE WITH GRIEF

The nurse can play a major role in assisting the patient
to work through the grieving process.
1. Identify stage of grieving.
2. Allow time for patient to verbalize feelings, hopes,
   and fears.
3. Support expressions of hope but avoid false reassurance.
4. Support patient and family through grief work.
   Recommend CF support groups as indicated.
5. Refer as appropriate for genetic counseling, career
   counseling, or social service.
6. Intervene for pathologic symptoms of grief such
   as anxiety, sleeplessness, and hallucinations.
7. Be aware of your own feelings of grief and share

these with peers or a support group for nurses and
other health care providers.

MONITORING FOR INFECTION

Because the adult with CF is very vulnerable to infection or superinfection, the nurse needs to be aware of
providing an environment that is as free of pathogens as
possible.
1. Monitor patient's temperature frequently.
2. Monitor color, volume, and consistency of sputum.
3. Collect sputum specimens correctly and send for
   culture and sensitivity as indicated.
4. Give antibiotics as prescribed and on time to
   maintain adequate blood level.
5. Keep all persons with upper respiratory infections
   away from patient.
6. Wash own hands frequently and encourage visitors to wash hands before touching the patient.
7. Provide frequent mouth care, especially after postural drainage.
8. Assist patient to wash hands after coughing.

PROMOTING ADEQUATE NUTRITION

Because the patient with CF often has difficulty in
maintaining nutrition, the nurse may need to be inge-
nious in promoting nutrition.
1. Perform baseline and periodic assessment of nutrition including food history, recording of daily intake, output, and daily weight.
2. Monitor blood glucose levels so that insulin can be
   given as prescribed according to blood glucose
   findings.
3. Provide small, frequent feedings.
4. Work with dietitian and patient to provide feedings that will appeal to patient.
5. Administer pancreatic enzymes and vitamins as
   ordered.

TEACHING AND COUNSELING

Because the adult patient has had CF for several years,
teaching is more in the form of review and reinforcement. In addition to the teaching guidelines for patients
with COPD on p. 930, the following areas should be addressed with the patient with CF:
1. Review daily nutrition requirements, vitamins,
   and the need to check weight daily.
2. Review daily pulmonary exercises and treatments.
   a. Postural drainage and clapping
   b. Aerosol medication before postural drainage
3. Review medications in terms of usual dose, expected effects, and side effects. In some sections
   of the United States, medications can be obtained
   at substantial discount through the local Cystic
   Fibrosis Foundation.

TABLE 33-23 Research in the prevention and treatment of cystic fibrosis

Subject	Topic	Findings	Future Goals
Prevention	CF gene	Gene identified in 1989—location, size mutations and defective protein	To define protein structure and function To treat or alter defective protein To identify and change sodium and chloride ion movement in CF cell To identify causes of CF
	Vaccinations		To develop vaccines to prevent lung infections
	Genetic counseling	Phosphatase and pancreatic trypsin for neonatal diagnosis	To identify CF carriers—prenatal and neonatal diagnosis
Treatment	Antibiotics	Prophylactic use Early use Aerosolized antibiotic Oral route effectiveness	To treat lung infections effectively To decrease side effects of frequent treatment To decrease hospitalizations
	Lung transplantation		To replace damaged lungs

4. Review clinical symptoms that indicate that the health care provider should be notified.
   a. Signs of an acute respiratory infection such as fever, increased fatigue, shortness of breath, increased production of sputum, or change in color of sputum
   b. Hemoptysis
   c. Sudden sharp chest pain
5. Assess patient's knowledge and understanding of fertility, genetic testing, and contraceptive methods
6. Assess patient and family knowledge of community and social resources for assistance with health care reimbursement programs, disability insurance, and finding an appropriate support group.

RESPIRATORY FAILURE

Patients with CF eventually succumb to progressive respiratory and cardiac failure.[32] Because these patients have a fatal disease they usually have do not resuscitate (DNR) orders and are not intubated or placed on mechanical ventilation. The patient and family have to be involved in the DNR decision, and nurses play an important role in supporting the patient and family in their decision. The median age of death of adults with CF is approximately 22 for women and 28 for men.

RESEARCH

There is considerable on-going research in CF. Table 33-23 summarizes research projects, findings, and future goals. The identification of the CF gene, in 1989, was a major breakthrough and has raised hope for future progress in preventing and treating CF.

RESPIRATORY INSUFFICIENCY AND RESPIRATORY FAILURE

The terms respiratory insufficiency and respiratory failure describe two states of altered lung function that differ primarily in their degree of severity. *Respiratory insufficiency* exists when the oxygen and carbon dioxide exchange is inadequate to meet the body's needs during normal activities and is usually accompanied by symptoms such as dyspnea. *Respiratory failure* exists when hypoxemia, hypercapnia, and respiratory acidosis exceed predetermined values.

EPIDEMIOLOGY/ETIOLOGY

Many disorders can lead to or are associated with both respiratory insufficiency and failure (Table 33-24).

PREVENTION

Prevention of both respiratory insufficiency and failure is focused on early identification of persons at high risk of developing either of these disorders. In the inpatient setting, a preventive plan of care should be developed for every person with an increased risk of developing either respiratory insufficiency or failure. A preventive plan of care should include but is not limited to:
1. Keeping airway clear
   a. Instituting regularly performed deep breathing and coughing maneuvers
   b. Nasotracheal suctioning if necessary
2. Optimal activity level
3. Judicious use of sedatives or analgesics
4. Assessing regularly for signs and symptoms indicating deterioration of respiratory status
Persons with COPD have an increased risk of developing respiratory insufficiency or failure as a complication

TABLE 33-24 Disorders associated with respiratory insufficiency and failure

Pulmonary Disorders	Nonpulmonary Disorders
Severe infection	CNS disturbance secondary to drug overdose, anesthesia, head injury
Pulmonary edema	
Pulmonary embolus	
COPD	Neuromuscular disorders (e.g., Guillain-Barré syndrome, myasthenia gravis, multiple sclerosis, poliomyelitis, muscular dystrophy, spinal cord injury)
CF	
ARDS	
Cancer	
Chest trauma	
Severe atelectasis	
Airway compromise secondary to trauma, infection, or surgery	Postoperative reduction in ventilation following thoracic and abdominal surgery
	Prolonged mechanical ventilation

of their chronic disease. They should be counseled to contact their physician if they experience any change in the following:

1. Sputum production
2. Degree of dyspnea
3. Activity tolerance
4. Changes in ability to think clearly, unexplained irritability, and so on
5. Any change in medications

PATHOPHYSIOLOGY

The respiratory system is made up of two basic parts: the gas exchange organ (the lungs) and the pump (the respiratory muscles and the respiratory control mechanisms). Any alteration in the function of the gas exchange unit or the pump mechanism can result in respiratory insufficiency or failure.

Regardless of the underlying condition, the resultant events or processes that occur in respiratory failure are the same. With inadequate ventilation, the arterial oxygen falls, and tissue cells become hypoxic. Carbon dioxide accumulates, leading to a fall in pH and respiratory acidosis.

Lung or gas exchange unit respiratory failure is usually seen in persons with underlying primary pulmonary disease such as COPD. In this situation, respiratory failure is a result of pathology directly affecting the respiratory unit.

Pump failure is associated with the extrapulmonary disorders that may precipitate respiratory failure. In this situation the underlying disorder decreases the ability of the lungs to move oxygen and carbon dioxide in and out of the lungs by altering either the central ventilatory control mechanism (drug overdose), neuromuscular

PHYSIOLOGIC CRITERIA FOR ACUTE RESPIRATORY FAILURE

Sudden onset of
PaO_2 60 torr or less (measured on room air)
$PaCO_2$ 50 torr
pH 7.35

function (Guillian-Barré syndrome), or chest wall movement (flail chest).

CLINICAL MANIFESTATIONS

As indicated earlier, respiratory failure is defined by predetermined physiologic criteria. Physiologic parameters that define acute respiratory failure are presented in the box above.

Hypercapnia and hypoxemia are present in chronic respiratory failure and respiratory insufficiency. In these disorders, the pH usually stays within the range of 7.35 to 7.40 because of compensation. Patients with chronic respiratory failure or respiratory insufficiency develop *acute respiratory failure* as a result of a secondary insult to their already compromised pulmonary system, usually in the form of a respiratory infection. The individual can no longer compensate for the altered lung function; and a dramatic decrease in pH (below 7.35), accompanied by severe hypoxemia, occurs. Because hypercapnia preexists in these individuals, the $PaCO_2$ is less relevant than pH and PaO_2 in determining respiratory status. In fact, these patients often display few clinical signs or symptoms, even though they may have major blood gas derangements.

Underlying blood gas alterations are the basis for the clinical signs and symptoms associated with respiratory failure. The common signs associated with hypoxemia, hypercapnia, and respiratory acidosis are presented in the box below. The signs and symptoms are presented together, because the blood gas derangements causing them usually occur simultaneously.

In acute respiratory failure, there is a marked decrease in vital capacity. However, pulmonary function testing is only useful if the patient is alert and able to

SIGNS AND SYMPTOMS ASSOCIATED WITH HYPERCAPNIA, HYPOXEMIA, AND RESPIRATORY ACIDOSIS

Headache	Cardiac dysrhythmias
Irritability	Tachycardia
Confusion	Hypotension
Increasing somnolence coma	Cyanosis
Asterixis (flapping tremor)	

TABLE 33-25 Normal function, primary pathology, and clinical picture in acute respiratory failure

Normal Function	Pathology	Clinical Picture
ALVEOLAR/CAPILLARY MEMBRANE		
Site of oxygen and carbon dioxide exchange	Interstitial and alveolar edema, airway obstruction from mucus and bronchoconstriction causing inadequate O_2 and CO_2 transport and exchange, with resultant hypoxemia, hypercapnia, and acidosis	Headache, cardiac arrhythmias, $PaCO_2$, ↓ PaO_2, and pH, irritability, cyanosis confusion, tachycardia, hypotension, asterixis (flapping tremor), increasing somnolence with eventual coma.
RESPIRATORY MUSCLES		
Expand and contract chest and lungs	Respiratory muscle strength and endurance unable to counterbalance mechanical load placed on muscles	Increased work of breathing, dyspnea, exhaustion, vital capacity
CENTRAL AND PERIPHERAL CHEMORECEPTORS		
Controls rate and depth of ventilation in response to pH and CO_2 in CSF (central) or low levels of PO_2 (peripheral)	Decreased or absent response to CO_2, pH, or PO_2 levels	Increasing somnolence progressing to coma if untreated, worsening hypoxemia, hypercapnia, and acidosis
RIGHT-SIDED CARDIAC OUTPUT		
Right side: receive unoxygenated blood from systemic circulation and carry deoxygenated blood to lungs for reoxygenation	Increased pulmonary vascular resistance from hypoxemia or lung pathology increases pressure on right side of heart, causing increased venous pressure	Peripheral edema, neck vein distention, hepatomegaly

cooperate. Vital capacity can be measured at the bedside with a Wright respirometer. It is important for the nurse to recognize that the signs and symptoms associated with hypoxemia and hypercapnia depend more on the rate of change in value than on absolute value. The patient with COPD may show few signs until severe acute respiratory failure occurs. The normal function, pathophysiology, and clinical picture of a person with acute respiratory failure are presented in Table 33-25.

MEDICAL MANAGEMENT

Medical management of respiratory failure is presented in the box at right.

■ ASSESSMENT
SUBJECTIVE DATA

Subjective data include the following:
1. History of past or present associated disorders (see Table 33-22).
2. Recent onset of change in respiratory status
   a. Change in sputum
   b. Increased dyspnea
   c. Change in mental status
   d. Complaints of chest tightness or pain
3. Current medications
   a. Any recent changes in medication regimen
4. Self-care modalities

If available, a family member or friend may be able to provide objective information about changes in the patient.

OBJECTIVE DATA

Objective data include the following:
1. Assess general appearance

MEDICAL MANAGEMENT OF RESPIRATORY FAILURE

1. Medical therapy is based on degree of severity
   a. Severe acute respiratory failure—focus on immediate oxygenation and ventilation
   b. Less severe acute respiratory failure—underlying cause determined and treated concurrently while treating hypoxemia and hypercapnia
2. Clinical evaluation
   a. Diagnostic studies
      (1) Arterial blood gases
      (2) Chest x-ray
      (3) Bedside pulmonary spirometry
      (4) Sputum for culture and sensitivity (C & S)
   b. Treatment
      (1) Oxygen therapy
      (2) Ventilation—may require intubation and mechanical ventilatory support (see Chapter 34)
      (3) Treatment of complications
      (4) Treatment of underlying cause

a. Mental status—may vary from agitation to somnolence
2. Assess vital signs
   a. Tachycardia
   b. Tachypnea, bradypnea, or apnea
   c. Hypotension
3. Pulmonary examination
   a. Select components of pulmonary examination that patient can tolerate. Findings will depend on underlying cause of respiratory failure.
   b. Assess laboratory findings
      (1) ABGs for blood gas derangements associated with acute respiratory failure
      (2) Sputum C&S—frequently positive
      (3) Bedside spirometry: vital capacity = less than 15 ml/kg ideal body weight

■ DATA ANALYSIS: NURSING DIAGNOSES

Possible nursing diagnosis for the person with respiratory failure may include but are not limited to, the following:

Diagnostic Title	Possible Etiologies
Cardiac output, decreased, alteration in	Increased pulmonary vascular resistance
Nutrition, altered: less than body requirements	Unable to maintain intake large enough to balance increased metabolic needs from increased work of breathing
Gas exchange, impaired	Ventilation/perfusion imbalance
Airway clearance, ineffective	Fatigue, tracheobronchial infection, airway obstruction
Knowledge deficit: prevention and treatment	Lack of exposure or recall, cognitive impairment

■ PLANNING: EXPECTED PATIENT OUTCOMES

Expected patient outcomes for the person with respiratory failure may include, but are not limited to, the following. The patient will be able to:
1. Describe signs and symptoms that should be reported to the physician
2. Demonstrate improved ventilation and oxygenation by
   a. Arterial blood gas pH and $PaCO_2$ that returns or stays within acceptable baseline limits
   b. PaO_2 at optimal level for individual
   c. Explains how and when to use oxygen therapy
   d. Sensorium returns to or is maintained at pre-respiratory failure level
   e. Respiratory rate within or near to normal levels, moderate tidal volume
   f. Absence of dyspnea or dyspnea returns to preacute illness level
3. Demonstrate effective airway clearance by
   a. Effective coughing maneuvers
   b. Appropriate use of nebulizers, humidifiers

4. Demonstrate adequate cardiac output
   a. Absence of pulsus paradoxus
   b. Blood pressure within acceptable limits
   c. Heart rate and rhythm within acceptable limits
   d. Pulses are equal and present in all extremities
   e. Urinary output exceeds 30 ml/hr
5. Demonstrate adequate nutritional intake to balance metabolic needs
   a. Weight stabilizes at preacute illness weight
   b. If preillness weight outside acceptable limits for patient's size and age, the patient's weight progresses toward an established goal weight

Patients with underlying COPD will also meet the outcome criteria for persons with COPD (see p. 921).

■ IMPLEMENTATION

The level of nursing interventions for acute respiratory failure will depend on the patient's immediate status. The patient's condition may vary from critically ill, requiring immediate life support measures (cardiopulmonary resuscitation), to less urgent, in which aggressive nursing interventions can prevent further deterioration of physical status. Nursing interventions for acute respiratory failure include the following.

IMPROVING GAS EXCHANGE

Oxygenation

Severe hypoxemia is incompatible with life. Thus it is imperative to rapidly initiate oxygen therapy if severe hypoxemia is present. General oxygen therapy is discussed in Chapter 34.

The effectiveness of oxygen therapy is evaluated with arterial blood gas measurements. Supplemental oxygen should be provided to maintain a PaO_2 or 60 to 90 torr. Persons without underlying pulmonary disease can receive oxygen by either high-flow or low-flow systems. There are hazards associated with prolonged exposure to high concentrations of oxygen, however.

Oxygen toxicity is the term used to describe the damage to lung tissue that results from prolonged exposure to high oxygen concentrations. Although the exact effects of oxygen in any one individual may depend on the person's underlying pathologic condition, it is believed that exposure to greater than 60% oxygen for a period of more than 36 hours or exposure to 100% oxygen for a period of more than 6 hours will result in atelectasis and alveolar collapse. Breathing very high concentrations of oxygen (80% to 100%) for prolonged periods (24 hours or more) is often associated with the development of ARDS. Thus it is a firm general principle that the lowest amount of oxygen that will achieve an acceptable PaO_2 is the amount that should be used.

Special precautions must be taken when administering oxygen to patients with COPD to avoid concurrent elevation of their $PaCO_2$ levels, resulting in carbon dioxide narcosis or coma (see the box on p. 946).

OXYGEN THERAPY FOR COPD PATIENTS

Oxygen therapy resulting in elevated PaO_2 levels may decrease the ventilatory drive in COPD patients who are chronically hypoxemic. Decreased ventilatory drive causes hypoventilation, which causes elevated $PaCO_2$ levels, respiratory acidosis, and, ultimately, carbon dioxide narcosis.

Patients with COPD must receive supplemental oxygen via a low-flow controlled oxygen therapy system. The Venturi mask provides oxygen at controlled ranges of 24% to 40% (see Figure 34-17). Low-flow oxygen can also be provided by nasal cannula. However, the actual concentration of oxygen delivered to the lungs by cannula depends on the patient's ventilatory pattern. Regardless of the oxygen delivery system used, the patient's response to oxygen therapy can only be accurately assessed by arterial blood gas measurements.

It must be remembered that adequate oxygenation is essential for life. Therefore, if adequate oxygenation cannot be maintained without concurrent hypercapnia, oxygen therapy must still be continued. In this situation, ventilatory support is instituted to combat the hypercapnia.

Although it is important to realize that CO_2 narcosis might be precipitated if a chronically hypoxemic person receives high concentrations of oxygen, research has failed to support this standard clinical practice. Medical research on the effect of administering high oxygen concentrations to patients with COPD who were in respiratory failure showed little change in their respiratory drive.[104] These findings can be balanced in care of the chronically hypoxemic patient in acute respiratory failure by basing practice on the principle that the first priority for survival in a person experiencing acute respiratory failure is to receive adequate oxygen. However, these patients may also be at risk of developing CO_2 narcosis; therefore, they must be monitored continuously during oxygen therapy in order to intervene if a loss of ventilatory drive should occur.

Ventilatory Support

Ventilatory support is focused on reversing hypercapnia caused by hypoventilation. Aggressive nursing interventions to improve ventilation can often be effective in preventing the need for intubation and artificial ventilatory support (see interventions to improve airway clearance following the discussion on mechanical ventilation.)

Mechanical Ventilation

If, despite all the measures discussed, the person is unable to maintain ventilation (as indicated by a rising arterial $PaCO_2$, mechanical ventilation is necessary. The basic use of respirators, endotracheal and tracheostomy tubes, and the suctioning procedure for an artificial airway are discussed in Chapter 34.

A volume-limited ventilator is the ventilator of choice for patients with respiratory failure. The ventilator is set for a predetermined degree of control on the basis of the patient's ventilatory adequacy. Table 33-26 presents the basic ventilator control modes and their functions.

Patients requiring mechanical ventilation for acute respiratory failure are placed in an intensive care unit. Intensive nursing care includes frequent monitoring of the patient's vital functions and maintenance of optimal physical and mental status during their critical illness (see Chapter 34).

IMPROVING AIRWAY CLEARANCE

Airways clogged with excess mucus are one of the most reversible components precipitating acute respiratory

TABLE 33-26 Control modes of volume-limited ventilators

Ventilatory Mode	Function	Respiratory Status
Control/assist	Cycles inspiration Controls rate and depth of breathing	Apnea Used for person requiring PEEP
Intermittent	Cycles inspiration at a rate lower than patient's respiratory rate; independent O_2 source maintains predetermined FiO_2 during spontaneous ventilation	Patients who have spontaneous but inadequate ventilatory drive; also used to wean patient from ventilator
PEEP	Increases volume of air in lungs at FRC, thus alveoli that would collapse are kept open to increase gas exchange; used either with control/assist or IMV mode	Used for patients who are hypoxemic; increases PaO_2 at lower FiO_2; effective with decreased lung compliance; can cause dangerous decrease in cardiac output in presence of increased lung compliance

FiO_2, fraction of impaired O_2; FRC, functional residual capacity; IMV, intermittant manditory ventilation (see Chapter 34)

failure. Nursing interventions that promote a patent airway and can prevent deterioration of respiratory status include:

1. Effective cough maneuvers (Chapter 34)
2. Frequent deep-breathing exercises
3. Position change every 2 hours
4. Elevate head and chest
5. Nasotracheal suctioning if patient is unable to cough effectively
6. Bronchodilator medication as ordered (Table 33-18)

IMPROVING BREATHING PATTERN

Nursing interventions for patients in acute respiratory failure must be implemented in a firm, assured, but emphathetic manner. The patient may be agitated or nearly exhausted from hypoxemia, hypercapnia, and the increased work of breathing. It is imperative that the patient be gently guided in respiratory maneuvers to improve breathing. The nurse must be alert for signs and symptoms indicating that the patient's condition has changed from acutely ill but adequately ventilating to critically ill with insufficient ventilation to maintain body function. Nursing interventions include the following:

1. Encourage forward leaning postures (see Figure 33-6).
2. "Coach" patient to a slow rapid respiratory rate and avoid gulping large quantities of air.
3. If ordered, assist with IPPB treatments. Although the therapeutic effect of IPPB has been questioned, the treatment, at least for the short term, helps to slow respiratory rate and decreases the work of breathing. Specific aspects of IPPB therapy are presented in Chapter 34.

IMPROVING CARDIAC OUTPUT

Decreased cardiac output may result as a complication of acute respiratory failure or may be a precipitating factor related to underlying *cor pulmonale*. Diminished cardiac output causes tissue hypoxia, which creates a metabolic acidosis in addition to the respiratory acidosis caused by the respiratory failure. Specific aspects of care include the following:

1. Limiting fluid intake as ordered
2. Monitoring for signs of inadequate tissue perfusion (urinary output less than 30 ml/hr, cool extremities with decreased peripheral pulses)
3. Administering medications as ordered

See Chapter 28 for detailed care of the patient with decreased cardiac output.

MAINTAINING ADEQUATE NUTRITION

Individuals with acute respiratory failure are at increased risk for nutritional deficits because of the in-

RESEARCH

Treoloar D and Stechmiller J: Pulmonary aspiration in tube-fed patients with artificial airways, Heart Lung 13(6):667-671, 1984.

Thirty patients in a surgical ICU with artificial airways and ventilated with IMV mode who were receiving continual enteral tube feedings via a Dobbhoff feeding tube regulated by an IMED infusion pump were studied for the occurrence of silent aspiration. Methylene blue dye (1%) was thoroughly mixed with each tube feeding. The presence of blue-tinged secretions suctioned from the tracheostomy or endotracheal tube was considered a sign of pulmonary aspiration of the tube feeding. Patients in the study were followed for an average of 8.1 days. None of the 30 participants demonstrated silent aspiration as defined in this study. The investigators concluded that assuming a safe procedure for administering enteral feeding is followed; supplemental enteral therapy using Dobbhoff feeding tubes in critically ill patients with artificial airways is a safer procedure than previously indicated in the literature. ■

creased work of breathing. Nursing interventions are the same as those for the patient with COPD (p. 903). Additional aspects of care must be considered for patients who require mechanical ventilatory support. The overall focus of nutritional interventions is to prevent or correct malnutrition. Nutritional intake affects ventilatory drive, respiratory muscle function, and the amount of oxygen consumed and carbon dioxide produced from metabolic processes. Persons who have fasted for a few days or have been maintained on 5% dextrose intravenously may have severely depleted glycogen stores necessary for adequate respiratory function. Thus nutritional status can have a major impact on the individual's ability to be successfully weaned from the ventilator. Actions must focus on providing appropriate nutrition to meet their specific metabolic needs while on the ventilator and during and after weaning from it. Nutritional support by either enteral supplementation or parenteral hyperalimentation may be necessary. Whenever feasible, the gastrointestinal route should be used rather than parenteral therapy because it poses fewer risks and is more economical. The research box above discusses aspiration of tube feedings by patients with artificial airways.

PATIENT TEACHING

Patients with respiratory failure who have underlying COPD require the same interventions as those listed in the box on p. 930.

If respiratory failure is a complication of a disease other than COPD, the patient's knowledge needs to be assessed as to causative and contributing factors. Appropriate teaching is then instituted. All patients need to be able to explain home-going medications and treatments and plans for follow-up care.

CHAPTER SUMMARY

- Pulmonary disorders can be classified by the way ventilation is altered. The three major categories of pulmonary disorders are restrictive, obstructive, and vascular.

- In restrictive diseases, lung volume and lung compliance are reduced.

- Restrictive lung diseases include acute bronchitis, pneumonia, tuberculosis, fungal infections, occupational-related lung diseases, ARDS/HPPE, and cancer of the lung.

- Regardless of the causative agent, pneumonia results in acute inflammation of lung tissue. Inflamed tissue often involves both the conducting airways and alveolar tissue; thus both airway clearance and gas exchange may be impaired.

- ARDS results in severe hypoxemia without hypercapnia. Patients with ARDS/HPPE usually require mechanical ventilation with PEEP in order to safely provide adequate oxygen.

- Pulmonary emboli are a common pulmonary vascular problem that usually occur in persons who have been immobile for prolonged periods or who have had a disruption of the vascular system from injury or surgery.

- Primary prevention of respiratory infections such as tuberculosis includes prevention of the spread of infection by teaching the infected person to cover nose and mouth when coughing or sneezing so that droplet nuclei are not released into the air.

- Tuberculosis rates are up and this is generally attributable to the result of TB in persons with AIDS.

- Histoplasmosis, coccidiodomycosis, and blastomycosis are three major fungal infections of the lungs. Amphotericin B is the standard therapy for mycotic infection.

- The cause of cancer of the lung is closely related to cigarette smoking. From available research data, it seems evident that curtailing smoking is a primary preventive measure.

- Efforts to detect malignant lesions of the lungs early while curative treatment may be possible are critical. The nurse should encourage all persons over the age of 40 to obtain a chest x-ray periodically in addition to a yearly physical examination.

- Cystic fibrosis is an inherited disease that causes airway obstruction. It usually develops in childhood.

- Because of better treatment, more patients with CF are living into their 20s.

- Obstructive lung diseases result in an obstruction to airflow, predominantly on expiration.

- COPD is an umbrella label for a variety of pulmonary disorders that cause a chronic limitation of airflow. The most common chronic airflow disorders are emphysema, chronic bronchitis, and asthma.

- Hypoventilation results in elevation of arterial carbon dioxide. Hyperventilation results in lowered arterial carbon dioxide.

- To facilitate breathing, the nurse teaches the person with COPD abdominal breathing, leaning-forward postures, inhalation-exhalation exercises, and muscle reconditioning exercises.

- Respiratory failure is defined by the physiologic criteria of $PaO_2 = 60$ torr or less, $PaCO_2 = 50$ torr or greater, and a pH = 7.35 or less.

- Persons with COPD who have chronically elevated carbon dioxide and low oxygen levels are considered to have chronic respiratory failure. These chronically ill people are at high risk of developing acute respiratory failure, in addition to their chronic failure.

QUESTIONS TO CONSIDER

- What is the quality of air in the community in which you reside? If air pollution is a problem, what are the major contributing factors (e.g., industries, automobile exhaust)? Are there community groups working to improve the problem? If so, what activities are they involved in and how might a nurse be helpful to their efforts?

- Where is the branch of the American Cancer Society and the American Lung Association nearest your community? What services do they provide for health professionals and for patients?

- What is the tuberculosis case rate in the area in which you live? Is this higher or lower than the national rate of 9/100,000 population? List the factors that contribute to a higher or lower case rate in your community.

- Develop a plan of self-care to assist Mr. Barr to control his intermittent attacks of severe dyspnea. Mr. Barr was diagnosed 2 years ago with COPD, with predominant chronic bronchitis. He is a 65-year-old widower who lives alone in a second floor apartment. He tells you that whenever he experiences shortness of breath, he becomes terrified that he will pass out and no one will find him.

- A newly admitted patient who has a history of acute asthma complains that her theophylline is making her "nervous." What information would you need to obtain in order to assess this person's response to her medication? What information would you give to this patient about self-administration of the theophylline?

- Mrs. Jones has just been admitted to your unit. She has a long-standing history of COPD with chronic respiratory failure. She recently developed a viral bronchitis. She arrives on your unit with ABGs of $PaO_2 = 55$, $PaCO_2 = 80$, pH = 7.30. She appears extremely short of breath and is very restless. What information do you need to obtain to assess this patient's current status? What is your immediate plan of care?

- Describe the unique developmental needs of young adults with CF.

- Considering the trend of increasing life expectancy for patients with CF, what moral and ethical developments may the nurse encounter when caring for them?

- Discuss the clinical manifestations of CF in adults.

- Explain current therapy used to treat adults with CF.

- Describe the nature of respiratory insufficiency and the care of the patient with an artificial airway or mechanical ventilation.

REFERENCES AND SELECTED READINGS

1. American Cancer Society, Cancer facts and figures—1989, Atlanta, 1989, The Association.
2. Alford RH: Histoplasmosis. In Conn HF: Current therapy, Philadelphia, 1982, WB Saunders, Co.
3. *American Lung Association: Occupational lung disease: an introduction, New York, 1979, The Association.
4. American Lung Association: Chronic obstructive pulmonary disease, New York, 1981, The Association.
5. American Lung Association: Facts in brief about lung disease, New York, 1983, The Association.
6. American Lung Association: The asthma handbook, New York, 1984, The Association.
7. American Lung Association: The Lung, research accomplishments and frontiers, New York, 1986, The Association.
8. American Lung Association of Northern Ohio: The pulmonary press, 1(2):1-5, 1989.
9. American Lung Association: Diagnostic standards and classification of tuberculosis, New York, 1981, The Association.
10. American Thoracic Society: Cigarette smoking and health 132:1133-1138, 1985, The Society.

11. Ayres SM: Mechanisms and consequences of pulmonary edema: cardiac lung, shock lung and principles of ventilatory therapy in adult respiratory distress syndrome, Am Heart J 103(1):97-111, 1982.
12. *Barry MA et al: Tuberculosis infection in urban adolescents: results of a school-based testing program, Am J Public Health 80:439-441, 1990.
13. *Barstow R: Coping with emphysema, PhD Dissertation, University of California, San Francisco, 1973, Dissertation Abstracts International 34:913B-1802B, 1973.
14. Bates D: Respiratory function in disease, ed 3, Philadelphia, 1989, WB Saunders, Co.
15. Bonomi P: Primary lung cancer. In Rakel RE, editor: Conn's current therapy 1990, Philadelphia, 1990, WB Saunders, Co.
16. *Borland R et al: Effects of workplace smoking bans on cigarette consumption, Am J Public Health 80(2):178-180, 1990.
17. Bradley RB: Adult respiratory distress syndrome, Focus on Critical Care, 14:48-59, 1987.
18. Brisette S, Zinman R, and Reidy M: Nursing care plans for lessons in young adults with advanced cystic fibrosis, Issues in contemporary pediatric nursing, 10(2): 87-97, 1987.
19. Bryan CL and Jenkinson SG: Oxygen toxicity, Med Clin North Am 65:455-471, 1981.
20. *Burrows B: An overview of C.O.L.D., Med Clin North Am 65:455-571, 1981.
21. Callahan M: A prudent pulmonary rehabilitation program, Am J Nurs 85:1368-1369, 1985.
22. Campbell NA et al: The effects of simple relaxation technique on oxygen consumption in patients with COPD, Am Rev Respir Dis 133:A354, 1986.
23. Carpenito L: Nursing diagnosis-application to clinical practice, ed 3, Philadelphia, 1989, JB Lippincott Co.
24. Carrieri VK, and Janson-Bjerklie S: Dyspnea. In Carrieri VK, Lindsey AM, and West CM: Pathological phenomena in nursing, Philadelphia, 1986, WB Saunders Co.
25. *Caruthers DD: Infectious pneumonia in the elderly, Am J Nurs 90(2):56-60, 1990.
26. *Centers for Disease Control, Cigarette smoking—behavorial risk factor surveilance system, 1988, MMWR 38(49):845-847, 1989.
27. Centers for Disease Control, Morbidity and Mortality Weekly Report—Summary of Notifiable disease United States 1988, MMWR 37(54):41-43, 1988.
28. Centers for Disease Control, Morbidity and Mortality Weekly Report: update: tuberculosis elimination—United States, MMWR 39(10):153-156, 1990.
29. Centers for Disease Control, Morbidity and Mortality Report: Cigarette smoking—behavorial risk factor surveilliance system, MMWR 38(49):845-848, 1989.
30. Centers for Disease Control, Decrease in lung cancer incidence among males: United States, 1973-1983, MMWR 35:495-596, 1986.
31. *Cornell C: Tuberculosis in hospital employees, Am J Nurs 88:484-486, 1988.
32. Cherniak R: Current therapy of respiratory disease-2, Toronto, 1986, BC Decker Inc.
33. Cosenza JJ and Norton LC: Secretion clearance: state of the art from a nursing perspective, Crit Care Nurs 6:23-37, 1986.
34. Davis PB: Pathophysiology of pulmonary disease in cystic fibrosis, Semin Respir Med 6(4):261-269, 1985.
35. Davis PB and diSant' AP: Diagnosis and treatment of cystic fibrosis—an update, Chest 85(6):802-808, 1984.
36. Doenges M, Jeffries M, and Morrhouse M: Nursing care plans—nursing diagnosis in planning patient care, ed 2, Philadelphia, 1989, FA Davis, Co.
37. Dolovich J and Hargreave FE: Strategies in the control of asthma, Med Clin North Am 65:1033-1043, 1981.

---

*References preceded by an asterisk are particularly well suited for student reading.

38. Donner C: The critical difference pulmonary edema, Am J Nurs 88:59, 1988.

39. Dougherty S: The malnourished respiratory patient, Crit Care Nurs 8:13-15, 18-22, 1988.

40. *Douglas RG: Prophylaxis and treatment of influenza, N Engl J Med 322(7):443-449, 1990.

41. Drugs for asthma, Med Lett Drugs Ther 24:83-86, 1982.

42. *Engelking C: CE lung cancer chemotherapy, Am J Nurs 87:1438-1439, 1987.

43. *Engelking C: Teaching, counseling and caring, Am J Nurs 87:1439-1440, 1987.

44. *Engelking C: CE lung cancer. The language of staging, Am J Nurs 87:1434-1437, 1987.

45. *Fiore MC et al: Trends in cigarette smoking in the United States: the changing influence of gender and race, JAMA 261:49-55, 1989.

46. Fletcher CM and Pride NB: Definition of emphysema, chronic bronchitis, asthma, and airflow obstruction: 25 years from the CIBA symposium, (editorial), Thorax 39:81-85, 1984.

47. Fraser RG et al: Diagnosis of disease of the chest vol III, ed 3, Philadelphia, 1990, WB Saunders Co.

48. Freedberg PD, et al: Effect of progressive muscle relaxation on the objective symptoms and subjective responses associated with asthma, Heart Lung 16:24-30, 1987.

49. Fulmer J: The interstitial lung disease, Chest 82(2):172-178, 1982.

50. *Glass L: Exercise therapy for the patient with pulmonary dysfunction, Topics Clin Nurs 3(2):87-93, 1981.

51. Godfrey S: Exercise-induced asthma. In Clark TJH and Godfrey S, editors: Asthma, ed 2, London, 1983, Chapman and Hall.

52. *Gold W: Restrictive lung disease, Phys Ther 48(5):455-466, 1982.

53. Hanley MV, and Tyler ML: Ineffective airway clearance related to airway infection, Nurs Clin North Am 22(1):135-149, 1987.

54. Hartman B et al: *Pneumocystis carinii* pneumonia in the acquired immunodeficiency syndrome (AIDS)—diagnosis with bronchial brushings, biopsy, and bronchoalveolar lavage, Chest 87:603-607, 1985.

55. *Haylock PJ: Radiation therapy, Am J Nurs 87:1441-1446, 1987.

56. Hendeles L, Maasanari M, and Weinberger M: Update on the pharmacodynamics and pharmacokinetics of theophylline, Chest 88:1035-1115, 1985.

57. Heslop AP, et al: A study to evaluate the intervention of a nurse visiting patients with disabling chest disease in the community, J Adv Nurs 13:71-77, 1988.

58. Hogg J: Structure and function of small airways, Chest 77(2):297-282, 1980.

59. *Hodgkin JE: Chronic obstructive pulmonary disease, Park Ridge, Ill, 1979, American College of Chest Physicians.

60. Howder CL: Respiratory care: know the facts, Philadelphia, 1989, JB Lippincott.

61. Ingersoll GL: Respiratory muscle fatigue research: implications for clinical practice, Appl Nurs Res 2:6-15, 1989.

62. Irwin M and Openbrier D: A delicate balance—strategies for feeding ventilated COPD patients, Am J Nurs 3:274-280, 1985.

63. James B: Adult respiratory distress syndrome, Nursing '84, 2(27):792-795.

64. Janson-Bjerklie S and Shnell S: Effect of peak flow information on patterns of self-care in adult asthma, Heart Lung 17:543-549, 1988.

65. Janz NK et al: Evaluation of a minimal-contact smoking cessation intervention in an outpatient setting, Am J Public Health 77:805-809, 1987.

66. Johnson A: The elderly and COPD, J Gerontol Nurs 14:20-24, 1988.

67. Katz S: Primary lung abscess. In Rakel RE, editor: Conn's current therapy 1990, Philadelphia, 1990, WB Saunders Co.

68. Kerston LD: Comprehensive respiratory nursing: a decision making approach, Philadelphia, 1989, WB Saunders Co.

69. Kravetz HM: Coccidioidomycosis. In Conn HF: Current therapy 1982, Philadelphia, 1982, WB Saunders Co.

70. *Krokosky NJ: Black lung and silicosis, Am J Nurs 85:883-886, 1985.

71. Laner M et al: The prone position in ARDS patients. A clinical study, Chest 94:103-107, 1988.

72. Lareau S and Larson J: Ineffective breathing pattern related to airflow limitation, Nurs Clin North Am 22:179-191, 1987.

73. Larson J and Kim MJ: Ineffective breathing pattern related to respiratory muscle fatigue, Nurs Clin North Am 22:207-224, 1987.

74. Larson J and Kim JJ: Respiratory muscle training with the incentive spirometer resistive breathing device, Heart Lung 13:341-345, 1984.

75. Lewis MI and Belman MJ: Nutrition and respiratory muscles, Clin Chest Med 9:337-348, 1988.

76. Lordi GM and Reichman LB: Tuberculosis and other myocobacterial disease. In Rakel RE, editor: Conn's current therapy 1990, Philadelphia, 1990, WB Saunders Co.

77. *Macklem P: Disease in small airways, Basics of R.D., 4:1-6, 1976.

78. *Madsen LA: Tuberculosis today, RN 53(3):44-51, March, 1990.

79. *Marx JL: The cystic fibrosis gene is found, Science 245:923-925, 1989.

80. Mascher L: Helpful exercises for your COPD patient, RN 6:33-35, 1984.

81. *Matthews LW and Drotar DD: Cystic fibrosis—a challenging long term chronic disease, Pediatr Clin North Am 31(1):133-152, 1984.

82. McCauley K and Weaver R: Cardiac and pulmonary diseases, nutritional implications, Nurs Clin North Am 18(1):81-95, 1983.

83. McDonald B: Validation of three respiratory nursing diagnoses, Nurs Clin North Am 20:697-710, 1985.

84. McGowan SE and Hunninghake GW: Neutrophils and emphysema, N Engl J Med 10:968-969, 1989.

85. *McNaull FW: CE lung cancer: tobaccism in America, Am J Nurs 87:1430-1432, 1987.

86. *McNaull FW: CE lung cancer: What are the odds? Am J Nurs 87:1428-1429, 1987.

87. Moser KM and Bordow RA: In Bordow RA, and Moser KM: Manual of clinical problems in pulmonary medicine with annotated key references, ed 2, Boston, 1988, Little, Brown & Co.

88. *Nocturnal Oxygen Therapy Trial Group: Continuous or nocturnal oxygen therapy in hypoxemic chronic obstructive lung disease: a clinical trial, Am Intern Med 93:391-398, 1980.

89. Norton LC et al: Common problems and state of the art in nursing care of the mechanically ventilated patient, Crit Care Nurs 6:23-37, 1986.

90. Openbrier DR, Hoffman LA, and Wesmiller SW: Home oxygen evaluation and prescription, Am J Nurs 88:192-197, 1988.

91. Openbrier DR Fuoss C, and Mall C: What patients on home oxygen therapy want to know, Am J Nurs 88:198-202, 1988.

92. Penn RL: Blastomycosis. In Conn HF: Current therapy 1982, Philadelphia, 1982, WB Saunders Co.

93. Peterson G: Application and assessment of oxygen therapy devices, Nurs Clin North Am 16:241-257, 1981.

94. *Pierce JP et al: Trends in cigarette smoking in the United States: educational differences are increasing, JAMA 261F:56-60, 1989.

95. *Pierce JP et al: Trends in cigarette smoking in the United States: projections to the year 2000, JAMA 261:61-65, 1989.

96. Preusser BA et al: Effects of two methods of preoxygenation on mean arterial pressure, cardiac output, peak airway pressure, and postsuctioning hypoxemia, Heart Lung 17:290-299, 1988.

97. Rakel RE: Conn's current therapy 1990, Philadelphia, WB Saunders Co.

98. Ramsdell JW: Bronchodilator drugs. In Bordow RA and Moser KM: Manual of clinical problems in pulmonary medicine, Boston, 1988, Little, Brown & Co.

99. Renfroe KL: Effect of progressive relaxation on dyspnea and state anxiety in patients with chronic obstructive pulmonary disease, Heart Lung 17:408-413, 1988.

100. Report of ATS-ACCP ad hoc subcommittee on pulmonary nomenclature, ATS News, 2, 1981.

100a. *Roberts SL: High-permeability pulmonary edema: nursing assessment, diagnosis and interventions, Heart Lung 19(3): 287-299, 1990.

101. Rochester D: Respiratory muscle function in health, Heart Lung 13:349-354, 1984.

102. Rogge JA et al: Effectiveness of oxygen concentrations of less than 100% before and after endotracheal suction in patients with chronic obstructive pulmonary disease, Heart Lung 18:64-71, 1989.

103. Roussos C: Function and fatigue of respiratory muscles, Chest 88:1245-1325, 1985.

104. Schmidt GA and Hall JB: Acute and chronic respiratory failure assessment and management of patients with COPD in the emergent setting, Concepts in Emergency and Critical Care 261:3444-3453, 1989.

105. *Selwyn PA et al: A prospective study of the risk of tuberculosis among intravenous drug users with human immunodeficiency virus infection, N Engl J Med 320(9):545-550, 1989.

106. Shekelton ME: Coping with chronic respiratory difficulty, Nurs Clin North Am 22(3):569-581, 1987.

107. Snider G: The pathogenesis of emphysema—twenty years of progress, Am Rev Resp Dis 124(3):321-324, 1981.

108. Snider G: Conference summary, Chest 85:845-895, 1984.

109. Spector N: Nutritional support of the ventilator-dependent patient, Nurs Clin North Am 24:407-414, 1989.

110. Stead WW et al: Racial differences in susceptibility to infection by *Mycobacterium tuberculosis*, N Engl J Med 322(7):422-427, 1990.

111. Tiep BL et al: Pursed-lip breathing training using ear oximetry, Chest 90:218-221, 1986.

112. Traver G: Measures of symptoms and life quality to predict emergent use of institutional health care resources in chronic obstructive airway disease, Heart Lung 17:689-697, 1988.

113. Treoloar D and Stechmiller J: Pulmonary aspiration in tube fed patients with artificial airways, Heart Lung 13:667-671, 1984.

114. Tuberculosis—new views of an old disease, N Engl J Med 312:1514-1515, 1986.

115. U.S. Environmental Protection Agency, Indoor air facts—environmental tobacco smoke, EPA #5, Washington DC, June 1989.

116. West JB: Pulmonary pathophysiology—the essentials, ed 3, Baltimore, 1987, Williams & Wilkins.

117. Wicklund S et al: Nurses drug alert, Am J Nurs 86:63-70, 1985.

118. Witkowski A: Pulmonary assessment—a clinical guide, Philadelphia, 1985, JB Lippincott Co.

119. Witta K et al: Myths and facts about mechanical ventilation, Nursing 18:25, 1988.

120. Wood RF, Boot TF, and Doershuk CF: Cystic fibrosis: state of the art, Am Rev Resp Dis 113:833-877, 1976.

121. York K: Clinical validation of two respiratory nursing diagnoses and their defining characteristics, Nurs Clin North Am 20:657-667, 1985.

122. Youmans GP, Patterson PY, and Sommers HM: The biologic and clinical basis of infectious disease, Philadelphia, 1975, WB Saunders Co.

123. Zabelbaum G, and Pare J: Manual of acute respiratory care, Boston, 1982, Little, Brown & Co.

CHAPTER 34

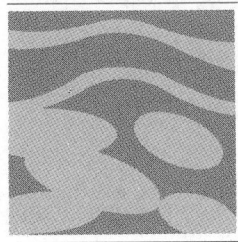

Common Interventions for Respiratory Problems

WILMA J. PHIPPS
JOSEPHINE BRUCIA

CHAPTER OBJECTIVES

After studying this chapter, the student should be able to:

1 Describe the factors that must be present for normal breathing and for oxygen-carbon dioxide exchange.
2 Describe primary and secondary prevention of respiratory problems.
3 Describe nursing care for the patient who has an endotracheal tube or tracheostomy.
4 Discuss the precautions to be observed when feeding the patient who is intubated.
5 Differentiate between a pressure-cycled and a volume-cycled ventilator.
6 Discuss the points to include in a teaching plan for the patient who is to have resectional surgery of the lung.
7 List precautions to be observed in care of chest tubes and water-sealed drainage and give the rationale for each.
8 Differentiate between a closed, open, and tension pneumothorax in terms of clinical manifestations and nursing management.

In order for breathing to take place normally, several factors are necessary: (1) an adequate supply of oxygen in the environment, (2) a patent airway, (3) normal functioning bellows motion of the chest wall and diaphragm, (4) an adequate number of functioning alveoli and capillaries that together form a terminal respiratory unit (TRU), (5) an adequate amount of hemoglobin to carry oxygen to the cells, (6) an intact circulatory system and an effective heart pump, and (7) a functioning respiratory center. Problems in one or more of the above can result in inadequate exchange of oxygen and carbon dioxide and, if severe enough, can cause death. Table 34-1 lists some of the conditions that can lead to inadequate oxygen-carbon dioxide exchange.

PREVENTION

Preventing conditions that impair oxygen-carbon dioxide exchange requires that health care providers be aware of the factors that cause problems and try to prevent their occurrence. Preventive activities include public or individualized education to decrease known pulmonary risk factors and interventions to prevent further deterioration of the individual's pulmonary status. Table 34-2 presents specific preventive nursing interventions.

INTERVENTIONS

MAINTAINING AN ADEQUATE SUPPLY OF OXYGEN IN THE ENVIRONMENT

The human pulmonary system functions at maximal efficiency within a relatively narrow range of atmospheric oxygen. As described in Chapter 31, oxygen moves from the atmosphere to the alveoli and from alveoli to arterial blood by simple gaseous diffusion. Thus any factor that alters the partial pressure of oxygen in the atmosphere will affect alveolar, arterial, and, ultimately, tissue oxygen levels.

Carbon monoxide poisoning is a relatively common cause of accidental injury and death or suicide. Carbon monoxide has 240 times greater affinity for hemoglobin than does oxygen. Thus, when an individual inhales carbon monoxide, hemoglobin becomes unavailable for oxygen transport, and tissue hypoxia results. In order to increase public awareness about possible sources of carbon monoxide poisoning, the points of emphasis outlined in the box on p. 955 should be included in any educational effort.

At high altitudes barometric pressure and, proportionately, oxygen partial pressure, decrease. Persons exposed to high altitudes, such as pilots, astronauts, mountain climbers, and those moving to high altitudes, will have various reactions, depending on the rate at which hypoxia develops, the cellular oxygen requirements related to physical exertion, and the duration of exposure.

The initial reaction to high altitudes results in the same signs and symptoms as seen in anyone experienc-

TABLE 34-1 Factors interfering with oxygenation and normal oxygen—carbon dioxide exchange

Necessary Component	Interference

Adequate supply of oxygen	Inhalation of air containing oxygen at subnormal pressure caused by:
	   Smoke inhalation
	   Carbon monoxide poisoning
	   High altitudes
	   Dilution of inspired air with inert gases (nitrogen, helium, hydrogen, methane, or anesthetic gases such as nitrous oxide)

Patent airway	Interference with the passage of oxygen from air through tracheobronchial tree to alveolar-capillary membrane caused by mechanical obstruction such as drowning, foreign bodies in tracheobronchial tree:
	   Children (aspiration of objects such as pennies, pins, jacks)
	   Unconscious adults (tongue obstructing airway, aspirated vomitus, loose dentures)
	   Mucus plug resulting in atelectasis
	 Allergic reactions resulting in bronchoconstriction, increased mucus secretions, and increased capillary permeability

Normally functioning bellows	Trauma to chest wall with possible sequelae of paradoxical breathing, pneumothorax, mediastinal shift Muscle or nerve trauma or impairment (quadriplegia, paraplegia, poliomyelitis, myasthenia gravis, Guillain-Barré syndrome, Landry ascending paralysis, muscular dystrophy)
Adequate functioning alveoli and capillaries to form TRU	Pulmonary edema Adult respiratory distress syndrome (high-permeability pulmonary edema) Physiologic shunts Damage to alveolar-capillary membrane secondary to conditions such as pulmonary emphysema
Adequate amount of hemoglobin	Severe anemia Carbon monoxide poisoning Methemoglobinemia
Intact circulatory system and pump	Congestive heart failure Hemorrhage
Functioning respiratory center	Depression of respiratory center by drugs (heroin, morphine, barbiturates, alcohol, or a combination of alcohol with a tranquilizer or barbiturates) Increased intracranial pressure (head injury or disease such as meningitis)

TABLE 34-2 Nursing interventions to prevent pulmonary system disease or deterioration

Primary Interventions	Secondary Interventions

Education about environmental inhaled irritants:
 1. Smoking/tobacco risks, cessation programs
 2. Air quality
 3. Activities to minimize risk in high exposure areas; (masks, air filters, promoting smoke-free work areas)
 4. Avoidance of repeated infectious agents
 Prompt treatment of pulmonary infections
	Patient education focused on recognition of signs and symptoms of pulmonary infection or deterioration:
	 1. When to initiate specific actions
	   a. Physician notification
	   b. Use of medications as needed
	 2. Correct use of home pulmonary equipment
	   a. O$_2$ therapy
	   b. IPPB*
	   c. Humidifiers
	   d. Suction machines
	   e. Ventilators
	 3. Self-care modalities
	   a. Postural drainage
	   b. Suctioning
	   c. Tracheostomy care
	   d. Pursed lip breathing, leaning forward postures, effective cough and relaxation techniques

*Intermittent positive-pressure breathing device.

PREVENTION OF CARBON MONOXIDE POISONING

1. Fire
   a. Fire prevention
   b. How to escape safely from a burning building
   c. Installation of smoke alarms
2. Safe use of home gas appliances
   a. Gas stoves and furnaces checked for leakage and improper combustion
3. Wood and kerosene stoves
   a. Ensure proper ventilation
4. Automobiles
   a. Hole in tail-pipe, allowing CO to enter car. Keep window open slightly when heater is on.
5. Signs and symptoms of carbon monoxide poisoning
   a. Headache, lethargy, tachycardia, and tachypnea

ing oxygen lack. Headache, dizziness, breathlessness, weakness, nausea, sweating, palpitation, dimness of vision, partial deafness, and sleeplessness occur with moderate hypoxia. With exertion, dyspnea and other symptoms worsen. At altitudes higher than 12,000 feet, the signs and symptoms intensify and may progress to convulsions and coma.

A person remaining in high altitudes for days or weeks will become acclimatized and will be able to work without becoming symptomatic. The five factors involved in acclimatization are: (1) increased pulmonary ventilation, (2) increased blood hemoglobin, (3) increased lung diffusing capacity, (4) increased tissue vascularity, and (5) increased cellular ability to use oxygen even at low arterial oxygen levels.[26]

Persons such as mountain climbers moving to high altitudes are advised to allow time for their bodies to adjust to changes in various altitudes. Trained climbers, especially those ascending to very high altitudes, allow themselves weeks or even months at base camps at various altitudes in preparation for their ascent.[26]

MAINTAINING A PATENT AIRWAY

An airway may be partially or completely obstructed. In partial airway obstruction the individual displays respiratory distress and produces sounds such as gurgling, snoring, or stridorous ventilations. When the airway is completely obstructed, the conscious person will have no breath sounds and will display signs of severe respiratory distress progressing to respiratory arrest. Airway obstruction is confirmed in the unconscious person when attempts to ventilate the person do not produce chest movement and no expiratory air passes from the individual's airway.

The type of intervention used to reestablish and maintain airway patency depends on the individual's level of consciousness, respiratory status, and the cause of airway obstruction. The conscious person with an obstructed airway must be assessed for adequacy of air exchange. If the individual can talk and cough, air exchange is adequate and interventions can be focused on the underlying cause. The conscious person with a completely obstructed airway will not be able to speak or cough and will soon lose consciousness if the obstruction is not relieved. Special maneuvers such as chest or abdominal thrusts and back blows are administered if the obstruction is caused by a foreign object blocking the airway. Organizations such as the American Heart Association and the American Red Cross offer training programs to certify proficiency in these basic life-saving techniques.

In the unconscious individual the tongue falls back, covering the glottis. By simply lifting the chin, the tongue is moved forward, opening the airway. An alternative position to keep the tongue from obstructing the unconscious person's glottis is to place the individual in a side-lying position.

When a person has a mechanical obstruction of the airway and is expected to be unconscious for some time, it may be necessary to use an artificial airway.

ARTIFICIAL AIRWAYS

Oral Airways

The simplest type of artificial airway is an oropharyngeal airway (see Chapter 22, Figure 22-12). The oropharyngeal airway keeps the tongue from falling back over the glottis. This type of airway is never used in a conscious individual, because it may cause vomiting or laryngospasm. An oropharyngeal airway must be inserted correctly to avoid pushing the tongue back against the glottis.

The esophageal gastric airway consists of a face mask with two ports. The lower port is for the esophageal tube, which is introduced into the esophagus to prevent gastric contents reflux. The upper port is used for ventilation. The esophageal gastric tube airway is never inserted into a conscious person.

Endotracheal and Tracheostomy Tubes

When a person is no longer able to maintain own airway, an endotracheal tube or tracheostomy is necessary. An endotracheal tube is usually chosen initially as a means of providing the airway; tracheostomy is only performed if airway maintenance is necessary for a prolonged period of time or if trauma to the airway prevents the use of an endotracheal tube. Although the tracheostomy has the *disadvantage* of a higher risk of infection, it is often elected for airway management because it is much more comfortable than an endotracheal tube and allows the person to eat.

In endotracheal intubation a tube is passed through either the nose or mouth into the trachea, whereas in a

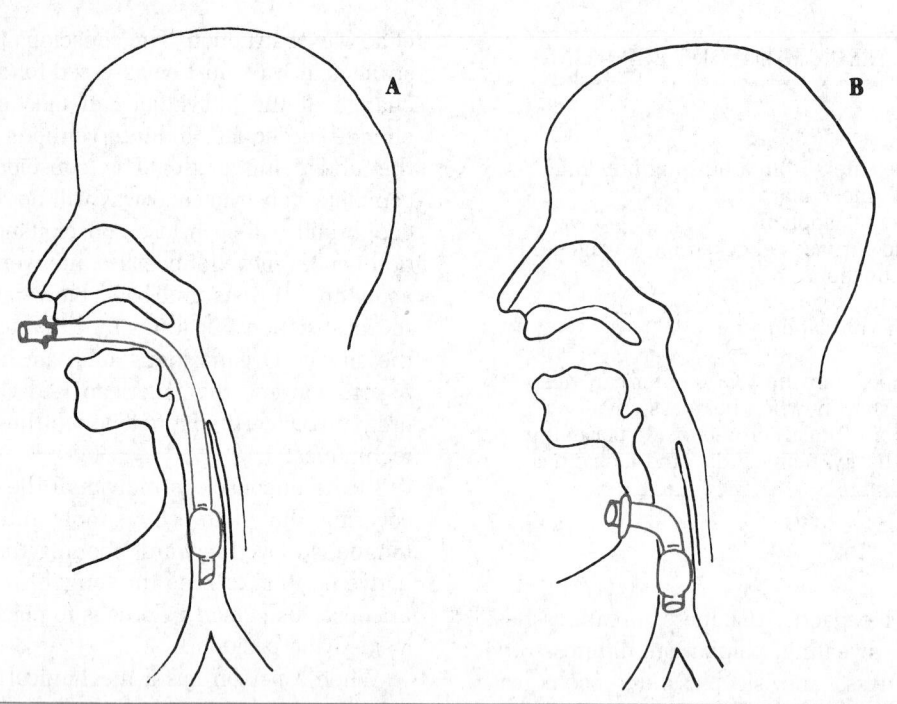

FIGURE 34-1 A, Position of endotracheal tube. **B,** Position of tracheostomy tube.

tracheostomy an artificial opening is made in the trachea into which a tube is inserted (Figure 34-1). These procedures are used (1) to establish and maintain a patent airway, (2) to prevent aspiration by sealing off the trachea from the digestive tract in the unconscious or paralyzed person, (3) to permit removal of tracheobronchial secretions in the person who cannot cough adequately, and (4) to treat the patient who requires positive pressure ventilation that cannot be given effectively by mask. Whether an intubation or a tracheostomy is performed initially depends on the facilities available and the wishes of the physician. Most physicians now consider it safer to do an emergency endotracheal intubation and then perform a tracheostomy as a nonemergency procedure in the operating room if prolonged support of the airway is needed. In this instance the endotracheal tube is not removed until after the tracheostomy opening is made.

A tracheostomy is necessary when an endotracheal tube cannot be inserted or when it is contraindicated, as in severe burns or laryngeal obstruction caused by tumor, infection, or vocal cord paralysis. Once the airway is secured, either by intubation or by tracheostomy, secretions are aspirated, and well-humidified oxygen is usually given. If the patient is unable to sustain respiration, a mechanical ventilator is attached to either the endotracheal tube or the tracheostomy tube. When mechanical ventilation is required, a cuffed tube is used. Usually an endotracheal tube is not left in place longer than 10 to 14 days. If the patient is unable to maintain a

free airway after this period of time, a tracheostomy is performed.

The endotracheal tube is made of plastic with an inflatable cuff so that a closed system with the ventilator may be maintained (Figure 34-2). The tube is inserted via the mouth or nose through the larynx into the trachea. If an oral endotracheal tube is used, a rubber airway or bite block is often necessary to prevent the patient from biting down on the tube and obstructing the airway.

Tracheostomy tubes are usually made of metal or plastic. They may have only a single lumen or may have both an inner and outer cannula (Figure 34-3). All adult-sized plastic tubes have a cuff that is inflated with air to fill the space between the outside of the tube and the trachea when a sealed airway is required for mechanical ventilation. Single-lumen tubes may need to be changed more often than tubes with an inner cannula that can be removed for cleaning. Usually tracheostomy tubes do not need to be changed more often than every 2 to 3 weeks; low-pressure cuffs are less likely to cause damage to the trachea (Figure 34-4). Single-lumen tubes are more difficult to clean and more likely to become plugged than are double-lumen tubes.

Silver tubes are commonly available in size 00 to 8 (no. 00 is used for the premature or newborn infant, whereas a no. 6 or 7 is used for most adults). The silver tracheostomy tube consists of two parts, an inner and an outer cannula. The outer cannula is removed only by the physician or a specially prepared nurse, whereas the

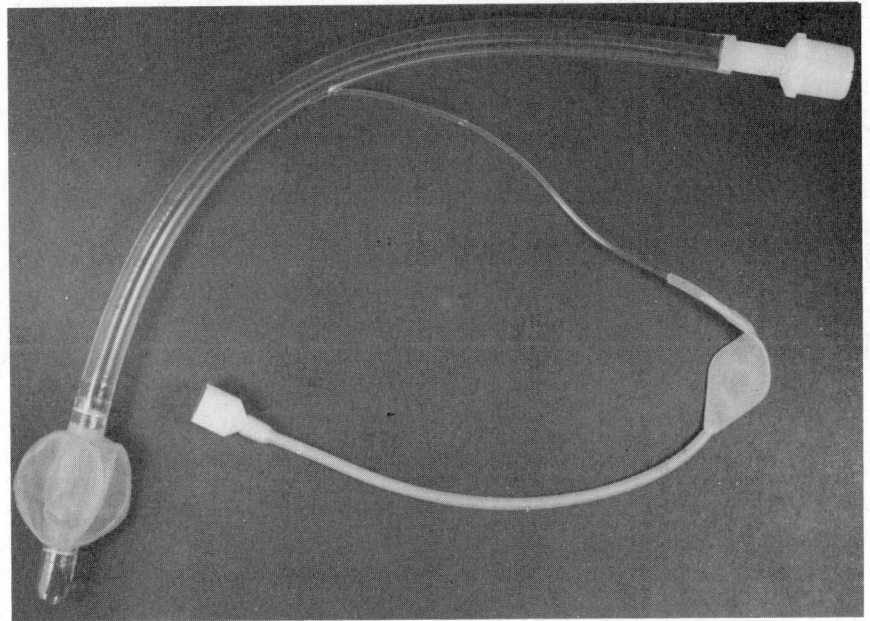

FIGURE 34-2 Forregar cuffed endotracheal tube. Cuff shown here is not inflated.

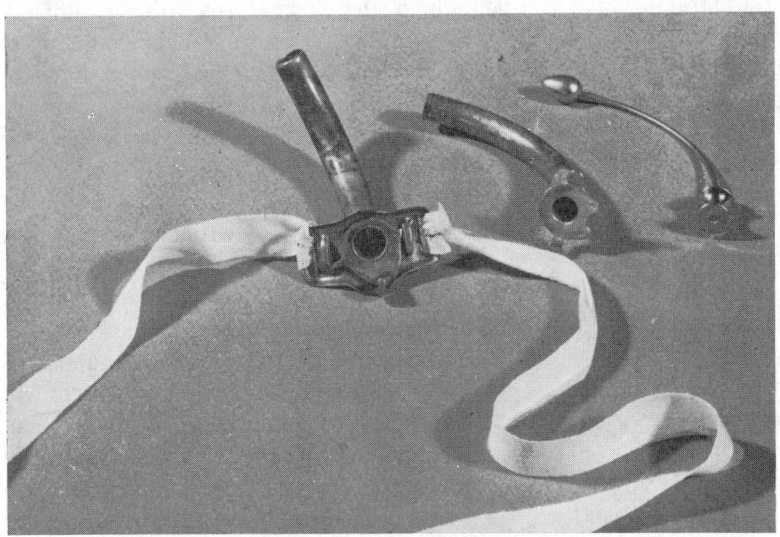

FIGURE 34-3 Parts of silver tracheostomy tube:outer tube with ties attached, inner tube, and pilot. (From DeWeese DD, and Saunders WH: Textbook of otolaryngology, ed 6, St Louis, 1982, The CV Mosby Co.)

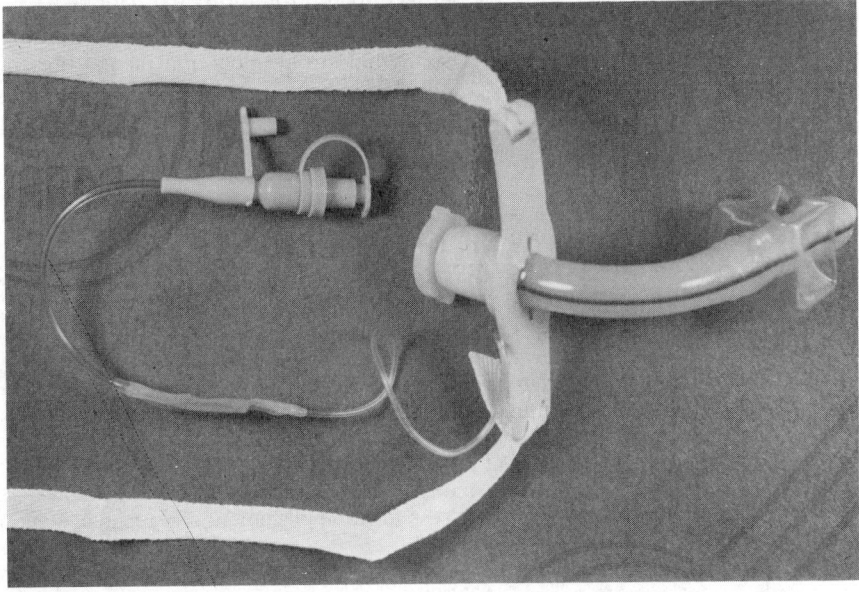

FIGURE 34-4 Portex cuffed tracheostomy tube.

inner cannula is removed regularly by the nurse for cleaning. The silver tracheostomy tube has a lock that must be turned to remove the inner cannula. The lock should be secured when the inner cannula is reinserted after cleaning. Twill tapes attached to either side of the tube (see Figure 34-3) are tied securely behind the neck to prevent the tube from becoming dislodged when the patient coughs or moves about.

Should the tube be coughed out, the opening may close, and the patient will be unable to breathe. Therefore, a tracheal dilator or curved hemostat is always kept at the bedside so that the opening can be held open if the tube is dislodged. Some surgeons prefer to place a retention suture on each side of the tracheostomy opening and tape the end of the suture to the skin. If the opening shows signs of closing, tension can be placed on the sutures to widen the opening.

The operative wound may be sealed with a plastic spray, or a small dressing may be placed around the tracheostomy tube. Although drainage should be minimal, the wound is inspected frequently for bleeding during the immediate postoperative period. The dressings are changed as they become soiled with mucus drainage. Occasionally, young children require elbow restraints to prevent them from removing the tube or putting objects into it.

Depending on the patient's condition, a tracheostomy can be either temporary or permanent; the person who has a laryngectomy will have a permanent tracheostomy. Any patient who has had a tracheostomy is apprehensive and is often fearful of choking. Thus when feasible, the procedure is thoroughly explained to the patient before surgery. Both patient and family need to understand that the *patient will be unable to speak* and that *constant attendance will be provided until the patient can give self-care safely.*

A fenestrated tracheostomy tube has an opening on the upper surface of the outer cannula that allows air inspired through the nose and mouth to pass through the tube. When the external opening is plugged, air can pass over the vocal cords, allowing the individual to talk. If ventilatory assistance is required, the inner cannula can be inserted so that the patient can be connected to a ventilator.

General care of the person with an endotracheal or tracheostomy tube. An endotracheal or tracheostomy tube provides a direct route for introduction of pathogens into the lower airway, increasing the risk of infection. It is essential that the following preventative nursing interventions be consistently implemented.

   1. Minimize infection risk
      a. Endotracheal airways irritate the trachea, resulting in increased mucus production. Assess the patient regularly for excess secretions, and

suction as often as necessary to maintain a patent airway. See the box on p. 960 for sterile suctioning procedure.
      b. Provide constant airway humidification. Endotracheal airways bypass the upper airway that normally humidifies and warms inspired air. An external source of warmed, humidified air must be provided to avoid thickening and crusting of bronchial secretions.
      c. All respiratory therapy equipment should be changed every 24 hours. In addition:
         (1) Replace any equipment that touches the floor.
         (2) Remove water that condenses in equipment tubing. Do not pour condensed water back into humidifier reservoir.
      d. Provide frequent mouth care. Secretions tend to pool in the mouth and in the pharynx, particularly if the cuff of the tube is inflated. There is an increased risk of ulceration or abrasion of the lips and oropharynx when an endotracheal tube or oral airway is present.
         (1) Gently suction oropharynx as needed.
         (2) Inspect the lips, tongue, and oral cavity regularly.
         (3) Clean the oral cavity with swabs soaked in saline.
         (4) Apply moisturizing agent to cracked lips.
      e. Maintain adequate nutritional levels.
         (1) The person with an endotracheal tube is allowed nothing by mouth. Nourishment will be given parenterally or by gastrointestinal feedings. Gastrointestinal supplemental feedings pose less infection risk and are more economical. See the box below for guidelines for administering gastrointestinal feedings to the intubated patient.
         (2) The patient with a tracheostomy tube is usually able to swallow and have a normal oral intake. Some experts prefer that the cuff on the tracheostomy tube be inflated

---

CARE OF THE INTUBATED PATIENT RECEIVING GASTROINTESTINAL FEEDINGS

1. Assess for the presence of bowel sounds.
2. Elevate the head of the bed at least 30 degrees.
3. Inflate the tube cuff.
4. Administer the gastrointestinal feeding to which methylene blue dye has been added.
5. Assess at regular intervals for aspiration. the presence of methylene blue in secretions indicates aspiration.
6. Regularly assess for tube placement and residual stomach contents.

while the patient is eating to prevent aspiration. Others believe that the inflated cuff bulges into the esophagus and makes swallowing more difficult, and they therefore prefer that the cuff be deflated. Nursing assessment will determine which technique to use. Methylene blue dye can be swallowed before each feeding or mixed with the tube feeding. If the dye does not appear in tracheal secretions, it is safe to proceed with the meal.

2. Ensure adequate ventilation and oxygenation.

    a. Assess lung sounds regularly. Unless the individual's underlying lung pathology alters lung ventilation, breath sounds should be heard bilaterally, and chest expansion should be symmetric. If a cuffed tube is inserted too far, it will slip into one of the main-stem bronchi (usually the right) and occlude the opposite bronchus and lung, resulting in atelectasis on the obstructed side. Even if the tube is still in the trachea, airway obstruction will result if the end of the tube is located on the carina (area at lower end of trachea at point of bifurcation of main-stem bronchi). This will result in dry secretions that obstruct both bronchi. Although these complications are more common with the use of an endotracheal tube, they can occur with a tracheostomy tube, especially in a small person with a short neck. In either case the tube is pulled back until it is positioned below the larynx and above the carina. The tube is then fastened securely in place.

    b. Turn and reposition every 2 hours for maximum ventilation and lung perfusion.

    c. Assess respiratory frequency, tidal volume and vital capacity.

    d. Perform postural drainage, cupping (clapping), and vibrating as appropriate.

3. Provide safety and comfort.

    a. Most endotracheal and tracheostomy tubes have cuffs for the following reasons:

        (1) To provide a sealed airway for positive pressure ventilation

        (2) To prevent aspiration in the unconscious person, during meals or during tube feedings

        (3) To exert pressure on bleeding sites following throat or neck surgery

    b. Assess tube placement at regular intervals.

        (1) The tube is secured around neck with tape or specially designed ties.

        (2) The endotracheal tube is marked to establish a landmark for position comparison and to measure and document the length of tube that extends beyond the patient's lips.

    c. Change tapes or ties whenever soiled to decrease skin irritation.

    d. Always keep a spare tube at the bedside.

    e. Minimize sensory deprivation.

        (1) Patients with endotracheal tubes or tracheostomy tubes with the cuff inflated cannot talk. Therefore an acceptable communication mode must be established.

            (a) Organize questions so that the patient can use a simple "yes" or "no" response, nodding head or using hand signals .

            (b) The patient may be able to use an erasable board (Magic Slate) or note pad to communicate.

            (c) Always talk to the patient and explain all procedures.

            (d) Reorient the patient frequently.

            (e) Encourage family and friends to talk with the patient.

            (f) Keep call light (or tap bell) within patient's reach.

            (g) Reinforce that the ability to speak will return when the tube is removed.

4. Observe special considerations during immediate extubation period.

    a. Monitor for signs such as increased respiratory distress, increased hoarseness, and laryngeal stridor, indicating upper airway obstruction secondary to laryngeal edema.

INFLATING AN ENDOTRACHEAL OR TRACHEOSTOMY CUFF

The cuff should be inflated to a volume that provides adequate occlusion around the tube without increasing the risk of tracheomalacia, tracheal stenosis, trancheoesophageal fistula, or erosion through a major blood vessel. Many experts recommend the "minimal leak technique," which follows.

1. Using a 10 or 20 ml syringe, slowly inject air into cuff.

2. As air is introduced, assess for air leak around tube. This is determined (1) by ability of patient to talk or make sounds, and (2) being able to feel air coming from patient's nose or mouth.

3. When the airway is sealed and no passage of air around the tube can be detected, remove 0.5 ml of air. This creates a "minimal leak" and assures that the lowest possible pressure is being exerted on the tracheal wall.

4. Auscultate over the trachea while ventilating the patient with either an Ambu bag or mechanical ventilator. A small amount of air should be heard gurgling past the cuff.

5. If an adequate seal cannot be obtained with 25 ml of air, notify the physician.

RESEARCH

Harris R and Hyman R: Clean versus sterile tracheostomy care and level of pulmonary infection, Nurs Res 33(2):80-84, 1984.

The purpose of this study was to determine if clean tracheostomy care was more effective than sterile technique as measured by the levels of postoperative pulmonary infection.

The sample consisted of 209 head and neck surgery patients from 10 hospitals. Hospitals were classified as using clean, sterile, or mixed aseptic techniques for tracheostomy care. An investigator-designed Pulmonary Infection Tool was used. Sterile technique and mixed aseptic technique resulted in higher infection rates than did clean technique.

The investigators caution that the hidden variable of the actual sterility of the individual nurse's sterile technique may have influenced the findings. As practiced in the participating hospitals, clean tracheostomy care was not associated with an increased infection rate in the patients studied. ∎

b. Assess for adequacy of cough and gag reflex.
c. After removal of a tracheostomy tube there is a temporary air leak at the incision site.
d. The stoma can be suctioned. However, frequent use of the stoma for suctioning can delay closure and healing of the tracheostomy incision.

Although the low-pressure cuffs used today reduce the risk of tracheal wall damage, it is important to inflate the cuff with the correct amount of air (see the box on p. 959).

The research box above summarizes a study of clean versus sterile tracheostomy suctioning and pulmonary infection.

Care of the person with a tracheostomy. Although nursing care of persons with either endotracheal or tracheostomy tubes is similar, patients with tracheostomies have additional nursing care needs. Analgesics and sedatives are given judiciously so as not to depress the respiratory center. The patient is suctioned as often as necessary, possibly every 5 minutes during the first few postoperative hours. The need for suctioning can be determined by the sound of the air coming from the tracheostomy tube, especially after the patient takes a deep breath. When respirations are noisy and pulse and respiratory rates are increased, the patient needs to be suctioned. Patients who are conscious can usually indicate when they need to be suctioned. With any sign of respiratory distress, the tube should be suctioned. If mucus is blocking the inner cannula of a silver tube and cannot be removed by suction, the inner cannula is removed to open the airway. When the mucus is thick, the inner

ROUTINE TRACHEOSTOMY CARE

Materials: Suction catheter, cleansing solutions (usually hydrogen peroxide and saline), tracheostomy care kit or two sterile basins, sterile applicators, sterile gloves, tracheostomy dressing (must be a nonshredding material), twill tape, disposable bag, and antibiotic ointment.

1. Wash hands and apply nonsterile gloves.
2. Explain procedure.
3. Suction mouth or oropharynx if needed.
4. Prepare sterile work field.
5. Remove soiled tracheostomy dressing and discard in disposable bag.
6. Put on *sterile gloves.* If tracheostomy has inner cannula, remove and clean it in hydrogen peroxide solution. Rinse with saline solution.
7. Inspect inner cannula lumen for patency before reinserting it.
8. Replace tracheostomy ties if soiled. Always hold tracheostomy in place with one hand while ties are being changed. If possible, a second nurse can assist to ensure that tube is not accidentally dislodged.
9. Tie end of twill tapes in a square knot on one side of neck.
10. Using sterile technique, clean tracheostomy incision. Apply antibiotic ointment.
11. Apply sterile tracheostomy dressing.

cannula should be cleaned and replaced at once because the outer tube may also become blocked. If, despite these measures, the patient becomes cyanotic, the physician should be summoned at once. A patient who is able to cough up secretions probably will require suctioning less frequently. The amount of mucus subsides gradually, and the patient eventually may go for several hours without being suctioned. However, even when secretions are minimal, the patient is apprehensive and needs constant attendance. The box above describes routine tracheostomy care.

See the box on p. 961 for the details of suctioning a person with an endotracheal or tracheostomy tube.

Care of the person discharged with a tracheostomy. Persons to be discharged with a tube in place are taught to care for and change the tube while in the hospital (Figure 34-5). A mirror will be necessary to perform his procedure, which may be begun a few days after surgery.

Patients who go home with the tracheostomy tube in place must be provided with necessary supplies or with instructions as to where to secure them and with knowledge of how to care for themselves. They should have suction equipment, which can be rented for home use or obtained in many communities through the local chapter of the American Cancer Society. Suction can be provided by attaching a suction hose to a faucet. Many hardware stores carry the necessary equipment. The amount of suction is controlled by the stream of water.

SUCTIONING A PERSON WITH AN ENDOTRACHEAL OR TRACHEOSTOMY TUBE

1. All persons with tubes require suctioning and should be suctioned as often as necessary. The frequency of suctioning is determined by auscultation. Much of the ability to produce an effective cough is lost, since it is impossible for the person who is intubated to build up the pressure needed to create an expulsive cough.

2. The mouth and oropharynx above the cuff are suctioned first. This catheter is discarded, and a *sterile catheter* is used to suction the trachea.

   It is not necessary to deflate the cuff each time the patient is suctioned. The nurse may wish to deflate the cuff once per shift to remove secretions pooled on top of the cuff and to ensure that it is properly sealed. Deflation should be performed when the nurse is ready to suction the trachea.

3. Suction as deeply as possible. In an adult, a catheter can be introduced through an endotracheal tube approximately 45 to 55 cm (18 to 22 in). The recommended depth through the tracheostomy tube is 20 to 30 cm (8 to 12 in). The catheter should be approximately one-half the diameter of the tube.

4. A fenestrated catheter with a whistle tip is attached to the suction outlet. The catheter is always inserted without suction. Once the catheter is in place, suction is applied by placing the thumb over the fenestration in the catheter.

5. Before beginning suctioning, the patient is hyperoxygenated with 100% oxygen. An Ambu, anesthesia, or Laerdal bag is used to deliver 6 to 10 breaths of 100% oxygen. Preoxygenation with 100% oxygen is necessary because oxygen will be removed during suctioning.

6. The suction catheter is lubricated with sterile water or a water-soluble lubricant. In the person with a tracheostomy, suctioning usually stimulates coughing. If the patient coughs, the catheter is removed because its presence obstructs the trachea and the patient must exert extra pressure to cough around it. As coughing occurs, the nurse or the patient should have tissues ready to receive mucus, which may be ejected with force.

7. If mucus is tenacious and difficult to remove, sterile saline solution may be instilled into the tube just before suctioning. From 5 to 15 ml is commonly used.

8. Although some clinicians recommend that the patient's head and shoulders be turned to the right when suctioning the left bronchus and vice versa, there is no objective evidence that this technique improves suctioning the desired bronchus. In most people the right main-stem bronchus is easier to enter anatomically and thus is suctioned more often than the left bronchus. The catheter is rotated as it is withdrawn with the suction on.

9. To prevent hypoxia, the patient must **not** be suctioned longer than 10 to 15 seconds at a time and should rest 1 to 3 minutes between aspirations, and 100% oxygen should be administered between suctioning. If secretions are interfering with breathing, suctioning may have to be more frequent.

10. The patient is monitored for signs of hypoxia such as tachycardia, bradycardia, or ectopic beats.

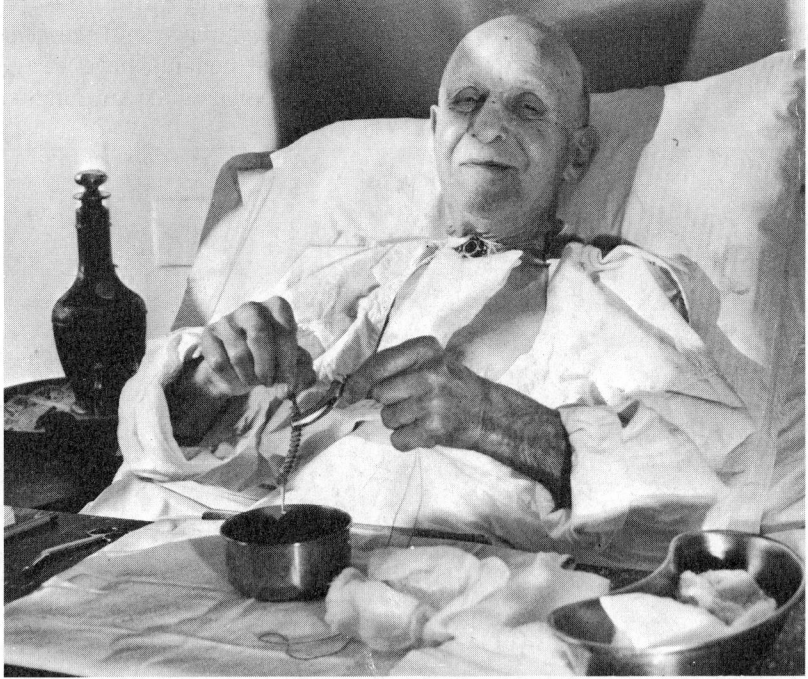

FIGURE 34-5 This 82-year-old man cares for his own tracheostomy tube. He is about to clean inner tube with small tube brush. (From Anderson HC: Newton's geriatric nursing, ed 5, St Louis, 1971, The CV Mosby Co.)

Persons who have a permanent tracheostomy must take some special precautions. They must not go swimming and must be careful while bathing or taking a shower that water is not aspirated through the opening into the lungs. They are advised to wear a scarf or a shirt with a closed collar that covers the opening, yet is of porous material. This material substitutes for some of the functions normally assumed by the nasal passages such as the warming of air and the screening out of dust and other irritating substances.

PROMOTING EFFECTIVE BREATHING PATTERNS
POSITION

Body position plays an important role in promoting optimal breathing patterns in persons with pulmonary dysfunction. Most persons with respiratory disease prefer a semi-upright or upright sitting position. The following modifications of the upright position maximize comfort and decrease ventilatory effort, while accommodating the individual's activity limitations.

1. A pillow placed lengthwise behind the person's back maximizes diaphragmatic movement. The overbed table with a pillow on top can be used as a support and a resting place for the head and arms (Figure 34-6).
2. A leaning forward posture can be achieved at the bedside with the overbed table and a pillow (see Chapter 33, Figure 33-6, A).
3. The patient can use a three-point leaning forward posture while sitting in a chair (see Chapter 33, Figure 33-6, B).
4. During ambulation a standing leaning forward posture can be used to optimize ventilatory effort (see Chapter 33, Figure 33-6, C).

RESPIRATORY ASSISTIVE DEVICES

A variety of devices may be used to help the patient breathe more effectively and to assist in raising secretions.

Because the diaphragm becomes flattened and less active in persons with chronically overinflated lungs secondary to an increase in residual volume, some people find that breathing is helped when an elasticized abdominal support is worn. The support is often made of a material similar to that used in elasticized girdles. Men may need to be persuaded to wear this kind of support, but after trying it they learn how much the support adds to their comfort and then accept it quite readily. Pressure from the girdle must be from below the umbilicus upward so that the flattened diaphragm is forced up into the thorax.

Incentive spirometry promotes alveolar gas exchange by voluntary sustained maximal inspiration. This is accomplished by taking a deep breath, thereby inflating even small, distal alveoli, and holding the breath for at least 3 seconds to allow time for gas exchange. Available in several models, this device consists of one or more small plastic balls in closed chambers, which are connected to tubing and a mouthpiece (see Chapter 22, Figure 22-14). The patient is instructed to inhale slowly and steadily through the tubing, thus creating vacuum in the chamber and raising the ball to the top. The number of times the person can raise the ball and the length of time the inspiration can be held reflects the effectiveness of the individual's effort.

Intermittent positive pressure breathing (IPPB) is a *controversial mode of treatment*. In recent years its therapeutic benefits have been questioned. Research has not demonstrated any long-term benefits from IPPB

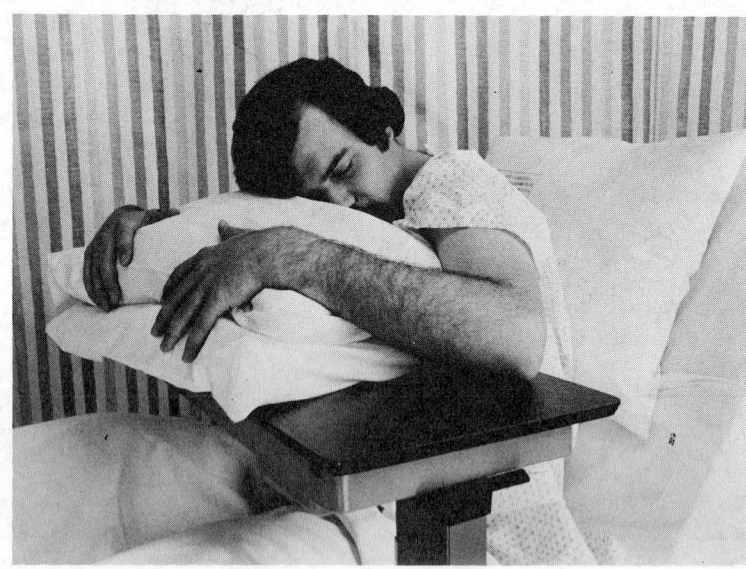

FIGURE 34-6 Pillows placed on overbed table provide comfortable support for patient who must sleep in upright position.

treatments. Additionally, it is an expensive modality that is probably no more effective than more cost-effective interventions such as incentive spirometry, hand-held nebulizers, and coughing and deep breathing. Many people, however, perceive a short-term relief from dyspnea after the use of IPPB.

With IPPB, a ventilator is used to deliver air or oxygen until a preset pressure is reached. The machine is cycled and controlled by the individual's respiratory rate. An IPPB treatment can be used to:

1. Prevent and reverse atelectasis
2. Clear secretions
3. Deliver medications
4. Slow breathing rates
5. Decrease the work of breathing

MECHANICAL VENTILATION

If the patient is unable to maintain ventilation (as indicated by a rising arterial PCO_2), mechanical ventilation is necessary. The ventilator will be attached either to an endotracheal or to a tracheostomy tube (p. 955). Because of the complexity of mechanical ventilation, the ideal place for these patients is in the intensive care unit where experienced nursing staff can care for them. Additionally, ventilators are constantly being improved and new models are introduced periodically. For this reason, an on-going staff development program is mandatory. The general principles for care of patients on ventilators follows. However, it must be stressed that a nurse can only become proficient in working with the patient after repeated experience under the preceptorship of more experienced nurses.

Many different kinds of ventilators are available. In general, there are two types, pressure-cycled and volume-limited. The Bird and Bennett (PR series) are pressure-limited ventilators. They are mainly used for IPPB treatments. Volume-cycled ventilators include (Figure 34-7), the Air Shields, Bennett MA-1 (Figure 34-8), Bennett 7200, Bear Emerson, Engstrom, Ohio 560, and Siemens's Servo. Table 34-3 lists the types of ventilators and their mode of function.

Volume-cycled ventilators are currently the most commonly used ventilators. They provide a wide range of flexibility to meet individual requirements for adequate oxygen and carbon dioxide exchange. The functions in that can be adjusted on the volume cycled ventilator are listed in the box at right.

With a *volume-cycled* machine a *constant volume* of air is delivered with each breath. The volume is preset and is delivered to the patient at whatever pressure is necessary to attain that volume. A volume-cycled machine should have a pressure cutoff valve. Such a mechanism allows a pressure limit to be set. If the pressure required to deliver the set volume exceeds the pressure limit, the machine will turn off before the en-

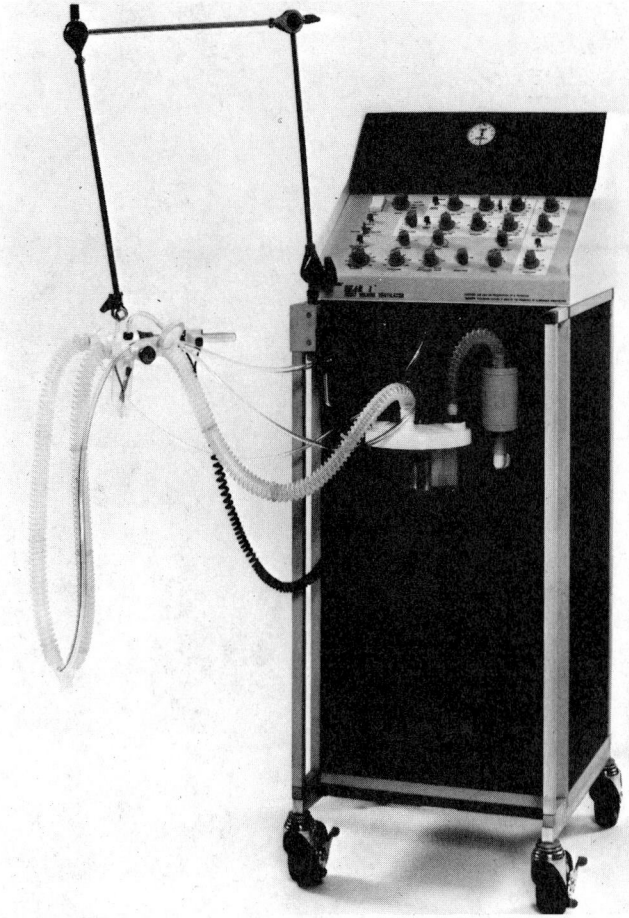

FIGURE 34-7 Bear volume-cycled ventilator. (From Abels LF: Mosby's manual of critical care, St Louis, 1979, The CV Mosby Co.)

FUNCTIONS THAT CAN BE ADJUSTED WITH VOLUME-CYCLED VENTILATORS

Tidal volume—volume of air in a normal breath

Sigh—periodic deep breath; used to prevent microatelectasis and decreased lung compliance; decreased need for sigh function due to ventilating with larger tidal volumes

FiO_2—oxygenation concentration delivered through the ventilator

Alarm systems—vary from machine to machine; basic alarms usually present are:

1. High-pressure alarm—increased resistance somewhere in system from lungs to machine
2. Low-pressure alarm—system not reaching minimal pressure required for ventilation
3. Low-volume alarm—when volume of ventilation does not equal the amount set

Control modes—Degree of ventilation that is controlled by the ventilator; can vary from complete ventilator control to almost total patient control (see Table 34-3)

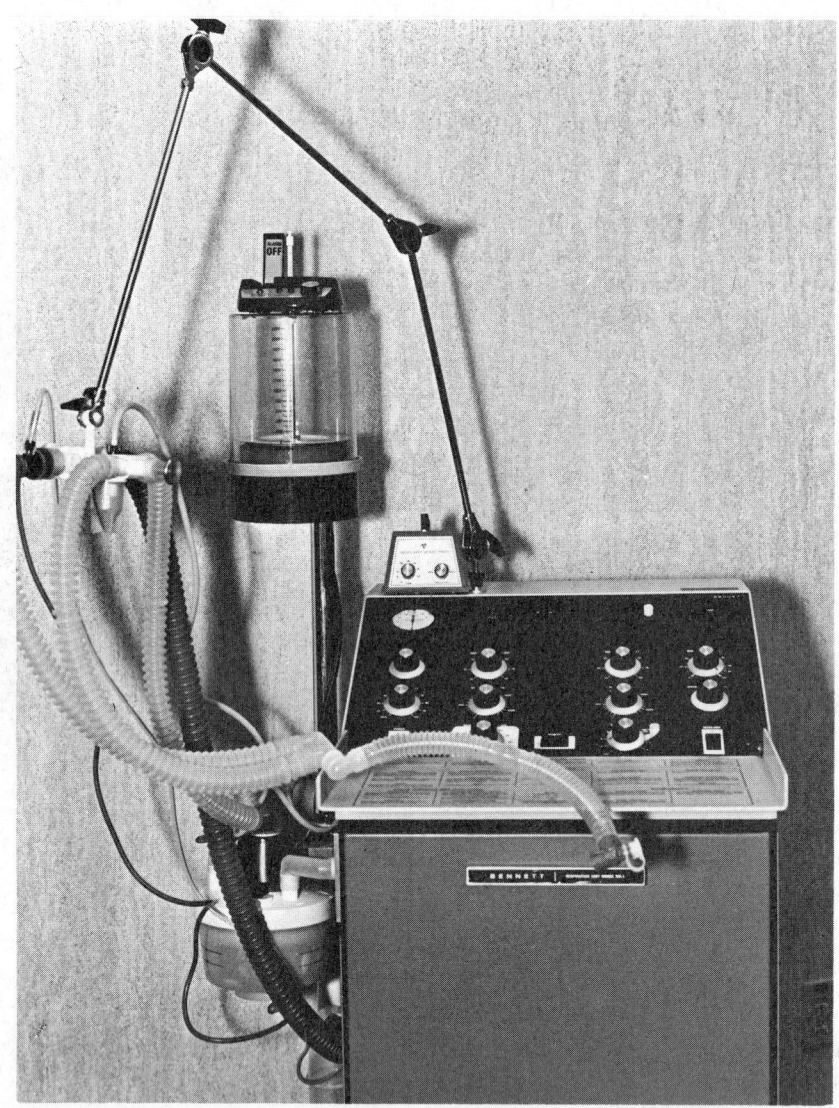

FIGURE 34-8 Bennett MA-1, volume-cycled ventilator. (From Abels LF: Mosby's manual of critical care, St Louis, 1979, The CV Mosby Co.)

TABLE 34-3 Types of mechanical ventilators

Types		Basic Function Mode
Positive pressure ventilator		Types of positive pressure ventilators are based on how inspiratory phase is ended.
Pressure-cycled ventilator		Inspiration ends at a preset pressure limit; time and volume are variable.
Time-cycled ventilator	(require intubation)	Inspiration is preset for a given time interval; volume and pressure are variable.
Volume-cycled ventilator		Preset volume of air is delivered. Time and pressure are variable. However, volume-cycled ventilators often have pressure- and time-cycled capacities.
Negative pressure ventilator (intubation not required)		Thorax, at least, is encapsulated. When ventilator expands, it creates negative pressure by pulling the thorax outward. Air rushes into the airways because of the pressure gradient created.
High-frequency ventilation (requires intubation)		System is still under clinical investigation. There are several variants of this system. All high-frequency ventilators use high respiratory rates to deliver small tidal volumes at low pressures.

tire volume is delivered. The pressure limit on a volume-cycled machine usually has an audible alarm. The nurse can set the limit slightly above (approximately 5 cm of water) the pressure required to ventilate the patient. The alarm will then go off if the patient coughs, accumulates secretion, or starts to resist the machine.

Regardless of which type of ventilator is used, mechanisms for various regulations are necessary if the machine is to be adjusted to each patient. It is preferable to have a respirator that can be used to assist or control the patient's breathing. "Assist" means that the patient's own inspiratory effort triggers (turns on) the machine. Most respirators have a *sensitivity control knob* that can be adjusted to respond to weak inspiratory efforts. "Control" implies the use of automatic cycling. The patient may be apneic and the machine set at the desired rate; the patient's own respiratory rate may be too slow, and the automatic cycling can be used to force an increase in the rate; or the patient's own respiratory efforts can be ignored and an automatic rate used to ventilate the patient. (Some machines with automatic cycling do not allow for the latter adjustment.) It is also helpful to be able to regulate the flow rates at which the gas is delivered to the patient. For example, patients breathing at rapid rates and high volumes need faster flow rates than those breathing slowly and at moderate volumes. A final necessity is the ability to regulate the inspired concentration of oxygen from 20% (room air) to 100%.

All mechanical ventilators must do the following:

1. Provide for the heating and humidification of inspired air
2. Provide a means for measurement of expired volumes
3. Be dependable for long periods of use
4. Be easily cleaned

Any patient on continuous mechanical ventilation should be "sighed" (given a deep breath) several times an hour. Some ventilators automatically "sigh" the patient, while with others the patient is "sighed" manually using a self-inflating (Ambu) or anesthesia bag. This periodic deep breathing is necessary to prevent alveolar collapse and resultant atelectasis.

POSITIVE-END EXPIRATORY PRESSURE

Positive end-expiratory pressure (PEEP) is a ventilator mode that has been shown to increase the effectiveness of mechanical ventilation in certain patients. PEEP involves the maintenance of positive pressure, at the end of expiration, rather than allowing airway pressure to return to normal (atmospheric) as usually occurs. By maintaining positive pressure, alveoli that would otherwise collapse on expiration are held open, thus increasing the opportunity for gas exchange across the alveolar-capillary membrane. This is accomplished by the increase in functional residual capacity. The result is a decrease in physiologic shunting and the ability to achieve a higher level of PaO_2 with lower concentrations of delivered oxygen (FiO_2). PEEP has its greatest use in the treatment of adult respiratory distress syndrome (ARDS), but is also used in treating any patient who would otherwise require unacceptably high concentrations of oxygen.

The hazards of PEEP are related to the increase in intrathoracic pressure. Most serious of the dangers related to this technique is the increased incidence of pneumothorax, particularly in those with friable lung tissue, as seen in persons with emphysema or lung cancer. The sudden disappearance of breath sounds on one side, in conjunction with signs of respiratory distress, in the patient being ventilated with PEEP *must be taken as an indication of a pneumothorax.* This can develop into a life-threatening episode if the pneumothorax is large, and the physician must be called immediately. Another less serious consequence of PEEP may be a reduction in venous return, which is impeded by the increased intrathoracic pressure, and a subsequent fall in cardiac output. This effect seems to be particularly common in patients who are relatively dehydrated and can sometimes be avoided by careful fluid administration.

General Care of the Person on a Ventilator

In planning care for the patient on a mechanical ventilator, it is imperative to know the patient's ability to breathe spontaneously in the event of accidental disconnection from the ventilator. In most facilities, respiratory therapists regularly monitor ventilator function and settings, but the nurse is also responsible for ensuring that the ventilator settings are maintained. Usually a checklist is used to verify the ventilator settings on an hourly basis.

The patient should be assessed on a regular basis and any time a ventilator alarm sounds. The cause of an alarm sounding can be a dysfunction anywhere from the person's lungs to the machine. Trouble-shooting should be carried out in a systematic fashion, starting with the patient and moving toward the machine. Assessment should include the following:

1. Patient assessment
    a. Inspection
        (1) Does the person appear to be in respiratory distress?
        (2) Is the person's chest moving with machine-cycled inspiration?
        (3) Is the chest moving bilaterally?
    b. Auscultation
        (1) Are breath sounds present?
        (2) Are adventitious sounds present?
        (3) Are breath sounds coordinated with ventilator inspiration?

2. Tubing to machine assessment
   a. Inspection
      (1) Is there an air leak around the endotracheal cuff?
      (2) Is there excess condensation in the tubing? (Always remove water from tubing system. Do not empty back into humidifier reservoir). Note: Not all ventilators have humidifiers.
      (3) Check all ventilator settings and readouts.

If the alarm continues to sound and the cause cannot be determined or the patient is in respiratory distress, the patient is disconnected from the machine and manually ventilated with an AMBU bag with oxygenated air until the problem can be resolved.

Weaning from the Ventilator

The decision to wean a person from the ventilator is based on clinical evidence of improved physical status. Weaning is most successful when performed by a nurse who has developed a trust relationship with the patient. Underlying pathology that compromised the patient's respiratory status must be stabilized. Weaning is initiated when the patient meets certain physiologic criteria such as:

1. Acceptable arterial blood gases
2. Tidal volume greater than 10 ml/kg
3. Vital capacity greater than 15 ml/kg

The weaning process should be individualized to meet the patient's needs. The *two major methods* of weaning are as follows:

1. T-piece weaning
   a. Place patient in upright sitting position.
   b. Deflate endotracheal or tracheostomy cuff.
   c. Disconnect patient from ventilator.
   d. Connect a T-piece (Figure 34-9) to endotracheal tube cuff to provide oxygenated humidified air.
2. Intermittent mandatory ventilation (IMV) weaning (particularly useful for the person who is difficult to wean from the ventilator)
   a. Patient remains connected to the ventilator. The number of mandatory breaths delivered by the machine is gradually reduced, allowing the patient to take an increasing number of breaths independently.

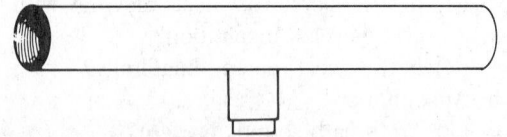

FIGURE 34-9 T-piece used for weaning from ventilator. (From Abels LF: Mosby's manual of critical care, St Louis, 1979, The CV Mosby Co.)

b. Patient is disconnected from the ventilator when predetermined physiologic criteria are maintained.

Nursing interventions during the weaning process include the following:

1. Before initiating weaning, prepare the patient. Teach effective breathing techniques. Inform the patient that weaning may take several attempts.
2. Obtain baseline vital signs, tidal volume, and vital capacity.
3. Stay with the patient during the initial weaning process.
4. Coach the patient as needed to breath slower and deeper.
5. Suction as needed.
6. Monitor for the clinical signs of hypoxemia and hypercapnia (tachycardia, dysrhythmias, increased blood pressure, agitation, diaphoresis, or increased somnolence).
7. If patient cannot breathe on own, reconnect to ventilator.
8. Weaning may require several attempts for longer periods of time before the ventilator can be disconnected.

Care of the Patient Discharged on a Ventilator

It is becoming more common for patients who cannot be weaned from the ventilator to be sent home on the ventilator. Before discharge, careful planning is required to assure that the home can accommodate the patient and the necessary equipment. Home care of patients such as these are discussed in detail in Chapter 78.

MAINTAINING AN ADEQUATE NUMBER OF TERMINAL RESPIRATORY UNITS TO AERATE THE ALVEOLI

The person with pulmonary disease may have impaired ability to aerate alveoli, which can be caused by the following types of pulmonary dysfunction.

1. Restrictive lung disorders—pulmonary diseases that limit full lung and thoracic expansion. Restrictive diseases are discussed in Chapter 33.
2. Obstructive airway disorders—airflow is limited primarily on expiration because of narrowing of the airways. These diseases can result from lung tissue changes or from excess secretions narrowing or blocking the airways (see Chapter 33).

NURSING MANAGEMENT

Nursing actions to facilitate alveolar aeration are divided into the following:

1. Interventions that promote optimal airway function
2. Interventions that manage pulmonary secretions

3. Interventions that promote effective breathing patterns

PROMOTING OPTIMAL AIRWAY FUNCTION

Environment

Proper ventilation, humidity, and room temperature will help the individual with pulmonary dysfunction breathe more easily. The patient should be taught about the following environmental aspects when planning for an optimal environment.

1. Humidity of 30% to 50% is ideal. This can be achieved by a humidifier as necessary.
2. An air conditioner may reduce dyspnea by controlling temperature and eliminating pollutants from outside air from entering. The cost of an air conditioner is a medically deductible expense for persons with chronic obstructive pulmonary disease (COPD) with a prescription from their physician.
3. Inhaled irritants, especially tobacco smoke, should be avoided.
4. A scarf or mask can be worn over the nose and mouth in cold weather to help warm the air and prevent bronchospasm.
5. Announcements on radio and television regarding pollution alerts should be heeded, and the person should avoid being outdoors when an alert is in effect.

Hydration

Individuals with respiratory problems often have a tenuous fluid balance. Congestive heart failure is commonly associated with pulmonary disease, thus increasing the risk of fluid overload. It is important for the individual to maintain a high enough fluid intake to liquify secretions, without fluid overload that could burden the already compromised cardiac function.

Humidification

Persons with a compromised respiratory system may benefit from humidification of their inspired air, particularly in a cold climate where heated air contains very little moisture.

In the home setting, environmental humidity can be increased by a furnace or room humidifier. Additionally, humidity in ambient air can be increased by placing pans of water over warm air furnace vents.

In recent years concern has been raised about cross-infection from room humidifiers. For this reason, the Centers for Disease Control (CDC) has issued the recommendations listed in the box above right.

When supplemental oxygen therapy is used, the gas is diffused through a bubble diffusion humidifier to increase inspired air humidity (Figure 34-10). Although the oxygen is humidified, the patient should be regularly assessed for nasal irritation, because the inspired

---

PRECAUTIONS WHEN USING HUMIDIFIER

1. Use only a **direct heated** humidifier or nebulizer with a **bacterial filter.** Cold vapor or cool mist humidifiers are not recommended because they cannot withstand daily sterilization.
2. Use only **sterile water** in the humidifier and drain remaining water each time the humidifier is refilled or at least every 24 hours. Tap water is not safe to use because it is frequently contaminated with *Pseudomonas, Flavobacterium, Acinetobacter,* or other organisms.
3. Establish a routine maintenance schedule.
4. Set medical guidelines to determine which patients should receive humidification and which should not. It may not be advisable to use humidifiers for immunosuppressed patients.
5. **Do not send** humidifying unit home with patients because of the concern about transporting highly resistant hospital organisms into the community.

---

gas is much dryer than ambient air. There are several types of humidifiers that can be used with high-flow oxygen therapy or a mechanical ventilator. Many of them have an adjustable heating element that allows the temperature of the water to be heated to provide up to 100% relative humidity (warmer air can hold more moisture than cooler air).

The person with increased sputum production often requires aerosol therapy, which provides deep deposition of moisture and medications into the airways. In order for liquids to penetrate deeper into the airways, the liquid must be suspended in a gas as very small particles. Aerosol therapy is delivered by a nebulizer that breaks aerosolized liquids into smaller particles and can deliver a specific percentage of oxygen. An ultrasonic nebulizer is an electrically driven unit that delivers smaller particles at higher humidity levels.

Nebulizer Therapy

Nursing management is as follows:

1. Never leave a person receiving ultrasonic nebulizer therapy unattended. Rehydrated and loosened secretions can obstruct an airway.
2. Bronchodilators and mucolytic agents delivered by a nebulizer must be *diluted* according to manufacturer's directions (see Chapter 33).
3. Dilute saline solutions are preferred as aerosols.
4. Encourage the patient to take slowed, deeper inhalations.
5. Instruct the patient in the correct use of hand-held metered-dose inhalers (see Chapter 33).

Pulmonary Physiotherapy

The person who has difficulty in breathing may be taught how to increase the efficiency of his or her

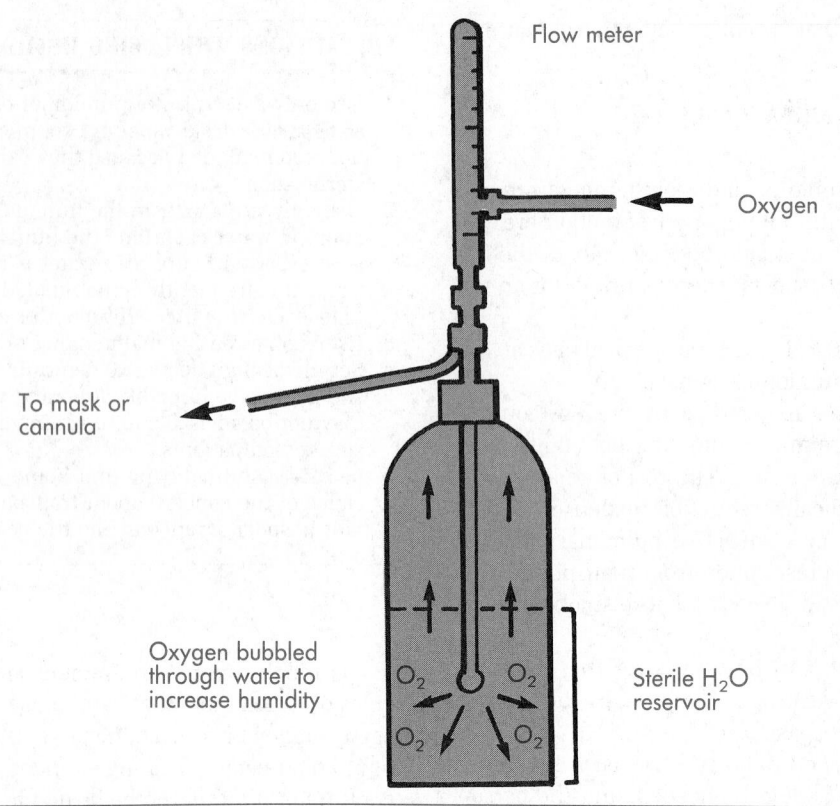

FIGURE 34-10 Bubble diffusion humidifier provides humidity to oxygen being administered by nasal cannula or mask.

breathing pattern. Breathing exercises are usually a part of pulmonary physiotherapy, which commonly includes *segmental postural drainage, clapping,* and *vibrating.* Although pulmonary physiotherapy activities may be performed by a physical therapist, they are often part of a nurse's responsibility. Regardless of where the primary responsibility lies, nurses must be familiar with the techniques so that they can demonstrate and reinforce them and be sure that the individual is doing them correctly. Also, the need for pulmonary physiotherapy may occur at a time when the physical therapy department is closed.

Segmental Postural Drainage

Segmental postural drainage with clapping and vibration is a technique used to combine the force of gravity with the natural ciliary activity of the small bronchial airways to move secretions upward toward the main bronchi and the trachea. From this point the patient can cough them up, or they can be suctioned. In the treatment of chronic obstructive pulmonary disease, drainage of all segments is usually accomplished by placing patients in various postural drainage positions (Figure 34-11). Treatment may also be directed at draining specific areas of the lung. While the patient is in each position, *clapping* with a cupped hand is done over the area

being drained. This maneuver helps to loosen secretions and stimulate coughing (Figure 34-12, *A*). After the area has been clapped for approximately 1 minute, the patient is instructed to breathe deeply. *Vibrating* (pressure applied with a vibrating movement of the hand on the chest) is performed during expiratory phase of the deep breath (Fig. 34-12, *B*). This helps the patient to exhale more fully. The procedure is repeated as necessary. When the patient cannot tolerate a head-down position, a modified position is used (Fig. 34-12, *C*).

Positions that provide gravity drainage of the lungs can be achieved in several ways, and the procedure selected usually depends on the age and general condition of the person as well as the lobe or lobes of the lungs where secretions have accumulated. A young person usually can tolerate greater lowering of the head than an elderly person whose vascular system adapts less quickly to change of position. A severely debilitated patient may only be able to tolerate slight changes in the position.

Postural drainage can be achieved in several ways. Electric hospital beds can be tilted into a head-down position with little difficulty. If an electric bed is not available (for example, in the home), blocks can be placed under the casters at the foot of the bed. If these are not available, the foot of the bed can be supported on the

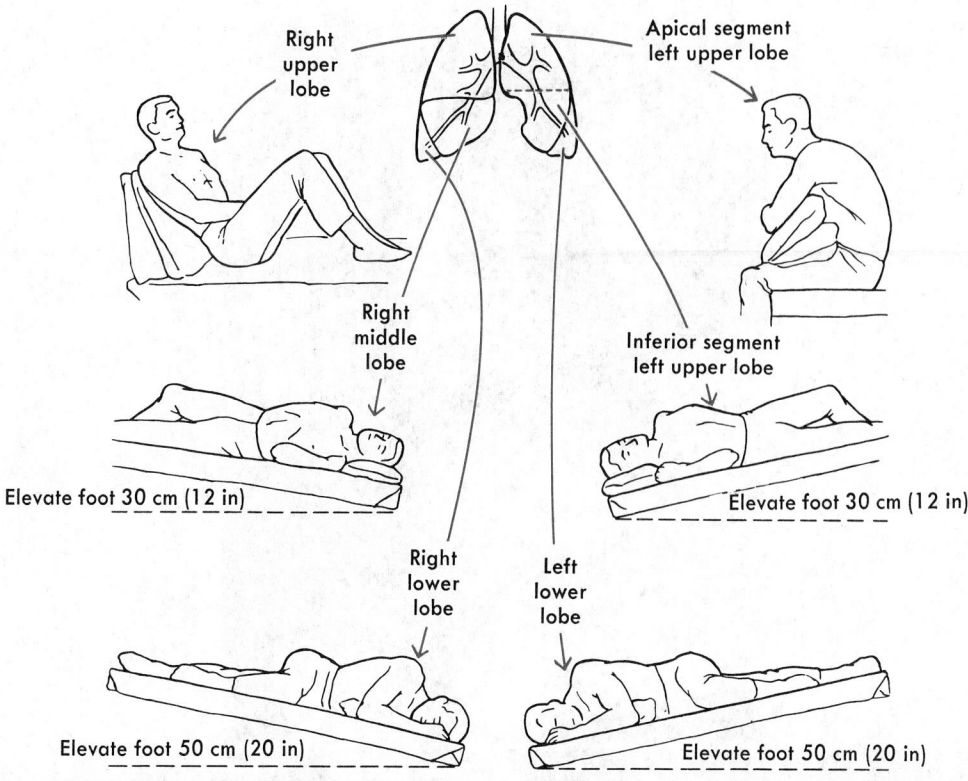

FIGURE 34-11 Postural drainage requires that patient assume various positions to facilitate flow of secretions from various portions of lung into bronchi, trachea, and throat so that they can be raised and expectorated more easily. Drawing shows correct positions to drain various portions of lung.

seat of a firm chair to provide a position in which the head is lowered.

The nurse needs to know the part of the lung affected and how to position the patient to drain that portion of the lung (Figure 34-11). For example, if the right middle lobe of the lung is affected, drainage will be accomplished best by way of the right middle bronchus. The patient should lie supine with the body turned at approximately a 45-degree angle. The angle can be maintained by pillow supports placed under the right side from the shoulders to the hips. The foot of the bed is raised about 30 cm (12 in). This position can be maintained fairly comfortably by most patients for half an hour at a time. On the other hand, if the lower posterior area of the lung is affected, the foot of the bed can be raised 45 to 50 cm (18 to 20 in) with the patient assuming a prone position for drainage. A summary of the positions for segmental postural drainage is given in Table 34-4.

Postural drainage and percussion should be planned so as to achieve maximal benefit. The best time is generally in the morning soon after arising and at night before retiring. Frequency of treatments will depend on each person's needs, but care should be taken to avoid exhaustion, which will result in shallow ventilation and negates the positive effects of the treatment.

Patients having postural drainage of any kind are encouraged to breathe deeply and to cough forcefully to help dislodge thick sputum and exudate that is pooled in distended bronchioles, particularly after inactivity. Humidity, bronchodilators, or liquefying agents often are given 15 to 20 minutes before postural drainage is started, since they facilitate the removal of secretions. The patient may find that sputum can best be raised on resuming an upright position even though no drainage appeared while lying down with the head and chest lowered.

Because some patients complain of dizziness when assuming positions for postural drainage, the nurse stays with the patient during the first few times and reports any persistent dizziness or unusual discomfort to the physician.

Postural drainage may be contraindicated in some persons because of heart disease, hypertension, increased intracranial pressure, extreme dyspnea, or advanced age. However, most people can be taught to assume the positions for postural drainage and can proceed without help after being supervised once or twice.

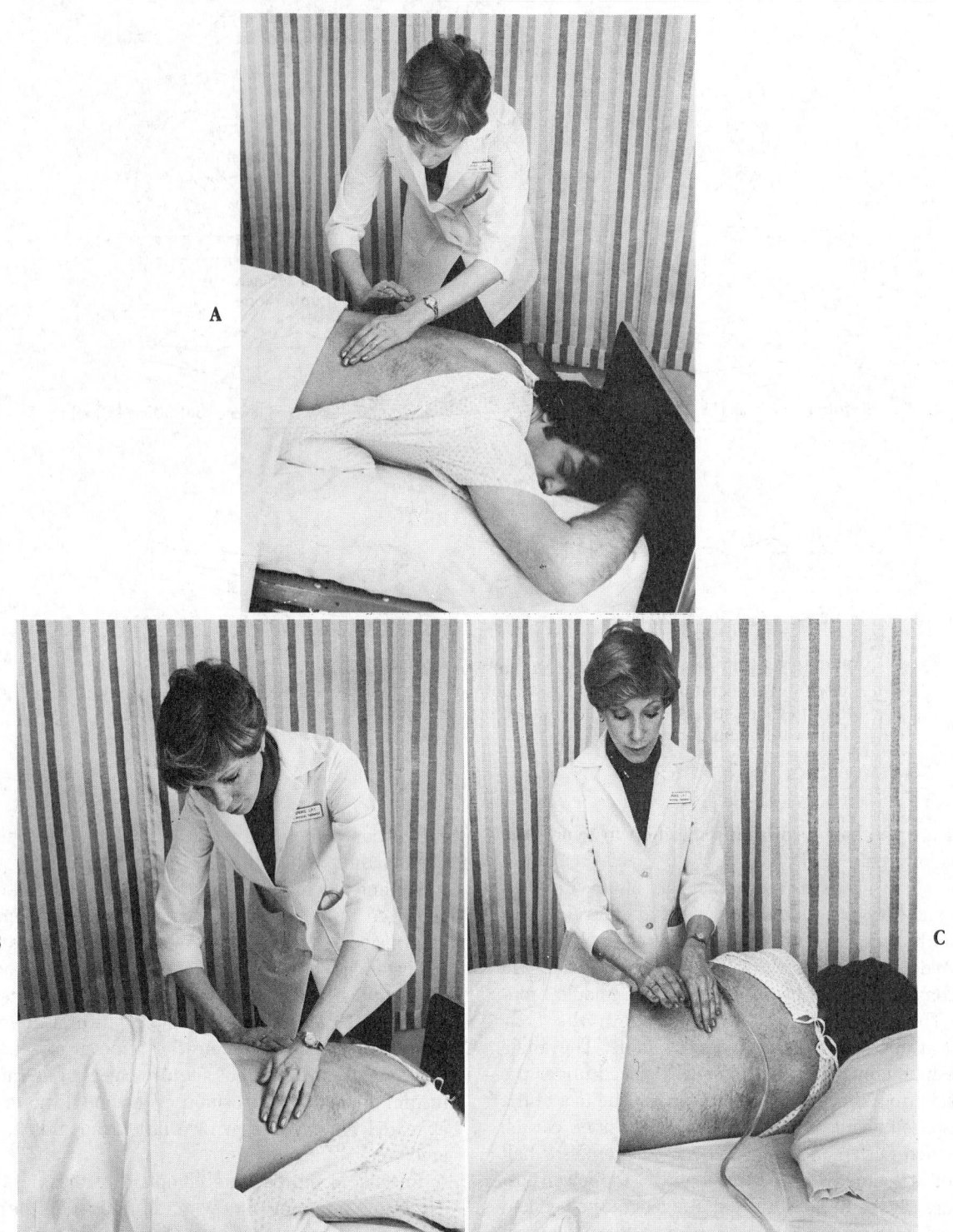

FIGURE 34-12 A, Patient is in supine position with head down at 15-degree angle for postural drainage of lower lobes. Note cupped position of physical therapist's hands as she claps patient. Patient's gown is pulled aside for purposes of illustration; ordinarily clapping is never performed on bare skin. **B,** Physical therapist follows clapping with vibrating, applying pressure during expiration. **C,** Even when patient cannot tolerate head-down position, such as after thoracic surgery, patient can still receive chest physiotherapy in modified positions.

TABLE 34-4 Positions for segmental postural drainage, clapping, and vibrating

Area of Lung	Position of Patient	Area To Be Clapped and/or Vibrated
Upper lobe		
Apical bronchus	Semi-Fowler's position, leaning to right, then left, then forward	Over area of shoulder blades with fingers extending over clavicles
Posterior bronchus	Upright at 45-degree angle, rolled forward against a pillow at 45 degrees on left and then right side	Over shoulder blade on each side
Anterior bronchus	Supine with pillow under knees	Over anterior chest just below clavicles
Middle lobe (lateral and medial bronchus)	Trendelenburg position at 30-degree angle or with foot of bed elevated 35-40 cm (14-16 in), turned slightly to left	Anterior and lateral right chest from axillary fold to midanterior chest
Lingula (superior and inferior bronchus)	Trendelenburg position at 30-degree angle or with foot of bed elevated 35-40 cm (14-16 in), turned slightly to right	Left axillary fold to midanterior chest
Lower lobes		
Apical bronchus	Prone with pillow under hips	Lower third of posterior rib cage on both sides
Medial bronchus	Trendelenburg position at 45-degree angle or with foot of bed raised 45-50 cm (18-20 in) on right side	Lower third on left posterior rib cage
Lateral bronchus	Trendelenburg position at 45-degree angle or with foot of bed raised 45-50 cm (18-20 in) on left side	Lower third of right posterior rib cage
Posterior bronchus	Prone Trendelenburg position at 45-degree angle with pillow under hips	Lower third of posterior rib cage on both sides

Chest percussion (clapping) is contraindicated in the case of pulmonary emboli, hemorrhage, exacerbation of bronchospasms, severe pain, and over areas of resectable carcinoma. Often patients with a chronic pulmonary problem need to be taught to do postural drainage independently so that they can continue at home. The position usually is maintained for 10 minutes at first, and the period of time is gradually lengthened to 15, 20, or even 30 minutes as the patient becomes accustomed to the position. At first, elderly persons usually are able to tolerate these positions only for a few minutes. They need more assistance than most other patients during the procedure and immediately thereafter. They should be helped to a normal position in bed and requested to lie flat for a few minutes before sitting up or getting out of bed. This helps to prevent dizziness and reduces the danger of accidents.

The patient may feel nauseated because of the odor and taste of sputum. Therefore, the procedure should be timed so that it comes at least 1 hour before meals. A short rest period after the treatment often improves postural drainage. Aromatic mouth washes should be available for frequent use by any patient who is expectorating sputum freely.

Breathing Exercises

Breathing exercises can both improve airway function and increase overall breathing effectiveness. These exercises are presented in detail in Chapter 33. The various breathing maneuvers include:

1. Improved breathing techniques, which include pursed lip breathing, slowed breathing, exhaling with activity, and abdominal breathing
2. Effective coughing techniques
3. Inspiratory muscle training
4. Muscle reconditioning

MANAGING PULMONARY SECRETIONS

The mucous glands lining the respiratory tract respond to inflammation by increased mucus secretion. Sputum that may contain mucus, cellular and foreign debris, microorganisms, blood and pus, is ejected from the lungs by coughing or clearing the throat. Sputum accumulates in the respiratory passages when the individual has excess sputum that cannot be effectively removed by coughing. The accumulated sputum provides an excellent medium for the growth of pathogens and can obstruct airways resulting in atelectasis, hypoxemia, and hypercapnia. Many of the interventions that assist patients to manage pulmonary secretions have been discussed under aerating the alveoli (p. 966).

In addition to adequate hydration, humidification, and postural drainage, additional measures to manage pulmonary secretions are, (1) administering medications as ordered, and (2) suctioning the airway.

Administering Medications

Medications may be ordered to increase secretions, decrease secretions, thin secretions, or to suppress a non-

TABLE 34-5 Medications used to treat cough

Desired Effect	Medications Prescribed
↑ Secretions	Expectorants
	Ammonium chloride
	Ammonium carbonate
	Sodium iodide
	Potassium iodide (saturated solution; SSKI)
	Ipecac
	Terpin hydrate
↓ Secretions	Anticholinergic agents
	Atropine
Thin secretions	Mucolytic agents
	Acetylcysteine (Mucomyst)
	Desoxyribonuclease (Dornavac)
Depress cough reflex	Antitussives
	Narcotic
	Codeine
	Nonnarcotic agents
	Benzonatate (Tessalon)
	Noscapine (Nectadon)
	Dextromethorphan hydrobromide (Romilar)
	Carbetapentane citrate (Toclase)
	Levopropoxyphene napsylate (Novrad)
	Chlophedianol hydrochloride (Ulo)

productive cough. Table 34-5 presents examples of common medications that may be prescribed for these purposes.

When pulmonary secretions cannot be managed effectively with the noninvasive interventions described above, oropharyngeal or tracheobronchial suctioning is performed to remove secretions and to stimulate a productive cough. The procedure is the same whether the suction catheter is introduced through the mouth or nose.

Tracheobronchial Suctioning

Tracheobronchial suctioning is carried out as follows:

1. The patient is prepared for suctioning by a thorough explanation of what is to be done. If coughing is painful, as after throacic surgery, for example, pain medication is administered 30 minutes before the procedure. Suctioning is *not* performed immediately before or after meals.
2. Proper positioning of the patient will assist with suctioning. The patient should be in a sitting position, with the head of the bed elevated. A pillow under the shoulders will help hyperextend the neck, which facilitates entry of the catheter into the trachea. It may also be helpful to elevate each shoulder in turn while having the patient turn the head to the opposite side in an attempt to direct

the catheter first into the right and then into left main-stem bronchi.

3. Nasotracheal suctioning is a *sterile procedure;* each piece of equipment, catheter, glove, water, lubricant, and basin are used only once. A suction source that is capable of creating a vacuum of −80 cm of water is necessary. For adults, a size 14 French catheter, 35 cm (14 in) in length, is usually used. A water-soluble lubricant should be applied to the outside of the catheter. The sequence of steps of the procedure is as follows:
   a. Preoxygenate the patient with a few breaths of a high concentration of oxygen (80% to 100%) from an anesthesia or Ambu bag. This helps prevent hypoxia during suctioning.
   b. Insert the lubricated catheter, without applying suction, through the nares. When the catheter reaches the posterior pharynx (a distance of about 10 to 12.5 cm [4 to 5 in]), the patient is asked to cough in order to facilitate entry into the trachea. If the tongue is obstructing passage of the catheter, have the patient stick the tongue out while coughing or have another person grasp the tongue with a piece of gauze and pull the tongue forward.
   c. Continue to insert the catheter until meeting resistance. At this point suction is applied intermittently while removing the catheter, rotating the catheter 360 degrees at the same time.
   d. Limit suctioning to 10 seconds.
   e. Administer a few breaths of 80% to 100% oxygen.
4. When secretions become tenacious, mucus plugs can form, causing airway obstruction. If tracheobronchial suctioning is unsuccessful in maintaining a clear airway, a fiberoptic bronchoscopy may be performed to remove impacted secretions. Care during a bronchoscopy is discussed in Chapter 33.

MAINTAINING TRANSPORTATION OF OXYGEN

The transportation of oxygen from the atmosphere to body tissues requires several interactive physiologic processes:

1. Ventilation
   a. Atmospheric oxygen must reach the alveolar-capillary membrane.
2. Diffusion
   a. Oxygen and carbon dioxide must move across the alveolar-capillary membrane.
3. Perfusion
   a. There must be sufficient pulmonary blood flow for diffusion to occur and to carry oxygen from the alveolar-capillary membrane to the body tissues.
4. There must be sufficient functional hemoglobin to carry oxygen (SaO_2) and dissolved oxygen (PaO_2).

a. The relationship between oxyhemoglobin and dissolved oxygen is represented by the oxyhemoglobin dissociation curve (see Chapter 31).

b. Normal total oxygen content in arterial blood is approximately 16 to 20 ml/100 ml of blood.

5. Cardiac output

a. There must be sufficient cardiac output to respond to changing tissue needs.

b. Normal resting cardiac output is approximately 5 L/minute.

The total amount of oxygen being transported to the tissues can be calculated by multiplying the cardiac output by total oxygen transported.

$$\frac{500 \text{ ml}}{\text{minute}} \times \frac{20 \text{ ml oxygen}}{100 \text{ ml blood}} = \frac{1000 \text{ ml}}{\text{minute}}$$

Respiratory dysfunction often results in or from alteration in one of the processes necessary for adequate tissue oxygenation. The resultant clinical manifestations may range from mild hypoxemia to severe life-threatening hypoxemia.

Medical management focuses on treating the underlying pathology and improving tissue oxygenation. The most common intervention to improve oxygenation is oxygen therapy.

OXYGEN THERAPY

In most acute care facilities the Respiratory Therapy Department is responsible for initiating and maintaining oxygen therapy. The nurse is responsible for monitoring the patient's response to the therapy, and in certain situations, must be capable of initiating oxygen therapy.

Thus it is important for the nurse to be familiar with the various types of oxygen delivery systems.

Oxygen delivery systems are divided into low-flow and high-flow systems. Low-flow or nasal cannula oxygen therapy devices (that is, the simple face mask or the partial rebreather mask) provide only part of the person's inspired air. During inspiration, room air mixes with the delivered oxygen to provide the total amount of inspired air. High-flow oxygen therapy devices (that is, nonrebreathing masks such as Venturi masks) provide the total amount of inspired air. Thus the oxygen concentration can be accurately controlled.

LOW-FLOW SYSTEMS

Nasal cannulas (Figure 34-13) are the most common devices for delivering oxygen. The cannula is less constricting than a face mask and can be used well for low oxygen concentrations in both the hospital and the home. The major disadvantages of a cannula are as follows: (1) oxygen concentration depends on the individual's respiratory pattern, and (2) the cannula may dry out the nasal membranes and cause nasal congestion. Nasal cannulas can deliver between 1 to 6 L of oxygen per minute (24% to 45% O_2).

A newer method of oxygen delivery is the *transtracheal* catheter, which is inserted directly into the trachea between the second and third tracheal cartilages. *Transtracheal* oxygen delivery was pioneered by Heimlich. It is used for persons with chronic pulmonary disease who require oxygen at home. One of its major advantages is that it does not interfere with talking, eat-

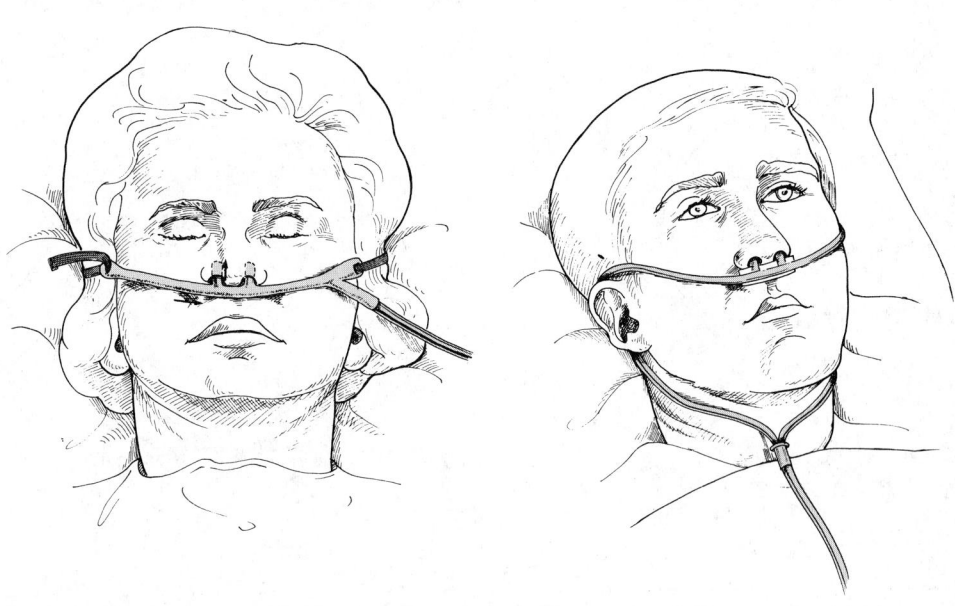

FIGURE 34-13 Two types of nasal cannulas. (From Abels LF: Mosby's manual of critical care, St Louis, 1979, The CV Mosby Co.)

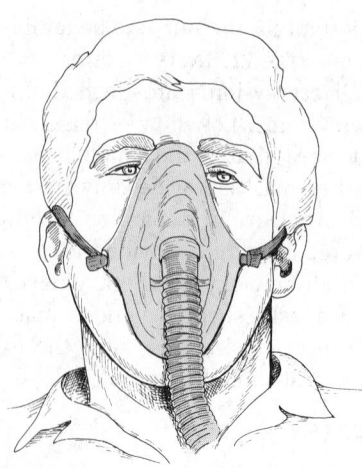

FIGURE 34-14 Simple face mask. (From Abels LF: Mosby's manual of critical care, St Louis, 1979, The CV Mosby Co.)

ing, or drinking. Also it delivers oxygen throughout the respiratory cycle, in contrast to a nasal cannula, which delivers oxygen on inspiration only. Thus, most patients can cut their resting flow rates in half. Those who require 2 L/min with a cannula will only need 1 L/min with a transtracheal catheter. For more information see reference 53.

The *simple face mask* delivers oxygen through an entry port (Figure 34-14). Room air, which mixes with the oxygen, enters through small holes at the side of the mask; and expired air leaves through the holes. The concentration of inspired oxygen will vary with the individual's respiratory pattern. At a flow rate of 4 to 6 L/min a face mask will deliver approximately 35% to 45%

oxygen. The face mask is less convenient and comfortable than the nasal cannula.

A *partial rebreather mask* consists of a face mask and a reservoir bag (Figure 34-15). The first one third of expired air mixes with the oxygen that is delivered into the reservoir bag. The individual thus inspires a mix of supplemental oxygen plus oxygen that was in the expired air. The expired air that is mixed with the oxygen is dead space air that does not contain carbon dioxide. The partial rebreather mask can deliver between 60% to 90% oxygen concentration.

HIGH-FLOW SYSTEMS

A *nonrebreathing mask* consists of a mask and a reservoir separated by a one-way valve that prevents expired air from mixing with the supplemental oxygen (Figure 34-16). Exhaled air is directed out of the mask through exhalation ports. If the mask conforms tightly to the face, a 100% oxygen concentration can be delivered. The mask becomes uncomfortable after a few hours and is only tolerable for short-term use.

Venturi (Venti) masks pass oxygen through a restricted port that increases velocity of gas flow and allows air to be pulled into the mask (Figure 34-17). The high flow of the inspired gas makes the concentration of inspired oxygen less dependent on the individual's respiratory pattern. Venti masks can deliver accurate low concentrations of oxygen between 24% and 50%. Thus this system is particularly useful for people with COPD who may lose their hypoxic respiratory drive at higher oxygen concentrations.

The patient's physiologic response to oxygen therapy can be accurately assessed only by evaluating arterial blood oxygen levels. Arterial blood oxygen can be as-

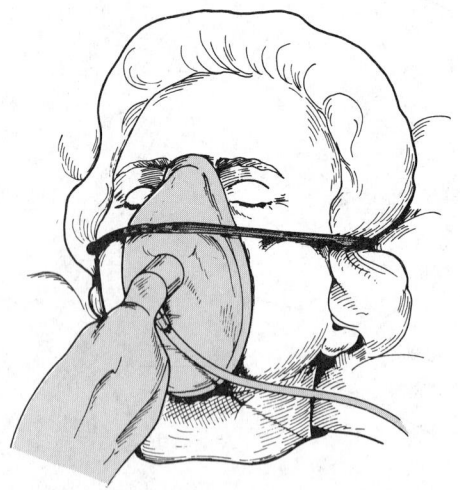

FIGURE 34-15 Plastic face mask with reservoir bag. (From Wade JF: Comprehensive respiratory care, ed 3, St Louis, 1982, The CV Mosby Co.)

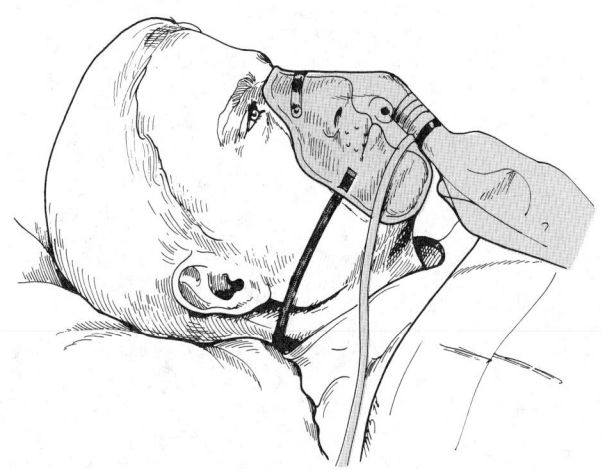

FIGURE 34-16 Nonrebreathing face mask. (From Abels LF: Mosby's manual of critical care, St Louis, 1979, The CV Mosby Co.)

sessed by obtaining an arterial blood sample or by less invasive techniques such as ear or finger oximetry.

It is important to determine early during the patient's hospitalization if home oxygen therapy will be required. Discharge education about home oxygen therapy should begin early during hospitalization and be coordinated with the selected home oxygen therapy provider (see Chapter 78).

MAINTAINING A FUNCTIONING RESPIRATORY CENTER

Hypoventilation or apnea can occur if there is depression of the respiratory center by general anesthesia, morphine, cocaine, heroin, barbiturates, or alcohol. Diseases of the central nervous system, such as bulbar poliomyelitis or meningitis, also will depress the respiratory center, as will an increase in intracranial pressure. In these situations the patient's respirations will have to be supported until the patient is able to maintain his or her own breathing. Intubation with an endotracheal tube, supplemental oxygen, and artificial respiration with a ventilator may all be required. The conditions causing depression of the respiratory center will need to be identified and treated while the person's ventilation is being maintained. Details of management of patients in respiratory failure are discussed in Chapter 33.

MAINTAINING BELLOWS FUNCTION OF THE CHEST WALL AND DIAPHRAGM

Whenever there is interference with the bellows function of the chest wall, there will be changes in the breathing pattern. The major cause of disruption of the bellows function is trauma to the chest. Chest surgery will also interfere with the bellows function of the chest. Chest trauma and its complications are discussed first.

CHEST TRAUMA

Epidemiology/Etiology

Trauma to the chest is a major problem most often seen first in the emergency department. Injury to the chest may affect the bony chest cage, pleurae and lungs, diaphragm, or mediastinal contents.

TABLE 34-6 Types of penetrating and nonpenetrating (blunt) chest injuries

Penetrating	Blunt (Nonpenetrating)
Open pneumothorax (sucking chest wound)	Closed pneumothorax
	Tension pneumothorax
Hemothorax	Tracheobronchial injury
Tracheobronchial injury	Flail chest
Pulmonary contusion	Diaphragm rupture
Diaphragm rupture	Mediastinal injury
Mediastinal injury	Fractured ribs

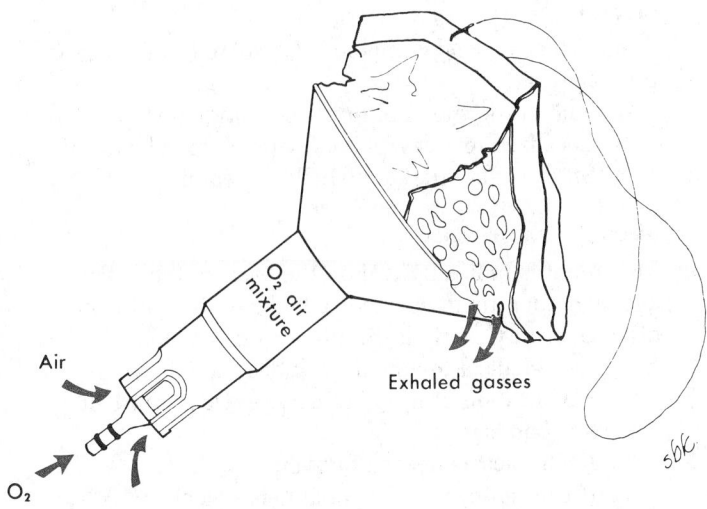

FIGURE 34-17 Ventimask allows air to be mixed with oxygen to provide diluted oxygen to patient. (From Wade JF: Comprehensive respiratory care, ed 3, St Louis, 1982, The CV Mosby Co.)

Injuries to the chest are broadly classified into two groups—blunt and penetrating (Table 34-6). *Blunt* or nonpenetrating injuries damage the structures within the chest cavity without disrupting chest wall integrity. *Penetrating* injuries disrupt chest wall integrity and result in alteration in intrathoracic pressures.

The leading cause of blunt chest injuries in the United States is motor vehicle steering wheel impaction in the person not wearing a seat belt. Blows to the chest with blunt objects or as a result of a fall also cause nonpenetrating chest injury. Penetrating wounds usually result from gunshot or stabbing injuries.

Prevention

Nurses can promote prevention of chest trauma through public education programs focused on safe practices in vehicle use and in the work place. The major preventable focus is promoting the use of seat belts when operating a motor vehicle.

RIB FRACTURES

Pathophysiology

Rib fractures are the most common blunt injury. Ribs 3 through 10 are most often fractured, because they are less protected by the chest muscles.[29] The ribs usually fracture at the point of maximum impact, but they may fracture at a distant site from impact. Rib fractures are caused by blows, crushing injuries, or *strain* caused by *severe coughing* or *sneezing spells*. If the rib is splintered or the fracture displaced, sharp fragments may penetrate the pleura and lung, resulting in a hemothorax or pneumothorax which are penetrating injuries.

Clinical Manifestations

Common signs and symptoms of rib fracture include the following:

1. Pain at the site of injury, increasing on inspiration
2. Localized tenderness and crepitus on palpation
3. Splinting of chest and shallow breathing

Medical Management

Treatment is individualized on the basis of the patient's age, whether there is preexisting chronic pulmonary disease history, and the number and location of ribs fractured. Medical treatment includes the following:

1. Stabilization of the fracture site with a rib belt or Ace bandage
2. Analgesics as needed for pain
3. If pain is severe, a regional nerve block

■ Assessment

Subjective data. Subjective data include the nature of the injury and when it occurred. If patient is unable to answer questions, data are obtained from those with the patient.

Objective data

1. Pain at site of injury that increases on inspiration
2. Area tender to the touch
3. Patient splints chest and takes shallow breaths

Diagnostic tests. Fractures are confirmed by chest x-ray findings.

■ Data Analysis: Nursing Diagnoses

Nursing diagnoses are determined from assessment of patient data. Possible nursing diagnoses for the person with rib fracture may include, but are not limited to, the following:

Diagnostic Title	Possible Etiologies
Ineffective airway clearance	Pain/trauma to rib cage
Anxiety	Threat to change in health status
Ineffective breathing pattern	Pain, musculoskeletal impairment
Pain	Trauma to rib cage
Knowledge deficit: condition and its treatment	Lack of exposure to information

■ Planning: Expected Patient Outcomes

Expected patient outcomes for the person with fractured ribs may include, but are not limited to, the following:

1. Pain is improved.
2. Patient is breathing effectively.
3. Patient maintains a patent airway.
4. Patient is less anxious.
5. Patient understands follow-up therapy.
6. Patient understands that physician is to be noti-

fied if shortness of breath, hemoptysis, or temperature elevation occur.

■ Implementation

Initial care for fractured ribs. If ribs are fractured and the rib has not penetrated the pleura, the chest is strapped with adhesive tape or an Ace bandage or chest binder is applied.

1. Check strapping to be sure it is secure.
2. Give analgesics as needed for pain and to slow respiratory rate in the patient who is anxious and may be hyperventilating.

Maintaining the airway. Persons with rib fractures may develop atelectasis secondary to their shallow breathing and their reluctance to expand their lungs fully. They should be assisted to periodically expand their lungs fully:

1. Administer analgesics to reduce pain
2. Coordinate lung-expanding maneuvers such as deep-breathing, coughing, sighing, or yawning to coincide with the analgesics' peak effect time.
3. Splint the fracture site to assist lung-expanding exercises
4. Reposition patient every 2 hours

Assisting with comfort and ADL

1. Place patient in position of comfort. May be able to breathe easier in Fowler's or semi-Fowler's position.
2. Give prescribed analgesics.
3. If pain persists despite analgesics, notify the physician, who may infiltrate the intercostal spaces above and below the fractured rib(s) with 1% procaine.

FLAIL CHEST

Pathophysiology

When multiple ribs or the sternum are fractured in more than one place, a portion of the chest wall becomes separated from the chest cage, resulting in a *flail chest*. Thus the chest wall no longer provides the rigid bony support that is necessary to maintain the bellows function required for normal ventilation. This causes *paradoxical respiratory* movement. Upon inspiration the dislocated segment is pulled inward by the subatmospheric intrapleural pressure. During expiration the dislocated segment bulges outward as intrapleural pressure becomes less negative (Figure 34-18, *A to D*).

Flail chest usually causes localized atelectasis secondary to decreased ventilation, resulting in hypoxemia. Because of the increased work of breathing, the individual may also develop hypercapnia and respiratory acidosis.

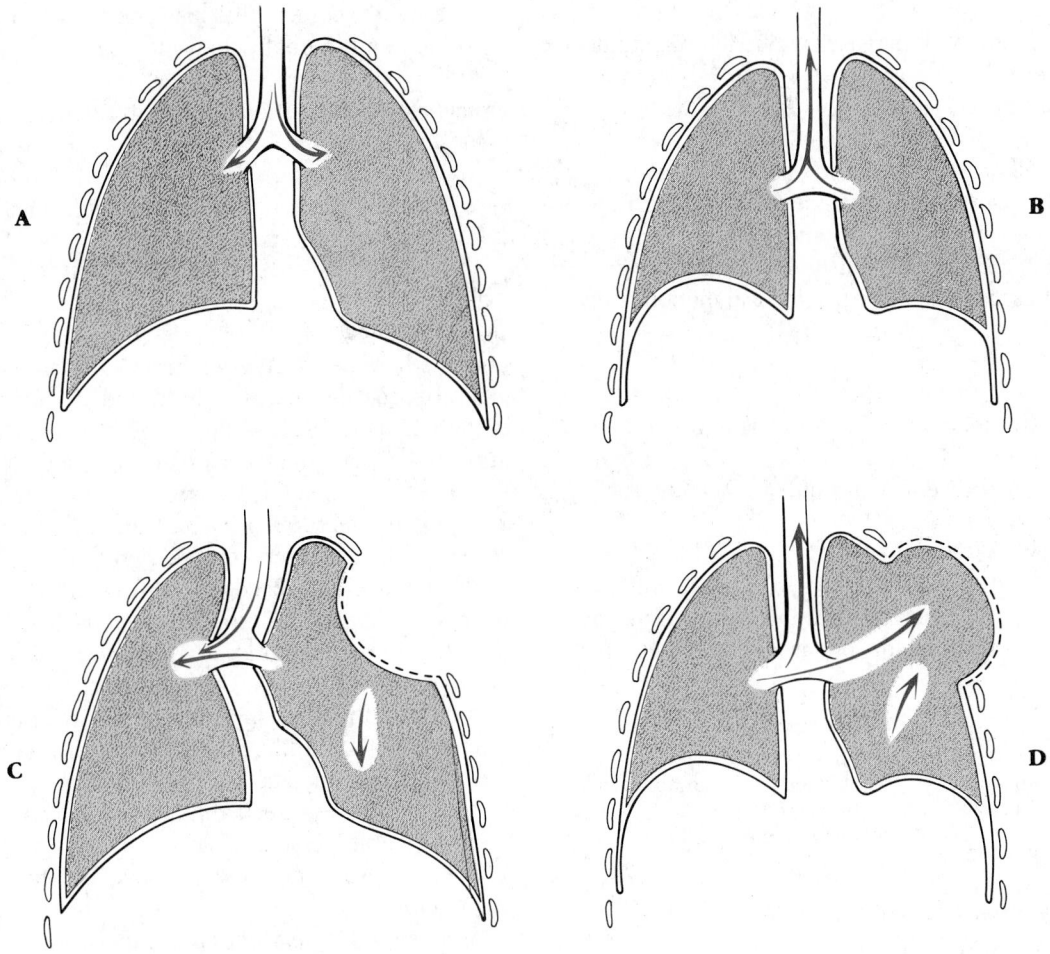

FIGURE 34-18 Normal respiration: **A,** inspiration; **B,** expiration. Paradoxical motion: **C,** inspiration, area of lung underlying unstable chest wall sucks in on inspiration; **D,** same area balloons out on expiration. Note movement of mediastinum toward opposite lung on inspiration.

Clinical Manifestations

The person with a flail chest will demonstrate the following signs and symptoms:

1. Severe chest pain
2. Paradoxical chest movement
3. Oscillation of mediastinum, with movement toward unaffected side with inspiration and returning toward midline on expiration
4. Increasing dyspnea
5. Tachypnea with shallow respirations
6. Accessory muscle breathing
7. Decreased breath sounds on auscultation
8. Anxiety related to above signs and symptoms

Medical Management

Treatment for flail chest includes the following:

1. Stabilize the flail segment. After initial stabilization the individual is usually intubated and placed on a *volume-cycled ventilator.* Positive-pressure mechanical ventilation provides internal stabilization of the chest, decreases the work of breathing, and initiates the bellows function normally provided by the intact bony chest cage. If prolonged ventilatory support is required, a tracheostomy is performed.
2. Provide supplemental oxygen.
3. Correct acid-base imbalance. Mechanical ventilation is used to correct *respiratory* acid-base imbalance.
4. Provide analgesics for pain control.

■ Assessment

Subjective data. Data to be collected includes nature of the injury and when it occurred. Often the patient is too badly injured to answer questions, and data are obtained from those accompanying the patient.

Objective data

1. Pain is severe and increases with each respiratory movement.
2. Mediastinum oscillates, or "flutters", with each respiration.
3. Decreased breath sounds on auscultation.
4. If there is severe interference with cardiac function, neck veins will be distended.
5. Vital signs: increased pulse and respiratory rate. Blood pressure will fall if paradoxical motion is not relieved.

Diagnostic tests

1. Chest x-ray examination to determine extent of trauma.
2. Arterial blood gases to determine PaO_2 and $PaCO_2$.

■ Data Analysis: Nursing Diagnoses

Nursing diagnoses are determined from assessment of patient data. Possible nursing diagnoses for the person with a flail chest may include, but are not limited to, the following:

Diagnostic Title	Possible Etiologies
Airway clearance, ineffective	Trauma to chest wall
Gas exchange, impaired	Ventilation/perfusion abnormality
Pain	Trauma to chest wall

■ Planning: Expected Patient Outcomes

1. Patient's airway is improved.
2. PaO_2 and $PaCO_2$ are improved.
3. Patient is more comfortable.

■ Implementation

Improving airway clearance. Nursing interventions focused on effective airway clearance are a critical component of care for the person with flail chest. Shallow breathing and the inability to cough effectively can result in a fatal pulmonary infection.

The following nursing actions are indicated:
1. Suction airway as needed to maintain patency.
2. Liquefy pulmonary secretions by providing adequate fluid intake and humidification of the respiratory tract.
3. After extubation, time coughing maneuvers to coincide with peak effect of analgesics.

Improving gas exchange. Nursing interventions to promote adequate oxygen and carbon dioxide exchange are aimed at stabilizing the flail segment and include the following:
1. Initially, provide direct support to the flail segment with the hands or sandbags.
2. After spinal injury is ruled out, turn the patient on to the affected side. This provides stabilization of the flail segment and also encourages lung expansion on the unaffected side

Promoting comfort. Interventions to promote comfort include the following:
1. Administering analgesics as needed
2. Splinting the flail segment with hands during coughing and movement (see Figure 34-23)

PNEUMOTHORAX

Pathophysiology

Pneumothorax is a condition in which there is air in the pleural space between the lung and the chest wall. It can occur as a result of penetrating or nonpenetrating injuries, or a pneumothorax can occur spontaneously.

A *closed pneumothorax* is caused by a blunt injury resulting in fractured ribs piercing the pleural membranes, or by a sudden compression of the rib cage. Air enters the pleural space, increasing intrapleural pressure that collapses the lung (Figure 34-19, B). A variant of a closed pneumothorax is a *spontaneous pneumothorax* that can result from the rupture of an emphysematous bleb on the lung surface, but it may also follow severe bouts of coughing in persons with a chronic pulmonary disease such as asthma. Rather frequently it occurs as a single or recurrent episode in an otherwise healthy young person. If large enough and left untreated, a closed pneumothorax can become a tension pneumothorax.

A *tension pneumothorax* occurs when air leaking into the intrapleural space cannot escape during expiration. Although usually a result of a closed pneumothorax, a tension pneumothorax can be caused by a penetrating chest injury. The accumulating air builds up positive pressure in the chest cavity resulting in:
1. Lung collapse on the affected side
2. Mediastinal shift toward the unaffected side
3. Compression of mediastinal contents (heart and great vessels) resulting in decreased cardiac output and venous return.

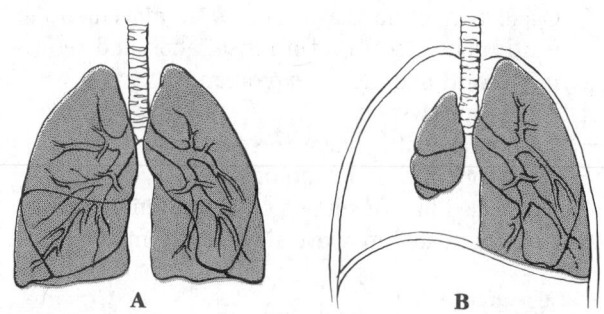

FIGURE 34-19 A, Normal expanded lungs. **B,** Complete collapse of right lung caused by air in pleural cavity (pneumothorax).

An *open pneumothorax* occurs when a *penetrating* chest wound opens the intrapleural space to atmospheric pressure. Each time the person inspires, air is sucked into the intrapleural space, increasing intrapleural pressure. An open pneumothorax is also called a sucking chest wound because the wound makes a sucking sound on inspiration and expiration. Blood also may leak into the pleural cavity creating a *hemothorax*.

Clinical Manifestations and Medical Management

The clinical manifestations and medical management of the various types of pneumothorax are presented in Table 34-7.

Nursing Management

Nursing diagnoses and interventions associated with the specific types of pneumothorax are presented in Table 34-8.

PULMONARY CONTUSION

Pathophysiology

Contusion of the pleurae or lung parenchyma is a penetrating injury. It usually results from sudden compression, followed by rapid decompression of the thoracic cavity, causing blood to extravasate into the pulmonary tissue. The contusion is usually self-limiting, since pulmonary vasculature is a low-pressure system. However, extensive contusion can precipitate pulmonary edema, with resultant hypoxemia, hypercapnia, and respiratory acidosis.

Clinical Manifestations

Pulmonary contusion may vary from total absence of symptoms to the full spectrum of symptoms associated with noncardiogenic pulmonary edema. The onset of signs and symptoms (some of which may be delayed) include the following:

1. Increasing dyspnea
2. Tachypnea
3. Increasing restlessness
4. Crackles noted on auscultation
5. Hemoptysis

Medical and Nursing Management

Medical treatment of pulmonary contusion depends on the severity of the injury. Treatment may vary from outpatient monitoring to intubation and mechanical ventilatory support when pulmonary edema is present.

TABLE 34-7 Clinical manifestations and medical management of pneumothorax

Pneumothorax	Clinical Manifestations	Medical Management
Closed or Spontaneous	A small or slowly developing pneumothorax may produce no symptoms. A larger or rapidly developing pneumothorax results in the following: 1. Sharp pain on inspiration 2. Increasing dyspnea 3. Increasing restlessness 4. Diaphoresis 5. Hypotension 6. Tachycardia 7. Absence of chest movement on affected side 8. Breath sounds absent on affected side 9. Hyperresonance on affected side	Observation on an outpatient basis Supplemental oxygen Needle aspiration of air from pleural space Insertion of chest catheter connected to water-sealed drainage system If frequent recurrences, tetracycline or talc instilled into pleural space to cause adhesions between pleurae; if this procedure fails, lung portion with defect resected and parietal pleura abraded
Open	1. Sucking sounds at wound site with respiration 2. Tracheal deviation (trachea moves toward unaffected side during inspiration and returns toward midline with expiration)	Occlude open wound Same as closed pneumothorax
Tension	1. Severe dyspnea 2. Agitation 3. Trachea deviated from midline toward unaffected side 4. Jugular venous distension 5. Absence of chest movement on affected side 6. Hypotension, tachycardia 7. Breath sounds absent on affected side 8. Hyperresonance on affected side 9. Diminished heart sounds	Same as open pneumothorax

TABLE 34-8 Nursing diagnoses and interventions for pneumothorax

Pneumothorax Type	Nursing Diagnoses	Nursing Interventions
Closed (spontaneous)	Knowledge deficit: condition and treatment	For outpatient or for patient after chest tube removal, instruct to: 1. Report any increased dyspnea to physician 2. Avoid strenuous exercise or activity that increases rate and depth of breathing 3. Avoid holding breath 4. Follow physician's instructions about resuming normal activity
	Impaired gas exchange	Perform the following: 1. Place in semi-Fowler's position 2. Administer oxygen 3. Obtain thoracentesis tray and water-sealed drainage equipment (see p. 987 for care of the patient with chest tubes)
Open	Knowledge deficit	Same discharge instruction as for closed pneumothorax
	Impaired gas exchange	Perform the following: 1. Occlude wound with nonporous covering 2. Same interventions as for closed pneumothorax
Tension	Knowledge deficit	Same discharge instruction as for patient with closed pneumothorax
	Impaired gas exchange	Tension pneumothorax—life-threatening event; imperative that interventions be carried out immediately to relieve increased intrapleural pressure; interventions same as those listed for closed pneumothorax
	Decreased cardiac output	Perform the following: 1. Monitor vital signs frequently 2. Observe for cardiac dysrhythmias 3. Palpate for subcutaneous emphysema in upper chest and neck

THORACIC SURGERY

Intelligent nursing care of patients undergoing thoracic surgery depends on knowledge of the anatomy and physiology of the chest, of the surgery performed, and of procedures and practices that assist the patient to recover from the operation. When endotracheal anesthesia became possible, surgery of the chest was given a great impetus.

Principles of Resectional Surgery

Principles of resectional surgery are as follows:

1. Endotracheal anesthesia is used for surgery involving the lung in which the pleural space is entered.
2. With endotracheal anesthesia it is possible to keep the uninvolved ("good") lung expanded and functioning when the chest is opened and atmospheric pressure enters the pleural space.
3. To understand resectional surgery and the purpose of chest tubes and water-seal drainage, an understanding of the following is necessary.
   a. *Physiology of breathing*
      (1) The pressure in the pleural space (the space between the visceral and parietal pleura) is subatmospheric (less than 760 mm Hg) and is referred to as *negative*.
      (2) The pressure in the pleural space is usually 756 mm Hg and goes down to 761 mm Hg

before inspiration. This change in pressure allows air (atmospheric pressure) to enter the lungs.

      (3) When the pleura is entered surgically or by trauma to the chest wall, atmospheric pressure enters the pleural space, and the lung collapses.
   b. *Purpose of chest tubes and water-seal drainage*
      (1) After resectional surgery of the lung (except pneumonectomy), one or two drainage tubes are inserted into the pleural space. Each tube is connected to a water-seal drainage bottle containing 1-2 cm of sterile water (see Figure 34-20).
      (2) The glass rod connected to the chest tube is under water. This "seals" the chest tube, allowing air and fluid to drain from the pleural space into the water-seal bottle and preventing air or fluid from entering the pleural space.
      (3) In all resectional surgery (except pneumonectomy), the remaining portions of the lung must overexpand and fill the space left by the resected portion.
      (4) The removal of air and fluid from the pleural space accomplishes two basic purposes. These are to (1) *aid in the expansion of the remaining portion of the lung as air (posi-*

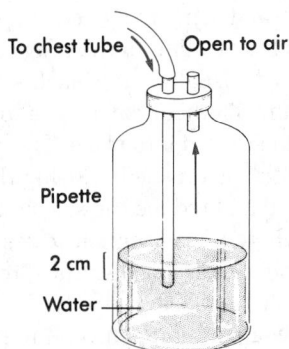

FIGURE 34-20 Water-sealed closed chest drainage showing type of tube under water. (From Abels LF: Mosby's manual of critical care, St Louis, 1979, The CV Mosby Co.)

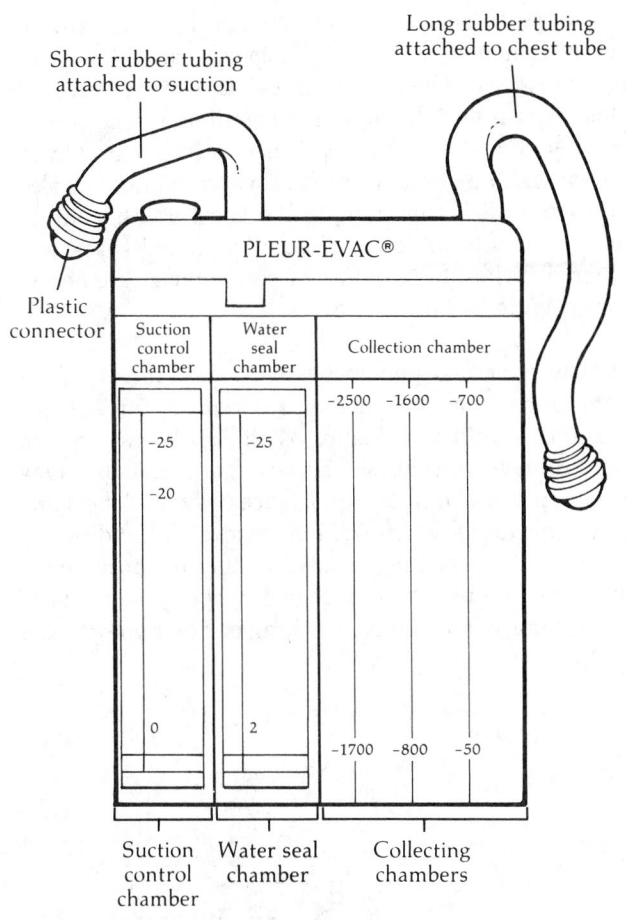

FIGURE 34-21 Pleurevac—one of several available brands of chest drainage systems. The system functions like a three-bottle system in that the unit collects drainage, maintains a seal to prevent air from entering pleural cavity, and prevents excessive build-up of negative pressure. (From Thompson et al: Mosby's Manual of Clinical Nursing, ed 2, St. Louis, 1989, The CV Mosby Co.)

tive pressure) *and fluid escapes through the drainage tubes,* and (2) *to reestablish negative pressure in the pleural space.*

(5) Nursing actions necessary to maintain the integrity of the chest tubes and water-seal drainage will be discussed under postoperative care.

(6) Other closed chest drainage systems such as Pleurevac may be used (Figure 34-21).

Types of Resectional Surgery

Table 34-9 presents the types of resectional surgery and the indications for the use of each type. A brief discussion of each type of resectional surgery follows.

Exploratory thoracotomy. An exploratory thoracotomy is performed to confirm a suspected diagnosis of lung or chest disease. The usual approach is by a posterolateral

TABLE 34-9 Types of thoracic surgery and indications for their use

Procedure	Indications
Exploratory thoracotomy	To confirm suspected diagnosis of lung or chest disease, especially carcinoma; to obtain a biopsy
Pneumonectomy (removal of a lung)	Bronchogenic carcinoma when lobectomy will not remove all of lesion; tuberculosis when other surgery will not remove all of diseased lung
Lobectomy (removal of lobe of lung)	Bronchogenic carcinoma confined to a lobe, bronchiectasis, emphysematous blebs or bullae; lung abscess, fungal infections, benign tumors; tuberculosis
Segmental resection (segmentectomy); (removal of one or more lung segments)	Bronchiectasis; lung abscess or cyst; metastatic carcinoma
Wedge resection (removal of pie-shaped section from surface of lung)	Well-circumscribed benign tumors, metastic tumors, or localized inflammatory disease
Decortication (removal of a fibrinous peel from the visceral pleura)	Chronic empyema
Thoracoplasty (removal of ribs)	Residual air space after surgery; chronic empyema space

parascapular incision through the fourth, fifth, sixth, or seventh intercostal space. Occasionally, an anterior approach is used. The ribs are spread to give the best possible exposure of the lung and hemithorax. The pleura is entered, and the lung examined; a biopsy usually is taken; and the chest is closed. This procedure may also be used to detect bleeding in the chest or other injury after trauma to the chest. Since the pleural space was entered, a chest tube and water-seal drainage are necessary (Figure 34-20).

Pneumonectomy. A pneumonectomy, the removal of an entire lung, is most commonly performed to treat bronchogenic carcinoma (Figure 34-22, *B*). It may also be used to treat tuberculosis. However, a pneumonectomy is only performed in those instances when a lobectomy or segmental resection will not remove all the diseased tissue. A thoracotomy is made in either the posterior or anterior chest using the method described under exploratory thoracotomy. Before the lung can be removed, the pulmonary artery and vein are ligated and then cut. The main-stem bronchus leading to the lung is clamped, divided, and sutured, usually with black silk. To ensure an airtight closure of the bronchus, a pleural flap is placed over it and sutured into place. The phrenic nerve on the operative side is crushed, causing the diaphragm on that side to rise and reduce the size of the remaining space. Because there is no lung left to reexpand, drainage tubes are not used. Ideally, the pressure in the closed chest is slightly negative. The fluid left in the space will consolidate in time, preventing the remaining lung and heart from shifting toward the operative side (mediastinal shift).

Lobectomy. In a lobectomy one lobe of the lung is removed (Figure 34-22, *C*). It is used to treat bronchiectasis, bronchogenic carcinoma, emphysematous blebs or bullae, lung abscess, benign tumors, fungal infections, and tuberculosis. For a lobectomy to be successful, the disease must be confined to one lobe, and the remaining

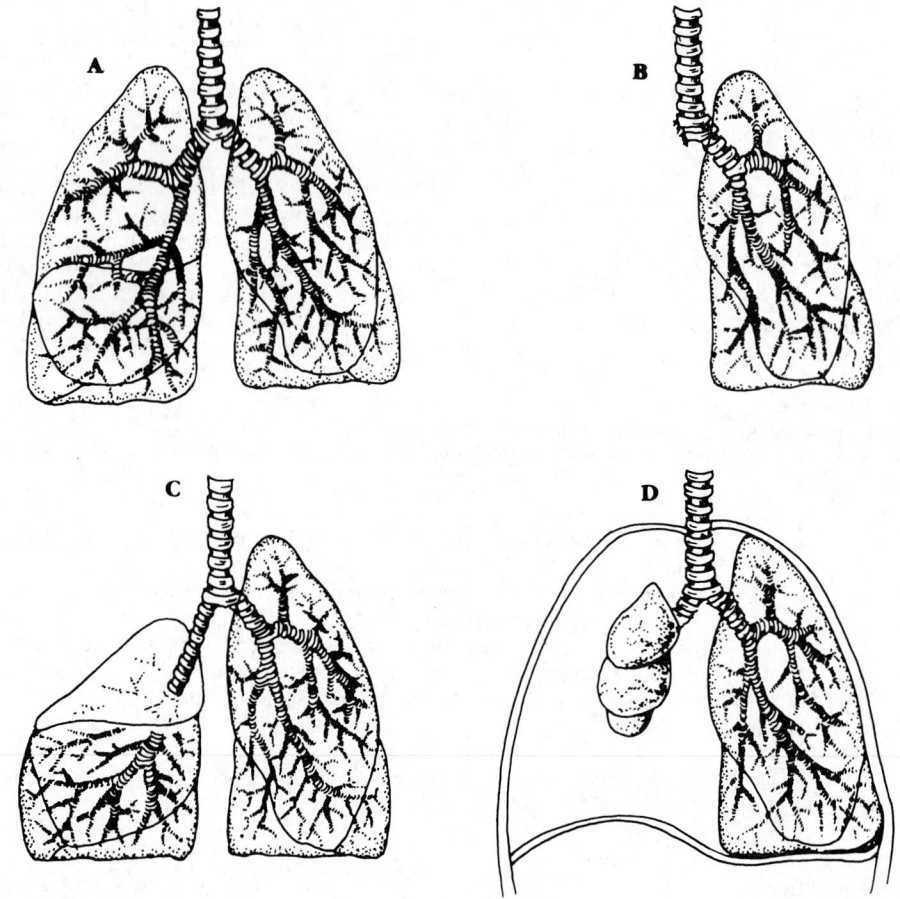

FIGURE 34-22 A, Normal lungs. **B,** Surgical absence of right lung after a pneumonectomy. **C,** Surgical absence of the right upper lobe after a lobectomy. **D,** Complete collapse of right lung as a result of air in the pleural cavity (pneumothorax).

lung tissue must be capable of overexpanding to fill the space of the resected lobe. One or two chest tubes are connected to water-seal bottles for postoperative drainage.

Segmental resection (segmentectomy). In a segmental resection, one or more segments of the lung are removed. This operation is used in an attempt to preserve as much functioning lung tissue as possible. It is a very taxing operation for the surgeon, since the dissection between segments must be performed very carefully and slowly, and the identification of the segmental pulmonary artery and vein and bronchus is more difficult than when a lobe is involved. Since there are 10 segments in the right lung and eight segments in the left lung, only a portion of a lobe or lobes may need to be removed. The most common indication for segmentectomy is bronchiectasis. It is also used to treat the other conditions listed in Table 34-9. Chest tube(s) and water-seal drainage are necessary postoperatively. Because of air leaks from the segmental surface, the remaining lung tissue may take longer to reexpand.

Wedge resection. In a wedge resection, a well-circumscribed diseased portion is removed without regard to the segmental planes. The area to be removed is clamped, dissected, and sutured. Chest tube(s) and water-sealed drainage are used postoperatively.

Decortication. In a decorticaton a fibrinous peel is removed from the visceral pleura, allowing the encased lung to reexpand and obliterate the pleural space. This procedure is discussed further under the treatment of empyema (Table 34-10). Chest tube(s) and chest suction are used to facilitate the reexpansion of the lung. If the lung has been encased for a long time, it may be incapable of reexpanding after decortication. In this situation thoracoplasty may be necessary.

PREOPERATIVE CARE AND EVALUATION

Special tests are required by a patient having chest surgery (see Chapter 31 for details about each test).

Radiologic Procedures
The following radiologic procedures are performed:
1. Posteroanterior (PA) and lateral chest films
2. Other x-ray examinations
   a. Laminograms (tomograms, planograms)
      (1) In this x-ray technique special layers of lung tissue are visualized. They are used to study neoplasms, cavities, and densities of the lung.
   b. CT scanning
      (1) CT scanning provides more accurate information than laminography in some instances.

Bronchoscopy
Bronchoscopy will be performed before any thoracic surgery. For the patient being considered for pneumonectomy, the evaluation will be even more precise, because it must be determined if the uninvolved lung will be able to maintain the patient's respiration after the diseased lung is removed.

Pulmonary Function Tests
Pulmonary function tests are usually used to determine the patient's ability to withstand pneumonectomy. In one center, patients who are being considered for pneumonectomy are evaluated on the basis of their forced expiratory volume in the first second (FEV_1) as follows:
1. If the FEV_1 is greater than 70% of the predicted normal level (approximately 2.5 L of flow), the patient's lung function is essentially normal, and the patient should be able to tolerate a pneumonectomy as long as cardiac status and arterial blood gas levels are acceptable.
2. If the FEV_1 is less than 35% of the predicted normal level (less than 1.1 L of flow), there is severe ventilatory impairment, and *surgical resection is not feasible.*
3. If the FEV_1 is between 35% and 70% of the predicted normal level (1.2 to 2.4 L of flow), there is mild-to-moderate ventilatory impairment, and further studies will be necessary to determine the maximal tolerable resection.

The nurse should be sure that the patient understands what tests are to be performed and the preparation for them. The person's significant others also are kept informed. Pulmonary function tests are described in Chapter 31.

Teaching
The proposed surgery is discussed with both patient and family. The goal of teaching is to prepare the patient for what he or she is expected to do postoperatively. In some hospitals nurses from the operating room, recovery room, or intensive care unit do the preoperative teaching. Even when this is so, the nurse caring for the patient is responsible for determining what the patient understands about the impending surgery and to be sure that preoperative teaching is completed.

Points to be discussed in teaching include:
1. Patient's knowledge of procedure
2. Explanation of procedure as necessary, including intubation for anesthesia, site of incision and chest tube(s) and drainage system
3. Where patient will go immediately following surgery
   a. To Recovery Room—for how long
   b. To Intensive Care Unit—for how long
4. Oxygen

5. Intravenous and/or blood administration
6. Pain medication
7. What patient will be asked to do
   a. Coughing and deep breathing
   b. Arm exercises
   c. Ambulation

POSTOPERATIVE CARE

The care of the patient after thoracic surgery centers on promoting ventilation and reexpansion of the lung by maintaining a clear airway, promoting comfort by pain relief, promoting reexpansion of the lung by proper maintainance of the water-seal drainage system, promoting arm exercises to maintain full use of the patient's arm on the operated side, promoting nutrition, and monitoring the incision for bleeding and subcutaneous emphysema.

In most hospitals the patient will go from the recovery room to the intensive care unit. The immediate postoperative nursing care is outlined here.

Oxygen Therapy

Oxygen is attached to the endotracheal tube. After extubation, oxygen is given by cannula usually at 6 L/min. An oxygen mask is not used because of a need to have the patient cough and raise secretions frequently.

Hemodynamic Monitoring

The patient is usually attached to a cardiac monitor and a Swan-Ganz catheter and central venous pressure line may be used for hemodynamic monitoring.

Position of Patient in Bed

The patient is kept flat in bed or with head elevated slightly (20 degrees) until blood pressure is stabilized to preoperative levels. Once blood pressure is stabilized, the patient can usually breathe best in semi-Fowler's position with a pillow under the head and neck but not under the shoulder and back because of the subscapular incision.

Monitoring Vital Signs

Vital signs are taken every 15 minutes until the patient is well recovered from anesthesia and then every hour until condition has stabilized. It is not unusual for blood pressure to fluctuate during the first 24 to 36 hours, and close monitoring of the patient is essential. A persistently low blood pressure is reported to the surgeon.

Initiating Coughing and Deep Breathing Exercises

The patient should be assisted to cough as soon as conscious. If the blood pressure is stable, the patient is assisted to a sitting position, and the incision is supported anteriorly and posteriorly by the nurse's hands. Firm, even pressure over the incision with the open palm of

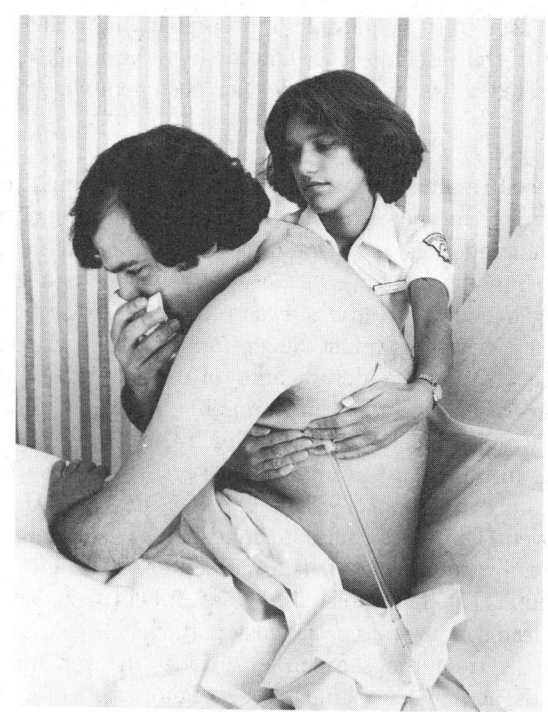

FIGURE 34-23 Nurse assists patient to cough by splinting incision with firm support from hands. This lessens muscle pull and pain as patient coughs. Note that nurse keeps her head behind patient while he coughs, and patient uses tissue to cover mouth.

the hands is a most effective method. The nurse's head should be behind the patient when the patient is coughing (Figure 34-23). The patient is encouraged to breathe deeply, exhale, and then cough. Sips of fluids, especially warm ones such as tea or coffee, often facilitate coughing. Mist therapy may be used to loosen secretions. Coughing *keeps the airway patent, prevents atelectasis, and facilitates reexpansion of the lung.* The patient should be assisted to cough every hour for the first 24 hours, and then every 2 to 4 hours. The patient should cough until the chest sounds clear. Otherwise, secretions will accumulate in the tracheobronchial tree.

When a patient is unable to cough effectively, tracheobronchial suctioning (p. 972) is performed. If suctioning fails to clear the airway, bronchoscopy may be necessary, since it is crucial that the airway is kept clear. In these situations, *bronchoscopy* is performed at the bedside with a *fiberoptic bronchoscope* (see Chapter 31).

Promoting Abdominal Breathing

Abdominal breathing exercises are a valuable adjunct to the care of the patient with chest surgery because they improve ventilation without increasing pain and assist in coughing more effectively (Figure 34-24). The exer-

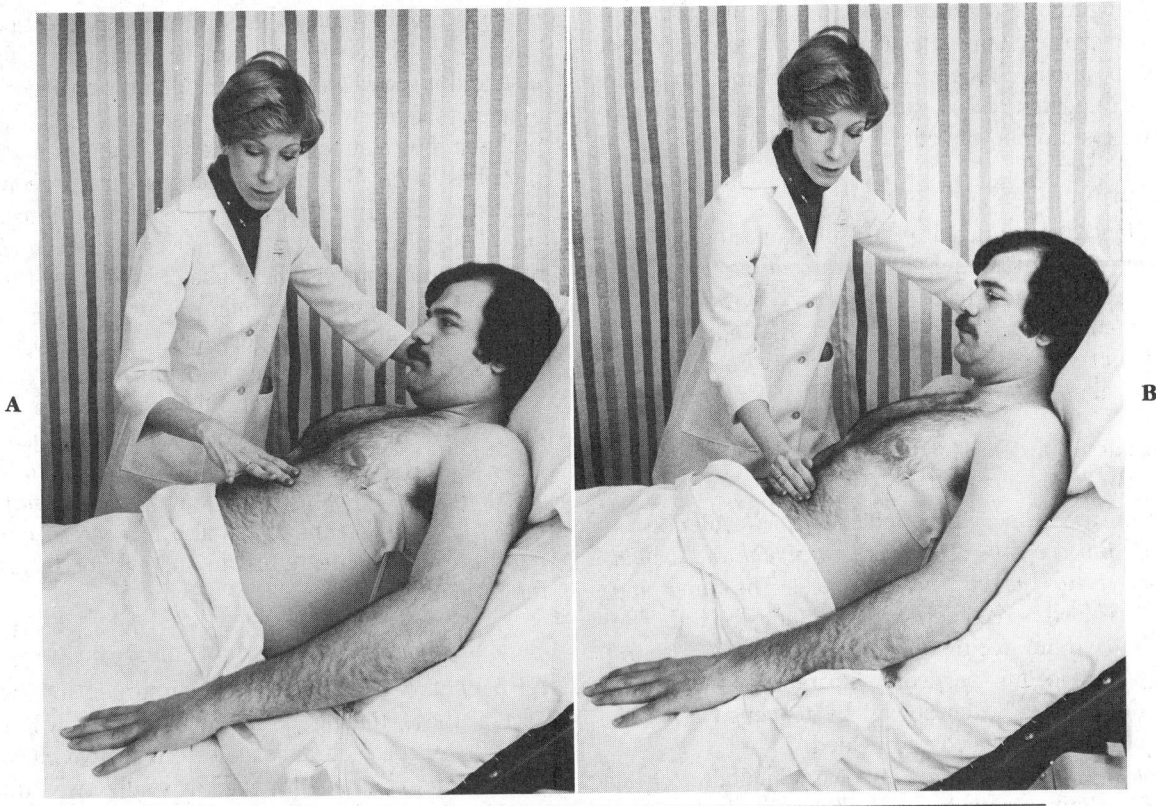

FIGURE 34-24 A, Physical therapist assists patient in learning augmented abdominal breathing. Patient is instructed to inhale through nose, using abdominal muscles and concentrate on moving lower ribs under therapists hand. This exercise improves ventilation of bases of lungs. **B,** Physical therapist places hand on upper abdomen in assisting patient to exhale fully.

cises should be *taught preoperatively* so that the patient has time to practice them before surgery. The patient can cough most effectively 20 to 30 minutes after receiving pain medication, and this should be capitalized on by the nursing staff.

Promoting Comfort by Pain Relief

Morphine or meperidine hydrochloride is usually ordered for pain. Medication for pain should be given as needed and may be required as often as every 3 to 4 hours during the first 48 to 72 hours. The patient is extremely uncomfortable and will not be able to cough or turn unless there is relief from pain. In some instances the dose of the narcotic is decreased so that it may be given more frequently and yet not depress respirations. The tubes in the chest cause pain, and the patient may attempt rapid, shallow breathing to splint the lower chest and avoid motion of the catheters. This impairs ventilation, makes coughing ineffective, and causes secretions to be retained. Thus it is a nursing responsibility to make the patient comfortable, because this facilitates deep breathing and coughing. *Pain medication*

should never be withheld without first consulting with the surgeon because undermedication is counterproductive. If, despite all efforts, and patient's discomfort is interfering with adequate chest excursion, an intercostal nerve block may be performed.

Promoting Arm Exercises

Passive arm exercises are usually started the evening of surgery. The purpose in putting the patient's arm through range of motion is to prevent restriction of function. Most patients are reluctant to move the arm on the operative side, but with proper preoperative instruction and postoperative follow-through they do so readily. It is important for both the patient and nurse to understand that the longer the arm is unexercised, the stiffer it will become. The patient should put both arms through active range of motion two or three times a day within a few days. The recommended exercises are similar to those done after mastectomy (see Chapter 59). The exercises are best performed when the patient is upright or lying on the abdomen. Exercises such as elevating the scapula and clavicle, "hunching the shoulders," bringing the scapulae as close together as possible, and hyperextending the arm can only be performed in these positions. Since lying on the abdomen may not be possible at first, these exercises are performed with the patient sitting on the edge of the bed or standing.

Promoting Nutrition

The patient is encouraged to take fluids postoperatively and to progress to a general diet as soon as it is tolerated. Forcing fluids helps to liquefy secretions and makes them easier to expectorate. A diet adequate in protein and vitamins (especially vitamin C) facilitates wound healing.

Monitoring the Incision for Bleeding or Subcutaneous Emphysema

Dressings are checked periodically for evidence of bleeding. *Blood on the dressings is unusual and should be reported to the surgeon at once.* The time and amount of blood is recorded in the patient's record. The surgeon may reinforce the dressing, and, in the rare instance when bleeding persists, the patient may be taken back to surgery. The chest will be reopened and the source of bleeding located and ligated.

Subcutaneous emphysema is not unusual after chest surgery. In subcutaneous emphysema, air leaks from the pleural space through the thoracotomy incision or around the chest tubes into the soft tissues. When palpating the chest, the presence of air under the skin is readily detected and has been described as feeling like "tissue paper" or "Rice Krispies" under the skin. Subcu-

taneous emphysema is most notable in the neck and chest, and, if considerable air is leaking, the patient's face and neck will become considerably enlarged. Small amounts of air will reabsorb over time and cause no problem; but if subcutaneous emphysema is worsening, the chest tube may be changed by the surgeon and a larger one inserted, because air is leaking into the tissues faster than it is being removed by the tube. Additional suction may also be applied to the chest tube(s) in an attempt to remove air more rapidly. Rarely a patient will need to return to surgery for closure of air leaks.

The patient with a pneumonectomy should have only a small amount (if any) of subcutaneous emphysema. *Progressive subcutaneous emphysema after pneumonectomy is very serious, and should be reported to the surgeon immediately because it could indicate a major leak in the bronchial stump.* This also is a rare occurrence, requiring immediate return to surgery for reclosure of the bronchial stump.

Maintaining Chest Tube(s) and Drainage

All patients who have resectional surgery of the lung, except those having a pneumonectomy, will require drainage of the pleural space by one or two chest tubes connected to closed drainage. Usually two tubes are used, although some surgeons may prefer only one tube. When two tubes are used, one catheter is inserted through a stab wound in the anterior chest wall above the resected area. This is referred to as the *anterior* or *upper tube.* It is used to remove air from the pleural space. The second tube is inserted through a stab

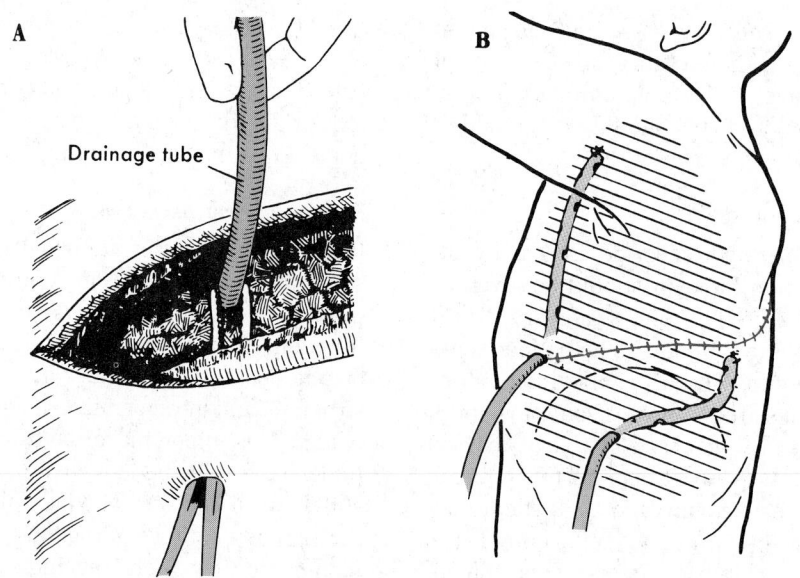

FIGURE 34-25 A, Drainage tube being inserted into pleural space. **B,** Note that upper and lower tubes are placed well into pleural space. (From Johnson J, MacVaugh H III, and Waldhausen JA: Surgery of the chest, a handbook of operative surgery, ed 4, Copyright 1970 by Year Book Medical Publishers, Inc, Chicago. Used by permission.)

wound in the posterior chest and is referred to as the *posterior* or *lower tube*. It is primarily for the drainage of *serosanguineous* fluid that accumulates as the result of the operative procedure. The lower tube may be of a larger diameter than the upper tube to prevent it from becoming plugged with clots. Figure 34-25 shows the placement of tubes within the pleural space. When only one chest tube is used, it is usually placed anteriorly above the resected area of the lung.

When initiating chest tube drainage, a 2 L clear glass bottle is usually used for each chest tube, although other commercial devices, such as the PleureVac system (Figure 34-21) are available. Approximately 300 ml of sterile water, or enough to fill the bottles 1 to 2 cm from the bottom, is then added. If considerable drainage accumulates in the bottle, this will increase the amount of subatmospheric (negative) pressure in the system, and it will be more difficult for the patient to expel air and fluid from the pleural space. In this instance, the glass rod may be pulled up so that less of it is under water; or the surgeon may order that the drainage bottle be changed. In this case a sterile setup is prepared. When the sterile bottle with sterile water and the tubing are ready, the chest tube is clamped as close to the patient's chest as possible. The chest tube is then disconnected from the drainage tubing, the sterile setup is connected, and the chest tube is unclamped. The amount of drainage in the bottle should be measured and usually is sent to the laboratory for examination.

As the patient breathes, there will be movement of fluid in the glass tube that is under water. This is known as *fluctuation* or *oscillation*, and the column will move up when the patient inhales or coughs, and it will fall when the patient is exhaling.

Some thoracic surgeons wish to have the chest tubes "milked" or "stripped" every hour to prevent formation of clots that could plug the tubes; the practice of routinely stripping chest tube(s) is becoming less common, however, because it increases the negative pressure exerted on the pleural space. A study by two clinical nurse specialists revealed the following: (1) The pressure generated by stripping was considerably higher than the suction pressures of −15 to −20 cm of water commonly applied to chest drainage systems; (2) the amount of pressure was directly related to the length of the tubing stripped; and (3) even stripping only a few centimeters produced pressures near −100 cm of water and stripping the entire tube produced pressures exceeding −400 cm of water.[12] They also found that higher negative pressures resulted when a roller was used to strip the tubes rather than the hands.[12]

Undesirable side effects of increased levels of negative pressure reported in the literature include (1) lung entrapment in the thoracic tube eyelets and focal tissue infarction and (2) persistent pneumothorax.[46] The per-

---

MAINTAINING CHEST TUBES AND CLOSED CHEST DRAINAGE

1. Mark water level in bottle with strip of adhesive tape so that amount of drainage can easily be determined. Write date and hour on tape.
2. Fasten tubing to the bed so that there are no dependent loops between the bottles and the bed (see Figure 34-16). Dependent loops allow fluid to collect in tubing and impede removal of air and fluid from pleural space.
3. Be sure that tip of chest tube is 1 to 2 cm under water so that if the bottle accidently tips over, the tube will remain under water.
4. Check the glass rod in the bottle for fluctuation frequently. If the column of water is not fluctuating:
   a. Be sure patient is not lying on tubes.
   b. Check connections to be sure chest tube system is intact.
   c. Ask patient to cough or change position to see if fluctuation is restored.
   d. Fluctuation will stop when lung is reexpanded. Call the surgeon if the tubes are not patent (column of fluid not fluctuating).
5. Keep two hemostats at the bedside so that the chest tube can be clamped if a bottle is accidentally broken.

When a bottle is broken, the chest catheter should be clamped and then reconnected to a sterile setup as soon as possible. Sterile water should be used in the bottle. As soon as the system is reconnected with the tip of the tube under water, the clamp should be removed. *Except in case of an emergency such as a broken bottle, most thoracic surgeons prefer that tubes not be clamped, and a specific order is written if clamping is desired.*

6. Never clamp chest tubes unless a bottle breaks (a rare occurrence) or without a written order. When chest tubes are clamped, air (positive pressure) may be trapped in the pleural space and further collapse the lung. If a patient is being transported from one place to another, such as to the x-ray department, tubes should not be clamped unless it is necessary for only a few minutes.
7. Never lift chest tube bottles above the level of the patient's chest, as this would allow fluid to be pulled into the pleural space.
8. The water-seal bottles should be placed on the floor so that they will not be broken by a lowered side-rail. When a Hi-Lo bed is being used, care is taken not to lower the bed onto the bottles.
9. If additional suction is being used, check frequently to be sure it is functioning at the prescribed level of negative pressure

sistent pneumothorax occurs when the pleural surface of lung, which normally has air leaks at the close of the operative procedure, does not "seal off." Usually fibrin will seal the air leaks; however, the presence of an increased amount of negative pressure may prevent the air leaks from sealing off and may even increase the size of the air leaks. This is the reason why some thoracic surgeons do not attach additional suction to the waterseal drainage system for the first 24 hours or more after surgery. They believe that this amount of time is sufficient in most instances to allow the pleural surface to seal off.

In view of these findings, the nurse should consult with the thoracic surgeon about the desirability of routinely stripping chest tubes. Because the anterior (upper) tube usually evacuates mainly air, there is less reason to believe that this tube will clot off. Posterior tubes, which are commonly inserted lower in the chest, usually drain more fluid and blood and are more likely to clot off. However, gentle squeezing of the tube is usually sufficient to move the bloody drainage along in the tubing. Special caution should be used in stripping tubes of patients with a known history of fragile tissue, such as occurs in emphysema.[12] The nursing measures necessary in maintaining chest tubes and closed drainage are listed in the box on p. 987.

Suction. Suction is usually used to speed reexpansion of the lung after surgery, using either wall suction (Figure 34-26, *A*) or an Emerson suction machine (Figure 34-26, *B*). Most often −30 cm of suction is applied, but this amount varies according to the surgeon's preference. When it is particularly important to regulate the exact amount of suction used, a "breaker" bottle may be added to the system between the suction source and the patient's drainage bottle. The use of a breaker bottle provides for control of the amount of suction that is applied to the water-sealed bottle and thus to the patient's pleural space. The stopper in the control bottle has three openings. One is connected to the water-sealed bottle, one is connected to the suction source, and the third contains a glass rod that is under water and open to the outside (Figure 34-27). The amount of suction produced will be determined by the distance between the

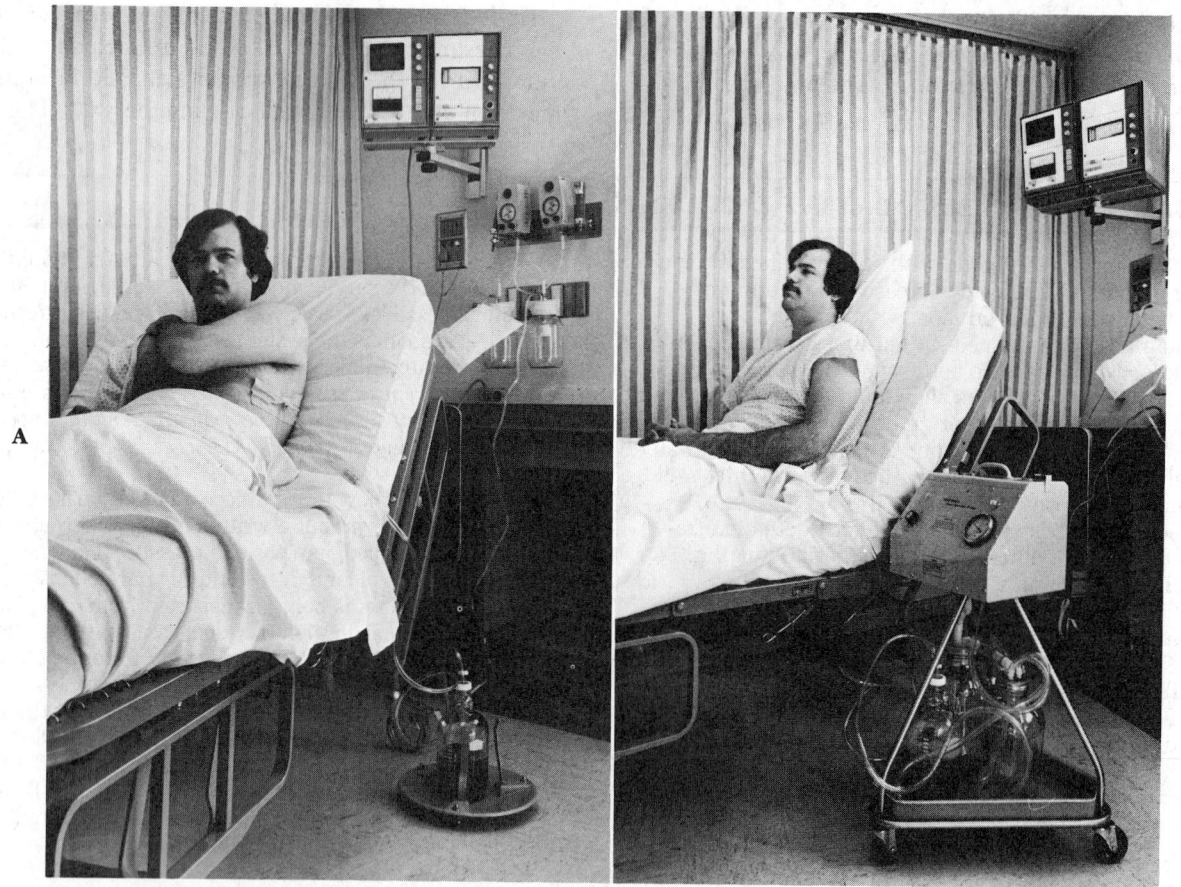

FIGURE 34-26 Chest tube with water-seal suction. **A,** Wall outlet provides source of suction. Note holder used to secure bottle in upright position. **B,** Emerson suction machine as source of vacuum.

surface of the water and the tip of this tube. When the suction source is turned on, the level of water in the open tube will sink in proportion to the amount of negative pressure in the system. Thus if there is 15 cm of water between the surface of the water and the tip of the tube, the amount of negative pressure in the system will be 15 cm of water pressure. Because the water will be at the bottom of the tube when this amount of pressure is reached, any increase in negative pressure will cause air to be drawn in from the outside, *breaking* the suction at this level. Therefore, it can be expected that the water in the breaker bottle will bubble almost continuously. If it fails to bubble at all, the desired level of suction is not being attained. When the water in the breaker bottle is not bubbling, the tubing should be checked for air leaks. If there are no leaks and bubbling still does not occur, the surgeon should be notified at once, since the air leak in the pleura may be so great that the amount of negative pressure is not sufficient to overcome it. In this instance water may be added to the breaker bottle to increase the distance between the surface of the water and the tip of the tube, thereby increasing the amount of negative pressure being exerted on the pleural space.

The distance the tube is placed under water in the breaker bottle is determined by the surgeon. A breaker bottle and suction may be attached to one or both tubes. Most commonly it is attached to the upper tube, as this is where air is most likely to be leaking from the pleural surface. A small empty trap bottle is usually attached by tubing between the breaker bottle and the suction source. The purpose of this bottle is to protect the suction motor from becoming wet should the breaker bottle overflow. See the box on p. 987 for summary of actions to maintain chest tubes.

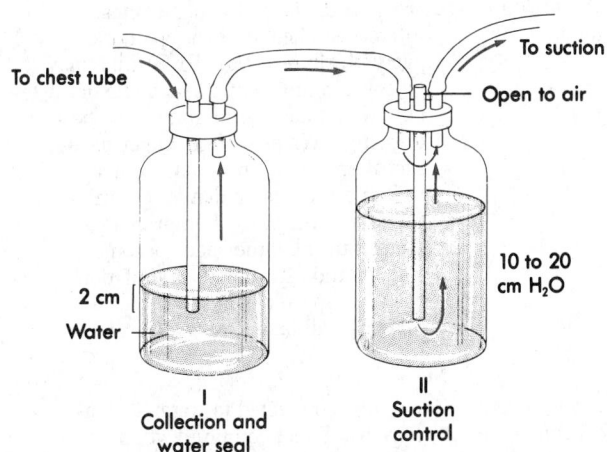

FIGURE 34-27 Water-sealed closed drainage system with suction control bottle. (From Abels LF: Mosby's manual of critical care, St Louis, 1979, The CV Mosby Co.)

Ambulation. There is no contraindication to ambulating with a chest tube in place. As long as the water-sealed bottle remains below the level of the chest, the patient may assume any position of comfort in bed or may be out of bed in a chair.

Removal of chest tubes. Chest tubes are removed when there is no fluctuation of fluid in the glass rod, and when x-ray films confirm the full reexpansion of the lung. Most patients have their chest tube(s) removed in about 72 hours postoperatively. If there is a persistent air space in the apex of the lung, the upper tube may be left in longer. *Surgeons are concerned about leaving tubes in very long because of the risk of an ascending tube track infection.* The patient should receive medication for pain 30 minutes before removal of the tube. Physicians vary in the exact procedure used to remove the tube, but generally a sterile scissors, 4 in × 4 in gauze squares, and adhesive tape are required. The suture holding the tube in place is cut, the patient is asked to exhale deeply, and the tube is removed. If a purse-string suture was used, it is retied, and a dry sterile dressing is placed over the site. Some physicians cover the site with a Telfa dressing instead of gauze squares to ensure an airtight dressing. The dressing is covered securely by three strips of 2-inch adhesive tape.

Care After Pneumonectomy

The postoperative care discussed in the box applies to all patients with resectional surgery except those having a pneumonectomy. The special care required after pneumonectomy is outlined in the box on p. 990.

Thoracoplasty

A thoracoplasty is an extrapleural procedure involving the removal of ribs to reduce the size of the chest cavity. Before the widespread use of resectional surgery, thoracoplasty was the basic surgical treatment for tuberculosis. Today thoracoplasty is used infrequently and then only to prevent or treat the complications of resectional surgery. When it is felt that a patient's lung may not be able to expand sufficiently after a resection to fill the space, a thoracoplasty is performed 2 to 3 weeks before the resection. It also may be performed before pneumonectomy, as this will reduce the chance of mediastinal shift after surgery. This type of thoracoplasty is often called a *preresection* or *tailoring* thoracoplasty; that is, the chest wall is tailored to reduce its size.

If the remaining portions of the lung fail to reexpand sufficiently after resection or if another complication such as empyema occurs, a thoracoplasty is performed. In general, it is used when there is a space in the chest that cannot be obliterated by other means. Usually no more than three ribs are removed; therefore, paradoxi-

SPECIAL CARE FOLLOWING PNEUMONECTOMY

1. Chest tubes are not necessary because there is no lung left to reexpand on the operative side.
2. Patient may lie on back or *operated side only*. Patient is not allowed to lie with operative side uppermost because of fear that the sutured bronchial stump may open, allowing fluid to drain into the unoperated side and drown the patient.
3. Pressure in the operative side will be checked in the operating room after the chest is closed. A pneumothorax apparatus (which can instill or remove air) will be used to check the pressure in the operative space, and air will be removed or instilled as necessary to bring the pressure to slightly negative (slightly less than 760 mm Hg).
4. The surgeon will palpate the patient's trachea at least daily to determine if it is in midline. Deviation of the trachea toward either the operated or unoperated side is a sign of *mediastinal shift*. If pressure builds up in the operated side, the trachea will deviate toward the unoperated side. The treatment is to remove air (positive pressure) with a pneumothorax apparatus. Mediastinal shift toward the "good" lung can seriously compromise ventilation and needs to be treated promptly. Deviation of the trachea toward the operated side indicates that more pressure (air) needs to be instilled into the empty space.
5. The patient with a mediastinal shift resembles the patient in congestive heart failure. Neck veins are distended, the trachea is displaced to one side, pulse and respirations are increased, and dyspnea is present.
6. Serous drainage will collect in the operated space and over time will congeal to the consistency of axle grease. This is often sufficient to keep the mediastinum from shifting toward the operative side. Persis-

tent mediastinal shift toward the operative side may have to be treated with *thoracoplasty* (removal of ribs) to reduce the size of the remaining space and assist in maintaining the mediastinum in midline. Thoracoplasty is described on p. 987.

7. It usually takes 2 to 4 days for the remaining lung to adjust to the increase in blood flow. For this reason the amount of fluids and blood given intravenously is monitored closely to prevent fluid overload. CVP monitoring is common. Rales are commonly heard over the base of the remaining lung, and vascular markings will be more prominent on x-ray films. Any increase in rales, in pulse or blood pressure, and in dyspnea may indicate circulatory overload and should be reported immediately. Treatment may include diuretics and/or digitalization along with discontinuing intravenous fluids.
8. Deep breathing, coughing, and arm exercises are the same as described earlier (p. 984 and 985).
9. Patients who have had a lung removed may have a lowered vital capacity, and exercise, and activity should be limited to that which can be performed without dyspnea. Because the body must be given time to adjust to having only one lung, the patient's return to work may be delayed.
10. If the diagnosis is cancer, radiation therapy is usually given, and it may be started before the patient leaves the hospital. (See Chapter 17 for further discussion of nursing care for patients receiving radiation therapy.)
11. The patient who has had a pneumonectomy for cancer is urged to report to the physician at once if hoarseness, dyspnea, pain on swallowing, or localized chest pain develop because these symptoms may be signs of complications.

TABLE 34-10 Long-term complications of resectional surgery

Complications	Signs and Symptoms	Treatment
EMPYEMA		
Pus in the pleural space is a dreaded complication of thoracic surgery. Pus may drain from chest tube(s) or if chest tubes are already removed can be obtained on thoracentesis (insertion of a needle attached to a syringe with a threeway stopcock used to remove fluid, blood, or pus from pleural space).	Unexplained elevation in temperature Evidence of pleural exudate on x-ray film	*Dependent drainage* by thoracentesis, intercostal chest tube, or open drainage with rib resection. Chest tube may be connected to water-seal bottle or cut off and allowed to drain into chest dressings. Water-seal no longer necessary if empyema space has a thick wall and there is no danger of lung collapse. Over time as empyema drains out tube, the space becomes smaller and fills in with granulation tissue. If space persists, a *thoracoplasty* will be necessary. (p. 987).
BRONCHOPLEURAL FISTULA		
Opening in the sutured bronchus that permits communication between bronchus and pleural space. Space usually becomes infected and empyema develops.	Cough (usually nonproductive), fever, leukocytosis, anorexia, expectoration of purulent sputum, and evidence of pleural exudate on x-ray film	Chest tube connected to water-seal, as there is a direct communication between bronchus (positive pressure being inspired) and the pleural space. A persistent bronchopleural fistula is treated by thoracoplasty and a muscle implant to seal off the bronchus.

cal motion after thoracoplasty is seldom seen anymore. Paradoxical motion is discussed under chest injuries (p. 976).

Complications of Chest Surgery

In the immediate postoperative period (24 to 48 hours) hypotension, cardiac dysrhythmia, pulmonary edema, and subcutaneous emphysema (p. 986) may occur. Long-term complications include a residual air space, which results from failure of the remaining portions of the lung to reexpand and fill the space. If this space is small, no treatment is indicated. Two major complications of chest surgery tend to occur later in the postoperative period and require treatment: empyema and bronchopleural fistula. The patient may have empyema alone or empyema and a bronchopleural fistula. The signs and symptoms and treatment of these two complications are outlined in Table 34-10.

CHAPTER SUMMARY

- ✔ Several factors that are involved in normal breathing: (1) adequate supply of O_2, (2) patent airway, (3) normal functioning bellows motion of chest wall and diaphragm, (4) adequate number of terminal respiratory units (alveoli and capillaries) for diffusion, (5) adequate amount of hemoglobin, (6) intact circulatory system and effective heart pump and, (7) functioning respiratory center.

- ✔ Primary prevention of pulmonary system disease includes education about environmental inhalants including the risk of smoking, air pollution, and avoidance of pulmonary infections.

- ✔ When a patient cannot maintain his or her own airway, intubation with an endotracheal or tracheostomy tube may be necessary. Endotracheal tubes are used for short periods of time. If longer intubation is required, a tracheostomy performed in the operating room is the treatment of choice.

- ✔ General care of the person with an endotracheal or tracheostomy tube includes measures to minimize infection including proper suctioning technique, humidification of the airway, proper care of respiratory therapy equipment, frequent mouth care, and adequate nutrition.

- ✔ To ensure adequate ventilation and oxygenation, the patient's lungs sounds are assessed frequently. Turning and repositioning every 2 hours, assessing respiratory frequency, tidal volume and vital capacity, and providing chest physiotherapy including clapping, vibrating, and postural drainage as essential.

- ✔ Precautions pertaining to endotracheal or tracheostomy tubes includs assessing tube placement at reg-

ular intervals, keeping a spare tube on hand for emergencies, minimizing sensory deprivation by developing a method of communication, talking directly to the patient and explaining all procedures, reorienting patient frequently, encouraging family and friends to talk with the patient, keeping call light within reach, and reinforcing that the patient will be able to speak after extubation.

- ✔ Precautions to be observed after extubation include frequent monitoring for respiratory distress, adequacy of cough and gag reflex, and care of stoma incision.

- ✔ Patients who are being discharged with an endotracheal or tracheostomy tube in place will need to be taught how to care for their own tubes before discharge. The home will need to be visited before discharge to be sure that the patient and equipment can be accommodated. The community source for equipment and supplies will need to be determined before discharge.

- ✔ Effective breathing patterns can be facilitated by proper positioning, and the use of respiratory assitive devices such as incentive spirometery, and possibly IPPB.

- ✔ When a patient is unable to maintain ventilation, the $PaCO_2$ will increase and mechanical ventilation will be necessary.

- ✔ There are two major types of ventilators, pressure-cycled and volume-cycled. Currently volume-cycled ventilators are more commonly used. Before attaching ventilator, the patient will be intubated with either an endotracheal or a tracheostomy tube.

- ✔ A volume-cycled ventilator delivers a constant volume of air at a preset pressure with each breath. These ventilators have a cutoff valve, which will stop the cycle if the pressure required to deliver the desired volume exceeds a preset level.

- ✔ All patients on continuous mechanical ventilation need to be sighed (given a deep breath) several times each hour. Newer models of ventilators have automatic sign mechanisms. Otherwise, the patient is sighed manually with a self-inflating anesthesia (Ambu) bag connected to oxygen. The purpose of this periodic deep breathing is to prevent alveolar collapse and atelectasis.

- ✔ The patient on a ventilator requires constant attendance and is best managed in an intensive care unit.

- ✔ After the patient's underlying pulmonary problem is improved, the patient will be weaned from the ventilator. Weaning is best carried out by a nurse who has developed a trust relationship with the patient.

↙ There are two major methods of weaning, T-piece weaning and intermittent mandatory ventilation (IMV) weaning. Several attempts for increasing periods of time may be necessary before the ventilator can be discontinued.

↙ Nursing management to facilitate aeration of alveoli requires interventions that promote optimal airway function, promote effective breathing patterns, and manage pulmonary secretions. Measures to achieve these include hydration, humidification of the airways, nebulizer therapy, segmental postural drainage, and breathing exercises.

↙ When the patient cannot manage secretions, tracheobronchial suctioning may be necessary. If this is not successful in clearing the airway, fiberoptic bronchoscopy may be used to remove impacted secretions.

↙ Maintaining transportation of oxygen to body tissues requires several interactive physiologic processes. These include ventilation, perfusion, and diffusion. Also required are sufficient hemoglobin and an adequate cardiac output.

↙ Several modes are used to deliver O_2 to the patient. These include nasal cannulae and several types of face masks that can deliver various concentrations of O_2.

↙ To assure an adequate functioning respiratory center, conditions that depress the respiratory center must be identified and treated.

↙ Interference with the bellows function of the chest wall and diaphragm can be caused by chest trauma or chest surgery.

↙ Chest trauma is divided into blunt and penetrating injuries. The most common blunt injury is fractured ribs.

↙ The major cause of chest trauma is automobile accidents in which the chest hits the steering wheel.

↙ Chest trauma is managed by stabilization of the fracture site and analgesics to reduce pain.

↙ When several ribs or the sternum are fractured in more than one place, the patient may develop a flail chest with paradoxical breathing.

↙ Nursing management of the person with a flail chest includes improving gas exchange and airway clearance and promoting comfort.

↙ A pneumothorax occurs when air enters the pleural space between the lung and chest wall. There are three main types of pneumothoraces: closed or spontaneous, open, and tension.

↙ If an open sucking wound of the chest has been sustained, the wound should be covered immediately to prevent air from entering the pleural cavity and causing a pneumothorax.

↙ After resectional surgery of the lung (except for pneumonectomy), one or two chest tubes are inserted into the pleural space and connected to water-sealed drainage.

↙ Postoperative nursing care of the patient after thoracic surgery centers on promoting ventilation and reexpansion of the lung by maintaining a clear airway, promoting comfort by pain relief, promoting reexpansion of the lung by proper maintenance of the water-seal drainage system, promoting nutrition, and monitoring the incision for bleeding and subcutaneous emphysema.

↙ Bronchopleural fistula and empyema are long-term complications of resectional surgery of the lung.

QUESTIONS TO CONSIDER

▪ How would you provide emotional support to the patient who is intubated?

▪ What can the nurse do to reduce the number of persons affected by respiratory problems?

▪ Would your nursing priorities be different for the 30-year-old having a lobectomy and a 60-year-old having the same procedure? If so, how would they differ?

▪ What plans would you make for a patient being sent home on a ventilator?

REFERENCES AND SELECTED READINGS

1. Acre S: Helping patients breathe more easily, Geriatr Nurs 7:230-233, 1984.
2. *Albanese A and Toplitz A: A hassle-free guide to suctioning a tracheostomy, RN 45(4):24-30, 1982.
3. Bates DV: Respiratory function in disease, Philadelphia, 1989, WB Saunders Co.
4. *Brown I: Trach care? Take care—infection's on the prowl, Nursing '82 12(5):44-45, 1982.
5. Byra C: High frequency ventilation, Crit Care Nurse 5,6:42-47, 1985.
6. Cameron TJ: Fiberoptic bronchoscopy, Am J Nurs 81:1462-1465, 1981.
7. *Carroll PL: Lowering the risks of endotracheal suctioning, Nursing '88 18:15:46-50, 1988.
8. Centers for Disease Control: Humidifiers: tips given on trimming hazards, Atlanta, 1979, The Centers for Disease Control.
9. *Chalikian J and Weaver T: Mechanical ventilation—where it's at, where it's going, Am J Nurs 84:1373-1379, 1984.
10. Cherniack RM: Current therapy of respiratory disease—two, Toronto, 1986, BC Decker Inc.

References preceded by an asterisk are particularly well suited for student reading.

11. *Chulay M and Graeber GM: Efficacy of a hyperinflation and hyperoxygenation suctioning intervention, Heart Lung 17:1:15-22, 1988.

12. *Duncan C and Erickson R: Pressures associated with chest tube stripping, Heart Lung 11:166-171, 1982.

13. Erickson R: To cough or not to cough, Nursing '82 12(6):124-126, 1982.

14. *Erickson R: Solving chest tube problems, Nursing '81 11(6):62-68, 1981.

15. *Erickson R: Chest tubes: they're really not that complicated, Nursing '81 11(5):34-43, 1981.

16. *Fuchs Carroll P: Caring for ventilator patients, Nursing '86 16(6):34-39, 1986.

17. *Fuchs PL: Streamlining your suctioning techniques, part 1, nasotracheal suctioning, Nursing '84 14(5):55-61, 1984.

18. Fuchs PL: Before and after surgery: stay right on respiratory care, Nursing '83 13(5):47-50, 1983.

19. *Greenwood BS: The before and after of good postop pulmonary care, Nursing '82 12(12):68-69, 1982.

20. Hagarty E: Weaning your COPD patient from the ventilator, RN 47(7):36-40, 1984.

21. Harris RB and Hyman RB: Clean vs. sterile tracheostomy care and level of pulmonary infection, Nurs Res 33:80-85, 1984.

22. *Hoffman LA: Airway management for the critically ill patient, Am J Nurs 87:1:39-43, 1987.

23. *Hoffman LA and Maskiewicz RC: The specifics of suctioning, Am J Nurs 87:1:44-53, 1987.

24. Hoyt SK: Chest trauma, Nursing '83 13(5):34-41, 1983.

25. *Hughes JM: Postoperative pulmonary care: past, present, and future, Crit Care Q 6:67, 1983.

26. Janowski S: Mechanical ventilation—bringing the patient into focus, Nursing '84 11:1384-1388, 1984.

27. Johnson DL Giovannoni RM, and Driscoll FA: Ventilator-assisted patient care, Maryland, 1986, Aspen Publishers Inc.

28. *Kersten LD: Comprehensive respiratory therapy, Philadelphia, 1989, WB Saunders Co.

29. Kryger M, editor: Pathophysiology of respiration, New York, 1981, John Wiley & Sons Inc.

30. *Landis K and Smith S: The mechanically ventilated patient: a comprehensive nursing care plan, Crit Care Q 6:43, 1983.

31. *Langston HT and Barker WS: The adult thoracic surgical patient. In Neville, WE, editor: Care of the surgical cardiopulmonary patient, ed 2, Chicago, 1983, Yearbook Medical Publishers Inc.

32. *Leininger BJ: Thoracic trauma. In Neville WE: Intensive care of the surgical cardiopulmonary patient, Chicago, 1983, Yearbook Medical Publishers.

33. Oermann M et al: After a tracheostomy—patients describe their sensations, Ca Nurs 6:361-366, 1983.

34. *Openbrier DR, Fuoss C, and Mall CC: What patients on home oxygen therapy want to know, Am J Nurs 88:2:198-202, 1988.

35. *Openbrier DR, Hoffman LA, and Weismiller SA: Home oxygen evaluation, Am J Nurs 88(2):192-197, 1988.

36. *Perdue P: Urgent priorities in severe trauma: life-threatening respiratory injuries, RN 44(4):27-33, 1981.

37. *Preucser BA et al: Effects of two methods of preoxygenation on mean arterial pressure, cardiac output, peak airway pressure, and post suctioning hypoxemia, Heart Lung 17:3:290-298, 1988.

38. *Rhodes M: Update on chest trauma, Crit Care Q 6:39, 1983.

39. *Rifas EM: How you and your patient can manage dyspnea, Nursing '80 10(6):34-41, 1980.

40. *Risser NL: Preoperative and postoperative care to prevent pulmonary complications, Heart Lung 9:57-67, 1980.

41. Roth Fromme L and Kaplow R: High frequency jet ventilation, Am J Nurs 84:1380-1383, 1984.

42. Rouses S: An illustrated guide to trach care, RN 47(7):48-50, 1984.

43. Schumann L and Parsons GH: Tracheal suctioning and ventilator tubing changes in adult respiratory distress syndrome: use of a positive end-expiratory pressure valve, Heart Lung 14:362-367, 1985.

44. *Slonim NB and Hamilton LH: Respiratory physiology, ed 5, St Louis, 1987, The CV Mosby Co.

45. Sporn PHS and Morganroth ML: Discontinuance of mechanical ventilation, Clin Chest Med 9:1:133-126, 1988.

46. Stahley TL and Tench WD: Lung entrapment and infarction by chest tube suction, Radiology 122:307, 1977.

47. *Stovsky B and Dragonette P: Comparison of two types of communication methods used after cardiac surgery with patients with endotracheal tubes, Heart Lung 17:3:281-289, 1988.

48. Sumner S and Lewandowski V: Guidelines for using artificial breathing devices, Nursing '83 13(10):54-57, 1983.

49. Traver G, editor: Respiratory nursing: the art and the science, New York, 1982, John Wiley & Sons Inc.

50. Treolar D and Stechmiller J: Pulmonary aspiration in tube-fed patients with artificial airways, Heart Lung 13:667-671, 1984.

51. *Vasbinder-Dillon D: Understanding mechanical ventilation, Crit Care Nurs 8:7:42-56, 1988.

52. Wade JR: Comprehensive respiratory care, St Louis, 1982, The CV Mosby Co.

53. Wesmiller SW, Hoffman LA, and Wiseman M: Understanding transtracheal oxygen therapy, Nursing '89 19(12):43-47, 1989.

54. Wilkins MA, Sheldon RL, and Krider SJ: Clinical assessment in respiratory care, 2nd ed. St Louis, 1985, The CV Mosby Co.

ALTERATIONS IN METABOLISM AND ENERGY BALANCE

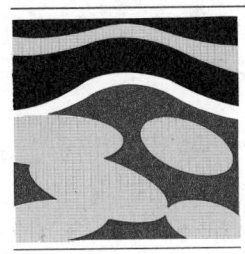

CHAPTER 35

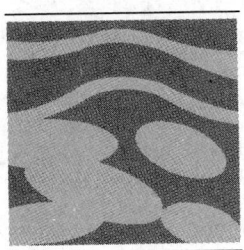

Assessment of the Endocrine System

VIRGINIA L. CASSMEYER

CHAPTER OBJECTIVES

After studying this chapter, the student should be able to:
1 Describe the locations of various endocrine glands in the body and the mechanisms that control hormone synthesis and release from these glands.
2 Describe the functions of the hormones secreted by the pituitary, thyroid, parathyroid, adrenal cortex, and adrenal medulla glands, and the endocrine pancreas.
3 Identify the physiologic changes that occur within the endocrine system with aging.
4 Identify subjective and objective data that should be collected on clients with actual or potential health problems of the endocrine system.
5 Describe the common diagnostic tests used to identify endocrine dysfunction and explain the meaning of results.

The complexity of the human body and the specialization of cells and tissues require an internal communication system that integrates processes so that several body parts can function as a unit to meet selected needs. Two systems, the endocrine and nervous systems, function together to coordinate body processes so that an appropriate response can be made to changes in the environment.

The endocrine system consists of the anterior and posterior pituitary, thyroid, parathyroid, adrenal cortex, adrenal medulla, pancreas, gonads, pineal body, and thymus. There are also specialized endocrine cells located in various parts of the gastrointestinal tract. The hormones from these endocrine glands are vital to the important life transactions of the organism, including differentiation, reproduction, growth and development, adaptation, aging, and senescence.[17] This is the first of three chapters that focus on the role in these processes of the anterior and posterior pituitary, thyroid, parathyroid, adrenal cortex and adrenal medulla glands, and endocrine pancreas. The neuroendocrine response to stressors, which involves the nervous system, the adrenal medulla, and other endocrine glands, is discussed in Unit III, Chapter 9. The gastrointestinal hormones are

discussed in Unit VIII, sections 2 and 3. The gonads are discussed in Unit IX.)

ANATOMY AND PHYSIOLOGY

GENERAL ENDOCRINE PROCESSES

The endocrine system integrates body functions by the synthesis and release of hormones. *Hormones* are chemical substances that are secreted into body fluids, usually blood, by a group of specialized cells, so that they may exert a physiologic effect at another site. Hormones can travel moderate to long distances, such as from the pituitary to the ovaries, or very short distances, such as from one cell group in the pancreas to another. When hormones influence cells close to the site of origin, this is referred to as *paracrine* functioning.

A hormone acts only on cells or tissues that have *re-*

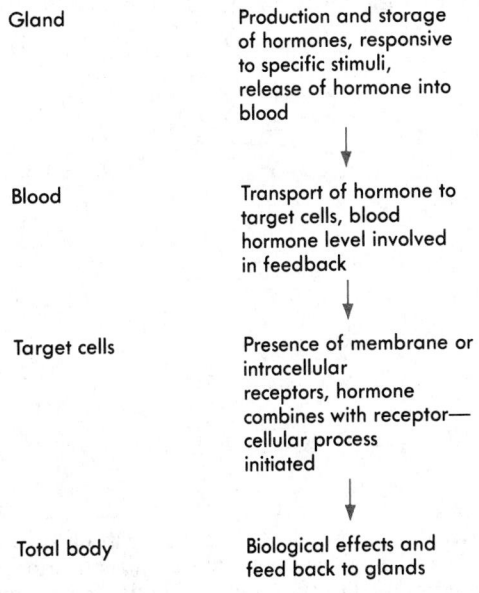

FIGURE 35-1 Summary of processes involved in the activity of endocrine glands and hormones.

ceptors for the specific hormone. The cell or tissue that responds to a particular hormone is called the *target cell* or *target tissue*. Hormones, when stimulating cells, set in motion various intracellular processes so that metabolic responses, growth and development changes, and response to stressors occur as needed by the body. Hormones themselves do not produce these responses; rather hormones set in motion a chain of events necessary to produce the desired and needed response. A summary of the processes involved in the activity of endocrine glands and their hormones is shown in Figure 35-1. Hormones can be classified by chemical structure into six groups as shown in the box at right.

CONTROL OF HORMONE LEVELS

The level of hormones must be kept within very definite limits, because the amount of hormone available to a tissue is critical for its health. One factor responsible for controlling levels is *feedback control*. A simple closed-loop negative feedback system is illustrated in Figure 35-2. This diagram reveals a basic type of feedback. Gland A is stimulated to produce hormone X. Hormone X stimulates organ B to change (increase or decrease) substance Y. The change in substance Y inhibits the production and secretion of hormone X. This simple system is an illustration of the negative feedback regulation of, for example, parathyroid hormone, antidiuretic hormone, and insulin (Table 35-1).

A more complex feedback mechanism controls the levels of other hormones. The most elaborate feedback mechanism is demonstrated by the interaction of the hypothalamus and the anterior pituitary with the thyroid gland, the adrenal cortex, and the gonads. The basic parts of this feedback loop are illustrated in Figure 35-3. When the level of hormone produced by the thy-

MAJOR CHEMICAL CLASSES OF HORMONES AND SPECIFIC HORMONES IN EACH CLASS

Biogenic amines	Dopamine, epinephrine, norepinephrine
Amino acids	Thyroxine (T_4), triiodothyronine (T_3)
Peptides	Antidiuretic hormone (ADH, vasopressin), oxytocin, corticotropin-releasing hormone (CRH), gonadotropin-releasing hormone (GnRH), growth hormone–releasing hormone (GHRH), growth hormone–inhibiting hormone (somatostatin, GHIH), thyrotropin-releasing hormone (TRH)
Proteins	Adrenocorticotropin (ACTH), calcitonin, glucagon, growth hormone (GH), insulin, prolactin (PRL), parathyroid hormone (PTH)
Glycoproteins	Follicle-stimulating hormone (FSH), luteinizing hormone (LH), thyroid-stimulating hormone (TSH)
Steroids	Adrenal androgens, aldosterone, estrogens (E_2, E_3), glucocorticoids, progesterone (P_4), testosterone (T), and vitamin D (cholecalciferol)

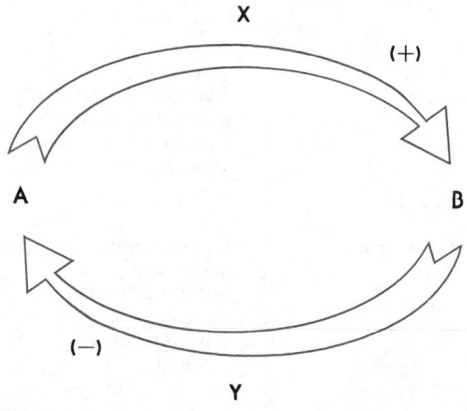

FIGURE 35-2 Closed-loop negative feedback system. This principle of control is applicable to all endocrine glands. (Redrawn from Harvey AM et al: The principles and practice of medicine, ed 18, Englewood Cliffs, NJ, 1972, Prentice-Hall, Inc.)

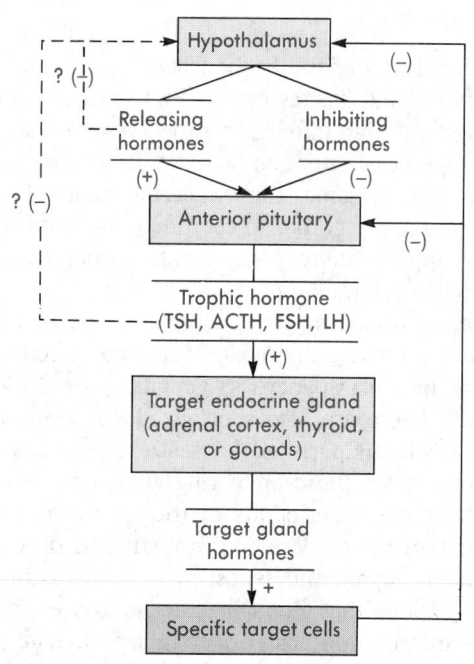

FIGURE 35-3 Complex feedback system between hypothalamus, anterior pituitary gland, target endocrine glands, and specific target cells. (Redrawn from Harvey AM et al: The principles and practice of medicine, ed 20, New York, 1980, Appleton-Century-Crofts.)

TABLE 35-1 Examples of negative feedback regulation of parathyroid hormone, antidiuretic hormone, and insulin

Stimulus		Gland A		Hormone X		Organ B		Substance Y
Decreased serum calcium	→ +	Parathyroid gland ↑ ⊖	→	Parathyroid hormone	⌐ ⌊→	Kidney, bone, gas- trointestinal tract	→	Increased serum calcium
Increased serum osmolality	→ +	Posterior pituitary ↑ ⊖	→	Antidiuretic hormone	→	Kidney	→	Reabsorption of water leads to decreased serum osmolality
Increased serum glucose	→ +	Beta cells of pancreas ↑ ⊖	→	Insulin	→	Fat cells, liver, muscle cells	→	Increased uptake of glucose leads to decreased serum glucose

roid gland, the adrenal cortex, or the gonads is adequate, the release of trophic hormones by the pituitary gland and/or of releasing hormone by the hypothalamus are inhibited by negative feedback. The level of trophic hormone and/or releasing hormone may, in turn, exert a negative feedback on the hypothalamus. Also, to control the level of selected hormones, the hypothalamus synthesizes and releases inhibiting hormones (Figure 35-3). The amounts of prolactin and growth hormone released by the anterior pituitary are in part controlled by a prolactin-inhibiting hormone (dopamine) and a growth hormone–inhibiting hormone (somatostatin, GHIH).

Although negative feedback control is a distinguishing feature of the endocrine system, not all hormones are controlled by it. For example, estrogen in males, testosterone in females, placental hormones, and hormones produced by ectopic tumors are not under feedback control.[20]

A second factor regulating hormone levels is *intrinsic rhythmicity*. These intrinsic rhythms can vary over minutes, days, or weeks. For example, adrenocorticotropic hormone (ACTH), cortisol, glucocorticoids, and growth hormone demonstrate daily circadian rhythms, whereas the reproductive hormones in females demonstrate a pattern that varies over several weeks.

These intrinsic rhythms are controlled by various factors. The environmental factor of sleep-wake patterns influences in some unknown way the circadian rhythms of growth hormone, ACTH, and cortisol. Age, growth, and development influence the intrinsic rhythmicity of gonadotropins and gonadal steroids. Neurogenic factors influence the intrinsic rhythm of other hormones such as prolactin.

Extrinsic factors such as pain, trauma, infection, and other stressors are a third factor influencing levels of selected hormones. These extrinsic factors can override the normal feedback mechanisms or intrinsic rhythmic-

ity and increase secretion of hormones above normal levels.

Last, the level of hormones is affected by excretion or metabolic inactivation. The liver and the kidneys are primarily responsible for hormonal inactivation and excretion, and diseases of these organs can result in increased hormone levels.

In summary, hormone levels are controlled by multiple mechanisms. Appreciation of these mechanisms helps to clarify the rationale for the various types of diagnostic testing used to assess pathologic conditions of the endocrine system.

RECEPTORS

The exact way in which hormones stimulate various cellular responses is not completely understood. No hormone is believed to initiate reactions in the cell de novo. The biochemical machinery of the cell responds to the presence of the hormone by increasing or decreasing the rate at which it carries out its functions, but all the equipment for the function of the cell is present in the cell.

It is hypothesized that hormones initiate cellular activity in one of two ways. The hormone initiates cellular activity by combining either with an intracellular receptor or a membrane receptor. Steroid hormones such as adrenal steroids, gonadal steroids, and active derivatives of vitamin D and thyroid hormone, which are lipid soluble, are believed to use intracellular receptors. These hormones freely cross the plasma membrane and combine with their specific intracellular receptor. The steroid-receptor complex is changed in size and conformation and is translocated to the nucleus, where it combines with acceptor sites located in the nucleus near the DNA sequences. The binding of the hormone-receptor complex initiates transcription of DNA, translation of RNA, and synthesis of protein. A summary of this model of hormone activation is shown in Figure 35-4.

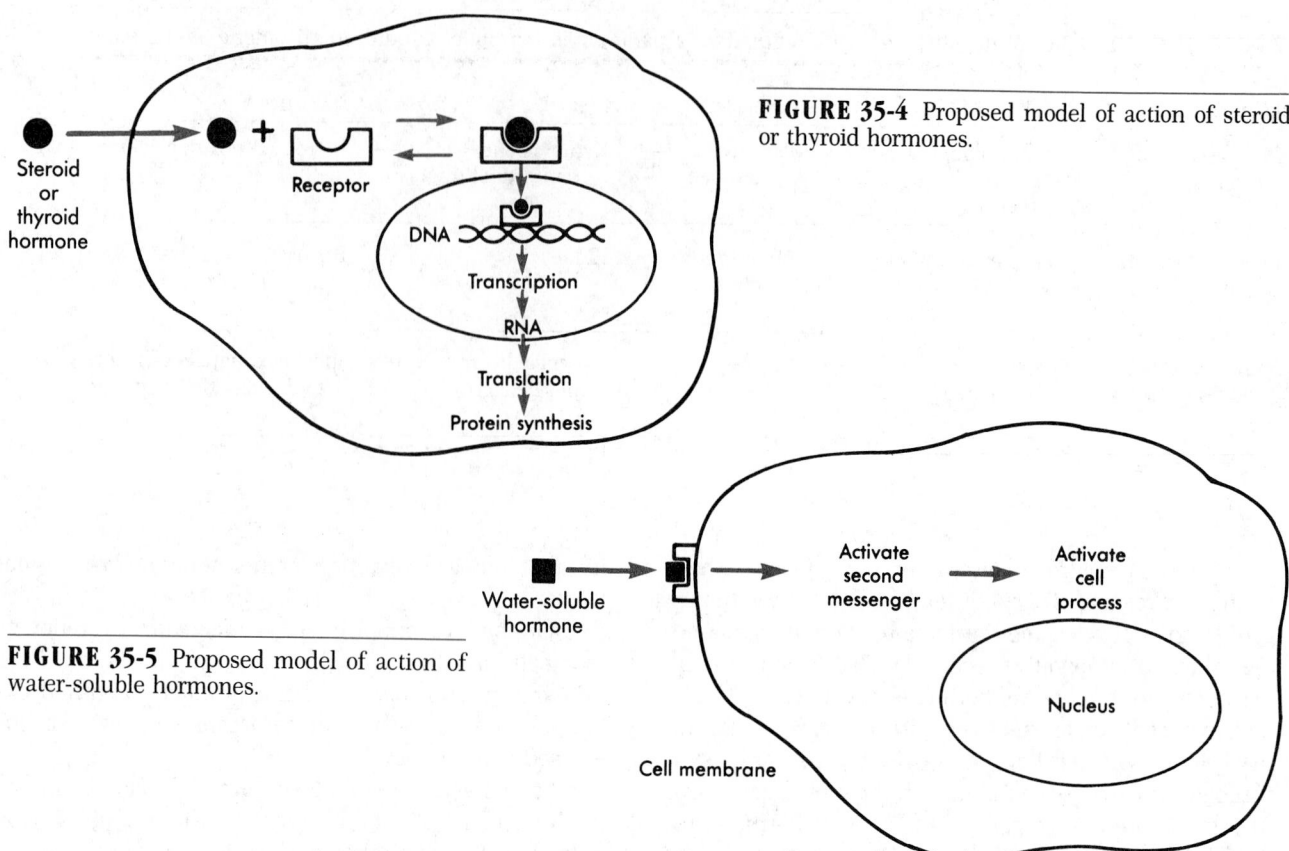

FIGURE 35-4 Proposed model of action of steroid or thyroid hormones.

FIGURE 35-5 Proposed model of action of water-soluble hormones.

Water-soluble hormones (hypothalamic-releasing hormones, anterior and posterior pituitary hormones, parathyroid hormone, calcitonin, insulin, glucagon, and biogenic amines) are believed to utilize membrane receptors. The hormone combines with its specific receptor on the plasma membrane, and this hormone-receptor combination activates a second messenger located inside the cell. The second messenger then initiates a sequence of events in the cytoplasm that results in altered cell function. Cyclic adenosine monophosphate (cyclic-AMP) has been identified as the second messenger for several hormones. It is hypothesized that the combination of the hormone with the receptor activates adenyl cyclase, which causes the formation of 3′, 5′-cyclic AMP from adenosine triphosphate (ATP). The cyclic AMP activates protein kinases. These activated kinases phosphorylate specific proteins in the stimulated cell and result in altered cell function.

Although cyclic AMP has been identified as a second messenger for several hormones, other compounds serve as second messengers. Calcium ions, calmodulin, adenosine, and prostaglandins are some of the other potential second messengers. A summary of this model of hormone activation is presented in Figure 35-5.

In summary, hormones initiate cellular activity by combining with specific receptors. Although hormonal-receptor interaction has been hypothesized to fall into

one of two major models, there may be hormones that use both models of hormone action.[10] Research on receptors is ongoing.

LOCATION OF GLANDS AND FUNCTION OF HORMONES

The various endocrine glands are located throughout the body (Figure 35-6). In addition to the glands depicted, there are endocrine cells throughout various parts of the gastrointestinal tract.

HYPOTHALAMUS AND PITUITARY GLAND

The hypothalamus, a part of the diencephalon, consists of numerous poorly defined nuclei. The hypothalamus forms the lower portion of the lateral walls and the floor of the third ventricle. It is bordered anteriorly by the optic chiasma. The hypothalamic sulcus and thalamus lie on the dorsal border; the internal capsule, subthalamic nuclei, and basis peduncle form the lateral boundaries. On its inferior surface the hypothalamus is continuous with the pituitary stalk. Figure 35-7 shows a sagittal section through the brain. The anterior, dorsal, and inferior boundaries are depicted. Although the hypothalamus is a very small area of the brain, it receives input directly or indirectly from almost every other part of the brain.

The *pituitary gland,* which is approximately 1 cm in

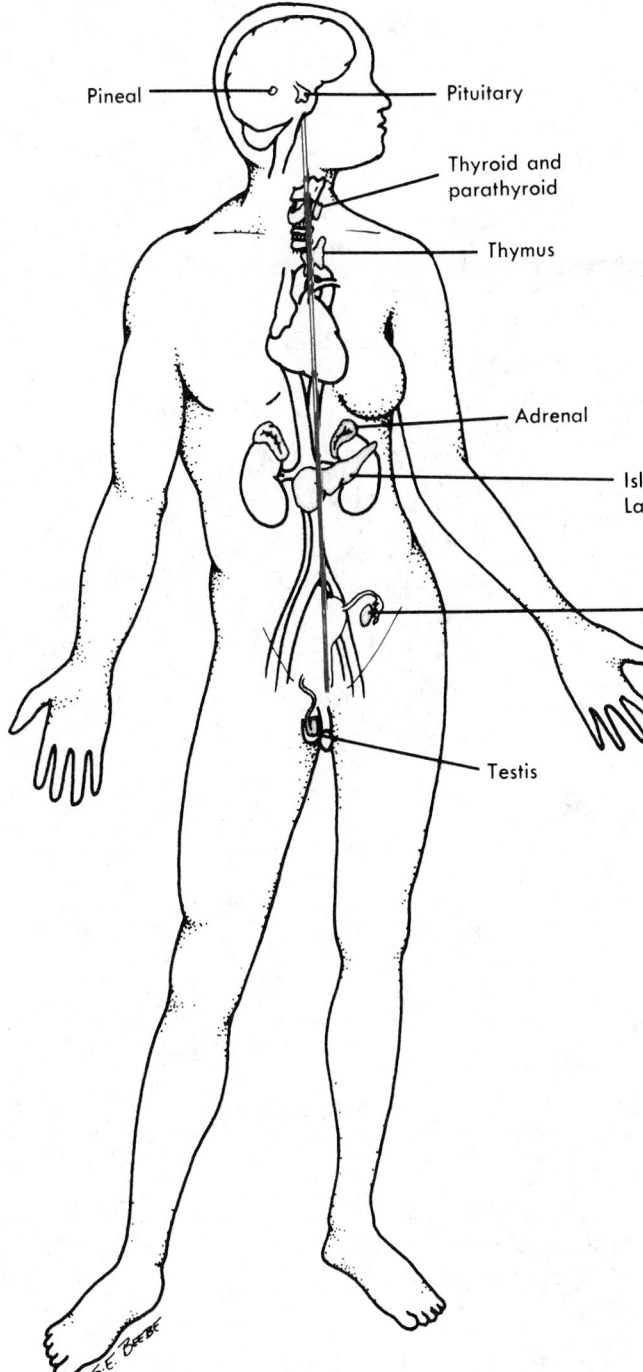

Pineal

Pituitary

Thyroid and parathyroid

Thymus

Adrenal

Islets of Langerhans

Ovary

Testis

FIGURE 35-6 Endocrine system. (From Tucker SM et al: Patient care standards, ed 4, St Louis, 1990, The CV Mosby Co.)

HYPOTHALAMIC-PITUITARY RELATIONSHIP

The hypothalamus serves as a critical link between the rest of the nervous system and the endocrine system. It controls both the posterior and anterior pituitary glands. By its control of the anterior pituitary gland, it controls other endocrine glands. Figure 35-8 depicts the connections between the hypothalamus and the pituitary gland. The hypothalamus is connected to the posterior pituitary gland by nerve tracts that originate in the paraventricular and supraoptic nucleus of the hypothalamus. Posterior pituitary hormones are actually synthesized in the hypothalamus and transported along nerve axons to the posterior pituitary gland where they are stored.

The hypothalamus and anterior pituitary gland are connected by the hypothalamic-hypophyseal portal blood supply. Blood entering the anterior pituitary gland has first passed through the hypothalamus. The hypothalamus regulates anterior pituitary function by the synthesis and secretion of releasing or inhibiting hormones into the hypothalamic-hypophyseal portal blood supply. These hormones are released in the anterior pituitary gland and stimulate the release of or inhibit the release of appropriate hormones.

The exact number and type of releasing and inhibiting hormones is unknown. Research has been extensive in this area. At present six releasing/inhibiting hormones have been identified: growth hormone–releasing hormone (GHRH), growth hormone–inhibiting hor-

size and weighs 500 mg, lies in the sella turcica of the middle cranial fossa. This gland is composed of two functionally distinguishable components: the adenohypophysis (anterior pituitary) and the neurohypophysis (posterior pituitary). The posterior pituitary is a continuation of the pituitary stalk. The anterior pituitary, which makes up 75% of the total gland, arises embryonically from an outpouching of ectoderm and fuses with the posterior pituitary.

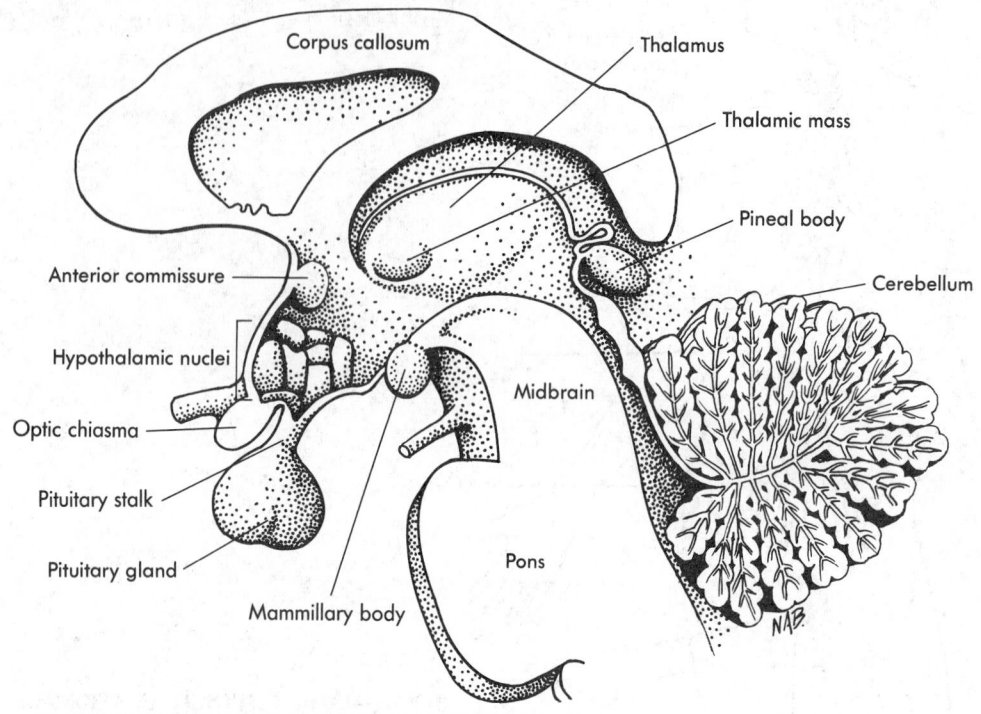

FIGURE 35-7 Sagittal section through the brain.

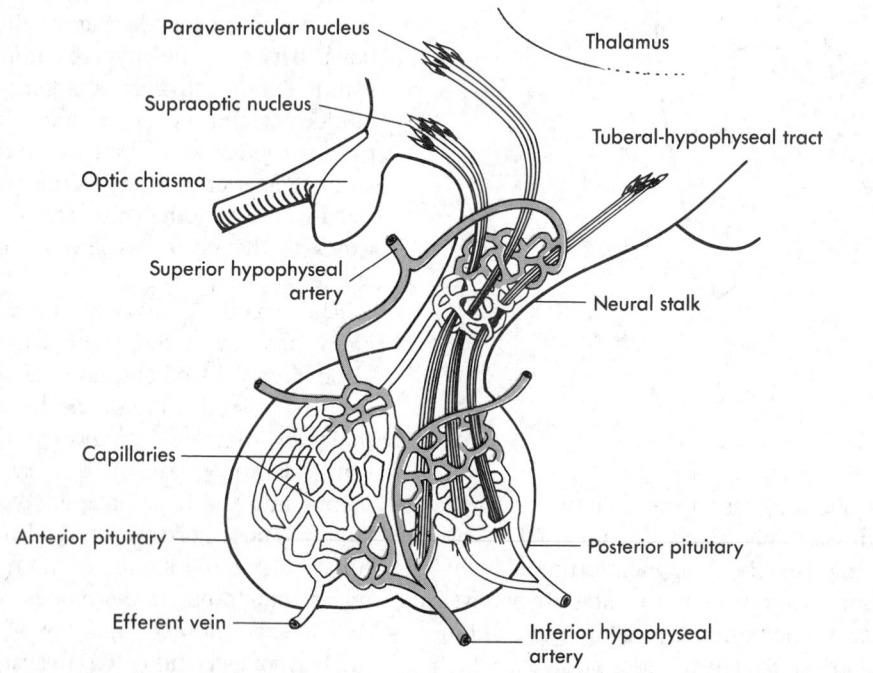

FIGURE 35-8 Hypothalamic pituitary connections. The hypothalamus connects to the posterior pituitary gland by nerve tracts. The connection between the hypothalamus and the anterior pituitary gland is vascular.

mone (GHIH, somatostatin), thyrotropin-releasing hormone (TRH), corticotropin-releasing hormone (CRH), gonadotropin-releasing hormone (GnRH), and dopamine (prolactin-inhibiting hormone).

Some researchers believe there is another PIH, as yet not chemically identified. There are also data to support the presence of a prolactin-releasing hormone, but this substance has not been identified. GnRH stimulates the release of both gonadotropins from the anterior pituitary gland.

PITUITARY HORMONES

The posterior pituitary gland stores and releases two hormones: antidiuretic hormone (ADH), or vasopressin, and oxytocin. Both of these hormones are synthesized in the paraventricular and supraoptic nucleus of the hypothalamus. The blood level of these two hormones is controlled by multiple factors that act either as stimulators or inhibitors. The regulation and function of antidiuretic hormone and oxytocin are outlined in Table 35-2.

The anterior pituitary gland produces six hormones. These hormones are produced in specific cells located throughout the anterior pituitary gland. The hormones and their regulation and functions are outlined in Table 35-3.

THYROID GLAND

The thyroid gland (Figure 35-9) is located in the anterior aspect of the neck just below the cricoid cartilage. It consists of two lobes connected by the isthmus that lies on the upper part of the trachea. The gland weighs approximately 20 gm and is composed of two distinct cell types: follicular cells and parafollicular cells. The follicular cells are responsible for thyroxine and triiodothyro-

TABLE 35-2 Posterior pituitary hormones, regulation, and function

Hormone	Regulation	Function

Antidiuretic hormone (ADH, vasopressin)	STIMULATORS
	Primary
	Increased serum osmolality (as little as 1% increase) via hypothalamic osmoreceptors
	Others
	Modest volume depletion via atrial volume receptors
	Modest hypotension via baroreceptors
	Stressors
	  Psychologic
	  Pain
	  Nausea and vomiting
	Chemicals
	  Cholinergic agonist
	  β-adrenergic agonist
	  Barbiturates
	  Morphine
	  Nicotine
	INHIBITORS
	Primary
	Decreased serum osmolality (as little as 1%) via osmoreceptors
	Modest increased volume and blood pressure via atrial volume receptors and baroreceptors
	Chemicals
	  Alcohol
	  α-adrenergic agonist
		Target organ: kidneys
		Major regulator of osmolality and body water volume
		Increases permeability of collecting ducts in kidney to water, resulting in increased H_2O reabsorption
		May stimulate H_2O intake by stimulating perception of thirst

Oxytocin	STIMULATORS
	Primary
	Suckling via neurogenic reflex conducted from afferent fibers in nipple to hypothalamus
	Others
	Uterine contraction via neurogenic reflex from afferent fibers in uterus
	INHIBITORS
	Stressors
	  Psychologic
	  Physical
	α-Adrenergic stimulation
		Target organ: breast tissue and uterus
		Results in milk "let-down" in lactating breast
		Causes increased uterine contraction after labor has begun; role in initiating labor unclear

TABLE 35-3 Anterior pituitary hormones, their regulation and function

Hormone	Regulation	Function

Growth hormone (GH)	Controlled by GHRH/GHIH
	GH shows episodic secretion with increases after eating (particularly a high-protein diet) and after onset of deep sleep (usually within 1-2 hours after sleep)
	Other stimuli that increase GH
	  Exercise (strenuous)
	  Hypoglycemia
	  Stressors
	  Chemicals
	    Arginine infusion
	    L-dopa
	    Clonidine
	    TRH in acromegaly
	    Adrenergic agonists
	    Beta-adrenergic antagonists
	Hyperglycemia decreases GH
		Target organ: whole body
		Possibly works on most tissue through action of somatomedin(s)
		Concerned with growth of cells, bones, and soft tissues
		Increases mitosis
		Affects carbohydrate, protein, and fat metabolism
		Increases blood glucose by decreasing glucose utilization; insulin antagonist
		Increases protein synthesis
		Increases lipolysis, free fatty acid levels, and ketone formation
		Increases electrolyte retention and extracellular fluid volume

Prolactin (PRL)	Controlled by prolactin-releasing hormone (PRH) and PIH; PRL chronically inhibited by hypothalamus
	PRL shows episodic secretions occurring during later hours of sleep
	Other stimulants
	  Stressors
	  Suckling
	  Chemicals
	    Estrogen
	    TRH
	    Dopamine antagonist
	    Chlorpromazine
	Chemicals that are dopamine agonists (L-dopa, bromocriptin) inhibit PRL
		Target organ: breast, gonads
		  Necessary for breast development and lactation
		  Regulator of reproductive function in males and females

Thyroid stimulating hormone (TSH)	Controlled by TRH and negative feedback from plasma T_4 levels.
	  Increase $T_4 \rightarrow$ decrease TSH
	  Decrease $T_4 \rightarrow$ increase TSH
		Target organ: thyroid gland
		  Necessary for growth and function of thyroid; controls all functions of thyroid

Adrenocorticotropin (ACTH)	Controlled by CRH and negative feedback by cortisol levels
	ACTH shows episodic secretion with rhythm that peaks between 6 and 8 AM
	Circadian pattern related to sleep-wake pattern and caused by increased CRH
	Physiologic and psychologic stressors (for example, hypoglycemia, infections, pain, anxiety) increase ACTH caused by increased CRH (override negative feedback); changes in cortisol influence ACTH
	  Increase cortisol $\rightarrow$ decrease ACTH
	  Decrease cortisol $\rightarrow$ increase ACTH
		Target organ: adrenal cortex gland
		  Necessary for growth and maintenance of size of adrenal cortex
		  Controls release of glucocorticoids (cortisol) and adrenal androgens
		  Minor role in release of mineralocorticoids (aldosterone)

Gonadotropins
  Follicle-stimulating hormone (FSH)
  Luteinizing hormone (LH) (also previously called interstitial cell–stimulating hormone (ICSH) in males)
	Secretion controlled by GnRH
	Amount of FSH secreted is decreased by inhibin in males
	Amount of LH secreted is decreased by testosterone in males
	Sex steroids in females exert a positive feedback on FSH and LH at certain times in the normal menstrual cycle and a negative feedback at other times
		Target organs: gonads
		  Stimulates gametogenesis and sex steroid production in males and females

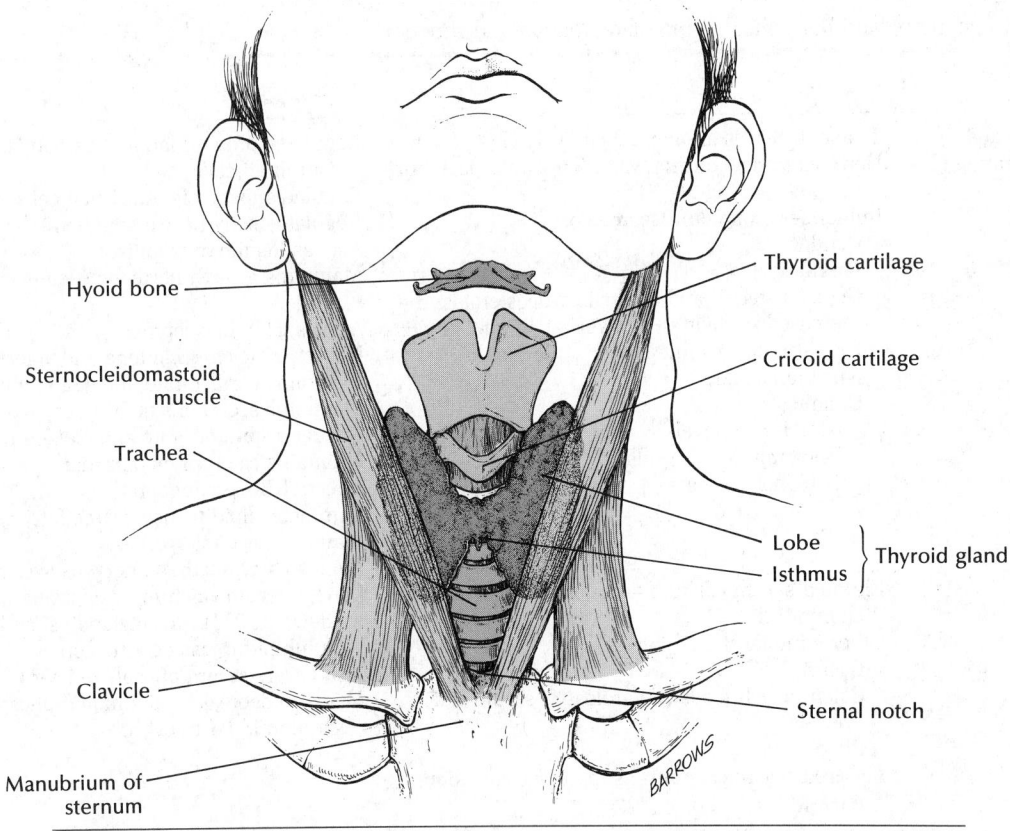

FIGURE 35-9 Midline neck structures; note the thyroid gland in the anterior neck. (From Malasanos L et al: Health assessment, ed 4, St Louis, 1990, The CV Mosby Co.)

nine hormone production. These processes are carried out under the control of thyroid-stimulating hormone (TSH) and TRH. Multiple steps are involved in the production of thyroid hormone (see the box below).

The parafollicular cells (C-cells) synthesize and secrete the hormone calcitonin that is involved with calcium metabolism. The thyroid hormones and their regulation and functions are outlined in Table 35-4.

PARATHYROID GLAND

The parathyroid gland consists of four minute glands, one each located on the posterior aspect of the upper and lower poles of each lobe of the thyroid. Occasionally, normal extra parathyroid glands are found. These may be on the thyroid gland, in the mediastinum, or behind the esophagus.

The parathyroid gland produces one hormone: parathyroid hormone (PTH). This hormone is continually synthesized. Figure 35-10 depicts the primary regulator of PTH and its function.

There are two factors related to parathyroid gland function that should be remembered. First, other factors like calcitonin levels and serum phosphate levels influence PTH secretion, probably by decreasing serum cal-

cium. Second, the biologic regulators probably never totally depress PTH secretion.[19]

ADRENAL GLAND

The adrenal glands are retroperitoneal abdominal organs that cap the upper pole of each kidney. Each gland consists of two glands: the outer gland is the *adrenal cortex,* and the inner core is the *adrenal medulla.* The cortex consists of three zones: the zona glomerulosa, zona fasciculata, and the zona reticularis.

PRODUCTION OF THYROID HORMONE

Steps in production of thyroid hormones by follicular cells
1. Uptake of iodide and oxidation of iodine
2. Production of thyroglobulin
3. Organification of thyroglobulin (iodine binds to tyrosine residues in thyroglobulin) to form 3-monoiodotyrosine and 3,5-diiodotyrosine
4. Coupling of mono- and di-iodo compounds to form thyroxine (T_4) or triiodothyronine (T_3)
5. Hormone stored in follicle attached to thyroglobulin
6. With appropriate stimulation, proteolysis cleaves T_4 and T_3 off thyroglobulin
7. T_3 and T_4 released and thyroglobulin recycled

TABLE 35-4 Thyroid gland hormones and their regulation and function

Hormone	Regulation	Functions

Thyroxine T_4 and Triiodothyronine (T_3)	T_4 and T_3 levels are controlled by TSH
	Hormones show diurnal variation with a peak during late evening
	Influences on amount secreted
	    Gender
	    Pregnancy
	    Gonadal steriod and adrenal corticosteroids; increased steroids = ↑ levels of T_4 and T_3
	    Exposure to extreme cold = ↑ levels
	    Nutritional state
	    Chemicals
	        GHIH = ↓ levels
	        Dopamine = ↓ levels
	        Catecholamines = ↑ levels
		Regulates protein, fat, and carbohydrate catabolism in all cells
		Regulates metabolic rate of all cells
		Regulates body heat production
		Acts as insulin antagonist
		Maintains growth hormone secretion, skeletal maturation
		Affects CNS development
		Necessary for muscle tone and vigor
		Maintains cardiac rate, force, and output
		Maintains secretions of GI tract
		Affects respiratory rate and oxygen utilization
		Maintains calcium mobilization
		Affects RBC production
		Stimulates lipid turnover, free fatty acid release, and cholesterol synthesis
		Regulates sympathetic nervous system activity

Calcitonin	Elevated serum calcium—major stimulant for calcitonin
	Other stimulants
	    Gastrin
	    Calcium-rich foods (regardless of serum Ca^{++} levels)
	    Pregnancy
	Lowered serum calcium—suppresses calcitonin release
		Lowers serum calcium by opposing bone-resorbing effects of PTH, prostaglandins, and calciferols by inhibiting osteoclastic activity
		Also lowers serum phosphate levels
		May also decrease calcium and phosphorus absorption in GI tract

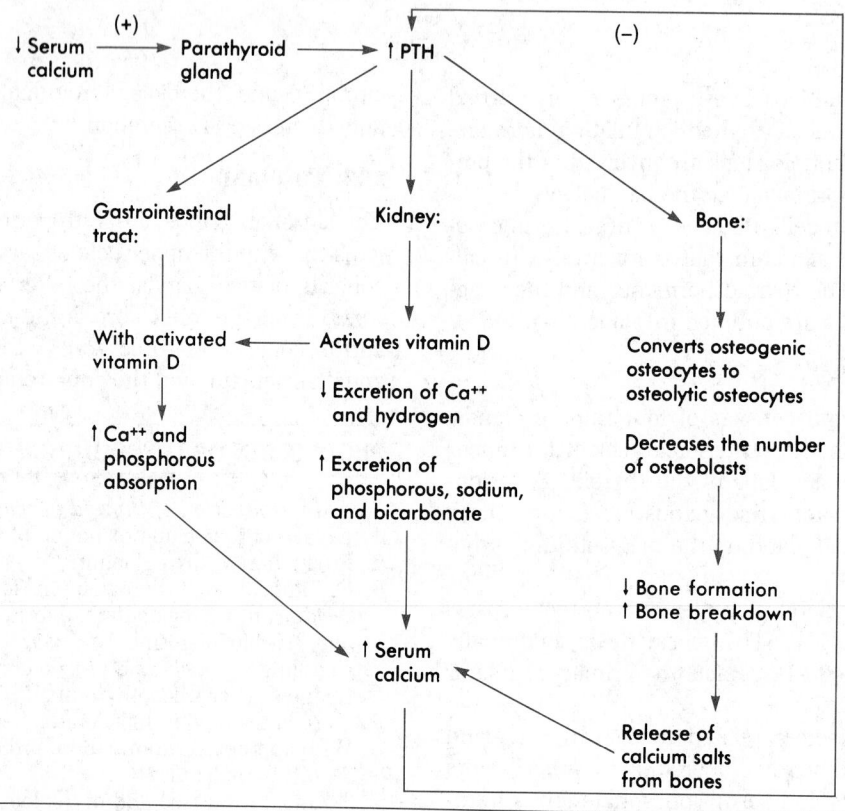

FIGURE 35-10 Regulation and function of PTH.

TABLE 35-5 Adrenal cortex hormones, their regulation and functions

Hormone	Regulation	Functions
Glucocorticoids (cortisol)	The level of cortisol is controlled by CRH/ACTH. Cortisol shows episodic secretion with a circadian rhythm that peaks between 6 and 8 AM; this circadian pattern follows the circadian pattern of CRH/ACTH. Physiologic and psychologic stressors (for example, hypoglycemia, hypoxia, pain, infection, trauma, anxiety) result in increased cortisol via increased CRH and ACTH. This stress response overrides the negative feedback cortisol normally exerts on ACTH.	Overall effect: maintain blood glucose level by increasing gluconeogenesis and decreasing rate of glucose utilization by cells. Increases protein catabolism Promotes lipolysis Antiinflammatory Degrades collagen Decreases T-lymphocyte participation in cellular-mediated immunity by decreasing circulating level of T-lymphocytes Increases neutrophils by increasing release and decreasing destruction Decreases new antibody release Decreases eosinophils, basophils, and monocytes Decreases scar tissue formation Increases RBC formation and possibly increases platelet formation Increases gastric acid and pepsin production Promotes sodium and water retention Maintains emotional stability
Mineralocorticoids (aldosterone)	Major regulator is renin-angiotensin system. When vascular volume or sodium is decreased, the renin-angiotensin system is activated (See Chapters 9, 23, and 47), and angiotensin II stimulates release of mineralocorticoids. Other regulators Increased serum potassium (K^+) directly stimulates adrenal cortex to release mineralocorticoids. CRH/ACTH system is a weak regulator	Maintains sodium and volume status Increases sodium reabsorption in distal tubules Increases potassium and hydrogen excretion in distal tubules
Adrenal androgens	Major regulator is CRH/ACTH system.	Responsible for some secondary sex characteristics in females; in males, work like gonadal steroids

Adrenal Cortex Hormones

The adrenal cortex produces three hormones: *mineralocorticoids* (aldosterone), produced in the zona glomerulosa; *glucocorticoids* (cortisol) and *androgens,* produced in the zona fasciculata and zona reticularis. The glucocorticoids and mineralocorticoids are not only secreted and used daily but are two major hormones that are secreted as part of the physiologic stress response to stressors, which is discussed in Chapter 9. The mineralocorticoids and glucocorticoids are necessary for life. Table 35-5 outlines the regulation and functions of the adrenal cortical hormones.

Adrenal Medulla Secretions

The adrenal medulla makes up approximately 10% of the total adrenal gland. The adrenal medulla arises embryonically from the neural crest and is really a modified sympathetic ganglion. The adrenal medulla is innervated by preganglionic splanchnic nerves. With stimulation of the sympathetic nervous system via the hypothalamus and medulla oblongata, the adrenal medulla is stimulated, and *catecholamines* (epinephrine and norepinephrine) are released. The catecholamines travel by blood to parts of the body and stimulate target cells. The catecholamine norepinephrine is also released from the terminals of postganglionic sympathetic fibers.

The adrenal medulla releases two different types of catecholamines, *epinephrine* and *norepinephrine*. The normal adrenal medulla secretes approximately 85% epinephrine and 15% norepinephrine. These catecholamines have different effects in the body because of the different receptors on body organs. These receptors are classified as α-adrenergic and β-adrenergic. β-receptors are subdivided into β_1- and β_2-receptors. β_1-receptors are located primarily in the heart, and β_2-receptors occur elsewhere in the body. α-receptors also can be subdivided into two types: α_1, which occur on target organs and are excitatory; and α_2, which occur at presynaptic sites and, when stimulated, inhibit release of the catecholamines. Much of what is known about adrenergic

TABLE 35-6 Effects of adrenal-medullary-sympathetic stimulation on body organs

Organ	Effect*
Heart	Increased conduction velocity, automaticity, contractility, rate, and stroke volume caused by β_1-stimulation
Blood vessels	
Coronary vessels, brain, lungs	Dilation caused by β_2-stimulation and autoregulatory phenomena
Skin, mucosa, abdominal viscera, renal and salivary gland vessels	Constriction caused by α_1-receptor stimulation; renal vessels have dopaminergic receptors also
Veins	Constriction caused by α_1-stimulation
Bronchial muscles	Relaxation caused by β_2-stimulation
Gastrointestinal tract	Inhibition of production of gastrointestinal secretions; decreased motility and contraction of sphincters
Gallbladder	Relaxation
Kidney	Increased renin secretion caused by β_2-stimulation
Urinary bladder	Relaxation of detrusor muscle and contraction of sphincter
Skin	Pilomotor muscle contraction and localized sweating
Liver	Glycogenolysis and gluconeogenesis caused by β_2-stimulation
Pancreas	Decreased secretion of exocrine cells; β_2-stimulation causes increased secretion of islet β-cells but α-stimulation causes decreased secretion of islet cells; α-effect predominates
Fat cells	Lipolysis
Brain	Increased alertness, restlessness
Eyes	Dilation of pupils and relaxation of ciliary bodies

*These total effects would be seen in the physiologic response to stressors as discussed in Chapter 9.

receptors is based on the effects of various pharmacologic agents.

Norepinephrine is a more potent stimulator of α-receptors, whereas epinephrine stimulates α- and β-receptors. The final effect on an organ of stimulation of the sympathetic nervous system and adrenal medulla depends on the type of receptors in a particular organ. Table 35-6 lists the effects of adrenal-medullary-sympathetic stimulation on body organs.

A small quantity of catecholamines is released at all times, and this helps to maintain homeostasis. In the presence of a major stressor, either physiologic or psychologic, increased amounts of catecholamines are released in an attempt to overcome the stressor and all

the effects listed in Table 35-6 may be seen. This increased adrenal-medullary-sympathetic stimulation is part of the *physiologic stress response*, which is discussed in more detail in Chapter 9.

PANCREATIC ENDOCRINE FUNCTIONS

The pancreas is both an exocrine and an endocrine gland. It lies retroperitoneally behind the stomach, with its head and neck in the curve of the duodenum, its body extending horizontally across the posterior abdominal wall, and its tail touching the spleen. The cells of the pancreas that serve the endocrine function are the *islets of Langerhans*. There are over 1 million islet cells spread throughout the total pancreas; these cells make up 1% to 2% of the pancreatic mass. The islets of Langerhans consist of four cell types: (1) α-cells, which make up 20% of the cells and secrete glucagon; (2) β-cells, which make up 70% of the cells and secrete insulin; (3) delta cells, which make up 10% of the cells and secrete somatostatin; and (4) F-cells, which secrete pancreatic polypeptide. The purposes of somatostatin and pancreatic polypeptide are unclear. The secretions of the α and β cells are discussed below.

INSULIN

Insulin is a protein hormone that is secreted as a prohormone. The removal of a connecting peptide (C-peptide) fragment results in the active hormone. Both insulin and C-peptide are secreted into the blood in equal amounts. Insulin has an unstimulated basal secretion that controls metabolism between meals. Insulin also shows meal-related increases. The major stimulus is glucose, but insulin secretion is also stimulated by the intake of amino acids. Acetylcholine increases insulin secretion, whereas catecholamines acting on α-adrenergic receptors inhibit insulin secretion.

Overall insulin is an anabolic hormone, and although it can affect every cell in the body, its major effects are seen on the liver, adipose tissue, and the muscle (see the box on the opposite page).

GLUCAGON

Glucagon, along with epinephrine, growth hormone, and glucocorticoids, functions as a counterregulatory hormone to insulin. Its overall function is to increase blood glucose. Glucagon is stimulated by a decreased blood glucose level and by increased amino acid levels. The purpose of glucagon is to increase blood glucose. The primary target of glucagon is the liver. In the liver, glucagon results in glycogenolysis. When the need for glucose is greater than can be provided by *glycogenolysis,* glucagon promotes amino acid transport from the muscle and stimulates *gluconeogenesis.* Glucagon also promotes lipolysis and ketone formation. Glucagon works with epinephrine, glucocorticoids, and growth

ACTION OF INSULIN

LIVER CELLS	ADIPOSE TISSUE	MUSCLE
Increases glycogenesis	Increases fatty acid synthesis	Increases glycogenesis
Increases fatty acid synthesis	Increases glycerol synthesis and formation of triglycerides	Increases amino acid uptake and protein synthesis
Decreases glycogenolysis, gluconeogenesis, and ketogenesis	Decreases lipolysis	Decreases protein catabolism

hormone in carrying out the metabolic functions designed to return the blood glucose to normal.

PHYSIOLOGIC CHANGES WITH AGING

Changes in the endocrine system are associated with normal aging. Endocrine dysfunction may result from cellular damage due to aging, wear and tear on the endocrine tissue from long-term use, or genetically programmed cellular changes.[12] Endocrine changes may result in altered synthesis and secretion of hormones, altered metabolism of hormones, altered circulatory levels of hormones, altered biologic activity, altered target cell and target tissue responsiveness, or altered intrinsic rhythms. Although findings are not consistent, the following is a summary of the major alterations in endocrine function that are most frequently reported.*

1. The most commonly seen change is decreased ovarian functioning, resulting in increased gonadotropins and changes in reproductive and sexual functioning. No similar change in males has been reported.
2. Impaired secretion of hypothalamic hormones or impaired response to feedback may influence endocrine system responsiveness to alterations in the internal environment, and thus to stressors.
3. The anterior pituitary gland shows morphologic changes with increased fibrosis and microadenoma formation, a decrease in basal levels of prolactin in females and a decrease in growth hormone and somatomedins.
4. Antidiuretic hormone secretion in response to changes in serum osmolality is increased, resulting in increased levels of ADH. However, elderly persons have alterations in renal function that decrease the ability to concentrate urine and can result in hyponatremia. Nocturia is commonly present.
5. Various changes in thyroid gland structure, including glandular atrophy, fibrosis, nodularity, and infiltrates have been found. The following changes in thyroid hormone levels have been reported:
   a. Decreased T_4 secretion and metabolism
   b. Decreased plasma T_3 levels
   c. Increased basal plasma TSH levels
   d. Decreased responsiveness in TSH secretion to TRH

Hypothyroidism is very common in the elderly. Whether all these changes in thyroid structure, function, or disease can be attributed to the aging process is unclear. Some of the early clinical manifestations of hypothyroidism, such as skin and hair changes, neurologic changes, or gastrointestinal change can be seen in elderly persons for other reasons, leading health care professionals to ignore or potentially misdiagnose the changes.

6. Calcium homeostasis is altered in the older adult. Changes found include decreased intake of calcium, negative calcium balance, bone loss, decreased intestinal adaptation to varied calcium intake, hypercalciuria, and decreased vitamin D levels. Age-related alterations in PTH may explain some of the changes in calcium homeostasis, but more research is needed.
7. The adrenal cortex gland, which is small and contains fibrous tissue, responds to feedback mechanisms and maintains circadian patterns of cortisol secretion in response to circadian patterns of ACTH. However, the amount of cortisol secreted is decreased because of decreased metabolic clearance and decreased usage. Thus increased blood cortisol levels result in decreased secretion. The amount of androgens secreted by the adrenal cortex is decreased, and the renin-aldosterone response to postural changes and volume depletion is depressed.
8. Impaired glucose tolerance in the elderly is multifactorial. Delayed glucose induced insulin secretion, altered hepatic handling of glucose, and impaired insulin-mediated glucose uptake are all part of the problem and result in elevated blood glucose levels after glucose loads such as eating. These changes may result in blood glucose values that are higher than what are usually considered normal but are not diagnostic for diabetes mellitus.
9. Non–insulin-dependent diabetes mellitus is one of the more common chronic diseases of the elderly.[21]

If the changes described in the preceding section are ignored, the elderly may be misdiagnosed. Particularly, they may be diagnosed as having diabetes mellitus when further assessment reveals this to be untrue, although diabetes mellitus does occur more frequently in the elderly. Changes in serum sodium and potassium must be carefully evaluated to differentiate changes re-

*References 1, 2, 4, 6, 9, 12, 16.

lated to aging from those that might be due to drugs such as diuretics, other diseases such as congestive heart failure, or diet. The potential role of changes in PTH in development of metabolic bone disease needs more exploration. It is important to remember that the hypothalamic-pituitary-adrenal axis and the hypothalamic-pituitary-thyroid axis, which are important in daily living and response to stressors, are intact but may be slower to respond.

Besides the changes listed above, changes in response to actual endocrine pathology have been reported. Some elderly persons with hyperthyroidism have subtle signs and symptoms that make diagnosis difficult. Elderly persons tolerate hypothyroidism better, and there may be a greater insufficiency of thyroid hormones when they are first diagnosed. Also, early signs of hypothyroidism may be overlooked because they can occur in normal aging in the absence of thyroid pathology.

SUBJECTIVE DATA

A review of the normal functions of all hormones as described on the preceding pages reveals that they influence four broad domains. These are: maintenance of a normal internal environment; energy production, storage, and utilization; growth and development; and reproductive and sexual function. Alterations in endocrine function lead to varied manifestations because of disruption in maintenance of a normal internal environment, inadequate energy production, stores and utilization, abnormal growth and development, and abnormal reproductive and sexual function. Systematic assessment of multiple parameters is necessary to define the healthiness of a person's endocrine system or needs. The anatomic location of endocrine glands precludes their direct assessment. A thorough history from the patient or significant others is absolutely necessary. Special attention should be paid to the patient's history regarding fluid/nutritional intake, elimination pattern, energy level, perception of changes in body characteristics, reproductive and sexual function, and tolerance to stressors.

FLUID/NUTRITIONAL INTAKE

Endocrine abnormalities can lead to alteration in fluid and food intake (increased or decreased) that may or may not be associated with weight loss or weight gain. Many of the endocrine problems are chronic and require long-term special diets, and—at times—fluid restrictions. Qualitative and quantitative assessment of food intake is necessary to determine the cause of weight loss or gain, adequacy of intake for normal metabolic needs, and adherence to any special diet. Having the patient list food and fluid taken on the previous day

is an excellent way to assess fluid/nutritional intake. The history must include alcohol and snacks. The preferences of the patient with regard to types of food, as well as times of eating, are important in providing a diet that meets nutritional needs. Elements such as a pleasant environment, mouth care prior to meals, and small meals to decrease anorexia and nausea may be necessary. Assessment of how the patient is tolerating foods and fluids must be ongoing.

ELIMINATION PATTERN

The endocrine system is involved in maintenance of water and electrolyte balance. The history should include information on the frequency, approximate amount, and color of urinary elimination. The presence of *nocturia* or *dysuria* is also noted. In endocrine disease, depending on the cause, there may be a history of increased output and increased thirst, or decreased output and increased weight. Some patients may be on diuretics, and their adherence to the therapy should be assessed. The frequency and color of bowel movements also are determined. Information concerning constipation or other changes in bowel habits that may be caused by changes in water balance, dietary intake, or sluggishness of the bowel may be elicited. Treatment of pathology may include changes in diet and fluid intake that will influence elimination. The patient's previous pattern of elimination will help the nurse teach about needed changes such as decreasing fluid intake after dinner to decrease nocturia.

ENERGY LEVEL

Because the endocrine system is directly involved in the metabolism (storage and utilization) of nutrients for energy, pathology will usually decrease the person's energy level. Many patients will complain of "not being able to do their normal things." It is important to assess the person's energy level and to use this as a guide for helping plan activities of daily living. Some persons need help in adjusting their activities to allow for rest periods; they may need assistance in eliminating activities or in changing the ways they do activities to conserve energy.

Most endocrine problems can be well controlled so that permanent changes in life-style will not be necessary. Recovery may be slow, however; and the patient's physical status may be so damaged that, although the energy level may be normal, additional time will be required for complete recovery.

PERCEPTIONS OF CHANGES IN BODY CHARACTERISTICS

Changes in hair distribution, body proportions, voice, skin pigmentation, and facial appearance may accompany problems of the endocrine system. A description of changes by patients or their significant others is very important, because characteristics of persons vary so greatly and changes may not be so extensive that observation alone will pick them up.

The collection of information regarding changes in body characteristics is important not only in helping to define the physiologic problem but also in identifying potential or present emotional or psychologic problems. Some of the changes that occur with endocrine problems are irreversible even when problems are controlled. Body characteristics are part of the identity of the person, and the person may have problems dealing with the changes. (See Chapter 18 for a detailed discussion of body image.)

REPRODUCTIVE AND SEXUAL FUNCTION

The endocrine system is very involved with reproductive functions. A thorough reproductive and sexual history must be obtained. Data regarding the menstrual cycle (onset, frequency of menses, duration, amount of flow), presence of problems with the cycle (for example, menorrhagia), presence of impotence, and any perceived problem with fertility should be obtained. The history should also include information about satisfaction with sexual relationships for two reasons. First, sometimes the first changes in reproductive functioning will manifest themselves as changes in sexual satisfaction. Second, reproductive changes may not be a problem for the patient if sexual satisfaction is maintained. For example, infertility may not be a concern if childbearing is not a desired outcome (see Chapter 51).

TOLERANCE TO STRESSORS

The endocrine system helps the body respond to all types of physical and psychologic stressors. The patient or significant others should be questioned in relation to the person's ability (or change in ability) to tolerate stressors. Such things as intolerance to heat and cold, increased frequency of infections, increased irritation, euphoria, depression, increased crying, or increased anger may be elicited. Depending on the person's ability to handle stressors, special environmental controls to decrease the chance of infection and to maintain a consistent physical and emotional environment may be necessary.

OTHER SUBJECTIVE INFORMATION

Each endocrine problem has unique clinical manifestations that will be described in Chapters 36 and 37. As part of the history for a patient with a known diagnosis, the patient should be asked if continued signs and symptoms associated with the specific uncontrolled pathology are still present. In addition, information regarding whether the patient is experiencing any signs and symptoms of any uncontrolled endocrine pathology is elicited. The last area to be assessed concerns the patient's teaching-learning needs. The person's learning style, adherence to the prescribed therapeutic regimen, difficulty in carrying out the regimen, and other self-management skills are determined.

OBJECTIVE DATA

The collection of objective data about the endocrine system may require a complete physical examination. The major areas in which abnormalities may be found are discussed next. Collection of this data requires a thorough inspection and use of the techniques of palpation and auscultation. (See the box below for outline of areas to be examined with a head-to-toe approach.)

Inspection should be used to assess the patient's growth and developmental status. Such things as height, weight, body proportions, amount and distribution of muscle mass, fat distribution, skin pigmentation, and hair distribution should be assessed. A great variation in these parameters exists in the general population, and often the changes will not be obvious. Inspection of family members for like characteristics will provide information as to whether the characteristics seen in the patient are caused by hereditary or pathophysio-

---

SUMMARY OF OBJECTIVE DATA TO BE COLLECTED USING A HEAD-TO-TOE APPROACH

General	General appearance, body proportions (normal for age), height, weight, general body characteristics, any skin abrasions, sores, wounds, temperature, respiratory rate, type of respiration
Skin	Pigmentation, turgor, presence of edema, sweating, flushing
Face/scalp	Hair distribution, change in amount of facial/scalp hair, presence of exopthalmos
Oral cavity	Mucous membrane moisture
Neck	Jugular veins, thyroid gland
Cardiovascular	Blood pressure and pulse, check for orthostatic changes; temperature; more extensive evaluation indicated if problem identified
Abdomen	Abdominal striae
Musculoskeleton	Muscle mass, strength
Nervous system	Alertness, responsiveness, mood, tremors; possible necessity of a more extensive evaluation if problem is evident

logic alterations. The patient's alertness, responsiveness, and speech patterns can be assessed when the history is being collected.

The endocrine system plays a major role in growth and development, metabolism of food products, and regulation of sex hormones. All of these functions, if affected, cause changes in body characteristics. Some examples of specific changes are (1) *dwarfism* caused by thyroid and pituitary problems; (2) changes in fat distribution, producing *buffalo hump* and *thickened girdle* from adrenocortical excess; (3) presence of *purplish striae* instead of white striae because of adrenocortical excess; (4) *muscle wasting* with a wide variety of endocrine problems; and (5) *change in sexual characteristics* because of abnormalities of hormonal levels. All of these changes can be identified during inspection.

Inspection and palpation are used to check skin turgor, mucous membrane moisture, and jugular vein distension (JVD), and to check for the presence of edema. All of these data will give information about the fluid and electrolyte status of the person, which can be changed with almost any endocrine problem.

Following are changes that may be found:

1. The finger should slide over the mucous membrane easily. In states of fluid depletion as would be seen in diabetes mellitus, adrenocortical insufficiency, and possibly diabetes insipidus the mucous membranes are sticky.
2. Edema as might be seen in adrenocortical excess can be graded from 1+ to 4+ (see Chapter 23).
3. Skin turgor can be checked on the forearm, on the forehead, or over the sternum.
4. Abnormal JVD may be present with fluid overload.

Assessment of cardiovascular status is imperative. A minimal assessment includes checking orthostatic blood pressure and pulse. If fluid volume or electrolyte problems are present, a more extensive evaluation of such things as rhythm and heart sounds will be necessary.

Of all the endocrine organs discussed, only the thyroid will be routinely examined. In disease states, sometimes the pancreas and parathyroid gland can be palpated. The thyroid gland is usually examined along with examination of the head and neck. Palpation of the thyroid provides information about the size, shape, and symmetry of the gland, and the presence of nodules or tenderness. Auscultation may be used to assess for bruits.

DIAGNOSTIC TESTS

Endocrine dysfunction can in most instances be classified as resulting from hypersecretion or hyposecretion. The excess or deficient secretion can result from primary dysfunction of the endocrine gland; abnormal functioning of the pituitary gland, resulting in second-

---

PREPARATION OF PATIENTS FOR DIAGNOSTIC TESTS

Physical preparation as ordered
Explain purpose of test
Explain what to expect prior to and during the test
Explain any special care after the test

---

ary thyroid, adrenal, or gonadal dysfunction; abnormal endocrine gland functioning secondary to a nonendocrine disease; ectopic secretion of hormones by nonendocrine tissue; or from iatrogenic causes. Although most diseases can be classified in one of these categories, endocrine dysfunction can result from abnormal receptor functioning or intracellular responses. Diagnostic tests are used to evaluate the level of hormones in the blood (both basal and cyclic changes); the adequacy of endocrine tissue in secreting hormone in response to exogenous stimulants; the interrelationships between the hypothalamus, anterior pituitary gland, and other endocrine glands controlled by the anterior pituitary hormones; and the various substrates controlled by the endocrine system.

In most potential disease states several tests are necessary. Most of the tests of the endocrine system require taking samples of blood; some cause discomfort, and some require fasting. The nurse is responsible for preparing the patient appropriately. The routine physical preparation for any test will vary from institution to institution. Besides carrying out the physical preparation, the nurse teaches the patient as appropriate (see the box above).

Because the endocrine system affects fluid and electrolytes, patients with suspected pathology or those being evaluated to establish total health status will have serum electrolytes evaluated. In this section specific diagnostic tests for evaluation of particular glands will be described. The diagnostic tests for each gland are discussed separately.

PITUITARY FUNCTION TESTING

Pituitary gland malfunction can lead to a wide variety of symptoms, depending on which hormone is in excess or in deficit. The pituitary gland, as described previously, is interrelated with functions of the thyroid, the adrenal glands, and the gonads. The tests for the function of the pituitary with regard to TSH, ACTH, and gonadotropins will be discussed when the diagnostic tests of these glands are discussed. Pituitary malfunction may be associated with pituitary tumors, and skull x-ray films to assess the size of the pituitary gland will be carried out. Computed tomography (CT) scanning or magnetic resonance imaging (MRI) may be used to demonstrate the presence of intrasellar masses. In some instances pneumoencephalograms may be necessary to define the size of the mass or to exclude empty sellar syndrome.

GROWTH HORMONE

The absence or deficit of growth hormone (somatotropin, [GH]) leads to dramatic changes in appearance. Diagnostic tests for somatotropin will include skeletal x-ray films to assess changes in bone structure. Assay of growth hormone is possible. GH release follows a diurnal pattern; basal levels can best be determined in the morning, but they are usually less than 3 μg/ml. Growth hormone secretion can be stimulated by L-dopa, bromocriptine, and hypoglycemia. The provocative tests are done as follows: (1) basal levels of GH are determined; (2) L-dopa (500 mg orally), bromocriptine (5 mg orally), or insulin (0.1 U/kg IV) is given; and (3) blood is drawn at intervals up to 120 minutes after stimulation. GH usually peaks at approximately 60 minutes after provocative stimulation.

PROLACTIN

Prolactin excess is seen in the presence of some pituitary tumors, or it may be idiopathic. Prolactin deficiency may result in failure of postpartum lactation. Levels of prolactin can be measured by radioassay; the normal level is 0 to 23 ng/ml. Provocative tests for prolactin with the use of chlorpromazine or thyroid-releasing hormone (TRH) are available. The tests are done as follows: (1) basal levels of prolactin are measured; (2) chlorpromazine (0.7 mg/kg IM) or TRH (400 μg IV) is given; and then (3) serum levels of prolactin are drawn at timed intervals up to 240 minutes.

ANTIDIURETIC HORMONE (ADH)

Absence of ADH leads to a disease called *diabetes insipidus*. The major symptom of this problem is an output of large quantities of dilute urine (greater than 7 to 11 L per day). Before diabetes insipidus can be conclusively diagnosed, the patient must be shown to have a deficiency in ADH, and the patient's kidney must be able to respond to ADH. Exogenous sources of ADH have no effect if the patient's kidney cannot respond. Exogenous ADH will increase the osmolality of the urine, whether the dilute urine is caused by excess intake of water or by diabetes insipidus. The differentiation is made between these two conditions by demonstrating response or lack of response to osmolality changes in the serum.

WATER DEPRIVATION TEST

Water is withheld for 4 to 18 hours, and the person's response to this deprivation is documented. A person without diabetes insipidus will respond with a rapid decrease in urine volume and an increase in urine osmolality. A patient with diabetes insipidus will have no decrease in volume and no increase in urine osmolality.

The person who can not produce ADH is susceptible to vascular collapse, because the massive output of urine will continue unabated. Close monitoring for impending collapse during the test is required. Monitoring should include hourly vital signs, urine output, and specific gravity. If a weight loss greater than three to five percent of body weight occurs, the test should be terminated. The patient with *psychogenic polydipsia* may have extreme behavioral problems associated with the deprivation of water and will need emotional support during this period of time.

THYROID FUNCTION TESTING

Testing for thyroid function can be made at the hypothalamic, pituitary, thyroid, or serum levels. The major tests and their procedures, preparations, and interpretations are presented in Table 35-7. The most commonly used tests are serum thyroxine (T_4), serum triiodothyronine (T_3), and free thyroxine index (FT_4I).

PARATHYROID FUNCTION TESTING

Because the maintenance of normal calcium and phosphorus metabolism involves multiple systems besides the parathyroid (skeletal, gastrointestinal, and urinary), when parathyroid function is being assessed, the patient will also have diagnostic tests of these other systems. This is necessary to determine whether the problem with calcium and phosphorus metabolism is caused by altered parathyroid metabolism or by other disease states. In addition, because calcium has a very important role in the maintenance of normal neuromuscular irritability and because hypocalcemia can be lethal, the patient will be assessed and continually monitored for the presence of Trousseau's and Chvostek's signs when hypoparathyroidism is suspected (see Chapter 23).

The specific tests of parathyroid function consist of serial lab determinations of serum calcium and phosphorus, urinary calcium, and serum alkaline phosphatase. Normally, serum calcium levels are 8 to 11 mg/100 ml, serum phosphorus levels are 2.5 to 4.5 mg/100 ml, urinary calcium excretion in 24 hours is 75 to 175 mg, and serum alkaline phosphatase measures 50 to 135 IU/L.

High levels of serum calcium with low levels of serum phosphorus and high urine calcium indicate *hyperparathyroidism*. Associated elevations of alkaline phosphatase indicate bone destruction. Low serum calcium with high serum phosphorus and low urine calcium indicate *hypoparathyroidism*. Parathyroid hormone levels can be measured by radioimmunoassay. Normal levels depend on the serum calcium level. High levels of PTH in the presence of high levels of calcium indicate hyperparathyroidism. Low levels of PTH in the presence of low levels of serum calcium indicate hypoparathyroidism.

TABLE 35-7 Tests of thyroid function

Function Test	Procedure and Preparation	Interpretation
HYPOTHALAMUS LEVEL TEST		
TRH stimulation test	TRH is given IV and then serum thyroid-stimulating hormone (TSH) levels are repeatedly measured. Patient may feel facial flushing, the urge to urinate, or nausea for 5 minutes after injection. These are self-limiting and not complications.	Normal serum TSH begins to rise at 10 min and peaks at 45 min, subnormal tests reflect diminished TSH reserve; supranormal response occurs in patients with hypothyroidism of thyroid origin; no response occurs in most patients with thyrotoxicosis except when it is caused by excess TSH.
PITUITARY LEVEL TESTS		
TSH radioimmunoassay	Blood sample is taken; no special preparation is needed.	Test directly measures TSH levels; measurement aids in differentiating primary and secondary hypothyroidism; values are elevated in primary hypothyroidism because of loss of negative feedback. Test may also be used to diagnose thyrotoxicosis. With the new assay methods, the presence of TSH in serum rules out thyrotoxicosis. If TSH is undetectable, thyrotoxicosis is confirmed.
TSH stimulation test	Baseline levels of radioactive iodine uptake (RAIU) and protein-bound iodine (PBI) are taken, TSH injection is given, and repeat RAIU and PBI levels are taken.	Test assists in differentiating between primary and secondary hypothyroidism; in primary hypothyroidism repeat level of RAIU and PBI stays the same; if they become normal, this indicates hypothyroidism caused by too little TSH (secondary).
THYROID LEVEL TESTS		
RAIU	A tracer dose of radioactive iodine is given by mouth. At 2, 6, and 24 hr following administration, scintillation detector is placed over neck in region of thyroid and amount of accumulated iodine is measured; excess iodine in any foods, cough medicine, x-ray media, other medications, and enriched iodine foods affect test by giving low readings. Diarrhea, causing decreased absorption of tracer dose, gives low readings. Renal failure, causing decreased excretion can cause elevated readings. No radiation precautions are necessary.	Normal thyroid will take up 5% to 35% of tracer dose. Increased uptake occurs in hyperthyroidism. Excess tracer dose is excreted in urine and can be measured. Urine is collected for 24 hr; decreased amounts in urine indicate hyperthyroid state.
Thyroid scan	Dose of radioactive iodine or labeled pertechnitate is given, and scintillation scan is done. Scanner is moved over thyroid, and a picture of distribution of radioactivity is recorded. No radiation precautions are necessary.	Size, shape, and anatomic function of gland are assessed; areas of increased or decreased uptake are noted.
Thyroid ultrasound	Thyroid is assessed by ultrasound.	Test is helpful in defining "cold" area as cystic or solid.
Thyroid suppression test	RAIU test and serum T_4 levels are done. Patient is given thyroid hormone for 7-10 days and RAIU and serum T_4 tests are repeated	If euthyroid (normal), repeat RAIU and serum T_4 levels will be low; failure of hormone therapy to suppress RAIU and serum T_4 indicates hyperthyroidism.

ADRENAL FUNCTION TESTING

The adrenal function tests can be divided into those designed to test *medullary* function and those designed to test *cortical* function.

ADRENAL CORTICAL FUNCTION TESTS

Since the adrenal cortex affects so many physiologic functions, tests that are diagnostic for many disorders may be ordered. Analysis of blood to ascertain electrolyte balance, a glucose tolerance test to determine the

TABLE 35-7 Tests of thyroid function—cont'd

Function Test	Procedure and Preparation	Interpretation
TESTS RELATED TO SERUM LEVELS OF THYROID HORMONE		
Thyroxine-binding globulin (TBG)	Blood sample is taken; no special preparation is needed.	Test measures levels of TBG; TBG can be elevated or depressed by other conditions unrelated to thyroid problems; it is helpful in determining amount of bound and active T_3 and T_4.
Serum T_4 concentration	Radioassay of blood is done; no special preparation is needed.	Test measures circulating thyroxine that is bound to TBG and free T_4; normal values are 4.7-11 μg/100 ml. Hyperthyroidism and increased TBG such as occurs in pregnancy and estrogen therapy causes increased T_4 values. Hypothyroidism and decreased TBG as seen with glucocorticoid therapy and hypoproteinemia causes decreased T_4 values.
Serum T_3 concentrations	Radioassay of blood sample is done; no special preparation is needed	Test measures circulating T_3 that is bound to TBG and free T_3; normal values are 70-170 ng/100 ml and are elevated in T_3 thyrotoxicosis; variations in TBG can influence test results as they do for serum T_4.
Triiodothyronine resin uptake (T_3U)	Blood sample is drawn; in laboratory, resin and radioactive T_3 are added to sample of blood. Radioactive T_3 will bind to unoccupied sites of TBG. Excessive radioactive T_3 will bind to resin. Radioactive counts are done on blood and resins to determine amount of T_3 (radioactive) bound to resin.	Normally 25% to 30% of radioactive T_3 will bind to resin; in hyperthyroidism, where there are increased amounts of endogenous thyroid hormone, value of amount binding to resin will be increased; in hypothyroidism, T_3 resin uptake will be low. This test is not a measure of the patient's endogenous T_3 level. Test is affected by total amount of TBG. In wasting diseases where amount of TBG may be decreased, reading may be falsely elevated. In conditions such as pregnancy and estrogen therapy, abnormal amounts of TBG may be available, and a false-low resin uptake may be obtained; phenytoin (Dilantin) and salicylates compete with thyroxine for TBG sites and may give false-negative T_3 resin uptake.
Free T_4 and free T_3 (FT_4 and FT_3)	Blood sample is taken; special laboratory procedures are required.	Test measures unbound metabolically active T_4 or T_3. These are difficult tests and are not used frequently. Instead FT_4I is calculated; FT_4I varies directly with FT_4.
Free T_4 index (FT_4I)	Serum T_4 and T_3U are measured.	Free T_4I is product of serum T_4 and T_3U; changes in TBG cause reciprocal alterations in serum T_4 and T_3U so that FT_4I stays normal.
Thyroid antibodies	Blood sample is taken. In laboratory, RBCs are latex-coated with thyroid globulin and mixed with blood.	Test may differentiate cause of thyroid enlargement; if antibodies are present, agglutination occurs.

ability of the patient to use carbohydrates, and a test of the ability of the renal tubules to concentrate and dilute urine will probably be done. In addition, x-ray films of the kidney area may be taken to ascertain the presence of adrenal tumors.

Diagnostic tests of adrenocortical function include tests of all three types of hormonal secretions. Plasma cortisol follows a diurnal pattern and is measured at 8 AM and 4 PM. Plasma aldosterone, angiotensin II, and renin are measured to evaluate the renin-angiotensin-aldosterone system. Plasma levels of aldosterone are increased by dietary potassium loading, sodium restriction, and assumption of an upright position. Aldosterone levels may be measured before and after manipulating these factors. Plasma levels of androgens are also measured to evaluate the adrenal androgen system. ACTH levels can also be measured.

Twenty-four–hour urine collections may also be ana-

TABLE 35-8 Tests of adrenocortical function

Function Test	Procedure and Preparation	Interpretation
ACTH stimulation test (various tests available)	Synthetic adrenocorticotropic hormone (ACTH) is given in 500-1000 ml of normal saline at 2 U/24 hr; then 17-OHCS and plasma cortisol levels are measured; alternative way is to infuse 25 units of ACTH over an 8-hr period on 2-3 days and measure 17-OHCS and plasma cortisol levels on these days.	Normally 17-OHCS excretion increases to 25 mg/24 hr, and plasma cortisol increases to 40 µg/100 ml or greater; in patients with secondary adrenal insufficiency, the 17-OHCS rate is 3-20 mg/24 hr, and the cortisol level is 10-40 µg/100 ml
Screening ACTH stimulation test	ACTH, 25 U, is given IM, and plasma cortisol level is measured before and 30 and 60 min after tests.	Normally plasma cortisol increases 7 µg/100 ml
Cortisone suppression test	Twenty-four-hour urine specimen for 17-OHCS is collected for baseline; dexamethasone, 0.5 mg, is given every 6 hr for 2 days; 24-hr urine is collected for these 2 days.	Dexamethasone suppresses pituitary secretion of ACTH and thus steroid levels; normally by second day of dexamethasone, 24-hr urinary level of OHCS should drop more than 50% below baseline. Patients with adrenocortical excess (primary) will not show decrease in 24-hour urine levels; patients with secondary adrenocortical excess will have drop, but less than 50%.
Screening suppression test	Dexamethasone, 1 mg, is given at 12 PM. At 8 AM cortisol level is drawn.	Normally cortisol should be less than 5 µg/100 ml.
Mineralocorticoid suppression test (various tests are available)	Saline, 500 ml/hr, for 4 hr is infused intravenously. An alternative is that patient is placed on normal sodium diet (100 mEq) or high sodium diet (200 mEq). After patient is in sodium balance, deoxycorticosterone acetate (DOCA) (10 mg q12h) is administered IM for 3-5 days.	Normally saline infusion depresses plasma aldosterone to <8 µg/100 ml if patient has been on a sodium-restricted diet and to <5 µg/100 ml if patient has been on a normal sodium diet. Normal persons on a sodium diet of 100 mEq/day will have a 70% decrease in aldosterone.

lyzed for 17-ketosteroids (17-KS), 17-ketogenic steroids (17-KGS), and 17-hydroxycorticosteroids (17-OHCS). These compounds are metabolites of the hormones produced by the adrenal gland. These 24-hour urine collections require special preservatives, and the nurse should know the institution's requirements and make sure the appropriate container is available.

In addition to the above studies, other definitive tests are available to determine whether hypofunction or hyperfunction of the adrenal cortex is present and to establish whether the malfunction is caused by a primary adrenal cortical problem or whether the malfunction is secondary to pituitary malfunction. These studies are described in Table 35-8.

ADRENAL MEDULLARY FUNCTION TESTS

The function of the adrenal medulla can be assessed by the assay of catecholamines and their metabolites in the urine. A 24-hour urine collection is carried out; catecholamines or the end product, 3-hydroxy-4-methoxymandelic acid, also called vanillylmandelic acid (VMA) is assayed.

Pressor tests to establish a diagnosis of *pheochromocytoma* (adrenal-medullary tumor) require manipulation of the blood pressure. In one test, histamine, 0.01 to

0.025 mg, is given intravenously. A dramatic rise in blood pressure of at least 50 mm Hg higher than the elevation provoked by the immersion of the patient's hand in cold water will be seen if the patient has pheochromocytoma. Urine collection after the test will contain increased catecholamines. The patient needs to be monitored closely for hypertensive crisis, and intravenous antihypertensive agents should be readily available.

Another test uses phentolamine (Regitine), which will cause a drop of at least 35 mm Hg in the systolic blood pressure and a drop of at least 25 mm Hg in the diastolic blood pressure if the elevated pressure is caused by excess catecholamines. A major hypotensive crisis can occur during this test, and the patient needs very careful monitoring.

PANCREATIC ENDOCRINE FUNCTION TESTING

The major endocrine disorder of the pancreas is caused by disturbance in production, action, or metabolic rate of utilization of insulin. The relative lack of insulin leads to elevated blood glucose levels and the presence of glucose in the urine. The majority of diagnostic tests of pancreatic endocrine function are based on assessment of blood or plasma glucose levels. Urine glucose is still

TABLE 35-9 Diagnostic blood tests for pancreatic endocrine function

Test	Procedure and Preparation	Interpretation
Fasting blood glucose	NPO after midnight	Normal level should be at 60 to 120 mg/100 ml; elevated level indicates a need for further study to rule out diabetes mellitus.
Two-hr postprandial blood glucose	Blood glucose measured 2 hr after heavy meal or 2 hr after receiving loading dose of 100 g of sugar	Blood glucose should be within normal limits; levels above 120 mg/100 ml should be investigated further.
Glucose tolerance test (GTT)	NPO after midnight; samples of blood and urine collected at beginning of test; patient given mixture of glucose to drink or a meal containing 150-300 g of carbohydrate; blood and urine collected at intervals of ½, 1 and 2 hr (2-hr GTT); samples may be collected at 3-, 4-, and 5-hr intervals (5-hr GTT); presence of gastrointestinal disorder that interferes with oral glucose absorption requires administration of intravenous glucose; test done in same manner as for oral GTT	Interpretation of results differs according to source of blood, method of analysis, and critical levels established by various authorities; Levels established by the National Diabetes Data Group (1979) as diagnostic for diabetes mellitus in nonpregnant adults are as follows: | Source	Fasting (mg/dl)	2 hr after glucose load (mg/dl)
Venous plasma	>140	>200
Venous whole blood	>120	>180
Capillary whole blood	>120	>200	
Cortisone-glucose tolerance test	Performed similar to GTT, except that cortisone is administered at start of test	Used when GTT results are inconclusive. Cortisone causes an abnormal increase in blood glucose, and decreased peripheral utilization of glucose in persons predisposed to diabetes; blood glucose level of 140 mg/100 ml at end of 2 hr is considered positive test

sometimes measured and thus the nurse still needs to be familiar with these tests. Insulin can be measured by radioimmunoassay; normal levels depend on glucose levels.

BLOOD TESTS

Common tests to assess blood glucose levels are described in Table 35-9, and a more detailed explanation of them can be found in Chapter 37.

URINE TESTS

Urine testing is familiar to most of the public. Testing of urine for sugar is part of a complete urinalysis, and although used less frequently, the urine of patients with known or suspected diabetes mellitus may be tested for sugar and acetone by one of the following methods.

Clinitest is a copper reduction method of testing the urine for sugar. It comes in a compact kit and is convenient for use, because it is small and easy to carry and store. The kit contains a test tube, a medicine dropper, caustic tablets, and a color chart. Either 2 or 5 drops of urine are placed in the test tube with 10 drops of water, and a Clinitest tablet is added. The tablet generates heat, and the color of the solution is graded by comparing it with the 2-drop or 5-drop color chart. Certain

drugs can affect the accuracy of this testing product. Large amounts of vitamin C, cephalosporin preparations such as cephalothin (Keflin), Gantrisin, L-dopa, Benemid, and Isoniazid can give false-positive ratings.

Tes-Tape, Clinistix, and *Diastix* are strip tests for glucose. Because color charts vary for each product, caution must be exercised in interpreting results. Also, test results must be read at specified time intervals to be accurate.

Acetest tablets may be used to test for acetone. Urine is dropped on the tablet. If acetone is present, varying shades of lavender will appear and can be compared with a color chart. *Ketostix* is a strip product that can also be used to detect the presence of ketones.

Single specimens of urine are frequently used to test the urine for the presence of sugar. If the physician desires to know the amount of sugar being excreted in the urine at a particular time, a *double-voided urine* is ordered. To obtain this type of specimen, the patient is asked to void, then is given water to drink, and voids again in 30 minutes. The second specimen is tested by one of the methods described above. If patients are taught to test their urine at home, usually the double-void technique is taught.

In some situations the physician may wish to find out what time of day the most sugar is excreted. To determine this, *fractional* or *group* urines may be collected. All the urine voided from before breakfast to just before lunch is collected, and a sample is tested for sugar. This is the first specimen; the second is collected from before lunch to just before dinner; the third, from dinner to before bedtime; and the fourth, from bedtime until the next morning.

Twenty-four-hour urine collections also may be obtained to determine the quantity of sugar excreted in a day. In this collection the first specimen of the morning is discarded. All urine excreted for the next 24 hours is collected in a gallon container and sent to the laboratory. It is important that patients know they must add the first urine voided the next morning to the specimen.

CHAPTER SUMMARY

- Normal differentiation of tissue, reproduction, growth and development, adaptation, aging, and senescence depend on a healthy endocrine system.

- The endocrine system integrates body functions so that appropriate body parts will respond as a unit to meet selected needs.

- Hormone levels are finely regulated by various types of feedback mechanisms.

- Many hormones display intrinsic rhythms that vary minute to minute, daily, or over longer periods.

- A hormone acts only on tissue that has an appropriate receptor for the hormone.

- Steroid hormones and thyroid hormones are lipid soluble and enter cells to combine with intracellular receptors.

- Other types of hormones (biogenic amines, small peptides, protein hormones and glycoproteins) are water soluble and combine with membrane receptors; the combination of hormone and membrane receptor stimulates a second messenger such as cyclic AMP.

- The hypothalamus serves as a major link between the rest of the nervous system and the endocrine system by its control of the pituitary gland, as well as its communication with other parts of the brain and the autonomic nervous system.

- Posterior pituitary hormones, antidiuretic hormone, and oxytocin are synthesized in the hypothalamus and stored in the pituitary.

- ADH controls serum osmolality, and oxytocin is involved in lactation and uterine contraction.

- The hypothalamus controls anterior pituitary gland function by synthesis of releasing or inhibiting hormones. The hypothalamus secretes prolactin-inhibiting and prolactin-releasing hormones, growth-hormone-releasing and growth-hormone-inhibiting hormone, corticotropin-releasing hormone, gonadotro-

pin-releasing hormone, and thyrotropin-releasing hormone.

- The anterior pituitary secretes six hormones, including growth hormone, prolactin, follicle-stimulating hormone, luteinizing hormone, thyroid-stimulating hormone, and adrenocorticotropin.

- Control of anterior pituitary secretion is regulated by the hypothalamus and by negative feedback.

- The thyroid gland consists of two cell types: follicle cells, which synthesize thyroid hormone; and C-cells, which synthesize calcitonin.

- Control of thyroid function is from the hypothalamus, the anterior pituitary gland, and external factors.

- Thyroid hormone alters protein, carbohydrate, and fat metabolism; calorigenesis; growth and development; cardiac, respiratory, musculoskeletal, neurologic, and reproductive function; and function of the sympathetic nervous system.

- Calcitonin is involved in calcium homeostasis.

- The parathyroid glands are four small glands lying on the posterior aspect of the thyroid; parathyroid hormone is responsible for maintaining serum calcium levels.

- The adrenal cortex gland secretes adrenal androgens, which are involved in development of secondary sex characteristics, aldosterone and glucocorticoids. Aldosterone is a major controller of sodium balance and volume status. Glucocorticoids are involved in gluconeogenesis, protein catabolism, and lipolysis, are antiinflammatory and suppress immune responsiveness, alter mood, and maintain emotional stability.

- Glucocorticoid production is controlled by the hypothalamus, the anterior pituitary gland, and external factors such as glucose level and physiologic and psychologic stressors. Aldosterone levels are controlled by the renin-angiotensin system, which responds to changes in sodium and volume, and by the serum potassium level.

- The adrenal medulla produces and secretes epinephrine and norepinephrine and works with the sympathetic nervous system in a coordinated response to stressors; all body systems are affected.

- The adrenal medullary sympathetic response is designed to stimulate organ systems that are necessary for life, such as the cardiovascular, respiratory, and neurologic systems, and to inhibit systems such as the gastrointestinal, hepatic, and pancreatic.

- The endocrine functions of the pancreas are carried out by the islet cells.

- The beta cells secrete insulin, which works on muscle, hepatic, and fat cells to lower blood glucose, store carbohydrates and fat, and synthesize protein.

- ✔ The alpha cells secrete glucagon, which elevates blood glucose and mobilizes fat. Glucagon works with cortisol, growth hormone, and epinephrine to counterbalance the effects of insulin.

- ✔ Aging alters endocrine functioning, specifically pituitary, adrenal, pancreatic, thyroid, and parathyroid functioning.

- ✔ Aging is associated with altered bone and calcium metabolism, hypothyroidism, and diabetes mellitus.

- ✔ Most disorders of the endocrine system result in hypersecretion or hyposecretion of hormones.

- ✔ Diagnostic tests of the endocrine system focus on hormone levels; the interrelationship between the hypothalamus, the anterior pituitary gland, and other endocrine glands; or the substrates controlled by the hormone.

- ✔ Endocrine dysfunction affects fluid intake, nutritional intake, elimination, energy level, body characteristics, reproductive and sexual functioning, tolerance to stressors, and almost every physiologic system.

- ✔ An entire endocrine system history must be completed, along with a thorough head-to-toe physical examination.

- ✔ Because many endocrine problems are chronic, the history must also focus on learning styles and needs and home care skills.

QUESTIONS TO CONSIDER

- ■ What are the roles of the hypothalamus, pituitary, thyroid, and adrenal cortex in response to stressors such as bleeding?

- ■ Contrast the major changes in fluid balance, nutritional intake, energy level, tolerance to stressors, body characteristics, elimination, cardiovascular function, and neurologic functions that you would expect in the presence of hypothyroidism with those you would expect in hyperthyroidism.

- ■ Which hormones influence the fluid and electrolyte status of the body?

- ■ Deficiencies of which hormones would cause changes in growth and development?

REFERENCES AND SELECTED READINGS

1. Blackman M: Pituitary hormones and aging, Endocrinol Metab Clin North Am 16(4):981-994, 1987.
2. Davis PJ and Davis FB: Endocrinology and aging. In Reichel W, editor: Clinical aspects of aging, Baltimore, 1983, Williams & Wilkins.
3. DeGroot L et al: Endocrinology, ed 2, New York, 1989, Grune and Stratton Inc.
4. *Ebersole P and Hess D: Toward healthy aging, ed 3, St Louis, 1990, The CV Mosby Co.
5. Evans R: The steroid and thyroid hormone receptor superfamily, Science 240:889-895, 1988.
6. *Feit H: Thyroid function in the elderly, Clin Geriatr Med 4:151-161, 1988.
7. *Gavin L: The diagnostic dilemmas of hyperthyroxinemia and hypothyroxinemia, Adv Intern Med 33:198-204, 1988.
8. Guyton AC: Human physiology and mechanisms of disease, ed 4, Philadelphia, 1987, WB Saunders Co.
9. Ingbar SH: The effects of aging on the thyroid hormone economy in man, Prog Clin Biol Res 74:135-145, 1981.
10. King RJB: Enlightenment and confusion over steroid hormone receptors, Nature 312:20, 1984.
11. *Lancaster LE: Renal and endocrine regulation of water and electrolyte balance, Nurs Clin North Am 22:761-772, 1987.
12. *McCance KL and Huether SE: Pathophysiology: the biological basis for disease in adults and children, St Louis, 1990, The CV Mosby Co.
13. National Diabetes Data Group, National Institutes of Health: Classification and diagnosis of diabetes mellitus and other categories of glucose intolerance, Diabetes 26:1034-1057, 1979.
14. *Poyss AS: Assessment and nursing diagnosis in fluid and electrolyte disorders, Nurs Clin North Am 22:773-783, 1987.
15. Segarnick DJ: Steroids, AAOHN Journal 35(6):286-289, 1987.
16. Spaulding S: Age and the thyroid, Endocrinol Metab Clin North Am 16(4):1013-1025, 1987.
17. Tepperman J: Metabolic and endocrine physiology: an introductory text, ed 5, Chicago, 1987, Year Book Medical Publishers Inc.
18. VanGilder JC: The hypothalamic anterior pituitary relationships and their tumors: a review, Surg Neurol 30:187-196, 1988.
19. West JB, editor: Best and Taylor's physiological basis of medical practice, ed 11, Baltimore, 1985, Williams & Wilkins.
20. Wilson J and Foster D: Williams' textbook of endocrinology, ed 7, Philadelphia, 1985, WB Saunders Co.
21. Wingard DL et al: Community-based study of prevalence of NIDDM in older adults, Diabetes Care 13(2):3-8, 1990.

---

*References preceded by an asterisk are particularly well suited for student reading.

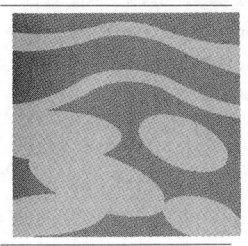

Management of Persons with Problems of the Pituitary, Thyroid, Parathyroid, and Adrenal Glands

VIRGINIA L. CASSMEYER

CHAPTER OBJECTIVES

After studying this chapter, the student should be able to:

1 Describe the pathophysiology of hyper- and hyposecretion of the anterior and posterior pituitary, thyroid, parathyroid, and adrenal glands.

2 Describe the clinical manifestations, including history, physical examination, and diagnostic test findings, associated with hyper- and hyposecretion of the anterior and posterior pituitary, thyroid, parathyroid, and adrenal glands.

3 Develop a nursing plan of care, including identification of appropriate nursing diagnosis, patient outcomes, and interventions, for a patient with hyper- or hyposecretion of the anterior or posterior pituitary, thyroid, parathyroid, or adrenal glands.

4 Identify reasons for surgery of the pituitary, thyroid, parathyroid, or adrenal glands.

5 Develop a nursing plan of care for an individual having surgery on the pituitary, thyroid, parathyroid, or adrenal glands.

6 Identify self-care skills needed by a patient on long-term hormonal replacement therapy for pituitary, thyroid, parathyroid, or adrenal cortex insufficiency.

7 Develop a teaching plan for a patient on long-term hormonal replacement therapy for pituitary, thyroid, parathyroid, or adrenal cortex insufficiency.

Alterations in function of the endocrine system results in a variety of physiologic changes. Dysfunction of the endocrine system is very serious and can be fatal because of the vital functions regulated by the hormones from the pituitary, thyroid, parathyroid, and adrenal glands. The end result of most pathologic processes affecting the endocrine glands is depression or elevation of blood levels of hormones.

Many types of pathologic processes can result in destruction of endocrine tissue and decreased blood levels of hormones. Selected types of problems that result in decreased blood hormone levels include:

1. Destruction of glands by infiltrative processes, in-

farction, infection, autoimmune and immunologic processes, and tumor

2. Abnormal embryonic development, resulting in structural problems or inadequate capacity for synthesis

3. Destruction of glands by surgical removal, radiation therapy, or trauma

The target cells for the selected hormones can become nonresponsive to the hormones. Although in this type of problem the blood hormone levels may be normal or even high, the condition mimics those seen with depression of blood hormones.

Selected types of problems that result in increased blood levels of hormones include:

1. Hyperplasia or hypertrophy of endocrine glands

2. Benign or malignant tumor growth with capacity to secrete hormone

3. Stimulation of glands by trophic factors liberated from ectopic nonendocrine sites

4. Secretion of hormones by ectopic nonendocrine tissues

5. Exogenous administration of hormones

6. Decreased metabolism of hormones, resulting in prolonged activity of hormones

For those endocrine glands controlled by the hypothalamus and pituitary gland, which include the thyroid and adrenocortical glands and the gonads, pathologic states resulting in hyper- or hyposecretion can be classified as primary or secondary. Primary problems occur when the thyroid gland, adrenal cortex gland, or gonads are diseased. Secondary dysfunction occurs when the problem results from hypothalamic or anterior pituitary dysfunction.

Benign and malignant cell growth of endocrine glands can occur. Although hormonal levels are often not immediately affected by the tumor growth, progressive growth can either destroy normal tissue, resulting in hyposecretion of hormones, or the tumor can be made up of secreting tissue, resulting in hypersecretion. Also, the treatment of the tumor by surgery, radiation, or drug therapy often results in *iatrogenic-induced* depressed blood levels of hormones.

PITUITARY GLAND

HYPERPITUITARISM: ANTERIOR PITUITARY GLAND
ETIOLOGY/EPIDEMIOLOGY

Hyperpituitarism of the anterior portion of the pituitary gland may involve only a single hormone or two or more hormones. The cause may be a primary problem in the pituitary gland or secondary to hypothalamic dysfunction. Pituitary adenomas are a common cause of hyperpituitarism. Pituitary adenomas of the anterior pituitary gland account for 6% to 18% of all intracranial tumors.[65] In most patients the cause is unknown and no family history exists. Pituitary adenomas are almost always *secreting* or *functioning* tumors. These tumors are usually benign, but some can grow very aggressively. Previously, adenomas were classified as chromophilic, eosinophilic, or basophilic based on the staining characteristics of the tumor cells, but this method has proved to be inadequate. Classification usually is now based on the specific hormone secreted, for example, prolactinoma, somatotroph tumors, corticotroph tumors, or gonadotroph adenomas. Tumors are also classified by size and invasiveness of the sella turcica (see the box below).

Prolactin-secreting tumors[65] (prolactinomas) account for 60% to 80% of all pituitary tumors. The next most frequently occurring tumor secretes growth hormone (GH) (somatotroph tumor). Tumors that secrete adrenocorticotrophic hormone (ACTH) (corticotroph tumors) are the third most frequently occurring tumors. Gonadotroph adenomas, reported in the past to be rare, may be more common than initially thought.[57] It is possible that adenomas once classified as nonsecreting actually secrete gonadotropins or their subunits.[58] Thyroid-stimulating hormone–(TSH-)secreting tumors are still considered to be rare. Pituitary adenomas can occur as part of multiple endocrine neoplasia, type 1 (MEN I). MEN I is a hereditary disorder that consists of primary hyperparathyroidism, pancreatic islet cell tumor, and pituitary adenoma. The pituitary adenoma in MEN I is secreting and usually secretes GH, but some have been found to secrete prolactin or ACTH.

Pituitary hyperfunctioning also can result from hyperplasia of pituitary tissue. The cause of hyperplasia is not always known, but one hypothesis is that altered feedback signals can cause the hypersecretion.[65] Diminished feedback from target organ secretions can result in hyperplasia and hypersecretion.

PATHOPHYSIOLOGY

The alterations in physiologic functioning that occur with pituitary tumors result from the presence of a space-occupying mass in the cranium and from the effects of the excessive secretion of hormones.

Neurologic Alterations

Neurologic alterations occur because the growing tumor presses on the dura, diaphragm sellae, or adjacent structures. The optic chiasm lies anteriorly and superiorly, and tumors that extend upward press on it. In some patients, cranial nerves III, IV, and VI also may be involved with lateral extension of tumors. The tumor may involve the neighboring bony structures or the temporal or frontal lobe, and very large tumors may compress or infiltrate the hypothalamus.

Hemorrhage into the tumor can result in a sudden increase in size, with rapid onset of various neurological signs and symptoms.

Endocrine Alterations

Depending on which hormone is being secreted by the tumor, a variety of effects may be seen. This section focuses on hypersecretion of prolactin, GH, and gonadotropins. The pathophysiologic factors associated with increased secretion of ACTH or TSH are the same as those seen with adrenocortical hormone or thyroid hormone excess and are discussed in later sections.

Prolactin hypersecretion. Prolactin excess usually results from pituitary tumors but can also result from pharmacologic agents such as psychotropics, antihypertensives, estrogens, and opiates or from central nervous system (CNS) disease that interferes with dopamine secretion. It also may be idiopathic. Prolactin hypersecretion interferes with the hypothalamic-pituitary-gonadal axis. It inhibits the normal release of gonadotropins and gonadal steroids is both females and males. Excessive secretion of prolactin stimulates breast development and milk production in persons with near-normal levels of ovarian steroids.

CLASSIFICATION OF PITUITARY ADENOMAS

Enclosed	No invasion into the floor of the sella turcica
Invasive	Destruction of part or all of the sella turcica
Microadenoma	Enclosed tumors < 10 mm in diameter
Macroadenoma	Enclosed tumors > 10 mm in diameter; these tumors may show suprasellar extension

Growth hormone hypersecretion. In conditions of GH excess, secretion remains episodic, but the number, duration, and amplitude of pulses are increased and occur randomly throughout the day. The excessive secretion of GH produces excessive amounts of somatomedins and the characteristic proliferation of bone, connective tissue, cartilage, and soft tissue resulting in gigantism or acromegaly. GH excess that occurs in childhood and adolescence before closure of the epiphysial plate produces proportional growth of the skeleton and *gigantism*. *Acromegaly* results when GH excess occurs in adult life. It involves overgrowth of soft tissue and terminal skeletal structures such as the nose, jaw, forehead, hands, and feet.

Excessive GH exaggerates the normal depression of carbohydrate metabolism, increasing insulin resistance and depressing glucose uptake. Changes in GH can alter fat metabolism and renal excretion of phosphorus and calcium.

Gonadotropin hypersecretion. Gonadotropin tumors occur most often in middle-aged persons and are found in males more frequently than in females. Hypersecretion of follicle-stimulating hormone (FSH) is most common, although the tumors can secrete leutenizing hormone (LH) or both hormones.[58] The hypersecretion occurs both basally and in response to stimulation. The hypersecretion of gonadotropins frequently causes no clinical changes, although hypersecretion of FSH without LH can result in secondary hypogonadism. Importantly, the patient gives a history of normal pubertal development and fertility even if hypogonadism is currently present.

CLINICAL MANIFESTATIONS

Clinical manifestations vary depending on the type of tumor and are summarized next.

1. Neurologic
   a. Microadenomas (enclosed)
      (1) Radiographic abnormalities on standard roentgenograms, computed tomography (CT) with or without contrast media, or magnetic resonance imaging (MRI)
      (2) No other neurologic signs and symptoms
   b. Macroadenomas (enclosed or invasive)
      (1) Radiographic abnormalities on standard roentgenograms, CT, or MRI
      (2) Visual defects often first seen as losses in superior temporal quadrants with progression to hemianopia or scotomas and finally to total blindness
      (3) Headache
      (4) Somnolence
      (5) Occasional signs of increased intracranial pressure (hydrocephalus, papilledema)
      (6) With very large tumors, disturbance in appetite, sleep, temperature regulation, and emotional balance because of hypothalamic involvement
      (7) Behavioral changes and seizures with expansion causing compression of the temporal or frontal lobe
2. Endocrine
   a. Prolactin hypersecretion
      (1) Females
         (a) Usually microadenomas
         (b) Menstrual disturbances such as irregular menses, anovulatory periods, oligomenorrhea or amenorrhea
         (c) Infertility
         (d) Galactorrhea
         (e) Manifestations of ovarian steroid deficit such as dyspareunia, vaginal mucosal atrophy, decreased vaginal lubrication, decreased libido
      (2) Males
         (a) Usually macroadenomas
         (b) Decreased libido and possible impotence
         (c) Reduced sperm count and infertility
         (d) Gynecomastia
      (3) Both males and females
         (a) Increased basal levels of serum prolactin (23 to >10,000 ng/ml)
         (b) Depressed levels of gonadal steroids
   b. GH hypersecretion
      (1) Macroadenomas with resultant radiographic findings, headache, and visual changes
      (2) Changes in facial features (coarsening of features; increased size of nose, lips, and skin folds; prominence of supraorbital ridges; growth of mandible resulting in prognathism and widely spaced teeth; soft tissue growth resulting in facial puffiness)
      (3) Increased size of hands and feet (Figure 36-1); weight gain
      (4) Deepening of voice from thickening of vocal cords
      (5) Increases in vertebral bodies resulting in thoracic kyphosis
      (6) Enlarged tongue, salivary glands, spleen, liver, heart, kidney, and other organs; cardiomegaly may result in increased blood pressure and signs and symptoms of congestive heart failure
      (7) Elevated blood pressure even without cardiac failure
      (8) Snoring, sleep apnea, and respiratory failure
      (9) Dermatologic changes: acne, increased

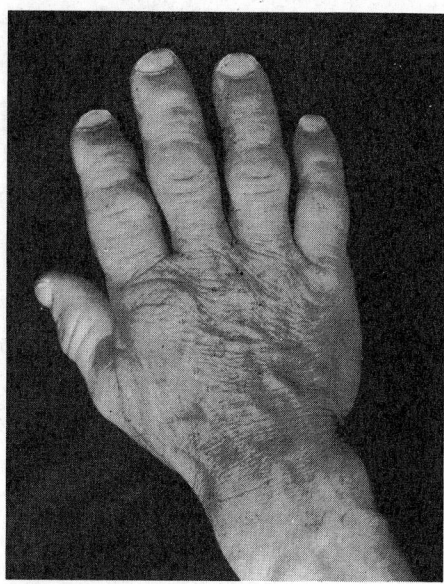

FIGURE 36-1 Hand showing characteristics of acromegalic condition. (From Schottelius B and Schottelius D: Textbook of physiology, ed 18, St Louis, 1978, The CV Mosby Co.)

sweating, oiliness, development of skin tags
(10) Hypertrophy progressing to atrophy of skeletal muscles
(11) Backache, arthralgia, or arthritis from joint damage and bony overgrowth
(12) Peripheral nerve damage such as carpal tunnel syndrome or neuropathies from bony overgrowth and changes in nerve size
(13) Impaired glucose tolerance progressing to diabetes mellitus with its manifestations
(14) Changes in fat metabolism resulting in hyperlipidemia
(15) General changes in mobility: presence of lethargy and fatigue
(16) Radiographic findings indicative of bony proliferation in hands, feet, skull, ribs, vertebrae
(17) Increased serum levels of GH
(18) Electrolyte changes: increased urinary excretion of calcium; elevated blood phosphate level
  c. Gonadotropin hypersecretion
(1) Usually no clinical manifestations
(2) If signs and symptoms present: secondary hypogonadism such as changes in secondary sexual characteristics or atrophy of external genitalia, with history of normal pubertal development and fertility
(3) Elevated levels of FSH, LH, or both hormones or of subunits of the gonadotropins

MEDICAL MANAGEMENT

Untreated GH-secreting tumors can result in major neurologic alterations as well as continual systemic changes if the hormone level is not returned to normal and if tumor growth is not inhibited. Treatment consists of surgery, radiation, or pharmacologic agents. The primary treatment is neurosurgery using a transsphenoidal approach. Radiation therapy may be used as an adjunct to surgery or as an alternative. Radiation lowers hormone levels much more slowly and is associated with a high incidence of hypopituitarism. Bromocriptine (Parlodel), a dopamine agonist, is effective in lowering GH levels but not always to the level needed, and therefore it is used mainly if surgery and radiation have not been effective.

A long-acting somatostatin analog (octreotide, [Sandostatin], SMS 201-995) is available and has been approved by the Food and Drug Administration (FDA) for use in treating carcinoid.[2] In experimental studies with persons with acromegaly, it has been found to be effective in reducing plasma GH levels as well as relieving some clinical manifestations of GH excess, such as headache, arthropathy, swelling of soft tissue, excess perspiration, sleep apnea, and neuropathy. Sandostatin must be given by subcutaneous injection three or four times daily. It also can be given by continous subcutaneous infusion. Side effects include pain at injection site, diarrhea, steatorrhea, abdominal cramps, and flatulence. This drug has also been used preoperatively and appears to improve the success of surgery. The routine use of somatostatin analogs for persons with acromegaly will depend on future research.

For prolactin-secreting tumors, some authorities[64] have recommended no treatment for persons with a microadenoma who have no annoying symptoms and if patients do not wish to become pregnant. Studies have shown that the incidence of microadenomas progressing to macroadenomas is very low.[40] However, the ovarian dysfunction and the low estrogen state that can be associated with elevated prolactin levels may result in premature osteoporosis; thus other experts recommend that all prolactin-secreting tumors be treated.

When treatment is recommended, the dopamine agonist bromocriptine (Parlodel) is used for enclosed tumors. Drug therapy effectively returns hormone levels to normal, restores fertility, and decreases tumor size in most patients. Transsphenoidal adenomectomy is still frequently used for invasive tumors and for some enclosed macroadenomas. Because the use of bromocriptine during gestation is very limited, patients who become pregnant after successful bromocriptine therapy are treated in various ways.[40] In persons with microadenomas, the drug may be stopped during pregnancy and the patient monitored for signs and symptoms of tumor enlargement. Visual testing is used to monitor for enlargement, and if enlargement is suspected, a CT scan or MRI is done. After delivery and if surgery was not done, bromocriptine is restarted. If signs and symptoms recur, the drug may be reinstituted. For larger tumors, pre-pregnancy surgery may be done. In some instances, bromocriptine may be continued throughout pregnancy.

■ ASSESSMENT

Assessment of the patient with potential hyperpituitarism of the anterior pituitary gland focuses on identification of manifestations of these problems, particularly as they relate to the patients' total health.

Subjective Data

Subjective data include the following:
1. History of sensory alterations, particularly vision, as well as other peripheral sensory changes
2. Discomforts—temporal or frontal headache of moderate intensity, arthralgia, backache
3. History of changes in body appearance—coarsening of facial features; increases in ring, glove, or shoe size; increase in sweating or oiliness of skin
4. History of change in energy level (lethargy, fatigue) or decrease in mobility
5. Psychosocial concerns—behavioral changes such as anxiety, irritability, concerns about self-image
6. History of menstrual changes in females, impotency in males, changes in libido; infertility concerns
7. Drug history—taking oral contraceptives, psychotropic drugs
8. Knowledge level related to disorder, treatment, potential outcome of treatment

Objective Data

Data about neurologic and endocrine effects include the following:
1. Functioning of cranial nerves II, III, IV, and VI (see Chapter 59)
2. Retinal changes indicative of papilledema or elevated blood pressure
3. Mental status—alertness, emotional status
4. Peripheral nerve functioning (see Chapter 59)
5. Body appearance, description
6. Mobility and joint functioning (see Chapter 68)
7. Vital signs—blood pressure, pulse, respirations, temperature
8. Body weight and height
9. Presence of organomegaly, particularly cardiac and hepatic, and signs associated with these changes

■ DATA ANALYSIS: NURSING DIAGNOSES

Nursing diagnoses are determined from assessment of patient data. Possible nursing diagnoses for the person with hypersecretion of the anterior pituitary gland associated with pituitary tumor include, but are not limited to, the following:

Diagnostic Title	Possible Etiologies
All patients with pituitary tumors—pretreatment	
Anxiety	Uncertainty about cause of problem and outcome of treatment
Knowledge deficit: disorder and treatment	New diagnoses and new treatment
Pain	Headache from intracranial mass
Self-esteem disturbance	Changes in body characteristics or functions associated with hormonal excess
Sensory/perceptual alterations: visual	Pressure on optic chiasma disrupting functioning of cranial nerve II or pressure on cranial nerves III, IV, and VI
Patients with prolactin-secreting tumors—pretreatment	
Knowledge deficit: disorder, treatment, and relationship of disorder to sexual functioning	New diagnoses and treatment
Sexual dysfunction	Alteration in menstrual cycle, decreased libido, or impotence associated with increased secretion of prolactin
Patients with GH-secreting tumors—pretreatment	
Knowledge deficit: disorder, treatment, and effect of treatment on signs and symptoms	Newly diagnosed disorder and new treatment
Mobility, impaired physical	Pain from pressure on nerve roots
Pain	Pressure on nerves associated with changes in joints and vertebrae associated with abnormal bone growth
Patients with any type of tumor treated with surgery	
Fluid volume deficit, potential	Disruption in normal antidiuretic hormone (ADH) secretion or adrenal cortex functioning associated with surgical trauma
Gas exchange, impaired	Lack of adequate deep breathing; instructions not to cough and nasal packing and drainage
Infection, potential for	Loss of barriers to organisms associated with disruption of external incision in mucous membrane from improper care; disruption of internal incision through dura associated with increased intracranial pressure (ICP) resulting in cerebrospinal fluid (CSF) leak

Diagnostic Title	Possible Etiologies
Knowledge deficit: procedure, expected outcomes, and expected complications	New treatment so no previous exposure to information

Patients with any type of tumor treated with radiation

Injury, potential for	Inability to maintain homeostasis, cardiac output, respiratory functioning, and fluid and electrolyte balance associated with ACTH and/or TSH deficiency
Knowledge deficit: procedure, expected outcomes, and potential complications	Newly prescribed treatment so no previous exposure to information
Sexual dysfunction	Impotency, decreased libido, change in menstrual cycles associated with long term loss of adequate synthesis and secretion of gonadotopins

Patients with any type of tumor treated with drug therapy

Knowledge deficit: drugs, self-administration techniques, expected results, and potential side effects	Newly prescribed treatment so no previous exposure to information

■ **PLANNING: EXPECTED PATIENT OUTCOMES**

Expected patient outcomes for the person with hypersecretion of the anterior pituitary gland associated with pituitary tumor may include, but are not limited to, the following:

All patients—pretreatment

1. Anxiety is controlled, as evidenced by patient's ability to sleep and carry on with other activities and by patient's statement.
2. Adequate knowledge is attained as evidenced by patient's and significant others ability to explain potential disorder, diagnostic tests and their purposes, and potential treatment.
3. Headache is controlled by prescribed interventions.
4. Self-esteem is improved as evidenced by patient's ability to talk positively about self, correctly identifies body characteristics and functions that are reversible and that will not change
5. Patient is able to function independently in the hospital or at home.

Patients with prolactin-secreting tumors—pretreatment

1. Adequate knowledge is attained as evidenced by the patient's and significant others ability to describe disorder, potential treatment, how the sexual dysfunction relates to prolactin excess, and the effects of treatment on sexual functioning.
2. Sexual dysfunction will cause no long term problems as evidenced by patient statements and explanation that treatment should resolve the problem.

Patient with GH-secreting tumors—pretreatment

1. Knowledge is adequate as evidenced by the patient's and significant others ability to describe the disorder, treatment, and effects of treatment on signs and symptoms.
2. The patient is independent in activities of daily living (ADLs) and states that he or she can participate in all activities enjoyed.
3. The patient states that interventions prescribed control back and joint discomfort and that discomfort does not limit activity.

Patients with any type of tumor treated with surgery

1. The patient does not develop fluid volume deficit, as evidenced by decreased blood pressure, poor skin turgor, unrelieved thirst, or hemoconcentration.
2. The patient maintains adequate gas exchange, as evidenced by clear breath sounds, arterial oxygen and carbon dioxide pressure (Pa_{O_2}, Pa_{CO_2}) and percentage of O_2 saturation within normal limits, no tachycardia, and appropriate response to interactions.
3. The patient remains free of infection and shows no evidence of CSF leak.

Patients with any type of tumor treated with radiation

1. No injuries occur because the patient's and significant others ability to state signs and symptoms they should monitor for and report immediately.
2. Knowledge is adequate as evidenced by the patient's and significant others ability to explain radiation procedure, expected outcomes, and potential complications.

Patients with any type of tumor treated with drug therapy

1. Knowledge is adequate as evidenced by the patient's and significant others ability to name drugs, state how to administer, and describe the expected results and potential side effects.

■ **IMPLEMENTATION**

Nursing Care Before Definitive Medical Treatment

The patient with a hormonal excess due to a secreting pituitary tumor will seek care for various reasons, including symptoms and signs such as frequent or persistent headache, visual changes, or changes in body characteristics or function. The major nursing need at this stage of the illness is patient education. The patient and significant others need to know:

1. How the symptoms present in the patient relate to a pituitary tumor and hormone excess.
2. What is meant by the term *tumor;* some people automatically assume that tumor means cancer. These tumors usually are not malignant.
3. What diagnostic tests are planned, including blood tests; skull roentgenogram, CT scan, or MRI; and visual assessment.

4. What treatment is available for the tumor. Based on the signs and symptoms, the physician has a high index of suspicion for the type of tumor and potential treatment. This is the information the physician shares at this time and which the nurse reinforces.

5. What outcomes are expected from the treatment, including reversibility or irreversibility of signs and symptoms.

This knowledge assists the patient in dealing with the physiologic changes and should help to relieve uncertainty and decrease anxiety. Usually this teaching is done in an outpatient setting. Thus the nurse must have a model of a brain available, which may be used to help the patient understand better what is happening, as well as written material for the patient to read after leaving the outpatient setting. The nurse should also provide the name and telephone number of someone (nurse, physician) who can be contacted if the patient thinks of more questions.

The patient may need immediate treatment for headache, such as mild nonnarcotic analgesics. Other helpful measures include sitting and lying with the head elevated. Relaxing in a dark room, listening to quiet music, meditation, and other types of relaxation may also help. The nurse needs to identify, in cooperation with the patient, measures that help relieve the headache. The patient with a GH-secreting tumor requires comfort measures to deal with joint and back pain and impaired mobility. These measures may include nonnarcotic analgesics, warm baths, range of motion (ROM) exercises, and moist or dry heat.

Nursing care related to *visual disturbances, self-esteem disturbances,* and *sexual dysfunction* is primarily educational at this stage of care. The patient and significant others need to know that changes in body characteristics and vision are not always reversible, but that progressive changes will be stopped and they will be helped to cope with irreversible changes. Sexual dysfunction associated with prolactin excess is usually reversible. The patient must be assessed for the ability to maintain a safe environment if visual disturbances are present. Although severe visual disturbances rarely occur, interventions such as those discussed in Chapter 65 for the person with blindness may be necessary.

Nursing Care After Surgery

Following a transsphenoidal adenectomy, the patient's care has four additional focuses: prevention of infection, fluid volume deficit, and respiratory complications and patient education. These are guided by the nursing diagnoses and expected patient outcomes described earlier. The patient continues to need care for pain and discomfort and visual problems, if these were present before surgery.

Preventing infection. With transsphenoidal adenectomy, the sella turcica is entered from below through the sphenoid sinus and the tumor is removed. An external incision is made between the upper gum and lip, and an internal incision is made through the sella turcica and dura. Care to prevent disruption of both these incisions and to prevent infection are nursing concerns. Care of the incision in the mouth consists of rinsing the mouth with saline or mouthwash and cleansing the teeth with a Toothette or cotton swab. Brushing the teeth is forbidden until the suture line heals.

Oral fluids and a clear liquid diet are given as soon as the patient is alert and no longer nauseated from the anesthetic. The diet can progress to solid foods as soon as tolerated, which is usually by the second or third meal after surgery. Because of the mouth incision, rough foods that could irritate the mucous membrane and disrupt the suture line must be avoided. The discomfort associated with eating rough food usually serves as a limiting guideline.

The major occurrence that can disrupt the incision made through the sella turcica and dura is increased CSF pressure. After the tumor is resected, the sella turcica is packed with muscle or fat from the abdomen or thigh. (*Note:* it is important that the patient be prepared for this additional incision.) The floor of the sella turcica is reconstructed with bone or cartilage. This patching, although strong, can be disrupted by increased ICP, which in turn increases pressure on the incisional site. Activities such as bending over, straining, coughing, sneezing, and blowing the nose are forbidden. The head of the patient's bed should be elevated at least 30 degrees when the patient is reclining. In most cases these interventions will prevent disruption of the patch and incision.

CSF leakage will occur if the patching and incision in the sella turcica are disrupted. The nurse monitors for signs and symptoms of such leakage. After surgery the patient's nose is packed for 24 to 48 hours, and a gauze sling is worn under the nose to absorb drainage (see Chapter 32). A CSF leak may be identified by:

1. Complaints of postnasal drip, even with packing in place
2. Observation that the patient is constantly swallowing or stating that he or she needs to swallow constantly.
3. Appearance of a halo on the gauze sling (CSF is clear and, when mixed with serous fluid on gauze, will form a halo surrounding the serous drainage.)

Nasal drainage can be differentiated from CSF based on glucose content. Although the nurse can assess the glucose content of nasal drainage with Tes-Tape, this is unreliable and fluid should be sent to a laboratory for accurate assessment. If a CSF leakage occurs or is suspected, bed rest with the patient's head elevated is reinstituted and maintained until the leakage is ruled out or clears. Occasionally, patients will have to return to surgery for repair of the site in the sella turcica.

If a CSF leak occurs and has been established as a CSF leak, the patient is at high risk for infection, including meningitis. Besides instituting restriction of activities to prevent or control a CSF leak, the nurse should begin careful monitoring to identify early signs of an infection. Monitoring includes temperature checks at least every 4 hours and evaluation for presence of nuchal rigidity (see Chapter 59) or headaches at the same time. Antibiotics should be administered as prescribed.

Preventing fluid volume deficit. Fluid volume deficit is a potential problem in any patient during the postoperative period. However, the patient who has had a transsphenoidal adenectomy is at higher risk because *diabetes insipidus* may be caused by inadequate release of ADH. Diabetes insipidus, if it does occur, is usually temporary because ADH is produced in the hypothalamus and adequate amounts can be released from it even if there is damage to the posterior pituitary gland.

Polyuria (urine output greater than 200 ml/hour) and continuously dilute urine (specific gravity of 1.000 to 1.005) are signs of diabetes insipidus. Intake and output measurements every 4 to 8 hours, specific gravity checks of each urine specimen, daily patient weighing, and assessment for complaints of thirst help to identify the presence of diabetes insipidus early. If a deficit in ADH does occur, treatment depends on the severity. If the deficit is mild and the patient can take in enough fluids to maintain fluid volume and still receive adequate rest during the night, replacement of fluids guided by the patient's thirst is the only treatment. The patient should have easy access to cold water. If the deficit of ADH is more severe, requiring frequent awakenings for urination and water intake and thus inadequate sleep, or if the patient is unable to take in adequate fluids, vasopressin is given. In the immediate postoperative period, aqueous vasopressin, given subcutaneously or intramuscularly, is the drug of choice if replacement therapy is necessary.

Although rare following adenectomy, ACTH deficiency resulting in glucocorticoid deficiency is a potential problem and can result in severe fluid volume deficit as well as other complaints and needs. All patients should be monitored for potential glucocorticoid deficiency. The monitoring should identify early signs and symptoms of adrenal insufficiency, as described on p. 1077. It includes that just described to assess for the adequacy of ADH, as well as vital signs every 4 hours and observation of energy level, alertness, patient's stated feelings of well-being, and appetite. If abnormalities in these data are found, serum sodium, potassium, and

glucose levels may be obtained. The presence of increased urine output, hypotension while lying or orthostatic hypotension, persistent nausea, vomiting, fatigue and tiredness, low sodium level, increased potassium level, hypoglycemia, and acidosis indicate inadequate ACTH and glucocorticoid secretion. Hydrocortisone (Cortef) or other high-potency corticoids and fluid replacement are provided. If the deficit in ACTH is permanent, the patient will have to be treated as discussed for persons with chronic adrenal insufficiency (see p. 1078).

Preventing respiratory complications. Because of the caution against coughing and the nasal packing necessitating mouth breathing, patients are at some risk for ineffective gas exchange. Patients should be instructed about mouth breathing and deep breathing exercises before surgery, have an opportunity to do a return demonstration, and then be monitored for compliance with deep breathing exercises at least every 2 hours for the first 1 to 3 postoperative days. Assessment of vital signs and breath sounds every 4 to 8 hours helps to identify any impairment of air exchange. Maintenance of adequate fluid intake helps to prevent drying of mucous secretions and the formation of mucous plugs.

Other physical care. Incisional discomfort and headache may occur after surgery and are treated with nonnarcotic analgesics or codeine. Persistent headaches may indicate meningitis and should be reported to the physician immediately. A firm mattress, ROM exercises, back massage, ambulation frequently throughout the day, and heat may be used to help decrease back and joint discomfort in persons with GH-secreting tumors. Ambulation as soon as possible helps to prevent deterioration in mobility and joint movement. Visual problems should be managed as they were preoperatively, and the patient's vision should be monitored for deterioration postoperatively. Rearranging the room so that needed articles are placed in line with intact vision or other interventions (see Chapter 65) may be necessary. Although visual complications following transsphenoidal resection are rare, the visual pathway can be damaged during surgery, or the muscle and fat graft placed at the conclusion of surgery may migrate upward and compress the optic nerve.[27,28]

Patient education. The first focus of patient education is similar to that for any patient during the postoperative period and includes preparing the patient for day-to-day care (see Chapter 22). The second focus of patient education in the postoperative period is to prepare the patient for resuming self-care and discharge and assuming responsibility for any special follow-up care. The patient should know when to return to see the physician (usually within 1 to 2 weeks), again in 1 month, and then every 6 to 12 months. The first follow-up visit allows for the assessment of the patient's general recovery from surgery and hormonal status. The other visits allow for assessment for recurrence of the tumor.

The third focus of patient education is to prepare the patient to manage any hormonal deficiencies that have occurred. If ADH or ACTH and glucocorticoid deficiency occurred postoperatively, diagnostic tests are done before the patient leaves the hospital to identify whether the deficiencies are permanent. If permanent, the patient needs the same education required by any patient with diabetes insipidus (see p. 1035) or adrenocortical insufficiency (see p. 1082).

If a deficiency of ACTH and glucocorticoid occurs, secretion of other hormones from the anterior pituitary gland, such as TSH or gonadotropins, may also be deficient. These deficiencies do not cause immediate postoperative concerns and may not even be evident in the immediate postoperative period. However, the adequacy of anterior pituitary secretion of these hormones is assessed before discharge or at the return visits. If the patient develops no deficiency during the postoperative period, approximately 4 to 6 weeks after surgery, diagnostic tests to evaluate the hormonal response to surgery and the adequacy of other hormone synthesis and secretions are completed.

The last focus of patient education is to reinforce care needs for irreversible changes in body appearance, joint and back pain, and visual problems. Information shared may include ways to minimize body changes with makeup and clothes, frequent showers to help control increased sweating and oily skin, pain management techniques (see Chapter 16), modification of activities to decrease stress and strain on the joints and back (Chapter 70), and referral to the Society for the Visually Impaired.

Nursing Care of Patients Receiving Radiation Therapy

Radiation therapy may be used as an adjunct or as an alternative to surgery. For patients receiving radiation, the major focus of care, in addition to that described for all patients before definitive medical treatment, is patient education. Radiation therapy is done on an outpatient basis. Radiation treatments are usually given over 4 to 6 weeks. The response to radiation is slow, and hypopituitarism develops in many patients. Deficiencies of ACTH and gonadotropins typically occur, although deficiency in TSH may also occur.[38]

Patient education should focus on how the procedure is done. A visit to the radiation therapy department should be planned. Patients need to know the number of visits required and when they will begin to see or experience effects. They also should be told of the possibility of hormonal deficits as a side effect. The nurse should emphasize that these do not occur until many years after the therapy.[38] Radiation therapy can cause damage to surrounding tissue and swelling of the tumor[22,38] and worsen neurologic signs and symptoms. The patient must know to report any worsening of signs and symptoms.

Nursing Care of Patients Treated With Drug Therapy

Patients treated with bromocriptine alone or as adjunctive therapy must know how to take the drugs. For prolactin-secreting tumors, 2.5 mg to 15 mg daily usually is effective. Higher doses may be necessary for GH-secreting tumors. The major side effects are mild nausea, vomiting, nasal stuffiness, postural hypotension, depression, nightmares, and cold-induced peripheral vasospasm. Continual hormonal analysis is carried out to monitor the effectiveness of therapy. Prolactin levels usually return to normal within a few days. Elevated GH levels take longer to decrease. If patients are placed on the somatostatin analog, they may need to be taught how to self-administer the drug by subcutaneous injection, how to prepare the injection site, how to prepare the subcutaneous injection, how to store the drug, how to care for syringes and needles, and so forth. The information is similar to that taught to persons with diabetes mellitus about subcutaneous injections (see Chapter 37).

HYPERPITUITARISM: SYNDROME OF INAPPROPRIATE ANTIDIURETIC HORMONE

ETIOLOGY

The causes of syndrome of inappropriate antidiuretic hormone (SIADH) are many (see the box below). This disorder is associated with various pathologic processes as well as with drug therapy.

PATHOPHYSIOLOGY

In SIADH, total body water increases because of water retention and a hypo-osmolar state results from hypona-

---

ETIOLOGIC FACTORS ASSOCIATED WITH SIADH

Pulmonary disorders: malignant neoplasms such as oat cell adenocarcinoma of the lung, tuberculosis, ventilator patients receiving positive pressure
Other malignancies: duodenum, pancreas, prostate lymphoma, sarcoma, leukemia
CNS disorders: tumors, infection, trauma
Endocrine disorders that result in hypovolemia and impaired free water excretion, particularly if associated with fluid replacement (adrenal insufficiency, anterior pituitary insufficiency)
Drugs such as clofibrate, chlorpropamide, thiazides, vincristine, cyclophosphamide, morphine
Stressors: fear, acute infections, pain, anxiety, trauma surgery

tremia (low serum sodium concentration). In SIADH the ADH release follows one of four patterns[49,65]:

1. ADH release is erratic and unrelated to plasma osmolality.
2. ADH release varies with the plasma osmolality, but the osmostat has been reset and ADH release occurs at a lower plasma osmolality.
3. ADH release is normal in response to a normal or elevated plasma osmolality, but ADH is not reduced as the plasma osmolality is lowered.
4. ADH release is normal, but the patient is more sensitive to the released ADH, or some "unmeasured factor" that increases water retention is released.

The abnormally released ADH or the increased sensitivity of cells to ADH increases the permeability of the distal renal tubules and collecting ducts to water, and water resorption by the kidney increases. Intravascular volume increases, but edema is not present, as would be seen in congestive heart failure (see Chapter 28) or cirrhosis (see Chapter 39). Edema does not occur because the volume expansion in SIADH results in *natriuresis* (urinary sodium excretion). The natriuresis results because of enhanced glomerular filtration and decreased proximal tubular sodium absorption, even with hyponatremia.

It is important to note that a reduction in plasma sodium level to 119 mEq/L from 139 mEq/L within 2 hours can result in death, whereas a reduction to as low as 99 mEq/L in 16 days results only in lethargy.[49] The following are some guidelines for understanding the potential changes that may occur in patients and for planning the monitoring that needs to be done[49]:

1. As serum sodium levels falls below 125 mEq/L, the patient complains of nausea and malaise.
2. At serum sodium levels between 115 and 120 mEq/L, headache, lethargy, and obtundation may appear.
3. Seizures and coma are not usually seen until the plasma sodium concentration falls below 110 to 115 mEq/L.

The hyponatremia results in hypo-osmolality and creates an osmolar gradient across the blood-brain barrier and other cellular membranes. This osmolar gradient results in water movement into the brain and other cells and cellular overhydration.

CLINICAL MANIFESTATIONS

Signs, symptoms, and diagnostic test results include the following:

1. Fluid and electrolyte changes
   a. Decreased plasma sodium and plasma osmolality
   b. Increased urinary sodium and urinary osmolality
   c. Decreased urinary volume
   d. Increased weight
   e. Absence of edema
2. Neurologic changes (depending on severity of serum sodium depression and the rapidity of the reduction in plasma sodium concentration)
   a. Lethargy, headache, mild disorientation that progresses to seizures
   b. Emotional/behavioral changes, such as anxiety, irritability, uncooperativeness, hostility
   c. Gastrointestinal (GI) changes: anorexia, nausea, vomiting

INTERVENTIONS

Medical Management

Medical management in acute SIADH focuses on treatment of the etiologic factor, such as carcinoma, infection, and so forth, and correcting, or at least restoring toward normal, the plasma sodium level and plasma osmolality. Water restriction is the first priority of management. Water may be restricted to as little as 500 ml/day. Oral salt intake is increased if the patient is able to take in oral nutrients.

If the patient's plasma sodium level is less than 120 mEq/L and the patient is exhibiting CNS manifestations such as nausea, vomiting, lethargy, and headaches, more rapid correction of the low plasma sodium is necessary. This severe *hyponatremia* is treated with hypertonic saline (3% sodium chloride) and a loop diuretic such as furosemide (Lasix) or ethacrynic acid.[13,63,65] The goal of this later therapy is not to return the plasma sodium level to normal, but to increase it to 125 to 130 mEq/L or to administer enough sodium chloride to relieve symptoms or increase the plasma sodium by 25 mEq/L.[63] This correction needs to be done cautiously because of potential complications from either too rapid or too slow correction. Verbalis[63] recommends that the plasma sodium should be increased as necessary but that the rate of increase should be no faster than 0.5 to 2 mEq/L/hour. Too slow a correction of plasma sodium can worsen the neurologic manifestations. Too rapid of an increase in the plasma sodium can produce a plasma solution that is relatively hypertonic compared to the intracellular compartment and a shifting of fluids from the intracellular to the extracellular compartment. A rapid shift of fluids can result in central pontine myelinolysis, which is demyelination of the pons. This demyelination results in dysfunction of the nerve tracts that travel through or originate in the pons. During treatment with hypertonic saline or loop diuretics, plasma osmolality and serum sodium are monitored every 2 to 4 hours.

Chronic SIADH and hyponatremia are treated at first by water restriction. If water restriction alone cannot prevent hypo-osmolality, pharmacologic treatment is added. Demeclocycline, a tetracycline derivative, blocks the action of ADH on the renal tubule and collecting duct cells and decreases urine osmolality. Diuretics may be used on a long-term basis, and a high-sodium diet may be continued.

Nursing Management

Nursing interventions are as follows:

1. Perform assessment.
   a. Identify patients at high risk.
   b. For high-risk patients, monitor daily weights, daily intake and output, daily serum and urinary sodium levels and osmolality, and vital signs and neurologic status every 4 hours. Report any decrease below normal in serum sodium (if the level is below 125 mEq/L, report laboratory results immediately), any signs of fluid retention (increased weight, decreased output), and any neurologic changes (complaints of headaches or nausea, decreased responsiveness).
   c. For patients with diagnosed SIADH being treated aggressively with hypertonic sodium or loop diuretics, the frequency of monitoring is increased to every 1 to 2 hours. Any deterioration in neurologic status is reported immediately.
   d. For patients with chronic SIADH, monitor weights daily to weekly and report any increases not attributed to dietary changes or any complaints of nausea, headaches, or lethargy. Monitoring by the nurse in the outpatient department is the same as that described for high-risk patients.
2. Provide supportive care.
   a. Restrict fluids as prescribed.
   b. Control discomfort from thirst.
      (1) Space fluids throughout 24-hour period.
      (2) Use ice chips, which allow more frequent relief of thirst with less fluid intake.
      (3) Provide frequent mouth care.

CAUSES OF HYPOPITUITARISM

Tumors: craniopharyngioma, primary CNS tumors, nonsecreting pituitary tumors
Ischemic changes: Sheehan's syndrome (ischemic changes following postpartum hemorrhage or infection resulting in shock)
Developmental abnormalities
Infections: viral encephalitis, bacteremia, tuberculosis
Autoimmune disorders
Radiation damage, particularly following treatment of secreting adenomas of pituitary gland
Trauma, including surgery

---

   c. Administer drugs or fluids as ordered.
3. Provide care appropriate to specific etiologic factor (varies).
4. Patient teaching
   a. Review purpose of fluid restriction and how to manage it.
   b. Review self-monitoring required on a long-term basis (intake and output measurement, weight change).
   c. Discuss drug therapy as appropriate.

HYPOPITUITARISM: ANTERIOR PITUITARY GLAND

ETIOLOGY

Several disorders can interfere with the function of the anterior pituitary gland and cause hyposecretion of one or more hormones (see box below, left). Panhypopituitarism (deficiency of all anterior pituitary hormones and of ADH from the posterior pituitary gland) may be present, or there may be isolated deficiency of one anterior pituitary hormone. If panhypopituitarism occurs, unless it results from surgical removal of the pituitary gland, the deficiencies of the anterior pituitary hormones usually do not appear simultaneously. Deficits of GH and gonadotropins usually occur first, followed by deficits of TSH and then ACTH.

PATHOPHYSIOLOGY

In hypopituitarism the symptoms vary widely depending on the cause and the endocrine dysfunction present. If a tumor is the cause, the patient may have some of the symptoms described for secreting pituitary tumors. These include symptoms resulting from growth of a space-occupying lesion in the cranium, effects resulting from pressure on the optic chiasm, and potential disturbances of cranial nerves III, IV, and VI. If the tumor arises from regions surrounding the pituitary such as Ratke's pouch (craniopharyngiomas), the hypothalamus, or the third ventricle, the neurologic signs and symptoms will be more severe and include manifestations of increased ICP.

The endocrine dysfunction may be the result of hypothalamic damage or primary pituitary disease. The most frequent pathophysiologic alteration results from lack of synthesis and secretion of gonadotropins. The second most frequently encountered problem is deficiency of GH synthesis and secretion. The symptoms associated with deficiency of individual anterior pituitary hormones are summarized in Figure 36-2. The patient with hypopituitarism exhibits all or only selected aspects of these deficiencies. Usually the pathologic alteration progresses slowly.

CLINICAL MANIFESTATIONS

Although the exact manifestation will vary depending on the cause of the anterior pituitary problem and the

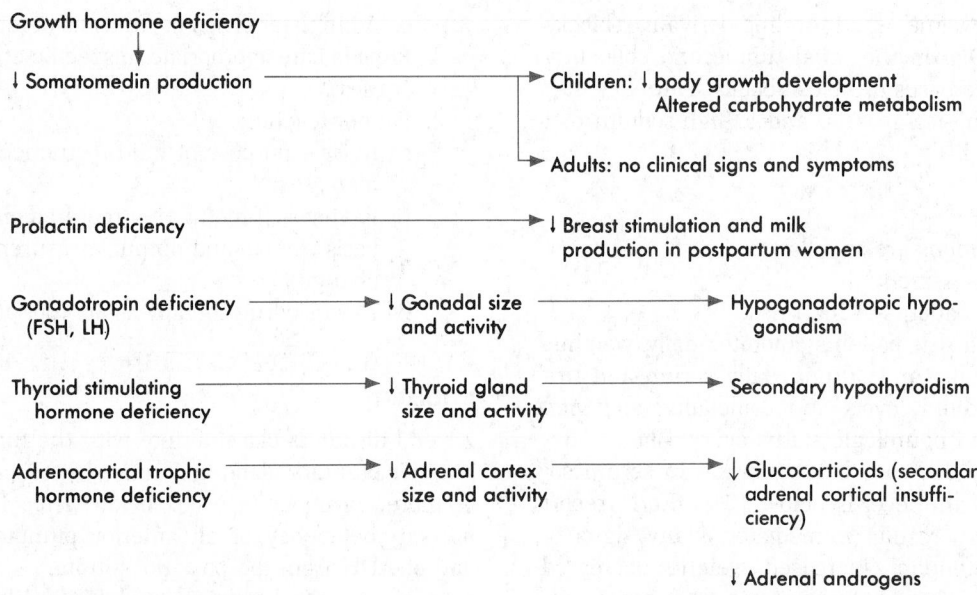

FIGURE 36-2 Pathophysiology associated with individual anterior pituitary hormone deficiency.

type of hormonal deficiency, the major manifestations include the following:

1. Manifestations based on cause such as bacteremia, viral hepatitis, autoimmune disorders, and trauma
2. Manifestations such as vision changes, papilledema, or hydrocephalus if cause is tumor
3. Manifestations of gonadotropin deficiency
   a. Decreased serum levels of FSH, LH, and gonadal steroids
   b. Children—delayed puberty
   c. Adults
      (1) Females—oligomenorrhea or amenorrhea, uterine and vaginal atrophy, potential atrophy of breast tissue, loss of libido, decrease in body hair
      (2) Males—loss of libido, decreased sperm count, possible impotence, decreased testicular size, decreased total body hair
4. Manifestations of GH deficiency
   a. Children
      (1) Stunted growth (below third percentile) with normal body proportions (Figure 36-3), excessive subcutaneous fat, poor muscle development
      (2) Immature facial features, immature voice
      (3) Slow growth of nails and thin hair
      (4) Delayed puberty but eventual normal sexual development
      (5) Decreased levels of GH

   b. Adults
      (1) No clinical manifestations
      (2) Decreased basal levels of GH or decreased response to provocative testing
      (3) Some persons may have normal GH levels with low levels of somatomedins
5. Manifestations of prolactin deficiency
   a. Failure to lactate in the postpartum female
   b. Decreased serum levels of prolactin
6. Manifestations of TSH deficiency
   a. Signs and symptoms of secondary hypothyroidism
   b. Decreased serum level of TSH and thyroid hormone
7. Manifestations of ACTH deficiency
   a. Signs and symptoms of secondary ACTH insufficiency; *no hyperpigmentation*
   b. Decreased serum levels of ACTH, glucocorticoids, and adrenal androgens (aldosterone levels may be normal)

MEDICAL MANAGEMENT

Medical management is directed toward identifying patients with deficiency syndromes, treating the underlying problem, and supplying the appropriate hormonal replacement. The target gland hormone (thyroid, cortisol, or gonadal steroids) is replaced as necessary. If a childbearing females desires fertility, gonadotropins must be replaced. However, prolactin does not need to be replaced.

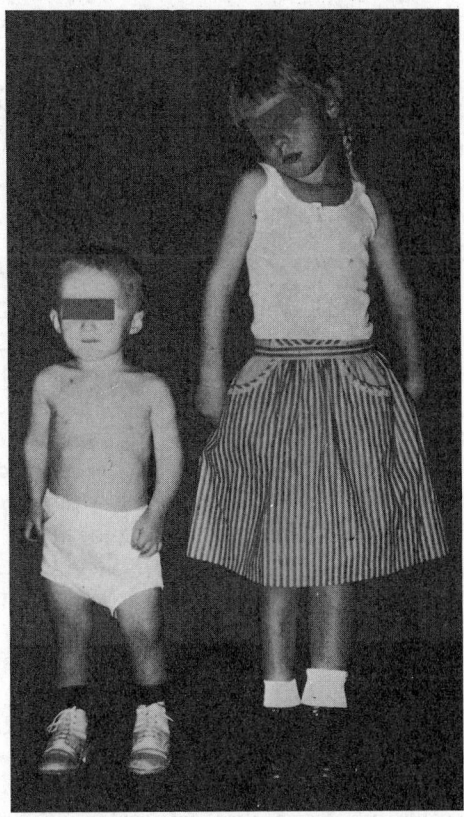

FIGURE 36-3 Hypopituitary dwarfism in 4-year-old boy whose height is 25 inches (62 cm). Girl is also 4 years old and has normal height of 39 inches (97 cm). Dwarf has a normal face, as well as head, trunk, and limbs of approximately normal proportions. (From Brashear HR and Raney RB: Shand's handbook of orthopaedic surgery, ed 9, St Louis, 1978, The CV Mosby Co.)

Replacement therapy of GH is used for all short children with GH deficiency. The source of GH in the past has been human cadaver pituitaries, but the occurrence of lethal infection in persons receiving this form of GH caused great concern and limited use. Biosynthetic human GH is now available. In the first year of treatment, there is a rapid catch-up pattern of growth, but the growth pattern then returns to normal. GH replacement also has been effective in some children with short stature who have normal GH levels.[21]

■ ASSESSMENT

Assessment focuses on identifying signs and symptoms of the hormonal deficiencies and etiologic factors. In addition, data are collected on how well the patient is dealing with the disorder. In this section, only data relevant to GH and gonadotropin deficiencies are described. (TSH and ACTH deficiencies are described later in the chapter.) Major areas for assessment include the following.

Subjective Data

1. History of changes in neurologic status, especially related to the presence of tumors (headache, vision changes)
2. History of previous pituitary damage, such as head or neck radiation or cranial surgery
3. In children, history of growth pattern and sexual development
4. In adults, history of sexual development and changes such as oligomenorrhea, amenorrhea, decreased libido, impotence, changes in secondary sex characteristics
5. History of generalized symptoms of deficiency, such as change in muscle strength, fatigue, lethargy, depression
6. Knowledge regarding disorder and proposed treatment

Objective Data

1. Visual changes: visual field, visual acuity
2. Facial features, body proportions
3. Distribution of fatty tissue and hair
4. Presence or absence of secondary sex characteristics

■ DATA ANALYSIS: NURSING DIAGNOSES

Nursing diagnoses are determined from assessment of patient data. Possible nursing diagnoses for the person with GH or gonadotropin deficiency include, but are not limited to, the following:

Diagnostic Title	Possible Etiologies
Body image disturbance	Lack of normal sexual development (child); lack of normal growth (child); change in sexual characteristics (adult)
Coping, ineffective individual	Lack of learned coping strategies; uncertainty about cause of problem
Knowledge deficit: disease procedures, treatment, nursing care needs	New disease and never being exposed to information
Sensory/perceptual alterations: visual	Growth of mass in cranium causing pressure on optic chiasm or cranial nerves III, IV, or VI
Sexual dysfunction	Alteration in desire or functioning associated with alterations in gonadotropin levels

■ PLANNING: EXPECTED PATIENT OUTCOMES

Expected patient outcomes for the person with deficiency of GH or gonadotropin may include, but are not limited to, the following:

1. Body image will improve as evidenced by the pa-

tient describing self in positive terms and describing ways to minimize body image changes.

2. Coping will improve as evidenced by the patient listing coping strategies helpful in dealing with the stressors related to hormonal deficiencies.

3. The patient describes the hormonal deficiency causing the problem, how it relates to the signs and symptoms, any tests planned, and the treatment planned.

4. The patient does not suffer any injuries related to the vision loss and maintains independence in ADLs.

5. The patient describes how therapy can reverse sexual dysfunction.

■ **IMPLEMENTATION**

One focus of care is helping the patient deal with disturbances or alterations in body image. The patient should know what changes are reversible. Treatment with sex steroids helps to initiate the development of sexual characteristics in the adolescent entering puberty. Treatment with sex steroids restores secondary sexual characteristics in adults, and treatment with gonadotropins restores fertility in the female with normal menstrual cycles. Replacement of GH increases growth in the child with short stature. The parents and child should know what growth outcome is expected so that unrealistic goals are not set. (Refer to Chapter 18 for additional information on how to assist persons with alterations in body images.)

Another focus of care is to help patients cope with signs and symptoms that are not reversible or that take a long time to reverse. Helping them see their positive attributes is one alternative. Another alternative is helping them develop positive coping strategies such as relaxation techniques and new hobbies. (See Chapters 10 and 11 for additional information on coping.)

Patient education is another focus of care. The patient must be prepared for various diagnostic tests, including blood tests and roentgenograms, CT scans, or MRI of the head. If a tumor is the cause of the deficiency, the tumor is removed. A transsphenoidal approach is usually used, or the tumor is treated by radiation. Hormonal replacement of GH in children and therapy with gonadal steroids and gonadotropins in adolescents and adults are individualized. The patient needs to be taught how to take the hormones. GHs are given subcutaneously. Gonadal steroids are given orally to restore sexual characteristics, and gonadotropin or clomiphene citrate is used in females to induce ovulation if pregnancy is desired. An important focus of teaching is for patients to realize the need for adequate steroids to prevent premature bone dimineralization. Patients who decline hormone therapy, particularly women, need to be monitored periodically

for accelerated bone loss and must take adequate calcium.[47]

If visual changes are present, care as described on p. 1040 is necessary. In relation to the sexual dysfunction, patient education about the cause of the problem and the replacement therapy described previously are the major interventions.

PITUITARY APOPLEXY

Persons with pituitary tumors may have a history of sudden onset of severe headache, vomiting, visual impairment, and altered mental and autonomic functioning (hypotension, hyperthermia). This syndrome, called *pituitary apoplexy,* is the result of a sudden enlargement of the tumor by hemorrhagic necrosis occurring from damage to the tumor's fragile vascular supply. Some other causes of pituitary hemorrhage include head injury, pregnancy and delivery, long-term ventilatory support, meningoencephalitis, estrogen drug therapy, anticoagulation, and radiation therapy.

Laboratory abnormalities include leukocytosis, xanchromic or bloody CSF, and increased CSF pressure. Radiographic examination may show an enlarged sella turcica.

The treatment of these patients is still controversial. Most authorities agree that corticosteroids should be given to correct any adrenal insufficiency and to decrease cerebral edema.[65] Most patients with visual or mental changes are treated with decompression surgery using a transsphenoidal approach. Many patients recover with normal endocrine function, but if deficiencies occur later, care is similar to that described on p. 1032.

HYPOPITUITARISM: POSTERIOR PITUITARY GLAND—DIABETES INSIPIDUS
ETIOLOGY

Pituitary diabetes insipidus (DI) results from a lack of sufficient ADH. The cause may be a brain or pituitary tumor, head trauma, encephalitis, meningitis, hypophysectomy, or cranial surgery. The cause is often idiopathic, although a rare hereditary form of the disease occurs. Nephrogenic DI is a second form of the disorder and results from failure of the renal tubules to respond to ADH.

PATHOPHYSIOLOGY

The lack of adequate ADH or ineffective kidney response to ADH results in insufficient water reabsorption by the kidney. The loss of excessive water from the body (polyuria) stimulates the perception of thirst (polydipsia). If the problem is longstanding, the kidney, pelvis, and urinary bladder may show changes caused by the large urine volume. When inadequate water replacement occurs, CNS and vascular changes from hyperosmolality and volume depletion can occur.

CLINICAL MANIFESTATIONS

Inadequate *water reabsorption* by the kidneys results in the following symptoms:

1. Polyuria—as much as 20 L urine/day may be excreted; urine is dilute with a specific gravity of 1.005 or less or an osmolality of 200 or less
2. Polydipsia secondary to increased thirst
3. Only slightly elevated serum osmolality because water intake is usually maintained
4. Abnormal results on tests for urine concentration
   a. Water deprivation test (see Chapter 35)—no increase in urine concentration with either pituitary or nephrogenic DI
   b. ADH replacement—increase in urine osmolality with pituitary DI but no response with nephrogenic DI
5. Sleep disturbances from polyuria
6. Inadequate *water replacement* results in:
   a. Hyperosmolality—irritability, mental dullness, coma, hyperthermia
   b. Hypovolemia—hypotension, tachycardia, dry mucous membranes, poor skin turgor

INTERVENTIONS

Medical Management

The person with pituitary DI is treated with vasopressin replacement. Temporary DI associated with head trauma or surgery is treated with aqueous vasopressin, 5 to 10 IU subcutaneously. For chronic DI, the most frequently used preparation is desmopressin (DDAVP), a synthetic analog of vasopressin. It is taken nasally in doses of 5 to 20 μg daily or 5 to 10 μg twice daily. Duration of action is 12 to 24 hours. DDAVP has very few of the smooth muscle or vascular side effects that may occur with vasopressin tannate. For persons who have some residual pituitary function, chlorpropamide and clofibrate (which stimulate the release of endogenous ADH) may be prescribed.

The most common treatment for persons with nephrogenic DI is a low-sodium, low-protein diet and thiazide diuretics. The low-sodium diet and thiazide diuretics induce a mild volume depletion. This volume depletion enhances sodium chloride and water reabsorption in the proximal part of the kidney tubule, resulting in less water being delivered to the collecting tubules where ADH should be; therefore less water is excreted. The diuretic also increases the osmolality of the medullary interstitial space and thus promotes more water resorption in collecting tubules that are less permeable because of inadequate ADH.[49] The protein restriction helps control water loss by decreasing solute excretion. A last therapy in nephrogenic DI is administration of nonsteroidal anti-inflammatory agents, which impair prostaglandin production in the kidney and increase urinary concentrating ability.[49]

If the patient is showing *hypernatremia* and clinical signs and symptoms such as mental changes and hyperthermia are present, replacement of water must be instituted. Water replacement must be done carefully over 48 hours[49] to avoid cerebral edema, seizures, or even death. Too rapid a correction of hypernatremia by fluid administration may result in the establishment of an osmotic gradient, with the plasma osmolality being less than the intracellular osmolality and the entry of water into the brain. The water deficit for a patient with hypernatremia is estimated, and this deficit, along with continual insensible water loss or dilute urinary loss, is replaced over 48 hours. The exact fluid administered will vary depending on the patient's needs. If pure water loss is present, free water is given orally or in the form of dextrose in water. If the patient is hypotensive as well as hypernatremic, isotonic saline is given until *vascular volume* is adequate, and then free water is given. If the patient has a slight deficit in sodium along with free water deficit, one-quarter strength sodium chloride is used. During fluid replacement, serial measurement of plasma sodium level and assessment of mental and circulatory status are required every 1 to 2 hours.

Nursing Management

Nursing interventions for the person with DI focus on maintenance of fluid and electrolyte balance, provision of rest, and teaching.

1. Maintain fluid and electrolyte balance.
   a. Assess intake and output, daily weights, urine specific gravity, vital signs (orthostatic), skin turgor, and neurologic status every 1 to 2 hours during the acute phase, then every 4 to 8 hours until discharge, and then on return to physician or outpatient clinic.
   b. Provide fluids; be sure that they are within reach of patient.
2. Provide daily rest periods during time when nocturia interferes with sleep.
3. Provide patient teaching.
   a. Diagnostic tests: purposes, procedures, and required monitoring (see Chapter 35)
   b. Self-management: drug therapy
      1. Administration: method and frequency
      2. Effectiveness: if nasal congestion occurs, drug effectiveness may decrease and polyuria and thirst occur
      3. Side effects: particularly signs of volume excess (weight gain, edema)

THYROID GLAND

Disorders of the thyroid gland are relatively common endocrine problems. They are second to diabetes mellitus in occurrence. Alterations in the thyroid gland may be associated with hypersecretion, hyposecretion, or normal secretion of thyroid hormone.

A goiter is a typical finding in many patients with

thyroid problems. Goiter is an enlargement of the thyroid gland that causes the gland to form a protuberance on the anterior aspect of the neck. Goiters occur because of hypertrophy of the gland when it is being stimulated by increased amounts of TSH or any substances that act as TSH. Goiter can be associated with hyperthyroidism, hypothyroidism, or euthyroidism.

HYPERSECRETION OF THYROID HORMONE: HYPERTHYROIDISM
ETIOLOGY/EPIDEMIOLOGY

Hyperthyroidism, also called thyrotoxicosis, is a condition that results when tissues are stimulated by excessive thyroid hormone. The numerous causes of hyperthyroidism are summarized in Table 36-1. The most common cause is toxic diffuse goiter (Graves', or Basedow's, disease). The second most common cause is toxic multinodular goiter.

Graves' Disease

Graves' disease is a disorder characterized by one or more of the following: *diffuse goiter, hyperthyroidism,* and *infiltrative ophthalmopathy.* Occasionally, *infiltrative dermopathy* is seen. It is important to note that ophthalmopathy or dermopathy can occur without hyperthyroidism. Graves' disease is most often seen in females under age 40.

Research supports the contention that Graves' disease is caused by stimulation of the gland by immunoglobulins of the IgG class. It is believed that the thyroid related immunoglobulins are a heterogenous group of antibodies directed at varying sites within the thyroid cell membrane. These immunoglobulins are called *thyroid-stimulating immunoglobulins* (TSIs).

The cause of the abnormal development of immunoglobulins is unknown. Heredity, gender, and perhaps emotions have a role.[64] The hereditary influence is manifested by the higher frequency of Graves' disease in persons with specific haplotypes and the higher rate in monozygotic twins. Graves' disease occurs 7 to 10 times more often in women than in men. The disease often occurs after severe emotional stress.[64] The exact incidence of Graves' disease is uncertain, but it is thought to occur in approximately 0.4% of the U.S. population.[64]

Toxic Multinodular Goiter

Toxic multinodular goiter is a disorder characterized by the presence of many thyroid nodules and a milder form of hyperthyroidism than that seen with Graves' disease. Toxic multinodular goiter usually occurs after age 50 in persons who have had multinodular goiter for many years. The multinodular goiter is probably caused by mild iodide deficiency.[16] Unlike Graves' disease, it does not have an autoimmune basis.

TABLE 36-1 Causes and definitions of types of hyperthyroidism

Cause	Definition
Toxic diffuse goiter (Graves' disease)	See discussion in text
Toxic multinodular goiter	See discussion in text
Toxic adenoma	Single or occasionally multiple adenomas of follicular cells that secrete and function independent of TSH
Thyroiditis	Increased amount of thyroxine (T_4) and triiodothyronine (T_3) released during acute inflammatory process; transient hyperthyroid state followed by return to euthyroid state, and eventually to hypothyroid state as gland is destroyed by the recuring inflammatory exacerbations; hyperthyroid state usually requires no treatment
T_3 thyrotoxicosis	T_3 level elevated but cause unknown; T_4 normal or low; should be suspected in patients who have normal T_4 but have signs and symptoms of thyrotoxicosis
Hyperthyroidism caused by metastatic thyroid cancer	Rare because thyroid cancer cells do not usually concentrate iodine efficiently; may occur with large follicular carcinomas
Pituitary hyperthyroidism	Rare; pituitary adenomas may secrete excess TSH; treatment involves removal of pituitary tumor
Chorionic hyperthyroidism	Chorionic gonadotropin has weak thyrotropin activity; tumors such as choriocarcinoma, embryonal cell carcinoma, and hydatiform mole have high concentrations of chorionic gonadotropins that can stimulate T_4 and T_3 secretion; hyperthyroidism disappears with treatment of tumor
Struma ovarii	Ovarian dermoid tumor made up of thyroid tissue that secretes thyroid hormone
Factitious hyperthyroidism	Results from ingestion of exogenous thyroid extracts
Iodine-induced hyperthyroidism (Jod-Basedow)	Overproduction of thyroid hormone resulting from administration of supplemental iodine to a person with endemic goiter

PREVENTION

Only two of the causes of hyperthyroidism are preventable: factitious (artificial) hyperthyroidism and iodine-induced hyperthyroidism. Prevention of factitious hyperthyroidism is possible by appropriate health teaching regarding safe measures for weight reduction and weight control. To prevent iodine-induced hyperthyroidism, persons with endemic goiter who are treated with supplemental iodine must be monitored very closely. Secondary preventive health care measures for persons with hyperthyroidism include early detection of signs and symptoms and early prompt treatment to prevent disease progression.

PATHOPHYSIOLOGY

In hyperthyroidism the normal regulatory control of thyroid function is lost, resulting in an increased concentration of thyroid hormone and increased peripheral manifestations of thyroid hormone excess. Thyroid hormone increases metabolic rate and calorigenesis; alters protein, fat, and carbohydrate metabolism; directly stimulates some body functions such as bone and bone marrow; and increases sympathetic (adrenergic) activity. The interaction of these various alterations results in changes in almost every body system. Enlargement of the thyroid gland (goiter) occurs because of increased stimulation of the thyroid gland by TSH or TSH-like substances in most causes of hyperthyroidism.

In Graves' disease, ophthalmopathy may precede, occur at the same time, or follow hyperthyroidism. In ophthalmopathy the retrobulbar connective tissue and extraocular muscle volume are expanded. This volume expansion occurs because of fluid retention resulting from the accumulation of glycosaminoglycans. The increase in tissue mass forces the eye forward (proptosis) up to the limits of the restraining action of the extraocular muscles. The pressure in retrobulbar space increases because of an increase in retrobulbar tissue and limited forward movement and causes periorbital and lid edema and pressure on the optic nerve.[20] The stretched enlarged extraocular muscles do not function well.

Glycosaminoglycans and fluid accumulation also occur in the connective tissue in other parts of the body. This accumulation is particularly seen in the pretibial area.

The pathophysiologic factors just described are related to specific clinical manifestations in Table 36-2. It must be remembered that the underlying pathophysiology of all manifestations of hyperthyroidism is not known.

CLINICAL MANIFESTATIONS

The typical patient with hyperthyroidism is nervous and has tremors, muscle weakness, weight loss, intolerance to heat, increased sweating, warm skin, increased fre-

quency of defecation, tachycardia, and widened pulse pressure resulting from increased systolic and decreased diastolic pressures. The patient usually demonstrates emotional lability and may give a history of amenorrhea. These symptoms may have been present for six or more months. A complete listing of all manifestations is given in Table 36-2.

A goiter is usually present. Goiters are seen in toxic diffuse goiter (Graves' disease), toxic multinodular goiter, pituitary hyperthyroidism (secondary hyperthyroidism), thyroiditis, triiodothyronine (T_3) thyrotoxicosis, and iodine-induced hyperthyroidism. Chorionic hyperthyroidism may or may not be associated with a goiter. In toxic adenomas small well-defined nodules occur, whereas with cancer there are ill-defined nodules. Persons with hyperthyroidism resulting from struma ovarii and persons with factitious hyperthyroidism do not have goiters.

When hyperthyroidism is suspected, various diagnostic tests are necessary to confirm the diagnosis. (See Chapter 35 for a complete description of tests used.) The first tests done are measurement of serum thyroxine (T_4) and free T_4 or free T_4 index. In most cases of hyperthyroidism, these levels are elevated. If these tests are not conclusive, a serum T_3 level and free T_3 is done. In T_3 thyrotoxicosis, these levels are elevated with normal T_4 and free T_4 index. Radioactive iodine uptake (RAIU) is elevated in all types of hyperthyroidism except thyroiditis, factitious thyrotoxicosis, and struma ovarii.

When serum thyroid hormone levels and RAIU tests are inconclusive, a thyroid-releasing hormone (TRH) test or thyroid suppression test is done. Patients with hyperthyroidism usually show blunted TSH response to TRH and no suppression of RAIU with exogenous thyroid therapy.

MEDICAL MANAGEMENT

Medical therapy is designed to reduce the output of thyroid hormone and to antagonize the effects of thyroid hormone on peripheral tissue. Two approaches that may be used to achieve these goals are (1) the use of drugs to antagonize the effects of thyroid hormone and to reduce the output of thyroid hormone or (2) ablation (therapy to remove or destroy tissue) of thyroid tissue by surgery or radioactive therapy. Drug therapy is usually used first to promote a euthyroid state before using ablation therapy. After the initial drug therapy, the drugs may be continued or surgery or radioactive therapy may be used. The choice of therapeutic measures is individualized based on age, size of goiter, severity of hyperthyroidism, duration of illness, reproductive status, and cause of hyperthyroidism.[25] The various therapies are discussed next. In adults with Graves' disease, radioactive iodine is the therapy of choice after short-term treatment with antithyroid drugs. Surgery is the treat-

TABLE 36-2 Pathophysiologic factors and clinical manifestations as a result of elevated thyroid levels (hyperthyroidism)

Pathophysiologic Factors	Clinical Manifestations	Pathophysiologic Factors	Clinical Manifestations
CENTRAL NERVOUS SYSTEM ALTERATIONS		**ALTERATION IN EYES**	
Result in part from increased adrenergic activity	Nervousness: restless, short attention span, compulsion to move Emotional lability: crying without apparent cause, loss of temper, severe psychic disturbance Hyperkinesia: cannot sit still, taps feet, drums fingers, shifts position; movements quick, jerky, rhythmic; tremors of hands, tongue, eyelids	Results from increased adrenergic activity	"Bright-eyed stare" results from retraction of upper eyelid (can see rim of sclera between lid and limbus) Lid lag (upper lid lags behind globe with slow downward gaze) Globe lag (globe lags behind lid with upward gaze) Lid movement: jerky and spasmodic Graves' disease: (ocular changes caused by infiltrative ophthalmopathy) (Figure 36-4) Early symptoms of infiltrative ophthalmopathy; sense of irritation and excessive tearing; injected conjunctivae; later: exophthalmos, feeling of pressure behind globe, sleep with eyes partly open; periorbital edema, vision blurred, double vision, eyes tire easily; extraocular muscle involvement, corneal ulceration and eventually optic nerve involvement (optic neuropathy)
CARDIOVASCULAR SYSTEM ALTERATIONS			
Result from increased adrenergic state as well as the hyperdynamic state stimulated by increased metabolism and increased heat production	Tachycardia (pulse > 90) even at rest Increased systolic and decreased diastolic pressures with increased pulse pressure, palpitations Loud heart sounds with possible murmurs at apex Dysrhythmias: supraventricular, atrial fibrillation Heart failure if underlying heart disease; poor response to digitalis preparations Edema: mild, present even without heart failure		
RESPIRATORY ALTERATIONS		**ALIMENTARY SYSTEM ALTERATIONS**	
Result from changes in muscle structure caused by altered metabolism	Dyspnea; may be present even without heart failure Reduced vital capacity caused by weak muscle Ventilation increased greater than oxygen uptake during exercise	Result in part from increased metabolism	Increased appetite at meals and between meals Weight loss because intake less than requirements Increased frequency of stools; stools less formed Hepatic dysfunction in severe cases (decreased serum albumin, increased serum enzymes, jaundice)
SKIN AND HAIR ALTERATIONS		**ALTERATION IN METABOLISM**	
Result in part from increased circulation seen with thyroid hormone excess associated with increased adrenergic activity	Skin: warm and moist because of vasodilation, texture smooth and pink, particularly noticeable over thorax, elbows Palmar erythema Hair: fine, friable, some falling out Nails: soft, friable If Graves' disease, infiltrative dermopathy: induration, thickening and hyperpigmentation of skin over pretibial area (pretibial myxedema) and over dorsum of feet; may have clubbing of digits and osteoarthropathy	Result from increased metabolic rate	Increased body temperature Intolerance to heat Muscle wasting caused by degradation of protein Increased degradation of insulin worsening diabetes mellitus Increased degradation of triglycerides (increased serum free fatty acids; decreased cholesterol and serum triglycerides)
		HEMATOPOIETIC SYSTEM ALTERATIONS	
		Result from increased erythropoietin and stimulatory effect of thyroid hormone on bone marrow	Increased RBC mass with normal indices (see Chapter 30) Decreased total WBC count caused by decreased granulocytosis
MUSCULOSKELETAL ALTERATIONS		**REPRODUCTIVE ALTERATIONS**	
Result in part from impaired ability to phosphorylate creatine and direct action of thyroid hormone in stimulating bone resorption	Weakness, fatigue, and generalized wasting most prominent in proximal muscles: difficulty climbing stairs or maintaining leg in extended position; difficulty in rising from sitting or lying position seen in extreme form Increased excretion of calcium and phosphorus ions sometimes associated with demineralization of bone and fractures Hypercalcemia may occur	Result from alteration in the secretion and metabolism of gonadotropins and gonadal steroids	Prepubertal: delayed sexual development Postpubertal: increased libido; menstrual alterations (change in intermenstrual interval, diminished menstrual flow); decreased fertility; increased incidence of spontaneous abortions

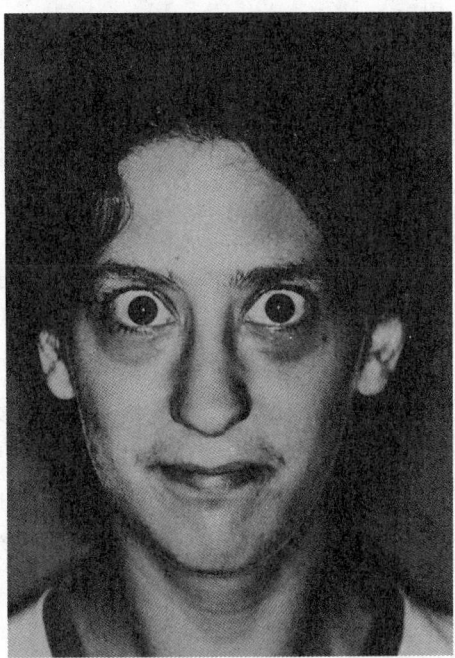

FIGURE 36-4 Ophthalmopathy of Graves' disease. Patient has typical noninfiltrative changes (stare with severe upper and lower lid retraction). (From Rose L and Kaye D: Fundamentals of internal medicine, St Louis, 1983, The CV Mosby Co.)

ment of choice for patients with Graves' disease who have large goiters and is frequently still used as primary therapy for children and adults of child-bearing age who have Graves' disease. Surgery is often the treatment of choice for patients with toxic multinodular goiter because of the poor iodine uptake of these goiters,[60] unless the patient is a poor surgical risk.

Drug Therapy

Thioamides. *Propylthiouracil* (PTU) and *methimazole* (Tapazole) are the most frequently used antithyroid drugs. The action of these drugs is slow, and it usually takes 2 to 4 weeks before improvement is noticeable. This is because these drugs block thyroid hormone synthesis and not the secretion of the hormone itself. The supply of hormone stored in the gland must be reduced before improvement is seen, and this takes from 2 to 4 weeks. The patient usually is started on a relatively large dose of the antithyroid drug (propylthiouracil, 300 to 450 mg/day in three divided doses; methimazole, 30 to 45 mg/day in three divided doses). Then the dosage is gradually reduced to a level sufficient to maintain the euthyroid state (propylthiouracil, 100 to 150 mg/day, or methimazole, 10 to 15 mg/day, both given in divided doses). When antithyroid drugs are used as the primary therapy, they usually are continued for 6 to 18 months or longer. Approximately one-half the persons with Graves' disease will develop a spontaneous remission of

their hyperthyroidism. Although it is impossible to predict which persons will go into remission, persons whose goiters decrease in size and who remain euthyroid as drug dosage is decreased are the most likely candidates. No guarantee exists that patients will remain in remission. In one study the remission rate 1 year after discontinuance of medications was only 38%.[25] The patient should see the physician regularly after drugs are discontinued so that early signs of recurrence can be detected. Patients who redevelop hyperthyroidism require drug therapy, radioactive iodine therapy, or surgery.

Antithyroid drugs must be taken several times a day to maintain an adequate blood level and drug effect. This administration schedule is a disadvantage to using drugs as a primary therapy.

Patients are instructed to look for toxic signs of the drugs, such as fever, sore throat, and skin eruptions or any signs of infection and to call their physician immediately if these signs appear. The signs of infection need to be reported immediately because they may indicate *agranulocytosis* (lack of production of granulocytes). If this occurs, the drugs are stopped immediately. Almost all patients' recover from agranulocytosis; however, the patient's hyperthyroidism must be treated with some alternative therapeutic measure, as discussed next.

Iodides. Preparations of iodine, such as *Lugol's solution,* are used in the treatment of hyperthyroidism. Iodides reduce the metabolic rate rapidly because they block the release and synthesis of thyroid hormone. However, these actions are not sustained, and iodides can only be used as the primary treatment of hyperthyroidism for 1 to 3 weeks. Iodides also may be reduce glandular vascularity and may be used preoperatively to prevent hemorrhage. When Lugol's solution is ordered, it is more palatable given in milk or fruit juice. It should be taken through a straw because it may stain the teeth. A brassy taste in the mouth and sore teeth and gums are signs of toxicity, but these complications rarely occur.

There are some disadvantages to the use of iodides, including (1) the patient cannot be treated for some time (weeks) with radioactive iodine (RAI) because the thyroid gland is saturated with iodide and the RAI will not be taken up; (2) some persons develop an exacerbation of their disease when RAI is given following iodide treatment; and (3) if iodide is given before treatment with other antithyroid drugs, this also may result in an exacerbation of hyperthyroidism.

Other drugs. The β-adrenergic blocking drugs, such as propranolol (Inderal), are used to treat symptoms from increased sympathetic nervous system stimulation, such as tachycardia, dysrhythmias, and angina. These drugs also improve tremors, restlessness, anxiety, and sometimes myopathy. Propranolol, 20 to 40 mg every 4 to 6 hours, may be given for symptom control, except in persons with congestive heart failure or bronchial asthma. Propranolol is used in all patients with *thyroid storm.*

Lithium has been found to block hormone release. However, it is used less often than other drugs and is saved for times when patients develop toxicity to other drugs or as an adjunct to other therapy during thyrotoxic crisis. Because lithium has the ability to block the release of thyroid hormone, hypothyroidism can occur as a side-effect of lithium therapy.

Radioactive Iodine Therapy

RAI therapy with ^{131}I is increasingly being used because it (1) can be given on an outpatient basis; (2) is safer for a wider range of patients, including the elderly, who are poorer surgical risks; (3) can result in faster improvement in thyroid function than antithyroid drug therapy; and (4) although still controversial, can be used in women of childbearing age. RAI is given orally in one dose. The dosage is individualized, but on the average it is 80 to 90 µCi/g of thyroid tissue or equivalent to 6000 to 7000 rad. Although symptoms of hyperthyroidism will decrease in approximately 3 weeks, *a euthyroid state will not be achieved for 6 months.* The treatment must be repeated in about 20% of patients.

The RAI is eliminated in a very short time after treatment, approximately 2 days. Because of this short excretion time, no tests are used to monitor RAI elimination from the body. RAI is excreted in urine, saliva, sweat, and feces. The major precaution to protect others is care with body secretions, particularly urine. The toilet should be flushed two or three times after each use. The patient should increase his or her intake of liquids to aid in the RAI's excretion. Other precautions include using separate eating utensils, separate towels and washcloths, washing these as well as underclothes and bed linens separately. Other precautions include rinsing bathroom sinks and tubs thoroughly after use, and washing hands carefully after using the bathroom. Although the amount of radiation in the patient's body is minimal, the patient should sleep alone for a few days and avoid kissing and sexual intercourse. Prolonged physical contact with anyone, including holding a baby, should be avoided. Breast-feeding is not allowed. The length of time these restrictions are required varies, but it is usually only for a few days, sometimes only 2 days.

RAI is not used in pregnant women because of the potential effect on the fetus; the placenta transports iodine easily. As stated previously, the use of RAI in women in their childbearing years is still controversial.

If used in this age group, pregnancy should be delayed for 6 months after therapy.[65]

The major side effect of RAI therapy is hypothyroidism. Although different authorities[25,65] report different figures for the percentage of persons developing hypothyroidism each year after ^{131}I therapy, eventually almost 100% of all persons become hypothyroid. Persons must be told about this complication before treatment. Patients are monitored for this complication and should know the signs and symptoms of hypothyroidism (see p. 1046) and report their onset to their physician.

Surgery

As previously mentioned, surgery is still used in selected patients with hyperthyroidism, including those with very large goiters, persons whose thyroid glands have a low uptake of iodine, children, and pregnant women. Thyroid surgery has the advantage over RAI therapy in that the incidence of hypothyroidism is much less. However, it is important to remember that the remaining thyroid tissue can hypertrophy and result in a recurrence of hyperthyroidism. The risks associated with thyroid surgery are very minimal in patients treated by experienced surgeons.[25] Thyroid surgery and care of the patient having thyroid surgery are discussed on pp. 1055-1057.

Care of the Eyes

Various ocular changes occur in Graves' disease. Patients usually have a staring gaze, lid lag on downward gaze, and globe lag on upward gaze, which are partly caused by increased activity of the sympathetic nervous system. In addition, more serious ocular conditions resulting from infiltrative changes may be present. The mild symptoms of lid lag and so forth cause no functional changes in vision and usually resolve with adequate treatment of the hyperthyroidism. The changes from infiltration of the extraocular muscles and retrobulbar space require other treatment and do not resolve with treatment of the hyperthyroidism. Treatment of eye changes is multifocal. For the mild changes of lid lag and so on, no additional treatment other then dark glasses may be necessary if the patient experiences photophobia and sensitivity to wind or cold. For periorbital and lid edema, the patient is instructed not to sleep in the prone position and to sleep with head elevated. Sometimes diuretics are used. If the patient experiences a gritty feeling with eyelid closure, 1% methylcellulose eye drops (artificial tears) may be used.

When proptosis or eyelid retraction prevents imperfect coverage of the globe of the eye, surgery such as section of Müller's muscle, scleral graft insertion in the eyelids and tarsorrhaphy may be done.[20] For persons who show severe inflammatory changes such as injection, pain, or chemosis of the conjunctiva, systemic or retrobulbar steroids are tried. Often glucocortocoid therapy halts the progression of the process and causes regression. The patient needs to be monitored for side effects of the steroid therapy.

If the disease progresses and the patient develops persistent diplopia, extraocular muscle surgery to correct dysfunction may be done. If proptosis and other problems are so severe that optic neuropathy, corneal ulcerations, and severe discomfort occur and are unresponsive to steroids, orbital decompression or supervoltage x-ray therapy may be used. The orbital decompression expands the orbital space. The radiation potentially shrinks the retrobulbar tissue. None of the therapy described here attacks the basic pathophysiologic process, that is the infiltrative changes directly. That is, the therapy does not inhibit the production of glycosaminoglycan in the retrobulbar tissue. Better understanding of this pathophysiologic process will add new treatment measures.[20] For a detailed discussion of the surgical procedures, the reader should consult Chapter 65.

■ ASSESSMENT

As described, hyperthyroidism can affect almost every system of the body and cause major physiologic and psychosocial problems.

Subjective Data
Subjective data include the following:
1. History of emotional and mental status changes
2. Complaints of palpitations or chest pain
3. Complaints of dyspnea, with or without exercise
4. History of changes in hair, skin, nails, or amount of sweating
5. Complaints of visual disturbances and irritations; reports of eyes tiring easily
6. Appetite, history of nutritional intake and weight changes
7. History of increased stool frequency and stool bulk
8. History of intolerance to heat
9. Complaints of weakness, fatigue, decreased ability to complete ADL
10. History of changes in menses or change in libido
11. Knowledge—disease, treatment, care needs

Objective Data
Objective data include the following:
1. Mental status changes—shortened attention span, emotional lability, hyperkinesia, tremor
2. Cardiovascular status changes—increased systolic blood pressure, decreased diastolic pressure, tachycardia at rest, dysrhythmias, murmurs

3. Skin and hair changes—warm, flushed, moist skin; dermopathy; fine, thinning hair
4. Eye changes—lid lag, globe lag, diplopia, injection of conjunctiva, decreased acuity
5. Nutritional/metabolic changes—decreased weight, increased appetite and intake, decreased serum triglycerides and cholesterol
6. Musculoskeletal changes—muscle weakness, decreased muscle tone, difficulty rising from sitting position
7. Thyroid changes—goiter, presence of bruits over thyroid, abnormal laboratory blood test results— elevated T_4 and free T_4 index; other tests may also be abnormal, but these are the major ones

■ DATA ANAYSIS: NURSING DIAGNOSES

Nursing diagnoses are determined from assessment of patient data. Possible nursing diagnoses for the person with hyperthyroidism include, but are not limited to, the following:

Diagnostic Title	Possible Etiologies
Activity intolerance, potential	Muscle weakness and wasting associated with altered metabolism
Cardiac output, decreased	Dysrhythmias associated with increased sympathetic activity
Coping, ineffective individual	Altered processing of sensory input, decreased attention span, emotional lability
Home maintenance management, impaired	Delay between initiation of therapy and return of euthyroid state
Hyperthermia	Increased heat production greater than dissipation
Knowledge deficit: disease, treatment, outcomes, self-monitoring needs	Never presented with new information
Nutrition, altered: less than body requirements	Increased metabolic needs
Sensory/perceptual alterations: visual	Disruption of function of optic nerves or extraocular muscles of eyes associated with infiltrative changes
Sleep pattern disturbance	Increased metabolic rate, restlessness

■ PLANNING: EXPECTED PATIENT OUTCOMES

Expected patient outcomes for the person with hyperthyroidism may include, but are not limited to, the following:
1. The patient demonstrates no further decrease in activity tolerance and shows, over 2 to 3 months, a gradual increase in activity.
2. The patient shows evidence of adequate tissue perfusion and cardiac output as evidenced by no

change in mental status, breath sounds clear, and no edema formation, the patient's heart rate stays within 20 beats of baseline, and a gradual decrease in resting heart rate occurs.

3. The patient shows effective coping as evidenced by rating self as less anxious or less stressed on a 1 to 10 scale, with 1 meaning no stress and 10 the worst stress; the patient lists three ways to cope with feelings.

4. The patient identifies home maintenance difficulties and states how these can be taken care of until health is stable.

5. The patient has normal body temperature and patient states that he or she is comfortable.

6. The patient is able to:
   a. Describe how hyperthyroidism causes the signs and symptoms present.
   b. List treatment options available.
   c. List expected outcomes of treatment with realistic time frames.
   d. List signs and symptoms requiring self-monitoring (signs and symptoms of hypothyroidism, hyperthyroidism, agranulocytosis).
   e. List precautions to be observed if RAI therapy is used.

7. Nutritional status is improved as evidenced by stable and gradual increase of weight.

8. The patient's visual acuity remains stable or improves; the patient does not complain of eye pain, diplopia, or a decrease in acuity that goes undetected.

■ **IMPLEMENTATION**

A nursing care plan for a specific patient is presented on pp. 1043 to 1044 and illustrates some of the care needs of persons with hyperthyroidism. Many patients with hyperthyroidism are managed outside the hospital setting. Possible interventions include the following:

1. Maintain and increase activity tolerance.
   a. Encourage short walks if cardiac output is stable.
   b. Space activity between rest periods.

2. Maintain cardiac output.
   a. Monitor cardiovascular status every 4 to 8 hours.
   b. Report any changes to the physician, such as increased tachycardia, dysrhythmias, or signs of congestive heart failure (see Chapter 28).
   c. Decrease cardiac workload by decreasing physical and emotional stressors.

3. Facilitate improved coping; offer patients interventions to help them relax, such as music, back rubs, and distraction.

4. Maintain home maintenance.

a. Work with the patient and significant others to identify problem areas related to home maintenance.
   b. Identify someone who can take on selected tasks.
   c. Help the patient plan schedule for doing tasks so that he or she has adequate rest.

5. Maintain normal body temperature.
   a. Monitor temperature every 4 hours; report any elevations.
   b. Use external cooling devices as ordered.
   c. Maintain room temperature in cool range.
   d. Encourage frequent showers and wearing cool clothes to help with comfort and heat dissipation.

6. Enhance patient knowledge.
   a. Describe the disease and how it causes signs and symptoms.
   b. Clarify treatment options.
   c. List the expected outomes, such as relief of symptoms in 4 weeks if receiving drug therapy, need for drug therapy for extended periods, and the potential complications of therapy.
   d. List signs and symptoms the patient must self-monitor.
   e. List precautions if the patient received RAI, such as how long he or she should sleep alone, refrain from intimate contact, limit physical contact with children, and handle own clothes and eating utensils separately.
   f. List planned follow-up care.

7. Maintain adequate nutrition intake.
   a. Monitor intake and output every 8 hours.
   b. Weigh daily.
   c. Monitor nutritional intake.
   d. Provide frequent high-protein, high-calorie meals.

8. Promote good eye care.
   a. Monitor cornea for damage, visual acuity, and patient complaints every shift.
   b. Initiate appropriate measures such as dark glasses, elevating head of bed, use of artificial tears, and taping eyelids closed at various intervals.
   c. Report any new complaints immediately.

9. Promote adequate rest.
   a. Provide quiet, comfortable environment.
   b. Provide back rubs.
   c. Use home remedies such as hot milk to assist in promoting sleep.
   d. Encourage quiet periods even if the patient does not sleep.

See research box (p. 1046) for a description of research supporting the effectiveness of different relaxation measures.

NURSING CARE PLAN

PERSON WITH HYPERTHYROIDISM

DATA: Mrs. Talbot, a 28-year-old housewife, is admitted for diagnostic evaluation before a thyroidectomy, which is scheduled to be performed in 2 weeks. Graves' disease was diagnosed 2 days ago; hospitalization was delayed until child-care arrangements were made for her 6-year-old stepson. (The marriage occurred 3 months ago.) Initial therapy, started 2 days ago, is Tapazole and Lugol's solution. The ECG report is sinus tachycardia (rate 132).

The nursing history identified the following about the patient:
- She feels overwhelmed, cries frequently, and fears losing control of temper.
- She has lost 15 lb in 2 months and is always hungry, although she is eating large amounts of food.
- She is bothered by heat, others' noisiness, and her own clumsiness.
- She expects medicine to make her feel better and dreads surgery.

The physical examination revealed the following:
- BP: 140/60; pulse: 132, R: 24
- Staring gaze of eyes with proptosis (equal bilaterally); lid lag and globe lag present; right eye slightly reddened
- Skin warm and perspiration present
- Increased muscle tone with weakness of lower extremities; quick muscle response to sudden noise; fine tremor of both hands
- Diffuse visible enlargement of thyroid
- *Bruit* present over thyroid

Collaborative nursing actions include those to prevent further environmental stressors that could make the patient more uncomfortable and increase her signs and symptoms.

Nursing actions include monitoring the following: temperature, pulse, respiration, blood pressure, weight, excessive hunger, and tremulousness.

NURSING DIAGNOSIS

Decreased cardiac output related to increased sympathetic stimulation

Expected Patient Outcomes	Nursing Interventions	Rationale
Patient's pulse rate is less than 20 above baseline during first 72 hr. Pulse rate decreases gradually after 72 hr. Undetected cardiac dysrhythmias do not occur.	Assess vital signs, especially heart rate and rhythm, at least q4h; if worsens, assess q1h. Instruct patient to report palpitations, chest pain, and dizziness. Assess daily weight, daily intake and output; assess for signs of edema, jugular vein distention, and pulmonary congestion q8h. Decrease known stressors; explain all interventions, and listen to patient. Balance periods of activity with rest. Administer prescribed drugs and monitor therapeutic response. Report any changes to physician.	The early detection of atrial fibrillation or thyroid storm allows prompt treatment and prevents cardiovascular crisis.

NURSING DIAGNOSIS

Ineffective individual coping related to personal vulnerability to environmental stimuli

Expected Patient Outcomes	Nursing Interventions	Rationale
Patient explains reason for change in behavior. Emotional lability is minimized. Patient identifies at least one coping mechanism that will help during periods of nervousness.	Discuss reasons for emotional lability. Maintain calm, relaxed environment. Encourage visitors who are calm and will not upset her. Provide privacy (such as a single room). Suggest that others avoid sharing distressing news with her. Explain all interventions. Avoid stimulants such as coffee, caffeine, and alcohol. Help her identify previous coping mechanisms or explore new ones. Offer measures to help her relax. Include family in discussions.	A supportive environment can reduce environmental stimuli and stressors and assist patient in coping.

Continued.

PERSON WITH HYPERTHYROIDISM—cont'd

NURSING DIAGNOSIS

Nutrition, altered: less than body requirements related to increased metabolic needs

Expected Patient Outcomes	Nursing Interventions	Rationale
Patient's normal weight is maintained. Patient gains at least 0.5 kg/wk, if weight is below normal.	Monitor weight qod to weekly. Monitor serum albumin, hemoglobin, and lymphocyte levels. Help her plan for high-calorie, high-protein, high-carbohydrate diet with selection from all food groups. Suggest six small meals per day or between-meal snacks.	Increase nutrient intake to meet increased metabolic demand.

NURSING DIAGNOSIS

Sensory/perceptual alterations (potential visual) related to infiltrative changes associated with Graves' disease

Expected Patient Outcomes	Nursing Interventions	Rationale
Patient's vision does not worsen. Patient can explain measures to protect eyes.	Assess visual acuity, ability to close eyes, and photophobia. Protect eyes from irritants: 1. Use patches or glasses when in high wind. 2. Use artificial tears, if prescribed. 3. Elevate head of bed at night. Instruct patient not to lie prone. If eyes do not close completely, check about using shields at night.	These measures can prevent corneal injury and minimize risk of loss of vision.

NURSING DIAGNOSIS

Hyperthermia related to increased heat production greater than dissipation

Expected Patient Outcomes	Nursing Interventions	Rationale
Patient states that she feels more comfortable. Patient has normal body temperature.	Control environmental temperature for comfort (fans may be helpful) Suggest that she take frequent showers. Encourage adequate fluid intake and monitor fluid losses. Monitor temperature q4h.	These measures keep her comfortable by increasing heat loss.

NURSING DIAGNOSIS

Activity intolerance related to generalized muscle weakness

Expected Patient Outcomes	Nursing Interventions	Rationale
Patient states fatigue is decreased. Patient maintains current activity level.	Assess activity schedule. Suggest ways to modify fatiguing activities. Identify activities than can be done by others until condition is controlled. Schedule rest periods between activities. Encourage activities that promote sleep at night. At present, keep activities at current level.	Reduction of energy expenditure is necessary to reduce fatigue in persons with increased metabolism until treatment decreases metabolism.

THROID CRISIS OR THYROID STORM

Thyroid crisis or *storm* is a medical emergency in which patients develop severe manifestations of the signs and symptoms of hyperthyroidism, including an elevated temperature; increased tachycardia or onset of dysrhythmias; worsening tremors and restlessness; worsening mental status, including a delirious or psychotic state or coma; and sometimes complaints of abdominal pain. Blood pressure and respiratory rate increase above baseline. This state is usually seen in persons with Graves' disease, and symptoms result from a severe increase in metabolism and are usually precipi-

NURSING CARE PLAN

PERSON WITH HYPERTHYROIDISM—cont'd

NURSING DIAGNOSIS

Home maintenance management, impaired, related to delay between initiation of therapy and stabilization of patient

Expected Patient Outcome	Nursing Interventions	Rationale
Patient states plan for home maintenance management.	Assist her to identify home maintenance difficulties. Assist her to identify persons who can provide temporary help. Make referrals as needed, such as to social services. Identify persons who can help monitor her compliance with medical regimen. Help patient plan own schedule to allow for rest.	These measures increase resources available to patient and reduce stress from inability to meet expectations of role.

NURSING DIAGNOSIS

Knowledge deficit (disease, treatment, expected outcomes) related to new information and no previous exposure to information

Expected Patient Outcome	Nursing Interventions	Rationale
Patient explains medical regimen and care needs.	Explain how and when to take prescribed medications. Describe symptoms of infection to be reported to physician, such as sore throat or fever. Describe ways to plan prescribed dietary intake. Provide required teaching about care needs (comfort, sleep, rest). Explain the reason for the delay before surgery.	These measures increase likelihood of compliance with therapy used to achieve euthyroid state and optimal physical status before surgery.

tated by a major stressor such as infection, trauma, or surgery. Thyroid crisis or storm can occur following thyroidectomy because as the gland is manipulated, hormone is released into the blood stream. Thyroid crisis also may occur in a person who has been inadequately treated.

Patients with thyroid storm must be hospitalized. The immediate focus of care is to lower the metabolic rate as fast as possible, remove the precipitating cause, and support physiologic functioning. The typical therapeutic regimen is outlined in the box on p. 1046.

HYPOSECRETION OF THYROID HORMONE: HYPOTHYROIDISM

ETIOLOGY/EPIDEMIOLOGY

Hypothyroidism is a metabolic state resulting from a deficiency of thyroid hormone that may occur at any age. Congenital hypothyroidism results in a condition called *cretinism*. Hypothyroidism may result from:

1. Loss or atrophy of thyroid tissue—autoimmune thyroiditis, ablative therapy for hyperthyroidism, thyrotoxic drugs, congenital agenesis, maldevelopment
2. Loss of trophic stimulation—pituitary dysfunction (pituitary or secondary hypothyroidism), hypothalamic dysfunction

3. Miscellaneous alterations—deficit in hormone biosynthesis, peripheral resistance to thyroid hormone, idiopathic factors, environmental factors (iodine deficiency)

The most frequent causes of hypothyroidism are autoimmune thyroiditis, ablative therapy, and idiopathic.[52] Hypothyroidism is estimated to affect 1% of the population, and it is believed to be particularly underdiagnosed in the elderly. (See Chapter 35 for a discussion of thyroid function and changes in function with aging.) In neonatal screening programs, hypothyroidism is detected in one of every 4000 to 5000 newborns.[64]

PREVENTION

Primary prevention is not possible for most causes of hypothyroidism. Preventive efforts should be directed toward secondary prevention so that early detection and treatment is instituted and sequelae of hypothyroidism are prevented. Newborns and the elderly, particularly elderly women, should be the major focus of screening programs.

PATHOPHYSIOLOGY

Regardless of the cause of hypothyroidism, the end result is a deficiency in the level of thyroid hormone. A

RESEARCH

Hyman RB, Feldman HR, Harris RB, Levin RF, and Malloy GB: The effects of relaxation training on clinical symptoms: A meta-analysis, Nurs Res 38:216-220, 1989.

Many clinical problems are associated with anxiety and tension. These states elicit a stress response. Several relaxation techniques have been proposed as useful treatments for these problems. This study was a meta-analysis to determine: (1) the overall effectiveness of relaxation techniques in relieving clinical symptoms and (2) the effectiveness of some techniques over others in relation to specific symptoms.

Relaxation training was defined as nonpharmacologic, nonmechanical-assisted techniques to facilitate a relaxed state and excluded Benson's relaxation technique, Jacobson's progressive muscle relaxation, rhythmic breathing, imagery, Lamaze, meditation, autogenic training, hypnosis, trancendental meditation (TM), yoga, and zen. Biofeedback-assisted relaxation was not included. Studies were used from 1970 that investigated relaxation training on adult subjects not hospitalized for psychiatric reasons. The literature search resulted in 100 studies, 48 of which fit the criteria.

The most common problems for which relaxation was prescribed included insomnia, acute pain, anxiety, and hypertension. Relaxation treatments often included more than one treatment. The analysis revealed that relaxation techniques do affect some clinical symptoms. The treatment worked better for nonsurgical subjects than for surgical subjects. All treatments, except Benson's relaxation, showed evidence of effectiveness. The problems most consistently improved were hypertension, headache, and insomnia. Effectiveness of techniques for pain and anxiety were low to moderate. The results for acute pain were very low. Research is still needed to study whether the effectiveness of relaxation techniques vary depending on symptoms as well as the acuteness or chronicity of the problem. ▪

---

lack of thyroid hormone results in a general depression of basal metabolic rate and alters the development or functioning of almost every system of the body. Alterations in the integumentary, cardiovascular, nervous, musculoskeletal, alimentary, and reproductive systems are often seen. One major change is an accumulation of hyaluronic acids and alteration of ground substances producing mucinous edema. The lack of thyroid hormone results in an increase in TSH and frequently a goiter in most persons with hypothyroidism.

The pathophysiologic changes usually occur very slowly. Thus the disease may be present for years before it is diagnosed.

CLINICAL MANIFESTATIONS

The manifestations of hypothyroidism vary with the severity of the deficiency and the age of onset. Manifesta-

THERAPEUTIC REGIMEN FOR PATIENT WITH THYROID CRISIS OR STORM

1. Initiate an intravenous line for medications and fluids.
2. Administer increasing doses of oral propylthiouracil as ordered (doses as great as 400 mg every 6 hours may be given).
3. Administer iodide preparations as ordered.
4. Administer cortisol, 50 to 100 mg, intravenously every 6 hours as ordered. Cortisol helps to inhibit the release of thyroid hormone.
5. Administer propranolol orally or intravenously as ordered. Propranolol (β-adrenergic blocker) can worsen asthma or congestive heart failure because it constricts bronchial smooth muscles and causes a decrease in cardiac output.
6. Initiate measures to lower body temperature, including external cooling devices, cold baths, and acetaminophen. Salicylates are contraindicated because they inhibit thyroid hormone binding to protein carriers and thus increase free thyroid hormone levels.
7. Initiate other support therapy as ordered, including oxygen, cardiac glycosides, and treatment measures for the precipitating event.
8. Monitor the patient's temperature, intake and output, neurologic status, and cardiovascular status every hour.
9. Maintain a quiet, calm, cool, private environment until crisis is over.
10. Maintain continuity of care.
11. Decrease stressors by use of patient education, comfort measures, or family support.
12. Decrease physical activity as much as possible.

---

tions of hypothyroidism in infants are not usually seen until several months after birth, when signs such as retardation of mental and physical development occur and are usually irreversible. Thus early recognition requires serum T_4 measurements. Figure 36-5, although an older picture, clearly shows the effect of severe untreated infantile hypothyroidism.

In adults, early signs and symptoms are vague and may go unrecognized. A typical clinical picture is as follows. Early complaints may consist of tiredness, lethargy, and weakness resulting in the inability to carry out a normal day's activities. Intolerance to cold and constipation develop. There may be alterations in menstrual cycles, menorrhagia, and inability to conceive. Loss of interest in sexual activity may be noted by men or women. As the disease progresses, mental dysfunction occurs, appetite decreases, changes in physical characteristics are noted, muscle and joint discomforts are present, and chest pain occurs. If not treated, myxedema coma will develop. The full spectrum of signs and symptoms of hypothyroidism are listed in Table 36-3.

The patient with hypothyroidism may or may not have a goiter. An enlarged thyroid gland is seen when the disease results from thyroiditis, defective hormone

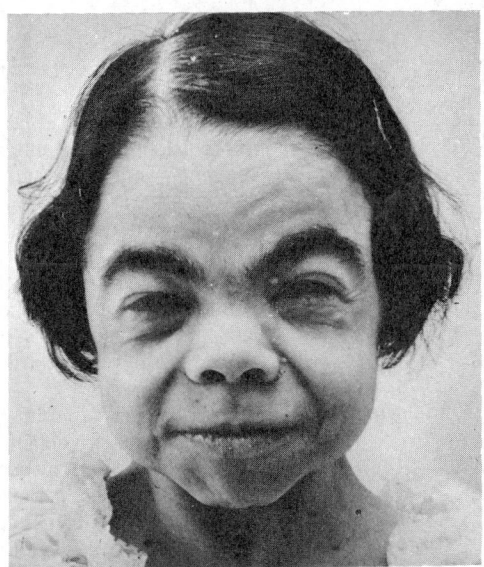
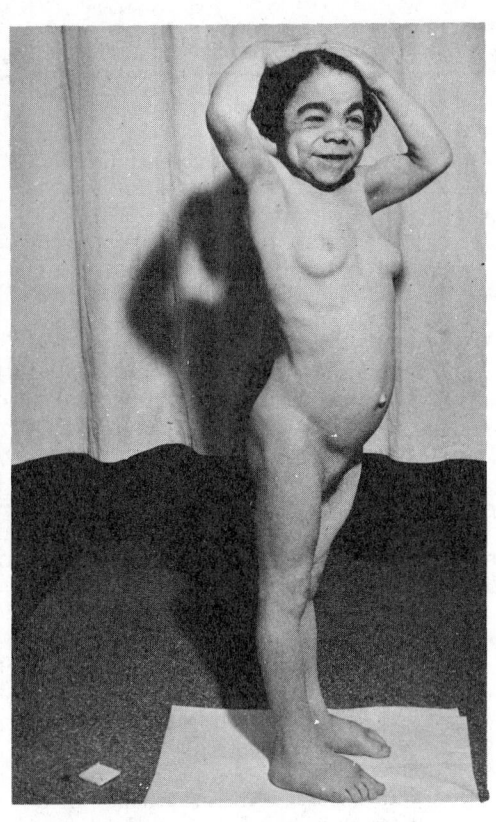

FIGURE 36-5 Adult cretin (33 years old, untreated). Note characteristic cretinoid features, dwarfism (height 44 inches [104 cm]), absent axillary and scant pubic hair, poorly developed breasts, truncal obesity, and small umbilical hernia. Patient has primary amenorrhea. (From Schneeburg NG: Essentials of clinical endocrinology, St Louis, 1970, The CV Mosby Co.)

biosynthesis, peripheral resistance to thyroid hormone, and environmental factors.

MEDICAL MANAGEMENT

Hypothyroidism is treated with replacement of thyroid hormone. Various preparations are available (Table 36-4). Most often, L-thyroxine is used. The major precaution is to initiate drug therapy slowly, particularly if the patient has heart dysfunction or is elderly. The initial daily dose usually should not exceed 12.5 to 25 μg of L-thyroxine. This dose is increased by increments of 25 to 50 μg every 2 to 4 weeks until a normal metabolic rate is attained.[64,65]

The optimal maintenance dose of replacement therapy varies and is determined by the clinical state. The earliest clinical responses are diuresis, resulting in weight loss and regression of puffiness. The pulse rate then increases, appetite improves, constipation is relieved, and mental and motor activity increase.[64]

The major side effects of thyroid replacement therapy are (1) inadequate treatment, with the patient continuing to show signs and symptoms of hypothyroidism; (2) excessive treatment, resulting in signs and symptoms of hyperthyroidism; (3) increases in drug dose at too fast a rate, resulting in cardiac problems such as angina, palpitations, tachycardia, or cardiac failure; and (4) bone loss and decreased bone density.[44] During the

initiation of therapy, the patient is seen every 2 to 4 weeks. After the patient is stable, thyroid hormone replacement should be monitored annually by such tests as serum free T_4 index, TSH level, and serum T_3 level.

■ ASSESSMENT

Subjective Data

Hypothyroidism affects every system of the body. The early manifestations will most likely be identified by a thorough history. The history should focus on assessing the following areas for changes:

1. Changes in physical energy level and activity or mental/neurologic status
2. Changes in skin, hair (head, body), nails
3. Presence of chest pain, occurrence of syncope
4. Changes in appetite and weight with a typical nutrition intake
5. Changes in bowel elimination
6. Presence of discomfort—headache, muscle or joint pain, intolerance to cold
7. Changes in sexual function
   a. Women—changes in menses, libido, difficulty conceiving
   b. Men—changes in libido
8. Knowledge level—dysfunction, diagnostic tests, treatment

TABLE 36-3 Clinical manifestations of hypothyroidism in adults

Body System	Signs and Symptoms	Body System	Signs and Symptoms
Integumentary	Puffy appearance and thickened features around eyes and of hands, feet, and tongue caused by mucinous edema (Figure 36-6); pallor and yellow tinged skin (anemia and hypercarotenemia); dry coarse skin (decreased sweat and sebaceous gland functioning); slow wound healing (altered protein metabolism); bruising (increased capillary fragility); skin cool (changes in circulation and decreased basal metabolic rate); hair of head, body shows decreased growth, is dry and brittle, falls out; eyebrows may also show loss; hoarse deep voice (thickening of vocal cords)	Respiratory	Pleural effusion, usually only seen on chest roentgenogram; lung volumes normal but decreased breathing capacity; alveolar hypoventilation with severe hypothyroidism
Cardiovascular	Enlarged heart and diminished heart sounds (effusion into the pericardial sac of protein and mucopolysaccharide and dilation of left ventricle); decreased cardiac output at rest (decreased stroke volume and heart rate); increased peripheral vascular resistance at rest and reduced blood volume; increased cardiac output and decreased vascular resistance with exercise; increased coronary artery disease (increased serum cholesterol); angina or worsening of angina with treatment; ECG changes including sinus bradycardia, prolonged PR interval, low amplitude, alteration of ST segment and flattened T wave; increased cardiac enzymes (CK, LDH, ALT)*	Gastrointestinal	Decreased appetite; modest increase in weight; decreased peristaltic activity; constipation; achlorhydria and low serum vitamin B_{12} with pernicious anemia (12% of patients)[64]
		Neurologic	Slowing of all intellectual functioning (loss of initiative, memory deficit, slowed slurred speech); somnolence, lethargy, dementia; headache; periods of confusion; syncope; coma precipitated by trauma, infection, respiratory failure, use of depressant drugs or sedatives; hearing loss; slowed, clumsy movements; numbness and tingling of extremities (mucinous deposits around peripheral nerves); decreased tendon reflexes
		Hematopoietic	Decreased production of erythropoietin (decreased oxygen requirements); decreased RBC count with mild normocytic, normochromic anemia; occasional macrocytic anemia from vitamin B_{12} deficiency; normal total and differential WBC counts; normal platelet count but decreased adhesiveness; Possible decrease in clotting factors VIII and IX, resulting in abnormal clotting
Musculoskeletal	Muscular stiffness and aching (delayed muscular contraction and relaxation); normal muscle strength, muscles firm, and normal to increased muscle mass; stiffness of joints and joint effusions	Metabolic	Decreased basal metabolic rate, heat production, and body temperature; decreased synthesis and degradation of protein; decreased absorption of glucose and uptake by cells and decreased degradation of insulin (thus diabetics usually need less insulin); decreased synthesis and degradation of lipids resulting in increased serum cholesterol, phospholipids, triglycerides and low-density lipoprotein; occasional alterations in adrenal and pituitary function (adrenal insufficiency, decreased secretion and effectiveness of GH, increased prolactin)
Renal	Decreased urine flow, decreased excretion of water load; decreased ability to concentrate urine; mild proteinuria; increased interstitial fluid		
Reproductive	Women: anovulation, inability to conceive, increased spontaneous abortions, menorrhagia, decreased libido; men: decreased libido, impotence, oligospermia		

*CK, Creatine phosphokinase; LDH, lactate dehydrogenase; ALT, alanine aminotransferase.

Objective Data

Data are collected using a head-to-toe approach, with particular emphasis on the following systems. The nurse is assessing to see if the typical signs of hypothyroidism are present.

1. Mental status: intellectual functioning; memory; speech pattern; presence of somnolence, lethargy, or confusion
2. Body weight and temperature
3. Skin: pigmentation, temperature, presence of nonpitting edema
4. Neck/hair: quality and quantity of head and body hair, thyroid examination
5. Cardiovascular: pulse rate, blood pressure at rest and with exercise, heart size
6. Respiratory: rate, breath sounds
7. Abdomen: bowel sounds
8. Motor: muscle strength, tone, and mass; range of motion; deep tendon reflexes; joint movement

TABLE 36-4 Replacement therapy in hypothyroidism*

Drug	Comments
Sodium L-thyroxine: levothyroxine (Synthroid, Levoid)	Synthetic T_4 only; T_3 levels increased by peripheral conversion of T_4 to T_3; parenteral and oral forms available; most commonly used drug; normal dosage, 1.8 μg/kg body weight
Sodium L-triiodothyronine (Cytomel, Trionine)	Synthetic T_3; therapeutic effects more difficult to monitor; may experience peaks in serum T_3 levels
Synthetic combinations of T_3 and T_4: liotrix (Euthroid, Thyrolar)	Synthetic T_4 and T_3; therapeutic effects more difficult to monitor; may experience peaks in T_3 levels
Natural combination of T_3 and T_4: thyroid extract	Natural preparation of T_3 and T_4 from animal thyroid; potency may vary

*Therapeutic equivalence: L-thyroxine 100 μg = L-triiodothyronine 25 μg = liotrix 1 unit = thyroid extract 60 mg.

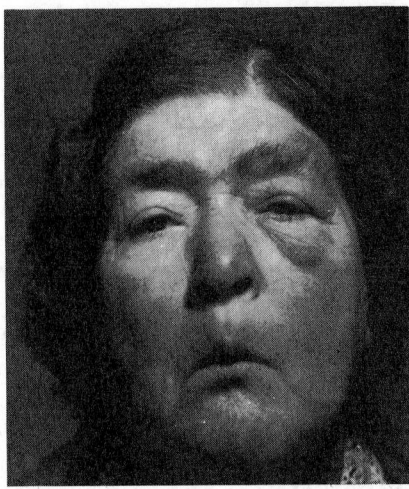

FIGURE 36-6 Adult with severe hypothyroidism showing typical puffiness around eyes. (From Schottelius B and Schottelius D: Textbook of physiology, ed 18, St Louis, 1978, The CV Mosby Co.)

■ DATA ANALYSIS: NURSING DIAGNOSES

Nursing diagnoses are determined from assessment of patient data. Possible nursing diagnoses for the person with hypothyroidism include, but are not limited to, the following:

Diagnostic Title	Possible Etiologies
Activity intolerance	Poor work capacity associated with poor cardiac function, decreased breathing capacity, and muscle stiffness
Body image disturbance	Change in appearance (weight gain, hair and skin changes) and change in functioning (decreased mental and physical function)
Constipation	Decreased peristaltic action, decreased physical activity
Hypothermia	Decreased heat production associated with decreased metabolic rate
Knowledge deficit: disease, treatment, expected outcomes, self-monitoring and follow-up care	New interventions with no previous exposure to information
Nutrition, altered: more than body requirements	Decreased metabolic rate
Pain	Headache and joint pain associated with chronic thyroid problems

Diagnostic Title	Possible Etiologies
Self-care deficit (varies), bathing/hygiene, dressing/grooming, feeding, toileting	Inability to do care associated with altered thought process and mental functioning
Sexual dysfunction	Alterations in menstrual cycle, ovulation, sperm production, and libido
Skin integrity, impaired	Mucinous deposits in skin, decreased circulation and immobility
Thought processes, altered	Slowing of intellectual functions associated with chronic deficit of thyroid hormone

■ PLANNING: EXPECTED PATIENT OUTCOMES

Expected patient outcomes for the person with hypothyroidism may include, but are not limited to, the following:

1. The patient shows a gradual increase in activity tolerance over 2 to 3 months.
2. The patient and significant others can relate body image changes to hypothyroidism and verbalize that most changes are reversible.
3. The patient maintains a bowel pattern that was typical for him or her before onset of illness.
4. The patient maintains a body temperature of 36° to 37° C.
5. The patient and significant others are able to:
   a. Explain the disease in simple terms.
   b. Explain that treatment is lifelong drug therapy.
   c. Explain that treatment should reverse most signs and symptoms.

d. Describe self-monitoring needs and planned follow-up.

6. Nutritional status will improve as evidenced by a gradual decrease in body weight.
7. The patient states pain is controlled.
8. The patient's self-care needs are met.
9. The patient and significant others can explain that sexual dysfunction will decrease as thyroid status is returned to normal.
10. The patient's skin remains intact.
11. Alteration in thought processes will not lead to injuries or loss of patient's dignity as evidenced by no injuries and patient's participation in decisions as much as possible.

■ IMPLEMENTATION

The nursing interventions required by the patient with hypothyroidism vary greatly depending on the severity of disease. Not every patient has all the nursing diagnoses previously listed. Many persons are treated as outpatients. The hypothyroid state is reversed slowly, so the patient will not return to the premorbid health state for 2 to 3 months. Potential nursing interventions include:

1. Promote activity to the level of patient tolerance.
   a. At first the patient will have a very limited tolerance and may only be able to move around in the room. Activities should be increased gradually.
   b. Monitor the cardiovascular response to new activities. If the patient complains of chest pain or develops an unacceptable heart rate above baseline, stop the activity and then restart at a slower rate.
   c. Monitor blood pressure; pulse, and respirations before, during, and after each new activity.
2. Promote positive body image.
   a. Provide information that helps the patient and significant others understand how body changes relate to the hypothyroidism.
   b. Educate about reversible body changes.
   c. Help the patient see the positive changes that have occurred.
3. Promote normal bowel elimination.
   a. Monitor bowel elimination.
   b. Maintain adequate fluid intake.
   c. Increase bulk in the diet.
4. Treat hypothermia.
   a. Monitor temperature every 4 hours.
   b. Maintain an environmental temperature that is comfortable for the patient.
   c. Use blankets to increase body temperature if necessary.
5. Teach patient about:
   a. Nature of the disorder, diagnostic tests, treatments; need for lifelong replacement therapy.

b. Medications—dosage, method of administration, side effects.
c. Self-monitoring of vital signs, body weight, any signs of skin breakdown, any signs of constipation.
d. Methods to prevent skin breakdown and constipation.
e. Need for periods of rest alternating with activity.
f. Need for continued follow-up care.
6. Facilitate intake of nutritional diet that is low in calories and includes food from all food groups.
7. Promote comfort.
   a. Use nonmedicinal comfort measures such as massage, cool or warm heat, and distraction to promote pain control.
   b. If medications are used, monitor patient carefully. Patient will have a lower tolerance for sedative and depressant medications.
8. Provide for self-care needs. At first patient may require complete care for hygiene, toileting, and dietary needs.
9. Facilitate patient's understanding of the relationship between the sexual problems and the hypothyroidism.
10. Maintain skin integrity.
    a. Monitor skin condition each shift.
    b. Institute preventive care measures such as an egg crate mattress, sheepskin pads, and soft sheets.
    c. If patient is unable to or does not turn by self, assist in turning every 2 hours.
11. Facilitate a safe environment and orientation to environment.
    a. Monitor neurologic status every shift.
    b. Incorporate into contacts with the patient information about date, place, time, current events, and current activities to facilitate orientation.
    c. Maintain a safe environment: remove any clutter, keep bed low, and keep bed rails up.
    d. Use frequent stimulation; at dusk, as well as at night, use nightlights to prevent confusion.
    e. Inform significant others of relationship between mental status and hypothyroidism.
    f. Involve patient, as possible, in decisions about care.

MYXEDEMA COMA

Myxedema coma represents the most severe form of hypothyroidism and can ultimately occur in any patient with untreated prolonged hypothyroidism. Precipitating factors include sedative drugs and narcotics, exposure to cold, surgery, infections, and trauma. The patient has all the classic symptoms of hypothyroidism and also is comatose, has severe hypothermia (temperatures below

23.3° C have been recorded), and dilutional hyponatremia. Respiratory insufficiency with carbon dioxide retention and respiratory acidosis may occur.

Therapy for patients with myxedema coma includes supportive care (cardiovascular, respiratory, and fluid balance support), treatment of the underlying precipitating factor, and administration of thyroid hormone. Thyroid hormone is given intravenously. Usually L-thyroxine, 2 μg/kg is given as the initial dose, with an additional 100 μg every 24 hours. Hydrocortisone (100 mg daily) is recommended by some authorities because adrenocortical insufficiency is frequently present.[65] The patient is kept warm enough to avoid additional heat loss without overwarming to avoid vascular collapse. Tracheal intubation and mechanical ventilation may be necessary. Improvement is seen in 3 to 24 hours.

Nursing interventions include care of the comatose patient, surveillance of respiratory, cardiovascular, and fluid status, care of the patient with respiratory insufficiency, preventive care for problems of immobility, and assistance with the institution of the medical regimen.

SIMPLE GOITER

Some problems of the thyroid, such as simple goiter, thyroiditis, and cancer of the thyroid, are not associated with consistent changes in thyroid hormone levels. Changes in thyroid levels, however, can occur with any of these problems.

ETIOLOGY/EPIDEMIOLOGY

Any enlargement of the thyroid gland is called a *goiter*. If this enlargement is not associated with hyper- or hypothyroidism, cancer, or inflammation, it is referred to as *simple goiter*. Goiter may also be described in terms of occurrence: endemic or sporadic. *Endemic goiter* refers to goiters that occur in a particular geographic region and from a common cause, such as iodine deficiency. *Sporadic goiter* describes goiters that occur sporadically in regions that are not the locus of endemic goiters.

Endemic goiter from environmental iodine deficiency is found in all continents except North America and is estimated to affect more than 200 million people. In the United States, regions such as the Great Lakes Basin, which previously had a high incidence of endemic goiter, no longer have this problem because of education about the use of iodized salt.

Simple, sporadic goiter may result from any of several factors that impair the ability of the thyroid to synthesize adequate quantities of hormone that is, act as goitrogens (see the box below, left). In most cases of simple goiter, no extrinsic factors or intrinsic problems can be identified.

Simple goiter is seen most frequently in females (3:1 ratio with males)[65] and occurs most often during pregnancy or adolescence. Heredity also plays a role because goiters occur in particular families.[64]

PATHOPHYSIOLOGY

The underlying pathophysiologic fact involved in simple goiter formation is an increase in TSH. It is believed that when factors inhibit normal thyroid hormone production, hypersecretion of TSH occurs because of a lack of negative feedback. The increase in TSH results in an increase in thyroid mass.

The increase in TSH increases the turnover of iodine, and the T_3 to T_4 ratio in thyroid secretion is increased.[65] *The patient remains euthyroid at the expense of the elevated TSH and an enlarged gland.*

CLINICAL MANIFESTATIONS

Thyroid enlargement, which varies greatly, is the cause of the signs and symptoms of simple goiter. The primary symptom may be disfigurement, or the person may complain of tightening of garments worn around the neck. If the goiter is very large, it may displace or compress the esophagus or trachea and cause dysphagia, choking sensation, or inspiratory stridor. Compression of the recurrent laryngeal nerve may lead to hoarseness, although this sign is more suggestive of cancer. Narrowing of the thoracic inlet decreases venous return from the head, neck, and upper limbs and results in venous engorgement. This obstruction is accentuated with elevation of the person's arms and results in dizziness and syncope (Pemberton's sign).[64]

INTERVENTIONS
Medical Management

Medical management is directed at removing the stimulus causing the increased thyroid mass. If extrinsic factors such as goitrogenic drugs or foods are the cause, they are eliminated. Iodine deficiency, although very rare, is ruled out and replacement is instituted if appropriate. Only small doses of iodide, such as saturated solution of potassium iodide (SSKI) or Lugol's solution are needed.

In most instances the cause of goiter is unknown and therapy is directed at supplying exogenous hormone, which will inhibit TSH secretion. Sodium L-thyroxine in doses of 150 to 200 μg is usually necessary. The adequacy of the dosage in suppressing TSH secretion is verified by a RAIU test that should have a value of less than 5%. Surgery is sometimes necessary if obstruction is not relieved with other therapy. Surgery will result in

---

GOITROGENIC FACTORS

Iodine deficiency
Foods with goitrogenic factors: cabbage, turnips, soybeans
Drugs: lithium, thiocarbamides, sulfonylureas
Intrinsic abnormality in thyroid hormone syntheses

the need for lifetime replacement therapy because the total thyroid gland is removed.

Nursing Management

Nursing care focuses on prevention of the problem and supportive care for active problems. The importance of adequate iodine in the diet is stressed. Persons with a family history of goiter should be monitored at regular intervals and educated regarding goitrogenic foods that should be avoided.

The patient with a large goiter may need help with altered body image related to disfigurement. An open and trusting relationship is necessary so that the patient can share feelings and concerns. The goiter may be concealed by the use of scarves, high collars, and makeup. Patient teaching includes:

1. Explanation of diagnostic tests and treatment
2. Medication regimen—method of administration, dosage, and side effects
3. Need for continual follow-up care

If surgery is necessary, nursing management will include care as described for thyroid surgery on pp. 1056 to 1057.

THYROIDITIS

There are three types of thyroiditis (inflammation of the thyroid): acute, subacute, and chronic. Hashimoto's thyroiditis, a form of chronic thyroiditis, is the most common form of thyroiditis and is described here. Major characteristics of the other forms of thyroiditis are summarized in Table 36-5.

ETIOLOGY/EPIDEMIOLOGY

Hashimoto's thyroiditis affects women more frequently than men and usually occurs between ages 30 and 50. It is increasing in frequency.

In Hashimoto's thyroiditis the thyroid is infiltrated with lymphocytes and antithyroid antibodies. These findings support the belief that Hashimoto's thyroiditis is an autoimmune disease, and it is generally believed that it is one of the triad of autoimmune thyroid disorders that include Graves' disease and primary thyroid atrophy. The mechanisms for the autoimmunity are not understood, although significant association exists between Hashimoto's thyroiditis and specific haplotypes as well as other autoimmune diseases.

PATHOPHYSIOLOGY

The lymphocytic infiltration in Hashimoto's thyroiditis results in obliteration of thyroid follicles and fibrosis. The destruction of the gland decreases the serum levels of T_4 and T_3 and thus increases TSH. The increased TSH causes hyperfunction of thyroid tissue and goiter formation. The increase in thyroid tissue is not usually associated with overproduction of thyroid hormone, although transient hyperthyroidism can occur. The increase in thyroid tissue and hyperfunction help to maintain a euthyroid state for some time, but eventually hypothyroidism will develop.

TABLE 36-5 Thyroiditis: types and characteristics

Type	Characteristics
ACUTE THYROIDITIS	
Acute pyogenic thyroiditis	Rare form of thyroiditis; results from infection of thyroid by pyogenic organism; symptoms include pain and tenderness in thyroid, dysphagia, fever, malaise; treated symptomatically
SUBACUTE NONSUPPURATIVE THYROIDITIS	
De Quervain's thyroiditis Granulomatous thyroiditis	Rare form of thyroiditis; results from viral infection of thyroid gland; may follow an upper respiratory infection; most commonly seen in 4th and 5th decades of life; symptoms include pain in thyroid, fever, hoarseness, dysphagia, feelings of palpitation, nervousness, lassitude, thyroid moderately enlarged; subsides in a few months; treatment usually symptomatic; aspirin for mild cases; glucocorticoids when disease is nonresponsive to other measures
SUBACUTE LYMPHOCYTIC THYROIDITIS	
Painless thyroiditis Lymphocytic thyroiditis	Form of thyroiditis increasing in frequency; etiologic factor unknown but possible autoimmune factor; symptoms include self-limiting form of hyperthyroidism and nontender enlarged thyroid gland, which may be followed by hypothyroidism; treatment symptomatic during hyperthyroidism phase and may include β-adrenergic blockers but not propylthiouracil (not effective); monitor annually for hypothyroidism
CHRONIC THYROIDITIS	
Hashimoto's thyroiditis	See text
Riedel's thyroiditis	Rare form of thyroiditis; cause unknown; extensive fibrosis of gland occurs; symptoms include insidious onset; symptoms from compression of trachea, esophagus, and recurrent laryngeal nerve; gland enlarged, hard; hypothyroidism can occur; treatment is symptomatic with surgery for symptoms of compression; thyroid replacement for hypothyroidism

CLINICAL MANIFESTATIONS

The major clinical finding in Hashimoto's thyroiditis is *diffuse thyroid enlargement,* found as a goiter on examination. The thyroid is firm and smooth, moves freely, and is usually painless. Both lobes are enlarged, but one lobe may be larger than the other. Some persons may experience dysphagia or choking. Other clinical signs and symptoms vary depending on the thyroid state. The person may have transient periods of hyperthyroidism early in the disease when an exacerbation occurs and functioning tissue is still present that releases increased amounts of hormone. The person may be euthyroid for several years. As the disease progresses, the gland is destroyed and signs and symptoms of hypothyroidism occur.

Laboratory test results vary depending on the stage of the disease. In early stages the serum TSH and RAIU are elevated, but serum T_4 and T_3 are normal. Over years the T_4 and T_3 levels will decrease. *Antithyroid antibodies are almost always present in the serum.* The diagnosis is usually based on the presence of serum antibodies. If the diagnosis is inconclusive, a needle aspiration biopsy or open biopsy is necessary.

INTERVENTIONS

Medical Management

The medical treatment depends on the signs and symptoms and may include the following:

1. No treatment for mild asymptomatic disease
2. Thyroid hormone replacement for goiter or hypothyroidism
3. Surgery if the goiter is unresponsive to thyroid hormone, is pressing on adjacent structures, or is disfiguring

Nursing Management

Nursing care focuses primarily on patient teaching related to the progress of the disorder, diagnostic tests, and treatment. The patient may need assistance in dealing with alterations in body image because of disfigurement from the goiter. Although Hashimoto's thyroiditis usually does not cause any discomfort, analgesics may occasionally be necessary.

CANCER OF THE THYROID
ETIOLOGY/PATHOPHYSIOLOGY

Cancer of the thyroid is less prevalent than other forms of cancer, and only a very small percentage of thyroid neoplasms are malignant. Two general types of malignant neoplasms are found: those arising from follicular epithelium (papillary, follicular, anaplastic) and those arising from parafollicular tissue. Non-Hodgkin's lymphomas can also develop in thyroid tissue. Table 36-6 presents characteristics for the five forms of primary thyroid malignant neoplasms.

CLINICAL MANIFESTATIONS

Cancer of the thyroid is usually associated with a painless single nodule in a normal gland. The nodules are usually firm, and normal thyroid function is present. Only 20% of "cold" nodules seen on thyroid scans are malignant.[64] The presence of other manifestations depends on whether metastasis is present.

INTERVENTIONS
Medical Management

Medical management of persons with cancer of the thyroid includes use of all modalities of cancer treatment: surgery, radiation, hormonal suppression, and chemotherapy. For occult papillary cancer, treatment consists of lobectomy and isthmectomy followed by thyroid hormone suppression therapy. (administration of thyroid hormone preparation to suppress TSH). For extrathyroidal papillary carcinoma and invasive follicular carcinoma, a total thyroidectomy followed by ^{131}I therapy is frequently done. Removal of the entire thyroid gland in follicular carcinoma increases the effectiveness of treatment of distant metastasis with [131]I. Follicular cancer does trap iodine, but not nearly as well as normal thyroid tissue. A total thyroidectomy allows for the metastatic tissue to trap the iodine without competition.

Treatment of intrathyroidal papillary carcinoma and noninvasive follicular carcinoma is more controversial. Some authorities recommend the conservative approach used for occult papillary carcinoma, and others recommend the approach used for extrathyroidal papillary and invasive follicular carcinoma.[29,34,65] For both papillary and follicular cancer, involved lymph nodes are resected during surgery. Also, these patients may be seen every 2 to 3 months, and any recurrence is treated with ^{131}I therapy. Suppressive thyroid hormone therapy and ^{131}I therapy are frequently used after surgery.

Anaplastic thyroid cancer may be treated aggressively with surgery, radiation therapy, and chemotherapy,[34] but frequently the cancer is too far advanced and only palliative surgery is done.[65]

Thyroid lymphoma usually is treated using radiation and chemotherapy; however, very small lymphomas may be treated surgically. Medullary carcinoma is treated with total thyroidectomy. These tumors do not respond to ^{131}I therapy or thyroid hormone suppression. Recurrence and metastatic lesions have been treated with surgery and sometimes radiation therapy. Calcitonin levels can be used to monitor for recurrence.

For some patients with certain tumors and lymph node involvement, a modified neck dissection is recommended by some authorities;[29] not all authorities recommend this procedure.[65] (See Chapter 32 for a discussion of neck dissection.)

TABLE 36-6 Characteristics of the four types of thyroid cancer

| Characteristic | Cancers of the Follicular Epithelium | | | Thyroid Lymphoma | Cancer of Parafollicular Tissue |
	Papillary	Follicular	Anaplastic		Medullary
Incidence of all thyroid cancers	65%	20%	5%	5%	5%
Age	Young persons	After 40	After 60	After 40	After 50
Female/male ratio	2-3:1	2-3:1	F > M	F > M	F = M
Metastasis	By intraglandular lymphatics; slow-growing tumor	By blood vessels to distant sites (bone, lung, liver); occurs early	By direct invasion to adjacent structures; highly malignant	By lymphatic system; gland fixed to other structures	By intraglandular lymphatics and blood vessels
Prognosis	Good; rarely causes death in young persons if occult or intrathyroidal	Good if minimally invasive lesion	Prognosis varies with cell type; for giant cell, very poor (<6 months from diagnoses); for small cell, better (5-year survival rate of 20% to 50%)	Good	Moderate; 10-year survival is estimated as 2 out of 3 persons
Symptoms	Asymptomatic	Goiter may have been present for years	Hoarseness, inspiratory stridor, dysphagia (signs of invasion of adjacent areas)	May have long history of previous goiter; rapid enlargement of goiter, hoarseness, dysphagia, pressure sensation, dyspnea, some pain	Because tumor produces hormones, possible paraendocrine manifestations such as carcinoid syndrome, watery diarrhea, Cushing's syndrome
Tumor	Occult (<1.5 cm in diameter), intrathyroidal (>1.5 cm in diameter but does not extend through thyroid surface), and extrathyroidal (extends through thyroid surface); well differentiated; psammoma body found in 40% of tumors and virtually diagnostic of malignant nature; tumors appear as "cold" spots on thyroid scan	Well differentiated to poorly differentiated; cyst formation and calcification possible; tumors may appear as "hot" areas on thyroid scan	Two cell forms: giant cell and small cell	Usually of nodular histocytic form	Tumor of C cells of thyroid; not encapsulated; some appear as "cold" spots on thyroid scan; may produce ACTH, prostaglandin, or carcinoembryonic antigen

TABLE 36-6 Characteristics of the four types of thyroid cancer—cont'd

| Characteristic | Cancers of the Follicular Epithelium | | | Thyroid Lymphoma | Cancer of Parafollicular Tissue |
	Papillary	Follicular	Anaplastic		Medullary
Other	Growth partially dependent on TSH; thyroid hormone can cause regression of metastatic lesions; ^{131}I may be used for non-resectable lesions; may have history of radiation therapy to head and neck	Suppressive thyroid therapy can cause regression of metastatic lesions; radiation therapy with ^{131}I may be used when vascular invasion or metastasis present	—	Strong association with Hashimoto's thyroiditis; may have lymphoma at other sites	Occurs as a familial form as part of multiple endocrine neoplasia (MEN) type 2a or MEN 2b; in MEN 2a, there is medullary carcinoma, adrenal medullary hyperplasia or bilateral pheochromocytomas and hyperparathyroidism; in MEN 2b, there is medullary carcinoma, bilateral pheochromocytomas; and an unusual phenotype with ganglioneuromas of eyelids, oral mucosa, tongue, and labia, marfanoid habitus, skeletal abnormalities, and prominent corneal nerves;[34] also occurs as a non-MEN familial form

Nursing Management

Care of the patient with a thyroid nodule first focuses on helping the patient through the diagnostic process. Thyroid nodules occur frequently, and most are not cancerous. No one diagnostic test is completely reliable. Depending on patient characteristics and physician philosophy, various tests may be performed. The nurse prepares the patient for each test, particularly focusing on education. These tests are described in Chapter 35. The diagnostic workup may consist of routine thyroid function tests to establish thyroid function. Although these tests are not conclusive for thyroid cancer, normal test results support a benign nodule.[34] Serum calcitonin and carcinoembryonic antigens (CEAs) may be measured and may be high in some patients with medullary carcinoma.[34] Other tests that may be used are ultrasound (aids in differentiating cystic nodules, which are usually benign, from solid nodules), thyroid hormone suppression (based on the belief that if the nodule decreases in size, it is benign), radionuclide imaging (based on the idea that cancer cells do not concentrate iodine and then are labeled as "cold" on scans), and fine-needle aspiration (which is relatively reliable for diagnosing all cancer types except follicular carcinoma). For potential follicular cancer, a hemithyroidectomy may be done.

Once a diagnoses of thyroid cancer is made, nursing care focuses on preparing the patient for surgery. Surgery of the thyroid is described in the next section. The person who is diagnosed with thyroid cancer has some of the same concerns as persons diagnosed with other types of cancer (see Chapter 17).

SURGERY OF THE THYROID

Surgery of the thyroid is used for patients who have hyperthyroidism that is not treatable by radioactive iodine therapy because of patient characteristics (pregnancy,

GUIDELINES FOR POSTOPERATIVE CARE FOLLOWING THYROID SURGERY

1. Monitor for and report signs of complications.
   a. Laryngeal nerve damage: hoarseness, weak voice
   b. Hemorrhage or tissue swelling
      (1) Bleeding on dressing: check back of dressing by slipping hand gently under neck and shoulders
      (2) Choking sensation
      (3) Difficulty in coughing or swallowing
      (4) Sensation of dressing being too tight even after it is loosened
   c. Calcium deficiency (tetany)
      (1) Early signs: tingling around mouth or of toes and fingers, decreasing serum calcium levels
      (2) Later signs: positive Chvostek's and Trousseau's signs (Chapter 23), grand mal seizures
   d. Respiratory distress associated with any of signs just listed
2. Provide emergency care.
   a. Keep emergency supplies readily available:
      (1) Tracheostomy set (for laryngeal nerve damage), oxygen and suction equipment, suture removal set (for respiratory obstruction from hemorrhage)
      (2) Intravenous calcium gluconate or calcium chloride (for tetany)
   b. For acute respiratory distress:
      (1) Call for immediate medical help.
      (2) Raise head of bed.
      (3) Loosen dressing over incision.
      (4) Give calcium as ordered, if signs and symptoms of tetany are present.
      (5) If loosening the dressing does not relieve symptoms of respiratory distress and if medical help is not readily available, remove clips or sutures as instructed.
3. Provide comfort.
   a. Avoid tension on suture lines; encourage patient to support head when turning by placing both hands behind neck.
   b. Give prescribed analgesics as necessary.
4. Maintain nutritional status.
   a. Start soft foods as soon as tolerated (only fluids may be tolerated initially).
   b. Encourage a high-carbohydrate, high-protein diet.
5. Teach patient:
   a. ROM exercises to neck when suture line is healed, to prevent permanent limitations
   b. Need for lifelong thyroid hormone replacement therapy following a total thyroidectomy
   c. Any special care measures related to the underlying disease
   d. Need for follow-up care

child, patient's preference) or that is not well controlled by antithyroid drugs. Surgery also is indicated for patients with large goiters that are compressing adjacent structures or are disfiguring, as well as for patients with cancer of the thyroid. Part (subtotal thyroidectomy, in which one lobe or 75% to 80% of the gland is removed) or all (total thyroidectomy) of the thyroid may be removed.

PREOPERATIVE CARE

The patient having surgery of the thyroid needs care directed toward producing and maintaining a euthyroid state (see earlier sections on hyperthyroidism or hypothyroidism), if this is not already present. Patients with both hyper- and hypothyroidism have been treated medically for varying lengths of time to induce the euthyroid state, and this care must be continued. Because patients who have recently experienced alteration in thyroid hormone levels may have an altered nutritional status, extra attention should be paid to promoting and maintaining positive nitrogen balance.

The patient with previous abnormal thyroid hormone levels may still be having difficulty coping effectively. The patient with a diagnosis of cancer may be experiencing major disruption in coping because of that diagnosis. Therefore the patient who is to have surgery of the thyroid requires a nonstressful environment (quiet room and calm, relaxed approach by staff). General measures to induce relaxation, such as back rubs, a consistent nurse, and a consistent schedule should be included in patient care.

Patient teaching regarding general preoperative and postoperative care (see Chapter 20) is given. The patient also needs to learn how to cough and to move the head and neck postoperatively without placing strain on the suture line. Thus the patient is taught preoperatively to support the neck by placing both hands behind the neck when moving the head or when coughing.

POSTOPERATIVE CARE

Immediate guidelines for postoperative care are listed in the box at left. In addition to routine monitoring, the patient is monitored for major complications that can occur following thyroid surgery: recurrent laryngeal nerve injury, hemorrhage, tetany, and respiratory obstruction. Signs of these complications are reported immediately to the surgeon. Although the signs of laryngeal nerve damage may be related to intubation during surgery, such hoarseness should clear gradually. If hoarseness persists or worsens, it is reported immediately to the surgeon. Hoarseness may be a first sign of laryngeal nerve damage, which can result in vocal cord spasm and respiratory obstruction. An emergency tracheostomy may be necessary, and equipment for this should be available on the nursing unit.

The patient is monitored for presence of hemorrhage for the first 12 to 24 hours postoperatively. Hemorrhage can result in incisional bleeding or in compression of the trachea or surrounding tissue. If hemorrhage causes compression, the patient will complain of signs of compression. If these signs should occur and if loosening of the dressing does not relieve respiratory distress and medical assistance is not immediately available, the nurse may be instructed to remove clips or sutures. The patient may need to be taken back to surgery for retying of the blood vessels and resuturing of the wound.

Although the occurrence of tetany is minimal, the parathyroid glands can be injured during surgery or inflammation may block the normal release of parathyroid hormone. If the level of parathyroid hormone drops, symptoms of calcium deficiency can occur. If not treated promptly, calcium deficiency can result in contraction of the glottis, respiratory obstruction, and death. Tetany may appear from 1 to 7 days postoperatively. Treatment for calcium deficiency is calcium chloride or calcium gluconate given intravenously. Oral calcium is then necessary until normal parathyroid function returns.

The nurse must know that respiratory obstruction can occur from (1) recurrent laryngeal nerve damage causing vocal cord spasms that close off the larynx, (2) tracheal compression from hemorrhage, (3) tissue swelling, or (4) tetany. The nurse should be prepared to deal with all these problems.

A patient who had surgery for hyperthyroidism, although treated to promote a euthyroid state before surgery, requires extra monitoring of cardiovascular and respiratory status after surgery to assist in identifying early any problems caused by the hyperthyroid state. During surgery with manipulation of the gland, extra hormone can be released and this may precipitate a thyroid storm or crisis. If a total thyroidectomy was done, the patient needs to be monitored for signs of hypothyroidism (see p. 1046) and started on replacement therapy.

PARATHYROID GLAND

HYPERSECRETION OF PARATHYROID HORMONE: PRIMARY HYPERPARATHYROIDISM

ETIOLOGY/EPIDEMIOLOGY

Primary hyperparathyroidism is being diagnosed with increased frequency, probably because of more frequent routine measurements of serum calcium levels. The exact number of persons requiring treatment for hyperparathyroidism based on elevated serum calcium levels is unknown because many of these persons have no other symptoms. Primary hyperparathyroidism occurs most frequently in adults between ages 20 and 50 and is two to four times more common in women.[65]

The most frequent cause of primary hyperparathyroidism is benign adenomas, although hyperplasia and malignant tumors may also be causes. The cause of adenomas, hyperplasia, or malignant tumors is not known, but a history of earlier radiation of the neck has been reported in some patients.[64]

Another theory is that the "set point" at which ionized calcium inhibits parathyroid gland tissue may be increased so that the normal negative feedback control between calcium and parathyroid gland function is lost. A genetic component is present in some persons who have primary hyperparathyroidism as part of the syndrome of MEN I (primary hyperparathyroidism is associated with islet cell tumors and pituitary adenoma) or part of MEN 2a (primary hyperparathyroidism is associated with medullary thyroid carcinoma and pheochromocytomas).

PATHOPHYSIOLOGY

The alteration in physiologic functioning associated with hyperparathyroidism is the result of one or two major problems:

1. The exaggeration of the normal effects of parathyroid hormone (PTH) on the skeletal, renal, and gastrointestinal (GI) systems
2. The associated hypercalcemia

The primary function of PTH is the maintenance of a normal serum level of calcium. Hypersecretion of PTH results in continual stimulation of target organs and elevates serum calcium. The normal negative feedback of serum calcium on PTH secretion is lost or ineffective. In the skeletal system, increased PTH increases bone resorption, resulting in osteopenia and, in very severe cases, cysts and fractures from *osteitis fibrosa cystica*. Joint changes also occur. In the renal system, increased PTH enhances the reabsorption of calcium from the glomerular filtrate, reabsorption of phosphate, and alteration in the excretion of bicarbonate. Production of activated vitamin D increases. Elevated PTH effects on the GI tract are indirect and occur through the action of vitamin D. The activated vitamin D results in increased calcium absorption through the GI tract.

The processes just described result in elevated serum calcium, which in itself leads to neurologic, musculoskeletal, cardiac, GI, and renal alterations. The alterations in the various systems caused by hypercalcemia result in most of the clinical manifestations. The relationship between the pathophysiology of hyperparathyroidism and the clinical manifestations is presented in Table 36-7.

Because calcitonin from the C cells of the thyroid opposes the effect of PTH, it would be logical to assume that in response to the increased serum calcium, calcitonin secretion would increase. This is not seen in primary hyperparathyroidism.

TABLE 36-7 Clinical manifestations of primary hyperparathyroidism and related pathophysiology

Body System	Signs and Symptoms	Body System	Signs and Symptoms
Skeletal	Bone pain; presence of osteopenia, increased bone resorption surface, cysts and cystlike areas, increased number of osteoclasts; unmineralized osteoid may be seen on bone biopsy and x-rays; bone formation is increased but resorption is greater than formation; results in increased osteoblasts and increased alkaline phosphatase levels; fractures; arthralgia, particularly of the joints of hands, synovitis, or pseudogout may result from the hypercalcemia; gout may also be present	Gastrointestinal	GI symptoms result from hypercalcemia; include anorexia; nausea and vomiting; constipation; peptic ulcer in some instances from increased gastrin secretion stimulated by increased calcium; pancreatitis
Renal	Early in disease: hypocalciuria in relation to increased serum calcium and increased phosphate clearance; later: elevated serum calcium level overwhelms reabsorptive capacity of kidney and hypercalciuria, polyuria, and polydipsia develop; nephrolithiasis with or without pyelonephritis; renal colic; nephrocalcinosis; metabolic acidosis (hyperchloremic acidosis) from ineffective bicarbonate reabsorption; renal insufficiency and failure may result from nephrolithiasis and nephrocalcinosis	Neurologic	CNS changes result from altered neurologic function caused by elevated calcium; calcium acts as a neurologic depressant; changes include impaired mentation and loss of memory, emotional lability, depression, apathy, somnolence, coma; peripheral nervous system changes include hypoactive reflexes, abnormal tongue movement resembling fasciculation, decreased vibratory sense in feet, glove and stocking sensory loss
		Muscular	Changes result from neuropathy rather than myopathy;[64] include weakness, aches, and pains; difficulty with climbing stairs and getting up from sitting position; changes in lower exremities before upper
		Cardiovascular	ECG changes related to effect of calcium on electrical activity of heart; include shortened QT interval, dysrhythmias; increased sensitivity to cardiac glycosides; hypertension; anemia
		Other areas	Pruritus; soft tissue calcification: band keratopathy; ectopic calcification in skin, arteries, lungs; all caused by increased calcium

CLINICAL MANIFESTATIONS

The patient with primary hyperparathyroidism may be asymptomatic, with only an increased serum calcium level. Other patients may have only nonspecific symptoms, such as weakness and easy fatigability; still others may have many manifestations (Table 36-7) caused by the increased PTH or hypercalcemia. Diagnostic findings include the following:

1. Laboratory tests
   a. Blood—elevated serum calcium, decreased serum phosphate, elevated PTH levels
   b. Urinary—elevated urinary cyclic adenosine monophosphate (AMP)
2. Radiographic—abnormalities particularly noticeable in the phalanges

MEDICAL MANAGEMENT

The first priority in medical management is to deal with the hypercalcemia. Hypercalcemia is discussed in detail in Chapter 23. The following is a brief review.

Hypercalcemia (serum calcium greater than 13 mg/100 ml) is treated immediately with normal saline infusion, intravenous or oral diuretics (furosemide or ethacrynic acid), restriction of calcium in the diet, restriction of drugs that increase serum calcium, and cardiac support. Once the calcium is in a safer range, the patient can be treated less aggressively, and oral fluid intake of 3 to 5 L/day and sodium chloride intake of 300 to 400 mEq/day should be instituted to help maintain urinary calcium excretion. Diuretics, either furosemide or ethacrynic acid, are continued. Potassium and magnesium need to be replaced. Dietary restrictions of calcium and restriction of drugs that can increase calcium are continued until surgery.

At the same time, diagnostic tests are implemented to identify the cause of the hypercalcemia. Other causes of hypercalcemia are listed in the box on p. 1059.

Once hyperparathyroidism is diagnosed and when the calcium level has been stabilized, surgery is the treatment of choice. In patients with only mild asympto-

CAUSES OF HYPERCALCEMIA (OTHER THAN HYPERPARATHYROIDISM)

Malignancy
Leukemia, lymphoma, multiple myeloma
Vitamin D intoxication
Hypervitaminosis A
Granulomatous diseases
Other endocrine disorders: thyrotoxicosis, adrenal insufficiency
Milk-alkali syndrome
Immobilization

matic hypercalcemia who have a normal renal function, urinary calcium excretion, and skeletal system, treatment may be delayed and the patient is observed regularly.

For patients with symptoms who are appropriate surgical risks, parathyroid surgery is performed.

If a single adenoma is the problem, it is removed. With hyperplasia, usually three complete glands and part of the fourth are removed. Sometimes in hyperplasia a total parathyroidectomy is performed, with transplantation of some parathyroid tissue into the muscle of the forearm to avoid loss of function of the residual tissue in the neck resulting from vascular failure, which is a complication of surgery.

If no abnormal glands are found during the exploration of the neck, the search may be extended into the retroesophageal and retropharyngeal spaces. Later surgical exploration may be necessary if no abnormal tissue is found during the initial surgery. This latter surgery is only carried out after instituting localizing procedures. Subsequent surgery may require mediastinal exploration.

Serum calcium levels decline within 24 hours after successful surgery, and subnormal levels may be present for 4 to 5 days. Severe postoperative hypocalcemia may occur. The hypocalcemia may result from "hungry bone syndrome," which causes an increase in new bone formation. This syndrome is treated with calcium replacement. Most patients develop hypocalcemia because of temporary hypoparathyroidism. This is also treated with calcium replacement and usually resolves in 1 week. If permanent hypoparathyroidism occurs, the patient is treated as described on p. 1064.

Medical treatment may be the only treatment used in some patients who are not suitable candidates for surgery. Medical treatment for these persons consists of the measures just described. In addition, mithramycin (Plicamycin) may be given intravenously to inhibit bone resorption. Some patients may be treated with phosphate replacement given orally or intravenously. Calcitonin has been used but has not been as effective as other therapy.[6,65] In combination with glucocorticoids, which is used for causes of hypercalcemia other then hyperparathyroidism, calcitonin may be more effective.[6] Dialysis has also been used.

■ ASSESSMENT

Subjective Data

Nursing assessment includes identifying the presence of signs and symptoms of hyperparathyroidism and the resultant hypercalcemia. The following areas should be assessed:

1. Mental status—history of change in mentation, personality, or alertness
2. Skeletal system—presence of bone or joint pain
3. Renal system
   a. Changes in urinary output, particularly polyuria or nocturia
   b. Symptoms of renal colic or pyelonephritis
4. GI system
   a. Normal 24-hour intake
   b. Symptoms of anorexia, nausea, vomiting
   c. Changes in bowel elimination
5. Neuromuscular system
   a. Symptoms of fatigue or weakness
   b. Changes in ability to carry out ADLs
   c. Presence of pruritus
   d. Presence or absence of flank pain

Objective Data

Objective data to be collected include the following:

1. Mental status—short-term memory, affect, alertness, orientation
2. Skeletal system—ROM, presence of excessive immobility
3. Renal system—urinary output, characteristics of urine
4. GI system—fluid/food intake, bowel movements, bowel sounds, weight
5. Neuromuscular system—muscle strength, peripheral sensory function, reflexes
6. Cardiovascular system—blood pressure, pulse (rhythm, rate), ECG

■ DATA ANALYSIS: NURSING DIAGNOSES

Nursing diagnoses are determined from assessment of patient data. Possible nursing diagnoses for the patient with primary hyperparathyroidism include, but are not limited to, the following:

Diagnostic Title	Possible Etiologies
For patients treated medically on long-term basis and acutely before surgery	
Activity intolerance	Muscular weakness, decreased cardiac output associated with changes in electrical activity of heart
Cardiac output, decreased	Dysrhythmias associated with altered electrical conduction
Constipation	Decrease in GI motility

Diagnostic Title	Possible Etiologies
Injury, potential for	Muscular weakness, altered mental status, bone demineralization
Knowledge deficit: immediate treatment, diagnostic tests, surgery, follow-up, long-term treatment	New problem and treatment with no previous exposure to information
Nutrition, altered: less than body requirements	Anorexia, nausea, vomiting
Pain	Bone changes, joint changes, potential renal colic and pruritus

For patients following surgery

Breathing pattern, ineffective	Tracheal obstruction associated with spasm of vocal cords or hemorrhage, laryngeal stridor associated with low serum calcium level
Injury, potential for	Hemorrhage, increased neuromuscular excitability associated with low serum calcium level
Knowledge deficit: follow-up care after surgery	No previous exposure to information

■ PLANNING: EXPECTED PATIENT OUTCOMES

Expected patient outcomes for the person with primary hyperparathyroidism may include, but are not limited to, the following:

For patients treated medically on long-term basis and acutely before surgery

1. Activity level does not decrease any further, and the patient gradually increases activity, as evidenced by more ambulation.
2. Cardiac output is maintained as evidenced by stable blood pressure; dysrhythmias or ECG changes are detected.
3. Normal patterns of bowel elimination (as established by assessment) are maintained.
4. Injury, such as from falls or dislodged arterial lines, does not occur.
5. The patient and significant others can:
   a. Describe the relationship between signs and symptoms and parathyroid dysfunction.
   b. Describe signs and symptoms that should disappear with treatment.
   c. List purpose and expectations for each diagnostic test.
   d. Explain purpose of treatment, signs of effectiveness, and symptoms to be reported.
   e. Describe plans for follow-up care, if appropriate.
6. Nutritional status is normal as evidenced by maintenance of weight or, if necessary, a return to normal weight, with a gain of 1 to 2 pounds per week; the patient eats 75% to 100% of every meal.

7. The patient states that pain reduction measures are effective; activities or self-care are not limited because of pain; signs of renal colic (bloody urine, pain, nausea) do not occur.
8. Output equals intake and is at least 2000 ml/day.

For patients following surgery

1. Patient maintains adequate air exchange, as evidenced by adequate breath sounds throughout lung field, arterial blood gases within normal range, and absence of signs of respiratory distress.
2. No injuries occur; the patient shows no undetected changes in vital signs or neuromuscular excitability.
3. The patient and significant others can:
   a. Describe reason for frequent vital signs and neurologic assessments.
   b. Describe symptoms they should report immediately.
   c. Describe plans for follow-up care.

■ IMPLEMENTATION

The care of the patient varies depending on the treatment. This section describes the care during the acute preoperative period or for patients treated medically.

Promoting Activity

The patient with hyperparathyroidism may have activity intolerance and needs to be involved in some weight-bearing activities that provide bone stress. This helps lower serum calcium levels. Thus a schedule of progressive activities is planned with the patient. Activities are spaced so fatigue is lessened. Goals should be identified with the patient to provide motivation and encourage increased activity. Activities such as bathing may require assistance to conserve energy for ambulation.

Maintaining Cardiac Function

Hypercalcemia associated with hyperparathyroidism presents a risk for decreased cardiac functioning. The patient is monitored frequently (every 2 to 4 hours) to detect early signs and is instructed to report any episodes of palpitations or vertigo. If dysfunction occurs, the patient may need to be placed on continuous cardiac monitoring. The patient receiving digitalis therapy is monitored closely for digitalis toxicity because the myocardium is unusually sensitive to digitalis in the presence of hypercalcemia. The dose may be decreased.

Promoting Bowel Elimination

The patient's bowel movements are monitored because constipation is a major problem. Fluids, dietary fiber, and ambulation are increased for prevention of constipation (see Chapter 44). If preventive measures are ineffective, stool softeners or laxatives may be prescribed by the physician.

Promoting Safety

Hyperparathyroidism may increase the likelihood of the patient being injured in a fall because of weakness or because of changes in mental status. If altered mental functioning is present, patients are placed in an environment where they can be observed closely, measures to increase orientation are used, and side rails are kept up. Soft restraints may be necessary but should be the last alternative.

If weakness is a factor, the patient must be assisted when up, have nonskid slippers for ambulation, and be provided with a room that is free of unnecessary equipment. A gradual increase in activity or the incorporation of isometric exercises may increase endurance. A physical therapist may be helpful in planning an exercise strengthening program.

Patient Teaching

Patient teaching includes information about diagnostic tests and how the various nursing diagnoses relate to the patient's altered physiologic condition. This may help the patient cope more effectively with changes that are occurring. Frequent reexplanations may be required by the person with altered mental functioning.

The family is included in the teaching. Because the patient's condition can be critical and may change rapidly, it may be helpful to plan with the family for daily formalized updates. Patients receiving medical therapy need instructions regarding comfort measures, safety, diet, activities, increased fluid intake, prevention of constipation, medications, and planned follow-up. Much of the care the patient required as an inpatient must be provided at home. Written as well as verbal instructions are helpful.

Patients treated with surgery need the general teaching described in Chapter 20.

Maintaining Nutrition

Nutritional needs for the person with hyperparathyroidism include a need to restrict calcium intake and control nausea and anorexia. The diet is monitored for foods high in calcium (see box above, right), and these foods are avoided. This may help decrease the hypercalcemia. The nurse should note that very few groups of food are high in calcium. Anorexia is often present, and measures such as environmental control of noxious stimuli, providing rest, and giving oral hygiene (see Chapter 42) are taken to encourage the person to eat. Referral to a dietitian may be helpful to patient and family. The patient also needs to increase fluid and sodium intake.

Promoting Comfort

The exact cause of patient discomfort must be identified. If bone or joint pain is present, proper positioning, support of joints and body parts, and gentleness in mov-

---

FOODS HIGH IN CALCIUM (MILLIGRAMS)

Almonds	332 mg/1 cup
Blackstrap molasses	137 mg/1 tbsp
Brazil nuts	260 mg/1 cup
Broccoli spears	132 mg/1 cup
Cabbage (cooked)	220 mg/1 cup
Canned mackerel	221 mg/3 ounces
Cheese (blue cheese, cheddar, American)	About 100 to 150 mg/1 ounce
Collards (cooked)	289 mg/1 cup
Custard	280 mg/1 cup
Dandelion greens (cooked)	252 mg/1 cup
Egg	27 mg/1 egg
Green beans	80 mg/1 cup
Ice cream	175 mg/1 cup
Ice milk	292 mg/1 cup
Kale (cooked)	147 mg/1 cup
Lima beans	75 mg/1 cup
Macaroni (enriched) and cheese, baked	398 mg/1 cup
Milk (whole, 2%, skim, buttermilk)	290 mg/1 cup
Mustard greens (cooked)	193 mg/1 cup
Oranges	50 mg/1 orange
Oysters	226 mg/1 cup
Peanut halves	107 mg/1 cup
Pizza (cheese)	107 mg/1 slice
Raisins, dried	124 mg/1 cup
Rhubarb (cooked)	212 mg/1 cup
Salmon, pink, canned	167 mg/3 ounces
Sardines	372 mg/3 ounces
Spinach (drained solids)	212 mg/1 cup
Turnip greens (cooked)	250 mg/1 cup
White sauce, medium	305 mg/1 cup
Yogurt	295 mg/1 cup

---

ing the patient are required. If renal colic is the cause of pain, the pain is severe and narcotics are necessary for relief; their effectiveness must be documented. Measures are taken to relieve pruritis as necessary (see Chapter 73); antihistamines or mild tranquilizers may be required.

Promoting Urinary Elimination

The first intervention for alteration in urinary elimination is to increase the patient's fluid intake, which will decrease the urinary mineral concentration and thus decrease urinary stone formation. A fluid intake of at least 3 L/day should be the goal unless other physiologic alterations such as cardiac or renal problems are present. Fluids are given throughout the 24 hours. The urine is strained through a gauze mesh to collect any small stones that pass, and the patient is monitored continually for recurrence of stone formation. Monitoring includes assessing intake and output and observing for presence of renal colic flank pain, hematuria, or nausea and vomiting. Immobility is avoided.

Other Care

The major medical therapy for patients with severe hypercalcemia is hydration. Large volumes of intravenous normal saline may be prescribed. The patient's tolerance of the large fluid volume is monitored every 2 to 4 hours and includes monitoring intake and output, weight, breath sounds, blood pressure, and pulse. Large doses of furosemide or ethacrynic acid are also usually prescribed. The patient must have adequate renal function to tolerate these therapeutic measures. Serum electrolytes, particularly potassium and magnesium, are monitored because hypokalemia and hypomagnesemia are potential complications along with fluid overload. The effectiveness of hydration therapy is observable within 24 hours and is evaluated by monitoring serum calcium levels and urinary calcium excretion.

Phosphates lower calcium levels by inhibiting bone resorption, and if an acute elevation of serum phosphate occurs, calcium phosphate salts precipitate out. Extensive precipitation of calcium phosphate salts can result in hypocalcemia and renal failure. Therefore the patient's intake and output, weight, and other measures of renal function must be monitored continuously along with serum phosphate levels. Monitoring also includes the side effects and signs of toxicity of other therapeutic agents.

Postoperative Care

Most patients with primary hyperparathyroidism are treated surgically. Postoperatively the care requirements are very similar to those required following thyroidectomy (see p. 1056). Potential physiologic complications include hemorrhage, hypocalcemia, and and airway obstruction. The patient's fluid volume, neurologic, respiratory, and cardiovascular states are monitored routinely. The serum calcium level will decrease within 24 hours, and the patient is monitored for tetany. Parathyroid function usually returns to normal within 5 to 7 days after a partial parathyroidectomy because the remaining tissue resumes normal functioning.

If mild hypocalcemia occurs, calcium is replaced orally. Severe hypocalcemia can occur if there has been tremendous bone demineralization. With the removal of the elevated PTH, the calcium-deficient bones extract larger-than-normal quantities of calcium from the extracellular fluids. For patients with severe hypocalcemia, calcium chloride or calcium gluconate is given intravenously. These calcium preparations should be readily available for immediate administration if necessary. If permanent hypoparathyroidism results because the remaining tissue does not resume normal secretion or because a total parathyroidectomy is done, the patient will need continual treatment.

A tracheostomy set should be kept on the nursing unit because respiratory obstruction from hemorrhage, edema, or vocal cord spasms is a potential complication. The patient is assessed initially every hour for adequacy of respiratory effort. A semi-Fowler's position will help to decrease edema and thus decrease risk of respiratory distress.

Patient teaching following surgery includes:
1. Planned medication regimen, if appropriate
2. Need for adequate exercise and diet
3. Any self-monitoring that is necessary
4. Signs and symptoms of hypocalcemia or recurrence of hypercalcemia that must be reported immediately
5. Need for follow-up care

HYPERSECRETION OF PARATHYROID HORMONE: SECONDARY AND TERTIARY HYPERPARATHYROIDISM

Secondary hyperparathyroidism is a disease characterized by excessive production of PTH resulting from chronic hypocalcemia. *Malabsorption* and *chronic renal failure* are two common causes of secondary hyperparathyroidism. In these conditions the calcium level is chronically low. In chronic renal failure the low calcium results from *hyperphosphatemia,* a decrease in production of activated vitamin D, and a decrease in calcium absorption. There also may be a decreased sensitivity of the bones to the action of PTH.[64] The low calcium level is a chronic stimulus to the parathyroid glands and results in their hyperplasia. The hyperplasia and excessive production of PTH is usually able to keep the calcium level close to normal, but at the expense of bone destruction. The bone lesions are characterized by osteomalacia, osteosclerosis, and osteitis fibrosa cystica.

Treatment for secondary hyperparathyroidism is directed at decreasing the chronic stimulation of the parathyroid gland by improving the calcium level. In patients with malabsorption, calcium supplements and vitamin D are used. In patients with chronic renal failure, the treatment is first directed toward (1) lowering the phosphorus level with a phophorus-depleting agent such as aluminum hydroxide and (2) increasing the calcium level with calcium and vitamin D supplementation (see Chapter 50). If medical therapy does not lower the phosphorus level and thus elevate the calcium level and halt the chronic stimulation of the parathyroid gland and the bone destruction, a subtotal parathyroidectomy may be done.

Tertiary hyperparathyroidism is the result of long-standing secondary hyperparathyroidism. It is characterized by the development of autonomous parathyroid gland functioning that is not under normal homeostatic control mechanisms. When tertiary hyperparathyroidism occurs, the patient with chronic renal failure or malabsorption syndrome will develop *hypercalcemia*. In many instances, with removal of the chronic stimulus of hypocalcemia to the parathyroid gland, the hyperplasia will regress. The usual treatment for tertiary hyperparathyroidism is to prevent complications of hypercalcemia by hydration, diuretics, and restriction of calcium intake, until the gland returns to normal. In some patients the glandular hyperplasia does not regress and a partial parathyroidectomy is necessary.

The care for patients who undergo partial parathyroidectomies for secondary or tertiary hyperparathyroidism is the same as for patients who have partial parathyroidectomies for primary hyperparathyroidism. Nurses have a major role in helping patients with malabsorption syndrome or chronic renal failure to follow prescribed regimens so that secondary or tertiary hyperparathyroidism is prevented.

HYPOSECRETION OF PARATHYROID HORMONE: HYPOPARATHYROIDISM

ETIOLOGY

The causative factors of true hypoparathyroidism may be classified into three major categories: surgically induced, idiopathic, and functional.[65] Hypoparathyroidism occurs mainly from trauma of the anterior neck during surgery, particularly thyroid surgery, parathyroid surgery, or radical neck surgery. In rare instances, hypoparathyroidism may result from radioactive iodine therapy for hyperthyroidism or thyroid cancer. Idiopathic hypoparathyroidism is deficient hormone production from unknown causes. It may be seen at an early age and is probably the result of a genetic defect. There may be an autoimmune basis for early-age idiopathic hypoparathyroidism because many of these persons have abnormal antibodies directed against the parathyroid gland.[65] Late-onset idiopathic hypoparathyroidism is has no known cause. Functional hypoparathyroidism is the result of chronic hypomagnesemia that may be seen in malabsorption or alcoholism and appears to impair PTH release.

In pseudohypoparathyroidism the secretion and release of PTH is normal, but there is target tissue resistance to PTH. The cause of the resistance is unknown.

PATHOPHYSIOLOGY

A deficiency of or tissue resistance to PTH results in decreased bone resorption, decreased activation of vitamin D (and thus decreased intestinal absorption of calcium), increased renal excretion of calcium, and decreased renal excretion of phosphorus. The end result is hypocalcemia and hyperphosphatemia. The major physiologic alterations result from the effects of low calcium levels on neuromuscular irritability. Nerves show decreased thresholds of excitation, repeated responses to a single stimuli, and, in severe cases, continuous activity. Car-

diac activity is altered. Calcification of basal ganglia and of the lens of the eye may occur.

CLINICAL MANIFESTATIONS

True Hypoparathyroidism

The severity of the hypocalcemia and the chronicity of the problem dictate the signs and symptoms seen with true hypoparathyroidism. In mild cases, which result in only mildly decreased serum calcium levels, the patient may be asymptomatic. In more severe cases, any or all of the following clinical manifestations may be seen.

1. Neuromuscular manifestations: changes in nerve activity affect peripheral motor and sensory nerves
   a. Numbness and tingling (paresthesia) around mouth, tips of fingers, and sometimes in the feet
   b. Tetany with positive Chvostek's and Trousseau's signs (see Chapter 23) spasms of wrists, fingers, and forearms, or feet and toes
   c. Convulsions that may consist of tonic spasms of the total body or the more typical tonic-clonic activity
   d. Laryngeal stridor and dyspnea
   e. Other neurologic signs: headache, papilledema, elevated CSF pressure, local signs that mimic a cerebral tumor; extrapyramidal neurologic signs and symptoms include gait changes, tremors, rigidity, and spasms; signs and symptoms of parkinsonism may occur (see Chapter 63)
2. Emotional-mental manifestations: irritability, depression, anxiety, emotional lability, memory impairment, confusion, frank psychosis
3. Cardiovascular manifestations (effect of hypocalcemia)
   a. Prolonged QT and ST intervals and occasional dysrhythmias
   b. Resistance to effects of digitalis preparations
   c. Decreased cardiac output from congestive heart failure
4. Eye manifestations (calcification of lens)
   a. Cataract formation
   b. Eventual loss of all sight
5. Dental manifestations (depending on age of onset)
   a. Enamel defects seen on the tooth crown
   b. Delayed or absent tooth eruption
   c. Defective dental root formation
6. Integumentary manifestations: fragile nails, thin patchy hair, dry scaly skin, skin infections (usually candidiasis), vitiligo
7. GI manifestations: malabsorption, steatorrhea

Diagnostic Tests

Laboratory tests for the patient with hypoparathyroidism may show the following findings (see Chapter 35):

1. Decreased serum calcium and increased serum phosphate levels
2. Low to undetectable levels of PTH by radioimmunoassay
3. Low basal levels of urinary cyclic AMP and increased levels after exogenous PTH administration

Pseudohypoparathyroidism

The patient with pseudohypoparathyroidism may have the same signs and symptoms as seen with true hypoparathyroidism. In addition, such patients may have skeletal and developmental abnormalities, including short stature, round face, short neck, stocky body, and discrete bone lesions. The most common bone lesion is unilateral or bilateral shortening of the fourth and fifth metacarpal and metatarsal bones. Mental retardation may also be present. The patient has low serum calcium and high serum phosphorus with a normal to high PTH level on radioimmunoassay.

MEDICAL MANAGEMENT

The first priority of treatment is correction of calcium levels to prevent tetany. This is achieved by giving intravenous calcium gluconate or calcium chloride. Airway patency must be maintained. Maintenance of a calcium level of about 7 mg/100 ml usually prevents signs and symptoms such as laryngeal stridor and convulsions.

The cause of hypoparathyroidism is then identified, and long-term therapy is started as soon as possible. Normal serum calcium levels are maintained by supplemental dietary and elemental calcium, by dietary phosphate restriction and phosphate-binding agents such as aluminum hydroxide, and by vitamin D therapy to increase GI absorption of calcium. Vitamin D preparations include ergocalciferol (Drisdol, Geltabs), dihydrotachysterol (Hytakerol), or the cholecalciferol metabolites calcifediol (Calderol) or calcitriol (Rocaltrol).

It takes several weeks before the full effect of vitamin D therapy is seen. Major complications of therapy are vitamin D toxicity and renal calculi formation. Renal calculi can occur in the hypoparathyroid patient even in the presence of normal serum calcium because the lack of PTH results in excessive urinary calcium excretion. The patient is monitored at 6- to 12-month intervals to evaluate the effectiveness of treatment and to assess for side effects.

■ ASSESSMENT

Assessment focuses on identifying signs and symptoms of hypocalcemia and on identifying the patient's and significant others' knowledge level regarding the altered health state.

Subjective Data

Major assessment for the person with hypoparathyroidism include the following focus.

1. Neuromuscular/emotional-mental status: history of paresthesia, episodes of spasms in extremities, convulsion, and changes in behavior, mood, memory, or orientation
2. Cardiovascular status: complaints of palpitations, syncope, edema
3. Eyes: history of visual changes
4. Integumentary status: changes in pigmentation, reports of skin dryness or hair loss
5. Knowledge level: disease process, relationship of signs and symptoms and functional changes to disease, medical therapy

Objective Data

The following objective data are collected.

1. Neuromuscular/emotional-mental status: Chvostek's and Trousseau's signs, affect, memory, orientation
2. Cardiovascular status: blood pressure, pulse rate and rhythms, heart sounds, presence of edema, weight
3. Eyes: visual acuity
4. Teeth: abnormal dentation (lack of eruption, enamel defects)
5. Integumentary status: pigmentation, presence of infection, hair loss
6. Musculoskeletal status: height, body proportions, hand defects (shortened fourth and fifth fingers)

■ DATA ANALYSIS: NURSING DIAGNOSES

Nursing diagnoses are determined from assessment of patient data. Possible nursing diagnoses for the person with hypoparathyroidism include, but are not limited to, the following:

Diagnostic Title	Possible Etiologies
Anxiety	Uncontrollability or alarming quality of signs and symptoms
Breathing patterns, ineffective	Obstruction to air exchange associated with laryngeal spasm
Cardiac output, decreased	Impaired electrical activity and contractility associated with low serum calcium level
Injury, potential for	Altered mental status associated with tetany
Knowledge deficit: disease, diagnostic tests, treatment, side effects, follow-up	New diagnoses and no previous exposure to information
Sensory/perceptual alterations: visual	Calcification of lens

■ PLANNING: EXPECTED PATIENT OUTCOMES

Expected patient outcomes for the person with hypoparathyroidism may include, but are not limited to, the following:

1. Signs of anxiety such as restlessness, constant motion, or jitteriness are not noted.
2. Adequate air exchange is maintained, as confirmed by adequate blood gases; stridor and dyspnea are absent.
3. Blood pressure is maintained; undetected dysrhythmias do not occur.
4. Injury does not occur from convulsions or undetected tetany.
5. Patient and significant others can explain planned diagnostic tests and treatments, long-term therapy and follow-up, and self-monitoring for signs of tetany or hypercalcemia.
6. Patient maintains independent activities.

■ IMPLEMENTATION

Nursing care is directed toward dealing with anxiety; monitoring and intervening to prevent respiratory distress, cardiac dysfunction, or injury; and patient education.

Controlling Anxiety

The alarming quality of the signs and symptoms of hypoparathyroidism and hypocalcemia can provoke great anxiety. A major intervention is to establish confidence in the patient that the nurse understands the patient's physical status, understands the symptoms, and is available. The patient should be placed in a room so the nurses' station is visible. The patient's call light should be answered promptly. The nurse needs to follow up on any patient complaint. Hyperventilation, which can accompany anxiety, worsens the hypocalcemia because hyperventilation causes respiratory alkalosis, which in turn causes more of the ionized calcium to bind to serum protein. The decrease in ionized calcium exacerbates symptoms of hypocalcemia. Thus the patient should be supported to prevent hyperventilation. Keeping patients informed of their serum calcium levels will also help them feel in control and may lessen anxiety.

Monitoring/Supporting/Preventing Injury

A routine schedule for monitoring is developed and monitoring may need to be done as frequently as every hour. Parameters to monitor include the following:

1. Chvostek's and Trousseau's signs (see Chapter 23)
2. Airway patency
3. Mental status—orientation
4. Emotional status—anxiety, irritability
5. Vital signs, particularly pulse rate and rhythm

Any abnormal changes that are detected are reported immediately so that treatment can be instituted and convulsions prevented. The initiation of maintenance therapy does not immediately correct the physiologic problem, and therapy will be adjusted to maintain a normal serum calcium level without complications. Monitoring is continued during this period of adjustment or with any future changes.

A high priority for care is the maintenance of a safe environment. Seizure precautions such as padded bed rails, suctioning equipment, a tracheostomy tray, and intravenous calcium must be readily available. The patient should be in a room that facilitates easy and frequent observation.

If visual changes are present, the environment is structured to allow the patient to function as independently as possible. If confusion or memory deficits are present, the patient is reoriented frequently. The room should be free of clutter. A chest restraint may be necessary.

Patient Education

The potential for convulsions and spasms and the necessity for diagnostic tests and frequent monitoring need to be explained to the patient and significant others. The nurse must explain the relationships between the signs and symptoms, tests, monitoring, the disease, and each new intervention.

Patient teaching includes the following:

1. Nature of the disease and need for long-term therapy
2. Medication administration
   a. Take prescribed calcium, phosphate-binding agents, and vitamin D daily
   b. Monitor for signs of:
      (1) Ineffective treatment—recurrence of tetany
      (2) Signs of hypercalcemia—thirst, polyuria, lethargy, decreased muscle tone, constipation
      (3) Complications—renal stones (flank pain or pain radiating down into groin)
3. Need for continual follow-up care every 6 to 12 months
4. Dietary changes—increased calcium and decreased phosphorus

ADRENAL GLAND

The adrenal cortex is essential to life. Without the hormones cortisol and aldosterone, the body's metabolic processes respond inadequately to even minimal physical and emotional stressors such as changes in temperature, exercise, or excitement. More severe stressors

HYPERFUNCTION (↑)　　　　　　　　　　HYPOFUNCTION (↓)

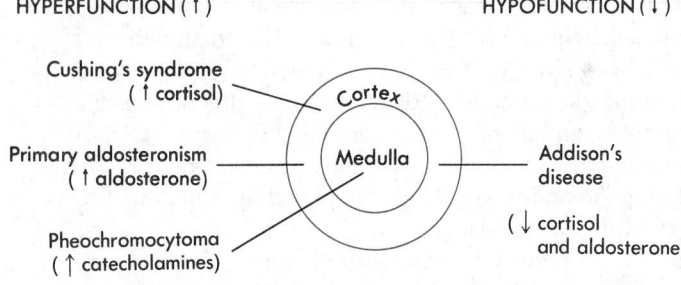

Cushing's syndrome
(↑ cortisol)

Primary aldosteronism
(↑ aldosterone)

Pheochromocytoma
(↑ catecholamines)

Cortex

Medulla

Addison's
disease

(↓ cortisol
and aldosterone)

FIGURE 36-7 Adrenal gland dysfunctions.

TABLE 36-8 Frequency of various causes of Cushing's syndrome[65]

Cause	Percent
Excessive pituitary secretion of ACTH	68
Adrenal adenomas and carcinoma	17
Ectopic secretion of ACTH	15

such as serious infections, surgery, or extreme anxiety may result in shock and death.

The adrenal medulla is not essential to life because the sympathetic nervous system produces similar although slower responses. Dysfunction of the adrenal gland can be manifested as an increased or decreased function of the cortex or increased function of the medulla (Figure 36-7).

HYPERFUNCTION OF THE ADRENAL CORTEX: CORTISOL EXCESS
ETIOLOGY/EPIDEMIOLOGY

Excessive levels of glucocorticoids, whatever the cause, result in a constellation of symptoms known as Cushing's syndrome. The causes of Cushing's syndrome may be divided into 3 major groups.

1. Primary Cushing's syndrome: excessive cortisol production resulting from adrenal adenomas or carcinomas; also called *adrenal Cushing's syndrome*
2. Secondary Cushing's syndrome: excessive cortisol production resulting from adrenal hyperplasia because of excessive ACTH production. The excessive ACTH production may result from either:
   a. Increased release of ACTH from the pituitary gland because of pituitary or hypothalamic problems; also called *Cushing's disease* or *pituitary Cushing's syndrome*
   b. Increased release of ACTH from ectopic nonpituitary sites such as bronchogenic carcinoma, pancreatic carcinoma, and bronchial adenoma; also called *ectopic Cushing's syndrome*
3. Iatrogenic Cushing's syndrome: excessive cortisol levels resulting from chronic glucocorticoid therapy. This is the most frequent cause of Cushing's syndrome seen in clinical practice and is discussed on p. 1071.

The frequencies of Cushing's syndrome from the various etiologies are presented in Table 36-8. Overall, Cushing's syndrome from pituitary disease is most often found in females in the second to fourth decades of life, although ectopic ACTH hypersecretion is found most frequently in males, probably because of the higher incidence of bronchogenic oat cell carcinoma.

PREVENTION

Most causes of excessive cortisol production are not preventable except for the ectopic secretion of ACTH from bronchogenic carcinoma. Elimination of smoking would decrease the occurrence of bronchogenic carcinoma.

Secondary preventive activities should be a major focus of nursing care. Nurses should help patients to deal with their chronic health problems, carry out self-monitoring practices to identify exacerbations early, and maintain their therapeutic regimens. These practices help to prevent progression of problems. One group of particular importance because of their large number is patients receiving long-term glucocorticoid therapy. Through their patient educator roles, nurses can help patients maintain their therapy in the safest manner possible.

PATHOPHYSIOLOGY

The major end result of Cushing's syndrome is excessive production of cortisol. Early in the noniatrogenic disorders, the most prominent alteration is loss of the normal diurnal secretory pattern. With loss of the diurnal pattern, the morning level of cortisol production may not be abnormally elevated, but levels during the day do not show the normal decrease below the morning peak. At later stages, cortisol is elevated at all times.

The pathophysiologic factors associated with cortisol excess primarily result from exaggeration in all the known actions of glucocorticoids and include alterations in the following:

1. Protein, fat, and carbohydrate metabolism
2. Inflammatory and immune response
3. Water and mineral metabolism
4. Emotional stability
5. RBC and platelet levels

Excessive cortisol may also disturb secretion of other anterior pituitary hormones (prolactin, thyrotropin, LH, GH) and alterations in sleep patterns. Some of these alterations may contribute to the clinical picture.[64]

In many instances, cortisol excess is also associated with excessive production of androgen; this results in virilization in females. Adrenal tumors may secrete cortisol, androgens, and mineralocorticoids in various proportions. Depending on which hormone is produced in excess, the patient will have (1) the clinical picture associated with Cushing's syndrome, (2) only the effects of androgen excess, (3) a clinical picture similar to that for hyperaldosteronism, or (4) any combination of these three.

CLINICAL MANIFESTATIONS

The manifestations are presented here according to the ways in which they alter the patient's normal adrenocorticol physiologic status.

Alteration in Protein, Fat, and Carbohydrate Metabolism

Altered protein metabolism. Excessive catabolism of proteins results in loss of muscle mass, causing the following symptoms:

1. Muscle wasting, particularly of the extremities, resulting in thin arms and legs, difficulty getting up from low chairs, difficulty climbing stairs, or generalized weakness and fatigue
2. Depletion of the protein matrix of bone, resulting in osteoporosis, compression fractures of the spine, backache, bone pain, and pathologic fractures
3. Loss of collagen support of the skin, resulting in thin, fragile skin that bruises easily, ecchymosis at trauma sites, and pink to purple cutaneous striae
4. Poor wound healing

Altered fat metabolism. Changes in fat metabolism cause obesity with abnormal deposition of fat in the face producing *moon face* (see Figure 36-8), in the intrascapular area producing the *buffalo hump,* and in the mesenteric bed producing *truncal obesity.* The redistribution of fat with these characteristic features may be seen in patients without obesity. Body weight usually is increased.

Altered carbohydrate metabolism. Increased hepatic gluconeogenesis and impaired insulin use results in postprandial hyperglycemia and occasionally frank diabetes mellitus with all its signs and symptoms (see Chapter 37). Patients with concurrent diabetes mellitus may have worsening of signs and symptoms of their diabetes mellitus.

Alteration in Inflammatory and Immune Response

Cortisol excess results in decreased lymphocytes, particularly T lymphocytes; decreased cell-mediated immunity; increased neutrophils; and altered antibody activity. These changes make the person particularly vunerable to viral and fungal infections. The depression in inflammatory and immune responsiveness results in opportunistic infections such as *Pneumocystis carinii* or other fungal infections. Early signs of infection, such as fever, may not be seen. Poor wound healing may also be related to infections.

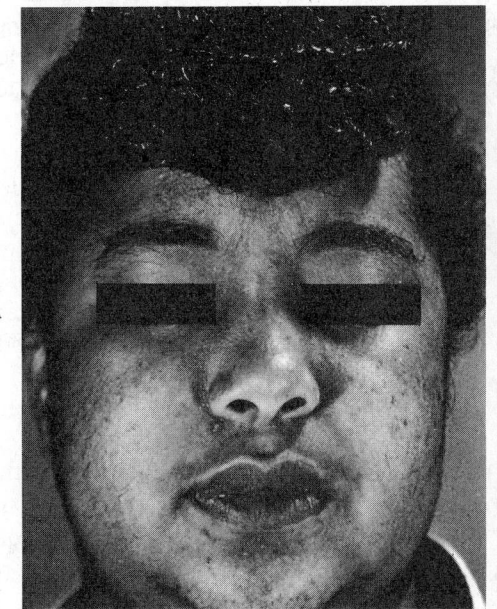
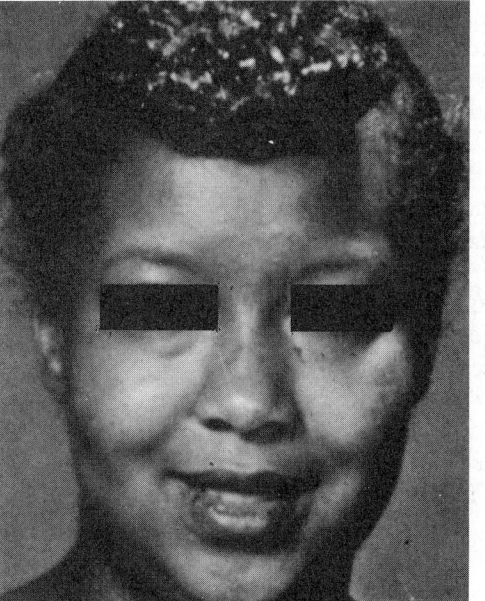

FIGURE 36-8 Facial changes characteristic of increased cortisol hormone. **A,** Before treatment. **B,** Six months after treatment. (From Thibodeau GA and Anthony CP: Structure and function of the body, ed 8, St. Louis, 1988, The CV Mosby Co.)

Alterations in Water and Mineral Metabolism

Cortisol itself possesses mineralocorticoid activity; therefore cortisol excess results in characteristic signs and symptoms of increased mineralocorticoid activity even though the level of aldosterone is normal. These include the following:

1. Sodium and water retention, which may accentuate body weight increase and may cause edema; serum sodium is usually normal
2. Hypertension, which is found in almost every patient with excessive cortisol and may be caused by increased volume or by increased sensitivity of arterioles to circulating catecholamines
3. Hypokalemia, hypochloremia, and metabolic alkalosis if cortisol excess is severe, because of increased excretion of potassium and chloride (most often seen with ectopic Cushing's syndrome)[64]
4. Increased calcium resorption from the bones and renal calculi from hypercalciuria (resulting in renal colic)

Alteration in Emotional Stability

Various emotional changes may occur. They range from irritability and anxiety, to mild depression and poor concentration and memory, to severe depression and psychosis. Euphoria and sleep disorders are frequently noted.

Hematologic Alterations

Various changes in blood components, which occur as the result of excessive cortisol, are:

1. High to normal RBC count, hemoglobin, and hematocrit (may account in part for facial plethora [appearance of increased facial circulation])
2. Leukocytosis, lymphopenia, and eosinopenia
3. Increases in various clotting factors and platelets, resulting in thromboembolic phenomena

Excessive Androgen Activity

If excessive androgens are present, the female patient will exhibit virilization, which includes the following signs:

1. Hirsutism, manifested as a fine downy coat of hair on the face and total body
2. Loss of scalp hair
3. Acne
4. Changes in menstrual cycle, varying from irregularities to oligomenorrhea to amenorrhea
5. Changes in libido

Other Findings

Hyperpigmentation may be present and indicates an elevation of ACTH, usually from an ectopic site. ACTH has melanotrophic activity. The hyperpigmentation is seen on the skin and mucous membranes.

Diagnostic Tests

Various diagnostic procedures are performed to confirm the diagnosis and differentiate among the various causes of cortisol excess. Positive test results, regardless of the cause, include the following (see Chapter 35 for a detailed discussion of these tests):

1. Elevated serum cortisol level or elevated excretion of urine-free cortisol
2. Elevated urinary levels of 17-ketogenic steroids (17-KGS) and 17-hydroxycorticosteroids (17-OHCS)
3. Loss of diurnal rhythms of cortisol production
4. Loss of suppression of endogenous cortisol with the normal and screening cortisone suppression tests
5. Abnormalities in serum electrolytes, chemistry, and hematology, as described earlier

Secondary Cushing's syndrome from either pituitary disease or diseases that cause ectopic ACTH secretion results in elevated plasma ACTH, whereas persons with primary Cushing's syndrome have ACTH levels too low to measure. Pituitary and ectopic Cushing's syndromes are differentiated by response to the high-level dexamethasone suppression test (2 mg dexamethasone given every 6 hours). Pituitary production of ACTH and thus of cortisol is suppressed with this high level of drug, whereas no suppression occurs in ectopic Cushing's syndrome. The presence of pituitary, ectopic, or adrenal tumors may be demonstrated by CT scans, ultrasound, and angiographic studies.

To analyze the results of the diagnostic tests accurately, various factors that cause false-positive results must be eliminated. These factors include the following:

1. Persons with acute or chronic illnesses; acute stressors may result in high cortisol levels and abnormal dexamethasone tests; these tests must be repeated after the patient is stable.
2. Obesity; results in high levels of urinary 17-OHCS and 17-KGS and abnormal screening suppression tests, but urine-free cortisol, serum cortisol, and response to normal suppression test are normal.
3. Pregnancy, estrogen therapy, and oral contraceptives; the elevated estrogen associated with these states can increase serum cortisol and give abnormal results on a screening cortisol suppression test, but urine-free cortisol and response to normal suppression test are normal.
4. Alcoholism; alcoholics may have both the clinical and diagnostic characteristics of Cushing's syndrome, but abstinence from alcohol reverses signs, symptoms, and abnormal test results.
5. Depression; endogenous depression results in increased cortisol levels, loss of diurnal rhythm, increased urine-free cortisol, increased urine 17-OHCS and 17-KGS, and abnormal suppression

tests; however, patients with depression will have an increase in cortisol in response to insulin-induced hypoglycemia, whereas patients with true Cushing's syndrome do not.

MEDICAL MANAGEMENT

Medical management is directed toward identifying the cause of the problem and removing the cause of cortisol excess, if possible. In iatrogenic Cushing's syndrome, care is directed toward control of signs and symptoms if the chronic therapy cannot be terminated.

For patients with pituitary Cushing's syndrome resulting in adrenal hyperplasia, six therapeutic options are available. (Table 36-9), although transsphenoidal removal of the pituitary tumor is the first line of therapy. When pituitary tumor removal is not possible or successful, other methods are used as adjunctive therapy.

For patients with the ectopic syndrome, the first line of therapy is to remove the source of the ectopic ACTH secretion. If this is not possible, drugs that inhibit cortisol production (Table 36-9) may be used. In some instances, when the site of ectopic ACTH cannot be found and the signs and symptoms cannot be controlled, bilat-

eral adrenalectomy may be done.

For adrenal tumors, the treatment of choice is tumor removal. If the tumor is localized to one gland, a unilateral adrenalectomy is done. When there has been excessive cortisol production by one gland, the negative feedback has caused a decrease in ACTH and subsequent atrophy of the unaffected gland. Thus the patient needs glucocorticoid replacement therapy for some time until normal function of the other adrenal gland returns. If the adrenocortical tumors are bilateral, bilateral adrenalectomy is done and the patient will receive lifetime hormone replacement therapy.

■ ASSESSMENT
Subjective Data

The following data are collected during the nursing history:

1. General data
   a. Changes noted in body proportions, weight, hair distribution, pigmentation, bruising, delayed wound healing
   b. History of discomfort, particularly back pain
   c. History of frequent infections: skin, respiratory

TABLE 36-9 Medical management of patients with pituitary Cushing's syndrome

Treatment	Comments	Complications
Transsphenoidal adenectomy	First approach for pituitary tumors; preserves normal pituitary function; very successful for microadenomas; less successful for macroadenomas or invasive tumors	Complete recovery of gland requires a year or so; patients may require glucocorticoids for some time
Transsphenoidal hypophysectomy	Gives 100% cure but removes total pituitary; may be used for invasive tumors or macroadenomas	Requires replacement therapy of glucocorticoids, thyroid hormone, gonadal steroids, and possibly ADH for life
Radiation therapy by conventional methods, heavy particles or implants	Implants successful if no evidence of exact tumor found; conventional and heavy particle therapy used as adjunct to surgery	Complete remission not always possible; may develop hypopituitarism or damage to visual system
Bilateral total adrenalectomy	Produces complete cure of signs and symptoms of cortisol excess; does not decrease ACTH	Replacement therapy of glucocorticoids and mineralocorticoids required for life; hyperpigmentation because ACTH still elevated; visual problems from a continually growing tumor (Nelson's syndrome)

Drug therapy (work at level of adrenal gland)
  Aminoglutethimide (inhibits cholesterol synthesis)
  Mitotane (inhibits cortisol production; can destroy gland)
  Metyrapone (partially inhibits adrenal cortex steroid synthesis)
	Used as adjunct to surgery of pituitary or radiation when complete remission not achieved; used for unresectable malignant tumors producing ACTH or unresectable adrenal carcinoma	All drugs have toxic effects; control symptoms but do not cure; can result in permanent adrenal insufficiency (mitotane); all patients require adrenal steroid replacement during therapy; patient can develop Nelson's syndrome because pituitary tumor remains

Drug therapy (work at level of pituitary gland) Cyproheptadine (serotonin antagonist that inhibits ACTH release)	Thus far used only in a few patients who have had recurrence after pituitary adenectomy	Effective only as long as drug is given; some patients show no response

2. Neurologic data: changes noted in behavior, concentration, memory
3. Nutritional data
   a. Usual 24-hour food/fluid intake
   b. History of increase in thirst
4. Musculoskeletal data: complaints of weakness, fatigue, or difficulty doing normal activities
5. Elimination data: changes in urinary output
6. Sexuality data
   a. Females: changes in menstrual history, secondary sexual characteristics, libido, or feelings about self
   b. Males: changes in libido, secondary sexual characteristics, feelings about self
7. Knowledge level: condition, treatment, diagnostic tests

Objective Data

Physical examination of the patient is directed toward the following data:

1. General: body appearance (presence of moon facies, buffalo hump, truncal obesity, thin arms and legs, hyperpigmentation, striae, bruises, ecchymoses, fragile skin, facial plethora, unhealed wounds)
2. Neurologic: affect and its appropriateness to situation, short-term memory, concentration
3. Cardiovascular: blood pressure, pulse, weight, presence of edema, jugular vein distention
4. Nutrition: intake of food and fluids
5. Musculoskeletal: muscle mass, strength, ability to stand up from a sitting position or do knee bends
6. Elimination: urinary output, presence of glycosuria
7. Sexuality: female secondary sexual characteristics, body hair distribution, scalp hair changes, presence of acne

■ DATA ANALYSIS: NURSING DIAGNOSES

Nursing diagnoses are determined from assessment of patient data. Possible nursing diagnoses for the person with cortisol excess include, but are not limited to, the following:

Diagnostic Title	Possible Etiologies
For patients during the acute period before definitive treatment or if definitive treatment is not possible	
Activity intolerance	Muscle weakness, abnormal carbohydrate metabolism, abnormal electrolyte balance
Body image disturbance	Changes in body characteristics, change in functioning
Coping, ineffective individual	Inability to mount a normal physiologic response to stressors, possible lack of learned coping strategies, emotional lability

Diagnostic Title	Possible Etiologies
Fluid volume excess	Abnormal retention of sodium and water
Infection, potential for	Inability to fight organisms because of depression of immune and inflammatory responsiveness
Injury, potential for	Falls associated with muscle weakness and bone changes
Knowledge deficit: disease, diagnostic tests, treatment, side effects, expected outcomes	New disease, new tests, never exposed to information previously
Nutrition, altered: more than body requirements	Increase in appetite with increased cortisol, alteration in metabolism
Pain	Demineralization of bone resulting in compression fractures

■ PLANNING: EXPECTED PATIENT OUTCOMES

Expected patient outcomes for the patient with cortisol excess may include, but are not limited to, the following:

For patients during the acute period before definitive treatment or if definitive treatment is not possible

1. Activity tolerance improves as evidenced by maintenance of current activity level and a weekly increase in activity.
2. Body image improves as evidenced by the patient speaking about self in positive terms.
3. Coping is adequate as evidenced by absence of signs of uncontrolled stress (restlessness, lack of attention, increased heart rate or blood pressure)
4. Fluid volume returns to normal as evidenced by elimination of signs of hemodilution or edema
5. Early signs and symptoms of infections are detected.
6. Falls do not occur.
7. The patient and significant others can:
   a. Explain the rationale and procedure for diagnostic tests.
   b. Explain the cause of the disease and how signs and symptoms relate to the disease.
   c. Describe the treatment and the expected effects.
   d. Describe replacement or other medication therapy (drug, dosage, frequency, side effects).
   e. Describe plans for follow-up care.
   f. State need for bracelet, necklace, or identification card if receiving replacement therapy.
8. Nutritional status is adequate as evidenced by a gradual decrease in weight and a decrease in caloric intake.

9. The patient states pain is controlled; activities are not limited because of pain.

■ IMPLEMENTATION

Physiologic Needs

The patient with excessive cortisol secretion needs skilled nursing care. The patient can be critically ill. During the acute period the primary focus of care is on the high-priority needs of supporting coping, restoring fluid balance, and preventing infections and injuries. In the more stable patient these needs are still a focus of care, but the focus will expand to the other needs described by the additional nursing diagnoses listed earlier.

Immediate Needs

1. Decrease controllable stressors.
   a. Provide continuity of care.
   b. Explain all procedures slowly and carefully.
   c. Spend time with patient and listen carefully.
   d. Avoid sudden noises, temperature changes, drafts, and unnecessary invasion of privacy.
   e. Promote relaxation.
2. Monitor physiologic coping ability.
   a. Ensure blood pressure and pulse remain stable.
   b. Take vital signs at least every 2 to 4 hours.
3. Control fluid volume excess.
   a. Restrict fluids as prescribed; distribute fluids throughout the 24 hours; use ice chips to prevent thirst.
   b. Provide a diet low in sodium as necessary.
   c. Provide potassium replacement as ordered and increase intake of foods high in potassium.
   d. Monitor daily weight, intake and output every 4 to 8 hours, and laboratory values of sodium, potassium chloride, bicarbonate, and pH.
4. Prevent infection and falls.
   a. Monitor temperature every 4 hours.
   b. Assess mouth, lungs, and skin every shift for early signs of infection; report signs immediately.
   c. Limit staff and visitors with signs and symptoms of upper respiratory infections.
   d. Institute preventive care: sterile technique for invasive procedures; routine turning, coughing, and deep breathing every 2 hours; oral hygiene before breakfast, after meals, and at bedtime.

Later Needs

Maintaining and increasing activity. The first goal is to maintain the patient's current activity level. This requires assisting with some activities that require energy, such as bathing. In addition, the nurse should space out activities and provide rest periods between them. When electrolyte and fluid balance and glucose metabolism have been stabilized, the patient's energy level will increase, and more activities can be added gradually on a week-by-week basis.

Promoting nutritional balance. Patients with cortisol excess are usually overweight. The nurse should provide a diet that restricts calories but is high in protein and that meets special needs based on glucose metabolism. Because cortisol excess can increase appetite, patients need assistance in controlling calories; the approach to this is individualized (see Chapter 19 for a discussion of techniques that can be used). The patient's nutritional status should be monitored by checking weight, actual food intake, and blood glucose level. Blood glucose levels should be monitored every 4 to 8 hours until the patient is stable.

Promoting comfort. Pain occurs because of demineralization of bones and compression fractures. Measures that can be used to promote comfort include (1) providing a mattress with good support, (2) instituting back rubs to promote relaxation, and (3) using pain medications as appropriate. If these measures are unsuccessful, the nurse should consult the physician and physical therapist about other alternatives, including braces. It is important to remember that pain must be controlled so that ambulation and activity can be maintained.

Promoting positive body image. Another major focus of care is helping the patient deal with changes in body image, sexuality, and self-concept. Patients should know that some body changes are reversible with treatment, and they are helped to accentuate positive attributes. To help increase their self-concept as they recover, they are assisted in setting realistic goals within their physiologic tolerance. Clear explanations about changes in sexual characteristics and changes that will occur with treatment help patients to cope better.

Patient teaching. Education of patients and significant others is ongoing. At first the patient needs basic information regarding the care being given and any restrictions such as diet and limitation of some visitors. Many diagnostic tests may be necessary, and careful explanations are given. Over time the patient needs information about the disease process and planned treatment, long-term care needs related to the disease process, and specific care for complications such as adrenal insufficiency, which can occur with some treatments.

IATROGENIC CUSHING'S SYNDROME

Iatrogenic Cushing's syndrome occurs when large doses of exogenous glucocorticoids are taken for their therapeutic antiinflammatory effects. As described in Chap-

THERAPEUTIC USE OF GLUCOCORTICOIDS: CLINICAL SITUATIONS

1. Eye surgery or trauma: usually given as drops, ointment, or intraorbital, so systemic effects are minimal
2. Dermatologic disorders: used as ointments; can have systemic effects if used over large part of body or used daily
3. Autoimmune diseases: rheumatoid arthritis, lupus erythematosus, scleroderma
4. Hematologic disorders: hemolytic anemia, thrombocytopenia, lymphomas, leukemias
5. Allergic reactions: anaphylaxis, contact dermatitis, transfusion reactions
6. GI disorders: ulcerative colitis, Crohn's disease, hepatitis
7. Nephrologic disorders: nephrotic syndrome
8. Neurologic disorders: head trauma and surgery to prevent cerebral edema and increased intracranial pressure
9. Cardiopulmonary disorders: asthma, chronic obstructive pulmonary disease, myocarditis
10. Transplantations: renal, liver, heart, and β-cell transplantation
11. Other: glucocorticoids are part of many protocols for various malignancies

---

ter 35, the glucocorticoids have profound antiinflammatory and immunosuppressive effects. Because of these effects, glucocorticoids are frequently prescribed in therapeutic doses to suppress undesirable inflammatory reactions and immune responses. Examples of clinical situations in which glucocorticoids might be used for their antiinflammatory and immunosuppressive effects are presented in the box above.

Clinical Manifestations

Regardless of the purposes, when glucocorticoids are given for any reason other than replacement therapy, the person will receive dosages that will elevate the serum glucocorticoid level above normal. Adrenocorticosteroids used in this manner can cause problems when they are prescribed for long-term, continuous use and when they are withdrawn following long-term use. The total dosage and the duration of therapy determine the side effects. The larger the dose and the longer the time during which glucocorticoids are used, the greater are the side effects.

Long-term therapeutic doses of glucocorticoids can result in the full clinical picture of Cushing's syndrome. However, at other times the clinical picture seen with iatrogenic Cushing's syndrome can be different. Suppression of growth in children can be more severe than in endogenous Cushing's syndrome, and it is irreversible. Bone changes may be greater in iatrogenic Cushing's syndrome, and patients often develop vascular ne-

crosis. Fluid and electrolyte disturbances may not be as severe because synthetic glucocorticoids possess less mineralocorticoid activity than natural glucocorticoids. Severe myopathy can occur. Peptic ulcers occurs more often in patients who receive glucocorticoid therapy for more than 30 days.[64] Patients receiving glucocorticoid therapy are very susceptible to cataract formation, which is not seen in endogenous Cushing's syndrome. It is important to remember that patients receiving long-term glucocorticoid therapy are very susceptible to all types of infection.

When glucocorticoids are given for a prolonged period, they must be withdrawn slowly. The reason for this is that the high blood levels of exogenous glucocorticoids cause negative feedback to the hypothalamus and anterior pituitary gland, and the production of corticotropin-releasing factor (CRF) and ACTH is suppressed. The lack of ACTH results in depression of the hypothalamic-pituitary-adrenal axis and adrenal atrophy. Thus, if glucocorticoids are stopped suddenly, the patient develops signs and symptoms of adrenal insufficiency because of an inability to produce the glucocorticoids internally. It has been found that it may take as long as 9 months for return of normal hypothalamic-pituitary-adrenal function.[64] In some instances after withdrawal, the patient may be able to produce enough glucocorticoids to meet body needs in nonstressful times but may need additional glucocorticoids during increased stress.

■ Implementation

Teaching and counseling. Patients on prolonged therapeutic glucocorticoids therapy need considerable teaching to be able to manage therapy and to identify signs and symptoms of complications (see the box on p. 1073). In addition, counseling is usually needed to help the patient cope with changes in appearance and behavior.

The disturbances associated with long-term therapeutic doses of glucocorticoids cannot be completely avoided, but they often can be minimized and complications avoided. The changes in body structure may not be avoidable. Patients should be aware of these side effects and be supported in dealing with these changes. Instructions on use of clothes, makeup, and so on may be incorporated into care.

The patient and significant others must be aware of potential changes in behavior that may occur. Usually patients adjust to the therapy, but if behavior changes occur, the physician should be notified immediately. Written and verbal instructions should be given (see the research box on p. 1073).

Promoting nutrition and fluid balance. Blood glucose levels may be monitored frequently, particularly if there is a family history of diabetes mellitus. If hyperglycemia develops, dietary control is necessary to control blood

TEACHING FOR PERSONS RECEIVING LONG-TERM THERAPEUTIC DOSES OF GLUCOCORTICOIDS

1. Take drugs as prescribed.
   a. Do not miss a dose or stop medication suddenly.
   b. Drug must be withdrawn slowly under a physician's supervision.
   c. If nausea and vomiting occur and drug cannot be taken, notify physician immediately.
   d. Keep sufficient tablets on hand to avoid missing a dose.
   e. Take drug with food or antacids.
   f. With alternate-day therapy, take twice the normal dose every other day at 8 AM.
   g. If traveling, *carry* medications (do not ship them).
2. Monitor self for and report side effects of weight gain, edema, behavior changes, GI bleeding, increased urination or thirst, or signs of infection.
3. Check blood glucose level if directed.
4. Prevent infections.
   a. Avoid persons with infections, especially children.
   b. Avoid crowded, poorly ventilated places.
   c. Care for wound carefully.
   d. Report signs of infection, which may include feelings of increased weakness, feeling poorly, and having less energy.
5. Maintain a nutritious diet, including foods from all food groups (see Chapter 40); follow directions for any prescribed diet (low calorie, high potassium, low sodium).
6. Carry out a regular exercise program; walking will help to strengthen muscles and decrease bone problems.
7. Have yearly eye examinations.
8. Consult physician regularly as instructed.

RESEARCH

Streiff LD: Can clients understand our instructions, Image 18:48-52, 1986.

Written instructions are an important tool for patient education. Twenty percent of people in the United States are functionally illiterate in that they are not able to read at a fourth to fifth grade level. This study was designed to determine whether clients in an ambulatory care setting read at a level that allowed them to comprehend the written materials. Interviews and assessment of reading level, using the Wide Range Achievement Test (WRAT), was performed on 106 adults. The last grade completed in school, and thus the reported level of reading skills, for the subjects ranged from 3 to 18 grades with a mean of 9.9. The actual reading skills ranged from 1.7 to 13.5 grades with a mean of 6.8.

The readability level of 28 different patient education materials was assessed by three methods. The mean readability level calculated from the averages of the three tests for each pamphlet was 11.2 grades.

In conclusion, most of the study participants read at a level that does not allow comprehension of this material. Several recommendations were made by the researcher:

1. Clients should be tested by use of the WRAT or some other method for their reading levels.
2. Written material should be assessed for readability level and this should be published with the material.
3. Materials developed by nurses should be written at lower readability levels. ■

glucose levels. Some patients may develop insulin-dependent diabetes mellitus (see Chapter 37).

Most persons experience an increase in appetite. If weight gain is a problem, a calorie-restricted diet may be necessary. To prevent GI problems, steroids should be taken with food or antacid. Stools should be guaiac-tested regularly to monitor for early signs of GI irritations.

If fluid retention becomes a problem, the patient is placed on a sodium-restricted diet. The patient is weighed frequently, and the extremities are observed for signs of edema; changes are reported as soon as possible because diuretic therapy may be necessary. To prevent hypokalemia, the person should be on a diet high in potassium, and a potassium replacement may be prescribed unless some underlying condition results in potassium retention.

Promoting activity. The effects of glucocorticoids on muscle wasting and bone demineralization can best be minimized by promoting a regular exercise regimen incorporating weight bearing, adequate dietary protein, and ambulation.

Preventing infection. The person receiving prolonged glucocorticoid therapy must avoid anyone with an infection. Because young children frequently have upper respiratory infections, close contact with them may have to be limited. Crowded, poorly ventilated environments should also be avoided. The patient is monitored constantly for signs of infection, and the primary health caregiver should be notified immediately if any signs of infection occur.

Preventing complications. To prevent adrenal insufficiency secondary to sudden withdrawal, patients taking glucocorticoids for a prolonged time must have the steroids withdrawn gradually to allow the hypothalamic-pituitary-adrenal axis to recover. During the time the drug is being withdrawn, these patients should be monitored for signs and symptoms of adrenal insufficiency. If symptoms occur, withdrawal is slowed. To prevent sudden withdrawal in emergency situations, the patient should wear an identification bracelet or carry an identification card that states the name and dosage of the prescribed glucocorticoid. If the patient is ill or injured and requires emergency care, those treating the patient will be able to determine if more glucocorticoids are needed because of the increase in stressors; additional glucocorticoids can be given intravenously if they cannot be tolerated by mouth.

To prevent depression of the hypothalamic-pituitary-adrenal axis, some physicians prescribe every-other-day glucocorticoid therapy. In these instances, *double the patient's daily dose is given at 8 AM every other day.* The benefit of this schedule is that it allows the serum glucocorticoid level to drop low enough every other day to prevent the negative inhibition of the hypothalamus and the anterior pituitary gland. Thus every other day the person has a normal secretion of endogenous CRF and ACTH and normal stimulation of the adrenal cortex. Thus atrophy of the adrenal cortex gland does not occur. Even though the glucocorticoid level drops low enough to prevent negative feedback, the antiinflammatory effect is not reduced. Even though every-other-day therapy should prevent hypothalamic-pituitary-adrenal axis depression, the dose of glucocorticoids is still tapered when they are withdrawn.

It may take some time for the adrenal cortex to recover sufficiently to respond to additional stressors after withdrawal of therapeutic doses of glucocorticoids. Therefore patients with a recent history of glucocorticoid therapy are monitored for manifestations of adrenal insufficiency, particularly at times of stress.

Although most of the emphasis in this section has been on care of patients receiving oral therapy, the information applies equally to those receiving prolonged steroids intravenously or topically.

HYPERFUNCTION OF ADRENAL CORTEX: ALDOSTERONE EXCESS
ETIOLOGY/EPIDEMIOLOGY

Aldosterone excess, aldosteronism, can be either primary (Conn's syndrome) or secondary. Primary aldosteronism results from bilateral nodular hyperplasia or from a single aldosterone-producing adenoma. Secondary aldosteronism results from the presence of exogenous conditions that stimulate the renin-angiotensin-aldosterone system (see the box above, right.)

Primary aldosteronism is a rare disorder affecting approximately 2% of the hypertensive population. It is twice as common in women as in men and occurs most frequently in the third to fifth decades of life.

PATHOPHYSIOLOGY AND CLINICAL MANIFESTATIONS

In primary aldosteronism, excessive aldosterone is secreted and stimulates the reabsorption of sodium in the kidney in exchange for potassium and hydrogen. The increased sodium retention is accompanied by water retention and results in volume expansion and hypertension. The hypertension may result in ECG and radio-

---

EXOGENOUS CAUSES OF SECONDARY ALDOSTERONISM

Cardiac failure
Liver disease
Nephrosis
Renal artery stenosis
Bartter's syndrome (hypertrophy and hyperplasia of the juxtaglomerular cells)
Idiopathic cyclic edema
Pregnancy
Hypovolemic states
Estrogen therapy

---

logic changes of left ventricular enlargement and in retinopathy. Although the extracellular volume is expanded, edema is not usually present. Headache is a typical clinical finding.

The loss of intracellular and extracellular potassium changes the excitability of muscle membrane, resulting in muscular weakness, intermittent paresthesia, and sometimes diminished deep tendon reflexes. Paralysis can also occur. Low potassium can result in ECG changes, dysrhythmias, and hypersensitivity to digitalis preparations. Severely low levels of potassium result in loss of the concentrating ability by the kidney tubules, leading to increased water loss, polyuria, nocturia, and polydipsia. The increased loss of water by the kidney can result in hypernatremia. Excessive loss of hydrogen ions results in hypokalemic alkalosis, producing signs and symptoms of tetany.

Aldosterone secretion is high with low plasma renin activity. The aldosterone level does not decrease in response to sodium loading and does not increase in response to volume and sodium depletion or assumption of the upright position. Laboratory test results are listed in the box on p. 1075.

Secondary aldosteronism results when increased renin secretion is stimulated by the various pathologic factors. Usually the increased renin activity results from decreased perfusion pressure or decreased effective plasma volume to the kidney. The increased aldosteronism leads to hypokalemia and alkalosis. Hypertension may or may not be present, and some of the patients have edema. Sodium concentration is normal or low.

MEDICAL MANAGEMENT

The major treatment for primary aldosteronism from an adenoma is surgical resection. The electrolyte imbalance and volume excess is corrected with sodium restriction, potassium replacement, and spironolactone or amiloride before surgery. Spironolactone is prescribed in doses as high as 200 to 400 mg/day and amiloride in doses of 20 to 40 mg/day. Spironolactone is a mineralo-

LABORATORY TEST RESULTS WITH PRIMARY ALDOSTERONISM

BLOOD TESTS

Low serum potassium level (hypokalemia)
High serum sodium level (hypernatremia)
Elevated serum bicarbonate level and pH (alkalosis)
Low serum magnesium level (hypomagnesemia)
Elevated plasma aldosterone with low plasma renin levels

URINE TESTS

Low specific gravity (dilute urine)
Increased urinary protein
Increased urinary aldosterone

---

corticoid antagonist. It blocks the effect of aldosterone on the kidney tubule, and thus blocks the abnormal reabsorption of sodium and potassium excretion. Potassium is conserved with spironolactone. Amiloride also is a potassium-sparing diuretic.

For bilateral hyperplasia, medical treatment with sodium restriction, potassium replacement, and spironolactone is the treatment of choice. If the hypertension is not controlled by this treatment, traditional antihypertensive therapy is used. Some patients respond to suppression of aldosterone secretion by glucocorticoids.[65]

In secondary aldosteronism, medical treatment for the abnormal sodium and water retention is sodium restriction, potassium replacement, and diuretics. In addition, treatment is directed toward the underlying pathologic factors.

■ ASSESSMENT

Subjective Data

The following information from the nursing history is pertinent for the person with aldosterone excess.

1. History of weakness, paresthesia, palpitations
2. History of visual changes, headaches
3. History of polyuria, nocturia, increased thirst, kidney infections
4. Nutritional intake
5. History of edema, weight change
6. Knowledge of the disease, planned tests, therapy

Objective Data

The following objective data are collected.

1. Vital signs, especially blood pressure
2. Heart sounds, point of maximal impulse (PMI)
3. Weight
4. 24-hour fluid intake and output
5. Visual acuity
6. Muscle strength, deep tendon reflexes, sensory perception
7. Edema

■ DATA ANALYSIS: NURSING DIAGNOSES

Nursing diagnoses are determined from assessment of patient data. Possible nursing diagnoses for the patient with aldosterone excess (before surgery or while being treated medically only) include, but are not limited to, the following:

Diagnostic Title	Possible Etiologies
Activity intolerance	Muscle weakness and fatigue associated with electrolyte imbalance, especially hypokalemia
Fluid volume excess	Abnormal retention of sodium and water associated with increased aldosterone
Knowledge deficit: disease, diagnostic tests, treatment, side effects, expected outcomes	New disease, new treatment, never given information previously
Pain	Headache associated with hypertension

■ PLANNING: EXPECTED PATIENT OUTCOMES

Expected patient outcomes for the patient with aldosterone excess (before surgery or while being treated medically only) may include, but are not limited to, the following.

1. Tolerance to activity improves as potassium level improves.
2. Fluid balance is maintained, as evidenced by normal serum sodium levels.
3. The patient and significant others can:
   a. Describe the disease and its relationship to patient problems.
   b. Explain the purpose and procedures of diagnostic tests.
   c. Describe planned treatments and expected effects.
   d. Explain the need for long-term care.
   e. Explain when the physician or nurse should be contacted.
4. Headaches are controlled.

■ IMPLEMENTATION

Nursing interventions are directed toward monitoring for potential complications, increasing activity tolerance, promoting fluid balance, patient teaching, and promoting comfort.

Monitoring for Complications

Potential complications include hypertension, hypokalemia, tetany, and alkalosis. Until the patient's condition is stabilized, vital signs are monitored at least every 4 hours. If hypertension is present, hourly vital signs may be necessary. Any increases are reported immediately and managed as directed. Cerebral dysfunction may indicate uncontrolled hypertension. Care is designed to prevent activities that increase blood pressure, such as Valsalva maneuver, straining at stool, or heavy exertion. If antihypertensive drugs are ordered, monitoring for side effects must be included.

Assessment of serum electrolytes (especially potassium), and the presence of weakness, cardiac dysrhythmias, and Chvostek's and Trousseau's signs should be ongoing.

Complications are present preoperatively, and hypertension remains a potential complication for some time after surgery. It may take as long as 1 month for the blood pressure to return to normal. In addition, hypoaldosteronism may occur postoperatively and result in sodium loss and potassium retention. A high sodium intake prevents sodium deficit in the postoperative period.[64]

Increasing Activity Tolerance

Care is spaced to allow for rest periods. Activity is increased gradually, and as potassium is returned and maintained at a normal level, strength should increase. A high-potassium diet, potassium replacement, and spironolactone are given as prescribed.

Maintaining Fluid Balance

The fluid volume status is monitored by checking daily weights, intake and output, and serum electrolytes. A sodium-restricted diet may be necessary preoperatively and a high-sodium diet may be necessary when surgery is performed. If the patient is treated medically, a long-term sodium-restricted diet is maintained.

Patient Teaching

Ongoing teaching is necessary and includes the following:

1. Preoperative
   a. Information about diagnostic tests and proposed surgery
   b. Need for long-term care
2. Postoperative
   a. Prescribed diet—may include a high-sodium diet to be followed for several weeks or longer
   b. Monitoring for unstable blood pressure and fluid volume deficit
3. Patient treated medically
   a. Medication (diuretics)—dosage, frequency, side effects
   b. Signs and symptoms of uncontrolled disease to be reported to physician
   c. Need for continued medical follow-up care

Promoting Comfort

Headache may be eased by use of cold packs, relaxation therapy, and analgesics. Polydipsia may be controlled by making sure the patient has ready access to ice water and receives good oral hygiene.

HYPOFUNCTION OF THE ADRENAL CORTEX: CORTISOL INSUFFICIENCY

ETIOLOGY/EPIDEMIOLOGY

Inadequate secretion of cortisol may occur as a result of (1) insufficient secretion of ACTH resulting from hypothalamic pituitary disease (secondary adrenocortical insufficiency); (2) insufficient secretion of ACTH and adrenal atrophy resulting from suppression of hypothalamic-pituitary function by long-term exogenous glucocorticoids given in therapeutic doses (seen only with abrupt drug withdrawal); or (3) destruction of the adrenal cortex itself (primary adrenocortical insufficiency). Primary insufficiency, also called Addison's disease, can result from several causes (see the box below).

The most common cause of adrenocortical insufficiency is idiopathic atrophy of the adrenal gland. Infiltration of the adrenal gland with carcinoma often occurs, but usually it does not lead to insufficiency.[64] Tuberculosis as a cause of adrenocortical insufficiency has decreased since the advent of antituberculosis chemotherapy.

Idiopathic adrenocortical insufficiency probably has a genetic component because it often occurs in families and is associated with specific haplotypes. It can be part of multiple endocrine defects caused by autoimmune processes, such as those associated with thyroid and parathyroid gland dysfunction.

PATHOPHYSIOLOGY

Adrenocortical insufficiency, whether primary or secondary, is a rare problem. When it occurs, however, it is life threatening because the adrenocortical hormones are necessary for existence. The disorder can occur abruptly, as with hemorrhage and infarction, or slowly, as with idiopathic insufficiency. With slow progressive destruction, the adrenal cortex initially may be able to meet the hormonal needs of daily living, but when a stressor occurs, insufficiency becomes evident as the gland cannot meet the extra needs associated with the stress response.

Primary adrenocortical insufficiency deprives the

CAUSES OF ADDISON'S DISEASE

Idiopathic atrophy, probably caused by an autoimmune abnormality
Infection of adrenal glands
Infiltration of adrenal glands with cancer
Impairment of blood flow from vasculitis or thrombosis
Hemorrhage and infarction secondary to septicemia (Waterhouse-Friderichsen syndrome)
Destruction of adrenal glands by chemicals, such as mitotane
Congenital hypoplasia
Surgical removal of adrenal glands

body of both mineralocorticoids and glucocorticoids. These hormonal losses decrease the body's ability to retain sodium and excrete potassium. The loss of sodium decreases extracellular electrolytes and fluid volume. The decreased volume, along with decreased vascular tone, diminishes cardiac output and decreases renal perfusion. Excretion of waste products is inhibited.

The loss of glucocorticoids in primary adrenocortical insufficiency decreases hepatic gluconeogenesis and increases tissue glucose uptake. Muscle strength is lost. Various GI disorders occur, and mental and emotional functioning and stability are impaired. The loss of negative feedback of glucocorticoids on pituitary secretion of ACTH results in uncontrolled ACTH release along with β-lipotropin. The β-lipotropin is hydrolyzed to β-melanocyte-stimulating hormone (β-MSH). Thus excessive amounts of ACTH and β-MSH are present in the serum. Various changes in sexual characteristics may be result from a decrease in adrenal androgen or from the general debility associated with the insufficiency.

Secondary adrenal insufficiency results in similar pathophysiologic disturbances, except that the fluid and electrolyte imbalances are not usually as severe because the adrenal cortex can still produce mineralocorticoids (aldosterone) in response to the renin-angiotensin system. In addition, because ACTH secretion is diminished, there is no increase in serum levels of β-MSH.

CLINICAL MANIFESTATIONS

In chronic insufficiency the earliest symptoms are vague and the clinical picture is not easy to recognize. Clinical signs of acute and chronic insufficiency include the following.

Mental and Emotional Changes

Mental and emotional changes are some of the earliest symptoms and may include lethargy, loss of vigor, depression, irritability, and loss of ability to concentrate. The patient can become increasingly apathetic and not be able to participate in any ADLs.

Hypoglycemia

Hypoglycemia is seen in about 50% of the patients with adrenocortical insufficiency. Periods of fasting may exacerbate the problem.

Change in Muscle Strength

Weakness and fatigue are some of the most common findings in adrenocortical insufficiency. At first this may be episodic but can progress to general prostration. The muscle changes may be associated with muscle pain.

Gastrointestinal Disturbances

Anorexia, nausea, and vomiting are very common manifestations. Diarrhea or constipation may be present. Abdominal pain occurs frequently, and all patients experience weight loss.

Fluid and Electrolyte Disturbances

Electrolyte changes include low serum sodium and high serum potassium levels. However, the total body potassium is low because potassium moves out of the cells in response to the extracellular hypo-osmolality. Some of the potassium is lost through the GI tract and the kidney and less potassium is taken in. The low serum sodium level can result in dizziness, confusion, and neuromuscular irritability; some patients give a history of salt craving. The high serum potassium level can result in ECG changes (a peaked T wave and broadened QRS complex) (see Chapter 27) and, if very severe, cardiac standstill. Muscles become weaker and flaccid paralysis can occur.[64] Occasionally, high serum calcium levels may be present because of increased protein concentration associated with volume deficit.

Along with the sodium deficit, a fluid volume deficit also occurs. Signs of dehydration, such as poor turgor, sunken eyeballs, and dry mucous membranes, are present. Hypotension is seen initially with postural changes but eventually is present all the time. Complete vascular collapse (shock) may occur.

Hyperpigmentation

Hyperpigmentation is seen only in primary adrenocortical insufficiency when ACTH and possibly β-MSH are elevated. It appears as a bronzing seen with a normal suntan in light-skinned persons or generalized darkening in dark-skinned persons. The hyperpigmentation affects both exposed and unexposed skin areas as well as mucous membranes. It is often exaggerated over pressure areas such as knuckles, knees, elbow, and ischial tuberosities. Palmar creases, thumbnails, and the dorsum of the tongue may also show the unusual pigmentation.

Changes in Sexual Characteristics

Most females experience loss of body and axillary hair and menstrual changes. The menstrual changes may be related more to the weight loss than to changes in adrenal androgens. Males experience impotence, probably related to the generalized debility associated with the adrenocortical insufficiency.

Diagnostic Tests

Diagnostic tests that will show abnormalities include the following:

1. Low serum sodium and glucose, high serum potassium levels
2. Increased serum blood urea nitrogen (BUN) from hemoconcentration and decreased renal perfusion
3. Normal basal levels of cortisol may be noted; low

TABLE 36-10 Comparison of antiinflammatory and mineralocorticoid potency of derivatives of adrenocorticosteroids

Drug	Antiinflammatory Potency*	Mineralocorticoid Potency†
Hydrocortisone (cortisol)	Potency = 1	Potency 0.03 times that of Doca
Cortisone acetate	Potency 0.8 times that of hydrocortisone	Potency 0.03 times that of Doca
Prednisone	Potency 4 times that of hydrocortisone	Potency 0.04 times that of Doca
Methylprednisolone	Potency 6 times that of hydrocortisone	Potency 0.02 times that of Doca
Triamcinolone	Potency 5 times that of hydrocortisone	No mineralocorticoid activity
Dexamethasone	Potency 30 times that of hydrocortisone	Only mild natriuretic effect
Desoxycorticosterone (DOC)	Zero antiinflammatory effect	Potency = 1
Fludrocortisone	Potency 10 times that of hydrocortisone	Potency 4.2 times that of Doca

*Potency relative to hydrocortisone, whose potency = 1.
†Potency relative to Doca (desoxycorticosterone acetate), whose potency = 1.

to normal levels during acute illness indicate adrenocortical insufficiency

4. Response to ACTH stimulation
   a. Low or no plasma cortisol with primary insufficiency
   b. Normal response to repeated stimulation with secondary insufficiency
5. Elevated ACTH serum levels with primary insufficiency
6. Abnormal ACTH response to metyrapone or hypoglycemia with secondary insufficiency

MEDICAL MANAGEMENT

Chronic adrenal insufficiency is treated by hormone replacement. In primary insufficiency a glucocorticoid, usually cortisone or hydrocortisone, 37.5 mg daily (25 mg on awakening and 12.5 mg before 4 PM), and a *mineralocorticoid,* usually fludrocortisone (0.1 to 0.2 mg daily), are prescribed. Other forms of these drugs may be prescribed. If a different adrenocortical derivative with glucocorticoid properties, such as prednisone, is prescribed, the dosage is equivalent to the antiinflammatory potency of hydrocortisone. For example, the dosage of prednisone is approximately 10 mg/day. Table 36-10 presents a comparison of the antiinflammatory potency of the adrenocortical steroids relative to the glucocorticoid potency of hydrocortisone and the mineralocorticoid potency of desoxycorticosterone acetate (Doca). In secondary insufficiency, only glucocorticoid replacement is necessary.

The dose of glucocorticoids or mineralocorticoids is adjusted until the patient has no symptoms. The dosage of glucocorticoids is temporarily tripled or doubled in situations such as psychologic stressors, vacations, infections, trauma, or dental work. When the stressors have dissipated, the dosage is returned to normal. Some physicians have the patient keep a parenteral form of cortisol at home and instruct significant others in its administration for emergency purposes.

■ ASSESSMENT

Subjective Data

Because the clinical manifestations are subtle and affect a variety of systems, a thorough assessment is necessary. The following subjective data are important for the patient with cortisol insufficiency.

1. General: history of weakness, fatigue, muscle pain, dizziness, changes in behavior, lethargy, depression, attention or ability to do work and activities
2. Appearance: history of changes in pigmentation
3. Nutrition: history of anorexia, nausea, vomiting, salt craving, weight loss, and abdominal pain; usual 24-hour food/fluid intake
4. Elimination: history of changes in bowel habits, urinary output
5. Sexual
   a. Females: menstrual history, history of changes in body-axillary hair
   b. Males: history of impotence
6. Knowledge: disease, treatment, expectations

Objective Data

The following data are collected during physical assessment.

1. Emotional-mental status: affect, attention, activity level
2. Integumentary status: hyperpigmentation, axillary-body hair distribution, skin turgor, eyeball softness
3. Cardiovascular status: blood pressure and pulse, especially with postural changes; heart rhythm
4. Gastrointestinal status: weight, 24-hour intake and output, abdominal tenderness
5. Musculoskeletal status: muscle strength; presence of wasting; ability to do ADL, get up from sitting position, or walking

■ DATA ANALYSIS: NURSING DIAGNOSES

Nursing diagnoses are determined from assessment of patient data. Possible nursing diagnoses for the patient with cortisol insufficiency include, but are not limited to, the following:

Diagnostic Title	Possible Etiologies
Activity intolerance	Muscle weakness, postural hypotension, electrolyte imbalance
Coping, ineffective individual	Inability to mount normal response to stressors, insufficient learned coping mechanisms
Fluid volume deficit	Sodium and water loss associated with deficiency of adrenal cortex hormones
Injury, potential for	Instability associated with weakness, electrolyte imbalance
Knowledge deficit: disease, diagnostic tests, treatment, side effects, expected outcomes	New disease, new treatment, no previous exposure to information
Nutrition, altered: less than body requirements	Decreased intake associated with anorexia, nausea, vomiting
Pain	Abdominal discomfort
Self-esteem disturbance	Change in functional ability, change in body characteristics

■ PLANNING: EXPECTED PATIENT OUTCOMES

Expected patient outcomes for the person with cortisol insufficiency may include, but are not limited to, the following:

1. Activity tolerance improves as evidenced by increased activity level.
2. Coping improves as evidenced by no signs and symptoms of stress; stressors are avoided when possible.
3. Fluid intake is approximately 3000 ml/day, and signs of fluid deficit decrease.
4. The patient experiences no injuries.
5. The patient and significant others can describe:
   a. Effect of stressors on the disease and measures to be taken to reduce them
   b. Home medication program, need for continued treatment if replacement is necessary, and situations that require an increase in medication dosage
   c. Medical follow-up plan
      (1) Symptoms indicating adrenal crisis and need for medical attention
      (2) Need for continual medical follow-up
      (3) Need to carry identification card with information concerning physician and current medication
6. Nutritional status improves as evidenced by increase in weight; the patient eats and retains 100% of prescribed diet.
7. The patient states pain is controlled.

■ IMPLEMENTATION

Preventing Complications

One focus of nursing intervention is the prevention and early detection of the potential complications of addisonian crisis, electrolyte imbalances, and hypoglycemia. A sample nursing care plan is presented on pp. 1080-1081.

Addisonian crisis. Acute adrenal insufficiency or addisonian crisis is a potential complication for any patient with adrenal insufficiency. The management for this condition is described on p. 1082.

Electrolyte imbalances. Until the patient is stabilized, serum values are monitored daily or more frequently as necessary. During the early phase of illness, a neurologic assessment is made at least every 4 hours for signs of hyponatremia (dizziness, confusion, neuromuscular irritability); this assessment can be incorporated with taking vital signs. Sodium replacement is given as prescribed. In the acute phase, sodium is given as normal saline infusion. The amount is determined by vascular volume assessment.

If serum potassium levels are elevated, the patient should be placed on a cardiac monitor to check for changes in T wave or QRS complexes or for changes in rhythm. The hyperkalemia usually disappears with cortisol and fluid therapy, and the patient may actually need potassium following the acute period. Until serum potassium level returns to normal, the nurse should make sure the patient does not inadvertently receive potassium in intravenous fluids or medications. Measures to prevent infections and trauma, which can increase cell death and the liberation of potassium into the extracellular space, are incorporated into the nursing care.

Hypoglycemia. Monitoring for signs and symptoms of hypoglycemia and monitoring of blood glucose levels are done on a routine basis, such as every 4 hours. Glucose is given in intravenous fluids as prescribed and, when food is allowed, snacks may be incorporated between meals to avoid long periods of fasting. If symptoms of hypoglycemia occur, the blood glucose is checked, if possible, and treatment initiated for the hypoglycemia (see Chapter 37).

Additional Nursing Activities

Nursing care that relates to identified nursing diagnoses includes the following.
1. Promote activity tolerance.
   a. Limit activities until vascular volume is stable and blood pressure is normal.

PERSON WITH ADRENAL INSUFFICIENCY

DATA: Mr. Jones is admitted from the emergency room with complaints of feeling so tired that he is unable to get out of bed. He also complains of nausea, vomiting, and diarrhea and having no appetite. He gives a history of feeling poorly for the last 2 months with increasing fatigue. Mr. Jones thought he just could not recover from the flu that had been prevalent in the winter. He is an accountant and had been working everyday; he also believed that his work partly caused his fatigue.

Physical examination reveals the following:
- 52-year-old white male with "good tan" (NOTE: patient denies sun exposure)
- looks ill
- Skin cool, sweaty
- Complains of lightheadedness when HOB elevated
- Lungs clear
- Heart rate—sinus tachycardia; jugular vein distention—flat when HOB elevated 15 degrees
- Skin turgor poor; mucous membranes dry
- Blood pressure: lying, 90/60; sitting, 70/50
- Pulse, 110
- Respirations, 20
- Temperature, 36.5°C
- Weight, 70 kg (lost 3 kg in last month)

Laboratory results were:
- WBCs, 16,000
- Blood glucose, 60 mg/100 ml
- Sodium, 130 mEq/L
- Chloride, 86 mEq/L
- Hct, 46%
- Hgb, 15 g/100 ml
- BUN, 39 mg/100 ml
- Creatinine, 0.8 mg/100 ml

NURSING DIAGNOSIS
Activity intolerance related to postural hypotension

Expected Patient Outcome	Nursing Interventions	Rationale
Activity level increases gradually.	Provide bed rest for first 24 hr. Avoid any unnecessary activities, such as bathing for first 12 hr. Explain that when hormone level returns to normal, he will feel stronger.	Activities should only be increased when serum glucocorticoid levels return to normal.

NURSING DIAGNOSIS
Coping, ineffective individual, related to inability to mount normal response to stressors

Expected Patient Outcome	Nursing Interventions	Rationale
Stressors and signs of stress decrease.	Decrease stressors from noise, lights, and temperature changes. Explain everything to patient. Maintain consistent persons caring for patient for first 24 hr. Pad door to prevent slamming. Set temperature to comfortable level. Keep stressful news from reaching patient. If family members are comforting, have one stay with patient. Make sure family members are calm.	Because of lack of glucocorticoids, patient can not respond physiologically to any stressor; nurse should limit stressors.

CHAPTER 36 Management of Persons with Problems of the Pituitary, Thyroid, Parathyroid, and Adrenal Glands **1081**

NURSING CARE PLAN
PERSON WITH ADRENAL INSUFFICIENCY—cont'd

NURSING DIAGNOSIS
Fluid volume deficit related to inability to conserve fluid

Expected Patient Outcomes	Nursing Interventions	Rationale
Fluid intake is approximately 3000 ml/day. Signs of fluid deficit decrease.	Monitor intake and output hourly. Monitor BP and pulse hourly until normal. Weigh daily. Monitor Hct, Hgb, and BUN daily. Administer intravenous fluids (usually D_5NS) as ordered. Administer cortisol as ordered.	Surveillance will identify any problems with replacement therapy early so that solutions can be changed. Fluid volume deficit results from excessive loss of sodium and water and lack of glucocorticoids.

NURSING DIAGNOSIS
Injury, potential for, related to weakness and hypoglycemia

Expected Patient Outcomes	Nursing Interventions	Rationale
Patient experiences no injury.	Keep bed low. Keep bed rails up. Maintain quiet environment with consistent nurse for 24 hr. Monitor blood glucose q4h. Instruct patient to stay in bed.	Hypoglycemia and weakness can lead to injury; nurse should provide safe environment.

NURSING DIAGNOSIS
Knowledge deficit related to new problem with no previous exposure to information

Expected Patient Outcome	Nursing Interventions	Rationale
Patient and significant others can explain what will happen over next 24 hr.	Explain all care to patient and family so that no unexpected event occurs. Focus only on care to be given for next 24 hr. Help patient and family know that patient will be much more stable in 24 hr.	Patient can only handle minimal knowledge, so limit to what must be provided in first 24 hr; knowledge helps to decrease stress.

b. Gradually increase activity and monitor for fatigue and weakness.
c. Schedule rest periods throughout the day.
2. Facilitate coping.
  a. Provide stressor-reduced environment: quiet private room, controlled temperature; limit visitors but promote visits by persons who have a calming effect.
  b. Avoid surprises; explain everything carefully before proceeding with care.
  c. Use preventive measures for infection or trauma, such as sterile technique, coughing and deep breathing, and good skin care.
  d. Provide continuity of care.
  e. Help patient identify daily stressors and ways to avoid and cope with these stressors.
3. Promote fluid balance.
  a. Monitor for fluid deficit:
    (1) Weigh every day

    (2) Intake and output every 1 to 8 hours
    (3) Laboratory values for signs of hemoconcentration every day
    (4) Skin turgor every 4 hours
    (5) Vital signs every 1 to 4 hours
  b. Report signs of increasing fluid deficit immediately.
  c. Maintain fluid intake at several liters a day.
  d. Provide diet with "normal" sodium (approximately 4g of sodium chloride) level.
4. Prevent injury from falls.
  a. Remove unnecessary equipment from room.
  b. Assist patient with ambulation.
  c. Use side rails as necessary and keep bed low to floor.
5. Promote good nutrition.
  a. After patient is stable, provide high-calorie diet incorporating foods from all food groups.
  b. Provide good oral hygiene before meals.

INSTRUCTIONS FOR PATIENTS ON REPLACEMENT DOSES OF GLUCOCORTICOIDS AND MINERALOCORTICOIDS

1. Follow medication regimen.
   a. Take drugs with meals or snacks.
   b. Glucocorticoids: take ⅔ of dose at approximately 8 AM and ⅓ of dose at approximately 4 PM.
   c. Mineralocorticoids: take medication in the morning.
   d. Do not omit a drug dose.
   e. Keep sufficient medication on hand.
   f. If unable to retain oral form of drug, take parenteral form as instructed.
   g. Carry drugs when traveling; do not ship drugs with luggage; make sure traveling companion knows how to give the injectable form of glucocorticoid.
2. Wear a Medic Alert bracelet or necklace that lists condition, drugs and dosage, and name and phone number of physician.
3. Monitor self for presence of increased stressors (fever, infections, dental work, accidents, family or personal crises) and increase dose of glucocorticoids as instructed or consult physician (normal dose covers only daily needs; does not provide for additional stressors).
4. Monitor self daily for signs and symptoms of insufficient drug therapy (anorexia, nausea, vomiting, weakness, depression, dizziness, polyuria, weight loss) and report immediately (larger drug dose may be necessary).
5. Monitor self daily for signs and symptoms of excessive drug therapy (rapid weight gain, round face, edema, hypertension) and report immediately (smaller drug dose may be necessary).
6. Eat a well-balanced diet, choosing foods from all food groups.
7. Maintain a regular schedule with adequate sleep, regular meals, and regular exercise (irregular health habits increase glucocorticoid needs).
8. Eliminate as many work and home confrontations as possible to decrease stress response that increases glucocorticoid needs.
9. See physician as instructed; consult as necessary if questions arise concerning therapy.

---

   c. Provide an environment conducive to eating (see Chapter 42).
6. Promote comfort: back rubs and relaxation techniques; promote stress reduction.
7. Improve self-esteem.
   a. Help patient and significant others understand relationship between changes in self and the disease process; explain that physical changes are reversible.
   b. Help patient set short-term realistic goals.
   c. Compliment patient on accomplishments.
   d. Involve patient in decision making, even if patient is unable to perform physical activities.

Patient Teaching

The initial teaching during the acute phase relates to proposed diagnostic tests and immediate interventions. After the patient is stable, information is given about the disease and long-term needs. Instructions about replacement therapy are similar to those given to patients taking therapeutic doses of glucocorticoids, but some important differences exist (see the box above).

ADDISONIAN CRISIS (ADRENAL CRISIS)
Etiology

Addisonian crisis is a severe exacerbation of adrenal insufficiency. It may occur in any person with chronic insufficiency regardless of the cause. It is usually seen in an undiagnosed person who undergoes a major stressor, in a person who has abrupt withdrawal of therapeutic glucocorticoids, or in a person who has been poorly controlled and enters a stressful situation. It may also be precipitated in a previously well person by adrenal hemorrhage associated with septicemia or anticoagulants.

Clinical Manifestations

The signs and symptoms of addisonian crisis are acute exaggerations of the manifestations seen with chronic adrenal insufficiency (see p. 1077) and may include severe hypotension, shock, coma, and vasomotor collapse.

Interventions

Medical management. When addisonian crisis occurs, the first line of therapy is replacement of glucocorticoids and fluids. A large dose of hydrocortisone hemisuccinate is given intravenously immediately and repeated as necessary. A continuous rapid infusion of normal saline is started, and 5% dextrose is usually added to the first liter to correct hypoglycemia. Soluble cortisol preparations may be added to the fluids. The first liter of solution may be given in as little as 30 minutes.[64] Hemodynamic monitoring, such as central venous pressure and arterial pressures, may be used to help decide the exact amount of fluids needed. The fluid deficit is usually corrected in 4 to 6 hours.

The large doses of glucocorticoids given initially provide sufficient mineralocorticoid activity; thus additional mineralocorticoids are not needed. If the vascular status does not improve with the glucocorticoid and fluid therapy, a sympathomimetic drug may be given. Treatment measures directed toward the precipitating cause, such as infection or trauma, are also included.

Nursing management. Nursing care is directed toward assisting with implementation of medical therapy, monitoring for effectiveness of therapy, monitoring for side effects of therapy (such as fluid overload), and preventing or detecting complications that may result from the patient's changed mental status (particularly respiratory depression). Monitoring for fluid status may include vital signs taken as often as every 15 minutes, hourly intake and output, and daily weights. Temperature is monitored hourly because hyperpyrexia is often present.

A second major focus of care is avoiding additional stressors. These patients should do absolutely nothing for themselves and should be protected from all stimuli and from exposure to infection. To decrease stressors, the same nurse should provide care for the first several hours, during which time the patient becomes stabilized. One-to-one care may be necessary. To prevent aspiration, the patient is given nothing by mouth until nausea and vomiting are relieved and until mental status is normal. After several hours, oral liquids may be given, and oral glucocorticoids may be started within 48 hours. The patient may experience a severe headache that may be relieved by an ice bag. After the patient's condition is stable, medical and nursing care as described for the patient with adrenal insufficiency will be required.

HYPERSECRETION OF THE ADRENAL MEDULLA: PHEOCHROMOCYTOMA
ETIOLOGY/EPIDEMIOLOGY

Pheochromocytoma is a catecholamine-producing tumor of the sympatheticoadrenal medullary system that causes hypertension. Although pheochromocytomas account for less than 1% of the cases of hypertension, it is important that they be diagnosed because these persons can be cured.

A single benign adrenal medulla tumor is the most common pathologic finding. They occur most frequently between the fourth and fifth decades of life and are slightly more common in females. The tumors are most frequently found in the abdomen around or in the adrenal medulla, but they can be found anywhere along the sympathetic nervous system trunk. The tendency to develop pheochromocytomas may be inherited and may be part of the MEN syndromes. Pheochromocytomas may be found in MEN 2a in association with hyperparathyroidism and medullary thyroid carcinoma or in MEN 2b in association with medullary thyroid carcinoma and multiple mucosal neuromas.

PATHOPHYSIOLOGY

Pheochromocytomas of the adrenal medulla release excessive amounts of catecholamines, both epinephrine and norepinephrine. A tumor of the sympathetic nervous system trunk releases excessive amounts of norepinephrine. The hormone release may be constant or episodic, producing constant or episodic clinical manifestations.

A paroxysm or crisis may be precipitated by any lifting, straining, bending, or exercise that increases intraabdominal pressure or moves abdominal contents. Palpation of the abdomen may also precipitate a paroxysm. Anxiety or stress does not usually precipitate an attack.[64] In some patients no precipitating factors can be identified. The frequency of paroxysms varies but usually increases as the disease progresses.

Release of norepinephrine causes an exaggeration of its effects on α-receptors, producing massive vasoconstriction. Release of epinephrine causes an exaggeration of its effects on β-receptors, producing cardiac stimulating effects and alterations in metabolism.

CLINICAL MANIFESTATIONS

The most common manifestation of pheochromocytoma is hypertension that is usually sustained. Blood pressure is usually very labile with superimposed paroxysms.[64] Occasionally patients show true paroxysms with elevation of blood pressure only present intermittently. The hypertension is resistant to treatment by traditional antihypertensive drugs. Along with the hypertension, orthostatic hypotension is frequently present, resulting from a decrease in plasma volume and loss of tone of postural reflexes.[12]

Other manifestations frequently present include the following.

1. Signs of cardiac stimulation: tachycardia, palpitation, chest pain, ECG changes, angina
2. Headaches that are throbbing, abrupt, and severe
3. Increased metabolic rate manifested by heat intolerance, sweating, fever, wasting of fat stores, and weight loss
4. Elevated blood glucose level
5. Nausea, vomiting, and epigastric pain
6. Tremors, weakness, and nervousness or anxiety
7. Flushing
8. Tachypnea

The diagnosis is confirmed by assays of catecholamines and their metabolites in urine (see Chapter 35). Only very occasionally are pharmacologic tests used; these tests either demonstrate the dependence of the hypertension on catecholamines by evaluating response to an α-receptor antagonist or provoke a paroxysm. Both types of tests are very hazardous. CT scans, arteriography, and venography, used to localize the tumor, are abnormal.

INTERVENTIONS
Medical Management

Before surgery, treatment consists in controlling hypertension and symptoms of cardiac stimulation. An α-adrenergic blocker such as phenoxybenzamine (usual dose, 10 to 20 mg every 6 to 8 hours) or prazosin (usual dose, 2 to 5 mg twice a day) is given to help control blood pressure and paroxysms and to increase blood volume. This therapy is started 1 to 2 weeks before surgery. Phentolamine may also be given if hypertension crisis occurs. A liberal salt diet is prescribed to restore blood volume. If necessary, saline and blood products are given 12 to 24 hours before surgery.

Tachycardia, dysrhythmias, sweating, and angina are controlled with a β-blocker such as propranolol. This is started only after α-adrenergic blockade is established.

Surgical resection of the tumor is the treatment of choice. Postoperative management is directed toward maintaining a normal blood pressure. Immediately after surgery the patient may be hypertensive; this hypertension is first managed with diuretics and then with phentolamine if necessary. Later the patient may need fluid replacement for hypotension.

Some tumors are not resectable because of disseminated malignancy or other illnesses. Pheochromocytomas do not respond to radiotherapy or chemotherapy. The tumors are slow growing, and morbidity results from excessive catecholamine secretion. The disease is controlled with α- and β-adrenergic blocking agents and α-methyl-para-tyrosine, which reduces the production of catecholamines.

Nursing Management

Preoperative management. Preoperatively, nursing care is directed toward instituting measures to help stabilize the patient's hemodynamic status, monitoring the clinical state, preparing the patient for tests and surgery, and preventing paroxysms. Patients experiencing hypertensive crisis should be in an intensive care unit because cardiac, blood pressure, and neurologic monitoring is required as frequently as every 15 to 60 minutes. If phentolamine infusion is necessary, the blood pressure is checked every 15 minutes, and the drug is given by controlled infusion at a rate to keep the blood pressure at a prescribed level. During this time the patient must be informed about planned diagnostic tests and planned treatment and is prepared for surgery. Activities that precipitate paroxysms, such as bending, Valsalva maneuver, and lifting, should be limited.

Postoperative management. The patient continues to need close monitoring of blood pressure, pulse, cardiac rhythm, neurologic status, and the effectiveness of treatment. Following the hypertensive period, hypotension may occur; thus nursing care is directed toward continual monitoring and administration of fluids or plasma expanders as prescribed.

Surgery results in complete remission of symptoms in 75% of patients;[12] therefore discharge teaching for most patients is directed toward helping the patient plan for resumption of normal activities, maintenance of an adequate diet, and follow-up care. For those who did not

have complete remission, discharge teaching is directed toward helping the patient arrange antihypertensive therapy.

Care of the nonsurgical patient. For patients treated medically, nursing care is directed toward helping the patient attain skills necessary for self-care. Patient teaching includes the following:

1. Knowledge about the disease and its relationship to the signs and symptoms
2. Medication regimen—purpose, dosage, expected effects, side effects
3. Blood pressure self-measurement
4. Methods to prevent paroxysms—preventing constipation, avoiding Valsalva maneuver, avoiding bending or flexion of the body
5. Importance of follow-up care

SURGERY OF THE ADRENAL GLAND

Adrenalectomy, either unilateral or bilateral, may be done for a variety of reasons (see the box below).

PREOPERATIVE CARE

The patient who has dysfunction of the adrenal glands is very fragile before surgery. Medical treatment will be used to stabilize the patient hormonally before surgery. The patient's nutritional status should be stabilized by a high-protein, high-calorie diet with adequate minerals and vitamins. Electrolyte imbalances (sodium, potassium, acid-base) are corrected. On the night before surgery, the morning of surgery, and during surgery, the patient is given a soluble preparation of cortisol. If hypotension occurs during surgery, additional cortisol and fluids are given as needed. Care is the same regardless of whether a unilateral or a bilateral procedure is performed.

POSTOPERATIVE CARE

The patient having an adrenalectomy is usually sent to the intensive care unit postoperatively because of the

---

DISORDERS THAT RESPOND TO ADRENALECTOMY

UNILATERAL

Single adenomas or carcinomas of adrenal cortex
Single tumors of adrenal medulla

BILATERAL

Bilateral adrenal hyperplasia if other forms of therapy are ineffective
Bilateral adrenal cortex adenomas or carcinoma
Bilateral adrenal medulla tumors
Removal of source of excessive cortisol secretion in response to ectopic ACTH secretions if ectopic site not controllable and Cushing's syndrome is severe

---

high risk of addisonian crisis and the careful monitoring needed to maintain fluid and electrolyte balance. Immediately after a bilateral adrenalectomy, the patient is depleted of both glucocorticoids and mineralocorticoids, and the patient who is not managed correctly will develop adrenal crisis (see p. 1082). Hemodynamic monitoring (central venous pressure, blood pressure, pulse, and at times pulmonary wedge pressure) is done continuously. In addition, daily serum electrolytes, blood glucose levels every 4 hours, daily weights, and hourly intake and output are monitored.

Intravenous cortisol replacement is continued for at least the first 24 hours postoperatively and usually for 48 hours. Fluids are given based on the clinical data and usually include saline/dextrose solutions. On the second day postoperatively, mineralocorticoids may be started. By the third day, the patient is usually able to tolerate oral glucocorticoids and a normal diet. If unusual weakness or anorexia, nausea, or vomiting occur, glucocorticoids are increased. If unusual hypotension occurs, mineralocorticoids and fluids are adjusted appropriately.

A major complication of surgery is poor wound healing and infection. Strict aseptic technique is used with wound care. Splinting the incision during coughing or turning prevents stress on the suture line and promotes comfort. Other postoperative needs are similar to those described for the patient with adrenal insufficiency (see

pp. 1079-1082). Replacement therapy is necessary throughout life.

For the patient who has had a unilateral adrenalectomy, monitoring, hormonal support, fluid therapy, and other care needs are the same during the immediate postoperative period as for the patient with a bilateral adrenalectomy. After the patient is stabilized and has successfully passed any physiologic and psychologic crises, the glucocorticoid support is slowly withdrawn because eventually a single gland can maintain enough hormonal secretion for both daily living and additional stressors. When glucocorticoids are withdrawn, monitoring for signs and symptoms of adrenal insufficiency and crisis must be continued because the remaining gland may have atrophied and may not have fully recovered. If signs and symptoms occur, glucocorticoids are restarted and then again slowly withdrawn.

It is important to remember that a patient who has chronic adrenal insufficiency and who requires surgery for an unrelated adrenal problem requires the preoperative and postoperative care just described.

See the box below for a summary of preoperative and postoperative care.

CHAPTER SUMMARY

✔ Various pathologic processes, including tumor growth, hyperplasia, atrophy, autoimmune processes, infections, and ischemic changes, can affect

---

NURSING CARE OF THE PATIENT UNDERGOING ADRENAL SURGERY

PREOPERATIVE

1. Provide supportive care.
2. Assist patient with usual preoperative care.
3. Maintain nutritional status with a high-protein, prescribed calorie diet with adequate minerals and vitamins.
4. Assist with correction of fluid and electrolyte imbalance.
5. Assist with hormonal therapy as prescribed.
6. Assist with measures used to prevent or treat crises of adrenal hormonal excess or deficit.
7. Administer prescribed intravenous fluids and glucocorticoids before surgery.

POSTOPERATIVE

1. Establish monitoring schedule to detect complications of surgery and:
   a. Adrenal crisis
   b. Blood pressure alterations
   c. Blood glucose alterations
   d. Fluid and electrolyte imbalances
2. Because the patient may have unusual activity intolerance, pace postoperative activities with alternate periods of rest and a gradual increase in self-care.

3. Provide measures to minimize effects of postural hypotension:
   a. Supply Ace bandages or elastic stockings.
   b. Assess effects of posture on blood pressure.
   c. Assist or accompany the patient during ambulation while blood pressure remains labile.
4. Provide measures to decrease risk of infection in the immunosuppressed patient (for instance, strict surgical asepsis, coughing and deep breathing, avoiding contact with persons with upper respiratory infections).
5. Administer cortisol replacement as typically prescribed:
   a. Intravenous route for the first 24 to 48 hours
   b. Oral route when patient is able to tolerate food by mouth
6. Administer mineralocorticosteroid (fludrocortisone) replacement, if prescribed; typically prescribed when cortisol replacement is less than 40 to 50 mg/24 hours in the patient with bilateral adrenalectomy.
7. Assist patient and family in learning about required hormonal replacement:
   a. Bilateral adrenalectomy—maintenance dose of cortisol and mineralocorticoids
   b. Unilateral adrenalectomy—doses of cortisol dependent on degree of suppression of hypothalamic-pituitary-adrenal axis

the endocrine glands. The pathophysiologic alteration that occurs in the endocrine glands can be classified as hypoactivity and hyposecretion or hyperactivity and hypersection.

✔ Endocrine dysfunction can also result from resistance to the action of hormone at the level of the target cell; this type of problem mimics those seen with hyposecretion of hormone.

✔ Cancer tumors of the endocrine glands can be made up of
  a. secreting cells that result in hypersecretion or
  b. nonsecreting cells that do not change hormone level or cause hyposecretion by depressing the function of normal tissue.

✔ Hypersecretion of the anterior pituitary gland is usually of one hormone: prolactin resulting in amemorrhea and galactorrhea or growth hormone resulting in gigantism in children and acromegaly in adults.

✔ Hypersecretion of the anterior pituitary gland is usually caused by an adenoma; these adenomas can cause neurologic problems, vision changes, headache, and changes in mentation by their compression on normal neural tissue.

✔ Prolactin-secreting tumors are controlled by drug therapy; growth hormone–secreting tumors are resected.

✔ Surgical removal of the pituitary tumor does not usually disrupt normal pituitary action.

✔ Nursing care for the patient with a pituitary adenoma consists of (1) helping the patient deal with the irreversible changes (growth changes, bone changes in acromegaly, possibly visual changes); (2) helping the patient achieve a stable metabolic status before surgery; (3) preparing the patient for surgery; (4) caring for the patient after surgery, with a particular focus on monitoring fluid and electrolytes status, monitoring for signs of hormonal deficit (ADH, adrenocortical hormones), preventing increases in intracranial pressure and stress on suture line, and preventing infection; and (7) preparing for home care.

✔ Syndrome of inappropriate antidiuretic hormone (SIADH) results from hypersecretion of the posterior pituitary gland.

✔ SIADH causes abnormal water reabsorption, as well as hyponatremia and hypo-osmolality, which cause fluid movement from the extracellular to the intracellular compartment and change electrical activity of nerves, potentially resulting in seizures.

✔ Nursing care in SIADH is focused on increasing osmolality and sodium by water restriction, monitoring for and reporting critical changes (sodium <120 mEq/L, neurologic changes), maintaining a safe environment, and patient education.

✔ Hyposecretion of the anterior pituitary gland can be of one hormone or all anterior pituitary hormones and ADH (panhypopituitarism).

✔ Hyposecretion of gonadotropins results in reproductive problems; hyposecretion of prolactin results in problems in lactation in postpartum patients; hyposecretion of TSH results in hypothyroidism; and hyposecretion of ACTH results in adrenocortical insufficiency.

✔ Diabetes insipidus, a deficiency of ADH, results from posterior pituitary gland insufficiency.

✔ Although diabetes insipidus can cause volume deficit and hypernatremia, it usually does not because the thirst precipitated will cause increased fluid intake.

✔ Vasopressin in a nasal spray is used to treat permanent diabetes insipidus.

✔ Hypersecretion of thyroid hormone most frequently results from Graves' disease, which is caused by an autoimmune process.

✔ Graves' disease can include hyperthyroidism, goiter, pretibial myxedema, and ophthalmopathy.

✔ Hyperthyroidism results in increased activity of the neurologic system, increased GI motility, increased metabolism, heat production and calorigenesis, increased cardiac activity, increased respiratory activity, and muscle wasting. Many of these changes result from hyperactivity of the sympathetic nervous system.

✔ Thyroid crisis results from worsening hyperthyroidism when critical increases occur in metabolism, calorigenesis, and sympathetic stimulation.

✔ Hyperthyroidism is treated with antithyroid drugs, radiation therapy, or surgical resection. Use of radioactive iodine after stabilizing the patient is the treatment of choice.

✔ The major nursing needs of the patient with hyperthyroidism include potential decrease in cardiac output, hyperthermia, activity intolerance, ineffective coping, home maintenance problems, nutritional problems, sleep pattern disturbances, and visual deficits.

✔ Except for surgery, treatment of hyperthyroidism does not result in immediate improvement; that is, the return to a euthyroid state may not be observed for 6 to 8 weeks.

✔ Hypothyroidism is seen most frequently in older women; has a slow, insidious onset; and causes neurologic, respiratory, cardiovascular, GI, and metabolic dysfunction.

- Untreated hypothyroidism in neonates can result in severe mental and physical retardation.

- Hypothyroidism requires lifelong hormonal replacement.

- Nursing interventions for patients with hypothyroidism need to address activity intolerance, body image disturbances, constipation, hypothermia, pain, self-care deficits, sexual dysfunction, impaired skin integrity, altered mental status, and knowledge deficits.

- The problems of patients with hypothyroidism vary from minimal dysfunction to severe dysfunction, in which the patient requires complete care, is unresponsive, and may have respiratory failure and diminished cardiac reserve.

- Myxedema coma is the diagnostic title given the condition in which the patient has critically depressed physiologic function resulting from hypothyroidism.

- Various processes, including infection and an autoimmune process, can result in an inflammatory process of the thyroid; this process can be acute, subacute, or chronic.

- Hashimoto's thyroiditis is the most frequently occurring form of thyroiditis. It is an autoimmune disease and has exacerbations and remissions.

- With Hashimoto's thyroiditis the thyroid is enlarged, smooth, and painless. With disease progression, the thyroid is eventually destroyed and hypothyroidism occurs. During acute exacerbations, before the gland is destroyed, the patient can experience episodes of hyperthyroidism.

- Cancer of the thyroid is more rare than other forms of cancer. It can be classified into one of five types: papillary, follicular, anaplastic, medullary, or thyroid lymphoma.

- The prognosis in thyroid cancer varies from very good for patients with papillary and follicular cancer to very poor (less than 6-month survival from diagnosis) for those with anaplastic tumors.

- Most cancers of the thyroid are treated with total thyroidectomy. Thus, following surgery, the patient requires hormonal replacement therapy.

- Nursing interventions for patients with thyroid cancer focus on preparing them for diagnostic tests, preparing them for surgery, helping them to cope with the diagnosis, and caring for them postoperatively.

- The major nursing needs following thyroid surgery relate to monitoring for respiratory distress or any of its etiologic factors: internal hemorrhage, which can cause compression on the trachea; laryngeal damage to the vocal cords and obstruction of the airway; or

- tetany, which can cause laryngeal spasms. Any signs of respiratory distress or its causes need to be reported immediately.

- The tetany results from damage to the parathyroid glands during thyroid surgery. The nurse should have an intravenous preparation of calcium available as well as a tracheostomy tray.

- A goiter is an enlargement of the thyroid gland. It can result from iodine deficiency, exposure to goitrogens, hypothyroidism, or hyperthyroidism.

- Hyperparathyroidism can be primary, secondary, or tertiary. Primary hyperparathyroidism results from adenomas and hyperplasia; secondary from chronic hypocalcemia, which causes chronic stimulation of the parathyroid gland; and tertiary from the development of an autonomous parathyroid gland chronically stimulated by a hypocalcemic state.

- In primary hyperparathyroidism, continual bone resorption and changes in renal and GI processing of calcium occur. The results are hypercalcemia and changes in neurologic, GI, and cardiac functioning. Renal stones can occur; bone density decreases.

- Secondary hyperparathyroidism is a compensatory process that maintains the plasma level of calcium at the expense of bones; chronic renal failure is a major cause.

- Hypercalcemia is treated before parathyroid surgery by hydration with normal saline and diuretics such as furosemide or ethacrynic acid; thiazide diuretics are not used because they inhibit calcium excretion.

- Primary hyperparathyroidism is treated by surgery; three to three and one-half glands are removed.

- The major complications following parathyroid surgery are hypocalcemia and laryngeal spasms from tetany and respiratory obstruction from compression of the trachea by hemorrhage or from laryngeal nerve damage.

- The calcium level declines within 24 hours after parathyroid surgery, and hypocalcemia may occur.

- Hypoparathyroidism can result from trauma or surgery or be idiopathic.

- Hypoparathyroidism results in hypocalcemia, which leads to cardiac and neurologic problems; the latter result from increased excitability of neurons.

- The treatment for hypoparathyroidism is vitamin D and calcium replacement.

- The adrenal cortex secretes glucocorticoids and mineralocorticoids that are essential for life and adrenal androgens.

- Glucocorticoid excess (Cushing's syndrome) can result from excessive production of ACTH by the pituitary gland, excessive production of ACTH by ectopic tumors, excessive production of glucocorticoids by the adrenal glands, or intake of large doses of exogenous steroids.

✔ Glucocorticoid excess results in increased protein breakdown and muscle wasting, abnormal metabolism of fats with changes in fat stores and increased serum lipid levels, and increased glucose production. Abnormal retention of sodium and water with increased excretion of potassium and hydrogen ions also occurs. Bone demineralization results. Suppression of the immune system and the inflammatory response is a major result of glucocorticoid excess.

✔ Patients with glucocorticoid excess have fluid volume excess, hypernatremia, hypocalcemia, alkalosis, infections, muscle wasting, osteoporosis, hyperglycemia, peptic ulcers, mental changes, body changes (thin extremities, truncal obesity, moon face, kyphosis), poor wound healing, and bruising.

✔ Nursing care for patients with Cushing's syndrome focuses on the nursing diagnoses of activity intolerance, disturbances in body image, ineffective coping, fluid volume excess, potential for infection and injury, nutrition excess, pain, and knowledge deficit.

✔ The most frequent cause of Cushing's syndrome is iatrogenic, and the treatment focuses on dealing with the signs and symptoms of glucocorticoid excess.

✔ When patients have been taking long-term steroids, drug therapy must be tapered as it is discontinued.

✔ Aldosterone excess results in sodium and water excess, volume expansion, hypokalemia, and hypertension.

✔ Treatment for aldosterone excess is designed to lower blood pressure using sodium restriction and spironolactone or amiloride diuretics or surgery.

✔ Adrenocortical insufficiency is a medical emergency because the person is not able to mount a compensatory response to a major stressor. When glucocorticoids are deficient and a stressor is present, the person is unable to retain needed water and sodium, maintain blood pressure, and produce energy substrates (glucose, fatty acids).

✔ Untreated glucocorticoid deficiency results in shock.

✔ Patients deficient in glucocorticoids require lifetime replacement therapy. They must know what to monitor to identify signs of a deficit or an excess, must know when to take additional hormones, and must wear or carry appropriate identification.

✔ Hyperpigmentation occurs in patients with Cush-

ing's syndrome resulting from increased ACTH and primary adrenocortical insufficiency, which is associated with increased ACTH.

✔ Tumors of the adrenal medulla cause excessive production of catecholamines and are called pheochromocytomas.

✔ Hypertension, constant or paroxysmal, is the major sign of pheochromocytoma.

✔ Activities such as increased abdominal pressure, Valsalva manuver, straining, and bending over can increase release of catecholamines and worsen hypertension in pheochromocytoma.

✔ Before surgery for pheochromocytoma, blood pressure is lowered using α-adrenergic blockers.

✔ Surgery is the treatment of choice for patients with pheochromocytoma. If bilateral tumors are present, after surgery the patient will be deficient in glucocorticoids and will need lifelong replacement therapy.

QUESTIONS TO CONSIDER

- Which endocrine gland dysfunction causes each of the following?
  1. Major problems in fluid status
  2. Major alterations in energy production and use
  3. Major alterations in mineral/electrolyte balance

- What are some techniques that can be used to help patients in complying with dietary restrictions that are a common part of the therapeutic regimen for many endocrine problems?

- What instructions should be given a person taking long-term glucocorticoids for their antiinflammatory effect?

- What are several techniques that can be used to help patients remember to take drugs on a regular schedule?

- What are 10 self-care activities that persons with immune suppression resulting from elevated glucocorticoid levels should learn and implement? Give a rationale for each activity.

- Differentiate the effects of elevated and depressed calcium levels on the neurologic system, cardiac system, and renal system.

- Contrast the abnormalities in the cardiac system caused by hypothyroidism and hyperthyroidism.

REFERENCES AND SELECTED READINGS

1. Barkan A: Acromegaly and giantism. In the Endocrine Society: 41st Post Graduate Annual Assembly syllabus, Bethesda, Md, 1989, The Society.
2. Barkan AL et al: Treatment of acromegaly with the long-acting somatostatin analogue SMS 201-995, J Clin Endocrinol Metab 66:16-23, 1988.
3. Barkan A et al: Preoperative treatment of acromegaly with long-acting somatostatin analog SMS 201-995: shrinkage of invasive pituitary macroadenomas and improved surgical cure rate, J Clin Endocrinol Metab 67:1040-1048, 1988.
4. Baumann G: Acromegaly, Endocrinol Metab Clin 16:685-703, 1987.
5. Baylin S: Familial and sporadic carcinoma of the thyroid. In the Endocrine Society: 41st Post Graduate Annual Assembly syllabus, Bethesda, Md, 1989, The Society.
6. Bilezikian JP: Therapy of hypercalcemia. In the Endocrine Society: 41st Post Graduate Annual Assemby syllabus, Bethesda, Md, 1989, The Society.
7. Braverman L: Use and abuse of iodides and thyroid hormones. In the Endocrine Society: 41st Post Graduate Annual Assembly syllabus, Bethesda, Md, 1989, The Society.
8. Brennan M: Adrenocortical carcinoma, CA 37:348-365, 1987.
9. Brunt LM and Wells SA: Advances in the diagnoses and treatment of medullary thyroid carcinoma, Surg Clin North Am 67:263-279, 1987.
10. *Cagno J: Diabetes insipidus, Crit Care Nurse 9(6):86-93, 1989.
11. Cannoni M et al: Hypoparathyroidism, Acta Otorhinolaryngol Belg 41:926-943, 1987.
12. Chernow B et al: Critical care endocrinology. In Shoemaker WC et al, editors: Textbook of critical care, ed 2, Philadelphia, 1989, WB Saunders Co.
13. Civetta JM, Taylor RW, and Kirby RR, editors: Critical care, Philadelphia, 1988, JB Lippincott Co.
14. Cooper DS: Antithyroid drugs. In the Endocrine Society: 41st Post Graduate Annual Assembly syllabus, Bethesda, Md, 1989, The Society.
15. Cryer P: Pheochromocytoma and adrenergic dysfunction. In the Endocrine Society: 41st Post Graduate Annual Assembly syllabus, Bethesda, Md, 1989, The Society.
16. DeGroot LJ: Complications of Graves' disease. In the Endocrine Society: 41st Post Graduate Annual Assembly syllabus, Bethesda, Md, 1989, The Society.
17. DeGroot LJ: Unusual forms of thyrotoxicosis. In the Endocrine Society: 41st Post Graduate Annual Assembly syllabus, Bethesda, Md, 1989, The Society.
18. Fujimoto Y and Obara T: How to recognize and treat parathyroid carcinoma, Surg Clin North Am 67:343-357, 1987.
19. *German K: Fluid and electrolyte problems associated with diabetes insipidus and syndrome of inappropriate antidiuretic hormone, Nurs Clin North Am 22:785-796, 1987.
20. *Gorman CA: Thyroid orbitopathy: the gravest problem in Graves' disease. In the Endocrine Society: 41st Post Graduate Annual Assembly syllabus, Bethesda, Md, 1989, The Society.
21. Grumbach MM: Evaluation of treatment of the child with short stature. In the Endocrine Society: 41st Post Graduate Annual Assembly syllabus, Bethesda, Md, 1989, The Society.
22. Gryfinski J: Amenorrhea galactorrhea syndrome in the prolactin secreting pituitary tumor: nursing implications, J Neurosurg Nurs 17:301-308, 1985.

23. Guerrier B: Cancer of the thyroid body: indications for surgery, Acta Otorhinolaryngol Belg 41:765-781, 1987.
24. Halberg FE and Sheline GE: Radiotherapy of pituitary tumors, Endocrinol Metab Clin 16:667-684, 1987.
25. Harada T et al: Current treatment of Graves' disease, Surgical Clin North Am 67:299-314, 1987.
25a. Hyman RB et al: The effects of relaxation training on clinical symptoms: A meta-analysis, Nurs Res 38:216-220, 1989.
26. Jagger P: Addison's disease, polyglandular deficiency syndrome. In the Endocrine Society: 41st Post Graduate Annual Assembly syllabus, Bethesda, Md, 1989, The Society.
27. Kruger LB: Complications of transsphenoidal surgery, J Neurosurg Nurs 17(3):179-183, 1985.
28. Laws ER: Pituitary surgery, Endocrinol Metab Clin 16:647-665, 1987.
29. Lennquist S: The thyroid nodule: diagnoses and surgical treatment, Surg Clin North Am 67:213-232, 1987.
30. *Lockhart J: Action stat, Nursing'88 18:33, 1988.
31. Loriauy DL: Cushing's syndrome. In the Endocrine Society: 41st Post Graduate Annual Assembly syllabus, Bethesda, Md, 1989, The Society.
32. Marx SJ: Familial multiple endocrine neoplasia type 1. In the Endocrine Society: 41st Post Graduate Annual Assembly syllabus, Bethesda, Md, 1989, The Society.
33. *Mathewson MK: Thyroid disorder, Crit Care Nurse 7(1):74-85, 1984.
34. Mazzaferri E et al: Solitary thyroid nodule: diagnoses and management, Med Clin North Am 72:1177-1211, 1988.
35. McCance K and Huether SE: Pathophysiology: the biologic basis for disease in adults and children, St Louis, 1990, The CV Mosby Co.
36. McKenzie JM: Thyroid autoimmunity—etiologies, pathogenesis and management. In the Endocrine Society: 41st Post Graduate Annual Assembly syllabus, Bethesda, Md, 1989, The Society.
37. Melen O: Neuro-ophthalmologic features of pituitary tumors, Endocrinol Metab Clin 16:585-608, 1987.
38. Melmed S: Acromegaly, New Eng J Med 322:966-975, 1990.
39. Miyagawa K et al: Multiple endocrine neoplasia type I with Cushing's disease, primary hyperparathyroidism, and insulin—glucagonoma, Cancer 61:1232-1236, 1988.
40. Molitch M: Lactation and prolactinomas. In the Endocrine Society: 41st Post Graduate Annual Assembly syllabus, Bethesda, Md, 1989, The Society.
41. Molitch ME: Pathogenesis of pituitary tumors, Endocrinol Metab Clin 16:503-527, 1987.
42. *Nabarro JD: Acromegaly, Clin Endocrinol 26:481-512, 1987.
43. *O'Neil J: Thyroid crisis, Nursing '87 17(11):335-338, 1987.
44. Paul T et al: Long-term L-thyronine therapy is associated with decreased hipbone density in premenopausal women, JAMA 295:3137-3141, 1988.
45. Pech A et al: Post-operative monitoring and treatment, Acta Otorhinolaryngol Belg 41:893-909, 1987.
46. Rahier J and Gerard R: Medullary carcinoma of the thyroid, Acta Otorhinolaryngol Belg 41:710-726, 1987.
47. Rebar R: Amenorrhea. In the Endocrine Society: 41st Post Graduate Annual Assembly syllabus, Bethesda, Md, 1989, The Society.
48. Roher HD and Goretzki PE: Management of goiter and thyroid nodules in an area of endemic goiter, Surg Clin North Am 67:233-249, 1987.
49. Rose, D.B.: Clinical physiology of acid-base and electrolyte disorders, ed 3, New York, 1989, McGraw-Hill Book Co.

*References preceded by an asterisk are particularly well suited for student reading.

50. Sakiyama R: Common thyroid disorders, AFP 38(1):227-238, 1988.

51. Sarsany S: Thyroid storm, RN 51(7):46-48, 1988.

52. Sawin CT: Hypothyroidism, Med Clin North Am 69:989-1003, 1988.

53. *Schira M: Steroid dependent states and adrenal insufficiency, Nurs Clin North Am 22:837-841, 1987.

54. Singer FR: Calcitonin: actions and therapeutic uses. In the Endocrine Society: 41st Post Graduate Annual Assembly syllabus, Bethesda, Md, 1989, The Society.

55. Sitges-Serra A and Caralps-Riera D: Hyperparathyroidism associated with renal disease, Surg Clin North Am 67:359-377, 1987.

56. Sivula A and Ronni-Sivula H: Natural history of treated primary hyperparathyroidism, Surg Clin North Am 67:329-341, 1987.

57. Snyder PJ: Gonadotroph cell adenomas of the pituitary, Endocr Rev 6:552-630, 1985.

58. Snyder PJ: The myth of the nonsecreting pituitary adenoma. In the Endocrine Society: 41st Post Graduate Annual Assembly syllabus, Bethesda, Md, 1989, The Society.

58a. Streiff LD: Can clients understand our instructions, Image 18:48-52, 1986.

59. Svec F: Steroid usage: too much of a good thing. In the Endocrine Society: 41st Post Graduate Annual Assembly syllabus, Bethesda, Md, 1989, The Society.

60. Thomas C and Groom RD: Current management of the patient with autonomously functioning nodular goiter, Surg Clin North Am 67:315-328, 1987.

61. Thompson N and Cheung P: Diagnoses and treatment of functioning and non-functioning adrenocortical neoplasms including incidentalomas, Surg Clin North Am 67:423-436, 1987.

62. Vance ML and Thorner MO: Prolactinomas, Endocrinol Metab Clin 16:731-753, 1987.

63. Verbalis JG: SIAD and other hyponatremic states. In the Endocrine Society: 41st Post Graduate Annual Assembly syllabus, Bethesda, Md, 1989, The Society.

64. Wilson JD and Foster DW, editors: Williams' textbook of endocrinology, ed 7, Philadelphia, 1985, WB Saunders Co.

65. Wyngaarden JB and Smith LH, editors: Cecil textbook of medicine, ed 18, Philadelphia, 1988, WB Saunders Co.

66. Young WF et al: Cushing's syndrome due to primary multinodular corticotrope hyperplasia, Mayo Clin Proc 63:256-262, 1988.

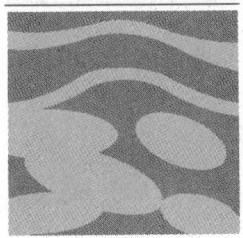

CHAPTER 37

Management of Persons with Diabetes Mellitus and Hypoglycemia

VIRGINIA L. CASSMEYER

CHAPTER OBJECTIVES

After studying this chapter, the student should be able to:

1. Differentiate between insulin-dependent diabetes mellitus (IDDM), non-insulin-dependent diabetes mellitus (NIDDM), gestational diabetes mellitus (GDM), malnutrition-related diabetes mellitus, and other types of diabetes mellitus.
2. Describe the epidemiology and etiology of IDDM and NIDDM.
3. Describe primary, secondary, and tertiary preventive interventions for persons with existing or potential diabetes mellitus.
4. Explain the pathophysiologic basis for IDDM, NIDDM, diabetic ketoacidosis (DKA) and hyperosmolar, hyperglycemic, nonketotic coma (HHNC).
5. Describe the common manifestations of IDDM, NIDDM, DKA, and HHNC.
6. Describe the medical management of IDDM, NIDDM, DKA, and HHNC.
7. Describe the major focus of dietary management for persons with IDDM and NIDDM and two systems for management.
8. Explain the role of exercise in management of IDDM and NIDDM.
9. Describe types of insulin, insulin regimens, and complications of the regimens.
10. Describe oral hypoglycemic agents: how they work, normal dosages, and side effects.
11. Describe chronic complications of diabetes mellitus, the relationship between the complications and metabolic control of the disease, and medical management of the complications.
12. Develop a nursing care plan, including nursing diagnoses; patient outcomes; and interventions for newly-diagnosed IDDM or NIDDM, acute complications of diabetes mellitus, or chronic complications of diabetes mellitus.
13. Describe precautions to be taken after an acute illness.
14. Explain special needs of the person who has diabetes mellitus and is undergoing surgery.
15. Describe the benefits and risks of pancreatic transplantation.
16. Define hypoglycemia.
17. Describe the various causes of fasting and reactive hypoglycemia.
18. Describe the medical and nursing management of hypoglycemia.

DIABETES MELLITUS

Diabetes mellitus does not have a single definition. It is a complex chronic disorder, characterized by disruption of normal carbohydrate, fat, and protein metabolism and the development over time of microvascular and macrovascular complications and neuropathies. It encompasses a heterogeneous group of anatomic and chemical problems predominated by an *absolute* or *relative* deficiency of insulin or its action and by glucose intolerance.

The professional nurse has a significant role in the care of persons with diabetes mellitus because the outcome of this major health problem almost completely depends on patients' self-management. Professional nurses have the responsibility of helping patients gain the knowledge, skills, and attitudes necessary for accurate self-management.

CLASSIFICATION

The need for uniform classification of glucose abnormalities encountered in clinical practice resulted in development, in 1979, in a classification system (Table 37-1) by an international work group, sponsored by the National Diabetes Data Group of the National Institute of Health.[62] This classification system clearly separated insulin-dependent diabetes mellitus (IDDM) and non-insulin-dependent diabetes mellitus (NIDDM) and was accepted by the World Health Organization.[90] It replaces diagnostic labels such as juvenile onset diabetes and maturity onset diabetes and provides for classification of impaired glucose tolerance, previous history of glucose abnormalities, and potential for glucose abnormalities, replacing terms such as *chemical diabetes, subclinical diabetes, latent diabetes,* and *prediabetes.* This system was modified by the World Health Organization in 1985, and malnutrition-related diabetes mellitus was added as a separate category.

Because the majority of cases of diabetes mellitus are either IDDM or NIDDM, this chapter will focus on

TABLE 37-1 Classification system for diabetes mellitus and other categories of glucose intolerance

Class	Characteristics
Insulin-dependent diabetes mellitus (IDDM): type 1	Persons are deficit in insulin (insulinopenic) and depend on exogenous insulin to prevent ketoacidosis and sustain life.
	Abrupt onset of symptoms, usually as a youth and almost always before age 30.
	With certain HLA types, an autoimmune mechanism and precipitation by an environmental factor, such as a viral infection, have been associated with susceptibility and onset.
Non-insulin-dependent diabetes mellitus (NIDDM): type 2	Persons do not depend on insulin to sustain life but may be treated with insulin; they are resistant to ketoacidosis except during periods of excessive stress.
	Onset is usually after age 40, without classic symptoms.
	Associated with endogenous insulin levels that may be mildly depressed, normal or high and with tissue insensitivity to insulin.
	Obesity and heredity have been associated with susceptibility and onset.
Gestational diabetes mellitus (GDM)	Person has onset of glucose abnormality during pregnancy.
	Women with known diabetes mellitus who become pregnant are not classified in this group.
	After delivery, the woman is reclassified on the basis of blood or plasma glucose testing.
Malnutrition-related diabetes mellitus	Persons require insulin.
	Diabetes mellitus found in tropical areas.
	It presents in young adults with histories of nutritional deficiencies.
	Ketosis is not usually present.
Other types of diabetes mellitus	Diabetes mellitus may be associated with other disorders such as pancreatic disease, other endocrine diseases, drugs, and genetic syndromes.
Impaired glucose tolerance (IGT) a. Obese b. Nonobese c. Associated with other conditions	Persons have glucose levels higher than normal but lower than those considered diagnostic for diabetes mellitus.
	It may be subclassified as obese or nonobese, or include persons with other conditions such as pancreatic disease, other endocrinopathies, or drug history.
Previous abnormality of glucose intolerance (PreAGT)	Persons have *past* history of glucose intolerance *but now have normal glucose levels.*
	It is designed for epidemiologic and research purposes.
Potential abnormality of glucose (PotAGT)	Persons have *no history of glucose intolerance* but have a *potentially higher risk* because of historical factors such as delivering large babies, obesity, or relatives with diabetes mellitus.

these two classifications. Most of the information, however, applies to the other classifications.

EPIDEMIOLOGY

Diabetes mellitus is a major health problem. There are now over 6 million persons with known diabetes mellitus, and it is likely that for every known case of diabetes, another remains undiagnosed.[68] IDDM accounts for approximately 10% of all cases, has a peak incidence in the age range of 11 to 14 years, affects boys somewhat more frequently than girls, and is more common in whites.[68] NIDDM accounts for 80% to 90% of all cases, shows a dramatic increase with age (see Chapter 35 for a discussion of the influence of aging on the incidence of diabetes mellitus), occurs more frequently in females, and has a higher incidence in nonwhite persons (particularly Hispanics, native Americans, and blacks). There has been some increase in the incidence of IDDM and NIDDM in the United States over the last few years. *Malnutrition-related diabetes mellitus* occurs primarily in young adults with histories of nutritional deficiencies

who live in tropical areas.[68] *Gestational diabetes mellitus* (GDM) occurs in 2% of all pregnant women. Occurrence increases with maternal age but is not affected by race.[68] Of persons with impaired glucose tolerance, 25% will eventually develop diabetes mellitus.[4]

ETIOLOGY

Just as the epidemiology of the different classes of diabetes varies, so do the etiologic factors (Table 37-2). Current information about the etiology of IDDM supports a genetic or inherited basis that has a permissive role in determining an individual's susceptibility to diabetes mellitus. Environmental factors can trigger onset in susceptible persons. In NIDDM the inherited or genetic factor is dominant, but environmental factors, especially obesity, have a major influence on the onset and the clinical course of the disease.

PREVENTION

Preventive health care for diabetes mellitus may be primary (prevention of the primary disease), secondary

TABLE 37-2 Etiologic factors in IDDM and NIDDM

Factors	IDDM	NIDDM
Genetic	Associated with HLA antigens located on chromosome 6 (particularly DR3 and DR4)	Not associated with HLA antigens except in three specific populations (Pimas, Xhosas and Fijians)[68]
Heredity	Unknown: familial aggregates rare; less than 50% concordance in monozygotic twins	Unknown except for the subclass of NIDDM in the young (also called maturity onset DM of the young (MODY), which is dominant[68]
		Probably multifactorial because familial aggregates are common, shows 55%-100% concordance in monozygotic twins
Autoimmune basis	Strong autoimmune basis as seen by: Presence (at diagnosis) of inflammatory cells around islet cells Occurrence of IDDM in patients with other autoimmune diseases or presence of lymphocytic insulitis Presence of islet cell antibodies and anti-insulin antibodies in high proportion of persons with IDDM	No strong autoimmune basis
Environmental factors	Frequent coincidence between IDDM and environmental factors such as acute viral infections	Obesity: urbanization and dietary habits that might be partially related to increased chance of obesity Decreased physical activity that accentuates obesity

(early detection and control of the disease), or tertiary (control of complications).

PRIMARY PREVENTION

Primary prevention is directed toward avoidance of obesity and weight reduction, if necessary, to prevent the onset of NIDDM. Although hereditary or genetic factors have a role in the development of IDDM and NIDDM genetic counseling is still not recommended because of the unknown nature of the pattern of transmission. This does not deny familial history as a risk factor particularly for NIDDM.

SECONDARY PREVENTION

It is estimated that there are 4 to 6 million persons with undiagnosed diabetes mellitus. Although mass screening has been carried out, many authorities believe screening of high-risk persons (see the box below) is a better use of resources than screening of the entire population. IDDM is not effectively identified with a screening approach because of its abrupt onset. Screening programs can be carried out in health departments, neighborhood clinics, hospital outpatient clinics, physicians' offices, industry and health fairs, or by mobile health units offering screening programs for diabetes and other

PERSONS AT RISK FOR DEVELOPING DIABETES MELLITUS

Obese persons
Elderly persons
Persons with a family history of diabetes mellitus
Women who give birth to babies weighing more than 9 pounds

health problems. Follow-up of all positive findings is essential.

Because of the number of persons with undiagnosed diabetes and the strong association between diabetes and hypertension, atherosclerotic heart disease, and peripheral vascular disease, health-seeking behaviors that diminish the risk for the latter will help diminish complications in persons with both known and undiagnosed diabetes. Health teaching programs should involve persons of all ages: those in schools, in industry, or in senior citizen groups.

Persons with known diabetes must have access to education, dietary support, social support systems, medical care, and nursing care so that prevention and early detection of complications is possible. Services include programs for hypertension detection and control, smoking cessation, eye care, and foot care.

TERTIARY PREVENTION

Because chronic complications are still common in diabetes mellitus, many nurses who work with those who have the disease will be involved in tertiary prevention. Major emphasis will be on (1) education about foot care to prevent ulcer formation, gangrene, and amputation; (2) yearly routine ophthalmology examinations to identify retinal changes early so that appropriate therapy can be instituted to prevent blindness; (3) monitoring for presence of albuminuria to identify the onset of potentially irreversible kidney disease; (4) helping patients control hypertension, improve control of metabolic status, and develop low protein diets to preserve kidney function; and (5) educating patients about tests or medications used to control complications. Tertiary preventive techniques may also help stop progression of gastrointestinal changes such as delayed emptying, diarrhea, and constipation, and sexual alterations.

PATHOPHYSIOLOGY

PATHOGENESIS OF DEFECTIVE INSULIN ACTION

In diabetes mellitus, there is an absolute or relative deficiency of insulin and its action. The pathogenesis of insulin deficiency is different in IDDM and NIDDM. It is important that nurses working with persons with diabetes understand the pathology underlying the deficiency, particularly as it relates to NIDDM. Persons with diabetes are exposed to new findings from news reports and will frequently question health team members about them. For example, common questions about NIDDM include, "How can I have diabetes when I have insulin in my blood?" and "Would a pancreatic or islet cell transplant help me?".

An absolute deficiency in insulin secretion usually occurs with IDDM and results from destruction of pancreatic β cells by the interaction of genetic, immunologic, and environmental factors. In the very early phases of IDDM, there is a reduction in the first phase or immediate plasma insulin response when patients are tested intravenously for glucose tolerance. (NOTE: The first phase of insulin release is a rapid, transient (10-minute) burst of insulin not related to the level of elevated glucose.)[68] The loss of the first phase of insulin release does not affect glucose homeostasis.

Overt IDDM appears when 80% or more of β-cell activity is lost.[3] At this stage, both the first and second phases of insulin release are disturbed. Not all persons with IDDM have the same level of β-cell dysfunction; this may account for differences in how well the IDDM can be controlled. Resistance to the peripheral action of insulin (endogenous or exogenous) may also be present in IDDM.[3]

In NIDDM, serum insulin levels may be depressed, normal, or high. Research indicates that the pathogenic sequence in NIDDM (culminating in a relative insulin deficiency) may be the result of one factor or a combination of factors:

1. An islet cell defect results in a slowed or delayed response in the release of insulin to a glucose load.[4,68] Although basal insulin levels are normal or high, the insulin secretion does not keep pace with glucose demands.
2. The number of insulin receptors is reduced because of "down regulation" from elevated insulin levels.[4] Although there is sufficient insulin, cells cannot be stimulated because the number of receptors available for activation is decreased (see Chapter 35).
3. There is a postreceptor defect.[3,68] Although insulin is present and binds to the receptor, the intra-

cellular activation necessary for normal cell stimulation does not occur.
4. There is an impairment in the suppression of hepatic glucose production and reduced peripheral uptake of glucose, both of which contribute to hyperglycemia.

ROLE OF GLUCAGON IN PATHOGENESIS OF DIABETES MELLITUS

Persons with diabetes have a defect in pancreatic α-cell function in addition to the β-cell dysfunction. Persons with diabetes show an insensitivity in the regulation of glucagon (secreted by the α cells) in response to hyperglycemia or hypoglycemia, resulting in a continual elevated glucagon level.[68] Controversy exists about whether (1) this is a primary defect associated with diabetes mellitus or secondary to a lack of insulin action, (2) elevation in glucagon is a necessary prerequisite for the alterations in metabolism seen in diabetes, or (3) treatment designed to suppress glucagon should be part of the regimen for persons with diabetes. At this time it is known that glucagon levels are elevated and they can worsen the metabolic alterations. In the following sections, only the effects of a deficiency in insulin secretion and its actions will be discussed. However, it is important to remember that hyperglucagonemia may also be involved.

EFFECTS OF DEFICIENCY OF INSULIN SECRETION OR ACTION

To understand the effects of an absolute or relative deficiency of insulin and its action, the normal functions of insulin must be understood (see Chapter 35).

A lack or deficiency of insulin or its action results in hyperglycemia. After a meal, because insulin levels are low or the action of insulin is impaired, *glucose is not taken up from the portal vein by the liver* (the normal process). Thus glucose enters the general circulation, and *glycogenesis* is *inhibited*. In addition, the *liver* continues to *synthesize glucose* (via glycogenolysis or gluconeogenesis) and to release glucose into the blood stream, worsening hyperglycemia. *Insulin-dependent peripheral tissues,* such as skeletal muscle and adipose tissue, *do not extract glucose from the blood* as they normally would; and muscle cells metabolize their own glycogen supply.

Amino acid transport into cells also requires insulin; thus, amino acid uptake and protein synthesis *are impaired.* In fact, proteins are actually catabolized and amino acids are liberated to provide the substrate necessary for gluconeogenesis.

The *metabolism* of *fatty acids, triglycerides,* and *glycerol is altered;* instead of lipogenesis, lipolysis is seen. The liver will continue the formation of ketone bodies (ketogenesis), which may occur at a very brisk

TABLE 37-3 Metabolic alterations seen in deficiency of insulin and its action

Cell Type	Substrate Metabolism		
	Carbohydrate	Protein	Fat
Liver cell	↑ Glycogenolysis ↑ Gluconeogenesis	↑ Protein breakdown	↑ Ketogenesis
Muscle cell	↑ Glycogenolysis liberating lactate and pyruvate ↓ Glucose uptake	↑ Protein catabolism ↑ Liberation of amino acids ↓ Amino acid uptake	
Fat cell	↓ Glucose uptake		↑ Lipolysis ↓ Lipogenesis

rate. Table 37-3 summarizes the metabolic alterations seen in insulin deficiency.

The increase in blood glucose results in more glucose being filtered than can be reabsorbed in the renal system, and *glucose is excreted* in the urine. This usually occurs when the serum glucose level is over 180 mg/100 ml, given that renal function is normal. The *glucose excretion results in an osmotic diuresis* and the loss of fluid and electrolytes. If the level of ketones is higher than the renal threshold, ketones are excreted in the urine, producing additional fluid and electrolyte losses.

The severity of the altered metabolism depends on the severity of insulin deficiency or its action. In mildly deficient states, altered glucose metabolism with hyperglycemia and glycosuria may occur only after meals. In the fasted state, glucose levels and protein metabolism may be normal. As the deficiency increases in severity, hyperglycemia, glycosuria, and protein catabolism will be present all the time. The altered lipid metabolism resulting in abnormally high production of ketones may be seen only in markedly insulin-deficient states and is usually present only in IDDM.

If the alterations described above are not corrected or are poorly corrected, acute and chronic complications can occur. Because many persons with diabetes will have signs and symptoms of either acute or chronic complications at the time of first diagnosis the pathophysiology associated with these complications is discussed next.

ACUTE METABOLIC CHANGES ASSOCIATED WITH SEVERE DEFICIENCY OF INSULIN OR ITS ACTION

Diabetic Ketoacidosis

Diabetic ketoacidosis (DKA) occurs with severe insulin deficiency. It can occur in the undiagnosed diabetic person; in the diagnosed person whose insulin needs become greater than the prescribed therapy because of infection, trauma, emotional upsets, or other stressors; or in the person who stops treatment. It is usually seen in persons with IDDM but can occur in those with NIDDM.

The pathophysiology of DKA (Figure 37-1) is a continuation of that described for the effects of a deficiency of insulin and its actions. However, an increase in the counterregulatory hormones (glucagon, growth hormone, cortisol, and catecholamines) is important in the pathogenesis of DKA. These four hormones accentuate the hyperglycemic state resulting from insulin deficiency and the lipolysis and ketogenesis. In DKA there is a constant state of hyperglycemia with its resultant osmotic diuresis, a constant state of protein breakdown with the liberation of potassium, increased urea nitrogen formation leading to more diuresis, and massive ketone formation.

The ketones are an acid source and use the body's alkali reserve for buffering, resulting in acidosis. Ketones are also excreted in the urine, increasing diuresis. The diuresis resulting from the excretion of glucose, urea, and ketones results in the loss of sodium, water, potassium, and phosphate. The sodium loss prevents the formation of bicarbonate, and the alkali reserve of the body cannot be replaced. When the alkali reserve is depleted, the pH of the blood decreases, and compensatory mechanisms to control the metabolic acidosis are stimulated (see Chapter 24). These responses cause the kidney to try to excrete even more acids, which worsens the fluid and electrolyte imbalance. The lungs try to compensate by excreting hydrogen ions as CO_2, but because acid is continually formed, complete compensation cannot occur and the pH remains low, altering cellular functioning.

The diuresis from all processes described above results in hyperosmolality, dehydration, hemoconcentration, and shock. The hyperosmolality causes fluids to move from the intracellular to the extracellular compartment, which also causes altered cellular functioning. Poor tissue perfusion from shock contributes to the altered cellular functioning. With shock and tissue hypoxia, lactic acidosis can occur and worsen the acidotic state. If this process is not interrupted, the patient will lapse into coma.

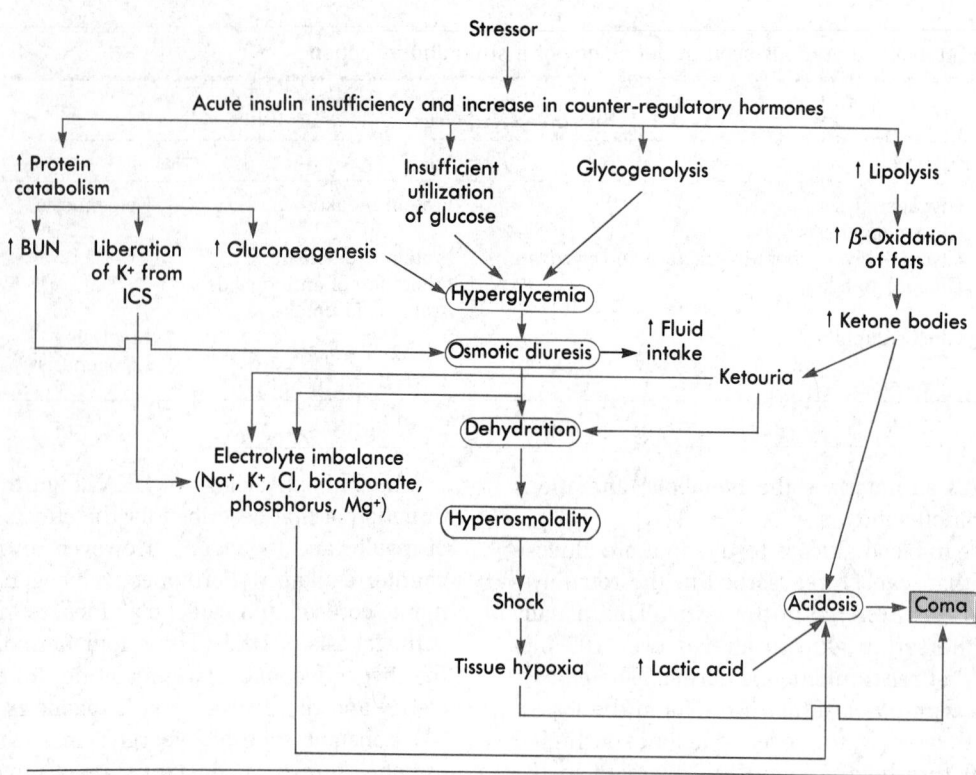

FIGURE 37-1 Summary of pathogenesis of diabetic ketoacidosis coma.

Hyperglycemic, Hyperosmolar, Nonketotic Coma (HHNC)

Hyperglycemic, hyperosmolar, nonketotic coma (HHNC) can occur when the action of insulin is severely inhibited. HHNC is seen in patients with NIDDM. It can occur in a person with undiagnosed NIDDM or in a poorly treated patient and is almost always precipitated by a specific factor (Table 37-4). HHNC is primarily seen in elderly persons with NIDDM.

The pathophysiology of HHNC is, in part, a continuation of that described previously for the effects of a deficiency of insulin and its action, but the serum glucose level becomes extremely high (≥600 mg/100 ml).[68] The reason for the high glucose level is that, although early in the pathogenesis of HHNC the patient has an osmotic diuresis from the hyperglycemia, which helps eliminate some of the excessive glucose, this diuresis is not maintained. The diuresis is inhibited, primarily because of a contraction of the extracellular fluid volume resulting from lack of adequate fluid intake. The lack of fluid intake may be due to failure to respond to the stimulus of thirst or inadequate administration of fluids. The patient may also be losing excess fluids from other processes such as vomiting or inability to concentrate urine. The contraction of extracellular fluid volume decreases the glomerular filtration rate and, therefore, the excretion of glucose.

Thus, glucose is not being lost from the vascular space through diuresis or by uptake into the cell, but is continually added because of the ineffective insulin metabolism. Glucose may actually be added in greater quantities because of the effects of glucagon, cortisol, growth hormone (GH), and epinephrine. These hor-

TABLE 37-4 Factors that precipitate HHNC[4,68]

Factor	Examples
Associated illnesses	Infections (gram-negative pneumonia, acute pyelonephritis, septicemia)
	Renal failure
	Lactic acidosis
	Myocardial infarction
	Cerebrovascular accidents
	Gastrointestinal (GI) hemorrhage
	Subdural hematoma
	Pancreatitis
	Arterial thrombosis
	Congestive heart failure
	Cognitive dysfunction resulting in lack of thirst perception
Therapeutic procedures	Dialysis: peritoneal, hemodialysis
	Total parenteral nutrition
	Hyperosmolar tube feedings
	Surgery
Drugs	Glucocorticoids, diuretics, diphenylhydantoin, β-adrenergic blocking agents, immunosuppressive agents, diazoxide

mones inhibit cellular uptake of glucose, which results in severe hyperglycemia and hyperosmolality.

The hyperosmolality initiates a major shift of fluids from the intracellular to the extracellular space, which may initially lead to additional diuresis. Eventually, both intracellular and extracellular dehydration occur. Intracellular fluid loss results in central nervous system (CNS) dysfunction. The extracellular fluid loss may be so severe that it results in shock and hypoxia. Cellular dysfunction and coma then occur.

A major difference between DKA and HHNC is that HHNC is not associated with ketosis and acidosis. Acidosis, if present, is usually very mild and occurs as a result of lactic acidosis from shock or other illnesses. The reason for the lack of ketosis is not fully understood. It is known that free fatty acid levels are usually lower in HHNC than in DKA, this decreases the availability of substrate for ketogenesis.[68] It was previously believed that higher insulin levels in NIDDM prevented lipolysis and thus inhibited ketogenesis, but peripheral insulin

levels have not been found to be higher in HHNC than in DKA. It is possible that the person with HHNC has higher hepatic insulin levels, even though peripheral insulin levels are low, and this would inhibit ketogenesis. It is also possible that extremely high hyperglycemia and hyperosmolality block the formation of ketones by inhibiting lipolysis.[68] A difference in the level or action of the counterregulatory hormones (glucagon, cortisol, GH, or epinephrine), all of which can influence the amount of lipogenesis, may be present in HHNC but not in DKA.[68] Figure 37-2 summarizes the pathogenesis of HHNC.

LONG-TERM CHANGES ASSOCIATED WITH INSULIN DEFICIENCY OR ITS ACTION

Alterations in structure and function of vessels and nerves are major pathophysiologic changes that occur in all types of diabetes. The role of uncontrolled alterations in carbohydrate, fat, and protein metabolism in vascular and nerve changes is still controversial. Re-

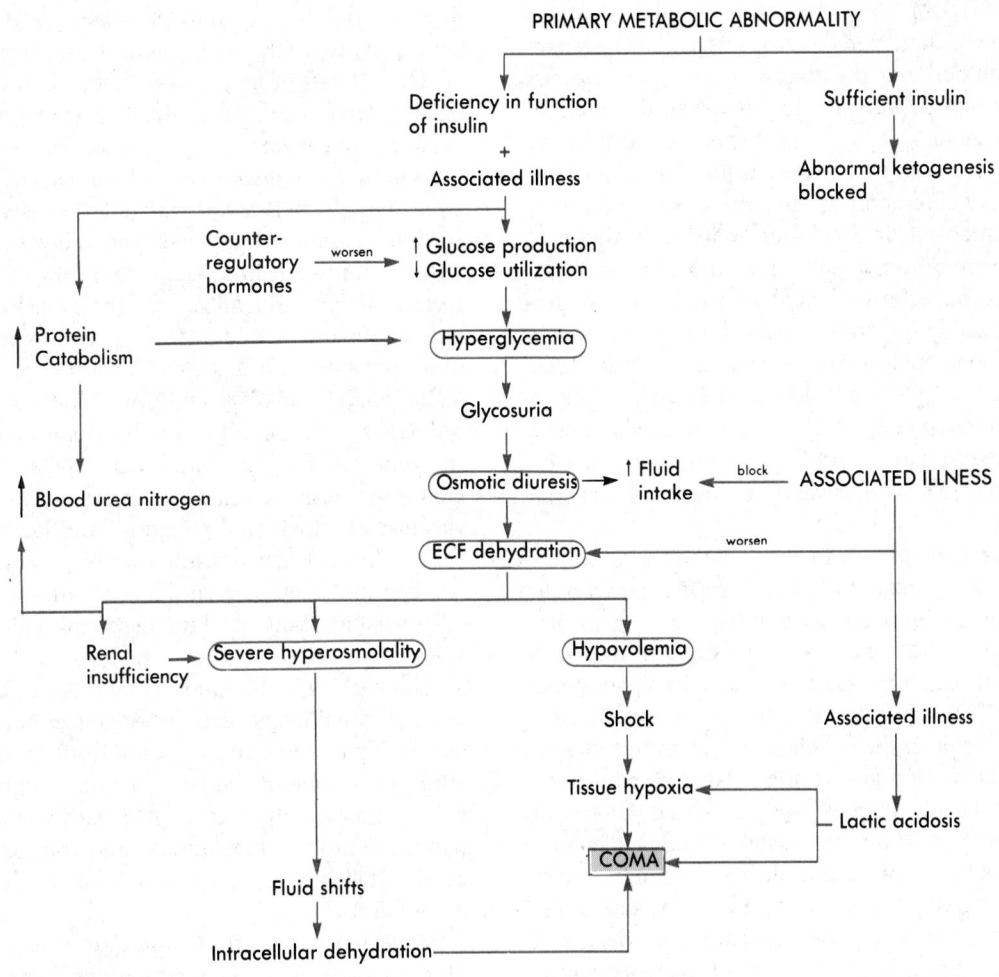

FIGURE 37-2 Pathogenesis of HHNC.

search continues in an effort to identify whether the altered metabolism associated with a deficiency of insulin or its action causes these problems or whether some pathologic process causes both the deficiency in insulin or its action and the vascular and nerve changes. *These changes occur at variable times during the disease and, although they rarely occur within the first 5 to 10 years after diagnosis of IDDM, many persons with NIDDM may first be diagnosed as having diabetes when they enter the health care system with complaints related to these long-term complications.* The resulting alterations are classified as *macrovascular changes, microvascular changes,* or *neuropathy.* Major problems include *cardiovascular disease, renal disease, blindness, autonomic neuropathy,* and *diabetic foot problems.*

Macrovascular Changes

Persons with diabetes mellitus develop macrovascular changes from *atherosclerosis* that are the same as those seen in persons without diabetes. However, it is well known that persons with diabetes are prone to develop atherosclerosis at an earlier age and that the disease progresses faster and is more severe and extensive. Persons with NIDDM develop macrovascular changes more frequently than persons with IDDM. The exact mechanism underlying the formation of *atheromatous lesions* is unknown, but probably involves the interaction of many factors. It has been hypothesized that the initial event involves endothelial injury, which is followed by the proliferation of smooth muscle cells with an accumulation of intracellular matrix. Endothelial lesions can result from mechanical and chemical factors, such as hypertensive lipid disorders, tissue hypoxia, and possibly hyperglycemia. The smooth muscle cell proliferation, lipid accumulation, and extracellular matrix formation that result are accelerated by various factors, such as presence of abnormal lipids, tissue hypoxia, platelet changes, and hormonal changes. Diabetes is associated with several of these atherogenic factors.

Insulin has a major role in the metabolism of lipids. Lipid disorders are frequently found in persons with diabetes mellitus. The *hyperlipoproteinemia* seen in diabetes is usually identified as *type IV* or *type V,* and is often the result of an excess of low density lipoproteins (see Chapter 40). Diabetes is also considered to be a contributing factor in the development of hypertension.

Macrovascular changes result in decreased lumen size, compromised blood flow, and decreased delivery of oxygen to tissues, resulting in tissue ischemia. The end result is usually cerebrovascular disease, coronary artery disease, renal artery stenosis, or peripheral vascular disease. Cardiovascular complications cause the deaths of many persons with IDDM or NIDDM. Diabetes mellitus is an independent risk factor for atherosclerotic cardio-vascular disease and 25% to 75% of all persons with diabetes have some lipid abnormality.[3]

Microvascular Changes

Microvascular changes seen in persons with diabetes do not occur in persons without diabetes. These changes are characterized by thickening of the capillaries and damage to the basement membrane and result in *diabetic nephropathy* and *retinopathy.* The causes of the changes are unknown but believed to be related to uncontrolled diabetes. Various factors, such as the role of protein fractions, glycoproteins, lipids, and lipoproteins have been studied; but no conclusive evidence is yet available about the relationship between these factors and the microvascular changes seen in persons with diabetes.

Diabetic nephropathy. One of the major results of microvascular changes is alteration in renal structure and function. Renal failure frequently results from the changes, and diabetic nephropathy may account for 30% of the persons receiving long-term renal dialysis.[3,68] Four types of kidney lesions can occur: (1) *glomerular lesions,* (2) *arteriosclerosis of the renal arteries,* (3) *tubular lesions,* and (4) *pyelonephritis.*

Three types of glomerular lesions can occur. *Diffuse glomerulosclerosis,* resulting in severe proteinuria and renal failure, is one type of glomerular lesion. A second type is *nodular glomerulosclerosis (Kimmelstiel-Wilson syndrome),* which involves nodular masses of laminated hyaline material that occur randomly throughout the kidney and result in a *nephrotic syndrome* with *proteinuria, edema,* and *hypertension.* This lesion is found only in persons with diabetes and occurs in 10% to 35% of all persons with diabetes. A third type of glomerular lesion is an exudative one in which *eosinophilic fibrinoid deposits* are found in the Bowman's capsule or over the outer surface of glomerular capillary loops. These glomerular lesions, along with arteriosclerosis, obliterate vascular channels and glomeruli and lead to *renal failure.* Tubular lesions result from deposits of glycogen, fat, and mucopolysaccharides within the epithelial cells of the distal tubules and the descending limb of Henle's loop.

Although renal abnormalities can be identified through renal biopsy early in the onset of diabetes, clinical problems are often not seen until 10 or more years after onset. One of the earliest visible signs is microalbuminuria, which is reversible with meticulous treatment. Eventually, intermittent and constant proteinuria occurs, followed by renal insufficiency progressing to renal failure.

Hypertension is the *factor that most often accelerates nephropathy associated with diabetes mellitus.* Aggressive treatment of the hypertension is necessary and blood pressure should be normalized (see Chapter 29). Obstructive nephropathy, repeated infections, and nephrotoxic drugs, such as contrast media used for x-rays, can also accelerate the progression of diabetic nephropathy to renal failure.

Diabetic retinopathy. Diabetic retinopathy is a leading cause of blindness in the United States. Retinopathy will affect 50% to 80% of all persons with diabetes 10 to 15 years after diagnosis.[4]

The primary lesion is the formation of microaneurysms in the retinal vessels, followed by hemorrhage and exudate formation. These early retinal changes, called background or simple retinopathy, may progress to a more serious stage, *proliferative retinopathy,* in which new blood vessels form on the retina. These new vessels bleed, causing vitreous hemorrhage and retinal detachment (see Chapter 64). The bleeding is usually repetitive and leads to permanent loss of vision.

There are *no symptoms of early retinal changes,* and persons with diabetes are encouraged to have yearly eye examinations by an ophthalmologist. Hypertension, which can worsen the retinopathy, should be screened for and adequately controlled.[3]

Cataracts also occur in persons with diabetes. Cataracts may be caused by prolonged hyperglycemia, resulting in polyol-increased metabolism via the polyol pathway, with increased sorbitol formation and intralens hyperosmolality, swelling, and opacity formation.

Neuropathy

Persons with IDDM or NIDDM usually have one or more alterations that affect peripheral nerves, the autonomic nervous system (ANS), the spinal cord, or the CNS. Symmetric peripheral neuropathy and autonomic neuropathy are by far the most common disorders and will be the focus of this discussion.

Neuropathies unique to diabetes may occur from increased metabolism via the polyol pathway that results from hyperglycemia. Metabolism via this pathway causes accumulation of sorbitol in nerve cells. Sorbitol accumulation can result in hyperosmolality, fluid shifts with swelling, and subsequent nerve dysfunction. Sorbitol accumulation can also lower nerve myo-inositol content, and this change disrupts sodium/potassium adenosine triphosphatase (ATPase) activity, decreases energy metabolism, and can result in nerve dysfunction and structural damage. The result of the nerve changes is altered nerve conduction.

Symmetric peripheral polyneuropathy. The most common type of neuropathy is symmetric peripheral polyneuropathy. Sensory changes and then loss in the distal lower extremities are the most common nerve involvement. Eventually motor loss in the lower extremities and sen-

AUTONOMIC NEUROPATHIC CHANGES WITH DIABETES MELLITUS

Bladder	Becomes hypotonic or atonic and empties poorly; neurogenic bladder
Sexual function	Inability to have an erection (male), change in lubrication (female)
GI system	Delayed gastric emptying, impaired gastric acid secretion, constipation or diarrhea
Sweating	May be inhibited or excessive; ANS response to changes in environmental temperature is lost or decreased
Cardiovascular reflexes	Impaired maintenance of blood pressure and cerebral blood flow during position changes or in response to other stimuli; heart rate may be high at rest because of loss of parasympathetic function but remains fixed with activity

sory and motor loss in the upper extremities can occur. The impairments occur slowly and are progressive.

Autonomic neuropathy. Autonomic neuropathy is also common. Alteration of the autonomic nervous system's control of the bladder, sexual functions, gastrointestinal tract, sweating mechanisms, and cardiovascular reflexes can occur (see the box above). The impairments occur slowly and arogressive. A patient may experience some or all of the dysfunctions.

The Diabetic Foot

The macrovascular and microvascular changes and the neuropathy all contribute to changes in the lower extremity called *the diabetic foot.* One major factor is sensory neuropathy, which may lead to painless trauma, ulceration, and infection. Sensory and motor neuropathy contribute to bone changes and deformed feet that change gait and pressure distribution and contribute to infection. Autonomic neuropathy can result in anhidroses with resultant cracking of the skin, which also contributes to infection. Macrovascular and microvascular changes produce tissue ischemia and skin changes that can cause ulcerations and infections and prevent healing. The interrelationship of all these factors, as they contribute to lesions that result in gangrene and ultimately amputation, is illustrated in Figure 37-3. It is important to note that the vascular changes (angiopathy) may actually worsen neuropathy and vice versa (shown by the ? in Figure 37-3). Either may contribute to the occurrence of foot lesions.

Gangrene can be either dry or wet. *Dry* gangrene occurs when tissue death is not associated with inflammatory changes. *Autoamputation* of affected toes is the

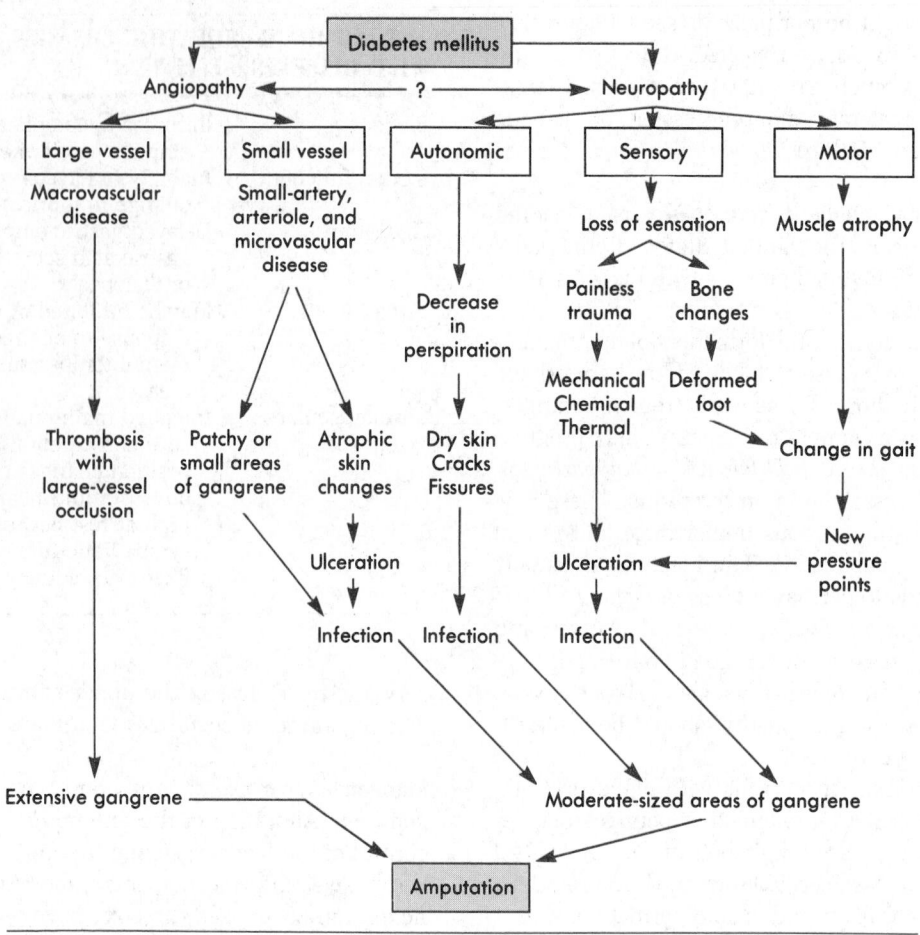

FIGURE 37-3 How foot lesions of diabetes can lead to amputation. (Adapted from Levin ME: Medical evaluation and treatment. In Levin ME, and O'Neal LW, editors: The diabetic foot, ed 2, St Louis, 1977, The CV Mosby Co.)

treatment of choice. The area must be kept dry, or wet gangrene can occur. *Wet* gangrene is gangrene coupled with inflammation; septicemia and septic shock may occur.

Prevention is the key to care of the diabetic foot. It is estimated that a 50% to 75% reduction in need for amputation is possible with prevention.

CLINICAL MANIFESTATIONS

Clinical manifestations of diabetes mellitus vary, depending on the type and stage of the disease.

COMMON INITIAL MANIFESTATIONS OF IDDM

In persons with IDDM there is usually a history of sudden onset, and patients have signs and symptoms resulting from the pathophysiologic changes discussed above under the effects of insulin deficiency. Signs and symptoms may include:

1. Increased urine output (*polyuria*) resulting from the glycosuria secondary to hyperglycemia

2. Increased thirst (*polydipsia*) secondary to osmotic diuresis and hyperosmolality

3. Increased appetite (*polyphagia*) secondary to cellular starvation

4. Loss of weight in the presence of polyphagia secondary to ineffective protein, fat, and carbohydrate metabolism

5. Weakness and lethargy secondary to inadequate energy production

6. Elevated fasting serum glucose; values greater than 140 mg/100 ml with a plateau of approximately 300 to 500 mg/100 ml

7. Glycosuria

The patient may exhibit various signs and symptoms related to extracellular volume deficit such as poor skin turgor, excessive weight loss, dry mucous membranes, soft or sunken eyeballs, tachycardia, orthostatic hypotension, or hypotension while supine. These manifestations occur if the patient is unable to take in enough fluids to replace losses from osmotic diuresis. The severity of the signs and symptoms depends on how dehydrated the patient becomes.

Some persons with IDDM exhibit more subtle manifestations such as presence of viral syndrome in infants and toddlers; recurrence of bed-wetting in school-aged children; or weakness, lethargy, and weight loss in any age group. Vaginitis may be an early symptom in females.

COMMON INITIAL MANIFESTATIONS OF NIDDM

The clinical manifestations initially seen in persons with NIDDM vary greatly. Some persons are *asymptomatic,* and the *diagnosis* is made when *hyperglycemia* or *glycosuria* is found on routine examination. Other persons may seek help because of subtle signs of hyperglycemia such as weakness, fatigue, and inability to carry out normal activities. Weight gain rather than weight loss is usually present. Some patients complain of recurrent infections. Sometimes the patient can have the same classic signs and symptoms seen in persons with IDDM. Frequently, persons with NIDDM are not diagnosed until they seek help for signs and symptoms associated with long-term changes associated with a deficiency of

insulin action. These patients may have manifestations of cerebrovascular disease, coronary artery disease, visual changes, peripheral neuropathy, or gangrene.

MANIFESTATIONS OF DKA

Signs and symptoms resulting from the pathogenesis of DKA may be the initial manifestations for some persons with IDDM, although DKA is most frequently seen in persons who have been previously diagnosed and experience additional stressors, such as an infection, or who stop taking their insulin or greatly increase their food intake. It has been reported that 20% of the episodes of DKA occur in undiagnosed persons with diabetes and 80% occur in previously diagnosed persons with diabetes.[68] Table 37-5 summarizes the clinical manifestations of DKA and compares these with HHNC. The onset can be gradual or relatively sudden.

MANIFESTATIONS OF HHNC

Signs and symptoms resulting from the pathogenesis of HHNC may be the initial manifestations for some persons with NIDDM. These manifestations are usually

TABLE 37-5 Signs and symptoms of DKA and HHNC

	DKA	HHNC
Onset	Gradual or sudden; classical symptoms of hyperglycemia usually present before DKA	Gradual
Precipitating factors	Infection, other stressors, stopping insulin in known IDDM	See Table 37-4
Symptoms	Polyuria and thirst from osmotic diuresis; nausea, vomiting, abdominal pain from acidosis; weakness, headache and fatigue from acidosis and electrolyte imbalance; dim vision	Polyuria from osmotic diuresis leading to oliguria from volume depletion or renal insufficiency. Poor fluid intake; history of lethargy or somnolence from hyperosmolality
Signs	Hypothermia; signs of dehydration and hypovolemic shock (tachycardia, hypotension, dry skin, weight loss, etc.); hyperpnea (Kussmaul's breathing) from respiratory compensation of metabolic acidosis; fruity odor to breath from respiratory elimination of acetone; lethargy to coma from effects of acidosis and dehydration; flushed face; weight loss	Normal to elevated temperature; signs of severe fluid deficit; usually no hyperpnea unless lactic acidosis is present; lethargy, confusion, coma, seizures, focal neurologic deficits (hemiplegia) and other signs (gastric distention, ileus, hematemesis) from hyperosmolality
LABORATORY VALUES		
Serum glucose	>250-350 mg/100 ml	Usually >600 mg/100 ml
Osmolarity	Between 300 and 350 mOsm/L	>350 mOsm/L
Serum acetone	Highly positive	Nondetectable or very slight
Bicarbonate	<15 mEq/L	Normal
Arterial pH	<7.2	>7.3
Serum Na$^+$ and Cl$^-$	Low, normal, or high, depending on proportion lost with water; total body level of Na$^+$ is deficient	Normal to high, depending on proportion lost with water; total body level of Na$^+$ is deficient
Serum K$^+$	Normal to high, but total body level is low; ECF level elevated from acidosis	Normal, but total body level is low
Serum phosphorus	High, but total body level is low	High, but total body level is low
Serum magnesium	High, but total body level is low	High, but total body level is low
Anion gap	Increased	Normal
Blood urea nitrogen (BUN)	Normal to slight elevation	High, about 87 mg/100 ml
Others	Elevated WBCs	Elevated WBCs, triglycerides and cholesterol

precipitated by one of the factors listed in Table 37-4. HHNC is seen slightly more frequently in persons who have been previously diagnosed and experience a precipitating factor, although it occurs very frequently in persons with undiagnosed NIDDM. Table 37-5 summarizes the signs and symptoms of HHNC and compares these with DKA. Onset is very gradual, and a precipitating factor is almost always present.

MEDICAL MANAGEMENT

Medical management of the person with IDDM or NIDDM has five major focuses: (1) diagnosing the presence of diabetes mellitus, (2) managing acute manifestations such as DKA or HHNC, (3) establishing goals related to level of daily control, (4) establishing day-to-day medical management plans for IDDM or NIDDM, and (5) managing manifestations associated with macrovascular and microvascular changes, neuropathy, and the diabetic foot.

DIAGNOSIS OF DIABETES MELLITUS

The diagnosis of diabetes is not always easy, and controversy has existed about what fasting plasma glucose level is really diagnostic. This is particularly true for the elderly. The diagnostic tests used for diabetes are described in Chapter 35. Guidelines for diagnosis are listed in the box at right.

MANAGEMENT OF DKA AND HHNC

The management of DKA and HHNC when present becomes a medical priority, whether these are part of the initial manifestations of diabetes mellitus or occur after the onset of diabetes. Management involves fluid and electrolyte replacement, insulin therapy, and other measures based on the original severity of the problem and continual assessment. Treatment also involves measures directed toward the precipitating factors. The management of DKA and HHNC are similar; generalized management guidelines for adults are presented in the box on p. 1103.

ESTABLISHING GOALS RELATED TO LEVEL OF CONTROL

Criteria for levels of metabolic control vary depending on (1) the philosophy of the health team about the benefits of meticulous control in avoiding the long-term manifestations of deficiency of insulin or its action, and (2) what the health team believes is realistic for an individual patient based on the patient's age, ability, other health problems, support and desires. It is important to remember that, although not conclusive, data suggest that long-term complications can be prevented or arrested by normalizing the metabolic environment; therefore, the goal frequently is to achieve good-to-excellent metabolic control. However, the achievement of excellent or ideal control increases the risk of hypogly-

METABOLIC CRITERIA FOR DIAGNOSIS OF DIABETES MELLITUS

IDDM AND NIDDM
Adult Men and Nonpregnant Women

1. Random plasma glucose ≥200 mg/100 ml plus presence of polydipsia, polyuria, polyphagia, and weight loss, *or*
2. Fasting plasma glucose ≥140 mg/100 ml on at least two occasions *or*
3. If fasting plasma glucose <140 mg/100 ml, perform oral glucose tolerance test; must have two tests showing plasma glucose ≥200 mg/100 ml at 2 hours and at least one other time between 0 and 2 hours after a 75 g dose of glucose

Children

1. Random plasma glucose ≥200 mg/100 ml plus presence of polydipsia, polyuria, ketonuria, and weight loss, *or*
2. Fasting plasma glucose ≥140 mg/100 ml on at least two occasions *and* plasma glucose ≥200 mg/100 ml at 2 hours and at least one other time between 0 and 2 hours after a glucose dose of 1.75 g/kg ideal weight (up to 75 g)

GDM: Pregnant Women

1. Two plasma glucose values ≥ to the following fasting or after 100 g of oral glucose:
   Fasting ≥ 105 mg/100 ml
   1 hour ≥ 190 mg/100 ml
   2 hour ≥ 165 mg/100 ml
   3 hour ≥ 145 mg/100 ml

IMPAIRED GLUCOSE TOLERANCE
Adult Men and Nonpregnant Women

1. Fasting plasma glucose <140 mg/100 ml, *and*
2. A 2-hour oral glucose tolerance test plasma glucose ≥140 mg/100 ml but <200 mg/100 ml, *and*
3. An intervening oral glucose tolerance test plasma glucose ≥200 mg/100 ml

Children

1. Fasting plasma glucose concentration < than 140 mg/100 ml, *and*
2. A 2-hour oral glucose tolerance test plasma glucose ≥140 mg/100 ml

cemia and can place a tremendous burden on the patient. The patient must participate in establishing the goals of therapy, and everyone involved must know what those goals are.

The level of control is evaluated in several ways. The indexes used to evaluate level of control and indications of good-to-excellent control in adults with IDDM or NIDDM can be found in Table 37-6. In addition to meeting the criteria of these indexes, the patient should be attaining or maintaining a normal weight.

MEDICAL MANAGEMENT GUIDELINES FOR ADULTS WITH DKA OR HHNC[3,4,68]

FLUIDS: MAJOR PRIORITY; ADEQUATE FLUID REPLACEMENT ALONE WILL DECREASE HYPERGLYCEMIA.

DKA Isotonic saline is fluid of choice unless patient has history of hypertension or congestive heart failure; give fluids at rate of 1 to 2 L for first hour, slow to 1 L/hr for next 2 to 3 hours, then slow to 500 ml/hr; total amount, type, and rate based on continual assessment of intake and output, weight, hemodynamic status, mental status, and laboratory determinations; dextrose added as 5% glucose in saline when plasma glucose reaches 250 mg to 300 mg/100 ml

HHNC Usually start with 0.5 normal saline because of hyperosmolality; give at rate of 1.5 L/hr for first hour, 1 L/hr for next 2 hours, then 500 to 750 ml/hr for next hour; when serum osmolarity is <320 mOsm/L switch to normal saline; add dextrose (5% in saline) when glucose is 250 to 300 mg/100 ml; monitor central venous pressure or pulmonary capillary wedge pressure (see Chapter 26), weight, intake and output, BP, pulse and respiration, mental status; laboratory determinations will guide treatment

INSULIN: PLASMA GLUCOSE LEVEL SHOULD FALL ABOUT 75 TO 100 MG/100 ML/HR IF ADEQUATE INSULIN IS GIVEN.

Insulin needs are very similar in DKA and HHNC

DKA Low-dose protocol most common; IV bolus of 5 to 10 U of regular insulin followed by continuous infusion, by controlled administration, of 5 to 10 U/hr (0.1 U/kg body weight) until plasma glucose level reaches about 250 mg/100 ml (which takes 4 to 6 hours) *and* pH = 7.30 *or* HCO_3^- is ≥18 mEq/L (which takes 8 to 12 hours), then switch to usual insulin regimen

Hourly IM injections of 5 to 10 U regular insulin may be used instead of IV route

HHNC Low-dose regimen similar to that for DKA; give 10 to 15 U regular insulin as IV bolus followed by 5 to 10 U/hr until plasma glucose level is 250 to 300 mg/100 ml, then decrease to 2 to 3 U/hour; when stable switch to usual insulin regimen

Hourly IM insulin injections may be used

POTASSIUM: REPLACEMENT IS INDIVIDUALIZED. THE MAJOR ELECTROLYTE NEEDED IS POTASSIUM.

Potassium is started after an adequate urine output is established, after obtaining serum for potassium level and an electrocardiogram (ECG); ECG can be used to monitor the serum potassium level (T-wave changes) (see Chapter 23)

DKA *Potassium* replaced based on plasma K^+ levels; guidelines for adults[68]: if serum K^+ is <3 mEq/L, give K^+ 40 to 60 mEq/hr; if serum K^+ is 3 to 4 mEq/L, give K^+ 30 mEq/hr; if serum K^+ is 4 to 5 mEq/L, give K^+ at 20 mEq/hour; if serum K^+ is 5 to 6 mEq/L, infuse K^+ at 10 mEq/hour; if serum K^+ is greater than 6 mEq/L, withhold K^+ until serum K^+ is less than 6 mEq/L

HHNC Recommended guidelines for *potassium* replacement in HHNC:[68] if serum K^+ is <3 mEq/L, give one dose of K^+ (60 mEq/hr) and recheck; if serum K^+ is 3 to 4 mEq/L, give 40 mEq/hr twice and recheck; if serum K^+ is 4 to 5 mEq/L, give K^+ at 20 mEq/hr; if serum K^+'s greater than 5 mEq/L do not give K^+

OTHER ELECTROLYTES INCLUDE:

DKA *Bicarbonate:* most experts do not recommend bicarbonate for routine use in DKA; if used, give only if arterial pH is <7.0 and patient has other problems such as hypotension, shock, or arrhythmia; give as an infusion of 1 to 2 mEq/kg over 2 hours

Phosphate: hypophosphatemia may occur during treatment; modest reduction in phosphate could result in changes in myocardial, diaphragmatic, and skeletal muscle function; outcome of care has not been shown to be affected by replacement, so not all authorities recommend replacement; if administered, give at rate of 1.5 mEq/kg/24 hr as potassium phosphate; *hyperphosphatemia can cause hypocalcemia*

Magnesium: no recommendation for routine replacement in DKA

HHNC *Phosphate:* phosphate replacement guidelines are the same as those listed for DKA

Magnesium: no recommendation for routine replacement in HHNC; give if serum level is low or signs of tetany are present; deliver 500 ml of 2% $MgSo_4$

OTHER MEASURES MAY INCLUDE:

Nasogastric intubation to prevent vomiting and aspiration if bowel sounds decrease and patient is obtunded; Maintain airway and oxygenation if patient is obtunded;

Monitor cardiovascular function with ECG to assess effects of K^+ on cardiac rhythm and adequacy of replacement and to assess for complications, such as myocardial infarction (MI) or cardiac ischemia, that may have been the precipitating event; monitor fluid status: central venous pressure (CVP), Swan-Ganz catheter, indwelling urinary catheter

TABLE 37-6 Laboratory indexes for evaluating level of control in adults with IDDM[3] or NIDDM[4]

Laboratory Indexes	IDDM: Desired Levels		NIDDM: Desired Levels	
	Adequate	Ideal	Adequate	Ideal
Fasting or premeal glucose	Self-monitored blood glucose (SMBG) 160-200 mg/100 ml	70 to 120 mg/100 ml	Plasma glucose (PG) PG ≤ 140 mg/100 ml	PG ≤ 115 mg/100 ml
2 hour or postmeal glucose	—	SMBG < 180 mg/100 ml	PG ≤ 200 mg/100 ml	PG ≤ 140 mg/100 ml
Glycosylated hemoglobin (GHb) (Normal = 5%-8%); Hemoglobin A_{1c} (HbA_{1c}) (Normal = 4%-6%)	GHb 10.0%-11.0%; HbA_{1c} 8%-9%	GHb 7%-9%; HbA_{1c} 6%-7%	GHb ≤ 10%; HbA_{1c} ≤ 8%	GHb ≤ 8%; HbA_{1c} ≤ 6%
Urine glucose or acetone	Intermittent positive glucose and rare positive ketones	No positive urine glucose or ketones	Essentially no positive urine glucose results	
Fasting plasma cholesterol	—	—	<240 mg/100 ml	<200 mg/100 ml
Fasting plasma triglycerides	—	—	≤200 mg/100 ml	≤150 mg/100 ml

ESTABLISHING DAY-TO-DAY MEDICAL MANAGEMENT PLANS FOR IDDM AND NIDDM

Long-term medical therapy for persons with IDDM or NIDDM consists of the following (in order of priority):

1. Appropriate diet (p. 1109)
2. Appropriate exercise regimen (p. 1113)
3. Appropriate insulin therapy for IDDM (p. 1114) and, if necessary, oral hypoglycemic agents or insulin for NIDDM.

These three phases of a patient's day-to-day management must be regulated together to prevent substantial variations in plasma or blood glucose levels.

MANAGING MANIFESTATIONS OF VASCULAR CHANGES AND NEUROPATHY

Prevention is the major focus of care for long-term manifestations associated with changes in the vascular bed and neuropathy. It is important to remember that for some patients with NIDDM, signs and symptoms of these changes may be the initial manifestations of diabetes mellitus. Table 37-7 summarizes some general medical treatment modalities used for various problems resulting from the vascular changes of neuropathies.

■ ASSESSMENT

Assessment of the patient with IDDM or NIDDM has several focuses, depending on the stage of illness and the reason the patient is seeking health care.

PATIENT WITH ACUTE MANIFESTATIONS

Data to be recorded for the patient with manifestations of acute metabolic alterations or at risk for developing these conditions (such as admitted with associated medical problems) are:

Subjective Data

1. *Neuromuscular:* history of tiredness, lethargy, weakness, headache, visual changes, seizures
2. *Circulation:* history of dizziness, palpitations
3. *Gastrointestinal:* history of polyphagia, nausea, vomiting, thirst, abdominal pain or bloating, weight changes (increases or decreases)
4. *Urinary:* history of polyuria, nocturia, oliguria preceded by polyuria, recurrence of bed-wetting in child
5. *Psychosocial:* perception of the problem, fears, anxieties
6. *Stressors:* history of recent physical or psychological stressors, recent life changes
7. *Others:* history of pruritus, vaginal itching, recurrent or recent infections

Objective Data

1. *Neuromuscular:* level of consciousness, sensory-motor status, reflexes, muscle mass and strength, presence of seizures or tremors, self-care ability
2. *Cardiovascular:* blood pressure (supine and orthostatic), pulse rate and rhythm, jugular vein distention
3. *Respiratory:* ability to maintain adequate airway, respiratory rate and depth, breath odor
4. *Gastrointestinal:* bowel sounds, abdominal distention, weight
5. *Fluid status:* intake and output, tongue appearance, moisture of mucous membranes, skin tur-

TABLE 37-7 Summary of medical treatment for problems related to vascular changes and neuropathies

Problems	Treatment
Cerebrovascular and cardiovascular dysfunction secondary to macrovascular changes (stroke, MI, hypertension)	Same treatment as that prescribed for persons without diabetes; metabolic control of diabetes must be attained for the most effective treatment of problems
Renal insufficiency or failure secondary to diabetic nephropathy	Rigorous control of hypertension to help prevent renal damage; same treatment as that prescribed for persons without diabetes; persons with diabetes placed on peritoneal dialysis may have difficulty with glucose regulation because of glucose in the dialysate Less insulin is usually needed in the presence of renal insufficiency because insulin is excreted more slowly
Pyelonephritis	Same treatment is prescribed as for persons without diabetes
Retinopathy secondary to microvascular changes	Photocoagulation and vitrectomy are prescribed (see Chapter 64); hypertension must be controlled
Cataracts secondary to increased polyol pathways	Same treatment as prescribed for persons without diabetes
Symmetric peripheral polyneuropathy	Treatment is primarily symptomatic, cold compresses at night or capsaicin 0.075% (Axsain) a topical analgesic cream has been used; nonnarcotic analgesics including phenytoin, carbamazepine, and amitriptyline also have been used Aldose-reductase inhibitors (sorbinol), which inhibit formation of sorbitol from glucose, are being tested[3,4,68] Myo-inositol supplements and B vitamins also have been used to prevent or reverse neuropathy, but data are inconclusive[68]
Autonomic neuropathies:	
Sudomotor dysfunction with resultant heat intolerance	Prevention of heatstroke and hyperthermia is necessary
Bladder dysfunction	Bladder is to be emptied regularly (every 3 to 4 hours while awake) Cholinergic stimulation with drug such as bethanechol chloride is advisable Resection of internal bladder sphincter to decrease resistance to emptying has been used
Sexual dysfunction	Females: for lack of lubrication, over-the-counter lubricants; to thicken vaginal walls and decrease dyspareunia, estrogen creams Males: for erection problems, injection of papaverine and phentolamine, which are injected directly into the corpus and cause luminescence for ½ to 2 hours if a rubber band is placed at the base of the penis after injection; yohimbine, an α2-adrenergic blocker, increases blood flow into the corpus and is effective when the problem is vascular in nature; suction (to draw blood into the corpus); penile prosthesis (simple or complex) that require surgery are available
Gastroparesis	For delayed gastric emptying; small, low fiber diets, metoclopramide (Reglan), or bethanechol chloride For constipation (the most frequent GI symptom); stool softeners, laxatives, cathartics, or metoclopramide For diarrhea (from decreased sympathetic inhibition, bacterial overgrowth, pancreatic insufficiency or bile salt malabsorption); antibiotics, bile salt sequestrants, or diphenoxylate hydrochloride and atropine (Lomotil)
Orthostatic hypotension	After identifying cause, therapy may include volume repletion, high salt diet, mineralocorticoid therapy, or waist-high Jobst stockings.
Hypoglycemic unawareness	Rigorous control of blood glucose, if possible; frequent blood glucose checks; avoid hypoglycemia-inducing activities
Diabetic foot	Prevention is the key. For dry gangrene: keep area dry, monitor for infection and extension of gangrene For wet gangrene: bed rest; antibiotic therapy; cleansing and debridement; application of platelet drive growth factors is being tested on many types of ulcers;[51] amputation (see Chapter 70) may be necessary if wet gangrene spreads.

gor, firmness of eyeballs, skin temperature and color, body temperature and weight

6. Others: presence of infection (pulmonary, vaginal, skin, etc.)

STABILIZED NEWLY DIAGNOSED PATIENT

For the stabilized person with newly-diagnosed diabetes, the following assessment data are necessary to establish baselines and for necessary teaching. Because many adults will first be diagnosed when they are already experiencing long-term complications of diabetes mellitus (macrovascular, microvascular, and neurologic changes that affect the cardiovascular system, eyes, gastrointestinal and urinary system, sexual function, feet, and peripheral nerves), the nursing assessment will include data relevant to these complications. (See pages 1097 to 1100 for a detailed discussion of these complications.)

Subjective Data

1. *Psychosocial/emotional:*
   a. Perception of meaning of diagnosis
   b. Expectation of treatment (may include patient's previous experience with persons with diabetes)
   c. Typical day (meal intake and times, work schedule, social activities, hours of sleep, daily exercise)
   d. Identified life stressors
   e. Coping strategies currently used
2. *Knowledge level:* concept of diabetes, manifestations of uncontrolled metabolic state, therapeutic regimen, self-monitoring skills, sick-day guidelines, travel guidelines
3. *Family patterns:* food buying and cooking
4. *Cardiovascular:* drugs, history of blood pressure problems, chest pain or leg pain with exercise
5. *Respiratory:* smoking history
6. *Neuromuscular:* history of changes in vision or speech, dizziness, confusion, headache, or symptoms of neuropathy (tingling, numbness, pain at rest that disappears with activity)
7. *Gastrointestinal:* history of indigestion, dysphagia, weight changes, changes in bowel habits or constipation
8. *Urinary:* history of changes in urinary frequency or incontinence
9. *Sexual function*
   a. Females: menstrual history, history of changes noted with intercourse (if sexually active)
   b. Males: problems with impotence or amount of ejaculate (if sexually active)
10. Insurance, financial security

Objective Data

1. *Emotional/mental:* emotional state, responsiveness, attention, alertness, comprehension, appropriateness of responses
2. *Neuromuscular:*
   a. Eyes: visual acuity (with or without glasses), appearance of retina
   b. Sensory: touch, temperature, pain, vibratory sense (especially of lower extremities), position sense
   c. Motor: range of motion, muscle strength (both upper and lower extremities)
   d. Coordination: dexterity, fine movements
3. *Cardiovascular:* blood pressure, all peripheral pulses
4. *Gastrointestinal:* bowel sounds, weight and height
5. *Urinary:* output and fluid intake
6. *Vagina:* discharge, irritation
7. *Skin:* intactness, temperature, presence of lesions, moisture, hair distribution, texture (especially on lower extremities)

PREVIOUSLY DIAGNOSED PATIENT

For the person with previously diagnosed diabetes who is seen during routine or home visits or is hospitalized, all or parts of the preceding data are collected. It is particularly important to assess for any patient reports consistent with the onset of long-term complications. The person's feet are examined at each visit, and weight is measured. The patient is assessed for presence of new stressors because these can influence diabetic control and management. The patient's adherence to the therapeutic regimen is also assessed. If nonadherence is a problem, it is important to identify the possible cause. Self-management skills may need to be evaluated, but most problems with adherence are the result of knowledge deficits or differences between patient and health team goals.

■ DATA ANALYSIS: NURSING DIAGNOSES

Nursing diagnoses are determined from assessment of patient data. The diagnoses for the person with diabetes mellitus will vary, depending on the stage of the disease. *Possible nursing diagnoses for the person with acute manifestations of diabetes mellitus* may include, but are not limited to, the following:

Diagnostic Title	Possible Etiologies
Activity intolerance	Bedrest; decreased vascular volume associated with increased loss
Cardiac output, alteration in: decreased potential	Electrolyte disturbances especially potassium associated with polyuria
Fatigue	Inadequate nutrients and electrolytes associated with impaired metabolism

Diagnostic Title	Possible Etiologies
Fluid volume deficit	Increased fluid loss and decreased fluid intake
Injury, potential for	Falls, dislodgment of lines, or trauma from seizures associated with altered consciousness
Self-care deficit: total	Impaired consciousness; extreme weakness

Possible nursing diagnoses for the stabilized newly diagnosed patient may include, but are not limited to, the following:

Diagnostic Title	Possible Etiologies
Constipation, potential for	Decreased motility associated with changes in autonomic control of GI tract
Diarrhea, potential for	Increased motility associated with changes in autonomic control of GI tract
Infection, potential for	Depressed immune competence in persons with diabetes
Injury, potential for	Decreased awareness of symptoms of low blood glucose
Knowledge deficit: disease, goals of care, treatment, self-monitoring and care needs	New diagnoses, no previous exposure to information
Nutrition altered: less than required	Alteration in metabolism associated with uncontrolled IDDM
Nutrition altered: more than required	Alterations in metabolism associated with NIDDM
Sensory/perceptual alterations: peripheral, potential	Loss of sensation and decreased circulation to lower extremities associated with uncontrolled hyperglycemia
Sensory/perceptual alterations: visual, potential	Retinal damage associated with uncontrolled hyperglycemia
Sexual dysfunction, potential	Impotence, impaired lubrication, painful intercourse associated with changes in neurologic control of genitalia
Skin integrity impaired, potential	Altered circulation and sensation in feet
Urinary elimination, altered patterns, potential	Changes in bladder control associated with neuropathy; changes in renal function associated with uncontrolled hyperglycemia or elevated blood pressure

If the patient has developed long-term manifestations of a deficiency in insulin or its action, nursing diagnoses identified as potential diagnoses become actual diagnoses. *Additional nursing diagnoses for the previously diagnosed person on follow-up or home visits or on*

readmission to the hospital may include, but are not limited to, the following:

Diagnostic Title	Possible Etiologies
Health maintenance, altered	Worsening physical condition; lack of understanding or acceptance of goals of therapy, lack of material resources
Noncompliance: diet, medication, self-monitoring, return appointments, exercise	Lack of knowledge; disagreement with goals of care; economic resources limited; inability to cope with diagnoses; denial of seriousness of illness
Powerlessness	Feelings inadequate in carrying out the therapeutic regimen
Self-esteem, disturbance	Change in appearance; change in role; change in social involvement

■ PLANNING: EXPECTED PATIENT OUTCOMES

Just as nursing diagnoses may vary, so may patient outcomes. Expected patient outcome for a patient with diabetes mellitus, at various stages, may include, but are not limited to, the following.

PATIENT ADMITTED WITH ACUTE MANIFESTATIONS OF DIABETES MELLITUS

1. Activity tolerance increases gradually; patient takes on one new activity each day
2. Cardiac output is maintained as evidenced by electrolytes returning to normal; blood pressure is maintained
3. Patient is less fatigued
4. Fluid status returns to normal as indicated by a stable blood pressure without orthostatic changes, moist mucous membranes, normal skin turgor
5. No injuries occur as indicated by no falls, line dislogement, or injury with seizures
6. Self-care needs are met

STABILIZED NEWLY DIAGNOSED PATIENT

1. Normal bowel elimination pattern is regained or maintained
2. Signs of infection, if they occur, are recognized early and reported immediately
3. No injuries occur because no undetected hypoglycemic episodes occur
4. An adequate level of knowledge is attained as evidenced by patient or significant others ability to:
   a. Explain the metabolic alterations that occur with diabetes mellitus
   b. Explain signs and symptoms of hyperglycemia and hypoglycemia and what to do when either of these occur
   c. Explain the daily plan of care

d. Describe the medication therapy: type of insulin or hypoglycemic agent, dose, frequency, method of administration, storage of insulin

e. Demonstrate correct technique for insulin administration

f. Test blood and urine accurately and state appropriate course of action based on findings

g. Demonstrate proper foot care

h. State need to carry diabetes identification card or wear Medic Alert bracelet at all times

i. State plan for regular follow-up care

5. For patient with IDDM, gain of 1 to 2 lb/week until at ideal body weight

6. For patient with NIDDM, nutrition is adequate as evidenced by loss of 1 to 2 lb/week until at ideal body weight

7. Undetected changes in peripheral nerve function or peripheral circulation do not develop (if problem occurs, patient can implement safe foot care practices)

8. Undetected changes in vision do not develop (if problem occurs, patient will contact endocrinologist for referral to ophthalmologist for treatment)

9. Undetected changes in sexual functioning do not develop (if sexual dysfunction occurs, patient can state therapeutic measures available)

10. Skin infections or ulcers do not occur (if skin problem occurs, patient can describe the necessary care)

11. Normal urinary elimination is maintained (if decrease occurs, patient will notify physician and can describe causes and care measures)

PREVIOUSLY-DIAGNOSED PATIENT

1. Patient demonstrates adequate health maintenance and compliance, as evidenced by:
   a. Adequate hygiene practices
   b. No signs of overexertion
   c. No episodes of wide fluctuation in recorded blood glucose
   d. Hemoglobin A_{1c} within goal range
   e. Weight that is normal or returning to normal
   f. Serum lipids within goal range
   g. No episodes of hypoglycemia
   h. Intact skin of feet
   i. Appointments kept for regular follow-up care

2. Patient participates in care, makes decisions and choices, and sets priorities, as pertinent

3. Patient demonstrates positive self-esteem

■ IMPLEMENTATION

The nursing care of persons with diabetes mellitus can be categorized into five broad areas: (1) assisting with restoration of metabolic stability in the acutely ill patient, (2) assisting with day-to-day management for the person with IDDM or NIDDM, (3) assisting with prevention of complications or management of complications if they occur, (4) assisting with attainment of self-management skills, and (5) managing the patient during surgery.

The priority of care for the restoration of metabolic stability is dealing with DKA and HHNC if these conditions are present. Assisting with day-to-day management requires that the nurse understand dietary management, principles of exercise, complications and medications. Assisting with prevention or management of complications requires consistent monitoring at follow-up visits and ongoing patient education. Assisting with self-management skills requires helping patients to gain information in ten areas: (1) definition of disease, (2) nutrition, (3) activity and exercise, (4) medication, (5) blood glucose self-monitoring, (6) care for hypoglycemia, (7) handling concurrent illnesses, (8) psychological adjustment, (9) hygiene and foot care, and (10) follow-up care. For these last areas of focus, the nurse will establish priorities for the information presented and help patients gain cognitive knowledge and psychomotor skills. Two more areas of concern to the nurse in assisting with self-management skills include being aware of teaching materials available and of economic issues that affect the person with diabetes mellitus.

The last area of care is related to managing the patient during surgery. Besides the needs discussed in Chapters 20 to 22, the patient with diabetes has special needs, which must be met, to maintain diabetic control.

Each of the above focuses of care is discussed below. There is also a small section about the status of pancreatic and islet transplantation in diabetes mellitus.

ASSISTING WITH ESTABLISHMENT OF METABOLIC STABILITY

For the first 24 to 48 hours, the patient with DKA or HHNC is acutely ill and requires intense nursing care, possibly in an intensive care unit. One of the major nursing strategies is surveillance of:

1. Vital signs at least every hour (more frequently if shock is present)

2. Intake and output every hour

3. Neurologic checks every hour: level of consciousness (LOC), appropriateness of response, and occurrence of other symptoms such as seizures

4. Signs of resolution of dehydration (improved skin turgor, increased moisture of mucous membranes, improved weight, improved urine output, increased blood pressure and decreased pulse) or hyperosmolality (increase in urine output, improved LOC, resolution of facial neurologic signs, lowered serum osmolality), and of acidosis (improved LOC, resolution of Kussmaul's breathing, and improvement in serum bicarbonate and arterial pH)

5. Signs of fluid overload that may occur if patient is overtreated: congested breath sounds, bounding pulse, blood pressure above desired range, decreased mental status

6. Signs of hypoglycemia that may become evident as patient recovers; tachycardia, anxiety, sweating, palpitations, incoherent speech

7. Assessment of CVP, pulmonary wedge pressures, and intra-arterial blood pressure (if these monitoring devices are used)

A flow chart that allows for clear, concise documentation of the assessed parameters needs to be implemented. This flow chart should also have spaces for documentation of laboratory tests (electrolytes, arterial pH, glucose, and ketones). Unexpected results are reported immediately.

The medical management of DKA and HHNC are described in the box on p. 1103. Prescribed fluids, electrolytes, and insulin are administered with care and precision. Any difficulties with maintaining the infusion are reported immediately. Frequent adjustments in the type and amount of fluids may be necessary.

Nursing care during the acute phase must be directed toward maintaining safety and preventing complications associated with the unconscious, immobilized state (see Chapter 60). A nasogastric tube may be inserted if abdominal distention, nausea, and vomiting are present. Any discomfort is usually related to abdominal distention and cramping, which is controlled by the fluid and electrolyte therapy and nasogastric suctioning. Additional care needs are dictated by the factors (such as pneumonia or myocardial infarction) that precipitated the acute crisis.

As soon as the patient is alert and stable, oral fluids are initiated, solid foods are given as tolerated, and normal insulin or oral agent regimen is implemented. The patient must be monitored carefully for tolerance and adequacy of intake and medication. Activities are increased gradually, and rest periods are scheduled between activities.

ASSISTING WITH DAY-TO-DAY MANAGEMENT
NUTRITION

Nutritional management is the keystone of therapy in all types of diabetes mellitus. The dietary needs of the patient are constantly evaluated, and changes are made in the recommendations for nutritional management.

Dietary Recommendations

The current dietary recommendations of the American Diabetes Association (ADA) include:

1. Sufficient calories to promote normal growth and activity in the child with diabetes and to maintain normal weight and activity in the nonobese adult with diabetes

2. Calorie restrictions to promote weight reduction in the obese adult

3. Calorie intake distributed as follows: carbohydrate, 50% to 60%; protein, 20%; fats, 30%

4. Saturated fats limited to 10% monosaturated fats 10% to 15%; polyunsaturated fats up to 10%

5. Dietary cholesterol restricted to < 300 mg/day

6. Limitations of refined sugar

7. Vitamins and minerals, as recommended for the persons without diabetes

Most persons need 25 kilocalories (kcal)/kg of ideal body weight to maintain their weight and meet basic metabolic needs. With this as the basis, kilocalories (kcal) are added or subtracted, based on activity level and need to lose weight (Table 37-8).

Another dietary component that is manipulated is fiber. A high-fiber, high-carbohydrate diet has been shown to decrease insulin requirements and cholesterol, fasting, and postprandial glucose serum levels. Fiber can increase satiety, which might help with weight reduction. Fiber delays gastric emptying and decreases peak blood glucose, so when it is introduced in the diet, blood glucose should be monitored and insulin or any oral agents may need to be adjusted.

This dietary manipulation requires that 15 to 40 g of plant fiber be added to the diet each day.[3,4] The fiber source should be a natural one; not a commercial fiber supplement. Some high-fiber foods are listed in the box on p. 1110. A review of this material reveals that in-

---

TABLE 37-8 Estimating caloric needs, for activity or weight reduction, in adults

Category	Activities	Changes to Basic Metabolic Need*
Light	Ambulating in hospital, washing clothes, walking at 2.5 to 3 miles/hr, carpentry, electrical work, golfing, sailing	Add 5 kcal/ kg of IBW†
Moderate	Weeding and hoeing, bicycling, dancing, tennis, walking 3.5 to 4 miles/hr, scrubbing floors, work involving loading and stocking	Add 10 kcal/ kg of IBW†
Heavy	Climbing, walking uphill with a full load, basketball, football, swimming	Add 15 to 25 kcal/kg of IBW†
Weight reduction		Subtract 5 kcal/ kg of IBW†

*Basic metabolic need = 25 kcal/kg of ideal body weight (IBW)
†Estimated ideal body weight: for *men,* add 6 pounds to 106 for each inch over 5 feet; for *women,* add 5 pounds to 100 for each inch over 5 feet (note: kg = pounds/2.2).

FIBER CONTENT OF SELECTED FOODS

FOOD	SERVING SIZE	FIBER (G)
Breads/Cereals		
100% bran cereal	½ cup	10
Kidney beans	½ cup	4.5
Peas	½ cup	5.2
Potatoes, white	1 small	3.8
Rice, brown	½ cup	1.3
Bread, whole-grain wheat	1 slice	2.7
Fruit		
Apple, uncooked	1 small	3.9
Orange	1 small	2.1
Strawberries	¾ cup	2.4
Peach	1 medium	1.0
Cooked Vegetables		
Beets	½ cup	1.7
Broccoli	½ cup	2.6
Carrots	½ cup	2.2
Lettuce, uncooked	½ cup	0.5

creasing fiber content to the 40 g range takes careful planning.

Research to fully define the benefits of a high-fiber diet[6] and its side effects is ongoing. Fiber should be added gradually to avoid abdominal discomfort, and water intake should be increased. For additional information about this diet, consult reference 6.

Future recommendations for nutritional management may be influenced by the knowledge that foods do not all cause the same rise in blood glucose levels. The term *glycemic index* is used to describe the change in blood glucose levels from ingestion of specific foods. With glucose given a glycemic index of 100%, potatoes, white rice, honey, and carrots have an index of 70% whereas peanuts, lentils, and kidney beans have an index below 30%.[34] The physical form of the food and the combination of nutrients are important factors in the glycemic index. At this time, information about the glycemic index of foods is applied on an individual basis only and has not been incorporated into general recommendations for diabetic diets.

Principles of Dietary Management

If the person with diabetes mellitus has a nutritional history that incorporates the dietary recommendations described in the preceding section, few dietary changes will be needed. The diabetic diet is one that all persons should follow; however, given the dietary habits of most Americans, some dietary changes are usually necessary. Recommendations need to be made with the awareness that eating habits are hard to change.

To be successful, dietary planning must consider:
1. Food preferences and lifestyle (see Chapter 40)
2. Other required dietary modifications such as food consistency or specific nutrient restrictions
3. Activity/rest patterns: amount, timing, and level of exercise; level of activity associated with work; sleep patterns
4. Actions of prescribed hypoglycemic agents (onset, peak, and duration of action)

Calories, carbohydrates, fats, and proteins must be distributed on a consistent basis so that the blood level of nutrients matches the blood level of insulin or any oral hypoglycemic agent. Consistency in timing of meals is also important for the person who needs to lose weight. Distribution of calories over 24 hours with frequent meals helps to prevent large increases in postprandial blood glucose and allows the blood glucose to return to the preprandial level before the next meal regardless of whether the patient is receiving a hypoglycemic agent.

Systems for Learning and Maintaining Dietary Plans

Once the goals of nutritional therapy are established, patients are taught one of several methods for manipulating calories and food.

Exchange system. The exchange system is the most frequently used method. Foods are grouped according to calories, carbohydrate, fat, and protein content into six major groups: milk and milk products, vegetables, fruits, breads and starchy vegetables, meats, and fats. The meats are subdivided, according to fat content, as lean, moderate-, or high-fat. A seventh group includes free foods (see Table 37-9).

The total number of exchanges for each day is determined from the total calorie, carbohydrate, fat, and protein prescription. The number of exchanges is divided into a meal/snack pattern that is consistent with lifestyle and medications. The person selects foods from the appropriate groups according to the distribution of the exchanges in the prescribed meal/snack pattern. Table 37-10 gives examples of meal plans using the exchange system.

Exchange-list values for items sold at popular fast food chains have been published, and there are special cookbooks available. Information about the exchange system is available from hospitals, clinics, physician offices, the local chapter of ADA, and diabetes education literature.

Other measured systems. Another method of dietary management is the *point system*. Foods are assigned points for calorie and carbohydrate, protein, and fat content. The total daily food allowance is written as number of calorie and carbohydrate points and the person is instructed to select foods according to a point distribution. Meat, milk, and fats are included at each meal. Other

TABLE 37-9 Examples of food exchanges[2]

Exchange	Calories	CHO (g)	Protein (g)	Fat (g)
MILK EXCHANGE	80	12	8	trace
1 C skim or nonfat milk				
1 C plain nonfat yogurt				
½ C skim powdered milk				
1 C skim buttermilk				
1 C lowfat 2% yogurt	120	12	8	5
1 C lowfat (2%) milk				
VEGETABLE EXCHANGE* (NONSTARCHY)	28	5	2	—
½ C cooked, 1 C raw				
beets, carrots, brussel sprouts, onions, sauerkraut, eggplant, asparagus, cabbage, celery, green or wax beans, or mustard greens				
1 medium tomato				
FRUIT EXCHANGE	60	15	—	—
1 small apple, orange, peach, tangerine, or pear				
½ C applesauce				
½ banana or grapefruit				
⅓ cantaloupe				
⅛ honeydew melon				
BREAD EXCHANGE (INCLUDES STARCHY VEGETABLES)	80	15	3	trace
1 slice bread				
½ bagel, 1 tortilla				
½ hamburger bun				
½ small baked potato				
⅓ C corn, ½ C peas				
½ C oatmeal				
½ C cooked pasta				
⅓ C rice				
6 saltines				
MEAT EXCHANGE				
Lean Meat	55	—	7	3
1 oz lean beef, pork, veal, or poultry without skin				
2 oz fish				
¼ C dry cottage cheese				
¼ C tuna, mackerel				
1 oz diet cheese (<55 calories/oz)				
Medium-Fat Meat	75	—	7	5
1 oz 15%-fat beef, boiled ham, or liver				
1 egg†				
High-Fat Meat	100	—	7	8
1 oz 20%-fat beef, ground pork, duck, or regular cheeses				
1 frankfurter				
1 oz lunchmeat				
1 T peanut butter (contains unsaturated fats)				
Fat Exchange‡	45	—	—	5
1 t margarine				
⅛ avocado				
1 t oil				
1 strip crisp bacon				
1 t regular mayonnaise				
1 T reduced-calorie mayonnaise				
1 T cream cheese				
Free Exchanges	—	—	—	—
Unsweetened gelatin				
Calorie-free beverages				
Coffee, tea, spices, bouillon				

*Some vegetables, such as lettuce, raw spinach, radishes, and watercress, can be used as desired.
†Eggs and other foods high in cholesterol need to be restricted.
‡Margarine and oil should be made from corn, cottonseed, safflower, soy, or sunflower oil.

TABLE 37-10 Sample of two menu plans using the exchange list*

Exchanges	Menu I	Menu II
	BREAKFAST	**BREAKFAST**
1 Fruit	½ Glass orange juice	½ Grapefruit
1 Milk (skim)	1 Glass skim milk	1 Glass skim milk
1 Meat (medium-fat)	1 Egg, poached	1 Scrambled egg
3 Bread	2 Toast, ½ C oatmeal	1 English muffin, ½ C bran flakes
2 Fat	2 t Margarine	2 t Margarine
	LUNCH	**LUNCH**
1 Fruit	½ Banana	1 Peach
1 Milk (skim)	1 Glass skim milk	1 Glass skim milk
2 Meat (lean)	Tuna salad sandwich (½ C water-packed tuna	1 MacDonald's cheeseburger (2 bread, 2 meat, 1
2 Bread	with celery, 2 slices of bread, 3 t mayonnaise	fat)
3 Fat	and lettuce)	1 Lettuce salad with 2 T French dressing
	AFTERNOON SNACK	**AFTERNOON SNACK**
1 Bread	6 Saltine crackers	¾ oz Pretzels
1 Fruit	1 Pear	15 Grapes
	DINNER	**DINNER**
1 Fruit	¾ C strawberries	½ C Applesauce
2 Vegetable (non-starchy)	1 C green beans	Sliced tomatoes
4 Meat (lean)	4 oz Round steak	4 oz Chicken
1 Milk (skim)	1 Glass skim milk	1 Glass skim milk
2 Bread	1 Small baked potato	⅓ C Rice
—	1 Roll	1 Slice bread
3 Fat	2 T Sour cream/2 t margarine	3 t Margarine
	EVENING SNACK	**EVENING SNACK**
1 Bread	3 Rye wafers	6 Saltine crackers
1 Milk	1 C Nonfat yogurt	1 Glass skim milk

*Distributed over three meals and two snacks. Diet based on 2100 calories with 48% CHO (253 g); 31% fats (71 g); 21% protein (112 g).

methods that may be taught are the *percent of carbohydrate system* and the *calculation of dietary intake from tables of food values system.*

Rigid menu plan. Some individuals who have difficulty with the systems described above are given a rigid menu plan that states the amount and type of food to eat or drink at each meal and snack. For example, the breakfast plan could be: ½ grapefruit, 1 C oatmeal, 1 slice toast with 1 t margarine, 1 C 2% milk, and coffee. This system is used until the person is ready for more independence.

Unmeasured diets. Some physicians prescribe unmeasured diets, particularly for young persons with diabetes. Guidelines for this approach include:
1. Distribute meals and snacks to meet requirements of lifestyle and medications.
2. Eat sufficient food to satisfy appetite.
3. Select foods from all food categories.
4. Restrict sweets; some sweets may be taken as prescribed.

Dietetic Foods, Sweeteners, and Alcohol

The diabetic diet does *not* require the use of special or dietetic foods. The unrestricted use of dietetic or diabetic candy or cookies cannot be allowed because, although these foods are sugar-free, they contain calories from other basic ingredients.

Various sweeteners other than sugar are available in the United States, including saccharin, fructose, sorbitol, and aspartame. All of these sweeteners, except saccharin, have a nutritive value of approximately 4 kcal/gm. *Aspartame,* because of its excessive sweetness, is used in such small quantities that its caloric value can usually be ignored. *Fructose* is a natural sugar found in many fruits. Because it is absorbed slowly and because part of its metabolism does not depend on insulin, it has been proposed as a sweetener for persons with diabetes mellitus. However, because part of its metabolism requires insulin and because it yields 4 kcal/g when metabolized, fructose must be calculated into the dietary prescription. *Sorbitol* may be found in certain prepared foods. It is metabolized to fructose in the liver; therefore, the precautions described for fructose apply. Excessive sorbitol can lead to diarrhea from slow gastrointestinal absorption.

Alcohol does not furnish carbohydrate, protein, or fat; but it yields 7 kcal/g when metabolized and must be included in caloric calculations if weight loss is necessary. Some alcohol may be permitted, but the patient must be instructed about the caloric value of pure alcohol; the high carbohydrate content of beer, cordials, wine, and mixed drinks; the inhibiting effect of alcohol on gluconeogenesis with the possible precipitation of hypoglycemia, and the alcohol-induced increase in triglyceride levels.[4] Hypoglycemia is especially common if alcohol is taken while fasting, particularly in the person with diabetes who may have insulin available from a prior injection.[3,4]

Additional Nursing Activities Related to Dietary Plan

Facilitating nutritional therapy for the hospitalized person with diabetes mellitus also includes:

1. Helping the patient eat according to the dietary plan.
2. Monitoring and recording food intake.
3. Providing substitutes for refused food.
4. Coordinating care so a patient's food is not delayed or omitted.
5. Obtaining foods the patient can tolerate if nauseous or vomiting.
6. Monitoring patient for effectiveness of dietary management (attainment or maintenance of weight goal, stable blood glucose, and patient satisfaction with diet).

EXERCISE

Exercise is as important for the person with diabetes as for the person without diabetes. In addition to cardiorespiratory conditioning, enhancement of work capacity, and improvement in sense of well-being, the person with diabetes may benefit from better blood glucose control. Exercise increases the uptake of glucose by active muscle cells without the need for insulin and can increase tissue sensitivity to insulin. Overall, exercise has a hypoglycemic effect. In obese persons, exercise can help in weight loss. Exercise by persons with diabetes, particularly if they are on insulin or an oral hypoglycemic agent, must consider the dietary plan and medications. Fair-to-good metabolic control should be achieved before starting an exercise program.[3,4]

Before the program is started, the person should have a complete cardiovascular examination, including a stress electrocardiogram (ECG) if over age 40 or if a history of cardiovascular disease is present. Working capacity should be evaluated to determine the level of exercise that can be instituted safely. Persons with diabetes mellitus should also be evaluated for presence of proliferative retinopathy, neuropathy, and hypertension,

---

GUIDELINES FOR EXERCISE PROGRAM OF THE PERSON WITH DIABETES MELLITUS

Exercise type: aerobic, start with light level
Exercise session: each session should include:
1. 5 to 10 minutes of warm-up stretching and limbering exercises
2. 20 to 30 minutes of aerobic exercise with heart rate in target zone (75% to 80% of maximal heart rate)
3. 15 to 20 minutes of light exercise and stretching to cool down

Exercise frequency: three to five times/week
Special precautions:
1. Carry ID card or wear bracelet identifying wearer as having diabetes mellitus and stating what to do if person is acting abnormally
2. Monitor self, during and after exercise, for hypoglycemia (may include blood glucose self-monitoring, at least at start of exercise program)
3. Carry a source of easily absorbed carbohydrate
4. Avoid dehydration
5. Consult professional (podiatrist) about footwear for planned exercise
6. Exercise when blood sugar is highest (1 to 3 hours after meals)
7. For regular, planned exercise, a decrease in insulin may be prescribed*
8. Consume extra carbohydrate before, during, or after exercise; need is dictated by blood glucose level, any reduction of insulin, length and level of exercise, presence of symptoms of hypoglycemia, and whether exercise was planned or spontaneous

Precautions for selected persons:
1. Persons with insensitive feet should avoid running and jogging and choose cycling or swimming
2. Persons with proliferative retinopathy should avoid exercises associated with Valsalva maneuver that cause jarring and jolting of head or exercises with head in low position
3. Persons with hypertension should avoid exercises associated with Valsalva maneuvers and exercises involving intense exercise of the torso and arms (exercises involving the lower extremities are preferred)

*Protocols on how to decrease insulin dose are described in references 3 and 4.

---

because special precautions are necessary for these persons. General guidelines for an exercise program are listed in the box above.

MEDICATIONS

Insulin is necessary for every person with IDDM; insulin or oral hypoglycemic agents may be necessary for some patients with NIDDM.

TABLE 37-11 Action of insulin preparations

Type of Insulin	Time of Onset (hr)	Peak of Action (hr)	Duration of Action (hr)	Insulin Appearance
RAPID-ACTING				
Regular	<1	2-4	4-6	Clear
Crystalline zinc	<1	2-4	4-6	Clear
Semilente	<1	4-7	12-16	Cloudy
INTERMEDIATE-ACTING				
NPH	1-4	8-14	16-20	Cloudy
Globin zinc	2-4	6-10	12-18	Clear
Lente	1-4	8-14	16-20	Cloudy
LONG-ACTING				
Protamine zinc	4-8	16-18	36+	Cloudy
Ultralente	4-8	8-20	36+	Cloudy

Insulin

Properties of insulin. Four properties of insulin preparations may be identified in the prescription: type of action, strength, species source, and purity.

Type of action. All insulins are hypoglycemic, but they differ in: speed of effect *(onset),* time of greatest action *(peak),* and how long they act *(duration).* Insulins are classified as rapid-, intermediate-, and long-acting (Table 37-11). Food and activity must be coordinated with insulin action so that (1) insulin is available when food is eaten and absorbed for optimal metabolism, and (2) food is available while insulin is acting to prevent hypoglycemic reactions.

Three principles are useful in coordinating food and hypoglycemic medications:
1. Food must be taken after insulin within the time of onset; for example, with regular insulin food must be taken within 1 hour after injection, but regular insulin should be given 30 minutes before meals so it is available with the food.
2. Intermediate- or long-acting insulin requires that a supplemental feeding be timed to match the peak action of the insulin; for example, a 4 PM feeding after a 7 AM injection of NPH insulin.
3. Intermediate- or long-acting insulin given at bedtime requires a bedtime snack.

Strength. Insulin preparations vary in the concentration of insulin units in 1 ml volume. The strength most frequently used is U-100 insulin, or 100 U/ml. A low-dose syringe that contains only a 0.3 or 0.5 ml volume is available for U-100 insulin. It is designed so that the outside length of the syringe is the same as that of 1 ml syringe, but the lumen is smaller; therefore, the lines for the individual units are easier to read. In *insulin resistance,* a rare condition in which daily insulin doses exceed 100 units, U-500 insulin may be ordered. It is very important that the insulin concentrations and the insulin syringe calibration match in units per milliliter to prevent errors in dosing (Figure 37-4).

Species. Insulin antigenicity can decrease insulin receptor effectiveness. In the past, most insulin was prepared from a combination of beef and pork pancreata. Single-species insulin (usually pork) could be obtained for patients with beef-insulin allergy or antibodies. Pork insulin most closely resembles human insulin and is considered the least antigenic animal insulin. Several single-species pork or beef preparations have been marketed and are used to decrease insulin antibody formation.

"Human" insulin is now available for use in the United States; it is either porcine (pork insulin modified enzymatically to structurally resemble human insulin) or bacterially produced, using recombinant deoxyribonucleic acid (DNA) techniques. Human insulin has less antigenicity than animal insulin, and it greatly expands the insulin resources of the world. Human insulin is available as regular, lente, NPH, and ultralente, but its onset, peak, and duration are slightly different than that of animal insulin, so the patient's insulin should not be changed from one species to another on a random basis.

The variety of short-acting insulins available are listed in Table 37-12. Many varieties of intermediate and long-acting insulins are also available.

Purity. Over time, manufacturers have improved the purity of insulin preparations, but standard (single-peak) insulins may contain small amounts of proinsulin-like substances and other antigenic substances (for example, glucagon-like, pancreatic polypeptides). Insulins labeled "highly purified" (single component) that are now being marketed contain less than 10 parts per million (PPM) of antigenic substances and are recommended for persons with newly diagnosed diabetes, insulin allergy, or insulin lipodystrophy and when intermittent insulin therapy is required.

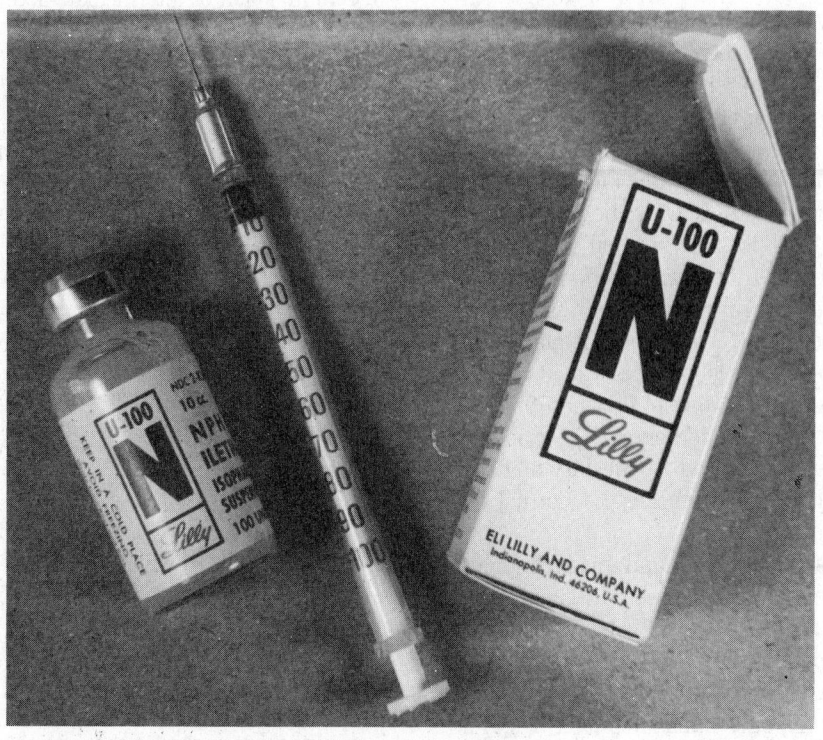

FIGURE 37-4 U-100 Iletin II NPH insulin and disposable U-100 insulin syringe.

TABLE 37-12 Species of regular insulins available in the United States

Product	Beef/Pork	Beef	Pork	Porcine	Human Recombinant DNA
Iletin II, Regular (Lilly)		√	√		
Regular Purified Pork (Squibb-Novo)			√		
Velosulin (Nordisk-USA)			√		
Semilente Purified Pork (Squibb-Novo)			√		
Iletin 1, Regular (Lilly)	√				
Regular (Squibb-Novo)			√		
Iletin 1, Semilente (Lilly)	√				
Semilente (Squibb-Novo)		√			
Humulin R (Lilly)					√
Novolin R (Regular) (Squibb-Novo)				√	
Velosulin Human (Regular) (Nordisk-USA)				√	

From Long B and Phipps WJ: Medical-surgical nursing, ed 2, St Louis, 1989, The CV Mosby Co.

Because of the many changes being made in insulin preparations, the nurse must clarify the insulin prescription if the type, strength, purity, or species is unclear. A change in any one of the properties may lead to differences in action. When the insulin prescription is changed, careful patient monitoring is necessary to identify the extent of clinical effect.

Insulin regimens. Insulin therapy may include various regimens.[61,80] In persons with IDDM, the goal is usually to mimic, as closely as possible, normal endogenous insulin secretion patterns. In persons without diabetes there is a meal-related increase in insulin secretion, with basal secretion between meals. There is also a tendency for glucose to reach its lowest peak at 3 to 4 AM and for basal insulin secretion to rise, between 5 and 8 AM, *before* breakfast (dawn phenomenon). Descriptions of various regimens are presented in the box at right, regimens 3 to 6 are designed to mimic the normal endogenous secretion pattern.

Each regimen has advantages and disadvantages. *Regimen 3* requires only two injections, but because intermediate-acting insulin peaks 8 to 12 hours after administration, it may peak during the night. This peak, along with the normal 3 to 4 AM drop in blood glucose, may cause nocturnal hypoglycemia. *Regimen 4* should lessen the chance of nocturnal hypoglycemia and provide better coverage for the normal pre-breakfast rise (dawn phenomenon) of blood glucose, but requires three injections. Neither of these regimens allow flexibility in *meal size* or *time;* the person must eat on time or hypoglycemia can occur. For example, the morning intermediate-acting insulin will begin working in 1 to 4 hours and peak in 8 to 14 hours so that, if food is not provided at lunchtime, a hypoglycemic reaction can occur.

Regimen 5 requires four injections per day, but allows flexibility in meal size because the dose of rapid-acting insulin can be increased or decreased on the basis of the planned meal. Meals should still be on a relatively consistent basis so that insulin is taken on a consistent basis because there is no basal insulin coverage during the day. The preprandial insulin must be taken an adequate time (usually 30 minutes) *before* meals to prevent postprandial hyperglycemia. *Regimen 6* allows the same flexibility in meal size as regimen 5. It also allows flexibility in meal time, because basal insulin coverage is provided between meals by the long-acting insulin. The preprandial insulin must still be taken an *adequate time before meals* to prevent postprandial hyperglycemia. With regimen 6 there can be a large subcutaneous depot of long-acting insulin available all the time; if something occurs that increases absorption or if a meal is missed completely, hypoglycemia can occur.

Regimens 3 through 6 (particularly 5 and 6) require

INSULIN THERAPY REGIMENS

1. One injection of intermediate-acting insulin per day
   a. Most frequently used in persons with NIDDM who are not controlled with diet and/or oral hypoglycemic agents
   b. Does not mimic the normal endogenous pattern
2. Two injections of intermediate-acting insulin per day
   a. Also used mostly in persons with NIDDM
   b. Does not mimic the normal endogenous pattern
3. Split and mixed insulin regimen: injection of rapid-acting insulin and intermediate-acting insulin at breakfast and supper
   a. Used in many persons with IDDM and some with NIDDM
   b. Theoretically, the morning rapid-acting insulin covers breakfast and early morning, the morning intermediate-acting insulin covers lunch and afternoon, the evening rapid-acting insulin covers the evening meal, and the evening intermediate-acting insulin covers the bedtime snack, the *basal level needed* during the night, and the normal prebreakfast rise (dawn phenomenon) in glucose
4. Split and mixed insulin regimens similar to no. 3 above, except that the evening intermediate-acting insulin is given at bedtime instead of at the evening meal
   a. Used in persons with IDDM and some with NIDDM
   b. Theoretically provides better basal nighttime coverage and provides coverage for the natural pre-breakfast glucose elevation (dawn phenomenon)
5. Multidosage regimen: three injections of rapid-acting insulin, one before each meal; one injection of intermediate insulin at bedtime
   a. The rapid-acting insulin provides coverage for each meal
   b. The bedtime intermediate-acting insulin provides the nighttime basal level and coverage for the natural pre-breakfast glucose elevation (dawn phenomenon)
6. Multidose regimen: three injections of rapid-acting insulin, one before each meal; one injection of long-acting insulin at breakfast or at supper, or split between breakfast and supper (provides the same coverage as no. 5 above)

---

frequent blood glucose self-monitoring, before and after meals, to determine how much insulin is needed. An algorithm is usually developed for the patient using regimen 5 or 6, and, although adherence to this algorithm will increase metabolic control, it requires a large investment of the patient's time and interest *every day.* Regimens 5 and 6, because they provide tighter control, also predispose the patient to hypoglycemia. Algorithms also may be developed for patients on regimens 3 and 4.

Insulin pump. Use of a portable infusion pump (Figure 37-5) to deliver insulin continuously can mimic a physiologic state. The pump is programed to deliver a basal level of *rapid-acting insulin continuously,* with the basal level varied so that it is lower from 12 midnight to

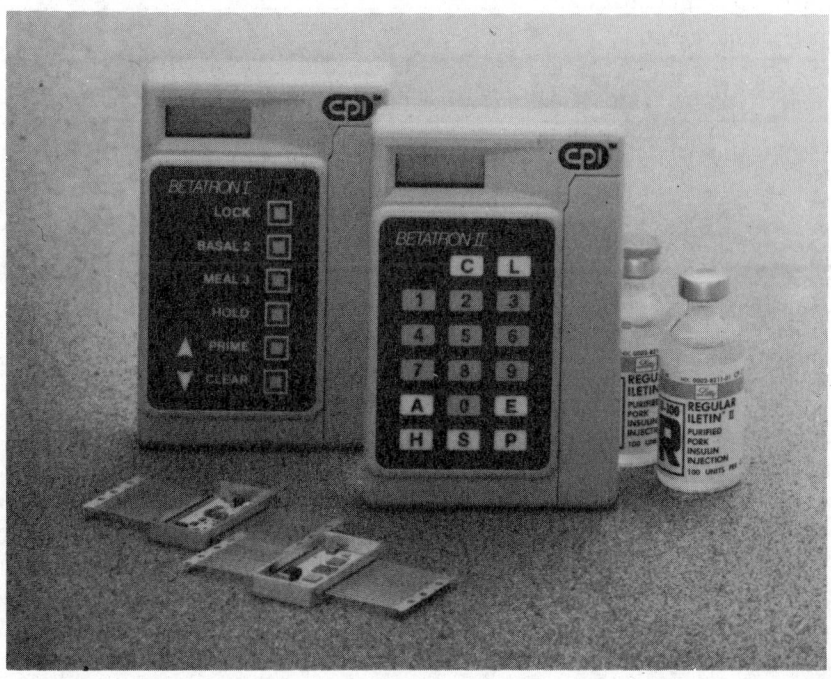

FIGURE 37-5 Insulin infusion pumps. (Courtesy Cardiac Pacemakers, Inc St Paul, Minn) (From Long B, and Phipps W: Medical surgical nursing, ed 2, St Louis, 1989, The CV Mosby Co.)

4 AM, when glucose is naturally dropping, and higher from 5 to 9 AM, when glucose is normally increasing, and is manually activated to deliver a bolus of rapid-acting insulin in the preprandial period (the bolus must be taken an adequate time *before* a meal).

The use of an insulin pump prevents multiple injections (injection site is changed every 48 hours) and prevents the subcutaneous deposit of insulin that provides 24-hour basal coverage with regimen 6.

The pump allows flexibility in meal size and time. It requires intensive self-monitoring of blood glucose, adherence to an algorithm that requires an intense investment of the patient's time and interest, and wearing of the pump at all times. Interest, time, and repeated practice are required to learn how to program the pump. The pump has an alarm that informs the person if the battery is low, if insulin is infusing too rapidly, or if there is an occlusion in the line. Pumps are expensive, but some insurance policies reimburse the expense.

Oral Hypoglycemic Agents

Oral hypoglycemic agents are used in treating persons with NIDDM who are not controlled by diet and exercise. These agents are not insulin; to refer to them as oral insulin is a misnomer.

Six oral hypoglycemic agents are currently used in the United States. The half-life, duration of action, and dose range vary (Table 37-13). These agents are all sulfonylureas, which are thought to help control hyperglycemia by (1) increasing the ability of the islet cells of the pancreas to secrete insulin, and (2) increasing the insulin sensitivity of extrapancreatic tissues.

Persons taking oral hypoglycemic agents need to adhere to the prescribed doses, and the prescribed diet, maintain the usual amount of exercise, carry out prescribed self-monitoring and take general health precautions.

Because of a study conducted in the 1970s by the University Group Diabetes Program (UGDP), much controversy has surrounded the use of these agents. The researchers in this study reported that the death rate from cardiovascular disease was two and one-half times higher in persons receiving tolbutamide than in those receiving a placebo. The results of the UGDP study have been challenged by numerous groups, but the FDA recommends that oral hypoglycemic agents be limited to persons with symptomatic NIDDM that cannot be adequately controlled by diet or weight loss alone, and in whom the addition of insulin to the therapeutic regimen is impractical or unacceptable.

Oral hypoglycemic agents are not to be used in treating persons with IDDM or GDM. The sulfonylureas are metabolized by the kidneys and liver; thus the person with liver and kidney dysfunction may be at higher risk for development of side effects, particularly hypoglycemia.

Complications of oral hypoglycemic agents, besides hypoglycemia, include allergic skin reactions, gastrointestinal distress, and hematologic disorders. Chlor-

TABLE 37-13 Oral hypoglycemic agents

Drugs	Trade Names	Half-Life (hrs)	Duration of Action (hrs)	Dosage Range
Acetohexamide	Dymelor	5-8	12-24	500 mg-1.5 gm
Chlorpropamide	Diabinese	36	24-48	100 mg-500 mg
Tolazamide	Tolinase	7	12-24	100 mg-1 gm
Tolbutamide	Orinase	4-6	6-12	500 mg-3 gm
Glipizide	Glucotrol	2-4	12-24	5 mg-40 mg
Glyburide	Micronase	10	24	2.5 mg-20 mg

propamide causes water retention and dilutional hyponatremia. These complications are rare, but hypoglycemic reactions that result from oral hypoglycemic agents may take several days to resolve because of the long duration of action of these drugs and the blood levels that will be present for some time.

Many drugs interact with oral hypoglycemic agents and can potentiate, prolong, or shorten the action of the agents. A pharmacist or physician is consulted if drug interactions are suspected.

Some patients with NIDDM may be treated with a combination of insulin and oral agents. Theoretically, the oral agents should increase the patient's tissue sensitivity to both endogenous and exogenous insulin. This therapeutic regimen is still experimental, but if proven to be effective, it may be used more frequently.[4]

Complications of Medications

Insulin hypersensitivity and resistance. Insulin hypersensitivity occurs in some patients. Most reactions are local, consisting of *wheals* at injection sites, but systemic symptoms and *anaphylactic reactions* can occur. The hypersensitivity may be the result of several factors, including improper injection technique, sensitivity to the alcohol used to prepare the skin, sensitivity to the modifying proteins in the insulin, or sensitivity to the species source.

Treatment for hypersensitivity varies depending on the cause. Improper technique or hypersensitivity to the alcohol is ruled out first, proper injection technique is ensured, then a more purified form of alcohol or a different antiseptic agent is used to prepare the skin. If the modifying protein in the insulin is thought to be the causative factor, the patient may be switched from NPH to lente insulin. If the species source is thought to be the cause, the patient is switched to another species source. Single-component insulin may also be used. If the hypersensitivity is severe, an antihistamine may be given to treat the symptoms until the allergic response disappears. Corticosteroids may be used for severe reactions. If the patient is found to be allergic to all types of insulin, desensitization may be necessary.

Insulin resistance, defined as an insulin requirement greater than 200 U/day for a period longer than 2 days in the absence of infection or other factors that would increase insulin need, can also occur. The etiology of insulin resistance is unknown, but is thought to be the result of the development of antibodies that render insulin inactive. All patients who have been on insulin for 6 weeks to 3 months develop some antibodies to insulin. Usually these antibodies are not sufficient to interfere with the response to insulin and the control of diabetes.

Insulin resistance may be treated by a different species of insulin or by single-peak and single-component insulin. In some instances, adrenocorticotropic hormone (ACTH) or adrenal glucocorticoids may be used for short-term treatment. In most instances, insulin resistance is self-limiting. For this reason, some physicians do not use adjunctive therapy such as steroids; instead, they treat the patient with higher doses of insulin during the period of resistance. When high doses of insulin are used to treat insulin resistance, the patient must be monitored carefully for hypoglycemia; the dose will need to be decreased when the resistance period passes.

Hypoglycemia. Hypoglycemia (frequently defined as a plasma glucose level < 50 mg/100 ml) is a major complication of insulin therapy or oral hypoglycemic agents. Hypoglycemia is caused by an excess of insulin or oral hypoglycemic agent in relation to food intake or energy expenditure (see the box below).

The signs and symptoms of hypoglycemia (see the

CAUSES OF HYPOGLYCEMIA FROM EXOGENOUS INSULIN OR ORAL HYPOGLYCEMIC AGENT

1. Excessive dose of insulin or oral hypoglycemic agent or prolonged action of these drugs
2. Too little food intake (meal delayed or skipped), delayed gastric emptying, vomiting, or diarrhea
3. Excessive exercise in relation to food intake and insulin or oral hypoglycemic agent doses
4. Unknown causes

SIGNS AND SYMPTOMS OF HYPOGLYCEMIA

SYMPATHETIC NERVOUS SYSTEM ACTIVITY

Pallor	Palpitation	Weakness*
Perspiration*	Nervousness*	Trembling
Piloerection	Irritability	Hunger
Tachycardia		

CENTRAL NERVOUS SYSTEM ACTIVITY

Headache	Fatigue
Blurred vision	Numbness of lips, tongue
Diplopia	Mental confusion*
Incoherent speech	Convulsions
Emotional changes	Coma

*Signs most commonly reported by patients.[64]

CARBOHYDRATES (10 TO 15 G) FOR RELIEF OF HYPOGLYCEMIA

½ C pure fruit juice
½ C sugar carbonated soda drink
½ C regular gelatin dessert
4 cubes or 2 packets sugar
2 squares graham crackers
2 to 3 pieces of hard candy

---

box above) can be related to two factors: increased sympathetic nervous system activity and the deprivation of CNS glucose supply. The exact signs and symptoms seen in a particular individual vary with the rapidity of the drop in blood glucose level and the duration of hypoglycemia. A *rapid* drop in plasma glucose results primarily in manifestations from increased sympathetic nervous system activity. In *slow-developing* hypoglycemia, as might be seen with long-acting insulin or with oral hypoglycemia agents, the CNS signs and symptoms predominate. If a rapid drop occurs and is allowed to persist, all signs and symptoms usually occur.

Hypoglycemia may occur during sleep, particularly in persons on multidose insulin regimens, and the only symptoms may be nightmares, sweating, and headache upon arising. Nighttime hypoglycemia may be part of the *Somogyi phenomenon*.

Patients with diabetes mellitus who are treated with β-adrenergic antagonists may be at special risk for hypoglycemia. The β-adrenergic agents block or inhibit the appearance of early signs and symptoms of hypoglycemia by blocking the sympathetic nervous system. In addition, these drugs prevent or block gluconeogenesis and glycolysis, thus inhibiting the normal endogenous response to hypoglycemia, making it harder to reverse the problem.

Signs and symptoms similar to those of hypoglycemia may occur when the blood glucose level is elevated and drops rapidly to a level that *is still in an elevated range*. The sudden rapid drop in blood sugar, regardless of the final level reached or the levels at which this occurs, is a stimulus for the physiologic neuroendocrine response to stressors to come into play. Thus, a patient whose glucose level drops from 500 mg/100 ml to 300 mg/100 ml very rapidly may demonstrate the same signs and symptoms as a patient whose glucose drops to 30 mg/100 ml. Patients with uncontrolled diabetes may complain of feeling hypoglycemic, even though their plasma glucose

levels are high. The patient is often labeled as "a malingerer" or "uncooperative" because health team members may believe that the patient is trying to obtain more food. The nurse who is aware of the above phenomena may be able to help others understand the patient's complaints and help avoid such labeling.

The treatment for hypoglycemia is fast-acting carbohydrates. If a question exists about the validity of the diabetic's feelings about an impending hypoglycemic reaction, blood should be drawn immediately for a blood glucose test and *sugar given at once*. The nurse should understand that, when in doubt, it is always safer to give sugar than to risk nervous system damage from hypoglycemia. Usually 10 to 15 g of carbohydrate will be sufficient to overcome hypoglycemia (see the box above). If the individual is already unconscious, 50% glucose will usually be given intravenously. *When the person's symptoms have cleared, a snack consisting of complex carbohydrates and proteins* such as cheese or peanut butter and crackers should be given. If the next meal is due soon, it can be eaten instead of the snack.

Glucagon, a pancreatic hormone that acts primarily by mobilizing hepatic glycogen, may be given to treat insulin reaction. The effects of this glycogen conversion last about 1½ hours; therefore, treatment with sugar, complex carbohydrates, and proteins will also be required to prevent a recurrence of the hypoglycemia. Glucagon is given intramuscularly, and some physicians instruct their patients to take it when an insulin reaction occurs. If the patient is unconscious, the family administers the drug and then seeks medical assistance.

The patient who develops hypoglycemia while taking oral hypoglycemic agents may need treatment for several days, and hospitalization may be mandatory. These patients may need dextrose infusion and glucocorticoids to promote gluconeogenesis along with the other therapy. The reason any hypoglycemic period is serious is that it interferes with the oxygen consumption of nervous tissue. Repeated or prolonged attacks can cause irreparable brain damage.

Somogyi phenomenon. The Somogyi phenomenon is a reaction characterized by alternating hypoglycemic re-

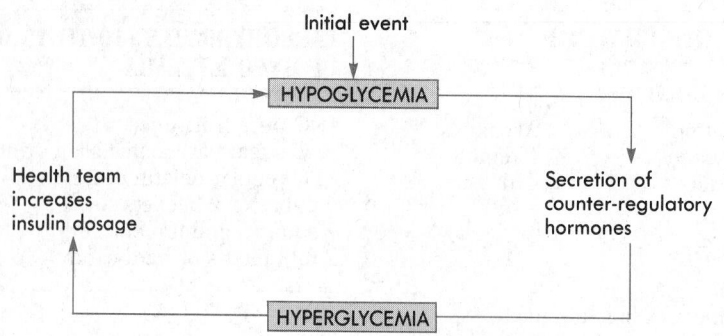

FIGURE 37-6 Sequence of events in the Somogyi phenomenon.

actions and periods of hyperglycemia. This phenomenon is most frequently seen during initial periods of blood glucose regulation. The person being treated with intermediate- or long-acting insulin may experience hypoglycemia at peak times of insulin activity. As is true with healthy persons without diabetes, hypoglycemia in persons with diabetes stimulates the production of counterregulatory hormones (glucagon, glucocorticoids, growth hormone, and epinephrine). These hormones promote glycogenolysis and gluconeogenesis. In normal persons the blood glucose level is brought only to the normal range because, as it is elevated, insulin secretion is stimulated and the blood glucose level lowered. In persons with diabetes, the blood glucose goes to abnormally high levels because insulin secretion does not respond in the normal way. In some instances, the signs and symptoms of hypoglycemia are not obvious enough to be detected. In some instances, the hypoglycemia occurs at night and is undetected; hyperglycemia following the hypoglycemia is recognized in the early morning and may be mistaken for the dawn phenomenon. The assumption is made that the patient needs higher doses of insulin, but this treatment worsens the problem. Figure 37-6 illustrates this cycle.

The signs and symptoms of the Somogyi phenomenon can be any of those normally associated with hypoglycemia, but frequently they consist only of nighttime sweats, nightmares, and a headache on arising. There may be weight gain in the presence of glycosuria, relatively normal blood glucose with positive ketones (remember that counterregulatory hormones stimulate lipolysis and β-oxidation of fats), and wide fluctuations in blood glucose unrelated to meals.

Treatment consists of decreasing insulin dose. A primary nursing role is to document complaints of hypoglycemia, glucose intake, and laboratory results, and to look for complaints of night sweats, nightmares, and early morning headaches. The nurse should also correlate these complaints and laboratory results with the times of meals. Such data will help to identify the phenomenon.

ASSISTING WITH MANAGEMENT OF VASCULAR CHANGES AND NEUROPATHIES

Nurses working with persons with diabetes mellitus will, at some time, assist with the institution of therapy needed for management of macrovascular or microvascular changes or neuropathies. Patients with these problems may be seen in an ambulatory setting or in various clinical areas of the hospital. Nursing activities for persons with these problems may include:

1. Teaching about and assisting with necessary diagnostic tests, such as eye examinations, nerve conduction studies, or vascular studies
2. Giving prescribed treatments
3. Assisting with incorporating new medications into daily care
4. Monitoring diabetic status (glucose control) carefully and assisting with changes in the therapeutic plan
5. Teaching self-management skills, as pertinent

The management goal is to keep the patient in "good" metabolic control, since this greatly influences recovery from complications such as foot ulcers and cardiovascular problems and may help to prevent progression of vascular changes and neuropathies.

ASSISTING THE PERSON TO GAIN SELF-MANAGEMENT SKILLS

A major responsibility of the professional nurse is helping persons gain self-management skills for any chronic health problem through teaching and counseling. Self-management skills are probably the major determinant of how well the health problem is controlled and the quality of life maintained. This is particularly true for persons with diabetes mellitus. Research supports that patient education has a positive effect on patient outcomes (see research box).

The American Association of Diabetes Educators have identified 10 components that should be incorporated into any quality educational program for persons

RESEARCH

Brown SA: Effects of educational interventions in diabetes care: a meta-analysis of findings, Nurs Res 37:223-230, 1988.

Meta-analysis techniques were used to analyze data from 47 studies about the effects of patient teaching on knowledge, self-care behavior, and metabolic control. The analysis was designed to answer the following research question:

What is the magnitude of the effect of patient teaching in diabetic adults?

In this analysis, patient teaching appeared to enhance patient outcomes and have a positive effect on knowledge, self-care behavior, and metabolic control. ■

TEN COMPONENTS OF DIABETIC EDUCATION*

1. Definition of disease
2. Nutritional skills
3. Exercise knowledge
4. Medications
5. Self-monitoring of metabolic status
6. Care for hypoglycemia in persons with diabetes
7. Managing concurrent illnesses
8. Psychological adjustment
9. Hygiene and foot care
10. Follow-up

*From a joint task force for the American Diabetes Association and the American Association of Diabetes Educators, Spring 1979, American Diabetes Association.

with diabetes mellitus (see the box above, right) and have proposed that programs be planned and organized in three phases:

1. *Initial management:* emphasis placed on knowledge and skills needed to survive
2. *Home management:* emphasis placed on knowledge and skills needed to be completely self-sufficient in daily management
3. *Improvement of lifestyle:* emphasis placed on knowledge and skills needed to gain flexibility in management, insight, and self-determination

The nurse can use these three phases to set priorities for patient teaching and avoid giving too much information at a time.

In the next section, each component will be discussed. Examples of knowledge and skills from the three phases will be given. Patient teaching and counseling take place in the hospital or in ambulatory settings such as clinic or home.

Definition of Disease

To gain the self-management knowledge and skills necessary to live with diabetes mellitus and maintain a high quality of life, a person must understand the disease process (pathophysiology, signs and symptoms, and roles of nutrition, exercise, and medications in management).

Survival knowledge and skills include:

1. A basic working definition of diabetes mellitus, including a statement that insulin is needed for normal metabolism
2. A basic description of what effects a deficiency in insulin and its action have on the body
3. A basic description of the roles of dietary manipulation, exercise regimen, and medications on disease control

As *self-sufficiency* is attained, knowledge of the actual signs and symptoms of diabetes mellitus and how the signs and symptoms relate to the absolute or relative de-

ficiency of insulin need to be attained. The person will be able to explain how diabetes is diagnosed and the relationship between nutritional state and insulin deficiency, whether absolute or relative.

As the person gains increasing *flexibility, insight,* and *self-determination,* areas of understanding will include:

1. The significance of continual hyperglycemia on the development of vascular changes and neuropathy with resultant visual, cardiac, renal, and foot problems
2. The difference between types of diabetes and the importance of heredity and genetic factors
3. The potential for other family members to develop diabetes mellitus and ways in which risk factors can be decreased.

Nutritional Skills

The registered dietitian who is part of the health team is usually responsible for the nutrition component of the educational program for the person with diabetes, but the nurse is also involved. A dietary history should be part of the nurse's initial assessment. Any pertinent data are shared with other health team members, particularly the dietitian.

Because of the difficulty in changing food habits, the patient should be involved in setting goals for dietary changes. Some of the compromises that may be necessary are:

1. Identifying an acceptable weight-loss schedule for the obese person
2. Incorporating an alcoholic beverage into the daily plan
3. Distributing food in a different pattern (e.g., a large noon meal and a small evening meal)
4. Adding desserts to some meals
5. Adding dietetic candies and cookies

Information about cultural or social food habits that are

identified in the dietary history into the dietary plan. For example, make accommodations for a vegetarian diet or for a large amount of fast food in the diet.

The system for maintaining the dietary plan will usually be identified by the patient and the registered dietitian. The selected system is documented in the nursing care plan so that everyone involved uses the same terminology and food groupings. The mutually established goals, including compromises and sociocultural practices, are also documented so the patient is not given conflicting information. Significant others should be included in the teaching.

After dietary goals are established, help the patient to apply dietary knowledge through:

1. Simulations in which the person chooses foods from the hospital menu, food models, or other learning tools
2. Patient participation in documenting food intake, blood and urine results, activity, and medications and in discussing how these interrelate.

Evaluate the patient's and significant other's satisfaction with the plan. Additional needs may be identified over time, and communicated to the dietitian, to be incorporated into the plan.

Survival skills that the patient should possess after the initial management period are: (1) ability to manage the diet, on a daily basis, for stable conditions over 1 week; (2) knowing who to contact if unusual events requiring adjustments occur and; (3) how to handle sick days.

As *self-sufficiency* is attained, patients will be able to:

1. Manage their diets on a daily basis, making adjustment for normal life changes
2. Select appropriate foods from restaurant menus or at social occasions
3. Handle dietary needs while traveling or for shift work
4. Handle dietary needs at unplanned social events (such as a "happy-hour" after work, unexpected business dinner, or unexpected company)
5. Evaluate their success in dietary management through evaluating weight changes and hemoglobin A$_{lc}$ levels, or blood glucose self-monitoring

As they gain skills for *improvement of lifestyle,* patients will incorporate other dietary principles into health habits:

1. Make a conscious effort to include adequate vitamins and minerals, eliminate excess salt, decrease saturated fat intake, decrease caffeine intake
2. Keep up-to-date on new findings about dietary management and consult health team members about the new recommendations
3. Avoid "quack" recommendations
4. Manipulate diet, exercise, and medications to-

gether to cover a vast number of daily situations
5. Work with others in the household to help them incorporate principles of healthy eating into the diet.

Exercise Knowledge

Exercise is another major area of patient education for persons with diabetes mellitus. In order of priority, nursing activities include: (1) obtaining an exercise history and (2) helping the person understand and obtain a preexercise examination to plan an enjoyable and safe exercise program. This includes:

1. Helping select an exercise that will not cause problems if conditions such as neuropathy or proliferative retinopathy are present
2. Referring to a podiatrist for correct footwear for the chosen exercise
3. Helping establish a regular exercise routine to reduce the risk of hypoglycemia
4. Explaining the components of a safe exercise program and special needs of the person with diabetes
5. Teaching how to monitor cardiovascular tolerance (such as by pulse rate and level of exertion)
6. Identifying the parameters to monitor before daily exercise (blood glucose level, ketone level, and environmental temperature)
   a. Patient should not exercise if blood glucose is >300 mg/100ml or if there are ketones in the urine
   b. If weather is hot, suggest exercising in an air-conditioned area, such as a shopping mall or gymnasium, or using an exercise bicycle to avoid dehydration

During the *initial management* period, the patient may be given an exercise prescription that states the type, amount, and frequency of exercise and strict guidelines on when not to exercise and on monitoring to be done before, during, and after exercise. As *self-sufficiency* is attained, the person will be able to carry out more spontaneous exercises safely, know how to cover glucose needs with extra carbohydrates, and be able to identify self-monitoring needs. As additional *flexibility* is gained, the person receiving insulin will learn how to adjust insulin dose to activity programs, have a larger selection of activities to choose from, and encourage exercise as a family activity.

Managing Medications

Insulin knowledge. Patients taking insulin should be able to name their prescribed type and species source of insulin, their dose and the peak effects, and how the exercise regimen and diet are coordinated with the insulin. They should know insulin measurement (units) and the need for a similarly calibrated syringe. In addition, they must know how to handle insulin needs on sick days.

SUMMARY OF PATIENT TEACHING ABOUT INSULIN USE

1. Know type, species, action, and dose of insulin.
2. Know relationship between insulin, diet and exercise.
3. Use disposable syringes.
4. In drawing up modified insulin, know vials must be rotated, not shaken, and air bubbles must be removed from syringe.
5. In mixing two insulins in one syringe, know to draw up regular insulin first, then modified insulin.
6. Use prefilled syringes if preparing syringes presents difficulties.
7. Rotate injection sites, using all sites in one geographic area before moving to another; document sites to facilitate rotation.
8. Insert needle, at 45- or 90-degree angle, into area under fatty tissue, not into muscle.
9. Store currently-used insulin vial at room temperature (avoid temperatures over 90° F).

MIXING TWO INSULINS IN ONE SYRINGE

1. Gather equipment.
2. Wash hands.
3. Roll bottle of modified insulin.
4. Cleanse tops of bottles.
5. Draw up *air equivalent* to dose of *modified* insulin, and inject the air into modified insulin vial. (Do not draw up this insulin.) Remove needle from vial.
6. Draw up *air equivalent* to dose of *regular* insulin, inject the air into the bottle, and withdraw the regular insulin to the correct dose. Remove all air, and readjust to correct dose.
7. Return to bottle of *modified* insulin, and draw up correct dose.
8. Discard insulin in syringe and start over if an error is made.

Insulin self-administration. For safe insulin administration, patients must know how to draw insulin into the syringe, mix two insulins (if pertinent), select and prepare the injection site, rotate sites, and inject insulin. The essential teaching points are summarized in the box above, left.

Most persons will have some fears related to self-injection and will want to delay learning this skill. Repeated practice may be necessary, so patients should be started on self-injections as soon as insulin treatment is deemed necessary.

Preparing insulin dose. The patient is taught to draw the required dose of insulin into the syringe using correct technique (consult a fundamentals of nursing textbook if necessary) and to rotate or roll the insulin bottle to return any precipitated particles to solution.

The procedure can be practiced using saline solution and a syringe. For the first injection, the nurse may elect to delay preparation and focus first on self-injection. Adults may be better able to focus on preparing the syringe after experiencing self-injection. If the patient has difficulty with preparation because of motor, sensory, or visual problems, a family member or friend may be taught to prepare the syringe. Prefilled syringes must be rotated to return precipitated particles to the solution.

Mixing two insulins. If the patient is using two insulins, they may be mixed in one syringe so only one injection is necessary (see box above, right). Regular insulin can be mixed with any other insulin. Lente insulins can be mixed with each other, but not with other insulins (except regular). Mixing two insulins in the same syringe is one of the more complex psychomotor skills the patient has to learn; therefore, learning this skill may be delayed.

A major complication with mixing two insulins in one syringe is that the two vials of insulin can be contaminated with the insulin from the other vial. Another concern is the dead space of the needle. The first insulin drawn up fills the dead space and is actually included in the measurement of the second insulin. New syringes with little or no dead space eliminate this concern for the most part, and, if the two insulins are always drawn up in the same sequence, the amount will always be the same.

If the patient has difficulty mastering this skill, several alternatives are available:

1. Take two separate injections each time.
2. Have a family member, friend, or community health nurse prefill the syringes; a week's supply can be drawn up at one time.
3. Premix a 4-week supply in one mixing bottle. For example, if the prescription is 16 U NPH and 8 U regular insulin, the ratio is 2:1; 10 ml of NPH could be mixed with 5 ml of regular insulin and a dose of 24 U is then measured from the mixing bottle. This alternative works if the patient is on a relatively fixed insulin regimen. The diaphragm on the mixing vial lasts for about 3 months.
4. Use commercially premixed insulin (Novolin 70/30 and Mixtard Human 70/30 are two such preparations).

Selection and preparation of injection sites. Any area of subcutaneous tissue can be used for injection. The recommended sites are illustrated in Figure 37-7. When selecting a site, the patient's ability to use it must be considered. Some patients have difficulty using arms and buttocks because of dexterity, and some have difficulty using the abdomen, so the thigh may be the easiest site to use for the *first* injection.

Although some recommend that the arms and legs be avoided if the person will be using the extremities in physical activities, the need for this is not clear. It is

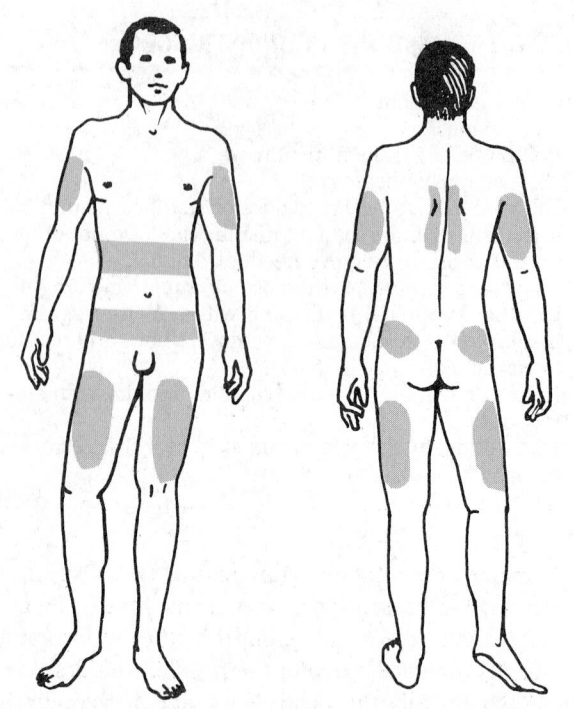

FIGURE 37-7 Rotations of sites for insulin injections.

known that insulin absorption from the different body areas varies (abdomen > arm > thigh), but an increase in absorption from the arms and thighs with exercise has not been supported by all researchers. What seems more important for preventing hypoglycemia during exercise is teaching the person to exercise at a time when the blood glucose should be highest.

If the patient exercises infrequently and has only one injection a day, it may be possible to avoid using the arms and legs. However, with daily exercise and a multiple injection regimen, avoiding the arms and legs is impractical; teaching should focus on the principles related to rotating sites. In preparing the site, all that is needed is to cleanse the area with alcohol.

Rotation of sites. Injection sites must be rotated to achieve proper absorption. *Lipodystrophy* can occur with repeated injections at the same site, causing poor absorption of the medications. Two forms of lipodystrophy can occur: hypertrophy and atrophy. *Hypertrophy* is thickening of an injection site due to development of fibrous scar tissue from repeated injections. A hypertrophic area is usually devoid of nerve endings, and the patient likes to reuse it because injections are painless, but absorption is erratic. *Atrophy* is loss of subcutaneous fat from unknown causes. Lipodystrophies may be partially caused by impurities in insulin; development of purified insulins have decreased this problem, but rotation of sites is still important.

The principles of site rotation are listed in the box

PRINCIPLES OF INSULIN INJECTION SITE ROTATION

Do not use a site more than once every 4 to 6 weeks.
Sites should be 1 to 1½ inches apart.
Use all sites in one geographic area, then move to next area.
Document site usage.

above. Each injection area has multiple sites, as indicated by the dots in Figure 37-7.

Injection of insulin. Insulin should be administered directly under the subcutaneous tissue (Figure 37-8). This can be achieved by pinching up the skin and injecting at a 45- to 90-degree angle. If the person has considerable fatty tissue (>1 inch) a 90-degree angle is safe. Use a 45-degree angle when the fatty tissue is less than 1 inch. The needle length may vary from ½ to ⅞ inches. (Consult a fundamentals of nursing text if necessary for principles of correct subcutaneous injection.) Jet spray injectors for insulin injection are available for insulin injection and are expensive, but may be helpful to persons in coping with multiple daily injections.

Storage of supplies and care of syringe. Patients need to develop a home storage system for equipment (syringes, alcohol, cotton balls) and currently used bottle of insulin (e.g., a box in a cool closet). Insulin need not be stored in the refrigerator, since it is stable for 1 year at room temperature. Temperatures below freezing and above 90° F should be avoided. The current recommendation is to keep the currently used insulin bottle, with the other supplies, at room temperature and store extra bottles in the refrigerator. Store prefilled syringes in the refrigerator.

Patients should always have an extra bottle of each type of insulin they use. Insulin has an expiration date, which should be checked at purchase; purchase only the amount that can be used before the expiration date. When traveling, insulin and supplies should be hand-carried to prevent loss.

Almost all patients use disposable syringes, and many patients reuse them. Although research has shown no infections on reuse of disposable syringes, normal flora was cultured from some reused syringes (see research box). Reuse of syringes is economically advantageous, but more research is needed, about the safety of this practice and how the syringes should be managed between uses.

A few persons still use glass reusable syringes, which are less expensive than others. These patients must learn one of two sterilization techniques: (1) immerse syringe and needle in 70% alcohol between injections and boil weekly for 10 minutes, or (2) boil syringe and needles daily for 10 minutes. A strainer placed in a

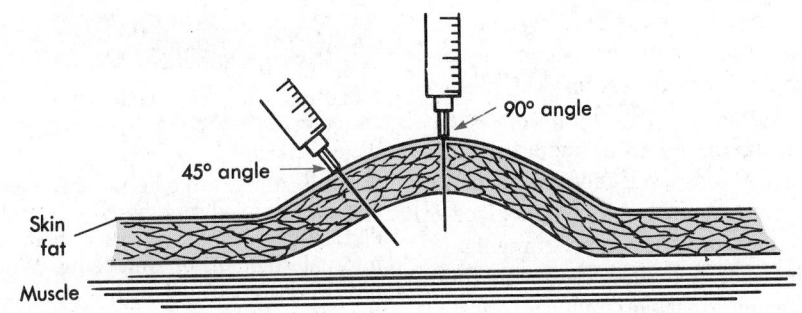

FIGURE 37-8 Insulin is injected into the pocket between subcutaneous fat and muscle, occurring when the skin is pinched up. The angle of injection may be 45 or 90 degrees.

saucepan simplifies draining and handling the boiled equipment. Because there are many things the patient and family must learn, disposable syringes may be used until the patient feels more comfortable with other skills before learning the sterilization methods.

Measures to assist the sensory-impaired person. Adaptation of equipment may be necessary for the sensory-impaired person. A number of aids available for the visually handicapped are advertised in diabetic publications or are available from the American Foundation for the Blind.* Special syringes with plunger locks, attachable devices for locking the plunger, and attachable needle and insulin bottle guides to facilitate entry of the needle into the bottle can be purchased. Persons who have failing vision may also use a small magnifying adapter that can be clipped to a syringe.

Persons with poor vision may draw air instead of insulin into the syringe. They must be cautioned to invert the bottle completely and insert the needle only a short

*American Foundation for the Blind, Inc, 15 West Sixteenth St, New York, NY 10011.

RESEARCH

Poteet GW, et al: Outcome of multiple usage of disposable syringes in the insulin-requiring diabetic, Nurs Res 36:350-352, 1987.

This study was designed to identify problems with reuse of disposable insulin syringes. The sample consisted of 166 persons with IDDM, 74 of whom reused syringes anywhere from 2 to 20 times. Reusers received a significantly higher number of injections, had lower incomes, and were female. Syringes from 44 of the reusers were cultured. Four of the cultures showed normal skin flora growth. No evidence of infection related to reuse was found. The seriousness of the contamination with normal flora needs more study. ▪

distance. They are often advised to use only about two thirds of a bottle of insulin. Some persons have a community health nurse or a friend draw the last doses from a bottle of insulin or go to a clinic for the last few injections.

Some individuals, though not able to prepare an insulin dose accurately because of motor or sensory problems, are still capable of giving their own injections. Prefilled syringes may be used. Automatic injectors may be used for some persons with physical handicaps.

Oral hypoglycemic agents. Although care is less complex, patients receiving hypoglycemic agents must be equally prepared to handle their medication. Each patient must know the name of the drug, dose, and peak effects, and how the diet and exercise regimen are coordinated with the drug therapy. Patients must know how to handle their drug on sick days. Oral hypoglycemic agents should be kept out of reach of children and in a place that is dark and cool. The medication should be hand-carried when traveling to prevent loss.

Self-monitoring of Metabolic Status

All patients need to do some self-monitoring. In the past, urine testing was the method patients used to assess metabolic control, but most persons are using blood glucose self-monitoring techniques.

Blood glucose self-monitoring. Various types of home tests for blood glucose self-monitoring correlate well with laboratory measurement of blood glucose level. A reflectance meter adds to the cost and inconvenience of monitoring, but gives a precise numerical value. Newer meters are smaller, some are the size of fountain pens and credit cards and thus are more convenient. Some test strips (Chemstrip bG, Visidex) do not require a meter, but instead indicate the range of blood glucose; for some patients, knowing the range is sufficient and thus a meter is not required.

Blood glucose self-monitoring has been found to facilitate attainment of glycemic control in IDDM (type 1) and in pregnant women. Its value in person with NIDDM has not been shown. It is always used by those with multiple-injection regimens or infusion pumps and by many on diet only, oral agent, or less frequent insulin injection regimens. Blood glucose self-monitoring can be used to validate subjective symptoms of hypoglycemia or hyperglycemia, and it provides more immediate feedback about the effects of nonadherence with the prescribed regimen. There is great variability in physicians' recommendations for frequency of blood glucose testing. Many patients are advised to test before and after meals and at bedtime for a short period, and, once they are stable, four times a day on only 1 day each week and whenever they feel sick. Persons who manipulate their insulin may need to test four or more times daily at all times. To test, the person sticks a finger and applies a drop of blood to a commercially prepared glucose oxidase stick. Timing of the reading and preparation of the specimen are very important in obtaining accurate results. Research has shown that, although most patients experience difficulty at first, especially sore fingers and inconvenience, these disappear for most persons.[33] Research also shows that most patients decrease their frequency of monitoring below that prescribed.[33] This may be appropriate for most, but if not, the nurse must reinforce the need for continual monitoring. Self-monitoring of blood glucose is expensive. Most insurance companies will reimburse for the reflectance meter, but not for the test strips.

Urine testing. Urine testing for glucose is not recommended. It can only be an effective method of monitoring if the patient has an accurate renal threshhold (which must be established), is not on a multiple-injection regimen or an insulin pump, and is not pregnant.

The nurse should know that there are still various tests available that might be used as part of a routine urinalysis. See Chapter 35 for a discussion of urine glucose testing technique.

Even patients who use blood glucose self-monitoring must do urine testing for the presence of ketone bodies. All patients are encouraged to test for ketones when they feel sick; other testing times are individualized.

Other types of patient self-monitoring. Although health professionals emphasize use of physiologic parameters to monitor glucose status, patients continue to use symptoms as guides for self-regulation.[43] In the presence of some chronic illnesses, when patients are told the disease may be asymptomatic, they report that symptoms guide them. One research study has shown that not only do patients use symptoms for self-regulation, but they take action on the basis of these symptoms (see the research box). Further studies are investi-

RESEARCH

Hamera E, et al: Self-regulation in individuals with type II diabetes, Nurs Res 37(6):363-367, 1988.

In this study, a model for self-regulation of diabetes was tested. The model proposed that individuals monitor their disease status by comparing their current status with an internal standard of well-being. When a discrepancy was noted and associated with a change in blood glucose, action was taken to relieve the symptom and thereby regulate blood glucose. Data from interviews with 173 persons with NIDDM were used to test the variables symptom-associating and action taking from the model. Most subjects did associate symptoms, and of those, most took action. Symptom-associating and action taking were not related to metabolic control. Women and persons who were currently on insulin were more likely to associate symptoms with high or low blood glucose, but insulin taking was not related to action taking. Actions taken included: (1) eating or drinking caloric foods, (2) taking fluids, and (3) resting. Not all actions were logical for the associated blood glucose level (such as exercise for symptoms associated with low blood glucose or eating for symptoms associated with high blood glucose). The authors suggest that potential use of this type of self-regulation must be considered in the care plans of persons with diabetes. ■

gating the accuracy of the symptoms in relation to actual blood glucose levels.[43] Results of this type of study have important implications for future patient education of the person with diabetes mellitus.

Patient teaching regarding self-monitoring. Techniques for appropriate monitoring must be part of the teaching plan. Teaching should include knowledge about testing procedures, demonstrations, return demonstrations by patients, and information about what to do with the collected data. All patients should use a diary or log to record date, time, and monitoring results. Other diary notations may include medications, food intake, activity level, and illnesses so the person can begin to see the relationship between blood glucose or urine ketone levels and their regimens.

In the *initial* stage of management, the patient may be asked only to record the results and call the health care professional every day for several days. As patients gain *self-sufficiency*, they may be given parameters to follow such as one of the following:

1. Repeat test.
2. Do a self-evaluation of how well diet, medications, and exercises have been followed.
   a. If any deviations have occurred, return to the regimen and continue monitoring for another day.
   b. If test results do not improve, call nurse/physician.
   c. If test results improve, continue regimen.

3. Call in results that are greater than a predefined level.

As patients gain *flexibility* and *self-determination*, they may manipulate insulin/diet/exercise independently on the basis of the monitoring results. Patients will progress toward more independence on the basis of ability and interest.

Care for Hypoglycemia in Persons With Diabetes

Patients receiving insulin or oral hypoglycemic agents must have information about hypoglycemia, also known as insulin shock, including:

1. Signs and symptoms associated with hypoglycemia
2. Assistance with recall of symptoms of a hypoglycemia reaction
3. Knowledge of appropriate treatment of hypoglycemia
4. How to get an identification card or Medic-Alert bracelet or necklace, and the importance of carrying or wearing it at all times
5. The importance of carrying a quickly absorbed glucose source
6. The importance of identifying why the hypoglycemic reaction occurred so it can be avoided in the future

Because hypoglycemia can occur suddenly, family members and friends should also learn the symptoms and how to handle a reaction. If a patient is too groggy to swallow, another person can be taught to place a teaspoon of corn syrup, honey, or cake icing in the patient's mouth between the gums and cheek. This will be absorbed through the oral mucosa, and the patient will usually arouse sufficiently to take a glass of juice, milk, or sweetened coffee or tea.

If glucagon is prescribed for hypoglycemic reactions, a family member is taught how to give the injection. Patients who receive glucagon or respond slowly to the carbohydrate must be taken to the hospital immediately. Some patients will need prolonged therapy for hypoglycemia, particularly if taking oral agents.

All information about hypoglycemia should be taught as part of the *survival* skills during the initial management phase.

Managing Concurrent Illnesses

All illnesses influence the status of diabetes control. In most instances, the person with diabetes needs increased insulin during a concurrent illness (especially infection), yet many mistakenly believe that if they cannot eat they do not need to take the prescribed insulin or oral hypoglycemic agent. Patients with IDDM (type I) who fail to take insulin when they are sick frequently develop ketoacidosis. These persons should take *carbohydrate* in some form.

Guidelines for the person with diabetes and a concurrent illness include:

1. Take all or part of the prescribed dose of insulin.
2. Spread 50% of the daily CHO allowance over 24 hours.
3. Increase fluid intake.
4. Include food items with more simple sugars than normally allowed such as custard, nondiet soft drinks, gelatin.
5. Advance toward the normally prescribed diet as soon as possible.
6. Institute blood glucose monitoring on a more frequent basis and monitor urine for ketones.

The person must know when to call the primary health care provider. Each person will receive individual instructions, but in general, the primary health care provider should be called if:

1. A full day's blood glucose levels are consistently elevated beyond a specified level
2. Ketone bodies persist in the urine
3. The person is not able to take *any* food or fluids for longer than 4 hours
4. The person is febrile

Patients should learn about contacting a health professional for instructions on illness days as part of their *initial home-management* teaching. As they gain *self-sufficiency* and *flexibility*, they will have mastered the necessary manipulations.

Psychological Adjustment

Adjustment to a chronic illness, such as diabetes, is ongoing. The degree to which persons with diabetes mellitus adjust, as evidenced by taking control of the disease management, often depends on how well they adapt emotionally to their diagnosis.

Helping the person begin to cope with the chronic illness must be one of the first nursing care priorities. Patients must have a chance to work through their feelings of loss, shock, disbelief or anger in response to the crisis. They need to feel accepted, regardless of their behavior.

Teaching and management are instituted in a manner to avoid overwhelming the patient. The patient must know that support is available at all times. Questions and concerns should always be listened to and handled professionally. The concerns may seem minute to the health team members, but they are great for the patient.

Giving the patient a chance to master a skill and take control is often very helpful because it increases the person's confidence and self-esteem. Patients master skills at different rates, so the nurse must always approach each patient as an individual and move at the patient's pace. Because patients are not hospitalized as long as they used to be, the community health nurse is often involved and must be informed before discharge of how well the patient is coping.

Family members and friends are included, as appropriate, to give them a better perspective of what the patient is dealing with. Local chapters of the ADA and the Juvenile Diabetes Association sponsor support groups in some communities. Patients and families may find these groups helpful, both initially and over time.

As patients deal with chronic illness, they may deviate from parts of their regimens as a means of testing importance, either because of the effect on their lifestyle or because they do not know if the regimen is really necessary. If this behavior occurs, it must be accepted without value judgment, and the cause of the deviation identified. It must not be assumed that knowledge deficit is the cause of nonadherence; adherence to the diabetic regimen requires a large investment of the patient's energy and time, which may be difficult to do every day. The patient needs support to get back on the regimen.

Ultimately, patients are the final decision-makers about self-care. The health team provides the teaching, the support, the guidance, and the counseling, but the patient makes the final decisions. Time for psychological counseling should be available in every follow-up visit.

Hygiene and Foot Care

Hygiene. Persons with diabetes are susceptible to infection. The effectiveness of the skin as a first line of defense is diminished. Uncontrolled diabetes leads to loss of fat deposits under the skin, loss of glycogen, and catabolism of body proteins. Protein loss can hamper inflammatory response and wound healing and impair leukocyte function, migration of leukocytes to site of infection, phagocytosis, and bacterial killing, all of which are involved in combating infection. Decreased circulation to selected body parts can also delay healing. The skin must be kept supple and as free of pathogenic organisms as possible. This is especially true in warm, moist areas that encourage growth of organisms (between the toes, under the breasts, and in the axillae and groin). It is very important that persons with diabetes carry out hygienic measures for prevention of infection daily, with special emphasis on foot care. They should also avoid persons with upper respiratory tract infections, and must seek medical attention immediately if an infection occurs.

Foot care. The need for foot care cannot be over-emphasized. The patient's feet should be visually assessed at every follow-up visit (see the box above, right). This action by health caregivers may reinforce the need for the person to practice preventive self-care at home.

The patient must practice preventive care on a daily

ASSESSMENT OF FEET OF PERSONS WITH DIABETES

Color: compare one foot with the other.
Temperature: compare both feet with upper legs; assess for line of demarcation.
Sensory function: test for pinprick and vibratory sense.
Reflexes: test Achilles tendon reflex.
Pulses: check dorsalis pedis and posterior tibialis.
Lesions: examine for calluses, cuts, bruises, cracks, or infection.
Self-care: discuss self-care regimen being used.

GUIDELINES FOR FOOT CARE IN PERSONS WITH DIABETES

1. Inspect feet daily for color changes, temperature changes, swelling, cuts, cracks, redness, blisters, or other signs of trauma; report changes immediately. (A mirror can be used to see bottom of feet.)
2. Wear well-fitting shoes and clean stockings when walking; never walk barefoot.
   a. Inspect shoes, before putting them on, for foreign objects, nail points, or wrinkles.
   b. There should be enough room in shoes to allow the toes to wiggle easily.
   c. Break in new shoes gradually.
3. Bathe feet daily and dry them well, paying particular attention to area between the toes.
4. Immediately after bathing, when toenails are soft, cut (or have someone else cut) nails straight across; smooth cut nails with an emery board.
5. If feet are dry, apply bland cream or petroleum jelly to heels and feet (but not toes).
6. Do not self-treat calluses, corns, or ingrown toenails; consult a podiatrist if these are present.
7. Bath water should be 30° to 32° C (85° to 90° F) and should be tested with a bath thermometer or elbow before immersing the feet.
8. Heating pads and hot-water bottles should not be used; wear socks if feet are cold.
9. Measures that increase circulation to the lower extremities should be instituted, including:
   a. Avoid smoking
   b. Avoid crossing legs when sitting
   c. Protect extremities when exposed to cold
   d. Avoid immersing feet in cold water
   e. Use socks or stockings that do not apply pressure to the legs at specific sites
   f. Institute an exercise regimen (p. ●●●)
10. Do not walk or jog in the dark; have a light source.
11. Obtain proper shoes before jogging.

basis. If neuropathy or bone changes occur, a podiatric consultation will be necessary. The podiatrist can help the patient by treating calluses and corns and by relieving pressure areas through custom-made shoes. Teaching about foot care (see the bottom box on p. 1128) is part of the *initial* management.

Follow-up

Follow-up of patient teaching may be accomplished in a clinic, physician's or nurse's office, home, hospital, or in an ambulatory education program. It must be continuous and meet the identified patient needs. It is often incorporated into routine return visits for assessment of disease control, and thus can be forgotten or missed when time is limited. The nurse responsible for this follow-up should identify the goals for each visit ahead of time so time is used effectively and teaching needs are met. Because of shortened hospital stays and because of the complexity of skills the patient with diabetes mellitus must master, a home health nurse may provide some of the follow-up nursing care.

Teaching Materials for Patient Education of Persons With Diabetes

The teaching needs described in preceding sections are summarized in the box below. In addition to planning

---

SUMMARY OF THE KNOWLEDGE AND SKILLS THE PERSON WITH DIABETES MELLITUS MUST LEARN FOR ADEQUATE SELF-CARE

Basic understanding of diabetes mellitus and how it changes metabolism

Therapeutic regimen prescribed and how it works to keep blood glucose normal

Diet (for example: calories, carbohydrates) ordered, how to calculate diet for each meal, how to incorporate personal preferences

Exercise and its effect on caloric and insulin needs; how to manage if exercise level is increased

If on insulin: type, amount, time to be administered, method of administration, ability to inject the insulin accurately, and ability to care for equipment

If on oral hypoglycemic agents: type, dosage, time schedule, potential side effects, and what to do if new or unexpected symptoms occur

Self-monitoring routine for monitoring glucose status or ketones (blood glucose monitoring or urine ketones); how to do the tests accurately; what to do if results show hyperglycemia, ketonuria, or hypoglycemia; and how to care for equipment and supplies

Signs and symptoms of hypoglycemia, how to treat them, and what to do if they occur frequently

Signs and symptoms of hyperglycemia and what to do when they occur

How to manage diabetes mellitus on days when usual diet cannot be maintained because of illness

How to prevent lower extremity trauma or injury

Type of follow-up care necessary

Who to contact with questions

---

and implementing an individualized teaching plan, the professional nurse is responsible for developing materials that can be used to complement or supplement any verbal exchanges. Written instructions should be provided for all parts of the diabetic education program so the patient has a resource to consult at home.

Many patient teaching materials are available from drug companies, private clinics, various diabetes education programs, and local chapters of the ADA. These materials were designed for the "typical" person; they must be evaluated for usefulness for a particular person. Streiff[62] found, from an evaluation of various printed materials for diabetic education, that a high school reading level was required; an evaluation of 106 adults revealed an average reading level of less than seventh grade (6.8). The patient's learning abilities must therefore be part of the initial assessment. Information about reading level and targeted population should be included when developing new materials.

Nurses working with persons with diabetes need to be aware of the characteristics of the elderly learner, because the incidence of type II diabetes (NIDDM) increases with age. Only a limited number of publications that focus on elderly persons with type II diabetes have been developed, and only one diabetes-related series[30] could be found that incorporated principles of learning for the elderly, such as large print, nonglare paper, or use of multimedia.

Economic Issues Related to Diabetes

Diabetes mellitus is an expensive disease, for the patient and for society. Even the very well controlled person with stable diabetes and no complications will be affected by economics. The cost of the medications, syringes, and self-monitoring equipment alone may be prohibitive. Nurses need to be aware of this and economize wherever possible. For example, limit blood glucose self-monitoring to what is necessary, continue to evaluate the possibility of reusing syringes, etc.

Another economic issue that nurses must be aware of is health insurance coverage. Many persons with diabetes do not have adequate coverage.[76] because (1) the cost of private insurance may be prohibitive and (2) some companies will not insure people with diabetes. Also, many large companies are self-insured; they use their own funds to pay claims.[76] This type of coverage is exempt from many of the laws regulating insurance companies, which could have a severe effect on the person with diabetes.[76] Prepaid capitation plans also have rules that may not adequately support the needs of persons with chronic illnesses. Therefore, even if a person is part of a group plan, the plan may be inadequate.

Nurses should either refer patients with diabetes to social workers or help them obtain information needed to evaluate insurance plans that may be available to them. Questions patients need to ask include:

1. Are routine visits to diabetes specialist, podiatrist, dietitian, and ophthalmologist covered?
2. Does the insurance cover reflectance meters or external infusion pumps?
3. Will the cost of glucose test strips be covered?
4. Are syringes, alcohol pads, insulin, or oral hypoglycemic agents covered?
5. Would special footwear be covered? Would procedures/medications for complications be covered?
6. Is diabetes education covered?

Nurses will indirectly help patients with the economic issues related to insurance through patient education. However, nurses should also work on a societal level to promote adequate reimbursement (particularly for diabetes education) and to promote formation of "Pooled Risk Plans" as insurance alternatives.

The patient with diabetes may also have trouble obtaining other types of insurance, such as disability and life. Often the premiums can be prohibitive.

A third economic issue affected by diabetes is employment. Persons with diabetes may not qualify for some jobs because of poor vision or presence of peripheral vascular disease, which would interfere with walking, but they may also face discrimination. Problem areas include: (1) the armed forces (diabetes makes the person ineligible; if onset occurs after acceptance, it may result in termination) and (2) law enforcement agencies, including the FBI.

Employment may also be limited because of inability to obtain necessary licenses. Individual driver's licenses are not automatically withheld because of diabetes, but most states require a physician's statement to confirm the person's ability to drive safely, and the state can place restrictions on driving despite the physician's recommendation. The few studies that have been conducted do not support a major increase in motor vehicle accidents among people with diabetes.[76]

Persons who have IDDM or NIDDM and are on insulin are prohibited from driving a commercial motor vehicle in interstate or foreign commerce.[76] Also, people who are being treated with medications for diabetes are, at present, prohibited from obtaining licenses to fly noncommercial airplanes. These restrictions may prevent persons from reporting their medications or cause them to avoid insulin, regardless of their clinical state. Saudek[76] reported no knowledge of restriction on obtaining retail or professional licenses. The terms prediabetes and chemical diabetes should not be used; they are not diagnoses but will cause problems for patients.

SPECIAL NEEDS OF THE PERSON WITH DIABETES HAVING SURGERY

Most nurses working in acute care centers will at some time work with a person with diabetes who is undergoing surgery. The presence of diabetes mellitus adds spe-

cial needs to the patient's care.

Surgery is a physical and psychological stressor for anyone. For the person with diabetes mellitus, there are added risks in surgery. The stressors of surgery can result in disruption of metabolic control. Persons with diabetes mellitus have a high risk of infection because of decreased resistance to infection and slower wound healing. Many persons with diabetes mellitus are elderly, and that also increases the risks associated with surgery. If the person has developed macrovascular or microvascular complications or autonomic neuropathies, the risks associated with surgery are further increased.

Effects of Surgery on Metabolic Control of Diabetes

The person with diabetes mellitus faces the risk of developing hypoglycemia or hyperglycemia during the perioperative period. To explain this, a brief review of factors that change insulin needs follows. During the perioperative period, persons are not usually given anything by mouth and are given intravenous fluids. This decreases total calorie intake and may also decrease insulin needs; however, the effects of surgery on counterregulatory hormones usually increases the need for insulin. The stressors of surgery cause the release of glucocorticoids and catecholamines, which elevate blood glucose.

There are many ways to manage the person with diabetes during periods of fasting. To minimize the disruption in metabolic control, the person should be thoroughly regulated before surgery, and the surgery should be scheduled for early morning to minimize variation from normal control measures. Persons with diabetes are kept on their normal food, fluid, and medication routines until the night before surgery if at all possible.

Management of Glucose Control, During Surgery, in Person Treated With Insulin

Various protocols may be used to maintain glucose control in the person on insulin. Neither hyperglycemia nor hypoglycemia should be allowed to occur. One of the most commonly used perioperative protocols is starting an intravenous infusion of glucose the morning of surgery and giving one-half the usual insulin dose subcutaneously. The IV glucose will usually cover this insulin during the intraoperative period and prevent hypoglycemia, and the insulin will cover, in part, the glucose needs. If the surgery is long, blood glucose levels may be checked during surgery; insulin or extra glucose can be given as needed.

During the postoperative period, the person is maintained by intravenous glucose infusion until food can be taken. Insulin is given either by dividing the normal daily dose equally over a 24-hour period and giving it subcutaneously or by adding regular insulin directly to the intravenous fluids. If the person is on a standard dose of insulin, extra insulin may be administered based on blood glucose checks. These checks must be performed every 4 or 6 hours. Some patients may receive no daily insulin dose and instead will be given insulin based on amount of blood glucose.

Management of Glucose Control, During Surgery, in Person Not Normally Receiving Insulin

Persons with diabetes who are not normally managed with insulin will receive an intravenous infusion of glucose on the morning of surgery, after fasting during the night. Such patients may be able to meet their usual insulin needs with their endogenous insulin supply, but in times of stress they may require exogenous insulin. After surgery, blood glucose and urine acetone levels are checked every 4 to 6 hours; if hyperglycemia is present, exogenous insulin may need to be given.

Management of the Person, During Surgery, Unable to Eat Prescribed Diet

All persons with diabetes, whether or not they are treated with insulin, should receive 125 to 250 g of carbohydrates per day until their normal diet is resumed. Fewer carbohydrates than this may result in *starvation ketosis*. The patient's normal diabetic regimen should be reinstituted as soon as possible. Blood glucose and urine acetone levels should be monitored frequently, even after the patient's usual diet and medication are resumed. The increase in catabolism because of the surgery will remain for some time, and additional insulin may still be needed. By the time patients are discharged, they should be back on their normal regimens. Other postoperative care measures are similar to those for all surgery patients (see Chapter 22). Initiation of these measures should prevent complications.

TRANSPLANTATION AS A MODALITY TO IMPROVE GLUCOSE CONTROL IN IDDM

Pancreatic transplantations have been performed since 1966. Cadaver and live donor pancreas, whole and segmental sections, have been transplanted. Over 1500 transplantations were performed from 1966 to 1988. The graft and patient survival rates have increased. In transplantations performed since 1985, the 1 year patient and graft survival rates were 88% and 55%, respectively.[85]

Pancreatic transplantation poses a unique problem; the exocrine function of the transplant is not needed, but it must be handled in some way. Digestive enzymes released from the exocrine ducts can be very irritating to tissue. Several approaches to solving this problem have been used, including injecting the exocrine duct with synthetic polymer or anastamosis of the ducts to bowel or bladder. The bowel anastomosis is the most physiologic because the GI tract will not be damaged by

the digestive enzymes, but the transplanted pancreas is exposed to GI bacteria. The bladder anastomosis can lead to bladder damage from the exocrine secretions, but it does allow for easy assessment of graft function through assessment of urine amylase.

The major issue about transplantation for treatment of diabetes mellitus is benefits versus risks. The documented benefits of transplantation are its favorable effects on neuropathy and progressive nephropathy. It has no influence on the progression of proliferative retinopathy, however. The risks are due to the immunosuppression necessary to prevent rejection.

Immunosuppressive therapy used at a transplantation site[85] includes cyclosporine, azathioprine, and prednisone for long-term therapy, and antilymphocyte globin or OKT3 monoclonal antibodies for induction of immunosuppression or rejection. The tremendous risk of infection, the side effects of these drugs, the cost of immunosuppression ($7000/year), the long hospitalization (2 to 3 weeks), and the frequent postdischarge clinic visits (twice a week)[93] must be considered when risks and benefits are weighed.

Currently, some of the risks are eliminated because most pancreas transplantations are performed in persons who have or are receiving a renal transplantation. Thus, these patients are already undergoing immunosuppressive therapy. Transplantation in a nonkidney transplanted person with IDDM has been performed infrequently. Interestingly, persons who have a renal transplant with the pancreatic transplant have survived the longest.

Another type of transplantation that could possibly be used in IDDM is islet transplantation, which is is still in an experimental stage. Techniques have been developed[54] to isolate islet cells from adult or fetal pancreatic tissue; the estimated 250,000 islets needed for a single transplantation can be obtained from one human pancreas.[54] Islet cells have been transplanted into various sites, including the kidney capsule, the liver (by injection into the portal vein), and the spleen. Research about whether the site of transplant influences graft survival is ongoing.

Islet transplantation is believed to offer several advantages over pancreatic transplantation. A major advantage relates to immunosuppression needs. In animal studies, pretreatment of islet cells to destroy leukocytes on the donor tissue allows for transplantation of the cells into a temporarily immunosuppressed recipient animal, and the graft survives after withdrawal of immunosuppressors.[54] Transplantation of islets in humans has been limited to persons who are immunosuppressed because of renal transplantation. A clinical trial is now in progress at one center[54] to transplant islets into persons with long-term IDDM and no kidney damage.[54] The results of this trial and others will provide definitive information on the role of islet transplantation in diabetes mellitus.

A second major advantage of islet transplantation is that there are no exocrine secretions to be dealt with.

Nursing Management

The success of pancreatic and islet transplantations are assessed by analyzing blood glucose response and C-peptide levels. A successful transplantation results in normoglycemia within 2 to 3 days. Insulin levels can also be measured, but the patient cannot be on exogenous insulin. If bladder anastomosis of the exocrine pancreatic ducts is used, the success of the transplantation can be analyzed through urine amylase levels. Rejection results in elevation in blood glucose level, decrease in C peptide level, and decrease in urine amylase level.

Pretransplantation nursing care focuses on helping with screening tests, psychological support (to help patient and family deal with the potential demands), referral, as necessary, for economic assistance, and education to prepare the family and patient for the burden they will have.

After the patient is selected for and elects to have a transplantation, then the decision is made whether to screen family members for a live donor or use a cadaver transplant. If a cadaver transplant is used, the patient is placed on a waiting list.

Tissue typing is performed to help match the patient with the donor. Each clinical transplantation center has its own immunosuppressive protocol, and the nurse will be involved in implementing it before transplantation and during the postoperative period.

Postoperatively, these patients are critically ill and need careful monitoring of hemodynamic status, fluid and electrolyte status, immune status, and graft status. Any signs of rejection must be identified as quickly as possible so that antirejection therapy can be initiated. The patient also needs all the care any patient would get during the postoperative period (see Chapter 22).

A major focus of nursing care is to prepare the patient for discharge. The patient must be able to self-monitor, know what to report, and know how to handle immunosuppressive therapy. The patient will be seen twice weekly for some time after transplantation.

Transplantation as a treatment in IDDM is still a relatively rare procedure, but as advances are made in understanding immunosuppression, more may be seen.

HYPOGLYCEMIC STATES

Hypoglycemia is the condition in which the plasma or blood glucose concentration falls below normal. It may be clinically serious because a sudden drop in blood glucose deprives the nervous system of its energy supply.

ETIOLOGY

Hypoglycemia is classified as either fasting or reactive. The former is seen after periods of fasting that range from a few to several hours; the latter occurs only after the intake of a meal.

Fasting hypoglycemia is most commonly seen as a side effect of insulin therapy or use of oral hypoglycemic agents, in persons with diabetes mellitus who take or accumulate too much insulin or oral hypoglycemic agent, who have decreased intake or decreased absorption of carbohydrate, or exercise more than usual. Fasting hypoglycemia also occurs from underproduction of glucose or overproduction of insulin (see the box below). With the autoimmune disease, antibodies against insulin bind up insulin, allowing a large inactive supply to be present in the blood. Antibodies then suddenly release insulin, resulting in relative overproduction, or the antibodies mimic insulin at the insulin receptor.[41]

Reactive hypoglycemia (also called functional) is the second most frequently diagnosed cause of hypoglycemia. True reactive hypoglycemia is seen in persons after surgery of the stomach or duodenum, such as gastrectomy or gastrojejunostomy, which result in rapid gastric emptying. Reactive hypoglycemia is idiopathic in most instances.

Reactive hypoglycemia may be overdiagnosed. Frequently, no abnormal decrease in blood glucose can be found except after a prolonged (5 hours) glucose tolerance test; this decrease does not correspond to the occurrence of symptoms. The term *idiopathic postprandial syndrome* has been used to differentiate this condition from true reactive hypoglycemia, where there is a documented decrease in blood glucose at the time of symptom occurrence.

PATHOPHYSIOLOGY

Regardless of the cause of fasting hypoglycemia or reactive hypoglycemia, the end result is an imbalance between the body's need for glucose and the blood glucose

---

CAUSES OF FASTING HYPOGLYCEMIA

BOTH AN INCREASE IN INSULIN AND A DECREASE IN GLUCOSE
Improper treatment of diabetes mellitus

UNDERPRODUCTION OF GLUCOSE
Hormonal deficiencies: ACTH, cortisol, glucagon and catecholamines
Acquired liver disease
Drugs: alcohol, propranolol, salicylates

OVERPRODUCTION OF INSULIN OR INSULIN-LIKE MATERIAL
Insulinoma
Extrapancreatic tumors
Autoimmune disease

concentration. Normally the blood glucose level is kept within fine limits; during fasting states insulin is decreased and counterregulatory hormones promote hepatic glucose production and decreased glucose use by tissues other than the nervous system.

This fine regulation is not maintained in either type of hypoglycemia because there is more insulin than normal or because glucose production is inhibited. The end result is low blood glucose; counterregulatory hormones are secreted to the extent possible but are not effective in bringing the glucose to normal. The epinephrine that is secreted produces symptoms by increasing the activity of epinephrine-sensitive organs or tissues (such as the heart or sweat glands). The CNS is deprived of its source of energy and dysfunction results.

CLINICAL MANIFESTATIONS

The signs and symptoms seen in fasting hypoglycemia and reactive hypoglycemia are the same as those described for hypoglycemia associated with diabetes mellitus. The diagnosis of *fasting* hypoglycemia is based on history, plasma insulin and plasma glucose levels, and identification of one of the listed etiologic factors. The patient may be admitted for fasting for up to 72 hours to see if hypoglycemia develops.

The diagnosis of *reactive* hypoglycemia should be based on a mixed-meal tolerance test. In this test, a standardized meal is ingested, and plasma glucose and symptoms are checked every 30 minutes for 5 hours. If the blood glucose level drops and the patient has symptoms, reactive hypoglycemia is diagnosed.[41] An oral glucose tolerance test should not be used to diagnose this problem.[41]

INTERVENTIONS
MEDICAL MANAGEMENT

Medical therapy consists of treating symptoms of hypoglycemia with glucose replacement (50% glucose solution, by infusion or orally. Oral therapy is the preferred method. After the cause is identified, treatment may include the following:

1. Surgery for insulinomas or extrapancreatic tumor
2. Diazoxide therapy for inoperable insulinomas to suppress insulin secretion
3. Discontinuance of drugs that induce hypoglycemia (alcohol, propanolol, salicylates)
4. Correction of hormonal deficiency
5. Correction of hepatic disease

The dietary control that is commonly recommended is a low-carbohydrate, high-protein diet, but its efficacy has not been established by research. The major medical therapy is avoidance of simple sugars and fasting.

NURSING MANAGEMENT

Nursing care of the person with hypoglycemia is directed toward the following nursing diagnoses:

1. Comfort, alteration in, related to sympathetic symptoms
2. Injury, potential for, related to CNS dysfunction
3. Knowledge deficit: disease, tests and treatments related to new diagnosis

During the early phase of illness the patient is monitored for the presence of changes in CNS function that might indicate hypoglycemia. A protocol for treatment of symptoms should be established and instituted; symptoms, such as sweating, trembling, and shakiness, which result with increased sympathetic stimulation, may cause considerable discomfort. Cool baths and a cool environment may relieve some discomfort. Relaxation therapy that includes backrubs, relaxation exercises, music, or distraction may also be helpful.

Patient teaching includes:

1. Diagnostic tests: purpose, procedures
2. Cause and treatment
3. Dietary management: avoidance of simple sugars and fasting
4. Preparation for surgery (see Chapter 20)

NURSING CARE PLAN

PERSON WITH DIABETES MELLITUS

DATA: Mrs. Forbes is an obese, 52-year-old married woman with NIDDM diagnosed 3 years ago. She was referred to a short-term ambulatory diabetes education program by her physician for instruction on insulin administration because blood glucose control had not been achieved with dietary measures alone or in conjunction with oral hypoglycemic agents.

The nursing history identified the following:
- She saw referral as necessary but perceived the need for insulin and her inability to control weight as personal failures.
- She maintained inconsistent sleep/activity schedule. (Worked as an LPN 8 PM to 8 AM Saturday and Sunday, with 2 to 4 hours sleep during those days; arose at 8 AM and retired at 11 PM on other days.)
- She had accurate knowledge about dietary modifications and had participated successfully in several weight reduction programs with 20- to 40-pound weight loss each time.
- She did regular checks of feet and wore proper shoes.
- She did not exercise consistently.
- She has performed blood glucose monitoring on others, and once or twice on self.

- She stated that work was important to her; satisfactions were derived from work group socialization and it "keeps me busy".
- She feared that her husband would die suddenly at home. Two years ago she had performed CPR when he had a cardiac arrest at home. Realized that she maintained work schedule "to keep me from worrying about husband".

Objective data included the following:
- Blood glucose, (fasting), 220 mg/100 ml
- Weight, 200 lb
- Height, 5'4"
- BP, 134/84
- Urine negative for ketones
- Urine negative for microalbuminuria
- Peripheral pulses present
- Legs warm and dry, color even with rest of body
- Patellar and Achilles tendon reflexes 3+ (on 1 to 4 scale)
- Identified touch in lower extremities
- Discriminated between sharp and dull in lower extremities
- Felt vibration in lower extremities
- Vision 20/20 on Snellen Chart eye examination.

Collaborative nursing actions included teaching Mrs. Forbes those measures that would help her achieve control of blood glucose (insulin, diet, and exercise) and teaching her to detect, prevent, and treat hypoglycemic reactions. The nurse reported Mrs. Forbes' work schedule to the physician and asked for insulin dose alterations on weekends. The physician was unaware of her work schedule and stated that blood glucose control could not be optimum with this schedule.

NURSING DIAGNOSIS

Knowledge deficit: self-injections, care of equipment, and self-monitoring blood glucose related to lack of exposure to information

Expected Patient Outcomes	Nursing Interventions	Rationale
Patient will independently administer injection to self	Support patient as necessary to self-inject insulin	Adults who perform this task have minimal discomfort and realize they are capable of giving own insulin
Patient will perform self monitoring blood glucose (SMBG) accurately	Observe patient's skill in SMBG; correct as necessary	Evaluation of patient technique is necessary to ensure accuracy
Patient will use measurements obtained by SMBG to achieve fasting blood glucose below 140 mg/dl	Review, with patient, effect of activity, dietary intake, and insulin on blood glucose. Instruct patient on frequency and timing of SBGM	SMBG gives almost immediate feedback about previous behaviors and reinforces value of therapeutic measures
Patient can describe symptoms of hypoglycemia and knows how to treat	Review, with patient, signs and symptoms and treatment measures for hypoglycemia	This knowledge assures that patient can safely give own insulin and decreases fear of reaction
	Review with patient information about care of insulin and supplies	This knowledge assures that insulin and equipment will be stable
Patient can describe how to care for insulin and supplies	Refer to dietitian for modification of diet necessary with insulin and verification of diet knowledge	The dietitian is appropriate person to teach about diet

NURSING CARE PLAN

PERSON WITH DIABETES MELLITUS—cont'd

NURSING DIAGNOSIS

Altered health maintenance: related to ineffective coping skill

Expected Patient Outcomes	Nursing Interventions	Rationale
Patient will state at least one change that will improve blood glucose control	Counsel patient about effects of stress, lack of exercise, and activity pattern on blood glucose	Patient's understanding of how stress impairs health is necessary before change
	Explore with Mrs. Forbes willingness and ability to change behaviors: sleep/activity, coping, and exercise	Goals are more likely to be achieved if patient makes realistic choices after considering cost and benefits
	Engage Mrs. Forbes in mutual problem solving; refrain from prescribing	Increasing patients' sense of control can help with self-esteem and enhance attitudes toward change
	Explore sources for long-term support in learning more effective coping skills. Suggest support groups: 1. For spouses of patients with MI 2. For weight loss *and maintenance* of weight loss 3. Available at work in health service program 4. For exercise	Changing lifestyle, eating behaviors, and coping skills is very difficult; support over long periods of time is usually required
	Suggest to Mrs. Forbes that she seek a trial period on day shift on weekends	Trial period can help person make informed choices about work schedule

CHAPTER SUMMARY

- Diabetes mellitus is a complex metabolic disorder, which may be clinically categorized in one of five different classifications. The two major classifications are non-insulin-dependent diabetes mellitus (NIDDM) and insulin-dependent diabetes mellitus (IDDM).

- Insulin deficit is a central feature of the disease; insulin deficit may be absolute, when β cells do not secrete insulin, or relative, when β cell defect and peripheral resistance to insulin is present.

- Glucagon excess and increase in other hormones counterregulatory to insulin contribute to hyperglycemia; these excesses are increased under stress.

- The classic signs and symptoms of IDDM are polyuria, polydipsia, polyphagia, weight loss, weakness, and fatigue. Patients with IDDM may have these symptoms or signs and symptoms of DKA; patients with NIDDM may have the same symptoms, except that they have weight gain instead of weight loss, or they may have signs and symptoms of HHNC or vascular changes and neuropathy.

- Taking measures to prevent and treat obesity is the focus of primary prevention of NIDDM; screening to detect undiagnosed cases (50%) is the focus of secondary prevention; detecting and preventing progression of complications is the focus of tertiary prevention.

- Insulin deficit and hyperglycemia lead to many immediate alterations in metabolism, including hyperosmolarity and osmotic diuresis, glycosuria, cellular starvation, calorie loss, and increased fat metabolism and catabolism.

- Diabetic ketoacidosis (DKA) and hyperglycemic, hyperosmolar, nonketotic coma (HHNC) are two life-threatening situations that occur in uncontrolled diabetes mellitus; they are usually precipitated by infection, stressors, or failure to follow regimen.

- Medical management of DKA and HHNC includes intensive fluid replacement, low-dose insulin infusion, and potassium replacement. The patient may also need phosphate and magnesium replacement.

- Hyperglycemia, from poorly controlled diabetes mellitus, seems to be a major predictor of the development of microvascular lesions (nephropathy, retinopathy), macrovascular lesions (atherosclerotic disease), and neuropathy (autonomic and peripheral).

- Amputation of a limb may be necessary because of alterations in blood vessels and nerves, tissue trauma, or infection occurring in persons with inadequate skin integrity and insensitivity to pain and pressure. Proper foot care, which helps to prevent an infection, can reduce the chance of amputation.

- Because patients must be responsible for diabetes management, nurses must assess the knowledge and coping skills of patients early in hospitalization so that appropriate education and counseling can proceed.

- A well-educated person will be assertive in describing special needs relating to patterns of food intake, exercise, monitoring, medications, and foot care.

- Assessment of the patient includes collecting objective data about metabolic status and assessing cardiovascular-renal status, vision, and nerve function. The lower extremities should be examined carefully.

- The major nursing focuses in patients with DKA or HHNC are (1) monitoring intake and output, weight, vital signs, mental status, ECG, blood glucose, urine ketones, serum electrolytes and osmolality; (2) implementing the medical plan; (3) reporting unexpected changes immediately; and (4) providing a safe environment.

- The three primary modalities of treatment for diabetes mellitus are diet, exercise, and hypoglycemic agents; education for self-management of these modalities is an integral part of nursing care.

- Dietary recommendations include calorie distribution of CHO (55% to 60%); fat, (20% to 30%) with restriction in saturated fat to 10%; protein (20%); limitation of cholesterol, sodium, and refined simple CHO; and increased use of complex, unrefined CHO.

- Exercise has a hypoglycemic action in most instances; it can increase hyperglycemia if blood glucose levels are above 300 mg/100 ml or if exercise is intense. Exercise does aid in cardiovascular fitness and weight reduction and maintenance, and it decreases peripheral resistance to insulin.

- Nurses and patients must be careful to use prescribed insulin: strength, species, length of action, purity.

- Oral hypoglycemic agents are used in NIDDM; they stimulate the pancreas and decrease peripheral resistance. They may induce hypoglycemia.

- Self-monitoring of blood glucose is always used by patients using insulin pump therapy or multiple injections. Patients treated in other ways use self-monitoring of blood glucose. This technology has made it possible to achieve normoglycemia in well-educated patients.

- Hemoglobin A_{IC} measures the amount of glycosyla-

tion of normal hemoglobin A; it correlates with the average blood glucose levels over the past 3 months.

- The treatment of hypoglycemia must be prompt; 10 to 15 g of simple CHO is given as soon as symptoms are detected. The first signs present are those of epinephrine excess; later signs are those of cerebral dysfunction. The signs and symptoms may be prolonged if the patient is on oral hypoglycemic agents.

- Insulin or oral hypoglycemic agents should not be omitted when short illness occurs; about 50% of normal daily CHO intake should be distributed over 24 hours.

- The impact of the diagnosis of diabetes mellitus and living with this chronic illness may be expressed by patients emotionally, in concerns about the future, in family conflicts, and in noncompliance.

- Patients fasting or undergoing surgery require modifications of insulin and food intake and increased monitoring of metabolic status.

- Foot care includes daily inspection, measures to maintain integrity of skin, and prevention of injury. Referral to podiatric services is highly recommended.

- Diabetes education must be individualized and planned over time. Initial instruction should be restricted to "survival skills" and beginning home management skills, with referral for continued education.

- An educational program for persons with diabetes mellitus has 10 components: these components include knowledge, skills, and attitudes for effective diabetes management.

- Evaluation of nursing interventions includes assessment of whether the metabolic balance is improved, whether the patient has the requisite knowledge and coping skills for self-management, and whether appropriate referrals were made.

- Diabetes treatment is expensive. Persons with diabetes may have difficulty getting health insurance and certain jobs.

- Pancreatic transplantation is a therapeutic modality used in selected persons with IDDM; the procedure offers the benefits of normoglycemia and control of neuropathy and nephropathy, but the risks of severe immunosuppression.

- Hypoglycemia can occur separately from diabetes mellitus.

- Hypoglycemia can be classified as fasting (includes excessive insulin production from insulinomas) or reactive (hypoglycemia after a meal).

- The signs and symptoms of fasting or reactive hypoglycemia are caused by the release of epinephrine and inadequate glucose for normal neurologic function.

✔ Reactive hypoglycemia can be inappropriately diagnosed if oral glucose tolerance testing is used; the diagnostic test of choice is a mixed-meal tolerance test.

✔ Insulinomas, which cause fasting hypoglycemia, are treated surgically; reactive hypoglycemia is treated with dietary manipulation.

QUESTIONS TO CONSIDER

- What physiologic parameters are monitored in a person with DKA? Make a flow chart indicating frequency. Are the parameters different for a person with HHNC?

- How is hypoglycemia treated? What is the rationale for each part of treatment?

- What skills/knowledge are included in a teaching plan to provide the patient with the survival skills discussed in this chapter?

- How would you determine whether poor control by a patient diagnosed with diabetes mellitus is due to knowledge deficit, noncompliance, ineffective coping, or lack of resources? Be specific.

- How would you determine whether a person with diabetes is developing problems associated with autonomic neuropathy? Be specific.

REFERENCES AND SELECTED READINGS

1. American Association of Diabetes Educators: Education for continuous subcutaneous insulin infusion pump users, Diabetes Educ 13:10, 1986.
2. *American Diabetes Association and American Dietetic Association: Exchange lists for meal planning, Alexandria, Va, 1986, The Association.
3. *American Diabetes Association: Physician's guide to insulin-dependent (type I) diabetes, diagnosis and treatment, Alexandria, Va, 1988, The Association.
4. *American Diabetes Association: Physician's guide to non-insulin-dependent (type II) diabetes, Diagnosis and Treatment, ed 2, Alexandria, Va, 1988, The Association.
5. American Diabetes Association: Principles of nutrition and dietary recommendations for individuals with diabetes mellitus 1986, Diabetes Care 10(1):126-132, 1987.
6. Anderson JW et al: Dietary fiber and diabetes, a comprehensive review and practical application, J Am Diet Assoc 87:1189-1197, 1987.
7. *Anderson J and Clark JT: The promise of fiber, Diabetes Forecast 40:47-48,50,52, 1987.
8. Ashley D: Surgery and the diabetic patient, Post Anesth Nurs 1:205-207, 1986. 8a. Atkinson MA and MacClaren NK: What causes diabetes? Scientific American 263:62-71, 1990.
8a. Atkinson MA and Maclaren NK: What causes diabetes? Scientific American 263:62-67, 1990.
9. Bach JF: Mechanisms of autoimmunity in insulin dependent diabetes mellitus, Clin Exp Immunol 72:1-8, 1988.
10. Baker DE and Campbell RK: The second generation sulfonylureas, glipizide and glyburide, Diabetes Educ 11:29-36, 1985.
11. *Ball P: The diabetic patient, AORN J 43:485-491, 1986.
12. Bantle JP et al: Rotation of the anatomic regions used for insulin injections and day-to-day variability of plasma glucose in type I diabetic subjects, JAMA 263:1802-1806, 1990.
13. Bernbaum M et al: Promoting diabetes self-management and independence in the visually impaired, a model clinical program, Diabetes Educ 14:51-54, 1988.
14. Bild DE et al: Lower extremity amputation in people with diabetes, epidemiology and prevention, Diabetes Care 12:24-31, 1989.
15. Brown SA: An assessment of the knowledge base of the insulin-dependent diabetic adult, J Community Health Nurs 4(1):9-19, 1987.
16. Brown SA: Effects of educational interventions in diabetes care: a meta-analysis of findings, Nurs Res 37:225-230, 1988.
17. Burnett KF et al: Computer assisted management of weight, diet, and exercise in the treatment of type II diabetes, Diabetes Educ 13:234-236, 1987.
18. *Butts DE: Fluid and electrolyte disorders associated with diabetic ketoacidosis and hyperglycemic hyperosmolar nonketotic coma, Nurs Clin North Am 22:827-836, 1987.
19. Byrnes CA: What's new in the diabetic diet, Nursing 17(8):58-59, 1987.
20. Callahan ME and Bradley DJ: Teaching your diabetic patient to chart, Nursing 18(3):48-49, 1988.
21. Campaigne BN and Gunnarson R: The effects of physical training in people with insulin-dependent diabetes, Diabetic Med 5:429-433, 1988.
22. *Christman C and Bennett J: Diabetes, new names, new test, new diet, Nursing 173:34-41, 1987.
23. Collier JH: The management of diabetes in orthopaedic patients, Orthop Nurs 7(2):11-18, 1988.
24. Daly AS and Soler NG: Nutrient intake of young adult women with diabetes mellitus, Diabetes Educ 13:198-202, 1987.
25. Davidson M: Pathophysiology and management of type II diabetes. In The Endocrine Society: 41st Post Graduate Annual Assembly Syallabus, Bethesda, Md, 1989, The Endocrine Society.
26. *DeFeo P et al: Somogyi and dawn phenomena: mechanisms, Diabetes Metab Rev 4:31-49, 1988.
27. DeFronzo R: The triumvirate, B-cell, muscle, liver: a collusion responsible for NIDDM, Diabetes 37:667-687, 1988.
28. Drell DW and Notkins AL: Multiple immunological abnormalities in patient with type I insulin-dependent diabetes mellitus, Diabetologia 30:132-143, 1987.
29. Dunn SM: Reactions to educational techniques, coping strategies for diabetes and learning, Diabetic Med 3:419-429, 1986.
30. Eaks GA, editor: The look, listen, and learn series, Kansas City, 1985, ADA Heart of America Affiliate.
31. Editor: Will surgery complicate your patient's drug therapy, Emerg Med 19(18):57-93, 1987.
32. Field JB: Catch a falling sugar, Emerg Med 17(20):16-36, 1985.
33. Fox MA et al: Blood glucose self-monitoring usage and its influence on patients' perceptions of diabetes, Diabetes Educ 10:27-31, 1984.
34. Franz MJ: Evaluating the glycemic response to carbohydrates, Clin Diabetes 11:127-130, 1986.
35. *Freeman WL: The dietary management of non-insulin dependent diabetes mellitus in the obese patient, Prim Care 15:327-352, 1988.
36. Freinkel R: Caring for your skin, Diabetes Forecast 41:76-81, 1988.
37. Frey MA and Denyes MJ: Health and illness self-care in adolescents with IDDM, a test of Orem's theory, Advances Nurs Sci 12:67-75, 1989.

*References preceded by an asterisk are particularly well suited for student reading.

38. Ganda OP: Hormones affecting the secretion and actions of insulin. In Marble A et al, editors: Joslin's diabetes mellitus, ed 12, Philadelphia, 1985, Lea & Febiger.

39. Germain CP and Nemchek RM: Diabetes self-management and hospitalization, Image 20:74-78, 1988.

40. Goldberg A and Coon P: Non-insulin dependent diabetes mellitus in the elderly, Endocrinol Metab Clin 16:843-865, 1987.

41. Gorden P: The clinical spectrum of hypoglycemia. In The Endocrine Society: 41st Post Graduate Annual Assembly Syllabus, Bethesda, Md, 1990, The Endocrine Society.

42. Gutherie DW: Diabetes patient education, nurse specialist approach, Diabetes Educ 12:131-134, 1986.

43. *Hamera E et al: Self-regulation in individuals with type II diabetes, Nurs Res 37:363-367, 1988.

44. Harati Y: Diabetic peripheral neuropathies, Ann Intern Med 107:546-559, 1987.

45. Harris G: Filling the gaps between patients and professionals, Diabetes Educ 13:133-136, 1987.

46. *Hernandez CM: Surgery and diabetes minimizing the risks, Am J Nurs 87:788-792, 1987.

47. *Herget MJ and Williams AS: New aids for low vision diabetics, Am J Nurs 89:1319-1322, 1989.

48. Holmes CS, editor: Neuropsychological and behavioral aspects of diabetes, New York, 1990, Springer-Verlag.

49. *Horton E: Role and management of exercise in diabetes mellitus, Diabetes Care 7:201-211, 1988.

50. Ivy J: Exercise and complications, Diabetes Forecast 43:46-49, 1990.

51. *Knighton DR: Treating diabetic foot ulcers, Diabetes Spectrum 3:51-56, 1990.

52. Koschinsky T et al: New approach to technical and clinical evaluation of devices for self-monitoring of blood glucose, Diabetes Care 11:619-629, 1988.

53. Lacey PE: Islet transplantation, Clin Chem 32(10B):B76-B82, 1986.

54. Lacy PE and Scharp DW: Islet cell transplantation. In Rifkin H and Porte D, editors: Ellenberg and Rifkin's diabetes mellitus, theory and practice, ed 4, New York, 1990, Elsevier.

55. Lagana D: The reuse of insulin syringes, Pract Diabetology 10(11):20-21, 1987.

56. Lefebvre PJ and Scheen AJ: Hypoglycemia. In Rifkin H, and Porte D, editors: Ellenberg and Rifkin's diabetes mellitus, theory and practice, ed 4, New York, 1990, Elsevier.

57. Lilienfeld D et al: Obesity and diabetes as risk factors for postoperative wound infections after cardiac surgery, Am J Infect Control 16:3-6, 1988.

58. Lumey W: Controlling hypoglycemia and hyperglycemia, Nursing 18(10):34-41, 1988.

59. Manley G: Diabetes and sexual health, Diabetes Educ 13:366-369, 1987.

60. McCance KL and Huether SE: Pathophysiology, the biological basis for disease in adults and children, St Louis, 1990, The CV Mosby Co.

61. *Nath C et al: Lessons in living with type II diabetes mellitus, Nursing 18(8):44-49, 1988.

62. National Diabetes Data Group: Classification and diagnoses of diabetes mellitus and other categories of glucose intolerance, Diabetes 28:1039-1057, 1979.

63. Nuttall F: The high-carbohydrate diet in diabetes management, Adv Intern Med 33:165-184, 1988.

64. Paulk LH: Hypoglycemic reactions from the diabetic's perspective, unpublished master's thesis, Kent, Ohio, 1983, Kent State University.

65. Perriello G et al: The dawn phenomenon, nocturnal blood glucose homeostasis in insulin-dependent diabetes mellitus, Diabetic Med 5:13-21, 1988.

66. *Poteet GW et al: Outcome of multiple usage of disposable syringes in the insulin-requiring diabetic, Nurs Res 36:350-352, 1987.

67. Prather RC: Sexual dysfunction in the diabetes female, a review, Arch Sex Behav 17:277-285, 1988.

68. Rifkin H and Porte D, editors: Ellenberg and Rifkin's diabetes mellitus, theory and practice, ed 4, New York, 1990, Elsevier.

69. Ritchie CM and Atkinson AB: Towards better management of the diabetic patient with raised blood pressure, Diabetic Med 3:301-305, 1986.

70. Robertson C: When your pregnant patient has diabetes, RN 50(11):18-22, 1987.

71. Rosenberg CS: Wound healing in the patient with diabetes mellitus, Nurs Clin North Am 25:247-261, 1990.

72. Rubin R et al: Effect of diabetes education on self-care, metabolic control, and emotional well-being, Diabetes Care 10:673-679, 1989.

73. *Sabo CE and Michael SR: Diabetic ketoacidosis: pathophysiology, nursing, diagnoses, and nursing interventions, Focus on Crit Care 16:21-28, 1989.

74. *Sabo CE and Michael SR: Managing DKA and preventing a reoccurrence, Nursing 19:50-56, 1989.

75. *Samanta A et al: Management of the acutely ill diabetic patient, Intensive Care Nurs 1:194-203, 1986.

76. Saudek CD and Segal-Polin S: Economic aspects: insurance, employment, and licensing. In Rifkin H and Porte D, editors, Ellenberg and Rifkin's diabetes mellitus, theory and practice, ed 4, New York, 1990, Elsevier.

77. *Schumann D: Post-operative hyperglycemia: clinical benefits of insulin therapy, Heart Lung 19:165-173, 1990.

78. Shoemaker WC et al: Textbook of critical care, ed 2, Philadelphia, 1989, WB Saunders.

79. Skeleton CW: Use of glycosylated hemoglobins in the long-term management of diabetes, Nurse Pract 11(3):42-51, 1986.

80. Soulier S et al: The prevention of plantar ulceration in the diabetic foot through the use of running shoes, Diabetes Educ 13:130-132, 1987.

81. Steffes MW: Complications of diabetes mellitus and factors affecting their progression, Clin Chem 32(10B):B54-B61, 1986.

82. *Streiff LD: Do clients understand our instructions?, Image 18:48-52, 1986.

83. Sutherland DER: Current status of transplantation of the pancreas, Adv Surg 20:303-304, 1987.

84. Sutherland DER et al: Pancreas transplantation, Clin Chem 32:(10B):B83-B96, 1986.

85. Sutherland DER et al: Pancreas transplantation. In Rifkin H and Porte D, editors: Ellenberg and Rifkin's diabetes mellitus, theory and practice, ed 4, New York, 1990, Elsevier.

86. Vasterling JJ: The role of aerobic exercise in reducing stress in diabetic patient, Diabetic Educ 14:197-201, 1988.

87. Wang JT et al: Effects of habitual physical activity on age related glucose intolerance, J Am Geriatr Soc 37:203-209, 1989.

88. Wilson JD and Foster DW, editors: Williams' textbook of endocrinology, ed 7, Philadelphia, 1985, WB Saunders.

89. World Health Organization Study Group: Diabetes mellitus, report of a WHO study group, Geneva, WHO Tech Rep Ser 727:1-113, 1985.

90. World Health Organization: WHO expert committee on diabetes mellitus, second report, Geneva, WHO Tech Rep Ser 646:1-80, 1980.

91. Wyngaarden J and Smith LH, editors: Cecil textbook of medicine, ed 18, Philadelphia, 1988, WB Saunders.

91a. Yeates S and Blaufuss J: Managing the patients in diabetic ketoacidosis, Foc Crit Care 17:240-248, 1990.

92. Zanella MT et al: Hypertension and diabetes, Drugs 35(suppl 6):135-141, 1988.

93. Zehrer J and Rode S: When your diabetic patient has a pancreas transplant, Nursing 18:108-109, 1988.

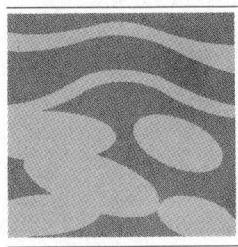

Assessment of the Liver

VIRGINIA L. CASSMEYER

CHAPTER OBJECTIVES

After studying this chapter, the student should be able to:
1 Describe the normal anatomy of the liver.
2 Describe the role of the liver in metabolism and maintenance of energy balance.
3 Explain the basis for subjective and objective data that must be collected to identify problems of the hepatic system.
4 Describe the various laboratory and diagnostic tests used in identifying the pathophysiologic states of the liver.
5 Develop a plan of care for patients undergoing the radiologic and special tests used in diagnosing hepatic dysfunction.

Because of its multiple functions, the liver is of prime importance in metabolism and in the maintenance of normal energy stores. Pathologic conditions of the liver can cause a variety of problems affecting the total body.

ANATOMY AND PHYSIOLOGY

ANATOMIC CONCEPTS

The liver, which weighs 1.3 to 1.8 kg, is one of the largest organs in the body. It consists of two lobes and is located in the right upper quadrant of the abdomen under the diaphragm. It extends up under the ribs and is 4 to 8 cm in height in the midsternal line and 6 to 12 cm in height in the midclavicular line. The liver normally extends from the fifth intercostal space to just below the right costal margin (Figure 38-1).

The liver receives 25% of the cardiac output from two sources, the portal vein and the hepatic artery. Most of blood flow (75%) is derived from the portal vein; thus the liver receives mostly unoxygenated blood (Figure 38-2). The liver is innervated by the sympathetic and parasympathetic nervous systems. Sympathetic fibers innervate the hepatic artery branches and the bile ducts. Parasympathetic innervation is supplied to the intrahepatic and extrahepatic biliary tract system. Stimulation of the sympathetic and parasympathetic nervous systems affects blood flow and the flow of bile within the biliary tract, but the function of the hepatic cells or parenchymal cells is not influenced.

The functional unit of the liver is the liver lobule (Figure 38-3). Each lobule is composed of multiple plates of hepatic cells. Between the individual cells of the cellular plate are biliary canaliculi. On each side of the cellular plate is a venous sinusoid, which receives blood from branches of the portal vein and hepatic artery. As blood flows through the sinusoids, substances can be exchanged between the hepatic cells and the blood.

The sinusoids are lined with phagocytic cells of the reticuloendothelial system (Kupffer cells). These cells cleanse the blood of bacteria and other foreign products. Because the portal blood originates in the gastrointestinal (GI) tract, some bacteria or other foreign products always need to be removed.

The blood from the venous sinusoids empties into the central vein and then into the hepatic vein. The hepatic vein empties into the inferior vena cava.

PHYSIOLOGIC CONCEPTS

The liver can be thought of as a metabolic factory and a waste disposal plant. As should be evident from the anatomic description of the blood and bile flow, the liver is ideally structured to carry out its multiple metabolic and waste disposal functions. The major functions of the liver are summarized in the box on p. 2042. Each of these functions is presented in more detail in the following sections.

CARBOHYDRATE, PROTEIN, AND FAT METABOLISM

The liver has a significant role in the metabolism of each of the three major food nutrients. The liver either oxidizes these components for energy, uses the nutrients to synthesize storage forms of substances for future use, or uses the nutrients to synthesize other essential compounds.

Carbohydrate

Immediately after meals, the liver extracts glucose, fructose, and galactose from the blood. These simple sugars are metabolized into glycogen (*glycogenesis*) to replenish liver stores. If the diet ingested is low in car-

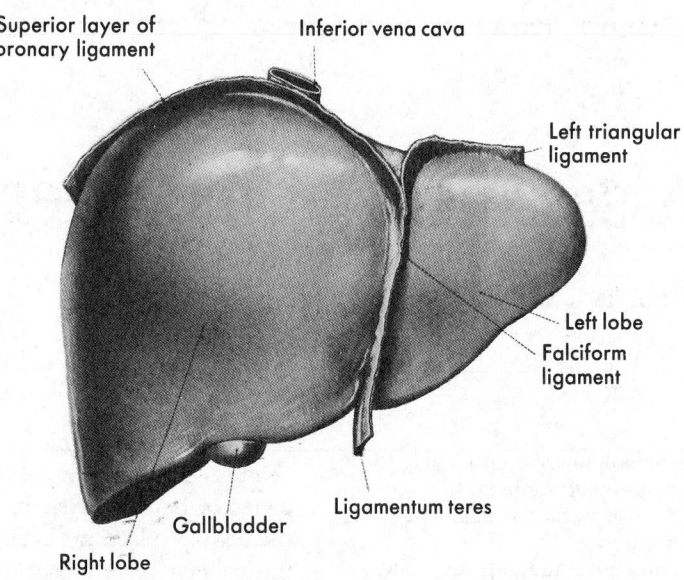

FIGURE 38-1 Anterior view of liver. (From Hamilton WJ, editor: Textbook of human anatomy, ed 2, St Louis, 1976, The CV Mosby Co. By permission of Macmillan, London & Basingstoke.)

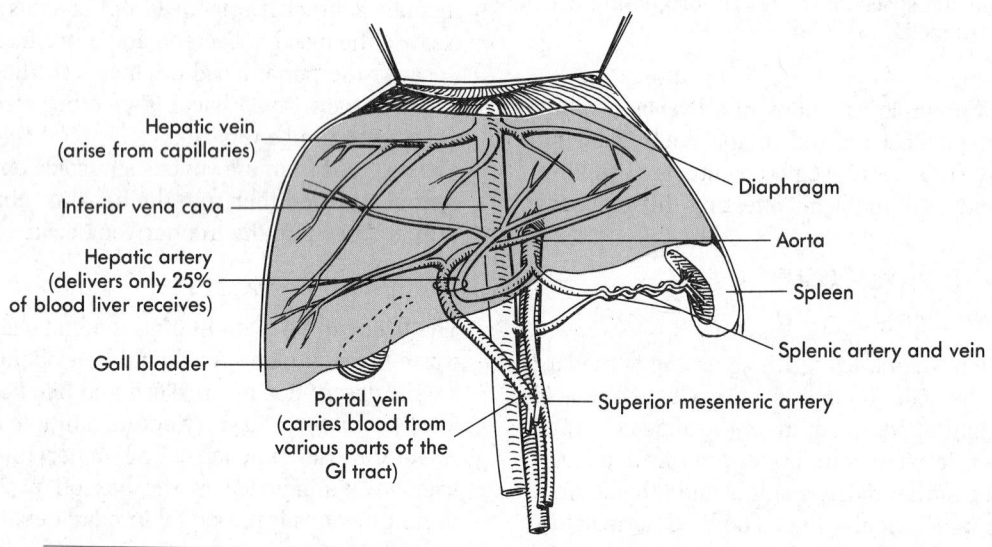

FIGURE 38-2 Diagram demonstrating circulation of liver. (Modified from Porth C: Pathophysiology: concepts of altered health status, Philadelphia, 1982, JB Lippincott Co.)

bohydrates, the liver converts protein to glucose to replenish glycogen stores. If more carbohydrate is ingested than is needed to replenish glycogen stores or to supply energy, the excess carbohydrate is converted to fat (*lipogenesis*). Between meals and during other fasting states, the liver assists in maintaining the blood glucose concentration. It does this by breaking down glycogen (*glycogenolysis*) or forming new glucose (*gluconeogenesis*). The new glucose is made from amino acids glycerol, and lactic acids. Through glycogenesis, lipogenesis, glycogenolysis, and gluconeogenesis, pro-

cesses, which are under hormonal control, the liver helps to maintain a normal blood glucose level, preventing high levels immediately after eating (postprandial) and hypoglycemia between meals or during other periods of fasting.

Proteins

The liver is vital to normal protein metabolism. It provides needed amino acids through the process of transamination. It also is the only source of some of the ma-

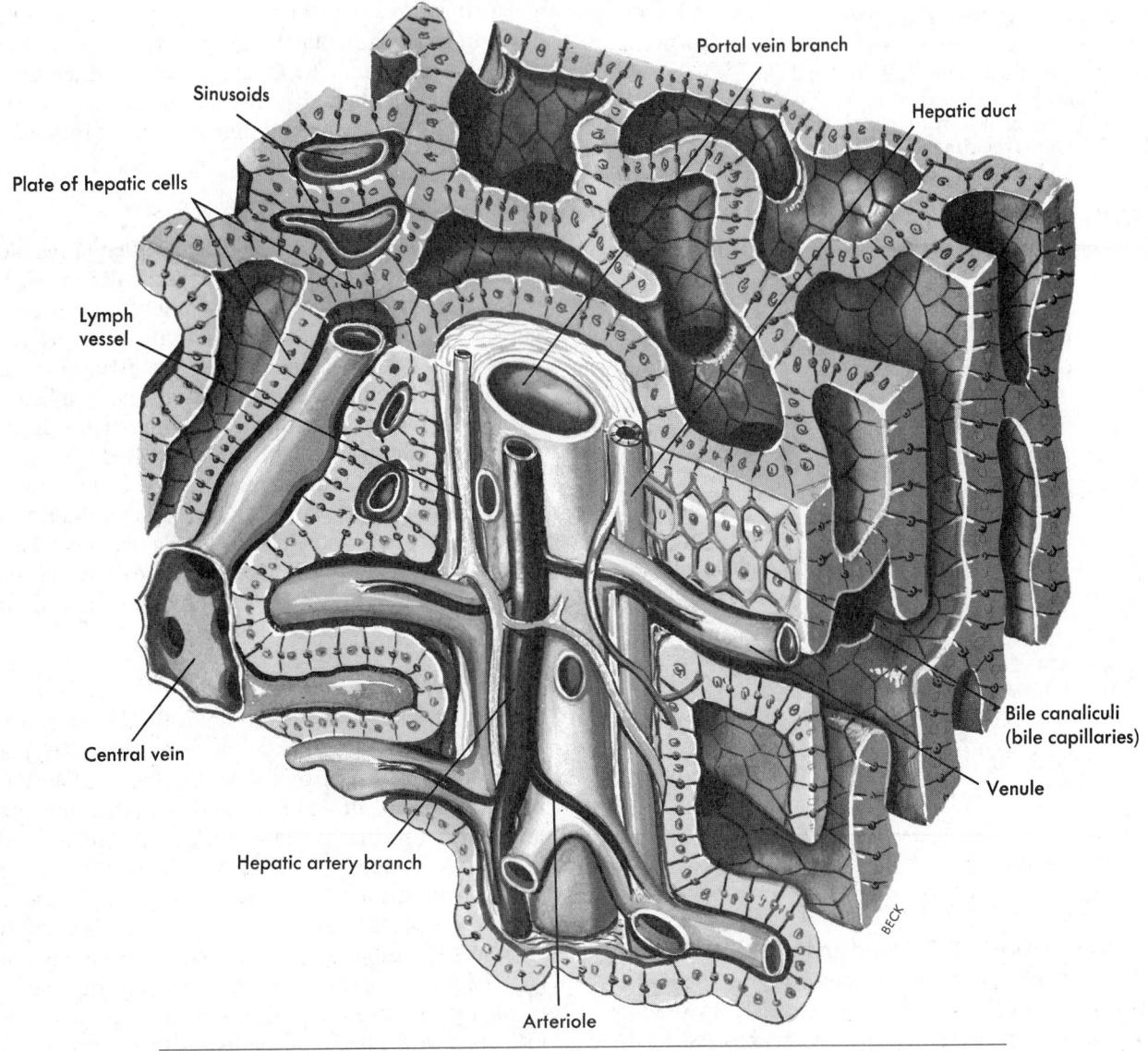

FIGURE 38-3 Liver lobule. Blood from branches of the portal vein and hepatic artery passes through sinusoids between plates of hepatic cells. Sinusoidal blood empties into the central vein, which leads to the hepatic veins. Bile canaliculi empty bile into bile ducts. (From Anthony CP and Thibodeau GA: Textbook of Anatomy and Physiology, ed 11, St Louis, 1983, The CV Mosby Co.)

jor plasma proteins. One of these major proteins is albumin, which is necessary for the maintenance of a normal internal environment and for fluid and electrolyte balance. *Albumin,* produced only in the liver, is responsible for maintaining colloid osmotic pressure and thus the proper distribution of fluids between the vascular and interstitial compartments.

The liver is the source of several clotting factors. It produces fibrinogen (factor I), prothrombin (factor II), factor V (proaccelerin), factor VII (serum prothrombin conversion accelerator), factor IX (Christmas factor), and factor X (Stuart, or Stuart-Prower, factor). The pro-

duction of factors II, VII, IX, and X requires vitamin K. Because vitamin K is a fat-soluble vitamin, it requires adequate production and excretion of bile for its absorption. In addition to protein synthesis, the liver catabolizes proteins as necessary for energy or glucose production.

Fats

The liver is involved in multiple aspects of fat metabolism. Triglycerides in the diet are absorbed in chylomicrons. The chylomicrons are taken up by the liver, and the triglycerides are metabolized to fatty acids. These

SUMMARY OF LIVER FUNCTIONS

1. Carbohydrate, protein, and fat metabolism
   a. Carbohydrate metabolism
      (1) Glycogen formation and storage
      (2) Glucose formation from glycogen (glycogenolysis) and from amino acids, lactic acids, and glycerol (gluconeogenesis).
   b. Protein metabolism
      (1) Protein catabolism
      (2) Protein synthesis
         (a) Albumin
         (b) alpha-(α) and beta-(β)Globulins
         (c) Clotting factors
         (d) C-reactive protein
         (e) Transferrin
         (f) Enzymes
         (g) Ceruloplasmin, and so on
      (3) Formation of needed amino acids
   c. Fat metabolism
      (1) Oxidation of fatty acids for energy
      (2) Ketone formation
      (3) Synthesis of cholesterol and phospholipids
      (4) Formation of triglycerides from dietary lipids and excessive dietary carbohydrates and proteins
      (5) Formation of lipoproteins
2. Production of bile salts
3. Bilirubin metabolism
4. Detoxification of endogenous and exogenous substances
   a. Ammonia
   b. Steroids
   c. Drugs
5. Storage of minerals and vitamins
6. Blood reservoir

---

fatty acids may be (1) oxidized and utilized for energy by the liver and other body tissues; (2) metabolized to ketones; (3) converted to phospholipids; (4) used to combine with cholesterol, which is synthesized in the liver, to form cholesterol esters; or (5) reesterified to triglycerides and combined with protein, cholesterol, and phospholipids to form lipoproteins. The liver also uses fatty acids released from adipose tissue storage sites for these same processes.

PRODUCTION OF BILE SALTS

Bile production is one of the major functions of the liver. Bile is a complex compound composed of cholesterol, phospholipids, bile salts, bile pigments (bilirubin), and very small amounts of proteins and electrolytes. Ninety-seven percent of bile is water. Metabolites of drugs and other substances that need to be excreted may also be found in bile. Bile salts are necessary for the absorption of fats, cholesterol, and fat-soluble vitamins. Bile is released from the liver and concentrated and stored in the gallbladder. The liver secretes approximately 700 ml of bile daily. The bile salts released during each meal are reabsorbed into the enterohepatic cir-

culation and recycled 2 or 3 times during a meal. Bile is reabsorbed along the total intestinal tract, but the terminal ileum has a major role in its active reabsorption. If the terminal ileum is diseased or resected, reabsorption of bile does not occur and abnormal fat absorption results.

BILIRUBIN METABOLISM

Bilirubin is a byproduct of the *heme* portion of red blood cells and is released when these cells are destroyed. The released bilirubin is not water soluble (unconjugated). Unconjugated bilirubin is carried in the blood bound to albumin and other proteins. The liver extracts the unconjugated bilirubin from the blood and combines it with glucoronide into a water soluble form (conjugated). The conjugated bilirubin is secreted into the bile and then enters the duodenum. In the GI tract, bilirubin is metabolized to urobilinogen. *Urobilinogen* is excreted in feces as stercobilin, giving feces its brown color, or it is reabsorbed. Most of the reabsorbed urobilinogen is extracted from the blood by the liver and recycled; some is excreted in the urine.

DETOXIFICATION

The liver has a prime role in detoxification of endogenous and exogenous substances. Ammonia (NH_3) is a major toxic product handled by the liver. Ammonia is produced in the gut and the liver from the deamination of amino acids, that is the removal of the amino group (NH_2) from amino acids. Bacteria in the GI tract are responsible for the ammonia formation in the gut. Peripheral blood ammonia levels are kept very low because the ammonia from the gut is extracted from the enterohepatic circulation by the liver and it, along with the ammonia produced in the liver, is detoxified by conversion into urea, which is then excreted by the kidneys.

Steroid hormones (estrogen, progesterone, testosterone, corticosterone, aldosterone) are inactivated by the liver. Liver diseases may depress this inactivation, resulting in pathologic levels of these hormones.

The liver detoxifies many drugs; all barbiturates (except phenobarbital and barbital) and many sedatives are inactivated by the liver. The status of the liver has an important role in the effectiveness or toxicity of these and other drugs.

STORAGE OF MINERALS AND VITAMINS

The liver stores reserves of various minerals and vitamins. This storage prevents abnormal internal levels from occurring, although the oral intake may be very irregular. Vitamins A, D, and B_{12} are stored in sufficient quantities to prevent deficiencies for months. Vitamins E and K are also stored. Iron in the form of *ferritin* is stored and can be used to resupply iron for hemoglobin formation as needed; copper is stored as well.

BLOOD RESERVOIR

The liver, because of its tremendous vascular supply and sinusoidal system, can act as a reservoir for blood. When the venous vascular volume becomes greater than can be handled by the right side of the heart, the excess blood can accumulate in the liver.

PHYSIOLOGIC CHANGES WITH AGING

The liver decreases in size with aging, and enzymes involved in metabolism of drugs have been found to be decreased in the aged.[9,13] However, common liver function tests are normal. The major effect of the hepatic changes of these enzymes is on the metabolism of such drugs as anticonvulsants, psychotropics, and oral anticoagulants.[4,13] The level of these drugs in the body may be increased because of slowed metabolism. The nurse should be alert to signs and symptoms that indicate drug toxicity.

SUBJECTIVE DATA

A thorough history is necessary to assess adequately the health status of persons with potential dysfunction of the hepatic system. These data assist in identifying immediate nursing needs and providing information necessary for helping patients to live with chronic problems of the hepatic system. The assessment focuses on comfort status; nutritional status; fluid and electrolyte status; elimination patterns; energy level; perception, motion, and cognition; and potential exposure to toxins.

COMFORT STATUS

Discomfort resulting from abdominal pain or *pruritus* (itching) may be one of the major problems of persons with hepatic dysfunction. The person may complain of continuous upper abdominal discomfort or a dull ache in the upper right quadrant. The discomfort does not usually alter normal functioning. The discomfort is most significant in that it provides verification for the underlying pathological process. Comfort status may be altered because of the general body aching associated with acute viral infections of the hepatic system. Most distressing to the patient is the pruritus usually associated with jaundice, which may cause significant discomfort. The history should include an assessment of factors that worsen itching and of measures that help to relieve it.

NUTRITIONAL STATUS

Persons with hepatic dysfunction often experience alterations in nutritional status. Some hepatic problems result in anorexia, nausea, and vomiting, and the patient should be questioned about the occurrence of such epi-

sodes. Assessment should include onset, precipitating factors, association with food or alcohol intake, and measures that provide relief.

Poor nutritional habits and malnutrition resulting from life-style patterns or food intolerances may be present. The person's normal daily intake should be ascertained. Alcohol use should also be assessed. Weight loss may have been noticed by the patient but can be hidden by water retention. The patient may have noticed changes in muscle mass, even though overall weight may have stayed the same. Also, alcohol, which provides calories but has no nutrient value, may hide the weight loss normally associated with malnutrition.

Persons with chronic problems of the hepatic system often require treatment with special diets, such as low sodium, altered protein intake, water restriction, and so forth. In anticipation of these needs, the history should include information about food intolerances and food preferences.

FLUID AND ELECTROLYTE STATUS

Hepatic dysfunction can be associated with volume deficit from nausea and vomiting or even from acute bleeding with cirrhosis. Fluid volume excess from abnormal sodium and water retention may also be present. Sometimes patients show interstitial fluid excess with vascular volume deficit. Levels of electrolytes particularly sodium, potassium, hydrogen, and bicarbonate, can be elevated or decreased.

To establish the patient's needs, the history collected should include information about:
1. Normal fluid and food intake and output
2. Abnormal fluid and electrolyte losses, such as vomiting, diarrhea, or bleeding
3. Changes in weight, both losses and gains
4. Occurence of signs and symptoms of fluid or electrolyte deficit, such as weakness, dizziness, and syncope
5. Occurence of signs and symptoms of fluid or electrolyte excess, such as edema in hands, feet, and legs and an increase in abdominal girth

ELIMINATION PATTERNS

Intestinal and urinary elimination may be altered in persons with liver problems. If obstruction of bile flow is present, the patient may give a history of clay-colored (grayish-white) stools or dark urine. Blood in the urine or stools may also be reported by persons with cirrhosis. A reported decrease in urine output or the occurence of nocturia may result from sodium and water retention.

ENERGY LEVEL

Because of altered nutrient intake, abnormal fluid and electrolyte status, and increased metabolic needs, persons with hepatic problems often complain of an inability to carry out normal activities or simply a decrease in energy. Some may give specific complaints of weakness. Although these complaints may occur in various situations, it is important to assess whether they are present so that complete nursing care can be provided. Although such complaints may resolve as the underlying problem is controlled, the patient and significant others must understand that restoration of energy level takes time to return to normal.

PERCEPTION, MOTION, AND COGNITION

Chronic health problems of the hepatic system can cause changes in neurologic functioning, particularily in relation to the peripheral nervous system and higher cognitive functions. The patient should be asked about alterations in sensation in extremities, any noticeable changes in memory, episodes of forgetfulness or blackouts, and alterations in coordination or in ability to do fine motor tasks. The *onset* of any alterations, *pattern* of changes (continuous or intermittent), and *duration* of any changes should be determined.

EXPOSURE TO TOXINS

Hepatic dysfunction can be caused by various agents, such as alcohol, drugs, industrial chemicals, and viruses. A history of exposure to any toxins must be elicited. A *drug and alcohol history* is necessary to determine whether the patient has been exposed to these two toxins. The drug history should focus on prescription, over-the-counter, and street drugs. The alcohol history should focus on normal amount of intake and time since last intake. An *occupational history* helps to identify potential toxins in the work environment. An *environmental/social history* might identify potential sources of viruses. (See box below for significant sources of contact with the hepatitis viruses.) The environmental/social history also can help identify particular persons, factors, or places associated with substance abuse, if

---

HEALTH HISTORY NECESSARY TO IDENTIFY EXPOSURE TO HEPATITIS VIRUSES

Contact with persons with jaundice
Travel or visits to environments with poor sanitation (camping trips, travel to less well-developed countries, and so on)
Ingestion of shellfish
History of recent ear piercing or tattooing
History of recent blood transfusions
Intravenous drug abuse (sharing of contaminated needles)
Occupational exposure (health service personnel with frequent blood contact, personnel in day care centers, personnel in centers of custodial care, and so forth)
History of active homosexual or bisexual lifestyle

---

this is a problem. Data about persons, factors, or places associated with substance abuse are needed for long-term management of drug and alcohol abuse (see Chapter 19).

OBJECTIVE DATA

To assess the functioning of the hepatic system completely, a thorough assessment of the total body will be required. First, examination of the overall appearance of patients will be necessary. Do they appear chronically or acutely ill? Are they attentive, restless, or lethargic? Do they appear nourished, or malnourished? Do they appear jaundiced? Are there any other signs of hepatic dysfunction, such as enlarged abdomen, palmar erythema, change in secondary sexual characteristics, bruises, muscle wasting, or edema?

After the general inspection, the assessment should focus on fluid status. Vital signs, including orthostatic changes, weight, temperature, skin turgor, mucous membrane moisture, presence of edema, and behavior, should be assessed. To assess energy level and nutritional status, the patient's total muscle mass and muscle strength should be examined.

While performing the assessment mentioned previously, the patient's mental status, affect, and alertness should be noted. Note changes in facial expression, responsiveness, and affect. Are there periods of confusion or disorientation? Is the affect appropriate for this situation? Because handwriting or the ability to draw a box, triangle, or square deteriorates with worsening of liver function, a sample of handwriting or a drawing of a geometric figure may be obtained from the patient.

After assessing the total person, the examination should focus on the abdomen. Inspection of the abdomen for enlargement, presence of distended or dilated periumbilical veins (*caput medusae*), and ascites, which is characterized by distention, tight glistening skin, and bulging flanks, should be performed.

Palpation or percussion of the abdomen to ascertain the presence of a fluid wave and shifting dullness, which are indicative of ascites, should be performed. Palpation and percussion are also used to assess for hepatic tenderness, size, and consistency and the presence of hepatic masses. The spleen is often enlarged in the patient with chronic hepatic dysfunction and should be palpated and percussed. Lastly, abdominal girth should be measured.

DIAGNOSTIC TESTS

Various tests help in assessing the status of the hepatic system. Many of the tests require taking samples of blood; other tests are more extensive and may cause discomfort; still others may require fasting. The nurse is

TABLE 38-1 Laboratory tests of liver function

Function and Test	Procedure and Preparation	Interpretation
Fat metabolism		
Serum total cholesterol and cholesterol esters	Blood drawn; fasting may be required	Normal level is 140-220 mg/100 ml of blood; approximately 70% is cholesterol ester; in hepatocellular disease, amount of total serum cholesterol and cholesterol ester may be decreased; in obstructive biliary tract disease, total serum cholesterol is increased, but amount of esterified cholesterol is decreased; normal cholesterol levels rise with age.
Serum phospholipids	Blood drawn; no special preparation	Normal level is 150-250 mg/100 ml; serum phospholipids tend to be low in severe hepatocellular disease and high in obstructive biliary tract disease.
Protein metabolism		
Total serum protein	Blood drawn; no special preparation	Normal level is 6-8 g/100 ml; measures all serum protein; may be normal in hepatocellular disease because increased serum globulin will replace decreased serum albumin; increased serum globulin is seen in chronic inflammatory disease, neoplastic diseases, and biliary obstruction.
Albumin	Blood drawn; no special preparation	Normal level is 3.4-5.0 g/100 ml; albumin made only in liver; in hepatocellular disease there may be a decrease in serum albumin level.
Protein electrophoresis	Blood drawn; no special preparation; protein fraction of blood will migrate in characteristic directions in electrical field; after separation of fractions, specimen stained, and densitometer used to measure amounts of various serum protein	Normal fractions in relation to total serum protein (100%) are albumin, 52%-68%; α-globulins, 12%-17%; β-globulins, 7%-15%; and immune serum globulins (γ-globulins), 9%-19%; in severe hepatocellular damage, amount of albumin may be decreased; inflammatory processes of the liver may produce increased amounts of α_1-globulins, neoplastic disease is associated with increased levels of α_2-globulins, and some patients with obstructive biliary tract disease may have high levels of β-globulins.
Immunoglobulins	Blood drawn; no special preparation	Five classes of antibodies; IgA, IgG, IgM, IgE, and IgD; IgA and IgG are often increased in the presence of cirrhosis; IgG is elevated in the presence of chronic active hepatitis; biliary cirrhosis and hepatitis A cause an increase in the IgM component.
Blood urea nitrogen (BUN)	Blood drawn; no special preparation	Normal is 10-20 mg/100 ml; in severe hepatocellular disease if portal venous flow is obstructed, level may decrease; varies with dietary protein intake and fluid volume.
Serum prothrombin time (PT)	Blood drawn; no special preparation; reflects activity of extrinsic and common coagulation pathways, including prothrombin, fibrinogen, and factors V, VII, IX, and X	Normal PT is 12-15 sec or 100%, as compared to control level; PT may be increased in hepatocellular disease because of the inability of liver to produce clotting factors or in obstructive hepatic or biliary tract disease because of the malabsorption of vitamin K; persistence of abnormal PT after parenteral administration of vitamin K indicates hepatocellular damage.
Serum partial thromboplastin time (PTT) and activated partial thromboplastin time (APTT)	Blood drawn; no special preparation; reflects activity of intrinsic and common coagulation pathways	Normal PTT is 68-82 sec with standard technique, APTT is 32-46 sec; PTT and APTT will be increased in hepatocellular disease because of the inability of liver to produce clotting factors.
Blood ammonia levels	Blood drawn; may require fasting	Normal level is less than 75 μg/100 ml; may be elevated in severe hepatocellular disease because of obstruction of portal blood flow and rarely because of decreased urea synthesis.

Continued.

TABLE 38-1 Laboratory tests of liver function—cont'd.

Function and Test	Procedure and Preparation	Interpretation
Bilirubin metabolism		

Total bilirubin
  Conjugated (direct)
  Unconjugated (indirect)
	Blood drawn; no special preparation	Total serum bilirubin measures both conjugated and unconjugated bilirubin; normal total serum bilirubin values range from 0.1-1 mg/100 ml; conjugated bilirubin acts directly with diazo reagents; unconjugated bilirubin requires addition of methyl alcohol; thus the terms *direct* and *indirect;* conjugated bilirubin increases in the presence of hepatocellular or obstructive biliary tract disease; unconjugated bilirubin is elevated in the presence of increased hemolysis of red blood cells or hepatocellular disease.

Urine bilirubin	Spot urine specimen; no special preparation	Normally no bilirubin is excreted in urine; urine with abnormal bilirubin is mahogany colored and has a yellow foam when shaken *(foam test);* unconjugated bilirubin even in excess is not excreted in urine because it is not water soluble; conjugated serum bilirubin levels greater than 0.4 mg/100 ml will lead to conjugated bilirubin being excreted in urine because it is not water soluble and indicates hepatocellular or obstructive biliary tract disease; bilirubinuria may be present before jaundice.
Urine urobilinogen	24-hr urine collection or 2-hr afternoon collection	Normally 0.2-1.2 units found in specimen; fresh urine urobilinogen is colorless; decreased amounts of urine urobilinogen found in obstructive biliary tract disease; increased amounts found in hepatocellular disease; alterations in intestinal flora by broad-spectrum antibiotics may change test.
Fecal urobilinogen	Stool specimen; no special preparation	Normally 90-280 mg/day; presence of fecal urobilinogen (stercobilin) gives stool brown color; absence of stercobilin causes stools to become clay (grayish-white) to white colored; increased amounts of stercobilin found with increased hemolysis of red blood cells; absence of fecal stercobilin indicates obstructive biliary tract disease.
Serum enzymes		
Asparate aminotransferase (AST), formerly called serum glutamicoxaloacetic transaminase (SGOT) alanine aminotransferase (ALT), formerly called Serum glutamicpyruvic transaminase (SGPT) Lactic dehydrogenase (LDH) Gamma-glutamyl transpeptidase (GGT) (γ-glutamyltransferase)	Blood drawn; no special preparation	Normal values vary depending on measurement used; these enzymes are present in hepatic cells, and with necrosis of hepatic cells, enzymes are released and elevated serum levels will be found; GGT is found in high levels in liver cells as well as kidneys; ALT is primarily present in liver cells; AST is also present in high levels in skeletal and heart muscle; LDH is also present in heart cells, kidneys cells, skeletal muscle cells, and erythrocytes, but in each tissue the LDH enzyme has a characteristic composition: thus the tissue source of elevated serum LDH levels can be determined by isoenzyme tests; with the other three enzyme tests, necrosis of other organs must be ruled out; GGT is elevated early in liver disease, and elevation persists as long as cellular damage continues; GGT is routinely elevated in alcohol-induced liver disease and increased levels are often seen before other abnormal test results occur.
Alkaline phosphatase	Blood drawn; no special preparation	Normal values vary depending on measurement used; this enzyme originates in liver, bone, intestine, and placenta; alkaline phosphatase is slightly to moderately elevated in hepatocellular disease but extremely elevated in obstructive biliary tract and bone disease.

TABLE 38-1 Laboratory tests of liver function—cont'd.

Function and Test	Procedure and Preparation	Interpretation
Antigens and antibodies of viral hepatitis	Blood drawn; no special preparation	Normally no hepatitis antigens are found in the serum or other body fluids; *hepatitis A virus (HAV)* can be found in the stool during the last part of the incubation period and early prodromal phase; *IgM-class anti-HAV* appears in the acute and early convalescent period and is used to diagnose hepatitis A; *IgG-class anti-HAV* becomes detectable during the convalescent period and confers enduring protection; hepatitis B has many associated serum particles; complete *hepatitis B virus (HBV)* is also called Dane particle; a *core antigen (HB$_c$Ag)* can be found in the liver, an *antibody (anti-HB$_c$)* can be found in the blood, and the presence of *anti-HB$_c$* indicates past infection with HBV at some undefined time; a *surface antigen (HB$_s$Ag)* and several subtypes and *antibody (anti-HB$_s$)* are also measurable; *HB$_s$Ag*, previously called Australia antigen, is one of antigens measured to diagnose hepatitis B, and its presence indicates infectivity; presence of *anti-HB$_s$* indicates past infection and immunity to HBV, presence of passive antibodies from HBIG, or immune response from HBV vaccine; *hepatitis B$_e$* antigen *(HB$_e$Ag)* indicates high infectivity and its *antibody (anti-HB$_e$)* chronic infectivity. A virus associated with non-A, non-B hepatitis has been identified and termed *hepatitis C virus (HCV)*; an assay for an *antibody* to hepatitis C virus *(anti-HCV)* has been developed. *Anti-HCV* has been found in approximately 50% of persons with non-A, non-B hepatitis.

responsible for preparing the patient for the tests. The physical preparation of the patient will vary from institution to institution, and the nurse needs to learn the routine preparation. In addition to the physical preparation, the nurse carries out appropriate teaching and monitoring of the patient before, during, and after the diagnostic tests.

LABORATORY TESTS

Multiple tests may be necessary to determine the extent and seriousness of hepatic disease. Many tests require serial readings to be of benefit. The procedure, special preparation, and interpretation of frequently used blood, stool, and urine studies for evaluation of liver function are summarized in Table 38-1. Bromsulphalein (BSP) excretion test measures the excretory capacity of the liver. This test is rarely used at this time. (See reference 12 for information on this topic.)

RADIOLOGIC TESTS

Roentgenologic tests are used to assist in identifying the cause of hepatic dysfunction. Besides the examinations described in the following section, abdominal films, barium swallow, barium enema, and gastroscopy may be ordered. These tests help to identify the presence of

pathologic GI conditions that may cause similar signs and symptoms as found in hepatic dysfunction or that may result from complications of hepatic dysfunction.

ULTRASONOGRAPHY

Ultrasonography of the liver may be done. This test helps to differeniate between causes of jaundice associated with increased serum bilirubin levels and to identify hepatic metastases, hematomas, and abscesses.

The preparation of the patient for ultrasonography is relatively simple. Usually the patient is not allowed to eat for 8 to 12 hours before the procedure, because bowel gas in the GI tract will interfere with the test. Any residual barium needs to be removed from the GI tract before the test. The patient must be well hydrated, because dehydration can decrease the ability of ultrasonography to distinguish between the liver and surrounding tissues. Ultrasound is used intraoperatively to identify hepatic tumors.[2]

COMPUTED TOMOGRAPHY (CT SCAN)

Computed tomography can also be used to assess patients with potential hepatic problems. It is helpful in identifying problems similar to those described for ultrasonography. Contrast medium can be used with the CT scan to intensify the appearance of vascular structures and hepatic parenchyma. The patient should eat nothing for 8 to 12 hours before the test; if contrast medium is to be used, the patient should be assessed for allergies to iodine or contrast media. Barium studies should be done at least 4 days before the CT scan or after the scan because the barium can interfere with test results.

RADIONUCLIDE IMAGING

The liver may be outlined by radionuclide imaging techniques. Selected radioisotopes are given intravenously. After the injection of the radioisotope, the patient is placed supine, and a scintillation detector is passed over the abdomen in the area of the liver. The radiation coming from the isotopes immediately beneath the probe of the scanner is detected, amplified, and recorded. Scanning helps to differentiate nonfunctioning areas from normal tissue and helps to identify hepatic tumors, cysts, and abscesses. Usually a nonfunctioning area will appear as an area of decreased activity. However, gallium-67 (^{67}Ga) is preferentially taken up by hepatocellular carcinomas and abscesses, and these areas will appear as areas of very heavy radioactivity. Adverse reactions to the radioisotopes used for radionuclide imaging are unusual, and the procedure is relatively safe. Discomfort is minimal and is related to the intravenous injection and the position on the x-ray table. Only small amounts of radioactive material are given, and radiation precautions are *not* necessary. Except for ^{67}Ga scanning, no special preparation is required. Gallium-67 is excreted by the GI tract. To avoid absorption of the radioisotope by the GI contents, cleansing of the bowel with laxatives and enemas is prescribed. The exact preparation will vary from institution to institution. Radionuclide imaging is being used less than other tests such as CT scan or ultrasonography in patients with potential hepatic dysfunction.[2]

ANGIOGRAPHY AND PORTAL PRESSURE MEASUREMENTS

Catheterization of the hepatic artery, portal venous system (by various routes), and the hepatic vein allows the injection of a contrast media and the visualization of the vascular supply of the hepatic system. The patency of the system and the presence of tumors, abscesses, collateral circulation, varices, and bleeding may be determined by use of angiography.

Portal and hepatic vein pressure (wedged hepatic vein pressure [WHVP]) can be measured. These readings may be done in conjunction with angiography or as a separate study. These measurements help in determining the degree of portal hypertension.

The presence of allergy to contrast media must be ascertained before angiography is done. After both angiography and pressure readings, the site of insertion is ob-

served for bleeding, and the patient's vital signs are checked frequently (such as every 15 minutes for one hour, every 30 minutes for one hour, every hour for 4 hours, and then if the patient is stable, every 4 hours). The patient is kept on bed rest for 24 to 48 hours and positioned on the left side to decrease the chance of bleeding.

SPECIAL TESTS
BIOPSY OF THE LIVER

A biopsy of the liver may be used to aid in establishing the cause of liver disease. In this procedure a specially designed needle is inserted through the chest or abdominal wall into the liver, and a small piece of tissue is removed for study. This procedure is contraindicated in a patient who has an infection of the right lower lobe of the lung, ascites, or a blood dyscrasia, as well as in any patient unable to cooperate by holding his/her breath. To avoid hemorrhage, vitamin K may be given parenterally for several days before and after the biopsy is taken. A biopsy usually is not done if the prothrombin time is below 40%. The physician should explain the procedure to the patient; for example, the importance of being able to hold one's breath and remain absolutely still when the needle is introduced. Movement of the chest may cause the needle to slip and to tear the liver covering. Most hospitals require that the patient sign a written permission form for the procedure to be done. Food and fluids may be withheld for several hours preceding the test, and a sedative usually is given about 30 minutes before the biopsy.

A liver biopsy is performed as follows: The patient lies supine; the skin over the area selected (usually the eighth or ninth intercostal space) is cleansed and anesthetized with procaine hydrochloride. A nick is made in the skin with a sharp scalpel blade. Then the patient is instructed to take several deep breaths and then to hold his or her breath while the needle is introduced through the intercostal or subcostal tissues into the liver. The special needle assembly is rotated to separate a fragment of tissue and then is withdrawn. The specimen is placed into an appropriate container, which is labeled and sent to the pathology laboratory. A simple dressing is placed over the wound.

The dangers of liver biopsy, which is done relatively "blind," are accidental penetration of blood vessels, causing hemorrhage, or accidental penetration of a biliary canniculi, causing a chemical peritonitis from leakage of bile into the abdominal cavity. After the procedure the patient's pulse rate and blood pressure should be taken every 30 minutes for the first few hours and then hourly for at least 24 hours. The physician may order pressure applied to the biopsy site to help stop any bleeding. An effective way to apply pressure is to have the patient lie on the right side with a small pillow or folded bath blanket placed under the costal margin for several hours after the biopsy. Bed rest is maintained for 24 hours after the test.

ENDOSCOPY

The hepatic system and gallbladder can be examined by endoscopy. Two types of endoscopic procedures can be done. The tube can be inserted through the peritoneum (*peritoneoscopy*), thus affording direct visualization of the abdominal organs and the taking of biopsies. An *esophagoscopy* or *gastroscopy* may be done to visualize esophageal varices or injection sclerotherapy. Fasting is required before the test, and the patient may be given a preprocedural sedative.

PARACENTESIS

A paracentesis, or peritoneal tap, can be done to remove peritoneal fluid (ascitic fluid) for cytology or other laboratory studies or to drain large volumes of ascitic fluid. When such conditions as respiratory distress, severe abdominal discomfort, or cardiac dysfunction, are present because of the ascites, a paracentesis may be necessary. It is important to note that repeated paracenteses are not the treatment of choice for controlling chronic, recurring ascites because of complications.

When paracentesis is performed, the skin is cleansed and the abdominal wall anesthesized. A long, aspiration needle is inserted, and fluid is aspirated for diagnostic tests or drained as necessary. In preparation for the procedure, the patient is given a complete explanation, a consent form is signed, and the patient should void immediately before the procedure to diminish the risk of puncturing the bladder. Sterile technique must be maintained during the procedure.

The complications of paracentesis include peritonitis, if sterility is not maintained, and peritoneal bleeding resulting from trauma to blood vessels. The patient's vital signs, including temperature, urine output, and skin temperature and moisture, should be monitored for signs of peritonitis or bleeding. The patient's abdomen should be assessed for rigidity and his or her sensorium for confusion.

Removal of large amounts of fluid from the peritoneal space can result in hypovolemia and shock because additional fluid can shift from the intravascular compartment into the peritoneal cavity, although this risk is minimal in the patient with cirrhosis and edema. Other substances that are lost with removal of large amounts of ascitic fluid are protein and potassium. Postprocedural monitoring of vital signs, mental status, urine output, skin temperature and moisture, mucous membrane moisture, and so forth should be instituted to monitor for hypovolemia. Laboratory studies should be monitored to determine whether protein and potassium levels are normal.

PERITONEAL LAVAGE

Peritoneal lavage may be used to assess damage to the liver from abdominal trauma in persons with altered states of consciousness who cannot give a satisfactory history. It may also be used in patients with abdominal trauma when unexplained hypotension is present, when unreliable physical examination results are present, or when the patient requires general anesthesia for other injuries.

Peritoneal lavage can be done by either the closed or open method. In the *closed method,* a peritoneal dialysis catheter is inserted, and the peritoneal space is aspirated for gross blood. If no gross blood is found, lavage is carried out with normal saline. In the *open method* the peritoneum is exposed completely and then opened enough to allow entry of a dialysis catheter. Again, gross blood is aspirated first, and if no blood is found, lavage is carried out.

Peritoneal lavage requires a complete explanation to the patient and significant others and informed consent. A nasogastric tube and Foley catheter are inserted before the procedure to prevent penetration of the intestines or bladder. In the closed method a local anesthetic is used, whereas in the open method general anesthesia is necessary. Postprocedural care involves monitoring for peritonitis and bleeding in patients who have closed peritoneal lavage. Patients who have open peritoneal lavage require general postanesthetic care (see Chapter 22).

CHAPTER SUMMARY

- ✓ The liver is important for adequate energy production and waste disposal.

- ✓ Pathophysiologic conditions of the liver result in discomfort, inadequate nutrition, fluid and electrolyte deficit or excess, bleeding, altered elimination, inadequate energy levels, and altered perception, cognitive, and motor functioning.

- ✓ Pathophysiologic conditions of the liver can result from exposure to various toxins, including drugs, alcohol, chemicals, and viruses.

- ✓ Liver dysfunction results in multiple abnormalities in blood studies, which are used to help to identify the pathophysiologic state or other nursing needs.

- ✓ Radiologic, endoscopic, and other invasive tests are used to help in identifying the exact pathophysiologic condition. These tests all require special preparation and postprocedural care.

QUESTIONS TO CONSIDER

- What functional abnormalities occur most often in persons with hepatic dysfunction?

- Think about ways to gain information about alcohol and illegal drug use. What information do you need to obtain? What are some questions you could use to ascertain this information?

- What laboratory tests can be used to differeniate hepatitis A infection from hepatitis B infection?

- How do the abnormal laboratory results commonly seen in hepatic dysfunction relate to the normal functions of the hepatic system?

REFERENCES AND SELECTED READINGS

1. Berne R and Levy M, editors: Physiology, ed 2, St Louis, 1988, The CV Mosby Co.
2. Clouse ME: Current diagnostic imaging modalities of the liver, Surg Clin North Am, 69(2):193-234, 1989.
3. *Coleman WH: Gastroscopy: a primary diagnostic procedure, Prim Care 15(1):1-11, 1988.
4. Conrad KA and Bressler R, editors: Drug therapy for the elderly, St Louis, 1984, The CV Mosby Co.
5. *Ebersole P and Hess P: Toward healthy aging: human needs and nursing response, ed 3, St Louis, 1989, The CV Mosby Co.
6. Hawkins ML et al: Diagnostic peritoneal lavage in blunt trauma, South Med J, 81(3):293-296, 1988.
7. Johnson LR: Gastrointestinal physiology, ed 3, St Louis, 1985, The CV Mosby Co.
7a. Mosley JW et al: Non-A, non-B hepatitis and antibody to hepatitis C virus, JAMA 263:77-78, 1990.
8. Reichling JJ and Kaplan MM: Clinical use of serum enzymes in liver disease, Dig Dis Sci, 33(12):1601-1614, 1988.
9. Steinberg FU, editor: Care of the geriatric patient, ed 6, St Louis, 1983, The CV Mosby Co.
9a. Stevens CE et al: Epidemiology of hepatitis C virus, JAMA 263:49-53, 1990.
10. *Tilkian SM, Conover MB, and Tilkian AG: Clinical implications of laboratory tests, ed 4, St Louis, 1987, The CV Mosby Co.
11. Waite WW: Clinical laboratories for the practicing pharmacist: liver function tests, Am Pharm NS28(12):51-55, 1988.
12. Widmann F: Goodall's clinical interpretation of laboratory tests, ed 10, Philadelphia, 1987, FA Davis Co.
12a. Witkin GB et al: Choosing liver function tests, Emergency Med 19(20):22-46, 1987.
13. Wyngaarden JB and Smith LH, editors: Cecil textbook of medicine, ed 18, Philadelphia, 1988, WB Saunders Co.

*References preceded by an asterisk are particularly well suited for student reading.

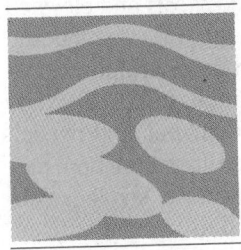

Management of Persons with Liver Problems

VIRGINIA L. CASSMEYER

CHAPTER OBJECTIVES

After studying this chapter, the student should be able to:

1. Describe the medical and nursing care needs of patients with liver abscesses, tumors, and trauma.
2. Contrast differences between pathophysiology and signs and symptoms of focal liver disease and diffuse hepatocellular liver disorders.
3. Differentiate between toxic and viral hepatitis.
4. Differentiate between hepatitis A, B, delta, and non-A, non-B.
5. Describe the pathophysiologic basis of the clinical manifestations in cirrhosis and the sequelae of cirrhosis.
6. Develop a plan of care for patients with viral or toxic hepatitis or cirrhosis.
7. Describe the common medical and nursing needs of a patient with ascites, esophageal varices, portal systemic encephalopathy, or hepatorenal syndrome.
8. Describe the common needs of a person before and after a hepatic transplantation.

The liver or hepatic system is affected by a variety of disorders that produce many physiologic and psychosocial needs for patients as well as many nursing care challenges. Some patients with liver problems are critically ill and will require intensive care nursing; some problems of the liver are chronic in nature and require nursing care that helps the patient make the changes necessary to control the problem and prevent its progression. Patients with chronic problems often have acute exacerbations, so there will be periods in which intensive, total care is required; as stabilization of the alteration occurs, emphasis on regaining self-management skills is required.

Severe liver problems can result from a variety of causes such as infective organisms, neoplastic growths, toxic agents, and trauma. The pathologic states that result can be classified in several ways. In this chapter, disorders will be classified as focal (localized to one portion of the liver) hepatocellular disorders and diffuse (spread through a major portion of the liver) hepatocellular disorders (see the box at right).

FOCAL HEPATOCELLULAR DISORDERS

Three of the more common focal hepatocellular disorders are discussed next.

LIVER ABSCESS
ETIOLOGY/EPIDEMIOLOGY

Liver abscesses may result from a variety of organisms, including *Escherichia coli, Staphylococcus, Streptococcus, Pseudomonas, Proteus,* and *Klebsiella.* In patients with depressed immune functioning, such as those with neutropenia or leukemia, systemic candidiases with multiple hepatic abscesses have been found. Many persons with abscesses have multiple bacteria involved.[59] *Entamoeba histolytica* is an important worldwide cause of amebic liver abscess and dysentery. It most frequently is found in tropical and subtropical regions, but it is also found in temperate zones and in many parts of the United States.

PATHOPHYSIOLOGY

Pyogenic abscesses can occur as either a singular large abscess or multiple small and/or microscopic abscesses. Amebic liver abscesses are typically large and singular.

COMMON LIVER DISORDERS

FOCAL HEPATOCELLULAR DISORDERS

1. Abscess of the liver
2. Trauma to the liver
3. Tumors of the liver

DIFFUSE HEPATOCELLULAR DISORDERS

1. Hepatitis
2. Cirrhosis
3. Sequelae of chronic diffuse hepatocellular disorders
   a. Portal hypertension
   b. Ascites
   c. Esophageal varices
   d. Portal-systemic encephalopathy
   e. Hepatorenal syndrome

Liver abscesses are usually a secondary site of infection. Pyogenic organisms originating in various areas of the body reach the liver through the biliary, vascular, or lymphatic systems. In addition, pyogenic organisms may be introduced by penetrating injuries to the liver or by direct contiguous extension. In amebic abscesses, the vegetative form of the organism moves from the gut to the small portal vessels and into the hepatic tissue, where it becomes activated and causes tissue destruction and abscess formation.

The abscess formation may disrupt hepatic function, but most of the altered physiologic function is caused by the presence of an acute infective process. If liver abscesses are not identified, they continue to increase in size and can perforate into the pleural cavity, the peritoneal cavity, or the pericardial cavity.

CLINICAL MANIFESTATIONS

Signs and Symptoms

The major manifestations of liver abscess are caused by the infection rather than by changes in hepatic functioning. There is usually a history of not feeling well for several weeks. Common manifestations of the infectious process include:

1. Temperature elevation ranging between 102° F (38.8° C) and 106° F (41.1° C)
2. Presence of cough
3. Presence of chills
4. Diaphoresis
5. Presence of difficult breathing or abnormal breath sounds from pleural involvement
6. Right upper abdominal quadrant pain and tenderness
7. History of anorexia, nausea, and vomiting
8. Weight loss
9. Signs and symptoms of peritonitis (see p. 1154), if there is rupture and leakage of abscess into the peritoneal cavity

Manifestations of altered hepatic function that may be present are:

1. Hepatomegaly
2. Jaundice and pruritis
3. Splenomegaly
4. Abdominal distention and ascites

The patient with *pyogenic abscesses,* particularly multiple small or microscopic abscesses, may have clinical manifestations of sepsis and septic shock. The patient with *amebic abscesses* may have signs and symptoms of intestinal amebiasis or give a history of previous intestinal signs and symptoms such as bloody, mucoid diarrhea; generalized abdominal pain; rectal tenesmus; dehydration; and hypotension. But many patients with amebic abscess report no previous history of intestinal signs and symptoms.

Diagnostic Tests

Diagnostic tests usually reveal leukocytosis and elevated erythrocyte sedimentation rate due to the infection and moderate elevation of serum alkaline phosphatase and minimal elevation of serum transaminases (AST, ALT) from liver cell damage. Hyperbilirubinemia and hypoalbuminemia resulting from impaired liver function may also be present. In amebic liver abscesses, serologic laboratory tests such as immunoglobulins against antigen, indirect hemagglutination (IHA) titers, complement fixation tests, and latex agglutination tests are highly diagnostic for the amebic infection. Hepatic radioisotope scans, ultrasonic scanning, and CT scans also are used in diagnosis and follow-up evaluation and reveal the presence of abscesses.

INTERVENTIONS

Medical Management

The medical management for the patient with liver abscesses includes the following:

1. Supportive measures—fluid and electrolyte replacement and control of temperature elevation
2. Surgical drainage of the abscess and antimicrobial therapy for pyogenic abscesses
3. Metronidazole (Flagyl), chloroquine, and dehydroemetine, or emetine for amebic abscesses. Needle aspiration or surgical drainage of amebic abscesses is only indicated in select patients because these abscesses respond very well to medication alone, and needle aspiration or surgical drainage have not demonstrated a greater therapeutic effectiveness.

Nursing Management

Nursing management is directed toward assisting with (1) the control of discomfort including dealing with pruritis if jaundice is present (see p. 1159 and 1170), (2) fluid and nutritional deficits, (3) the medical regimen (diagnostic tests and therapeutic measures), and (4) assisting the patient to attain appropriate knowledge for self-management. In the very acute situation, nursing management may incorporate the care needs described for a patient with sepsis and septic shock (see Chapter 25) or severe intestinal colitis, appendicitis, and megacolon (see Chapter 44). Some potential nursing diagnoses for persons with the less acute form of liver abscesses are presented in the box on p. 1153. The first priority of care is to help with treatment of fluid volume deficit or shock, if present. The next priority is to provide comfort measures. The high temperature, episodes of chills and diaphoresis, pruritus, anorexia, and abdominal pain all cause discomfort. During periods of chills, adequate blankets to provide comfort without increasing temperature will be necessary. Drafts should be eliminated. Cool sponge baths may help lower the temperature. Linens and gowns should be changed if diaphore-

POTENTIAL NURSING DIAGNOSES FOR LESS ACUTE FORM OF LIVER ABSCESSES

Fluid volume deficit: actual (2) related to fever, nausea, and vomiting; diaphoresis; and decreased intake

Nutrition, altered: less than body requirements related to anorexia and increased metabolic needs

Knowledge deficit: immediate needs and long-term needs related to new disease and no previous exposure to information

Pain related to stretching of liver capsule, muscle aches with febrile illness, and pruritis associated with jaundice

---

sis occurs. Pruritus, as summarized in the following discussion and described in more detail on p. 1170, can be controlled with cool sponge baths, use of soft linens, prevention of dry skin, and provision of a cool environment.

Another aspect of care is to provide adequate fluids and nutrition. At first the patient may only tolerate intravenous fluids or at least need intravenous fluids to replace deficits. The nurse is responsible for seeing that the fluids are administered as ordered and for monitoring therapy effectiveness (patient shows no signs of dehydration, regains and maintains weight, and shows no hemoconcentration in laboratory values) and potential side effects of therapy (patient shows no signs of fluid overload). Oral fluids and food will be given as tolerated. The goal is to provide adequate calories, nutrients, vitamins, and minerals for the patient's size, age, and metabolic needs. Food should be given in small amounts, and the patient's preferences should be incorporated to help overcome anorexia. Frequent oral hygiene (at least once every eight hours) is necessary because fever and fluid loss cause drying of the mucous membranes and may worsen anorexia. The environment should be clean, free of odors, and relaxed.

In assisting with the medical regimen, the nurse will be primarily involved with preparing patients physically for tests (instituting nothing by mouth status or other preparations as necessary as described in Chapter 38 for specific test). The patient will also need appropriate education about the various tests (what will be done, purpose of test, and special care necessary as described in Chapter 38). The nurse will be involved in preparing those patients having surgical drainage of abscesses for surgery and providing appropriate postoperative care similar to that needed by any patient (see Chapter 22). The nurse will also be involved in administering the prescribed antimicrobials and amebicidal agents. This involves not only appropriate administration, but also monitoring for side effects.

Patient education for long-term care is also a major nursing responsibility. For some patients with liver ab-

scesses the medication may need to be taken for some time (several weeks to several months). The patient must be instructed about the importance of continual compliance with medications. In addition, the patient should be instructed to report immediately any signs and symptoms of recurrence of infection (recurring chills, fever, and diaphoresis), of spread of infection (worsening abdominal pain or increased difficulty breathing), or of worsening of hepatic functioning, for example, cirrhosis (see p. 1173), as well as any side effects of the medication. Instructions about the need for continual follow-up should be emphasized.

For the person with amebic abscesses, prevention of recurrence is important. The nurse should help the patient identify potentially contaminated sources of food and water and help to identify ways to decontaminate or avoid these sources, such as using iodine-releasing tablets in water and scalding of vegetables or not eating peelings of fresh fruits.

LIVER TRAUMA

Because of its location and size, the liver is frequently subjected to trauma, which may be either penetrating (gunshot wounds, stab wounds) or blunt (collision with steering wheel during automobile accidents, falls). If the injury is severe, rupture of the liver may occur with severe internal hemorrhage.

PATHOPHYSIOLOGY

The pathophysiology seen varies with the types of injury. Liver injuries are graded on a scale of one to five.[49a] In grade one there is laceration and capsular tear with minimal damage to the parenchyma. In grades two through five there is increasing parenchymal damage with fractures of the liver. In grade five, the damage extends into the retrohepatic vasculature. The liver is a highly vascular organ, and severe hemorrhage that results in hypovolemic shock may occur. Stab wounds often make a relatively superficial incision and may do no more damage than a needle biopsy of the liver. Gunshot wounds and blunt trauma often result in significant hemorrhage that results in hypotension or shock and leakage of bile from the biliary canniculi. Hypovolemic shock may occur. If the peritoneal cavity has been contaminated by blood or bile, *peritonitis* occurs (see box on p. 1154). Less severe blunt trauma may result in subcapsular hematoma only.

Late complications of liver trauma may include the following:

1. Severe hemorrhage, resulting from disseminated intravascular coagulation that often accompanies shock during the total course of treatment
2. Degeneration and sloughing of segments of the liver that have had disruption in circulation with resultant hemorrhage

3. Intrahepatic abscess formation
4. Traumatic hepatic cyst formation
5. Infections of other areas of body following hepatic trauma
6. Subphrenic abscess formation
7. Biliary fistulas

The mortality rate for liver trauma has decreased over the years. The mortality rate depends on type of injury (highest for blunt trauma because of the larger portion of liver damaged and because of other associated injuries), severity of the injury (highest for those requiring resection of a large amount of liver), and the presence of associated injuries (increasing mortality with each additional injury to another organ).

CLINICAL MANIFESTATIONS

Signs and Symptoms

The manifestations of liver trauma vary with type of injury. If the trauma is associated with a *penetrating injury,* an entry and sometimes exit wound or wounds on the anterior, lateral, or posterior aspects of the body may be present. In *blunt trauma* there will be no external injury, and pain is the most common symptom. Pain may be accentuated with respiration and referred to the shoulder as the result of irritation of the diaphram. Signs and symptoms of shock may be present (see Chapter 25). If peritoneal contamination from hemorrhage or bile has occurred, signs and symptoms of *peritonitis* may be present (see the box below, left).

Diagnostic Tests

In some instances the only sign of hepatic trauma is the presence of blood in peritoneal lavage (see Chapter 38 for a description of this test). Laboratory studies may reveal a decreasing hematocrit and hemoglobin from blood loss and leukocytoses from peritoneal infection and inflammation.

INTERVENTIONS

Medical Management

The immediate medical management for patients with suspected liver trauma is the same as that for any patient with intraabdominal trauma and includes the following:

1. Maintenance of airway
2. Intravenous therapy

SIGNS AND SYMPTOMS OF PERITONITIS

Abdominal tenderness
Rebound tenderness
Muscle rigidity or spasms
Decreased or absent bowel signs
Sometimes a fluid wave is present

---

3. Type and crossmatch for blood replacement
4. Drawing blood for laboratory tests
5. Urinary output monitoring
6. Central venous pressure (CVP) monitoring
7. Treatment of shock with fluids, dextran, and blood components (see Chapter 25)
8. Immediate surgical exploration of the abdomen to detect the presence of abdominal hemorrhage, trauma to liver or other organs, presence of necrotic tissue or presence of bile drainage
9. Treatment of peritonitis

Nursing Management

The *first* major nursing focus for the patient with suspected liver trauma is to establish and implement a system of monitoring that focuses on cardiovascular and volume status, neurologic status, and signs and symptoms of peritonitis (see the box below). This monitoring is required from the moment the patient is first seen through the postoperative period.

The *second* major focus for the nurse is to assist with the initiation of monitoring devices such as the Foley catheter and CVP lines, administration of fluids and blood, and collection of specimens for laboratory tests. The nurse will also be helping to prepare the patient for surgery if this is necessary.

The *third* major nursing focus is to assist the patient who is alert to control anxiety and fear. A major intervention that helps with the control of fear and anxiety is complete, simple explanations of everything that is going on. The nurse should strive to maintain a calm environment while carrying out interventions efficiently and rapidly. Maintaining continuity of care is essential.

The *fourth* major nursing focus is to assist the family or significant others. They need to be kept informed, given time to ask questions and to share fears, and of-

---

ASSESSMENT PARAMETERS FOR THE PATIENT WITH SUSPECTED LIVER TRAUMA

Vital signs every 15 minutes (blood pressure, pulse)
CVP every hour
Other hemodynamic monitoring, such as intra-arterial pressure monitoring, cardiac output measurements, etc as ordered
Urinary output and other fluid losses documented hourly
Intake documented hourly
Serum and urinary electrolytes and osmolality at least daily
Hematocrit and hemoglobin daily
Neurologic checks for alertness, responsiveness, and motion every hour
Respiratory status (rate, breath sounds, blood gases)
Skin temperature, color, and moisture every hour
Bowel sounds, pain, abdominal tenderness

fered spiritual support. During a critical situation, family members can easily be forgotten.

After the acute/critical period, which includes the postoperative period for some patients, continual monitoring as described above plus provision of emotional support for the patient and family are still needed. The patient will also need help with self-care, gradual increase in activity, and comfort measures. Over the long term, the patient needs to be able to do self-monitoring for signs and symptoms of residual liver damage that result from a decrease in the normal function of the liver and to be aware of the importance of continual follow-up for several months.

LIVER TUMORS

Liver neoplasms or tumors may be either benign or malignant. Benign lesions include hemangioma, cysts, and, rarely, adenoma. Most benign tumors are asymptomatic, but occasionally they enlarge enough to become symptomatic. If they become symptomatic, surgical intervention may be required. The care would be the same as that described later for the patient having surgical resection for malignant neoplasms. The focus of this section will be on malignant neoplasms.

ETIOLOGY/EPIDEMIOLOGY

Malignant tumors may be either primary or metastatic. Primary hepatic carcinomas may arise within the liver cell (hepatocellular) or the bile duct cell (cholangiocellular) or may be of mixed origin. *Hepatocellular* tumors are the most common. Primary liver cancer accounts for only 1% to 2% of malignant tumors found at death in the United States but is much more common in areas of Africa. Primary liver tumors are more common in men than in women and usually occur in the fifth and sixth decades of life. Chronic liver disease from hepatitis B, cirrhosis, hemochromatosis, or any other cause appears to predispose individuals to the development of primary liver cancer.

Metastatic tumors are common. They occur 20 times more frequently than primary tumors and rank second to cirrhosis as a cause of fatal liver disease. The liver most commonly receives metastatic cells from the gastrointestinal tract, the lungs, the breasts, the kidneys, and melanomas of the skin, although virtually any neoplasm can metastasize to the liver.

PATHOPHYSIOLOGY

Primary tumors may arise from liver cells or bile ducts or from both. The lesions may be multiple or singular, diffuse or nodular, and may spread to only a lobe or to the entire liver. The cancerous cells appear to compress the surrounding normal liver cells and may spread by invading the portal vein branches. Some cells infiltrate the gallbladder, mensentery, peritoneum, and dia-

phragm by direct extension. Primary cancers also tend to cause hemorrhage by extension into the vascular tissue of the liver and necrosis by depriving normal hepatic tissue of adequate circulation. The most common site for metastasis of the primary liver lesion is the lung, but it may also metastasize to the adrenal glands, spleen, vertebrae, kidney, ovary, or pancreas. Primary lesions tend to grow rapidly, sometimes without signs or symptoms, and the patient may live only a short time after the diagnosis.

Metastatic carcinoma of the liver varies from a few small nodules to large nodules. Adjacent nodules may eventually grow together and compress the surrounding liver tissue. Usually different parts of the liver are uniformly involved; thus liver biopsy may be a useful diagnostic aid.

CLINICAL MANIFESTATIONS

Signs and Symptoms

Early signs and symptoms of *primary* liver tumors may be absent, minimal, or severe. In a small number of cases the tumor is only an incidental finding at surgery. The signs and symptoms seen depend on the extent of tumor growth, hepatocellular damage, and liver failure.

The most common early signs and symptoms are enlarging right upper quadrant masses that result in complaints of epigastric fullness, pain, or discomfort. Other signs and symptoms that may be seen include weight loss and changes in liver function tests. Ascites, hepatic failure, variceal bleeding, fever, hepatic bruits, and jaundice may also be seen. In patients with cirrhosis, primary malignant tumors often cause a severe worsening of hepatic function (with onset of ascites, mental changes, variceal bleeding). With metastatic liver tumors the patient may have anorexia, weakness, weight loss followed by weight gain with ascites, hepatomegaly, hepatic bruits, and jaundice.

Diagnostic Tests

Diagnostic tests include blood studies, radioisotope scans, liver biopsy, ultrasonography, and CT scans. The blood studies may show increased erythrocyte sedimentation rate associated with generalized inflammation of the liver, anemia resulting from increased metabolism and decreased food intake, hyperbilirubinemia, elevated alkaline phosphatase, aspartate aminotransferase (AST), and alanine aminotransferase (ALT), decreased blood glucose, and hypoalbuminemia from impaired liver function. The number of abnormalities depends on the severity of hepatocellular damage. A special blood test that may be used to help diagnose primary liver carcinoma is serum concentrations of α-fetoprotein (AFP). AFP in concentrations of 500 ng/ml to 5 mg/ml is found in up to 70% of patients with hepatocellular cancer. It is also found in a small percentage of patients with metastatic carcinoma or viral hepatitis, but rarely is the level elevated as high as it is with hepatocellular carcinoma. High levels that occur in any adult without obvious gastrointestinal tract tumors strongly suggest the presence of primary liver cancer.

Radioisotope and CT scans and ultrasonography may reveal lesions in the liver. A liver biopsy is necessary to establish a definitive diagnosis of cancer.

INTERVENTIONS
Medical Management

For many hepatic tumors, both primary and metastatic, there is no medical and surgical treatment, because the lesion is too far advanced at the time of diagnosis. Treatment is supportive and similar to that used in cirrhosis; for example, control of pain and other discomforts, paracentesis and a low sodium diet for control of ascites, and restriction of protein intake if the patient is having difficulty in handling ammonium or is unable to detoxify the ammonium removed from amino acids during deamination.

For solitary primary tumors and some metastatic solitary tumors, surgery may be performed. The remarkable regenerative capacity of the liver permits resection of as much as 90% of it. Orthotopic transplantation (removal of recipient's liver and replacement with a graft liver) have been carried out in some patients, but the survival rate is poor.[59]

Chemotherapy has been used in an effort to induce regression of primary and metastatic tumor growth. Chemotherapeutic agents have been given systemically or by infusion into the hepatic artery. Theoretically arterial infusion allows more drug to be delivered directly to the tumor and decreases systemic side effects. Regional chemotherapy results have been promising.[56] 5-fluorouracil (5-FU), 5-fluorodeoxyuridine (FUDR), and doxorubicin are agents that have been used in combination with radiation. Doxorubicin, 5-FU, methyl CCNU, carmustine, streptozotocin, and mitomycin have been given systemically alone or in combination. 5-FU and FUDR are the drugs most frequently given by hepatic artery infusion.

Radiation therapy may occasionally be used to control pain. It does not contribute to survival. Immunoradiotherapy, which combines specific immunoglobulins directed toward an antigen of a primary hepatic tumor with an isotope for therapeutic radiation, is being tested experimentally and clinically.[51] The primary hepatic tumor has two antigens, ferritin and alphafetoprotein, for immunoradiotherapy targeting.[51] Hepatic dearterialization is also used as a palliative measure. Hepatic dearterialization, which decreases the oxygen delivered to the tumor, can decrease tumor mass and may help control some symptoms such as pain.[10,56]

COMMON NURSING DIAGNOSES FOR PATIENTS WITH HEPATIC TUMORS

Anxiety related to uncertain outcome of tests or prognosis

Coping, ineffective related to crisis situation

Fear related to diagnosis of cancer

Grieving, anticipatory related to prognosis

Home maintenance management, impaired, related to fatigue and weakness associated with cancer and the treatment or the progression of the disease

Knowledge deficit: diagnostic tests, treatment, expected outcomes related to new information with no previous exposure to information

Nutrition, altered: less than body requirements, related to increased metabolic needs with decreased intake

Pain related to stretching of liver capsule by growth of tumor or metastasis to other body areas

Self-esteem disturbances related to changes in role and appearance and the illness

Nursing Management

The nursing management for the patient with hepatic tumors will be guided by nursing diagnoses. See the box above for common nursing diagnoses.

General needs. The nursing management of patients with hepatic tumors will vary some, depending on the stage of the illness and the treatment modalities being used. All patients will need help coping with the anxiety and fear associated with the diagnoses of cancer and will require education regarding diagnostic tests and treatment. In addition, the patient and significant others may need assistance in dealing with the psychosocial and physiologic alterations associated with cancer, such as grieving, changes in home maintenance management, changes in self-esteem, pain, and alteration in nutrition (see Chapter 17).

When no surgical or medical treatment is possible, the care will be directed toward the needs arising from the diagnosis of cancer as listed previously. Other interventions will be needed to manage physiologic changes that occur as liver failure progresses, such as fluid volume excess, alteration in thought processes, and pain associated with pruritus. Interventions for these needs associated with liver failure are discussed in detail on pp. 1177-1182.

Care of the patient having hepatic resection
Preoperative care. For the patient having surgical resection of a hepatic tumor, skilled preoperative and postoperative care is necessary. Preoperative teaching about the preoperative preparation, the procedure itself, and postoperative care will be needed. The patient may need vitamin K for defects in clotting factors as well as other

vitamins if deficits are present. Preparation of the bowel is the same as for intestinal surgery (see Chapter 44). If blood volume deficit is present, blood will be given. The goal is to make the patient as physically stable as possible before surgery.

Postoperative care. Postoperatively the patient will be in an intensive care unit, because close monitoring is necessary. Hypovolemia from blood loss is a complication. Sepsis is the most common complication. Vital signs should be monitored every 15 minutes until stable and then every hour. Dressings should be checked for oozing or bleeding. Intake and output, serum electrolytes, and hematocrit or hemoglobin levels are carefully monitored. Weights should be recorded daily. Assessment of the cardiorespiratory system (cardiac rhythm, breath sounds, and blood gases) is also necessary. Temperature should also be monitored at least every 4 hours.

Assessment not only focuses on the potential for sepsis, hypovolemic shock, and cardiorespiratory complications, but it should also include assessment related to decreased liver function (blood glucose, coagulation status, serum albumin levels and neurologic status). The patient may need glucose, albumin, and blood replacement. Restriction of protein may be necessary if the patient is not able to adequately metabolize the ammonium released during the breakdown of proteins.

The patient may have a chest tube attached to water-seal drainage, because the surgery can be performed through a thoracoabdominal incision. The care of patients with water-seal chest drainage is discussed in Chapter 34. To promote turning and coughing, adequate pain control must be provided with pain medications, splinting of the incision, and proper positioning (upright).

The patient will be NPO for several days and will have a nasogastric tube attached to suction. Frequent mouth care every 4 hours and monitoring of the nasogastric suction are indicated. Food will be started on approximately the fifth postoperative day. At first, liquids will be given, and then the diet will be advanced as tolerated based on appetite. The patient needs adequate calories, protein, vitamins, and minerals. The nurse must monitor the patient for adequacy of intake by monitoring caloric intake. The patient's tolerance to protein nitrogenous waste products must be monitored. If the patient can not metabolize protein adequately because of loss of liver tissue, a low-protein diet (as used for portal-systemic encephalopathy see p. 1192) is necessary. If the patient can adequately detoxify ammonium, then a high-protein diet is given.

After surgery the patient may sit on the side of the bed or be out of bed by the third postoperative day. Close monitoring of vital signs, tolerance for activity, and respiratory status are required.

Discharge care. In preparation for discharge the patient should receive instructions concerning dietary restrictions, if necessary. The patient's liver function will be limited for up to 6 months following surgery, and protein and sodium restrictions may be necessary. Corticosteroids may be given to enhance regeneration and prevent fibrosis, and if they are to be continued after discharge the patient needs to receive written and verbal instructions regarding dosage, purpose, how to take, and side effects that need to be reported to the physician. The patient's activity tolerance will gradually increase. The patient will need instruction on activities that are permitted and activities to avoid. Activity restrictions vary from patient to patient. The patient needs to know how to monitor himself or herself in relation to activity tolerance. Usually the patient uses his/her feeling of fatigue and tiredness as indicators of what can or can not be done. The patient will not be able to assume all ADL immediately because of fatigue, and the nurse must assess whether self-care and home care needs can be met by the family or if outside help is necessary. Appropriate referrals should be made if necessary for home health care.

Care of the patient having chemotherapy. Chemotherapy is increasingly being used to treat primary and metastatic tumors of the liver. It may be given systematically or by perfusion into the hepatic artery. All chemotherapeutic agents have major side effects, and one of the major focuses of nursing will be to help the patient and family deal with these side effects (see Chapter 17). In addition, patients may need to learn to care for an external infusion pump, as shown in Figure 39-1, or an internal pump, as shown in Figure 39-2.

Hepatic arterial infusion. Patients receiving chemotherapy through the hepatic artery have additional needs. Hepatic arterial infusion can be accomplished by one of two methods. In the first method, a percutaneous catheter is inserted into the hepatic artery using fluoroscopy. The catheter is attached to an external infusion pump that is filled with the appropriate chemotherapeutic agent and programmed to deliver the agent over a desired period of time. The catheter is removed after each drug treatment cycle. In the second method, a catheter is surgically inserted into the hepatic artery and connected to an implanted infusion pump (see Figure 39-2). Characteristics of the infusaid pump (an internal pump) are described in the box on p. 1158.

The implanted pump can be filled with the correct amount of drug and programmed to deliver the chemotherapeutic agent over a desired time interval and at a desired dosage. In chemotherapy-free intervals the pump is filled with a heparin solution, so that patency of the hepatic artery catheter is maintained. Depending on flow rates and drug schedule, the chamber is refilled at

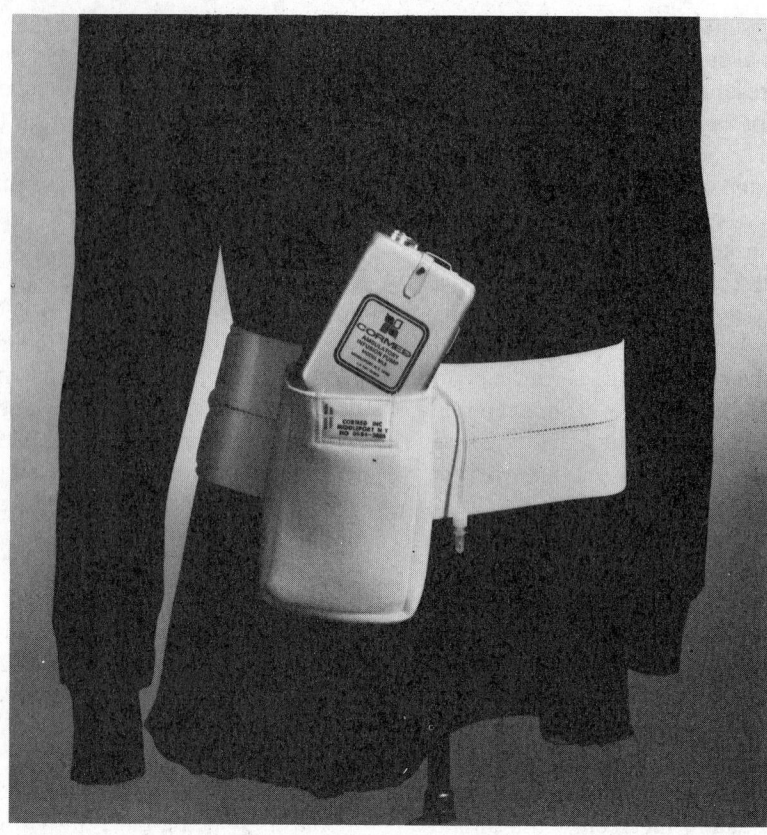

FIGURE 39-1 External infusion pump. Lightweight, battery-operated infusion pump for ambulatory patient. Flow rate is adjustable; power pack operates for 7 days before needing recharging. (Courtesy CORMED, Inc., Middleport, NY.)

CHARACTERISTICS OF INFUSAID PUMP[24]

1. The pump has two chambers: one for the drug solution and one that contains a fluorocarbon fluid.
2. The two chambers are separated by a flexible metal bellows.
3. The drug reservoir has a capacity of approximately 50 ml (model 400) and is refilled every 2 weeks by percutaneous injection into the insertion site with the use of a special needle.
4. The fluorocarbon is temperature sensitive and converts from a liquid to vapor at body temperature.
5. The vapor exerts pressure on the bellows, forcing the drug solution from its reservoir into the catheter. This occurs at a constant preset rate, and typically 2 to 3 ml/day of solution is delivered.
6. *Drug dosage* is controlled by manipulating the concentration of the chemotherapeutic agent.
7. The fluorocarbon vapor is reliquefied as the drug chamber is refilled; vaporization again occurs, and the next dosage is delivered.

INSTRUCTIONS REGARDING SELF-CARE FOR PATIENTS WITH IMPLANTED PUMPS

1. Avoid deep-sea diving, mountain climbing, or long-distance airplane trips. These activities change atmospheric pressure and can change vaporization of the fluorocarbon and thus the delivery rate.
2. Monitor body temperature daily, and report elevations immediately.
3. Avoid long hot baths, saunas, and spas. These activities can change the flow rate.
4. Avoid contact sports because they can damage the pump.
5. Wear a Medic Alert bracelet or necklace that indicates the presence of an implantable pump and gives information such as the physician's name.
6. Return for follow-up care as prescribed—usually every 2 weeks.
7. Contact the nurse/physician/outpatient department any time questions arise.
8. Individualized instructions about side effects of the specific chemotherapeutic agents that need to be monitored for and reported.

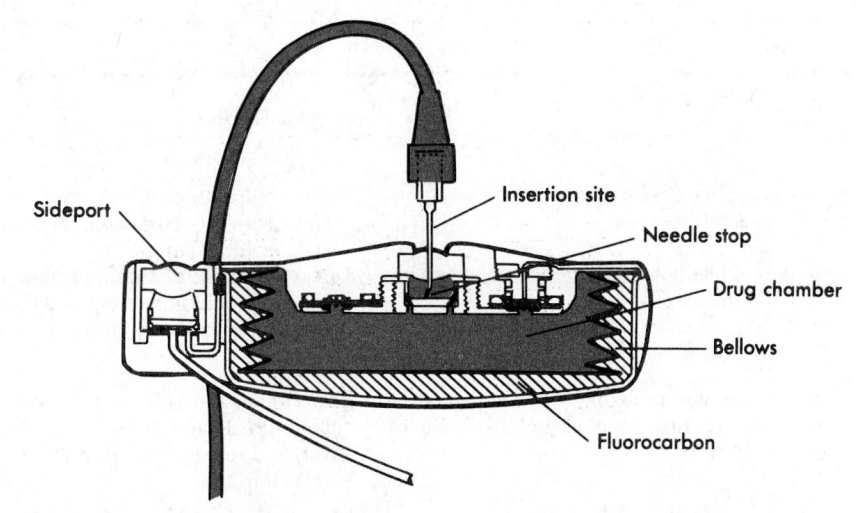

FIGURE 39-2 Implantable infusion pump. Infusaid pump.

various intervals that are scheduled so that the chamber never empties completely.

The implanted infusion pump allows the patient to be treated at home.[29] The patient comes into an outpatient site at prescribed times for addition of drugs or heparin solution and a recheck of pump flow rate. The patient will need physical care before and after surgery are similar to that of any patient having surgery (Chapters 20-22) and instructions regarding self-care and needs related to the chemotherapeutic agent being used (see Chapter 17 and a pharmacology text). The nurse will also be involved in refilling the pump at the prescribed intervals.

DIFFUSE HEPATOCELLULAR DISORDERS

Regardless of the type of diffuse hepatocellular disorder, jaundice is a major problem. Jaundice is a group of symptom caused by a disturbance of the physiology of bilirubin (see Chapter 38 for an explanation of bilirubin metabolism). Regardless of the cause of jaundice, there is an excess of bilirubin in the blood that eventually is distributed to the skin, mucous membranes, and other body fluids and tissues, giving them a yellow discoloration. If the bilirubin has been processed by the liver (extracted, conjugated, and secreted), it is water soluble and can be excreted in urine, which will be darker than usual. The presence of bilirubin in the skin causes pruritus (itching) in about 20% to 25% of the patients who have jaundice. Regardless of the type of jaundice, there will be an increase in the total serum bilirubin (normal: 0.5 to 1.0 mg/dl). Jaundice can usually be detected when bilirubin concentrations exceed 2.5 mg/dl. The changes in concentration of bilirubin and bilirubin metabolites in the serum, urine, or stool (see Chapter 38)

help in determining the type of jaundice. Serum bilirubin levels must be combined with other laboratory and diagnostic tests and interpreted in view of the history and clinical findings.

Jaundice can result from hemolysis and obstruction of extrahepatic and intrahepatic biliary ducts. Table 39-1 compares the different causes of jaundice. A common cause of *intrahepatic cholestasis* (stasis of bile within the small biliary canniculi of the liver) is drug reactions such as from phenothiazines. Clay-colored (grayish-white) stools indicate that bile is not reaching the intestine and suggest *extrahepatic obstruction* (Obstruction of hepatic, gallbladder, or common bile duct). An absence of urobilinogen in the urine supports this inference because bile and bilirubin must reach the intestines for the normal formation of urobilinogen, some of which is usually excreted in the urine. Frequent causes of extrahepatic obstruction are gallstones lodged in the common bile duct, pancreatitis, and carcinoma of the head of the pancreas, all of which are discussed in Chapter 46.

In hepatocellular damage, there is interference with uptake, conjugation, and excretion of bilirubin into bile. Excretion is the most profoundly affected process and a predominantly conjugated hyperbilirubinemia is seen. The level of jaundice does not correlate with the severity in hepatitis; but in cirrhosis, jaundice suggests a poorer prognosis.

HEPATITIS

Hepatitis may be defined as any acute inflammatory disease of the liver. Although the term *hepatitis* is most commonly used in conjunction with viral hepatitis, the disease can be caused by viruses, bacteria, or toxic injury to the liver.

TABLE 39-1 Types of jaundice

Category	Pathology	Possible Findings
OBSTRUCTIVE		
Intrahepatic	Suppression of bile flow in canaliculi or small biliary ductiles (cholestasis)	Direct* bilirubin elevated; alkaline phosphatase elevated; no enlargement of bile ducts seen on scan or ultrasound
Extrahepatic (bile duct obstruction)	Obstruction of bile flow in large bile ducts, as in gallbladder disease	Direct* bilirubin elevated; alkaline phosphatase elevated; enlargement of bile ducts documented by scan, ultrasound; absence of urobilinogen in urine
HEPATOCELLULAR	Hepatocyte injury from toxins (toxic hepatitis), viruses (viral hepatitis) or as part of syndrome of cirrhosis (all types)	Transaminases (ALT, AST) elevated 10- to 15-fold; both direct* and indirect† bilirubin may be elevated (direct more than indirect); prolonged prothrombin time
HEMOLYTIC	Excessive amounts of bilirubin are released from RBCs as would be seen in sickle-cell anemia or other hemolytic anemias; liver is unable to excrete bilirubin as rapidly as it forms	Usually mild elevation of total bilirubin (indirect more than direct)

*"Direct" measures conjugated bilirubin.
†"Indirect" measures unconjugated bilirubin.

Although there are some differences in the pathologic and clinical phenomena of viral, bacterial, and toxic hepatitis, the clinical management of the person with any of these types of hepatitis is quite similar. The particular aspects of care for toxic and viral hepatitis are discussed next. It should be pointed out that any form of hepatitis can result in *postnecrotic cirrhosis* (p. 1171), unless the hepatitis responds to treatment.

TOXIC HEPATITIS
Etiology/Epidemiology
Because the liver has a primary role in the metabolism of foreign substances, many agents, including drugs and alcohol, industrial toxins, and plant poisons can cause toxic hepatitis (Table 39-2). Many health care workers are concerned about hepatic injury caused by adverse drug reactions from the drugs they handle (especially those needing to be mixed from powder). However, only a minor number of the cases of acute hepatic disease in health care workers are the result of adverse drug reactions. However, up to 25% of all cases of fulminant hepatic failure are the result of adverse drug reactions.[60]

Classification of the Hepatotoxins
The agents that produce hepatic injury can be categorized into two major groups: *predictable (intrinsic)* hepatotoxins and *nonpredictable (idiosyncratic)* hepatotoxins. The predictable hepatotoxins are further divided into two subgroups: *direct* and *indirect* (see the box at right). The selected agents listed in Table 39-2 have

CLASSIFICATION OF HEPATOTOXINS

PREDICTABLE HEPATOTOXINS
Agents cause toxic hepatitis with predictable regularity and produce injury in a high percentage of persons exposed to them; occurrence of toxic hepatitis is dose-dependent.

NONPREDICTABLE HEPATOTOXINS
Agents produce hepatic injury only in unusually susceptible persons and in only a small percentage of persons exposed to them; occurrence is not dose-dependent.

DIRECT PREDICTABLE HEPATOTOXINS
Agents have direct effect on hepatic cells and organelles producing structural changes that lead to metabolic defects.

INDIRECT PREDICTABLE HEPATOTOXINS
Agents first interfere with normal metabolic function, and this alteration in metabolic function produces structural changes.

been classified according to type of hepatotoxin. As should be noted, most drugs are nonpredictable (idiosyncratic) hepatotoxins. Acetaminophen, which is a predictable hepatotoxin, produces injury at high doses only and has been increasingly used in suicide attempts.[60]

Pathophysiology
The morphologic changes produced in the liver by the toxins will vary, depending on the specific hepatotoxin.

TABLE 39-2 Selected hepatoxins and class of hepatotoxins

Agents	Type of Hepatotoxin
INDUSTRIAL TOXINS	
Carbon tetrachloride and other chlorinated hydrocarbons	Predictable; direct
Yellow phosphorus	Predictable; direct
PLANT POISONS	
Mushroom poisoning (*Amanita phalloides* and related poisons)	Predictable; direct
DRUGS	
Ethanol	Predictable; indirect
Tetracycline	Predictable; indirect
Methotrexate	Predictable; indirect
L-Asparaginase	Predictable; indirect
Puromycin	Predictable; indirect
6-Mercaptopurine	Predictable; indirect
Acetaminophen	Predictable; indirect
Mithramycin	Predictable; indirect
Urethane	Predictable; indirect
Cholecystographic dyes	Predictable; indirect
Rifamycin B	Predictable; indirect
Phenytoin	Nonpredictable
Para-aminosalicylic acid (PAS)	Nonpredictable
Isoniazid (INH)	Nonpredictable
Chlorpromazine	Nonpredictable
Androgens and anabolic steroids	Nonpredictable
Chlorpropamide	Nonpredictable
Imipramine	Nonpredictable
Methyldopa	Nonpredictable
Monoamine oxidase inhibitors	Nonpredictable
Oral contraceptives	Nonpredictable
Sulfonamides	Nonpredictable
Allopurinol	Nonpredictable
Clindomycin	Nonpredictable
Trythromycen estolate	Nonpredictable
Nitrofurantoin	Nonpredictable
Oxacillin	Nonpredictable

For example, carbon tetrachloride, tetracycline, and ethanol cause fatty infiltration and/or necrosis. Oral contraceptives, cholecystographic dyes, and chlorpromazine produce cholestasis and portal inflammation. Regardless of the morphologic changes, some alteration in liver function occurs. The alteration may result in only minimal manifestations of altered liver function such as slightly elevated serum enzymes or major manifestations associated with terminal liver failure (see pp. 1173-1174).

Prevention

The nurse can assist in the prevention of toxic hepatitis by teaching the danger of injudicious use of materials that are known to be injurious to the liver and by emphasizing the need for a diet (well-balanced diet with recommended dietary requirements of nutrients and with minimal or no alcohol) that is protective to the liver.

Because cleaning agents, solvents, and related substances sometimes contain products that are harmful to the liver, the public should read instructions on labels and should follow them explicitly. Dry-cleaning fluids may contain carbon tetrachloride, which can cause liver injury if warnings to avoid inhalation of the fumes and to keep windows open are not heeded. If people must use these agents inside the home, a good practice is to open the windows wide; use the cleaning materials as quickly as possible; and then vacate the room, the apartment, or the house for several hours, leaving the windows open.

Many solvents used to remove paint and plastic material and to stain and finish woodwork contain injurious substances and should be used outdoors and not in the basement, since dangerous fumes may spread throughout the house. Cleaning agents and finishes for cars should be applied outdoors or in the garage with the door open. Nurses in industry have a responsibility to teach the importance of observing regulations to avoid industrial hazards. Nitrobenzene, tetrachloroethane, carbon disulfide, and dinitrotoluoyl are examples of injurious compounds used in industry.

Some drugs that are known to cause mild damage to the liver must be used therapeutically. However, the nurse should warn the public about the use of preparations that are available without prescription that may be injurious. Many drugs, prescription and nonprescription, reach the market before dangers resulting from their extensive use have been conclusively ruled out; for example, the prescription drug chlorpromazine, which was being widely used as a tranquilizer, has been found to cause stasis of bile in the canaliculi of the liver, which can lead to serious hepatic damage. A safe rule to follow is to avoid taking any medication except that specifically prescribed by a physician for a specific ailment.

Clinical Manifestations

Signs and symptoms. Anorexia, nausea, vomiting, and lethargy are common early symptoms of toxic hepatitis and may be mistaken for flu symptoms. Icterus, hepatomegaly, and hepatic tenderness follow. Removal of the hepatotoxin may result in rapid recovery, but toxic hepatitis may be fatal or cirrhosis may develop rapidly with all the signs and symptoms described on pp. 1173-1174.

Diagnostic tests. Various abnormalities in blood and urine tests may occur. The serum enzymes (ALT, AST), which are elevated because of cell necroses, are particularly valuable in evaluating the severity of the injury. The higher the enzyme levels, the more severe the cellular damage to the liver. Total, conjugated, and unconjugated bilirubin will be elevated if jaundice is present.

Bilirubin also can be found in the urine. Other abnormalities in laboratory tests consistent with impaired liver function, such as prolonged prothrombin time, low albumin, elevated globulin, will be found if the toxic hepatitis results in cirrhoses.

Interventions

Medical management. Attention is directed toward identifying the toxic agent and removing or eliminating it. Gastric lavage and cleansing of the bowel may be indicated to remove the hepatotoxin(s) such as drugs from the intestinal tract. In some instances there may be a specific treatment for a particular hepatotoxin. For example, the toxic effects of acetaminophen depend on tissue levels of glutathione. In certain cases of acetaminophen toxicity, acetylcysteine, which can serve as a surrogate for glutathione, may be given. However in most instances, medical treatment is supportive and directed toward particular manifestations, such as treatment of cirrhosis, portal-systemic encephalopathy coma, or accompanying renal failure.

Nursing management. The major focus for nursing management occurs in the community or other outpatient setting and is directed toward the nursing diagnosis, potential for injury related to improper use of chemicals at home, exposure to chemicals in the work environment, or injudicious use of drugs or other materials. The nursing care involves patient education as discussed in the section on prevention (see p. 1161).

For the patient with acute toxic hepatitis the nursing management in the acute care setting will be directed toward promoting comfort, maintaining normal fluid and electrolyte balance, promoting a well-balanced diet when food and fluid are allowed, and promoting rest as discussed in the section on viral hepatitis (see pp. 1168-1169). The nurse will also be assisting with the implementation of any medical regimen. If cirrhosis develops or portal-systemic encephalopathy occurs, the patient may require all the interventions described for the patient with cirrhosis (p. 1177-1183).

VIRAL HEPATITIS

Viral hepatitis is by far the most important infection that affects the liver. It is a major health problem in the United States and in many other countries. The term *viral hepatitis* is used to refer to several clinically similar but etiologically and epidemiologically distinct infections.

Etiology/Epidemiology/Transmission

There are currently four types of hepatitis: hepatitis A; hepatitis B; non-A, non-B hepatitis; and delta hepatitis. Research indicates that there is more than one type of non-A, non-B hepatitis. One virus, labeled as hepatitis C virus, has been identified as possibly responsible for pa-

rentally transmitted non-A, non-B hepatitis. A virus responsible for enterically transmitted non-A, non-B hepatitis has not been identified. Delta hepatitis, the most recently characterized hepatitis, is an infection caused by a defective virus that is only active in the presence of hepatitis B.[27]

Viral hepatitis is a reportable disease in all states. Statistics from the Center for Disease Control (CDC) indicate that viral hepatitis is one of the most frequently reported infectious diseases in the United States. In 1988 the total number of reported cases was 56,790. There were 28,500 cases of hepatitis A; 23,200 cases of hepatitis B; 2620 cases of non-A, non-B hepatitis; and 2470 cases of unspecified type of hepatitis. It is well accepted that the figures for any given year may be grossly underestimated, because reporting from some areas is incomplete and carriers with subclinical manifestations are often not reported as having active disease.

The vast majority of cases of hepatitis that are seen clinically are caused by hepatitis A or hepatitis B. Most cases of all types of hepatitis occur in young adults. Factors such as the viral agent, transmission, and high-risk groups vary for the four types of hepatitis. Table 39-3 summarizes the difference between the four types of hepatitis.

Prevention

Prevention of viral hepatitis is one of the major focuses of nursing. Preventive care can be categorized into three groups: general measures that help to prevent the spread of many infectious diseases, measures used with patients with known hepatitis, and prophylactic preventive measures for persons exposed to hepatitis or for persons in high-risk groups.

General preventive measures. The major activity that can assist in the general prevention of hepatitis is thorough handwashing by all persons. All feces, urine, blood and other body fluids should be considered potentially infectious for a wide variety of organisms and disposed of properly. Nurses should be involved in the promotion of the development of adequate sewage disposal systems to prevent contamination of food and water supplies that may result in endemic forms of hepatitis A.

Because hepatitis B; parentally transmitted non-A, non-B hepatitis; delta hepatitis; and possibly hepatitis A as well as carrier states of some types of hepatitis can be spread by contaminated needles and other equipment that comes in contact with infected blood and body fluids, disposable and nondisposable needles, syringes, and other equipment used in patient care must be handled with great care. *All equipment should be treated as if it had been used on an infected person and handled using universal precautions no matter who the patient.*

Needles should *not be recapped.* They should be discarded in puncture-resistant containers designated for

TABLE 39-3 Etiologic/epidemiologic/transmission characteristics of hepatitis

	Hepatitis A	Hepatitis B	Non-A, Non-B	Delta Hepatitis
Age group	Older children and young adults	Young adults because of life-style	All age groups but highest in adults because of more frequent blood transfusions	Same as for hepatitis B
Transmission	Primarily person-to-person through fecal contamination; common source epidemics from contaminated food and water; rare transmission by blood; *not* transmitted by shared utensils and kissing	Percutaneous or permucosal routes through infective blood or body fluids introduced by contaminated needles and sexual contact; spread by personal contact in households and among children; rare transmission by blood transfusion, since screening of blood for presence of hepatitis B surface antigen (HB$_s$Ag); *not transmitted* fecal-oral route or by contaminated H$_2$O	Parentally transmitted form is spread percutaneously through infected blood transfusion and parenteral drug abuse; enterically transmitted form of non-A, non-B found in Southeast Asia, North Africa, and Mexico is spread by contaminated water and close personal contact	Routes same as those for hepatitis B
Incubation period	15-50 days; average 28-30 days	45-160 days, average 60-120 days	Variable—14-150 days; 50 days average	Unknown
Secretions that have been found to contain infective agent	Stools of infected persons	Highest in blood and serous fluids; also found in saliva, semen, urine, nasopharyngeal washings, feces, and pleural fluid	Blood	Blood
Greatest infectivity	2 weeks before onset of jaundice	—	—	Infections occur as either coinfection with hepatitis B or superinfection in hepatitis B carrier
Clinical onset	Abrupt	Insidious	Insidious	Insidious
Diagnostic serologic tests	Confirmed by presence of immunoglobin against hepatitis A virus (IgM-class anti-HAV) in serum (found during acute and early convalescent period)	Confirmed by HB$_s$Ag, hepatitis B$_e$ antigen (HB$_e$Ag), antibody against hepatitis B$_e$ antigen (anti-HB$_e$), antibody against core antigen (anti-HB$_c$) (see Chapter 38 for discussion)	An antibody to hepatitis C virus (anti-HCV) has been found in approximately 50% of persons in one study who developed parentally transmitted non-A, non-B hepatitis; Some authorities[54a] recommend that this serological test be used for donor screening for blood donations	Delta antigen in serum during early infection; delta antibodies during or after infection (first test for antigen not available for routine use)
Indication of protective immunity	IgG-class anti-HAV appears during the convalescent period and indicates immunity	Antibody against hepatitis$_s$ antigen (anti-HB$_s$) indicates immunity	No tests available; people have had repeated infections	No test available but can only occur if hepatitis B virus is present

From Advisory Committee on Immunization Practices (ACIP): Morbid Mortal Week Rep 39(52):1-26, 1990.

Continued.

TABLE 39-3 Etiologic/epidemiologic/transmission characteristics of hepatitis—cont'd

	Hepatitis A	Hepatitis B	Non-A, Non-B	Delta Hepatitis
Chronic carriers	None demonstrated	Frequent—6% to 10% of adult persons with HBV become carriers; 90% of infected infants and 25% to 50% of infected children become carriers	8% of persons with non-A, non-B hepatitis become carriers	80% of those persons who have superinfection with delta hepatitis become carriers with superinfection
Mortality	Infrequent (<0.6%)	1%-2%	Unknown	Unknown
Subsequent chronic disease	Virtually absent	About 10% develop chronic disease	High—20% to 70% develop chronic disease	Frequent in persons who contact a superinfection of delta hepatitis
High-risk groups	Staff and children at day-care centers where children in diapers are cared for; staff and persons in institutions for custodial care (prisons, institutions for developmentally disabled); international travelers to developing countries	Immigrants/refugees from areas of high HBV endemic areas; clients and staff in institutions for developmentally disabled; users of illicit parenteral drugs; fetuses of infected mothers; homosexually active men; household and sexual partners of HBV carriers; patients on hemodialysis; male prisoners; health care workers with frequent contact with blood	Persons receiving frequent blood transfusions; international travelers to endemic area	Same as for hepatitis B

this purpose. Other disposable equipment should also be discarded in appropriate containers; the containers are marked contaminated to alert persons handling the rubbish.

Nondisposable equipment should be rinsed, packaged so sharp objects do not accidentally puncture someone, and sterilized by dry heat and steam under pressure (autoclaving) or by gas sterilization. If invasive reusable equipment is used in an environment in which autoclave sterilization is not available and boiling is the only available way to sterilize, the nurse should see that everything placed in the water sterilizer is covered completely and boiled for at least 30 minutes. The nurse should realize that the boiling time needed to destroy hepatitis viruses is unknown and that water sterilization of invasive equipment, such as catheters, to be used for another patient is *not* an acceptable method for preventing the transmission of hepatitis.

Preventive measures used with persons with known hepatitis. Patients with known hepatitis A should be placed on *enteric precautions* during the time of infectivity which is part of universal precautions. Children should be in private rooms, but responsible adults do not require one.

Good handwashing after fecal and urine elimination is the major isolation measure. Anyone who must handle feces or potentially contaminated articles (bedpan, diapers, rectal thermometer) should wear gloves and gowns and wash hands thoroughly after completing care (see research box on p. 1165). Separate toilet facilities are sometimes used, but this is not necessary if fecal contamination, which might occur in a person who is confused, is not a problem. The toilet should be cleansed thoroughly daily. All disposable and nondisposable equipment and linens should be bagged properly and labeled correctly before being removed from the patient's room.

For patients with hepatitis B; non-A, non-B hepatitis; and delta hepatitis; good handwashing and blood/body fluid precautions (also part of universal precautions) are used. Any time blood or body fluids are handled, gown and gloves should be worn when the amount of potential contamination with blood or body fluids is great (such as in the operating room or in intensive care) double-gloving is used. The benefit of this is unknown (see research box). If splattering of contaminated blood and body fluids is likely, goggles and a mask are worn. Care must be taken to avoid contact between the blood

RESEARCH

Korniewicz DM, Laughon BE, Butz A, and Larson E: Integrity of vinyl and latex procedure gloves, Nurs Res 38:144-146, 1989.

The use of protective gloves in the delivery of nursing care is a critical component in preventing the spread of hepatitis B virus (HBV) and human immunodeficiency virus (HIV). The risk of transmission of HBV exceeds that for HIV. The effectiveness of gloves in preventing transmission of HBV or HIV is dependent on the integrity of the gloves during use. This study was designed to determine the integrity of vinyl and latex procedure gloves under in-use conditions that are present in clinical practice.

In this study, 645 latex and vinyl gloves from 28 lot numbers and five manufacturers were first tested for presence of visible defects when filled with water and allowed to hang vertically for 2 minutes. Next, 90 vinyl and 90 latex gloves with no visible defects were checked for permeability to dye after being worn by one of 28 subjects during one of three levels of hand manipulation, some of which mimicked activities performed during routine patient care. The permeability of the gloves to *Serratia marcescens* was also tested using fifty of each type of glove.

Visible defects were present in 4.1% of the vinyl gloves and 2.7% of the latex gloves. Fifty-three percent of vinyl and 3% of the latex gloves showed dye penetration, and 20% of latex gloves and 34% of vinyl gloves that were water tight allowed for penetration of *S. marcescens*.

Glove standards set by the American Society for Testing and Materials (ASTM) allow for a failure rate of 1.5% for sterile surgical latex gloves and 2.5 for non-sterile latex gloves by the water-tight method. When the water-tight test was used in this study, the latex glove failure rate was equal to the standards established by ASTM, whereas the vinyl glove failure rate was much higher. When more sensitive tests were used to examine the gloves, both the latex and the vinyl gloves showed failure rates higher than the standard.

Latex gloves maintained better integrity when tested after in-use conditions than did vinyl gloves in all tests. Because all gloves showed leakage, this finding re-emphasizes the need for excellent handwashing before and after all patient care activities, the importance of not reusing gloves, and the importance of not just washing the gloved hands between patient contacts. Additionally, in situations where high stress is placed on the gloves during patient care, gloves may need to be changed. ▪

---

and body fluids of an infected person and open cuts, the mucous membranes, or eyes of another person. All invasive equipment such as needles, lancets, and dental drills should be disposed of properly or sterilized properly. All contaminated linens and other items should be bagged and labeled correctly. Persons who have had viral hepatitis should not be blood donors. The patient with acute hepatitis B; non-A, non-B hepatitis; or delta hepatitis should not have intimate sexual contact during the period of infection. Protection of household and sexual contacts of persons who become hepatitis B carriers is discussed later in this chapter.

Prophylaxis

Prophylaxis can be instituted either before exposure for persons at high risk and/or after exposure. The recommendations for prophylaxis vary for the different types of hepatitis and are reevaluated on a continual basis by the CDC.

Hepatitis A. For hepatitis A, the following recommendations have been made by CDC.[1]

Preexposure prophylaxis is recommended for travelers to developing countries who will be eating in settings of poor or uncertain sanitation or visiting extensively with local persons. The recommended therapy is immune globulin, 0.02 ml/kg, for persons traveling for less than 3 months and 0.06 ml/kg every 5 months for those traveling for prolonged periods.

Postexposure prophylaxis is recommended for selected persons who have had contact with a person known to be positive for hepatitis A, if the prophylaxis is given *within* 2 weeks of exposure. Postexposure prophylaxis for the following people is recommended:

1. Close household and sexual contacts of persons with hepatitis A
2. *Staff* and *attendees* of day-care centers, if hepatitis A cases are recognized among attendees or employees, or two or more households of center attendees have recognized cases; household members of families with children in diapers, if three or more families of attendees report cases
3. Residents and staff in institutions for custodial care who have close contact with person, with hepatitis A
4. Hospital staff who have close contacts with patients with hepatitis A (only if outbreaks occur)
5. Persons exposed to a common source of infection (infected food or water), if identified within 2 weeks of exposure
6. Food handlers working with a food handler diagnosed as having hepatitis A; patrons of food establishments only treated in rare instances

Hepatitis B. For hepatitis B, there is a vaccine available that provides active immunity (hepatitis B vaccine) and an immune globulin with high amounts of anti-HB$_s$ (HBIG). The hepatitis B vaccine is used in both preexposure and postexposure prophylaxis. HBIG is used in only certain postexposure situations.

Hepatitis B vaccine is given as a series of three intramuscular injections (deltoid in adults and children; anterolateral thigh muscles in infants and neonates), with the second and third doses given 1 and 6 months after the first dose. The vaccine has shown an efficacy of 85% to 95%.[49] The effect of the vaccine on the developing fetus is not known. Because hepatitis B infection in pregnant women results in a severe infection in the mother and chronic infection in the infant and because the vaccine contains only noninfectious HB_sAg particles, pregnancy should not be considered a contraindication for its use if necessary.[1] Soreness at injection site is the most common side effect.[1]

Hepatitis B vaccine causes *no adverse effects or benefits* in HBV carriers.[14] Because hepatitis B vaccine has no benefits for HBV carriers and because of the cost of the vaccination (approximately $110/person), prevaccination serologic screening for anti-HB_c and anti-HB_s may be done to identify both carriers and previously infected noncarriers who have adequate immunity. The cost of screening will be weighed against the cost of unnecessary but harmless vaccination to identify whether screening before vaccinating should be performed.

Preexposure vaccination is recommended for the following[1]:

1. Health care workers at high risk for exposure (medical technologists or staff, phlebotomists, most nurses in acute and critical care settings surgeons, pathologists, oncology and dialysis unit staff, dentists, oral surgeons, dental hygienists, laboratory and blood bank technicians, emergency medical technicians, and morticians)
2. Clients and staff of institutions for developmentally disabled
3. Hemodialysis patients
4. Sexually active homosexual men
5. Users of illicit injectable drugs
6. Recipients of frequent blood products, particularly patients with clotting disorders who receive frequent transfusions of clotting factors
7. Household and sexual contacts of HBV carriers
8. Some American populations, including infants, such as Alaskan Eskimos, native Pacific islanders, and immigrants and refugees and their infants from areas where hepatitis B is endemic, such as Eastern Asia; adoptees from countries of high HBV endemicity and families of adoptee with positive HB_sAg tests
9. Long-term correctional facility inmates
10. Heterosexually active persons with multiple sexual partners
11. International travelers who plan to reside in areas with a high endemic incidence of hepatitis B for 6 months or longer

Postexposure prophylaxis for hepatitis B should be considered for the following[1]:

1. Infants born to HB_sAg-positive mothers
2. Persons who have percutaneous or permucosal exposure to HB_sAg-positive blood
3. Persons who have sexual contact with HB_sAg-positive persons
4. Infants <12 months exposed to primary care giver who has acute hepatitis B

Infants exposed perinatally are given HBIG at birth, and the hepatitis B vaccination series is started at the same time, if possible. Persons who have percutaneous or permucosal exposure and are unvaccinated are also treated with HBIG, and the hepatitis B vaccination series is started. If the exposed person has been vaccinated, he/she is checked for anti-HB_s and given HBIG immediately plus a booster dose of hepatitis B vaccination. The CDC also makes recommendation about prophylaxis after percutaneous or permucosal exposure from a source with unknown hepatitis B virus status.[1]

Booster immunization doses, described previously, are recommended for previously vaccinated persons who experience percutaneous or needle exposure to HB_sAg-positive blood. In addition, it is recommended that patients on hemodialysis be assessed semiannually by antibody testing, and if their antibody level declines below 10 mlU/ml, they should be given a booster dose.[1] For persons with normal immune status, booster doses and routine serologic testing to assess antibody level are not necessary.[1]

Although the hepatitis B vaccine has been available since 1981, the incidence of the disease has not decreased.[26,42,43] This lack of decrease may be due to health care workers who are uninformed about who should be vaccinated, the inability of health care workers to reach high-risk groups, unfounded patient concerns about the safety of the vaccine, and incomplete identification of high-risk persons. With regard to this last factor, it has been shown that 30% of persons with acute hepatitis B infection do not indicate any source of contact or definable risk even when questioned thoroughly.[1]

One major factor that is a real impediment to universal vaccination is the cost ($110 to $120 per adult). Unless this cost can be decreased, universal vaccination will not be possible without a major increase in health care costs. In developing countries, vaccines have been made available at cost (approximately $1.00 a dose).[26]

Non-A, non-B hepatitis. Prophylaxis for non-A, non-B hepatitis is not as effective as that for hepatitis B. For travelers to countries where a fecal-oral form of non-A, non-B hepatitis occurs in endemic proportions, preventive health teaching is the best prophylactic measure. The value of immunoglobulin in this situation is unknown.[1] For postexposure prophylaxis in persons exposed through breaks in the skin to blood from a patient with non-A, non-B hepatitis, immunoglobulin may be given, but its value is uncertain.[1]

Delta hepatitis. Delta hepatitis requires the presence of hepatitis B virus; thus the preexposure and postexposure prophylaxes that are recommended for hepatitis B should suffice to prevent delta hepatitis.[1] Currently there is no prophylaxis for preventing HDV infection in HBV carriers except health teaching.

Pathophysiology

Viral hepatitis causes diffuse inflammatory infiltration of hepatic tissue with mononuclear cells and local, spotty, or single cell necrosis. The liver cells may be very swollen. With typical viral hepatitis, there is no collapse of lobules, no loss of lobular architecture, and minimal or no fibrosis. Inflammation, degeneration, and regeneration may occur simultaneously, distorting the normal lobular pattern and possibly creating pressure within and around the portal vein areas. These changes may be associated with elevated serum transaminase levels, prolonged prothrombin time, and slightly elevated serum alkaline phosphatase level.

The outcome of viral hepatitis may be affected by such factors as the following:

1. Virulence of the virus
2. Amount of hepatic damaged sustained
3. Natural individual barriers to damage and disease of the liver, such as nutritional status and overall health of individuals
4. Supportive individual care the patient receives

The majority of patients recover normal liver function, but the disease can progress to atypical life-threatening variants (see the box at right). Chronic sequelae can occur with all types of hepatitis but are virtually absent with hepatitis A. Because of the continual destruction of the liver in *chronic active hepatitis* there are continual signs and symptoms of liver impairment and histopathologic changes on a liver biopsy. Chronic active hepatitis is usually indicative of a poor prognosis but can revert to an inactive form. *Chronic relapsing hepatitis* is characterized by the reappearance of symptoms and signs after recovery from an acute episode is believed to have occurred (usually within 6 months). *Chronic persistent hepatitis* refers to cases of hepatitis with a benign course where all the signs and symptoms do not resolve in the usual time frame. The patient may be asymptomatic, except for minimal abnormalities in serum transaminase levels. There is no indication of progression to severe hepatic dysfunction, and eventually full recovery occurs.

Clinical Manifestations

Manifestations of the various forms of hepatitis are not clinically distinct from each other, except that, with hepatitis A, the manifestations may be more abrupt in onset. The signs and symptoms and abnormal diagnostic tests can be grouped into three phases: preicteric, icteric, and posticteric phases.

Preicteric (prodromal phase). The preicteric or prodromal phase lasts for approximately 1 week. During this phase the patient may have the following: elevated temperature and chills; nausea, vomiting, dyspepsia, and anorexia; headache, arthralgia, and tenderness in right

---

ATYPICAL LIFE-THREATENING VARIANTS OF HEPATITIS

Fulminant viral hepatitis	Sudden, severe degeneration and atrophy of liver, resulting in hepatic failure
Subacute fatal viral hepatitis	Severe but slower degeneration of the liver
Confluent hepatic necrosis— submassive or massive	Destruction of substantial groups of adjacent cells with necrosis of portions of a lobule (submassive) or entire lobule (massive); can result in chronic active disease or cirrhosis, but most patients will recover

---

upper abdominal quadrant; weakness and general malaise; and loss of desire to smoke.

The *major manifestation* is *anorexia*. Other signs are loss of weight, enlarged liver, and enlarged lymph nodes.

Icteric phase. The icteric phase starts with the onset of jaundice. The icteric phase reaches its intensity in 2 weeks and lasts from 4 to 6 weeks. During this phase the signs and symptoms present during the preicteric phase may decrease, although the anorexia, nausea, vomiting, dyspepsia, weakness, and malaise may worsen. Liver tenderness usually increases.

Jaundice occurs because bilirubin metabolism is disrupted. Signs of impaired bilirubin metabolism and jaundice in patients include the following: yellow sclera and skin most noticeable on the palms of hands and soles of feet in non-white persons; dark amber urine (conjugated bilirubin being excreted into urine); elevated total, unconjugated, and conjugated bilirubin; bilirubinuria and increased urine urobilinogen, and light brown- to clay-colored (grayish-white) stools (stool color depends on the amount of bile with bilirubin pigment that is emptied into the GI tract). If the biliary canaliculi are completely blocked, clay-colored stools will be seen. Normally only partial obstruction occurs, and stools are light brown.

Other laboratory abnormalities may also be present and include the following: elevated serum transaminases (ALT and AST), elevated alkaline phosphatase, and abnormal serologic tests (blood tests for various hepatitis antigens and antibodies). If an *atypical form* of acute viral hepatitis occurs, other blood abnormalities demonstrating impairment of the metabolic function of the liver may be seen and include prolonged prothrombin time, prolonged partial thromboplastin time, and decreased serum albumin levels.

Posticteric phase. The posticteric or convalescent phase begins with the disappearance of jaundice and normally lasts for several weeks. But it may take as long as 4 months. The development of chronic forms of hepatitis may be seen during this phase.

Medical Management

Medical management focuses on making an appropriate diagnosis and then providing general support. There is no specific medical treatment for viral hepatitis. General support includes fluid and electrolyte replacement, vitamin K replacement if the prothrombin time is prolonged, and antihistamines for pruritus associated with jaundice, and antiemetics. The use of drugs for restlessness and abdominal discomfort is avoided because most sedatives and pain medications are detoxified in the liver. Corticosteroid therapy may be used for some forms of fulminant *viral hepatitis* that are life threatening, but its use is controversial. For some persons who have chronic hepatitis B with progressive liver damage, interferon alfa-2b given subcutaneously daily for 16 weeks has been shown to be effective in promoting remission.[47]

■ Assessment

Nursing assessment focuses on identifying the physiologic and psychosocial changes related to viral hepatitis and identifying the potential source of transmission that may be controllable.

Subjective data. Subjective data include the following:
1. Presence of discomfort: history of headache, right upper abdominal quadrant tenderness, arthralgia, itching
2. Presence of GI alterations: history of anorexia, nausea, vomiting, dyspepsia
3. Changes in nutritional intake of food and fluids
4. History of changes in weight
5. History of episodes of temperature elevations, chills, or lymph node tenderness
6. Complaints of weakness/malaise not relieved by rest
7. History of potential exposure to hepatitis virus: work environment, child-care facilities, recent international travel, injections of illegal drugs, recent blood transfusions, contaminated food and water, recent sexual contact with infected person, homosexual or bisexual lifestyle
8. Knowledge about the disease
9. Length of time since onset of symptoms

Objective data. Objective data include the following:
1. Skin/sclera—adequacy of skin turgor, presence of jaundice or lesions from scratching; if jaundice is present, the nurse should assess the patient for the presence of petechiae or bruises
2. Lymph nodes: enlargement
3. Abdomen: liver enlargement, guarding in right upper quadrant
4. Documented nutritional and fluid intake and output
5. Temperature
6. Weight/height
7. Musculoskeletal: strength, ability to do activities

■ Data Analysis: Nursing Diagnoses

Nursing diagnoses are determined from the assessment of patient data. Possible nursing diagnoses for the person with viral hepatitis may include, but are not limited to, the following:

Diagnostic Title	Possible Etiologies
Fatigue	Imbalance between energy level and demand; decreased rest; feeling of malaise
Fluid volume deficit, potential for	Vomiting; sweating; decreased intake; elevated temperature
Infection, potential for spread	Length of infectivity and transmission to others through blood and/or body fluids
Injury, potential for	Altered clotting or prothrombin time
Knowledge deficit: diagnostic tests, manifestations, isolation, prophylaxis for others, treatment, prevention of future cases	Anxiety; new diagnosis; multiple tests
Nutrition, altered: less than body requirements	Anorexia; inadequate intake; increased metabolic needs
Pain	Arthralgia, itching, headaches, abdominal tenderness
Skin integrity, impaired, potential	Jaundice, itching, and scratching
Social isolation	Physical isolation; fear of others catching disease

For persons with hepatitis B who have a homosexual or bisexual lifestyle or a history of illegal drug use, the diagnosis of health maintenance, altered, related to lack of use of safe sex practices or to illegal drug use with shared equipment would also be appropriate.

■ Planning: Expected Patient Outcomes

Expected patient outcomes for the person with viral hepatitis may include, but are not limited to, the following:
1. Patient will be able to explain why fatigue occurs and will indicate a decrease in fatigue as evi-

denced by giving it a lower rating on a scale of 1 to 5, with 1 indicating no fatigue.

2. Patient will maintain good skin tone, stable weight, adequate and balanced intake and output and demonstrate no significant orthostatic postural changes in BP (decrease in systolic BP between lying and standing of ≤10 mm Hg) or pulse (increase in pulse between lying and standing of ≤10 beats/min).

3. Patient will not experience undetected bleeding.

4. Patient will be able to demonstrate adequate isolation precautions while hospitalized and describe appropriate isolation precautions for use at home.

5. Patient will be able to list the diagnostic tests prescribed, explain why isolation precautions are necessary, list significant others who require prophylaxis, describe the purpose of all treatments, and describe care necessary for prevention of future infections.

6. Patient will increase food intake until adequate in amount and content for body size.

7. Patient will verbalize that pain is controlled and/or rate pain on a scale from one (no pain) to ten (severe pain).

8. Patient's skin remains intact and free of lesions.

9. Patient will express that isolation is not distressing and will share information that reveals he or she is being kept up to date about family affairs.

■ Implementation

The patient with hepatitis needs general supportive care that promotes rest, fluid balance, prevention of injury, prevention of spread of disease, adequate knowledge, adequate nutrition, comfort, prevention of impairment of skin integrity, and prevention of social isolation. If the patient with hepatitis B or delta hepatitis has a history of a homosexual or bisexual lifestyle, counseling and patient education about safe sex practices, as described in Chapter 77, will be necessary. If a history of illegal drug use is elicited the patient needs the care described in Chapter 19. The spread of the human immunodeficiency virus (HIV) and the hepatitis virus can be stopped in users of illegal drugs if the practice of sharing equipment ceases. Some persons have suggested that sterile needles/syringes should be distributed to persons who are addicted to intravenous drugs.

Monitoring fatigue. The patient with hepatitis will need considerable rest during the acute phase of the illness. The level of physical activity allowed will be individually determined on the basis of the amount of fatigue and severity of the disease. Rest periods should be interspersed throughout the day, and patient care should be scheduled to allow for uninterrupted periods for napping and relaxation. If hepatic enzyme levels increase with resumption of near normal activities, limitations on activity will be reimposed.

Maintaining food and fluid intake. During the acute phase of the illness the patient needs 3000 ml/day of fluids because of the increased fluid needs associated with febrile illness and vomiting. The fluid can usually be given orally if nausea and vomiting are not severe. When nausea and vomiting are severe, intravenous infusions are given. Intake, output, and weight should be monitored to assess the patient for adequacy of intake. Fluids such as fruit juices and carbonated beverages that provide both volume and nutrients are encouraged. Because patients with impaired liver function may not produce adequate levels of albumin and may not metabolize aldosterone, abnormal fluid retention can occur. Although abnormal retention of fluids is rare in acute viral hepatitis, the patient should be monitored for abnormal fluid retention.

No special dietary restrictions are required in most patients. The diet should be well balanced and provide adequate nutrients and calories based on the patient's size and age. The diet should be planned with the patient so that it is appealing. Frequent, small meals are usually better tolerated than larger meals. Fats may need to be restricted if poorly tolerated. Intolerance to fatty foods can occur if bile obstruction is severe. Good oral hygiene and the maintenance of a clean, pleasant environment may enhance appetite. Antiemetics may be used and should be given ½ hour before meals. Alcoholic beverages should be avoided, since they are metabolized in the liver and can damage it.

Preventing injury. In a patient with a prolonged prothrombin time, bleeding may be a major problem. The patient should be assessed carefully for signs of bleeding. This includes monitoring the urine and stools for fresh or old blood, monitoring any incisions for recurrent bleeding, monitoring the skin for petechiae, monitoring vital signs, and monitoring prothrombin time, hematocrit, and hemoglobin. Minor procedures such as drawing of blood can result in hematoma formation, if precautions are not instituted. Care to prevent hematoma formation includes the following:

1. Planning so that all blood samples are collected at one time to avoid several punctures

2. Avoiding intramuscular and subcutaneous injections, if possible

3. Applying of pressure to injection sites and venapuncture site for 5 minutes after the procedure

4. Using of soft toothbrushes or swabs to avoid injury to gums and resultant bleeding

If prothrombin time is prolonged, vitamin K may be administered.

Isolation. All patients with hepatitis require isolation to prevent spread of the virus. For patients with hepatitis A, the following *enteric precautions* or universal precautions will be necessary:

1. Good handwashing by patient and staff
2. Wearing gloves when handling feces/urine
3. Wearing a gown when soiling of uniform is likely
4. Cleansing of toilet daily and use of private toilet
5. Private room is necessary only if patient cannot take care of himself or herself regarding proper disposal of feces and urine
6. Proper cleansing, bagging, and labeling of contaminated items such as bed linens and bedpans
7. Discarding contaminated items such as rectal thermometers if possible

For the patient with hepatitis B, *blood and body fluid precautions* are necessary. Universal precautions are usually used and include the following:

1. Good handwashing by patient and staff
2. Wearing gloves when handling blood or body fluids
3. Wearing a gown, goggles, and/or mask when splattering of blood or body fluids is likely
4. Proper cleansing, bagging, and labeling of contaminated equipment and linens
5. Proper disposal of needles or any items exposed to the patient's blood or body fluids
6. Careful labeling of blood specimens to protect personnel working with them
7. Avoidance of contamination of open cuts and mucous membranes with patient's blood or body fluid
8. Teaching patients to avoid intimate sexual contact with others until liver function tests have returned to normal

The nurse in the hospital at times and particularly the nurse in the community will also be involved in identifying patient contacts who will require prophylaxis. Prophylactic therapy should be administered to contacts as described on p. 1165.

Providing comfort measures. During the early phase of the illness the patient may have headaches and arthralgia, resulting in discomfort. The use of general comfort measures, relaxing baths, backrubs, fresh linen on the bed, and a quiet, dark environment may help make the patient more comfortable. During the icteric phase of the illness, the presence of bile pigments in the skin may cause severe *pruritus* (itching). The cause of pruritus is unknown, but it is known to be aggravated by the presence of bile pigments in the skin and by tissue anoxia and dilation of capillaries. Pruritus can be ex-

hausting and demoralizing to the patient.

Measures to control pruritus include the following:

1. Use of cool, light, nonrestrictive clothing and avoidance of clothes or blankets made of wool
2. Use of soft, dry, clean bedding; use of warm, not hot, tub baths
3. Application of emollient creams and lotions to dry skin
4. Avoidance of activities that promote sweating and increase body temperature
5. Maintenance of a cool environment
6. Administration of antihistamines as ordered
7. Use of diversional activities such as reading, television, and radio to reduce the patient's perception of pruritus

The major aim of care is to prevent scratching with resultant injury to the skin. It is impossible for people with pruritus not to scratch. Sometimes the person may be given a soft cloth with which to rub the skin. The patient's fingernails should be kept short, and the patient's hands should be kept clean to decrease the likelihood of excoriation or infection, if scratching occurs.

Avoidance of social isolation. The nurse must work with the patient and significant others so that they understand that the needed isolation does not prohibit social interaction and visiting. Fear of spread of the infection can lead others to avoid the patient. Proper teaching can ensure that both isolation and the patient's need for support from significant others are maintained.

Patient teaching. A major focus of care is patient education. A majority of patients will be treated at home for the duration of their illness. The nurse must prepare these persons for adequate home care by teaching them about the measures described above for the provision of adequate rest, provision of adequate fluid and nutritional intake, relief of discomfort, identification of signs and symptoms of bleeding, and maintenance of adequate isolation. The patient must be able to detect changes indicating a worsening of his or her condition (for example, increasing fatigue, uncontrolled nausea and vomiting, onset of bleeding, worsening of upper quadrant discomfort, and water retention) and be instructed to report these changes immediately.

All patients, whether treated in the hospital or at home, should understand that it may take several months or longer for complete recovery and that they must be evaluated frequently for repeated assessment of blood studies to monitor their progress. Blood studies may be performed weekly for several weeks and then monthly until they return to normal. If blood studies do not show the expected improvement from the care being given, more invasive procedures, such as a liver biopsy, will be necessary to identify why. The patient will be followed for at least 1 year after liver function tests have returned to normal to ensure that relapse does not occur.

CIRRHOSIS OF THE LIVER

Cirrhosis of the liver is the term applied to chronic disease of the liver characterized by diffuse inflammation and fibrosis of the liver resulting in drastic structural changes and significant loss of liver function. The basic changes in cirrhosis are liver cell death and replacement of normal tissue by regeneration of cell mass and scar tissue that results in nodules of normal liver parenchyma surrounded by fibrous tissue. These changes result in loss of function and distortion of the structure with a resultant obstruction of hepatic blood flow.

Cirrhosis of the liver can be classified in various ways. Table 39-4 lists the major types of cirrhosis based on a pathologic classification.

ETIOLOGY/EPIDEMIOLOGY

As can be seen from Table 39-4, cirrhosis can result from liver disease secondary to intrahepatic and extrahepatic cholestasis, viral hepatitis, and other hepatotoxins (drugs, chemicals). Alcoholism and malnutrition are two major predisposing factors for development of Laënnec's cirrhosis. Less common causes of cirrhosis are right-sided congestive heart failure, hemochromatosis, Wilson's disease, glycogen storage disease, cystic fibrosis, and small bowel bypass. In some patients the cause is not identifiable.

Postnecrotic cirrhosis from hepatotoxins is the most common type of cirrhosis on a worldwide basis. Laënnec's cirrhosis is the most common type in North America and accounts for 75% of all cases of cirrhosis.

The role of alcohol in the development of cirrhosis is still under study. It is known, however, that approximately 15% of all alcoholics will develop cirrhosis and that the volume of alcohol rather than the type of alcohol is the important factor. Most persons with Laënnec cirrhosis give a history of consumption of the equivalent of a pint of whiskey a day for 15 years.

Cirrhosis as a cause of death in the United States now ranks fourth in middle-aged men and women, accounting for 350,000 deaths each year. Cirrhosis can occur in any age group, but in the United States it is more common in 45- to 64-year-old white men and in nonwhites of both sexes.

PREVENTION

In the United States, programs aimed at the prevention of cirrhosis are designed primarily to control the ingestion of alcohol. The loss of time from work related to alcoholism is estimated to cost billions of dollars annually. Many large corporations have or are organizing programs to help employees control their alcoholic intake (see Chapter 19).

PATHOPHYSIOLOGY

In Laënnec's cirrhosis secondary to alcoholism and in other types of cirrhosis, fatty infiltration of the liver is the first alteration seen. This fatty infiltration is usually reversible if the causative factor (alcohol, malnutrition, or biliary obstruction) is halted or reversed. If the degenerative process continues, acute inflammation (alcoholic hepatitis) and cirrhosis result.

The end result of cirrhosis is loss of liver function and obstruction of hepatic portal blood flow. Alterations in physiology are usually seen late in the progression of

TABLE 39-4 Types of cirrhosis

Type	Etiology	Description
Laënnec's cirrhosis (nutritional, portal, or alcoholic cirrhosis)	Alcoholism, malnutrition	Massive collagen formation; liver in early fatty stage is large and firm; in late state it is small and nodular
Postnecrotic cirrhosis	Massive necrosis from hepatotoxins, usually viral hepatitis	Liver is decreased in size with nodules and fibrous tissue
Biliary cirrhosis	Biliary obstruction in liver and common bile duct	Chronic impairment of bile drainage; liver is first large then becomes firm and nodular; jaundice is major symptom
Cardiac cirrhosis	Right-sided congestive heart failure (CHF)	Liver is swollen and changes are reversible if CHF is treated effectively; some fibrosis occurs with long-standing CHF
Nonspecific, metabolic cirrhosis	Metabolic problems, infectious diseases, infiltrative diseases, gastrointestinal diseases	Portal and liver fibrosis may develop; liver is enlarged and firm

TABLE 39-5 Relationship between normal liver functions and altered functions associated with cirrhosis

Normal Functions of the Liver	Altered Physiological Functions
Maintenance of normal size and drainage of blood from GI tract	Liver inflammation ↓ Venous congestion of gastrointestinal tract → Altered GI function ↓ GI symptoms
Metabolism of carbohydrates	Increased glycogenesis and decreased glycogenolysis and gluconeogenesis ↓ Altered glucose metabolism ↓ Decreased energy
Metabolism of fats	Increased fatty acid and triglyceride synthesis and decreased fatty acid oxidation and triglyceride release Fatty liver Decreased energy production; weight loss ↓ Hepatomegaly
Protein metabolism	Decreased production of albumin → decreased colloidal osmotic pressure → edema and ascites Decreased production of clotting factors ↓ Altered clotting studies ↓ Bleeding tendencies ↓ Blood loss → Anemia Decreased protein synthesis in general ↓ Alteration in immune function and alteration in healing
Detoxification of endogenous substances	Decreased metabolism of sex steroids (estrogen, progesterone, testosterone) ↓ ↓ Male Female ↓ ↓ Loss of masculine characteristics and development of some feminine characteristics from excessive estrogen Loss of feminine characteristics and development of some masculine characteristics from excessive testosterone Decreased metabolism of aldosterone ↓ ↓ Sodium and water retention Increased potassium and hydrogen excretion ↓ ↓ Edema, ascites Hypokalemia and alkalosis Decreased metabolism of ammonia (usually resulting from blood bypassing liver rather than loss of parenchymal cell function)→Increased ammonia levels Hepatic encephalopathy ←⏋ ↓ Neurologic changes in coordination, memory, orientation, etc

TABLE 39-5 Relationship between normal liver functions and altered functions associated with cirrhosis—cont'd

Normal Functions of the Liver	Altered Physiological Functions
Detoxification of exogenous substances	Decreased metabolism of drugs ↓ Altered drug effects and potential increase in toxicities and side effects
Metabolism and storage of vitamins and minerals	Decreased stores of vitamins and minerals ↓ ↓ Decreased RBC production Decreased energy production ↓ anemia
Bile production and excretion	Obstruction to bile flow ↓ Decreased fat absorption ↓ Decreased vitamin K absorption ↓ Decreased clotting factors ↓ Bleeding/blood loss
Bilirubin metabolism	Decreased uptake of bilirubin from circulation → Increased unconjugated bilirubin → Jaundice, pruritus, scratching, and skin lesions Decreased conjugation and release of bilirubin → Increased conjugated bilirubin and increased urine bilirubin → jaundice, pruritus, scratching, and skin lesions Decreased excretion of bilirubin to bowel → light-colored stools (clay or grayish-white) Decreased reuptake of urobilinogen → urine urobilinogen → dark urine

the disease because of the large reserve capacity of the liver. As much as three fourths of the liver can be destroyed before physiologic function is altered.

In the United States the pathophysiology seen most often is a result of both cirrhosis and long-term alcohol abuse. The relationship between normal functions of the liver and alterations seen in cirrhosis are presented in Table 39-5.

The fibrosis in the liver that results from continual destruction distorts the hepatic structures and results in obstruction of splanchnic veins and portal blood flow. This obstruction can result in additional problems with fluid retention, including worsening edema, ascites, and hypothorax. Increased portal pressure and splanchnic vein congestion result in splenomegaly and altered spleen function, which can cause leukopenia, thrombocytopenia, and anemia. Portal hypertension causes increased venous pressure, vascular hemostasis, varicose veins hemorrhoids, and esophogeal varices. (Figure 39-3, A, depicts the venous drainage of splanchnic organs,

and Figure 39, B, depicts the massive ascites and dilated vasculature that can be seen in cirrhosis.)

CLINICAL MANIFESTATIONS

Signs and Symptoms

A wide variety of signs and symptoms can be seen in persons with cirrhosis. The patient may exhibit any or all of the signs and symptoms. Most manifestations can be directly related to the pathophysiology (Table 39-5 and Figure 39-4).

It is important for the reader to note the long history and the vague, nonspecific early symptoms. Usually the patient gives a history of failing health with symptoms such as nausea, vomiting, anorexia, indigestion, flatulence, and constipation. Weight loss or the severity of malnutrition may be hidden because of abnormal water retention. Also, the severity of malnutrition may not be obvious because of the calories obtained from alcohol, which maintains weight but does not provide proper nutrients. Abdominal pain may be present and is variable

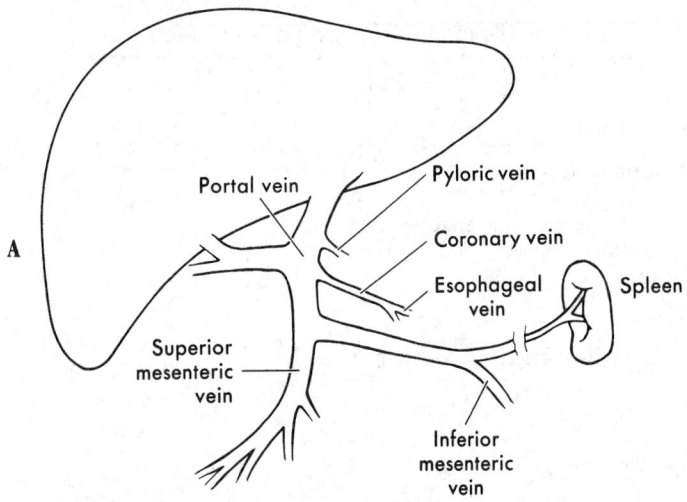

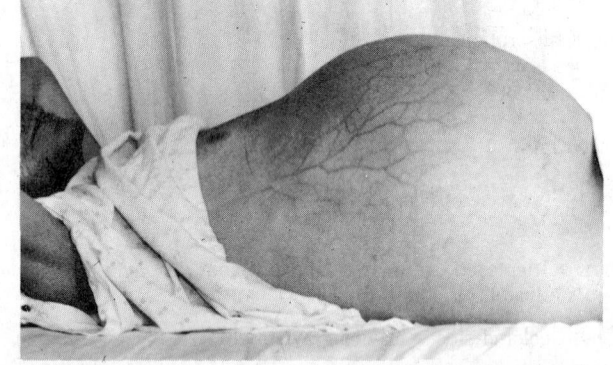

FIGURE 39-3 A, Splanchnic veins. Venous drainage of splanchnic organs. When portal hypertension develops, other vessels can become engorged, leading to stasis and hypoxia of respective organs. **B,** Massive ascites. Note the bulging flanks, dilated upper abdominal veins, and everted umbilicus. (*A,* from Groer ME and Shekleton, ME: Basic pathophysiology: a conceptual approach, ed. 2, St. Louis, 1983, The C.V. Mosby Co.; *B,* from Prior JA, Silberstein JS, and Stang JM: Physical diagnosis: the history and examination of the patient, ed 6, St Louis, 1981, The CV Mosby Co.)

in character. It may be dull, mild, sharp, steady, or wavelike. It may be confined to the liver area (right upper quadrant) or referred to the lower abdomen.

Later signs and symptoms, such as jaundice, ascites, and edema, usually occur gradually. Many of the late signs of cirrhosis are caused by the development of sequelae of cirrhosis that are discussed later in this chapter. It is important for the reader to note that many of the signs and symptoms listed in Figure 39-4 have multiple causes. Examples of signs and symptoms shown in Figure 39-4 that have multiple causes are fatigue,

edema and ascites, bleeding, and anemia. The potassium changes (hypokalemia) and sodium changes seen in persons with cirrhoses also result from multiple etiologies including abnormal excretion as well as changes in oral intake.

Diagnostic Tests

The patient with cirrhosis will have various abnormalities in blood and urine laboratory data as depicted in Figure 39-4, such as increased levels of total, unconjugated, and conjugated bilirubin; increased urine bilirubin; increased urine urobilinogen; increased prothrombin time; decreased platelets, white blood cells, and red blood cells; decreased serum albumin and serum glucose; hypokalemia; hyponatremia; and elevated levels of serum enzymes (ALT, AST, LDH, and alkaline phosphatase). Other studies such as liver biopsy, CT scan, endoscopy, barium contrast, angiography, and so on may be done if the clinical manifestations are vague or inconsistent. The results of these later diagnostic tests will depend on what sequelae the patient has developed.

MEDICAL MANAGEMENT

There is no specific medical management for the treatment of cirrhosis. Management is directed toward removal or treatment of causative factors such as alcoholism, biliary obstruction, infections, and cardiac problems and toward preventing additional liver damage. Because alcoholism and malnutrition are major factors in the development of cirrhosis, extra attention must be given to supplying an adequate diet (well-balanced, normal nutrients) and to helping the patient control alcohol intake.

Other therapy will depend on the signs and symptoms the patient exhibits and may include the following: antihistamines for pruritus; potassium for hypokalemia; diuretics (particularly aldosterone antagonists for edema because the patient with cirrhosis does not catabolize aldosterone appropriately and has hyperaldosteronism); and folic acid, thiamine, and other vitamins and minerals for vitamin deficiency and anemia. Persons with alcoholism are particularly deficient in thiamine and folic acid because these water-soluble vitamins have been depleted and thus deficits occur rapidly with lack of intake of nutrients. Sodium and fluids are also usually restricted. Occasionally albumin may be given for hypoalbuminemia, however its effects last only a short time. If ascites causes severe distress, paracentesis may be done. Additional therapy will be used to treat sequelae of chronic liver disease and is described later.

■ ASSESSMENT

A thorough nursing assessment is necessary to adequately define the multiple nursing diagnosis that can occur.

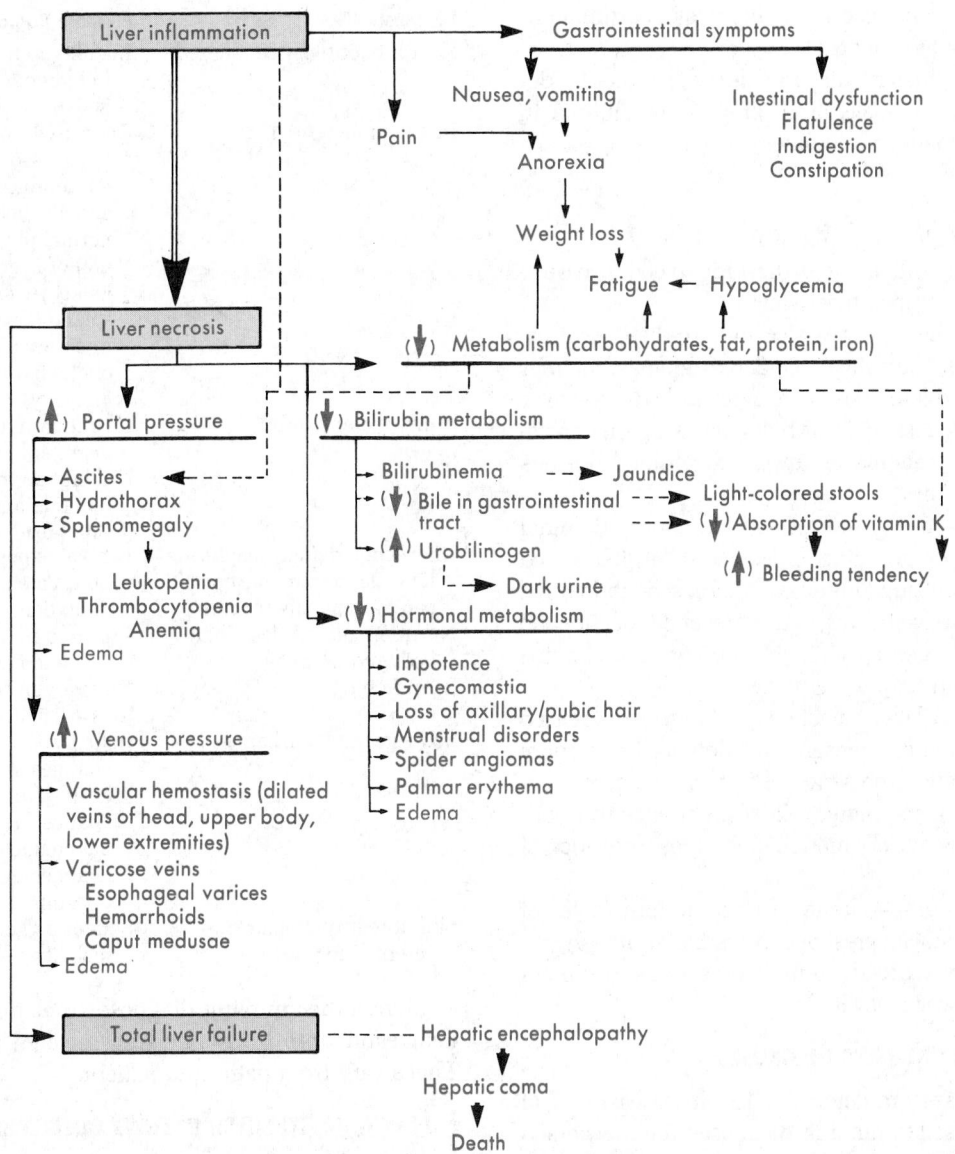

FIGURE 39-4 Progression of liver cell failure. Pathophysiology of signs and symptoms that occur in cirrhosis. NOTE: Process can be arrested if adequate liver regeneration occurs. Regeneration is rarely complete, and there is always some liver cell deficiency.

Subjective Data

Subjective data include the following:

1. Overview of patient's complaints, including length of time patient has had them, a history of temperature elevations; history of frequent infections
2. General body characteristics: history of changes in color of skin or sclera or history of skin marks such as bruising and hematomas; history of changes in secondary sex characteristics (external genitalia, body hair distribution, breast tissue); history of increase in abdominal size (belt size): history of edema; any complaints of itching
3. Social habits: drug and alcohol use, amount, fac-

tors that precipitate use, any attempts to quit, limitations on success, reasons for failure; last time patient had a drink; work environment
4. Nutritional history—daily 24-hour intake for past 1 to 3 days, history of recent change in appetite
5. GI system—complaints of nausea, vomiting, anorexia, indigestion, flatulence or abdominal tenderness
6. Elimination—history of any changes in amount or color of urine, changes in bowel movements, or changes in color of feces
7. Neuromuscular—any complaints of weakness, fatigue, history of decreased ability to do work; his-

tory of any changes in memory or coordination; any history of tremors

8. Sexuality—history of impotence (males), decreased libido (males and females) or change in menstrual patterns (females)

Objective Data

Objective data include the following:

1. Vital signs, including orthostatic blood pressure and pulse, temperature, weight
2. Skin and sclera—presence of jaundice, bruises, hematomas, petechiae, spider angiomas, palmar erythema, dilated vessels on upper body or lower extremities, loss of chest hair (males), gynecomastia (males), edema of lower extremities, lesions from scratching
3. Abdomen—bowel sounds, presence of abdominal distention or guarding, presence of ascites (fluid wave or shifting dullness), increased abdominal girth, increased liver size, presence of hepatic bruits, enlarged spleen, presence of dilated veins on abdomen (*caput medusae*)
4. Neuromuscular—muscle wasting, decreased muscle strength, presence of deficits in memory or coordination, presence of tremors, asterixis, exaggerated deep tendon reflexes, changes in orientation, behavior or emotional changes, presence of apraxia
5. GI/elimination—volume of urine output, color of urine and stools, presence of testicular atrophy
6. Respiratory—breath sounds, presence of dullness in right lower lobe (RLL)

■ DATA ANALYSIS: NURSING DIAGNOSES

Nursing diagnoses are determined from assessment of patient data. Possible nursing diagnoses for the person with cirrhosis may include, but are not limited to, the following:

Diagnostic Title	Possible Etiologies
Breathing pattern, ineffective	Increased restriction of chest movement from ascites or hydrothorax; decreased depth of breathing from limited mobility
Fatigue	Energy needs greater than energy production associated with anemia, altered metabolism, and poor food intake; electrolyte imbalance
Fluid volume, excess	Abnormal fluid retention associated with increased circulating aldosterone, decreased colloidal osmotic pressure or hepatorenal syndrome
Health maintenance, altered	Inability to make appropriate judgments because of alcoholism
Infection, potential for	Decreased immune competence associated with altered protein metabolism and alcoholism; loss of normal phagocytic function of liver or decreased leukocytes secondary to splenomegaly; alterations in external immune barriers (skin and GI mucosal integrity)
Injury, potential for	Alteration in clotting mechanism, enhancing bleeding; alteration in neurologic function and strength that could lead to falls
Knowledge deficit: diagnostic tests, treatment, home care, and follow-up care	Lack of exposure to information; potential cognitive limitations
Nutrition altered: less than body requirements	Impaired metabolism, nausea, and decreased intake
Pain: itching	Enlarged liver and pruritis associated with jaundice
Self-esteem disturbances	Inability to accept physical changes of abdominal girth, jaundice, and change in secondary sexual characteristics; changes in roles and relationships
Skin integrity, impaired, potential for	Scratching, edema, impaired mobility

Many other nursing diagnoses that might be identified result from the sequelae associated with cirrhosis. These vary from patient to patient.

■ PLANNING: EXPECTED PATIENT OUTCOMES

Expected patient outcomes for the person with cirrhosis may include, but are not limited to, the following:

1. The patient shows no increase in dullness on percussion of thorax and has normal breath sounds and normal chest x-ray films.
2. The patient demonstrates a gradual increase in activities, is able to meet self-care needs, and ambulates an increased amount each day.
3. The patient has an output of urine that is greater than fluid intake until excess fluids are excreted, has a daily decrease in weight, has resolution of edema, has a decrease of abdominal girth, and return of electrolytes to normal.
4. The patient verbalizes that alcohol is a problem, states that alcohol has caused his or her problem, lists resources available for assisting with alcohol problem, and contacts one resource (alcohol counselor, Alcoholics Anonymous, inpatient center).

5. The patient develops no new infection(s), and has a return to normal temperature.

6. The patient does not develop any undetected bleeding, maintains normal vital signs, and has no falls or injuries.

7. The patient or significant other can perform the following:
   a. List prescribed diagnostic tests
   b. Describe the planned treatment regimen and the patient's long-term role in treatment
   c. Explain the dietary plan to be followed at home
   d. Explain prescribed fluid restrictions
   e. Explain prescribed medications, such as diuretics and vitamins, (dosage, expected effects, and side effects to report)
   f. Explain ways to prevent bleeding, infections, and progression of disease
   g. Explain plans for follow-up care and signs and symptoms (weight gain, increased temperature, bleeding, or change in behavior) that should be reported to physician

8. The patient eats food from all food groups (unless restricted) in adequate amounts to meet caloric needs and experiences a decrease in signs of muscle wasting.

9. The patient describes that itching is controlled and is not observed scratching.

10. The patient describes self in positive terms, discusses accomplishments, and sets realistic goals.

11. Patient's skin maintains intact skin, and shows healing of any lesions.

■ IMPLEMENTATION

The patient with cirrhosis may be acutely ill and may require intensive care nursing or may be relatively free of acute problems and require teaching, counseling, and support. The nurse must set priorities for care on the basis of the patient's needs. Care for the various patient outcomes are described next and in the nursing care plan on pp. 1178 to 1181.

Supporting Respiration

The patient with cirrhosis has decreased resistance to infection and may be particularly prone to respiratory infection, because of the presence of a hydrothorax and/ or shallow breathing. The patient may experience dyspnea because of pressure on the diaphragm from ascites.

A high Fowler's position may assist respiratory exchange. The patient who is on bed rest should be encouraged to turn frequently and to take deep breaths to prevent stasis of secretion. Hydrothorax is sometimes treated with thoracentesis (see Chapter 34). The nurse should prepare the patient for this procedure, assist with the procedure, and monitor the patient's response during the procedure and afterwards.

Controlling Fatigue

Patients with cirrhosis will have various levels of fatigue. The amount and type of activity encouraged will depend on the individual's energy level, level of consciousness and coordination, and whether any sequelae to cirrhosis are present. If the patient has severe fluid excess and ascites or signs and symptoms of other sequelae, bed rest is usually required. When bed rest is required, special attention to skin care is necessary, particularly if the patient also has severe peripheral edema. Alternating pressure mattresses, flotation pads, or egg crate mattresses may be helpful. If bedrest is not required, the patient should be gotten up and ambulated within the room or hall as tolerated. Level of tolerance is based on the patient's statement about the level of fatigue and/or pulse changes (pulse should not increase by more than 10 beats above baseline).

Maintaining Fluid and Electrolyte Balance

Most patients with cirrhosis will have sodium retention and hypokalemia. A great majority of patients will have ascites, and some will also have peripheral edema. The exact management of these will vary, depending on the patient's needs.

Potassium replacement will be given for *hypokalemia*. It is usually given orally, and the nurse should monitor the patient's serum K^+ values to verify that the patient is not developing hyperkalemia. Some patients with cirrhosis have decreased renal function, which impairs the excretion of potassium and can develop hyperkalemia quite rapidly.

Sodium imbalance and ascites are treated in several ways. Restriction of sodium aids greatly in limiting the formation of ascitic fluid. The basis for determining the amount of dietary restriction necessary to reduce sodium and water retention may initially be a collection of urine for 24 hours to determine sodium loss. Sodium is generally restricted to 1 g daily. The sodium restriction along with bed rest may be enough to relieve the ascites and edema.

If bed rest and sodium restriction do not improve ascites, diuretics may be used. Spironolactone A (aldactone A), which inhibits the reabsorption of sodium in the distal tubules and promotes potassium retention by inhibiting the synthesis and renal effects of aldosterone, is frequently used. The therapy will be adjusted on an individual basis. Sometimes furosemide (Lasix) or another diuretic will be used with spironolactone. Because furosemide causes potassium excretion and can worsen hypokalemia, the patient's serum potassium level is monitored frequently and the patient is observed for signs and symptoms of hypokalemia such as abdominal distention, nausea, vomiting, anorexia, decreased bowel sounds, weakness, or irregular pulse.

NURSING CARE PLAN
PERSON WITH CIRRHOSIS

DATA: Mr. S. is a 55-year-old salesman with portal hypertension who is admitted to the hospital with upper gastrointestinal bleeding. Endoscopy revealed enlarged esophageal and upper gastric veins and a bleeding ulcer. Gastric lavage with iced saline controlled bleeding; 1 U of packed red blood cells was given. Treatment orders included protein (20 g/day) and sodium (1000 mg/day) restrictions, fluid (1000 ml/day) restriction, neomycin 1 g every 4 hours, thiamine 1 ml intramuscularly, vitamin K subcutaneously 1 time a day, and spironolactone 25 mg twice a day. A physical exam revealed slight jaundice of sclera and skin; ascites and peripheral edema; thin legs and arms and poor musculature; signs of increased estrogen; orientation to person, place, and time; and coherence; blood pressure of 116/60 mm Hg; pulse of 90 beats/min; and respiration rate of 32.

The nursing history identified the following:
■ Mr. S. has participated in Alcoholics Anonymous (AA) for 1 year; he has not been drinking since then.
■ Mr. S. has had influenza-like symptoms the past 2 weeks but continued with his busy schedule. He complains of fatigue, anorexia, and itching.

Collaborative nursing actions include interventions to prevent further impairment of physical status from hemorrhage and ammonia toxicity and to assist in treatment of the gastric ulcer and fluid excess. Nursing actions include monitoring for the following:
■ Signs of hemorrhage: hematemesis, decreased blood pressure, tachycardia, restlessness, stools testing positive for guaiac, and cool, moist skin
■ Signs of hepatic encephalopathy: change in mental status, asterixis, and change in handwriting, tremors

NURSING DIAGNOSIS

Fatigue related to muscle wasting, blood loss, and potential anemia

Expected Patient Outcomes	Nursing Interventions	Rationale
Mr. S. will indicate on a weekly basis that he is less fatigued. He will show improved rating of fatigue on a scale of one (no fatigue) to ten (severe fatigue). Patient will show a gradual increase in activities on a weekly basis.	Ensure or maintain bed rest as prescribed during the acute phase. After acute phase, encourage increasing activity interspersed with rest periods as tolerated. Intervene if patient shows fatigue after or during visits by family or friends. Make sure diet is well balanced nutritionally and that patient takes calories, protein, and sodium within proper restrictions.	Graduated increase of activity is important so as not to overtax patient who has poor nutritional status and activity intolerance.

NURSING DIAGNOSIS

Nutrition, altered: less than body requirements related to anorexia and flu-like symptoms

Expected Patient Outcomes	Nursing Interventions	Rationale
Mr. S. ingests required nutrients and adequate calories on a daily basis; signs of muscle wasting lessen.	Assess knowledge of nutrient needs. On a daily basis, plan and implement well-balanced, high carbohydrate, low-protein diet with adequate vitamins. Decrease roughage in diet. Encourage use of salt substitute or alternative seasonings such as Mrs. Dash. Give antiemetics as prescribed and mouth care if nausea is present. Suggest small, frequent meals, 6 meals/day. Use measures that encourage eating such as a clean environment and making sure patient is rested and comfortable. Support continuation of AA activities while patient hospitalized.	Food intake within prescribed limitation can influence liver regeneration; nursing measures can influence amount of intake in anorectic patient. Low-roughage diet is necessary because of esophageal varices. It is important that patient continue AA participation as he has for past year. AA representatives should be allowed to see patient as condition permits.

NURSING CARE PLAN

PERSON WITH CIRRHOSIS—cont'd

NURSING DIAGNOSIS

Fluid volume excess related to impaired metabolism of aldosterone and hypoalbuminemia

Expected Patient Outcomes	Nursing Interventions	Rationale
Mr. S.'s weight and abdominal girth decrease daily. Edema resolves. Serum sodium and potassium levels remain within normal limits.	Monitor weight daily, blood pressure q4h, assess edema every shift, and measure abdominal girth daily. Monitor intake and output on every shift until excess fluid is excreted. Teach patient the rationale for sodium restriction as the patient shows interest. Provide bed rest for ascites. Give the patient prescribed diuretics. Restrict fluids; provide those that are best tolerated, and space the fluids throughout 24 hours.	Diuresis in cirrhosis is undertaken slowly using very conservative measures because of the contracted intravascular fluid volume. Diuresis in excess can jeopardize renal perfusion and precipitate portal-systemic encephalopathy so careful monitoring is necessary.

NURSING DIAGNOSIS

Breathing pattern, ineffective related to ascites and immobility and potential status of secretions

Expected Patient Outcomes	Nursing Interventions	Rationale
Mr. S.'s dyspnea is decreased or does not worsen as indicated on a scale of one (no dyspnea) to five (severe dyspnea). Breath sounds are clear.	Monitor respirations and breath sounds q4h. Place in high Fowler's position. Encourage patient on bed rest to turn frequently, q2h. Encourage deep breathing q2h.	Nursing measures to encourage deep chest excursions are important when ascites and immobility are present. High Fowlers position can relieve pressure on diaphragm, which can decrease chance of stasis of secretions.

NURSING DIAGNOSIS

Impaired, skin integrity, potential related to immobility, poor nutrition, edema, and jaundice

Expected Patient Outcomes	Nursing Interventions	Rationale
Mr. S.'s skin remains intact.	Assess patient's skin daily for signs of possible breakdown. Use measures such as egg crate mattress and routine turning schedule to prevent skin breakdown. Keep skin clean and moisturized. Clean and apply lotion every shift. Keep nails short and clean. Provide soft cloth to rub skin.	Patient has poor nutrition, edema, immobility; all of these are risk factors for decubitus ulcers requiring preventive care. Jaundice could lead to scratching and requires preventive care.

NURSING DIAGNOSIS

Pain: itching related to jaundice and environmental stimuli

Expected Patient Outcomes	Nursing Interventions	Rationale
Patient states that he feels more comfortable and that itching is decreased. Patient not observed scratching.	Avoid heat and heavy clothing; provide a cool environment. Apply antipruritic lotion as prescribed to skin as needed at least every shift. Give patient prescribed antihistamines. Use diversional activities such as music. Keep patient's fingernails cut short and clean. If patient must scratch, provide soft cloth to prevent excoriations. Use tepid water for bathing.	Nursing measures relieve or lessen the effects of environmental stimuli, reduce itching, and promote comfort.

Continued.

NURSING CARE PLAN

PERSON WITH CIRRHOSIS—cont'd

NURSING DIAGNOSIS

Infection, potential for related to immunosuppression

Expected Patient Outcomes	Nursing Interventions	Rationale
Mr. S. develops no infections; temperature remains normal.	Monitor patient for signs of infection every shift. Use sterile technique for all invasive procedures. Encourage pulmonary hygiene such as turning and deep breathing every 1 to 2 hr. Restrict exposure to persons with infections.	Infection in patient with cirrhosis can be life threatening because they can cause sepsis and can precipitate failure, which may result in hepatic encephalopathy and septicemia. Measures to prevent infection are essential in persons whose immune systems are suppressed. Early detection is important for early treatment.

NURSING DIAGNOSIS

Coping, ineffective individual related to health crisis

Expected Patient Outcomes	Nursing Interventions	Rationale
Mr. S. will describe at least one coping mechanism to deal with health crisis.	Assess patient's perception of health and present illness. Identify and support patient's coping strategies such as prayer, music, conversation, etc. Listen actively if patient expresses feeling of powerlessness, fears, or spiritual distress. Plan time daily for listening. Assess and facilitate family support. Meet with family or significant other on a scheduled basis.	Support of patient undergoing a health crisis can facilitate use of intrapersonal family resources. One can expect this patient to be discouraged and fearful.

NURSING DIAGNOSIS

Injury, potential for bleeding and falls related to decreased metabolic function of liver

Expected Patient Outcomes	Nursing Interventions	Rationale
No undetected bleeding occurs. Vital signs return to normal.	Monitor the following for bleeding: urine, stool, Skin, and mucous membranes. Check patient's vital signs q4h and prothrombin and PTT levels and thrombocytes daily. Avoid injections if possible; apply pressure at all puncture sites for 5 min. Give prescribed vitamin K. Teach patient to use soft toothbrush and to avoid straining or coughing.	Patient's esophageal varices and cirrhosis make him a candidate for bleeding and falls; surveillance is the major nursing focus, as well as decreasing precipitating factors.
No falls occur.	Provide support when patient is ambulating to prevent falls. Maintain safe environment.	

Removal of fluid through the kidneys has the advantage of not removing essential body protein such as occurs when fluid is removed from the abdominal cavity by paracentesis. However, diuretic therapy may cause serious side effects for the patient with cirrhosis. An extremely rapid diuresis can precipitate *oliguria* and *uremia* caused by the rapidly diminished blood volume. According to one expert, ascites cannot be mobilized at rates greater than 500 ml/day or approximately 1 lb/day.[5] If the patient has a fluid loss that is greater than 400 to 500 ml greater than intake unless the patient has peripheral edema, which could contribute to a fluid loss greater than 400-500 ml/day, nonascitic extracellular fluid is being lost.[5] Infusions of albumin in 25 g units to

NURSING CARE PLAN

PERSON WITH CIRRHOSIS—cont'd

NURSING DIAGNOSIS

Self-esteem disturbance related to inability to accept physical changes of increased abdominal girth, jaundice, and change in secondary sexual characteristics and potential changes in role

Expected Patient Outcomes	Nursing Interventions	Rationale
Mr. S. describes self in realistic terms, which include positive characteristics.	Encourage patient to participate in goal setting and decision making. Help patient identify personal strengths and give positive feedback. Assist family to understand patient's need for a positive self-concept and how they can help. Assist patient to explore ways to diminish overt signs of jaundice and ascites and thus help body image.	Poor self-esteem can lead to poor coping, causing the patient to resume alcohol consumption.

NURSING DIAGNOSIS

Knowledge deficit: follow-up care and home care related to change in health status and previous inability to cope with information

Expected Patient Outcomes	Nursing Interventions	Rationale
Mr. S. describes nature of cirrhosis and therapeutic regimen.	Assess patient's knowledge and clarify the following, as necessary: basis of signs and symptoms and therapeutic regimen, dietary and fluid restrictions, medication therapy, avoidance of infection and bleeding, and signs (increased temperature, bleeding, worsening jaundice, change in mental status, etc) requiring immediate medical follow-up.	Patient has had the problem for some time, so first assess his knowledge; he may not need teaching.

promote retention of an adequate vascular volume may be given to prevent *azotemia* and *encephalopathy* by maintaining adequate perfusion to the kidneys and the brain and to promote diuresis. The administration of salt-poor albumin may expand the blood volume rapidly, and the patient should be monitored carefully for signs of congestive heart failure and *pulmonary edema* during and after administration.

Fluid restriction will be used if hyponatremia secondary to fluid retention is present. Fluid restriction is monitored closely, because it may lead to decreased output and the *hepatorenal syndrome* (see p. 1192). When fluids are restricted, the nurse must work with the patient to provide fluids that are tolerated best and to spread the allotted fluids throughout the total 24 hours. Fluids will have to be distributed to provide some at each meal and some for required medicine. Some fluids should be given on all three shifts while the patient is hospitalized. At home the patient should distribute fluids over the waking hours.

To further evaluate the effectiveness of therapy, daily weights are required. Measurements of abdominal girth assist in determining the gross amount of abdominal swelling. Patients need to be taught the importance of monitoring and reporting weight gain or rapid increase in abdominal girth after discharge. When ascites is intractable to the above therapies, other procedures such as a peritoneal venous shunt may be used. Peritoneal venous shunts are described in the section on sequelae (p. 1184).

Assisting the Patient to Avoid Alcohol

A major nursing focus for many patients is helping them to deal with alcoholism. Helping the patient cope with alcohol requires that the patients trust that the health team is interested in their well-being. The patient must admit that he or she has a drinking problem. Confrontation may sometimes be used to help the patient recognize the problem. See Chapter 19 for a discussion of various techniques and support systems to assist persons with alcohol problems.

Preventing Infection

The loss of the normal phagocytic function of the liver and the leukopenia and malnutrition associated with cirrhosis require that precautions be taken to avoid in-

MONITORING TO DETECT BLEEDING

1. Monitor urine and stool for blood.
2. Check the patient's body daily for purpura, hematomas, and petechiae.
3. Check mouth, especially gums, carefully for signs of bleeding.
4. Check vital signs at least every 4 hours.
5. Monitor prothrombin time, partial thromboplastin time, and thrombocyte count frequently.

MEASURES TO DECREASE RISK OF BLEEDING IN PERSONS WITH CIRRHOSIS

1. Avoid all intramuscular and subcutaneous injections, if possible.
2. Use the smallest gauge needle possible when giving an injection.
3. Apply pressure to injection sites and venous puncture sites for at least 5 minutes and to arterial puncture sites for at least 10 minutes.
4. Give vitamin K as ordered.
5. Use or instruct patient to use a soft-bristled toothbrush or cotton swabs for oral hygiene.
6. Instruct patient not to strain at stool and to avoid vigorous blowing of nose or coughing.
7. Instruct patient to avoid foods (for example, spicy, hot, raw) that can traumatize esophageal varices.
8. Provide assistance to avoid falls.
9. Make sure that room is free of clutter, that floors are dry, and that shoes or slippers are worn to avoid injuries.

fection. These precautions involve proper handwashing, observing sterile technique with all invasive procedures, respiratory preventive care, and avoidance of contact with persons with infections. The patient must be monitored carefully for presence of infection, and any increase in temperature should be reported immediately so that appropriate measures can be taken.

Preventing Bleeding and Falls

The patient with cirrhosis is at great risk for bleeding because of poor vitamin K absorption, impaired production of clotting factors, and thrombocytopenia. In addition, the patient may have gastritis, esophageal varices, and hemorrhoids that are easily injured by any substance that comes in direct contact with these dilated vessels. Nursing care should focus on monitoring for the presence of bleeding (see the box above) and instituting measures that decrease the risk of bleeding from trauma or injury to varices (see the box at right). The information to be shared about diagnostic tests is described in Chapter 38. Treatment measures that will need to be explained include the dietary restrictions (sodium and protein), the fluid restrictions, the diuretics potassium supplements, and vitamin and mineral supplements. If bedrest is prescribed, the reason this is necessary must also be explained.

Promoting Nutrition

Most patients with cirrhosis will require a well-balanced high-protein, high-carbohydrate diet with adequate vitamins to provide nutrients for repair of the liver. When nausea is a problem, antiemetics should be given 30 minutes before meals to help increase food tolerance. Sodium restriction is frequently necessary, and this restriction can make finding a palatable diet more difficult. Salt substitutes and information on alternative seasonings may help. The liver dysfunction and the presence of portal hypertension, which results in blood flowing through the portal vascular system being shunted around the liver, result in an impairment in the metabolism of ammonia. Ammonia, which originates from deaminiation of protein, is very toxic to the body.

Protein restriction will be necessary for the patient with cirrhosis who can not metabolize ammonia, which would be evident by the onset of signs and symptoms of portal systemic encephalopathy (p. 1190).

Frequent oral hygiene and a pleasant environment should be provided to help increase food intake. The patient's food preferences should be incorporated into the diet. Food should be served in small, frequent amounts. Because persons with cirrhosis need increased calories but often have poor appetites, measures to increase calories without increasing the amount of food should be used. These measures include use of butter as a seasoning, adding dry milk to appropriate foods, and using gravies and sauces. The patient with cirrhosis has the same nutritional needs after discharge, and the person who shops and cooks for the patient must be included in the teaching. The patient's economic situation should be assessed to determine his or her ability to purchase the food required for the prescribed diet. A social service referral may be necessary to help the patient obtain financial assistance. For the person who eats out frequently, instruction on how to select appropriate meals from a restaurant menu will be necessary. If the patient's meals are obtained through a service such as Meals on Wheels, arrangements can be made for some special dietary requirements.

Controlling Pruritis

The management of pruritis will be similar to that discussed under care of patients with hepatitis on p. 1170.

Promoting a Positive Self Esteem

The patient with cirrhosis may experience changes in body appearance and in roles and relationships. If the

RESEARCH

Muhlenkamp AF and Sayles JA: Self-esteem, social support, and positive health practices, Nurs Res 35:334-338, 1986.

This study was designed to identify the relationships among perceived social support, self-esteem, and positive health practices. Ninety-eight adults living in a selected apartment complex completed three different questionnaires that assessed personal resources, self-esteem, and life-style activities. A simple correlation matrix revealed significant positive relationships between self-esteem, social support, and life-style. A theoretic causal model was developed and tested using path analytic techniques. Twenty-eight percent of the variance in life-style was accounted for by the variables in the model. Self-esteem had a significant direct effect on life-style, and social support had a significant direct effect on self-esteem resulting in an indirect effect on life-style.

This study revealed that persons with high self-esteem perceived their social support to be very adequate and, most importantly, they maintained more positive health practices than those with lower levels of self-esteem. Although from only one study, if replicated in other studies, these results reveal that a major way to promote positive health practices is to improve self-esteem and social support. ■

patient isn't helped to establish or maintain positive self-esteem, this can add to the problem of alcoholism. The nurse is in a prime position to help promote positive self-esteem by giving the patient as much control as possible (see research box above). Positive self esteem can be facilitated by:

1. Involving the patient in goal setting
2. Allowing the patient to make as many decisions as possible
3. Giving positive feedback for accomplishments
4. Supporting the patient in times of failure whatever the failure might be, including conflicts with family or friends or participation in drinking
5. Helping the patient recall past accomplishments
6. Helping significant others provide positive feedback
7. Helping the patient learn ways to disguise jaundice or ascites

Providing Skin Care

Because of pruritus, malnutrition, and the edema often associated with cirrhosis, the patient is prone to skin lesions and decubitus formation. Preventive nursing care to avoid skin breakdown, such as air mattresses, frequent turning, backrubs, and massage of bony prominences should be instituted. Measures to prevent pruritus will assist in preventing damage to the skin resulting from the patient's scratching.

SPECIFIC TEACHING CONTENT FOR THE PATIENT WITH CIRRHOSIS

1. Avoidance of further hepatic damage: abstain from alcohol; any drugs not prescribed by physician, including over-the-counter drugs, such as analgesics or cold remedies; work environment hazards; home hazards
2. Dietary regimen (may include sodium and/or protein restrictions) but usually should be well balanced and include sources high in protein such as milk, eggs, fish, and poultry
3. Fluid restriction if required; how to incorporate restrictions throughout the day
4. Signs and symptoms requiring immediate follow-up: weight gain, increased abdominal girth, recurrence of edema, fever, bleeding (blood in urine, stool, or vomitus; epistaxis; cuts that continue to bleed), change in mental function or behavior
5. Measures that lessen chance of bleeding
6. Drug therapy (diuretics, potassium, antihistamines)
7. Activity plan that promotes adequate rest
8. Care measures that help to control pruritus

Patient Teaching

All patients will need to be prepared for diagnostic tests, to understand their treatment, and to learn to meet long-term care needs. Information should be given verbally and supplemented with written information, depending on the patient's physical status; the information may need to be repeated several times and given in small amounts. Family members or significant others should be included so that they can help reinforce the information or help to participate in the patient's care. Long-term care usually requires major changes in lifestyle (diet, fluid intake, and alcohol intake), and thus continual support is necessary. Specific information that the nurse may want to include in the teaching plan is highlighted in the box above.

SEQUELAE OF CIRRHOSIS

Persons with cirrhosis very frequently develop portal hypertension that can result in ascites, esophageal varices, and/or portal-systemic encephalopathy. Each of these major complications is discussed below.

PORTAL HYPERTENSION

As structural damage occurs, the portal vascular system may become obstructed. This obstruction to blood flow causes a rise in portal venous pressure and results in portal hypertension. The obstruction to portal blood flow can cause splenomegaly because of increased vascular pressure and venous congestion in the spleen, contribute to ascites by causing leakage of albumin and fluid from the vascular compartment of the liver into the peritoneal cavity, and cause the development of collateral channels of circulation that bypass the obstruction. Collateral channels are most likely to occur in the paraumbilical and the hemorrhoidal veins, and at the cardia of the stomach extending into the esophagus.

Management

The nursing and medical management of portal hypertension is directed first to treatment of the consequence of portal hypertension: ascites and esophageal varices. The only way to achieve permanent lowering of portal pressure is surgical treatment to reduce blood flow through the obstructed portion of the portal system (see p. 1189). Because of the risks of the surgery and the frequent fatalities from hepatic failure after surgical treatment with a portacaval shunt, the shunt procedure is used only in persons who have esophageal varices (see p. 1185), have bled from the varices, and do not respond to other therapy. Surgical care will be discussed later in this chapter.

ASCITES

As mentioned earlier, ascites is one of the most frequent complications of cirrhosis of the liver and results in

part from the portal hypertension. Other contributing factors are decreased hepatic synthesis of albumin, increased levels of aldosterone, and obstruction of hepatic lymph flow. Ascites may occur with or without peripheral edema. Because ascites is so frequently seen, the required therapy and nursing care were discussed in the section related to general care needs of patients with cirrhosis (pp. 1177-1183). In this section, care related to use of a peritoneal venous shunt will be described.

PERITONEAL VENOUS SHUNT

In chronic and resistant ascites caused by cirrhosis, a LeVeen or Denver peritoneal venous shunt may be used (Figure 39-5). The shunt allows for the continuous reinfusion of ascitic fluid back into the venous system through a silicone catheter with a one-way pressure sensitive valve. One end of the catheter is implanted in the peritoneal cavity, and the tube is channeled through subcutaneous tissue to the superior vena cava where the other end is implanted. The valve opens when there is a pressure differential greater than 3 mm of water between the peritoneal cavity and the vein in the thoracic

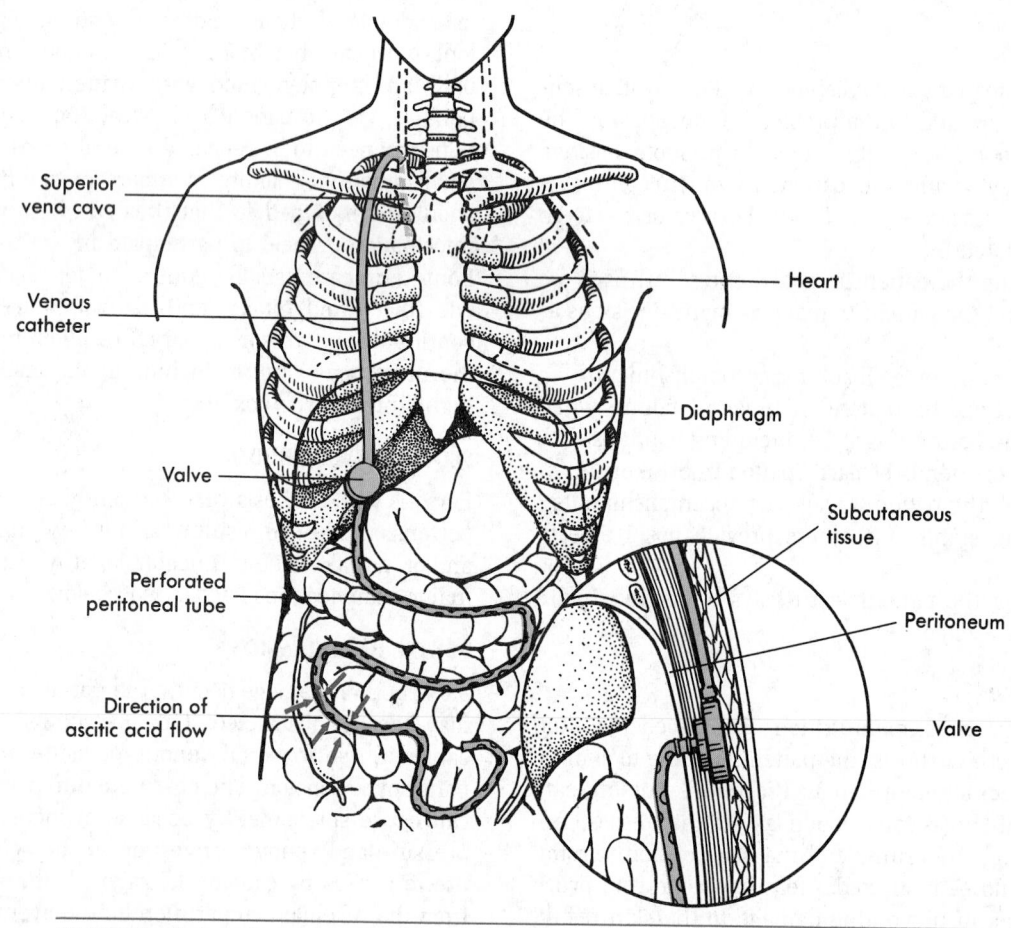

FIGURE 39-5 LeVeen shunt, showing placement of catheter.

cavity, allowing fluid to move from the peritoneal cavity into the superior vena cava.

Persons treated with a shunt may also receive furosemide therapy, and the two together have been successful in relieving ascites in some patients. Persons who have a shunt may still have severe problems, including disseminated intravascular coagulation (DIC), bleeding esophageal varices, and congestive heart failure.[5]

A modification of the original LeVeen peritoneal venous shunt, the Denver shunt, is sometimes used when ascites is marked and is the result of malignancy. Malignant ascites may contain particulate matter that can stop the flow of ascitic fluid through the tubing. The Denver shunt has a subcutaneous pump that can be compressed manually to irrigate the tubing. Increased comfort and improvement of renal and respiratory function have been reported when the Denver pump is used.[31]

When shunts are first implanted and functioning, there can be dramatic changes such as hemodilution of intravascular fluid, decrease in abdominal girth, and increase in renal output. As peritoneal fluid is removed, less of a pressure gradient exists between the peritoneal cavity and the superior vena cava, and thus less fluid will be removed. To force the valve open, deep breathing is encouraged at regular intervals (every 1 to 2 hours) with the patient in the supine position.

ESOPHAGEAL VARICES
PATHOPHYSIOLOGY

Bleeding esophageal varices are the most dangerous consequence of portal hypertension. The mortality rate associated with variceal hemorrhage is 50%.[5] In portal hypertension, the azygos and vena cava veins become distended where they join the smaller vessels of the esophagus. This distention occurs because of the greater volume of blood flowing through these vessels as a result of higher pressure within the portal system. The higher portal venous pressure causes the blood, which would normally flow through the liver, to be forced into these other vessels (see Figure 39-3A for a diagram of the relationship between these various blood vessels.) These small vessels were not designed to carry much blood and become tortuous and fragile. The changes in the structure of these vessels make them prone to injury by mechanical trauma from ingestion of coarse foods and acid pepsin erosion, which may result in bleeding. Bleeding may also occur as a result of coughing, vomiting, sneezing, straining at stool (Valsalva maneuver), or any physical exertion that increases abdominal venous pressure. Bleeding is frequently abrupt and without pain. Severe hematemesis and resultant shock may follow, requiring emergency treatment.

CLINICAL MANIFESTATIONS
Signs and Symptoms

The major manifestation of bleeding esophageal varices is upper GI bleeding that might be seen as blood in vomitus, melana, or massive hemorrhage. The patient may have signs and symptoms of hypovolemic shock (see Chapter 25) or may exhibit signs and symptoms of portal-systemic encephalopathy (see p. 1190).

Diagnostic Tests

Various diagnostic tests will be used to establish the diagnosis of esophageal varices. These include routine liver function tests such as serum enzymes, bilirubin, and albumin to establish the presence of cirrhosis and esophagoscopy, angiography, or barium studies to identify the presence of esophageal varices.

INTERVENTIONS
Medical Management

The first priority in medical management is to establish the source of gastrointestinal bleeding. *Esophagoscopy* is the major diagnostic tool, and, if this isn't possible, *angiography* is used. If severe hemorrhage is not present, barium studies or scans may be used. It must be remembered that, in patients with cirrhosis, bleeding may be from other causes such as peptic ulcers and gastritis.

After diagnosis, the first line of therapy is to control bleeding and replace blood volume. Bleeding may be controlled with:
1. Gastric lavage
2. Pharmacological therapy
3. Injection sclerotherapy
4. Balloon tamponade of varices
5. Surgery—ligation and shunts

Each of these medical interventions are described in more detail in the next section as well as a description of the nursing care involved in assisting with the implementation of these medical interventions.

Nursing Management

The first priority of nursing care in the management of patients with esophageal varices is to establish monitoring parameters of cardiac output; adequacy of vascular volume; effectiveness of tissue perfusion; adequacy of hemostasis treatment; and adequacy of fluid and electrolyte, respiratory, renal, and neurologic status. Surveillance must be instituted immediately upon admission of the patient and continued on a frequent basis (every 15 to 60 minutes), because the patient can loose several units of blood within one hour if hemorrhage is severe. The nurse in collaboration with the physician decides what physiologic parameters to measure and what minimum and maximum values are acceptable.

If the hemorrhage is considered to be minor, introduction of a nasogastric tube by the nurse or physician and administration of an antacid through the tube may be sufficient to control the hemorrhage. The nasogastric tube removes gastric secretions, and the antiacids neutralize gastric acids that may irritate esophageal varices. If hemorrhage is more severe, pharmacologic therapy will be started. Pharmacologic therapy includes vasopressin administration and sometimes use of propranolol (Inderal).

Pharmacologic therapy. Vasopressin is given intravenously mixed in 120 to 200 ml of Dextrose either on an intermittent basis or as a continuous infusion. It lowers portal pressure by causing splanchnic vasoconstriction and can thus stop or control esophageal bleeding. Side effects, which the nurse will monitor for and report immediately, include abdominal cramping and pallor. Coronary artery vasoconstriction can occur, as well as mesenteric artery vasoconstriction; thus vasopressin must be used with caution in persons with coronary artery disease and in the elderly.[5,30]

Propranolol (Inderal), a β-adrenergic blocking agent, has been shown to decrease esophogeal bleeding in some patients, but not all, studies support this finding.[5,30] Thus it is still used experimentally to treat variceal bleeding. If pharmacologic therapy is not effective in controlling bleeding, sclerotherapy will be used.

Injection sclerotherapy. For emergency treatment of varices and longer-term control or for control and prevention of rebleeding in patients who may not be candidates for surgery, injection sclerotherapy may be used. In this procedure a fiberoptic endoscope is introduced into the esophagus by the physician; and, once the bleeding site is identified, a sclerosing agent (sodium morrhuate, 5 ml) is injected into the varices. This agent causes thromboses and sclerosis of the vessel and should result in hemostasis in 3 to 5 minutes. If hemostasis does not occur, a second injection may be given. The procedure may be repeated as necessary and can be while the patient is bleeding or as an elective procedure. Before the procedure the patient and significant others need an explanation of the procedure, and the patient should receive nothing by mouth for at least 6 hours. A mild sedative and a local anesthetic will be given. After the procedure the nurse will monitor the patient for complications (perforated esophagus, aspiration pneumonia, pleural effusion, and worsening of ascites). Respiratory support to ensure adequate air exchange must be provided. *Retrosternal pain* is often present and is treated with analgesics; fever is common for several days. The procedure has shown very favorable results in some patients.

Esophageal tamponade. If bleeding is not controlled by the preceding methods, balloon tamponade of varices

may be instituted. The esophagogastric tube (Sengstaken-Blakemore) is a three-lumen tube with two balloon attachments. One lumen serves as a nasogastric suction tube, the second is used to inflate the gastric balloon, and the third is used to inflate the esophageal balloon (Figure 39-6). The tube is passed by the physician through the nose into the stomach with the balloons deflated. When the tube is in the stomach, the gastric balloon is inflated, and the lumen is clamped; the tube is then pulled out slowly so that the balloon is held tightly against the *cardioesophageal junction*. A "football helmet"-shaped device is used to provide traction on the tube, which keeps it in the proper position.

If bleeding continues after the gastric balloon is inflated, the esophageal balloon, which is connected by a Y-tube to a manometer, is inflated to the desired amount of pressure as determined by the physician and then clamped. To stop the bleeding, the pressure must be greater than the patient's portal venous pressure. If bleeding is from esophageal varices rather than from the gastric mucosa, blood will no longer be aspirated from the stomach. If blood is still present, the stomach may be lavaged with a small amount of ice water, or a solution of iced alcohol and water may be circulated through gastric the balloon to provide vasoconstriction as well as pressure.

The nasogastric lumen is usually connected to intermittent gastric suction, which permits easy appraisal of cessation of bleeding and also keeps the stomach empty. It is important to remove all blood from the stomach, because its presence may precipitate portal-systemic encephalopathy from ammonia produced from the digestion of protein in the blood.

The esophageal balloon can be left inflated for up to 48 hours without tissue damage or severe discomfort. The fully inflated gastric balloon with traction exerted on it, however, compresses the stomach wall between the balloon and the diaphragm, causing ulceration of the gastric mucosa and severe discomfort. To offset the possibility of necrosis, the physician may release the traction on the gastric balloon and deflate the gastric balloon pressure periodically. If the gastric balloon ruptures (and the patient is not intubated), the entire tube may move up and obstruct the airway; if the tube is dislodged the esophageal balloon is deflated at once by the nurse, and the entire tube is removed. The major complication of the tube is ulceration.

Nursing care of the patient with esophageal tamponade includes the following:

1. Explain procedure and provide continued support to patient during the procedure.
2. Monitor vital signs every 15 minutes until blood pressure is stable and then monitor hourly or every 2 hours.
3. Measure and record pressures in the esophageal

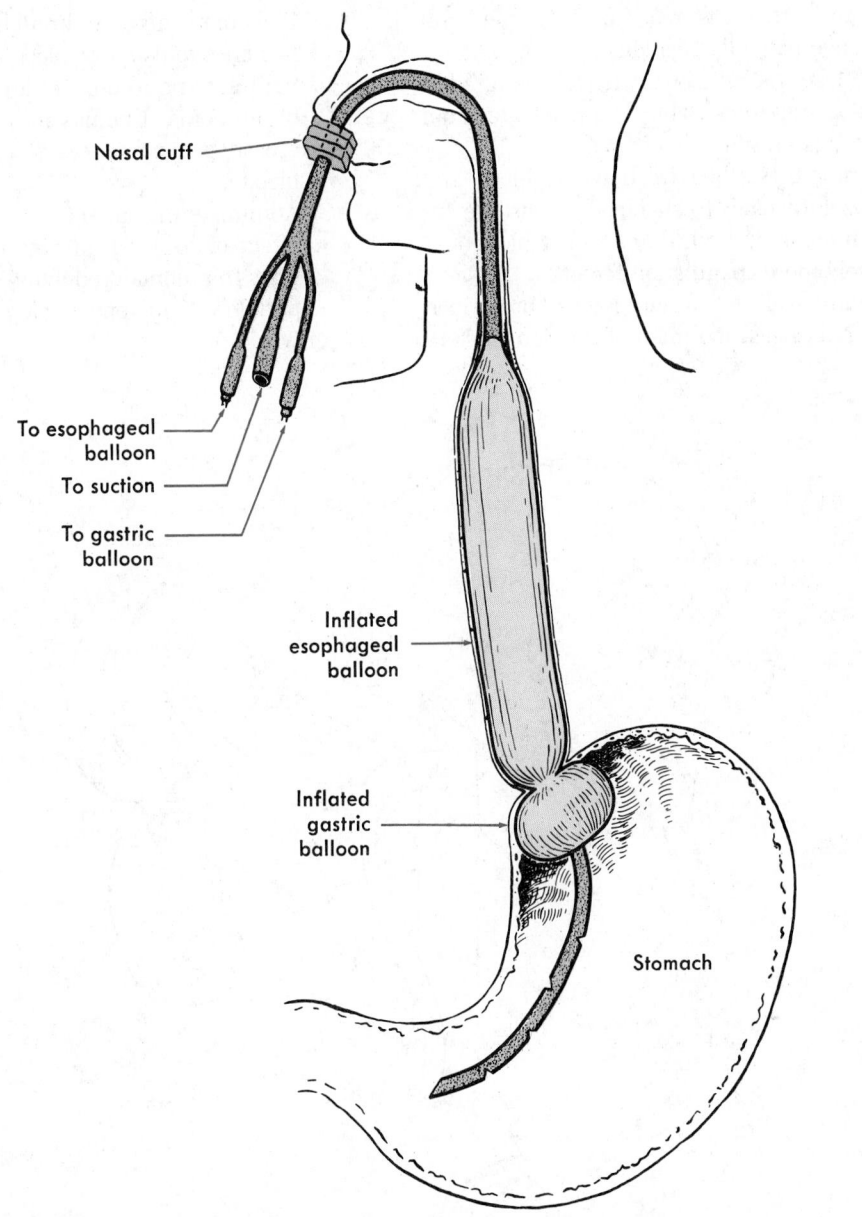

FIGURE 39-6 Sengstaken-Blakemore tube with esophageal and gastric balloons inflated. (Redrawn from Rubber appliances in surgery and therapeutics, Providence, RI, Davol, Inc.)

balloon every hour; maintain pressure at prescribed level.

4. Ensure that patient does not pull on the tube.
5. Provide care to mouth and nares every 1 to 2 hours.
   a. Provide patient with tissues, and encourage spitting of saliva into tissues.
   b. Have patient rinse mouth well to remove any old blood; a Water Pik under low pressure may be helpful.
   c. *Gently* suction mouth and throat if patient is too weak to expectorate secretions on own.
   d. Keep nostrils clean and lubricated with water-soluble jelly.
6. Maintain transfusions and infusions at prescribed rates.
7. If iced solutions are used in the balloons, report patient chilling to the physician who may then order a warming blanket.
8. Record intake and output; test gastrointestinal output for occult blood (guaiac).
9. Consult physician concerning permissible patient movement; passive range of motion is usually allowed.

10. Provide comfort measures (for example, rub back, change patient's position).

The nurse will be assisting with the following additional therapeutic measures when hemorrhage from esophageal varices is present:

1. Administering prescribed fresh whole blood and intravenous infusions; fresh blood avoids the increased ammonia and citrate of stored blood and has relatively more coagulation factors

2. Administering saline cathartics as prescribed through the nasogastric lumen of the Sengstaken-Blakemore tube or through a nasogastric tube to hasten expulsion of blood from the gastrointestinal tract and to prevent an increase in production of ammonia. Enemas may also be ordered to decrease gut content and bacterial action on the blood

3. Administering lactulose or neomycin to decrease effect of bacteria on digested blood in the intestines (ammonia production) in an effort to prevent portal-systemic encephalopathy

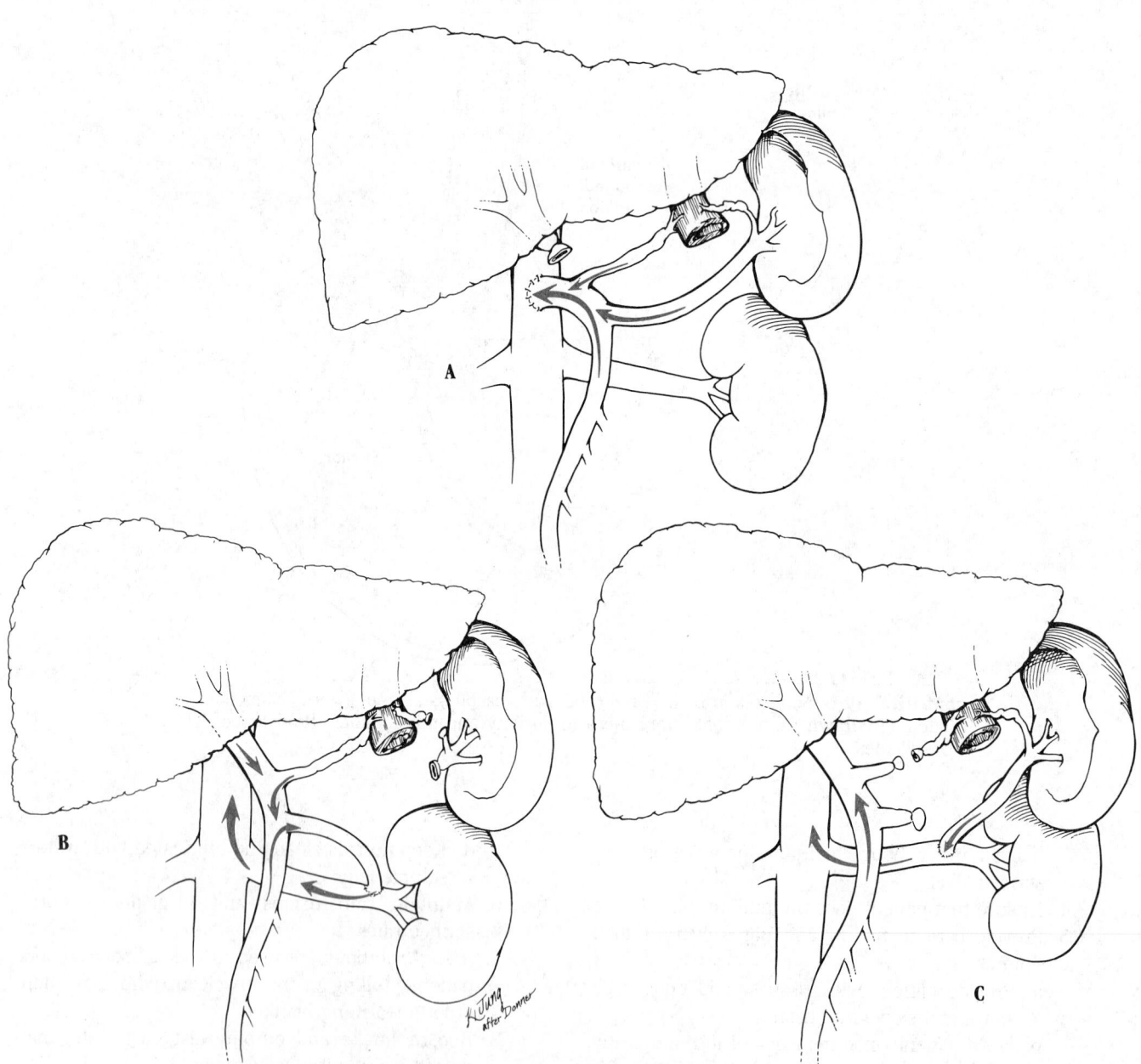

FIGURE 39-7 Decompression operations for portal hypertension. **A,** End-to-side partacaval shunt. **B,** Splenorenal shunt. **C,** Distal splenorenal shunt.

Shunt procedures. Shunt procedures are one of the last measures used to treat esophageal bleeding. The mortality rate for emergency surgical interventions is 50%.[11] When performed in a stable patient who has a bilirubin below 2 mg/100 ml, a serum albumin greater than 3.5 g/100 ml, no ascites, no neurologic disorders, and excellent nutrition, the mortality rate decreases to 10%.[52] It is important to remember that, because of the risk of surgery and the frequent fatalities from hepatic failure after surgery, a prophylactic shunt is not recommended. Shunts are only recommended in patients who have had at least one episode of bleeding from varices and who do not respond to other therapy.

Depending on the location of the obstruction, various operative procedures may be used (Figure 39-7). The purpose of all procedures is to decrease the blood flow through the portal vascular system and thus decrease portal hypertension. Portal hypertension is lowered by shunting blood around the liver. The lowering of portal hypertension will decrease the pressure in the esophageal vessels and the bleeding from the varices. Preoperatively the patient's vascular volume will be stabilized with fluids and blood as necessary. Vitamin K may be given to correct coagulation problems, antibiotics may be given prophylactically, and nutritional status will be improved as much as possible.

Postoperatively, the patient needs intensive care and constant attention regarding the following:

1. Narcotics for pain (the amount given is usually guarded because most narcotics are metabolized in the liver)
2. Avoiding sedative drugs because of their toxic effects on the diseased liver
3. Observing carefully for impending portal-systemic encephalopathy (beginning signs include mental confusion, slowness in response, generally inappropriate behavior)
4. Encouraging deep breathing hourly
5. Recording fluid intake and output accurately, and reporting any lessening of output (renal function sometimes decreases for a time after surgery)
6. Monitoring for hemorrhage (signs of shock)
7. Monitoring for signs of thrombosis at site of anastomosis (pain, distention, fever, nausea)
8. Encouraging activity within the prescribed limits; leg and arm exercises are often started on the first postoperative day
9. Monitoring the lower extremities for signs of edema; elevation of the lower extremities may be ordered to prevent edema formation (edema may form from the sudden increase of blood flow into the inferior vena cava)

All patients who have had a portal-systemic shunt are at risk for *portal-systemic encephalopathy*. Some patients will require lifelong restriction of protein, because the shunted blood bypasses the liver and thus limits ammonia detoxification.

PORTAL-SYSTEMIC ENCEPHALOPATHY

Portal-systemic encephalopathy (PSE), also called hepatic encephalopathy or hepatic coma, is one of the major sequelae of cirrhosis. The onset of the condition may be acute or chronic.

PATHOPHYSIOLOGY

Portal-systemic encephalopathy is a metabolic encephalopathy of the brain associated with liver failure. Portal-systemic encephalopathy results from several metabolic derangements. A major cause is increased blood ammonia levels. Normally ammonia, which is formed in the intestine from the breakdown of protein by intestinal bacteria, is carried directly to the liver and converted to urea through the *Krebs-Henseleit* cycle in the liver. In liver failure, ammonia levels may be increased at the same time that the detoxification ability of the liver is decreased or when blood is shunted past the liver. There are many factors that can increase ammonia levels.

A second hypothesis related to the onset of portal-systemic encephalopathy has been called the false-neurotransmitter hypothesis. It has been shown that patients with portal-systemic encephalopathy have increased levels of aromatic or short-chain amino acids and a decrease in branched-chain amino acids. Normally short-chain amino acids are cleared by the liver. With liver failure they are not cleared and the levels are increased. These short-chain amino acids cross the blood-brain barrier. The short-chain amino acids such as phenylalanine, tryptophan, and tyrosine act as weak neurotransmitters and compete with regular neurotransmitters, resulting in an impairment of normal neurologic function.

A third major cause in the onset of portal-systemic encephalopathy is presence of any of a number of metabolic derangements that may indirectly increase ammonia levels or depress liver function. *Hypokalemia* is a major metabolic factor precipitating portal-systemic encephalopathy. As serum potassium decreases, it shifts from the cells in exchange for sodium and hydrogen. The shift of hydrogen ion into the intracellular compartment increases the acid level in the intracellular compartment, decreases the pH, increases the base in the extracellular compartment, and increases the pH. The extracellular alkalosis increases liberation of H^+ from ammonium (NH_4) and the formation of ammonia (NH_3), which is gaseous and crosses readily into cells where it accumulates and exerts toxic effects. Increased accumulation of base in the extracellular compartment from other causes can precipitate the same type of response.

Constipation may also increase formation and absorp-

TABLE 39-6 Stages of portal-systemic encephalopathy

Stage 1 (Prodromal)	Stage 2 (Impending)	Stage 3 (Stuporous)	Stage 4 (Coma)
Change in sleep pattern	Lethargy	Confused, somnolent	Unconscious
Slow response	Disorientation to time	Stupor, but arousable	No intellectual functioning
Shortened attention span	Impaired computation	Disorientation to place	Loss of deep tendon reflexes
Depressed or euphoric	Decreased inhibition	Anger, rage, paranoia	If responsive, it is only to deep pain
Irritable	Anxiety or apathy	Increased reflexes	
Tremors	Inappropriate behavior	Clonus	
Some incoordination	Speech slurred	Babinski reflex	
Writing impaired	Decreased reflexes		
	Ataxic		
	Asterixis		

tion of ammonia from the gut, or it may induce straining and thus precipitate bleeding from esophageal varices or hemorrhoids. Other metabolic factors such as exercise and infection may precipitate portal-systemic encephalopathy by causing increased ammonia formation or decreased liver function.

A fourth major causative event in the onset of portal-systemic encephalopathy is increased cerebral nervous system sensitivity to depressants. Any hypoxic insult or sedative, which can increase the sensitivity of the central nervous system to any substance, can precipitate portal-systemic encephalopathy.

Common factors found in the clinical setting that can precipitate PSE are summarized in the box below.

CLINICAL MANIFESTATIONS

Signs and Symptoms

The manifestations of portal-systemic encephalopathy vary and may occur quickly or gradually over the course of a few days. Portal-systemic encephalopathy results in alterations in the state of consciousness, in intellectual function, in behavior and personality, and in neuromuscular function. The state of consciousness may fluctuate from hypersomnia, to slow responses, to unconsciousness. Alterations in intellectual functioning such as shortened attention span or loss of recognition of self may be seen. Personality and behavior changes may vary from exaggeration of normal behavior to rage. Neuromuscular abnormalities such as metabolic tremor and ridigity may occur. These intellectual, personality, and behavioral changes have been graded in four stages (see Table 39-6).

Other associated findings are the occurrence of asterixis (liver flap) that may be elicited when the patient is asked to dorsiflex the hand while the rest of arm is extended and resting on the bed. Asterixis appears at the beginning of stage 2. A peculiar sweetish odor can frequently be detected on the breath (*fetor hepaticus*). Changes may also be seen on encephalography (EEG). During the latter stages of portal-systemic encephalopathy, hyperventilation may be present. The temperature rises, and the pulse rate increases.

COMMON FACTORS ASSOCIATED WITH PORTAL SYSTEMIC ENCEPHALOPATHY

FACTORS DEPRESSING CNS OR LIVER FUNCTION

Hypoxia
  Secondary to hemorrhage and hypovolemic shock
  Secondary to morphine and other sedatives
Infections

Exercise
  In patients with chronic liver disease who are in impending coma
Sedatives
Abdominal paracentesis
  Resulting in reduction of plasma volume

FACTORS INCREASING LEVEL OF AMMONIA

Gastrointestinal ammonia (old blood in bowel from gastrointestinal hemorrhage)
High-protein intake
Transfusions, especially with stored blood because it contains more ammonia
Hypokalemia
  Secondary to thiazide diuretics
  Secondary to potassium loss from the bowel
Alkalosis secondary to hyperventilation or hypokalemia
Shunting of blood into systemic circulation without passing through hepatic sinusoids
  Natural collateral bypass of liver
  Surgical bypass of liver
Constipation

Diagnostic Tests

Patients with portal-systemic encephalopathy will have the abnormal liver function as described for patients with cirrhosis (p. 2074). An elevated serum NH_3 level provides the definitive diagnosis, but not all patients show any an increase in NH_3. Therefore treatment is determined by the signs and symptoms and not the serum NH_3 level.

MEDICAL MANAGEMENT

Medical management of portal-systemic encephalopathy is threefold and includes the following:

1. Identification of precipitating factors and treating them (hypokalemia, hemorrhage, hypoxia).
2. Instituting a program to lower ammonia level. This can be achieved by:
   a. Decreasing the substrate necessary for protein, the production of ammonia
      (1) Decreasing protein in diet (usually between 20 to 40 cm/day, and protein may be eliminated completely in several days)
      (2) Removing blood from GI tract
   b. Decreasing formation of ammonia by bacteria in GI tract by giving antibiotics to sterilize the GI tract
   c. Increasing elimination of ammonia from the body by giving lactulose.
3. Providing supportive care.

NURSING MANAGEMENT

Nursing management is directed toward the following four goals:

1. Providing continual, regular monitoring of patients at high risk of portal-systemic encephalopathy
2. Assisting with the therapeutic regimen
3. Providing supportive care
4. Providing long-term care

Providing Continual Monitoring

As can be seen from a review of Table 39-6, the early indications of portal-systemic encephalopathy are very subtle and can easily be missed if regular, objective assessments are not made. The nurse must (1) be as descriptive as possible, (2) assess skills such as handwriting or the ability to draw a circle, box, or square, and (3) maintain continuity of care so that the staff becomes familiar with the patient's behavior. Early detection of symptoms allows for more rapid treatment and consequently improves the patient's chance of recovery.

The continual monitoring should also focus on the patient's vital signs (particularly pulse, respiration, and temperature) and on the patient's total cirrhotic status to identify worsening of the patient's basic condition, which could be seen by the onset of fever or worsening of laboratory studies (such as serum enzymes [ALT, AST], prothrombin time, bilirubin, and albumin) and can increase the risk of portal-systemic encephalopathy.

Assisting with Therapeutic Regimens

If encephalopathy is present, a major focus of nursing will be to implement the prescribed regimen. The first treatment may be directed toward eliminating the causes of portal-systemic encephalopathy such as GI bleeding or hypokalemia, if known.

The second approach will be directed toward decreasing ammonia levels. Interventions will include the following:

1. Eliminating protein intake or severely restricting it
2. Increasing carbohydrate intake to decrease metabolism of endogenous proteins
3. Administering oral cathartics or enemas to empty the bowel and decrease ammonia formation
4. Administering intestinal antibiotics such as neomycin to kill bacteria in the gastrointestinal tract
5. Administrating of lactulose
   a. Lactulose is a synthetic disaccharide that is degraded by bacteria in the lower intestines, causing acidification of the intestinal lumen and increased formation of NH_4 and the GI elimination.
   b. Lactulose also acts as an inhibitor of coliform growth and stimulates fecal excretion.
   c. Lactulose can be given orally or as an enema, and it is often one of the first agents used.

Providing Supportive Care

The patient with portal-systemic encephalopathy is very ill and requires excellent care directed toward prevention of respiratory problems. This includes turning and deep breathing and may include administration of oxygen, suctioning, or even ventilatory support. Coughing is prohibited if the patient has esophageal varices. The patient also needs care to prevent skin breakdown that may be worsened by malnutrition, ascites, and frequent or incontinent stools. Infections must also be prevented.

Many patients with portal-systemic encephalopathy die of renal failure secondary to an inadequate circulating blood volume (hypovolemia). In some patients, renal function progressively deteriorates without any apparent cause. The treatment of portal-systemic encephalopathy requires a careful balancing of fluid administration to maintain adequate perfusion of the kidney without creating an excessive load on the cardiovascular system. Therefore when intravenous solutions are being administered, the desired flow rate is monitored very closely, and the patient is observed for signs of cardiovascular overload. To adequately monitor renal function, an indwelling catheter is often inserted, especially if the patient is being maintained on intravenous fluids. Central venous pressure (CVP) monitoring is also commonly used. The nurse is alert to changes in the CVP readings suggestive of either hypervolemia or hypovolemia. The supportive nursing care required by any patient with hepatic disease as well as by any unconscious patient should be given.

Because most narcotics and sedatives must be detoxified by the liver, they are contraindicated in patients with impaired liver function. If a sedative must be used, drugs such as chlordiazepoxide (Librium), barbital, or phenobarbital, which are excreted by the kidney, are prescribed. If any sedatives, analgesics, or hypnotics are used, they should be given in smaller than normal doses, and the patient's response in terms of development of signs and symptoms of portal-systemic encephalopathy such as behavioral or mental changes and asterixis should be evaluated carefully.

Maintenance of adequate nutrition is a major nursing focus. A low-protein diet is often less palatable. Providing good oral hygiene, maintaining a pleasant clean environment, and serving small attractive meals may help increase appetite. If proteins need to be severely restricted for some time, the use of a dietary or intravenous supplement that provides selected branched-chain amino acids and is lower in short-chain amino acids may be used. Commercial oral preparations and intravenous preparations are available. These supplements also provide carbohydrates. Vitamins and minerals are added as necessary.[4]

Providing Long-Term Care

Some patients may always be under the threat of developing portal-systemic encephalopathy and may be kept on a low-protein diet (20 to 40 g/day) indefinitely. Lactulose and neomycin may also be used indefinitely. The patient and family will need instructions regarding the dietary restrictions and how to take medications. They also must be taught to be alert for subtle changes in the patient's behavior that indicate worsening or onset of portal-systemic encephalopathy and to seek medical attention immediately if the patient shows any behaviors indicative of worsening portal-systemic encephalopathy. In addition to the above needs, the patient and family will have all the other needs as other patients with cirrhosis (p. 1177-1183).

HEPATORENAL SYNDROME

Hepatorenal syndrome is a poorly understood sequalae of cirrhosis. It is characterized by sudden renal failure for no known cause in a patient with progressively worsening liver failure.

The pathogenesis of hepatorenal failure is uncertain but includes a marked decrease in renal cortex blood flow due to intrarenal vasoconstriction. The intrarenal vasoconstriction can possibly result from the following[30,44]:

1. An increase in renin

2. A decrease in prostaglandin production by the kidney
3. The release of endotoxin in the body because of liver failure
4. A change in sympathetic activity, causing vasoconstriction
5. The production of a vasoconstriction by the diseased liver

The patient with hepatorenal failure has oliguria and azotemia. Blood pressure may be elevated or decreased. The patient complains of anorexia, fatigue, and weakness. Fluid retention leads to hyponatremia and a decrease in urine osmolality. The continual accumulation of waste products and alterations in fluid and electrolytes cause neurologic changes that can resemble those of portal-systemic encephalopathy. Blood pressure continues to drop. Hepatorenal failure carries a very poor prognosis.

The first focus of medical management is to identify whether the oliguria is due to decreased cardiac output, hepatorenal syndrome, or acute tubular necrosis. Any of these processes can happen in the person with cirrhosis. Once the diagnosis of hepatorenal syndrome is made, the management is designed to improve hepatic function and support renal function. Fluid and electrolytes are given to maintain hemodynamic status. Potentially nephrotoxic drugs such as neomycin are stopped. Some patients have shown improvement after a portacaval shunt has been implemented for other reasons, and others have shown improvement with a decrease in ascites. Liver transplantation is the major intervention for most patients.[44] Hemodialysis has been successful in treating hyperkalemia. Continuous arteriovenous hemodialysis or ultrafiltration may be used to treat fluid overload and pulmonary edema. Note that these last treatments only improve symptoms and not the hepatorenal syndrome itself, because the basic problem is in the liver and not in the kidney.

HEPATIC TRANSPLANTATION

Hepatic transplantation is performed for various reasons, including biliary atresia, chronic active hepatitis, fulminant hepatitis, end-stage cirrhosis with sequelae, metabolic diseases of the liver, and hepatic malignancy. One problem with using transplants in malignancy is the excessively high recurrence rate.[34]

Transplantation of the liver is performed only at selected centers, and the patient must usually meet the following selected criteria:

1. Being free of infection outside liver
2. Being free of coexisting cardiopulmonary disease
3. Usually being no older than 55 years of age
4. Being able to meet care needs after transplantation

Most organs are obtained from brain-dead donors whose

livers are free of disease and who have had adequate maintenance of blood pressure and blood volume, though organ transplantation from live donors has been performed in children. The recipient of live donor transplant is matched for human lymphocytic antigens and blood group. The recipient receiving a cadaver organ is usually matched for blood group and may be matched for human lymphocytic antigen, but not always. Transplants, using cadaver organs, have been performed despite the presence in the recipient of cytoxic antibodies against the donor organ and incompatible blood groups.[54] Both vascular and biliary drainage system reconstruction is necessary.

PREOPERATIVE CARE

Preoperatively the patient undergoes extensive evaluation to determine if:
1. He/she is a candidate for transplantation.
2. He/she has contraindications to transplantation such as advanced cardiopulmonary or cerebrovascular disease, sepsis, active drug or alcohol abuse, malignant disease outside the liver, or a positive human immunodeficiency virus (HIV) test or the inability to manage an immunosuppression regimen.

The patient will have many blood tests performed to establish blood type, as well as presence of HIV; proper liver function; normal cholesterol, triglyceride, electrolyte, and ammonia levels; and normal renal function (blood urea nitrogen or creatinine). Other tests include chest x-ray, electrocardiogram, pulmonary function test, and a test to assess the portal and hepatic vascular system function.

The patient will be seen by a financial coordinator because postoperative transplantation requires extensive home management and financial resources. The patient is also seen by other health team members such as a cardiologist, psychiatrist, dentist, and nutritionist to establish that the patient's overall health status is the best possible and any impairments are controlled. Much of this preoperative care is coordinated by a transplant coordinate, who is often a registered nurse. Once the patient is accepted for transplantation, he/she is placed on a recipient list and then must wait for an appropriate organ.

POSTOPERATIVE CARE
General Physical Care

The major physiologic complications postoperatively include rejection, infection, and occlusion of vessels. In addition, because of the patient's preoperative illness and the surgery itself, all patients are at increased risk for any of the common postoperative complications described in Chapter 22.

Postoperatively the patient will be in an intensive care unit. Constant monitoring of hemodynamic, cardiovascular, neurological, and respiratory status; fluid and electrolyte balance; and liver function is necessary. Bed rest is maintained for several days. Measurements of liver function should show improvement immediately (within 24 hours) if a complication does not occur. Immunosuppression, with cyclosporine and prednisone and some times other agents, is started before surgery and must be given on a very regular schedule after the operation.

Immunosuppression/Rejection

Immunosuppression is usually maintained with cyclosporine and corticosteroids. Because of the nephrotoxicity of cyclosporine, various centers have looked at ways to decrease the dosage of cyclosporine. One approach is to include azathioprine, which had been used previously with other types of transplants, so the dose of cyclosporine can be decreased.[34]

The amount of immunosuppressive therapy will be altered on the basis of the appearance of signs of rejection that are listed below.
1. Increased temperature ($\geq 38°$ C), tachycardia malaise, hypertension, fluid retention
2. Enlargement of the liver
3. Tenderness over the transplant site
4. Recurrence of abnormal liver function tests (enzymes, bilirubin, albumin, and clotting factors)
5. Altered functioning seen on hepatic scan or hepatic perfusion studies or abnormalities on liver biopsy

If signs of rejection occur, the dosage of immunosuppressive agents may be increased, or additional agents, such as monoclonal antilymphocyte antibodies (OK T3), are added. Acute rejection episodes are treated with bolus corticosteroids and those episodes unresponsive to regular therapy are treated with OKT3 or antilymphocyte globulin. The nurse must always be aware that these drugs will increase the risk of infection.

Providing Psychosocial Care

While instituting the tremendous physical care needed, the nurse must deal with the psychosocial needs of the patient and family. The patient and family must be kept aware of the status of the transplant. They will have been informed of the risks of the procedure before surgery, and keeping them informed will help them deal with the uncertainty. The patient and family need time to express fears and concerns. They also need help coping with the physical isolation that is instituted because of the increased risk of infection, the social isolation, and the separation that can occur with the long hospitalization (several weeks to a month) that is sometimes involved.

The nurse can help the patient and family stay up-to-date. Short frequent meetings between health team members and the patient and family can result in patients and families getting answers to many of their questions and an established time during each day for longer meetings can be set aside as necessary. If family members cannot visit often, the nurse can decrease the patient's homesickness and isolation by encouraging telephone calls and communications by audiotapes or letters. The nurse can help the patient cope with the long isolation by encouraging hobbies such as reading, crossword puzzles, needlework, and television.

Patient Teaching

A major focus of care will be on patient education. The patient and family must receive education before surgery, immediately after surgery, and in preparation for discharge. They will need considerable education about the immunosuppressive agents. They must be taught how the medications are to be taken, (see a pharmacology textbook) the importance of never missing a dose of immunosuppressive therapy, and how to monitor for signs of infection or rejection. The patient must learn ways to avoid infections (for example, avoid persons with upper respiratory infections and avoid large crowds). Follow-up care must be understood, and there should be a way for the patient to contact some member of the health team (either the nurse or physician) at all times.

CHAPTER SUMMARY

- Liver abscesses may be pyogenic and treated with broad-spectrum antibiotics and surgery, or they may be amebic and treated with amebicidal drugs.

- Metastatic tumors of the liver are 20 times more prevalent than primary tumors of the liver. Symptoms occur late; jaundice, ascites, and weakness are common.

- Malignant lesions of the liver are treated with resection, palliative use of radiation, and chemotherapy by systemic routes or hepatic arterial infusion.

- New forms of treatment such as immunoradiotherapy and hepatic dearterialization for malignant lesions of the liver are being experimentally tested.

- Injury to the liver, which frequently results from trauma, can lead to major hemodynamic changes.

- The incidence of toxic hepatitis may be reduced by decreased use or proper use of toxins such as petroleum distillates.

- There are four known types of viral hepatitis. Measures to control hepatitis A are directed toward handwashing, thus interrupting the fecal-oral route of transmission. The other three types are spread through blood and body fluid routes.

- There are many tests that use serologic markers (antigens, antibodies) for differentiating the type of hepatitis; HBsAg is one test for hepatitis B. Hepatitis A is detected by the presence of IgM-class anti-HAV.

- The Centers for Disease Control considers hepatitis B to be the greatest occupational hazard for health care workers. Measures to decrease risk include hepatitis B vaccination, handwashing, and blood/body fluid precautions used with all patients.

- Preexposure and postexposure prophylaxis for hepatitis A and B include immune globulin (passive immunity for hepatitis A) and HBIG (passive immunity for hepatitis B) and hepatitis B vaccine (active immunity for hepatitis B).

- Anorexia and influenza-like symptoms are often more acute in hepatitis A, but these symptoms occur in all types of hepatitis. They occur before icterus (jaundice) appears.

- Most persons with viral hepatitis recover within 6 months and have no residual liver damage. Hepatitis B and non-A, non-B hepatitis may lead to a carrier state, atypical course of illness, chronic hepatitis, or cirrhosis.

- All types of jaundice involve increased serum levels of bilirubin. Hemolytic jaundice is a problem of excessive red blood cell breakdown; obstructive jaundice is associated with an elevation of conjugated bilirubin (direct) and an absence of urinary urobilinogen, and hepatocellular jaundice is often associated with elevated serum transaminases.

- In the United States, cirrhosis is most commonly a result of chronic alcoholism and is characterized by multiple abnormal hepatic function tests. Portal hypertension and bleeding esophageal varices are two life-threatening problems.

- Patients with cirrhosis can have a long history of vague gastrointestinal complaints and failing health.

- Cirrhosis eventually leads to fatigue, hypoglycemia, fluid and electrolyte disturbances, bleeding, immune incompetence, poor wound healing, ascites, edema, muscle wasting, jaundice, and changes in secondary sexual characteristics if the process is not stopped. The major focus of nursing care is on supporting the patient by dealing with problems related to altered liver function and helping patients deal with the alcoholism that is frequently the cause.

- The major sequelae of cirrhosis are portal hypertension, varices, ascites, portal-systemic encephalopathy, and hepatorenal syndrome.

- Varices are treated pharmacologically, with sclerosis, with balloon tamponade, and in some instances, with surgery for shunting procedure.

✔ Ascitic fluid must be decreased slowly at a rate of no greater than 500 ml/day to prevent hypokalemia, elevated BUN, oliguria, and hepatic encephalopathy.

✔ Resistant ascites may be treated with use of peritoneal venous shunt.

✔ Hepatic encephalopathy causes subtle neurologic changes that can be missed unless assessment focuses on collecting objective neurologic data.

✔ Hepatic encephalopathy can be precipitated by increased ammonia from GI bleeding or increased protein in the diet, by electrolyte imbalances such as hypokalemia and alkalosis, and by CNS depressants such as hypoxia and sedation.

✔ Hepatic encephalopathy is treated with neomycin, lactulose, and a low-protein diet.

✔ Hepatorenal syndrome is renal failure from no known cause in persons with hepatic failure; it has a very poor prognosis.

✔ Liver transplantation is increasingly being performed for a variety of liver problems.

✔ Cyclosporine and glucocorticoids are the major immunosuppressive agents used in liver transplantation.

✔ Patient education is a major nursing intervention for most patients with diffuse liver disease because of the chronicity of the liver problems.

QUESTIONS TO CONSIDER

■ How do patients who have developed a chronic carrier state for hepatitis B need to change their life-styles to prevent the spread of hepatitis B?

■ What questions should you incorporate in your assessment that would identify persons at high risk for exposure to hepatitis B?

■ How do neomycin, lactulose, a low-protein diet, and prevention of constipation and gastrointestinal bleeding prevent hepatic encepalopathy?

■ What are the major signs of hepatic transplant rejection?

■ What factors play a role in increasing the chance of bleeding or infections in a person with cirrhosis?

REFERENCES AND SELECTED READINGS

1. *Advisory Committee Immunization Practices (ACIP): Recommendation for protection against viral hepatitis, MMWR 39(S-2):1-26, 1990.

2. *Adinaro D: Liver failure and pancreatitis: fluid and electrolyte concerns, Nurs Clin North Am 22:843-852, 1987.

3. Alter MJ et al: The changing epidemiology of hepatitis B in the United States, JAMA 263:1218-1222, 1989.

4. *Anderson FP: Portal-systemic encephalopathy in the chronic alcoholic, Critic Care Quart, 8(4):40-52, 1989

5. Arora S and Kaplan MM: Cirrhosis. In Rakel RE, editor: Conn's current therapy, ed 28, Philadelphia, 1989, WB Saunders Co.

6. Arroyo V et al: Pathophysiology of ascites and functional renal failure in cirrhosis, Journal of Hepatol 6:239-257, 1988.

7. Barry RE and Williams AJK: Metabolism of ethanol and its consequences for the liver and gastrointestinal tract, Digest Dis 6:194-202, 1988.

8. Black M: Primary biliary cirrhosis. Hosp Med 21(6):184-205, 1986.

9. *Brown M: Gastroesophageal varices, Prim Care 15:175-186, 1988.

10. Clouse ME: Hepatic artery embolization for bleeding and tumors, Surg Clin North Am: 69:419-432, 1989.

11. Cutler BS et al: Manual of clinical problems in surgery, Boston, 1984, Little, Brown & Co.

12. Davis M: Alcoholic liver injury, Proc Nutr Society 47:115-120, 1988.

13. DiBisceglie A et al: Hepatocellular carcinoma, Ann Intern Med 108:390-401, 1988.

14. Dienslag JL et al: Hepatitis B vaccine administered to chronic carriers of hepatitis B surface antigen, Ann Intern Med 96:575-579, 1982.

15. Dindzans VJ et al: Medical problems before and after transplantation Gastroenterology Clin North Am 17:19-31, 1988.

16. *Dobberstein K: The liver: to know it is to love it, Am J Nurs 87:74, 1987.

17. *Dodd RP: Ascites: when the liver can't cope, RN 47(10):26-30, 1984.

18. Erikson I and Mitchell C: Which child gets the transplant? Am J Nurs 88:287-288, 1988.

19. Falkson G et al: Prognostic factors for survival in hepatocellular carcinoma, Cancer Res 48:7314-7318, 1988.

20. Feliciano DV: Surgery for liver trauma, Surg Clin North Am 69:273-284, 1989

21. Franks AL et al: Hepatitis B virus infection among children born in the U.S. to Southeast Asian refugees, New Engl J Med 321:1301-1305, 1989.

*References preceded by an asterisk are particularly well suited for student reading.

22. Freditti SL: When the liver fails, Am J Nurs 84:64-67, 1984.

23. Frey CF et al: Liver abscesses, Surg Clin North Am 69:259-271, 1989.

24. *Gullate MM and Foltz AT: Hepatic chemotherapy via implantable pump, Am J Nurs 83:1674-1678, 1989.

25. Henderson JM: Surgical methods for the prevention of first and recurrent variceal bleeding, Z Gastroenterol 26(suppl 2):49-53, 1988.

26. Hoofnagle JH: Toward universal vaccination against hepatitis B virus, New Engl J Med 321:1333-1334, 1989.

27. Hoofnagle JH: Type D (Delta) hepatitis, JAMA 261:1321-1325, 1989.

28. Jenkin RL and Fairchild RB: The role of transplantation in liver diseases, Surg Clin North Am 69:371-382, 1989.

29. Jensen DM: Portal-systemic encephalopathy and hepatic coma Med Clin North Am 70:1081-1092, 1986.

30. *Keith JS: Hepatic failure: etiologies, manifestation, and management. Crit Care Nurse 5(1):60-86, 1985.

31. *Klopp A: Shunting malignant ascites, Am J Nurs 84:212-213, 1984.

31a. Korniewicz DM, Laughon BE, Butz A, and Larson E: Integrity of vinyl and latex procedure gloves, Nurs Res 38:144-146, 1989.

32. Longley DG, Skolnick ML, and Sheahan D: Acute allograft rejection in liver transplant recipients: lack of correlation with loss of hepatic artery diastolic flow, Radiology 169:417-420, 1988.

33. Ludwig J: Etiology of biliary cirrhosis: diagnostic features and a new classification, Zentralbl Allg Pathol 134:132-141, 1988.

34. Maddrey WC and Thiel DHV: Liver transplantation: an overview, Hepatology, 8:948-959, 1988.

35. Mattsson L, Weiland O, and Glaumann H: Long-term follow-up of chronic post-transfusion non-A, non-B hepatitis: clinical and histological outcome, Liver 8:184-188, 1988.

36. Maxwell AJ, and Mamtora H: Fungal liver abscesses in acute leukemia—a report of two cases, Clin Radiol 39:197-201, 1988.

37. *McCormack A, Itkin J, and Cloud C: The patient with liver failure, RN 47(10):32-33, 1984.

38. Metzger U: Intraportal chemotherapy for colorectal hepatic metastases, Antibiot Chemother 40:51-60, 1988.

39. Meller H: Liver transplantation: post operative ICU care, Crit Care Nurse 8(6):19-31, 1988.

40. *MMWR: Hepatitis A among drug abusers, MMWR 37:297-305, 1988.

41. *MMWR: Hepatitis B among parenteral drug abusers—North Carolina, MMWR 35:481-483, 1986.

42. MMWR: Changing patterns of groups at high risk for hepatitis B in the United States, MMWR 37:429-437, 1988.

43. MMWR: Update on hepatitis B prevention, MMWR 36:353-366, 1987.

43a. Mosley JW et al: Non-A, non-B hepatitis and antibody to hepatitis C virus, JAMA 263:77-78, 1990.

43b. Muhlenkamp AF and Sayles JA: Self-esteem, social support, and positive health practices, Nurs Res 35:334-338, 1986.

44. Munoz SJ and Maddrey W: Major complications of acute and chronic liver disease. Gastroenterol Clin North Am 17:267-287, 1988.

45. O'Mary SS: Liver cancer: primary and metastatic disease, Semin Oncol Nurs 4(4):265-273, 1988.

46. Patt Y: Hepatic arterial infusion of chemotherapy for metastatic colorectal cancer in the liver: why, how, and what, Antibiot Chemother 40:1-11, 1988.

47. Perillo RP et al: A randomized, controlled trial of interferon alfa-2b alone and after prenisone withdrawal for the treatment of chronic hepatitis B, New Engl J Med 323(5):295-301, 1990.

48. Pessayre D and Larrey D: Acute and chronic drug-induced hepatitis, Baillieres Clin Gastroenterol 2:385-422, 1988.

49. Schreeder M: Viral hepatitis, Prim Care 15:157-173, 1988.

49a. Semonin-Holleran R: Critical nursing care for abdominal trauma, Crit Care Nurse 8(3):48-58, 1988.

50. *Sheets L: Liver transplantation, Nurs Clin North Am, 24(4):881-889, 1989.

51. Sitzman J and Order SE: Immunoradiotherapy for primary nonresectable hepatocellular carcinoma, Surg Clin North Am 89:393-400, 1989.

52. Smith GS: Evaluation of patients with portal hypertension. In Rutherford RB, editor: Vascular surgery, Philadelphia, 1984, WB Saunders Co.

53. Solomon J, Harrington D, and Gogel HF: When the patient suffers from esophageal bleeding, RN 50(2):24-27, 1987.

54. Starzel TE and Iwatsuki S: Transplantation of the liver. In Schiff L and Schiff ER, editors: Diseases of the liver, ed 6, Philadelphia, 1987, JB Lippincott Co.

54a. Steven CE et al: Epidemiology of hepatitis C Virus, JAMA 263:49-53, 1990.

55. Stone MD and Benotti PN: Liver resection: preoperative and postoperative care, Surg Clin North Am 69:383-391, 1989.

56. Vitale G, Heusen LS, and Polk H: Malignant tumors of the liver, Surg Clin North Am 66:723-741, 1986.

57. Wall WS: Liver transplantation: current concepts. Can Med Assoc J 139(7):21-28, 1988.

58. Williams NN: Infusional versus systemic chemotherapy for liver metastases from colorectal cancer, Surg Clin North Am 69:401-410, 1989.

59. Wyngaarden JB and Smith LH, editors: Cecil textbook of medicine, ed 18, Philadelphia, 1988, WB Saunders Co.

60. Zimmerman HJ and Maddrey WC: Toxic and drug-induced hepatitis. In Schiff L and Schiff ER, editors: Diseases of the liver, ed 6, Philadelphia, 1987, JB Lippincott Co.

ALTERATIONS IN NUTRITION AND ELIMINATION

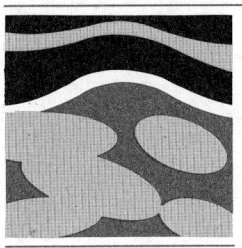

CHAPTER 40

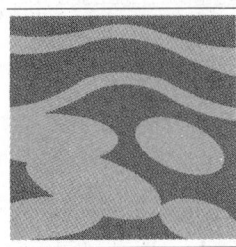

Assessment of Nutritional Status and Dietary Counseling

JANICE NEVILLE

CHAPTER OBJECTIVES

After studying this chapter, the student should be able to:
1 Identify nutritional requirements for health.
2 Describe data collection for assessment of nutritional status and signs of nutritional deficiency.
3 Explain use of the Daily Food Guide as an assessment tool.
4 Describe different types of diet modifications and principles of therapeutic diets.
5 Describe patient teaching in terms of food costs, food labeling, and food additives.

Nutritional needs and nutritional care are major concerns of the general public, government agencies, and health professionals. Malnutrition is a major problem in hospitalized patients. Nurses, physicians and dietitians have been challenged to identify the nutritional needs of patients and to improve the quality of care. The patient also has responsibilities, whether hospitalized or at home, but should be able to expect nutritional care as an integral component of health care.

Nutrition is a health issue. In 1976 the relative contributions to death and disease were assessed by the Surgeon General. At that time, as much as 50% of the U.S. mortality was attributed to unhealthy behavior or life styles, 20% to human biologic factors, and only 10% to inadequacies in health care. National goals for 1990 were identified. The data were used to develop a national strategy for health improvement. Nutrition objectives included specific goals for the improvement of health status, reduction of risk factors, and improvement of services.[32] The process of establishing national disease prevention and health promotion objectives for the year 2000 has been in progress since 1987. The working draft identifies five areas in which specific, measurable objectives are being developed. The areas are health status, risk reduction, public awareness, professional education and awareness, and services and

protection. For example, an objective in public awareness is "increase to at least 80% the proportion of people age 21 and older who use food labels to make food selections." An objective in professional education and awareness is "increase to at least 50% the proportion of primary care providers who provide nutrition counseling and/or referral to qualified nutritionists and/or dietitians."[42]

The emphasis in the national objectives is twofold—promoting health and preventing disease. Individuals with good nutritional status are less likely to get sick, and they are generally less seriously ill if sickness does occur. They are better able to withstand trauma and stress. Recovery is significantly affected, and it can be enhanced by appropriate nutrition therapy.

Many persons enter the hospital in poor nutritional status, and nutritional status may deteriorate during hospitalization.[7,9,15] Studies of general populations in the United States have identified very few cases of frank deficiency disease, but a significant proportion of the population is either malnourished or at significant risk of developing nutritional problems. Obesity is a major health problem in the United States and is present in the population at all age levels. Adolescents have the highest prevalence of unsatisfactory nutritional status, and many persons over 60 years of age present evidence of poor status. People are adopting new eating styles that have been identified as a critical public health concern.

Maintenance of good nutrition is a major nursing objective. Nutritional evaluation is an important part of total patient assessment and provides essential information for differential diagnosis and for planning appropriate interventions. An awareness of nutritional deficits, excesses, or imbalances that may exist can be of particular importance in determining management of the person. Monitoring the nutritional well-being of the person throughout hospitalization or on an ongoing basis to assure maintenance of or improvement in status is as important as the initial assessment.

NUTRITION: A NATIONAL HEALTH PRIORITY

In 1988 the first *Surgeon General's Report on Nutrition and Health* was published.[37] The report is considered as significant an event in the history of public health as the 1964 *Surgeon General's Report on Smoking and Health.* The report is meant for use by policymakers, and it has already had a significant impact on the formulation of nutrition objectives for the year 2000 because it reviews the research on the role of diet in disease prevention and health promotion. Changes in food behavior are clearly identified as a national priority: "For the two out of three adult Americans who do not smoke and do not drink excessively, one personal choice seems to influence long-term health prospects more than any other; what we eat."[37]

A major health challenge to the adult population is the presence of chronic disease. Recent statistics reveal the first three causes of death to be diseases of the heart (35.8%), malignant neoplasms (22.5%), and cerebrovascular diseases (7.1%). These account for 65.4% of total deaths. Diabetes mellitus (seventh in rank), chronic liver disease and cirrhosis (ninth), and atherosclerosis

(tenth) account for 1.8%, 1.2%, and 1.1% of all deaths respectively. Another 3.7% of deaths are caused by chronic obstructive pulmonary disease.[23] The 1964 and 1988 reports from the Surgeon General indicate that basic changes in diet and smoking behavior would significantly change these figures. Findings reinforced the importance of the dietary guidelines issued in 1985. Recommendations are presented in Table 40-1; they are qualitative and specify certain changes in food choice.

Risk factors of excessive body weight, elevated blood pressure, elevated blood lipids, and/or glucose are associated with eating styles that reflect the relative availability of food in this culture. Excessive intakes of calories, sodium, fats, and alcohol have all been documented as increasing the risk of chronic disease. In addition, there is concern that the public has substituted sweets and added sugars for the vegetables, fruits, and grains containing the complex carbohydrates, starch, and fiber.

In an effort to encourage the American adult to prevent or slow down the development of chronic disease, dietary guidelines have been established.[40] The center sheet for the second edition of the Dietary Guidelines for Americans is shown in Figure 40-1. The guidelines are quite general, providing the concepts and rationale for change without portion sizes or menus, which are

TABLE 40-1 Dietary recommendations from the Surgeon General[37]

Category	Recommendations
ISSUES FOR MOST PEOPLE	
Fats and cholesterol	Reduce consumption of fats (especially saturated fats).
	Choose foods relatively low in fats and cholesterol, such as vegetables, fruits, whole grain foods, fish, poultry, lean meats, and low-fat dairy products.
	Use food preparation methods that add little or no fat.
Energy and weight control	Achieve and maintain a desirable body weight.
	Choose a dietary pattern in which energy (caloric) intake is consistent with energy expenditure.
	Limit consumption of foods high in calories, fats, and sugars, and minimize alcohol consumption.
	Increase energy expenditure through regular, sustained physical activity.
Complex carbohydrate and fiber	Increase consumption of whole grain foods and cereal products, vegetables (including dried beans and peas), and fruits.
Sodium	Choose foods low in sodium, and limit the amount of salt added in food preparation and at the table.
Alcohol	To reduce risk for chronic disease, take alcohol only in moderation (no more than two drinks a day) if at all.
	Avoid drinking any alcohol before or while driving, operating machinery, taking medication, or engaging in any other activity requiring judgment.
OTHER ISSUES FOR SOME PEOPLE	
Fluoride	Community water systems should contain fluoride at optimal levels for prevention of tooth decay.
	If such water is not available, use other appropriate sources of fluoride.
Sugars	Those who are particularly vulnerable to dental caries, especially children, should limit their consumption of foods high in sugars.
Calcium	Adolescent girls and adult women should increase consumption of foods high in calcium, including low-fat dairy products.
Iron	Children, adolescents, and women of childbearing age should consume foods that are good sources of iron, such as lean red meats, fish, certain beans, and iron-enriched cereals and whole grain products. This issue is of special concern for low-income families.

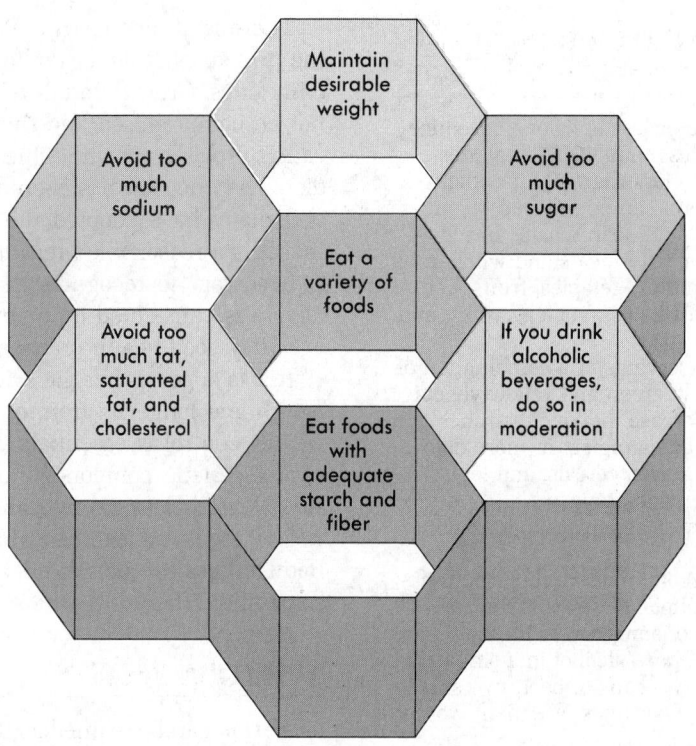

FIGURE 40-1 Dietary guidelines for the American public. (From US Department of Agriculture and the US Department of Health and Human Services, Washington DC, 1985.)

available from other sources. They are meant to reduce the risk of nutritional deficiencies and chronic disease in healthy Americans. The guidelines are similar to many of the dietary modifications prescribed for patients with heart disease or diabetes mellitus. The difference is one of degree.

The American Cancer Society released a leaflet for the public recommending "ten steps to a healthier life and reduced cancer risk".[2] The factors are divided into protective and risk groups.

Protective factors
1. Eat more cabbage-family vegetables (broccoli, cauliflower, brussel sprouts, cabbage, kale— sometimes called "cruciferous" vegetables).
2. Add more high-fiber foods.
3. Choose foods with vitamin A.
4. Do the same for vitamin C.
5. Add weight control.

Risk factors
6. Trim fat from your diet.
7. Subtract salt-cured, smoked, nitrite-cured foods.
8. Stop cigarette smoking.
9. Drink alcohol moderately.
10. Respect the sun's rays.

The recommendations are based on an array of animal research and epidemiologic findings that suggest that

the nutritionally adequate diet long recommended for the public has long-term benefits in disease prevention and health promotion.[12]

In 1989 the National Research Council published the report of the Committee on Diet and Health that reviewed all of the evidence on dietary risk factors and chronic disease.[26] The report assesses risks and benefits and makes quantitative recommendations (see the box on p. 1204). In 1985 a consensus panel from the National Institutes of Health recommended that the public (except for children under the age of 2 years) be advised to adopt a diet that reduces total dietary fat intake to 30% of total calories, reduces saturated fat intake to less than 10% of total calories, and reduces cholesterol intake to 300 mg or less.[24] In 1988, an expert panel recommended Step 1 and Step 2 diets for adults with high blood cholesterol. The Step 1 diet (30% of calories or less from total fat, not more than 10% from saturated fat, and up to 10% from polyunsaturated fat; less than 300 mg of dietary cholesterol) was identified as a treatment regimen and was confirmed as appropriate for the general population.[14] It was suggested that further reductions in total fat and cholesterol intake might be beneficial. Because heart disease is the leading cause of death for women, as well as men, all adults are being urged to consume a more healthful diet.[34]

DIETARY RECOMMENDATIONS FROM THE NATIONAL RESEARCH COUNCIL

Reduce total fat intake to 30% or less of calories. Reduce saturated fatty acid intake to less than 10% of calories, and the intake of cholesterol to less than 300 mg. daily. The intake of fat and cholesterol can be reduced by substituting fish, poultry without skin, lean meats, and low-fat or nonfat dairy products for fatty meats and whole-milk dairy products; by choosing more vegetables, fruits, cereals, and legumes; and by limiting oils, fats, egg yolks, and fried and other fatty foods.

Every day eat five or more servings of a combination of vegetables and fruits, especially green and yellow vegetables and citrus fruits. Also, increase intake of starches and other complex carbohydrates by eating six or more daily servings of a combination of breads, cereals, and legumes.

Maintain protein intake at moderate levels.

Balance food intake and physical activity to maintain appropriate body weight.

The committee does not recommend alcohol consumption. For those who drink alcoholic beverages, the committee recommends limiting consumption to the equivalent of less than 1 oz of pure alcohol in a single day. This is the equivalent of two cans of beer, two small glasses of wine, or two average cocktails. Pregnant women should avoid alcoholic beverages.

Limit total daily intake of salt (sodium chloride) to 6 g or less. Limit the use of salt in cooking and avoid adding it to food at the table. Salty, highly processed salty, salt-preserved, and salt-pickled foods should be consumed sparingly.

Maintain adequate calcium intake.

Avoid taking dietary supplements in excess of the RDA in any one day.

Maintain an optimal intake of fluoride, particularly during the years of primary and secondary tooth formation and growth.

From National Research Council: Diet and health: implications of reducing chronic disease risk, report of the Committee on Diet and Health, Food and Nutrition Board, National Academy Press, Washington, DC, 1989.

The National Research Council recommendations are consistent with dietary guidelines published from 1985 to date.[14,29,37] Per capita use of food in this country has changed over the years. Recent data on food intake by adults shows 37% of calories from dietary fat.[27] The diet with no more than 30% of calories from fat is best described as a moderate-fat diet, although it is popularly called a low-fat diet. Public education projects in print and video will encourage people to reduce intake of dietary fat, cholesterol, and sodium.

There is some argument about providing guidelines such as these to the public. Some believe that the evidence clearly identifies a high-risk situation and that a public education drive is justified. Others believe that the education should be given only by a physician to persons diagnosed as ill or at risk.

There is also concern that too rigid an application of the principles at either end of the life span could cause difficulties. Growth and development of children should not be compromised and the elderly may have complicating problems or difficulties in obtaining an adequate diet. The question has been debated in the public press and many have adopted the pattern with the thought that it is a reasonable precaution. Whatever the view, it is necessary to recognize that control of these dietary factors is considered by many people to be a matter of everyday good health practice.

It also appears that the evidence of adverse effects on health and longevity from obesity is overwhelming and weight control is essential.[25] Recent evidence shows a strong genetic component to the development of obesity. Nevertheless, there is an element of individual control of food and exercise that should be encouraged. Body fatness can be altered, although it may be easy for some and difficult for others.

NUTRITION PROCESS

Nutrition can be defined as the sum of the processes by which a living organism ingests, digests, absorbs, transports, uses, and excretes nutrients and their metabolites. With adequate supplies of the proper nutrients, the organism can grow, function, and reproduce. When supplies are limited, growth, function, or reproduction may be impaired. Since the body exists in a state of dynamic equilibrium, tissue building and breakdown are continuous. Muscles, organs, bones, fat, and the blood participate in the constant exchange of materials, with some tissues more active than others. There is some loss; therefore replacement from food is necessary throughout life. Periods of growth increase requirements for nutrients and energy.

Homeostatic mechanisms tend to protect the body against minor or temporary changes in nutrient status as nutrient reserves are mobilized to meet needs. With nutrient *deficits*, adaptations occur to conserve body resources. For example, when energy supplies are limited, physical activity and then basal metabolism are reduced. Over time, gradual tissue loss of the nutrients occurs. Reductions in enzyme activity and alterations in metabolite levels develop. If this process is permitted to continue long enough, lesions such as those listed in Table 40-2 become evident. The classical deficiency diseases such as scurvy, beriberi, and pellagra are results of depletions of vitamin C, thiamin, B-complex vitamins, and niacin that are continued long enough for identifiable lesions in skin, tongue, and organs to develop as clinical signs of malnutrition. If untreated, progressive depletion results in death.

Nutrition *excesses* can also produce malnutrition.[1,13,28] Mechanisms tend to protect the body by ac-

TABLE 40-2 Physical signs indicative or suggestive of malnutrition

Body Area	Normal Appearance	Signs Associated with Malnutrition
Hair	Shiny, firm, not easily plucked	Lack of natural shine; hair dull and dry, thin and sparse; hair fine, silky, and straight; color changes (flag sign); can be easily plucked
Face	Skin color uniform; smooth, pink, healthy appearance; not swollen	Skin color loss (depigmentation); skin dark over cheeks and under eyes (malar and supraorbital pigmentation); lumpiness or flakiness of skin of nose and mouth; swollen face; enlarged parotid glands; scaling of skin around nostrils (nasolabial seborrhea)
Eyes	Bright, clear, shiny; no sores at corners of eyelids; membranes a healthy pink and moist. No prominent blood vessels or mound of tissue or sclera	Eye membranes are pale (pale conjunctivae); redness of membranes (conjunctival injection); Bitot's spots; redness and fissuring of eyelid corners (angular palpebritis); dryness of eye membranes (conjunctival xerosis); cornea has dull appearance (corneal xerosis); cornea soft (keratomalacia); scar on cornea; ring of the blood vessels around cornea (circumcorneal injection)
Lips	Smooth, not chapped or swollen	Redness and swelling of mouth or lips (cheilosis), especially at corners of mouth (angular fissures and scars)
Tongue	Deep red in appearance; not swollen or smooth	Swelling; scarlet and raw tongue; magenta (purplish color) tongue; smooth tongue; swollen, sore; hyperemic and hypertrophic papillae; atrophic papillae
Teeth	No cavities; no pain; bright	May be missing or erupting abnormally; gray or black spots (fluorosis); cavities (caries)
Gums	Healthy; red; do not bleed; not swollen	"Spongy" and bleed easily; recession of gums
Glands	Face not swollen	Thyroid enlargement (front of neck); parotid enlargement (cheeks become swollen)
Skin	No signs of rashes, swellings, dark or light spots	Dryness of skin (xerosis); sandpaper feel of skin (follicular hyperkeratosis); flakiness of skin; skin swollen and dark; red, swollen pigmentation of exposed areas (pellagrous dermatosis); excessive lightness or darkness of skin (dyspigmentation); black and blue marks from skin bleeding (petechiae); lack of fat under skin
Nails	Firm, pink	Nails are spoon shaped (koilonychia); brittle, ridged nails
Muscular and skeletal systems	Good muscle tone; some fat under skin; can walk or run without pain	Muscles have "wasted" appearance; baby's skull bones are thin and soft (craniotabes); round swelling of front and side of head (frontal and parietal bossing); swelling of ends of bones (epiphyseal enlargement); small bumps on both sides of chest wall (on ribs), beading of ribs; baby's soft spot on head does not harden at proper time (persistently open anterior fontanelle); knock-knees or bowlegs; bleeding into muscle (musculoskeletal hemorrhages); person cannot get up or walk properly
Internal systems		
Cardiovascular	Normal heart rate and rhythm; no murmurs or abnormal rhythms; normal blood pressure for age	Rapid heart rate (above 100, tachycardia); enlarged heart; abnormal rhythm; elevated blood pressure
Gastrointestinal	No palpable organs or masses (in children, however, liver edge may be palpable)	Liver enlargement; enlargement of spleen (usually indicates other associated diseases)
Nervous	Psychologic stability; normal reflexes	Mental irritability and confusion; burning and tingling of hands and feet (paresthesia); loss of position and vibratory sense; weakness and tenderness of muscles (may result in inability to walk); decrease and loss of ankle and knee reflexes

From Christakis G: Am J Public Health 63(suppl.): 1-82, 1973.

TABLE 40-3 Recommended dietary allowances,[a] revised 1989
Designed for the maintenance of good nutrition of practically all healthy people in the United States

		Weight[b]		Height[b]		Protein	Fat-Soluble Vitamins			
Category	Age (yrs) or Condition	(kg)	(lb)	(cm)	(in)	(g)	Vita-min A (μg RE)[c]	Vita-min D (μg)[d]	Vita-min E (mg α-TE)[e]	Vita-min K (μg)
Infants	0.0-0.5	6	13	60	24	13	375	7.5	3	5
	0.5-1.0	9	20	71	28	14	375	10	4	10
Children	1-3	13	29	90	35	16	400	10	6	15
	4-6	20	44	112	44	24	500	10	7	20
	7-10	28	62	132	52	28	700	10	7	30
Males	11-14	45	99	157	62	45	1000	10	10	45
	15-18	66	145	176	69	59	1000	10	10	65
	19-24	72	160	177	70	58	1000	10	10	70
	25-50	79	174	176	70	63	1000	5	10	80
	51+	77	170	173	68	63	1000	5	10	80
Females	11-14	46	101	157	62	46	800	10	8	45
	15-18	55	120	163	64	44	800	10	8	55
	19-24	58	128	164	65	46	800	10	8	60
	25-50	63	138	163	64	50	800	5	8	65
	51+	65	143	160	63	50	800	5	8	65
Pregnant						60	800	10	10	65
Lactating	1st 6 months					65	1300	10	12	65
	2nd 6 months					62	1200	10	11	65

From Food and Nutrition Board, National Academy of Sciences—National Research Council, 1989.
[a]The allowances, expressed as average daily intakes over time, are intended to provide for individual variations among most normal persons as they live in the United States under usual environmental stresses. Diets should be based on a variety of common foods in order to provide other nutrients for which human requirements have been less well defined.
[b]Weights and heights of Reference Adults are actual medians for the U.S. population of the designated age, as reported by NHANES II. The median weights and heights of those under 19 years of age were taken from Hamill et al. (1979) (see pages 16-17). The use of these figures does not imply that the height-to-weight ratios are ideal.
[c]Retinol equivalents. 1 retinol equivalent = 1 μg retinol or 6 μg β-carotene.
[d]As cholecalciferol. 10 μg cholecalciferol = 400 IU of vitamin D.
[e]α-Tocopherol equivalents. 1 mg d-α tocopherol = 1 α-TE.

cumulating reserves or, for some nutrients, by increasing the rate of excretion from the body or decreasing efficiency of absorption. When excesses are large or prolonged over time, increased concentrations of nutrients and alterations in enzyme activities and levels of metabolites develop. Over time, clinical signs and symptoms develop. The most common example of this type of malnutrition in the U.S. population is obesity. Consumption of energy-yielding compounds (for example, protein, fat, carbohydrate, and alcohol) in amounts greater than needed for energy expenditure results in storage of energy as body fat. Eventually, the stores of body fat become large enough to affect body functioning, physical mobility, and health.[25,42]

NUTRITION REQUIREMENTS

Good nutritional status exists when protein, fat, carbohydrate, minerals, vitamins, and water are consumed in sufficient amounts and are used appropriately by the body to meet needs regardless of age, sex, life-style, or state of health. All persons need the same basic nutrients throughout life. The amounts required vary in predictable patterns. Growth, basal metabolic needs, and

physical activity are the major factors responsible for changing nutrient needs. Disease, trauma, variations in metabolism (normal and abnormal), medications, and treatments can also affect needs.[30]

Since 1940, the Food and Nutrition Board of the National Academy of Sciences has periodically reviewed existing nutrition knowledge and research to formulate recommendations for the amounts of the different nutrients to be used as a basis for planning nutritionally adequate diets. Table 40-3 illustrates the changes in amounts of nutrients recommended from infancy throughout life. The level of iron intake recommended for women during the reproductive years is high because many young women do not include iron-rich foods in their diets and their iron stores are poor.

Nutrient recommendations now include information about safe and adequate levels for two vitamins, five trace elements, and three electrolytes (see Tables 40-4 and 40-5). Note that since the toxic levels for many trace elements may be only a few times usual intakes, the upper levels for the trace elements should not be habitually exceeded. Safe intake levels vary considerably. For example, rather small but constant consumption of energy (kilocalories [kcal]) will produce excess fat. Pro-

Water-Soluble Vitamins							Minerals						
Vita-min C (mg)	Thia-min (mg)	Ribo-flavin (mg)	Niacin (mg NE)^f	Vita-min B$_6$ (mg)	Fo-late (μg)	Vitamin B$_{12}$ (μg)	Cal-cium (mg)	Phos-phorus (mg)	Mag-nesium (mg)	Iron (mg)	Zinc (mg)	Iodine (μg)	Sele-nium (μg)
30	0.3	0.4	5	0.3	25	0.3	400	300	40	6	5	40	10
35	0.4	0.5	6	0.6	35	0.5	600	500	60	10	5	50	15
40	0.7	0.8	9	1.0	50	0.7	800	800	80	10	10	70	20
45	0.9	1.1	12	1.1	75	1.0	800	800	120	10	10	90	20
45	1.0	1.2	13	1.4	100	1.4	800	800	170	10	10	120	30
50	1.3	1.5	17	1.7	150	2.0	1200	1200	270	12	15	150	40
60	1.5	1.8	20	2.0	200	2.0	1200	1200	400	12	15	150	50
60	1.5	1.7	19	2.0	200	2.0	1200	1200	350	10	15	150	70
60	1.5	1.7	19	2.0	200	2.0	800	800	350	10	15	150	70
60	1.2	1.4	15	2.0	200	2.0	800	800	350	10	15	150	70
50	1.1	1.3	15	1.4	150	2.0	1200	1200	280	15	12	150	45
60	1.1	1.3	15	1.5	180	2.0	1200	1200	300	15	12	150	50
60	1.1	1.3	15	1.6	180	2.0	1200	1200	280	15	12	150	55
60	1.1	1.3	15	1.6	180	2.0	800	800	280	15	12	150	55
60	1.0	1.2	13	1.6	180	2.0	800	800	280	10	12	150	55
70	1.5	1.6	17	2.2	400	2.2	1200	1200	320	30	15	175	65
95	1.6	1.8	20	2.1	280	2.6	1200	1200	355	15	19	200	75
90	1.6	1.7	20	2.1	260	2.6	1200	1200	340	15	16	200	75

^{f}1 NE (niacin equivalent) is equal to 1 mg of niacin or 60 mg of dietary tryptophan.

TABLE 40-4 Estimated safe and adequate daily dietary intakes of selected vitamins and minerals*

Category	Age (yr)	Vitamins		Trace Elements†				
		Biotin (μg)	Pantothenic Acid (mg)	Copper (mg)	Man-ganese (mg)	Fluoride (mg)	Chromium (μg)	Molybdenum (μg)
Infants	0-0.5	10	2	0.4-0.6	0.3-0.6	0.1-0.5	10-40	15-30
	0.5-1	15	3	0.6-0.7	0.6-1.0	0.2-1.0	20-60	20-40
Children and adolescents	1-3	20	3	0.7-1.0	1.0-1.5	0.5-1.5	20-80	25-50
	4-6	25	3-4	1.0-1.5	1.5-2.0	1.0-2.5	30-120	30-75
	7-10	30	4-5	1.0-2.0	2.0-3.0	1.5-2.5	50-200	50-150
	11+	30-100	4-7	1.5-2.5	2.0-5.0	1.5-2.5	50-200	75-250
Adults		30-100	4-7	1.5-3.0	2.0-5.0	1.5-4.0	50-200	75-250

From Food and Nutrition Board, National Academy of Sciences—National Research Council, 1989.
*Because there is less information on which to base allowances, these figures are not given in the main table of RDA and are provided here in the form of ranges of recommended intakes.
†Since the toxic levels for many trace elements may be only several times usual intakes, the upper levels for the trace elements given in this table should not be habitually exceeded.

TABLE 40-5 Estimated sodium, chloride, and potassium minimum requirements of healthy persons*

Age	Weight (kg)*	Sodium (mg)*†	Chloride (mg)*†	Potassium (mg)‡
Months				
0-5	4.5	120	180	500
6-11	8.9	200	300	700
Years				
1	11.0	225	350	1000
2-5	16.0	300	500	1400
6-9	25.0	400	600	1600
10-18	50.0	500	750	2000
>18§	70.0	500	750	2000

From Food and Nutrition Board, National Academy of Sciences—National Research Council, 1989.
*No allowance has been included for large, prolonged losses from the skin through sweat.
†There is no evidence that higher intakes confer any health benefit.
‡Desirable intakes of potassium may considerably exceed these values (~3,500 mg for adults—see text).
§No allowance included for growth. Values for those below 18 years assume a growth rate at the 50th percentile reported by the National Center for Health Statistics (Hamill et al., 1979) and averaged for males and females.

tein and sodium are nutrients with intermediate ranges. Intakes of protein and sodium two or three times recommendations produce chronic, subtle, adverse effects. The range is relatively wide for most vitamins and some trace elements in which intakes ten times or more produce undesirable effects.

All nutrients are of equal importance, although they are not required in equal amounts (Figure 40-2). The nutrients providing energy (protein, fats, carbohydrates) and water are required in much larger quantities than vitamins that regulate body processes. The differences in the quantities of various nutrients required by an individual are much greater than the change in amounts of any one nutrient over the life cycle. If a person consumed vitamin A in the quantities recommended for calcium or phosphorus, toxicity would result. When food is used as the source for nutrients, such imbalances are unlikely to occur; however, nutrients are available in concentrated forms as dietary supplements, over-the-counter preparations, and prescription drugs. Should these concentrated nutrients be prescribed for the person, the nurse handles them with the same care as any other medication. There is an unsupported intuitive feeling that nutrient supplements are essential. Response to these supplements occurs only when persons have been relatively nutrition deficient, eating foods

TABLE 40-6 Median heights and weights and recommended energy intake

		Weight		Height			Average Energy Allowance (kcal)*		
Category	Age (yrs) or Condition	(kg)	(lb)	(cm)	(in)	REE† (kcal/day)	Multiples of REE	Per kg	Per Day‡
Infants	0.0-0.5	6	13	60	24	320		108	650
	0.5-1.0	9	20	71	28	500		98	850
Children	1-3	13	29	90	35	740		102	1300
	4-6	20	44	112	44	950		90	1800
	7-10	28	62	132	52	1130		70	2000
Males	11-14	45	99	157	62	1440	1.70	55	2500
	15-18	66	145	176	69	1760	1.67	45	3000
	19-24	72	160	177	70	1780	1.67	40	2900
	25-50	79	174	176	70	1800	1.60	37	2900
	51+	77	170	173	68	1530	1.50	30	2300
Females	11-14	46	101	157	62	1310	1.67	47	2200
	15-18	55	120	163	64	1370	1.60	40	2200
	19-24	58	128	164	65	1350	1.60	38	2200
	25-50	63	138	163	64	1380	1.55	36	2200
	51+	65	143	160	63	1280	1.50	30	1900
Pregnant	1st trimester								+0
	2nd trimester								+300
	3rd trimester								+300
Lactating	1st 6 months								+500
	2nd 6 months								+500

From Food and Nutrition Board, National Academy of Sciences—National Research Council, 1989.
*In the range of light to moderate activity, the coefficient of variation is ±20%.
†Resting energy expenditure.
‡Figure is rounded.

marginal in nutrient value, and when the supplement provides the specific nutrient or nutrients that are deficient. There is a point beyond which supplementation does not help the person and *may actually cause harm*. Continued intake of vitamins and minerals at levels from 10 to 100 times the recommended daily allowance

(RDA) is associated with chronic toxicity. As a guide, recommended levels of energy intake for the public are published (Table 40-6). There can be great differences in the amount of energy needed to maintain appropriate body weight depending on mass and physical activity.

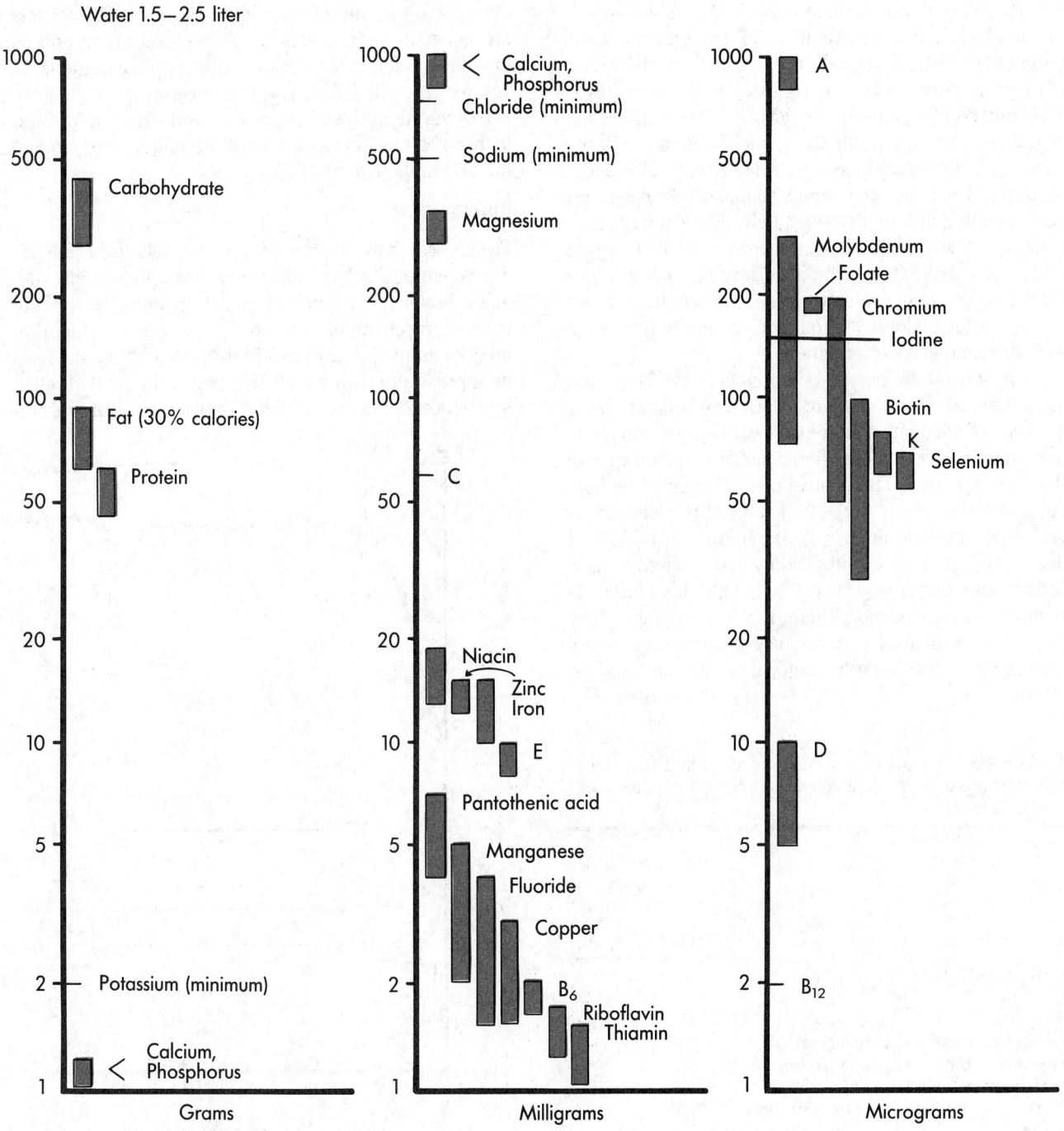

FIGURE 40-2 Recommended dietary allowances. From the National Research Council—National Academy of Sciences, 1989. Carbohydrate and fat vary with energy needs and are calculated from the average kilocalories for men and women.

ENERGY NEEDS

Energy needs can be predicted from patterns of growth and body size and from physical activity. There is a constant need for energy to maintain circulation, respiration, muscle tone, and body temperature. People of similar size have similar basal energy requirements, since the requirement is related to the amount of muscle tissue and can be predicted from body weight (excluding excess body fat, since adipose tissue is relatively inert). The total energy requirement may vary widely depending on physical activity (Table 40-7). Recommendations for caloric intake are based on the growth, activity, and life style of most Americans (Figure 40-3). Since this is a sedentary life pattern, the levels recommended are moderate, particularly for the adult. To emphasize the differences in energy needs associated with differences in physical activity, the range of kilocalorie needs for persons doing different types of light physical work is illustrated. The range of energy needs is wide. The best method for determining the adequacy of energy intake for the person is to evaluate weight for height (and rate of growth for children) in relation to energy intake assessed from dietary information.

A person's daily energy requirements are large and are measured in thousands of calories. In addition to the question of adequate but not excessive energy supply to meet patient needs is the question of the importance of the energy source. The relative contributions of protein, fat, and carbohydrate to the fuel value of the diet can be varied within wide limits without harm. Up to 80% of dietary calories may be supplied by carbohydrate in persons whose major food staple is grain. This pattern is seen in some persons, although it is not typical. The usual American food pattern includes generous use of animal foods (particularly beef), fats, oils, and sugars.

TABLE 40-7 Comparison of calories used in 1 hour for different types of physical activity (exclusive of basal energy needs)

| Activity | Calories Expended per Hour | |
	Woman (121 lb)	Man (143 lb)
Lying quietly	6	7
Sitting	22	26
Standing	28	32
Ironing, dishwashing, driving car	55	65
Working in office, painting furniture	82	98
Walking, waltzing, bicycling	138	162
More active walking, skating, doing fox-trot	220	260
Running, climbing stairs, sawing wood	358	422
High-speed walking, swimming	468	552

As much as 25% of total calories may come from protein in self-selected diets. Levels above this are rare, since the diet becomes unpalatable and expensive. Provision of 10% of required calories as protein from a variety of foods (animal and plant) is generally sufficient to meet needs for protein of good quality, that is, containing the essential amino acids and sufficient nitrogen for body needs. Some fat in the diet is needed to provide the essential fatty acids and to ensure adequate supplies and efficient absorption of fat-soluble vitamins. Dietary fats are concentrated sources of energy and are useful in providing calories for persons unable to consume large volumes of food. There is a basic requirement for some carbohydrate in the diet as starch and sugar (to prevent ketosis) and as fiber. Most foods are mixtures of protein, fat, and carbohydrate (Figure 40-4).

PROTEIN

Protein is widely distributed in foods. When these foods are consumed in quantities sufficient to provide adequate protein, the fats and carbohydrates are also provided to meet minimum needs. As a general rule, proteins of animal origin provide the essential amino acids in appropriate quantities. Plant proteins may be limited in one or more of the essential amino acids, but few per-

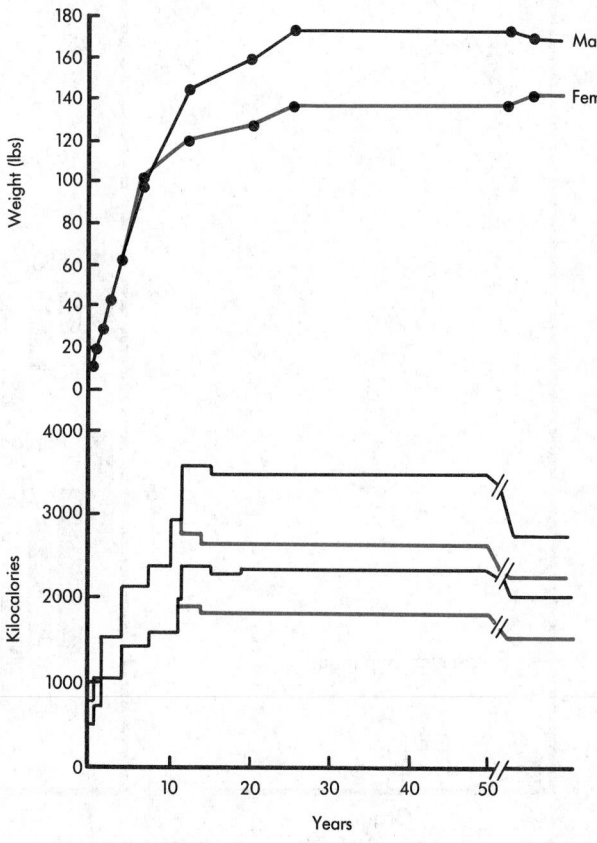

FIGURE 40-3 Recommended daily dietary allowances for kilocalories over the life cycle. The range is ± 20% of the average in Table 40-6.

sons limit their intake to only one protein source even if they eliminate meat. The quality of dietary protein is a function of the amino acid supply provided by the combination of foods eaten at one feeding. A mixture of plant-animal protein or of plant-plant protein can provide the full range of essential amino acids. The protein status of the patient is more often at risk because total food intake is limited in quantity than because of poor quality of protein. An exception to this is the patient being maintained too long on a clear-liquid diet or intravenous saline or dextrose as the sole source of nourishment.

For both men and women the RDA of protein is 0.75 g/kg of body weight. The average man needs more protein per day than the average woman because of his larger body size. The pregnant woman should be supplied with extra protein for fetal growth. The recommendations exceed actual protein requirements for most persons. The protein not needed for synthesis is used as energy or converted to body fat. If energy intake is not sufficient to meet needs, protein may be used for fuel rather than for synthesis of new tissue. Scrimshaw has said:

There is no doubt that good nutrition requires a balanced complement of protein and calories, and neither can be neglected in the diets of the underprivileged and the vulnerable. To the extent that the pendulum swung too far in emphasizing protein in the 1960s, and too far in emphasizing calories in the 1970s, it must come to a more appropriate intermediate position for the 1990s and beyond.[36]

This is true when considering nutritional needs of individuals as well as needs of populations. Severe limitations in protein supply (50% or less RDA) can stunt growth and reduce body protein content. Adequate protein supplies in a diet of insufficient fuel value help set the stage for protein-calorie malnutrition (Chapter 52). Generous supplies of protein will not result in increased body protein or muscle mass without exercise or physical activity. Body protein (and body calcium) may be lost despite adequate dietary intake in the absence of physical activity. Early patient ambulation, bed exercises, and physical therapy may contribute to improved nutritional status.

VITAMINS AND MINERALS

One might judge any food that provides one tenth of the day's recommended vitamin intake as being an important source. Note in Figure 40-5 that for the range of vitamins provided by each food, none provides 10% or more of each of the 13 vitamins. Milk comes closest in that all vitamins are provided. Of plant foods, vegetable leaves and stems are consistent in providing important quantities of many, but not all, vitamins. Milk also provides high-quality protein, significant calcium, and other minerals and is readily available at reasonable cost. For these reasons it is a basic food in most hospital diets and is recommended in most nutrition education materials. The green leafy vegetables are superior sources of vitamins A and C and of iron as well as other minerals, thus complementing milk and improving the nutritional quality of the diet.

Vitamins are not equally distributed in foods. Note in the column for vitamin C in Figure 40-5 that foods appear to be either rich sources of the vitamin or severely limited. This is also true for vitamins A, B_{12}, and D. Certain fruits or vegetables must be selected to assure adequate intake of vitamins C and A. Animal products contribute vitamins B_{12} and D, although some ready-to-eat breakfast cereals and some soy-milk products may be fortified with these vitamins. Sunshine provides addi-

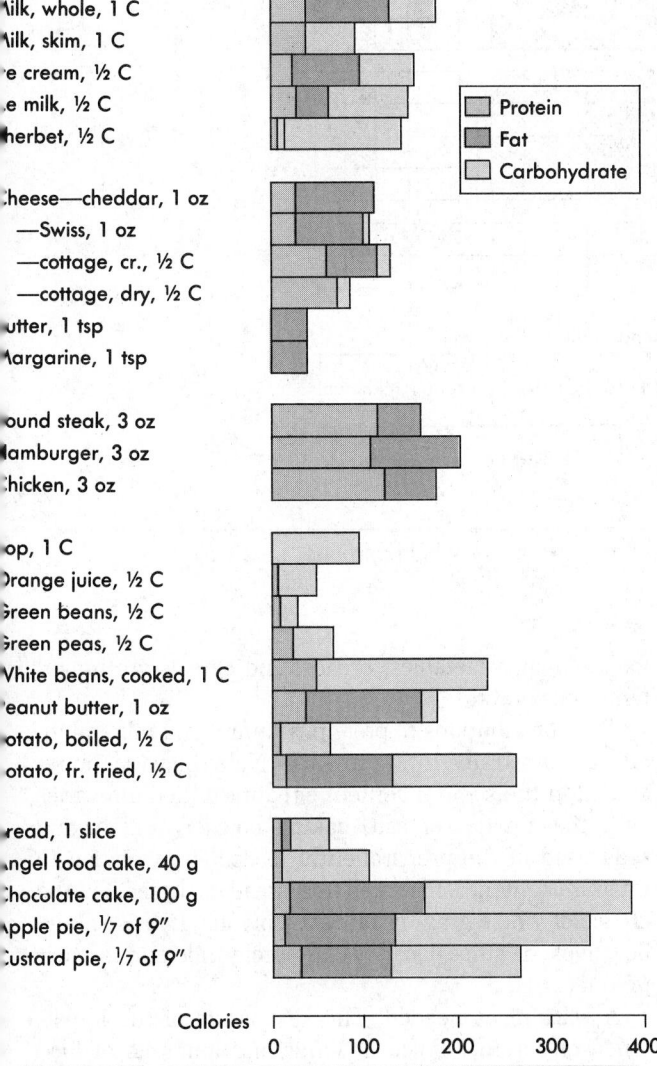

FIGURE 40-4 Protein, fat, and carbohydrate concentrations in some common foods, presented as calories contributed by each and total calories in ordinary portions.

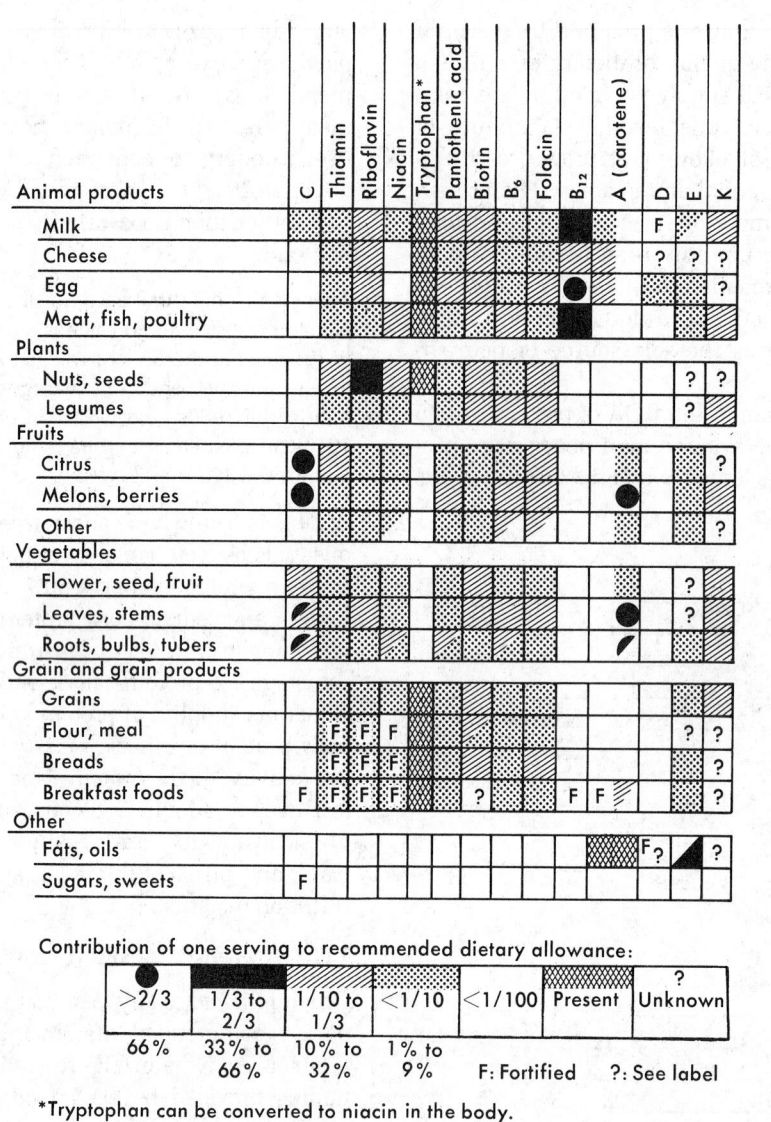

FIGURE 40-5 Foods as sources of vitamins. Serving size is household portion.

tional vitamin D, and our symbiotic relationship with intestinal flora appears to provide biotin and vitamin K. Deficiencies in these nutrients are rare, as are deficiencies in vitamin E. In contrast to vitamin C, thiamin is found in most foods, but no one food is superior in content. When persons substitute sugars and sweets (including honey) or alcohol for other foods, they obtain concentrated sources of energy that yield small levels of vitamins or minerals.

A similar illustration could be presented for many of the minerals, but complete analyses of food for all the mineral elements are not yet available. Table 40-8 illustrates the contributions of calcium and iron of various foods in relation to their energy value. The contributions of calcium from milk and green leafy vegetables are obvious. Calcium and iron are not evenly distributed in

foods. Meat, vegetables, breads, and cereals are important contributors.

The contributions to protein, vitamin, and mineral intake are illustrated in Figure 40-6. Note the variation recorded in the sodium content of oatmeal. Sodium varies with the amount of salt, baking powder, and baking soda used in the preparation of foods. The variation in thiamin content illustrated for bread is based on the choice of whole grain or enriched breads. Labels should be checked, since local bakeries may not enrich their products.

A warning is needed. This discussion of the importance of careful choice in kinds and amounts of food might tempt one to conclude that it is simpler to rely on vitamin and mineral supplements. These drugs, when subjected to the same rigorous examination for the

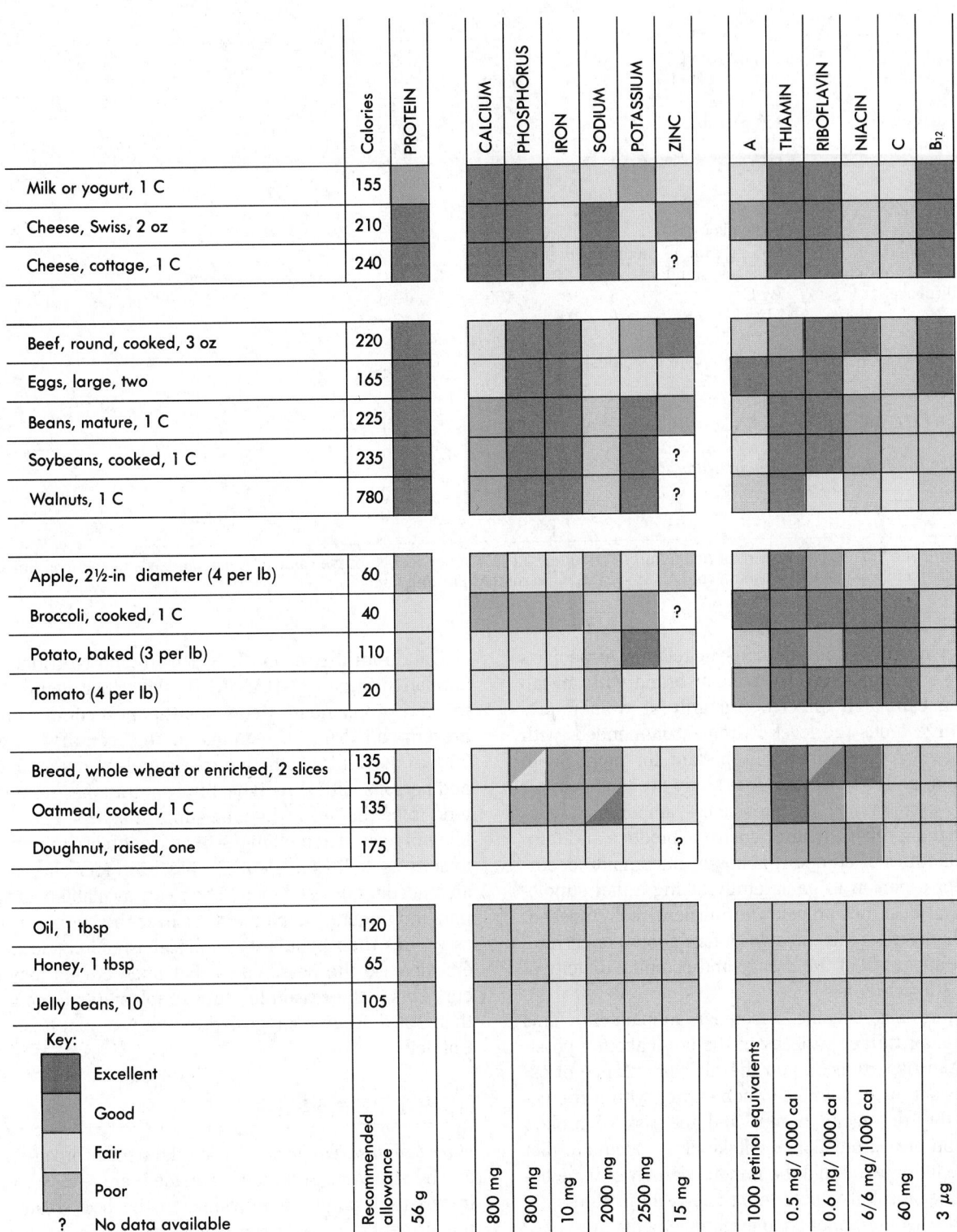

FIGURE 40-6 Foods as sources of nutrients. Serving size is household portion, and recommended allowance is for adult men.

TABLE 40-8 Nutrient densities of foods: calcium and iron contributions of common foods yielding 1000 calories

Food	Amount	Calcium (mg)	Iron (mg)
Milk (regular, whole)	190 ml (6⅓ C)	1814	0.6
Milk (fluid, skim)	340 ml (11⅓ C)	3362	1.1
Cheese	220 g (½ lb)	1701	2.3
Beef (lean, cooked)	450 g (1 lb)	54	15.9
Eggs (large)	12	324	14.4
Almonds	1¼ C	380	7.6
Kidney beans	4⅔ C	327	20.5
Orange juice	9 C	243	4.5
Lettuce	14 heads	1512	37.8
Potatoes	1.35 kg (3 lb [9 medium])	91	7.2
Bread, (white, enriched)	16 slices, standard	348	9.0
Oatmeal (cooked)	7½ C	165	10.5
Honey	1 C	17	17
Margarine	150 g (5 oz)	29	0
Beer	2.4 L (80 oz [6 ⅔ bottles])	120	Trace
Whiskey	450 ml (15 oz)	0	0
Apple pie	⅔ of pie	33	1.1
Chocolate cake with icing	⅓ of cake	216	3.1
Recommended dietary allowance for 1 day			
Man		800	10.0
Woman		800	18.0

Data from United States Department of Agriculture, Agriculture Research Service: Nutritive value of American foods in common units, Agriculture handbook no 456, Washington, DC, 1975, U.S. Government Printing Office.

range of nutrients and amounts in relation to people's needs are no panacea. One popular brand with an advertising campaign directed primarily at women provides three times the level of iron recommended, with none of the other minerals important for hemoglobin formation, and "some" vitamins. Many over-the-counter vitamin preparations provide excess amounts of vitamins that are relatively inexpensive to produce and minimal quantities of others. It is not an uncommon occurrence for a person to be carefully taking a diet supplement that does not provide the nutrient really needed. The pharmacist can provide information concerning content adequacy of the dosage and potential toxicity of dietary supplements.

Calcium has become a popular supplement. This comes as a result of publicity in the press about a possible role in hypertension and the high prevalence of osteoporosis in older women, which carries with it the potential for "dowager's hump" and the risk of broken hips. The best protection is intake of an adequate diet over the lifetime to build the mineral density of bone before menopause, at which time there is mineral loss associated with hormonal change. Supplements are being widely recommended without any warning that too much calcium carries a penalty as does too little.[8] There is little publicity given to the fact that males too are at risk from osteoporosis because they are now living longer.

Data from the second U.S. Health and Nutrition Examination Survey (NHANES II) show that vitamin and mineral supplements are among the most common nonprescription drugs consumed in this country. Almost 35% of the adult population take supplements regularly, and persons with the highest nutrient intakes from food tend to be the ones who take supplements.[19] The possibility of age-related changes in susceptibility to nutrient toxicity as well as inadequacy has been identified as an area needing investigation. The ready availability of vitamin and mineral supplements as over-the-counter drugs as well as their popularity as placebos or miracle workers increase the possibilities that toxic effects may occur. This is the reason limiting supplements to no more than 100% RDA is suggested by the National Research Council.

NUTRITIONAL STATUS

Nutritional impairment can be defined in broad terms as any situation in which an inadequate, excessive, or imbalanced supply of nutrients to the body results in impairment of growth or productivity, increased susceptibility to infection or chronic disease, or impairment in functioning in the day-to-day activities of life. A child consuming a diet with marginal levels of iron and zinc may grow and function at relatively normal rates until challenged by one of the common infectious diseases of childhood. The obese person pays a price for excessive energy intake in the large deposits of adipose tissue that create increased risks of diabetes mellitus, coronary artery disease, or gallbladder disease and interfere with functioning of organs and ordinary activities such as walking or running or finding attractive clothing at a reasonable price. The adolescent girl who has maintained a slim and attractive appearance by limiting caloric intake without considering the vitamin and mineral content of foods has set the stage for nutritional impairment both of herself and of the child she bears. The middle-aged woman whose diet is low in calcium and vitamin D because of diet or lack of exposure to the sun has increased risk of osteoporosis and bone fracture, conditions for which postmenopausal women are already at considerable risk. The person who takes large doses of protein or vitamin or mineral supplements can produce imbalances that may result in physical impairment, symptoms mimicking serious disease, impairment of growth (in children), or deficiencies of other nutrients.

Management of nutritional impairment requires assessment of the nutritional status of the individual so that the nutritional needs of the person are identified and the appropriate interventions to meet the needs are devised. This includes seeing that hospitalized patients receive and eat the foods they need, whether a regular or modified diet is prescribed, and that persons learn how to meet their nutritional needs at home. The nurse serves as a liaison between the patient and other professional persons in interpreting the patient's nutritional and dietary problems. Explanation to family and friends is often needed as well.

To assess nutritional status, it is necessary to determine the nutrient supply to the body, availability for stores and metabolic processes, body size and composition, and physical signs. The basic principles are those used in general evaluation: (1) observing the person's general appearance, and (2) obtaining careful medical and dietary histories, physical examination, and selected laboratory measurements. There is no one simple test of a person's nutritional state. Furthermore, long periods of time may elapse from the initial limitation of nutrient supply until malnutrition becomes clinically obvious. A person with good body stores of a nutrient as a result of consuming a nutritionally sound diet can tolerate relatively long periods of deprivation of that nutrient. The rate at which depletion progresses will be affected by the stores available and the rate of body utilization or excretion of the nutrient. The time elapsing between the insult to nutrient supply and the actual appearance of clinical signs obvious on physical examination can be as little as a week or as long as several years. For this reason, it is important to remember that dietary, laboratory, and clinical data may appear to be poorly corre-

lated. This lack of correlation has been interpreted by some persons as demonstrating the impossibility of making an assessment and by others as evidence that one type of data is superior or more reliable than another. Actually, these data measure different points along a continuum of deprivation or excess. It is hoped that attention to the nutritional needs of the person, assessment, and appropriate interventions will protect the person and reduce the risk of impaired growth and body function. Prevention or alleviation of malnutrition requires identification of its degree and cause so that appropriate remedies may be instituted.

The nurse has the opportunity to incorporate questions and observations relevant to nutritional needs in the health assessment. Not only does this identify nutrition-related nursing diagnoses, but it also identifies persons at risk who require more extensive evaluation. As stated previously, the person's nutritional well-being is a shared responsibility and frequently requires the knowledge and skills of nurse, dietitian, physician, and others. The initial assessment is important, but nursing responsibility does not end there, since the patient's condition may improve or regress and changes need to be identified. If problems are identified early, the appropriate interventions can be promptly formulated, and the person can be protected from serious sequelae.

ASSESSING NUTRIENT SUPPLY

The adequacy of the diet, in terms of quality and quantity, can be quickly estimated by comparing it with recommended patterns of food intake. A good, or balanced, diet consists of any combination of foodstuffs that yields needed nutrients in sufficient amounts to promote growth and metabolism. For most persons a good diet is one that is tasty, filling, refreshing, or desirable for some special reason important to that person. Persons may believe that a particular food or nutrient has special properties to improve or harm health. The terms "normal," "usual," or "average" diet are ambiguous and uninformative.

Diagnoses of malnutrition are of five general types:

Quantity	Quality
Excessive	Satisfactory
Inadequate	Satisfactory
Satisfactory	Inadequate
Inadequate	Inadequate
Excessive	Inadequate

Quantity refers to volume of food intake and particularly to the energy intake. Quality relates to the protein, vitamin, and mineral content.

TAKING DIETARY HISTORY
Methods

Information about nutrient supply obtained during the initial assessment is necessarily subjective. It must be obtained from the patient or family by interview. Since both kinds and amounts of nutrients are important, intake data must be both qualitative and quantitative.[33] Skill in interviewing is required, since biases can be introduced or "proper" answers supplied by leading questions. The following questions should be considered, one at a time:

When did you first have something to eat or drink yesterday?

Did you eat breakfast yesterday?

Did you have orange juice for breakfast yesterday?

Notice that the first question makes no assumptions. The second question reminds one that breakfast is desirable and tempts one to provide information about breakfast, whether real or imaginary. The third question restricts freedom to answer even more and includes the interviewer's perception of an appropriate food choice. Further it implies that orange juice at breakfast is essential, in effect misinforming the patient.

Directing specific questions about food consumption to the day preceding the interview is a technique frequently used in nutrition surveys designed to assess the nutritional status of groups. It is simple and rapid and takes about 15 minutes. Although the 24-hour recall is useful as a device for continued monitoring, it should not be used for initial assessment. Food intake on a single day is a poor indicator of nutrient supply for an individual. Not only does food intake vary over the week according to work, school, and family schedules, but intake immediately preceding hospitalization or appointments for care is often atypical.

Usual Eating Patterns and Changes

It is more useful to ask the person to describe his or her *usual eating patterns,* including when, what, and how much foods or liquids are consumed, with gentle probing to obtain details about food preparation, use of seasonings, and so forth. Far too often the questions about diet provide a social rather than information exchange:

"Has the baby been eating well?" "Yes."

"How's your diet?" "Fine."

Unfortunately, exchanges such as these may be charted as "Nutrition no problem" or "Patient well nourished." Any problems the patient may have are unidentified and are likely to remain so.

Questioning should elicit a picture of total food consumption for the day. Designation of meals and snacks is not really necessary and may bias answers by implying value judgments. The following approach is more likely to provide useful information:

What is the first thing you usually eat or drink? When? How much? What else? You said you usually have 2 slices of toast; do you put anything on your toast? When do you eat or drink again? Let's review this now. You said you usually have a cup

of soup for lunch at work; what do you have on the days when you're not working? What kind of milk do you buy?

The interviewer should make no assumptions. Some people put cream, milk, or sugar in coffee or tea, and some do not. Some people put dressing on their salads, and some do not. Find out what the person does by asking.

Portion sizes are important and are difficult to estimate without some visual reference. A hamburger can vary from 42 g (1.5 oz) to 168 g (6 oz) or more, making a significant difference in determining whether nutrient supply is adequate. The glass used at home may hold 90, 240, 300, 360, or even 480 ml (3, 8, 10, 12, or 16 oz) of fluid. Dietitians frequently use food models, measuring cups, spoons, and other aids for obtaining intake data. For the hospitalized patient, the equipment and portions on the tray can be used as a basis for comparison.

Food and fluid *preferences* and *dislikes* should be identified. This information is most frequently asked to be sure a patient is satisfied with hospital meals. It is also useful in determining fluid intake, potential inadequacies or excesses, and food intolerances. If a person reports not eating a particular food, it is important to determine if taste, intolerance, or allergy is a determinant.

When the usual eating pattern has been determined, any *recent changes* from the pattern should be identified and described together with any explanations. Changes may be the result of illness (for example, anorexia, nausea, vomiting, and diarrhea), self-imposed dietary regimens, or emotional or physical stress. Experience with special or prescribed diets should be recorded.

Use of Supplements

Since nutrient supply is affected by use of *supplements, medications,* and *drugs,* the person is asked about any intake of these items and whether they have been prescribed by a physician or not. Whenever possible, the product, content, and size of the dose should be recorded.

Additional Data

Information about *financial resources* for food, *facilities* for purchasing, storing, and preparing food, as well as occupation and *daily activities* provides information about nutritional needs and the ease with which needs are met.

The person should be invited to describe any *problems with diet.* These can include problems resulting from a lack of information about a diet previously prescribed; concerns or fears about food, which may generate from the media or from ideas of others; and physical difficulties with sight, taste, chewing, movement, or pain, which may affect intake. Does the person need help with eating? What kind of help?

It is also useful to have the person describe *weight* and *nutrition status*. Does the person perceive body weight as normal, excessive, or low? Have there been major fluctuations in body weight over the last year? Does the person consider diet or nutritional state a problem?

An important source of objective information about intake of the institutionalized patient is frequently ignored, that is, the choice of food the patient makes from menus and the food actually consumed from the tray, snack bar, and gifts, as well as from other modes of nutrient supply such as medications, intravenous or tube feedings, and fluids kept at the bedside. Not only can the patient be asked about these, but also direct observations can be made. Unexpected or inappropriate response to nutrition therapy may be explained by the difference between plans and implementation, if someone takes the time to observe what is happening and intervenes. For example, two women were admitted to the hospital for evaluation and treatment of heart disease. Both women had severe hypertension and were obese; both were prescribed 1000 calorie, limited-sodium diets. After one week, the physician noted that one patient was responding well, with significant weight loss recorded, while the other was gaining weight, both as body fat and increased edema, despite eating only half the food on the tray. The dietitian, when called, determined that the second patient was consuming a high-calorie, high-sodium diet consisting primarily of candy and other items brought daily by visitors at the patient's request.

The information gathered by the nurse about usual dietary patterns and changes provides basic data that can be evaluated rapidly to estimate adequacy of intake and to identify current and potential problems. For more complete and detailed study of intake and analysis, the dietitian can offer special expertise and assistance.

EVALUATING NUTRIENT INTAKE

Individuals need energy, nitrogen, essential amino acids, at least 17 mineral elements, and 13 vitamins. Foods are mixtures of these nutrients. No one food provides the full range of nutrients in proper proportions to meet needs. It is important to know whether the patient is consuming a sufficient variety of different foods to provide the full spectrum of nutrients. The system of food grouping is based on analysis of foods to determine their nutrient concentration. The recommended numbers of servings from different classes of foods are designed to provide the range of nutrients needed in amounts relative to body needs. Persons who eliminate one or more types of food from the diet are likely to have diets of poor quality.

The food guides that have been developed to help people choose the kinds and amounts of food to eat for

---

DAILY FOOD GUIDE[40]

FOOD GROUP	SERVINGS RECOMMENDED (ADULTS)
Vegetables and Fruits	4 servings total
Vitamin A rich: dark green or deep yellow (e.g., broccoli, kale, carrots, squash, turnips, mustard greens)	1 serving (½ C) at least every other day
Vitamin C rich: citrus fruits and juices, cantaloupe, tomato, cabbage, pepper, strawberries	1 serving (½ C or usual portion)
Other fruits and vegetables	2 or more servings (½ C or usual portion; i.e., medium potato or apple)
Bread and Cereal (whole grain or enriched)	4 or more servings (1 slice bread, 30 g dry cereal, ½ -¾ C cooked cereal, rice, macaroni, noodles, spaghetti)
Milk Fluid milk: whole, skim, cultured, evaporated; milk solids may be in beverage or mixtures fortified with vitamin D	2 or more glasses
Meat, Poultry, Fish, and Beans	2 or more servings (60-75 g meat, fish, poultry, liver; 2 eggs; 1 C beans, peas, lentils; 4 tbsp peanut butter)
Caution	Fats, sweets, alcohol

---

health can be used for a rapid evaluation of adequacy of the diet eaten at home or food intake in the hospital. There are many different food guides, since to be effective they must be devised for a specific country or culture and feature the foods readily available and acceptable to the people being evaluated.

A daily food guide used in the United States is shown in the box above. The guide groups staple food items rich in protein, vitamins, and minerals into four major classes according to their major nutrient contributions. Recommendations are made for the number and size of servings to be selected from each food group. One can evaluate a diet quickly by checking to see if the recommended types of food and servings are included in the usual dietary pattern.

Since foods are mixtures of nutrients, the protein, vitamin, and mineral requirements are substantially met when the daily intake includes the recommended servings from each group. The calorie level of the basic diet is low (Table 40-9) but is approximately sufficient for adult basal metabolism. Adequacy of energy intake is best judged by evaluation of body weight. In this

TABLE 40-9 Protein and calorie values of basic diet selected to meet recommendations outlined in food guide for an adult

Group and Food Chosen	Protein (g)	Calories
Milk, ½ L (1 pint) Whole (skim)	18	330 (180)
Vegetable-fruit, 4 servings Broccoli (½ C) Potato, 1 medium Lettuce, ⅙ head Apple, 6 cm (2½-in) diameter	6	190
Meat, 2 or more servings Cheese, 30 g (1 oz) Beef, 75 g (2½ oz) Poultry, 75 g (2½ oz)	56	341
Bread-cereal, 4 servings Cornflakes, 30 g (1 oz) Bread, 3 slices	8	290
TOTAL	88	1151 (1001)

MILK EQUIVALENTS (BASED ON CALCIUM CONTENT)

1 C (8 oz) fluid milk =
5 level tbsp dried milk solids
1 C yogurt
1¾ C ice cream
1½ C cottage cheese
40 g (1½ oz) cheddar, American, or Swiss cheese
1 C pudding

method of evaluation, fats, oils, and sweets are not tabulated, since they provide primarily energy.

Each food grouping contributes particular nutrients to the total diet. The absence of any one food group from the diet or over consumption of particular types of food should alert the nurse that the patient has a potential nutrition problem.

Milk and Milk Products

Milk and milk products and foods from the *meat group* are excellent sources of high-quality protein. In contrast to the meat group, milk provides calcium, phosphorus, and riboflavin abundantly as well as other minerals and vitamins. Milk is not a rich source of iron or vitamin C and should not be used as the sole protein food in the diet. There are many different types of milk: homogenized, 2%, skim milk, buttermilk, yogurt, and powdered, evaporated, and condensed milk. Use of milk fortified with vitamin D is desirable, especially for children, pregnant or lactating women, and persons with limited exposure to sunlight as a result of their life-style. Therefore the person should be questioned to determine if fortified milk is used. Skim milk may be fortified with vitamin A as well as vitamin D, since that fat-soluble vitamin is removed when milkfat is removed. Cheese is included in this group because of its calcium value. When evaluating the diet, all milks and cheeses used should be considered. There is a tendency to consider only milk used as a beverage, but it is an important ingredient in soups, puddings, ice cream, and frozen desserts (see the box above).

Vegetables and Fruits

Vegetables and fruits are important primarily as sources of vitamins and minerals. They contribute some protein depending on their type, but cereal grains and the plant foods in the meat group contribute more. Fruits and vegetables are low in calories unless prepared with additional fats or sugars; they are high in nutritional value. Since vitamins A and C are not evenly distributed in all fruits and vegetables, the diet should be checked to be sure that a food rich in vitamin C is included daily and a food rich in vitamin A is included at least every other day. Foods rich in vitamin C include citrus fruits and juices, melons, berries, dark green leafy vegetables, broccoli, cabbage, green peppers, and tomatoes. Foods rich in vitamin A include dark green or deep yellow vegetables. As a general guide, foods with the deeper colors are richer sources of vitamins. Other fruits and vegetables may contribute varying amounts of vitamins C and A, but the choices described above are needed to ensure adequate intake. In addition, fruits and vegetables contribute a wide range of other vitamins including folacin (folic acid) and minerals including potassium. They are quite low in sodium unless salt is added in preparation. They also contribute fiber to the diet.

Meat Group

The *meat* group includes animal and plant products that are rich in protein. Meat, fish, poultry, and eggs contribute protein, fat, and vitamin B complex, including B_{12}, and minerals (for example, iron and copper). Nuts and seeds contribute protein and fat, while the legumes contribute protein and starch. The plant products also contribute vitamins and minerals except vitamin B_{12}. The meat-plant group described here is primarily important for protein content, trace minerals, thiamin, and niacin.

Bread and Cereals

Bread and cereals should be whole grain or enriched. They contribute some protein, but most of their energy value is supplied as complex carbohydrates. The whole grain forms are important sources of fiber. These foods are important as sources of many vitamins and miner-

TABLE 40-10 A pattern for daily food choices[39]

Food Group	Suggested Daily Servings
Breads, cereals and other grain products	6 to 11 Include several servings of whole grain products
Fruits Citrus, melon, berries Other fruits	2 to 4
Vegetables Dark-green leafy Deep-yellow Dry beans and peas Starchy Other vegetables	3 to 5 Include all types regularly; use dark-green leafy vegetables and dry beans and peas several times a week
Meat, poultry, fish and alternates	2 to 3 Total 5 to 7 oz lean
Milk, cheese, and yogurt	2 (3 for teens and women who are pregnant or breast feeding; 4 for pregnant or breast feeding teens)
Fats, sweets, and alcoholic beverages	Avoid too many fats and sweets; drink alcoholic beverages in moderation

als, especially because they are inexpensive in comparison with most food items. In surveys it has been noted that these foods provide important amounts of iron in the diet for many people. They are not good sources of vitamins A and C, however, although they contribute valuable levels of thiamin, riboflavin, and niacin. Desserts (for example, cookies, cake, and doughnuts) are grain foods of high caloric value because of added fats and sugars.

The National Dairy Council* publishes a colorful *Guide to Good Eating* that provides information similar to the *Daily Food Guide*. Additional information is given about combination foods such as pizza and other food items (such as condiments, chips, fats, oils, sweets, and beverages). The *Diet and Health Report* recommends more servings of breads and cereals, vegetables, and fruits for increased levels of fiber and vitamins A and C (Table 40-10).

USE OF THE DAILY FOOD GUIDE

The box on p. 1220 is an assessment of a diet history. The individual is a 45-year-old woman with obesity and hypertension; her meals are eaten at home.

When using the *Daily Food Guide* for rapid screening of nutrient supply, remember that the food group system is not a complete diet, but it is the foundation for meal planning. Additional servings from the groups, as well as fats, oils, and sweets, are used to meet energy and growth needs. Alcoholic beverages may be used by the person as well, thus increasing caloric intake with little contribution of protein, vitamins, or minerals. Levels of folacin and magnesium are likely to be low unless the diet includes green leafy vegetables. Levels of vitamin E might be low if vegetable oils are not used in food preparation or as salad dressings. The diet histories of girls and women should be checked to see if iron-rich foods are included, because menstruation and childbearing increase iron needs. Iron-rich foods include green leafy vegetables, meat, liver, seafood, egg yolks, nuts, legumes, and whole and enriched grains and cereals.

The *Daily Food Guide* can also be used for evaluating *vegetarian* diets. Many people are vegetarians, and their reasons vary (for example, religion, food cost, and philosophy). The diets vary as well. Some persons eliminate only red meat such as beef, lamb, veal, and pork but do eat fish. Others eliminate all muscle meats including fish and poultry. Still others use animal products such as milk, cheese, and eggs; these persons are called lacto-ovo-vegetarians. There are some who eliminate all foods of animal origin from the diet and some who choose from a very limited list of plant products. Some eat only cereal grains, others only fruits or seeds. Generally, the lacto-ovo-vegetarian diet is nutritionally sound when a variety of foods is included.[6,22] Persons on more restricted vegetarian (vegan) diets should be considered at nutritional risk and candidates for more detailed study. One potential problem is vitamin B_{12} insufficiency unless fortified cereal or a dietary supplement is taken. The young adult who has changed to a vegan diet may use body stores of B_{12} for a time (a 5-year store is possible) but is at potential risk especially if intake of folacin in vegetables is high, masking the signs of megaloblastic anemia.

Other dietary guides could be used in the same manner if the population served represents a particular ethnic or cultural group with a different pattern of food use. The pattern described here is applicable for the majority of the U.S. population. Hospital diet manuals also provide food patterns that can be used as evaluation tools. In addition to describing regular or normal diets, the manuals provide patterns for modified diets prescribed as therapeutic regimens. When these patterns are used for evaluation, they provide a mechanism for separating quickly those persons who are most likely consuming an adequate nutrient supply from those who are not. When an individual's food intake does not adhere to a recommended pattern, he or she may or may not be obtaining adequate nutrients. The evaluation of the diet must be extended, and the evaluation becomes more arduous. Tables of food composition can be used and nutrient intake estimated through calculation of the

*Rosemont, IL 60018-4233

ASSESSMENT OF A DIET HISTORY

DIET

45-year-old woman with obesity and hypertension; meals eaten at home

7:00 AM

1 C cooked oatmeal
2 tsp sugar
1 C skim milk (fortified)
3 C coffee, plain

10:15 AM

2 C coffee, plain

1:00 PM

Sandwich
    2 slices white bread, enriched
    ½ tsp margarine
    ½ tsp mayonnaise
    60 g (2 oz) meatloaf or luncheon meat
4 cookies (fig bars, gingersnaps)
3 C coffee, plain

4:00 PM

7 cookies
½ C unsweetened fruit (canned, frozen, or fresh)
2 C tea, plain

10:00 PM

8 soda crackers
60 g (2 oz) American cheese
360 ml (12 oz) cola (sweet)
½ C homemade bread-and-butter pickles

Midnight

2 aspirin
1 C tea, plain

ASSESSMENT

Food Group	Servings	Evaluation
Milk		Choice from milk group adequate. Fruit and vegetable intake low; choice of items rich in vitamin C or A happenstance. Meat intake low. Bread intake is 6 servings. Intake of sweets, particularly cookies, high. Use of pickles and soda crackers questionable, since patient reports that low-sodium diet was prescribed for her several years ago.
Skim milk	1	
Cheese	1	
Fruits, vegetables		
Fruit	1	
Vegetable	1	
Meat-protein		
Meatloaf	1	
Bread, cereal		
Oatmeal	2	
Bread, enriched	2	
Crackers	2	
Sweets		
Cookies	11	
Cola (360 ml [12 oz])		
Pickles, cucumber		Dietitian was asked to check caloric value. Intake is 1500-1600 cal/day, which includes about 800 cal from basic food items; remainder from sweets and fat. Protein levels adequate, although source of protein could be improved.
Fats		
Margarine		
Mayonnaise		

NOTE: Identify nutritional risks for this person; identify appropriate interventions and behavioral goals for her.

nutrient value of each food.[31] Referral to the dietitian is appropriate.

ASSESSING NUTRITIONAL DEFICIENCY

At one time, a great deal of emphasis was placed on looking for specific signs of nutritional deficiency as part of the clinical examination. This was based on the observation made of populations with classic deficiency diseases. One can find lists of the signs in most nutrition textbooks. One need not be a physician to recognize major signs of nutritional deprivation. It is hoped that nutrition problems can be identified before major signs and symptoms appear.

Signs of malnutrition may be caused by a nutrient lack or nonnutritional factors such as poor hygiene (for example, bleeding gums and bad teeth). They may be the result of inadequate nutrient intake or a disease or condition that interferes with the body's ability to digest,

absorb, or metabolize nutrients. It is important to make these differentiations.

SUBJECTIVE DATA

The patient's (or family's) description of the current illness, previous illness and surgery, pregnancy, weight, weight change, growth, and use of prescribed and over-the-counter medications provides information, most of which can be checked by examination, measurements, and appropriate laboratory studies. The history provides data for determining likely problems and defining the priorities for testing.

OBJECTIVE DATA

The World Health Organization (WHO) has published classifications of the physical signs most often associated with malnutrition, and these have been adapted for use in the United States.[17] Table 40-2 lists the signs associated with normal appearance and with malnutrition. Evaluation also includes height, weight, and growth patterns.

Height and Weight

Height and weight are easily measured and are important data to obtain and use. Weight and height can be compared with tables of recommended values as a guide. A useful item of historical information is the weight of the adult at age 25 and the person's perception of desirable body weight. The first provides data about a good weight for the person (if not obese at 25), and the second helps predict the person's response to attempts to change weight (Table 40-11).

For all persons, periodic recording of weight changes can provide valuable data about health status and response to therapy and can serve as an early warning of problems. Even in hospitals where weight is measured, the data usually are not used as they should be.

The nurse should review the methods for obtaining accurate measurements of height or length. Errors of up to 5 cm have been recorded in measurements made on the commonly used type of clinical scale with a measuring rod. The most reliable measurement of weight is made in the morning after voiding and before food or drink are taken.

Interpretation of weight requires some knowledge of body fluid compartments (see Chapter 23). Very rapid fluctuations in weight (possibly as much as 5 kg in 24 hours) are usually caused by body fluid changes and may signal difficulties with edema or dehydration. A steady downward course in weight may signal that the person is catabolizing body protein or possibly body fat. For some persons this weight loss represents significant deterioration and should be stopped if possible. If loss of fat is the goal, the record represents progress. In general, loss of body fat is a slower process (about 0.5 to 1 kg/wk), since fat is a concentrated source of energy.

Body fatness can be estimated from weight for height. Generally a weight of 15% to 20% above the standard tables represents excessive body fat, although some persons can be overweight but not overfat because of muscle development. The person's general appearance gives one a rapid estimate of overweight or underweight. Fatness can be checked with the use of calipers.

Mouth and Teeth

Although all of the physical signs listed in Table 40-2 should be considered, evaluation of the mouth and teeth are especially important. Persons with missing or decayed teeth or dentures that are uncomfortable may have poor nutritional status because eating is painful and unpleasant. They may have problems with appropriate oral hygiene as well. Not only may these difficulties be present at the initial contact, but further problems may develop such as increased pain, bleeding, and infection. Identification of these problems and care directed toward them are essential to the person's well-being. The mouth is checked for cleanliness, odor, evi-

TABLE 40-11 Height and weight tables for adults; desirable weights for persons age 25 and over

Men*				Women*†				
Height	Small Frame	Medium Frame	Large Frame	Height	Small Frame	Medium Frame	Large Frame	
ft in	(lb)	(lb)	(lb)	ft in	(lb)	(lb)	(lb)	
5 2	112-120	118-129	126-141	4 10	92-98	96-107	104-119	
5 3	115-123	121-133	129-144	4 11	94-101	98-110	106-122	
5 4	118-126	124-136	132-148	5 0	96-104	101-113	109-125	
5 5	121-129	127-139	135-152	5 1	99-107	104-116	112-128	
5 6	124-133	130-143	138-156	5 2	102-110	107-119	115-131	
5 7	128-137	134-147	142-161	5 3	105-113	110-122	118-134	
5 8	132-141	138-152	147-166	5 4	108-116	113-126	121-138	
5 9	136-145	142-156	151-170	5 5	111-119	116-130	125-142	
5 10	140-150	146-160	155-174	5 6	114-123	120-135	129-146	
5 11	144-154	150-165	159-179	5 7	118-127	124-139	133-150	
6 0	148-158	154-170	164-184	5 8	122-131	128-143	137-154	
6 1	152-162	158-175	168-189	5 9	126-135	132-147	141-158	
6 2	156-167	162-180	173-194	5 10	130-140	136-151	145-163	
6 3	160-171	167-185	178-199	5 11	134-144	140-155	149-168	
6 4	164-175	172-190	182-204	6 0	138-148	144-159	153-173	

From Metropolitan Life Insurance Company, New York.
*Height for men with shoes with 1 in heels; height for women with shoes with 2 in heels.
†For women 18-25 years old, subtract 1 lb for each year under 25.

dence of irritation or lesions, soreness, paralysis, and ability to chew. Although bleeding gums usually are associated with vitamin C deficiency, they are more frequently associated with poor oral hygiene and periodontal disease in the U.S. population.

DIAGNOSTIC TESTS

The blood and urine analyses routinely done for patients contain data useful in the evaluation of nutritional status. There are also special tests that can be used to confirm impressions obtained from evaluation of nutrient supply and the clinical examination.

ROUTINE TESTS

Urinalysis routinely includes tests of pH, protein, glucose, and acetone. Urine can also be tested for creatinine and certain vitamins (see Table 40-12). If these tests are ordered, a protocol for collecting and handling the specimens should be requested from the laboratory.

Blood is frequently tested for hemoglobin, hematocrit, serum protein, and cholesterol. The values will be influenced by recent blood loss, so one should determine whether the person was a recent blood donor as well as checking for loss from bleeding. The values may also be affected by blood transfusions or intravenous solutions; therefore timing of the sample is important.

Low levels of *hemoglobin* most frequently are associated with iron or protein deficiency; however, a variety of nutritional and nonnutritional factors may be involved. About 10% of the U.S. population is estimated to have some degree of anemia related to low *iron* intake. Elevated hemoglobin levels are also seen with dehydration and polycythemia. Hematocrit values are indicative of anemias resulting from low intake of iron and are elevated in polycythemia. More specific evidence of iron deficiency is obtained from tests of serum iron and transferrin; these tests detect reduced stores before anemia develops. If these are normal, another explanation for the anemia must be sought.

Protein deficiency is uncommon in the United States but not necessarily in the hospitalized patient. The patient's appearance, muscle mass, and body weight are indicative of protein status. The serum protein level, and especially albumin in relation to globulin, falls with protein deficiency but is not considered particularly sensitive or specific for protein. Serum protein levels may be maintained for some time even with limited protein intake. Nitrogen-creatinine ratios in the urine and ratios of specific amino acids in plasma have been used but are not standard procedures as yet for determination of protein deficiency.

SPECIAL TESTS

Other blood tests are available to test nutritional status. Some tests measure the stores of a nutrient, some measure the circulating nutrient, and others measure the activity of enzymes dependent on the nutrient for activity. These are not routine tests and may be costly to the patient in terms of laboratory fees or discomfort. The decision to request such tests is based on the evaluation of the patient's nutrient intake and physical condition and identification of the possible nutrient problem and the proper test to verify it. For many nutrients, especially the trace elements, laboratory methods have not been standardized and criteria for interpretation of results have not been developed. When the information is essential for patient care, the knowledge and skills of nurse, physician, dietitian, and laboratory personnel are needed.

Tests for levels of *glucose, cholesterol,* and *triglycerides* are often part of the regular series of studies. These levels have implications for nutritional status and for health status, particularly as related to the development of diabetes mellitus and coronary heart disease. They are discussed in the chapters describing these diseases.

Inadequacies of *thiamin* are frequently found in chronic alcoholics, and since there is a high index of suspicion adequate thiamin is provided. A recent review of thiamin intake in the elderly revealed that about 5% of those over the age of 60 had impaired thiamin status. This was seen in those confined in institutions and in ill persons. The combination of poverty and old age in-

TABLE 40-12 Tests for nutritional status

Nutrient	Laboratory Test
Iron	Hemoglobin, hematocrit
	Serum iron, transferrin, ferritin
	Total iron-binding capacity
Protein	Serum protein, albumin, hemoglobin
	Nitrogen balance studies
Calcium	Bone density
Copper	Serum copper
Zinc	Serum zinc
Vitamin C	Serum ascorbic acid
Thiamin	Urinary thiamin
	Erythrocyte transketolase—thiamin pyrophosphate (TPP) effect
Riboflavin	Urinary riboflavin
	Erythrocyte glutathione reductase—flavin adenine dinucleotide (FAD) effect
Niacin	Urinary N′-methylnicotinamide
Folacin	Serum folate
Vitamin B$_{12}$	Serum vitamin B$_{12}$
Vitamin A	Plasma vitamin A
	Plasma carotene
Vitamin D	Serum alkaline phosphatase
	Serum 25-OH vitamin D
Vitamin E	Serum tocopherol
Vitamin K	Prothrombin time
	Abnormal prothrombin

creases the risk.[16] These persons respond promptly to ordinary levels of thiamin, which suggests that there may be inadequate ingestion. Alcohol does interfere with the absorption of thiamin when the two are consumed together, but this has not been documented for the elderly.

Niacin status has been of particular interest in the United States since pellagra was a major public health problem in the Southwest in the early 1900s. It is rare now, but it occurs occasionally in chronic alcoholics or persons on severely limited diets. Its rarity is in part the result of enriched grain and bread products, but is probably more attributable to the generous protein level of most American diets. In addition to obtaining preformed niacin from food, the body can obtain the vitamin from the amino acid tryptophane. When evaluating intake, one considers the protein content of the diet as well as the niacin content.

Of all the vitamins, *folacin* is probably the most frequently tested in patients. This is because deficiency has been reported as common in pregnant women and in women taking estrogens. In addition, megaloblastic anemia can be identified readily in standard clinical blood examinations.

Vitamin B$_{12}$ status can also be checked by measuring serum levels. Since B$_{12}$ deficiency may be caused by inadequate intake or by an inability to absorb the vitamin from food (pernicious anemia), a series of tests is used by the physician for differential diagnosis. Megaloblastic anemia is a clinical sign of folacin or B$_{12}$ inadequacy. When folacin intake is very high in relation to B$_{12}$ supplies in the body, megaloblastic anemia may not be apparent, and permanent damage to the body may occur if one waits until clinical signs appear. This can happen in persons whose diet appears adequate in B$_{12}$ but who cannot absorb it. It may occur in persons whose diet is inadequate in B$_{12}$ (for example, vegans) but whose folacin intake is high because of good intakes of foods such as green leafy vegetables or, more frequently, because of folic acid supplements that may be self-chosen.

Assessment of *vitamin A* nutriture is important for two reasons. Repeated studies of the American population show significant numbers of people with inadequate vitamin A intake and low vitamin reserves in the liver. Persons with impaired fat absorption or other absorption problems such as gluten enteropathy will have impaired absorption of fat-soluble vitamins. In addition, vitamin A is a popular dietary supplement for persons concerned about their skin or health, and they frequently take very large doses of the vitamin over long periods. Vitamin A is toxic when taken in excess and may result in either acute or chronic, hard-to-identify symptoms. Persons taking isoretinine, a form of vitamin A, for treatment of acne are also at risk for toxicity.

Plasma levels of vitamin A and the provitamin carotene can be measured. An individual may maintain acceptable levels (20 μg/100 ml) even with low intake, if liver stores are available for mobilization. Plasma carotene levels reflect one form of vitamin intake: that from green leafy and yellow vegetables. A low plasma carotene level would be expected in persons not including these foods, just as a high level would be expected in persons eating generous amounts. The high intake of carotenes does not pose the same hazard of toxicity as does high intake of vitamin A.

DIET MODIFICATIONS

The modification needed by the person may be simply assistance in changing the usual food intake pattern to the normal pattern recommended for health. It may involve adjustments to meet special dietary problems imposed by disease, trauma, or metabolic abnormalities. For this reason dietary modifications must be considered before determining intervention. Therapeutic diets should not be imposed on the person without good reason. Principles basic to prescribing diets are listed in the box on p. 1224.

A diet prescription is based on the determination of each patient's nutrient needs. When no constraints have been imposed by temporary or permanent alterations in nutritional processes (for example, digestion or absorption) or body functioning by illness or trauma, the "normal" ("house") diet is prescribed. This is not considered a "modified diet," since the term "modified" is used to describe diets different in some way from normal. Meeting the prescription for a "normal" diet does require modification of usual food behavior for those persons whose food practices are poor. The diet prescription may consist of one or many modifications to be followed for varying lengths of time—from one day to a lifetime. The person with chronic disease is often faced with the necessity for permanent changes in food habits. In some instances dietary modification does not necessitate a change in food behavior because the person's usual diet actually meets the prescribed modification. A brief discussion of diet modifications and possible applications is included here to illustrate the scope of diet therapy. Consult this text and suggested reading lists for details.

MODIFICATIONS IN NUTRIENTS
PROTEIN MODIFICATION

Protein may be increased to levels twice those usually recommended for persons with protein losses from tissue catabolism, bleeding, and exudates. On the other hand, protein may be decreased to levels one half to one third those recommended. In chronic renal failure diet management involves providing sufficient protein to

PRINCIPLES OF THERAPEUTIC DIETS

In deciding on the dietary management of a disease certain general principles should govern the prescription and formulation of any special diet.

1. The diet should provide all essential nutrients as generously as its special characteristics permit.
2. The special therapeutic regimen should be patterned as much as possible after a normal diet.
3. The special diet should be flexible; it should consider the patient's gustatory habits and preferences, his economic status, and any religious rules that may govern his food intake.
4. A diet should be adapted to the patient's habits with regard to work and exercise.
5. The foods that are included in the special diet must agree with the patient.
6. The diet should emphasize natural, commonly used foods that are readily available and easily prepared at home.
7. A simple and clear explanation of the purpose of the diet and reason for it should be given to the patient and to the members of his family who are responsible for the preparation of his meals.
8. Except for cases where a maintenance diet must be adhered to for life, patients should be taken off special diets as soon as possible. Practically anybody required to follow a therapeutic diet feels conspicuous and set apart; this is especially important in the case of young children, who are more impressionable and for whom a prolonged special diet may be the making of an emotional problem.
9. The diet must be absolutely justified and defensible. Hospitals, patients, and patients' families alike will benefit if the number of special diets is reduced to those that are really necessary.
10. Feeding by mouth is always the method of choice; only when the patient is incapable or will not eat and drink enough should tube feeding or, if this is contraindicated, parenteral feeding be resorted to.

From Burton, B and Foster, W: Human nutrition, ed 4, Copyright © 1988, McGraw-Hill Book Co. Used with permission of McGraw-Hill Book Co.

prevent tissue protein catabolism and yet avoid accumulations of urea. In hepatic coma dietary protein is adjusted to individual tolerance. In some instances control of the amino acid content of the diet may be required. Children with phenylketonuria need the same nutrients for growth as the healthy child. Their diet must be modified, however, because they cannot convert phenylalanine to tyrosine and subsequent normal metabolites. The diet should provide sufficient phenylalanine for growth but not enough to raise serum levels to those causing central nervous system damage. Phenylalanine cannot be eliminated from the diet as it is an essential amino acid. Tyrosine becomes an essential amino acid for this child as his body cannot convert phenylalanine to tyrosine. Specific proteins may be eliminated with gluten-induced enteropathy or allergies.

FAT MODIFICATION

Fat modifications include increasing or decreasing total fat intake, altering the proportion of dietary calories obtained from fat, and altering the fatty acid composition of the diet. Total fat may be increased to provide essential calories in a concentrated form. Total fat may be decreased for patients with gallbladder disease to reduce pain and contraction of the gallbladder. Alterations in the proportion of dietary calories from fat may be used for patients with primary or secondary disorders of lipid metabolism or to induce ketosis. The prescription should specify the proportions desired for the patient: 10% to 15% of total calories ("low"); 25% to 30% of total calories ("moderate"); 40% to 45% of total calories ("usual"); 60% to 80% of total calories ("ketogenic"). Modifications may also be made in the kind of fat in the diet: short-chain, medium-chain, or long-chain triglycerides or saturated, monounsaturated, and polyunsaturated fatty acids. Modifications in chain length may be prescribed for patients with disorders of digestion and absorption. Modifications in saturated and unsaturated fatty acids may be prescribed to alter serum lipid levels.

CARBOHYDRATE MODIFICATION

Carbohydrate modifications include increasing or decreasing total carbohydrate intake, altering the proportion of dietary calories obtained from carbohydrate, controlling the type of carbohydrate, and eliminating or reducing specific carbohydrate components. The dietary prescription for a patient with diabetes mellitus might include a decrease in total carbohydrates, a change in the ratio of simple to complex carbohydrates, and substitution of carbohydrate derivatives such as hexitols or dextrins for sucrose. Lactose may be eliminated from the diet of patients with lactase insufficiency and sucrose from the diet in patients with invertase insufficiency. Fructose and sucrose are excluded from the diet of persons with hereditary fructose intolerance and galactose and lactose from the diet of patients with galactosemia.

CALORIE MODIFICATION

A modification frequently ignored is that of calories. So much attention has been given to obesity that underweight and emaciation resulting from the intake of foods in amounts insufficient to meet body needs may be overlooked. Surgical patients, the elderly, and patients on long-term therapies such as chemotherapy or radiation are likely to become severely emaciated while receiving therapy. This creates a situation in which the patient cannot heal or benefit from treatment. It is essential to remember that weight gain or loss is related to energy balance (see Chapter 42).

VITAMIN MODIFICATION

Modifications in vitamin concentrations are generally limited to increasing dosage or providing the vitamin in an alternate form to enhance absorption or utilization. Medicinal sources are frequently used. A diet low in vitamin A and carotene is prescribed for patients with vitamin A toxicity.

SODIUM AND POTASSIUM MODIFICATIONS

Often the mineral content of a diet must be controlled. *Sodium* restriction is one of the most common dietary modifications prescribed and is frequently combined with modifications in calories, sources of carbohydrate, and other minerals. Persons with hypertension, fluid retention, or kidney disease are usually expected to control the amount of sodium they eat. The term "control" is used here deliberately, since the goal is to balance sodium intake with sodium need, with the body's ability to handle sodium, and with the physiologic effects of drugs or medications. The level of sodium recommended may vary from 250 mg to 2 g or more per day. Elimination of sodium from the diet can precipitate dehydration.

Potassium levels may be specified for patients with kidney disease and for those with electrolyte imbalance. Other mineral modifications include diets low or high in calcium and diets low in copper. Medicinal sources of minerals are frequently prescribed.

MODIFICATIONS IN CONSISTENCY AND AMOUNTS

Liquid (clear and full), *puréed,* and *soft* diets represent modifications in consistency. They may be used when the patient has difficulties in chewing or swallowing or when the patient has lesions of the gastrointestinal tract. They may be used serially for the postoperative patient. Modifications in fiber or residue content of the diet are often prescribed.

Meal size and *frequency* may be modified for treatment of appetite disorders, diabetes mellitus, dumping syndrome, hypoglycemia, peptic ulcer, and other disorders. Modifications in the *method of feeding* include tube feeding, parenteral or intravenous infusions, and sterile food service.

In some cases the prescription may specify *elimination of specific foods* or beverages from the diet. This approach is used in food allergy. Food elimination may lead to rather bizarre and unusual dietary patterns that should be checked closely for adequacy. Sometimes the diet order specifies foods that may be served to the patient. This is usually a list of bland items such as gela-

tin, soft-cooked egg, farina, and mashed potato. Patient distress and boredom may be alleviated by asking the physician to change the order to "diet as tolerated."

Any diet modification, when imposed, should be justified. Theories of the appropriate nutritional therapy in some diseases vary depending on the interpretation of indirect evidence. Carefully controlled studies are needed to determine the efficacy of modifications, including some that have been used for years (for example, the elimination of "gas-forming" or strong-flavored foods). At times it appears as though folklore rather than scientific method fathered some diet and food restrictions. In recent years there has been a trend toward liberal interpretation of dietary therapy. In part this has been the result of a recognition that many restrictions were without basis in fact and that life lived according to these restrictions was so onerous that emotional well-being was lost without a compensating increase in physical well-being.

METHODS OF FEEDING

Oral feeding is the method of choice; however, when patients cannot take food by mouth, alternative methods are employed. The time period may be short or long. The same considerations governing oral nourishment apply to nourishment by tube or vein. Are all of the nutrients being supplied? For short-term care, patient stores may provide missing nutrients. For long-term care or for persons without stores (infants, debilitated persons), adequacy of all nutrients should be checked, or deficiencies may occur. Providing sufficient calories without unfavorable reactions in a patient may present a problem.

An alternative route for nourishing patients who cannot be fed by mouth or through the digestive tract is by intravenous infusion. The nutrients and fluid may be delivered into a peripheral vein (intravenous feeding) or into the vena cava (total parenteral nutrition [TPN]) (see Chapter 42). The supply of calories and amino acids that can be delivered by the intravenous route is limited. TPN has made it possible to deliver a slow, continuous infusion of hyperosmolar fluid without damage to the vein. The benefits of TPN, however, have their costs as well, such as complications related to the central venous catheter, electrolyte imbalance, metabolic disturbances, and occasionally allergic reactions following administration of protein hydrolysates. The composition of the infusate varies. Certain vitamins and minerals may be absent and others may be provided in concentrations high enough to produce overload if continued for long periods. The ingestion of foods and fluids by way of the gastrointestinal tract is a far more efficient and effective method of meeting the body's nutrition needs.

DIET/DRUG MODIFICATIONS

Various drugs and medications that a person is taking may affect body functions in such a way that diet modification is needed. The obvious illustration of this phenomenon is the treatment regimen for persons with diabetes mellitus: diet, exercise, insulin activity, and hypoglycemic drugs. Moderate to severe elevations in blood pressure may be experienced by patients taking monoamine oxidase inhibitors when they consume large quantities of foods such as aged cheddar cheese, herring, or wines. These foods are rich in tyramine, and metabolism of tyramine is dependent on monoamine oxidase. Some persons receiving penicillamine therapy may experience a subjective loss of taste for salt and sweet. The diarrhea commonly associated with high-dosage neomycin therapy reflects an induced malabsorption syndrome. Some persons being maintained on barbiturates or anticonvulsants may develop folic acid deficiency, and some taking large doses of isoniazid may show signs of vitamin B_6 deficiency. Thiazide diuretic therapy may deplete cellular potassium. Some medications or products may yield so much sodium as to negate any benefit from a sodium-controlled diet; some products contain lactose as a filler. Since new and more powerful drugs are constantly being developed, this list is certain to grow. A diet prescription must be translated into a diet plan or food pattern that will meet the person's physical needs and yet provide enough flexibility that the patient will enjoy the food. If a modification is required for only a short time, it may not be difficult to plan. However, if the modification is one to be followed at home after discharge from the hospital, such things as cost, availability, ease of preparation, and relationship to family food requirements must be taken into account.

CONSIDERATIONS WHEN MAKING DIETARY MODIFICATIONS

An unwritten but essential part of each diet order is that the diet should provide all nutrients as generously as its special characteristics permit. If the modification is so restrictive that the food plan will not provide adequate supplies, the physician should be notified so that appropriate adjustments in diet or medication can be made. Clear liquid diets, for example, supply important fluids, some calories, and some sodium and chloride, but they have little other nutrient value. When milk must be eliminated from the diet, it is necessary to identify and eliminate all food items containing milk and replace the calcium, phosphorus, riboflavin, and protein value of milk by incorporating other foods into the food plan. Alterations in the diet—changes in the proportions of calories from protein, fat, and carbohydrate—may in themselves change nutrient requirements. For example, increased polyunsaturated fat should be accompanied by increased dietary levels of vitamin E and increased protein accompanied by increased vitamin B_6. This is accomplished by including foods rich in the desired components in the patient's diet. For example, the polyunsaturated fat may be provided by corn oil or safflower oil, which contain both the desired fat and vitamin E.

Vigorous therapeutic measures aimed at treating one condition may precipitate others when care is disease focused. For example, the traditional regimen for peptic ulcer emphasized maintaining the patient on a diet of milk, cream, and foods high in calories and fat for months or years. Gain in weight and particularly in body fat was not unusual. Ulcers are most prevalent in middle-aged men, the group most at risk from coronary artery disease.

Foods contain a variety of nutrients in varying proportions. The diet plan should guide selection of the kinds of foods in the amounts dictated by the diet prescription. Calorie, protein, fat, and carbohydrate concentrations of some common foods are shown in Figure 50-4. Notice how many of the foods contain protein. Intake of all these foods would have to be limited if protein is restricted. Calorie needs would have to be supplied by foods consisting primarily of carbohydrate or fat.

Some dietary prescriptions can be met only by using different or unusual food items such as casein hydrolysate (low in phenylalanine or starches) made from wheat or corn or other plant sources. These cannot be handled in the same way as the foods they replace. New techniques and recipes must be developed. The final products differ in appearance, texture, and taste from those they replace. Patients whose diets require such products should have help in learning how to cook the products and use them in the diet. Since information about staple food items is the best available, food plans for diet modifications tend to emphasize staple foods and do not include many new items on the food market.

Interest in dietary fiber is high, although there is disagreement regarding the definition of fiber, conflicting data about the values of high- and low-fiber diets, and disagreements as to the relative merits of fiber from grains, vegetables, and fruits. Bran may be prescribed as an adjunct to diet together with increased use of foods containing complex carbohydrate. Sufficient fiber in the diet has been recommended for many years for proper elimination of waste products.

DIETARY COUNSELING

The quality of the diet is most easily judged by determining whether the person is consuming the recommended amounts of the different types of foods. Intervention can be of two different types: (1) working with the person to include the missing items in dietary intake or (2) finding an acceptable alternate food that provides the missing nutrients.

ASSESSMENT

The dietary history of a person serves as a useful screening device. The adequacy of the diet in terms of quality and quantity can be quickly estimated by comparing it with recommended patterns of food intake. It may also provide information about unusual or bizarre uses of food, which in turn may be a key factor in the health problem. Examples are hypokalemia associated with excessive intake of licorice or cathartics and fever associated with consumption of a gallon of coffee. These imbalances are rare. Identification of factors affecting nutrition status (for example, faulty dietary habits, inadequate intake, poor absorption, decreased utilization, increased excretion, increased destruction, increased requirements) permits designing an effective treatment program. Treatment may require dietary modifications, medications, and changes in living patterns.

PLANNING

The goals for dietary counseling are determined by the results of the nutritional assessment and the diet prescribed while the patient is hospitalized or to be followed at home.

The definition of "good" food is very personal and is a product of all the experiences associated with food over a lifetime. The major challenge in diet therapy can be summarized as providing "good" food for the person within the limits imposed by health and nutrient needs. One basic principle of learning is that persons learn by building on what they already know. People know about their present dietary intake and are much more likely to learn when taught about how to make changes in their current dietary pattern to meet the diet prescription. Too often diets are imposed on people as though they had no previous experience with food. Instructions for diet modifications should *begin with the person's current food habits* and should *stress the necessary changes to be made.*

The person's history of usual food intake is compared with the appropriate guide for food choice (basic food pattern or therapeutic regimen as described in the diet manuals or nutrition texts). The patient's food consumption in the hospital is observed. Good food practices that should be continued, practices that are neither particularly valuable nor harmful, and practices that need to be changed are identified. Treatment and medications are checked to determine if these affect appetite, nutrient need, meal composition, or frequency. It is determined whether the diet to be followed at home is the same as or different from the current diet.

The special services the person requires need to be coordinated so that schedule conflicts are avoided. For example, some laboratory studies require that patients fast; others require that they eat a special type of test meal. Coordination of laboratory, dietary, and nursing care schedules in such situations is essential to the accuracy of the results and to the patient's comfort. Quite often the need for consultation can be identified by the nurse early in the patient's hospital stay. The consultation can then be scheduled and provided before the day of discharge. The so-called discharge diet instruction is often omitted or rendered useless because it is left until the last minute when the patient's major interest is to get home as quickly as possible.

INTERVENTIONS

The nurse serves as an interpreter to the patient by providing brief and easily understood explanations about the diet, any modifications in it, and the food selections on the tray. The nurse also serves as an interpreter by providing pertinent information about the patient to the physician, dietitian, or food service unit so that the diet prescription or food on the tray provides not only nutrients but also conforms insofar as possible to ethnic, religious, or personal preferences and provides eating pleasure.

APPROACH IN PATIENT TEACHING

One goal of patient education is to provide information so that the person can make informed choices. The final goal, however, is a change in behavior related to food so that the person is well nourished. Even small changes in food behavior can benefit the person. An obese person who reduces caloric intake from 3000 to 2500 calories/day has made a significant behavior change, although one cannot credit the person with complying to a dietary prescription of 1000 calories. The person with inadequate calcium intake may be willing to use milk instead of cream substitutes in coffee. The final goal of dietary adherence is more obtainable when changes are taken in small steps, one at a time. In part this is because the goal is realistic and progress can be measured. In addition, the patient has been involved in setting the goals, and the patient, not the nurse, is the one who must implement the goal.

This approach to patient teaching is more efficient for the therapist and less frustrating for the patient. It is irritating to be lectured on the importance of including milk in the diet when milk and cheese are favorite foods. It can be boring to listen to a description of the evils of salt and calories in potato chips or french-fried potatoes when one never eats them. A patient can say, "Yes, I understand" aloud and in many instances truly understand but not accept the recommendations. Consideration must be given to social, cultural, and economic factors as well as to the person's knowledge of and beliefs about nutrition.

EATING INTERVALS

The convention of three meals a day is just that—a convention and a convenience. For many it is a fiction. Most people eat more often, while the economically deprived may eat only once a day. There may be some advantage to eating smaller meals at shorter intervals as long as total nutrient needs are met. Although physiologic evidence does not support a rigid pattern of three feedings a day, there is evidence that omitting breakfast impairs physiologic and mental efficiency. Except in special circumstances (insulin-dependent diabetes, for example), the number of feedings a day can be determined by the person's desires and life style. If no breakfast is eaten, however, consumption of some food at the beginning of the day should be considered as a desirable goal. Since breakfast is generally the meal most enjoyed by hospitalized patients, this can be a useful mechanism for initiating breakfast as a meal at home as well. Each feeding, whether called a meal or snack, should include a mixture of nutrients.

FOOD COSTS

Cost is an important factor in family food patterns. The nurse, when attempting to teach a person about diet, is frequently challenged about food cost. Vague generalities such as "use cheaper cuts of meat" are not particularly helpful. Suggestions should be specific, based on the person's diet and income. They should provide enough information to serve as a basis of action. The price of an envelope of flavored sugar used by many low-income families to make a beverage is equivalent to the price of enough dried skim milk solids for 1 L of milk. Which is the better buy? Where and how can a person get food stamps? The nurse with personal experience in managing food budgets, purchasing, cookery, and so forth, is in a position to offer practical advice. There are many useful materials available on food purchasing, storage, and preparation. The dietitian will be able to help select the materials that are best for the patient.

In most cases, money spent for food can be reduced and the nutritive value of the diet improved by (1) planning the menu at home, (2) listing kinds and amounts of food to be bought, (3) purchasing items on the list, and (4) controlling waste caused by preparing more food than is needed or from foods spoiling before use.

FOOD LABELING

Food labels can be used as a basis for food choice. Currently many changes are being made in food-labeling practices and regulations governing the use of certain terms describing foods. These changes are designed to improve the nutrition information given on food labels and to provide meaningful information to the public. The nutrition-labeling program is voluntary for most foods; however, if a nutrient is added to any product or if a nutritional claim is made either on the label or in advertising, the product label must have full nutrition labeling. On food labels the levels of vitamins and minerals will be listed as a percentage of the United States recommended daily allowance (US-RDA). To meet the regulations the label must include size of serving, number of servings per container, calories, protein, carbohydrate, fat, and the percentage of the US-RDA for vitamin A, vitamin C, thiamin, riboflavin, niacin, calcium, and iron. Another 12 vitamins and minerals may be listed at the option of the food producer. The US-RDA is based on the standard RDA but is condensed to four categories: infants, children under 4 years of age, adults and children over 4 years of age, and pregnant or lactating women. Consumer memos describing the regulations are available from the Food and Drug Administration. The regulation allows for a statement on the label of cholesterol, total fat, and polyunsaturated and saturated fat. This is helpful for persons on fat-modified diets.

The data in Table 40-13 were taken directly from food labels. One advantage to the system is that information on the label is based on the analysis of the specific brand so that differences in an item such as tuna packed by several different companies can be identified by comparing the labels. The labeling system may be changed, but the concept of nutrition labeling has apparently been accepted. The advantages to persons attempting to control energy intake or modifying protein, fat, or carbohydrate intake are obvious. For those concerned with cost, the attraction of getting more nutritional value for the money may provide motivation for reading labels.

Nutrition labeling does not include the listing of the ingredients. Lists of ingredients are not required on foods covered by "standards of identity" such as mayonnaise, ice cream, or peanut butter. Current regulations require that ingredients be listed in descending order by weight. This does help, although general terms such as "spices," "vegetable oil," or "starch" offer insufficient information for someone who must avoid a particular spice or choose food high in polyunsaturated fat.

Many new products are specifically designed by intent and advertising to replace staple items. Several breakfast drinks are being marketed that look and taste like orange juice and that have been enriched with ascorbic acid so that they may have as much or more ascorbic acid as orange juice. But these breakfast drinks are *high in sodium and low in potassium*, whereas orange juice is low in sodium and high in potassium. A wide variety of substitutes for coffee cream, sour cream, and whipped cream are on the market. They are convenient to use, easy to store, and acceptable in flavor to most people. Can they be used by persons on restricted diets? Many of these products are made from coconut oil, which is a highly saturated fat. Such products can-

TABLE 40-13 Nutrition label as a guide for choosing food

	Tuna Packed in Oil	Chocolate Bar	Skim Milk	Gelatin Dessert
Serving	3¼ oz	1½ oz	1 C	½ C
Servings per container	2	1	4	4
Required				
Calories	230	230	90	80
Protein (g)	22.5	3	8	2*
Fat (g)	15	4	1	0
Carbohydrate (g)	0.5	12	11	18
US-RDA	%	%	%	%
Required listing				
Protein	100	4	20	†
Vitamin A	†	†	10	†
Vitamin C	†	†	4	†
Thiamin	2	2	6	†
Riboflavin	8	6	25	†
Niacin	120	†	†	†
Calcium	†	8	30	†
Iron	8	2	†	†
Optional listing				
Vitamin D			25	
Vitamin B$_6$	25		4	
Vitamin B$_{12}$	45		15	
Vitamin E	10			
Pantothenic acid			6	
Phosphorus			20	
Magnesium			8	
Zinc			4	

*Not a significant source of protein.
†Contains less than 2% of the U.S. recommended daily allowance.

not be recommended as a source of polyunsaturated fat. They are excellent calorie sources, however.

Notice the difference in protein, fat, and carbohydrate in ice cream, ice milk, and sherbet in Figure 40-4. The fat of ice cream is butterfat; that of ice milk is vegetable fat; sherbet is essentially fat free. All contain sucrose. "Diabetic" ice creams substitute other carbohydrates for sucrose and usually have a high fat level to provide good texture. As a result the calorie content of "diabetic" ice creams is often higher than that of conventional ice cream.

The recent renewed interest in nutrition and health has resulted in health claims in labeling and advertising for certain foods. For example, some assert that various foods will prevent disease.[18,20] Some claims focus on fiber intake in relation to cancer and serum cholesterol. Others emphasize low fat–low cholesterol or cholesterol-free diets and low sodium intake in relation to heart disease. Site-of-purchase information on fast

foods, which are generally high in fat and sodium, has also been provided.[21]

FOOD ADDITIVES

The public has become more interested in food and nutrition. The consumer movement has, among other things, focused attention on food processing and food additives. Additives may be foods, derived from foods, or products created in the laboratory. The most widely used food additive is sucrose, ordinary table sugar. Sodium chloride, table salt, is the second. Monosodium glutamate, mustard, and black pepper are food additives used in large quantities also. Most of the current concern about food additives relates to safety. Excessive intake of sugar has been related to obesity, tooth decay, and coronary artery disease; excessive intake of salt has been related to hypertension. Questions have been raised about the safety of nonnutritive sweeteners, nitrates used in curing meats, and antioxidants such as BHT used to keep fat from becoming rancid. The food industry's use of additives is regulated by the Food and Drug Administration. In 1958, the food additives amendment to the Food, Drug, and Cosmetic Act of 1938 was passed; it requires proof of safety before a substance may be added to food. In 1960, the color additive amendment was enacted to control all color additives, natural and synthetic.

Generally recognized as safe (GRAS) substances have been classified by technical effect, and each group is being reviewed for use and safety. One such group is Technical Effect Code 16, leavening agents that include yeast and baking powder. The review for each group is published as completed.

Concern with pesticide residues (as well as food additives) has caused some people to turn to a "natural" or "organic" diet. Some believe that the body can use only nutrients from a natural source despite evidence to the contrary. Others want food that has been grown without the use of chemical fertilizers or pesticides and processed without additives. Foods labeled "organic" or "natural" usually cost more. The terms are not defined by law, and values are being claimed for products without evidence to support them. Current concern with food additives and pesticides has obscured other issues of food safety. It is just as important to be sure that food is free from microbiologic and insect contamination. Foods themselves contain natural substances that can be harmful. Legislation cannot protect the individual from poor food choices or ensure good food handling practices in the home.

MALNUTRITION IN HOSPITALIZED PATIENTS

Malnutrition was identified as the "skeleton in the hospital closet" in 1974.[7] Prevalence was as high as 50% in hospitalized patients, both medical and surgical. The situation has not improved.[15] There is a real possibility that current trends in short-term acute care admissions have increased the number of patients admitted at a severe nutritional advantage because of inadequate nutritional preparation for surgery. The extensive use of TPN does not seem to solve the problem, and it is costly. In addition, DRG (diagnosis related group) practices result in earlier patient discharge. The problem has been attributed to lack of physician awareness and inadequate nutritional education. One solution is a program of physician education, greater nutrition risk screening, and greater use of dietitians for monitoring and education.

The nurse should be alert to the risk of malnutrition in patients. Good nutritional status is essential. It enables the patient to withstand debilitation from illness and trauma, and it provides the raw materials required by the body for healing. Many hospital practices actually reduce body stores of nutrients and impair status. Every time blood is drawn for tests or lost by bleeding, the need for iron, protein, copper, folate and so forth is increased. Every time a patient is held NPO for tests or procedures, needed nutritional supplies are not being replenished. The patient nauseated from illness, medication, or radiation has an increased need for nutrients from the food that is not eaten. Loss of appetite is a common effect of surgery.

Hospitals use many different protocols to calculate body compartments of muscle and fat and degrees of malnutrition.[9] In spite of this, some patients still enter the hospital reasonably well-nourished and then develop malnutrition. Esoteric tests are not always needed. The observant nurse can determine the patient's risk. Look at the patient. Is weight appropriate for height? Is weight being lost or gained? Is the patient being served enough food to meet needs? Is the patient eating the food? If a tube feeding is used, is it being administered at an appropriate rate? Is the diet order more restrictive than necessary? One cause of malnutrition could be due to the patient's inability to read and mark a selective menu.

Nutrition promotion and malnutrition prevention are concepts that can make a profound difference in a patient's ability to recover from trauma and illness. The nurse can help make that "skeleton in the hospital closet" disappear.

CHAPTER SUMMARY

- National nutrition objectives include specific goals for improvement of health status, reduction of risk factors, and improvement services.

- Dietary recommendations include reducing fats (especially saturated), cholesterol, sodium, and alcohol; increasing intake of complex carbohydrates (CHO), fiber, vegetables, and fruits; and maintaining protein

and calcium intake (increasing calcium intake in adolescent girls and women).

- All persons need the same nutrients throughout life; the amounts required vary in predictable patterns.

- Excess dietary supplementation of vitamins and minerals may cause harm; continued intake at levels from 10 to 100 times the RDA is associated with chronic toxicity.

- People of similar size have similar basal energy requirements; the total energy requirement varies depending on physical activity.

- Good nutrition requires a balanced complement of protein and calories. Protein not needed for synthesis is used for fuel; protein may be used for fuel rather than for synthesis if energy intake is insufficient.

- A dietary history includes the person's usual eating patterns (including likes and dislikes) and changes; financial resources; facilities for purchasing, storing, and preparing food; daily activities; problems with diet; and weight perception and changes.

- Daily food guides are good tools for a rapid evaluation of nutrient intake. Food groups include vegetables and fruits; bread, cereals, and other grain products; milk and other dairy products; and meat, poultry, fish, and beans.

- Signs of malnutrition can be noted in the hair, face, eyes, lips, tongue, teeth, gums, glands, skin, nails, muscular and skeletal systems, and weight-for-height changes.

- Routine tests that may be used in the diagnosis of malnutrition include urinalysis for protein, glucose, and aceteone; and serum level tests of hemoglobin (iron), hematocrit, protein, and cholesterol.

- Therapeutic diets should provide all essential nutrients and be flexible, designed around the person's usual patterns of daily living. Feeding by mouth is always the method of choice when possible.

- Prescribed protein intake is increased for persons with protein losses from tissue catabolism, bleeding, and exudates; it is decreased when the kidney is in failure and cannot process waste products. Certain conditions require control of specific amino acids in the diet.

- Fat intake is decreased for the patient with gallbladder disease. Modifications in saturated and unsaturated fatty acids may be prescribed to alter serum lipid levels.

- Carbohydrate intake is modified for persons with diabetes mellitus. Lactose may be eliminated from the diets of persons with lactase deficiency.

- A sufficient calorie intake is important for surgical

patients, the elderly, and patients on long-term therapies such as chemotherapy or radiation.

✔ Sodium restriction is one of the most commonly prescribed dietary modifications for persons with hypertension, fluid retention, congestive heart failure, or kidney disease.

✔ Potassium intake may be modified for persons with electrolyte imbalances.

✔ Dietary prescriptions may include modifications in food consistency (liquid, pureed, soft), amounts of foods, and methods of administration.

✔ The goal of nutritional education is to provide information so the patient can make informed choices. Topics include (in addition to dietary modifications) frequency of eating, costs of food, and the need to read food labels.

✔ Malnutrition is a major problem for hospitalized patients. Many hospital practices actually reduce body stores of nutrients and impair status.

QUESTIONS TO CONSIDER

- How could the Daily Food Guide be used to plan meals for persons of different ethnic origins, such as Italian, Mexican, Greek, or Vietnamese?

- Examine the charts of several hospitalized patients. In what ways has their nutritional status been threatened? For what potential problems does this place each patient at risk?

- Examine dietary resources on your hospital division. What information is available for your use in patient care and for patient teaching?

REFERENCES AND SELECTED READINGS

1. *Alhadeff L et al: Toxic effects of water-soluble vitamins, Nutr Rev 42:33-40, 1984.
2. American Cancer Society: Taking control: ten steps to a healthier life and reduced cancer risk, Publ 85-2MM, no 2019.05, New York, 1985, The Society.
3. American Dietetic Association: Position paper on identifying food and nutrition misinformation, J Am Diet Assoc 88:1589-1591, 1988.
4. *American Dietetic Association: Position paper on issues in feeding the terminally ill adult, J Am Diet Assoc 87:78-85, 1987.
5. *American Dietetic Association: Position paper on nutrition, aging, and the continuum of health care, J Am Diet Assoc 87:344-347,1987.
6. *American Dietetic Association: Position paper on vegetarian diets, J Am Diet Assoc 88:351-355,1988.
7. †Butterworth CE: The skeleton in the hospital closet, Nutr Today 9:4-8, 1974.
8. *Calcium: how much is too much? Nutr Rev 43:345-346, 1985.
9. Cerra FB: Pocket manual of surgical nutrition, St Louis, 1984, The CV Mosby Co.
10. †Christakis G: Nutritional assessment in health programs, Am J Public Health 63(suppl):1-82, 1973.
11. Copper deficiency induced by megadoses of zinc, Nutr Rev 43:148-149, 1985.
12. Creasy WA: Diet and cancer, Philadelphia, 1985, Lea & Febiger.
13. †Deutsch RM: The new nut among the berries, Palo Alto, Calif, 1977, Bull Publishing Co.
14. *Expert Panel: Report of the National Cholesterol Education Program Expert Panel on Detection, Evaluation and Treatment of High Blood Cholesterol in Adults, Arch Intern Med 148:36-69, 1988.
15. Hospital malnutrition still abounds, Nutr Rev 46:315-317, 1988.
16. *Iber FL et al: Thiamin in the elderly: relation to alcoholism and neurological degenerative disease, Am J Clin Nutr 36:1067-1082, 1982.
17. †Jellife DB: The assessment of the nutritional status of the community, WHO memograph no 53, Geneva, 1966, World Health Organization.
18. Kessler DA: The federal regulations of food labeling: promoting foods to prevent disease, New Eng J Med 321:717-725, 1989.
19. Koplan JP et al: Nutrient intake and supplementation in the United States (NHANES II), Am J Public Health 76:287-289, 1986.
20. Marwick C: Changes brewing for food labels as national concern about diet and health continues to grow, JAMA 262:2354-2355, 1989.
21. *Massachusetts Medical Society Committee on Nutrition: Fast-food fare: consumer guidelines, New Eng J Med 321:752-755, 1989.
22. *Mutch PB: Food guides for the vegetarian, AM J Clin Nutr 48:913-919, 1988.
23. National Center for Health Statistics: Advance report of final mortality statistics, 1987, Monthly Vital Statistics Report 38 (suppl 5):1, Sept 26, 1989.
24. National Institutes of Health: Lowering blood cholesterol to prevent heart disease, National Institutes of Health Consensus Development Conference Statement, vol 5, no 7, Washington, DC, 1985, NIH.
25. National Institutes of Health: Health implications of obesity, National Institutes of Health Consensus Development Conference Statement, vol 5, no 9, Washington, DC, 1985, NIH.
26. National Research Council: Diet and Health: Implications of reducing chronic disease risk, report of the Committee on Diet and Health, Food and Nutrition Board, National Academy Press, Washington, DC, 1989, The Council.
27. National Research Council: Recommended dietary allowances, ed 10, National Academy Press, Washington, DC, 1989, The Council.
28. Nutrient toxicity: special report, Nutr Rev 39:249-256, 1981.
29. Nutrition Committee: Position statement: dietary guidelines for healthy American adults; a statement for physicians and health professionals, Pub No 71-1003, Dallas, 1988, American Heart Association.
30. Nutritional requirements of man: a conspectus of research

*References preceded by an asterisk are particularly well suited for student reading.
†References preceded by a dagger are classic readings.

from the Journal of Nutrition, Washington, DC, 1980, The Nutrition Foundation.

31. Pennington JAT: Bowes and Church's food values of portions commonly used, ed 15, Philadelphia, 1989, JB Lippincott Co.

32. Promoting health/preventing disease: objectives for the nation, Washington, DC, Fall 1980, Public Health Service, Department of Health and Human Services.

33. Promoting health/preventing disease: year 2000 objectives for the nation, draft for public review and comment. Washington, DC, September 1989, Department of Health and Human Services.

34. Sandmaier M: The healthy heart handbook for women, National Institutes of Health Pub No 87-2720, Washington, DC, 1987, NIH.

35. Schneider EL et al: Recommended dietary allowances and the health of the elderly, N Eng J Med 314:157-160, 1986.

36. †Scrimshaw NS: Through a glass darkly: discerning the practical implications of human dietary protein-energy interrelationships, Nutr Rev 35:321-337, 1977.

37. Surgeon General's report on nutrition and health, DHHS (PHS) Pub No 88-50210, Washington, DC, 1988, Department of Health and Human Services.

38. US Department of Agriculture: The hassle-free daily food guide, Washington DC, 1980, US Superintendent of Documents.

39. US Department of Agriculture, Human Nutrition Information Service: Nutrition and your health: dietary guidelines for Americans; eat a variety of foods, Home and Garden Bulletin No 232-1, Washington DC, 1986, US Superintendent of Documents.

40. US Department of Agriculture and the US Department of Health and Human Services: Nutrition and your health: dietary guidelines for Americans, ed 2, Washington, DC, 1985, US Superintendent of Documents.

41. Welsh SO and Marston RM: Review of trends in food use in the United States, 1909 to 1980, J Am Diet Assoc 81:120, 1982.

42. †Wishnofsky M: Calorie equivalents of gained or lost weight, Am J Clin Nutr 6:542-546, 1958.

43. Wright RA, Heymsfield S, and McManus CB: Nutritional assessment, Boston, 1984, Blackwell Scientific Publications Inc.

44. †Young, CM et al: Comparison of dietary study methods: dietary history vs seven-day records vs 24-hr recall, J Am Diet Assoc 28:218-221, 1952.

CHAPTER 41

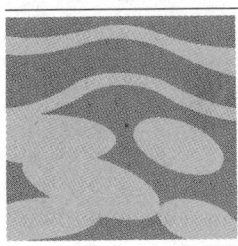

Assessment of the Gastrointestinal System

BARBARA C. LONG

CHAPTER OBJECTIVES

After studying this chapter, the student should be able to:
1 Describe the functions of the mouth, esophagus, stomach, and intestines.
2 Identify secretions of the gastrointestinal tract involved in the digestion of carbohydrates, fats, and proteins.
3 Describe the gastrointestinal changes that occur with aging.
4 Recognize subjective and objective data pertinent to nursing assessment of the gastrointestinal system.
5 Identify useful data that is obtained from diagnostic tests for problems of the gastrointestinal tract, and describe nursing responsibilities associated with the tests.

Maintenance of adequate nutrition and elimination requires a functioning gastrointestinal tract. Normally, food and fluids are placed in the mouth, pushed to the pharynx by the tongue, and swallowed by automatic reflex activity down the esophagus into the stomach. Digestion starts in the mouth and terminates in the small intestine, although fluids continue to be reabsorbed in the colon. Abnormalities that interfere with passage of food will interfere with nutrition; therefore assessment of nutrition requires assessment of the gastrointestinal tract. Healthy functioning also requires elimination of the waste materials without loss of excessive fluid or electrolytes.

This chapter provides a brief review of the anatomy and physiology of the gastrointestinal (GI) tract, subjective and objective data that are pertinent to GI functioning, and diagnostic tests.

ANATOMY AND PHYSIOLOGY

The upper gastrointestinal tract consists of those structures that aid in the ingestion and digestion of food, namely, the mouth, esophagus, stomach, and duodenum (Figure 41-1). The subconscious or actively conscious thought of food initiates the physiologic re-

sponses of the body that are ultimately responsible for delivery of a particular nutrient to the individual cell. The hypothalamus is responsible for notifying the body that it is satisfied or has received sufficient food.

The lower gastrointestinal tract consists of the small and large intestines. Digestion is completed in the small intestine and most of the nutrients are absorbed in this organ. The large intestine serves primarily to absorb water and electrolytes and to eliminate the waste products of digestion.

MOUTH
SALIVATION

The cortical thought regarding "food" initiates saliva production from the parotid, submaxillary, buccal, and sublingual glands. The salivary secretions are made up of *serous* secretion, containing ptyalin for starch digestion (produced by the parotid and submaxillary glands), and *mucous* secretion for lubrication (produced by the buccal, sublingual, and submaxillary glands). These two secretions account for one half of the upper gastrointestinal tract secretions.

MASTICATION

The teeth serve the function of initial food breakdown. No other part of the gastrointestinal tract can perform this function if the teeth are missing. Enzymes can act only on the exposed surfaces of the food particles. Very fine particulation prevents excoriation of the lining of the tract, and the rate of digestion depends on the total surface area of food particle exposed.[5] General health teaching for children and adults should stress the reason behind thorough mastication of all food substances that are ingested.

The structures of the mouth are illustrated on p. 1239. The major structures that aid ingestion and digestion are the teeth, to grind the food; the salivary glands, to moisten food and mucous membranes and begin carbohydrate digestion; and the tongue, to push the food to the pharynx to initiate swallowing.

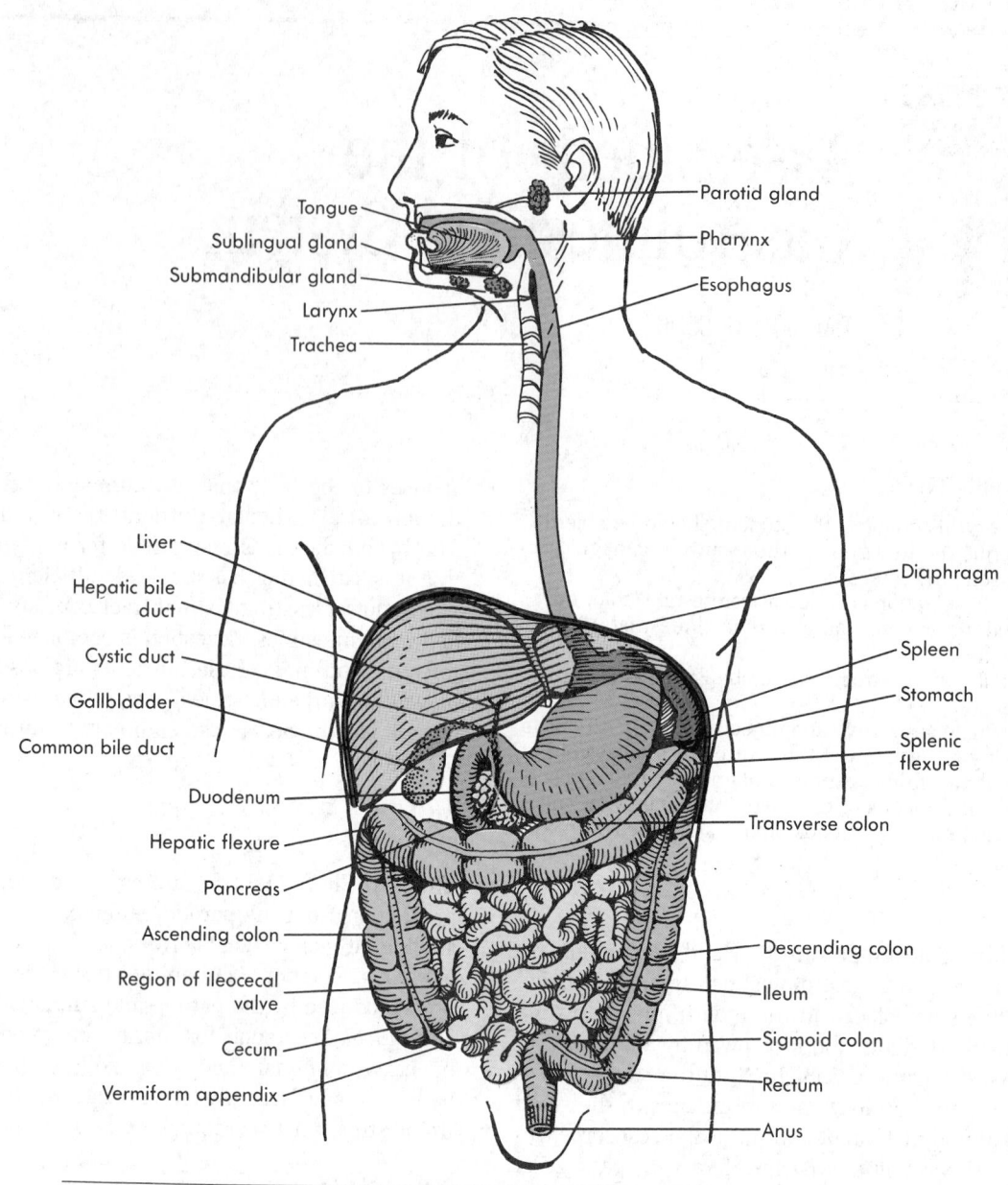

FIGURE 41-1 Organs of the digestive system and various structures.

ESOPHAGUS
STRUCTURE

The esophagus is a hollow tube, the upper one third is composed of skeletal muscle and the remainder is smooth muscle. It is lined with mucous membrane, which secretes a mucoid substance for protection. The bolus of food arrives at the cardiac sphincter of the stomach within 5 to 10 seconds of ingestion.[5]

The cardiac sphincter prevents reflux of stomach contents back into the lower esophagus. This area is heavily layered with mucoid glands. The secretions adhere to the food particles and prevent actual contact

with the wall mucosa. The coated particles adhere to each other, forming a bolus for digestion. These secretions act as a protective mechanism for the sphincter zone because they themselves are strongly resistant to digestion.

DEGLUTITION

Swallowing (deglutition) must be accomplished without compromising respiration. It consists of three phases: a voluntary phase in which the tongue forces the bolus of food into the pharynx, an involuntary pharyngeal phase in which the food moves into the upper esophagus, and an esophageal phase during which food moves from the pharynx down into the stomach. Food is prevented from passing into the trachea by the closing of the trachea and the opening of the esophagus.

STOMACH
STRUCTURE

The stomach and remainder of the gastrointestinal tract are made up of five layers of smooth muscle. This smooth muscle has two types of contractions: (1) *tonus* contractions, which are continuous and which determine both the amount of steady pressure exerted within the area and the degree of resistance to the movement of food at the sphincter, and (2) *rhythmic* contractions, which may be either as slow as every 2 to 3 minutes or very rapid and which are responsible for the mixing of the food and for peristaltic propulsion.

The entire tract is innervated through the intramural plexus, which begins in the wall of the esophagus and extends through the anus. The plexus is composed of two layers, *Auerbach's* plexus and *Meissner's* plexus. Stimulation to the plexus increases the tonic contractions and the intensity and rate of rhythmic contractions.[5] Innervation is accomplished through the vagus nerve and comprises both sympathetic and parasympathetic fibers.

MOVEMENT

The food bolus enters the stomach, the largest dilated portion of the tract. There is relatively little muscular tone, allowing for increased distention. Movement of food through the stomach and intestines is by *peristalsis*, the alternate contraction and relaxation of muscle fibers that propels the substance in a wavelike motion. The mucous membrane lining of the stomach is arranged in thick folds known as *rugae*. These rugae provide an increased surface area for exposure and contain the gastric pit openings from the fundic, pyloric, and cardiac glands.

As the food moves toward the pyloric sphincter, peristaltic waves increase in force and intensity. The fluid mass now becomes known as *chyme* (Figure 41-2). Chyme is pumped through the pyloric sphincter into the duodenum. Emptying of stomach contents is regulated by two factors: *consistency* of the fluid chyme and the *receptiveness* of the duodenum.[5] The pyloric sphincter activity stops with vagal stimulation of the *enterogastric* reflex. This sphincter activity is also slowed when the chyme requires an increased time for digestion (as in the case of fatty foods or high levels of protein).

SECRETION

The digestive function of the stomach is controlled by two hormones, gastrin and enterogastrone (Table 41-1). Gastrin secretion is activated by the smell or taste of food and by protein foods entering the stomach. It stimulates the flow of gastric juice, which has a high pepsin and hydrochloric acid content. The production of gastric secretions decreases when the pH falls and as enterogastrone is released from the small intestine. Protein digestion begins in the stomach.

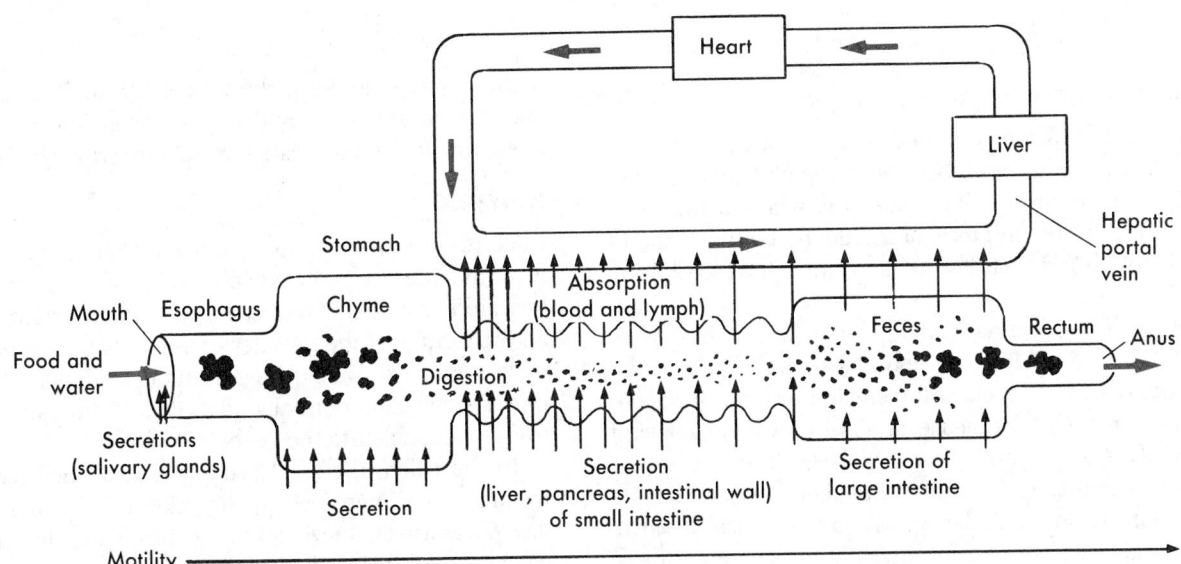

FIGURE 41-2 Summary of gastrointestinal activity involving motility, secretion, digestion, and absorption. (From Vander AJ et al: Human physiology, ed 4, Copyright © 1985 by McGraw-Hill Book Co, New York. Used with the permission of McGraw-Hill Book Co.)

TABLE 41-1 Gastrointestinal secretions

Secretion	Type	Action
ENTIRE GASTROINTESTINAL TRACT		
Mucus		Increases food adhesion Prevents contact of food with mucosal wall Enhances free passage of food Neutralizes small amounts of acids and alkali Makes some food particles more resistant to digestion
MOUTH		
Salivary amylase (ptyalin)	Enzyme	Catalyzes hydrolysis of starch into dextrins (first step in carbohydrate digestion)
STOMACH		
Gastrin	Hormone	Stimulates flow of gastric acid and pepsin
Pepsin	Enzyme	Catalyzes hydrolysis of protein into polypeptides (first step in protein digestion)
Renin	Enzyme	Catalyzes conversion of soluble casein in milk to insoluble form
SMALL INTESTINES		
Enterogastrone	Hormone	Inhibits gastric secretion and mobility
Secretin	Hormone	Stimulates pancreatic exocrine secretion Stimulates (weakly) production of bile and other intestinal secretions
Cystokinin-pancreozymin (CCK-PZ)	Hormone	Stimulates pancreatic exocrine secretion Stimulates bile flow into duodenum
Enterokinase	Enzyme	Converts pancreatic trypsinogen into trypsin, which splits proteins into peptides and amino acids
INTESTINAL JUICE (INTESTINAL MUCOSA)		
Lactase	Enzyme	Hydrolyzes lactose (milk sugar) into glucose and galactose
Maltase	Enzyme	Hydrolyzes maltose (malt sugar) into glucose
Sucrase	Enzyme	Catalyzes splitting of sucrose (cane sugar) into glucose and fructose
PANCREAS (EXOCRINE)		
Amylase	Enzyme	Hydrolyzes starch into maltose, lactose, and sucrose
Lipase	Enzyme	Catalyzes splitting of fats into glycerol and fatty acids

INTESTINES
STRUCTURE

The small intestine is about 2.5 cm (1 inch) wide and 6 m (20 feet) long and fills most of the abdomen. It consists of three parts—the *duodenum*, which connects to the stomach; the *jejunum* or middle portion; and the *ileum*, which connects to the large intestine (see Figure 41-1).

The large intestine is about 6 cm (2½ inches) wide and 1.5 (5 feet) long. It consists of three parts—the *cecum*, which connects to the small intestine; the *colon*; and the *rectum*. The ileocecal valve prevents backward flow of fecal contents from the large intestine to the small intestine. The vermiform appendix, which has no function, is an appendage close to the ileocecal valve. The *colon* consists of four parts—the ascending, transverse, descending, and sigmoid colons. The points at which the colon changes direction are named for adjacent organs—the liver (hepatic flexure) and the spleen (splenic flexure). The *rectum* is 17 to 20 cm (7 to 8 inches) long, ending in the 2 to 3 cm anal canal. The opening (anus) is controlled by a smooth muscle internal sphincter and a striated muscle external sphincter.

MOVEMENT

Contents of the small intestine (*chyme*) are propelled toward the anus by peristaltic movement, that is, wavelike forward movements produced by alternating contraction and relaxation of the muscles of the intestinal wall. This movement also mixes the intestinal contents. Chyme moves slowly and normally takes 3 to 10 hours to move from the stomach to the ileocecal valve.

In the colon, the fecal contents are pushed forward by mass movements occurring only a few times each day. These mass movements are stimulated by gastrocolic reflexes initiated when food enters the duodenum from the stomach, especially after the first meal of the day. This is therefore the most frequent time of the day for defecation to occur.

The *defecation* reflex occurs when feces enter the

rectum. Afferent impulses are transmitted to the sacral segments of the spinal cord from which reflex impulses are transmitted back to the colon, sigmoid, and rectum, initiating relaxation of the internal anal sphincter.

SECRETION AND DIGESTION

The major portion of digestion occurs in the small intestines by the action of pancreatic and intestinal secretions and by bile. These secretions are stimulated by the hormones secretin and cystokinin-pancreozymin (CCK-PZ) (Table 41-1).

The digestion of *carbohydrate* begins in the mouth, where the breakdown of polysaccharides to disaccharides occurs by the action of amylase. The disaccharides are then broken down into monosaccharides (glucose, galactose, and fructose) by the action of the enzymes within the intestinal mucosa and by pancreatic amylase.

Protein digestion begins in the stomach with the breakdown of proteins into polypeptides (an intermediate step) by the action of pepsin. In the small intestines, the polypeptides are further broken down by trypsin (which has been converted from pancreatic trypsinogen by enterokinase) into peptides and amino acids.

Fat requires emulsification into small droplets before it can be broken down into glycerol and fatty acids. Some fats that are already emulsified, such as cream and butter, may begin to be digested by a small amount of lipase in the stomach. Most fat digestion, however, occurs in the small intestines with the emulsification by bile and action of pancreatic lipase.

ABSORPTION

The intestinal wall has many folds, which are covered by fingerlike projections (villi). Epithelial cells cover the surface of each villus, and each cell has several microvilli projecting from its surface. The intestinal folds, villi, and microvilli thus greatly increase the absorptive area of the small intestine. In the center of each villi is a blind-end lymph vessel (lacteal) for absorption into the lymphatic system. The lacteal is surrounded by capillaries, venules, and arterioles for absorption into the portal blood system (Figure 41-3).

Ninety percent of absorption occurs within the small intestine either by active transport or diffusion. Many nutrients, such as amino acids, monosaccharides, sodium, and calcium, are transported by active transport, requiring metabolic energy expenditure. Other nutrients, such as fatty acids and water, diffuse passively across the cell membrane. Pancreatic lipase and conjugated bile salts must be present in the intestinal lumen for hydrolysis of fats into fatty acids to permit diffusion across the cell membranes of the villi.

Approximately 450 ml of chyme reaches the cecum per day. The transit time in the large bowel is slow, taking about 12 hours for material to reach the rectum. Re-

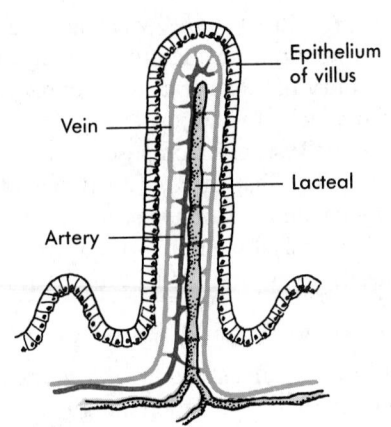

FIGURE 41-3 Intestinal villus. Note the circulatory vessels surrounding the lacteal, which drains into the lymphatic system.

absorption of water, electrolytes, and bile salts occurs predominantly in the ascending colon. The colon has the capacity to absorb six to eight times more fluid than is delivered to it daily. Approximately 100 ml of fluid contents remains to be mixed with the residue of feces. Normally, this residue (*feces*) is evacuated on a fairly regular schedule. This schedule differs for each individual and may vary from daily evacuation to evacuation every 3 to 4 days.

FLUID AND ELECTROLYTE BALANCE

The gastrointestinal tract secretes approximately 8 L of fluid daily, most of which is normally absorbed. These secretions have a high electrolyte content; for example, gastric juice contains ten times, and intestinal secretions two times, the amount of potassium found in serum. Severe fluid and electrolyte imbalances may occur with excessive losses of gastrointestinal fluids (see Chapter 23). The deficits most commonly encountered include the following:

1. Sodium and potassium deficits: vomiting, diarrhea, gastric suctioning, intestinal fistulas
2. Calcium and magnesium deficits: malnutrition (malabsorption), intestinal fistulas
3. Metabolic alkalosis: loss of gastric acid by gastric suctioning or persistent vomiting
4. Metabolic acidosis: loss of bicarbonate-rich intestinal secretions by severe diarrhea or intestinal fistulas

OTHER FUNCTIONS OF THE GI TRACT

In addition to its role in nutrition and fluid balance, the GI tract supports bacterial growth and has a role in antibody formation. Intestinal bacteria synthesize vitamin K which, in addition to dietary vitamin K, is required for production of clotting factors II (prothrombin), VII, IX, and X (Chapter 30). Patients who have severe malabsorption or who are receiving antibiotic enemas that destroy the intestinal bacteria may experience severe bleeding from lack of vitamin K.

The immune system is composed of two elements, B cells and T cells (Chapter 8). The B cells, from which the immunoglobulins (antibodies) develop, are manufactured in organized lymphoid tissue located in lymph nodes, spleen, lungs, and the *GI tract*.

PHYSIOLOGIC CHANGES WITH AGING

Gastrointestinal changes occur with aging but do not necessarily interfere with functioning.

In the mouth, aging teeth become darker and may loosen from loss of supporting bone and gums. Teeth may become uneven or develop fractures, and circulation of the gums is reduced. Gum changes affect the fit of dentures. Salivary gland output decreases, leading to increased dryness of mucous membranes and making them more susceptible to breakdown. Dryness of the mouth may also interfere with chewing.

Changes in the ability to digest and absorb foods are related to decreased secretion of most digestive enzymes and bile production. Absorption of fats and fat-soluble vitamins becomes impaired. The increased residue resulting from decreased digestion and absorption may lead to increased flatulence. Gas-forming foods may be less well tolerated than they were when the person was younger.

Decreased intestinal motility may result from decreased peristalsis, decreased muscular tone of the intestinal wall, and decreased abdominal muscle strength. Decreased anal sphincter tone may also be present. These changes contribute to the increased occurrence of constipation in the older person.

SUBJECTIVE DATA

Data from the health history that are pertinent to gastrointestinal functioning are listed in the box. Because people may feel more comfortable about answering embarrassing questions after some rapport has been established, questions about bowel habits are usually placed in the latter part of a total health history.

DENTAL PROSTHESES

All persons should be asked about the presence of dental prostheses. It is important to ascertain if the person has any artificial dentures (bridges or partial or full plates), if the prosthesis is being worn, and if it fits and is comfortable. Chewing and digestion can be impaired if the person does not wear the prosthesis. If the teeth are noted to have caries during the physical inspection of the mouth, data are obtained concerning regularity of dental checkups for use in health teaching.

NURSING HISTORY: GASTROINTESTINAL DATA

1. General data
   a. Presence of dental prosthesis, comfort
   b. Difficulty eating or digesting food
   c. Nausea or vomiting
   d. Weight loss
   e. Pain
2. Specific data if symptoms are present
   a. Situations or events that affect symptoms
   b. Onset, possible cause, location, duration, character of symptoms
   c. Relationship of specific foods, smoking, or alcohol to severity of symptoms
   d. How the problem was managed before seeking assistance of a health care provider
3. Normal pattern of bowel elimination
   a. Frequency and character of the stool
   b. Use of measures to encourage evacuation (for example, specific food, laxatives, and enemas)
4. Recent changes in normal pattern
   a. Changes in character of stool (for example, constipation, diarrhea, or alternating constipation and diarrhea)
   b. Changes in color of stool (if bleeding is present: stool mixed or streaked with blood, amount, rectal bleeding after evacuation, menstruation present)
   c. Drugs or medications being taken, if changes in elimination are present
   d. Measures taken to relieve symptoms

NAUSEA AND VOMITING

Nausea and vomiting may be caused by a gastrointestinal problem such as gastritis or by a number of other factors unrelated to pathologic conditions of the upper gastrointestinal tract. These may include side effects of drugs, fluid and electrolyte imbalances, or radiation effects.

WEIGHT LOSS

Weight loss may be caused by a pathologic condition, nausea and vomiting, anorexia, or deliberate action on the part of the person to lose weight. Gradual weight loss and lack of appetite in the older person are not necessarily abnormal findings but are worth investigating.

PAIN

Pain is frequently the reason given when people seek medical attention, despite the fact that pain by itself is not an early or common symptom of gastrointestinal disease. Pain may be reported in the mouth, throat, upper abdomen, or rectal area. Abdominal pain may be specifically directed to one particular quadrant or may be referred to another somatic or skeletal part that shares the same innervation. (See Chapter 16 for a description of referred pain sites.) The pain sensation is thought to arise from the distention or sudden contraction of a hollow viscus; therefore local stretching or traction on pain-sensitive structures will elicit the pain stimulus. The painful area may demonstrate local muscle guarding, which serves as a protective mechanism as the overlying muscles contract.

Abdominal pain or discomfort may be reported as heartburn, indigestion, or stomach ache and requires further clarification. The pain may interfere with chewing or swallowing food. Specific foods, such as spicy foods or very hot or cold foods, alcohol, or smoking may initiate or aggravate the pain. Abdominal pain may have been self-treated with commercial antacids.

BOWEL PATTERNS

Normal patterns of evacuation vary greatly. Problems may exist without the person's awareness; therefore all persons are asked what their normal pattern is, if they take anything to maintain this pattern, and if they have noticed any changes in this pattern.

Constipation is identified by small, hard dry stools passed with difficulty and usually at infrequent intervals, although a person may pass a constipated stool every day. Data concerning the frequency of bowel elimination are obtained from all hospitalized persons at the time of admission; this serves as a baseline against which subsequent elimination is compared. Continued assessment of frequency is also indicated for all persons

who are inactive or who have fluid or diet restriction, because they have a high potential for developing constipation or fecal impaction. Information concerning measures used frequently by the person to help maintain normal bowel elimination will provide data for health teaching.

Changes in the normal pattern of bowel elimination may indicate a physiologic deviation, such as constipation, or a pathologic deviation, such as enteritis (inflammation of the bowel) or cancer. Diarrhea and stools containing mucus, pus, and possible undigested food may indicate enteritis or invasion by a parasite. Alternation of diarrhea and constipation may occur as a result of cancer of the colon. Partial obstruction of the descending colon may produce small ribbon-shaped stools, whereas no stool will be passed if obstruction is complete. Diarrhea and constipation may also occur as a result of medical therapy or surgical intervention.

Bright red blood in the stool indicates lower gastrointestinal bleeding. Blood from the upper gastrointestinal tract is changed by digestive secretions, and the stool appears black and sticky (tarry). Blood in the stool (*melena*) may be a recent or a chronic symptom and may result from erosion of the mucosa, leading to perforation of the muscle wall or rupture of a blood vessel.

OBJECTIVE DATA

MOUTH AND PHARYNX

Physical examination of the mouth (Figure 41-4) will provide data indicating ability to salivate, masticate, and swallow, as well as signs of local or systemic disease that can interfere with nutrition. A tongue blade and flashlight are needed for the examination of the oral cavity. The person should be seated comfortably on a level with the examiner and should remove any dental appliances and makeup.

LIPS

The lips are observed for symmetry in form and function and for color, moisture, swelling, cracks, or lesions. Asymmetry is often accompanied by drooling and may be the result of facial nerve paralysis from peripheral or central nervous system involvement. If asymmetry is noted, the ability to masticate and swallow is assessed.

The lips are normally reddish in color and are good indicators of pallor or cyanosis. Dryness may indicate dehydration. Swelling is usually the result of edema of the inflammatory response such as with allergy. Cracks or fissures can occur with overdryness or exposure to cold or, if in the corners of the mouth (*angular stomatitis*), from lack of dentures, poorly fitting dentures, or a riboflavin deficiency.

Lesions may be benign or malignant. A frequently encountered benign lesion is *herpes simplex* (cold sore,

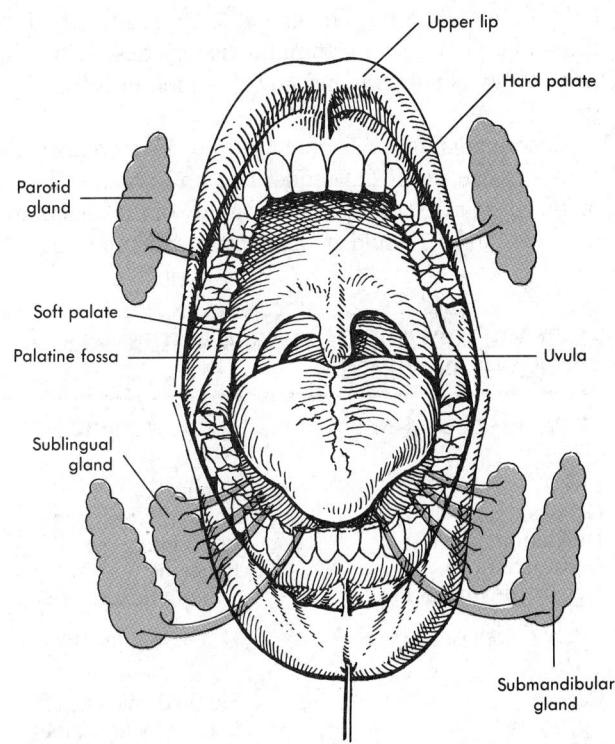

Upper lip

Hard palate

Parotid gland

Soft palate

Palatine fossa

Uvula

Sublingual gland

Submandibular gland

FIGURE 41-4 Structures of the mouth.

fever blister), which is caused by a virus and which can create enough discomfort to limit mastication. Any lesion on the lip that does not heal should be referred to the physician for tests for possible malignancy.

TEETH

A full set of teeth consists of 20 teeth in children and 32 teeth in adults. The enamel surface should be white but will darken with surface stains (tea, coffee, tobacco). Commonly found abnormalities include caries; loose teeth; absence of some or all teeth; failure of a tooth to erupt, resulting in swelling and possible discomfort; and worn crown surfaces. These conditions may impair adequate mastication.

GUMS

The gums, or *gingivae,* are normally pink in color, attach to the teeth, and fill the interdental surfaces. If the person is edentulous, the gingivae are examined for areas of redness caused by improperly fitting dentures. The person is then asked to insert the dentures to assess correct fit and comfort for adequate mastication. Recession of the gum line is not uncommon in older individuals. Bleeding of the gums may occur with improper tooth brushing, dental calculus, aspirin (because of anticoagulant properties), oral infections, or blood dyscrasias. Painful gums may interfere with mastication.

MUCOSA

The mucosa is light pink, although patchy pigmentation is seen in black individuals.[1] In the older person the mucosa may appear shiny as a result of a thinner, less vascular surface. The mucosa is examined for moisture, white spots or patches, debris, areas of bleeding, or ulcers. Dryness and debris may indicate dehydration. White curdy patches, which are removable with some effort, may be caused by *candidiasis* (thrush). White nonremovable patches (leukoplakia), white plaques within red patches, or red granular patches may be premalignant lesions and should be reported to the physician. A round or oval white ulcer surrounded by an area of redness is indicative of an *aphthous ulcer* (canker sore). The orifice of the parotid gland can be observed on the buccal mucosa near the upper second molar; inflammation of the parotid gland occurs with mumps.

PHARYNX

When the tongue is depressed with a tongue blade and the person says "Ah," the soft palate is observed for symmetry (necessary for effective swallowing). The uvula, soft palate, tonsils, and posterior pharynx are observed for signs of inflammation (redness, edema, ulceration, thick yellowish secretions). The size of the uvula is also noted; a swollen uvula can cause pain and can limit swallowing.

TONGUE

Tongue mobility and function are essential to mastication, taste, and swallowing. Normally, there is no limitation in movement in any direction, but the tongue will deviate to the paralyzed side with paralysis of the twelfth cranial (hypoglossal) nerve. A thin white coating and presence of large papillae on the dorsum of the tongue are normal findings. A thick coating indicates poor oral hygiene, and a smooth red surface suggests a nutritional deficiency. The ventral surface is examined for leukoplakia, ulceration, or nodules, any of which may indicate malignancy.

BREATH

Any distinctive odor of the breath is noted. A foul odor, *fetor oris,* may occur with poor hygiene or with dental or oral infections. Odor may occur after the ingestion of certain foods, such as garlic or alcohol, or with some systemic diseases (odor of acetone with diabetes, ammonia with liver disease).

JAWS

Normally the mandible will slide forward and down with ease. A normal "cracking" sound may be heard when the mouth is opened widely. Limitation of motion will affect mastication.

ABDOMEN

Examination of the abdomen may vary with different individuals because signs are often found that require alteration in technique. The examination is supported by the attainment of a meaningful history describing the nature and site of pain and any alteration in bowel habits.

Examination of the abdomen will determine the presence or absence of (1) tenderness, (2) organ enlargement, (3) masses, (4) spasm or rigidity of the abdominal muscles, and (5) fluid or air in the abdominal cavity.

ANATOMIC LOCATION OF VISCERA WITHIN EACH ABDOMINAL QUADRANT

RIGHT UPPER QUADRANT (RUQ)	**LEFT UPPER QUADRANT (LUQ)**
Liver	Stomach
Gallbladder	Spleen
Duodenum	Left kidney
Right kidney	Pancreas
Hepatic flexure of colon	Splenic flexure of colon

RIGHT LOWER QUADRANT (RLQ)	**LEFT LOWER QUADRANT (LLQ)**
Cecum	Sigmoid colon
Appendix	Left ovary and tube
Right ovary and tube	

The procedure requires knowledge of the terms used to designate the divisions of the abdomen (Figure 41-5) and the location of its anatomic structures (see the box on the opposite page). Physical examination of the abdomen is performed in the following order: inspection, auscultation, percussion, and palpation. Auscultation is performed before percussion and palpation because the latter two may alter the frequency and intensity of bowel sounds.

INSPECTION

Light is shined across the abdomen. The skin is inspected for color and texture, scars, engorged veins, visible peristalsis, masses, and abnormal contour.

Finding	Interpretation
Scars or striae	May be result of pregnancy, obesity, ascites, tumors, edema, surgical procedures, or healed burned areas
Engorged veins	May be caused by obstruction of vena cava or portal vein and circulation from abdomen
Skin color	Observe for evidence of jaundice or inflammation (redness)
Visible peristalsis	May be caused by pyloric or intestinal obstruction; normally peristalsis not visible except for slow waves in thin persons

Finding	Interpretation
Visible pulsations	Normally slight pulsation of aorta, visible in epigastric region
Visible masses and altered contour	Observe for hernias, distention of ascites, and obesity; instructing patient to cough may bring out hernia "bulge" or elicit pain or discomfort in the abdomen; marked concavity may be caused by malnutrition

A normal finding is an *umbilical calculus*, which is an accumulated hard mass of debris and desquamated skin within the umbilicus, causing inflammation and resulting from poor hygiene. The integrity and turgor of the skin are reliable indicators of total body hydration. Measurement of abdominal girth provides a baseline for the evaluation of increase or decrease in size because of distention. A measuring tape is placed around the abdomen at the level of the umbilicus or 2.5 cm below, and the reading is taken. It is important that all subsequent measurements be taken at the same level for accurate evaluation.

Abdominal distention may be caused by air or fluid in the gastrointestinal tract or fluid in the peritoneal spaces (ascites). *Air* collects from the air that is swallowed, from gas formed by bacterial action, or from gas that has diffused from the blood. Decreased peristalsis

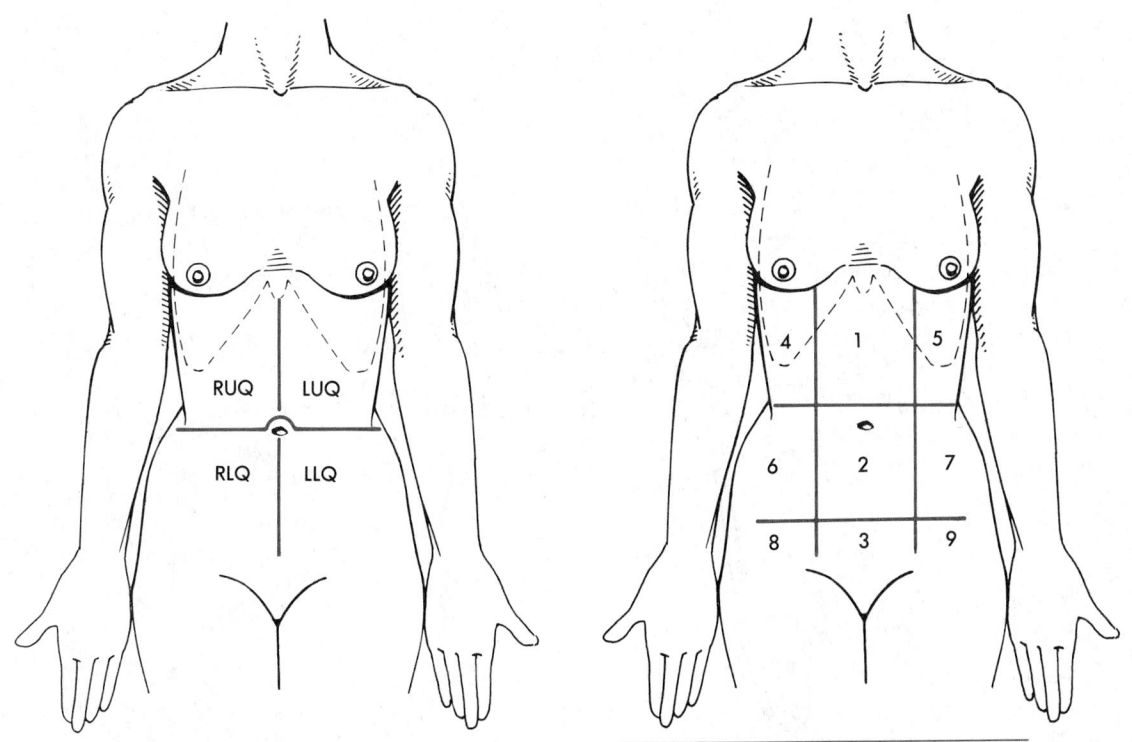

FIGURE 41-5 Topographic division of the abdomen commonly used to localize signs and symptoms and anatomic location of viscera within the abdomen. *1*, Epigastrium; *2*, umbilical; *3*, suprapubic (bladder and uterus); *4* and *5*, right and left hypochondrium; *6* and *7*, right and left lumbar or flank; *8* and *9*, right and left iliac or inguinal.

permits the air to collect in one portion of the gastrointestinal tract. *Fluid* accumulates in the tract as it becomes obstructed. Ascites usually results from increased portal hypertension secondary to liver or heart disease.

AUSCULTATION

Auscultation is used primarily to determine the presence or absence of peristalsis and is done before percussion and palpation to avoid an increase or decrease of peristalsis secondary to disturbing the viscera and causing abnormal activity. Other sounds such as friction rubs or murmurs may be heard (Figure 41-6). Most intestinal sounds occur at a rate of 5 to 34 per minute (although some may not be audible for up to 5 minutes) and are high pitched and gurgling in quality. A normal peristaltic wave produces audible sounds of air and fluid movement through the intestine. The sounds are the loudest to the right and below the umbilicus.

Finding	Interpretation
Absence of sounds	Peritonitis, paralytic ileus, pneumonia, and hypokalemia
Repeated, high-pitched sounds occurring at frequent intervals	Increased peristalsis heard in gastroenteritis, early pyloric obstruction, early intestinal obstruction, and diarrhea

Finding	Interpretation
Bruit	Presence of abnormal sounds (turbulence of blood flow through partially occluded or diseased aorta or renal artery)
Hum and friction rub	Heard over liver and splenic areas, indicating peritoneal inflammation

PERCUSSION

Percussion of the abdomen has relatively limited value. It is used primarily to confirm the size of various organs and to determine the presence of excessive amounts of fluid or air. Normally, percussion over the abdomen is tympanic because of the presence of a small amount of swallowed air within the gastrointestinal tract. A dull or flat percussion note will be found over a solid structure, such as a distended bladder or enlarged uterus, and over the lower border of the liver in the seventh interspace. Tympanic sounds should be heard beginning at the ninth interspace in the left upper quadrant of the abdomen (Traube's space). Dullness or flatness of tone in this area may be caused by some enlargement of the spleen or the left kidney.

The four quadrants are percussed beginning with the thorax area and moving downward systematically. The

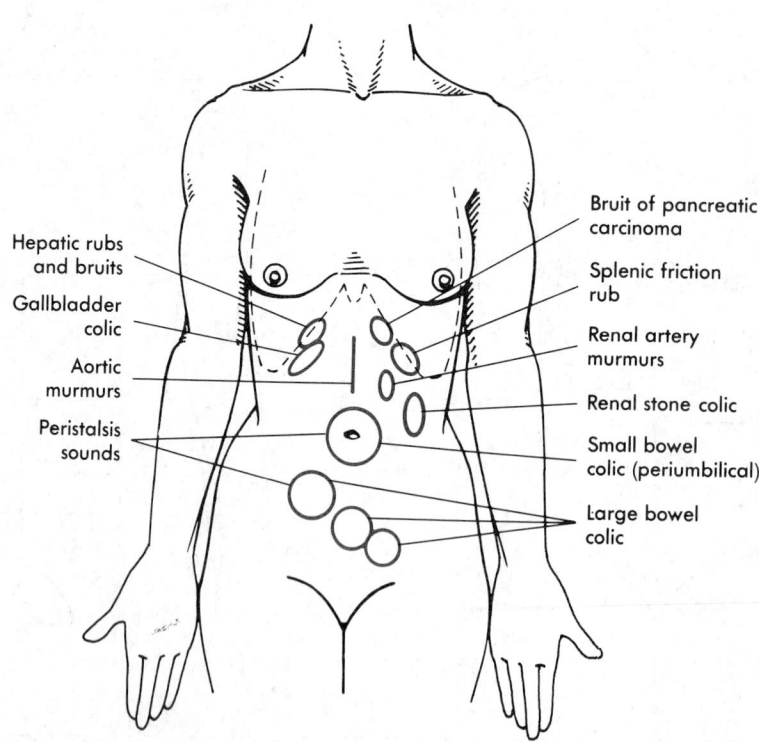

FIGURE 41-6 Optimal areas for auscultation of various sounds in the abdomen, and localization of some types of pain.

degree of tympany, from soft to pronounced, determines gaseous bowel distention.

PALPATION

Palpation aids in confirming the findings of inspection and history data. Palpation is of value in determining the outlines of the liver, spleen, kidneys, uterus, and bladder when these organs are enlarged and in determining the presence and characteristics of abdominal masses and the degree of tenderness or muscle rigidity.

Abnormal findings may include (1) direct tenderness over an organ capsule, (2) rebound tenderness (Blumberg's sign), (3) muscular rigidity, or (4) masses that may be felt if they are large enough or close enough to the surface. Distinction should be made between a distended abdomen that is firm to the touch (indicating an active obstruction with fluid and gas accumulation) and an abdomen that is soft to the touch (indicating a resolving obstruction or a normal occurrence).

RECTUM

The normal perineal skin and perianal area resembles the skin on the remainder of the body with no breaks in its integrity. Abnormal findings may include pruritus ani, coccygeal or pilonidal sinus tract openings, fistulas, fissures, external hemorrhoids, or rectal prolapse. Internal hemorrhoids may appear when the patient strains down.

DIAGNOSTIC TESTS

Many of the examinations and tests performed for diagnosis of problems of the upper gastrointestinal system are both time consuming and vaguely unpleasant. Several of the tests are intrusive procedures and as such may present added stress for the individual and family.

The individual may already be physically debilitated because of poor nutritional intake and may be vomiting and experiencing acute or chronic pain. These data are used to plan for thorough and complete explanation of the tests and examinations to be done so that the patient or significant others may offer optimal cooperation.

In many institutions the responsibility for explaining the procedures to the patient has been assumed by representatives from the radiology department or laboratory. Prepared literature that explains the procedures is also available for the patient and family. This approach, however, does not relieve the nurse of the responsibility to understand the rationale and technique for each procedure, assess the patient's understanding, and answer questions that the patient or family may have. The various tests and procedures are scheduled so that the time expended by the patient is best utilized; for example, a gastric analysis should be scheduled before a barium swallow, because the stomach must be empty for the gastric analysis.

The person's ability to tolerate discomfort before and during the examination is assessed. Narcotics and many sedatives will depress gastric emptying; therefore a notation to the radiologist or physician is made if these drugs are given before diagnostic tests of the stomach. If the radiologist is aware that a narcotic has been given within 2 hours before the ingestion of barium, the decreased emptying time of the stomach will not necessarily be attributed to a definite pathologic problem. In this way inadvertent errors and unnecessary repetition of time-consuming and expensive examinations may be avoided.

LABORATORY TESTS
STOOL EXAMINATION

Gross, microscopic, chemical, and bacterial examinations of the stool supply information that is helpful in establishing a diagnosis of gastrointestinal disease. Stools that are abnormal in color (Table 41-2), odor, amount, consistency, and number are significant. Abnormal stools should be accurately described, and a specimen should be saved for examination by the physician. The physician may order further laboratory studies to be performed. Stool examinations are required for the complete evaluation of all patients with gastrointestinal complaints.

Detection of *occult blood* in the stool is useful in identifying bleeding of the gastrointestinal tract, which is commonly seen in gastrointestinal diseases such as carcinoma of the stomach and colon, ulcerative colitis, and diverticulitis. Occult blood may be identified by one of three tests—guaiac (Hemoccult), benzidine, or orthotoluidine (Occultest). The guaiac test is the least sensitive and does not require special preparation. Meat, poultry, or fish can cause a false-positive test, and vitamin C in quantities greater than 500 mg/day may cause a false-negative test; therefore these substances must be omitted from the diet for 3 days before testing with benzidine or orthotoluidine.[6]

TABLE 41-2 Interpretation of feces color

Color	Interpretation
White	Barium
Gray, tan (clay)	Lack of bile, biliary obstruction
Red	Lower gastrointestinal bleeding
	Beets
Black	
Tarry	Upper gastrointestinal bleeding
Dry	Iron

The nurse is responsible for seeing that specimens are collected. A person who is ambulatory may be given a specimen box and spatula and instructed in obtaining a specimen. Otherwise, the specimen is collected by the nursing personnel. The nurse should be familiar with and also should inform auxiliary staff of any special techniques that are required to preserve stools for special examinations. For example, a specimen to be examined for amebae must be kept warm if the stool is liquid and taken immediately to the laboratory for examination. It can be kept warm by placing the specimen box in a pan of warm water. If an enema must be given to collect a stool specimen, it is important that plain tap water or normal saline solution be used, because soaps or hypertonic solutions may change the consistency of the stool and alter any abnormal contents.

At any time during hospitalization that any abnormality in the color of the stool is noted, a specimen is collected and retained for physician inspection. This applies to all patients regardless of their primary medical diagnosis.

CARCINOEMBRYONIC ANTIGEN MONITORING

Carcinoembryonic antigen (CEA) is an antigen seen in fetal life. It was originally isolated in patients with colonic cancer but it is also seen in persons with ulcerative colitis, cirrhosis, in other forms of cancer and in chronic cigarette smokers.

The CEA test is not useful as a screening test for colonic and pancreatic cancer; however, it is useful as an indicator of the effects of therapy. For example, a drop in CEA level would suggest effectiveness of therapy. A continued high level or rise in level would suggest recurrence or spread of the tumor.

No preparation is required for the CEA test. However, heparin may interfere with test results; therefore heparin is withheld, if possible, for two days before the test. A blood sample is drawn.

EXFOLIATIVE CYTOLOGY

Exfoliative cytology is the study of the individual cells or clumps of cells to identify or to exclude the presence of malignancy. Because malignant cells tend to exfoliate (separate from the tumor), methods of accelerating exfoliation are used. This is accomplished by passing a Levin tube and lavaging the stomach vigorously with quantities of saline solution. *Chymotrypsin* may be administered to digest the overlying protective coat of mucus and thereby expose the mucosa to the irrigating solution. All the aspirated irrigating solution, cells, and bits of tissue obtained are sent to the laboratory for study.

Exfoliative cytology may also provide data concerning pernicious anemia, gastritis, and granulomatous diseases. Barium may interfere with cell evaluation; there-

fore no barium studies with oral barium should be planned within 24 hours before exfoliative cytologic testing.

RADIOLOGIC TESTS

Visualization of the GI tract may be performed by barium swallow, upper GI series, or barium enema. Barium is a radiopaque substance that, when ingested or given by enema in solution, outlines the passageways of the GI tract for viewing by fluoroscopy or x-ray films.

BARIUM SWALLOW

The purpose of barium swallow is identification of esophageal lesions, hiatal hernia, or esophageal reflux. The patient swallows a flavored barium solution, and the radiologist observes the progress of the barium through the esophagus and takes films. The test lasts approximately 15 minutes.

GASTROINTESTINAL SERIES: (UPPER GI SERIES)

The purpose of an upper GI series is visualization of the structure and motility of the stomach and small intestinal tract to detect tumors, ulceration, or inflammation of the stomach and duodenum and to reveal any abnormal anatomy or malposition of these organs. The procedure is similar to the barium swallow. The barium outlines the stomach wall and flows by gravity into the intestinal loops as the radiologist watches the television monitor and takes the radiograms. The test takes approximately 45 minutes. If the person has a spastic duodenal bulb or increased peristalsis in the duodenum, atropine, glucagon, or probanthine may be administered before the radiogram to slow the action of the small intestine, permitting better visualization of the area. This procedure is called hypotonic duodenography.

Following an upper GI series, the patient is often prescribed a laxative to hasten elimination of the barium; barium that remains in the colon may become hard and difficult to expel, leading to fecal impaction. The stool should return to the normal color (barium is white) after the barium is expelled.

BARIUM ENEMA

If both an upper GI series and a barium enema are to be performed, the barium enema is done first, before barium from the upper GI series reaches the colon. The purpose of the barium enema is visualization of the colon to detect colonic polyps, tumors, and chronic inflammatory bowel disorders. Cleansing of the colon by enemas precedes the procedure. Barium is instilled rectally through a rectal tube with an inflatable balloon to retain the barium in the colon. The patient is then placed in various positions while the radiologist observes on the monitor the barium flow through the colon. Air insufflation may be used to outline lesions or polyps. Because the procedure takes about 30 minutes and the retention of barium and air in the colon produces some discomfort, the patient may become exhausted and require a rest period. A laxative or enema may be prescribed for expulsion of the barium; the stools may be white-tinged for 2 to 3 days. Assess the patient for fecal impaction if stools do not return to normal during this time.

SPECIAL TESTS

TESTS OF GASTRIC FUNCTION

Gastric Analysis (Tube Method)

Examination of the fasting contents of the stomach may be used in establishing a diagnosis of gastric disease. The purpose is to quantify gastric acidity in the fasting and stimulated states. The normal level of basal acid output is 1 to 5 mEq/hr. In the person with symptoms of gastric disease, the gastric analysis test results may suggest the following:

1. Decreased gastric acid: gastric malignancy, pernicious anemia
2. Increased gastric acid: duodenal ulcer, Zollinger Ellison syndrome
3. Normal gastric acid: gastric ulcer

A nasogastric tube is inserted, and gastric contents are aspirated. The flow of gastric acid is then stimulated by betazole hydrochloride, histamine phosphate, or pentagastrin given subcutaneously. The person may experience side effects of the medication, including flushing, feeling of warmth, slight headache, or itching. Epinephrine is given to counteract effects of histamine if sensitivity occurs. If Zollinger-Ellison syndrome is suspected, secretin may be given; if the syndrome is present, acid secretion (which normally should decrease) will increase, and serum gastrin level will rise.

Tubeless Gastric Analysis

Tubeless gastric analysis may be used for detection of gastric achlorhydria. The test will indicate the presence or absence of free hydrochloric acid but cannot be used to determine the *amount* of free hydrochloric acid if any is present. For a tubeless gastric analysis, a gastric stimulant such as caffeine is given. One hour later, a cation exchange resin containing azure A is given orally with water on an empty stomach. If there is free hydrochloric acid in the stomach, on the introduction of this resin, a substance will be released in the stomach that will be absorbed from the small intestine and excreted by the kidneys within 2 hours. Absence of detectable amounts of blue dye in the urine indicates that free hydrochloric acid probably was not secreted.

BIOPSY

UPPER GASTROINTESTINAL BIOPSY

A biopsy of the oral cavity or tongue may be done on any lesion or ulcerated area that requires a differential diagnosis. This procedure is most generally carried out with the patient under local anesthesia. Following the biopsy, the biopsy site is assessed for bleeding. Planned oral hygiene using a neutral mouth wash solution is implemented at least every 4 hours until drainage from the site has ceased and at least three times a day thereafter. Biopsy of the stomach is performed during fiberoptic endoscopy.

RECTAL BIOPSY

Biopsy of lesions, polyps, or tumors of the lower sigmoid colon, rectum, and anal canal is generally done at the time of the sigmoidoscopic examination. A knife blade or snare is used to obtain the tissue sample. The sample is placed on a slide or in a fixative solution and sent to the laboratory for analysis. The procedure is not generally painful, although a feeling of pressure may be experienced. Bleeding from the site of the biopsy is uncommon. The person is instructed to report immediately any signs of rectal bleeding and to curtail physical activity until examined by a physician.

ENDOSCOPY

The entire gastrointestinal mucosa may be visualized directly by endoscopy. Disease processes may be located and inspected and a specimen of tissue (biopsy) may be obtained for microscopic study. The upper gastrointestinal tract may be visualized as far as the duodenum by insertion of a fiberscope through the mouth. A fiberscope inserted through the rectum is also used for visualization of the entire colon during a colonoscopy. The mucosa of the lower colon (sigmoid) and rectum may be observed by sigmoidoscopy or proctoscopy, both of which are more simple procedures. The nursing care for each of these procedures is summarized in Table 41-3.

The *fiberscope* (Figure 41-7) has a thin, flexible shaft that can pass around bends in the gastrointestinal tract. Glass fibers incorporated into the shaft of the instrument transmit light to the mucosa and transmit the image back to the examiner. Cameras may be attached for the purpose of taking pictures of abnormalities during the examination. A larger, rigid tube may be used for examination of the rectum.

UPPER GI ENDOSCOPY

Upper GI endoscopy includes *esophagoscopy, gastroscopy,* and *duodenoscopy,* either singly or combined, depending on the area to be observed. Upper GI endoscopy is especially useful for identifying upper gastrointestinal bleeding and for differentiating gastric malignancies from benign ulcers and gastric ulcers from duodenal ulcers. Other uses include visualization of esophageal strictures, varices and tumors, achalasia, and hiatal hernias, and surgical removal of gastric polyps. The patient is premedicated with valium, and the

TABLE 41-3 Gastrointestinal endoscopy

	Gastroscopy	Colonoscopy	Sigmoidoscopy
Visualization of	Esophagus and stomach	Entire colon	Sigmoid colon
Time	15-30 min	30-120 min	10-15 min
Sensation	Pressure but no pain	Pressure; analgesic given	Urge to defecate; some abdominal cramping
Diet	Nothing orally for 6-8 hrs before examination	Clear liquids for 3 days; Nothing orally for 8 hr before examination	Light supper, light breakfast
Patient teaching	Explanation of procedure: speaking not possible during procedure, hoarseness present for several days	Explanation of procedure	Explanation of procedure
POSTPROCEDURE CARE			
Special care	No food/fluids until gag reflex returns Safety precautions until sedative wears off	Plan rest period	Plan rest period
Vital signs	q30 min for 2 hrs	q4-6h	None
Monitor	Dyspnea, dysphagia, abdominal pain, fever, bleeding	Sudden abdominal pain, rise in body temperature Stools for gross blood	Sudden abdominal pain

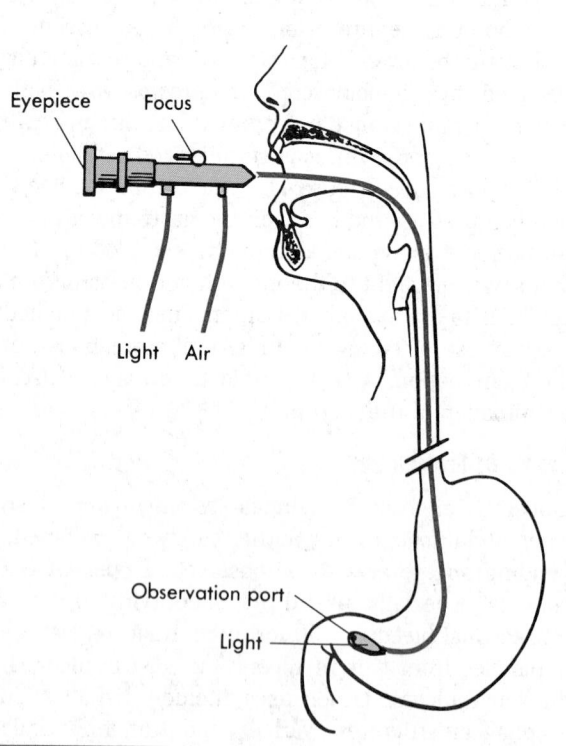

Eyepiece Focus

Light Air

Observation port

Light

FIGURE 41-7 Stomach may be visualized by means of a fiberscope.

throat is anesthetized with a topical anesthetic before the scope is introduced.

COLONOSCOPY

Fiberoptic colonoscopy is recommended for abnormalities of the colon that cannot be diagnosed by the usual means, for reexamination of anastomosis of the colon following surgery for colonic cancer or for surgical removal of colonic polyps. It is contraindicated when acute bleeding or inflammatory disease of the colon is present. The colonoscope (Figure 41-8) is 105 to 185 cm in length, and its use requires the skill of a specialist; however, it has the advantage of permitting more extensive visualization than the sigmoidoscope. Before colonoscopy the patient is premedicated with an intravenous infusion of diazepam (Valium) and meperidine (Demerol).

SIGMOIDOSCOPY AND PROCTOSCOPY

Sigmoidoscopy includes examination of the sigmoid colon, rectum, and anus, whereas proctoscopy is limited to the rectum and anus. Sigmoidoscopy is the most commonly used endoscopic procedure and is indicated for the screening of men over 40 years of age, persons with a familial history of colonic cancer, and persons with symptoms of lower gastrointestinal bleeding or inflammatory disease of the colon. The sigmoidoscopic examination permits inspection of a segment of the bowel that is particularly difficult to examine satisfactorily with contrast media. Approximately 75% of all polyps and tu-

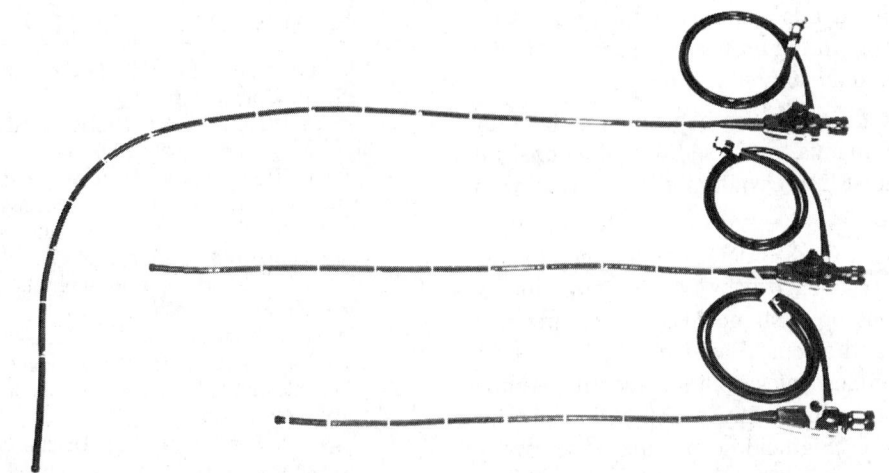

FIGURE 41-8 Flexible colon fiberscopes. (From Given BA and Simmons SJ: Gastroenterology in clinical nursing, ed 4, St Louis, 1984, The CV Mosby Co.)

mors of the large bowel are within the range of visualization of the sigmoidoscope.

Normal variations that may be seen during sigmoidoscopy include (1) temporary hyperemia caused by the irritation of enema solutions, (2) increased mucus production caused by inflammation, emotional disturbances, or commercial enema preparations, and (3) decreased mucus production resulting from habitual laxative ingestion.

CHAPTER SUMMARY

✔ Functions of the gastrointestinal tract include salivation and mastication in the mouth; swallowing in the esophagus; digestion of carbohydrates in the mouth, stomach, and intestines; digestion of protein in the stomach and small intestines; digestion of fat primarily in the small intestines; and absorption in the intestines.

✔ Disorders that interfere with gastrointestinal function alter nutritional status.

✔ Loss of gastrointestinal secretions causes fluid and electrolyte imbalances because of losses of fluid, sodium, potassium, calcium, magnesium, hydrogen ions, and bicarbonate.

✔ Intestinal bacteria synthesize vitamin K, which is necessary for coagulation.

✔ The GI tract is one of four sources involved in the production of B cells from which immunoglobulins develop.

✔ Gastrointestinal changes that may occur in elderly persons include gum and teeth changes, decreased secretion of most digestive enzymes and bile, and decreased intestinal motility and anal sphincter tone. These changes may interfere with chewing and ab-

sorption of fats, may increase residue that can cause flatulence, and may cause constipation.

✔ Subjective data for GI assessment include information about teeth; nausea and vomiting; weight loss; pain of the mouth, throat, abdomen, or rectal area; and bowel patterns.

✔ Objective data include assessment of the mouth and pharynx, jaws, abdomen, and rectum.

✔ The abdomen is generally divided into four quadrants for assessment: right and left upper and lower quadrants. Auscultation precedes percussion and palpation because these may alter the frequency and intensity of bowel sounds.

✔ Normal bowel sounds occur about 5 to 34 per minute, although some may not be audible for up to 5 minutes.

✔ Laboratory tests include stool examination for blood or parasites, carcinoembryonic antigen monitoring (as an indicator of effectiveness of cancer therapy), and exfoliative cytology of the stomach for malignant cells.

✔ The major radiologic tests include barium swallow, upper GI series, and barium enema. Retained barium in the colon may lead to fecal impaction. An upper GI series may alter the results of a barium enema, therefore if both tests are to be done, the barium enema should be done first. A barium enema can be uncomfortable and exhausting for the patient.

✔ A gastric analysis assesses the quantity of gastric acid in both fasting and stimulated states; a nasogastric tube is inserted to remove the gastric secretions. In a tubeless gastric analysis a cation exchange resin containing a blue dye is administered after a gastric stimulant is given; in the presence of gastric acid the dye is absorbed and excreted in the urine.

✔ Gastric acid is decreased with gastric malignancy and pernicious anemia, increased with duodenal ulcer and Zollinger-Ellison syndrome, and normal with gastric ulcer.

✔ Diagnosis of many GI disorders is often made following endoscopy (esophagoscopy, gastroscopy, duodenoscopy, colonoscopy, sigmoidoscopy, or proctoscopy). Valium and a topical anesthetic are used for the upper GI endoscopies; valium and meperidine are given before colonoscopy which is a more involved procedure. Sigmoidoscopy and proctoscopy are common procedures and do not require medication.

QUESTIONS TO CONSIDER

- What data would be most important from a nursing standpoint for a 20-year-old college student admitted for a second episode of abdominal pain with a tentative diagnosis of Crohn's disease (a chronic inflammatory bowel disease)? For a 30-year-old man admitted for an acute episode of Crohn's disease, which he has had for 8 years?

- Your best friend is scheduled to have a barium enema; what assistance can you give?

- Your patient is assigned to have a gastroscopy; she appears very anxious and tells you that she is afraid of gagging and throwing up during the examination. What should you tell her?

REFERENCES AND SELECTED READINGS

1. *Bates B: A guide to physical examination, ed 4, Philadelphia, 1987, JB Lippincott Co.
2. *Becker KL and Stevens SA: Performing in-depth abdominal assessment, Nursing '88 18(6):59-63, 1988.
3. DeVita VT Jr: Endoscopy in cancer diagnosis and management, Hosp Pract 19(11):111-122, 1984.
4. Fischbach FT: A manual of laboratory diagnostic tests, ed 3, Philadelphia, 1988, JB Lippincott Co.
5. Guyton A: Textbook of medical physiology, ed 7, Philadelphia, 1986, WB Saunders Co.
6. *Kee JL: Laboratory and diagnostic tests with nursing implications, Norwalk, Conn, 1983, Appleton Century-Crofts.
7. *Malasanos L et al: Health assessment, ed 4, St Louis, 1990, The CV Mosby Co.
8. *Pagana KD and Pagana TJ: Diagnostic testing and nursing implications: a case study approach, ed 2, St Louis 1986, The CV Mosby Co.
9. *Pagana KD and Pagana TJ: Pocket nurse guide to laboratory and diagnostic tests, St Louis, 1986, The CV Mosby Co.
10. Schroeder SA et al: Current medical diagnosis and treatment, Norwalk, Conn, 1989, Appleton & Lange.
11. Seidel HM et al: Mosby's guide to physical examination, St Louis, 1987, The CV Mosby Co.
12. *Smith CE: Assessing bowel sounds, Nursing '88 18(2):42-44, 1988.
13. Tilkian SM, Conover MB, and Tilkian AG: Clinical implications of laboratory tests, ed 4, St Louis, 1987, The CV Mosby Co.
14. Vander AJ et al: Human physiology, ed 4, New York, 1985, McGraw-Hill Book Co.
15. Way LW: Current surgical diagnosis and treatment, ed 8, Los Altos, Calif, 1988, Appleton & Lange.

*References preceded by an asterisk are particularly well suited for student reading.

CHAPTER 42

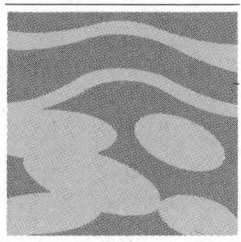

Management of Persons with Problems of Ingestion

BARBARA C. LONG
JANICE NEVILLE

CHAPTER OBJECTIVES

After studying this chapter, the student should be able to:
1. Describe etiology, pathophysiology, and interventions for obesity, including surgical approaches.
2. Describe etiology, pathophysiology, and interventions for protein-calorie malnutrition, including alternative feeding methods.
3. Describe etiology, clinical manifestations, and interventions for infections and tumors of the mouth.
4. Identify common esophageal disorders, their pathophysiology and interventions, including care of the surgical patient.

The person with good nutritional status has less risk of developing a pathophysiologic disorder and possesses resources to regain optimal functioning more quickly if illness or disease does occur. Good nutrition involves the ingestion of an adequate quantity, as well as quality, of food. Ingestion of excess quantities of highly caloric foods leads to obesity; underweight results from decreased food intake.

This chapter discusses problems related to excessive and inadequate ingestion of food, as well as conditions of the mouth or esophagus that may limit ingestion.

OBESITY

Obesity is the most frequently encountered type of malnutrition in the United States. Severe and morbid obesity places the person at a high health risk.

Obesity is generally defined as weight 20% greater than the desirable weight for adults of a given sex and height. The "desirable weight" is obtained from standard height/weight tables that contain arbitrary figures determined from pooled life insurance data. The greater the obesity, the greater the health risk. Persons who are 160% or more of the desirable weight have a higher mortality and morbidity. *Massive* or *morbid obesity,* which is often defined as 45 kg (100 lbs) over desirable weight, is extremely hazardous to health.

ETIOLOGY

Obesity does not usually have a single cause but results from a complex interrelationship of numerous physiologic, psychologic, or social factors. Old age is not a factor; most elderly persons are not severely obese.[14] Mild overweight is considered to be beneficial for elderly persons, because it provides an available source of nutrients during periods of stress or illness.[60]

GENETIC

Eighty percent of children born of two overweight parents will also be overweight.[1] It has been difficult, however, to determine if this results from genetic or social factors (such as overeating patterns). Strains of overweight mice have been developed, and studies of twins reared by normal and overweight parents have implicated heredity as a factor.

CENTRAL NERVOUS SYSTEM (CNS) DISTURBANCES

Eating activity is regulated by the appetite and satiety centers in the hypothalamus. Lesions in the ventromedial hypothalamus induce obesity.[1]

HORMONES

Selected hormones can influence the use of ingested calories. Thyroid hormones stimulate basal metabolism, requiring energy and calorie expenditure; thus the person who has a thyroid deficiency may experience weight gain. Decreased insulin in diabetes mellitus and increased cortisone production with Cushing's syndrome also lead to overweight.

SODIUM-POTASSIUM PUMP

The sodium-potassium pump uses 20% to 50% of calories ingested.[1] A functioning sodium-potassium pump requires action by the enzyme sodium-potassium-adenosine triphosphatase. Obese mice have been found to be deficient in this enzyme.

ACTIVITY

Because of their large body mass, persons who are very obese tend to be more sedentary and unable to expend energy to burn off some of their calories. When caloric input exceeds caloric output in terms of basal metabolism and physical activity, weight gain results.

SOCIAL FACTORS

Eating is a social custom. Some ethnic groups perceive that "fat is beautiful" and encourage the eating of large amounts of food. Parents who are socialized to eat large quantities of food pass on this practice to their children. Western societies often feed their infants high-caloric milk and cereals at a time when there is a greater chance for an increased number of fat cells to be produced.

Social gatherings usually involve eating or drinking high-calorie foods. In recent years there has been greater emphasis on serving low-calorie foods such as sliced raw vegetables at social functions. Diet drinks have also increased in popularity.

PSYCHOLOGIC FACTORS

Symbolic meanings may be attached to foods as a result of experiences from infancy and childhood. During times of stress, some people eat more food or more highly caloric foods and thus gain weight. Compulsive eating may occur, leading to severe obesity.

Obese persons who have tried many times unsuccessfully to lose weight may become sensitive to other persons' suggestions to eat low-caloric foods. Some have reported deliberately choosing high-caloric foods as a means of establishing control of their own identity. Body image is an important factor in obesity and may help to prevent weight gain by motivating a person to lose weight.

PATHOPHYSIOLOGY
TYPES OF OBESITY

Obesity results from the intake of foods in amounts exceeding body needs; the excess is stored as fat. In persons of normal weight who gain weight, fat is deposited by *hypertrophy* of existing fat cells in adipose tissue. These people respond well to weight reduction regimens. Fat cells can also increase in number (*hyperplasia*); this is seen primarily in children up to the age of 2, between the ages of 7 and 11, and during adolescence, but it may also occur in adulthood. Excessive food intake has been shown to be a stimulus for hyperplasia. Hyperplasia is irreversible and conditions persons to be overweight throughout their life.[21] Weight reduction in persons with hyperplastic obesity is difficult to achieve and to maintain.

ENERGY EFFICIENCY

Some persons can eat large quantities of caloric foods and not gain significant weight. Other persons gain weight with only slight increases in caloric intake. The difference is apparently the result of the ability to use the calories more or less efficiently.

METABOLIC CHANGES

Metabolic abnormalities have been noted in persons with severe or massive obesity (Table 42-1). Triglycerides are stored in fat deposits in adipose tissue. When the fatty acid is needed for energy, the triglycerides are released and circulated in the bloodstream. The obese person has increased amounts of serum triglycerides that may predispose the person to atheromatous plaques. Cholesterol is also formed by the release of triglycerides and may precipitate with bile salts to form gallstones.

Obese persons have a high risk of diabetes. The increased glucose intake places a stress on the pancreas to produce more insulin, and hyperinsulinism occurs. The pancreatic islet cells may first exhibit hyperplasia but then fail. An increased *resistance-to-insulin* effect also results from the large number of fat cells with a diminished number of insulin receptors.[14]

■ ASSESSMENT
SUBJECTIVE DATA

Weight reduction is not possible unless the person desires to lose weight and wishes to participate in a weight reduction program. Subjective data must therefore be collected before a program can be planned with the person. Data collected include the following:

1. Person's perception of his or her weight:

TABLE 42-1 Physiologic effects of obesity

Parameter	Metabolic Effect	Associated Disorder
Increased fatty acid utilization	Hypertriglyceridemia	Atherosclerosis, hypertension, emboli
	Increased cholesterol synthesis	Gallstones
Increased glucose	Hyperinsulinism leading to pancreatic β-cell failure	Diabetes mellitus
Increased body mass	Cumulative trauma to weight-bearing joints	Osteoarthritis
	Increased workload for heart	Angina, sudden death
	Decreased thorax expansion with decreased tidal volume	Respiratory insufficiency

Many persons who are slightly overweight perceive that they are moderately or severely overweight[50]; severely overweight persons who do not perceive their status may not be motivated to lose weight

2. Duration of weight gain:
   A person with a recent weight gain will respond more positively to a weight reduction program than one with a lifelong pattern of obesity
3. Perception of the cause of weight gain
4. Family history of obesity
5. Person's reasons for losing weight and the weight goal:
   The goals may or may not be realistic and may indicate a lack of knowledge about obesity
6. Weight reduction approaches used in the past, effectiveness of the approaches, and ideas about present approaches to be used
7. Eating patterns (meals and snacks)
8. Exercise patterns
9. Stressors that may be present (home, job, community, or personal)
10. Medications currently taken:
    Some medications cause weight gain (see the box at right).
11. Perceptions of self-worth:
    (Example: "What do you think about yourself as a person?")

OBJECTIVE DATA

Because of the increased health risks for the severely or morbidly obese person, it is important to differentiate among mild to moderate obesity (110% to 130% of desirable weight), severe obesity (130% to 200% of desirable weight), and morbid obesity (45kg [100 lb] over desirable weight).

Numerous formulas have been developed to try to determine body mass. It is necessary to differentiate fat from muscle. A person with overdeveloped muscles may weigh more than a fat person but not be obese (muscle weighs more than fat). Skin fold measurements (Chapter 40) are often used to determine the degree of fat.

A quick method for assessing the degree of obesity that correlates well with indexes that include skin fold measurements is the *body mass index*. To obtain a person's body mass index, the nude weight in kilograms is divided by the square of the barefoot height in meters:

$$\text{Body mass index} = \frac{\text{Weight (kg)}}{\text{Height (m)}^2}$$

For example, a woman who is 168 cm (1.68 m) tall and who weighs 60 kg will have a body index of 21.28 ($60/1.68^2$). The body mass index range for normal weight is 20 to 25 for men and 19 to 24 for women. Once body mass index exceeds 30, morbidity and mortality increase. When an index exceeds 40, the risk for

---

DRUGS THAT MAY CAUSE WEIGHT GAIN

Glucocorticoids
Estrogen, progestins, oral contraceptives
Antihypertensives that interfere with release of norepinephrine: reserpine, guanethidine
Monoamine oxidase (MAO) inhibitors
Tricyclic antidepressants
Phenothiazines
Antithyroid preparations
Valproic acid (Depakene)—an anticonvulsant
Cyproheptadine—an antihistamine

---

cardiovascular disease is comparable to that resulting from other major factors such as smoking, hypertension, and hypercholesterolemia.[1]

■ DATA ANALYSIS: NURSING DIAGNOSES
NUTRITION, ALTERED: MORE THAN BODY REQUIREMENTS

Etiological factors for this diagnosis will depend on the collected data and may include such factors as inappropriate eating patterns, job stress, and lack of exercise. In some instances, the cause will not be known but the person will have sought help in reducing weight.

■ PLANNING: EXPECTED PATIENT OUTCOMES

The person must be involved in the planning if expected outcomes are to be accomplished. The person is guided to set realistic outcomes. Therapy for the obese person should have three objectives: (1) reduction of the body fat component, (2) reduction of total body weight when indicated, and (3) maintenance of desirable body size and composition. Far too often, both patient and therapist look only at the pounds of weight lost or the rate of loss. No differentiation is made as to whether the pounds represent water, muscle, or fat. Very rapid weight loss is satisfying to both patient and therapist, whether the loss is in body fat or water and whether the loss is permanent or not. Rapid weight loss is usually the result of loss of water rather than fat.

Weight reduction is not achieved simply by lowering the fuel value of the person's diet. A deficit must be produced between energy expenditure and fuel intake so that body stores of fuel will be mobilized. The deficit may be achieved by increasing energy expenditures or decreasing caloric intake, as shown in Figure 42-1.

It is useful to set short-term, as well as long-term outcomes. Examples of long-term outcomes include:
Loses x kg by the end of 1 year
Maintains weight at x kg
Wears a size 12 dress
Plays 18 holes of golf, walking fast without shortness of breath

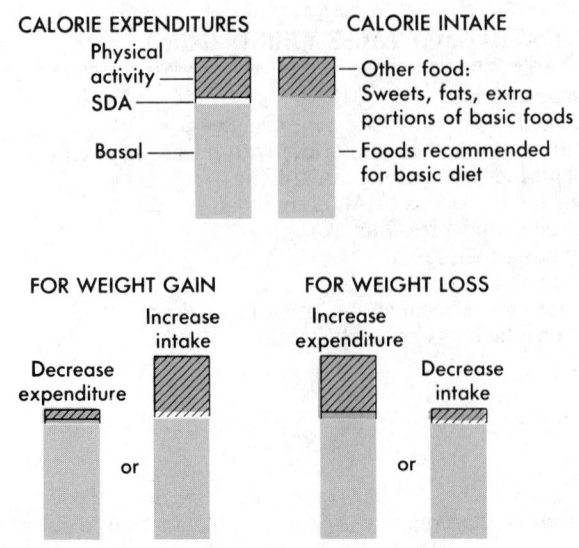

CALORIE EXPENDITURES

Physical activity
SDA
Basal

CALORIE INTAKE

Other food: Sweets, fats, extra portions of basic foods

Foods recommended for basic diet

FOR WEIGHT GAIN

Decrease expenditure

Increase intake

or

FOR WEIGHT LOSS

Increase expenditure

Decrease intake

or

FIGURE 42-1 Calorie balance in an average adult.

Short-term outcomes might include the following:
Loses 2 kg in 4 weeks
Walks x miles per day for 4 weeks
Swims 10 laps every other day
Wears a size 18 dress

■ IMPLEMENTATION

Effective weight loss or weight maintenance programs are usually a combination of several approaches. Dietary control and exercise are usually included in all programs. The purpose of therapy for obese persons is *weight control throughout the life span;* therefore most obese persons have to learn new patterns of eating and exercise. Physicians may prescribe medication as part of a weight reduction program. Surgery may also be performed for the massively obese person when all other methods fail.

DIET

Diet is the most important method of weight reduction. Dieting has been widely reported, even among those who are not overweight.[27] However, diet plans vary from balanced, low-calorie diets to nutritionally poor fad diets (Chapter 40). Books are written favoring various plans, not all of which are either appropriate or nutritionally sound. Many persons have tried different approaches but do not keep to one diet for any period of time. In general, the number of pounds lost by obese persons when dieting is 15 to 30 pounds; this weight is usually regained within 1 to 2 years unless eating patterns have changed.[1,46]

Persons consuming high levels of calories before weight reduction therapy are likely to be successful in achieving rapid weight loss, because the calorie deficit

between need and the recommended diet is large. Men have a reputation for being more cooperative than women because they lose weight more rapidly. If both a man and a woman are instructed to adhere to a 1000 calorie intake, however, the man would be expected to lose at a faster rate because his calorie deficit is larger.

Weight loss for some persons may be achieved by eating three regular balanced meals a day, including the four basic food groups, and avoiding fried foods, sweets, and between-meal snacks. Some persons achieve better results with planned, frequent small meals. Some obese persons omit breakfast but then snack frequently and thus ingest more calories and fewer required nutrients. Changes in eating patterns are therefore usually required for permanent weight loss.

One pound of adipose tissue has an energy potential of 3500 calories. To lose 1 pound of adipose tissue per week, a calorie deficit of 500 calories per day must be induced. If a person requires only 1500 calories to maintain current weight, that person should not be expected to lose more than 1 pound of body fat per week when adhering to a 1000 calorie diet. Weight loss is more rapid when lean body tissue is catabolized, because lean tissue has an energy potential of about 1850 calories. If a deficit of 500 calories per day were met by catabolizing lean tissue, the rate of loss would be about 2 pounds per week. Dehydration produces very rapid weight loss from loss of water. Water has no calorie value per se, but 1 L of water weighs approximately 1 kg.

When caloric intake is severely reduced, there is often a large initial weight loss as a result of loss of water. A plateau in observable weight loss is then reached when fat (which weighs less than water) is being lost. This plateau usually lasts 7 to 10 days and may lead to discouragement by the dieter. Observable weight loss will then be noted after this period but will not be as rapid because of the body's adaptation by decreased metabolic rate and fuel utilization.

Adhering to a diet plan is often difficult (Figure 42-2). The dieter often becomes preoccupied with food. There may be social pressures to eat, and it is difficult to resist available calorie-rich foods. Support from others is important and is the basis for more positive results when a person joins a weight-control group such as Weight Watchers.

Diets are planned on an individual basis, with the caloric intake planned at a level below the person's caloric need for maintaining weight. The calorie intake should come from complex carbohydrates and proteins. A protein intake of about 1 g/kg of ideal body weight should be maintained. Fats must be decreased. Salt-free diets are of no permanent value because the weight loss relates to water loss, and the weight will return when salt is added to the diet.

Fasting diets are controversial. Rapid weight loss

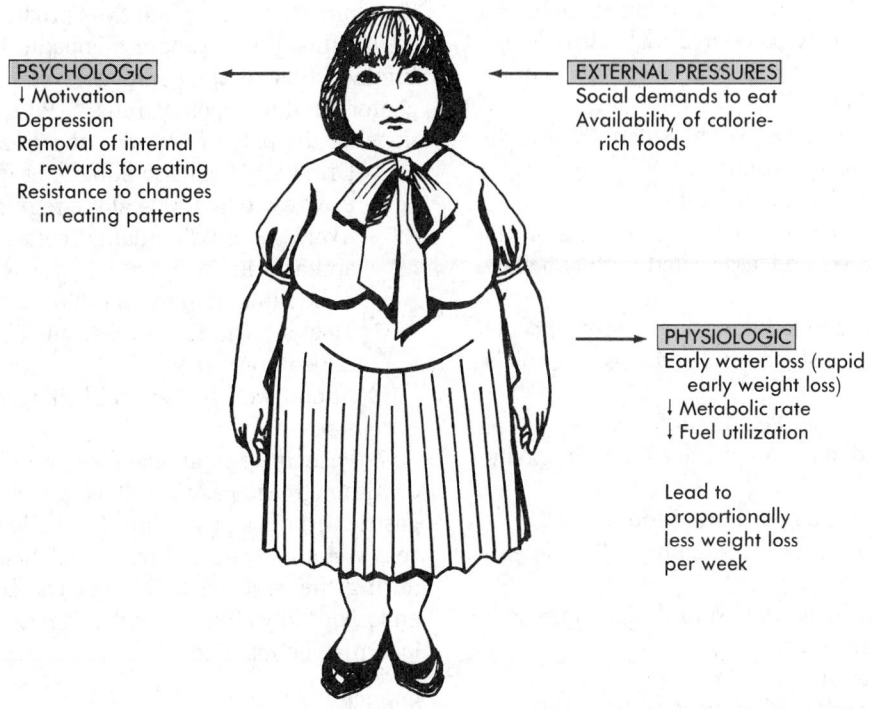

FIGURE 42-2 Factors influencing a person's ability to maintain a weight reduction program.

---

may be necessary in some instances; however, weight gain following the fasting period is a common occurrence. Most fasting programs use a high-protein liquid; some commercial products use hydrolyzed collagen that is low in nutritional value. Close medical supervision is imperative for fasting diets because risks are high (see the box below).

EXERCISE

Exercise is the second part of every weight reduction program. Although the actual number of calories used will be few, the combination of diet and exercise promotes loss of fat rather than lean tissue.[1] Exercise has added benefits, which include influencing plasma insulin and lipid levels, promoting muscle tone, increasing coronary perfusion, and creating psychologic well-being. The type and amount of exercise is planned with each person, depending on ability and preferences. *Brisk* walking is encouraged and is more easily tolerated

if done with another person. The distance walked is progressively increased. Group exercise and swimming programs designed for obese persons are also effective.

MEDICATION

The use of appetite suppressants is controversial because of long-term inefficiency and in some cases, such as with amphetamines, possible drug abuse.

Most over-the-counter dietary aids contain phenyl-propanolamine and bulk-producing agents.[13] Phenyl-propanolamine is a sympathomimetic with anorectic action similar to amphetamine but with no untoward CNS effects. Its usefulness as a weight control drug in humans has been questioned, however. The drug should not be used for more than 3 months and should not be taken concurrently with antihypertensive drugs or with monoamine oxidase (MAO) inhibitors. Nervousness, restlessness, insomnia, headache, nausea, and hypertension may be side effects of phenylpropanolamine.

Bulk-producing agents, such as methylcellulose, expand the stomach and provide a sense of fullness. The same effect can be produced by drinking 2 to 3 glasses of water before each meal.[13] Bulk-producing agents have a laxative effect.

BEHAVIOR MODIFICATION

The purpose of behavior modification is to help the person achieve a change in eating patterns, which is neces-

---

RISKS OF FASTING DIETS

Ketosis	Hepatic impairment
Metabolic acidosis	Polyneuritis
Hypokalemia	Wernicke's syndrome
Hyperuricemia	Ulcerative colitis
Hypotension	Renal insufficiency and death
Nephrolithiasis	in some instances

sary if weight reduction is to be maintained. Behavior modification programs may be offered by health clinics, self-help groups, or by commercial programs. Group sessions are more effective.

The technique of behavior modification for weight control is based on four approaches:

1. Self-monitoring of eating behavior
    a. Purpose is to increase dieter's awareness of calories consumed and associated eating behaviors
    b. Recording of all food/fluids consumed and the time and circumstances related to eating (daily log)
2. Control of environmental stimuli for eating
    a. Elimination of enticements to eating; for example:
        1. Eliminating snacks around the house
        2. Avoiding reading or watching TV while eating
    b. Replacement by positive stimuli; for example:
        1. Eating only at the table
        2. Using special dishes for eating
3. Teaching to enhance behavior change in eating to decrease intake
    a. Putting fork down between bites
    b. Taking smaller bites
    c. Eating chewy rather than soft foods to prolong the eating period but not the intake
    d. Drinking water with meals
4. Rewards for progress
    a. Short-term rewards: points or coins directed toward long-term goals or a small treat
    b. Long-term rewards: special big treat, such as new wardrobe or travel

Emphasis of the therapist should be on what the individual has chosen as the outcome of the weight reduction plan. "Better health" has not been shown to be a motivator for weight reduction.[55]

GASTRIC BALLOON

The Garren-Edward gastric balloon is a *temporary* method that may be used in conjunction with dietary control and behavior modification. Persons indicated for the procedure are those more than 20% above ideal body weight who have failed to achieve weight loss by serious dietary and behavior modification alone. Contraindications include a history of peptic ulcer, hiatal hernia, GI surgery, or concurrent use of antiinflammatory agents, anticoagulants, or drugs that cause gastric irritation.[20,46]

The gastric balloon is a polyurethane balloon with a hollow central channel that is inserted by endoscopy into the stomach. The balloon is then inflated with approximately 200 ml of air through a catheter attached to a self-sealing valve. The balloon occupies about 25% of

the stomach capacity and thus produces early satiety. It is also thought to suppress appetite by stimulating the fundus, thus sending inhibitory stimuli to the appetite center in the hypothalamus.[46] Postprocedure instructions for the patient include the following:

1. Drink a 500-calorie liquid diet for 1 week.
2. Progress to a 1000-calorie regular diet.
3. Avoid gastric stimulants (coffee, alcohol, tobacco) and aspirin.
4. Take multivitamin and mineral supplements.
5. Take antacid four times daily (between meals and at bedtime).
6. Attend weekly diet and behavior modification sessions.
7. Participate in an exercise program.

Although the gastric balloon procedure has low risks, gastric ulcer is a possibility. The balloon may cause nausea, vomiting, crampy pain, and heartburn, especially during the first week. The gastric balloon is removed endoscopically after 4 months. If necessary, another balloon may be inserted.

SURGERY

Surgery for obesity is reserved for persons with massive or morbid obesity who have diligently tried other meth-

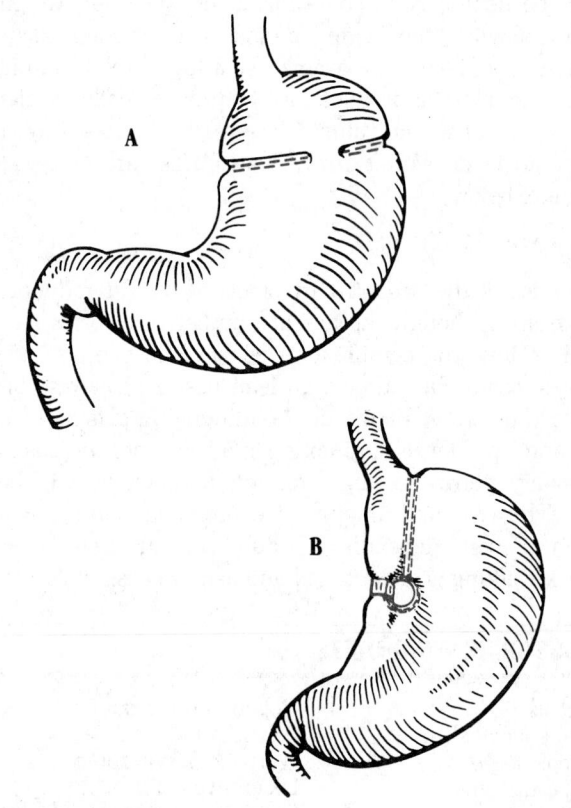

FIGURE 42-3 Gastric partitioning. **A,** Horizontal stapling. **B,** Vertical stapling.

ods and have failed. Obese persons are a high surgical risk, and the surgeries themselves add additional risks. Criteria for surgery include the following: (1) age 18-55, (2) body weight at least 100 pounds over ideal weight, (3) morbid obesity for at least 5 years, (4) evidence of serious dieting efforts, and (5) no major illnesses.

Gastroplasty (Gastric Stapling, Tucking, Partitioning)

In this procedure, the stomach is made smaller by placement of horizontal or vertical suture lines through the stomach walls (Figure 42-3). A small pouch is thus formed that limits the amount of food the person can take without experiencing pain and vomiting. The vertical suture line is preferred, because it results in fewer instances of subsequent dilation of the pouch and disruption of the suture line.[46] Gastroplasty has fewer consequences than does bypass surgery, because the GI tract is not opened and therefore remains intact.

Drainage from a nasogastric tube inserted postoperatively is small (approximately 300 ml). If irrigation is necessary, only a small amount of fluid (30 ml) is used. Clear fluids are introduced on about the third day and, when they are tolerated, the patient is advanced to a diet of pureed foods. A blenderized diet is followed for 8 weeks, at which time small amounts of soft, bland foods are introduced gradually. Supplemental B vitamins are given postoperatively. The patient is monitored postoperatively for perforation of the stomach by the staples, which is evidenced by upper abdominal pain radiating to the left shoulder. Pink urine, resulting from increased uric acid secretion, may be noted for the first 48 hours after surgery.

Gastric Bypass

A Roux-en-Y gastric bypass consists of a gastrojejunostomy with the jejunum attached to a closed-off pouch of the upper stomach (Figure 42-4). The food then bypasses most of the stomach and duodenum. This procedure involves intrusion of the gastrointestinal tract, and the care of the patient is similar to that for other gastric surgeries (Chapter 43). Complications include dumping syndrome, uncontrolled vomiting, leaks in the anastomosis, and pulmonary infections.

Intestinal Bypass

In the jejunoileal bypass procedure, approximately 14 inches of the jejunum and 4 inches of the ileum are preserved for bypass anastomosis (Figure 42-5). This procedure is now rarely performed because of its extensive complications, including malabsorption of fats and fat-soluble vitamins, protein malnutrition, hepatic dysfunction, prolonged severe diarrhea, polyarthritis, intestinal inflammation, osteomalacia, and renal stones.

PROTEIN-CALORIE MALNUTRITION
ETIOLOGY

Approximately 20% of hospitalized patients have protein-calorie malnutrition resulting from decreased nutrient intake, increased nutrient losses, or increased nutrient requirements (see the box on p. 1256). In developing countries, protein-calorie malnutrition is a major health problem. It may occur in two forms, *kwashiorkor* (protein deficiency when calorie intake is adequate) and

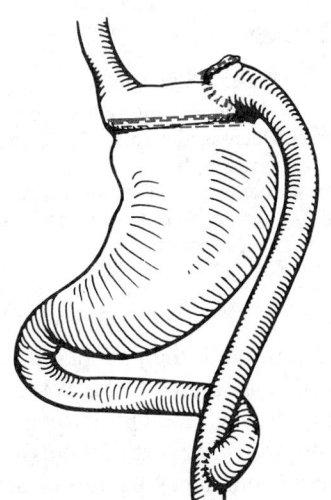

FIGURE 42-4 Roux-en-Y retrocolic gastric bypass. Stomach is completely stapled horizontally; jejunum is resected from duodenum and connected to stomach entrance, and distal duodenal stump is connected to jejunum to permit drainage of intestinal secretions.

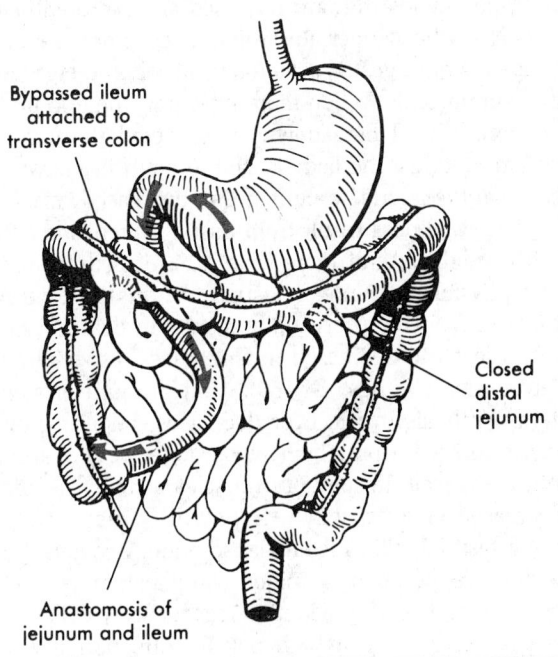

Bypassed ileum attached to transverse colon

Closed distal jejunum

Anastomosis of jejunum and ileum

FIGURE 42-5 Intestinal bypass.

CAUSES OF PROTEIN-CALORIE MALNUTRITION

DECREASED NUTRIENT INTAKE

Anorexia	Financial distress
Nausea	Inability to shop or cook
Dysphagia	Decreased desire to cook
Mouth disorders	Depression
Pain	Substance abuse

INCREASED NUTRIENT LOSSES

Vomiting	Diarrhea
Malabsorption	Immobility

INCREASED NUTRIENT REQUIREMENTS

Surgery	Infection
Fever	Cancer

marasmus (deficiency of both proteins and calories). The typical child with kwashiorkor has thin extremities and ascites of the abdomen.

PATHOPHYSIOLOGY

If diets contain sufficient carbohydrates and fats, these nutrients will be used for energy needs. When the caloric intake is reduced, however, increased amounts of body proteins will be used for energy. The body will meet energy requirements at the expense of protein needs.

A deficiency of both calories and protein is characteristic of protein-calorie malnutrition in adults. Proteins are constantly being synthesized and broken down into amino acids in the body to be reformed into other proteins. Amino acids that are not used are excreted. The body can synthesize certain amino acids (nonessential) but depends on ingested proteins to supply the eight essential amino acids. When more nitrogen (the end product of amino acid breakdown) is excreted than is ingested in proteins, the body is said to be in *negative nitrogen balance*, and weight loss, decreased muscle mass, and weakness result from tissue catabolism.

With weight loss of more than 10% of body weight, loss of physiologic function usually begins to develop, and loss of 35% to 40% usually results in death.[46] Protein loss leads to decreased muscle mass, especially in the liver, heart, lungs, GI tract, and immune system. Protein synthesis in the liver decreases, resulting in a decrease in serum proteins (hypoproteinemia). Cardiac output decreases. Respiratory muscles atrophy, leading to decreased vital capacity. Atrophy of GI mucosa and loss of intestinal villi cause malabsorption. Because lymphocytes are proteins, a major complication is a decrease in lymphocyte production, especially T cells; this places the individual at high risk for infection. Hemoglobin levels may also decrease, because both hemoglo-

bin and transferrin (which binds iron in hemoglobin) are proteins.

■ ASSESSMENT
SUBJECTIVE DATA

The following information is obtained from the person:
1. Patient's perceptions about the weight loss
2. Dietary history
3. Foods that can be tolerated; likes and dislikes
4. Ability and desire to eat
5. Facilities and ability for purchasing, storing, and preparing food
6. Financial resources, if appropriate

OBJECTIVE DATA

Objective data include the following:
1. Weight and height
   Underweight is considered to be less than 90% of desirable weight (Chapter 40); severe weight loss is less than 75% of desirable weight
2. Signs of infection or skin breakdown
3. Laboratory data
   a. Low hemoglobin levels in absence of blood loss
   b. Plasma albumin level of less than 3.0 g/100 ml on two or more determinations, indicating decreased protein synthesis
   c. Urinary creatinine of less than 20 mg/kg in 24 hours for males or less than 16 mg/kg in females, with a normal plasma creatinine level, indicating decreased muscle mass

■ DATA ANALYSIS: NURSING DIAGNOSES

Nursing diagnoses are determined from assessment of patient data. Possible nursing diagnoses for the person with protein-calorie malnutrition may include, but are not limited to, the following:

Diagnostic Title	Possible Etiologies
Fatigue	Muscle weakness, inadequate nutrition
Infection, potential for	Decreased nutrition, decreased immune response
Nutrition, altered: less than body requirements	Inadequate nutrient intake, increased nutrient losses, increased nutrient requirements

■ PLANNING: EXPECTED PATIENT OUTCOMES

If oral intake is permitted, the patient's fullest cooperation will be needed to increase the possibility of adequate nutritional intake. Patient participation in the planning is therefore a vital part of the care.

Expected patient outcomes for the person with protein-calorie malnutrition may include, but are not limited to, the following:
1. The patient includes rest periods in the day's activities
2. Infection does not occur

3. If eating is permitted, the patient:
   a. Participates in menu selection.
   b. Eats all food on tray, if hospitalized.
   c. Eats six small meals per day plus supplementary foods and vitamins, as planned, at home.
4. If tube feedings are given:
   a. Feedings are given at a slow, constant rate.
   b. Patient is hydrated.
   c. Patient states feeling comfortable.
   d. Complications do not occur or are quickly corrected.
5. If total parenteral nutrition (TPN) is given:
   a. Fluid and electrolyte balance is maintained.
   b. Hypoglycemia or hyperglycemia do not occur.
   c. Infection and air embolism do not occur.
   d. Patient states feeling comfortable.

■ IMPLEMENTATION

PREVENTING FATIGUE

The loss of muscle mass and the decreased utilization of nutrients lead to decreased energy production and fatigue. It is essential, therefore, that rest periods be planned to decrease energy expenditure. Dyspnea with exertion and pulse rates that take longer than 5 minutes to stabilize are signs that activities need to be modified.

PREVENTING INFECTION

Maintenance of medical and surgical asepsis is particularly important for the person with protein-calorie malnutrition. These individuals should avoid any person with upper respiratory infections. If the patient is relatively immobile in chair or bed, good skin care is essential to prevent skin breakdown and subsequent infection. Surgical wounds may heal more slowly, and they require strict surgical asepsis.

ENCOURAGING ORAL INTAKE

Adequate nutrients to meet nutritional requirements can be taken by oral, enteral (tube feedings, gastrostomy), or TPN. The best way to receive nutrients is the oral route. Persons with inadequate nutrition stores need encouragement to eat, although forced feeding may lead to frustration or nausea and vomiting. Motivating a person with anorexia to eat can be a challenge. Interventions that can correct the cause will lead to improved appetite. Providing an environment conducive to eating and providing several small meals rather than three large meals per day may facilitate an adequate nutritional intake.

A high-calorie, high-protein diet is indicated if the patient can eat. The diet is essentially a normal one with added protein and supplementary high-calorie feedings. High-protein diets are contraindicated if there is liver disease.

RESEARCH

Metheny N, Eisenberg P, and McSweeney M: Effect of feeding tube properties and three irrigants on clogging rates, Nurs Res 37(3):165-169, 1988.

The purpose of this study was to examine the effect of polyurethane and silicone feeding tubes of sizes 8 Fr, 10 Fr, and 12 Fr on the incidence of tube clogging and the efficacy of water, Coca-Cola, and cranberry juice in preventing tube clogging. In a laboratory setting, the tubes were divided equally among the 54 polyurethane and 54 silicone tubes connected to gravity flow feeding bags containing isotonic enteral formulas. On each of 3 days, one set of tubes at each station was irrigated periodically with one of the three irrigating fluids. The polyurethane tubes were significantly superior to silicone tubes in promoting flow of enteral formula. There was no significant difference in flow rates in tubes of varying diameters (although the 8 Fr tubes were significantly more difficult to aspirate). Both Coca-Cola and water were significantly superior to cranberry juice in maintaining tube patency. ■

TUBE FEEDINGS

When the person cannot swallow because of dysphagia, paralysis, or unconsciousness, enteral feedings are given. Tube feedings do not require surgery; therefore they are practical for moderate time periods.

Enteral Feeding Tubes

The most common types of feeding tubes are constructed of polyurethane or silicone; the polyurethane tubes have a larger inside diameter and have been shown to facilitate greater fluid flow (see the research box above). Enteral feeding tubes come in different sizes: 8 Fr (small bore), 10 Fr, 12 Fr, and 14 Fr (large bore). Some tubes have a monofilament or stainless steel stylet for easy passage. A tube with a weighted end may be used to help pass the tube through the pylorus into the duodenum or jejunum. Small bore tubes are more easily tolerated, but certain types of feedings may coagulate and block these tubes (Table 42-2). Small bore tubes also collapse with suction; therefore, aspiration of stomach contents for residual feedings cannot be done.

Technique

Administration of tube feedings may be by bolus, gravity drip, or infusion pump. *Bolus* delivery consists of infusing 300 to 400 ml of formula over several minutes four to six times daily.[24] It is appropriate only for persons who can eat and are receiving supplemental tube feedings. The sudden influx of the feeding may cause nausea, cramping, diarrhea, or aspiration. The *gravity* method consists of placing the fluid in a fluid bag at-

TABLE 42-2 Tube feedings

	Elemental	Supplemental	Liquid Whole Foods
Examples	Vivonex Flexical Pregestimil	Precision Vital	Ensure Sustacal Isocal
Content	Simple carbohydrates, amino acids	Complex carbohydrates, peptides	Complex carbohydrates, proteins
Osmolality	500-800 mOsm	450-600 mOsm	300-600 mOsm
Advantages	Given through small-bore tube Well tolerated for prolonged use	Can be given through small-bore tube More effective protein content than elemental	Lower osmolality Moderate price Acceptable flavor More nutritionally complete
Disadvantages	Unpalatable High osmolality Not well tolerated by bolus feeding Excellent culture media for bacteria Expensive Require monitoring of blood glucose and electrolytes	More expensive than liquid whole foods Tend to coagulate in tube Require monitoring of blood glucose and electrolytes	High fat content Tend to coagulate in tube May require a large-bore tube

tached to the nasoenteral tube and allowing the fluid to run in by gravity. Disadvantages of this method include erratic fluid flow and greater potential of tube blockage. The gravity method may be used for intermittent or continuous administration. Most persons can tolerate 250 to 400 ml per feeding given over 20 to 30 minutes. The *infusion pump* is the preferred method for more constant administration rate and less probability of tube blockage or of diarrhea; however, it is more expensive. Pump accuracy must be checked routinely by comparing the actual drop count with the preestablished rate.

Solutions

Different types of fluids may be given by tube feedings (Table 42-2). Blenderized whole foods may be used; these are nutritious and less expensive, but they require large-bore tubes and are good culture media for bacteria. Elemental and semielemental feedings are more easily digested and can be given through smallbore tubes, but they are more expensive and less nutritionally complete than liquid whole foods.

Preventing Complications

Methods of preventing complications include the following:

1. **Regurgitation with aspiration:** keep head elevated to at least 30 degrees at all times.
2. **Tube dislodgement:** tape tube to nose.
3. **Tube clogging**
   a. Give fluid at a constant rate (by pump, if possible).
   b. Give water before and after intermittent feedings.

4. **Nausea**
   a. Give feedings at lukewarm (room) temperature.
   b. Stop feeding if nausea is present, and notify physician.
   c. When restarting feeding, administer it more slowly until tolerated.
5. **Bacterial contamination**
   a. Do not let feeding hang for more than 6 hours.
   b. Change equipment every 24 hours.
6. **Dehydration**
   a. Give water as necessary; total fluid intake should equal urinary output.
   b. Isoosmolality is 300 mOsm; the greater the osmolality of the feeding, the more water is needed.
   c. Give extra water if the need is increased, such as with fever.
   d. Monitor for decreased skin turgor, thirst, and dry mucous membranes.
7. **Diarrhea**
   a. Initiate feedings slowly at half strength.
   b. Increase concentration and rate gradually (do not change both concentration and rate at the same time).
   c. If diarrhea occurs:
      (1) Decrease rate of fluid flow.
      (2) Administer prescribed antidiarrheal medication through tube.
8. **Hyperglycemia**
   a. Monitor urine for glucose and acetone.
   b. If urine tests positively, decrease rate of feeding flow and notify physician.

Home tube feedings

Home tube feedings can be maintained by persons after receiving instruction in insertion and care of the tube, in formula care and insertion, and in monitoring for complications. An enteral infusion pump may be rented or purchased. The person needs to know where in the community to purchase materials (tubes, administration sets, and formula bags).

GASTROSTOMY

Method

Gastrostomy is an alternative approach to nasogastric tube feedings when the person is unable to swallow for a long period. The procedure is performed under local or general anesthesia and involves the creation of an opening into the abdomen and insertion of the catheter through the stomach wall.

The *percutaneous endoscopic gastrostomy* (PEG) does not require incision into the abdominal cavity and is a safer and more rapid method. It is performed under local anesthesia; the patient is mildly sedated. A small incision is made on the skin of the abdomen, and a cannula is pushed through the adjacent abdominal and gastric walls while the site is observed through a gastroscope. A long silk suture is threaded through the cannula, grasped through the endoscope, and pulled up through the endoscope, which is then removed. The exit end of a specially prepared mushroom catheter is attached to the thread, and the catheter is then pulled in retrograde fashion through the esophagus and stomach and out the abdominal wall. Internal and external dams hold the catheter in place. A jejunostomy tube may be inserted by the same method.

Food and Fluids

After gastrostomy tube insertion, the physician may order the tube to be attached to low intermittent suction for 24 hours, or fluids may be started the first day. The following method may be used for giving the initial feedings, as tolerated:[11]

Day 1: One half concentration of feeding solution at 25 ml/hr by continuous drip

Day 2: Full-strength feeding solution at 50 ml/hr by continuous drip

Day 3: Full-strength solution at 75 ml/hr by continuous drip

After day 3, as tolerated: Change to bolus feeding of 500 ml every 4 to 6 hours for gastrostomies; jejunostomies require continuous infusions

Principles of administration are the same as for tube feedings. A dressing is not generally used to prevent the possibility of skin maceration, breakdown, or infection. The skin may be cleaned with hydrogen peroxide solution to remove crusts and rinsed with normal saline or water.

The psychologic trauma of not being able to eat normally is usually severe. The patient may become depressed and needs a great deal of encouragement. However, as most patients become proficient in feeding themselves, they gradually accept this method of obtaining nourishment as inevitable and adjust remarkably well. (A nursing care plan can be found on pp. 1260-1261).

Continent Tubeless Gastrostomy

A different type of gastrostomy does not require a tube and therefore lessens the chance of complications from tube irritation or obstruction. A small tube is formed of stomach wall and then pushed in to form an intussuception valve.[44] The "valve" is brought out flush with the skin surface to form a flat stoma. The valve prevents leakage of stomach contents; therefore no skin care or dressings are needed. A feeding tube is inserted through the valve for feedings. The stoma can be closed at a later date.

TOTAL PARENTERAL NUTRITION

Total parenteral nutrition (TPN) is a method of giving highly concentrated solutions (1800 to 2200 mOsm/L) intravenously to maintain protein synthesis when enteral nutrition is not possible. Indications for this therapy include (1) major gastrointestinal diseases, fistulas, or inflammatory diseases, (2) extensive negative nitrogen balance such as occurs with major body burns, trauma, or starvation, and (3) gastrointestinal side effects from radiation therapy.

Method

A small incision is made below the clavicle, and a Hickman catheter is inserted directly into the subclavian vein and threaded through the innominate vein into the superior vena cava (Figure 42-6) under strict aseptic conditions. The large amount of blood in the superior vena cava helps to dilute the highly concentrated solution rapidly and thus prevent phlebitis or vein occlusion. Catheters are designed so the end of the catheter can be capped between infusions. At the completion of an infusion, the catheter is filled with heparinized saline to prevent clotting and is capped until time for the next infusion.

The catheter is secured with one suture and covered by an air-occlusive dressing. The dressing may be transparent (Op-Site) or a gauze dressing covered entirely with adhesive tape. The infusion is started with a standard intravenous fluid (5% dextrose) until a radiograph confirms the location of the catheter tip in the superior vena cava.

Solutions

Solutions for TPN are good culture media, therefore they are prepared under strict aseptic conditions in the

NURSING CARE PLAN

PERSON WITH PROTEIN-CALORIE MALNUTRITION AND GASTROSTOMY

DATA: Mr. P. is a 67-year-old retired salesman who experienced progressive dysphagia for many months. He was diagnosed as having cancer of the upper esophagus and given a series of radiation treatments. He was admitted for a gastrostomy to be performed today.

The nursing history identified the following:
- Mr. P. cannot swallow solids and can swallow only small sips of liquid.
- Mr. P.'s mouth feels very dry, and tastes foul.
- Mr. P. has lost 50 pounds in the past 18 months and tires easily.

- Mr. P. states that he knows he will probably not live much longer and has his personal effects in order; his wife is very supportive.
- Mr. P. knows that he will be feeding himself through the gastrostomy at home.

Physical examination data included the following:
- Height 178 cm (70 in), weight 54 kg (120 lbs)
- Skin and mucous membrances dry; poor skin turgor; no signs of infection
- Respirations shallow
- Muscle strength of extremities weak, poor muscle tone

NURSING DIAGNOSIS

Nutrition, altered: less than body requirements related to inadequate nutrient intake and increased nutrient requirements

Expected Patient Outcomes	Nursing Interventions	Rationale
Mr. P.'s weight is not less than 54 kg.	Give gastrostomy feeding at constant drip	Because Mr. P. has not had food in a long time, sluggish peristalsis may be present.
	Monitor for nausea or abdominal fullness; give prescribed antiemetic if necessary.	Vomiting could lead to choking and aspiration because of narrowed esophagus.
	Give gastrostomy feeding while patient is in a sitting position.	Sitting position prevents reflux of feeding into the esophagus.

NURSING DIAGNOSIS

Fluid volume deficit related to decreased fluid intake

Expected Patient Outcomes	Nursing Interventions	Rationale
Mr. P.'s skin shows less dryness, improved turgor.	Flush tube with 60 ml water q2h, if tolerated.	Flushing tube increases hydration, as well as keeping tube patent, so Mr. P. receives prescribed amount.
Mr. P. has balanced intake and output.	Monitor intake and output each shift.	This ensures that fluid intake equals output, thus achieving fluid balance.

NURSING DIAGNOSIS

Oral mucous membranes, altered, related to radiation treatments and lack of oral fluid intake

Expected Patient Outcomes	Nursing Interventions	Rationale
Mr. P.'s mucous membranes of mouth are moist. Mr. P. states that mouth feels better.	Encourage Mr. P. to brush teeth 2×/day and to rinse mouth well with water or desired mouthwash every 1 to 2 hours.	Mr. P. may be bringing up discharge from esophagus. Keeping mouth clean will prevent debris from forming and giving mouth a bad taste; frequent rinsing will keep membranes moist.

NURSING DIAGNOSIS

Fatigue related to inadequate nutrient intake, increased nutrient demands, and muscle weakness

NURSING CARE PLAN

PERSON WITH PROTEIN-CALORIE MALNUTRITION AND GASTROSTOMY—cont'd

Expected Patient Outcomes	Nursing Interventions	Rationale
Mr. P. states feeling more rested.	Help Mr. P. plan for rest periods between planned activities. As Mr. P. feels stronger, encourage leg exercises; monitor pulse and respiration during activity.	Rest decreases energy expenditure and allows ATP to be stored for activity. Gastrostomy feedings will provide carbohydate (CHO) and fat for energy; exercises increase muscle tone; dyspnea on exertion and pulse that does not stabilize in 5 min indicate need to modify activity.

NURSING DIAGNOSIS
Infection, potential for, related to decreased protein intake

Expected Patient Outcomes	Nursing Interventions	Rationale
Infection of the skin, especially around gastrostomy tube, does not occur.	Wash hands well before giving patient care Encourage Mr. P. to be as active as possible within fatigue limits. Clean area around gastrostomy tube with hydrogen peroxide and water. Instruct Mr. P. to avoid persons with upper respiratory infections; encourage deep-breathing exercises 3 to 4 times a day.	Mr. P. is at high risk for infection because of decreased lymphocytes from lack of protein. Activity prevents pressure areas on skin and promotes circulation, thus helping to prevent infection. Cleaning removes crusts and debris that could lead to skin maceration and infection. Mr. P. is at high risk of pulmonary infections because of site of esophageal cancer, history of smoking, and decreased immune response.

NURSING DIAGNOSIS
Knowledge deficit related to lack of exposure

Expected Patient Outcomes	Nursing Interventions	Rationale
Mr. and Mrs. P. demonstrate gastrostomy feeding and care of tube.	Teach Mr. P. and wife how to give the feedings and care of the tube; assist in giving feedings before discharge.	Doing the feedings before discharge provides chance to feel comfortable doing the procedure.
Mr. and Mrs. P. describe formula care.	Explain reasons for formula care and ask for feedback.	If rationale known, Mr. P. is more likely to carry out the care correctly.
Mr. and Mrs. P. describe plans for feedings related to family meal times.	Help Mr. P. and wife to work out a feeding schedule so Mr. P. can be part of meal activities.	Keeping usual meal activities with the accompanying socialization that occurs will help patient digest feedings.
Mr. and Mrs. P. describe community resources for supplies and assistance.	Discuss where supplies can be obtained; suggest Mrs. P. get initial supplies before Mr. P. is discharged. Evaluate need for services of community health nurse.	If Mrs. P. is prepared and organized before Mr. P. is discharged, the first feedings will go more smoothly. A community health nurse can help the family adjust to home care.

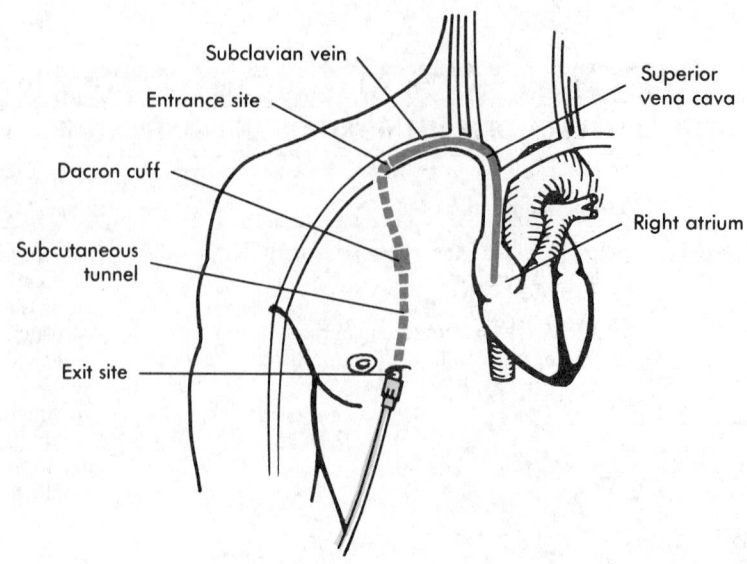

FIGURE 42-6 Placement of Hickman catheter for administration of TPN solutions.

pharmacy under a laminar airflow hood. The physician orders the solution contents based on the patient's nutritional needs. The solutions are kept refrigerated until ready for use and are then warmed to room temperature before infusion. Prepared formulas should be used within 24 to 36 hours to prevent contamination.

TPN solutions usually consist of 25% to 35% dextrose, 3% to 5% amino acids, electrolytes, minerals, and vitamins. Intravenous fat may also be added. Dextrose and fat are given for caloric value so that the proteins are saved for anabolism. Fat provides twice the caloric value of dextrose, exerts minimal osmotic pressure, and prevents fatty acid deficiency. Regular insulin may be added to the solution or given by injection for glucose utilization.

Complications

Complications of TPN may be mechanical, infectious, or metabolic. *Mechanical* problems may include pneumothorax, hemothorax, air embolism, catheter misplacement, brachial plexus injury, and thromboembolism. These complications are rare with correct catheter insertion and maintenance. *Infection* is a serious complication but can be prevented by conscientious aseptic technique during catheter insertion and subsequent care. The techniques of catheter care are described in detail in texts teaching the fundamentals of nursing.

The major *metabolic* alterations are hyperglycemia or hypoglycemia. Other possible alterations include fluid imbalances; electrolyte imbalances in sodium, potassium, calcium, magnesium, and phosphates; and acid-base imbalances (primarily acidosis). Vitamin D deficiency and vitamin A excess may also occur. Serum levels are monitored several times a week. Urine is tested

for sugar and acetone. The patient is weighed daily for the first 2 weeks and three times a week thereafter. Early satiety may occur for several days after TPN is discontinued (see the research box on the opposite page).

Patient Care

Care of the patient receiving TPN consists of preventing infection and air embolism, maintaining fluid and electrolyte balance, encouraging ambulation and activities of daily living, and promoting comfort (see the box on the opposite page). Hypoglycemia may occur with a very slow rate of administration; hyperglycemia and overhydration may occur with a very fast rate.

NAUSEA AND VOMITING
ETIOLOGY

Nausea and vomiting often are part of the body's response to insults to its integrity. They usually occur together, but occasionally, if the mechanism for vomiting is touched off by local pressure in the medulla, vomiting may be sudden and not preceded by nausea or any other warning sensation. Vomiting that occurs early in the morning may be related to pregnancy, metabolic states such as uremia, or chronic alcoholism.[59] Vomiting after meals is more likely to be associated with a gastric disturbance such as gastritis, food allergies, or food poisoning. Postoperative vomiting may occur at any time after surgery.

PATHOPHYSIOLOGY

There are two centers in the medulla involved with vomiting: the chemoreceptor emetic trigger zone and

RESEARCH

Martyn PA, Hansen BC, and Jen KC: The effects of parenteral nutrition on food intake and gastric motility, Nurs Res 33(6):336, 1984.

Persons being given parenteral nutrition (PN) have reported ravenous appetites while receiving PN but then have demonstrated early satiety when oral intake was resumed.

The purpose of this study was to investigate the effects of parenteral nutrition on food intake and gastric motility. Catheters to infuse parenteral nutrition and cannulas to measure gastric motility were surgically implanted into four healthy rhesus monkeys. The monkeys were allowed to continue eating on demand after surgery, while being administered PN in amounts ranging from 25% to 100% of the normal daily caloric intake. The monkeys ate beyond their caloric demands during the first 2 days, but then oral intake decreased directly proportional to the percent of calories infused. After cessation of PN, satiety continued for 8 to 14 days, indicating a physiologic basis for post-PN satiety. ∎

---

the vomiting center. The *vomiting center* may be stimulated directly through the vagal or sympathetic nerves. Gastrointestinal irritants, distention or injury of any of the viscera, pain, and psychic trauma cause nausea and vomiting in this manner. Increased intracranial pressure may stimulate vomiting by direct local pressure. The vomiting center also may be stimulated indirectly through the *chemoreceptor emetic trigger zone*. Emetic agents such as morphine sulfate, meperidine hydrochloride (Demerol), ergot derivatives, digitalis preparations, and metabolic emetic substances resulting from uremia, infection, and radiation stimulate the chemoreceptor center to produce vomiting. Labyrinthine stimulation, the primary factor in the nausea and vomiting of motion sickness (seasickness, airsickness), is also believed to pass through the trigger center. It still is not clear by what route irritating gasses such as those used in anesthesia affect the vomiting center or what specifically causes some women to vomit during the first trimester of pregnancy.

Nausea and vomiting are distressing to most people, but vomiting also causes serious effects. Prolonged and severe vomiting will interfere with nutrition and cause fluid and electrolyte imbalance, specifically dehydration and metabolic alkalosis with loss of potassium, chloride, and hydrogen ions (Chapter 24). The act of vomiting produces a strain on the abdominal muscles, and in some postoperative patients it may cause wound separation, wound dehiscence, or bleeding. Vomiting is especially dangerous for anesthetized patients, persons in coma, and infants because they are likely to aspirate the vomitus into the lungs. Aspiration may cause asphyxia, atelectasis, or pneumonitis, especially in the elderly per-

GUIDELINES FOR TOTAL PARENTERAL NUTRITION

1. Prevention of infection
   a. Maintain strict aseptic technique
   b. Keep solutions cold until ready for use; use within 24-36 hours
   c. Change dressings 3 times a week for gauze dressings, once a week for polyurethane dressings[45]
2. Prevention of air embolism
   a. Tape all connections of the system
   b. Clamp catheter when opening system
   c. Cover insertion site with an air-occlusive dressing (covered with adhesive tape) or transparent polyurethane (Op-Site) dressing
3. Maintain fluid and electrolyte balance
   a. Maintain a continuous uniform infusion rate
   b. If rate is too *slow:*
      1. Return rate to prescribed rate
      2. If prescribed rate does not resume, ask person to change position
      3. Monitor and report to physician signs of *hypoglycemia* (pallor, diaphoresis, tachycardia, hunger, trembling, behavioral changes)
   c. If rate is too *fast:*
      1. Slow infusion to prescribed rate
      2. Monitor for signs of *overhydration* (neck vein distention, cough, weight gain)
      3. Monitor for signs of *hyperglycemia* (sugar in urine, nausea, weakness, thirst, headache)
   d. Monitor daily weights and intake and output
   e. Monitor serum electrolyte, glucose, and blood urea nitrogen (BUN) levels
4. Encourage ambulation and activities of daily living
5. Promote comfort
   a. Provide for good oral hygiene
   b. Provide emotional support to enhance coping

---

son whose nasopharyngeal reflexes are less acute than those of a younger person.

NURSING ASSESSMENT

Subjective data include the onset and duration of the nausea and vomiting and the person's feelings of discomfort. The person may be experiencing "retching" or dry emesis.

Objective data consist of testing for skin turgor and examination of the mucous membranes for signs of dehydration if the vomiting has been prolonged.

The color of the vomitus may be greenish-yellow, red, or brownish. A greenish-yellow color is caused by gastric juice mixed with bile that has been forced back into the stomach. Bright red vomitus indicates overt bleeding of recent origin. It is important to ascertain whether the contents expelled from the mouth have been vomited from the stomach or coughed up from the lungs. Bloody sputum usually has a more frothy appear ance than hematemesis. Blood that has been in the stomach for a period of time becomes partly digested by the gastric juices and has a dark brown, "coffee-grounds" appearance. This blood may have originated in the stomach, or it may have been swallowed from the nose, mouth, or throat. Vomitus with a fecal odor indicates lower gastrointestinal obstruction.

IMPLEMENTATION

Treatment of nausea and vomiting depends on the cause. Medications or other substances known to cause nausea and vomiting are stopped, and fluid and electrolyte imbalances are treated. Fluids may be given intravenously if the vomiting persists. Most persons will have less vomiting if the emotional components of its cause are removed; therefore measures to reduce anxiety should be instituted. Sedation may help to quiet the patient. Nausea and gagging sometimes are relieved if the patient takes deep breaths through the mouth. Ginger ale and other effervescent drinks seem to have a remarkable effect in controlling postoperative nausea and vomiting and often can be taken and retained long before other fluids are tolerated. Effervescent fluids also may be effective in controlling vomiting from other causes such as motion sickness. Bland foods, such as a baked potato or crackers, may be more easily tolerated.

Antiemetic medications (Table 42-3) may be prescribed orally if the patient is able to retain the tablets. In many instances, however, the medication must be given by rectal suppository or by *deep* intramuscular injection to be effective. Medications to counteract motion sickness are effective prophylactically when taken about 30 minutes before the initial motion and then continued at regular intervals. Any of the antihistaminic drugs may cause drowsiness and dizziness, and the possibility of these reactions is pointed out to persons who are taking them when traveling. These medications are especially hazardous to use when driving. Very few antiemetics are significantly effective against nausea and vomiting induced by chemotherapeutic agents, although prochlorperazine (Compazine) does offer some relief. Some persons have obtained relief by the use of delta-9-tetrahydrocannabinol (THC), the active ingredient of marijuana.

It must be recognized that certain odors or sights can cause the nurse to experience nausea while caring for a patient, especially one who is vomiting. The nurse's own sensations can be diminished by taking slow deep breaths through the mouth rather than the nose. Swallowing repeatedly helps to prevent gagging.

The patient's comfort is facilitated by keeping the emesis basin within easy reach, preferably out of sight,

TABLE 42-3 Antiemetic medications

Generic Name	Trade Name	Dosage	Usage for Nausea and Vomiting
ANTIHISTAMINES			
Buclizine hydrochloride	Bucladin-S	50 mg	Motion sickness, Ménière's syndrome
Cyclizine hydrochloride	Marezine	50 mg	Motion sickness, postoperative nausea and vomiting, vertigo
Dimenhydrinate	Dramamine	50 mg	Motion sickness, vertigo
Hydroxyzine hydrochloride	Atarax, Vistaril	25-100 mg	Upper gastrointestinal disturbances, Ménière's syndrome, postoperative nausea and vomiting
Meclizine hydrochloride	Bonine, Antivert	25-50 mg	Motion sickness, vertigo, postradiation nausea and vomiting
PHENOTHIAZINES			
Chlorpromazine	Thorazine	10-25 mg	General use
Perphenazine	Trilafon	5 mg, IM	Severe nausea and vomiting
Prochlorperazine	Compazine	5-10 mg	General use
Promethazine hydrochloride	Phenergan	12-25 mg	Motion sickness, postoperative nausea and vomiting, vertigo
Triethylperazine	Torecan	10 mg	Postoperative or postradiation nausea and vomiting or chemotherapy
Triflupromazine hydrochloride	Vesprin	5-10 mg, IM	Severe nausea and vomiting
MISCELLANEOUS			
Benzquinamide hydrochloride	Emete-Con	50 mg, IM	Postoperative nausea and vomiting
Diphenidol hydrochloride	Vontrol	20-50 mg	Labyrinthine disturbances, postoperative nausea and vomiting
Trimethobenzamide hydrochloride	Tigan	200-250 mg	General use
Metoclopramide hydrochloride	Reglan	2 mg/kg IV q2h × 5 doses	Before chemotherapy

and emptying the basin immediately after vomiting has ceased. The patient usually appreciates the opportunity to rinse the mouth after vomiting; a flavorful mouthwash is often preferred. The room is kept well ventilated, because disagreeable odors can precipitate further emesis.

DISORDERS OF THE MOUTH

The mouth is an excellent barometer of general health, reflecting general disease and debility, as well as good health. Specific diseases of the mouth most often occur when general nutrition and oral hygiene are poor, when smoking is excessive, and when broken teeth irritate the tissues. The major disorders of the mouth are infections and tumors.

INFECTIONS OF THE MOUTH

Any of the structures of the mouth may develop infections, including the teeth which may develop caries, periapical abscess, or periodontal disease (inflammation of the structures supporting the teeth). These conditions are summarized in Table 42-4 but are not discussed in the text.

ETIOLOGY AND PATHOPHYSIOLOGY

Infections can occur in the buccal mucosa or the salivary glands. The etiology, clinical manifestations, and medical therapy for common mouth infections are described in Table 42-5. *Aphthous stomatitis* (the common canker sore) is a small ulcer on the oral mucosa that often occurs for unknown reasons but may also be associated with inflammatory bowel disease, prolonged fever, or infectious mononucleosis. *Herpetic stomatitis* (cold sore, fever blister) commonly occurs after physical trauma or with stress; the lesions are vesicular and ulcerative. *Vincent's infection* is a necrotic ulcerative inflammation of the gums (gingivitis); it may result from

poor mouth hygiene, inadequate diet and sleep, alcoholism, or other infectious diseases. *Candidiasis* is caused by a fungus and is commonly seen after prolonged administration of antibiotics. It is thought that the antibiotic eliminates the bacteria, permitting the existing fungus to flourish. It also frequently occurs after corticosteroid, radiation, or immune therapy or with AIDS.

Parotitis is an inflammation of the parotid gland, a salivary gland. Acute communicable parotitis (epidemic mumps) is caused by a virus that is transmitted by direct contact with the saliva. Noncommunicable parotitis occurs in debilitated persons whose oral hygiene is poor, whose mouths have been permitted to become dry, and who have not chewed solid foods regularly. Elderly persons are more susceptible than younger ones. Usually the *Staphylococcus* organism is not present.

PREVENTION

Infections of the mouth can be prevented in many instances by adequate nutrition, maintenance of moist mucous membranes, and good oral hygiene. Excessive use of tobacco is discouraged for persons who have an increased risk of developing stomatitis. Prevention of nutritional deficiencies, especially vitamin deficiencies, will help prevent stomatitis, and emphasis on restoring nutritional balance of the debilitated patient will decrease the incidence of mouth infections.

In addition to maintaining the nutrition of the cells, the mucous membranes must be kept moist to prevent infection. Adequate hydration is therefore important. Mouth breathing and oxygen administration may lead to dry mucous membranes. Patients who are not permitted to drink fluids should have frequent mouth care to keep the mouth clean and the mucous membranes moist. Persons whose normal habits include poor mouth or dental care need health education.

The importance of good mouth care cannot be overemphasized. If self-care is inadequate, the nurse must

TABLE 42-4 Disorders of the teeth

Disorder	Characteristics	Clinical Manifestations	Management
Dental caries	Tooth decay	Asymptomatic early; toothache later	Tooth refilled by dentist; patient taught to brush teeth regularly with fluoride toothpaste, avoid refined sugars, and see dentist regularly
Periapical abscess	Abscess around root of tooth; may spread to palate or soft tissues	Severe local pain, malaise, nausea, fever	Root canal therapy or tooth extraction, antibiotics, warm saline mouthwashes
Periodontal disease	Loss of tooth support from inflammation, or degeneration of supporting tissues from accumulation of microorganisms or plaque	Gingivitis, loosening of teeth, pain in tooth pockets	Patient teaching of good oral hygiene, flossing teeth, and dental follow-up in early stages; curettage, gingivectomy, or tooth extraction in later stage

TABLE 42-5 Mouth infections

Type	Etiology	Clinical Signs	Management
Aphthous stomatitis (canker sore)	Autoimmune disorder	Painful small ulceration on oral mucosa; heals in 1 to 3 weeks; is recurrent	Hydrocortisone-antibiotic ointment; Fluocinonide (Lidex) ointment in Orabase
Herpetic stomatitis (cold sore, fever blister)	Herpesvirus type I	Painful vesicles and ulcerations of mouth, lips, or edge of nose; fever, malaise, lymphadenopathy may occur	Palliative: mouthwashes, fluids, soft diet, topical acyclovir (Zovirax)
Vincent's gingivitis (trench mouth)	May be caused by *Borrelia vincentii* or a fusiform bacillus	Painful hemorrhagic gums with ulceration, fever, lymphadenopathy	Oral penicillin, topical hydrogen peroxide, good oral hygiene, referral to dentist for removal of plaque or tartar
Candidiasis (thrush)	*Candida albicans*	Creamy white, curdlike patches closely adherent to mucosa; bleeds and ulcerates when it is scraped off	Oral nystatin, ketoconazole, clotrimazole; amphotericin B for the immunocompromised person

intervene. In situations where the mouth is in poor condition and a fetid odor is present, the task is disagreeable and thus unfortunately is often not carried out as frequently as is needed. Patients who are at high risk of developing infections need mouth care several times a day, and those whose mouths are in poor condition and who are on the verge of developing stomatitis may need attention to oral hygiene as often as every 1 to 2 hours while awake.

■ ASSESSMENT

In patients at high risk of developing infections, the mouth is assessed daily for developing or healing inflammations.

Subjective Data

The patient is questioned about the presence and extent of the following symptoms: pain in the mouth, loss of appetite, nausea, foul taste, and change in salivation. The pain is caused by the inflammatory response, and it restricts ability or desire to keep the teeth and mouth clean, leading to anorexia. Swallowing of inflammatory debris may produce nausea.

Objective Data

The mouth is inspected for the following:
1. Cleanliness
2. Condition of teeth (caries, loose teeth, debris)
3. Signs of inflammation (redness, edema, ulceration, or white curdlike patches of thrush)
4. Bleeding of mucous membranes or gums

Assessment of the patient's ability to carry out oral hygiene measures includes assessment of mental status (decreased consciousnes or confusion), ability to open

mouth (may be restricted because of pain), and cleanliness of the mouth after oral hygiene measures are performed. The ability of the patient to ingest and swallow food is also assessed.

■ DATA ANALYSIS: NURSING DIAGNOSES

Nursing diagnoses are determined from assessment of patient data. Possible nursing diagnoses for the person with a mouth infection may include, but are not limited to, the following:

Diagnostic Title	Possible Etiologies
Knowledge deficit	Lack of exposure/recall
Nutrition, altered: less than body requirements	Difficulty chewing, foul taste, mouth discomfort
Oral mucous membrane, altered	Poor oral hygiene, inflammation
Pain: mouth	Inflammation

■ PLANNING: EXPECTED PATIENT OUTCOMES

Expected patient outcomes for the person with a mouth infection may include, but are not limited to, the following:
1. The patient's mouth is clean; mucosa is pink and moist.
2. Weight remains stable; patient eats a balanced diet.
3. Patient states mouth feels comfortable.
4. Patient can describe risk factors to be avoided to prevent recurrence of oral inflammation.

■ IMPLEMENTATION
Giving Medications

If antibiotics are ordered, they are given on time on a regular schedule to maintain blood levels. If the patient has difficulty swallowing tablets, the tablets are crushed, if possible, or the antibiotics may be given intramuscularly. If nystatin is prescribed for oral thrush, the suspension should be held and swished through the mouth for as long as possible before being swallowed.

Facilitating Eating

If the mouth is very sore and painful, eating may be difficult and the patient may need considerable encouragement. Soft foods, including pureed vegetables and fruits (except citrus, which are irritating to the mucous membranes), cooked cereals, soups, flavored gelatin, and ice cream are best tolerated. Hot, spicy foods that increase pain are to be avoided; cold drinks may be more soothing. High-protein, high-caloric drinks such as eggnog serve both nutritional and fluid needs.

Providing Mouth Care

Thorough and frequent mouth care is very important and includes the following:
1. Frequency of treatment
   a. Mild stomatitis: at least every 4 hours
   b. Severe stomatitis: at least every 2 hours
2. Types of solutions
   a. Alkaline mouthwashes, such as sodium bicarbonate (½ teaspoon in large glass of warm water) or sodium perborate
   b. Hydrogen peroxide diluted 1:4 with normal saline (mix just before using to prevent decomposition)
   c. Lidocaine rinses may be prescribed for stomatitis resulting from chemotherapy
3. Remove dentures if causing pain
4. Use foam/sponge toothbrushes, such as toothettes.
5. Wipe gums and teeth with moistened gauze wrapped around a tongue blade if a toothbrush causes pain; rinse with solution followed by water

Relieving Pain

Pain may be partially relieved by good oral hygiene. Smoking is contraindicated. Cold drinks or sucking on frozen Popsicles may be soothing. Analgesic drugs may be necessary, and lidocaine may be applied to provide topical anesthesia.

Patient Teaching

Persons at high risk of developing recurrent oral infec- contributing factors that can cludes maintaining good nu- st regularly, avoiding foods n, avoiding smoking, and us- chniques to decrease effects

TUMORS OF THE MOUTH
EPIDEMIOLOGY AND ETIOLOGY

The lips, the oral cavity, and the tongue are prone to develop malignant lesions. The largest number of these tumors are squamous cell carcinomas that grow rapidly and metastasize to adjacent structures more quickly than do most malignant tumors of the skin. In the United States oral cancer accounts for 4% of the cancers in males and 2% in females.[2] Over 90% occur in persons age 45-70. There is a higher incidence of cancers of the mouth and throat among persons who are heavy drinkers and smokers. The combination of high alcohol consumption and smoking causes an apparent breakdown in the body's defense mechanism, as evidenced by an increase in the levels of immunoglobulin A (IgA) in saliva.

The cure rate for cancer of the *lips* is high, because the lesion is easily apparent to the patient and to others. Metastasis to regional lymph nodes has occurred in only 10% of persons when diagnosed. In some instances, a lesion may spread rapidly and involve the mandible, and the floor of the mouth by direct extension. Occasionally, the tumor may be a basal cell lesion that starts in the skin and spreads to the lip.

Cancer of the *anterior tongue* and *floor of the mouth* may seem to occur together because their spread to adjacent tissues is so rapid. Metastasis to the neck has already occurred in over 60% of patients when the diagnosis is made because of the tongue's abundant vascular and lymphatic drainage. The mortality is high. Lesions about the base of the tongue may go unnoticed by the patient and may be far advanced when treatment is started.

Tumors of the *salivary glands* occur primarily in the parotid gland and are usually benign. Tumors of the submaxillary gland have a high incidence of malignancy. The malignant tumor grows more rapidly and may be accompanied by pain and impaired facial function.

Kaposi's sarcoma, seen in persons with AIDS, may occur in the mouth (Chapter 72). The lesion may be flat or nodular.

PREVENTION

Avoidance of predisposing factors may decrease the potential for developing cancer of the mouth. This includes avoidance of excess exposure to sun and wind on the lips, elimination of smoking or chewing tobacco or betel leaf, and maintenance of good oral and dental care. There is a high correlation between the incidence of cancer of the mouth and cirrhosis of the liver associated with alcohol intake. Early detection of oral cancer can help increase the patient's chance of survival. Any person with a mouth lesion that does not heal within 2 to 3 weeks is urged to seek immediate medical care.

CLINICAL MANIFESTATIONS

Malignant lesions of the mouth are usually asymptomatic. Early lesions are difficult to detect because there may be an initial inflammatory response that frequently disappears, leaving only a small ulcer or growth. Premalignant lesions (that may or may not become malignant) include *leukoplakia* (white patches), *erythroplasia* (red granular patches), and *erythroplakia* (white plaques within red patches). The red patches have a higher potential for malignancy than leukoplakia.[46]

Cancer of the *lips* usually occurs on the lower lip as a fissure or a painless indurated ulcer with raised edges. Cancers of the *anterior tongue and floor of the mouth* occur as hard plaquelike or ulcerated areas that do not heal. Lesions are usually unilateral, and multiple lesions may occur.

Parotid tumors occur as painless lumps that can be palpated anterior to or directly below the ear. Biopsy of the parotid gland is not recommended because of the potential for tumor seeding; therefore the entire gland is usually removed for examination.

MEDICAL MANAGEMENT

Treatment depends on the location and staging (Table 42-6) of the malignant tumor. Stages I and II oral cancers are treated by surgery or radiation. Stage III cancers require both surgery and radiation. Treatment for stage IV cancer is usually palliative.

Small, accessible stage I tumors can be excised surgically, but large tumors often require more extensive surgery. The tongue may be partially excised (hemiglossectomy) or totally excised (glossectomy). In a *functional* neck dissection on neck cancer with no growth in the lymph nodes, the lymph nodes are removed but the jugular vein, sternocleidomastoid muscle, and spinal accessory nerve are preserved; in a *radical* neck dissection (see Chapter 32) all of these structures are removed.[53] Reconstructive surgery is performed following tissue resection in a neck dissection.

Radiation may be in the form of external radiation by use of roentgenograms or other radioactive substances or in the form of internal radiation by means of needles or seeds (see Chapter 17). If both radiation and surgery are to be performed, radiation will usually be done *after* surgery because radiated oral tissue is more susceptible to infection and tissue breakdown from bacterial contamination by saliva.

■ ASSESSMENT

Subjective data include the following:
1. Knowledge about the effects of surgery or radiation
2. Concerns about possible physical changes
3. Concerns about impairments in eating and speaking
4. Pain or discomfort

Objective data include the following:
1. Condition of the patient's mouth (infection, tissue breakdown) during and following therapy
2. The patient's ability to eat and speak
3. Extent of the patient's interaction with other people

■ DATA ANALYSIS: NURSING DIAGNOSES

Nursing diagnoses are determined from assessment of patient data. Possible nursing diagnoses for the person with oral cancer include, but are not limited to, the following:

Diagnostic Title	Possible Etiologies
Body image, disturbance	Actual or threat of, facial/head disfigurement; foul breath
Communication, impaired verbal	Resection of oral tissue
Knowledge deficit	Lack of exposure/recall
Nutrition, altered: less than body requirements	Chewing or swallowing difficulties, anorexia, foul taste
Oral mucous membranes, altered	Oral cavity radiation, decreased salivation, mouth dryness

■ PLANNING: EXPECTED PATIENT OUTCOMES

Expected patient outcomes for the person after surgery for cancer of the mouth may include, but are not limited to, the following:
1. Incision heals without infection; patient states mouth feels better

---

TABLE 42-6 Staging of oral cancer

Stage	Tumor (T)	Lymph Node (N)	Metastasis (M)
I	$T_1 < 2$ cm	N_0 no growth	M_0 no metastasis
II	T_2 2-4 cm	N_0 no growth	M_0 no metastasis
III	$T_3 > 4$ cm	N_0 no growth	M_0 no metastasis
	$T_1, T_2,$ or T_3	N_1 palpable homolateral node	M_0 no metastasis
IV	$T_4 > 4$ cm with deep invasion	N_0 or N_1	M_0
		Any N_3 fixed nodes	Any M_1 metastasis to liver or lungs

2. Patient feeds self by appropriate means and consumes a nutritionally balanced fluid or soft diet
3. Patient has a means of communication and is working on improving speech
4. Patient interacts with others and states plans for gradual resumption of activities with others
5. Patient states plans for follow-up care
   a. Describes plans to stop smoking, if appropriate
   b. States time for next medical appointment
   c. States signs indicating need for medical attention (pain, bleeding, infection) and follow-up dental care
   d. Describes available community resources

■ IMPLEMENTATION
Facilitating Adaptation of Body Image
Treatment for cancer of the mouth interferes with major oral functions such as eating and speaking and thus creates major changes in the person's life. Changes in

the patient's ability to speak will vary from some limitation to complete inability to speak, depending on the amount of tissue resected or destroyed. Eating patterns will be changed in terms of the consistency of foods, as well as methods of ingestion. The patient may also have problems with choking and aspiration and with nasal returns and drooling. In addition, the person's facial appearance will change depending on the extent of tissue removed or destroyed, and even with reconstructive surgery, noticeable changes will be present.

Therefore one of the major problems that the person will have to cope with and adapt to is the change in body image. Patients need to know in advance the changes that will occur and the measures that will be taken to assist them during the adjustment period. The impact of the loss may be slightly minimized when the grieving process begins early. The full emotional impact of the loss, however, occurs after therapy. (See Chapter 18 for further discussion on body image.)

NURSING CARE OF THE PATIENT AFTER MOUTH SURGERY FOR CANCER

PREOPERATIVE CARE

1. Clarify patient's knowledge of expected changes after surgery
2. Explain expected postoperative measures (including suctioning, nasogastric tube)
3. Provide opportunities for patient to begin to express feelings about changes in body image

POSTOPERATIVE CARE

1. Monitoring
   a. Assess facial movement for facial nerve damage (if parotid gland excised): ask patient to raise eyebrows, frown, smile, show teeth, pucker lips
   b. Assess degree and character of drainage
      (1) Amount of drainage and presence of blood should be minimal
      (2) Hemorrhage may occur with wide resection of tongue
2. Maintaining adequate airway
   a. Place patient in side-lying position initially
   b. Place patient in Fowler's position when fully alert
   c. Suctioning of mouth (except for lip surgery)
   d. Gauze wick may be used to direct saliva into an emesis basin
   e. Maintain patency of drainage tubes, if used
3. Promoting oral hygiene and comfort
   a. Clean involved areas of mouth with cotton applicator moistened with hydrogen peroxide and saline
   b. Mouth irrigations
      (1) Use sterile equipment
      (2) Use solution of sterile water, diluted hydrogen peroxide, normal saline or sodium bicarbonate (avoid commercial mouthwashes)
      (3) Protect any dressings from getting wet

      (4) A catheter may be inserted along the side of cheek and the solution injected with gentle pressure; a spray may also be used
      (5) Give analgesics as indicated (pain is *not* usually severe)
4. Promoting nutrition
   a. Tube feedings will be used initially with hemiglossectomy
   b. Oral fluids: place in back of throat with aseptic syringe or feeding cup with attached tubing
   c. Eating soft foods
      (1) Encourage patient to feed self when possible
      (2) Teach patient to drink clear water after all meals to cleanse mouth
      (3) Avoid using fork, which may traumatize new tissue
   d. Foods
      (1) Avoid long-term use of commercial preparations such as instant breakfast drinks (may cause diarrhea or constipation)
      (2) Give fruit-flavored yogurt preparations which are less irritating than gelatin preparations and are easier to swallow
      (3) Avoid very hot or cold foods (hot foods irritate new tissue; cold foods may cause facial pain or paralyze oral functions)
5. Promoting speech
   a. Limit patient responses initially to *yes* or *no*, which can be answered by gestures
   b. When speech returns, encourage patient to speak slowly
   c. Listen carefully and validate communication before initiating action on requests
   d. Speak in a soft, clear voice
   e. Refer patient to speech therapist if necessary
6. Encourage socialization with others

Surgical Care

Oral prophylactic treatment is given and antibiotics may be administered *preoperatively* to decrease the number of bacteria present in the mouth at the time of surgery. Prostheses of the palate and jaw may be designed to replace portions of tissue that have been resected. If a prosthesis is to be made, impressions will be taken during the preoperative period; the prosthesis will be fitted when healing has occurred postoperatively.

Postoperative care of the patient is focused on promoting an adequate airway, mouth drainage, oral hygiene, comfort, nutrition, and speech (see the box on p. 1269).Good mouth care is essential for comfort, prevention of infection, and promotion of healing. Teeth brushing is usually contraindicated because of discomfort and potential trauma. Sterile equipment is used to prevent introduction of exogenous organisms. Patients are encouraged to assist in their oral hygiene as soon as possible.

The method used to feed the patient will depend entirely on the extent and nature of the therapy. Most patients can suction and feed themselves a few days following mouth surgery and are happier doing so. Through practice, the patient develops confidence in self-care and is often more adept than the nurse in placing the catheter or tube in a position where fluids can be received into the mouth and swallowed without difficulty. A mirror often helps. Privacy is essential during the initial period. The patient should not be hurried and is observed very carefully to determine how much assistance is needed.

Chewing is difficult without the tongue, and the person has a problem getting the food to the posterior pharynx. Sensation in the mouth is decreased, and the patient has difficulty locating the position of the food in the oral cavity. One method of eating is for the person to use the forefinger to push the food to the posterior pharynx.

The ability to speak is commonly lost for short or long periods after surgery, but if the vocal cords are intact, speech will eventually return. Loud noises are disturbing to the patient because the oral tissue loss may create a channel that amplifies sound; the person should therefore be addressed in a soft, clear voice. As speech begins to return, the patient is encouraged to speak slowly and to use the throat rather than the lips to achieve clarity. Speech retraining may be necessary, and a tape recorder may be useful so that the person can hear his or her own voice and work on improvements.

Because of difficulties with eating or talking or with disfigurement in the event of radical surgery, some persons may hesitate to interact with strangers. The person is encouraged to mingle with others as soon as clues indicating readiness are observed. Men are encouraged to shave using an electric razor as soon as this is permitted. Members of the family and close friends are encouraged to visit.

Care During Radiation Therapy

Methods of radiation treatment need to be explained fully to the patient (Chapter 17). Care of the patient with radioactive *needles* embedded in oral tissue includes the following directives:

1. Do not pull strings (to prevent alteration of dosage or direction of radiation or loss of the needles)
2. Check needles several times a day
3. Use alternative methods of communication because talking with needles in place is difficult or impossible
4. Monitor linen or equipment such as emesis basins for needles that may have been dislodged

Secondary effects of radiation therapy of the mouth include mucositis, xerostomia (dryness), and dental decay. Some of the changes may be permanent. *Mucositis,* inflammation of the mucous membranes, is an early reaction. Sloughing of the tissues may occur and cause a fetid odor. Dentures are not tolerated for some time thereafter because of the sensitivity of the tissues. Care of the patient with mucositis includes the following actions:

1. Good oral hygiene
2. Dentures that are worn are checked frequently for fit and removed at night
3. Avoidance of smoking (smoke is irritating to mucous membranes)
4. Avoidance of hot and cold foods or fluids (membranes are sensitive to changes in temperature)
5. Viscous lidocaine (Xylocaine) mouthwashes or lozenges if discomfort seriously interferes with eating

Dryness of the mouth begins 1 to 2 weeks after radiation is started and may persist throughout life. The dryness makes the mouth feel uncomfortable and gives an unpleasant taste. Frequent drinks of water, mouthwashes, and increased humidification of the air contribute to added moisture and comfort.

Dental decay, especially at the gingival margins, results from decreased salivary secretion and altered pH of the saliva. An active control program is started before radiation therapy is initiated and includes a conscientious tooth-brushing regimen using fluoride toothpaste, a soft toothbrush, and dental floss. Fluoride treatments for the teeth may also be given.

Palliative Care

Tissue necrosis and severe pain occur in advanced cancer of the mouth, either from failure of treatment or from death of tissue as a result of radiation. The patient usually experiences difficulty in swallowing, fear of choking, and the constant accumulation of foul-smelling secretions. The danger of severe and even fatal hemorrhage must always be considered. It is very difficult to induce these patients to take sufficient nourishing fluids. A gastrostomy may be done to permit direct introduction of food into the stomach. Family members caring for the person at home need considerable support from hospice or other community health nurses.

TRAUMA OF MOUTH AND JAW
ETIOLOGY

Injuries to the mouth usually result from blows to the face or pressure of foreign objects, such as occur with vehicular accidents. The soft tissue of the mouth may be bruised or lacerated, and the jaw may be fractured.

INTERVENTIONS
Medical Management

Lacerations of the mouth are cleansed or sutured if their extent and location warrant these measures. Antibiotics are usually prescribed for major lacerations because of the large numbers of bacteria found in the mouth.

Fractures of the jaw are treated by closed or open reduction and intermaxillary fixation. The teeth are wired, and then the upper and lower teeth are connected by rubber bands or tie wires to immobilize the jaw. Because of the excellent blood supply to the jaw, fractures usually heal in 5 to 8 weeks.

Nursing Management

Edema may be pronounced following trauma to the mouth and may interfere with respirations. Usually the head of the bed is elevated in semi-Fowler's position to aid in venous drainage from the area and thereby to lessen edema. Tight dressings about the face must be checked carefully because they may contribute to development of edema and may cause headache.

Immediately following wiring of the teeth, the nurse observes the patient for nausea and vomiting resulting from blood or other swallowed material, anesthetic, or emotional trauma. Care must be taken to prevent aspiration of vomitus. Vomitus and secretions must be removed by suction because the patient cannot expectorate them through the mouth. Usually a catheter can be inserted through the nasopharynx or into the mouth through a gap created by missing teeth or in the space behind the third molar. Scissors or a wire cutter should be at the bedside so that the wires can be cut or the elastic bands released if necessary. Specific orders should state the circumstances under which wires or rubber bands should be released.

Persons who have fixation by wiring must often subsist on liquids and must learn to take a high-calorie liquid diet through a catheter or straw. They need instruc-

tions about mouth hygiene, and they must be instructed to report any sudden swelling or pain that may occur after dismissal from the hospital.

ESOPHAGEAL DISORDERS
DYSPHAGIA
ETIOLOGY

Some persons have problems ingesting necessary nutrients because of difficulty in swallowing (*dysphagia*). The underlying cause of the dysphagia influences the person's ability to swallow either solids or liquids. Esophageal dysphagia may be of motor or of obstructive origin (see the box below). Some persons with an anxiety or conversion reaction may experience dysphagia without signs of organic lesions.

PATHOPHYSIOLOGY

Failure of coordination of the voluntary steps necessary to get the food to the esophagus may lead to dysphagia. There may be difficulty moving the food to the back of the throat and initiating the motion of swallowing.

Pharyngeal muscles may be severely weakened, resulting in difficulty moving the food from the oropharynx into the esophagus. Some function may be present so that swallowing can occur with difficulty. Pharyngeal dysphagia is associated with immediate regurgitation.[59] Fluids are more difficult to swallow than soft foods, and there may be regurgitation of fluids through the nasal passages. Aspiration of feedings may occur from failure of the glottis to close.

If the esophageal muscles are involved, esophageal peristaltic waves will be decreased and the lower esophageal sphincter may become incompetent, resulting in

---

CAUSES OF DYSPHAGIA

INCOORDINATION OF SWALLOWING
Upper motor neuron lesions

PHARYNGEAL WEAKNESS
Disease or trauma of cranial nerves V, IX, and X
Brainstem disorders causing bulbar palsy (poliomyelitis, amyotrophic lateral sclerosis, multiple sclerosis)
Diseases affecting neuromuscular transmission (myasthenia gravis, botulism)
Diseases affecting striated muscle (muscular dystrophy, polymyositis)

ESOPHAGEAL DISORDERS
Obstructive disorders
    External compression by enlarged thyroid
    Internal narrowing by tumors or strictures
Motor esophageal disorders
    Achalasia, esophageal spasm

heartburn. Difficulty in swallowing both solids and liquids is experienced.

Obstruction of the esophagus causes a decrease in the esophageal lumen. The patient has difficulty swallowing solids around the partial obstruction.

NURSING ASSESSMENT

A person who gives a history of difficulty in swallowing is questioned as follows concerning the nature and circumstances of the dysphagia:

Is there greater dysphagia with liquids or with solids?

Is dysphagia intermittent or does it occur each time swallowing is attempted?

Are there other associated symptoms, such as pain with swallowing?

What approaches to eating has the person found most useful?

If dysphagia is suspected, a physical assessment is made of the person's ability to swallow. The mouth is observed for signs of drooling, as occurs with facial paralysis seen in the patient with a cerebrovascular accident or with Bell's palsy. The gag reflex is elicited by touching the posterior tongue or pharynx with a tongue blade. The person is asked to swallow, and movement of the larynx is observed. A finger can be placed lightly over the thyroid cartilage of the larynx (Adam's apple) to facilitate detection of movement. If movement is limited and the gag reflex weak, a further assessment is made by placing 1 to 2 ml of water in the oropharynx and asking the patient to swallow.

NURSING MANAGEMENT

If the dysphagia results from *incoordination of swallowing,* the patient may chew a mouthful of food for a period of time and then accept a second mouthful, unaware that swallowing has not occurred. Considerable amounts of food can collect between the cheek and gums. The patient may need to be directed to close the mouth when swallowing, because it is difficult to swallow with an open mouth. Directions must be kept simple and extraneous conversation omitted so that the person can concentrate on swallowing.

The person with *pharyngeal weakness* can often tolerate solids more easily than liquids. The *double-swallow* technique may help the person who retains food in the pharynx. The person is instructed to (1) inhale, (2) put food bolus in pharynx and swallow, (3) exhale, and (4) swallow again. This helps to minimize the possibility of aspiration. The severely dysphagic person is closely supervised during feedings, and suction equipment should be available. A feeding syringe may be helpful when facial paralysis is present. The head-elevated position is the position of choice; if this is impossible, the patient is positioned on the *unaffected* side during feeding to ensure better control. If the ability to swallow is absent, tube feedings are usually instituted.

If *esophageal weakness* is present, frequent small feedings are suggested. Eating with the head elevated encourages movement of food through the esophagus by gravity. Regurgitation of food may occur several hours after eating, especially at night when the body is horizontal.

Persons with partially obstructive lesions may be able to eat solids cut into very small bites. Some persons can swallow only liquids; oral nutritional formulas or blenderized foods are given. Diarrhea may result from the lack of fiber.

GASTROESOPHAGEAL REFLUX DISEASE
ETIOLOGY

Gastroesophageal reflux disease (GERD) refers to a group of conditions that cause reflux of gastric and duodenal contents into the esophagus. Causes of GERD include an idiopathic incompetent lower esophageal sphincter, pregnancy, obesity, ascites, hiatal hernia, or postoperative resection of the lower esophagus for cancer. The major cause is a sliding hiatal hernia.

PATHOPHYSIOLOGY

At the junction of the esophagus and stomach, the esophagus is slightly hypertrophied and has a high resting wall tension as a result of its usual contracted state. The muscle at this point is called the lower esophageal sphincter (LES). When food enters the pharynx and esophagus, the LES relaxes to permit the food to pass into the stomach. At all other times, the LES is contracted to prevent reflux of gastric material back into the esophagus.

When LES pressure is lower than it should be, reflux occurs. LES pressure is increased by gastrin release in the stomach and is decreased by secretin and cholecystokinin from the small intestine. Other substances that decrease LES pressure include anticholinergics, caffeine, theobromine, ethyl alcohol, and smoking. Reflux is more likely to occur when gravitational pull is decreased, such as when the person is lying down.

Hiatal hernia refers to a protrusion of part of the stomach through the diaphragmatic hiatus into the thoracic cavity. The herniation may include the esophagogastric junction (sliding hiatal hernia or a separate portion of the stomach excluding the esophagogastric junction (paraesophageal hiatal hernia) (Figure 42-7). Factors contributing to the development of these hernias include obesity, trauma, and a general weakening of the supporting structures as a result of aging.

CLINICAL MANIFESTATIONS

The major symptom of GERD is *heartburn* (pyrosis). Persons with heartburn experience a substernal "burning" sensation that may be referred to the neck or back if severe. It is frequently accompanied by a sour regur-

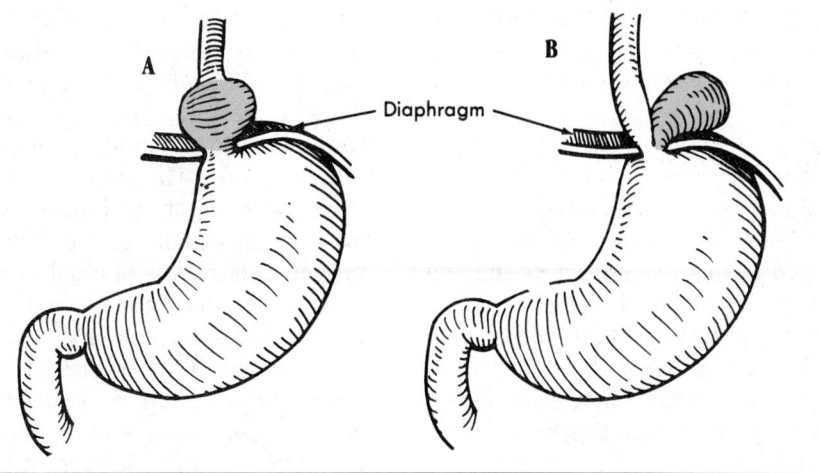

FIGURE 42-7 Hiatal hernia. **A**, Sliding hernia. **B**, Paraesophageal hernia.

gitation of gastric contents into the mouth but is not accompanied by nausea.

An incompetent LES can be diagnosed by roentgenograms in Trendelenburg's position or by fluoroscopy. A water siphon test is a fluoroscopic examination in which barium is swallowed, followed by plain water. If the LES is incompetent, the barium will be seen to reflux back into the esophagus. Overnight pH recordings measured from swallowed glass electrodes will demonstrate periods of increased gastric reflux. Scanning of the esophagus after ingestion of a radioisotope, technetium-99m, may also be used to measure reflux.[59] If a hiatal hernia is present, it may be diagnosed by roentgenogram (upper gastrointestinal series).

INTERVENTIONS

Medical Management

Gastric acidity can be decreased by administration of 30 ml of a liquid antacid taken 1 and 3 hours after meals, at bedtime, and whenever heartburn occurs. Gaviscon, which is a mixture of antacids with alginic acid, has been found to be effective in producing a viscous antacid foam that coats the esophagus and floats on the gastric contents. It is supplied in the form of liquid or tablets (that must be chewed well before swallowing).

If antacids are not effective, medications that increase LES contraction may be prescribed; these include bethanechol chloride (Urecholine) or metoclopramide hydrochloride (Reglan), to be taken 30 minutes before meals and at bedtime. Cimetidine, ranitidine, or famotidine (histamine H_2 receptor blockers) may be used for severe reflux. These drugs act by reducing gastric secretions, thereby decreasing the irritating effects.

Surgery may be indicated if a hiatal hernia is present that does not respond to medical therapy. Surgery may consist of (1) a posterior gastropexy (returning the stomach to the abdomen and suturing it in place) (Hill repair), (2) transabdominal or transthoracic fundoplica-

tion (wrapping the fundus around the lower part of the esophagus and suturing it in place, or the Nissen procedure), or (3) placing a doughnut-shaped silicone prosthesis around the intraabdominal esophagus (Angelchik prosthesis).[46] Care of the patient after surgery is similar to that after gastric surgery (Chapter 43) or thoracic surgery (Chapter 34), depending on the procedure performed.

Nursing Management

Patient teaching for GERD includes the following:
1. High-protein, low-fat diet (to stimulate release of gastrin and cholecystokinin)
2. Avoidance of foods containing caffeine (coffee, tea, colas), theobromine (chocolate), and alcohol, which decrease LES pressure
3. Small, frequent meals (to prevent gastric distention with resulting gastric acid secretion)
4. *Avoidance* of:
   a. Smoking (decreases lower esophageal sphincter [LES] pressure)
   b. Supine position for 2 to 3 hours after eating
   c. Bending over (increases intraabdominal pressure)
   d. Lifting heavy objects and wearing tight belts or girdles after eating (to prevent increased abdominal pressure)
5. Sleeping with the head slightly elevated (head of bed may be raised on 15 cm blocks) to prevent nocturnal regurgitation

ACHALASIA
ETIOLOGY

Achalasia, also called cardiospasm or aperistalsis, is a condition in which there is an absence of peristalsis in the esophagus and in which the esophageal sphincter fails to relax after swallowing. The cause is unknown, but the disorder is a direct result of disruption of the normal neuromuscular mechanisms of the esophagus. The disease may occur in persons of any age, but it is more prevalent in persons between 20 and 50 years of age.

PATHOPHYSIOLOGY

In the early phases of achalasia there is no gross lesion, but as the disease persists, the portion of the esophagus around the constriction dilates (Figure 42-8) and the muscular walls become hypertrophied. The dilated area becomes atonic, and esophageal peristalsis may be absent so that little or no food can enter the stomach. Although varying degrees of the condition exist, in extreme cases the esophagus above the constriction may hold a liter or more of fluid.

CLINICAL MANIFESTATIONS

Clinical manifestations of achalasia include the following:

1. Gradual onset of dysphagia for both liquids and solids (months to years)
2. Loss of weight; avitaminosis
3. Possible occurrence of substernal chest pain
4. Regurgitation of esophageal contents onto pillow at night
5. Diagnostic tests: barium swallow roentgenograms, esophagoscopy

INTERVENTIONS

Medical Management

Conservative temporary pharmacologic treatment consists of nitrates (isosorbide dinitrate) and calcium-channel blockers (nifedipine) to reduce LES pressure, but these drugs are only partly effective. The treatment of choice is forceful dilation of the LES by *pneumatic dilators*. In this procedure, the esophageal contents are first emptied; then a dilator with a deflated balloon is passed down to the LES. The person usually experiences retrosternal pain when the balloon is inflated for a 1-minute period. The balloon may be reinflated two or three times. Esophageal motility is not restored, but the open sphincter relieves the dysphagia in about 80% of persons and the size of esophageal lumen is reduced.

Surgical intervention, consisting of *cardiomyotomy*, may be necessary if sphincter dilation is unsuccessful. The muscular layer is incised longitudinally down to, but not through, the mucosa. Two thirds of the incision is in the esophagus, and the remaining one third is in the stomach; this permits the mucosa to expand so that food can pass more easily into the stomach. A fundoplication (p. 1273) is often performed concurrently to prevent postoperative gastric reflux.

Nursing Management

Until treatment can be initiated, the person is encouraged to drink fluids with meals and use the Valsalva maneuver (bearing down with a closed glottis) while swallowing, to increase LES pressure and to help push the food beyond the LES. A soft diet will encourage more rapid esophageal emptying.[33] Elevation of the head at night will help to prevent nocturnal regurgitation. One method for the patient to elevate the head of the bed at home is to fill two large cans with sand or soil to within 2 inches of the top, place the removed metal can tops over the sand/soil, and then put the cans under the legs of the head posts.

Care of the patient after esophageal surgery is described on p. 1273. The patient is monitored for signs of

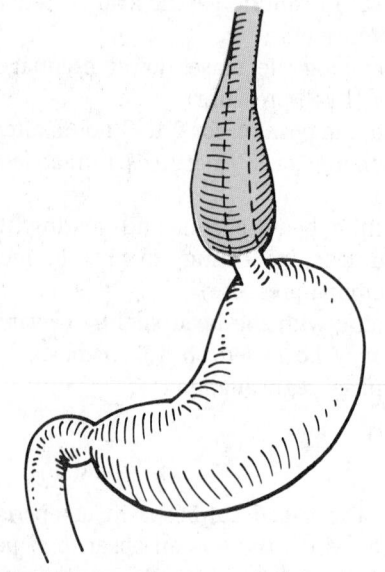

FIGURE 42-8 Achalasia.

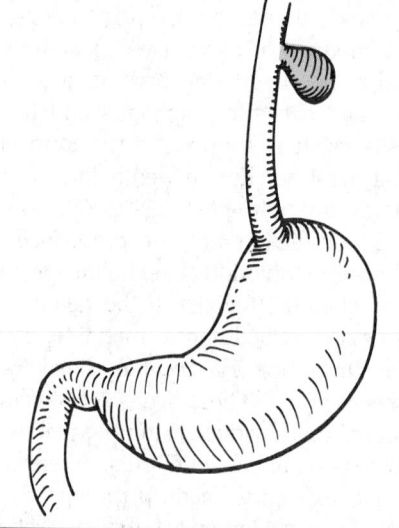

FIGURE 42-9 Esophageal diverticulum.

esophageal perforation as evidenced by chest pain, shock, dyspnea, and fever. Regurgitation occasionally occurs after surgery but can usually be controlled by antacid medications. Because regurgitation may still occur at night, the patient is advised to refrain from ingesting food or fluid for several hours before retiring and to sleep with the head elevated.

ESOPHAGEAL DIVERTICULUM
PATHOPHYSIOLOGY

An esophageal diverticulum is the outpouching of the esophageal mucosa and submucosa through a weakened portion of the muscular layer of the esophagus (Figure 42-9). It is most commonly found at the pharyngoesophageal junction. As food is ingested, some of it may pass into the diverticulum. After a sufficient amount has accumulated in the pocket, it overflows into the esophagus and is regurgitated. There is always danger that some of the regurgitated material may be aspirated into the trachea and lungs during sleep or that the diverticulum may enlarge and cause esophageal obstruction.

CLINICAL MANIFESTATIONS

The patient may complain of pain on swallowing, regurgitation, gurgling noises over the esophagus where the diverticulum is located, and a cough caused by tracheal irritation. Decomposition of food in the diverticulum may cause foul breath. The odor can be alleviated somewhat by frequent brushing of the teeth and the use of aromatic mouthwashes. Weight loss, weakness, and anemia are common. Esophageal diverticulum is diagnosed by barium swallow.

INTERVENTIONS

If the symptoms become severe, surgery is performed. The herniated sac is excised. Myotomy of the cricopharyngeal muscle (upper esophageal sphincter) may be sufficient for small pharyngoesophageal diverticulum. These procedures are well tolerated, and the administration of antibiotics makes postoperative infections rare. A temporary fistula may develop postoperatively, but this usually heals spontaneously. Nursing care of the patient after esophageal surgery is discussed on page 1276.

ESOPHAGEAL STRICTURE
ETIOLOGY AND PATHOPHYSIOLOGY

Strictures of the esophagus may result from ingestion of corrosive substances (alkaline or acid), scleroderma, reflux esophagitis, or prolonged nasogastric intubation. Irritation of the esophageal walls leads to formation of an anular stricture that decreases the esophageal lumen and leads to dysphagia. Food may collect and partially or totally obstruct the esophagus; fluids are easier to swallow than solids.

INTERVENTIONS

Treatment of esophageal strictures is accomplished with graduated dilation by mechanical dilators (bougies) or balloons. Rubber or metal *mechanical dilators* of increasing sizes are passed through the area of stricture, producing mild discomfort. Deflated *balloons* are passed through an endoscope to the stricture site and inflated with water to create pressure. The dilation procedure may be repeated every 3 to 4 weeks for severe strictures or every 4 to 6 months for mild strictures. The person takes nothing by mouth for 8 hours before the dilation procedure. Premedication may be given for highly anxious persons. The person should report to the physician any signs of esophageal perforation (chest pain, dyspnea, fever, shock).

If a satisfactory esophageal lumen cannot be maintained, surgery may be peformed. The stricture may be resected or bypassed with a segment of jejunum or colon.

ESOPHAGEAL CARCINOMA
EPIDEMIOLOGY

Carcinoma is the most common condition causing obstruction of the esophagus and accounts for about 2% of all deaths from cancer in the United States. The incidence is increasing among nonwhite females, persons with achalasia, smokers, and alcoholics. The tumor may develop in any portion of the esophagus but is most common in the middle and lower thirds. Most tumors are squamous cell carcinomas.

The only possible hope for successful treatment lies in very early diagnosis and treatment. Any person who has difficulty in swallowing, no matter how trivial it may seem, should be urged to seek medical advice at once. This applies particularly to persons over 40 years of age, because cancer of the esophagus occurs most often during ages 40 to 70. The incidence of cancer of the esophagus is more than twice as high in males than in females.

CLINICAL MANIFESTATIONS

The cancer is often well established before the first symptoms appear. The most common symptom is progressive dysphagia, first with solid food and eventually with liquids. As the esophagus becomes progressively obstructed, regurgitation may occur, and aspirated fluids may cause coughing and pneumonitis. The patient may have foul breath and a foul taste in the mouth.

Spread of the carcinoma is by local invasion, or through the blood stream or lymphatics. Neoplasms of the upper and middle esophagus may extend into the pulmonary system, and those of the lower esophagus into the diaphragm, vertebrae or heart. Metastasis is present in about 80% of esophageal cancers at the time of diagnosis.[53] Symptoms will depend on the area and extent of metastasis. Diagnosis is made by barium swallow and by biopsy through endoscopy. Computed tomography (CT) scans may be done to determine extent of surgery.

INTERVENTIONS

Medical Management

Esophageal carcinoma may be treated with surgery, radiation, chemotherapy, or a combination of these procedures. Surgery of resectable tumors usually consists of esophagogastrostomy (removal of the lower part of the esophagus and part of the stomach) and pyloroplasty (Chapter 43). Radiation and chemotherapy (cisplatin, fluorouracil, vincristine) 3 to 4 weeks before surgery reduces tumor size and facilitates surgery and length of survival. Radiation may be used alone for lesions in the upper esophagus. For nonresectable tumors, palliative relief may be obtained by YAG laser therapy (in which the laser "vaporizes" part of the tumor) to open the esophagus temporarily, or by inserting an esophageal tube (stent) in the tumor area to permit passage of food.

The prognosis for esophageal cancer is poor, and only a small percentage of persons live more than 5 years after surgery. Many persons are chronic invalids until death occurs.

Nursing Management

The care of the person experiencing surgery is described in the box at right. Special mouth care is important preoperatively because the patient may be spitting up a mixture of pus, blood, and decomposed food. *Mouthwashes* are useful in making the mouth feel fresher and are offered to the patient before eating. They are varied from time to time unless the patient has a preference, because sometimes the flavor of the solution becomes identified with the unpleasant throat secretions and becomes almost as distasteful as the secretions.

Postoperatively the nasogastric tube is usually left in place until complete healing of the esophageal anastomosis has occurred, because esophageal tissue is very friable and because the anastomosis may be under tension. If part of the stomach has been pulled up into the thoracic cavity, the patient may complain of a feeling of fullness in the chest or difficulty in breathing when eating is resumed. Smaller, more frequent meals may alleviate this problem.

Considerable psychologic support is usually required as the patient and family begin to cope with the diagnosis, prognosis, and physical debility of the patient. The person is taught to stop smoking (if applicable), to avoid others with upper respiratory infections and to seek medical help for even minor illnesses. Palliative and supportive care, as described in Chapter 17, are given as indicated.

NURSING CARE OF THE PERSON EXPERIENCING ESOPHAGEAL SURGERY

PREOPERATIVE CARE

1. Encourage improved nutritional status
   a. High-protein, high calorie diet if oral diet is possible
   b. TPN may be necessary for severe dysphagia or obstruction
2. Give good mouth care (p. 1267); breath may be foul
3. Give preoperative preparation appropriate for thoracic surgery (Chapter 34)
4. Give prescribed antibiotics before esophageal resection or bypass

POSTOPERATIVE CARE

1. Promote good pulmonary ventilation
2. Maintain chest drainage system as prescribed
3. Maintain gastric drainage system
   a. Small amounts of blood may drain from nasogastric tube for 6 to 12 hours after surgery
   b. Do not disturb nasogastric tube (to prevent traction on suture line)
4. Maintain nutrition
   a. Start clear fluids at frequent intervals when oral intake is permitted
   b. Introduce soft foods gradually to several small meals of bland foods
   c. Have patient keep head elevated for 2 hours after eating and while sleeping if heartburn occurs

CHAPTER SUMMARY

- Obesity does not have a single cause but results from a complex interrelationship of factors, including genetics, CNS disturbances, hormones, sodium-potassium pump efficacy, activity patterns, and social and psychologic factors.

- Persons of normal weight gain weight by hypertrophy of existing fat cells; obese persons have an increased number of fat cells (hyperplasia). Weight reduction in obese persons is difficult to achieve and maintain.

- Because of increased fatty acid utilization, increased glucose, and increased body mass, obese persons are at risk for atherosclerosis, hypertension, emboli, gallstones, diabetes mellitus, osteoarthritis, angina, and respiratory insufficiency.

- Effective weight loss programs combine several approaches, including dieting, exercise, and behavior modification.

- Surgery for morbid obesity usually consists of gastroplasty (most effective) and gastric bypass.

- Protein-calorie malnutrition in hospitalized patients results from persons who have difficulty or disinterest in eating, have nutrient losses through the GI tract, or have cancer or prolonged infection or fever.

- Signs of severe protein-calorie malnutrition include hypoproteinemia, decreased vital capacity, anorexia, and hemoglobinemia. These persons are at high risk for infection.

- Tube feeding solutions differ in terms of carbohydrate (CHO) or protein content, osmolality, consistency, palatability, flavor, and expense.

- Persons with protein-calorie malnutrition may be fed orally, enterally (tube feedings, gastrostomy), or by total parenteral nutrition (TPN).

- Gastrostomy may be performed surgically through the abdomen or by percutaneous endoscopy.

- TPN solutions are deposited into the superior vena cava to provide greater dilution of the highly concentrated solutions.

- Complications of TPN include infection, air embolism, electrolyte imbalances, overhydration, hyperglycemia, hypoglycemia, vitamin D deficiency, and vitamin A excess.

- Common infections of the mouth include aphthous stomatitis (canker sore), herpetic stomatitis (cold sore, fever blister), Vincent's gingivitis, thrush, and parotitis.

- Mouth infections may be prevented by adequate nutrition, maintenance of moist mucous membranes, good oral hygiene, avoidance of excessive tobacco and alcohol, and dental care.

- Mouth care for mouth infections includes frequent rinsing with alkaline mouthwash or diluted hydrogen peroxide and cleaning gums and teeth with a toothette or a gauze-wrapped tongue blade if a toothbrush causes pain. Hot, spicy, or irritating foods should be avoided.

- Contributing factors to cancer of the mouth and esophagus include alcohol and heavy smoking or chewing tobacco.

- Carcinoma of the mouth can occur on the lips, on the anterior tongue and floor of the mouth, and in the salivary glands. Kaposi's sarcoma may occur in the mouth of persons with AIDS. Treatment is by surgery and/or radiation.

- After surgery of the mouth for cancer, the patient may have problems with body image, verbal communication, eating, and mouth discomfort.

- Common esophageal disorders include gastroesophageal reflux, achalasia, diverticuli, and strictures. Dysphagia is a common symptom of esophageal disorders.

- Gastroesophageal reflux may occur with an idiopathic incompetent lower esophageal sphincter (LES), pregnancy, obesity, ascites, hiatal hernia, or after resection of the lower esophagus. Heartburn is a major symptom. Management includes medications (antacids, cimetidine, Reglan); surgery for hiatal hernia; high-protein, low-fat diet; avoidance of foods and beverages containing caffeine, theobromine, and alcohol; avoidance of activities that increase abdominal pressure; and sleeping with the head elevated to prevent reflux.

- Achalasia is aperistalsis of the esophagus with resulting dilation; treatment consists of dilation with pneumatic dilators or cardiomyotomy.

- Esophageal diverticula are outpouches of the esophagus where food collects, causing regurgitation and possible obstruction; treatment is by surgical excision or myotomy.

- Risk factors for cancer of the esophagus include smoking, alcohol, and achalasia. Any person with dysphagia should be urged to consult a physician.

- Cancer of the esophagus has a poor prognosis, because metastasis is usually present when the diagnosis is made. Treatment is by surgery, radiation, and chemotherapy.

- Postoperative care for esophageal cancer includes promotion of pulmonary ventilation, maintenance of gastric drainage systems, encouragement of good nutrition when eating is permitted, and good mouth care.

QUESTIONS TO CONSIDER

- Compare various weight loss programs from books or by visiting weight loss clinics in your community. Compare the probable effectiveness of the programs based on the principles described in this chapter.

- Examine the data of the case study described in this chapter. Explain the pathophysiologic bases of the patient's symptoms.

- Examine the latest issue of *Cancer Facts and Figures* (may be obtained from your local chapter of the American Cancer Society). What have been the trends in deaths from cancer of the mouth and esophagus during the past 30 years?

REFERENCES AND SELECTED READINGS

1. *Ackerman S: The management of obesity, Hosp Pract 18(3):117-135, 1983.
2. American Cancer Society, Inc: 1989 Cancer facts and figures, New York, 1988, The Society.

*References preceded by an asterisk are particularly well suited for student reading.

3. American College of Surgeons: Manual of pre-and postoperative care, ed 3, Philadelphia, 1983, WB Saunders Co.

4. *Anderson BJ: Tube feeding: is diarrhea inevitable? Am J Nurs 86:705-706, 1986.

5. *Atkins JM and Oakley CW: A nurse's guide to TPN, RN 49(6):20-24, 1986.

6. *Backer CI and LoCicero J: Surgical management of esophageal disorders, CCQ 9(3):12-19, 1986.

7. *Baker DJ: Ten years of TPN at home, Am J Nurs 84:1248-1249, 1984.

8. *Birdsall C: When is TPN safe? Am J Nurs 85:73, 1985.

9. Bengoa JM and Rosenberg IH: Parenteral nutrition therapy in gastrointestinal disease, Adv Int Med 28:363-385, 1983.

10. Bongiovanni GL: Essentials of clinical gastroenterology, ed 2, New York, 1988, McGraw-Hill Book Co.

11. *Bruckstein DC: Percutaneous endoscopic gastrostomy, Geriatr Nurs 9(2):32-33, 1988

12. *Carr P: When the patient needs TPN at home, RN 49(6):25-30, 1986.

13. Clark JB, Queener SF, and Karb VB: Pharmacological basis of nursing practice, ed 2, St Louis, 1986, The CV Mosby Co.

14. Drenick EJ: Definition and health consequences of morbid obesity, Surg Clin North Am 59(6):963-976, 1979.

15. Elliot D, Goldberg L, and Girard DE: Obesity: pathophysiology and practical management, J Gen Intern Med 2:188-196, 1987.

16. Fleming CR, and McGill DB: Total parenteral nutrition. In Berk JE, editor: Bockus' gastroenterology, ed 4, Philadelphia, 1985, WB Saunders Co.

17. *Foltz AT: Nutritional factors in the prevention of gastrointestinal cancer, Sem Oncol Nurs 4:239-245, 1988.

18. *Freeman JB and Fairfull-Smith RJ: Current concepts of enteral feeding, Adv Surg 16:75-112, 1983.

19. *Frogge MH: Future perspectives and nursing issues in gastrointestinal cancer, Sem Oncol Nurs 4:300-302, 1988.

20. Gastric balloon for treatment of obesity, Med Lett 28:77-78, 1986.

21. Groer MW and Sheckleton ME: Basic pathophysiology: a conceptual approach, ed 3, St Louis, 1989, The CV Mosby Co.

22. *Guiness R: How to use the new small-bore feeding tubes, Nursing 86 16(4):51-56, 1986.

23. *Hennessy KA: Now TPN therapy begins at home, RN 51(6):81-84, 1988.

24. Heymsfield SB and Andrews JS: Enteral nutritional support. In Berk JE, editor: Bockus' gastroenterology, ed 4, Philadelphia, 1985, WB Saunders Co.

25. *Hutchinson MM: Administration of fat emulsions, Am J Nurs 82:275-277, 1982.

26. Irwin M: Managing leaking gastrostomy sites, Am J Nurs 88:359-360, 1988.

27. Jeffrey RW et al: Prevalence of overweight and weight loss behavior in a metropolitan population: the Minnesota Heart Survey experience, Am J Public Health 74:349-352, 1984.

28. *Johndrow PD: Making your patient and family feel at home with TPN, Nursing 88 18(10):65-69, 1988.

29. *Johnson S: A safer gastrostomy for the high risk patient: percutaneous endoscopic gastrostomy, RN 49(3):29-32, 1986.

30. *Kagawa-Busby KS et al: Effects of diet temperature on tolerance of enteral feedings, Nurs Res 29:276-280, 1980.

31. Kennedy-Caldwell C: The morbidly obese surgical patient, Crit Care Nurse 7(5):87-89, 1987.

32. Martyn PA, Hanson BC, and Jen KC: The effects of parenteral nutrition on food intake and gastric mobility, Nurs Res 33(6):336-342, 1984.

33. McCallum RW: The management of esophageal motility disorders, Hosp Pract 23(2):239-250, 1988.

34. *McNamara JR: Esophageal cancer, Nursing 82 12(3):64-65, 1982

35. *Medvec BR: Esophageal cancer: treatment and nursing intervention, Sem Oncol Nurs 4:246-256, 1988.

36. *Metheny NM: Twenty ways to prevent tube-feeding complications, Nursing 85 15(1):47-50, 1985.

37. *Mogan J: Behavioral treatment of obesity, Occup Health Nurs 32:312-314, 1984.

38. Moore MC: Do you still believe these myths about tube feedings? RN 50(5):51-55, 1987.

39. *Podiasky P and Rudzinski HM: Percutaneous endoscopic gastrostomy, AORN J 45:1403-1411, 1987.

40. Ponsky JL and Aszodi A: Percutaneous endoscopic jejunostomy, Am J Gastroenterol 79:113-116, 1984.

41. Ponsky JL, Gauderer WL, and Stellato TA: Percutaneous gastrostomy, Arch Surg 118:913-914, 1983.

42. Preventing antineoplastic-induced vomiting, Am J Nurs 85:173-174, 1985.

43. *Ramos LY: Oral hygiene for the elderly, Am J Nurs 81:1468-1469, 1981.

44. Rosado IR and Gilsdorf RB: Creating a continent tubeless gastrostomy, Am J Surg 146:820-822, 1983.

45. Schreiber H and Guyton DP: Gastric bubble: therapy for obesity, Ohio State Med J 82:476-479, 1986.

46. Schroeder SA et al: Current medical diagnosis and treatment, Norwalk, Conn, 1989, Appleton & Lange.

47. *Schulmeister L: Join the fight against oral cancer, Nursing 87 17(5):66-67, 1987.

48. *Starkey JF, Jefferson PA, and Kirby DF: Taking care of a percutaneous endoscopic gastrostomy, Am J Nurs 88:42-45, 1988.

49. Steinhard AJ, Foster GD, and Grossman RF: Surgical treatment of obesity, Adv Psychosom Med 15:140-166, 1986.

50. Stewart AL and Brook RH: Effects of being overweight, Am J Public Health 73:171-178, 1983.

51. Sweet K: Hiatal hernia: what to guard against in postoperative patients, Nursing 83 13(12):39-45, 1983.

52. Van Itallie TB and Kral JG: The dilemma of morbid obesity, JAMA 246:999-1003, 1981.

53. Way LW: Current surgical diagnosis and treatment, ed 8, Norwalk, Conn, 1988, Appleton & Lange.

54. Waye JD: Expanding uses of therapeutic endoscopy, Hosp Pract 22(8):143-159, 1987.

55. White JH: The relationship of clinical practice and research, J Adv Nurs 9:181-187, 1984.

56. *White JH: Behavioral intervention for the obese client, Nurs Pract 11:27-34, 1986.

57. White JH and Schroeder MA: When your client has a weight problem: nursing assessment, Am J Nurs 81:550-563, 1981.

58. *Wilhelm L: Helping your patient "settle in" with TPN: Nursing 85 15(4):60-64, 1985.

59. Wyngaarden JB and Smith LH: Cecil textbook of medicine, ed 18, Philadelphia, 1988, WB Saunders Co.

60. Yen PK: A new look at obesity, Geriatr Nurs 4(3):184-189, 1983.

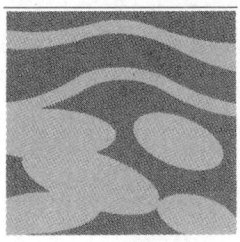

CHAPTER 43

Management of Persons with Problems of Digestion

BARBARA C. LONG

CHAPTER OBJECTIVES

After studying this chapter, the student should be able to:

1 Describe the etiology, pathophysiology, clinical manifestations and management of gastritis, peptic ulcer, cancer of the stomach, paralytic ileus, and malabsorption syndromes.

2 Compare and contrast the pathophysiology of gastric and duodenal ulcers, Zollinger-Ellison syndrome, and stress ulcers.

3 Describe the different effects of commonly used drugs for peptic ulcer.

4 Identify special preoperative and postoperative needs of patients undergoing gastric surgery.

5 Describe the effects of gastrointestinal changes on drug absorption.

Most digestion takes place in the stomach, duodenum, and jejunum. Gastritis, peptic ulcer, cancer of the stomach, and malabsorption syndrome are the major disorders of the digestive organs, whereas cancer of the small intestines is rare. Paralytic ileus (cessation of the peristalsis) may also affect digestion.

GASTRITIS

ETIOLOGY

Gastritis is an inflammation of the gastric mucosa and is the most common pathologic condition of the stomach. It may be acute or chronic, based on histologic criteria. Gastritis may be caused by exogenous or endogenous factors (see the box at right).

PATHOPHYSIOLOGY

Drugs, alcohol, bile salts, or pancreatic enzymes may damage the gastric mucosa *(erosive gastritis)*, disrupting the gastric mucosal barrier and allowing back-diffusion of acid and pepsin into the gastric tissue, which causes inflammation. The mechanism of stress-related gastritis seen with severe disorders is unknown but may result from mucosal ischemia. The gastric mucosa responds to most irritating agents by regeneration of the mucosa; therefore the disorders are often self-limiting.

With continued irritation, the tissue becomes inflamed and there may be bleeding.

Ingestion of corrosive acids or alkalies can result in inflammation and necrosis of the stomach wall *(corrosive gastritis)*. The necrosis may lead to perforation of the stomach wall with subsequent hemorrhage and peritonitis.

Chronic gastritis may be associated with atrophy of gastric glands and the appearance of patches of thin, gray, or greenish-gray mucosa *(atrophic gastritis)*. The loss of gastric mucosa will result in eventual diminution of gastric secretion and the development of pernicious anemia. Atrophic gastritis may be a precursor to gastric carcinoma. Chronic gastritis may also be associated with reflux of bile and bile acids from the duodenum into the stomach *(antral gastritis)*, usually observed in persons with peptic ulcer disease or following gastrojejunostomy.[22]

CLINICAL MANIFESTATIONS

Symptoms depend on the cause of the gastritis and its severity. Some gastritis is asymptomatic and requires no

---

CAUSES OF GASTRITIS

EXOGENOUS FACTORS

Bacterial infections, especially staphylococcal toxins
Drugs: nonsteroidal anti-inflammatory agents (including aspirin), sulfonamides, steroids
Alcohol
Ingestion of corrosive alkalies or acids
Irritating foods
Radiation

ENDOGENOUS FACTORS

Certain infectious diseases: typhoid fever, viral hepatitis, allergies
Bile salts and pancreatic enzymes
Severe disorders such as respiratory or renal failure, sepsis, major trauma

---

treatment. In other cases, anorexia is a common symptom. Some persons have only mild gastric discomfort or pain; belching and defecation often relieve the symptoms. Other persons have abdominal pain and severe nausea and vomiting, leading to severe dehydration that can have serious consequences in infants and in debilitated or elderly persons. Bleeding may occur in the form of hematemesis or melena (blood in the stools). There may be a severe drop in the hemoglobin and hematocrit levels.

In gastritis caused by corrosive acid or alkalies, there will be bloody vomitus and stools, and shock may occur. Death may result secondary to blood loss or perforation of a viscus. Those who recover will develop an obstruction. Endoscopy may confirm the diagnosis.

INTERVENTIONS
MEDICAL MANAGEMENT

Medical management of the patient with gastritis is as follows:

1. Mild gastritis: antacid, rest
2. Severe gastritis
   a. Intravenous replacement of fluid and electrolytes
   b. Antiemetics such as prochlorperazine (Compazine) or trimethobenzamide (Tigan), parenterally or by suppository
3. Erosive gastritis
   a. Antacids and histamine H₂ receptor antagonists (p. 1286) to inhibit gastric acid formation
   b. Sucralfate (Carafate) to coat the mucosa and prevent back-diffusion of acid and pepsin
4. Gastritis caused by bacterial agents: antibiotics
5. Atrophic gastritis
   a. Anticholinergics (for example, Pro-Banthine)
   b. Vitamin B₁₂

NURSING MANAGEMENT

When nausea and vomiting are present, the person is given nothing by mouth until symptoms subside. Tea, broth, and ginger ale are then given orally at frequent intervals. Bland feedings of custard, gelatin, and cream soups are usually tolerated after 12 to 24 hours, and then other foods are added gradually. Monitoring of fluid and electrolyte balance is important with excessive vomiting.

Persons with chronic superficial gastritis will usually respond to a diet that avoids highly seasoned or greasy foods. Carbonated liquids are well tolerated. Antacids may be required for a long period of time.

PEPTIC ULCER

A peptic ulcer is an ulceration involving the mucosa and deeper structure of the upper gastrointestinal tract. Pep-

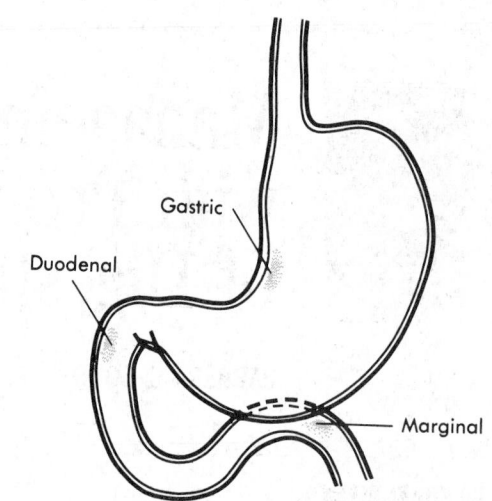

FIGURE 43-1 Most common sites for peptic ulcers.

tic ulcers may occur in the esophagus, stomach, duodenum, or jejunum (Figure 43-1), but the term usually refers to gastric and duodenal ulcers. An ulcer (usually of the jejunum) occurring near the site of an anastomosis is termed a *marginal* ulcer. Peptic ulcer disease is a *chronic* illness. Acute episodes may occur between periods of quiescence.

EPIDEMIOLOGY

Peptic ulcer is a common disorder that occurs with varying frequencies in different geographic locations. In the United States, peptic ulcer disease occurs in about 5% to 10% of the population,[23] and millions of dollars are lost annually from loss of work. The incidence of peptic ulcer has been declining, but it still remains a common disorder. Although the incidence of duodenal ulcers is about four times that of gastric ulcers, the mortality rate of gastric ulcers equals or exceeds that of duodenal ulcers.[6,38] Duodenal ulcers are more common in males than in females. Peptic ulcer recurrences often occur in the spring and fall.

ETIOLOGY

The causes of chronic peptic ulcer disease are still uncertain despite considerable research.[38] Cigarette smoking and regular use of aspirin are strongly associated with chronic peptic ulcers. Heredity also plays a major role. The role of stress is more obscure except in the development of stress ulcers (p. 1291).

ENVIRONMENTAL FACTORS

Although the relationship between *smoking* and ulcer development is not clearly understood, cigarette smokers have a higher incidence of peptic ulcers, delayed healing of gastric ulcers, and increased recurrence rate. There has been *no* evidence linking foods, coffee, or alcohol with peptic ulcers.

Ulcerogenic *drugs* such as corticosteroids, salicylates, ibuprofen, indomethacin, and phenylbutazone (Butazolidin), when given in massive doses, may cause acute ulcers; however, with the exception of aspirin, there is no conclusive evidence that they cause chronic peptic disease. The mechanisms of these ulcerogenic drugs vary. With the antiinflammatory steroids, there is mucosal injury secondary to increased gastric secretion and reduced gastric mucus secretion. The latter results from the steroid antiprotein synthetic action. With aspirin there is an increased exfoliation of mucous cells and a decrease in mucus production. Ulcerogenic drugs may exacerbate an already existing chronic peptic ulcer.

GENETIC FACTORS

There appear to be certain intrinsic factors that are not related to environmental factors. The tendency for gastric or duodenal ulcers is inherited independently; that is, gastric ulcers occur three times more often when there is a family history of gastric ulcers, and duodenal ulcers occur three times more often with a family history of duodenal ulcers. Duodenal ulcers also occur more often in people with type O blood and in those who do not secrete blood group substances in their saliva. Gastric ulcers occur more often in people with type A blood.

PATHOPHYSIOLOGY

Gastric acid is secreted in parietal cells of the fundus of the stomach, as a result of stimulation by acetylcholine (from the vagus nerve), by gastrin (secreted by cells in the pyloric area of the stomach), and by histamine (found in cells throughout the gastric mucosa) (Figure 43-2). There are two types of cellular receptors to histamine in the body, H_1 and H_2. H_1 receptors are found in cells of smooth muscle and capillaries and mediate contraction of smooth muscle and capillary dilation; these receptors can be blocked by antihistamine drugs. H_2 receptors are found in cells of the stomach and mediate secretion of HCl; these receptors are blocked by histamine H_2 receptor antagonists (p. 1286).

GASTRIC ULCERS

Most persons with gastric ulcers have a normal gastric secretion and a normal emptying rate of the stomach. Ulceration appears to occur because of a decreased resistance of the gastric mucosa to acid-pepsin injury (Table 43-1). Gastritis is usually present, resulting in shedding of the protective cells from the mucosal wall. A major causative factor in gastric ulcers appears to be increased *back diffusion* of gastric acid from the gastric lumen into the gastric mucosa (Figure 43-3). Free acid that has been secreted into the gastric lumen normally

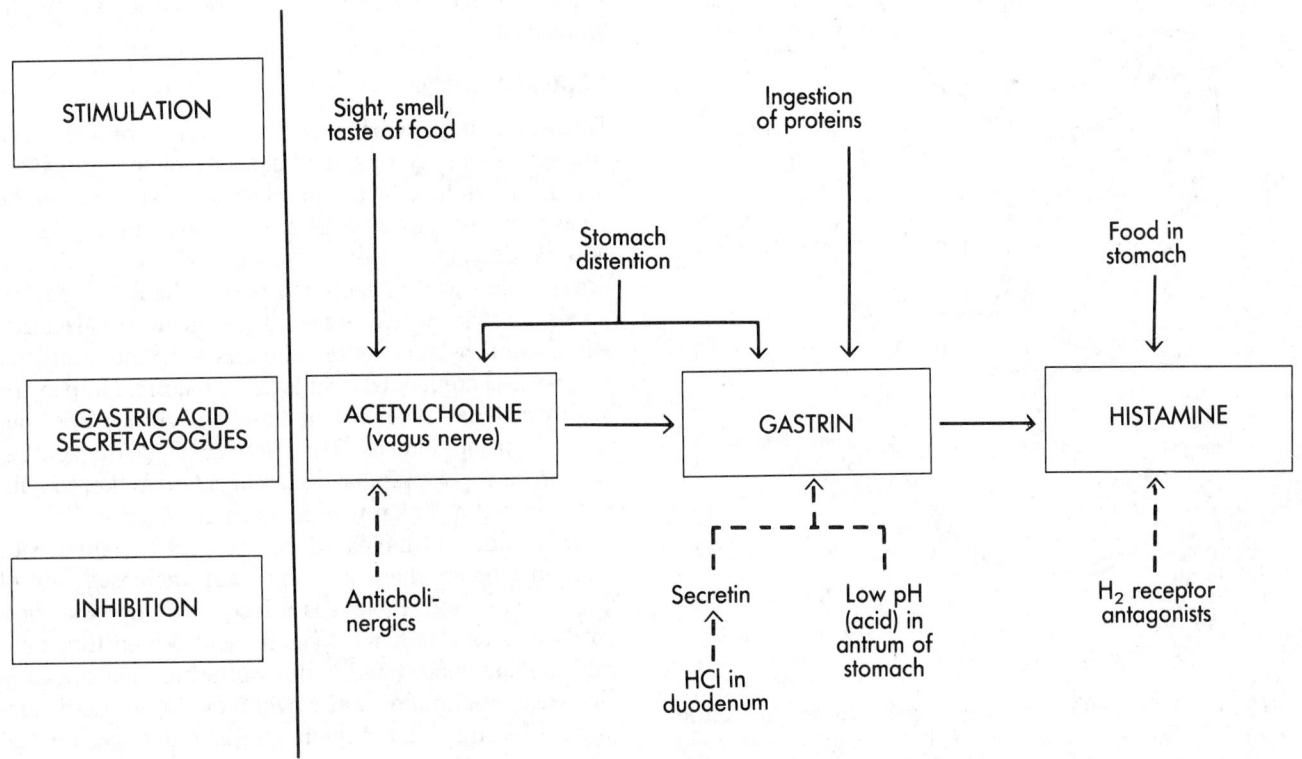

FIGURE 43-2 Stimulation and inhibition of gastric acid.

TABLE 43-1 Normal function, pathophysiology, and clinical picture in peptic ulcer

Normal Function	Pathophysiology	Clinical Picture
Thick gastric mucosal layer: barrier to back diffusion of HCl into tissues	*Gastric ulcer:* Breakdown of mucosal barrier, leading to increased back diffusion of acid through tissues; causes ulceration in gastric wall	Pain in epigastric area (where pain of both stomach and duodenum are localized) Pain described variously (often as gnawing or burning) because of visceral origin
Gastric acid increases with ingestion of food and decreases as food enters duodenum; alkaline secretions in duodenum buffer gastric HCl	*Duodenal ulcer:* Increased gastric HCl and increased rate of gastric emptying; the HCl in duodenum overwhelms the alkaline buffer and causes ulceration in duodenal wall	Pain is relieved by food and antacids
Basal gastric HCl peaks in evening and is low in morning	Basal gastric HCl level does not change	Pain is most severe during night

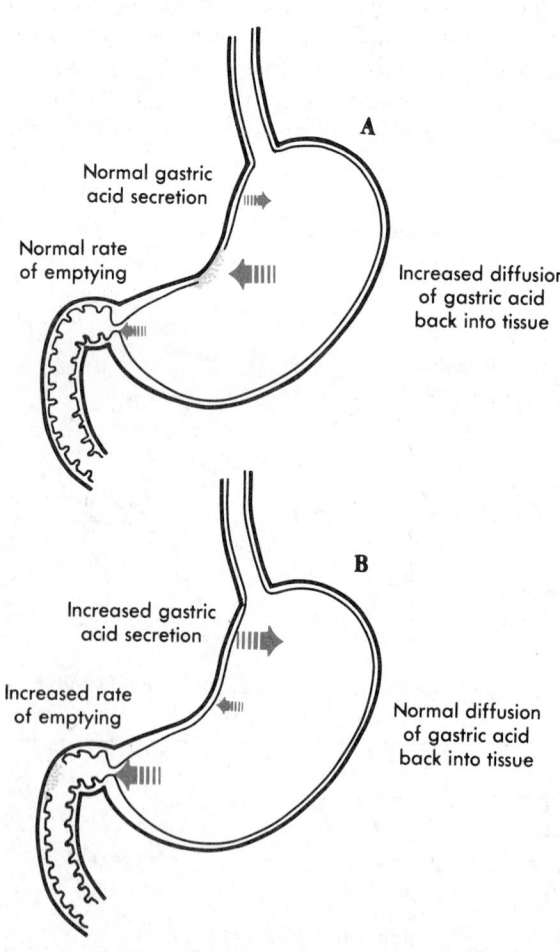

FIGURE 43-3 Pathophysiology of peptic ulcer. **A,** Gastric ulcer. **B,** Duodenal ulcer. Note that the major alteration with gastric ulcer is increased back diffusion, whereas with duodenal ulcer acid secretion and gastric emptying is increased.

diffuses back into the tissues at a very slow rate, if at all. Rapid diffusion causes local histamine release with a subsequent inflammatory reaction, resulting in leakage of interstitial and plasma fluid into the gastric lumen, bleeding, and tissue damage. The natural barriers to back diffusion of gastric acid can be broken down by bile acids, alcohol, and salicylates. The greater reflux of bile-containing duodenal contents seen with gastric ulcers may be caused by deficient contractile response of the pylorus to cholecystokinin and secretin.[15] Cigarette smoking has been shown to increase bile reflux into the stomach.[38]

DUODENAL ULCERS

Persons with duodenal ulcers have an increase in gastric acid secretory rate. The capacity to secrete gastric acid is determined by the number of parietal cells in the gastric mucosa; these cells are increased in the person with a duodenal ulcer. A second reason for the increased gastric acid secretion is the change in gastrin levels. Gastrin, which is peptide hormone released into the antrum by vagal stimulation, is a potent stimulator of gastric secretion. Gastrin levels are normal in persons with duodenal ulcers when the stomach is empty but increase postprandially. Thus both basal gastric acid secretion and postprandial gastric acid secretion are increased in the person with a duodenal ulcer.

In addition to increased gastric acid secretion with duodenal ulcer, there is a markedly increased rate of gastric emptying. Protein is a food substance that normally acts as a buffer for gastric acid. When the stomach empties more rapidly, this buffering mechanism is decreased and more gastric acid moves into the duodenum. The end result of the increased rate of gastric acid secretion and gastric emptying is an increased amount of acid content propelled into the duodenum, causing irritation and breakdown of the duodenal mucosa.

TABLE 43-2 Drug therapy for peptic ulcer

Drug	Action	Comments
Antacids	Neutralize gastric acid	Generally heal ulcers in 4-6 weeks Side effects limited to diarrhea or constipation Lack of adherence to regimen by many patients
Histamine H_2 receptor antagonists	Inhibit acid secretion	Generally heal ulcers in 4-6 weeks Side effects may interfere with administration
Sucralfate	Coats ulcer; prevents action of acid and pepsin on ulcer	Generally heals ulcers in 4-6 weeks Longer time span before recurrence Large capsule; may be difficult to swallow

CLINICAL MANIFESTATIONS

Clinical manifestations of peptic ulcer include the following:
1. Pain is a characteristic symptom.
   a. Located in upper abdomen near midline (epigastrium); may radiate around costal border to back
   b. Described as gnawing, aching, or burning
   c. Starts 1 to 2 hours after eating when the stomach begins to empty
   d. May disappear spontaneously after ingestion of food or antacid
   e. Often occurs at night when stomach is empty and gastric secretions are at a peak
   f. There are periods of exacerbation and recurrence
2. Some persons never experience pain, and the ulcer may be discovered accidentally by roentgenogram or postmortem examination.
3. Nausea and excessive salivation may be present.
4. Occult blood may be noted in stools if the ulcer erodes a small blood vessel.
5. Diagnostic tests are as follows:
   a. Upper gastrointestinal series roentgenograms to demonstrate ulceration
   b. Gastroscopy and duodenoscopy to observe the mucosa; biopsy is done for gastric ulcer to diagnose benign status
   c. Gastric analysis used under certain circumstances

MEDICAL MANAGEMENT

Medical treatment is directed toward relief of symptoms, healing of the ulcer, prevention of complications, and prevention of recurrence. The majority of peptic ulcers heal with drug therapy. Surgery is used most often following a second or third recurrence and in the treatment of complications.

DRUG THERAPY

The three different types of drugs given most commonly in the treatment of peptic ulcers are described in Table 43-2. *Antacids* are weak bases that neutralize the free hydrochloric acid (HCl) to prevent the continuous irritation of the exposed mucosa and to permit healing. *Histamine H_2 receptor antagonists* inhibit HCl secretion by binding to the histamine H_2 receptors on stomach cells and thus blocking release of histamine, which is a secretagogue (causing secretion flow) of HCl. Histamine H_2 blockers include cimetidine, ranitidine, and famotidine. *Sucralfate* is a drug that forms a protective barrier over the ulcer to prevent further irritation and to promote healing. It is used primarily for duodenal ulcers.

Anticholinergic drugs have theoretic value for duodenal ulcers by decreasing gastric acid secretion and delaying gastric emptying. They are now rarely used, however, because of side effects from the required high dosages and decreased effectiveness, compared with antacids and H_2 receptor blockers. Pirenzepine may be given to enhance the effect of cimetidine.

New drugs include the following:
1. Omeprazole (a proton pump blocker): blocks secretion of HCl
2. Prostaglandins: inhibit HCl secretion and enhance mucosal defenses
3. Colloidal bismuth subcitrate (De-Nol): coats and protects ulcer by binding with protein; may inhibit the growth of *Campylobacter pylori*, a bacteria frequently found in persons with peptic ulcer

SURGERY

Surgery may be performed when recurrent peptic ulcers do not respond to medical therapy or when a peptic ulcer perforates (p.1290), causing peritonitis, or erodes a blood vessel causing hemorrhage. Various types of surgery may be performed. The nursing care for persons undergoing gastric or duodenal surgery is described on p. 1292.

Vagotomy and Drainage

Vagotomy refers to the severing of the vagus nerve innervating the stomach. Recall that the vagus nerve is a secretagogue for HCl. The vagus nerve may be severed

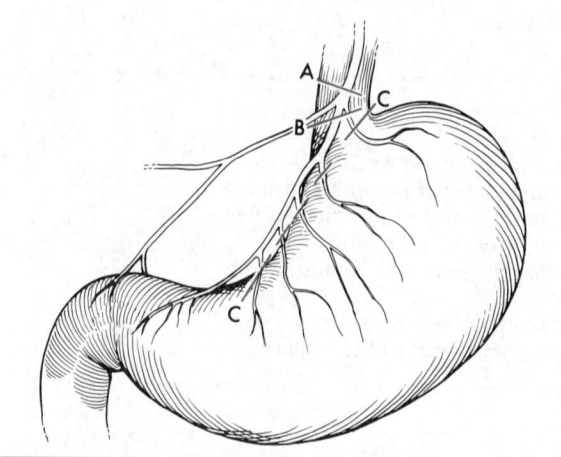

FIGURE 43-4 Different types of vagotomies: truncal (*A*), selective (*B*), and proximal (or parietal) cell (*C*).

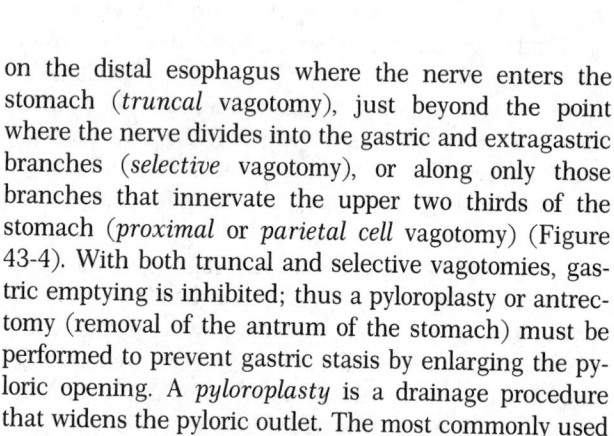

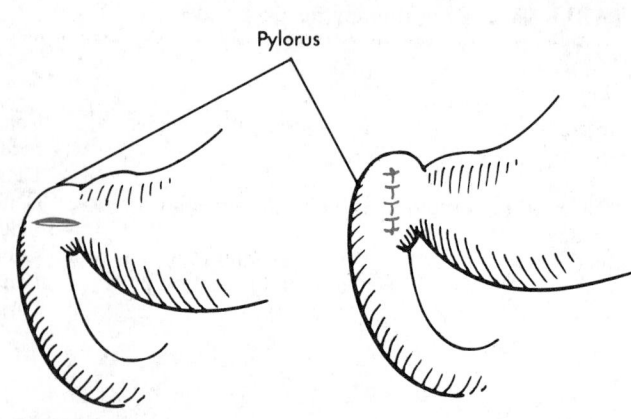

FIGURE 43-5 Heineke-Mikulicz pyloroplasty. Longitudinal incision across pylorus is pulled apart and closed in transverse position to widen pyloric outlet.

on the distal esophagus where the nerve enters the stomach (*truncal* vagotomy), just beyond the point where the nerve divides into the gastric and extragastric branches (*selective* vagotomy), or along only those branches that innervate the upper two thirds of the stomach (*proximal* or *parietal cell* vagotomy) (Figure 43-4). With both truncal and selective vagotomies, gastric emptying is inhibited; thus a pyloroplasty or antrectomy (removal of the antrum of the stomach) must be performed to prevent gastric stasis by enlarging the pyloric opening. A *pyloroplasty* is a drainage procedure that widens the pyloric outlet. The most commonly used procedure is the Heineke-Mikulicz pyloroplasty (Figure 43-5).

Advantages of vagotomy with pyloroplasty include the following:

1. Removal of vagal stimulation to acid-pepsin secretion
2. Reduction of the responsiveness of the parietal cells of the stomach
3. Low operative mortality and morbidity
4. Selective vagotomy preserves vagal innervation of viscera other than stomach and has fewer side effects than truncal vagotomy

Disadvantages include the following:

1. Higher ulcer recurrence rate than with antrectomy with vagotomy
2. Selective vagotomy is more difficult to perform than truncal vagotomy

Proximal (parietal cell) vagotomy. Proximal vagotomy is useful for treatment of chronic duodenal ulcers, but has a higher recurrence rate with gastric ulcers. It may be performed with other forms of surgery. Advantages of proximal vagotomy includes the following:

1. Preservation of gastric emptying; therefore pyloroplasty is not necessary
2. Fewer side effects than occur with other surgeries
3. No intrusion into gastrointestinal tract

Disadvantages include the following:

1. Requirement of greater expertise on the part of the surgeon
2. Higher ulcer recurrence rate than with antrectomy with vagotomy
3. Dumping syndrome and diarrhea are more frequent

Antrectomy and Vagotomy

An antrectomy consists of removal of 50% of the lower part of the stomach with anastomosis of the remaining segment to the duodenum (Billroth I) or to the side of the proximal jejunum (Billroth II) (Figure 43-6). Recall that the antrum (lower part) of the stomach is the site where the gastrin cells that stimulate secretion of HCl are located. The Billroth I is the traditional procedure for a gastric ulcer, whereas the Billroth II procedure is usually preferred for a duodenal ulcer. The duodenal stump is preserved in the Billroth II to permit bile flow into the jejunum to mix with food. A truncal vagotomy is performed in conjunction with the antrectomy to prevent ulcer recurrence.

Advantages of antrectomy with vagotomy includes the following:

1. Elimination of source of gastrin in stomach
2. Lower incidence of ulcer recurrence than with other surgical procedures
3. Low incidence of marginal ulceration

Disadvantages include the following:

1. Blind duodenal loop infection from stasis may occur in the Billroth II procedure

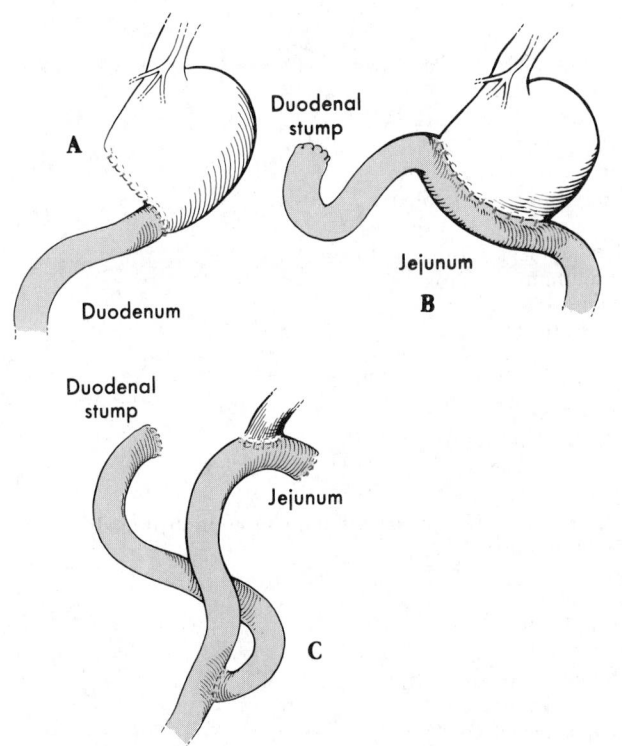

FIGURE 43-6 Types of gastric resections with anastomoses. **A,** Billroth I. **B,** Billroth II. **C,** Total gastrectomy.

2. More extensive surgery than vagotomy with drainage
3. Increased risk of anastomosis leakage

■ ASSESSMENT
SUBJECTIVE DATA

Subjective data to collect in assessment of the person with peptic ulcer include the following:
1. Pain: presence, location, character, time of occurrence in relation to eating and sleeping
2. Medications
   a. Drugs used for ulcer pain relief: when taken, effectiveness
   b. Drugs used frequently that contain aspirin or other nonsteroidal analgesics (aggravate the ulcer)
3. Meal patterns (to be used in patient teaching)
4. Smoking and alcohol consumption habits (both are contributing factors to ulcer formation and recurrence)
5. Knowledge of peptic ulcer: what it is, aggravating factors, therapy
6. Perceived stressors and concerns
7. General life-style: nature and hours of work and rest, sources of recreation and pleasure, and usual coping measures (obtain data regarding stress)

OBJECTIVE DATA

Objective data include monitoring for signs of complications of peptic ulcer that include: (1) gastric bleeding (hematemesis, occult blood in stools), (2) gastric perforation (severe abdominal pain with rigidity), and (3) pyloric obstruction (epigastric pain relieved by vomiting, weight loss).

■ DATA ANALYSIS: NURSING DIAGNOSES

Nursing diagnoses are determined from assessment of patient data. Possible nursing diagnoses for the person with peptic ulcer may include, but are not limited to the following:

Diagnostic Title	Possible Etiologies
Coping, ineffective individual	Situational stressors
Health maintenance, altered	Lack of knowledge
Knowledge deficit	Lack of exposure/recall
Pain: epigastric	Peptic ulceration

■ PLANNING: EXPECTED PATIENT OUTCOMES

Because peptic ulcer is primarily a chronic illness, it is vital that the patient be involved in the determination of outcomes and planning for necessary care. Expected patient outcomes for the person with a peptic ulcer may include, but are not limited to, the following:
1. Pain is decreased, minimal, or absent.
2. The patient identifies life stressors and uses stress management techniques.
3. The patient modifies health-risking behaviors (smoking, drinking alcohol) if pertinent.
4. The patient describes health-seeking behaviors (good nutrition, adequate rest, exercise) to be achieved to help prevent ulcer recurrence.
5. The patient describes the following:
   a. Factors that contribute to the healing of ulcers and to decreased occurrence
   b. Medication plan to be followed
   c. Plans for follow-up care.

■ IMPLEMENTATION

Nursing care centers on relieving the pain, counseling to help the person cope with life stressors, and teaching the patient about peptic ulcers and health maintenance.

RELIEVING PAIN
Medications

Taking medications appropriately is the major approach for relief of ulcer pain. The patient will be responsible for taking the medications at home and needs to understand the rationale for taking the drugs to ensure complete compliance of administration for maximum effectiveness.

Antacids. Antacids are mild bases that neutralize the gastric acid. The commonly used antacids are described

TABLE 43-3 Commonly used antacids

Generic Name	Trade Name	Comments
Aluminum hydroxide	Amphojel	Slow buffering effect
	ALternaGEL	Constipating
	Alu-Cap	Decreased absorption of phosphates
	Dialume	Contains sodium
		Edema of feet and legs with large doses
Aluminum carbonate	Basaljel	Same as for aluminum hydroxide
Aluminum and magnesium hydroxide	Maalox	A preferred antacid
		Good buffering effect
		Good taste
		Nonconstipating
		Low sodium content
Aluminum hydroxide and magnesium trisilicate	Gaviscon	Slower buffering effect
		Coats and protects ulcer
		Nonconstipating
Magaldrate	Riopan	A chemical combination of magnesium and aluminum hydroxide
		Intermediate buffering action
		Nonconstipating
		Low sodium content
		No acid rebound
Calcium carbonate	Alka-2	Rapid buffering effect
		Constipation may be severe
		May cause acid rebound
		May cause hypercalcemia
		Not suitable for long-term therapy
Magnesium and calcium carbonate	Marblen	Slow buffering effect
		Neutralizes more acid than do other antacids
		Nonconstipating
		Low sodium content
ANTACIDS WITH SIMETHICONE		
Aluminum and magnesium hydroxide, with simethicone	Mylanta	Same actions as aluminum and magnesium hydroxide alone
	Maalox Plus	Simethicone is non–gas-forming: lowers the surface tension of
	Gelusil	gas bubbles

in Table 43-3. The antacids of choice are the nonsystemic antacids, which are poorly absorbed from the stomach and therefore do not alter the pH of the blood or interfere with normal acid-base balance.

Aluminum hydroxide is a major ingredient because, in addition to its acid-neutralizing effect, it is thought to decrease pepsin activity, stimulate prostaglandin synthesis, and coat the ulcer surface.[35] Aluminum hydroxide also binds phosphates in the GI tract, leading to excretion of the phosphates; therefore prolonged ingestion of aluminum hydroxide may lead to phosphate depletion and osteoporosis. Aluminum hydroxide may cause constipation so it is usually combined with magnesium hydroxide, which has a laxative effect.

When given to a person in the fasting state, the buffering effect of the antacid is transitory; therefore, for maximal effectiveness, antacids should be taken *1 and 3 hours after meals*. For severe pain, antacids may be given at frequent intervals (every 30 minutes). Because of interference with absorption, antacids should not be given concurrently with cimetidine (a histamine H_2 receptor blocker) or with tetracycline.

Histamine H_2 receptor antagonists. Histamine is a stimulant for acid secretion in the stomach (p. 1281). H_2 receptor antagonists attach to H_2 receptors on histamine-secreting cells in the stomach and inhibit histamine secretion, thereby decreasing gastric acid secretion. About 60% of a person's daily gastric acid is secreted at night; suppression of nocturnal gastric acid is, therefore, an important factor in the effectiveness of these drugs to promote ulcer healing.[6] The drugs are given with meals and bedtime dose is often prescribed. Histamine H_2 receptor antagonists that are available for peptic ulcer therapy include cimetidine (Tagamet), ranitidine (Zantac), famotidine (Pepcid), and the newer drug nizatidine (Axid). The overall side effects are low but may include confusion, dizziness, and weakness (most common in elderly persons); diarrhea and abdominal cramps; bradycardia or tachycardia; impotence and gynecomastia; itching and rash; and thrombocytopenia. The patient needs to know about the possibility of a decreased libido and to monitor for signs of bleeding (from the thrombocytopenia). Cimetidine has increased toxicity when given concurrently with benzodiazepine, metoprolol, propanolol, phenytoin, theophyline, and tricyclic antidepressants.

Sucralfate. Sucralfate (Carafate) coats the ulcer to prevent irritation and thus promotes healing. The only major side effect is constipation. Because sucralfate decreases the absorption of tetracycline, phenytoin, cimetidine, and antacids, administration of sucralfate should be spaced apart from these drugs by at least 1 hour. Sucralfate should be given 1 hour *before* meals and at bedtime.

FOOD

There is no evidence that modifying the diet accelerates healing of an uncomplicated peptic ulcer. Diet is therefore based on promotion of comfort. Food in the stomach, especially protein, buffers gastric acid; however, food is also a stimulant for gastric acid secretion that may irritate the ulcer, thus causing pain. Controversy exists concerning whether relief of ulcer pain is better effected by three regular meals or six small meals a day. The person can best judge which approach provides the maximum comfort. Eating meals slowly helps to prevent overdistention and reflux of gastric contents back into the esophagus. If pain occurs between meals, snacks may help. Bedtime snacks may lead to pain during the night and thus should probably be omitted.

If foods that are thought to increase gastric acid (coffee, tea, or cola) lead to discomfort for an individual, they are best avoided. Milk should be avoided because of its secratogogue effect on HCl. Most persons with peptic ulcer learn early to avoid any food that increases their discomfort.

Alcohol can stimulate gastric acid secretion and break down the gastric mucosal barrier leading to gastritis, but there is no evidence to date that it is ulcerogenic. If alcohol is consumed, it should be taken in moderate amounts and not on an empty stomach.

COUNSELING

Stress plays a role in the pathogenesis of peptic ulcers, probably by means of the increased acid secretion from vagal stimulation.[29] Thus actions that avoid stressful situations or minimize the effect of stress can be beneficial for healing or for prevention of a recurrence.

The person first needs to identify the possible sources of stress at work or at home and the relationship of the ulcer pain to specific situations. Activities that promote relaxation for the individual (recreation or hobbies) are encouraged. A regular exercise program can

contribute to feelings of well-being and thus facilitate coping with stress. If removal from stressful environmental influences is impossible, the person must learn to cope with the stressful situations without reactivating the ulcer. Usual coping mechanisms are explored to determine effectiveness, and alternate approaches can be identified (Chapter 10). Stress management techniques, such as relaxation techniques, can be learned (Chapter 11). Occasionally the person is advised to obtain psychologic counseling for better understanding of the problems and for development of more effective coping behaviors.

PATIENT TEACHING

Important points to consider in teaching the person with peptic ulcer are summarized in the box below. Some of the teaching involves health maintenance (eat-

---

TEACHING THE PERSON WITH A PEPTIC ULCER

MEDICATIONS
1. Know dosage, administration, action, and side effects
2. Continue drug for prescribed time, even when symptoms abate
3. Keep antacids available at all times
4. Anticipate increased need for antacids during periods of stress
5. Avoid self-medication with systemic antacids (such as bicarbonate of soda) that alter acid-base balance
6. Avoid ulcerogenic drugs such as salicylates, ibuprofen, corticosteroids
7. Use acetaminophen (Tylenol) or buffered aspirin (if tolerated) for relief of pain

EATING
1. Eat three balanced meals a day
2. Eat between-meal snacks if this helps to relieve pain
3. Avoid any foods that increase discomfort
4. If alcohol is taken, drink minimally and not on an empty stomach
5. Avoid stress at mealtimes and plan for a quiet time after eating

SMOKING
1. Stop smoking if possible
2. If complete abstinence causes increased discomfort from stress, try to decrease number of cigarettes smoked

RELAXATION AND REDUCTION OF STRESS
1. Participate in recreation and hobbies that promote relaxation
2. Provide for a good night's sleep on a regular basis
3. Use relaxation techniques to decrease effects of stress
4. Participate in a reasonable exercise program for promotion of well-being
5. Structure home and work environment to keep stressors at a reasonable level
6. Avoid factors found to increase symptoms, if possible

NURSING CARE PLAN

PERSON WITH PEPTIC ULCER

DATA: Mr. Jones who is single is a 42 year old computer operator with a history of duodenal ulcer 4 years ago. He has had periods of epigastric distress for the past month with partial relief from Maalox. He was admitted 2 days ago with hematemesis, tarry stools, faintness, and a blood pressure of 96/54 mm Hg (usual 124/84 mm Hg). Intravenous fluids were initiated. Endoscopy revealed a bleeding duodenal ulcer. A nasogastric tube was inserted, and antacids were prescribed hourly per tube. Cimetidine was started by IV push. His BP is now stable, and the N/G tube was removed early today. Mr. Jones is taking oral fluids and has been started on a soft diet. The cimetidine has been changed to 300 mg with meals and at bedtime and Maalox 30 ml qlh and q3h pc.

The nursing history identified the following:

■ Mr. Jones is vague about the nature of peptic ulcer or possible complications.

■ Mr. Jones takes aspirin for headaches "from computer eyestrain."
■ Mr. Jones smokes 1½ packs of cigarettes a day; he has tried several times unsuccessfully to quit.
■ Mr. Jones spends two to three evenings a week at a local bar and "puts down quite a few beers."

Collaborative nursing actions include those to prevent further injury from hemorrhage or perforation. Immediate reporting of and treatment of early signs may prevent serious effects (loss of blood, peritonitis, or death). Nursing actions include *monitoring* for the following:

■ Signs of further hemorrhage: hematemesis, decreased blood pressure, restlessness, cool moist skin, stools that test positive for guaiac.
■ Signs of perforation: severe, sudden, sharp abdominal pain.

NURSING DIAGNOSIS

Pain: epigastric related to irritation of gastric acid on duodenal ulcer

Expected Patient Outcomes	Nursing Interventions	Rationale
Mr. Jones states that epigastric pain is decreased.	Give prescribed cimetidine with meals and at bedtime (8:00, noon, 5:00, and 10:00).	Cimetidine encourages healing by decreasing gastric acid secretion; give with meals to inhibit food-stimulated HCl secretion.
	Give prescribed antacid 1 and 3 hours after meals (9:00 AM, 11:00 AM; 1:00, 3:00, 6:00, and 8:00 PM).	Antacids neutralize HCL; they interfere with absorption of cimetidine if given concurrently.
	Teach relaxation measures as appropriate.	Relaxation facilitates rest to promote healing, thus decreasing pain.

NURSING DIAGNOSIS

Health maintenance, altered, related to lack of knowledge

Expected Patient Outcomes	Nursing Interventions	Rationale
Mr. Jones states plans to decrease smoking and drinking and to avoid aspirin.	Teach effects of aspirin, smoking, and alcohol on ulcer formation.	Aspirin is ulcerogenic; smoking delays healing; alcohol is a HCl secretagogue and may further irritate the ulcer.
	Discuss previous efforts at discontinuing smoking; explore additional ways, especially group programs such as those provided by the American Cancer Society, American Lung Society, or American Heart Association.	Programs that include group support are often more successful than a person trying to quit smoking alone.
	Explore with patient reasons for frequent visits to bars, then explore other ways of meeting his needs (such as nonalcoholic drinks or substituting other social activities).	Assisting Mr. Jones to think through for himself the reasons and alternate approaches will increase the potential for a behavioral change.
	Suggest Mr. Jones get his eyes examined (if appropriate); describe analgesics that do not contain aspirin (such as Tylenol or Anacin).	Headaches may be due to strain from decreased vision; fewer headaches will decrease need for analgesics.

NURSING CARE PLAN

PERSON WITH PEPTIC ULCER—cont'd

NURSING DIAGNOSIS
Knowledge deficit related to lack of recall or exposure

Expected Patient Outcomes	Nursing Interventions	Rationale
Mr. Jones describes nature of and therapy for peptic ulcer.	Review nature of peptic ulcer and possible recurrence, factors that contribute to healing, methods of pain relief (including administration and side effects of cimetidine and antacids), and need to report symptoms of bleeding, perforation, or pyloric obstruction to physician immediately.	Recall or reinforcement of earlier teaching will help promote retention.

ing, sleeping, exercise, and reduction of stress). For some persons, this may involve changes in life-style and they may need support over a period of time to reach their goals.

Because smoking and alcohol may be implicated in the healing or discomfort of ulcers, their use is discouraged. Trying to give up smoking may actually increase ulcer pain for some persons because of the effects of stress. These persons are encouraged to decrease the number of cigarettes smoked.

A nursing care plan for a person with a peptic ulcer can be found on the opposite page.

COMPLICATIONS OF PEPTIC ULCER

The major complications of peptic ulcer are perforation of a blood vessel causing hemorrhage, perforation of the muscular wall, or obstruction of the pyloric outlet.

HEMORRHAGE

Pathophysiology and Epidemiology

Bleeding occurs in about 15% to 20% of ulcer patients and occurs two to three times more often than perforation or outlet obstruction.[38] Erosion of larger blood vessels may cause gastric hemorrhage; erosion of smaller vessels or granulation tissue cause lesser bleeding. Other common causes of upper GI bleeding include esophageal varices (Chapter 39) and gastritis (p. 1279). Bleeding gastric ulcers are more likely to result in death than are bleeding duodenal ulcers, because the bleeding from gastric ulcers tends to be more severe and persons with gastric ulcers are usually older than those with duodenal ulcers. Rebleeding occurs in about 25% to 40% of patients.

Clinical Manifestations

The extent of clinical signs and symptoms depends on the extent of the upper GI bleeding, ranging from minimal signs (occult blood in stools) to frank bleeding and shock. Clinical manifestations may include the following:

1. Dizziness, faintness, restlessness, orthostatic hypotension, and finally, shock
2. Signs of bleeding
   a. Vomiting blood (hematemesis); the emesis may contain bright red blood from active bleeding or coffee-ground material from blood that has been digested by the gastric acid
   b. Aspiration of blood through nasogastric tube (similar in appearance to the blood in hematemesis)
   c. Tarry stools (melena) from degradation of hemoglobin in the digestive process

Diagnostic tests include endoscopy to identify the bleeding site. Angiography may be done if bleeding persists.

Interventions

Medical management. Medical management is as follows:
1. Hemodynamic stabilization of shock (Chapter 25)
2. Insertion of a nasogastric tube, followed by lavage with tap water or saline; iced saline is not necessary,[5,6] but if used, bags of normal saline can be refrigerated and the cold solution infused through the nasogastric tube
3. Antacids given hourly through nasogastric tube to neutralize gastric acids not removed by suction and to prevent acid reflux
4. Nothing by mouth until shock and bleeding are controlled, then liquid diet followed by soft diet
5. Medications
   a. Intravenous cimetidine when nothing by mouth is permitted, then orally
   b. Sucralfate may be given for duodenal ulcer
   c. Antacids continued every 1 and 3 hours after meals and at bedtime
6. Surgery if bleeding persists

Nursing management. Nursing care consists of monitoring for effectiveness of therapy and of promoting comfort.

1. Monitor:
   a. Vital signs and urinary output for response to shock therapy
   b. Nasogastric drainage, emesis, and stools for amount of blood loss
2. Provide special mouth care after vomiting (a weak solution of hydrogen peroxide will help remove blood from the oral mucosa)
3. Remove all evidence of bleeding as quickly as possible
4. Tell patient that rest and quiet will help stop the bleeding
5. Maintain a calm approach
6. Restrict activities only to those deemed necessary until massive bleeding has slowed down or stopped
7. Prepare patient for surgery, if necessary.

PERFORATION

Pathophysiology

Perforation is an erosion of a peptic ulcer through the muscular wall with spillage of gastrointestinal contents into the abdominal cavity. If the erosion is sealed before spillage occurs, the ulcer is said to have *penetrated*. About 10% of ulcers perforate; most are duodenal ulcers. The incidence of perforation increases with age.[38] Hemorrhage occurs concurrently with perforation about 10% of the time. Immediately on perforation, a chemical peritonitis results from contact with the gastrointestinal contents, and bacterial peritonitis follows within 12 hours.

Clinical Manifestations

Perforation of the peptic ulcer has the following clinical manifestations:

1. Severe, sharp abdominal pain
   a. Patient bends over and draws up knees to prevent pull on abdominal wall
   b. Abdomen becomes rigid, with rebound tenderness from peritonitis
2. Patient reluctant to move; holds body tense
3. Diaphoresis, rapid pulse, and shallow respirations
4. Diagnostic test: abdominal roentgenogram to visualize air beneath diaphragm with patient standing

Interventions

Medical management. The immediate care of the person with a perforated ulcer consists of (1) *parenteral fluids* to maintain fluid and electrolyte balance, (2) *nasogastric suction* (p. 1296) to empty stomach contents and prevent further contamination of the peritoneum, and (3) large doses of *antibiotics* to prevent sepsis. Most pa-

tients require surgery. A closure of the perforation through a laparotomy may be done; however, because about three fourths of persons with chronic ulcer disease who sustain a perforated ulcer continue to have severe ulcer disease, more definitive surgery to treat the ulcer (p. 1283) is usually done.

Nursing management. Nursing care includes the following:

1. Keep patient in low Fowler's position to pool escaped stomach contents in pelvic cavity
2. Provide emotional support to apprehensive person
3. Prepare patient for surgery, if necessary (p. 1292)
4. Postoperative:
   a. Monitor for signs of continuing peritonitis or abscess formation (fever, respiratory distress, abdominal pain)
   b. Monitor for paralytic ileus (distention, hyperactive or absent bowel sounds) that may result from peritoneal irritation (p. 1295).

PYLORIC OBSTRUCTION

Pathophysiology

Repeated cycles of inflammation and healing during recurrences of peptic ulcers can lead to obstruction of the gastroduodenal junction (pylorus) because of muscle spasm, edema, and scarring. Pyloric obstruction may also result from decreased gastric motility secondary to inflammation around an ulcer or to dilation of the stomach. Initially the obstruction is only partial, but it develops insidiously over days or weeks to complete obstruction. It occurs in 5% to 10% of persons with peptic ulcer, primarily with duodenal ulcers.

Clinical Manifestations

Initially, there will be symptoms of ulcer pain, epigastric fullness, anorexia, and nausea from partial obstruction of the pylorus that does not permit the stomach to empty fully. As the obstruction progresses, weight loss and malnutrition may develop if the person delays seeking medical attention. *Vomiting* copious amounts of undigested food results from the inability of the chyme to pass into the duodenum. Fluid and electrolyte imbalances occur as a result of the vomiting, especially loss of HCL, sodium, and potassium resulting in metabolic alkalosis, hypokalemia, and hyponatremia.

Diagnostic tests include plain abdominal radiographs that show large gastric fluid levels, and gastric aspiration after fasting to determine extent of gastric retention. Gastroscopy may be done to rule out an obstructing tumor.

Interventions

Obstruction from muscle spasm and edema can usually be treated by nasogastric suction for 48 to 72 hours to provide rest to the pylorus and ulcer therapy to treat the peptic ulcer. Parenteral fluids are given during this period; TPN may be necessary for the person with severe malnutrition. Before the nasogastric tube is withdrawn, a *saline load test* is performed: 700 ml of normal saline is instilled through the tube, which is then clamped. After 30 minutes, the stomach is aspirated; if less than 200 ml is aspirated, liquid feedings are initiated. If feedings are to be given before the tube is removed, aspirate and measure the residual before giving the feedings. Sedatives or tranquilizers are usually prescribed to ensure rest and relief of anxiety. Solid foods are introduced slowly, as tolerated.

If the obstruction is due to scarring of the pylorus, or if conservative treatment does not show improvement in 5 to 7 days, surgery (p. 1283) is performed to relieve obstruction.

OTHER ULCERATIVE DISORDERS

STRESS ULCERS

PATHOPHYSIOLOGY

Acute ulcers that are distinct from peptic ulcers may result when persons are experiencing life-threatening events such as severe trauma, burns, shock, sepsis, advanced carcinoma, or acute respiratory distress syndrome (ARDS). Stress ulcers are believed to be the result of decreased mucosal resistance and renewal. Two thirds of stress ulcer are benign gastric ulcers; the remainder are duodenal ulcers. The ulcers are shallow, discrete lesions with edema but little inflammatory reaction. The ulcers bleed easily.

CLINICAL MANIFESTATIONS

Because pain is usually absent, the presence of a stress ulcer is usually unknown until complications of upper gastrointestinal hemorrhage or perforation of the ulcer occur.

PREVENTION

Prevention is the key to management of stress ulcers. Histamine H_2 receptor antagonists (primarily ranitidine) are given to persons who are experiencing life-threatening events to keep the intragastric pH at >4.0. A nasogastric tube may be inserted to monitor the pH of the gastric secretions. The secretions are monitored every hour for the first 24 hours. If the pH is <4, ulcer treatment is initiated; if the pH is >4 after 24 hours, testing is reduced to every 4 hours.[25]

INTERVENTIONS

Measures to treat upper gastrointestinal hemorrhage and perforation are carried out (p. 1289). If bleeding persists, the bleeding site may be treated by electrocoagulation or photocoagulation (laser) through endoscopy. Surgery may be necessary.

ZOLLINGER-ELLISON SYNDROME

PATHPHYSIOLOGY AND ETIOLOGY

Zollinger-Ellison syndrome is an ulceration syndrome of the duodenum or jejunum caused by a *gastrinoma* (gastrin-producing tumor) found primarily in the non–insulin-producing islet cells of the pancreas. Gastrinomas may also occur in the submucosa of the duodenum or stomach, hilum of the spleen, or regional lymph nodes. Most of the patients have single tumors (although multiple tumors may occur), and 50% to 70% of the tumors become malignant. The syndrome occurs more often in males than in females and may occur at any age, although it is more common in ages 20 to 50 years.

The tumors produce an enormous quantity of gastrin that are responsible for stimulation of excessive gastric acid. The ulcers may not respond to conventional treatment, and complications are frequent. The syndrome may be accompanied by diarrhea, which is a result of the large quantities of acid passing into the duodenum, and by steatorrhea, a result of the lack of pancreatic lipase needed for fat digestion. Diarrhea of long duration can cause serious loss of electrolytes, particularly potassium and sodium.

CLINICAL MANIFESTATIONS

Abdominal pain, similar to that of a duodenal ulcer, is the chief characteristic of Zollinger-Ellison syndrome. Diarrhea and steatorrhea may also be present. The diagnosis is differentiated from duodenal ulcers by radioimmunoassay measurement of high serum gastrin levels. A computed tomography (CT) scan may be done for localization of a pancreatic tumor.

INTERVENTIONS

Medical interventions include replacement of nutrients; TPN may be necessary. Histamine H_2 receptor blockers are given to reduce acid secretion; large doses may be required. A newer drug, omeprazole (a proton pump blocker), may be prescribed. If a pancreatic tumor is located, a distal pancreatectomy (not a Whipple procedure) is performed. If the gastrinoma cannot be located or removed and if treatment is ineffective, a total gastrectomy (esophagojejunostomy) (p. 1295) may be necessary.

CANCER OF THE STOMACH

EPIDEMIOLOGY AND ETIOLOGY

Almost all gastric tumors are malignant. The incidence of cancer of the stomach has decreased dramatically for unknown reasons over the past 50 years; nevertheless, gastric cancer accounts for approximately 14,500 deaths each year in the United States.[2] The incidence is highest in Japan. Gastric cancer affects men twice as often as women. It rarely occurs under the age of 40 and is most frequent between the ages of 50 and 70.

The cause of gastric cancer remains unknown. Genetic and environmental factors are thought to be predisposing influences. Abnormalities related to gastric carcinoma include achlorhydria of the stomach and atrophic gastritis. Pernicious anemia is associated with a high incidence of gastric carcinoma, but it may result from a concurrent atrophic gastritis. The remaining gastric stump after a partial gastrectomy, usually a Billroth II procedure, may develop cancer at a later time.

PATHOPHYSIOLOGY

Cancer may develop in any part of the stomach but is found most often in the distal third. Most gastric cancers are adenocarcinomas and occur either in polypoid, ulcerative, or infiltrative forms. Growth of the tumors is either by expansion, forming discrete tumor nodules, or by individual cell infiltration. Gastric cancer may spread directly through the stomach wall into adjacent tissues; to the lymphatics; to the regional lymph nodes of the stomach; to the esophagus, spleen, pancreas, and liver; or through the bloodstream to the lungs or bones. Involvement of regional lymph nodes occurs early. There is a tendency toward intraperitoneal seeding, particularly to the peritoneal cul-de-sac. Prognosis depends on the depth of invasion and extent of metastasis. Three fourths of patients with gastric carcinoma have metastasis at the time of diagnosis.

CLINICAL MANIFESTATIONS

Unfortunately, the person with cancer of the stomach usually has no symptoms until the growth spreads to adjacent organs. Vague and persistent symptoms of gastric distress, flatulence, loss of appetite, nausea, gradual weight loss, and loss of strength may be the only complaints of the patient. These vague symptoms should never be ignored, and the person is encouraged to seek immediate medical advice. However, these symptoms are not necessarily symptoms of cancer. Pain does not usually appear until late in the disease, and the absence of this symptom is often the reason for the delay in seeking medical help. If the disease progresses untreated, marked cachexia develops, and eventually a palpable mass can often be felt in the region of the stomach. Often no early gastric symptoms appear, and fatigue, persistent anemia, and weight loss may be the only signs.

Most gastric cancers can be located by upper GI series x-ray examinations. This is usually followed by endoscopy with biopsy and cytologic examination.

MEDICAL MANAGEMENT

Surgery is the primary therapy for gastric cancer. If the tumor has not spread beyond the stomach, an antrec-

---

STAGES OF GASTRIC CANCER

Stage I	Tumor limited to mucosa (A) or submucosa (B), no lymph node or distant metastases
Stage II	Tumor involves gastric wall but not serosa, no metastases
Stage III	Tumor similar to Stage II, positive lymph nodes but no distant metastases
Stage IV	Tumor may extend beyond gastric walls, positive lymph nodes and distant metastases

---

tomy and a vagotomy are usually performed with removal of regional lymph nodes. Tumors high in the cardia of the stomach, however, require a total gastrectomy (esophagojejunostomy). Palliative surgery may be performed when there are complications such as hemorrhage or obstruction. Chemotherapy and radiation therapy have little effect on the outcome. The overall 5-year survival rate of gastric carcinoma in the United States is about 12%, but is much higher with stages I (70%) and II (30%).[35] The stages of gastric cancer are listed in the box above.

SURGERY OF THE STOMACH

Care of the patient having gastric surgery is summarized in the box on the opposite page.

PREOPERATIVE CARE
Nutrition

Patients with cancer of the stomach or with prolonged pyloric obstruction are often malnourished and require correction of the nutritional deficits before surgery. TPN may be given for 5 to 10 days before surgery.

Patient Teaching

The high abdominal incision that limits respiration places the person having gastric surgery at high risk for postoperative respiratory complications. Therefore preoperative teaching of ventilatory techniques takes a high priority.

Most patients having gastric surgery have a nasogastric tube in place for several days postoperatively, because of decreased peristalsis from manipulation of the gastrointestinal tract organs during surgery and for prevention of trauma or pressure on suture lines. Patients need to learn preoperatively that a nasogastric tube will be inserted and that they will be receiving fluids and nourishment intravenously for several days until peristalsis is reestablished.

POSTOPERATIVE CARE
Respiratory Care

The patient with gastric surgery tends to lie still and breathe shallowly to limit incisional pain. Pain medica-

NURSING CARE OF THE PATIENT AFTER GASTRIC SURGERY

INTERVENTION	RATIONALE
Preoperative Care	
1. Teach breathing exercises.	Exercises learned preoperatively have a greater probability of being performed postoperatively.
2. Explain special postoperative measures: nasogastric tube and parenteral fluids until peristalsis returns.	Knowing what to expect may decrease anxiety.

Postoperative Care

1. Promote pulmonary ventilation.
   a. Encourage patient to turn, breathe deeply, and cough at least q2h (or less until ambulating well); splint or support incision during coughing

   The high abdominal incision will cause patient to splint chest and breathe shallowly supporting incision will help patient cough more deeply

   b. Give pain medication before activities.

   Patient will be more active if feeling comfortable; activity will increase ventilation.

   c. Position patient in mid- or high-Fowler's position.

   Position promotes chest expansion.

2. Promote nutrition.
   a. Measure N/G drainage accurately.

   Drainage measured for maintenance of fluid and electrolyte balance; the amount of fluid lost by gastric drainage will be replaced by IV fluids.

   b. Monitor for signs of leakage of anastomosis (dyspnea, pain, fever) when oral fluids are initiated.

   Anastomotic leakage will be most evident when fluids first pass anastomosis site.

   c. Add food in small amounts at frequent intervals until well tolerated.

   Edema from surgery will further decrease stomach reservoir.

   d. Monitor for early satiety and regurgitation.

   Contents from a very full stomach may be regurgitated into esophagus, causing discomfort and esophagitis.

   e. If regurgitation occurs, tell patient to eat less food at a slower pace.

   This gives stomach time to adapt and prevents early satiety and distention.

   f. Report signs of dumping syndrome (weakness, faintness, palpitations, diaphoresis, nausea, diarrhea).

   Diet will need to be changed to low carbohydrate, high fat, high protein.

   g. Monitor weight.

   Slow weight loss can be expected from decreased intake; weight gain indicates fluid retention.

3. Provide comfort.
   a. Provide good mouth care until oral fluids can be resumed.

   Oral dryness and debris result from being NPO.

   b. Provide adequate analgesics during first few days; patient-controlled anesthesia (PCA) is effective

   Pain is to be expected; giving analgesics before pain becomes severe will increase effectiveness of analgesic.

   c. Splint incision with hands or towel before patient coughs.

   A pulling sensation on incision will make patient hesitant to cough; splinting supports the incision.

   d. Encourage ambulation.

   Encourages ventilation, comfort, and improved morale (Chapter 22).

4. Provide patient teaching.
   a. Gradually increase amount of food each meal until able to eat 3 to 6 meals/day, if possible.

   The stomach will expand and adapt slowly.

   b. If discomfort occurs after eating, decrease size of meals and amount of fluids with meals; eat more slowly.

   Ingestion of fluids leads to early satiety; eating too fast promotes air swallowing and gaseous feeling.

   c. Avoid stress during and immediately after meals; plan a rest period after eating.

   Stress stimulates blood flow to vital organs and away from stomach (decreases digestion); activity redirects blood flow to muscles.

   d. Elevate head when lying down (if cardia of stomach removed).

   This prevents gastroesophageal reflux (heartburn) by gravity flow.

   e. Teach relaxation exercises, if pertinent (Chapter 11).

   Relaxation exercises modify effects of stress.

   f. Monitor weight regularly.

   Weight loss >10% should be reported to physician; this may indicate partial obstruction.

   g. Report signs of complications: vomiting after meals, increasing feelings of abdominal fullness or weakness, hematemesis, tarry stools, persistent diarrhea.

   Facilitates early treatment of complications.

tions are given routinely, and breathing exercises are especially encouraged in the 30- to 90-minute period when the pain medication is at its peak effectiveness. A semi-Fowler's position assists with chest expansion. Ambulation is encouraged when permitted.

Gastric Drainage

Drainage from the nasogastric tube (p. 1296) after surgery usually contains some blood for the first 6 to 12 hours, but bright red blood, large amounts of blood, or excessive bloody drainage is reported to the surgeon at once. If the nasogastric tube stops draining, the surgeon is also notified immediately because a build-up of gas or fluid can cause pressure on the suture line, resulting in rupture or dislodgement of the sutures. It is the responsibility of the surgeon to adjust the placement of the nasogastric tube so that inadvertent dislodgement of the sutures is prevented.

Food and Fluids

While the nasogastric tube is used and until peristalsis resumes, fluids by mouth are restricted. Mouth care is therefore needed frequently to keep the mucous membranes of the throat and mouth moist and clean.

Until the tube is removed and until the patient is able to drink enough nutritious fluids, fluids are given parenterally. The average patient is given about 3500 ml of fluids intravenously each day (2500 ml for normal body needs plus enough to replace fluids lost through the gastric drainage). It is important for gastric drainage and urinary output to be accurately measured and recorded.

Fluids by mouth are restricted for about 12 to 24 hours after the nasogastric tube is removed. Small amounts of fluid are then given frequently, and the patient is observed for signs of leakage such as difficulty in breathing, pain, or rise in temperature. Foods are then added as tolerated by the patient. The dietary regimen must be adapted to the individual, because some persons tolerate increasing amounts of food and fluids better than others.

When the cardia of the stomach has been removed, some patients complain of nausea and vomiting. This difficulty is usually caused by irritation of the esophageal mucosa by the gastric juices that reflux into the esophagus when the patient lies flat. The patient is advised to elevate the head when lying down.

Early satiety is a common problem after gastric surgery. Regurgitation after meals also occurs and may be caused by eating too fast, eating too much, or postoperative edema around the suture line that prevents the food from passing into the intestines. If regurgitation occurs, the patient is encouraged to eat more slowly and decrease the size of the meal temporarily.

POSTOPERATIVE COMPLICATIONS

Early complications following gastric surgery include bleeding, duodenal stump leakage, and gastric retention. Later complications include dumping syndrome, anemia, and fat malabsorption.

Bleeding

Bleeding occurs at the anastomotic suture line and may or may not stop spontaneously. It can be noted during the first 24 hours and again between the fourth and seventh postoperative days. Endoscopy may be done to evaluate the bleeding. The care given is the same as that for upper gastrointestinal hemorrhage (p. 1291).

Duodenal Stump Leakage

Leakage may occur from the blind end duodenal stump of the Billroth II anastomosis. This usually occurs during the third to sixth postoperative day. The patient experiences severe upper abdominal pain that may radiate to the shoulder, abdominal rigidity, high fever, and leukocytosis. Bile-stained drainage may appear on the dressing. The patient is returned to surgery for insertion of a sump drainage tube. If spontaneous closure does not occur, surgery is scheduled in 4 to 6 weeks.

Gastric Retention

Retention of food in the stomach stump may result from edema of the anastomotic site, inversion of the tissue at the anastomosis, or a small anastomotic leak. The person complains of abdominal fullness and nausea and may vomit. Nasogastric suction is reestablished for 48 hours; then feedings are resumed slowly. Balloon dilatation by endoscopy may be performed. Surgery may be required if no improvement results.

Dumping Syndrome

The dumping syndrome is a group of symptoms that may occur a few weeks after surgery. The onset may occur during the meal or from 5 to 30 minutes after the meal. The attack may last 20 to 60 minutes. The patient complains of weakness, faintness, palpitations of the heart, and diaphoresis. Feelings of fullness, discomfort, and nausea often occur, and diarrhea may also develop.

The symptoms are thought to be caused by the rapid entry of hypertonic food directly into the jejunum without undergoing usual changes and dilution in the stomach. The chyme, more hyperosmolar than the jejunal secretions, causes fluid to be drawn from the bloodstream into the jejunum, decreasing blood volume leading to hypotension. The reaction appears to be greater after the ingestion of sugar, because sugar is the most osmotically active food. There is a sudden rise in blood sugar (hyperglycemia) with the entrance of glucose into the bloodstream, followed by a fall in blood sugar to subnormal levels (hypoglycemia). The rapid gastric emptying and the propulsion of chyme into the small intestine are thought to initiate an intensive gastrocolic reflex and to cause diarrhea and a feeling of fullness and discomfort.

Therapy for the dumping syndrome consists of a low-carbohydrate, high-fat, high-protein diet with fluids restricted to the times between meals. Anticholinergic drugs and serotonin antagonists may be helpful.

Weight Loss

After gastric surgery, the patient usually loses 5% to 10% of total body weight, because of decreased intake, and of decreased digestion and absorption from the smaller gastric reservoir. Eating six small meals a day may lead to increased intake.

Anemia

Iron-deficiency anemia can develop from the rapid gastric emptying that prevents mixing of the food with hydrochloric acid for release of the iron.[21] There is also less time for absorption. In addition, pernicious anemia may occur because the parietal cells do not release intrinsic factor for vitamin B_{12} metabolism. Therapy for anemia is discussed in Chapter 30.

Malabsorption and Blind Loop Syndrome

Malabsorption of fat may result from decreased acid secretion, decreased pancreatic enzymes, and increased upper gastrointestinal motility (p. 1298). Following a Billroth II gastrectomy, there may be stasis in the blind loop that fosters bacterial proliferation (blind loop syndrome). The bacteria deconjugate bile salts, making them unavailable for fat digestion.

The patient experiences steatorrhea, diarrhea, and weight loss. Deficiencies in fat-soluble vitamins may occur. Antibiotics are given to decrease the bacterial concentration in the blind loop. Pancreatic enzyme replacement may also be given. In some instances, surgery to change the Billroth II anastomosis to a Billroth I may be necessary.[35]

SPECIAL NEEDS AFTER TOTAL GASTRECTOMY

The nursing care of the patient who has had a total gastrectomy (esophagojejunostomy) differs in some ways from that of patients undergoing other types of gastric surgery. A thoracic approach is used, and the nursing care will be that for the patient who has had chest surgery (Chapter 34). Drains are usually inserted from the site of the anastomosis, and there may be serosanguineous drainage. There is little or no drainage from the nasogastric tube because there is no longer any reservoir in which secretions may collect, and there is no stomach mucosa left to secrete.

Following a total gastrectomy, the maintenance of good nutrition is difficult, because the patient can no longer eat regular meals and because the food that is taken is poorly digested and therefore poorly absorbed from the intestines. Because the patient also becomes anemic, ferrous sulfate, folate, and vitamin B_{12} are often prescribed. Patients who have had a total gastrectomy rarely regain normal strength. Most of them are semi-invalids as long as they live.

PARALYTIC ILEUS

ETIOLOGY

Paralytic, or adynamic, ileus is cessation of peristalsis (ileus) as a result of neurogenic impairment. Paralytic ileus commonly results from direct irritation of the gastrointestinal tract (occurring during surgery); from peritoneal irritation; and with some thoracic diseases (pneumonia or myocardial infarction), major trauma, sepsis, and electrolyte abnormalities (particularly hypokalemia).

PATHOPHYSIOLOGY

When peristalsis ceases, the stomach or small intestine (depending on the site of obstruction) becomes distended from large quantities of fluids and gas. The secreted fluid has a high electrolyte content and is acidic if in the stomach or alkaline if in the small intestine. Gas in the stomach occurs primarily from swallowed air. Gas in the small intestine may result from swallowed air or from gas that has diffused from blood vessels of the gastrointestinal tract. As the fluid and gas collect, the resulting distention causes edema of tissues of the gut wall with subsequent impairment of circulation and, if the fluid and gas are not removed, may cause rupture of the stomach or intestine. Shock occurs from excessive protein loss.

CLINICAL MANIFESTATIONS

Signs and symptoms of paralytic ileus include the following:

1. Abdominal distention with tympani
2. Obstipation (cessation of bowel movements)
3. Bowel sounds are decreased or absent
4. Vomiting that is frequent but not profuse
5. Signs of dehydration from persistent vomiting
6. Diagnostic tests
   a. Roentgenogram of abdomen shows gas-filled loops of distended bowel
   b. Laboratory test results: hemoconcentration, decreased serum chloride and potassium

INTERVENTIONS

The following are the medical and surgical treatments of paralytic ileus:

1. Gastrointestinal intubation until peristalsis resumes (see the following discussion)

2. Parenteral fluids and electrolytes until peristalsis resumes

3. Gradual resumption of fluids and food when bowel function returns

4. Surgery if medical management fails: decompression of bowel by enterostomy

GASTROINTESTINAL INTUBATION
PURPOSE AND TYPES OF TUBES

Nasogastric Tubes

Nasogastric tubes are inserted primarily for decompression of the stomach during paralytic ileus. They may also be used for (1) tube feedings (Chapter 42), (2) tests of gastric analysis (Chapter 41), or (3) lavage of gastric contents following gastric hemorrhage or perforation (pp. 1289-1290).

The *Levin* tube (Figure 43-7) is the most commonly used nasogastric tube. Because it is a single lumen tube, mucosal damage may result even with intermittent suction. Small-bore flexible tubes (such as Vivonex, Dobhoff, Duo) are used for certain types of tube feedings. The *Salem sump* tube is a double-lumen tube that has less potential for injury. The larger lumen of the sump tube drains the stomach; the smaller lumen provides a continuous air flow at atmospheric pressure, preventing adherence of the tube with the mucosa.

Intestinal Tubes

Intestinal tubes are inserted for decompression of the intestinal tract. These tubes are longer than nasogastric tubes to permit passage into the intestinal tract. There is a small balloon on the tip of each tube that, when inflated with air or injected with water or mercury, acts like a bolus of food. This balloon stimulates peristalsis that advances the tube along the intestinal tract. If peri-

stalsis is absent, the weight of the mercury in the balloon will usually carry it forward.

The *Miller-Abbott* tube is a double-lumen tube. One lumen leads to the balloon, and the other has openings along its course, permitting drainage of intestinal contents and irrigation. The mercury is inserted into the balloon of the tube after the tube is passed. The external end of the tube contains two openings, one for drainage of secretions (marked "suction") and the other for inflating the balloon (Figure 43-8). The balloon outlet should be clamped off and labeled "do not touch."

The *Cantor* intestinal tube, which is used less often, is a single tube with only one opening used for drainage. Before the tube is inserted, the balloon is injected with mercury with a needle and syringe. The needle opening is so small that the globules of mercury cannot escape through it. The mercury can be pushed so that it elongates the balloon for easy insertion.

Intestinal tubes are inserted in the same manner as nasogastric tubes; however, passage along the remainder of the gastrointestinal tract is dependent on gravity and peristalsis and may be facilitated as follows:

1. Encourage the following patient positions:
   a. Right side for 2 hours, then
   b. Supine with head elevated for 2 hours, then
   c. Left side for 2 hours

2. Encourage patient ambulation after passage of tube into pylorus (often assessed by roentgenogram)

3. Advance tube 2 to 10 cm (1 to 4 inches) at specified intervals to provide slack for peristaltic action

4. Secure tube to face when desired point has been reached; coil extra tubing on bed or pin to clothing

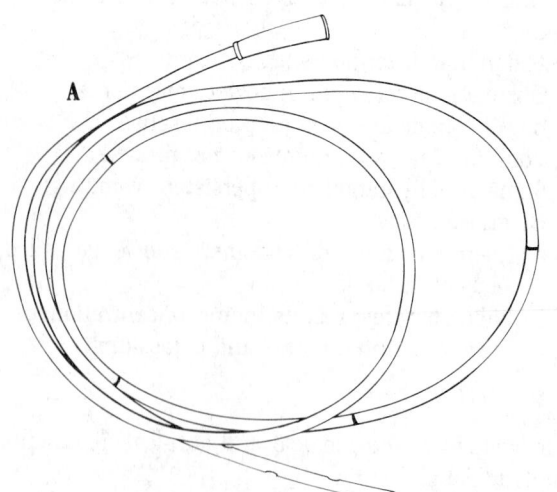
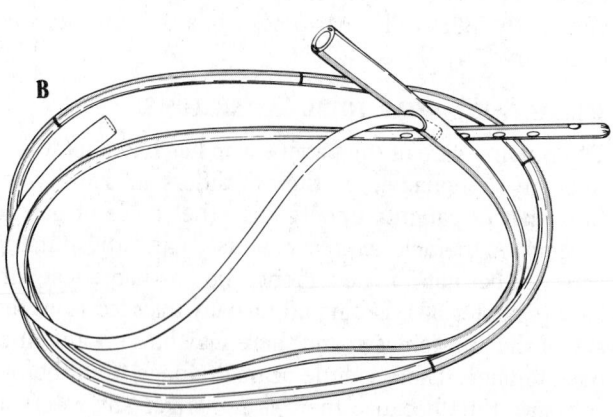

FIGURE 43-7 Nasogastric tubes. **A,** Levin tube. **B,** Salem sump tube.

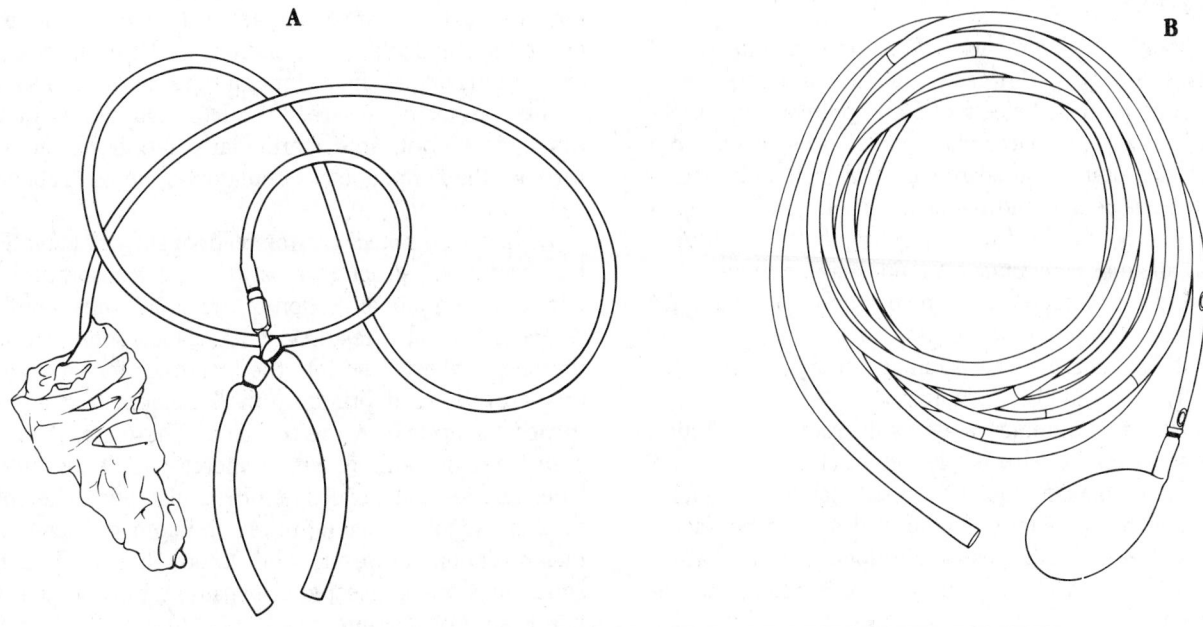

FIGURE 43-8 Intestinal tubes. **A,** Miller-Abbott tube. **B,** Cantor tube.

The intestinal tube is usually monitored daily by roentgenogram for signs of coiling or telescoping of the tube. Telescoping is movement of bowel along with the tube, resulting in intussusception (Chapter 44), a serious complication.

FACILITATING DRAINAGE

Because the gastric or intestinal fluid must move against gravity to be removed, suction is required. *Intermittent suction* is used for single-lumen tubes; constant suction could damage the mucosal wall if a section of the wall were to be pulled continually against the drainage holes of the tube. Intermittent suction permits the wall to drop away from the tube when suction is not occurring. A *low* suction pressure is used for the Levin and the intestinal tubes; high suction is used only with the sump tube. Constant suction is usually preferred for the sump tube.

Functioning of the suction apparatus is checked if no visible drainage is occurring or if the patient has nausea, vomiting, or abdominal discomfort. Normal saline solution is used to *irrigate* the tube, because a hypotonic solution such as water would increase electrolyte loss. It is difficult to aspirate irrigating solution from intestinal tubes because of the tubes' length. If no return flow can be obtained, only a small amount of fluid is used, and the amount instilled is recorded.

PREVENTING INJURY

Methods to prevent injury from gastric intubation include the following:

1. Tape tube securely to nostril so that it does not press against nostril
2. Pin tube loosely to clothing to support weight of tube and permit free head movement
3. Prevent oral inflammations (mucositis, parotitis) from dry mucous membranes or from bacterial movement up the tube
   a. Keep oral mucous membranes moist
   b. Give frequent mouth care
   c. Use ice chips sparingly (ingesting large amounts of hypotonic water from melted ice may produce electrolyte loss through suction)
   d. Provide hard candy (sour balls) for sucking to stimulate flow of saliva

PROMOTING COMFORT

The presence of the tube in the nasopharynx causes local discomfort, and the patient may complain of a lump in the throat, difficulty in swallowing, sore throat, hoarseness, earache, or irritation of the nostril. Methods to promote comfort include the following:

1. Remove excess secretions around nares
2. Apply *water-soluble* lubricant (K-Y jelly) to tube at nostril to prevent secretion build-up
3. Provide for relief of sore throat through the use of warm saline gargles, ice bag to neck, prescribed throat lozenges, or frequent position changes to relieve pressure of tube on throat
4. Use low- or mid-Fowler's position (unless contraindicated) to prevent esophageal reflux (heartburn) (Chapter 42)

MONITORING FOR COMPLICATIONS

In addition to inflammations of the mouth and parotid glands, the person with gastrointestinal intubation may experience fluid and electrolyte and pulmonary complications. *Fluid and electrolyte imbalances* result from loss of gastrointestinal secretions and include dehydration, hyponatremia, and hypokalemia. Loss of acid *gastric* contents may lead to metabolic *alkalosis,* whereas loss of alkaline *intestinal* contents may produce metabolic *acidosis* (Chapter 24). The person is monitored for signs and symptoms of these imbalances, and the amount and character of drainage from the tubes is carefully recorded every 8 hours.

Aspiration pneumonia may result from regurgitation of the stomach contents or placement of fluids in an incorrectly positioned tube. The breath sounds are monitored, and the person is encouraged to breathe deeply and cough on a regular basis. Positioning of nasogastric tubes in the stomach is ascertained before fluids are introduced.

MALABSORPTION SYNDROME

Malabsorption syndrome is a group of signs and symptoms resulting from inadequate absorption of fat in the small intestine. Because fat-soluble vitamins (A, D, E, and K) require fat for absorption, decreased absorption of these vitamins usually accompanies fat malabsorption. In addition, fat malabsorption often is accompanied by decreased absorption of protein, carbohydrate, and minerals. Different signs and symptoms specific to various nutrients result from malabsorption of nutrients other than fat.

ETIOLOGY AND PATHOPHYSIOLOGY

Malabsorption results when there are (1) alterations of digestion so that nutrients are not broken down into a form that can be transported across the cell membranes of the intestinal villi, (2) alterations in the transportation of nutrients across the cell membranes of the villi so nutrients cannot be absorbed, and (3) alterations in the transport of nutrients, particularly fat, from the villi through the lymphatic or circulatory systems (Table 43-4).

As has been noted, gastrointestinal surgery can affect fat absorption. Although most of the fat absorption occurs in the proximal portion of the small intestine, ileal resection can also result in fat malabsorption. Most of the bile salts excreted into the intestines for fat absorption are absorbed primarily in the ileum and are returned to the liver for reexcretion. Therefore, if the ileum is removed, there will be increased bile loss in the feces and less bile available for fat absorption. Removal of short segments of jejunum or ileum do not cause malabsorption; however, when more than 50% of the small intestine is resected or bypassed, nutrient absorption is severely compromised.

CLINICAL MANIFESTATIONS

The characteristic sign of malabsorption syndrome is *steatorrhea,* or excessive loss of fat in the stool. The fat gives the stool a light, greasy, bulky, mushy appearance and a foul odor. The stools float because of their low specific gravity and because of gas produced by action of intestinal bacteria on the undigested fat. Stools may be limited to one bulky stool a day or may be frequent. Steatorrhea causes flatulence with borborygmi (loud bowel sounds) and abdominal distention. The decreased fat absorption leads to weight loss, weakness, fatigue, and anorexia.

Signs and symptoms of vitamin deficiencies include bleeding (ecchymoses, hematuria), bone pain, fractures, hypocalcemia, anemia, glossitis, cheilosis, muscle ten-

TABLE 43-4 Causes of intestinal malabsorption

Factors Affecting Absorption	Mechanism	Examples
Altered digestion (intraluminal phase)	Decreased gastric function	Subtotal gastrectomy
	Decreased pancreatic lipase	Pancreatic insufficiency, pancreatitis, cancer of pancreas, cystic fibrosis, Zollinger-Ellison syndrome
	Decreased conjugated bile salts	Liver disease, biliary tract obstruction, enteric fistulas
		Drugs that precipitate bile salts (neomycin, cholestyramine)
Altered mucosal cell transport (mucosal phase)	Genetic abnormalities	Lactase deficiency
	Small bowel disease	Crohn's disease, celiac disease, tropical sprue, Whipple's disease, infectious or allergic enteritis, parasitic infections, small bowel ischemia
	Inadequate surface	Intestinal resection or bypass
	Drugs	Para-aminosalicylic acid, colchicine, irritant laxatives, neomycin
	Radiation	Radiation enteritis
Altered lymph/blood transport (transit phase)	Lymphatic obstruction	Lymphoma
	Altered blood supply	Superior mesenteric thrombosis

derness, peripheral neuritis, and dermatitis.[38] Protein deficiency results in edema, hypoalbuminemia, and loss of muscle mass. The person with malabsorption syndrome appears pale and emaciated and has dry, scaly skin that may be hyperpigmented.

INTERVENTIONS

Medical treatment is based on the underlying cause of the malabsorption syndrome. Some specific malabsorption diseases are discussed below; other conditions leading to malabsorption are discussed elsewhere in the text.

Nutrition is a major problem with malabsorption syndromes; therefore enteral or parenteral (TPN) feedings may be necessary. Enteral feedings are more economic and present fewer complications than TPN, but there is greater probability of diarrhea with enteral feedings. The severely malnourished person requires good mouth care for comfort and prevention of oral inflammations and good skin care to prevent skin breakdown.

ADULT LACTASE DEFICIENCY
EPIDEMIOLOGY AND ETIOLOGY

Lactase deficiency is a common disorder found among most populations of the world with the exception of Northern European Caucasians and their descendants. In North America, Blacks, Jews, Orientals, American Indians, Eskimos, and Mexicans are frequently affected. Lactase deficiency is usually a congenital disorder, although symptoms may not occur immediately. It also occurs occasionally after a subtotal gastrectomy. It may occur secondary to celiac sprue, Crohn's disease, or gastroenteritis.

PATHOPHYSIOLOGY

Lactose, a disaccharide found in milk, is hydrolyzed by action of the enzyme *lactase* into glucose and galactose for absorption into the bloodstream. When insufficient lactase is present, the undigested lactose remains in the gut and acts as (1) an osmotic agent drawing water into the intestinal lumen and (2) a substrate for bacterial fermentation, generating lactic and other organic acids, carbon dioxide, and hydrogen gas. The increased fluid load leads to increased peristalsis, resulting in malabsorption of other nutrients.

CLINICAL MANIFESTATIONS

The person with lactose intolerance has a history of gastrointestinal symptoms after the ingestion of milk. Symptoms include abdominal distention, discomfort or cramps, borborygmi, and a watery fermentive diarrhea. Diagnosis is made by a lactose tolerance test, a breath test, or jejunal biopsy specimen. In the lactose tolerance test, a rise in the blood glucose level of less than 20 mg/100 ml after the oral ingestion of 50 to 100 g of lactose following an overnight fast suggests lactose intolerance.

The breath test measures an increase in exhaled hydrogen.

INTERVENTIONS

All lactose-containing foods are removed from the diet until symptoms disappear. Some persons can tolerate some cheeses and yogurt, and these foods can be introduced slowly to determine the tolerance.

Teaching the person with lactase deficiency includes the following:
1. Avoid all foods containing lactose
   a. Milk and all other dairy products
   b. Baked foods that contain milk, butter, or added lactose
   c. Commercially prepared foods (including some fruits and vegetables) that are processed with lactose
   d. Margarines prepared with lactose
   e. Instant coffee
   f. Chocolates
   g. Cold cuts, hot dogs
2. Use vegetable oil based margarine
3. Use milk substitutes (for example, Ensure-Plus, Isocal)
4. Carefully read the labels of all commercially prepared foods
5. Take calcium supplements
6. Follow a lactose-free diet for life
7. Reevaluate diet if symptoms recur (abdominal distention, abdominal discomfort, watery diarrhea)

CELIAC SPRUE
ETIOLOGY AND PATHOPHYSIOLOGY

Celiac sprue (also known as gluten enteropathy and nontropical sprue) results from an intolerance to the gliadin fraction of grains (wheat, rye, barley, oats), causing an atrophy of the intestinal villi and microvilli. The proximal jejunum is the area most affected. The disease is thought to be a hypersensitivity response and is familial with a high incidence of childhood celiac disease or evidence of disease in relatives.[38] Symptoms disappear during adolescence but reappear in middle adulthood.

CLINICAL MANIFESTATIONS

Symptoms may vary from mild diarrhea and hypochromic, microcytic anemia to severe signs typically seen in malabsorption syndrome. Hypotension and abdominal distention frequently occur. Diagnosis is made by a symptom-abating response to a gluten-free diet.

INTERVENTIONS

The anatomic and clinical changes of celiac sprue can be reversed by a well-balanced, gluten-free diet. During the initial treatment, secondary vitamin and mineral deficiencies are treated with replacement therapy. Symptoms will recur with dietary indiscretions; thus the person must plan for a permanent change in dietary habits. The Celiac Sprue Association/United States of America* can provide information on celiac sprue and on availability of local chapters.

Teaching the person with celiac disease includes the following:

1. Avoid all foods containing gluten
    a. All food containing wheat, rye, oats, barley
    b. Commercially baked goods, pastas
    c. Commercial salad dressings
    d. Ice cream, candies
    e. Beer, ale (tea, carbonated beverages, and whiskey are permitted)
    f. Some instant coffees containing wheat flour as a filler
2. Use corn, soybean, or gluten-free flour for baking and cooking
3. Read carefully the labels of prepared foods
4. Follow a gluten-free diet for life
5. Eat a high-calorie, high-protein, low-fat diet in addition to the gluten-free foods
6. Reevaluate diet if symptoms occur (steatorrhea, flatulence with abdominal distention, diarrhea)

TROPICAL SPRUE

Tropical sprue differs from celiac sprue. It is endemic to the Caribbean, Southeast Asia, and India. The cause is unknown but appears to have both a nutritional and infectious basis. The initial symptoms are fatigue, diarrhea, and anorexia, followed by further signs of malabsorption syndrome after weeks to months. Symptoms are variable. Remission of symptoms occurs with treatment by tetracycline, folic acid therapy, and a balanced diet high in protein and normal in fat. Folic acid is usually continued as maintenance therapy after symptoms have abated.[38]

EFFECTS OF UPPER GASTROINTESTINAL CHANGES ON DRUG ABSORPTION

The presence or absence of food in the stomach can affect the absorption of medications taken by the oral route. Foods can interfere with drug absorption through changes in gastrointestinal motility and pH, changes in ionization or solubility of the drug, or interaction of a food component with the drug.

Drugs are absorbed more readily if the gastrointestinal tract is free of food. Drugs taken with water when the stomach is empty move rapidly into the small intestine, where much drug absorption takes place. Fatty foods delay gastric emptying for as much as 2 hours; therefore drugs that are absorbed in the small intestine have delayed absorption if taken with a meal high in fats. Whenever drug absorption is reduced by food, se-

*CSA/USA, 2313 Rocklyn Dr, No. 1, Des Moines, IA 50322.

MEDICATIONS TO BE TAKEN WITH FOOD

Aminophylline
Chlorothiazide (Diuril)
Ferrous sulfate
Indomethacin (Indocin)
Mitronidazole (Flagyl)
Nitrofurantoin (Macrodantin)
Phenylbutazone (Butazolidin)
Phenytoin (Dilantin)
Prednisolone
Reserpine (Serpasil)
Triamterene (Dyrenium)

---

rum therapeutic levels of the drug may not be achieved, or there may be a sustained release, thus prolonging the drug effects. Food particularly delays the absorption of antimicrobial drugs, specifically the tetracyclines, the penicillins, and the sulfonamides. On the other hand, medications that have a gastric irritant effect may be enhanced if taken with food (see the box above).

Drugs that are normally slightly acidic, such as aspirin or barbiturates, usually ionize and are absorbed in the stomach. If the stomach pH is increased, such as by milk or antacids, the rate and extent of absorption of these drugs will be decreased. Alteration in stomach acidity may also break down the protective coating of spansules or enteric-coated tablets, resulting in premature release of the contents. Acid liquids such as lemon, pineapple, or cranberry juices, or dry ginger ale may inactivate acid-unstable drugs such as ampicillin, penicillin G, cloxacillin, and erythromycin.

Food components can interact with oral medications by the chemical or physical binding of one substance on another (complexation), thus interfering with absorption of either the food component or the drug. Tetracycline becomes bound with calcium, aluminum, or magnesium ions when taken with milk or antacids, resulting in decreased absorption of tetracycline. Foods containing tyramine (cheeses, wines) may interact with monoamine oxidase (MAO) inhibitors, such as phenelzine (Nardil) or tranylcypromine (Parnate), which are depressants, causing hypertensive reactions.

CHAPTER SUMMARY

🖝 Gastritis may be caused by drugs, alcohol, or bile that damage the gastric mucosa (erosive gastritis) or by strong acids or alkalies that cause inflammation and necrosis of the stomach wall (corrosive gastritis). Chronic gastritis leads to loss of gastric mucosa and decreased secretion (atrophic gastritis).

🖝 The causes of peptic ulcer are still uncertain; cigarettes, aspirin, and heredity have been implicated as etiologic factors.

✔ Gastric acid secretion results from gastrin, histamine, and stimulation of the parietal cells in the fundus of the stomach from acetylcholine from the vagus nerve.

✔ Gastric ulcers result from breakdown of the gastric mucosal barrier, leading to increased back diffusion of HCl into the tissue; duodenal ulcers result from increased gastric acid secretion and increased rate of gastric emptying, which dump excess acid into the normally alkaline duodenum.

✔ Pain of peptic ulcers is generally located in the epigastrium, is relieved by food or antacids, and is worse at night when the stomach is empty and gastric secretions are at a peak.

✔ Medical therapy for peptic ulcers is by antacids (which neutralize the acid), histamine H_2 receptor antagonists (which prevent release of histamine), and sucralfate (which coats the ulcer, thus preventing acid irritation).

✔ Antacids containing aluminum hydroxide cause constipation unless given with magnesium hydroxide, which has a laxative effect. They should be given 1 and 3 hours after meals for maximum effectiveness. Antacids interfere with absorption of tetracycline and histamine H_2 blockers.

✔ Surgical treatment for peptic ulcers may consist of severing of the vagus nerve in one of three places, innervating the stomach and widening the pyloric outlet (vagotomy and drainage), or removing the lower half of the stomach and severing the vagus nerve where it enters the stomach (antrectomy with vagotomy).

✔ Nursing care of the patient with a peptic ulcer consists of relieving pain by giving medications and avoiding foods that aggravate ulcer pain, counseling the patient on avoidance of stress, and teaching the patient about peptic ulcers and health maintenance to help prevent further recurrences.

✔ The most common complication of peptic ulcer is hemorrhage; treatment consists of stabilization of shock, gastric lavage, and drugs for peptic ulcer therapy, but surgery may be needed if bleeding persists.

✔ Perforation of an ulcer through the stomach wall is treated with parenteral fluids, nasogastric suction, antibiotic therapy, and surgery.

✔ Peptic ulcers may result in pyloric obstruction; treatment consists of resting the stomach by providing nasogastric suction with fluids. Food may be initiated slowly when edema or muscle spasms subside. Surgery may also be necessary for tissue scarring.

✔ Stress ulcers may occur in the stomach when persons are experiencing life-threatening events; symptoms rarely occur until hemorrhage or perforation result. Prevention with ulcer therapy for high-risk persons is the best treatment.

✔ Zollinger-Ellison syndrome is one or more gastrinomas (usually found in the pancreas) that secrete large amounts of gastrin, thus stimulating gastric acid secretion, and causing duodenal or jejunal ulcers. Treatment consists of nutrient replacement, histamine H_2 blockers, removal of pancreatic tumor (if located), and possibly a total gastrectomy.

✔ Almost all gastric tumors are malignant; the cause is unknown but is related to gastric achlorhydria. Symptoms rarely occur until there is metastasis; therefore prognosis for 5-year survival is poor. Surgery is the primary treatment.

✔ Postoperative care after gastric surgery focuses on promoting pulmonary ventilation, promoting nutrition, providing comfort, and teaching.

✔ Dumping syndrome is a postoperative complication that results from rapid entry of hypertonic chyme directly into the jejunum, causing fluid from the bloodstream to be drawn into the jejunum. There is a sudden rise in hyperglycemia (from absorbed glucose) followed by hypoglycemia. Therapy consists of a low-carbohydrate, high-fat, and high-protein diet with fluids restricted between meals.

✔ Blind loop syndrome is a complication of Billroth II surgery, in which there is bacterial proliferation in the "dead-end" stump of the duodenum; the bacteria deconjugate bile salts, making them unavailable for fat digestion.

✔ Paralytic ileus is cessation of peristalsis from neurogenic impairment, usually as a result of irritation of the GI tract during surgery, or with some thoracic diseases or as a result of irritation to the peritoneum. Gastrointestinal intubation with suction provides removal of excess fluid and gas until peristalsis returns; surgery to decompress the bowel is sometimes necessary.

✔ Malabsorption syndrome results from inadequate absorption of fat in the small intestine; it is often accompanied by decreased absorption of protein, carbohydrates, and minerals. It results either from alteration in digestion or alteration in the transport of nutrients into the villi or from the villi into the lymphatic or circulatory systems.

✔ Adult lactase deficiency results in undigested lactose (from deficiency of lactase); the lactose acts as an osmotic agent in the intestinal lumen and as a substrate for bacterial fermentation, leading to gas collection and a watery fermentive diarrhea. Treatment consists of a lactose-free diet.

✔ Celiac sprue results from an intolerance to gluten

found in grains, causing atrophy of intestinal villi in the proximal jejunum; treatment consists of a gluten-free diet.

✓ Tropical sprue is a malabsorption disorder that appears to have both nutritional and infectious bases; treatment is with tetracycline, folic acid, and diet high in protein but normal in fat.

✓ Foods can interfere with drug absorption through changes in GI motility and pH, changes in solubility of the drug, or interaction of a food component with the drug.

QUESTIONS TO CONSIDER

- Compare and contrast the differences between gastric and duodenal ulcers in terms of etiology, pathophysiology, and surgical procedures.

- What changes would you have to make in your life if you were diagnosed as having a duodenal ulcer? A lactase deficiency? Celiac sprue?

- Compare the costs of the different antacids in your neighborhood pharmacy. Based on the comments in Table 43-3, which antacid would you select if you had a stress-related gastritis and why?

REFERENCES AND SELECTED READINGS

1. Altman DF: Gastrointestinal diseases in the elderly, Med Clin North Am 67(2):433-444, 1983.
2. American Cancer Society, Inc: 1989 Cancer facts and figures, New York, 1989, The Society.
3. American College of Surgeons: Manual of pre- and postoperative care, ed 3, Philadelphia, 1983, WB Saunders Co.
4. Baron JH: Current views of pathogenesis of peptic ulcer, Scand J Gastroenterol 80(suppl):1-10, 1982.
5. Berk JE: Bockus gastroenterology, ed 4, Philadelphia, 1985, WB Saunders Co.
6. Bongiovanni GL: Essentials of clinical gastroenterology, ed 2, New York, 1988, McGraw-Hill Book Co.
7. *Burkhart C: Upper GI hemorrhage: the clinical picture, Am J Nurs 81:1817-1820, 1981.
8. Clark JB, Queener SF, and Karb VB: Pharmacological basis of nursing practice, ed 2, St Louis, 1986, The CV Mosby Co.
9. Current status of maintenance therapy in peptic ulcer disease, Am J Gastroenterol 83:607-617, 1988.
10. Donaldson RM, Jr: Dyspepsia: the broad etiologic spectrum, Hosp Practice 22(9):41-49, 1987.

11. *Eastwood GL: Gastrointestinal problems in the elderly, Cancer 39(5):59-82, 1984.
12. *Englert DM and Guillory JA: For want of lactase . . ., Am J Nurs 86:902-906, 1986.
13. *Feickert DM: Gastric surgery: your crucial pre- and postop role, RN 50(1):24-35, 1987.
14. *Feickert DM, Jillson E, and Palazzo T: Gastrectomy for stomach carcinoma, AORN J 47:1396-1406, 1988.
15. Ganong WF: Review of medical physiology, ed 14, Norwalk, Conn, 1989, Appleton & Lange.
16. Given B and Simmons S: Gastroenterology in clinical nursing, ed 4, St Louis 1984, The CV Mosby Co.
17. Groer MW and Shekleton ME: Basic pathophysiology: a conceptual approach, ed 3, St Louis, 1989, The CV Mosby Co.
18. Gustavsson S et al: Trends in peptic ulcer surgery, Gastroenterol 94:688-694, 1988.
19. Hanson GS: Acute stress erosions: can they be prevented? Brit Med J 295:348, 1987.
20. Heppell J et al: Surgical treatment of recurrent peptic ulcer disease, Ann Surg 198:1-4, 1983.
21. *Hoppe MC, Descalso J, and Kapp SR: Gastrointestinal disease: nutritional implications, Nurs Clin North Am 18(1):47-55, 1983.
22. Jones FA: Prospects for peptic ulcer prevention, Postgrad Med J 63:323-326, 1987.
23. Kaye D and Rose LF: Fundamentals of internal medicine, St Louis, 1983, The CV Mosby Co.
24. Knight CD, Van Heerden JA, and Kelly KA: Proximal gastric vagotomy, Ann Surg 197:22-26, 1983.
25. *Konopad E and Noseworthy T: Stress ulceration: a serious complication in critically ill patients, Heart Lung 17(4):339-348, 1988.
26. *Lamphier RA and Lamphier RA: Upper GI hemorrhage: emergency evaluation and management, Am J Nurs 81:1815-1817, 1981.
27. Logan R: Non-steroidal anti-inflammatory drugs and peptic ulceration, Brit Med J 297:1130, 1988.
28. Marshall B: Peptic ulcer: an infectious disease? Hosp Pract 22(8):87-96, 1987.
29. Price SA and Wilson LM: Pathophysiology, ed 3, New York, 1986, McGraw-Hill Book Co.
30. Schroeder SA: Current medical diagnosis and treatment 1989, Norwalk, Conn, 1989, Appleton & Lange.
31. Sleisenger MH and Fortran JS: Gastrointestinal disease: pathology, diagnosis and management, ed 4, Philadelphia, 1988, WB Saunders Co.
32. Spiro HM: Clinical gastroenterology, ed 3, New York, 1982, Macmillan Co.
33. Tuyns AJ et al: Cancers of the digestive, alcohol, and tobacco, Int J Cancer 30:9-11, 1982.
34. Wang JF: Stomach cancer, Sem Oncol Nurs 4:257-264, 1988.
35. Way LW: Current surgical diagnosis and treatment, ed 8, Norwalk, Conn, 1988, Appleton & Lange.
36. Welch CE and Malt RA: Abdominal surgery, N Engl J Med 308(11):624-632, 1983.
37. Williams SR: Basic nutrition and diet therapy, ed 8, St Louis, 1988, The CV Mosby Co.
38. Wyngaarden JB and Smith LH: Cecil textbook of medicine, ed 18, Philadelphia, 1988, WB Saunders Co.

*References preceded by an asterisk are particularly well suited for student reading.

CHAPTER 44

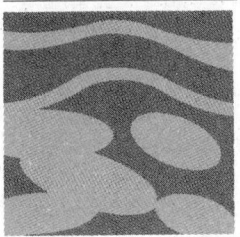

Management of Persons with Problems of Intestinal Elimination

BARBARA C. LONG
REBECCA ANNE ROBERTS

CHAPTER OBJECTIVES

After studying this chapter, the student should be able to:
1. Describe the etiology, pathophysiology, and management of constipation, diarrhea, flatulence, and fecal incontinence.
2. Describe the management of patients with appendicitis and peritonitis.
3. Differentiate ulcerative colitis, Crohn's disease, and diverticular disease and the care required for each.
4. Differentiate anorectal lesions and describe care following rectal surgery.
5. Describe the pathophysiology, prevention and management of parasitic intestinal infections.
6. Describe the nature and care of the patient with intestinal obstruction and hernias.
7. Describe the epidemiology, risk factors, pathophysiology, and preventive measures for colorectal cancer.
8. Describe care of the patient experiencing bowel surgery and a stoma for fecal diversion.

Health maintenance includes regular elimination of waste products from the bowel without loss of excessive amounts of fluids and electrolytes. Disorders of the large intestines often interfere with normal bowel elimination. Problems of elimination discussed in this chapter include the following:
1. Common bowel dysfunctions
2. Acute abdominal inflammations: appendicitis, peritonitis
3. Chronic inflammations: ulcerative colitis, Crohn's disease, diverticular disease of the colon
4. Anorectal disorders
5. Parasitic infections of the colon
6. Irritable bowel syndrome
7. Intestinal obstruction
8. Tumors of the bowel
9. Interventions for fecal diversion: ostomies

COMMON BOWEL DYSFUNCTIONS

Many people, especially the elderly, experience common bowel dysfunctions that interfere with normal elimination. Some of these common dysfunctions include constipation, diarrhea, flatulence, and fecal incontinence.

CONSTIPATION
ETIOLOGY AND PATHOPHYSIOLOGY

Constipation may be associated with disorders of the bowel, hypometabolism, and neurogenic or psychogenic disorders. In many instances, however, it may result from numerous secondary factors that can be prevented (Table 44-1).

Physiologically, constipation may result from decreased motility of the colon or from retention of feces in the lower colon or rectum. In either case, the longer the feces remains in the colon, the greater is the amount of water that is reabsorbed and the drier the stool becomes. The stool is then more difficult to expel.

Lack of dietary fiber and inadequate fluid intake lead to infrequent, dry stools. Dietary fiber increases the water content of the stool, and bacterial degradation of the fiber enhances colonic motility. If the body lacks fluid (dehydration), the colon will reabsorb an increased amount of water from the stool, leading to a hardened stool.

Defecation, which is initiated when the feces enters the rectum, can be voluntarily controlled by contraction of the external anal sphincter. If the defecation urge is not heeded, it soon disappears, and the feces remains in the rectum. The defecation urge occurs most frequently following meals, particularly breakfast, as a result of stimulation of the gastrocolic reflex from food entering the stomach. Most people defecate on a regular pattern, but this pattern varies among persons, from three times a day to once every 2 or 3 days.

TABLE 44-1 Etiology of constipation and diarrhea

	Constipation	Diarrhea
Pathologic conditions	Cancer of the bowel Structural bowel abnormalities Ileus Irritable bowel syndrome Diverticulosis Hypothyroidism Spinal cord disorders Cerebral disorders	Intestinal infections (viral, bacterial, parasitic) Inflammatory bowel disease Irritable bowel syndrome Gastrocolic fistula Cancer of the bowel Malabsorption syndrome Biliary obstruction Pancreatic insufficiency Neurologic disease; diabetic neuropathy, tabes dorsalis Hyperthyroidism Food allergies Reflex from pelvic disease Postvagotomy
Secondary factors	Low-fiber diet Inadequate food intake Physical inactivity Prolonged bed rest Poor bowel habits Stress Barium ingestion (x-ray films) Hypokalemia Hypercalcemia Hyperglycemia Pregnancy	Excessive fresh fruit intake Laxative habituation Stress
Drugs	Antacids (aluminum and calcium salts) Anticholinergics Antidepressants Antihistamines Antipsychotics Belladonna and derivatives Calcium channel blockers Diuretics Narcotics Salts of bismuth, calcium, and iron	Antacids (magnesium) Antibiotics Antihypertensives (antiadrenergic) Antineoplastics Cocaine Digitalis Laxatives

Occasional constipation per se is not detrimental to health although it can cause a feeling of general discomfort or abdominal fullness, anorexia, and anxiety in some persons. Habitual constipation leads to decreased intestinal muscle tone, increased use of Valsalva's maneuver as the person bears down in the attempt to pass the hardened stool, and an increased incidence of hemorrhoids. Chronic laxative use leads to hypokalemia, sodium depletion, and dehydration.

INTERVENTIONS

Constipation may be prevented by the following:
1. Patient teaching
   a. Good bowel habits
      (1) Plan the daily schedule to allow time for defecation when it usually occurs (usually after breakfast or dinner)
   b. Diet
      (1) Eat a high-fiber diet: whole grain cereals

and breads, fresh fruits and vegetables, nuts, and seeds (sunflower, sesame)
      (2) Avoid highly refined cereals and breads, pastries, pastas (unless made with whole grains), and ice cream
   c. Bran
      (1) If taken as a supplement, it must be used in moderation
      (2) It may cause flatulence, diarrhea, or intestinal blockage if taken in excess
      (3) Begin with a low dose (6 to 10 tsp/day) and increase gradually
   d. Fluids
      (1) Drink at least 2000 ml/day (8 glasses, 240 ml each)
   e. Activity
      (1) Participate in a daily exercise program such as brisk walking, exercises, sports
   f. Laxatives

(1) Avoid chronic use of laxatives, if possible; use only when other methods listed above fail

(2) If a laxative is necessary, a bulk laxative or stool softener is preferred

2. Regulation of hospitalized patients
  a. Monitor stools for constipation
  b. Take early preventive measures for high-risk patients (see the box at right)
  c. Encourage full diet as soon as permitted
  d. Encourage ambulation for all patients as permitted
  e. Provide privacy for defecation
  f. Facilitate exchange of constipating antacid with one that has a laxative effect

FECAL IMPACTION

If the stool is permitted to remain in the colon until it becomes exceedingly hard, a fecal impaction occurs. The impaction blocks the rectum and must be removed. If it cannot be softened and removed by oil retention and cleansing enemas, digital removal with a gloved finger may be necessary. This is an uncomfortable experience for the patient, and gentleness is required. Vagal stimulation with slowing of the heart may occur with digital removal. Preventive measures for fecal impaction include identification and assessment of high-risk persons and carrying out measures to increase peristalsis.

DIARRHEA
ETIOLOGY AND PATHOPHYSIOLOGY

Diarrhea occurs primarily as a result of diseases of the gastrointestinal tract, hypermetabolism, and food allergies, or as a reflex from adjoining pelvic organs or following vagotomy surgery (Table 44-1). Therefore it is more difficult to prevent diarrhea than constipation.

The definition of diarrhea is based on the consistency of the stool (watery) and not necessarily the number expelled per day although frequency may occur. Diarrhea may be caused by changes in the fecal contents (solutes

PERSONS AT HIGH RISK FOR CONSTIPATION AND FECAL IMPACTION

Nutritionally depleted
Dehydrated
Receiving constipating medications (see Table 44-1)
Undergoing barium studies
On prolonged bed rest
Confused, disoriented
Aged

exerting an osmotic effect or a fluid content increase) or by an increase in intestinal transit time so that less fluid is reabsorbed (Table 44-2). The final result is passage of feces high in water content.

Fluid and electrolyte imbalances may result from diarrhea, depending on its extent (see Chapter 23). Mild diarrhea in adults may lead to losses of sodium and potassium (leading to a metabolic alkalosis). Severe diarrhea leads to dehydration, hyponatremia, hypokalemia, and metabolic acidosis (from the loss of large amounts of bicarbonate). Malnourished or elderly persons tolerate severe diarrhea less well than do younger or well-nourished persons.

CLINICAL MANIFESTATIONS

Diarrhea can be distressing to the patient, because it reflects loss of control of body function, interferes with other activities, and may lead to skin breakdown. It may be accompanied by abdominal cramping, abdominal distention, and borborygmi (loud bowel sounds). It may also be painless, particularly if it is a result of stress. Defecation may be precipitated by the intake of food or may occur irrespective of time or situation.

INTERVENTIONS

Since diarrhea is usually caused by a pathologic condition or as a side effect of medications, medical treatment consists primarily of correcting the underlying cause.

TABLE 44-2 Types of diarrhea

Type of Diarrhea	Pathophysiology	Etiology
Secretory	Hypersecretion of water and salts in small or large intestine	Bacterial toxins (*E. coli,* cholera); increased bile acids after ileal resection; caffeine
Exudative	Abnormal mucosal permeability with intestinal loss of serum proteins, plasma, and mucus.	Crohn's disease; ulcerative colitis
Osmotic	Increased nonabsorbable solutes in bowel producing an osmotic effect	Saline laxatives; lactose intolerance, fat malabsorption; postgastrectomy syndrome
Rapid intestinal transit	Increased propulsive activity in colon leading to decreased water absorption	Irritable bowel syndrome, gastric and intestinal resection; surgical bypass; antibiotics, stress

Other measures include providing electrolyte replacement, allowing the bowel to rest, giving antidiarrheal medications, and providing for patient comfort.

1. Fluid and electrolyte replacement
   a. Oral fluids that may be taken at home
      (1) Gatorade, which contains 23 mEq of sodium, 17 mEq of chloride, 3 mEq of potassium, and 7 mEq of phosphate in a 5% glucose solution, is recommended
      (2) A home preparation of 1 tsp of salt, 1 tsp of bicarbonate of soda, and 4 tsp of sugar added to 1 L of drinking water is effective (this solution lacks potassium)
      (3) Avoid beverages containing caffeine or ethanol
2. Food intake
   a. Withhold food for 24 hours for severe diarrhea
   b. Restart diet with low-fiber, high-protein, high-carbohydrate foods, preferably cooked
   c. Give small, frequent feedings until diarrhea is stabilized
3. Antidiarrheal medications
   a. Motility-inhibiting drugs
      (1) Loperamide (Imodium), a narcotic analog with no physical dependence, is rapidly effective. It is contraindicated in persons with liver disease, or acute infectious diarrhea
      (2) Diphenoxylate hydrochloride with atropine (Lomotil), a narcotic analog with lower potential for dependency than narcotics, is very effective for control of diarrhea
      (3) Camphorated opium tincture (paregoric), a narcotic, may be prescribed
   b. Drugs that bind bacterial toxins: bismuth subsalicylate (Pepto-Bismol), is good for traveler's diarrhea, but turns stool black
   c. Antibiotics: doxycycline (a tetracycline) or trimethoprim and sulfamethoxazole (sulfonamides) may be prescribed for infectious diarrhea
4. Comfort measures
   a. Provide for personal hygiene after *each* stool; avoid rubbing anus with toilet paper
   b. Keep perineal area clean and dry to prevent skin breakdown
   c. Provide sitz baths three times a day for excoriated anus
   d. Use a protective ointment (such as zinc oxide) on perianal area
   e. Keep environment odor free with deodorizers as necessary

FLATULENCE
ETIOLOGY AND PATHOPHYSIOLOGY

One of the most common gastrointestinal discomforts is abdominal distention or pain resulting from the presence of intestinal gas (flatus). This gas results from swallowed air, from gas formed by the action of intestinal bacteria, and from carbon dioxide formed by the action of bicarbonate with hydrochloric acid or fatty acids. Swallowed air that is not belched passes into the intestines and diffuses passively between the intestinal lumen and the bloodstream depending on the partial pressure difference of the gas; thus different quantities of gas will be present in the intestinal lumen at different times.

Bacterial flora produces hydrogen through the action of the bacteria on ingested fermentable matter. Some vegetables (for example, legumes), fruits (for example, raw apples or melons), or whole grains contain some polysaccharides that cannot be digested; thus they serve as a substrate for bacterial action with the production of hydrogen.[69] Carbon dioxide can be produced during bacterial metabolism. Methane is also produced by bacteria in about one third of the adult population, and this appears to be a familial trait resulting from early environmental factors.[69] Persons who produce large amounts of methane or who eat high fiber diets have stools that float in water. Floating stools are also seen in persons with malabsorption syndromes because of the carbon dioxide and hydrogen produced from the unabsorbed food.

Persons experiencing abdominal distention or discomfort from gas may have problems with altered gastrointestinal motility or malabsorption syndromes, and these conditions need to be ruled out if the person experiences marked discomfort. The distention or "bloating" may be functional, and pain may be experienced by persons who have an increased pain response to intestinal distention.

INTERVENTIONS

Some of the following interventions may help to decrease the intestinal gas volume when a pathologic condition is not present:

1. Avoid activities that increase repetitive swallowing of air (such as gum chewing or talking while eating).
2. Maintain an erect position after meals to facilitate gas rising to the fundus of the stomach and being expelled.
3. Eat a low-fat diet to decrease carbon dioxide production.
4. Take antacids containing hydroxide and simethicone 1 hour after meals in order to neutralize hydrochloric acid and disperse the gas.

5. Avoid gas-forming carbohydrates identified as producing more discomfort.
6. Ambulate to increase peristalsis to move the gas through the intestinal tract if discomfort is present.

FECAL INCONTINENCE
PATHOPHYSIOLOGY

Normally, the contents of the bowel are moved by mass movements to the rectum. The rectum then stores this material until defecation occurs. Defecation may occur reflexly because of distention of the rectal musculature, or it may be inhibited voluntarily. Distention of the rectum initiates nerve signals that are transmitted to the spinal cord and then back to the descending colon, initiating peristaltic waves, which force more feces into the rectum. The internal anal sphincter relaxes and, if the external sphincter is also relaxed, defecation results. Voluntary regulation is under cortical control. Voluntary emptying of the rectum occurs when the external anal sphincter (under cortical control) is relaxed and the abdominal and pelvic muscles contract.

Defecation continues to occur even in the presence of most upper or lower motor neuron lesions because musculature of the bowel contains its own nerve centers that respond to distention through peristalsis. Peristalsis therefore persists or can be stimulated even when somatic paralysis is present. Defecation does not occur continually over 24 hours but occurs primarily during mass peristaltic movements following meals or whenever the rectum becomes distended.

ETIOLOGY

There are several causes of fecal incontinence. The external anal sphincter may be relaxed, the voluntary control of defecation may be interrupted in the central nervous system, or messages may not be transmitted to the brain because of a lesion within the cord or external pressure on the cord. The disorders causing breakdown of conscious control include cortical clouding or lesions, spinal cord lesions or trauma, and trauma to the anal sphincter (for example, fistula, abscess, or surgery). Perineal relaxation and actual damage of the anal sphincter are often caused by injury during childbirth or during perineal operations. Relaxation usually increases with the general loss of muscle tone in aging.

ASSESSMENT

The nature of the incontinence and the ability and willingness of the person and family to participate in a bowel-training program are assessed. Data include the following:

1. Nature of incontinence
   a. Frequency of defecations
   b. Nature of stool
   c. Time of defecation in relation to meals
2. Ability and motivation of person
   a. Awareness of need to defecate
   b. Degree of sphincter control
   c. Ability to contract abdominal and perineal muscles
   d. General physical condition
   e. Desire to learn bowel control
3. Willingness and ability of family to assist person in regular bowel-control program

INTERVENTIONS
Bowel Training

Many persons with fecal incontinence who are conscious and can sit on a toilet or commode can be taught *automatic* defecation; that is, they can carry out certain activities that permit them to defecate at regular times on a toilet or commode and remain continent for the remainder of the day. An effective bowel-training program must be consistent, and it requires cooperation and diligence on the part of the staff as well as the individual and family.

1. Carry out a bowel-training program (see the box below) on the basis of the person's pattern of defecation.
2. Promote a soft formed stool.
   a. Provide a high-fiber diet.
   b. Provide a fluid intake of 2500 to 3000 ml/day.
   c. Administer a stool softener if necessary.
3. Plan activities in conjunction with bladder training activities (see Chapter 49) if indicated (bladder incontinence often accompanies fecal incontinence).
4. Counsel and teach.
   a. Provide empathic communication and support

BOWEL TRAINING PROGRAM

1. Include person and the family or a friend in the planning.
2. Determine when bowel evacuation usually occurs; most frequent times are after breakfast or dinner.
3. Determine whether a morning or evening program is more suitable for the person.
4. Insert a glycerine or bisacodyl (Dulcolax) *suppository* 30 minutes before expected time of defecation; give suppository at *same time every day*.
5. If possible, have person sit on toilet for defecation.
6. If necessary, massage abdomen toward the sigmoid (left lower quadrant) to encourage defecation; digital rectal stimulation may also stimulate defecation.
7. Keep a daily record to determine whether program is producing desired results.

---

if incontinence occurs during the training program; this may only be temporary.

b. Encourage persons to participate in all or some of their own management to the extent possible, thus providing them with a sense of control.

c. Teach rationale for dietary and fluid intake.

d. Teach perineal exercises for *weak* perineal muscles (see Chapter 49).

Uncontrolled Fecal Incontinence

If none of the measures discussed is appropriate or successful, measures are taken to maintain the person's integrity, both psychologic and as physical. Loss of control over intestinal elimination may be associated with feelings of regression, inadequacy, guilt, and uncleanliness. The person needs to feel accepted as an adult and to have the condition accepted by others as a situational physical condition and not as a personal inadequacy. These persons are treated as adults, not as children; they are not made to feel that they are the cause of the incontinence.

Protective disposable pants are available and provide the persons with a sense of security and dignity. Cleansing of the anal and perineal area as soon as possible after fecal incontinence helps to maintain skin integrity and removes a source of discomfort and odor.

The person's usual defecation pattern is monitored, and plans can be made to place the patient on a commode, toilet, or bedpan at times that defecation is most likely to occur. Adequate intake of fiber foods and fluids, when possible, assists in defecation of a normal stool at less frequent intervals.

ACUTE ABDOMINAL INFLAMMATIONS

APPENDICITIS

EPIDEMIOLOGY/ETIOLOGY

Appendicitis is more common among males, and it occurs most frequently between the ages of 10 and 30 years, although it may occur at any age. Although there is no certain cause of the disease, occlusion of the lumen of the appendix by hardened feces (fecaliths), by foreign objects, or by kinking of the appendix may impair circulation and lower resistance to organisms within the body such as the colon bacilli or streptococci.

PATHOPHYSIOLOGY

Appendicitis is an inflammatory lesion of the vermiform appendix, located near the ileocecal valve. A small part of the appendix may be edematous or necrotic, or the entire appendix may be involved. An abscess may develop in the appendiceal wall or in the surrounding tissue. The serious danger is that the appendix will rupture and cause peritonitis.

CLINICAL MANIFESTATIONS

The typical symptoms of acute appendicitis are pain about the umbilicus and throughout the abdomen (which may soon become localized at a point known as *McBurney's point,* exactly halfway between the umbilicus and the crest of the right ilium) and nausea, anorexia, and vomiting. Light palpation of the abdomen will elicit pain in the right lower quadrant. Rebound tenderness is a common finding. The abdominal musculature overlying the area may feel tense as a result of voluntary rigidity. Rigidity noted over the entire abdomen is generally an indication of rupture of the appendix with resultant peritonitis. The person will often be noted to be lying on the side or back with knees flexed in an attempt to decrease muscular strain on the abdominal wall.

Acute appendicitis is remarkable for the suddenness of its onset. The person may have felt quite well an hour or two before the onset of severe pain. Approximately 90% of these persons will have a WBC count above $10,000/mm^3$, and approximately three fourths will have a neutrophil count above 75%. The temperature usually ranges from 38° to 38.5° C (100.5° to 101.5° F) and is accompanied by an increase in pulse. These symptoms are present in about 60% of persons with acute appendicitis.

There will be an area of hyperesthetic skin over the inflamed appendix before perforation. This response may be elicited by stroking the skin surface over the right lower quadrant with the point of a pin or by lightly grasping the skin over the right lower quadrant between the thumb and forefinger and gently pulling the fold upward. Both measures will elicit a verbal or facial pain response.

Other persons have less well-defined local symptoms because of the location of the appendix. It may be retrocecal, or it may lie adjacent to the ureter. If the symptoms are questionable, urinalysis and an intravenous pyelogram may be performed to rule out acute pyelitis or a ureteral stone. Many other diseases produce symptoms similar to appendicitis, and they sometimes need to be ruled out before a positive diagnosis can be made. Some of these are acute salpingitis, regional ileitis, mesenteric lymphadenitis, ovarian cyst, mittelschmertz, and biliary colic.

INTERVENTIONS

Medical Management

The appendix is removed surgically (appendectomy) as soon as possible to prevent rupture with subsequent peritonitis. The appendix is removed through a small incision over McBurney's point or through a right paramedial incision. The incision usually heals with no drainage. Drains are used when an abscess is discovered, when the appendix has ruptured, and sometimes when the appendix was edematous and ready to rupture and was surrounded by clear fluid. Bowel function is usually normal soon after surgery, and convalescence is short.

Nursing Management

Nursing interventions includes the following:

1. Preoperative care
   a. Bed rest (to localize infection if peritonitis occurs)
   b. Nothing by mouth during the diagnostic period in anticipation of early surgery
   c. Intravenous fluids as prescribed to maintain fluid and electrolyte balance
   d. No narcotics during diagnosis to prevent masking of symptoms; sedatives given if necessary
   e. An ice bag may help relieve pain; no heat is applied because this may increase circulation to the appendix and lead to rupture
2. Postoperative care
   a. General postoperative care (see Chapter 22)
   b. Food permitted as tolerated

PERITONITIS
ETIOLOGY

Peritonitis may be primary or secondary, aseptic or septic, and acute or chronic. Peritonitis is an inflammation of the peritoneum caused by trauma or by rupture of an organ containing bacteria, which are then introduced into the abdominal cavity. Some of the organisms found are *E. coli*, streptococci (both aerobic and anaerobic), staphylococci, pneumococci, and gonococci. Peritonitis also can be caused by chemical response to irritating substances that might be present following rupture of the fallopian tube in an ectopic pregnancy, perforation of a gastric ulcer, or traumatic rupture of the spleen or liver. Inflammation from chemical causes, however, is so closely followed by invasion of blood-borne bacteria that it is only a few hours before organisms may be isolated from most fluids that accumulate in peritonitis.

PATHOPHYSIOLOGY

Natural barriers are used in the body's attempt to control the inflammation. Adhesions quickly form in an attempt to wall off the infection, and the omentum helps to enclose areas of inflammation. These processes may result in involvement of only part of the abdominal cavity and may finally narrow the infected area to a small, enclosed one (abscess). As healing occurs, fibrous adhesions may shrink and disappear entirely so that no trace of infection can be found on surgical exploration of the abdomen at a much later date, or they may persist as constrictions that may permanently bind the involved structures together. Sometimes adhesions cause an intestinal obstruction by occluding the lumen of the bowel. If abscesses form, they are usually in the lower abdomen; however, they may be walled off in another area. For example, formation of an abscess following a ruptured appendix may develop under the diaphragm and may even perforate that structure and cause empyema.

Local reactions of the peritoneum include redness, inflammation, and the production of large amounts of fluid containing electrolytes and proteins. Hypovolemia, electrolyte imbalance, dehydration, and finally shock develop as a result of the loss of the fluid, electrolytes, and proteins into the peritoneal cavity. The fluid usually becomes purulent as the condition progresses and as the bacteria become more numerous. Peristalsis is halted by the severe peritoneal infection, and all the symptoms of acute intestinal obstruction (p. 1326) may be present.

CLINICAL MANIFESTATIONS

Clinical manifestations of peritonitis depend on the site and extent of inflammation but may include the following:

1. Abdominal pain and tenderness (local or diffuse, often rebound), abdominal rigidity
2. Nausea and vomiting
3. High fever, high leukocytosis
4. Weakness, diaphoresis, pallor, shock
5. Later signs: paralytic ileus, abdominal distention
6. Masked symptoms, possibly, in elderly persons or in those receiving corticosteroids

INTERVENTIONS
Medical Management

Postoperative medical management of peritonitis includes the following:

1. Nasogastric intubation to prevent gastrointestinal distention
2. Intravenous fluids and electrolytes to prevent or correct imbalances
3. Antibiotics to control infection
4. When the patient's condition is stabilized, surgery to close perforations or to drain abscesses

Nursing Management

Nursing management for the person with peritonitis includes the following:

1. Place patient on bed rest in semi-Fowler's position to help localize pus in lower abdomen or pelvis.
2. Give mouth care to patient to prevent drying of mucous membranes and cracking of lips from dehydration.
3. Monitor fluid and electrolyte replacement.
4. Encourage deep-breathing exercises; patient tends to have shallow respirations from abdominal pain or distention.
5. Use measures to reduce the patient's anxiety (see Chapter 10).

TABLE 44-3 Comparison of ulcerative colitis and Crohn's disease

	Ulcerative Colitis	Crohn's Disease
Usual area affected	Left colon, rectum	Distal ileum, right colon
Extent of involvement	Diffuse areas, contiguous	Segmental areas, noncontiguous
Inflammation	Mostly mucosal	Transmural
Mucosal appearance	Ulcerations	Cobblestone effect, granulomas
Character of stools	Blood present	No blood present
	No fat	Steatorrhea
	Frequent liquid stools	Three to five semisoft stools per day
Abdominal pain	May occur, mild	Right lower quadrant pain, cramping
Abdominal mass	No	Common in right lower quadrant
Complications	Toxic megacolon	Fistulas
	Pseudopolyps	Perianal disease
	Hemorrhoids	Strictures
	Hemorrhage	Abscesses
		Perforation
Extraintestinal manifestations	Anemia	Anemia
	Erythema nodosum	Malabsorption of fat and fat-soluble vitamins
	Pyoderma gangrenosa	Arthritis
	Arthritis	Hepatobiliary disease
	Liver disease	Iritis, conjunctivitis
	Iritis, conjunctivitis	Renal stones, obstructive uropathy
	Stomatitis	
	Thrombophlebitis	
Reasons for surgery	Poor response to medical therapy	Presence of complications
	Complications	
Response to surgery	Curative	Noncurative, high recurrence rate

CHRONIC INFLAMMATIONS

Chronic inflammations of the intestines include inflammatory bowel diseases (Crohn's disease and ulcerative colitis), and diverticulitis.

INFLAMMATORY BOWEL DISEASE

The inflammatory bowel diseases, ulcerative colitis and Crohn's disease, have many common features. Since the nursing care of these persons is fairly similar, these conditions are discussed together. Differences between ulcerative colitis and Crohn's disease are noted in Table 44-3.

EPIDEMIOLOGY/ETIOLOGY

Although inflammatory bowel diseases (IBD) can be found worldwide, there is a higher incidence in Western Europe and the United States. White persons are affected five times more often than black persons. It occurs frequently among Ashkenazi Jews[34] and has a higher incidence among American Jews than those living in Israel. The incidence of ulcerative colitis is twice that of Crohn's disease, but the incidence of the latter is increasing. Although inflammatory bowel disease can occur at any age, it is seen primarily in young adults, with the highest rate of onset between the ages 15 and 20.[69]

The cause of inflammatory bowel disease is unknown. Both *genetic* and *environmental* factors have been implicated. Controversy exists concerning the relationship of smoking and ulcerative colitis. Some reports indicate that smoking may provide some protection against ulcerative colitis.[38] An *infectious* origin by *Pseudomonas* or a "slow virus" has been suggested, but it may be possible that infection is actually a secondary rather than causative effect. Altered *immune* status may also be a factor. Emotional events have been shown to be related to exacerbations of the diseases, but a psychogenic cause of inflammatory bowel disease has not been established.

PATHOPHYSIOLOGY

Ulcerative colitis and Crohn's disease differ in their effect on the intestinal tract (see Table 44-3). Ulcerative colitis affects primarily the distal colorectal area; the involved areas are contiguous, and the mucosa becomes ulcerated with bleeding. Crohn's disease may occur in any part of the distal small intestine or the colon but affects primarily the ileum and ascending colon. The lesions may be separated by normal tissue, are granulomatous, and affect the intestinal wall.

In the early stages of *ulcerative colitis*, only the rectum or rectosigmoid colon is affected: the rectal mucosa

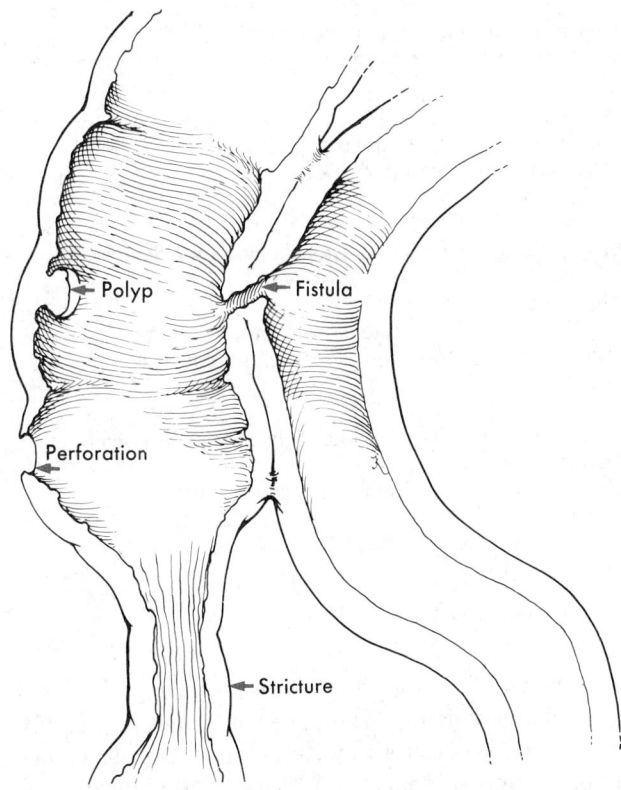

FIGURE 44-1 Selected complications of chronic inflammatory bowel disorders.

contains many superficial bleeding points. As the disease progresses, advancing up the colon, the bowel mucosa becomes edematous and thickened. The superficial bleeding points gradually enlarge and become ulcerated. The ulcers may bleed or perforate. The edematous mucosa may undergo changes and form pseudopolyps that may become cancerous. The continuous healing process, and the formation of scar tissue that accompanies it, may cause the colon to lose its normal elasticity and its absorptive capability. Normal mucosa is replaced by scar tissue, and the colon becomes thickened, rigid, and pipelike.

Crohn's disease is characterized by cobblestone granulomas along the mucosa, a thickening of the intestinal wall, and the formation of scar tissue. The lesions are likely to perforate and form fistulas that connect with the colon (Figure 44-1), bladder, or vagina. Scar tissue may form as the lesions heal, preventing the normal absorption of food, and strictures may form causing intestinal obstruction. Mesenteric lymph nodes are enlarged and firm.

CLINICAL MANIFESTATIONS

Signs and Symptoms

Inflammatory bowel disease is characterized by exacerbations and remissions. *Diarrhea* is a predominant symptom (Table 44-4). In *ulcerative colitis* there may be as many as 15 to 20 liquid stools a day containing blood, mucus, and pus. Abdominal cramps may or may not occur before the bowel movement. As the scarring within the bowel progresses, the feeling of the urge to defecate is lost, leading to involuntary leakage of stool. With severe diarrhea there may be losses of sodium, postassium, bicarbonate, and calcium ions. In *Crohn's disease* the diarrhea may consist of three to five large semisolid stools daily containing mucus and pus but no blood. Steatorrhea may also be present if the ulceration extends high in the small intestine. The abdominal colicky pain is relieved with a bowel movement. Fat-soluble vitamins, that is, A, D, E, and K, may be poorly absorbed with marked steatorrhea.

Right lower quadrant *abdominal pain* is characteristic of Crohn's disease and may be accompanied in the same area by a tender mass of thickened intestines. During an acute episode, the symptoms closely resemble those of appendicitis.

Other signs and symptoms include:
1. Anorexia, malaise, weakness from the chronic inflammation
2. Weight loss from malabsorption
3. Fever and leukocytosis (a high fever and WBC > 15,000/mm^3 suggests an abscess)
4. Iron-deficiency anemia (from bleeding and poor iron absorption and utilization)

Extraintestinal Manifestations

Inflammatory bowel disease may also exhibit the following symptoms:
1. Skin and mucous membranes
   a. Pyoderma gangrenosa: painful, necrotizing, indurated areas surrounded by denuded skin; seen on legs
   b. Erythema nodosum: painful red nodules on anterior leg surfaces; more common in women
   c. Stomatitis
2. Eyes: conjunctivitis, iritis
3. Joints
   a. Arthritis of large joints: minor, nondeforming
   b. Ankylosing spondylitis
   c. Sacroiliitis: mild sacroiliac pain
4. Liver and gall bladder
   a. Fatty infiltration of liver
   b. Pericholangitis, hepatitis
   c. Gallstones
   d. Cirrhosis
5. Kidney
   a. Kidney stones
   b. Fistulas to urinary tract
   c. Obstructive hydronephrosis
   d. Perinephric abscess

TABLE 44-4 Normal function, pathophysiology, and clinical picture of chronic inflammatory bowel disease

Normal Function	Pathophysiology	Clinical Picture
Chyme is liquid upon entering colon; water is absorbed in colon; blood is not a normal finding in stools	UC*: Hemorrhagic ulcerations in lower colon walls interfere with reabsorption of water from the chyme; stool remains liquid	UC: frequent liquid stools; bloody with severe disease
	CD†: Lesions are in ileum or ascending colon; some water is reabsorbed in the nonaffected colon; no bleeding	CD: 3 to 5 semisoft stools per day
Nutrients are absorbed in the small intestines	UC: Loss of fluid and blood by diarrhea	UC: anorexia, weight loss, anemia
	CD: Inflamed and scarred walls interfere with absorption of nutrients; fat is excreted in the stools	CD: same as for UC; steatorrhea
Chyme flows freely through intestinal lumen	CD: Edema and inflammation of intestinal wall cause narrowing of intestinal lumen leading to partial obstruction	UC: occasional mild abdominal discomfort
		CD: Cramping abdominal pain

* UC: ulcerative colitis.
† CD: Crohn's disease.

Diagnostic Tests

Diagnostic tests for inflammatory bowel disease may include one or all of the following:
1. X-ray films: barium studies, except in acutely ill persons; use of cathartics that may aggravate an electrolyte imbalance and may cause shock are avoided[34]
2. Endoscopy
   a. Sigmoidoscopy to help differentiate ulcerative colitis from Crohn's disease
   b. Colonoscopy to help in the diagnosis of Crohn's disease; used rarely for ulcerative colitis because of the possible complications of hemorrhage and perforation (limited data obtained)
3. Stool examination for occult blood (guaiac), fat, mucus, and pus
4. Blood tests for anemia

MEDICAL MANAGEMENT

Therapy for inflammatory bowel disease during exacerbations is primarily supportive and includes nutritional therapy and rest. Medications include the following:
1. Sulfasalazine (Azulfidine): the most commonly prescribed drug given in doses of 2 to 8 g/day for antiinflammatory therapeutic effect
2. Corticosteroids: suppression of inflammation but have no effect on cure
3. Antibiotics for acutely ill patients with signs of peritoneal irritation or with a fistula
4. Bulk hydrophilic agents such as psyllium (Metamucil) in preference to the antimotility drugs for diarrhea

Vitamin supplements are frequently necessary, particularly when anorexia and nausea are present. Replacement of vitamin B_{12} is given when there is a marked loss of ileum. When anemia is present, irondextran (Imferon) is given by Z-track injection, since oral intake of iron is ineffective because of the intestinal ulceration. Surgery may be performed for complications.

Surgery

Ulcerative colitis. Surgery is indicated for the person with ulcerative colitis when the person does not respond to medical management or when complications such as persistent hemorrhage, perforation or strictures of the colon, or toxic megacolon are present. Most surgeries are curative, and recurrences are few. Types of surgery that may be performed include the following:
1. Total proctocolectomy through an abdominal incision with *permanent ileostomy* (p. 1338)
2. Total proctocolectomy with a *continent ileostomy* (Kock pouch) (Figure 44-2)
   a. An intraabdominal reservoir with a "nipple valve" is formed from the distal ileum to provide continence for the ileostomy.
   b. The pouch eventually can hold approximately 500 ml.
   c. Contents of the pouch are removed several times a day by catheterization.
   d. Problems may result with the nipple valve or with thick ileal contents that may plug the stoma.
3. Total colectomy with *ileorectal anastomosis*: resection of the colon with anastomosis of the ileum with the *rectum*
   a. Residual rectal inflammation may lead up to a 50% failure rate.
   b. Recurrent diarrhea is a problem.

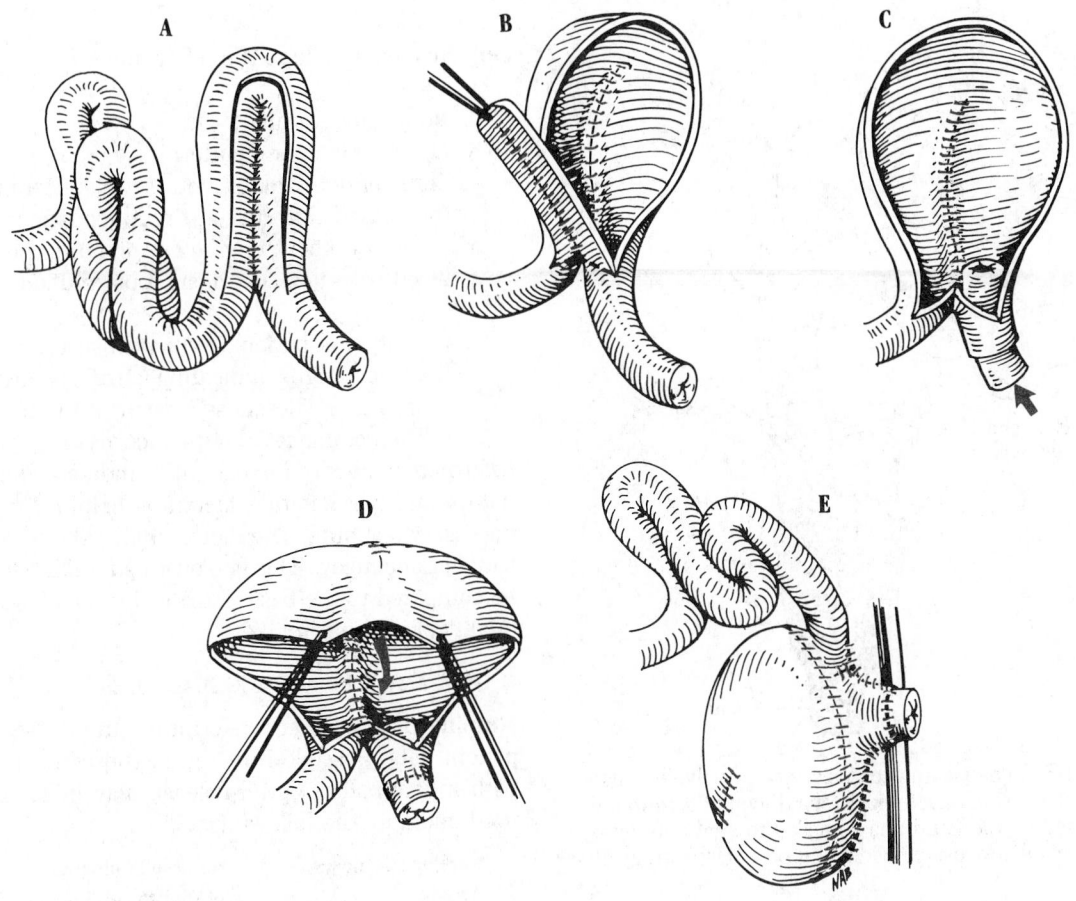

FIGURE 44-2 Continent ileostomy. **A**, Loop of bowel sewn together. **B**, Removal of anterior portion. **C**, Nipple valve made by pushing bowel back on itself. **D**, Pouch formation. **E**, End brought through stoma.

4. Total colectomy and mucosal proctectomy with *ileoanal anastomosis* (with or without a valveless pouch): resection of colon, removal of rectal mucosa leaving rectal muscle intact, and anastomosis of ileum with the *anal sphincter*. This type of surgery is now used more frequently than the continent ileostomies.
   a. A J-pouch may be created by a side-to-side anastomosis of a folded loop of the distal ileum; the apex of the pouch is incised and anastomosed to the anus (Figure 44-3).[52,65] W- and S-pouches (different looping of the distal ileum) are also being used.
   b. A 2-month temporary ileostomy is performed to permit healing of the anastomosis.
   c. Bowel incontinence may be a sequela.

Crohn's disease. Surgery is performed only in selected instances for Crohn's disease because of a high rate of recurrence. Surgery is indicated for bowel obstruction, fistulas, and intraabdominal abscess. Persons who respond poorly to medical management may undergo resective surgery to alleviate symptoms, with the knowledge of the likelihood of recurrence.

Two types of surgery may be performed, resection or bypass. Resection is preferred because bypass has a greater failure rate for control of the disease.[34]
   1. Segmental *resection* of diseased bowel with anastomosis of ileum with the remaining ascending or transverse colon is performed. Complications include *short bowel syndrome* (decreased absorptive surface) with malabsorption of vitamin B_{12} and of fat from loss of bile reabsorption (see Chapter 43).
   2. The diseased bowel is bypassed by anastomosis of ileum to the colonic area free of disease, leaving the diseased bowel intact. Complications include *blind loop syndrome* with possible bacterial overgrowth and malabsorption in the inactive loop.

■ ASSESSMENT
Subjective Data

Subjective data for the person with inflammatory bowel disease include the following:
   1. Patient's understanding of the disorder

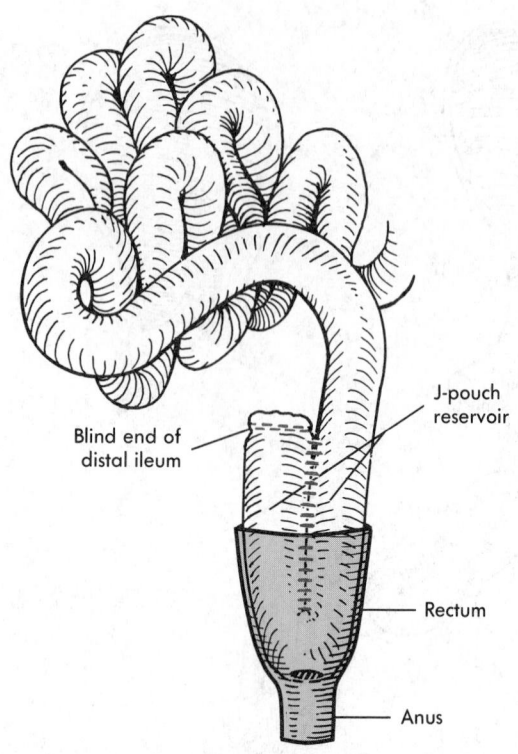

FIGURE 44-3 Ileoanal anastomosis with a valveless ileal reservoir. Side-to-side anastomosis of a J-loop of terminal ileum is incised at apex and anastomosed to anal sphincter; remaining rectal mucosa provides support. Defecation occurs through anus.

2. Patterns of bowel elimination: frequency, character, amount; presence of bleeding, fat, mucus, or pus; color and odor
3. Pain: location, character, frequency, relief with passage of stools, relief measures taken
4. Nutritional status
   a. Intolerance of certain foods
   b. Intake of caffeinated drinks, alcohol
   c. Appetite, presence of nausea
   d. Usual weight, recent weight loss
   e. Weakness, fatigue
5. Sleep: interference because of diarrhea or pain
6. Stress
   a. Perceived sources of stress in daily life
   b. Occupation: nature, hours of work, job satisfaction
   c. Usual coping methods and present effectiveness
7. Social relationships
   a. Extent of social activities, and interferences as a result of illness
   b. Availability and perceived support of significant others
8. Sexual: effect of illness on sexual relationships
9. Medications taken at home: type, dosage, effect

Objective Data

Objective data include the following:
1. Weight
2. Body temperature
3. Observable eating patterns
4. Signs of dehydration with severe ulcerative colitis (decreased skin turgor, dry mucous membranes)
5. Stool: number, character, amount, presence of blood (overt, guaiac test), pus, mucus, color and odor
6. Condition of perianal skin with severe diarrhea
7. Behavior: signs indicating stress or anxiety (for example, restlessness, pacing, twisting hands, verbal comments about concerns)

Information about the patient's understanding of the nature and precipitating factors is helpful for planning necessary teaching. The diet is analyzed in terms of nutritional adequacy. The person's usual daily intake can be compared to the basic four food groups to determine quality of nutrient intake.

■ DATA ANALYSIS: NURSING DIAGNOSES

Nursing diagnoses are determined from assessment of patient data. Possible nursing diagnoses for the person with inflammatory bowel disease may include, but are not limited to, the following:

Nursing Diagnoses	Possible Etiologies
Anxiety	Threat to self-concept, threat to/change in health status
Coping, ineffective, individual/family	Prolonged disability, situational crises
Diarrhea	Chronic bowel inflammation
Fatigue	Anemia, decreased nutritional intake, stress
Fluid volume deficit	Diarrhea, inadequate fluid intake
Knowledge deficit	Lack of exposure/recall
Nutrition, altered: less than body requirements	Anorexia, loss of nutrients by diarrhea
Pain: abdominal, rectal	Bowel disease, diarrhea
Sexual dysfunction, potential	Malnutrition, diarrhea, fatigue
Skin integrity, impaired, potential	Chronic diarrhea

■ PLANNING: EXPECTED PATIENT OUTCOMES

Expected patient outcomes for the person with inflammatory bowel disease may include, but are not limited to, the following:
1. Signs of anxiety decrease; patient sleeps for longer periods
2. Patient describes alternative coping measures, if appropriate
3. Family and significant others can describe:
   a. Approaches to promote patient's independence and control of own daily activities

b. Approaches to cope with their own feelings regarding patient's illness
4. Frequency of defecation decreases
5. Patient schedules activities to permit rest periods when fatigue is present
6. Patient is hydrated (moist skin and mucous membranes, good skin turgor)
7. Patient eats a high protein, high-calorie, high-vitamin well-balanced diet
8. Patient states feeling more comfortable and that abdominal discomfort is decreased; skin of elbows, sacrum and rectal area is intact
9. Patient expresses concerns regarding sexuality and explores alternative ways of meeting sexuality needs, if appropriate
10. Patient describes:
    a. Nature of illness and prescribed therapy
    b. Diet to be followed
    c. Measures to decrease bowel motility
    d. Measures to promote relaxation and rest
    e. Plans for participating in social activities
    f. Plans for following prescribed medical regimen
    g. Symptoms requiring medical attention (changes in nature of diarrhea or abdominal pain, persistent anorexia or nausea) and plans for regular medical follow-up

■ IMPLEMENTATION

Promoting Nutrition

During acute exacerbations of inflammatory bowel disease, the patient is usually malnourished from anorexia, inflammation of the bowel, and malabsorption. The method of feeding depends on the type and extent of the disorder. With severe or extensive disease, especially in Crohn's disease where absorption is decreased or when complications are present, TPN may be necessary. TPN also provides for rest of the inflamed bowel.

Elemental feedings similar to that given in tube feeding (Chapter 42) are started as soon as possible; these feedings are absorbed rapidly in the upper GI tract, causing minimal exertion load on the colon. Palatability is a problem with the oral intake of elemental diets. Serving the fluids chilled and offering a variety of flavors increases patient acceptance. A low-residue, high-protein, high-calorie diet is then gradually introduced.

During periods of remission, patients are advised to continue to eat a well-balanced, high-protein, high-caloric diet. Only those foods that cause problems are eliminated. The person with ulcerative colitis often needs to avoid intestinal stimulants such as alcohol, caffeinated beverages, high-fat foods, and very high-fiber foods such as *raw* fruits and vegetables (cooked fruits and vegetables are usually better tolerated). Milk is poorly tolerated by some persons. The services of a dietitian or nutritionist are used for diet planning and teaching.

Promoting Fluid Balance

Profuse diarrhea leads to loss of fluids and electrolytes (p. 1305). Fluids to 2500 ml/day are encouraged in persons on oral diets. The mouth is kept moistened, and lotion is applied to the skin. Weight is monitored for marked changes resulting from fluid losses or gains. Fluid intake and output are monitored daily.

Promoting Comfort

Patients are encouraged to use the toilet or commode whenever possible, but a weak, acutely ill person usually wants the bedpan accessible at all times. The bedpan should be emptied as often as it is used, which may be frequently for ulcerative colitis. Room deodorizers may be necessary. Patients who brace themselves on the bedpan by leaning on their elbows may develop pressure areas; these areas will need to be protected and massaged frequently.

The anal region often becomes excoriated from the frequent stools. Painful anal fissures and fistulas (p. 1320) may also develop. The anal area needs to be kept clean and dry. Medicated wipes (such as "Tucks") can provide greater comfort than toilet tissue. Sitz baths three times a day also promote comfort and cleanliness. Ointments such as Desitin or zinc oxide may be used to protect the perianal skin.

Promoting Healing: Giving Medications

Sulfasalazine (Azulfidine), the most commonly used medication, may be prescribed for therapeutic purposes and for maintenance. Instructions to the patient include the following:
1. Take sulfasalazine in equally divided doses.
2. Take medication with a full glass (240 ml) of water to maintain hydration.
3. If gastric upset occurs, take medication after meals or with food.
4. Maintain a fluid intake adequate to provide a urinary output of at least 1500 ml/day, to prevent crystallization in kidneys.
5. Avoid sunlight or use sunscreen because of photosensitivity.
6. Report to the physician side effects such as continuous headache, rash or peeling of skin, aching of joints, unusual bleeding or bruising (blood dyscrasias), jaundice, continuous nausea and vomiting.
7. Male infertility may occur.

For severe disease, *corticosteroids* are given in high dosages over a limited period to suppress inflammation. Dosages are then decreased and given on an alternate-day schedule; the corticosteroids are discontinued when

DATA: John Peters is an 18-year-old freshman college student with a history of ulcerative colitis diagnosed 1 year ago. He was admitted 3 days ago with severe bloody diarrhea and recent weight loss of 7 kg (15.5 lbs). He has felt fatigued for several weeks and had loss of appetite. Physical examination on admission indicated dry mucous membranes and decreased skin turgor. His height is 70 cm (5 ft 10 in) and weight is 59 kg (130 lbs). Admission blood count was: RBC, 3.5; hemoglobin, 9 g/dl; hematocrit 35%; WBC, 20,000/mm³. Serum sodium, potassium, calcium, and bicarbonate were all below normal levels. IV fluids with electrolytes were given for 48 hours to replace fluids and correct electrolyte imbalances, and to rest the colon. Stools have decreased from about 20 to 15 a day but are still liquid. Current physician's orders include bed rest with BRP, Ensure feedings orally six times a day, ampicillin 250 mg q6h po, prednisone 15 mg qid po, and Imferon 100 mg IM by Z-track qd.

The nursing history identified the following:

- John did not seek medical attention when the diarrhea started because he thought it was a "virus" and would stop with Lomotil.
- He knows that ulcerative colitis is a chronic disease but had hoped that it would not recur after the initial episode. He stopped taking prescribed sulfasalazine after he felt better and was starting college (he didn't want to appear "different").
- He states he's worried about failing his courses because he has missed numerous classes; if he fails, he loses his small scholarship.
- His parents, who live 200 miles away, are coming to see him this weekend.
- He states his "bottom" is sore from the diarrhea. (Inspection showed reddened areas but no skin breakdown.)
- When asked if his illness had interfered with his social life, he said "No," and quickly changed the subject.

NURSING DIAGNOSIS

Nutrition, altered: less than body requirements related to anorexia and loss of nutrients through diarrhea.

Expected Patient Outcomes	Nursing Interventions	Rationale
John's weight does not drop below 59 kg; shows signs of increasing to at least 60 kg.	Give prescribed Ensure feeding.	Ensure is an elemental diet; it provides necessary nutrients while decreasing the work load on the colon.
	Chill Ensure before giving, and offer a variety of flavors (if available).	Feedings are more palatable when chilled.
	When foods are permitted, encourage foods high in protein, calories, and vitamins.	Protein is necessary for healing, calories for weight gain, vitamins to replace losses.

NURSING DIAGNOSIS

Fluid volume deficit related to fluid loss from diarrhea

Expected Patient Outcomes	Nursing Interventions	Rationale
Skin turgor is improved. Mucous membranes are moist.	Monitor intake and output daily. Encourage John to drink at least one glass of water between feedings.	Intake equals output in a hydrated patient. At least 2500 ml is lost per day through perspiration, respiration, defecation, and urination.
	Encourage mouth care as necessary.	Good oral hygiene keeps mucous membranes moist and encourages eating.

NURSING DIAGNOSIS

Diarrhea related to exacerbation of ulcerative colitis

Expected Patient Outcomes	Nursing Interventions	Rationale
Stools become soft, formed, and less frequent.	Monitor stools for consistency and frequency. Give prescribed prednisone and ampicillin.	Progress is evaluated. Antiinflammatory and antibiotic agents promote healing.
	Provide medicated wipes for cleaning anus.	These are less abrasive than toilet tissue.
	Consider sitz baths if perineal discomfort continues.	Sitz baths provide warm, moist heat that increases circulation to perineum, thus decreasing discomfort.
	Apply a water insoluble ointment to perianal area.	Helps to prevent further irritation from frequent stools.

NURSING DIAGNOSIS

Anxiety related to inability to meet school requirements and possible threat to self-concept

Expected Patient Outcomes	Nursing Interventions	Rationale
John describes realistic plans for the immediate future.	Discuss the effects of stress on exacerbation of ulcerative colitis.	Colonic motor activity is increased with stress, leading to exacerbations.
	Help John explore: 1. Concerns related to school work 2. Probability of completing semester 3. Alternative approaches to immediate return to class 4. Support persons to facilitate decision making	Identification of specific concerns, support persons, and alternative approaches will make the "unknown" become "known" and give him a sense of control, thus decreasing anxiety. Support persons may include parents, school friends, academic school services advisor, personnel at student health center.
John discusses his concerns related to the ulcerative colitis.	Help John explore other concerns he may have.	John has stated he does not want to be "different;" his disease may be a threat to his self-concept.

NURSING DIAGNOSIS

Fatigue related to decreased nutrient intake and anemia

Expected Patient Outcomes	Nursing Interventions	Rationale
John states he feels less tired Pulse returns to baseline within 5 min after activity.	Give prescribed imferon (iron-dextran).	Decreased iron in RBC decreases oxygen carrying capacity; less oxygen is available for energy production (ATP).
	Schedule rest periods between activities.	Rest decreases energy demands.
	Use stabilization of pulse rate to determine the extent of allowed activity.	If baseline pulse rate does not occur within 5 min, the activity is demanding too much oxygen.

NURSING DIAGNOSIS

Knowledge deficit related to lack of information/recall pertaining to ulcerative colitis

Expected Patient Outcomes	Nursing Interventions	Rationale
John describes the nature or ulcerative colitis and self-care	Review the nature of exacerbations and recurrences of ulcerative colitis and the effect of sulfasalazine for maintenance therapy.	Knowing that exacerbations will probably occur but may be less severe with maintenance therapy may increase compliance.
	Relate recent inadequate fluid and nutrient intake to his present severe symptoms.	A well-balanced diet and adequate fluid intake may help decrease severity of future exacerbations.
	Reemphasize the effects of stress on exacerbations.	Stress is a major factor in exacerbations.
	Emphasize planning for rest periods; teach John how to take and and evaluate his pulse rate following activity.	John is provided with a means of control over fatigue.
	Provide information about the medication therapy.	Provide John with essential information he needs to control his ulcerative colitis.
	Explain the effect of unprescribed intestinal drugs on ulcerative colitis; recommend using Metamucil to help keep stools solid.	Drugs can irritate inflamed colonic wall; Metamucil provides bulk to stool without affecting the colon wall.
	Review any signs requiring medical attention; suggest he schedule a visit to the student health center for follow-up care.	John delayed seeking early medical help for the diarrhea; the college physician and nurse can facilitate ongoing health care and support.

remission can be maintained by sulfasalazine. Patients undergoing surgery require increased dosages of steroids before and after surgery because their own adrenal response has been suppressed.[34]

Decreasing Anxiety and Facilitating Coping

The inflammatory bowel diseases are lifelong illnesses with periods of exacerbation and remission that can disrupt the person's life situation. Emotions and stress have been noted to play a role in exacerbations. If the disease is of long duration, the patient is usually thin, nervous, and apprehensive and is inclined to be preoccupied with physical symptoms. Insecurity, dependency, and depressed or hostile behavior may be present. Family and friends may take over control of the person's life, adding to the person's feelings of loss of self-control.

The person caring for the patient may also experience feelings of frustration and dissatisfaction. Empathic communication over time is usually needed to establish a helping relationship. It may be necessary to plan to spend time with the person and with the family on a regular basis.

The person with inflammatory bowel disease can be helped to identify possible sources of life stressors and to examine ways to possibly reduce or modify the stress. The person's usual coping mechanisms can be assessed for effectiveness, and alternate coping strategies can be discussed as appropriate (see Chapter 10). Knowledge about the illness, diagnostic tests, and therapeutic modalities may help to decrease anxiety. Patients need to be included in planning of activities to gain some control over their lives.

Promoting Rest

Fatigue is common because of increased energy demands from the inflammatory process and decreased energy supply from inadequate nutrition and anemia. Planned rest periods should be included in the daily activities. The patient's complaints of fatigue and an evaluation of pulse stabilization following activity are criteria used to determine the amount of rest necessary. When the acute episode begins to subside, progressive activity is encouraged. During periods of remission, the person is encouraged to participate in social activities but must not overextend to the point of fatigue.

Promoting Sexuality

Sexual response may be decreased by inflammatory bowel disease, and this may interfere with sexual relationships. Malnutrition and frequent diarrhea lead to decreased libido. The person is given an opportunity to discuss any sexual concerns, and the nurse assists the person to communicate these concerns with the involved party. Alternate ways of meeting sexuality needs can be explored (see Chapter 52).

TEACHING THE PATIENT WITH INFLAMMATORY BOWEL DISEASE

1. Diet and fluids
   a. Eat a high-protein, high-vitamin diet
   b. Avoid any foods that increase symptoms (such as milk, alcohol, raw fruits and vegetables, beverages containing caffeine, fats)
   c. Take vitamin supplements if oral intake is reduced or following surgery for Crohn's disease
   d. Drink fluids to maintain a urinary output of at least 1500 ml/day
2. Elimination
   a. Take medications as prescribed
   b. Keep rectal area clean and dry; use analgesic rectal ointment or sitz baths for rectal discomfort
3. Rest and relaxation
   a. Use relaxation measures such as breathing exercises when emotional tension is present
   b. Identify a source for an ongoing supportive relationship
   c. Maintain a regular sleep schedule
   d. Schedule daily activities to avoid fatigue; take rest periods as necessary
   e. Participate in social activities, as appropriate
4. Health maintenance
   a. Report signs requiring medical attention (changes in severity of diarrhea or abdominal pain, persistent anorexia or nausea)
   b. Plan for regular follow-up care

Patient Teaching

Because inflammatory bowel diseases are lifelong illnesses, ongoing patient teaching is important to help the person learn effective self-care. Main points to be included in teaching are listed in the box above. Pamphlets to be used in patient teaching about inflammatory bowel disease can be obtained from the National Foundation for Ileitis and Colitis.* Local support groups are available in some communities.

A sample nursing care plan for a person with ulcerative colitis can be found on p. 1316.

DIVERTICULAR DISEASE OF COLON
EPIDEMIOLOGY/ETIOLOGY

Diverticula are small mucosal outpouchings or sacs through defects in the muscular wall of the colon (Figure 44-4). The presence of diverticula is termed *diverticulosis;* symptomatic diverticula are referred to as *diverticulitis.*

Diverticulosis rarely occurs before age 35; then probability increases progressively with age to about a 60% incidence in older persons. The number of persons who have diverticulosis of the colon is unknown, since many persons with diverticulosis are asymptomatic. The incidence of *diverticulitis* (inflammation of diverticula),

---

*444 Park Ave S., New York, NY 10016.

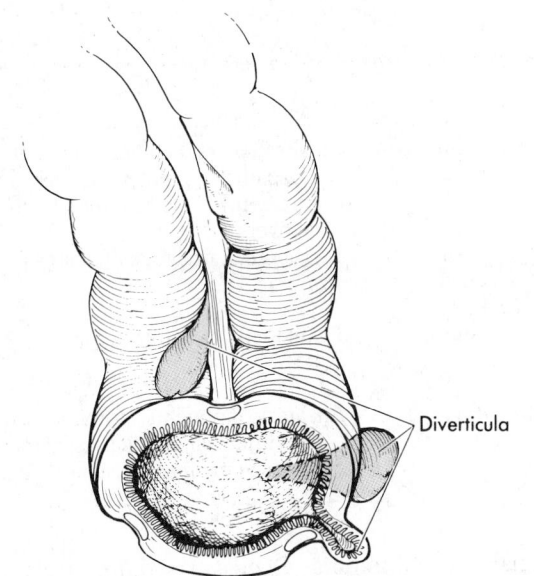

FIGURE 44-4 Diverticuli of colon.

however, peaks in middle age between the fifth and seventh decades of life.[52]

Diverticulosis has been described as a disease of Western civilization because of the high incidence in Western developed countries and the low incidence in nonindustrialized countries and Japan. The cause is thought to be the low intake of dietary fiber foods in most developed countries. Symptoms appear when diverticula become inflamed, when painful spasms associated with the diverticula occur, or when complications such as perforation, obstruction, or hemorrhage occur.

CLINICAL MANIFESTATIONS

Clinical manifestations include the following:
1. Diverticulosis
   a. Usually asymptomatic
   b. Possible massive bleeding; self-limiting
2. Diverticulitis
   a. Left lower quadrant abdominal pain (caused by muscular spasms of sigmoid colon)
   b. Constipation, or constipation alternating with diarrhea
   c. Fever and leukocytosis (may be absent or minimal in elderly persons)
3. Diagnostic tests
   a. Technetium-99m scintigraphy or selective angiography when hemorrhage occurs
   b. Barium enema *after* inflammation from diverticulitis subsides

INTERVENTIONS

Medical Management

The following treatments may be included in medical management:

1. Antibiotic therapy for diverticulitis
2. For hemorrhage
   a. Bed rest
   b. Blood replacement
   c. Infusion of epinephrine or vasopressin (Pitressin) may be given through a selectively placed catheter to stop the bleeding[52]
3. Surgical resection of involved portion of colon with an end-to-end anastomosis for *recurrent* episodes of diverticulitis for complications: perforation, fistulas, abscess
4. Temporary colostomy (6 to 8 weeks)

Nursing Management

During an *acute* episode, rest is encouraged. Bowel rest may be achieved by a soft or liquid diet; for severe episodes, intravenous fluids may have to be given. Pain medications are given as prescribed, and heat may be applied to the abdomen for relief of pain. But because appendicitis may have similar symptoms, and because heat application is contraindicated for appendicitis, it is imperative that the physician rule it out before heat is applied.

Teaching the person with nonsymptomatic diverticulosis centers on methods to increase the bulk of the stool and thus the diameter of the colon, resulting in decreased intraluminal pressure.
1. Diet high in vegetable fiber (fruits and vegetables, whole grain cereals)
2. Possible addition of unprocessed wheat bran to foods
   a. Small amount at first (in fruit juice or muffins)
   b. Slow increase over 4- to 6-week period to 10 to 25 g/day
   c. May initially cause abdominal distention and excessive flatus
3. Use of bulk-forming agents such as methylcellulose or psyllium

Since emotional tension often precipitates diverticular disease, the person may need assistance in learning how to reduce emotional tension. Relaxation techniques, planned rest periods, and regular sleeping hours may prove helpful.

MECKEL'S DIVERTICULUM

Meckel's diverticulum is a congenital outpouching of the *ileum* about 60 to 90 cm from the ileocecal valve. It occurs in about 2% of persons, more frequently in males.[53] Inflammation and perforation may occur, causing symptoms closely resembling those of appendicitis. Hemorrhage may also occur. Adhesions may lead to intestinal obstruction or intussusception (p. 1325). Meckel's diverticulum is the most frequent cause of ileal obstruction in young persons.[43] Surgical excision is done at any time that Meckel's diverticulum is discovered during surgery for other reasons or when symptoms of inflammation or obstruction or bleeding occur.

TABLE 44-5 Common anal lesions

Lesion	Description	Symptoms	Treatment
Anal fissure	Slitlike ulceration in epithelium of anal canal	Pain with defecation; bleeding; constipation	Stool softeners; analgesic ointments; sitz baths; sphincterotomy or fissurectomy if medical therapy ineffective
Anal abscess	Abscess in tissue around anus	Persistent throbbing anal pain with walking, sitting, defecation; systemic signs of infection	Incision and drainage of abscess
Anal fistula	Hollow track leading through anal tissue from anorectal canal through skin near anus	Purulent discharge near anus	Fistulotomy or fistulectomy
Hemorrhoids	Varicosities of lower rectum and anus	Bleeding with defecation; pain if thrombosed	Analgesic ointments for mild discomfort; injection, ligation, or hemorrhoidectomy for severe discomfort

ANORECTAL DISORDERS

INFLAMMATORY LESIONS

ETIOLOGY AND PATHOPHYSIOLOGY

Common inflammatory lesions of the anorectal area include anal fissures, anal abscesses, and anal fistulas (Table 44-5). Anal *fissures* usually result from trauma caused by passage of hard-formed stool that overstretches the anal lining. The fissure does not heal readily. Defecation initiates spasm of the anal sphincter, causing severe pain that lasts for some time. Slight bleeding may occur, and constipation is usually caused by restraining bowel movements to avoid pain.

An anal *abscess* is caused by infection from the anal canal and may follow an anal fissure. If the abscess involves the anal, paraanal, or perineal tissues, there is throbbing local pain caused by pressure on the somatic sensory nerves in the perineum, and there are local signs of inflammation. Any position is uncomfortable, because reflected pain is common. The abscess may also be located deep in the ischiorectal tissue.

An anal *fistula* results from the rupture or drainage of an anal abscess. It is usually a chronic condition, and unfortunately many persons attempt to treat themselves with over-the-counter medications before they seek competent medical care.

CLINICAL MANIFESTATIONS

Pain in the rectal area, especially with defecation, is the primary symptom of anal fissure and anal abscess. A person with an ischiorectal abscess is usually very ill; leukocytosis, fever, chills, and malaise are present. With an anal fistula, the person has periodic drainage that stains underclothing.

INTERVENTIONS

Local pain and spasms of anal *fissures* can sometimes be relieved by warm compresses, sitz baths, and the use of analgesic ointments. Docusate sodium (Colace) is usually prescribed to lubricate the canal and to soften the stool. Suppositories containing hydrocortisone may be prescribed for 2 weeks. Directions for insertion of the suppository for anal fissure include:

1. Lie down on left side in Sims' position
2. Insert suppository ½ *inch* into *anus*
3. Maintain position for 15 to 20 minutes
4. Push into the rectum the remaining suppository that has not melted[43]

Surgery is performed for anal fissures if medical therapy is ineffective, and it is the primary therapy for anal abscess and anal fistula (see Table 44-5). In a *sphincterotomy*, the internal sphincter is incised for sphincter relaxation. A *fistulotomy* is an incision into a superficial fistula to open it up for healing. Removal of a fissure (*fissurectomy*) or of a fistula (*fistulectomy*) may be necessary if the other surgeries are ineffective. Complicated fistulectomies may require hospitalization, but the other surgeries are often performed as ambulatory surgery.

Postoperative care includes sitz baths and stool softeners. The person is usually more comfortable with the use of a protected pillow or foam pad when sitting. When an abscess is incised and drained (I&D), there is usually a large amount of seropurulent drainage from the wound, and dressings will be required. The wound should heal from the bottom outward.

HEMORRHOIDS

ETIOLOGY AND PATHOPHYSIOLOGY

Hemorrhoids can be thought of as "varicose veins of the rectum." They result from venous congestion and interference with venous return from the hemorrhoidal veins. Hemorrhoids may be *external*—that is, distal to the anal sphincter—or *internal*—that is, proximal to the anal sphincter. Both types may be present at the same time. External hemorrhoids may be acute or chronic. The acute form is usually referred to as a

PREDISPOSING FACTORS FOR HEMORRHOIDS

Heredity
Long periods of standing or sitting
Prostatic enlargement
Chronic liver disease (backflow from portal hypertension)
Increased intraabdominal pressure
    Constipation
    Straining at defecation
    Pregnancy

---

thrombosed hemorrhoid and is actually a hematoma.[50] The chronic form is a skin tag consisting of folds of anal skin and a few blood vessels. The cause is not definitely known, but many factors seem to be involved (see the box above).

CLINICAL MANIFESTATIONS

Internal hemorrhoids are not apparent to the individual unless they become so large that they protrude through the anus, where they may become constricted and painful. They often bleed on defecation, and although the amount of blood lost may be small, continuous oozing over a long period of time may cause iron-deficiency anemia.

External hemorrhoids can be noted by the individual. They rarely bleed and seldom cause pain unless a hemorrhoidal vein ruptures and becomes thrombosed and inflamed.

Constipation often becomes worse after the hemorrhoids occur, because the person tries to restrain bowel movements that produce pain or bleeding. Although hemorrhoids rarely undergo malignant degeneration, constipation and bleeding are symptoms of cancer of the rectum. For this reason, all persons with these symptoms should have a medical examination to rule out cancer.

INTERVENTIONS
Local Treatment

The local application of ice, warm compresses, or analgesic ointments such as dibucaine (Nupercaine) gives temporary relief from pain and reduces the edema around external or prolapsed internal hemorrhoids. Sitz baths are also extremely helpful in relieving pain. Stool softeners prevent constipation and decrease irritation of the hemorrhoids during defecation.

Ligation

Internal hemorrhoids may be treated by ligating with latex bands. The hemorrhoid is grasped with forceps and pulled down into a special instrument which, when the trigger handle is pressed, slips a latex band over it. The band constricts the circulation and causes necrosis; the destroyed tissue usually sloughs off within a week. An enema is given before the treatment to prevent a bowel movement for 24 hours and thus prevent straining that would cause the band to break or slip off. No anesthesia is required. Local discomfort is minimal and usually is relieved by aspirin or acetaminophen.

Injection

The injection method is effective for bleeding and early prolapse of internal hemorrhoids. It is not effective for external hemorrhoids.[65] A sclerosing solution such as 5% phenol in oil is injected into the submucous areolar tissue in which the hemorrhoidal veins lie, producing an inflammatory reaction. Fibrous induration, which surrounds and constricts the veins, occurs at the site of the injection in 2 or 3 weeks. Bleeding from the hemorrhoids usually stops within 24 to 48 hours.

Infrared Photocoagulation

The physician inserts an infrared photocoagulator probe through an anoscope and applies radiation to each involved area for 1.5 seconds. The hemorrhoidal tissue then becomes necrotic and sloughs off. The procedure is repeated in three or four adjacent areas to completely destroy the hemorrhoid. A second treatment, if needed, may follow in 7 to 10 days.

Thrombosed External Hemorrhoids

A thrombosed external hemorrhoid usually occurs suddenly after some form of vigorous activity or severe diarrhea or constipation. It is characterized by an extremely painful anal lump. Treatment consists of excision of the entire mass; sutures are avoided if possible, since they increase the pain. A pressure dressing and ice packs are applied to lessen bleeding. Stool softeners and sitz baths are suggested until the wound heals.

Surgery

Surgical excision (hemorrhoidectomy) is the treatment used for external or internal hemorrhoids that do not respond well to more conservative treatment. Care of the patient is summarized in the box on p. 1322.

PARASITIC INFECTIONS
AMEBIASIS
ETIOLOGY AND PATHOPHYSIOLOGY

Amebiasis is caused by the protozoan parasite *Entamoeba histolytica,* which primarily invades the large intestine and secondarily the liver, forming abscesses. The active, motile form of the protozoa, the trophozoite, is not infectious and, if ingested, is easily destroyed by digestive enzymes. However, the inactive form (*cyst*) is highly resistant to extremes in temperature, most chemicals, and the digestive juices. When the cyst is swal-

NURSING CARE OF THE PERSON EXPERIENCING ANORECTAL SURGERY

1. Preoperative care
   a. An enema may not be prescribed if rectal pain is acute
   b. Stool softeners may be given to promote a soft stool postoperatively
2. Postoperative care
   a. Promotion of comfort
      (1) Give analgesics as prescribed (considerable rectal discomfort may be present)
      (2) Suggest side-lying position
      (3) Give sitz baths (monitor for hypotension secondary to dilation of pelvic blood vessels in early postoperative period)
   b. Promotion of elimination
      (1) Give prescribed stool softeners
      (2) Encourage patient to defecate as soon as the inclination occurs (prevents strictures and preserves the normal anal lumen)
      (3) Give an analgesic a short time before initial defecation
      (4) Monitor for hypotension (dizziness, faintness, rapid pulse) during first defecation
      (5) If an enema must be given, use a small-bore rectal tube
   c. Patient teaching
      (1) Clean rectal area after each defecation until healing is complete (sitz bath is recommended)
      (2) Avoid constipation with a high-fiber diet, high fluid intake, regular exercise, and regular time for defecation
      (3) Use stool softeners until healing is complete
      (4) Seek medical consultation for rectal bleeding, suppurative drainage, continued pain on defecation, or continued constipation despite preventive measures

lowed in fecally contaminated food or water, it easily passes into the intestines, where the active trophozoite is released and enters the intestinal wall. Here it feeds on the mucosal cells, causing ulceration of the intestinal mucosa.

Although the disease exists chiefly in tropical countries, it also prevails wherever sanitation is poor. The cyst can survive for long periods outside the body, and it is transmitted by direct contact from person to person, by insects, and by contaminated water, milk, and other foods. Sexual transmission accounts for a high incidence rate among homosexual men in some urban communities.

PREVENTION

Amebiasis can be prevented by control of the fecal contamination of water and food through good water treatment and sewage disposal systems. Persons traveling in countries where the incidence is higher should avoid eating fresh or other uncooked foods or drinking milk or unbottled water. Ice cubes can be a source of contamination, because cold does not eradicate the cysts. Boiling water for 10 minutes kills both trophozoites and cysts.[34]

CLINICAL MANIFESTATIONS

Symptoms usually begin from 1 week to several months after infection and depend on the extent of tissue invasion.

1. Mild: abdominal cramps, intermittent diarrhea and constipation, flatulence
2. Severe: frequent semiliquid or liquid stools containing blood and mucus; fever, colicky abdominal pains, tenesmus
3. Liver abscess: severe right upper quadrant pain, enlarged and tender liver, fever, rapid weight loss, prostration

Diagnosis is made by identification of the parasite in the stool during the acute stage of the disease. Immediately after defecation, a warm stool is sent to the laboratory for examination. If the laboratory is at a distance, the specimen container should be transported on a hot-water bottle or in a pan of warm water so that the organisms are to be found in the active stage. Several stool specimens from successive bowel movements may be requested. ELISAs have recently been developed for detection of the parasite.[9]

INTERVENTIONS

Medical Management

Amebicides may be effective against the parasite within the intestinal lumen (luminal amebicide) or only on the trophozoites within the intestinal wall. The drug of choice that is effective for mild or moderate amebiasis in both areas is *metronidazole* (Flagyl). The usual dosage is 750 mg three times daily for 5 to 10 days. Drinking alcohol while taking metronidazole may make the patient very ill. The drug also interacts with disulfiram and with oral anticoagulants. For severe infection, additional luminal amebecides must be given and may include diiodohydroxyquin (Iodoquinol), diloxanide furoate, chloroquine, dehydroemetine, or tetracycline.

During acute exacerbations the person may become dehydrated, exhausted, or anemic and require hospitalization. Infusions and blood transfusions may be necessary. A bland low-residue, high-protein diet is commonly prescribed. Opiates may be necessary to reduce bowel motility.

Nursing Management

Nursing management includes the following:
1. Encourage oral fluids to replace fluids lost by diarrhea
2. Monitor fluid and electrolyte balance

3. Record intake and output
4. Record number and character of stools
5. Use enteric isolation precautions
6. Teach patient:
   a. Rationale for washing hands after using the toilet and before eating to avoid reinfection
   b. Avoidance of alcohol when taking amebicides
   c. Taking amebicide after meals to prevent gastrointestinal side effects
   d. Importance of taking medication for prescribed time, even when feeling well
   e. Importance of follow-up stool examinations (weekly for 3 weeks)

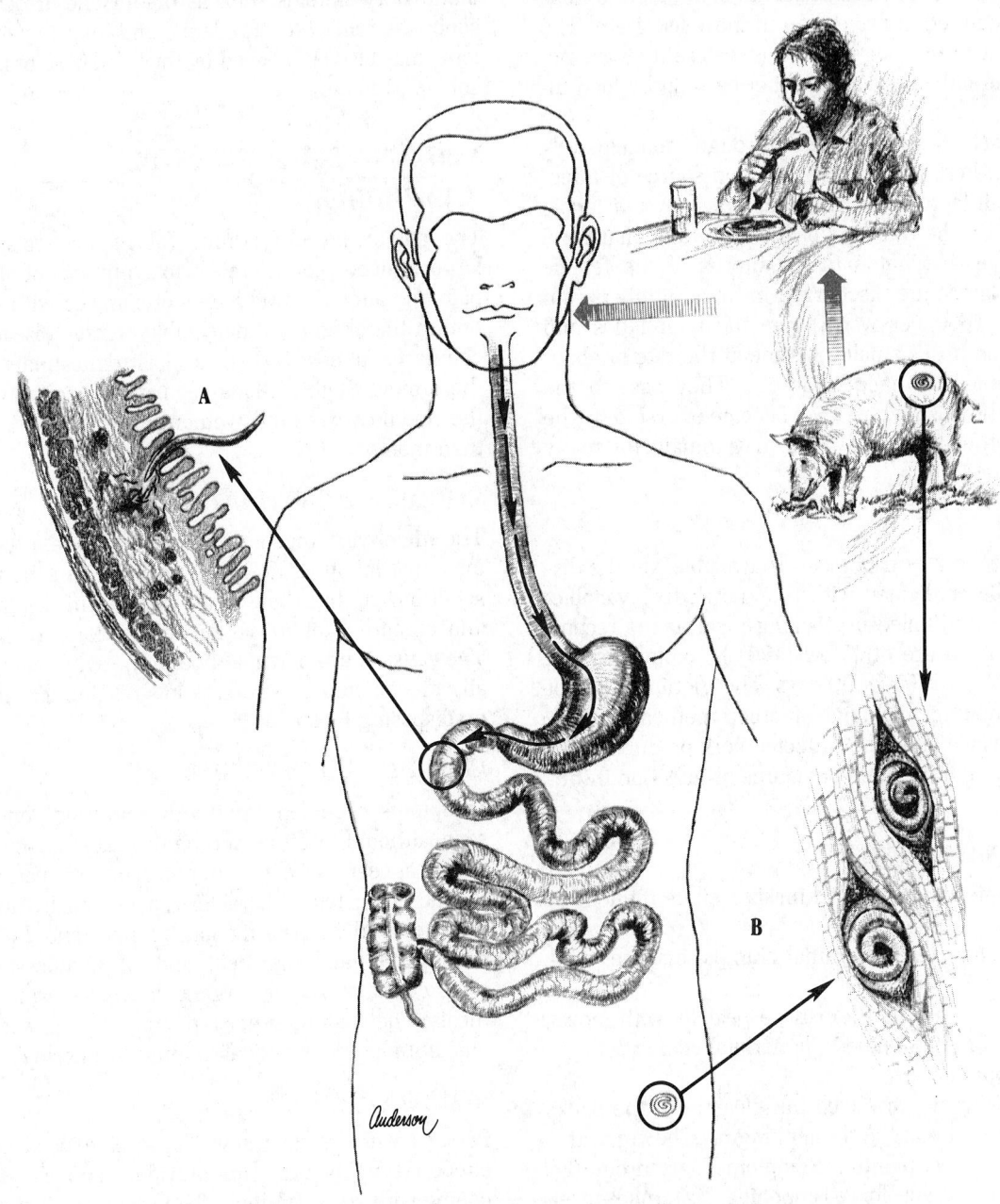

FIGURE 44-5 Life cycle of *Trichinella spiralis*. Infective larvae, encysted in pork and other meat when ingested, become adult worms in the small intestine. *A*, Female burrows into mucosa and deposits larvae into lacteals and blood vessels. *B*, Circulating larvae eventually penetrate skeletal muscle and become encysted. In humans these larvae are at a dead end, but in the pig and other animals they become a source of infection. (From Beck JW and Davies JE: Medical parasitology, ed 3, St Louis, 1981, The CV Mosby Co.)

TRICHINOSIS

ETIOLOGY AND PATHOPHYSIOLOGY

Trichinosis (trichinellosis, trichiniasis) is caused by the larvae of a species of roundworm, *Trichinella spiralis*, which become encysted in the striated muscles of humans, hogs, and other animals (rodents) that eat infected pork in garbage. Trichinosis has a worldwide distribution with the highest incidence occurring in Europe and the United States. It occurs more often in hogs that have been fed garbage than in those fed grain. The larvae do not form cysts in pork; therefore they are not visible to the naked eye and cannot be seen by food inspectors.

Trichinosis is transmitted through inadequately cooked food. Pork is the most common source of infection. When infected food is eaten, live encysted larvae develop within the intestine of the host; they mate and produce eggs that hatch in the uterus of the female worm. The larvae are discharged in huge numbers (approximately 1500 per worm) into the lymphatics and lacteals of the host's small intestine at the rate of about two every hour for about 6 weeks. They pass to the muscles of the host, where they become encysted by the reaction of the host's body and may remain for many years (Figure 44-5).

PREVENTION

No immunization for trichinosis is available, yet the disease could be eradicated with the knowledge available. Trichinae can be killed by cooking meat at the recommended temperature of 77° C (170° F) or by freezing meat at −15° C (5° F) for 20 days. The trichinae are not killed by smoking, pickling, or other methods of processing. Sausage and other infected pork products carelessly prepared are a common source of infection in humans.

CLINICAL MANIFESTATIONS

Clinical manifestations of trichinosis include the following:
  1. Early: diarrhea, abdominal cramps, malaise, nausea
  2. Weeks 2 to 8: muscle pain (especially with movement), fever, weakness, periorbital edema
  3. Eosinophilia

The more commonly involved muscles are in the back, eyeballs, jaw, throat, and diaphragm. Chewing and breathing may be painful. Symptoms vary from (1) asymptomatic except for eosinophilia, (2) mild fever with one or more mild symptoms, to (3) high fever with more severe symptoms. Infection may spread to the meninges, cardiac muscle, lungs, and kidneys in severe cases. Convalescence usually begins the second month but may be prolonged after severe illness. Vague muscle pains and malaise may persist for many months.[53]

The diagnosis is confirmed by the finding of larvae in a biopsy specimen taken from the deltoid or gastrocnemius muscle in the fourth week of infection.

INTERVENTIONS

Treatment is primarily symptomatic. Usually the person is placed on bed rest and a high-calorie, high-protein diet. Analgesics are given for muscle pain, and antiinflammatory steroids such as prednisone or dexamethasone may relieve fever, edema, and muscle pain. Symptoms may also be relieved by thiabendazole or mebendazole for 3 to 5 days.

IRRITABLE BOWEL SYNDROME

EPIDEMIOLOGY

The irritable bowel syndrome (also known as spastic colon or mucous colitis) refers to symptoms of abdominal pain and altered bowel habits of diarrhea with constipation in the absence of detectable organic disease. It accounts for almost 50% of all gastrointestinal illness in the United States.[69] It is seen most frequently during the middle years, and women are affected more often than men.

ETIOLOGY AND PATHOPHYSIOLOGY

The underlying mechanism appears to be a disorder of intestinal motility. Motility is increased in the proximal small bowel, and there is an increase in the frequency and amplitude of muscular contractions in the colon. The cause is unknown, although the symptoms are usually precipitated by stress. A low-residue diet may be a predisposing factor.[53]

CLINICAL MANIFESTATIONS

Symptoms occur intermittently and vary among persons, although each person has a characteristic pattern. There appear to be two major symptom patterns: (1) spastic colon type, characterized by colicky abdominal pain relieved by passing gas or stool and by periodic constipation and diarrhea; and (2) painless diarrhea type, characterized by urgent diarrhea during or after meals. The stool of either type may contain excess mucus, but all other physical findings are normal.

INTERVENTIONS

Persons with irritable bowel syndrome need empathic support from health care providers and assistance in coping with stress in their life experiences that may precipitate symptoms. Since the need for control is important to them, they should be included in decision making regarding their care. The irritable bowel syndrome diagnosis is made by the physician after ruling out other pathologic conditions, and the person needs to know that the condition is benign and is related to bowel irritability induced by stress. A planned schedule of regular physical activity and relaxation periods may be helpful.

The person is encouraged to eat a well-balanced diet. Some persons may respond to an increase in dietary fiber, but no direct benefits from addition of bran to the diet have been shown. Heat may be applied to the abdomen to relieve pain; analgesics are not useful. Psyllium (Metamucil, Hydrocil) may be helpful to add bulk to the stool.

INTESTINAL OBSTRUCTION OR INFARCTION

ORGANIC INTESTINAL OBSTRUCTION

ETIOLOGY

Intestinal obstruction refers to blockage in movement of intestinal contents through the small or large intestines. Obstruction may occur from *organic* (mechanical) causes that physically impede passage of intestinal contents or from *paralytic* causes (see Chapter 53) in which the passageway is open but peristalsis ceases.

Many different conditions may cause mechanical obstruction (see the box at right), but the most common causes are adhesions, strangulated hernias (p. 1327), or neoplasms (p. 1329). Neoplasms may be within the in-

CAUSES OF MECHANICAL INTESTINAL OBSTRUCTION

INTRALUMINAL
Foreign bodies, gallstones
Intussusception
Tumors

EXTRAMURAL
Adhesions
Hernias
Volvulus
Extrinsic masses

INTRAMURAL
Congenital strictures
Strictures secondary to
  Crohn's disease
  Radiation enteritis
  Bowel ischemia
  Hirschsprung's disease

testines (intraluminal) or extrinsic, entrapping loops of the bowel. *Volvulus,* a twisting of the bowel (Figure 44-6), usually results from congenital anomalies or from adhesions. *Intussusception* is a telescoping of a segment of the bowel within itself.

PATHOPHYSIOLOGY

When intestinal obstruction occurs, there is an increase in peristaltic waves proximal to the area of temporary

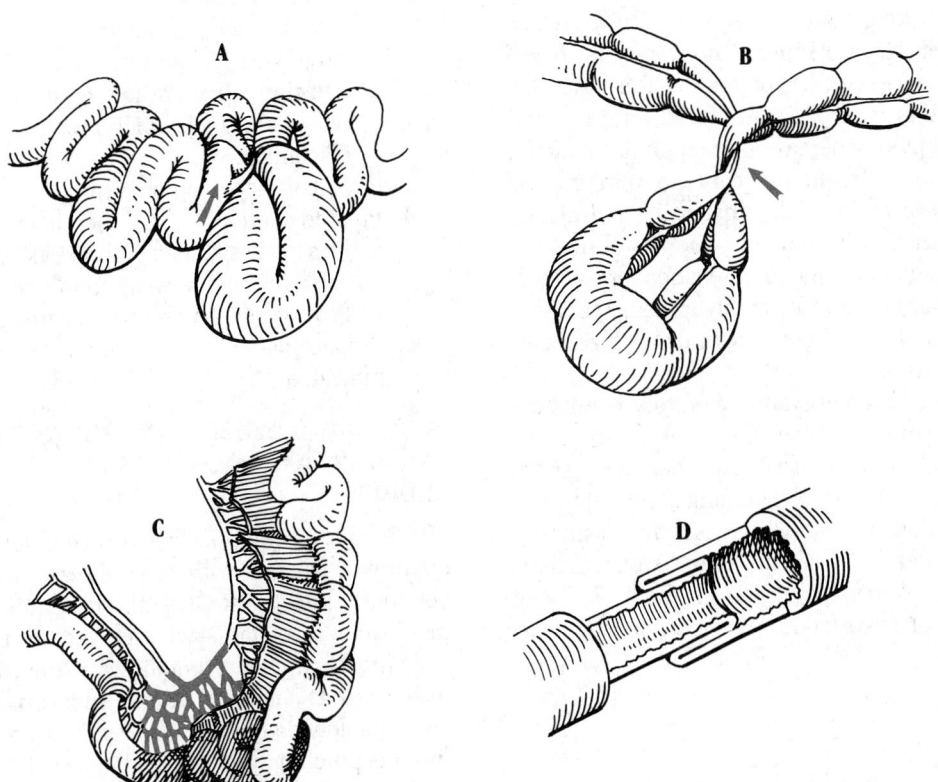

FIGURE 44-6 Some causes of intestinal obstruction. **A**, Constriction by adhesions. **B**, Volvulus. **C**, Mesenteric thrombosis. **D**, Intussusception.

obstruction in an effort to move the intestinal contents past the area of obstruction. Intraluminal pressure increases, the proximal intestine dilates, the smooth muscle becomes atonic, and peristalsis ceases. Large amounts of isotonic fluid move from the plasma and intestinal spaces into the distended gut, and the normal reabsorption of intestinal fluid and gas is impeded by edema of the tissues and decreased mucosal blood flow from the increased intraluminal pressure. Large amounts of gas collect in the distended area from swallowed air or from gas produced by bacteria that multiply as a result of stasis of intestinal contents. The net result is loss of large amounts of fluids and electrolytes producing severe dehydration, hypovolemia, and electrolyte imbalances.

Complications of a distended gut include perforation with peritonitis, and strangulation or volvulus that further compromises blood flow to the intestine, resulting in gangrene of the tissue. A gangrenous intestine will bleed into both the intestinal lumen and the peritoneal cavity and eventually will perforate. Some of the toxic fluid may be absorbed into the bloodstream, causing septic shock.

CLINICAL MANIFESTATIONS

The symptoms of intestinal obstruction vary with the site and degree of obstruction. During partial or early phases of mechanical obstruction, auscultation of the abdomen will reveal loud, frequent, *high-pitched* sounds, but when smooth muscle atony occurs, bowel sounds will be absent. Obstruction of the *proximal* small bowel results in profuse nonfecal vomiting and upper abdominal pain, whereas obstruction of the *distal* bowel results in less frequent fecal-type vomitus and cramping, poorly localized abdominal pain, and distention. When obstruction is complete, the bowel distal to the obstruction remains empty, and obstipation (no passage of stool or gas) results. In paralytic ileus, vomiting occurs less frequently, and bowel sounds are decreased or absent.

In early stages, vital signs and laboratory results are normal. As dehydration ensues, urinary output decreases; temperature increases; and hemoconcentration, leukocytosis, and electrolyte changes including hyponatremia, hypokalemia, and increases in plasma bicarbonate, pH, and BUN occur. Later signs include tachycardia, fever, and hypotension or shock. Air- and fluid-filled areas of obstruction are visualized by x-ray film examination.

INTERVENTIONS

Medical Management

The treatment for intestinal obstruction is nasogastric or intestinal intubation to relieve vomiting and reduce intestinal distention, the administration of fluids and elec-

trolytes by infusion to correct fluid and electrolyte imbalance, and the relief of mechanical obstruction by surgery. The operative procedure varies with the cause and location of the obstruction and the general condition of the patient. Constricting bands or adhesions are cut, and it may be necessary to resect the occluded bowel and to anastomose the remaining segments.

Nursing Management

The following activities are included in nursing management:

1. Monitor
   a. Fluid and electrolyte balance: fluid deficit, fluid overload with intravenous fluid replacement (monitor CVP), hyponatremia, hypokalemia
   b. Vital signs : an increase may indicate further obstruction, strangulation, or peritonitis
   c. Urinary output
      (1) Decreased urine production if shock is present
      (2) Urinary retention from pressure on bladder
   d. Gastric output
   e. Abdominal girth: increased girth from abdominal distention
   f. Bowel sounds: return of peristalsis
2. Maintain nasogastric or intestinal intubation (Chapter 43)
3. Promote ventilation
   a. Use Fowler's position for greater diaphragm expansion
   b. Encourage patient to breathe through nose and not swallow air which increases distention and discomfort
   c. Encourage deep breathing
4. Provide comfort
   a. Provide assistance with activities of daily living (patient may be weak from pain and vomiting)
   b. Provide mouth and nares care (patient is NPO)
5. Prepare patient for surgery (p. 1332) if surgery is indicated

ACUTE BOWEL INFARCTION: MESENTERIC VASCULAR OCCLUSION
ETIOLOGY

Mesenteric vascular occlusion is common. It occurs frequently in persons with heart disease, resulting in emboli to the intestines. Often the patient is elderly. It also may occur in patients who are recovering from recent abdominal surgery. Thrombosis of the mesenteric vein may occur as a complication of cirrhosis of the liver, following splenectomy, or as a result of an extension of a thrombophlebitic process in the ileocolic veins. The superior mesenteric arteries usually are occluded. Causes other than atherosclerosis or intravascular thromboses of the mesenteric vessels include vasculitis and connective tissue disorders.

PATHOPHYSIOLOGY

The blood supply to the lower part of the jejunum and ileum is usually interrupted by mesenteric vascular occlusion (see Figure 44-6). The walls of the intestine become thickened and edematous, then reddened, and finally black and gangrenous. Infarction of the small bowel may develop over a period of several weeks or may appear suddenly.

CLINICAL MANIFESTATIONS

In partial blockage of the superior mesenteric artery by an atherosclerotic plaque, pain is crampy and colicky in nature and may last for several hours after a meal. The pain is associated with the demand for oxygen that is necessary for the increased intestinal muscular activity. In the event of sudden occlusion, the patient complains of nausea, vomiting, and an acute onset of sharp abdominal pain between the xiphoid process and umbilicus. There is disturbed bowel function. The WBC count is elevated. Occasionally, a tender mass may be palpable in the epigastrium. The abdomen may be distended, and there will be an absence of bowel sounds. If there has been hemorrhage into the peritoneal cavity, generalized abdominal rigidity will be noted. The patient may be in shock when first seen, even when the condition is reported at the onset of symptoms.

INTERVENTIONS

Immediate hospitalization is required. Nothing is given orally, and a nasogastric tube is inserted and attached to suction. Parenteral fluids are started. Treatment depends on the suddenness and cause of the occlusion. If a clot can be found and removed after opening the superior mesenteric artery, the blood flow will be restored. If

necessary, damaged bowel tissue is removed surgically. Chronic occlusion may be corrected by endarterectomy or a bypass procedure. Antispasmodic drugs such as papaverine may also be given. The patient may be very ill both preoperatively and postoperatively and may need constant nursing care. The mortality from mesenteric vascular occlusion is high, particularly among elderly persons.

HERNIA
PATHOPHYSIOLOGY

A hernia is a protrusion of an organ or structure from its normal cavity through a congenital or acquired defect. Depending on its location, the hernia may contain peritoneal fat, a loop of bowel, a section of bladder, or a portion of the stomach. If the protruding structure of the organ can be returned by manipulation to its own cavity, it is called a *reducible* hernia. If it cannot, it is called an *irreducible* or an *incarcerated* hernia. The size of the defect through which the structure or organ passes (the neck of the hernia) determines largely whether the hernia can be reduced. When the blood supply to the structure within the hernia becomes occluded, the hernia is said to be *strangulated;* if the intestines are involved, it leads to intestinal obstruction.

TYPES OF HERNIAS

An *indirect inguinal hernia* is one in which a loop of intestine passes through the abdominal ring and follows the course of the spermatic cord into the inguinal canal (Figure 44-7). The descent of the hernia may end in the inguinal canal, or it may proceed into the scrotum (and occasionally in the labia). It is caused by the intestines being forced by increased intraabdominal pressure into

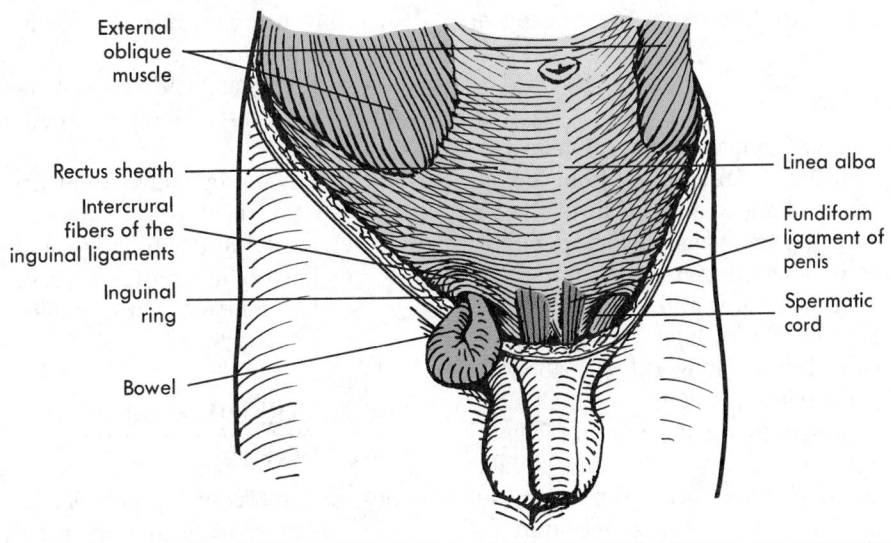

FIGURE 44-7 Inguinal hernia.

a congenital defect resulting from failure of the processus vaginalis to close after the descent of the testes in the male and after fixation of the ovaries in the female. Indirect hernias are much more common in men than in women. This higher incidence in men may be explained by the size of the testes, which must pass through the inguinal ring during fetal life.

A *direct inguinal hernia* is one that passes through the posterior inguinal wall. It is caused by increased intraabdominal pressure against a weak posterior inguinal wall. These hernias are more common in men. They are the most difficult to repair and are likely to recur after surgery.

A *femoral hernia* is one in which a loop of intestine passes through the femoral ring and down the femoral canal. It appears as a round bulge below the inguinal ligament and is thought to be caused by a congenital weakness in the femoral ring. Increased intraabdominal pressure as a result of pregnancy or obesity probably causes the herniation through weakened muscle. Femoral hernias are more common in women than in men, and the incidence of strangulated hernia is high. This is thought to be because of the inclination of the female pelvis.

An *umbilical hernia* is one in which a loop of intestine passes through the umbilical ring. It is caused either by the failure of the umbilicus to close at birth or by a defect in the umbilical scar, which opens in adult life when there is increased intraabdominal pressure such as occurs in pregnancy, intestinal obstruction, chronic cough, or COPD.

An *incisional hernia* is one that occurs through an old surgical incision. It is caused by the failure of the resected and approximated muscles and fascial tissues to heal properly because of wound infections, drains, or poor physical condition. As a result of increased intraabdominal pressure, a portion of the intestine or other organs and tissues may protrude through the weakened scar.

CLINICAL MANIFESTATIONS

The person with a hernia complains of a lump in the groin, around the umbilicus, or protruding from an old surgical incision. The swelling may have always been present, or it may have appeared suddenly after coughing, straining, lifting, or other vigorous exertion.

Palpation of the herniated area will reveal the contents of the sac as soft and nodular (omentum) or smooth and fluctuant (bowel). Fingertip palpation is used to feel the edges of the ring and its contents by inserting the examining fingertip into the ring and feeling for the impulse as the person coughs. At no time should the examiner attempt to replace (reduce) the sac in the ring, since the result may be the rupture of the strangulated contents or a reduction in the mass without relief of strangulation.

A femoral hernia may be palpated by placing the index finger over the femoral artery. The middle finger will then overlie the femoral vein, and the ring finger will overlie the femoral canal. As the person coughs, the examiner's fingertips will feel the sensation if the herniated sac is in the canal area.

A hernia may cause no symptoms except swelling that disappears when the person lies down and reappears on standing or coughing. If pain is present it may be caused by local irritation of the parietal peritoneum or by traction on the omentum. An incarcerated hernia may become strangulated, causing severe pain and symptoms of intestinal obstruction such as nausea, vomiting, and distention. These complications require emergency surgery, and a portion of bowel may have to be resected if it has become gangrenous from impairment of its circulation.

INTERVENTIONS

Medical Management

The only cure for a hernia is surgery. Surgery is postponed if the patient is coughing or sneezing; this may weaken the repair before healing occurs. Surgery is now often performed in ambulatory surgical centers, and local, spinal, or general anesthesia may be used. The herniating tissues are returned to the abdominal cavity, and the defect in the fascia or muscle is closed with sutures (*herniorrhaphy*). To prevent recurrence of the hernia and to facilitate closure of the defect, a *hernioplasty* may be performed using fascia or a variety of materials to strengthen the muscle wall.

Nursing Management

Postoperative nursing management includes the following:

1. Give food and fluids as tolerated
2. Monitor postoperative urinary elimination
3. Apply ice bags if scrotal edema occurs
4. Teach patient
   a. Report any early signs of wound infection (redness, discomfort) that may weaken the surgical repair
   b. Any postoperative ecchymosis will disappear in a few days
   c. Sexual functioning is not affected by surgery
   d. Restrict driving for 2 weeks
   e. Avoid heavy lifting, pulling, or pushing for 6 weeks

TUMORS OF THE BOWEL

BENIGN TUMORS

The most frequent tumors of the bowel are polyps (small tissue masses that protrude into the bowel lumen). Polyps may be single or multiple (most common), and they may be pedunculated (stemlike base) or sessile

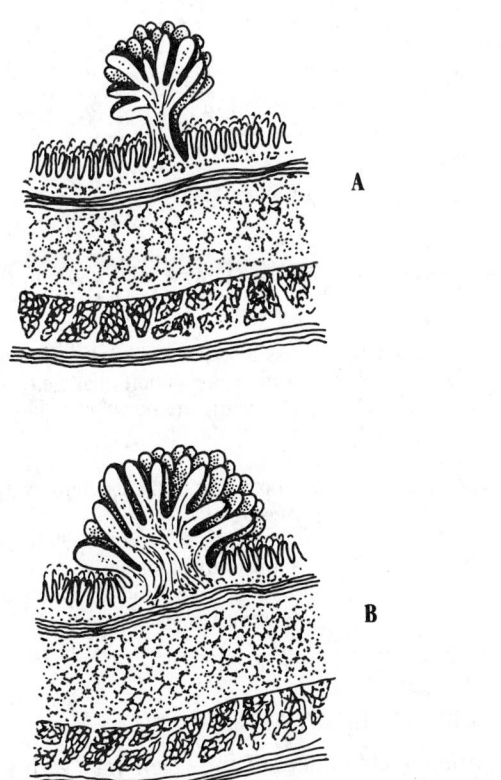

FIGURE 44-8 Colon polyps. **A**, Tubular adenoma (note pedicle) **B**, Villous adenoma.

(broad base). They may also be of two major types, hyperplastic or neoplastic. Hyperplastic polyps account for 25% of all polyps and are not premalignant.[58] The neoplastic polyps may be adenomatous or villous adenomas (Figure 44-8). The villous adenomas have a high probability of becoming malignant. The incidence of malignancy for neoplastic polyps ranges from 1% in adenomas <1 cm to 50% in adenomas >2 cm in size.[69] Adenomatous polyps may cause bleeding but are rarely painful. Polyps have a high recurrence rate. Pedunculated or small sessile polyps are usually removed by electrocautery and fulguration. Large sessile polyps are excised surgically.

Familial intestinal polyposis is a rare genetic disorder characterized by numerous adenomatous polyps in the lower bowel that usually become malignant. For persons with this disorder, removal of the colon leaving the rectum intact is recommended before malignancy occurs. The rectum is then examined on a regular basis, and suspicious lesions are excised.

CANCER OF THE BOWEL
EPIDEMIOLOGY

Malignant tumors of the colon and rectum are among the most commonly occurring malignancies in the United States, third to cancer of the lung and prostate

---

RISK FACTORS FOR COLORECTAL CANCER

Age >40
Past history
    Colon polyps (adenomas)
    Colorectal cancer
    Breast or genital cancer
    Inflammatory bowel disease
    Polyposis syndromes
Family history
    Colorectal cancer
    Polyposis syndromes

---

in men and second to cancer of the breast in women. Each year over 140,000 Americans develop cancer of the colon and rectum, and 60,000 will die. There have been only small changes in the incidence of death rates in recent years.

The incidence of bowel cancer is significantly higher in developed countries where the inhabitants are of Northern European descent, and it is lower in Africa, Asia, and South America. The incidence increases with age and reaches a peak in persons in the late 70s. Of the malignancies of the colon and rectum, 50% occur in the lower portion of the colon and rectum (Table 44-6). Cancer of the colon occurs more frequently in women, whereas rectal cancer is seen more often in men.

ETIOLOGY

Although the cause of cancer of the bowel remains unknown, environmental and genetic factors and preexisting disease appear to be influential (see the box above). The high incidence of colorectal cancer in industrial countries relates to a diet high in animal fat, protein, and refined carbohydrates that are low in dietary fiber. A direct causative relationship has not been established. Low-fiber diets decrease colonic transit time and potentially increase contact of endogenous or exogenous carcinogens with the bowel mucosa. Popular literature often suggests that certain foods are carcinogenic; however, research has not yet identified specific foods as carcinogenic for bowel cancer. Genetically, some "cancer families" have been identified in which cancers of certain body areas, including the bowel, are transmitted as dominant traits.

PATHOPHYSIOLOGY

Cancer of the colon may develop in one of two ways. In the *cecum* and *ascending colon,* the lesions tend to develop as polyps that grow as cauliflower-like masses protruding into the lumen of the colon (Figure 44-8). These lesions may ulcerate, but obstruction of the colon is uncommon. Eventually, the lesions penetrate the colon wall and extend into surrounding tissue.

TABLE 44-6 Comparison of cancer of colon by site

Ascending Colon	Descending Colon	Sigmoid Colon and Rectum
TYPE OF LESION		
Polypoid	Annular	Annular
INCIDENCE		
30%	20%	20% in sigmoid colon; 30% in rectum
SYMPTOMS		
Occult blood in feces; anemia; right upper quadrant pain; palpable mass; diarrhea	Gross blood in feces; progressive constipation; pencil-shaped stools	Gross blood in feces; altered bowel pattern (constipation, diarrhea): sensation of incomplete bowel evacuation
SURGERY		
Right hemicolectomy with anastomosis	Left hemicolectomy with anastomosis	Sigmoid: left hemicolectomy with anastomosis Upper rectum: resection with sutured or stapled anastomosis Lower rectum: abdominoperineal resection with colostomy

In the *descending* colon, especially the *rectosigmoid* portion, an annular lesion is more common. The early lesion is a small polypoid mass that becomes plaquelike. The plaque grows circumferentially, encircling the colon wall, and then contracts, causing narrowing of the lumen. Obstruction may result from formed stool on the left side unable to pass through the narrowed lumen. These lesions also eventually penetrate the colon wall and extend into adjacent tissue.

Cancer of the colon may spread by direct extension or through the lymphatic or circulatory systems, seeding at distant points in the peritoneum or at distant points in the colon. The liver is the major organ of metastasis. Most of the colorectal cancers are adenocarcinomas.

PREVENTION

No primary prevention measures are known to be effective for colorectal cancer. Low-fiber, high-fat diets have not been established as a cause; therefore, high-fiber, low-fat diets cannot be considered preventive measures.

Secondary prevention involves early detection. Anyone who develops a change in bowel patterns such as alternating constipation and diarrhea, a change in the shape of the stool, or the passing of blood should consult a physician. The American Cancer Society has recommended guidelines for screening of persons over age 40 (see the box at right). Other high-risk persons should also have regular screening by a physician. Regular occult blood testing of the stool, which is more acceptable to clients than endoscopy, is a minimum requirement. Proctoscopic examinations, however, should also be performed at selected intervals.

CLINICAL MANIFESTATIONS

Symptoms of cancer of the colon vary with the location of the growth (see Table 44-6). Adenocarcinoma of the *ascending* colon often has no symptoms. There are no symptoms of obstruction as a rule because the fecal contents in this portion of the colon are still liquid and able to flow past the growth. Diarrhea may occur. Cancer of the *descending* colon often produces symptoms of partial obstruction, because the formed stool has difficulty passing by the tumor and through the stenosed area. Progressive constipation occurs, and the stool may be small or flattened, pencil-shaped, or ribbon-shaped. Diarrhea may be alternated with constipation. Alteration of bowel patterns also occurs with cancer of the *rectum*.

Bleeding is a common sign of colorectal cancer. There is occult blood in the stool with cancer of the ascending colon, whereas gross blood in the stools can be noted with cancer of the descending colon and rectum. Weakness, malaise, anorexia, anemia, and weight loss are nonspecific symptoms that occur frequently with all colorectal cancers. Occasionally the tumor perforates into the peritoneal cavity, and peritonitis occurs before

AMERICAN CANCER SOCIETY RECOMMENDED GUIDELINES FOR EARLY DETECTION OF COLORECTAL CANCER

1. Digital rectal examination yearly after age 40
2. Occult blood stool test yearly after age 50
3. Proctosigmoidoscopy every 3 to 5 years after age 50, following two negative yearly examinations

any other signs of illness have been noticed by the individual.

DIAGNOSTIC TESTS

Diagnosis of cancer of the colon is made by physical examination, sigmoidoscopy, colonoscopy, and barium enema examination (see Chapter 41). Because 50% of colonic neoplasms occur in the sigmoid colon and rectum, many can be detected by flexible sigmoidoscopy. Colonoscopy is reserved for persons at high risk. Air-contrast barium enemas are more effective than single-contrast barium enemas in detecting neoplastic colonic lesions. Cancer of the rectum can be accurately diagnosed by pathologic examination of a biopsy specimen of the lesion taken during an endoscopic examination.

Carcinoembryonic antigen (CEA) (see Chapter 41) is not useful as a screening test for colorectal cancer, but it is a useful test to identify early recurrence and gauge the effectiveness of therapy.

INTERVENTIONS

Medical Management

Surgery. The treatment of cancer of the colon is always surgical, and the tumor, surrounding colon, and lymph nodes are resected. The location and amount of colon resected depends on the site of the cancer. *Resection and anastomosis* can be performed for cancer of the ascending, descending, or sigmoid colon and upper rectum (see the box below). These surgeries are performed through abdominal incisions, and natural defecation is maintained. The anastomosis may be done by suturing or stapling techniques. A greater amount of rectal tissue can be removed by the use of the stapling technique for anastomosis. After abdominal resection of the diseased

---

SURGERIES FOR COLORECTAL CANCER

RIGHT HEMICOLECTOMY
Resection of ascending colon and hepatic flexure (Figure 44-9,*A*)
Ileum anastomosed to transverse colon

LEFT HEMICOLECTOMY
Resection of splenic flexure, descending colon, and sigmoid colon (Figure 44-9,*B*)
Transverse colon anastomosed to rectum

ANTERIOR RECTOSIGMOID RESECTION
Resection of part of descending colon, the sigmoid colon, and upper rectum (Figure 44-9,*C*)
Descending colon anastomosed to remaining rectum

ABDOMINOPERINEAL RESECTION
Resection of sigmoid colon and rectum (Figure 44-9,*D*)
Proximal end of descending colon brought through abdominal wall to form colostomy (p. 1337)

---

colon, a "stapler gun" is inserted through the rectum to staple the end-to-end anastomosis.

Growths in the lower portion of the rectum require removal of the entire rectum (*abdominoperineal resection*). The operation is performed through two incisions: a low midline incision of the abdomen and a wide elliptic incision about the anus. Through the abdominal incision the sigmoid colon is resected, freed from its attachments, and temporarily left beneath the peritoneum of the pelvic floor. The proximal end of the descending colon is then brought out through a small stab wound on the abdominal wall and becomes the permanent colostomy. Through the perineal incision the anus and rectum are freed from the perineal muscles, and the anus, rectum, and sigmoid colon are removed. The perineal wound may be closed around Penrose drains, or it may be left wide open and packed with gauze and a rubber dam to cause it to heal slowly from the inside outward (Figure 44-10).

Obstruction or perforation of the colon usually requires a temporary colostomy, followed later by closure of the colostomy. Prognosis after surgery depends on the stage (see box below) and location of the growth. Low-lying stage C rectal cancers have a lower patient survival rate than a similar-staged colonic cancer.[69]

Radiation. In selected doses, radiation may be used as a *primary* treatment for rectal cancer. *Intraoperative* radiation therapy (IORT) may be used for treatment of local recurrences. Radiation from a linear accelerator or betatron is administered to the site during an operative procedure.[29] Adjoining structures are either removed or shielded from the beams. Radiation also may be used as an *adjunct* to surgery. It may be given *preoperatively* to shrink the tumor, to decrease the likelihood of cancer cell implantation at time of surgery, and to decrease lymphatic involvement. Surgery may be scheduled 2 weeks after low- to moderate-dose therapy and 6 weeks after high-dose therapy.[29] *Postoperative* radiation may be used to treat patients at high risk for local recurrence (stages B and C).

Chemotherapy. Chemotherapy is used for metastatic disease and for persons with a high risk of recurrence.[69] It is most effective for liver metastasis. The chemotherapeutic agent of choice is 5-fluorouracil (5-FU), either alone or in combination with other agents.

DUKES' CLASSIFICATION OF COLORECTAL CANCER

A—Confined to bowel mucosa
B—Invading muscle wall
C—Lymph node involvement
D—Metastases or locally unresectable tumor

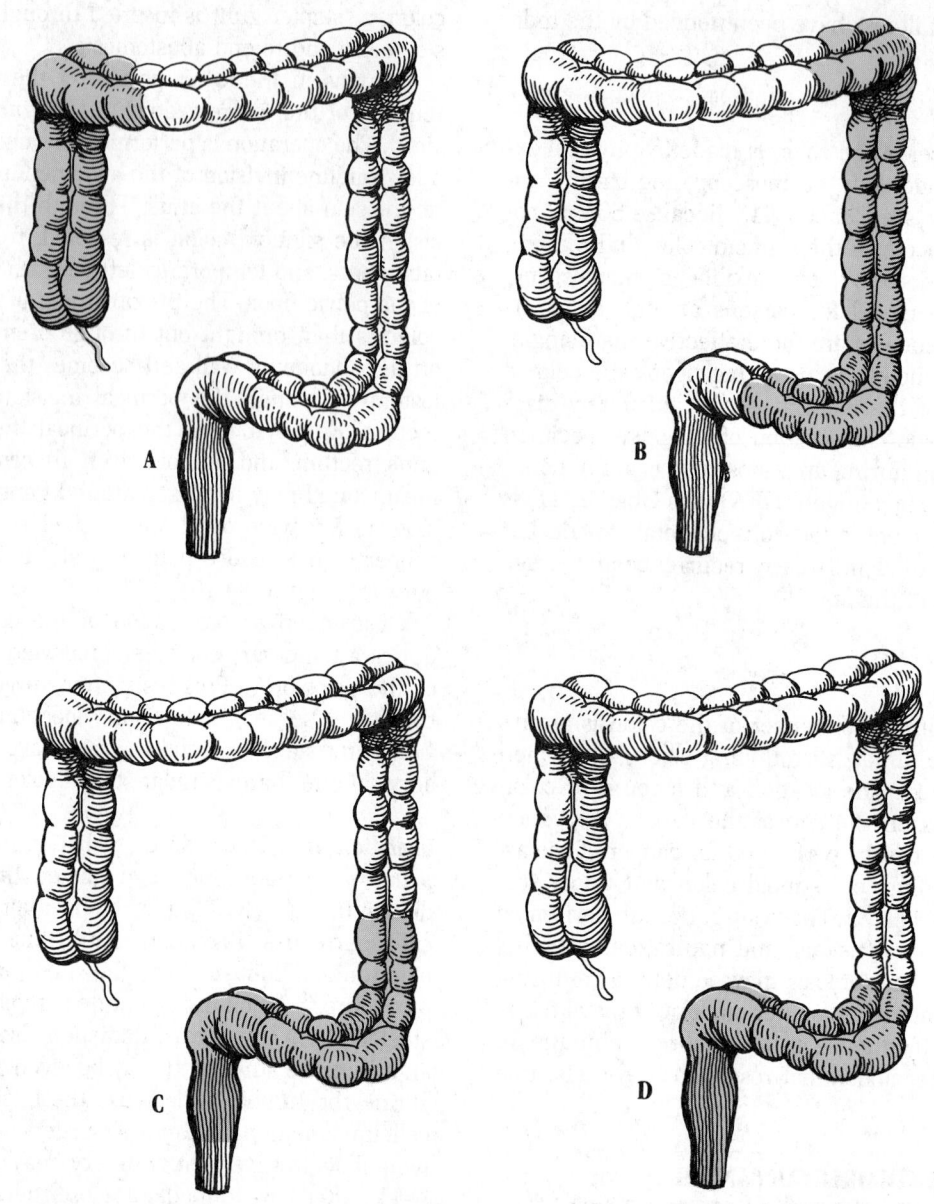

FIGURE 44-9 Bowel resection. **A**, Right hemicolectomy. **B**, Left hemicolectomy. **C**, Anterior rectosigmoid resection. **D**, Abdominoperineal resection.

Nursing Management

Teaching the general population, particularly high-risk persons, about *early detection* of colorectal cancer (see the box on p. 1330), is an ongoing nursing responsibility. Because of the lack of early warning symptoms, many persons do not seek treatment until the lesion is in a Dukes' C or D stage. The person must then deal with a prognosis that is less than favorable for a 5-year survival. Helping the patient and family to cope and to maintain hope becomes a major nursing challenge.

The general care of the person with colorectal cancer is the same as that for other types of cancer (see Chapter 17). Most patients will be experiencing surgery.

BOWEL SURGERY

The care of the person experiencing bowel surgery is summarized in the box on p. 1334.

Preoperative Care

Diet. A low-residue diet is given to diminish fecal matter in the bowel at the time of surgery. The diet may be supplemented with vitamins K and C that may be poorly absorbed because of the bowel preparation. Intestinal bacteria are a source of vitamin K; therefore the amount of available vitamin K is decreased when intestinal bacteria are reduced. Clear liquids are given the day before surgery, and intravenous fluids are usually started the evening before surgery.

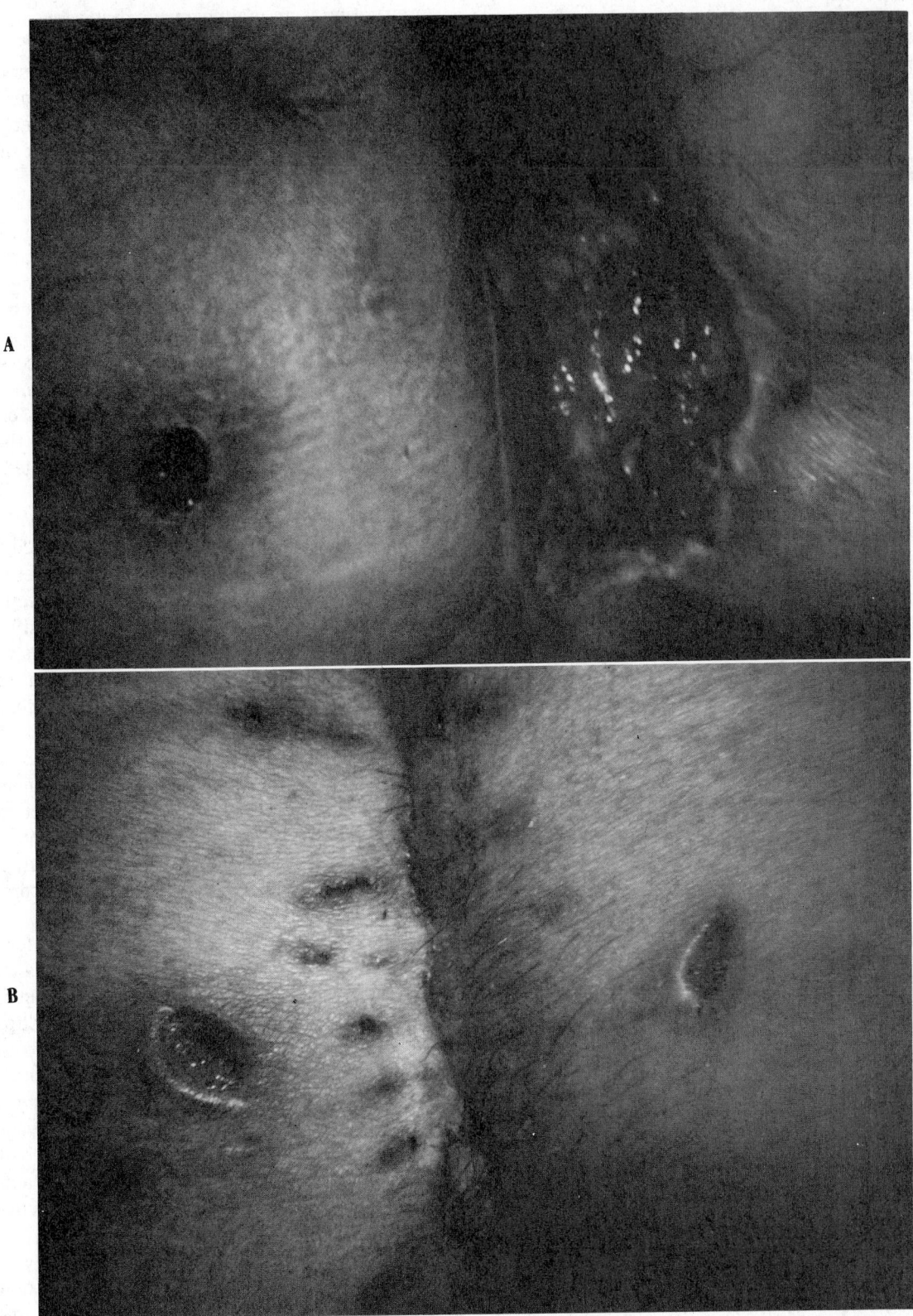

FIGURE 44-10 Perineal wound following an anteroposterior resection for cancer in rectum. **A**, Postsurgical wound; note site of the sump drain to the left of the wound. **B**, After healing; the perineum is completely closed, and the shape of the buttocks looks normal.

NURSING CARE OF THE PATIENT EXPERIENCING BOWEL SURGERY

PREOPERATIVE CARE

1. Preventing infection
   a. Give low-residue diet several days before surgery
   b. Give clear liquids on day prior to surgery
   c. Give prescribed antibiotic
   d. Give prescribed enemas and laxatives
2. Teaching
   a. Describe deep-breathing and coughing exercises
   b. Explain use of side rails to facilitate turning in bed without exerting pull on abdomen

POSTOPERATIVE CARE

1. Promoting oxygenation
   a. Encourage turning and deep-breathing exercises
   b. Encourage patient to be active
2. Maintaining fluid and electrolyte balance
   a. Maintain patency of gastrointestinal tube and record amount of drainage accurately, if NG tube is present
   b. Maintain prescribed flow of parenteral fluids
   c. Monitor for signs of fluid loss (dry skin and mucous membranes, decreased skin turgor)
3. Promoting elimination
   a. Monitor for signs of returning peristalsis (passage of flatus, return of bowel sounds)
   b. Encourage increasing ambulation
   c. Monitor character of initial stools
4. Promoting comfort
   a. Give good oral hygiene until oral fluids are taken freely
   b. Give analgesics on a fairly regular basis during the first 48 hours to prevent severe pain
5. Teaching
   a. Drink at least 2000 ml of fluid daily to avoid constipation
   b. Avoid use of laxatives without medical approval. Stool softeners or psyllium may be used
   c. Avoid heavy lifting for at least 6 weeks after surgery

Bowel preparation. Preparation of the bowel for surgery may be initiated several days before surgery, and a variety of mechanical (enemas) or chemical (drugs) approaches may be used. The purpose of bowel preparation is to cleanse the colon of fecal matter and to suppress bacterial growth in the colon to prevent postoperative infection.

Mechanical preparation usually consists of a program of laxatives and enemas for several days before surgery. It is contraindicated for persons with intestinal obstruction, and it may be poorly tolerated by acutely ill or elderly persons. An alternative approach is *whole gut lavage* that consists of ingestions (orally or by nasogastric tube) of large amounts of isotonic saline to clear out the fecal matter. A solution containing sodium sulfate and polyethylene glycol (GOLYTELY) may be used in place of the isotonic saline.[65]

Systemic antibiotics or oral nonabsorbable antibiotics may also be used to reduce colonic bacteria. A common preparation is an oral neomycin-erythromycin base.

Intubation. A nasogastric tube may be inserted before surgery to maintain gastrointestinal decompression until peristalsis returns. The tube may be inserted on the unit before the patient goes to surgery or at the time of surgery.

Postoperative Care

Fluid and electrolyte balance. If a nasogastric tube is inserted, special attention is given to keeping the tube draining and to maintaining fluid and electrolyte balance. The daily output from gastric drainage is recorded accurately; this amount influences the necessary fluid and electrolyte replacement. Nothing is given by mouth until the tube is removed. Food is withheld for the first 24 hours after the tube is removed; then the patient progresses rapidly to a regular diet as tolerated.

Oxygenation. Incisional pain may interfere with full respiratory excursion. Narcotics are administered as necessary, and active ventilatory measures are encouraged. Pulmonary embolism and infarction may occur 7 to 10 days after surgery. A miniheparin regimen, that is, 5000 units (50 mg) of heparin given subcutaneously every 12 hours, may be started preoperatively and continued postoperatively for prophylactic anticoagulation.[5]

Elimination. Ambulation is encouraged to promote return of peristalsis. Prolonged ileus may indicate an abdominal abscess from leakage of a left colectomy or anterior resection, or it may be caused by intestinal obstruction. The passage of gas or stool rectally indicates the beginning return of peristalsis and is reported to the physician.

After a bowel resection, it is not unusual for diarrhea to occur after peristalsis returns. Usually it is temporary and soon disappears. When the stool becomes normal, the person is advised to avoid becoming constipated, because a hard stool and straining to expel it could possibly injure the anastomosis, depending on its location. Persons who have a tendency to develop constipation are advised to try drinking fruit juice and water before breakfast or to take a glass of prune juice daily. They should not take laxatives, without medical approval. A stool softener or a mild bulk laxative such as psyllium is frequently prescribed.

Care following abdominoperineal resection. Abdominoperineal resection involves removal of greater amounts of tissue and formation of a colostomy. Therefore additional considerations are required for patients who have had general bowel surgery. Postoperative shock occurs frequently, and measures to prevent, monitor, and treat shock are instituted (see Chapter 25). The care of the patient is summarized in the box at right. Care of the person with a colostomy is discussed in a separate section to follow.

Urinary retention is a common occurrence following rectal excision, with approximately 50% of men experiencing some degree of adynamic bladder paralysis after the Foley catheter is removed. Factors that influence urinary retention include loss of pelvic support, chronic urinary tract infection, enlarged prostate, or nerve injury. Loss of pelvic support increases problems with micturition when the patient is supine; thus micturition may improve with ambulation. If nerve injury is present, problems with urinary retention and urinary tract infections may persist for 6 to 8 months, with partial resolution of retention but with urinary incontinence experienced at night.

Wound care depends on whether the rectal incision is closed or open. An open wound is irrigated until the person can take sitz baths. A catheter may be inserted into the wound for irrigation, or a handheld shower massage or Water Pik with the jet on lowest pressure may be used. Precise directions for irrigations are recorded on the nursing care plan. Wound drainage during the early postoperative period is serosanguineous and profuse, requiring frequent dressing changes.

Many patients complain of *phantom rectal sensations* and of feeling the necessity to defecate. An explanation of cortical perception and transmission of nerve impulses often helps the patient cope with these sensations.

Sexual difficulties may occur in about 40% of males following abdominoperineal resection. Difficulty with ejaculation is more commonly seen than impotence (difficulty with erection), but they may occur together. Females of childbearing years may require sterilization if the lesion involves the anterior rectal wall.

Convalescence after an abdominoperineal resection is prolonged and may require many months. During this time, the person should remain under close supervision.

INTERVENTIONS FOR FECAL DIVERSION: OSTOMIES

Diversion of the fecal stream may be indicated for managing congenital problems, traumatic injuries, and diseases in or adjacent to the gastrointestinal tract. The diversion may be temporary or permanent. In a temporary diversion, the fecal stream is rerouted to allow the gastrointestinal tract an opportunity to heal or to provide an outlet for the stool when an obstruction is present. A permanent diversion implies that the intestine cannot or will not be reconnected; thus a return to the usual elimination mode will not occur.

NURSING CARE OF THE PATIENT WITH AN ABDOMINOPERINEAL RESECTION

PREOPERATIVE CARE

1. Prepare patient as for other bowel surgery.
2. Prepare patient for a stoma (p. 1339).
3. Prepare patient for a perineal incision: wound may be open and, if so, it will take longer to heal.

POSTOPERATIVE CARE

1. Provide care as for other bowel surgery.
2. Preventing complications
   a. Shock
      (1) Monitor for early signs and institute shock measures.
   b. Hemorrhage
      (1) Check perineal dressing frequently: initial drainage is profuse and serosanguineous.
      (2) Reinforce initial dressings as necessary.
      (3) Report excessive bleeding to physician.
   c. Thrombophlebitis/pulmonary embolism
      (1) Encourage leg exercises (Chapter 24) until patient is ambulatory.
      (2) Encourage use of elastic stockings with elderly patients or those with poor leg circulation.
      (3) Encourage ambulation when permitted.
3. Promoting healing
   a. Maintain low continuous suction of sump catheters, if present.
   b. Change perineal dressing frequently as needed after first 24 hours.
      (1) Record precise directions for dressing change on nursing care plan.
      (2) Irrigate wound with normal saline solution by use of catheter, handheld shower massage, or Water Pik.
      (3) Cover with dry dressings, and hold in place with a T-binder. (The T "top" is wrapped around the waist and the T strap is brought up between the legs.)
   c. Substitute sitz baths for irrigation when patient is ambulatory. Maintain free flow of water on perineal wound in sitz tub (rubber ring may be helpful.)
   d. Provide stoma care (p. 1343).
4. Promoting urinary elimination
   a. Maintain patency of indwelling catheter.
   b. Monitor for residual urine when catheter is removed.
      (1) Keep accurate intake and output records.
      (2) Monitor for lower abdominal distention, patient discomfort, and restlessness.
   c. Use measures to encourage voiding if patient has inability to initiate stream.
5. Promoting comfort
   a. Assist patient to find a comfortable position in bed: side-lying is usually preferred.
   b. Assist patient to turn frequently.
   c. Try a foam pad under buttocks for supine position.
   d. Give narcotics at regular intervals until severe pain decreases (about 3 days postoperatively).

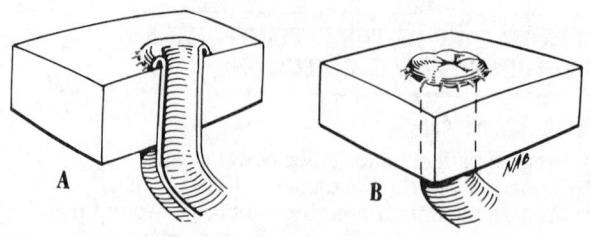

FIGURE 44-11 End sigmoid colostomy with a flush stoma. **A**, Cross section. **B**, Exterior view.

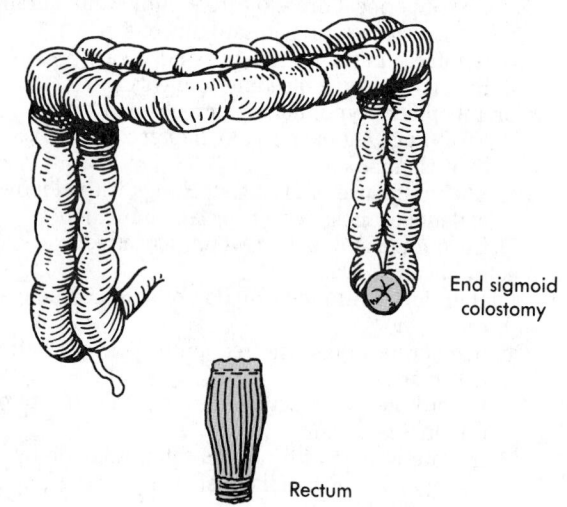

FIGURE 44-12 End sigmoid colostomy with an oversewn rectum left intact (Hartmann's pouch).

Whether it is temporary or permanent, the diversion results in the formation of an ostomy or stoma. This new opening is created by bringing the intestine to the skin surface and suturing it into place.

TYPES OF STOMAS

There are three types of functioning stomas: an end stoma, a loop stoma, and a loop-end stoma. A nonfunctional end stoma is referred to as a mucous fistula.

When an *end stoma* is created surgically, the proximal bowel is brought out through an incision in the abdominal wall, folded over on itself (forming a cuff), and sutured to the skin. The stomal surface is the mucosal lining layer of the intestinal wall (Figure 44-11). The remaining distal bowel can be surgically removed (p. 1331), oversewn to form a Hartmann's pouch (Figure 44-12), or brought to the skin surface to form another stoma, the *mucous fistula*. This distal stoma secretes mucus and requires dressings rather than pouches (see the box on p. 1337). It can be located at the base of the incision, adjacent to the proximal stoma (described as a double-barrel ostomy) Figure 44-13, or at a distance from it (Figure 44-14).

The *loop stoma* is created by bringing the bowel through an abdominal incision, sliding a support under the bowel, and opening the upper wall of the bowel. The posterior wall remains intact. There is one stoma, but there are two openings—proximal and distal (Figure 44-15). The loop ostomy is generally a temporary procedure and is often performed in an emergency situation (such as for gunshot or stab wounds or intestinal obstruction).

The *loop-end stoma* is similar to the end stoma in

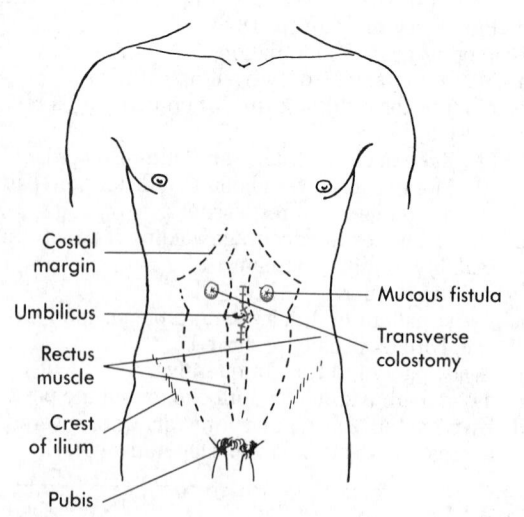

FIGURE 44-13 Transverse colostomy with adjacent mucous fistula.

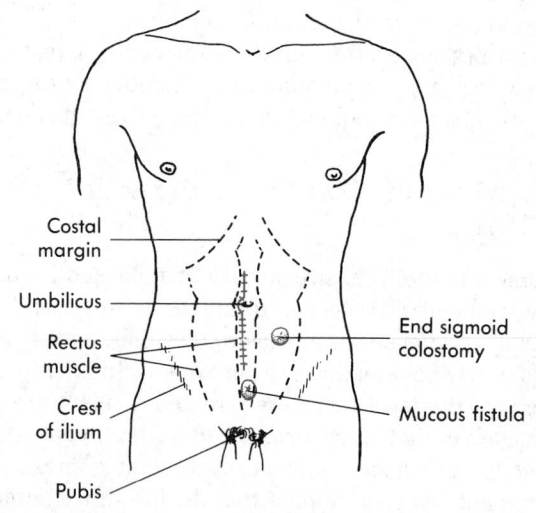

FIGURE 44-14 End sigmoid colostomy and mucous fistula.

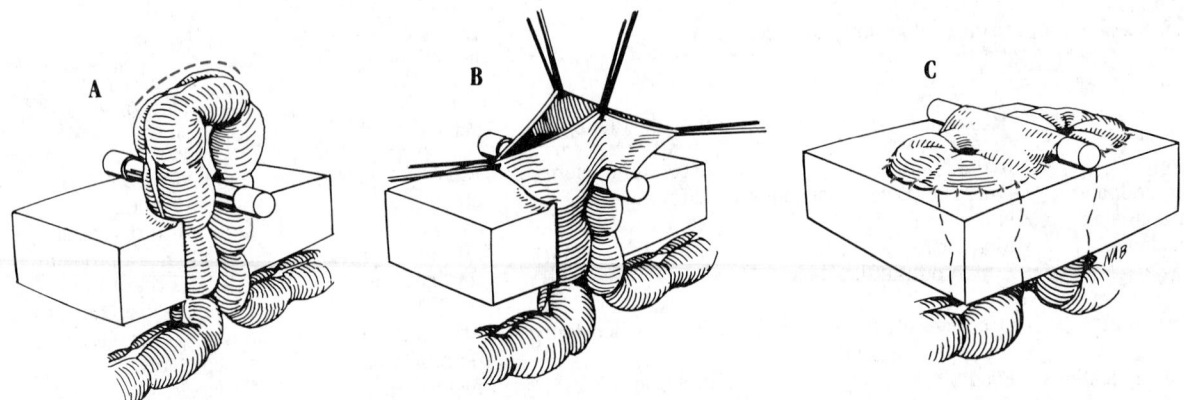

FIGURE 44-15 Loop colostomy. **A**, Bowel is brought through the incision and supported with the rod. **B**, Incision in anterior wall. **C**, Edges are folded over to make two openings in one stoma.

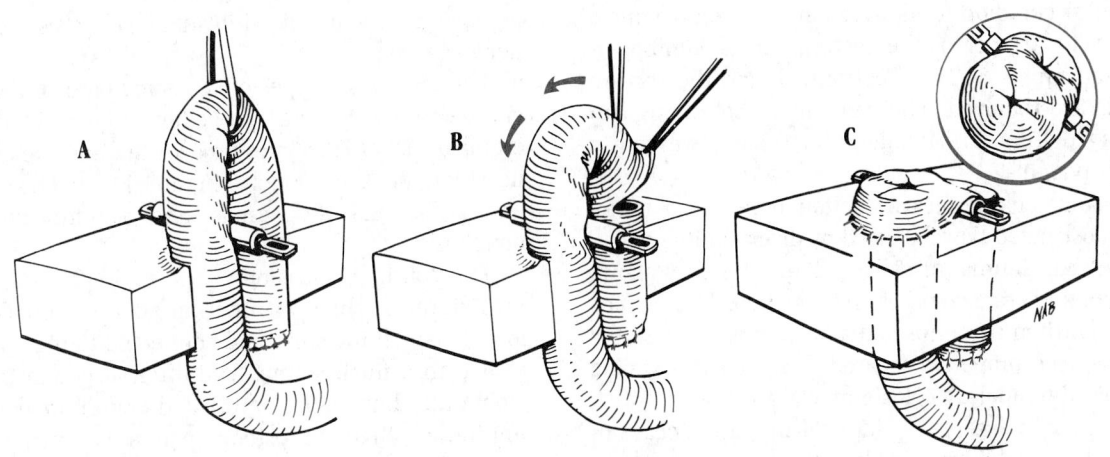

FIGURE 44-16 Loop-end stoma. **A**, Bowel end is oversewn; bowel is brought through the incision and supported with the rod. **B**, Incision in anterior wall close to end. **C**, Edges are folded over; distal end is a blind end.

that the bowel is resected and the stoma made from the proximal portion. It differs in that the divided end is oversewn and the stoma is made from a loop of the intestine just proximal to the end. This loop is supported on the skin surface by a small rod placed under the loop but on top of the skin. The loop is opened, and the edges are sutured to the skin at the time of surgery (Figure 44-16).

TYPES OF SURGERY
COLOSTOMY SURGERY

The surgical diversion of the large intestine will result in a colostomy. The anatomic location of the ostomy determines the name, such as *ascending, transverse, descending,* or *sigmoid* colostomy. The nursing care and patient needs differ for each type of colostomy (Table 44-7).

CARE OF THE MUCOUS FISTULA

1. Remove soiled dressing over mucous fistula.
2. Wash mucous fistula gently with soap and water (can be done during bath or shower); rinse and pat dry.
3. If necessary, place Vaseline gauze over mucous fistula to keep dressing from sticking.
4. Place one or two small dressings over opening.
5. Tape dressings *lightly* in place.
6. Report any rectal bleeding to physician (passing mucus from rectum is normal).

TABLE 44-7 Comparison of ileostomy and colostomies

	Ileostomy	Ascending Colostomy	Transverse Colostomy	Descending or Sigmoid Colostomy
Location	Ileum	Ascending colon	Transverse colon	Sigmoid colon
Type of drainage	Liquid-to-paste consistency	Liquid-to-soft	Soft	Soft-to-formed
Bowel regulation	No	No	No	Only with irrigations
Fluid balance	Monitor for dehydration if high output diarrhea	Same as ileostomy	May occur with bouts of diarrhea	Usually not a problem unless there were previous resections
Skin irritation	Occurs easily because of digestive enzymes	Same as ileostomy	Can occur from exposure to stool	Same as transverse colostomy
Other complications	Food blockage Prolapse of stoma Stricture Peristomal hernia	Prolapse Stricture Peristomal hernia	Prolapse Stricture Peristomal hernia	Prolapse Stricture Constipation Peristomal hernia

The most common fecal diversion is the end sigmoid colostomy for cancer of the rectum. An abdominoperineal resection (p. 1331) is performed, and the rectum and anus are removed. This permanent colostomy can be managed through irrigations or through wearing a drainable pouch.

Temporary colostomies are often done for a perforated or obstructed bowel caused by diverticulitis, volvulus, ischemia, trauma, or cancer. The colostomy allows for healing and eradication of any infection. The reanastomosis can then be performed at a later date when the bowel has been properly prepared. The length of time a person has a temporary colostomy will vary.

The person is assessed before closure, and occasionally the closure is postponed. In a person with an inoperable tumor, a colostomy is performed as a permanent diversion to alleviate or prevent obstruction.

ILEOSTOMY SURGERY

When the small bowel (ileum) is the site of the diversion, the ostomy is referred to as an ileostomy. The most frequent indications for an ileostomy are mucosal ulcerative colitis and Crohn's (granulomatous) colitis. Other indications are familial intestinal polyposis and Gardner's syndrome.

The three main types of ileostomy procedures are the end ileostomy (Brooke's procedure, Figure 44-17), loop-end ileostomy (Turnball's procedure), and the continent ileostomy or Kock pouch (Figure 44-2). The loop and end ileostomies are similar and require the use of pouches.

The continent ileostomy (see p. 1312) is a surgical procedure in which an internal pouch is created from loops of small intestine and connected to the abdominal wall with a flush stoma. The internal pouch holds the stool until the pouch is intubated and drained. A dressing rather than an ostomy pouch is worn over the stoma. This procedure can be performed in some patients with ulcerative colitis or familial polyposis.

A more popular procedure for persons with ulcerative colitis or familial polyposis is ileoanal anastomosis with an ileal reservoir.[49] An internal pouch is created from loops of intestine and connected to the anus (Figure 44-3). A temporary loop ileostomy is formed to allow the diversion of stool while the newly formed pouch heals. In 6 to 8 weeks after the initial surgery, the ileostomy is taken down and the person can pass stool through the anus. The person has several semisoft bowel movements per day.

PREOPERATIVE CARE

When the physician first tells the patient of the probable need for an ostomy, the immediate reaction is likely to be shock and disbelief. Whether the ostomy is to be temporary or permanent, it is difficult for most people to accept. Knowledge that it is a lifesaving or life-prolonging measure, confidence in the surgeon, and explanation and acceptance of the proposed operation by significant others may help the patient decide to have the operation. It is not unusual for the patient to be sad, with-

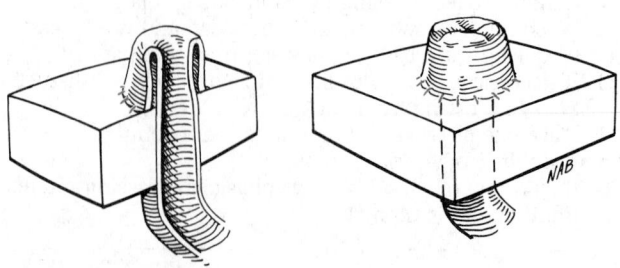

FIGURE 44-17 Ileostomy stoma (Brooke's procedure) with 1-inch stoma.

drawn, and depressed after learning of the need for ostomy surgery.

PREOPERATIVE TEACHING

The nurse should know what the patient has been told by the physician and should be prepared to supplement this and to assess how much more information to give the patient preoperatively. Some patients are very upset by the impending surgery and want little information. However, each patient should at least know what is meant by ostomy surgery and what type of management it will require (such as the need to wear a pouch). Many persons have misconceptions about the ostomy that add to the preoperative anxiety. Dispelling these myths and giving correct information can lessen fears concerning the ostomy. An enterostomal therapy nurse who has specialized in the care of persons with ostomies can assist with preoperative preparation and instruction.

After assessing the patient, the nurse can begin the preoperative instruction by eliciting the patient's questions or concerns. Patients may feel they do not know enough to ask questions. The following are some general guidelines for the nurse to use:

1. Provide a brief explanation of the gastrointestinal tract.
2. Using a simple drawing, explain which portions of the intestine will be removed, how the stoma will be formed, and where it will be located.
3. Describe briefly the appearance of the stoma, the sensation, and the type of bowel function.
4. Define terms such as ileostomy or colostomy, stoma, and pouch.
5. Describe briefly the management of the ostomy.
6. Describe the teaching plan for the patient, providing reassurance that, immediately after the surgery, care will be provided, and teaching will be started when self-care is resumed.
7. Offer to arrange for a visitor from the Ostomy Association.
8. Leave written information as desired for the patient and significant others to use as reference material.

During preoperative teaching, the nurse constantly observes the patient and is careful not to overwhelm with deep explanations that the patient does not require. If it is possible, significant others should be present during the instruction and encouraged to ask questions. Significant others who provide support, acceptance, and reassurance will enhance the patient's acceptance of the ostomy.

During the preoperative talk, the nurse should mention that the ostomy can be managed. Usually a normal life-style can be resumed, depending upon the prognosis and indication for the ostomy. Many well-written pamphlets echo this theme and show pictures of persons who have learned to manage well with an ostomy.

STOMA SITE

The potential stoma site is selected and marked by the surgeon or the enterostomal therapy nurse. It should be visible to the patient when sitting or standing, within the rectus muscle, and away from scars, bony prominences, and folds (Figure 44-18). The belt line should also be avoided. The stoma site influences the patient's ability to keep a good pouch seal and to manage the ostomy independently after surgery. The marking of the site can be overwhelming to the patient as the proposed surgery becomes more real. The nurse should anticipate the patient's need for support at this time.

INTRAOPERATIVE CARE

At the close of the operation, a pouch is applied over the stoma opening. A clear, disposable pouch is preferred to allow easy visualization of the new stoma.

The loop colostomy stoma may be opened in the operating room, or the surgeon may choose to open the loop of bowel in the patient's room within 72 hours postoperatively. A cautery is used to make an incision into the teniae coli on the external wall of the bowel. The bowel is then opened, and both proximal and distal bowel can be visualized. There are two pathways or openings in one stoma. The patient should be reassured that there will be no feeling of pain during the procedure, since there are no sensory (only motor) nerves in the stoma. There is, however, a very distinctive burning odor, and adequate ventilation during and following the procedure is required. The supporting rod of a loop stoma is removed 7 to 10 days after surgery. At this time, adhesions have formed that prevent the loop from retracting through the incision.

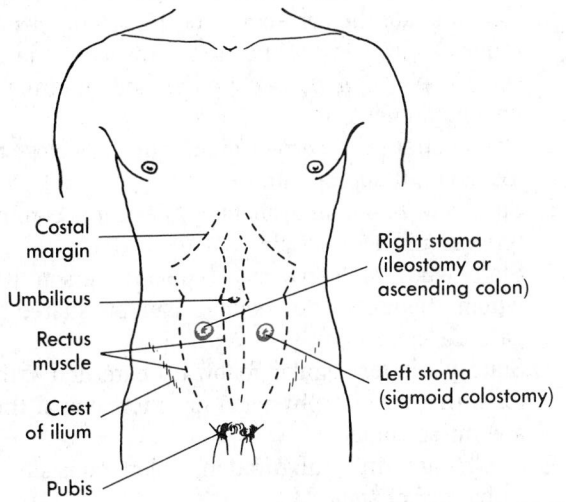

FIGURE 44-18 Best sites for ostomies.

GUIDELINES FOR CARE OF THE PERSON WITH A COLOSTOMY OR ILEOSTOMY

1. Prepare the person for surgery by describing the ostomy, answering questions, and dispelling misconceptions.
2. Monitor the stoma postoperatively for swelling, color, function, and intactness of mucocutaneous suture line.
3. Assess the readiness of the person to view the stoma and to begin learning about care of the ostomy.
4. Promote acceptance of the change in the body through own facial expressions and empathic interactions.
5. Instruct the person in the care of the ostomy through use of a detailed and individualized care plan.
6. Provide the person with written instructions and supplies.
7. Provide necessary follow-up care.
8. Inform the person of support services such as the United Ostomy Association and the American Cancer Society.

POSTOPERATIVE CARE

The immediate postoperative care for the colostomy or ileostomy patient follows the guidelines for bowel surgery (p. 1334). Hemorrhage through or around the stoma is rare; if it occurs, it is reported immediately. Specific guidelines for the ostomy patient are listed in the box above.

■ ASSESSMENT

Subjective Data

Subjective data include the person's knowledge of ostomy care, feelings about self and loss of a body part (see Chapter 18), usual coping strategies (see Chapter 10), and concerns about sexual activity (see Chapter 51). Data are collected over a period of time as the person becomes aware of the stoma presence.

Objective Data

The stoma is observed regularly for redness, edema, intactness of mucocutaneous suture line, and function. Redness reflects the circulation to the stoma, thus denoting viability. A dark, dusty, or black stoma is reported to the surgeon. A necrotic stoma may need to be revised.

Postoperative edema of the stoma is normal and results from manipulation during surgery. The pouch is changed within 24 to 48 hours after surgery to allow adequate clearance (⅛ to ¼ inch) for the enlarging stoma. A snug skin barrier or pouch that does not stretch can impede circulation to the stoma mucosa. Swelling begins to lessen within a week after surgery.

The sutures anchoring the stoma mucosa to the skin are inspected for intactness. Occasionally some of the stoma mucosa pulls away from the skin before healing has occurred. This *mucosal separation* is documented and monitored. It is of concern if more than the subcutaneous tissue levels are involved. Superficial separations heal by granulation. Deeper separations may need resuturing or packing with gauze dressings.

The stoma drainage initially is mucus and serosanguineous secretion. Stool may be present in the pouch if the intestines are being decompressed. Then, as the intestinal function returns, flatus is produced. Flatus and fecal drainage usually begin within 2 to 3 days for an ileostomy and 4 to 7 days for a colostomy. The initial drainage is liquid and becomes thicker as the diet progresses.

■ DATA ANALYSIS: NURSING DIAGNOSES

Nursing diagnoses are determined from assessment of patient data. Possible nursing diagnoses for the person who has had a colostomy may include, but are not limited to, the following:

Diagnostic Title	Possible Etiologies
Body image, disturbance	Change in body appearance
Constipation, colonic	Paralytic ileus following surgery
Coping, ineffective, individual	Adjustment to the new ostomy
Grieving	Loss of control over bowel function
Knowledge deficit	Lack of exposure/recall
Skin integrity, impaired	Irritation from stool or adhesive
Sexual dysfunction	Changed body structure or physiologic/psychologic factors

■ PLANNING: EXPECTED PATIENT OUTCOMES

The patient or significant others can do the following:
1. Demonstrate the correct use of the ostomy pouch: removal, cleansing of the stoma, inspection of the skin, application of the pouch, and ordering of new equipment.
2. Demonstrate the correct technique for colostomy irrigation, if appropriate.
3. State how to obtain available professional community resources
4. State who will serve as a support person with whom thoughts and feelings can be shared regarding the ostomy.
5. State plans for regular follow-up care and symptoms that require physician or enterostomal therapy nurse contact.
   a. Changes in configuration, color, consistency, or odor of stool
   b. Bleeding through stoma or rectum
   c. Persistent diarrhea or lack of stool evacuation

despite medications, treatment, fluids, diet, and exercise program

   d. Persistent skin irritation despite treatment

   e. Changes in contour of the stoma (for example, prolapse)

   f. Persistent leakage around the pouch

   g. Signs of dehydration and electrolyte imbalance

   h. Signs and symptoms of a food blockage with an ileostomy

■ IMPLEMENTATION

Initial Teaching

Teaching the patient about care of the colostomy or ileostomy begins in the immediate postoperative phase and continues until the patient leaves the hospital or is independent of care. A visiting nurse referral may be initiated to continue instruction.

It is most desirable for the patient to learn to care for the ostomy. This learning enhances the process of accepting the ostomy as being a part of oneself. Occasionally the location of the stoma or physical condition of the patient requires that a spouse, relative, or friend be taught the procedure. The patient should be involved whenever or in whatever way possible.

Teaching begins with the first pouch change. The patient may or may not be ready to observe the stoma and is not required to do so. The patient is informed that the stoma itself has no touch sensation and will not hurt during the procedure. However, removing the pouch may be painful since the entire abdomen is generally sore from surgery. Therefore premedicating the patient is preferable.

Viewing of the stoma is better received if the nurse first cleanses the skin and stoma of any blood, mucus, or stool. The nurse then carefully changes the pouch, explaining the steps briefly. The patient is not expected to remember the procedure steps at this time.

Patient Feelings

With each pouch change, the nurse allows the patient to express feelings or reactions to the stoma. Frequently patients will have a facial expression indicating disgust or will remark on the unsightliness of the stoma. The nurse must allow the patient to make these comments without attempting to diminish the importance of expressing these thoughts by giving false assurances. Nurses must also monitor their own expressions. Patients watch every facial expression or gesture of the nurses and are extremely sensitive to evidence of distaste.

Removal of any part of the body involves a sense of loss; therefore the patient may experience grief and mourning, which include shock, denial, anger, and depression. (See Chapter 14 for a discussion of these reactions). In addition, because the surgery results in the expelling of fecal contents through a new opening in

RESEARCH

Watson PG: The effects of short-term postoperative counseling on cancer/ostomy patients, Cancer Nurs 6:21-28, 1983.

The purpose of this study was to determine whether four counseling sessions during the postoperative period would have a favorable effect on the ostomy patient's self-esteem and self-concept. Of the subjects who were to have ostomy surgery for colorectal or bladder cancer, 31 were selected. All were asked to complete the Tennessee Self-Concept Scale and the Rosenberg Self-Esteem Inventory on the fourth to the seventh postoperative day and on the day before discharge. All were interviewed by the telephone 1 month after discharge and asked to answer questions about physical well-being, care of the ostomy, and involvement in activities. Of the 31 subjects, 17 participated in three or four counseling sessions with a rehabilitative counselor; these sessions started after the first day of testing and concluded before the last testing in the hospital. All other care and teaching remained the same for both groups.

The subjects who received counseling had more positive changes in self-concept and self-esteem than those who did not. The counseled subjects also reported greater levels of involvement in outside activities and independence 4 weeks after discharge. Short-term counseling had a favorable effect on the treatment group. ■

the abdomen, the patient will experience changes in body image and may have feelings of guilt, shame, disgust, and social withdrawal. These are discussed in Chapter 18. Counseling helps to facilitate increased self-esteem (see the research box above).

Usually the formation of the stoma is viewed as mutilating surgery, but for some individuals the surgery may be a relief or a release from coping with chronic pain, diarrhea, or debility. No matter what reaction is expressed, patients need time and the support of others to work through their feelings.

Formal Instruction

A planned systematic teaching protocol (see the box on p. 1342) enhances the patient's ability to learn to manage the ostomy. Teaching self care of the ostomy is usually begun once the nasogastric tube has been removed and the patient is feeling more comfortable physically. Teaching is planned over several days to allow the patient time to assimilate the information. At least three lessons are generally needed. Pouches are changed more often than necessary to allow for teaching and practice. During the first lesson the patient observes the steps of the procedure. During the second lesson the patient should assist with preparing the pouch, cleansing the skin and stoma, and centering the pouch around the stoma. The patient changes the pouch with supervision for the third lesson. Some persons need more practice, and additional sessions may be scheduled. Written in-

TEACHING PLAN FOR OSTOMY CARE

1. Start teaching with the first pouch change by explaining steps briefly; explain that the stoma has no touch sensation
2. Begin planned instruction when the patient is receptive to learning
3. Lesson 1
   a. Review each step of the procedure while patient observes
   b. Discuss the following conditions:
      (1) Redness of the stoma is a result of good circulation
      (2) Edema is normally present; it results from manipulation during surgery and will decrease within a week of surgery
   c. Demonstrate how to empty pouch, how to cleanse bottom edge, and how to apply clamp
   d. Demonstrate how to rinse pouch with tepid water using a bulb (asepto) syringe as needed to remove thick stool
   e. Give patient written instructions
   f. Plan for next lesson
4. Lesson 2
   a. Change pouch
   b. Have patient assist with preparing pouch, measuring stoma, and cleansing skin
   c. Discuss the following tasks:
      (1) Check for wear of pouch and frequency of pouch change
      (2) Observe skin for irritation
      (3) Clip hair around stoma or shave with an electric razor to prevent folliculitis (males)

5. Lesson 3
   a. Have patient assemble equipment, cleanse skin and stoma, and apply pouch following written instructions as needed
   b. Discuss the following information:
      (1) Dietary concerns, with emphasis on foods that cause odor and gas and foods that can cause blockage (ileostomy)
      (2) Maintenance of fluid and electrolyte balance
      (3) Resumption of normal activities, for example, bathing, clothing, traveling, sexual relationships
      (4) Purposes of the United Ostomy Association
      (5) Insurance coverage of supplies (refer to social worker as necessary)
6. Before discharge
   a. Have patient demonstrate pouch change without assistance; evaluate technique
   b. Have patient empty pouch in bathroom, rinse pouch, and apply clamp
   c. Review list of suppliers
   d. Ask patient to describe what to observe when changing pouch and what actions to take
   e. Ask patient to describe plans for follow-up care

Courtesy University Hospitals of Cleveland, Cleveland, Ohio.

structions and resource materials are imperative as a supplement to instruction. A visiting nurse referral may be needed for assessment of the patient's ability to adapt to the ostomy in the home environment.

The nursing care plan includes detailed information regarding the approaches and techniques used so that consistency of approach is used by all nurses caring for the patient. The care plan includes fluid and electrolyte balance, skin care, pouch selection and application, diet, colostomy irrigation (as appropriate), activity, sexuality, community resources, and complications.

Fluid and Electrolyte Balance

During the postoperative period attention to fluid and electrolyte balance is important for any person with an ostomy, but it is especially important for the person with an ileostomy. After surgery, the fecal drainage from the ileostomy is liquid and may be constant. Patients will have outputs ranging from 1000 ml to 1500 ml per 24 hours. Within 10 to 15 days this amount should decrease as the terminal ileum begins to absorb more water and the stool becomes thicker.

Exceptions are seen in patients who have had previ-

ous bowel resections or resections of the ileum for Crohn's disease. The more intestine that has been resected, the greater the chance for a high volume output of very liquid stool. Some patients need medications to help decrease the output and control the loss of fluid.

Diarrhea for a person with an ileostomy is watery and requires pouch emptying every 1 to 2 hours. The fluid may feel warm in the pouch. Volumes over 1500 ml are considered high output. Diarrhea accompanied by nausea and vomiting can rapidly progress to dehydration. Patients are taught to observe signs of dehydration and electrolyte imbalance. They should know how to replace fluids and electrolytes, as well as when to seek medical attention.

Persons with ileostomies may become dehydrated if given laxatives or routine preparations for diagnostic procedures. The ileostomy stoma is not irrigated as is a colostomy stoma.

Enteric-coated, time-released medications or hard tablets may not be absorbed in a patient with an ileostomy. Liquid or chewable forms of medications are preferred. The remaining ileum does develop a bacterial flora, so antibiotic therapy can also cause diarrhea.

Persons with ascending colostomies or colostomies following previous multiple resections may also have liquid stool and need instruction in maintaining fluid and electrolyte balance.

Skin Care

Skin irritation or infection. The skin around the stoma should appear as normal and healthy as any other abdominal skin. Any change from the normal skin should be considered a problem, and it requires proper identification of the cause and treatment. Prevention of skin breakdown is easier, less expensive, and less painful than treatment.

Skin irritation can be caused by an allergic reaction to the tape or skin barrier product, exposure of the peristomal skin to stool, rough or frequent removal of pouch adhesives, and/or a skin infection. Allergic reactions are treated by changing the type of adhesive or barrier and, if necessary, by the use of a steroid spray to decrease inflammation. Skin patch testing can help determine which products should be avoided.

Skin exposure to stool can be a major problem for someone with an ostomy. Ileostomy drainage contains residual digestive enzymes that will quickly break down the skin. Ascending colostomies also contain some residual enzymes. Any ostomy with very liquid drainage can lead to skin irritation if the skin is not properly protected. In addition to the irritation from the stools, the skin may be damaged from frequent removal of pouch adhesives from the skin.

Peristomal skin infections may be bacterial or fungal. The most common is a yeast infection from *Candida albicans*. The skin becomes bright red with papular lesions in an irregular area; secondary skin changes occur as the process continues, and dry, scaling areas develop. The skin lesion may be diagnosed by a potassium hydroxide stain (see Chapter 71). Treatment involves the use of nystatin (Mycostatin) powder sealed with a skin sealant.

Skin protection. An important means of protecting the peristomal skin is using a *skin barrier* with the pouch. Skin barriers include such products as karaya, Stomahesive (Squibb), Hollihesive (Hollister) Crixilene (Bard) Secure-Life (Coloplast), and Colly-Seel (Mason). Skin barriers attached to the pouches are available as one- or two-piece systems and as single-use items that can be used with any pouch.

There are several basic forms in which one may obtain skin barriers: powder, paste, washer, or wafers (Figure 44-19). A pouch will not adhere to powder, cream, or ointment; therefore if powder is applied to the skin, it must be sealed in before the pouch can be applied. Karaya *powder* releases acetic acid when applied to irritated skin and may result in a temporary stinging

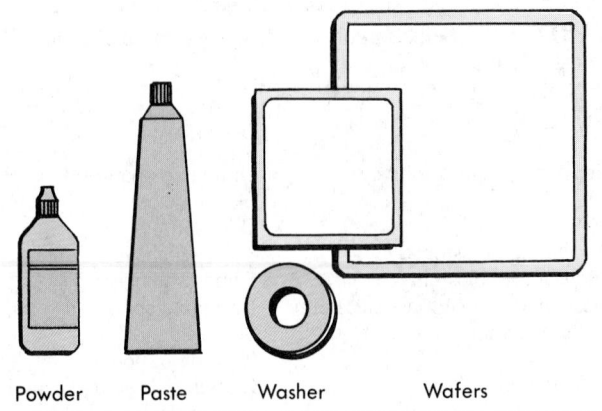

Powder   Paste   Washer   Wafers

FIGURE 44-19 Skin barriers.

of the skin. Stomahesive powder works well on irritated skin.

Paste (karaya, Stomahesive, or Premium) is available for use around the stoma, to fill in creases or folds, and to supplement skin barriers for a longer seal. The use of paste has made it easier to keep a pouch seal intact in poor locations.

Skin barrier wafers have provided an innovative method of skin protection. The wafers may be used with a variety of pouches and protect the skin from the stool. The opening in the wafer is carefully prepared so that it fits at the base of the stoma without rubbing into or onto the stoma.

Skin sealants come in sprays, liquids, gels, and wipes. These products coat the skin with a clear film. They are useful under pouch adhesives. When tape is removed from the skin, it removes the stratum corneum layer of the skin. When a skin sealant is used under the tape, the removal of tape removes the skin sealant and thus leaves the skin intact.

There are several basic principles for protecting skin and limiting peristomal skin irritation.

1. When a pouch seal leaks, the pouch should be immediately changed, not taped. Stool held against the skin can quickly result in severe irritation.
2. Pouches are removed gently, with one hand holding the skin in place to decrease pulling.
3. The skin should be gently but thoroughly cleansed, rinsed, and patted dry.
4. Peristomal hair (males) should be trimmed to prevent folliculitis.
5. A skin barrier should be used to protect the peristomal skin from liquid stool.
6. A skin sealant should be used under all tapes applied to skin.
7. The patient should be taught to change pouches whenever possible *before* leakage occurs.

TABLE 44-8 Selection of pouching system on the basis of ostomy type

Type of Ostomy	Pouching System
lleostomy, jejunostomy	Drainable open-end
	Skin barrier
	Odor-proof pouch
Ascending colostomy	Same as above
Transverse colostomy	Same as above
Descending or sigmoid colostomy	Drainable open-end
No irrigation	Skin sealants
	Odor-proof pouch
Irrigation	Closed-end security pouch
	Skin sealants
	Gas-release valve

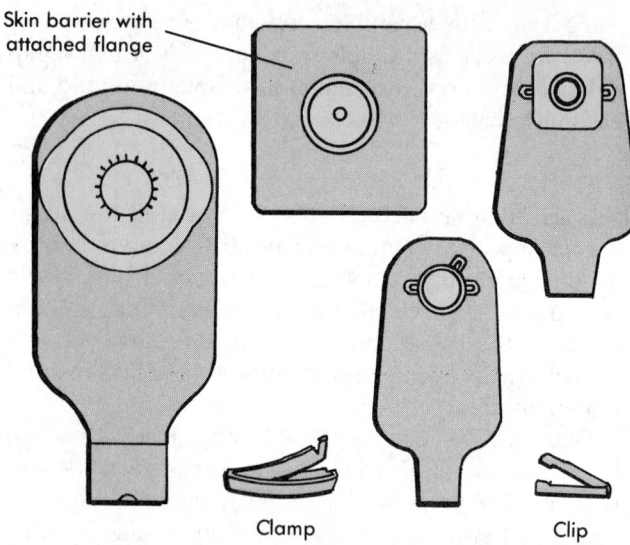

FIGURE 44-20 Drainable pouches.

Interventions for skin breakdown. If the skin does become irritated, careful and systematic treatment should begin. The use of antacids on the skin should be avoided, since they change the skin pH and may result in a secondary bacterial infection. Also, products containing large quantities of alcohol (for example, benzoin) should be omitted.

Skin barrier powders can be used to help dry moist skin irritations so that a skin barrier wafer and the pouch will adhere to the skin. In many instances, adding the powder and/or skin barrier wafer to the skin management system results in rapid improvement of the skin. Severe skin irritations should be treated by the enterostomal therapy nurse or physician.

Selection and Application of Pouches

Pouch selection. The most important phase of nursing care is the careful selection and application of an effective pouching system. An effective pouch system protects the skin, contains the stool and odors, molds to the body contour, allows comfortable bending and movement, and is inconspicuous under clothing. When the pouching system does not work, other processes of rehabilitation are often halted. Patients find it difficult to resume life activities when the pouch leaks constantly.

In an effective pouching system, there is no odor except when emptying. An odor-proof pouch contains the flatus and stool, which is· regularly emptied from the bottom of the pouch. Pinholes in a pouch will destroy the odor-proof quality of the material and should not be used for releasing the gas. Odor is normal when a pouch is emptied. This should be explained so that, as the flatus or stool is released from the pouch, the patient is aware that the odor is controlled at other times. If odor persists, it is usually because the pouch seal is not intact or the opening spout of the pouch has not been cleansed well.

The basic issues of selecting equipment include the type of ostomy; the size and contour of the abdomen; the peristomal skin condition; and the patient's physical and mental status, physical activities, financial situation, and personal preference. Table 44-8 outlines the selection of a pouching system on the basis of the type of ostomy.

Products for ostomy care are available in a variety of styles, shapes, and sizes. Disposable pouches are available in one- and two-piece systems, with skin barriers attached, and in a variety of materials (Figure 44-20). Reusable pouches are those that are worn, cleansed, and worn again. They are also available in one- and two-piece systems in a variety of materials. Pouch covers are available that make the wearing of a pouch more comfortable. Pouch covers can also be made simply and inexpensively. (Figure 44-21).

Pouch application. Once a pouching system (pouch and skin barrier) has been selected, the stoma is carefully measured. Skin barriers should be cut slightly larger than the stoma (3 mm [⅛ inch]). This allows room for the stoma to expand during peristalsis. The pouch opening should be slightly larger than the opening in the skin barrier (see box on the opposite page).

The patient is taught how to measure the stoma, since it will take approximately 6 months to reach "permanent" size. This size, however, can change with increases or decreases in body weight and changes in body contour. By knowing how to measure, the patient can select the correct size of pouches and cut skin barriers accordingly.

Before discharge, the patient needs a temporary supply of pouches and skin barriers, a list of what supplies

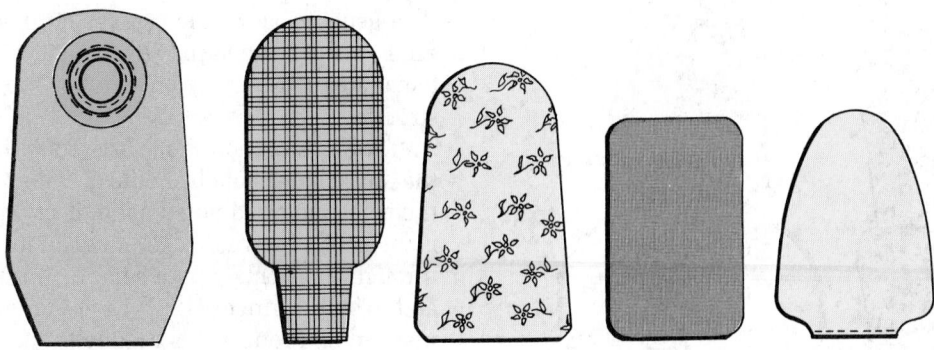

FIGURE 44-21 Pouch covers.

to order, and a list of local surgical supply stores. A prescription for ostomy supplies may be needed for the patient to receive Medicare or insurance reimbursement.

If a person with an ostomy is readmitted, the nurse identifies any assistance needed with ostomy care and maintains the pattern of care that is effectively working.

Diet

Anyone with an ostomy should eat balanced meals at regular intervals and chew foods slowly and thoroughly. Patients need to be informed that certain foods such as seeds, kernels, and other undigested residue will be visible in the stool.

A restricted diet is not required for these persons. However, many patients develop their own food preferences. They should be informed which foods tend to cause gas so that they can avoid these foods as they desire. Some pouches are available with gas relief valves that reduce the gas problem.

Persons with an ileostomy need to avoid high-fiber or high-residue foods for 4 to 6 weeks after surgery. These foods may then be added one at a time in small amounts. If cramping or a problem passing the food occurs, the person should wait a few weeks and try again. If unable to tolerate the food after two or three trials, the person should eliminate it from the diet.

Ileostomy patients must be aware of the potential for a food blockage. This is a large mass of undigested food, especially high-fiber food, that becomes lodged at a narrowing in the bowel and blocks the intestinal lumen. Blockage most commonly occurs when a person eats several high-fiber foods in one meal or does not chew the foods properly. Following ileostomy surgery some persons will discover they can eat only coconut, corn, celery, or Chinese foods in limited amounts.

If the ileostomy becomes blocked, the person should get into a knee-chest position and gently massage the area below the stoma. Stomal edema will develop with a food blockage; the pouch should be changed and the opening enlarged to accommodate the swelling. Diar-

POUCH CHANGE PROCEDURE

PATTERN

1. The pattern should be ⅛ inch larger than the stoma.
2. Always label the pattern for "top" or "skin" side.

SKIN BARRIER

1. Use ¼, ½, or full wafer depending on the size of the stoma and the abdomen.
2. Round the corners to conform to the shape of the adhesive on the pouch.
3. Trace the pattern on the paper side.
4. Cut hole on pattern line; line will not be visible when it is cut.
5. Smooth sides of the opening with finger.

POUCH

1. Pouch opening should be slightly larger than the opening of the skin barrier (paper can cut the stoma).
2. Trace pattern on the paper side of the pouch (use the opening from the skin barrier that has already been cut).
3. Cut the hole larger than the line of the pattern (cut outside the line).
4. The edges around the opening should be smooth.
5. Remove paper backing from the pouch, center the openings, and apply the shiny side of the skin barrier to the pouch.

APPLYING THE SYSTEM

1. Remove the pouch and skin barrier carefully.
2. Cleanse the skin with warm water.
3. Pat the skin dry.
4. Warm the skin barrier (the pouch is already attached).
5. Remove the backing; save this paper, because it can be used as a pattern in the future.
6. Center opening with the stoma; press and seal to the skin; hold hand against the pouch to help seal the skin barrier to the skin.
7. Close the bottom.

From Broadhurst BB and Broadwell DC: Ostomy care for children. Copyright © 1981 by Debra C Broadwell.

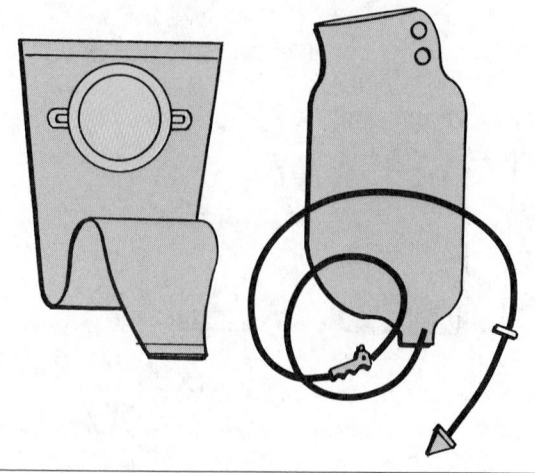

FIGURE 44-22 Colostomy irrigating sleeve and irrigating bag with cone attachment.

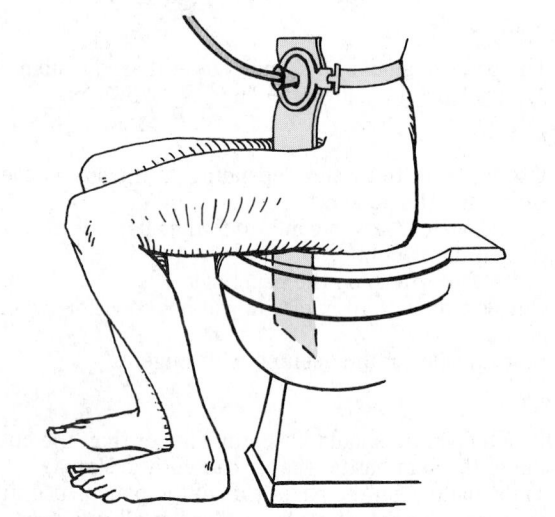

FIGURE 44-23 Colostomy irrigation with person sitting on the toilet; irrigating sleeve drains into the toilet.

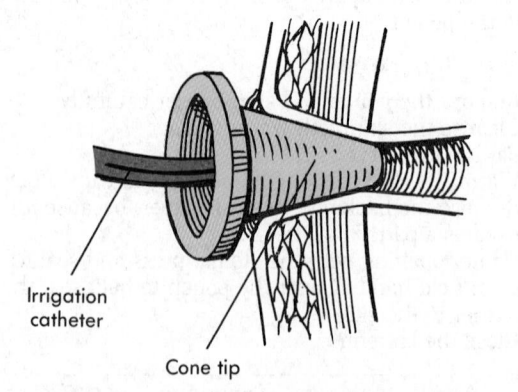

Irrigation catheter

Cone tip

FIGURE 44-24 Cone irrigating tip inserted in the stoma.

rhea usually follows the passage of the obstruction, and fluids must be replaced. Abdominal pain in the peristomal area is generally present for 3 to 5 days after obstruction.

If the obstruction is not passed within a few hours, the physician should be notified. It may be necessary for the person to be admitted for an ileostomy lavage, which is the gentle insertion of 30 ml to 50 ml of normal saline through the stoma with a small 14 Fr or 16 Fr catheter and a bulb syringe. Careful measurement of the fluid inserted and returned is required. This procedure is repeated until the obstruction is released. If the patient has had the food blockage for a long time, nasogastric suctioning and intravenous fluids may be required.

Colostomy Irrigation

Persons with sigmoid or descending colostomies may decide to manage the colostomy with regular irrigations. A colostomy irrigation is an enema given through the stoma for the purpose of stimulating the bowel to empty at a convenient and regular time. A patient who is free of stool between irrigations can wear a closed-end pouch with a gas relief valve or a stoma "cap," a small adhesive square pouch with an absorbent dressing. The stoma will continue to secrete mucus and expel flatus, so an ostomy covering with a gas filter is desirable.

The decision to irrigate a colostomy should take into consideration the following factors: whether the colostomy is temporary or permanent, the length of bowel above the colostomy, stomal complications, personal preference of the patient, and physical and mental status of the patient. Persons who respond unfavorably to colostomy irrigation include those who respond to stress with diarrhea, have had radiation therapy, have a poor prognosis, have a previous history of inflammatory bowel disease or radiation enteritis, or have a peristomal hernia.

Persons who have irrigated their colostomies successfully for years may develop irregular results with irrigation secondary to aging. As one ages, there is a decrease in mucus production and peristalsis. This is often frustrating for persons who may feel they have failed, because the elimination pattern is unpredictable.

Various types of commercial irrigation sets are available, and they all require similar supplies: an irrigation sleeve (Figure 44-22) which fits over the stoma and is long enough to drain into the toilet (Figure 44-23); a cone tip for the insertion of water into the stoma; an enema bag to contain the solution; and clips to close the top and bottom of the sleeve. A cone is used almost universally for insertion of the irrigation solution (Figure 44-24). Bowel perforations of the colon during colostomy irrigations are rarely seen because of the advancements of the cone.

When they are prescribed, irrigations are begun after

TABLE 44-9 General guidelines and tips for colostomy irrigation procedure

Guidelines	Tips
Assemble all equipment.	Try to keep all equipment together to facilitate daily routine.
Water container and water	
Irrigating sleeve and belt	
Items to clean skin and stoma	
Way to dispose of old pouch	
Clean, prepared pouch to reapply	
Skin-care items	
Remove old pouch and dispose of it.	Plastic bag is odor proof and handy to put pouch in.
Clean skin and stoma with water; let dry (NOTE: Observe condition and color of skin and stoma.	May use washcloth, toilet paper, or tissue.
Apply irrigating sleeve and belt securely (not too tight) (NOTE: If using karaya washer, dampen and apply this first).	Sleeve should be long enough to reach toilet; excess may be cut off.
Fill irrigating container with about 1 quart tepid water when ready to begin. (NOTE: Hot water traumatizes [burns] bowel and cold water causes cramping).	
Suspend irrigating container so bottom of container is even with top of shoulder. (NOTE: At lower height, water may not flow easily, and higher height will give too much force to water and cause cramping or incomplete results.)	Hang container on side of dominant hand; it will drape easily and be more manageable; hook or coat hanger can be used to get proper height.
Remove air from tubing (NOTE: This helps prevent air from increasing gas pains).	Do not use large amount of irrigating water, or irrigation container will need to be refilled.
Gently insert irrigating cone into stoma, holding it parallel to floor; start water slowly. NOTE: If water does not flow easily, try or check following:	Cone should fit snugly enough to block water in bowel; do *not* try to force it.
Slightly change position or angle of cone	Cone opening may be blocked by loop of bowel.
Check for kinks in tubing from irrigating container	
Check height of irrigating container	
Have patient take deep breaths	Deep breaths will relax abdominal muscles.
Stool immediately under skin level may be slightly hard and blocking water flow; instill *small* amount of water to loosen it.	Introduce water at slow rate, so it can penetrate behind stool and propel it out; fast rate of flow will spill out as it meets resistance of stool.
Water for irrigations will vary.	
People vary in amount of water they can hold at one time; some can take all at once, and others can tolerate small amount at one time.	Use approximately 500 ml for first irrigation and increase by 250 ml until 1000 ml (1 quart) of irrigation is reached.
Amount of water used can vary daily.	
Cleanse as much of fecal matter out as possible without making patient uncomfortable.	Ask patient to identify "full" feeling or need to expel stool.
Do *not* force water into bowel if (1) cramping occurs, (2) flow of water stops, or (3) water is forcefully returning around irrigating cone or catheter. Stop flow of water.	
If patient complains of feeling bloated or constipated, irrigate with additional 500 ml of water in same day or provide mild laxative.	People who have always had problems with constipation will continue to have; diet (fruits), high fluid intake, stool softeners, or laxatives may be used.
Majority of stool will return in about 15 minutes.	Patient should remain seated on toilet.
When most of stool has been expelled, rinse sleeve with water, dry bottom edge, roll out, close up end, and encourage activities for about 30-45 minutes to allow bowel adequate time to finish emptying.	Activity will stimulate peristalsis and allow for thorough results.
When irrigation is complete, assemble and apply clean pouch and skin barrier.	
Rinse out irrigation sleeve, hang it up to dry, and put away other equipment.	Rinse out with warm water to decrease odor; water may be run through sleeve by using irrigation container and tubing; sleeve could also be sprayed with cleansers (Peri-Wash or Uni-Wash) that help stool slide through sleeve, make cleaning easier, and decrease odor.
Check supplies and reorder as necessary.	Do not wait until supplies are depleted to reorder; it will take time for them to come.
Try to irrigate within same 2- or 3-hour period each day so patient can become regulated; if possible, try to irrigate close to time bowels moved before surgery.	

From Broadwell DC and Sorrells SL: Summary of your colostomy care. Copyright © 1976 by Debra C Broadwell.

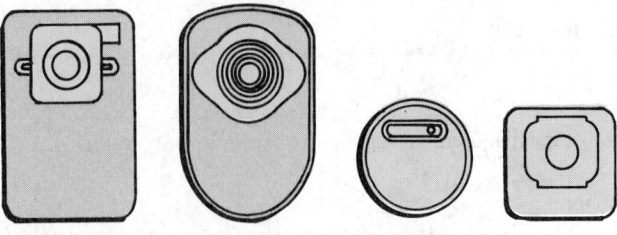

FIGURE 44-25 Closed end pouches and patches for regulated colostomies.

the bowel has begun to function and the stool is beginning to become soft, usually around the seventh day following surgery. The procedure is described in Table 44-9. Preferably, it is taught in the bathroom where the patient can either sit on the commode or on a chair (with a pillow) facing the commode. Once the perineal wound heals, the patient usually sits on the commode.

Cramping during an irrigation may be caused from inserting water too rapidly, from peristalsis, or from water that is too cold. The instillation of water should be stopped until the cramping subsides. When the irrigation is completed, a pouch is applied (Figure 44-25).

Activity

For persons whose condition warrants it, optimal recovery is achieved within 3 months, and they can return to their normal activities, including work. During the postoperative period, patients are usually first concerned about bathing and clothing. Most pouches hold very well in baths or showers. Once the incision(s) is healed, normal bathing habits can be resumed. Patients are informed that regular clothing can be worn. The only exceptions are the wearing of *tight* belts or restrictive waist bands directly over the stoma.

The person may participate in sports, although it is advisable to avoid direct-contact sports such as football. People find ways to return to those activities they enjoy. A young man who played professional football before surgery was able to return to professional football by playing a limited contact position as a placekicker. Swimming, playing tennis, and participating in planned exercise programs are all possible. The person is encouraged to socialize and continue those activities that resulted in satisfaction before the surgery (see the research box). No one knows who has an ostomy unless they are informed. Proper pouching systems are not evident.

For *traveling*, ostomy supplies should be carried by hand on airplanes or trains (rather than checked through with luggage) to facilitate maintenance of regimens if luggage should become delayed or misplaced. Plastic bags are useful for disposal of used supplies. Extra supplies should be taken for unanticipated events re-

RESEARCH

Kelman G and Minkler P: An investigation of quality of life and self-esteem among individuals with ostomies, J Enterost Ther 16:4-11, 1989.

In this study 50 persons who returned questionnaires made up the sample. Most (62%) had their ostomies for 5 years or longer. The subjects completed a demographic questionaire, a Quality of Life Index, and Morris Rosenberg's Self-Esteem Scale. The data indicated a significant relationship between self-esteem and quality of life. Mean scores on the self-esteem scale and the quality of life index indicated that most persons in the study had a positive outlook toward the ostomy and its management. ∎

quiring extra days or increased use. Eating moderately and using restraint when eating different foods are suggested. The person with an ostomy needs to be especially careful about water intake, particularly when traveling in areas where "traveler's" diarrhea is a high risk. A physician needs to be consulted if diarrhea develops that cannot be controlled.

Sexuality

The patient is provided with opportunities to ask questions regarding the return to normal sexual functioning. Many persons will not verbalize their concerns about sexuality so that a deliberate meeting must be planned to facilitate expression of these concerns. Arrangements can be made, if desired by the patient, for the significant other to be present when a frank discussion of sexual functioning is carried out by the nurse or physician. The patient and sexual partner can be assisted to consider sexual positions that may be more facilitating and less problematic if a pouch is worn. The pouch is emptied prior to sexual activity, and in some instances can be switched to a smaller pouch or covered with a pouch cover. A binder or special underwear can be used to hold the pouch in place.

About 15% of male ostomates have decreased sexual activity that may be related either to nerve injury or to psychologic reasons. Counseling may be helpful if nerve injury is not present and sexual difficulties are being experienced. A penile prosthesis may be an option for the male with nerve damage. Females have a decreased incidence of nerve injury because of the larger pelvis. Ostomy surgery does not interfere with contraception, pregnancy, or delivery; and pregnancy seldom produces complications with stoma care. A pamphlet entitled *Sex and the Ostomate* is available from the United Ostomy Association.*

---

*United Ostomy Association, Inc., 36 Executive Park, Suite 120, Irvine, CA 92714.

RESEARCH

Trainor MA: Acceptance of ostomy and the visitor role in a self-help group for ostomy patients, Nurs Res 31:102-106, 1982.

The purpose of this study was to determine whether members of the ostomy association who visited persons with new ostomies had a greater level of acceptance of the ostomy than ostomy club members who did not make visits. The effects that length of time (1) since surgery and (2) as a visitor had on the acceptance of the ostomy were also studied.

The sample consisted of 318 United Ostomy Association members. Of this sample, 54% were visitors and 46% were nonvisitors. The subjects filled out a personal information sheet as well as Linkowski's Acceptance of Disability Scale (the term "ostomy" was used in place of "disability.")

The results indicated that the ostomy visitors showed a greater level of acceptance of the ostomy than nonvisitors. The length of time as a visitor also affected acceptance. Time since surgery did not significantly affect acceptance in this sample. ■

Community Resources

During and after hospitalization, the patient and significant others have additional resources available to help them adapt to and cope with the ostomy. A representative from the local chapter of the United Ostomy Association can be requested to visit the patient either preoperatively or postoperatively. This visitor can share how he or she has learned to live well with the ostomy. The patient may wish to become a member and through meetings learn how others in the community are effectively dealing with the ostomy (see the research box above).

The enterostomal therapy nurse should be consulted preoperatively (if available) and can then coordinate instruction postoperatively. The social worker, clinical nurse specialist, dietitian, and clergy are consulted as needed.

In certain locations, the American Cancer Society will assist with providing ostomy supplies to persons with financial need. They also can provide assistance with information about home supplies, medications, and transportation.

Complications

Before hospital discharge, the patient or significant other is taught what to observe when changing the pouch and when to call the physician or enterostomal therapy nurse (see the box above right). Each time the pouch is changed, the patient should observe the color and shape of the stoma and the condition of the skin. Dramatic changes in stoma color, shape, or function, or bleeding from the stoma should be reported at once to

PATIENT REQUIREMENTS BEFORE DISCHARGE

1. Written information about the ostomy
2. Written instructions for application of the pouch
3. A list of supplies to order
4. A temporary supply of items needed for pouch changes
5. A measuring guide and instructions for determining the size of pouches to order
6. List of surgical supply stores in the area
7. Information about the United Ostomy Association and the local chapter
8. Phone numbers of the primary nurse, the enterostomal therapy nurse, the physician, and the visiting nurse service

the physician. Changes in function include prolonged diarrhea or constipation. An enterostomal therapy nurse should be consulted for pouching or skin problems.

Complications that may occur with an ostomy include narrowing or stricture of the stoma opening, prolapse of the stoma, peristomal hernia, lacerations of the stoma because of poorly fitting equipment, and recurrence of disease such as tumor or Crohn's disease.

CLOSURE OF THE COLOSTOMY

If the colostomy was performed to relieve obstruction or to divert the fecal stream to permit healing, the person will be readmitted to the hospital at a later date for a further examination and for possible resection of any diseased portion of the bowel. The ostomy may subsequently be closed.

In preparation for a resection of the bowel and closure of the colostomy, the physician may order irrigations of the colostomy, and probably both openings of a loop colostomy. Fluid, usually normal saline solution, is instilled into each opening through a catheter or cone. For this irrigation, the patient should sit on the bedpan or on the toilet. Unless there is complete obstruction, the solution into the distal loop will be expelled through the rectum. Mucus and shreds of necrotic tissue may be passed. The returns should be inspected before being discarded.

CHAPTER SUMMARY

✔ Common bowel dysfunctions include constipation, diarrhea, flatulence, and fecal incontinence.

✔ Pain from acute appendicitis may be localized at McBurney's point. Heat and laxatives are avoided preoperatively since they may precipitate appendiceal rupture.

✔ Peritonitis is an inflammation of the peritoneum from trauma or rupture of an organ. Loss of fluids into the peritoneal cavity leads to dehydration and shock; peristalsis may cease. Treatment consists of fluid replacement and antibiotic therapy; surgery may be necessary.

✓ Ulcerative colitis affects primarily the left colon with a continuous area of mucosal involvement; the liquid stools contain blood but no fat. Crohn's disease affects segmental areas of the ileum, cecum, and right colon, and involves submucosal layers; the frequent semisoft stools contain fat but no blood.

✓ Care of the person with ulcerative colitis or Crohn's disease includes a low-residue, high-protein, high-calorie diet, medications (corticosteroids, sulfasalazine), comfort measures to protect skin following diarrhea; facilitation of coping with life stresses, and promotion of sexuality.

✓ Surgery may be curative for ulcerative colitis but not for Crohn's disease; however, surgery to relieve obstruction or to evacuate fistulas may be life-saving for the patient with Crohn's disease.

✓ Diverticular disease involves outpouching of the colon wall; diverticulitis is the inflammatory condition, diverticulosis the quiescent phase. A high-fiber diet is encouraged to increase bowel transit time and stool bulk for diverticulosis.

✓ Inflammatory anorectal lesions include anal fissures, anal abscesses, and anal fistulas; hemorrhoids are varicose veins of the rectum. Relief of discomfort from anal lesions may include measures to prevent constipation (which irritates the lesions) and sitz baths.

✓ Care following anorectal surgery includes giving prescribed analgesics and sitz baths for comfort, stool softeners to promote early defecation with less trauma, and teaching the patient measures to prevent constipation.

✓ Amebiasis is an intestinal infection by a protozoan parasite, primarily ingested from fecally contaminated food or water. Treatment is by an amebicide such as metronidazole. The patient is taught measures to prevent reinfection.

✓ Trichinosis is an intestinal infection by a roundworm transmitted primarily by inadequately cooked pork. Encysted larvae develop within the intestinal wall.

✓ Intestinal obstruction may result from inhibition of peristalsis (paralytic ileus) or from mechanical obstruction such as by adhesions, volvulus, intussusception, hernias, or cancer. Large amounts of fluid and electrolytes are lost from the circulation into the intestinal lumen, resulting in fluid and electrolyte imbalances and finally shock. Therapy consists of inserting an NG tube, restricting oral intake, and removing the source of obstruction, if possible.

✓ Bowel infarction may result from interruption of blood flow in the mesenteric blood vessels, leading to interruption of bowel function. Surgery to remove the gangrenous bowel is usually indicated.

✓ Hernias may occur in the inguinal, femoral, or umbilical areas from mural defects or in weakened scars from previous abdominal surgeries. Of concern is the possible entrapment (incarceration) of a loop of bowel. The treatment is surgical repair.

✓ Colon polyps (adenomas) are benign growths that are premalignant; the villous adenomas are more likely than the pedunculated tubular adenomas to become malignant.

✓ Risk factors for bowel cancer (the second most common form of cancer) are age 40 or more; past history of colon polyps, colon cancer, cancer of the reproductive organs, or ulcerative colitis; or a family history of colorectal cancer or polyposis disorder.

✓ Recommendations for early detection of colorectal cancer include a digital rectal examination yearly after age 40; occult blood stool test yearly after age 50; and proctosigmoidoscopy every 3 to 5 years after age 50, following two negative yearly examinations.

✓ Cancers of the ascending colon are of the cauliflower-like mass type, and because the chyme is liquid at that point, there is less probability of obstruction. Cancer of the descending colon is usually characterized by an anular lesion, which may narrow the lumen and obstruct the more solid feces.

✓ Half of the colorectal cancers occur in the sigmoid and rectum.

✓ Surgery for cancer of the colon and upper rectum usually consists of resection with anastomosis; surgery for the lower rectum consists of an abdominoperineal resection with a colostomy.

✓ Care of the patient following bowel surgery includes breathing exercises to promote oxygenation, ensuring adequate fluid intake, monitoring for return of peristalsis, giving analgesics for pain, and teaching to avoid constipation and laxative use.

✓ Care of the patient following abdominoperineal resection includes monitoring for shock, hemorrhage, and pulmonary embolus; providing wound care and stoma care; providing sitz baths; promoting urinary elimination; and promoting comfort by positioning, foam pads for sitting, and analgesics.

✓ Types of stomas include end stoma (end of bowel brought out abdominal wall to form a single stoma), loop stoma (loop of bowel brought out abdominal wall and opened to create one stoma with two openings), and loop-end stoma (end of bowel oversewn and stoma made from intestinal loop close to end).

✓ Care of a person with a colostomy or ileostomy includes preparing the person for the surgery, monitoring the stoma, assessing readiness of the person to view the stoma, promoting acceptance of body changes, teaching the person stoma care, and informing the person of community support services.

✔ Teaching the person with a colostomy includes promoting nutrition and elimination, promoting return to normal activities and sexuality, and preventing complications.

✔ Stoma care includes cleaning of the skin to prevent skin breakdown, early treatment of excoriated skin, and application of pouches to prevent leakage.

✔ Persons with a descending or sigmoid colostomy may be able to regulate elimination by colostomy irrigation.

QUESTIONS TO CONSIDER

■ Compare and contrast ulcerative colitis, Crohn's disease, and diverticular disease.

■ Suppose you have recently been diagnosed as having ulcerative colitis. Your weight is 110 pounds, down from your normal 130 pounds. You have diarrhea about once every hour with occasional leakage. You feel tired and listless and have lost your appetite. What changes would you have to make in your life? What particular concerns do you think you might have? What kind of help would you seek?

■ Compare and contrast small and large bowel obstruction.

■ Obtain a copy of the most recent issue of *Cancer Facts and Figures* from your local chapter of the American Cancer Society. How does the incidence of colorectal cancer compare with other cancers among men and women? What are the recent trends?

■ What resources are available in your community for persons with a colostomy? Where can supplies be purchased? What would be the average monthly cost? Discuss with an enterostomal therapist common problems experienced by persons with ostomies.

REFERENCES AND SELECTED READINGS

1. *Alterescu KV: Colostomy, Nurs Clin North Am 22:281-290, 1987.
2. *Alterescu VA: The ostomy: what do you teach the patient? Am J Nurs 85:1250-1253, 1985.
3. Altman DF: Gastrointestinal diseases in the elderly, Med Clin North Am 67(2):433-444, 1983.
4. American Cancer Society: 1990 Cancer facts and figures, New York, 1989, The Society.
5. American College of Surgeons: Manual of preoperative and postoperative care, ed 3, Philadelphia, 1983, WB Saunders Co.
6. *Bates-Jensen B: Psychological response to illness: exploring two reactions to ostomy surgery, Ostomy/Wound Manage 23(3):24-30, 1989.
7. *Benedict P and Haddad A: Postop teaching for the colostomy patient, RN 52(3):85-90, 1989.
8. Berk JE, editor: Bockus gastroenterology, ed 4, Philadelphia, 1985, WB Saunders Co.
9. Bongiovanni GL: Essentials of clinical gastroenterology, ed 2, New York, 1988, McGraw-Hill Book Co.
10. *Broadwell D: Peristomal skin integrity, Nurs Clin North Am 22:321-332, 1987.
11. Broadwell DC and Jackson BS: Principles of ostomy care, St Louis, 1982, The CV Mosby Co.
12. Burkitt DP: Etiology and prevention of colorectal cancer, Hosp Pract 19(2):67-77, 1984.
13. *Bustin MP and Iber FL: Management of common nonmalignant GI problems in the elderly, Geriatrics 38(3):69-75, 1983.
14. Collins SM: The irritable bowel syndrome, Can Med Assoc J 138:309-316, 1988.
15. Crohn BB, Ginzburg L, and Oppenheimer GD: Regional ileitis: a pathologic and clinical entity, JAMA 251:73-79, 1984.
16. Crooms JW and Kovalcik PJ: Obstructing left-sided colon carcinoma, Am Surg 50:15-19, 1984.
17. *Dobkin KA and Broadwell DC: Nursing considerations for the patient undergoing colostomy surgery, Semin Oncol Nurs 2:249-255, 1986.
18. *Doughty DB: Colorectal cancer: etiology and pathophysiology, Semin Oncol Nurs 2:235-241, 1986.
19. Dozois RR et al: Newer operations for ulcerative colitis and Crohn's disease, Surg Clin North Am 68:1339-1352, 1988.
20. Eastwood GL: GI problems in the elderly, Cancer 39(5):59-82, 1984.
21. *Edwards J and Krause S: Helping the emergency colostomy patient through reality shock, Nursing '87 17(7):63-64, 1987.
22. *Erickson P: Ostomies: the art of pouching, Nurs Clin North Am 22:311-320, 1987.
23. Farraye FA et al: Infectious bowel disease: advances in the management of ulcerative colitis and Crohn's disease, Consultant 28(10):39-47, 1988.
24. Ferguson E Jr: Operations of choice of cancers of the colon and rectum, Am Surg 50:121-127, 1984.
25. *Gillies DA: Body image changes following illness and injury, J Enterost Ther 11:186-189, 1984.
26. *Given B and Simmons S: Gastroenterology in clinical nursing, ed 4, St Louis, 1983, The CV Mosby Co.
27. *Greitzu S: Close up on cancer care: colorectal cancer, when a polyp is more than a polyp, RN 49(9):22-30, 1986.
28. *Grunberg KJ: Sexual rehabilitation of the cancer patient undergoing ostomy surgery, J Enterost Ther 13:148-152, 1986.
29. *Hassey KM: Radiation therapy for rectal cancer and the implications for nursing, Cancer Nurs 10:311-318, 1987.
30. *IAET: Standards of care: patient with colostomy, IAET, 1989, Irvine, Calif.
31. *Jackson BS and Broadwell DC: Ostomy surgery: an overview of historical, current, and future perspectives, Semin Oncol Nurs 2(4):227-2334, 1986.
32. *Joachim G: An update on inflammatory bowel disease, AAOHN 34(4):171-173, 1986.
33. *Joachim G et al: Inflammatory bowel disease: effects on lifestyle, J Adv Nurs 12:483-487, 1987.
34. Kaye D and Rose LF: Fundamentals of internal medicine, St Louis, 1983, The CV Mosby Co.

*References preceded by an asterisk are particularly well suited for student reading.

35. Kelman G and Minkler P: An investigation of quality of life and self-esteem among individuals with ostomies, J Enterost Ther 16:4-11, 1989.

36. *Khan AH: Colorectal carcinoma: risk factors, screening, early detection, Geriatrics 39(1):42-48, 1984.

37. *Kinash RG: Inflammatory bowel disease: implications for patients, challenges for nurses, Rehab Nurs 12:82-89, 1987.

38. Logan RF et al: Smoking and ulcerative colitis, Br Med J 288:751-753, 1984.

39. *McConnell EA: Meeting the challenge of intestinal obstruction, Nursing '87 17(7):34-41, 1987.

40. McLeod RS and Fazio VW: The continent ileostomy: an acceptable alternative, J Enterost Ther 11:140-146, 1984.

41. Mendeloff AI: Diet and colorectal cancer, Am J Clin Nut 48:780-781, 1988.

42. *Messner RL, Gardner SS, and Webb DD: Early detection: the priority of colorectal cancer, Cancer Nurs 9(1):8-14, 1986.

43. *Metheny NM: Fluid and electrolyte balance: nursing considerations, Philadelphia, 1987, JB Lippincott Co.

44. *Myer SA: Overview of inflammatory bowel disease, Nurs Clin North Am 19(1):3-10, 1984.

45. Neilan BA: Colorectal cancer, Clin Geriatr Med 3:625-635, 1987.

46. *Neufeldt J: Helping the inflammatory bowel disease patient cope with the unpredictable, Nursing '87 17(8):47-49, 1987.

47. Nord HJ: Complications of inflammatory bowel disease, Hosp Pract 22(11):65-72, 1987.

48. Porter JA et al: Complications of colostomy, Dis Colon Rectum 32:299-303, 1989.

49. Postier RG, O'Malley V, and Pruitt L: Continence-preserving operations for ulcerative colitis and multiple polyposis, J Enterost Ther 11:237-239, 1984.

50. Price SA and Wilson LM: Pathophysiology: clinical concepts of disease processes, ed 3, New York, 986, McGraw-Hill Inc.

51. *Rideout BW: The patient with an ileostomy: nursing management and patient education, Nurs Clin North Am 22(2):253-262, 1987.

52. *Rubin DM: New hope for colitis patients, AORN J 38:783-793, 1983.

53. Schroeder SA et al: Current medical diagnosis & treatment, Norwalk, Conn, 1989, Appleton & Lange.

54. *Shipes E: Psychosocial issues: the person with an ostomy, Nurs Clin North Am 22:291-302, 1987.

55. *Simmons MA: Using the nursing process in treating inflammatory bowel disease, Nurs Clin North Am 19(1):11-26, 1984.

56. Sleisinger M and Fordtran JS: Gastrointestinal disease: pathophysiology, diagnosis, and management, ed 4, Philadelphia, 1988, WB Saunders Co.

57. *Smith DB: The ostomy: how is it managed? Am J Nurs 85:1246-1249, 1985.

58. Smith LE: Surgical therapy in ulcerative colitis, Gastroenterol Clin North Am 18(1):99-110, 1989.

59. Steiner R, Banks PA, and Present DH: People, not patients: a source book for living with inflammatory bowel disease, New York, 1985, National Foundation for Ileitis and Colitis, Inc.

60. *Stotts NA, Fitzgerald KA, and Williams KR: Care of the patient critically ill with inflammatory bowel disease, Nurs Clin North Am 19(1):61-70, 1984.

61. Turnball GB: Dealing with sexuality after ostomy surgery, Progressions 1(1):15-18, 1989.

62. Watne AL, Boyd JB, and Bradford B: The elderly patient and colon surgery for cancer or diverticular disease, Am Surg 50:460-464, 1984.

63. *Watson PG: Meeting the needs of patients undergoing ostomy surgery, J Enterost Ther 12:121-124, 1985.

64. *Watts RC: The ostomy: how is it created? Am J Nurs 85:1242-1243, 1985.

65. Way LW: Current surgical diagnosis and treatment, ed 8, Norwalk, Conn, 1988, Appleton & Lange.

66. *Wicks LJ: Treatment modalities for colorectal cancer, Semin Oncol Nurs 2:242-248, 1986.

67. *Wilson C: The diagnostic work-up for the patient with inflammatory bowel disease, Nurs Clin North Am 19(1):51-60, 1984.

68. *Witt ME et al: Adjuvant radiotherapy to the colorectum: nursing implications, Oncol Nurs Forum 14(3):17-21, 1987.

69. Wyngaarden JB and Smith LH: Cecil textbook of medicine, ed 18, Philadelphia, 1988, WB Saunders Co.

70. *Young ME and Flynn KT: Third-spacing: when the body conceals fluid, RN 51(8): 46-68, 1988.

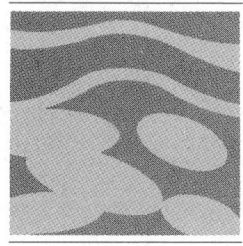

CHAPTER 45

Assessment of the Gallbladder and Exocrine Pancreas

VIRGINIA L. CASSMEYER

CHAPTER OBJECTIVES

After studying this chapter, the student should be able to:
1 Describe the basic anatomy of the gallbladder and pancreas.
2 List the stimuli for bile secretions.
3 List the stimuli for pancreatic enzyme and pancreatic electrolyte secretions.
4 Describe the functions of bile and pancreatic secretions in digestion and absorption.
5 Identify history data indicating gallbladder or exocrine pancreatic dysfunction.
6 Describe the various diagnostic tests used to identify pathophysiologic conditions of the gallbladder, the biliary ductal system, and the exocrine pancreas.
7 Develop a plan of care for the patient with a suspected gallbladder or exocrine pancreatic problem that focuses on the patient's needs in preparation for and after the various diagnostic tests.

The gallbladder and its associated ductal system and the exocrine pancreas are accessory organs of the gastrointestinal tract. Secretions essential to digestion and absorption of nutrients are supplied by the gallbladder and biliary system and the exocrine pancreas.

ANATOMY AND PHYSIOLOGY

GALLBLADDER AND BILIARY DUCTAL SYSTEM

The gallbladder and biliary ductal system are diagrammed in Figure 45-1.

The gallbladder is a pear-shaped organ that lies on the inferior surface of the liver. It is composed of serous, muscular, and mucous coats and has a usual capacity of 50 ml, although it can increase in size under normal conditions. The gallbladder is supplied by the superior and inferior cystic arteries, which originate from the hepatic artery. The venous blood leaves the gallbladder by superficial veins that empty into the liver. The gallbladder has a very good lymphatic system. Innervation of the gallbladder is from the parasympathetic and sympathetic nervous system.

The biliary ductal system consists of the hepatic duct, the cystic duct, and the common bile duct. The gallbladder is connected to the biliary ductal system by the cystic duct. The biliary ductal system is also innervated by the parasympathetic and sympathetic nervous systems.

The major function of the gallbladder is to concentrate and store bile. Bile, formed in the liver, is excreted into the hepatic duct and then passes through the cystic duct into the gallbladder. Here bile is concentrated fivefold to tenfold. The mucosa layer lies in multiple, irregular folds, which increase the absorptive capacity of the gallbladder appreciably. The biliary duct system provides a passageway for bile to be transported from the liver to the gallbladder or from the liver or gallbladder to the gastrointestinal tract. It is important to note that bile can be released directly from the liver; thus the gallbladder is not necessary for life.

Bile is primarily water (97%) with cholesterol, phospholipids, bile salts, bile pigments (bilirubin and biliverdin), and a small amount of protein and electrolytes. Metabolic end-products from metabolism of such substances as hormones and drugs are excreted in bile.

The release of bile from the gallbladder or liver is controlled by cholecystokinin (CCK), also sometimes referred to as cholecystokinin-pancreozymin. CCK is released from the walls of the duodenal intestinal mucosa when lipids, amino acids, and hydrogen ions enter the duodenum from the stomach. CCK travels by the blood to the gallbladder and causes contraction of the gallbladder's smooth musculature and relaxation of the spincter at the end of the common bile duct (the spincter of oddi). Parasympathetic stimulation, as well as other intestinal hormones (secretin, gastrin, glucagon, and vasoactive intestinal peptide), causes the same responses.

Gallbladder contraction and the simultaneous relaxation of the spincter of oddi allow bile to enter the duodenum and participate in digestive and absorptive processes. Bile salts are necessary for the absorption of lip-

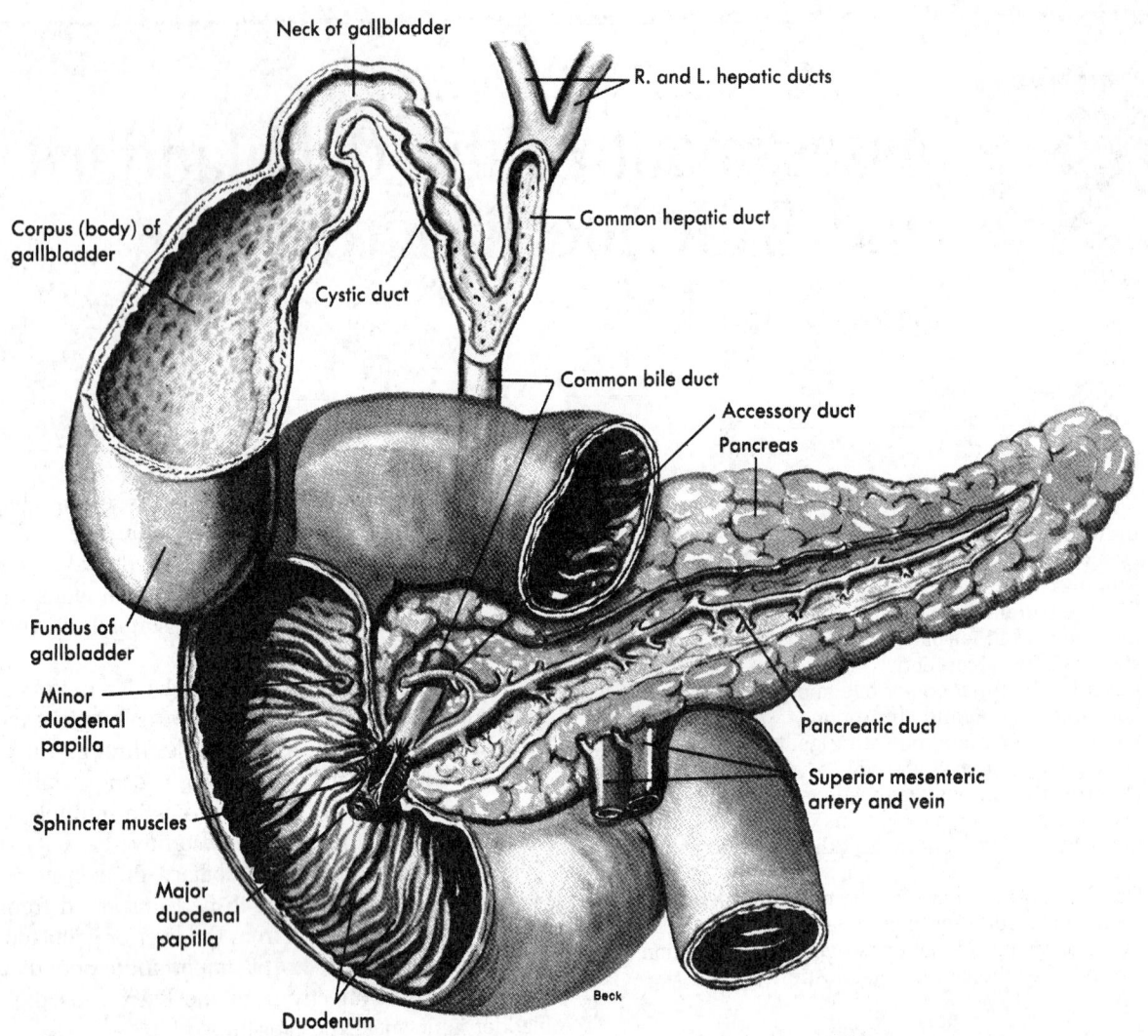

Neck of gallbladder

R. and L. hepatic ducts

Common hepatic duct

Corpus (body) of gallbladder

Cystic duct

Common bile duct

Accessory duct

Pancreas

Fundus of gallbladder

Minor duodenal papilla

Pancreatic duct

Sphincter muscles

Superior mesenteric artery and vein

Major duodenal papilla

Duodenum

Beck

FIGURE 45-1 Anatomic schemata of biliary and pancreatic ductal systems. Note head of pancreas surrounds common bile duct. (From Anthony CP and Thibodeau GA: Textbook of anatomy and physiology, ed 12, St Louis, 1987, The CV Mosby Co.)

ids and other fat substances. Bile salts facilitate fat digestion by emulsifying fats for action by intestinal lipases and facilitate the absorption of fats, fat-soluble vitamins, and cholesterol.

Most of the bile salts that are secreted into the duodenum are absorbed into the enterohepatic circulation by passive processes throughout the intestinal tract or by active reabsorption in the terminal ileum, returned to the liver, and then recirculated. Bile salts are recirculated six to nine times a day (two to three times per meal). Most of the bile salts are reabsorbed from the small intestines; the bile salts that enters the colon are acted upon by bacterial enzymes and partially deconjugated so that reabsorption can occur. The reabsorption from the intestinal tract is so efficient that only 15% to 25% of the bile salt pool has to be replaced per day. This

recirculation is necessary for the maintenance of an adequate amount of bile salts for fat digestion and absorption. Disease of the terminal ileum or disturbances in the enterohepatic circulation of bile salts, both of which can interfere with the recirculation of bile, can result in problems with fat absorption.

PANCREAS

The pancreas is an elongated, flattened organ located in the posterior abdomen with its head lying within the curvature of the duodenum and its tail resting against the spleen (Figure 45-1). The pancreas has both exocrine and endocrine functions. The exocrine functions are carried out by the acinar cells and duct system, and the endocrine functions are carried out by islets of Langerhans cells. This chapter focuses on the exocrine

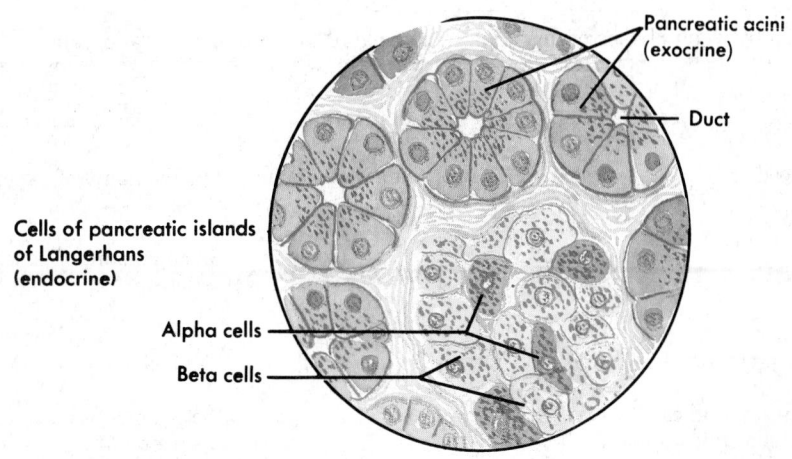

FIGURE 45-2 Exocrine pancreatic cells surrounding ductule. Note the interspersed endocrine cells. (From Thibodeau GA: Anthony's textbook of anatomy and physiology, ed 13, St Louis, 1990, The CV Mosby Co.)

functions. The pancreas receives arterial blood from the superior and inferior pancreaticoduodenal arteries and from branches of the splenic vein or the portal vein. The pancreas has an abundant lymphatic system and is innervated by the parasympathetic and sympathetic nervous systems. The parasympathetic nervous system is involved in the control of pancreatic exocrine secretions, and the sympathetic nervous system is involved in the control of blood flow.

The pancreas is divided into lobules. Individual lobules are groups of acini that drain into ductules. The ductules merge to form intralobular ducts that merge to form interlobular ducts. The interlobular ducts merge to form the main pancreatic duct (duct of Wirsung). In most persons the duct of Wirsung merges with the common bile duct and enters the duodenum at the ampulla of Vater. The spincter of Oddi controls the opening to these two merged ducts and prevents reflux from the duodenum. In most persons there is an accessory pancreatic duct that has a separate opening into the duodenum (lesser duodenal papilla). Interspersed between acini are the islets of Langerhans or endocrine cells (Figure 45-2).

The exocrine pancreas produces approximately 2000 ml of secretions daily. Two types of secretions are produced. One is an isoosmolar electrolyte solution with a high concentration of bicarbonate that is secreted by the

ductal epithelial cells. The other is rich in digestive enzymes (see the box below) and is secreted by the acinar cells.

The proteolytic enzymes are synthesized and secreted as inactive precursors to prevent autodigestion. After being released into the duodenum, trypsinogen is converted by enterokinase to trypsin. Once activated, trypsin can activate more trypsinogen and the other proteolytic enzymes. The pancreatic juices and pancreas also contain protease inhibitors, which provide additional protection against autodigestion.

Pancreatic secretions are primarily controlled by the hormones released from the duodenum during the intestinal phase of digestion. But the parasympathetic nervous system, which is stimulated during the cephalic and gastric phase of digestion and gastrin, which is released during the gastric phase of digestion, can stimulate release of pancreatic secretions. In Table 45-1, the phases of digestion are related to the hormonal or nervous stimuli and then to the types of pancreatic secretion released.

PHYSIOLOGIC CHANGES WITH AGING

The gallbladder and ductal system do not show changes with aging. The composition of bile has been shown to be increasingly lithogenic, which may be related to an increase in biliary cholesterol.[9] Cholelithiasis and cholecystitis increase in the aged. The pancreas shows anatomic and physiologic changes with aging. Ductal hyperplasia and fibrosis occur. These anatomic changes are not always associated with altered physiologic function, although the volume of stimulated pancreatic secretion decreases after age 40 and the enzyme output and the activity of lipase decrease.[9] One last change in pancreatic function noted in the elderly is an increase in pancreatitis following surgery.[7]

PANCREATIC ENZYMES

Proteolytic	Trypsinogen, chymotrypsinogen, procarboxypeptidase
Amylotic	Amylase
Lipolytic	Lipases
Nucleolytic	Ribonuclease, deoxribonuclease

TABLE 45-1 Relationship between phases of digestion, hormonal or nervous stimuli, and pancreatic secretions

Phase of Digestion	Hormonal or Nervous Stimuli	Type of Pancreatic Secretions
Cephalic Phase		
See, smell, taste, chew food	Vagal stimulation (parasympathetic)	Small amount of pancreatic enzyme secretions
Gastric Phase		
Food in stomach	Gastrin release	Small amount of pancreatic enzyme secretions
Distention of stomach		
Vagal stimulation		
Intestinal Phase		
Distention of intestine or protein in duodenum	Intestinal gastrin	Pancreatic enzyme-rich secretion
Amino acids in intestines, fat in intestines, hydrogen ions in intestines	Cholecystokinin	Large amount of pancreatic enzyme-rich secretion
Hydrogen ion in intestines	Secretin	Large amount of bicarbonate-rich secretion

SUBJECTIVE DATA

A thorough history is necessary to adequately assess the health status of persons with potential dysfunction of the gallbladder and biliary ductal system or the exocrine pancreas. These data assist in identifying immediate nursing needs and provide information necessary for assisting patients to live with chronic problems. The assessment focuses on comfort status, nutritional status, fluid and electrolyte status, elimination patterns, and presence of fatigue or weakness.

COMFORT STATUS

Discomfort resulting from pain or *pruritus* (itching) may be one of the major problems of persons with gallbladder and biliary ductal system dysfunction or pancreatic problems. Persons with gallbladder and biliary ductal system dysfunction often have very significant pain. The pain may be continuous or associated with meals. It may be colicky in nature. It is usually localized to the upper right quadrant and sometimes radiates to the subscapular shoulder area. In the presence of pancreatic problems, pain is also very significant. At first it may be localized to the epigastrium or to the right or left quadrant, but eventually it becomes diffuse. It may also be associated with food or alcohol intake. The patient must be asked about onset, precipitating factors, location, quality, associated symptoms, and relief measures.

If jaundice (yellow discoloration of skin, sclera, and excretions due to deposition of bile pigments associated with elevated serum bilirubin) is present, pruritus or itching, which is caused by jaundice, may cause significant discomfort. The patient must be asked about the presence of pruritus and measures that help to relieve it.

NUTRITIONAL STATUS

Persons with gallbladder and biliary ductal system dysfunctions and exocrine pancreatic problems frequently experience anorexia, nausea, and vomiting. They may also lose weight. Chronic problems may require treatment with a special diet. When the history is taken, both the quality and quantity of food intake should be evaluated. The person's normal daily food intake, food intolerances, and food preferences should be ascertained. A 24-hour diet recall is one way to assess food intake. The nutritional assessment should also focus on the use of alcohol and coffee. Questions about alcohol use, if necessary, may be very threatening and may be best assessed after the nurse-patient relationship has been established.

FLUID AND ELECTROLYTE STATUS

Because of the nausea and vomiting associated with pathologic conditions of the gallbladder and biliary ductal system or pancreatic problems, and because bleeding may occur with *acute pancreatitis,* it is very important to assess the patient's fluid and electrolyte status. The history should include information about the patient's usual intake and output. It is important to record any history of abnormal losses. Symptoms of fluid deficit such as complaints of weakness, weight loss, syncope, and dizziness should be assessed.

ELIMINATION PATTERNS

Intestinal and urinary elimination may be altered in persons with gallbladder and biliary ductal system problems or pancreatic problems. If biliary obstruction is present the patient may give a history of clay-colored (grayish) stools or dark (amber-colored) urine. When fat absorption is abnormal, as can occur with biliary obstruction or pancreatitis, *steatorrhea* (bulky, foul, fatty stools) may occur. The fluid deficit that may occur with acute gallbladder and pancreatic problems may result in a decrease in urine output.

FATIGUE AND WEAKNESS

Because of inadequate nutrient intake, abnormal fluid and electrolyte status, or increased metabolic needs, persons with gallbladder and biliary ductal system problems or pancreatic problems often complain of weakness, fatigue, or lassitude. Although these complaints may be present in a variety of situations, it is important to assess whether they are present in persons with gallbladder or pancreatic problems so that complete nursing care can be provided. Although these complaints may resolve as the underlying problem is controlled, the patient and significant others must understand that resolution of the problem will usually take time (in some cases, up to 8 weeks after effective treatment).

OBJECTIVE DATA

To completely assess the functioning of the gallbladder and biliary ductal system or the pancreas, a thorough assessment of the total body is required. Particular attention should be directed to (1) assessing vascular volume, (2) observing for characteristic signs of dysfunction, and (3) examining the abdomen.

In acute gallbladder and biliary ductal system dysfunction or pancreatic problems the vascular volume is assessed for signs of insufficiency. Vital signs including orthostatic changes, temperature and moisture of the skin, skin turgor, mucous membrane moisture, and behavior are evaluated immediately. Decreased blood pressure; elevated pulse, respiration, and temperature; dry skin; poor skin turgor; dry mucous membranes; restlessness; and complaints of thirst are signs of vascular volume deficit.

INSPECTION

After the vascular volume is assessed, the patient should be inspected for characteristic signs of gallbladder, biliary ductal system and pancreatic dysfunction. During this time, as well as during the taking of the history, the patient's mental status and alertness should be documented. Mental status changes may occur as a result of vascular volume deficit, the use of alcohol or drugs, or because of complications of the dysfunctions. The patient is weighed to determine weight loss or gain. Jaundice, a very common problem in gallbladder, biliary tract, and sometimes pancreatic problems, is also found in hepatic disease and hemolysis. Inspection will incorporate assessment for the presence of jaundice. The presence of jaundice can best be seen in the sclera or on the palms of the hands and soles of the feet. Differeniating between causes of jaundice requires laboratory tests that distinguish changes in different components of bilirubin metabolism. Information pertinent to this discussion is shown in Table 45-1 and in more detail in Chapters 38 and 39. Muscle wasting can accompany chronic pancreatic pathologic conditions, and the status of the muscle mass is evaluated. The abdomen should be inspected for distention, which may be found in gallbladder and pancreatic dysfunction. Abdominal girth is measured to assess for *ascites* (accumulation of fluid in the peritoneal cavity), which can occur with pancreatic dysfunction.

PALPATION AND PERCUSSION

The abdomen must be examined with light and deep palpation to assess for tenderness and guarding. If bowel sounds are to be assessed they should be auscultated before carrying out palpation and percussion. Light and deep palpation will assist in identifying the presence of direct tenderness, guarding, rebound tenderness, or muscular rigidity. These signs may all be present. It is important to note the location of any of them. In chronic pancreatitis, ascites can be present, and palpation to assess for fluid wave as described in Chapter 38 may be necessary.

DIAGNOSTIC TESTS

Various tests will help in assessing the status of the gallbladder and biliary ductal system and the pancreas. Many of the tests require taking samples of blood; other tests are more extensive and may cause discomfort; still others may require fasting. The nurse is responsible for preparing the patient for the tests. The physical preparation of the patient will vary from institution to institution and the nurse will need to learn the routine preparation. In addition to the physical preparation of the patient, the nurse carries out appropriate teaching and monitoring of the patient before, during, and after tests.

LABORATORY TESTS

The common laboratory tests to assess the status of the gallbladder and biliary ductal system are studies of bilirubin metabolism (total, conjugated, and unconjugated bilirubin; urine bilirubin and urobilinogen; and fecal urobilinogen), studies of clotting status (prothrombin time), and alkaline phosphatase. These tests are described in Table 45-2. Bilirubin is excreted in bile and thus obstruction of bile flow will cause abnormal test results of bilirubin metabolism. (The steps in bilirubin metabolism are described in Chapter 38.) If hepatic dysfunction, which can occur with gallbladder problems, is

TABLE 45-2 Laboratory tests of gallbladder and biliary ductal system function

Function and Test	Procedure and Preparation	Interpretation

Bilirubin metabolism
Total bilirubin
  Conjugated (direct)
  Unconjugated (indirect)
	Blood drawn; no special preparation	Total serum bilirubin measures both conjugated and unconjugated bilirubin; normal values range from 0.1-1 mg/100 ml; conjugated bilirubin acts directly with diazo reagents, unconjugated bilirubin requires addition of methyl alcohol; thus the terms *direct* and *indirect;* conjugated bilirubin is increased in presence of obstructive biliary tract disease and hepatocellular disease; unconjugated bilirubin is elevated with increased hemolysis of red blood cells or with hepatocellular disease

Urine bilirubin	Spot urine specimen; no special preparation	Normally no bilirubin is excreted in urine; urine with abnormal bilirubin is mahogany colored and has a yellow foam when shaken (foam test); unconjugated bilirubin even if in excess is not excreted in urine because it is not water soluble; conjugated serum bilirubin levels greater than 0.4 mg/100 ml will lead to conjugated bilirubin being excreted in urine because it is water soluble and indicates obstructive biliary tract or hepatocellular disease; bilirubinuria may be present before jaundice
Urine urobilinogen	24-hr urine collection or 2-hr afternoon collection	Normally 0.2-1.2 units found in specimen; fresh urine urobilinogen is colorless; decreased amounts of urine urobilinogen found in obstructive biliary tract disease; increased amounts found in hepatocellular disease; alterations in intestinal flora by broad-spectrum antibiotics may change test
Fecal urobilinogen	Stool specimen; no special preparation	Normally 90-280 mg/day; presence of urobilinogen gives stool brown color; absence of urobilinogen causes stools to become clay (grey) to white colored; increased amounts found with increased hemolysis of red blood cells; absence of fecal urobilinogen indicates obstructive biliary tract disease
Alkaline phosphatase	Blood drawn; no special preparation	Normal values vary depending on measurement used; this enzyme originates in liver, bone, intestine, and placenta; alkaline phosphatase is slightly to moderately elevated in hepatocellular disease but extremely elevated in obstructive biliary tract and bone disease
Serum prothrombin time (PT)	Blood drawn; no special preparation; reflects activity of prothrombin, fibrinogen, and factors V, VII, IX, and X, which are involved in the extrinsic pathway and the common pathway of clotting	Normal prothrombin time is 12-15 sec or 100%, as compared to control level; *prothrombin time* may be increased in obstructive biliary tract disease because of malabsorption of vitamin K or in hepatocellular disease because of inability of liver to produce clotting factors; persistence of abnormal prothrombin time after parenteral administration of vitamin K indicates hepatocellular damage

also believed to be present, some of the other laboratory tests listed in Table 38-1 may be used.

Pancreatic dysfunction causes characteristic changes in laboratory tests; identification of these changes helps in the diagnosis. These tests are described in Table 45-3. In addition to these tests, if biliary tract dysfunction is present, test results of bilirubin metabolism and alkaline phosphatase may be altered. Fecal fat levels may also be determined.

RADIOLOGIC TESTS

Roentgenologic tests are used to assist in identifying the cause of gallbladder and biliary ductal system problems or pancreatic dysfunction. Besides the examinations described in the following section, abdominal films, barium swallow, barium enema, and gastroscopy may be ordered. These tests help to identify the presence of pathologic gastrointestinal conditions that may cause similar signs and symptoms to those seen with problems of the gallbladder, biliary ductal system, or pancreas. These tests are described in Chapter 41.

ULTRASONOGRAPHY

Ultrasonography of the gallbladder, biliary ductal system and pancreas may be done. These tests help to differentiate between various causes of jaundice, to confirm cholelithiasis and cholecystitis, and to identify pancreatic pseudocysts and carcinoma, as well as other problems.

The preparation of the patient is relatively simple. Usually the patient is not allowed to eat for 8 to 12 hours before the procedure, because bowel gas in the

TABLE 45-3 Laboratory tests used for evaluating pancreatic disease

Test	Sample	Interpretation
Amylase	Serum or whole blood	Normal = 80-150 Somogyi units; in acute pancreatic damage level usually is elevated in 24-48 hr; in very acute damage level may rise to 600 Somogyi units within 4 hr of onset, reaching levels up to 2000 units in short time; decrease also occurs rapidly, and values may return to normal within 48-72 hr; chronic pancreatitis produces variable elevations that are less marked, and carcinoma of pancreas does not usually affect amylase levels; serum isoamylase can be measured although a technically more difficult test and not yet routinely done
	Urine (single specimen)	Normal = 2-50 Wohlgemuth units/ml
	Urine (24-hr specimen)	Normal = 6-30 Wohlgemuth units/ml and up to 5000 Somogyi units/24 hr; because amylase is excreted in urine, urine level is dependent on serum level; if serum level has already declined, urine level may be diagnostically useful since it may remain elevated up to 7 days after acute attack
Lipase	Serum	Normal = 0-1.5 units; in acute pancreatitis, lipase levels usually parallel serum amylase levels; level rises somewhat slower (peaks in 72-96 hr) but may remain elevated for 5-7 days
Calcium	Serum	Normal = 4.5-5.75 mEq/L (9.0-11.5 mg/100 ml); in severe cases of pancreatitis and steatorrhea, level may be low because calcium soaps are formed from sequestration of calcium by fat necrosis
Proteins (total)	Serum	Normal = 6-8 g/100 ml; may be decreased in acute pancreatitis caused by vascular colloid loss
Glucose	Whole blood or serum	Normal = 60-120 mg/100 ml; in severe, acute, or chronic pancreatic disease level may be elevated as a result of beta (β-) cell destruction causing decreased insulin production; stress can cause elevations and thus additional assessment is necessary when an elevation is found
White blood cells	Whole blood	Normal = 4.5-10.0 $\times$ 10^3 cells/mm^3; elevated count is usually found in the presence of acute pancreatitis
Methemalbuminenia	Peritoneal fluid	Normal = absent; results from destruction of hemoglobin in extravascular compartment and directly indicates hemorrhage of the pancreas
Antigens associated with cancer	Whole blood	Normals vary for specific marker; various serologic markers for pancreatic cancer are available including carcinoembryonic antigen (CEA), galactosyltransferase isoenzyme II (GT-II), and antibody CA-19-9. None are specific; elevations provide support for diagnosis but are not conclusive. Absence does not exclude diagnosis. Most useful in following patients after definitive treatment for recurrence

gastrointestinal tract will interfere with the test. Any residual barium needs to be removed from the GI tract before the test. The patient must be well hydrated, because dehydration can decrease the ability of ultrasonography to distinguish between organs and surrounding tissues.

COMPUTED TOMOGRAPHY (CT SCAN)

Computed tomography can also be used to assess patients with gallbladder, biliary ductal system, or pancreatic problems. It is helpful in identifying problems similar to those described for ultrasonography. Contrast medium can be used with the CT scan to visualize the biliary tract or to accentuate differences in tissue density of the pancreas.

The patient should eat nothing for 8 to 12 hours before the test. If contrast medium is to be used, the patient should be assessed for allergies to iodine or con-

trast media. Barium studies, if necessary, should be done at least 4 days before the CT scan or after the scan, because the barium can interfere with test results.

RADIONUCLIDE IMAGING

Radionuclide imaging may be used to assess the gallbladder or biliary ductal system. An intravenous injection of a ^{99m}Tc labeled derivative of iminodiacetic acid is given and provides a high-resolution image. The patient must be in a fasted state. This test is becoming the procedure of choice in verifying acute cholecystitis.[15]

CHOLECYSTOGRAPHY

A normal liver will remove radiopaque drugs such as iodoalphionic acid (Priodax), iopanoic acid (Telepaque), and iodipamide methylglucamine (Cholografin Meglumine) from the bloodstream and store and concentrate them in the gallbladder. The dye-filled gallbladder

PREPARATION OF PATIENT FOR CHOLECYSTOGRAPHY

1. Explain procedure.
2. Check for iodine or contrast media allergies.
3. Give a dose of radiopaque drug as ordered (usually 3 g).
4. Monitor for nausea, vomiting, diarrhea, and toxic signs. If vomiting occurs, the radiopaque substance may be repeated. If patient cannot tolerate anything by mouth, the drug is given intravenously in radiology.
5. Provide proper diet
   a. Fat-free evening meal
   b. No food after the evening meal
   c. May have black coffee, tea, or water morning of test
6. Give prescribed laxative as ordered in preparation for cholecystogram.

shows up as a dense shadow on x-ray examination (cholecystogram, gallbladder series). A functioning gallbladder shows up as a very well-defined shadow. If no shadow is seen, this indicates a nonfunctioning gallbladder. A preparation high in fat content is sometimes given after the first set of films to cause contraction of the gallbladder and excretion of the dye through the common bile duct. X-ray examination at this point would outline the bile ducts. Stones, which are not radiopaque, show up as dark patches on the film. Visualization of the gallbladder depends on absorption of the dye through the intestinal tract, isolation of it by the liver, and a free passageway from the liver to the gallbladder. If the results show a nonfunctioning gallbladder, sometimes the test is repeated to be sure that failure to visualize the gallbladder by x-ray examination was not caused by insufficient dye.

CHOLANGIOGRAPHY

Cholangiography is the x-ray examination of bile ducts to demonstrate the presence of stones, strictures, or tumors. The radiopaque substance may be administered intravenously or injected directly into the common bile duct with a needle or catheter at the time of surgery. Following operations on the common bile duct, the radiopaque drug, usually iodipamide methylglucamine, may be instilled through a drainage tube such as the T tube to determine the patency of the duct before the tube is removed. This dye also may be injected through the skin and abdominal wall into a bile duct within the main substance of the liver (*percutaneous transhepatic cholangiography*). This technique is useful in visualizing the location and extent of a pathologic process, such as obstructive jaundice. It permits decompression of the liver for improved function. The procedure helps the surgeon identify the location of pathologic processes before surgery, or it may indicate that surgery is not nec-

essary. The hazards of the examination occasionally may include bile leakage leading to bile peritonitis or bleeding caused by accidental rupture of a blood vessel.

SPECIAL TESTS

ENDOSCOPY

The gallbladder, biliary ductal system, and pancreas can be examined by endoscopy. Two types of endoscopic procedures can be done. The tube can be inserted through the peritoneum (peritoneoscopy), thus affording direct visualization of the abdominal organs and the taking of biopsies. Also the tube can be passed through the oral pharynx to the duodenum and into the biliary or pancreatic ductal system. This is known as endoscopic retrograde cholangiopancreatography (ERCP). Direct visualization is possible, dye can be injected through the scope, and biopsies can be taken.

Endoscopy is an invasive procedure that requires written consent of the patient. It is not without risk. Fasting is required prior to the test, and the patient may be given a sedative before the procedure.

GUIDED ASPIRATION CYTOLOGY

In suspected pancreatic cancer guided fine-needle aspiration cytology may be done. The aspiration is guided by ultrasound or CT scan.[15] Written consent is required.

CHAPTER SUMMARY

✔ The gallbladder, biliary ductal system, and pancreas are important for adequate digestion and absorption.

✔ Secretions from the gallbladder and pancreas are controlled primarily by the parasympathetic nervous system and intestinal hormones.

✔ Pathophysiologic conditions of the gallbladder, biliary ductal system, and pancreas result in discomfort and pain, inadequate nutrition, fluid and electrolyte deficits, alteration in elimination, and weakness and fatigue.

✔ Multiple abnormalities in blood studies can help in identifying pathophysiologic conditions of the gallbladder, biliary ductal system, and pancreas.

✔ Endoscopic examination and radiographic studies allow for visualization of the gallbladder, biliary ductal system, and pancreas.

QUESTIONS TO CONSIDER

- Think about the major areas you would need to assess during your history to accurately evaluate the functioning of the gallbladder, biliary tract system, and pancreas. What is the best way to evaluate nutritional status in the history? What are some physical assessment techniques or laboratory tests that can be used to evaluate nutritional status?

- The same laboratory tests of bilirubin metabolism are used in diagnosis of hemolysis, hepatic dysfunction, and dysfunction of the gallbladder or biliary tract. What differences in results would be seen in hemolysis versus hepatic dysfunction versus dysfunction of the gallbladder or biliary tract?

- Why can gallbladder disease result in pancreatic disease or vice-versa?

REFERENCES AND SELECTED READINGS

1. Anthony CP and Thibodeau GA: Textbook of anatomy and physiology, ed 12, St Louis, 1987, The CV Mosby Co.
2. Axon AT: Endoscopic retrograde cholangiopancreatography in chronic pancreatitis: Cambridge Classification, Radiol Clin North Am 27(1):39-50, 1989.
3. Balthazar EJ: CT diagnosis and staging of acute pancreatitis, Radiol Clin North Am 27(1):19-37, 1989.
4. Berne R and Levy M, editors: Physiology, ed 2, St Louis, 1988, The CV Mosby Co.
5. Gilinsky NH: The role of pancreatic function testing in the 1980's, South African Med J 71(4):235-238, 1987.
6. Jeffrey RB: Sonography in acute pancreatitis, Radiol Clin North Am 27(1):5-17, 1989.
7. *Knudsen F: Gastrointestinal and metabolic problems in older adults. In Steffle B, editor: Handbook of gerontological nursing, New York, 1984, Van Nostrand Reinhold Co.
8. *Marta MR: Endoscopic retrograde cholangeopancreatography: its role in diagnosis and treatment, Focus on Crit Care 14(5):62-63, 1987.
9. Sleisenger MH and Fordtran JS, editors: Gastrointestinal Disease: pathophysiology, diagnosis, management, ed 4, Philadelphia, 1989, WB Saunders Co.
10. Steinberg WM et al: Diagnostic assays in acute pancreatitis, Ann Intern Med 102:576-580, 1985.
11. Taylor EL and Harrington TM: Cholecystitis and cholelithiasis, Primary Care 15(1):147-157, 1988.
12. Thompson JM et al: Mosby's manual of clinical nursing, ed 2, St Louis, 1989, The CV Mosby Co.
13. vanSonnenberg E et al: Imaging and interventional radiology for pancreatitis and its complications, Radiol Clin North Am 27(1):65-72, 1989.
14. *Widmann F: Goodall's clinical interpretation of laboratory tests, ed 10, Philadelphia, 1987, FA Davis Co.
15. Wyngaarden JB and Smith LH, editors: Cecil textbook of medicine, ed 18, Philadelphia, 1988, WB Saunders Co.

*References preceded by an asterisk are particularly well suited for student readings

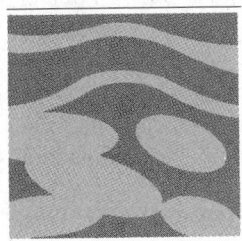

CHAPTER 46

Management of Persons with Problems of the Gallbladder and Exocrine Pancreas

VIRGINIA L. CASSMEYER

CHAPTER OBJECTIVES

After studying this chapter, the student should be able to:
1 Describe the pathogenesis and clinical manifestations of cholecystitis and cholelithiasis and cancer of the biliary tract.
2 Describe the nursing care needs of patients with disorders of the biliary system.
3 Develop nursing diagnosis, patient outcomes, and plans of interventions for patients with cholecystitis, cholelithiasis, and cancer of the biliary tract.
4 Explain the pathophysiologic basis for signs and symptoms of acute and chronic pancreatitis and pancreatic tumors.
5 Develop nursing diagnosis, patient outcomes, and plans of interventions for patients with acute or chronic pancreatitis, cancer of pancreas, or pancreatic surgery.

DISORDERS OF THE BILIARY SYSTEM

The biliary system is affected by inflammation and infection, stones and obstruction, and cancer. Each of these is described in the next section.

CHOLELITHIASIS/CHOLECYSTITIS

Cholelithiasis is stone formation in the gallbladder. *Cholecystitis* is an inflammation of the gallbladder that can be acute or chronic and is usually precipitated by gallstones.

EPIDEMIOLOGY

Cholelithiasis is a very common health problem affecting 20 million Americans with an estimated one million new cases per year.[33] Gallstones rank fifth as a cause of hospitalization for adults, and removal of the gallbladder is the third most common surgery performed.[33]

Cholelithiasis is two to three times more common in women, occurs most frequently in the middle and older age group, affects American Indians, Mexican-Americans, and whites more frequently than blacks or Orientals, is more common in persons who have sedentary life-styles, and occurs more frequently in multiparous women. In addition, women who take birth control pills have an accelerated onset of gallstone disease.[33] Cholelithiasis is more common in obese persons; in persons with a history of ileal disease and resection; in persons with diabetes mellitus; in persons with other endocrine problems; in persons with cirrhosis; in persons with hemolytic processes such as sickle cell anemia; and in persons with hyperlipidemia, persons on a cholesterol-lowering diet or a high-caloric diet, and those taking clofibrate.

Two thirds of the persons who have cholelithiasis have chronic cholecystitis.

ETIOLOGY/PATHOPHYSIOLOGY

Gallstones are composed primarily of cholesterol, bile salts, calcium, bilirubin, and proteins. *Three specific factors appear to contribute to the formation of gallstones: metabolic factors, stasis, and inflammation.* An increased concentration of one of the three substances present in bile (bile acids, bile pigments, and cholesterol) may result in their precipitation, giving rise to the formation of stones. An increased serum cholesterol level is a *metabolic* disorder occurring in the presence of such clinical situations as obesity, pregnancy, diabetes, and hypothyroidism. About 75% of gallstones in western cultures are cholesterol stones. The remaining 25% consist of bilirubin pigment stones and occurs in persons with hemolytic disease. Cholesterol stones are firm and radiolucent, but pure cholesterol stones are uncommon. Bilirubin stones are small and soft and are found mostly in the ducts. Calcium salts usually contribute to the composition of both types of stones and make them radiopaque.

Biliary *stasis* leading to stagnation of bile in the gallbladder leads to excessive absorption of water, which allows the salts to precipitate and form mixed stones. These stones may be quite variable in size and are sometimes small enough to have a gravel-like appearance on gallbladder x-ray films.

The third contributing factor to stone formation is *inflammation* of the biliary system. This condition causes the bile constituents to become altered, and the inflamed gallbladder mucosa absorbs more of the bile acids with a resultant reduction of the solubility of cholesterol.

Stones may lodge anywhere along the biliary tract where they may cause an obstruction that, if unrelieved, leads to jaundice and poor absorption of fats (Figure 46-1). They may cause pressure, subsequent necrosis, and infection of the walls of the biliary ducts; or they may stimulate spasms and pain. Occasionally, because of its location, a stone can block the entrance of pancreatic fluid and bile into the duodenum at the ampulla of Vater and can cause *pancreatitis*. It is difficult to differentiate this condition from obstruction caused by malignancy.

Cholecystitis may be acute and results from a blockage of the cystic duct secondary to stones or blockage of the duct secondary to edema and spasm initiated by the passage of the gallstone. The blockage results in distention of a gallbladder with edema of its walls. This leads to inflammation and ischemia; the inflamed wall allows

absorption of bile salts from the lumen, further increasing the inflammation. *A secondary infection* with one of several organisms that can reach the gallbladder through blood, lymph, or the biliary duct may occur. In acute cholecystitis the gallbladder is enlarged and tense. The walls may become friable and necrotic, and perforation may occur, resulting in peritonitis. The gallbladder may adhere to surrounding structures.

Cholecystitis may be chronic and follow several acute attacks. But most frequently chronic cholecystitis is the result of mechanical and chemical injuries precipitated by stones that result in scarring, thickening, and ulceration of the gallbladder wall. A secondary bacterial infection may be present in chronic cholecystitis. The gallbladder is pearly white in appearance and contains turbid bile and debris.

The inflammation associated with acute and chronic cholecystitis stimulates a *generalized inflammatory response* in the body. The blockage of bile flow results in *spasms* and *colicky pain*. The inflamed gallbladder can cause *pain* and *tenderness* in the *right upper quadrant.* Persons with chronic cholecystitis may have long-term obstruction that can result in disruption of normal GI functioning and jaundice. The relationship between normal physiology of the gallbladder and pathophysiology and clinical manifestations of gallbladder problems are depicted in Table 46-1.

PREVENTION

The major focus of preventive care is directed toward secondary prevention that prohibit complications in the presence of disease of the gallbladder. Nurses should be aware of populations at high risk for cholelithiasis and work toward early detection. Prevention of obesity and sedentary lifestyles, because these situations are associated with increased serum cholesterol, are primary preventive techniques that may help to decrease the occurrence of gallstones and thus cholecystitis. Control of chronic health problems such as diabetes mellitus, sickle cell anemia, and hyperlipidemia could help prevent cholelithiasis in persons with these three conditions.

CLINICAL MANIFESTATIONS
Signs and Symptoms

The patient with cholelithiasis and/or cholecystitis may have various manifestations. Cholelithiasis may cause no signs and symptoms until a stone becomes lodged in a biliary duct or until inflammation occurs, although a history of indigestion after consuming high caloric, fatty foods, occasional discomfort in the right upper quadrant of the abdomen, and more trouble than the normal person has with gaseous eructation after eating are common complaints.

If a stone lodges in the duct system, *gallstone colic or*

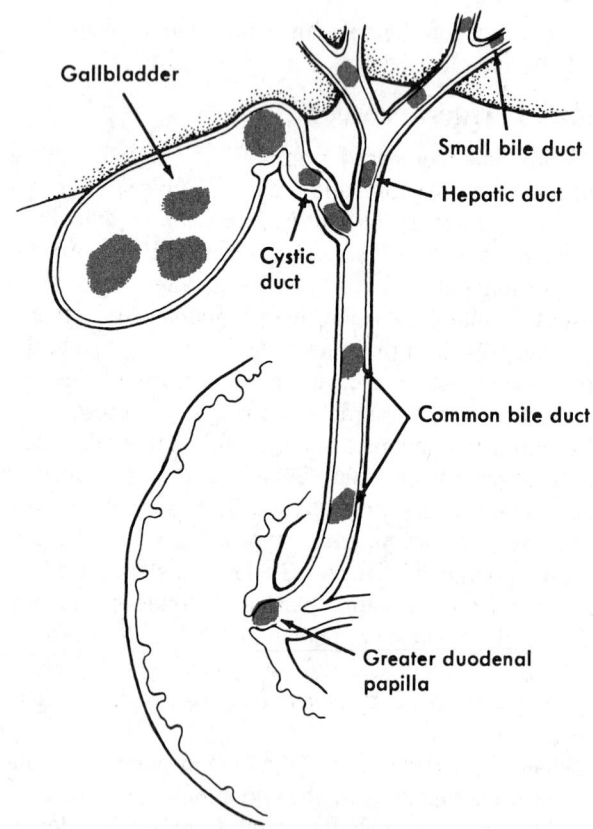

FIGURE 46-1 Common sites of gallstones.

Gallbladder

Small bile duct

Hepatic duct

Cystic duct

Common bile duct

Greater duodenal papilla

TABLE 46-1 Relationship of *normal function* of the gallbladder to *pathophysiology* and *clinical manifestations* of gallbladder disease

Normal Function	Pathophysiology	Clinical Manifestations
Concentration and storage of bile	Stasis of bile → stone formation → obstruction of bile flow ↓	↑ total and conjugated serum bilirubin, ↑ urinary bilirubin and ↓ urine urobilogen; jaundice; pruritus; clay-colored (grey) stools; impaired vitamin K absorption → prolonged prothrombin time
	Smooth muscle contractions	Biliary colic and generalized symptoms from severe pain
	Impairment of fat absorption	Intolerance of fatty foods, indigestion, eructation, nausea, and vomiting → hypovolemia → ↓ blood pressure, tachycardia, tachypnea, and diaphoresis; hypokalemia
	Acute or chronic inflammation of gallbladder	Chills, fever, and elevated white blood cells

biliary colic can occur. The pain comes on suddenly and may start in the midepigastrium, spread to the right upper quadrant of the abdomen, and radiate through to the back under the scapula and to the right shoulder. The pain may be extremely severe and is usually associated with tachycardia, diaphoresis, and nausea and vomiting. Frequently the patient paces or moves and turns constantly when laying in bed. Occasionally complete prostration occurs. If inflammation is present, the patient may have chills and fever. If the obstruction occurs in the common bile duct (choledocholithiasis), bile will be inhibited from reaching the GI tract, total and conjugated serum bilirubin will increase, and jaundice will occur. The excessive conjugated bilirubin will be excreted in the urine. Because no (or less) bile reaches the GI tract, urine urobilinogen will be decreased, and clay-colored (grey) stools will result. The absorption of fat and fat soluble vitamins will also be impaired. If vitamin K absorption is disrupted, a prolonged prothrombin time will occur.

Persons having an acute attack of cholecystitis may be very ill. With severe inflammation, chills and fever will be present along with an elevated WBC count. The major symptom of pain from biliary colic is described above. If perforation and peritonitis occur, the patient may have signs and symptoms of peritonitis, which includes sudden severe abdominal pain, distention, and rigidity; extreme tenderness; decreased or absent bowel sounds; tachypnea; tachycardia; and leukocytosis. In some patients the gallbladder may be palpable.

The patient with chronic cholecystitis usually has a history of several previous attacks of acute cholecystitis or a history indicative of cholelithiasis. There is usually a history of intolerance to fatty foods. Pain may be severe and is usually limited to the right upper quadrant. Nausea and vomiting may be present. Very frequently patients with chronic cholecystitis do not seek help until jaundice or an acute obstruction occurs. Figure 46-2 de-

picts the relationship between cholelithiasis and cholecystitis and other complications.

MEDICAL MANAGEMENT

Patients with an established diagnosis of cholelithiasis and cholecystitis may need the following medical treatment before definitive therapy:

1. Narcotic analgesics for colic pain; Meperidine hydrochloride (Demerol), thought to be less spasmogenic than morphine sulfate
2. Nothing by mouth and nasogastric suction for nausea and vomiting
3. Intravenous fluids to replace fluid and electrolytes

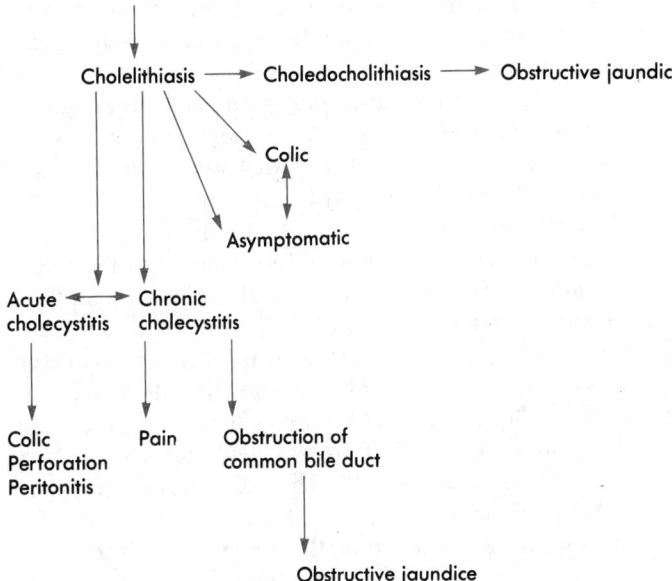

FIGURE 46-2 Relationship between cholelithiasis/cholecystitis and other complications of biliary system disease.

4. Antibiotics, if an infection is present
5. Vitamin K, if jaundice is present and prothrombin time is prolonged

Following stablization of the patient's physical status, diagnostic tests will be initiated to determine whether surgical or medical intervention is the treatment of choice. Although extracorporeal shock wave lithotripsy (ESWL) and dissolution therapy is currently used in 10% of patients with cholelithiasis, the intervention of choice for most patients is still surgery.[13] Gallstone lithotripsy is still being implemented under rigidly defined protocols as described in the following discussion. As more experience is gained, it may be applied to a larger number of patients.[2]

Dissolution Agents

Chenodeoxycholic acid and ursodeoxycholic acid (UDCA) now are being used to dissolve small ($\leq$ 20 mm in diameter) cholesterol stones. These two compounds are bile acids and increase cholesterol solubility. The drugs, which are taken daily for up to 2 years, can cause elevated liver enzymes and diarrhea. Also, gallstones can reoccur after the drugs are discontinued.

GALLSTONE LITHOTRIPSY

Lithotripsy involves the use of shock waves to disintegrate gallstones. Shock waves are applied to the gallstones located in the gallbladder or common and hepatic bile ducts, which are located by use of ultrasound. The shock waves are usually passed through a water medium, although some machines are "dry" lithotripters and use liquid couplers contained by membranes between the shock wave source and the patient's skin.[2] Approximately 1500 shocks are delivered over 1 to 2 hours. The fragments of the disintegrated stones are excreted through the common bile duct into the small intestines.

Use of lithotripsy for patient's with bile duct stones requires that the patient have an endoscopic spincterotomy or percutaneous transhepatic catherization at least 5 days before the lithotripsy.

At this time lithotripsy can be used only: (1) on patients who have fewer than three stones that are < 3.0 cm in diameter, (2) in patients with no acute complications of gallstone disease, (3) in patients with no acute cholecystitis, (4) in patients with no allergy to iodine or bile acids, (5) in patients with normal coagulation profiles, (6) in patients with normal liver and pancreatic function tests, and (7) in patients with no pacemaker or artificial heart valves.[2,13,20] The gallstones must be located so that the shock waves, which disintegrate the gallstones, do not penetrate the lung or head of the pancreas.[20] Lithotripsy is usually used in combination with dissolution agents. Modifications in the lithotripters have altered the body surface area over which the shock wave enters the patient. Some lithotripters allow the

waves to penetrate a larger body surface area, decreasing the pain.[2] Also, lithotripters vary in the actual pressure delivered to the body surface.[2] Currently, most lithotripters can be applied to patients using no anesthesia or only light IV sedation.[2]

■ ASSESSMENT

Although some patients are admitted in a relatively stable state for surgery or lithotripsy, other patients are acutely ill. Nursing assessment will provide direction for nursing care.

Subjective Data

Subjective data include the following:

1. Presence of discomfort or pain; onset, severity, location, precipitating factors
2. GI symptoms—nausea, vomiting, anorexia, eructation, fat intolerance, recent food intake, change in urine and stool color
3. History of fever and chills, previous attacks, jaundice
4. Knowledge of problem, treatment, and expectations of treatment

Objective Data

Objective data include the following:

1. Vital signs—blood pressure, pulse, respiration, temperature
2. Fluid status—weight, skin turgor, mucous membrane moisture, intake and output
3. Presence of jaundice
4. Abdomen—distention, tenderness, and guarding in right upper quadrant
5. Dark-colored urine, clay-colored (grey) stools

The patient who is to have surgery or lithotripsy requires additional assessment of the cardiovascular, neurologic, and respiratory systems similar to that required by all patients having surgery (see Chapter 20).

■ DATA ANALYSIS: NURSING DIAGNOSES

Nursing diagnoses are determined from assessment of patient data. Possible nursing diagnoses for the person with cholelithiasis/cholecystitis during the preoperative or prelithotripsy period include, but are not limited to, the following:

Diagnostic Title	Possible Etiologies
Fluid volume deficit, potential	Nausea and vomiting; decreased intake; fever
Injury, potential for bleeding	Impaired vitamin K absorption, which may result in bleeding
Knowledge deficit: illness, treatment	New diagnosis; no previous exposure to information
Pain	Inflammation of gallbladder, obstruction of bile flow, and spasms of bile ducts; itching
Self-care deficit: variable	Pain, fever, weakness

Possible nursing diagnoses after surgery or lithotripsy include, but are not limited to, the following:

Diagnostic Title	Possible Etiologies
Breathing pattern, ineffective	High surgical incision; abdominal distention
Fatigue	Surgical procedure; malnourishment before surgery
Fluid volume deficit, potential	Nausea and vomiting after surgery or lithotripsy; bleeding; loss of fluids through external drainage tubes.
Injury, potential for	Obstruction of T-tube after surgery or obstruction of bile duct by fragment of stone after lithotripsy
Knowledge deficit: needs immediately after treatment and at discharge	No previous exposure to information
Nutrition, altered: potential for less than body requirement	Nausea and vomiting after treatment
Pain	Incisional; spasms of ductal system associated with obstruction of T-tube or of cystic or common bile ducts
Skin integrity, impaired	Incision; potential long-term drainage tubes; potential bile drainage irritating the skin

■ PLANNING: EXPECTED PATIENT OUTCOMES

Expected patient outcomes for the person with cholelithiasis/cholecystitis during the preoperative or prelithotripsy period may include, but are not limited to, the following:

1. The patient will show improvement in skin turgor, and mucous membrane moisture and weight will stabilize; intake and output will be balanced.
2. The patient will not have any undetected bleeding.
3. The patient or significant other can:
   a. Explain the pathophysiology and how the signs and symptoms are related to the gallbladder problems.
   b. Explain the planned treatment and expected effects.
   c. Describe care needs for before and after diagnostic tests and treatment.
4. The patient will state pain is relieved.
5. The patient will have self-care needs met.

Expected patient outcomes for the person with cholelithiasis/cholecystitis during the postoperative period or the period after lithotripsy may include, but are not limited to, the following:

1. The patient's breath sounds will be clear and present in all lobes.
2. The patient will state fatigue is gradually improved and will rate fatigue as lessened on a 1 to 5 scale (1=no fatigue, 5=severe fatigue).
3. The patient will maintain normal fluid volume as evidenced by stable weight, moist mucous membranes, adequate skin turgor, and balanced intake and output.
4. The patient will have no undetected obstruction of T-tube drainage; the patient will report immediately recurrence of severe pain, jaundice, nausea and vomiting, or fever.
5. The patient or significant others can explain immediate care needs, pain relief methods, activity allowed, dietary requirements, signs and symptoms to report immediately, and follow-up care.
6. The patient will consume a balanced diet with food from all food groups and restricted in fat if the patient had lithotripsy.
7. The patient will state pain is controlled; the patient's activity will not be inhibited because of pain.
8. The patient's incision will heal without complications.

■ IMPLEMENTATION

The care needs before lithotripsy include:

1. Patient is educated about procedure.
2. Intravenous line is inserted.
3. Patient must lie prone on treatment table during the procedure. (This lets the gallbladder fall forward for better visualization). A comfortable position is promoted to facilitate maintenance of the position.
4. Hemodynamic status—blood pressure, EKG, and pulse oximetry—is assessed. These parameters are monitored during the total procedure because positioning can interfere with respiratory effort.
5. Oxygen may be given.
6. The stone is located by ultrasound; lithotripsy is started slowly at first and then increased.
7. Sedatives may be given if the patient complains of pain, discomfort, or anxiety.

Care needs after lithotripsy include:

1. Pain control (biliary colic may occur as a normal reaction as the disintegrated stones are passed to the duodenum) with dicyclomine HCL (Bentyl) or meperidine (Demerol).
2. Maintenance of adequate intake and output; a low-fat diet is given to prevent pain. This is usually continued only during the hospital stay. Nausea and vomiting may occur immediately after the procedure and if not prolonged, is treated symptomatically. Hematuria may be seen for 24 hours and if not prolonged, is not of concern.
3. Self-monitoring and reporting occurrence of fever, jaundice, abdominal pain, or severe nausea or vomiting.

TABLE 46-2 Surgeries of the gallbladder and biliary system

Procedure	Definition
Cholecystectomy	Removal of the gallbladder
Cholecystostomy	Creation of an opening into the gallbladder for decompression and drainage
Choledochostomy	Surgical incision into common bile duct
Choledocholithotomy	Removal of a stone from the common bile duct
Choledochoduodenostomy	Anastomosis between the bile duct and the duodenum
Choledochojejunostomy	Anastomosis between the bile duct and the jejunum
Cholecystogastrostomy	Anastomosis between the gallbladder and the stomach

MEASURES TO DECREASE RISK OF BLEEDING IN PERSONS WITH JAUNDICE AND LOW PROTHROMBIN LEVELS

1. Avoid all intramuscular or subcutaneous injections if possible.
2. Use the smallest gauge needle possible when giving an injection.
3. Apply pressure to injection sites and venous puncture sites for at least 5 minutes and to arterial puncture sites for at least 10 minutes.
4. Give vitamin K as ordered.
5. Use a soft-bristled toothbrush or cotton swabs for oral hygiene.
6. Instruct patient not to strain at stool and to avoid vigorous blowing of nose or coughing.
7. Provide assistance when patient is up to avoid falls.
8. Make sure that room is free of clutter, that floors are dry, and that patient wears shoes or slippers to avoid injuries.

4. Ultrasound and laboratory tests (lipase, amylase, bilirubin, creatinine, prothrombin time, partial thromboplastin time, hemoglobin, hematocrit, and serum enzymes) at 6 weeks, 3 months, and 6 months after the procedure.

Various surgical procedures can be carried out. Definitions of the various surgeries are described in Table 46-2.

Preoperative Care

Maintaining hydration. Some patients will be admitted with a fluid deficit because of nausea and vomiting and temperature elevation. They will require intravenous fluids that will need to be monitored closely for rate of infusion. The patient's responses to hydration (weight, intake and output, mucous membrane moisture, and skin turgor) will need to be checked frequently. Any increase in signs and symptoms of fluid deficit will need to be reported immediately. The patient will need to be monitored for potential fluid overload.

Preventing injury. If jaundice is present, the prothrombin level usually is low; and vitamin K preparations such as phytonadione (vitamin K_1, Mephyton) may be given before surgery. Occasionally, when the prothrombin level is very low but surgery is imperative, transfusions of whole blood or packed cell may be given immediately before the operation to provide prothrombin, which is essential for blood clotting. Until the prothrombin level returns to normal the nurse should monitor the patient for bleeding (bleeding gums, blood in urine or feces, occurrence of purpura or hematoma) and implement the measures listed in the following box.

Patient teaching. Teaching is implemented to prepare the patient for diagnostic tests and to help her or him understand the proposed treatment, including preoperative and postoperative care.

A general medical examination is done before biliary surgery, and includes a chest x-ray, x-ray study of the gallbladder, and examination of the urine and stools. Usually an ECG is ordered. Various tests of hepatic function may be made if disease of the liver is suspected; and if the patient is jaundiced, he or she is tested to determine the cause. The prothrombin level usually is determined. The patient must be taught about all these tests. Increasingly, stable patients scheduled for cholecystectomy are admitted the morning of surgery. This means that preoperative and postoperative teaching is given before admission or on the morning of surgery. The nurse must be prepared to give the necessary information in a very short period of time. Because of the high abdominal incision, patients undergoing gallbladder surgery are at high risk for developing atelectasis following surgery. Thus, major emphasis is given to teaching the patient how to breathe deeply and cough effectively after surgery, the way to splint the incision to reduce pain with coughing, and the best position to facilitate coughing.

Promoting comfort. Before surgery the nurse must focus on maintaining comfort. Analgesics should be given as ordered and evaluated for their effectiveness. The patient with a nasogastric tube requires frequent oral hygiene to avoid discomfort from not being allowed anything by mouth. Side-lying position, back massages, and relaxation technique may help to promote comfort.

Promoting self-care. Some patients are acutely ill; and, because of fever and chills, fluid imbalance, and pain, they will require assistance with hygiene, grooming, toileting, and other needs. Nursing care is scheduled around comfort measures so that the patients can participate in their care as much as possible. The nurse should help patients understand that their self-care deficits are temporary.

Postoperative Management

Postoperative care is focused on the potential nursing diagnoses. In the immediate postoperative period care focuses on comfort measures, maintenance of fluid status, and prevention or detection of complications such as respiratory problems or obstruction of T-tube or bile duct. Other care needs relate to reducing fatigue and promoting normal activity, providing a palatable diet, promoting skin integrity and preparing the patient for discharge (see nursing care plan on pp. 1370-1371).

Immediate care. On recovery from anesthesia the patient is usually placed in a low Fowler's position. Because breathing is painful, the patient may take shallow breaths to splint the incision and lessen pain. Following and based on on-going pain assessment medications for pain should be given fairly liberally during the first 48 to 72 hours, and the patient must be urged to cough and to breathe deeply at regular intervals (every 1 to 2 hours) to avoid atelectasis. The patient must also be helped and encouraged to change position and to move about in bed frequently. If a nasogastric tube is in use, it is attached to suction. Because essential electrolytes and abdominal gas are removed by this procedure, it is discontinued as soon as possible, usually within 24 hours if bowel sounds are normal and abdomen is soft and not distended. An infusion of 5% glucose in distilled water or in some concentration of saline is usually administered. When the nasogastric tube is removed, the patient is given clear fluids by mouth. Sweet, effervescent drinks such as ginger ale usually are tolerated best at first. Within a few days the patient usually is able to eat a soft, low-fat diet. Appetite will probably remain poor if bile is not flowing into the duodenum. The patient should be assessed for tolerance of oral fluids and foods. Tolerance is indicated by absence of nausea and vomiting, maintainence of soft abdomen, and lack of abdominal distention.

Dressings are checked frequently for the first few hours after surgery because, although hemorrhage from the wound is rare, it can occur. Occasionally, internal hemorrhage follows surgery of the gallbladder and bile ducts, particularly if the inflamed gallbladder was adherent to the liver. A decrease in blood pressure, increase in pulse rate, tachypnea, decreased urine output, restlessness, complaints of thirst, poor skin turgor, and so forth potentially indicate internal hemorrhage and are reported to the surgeon at once.

Promoting activity. Patients are usually permitted out of bed the evening of or the day after surgery. If a T-tube or a cholecystostomy tube is present, it may be attached to a small drainage bottle or plastic bag to permit greater freedom of movement. It may be placed in a pocket of the patient's bathrobe or attached to the robe below the level of the common duct. Patients may need help and encouragement because dressings are uncomfortable and they fear spilling the drainage when moving about. Patients benefit from a regular schedule of getting up and walking with assistance. This activity helps the patient to cope with fatigue. In preparation for discharge the patient should be given a schedule that incorporates a gradual increase in activity with rest periods. Heavy lifting must be avoided for some time after discharge, and plans must be made with family members so that they perform activities requiring heavy lifting.

Maintaining T-tube drainage. If the gallbladder is removed, the cystic duct is ligated, and a drain usually is inserted near its stump and brought out through a stab wound on the abdomen. This drain allows drainage of bile and small amounts of blood and other serous fluid or exudates onto the dressings. It is usually removed within 5 to 6 days when drainage has largely subsided.

If a *cholecystostomy* has been performed, a self-retaining catheter is inserted through an opening in the gallbladder and is attached to straight drainage. Bile will drain out through this catheter until it is removed, usually between 6 weeks and 6 months.

After exploration of the common duct, a T-tube with the short end placed into the common duct will probably be used. The long end of the soft rubber tube is brought out through a stab wound and sutured to the skin. The section of the T-tube emerging from the stab wound may be placed over a roll of gauze anchored to the skin with adhesive tape to prevent it from occluding (Figure 46-3). The T-tube is inserted to preserve patency of the common duct and to ensure drainage of bile out of the body until edema in the common duct has subsided enough for bile to drain into the duodenum normally. If the T-tube was clamped while the patient was being transported from the recovery room, it must be released *immediately* on arrival in the patient's room. The nurse should check the operative sheet carefully and seek clarification if the physician's written directions are not clear. The tube is usually connected to closed-gravity drainage similar to that used to drain the urinary bladder. Sufficient tubing should be attached so that the patient can move without restriction. The purpose of the tube should be explained, and the patient

NURSING CARE PLAN

PERSON EXPERIENCING CHOLECYSTECTOMY WITH EXPLORATION OF COMMON BILE DUCT

DATA: Mrs. C. is a 70-year-old female admitted with severe right upper quadrant pain, jaundice, low blood pressure, tachycardia, cool, sweaty skin, and fever. Her skin turgor is poor, and mucous membranes are dry. Her abdomen is tender to palpation. She gives a 2-week history of nausea and vomiting of bile-tinged secretions. Her laboratory values show hypernatremia (Na+= 150 mEq/L), hypokalemia (K+ = 3.0 mEq/L), elevated total (7.3 mg/100 mL) and direct (7 mg/100 mL) bilirubin and elevated alkaline phosphatase. Prothrombin time is prolonged (30 sec).

She is diagnosed as having acute cholecystitis and cholelithiasis. A nasogastric tube is inserted, she is placed on NPO, and an IV of D5NS with 40 mEq/kcal at 125 mL/hour is started. Vitamin K is given by injection, and Demerol is ordered for pain. Twenty-four hours after admission, when her hemodynamic status and fluid and electrolyte status are stabilized, she has a cholecystectomy. The following is a proposed plan of care for the postsurgical period.

NURSING DIAGNOSIS

Breathing pattern, ineffective related to high surgical incision

Expected Patient Outcomes	Nursing Interventions	Rationale
Breath sounds are clear. Respirations are within baseline range.	1. Monitor respirations and breath sounds (especially RLL) q2h to q4h for 24 hr then q4h while awake until patient is ambulating well. 2. Place patient in low Fowler's position and encourage patient to change position frequently. 3. Encourage deep breathing and coughing exercises at least q1h to q2h for 24 hr then q2h to q4h while awake until patient is ambulating well. 4. Splint incision to encourage deep coughing. 5. Encourage use of incentive spirometer q1h to q2h until ambulating well. 6. Encourage ambulation as permitted. 7. Give analgesics prior to ambulation based on assessment.	This monitoring will help the nurse identify early any respiratory problems; coughing, deep breathing, and ambulation will prevent atelectasis, a major respiratory complication. Incentive spirometer helps the client increase deep breathing efforts.

NURSING DIAGNOSIS

Fatigue related to surgical procedure

Expected Patient Outcomes	Nursing Interventions	Rationale
Patient will say fatigue is lessening	1. Space activities between rest periods and evaluate tolerance before increasing activity. 2. Assist patient with activities like bathing to conserve energy for ambulation. 3. Teach patient about need to continue to get adequate rest after discharge.	Fatigue is a common problem and is self-limiting. This care will prevent fatigue from becoming so severe that the patient does not participate in ambulation

NURSING DIAGNOSIS:

Fluid volume deficit, potential related to nausea and vomiting

Expected Patient Outcomes	Nursing Intervention	Rationale
The patient will maintain normal fluid volume as evidenced by stable weight, moist mucous membranes, adequate skin turgor, and balanced intake and output.	1. Monitor intake and output and N/G and T-tube drainage every shift, daily weight, daily laboratory values, and blood pressure and pulse q4h. 2. Administer fluids and electrolytes as ordered. 3. Provide oral fluids as tolerated after establishing presence of normal bowel sounds.	The monitoring will allow for detection of early signs of volume deficit and to assure that adequate fluid volume is maintained

NURSING CARE PLAN

PERSON EXPERIENCING CHOLECYSTECTOMY WITH EXPLORATION OF COMMON BILE DUCT—cont'd

NURSING DIAGNOSIS

Injury, potential for related to obstruction of T-tube or hemorrhage

Expected Patient Outcomes	Nursing Interventions	Rationale

The patient will have no undetected obstruction of the T-tube; The patient will have no undetected hemorrhage.	1. Monitor vital signs and for signs of shock q4h.
	2. Inspect dressing every 15 min for first few hours postoperatively for signs of bleeding or copious drainage.
	3. Monitor for decreased hematocrit (bleeding) daily or for jaundice associated with increased serum bilirubin (biliary obstruction).
	4. Maintain patency of T-tube:
	  a. Connect tube to closed gravity drainage.
	  b. Provide sufficient tubing to facilitate patient mobility.
	  c. Explain to patient importance of avoiding kinks, clamping or pulling of tube.
	5. Monitor amount and color of drainage from T-tube q8h.
	6. Monitor color of urine and stool q8h.
	7. Report signs of peritonitis (abdominal pain or rigidity, fever) immediately.
	8. If clamping of T-tube is prescribed before removal, monitor patient for signs of distress; if this occurs, unclamp tube and notify physician.
		Early detection of obstruction or bleeding will allow intervention before a crisis occurs.

NURSING DIAGNOSIS

Knowledge deficit: Self-care after discharge related to new needs and no previous exposure to information

Expected Patient Outcomes	Nursing Interventions	Rationale

Patient describes self-care needs.	1. Teach patient:
	  a. Techniques of dressing change if drainage is still occurring at time of discharge.
	  b. Any prescribed dietary changes such as low fat or low calories.
	  c. Signs to report to physician (excessive drainage, recurrence of jaundice, recurrence of light-colored stools).
	  d. Resumption of normal activities by 4 weeks, but avoidance of heavy-lifting activity until 6 weeks.
		Adequate knowledge will help the patient to take care of self.

NURSING DIAGNOSIS

Pain related to incisional discomfort or T-tube obstruction

Expected Patient Outcomes	Nursing Interventions	Rationale
The patient states pain is relieved.	1. Assess type and quality of pain. 2. Give analgesics fairly liberally for 48 to 72 hr after surgery based on assessment. 3. If nasogastric tube is present, give mouth and nose care as needed. 4. Encourage activity. 5. Use other pain-relieving measures, as appropriate. 6. Maintain T-tube patency as described above.	Pain can interfere with coughing, deep breathing, ambulation or nutrition when not controlled. The pain is also very debilitating for the patient.

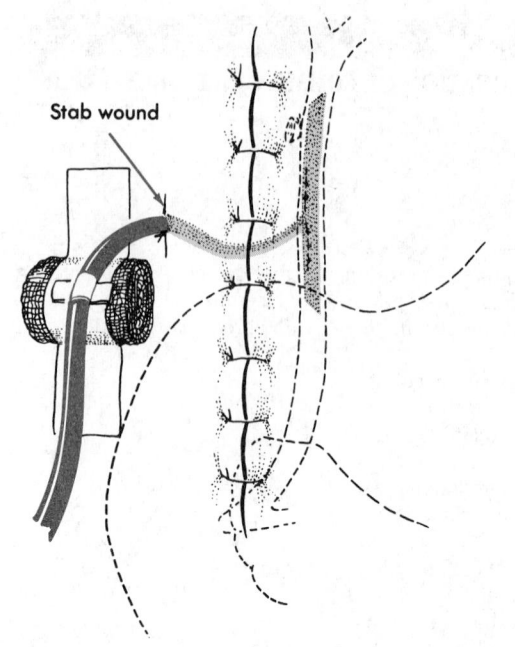

Stab wound

FIGURE 46-3 Section of T-tube emerging from stab wound may be placed over roll of gauze anchored to skin with adhesive tape to prevent its lumen from being occluded by pressure.

should be told why it must not be kinked, clamped, or pulled. The drainage should be checked for color and amount at least every 2 hours on the operative day. Some blood and blood-stained fluid may have drained from the tube during the first several hours, but drainage of more than a small amount of blood should be reported to the surgeon at once. The amount of drainage is measured and recorded daily. At first the entire amount of bile produced (normally 500 to 1000 ml/day) may flow through the tube, but within 10 days most of the bile should be flowing into the duodenum.

Before the T-tube is removed, the patency of the common bile duct must be assessed. The tube is clamped for variable intervals, and the patient is monitored for signs of distress. If distress occurs, the tube is unclamped immediately, and the surgeon is informed. A cholangiogram (Chapter 45) is usually performed to confirm the patency of the duct before the tube is removed. Following the removal of the T-tube, the patient may have chills and fever that usually subside within 24 hours. They are caused by edema and a local reaction to the bile. Occasionally flow of bile into the abdominal cavity causes *peritonitis*, and therefore any abdominal pain should be reported at once. The T-tube removal occurs at no specific time. Removal follows an x-ray examination that reveals no stones and the free flow of injected dye and a 5 to 7 day asymptomatic period in which the T-tube is clamped.[13] Also, the patient should

be reporting an improved feeling of well-being and having stools that have returned to a brown color.[13]

Following surgery the bile should either drain out through the drainage tube or flow into the intestine. If it does not do so, it can be assumed that the flow of bile is obstructed and that bile is being forced back into the liver and into the bloodstream. The nurse should observe the patient closely for jaundice, particularly in the sclerae. Urine should be examined for the brown color that is indicative of bilirubin: specimen should be saved for the surgeon's inspection when bilirubin is observed in the urine. The nurse may observe the patient's progress by noting the appearance of the stools. A light grey color is usual if all the bile is flowing out through the drainage tubes (unless bile salts are being given by mouth). The normal brown color of the stool should gradually reappear as bile drainage diminishes and finally disappears.

Patients should be told about any drainage tubes, and they should know if much bile is expected on the dressings so that they will not become alarmed by soiling of dressings, gowns, or bedclothes. Outer dressings usually should be changed frequently when there is excessive drainage, since the drainage is irritating to the skin, and wet dressings interfere with the patient's comfort and rest. Soap and water will remove bile from the skin. Montgomery straps make the changing of dressings much easier. Occasionally patients will be discharged with a T-tube in place. They must be taught how to care for it and how to monitor for complications that need to be reported to the surgeon.

Discharge teaching. The patient will need teaching similar to that given any patient having abdominal surgery with special emphasis on activity restriction, avoidance of heavy lifting, and diet. A patient who goes home with a T-tube in place, will need special instructions for care of the T-tube (see the box on the opposite page). The patient also needs instructions regarding expected follow-up care and the fact that a repeat cholangiogram may be performed before the tube is removed.

Promoting nutrition. Special diets are seldom prescribed following biliary tract surgery, but patients are advised to avoid excessive fat. The patient is taught the essentials of good nutrition, with emphasis on foods that are low in fat. Some patients will need to increase caloric intake to replace deficits caused by preoperative nausea and vomiting.

Maintaining skin integrity. The surgical incision for the T-tube is treated the same as most incisions (see Chapter 22). The nurse should remove any soiled dressing and cleanse the skin around the drains or tubes to remove any bile. If the T-tube is left in place for a prolonged pe-

DISCHARGE TEACHING REGARDING CARE OF THE T-TUBE

1. The patient must have instruction about whether the tube should be connected to continuous drainage, clamped continuously, or drained intermittently.
   a. If it is drained continuously, the patient must know how to empty the bag, the importance of keeping the bag below the level of the T-tube insertion site, and ways to maintain mobility with a continuous drainage system.
   b. If it is drained intermittently, the patient must know how to unclamp the tube and attach it to a drainage bag, how long to drain the tube, how to reclamp the tube, and how to measure drainage.
   c. If it is kept clamped, the tube and insertion site can be covered with a dry, sterile dressing.
2. The patient must have instructions about cleansing the insertion site. Usually a daily shower is all the cleansing that is necessary. A dry sterile dressing is reapplied every day.

3. The patient should be instructed on techniques that can be used to protect the skin such as zinc oxide or karaya gel.
4. The patient must be instructed about the self-monitoring that will be necessary:
   a. Assessment for infection (redness, warmth, and swelling at insertion site, temperature elevation, or purulent drainage from T-tube site)
   b. Assessment for obstruction (recurrence of pain in right upper quadrant, bile drainage *around* T-tube, recurrence of nausea and vomiting, clay-colored stools, brown urine, or jaundice)
   c. Assessment for tube dislodgement (sudden decrease in drainage or evidence that tube has shifted)
5. The patient should be instructed to report signs and symptoms of complications immediately.

---

riod, the patient must institute care as described in the box.

CARCINOMA OF THE BILIARY SYSTEM
ETIOLOGY/EPIDEMIOLOGY

Cancer of the biliary system is the fifth most common cancer of the alimentary tract and accounts for 6500 deaths per year.[24] It is more common in women and occurs in the sixth decade of life. The cause is unknown, but a very high percentage of these patients have gallstones.

PATHOPHYSIOLOGY/CLINICAL MANIFESTATIONS

Carcinoma can occur anywhere in the biliary system. It has a very insidious onset and can metastasize by direct extension, through the lymphatics, and through the blood system. Many patients have no symptoms that are referable to the gallbladder. Other patients have symptoms similar to those seen with cholelithiasis and cholecystitis. Pain that is intermittent and in the upper abdomen is the most common symptom. Anorexia, nausea, vomiting, weight loss, and jaundice may also be present. The patient may have a palpable abdominal mass. Signs and symptoms indicative of metastasis to liver or pancreas may also be present.

Various tests used to diagnose other diseases of the gallbladder (Chapter 45) may be used but are often not definitive.

INTERVENTIONS
Medical management

The major treatment for carcinoma of the biliary system is surgical, and surgery is performed as soon as the patient's condition warrants it in the hope that complete surgical removal of the lesion is possible. Surgery may involve resection of part of the liver and the gallbladder. Patients often benefit from surgery even when cure of the carcinoma is impossible, because various surgical procedures that help to restore the flow of bile into the gastrointestinal tract produce remarkable relief of symptoms and patients may feel relatively well for a time. Percutaneous insertion of tubes or catheters to by-pass obstructions will also be used. Other medical treatment is directed toward generalized support.

Nursing Management

One focus of care will be preoperative and postoperative management similar to that described for the patient with cholecystitis and cholelithiasis (pp. 1368-1372). If resection to the liver is also done the patient will need care as described in Chapter 39. Another focus of care will be that required for any patient with the diagnosis of cancer (see Chapter 17).

In addition, the patient will often need teaching with regard to dealing with an external or internal-external bile drainage system. For an external drainage system, teaching will be the same as that for a patient who is discharged with a T-tube (see the box above). For an internal-external drainage system, a multiperforated catheter is passed through the liver past the obstruction and into the duodenum. The catheter is attached at first to continuous drainage and then plugged if no complications such as fever, chills, or leakage are present. The patient must learn how to care for the skin around the tube, how to monitor for signs and symptoms of obstruction, and how to irrigate the tube. The tube must be irrigated daily to keep the perforations open.

DISORDERS OF THE PANCREAS

PANCREATITIS

Pancreatitis is a serious inflammatory disorder of the pancreas that can be *acute* or *chronic*. Because patient needs are different in acute and chronic pancreatitis, the disorders are discussed separately.

ACUTE PANCREATITIS

Acute pancreatitis can occur as a single episode or as recurrent attacks (recurrent acute pancreatitis). The unique morphologic feature of acute or recurrent acute pancreatitis is that, except in cases of alcohol-induced pancreatitis, the pancreas returns to normal after successful treatment.[35]

ETIOLOGY

Numerous factors have been identified as causative agents of acute pancreatitis (see the box below, left). In the United States the most common factor is alcoholism. The second most common cause is biliary tract disease. It has been estimated that there are approximately 5000 new cases of acute pancreatitis diagnosed each year in the United States.

PATHOPHYSIOLOGY

Although there are many known causes of pancreatitis, the manner in which they result in acute inflammation is unknown. The currently favored pathologic factor leading to the acute inflammation is *autodigestion*. This theory proposes that proteolytic enzymes, particularly trypsinogen, are activated within the pancreas itself. Once it is activated to trypsin, trypsinogen can activate itself and other enzymes. The activated proteolytic en-

zymes digest pancreatic and surrounding tissues and cellular membranes. This autodigestion results in edema, interstitial hemorrhage, vascular drainage, coagulation necrosis, fat necrosis, and parenchymal cell necroses. The injured tissue releases histamine and bradykinin, which increase vascular permeability and vasodilation and cause more edema. The initiation of activation of the proteolytic enzymes is thought to result from reflux of bile, obstruction of the pancreatic duct or ampulla of Vater, ischemia, anorexia, trauma, endotoxins, and exotoxins.

Regardless of the cause, the acute inflammatory process and autodigestion result in a spectrum of physiologic alterations that can occur as a mild to a very critical event. Figure 46-4 depicts some of the major pathophysiologic events seen in acute pancreatitis.

The majority of patients (80% to 90%) with acute pancreatitis recover without any residual dysfunction. The mortality rate is approximately 10%.[5] The following factors increase the risk of death from acute pancreatitis:

1. Hypotension
2. Need for massive fluid and colloid replacement
3. Respiratory failure associated with adult respiratory distress syndrome
4. Hypocalcemia

CAUSES OF ACUTE PANCREATITIS

Alcoholism
Biliary tract disease
Postoperative—abdominal or nonabdominal surgery
Post endoscopic retrograde cholangiopancreatography
Blunt abdominal trauma
Metabolic problems (increased serum calcium [hyperparathyroidism and postrenal transplant patients], hypertriglyceridemia)
Infections (especially viral)
Connective tissue disease with vasculitis such as systemic lupus erythematosus
Drugs (antihypertensives, diuretics, antimicrobials, immunosuppressives, and oral contraceptives)
Intestinal diseases such as regional enteritis and penetrating duodenal ulcers
Unknown

Adapted from Toskes PP and Greenberger NJ: Acute and chronic pancreatitis, Disease-a-Month 29:5-81, 1983; and Toskes PP: Recurrent acute pancreatitis, Hosp Pract 20:85-88, 90-92, 1985.

MAJOR COMPLICATIONS OF ACUTE PANCREATITIS

Cardiovascular
  Hypotension/shock from hypovolemia or hypoalbuminemia
Hematologic
  Leukocytosis from generalized inflammation or secondary infections, anemia from blood loss, disseminated intravascular coagulation (DIC) from unknown causes
Respiratory
  Atelectasis, pneumonitis, pleural effusion, adult respiratory distress syndrome (ARDS)
Gastrointestinal
  Hemorrhage from peptic ulcers, gastritis
Pancreatic/liver
  Hemorrhage from varices; pancreatic pseudocysts, abscesses, or pancreatic ascites
Renal
  Oliguria and increased blood urea nitrogen (BUN) from hypovolemia
Metabolic
  Increased blood glucose from decreased insulin release associated with the stress response or destruction of beta cells of pancrease; increased triglycerides from the stress response and changes in insulin release or secretion; decreased calcium associated with low albumin, precipitation of calcium with free fatty acids to form calcium soaps, and unknown causes.
Neurologic
  Encephalopathy

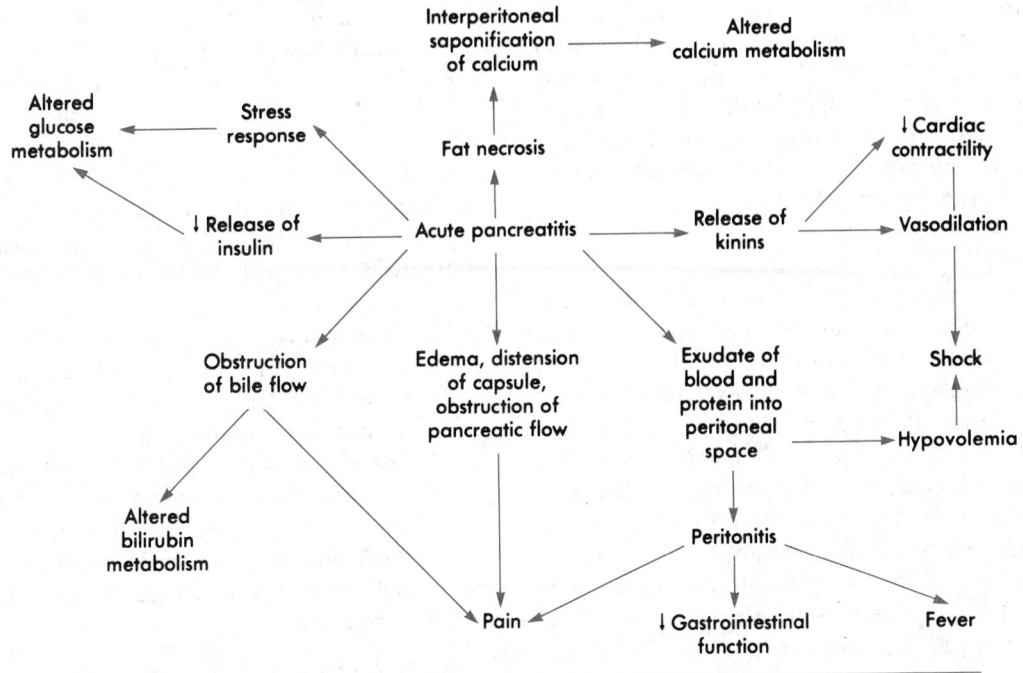

FIGURE 46-4 Summary of major pathologic events that occur in acute pancreatitis.

Multiple complications can occur as a result of acute pancreatitis. These complications can affect all systems. The right box on the opposite page lists some of the major complications.

CLINICAL MANIFESTATIONS

Signs and Symptoms

The major symptom of acute pancreatitis is *pain.* The pain varies from *mild* to *severe,* is *constant,* and is *incapacitating.* The pain may be experienced in the epigastrium and other parts of the abdomen, and it may radiate to the back, flanks, and substernal area. It is usually more intense when the person is lying supine. Other common symptoms are nausea, vomiting, and abdominal distention.

The patient with acute pancreatitis normally has a low-grade fever and signs and symptoms of fluid deficit (poor skin turgor, dry mucous membranes, tachycardia, and weight loss). Sometimes all the signs and symptoms of shock will be present. Abdominal tenderness and rigidity and diminished bowel sounds are present. Ten to twenty percent of patients develop respiratory problems, and decreased breath sound or rales may be auscultated. Other signs that might be present are jaundice from obstruction of common bile duct, purplish discoloration of the flanks (Grey Turner's sign) or the periumbilical area (Cullen's sign) from hemorrhagic necrosis of the pancreas, or tetany from low calcium.

Diagnostic Tests

Diagnostic tests of the greatest value in establishing a diagnosis are serum enzyme levels. A *serum amylase* level of greater than 300 Somogyi units in the presence of the symptoms outlined above usually establishes the diagnosis of acute pancreatitis. *Serum amylase* levels usually become elevated within 24 to 48 hours of the onset of acute pancreatitis and may range from 300 to 800 U. There is no apparent relationship between the severity of the disease and the height of the enzyme levels. Isoenzymes of amylase can be measured and provide even more specificity in diagnosing pancreatitis. Assays for isoenzymes are not yet widely available so that they are not routinely measured. *Serum lipase* also rises in pancreatitis and reaches its peak in 72 to 96 hours after the onset of the acute pancreatitis. In the absence of kidney failure, *urinary amylase* levels may also be used to diagnose acute pancreatitis.

Other laboratory findings include leukocytosis, anemia, increased serum bilirubin, altered laboratory values consistent with dehydration, and hyperglycemia. In severe cases hypocalcemia may be present. Elevation of ALT, AST, or alkaline phosphatase may be present and suggest gallstones as a cause of the pancreatitis, if no history of excessive alcohol consumption or other etiologic factors responsible for elevation of these enzymes are present.

Other diagnostic tests that may be used are: (1) abdominal x-ray examination that will reveal GI changes, such as distention associated with pancreatitis, (2) chest x-ray that may be done to identify respiratory changes, such as atelectasis, plural effusion, or pulmonary infiltrates; (3) ultrasonography that may be used to rule out an edematous pancreas and pseudocyst, and (4) endoscopic retrograde cholangiopancreatography (ERCP) to identify obstructions.

MEDICAL MANAGEMENT

Medical management is directed toward decreasing the secretions of the exocrine pancreas cells and resting it, replacing fluids and electrolytes, and treating the pain. Because exocrine secretions of the pancrease are released under the influence of stimuli from the gastrointestinal tract, to rest the exocrine pancreas, taking nothing by mouth is the major intervention. Nasogastric suctioning also is used in a majority of patients to decrease gastrin release, which stimulates gastric secretions and entry of gastric contents into the small intestines. Drug therapy to decrease exocrine pancreatic secretion has been used in the past, and new therapeutic agents are being tested, but currently no particular drugs to treat pancreatitis are recommended (see the box below). The medical management to *decrease exocrine pancreas* secretion *does not effect the endocrine pancreas functioning and insulin release.*

Intravenous fluids and colloids are used to return vascular volume to normal and maintain it. Intravenous or intramuscular analgesics (usually meperidine) are used to treat the pain. For selected patients with severe acute pancreatitis, peritoneal lavage to remove peritoneal toxic chemicals has provided some improvement in symptoms but not in survival or prevention of complications.[5]

■ ASSESSMENT

The patient with acute pancreatitis requires a thorough nursing assessment.

Subjective Data

Subjective data include the following:
1. Presence of discomfort: location, severity, precipitating factors, relief measures
2. GI complaints: nausea, vomiting, recent food and liquid intake
3. History of causes: alcoholism, gallbladder disease, recent trauma, recent surgery

---

DRUGS BEING TESTED FOR USE IN ACUTE PANCREATITIS

Somatostatin
Prophylactic systemic antibiotics
Phospholipase α_2 inhibitors

---

4. Respiratory complaints: any dyspnea, shortness of breath, pain with breathing
5. Miscellaneous: any episodes of temperature elevation

Objective Data

Objective data include the following:
1. General: affect—patient looks distressed, posture—sits with knees pulled towards abdomen, temperature
2. Fluid status: weight, intake and output, skin turgor, mucous membrane moisture
3. Cardiovascular status: blood pressure, including orthostatic changes, pulse
4. Respiratory status: respiratory rate, breath sounds
5. Abdomen: presence of tenderness or rigidity, presence of bowel sounds, presence of cyanotic or greenish yellow-brown discoloration on abdominal wall, Grey Turner's sign, Cullen's sign, and presence of ascites

■ DATA ANALYSIS: NURSING DIAGNOSES

Nursing diagnoses are determined from assessment of patient data. Possible nursing diagnoses for the person with acute pancreatitis may include, but are not limited to, the following:

Diagnostic Title	Possible Etiologies
Fluid volume deficit	Vomiting; lack of intake; pancreatic hemorrhage
Health maintenance, altered	Unhealthy life-style patterns, including alcoholism, poor nutrition, and obesity
Knowledge deficit: disease management	New diagnosis; no previous exposure to information
Nutrition, altered: less than body requirements	Nausea and vomiting; pain; life-style patterns
Pain	Inflammation of pancreas or peritoneum
Self-care deficit: variable	Weakness; pain

Potential complications that might occur and should be a focus of nursing are respiratory failure, shock, hypocalcemia, and hyperglycemia.

■ PLANNING: EXPECTED PATIENT OUTCOMES

Expected patient outcomes for the person with acute pancreatitis may include, but are not limited to, the following:
1. The patient will have adequate fluid volume as demonstrated by normal blood pressure, absence of othostatic changes, normal skin turgor, and moist mucous membranes
2. The patient will assume safe and adequate health practices (for example, improve diet, control obesity, or control alcoholism, if present as an etiologic condition of acute pancreatitis)
3. The patient and significant others will be able to:

a. Describe the disease, the need for specific tests, and the purpose of various interventions
b. Explain the relationship between the etiologic factor (alcoholism, biliary disease, and so on) and pancreatitis
c. Describe dietary restrictions
d. Explain plans for follow-up care
4. The patient will consume a diet high in protein and carbohydrates and show an increase in weight when able to eat
5. The patient states that pain is controlled and does not appear to be in pain (does not display distressed appearance, limited body movement, or limited activity)
6. The patient will have self-care needs met

■ **IMPLEMENTATION**

The patient with acute pancreatitis may be acutely ill and require intensive care. The priorities of care are control of pain, managing fluids and electrolytes, and monitoring for complications. Interventions for these and other needs are described next.

Maintaining Fluid and Electrolyte Balance

As soon as the patient is admitted, the nurse should institute monitoring related to fluid and electrolyte status, cardiac output, and renal status. This is a critical need. Monitoring includes intake and output; vital signs; daily weights; daily electrolytes; and as necessary, blood urea nitrogen (BUN), creatinine, and hemodynamic measurements. An indwelling catheter may be necessary, since decreased renal function can occur in association with hypotension and shock. Monitoring parameters and frequency of monitoring will depend on the stability of the patient's condition. Fluids, electrolytes, colloids, or blood will be given as necessary. The nurse is responsible for administering these and for monitoring the patient's response to them. Frequent adjustments in therapy may be necessary in relation to the patient's response to fluid therapy. If the patient develops shock, all the care described in Chapter 25 will be necessary.

Promoting Healthy Life-style Patterns

If unhealthy life-style patterns such as diet, obesity, or alcoholism are indicated as a cause of acute pancreatitis, the nurse must work with the patient on these problems. This care will not be instituted until the patient is stabilized, but it must be introduced before the patient leaves the hospital. See Chapters 19 and 40 for further information on coping with obesity or alcoholism.

Patient Teaching

Teaching the patient and significant others will be ongoing. At the beginning of hospitalization, the patient and significant others need basic instructions about the disease, the diagnostic tests, and the treatment. Because of the pain and the distress it causes and because of potential fluid status and cardiovascular instability, the patient and family may be experiencing tremendous stress and anxiety. Therefore explanations and instructions should be brief and as simple as possible and may need to be repeated. Support and continuity of care also need to be instituted to help decrease anxiety. Long-term education will be directed toward prevention of future attacks by avoiding alcohol, maintaining a nutritious diet, and continuing medications as prescribed. The patient must know that any recurrence of signs and symptoms should be reported immediately. Follow-up care must be explained in detail.

Promoting Nutrition

The patient will be placed on NPO and often has a nasogastric tube in place. Institution and maintenance of the NPO status is a major intervention. Good oral hygiene will be necessary to decrease discomfort from being placed on NPO and from the nasogastric tube. When the acute symptoms decrease (3 to 5 days), oral fluids and food are restarted. The patient is started on clear liquids and then advanced to a low-fat, bland diet, distributed over five to six small feedings daily. When refeeding starts, the patient must be observed carefully for pain, nausea, and vomiting, all of which indicate continuing inflammation. If these occur, the physician should be notified and the methods described previously for inhibition of pancreatic activity will be reinstituted. If food is restricted for long periods, parenteral hyperalimentation may be necessary. Following discharge from the hospital, patients are advised to avoid alcohol and other gastric stimulants, such as caffeine, and to remain on a low-fat, bland diet with several small feedings daily. High protein and fat foods must sometimes be avoided to keep pancreatic secretions at a minimum. The dietitian may need to work with the patient to help plan an appropriate diet.

Controlling Discomfort

Control of pain is a major priority. Meperidine hydrochloride, 75 to 100 mg every 3 to 4 hours, may be necessary to reduce pain. Morphine and codeine are not used because of their spasmogenic effects. Some patients find that the pain is decreased if they assume a sitting position with the trunk flexed or with their knees drawn up to the abdomen in a side-lying, knee-chest position. Sympathetic nerve blocks and epidural anesthesia can be used if pain is persistent and not relieved by meperidine.

The measures used to rest the pancreas (NPO status, and nasogastric suctioning) will also assist with pain control by decreasing the continual autodigestive process and associated edema and inflammation. In addition, the nurse should help the patient initiate relaxation techniques, such as deep breathing and imagery, and distraction techniques such as music, TV, and sewing, to help with pain control (see Chapter 16). These measures should be introduced after the patient has adequate pain control from analgesic drugs. If the patient is highly distressed, these techniques are not easily used. Importantly, comfort measures such as backrubs and purposeful touch should be implemented.

Providing Self Care

During the acute phase of the illness the patient will need assistance with all care. Dehydration and potential malnutrition make the patient particularly prone to skin breakdown. Because of the amount of monitoring and the total care that is necessary, a schedule must be established that provides for the necessary monitoring, meeting care needs, and rest periods.

Monitoring for Potential Complications

In addition to monitoring fluid and electrolyte, cardiovascular, and renal status as mentioned earlier, the patient must be monitored for the onset of respiratory problems, hypocalcemia, and hyperglycemia. Breath sounds should be monitored at least every shift. If any signs of respiratory distress are present, blood gases and a chest x-ray examination will be necessary. Preventive respiratory care, including routine turning, coughing, and deep breathing are essential. The serum calcium level is checked frequently, and the patient is monitored for signs of hypocalcemia (tetany, positive Trousseau's and Chvostek's signs, muscle twitching, jerking, and irritability). If any of these occur, they must be reported immediately because calcium replacement will be necessary. The patient also is monitored for hyperglycemia, and frequent checks of blood glucose should be carried out. If hyperglycemia occurs, it may be treated with insulin.

CHRONIC PANCREATITIS

In chronic pancreatitis there is permanent and progressive destruction of the pancreas, with normal tissue being replaced by fibrous tissue. Chronic pancreatitis can eventually lead to chronic insufficiency of pancreatic hormones.

ETIOLOGY

The major cause of chronic pancreatitis in adults in the United States is alcoholism. A major cause in children is cystic fibrosis; approximately 85% of patients with cystic fibrosis have impaired pancreatic exocrine function.[31] Other causes include the following: trauma; gastric or pancreatic surgery; neoplasms of the pancreas, islet cells, or duodenum; and severe protein and calorie malnutrition.

PATHOPHYSIOLOGY

The organ destruction that occurs in chronic pancreatitis is caused by the same factors as those described for acute pancreatitis (p. 1374); that is, autodigestion.

In chronic pancreatitis due to alcohol abuse the pancreatic juices secreted contain decreased bicarbonate, increased protein, and a decreased amount of substances that inhibit trypsin activation.[31] In addition, the pancreatic juices of persons with chronic pancreatitis may be altered in other ways that allow for calcium precipitation. The changes described above would allow for formation of protein plugs that block the pancreatic ducts and precipitate inflammation, fibrosis, and stenosis with loss of normal cell function.

The loss of normal cellular mass results in a deficiency of pancreatic exocrine secretion. Ductal obstruction and dilation have been thought to be the cause of the pain associated with chronic pancreatitis, but they cannot always be identified as a cause. The relationship between normal pancreatic function and the pathophysiology and the clinical manifestations of chronic pancreatitis are depicted in Table 46-3.

CLINICAL MANIFESTATIONS

Signs and Symptoms

The patient with chronic pancreatitis may initially have signs and symptoms identical to those described for the patient with acute pancreatitis, with *pain* being the *major manifestation*. The pain occurs in the right or left upper quadrant, in the back, or throughout the total abdomen. It is severe and constant and does not respond to normal food ingestion or antacids. It may be worsened by alcohol or high fat intake. Nausea, vomiting, and abdominal distention may be present, but they are usually secondary to the pain and its treatment. The patient also has a history of weight loss, diarrhea, steatorrhea, and malnutrition. Mild fever may be present, and jaundice is frequent. Ascites and abdominal mass may be seen. Signs and symptoms of diabetes mellitus may also be present.

Diagnostic Tests

Laboratory tests reveal leukocytosis. Bilirubin and alkaline phosphatase levels may be elevated if obstruction of the common bile duct is present. Serum lipase and amylase are usually not helpful in diagnosing chronic pancreatitis because of acinar cell atrophy and replacement of cells by fibrous tissue. Other specialized diagnostic tests that may be abnormal in chronic pancreatitis are tests of pancreatic secretion of bicarbonate-rich fluid or enzymes in response to the administration of secretin or CCK-pancreozym. Patients with chronic pancreatitis will show decreased amounts of bicarbonate-rich fluids or enzymes in response to these tests. The Bentiromide test is an indirect test of pancreatic secretory capacity.

TABLE 46-3 Relationship between normal physiology of the pancreas and pathophysiology and clinical manifestations of chronic pancreatitis

Normal Function	Pathophysiology	Clinical Manifestations
Production and secretion of digestive enzymes	Alteration in pancreatic secretions ↓	Pain → nausea, vomiting, and abdominal distention; fever
Production and secretion of bicarbonate-rich isoosmolar solution	Plugging of pancretic ducts ↓ Inflammation ↓ Stenosis and fibrosis ↓	
	Acinar cell mass diminished → Decreased enzyme and isoosmotic secretions to duodenum	Steatorrhea, diarrhea, weight loss, and malnutrition; dehydration and electrolyte imbalance
	Obstruction of biliary drainage	Increaed Bilirubin, jaundice, increased alkaline phosphatase
	Islet cells destroyed → Decreased insulin	Hyperglycemia and all other symptoms of diabetes mellitus

This compound requires chymotrypsin for its digestion before absorption. The amount of metabolic product excreted in urine after a 500 mg dose will be decreased in chronic pancreatitis. A D-xylose test will be used to rule out small bowel disease as the cause of malabsorption. Other abnormal findings include increased amounts of undigested meat fibers and split and neutral fat in the stool and elevated stool fat. Plain films of the abdomen, ultrasound examination of the abdomen, or CT scan of the abdomen may reveal pancreatic calcification. Endoscopic retrograde cholangiopancreatography (ERCP) of the pancreas may also show calcification and distortion of the pancreatic duct system.

INTERVENTIONS
Medical Management
The initial focus of treatment during an acute exacerbation of chronic pancreatitis may be the same as that for acute pancreatitis: analgesics for pain, nothing by mouth and nasogastric intubation to rest the pancreas, fluid and electrolyte replacement for fluid deficit, and supportive care for complications such as respiratory problems.

Once the patient is stabilized or for the less critically ill patient, a major focus of medical care is to confirm the diagnosis if it is not clear. Then the focus is to control pain, diarrhea, steatorrhea, weight loss, and diabetes mellitus.

For severe pain, narcotic analgesics will be used at first. Chronic control of pain and control of exocrine insufficiency is achieved with pancreatic extract replacement. In patients in whom this therapy is ineffective in controlling pain, an ERCP (see Chapter 45) will be used to identify the presence of duct obstruction or pseudocysts that may require surgery. Sometimes antacids and cimetidine may be used to decrease gastric acid secretion and thus pancreatic stimulation. Dietary manipulation, including avoiding high-protein foods, caffeine, and alcohol that increase gastric secretions and pancreatic stimulation, will often be necessary to help control pain. As stated previously, diarrhea, steatorrhea, and malabsorption will be treated with pancreatic enzyme replacement. If it is present, diabetes mellitus is treated as described in Chapter 37.

Nursing Management
For patients with chronic pancreatitis, the nursing assessment is the same as that described for acute pancreatitis (p. 1376). In some instances the nursing diagnoses, outcomes, and interventions are the same. But for the more typical patient with chronic pancreatitis, four major nursing diagnoses are the focus of nursing care (see box on p. 1380). The nurse must focus first on the patient's priority, which usually is the pain. This requires that the pain be adequately controlled, possibly with analgesics at first so that the patient is open to alternative therapeutic measures such as relaxation or massage. The patient must believe that dietary manipulations, pancreatic extract, and abstinence from alcohol will be effective to help control pain. In some instances the patient has had negative experiences with pain management during previous hospitalizations for exacerbations and thus believes that analgesics are not being given because the health team does not care about him or her. Thus it is very important that a trusting relationship be established between the patient and the nurse.

The patient must take large quantities of pancreatic extract with each meal. The patient must also learn to

POTENTIAL NURSING DIAGNOSIS FOR THE PATIENT WITH CHRONIC PANCREATITIS

Health maintenance, altered related to alcohol abuse or other unhealthy lifestyle pattern
Knowledge deficit: disease and treatment related to new diagnosis, lack of previous exposure to information, inability to accept information at earlier exposure
Nutrition, altered: less than body requirement related to malabsorption
Pain related to chronic inflammation of pancreas

manipulate necessary dietary changes (avoiding caffeine, high-protein foods, occasionally spicy foods, and large meals). And of course the patient must be helped with the alcoholism problem, if present, as described in Chapter 19.

If the therapy is effective, the patient should have adequate pain control, regain weight, and have less or no diarrhea. The patient needs to understand that it may take some time to achieve complete control of symptoms. Signs and symptoms that require immediate follow-up (recurrence of pain, occurrence of nausea and vomiting, occurrence of abdominal distention, recurrence or worsening of steatorrhea and diarrhea, and occurrence of signs and symptoms of diabetes mellitus) must be understood by the patient. If surgery is required, the nursing needs will be similar to those described on pp. 1381-1382.

PANCREATIC PSEUDOCYSTS

A pancreatic pseudocyst is a potential complication of acute and chronic pancreatitis, pancreatic trauma, or carcinoma. A pseudocyst is a collection of tissue, fluid, debris, and blood that fills a cavity contiguous with or surrounding the pancreas. The pseudocyst frequently disrupts the duct system of the pancreas. The signs and symptoms of pseudocysts are similar to those seen in acute pancreatitis, with pain being the most common symptom. An epigastric mass may be palpable.

Pseudocysts are serious for the following reasons: they worsen pain; they may rupture with or without bleeding; they may result in gastrointestinal bleeding because of erosive gastritis, peptic ulcer, or esophageal varices; they may result in pancreatic abscess formation; and they may cause ascites. Pancreatic pseudocysts may resolve spontaneously over six weeks. If no signs of complications are present, they are usually monitored by serial ultrasound examinations. If resolution does not occur, if the cyst increases in size, or if complications are present, surgery to drain the pseudocyst will be necessary. The care needs of the patient having surgery of the pancreas are described on pp. 1381-1382.

CANCER OF THE PANCREAS
EPIDEMIOLOGY/ETIOLOGY

Cancer of the pancreas is the fifth leading cause of death from cancer. Pancreatic cancer affects men more than women. It usually occurs after middle age. The cause of cancer of the pancreas is unknown, but it is diagnosed more often in smokers. Cancer of the pancreas also is associated with diets high in meat and fat, high coffee consumption, high alcohol consumption, and exposure to chemicals.[10]

PATHOPHYSIOLOGY

Most malignant tumors of the pancreas appear to begin in the ductal areas, causing eventual blockage and resulting in chronic pancreatitis. Direct extension of the lesion may cause its spread to the posterior wall of the stomach, the duodenal wall, the colon, and the common bile duct. The tumor may be diffusely spread over the entire gland, or it may be a well-defined growth. It commonly grows in a rapid manner and is highly invasive, and vascular, and lymphatic, and perineural metastases frequently occur. Many patients live only 3 to 6 months after diagnosis is confirmed.

CLINICAL MANIFESTATIONS
Signs and Symptoms

Symptoms of pancreatic malignancies are not usually detectable until late in the course of the disease. Pain occurs in about 85% of the patients. This may be preceded by vague anorexia, nausea, and weight loss over a period of months. Jaundice frequently occurs because of common duct obstruction but is seldom a primary sign. Changes in stools may occur if the pancreatic ducts are obstructed. Pain may be colicky or intermittent and often radiates to the back, abdomen, and chest. About half of the patients develop diabetes mellitus.

Diagnostic Tests

Definitive diagnosis before surgery is difficult. Diagnostic studies include CT scan, ERCP, duodenal cytology, pancreatic scans, and arteriography.

INTERVENTIONS
Medical Management

The primary treatment of the patient with pancreatic cancer is surgery, although the prognosis is usually poor. Surgery may be used for its curative effect in only a small percentage of cases. One procedure used for tumors of the head of the pancreas is pancreatoduodenal resection (Whipple's procedure) (Figure 46-5). Another procedure is total pancreatectomy with resection of parts of the gastrointestinal tract. Other procedures to help restore normal bile flow and the maximum pancreatic flow possible may be used.

Nonsurgical treatment with radiation and chemo-

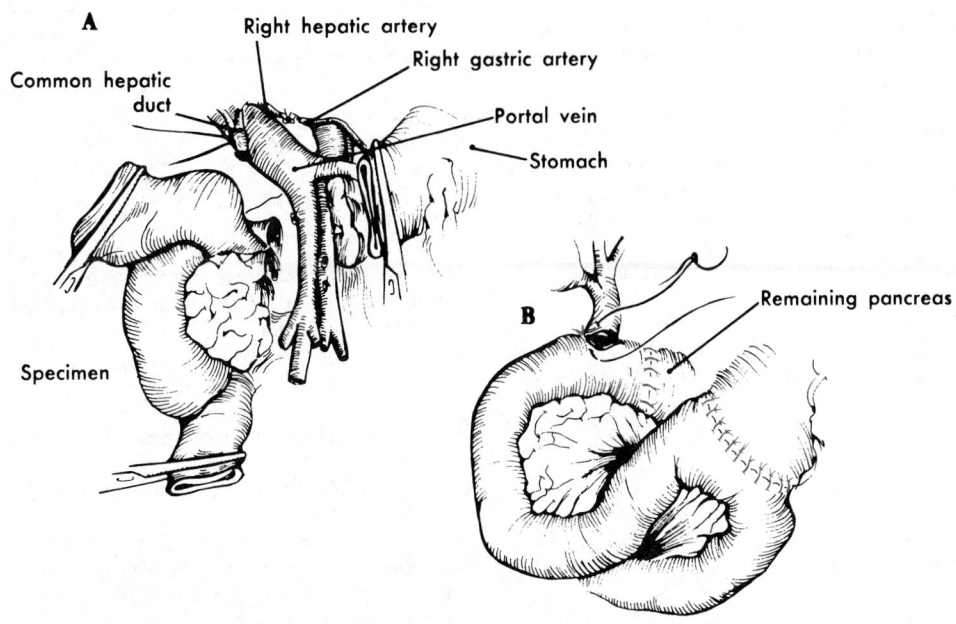

FIGURE 46-5 A, Radical one-step pancreatoduodenectomy (Whipple's procedure). Anastomosis and transresection completed. **B,** Reconstruction of gastrointestinal canal completed by means of three anastamoses: establishment of continuity with pancreas and jejunum, or duodenum, with gallbladder and jejunum, and with stomach and jejunum. (From Grundemann BJ and Meeker MH: Alexander's care of the patient in surgery, ed 7, St Louis, 1983, The CV Mosby Co.)

therapy may be used. Other medical care focuses on general supportive measures such as nutritional support, comfort measures, and maintenance of physical functioning.

Nursing Management

The nursing care for patients with cancer of the pancreas varies. In some patients, the focus will be related to care needs related to the surgery (see next section). In many patients the cancer is not resectable; thus care will be related to the needs induced by chemotherapy, radiation therapy, and the diagnosis itself as described in Chapter 17. This care includes the following: pain relief measures; nutritional, fluid, and electrolyte support; other comfort measures; promotion of maximum functioning and activity; and dealing with the grief, fear, and anxiety of the patient and the family.

SURGERY OF THE PANCREAS

Surgery of the pancreas may be used to treat pseudocysts, cancer, intractable pain, and calcification associated with chronic pancreatitis, traumatic injuries, and acute fulminant pancreatitis. The various surgical procedures are described in Table 46-4. The preoperative and postoperative care described below applies to patients undergoing partial or total pancreatectomy or the Whipple's procedure.

PREOPERATIVE CARE

Before surgery the patient should be as stable and as physically strong as possible. Fluid and vascular status should be normal. Nutritional status may be improved before surgery with hyperalimentation. If jaundice is present, the prothrombin time may be prolonged. This problem, if present, must be corrected with vitamin K or clotting factors. Before surgery the patient also needs the routine care described in Chapter 20. This includes collection of adequate baseline data, patient and family education, physical preparation, and emotional support of patient and family.

POSTOPERATIVE CARE

Following surgery the patient will be in an intensive care unit. The nurse must immediately establish the parameters that should be monitored continuously. Vital signs, output (for example, urinary and drainage tubes), intake, and hemodynamic parameters (CVP and arterial blood pressure) need to be monitored at least hourly. Laboratory measurements of hematocrit, blood gases, albumen, glucose, electrolytes, and serum and urine osmolality may be made at least daily or more frequently.

A major focus following surgery is *maintenance of adequate tissue perfusion.* Hypotension is a frequent occurrence and is treated with adequate replacement of fluids and electrolytes and blood. Vasopressors may be

TABLE 46-4 Selected surgical procedures of the pancreas

Procedures	Uses
Drainage procedures: drainage systems possibly established to drain fluid and debris from pancreas into adjacent structures such as stomach (cystogastrostomy) or jejunum (cystojejunostomy); also may involve placement of tube for external drainage	For pseudocysts
Resection of tail of pancreas and adjacent organ (spleen)	Cancer of tail of pancreas, chronic pancreatitis
Pancreatoduodenectomy (Whipple's procedure): removal of pancreas, ampulla of Vater, lower end of common bile duct, duodenum, and distal portion of stomach with anastomoses of stomach and pancreas and common bile duct to jejunum (Figure 46-5)	Carcinoma of the head of the pancreas, ampulla of Vater, duodenum, or common bile duct
Total pancreatectomy	Resectable cancers, trauma, intractable pain of chronic pancreatitis
Pancreatojejunostomy	Decompression of main pancreatic duct (palliative therapy for cancer of pancreas)
Cholecystoenterostomy	Decompression of biliary tract obstructed by pancreatic cancer
Partial pancreatectomy	For removal of portions of pancreas severely diseased with chronic pancreatitis; for liver donor tissue for transplantation for diabetes mellitus

needed for 24 to 48 hours. Signs and symptoms of hemorrhage must be continuously monitored for because of the massive resection and potential vascular bleeding or because of continual clotting factor defects.

A *second major focus* is *monitoring renal function*. A decrease in blood pressure or inadequate vascular volume can result in decreased glomerular filtration rate (GFR) and output. Maintenance of adequate vascular volume also helps prevent this potential problem. The fluid needs and/or drug needs are assessed on the basis of the continual monitoring carried out by the nurse. The importance of this surveillance cannot be overstated. An output of 20 to 50 ml/hr of urine is considered normal.

A *third major focus* is *prevention of respiratory complications*. Because of the high abdominal incision, respiratory efforts may be hampered, and atelectasis and pneumonia can occur. Preventive respiratory measures must be incorporated into the care plan. The patient who has a pancreatic resection may be on bed rest longer than other surgery patients, and this increases the possibility of respiratory complications.

The *patient may have various drainage tubes*. It is important that the *output from these tubes be measured carefully* so that *fluid* and *electrolyte balance* is *maintained*. Excellent skin care around T-tubes or other drainage tubes must be instituted. These patients may be malnourished before surgery; and bile, pancreatic, and gastric drainage are extremely irritating to the skin, and breakdown can easily occur.

The nurse must *monitor* the patient for *wound infection* and *infection* at *insertion sites* of *invasive* lines. The tubing and dressing for IV lines and wound dressings must be managed with aseptic technique. Temperature should be monitored carefully. Any signs of infection should be reported immediately.

Pain control is *another major focus* of *care*. Adequate pain control is necessary so that the patient is able to turn, cough, and deep breathe.

Maintenance of *nutritional status* is a *focus of care during* both the *preoperative and postoperative periods*. The poorly nourished patient will often start on hyperalimentation before surgery, and this will be continued after surgery. When oral food and fluids are allowed, clear fluids will be started first and advanced as tolerated. If a total pancreatectomy was performed, the patient will require pancreatic exocrine enzyme replacement. This may also be necessary if a large amount of the pancreas is removed during a partial resection. The patient's stools should be monitored for the presence of steatorrhea, which is used to assess the adequacy of exocrine replacement or the need for replacement. Weight changes will also help identify nutritional status. Also, if a portion of the stomach was removed, the *dumping syndrome* as described on pp. 1294-1295 may occur and is managed as described on p 1295. Management of the patient's nutritional status is an ongoing need.

Glucose metabolism must also be assessed. With a partial pancreatectomy in association with chronic pancreatitis, the islet cell mass will be decreased and may be insufficient to maintain normal glucose metabolism. If a total pancreatectomy is performed, insulin replacement will be necessary. At one institution, to minimize insulin insufficiency or to prevent it, islet cell autotransplantation is being performed along with total pancreatectomy. With this procedure, after removal of the pancreas, the islet cells are recovered and reinjected into the portal vein. This procedure helps to eliminate or minimize the diabetes mellitus associated with total pancreatectomy.[18] After partial or total pancreatectomy, all patients should have blood glucose monitored routinely, and insulin replacement should be given as needed. If insulin deficiency is present, it is treated as type I diabetes mellitus is treated (see Chapter 37).

Psychologic support will also be a major need because of the diagnosis, the acuity of the problem, the need for long-term dietary and drug management, and the physical debility that might have been present preoperatively and will be present after surgery. Support and encouragement must be provided during patient care. The patient needs help in recognizing progress and also must be helped to set realistic goals. The patient and family must be kept informed about all care measures.

An additional problem for the patient who is having pancreatic resection for intractable pain from chronic pancreatitis is potential narcotic addiction. The narcotic addiction may have occurred as a result of the previous management of the pain associated with chronic pancreatitis and must be dealt with. Immediately after surgery, the patient will continue to need narcotics for pain control, but once physical recovery is established, the patient and health team should work at decreasing and eliminating narcotic use. Some patients may need the assistance or support and counseling available in specialized hospital units or hospitals that treat the chemically dependent person (see Chapter 19). It is crucial to remember that adequate pain control with narcotic analgesics will be necessary during the immediate postoperative period, and that the patient's addiction will not be addressed until he or she is physiologically stable and physical sources of pain are thought to be controlled.

CHAPTER SUMMARY

- Cholecystitis and cholelithiasis are common health problems that could be decreased in incidence by decreasing obesity and controlling health problems such as diabetes mellitus.

- Biliary tract surgery is the treatment of choice for gallbladder disease even though lithotripsy and dissolving agents are available and used for some persons.

- Nursing needs before medical or surgical treatment of gallbladder disease focus on fluid volume deficit, bleeding, pain, self-care deficits, and knowledge deficits.

- Patient problems requiring nursing attention after medical or surgical treatment of gallbladder disease include ineffective breathing patterns, fatigue, fluid volume deficits, obstruction of T-tube or bile duct, knowledge deficit, and pain.

- Carcinoma of the biliary system is insidious and can be asymptomous until late in the disease.

- Care needs of the patient with biliary carcinoma may vary and may be focused on care after surgery, care to provide comfort, and care for a person with a terminal illness.

- Pancreatitis may be acute or chronic.

- Acute pancreatitis can result in severe fluid and electrolyte problems, metabolic disturbances, and pain. It is reversible.

- Chronic pancreatitis is progressive and usually results from alcoholism. It is not reversible.

- The patient with chronic pancreatitis will have acute exacerbations.

- Chronic pancreatitis results in pain, malnutrition, possibly diabetes mellitus, and variable fluid and electrolyte problems.

- Pain control measures, and measures to prevent malabsorption are the major focus of nursing care for all persons with chronic pancreatitis; many patients with chronic pancreatitis will also need measures to assist them in dealing with alcoholism.

- Cancer of the pancreas is insidious and has a very poor prognosis.

- Pancreatic cancer may result in chronic pancreatitis, jaundice, and pain.

- In rare instances of pancreatic cancer, a pancreatoduodenectomy may be performed.

- Postoperative care for the patient who has a pancreatoduodenectomy should focus on maintaining tissue perfusion, renal function, vascular volume, respiratory function, and skin integrity; preventing infections, controlling pain, and maintaining glucose metabolism and nutritional status.

QUESTIONS TO CONSIDER

- Differentiate the priority nursing needs of patient with acute pancreatitis from those for a patient with chronic pancreatitis.

- How do the nursing diagnoses relate to the pathophysiology of a patient with cholecystitis?

- What are some pain control measures that can be employed in chronic pancreatitis, cancer of the pancreas, or cancer of the biliary system?

REFERENCES AND SELECTED READINGS

1. *Adinaro D: Liver failure and pancreatitis: fluid and electrolyte concerns, Nurs Clin North Am 22(4):843-852, 1987.
2. Adwers JR: Clinical trials of gallstone lithotripsy, Hosp Pract 24(7):83-90, 1989.
3. *Bagg AM: Whipple's procedure: nursing guidelines, Crit Care Nurse 8(5):34-45, 1988.
4. *Birdsall C and Fiore-Lopez N: How do you manage pancreatic sump tubes, Am J Nurs 87:770-771, 1987.
5. *Blake RL: Acute pancreatitis, Primary Care 15:187-199, 1988.
6. Bradley EL: Complications of chronic pancreatitis, Surg Clin North Am 69:481-497, 1989.
7. Crist D and Cameron JL: The current management of acute pancreatitis, Adv Surg 20:69-124, 1987.
8. DiMagno EP: Early diagnosis of chronic pancreatitis and pancretic cancer, Med Clin North Am 72:979-992, 1988.
9. Fain JA and Amato-Vealey E: Acute pancreatitis: a gastrointestinal emergency, Crit Care Nurse 8(5):47-63 1988.
10. Fontham E and Correa P: Epidemiology of pancreatic cancer, Surg Clin North Am 69:551-567, 1989.
11. Frey CF, Bradley EL, and Beger HG: Progress in Acute Pancreatitis; Surgery, Gynecology and Obstetrics. 167:282-286, 1988.
12. Frey, C.F., et al: Pancreatic resection for chronic pancreatitis, Surg Clin North Am 69:499-527, 1989.
13. Glassman JA: Biliary tract surgery: tactics and techniques, New York, 1989, Macmillan Publishing Co Inc.
14. Holzbach RT: Pathogenesis and medical treatment of gallstones. In Sleisenger MH and Fordtran JS editors: Gastrointestinal disease, ed 4, Philadelphia, 1989, WB Saunders Co.
15. Ihse I and Lankisch PG: Treatment of chronic pancreatitis—current status, Acta Chir Scand 154:553-558, 1988.
16. Jeffres C: Complications of acute pancreatitis, Crit Care Nurse 9(4):38-46, 1989.
17. Jordan GL: Pancreatic resection for pancreatic cancer, Surg Clin North Am 69:569-597, 1989.
18. Kosel K et al: Total pancreatectomy and islet cell autotransplantation, Am J Nurs 82:568-571, 1982.
19. Lamb C: Abdominal pain: tracking and treating acute pancreatitis, Patient Care 20(1):76-79, 82, 87-88, 1986.
20. *Lancaster S and Biaro-Marshall D: Gallstone lithotripsy, Am J Nurs 88:1629-1630, 1988.
21. Moody FG: Pancreatitis as a medical emergency, Gastroenterol Clin North Am 17:433-443, 1988.
22. *Munn NE: When the bile duct is blocked, RN 20:50-57, 1989.
23. Potts JR: Acute pancreatitis, Surg Clin North Am 68:281-299, 1988.
24. Roberts JW: Carcinoma of the extraheptic bile ducts, Surg Clin North Am 66:751-756, 1986.
25. Roberts JW and Daugherty ST: Primary carcinoma of the gallbladder, Surg Clin North Am 66:743-749, 1986.
26. Rottenberg R: An update of pancreatic cancer, Patient Care 20(3):144-146, 151, 154-156, 158, 162, 1986.
27. Rowland GA, Marks DA, and Torres W: The new gallstone destroyers and dissolvers, Am J Nurs 89:1473-1478, 1989.
28. Sabesin S: Countering the danger of acute pancreatitis, Emer Med 19(17):71-73, 81-83, 87-89, 91-92, 95-96, 1987.
29. Sirinek KR and Aust JB: Pancreatic cancer: continuing diagnostic and therapeutic dilemma, Surg Clin North Am 66:757-776, 1986.
30. Sitges-Serra A et al: Pancreatitis and hyperparathyroidism, Br J Surg 75:158-160, 1988.
31. Steer ML: Classification and pathogenesis of pancreatitis, Surg Clin North Am 69:467-480, 1989.
32. Sievert W and Vakel N: Emergencies of the biliary tract, Gastroenterol Clin North Am 17:245-264, 1988.
33. Way LW and Sleisenger M: Cholelithiasis; Chronic and Acute Cholecystitis. In Sleisenger MH and Fordtran JS editors: Gastrointestinal disease, ed 4, Philadelphia, 1989, WB Saunders Co.
34. *Weinstein ND: Reactions to life-style warnings: coffee and cancer, Health Ed Qrtly 12(2):129-134, 1985.
35. Wyngaarden JB and Smith LH, editors: Cecil textbook of medicine, 18 ed., Philadelphia, 1988, WB Saunders Co.

*References preceded by an asterisk are particularly well suited for student readings.

CHAPTER 47

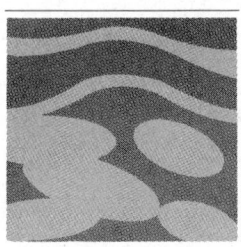

Assessment of Urinary Function

H. FRED FARLEY, JR.

CHAPTER OBJECTIVES

After studying this chapter, the student should be able to:
1   List seven major functions of the kidneys.
2   Describe the importance of impaired renal function-
    ing on the excretion of drugs.
3   Identify subjective and objective data for assess-
    ment of persons with impaired renal functioning.
4   List seven symptoms related to urination and the
    possible urinary problems they may indicate.
5   Describe the nursing implications of eight common
    radiologic examinations of the urinary tract.

An essential process for living tissue is *metabolism*, the process by which an organism is able to convert raw materials into energy. During metabolism, toxic waste products are formed. Maintaining *homeostasis*, or the state of equilibrium of the internal cellular environment, becomes essential for the continuation of life. There must be a means by which metabolic wastes are removed from living cells. Furthermore, the body must regulate fluid volume, electrolyte composition, and acid-base balance. The kidneys and other structures of the urinary system (Figure 47-1) play major roles in the regulation of the internal environment. Besides the role the kidneys play in maintaining the composition of body fluids and electrolytes within critical limits, providing a vehicle by which metabolic wastes are excreted from the body, and regulating the acid-base balance, these organs serve several other functions (see the box below).

ANATOMY AND PHYSIOLOGY

ANATOMY

UPPER URINARY TRACT

The *kidneys* are two bean-shaped organs that lie behind the parietal peritoneum at the costovertebral angle. The organs are composed of nephrons, a complex vascular system, an interstitium, and the urine collection system that begins with a tubular collection system and terminates with the renal pelvis. The *nephron* is referred to as the functional unit of the kidney. Each kidney contains approximately 1 million nephrons. The structures of the nephron involved in the process of urine formation include the glomerulus and Bowman's capsule, the proximal convoluted tubule, the loop of Henle, the distal convoluted tubule, and the collecting tubule (Figure 47-2). The kidneys are segmented into two distinctive regions: the cortex and medulla (Figure 47-3). Bowman's capsule and the convoluted tubules are located within the cortex, whereas the loop of Henle and the collecting tubules are in the medulla. As urine is formed, it drains into the convoluted tubules and flows into the collecting tubules and finally into the renal pelvis.

The *ureters* (Figure 47-1) arise as extensions of the pelvis and empty into the bladder in an area known as the *trigone* (Figure 47-4). The ureters are composed of smooth muscle and are innervated by the sympathetic nervous system. The function of the ureters is to propel urine from the renal pelves to the bladder.

LOWER URINARY TRACT

The *bladder,* located behind the symphysis pubis in the pelvic region (Figure 47-1), serves as a collecting bag for the urine. The mucous membrane is arranged in folds called *rugae* that, together with the elasticity of the muscular walls, can distend the bladder considerably to

MAJOR FUNCTIONS OF THE KIDNEYS

HOMEOSTASIS OF INTERNAL ENVIRONMENT

Fluid volume control
Electrolyte regulation
Acid-base balance
Excretion of metabolic wastes, toxins, and drugs

REGULATION OF BODY PROCESSES

Regulation of blood pressure
Stimulation of red blood cell production
Regulation of calcium-phosphate metabolism

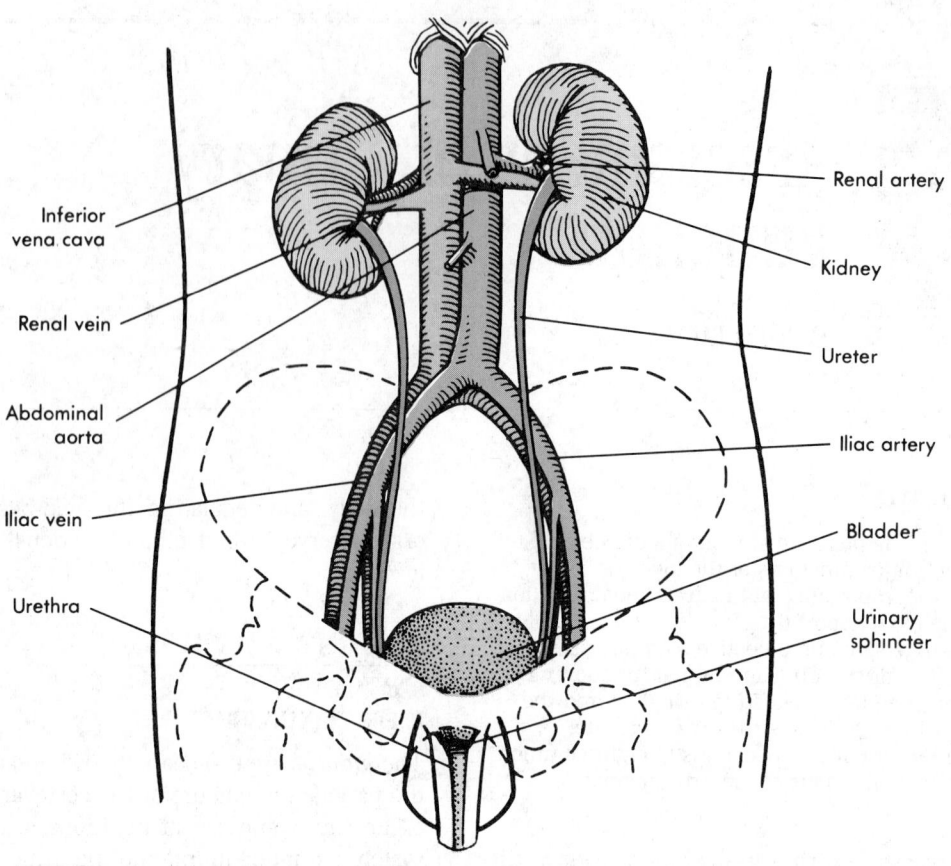

FIGURE 47-1 Organs and structures of urinary system.

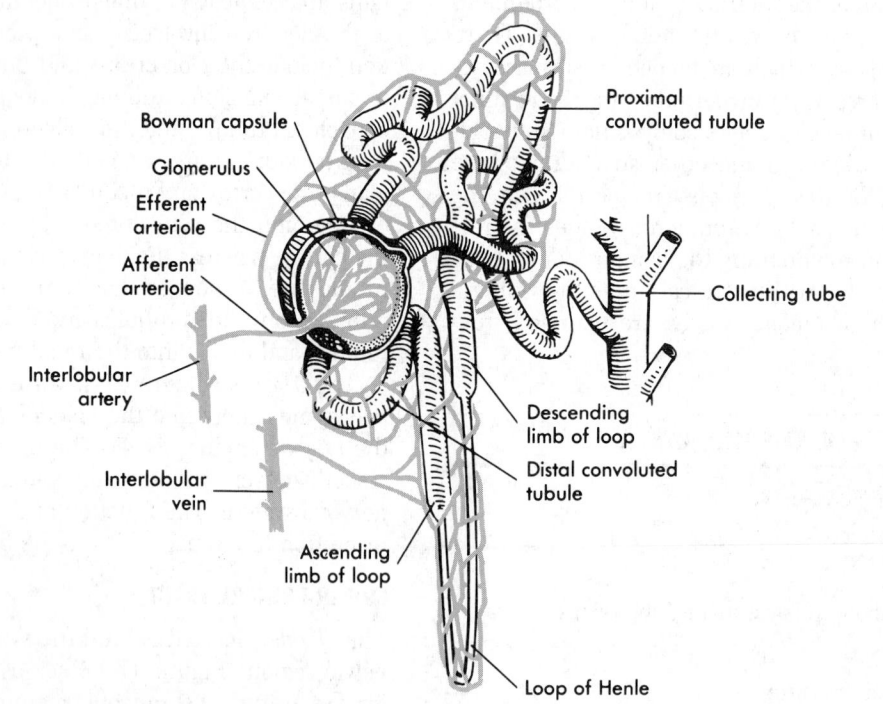

FIGURE 47-2 Nephron.

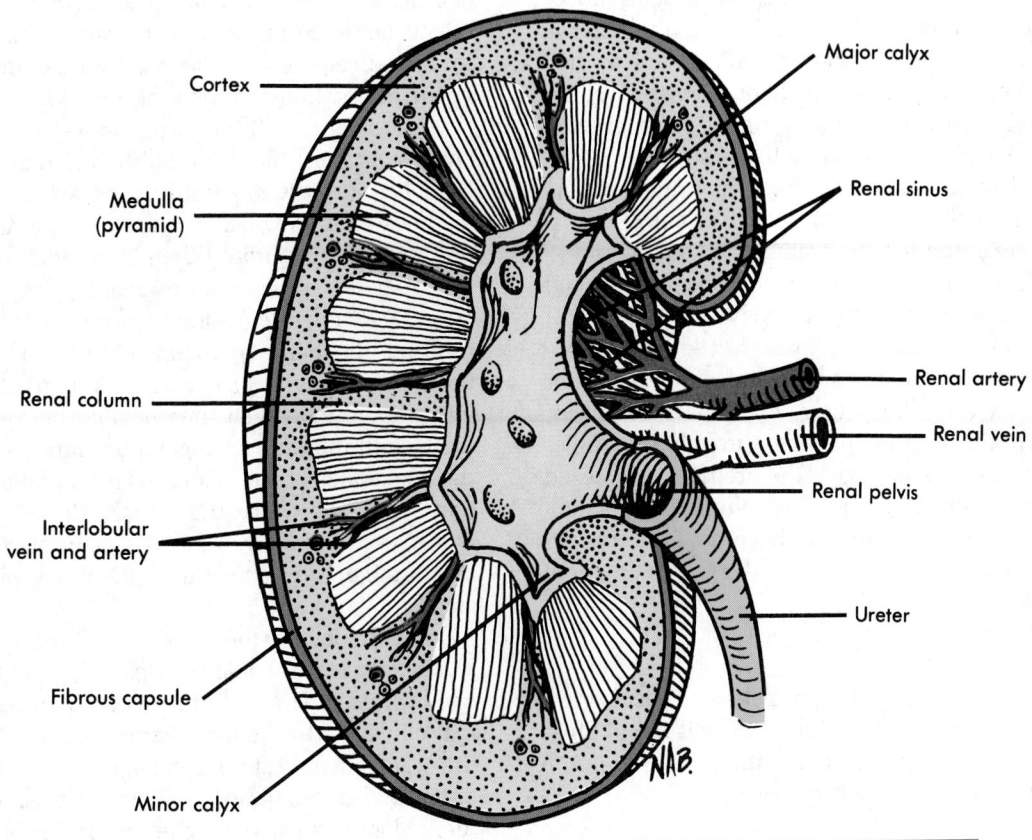

FIGURE 47-3 Frontal section of kidney.

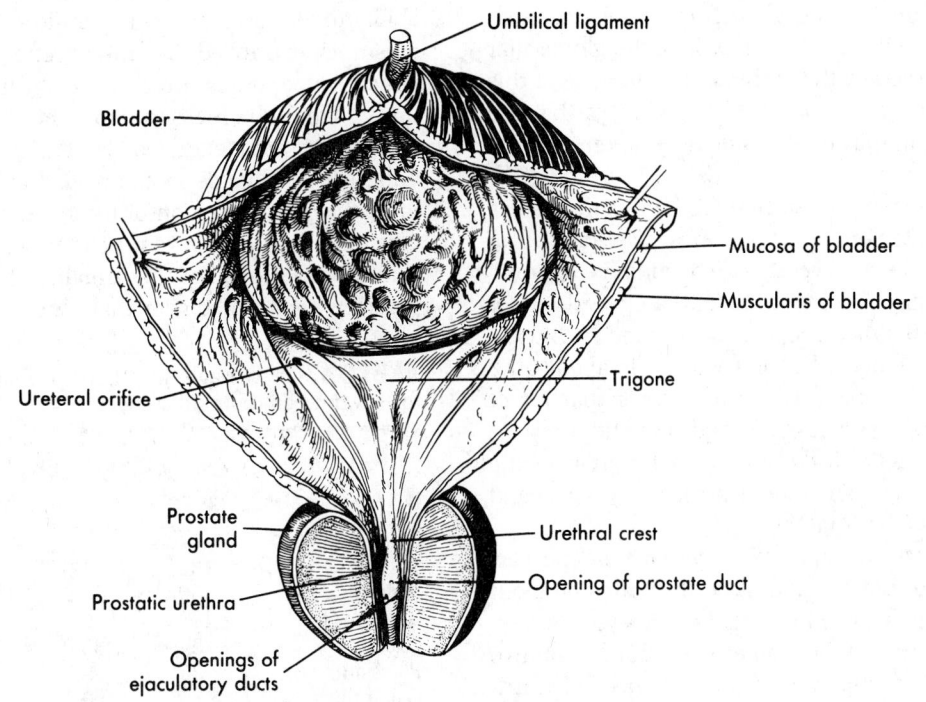

FIGURE 47-4 Interior of urinary bladder and some associated structures. (From Mc-Clintic, JR: Human anatomy, St Louis, 1983, The CV Mosby Co.)

hold large amounts of urine. A layer of skeletal muscle encircles the base of the bladder, forming the *external urinary sphincter*. The bladder is innervated by both the sympathetic and parasympathetic nervous systems. The urethral sphincter, operating under voluntary control, allows the urine to pass into the urethra.

The *urethra* serves as the outlet for urine from the bladder. The male urethra is about 20 cm (8 in) in length, whereas the female urethra is about 4 cm (1.5 in) long. The urinary meatus is the opening through which urine is excreted from the body.

The *prostate gland* is a male reproductive gland about the size of a walnut that encircles the upper portion of the male urethra (Figure 47-4). It is doughnut-shaped with the urethra passing through the "hole." When the prostate is enlarged, the urethra is squeezed, causing obstruction of urinary flow. Numerous prostatic ducts empty into the urethra. Bacteria from urinary tract infections may travel up these ducts, causing prostatic infection.

RENAL PHYSIOLOGY

A clear understanding of the physiology of the kidneys is essential to the mastering of the constellation of physiochemical changes that occur with renal failure. A short review of renal physiology follows.

ULTRAFILTRATION

As blood passes through the capillary bed of the glomerulus, filtration of the plasma occurs. In this process of *ultrafiltration,* primitive urine (*glomerular filtrate*) is formed. The volume of the glomerular filtrate approximates 180 L/day. Of this volume, 99% of the glomerular filtrate is reabsorbed by the kidneys. It is because of this tremendous reabsorptive power of the kidneys that the average urinary output of an adult is between 1 and 2 L/day.

Ultrafiltration is measured as GFR. GFR is defined as the amount of glomerular filtrate in a given period of time. The GFR in an average-sized adult is approximately 125 ml/min (7.5 L/hr). At this rate, a volume of approximately 60 times the plasma volume is filtered each day. The average GFR of a woman is about 10% less than that of a man. The same forces that affect fluid transport between vascular and interstitial spaces in other tissues of the body also affect filtration in the nephron. These factors include hydrostatic pressure and oncotic pressure (see Chapter 23).

The kidneys receive approximately 25% of the cardiac output, resulting in renal blood flow rates of about 600 ml/min. This blood supply to the kidneys is essential for the formation of the glomerular filtrate (primitive urine).[3] The blood supply also provides needed nutrients and oxygen to the cells of the kidneys. Severe or prolonged interruptions in cardiac output or renal perfu-

sion as a result of vascular obstruction have profound effects on the formation of urine as well as on the viability of the cells responsible for maintaining consistency in the internal environment of the body.

After passing through a series of progressively smaller arteries, blood enters the afferent arteriole that branches into the glomerular capillaries. The glomerulus, located in Bowman's capsule, is the first functional portion of the nephron. When blood enters the glomerular capillaries at a pressure greater than 60 to 70 mm Hg, an *ultrafiltrate* (primitive urine) is formed. The ultrafiltrate contains approximately the same concentration of elements as plasma. It is important to note that in a normal individual there should not be any plasma in the ultrafiltrate. As the ultrafiltrate passes through the remainder of the nephron, reabsorption and secretion occur to produce the actual urine that is then excreted from the body. Table 47-1 summarizes the average filtration rates and reabsorption rates of several substances.

Were it not for the conserving mechanisms in the kidneys, a person would be depleted of fluid and electrolytes within a period of only 3 to 4 minutes. The proximal convoluted tubule reabsorbs up to 85% to 90% of the water in the ultrafiltrate; up to 80% of filtered sodium; and the majority of filtered potassium, bicarbonate, chloride, phosphate, glucose, and amino acids. It is in the distal convoluted tubule and collecting tubule that the final development of the urine takes place.

Dehydration would still occur if the body did not have as an additional mechanism within the kidneys the ability to conserve water in the ultrafiltrate. This mechanism is controlled by antidiuretic hormone (ADH), which concentrates urine to 1% of the daily filtered volume. Through reabsorption, the kidneys vary the amount of fluid excreted so that intake over the required fluid balance is excreted. Reabsorption, leading to further concentration of urine, occurs when fluid intake falls short of that required for normal fluid balance. The kidney can vary the amount of fluid excreted so precisely that intake over that required for normal fluid

TABLE 47-1 Average filtration and reabsorption values for several common substances

Substance	Amount Filtered (per day)	Amount Excreted (per day)	Percent Reabsorbed
Water (L)	180	1.8	99.0
Sodium (g)	630	3.2	99.5
Glucose (g)	180	0.0	100.0
Urea (g)	54	30.0	44.0
Potassium (g)	35	2.0	94.0
Calcium (g)	5	0.2	96.0
Amino acids (g)	10	0.3	97.0

balance is excreted and intake under that required for normal fluid balance leads to further concentration of the urine. The mechanisms responsible for this increased urine-concentrating ability and precision in excreting appropriate urine volume are found in the *loop of Henle* and the distal convoluted and collecting tubules. The loop of Henle reaches into the medullary portion of the kidney, which is highly hypertonic in comparison to the filtrate. In the descending portion of the loop, sodium diffuses into the filtrate as the tubule passes deeper into the medullary area, and water moves out of the primitive urine in response to the high sodium concentrations. The results are a reduction in volume of the glomerular filtrate and a dramatic increase in its osmolality. In the ascending limb of the loop of Henle, sodium is reabsorbed into the interstitial tissues, but the loop is impermeable to the movement of water either into or out of the tubule. The primitive urine now presented to the distal convoluted and collecting tubules is greatly reduced in volume but is hypotonic because of the reabsorption of sodium. The influence of ADH on these last two segments of the tubules allows water to be reabsorbed into the interstitial tissue in an amount compatible with maintenance of proper fluid balance. The reabsorption of water from the ultrafiltrate increases osmolality and results in the excretion of hypertonic urine.

ELECTROLYTE BALANCE

Electrolyte balance is achieved mainly in the distal and collecting tubule portions of the nephron. As with fluid, the major conservation site for electrolytes is the proximal convoluted tubule where the vast majority of all filtered electrolytes are reabsorbed, thus preventing the depletion of these substances. The precise regulation of body electrolyte composition occurs in the distal tubular segments. Depending on the concentrations of electrolytes presented to the tubule cells in the primitive urine and the concentrations of these substances in the interstitium, tubular cells secrete or further reabsorb electrolytes into the urine. This regulation is by both *passive* and *active* mechanisms. Passive movement of electrolytes occurs across a concentration gradient; that is, electrolytes move from an area of higher concentration to an area of lower concentration. Active movement of electrolytes occurs by ion transport mechanisms and, therefore, can move electrolytes without respect to concentration gradients. Active transportation requires the expenditure of energy. Table 47-2 summarizes reabsorption and secretion by the nephron.

ACID-BASE BALANCE

The metabolic processes of the body generally produce excess acid. The body uses two major mechanisms for the maintenance of acid-base balance within a narrow range: respiratory and renal. Acid-base balance is maintained partially through the reabsorption of bicarbonate in the proximal tubule. More precise control of acid-base status is achieved through the regeneration of bicarbonate and secretion of hydrogen ions into the urine. Hydrogen ions are passively secreted in the proximal tubule and actively secreted in the distal tubule in exchange for sodium ions.

EXCRETION

Metabolic wastes are excreted in the glomerular filtrate. Creatinine contained in the glomerular filtrate is excreted unchanged in the urine. Other wastes, such as urea, are excreted unchanged in the glomerular filtrate but undergo reabsorption during passage through the nephron. The amount of waste material excreted in urine is only a portion of that which was originally contained in the glomerular filtrate. As electrolytes are reabsorbed by the nephron, so are most waste materials. It is important to remember that most drugs are either excreted directly by the kidneys, or they are metabolized by the liver to inactive forms, then excreted by the kidneys. Because of this role of the kidneys, some drugs are contraindicated, and the dose of others must be adjusted when renal function is impaired. Examples of drugs that are affected by renal failure include many classes of antibiotics, digitalis, salicylates, and long-acting barbiturates.

BLOOD PRESSURE REGULATION

The kidneys play an active role in the regulation of blood pressure. Four mechanisms have been identified

TABLE 47-2 Major sites of reabsorption and secretion within the nephron

Reabsorption	Secretion	Location
Glucose	Creatinine	Proximal tubule
Amino acids	Hydrogen ions	
Uric acid	Penicillin	
Sodium		
Potassium		
Calcium		
Magnesium		
Bicarbonate		
Phosphate		
Chloride		
Water		
Urea		
Sodium chloride		Loop of Henle
Chloride	Ammonium	Distal tubule
Water	Hydrogen ions	
Bicarbonate	Potassium	
Water		Collecting duct
Urea		

by which the kidneys regulate blood pressure: regulation of plasma volume, aldosterone, renin-angiotensin-aldosterone system, and prostaglandins.

The kidneys play a role in the regulation of plasma volume in two ways. The first of these is through the direct reabsortion of water to maintain plasma volume. The kidneys also regulate plasma volume by controlling the composition of extra cellular fluids. Aldosterone conserves body sodium by stimulating renal tubular reabsorption. This results in the conservation of water.

Renal regulation of blood pressure is also controlled by the renin-angiotensin-aldosterone system. *Renin* is a hormone released by the juxtaglomerular apparatus of the nephron in response to sodium depletion, renal artery hypoperfusion, or stimulation of the renal nerves through the sympathetic pathway. *Angiotensinogen,* which is produced in the liver, is activated to *angiotensin I* in the presence of renin. An enzyme in the lungs converts *angiotensin I* to the active form, *angiotensin II.* Angiotensin II is a powerful vasoconstrictor and also stimulates the release of aldosterone. The combined effect of these two mechanisms is an elevation in blood pressure. The systemic hypertension associated with renal disease (that is, renal artery occlusion, chronic renal failure, and acute renal rejection) results from the inappropriate activation of the renin-angiotensin-aldosterone system. In these conditions, the circulating blood volume is adequate, but renal perfusion is diminished, resulting in activation of the renin-angiotensin-aldosterone system.

In addition, renal prostaglandins seem to be locally active vasodilators and constrictors that serve to maintain renal blood flow and GFR in response to a variety of perfusion and endocrine changes.[8] The actual mechanism of action of prostaglandins is not completely understood.

ERYTHROPOIESIS

RBC production is controlled by the kidneys. *Erythropoietin* stimulates bone marrow to produce RBCs and prolongs the life of existing RBCs. Erythropoietin is produced in response to decreased oxygen delivery to the cells of the kidney. Persons with chronic renal failure often have serum hematocrit values of 18% to 30% (normal values are 42% to 47%). This decrease in hematocrit values is the result of decreased secretion of erythropoietin from the diseased kidneys compounded by bone marrow toxicity, decreased life span of RBCs, and increased bleeding, all of which are associated with the altered metabolic state present in chronic renal failure.

REGULATION OF PHOSPHATE AND CALCIUM

The kidneys also control calcium and phosphate metabolism. Vitamin D prohormone is converted to its active form by the kidneys. Active vitamin D regulates not only gastrointestinal (GI) absorption of calcium but also its deposition within the bone matrix as well as the metabolism of calcium and phosphorus. Parathyroid hormone (PTH) stimulates the tubular reabsorption of calcium and excretion of phosphate.

A constellation of signs and symptoms arises in patients with chronic renal failure that cannot as yet be explained. This leads to the belief that there may be some functions of the kidneys of which we are not yet aware. Because of this, nephrology remains an area rich with research questions.

MICTURITION

Urine flows out the kidney pelves and is propelled through the ureters by peristaltic action. About 200 to 300 ml of urine can collect in the bladder before the urge to void is initiated. Baroreceptors in the bladder wall are triggered by the stretching of the bladder walls, which causes reflex stimulation of parasympathetic nerves to the bladder, resulting in bladder contractions. When the motor nerves to the external urinary sphincter are inhibited, the muscle relaxes, opening the sphincter and permitting urine to be expelled. Stimulation of the sphincter muscles can keep the sphincter contracted against strong bladder contractions. Voluntary control over micturition can be exerted by a stimuli transmitted over descending spinal pathways from the brain stem.

Use of a large balloon (30 ml) indwelling catheter (such as after a transurethral resection of the prostate) can stimulate the parasympathetic nerves, causing uncomfortable bladder contractions. Pressure on the sphincter by the balloon can also create an urge to void, although the bladder has been emptied by the catheter.

PHYSIOLOGIC CHANGES WITH AGING

A direct relationship exists between blood supply to the kidneys and renal function. The rate of blood flow to the kidneys is about five to ten times greater than that to the heart, liver, and brain. Glomerular capillary pressure, which is the force that promotes ultrafiltration, is controlled by blood flow to the kidneys. Therefore physiologic alterations in the vascular bed can lead to changes in renal function.

Arteriosclerotic changes in renal arteries are the most common form of renal vascular pathology.[12] Arteriosclerotic changes occur to some extent in most normal individuals with aging. The degree of morphologic change experienced depends on the specific arteries affected and the extent of involvement within those arteries.

Aging is also known to cause predictable increases in both systolic and diastolic blood pressure.[20] This slow increase in blood pressure begins early in life and continues through adulthood. This relationship between aging and increasing blood pressure is so well accepted that normal blood pressure is commonly described as 100 mm Hg plus the age of the individual. Although this definition is not entirely accurate, it does emphasize the effect of aging on blood pressure. Untreated hypertension further accelerates the development of atherosclerosis, which can lead to renal failure.

Prostatic hypertrophy is a common physiologic change associated with aging that will be discussed in detail in Chapter 48. Prostatic hypertrophy that goes untreated will result in urinary obstruction that can lead to renal failure.

SUBJECTIVE DATA

URINATION

Obtaining baseline data concerning the person's usual voiding patterns, such as the frequency and general amount of urine voided, is helpful when changes are anticipated. Persons who are admitted to a hospital or other nursing facility are questioned about their ability to carry out toileting independently. All persons should be asked initially if any changes have been noted in voiding patterns. If changes have occurred, further data are obtained pertaining to onset, duration, and any measures that the person has taken to deal with these problems.

When asking questions about urination, it is important to recognize that some persons may be somewhat reluctant to answer, either because of embarrassment or misunderstanding. A calm, matter-of-fact approach by the interviewer will assist in putting the person at ease. Many persons are not familiar with terms such as "voiding" or "urination," and more colloquial words may need to be used in certain situations. The interviewer should be sure to validate that the person understands the questions so as to ensure that valid responses are obtained to questions.

Specific questions are directed at eliciting the presence of abnormal findings (Table 47-3). *Dysuria* (painful urination) is usually described as "burning with urination" and is usually associated with frequency and urgency when urinary tract infection is present. *Frequency* of urination is voiding at frequent intervals, either in small or large amounts; therefore, the approximate amount must be ascertained when this symptom is present. Voiding in small amounts may be caused by infection. Voiding in large amounts may be the result of an increased fluid intake or the effect of diuretics. If frequency is associated with suprapubic discomfort and the sense of fullness of the bladder but not with dysuria, the cause may be retention of urine in the bladder with frequent overflow of the excess amounts. *Urgency* refers to the need to void immediately. It commonly accompanies frequency in persons with urinary tract infections. A person with *nocturia* awakens at night with the need to urinate. Additional data that are collected when a person complains of nocturia include the num-

TABLE 47-3 Possible causes of urinary symptoms

Symptom	Problem	Question
Dysuria	Urinary tract infection	"Do you experience pain or burning on urination?"
Frequency on urination	Urinary tract infection Retention with overflow Excess fluid intake	"How frequently do you void?"
Urgency	Bladder irritation as result of inflammation Trauma Tumor	"Do you experience urgency or the need to void immediately?"
Nocturia	Increased fluid intake Diuretics Enlarged prostate Early renal failure	"Are you awakened at night with the need to void?" "If so, how often?"
Hesitancy	Partial urethral obstruction	"Do you have difficulty starting or maintaining your stream of urine?"
Decreased force and flow of urinary stream	Partial urethral obstruction Weakened perineal muscles	"Has the force of your stream of urine changed?"
Urinary incontinence	Stress Spinal cord injury CNS disease Urinary tract infection Partial urethral obstruction Trauma Prostatectomy	"Do you have difficulty controlling voiding?" "Do you dribble urine?"

ber of times this occurs at night, the amount of fluid intake in a 24-hour period, and whether this is a change in the usual voiding pattern.

Hesitancy refers to difficulty in initiating voiding. This is often accompanied by a decrease in the force and flow of the urinary stream. Persons with difficulties initiating voiding are asked if they have to strain to start or maintain the urinary flow. In men the most common partial obstruction is an enlarged prostate, whereas in women there may be weakened perineal muscles or meatal stenosis.

Urinary incontinence is the lack of control over voiding. Incontinency is assessed by determining the specific nature of the problem: occurrence continually or only with stress (such as exercise or coughing), the presence or absence of a sensation of fullness before voiding, health conditions associated with the incontinence, and the person's feelings about incontinence. Many persons are unwilling to admit that they have this problem, and assessment can be difficult. Any methods the person or family use to control the incontinence must also be identified.

PAIN

Pain resulting from urinary disorders is located in different areas of the body, depending on the organ involved. Referred pain is also fairly common with some urinary disorders. Pain from the kidney is usually experienced over the kidney site in the back between the twelfth rib and the iliac crest (costovertebral angle). Pain from the ureters may begin over the kidney area but radiate to the front along the course of the ureter and down the groin. Pain from the bladder is usually perceived in the suprapubic area. Any discomfort from prostatic disease is usually felt in the perineum. Data are collected regarding characteristics of the pain (see Chapter 16).

RENAL DISEASE

Whenever a urinary tract disorder is suspected, a complete assessment of renal history and functioning must be made. The following subjective data are useful guidelines for making a nursing assessment of a person with renal disease:
1. Person's perception of illness
   a. Factors leading person to seeking health care
   b. Expectations about current health care
2. Previous or concurrent illness
   a. Other chronic health problems
   b. Medication currently taken
3. Social needs
   a. Availability of supporting others
   b. Current occupation; capacity to continue present work
4. Fluid balance: dyspnea, visual changes, headaches

5. Electrolyte balance: lethargy, memory function, muscle weakness
6. Nutrition: anorexia, nausea and vomiting, history of special diets, knowledge of dietary restrictions, usual eating pattern
7. Elimination: Bowel pattern, laxative use, urinary pattern
8. Comfort: pruritus (extent, relief measures), sleep pattern, pain (nature, extent), mouth discomfort (odors, debris)
9. Mobility: fatigue, weakness, numbness, tingling, usual activity pattern
10. Sexuality: menses pattern (if appropriate), concerns about reproduction or sexuality

OBJECTIVE DATA

URINARY OUTPUT

Most persons have a urinary output approximately equal to their fluid intake. *Polyuria* (urinary output greater than 2500 ml/day) may occur with an intake greater than 2500 ml/day, uncontrolled diabetes mellitus, or renal disease. *Oliguria* (urinary output less than 400 ml/day) may be the result of suppression of urine formation by the kidneys or retention of urine in the bladder. When urinary retention is present, the person experiences suprapubic discomfort, and the enlarged bladder may be palpated above the symphysis pubis. Percussion usually reveals a tympanic sound. The frequent voiding of small amounts of urine is often a sign of retention with overflow. *Anuria* (urinary output less than 100 ml/day or the cessation of urinary output) is associated with renal failure.

Obtaining an accurate assessment of urinary output is often difficult in a hospital setting. Urine may be inadvertently discarded, or the patient may void into the toilet. The nurse should explain the importance of accurate urine collection to the patient. A communication system should be implemented to alert all staff members to patients whose output is being measured. In some cases, such as with shock or acute renal failure, when it is essential to accurately assess urinary output, an indwelling urinary catheter may be inserted. The risks and benefits of inserting an indwelling urinary catheter should always be assessed before placement of the catheter.

URINE CHARACTERISTICS

The urine is inspected for gross variations from normal. Normal urine varies in color from pale to deep yellow, depending on specific gravity. A very dark shade suggests that urine may be concentrated (high specific gravity) or that there may be an increased excretion of bilirubin. Certain medications and foods may also change the color of urine.

Hematuria (blood in the urine) may be detected overtly or may be present microscopically. In gross hematuria the urine may be pink-tinged to cherry red in color. If blood is observed in the urine of a woman having her menstrual period, the vaginal orifice can be blocked with cotton balls and another specimen obtained to ascertain the source of the blood. Hematuria with pain may be the result of calculi, a clot from renal bleeding, or bladder infection.

Cloudy urine may result from precipitation of phosphate salts in an alkaline urine or from bacterial growth. A urinary or vaginal discharge may also give the urine a cloudy appearance. Urine collection methods will be discussed in the section on diagnostic tests.

RENAL DISEASE

Objective data pertinent to specific renal diseases and to renal failure are discussed in Chapters 48 and 50, respectively. Some general data parameters are listed below:

1. Behavior: behavioral changes, level of alertness and orientation, apprehension, scratching, sleeping during day, grimacing, or showing other signs of pain
2. Vital signs
   a. Respirations: rate, depth
   b. Pulse: irregularities
   c. Blood pressure: postural
   d. Temperature (fever)
3. Weight: direction and rate of change
4. Skin and mucous membranes: lesions, moisture
5. Mouth: odor, presence of debris, condition of teeth
6. Chest: breath sounds (wheezing, rhonchi), pericardial friction rub
7. Extremities: peripheral edema, decreased muscle tone, decreased sensation, decreased balance
8. Urinary output: amount/hr, amount/day in relation to intake
9. Laboratory values
   a. Urine: urinalysis, specific gravity, culture
   b. Blood: electrolytes, pH, creatinine, BUN

ASSESSMENT OF THE ELDERLY

It is particularly important to recognize the physiologic changes that occur with aging so that normal variations can be distinguished from those due to aging. Of all age groups, the elderly show the greatest diversity.[1] Therefore, each elderly person who is assessed will show a different profile of physiologic changes. Important changes occurring with aging that affect the assessment of urinary function include nocturia, frequency, and urgency, resulting from decreased tone of bladder and pelvic muscles. Sphincter muscles also become weakened; however, urinary incontinence is not a nor-

mal part of aging and its presence should always be thoroughly evaluated.

Glomerular filtration rate is also affected by aging. In addition, decreased reabsorption results in less efficient urine concentration. As a result of these physiologic changes, serum creatinine and BUN are slightly elevated. Glucose reabsorption may also be decreased, resulting in normal serum values (for elderly persons) of 52 to 135 mg/dl (compared with standard values of 70 to 110 mg/dl).

DIAGNOSTIC TESTS

Special examinations of the urinary system are performed to identify the location and nature of existing disease. The accuracy of findings in many of the following tests depends on the assistance of the person in restricting or augmenting intake of fluids or in collecting specimens at designated time intervals. The person should be given clear, precise directions; written instructions are a valuable supplement to verbal directions.

Many of the diagnostic tests used to assess renal function are performed on an ambulatory basis. Therefore, it is important to assess the understanding of the patient about all instructions in preparation for the test. Some examinations must be performed under sedation; if so, the patient is instructed to make prior arrangements for someone to provide patient transportation after the procedure.

EXAMINATION OF THE URINE
URINALYSIS

In identifying disease of the urinary tract, one of the first tests performed is urinalysis. This test yields information about probable locations and causes of urinary disease and some information as to the extent of the illness. Urinalysis is a test that assists in establishing tentative diagnoses and predicting additional tests and observations required to make precise diagnoses. Urinalysis also indicates abnormalities of nonrenal and nonurologic origin (for example, diabetes mellitus). Table 47-4 indicates possible normal and abnormal findings.

CLEAN-CATCH SPECIMENS

Ideally, the urine specimen is collected from the first voiding of the day. This sample is preferable because it is concentrated and abnormal constituents are more likely to be present. The person is given a clean container in which to catch urine. Cleansing the meatus before collecting the specimen decreases the likelihood of external contamination; mild soap followed by water or a special antiseptic solution may be used. At least 50 to 100 ml of urine is collected for the test to ensure a sufficient amount to determine specific gravity and to

TABLE 47-4 Urinalysis

Test	Normal	Abnormal
Color	Amber-yellow	Red indicates hematuria (possible urinary obstruction, renal calculi, tumor, renal failure)
Clarity	Clear	Cloudy: debris, bacterial sediment (urinary infection)
pH	4.6-8.0 (average 6.0)	Alkaline on standing or with urinary tract infection Increased acidity with renal tubular acidosis
Specific gravity	1.003-1.035	Usually reflects fluid intake; the less the fluid intake, the higher the specific gravity If specific gravity remains low (1.010-1.014), renal disease is suspected
Protein	0-8 mg/dl	Proteinuria may occur with high-protein diet and exercise (particularly prolonged) Seen in renal disease
Sugar	0	Glycosuria occurs after a high intake of sugar or with diabetes mellitus
Ketones	0	Ketonuria occurs with starvation and diabetic ketoacidosis
RBCs	0-4	Injury to kidney tissue (see hematuria)
WBCs	0-5	UTI
Casts	0	UTI, renal disease

perform microscopic analysis. If analysis of the urine cannot be performed immediately, the specimen must be refrigerated to retard bacterial growth.

COMPOSITE SPECIMENS

A specimen of all the urine excreted over a specific period of time is often required for urologic diagnosis. The duration of urine collections may vary from 2 to 24 hours. Specimens are examined for sugar, protein, sediment (blood cells and casts), 17-ketosteroids, electrolytes, catecholamines, and breakdown products of protein metabolism. These tests provide information on (1) the ability of the kidneys to excrete and conserve various solutes, (2) the production in the body of excessive hormones that are excreted in the urine, (3) changes in the body's regulation of glucose metabolism, (4) identification of organisms difficult to recognize through routine urine cultures, and (5) presence of abnormal cells and debris in the urine.

The accuracy of findings in this type of test in most instances depends entirely on cooperation of the patient. Whether the specimen is to be obtained in the hospital or in the home, the person needs to be told exactly how to collect it. Instructions for a composite urine specimen are found in the box at right.

Composite urine tests may also involve collecting urine from multiple sources from the body. For instance, the person may pass urine from the urethra and also have a nephrostomy tube from which urine drains. Ureteral catheters may also be in place, with urine being collected from each kidney separately. Depending on the function of the test, whether the purpose is to measure the identified element in the urine as a whole or to measure separately the excretion of this element from each source, the urine collected from each source may be combined into one specimen container or collected into separate appropriately labeled containers.

URINE CULTURE

Urine cultures are used to confirm suspected infections, to identify causative organisms, and to determine appropriate antimicrobial therapy. Cultures are also obtained for periodic screening of urine when the threat of urinary tract infection (UTI) persists.

Urine in a properly collected and stored sample is considered to be normal if it contains 10,000 or fewer organisms per milliliter. Organisms of this magnitude are the result of normal urethral flora and do not signify UTI. A UTI is diagnosed when bacterial counts in a properly collected and stored sample reach 100,000 or more organisms per milliliter and the organisms are of one or very largely one bacterial type.[26] It is most likely that contamination of the urine specimen during collection has occurred when bacterial counts include predominant colonies of *Staphylococcus*, *Streptococcus*,

INSTRUCTIONS FOR COMPOSITE URINE SPECIMEN

1. The bladder is emptied and the urine *discarded* at the appointed time to start the test.
2. Urine from *all* subsequent voidings is saved.
3. Specific directions for storing the urine should be given. Some specimens need to be kept cold during the collection period; some need preservatives added: some need no special care.
4. The person should void into a separate receptacle before defecation to prevent contamination of the specimen.
5. The bladder is emptied, and the urine *added* to the collection at the appointed time to end the test.
6. The designated amount (properly labeled) is sent to the laboratory.
7. If an aliquot (5 to 10 ml sample of the total specimen) is the designated amount, the total amount collected is (1) measured and recorded on the specimen requisition and (2) mixed well before the aliquot is selected.

DIRECTIONS FOR COLLECTING A MIDSTREAM URINE SPECIMEN

EQUIPMENT NEEDED
Sterile container for the urine
Three sponges (cotton or gauze) saturated with cleansing
    solution

GENERAL DIRECTIONS
Only outside of collecting container is touched
Urine is collected in container well after urinary stream is
    started

SPECIAL DIRECTIONS
Female

Labia are kept separated throughout procedure
Meatus is cleansed with one front-to-back motion with
    each of the three cleansing sponges

Male

Foreskin is retracted if man is uncircumcised
Glans is cleansed with each of the three cleansing
    sponges

---

and diphtheroids; when two or more organisms contribute significantly to the total bacterial count; or when repeated cultures yield differing results. All of these results indicate a need to repeat the culture, paying particular attention to the collection of the specimen and to its handling.

Specimens for urine culture may be obtained either by catheterization or by midstream voiding (see the box above). It should be made clear, however, that *urethral catheterization should never be used routinely in collecting urine for culture because of the risk of introducing additional bacteria into the bladder*. Catheterization may be necessary to obtain a sterile urine specimen when the person is unable to void after being adequately hydrated or if the person is incontinent of urine. When a catheter is passed, meticulous attention is given to nontraumatic aseptic technique. After urine flow from the catheter is established, 5 to 10 ml of urine should be collected directly into a sterile specimen container. Care must be taken to ensure that the rim and the inside of the container are not touched by the catheter or by the hands. If a culture tube with a cotton plug is used as a specimen container, care must be taken to keep the tube upright to prevent moistening the cotton and thereby contaminating the specimen. Cultures may also be ordered on the urine taken from the renal pelvis during ureteral catheterization or when ureterostomy or nephrostomy tubes are in place.

In collecting a voided specimen for culture, the nurse must decide if the patient is capable of independently obtaining the specimen or if nursing or medical personnel will need to collect a midstream specimen. Most persons who are ambulatory and are given precise and unhurried directions will be able to collect their own midstream urine specimen.

The first voided specimen of the day should be used whenever possible, because bacteria will be more numerous. If the specimen is not cultured immediately, refrigeration is mandatory to prevent growth of organisms in the specimen.

EVALUATION OF BLADDER FUNCTION
MEASUREMENT OF RESIDUAL URINE

Normally, the bladder contains little or no urine after voiding; however, certain disease states inhibit the bladder from emptying completely. Some common conditions in which incomplete emptying of the bladder occurs are benign prostatic hypertrophy, urethral strictures, and interruptions in bladder innervation. Urine left in the bladder after voiding is called *residual urine*.

One way to determine the amount of residual urine is to *catheterize* the person immediately after voiding. This may be ordered by the physician on a one-time or on a repeated basis. Before catheterizing the person, the physician is consulted about the plan for establishing urinary drainage. If a large amount of residual urine is suspected, the physician may wish the catheter to be left in place in the bladder. *Residual urine volumes of 50 ml or less indicate near normal or returning bladder function.*

To avoid passing a catheter to measure residual urine volumes, x-ray film examination of retained urine may be performed. In this procedure a radiopaque substance excreted by the kidneys is injected intravenously. As the dye is excreted in the urine, it passes into the bladder. A sufficient amount of urine containing the radiopaque material is allowed to accumulate in the bladder before the person is instructed to void. Immediately after voiding, an x-ray film is taken. Any urine retained in the bladder will be visualized on the x-ray film. This means of determining residual urine is used in conjunction with other studies requiring visualization of the urinary tract.

CYSTOMETROGRAM

Cystometric examination is performed to evaluate bladder tone. In general, the examination is indicated when incontinence is present or when there is evidence of neurologic dysfunction of the bladder. A Foley catheter is inserted before the examination. After the person assumes a supine position, a liter bag of normal saline or sterile distilled water and a cystometer are connected to the catheter. Fluid is instilled at a constant and specified rate; measurements of the pressure exerted on the fluid by the bladder musculature are recorded after the instillation of every 50 ml of fluid. The person is asked to report feelings of fullness, the need to void, and any

TABLE 47-5 Selected renal function tests

Test	Normal Results	Purpose-Significance	Nursing Implications
Specific gravity of urine	1.010-1.026	Test measures ability of kidneys to concentrate urine.	First morning void is usually in the high normal range in healthy individual. False high is caused by presence of radiographic dyes.
Osmolality of urine	400-600 mOsm/kg	Test is excellent indication of renal function. Osmolality is total concentration of particles in solution.	No special preparation needed.
Fishberg concentration test	Urine volume 300/ml/12 hr Specific gravity of 1.024 or greater Urine osmolality of 850 mOsm or greater	Test is used to determine ability of kidney to conserve fluid, and as differential diagnosis for diabetes insipidus and psychogenic polydipsia.	No fluid can be taken during test period. Test period is 8 to 12 hr, usually during night First morning void assures maximum concentration. Three hourly urine specimens are collected for volume, specific gravity, and osmolality following test period. Patient should be observed for signs of vascular collapse.
Urine chemistries	Sodium: 130 to 220 mEq/L Potassium: 39 to 90 mg/24 hr Calcium: 100 to 300 mg/24 hr	Urine electrolytes reflect ability of kidney to excrete and reabsorb electrolytes.	Abnormal results may be caused by diseased processes other than renal disorders; for example, elevated urine calcium in hyperparathyroidism or prolonged immobilization.
Creatinine clearance	Men: 100 to 150 ml/min Women: 85 to 125 ml/min	Clearance is rate at which a substance is excreted in terms of plasma concentration. Because diet and metabolic state have little influence on it, serum creatinine is excellent for determining glomerular filtration rate.	Procedure 1. Patient empties bladder and time is noted. 2. *All* urine is saved for 24 hr. 3. Exactly 24 hr after start of procedure the patient voids, and specimen is saved. 4. Total urine volume and urine creatinine are measured. 5. Serum creatinine is determined at end of 24-hr period. 6. Creatinine clearance is then calculated by formula: $$\text{Clearance} = \frac{UV}{P}$$ U = Urine creatinine concentration V = Urine volume P = Plasma creatinine concentration
Serum creatinine	Men: .85 to 1.5 mg/100 ml Women: .7 to 1.25 mg/100 ml	Test indicates ability of kidneys to excrete nitrogenous wastes.	No specific preparation is needed for test. Diet and metabolic rate have little effect on serum creatinine.
Blood urea nitrogen (BUN)	5 to 20 mg/100 ml	Test indicates ability of kidneys to excrete nitrogenous wastes BUN gives a rough estimate of GFR.	BUN can be affected by high-protein diet, blood in GI tract, and catabolic state (injury, infection, fever, poor nutrition).

TABLE 47-5 Selected renal function tests—cont'd

Test	Normal Results	Purpose-Significance	Nursing Implications
Phenosulfonphthalein excretion test (PSP)	30% to 50% of PSP dye excreted in 15 min	Test measures tubular secretion rates.	Procedure 1. Patient drinks 8 to 10 glasses of water. 2. 1 ml PSP dye is given intravenously. 3. Urine specimens are collected at 15-, 30- and 60-min intervals. 4. The exact time the urine specimen is collected must be recorded to calculate excretion rates.

urgency or discomfort. Fluid is instilled until urgency occurs or it is determined that the sensation is absent. During cystometric examination, bethanechol chloride (Urecholine) may be administered to determine its effect on enhancing the tone of a flaccid bladder, or an anticholingeric medication may be given to assess relaxation in a hyperactive bladder. There is no specific care required after cystometric examination.

Electromyography may be used to evaluate sphincter tone and intactness of nerve pathways.

EVALUATION OF RENAL FUNCTION

When findings of the general physical examination or urinalysis suggest renal disease, tests of renal function are conducted. A summary of renal function tests is found in Table 47-5. It should be remembered that the best overview of the patient's clinical condition is obtained by comparing the results of a number of tests. Therefore, it is common for a series of renal function tests to be ordered for an individual.

Serum electrolytes do not give conclusive results in terms of renal function. Many factors influence serum electrolytes. In renal failure, the serum electrolytes may be normal, elevated, decreased, or any combination of these. Serum electrolyte levels are monitored closely in patients with renal failure so that their level can be adequately regulated. The normal ranges for the most commonly measured electrolytes are shown in the box below.

NORMAL VALUES OF SELECTED SERUM ELECTROLYTES

Sodium	135 to 140 mEq/L
Potassium	3.5 to 5.0 mEq/L
Chloride	98 to 102 mEq/L
Bicarbonate	24 to 28 mEq/L
Calcium	9 to 22 mg/100 ml

CLEARANCE TESTS

When renal disease is suspected, the physician will want to determine the amount of damage, if any, that has already occurred. The most practical and efficient way to identify losses in renal function is by means of clearance tests. These tests measure the amount of blood that an individual's kidneys can "clear" of a substance in a given amount of time. When the person's values are compared to normal values, changes in renal function become apparent. Clearance tests are also used to monitor the direction of change and the rate of change in renal function over time.

The *creatinine clearance* test is the most practical and widely used of all clearance tests. Creatinine is a substance that results from the breakdown of muscle tissue. It is produced at a relatively fixed and uniform rate throughout the day, it can be measured readily in the blood, and it is not influenced by dietary intake. Creatinine is excreted through the kidneys; it is filtered in the glomerulus and passes practically unchanged through the renal tubules. It is an ideal naturally occurring substance that, when blood and urine values are compared, allows one to estimate changes in glomerular filtration rates and overall kidney function. The creatinine clearance value for an individual is expressed in terms of milliliters per minute and is determined according to the following formula:

$$\text{Creatinine clearance (ml/min)} = \text{Urine volume (ml/min)} \times \frac{\text{Urine creatinine concentration (mg/ml)}}{\text{Plasma creatinine concentration (mg/ml)}}$$

For this test, a morning-to-morning 24-hour urine collection is obtained. (Refer to collection of composite urine specimens on p. 1394.) Immediately after the final urine specimen is collected, a blood specimen is drawn to determine the serum creatinine level. Both blood and urine specimens are sent together for analysis. Analysis of the total urine volume for the test period is essential for accurate determination of renal function. If one voiding is accidentally discarded, the test must be repeated. The nurse must ensure accurate collection of all urine in the prescribed time. A shorter period of time may be used in instances when collection of accurate urine collections over a 24-hour period is next to impossible.

The *sodium excretion* test measures tubular function. Specifically, this test provides information as to the kidney's ability to appropriately excrete or conserve this electrolyte; in chronic renal failure either inappropriate retention or excretion of sodium can occur. Knowledge of urinary excretion of this electrolyte is helpful in calculating sodium intake requirements of the patient. To determine change in direction and degree of tubular functions, comparison of current and past sodium excretion studies should be made. The test is performed by analyzing the sodium content of a 24-hour urine collection.

VISUALIZATION OF THE URINARY TRACT

Technologic advances in the last several years have made it possible to visualize the urinary tract by both direct and indirect means. These tests allow for assessment of both structure and function of the organs and tissues of the urinary tract. Visualization of the urinary tract is used not only for diagnosis but also to evaluate the patient's response to therapy over a period of time.

CYSTOSCOPY

Cystoscopy is the direct examination of the bladder using an instrument called a cystoscope (Figure 47-5). The cystoscope relies on a flexible optic fiber to provide illumination into the urinary tract. The instrument is attached to the illuminating source and then slowly passed through the urinary tract, thus enabling direct visualization of the urethra, ureteral orifices, and bladder.

Most hospitals require a signed permit before cystoscopy is performed after the person is given an explanation of what is to occur. Fluids are usually forced for several hours before the procedure. This ensures a continuous flow of urine in the event specimens need to be collected and aids in preventing multiplication of bacteria that may be introduced during the procedure. If general anesthetic is to be used, fluids may be administered intravenously. If x-ray films are to be taken during the procedure, bowel preparation may be ordered.

The cystoscopic examination may be performed with or without anesthesia. General anesthesia is required for cystoscopy when the person is quite apprehensive or when much manipulation is anticipated. In these instances, anesthesia reduces the possibility of trauma to the urethra or perforation of the bladder caused by sudden vigorous movement of the patient during the examination. Children are usually given a general anesthetic for this procedure.

Much of the discomfort felt during this procedure is the result of contraction or spasm of the bladder sphincters; this can be decreased through deep-breathing exercises and general relaxation on the part of the patient. A sedative such as diazepam (Valium) and a narcotic such as morphine or meperidine hydrochloride (Demerol) are usually given an hour before the examination.

If the patient is relatively comfortable, the cystoscope should be passed with little pain, provided there is no obstruction in the urethra. A local anesthetic such as procaine (usually 4%) may be instilled into the urethra before insertion of the cystoscope.

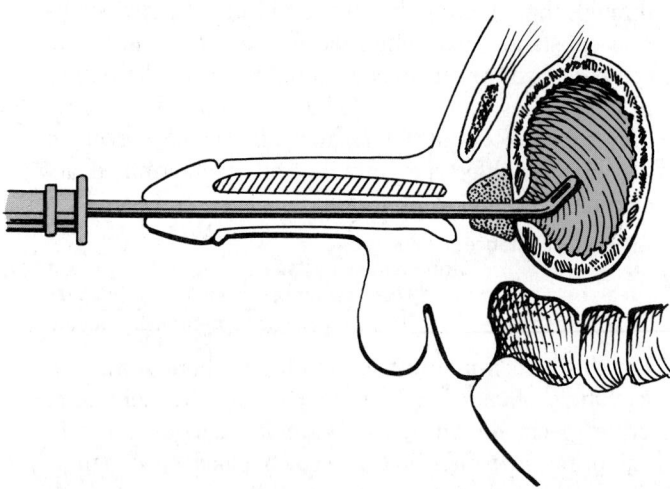

FIGURE 47-5 Cystoscope inserted for examination of bladder.

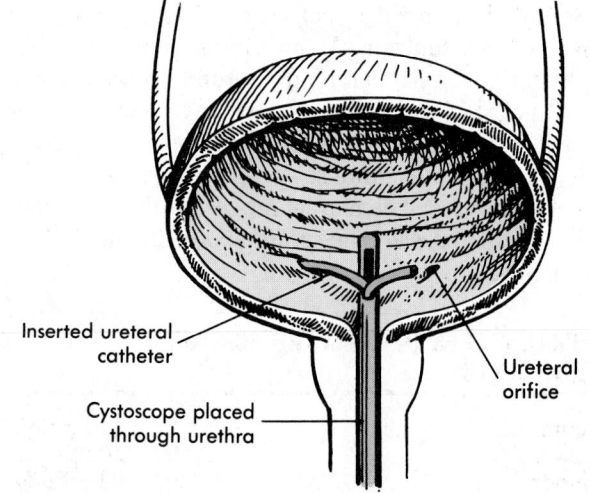

FIGURE 47-6 Ureteral catheterization through cystoscope. Note ureteral catheter inserted into left orifice. Right ureteral catheter is ready to be inserted.

When the patient is awake, passing the instrument will be followed immediately by a strong desire to void. This occurs as a result of the pressure the instrument exerts against the internal sphincter. During the examination, the bladder is distended with distilled water to make visualization more effective. As the bladder becomes increasingly distended, the urge to void increases.

During cystoscopy a number of tests may be performed on the urinary system. *Cystography* involves the injection of a radiopaque dye such as methiodal (Skiodan) or air as a contrast medium to visualize the bladder and determine its size, shape, and any irregularities. Bladder capacity may be measured through instillation of distilled water. A *voiding cystourethrogram* can reveal reflux of urine into the ureters on voiding, a bladder malfunction that can lead to pyelonephritis.

Ureteral catheterization (with a nylon, radiopaque, size 4 to 6 Fr catheter) can be performed through the cystoscope. The catheter is inserted into the ureteral opening in the bladder, into the ureter, and into the renal pelvis (Figure 47-6). This procedure may involve one or both ureters. It is performed (1) when culture and analysis of urine from individual kidneys is required; (2) when tests of renal function are to be performed on the kidneys separately; and (3) when visualization of the urinary tract is desired and intravenous pyelogram visualization has been inadequate, obstruction is present, or sensitivity to intravenous radiopaque material is noted.

The nurse validates the person's understanding of the procedure as part of the preoperative teaching. If local anesthesia is to be used, be certain to describe what the patient can expect during the procedure. The pa-

---

NURSING CARE PLAN

PERSON FOLLOWING CYSTOSCOPY

DATA: Mr. King is a 64-year-old retired accountant. He reports that up until last month he was in good health. He has no significant medical history and has never been hospitalized. He is currently taking no prescription medications. Mr. King visited his family physician 2 weeks ago and complained of urinary dribbling, which has increased significantly in the past several days. On further questioning, he states he has experienced nocturia for the last several months. He also has experienced increasing difficulty in initiating urination. On physical examination the physician noted a grossly enlarged prostate. Mr. King was admitted for cystoscopy.

NURSING DIAGNOSIS

Altered patterns of urinary elimination (nocturia) related to anatomic obstruction.

Expected Patient Outcomes	Nursing Interventions	Rationale
Patient does not complain of nocturia.	Limit fluid intake in evening hours; have patient empty bladder before going to bed.	Reduce urine production at time of sleep; empty bladder will reduce need to wake during night.

NURSING DIAGNOSIS

Knowledge deficit (cystoscopy) related to lack of exposure to information.

Expected Patient Outcomes	Nursing Interventions	Rationale
Patient can describe what to expect during and after cystoscopy.	Teach patient about procedure, stress sensations he may experience. Describe post-procedure routine. Instruct patient about post-procedure limitations.	Understanding procedure will reduce anxiety and facilitate compliance and relaxation. Providing information on restrictions may prevent post-procedure injury.

NURSING DIAGNOSIS

Pain related to diagnostic tests (cystoscopy)

Expected Patient Outcomes	Nursing Interventions	Rationale
Patient does not complain of pain after cystoscopy	Provide pain medication as prescribed. Encourage warm tub baths.	Analgesics to relieve pain; warm tub baths relax muscles, thereby relieving pain.

TABLE 47-6 Common radiologic examinations of the urinary tract

Test	Purpose	Procedure	Nursing Implications
Retrograde pyelography	Visualization of urinary tract	1. Ureteral catheterization required 2. Radiopaque material (Hypaque, Renografin) gently injected 3. X-ray films taken of renal collecting structures	Patient may experience discomfort in region of kidneys as dye is injected. Pain may be experienced if too large a volume of dye is injected and renal pelvis becomes distended.
Intravenous pyelography (IVP)	Determine size and location of kidneys Demonstrate presence of cysts or tumors Outline filling of renal pelvis Outline ureters and bladder	1. X-ray film of abdomen (KUB) taken to identify size and position of kidneys 2. Radiopaque dye given intravenously 3. X-ray films of kidneys taken at 3-, 5-, 10-, and 20-min intervals	Bowel cleansing is required. Fluids are often withheld for up to 8 hr to produce slight dehydration. The patient should be informed that a feeling of warmth, flushing of the face, and a salty taste in the mouth may occur as the dye is injected. The patient should be observed for signs and symptoms of a reaction to the dye, including respiratory distress, diaphoresis, urticaria, instability of vital signs or unusual sensations. CPR equipment and emergency medications should always be available for immediate use.
Kidney, ureters and bladder (KUB) x-ray films	Gross visualization of KUB Location of calcifications and stones possible	X-ray film of abdominal region obtained	Bowel cleansing may or may not be ordered.
Urethrography	Visualization of urethral size and shape	X-ray films of urethra taken after instilling 20 ml of radiopaque water-soluble lubricant	No special preparation is needed.
Computed tomography (CT)	Visualization of kidneys and renal circulation	Whole body CT scanner segments kidneys Can be done with IV contrast dye	If dye is used, the same implications apply as listed for IVP.
Renal angiography	Visualization of renal circulation Particularly useful in evaluating renal artery stenosis	Similar to IVP; however, contrast dye often injected directly into femoral artery by passing a catheter through artery to level of renal arteries	Nursing implications are the same as in IVP. Patient must be observed for bleeding at arterial puncture site, especially within first 4 hours. The pressure dressing should be checked for fresh bleeding. The puncture site should be checked for tenderness or swelling. Vital signs and distal pulses must be assessed frequently (q 15 min × 4 hr). Bed rest should be maintained for 8 hr after the procedure.
Renography	Visualization of urinary tract Measures renal blood flow Measures renal tubular and excretory function	Involves scintillation scanning or photography Radioactive isotope such as iodohippurate sodium tagged with iodine-125 or iodine-131 injected intravenously Scintillating probes placed over kidneys record photographs	Since only trace doses of bound isotopes are used, no special precautions are necessary.
Ultrasound	Used to distinguish between abnormal fluid collections and solid masses; used to identify obstructions and detect abscesses; often used to diagnose abscesses, ureteral leaks, and obstructions in renal transplant recipients	Sound waves used to outline internal body structures; procedure accomplished by computer interpretation of tissue densities	Procedure is painless and noninvasive. A full bladder assists in outline structures.

tient should not stand or walk alone immediately after cystoscopy because blood that has drained from the leg while in the lithotomy position will flow back into the vessels of the feet and legs as standing is assumed. Accidents caused by dizziness and fainting can occur from the sudden change in distribution of blood.

Three complications of cystoscopy that need to be monitored are bleeding, perforation of the bladder, and spread of infection throughout the urinary tract or into the bloodstream (sepsis). Observation for frank bleeding (pink-tinged urine is normal) is necessary. Urinary output and voiding pattern are monitored to detect obstruction, and fluid intake is increased to prevent stasis. Mild analgesics are given for discomfort, and warmth is provided if the patient complains of being chilly. Vital signs are monitored as necessary. The patient should be instructed that the first void after cystoscopy can be uncomfortable. Warm tub baths may provide comfort. (See sample nursing care plan on p. 1399).

RADIOLOGIC EXAMINATION

A number of radiologic examinations are used to visualize the urinary tract (Table 47-6). Since the kidneys lie retroperitoneally, any accumulation of flatus or feces in the intestine can obstruct the view on the x-ray film. To assure adequate visualization, bowel evacuation is necessary before the x-ray films are taken.

X-ray films of the urinary tract may be ordered in conjunction with other abdominal studies. Problems may arise in visualizing the urinary system if barium studies have been recently carried out. This problem can be prevented by scheduling tests so that examination of the urinary tract precedes barium contrast x-ray films of the GI tract.

RENAL BIOPSY

Renal biopsy is potentially the most accurate diagnostic tool for determining the type and stage of progression of renal pathology. Specifically, this test aids in differentiating diagnoses, following the progression of disease processes, assisting in selection of therapy most beneficial to the patient, and determining prognosis of the illness. The biopsy can be performed either through a skin puncture (closed biopsy) or through an incision (open biopsy) over the kidney.[6]

Inherent in taking a biopsy specimen of the vascular tissues of the kidney is a potential threat of hemorrhage. Throughout the procedure, care is given to prevent and detect early loss of blood. Before biopsy is performed, a thorough medical evaluation with particular attention to detection of any abnormality in bleeding or coagulation time is carried out. The patient's blood is usually typed and crossmatched with two units of blood; the blood is held for the patient until any threat of bleeding has passed.

An open biopsy carries less risk of hemorrhage and provides better visualization of the kidney; however, the risk of infection is increased. A longer time is also required for recovery.

Preparation before biopsy includes discussing the procedure with the patient. Topics covered should include the necessity for the examination, the procedure itself, and the care to be anticipated after the procedure. The patient is also encouraged to ask any questions regarding the procedure. The preparation of the patient is shared by the physician and the nurse. In most institutions it is necessary to have the patient sign a special permit before having the biopsy performed. The biopsy may be performed in the patient's room, the operating room, or in the radiology department.

The procedure for *percutaneous* (closed) *biopsy* is as follows: Before the biopsy, the patient is taken to the radiology department for localization of the kidney. This is accomplished with a plain film, a dye contrast film, or fluoroscopic location. The position of the kidney in relationship to body landmarks is marked on the skin in ink. The lower pole of the kidney is located, since this is the site for obtaining the biopsy specimen, because it contains the fewest number of large vessels. The patient is then transported to the area where the biopsy will be performed. The procedure may be accomplished by computed tomography (CT) actually guiding the placement of the biopsy needle. Sedation is usually not required except for patients who are restless and unable to relax sufficiently to follow necessary instructions during the procedure. The patient is placed in a prone position over a sandbag or firm pillow and an additional soft pillow. The physician identifies the location for biopsy, and a local anesthetic agent is injected. As the biopsy needle is inserted, the patient is instructed to take a

---

POSTPERCUTANEOUS RENAL BIOPSY PRECAUTIONS

1. Patient must remain on bed rest, flat, in a supine position, and motionless for 4 hours after the biopsy.
2. Cough must be avoided for first 4 hours after the biopsy.
3. Blood pressure and pulse should be taken by the following routine.
   a. Every 15 minutes for 1 hour
   b. Every 30 minutes for 1 hour, and
   c. Every hour for additional 2 hours or until stable
   The responsible physician should be notified of increases in pulse of more than 10 to 20 beats per minute above the baseline or decreases in blood pressure of more than 10 mm Hg, unless otherwise instructed by the physician.
4. Patient should remain on bed rest for 24 hours.
5. Patient may experience hematuria for first 24 hours after the biopsy.
6. Patient should avoid heavy lifting for 10 days after the biopsy.

breath and hold it. Pain may be felt in the kidney region as the tissue sample is taken. The needle is withdrawn immediately, and direct pressure is applied to the site for 20 minutes. A pressure dressing is then applied, and the patient is turned supine and kept flat for at least 4 hours. The nursing care requirements for the period immediately after the procedure are summarized in the box on p. 1401.

The procedure for an *open* biopsy is similar to other kidney surgery. The nursing care for this type of surgery is discussed in Chapter 49. The vast majority of biopsies are currently being performed by the percutaneous method.

CHAPTER SUMMARY

✔ The kidneys play an essential role not only in maintaining homeostasis but also in the excretion of drugs.

✔ The major functions of the kidneys include fluid and electrolyte regulation; acid-base balance; excretion of metabolic wastes, toxins, and drugs; regulation of blood pressure; RBC production and regulation of calcium and phosphate.

✔ In gathering data about urinary function, it is important to validate that the person understands all the questions asked, since many euphemisms exist about body elimination.

✔ The nurse must have a clear understanding of diagnostic tests to appropriately support the patient.

✔ The nurse must validate that the person understands all instructions related to diagnostic testing. Provide written information whenever possible.

QUESTIONS TO CONSIDER

- Why must the physician consider altering the medication dose of many drugs when the patient is in renal failure?
- What are the characteristics of normal urine?
- What objective data must the nurse collect in evaluating the person's renal function?
- What nursing care might be required after cystoscopy?

REFERENCES AND SELECTED READINGS

1. *Andreesen G: A fresh look at assessing the elderly, RN 52(6):28-40, 1989.
2. Black DAK: Renal disease, ed 4, Oxford, England, 1979, Blackwell Scientific Publications Ltd.
3. Brenner BM and Rector FC, Jr, editors: The kidney, ed 3, Philadelphia, 1986, WB Saunders Co.
4. †Dunn M: Renal prostaglandins' influences on excretion of sodium and water, the renin-angiotensin system, renal blood flow, and hypertension. In Brenner B and Stein J: Hormonal function and the kidney, Edinburgh, 1979, Churchill Livingstone Inc.
5. †Fennell S: Percutaneous renal biopsy, Am J Nurs 75:1292-1294, 1975.
6. French R: Guide to diagnostic procedures, ed 5, New York, 1980, McGraw-Hill Inc.
7. Goldberger E: A primer of water, electrolyte, and acid-base syndromes, ed 7, Philadelphia, 1986, WB Saunders Co.
8. Herman JR: Handbook of urology, Philadelphia, 1983, JB Lippincott Co.
9. †Juliani L: Assessing renal function, Nursing 78 8(1):34-35, 1978.
10. Kee JL: Laboratory and Diagnostic tests with nursing implications, ed 2, Norwalk, CT, 1986, Appleton-Century-Crofts.
11. Kunin CM: Detection, prevention and management of urinary tract infections, ed 4, Philadelphia, 1987, Lea & Febiger.
12. Leaf A and Cotran R: Renal pathophysiology, Oxford, 1985, Oxford University Press Inc.
13. Malasanos L et al: Health assessment, ed 4, St Louis, 1989, The CV Mosby Co.
14. *Marshall S: Flank pain, hematuria, and allergy to intravenous pyelogram dye; real or contrived? JAMA 245:1557, 1981.
15. Metheny N and Snively W: Nurses' handbook of fluid balance, ed 4, Philadelphia, 1983, JB Lippincott Co.
16. *Metheny N: Fluid balance: nursing considerations, ed 3, Philadelphia, 1987, JB Lippincott Co.
17. Munzig NC: Why physical assessment? Nephrol Nurse 2:56, 1980.
18. Pagana KD and Pagana TJ: Diagnostic testing and nursing implications, ed 2, St Louis, 1985, The CV Mosby Co.
19. †Papper S: The effects of age in reducing renal function, Geriatrics 28:83-87, 1973.
20. Porth C: Pathophysiology, ed 2, Philadelphia, 1986, JB Lippincott Co.
21. †Roberts SL: Renal assessment: a nursing point of view, Heart Lung 8:105-113, 1979.
22. Schrier R and Gottschalk C: Diseases of the kidney, ed 4, Boston, 1988, Little, Brown & Co Inc.
23. Smith DR: General urology, ed 12, Norwalk, CT, 1988, Appleton & Lange.
24. Tilkian SM, Conover MB, and Tilkian AG: Clinical implications of laboratory tests, ed 4, St. Louis, 1987, The CV Mosby Co.
25. Vander A: Renal physiology, ed 3, New York, 1985, McGraw-Hill Inc.
26. Weber J: Nurses' handbook of health assessment, Philadelphia, 1988, JB Lippincott Co.
27. Wyngaarden JB and Smith LH: Cecil textbook of medicine, ed 18, Philadelphia, 1988, WB Saunders Co.

*References preceded by an asterisk are particularly well suited for student reading.
†References preceded by a dagger are classic readings.

CHAPTER 48

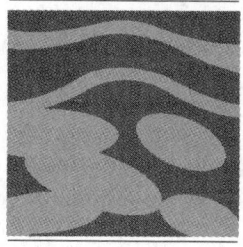

Management of Persons with Urinary Tract Problems

H. FRED FARLEY, JR.

CHAPTER OBJECTIVES

After studying this chapter, the student should be able to:
1 Identify six major health problems of the urinary system.
2 Describe the pathophysiology and management of polycystic kidney disease.
3 Describe etiology, pathophysiology, and management of lower urinary tract infections and pyelonephritis, including the importance of public awareness and patient teaching.
4 Compare glomerulonephritis and the nephrotic syndrome in relation to pathophysiology, clinical manifestations, and management.
5 Describe the pathophysiology and interventions for renal calculi.
6 Compare different approaches to prostatectomy and describe the related nursing interventions.
7 Differentiate types of urinary incontinence and describe appropriate management.

A major cause of morbidity and a significant cause of mortality in the United States is disease of the urinary system. Mortality from disease of the urinary system is generally associated with damage of interstitial tissues of the kidneys. When a disease process involves the tissues of the kidneys, renal function is directly threatened. If disease is present in the urinary drainage system, it not only affects tissues at the site of the disease but can also threaten renal function by two mechanisms: spread of the disease process or destruction of renal tissue from obstruction of urine flow. The primary objective for treatment of disease in any part of the urinary tract should be early detection and adequate therapy directed toward preserving or improving renal function; without renal function life can be maintained for only a few days.

During the last two decades some of the most striking developments in the treatment of urinary system diseases have evolved in both diagnosis and treatment of renal disease. Advances in computer tomography and ultrasound have made major contributions to diagnosis. New technologies in membrane development have pro-

vided improved dialysis while surgical and immunologic advances have greatly improved the success of transplantation.

Nurses can provide valuable assistance in significantly reducing morbidity related to the urinary system. This can be achieved by (1) increasing public awareness of preventive measures, (2) assisting in early detection of signs and symptoms of renal disease, (3) providing on-going health teaching for persons with renal disease, and (4) providing long-term care to the growing population of chronically ill individuals with urinary tract disease. This chapter describes common disorders of the urinary system and their management.

Major health problems of the urinary system can be divided into six categories as follows:
1. Congenital disorders
   a. Structural malformations of the urinary system
   b. Polycystic disease
2. Inflammatory disorders
   a. Urinary tract infection
   b. Pyelonephritis
   c. Chemical induced nephritis
   d. Glomerulonephritis
   e. Nephrotic syndrome
3. Vascular disorders
   a. Nephrosclerosis
   b. Renal artery stenosis
   c. Diabetic nephropathy
4. Obstructive disorders
   a. Calculi
   b. Neoplasms
   c. Prostatic hypertrophy
   d. Urethral strictures
5. Urinary incontinence
6. Trauma

CONGENITAL DISORDERS

Structural malformation of the urinary collecting system occurs in about 10% to 15% of the population.[26] These

CONGENITAL MALFORMATIONS OF URINARY TRACT

Duplication of ureters (partial or complete)
Hydroureters: dilation of ureters
Exstrophy of urinary bladder: eversion of bladder on outer abdominal wall
Epispadias: opening of urethra on dorsum of penis (Figure 48-1, *B*)
Hypospadias: opening of urethra on underside of penis (Figure 48-1, *A*)

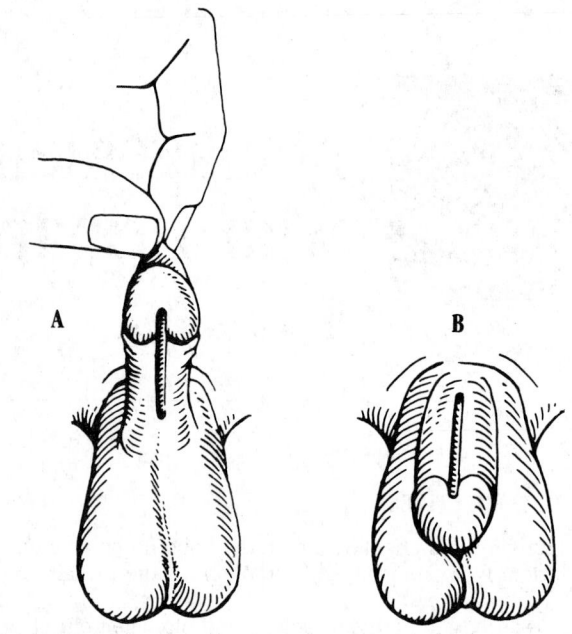

FIGURE 48-1 A, Hypospadias. **B,** Epispadias.

deviations range in severity from minor anomalies that do not require correction to those that are incompatible with life. Some of the congenital malformations that have a potential influence on urinary function in adult life are listed in the box above.

Details about the management of congenital disorders can be found in most pediatric nursing textbooks. However, polycystic disease is discussed in this chapter because it has significant adult morbidity.

POLYCYSTIC DISEASE
EPIDEMIOLOGY/ETIOLOGY

Polycystic disease is an inherited disease that involves the kidneys bilaterally. The kidneys are usually enlarged and filled with cysts. Polycystic disease is categorized into two groups: infantile and adult. Infantile polycystic disease is an autosomal recessive trait. The infant usually develops symptoms and dies within a few months after birth. Adult polycystic disease is an autosomal dominant trait affecting one in 500 persons. It affects both kidneys and symptoms generally develop in the third to fourth decade of life. End-stage renal disease is usually reached 10 to 15 years after the first symptoms arise.

PREVENTION

There is no preventive care for polycystic disease. However, early detection and medical care can prevent and control infection of diseased kidneys and retard the development of end-stage renal disease.

PATHOPHYSIOLOGY

As polycystic disease progresses, cysts in the kidneys enlarge and rupture (Figure 48-2). The ruptured cysts become infected and scar tissue develops. As scarring occurs, the number of functional nephrons decrease. The size of the cysts also increase gradually, creating pressure on surrounding parenchyma and causing ischemic atrophy.

CLINICAL MANIFESTATIONS

Persons with active polycystic disease present with abdominal or flank pain. Hematuria and hypertension are each present independently in approximately 50% of all cases of polycystic disease, although it is common for both hematuria and hypertension to be present in the same individual. The enlarged kidneys may be palpable either unilaterally or bilaterally. Recurrent urinary tract infections with chills and fever are common and frequent urine cultures are performed. A retrograde pyelograph, KUB (kidneys, ureters, bladder) x-ray, CT scan, and echography provide data about the size of the kidneys. Intravenous pyelogram (IVP) is most often used to confirm the diagnosis. Serum and urine electrolytes, as well as creatinine clearance tests, provide data about renal function.

INTERVENTIONS
Medical Management

No specific treatment is available and therapy is directed toward control of symptoms and prevention of infection. Hypertension is closely monitored and controlled. Infections are treated vigorously because the scarring leads to further progression of the disease process. Infection is difficult to eradicate and can lead to further destruction of kidney tissue. Antibiotic therapy is often instituted and should be given on time to ensure adequate blood levels. Urinary output is closely monitored. Symptoms of uremia may be present when renal function has deteriorated to the point of end-stage renal disease.

Nursing Management

Analgesic drugs may be necessary for control of flank pain associated with enlarged kidneys. Tepid baths will

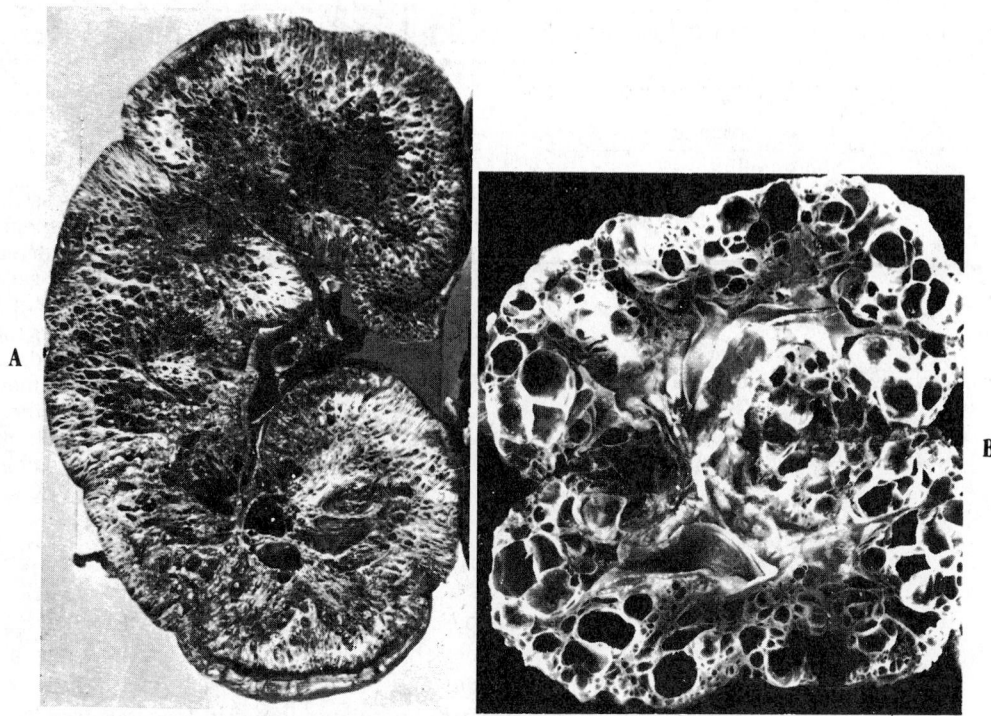

FIGURE 48-2 Polycystic disease of kidney. **A,** Newborn infant. **B,** Adult. (From Anderson WAD, and Kissane, JM: Pathology, ed 7, St Louis, 1977, The CV Mosby Co.)

also provide comfort during infections. When urinary bleeding from ruptured cysts becomes severe, bed rest is often instituted. Because polycystic disease is bilateral and leads to chronic renal failure, on-going support and health teaching are essential nursing interventions.

Patient Teaching

The patient is instructed to be alert to signs and symptoms of infection and bleeding. The emotional overtones of this illness can be severe for both the individual and the family. Challenges exist in helping the person deal with an illness on an individual basis when relatives have died of the same disease and children have not yet developed symptoms. Counseling may be required about family health care and the individual's role in passing on a potentially fatal disease to children. Patients are instructed to monitor urinary output and report changes to their physician.

INFLAMMATORY DISORDERS

The kidneys are susceptible to inflammation caused by bacterial infection, altered immune response, drugs and other chemicals, toxins, and radiation. Inflammation may be acute or chronic. This section will address the most common inflammatory disorders of the urinary system.

LOWER URINARY TRACT INFECTIONS

Urinary tract infections (UTIs) are a significant source of morbidity in the United States. These infections contribute to illness during the acute infection and also are significant in the development of chronic renal failure. Infection occurs in both acute and chronic stages in all portions of the urinary tract.[25]

EPIDEMIOLOGY AND ETIOLOGY

Table 48-1 is a summary of factors contributing to infection of the urinary tract. Although the great majority of uncomplicated urinary tract infections are asymptomatic and clear spontaneously, there remains a portion significant enough to warrant consideration as a health problem. Because untreated UTIs can lead to more significant problems they must be taken seriously. There is no controversy among those practicing preventive health care about the need for screening for asymptomatic infections; however, it is difficult to identify the specific groups at risk in which the detection and treatment of these infections yield significant improvement in the person's health. As the health care of our population becomes more oriented toward prevention of health problems, specific target populations will be better defined, and the number of screening programs for asymptomatic urinary tract infections should increase.

Urinary tract infection occurs more frequently in fe-

TABLE 48-1 Risk factors associated with development of urinary tract infections

Risk Factors	Common Examples
Female	Short urethra
Structural abnormality	Strictures
	Incompetent ureterovesical junction anomalies
Obstruction	Tumors
	Prostatic hypertrophy
	Calculi
	Iatrogenic causes
Impaired bladder innervation	Congenital spinal cord malformation
	Spinal cord injury
	Multiple sclerosis
Chronic disease	Gout
	Diabetes mellitus
	Hypertension
	Sickle cell disease
	Polycystic kidney disease
	Multiple myeloma
	Glomerulonephritis
Instrumentation	Catheterization
	Diagnostic procedures

males than males. Contributing factors include a shorter urethra with a close proximity to the vagina and rectum (see research box) and the lack of prostatic fluid that provides protection from UTI for males. Infection rates for females are approximately 1% in school-aged girls. This rate increases to approximately 4% for women in the child-bearing years, and 10% in women aged 70.[40] There is also increased risk of infection with increased sexual activity. Pregnancy does not seem to increase UTI rates, although spontaneous clearing of infections is decreased during pregnancy. Infection of the lower urinary tract also increases the incidence of acute kidney infections as a result of ascending microorganisms.

Structural and functional abnormalities of the urinary tract, obstruction to the flow of urine, and impaired bladder innervation promote infection of the urinary tract. Mechanisms that result in infection include stasis of urine that promotes a culture medium for bacterial growth, reflux of infected urine higher into the urinary tract, and increasing hydrostatic pressure.

Several chronic health problems (Table 48-1) predispose an individual to UTI by changing the metabolism of tissues, creating extrarenal obstruction, and altering the function and structure of kidney tissue.

Instrumentation of the urinary tract is also associated with high rates of urinary tract infection. Catheterization, even when performed without break in aseptic technique, results in a significant rate of infection of the bladder. Nosocomial infections account for a sizable

RESEARCH

Foxman B and Fredrichs RR: Epidemiology of urinary tract infection: diet, clothing and urination habits, Am J Public Health 75:1314-1317, 1985.

The purpose of this study was to assess the association between UTI and behaviors commonly mentioned as risk factors (urination habits, diet, laundry detergents). Subjects were female students at a student health service (44 with UTI and 181 control subjects). Use of tampons and drinking soft drinks were the only factors that were even moderately associated with both initial and recurrent UTI. It was hypothesized that inserting and removing tampons might spread bacteria from the vagina to the uretral opening. Soft drinks increase urinary pH, which might facilitate bacterial growth. On the other hand, cranberry juice, which has an acidifying effect on urine, also showed a slight relationship to UTI. ■

percentage of all urinary tract infections and should be closely monitored. Drug-resistant strains of *Staphylococcus* and *Pseudomonas,* along with various other organisms commonly found in hospitals, are frequently those involved in nosocomial UTI. Prevention and control of all UTIs can be most significantly influenced through a lowering of the rate of nosocomial infection.

Infections of the lower urinary tract involve the urinary bladder (*cystitis*) and the urethra (*urethritis*). In the upper urinary tract, infection may involve the kidney (*pyelonephritis*). The etiologic factors and general preventive and management principles are the same for infection elsewhere in the urinary tract. Pyelonephritis is discussed in greater detail on p. 1408.

PREVENTION

The most important defenses against UTI are large urine volume, free urine flow, and complete emptying of the bladder to prevent urinary stasis. Three considerations are important in preventing infection of the lower urinary tract: (1) preventing or minimizing morbidity that can accompany these infections, (2) preventing recurrence of the infection, and (3) preventing renal damage from untreated or inadequately treated ascending infections. Persons with lower urinary tract infections seek medical attention as a result of symptoms or are identified through routine urinalysis or screening of populations at high risk. Both education of the public and health care community assist in decreasing UTI and its complications. The box on the opposite page highlights information that should be included in public education programs.

PATHOPHYSIOLOGY

Most infections of the urinary tract result from gram-negative organisms, such as *Escherichia coli, Klebsiella,*

INFORMATION TO BE INCLUDED IN PUBLIC EDUCATION PROGRAMS ABOUT URINARY TRACT INFECTION

Symptoms of UTI
Need for prompt medical attention when symptoms of UTI occur
Need to continue drug therapy even though symptoms abate
Importance of follow-up care and repeat urine cultures
Maintenance of fluid intake of 3 to 4 L/day if the person's health permits

---

TABLE 48-2 Normal function, pathophysiology, and clinical picture in lower urinary tract infection

Normal Function	Pathophysiology	Clinical Picture
Urine produced in kidneys flows unobstructed through urinary tract. Urine is sterile until it reaches the urethra.	Urine stasis promotes bacterial growth. Bacteria may ascend urethra into bladder and ureters, leading to infection. Inflamed tissues may bleed.	Frequency, urgency, dysuria Fever and chills Hematuria Bacteriuria

Proteus, or *Pseudomonas*, that originate in the person's own intestinal tract and ascend through the urethra to the bladder. During micturition, urine may flow back up the ureters (vesicoureteral reflux) and carry bacteria present in the bladder up through the ureters to the kidney pelvis (Table 48-2). Whenever stasis of urine occurs, such as with incomplete emptying of the bladder, renal calculi, or genitourinary obstructions, the bacteria have a greater opportunity to grow. Urinary stasis also promotes a more alkaline urine, which also facilitates bacterial growth.

Urinary tract infections occur primarily when host resistance is impaired. The major factors preventing UTI are tissue integrity and blood supply.[10] A break in the surface of the mucous membrane lining of the urinary tract permits the bacteria to invade tissue and cause infection. Breaks in tissue integrity result from erosions caused by tips from indwelling catheters, trauma, or rough-edged renal stones; from neoplasms; or from invasion of the tissue by parasites such as *Schistosoma*. In the bladder, blood supply to tissues can be compromised when the pressure within the bladder is markedly increased, as may occur with overdistention of the bladder, contracture of the bladder neck; or obstruction of the urethra by an enlarged prostate, metastatic growth, or urethral stricture.

CLINICAL MANIFESTATIONS

The symptoms that bring the person with UTI to seek medical attention typically include frequency, urgency, burning on urination (dysuria), and possibly slight to gross hematuria. Most persons, however, are asymptomatic or minimally symptomatic. In these cases the UTI is identified only on routine examination of the urine. Bacteriuria and positive urine cultures serve as the basis for diagnosing lower urinary tract infections. Infection is indicated by growth of a single pathogen in excess of 1×10^5 organisms/ml of urine in a properly obtained and stored midstream specimen (Chapter 47).

MEDICAL MANAGEMENT

Treatment goals for lower UTI include sterilizing the urine and identifying any illness or urinary tract abnor-

mality that may be contributing to infection. After culture and sensitivity studies are performed, a 7- to 10-day course of antibiotic therapy is instituted. It is crucial that urine cultures be obtained before initiating drug therapy to ensure appropriateness of antimicrobial medication and to decrease the development of resistant strains of organisms. The urine should be recultured every few months during the following year to reconfirm urine sterility.

A more extensive urologic work-up including IVP and voiding cystogram may be performed for men and young children after a repeated, or even first, UTI or when infection does note abate. This work-up is performed on women when infection occurs repeatedly or cannot be cleared up with treatment. The rationale for this extensive work-up is that UTIs are not common in men and children and that a significant portion of infection in these populations, and in women with persistent infection, involves abnormality of the urinary tract.

Medications commonly used in the treatment of UTI include urinary antiseptics such as sulfisoxazole (Gantrisin) or nitrofurantoin (Furadantin). Systemic antibiotics are also frequently prescribed. Sulfonamides are widely used and are usually effective against the organisms causing a large percentage of UTIs. Sulfonamides are relatively safe and are less likely than most systemic antibiotics to contribute to growth of resistant organisms.

Additional treatment includes increasing fluid intake to 3 to 4 L/day unless contraindicated. Increased fluid helps to dilute the urine, lessen irritations and burning, and provide a continual flow of urine to discourage stasis and multiplication of bacteria in the urinary tract. Sitz baths may provide comfort for individuals with urethritis.

For persons with chronic bacteriuria, urine-acidifying agents may be prescribed. The effect of these medications is to provide a less suitable environment for bacterial growth and to enhance the effectiveness of antibiotic and urinary antiseptics. When bacteriuria becomes constant, prophylaxis may be undertaken with antimicrobial drugs.

■ ASSESSMENT

Subjective Data

The subjective data should include assessment of symptoms of frequency, urgency and burning on urination (dysuria). Chills and fever may be present. Data should be collected on predisposing factors, such as use of bubble baths or contraceptive jellies and a history of previous infections.

Objective Data

A urine culture is obtained because bacteriuria serves as the basis for diagnosis of lower UTI. The urine should also be tested for occult blood.

■ DATA ANALYSIS: NURSING DIAGNOSES

Nursing diagnoses are determined from assessment of patient data. Possible nursing diagnoses for the person with UTI may include, but are not limited to, the following:

Diagnostic Title	Possible Etiologies
Knowledge deficit	Lack of exposure/recall, information misinterpretation
Pain	Inflammation
Urinary elimination, altered patterns	Urinary infection

■ PLANNING: EXPECTED PATIENT OUTCOMES

Expected patient outcomes for the person with UTI may include, but are not limited to, the following:
1. Patient states relief of symptoms
2. Patient shows no further damage in kidney function; current damage is arrested
3. Sterile urine or urine bacteria count is less than 1×10^4 to 1×10^5

The person or significant other can state or describe the following:
1. Signs and symptoms of UTI
2. When and how to take prescribed medications
3. Plan for follow-up care including urine cultures
4. Rationale and means of increasing fluid intake to 3 to 4 L/day
5. Risk factors for UTI

■ IMPLEMENTATION

Antibiotic therapy must be given on time on a regular schedule to ensure adequate blood levels. If the patient is to undergo instrumentation, the nurse reinforces instructions about the specific procedure. Knowledge about potential sensations during instrumentation and deep breathing exercises during the procedure may assist in relaxing the patient.

Individuals with urethritis may experience pain or itching in the perineum. Sitz baths may provide relief of symptoms.

Patient Teaching

Patient education concerning the specific problem, the requirements for drug therapy, and follow-up care should facilitate completion of drug regimens for eradication of bacteria and early identification of recurrence of infection. Success in both of these areas depends directly on patient understanding and compliance and allows the patient to assist in overcoming this health problem. Female patients should be instructed in good perineal hygiene and to void after intercourse.

PYELONEPHRITIS

EPIDEMIOLOGY/ETIOLOGY

Pyelonephritis refers to bacterial infection of kidney tissue. This infection usually begins in the lower urinary tract and ascends into the kidneys. Lower urinary tract infection may be asymptomatic, and kidney involvement may be the first indication of lower urinary tract disease. Often diagnostic work-up of a person with pyelonephritis reveals previously unknown urinary tract obstruction or the presence of another chronic kidney disease. *Escherichia coli* is the most common organism identified in pyelonephritis, and resistance to antibiotic therapy rarely results. Pyelonephritis is most commonly associated with: (1) cystitis; (2) pregnancy; (3) obstruction, instrumentation, or trauma of the urinary tract. Other risk factors include septicemia and chronic health problems including diabetes, analgesic abuse, polycystic kidney disease, and hypertensive kidney disease.

PREVENTION

The most significant efforts in preventing pyelonephritis are through early detection and adequate treatment of lower urinary tract infections.

PATHOPHYSIOLOGY

Infection of the kidney occurs in both acute and chronic forms. Although *acute* pyelonephritis may temporarily affect renal function, rarely does this progress to the level of renal failure. *Chronic* pyelonephritis destroys renal tissue permanently through repeated inflammation and scarring (Table 48-3). The process of developing chronic renal failure from repeated kidney infections occurs over a number of years or after several extensive and fulminant infections. It is estimated that pyelonephritis represents the original diagnosis in one third of all persons with chronic renal failure.[10]

CLINICAL MANIFESTATIONS

The signs and symptoms of acute pyelonephritis may include those of lower urinary tract infection in addition to the following typical signs of inflammation: chills and fever, malaise, flank pain, costovertebral tenderness,

TABLE 48-3 Normal function, pathophysiology, and clinical picture in pyelonephritis

Normal Function	Pathophysiology	Clinical Picture
Fluid regulation Electrolyte regulation Blood pressure regulation Excretion of metabolic wastes	Acute inflammation results in hyperemia and suppuration of tissues (inflammatory response). Chronic inflammation results in scarring and atrophy, leading to chronic renal failure	*Acute:* flank pain, fever, chills, malaise, leukocytosis, WBC and bacteria in urine *Chronic:* persistent bacteriuria; hypertension, ↑BUN, ↓creatinine clearance in late stages

and leukocytosis. Urinalysis indicates presence of white blood cells (WBC), casts, and bacteria. In chronic pyelonephritis, the only symptoms may be persistent bacteriuria until sufficient cells have been destroyed to show signs of renal insufficiency (hypertension, increased BUN, and decreased creatinine clearance).

INTERVENTIONS
Medical Management

Optimal treatment of pyelonephritis includes early detection of the illness, antibacterial therapy based on urine cultures, and detection and treatment of any underlying systemic disease or urinary abnormality.[36] The course of antibiotic therapy may extend over weeks. The urine is recultured 2 weeks after drug therapy has been discontinued and monthly for several months thereafter. Should infection become chronic, maintenance drug therapy may continue indefinitely; the goal is to reduce and control the bacterial population of the urinary tract to prevent renal damage.

Nursing Management

It is important to maintain sufficient urinary flow to remove byproducts of the inflammation and to prevent urinary stasis with further bacterial growth. Fluid intake is encouraged to 3 L/day in persons capable of excreting this amount. Excessive fluids are contraindicated when the disease is complicated by renal failure.

During the acute phase, the patient is encouraged to rest. Prescribed analgesics may be given for flank pain. Back massage often provides short-term relief of discomfort. Pain eases as the inflammation resolves.

Patient Teaching. Persons with pyelonephritis may be treated at home; therefore, patient teaching is important. Instruct the patient to:

1. Continue antibiotic therapy even after symptoms resolve.
2. Drink 3 L/day of fluids unless otherwise instructed.
3. Monitor urinary output; report to physician a urinary output considerably less than fluid intake.
4. Weigh self daily; report a sudden weight gain to physician.
5. Take measures to prevent infection; report signs of urinary infection (flank pain increased, fever, chills, frequency, and urgency) to physician.
6. Continue with medical follow-up and get follow-up urine cultures as instructed.

TUBERCULOSIS OF THE KIDNEY
EPIDEMIOLOGY/ETIOLOGY

Renal tuberculosis is caused by *Mycobacterium tuberculosis*. Renal tuberculosis is an example of a kidney infection that is secondary to an infection in a different site (pulmonary tuberculosis). Tuberculosis of the kidney is acquired by hematogenous spread of the mycobacterium and is most common in men between 20 and 40 years of age.

PREVENTION

Prevention is primarily through the control of pulmonary tuberculosis by early detection and treatment.

CLINICAL MANIFESTATIONS

Signs and symptoms of renal tuberculosis are mild and usually include loss of appetite, unexplained weight loss, and intermittent fever. Hematuria may also be present. Diagnostic tests usually include screening for pulmonary tuberculosis. Urine samples are also obtained and screened for the presence of *Mycobacterium tuberculosis*.

INTERVENTIONS
Medical Management

Treatment is usually through the institution of antituberculosis medication, alone or in combination (see Chapter 33). Medications commonly used include isoniazid, rifampin, and ethambutol. Drug therapy is usually given for 9 to 18 months.

Nursing Management

Nursing interventions are the same as those for pyelonephritis (increased fluid intake, medications, rest).

CHEMICAL-INDUCED NEPHRITIS
EPIDEMIOLOGY/ETIOLOGY

Chemical-induced nephritis is an idiosyncratic reaction that results in damage to the tubules and interstitium of the kidneys. This disease process was first noted in patients who were sensitive to the sulfonamide drugs. Many other substances are now associated with chemi-

TABLE 48-4 Substances associated with chemical-induced nephritis

Category	Substance
Solvents	Carbon tetrachloride
	Methanol
	Ethylene glycol
Heavy metals	Lead
	Arsenic
	Mercury
Antibiotics	Kanamycin
	Gentamicin
	Amphotericin B
	Calistin
	Neomycin
	Phenazopyridine
Pesticides	
Poisonous mushrooms	

cal-induced nephritis, including those listed in Table 48-4.

PREVENTION

Prevention of chemical-induced nephritis is best managed by identifying causative agents and removing them from the environment. Many people are exposed to these agents as a result of their medical regimen. The health care professional must be aware of these agents as well as the signs and symptoms associated with chemical induced nephritis. With early detection and removal of the causative agent as soon as possible, the prognosis is improved.

A major risk factor is industrial exposure to chemicals. Occupational health professionals should be aware of potential risks and should educate employees as to appropriate preventive measures.

PATHOPHYSIOLOGY

Chemical-induced nephritis usually begins within 15 days of exposure to the chemical. The inflammatory process disrupts the ability of the glomeruli to filter. Furthermore, the capillary membrane is altered to the extent that it becomes permeable to plasma proteins and blood cells resulting in proteinuria and hematuria.

CLINICAL MANIFESTATIONS

Signs and symptoms of nephritis include fever, eosinophilia, hematuria, mild proteinuria, and rash. Oliguria or urine output of 400 ml or less in a 24-hour period occurs in approximately 50% of all cases. Urinalyses are obtained to assess for protein or blood cells. Serum toxicology screening may identify the source of the nephritis.

INTERVENTIONS

Medical Management

Medical management usually includes immediate withdrawal of the suspected chemical. Hemodialysis may be instituted to facilitate the removal of nephrotoxins from the blood. Steroids may be administered for their anti-inflammatory response. A sodium-restricted diet may be necessary to maintain fluid balance. Proteins may also be restricted if renal function is severely compromised.

Nursing Management

The patient is assessed for fluid and electrolyte status, including the presence of edema, blood pressure changes, and adventitious breath sounds. The person needs to know the rationale for maintenance of fluid balance and any sodium restrictions. The care of the person is similar to that for acute renal failure (see Chapter 50).

GLOMERULONEPHRITIS

Glomerulonephritis is a disease that affects the glomeruli of both kidneys. Etiologic factors are many and varied; they include immunologic reactions (lupus erythematosus, streptococcal infection), vascular injury (hypertension), metabolic disease (diabetes mellitus), and disseminated intravascular coagulation (DIC). Glomerulonephritis exists in acute, latent, and chronic forms.

ACUTE GLOMERULONEPHRITIS

Epidemiology/Etiology

The most common form of *acute glomerulonephritis* occurs 2 to 3 weeks after a streptococcal infection. Common sites of the primary infection include the throat (tonsillitis, strep throat) and the skin (impetigo). Children of preschool and grade-school age are most likely to develop the illness. Of all individuals developing acute poststreptococcal glomerulonephritis, approximately 1% to 2% will develop end-stage renal failure in which dialysis or transplantation is required to prevent death. Approximately 90% of children and 50% of adults with acute glomerulonephritis attain full recovery from illness, although recovery may require up to 2 years.[8] Little can be inferred from the severity of the acute episode regarding prognosis. Persons with mild illness may develop chronic disease, and those with severe illness may completely recover and have no recurrence of the illness.

Prevention

Prevention of acute poststreptococcal glomerulonephritis involves prompt medical treatment of sore throats and upper respiratory infections. Cultures should be obtained, and when indicated appropriate antibiotics should be prescribed.

Pathophysiology

Acute poststreptococcal glomerulonephritis is a result of an *antigen-antibody reaction* with glomerular tissue that produces swelling and death of capillary cells of glomerular tissue. The antigen-antibody reaction activates the complement pathway (see Chapter 8) resulting in chemotaxis of polymorphonuclear (PMN) leukocytes with release of lysosomal enzymes that attack the glomerular basement membrane (GBM). The response in the membrane is an increase in the three types of glomerular cells (endothelial, mesangial, and epithelial) causing an *increase in membrane porosity* with resultant proteinuria and hematuria. Renal function is depressed by scarring in the glomerulus causing oliguria and retention of water, sodium, and nitrogenous waste products, leading to edema and azotemia.

Clinical Manifestations

Complaints commonly voiced by the patient include shortness of breath, mild headache, weakness, anorexia, and flank pain. The usual signs associated with acute glomerulonephritis are the following:

1. Proteinuria
2. Hematuria
3. Increased urine specific gravity
4. Mild generalized edema
5. Elevated antistreptolysin O titer
6. Hypertension
7. Decreased urinary output
8. Elevated serum urea nitrogen
9. Elevated serum creatine levels

Signs and symptoms reflect damage to the glomeruli with leaking of protein and red blood cells into the urine, varying degrees of decreased glomerular filtration with retention of metabolic waste products, and fluid overloading of varying severity.

Urinalysis provides important data such as the presence of proteinuria, hematuria, and cell debris.

Medical Management

Persistent infection is treated promptly to help prevent further decrease in antigen-antibody complex formation. Persons with poststreptococcal glomerulonephritis are given a course of prophylactic antibiotic therapy; the drug of choice is penicillin. Prophylactic therapy may be continued for months after acute phase of the illness. Exposure to any infection must be avoided, since even mild infection may reactivate nephritis.

Bed rest is usually instituted until clinical signs of nephritis have resolved. Fluid retention is often a problem and is managed by initiating dietary sodium restrictions. Diuretic therapy is implemented when severe fluid overload develops. Elevated blood pressure is controlled by utilization of antihypertensive drugs only after fluid control has proved to be unsuccessful. Dietary protein is reduced when blood urea nitrogen and creatinine levels are elevated. It is important that the diet contain sufficient carbohydrates to prevent protein being used by the body for energy, resulting in muscle wasting and nitrogen imbalance.

■ Assessment

Subjective data. General questions to ask the patient include: (1) Have you experienced shortness of breath, headaches, weakness, or anorexia? (2) Have you noticed a change in your pattern of urination, either frequency or volume? (3) Do you recall a recent infection or symptoms of a virus?

Objective data. Objective data to gather should include the following:
1. Frequent assessment of vital signs
2. Daily assessment for edema
3. Intake and output
4. Daily weights

■ Data Analysis: Nursing Diagnoses

Nursing diagnoses are determined from assessment of patient data. Possible nursing diagnoses for the person with acute glomerulonephritis may include, but are not limited to, the following:

Diagnostic Title	Possible Etiologies
Knowledge deficit	Lack of exposure/recall, cognitive limitation
Nutrition, altered: less than body requirements	Anorexia, nausea
Fluid volume excess	Compromised regulatory mechanism, renal impairment
Urinary elimination, altered patterns	Urinary infection, decreased urinary output

■ Planning: Expected Patient Outcomes

Expected patient outcomes for the person with acute glomerulonephritis may include, but are not limited to, the following:
1. Fluid balance is achieved; edema is decreased
2. The person or significant other can explain the following:
   a. The rationale for therapy (prolonged bed rest, maintenance of fluid balance)
   b. Dietary changes (decreased sodium intake, adequate caloric intake, controlled protein intake as prescribed)
   c. Medication program to be followed at home (prophylactic antibiotic therapy, diuretic, antihypertensive therapy)
   d. Health maintenance program
      (1) Measures to prevent further infection

(2) Signs and symptoms that require immediate medical attention

(3) Plans for follow-up health care

■ Implementation

Activity. Bed rest is instituted until clinical signs disappear; this may involve a period of several months. Ambulation is allowed when blood sedimentation rates and blood pressure are normal and edema abates. If ambulation causes an increase in proteinuria or hematuria, bed rest is reinstituted. Since the period of bed rest may be extensive, the nurse may need to continue to reinforce the importance of bed rest as the patient starts to feel better. The importance of diversional activities should not be ignored. When bed rest is reinstituted after a period of ambulation, the person may become depressed as a result of the perceived setback in recovery. Helping the patient to express concerns and feelings can serve as a basis for helping make realistic plans about the illness and its sequelae.

Maintenance of fluid balance. Edema and fluid overloading are anticipated and treated initially with dietary sodium restrictions. The amount of sodium restriction depends on the severity of fluid retention and is maintained until dependent edema and circulatory overload are no longer a problem. The nurse is constantly alert and assessing for signs and symptoms of fluid overload. Antihypertensive therapy is implemented when fluid control measures have been unsuccessful.

Long-term care. The recovery period for acute glomerulonephritis may take up to 2 years. During this time proteinuria, hematuria, and cellular debris may exist microscopically, however, the patient generally exhibits normal renal function. Normal activity is resumed during the extended recovery phase, although fatigue, trauma, and infection must be avoided as they may exacerbate the nephritis. Since these persons usually feel well, they must be instructed by the nurse about the need to continue prescribed treatment and to maintain routine follow-up health care.

Patient teaching. Major components of patient teaching center around the topics listed above. Particular emphasis must be placed on signs and symptoms that require immediate attention (hematuria, hypertension, edema, headaches.) The person must also be instructed about the prescribed medication regimen.

CHRONIC GLOMERULONEPHRITIS

Epidemiology/Etiology

Although chronic glomerulonephritis (CGN) may follow the acute disease, the majority of persons give no history of the disease. In most instances, no evidence of predisposing infection can be found. The course of chronic glomerulonephritis is extremely varied. Some persons with minimal impairment in renal function continue to feel well and show little progression of disease. With other individuals, the progression of renal deterioration may be slow but steady, resulting in end-stage renal disease. In still other individuals the progression to end-stage disease is rapid.

Prevention

Since predisposing factors have not been identified for CGN, no preventive measures can be identified. Known infections should be treated promptly, as discussed under acute glomerulonephritis, to reduce the possibility of the acute disease progressing to CGN. Chronic diseases should be treated and controlled.

Pathophysiology

CGN is characterized by *slow progressive destruction* (sclerosis) of glomeruli and gradual loss of renal function. The glomeruli have varying degrees of hypercellularity and become sclerosed (hardened). The kidney decreases in size. Eventually there is tubular atrophy, chronic interstitial inflammation, and arteriosclerosis (Figure 48-3).

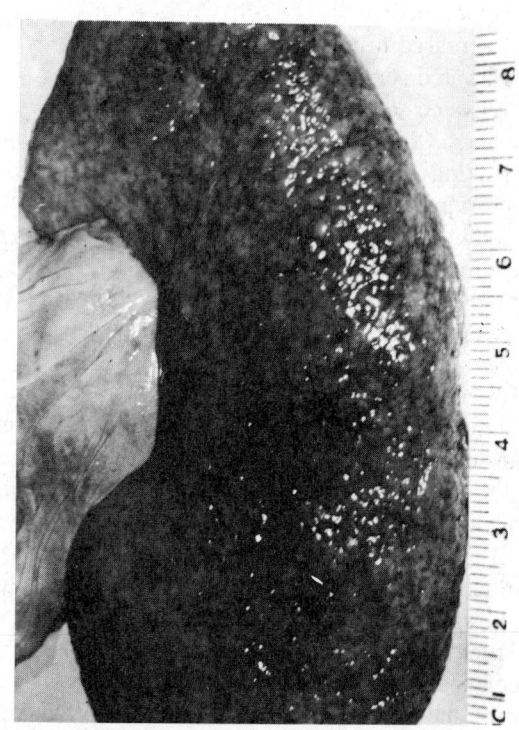

FIGURE 48-3 End-stage chronic glomerulonephritis. Note pebbly surface corresponding to surviving hypertrophied nephrons amid atrophy. (From Anderson WAD and Kissane JM: Pathology, ed 7, St Louis, 1977, The CV Mosby Co.)

Clinical Manifestations

Various symptoms of failing renal function may lead the person to seek health care. These include headache, especially in the morning; dyspnea on exertion; blurring of vision; lassitude; and weakness or fatigue. Signs of CGN may also include edema, nocturia, and weight loss.

Early in the disease process, urinalysis may show albumin, casts, and blood, despite normal renal function tests. The ability of the kidneys to regulate the internal environment will begin to decrease as more glomeruli become scarred, resulting in fewer functional nephrons. When few nephrons remain intact, hematuria and proteinuria decrease, the specific gravity of the urine becomes fixed at 1.010 (same as plasma), and nonprotein nitrogen level in the blood increases.

Interventions

No specific therapy exists to arrest or reverse this disease process. Care involves teaching the client to live healthfully, to avoid infections, to eat a balanced diet within prescribed limits, to take prescribed medications appropriately, to maintain follow-up health care, and to report to the physician any exacerbation in signs or symptoms. Treatment of renal failure begins when the illness progresses to end stage (see Chapter 50).

With any exacerbation of hematuria, hypertension, and edema, the client is returned to bed rest; and treatment similar to that for acute glomerulonephritis is administered. Signs of pulmonary edema and congestive heart failure are closely monitored. Specific treatment is symptomatic and supportive.

Women with CGN who become pregnant appear to be susceptible to toxemia and to spontaneous abortion. The woman who has had nephritis of any nature should be urged to see a physician if she plans on pregnancy. When pregnancy does occur, she should remain under close health supervision.

NEPHROTIC SYNDROME

Nephrotic syndrome (nephrosis) is not a single disease entity but a constellation of symptoms. In nephrotic syndrome there is damage to the glomeruli and quantities of protein are lost in the urine, resulting in the range of symptoms associated with this disorder.

EPIDEMIOLOGY/ETIOLOGY

Nephrotic syndrome has been associated with allergic reactions (insect bites, pollen, acute glomerulonephritis), infections (herpes zoster), systemic disease (diabetes mellitus, sickle cell disease), circulatory problems (severe congestive heart failure, chronic constrictive pericarditis), and pregnancy. Known glomerular disease is the most common precipitating event in adults. In 50% to 75% of adults who develop nephrosis, the dis-

ease progresses to renal failure within 5 years.[6] In many individuals, there will be periods of remission and exacerbation. Nephrosis may also exist in chronic forms.

PREVENTION

Other than treating the underlying illness, little can be done to prevent occurrence or recurrence of nephrosis.

PATHOPHYSIOLOGY

The initial physiologic change in nephrotic syndrome is a derangement of cells in the glomerular basement membrane, resulting in increased membrane porosity with loss of large amounts of protein in the urine (proteinuria). As protein continues to be excreted, serum albumin is decreased (hypoalbuminemia), thus decreasing the serum osmotic pressure (Table 48-5). The capillary hydrostatic fluid (push) pressure in all body tissues becomes greater than the capillary osmotic (pull) pressure, and generalized edema results (Figure 48-4). As fluid is lost into the tissues the plasma volume decreases, stimulating secretion of aldosterone to retain more sodium and water, thereby decreasing the glomerular filtration rate to retain water. This additional fluid also passes out of the capillaries into the tissue, leading to even greater edema.

CLINICAL MANIFESTATIONS

Clinical manifestations of nephrotic syndrome include severe generalized edema, pronounced proteinuria, hypoalbuminemia, and hyperlipidemia. Urine volumes and renal function may be either normal or markedly altered. Altered renal function and development of symptoms of renal failure occur as a result of progressing glomerulonephritis. Loss of appetite and fatigue are common. Women usually experience amenorrhea or other disturbances in the reproductive cycle.

Diagnosis is often made on the basis of clinical and

TABLE 48-5 Normal function, pathophysiology and clinical picture in nephrotic syndrome

Normal Function	Pathophysiology	Clinical Picture
Glomerular capillaries are impermeable to serum proteins. Plasma proteins create colloid osmotic pressure to retain intravascular fluid.	Glomerular capillaries become permeable to serum proteins, resulting in proteinuria and decreased serum osmotic pressure. Glomerular filtration rate decreases.	Severe generalized edema; pronounced proteinuria; hypoalbuminemia; hyperlipidemia

laboratory findings. However, renal biopsy is sometimes used as a means of a definitive diagnosis.

MEDICAL MANAGEMENT

Treatment of nephrotic syndrome is directed toward reducing albuminuria, controlling edema, and promoting general health. Corticosteroids may be useful in controlling the illness, but the response will vary from remission of nephrosis to no response at all. Prednisone is the steroid preparation most frequently prescribed. The diet should contain normal to increased amounts of protein (1g/kg body weight/day) and calories. Periodic determination of proteinuria and measures of renal function enable the physician to monitor response to treatment and level of kidney function.

To control edema, sodium intake is reduced and diuretics are given to increase fluid excretion. When diuretics are administered over prolonged periods, hy-

pokalemia often results. Potassium may be supplemented through dietary intake; medication supplements are initiated only after attempts to increase serum potassium through dietary means have failed. Bed rest is usually ordered when edema is severe; however, immobility is contraindicated for prolonged periods.

Persons with nephrosis need to direct particular attention toward preventing infection, because body defenses are impaired by protein losses and edematous tissues are particularly susceptible to injury. Culture and sensitivity studies are performed and appropriate antibiotic therapy instituted.

▪ ASSESSMENT

The subjective data are the same as those collected for glomerulonephritis (p. 1411). Specific assessment should include the following objective data:

1. Edema: amount, location, and degree of pitting
2. Intake and output
3. Daily weight
4. Abdominal girth
5. Condition of skin (severe edema may lead to skin breakdown)
6. Respiratory status: signs of pulmonary edema
7. Signs and symptoms of infection

▪ DATA ANALYSIS: NURSING DIAGNOSES

Nursing diagnoses are determined from assessment of patient data. Possible nursing diagnoses for the person with nephrosis may include, but are not limited to, the following:

Diagnostic Title	Possible Etiologies
Knowledge deficit	Lack of exposure/recall, information misinterpretation, cognitive limitation
Pain	Immobility, edema
Breathing pattern, ineffective	Ascites
Skin integrity, impaired, potential	Immobility, edema
Urinary elimination, altered patterns	Decreased urine production
Fluid volume excess	Compromised regulatory mechanism
Body image, disturbance	Change in body appearance (generalized edema, ascites)

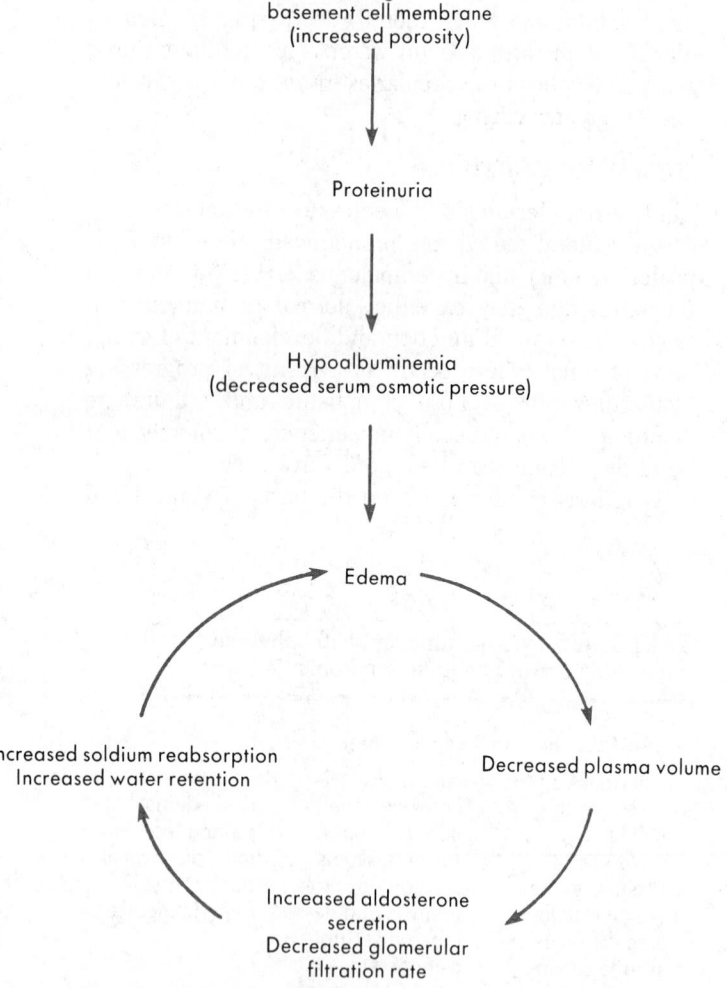

FIGURE 48-4 Pathophysiologic changes in nephrotic syndrome.

▪ PLANNING: EXPECTED PATIENT OUTCOMES

Expected patient outcome for the person with nephrotic syndrome may include, but are not limited to, the following:

1. The person maintains independence in activities of daily living (ADL)
2. The person remains free of infection
3. Edema and blood pressure are controlled: pulmo-

nary edema and congestive heart failure do not occur

4. The person or significant other can describe or state the following:
   a. Measures to prevent infection
   b. Name, dose, frequency, and side effects of prescribed medications (steroids, diuretics)
   c. Dietary prescription and plans for appropriate meals
   d. Signs and symptoms requiring immediate attention
   e. Plans for follow-up health care

■ IMPLEMENTATION

Assisting with Comfort and ADL

The patient may tire easily, requiring assistance with ADL. The patient is encouraged to be independent but not to the extent of fatigue.

As edema increases, the patient becomes increasingly uncomfortable. Careful positioning and frequent changes in position may increase comfort while also protecting the skin. An air or water mattress may increase comfort and prevent skin breakdown. Males may develop edema of the scrotum, which is particularly uncomfortable. A sling to support the scrotum will not only provide comfort but will also aid in reducing swelling. (See Chapter 23 for care of the person with edema.)

Promoting Nutrition

Usually a sodium and protein-restricted diet is prescribed[46] that is often not appetizing to the patient. Appetite may also be diminished as a result of fluid overload with the potential for inadequate nutrition. The nurse encourages adequate dietary intake through small, frequent feedings.

Medications

Steroids and diuretics are often administered to the person with nephrotic syndrome. Nursing assessment must include observing for side effects. Assess the person's response to diuretics and observe for signs and symptoms of overdiuresis and potassium imbalance.

Patient Teaching

As the person begins to convalesce, the teaching plan should include the following:

1. Medications: name, dose, actions, side effects
2. Nutrition: increased calories, adequate protein, decreased sodium
3. Self-assessment of fluid status, including edema and weight gain
4. Signs and symptoms requiring medical attention: increased edema, dyspnea, fatigue, headache, infection

VASCULAR DISORDERS

Vascular renal disease results from one of two processes: (1) disease of the main renal arteries or renal stenosis and (2) sclerosis of renal arterioles or nephrosclerosis.

RENAL ARTERY STENOSIS
EPIDEMIOLOGY/ETIOLOGY

Renal artery stenosis is the cause of approximately 5% of all cases of hypertension.[11] Stenosis of the renal artery is usually classified as either arteriosclerosis or fibromuscular dysplasia. In either case, the end result is a narrowing of the lumen of the arteries supplying the kidneys. Obstruction of the renal arteries can be caused by aneurysm, thrombosis, and emboli.

PREVENTION

Prevention centers around the underlying disease entities that may lead to thrombosis and emboli. Measures may also be taken to reduce risk of arteriosclerosis (see Chapter 28).

PATHOPHYSIOLOGY

Renal artery stenosis results in a major reduction in blood flow to the kidneys.[26] This change in renal perfusion causes increased secretion of renin and activation of the renin-angiotensin-aldosterone system. The end result is acceleration of hypertension, which, if untreated, leads to further pathologic changes in the kidneys.

CLINICAL MANIFESTATIONS

The signs of renal artery stenosis include:

1. Hypertension
2. Disparity in size of kidneys
3. Delayed appearance of contrast medium in renal arteriograph
4. Hyperconcentration of contrast media in the kidney's calyceal system on IVP
5. Lesion evidenced on renal arteriograph

INTERVENTIONS

Medical treatment includes vigorous antihypertensive therapy to control blood pressure. When a well-defined lesion exists in the renal artery, vascular surgery may be performed to improve circulation.

NEPHROSCLEROSIS
EPIDEMIOLOGY/ETIOLOGY

Whereas renal artery stenosis results in hypertension, hypertension can cause nephrosclerosis. Hypertension is a major precipitating factor in renal disease. It is estimated that approximately 10% of individuals with essential hypertension develop severe renal damage, and approximately 1% will develop end-stage renal disease and die unless supportive care is provided.[10]

PREVENTION

Prevention is best effected by improved screening to detect persons with hypertension and providing adequate treatment and follow-up care. Yearly blood pressure screening of persons with elevated blood pressure is a minimal preventive measure.

CLINICAL MANIFESTATIONS

Signs and symptoms of nephrosclerosis are the same as those listed for chronic renal failure (see Chapter 50). By the time the signs and symptoms have developed, the disease has progressed to an extreme point. Deterioration in renal function progresses gradually. However, if an acute or malignant phase of hypertension occurs, the process may accelerate.

INTERVENTIONS

Treatment of nephrosclerosis is directed toward early detection and treatment of hypertension. Causative factors are sought, and treatment to lower blood pressure is begun (see Chapter 29). When significant renal damage exists, stabilizing the person's current level of function or slowing deterioration of kidney tissue is the goal. Control of hypertension is continued, and management of end-stage renal disease and uremic symptoms provides for comfort and increased independence in daily living, although renal function may not improve.

The nursing assessment and implementation for patients with nephrosclerosis are the same as those outlined for chronic renal failure (see Chapter 50).

DIABETIC NEPHROPATHY
EPIDEMIOLOGY/ETIOLOGY

Persons with diabetes develop vascular changes at a more accelerated rate than nondiabetic persons. The end result of these vascular changes can be diabetic nephropathy.

PREVENTION

The most effective preventive measure is adequate control of patients with diabetes. They should have routine monitoring of renal function to detect the first signs of change in renal function.

PATHOPHYSIOLOGY

Vascular changes have been identified as a normal component of the aging process. A process of accelerated vascular change is most evident in the patient with type I diabetes, which often develops in childhood. In controlling the carbohydrate intake of the person with diabetes, abnormal metabolism of fat occurs, resulting in elevated serum cholesterol levels. Immunofluorescent and electron microscopic studies of the renal vasculature suggest that large quantities of lipids leak into these blood vessels and precipitate on the vessel walls. The vasculature changes caused by diabetes result in two distinct processes: glomerulosclerosis and nephrosclerosis. As described earlier, nephrosclerosis develops from sclerosing of the renal arterioles. Glomerulosclerosis is the scarring of the capillary loops in the glomerulus. Pathologic changes occur in the basement membranes of the kidneys. The first indication of renal involvement in the person with diabetes is usually proteinuria.

CLINICAL MANIFESTATIONS

The signs and symptoms of diabetic nephropathy are the same as those for chronic renal failure (see Chapter 50).

INTERVENTIONS

The medical management of the patient with diabetic nephropathy is the same as that listed for nephrosclerosis. Adequate control of the diabetes is essential.

The nursing assessment and implementation for persons with diabetic nephropathy are the same as those outlined for chronic renal failure.

OBSTRUCTIVE DISORDERS

Urinary tract obstruction can occur in any portion of the urinary tract from the urinary calyces to the meatus. Patients with obstructions have characteristic signs and symptoms, depending on the location and extent of the obstruction. If urinary obstruction is not corrected, renal failure may eventually develop. This section is a description of the major concepts related to obstruction of the urinary system and the care of patients with obstructive disorders. In subsequent sections specific obstructive disorders will be discussed.

HYDRONEPHROSIS
ETIOLOGY

Hydronephrosis is the dilation of the renal pelves and calyces with urine. Hydronephrosis may occur either unilaterally or bilaterally. Causes of obstruction of the urinary tract are summarized in Table 48-6.

PATHOPHYSIOLOGY

Obstruction of any part of the urinary system from the kidney to the urethra will generate pressure that may cause functional and anatomic damage to the renal parenchyma. When any part of the urinary tract is obstructed, urine collects behind the obstruction, producing a dilation of the urinary collecting structures. Muscles of the affected area contract in an effort to push the

TABLE 48-6 Causes of urinary tract obstruction

Location	Major Causes
Lower urinary tract	Bladder neoplasms
	Urethral strictures
	Calculi
	Tumors
	Benign prostatic hypertrophy (BPH)
Ureteral obstruction	Calculi
	Trauma
	Nephroptosis ("floating" or "dropped" kidney)
	Enlarged lymph nodes
	Lymphosarcoma
	Reticulum cell sarcoma
	Hodgkin's disease
	Congenital anomaly
Kidney	Calculi
	Ptosis
	Polycystic disease

urine around the obstruction. Partial obstruction may produce slow dilation of structures above the obstruction without functional impairment. As the obstruction increases, however, pressure builds up in the tubular system behind the obstruction, causing a backflow of urine and dilation of the ureter (*hydroureter*). The urine backup eventually reaches the kidney, causing dilation of the kidney pelvis (*hydronephrosis*). Pressure build-up in the renal pelvis leads to destruction of kidney tissue and eventually renal failure.

With obstruction, urine flow is decreased even to the point of stagnation. This stagnant urine provides a culture medium for bacterial growth, and rarely is obstruction seen without some infection. The specific effects that occur with obstruction will depend on the location of the obstruction, the extent of obstruction (partial or complete), and the duration. Obstruction in the lower urinary tract causes bladder distention. If this is prolonged, muscle fibers become hypertrophied and *diverticuli* (herniated sacs of bladder mucosa) develop between the hypertrophied muscle bands. Since the diverticulum holds stagnant urine, infection often occurs and bladder stones may form.

Obstruction of the upper urinary tract leads even more quickly to hydronephrosis because of the small size of the ureters and kidney pelvis. Increased pressure causes partial ischemia of arteries between the renal cortex and medulla and dilation of the renal tubules leading to tubular damage. Stasis of urine in the dilated pelvis predisposes to infection and calculi, which add to the renal damage. Some urine can flow back up the renal tubules into the veins and lymphatics as a compensatory mechanism. The unaffected kidney then takes on increased elimination of waste products. With prolonged

obstruction, the unaffected kidney hypertrophies and may function almost (80%) as effectively alone as both kidneys did before the obstruction. Obstruction of both kidneys leads to renal failure.

CLINICAL MANIFESTATIONS

Hydronephrosis can occur without any symptoms as long as kidney function is adequate and urine can drain. An acute upper urinary tract obstruction will cause pain, nausea, vomiting, local tenderness, spasm of the abdominal muscles, and a mass in the kidney region. The pain is caused by stretching of the tissues and by hyperperistalsis. Since the amount of pain is proportional to the rate of stretching, a slowly developing hydronephrosis may cause only a dull flank pain; whereas a sudden blockage or the ureter, such as may occur from a stone, causes a severe stabbing (colicky) pain in the flank or abdomen. The pain may radiate to the genitalia and thigh and is caused by the increased peristaltic action of the smooth muscles of the ureter in an effort to dislodge the obstruction and force urine past it.

The nausea and vomiting frequently associated with acute obstruction are caused by a reflex reaction to the pain and will usually be relieved as soon as the pain is relieved. A markedly dilated kidney, however, may press on the stomach causing continued gastrointestinal symptoms. If renal function has been seriously impaired, nausea and vomiting may be symptoms of impending uremia. (See Chapter 50 for discussion of uremia and renal failure.)

When the bladder is distended from lower urinary tract obstruction, the person will experience lower abdominal discomfort and a feeling of the need to void although voiding may not be possible. The bladder may be palpated above the symphysis pubis. With partial obstruction, such as that often seen in benign prostatic hypertrophy, the patient first complains of increasing urinary frequency because the bladder fails to empty completely at each voiding and therefore refills more quickly to the amount that causes the urge to void (usually 250 to 500 ml). Nocturia may also be present.

Diagnostic Tests

Table 48-7 provides a summary of the specific diagnostic tests used in the diagnosis of obstructive disorders. In addition to these diagnostic procedures, urinalysis and serum renal function studies will be obtained.

INTERVENTIONS
Medical Management

The medical management is specific to the cause of the urinary obstruction. When obstruction occurs, treatment centers around reestablishing adequate drainage from the urinary system, such as by placing a ureteral catheter above the point of obstruction. Strictures may

TABLE 48-7 Summary of tests used for diagnosis of obstructive disorders

	Renal Calculi	Renal Neoplasms	Prostatic Hypertrophy	Urethral Strictures
Cystoscopy	X	X	X	X*
Retrograde pyelography	X	X		
IVP	X	X	X	X*
KUB	X	X		
Urethrography			X	X
Computed tomography (CT)		X		
Renal angiography		X		
Renography				
Ultrasound		X		
Renal biopsy		X		

*Not always completed.

be successfully dilated. Sometimes surgery must be performed to insert a catheter into the kidney or bladder (nephrostomy, ureterostomy, suprapubic cystostomy).

The person with a sudden obstruction is frequently acutely ill and may have severe colic but will not be able to remain in bed until the pain has been relieved. Narcotics, such as morphine and meperidine, in combination with antispasmodic drugs, such as propantheline bromide (Pro-Banthine), and belladonna preparations are usually necessary to relieve severe colicky pain.

NURSING MANAGEMENT

Nursing interventions for the person with urinary obstruction are specific for the underlying cause and are described in the following sections describing calculi, tumors, prostatic hypertrophy, and urinary strictures. Some general principles of care for the person with a urinary obstruction are listed below:

1. Monitor
   a. Presence of pain: location, intensity, character, aggravating and alleviating factors
   b. Urine: output, hematuria, dysuria
   c. Nausea and vomiting
2. Assist in the maintenance of fluid and electrolyte balance
   a. Assess intake and output at least every 8 hours
   b. Administer and monitor prescribed intravenous fluids
   c. Encourage appropriate diet
3. Prevent urinary complications
   a. Maintain urinary drainage systems
   b. Use aseptic technique when working with urinary drainage systems

   c. Assess for bladder distention at least every 8 hours
   d. Assess for hematuria
   e. Assess for signs of renal failure (oliguria, proteinuria, anorexia, lethargy)
   f. Encourage activity, as tolerated, to prevent urinary stasis
4. Promote comfort
   a. Maintain a calm environment to decrease anxiety
   b. Administer analgesic or antispasmodic as necessary
   c. Assist with ADL as necessary
   d. Encourage self-care and independence as tolerated
5. Patient teaching
   a. Prescribed diet and fluid restrictions
   b. Necessary care if patient is discharged with an indwelling catheter
   c. Desired action, side effects, dosage, and frequency of prescribed medications
   d. Need for following the prescribed medical regimen to prevent further problems

RENAL CALCULI

Urinary stones (*urolithiasis*) may develop at any level in the urinary system but are most commonly found within the kidney (*nephrolithiasis*). Figure 48-5 illustrates the most common locations of calculi formation.

EPIDEMIOLOGY/ETIOLOGY

It is estimated that at least 1% of all people in the United States will develop urolithiasis. About one third of the individuals that have recurrent upper urinary tract calculi will eventually have the affected kidney removed.

Renal calculi (stones) are crystallizations of minerals around an organic matrix such as pus, blood, or devitalized tissue. The mineral composition of renal calculi varies. Most stones consist of calcium salts (oxalates, phosphates) or magnesium-ammonium phosphate; the remainder are cystine or uric acid stones.

No demonstrable cause can be found for over half of the renal stones that occur (*idiopathic*). A major predisposing factor is the presence of UTI. Infection increases the presence of organic matter around which the minerals can precipitate and increases the alkalinity of the urine (by the production of ammonia). This results in precipitation of calcium phosphate and magnesium ammonium phosphate. Stasis of urine also permits precipitation of organic matter and minerals.

PATHOPHYSIOLOGY

Because most stones are calcium oxalates, anything that leads to hypercalciuria is a predisposing factor to

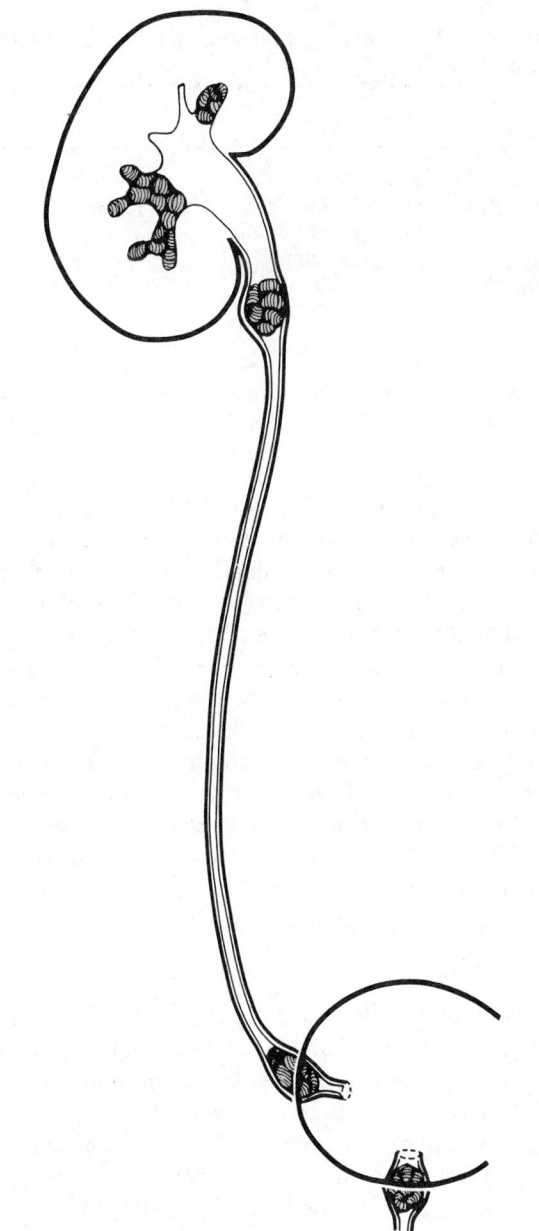

FIGURE 48-5 Most common locations of renal calculus formation.

TABLE 48-8 Renal calculus composition and contributing factors

Composition of Stone	Factors Contributing to Stone Formation
Calcium (oxalate and phosphate)	Hypercalcemia and/or hypercalciuria resulting from: hyperparathyroidism, vitamin D intoxication, multiple myeloma, immobilization, severe bone disease, renal tubular acidosis, and prolonged intake of steroids
Uric acid	High purine diet, gout
Cystine	Cystinuria resulting from genetic disorder of amino acid metabolism

ing's syndrome or prolonged intake of corticosteroids (loss of bone calcium); and renal tubular acidosis (increased calcium secondary to defective ammonia formation). Increased uric acid in the urine leading to uric acid stones may be seen with gout, with some leukemias, or in patients treated with cancer chemotherapeutic agents. Cystine stones usually result from a genetic defect. Both uric acid and cystine precipitate in acid urine.

PREVENTION

Measures can be taken to decrease the potential for renal stones in persons at high risk. Adequate hydration (intake of 2500 ml/day or more unless contraindicated) will help to prevent urinary stasis that can lead not only to stone formation but also to urinary tract infection. Persons restricted to bed should be encouraged to turn and move frequently, exercising arms and legs whenever possible. Urinary stasis can be prevented by sitting up in a chair or by changing the body position of an immobile bedfast patient. Even with exercises and the use of sitting in a chair, paraplegics and quadriplegics often develop renal calculi. Persons with indwelling catheters need scrupulous aseptic technique in catheter care to prevent infection and require adequate hydration and good catheter drainage to wash away minerals that can deposit at the tip of the catheter.

Renal stone formation can often be controlled by regulating urinary pH. Table 48-9 provides a summary of diet principles applied to renal calculi. Persons at risk for developing calcium oxalate, calcium phosphate, or magnesium-ammonium phosphate stones may be placed on an acid ash diet (Table 48-10) to promote excretion of an acid urine. Catheter irrigations using acetic acid solution or hemiacidrin (Renacidin) help provide an acid environment and thus decrease precipitation of calcium and phosphate. Persons at risk for developing uric acid or cystine stones may be placed on an alkaline-ash diet because uric acid and cystine are soluble in an alkaline urine.

renal stones.[35] (see Table 48-8). In persons for whom no underlying pathology can be identified, hypercalciuria may result from increased calcium absorption from the intestine or from decreased reabsorption of calcium by the kidney tubules. These persons do not have hypercalcemia because the calcium is eliminated in the urine. Hypercalcemia leading to hypercalciuria may be present with an increased calcium intake (milk, alkali); prolonged immobilization (loss of bone calcium); hypervitaminosis D (increased calcium absorption from the intestines); hyperparathyroidism, multiple myeloma, Paget disease, or cancer (loss of bone calcium); Cush-

TABLE 48-9 Summary of diet principles in renal stone disease.*

Stone Chemistry	Nutrition Modification	Diet Ash Urinary pH
Calcium Phosphate Oxalate	Low calcium (400 mg) Low phosphorus (1-1.2 g) Low oxalate	Acid ash
Struvite ($MgNH_4PO_4$)	Low phorphorus (1-1.2 g) (Associated with UTI)	Acid ash
Uric acid	Low purine	Alkaline ash
Cystine	Low methionine	Alkaline ash

*From Williams, SR: Nutrition and diet therapy, ed 6, St Louis, 1989, The CV Mosby Co.

TABLE 48-10 Acid and alkaline-ash food groups used to control pH of urine

Acid Ash	Alkaline Ash	Neutral
Meat	Milk	Sugars
Whole grains	Vegetables	Fats
Eggs	Fruit (except cranberries,	Beverages
Cheese	prunes, plums)	Coffee
Cranberries		Tea
Prunes		
Plums		

From Williams, SR: Nutrition and diet therapy, ed 6, St. Louis, 1989, The CV Mosby Co.

CLINICAL MANIFESTATIONS

Pain (*renal colic*) is the primary symptom in an acute episode of renal calculi. The location of the pain depends on the location of the renal stone. If the stone is in the pelvis of the kidney, the pain is caused by hydronephrosis and is more dull and constant in character, occurring primarily in the costovertebral angle. As the stone moves along the ureter the pain can be excrutiating and is intermittent in character. It is caused by spasm of the ureter and anoxia of the wall of the ureter from the pressure of the stone. The pain follows the anterior course of the ureter down to the suprapubic area and radiates to the external genitalia. Nausea and vomiting often accompany renal colic.

Patients frequently have two or three attacks of acute renal colic before the stone passes. This is probably because the stone gets lodged at a narrow point in the ureter causing temporary obstruction. The ureters are normally narrower at the ureteropelvic and ureterovesical junctions and at the point where they pass over the iliac crest into the pelvis. If the stone is to pass along the ureter by peristaltic action, the patient will have some pain.

Gross hematuria may occur if the stone has rough edges. Microhematuria is almost always present. Signs and symptoms of UTI (p. 1407) may also be present. Often a stone is "silent," causing no symptoms for years. This is especially true of very large stones that develop over a long period of time before resulting in symptoms. Extremely small smooth stones may be passed asymptomatically.

Diagnostic Tests

The diagnostic tests performed to determine the presence of renal stones include KUB, intravenous or retrograde pyelography, ultrasound, tomography, cystoscopy, and urinalysis.

Because recurrence of renal calculi is common, additional studies are carried out after the acute episode has subsided. Successive determinations of serum calcium, phosphorus, protein, electrolytes, and uric acid are performed to determine presence of underlying disease that can influence stone formation. The urinary pH is measured with pH paper each time the patient voids to determine the urine acidity or alkalinity. A *nitroprusside urine test* may be performed to check the presence of cystine. An accurate 24-hour urine collection is made to measure calcium, oxalate, phosphorus, and uric acid levels. The 24-hour urine collection may be made with the patient eating a normal diet or following a 3-day low-calcium, low-phosphorus diet.

INTERVENTIONS
Medical Management

Acute care. About 90% of urinary calculi are passed spontaneously. A person who is up and about is more likely to pass a stone than one who is in bed. The urine is strained and observed closely for passage of the stone and the person is permitted to carry out usual activities. If there is no infection or obstruction, the stone may be left in the ureter for several months. Fluids are prescribed for 2500 ml/day or more to promote passage of the stone and to prevent infection.

If some obstruction is present and the stone fails to pass, one or two ureteral catheters may be passed through a cystoscope up the ureter and left in place for 24 hours. The catheters dilate the ureter, and when they are removed the stone may pass into the bladder. If there are signs of infection, an attempt is made to pass a ureteral catheter past the stone into the renal pelvis. The catheter is left as a drain since pyelonephritis will quickly follow if adequate urinary drainage is not reestablished. Patients with ureteral catheters are usually confined to bed to prevent possible dislodgement of the catheters.

Stones in the lower ureter may be removed by cystoscopic manipulation. General anesthesia may be re-

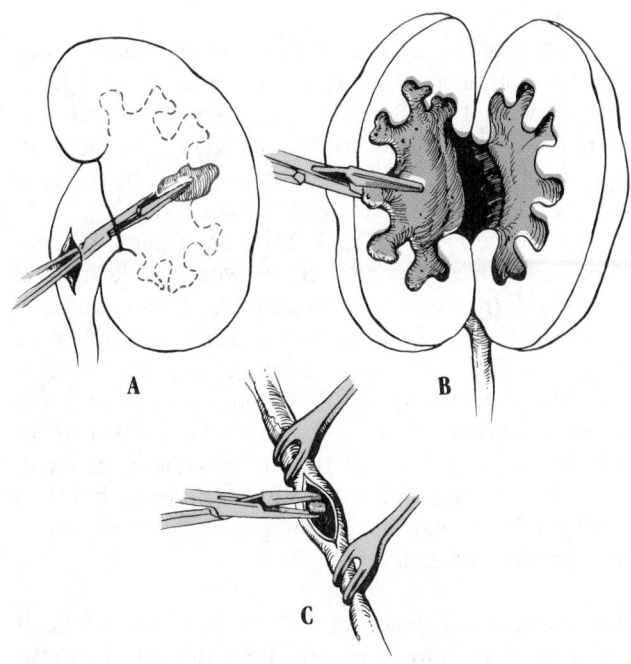

FIGURE 48-6 Location and methods of removing renal calculi from upper urinary tract. **A,** Pyelolithotomy, removal of stone through renal pelvis. **B,** Nephrolithotomy, removal of staghorn calculus from renal parenchyma (kidney split). **C,** Ureterolithotomy, removal of stone from ureter.

quired and care is similar to that after cystoscopy (see Chapter 47).

Surgery. Surgical intervention is indicated when a large stone (greater than 1 cm) is producing pain, obstruction, or infection. The operation for removal of a stone from the ureter is a *ureterolithotomy* (Figure 48-6, *C*). A radiograph is taken immediately preceding surgery, since the stone may have moved, and it is desirable to make the incision into the ureter directly over the stone. If the stone is in the lower third of the ureter, a rectus incision is made. If it is in the upper two thirds, a flank approach is used. If the patient has a ureteral stricture that causes stones to form, a plastic surgery procedure to relieve the stricture may be carried out as part of the operation.

Removal of a stone through or from the renal pelvis is known as a *pyelolithotomy* Figure 48-6, *A*). Removal of a stone through the parenchyma is a *nephrolithotomy* (Figure 48-6, *B*). Occasionally, the kidney may have to be split from end to end (a kidney split) to remove the stone. Patients in whom such a split is performed may develop severe hemorrhage after surgery.

Bladder stones may be removed through a suprapubic incision, or they may be crushed with a lithotrite (stone crusher) that is passed transurethrally. This procedure is known as a *litholapaxy*. After bladder stone

removal, the bladder may be irrigated (intermittently or constantly) with an acid solution such as magnesium and sodium citrate (G solution) or Renacidin to counteract the alkalinity caused by the infection and to help wash out the remaining particles of stone. If there has been a suprapubic incision, the care of the incision is similar to that after a suprapubic prostatectomy. (See Chapter 49 for care of the patient requiring urologic surgery.)

Percutaneous lithotripsy. Percutaneous lithotripsy is a technique that requires a percutaneous nephrostomy tract created through an incision of ¼ to ½ inch over the region of the kidney. An endoscope is then passed through the tract, and a snare basket is used to retrieve the calculi. If the calculi cannot be removed, ultrasonic lithotripsy is used to disintegrate the stone. Complications of the surgery are rare; however, hemorrhage, urinoma, sepsis, and abscess may develop.[30] Postoperatively the patient usually will experience pain similar to renal colic caused by the presence of calculi. Pain is controlled by administering meperidine hydrochloride. The patient may also experience copious drainage from the nephrostomy tract. Dressings should be changed frequently to prevent infection. Urinary drainage from the incision may be experienced for 3 to 4 days after the procedure. Patients are usually prescribed a 2-week course of antibiotic therapy after surgery.

Transcutaneous shock wave lithotripsy. Transcutaneous shock wave lithotripsy is a technique developed in Germany that has been used in the United States since early 1985. With this procedure, the patient is submerged in a large tub of warm water and ultrasonic waves are aimed by fluoroscopy over the area of the renal calculi. This aiming is best accomplished when the patient is able to control both breathing and movement while in the water bath. The water bath is necessary to allow for the passage of the shock waves into the body. Repeated firing of the ultrasonic waves results in disintegration of the calculi. It may require 1500 or more shock waves to break up a large stone. The patient may be sedated with Valium during the procedure. Pain of moderate intensity may be experienced during the passage of each sound wave; therefore, an epidural (preferred) or general anesthesia may also be used.

After the lithotripsy, the patient is observed for signs of bleeding. Blood pressure is monitored frequently for the first several hours after the procedure. Urinary output is also closely monitored for both quantity and quality. Blood initially may turn the urine cherry red to pink for the first several hours. The urine should then clear. Immediately after the procedure, the patient may experience redness or bruising on the skin at the site of the lithotripsy. Pain may also be experienced in this region from the force of the ultrasonic shock waves. Pain is usually localized to the skin as a result of the shock waves entering the body. The patient can be discharged within a few days after the procedure if complications, which have been rare, are not experienced.

The patient may also experience pain similar to renal colic after lithotripsy. This is usually a result of the passage of fragments of the pulverized renal stone through the lower urinary tract. Renal colic is usually controlled by use of narcotic analgesics. Since renal colic often occurs 3 or more days after lithotripsy, the patient should be made aware of this potential complication and informed about use of pain medications and signs requiring physician notification.

Occasionally urinary obstruction may occur as a result of stone fragments blocking the flow of urine. The patient is instructed to observe the volume of urine output for several days after discharge. The patient is weighed daily for several days following lithotripsy to detect urinary retention. Flank pain may also indicate urinary obstruction. When these symptoms are present, the patient should contact the physician immediately.

Candela laser therapy. The Candela laser is a pulsed-dye laser system designed to break up calculi that have migrated to the lower ureters. The laser probe is inserted through a ureteroscope. A new 2.4 mm flexible probe is expected to decrease the minor ureteral injury often caused by a wider probe and ureteroscope. An advantage of the Candela laser system is that is spares the patient the discomfort and cost of lithotripsy or surgery.[18]

Long-term care. Persons who have recurrent renal calculi benefit from ongoing prophylactic therapy determined by the type of stone being produced. For *calcium* stones, foods high in calcium are sometimes restricted, but a very low-calcium diet is usually unsatisfactory because it is unpalatable. Sodium or potassium phosphate may be prescribed to decrease urinary calcium; these drugs are contraindicated if the kidney is infected. Thiazide diuretics, particularly hydrochlorothiazide (HCTZ) decrease the calcium content in the urine by increasing reabsorption of calcium in the renal tubules.

Phosphate calculi develop in alkaline urine; therefore, their prevention depends on keeping the urine acidic and preventing urinary tract infections. Cranberry juice can be taken (200 ml 4 times daily) to keep the urine acidic. Ascorbic acid may also be prescribed to acidify the urine.

Prophylaxis for *uric acid* stones consists in alkalinizing the urine by the administration of sodium bicarbonate or citrate solution. Allopurinol (Zyloprim) is usually prescribed to inhibit synthesis of uric acid.

Nursing Management

The urine of all persons with relatively small stones should be strained. Urine can be strained easily by placing two opened 4 × 8 inch gauze sponges over a funnel. Stones vary in size and may be no bigger than the head of a pin. The stones are saved for inspection by the physician and sent to the laboratory for analysis.

Renal colic is an excruciating type of pain. The patient is involved in determining when medication is needed. Morphine or other opiates are given in doses to control the pain. Antispasmodics, such as atropine or methantheline bromide (Banthine), may also be prescribed to depress the smooth muscles of the ureter and lessen pain from spasm. Other methods for pain relief may be tried (see Chapter 16) but may not be effective.

Monitor intake and output and encourage fluids to 2500 ml/day or more to promote passage of the stone and prevent infection.

Patient teaching. The person who has had urinary calculi needs to know how to prevent development of further stones. Patient teaching includes the following:
1. Prevent urinary tract infections
   a. Drink at least 2500 ml fluids/day
   b. Avoid situations that lead to urinary stasis, if possible (for example, long periods of inactivity)
2. Follow any dietary prescriptions
3. Know name, dosage, and side effects of medications prescribed to acidify or alkaline the urine
4. Report to physician signs of recurrence of calculi (costovertebral pain or pain radiating to external genitalia)
5. Report to physician signs of urinary tract infection (burning on urination, frequency, urgency, fever)

TUMORS OF THE KIDNEY
EPIDEMIOLOGY/ETIOLOGY

Malignant renal tumors, primarily adenocarcinomas, account for 3% of all cancers. Small benign tumors (adenomas) may occur without causing significant damage or symptoms. Renal cell carcinomas rarely occur before the age of 30 years, are more commonly seen in the 50- to 70-year age range, and occur twice as often in men as in women.

PATHOPHYSIOLOGY

Renal carcinomas usually develop unilaterally but may occur bilaterally. In stage I the tumor margins are well defined (encapsulated) and compress the kidney parenchyma during growth rather than infiltrating the tissue. The upper pole of the kidney is usually involved, and the tumor is usually large at the time of diagnosis. In stage II the tumor invades the fat surrounding the kidney. Stage III consists of local metastasis either through direct extension or through the renal vein or lymphatics (lymph node involvement). Distant metastases during stage IV are primarily in the lungs or bone; but other areas, such as the liver, spleen, or brain, may also be involved.

CLINICAL MANIFESTATIONS

Hematuria is the most frequent sign of renal cell carcinoma. Unfortunately, the hematuria is often intermittent, lessening the person's concern and causing procrastination in seeking medical care. Any person with hematuria should have a complete urologic examination, since it is only by immediate investigation of the first signs of hematuria that there is any hope of cure. Other signs and symptoms include dull flank pain, flank mass, unexplained weight loss, fever, and polycythemia. Hypertension may also be present as a result of stimulation of the renin-angiotensin system.

An intravenous pyelogram may show a distortion of renal outline suggesting a kidney tumor. Small tumors in the parenchyma may not be apparent on a routine pyelogram but may be identified by a computed tomography (CT) scan (see Chapter 47) or by magnetic resonance imaging (MRI). CT is also useful in differentiating between renal cell carcinoma and a renal cyst. Angiography may also be performed to differentiate a cyst from a tumor.

INTERVENTIONS

Unless the person is a poor surgical risk or has extensive metastases, the diseased kidney is removed (*nephrectomy*) through transabdominal, thoracoabdominal, or retroperitoneal approach. The first two approaches are preferred to secure the renal artery and vein and to prevent any spread of malignant cells. (See Chapter 49 for care of the person requiring urologic surgery.)

Radiation has not proved to be beneficial, except for symptomatic bone metastases, and chemotherapy is also of limited value. Therapy with interferon-α appears to be promising.[40] Five-year survival rates after treatment of stages I, II, and IIIA are 70%.[41]

TUMORS OF THE BLADDER

EPIDEMIOLOGY/ETIOLOGY

The bladder is the most common site of cancer in the urinary tract. Cancer of the bladder occurs three times more often in males than in females and multiple tumors are common. About 25% of patients have more than one lesion at the time of diagnosis. This figure increases to about 50% in persons with papilloma grade I carcinoma over a 5-year period. Approximately 40% of all tumors involve the trigone, and an additional 45% involve the posterior and lateral walls of the bladder.

PREVENTION

Known factors predisposing to bladder cancer are exposure to the chemicals β-naphthylamine and xenylamine, infestation with *Schistosoma haematobium,* and cigarette smoking. Therefore exposure to these substances should be avoided.

PATHOPHYSIOLOGY

Tumors of the bladder range from small benign papillomas to large invasive carcinomas. Most of the neoplasms are of the transitional cell type since the urinary tract is covered with transitional epithelium. These neoplasms begin as papillomas; therefore, all papillomas of the bladder are considered premalignant and are removed when identified. Squamous cell carcinoma occurs less frequently and has a poorer prognosis. Other neoplasias include adenocarcinoma (which is often inoperable) and rhabdomyosarcoma (seen most frequently in infants).

Carcinomas of the bladder are graded and staged according to the definitions in the box below. Grade I and II bladder tumors are usually superficial, whereas grade III and IV tumors are usually invasive in nature.

CLINICAL MANIFESTATIONS

Painless hematuria is the first sign in the majority of patients with bladder tumors. It is usually intermittent resulting in the individual delaying in seeking early health care. Painless hematuria may also be seen in nonmalignant urinary tract disease and in cancer of the kidney; therefore, any hematuria should be investigated. Cystitis may provide the first symptoms of a bladder tumor, because the tumor may act as foreign body in the bladder. Symptoms of renal failure resulting from obstruction of the ureters sometimes is the reason given for seeking medical care. Vesicovaginal fistulas may occur before symptoms develop. The presence of renal failure

---

GRADING AND STAGING OF ADVANCEMENT OF CARCINOMAS OF THE BLADDER

GRADES	DIFFERENTIATION
Grade I	Well differentiated
Grade II	Medially differentiated
Grade III	Poorly differentiated
Grade IV	Anaplastic

STAGES	TISSUE INVOLVEMENT
Stage O	Mucosa
Stage A	Submucosa
Stage B	Muscle
Stage C	Perivesical fat
Stage D	Lymph nodes

or vesicovaginal fistulas indicate a poor prognosis since they usually occur after the tumor has infiltrated widely.

Cytologic examination of the urine may identify malignant cells before the lesion can be visualized by cystoscopy. The diagnosis is established by cystoscopic visualization and biopsy of the bladder. Clinical determination of the invasiveness of the tumor is important in establishing a therapeutic regimen and in predicting the prognosis. Any person who has had a papilloma removed should have a cystoscopic examination every 3 months for 2 years and then at less frequent intervals if there is no evidence of a new lesion. Repeated cystoscopies may seem unacceptable to persons who dread them; the necessity for frequent examination should be fully explained by the urologist and the explanation reinforced by the nurse. Emphasis is placed on the necessity for repeated cystoscopies, since papillomas tend to recur without symptoms until they are far-advanced tumors.

INTERVENTIONS

The treatment of bladder tumors depends on the size of the lesion and the depth of the tissue involvement.

Surgery

Small tumors with minimal tissue layer involvement may be adequately treated with *transurethral fulguration* or *excision*. A Foley catheter may or may not be inserted after surgery. The urine may be pink tinged, but gross bleeding is unusual. Burning on urination may occur and is relieved by drinking increased fluids to dilute the urine. Heat applied over the bladder and sitz baths may also provide relief. The patient is usually discharged within 1 to 2 days after surgery.

If the tumor involves the dome of the bladder, a segmental resection of the bladder may be performed. Over half of the bladder may be resected. A *cystectomy* (complete removal of the bladder) usually is performed only when the disease appears curable. Complete removal of the bladder requires permanent urinary diversion. Urinary tract surgery is discussed in Chapter 49.

Radiation

External cobalt radiation of large invasive tumors may be given before surgery to retard tumor growth. Supervoltage irradiation can be given when the patient physically cannot tolerate surgery. Radiation is not curative and has little value in patient management if the tumor is deemed inoperable. Internal radiation (radioisotopes or radon seeds) is rarely used since the introduction of better methods of external radiation.

Chemotherapy

Chemotherapy is primarily palliative. CMV (cisplatin, methotrexate, vinblastine) with or without doxorubicin

hydrochloride (Adriamycin) are the most commonly used agents. Thiotepa may be instilled into the bladder as a topical treatment. The patient is dehydrated 8 to 12 hours before Thiotepa treatment, and the drug remains in the bladder for 2 hours.

BENIGN PROSTATIC HYPERTROPHY
EPIDEMIOLOGY/ETIOLOGY

Benign prostatic hypertrophy or hyperplasia (BPH) is an adenomatous enlargement of the prostate gland. The prostate is an encapsulated gland weighing about 20 g that encircles the male urethra below the bladder neck. When the middle lobe of the gland enlarges, it causes narrowing of the urethra. More than half of all men over 50 years and 75% of men over 70 have some symptoms of prostatic enlargement. The cause is not known but seems to be related to the presence of male hormones.

PREVENTION

No preventive measures are known for BPH. However, early detection and adequate treatment can prevent complications that would result from obstruction if left untreated. The prostate should be palpated on yearly physical examinations for all men over age 30 to 35.

PATHOPHYSIOLOGY

The cause of BPH is not known. However, it is thought to be related to changing hormone levels. The signs and symptoms associated with BPH are a result of the prostate enlarging and causing partial or complete obstruction of the urinary tract.

CLINICAL MANIFESTATIONS

One of the early symptoms of BPH is *nocturia* (awaking at night to void) and urinary frequency in general. The man may notice that the urinary stream is smaller and more difficult to start (*hesitancy*). The bladder muscle must contract more forcibly to push the urine past the obstruction, and the overworked muscles hypertrophy. Stagnant urine is held in trabeculae, or cellules, formed by sagging of the atonic mucous membranes between hypertrophied muscle bands. The bladder will not empty completely at each voiding (*residual urine*); this urine becomes alkaline from stasis and is fertile medium for bacterial growth. The man will then complain of symptoms of cystitis (frequency, urgency), and bladder stones may occur. Some men develop hematuria from rupture of blood vessels that have been overstretched. Destruction of renal function can eventually occur from back pressure up the ureter to the kidney. Acute urinary retention is not uncommon.

Enlargement of the lateral lobes of the prostate gland may be palpated by digital rectal examination. Enlargement of the middle lobe is diagnosed by signs of partial obstruction of the urethra and visualization of the ob-

TABLE 48-11 Comparison of types of prostatic surgery

	Transurethral Resection	Suprapubic Resection	Retropubic Resection	Perineal Resection	Radical Perineal Resection
Reason for surgery	Enlargement of medial lobe surrounding urethra	Extremely large mass of obstructing tissue	Large mass located high in pelvic area	Large mass located low in pelvic area	Cancer of prostate gland
Location of incision	No incision; removal by way of urethra	Low midline abdominal incision through bladder to prostate gland	Low midline abdominal incision into prostate gland (bladder not incised)	Incision between scrotum and rectum	Large perineal incision between scrotum and rectum
Drainage tubes	Three-way Foley catheter with 30 ml bag in urethra, constant irrigation for 24 hr	Cystotomy tube or drain through incision; Foley catheter with 30 ml bag in urethra	Foley catheter with 30 ml bag in urethra, constant irrigation for 24 hr	Foley catheter with 30 ml bag in urethra	Foley catheter with 30 ml bag in urethra; drain in incision
Bladder spasms	Yes	Yes	Few	Few	Few
Dressing	None	Abdominal dressing easily soaked with urinary drainage	Abdominal dressing; no urinary drainage	Perineal dressing; no urinary drainage	Perineal dressing; urinary drainage
Complications	Hemorrhage; water intoxication; incontinence	Hemorrhage; wound infection	Hemorrhage; wound infection	Hemorrhage; wound infection	Urinary incontinence; wound infection; impotence; sterility

struction and bladder trabeculae by cystoscopy. Other diagnostic tests include IVP and occasionally urethrogram.

INTERVENTIONS

Surgery is the primary treatment for benign prostatic hypertrophy. During surgery the capsule of the prostate gland is left intact, and the adenomatous soft tissue is removed by one of four surgical routes: transurethral, suprapubic, retropubic, or perineal. See Table 48-11 for a comparison of the different approaches.

Transurethral Prostatectomy

Technique. Transurethral prostatic resection (TURP) is performed when the major enlargement exists in the medial lobe that directly surrounds the urethra. There must be a relatively small amount of tissue requiring resection so that excessive bleeding will not occur and the time required to complete the surgery will not be prolonged. A resectoscope (an instrument similar to a cystoscope but equipped with a cutting and cauterization loop attached to electric current) is passed through the urethra. The bladder is irrigated continuously during the procedure. The patient is grounded against electric shocks by a lubricated metal plate placed under his hips. Tiny pieces of tissue are cut away, and the bleeding points are sealed by cauterization (Figure 48-7). A

transurethral prostatectomy may be performed with the patient under general or spinal anesthesia.

Postoperative care. Following a TURP, a large (24 Fr) three-way Foley catheter with a 30 ml balloon is usually inserted into the bladder. After the retention balloon of the catheter is inflated, the catheter is pulled down so that the balloon rests in the prostatic fossa and provides hemostasis. Traction may be applied to the Foley catheter to increase pressure on the operative area to control bleeding. The large-size catheter (24 Fr) is used to facilitate removal of clots from the bladder. Since the catheter retention balloon exerts pressure on the internal sphincter of the bladder, the patient continually feels the urge to void. If the catheter is draining properly, the strongest of these sensations usually passes momentarily. Attempting to void around the catheter causes the bladder muscles to contract and results in a painful "bladder spasm."

The nurse should discuss the physiology of the "need to void" with the patient preoperatively so that spasms will be seen as an expected event and not an abnormal complication. The patient is taught that the catheter produces the sensation of fullness; the patient should not strain to pass urine around the catheter and should drink large amounts of fluids to reduce irritation and spasm. Narcotics are given to lessen the pain sensation;

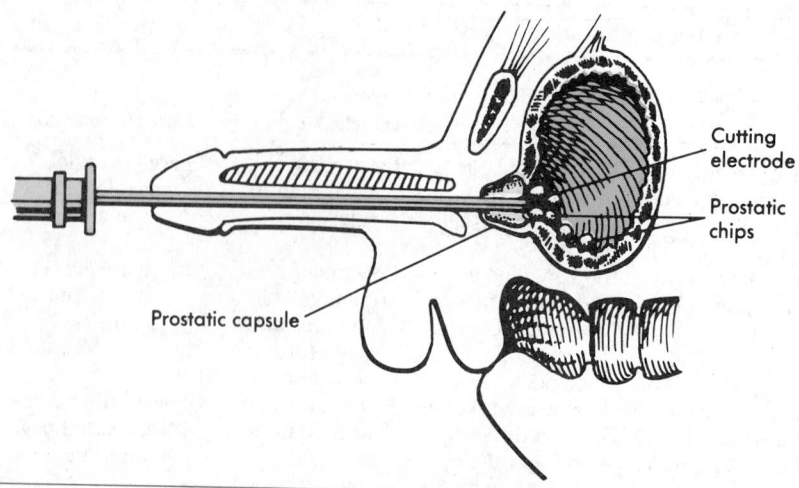

FIGURE 48-7 Transuretheral resection of prostate gland by means of resectoscope. Note enlarged prostate gland surrounding urethra and tiny pieces of prostatic tissue that have been cut away.

belladonna and opium suppositories are prescribed to relieve bladder spasms. As the nerve endings become fatigued, the frequency and severity of spasms decrease. This usually occurs by the end of 24 to 48 hours.

The bladder is constantly irrigated by a three-way drip apparatus with normal saline or another solution prescribed by the surgeon. The purpose of constant irrigation is to keep the bladder free of clots that would block the drainage of urine.

A full bladder increases pressure on the outside of the prostatic fossa "milking" the bleeding vessels. Straining to have a bowel movement may also cause prostatic hemorrhage as can enemas, rectal tubes, and rectal thermometers, all of which are avoided for about a week postoperatively.

Persistent bladder discomfort, bladder spasms, or failure of a catheter to drain properly usually signifies one of the following serious complications, which require immediate medical attention: (1) hemorrhage and clot retention, (2) displacement of the catheter, or (3) unsuspected perforation of the bladder during surgery.

Sometimes patients develop *water intoxication,* formerly known as transurethral resection (TUR) syndrome, as a result of excessive irrigating solution being absorbed into the venous sinusoids during surgery. Cerebral edema may result. Confusion and agitation on the part of the patient may be the first signs of this condition.

Constant bladder irrigation is usually discontinued after 24 hours if no clots are draining from the bladder. After catheter removal, the patient should measure and record the time and amount of each voiding. The patient may not be able to void after removal of the catheter because of urethral edema. When this occurs, the catheter may need to be reinserted. Continence is also

assessed since the internal and external sphincters lie above and below the prostate, close to the operative area, and may have been disturbed during surgery.

About 2 weeks after TURP when desiccated tissue is sloughed out, there may be a secondary hemorrhage. The patient, who probably is home at this time, must contact the physician immediately should there be any bleeding.

Suprapubic Prostatectomy

The alternate methods of prostatectomy are open operations. In the *suprapubic resection* the prostate gland is removed from the urethra by way of the bladder; this type of resection is performed when a large mass of tissue must be resected. The usual method of draining urine after surgery is illustrated in Figure 48-8, *A.* Some type of hemostatic agent will be placed in the prostatic fossa and urine will be drained by Foley catheter or cystotomy tube or both.

Hemorrhage is a possible complication, and the precautions are the same as those taken after TURP. Since there is some oozing of blood from the prostatic fossa, continuous bladder irrigations are usually ordered for the first 24 hours.

Cystotomy tubes are usually removed 3 to 4 days postoperatively; urethral catheters generally remain until the suprapubic wound is well healed. After the urethral catheter has been removed, the nursing care of the patient is similar to that for the patient undergoing transurethral resection. If the suprapubic wound should reopen and drain, a urethral catheter is usually reinserted.

Retropubic Prostatectomy

In a retropubic prostatectomy a low abdominal incision similar to that used for suprapubic prostatectomy is

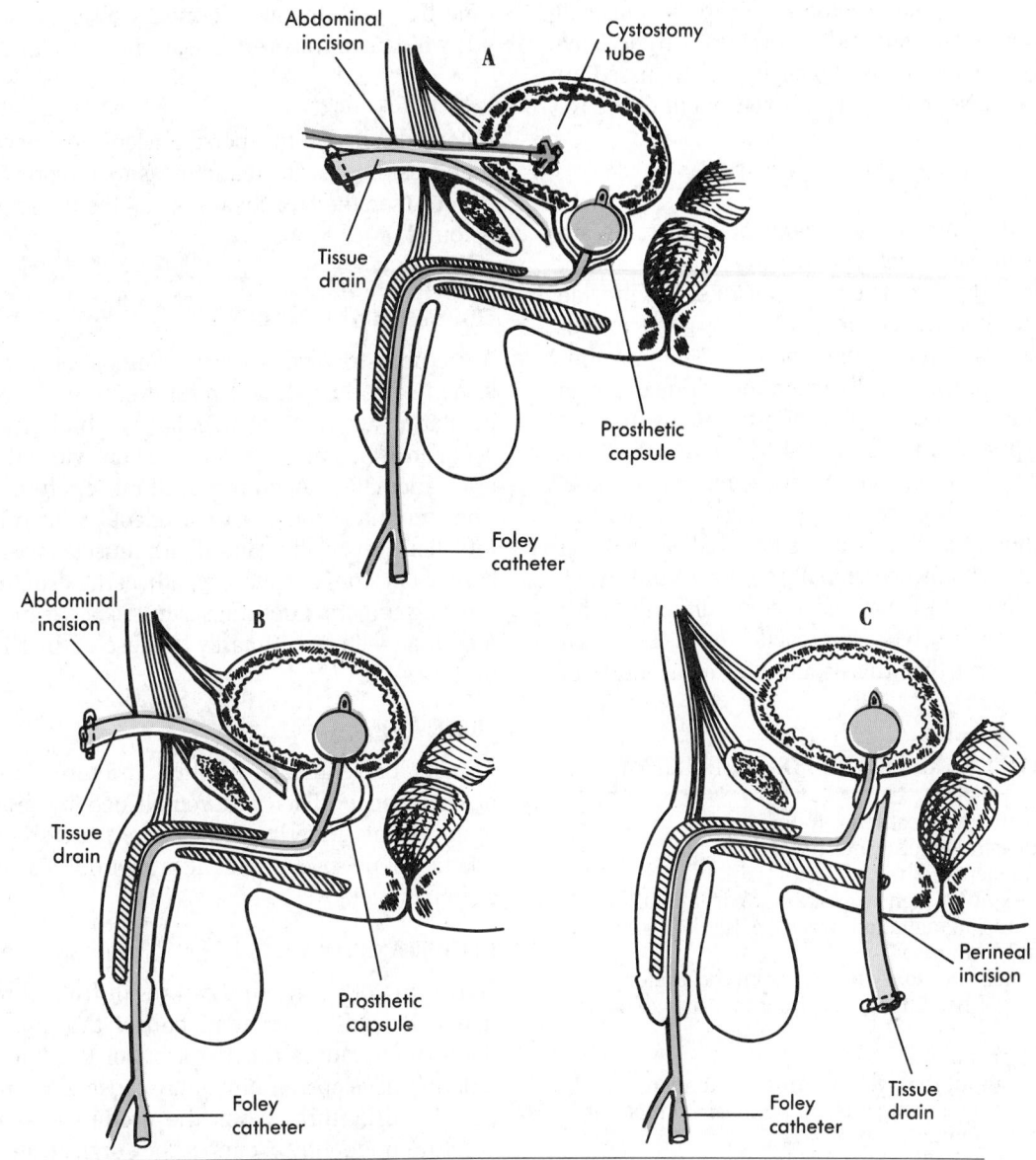

FIGURE 48-8 Three types of prostatectomies. **A,** Suprapubic; note placement of inflated Foley catheter in prostatic fossa. **B,** Retropubic. **C,** Radical perineal; note tissue drain placed in incision between scrotum and rectum.

made, but the bladder is not opened. Rather, it is retracted and the adenomatous prostatic tissue is removed through an incision in the anterior prostatic capsule (Figure 48-8, *B*).

Sphincter muscles are seldom damaged by retropubic prostatectomy, and there is no urine fistula. A large Foley catheter is inserted postoperatively, but bladder spasms are not usually a problem. When the Foley catheter is removed, the patient seldom has difficulty voiding. Hemorrhage from the prostatic fossa and wound infection may complicate the surgery; therefore, precautions are taken to prevent bleeding as discussed under TURP. No urinary drainage should be on the abdominal

dressing. If urine, purulent drainage, fever, or increased pain with ambulation occurs, the physician should be notified since these symptoms may indicate deep wound infection or pelvic abscess. Hospitalization generally is required for about 1 week after a retropubic prostatectomy.

Perineal Prostatectomy

The perineal approach is used primarily for confirmed or suspected cancer of the prostate (Figure 48-8, *C*). The incision is made between the scrotum and rectum. In addition to removal of the adenomatous prostate tissue, adjacent tissue may be excised when cancer is confirmed. Preoperative and postoperative care is similar to that given a patient having radical perineal surgery (see Chapter 56). Cancer of the prostate is discussed in Chapter 56 because of its greater involvement of the reproductive tract.

Patient Concerns

Common to all patients undergoing prostatectomy are concerns regarding *sexual functioning* and the *ability to be continent of urine.* The nurse may need to provide opportunity during interactions with the patient to promote expressions of these concerns by the patient. Impotence occurs physiologically when the perineal nerves are cut during a radical perineal prostatectomy and not with other types of prostatectomies. If the man believes that the surgery will or may produce impotence, however, it may occur because of psychological influences. Urinary incontinence frequently follows radical perineal prostatectomy but only occasionally after the other types of prostatectomy. Most men have some difficulty with continence after any type of prostatectomy. The man should understand that this is normal for a period of

---

POSTOPERATIVE CARE FOR PROSTATIC SURGERY

1. Maintain patency of catheter system
2. Monitor appearance of urine: red to light pink (24 hours) to amber (3 days)
3. Monitor patient for signs of water intoxication after TURP (confusion, agitation, warm moist skin, anorexia, nausea, and vomiting)
4. Instruct patient not to try to void around catheter; explain feeling of needing to void from pressure of catheter
5. After catheter removal:
   a. Monitor output for signs of urinary retention
   b. Monitor for continence; teach perineal exercises if dribbling occurs
6. Give prescribed medications (analgesics, antispasmodics) as needed; tell patient spasms will decrease in intensity and severity within 24 to 48 hours
7. Change dressings frequently around suprapubic wounds after suprapubic prostatectomy to prevent skin maceration
8. Give patient opportunities to discuss feelings about sexuality and possible incontinence
9. Teach patient to:
   a. Avoid vigorous exercises, heavy lifting (over 20 lbs), and sexual intercourse for at least 3 weeks after returning home
   b. Avoid driving for 2 weeks
   c. Avoid straining with defecation; use stool softeners or mild laxatives if needed
   d. Drink at least 2500 ml fluids/day to prevent urinary stasis and infection and to keep stools soft
   e. Notify physician if urinary stream diminishes or if bleeding occurs
   f. Report for medical postoperative visit; urinary stream will be checked at this time

---

time but will improve. Perineal exercises (see Chapter 49) will hasten recovery of control of voiding.

Patient Teaching

Before discharge the person needs to know activities that must be restricted and measures to prevent complications (see the box below). A sample nursing care plan is found on p. 1430.

URETHRAL STRICTURES
EPIDEMIOLOGY/ETIOLOGY

A urethral stricture is a narrowing or constriction of the lumen of the urethra. Urethral strictures can be congenital or acquired. Congenital urethral strictures can occur in isolation or in combination with other urinary tract anomalies. Acquired urethral stricture can result from trauma secondary to accident or instrumentation, infection (especially gonorrhea), muscle spasm, or pressure from the outside, by adjacent structures or by growing tumors. Urethral strictures occur more often in men than women, primarily because of the length of the urethra.

PREVENTION

Primary prevention of urethral strictures is prevention of occurrence. This is accomplished by prompt treatment of any underlying infection. Care should also be taken whenever the patient is to undergo urethral instrumentation.

PATHOPHYSIOLOGY

Narrowing of the urethra can result from chronic infection that leads to inflammation of the lining. The inflammation causes a hyperplasia of the lining and the stricture develops. Trauma may cause a complete severing of the urethra. When the urethra is anastomosed, stricture frequently occurs at the surgical site. The third leading cause of urethral stricture is the growth of a tumor that puts pressure against the exterior of the urethra, resulting in a stricture of the lumen.

CLINICAL MANIFESTATIONS

The first symptom of urethral strictures is usually a reduction in the size of the stream of urine. It may also be difficult to start the stream of urine. Other symptoms are those of urinary tract infection and urinary retention. Severe urethral strictures result in complete urinary obstruction leading to the signs and symptoms of hydronephrosis (p. 1417).

INTERVENTIONS

Urethral strictures are often repaired with urethroplasty (see Chapter 49). Strictures may also be corrected by dilation of the urethra. Dilation is accomplished by inserting splinting catheters into the urethra past the area of the stricture. The size of the splinting catheters can then be increased to cause gradual dilation of the urethra.

URINARY INCONTINENCE

EPIDEMIOLOGY/ETIOLOGY

Urinary incontinence is the involuntary expulsion of urine from the urinary tract. Urinary incontinence is encountered in a number of temporary and permanent conditions (Table 48-12). Inability to control urination is a problem that frequently leads to emotional distress and can seriously impair a person's socialization pattern if not appropriately handled. Incontinence must be managed either by the person or by others in a way that makes the person feel both physically and emotionally comfortable and socially acceptable.

More than 10 million Americans suffer from urinary incontinence. It is estimated that over 10 billion dollars a year is spent in managing patients with incontinence. As the population in the United States continues to age, incontinency will grow as a health care problem. Changes that occur with aging lead to decreased sensation and bladder muscle control that can result in urinary incontinence. Because persons are often embarrassed about the loss of bladder control, they do not seek assistance and often become isolated from social interactions. Because of this factor, it is not known how widespread this urinary problem may be.

TYPES OF INCONTINENCE

Four distinct types of urinary incontinence are described in the nursing literature.[23] The exact pattern of incontinence may vary among patients; however, incontinence generally can be categorized into one of these four types: stress, urge, overflow, or functional.

Stress incontinence typically results from the sudden increase in intra-abdominal pressure on the bladder that expels urine from the bladder. Causes can include lifting, exercising, coughing, sneezing, and laughing.

Urge incontinence occurs when the person perceives the need to void but urine leaks from the bladder before the person reaches the toilet. Urge incontinence results from decreased bladder capacity, bladder infection, or overdistention of the bladder. It is seen most often in older adults.

Where there is a constant dribbling of urine resulting from incomplete emptying of the bladder, it is called *overflow incontinence*. This type of incontinence can result from spinal cord injury, stroke, and diabetic neuropathy.

Functional incontinence occurs when the person is unable to reach the bathroom before voiding. It can result from impaired mobility, dementia, or severe depression.

The North American Nursing Diagnoses Association (NANDA) recognizes two additional nursing diagnoses, reflex and total incontinence.[31] *Reflex incontinence* occurs when the individual has involuntary loss of urine,

---

TABLE 48-12 Major causes of urinary incontinence

Cause of Urinary Incontinence	Factors Involved				
	Awareness of Need to Void	Cortical Ability to Inhibit Voiding	Reflex Arc	Bladder Response to Filling	Result
Cerebral clouding	Impaired	Impaired	Intact	Normal	Uncontrolled voiding because of reflex response
Infection	Intact	Intact, but overcome by strong reflex response	Abnormally stimulated	Heightened	Voiding because of strong reflex response (urgency)
Disturbance of CNS pathways (cortical lesions)	Diminished	Impaired	Intact	Heightened	Voiding because of reflex response
Disturbance of urethro-bladder reflex					
Upper motor neuron lesion	Destroyed	Destroyed	Intact but deranged	Heightened	Voiding because of reflex response
Lower motor neuron lesion	Destroyed	Destroyed	Destroyed or impaired	Diminished to absent	Distention or incomplete emptying
Tissue damage	Intact	Intact, but not functional because of poor muscle response	Intact	Normal	Loss of control of voiding because of muscular impairment

NURSING CARE PLAN

PERSON WITH TUR PROSTATECTOMY FOR BENIGN PROSTATIC HYPERTROPHY

DATA: Mr. Jones is a 67-year-old retired married automobile mechanic. He has been diagnosed by his physician as having benign prostatic hypertrophy. Mr. Jones has undergone medical examinations on an outpatient basis and has never been admitted to the hospital. He is slightly obese. On admission his blood pressure is 140/90. He denies any history of hypertension. Mr. Jones takes aspirin three to four times a day for control of what he describes as chronic headaches. He had a TURP performed today.

NURSING DIAGNOSIS

Urinary elimination, alteration in pattern related to surgery

Expected Patient Outcomes	Nursing Interventions	Rationale

Mr. Jones' urinary output equals his fluid intake.	1. Monitor urinary output and characteristics.
	2. Maintain constant bladder irrigation (CBI) as prescribed during first 24 hr.
	3. Maintain patency of indwelling urinary catheter:
	  a. Irrigate manually as prescribed to keep catheter free of clots.
	  b. Maintain straight line closed drainage system
	4. Encourage high fluid intake (2500 to 3000 ml/day) to promote increased urinary flow.
	5. After catheter is removed, monitor for signs of retention.
		Insure adequate bladder emptying. There is a potential for reabsorption of water from the bladder so output must be carefully assessed. Clots may also obstruct drainage catheter and must be detected early.

NURSING DIAGNOSIS

Pain related to bladder spasm

Expected Patient Outcomes	Nursing Interventions	Rationale
Mr. Jones states feeling more comfortable.	1. Teach him not to try to void around catheter. 2. Monitor him at regular intervals for 48 hr to identify early signs of bladder spasms. 3. Give prescribed medications (analgesics, antispasmodics). 4. Tell him spasms will decrease in intensity and frequency within 24 to 48 hr.	Bladder spasm frequently follows urologic procedures. Forcing voiding will encourage spasms. Antispasmodics may offer best relief by elimination or reduction of spasm.

NURSING DIAGNOSIS

Fluid volume excess, potential, related to irrigating fluid

Expected Patient Outcomes	Nursing Interventions	Rationale
Mr. Jones will not exhibit signs of water intoxication.	1. Monitor patient for signs of water intoxication during first 24 hours: confusion, agitation, warm moist skin, anorexia, nausea and vomiting. 2. Monitor fluid intake (oral, IV, CBI) and output	Irrigation fluid may be reabsorbed through bladder wall, resulting in water intoxication.

NURSING CARE PLAN

PERSON WITH TUR PROSTATECTOMY FOR BENIGN PROSTATIC HYPERTROPHY—cont'd

NURSING DIAGNOSIS

Infection/injury (hemorrhage), potential for, related to surgery

Expected Patient Outcomes	Nursing Interventions	Rationale
Mr. Jones does not exhibit signs of infection or hemorrhage.	1. Monitor vital signs; report signs of shock or fever. 2. Monitor appearance of urine for persistent bright red color rather than expected dark red beyond first few hours postoperatively. 3. Teach patient to avoid Valsalva's maneuver that may initiate prostatic bleeding. 4. Avoid use of rectal thermometers, rectal examinations, or enemas for at least 1 week. 5. Maintain strict asepsis of urinary drainage system; irrigate only when necessary. 6. Encourage high fluid intake.	Change in vital signs may alert nurse to infection. Bleeding is common after TURP, but must be closely monitored.

NURSING DIAGNOSIS

Incontinence, stress or urge, potential, related to catheter use

Expected Patient Outcomes	Nursing Interventions	Rationale

Mr. Jones achieves urinary continence.	1. Assess patient for dribbling after catheter is removed.
	2. If dribbing occurs:
	  a. Tell patient this is a common occurrence but that continence will return.
	  b. Teach patient perineal exercises.
		Dribbling is not uncommon after TURP but should resolve. Perineal exercises strengthen sphincter tone.

NURSING DIAGNOSIS

Sexual dysfunction, potential related to surgery

Expected Patient Outcomes	Nursing Interventions	Rationale

Mr. Jones describes effects of TURP on sexual functioning.	1. Give patient opportunities to discuss feelings about the effects of prostatectomy on sexual intercourse.
	2. Provide information as necessary:
	  a. Probable return of previous level of functioning.
	  b. Occurrence of retrograde ejaculation (first urine after intercourse may have a milky appearance).
	  c. Avoid sexual intercourse for 3 to 4 weeks after surgery.
		Sexual functioning usually returns to presurgical level. Patients often need to be encouraged to discuss their feeling about sexual intercourse.

NURSING DIAGNOSIS

Knowledge deficit (activity restriction, prevention of complications) related to lack of information

Expected Patient Outcomes	Nursing Interventions	Rationale

Mr. Jones describes activity restrictions and medical follow-up.	1. Teach patient:
	  a. Avoidance of heavy activities for 3 to 4 weeks.
	  b. Avoidance of straining at stool for 4 to 6 weeks; use stool softeners or laxatives as necessary.
	  c. Fluid maintenance of at least 2500 ml/day to prevent complications.
	  d. Instructions for medical follow-up.
		By adequately educating patient about postsurgical routine and restrictions the nurse can help ensure compliance with the medical regime.

occurring at a somewhat predictable interval when a specific bladder volume is reached. The person has no urge to void or awareness of bladder fullness. This type results from neurologic impairment and includes overflow incontinence.

Total incontinence occurs when an individual experiences a continuous and unpredictable loss of urine. This type of incontinence is the result of neurologic dysfunction.

PATHOPHYSIOLOGY
PHYSIOLOGY OF URINARY CONTINENCE

Bladder sphincter control is necessary to have urinary continence. Such control requires normal voluntary and involuntary muscle action coordinated by a normal urethrobladder reflex. As the bladder fills, the pressure within the bladder gradually increases. The detrusor muscle within the wall of the bladder responds by relaxing to accommodate the greater volume. When the bladder has filled to capacity, usually between 150 and 250 ml of urine, the parasympathetic stretch receptors located within the bladder wall are stimulated. The stimuli are transmitted through afferent fibers of the reflex arc for micturition. Impulses are then carried through the efferent fibers of the reflex arc to the bladder, causing contraction of the detrusor muscle. The internal sphincter, which is normally closed, reciprocally opens, and urine enters the posterior urethra. Relaxation of the external sphincter and perineal muscles follows, and the bladder content is released. Completion of this reflex arc can be interrupted and voiding postponed through release of inhibitory impulses from the cortical center, which results in voluntary contraction of the external sphincter. If any part of this complex control system is interrupted, urinary incontinence will result.

DISTURBANCES OF CEREBRAL CONTROL

Cerebral clouding is most common in the aged. In many instances the elderly person is incontinent because of a lack of awareness of a full bladder. This type of incontinence is often not associated with any definite pathologic problem at the cerebral level. Cerebral clouding also occurs in acutely ill persons—a result of dulled cerebration as a function of the illness. These patients may not have the energy to exercise voluntary control of bladder function. Likewise, a comatose patient is incontinent because of loss of ability to control voluntary use of the external sphincter. As soon as urine is released into the posterior urethra upon bladder filling, the bladder contracts and empties. This is why voiding sometimes occurs when a patient is under anesthesia.

Disturbance of the central nervous system pathways may occur in diseases such as cerebral embolus, cerebral hemorrhage, brain tumor, meningitis, or traumatic injury of the brain. Adequate voluntary (cortical or cere-

bral) control of bladder function is prevented in these situations. Urgency incontinence may be present as a result of the inability to inhibit completion of the urethrobladder reflex by the higher centers.

DISTURBANCES OF URETHROBLADDER REFLEX

Disturbance of the urethrobladder reflex may result from lesions of the spinal cord or damage to peripheral nerves of the bladder. This form of incontinence may be seen in persons with spinal cord malformations, injuries, or tumors, and those with compression of the spinal cord caused by fractures of the vertebrae, herniated disk, metastatic tumor, or postoperative edema of the spinal cord. This type of difficulty can result in two types of responses known as *neurogenic bladder: automatic* and *flaccid*. The person with a neurogenic bladder has no control over bladder function.

Lesions above the S2 level of the spinal cord or impairment of the cerebrocortical centers do not destroy the reflex arc for voiding, although they may affect control. Such lesions destroy the potential for cortical control to inhibit the reflex. The result is an "upper motor neuron" or "automatic" bladder. The bladder is hypertonic and has a small capacity of usually less than 150 ml. The increased detrusor tone and increased sensitivity to small amounts of urine present in the bladder result in precipitous voiding and the potential for vesicoureteral reflex.

Damage to nerves in the cauda equina or sacral segments of the spinal cord may cause destruction of the reflex arc by interruption of the afferent, efferent, or central components. The result is a "lower motor neuron" or "flaccid" bladder. The bladder is hypotonic with large capacities, sometimes of 500 ml or more. Overflow incontinence, retention of residual urine, and the potential for vesicoureteral reflux are problems imposed by a hypotonic bladder.

BLADDER DISTURBANCES

Overflow incontinence is considered to be caused by pressure exerted on the distended bladder by the abdominal muscles. Residual urine remaining in the bladder after incomplete emptying provides a medium for growth of bacteria, and UTI is common.

Infection anywhere in the urinary tract may lead to incontinence, since bacteria in the urine causes irritation of the mucosa of the bladder. The resulting inflammation stimulates the urethrobladder reflex abnormally.

Tissue damage to the sphincters of the bladder from instrumentation, surgery, trauma, scarring from urethral infection, lesions involving the sphincter, or relaxation of the perineal structures may cause urinary incontinence. The latter cause of incontinence is seen occasionally after childbirth. The problem is local in nature and does not involve the nervous system.

RELAXED MUSCULATURE

Stress incontinence is seen primarily in women who have relaxed pelvic musculature, but it may also occur in men after prostatectomy. When bladder pressure is suddenly increased, urine enters the proximal third of the urethra then returns to the bladder when pressure is decreased after exertion. Some of the urine escapes through the urethra.

MEDICAL MANAGEMENT

Medical management of incontinence includes treatment of any underlying disorders.

SPHINCTER DYSFUNCTION

Repair of a sphincter that has been cut is almost impossible. When the *external sphincter* has been damaged, the person will be incontinent on urgency. A voiding schedule can be planned so that voiding occurs before the bladder is full enough to exert sufficient pressure to open the internal sphincter involuntarily. When the *internal sphincter* is damaged, there may be no acute feeling of the need to void. Here the problem is not one of incontinence but of retention. To assure regular emptying of the bladder, a regular voiding schedule is necessary. *If both sphincters are damaged, there will be total incontinence.*

STRESS INCONTINENCE

Surgery may be indicated for severe stress incontinence. A *vesicourethropexy* (Marshal-Marchetti operation) consists of fixation of the urethra to the fascia of the rectus muscle of the abdomen with support given to the neck of the bladder. A suprapubic incision is usually made, but a transvaginal repair may be carried out if there is scar tissue around the urethra from vaginal surgery. A urethral catheter is inserted postoperatively and maintained for 5 to 6 days. The urine may be pink, but the urethral catheter is not irrigated as a rule. It is not uncommon for difficulty in voiding to be experienced immediately after the indwelling catheter is removed. The woman is observed for signs of vaginal bleeding. Straining and use of Valsalva's maneuver should be avoided until healing has occurred, and mild laxatives may be given to prevent straining from constipation. Surgeons differ in the amount of activity permitted in the early postoperative period.

Less invasive is the newer *Stamey* procedure, a suspension of the bladder neck by sutures passed adjacent to the ureterovesical junction.[17] A small incision is made above and lateral to the symphysis pubis. The needles are introduced suprapubically by endoscopy, and the positions are checked by cystoscopy before suturing. The procedure is then repeated on the opposite side. A percutaneous suprapubic catheter is inserted after the suturing; the catheter is removed when spontaneous voiding occurs, which may take several days. There is minimal postoperative discomfort. Antibiotics are given for 2 weeks postoperatively. The patient should refrain from sexual activity until permitted (usually 1 to 2 months).

URGENCY

Incontinence caused by urinary tract infection is generally temporary, responding to treatment of the infection by systemic antibiotics. Specific causes of infection such as obstruction must be identified and corrected where possible. Provision must be made for adequate fluid intake of 3000 ml or more per day unless contraindicated by the person's medical condition.

The person who has a brain tumor, meningitis, or traumatic injury to the brain that prevents adequate voluntary control of bladder function and causes urgency incontinence by inhibiting cortical control over the urethrobladder reflex may respond to a bladder retraining program. If the person's condition or response prohibits such a program, an internal or external drainage device should be used.

NEUROGENIC BLADDER DYSFUNCTION

Persons with injuries of the spinal cord experience a transitory period of "spinal shock" in which urinary retention occurs (see Chapter 63). This is treated with continuous or intermittent catheter drainage that aims to prevent urinary tract infection and overdistention of the bladder. After this acute stage, further management depends on the exact nature of any residual neurogenic bladder dysfunction. Persons with a lesion *above the sacral segments* and who have an intact urethrobladder reflex may initiate voiding by pinching or stroking trigger areas of the thighs or suprapubic area. In persons with a *lower motor neuron lesion* the use of the *Credé method*, which consists of exerting manual pressure over the bladder, may provide for more complete bladder emptying. The appropriateness of this technique must be determined by the physician based on the person's complete urologic status. An increasing number of persons with neurogenic bladder dysfunction are being taught intermittent self-catheterization using clean technique to prevent infection and manage incontinence (see Chapter 49). Maintenance of a regular schedule is stressed, and the frequency of catheterization is determined on an individual basis.

Certain medications are sometimes given alone or in conjunction with an intermittent catheterization program in the management of incontinence related to neurogenic bladder dysfunction. α-Adrenergic drugs such as ephedrine sulfate are used to increase urethral resistance. Anticholinergic drugs such as propantheline (Pro-Banthine) are prescribed to control the reflex bladder activity.

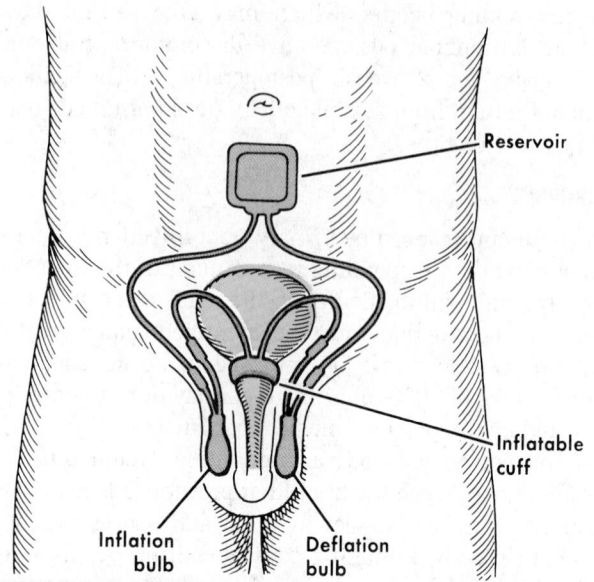

FIGURE 48-9 Artificial bladder sphincter. Compression and release of inflation pump bulb inflates cuff surrounding urethra stopping urine flow. Compression and release of deflation pump bulb deflates inflatable cuff, returning fluid to storage reservoir. This releases urethral constriction, permitting urine to flow.

ARTIFICIAL SPHINCTER

Implantation of an artificial urinary sphincter may be used to achieve continence when other methods have failed. In this procedure, a hydraulically activated sphincter mechanism is placed around the urethra or bladder neck. The sphincter is made to open and close at will by squeezing one of two bulbs implanted under the skin of the labia or scrotum (Figure 48-9). Postoperative nursing care of the person with such an implant includes observation for and reporting of fever or pain on inflation of the device, swelling of the genitalia, and recurrence of incontinence. Complications of the procedure include erosion of the urethra, abscess, cellulitis, and mechanical malfunctions in the system. Men have had more success with the artificial sphincter than have women.

■ ASSESSMENT

SUBJECTIVE DATA

The following questions should be asked when assessing for urinary incontinence:
1. What is the frequency of incontinence?
2. Can anything be associated with precipitating incontinence (stress, fear, coughing, sneezing, laughing, exercise)?
3. Is pain or burning present with incontinence?
4. Is there a state of awareness to void before incontinence?

OBJECTIVE DATA

The following objective data should be collected:
1. Volume of output
2. Characteristics of urine
3. Patient's ability to follow directions
4. Physiologic reason for incontinence (for example, spinal cord injury)

■ DATA ANALYSIS: NURSING DIAGNOSES

Nursing diagnoses are determined from assessment of patient data. Possible nursing diagnoses for the incontinent patient may include, but are not limited to, the following:

Diagnostic Title	Possible Etiologies
Knowledge deficit	Lack of exposure/recall
Coping, ineffective individual	Situational crises, personal vulnerability
Home maintenance management: impaired	Insufficient family resources, inadequate support systems
Mobility, impaired physical	Depression, anxiety
Self-care deficit: hygiene, toileting	Depression, anxiety, neuromuscular impairment
Self-esteem, disturbance performance	Change in social involvement
Skin integrity, impaired	Irritation, moisture
Urinary elimination, altered patterns	Sensorimotor impairment
Incontinence, functional	Altered environment, cognitive deficit, mobility deficit
Incontinence, reflex	Neurologic impairment
Incontinence, stress	Relaxed pelvic muscles, incompetent bladder outlet, overdistention between voids
Incontinence, total	Neurologic dysfunction
Incontinence, urge	Decreased bladder capacity, bladder infection, alcohol, caffeine, overdistention of bladder, bladder spasms

■ PLANNING: EXPECTED PATIENT OUTCOMES

Expected patient outcomes for the person with urinary incontinence may include, but are not limited to, the following:
1. The person is free of perineal skin irritation.
2. The person is free of urinary odor.
3. The person or significant others can describe or state the following.
   a. The relationship of adequate hygiene to the maintenance of skin integrity
   b. The relationship of adequate fluid intake to facilitate bladder training
   c. The bladder training program
   d. How to care for minor skin problems if they occur
   e. How to use professional and community resources
      (1) Available agencies

(2) How to obtain and maintain any needed supplies and equipment (drainage systems, commodes, protective padding, special beds)
  f. Plans for follow-up care
  g. Dose, desired action, and side effects of any prescribed medications

■ IMPLEMENTATION

No program of management of uncontrolled incontinence is likely to be successful without the cooperation of the individual involved. The person often becomes discouraged by recurring accidental voiding and needs a great deal of encouragement. Self-care of incontinence is encouraged whenever possible.

The person with urinary incontinence often experiences alterations in body image, and counseling may be needed to help deal with this problem (see Chapter 18). The person is encouraged to live as active a lifestyle as possible. Adult disposable waterproof pants are available for protection and to help give the person a feeling of security.

General interventions for the person with incontinence include perineal exercises, bladder retraining, or use of external urinary drainage.

PERINEAL EXERCISES

Perineal exercises are helpful in controlling mild stress incontinence or strengthening muscles after withdrawal of an indwelling catheter. The exercises consist in tightening and relaxing perineal and gluteal muscles and can be performed in a number of ways (see the box below). Much of the problem of incontinence caused by a relaxed perineum in women can be prevented if perineal exercises are taught before and after childbirth. These exercises also may be included as part of the health teaching of any woman.

BLADDER RETRAINING

When incontinence is caused by dulled cerebration in the elderly, by confusion, or by acute illness, control can usually be established if a persistent retraining schedule

---

PERINEAL EXERCISES

1. Tighten the perineal muscles as if to prevent voiding; hold for 3 seconds, then relax.
2. Inhale through pursed lips while tightening perineal muscles.
3. Bear down as if to have a bowel movement. Relax then tighten perineal muscles.
4. Hold a pencil in the fold between the buttock and thigh.
5. Sit on the toilet with knees held wide apart. Start and stop the urinary stream.

---

is carried out. A voiding schedule is developed and strictly adhered to until the person gradually relearns to recognize and react appropriately to the feeling of having to void. A successful program of this type, leading to complete rehabilitation, or continence, requires mental competence of the individual. Otherwise someone else must always remind the person to follow the schedule.

People ordinarily void on awakening, before retiring, and before or after meals. If a diuretic such as coffee has been taken, it is usually necessary to void about 30 minutes later. Using this knowledge, the nurse can begin to set up a schedule for placing the person on a bedpan or taking the person to the toilet. Then, if a record is kept for a few days of the times the person voids involuntarily, it is usually possible to determine the normal voiding pattern. If the schedule based on the pattern of incontinence is not successful, toileting every 1 to 2 hours should be carried out on a 24-hour basis.

During the retraining program, *mobilization* of the individual, attention to the *position* assumed for voiding, and adequate *fluid intake* contribute to reduction of the possibility of infection. Complete emptying of the bladder eliminates the possibility of residual urine acting as a medium for bacterial growth, whereas a high fluid intake provides for internal bladder irrigation.

Elderly persons isolated from their families and familiar surroundings, confused by institutionalization, or suffering feelings of loss of self-esteem frequently respond well to mobilization in bladder retraining programs. Their circulation is enhanced by the imposed mobility, their awareness is increased, and they respond to the attention given them. In instances in which nurses believe that it is easier to change bed linen than it is to establish an appropriate bladder retraining program a disservice is done to the individual and more work is actually created for the nurse. The person becomes subject to urinary tract infection and skin breakdown, and feelings of worthlessness are increased. For those who can be continent, incontinence is an indignity.

When it is possible, *toileting* should be carried out in surroundings that will remind the person of the voiding function; that is, the person should be taken to the bathroom where the toilet can be used. If this is not possible, a bedside commode can be an adequate substitute. Many men can void into a urinal more easily if allowed to stand at the bedside. The use of a bedpan is unfamiliar and distasteful to most persons, but in instances where women must remain in bed, voiding into a bedpan can be facilitated if the head of the bed is rolled up as high as allowed. This kind of positioning is more consistent with the position normally assumed for voiding and facilitates complete emptying of the bladder. Few persons can void adequately in the supine position.

Providing adequate amounts of *fluids,* a minimum of 3000 ml per day, is necessary to ensure that there will be adequate amounts of urine produced and present in the bladder to stimulate the voiding reflex at the proper times. Fluids may be given at scheduled times, the largest portion being given during the day *before 4:00 PM* to decrease the frequency of voiding through the night. Persons on fluid restriction because of medical problems should, of course, receive no more fluids than the amount prescribed.

EXTERNAL URINARY DRAINAGE

Occasionally there are justifications for the use of an indwelling catheter for the incontinent patient. Such reasons include the need to protect a surgical incision or to permit healing of a decubitus ulcer in the area. Indwelling catheterization, however, presents many potential dangers such as urinary tract infection, urethritis, epididymitis, and urethral fistulas. All other means to manage the incontinence should be tried before resorting to catheterization. (See Chapter 49 for details of catheter management.)

For the man, external drainage can be easily accomplished by applying a watertight apparatus to the penis. A number of commercial products are available for external urinary drainage and should be used whenever possible. The following is an alternative method. Select a condom of the correct size. Puncture a hole in the closed end of the condom with an applicator stick. Attach the punctured end of the condom to a firm rubber or plastic drainage tube with either a 3 mm (⅛ inch) piece of rubber tubing or a strip of adhesive tape (Figure 48-10). Before applying the condom, clean and dry the penis thoroughly and check it for edema, skin breaks, or discoloration. Invert the condom and roll it onto the penis. There should be no roll at the top that could cause constriction. At least 2.5 cm (1 inch) of the condom should remain between the meatus and drainage tube to allow for penile erection. There should not be so much slack as to cause twisting and subsequent interference with drainage. Elastoplast is then applied over the condom and around the penis (never touching the skin). *Under no circumstances should adhesive tape be used.* The Elastoplast must not be constricting.

The external catheter should be removed daily and the skin washed and checked. Frequent checking is necessary to determine whether edema or irritation is present and to ensure proper drainage. This is especially important in men with loss of sensation. The external device is attached to straight drainage or to a leg bag.

For persons who need external catheter drainage indefinitely, a rubber urinary appliance (sometimes called an *incontinence urinal*) may be used (Figure 48-11). Several models are available, and the one best suited to the person's needs is selected. Two appliances are recommended to allow for cleaning and drying. They

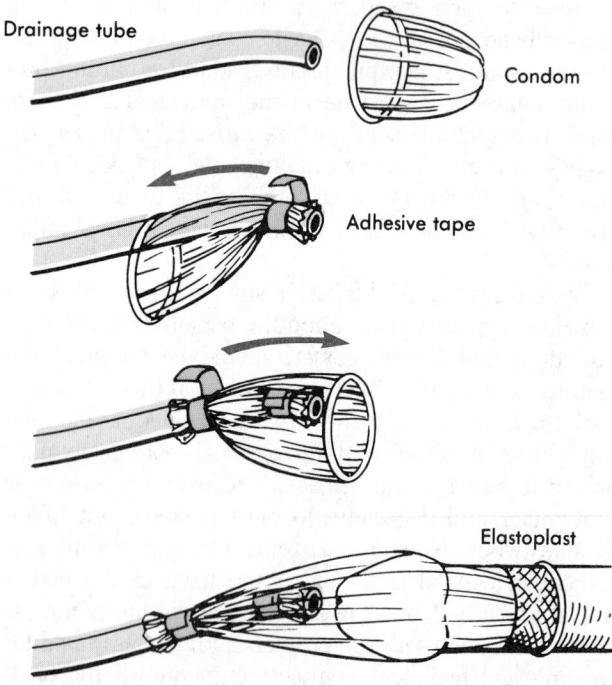

FIGURE 48-10 One method of making an external drainage apparatus.

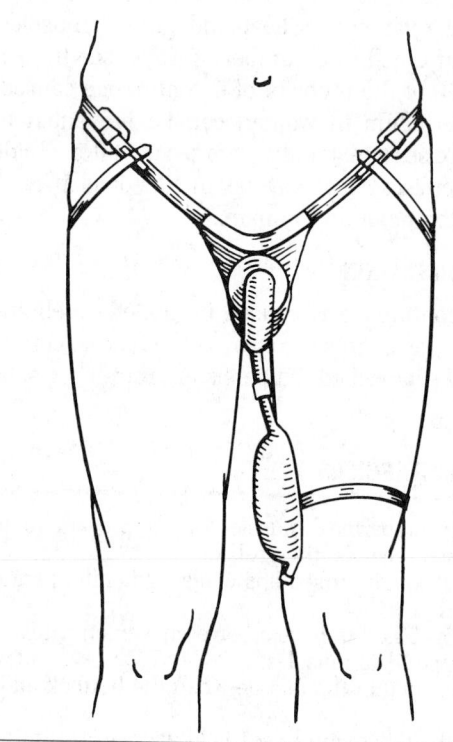

FIGURE 48-11 Rubber urinary appliance. Bag is emptied by drain valve at bottom bag.

should be washed in mild soap, turned inside out, and thoroughly dried before application.

Most persons prefer to manage their own incontinence if they are at all able to do so. The nurse supports and encourages this, offering assistance as necessary and instruction in basic principles of skin care, equipment selection, and maintenance. The choice of management method should take into account the person's ability to manage as independently as possible.

UNCONTROLLED URINARY INCONTINENCE

If none of the above measures are appropriate or successful, nursing goals of assisting the person to remain clean, free of odor, and free of ducubiti may require external urinary protection. The type varies with the sex, functional status, and physical status of the person.

Those who are incapacitated by critical illness or unconscious are dependent on the nursing staff to manage their incontinence by protective pants or external catheter drainage. Others may be capable of some or all of their own management. Men and women may wear protective waterproof pants lined by disposable or washable absorbent pads. A resourceful person may be able to improvise equipment that is as comfortable and is less costly than commercially available pants. Zippers, Velcro, elastic, and a variety of waterproof materials may be used. Bedding and furniture can be protected with waterproof materials such as commercially available squares of absorbent cellucotton backed with light plastic.

Whatever the type of padding, liners, or pants used, frequent changing is required for skin protection and comfort. The perineal and genital areas are thoroughly washed with soap and water and dried well at each changing. If possible, the person is bathed in a tub of warm water at least once a day. Periodic exposure of the perineal area to air is beneficial. A moisture barrier product (such as A&D ointment) helps protect the skin. Zinc oxide powder can be applied to lessen irritation. Excess amounts of powder are avoided, as this will cake

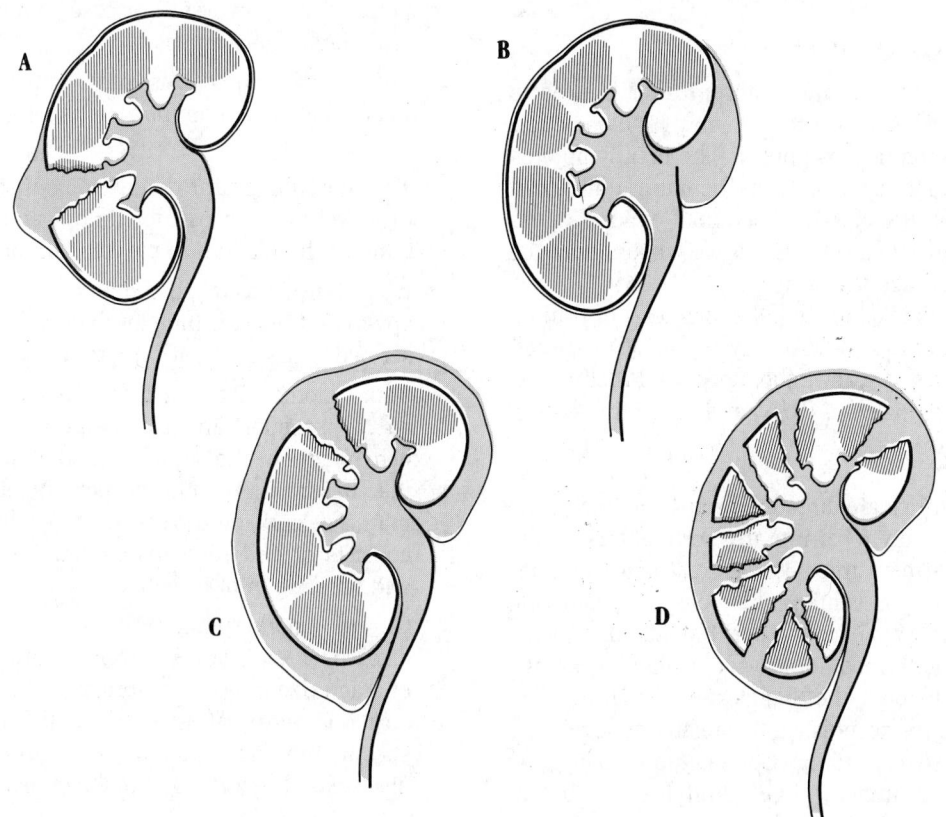

FIGURE 48-12 Four degrees of renal trauma. **A,** Urine is extravasating from split in renal parenchyma but confined under renal capsule. **B,** Urine is extravasating through tear in renal pelvis. **C,** Urine is extravasating through rent in kidney and capsule and surrounds kidney and renal pelvis. **D,** Kidney is shattered and urine is extravasating in all areas. (From Winter CC, and Morel A: Nursing care of patients with urologic diseases, ed 4, St Louis, 1977, The CV Mosby Co.)

on the skin and cause irritation. Deodorant sprays for use on dressings and liners are valuable, but they may cause skin irritation in persons who develop a hypersensitivity to them. Deodorant room fresheners may be helpful if the odor is strong.

If the person can be up, a favorite chair can be equipped with a commode seat. Special commode wheelchairs are also available, making it possible for the person to be more comfortable and to mingle socially with others.

TRAUMA TO URINARY TRACT

Assessing intactness of the urinary tract must be part of the evaluation of any person with traumatic injury to the lower trunk. Injuries particularly related to urinary tract damage include fractures of the pelvis and sharp blows to the body.

EPIDEMIOLOGY/ETIOLOGY

Pelvic fractures may result in *bladder perforation* and *urethral tearing*. A sharp blow to the body, particularly to the lower back, may result in *contusion, tearing,* or *rupture of a kidney* (Figure 48-12).

CLINICAL MANIFESTATIONS

Urinary output may be scant or absent after trauma to the urinary tract. Urine, if present, may be bloody and symptoms of peritonitis may appear. The first symptoms of trauma to the kidney usually are hematuria and pain or tenderness of the upper abdominal quadrant and flank on the involved side. Signs of shock may be present if hemorrhage is extensive.

Diagnostic tests used to facilitate diagnosis of trauma to the urinary tract include KUB, cystogram, IVP, renal-angiography, and CT scan. Laboratory tests include serial urinalysis, hemoglobin, BUN, and creatinine levels.

INTERVENTIONS

Treatment of injuries are directed toward stabilizing the patient and surgically repairing any perforations or lacerations of the urinary tract. Initial treatment includes control of bleeding, prevention of shock, and promoting drainage of urine. While stabilizing the patient, a cystotomy may be performed to provide urinary drainage when injuries involve the bladder or urethra. Vital signs, fluid balance records, and hematocrit levels are monitored to assess bleeding. Complaints of pain may indicate developing ureteral colic, signifying obstruction of the ureter by a clot. Surgical intervention is required to control severe hemorrhage; spontaneous healing of the kidney is otherwise permitted. Bed rest is maintained until gross hematuria clears; thereafter activity is progressed according to tolerance and continued absence of hematuria.

When urethral injuries are suspected, great care must be taken when inserting urinary catheters to prevent further injury to the urethra. It may be necessary for a urologist to insert the catheter during a retrograde urethrogram or cystogram[22] (see Chapter 47).

A kidney may become loosened and "float" or become displaced (*nephroptosis*). If symptoms of obstruction occur, the kidney may be sutured to its anatomic site (*nephropexy*). Postoperatively, the patient is positioned with the hips elevated to prevent tension on the suture line.

CHAPTER SUMMARY

✔ The major health problems of the urinary system include congenital, inflammatory, vascular, and obstructive disorders; urinary incontinence; and trauma to the urinary tract.

✔ Polycystic disease is an inherited disease in which cysts form in the kidneys and enlarge and rupture, causing scarring with loss of kidney function. Treatment is symptomatic with control of infection.

✔ Chronic health problems predisposing to urinary tract infections include diabetes mellitus, gout, hypertension, polycystic disease, multiple myeloma, and glomerulonephritis.

✔ Urinary tract infections may occur in the lower urinary tract (most common) or ascend into the kidney (pyelonephritis).

✔ The most important defenses against UTI are large urine volume, unobstructed flow, and complete emptying of the bladder to prevent urinary stasis.

✔ It is essential to teach the patient on antibiotic therapy for UTI to continue antibiotics for the entire prescribed course even if symptoms resolve.

✔ Acute glomerulonephritis usually follows a streptococcal infection and is a result of an antigen-antibody reaction; the significant effect is loss of glomerular basement membrane porosity. Proteinuria, hematuria, and fluid retention result. Management consists of bed rest, maintenance of fluid balance, and prevention of infection.

✔ Chronic glomerulonephritis may follow the acute disease or may develop from unknown cause; it is characterized by slow, progressive glomerular destruction terminating in renal failure. There is no specific therapy; patients are taught to live with their disease and report signs of exacerbation.

✔ Nephrotic syndrome is a constellation of symptoms (severe generalized edema, pronounced proteinuria, hypoalbuminemia, hyperlipidemia) resulting from kidney damage; it often progresses to kidney failure. Management consists of administering steroids and diuretics, promoting comfort (because of fatigue and massive edema), encouraging a restricted protein and sodium diet, and teaching the patient self-care.

✔ Vascular disorders include renal artery stenosis characterized by hypertension and nephrosclerosis caused by hypertension; treatment consists of control of hypertension and correction of the stenosis.

✔ Disorders that may obstruct the urinary tract include urinary calculi, tumors of the kidney or bladder, prostatic hypertrophy, or urethral strictures. Backup of urine causes hydronephrosis leading to kidney damage. General interventions include monitoring for signs of additional obstruction, promoting fluid balance and comfort, preventing urinary complications, and patient teaching.

✔ The most common urinary stones are calcium oxalates; the stones cause renal colic from urine backup or from irritation or stretching of the ureters. If the stone does not pass spontaneously and is causing symptoms or damage, it must be removed surgically or broken up by lithotripsy or laser treatment.

✔ Recurrence of some renal stones can be controlled by an alkaline or acid-ash diet (depending on the type of stone).

✔ Bladder cancer is more common than malignant renal tumors; both are removed surgically. If the entire bladder is removed, permanent urinary diversion is necessary.

✔ Benign prostatic hypertrophy is common in older men; the prostate enlarges and presses on the urethra causing urinary retention. The prostate may be removed by transurethral (preferred), suprapubic, retropubic, or perineal resection (the last three are open resections).

✔ A large three-way indwelling catheter with a 30 ml balloon is used to drain the bladder after prostatectomies; the catheter is pulled down in the prostatic fossa for hemostasis. Bladder spasms can be controlled with medication.

✔ Urinary incontinence is not a normal part of aging; whenever urinary incontinence is present, the cause should be thoroughly investigated.

✔ Major types of urinary incontinence include stress, urge, overflow, and funtional incontinence; two other forms are reflex and total incontinence. Control largely depends on cause. Stress incontinence may be controlled surgically. Nursing interventions include teaching perineal exercises and bladder retraining. Keeping the person dry is of utmost importance; waterproof pants or external urinary drainage may be used when control is inadequate.

QUESTIONS TO CONSIDER

- Why is it important to stress prevention of UTIs to patients at risk for infection?
- What nursing interventions should be considered for the patient with a urinary obstruction?
- Where and how do renal calculi develop? What can be done to prevent formation of the stones?
- What are major causes of urinary incontinence?

REFERENCES AND SELECTED READINGS

1. American Kidney Fund: Forum annual report highlights the accomplishments of ESRD networks, AKF Newsletter 2(2):4-5, 1985.
2. Analgesic abuse and the kidney, Kidney Int 17:250-260, 1980.
3. *Autry D, Lauzon F, and Holliday P: The voiding record, an aid to decreasing incontinence, Geriatr Nurs 5(1):22-25, 1984.
4. *Beber CR: Freedom for the incontinent, Am J Nurs 80:482-484, 1980.
5. Bennett WM: Consultation in nephrology, St Louis, 1989, The CV Mosby Co.
6. Black DAK: Renal disease, ed 4, Oxford, England, 1979, Blackwell Scientific Publications Ltd.
7. Brink CA et al: A digital test for pelvic muscle strength in older women with urinary incontinence, Nurs Res 38:196-199, 1989.
8. Brundage D: Nursing management of renal problems, ed 2, St Louis, 1980, The CV Mosby Co.
9. *Cain L and Bigongiari LF: The percutaneous nephrostomy tube, Am J Nurs 82:296-298, 1982.
10. Campbell M and Harrison J, editors: Urology, ed 5, Philadelphia, 1985, WB Saunders Co.
11. Cass AS: Immediate radiologic and surgical management of renal injuries, J Trauma 22:361-363, 1982.
12. *Chambers J: Save your diabetic patient from early kidney damage, Nursing '85 15(5):58-63, 1985.
13. *Chambers JK: Fluid and electrolyte problems in renal and urologic disorders, Nurs Clin North Am 22:815-816, 1987.
14. *Conti MT and Eutropius L: Preventing UTIs: what works? Am J Nurs 87:307-309, 1987.
15. *Doyle JE: Treating renovascular hypertension: bypass graft surgery, Am J Nurs 82:1559-1561, 1982.
16. *Folk-Lighty M: Solving the puzzles of patients' fluid imbalances, Nursing '84 14(2):34-41, 1984.
17. *Fowler JE and Crowley JL: Stress incontinence: endoscopic suspension of the vesical neck, AORN J 45:922-933, 1987.
18. Gibbs T: Nurse review: genitourinary problems, Springhouse, Penn, 1986, Springhouse Corp.
19. *Glass LF and Jenkins CA: The ups and downs of serum pH, Nursing '83 13(9):34-41, 1983.
20. *Harwood C: Pulverizing kidney stones: what you should know about lithotripsy, RN 48(7):32-37, 1985.
21. Herman JR: Handbook of urology, Philadelphia, 1983, JB Lippincott Co.
22. Janusek LW: Metabolic acidosis: physiology, signs and symptoms, Nursing '84 14(7):44-45, 1984.
23. *Kidd P: Ruptured bladder, Nursing '89 19(1):33, 1989.

*References preceded by an asterisk are particularly well suited for student reading.

24. *Killion A: Reducing the risk of infection from indwelling urethral catheters, Nursing '82 12(5):84-88, 1982.

25. Kunin C: Detection, prevention and management of urinary tract infections, ed 4, Philadelphia, 1987, Lea & Febiger.

26. Lancaster L: The patient with end stage renal disease, ed 2, New York, 1984, John Wiley & Sons Inc.

27. Lanners J and Bush I: Urology handbook for nurses and urology technicians, St Louis, 1988, Green Publishing.

28. Licina MG, Adler S, and Burns FJ: Acute renal failure in a patient with polycystic kidney disease, JAMA 245:1664-1665, 1981.

29. Lu L: Incontinence stress index: measuring psychological impact, J Gerontol Nurs 3(7):18-25, 1987.

30. *McCormick KA, Scheve AA, and Leaky E: Nursing management of urinary incontinence in geriatric inpatients, Nurs Clin North Am 23:231-264, 1988.

31. McLane AM: Classification of nursing diagnoses: Proceedings of the 7th conference (NANDA), St Louis, 1987, The CV Mosby Co.

32. *Metheny N: Renal stones and urinary pH, AM J Nurs 82:1372-1375, 1982.

33. *Moriarty MB: The NIH puts the spotlight on incontinence, RN 52(3):44-45, 1989.

34. *Newman D and Smith D: Incontinence: the problem patients won't talk about, RN 52(3):42-43, 1989.

35. *Orr ML: Drugs and renal disease, Am J Nurs 81:969-971, 1981.

36. Papper S: Clinical nephrology, ed 2, Boston, 1981, Little, Brown & Co Inc.

37. *Palmer MH: Incontinence: the magnitude of the problem, Nurs Clin North Am 23:139-158, 1988.

38. Percutaneous lithotripsy for renal calculi, Am J Nurs 85:772-773, 1985.

39. *Ruge CA: Shock (wave) treatment for kidney stones, Am J Nurs 86:400-401, 1986.

40. Prevention and treatment of kidney stones (Kidney Stone Consensus Conference), JAMA 260:977-981, 1988.

41. Schroeder, SA, et al: Current medical diagnosis and treatment, Norwalk, Conn, 1989, Appleton & Lange.

42. *Smith DAJ: Continence restoration in the homebound patient, Nurs Clin North Am 23:207-218, 1988.

43. Smith DR: General urology, ed 12, Norwalk, Conn, 1988, Appleton & Lange.

44. Taylor D: Renal hypertension; physiology, signs, and symptoms, Nursing '83 13(10):44-45, 1983.

45. Tower M: Urinary obstruction: the hidden threats in treatment, RN 45(5):58-63, 1982.

46. Way LW: Current surgical diagnosis and treatment, Norwalk, CT, 1988, Appleton & Lange.

47. Williams SR: Nutrition and diet therapy, ed 6, St Louis, 1989, The CV Mosby Co.

48. Wyngaarden JB and Smith LH: Cecil textbook of medicine, ed 18, Philadelphia, 1988, WB Saunders Co.

CHAPTER 49

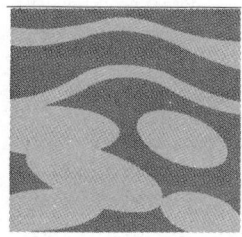

Common Interventions for Urinary Problems

H. FRED FARLEY, JR.
REBECCA ANNE ROBERTS

CHAPTER OBJECTIVES

After studying this chapter, the student should be able to:
1 Describe etiology and management of urinary retention.
2 Describe management of persons requiring assisted urinary drainage.
3 Identify measures to prevent fluid imbalances in persons with urinary problems.
4 Describe general guidelines for the care of patients after urologic surgery.
5 Define four types of urinary diversion procedures and the purpose of each type.
6 Describe nursing management for urinary stomas.

This chapter includes some common problems experienced by persons who have urinary disorders. Topics discussed in this chapter include the following:
1. Urinary retention
2. Assisted urinary drainage
3. Fluid imbalances in persons with urinary problems
4. Urologic surgery, including general preoperative and postoperative care and care of patients with urinary diversions

URINARY RETENTION

Urinary retention is the inability to empty the bladder. The kidney is producing sufficient urine, but the person is unable to expel the urine from the bladder.

CAUSES OF URINARY RETENTION

Causes of urinary retention may be categorized as mechanical or functional. Mechanical causes may be congenital or acquired and include anatomic blockage of urine flow in the lower urinary tract. Functional causes include impairment of urine flow in absence of mechanical obstruction. Causes of urinary retention are summarized in Table 49-1.

■ ASSESSMENT

Persons experiencing urinary retention may be unable to void any urine (retention) or may void small amounts of overflow urine but be unable to empty the bladder (retention with overflow). Urine remaining in the bladder is a good medium for bacteria to flourish leading to urinary tract infection (UTI).

SUBJECTIVE DATA

Subjective data to obtain from the person with urinary retention include the following:
1. Voiding pattern
2. Pain or burning on urination (probable UTI)
3. Sense of need to void or bladder fullness immediately after voiding (retention with overflow)

TABLE 49-1 Causes of urinary retention

Type of Retention	Cause
Mechanical causes	
Congenital	Urethral stricture
	Urinary tract malformation
	Spinal cord malformation
Acquired	Calculus
	Inflammation
	Trauma
	Tumor
	Hyperplasia
	Pregnancy
Functional causes	Neurogenic bladder dysfunction
	Ureterovesical reflux
	Decreased peristaltic activity of the ureter
	Detrusor muscle atrophy
	Anxiety, i.e., fear of pain after surgery
	Medications, i.e., anesthetics, narcotics, sedatives, and antihistamines

OBJECTIVE DATA

The following objective data should be collected:

1. Frequency of voiding (voiding frequently in small amounts is suggestive of UTI or retention with overflow)
2. Volume of each void
3. Characteristics of urine (color, clarity)
4. Palpation of bladder above symphysis pubis after voiding (for urine remaining in the bladder)
5. Comparison of fluid intake versus output

■ DATA ANALYSIS: NURSING DIAGNOSES

Nursing diagnoses are determined from assessment of patient data. Possible nursing diagnoses for the person with urinary retention may include, but are not limited to, the following:

Diagnostic Title	Possible Etiologies
Dysreflexia	Distended bladder
Knowledge deficit	Lack of exposure/recall, cognitive limitations
Urinary retention	Obstruction, position for voiding, immobility, inability to initiate stream

■ PLANNING: EXPECTED PATIENT OUTCOMES

Expected patient outcomes for the person with urinary retention may include, but are not limited to, the following:

1. Patient can state need to maintain fluid intake of 1500 to 2400 ml/day unless otherwise restricted.
2. Patient will void several times a day in volumes of 150 ml to 400 ml/void.
3. Bladder is not palpable after voiding.
4. Patient can describe signs and symptoms of urinary tract infection (UTI).

INTERVENTIONS
MEDICAL MANAGEMENT

Urinary retention is a urologic emergency and, if untreated, can lead to kidney damage. Interventions for urinary retention are aimed at reestablishment of urine flow. Some mechanical obstructions must be corrected by surgical intervention; others, such as that caused by an enlarged prostate, may require temporary urethral catheter drainage. Bethanechol chloride (Urecholine) may be prescribed to initiate voiding by stimulation of the detrusor muscle of the bladder. Intermittent catheterization may be used for long-term problems rather than maintaining an indwelling catheter.

NURSING MANAGEMENT

If the patient is having difficulty eliminating urine from the bladder in the absence of mechanical obstruction, measures that encourage voiding are attempted before catheterization is instituted. These measures may include ensuring a position that facilitates voiding (posi-

---

PATIENT TEACHING FOR RECURRENT URINARY RETENTION

1. Monitor for signs of retention or UTI
   a. Discomfort and distention over symphysis pubis
   b. Urinary output markedly less than fluid intake
   c. Voiding of cloudy urine
   d. Signs of UTI (burning on urination, frequency with urgency, fever)
2. Prevention of UTI
   a. Maintain adequate fluid intake (1500 to 2400 ml/day)
   b. Report early signs of UTI to physician

---

tional stimuli—male standing upright, female sitting upright), running water (auditory stimuli), or pouring water over the perineum or placing the patient's hands in water (tactile stimuli). Sitting in lukewarm water may help relax the urinary sphincters. Providing privacy and encouraging use of the bathroom whenever possible also help to promote voiding.

Urinary stasis in the bladder provides a medium for bacterial growth. The person with recurrent urinary retention needs to know how to monitor for and prevent urinary tract infection (UTI) (see the box above).

ASSISTED URINARY DRAINAGE
CATHETER USE

Assisted urinary drainage is used in a variety of clinical situations in both acute and chronic care. Following are major reasons for catheter drainage of some part of the urinary system:

1. Relieve temporary anatomic or physiologic obstruction
2. Permit healing of various parts of the urinary system postoperatively
3. Permit accurate measurement of urinary output in severely ill patients
4. Relieve inability to void
5. Achieve continence
6. Prevent retention of urine in certain persons with neurogenic bladder dysfunction
7. Permit irrigation to prevent obstruction of urine flow

Reestablishment of the flow of urine is an immediate treatment goal. The type of catheter used to provide drainage in the presence of obstruction will depend on the location of the blockage. The use of specific types of catheters is summarized in Table 49-2.

Catheters are used in urinary tract surgery to facilitate healing of some portion of the urinary tract by diverting urine from above the operative site or by "splinting" a narrow portion of the tract to prevent stricture

TABLE 49-2 Types of catheters

Type of Catheter	Description	Use
Whistle-tip	Open slant end	Hematuria or blood clots in urine
Robinson	Close end, many "eyes"	Intermittent catheterization
Foley	Balloon (5 or 30 ml) to secure catheter in bladder	Constant drainage
Coudé	Tapered curved end	Suspected prostatic hypertrophy
Ureteral	4 to 6 Fr size (urethral catheters are usually 14 to 16 Fr)	Drain ureters
Malecot	"Batwing" shaped-tip	Drain renal pelvis, nephrostomy drainage
Pezzar	Mushroom-shaped tip	Drain renal pelvis, nephrostomy drainage

until healing occurs. In critical care settings where hourly fluid balance assessments are necessary, urethral catheter drainage may be used until the patient's condition has stabilized.

Temporary inability to void may accompany spinal cord injury. After the use of general anesthetics, patients may also experience temporary urinary retention and may require intermittent urethral catheterization until the usual voiding pattern is resumed. Persons who have undergone urogenital surgery and some women following childbirth may have urinary retention secondary to edema of tissues surrounding the urethra.

In certain circumstances, urethral catheterization may be used to control urinary incontinence. Incontinence itself is not adequate reason for continuous catheter drainage unless urine retention is present or the integrity of the skin is threatened despite all possible nursing measures to manage the incontinence. Generally, the dangers of catheterization (infection) outweigh the advantages. Intermittent catheterization, however, is used as a means of continence for certain persons with neurogenic bladder dysfunction associated with birth defects, chronic illness, and spinal cord trauma. Not only can it offer continence to these persons, but it also can decrease urinary tract infections in persons who otherwise retain large amounts of residual urine in the bladder.

The techniques of urethral catheterization and bladder irrigation are described in fundamentals of nursing texts. Complete emptying of the bladder may be accomplished in most instances without side effects (see research box). Bladder irrigation is generally performed

RESEARCH

Bristoll SL et al: The mythical danger of rapid urinary drainage, Am J Nurs 89:344-345, 1989.

The purpose of this study was to investigate the question of how complete urinary drainage and threshold clamping affect the blood pressure, pulse, and blood loss of patients catheterized for urinary retention. Adult patients that appeared likely to have more than 1000 ml of urine in their bladders were eligible for the study. Six patients were randomly assigned to each of two groups. Group I underwent complete bladder drainage, and group II underwent threshold clamping. Blood pressures and pulse were obtained before, during, and 30 minutes after catheterization. The patients in group I experienced no unexpected changes in blood pressure or pulse after complete urinary drainage. Patients in group II experienced a rise in diastolic blood pressure and slight decreases in heart rate that were statistically but not clinically significant. No significant blood was found in the urine samples. It was concluded that complete drainage of a distended bladder is as safe as threshold clamping and likely to be more comfortable. ▪

when bleeding is present to prevent catheter obstruction by clots. Irrigation may be ordered intermittently or continuously. A three-way irrigation system is used for continuous irrigation.

DRAINAGE OF THE KIDNEY, PELVIS, AND URETERS

If a ureter becomes obstructed, a catheter must be placed directly into the renal pelvis. This prevents renal damage that otherwise would occur as pressure in the kidney increases because of continued urine formation. When there is complete obstruction of a ureter, a *nephrostomy* or *pyelostomy* tube may be inserted surgically into the renal pelvis (Figure 49-1). The surgical incision is located laterally and posteriorly in the kidney region. Catheters used as nephrostomy or pyelostomy tubes are usually of the Pezzar (mushroom) or Malecot (batwing) types. An alternate form of drainage for a ureteral obstruction is the surgical placement of a ureterostomy tube (a whistle-tip or many-eyed Robinson catheter, size 6 or 8 Fr) that is passed through an incision in the upper outer quadrant of the abdomen into the ureter above the obstruction. The catheter is then passed through the ureter to the renal pelvis.

If the ureter is unobstructed or partially obstructed, the renal pelvis may be drained by a ureteral catheter, which is passed up the ureter to the renal pelvis by means of a cystoscope (see Figure 47-6). Ureteral catheterization is performed before gynecologic and lower abdominal surgery when there is danger of not recognizing and accidentally injuring the ureter during the operation. Ureteral catheterization is also used after sur-

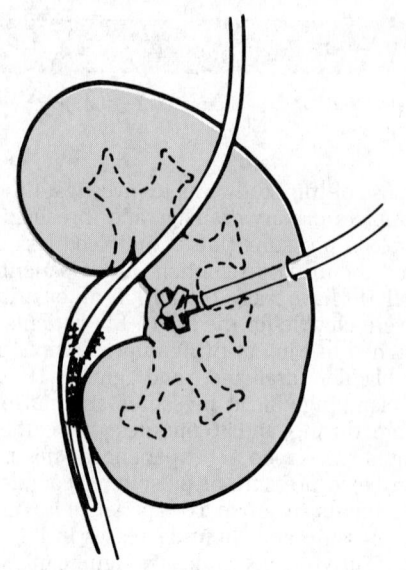

FIGURE 49-1 Placement of splinting catheter after repair of ureteropelvic stricture. Note use of nephrostomy tube for urinary drainage during healing of anastomosis.

gery involving the ureters in order to prevent stricture as the ureter heals. When used for this purpose, the catheter is referred to as a *splinting catheter* (Figure 49-1). Whether it is expected to drain urine will depend on its relation to other catheters used.

Adequate anchorage of *nephrostomy* and *ureteral* catheters must be provided to prevent accidental dislodgment and trauma to the tissues in which they lie. The openings made for these tubes are essentially fistulas that rapidly decrease in size on removal of the catheter. Even 30 minutes after removal of this type of catheter it is often impossible to reinsert a similar-sized tube. When a catheter is inserted during surgery, it is usually sutured in place. In this case, additional anchorage consists of affixing the tube to the skin with adhesive tape after the skin has been cleansed. When the tube is not sutured in place, it should be anchored to the skin at *two points* using adhesive—with some slack in the tubing between the anchor points.

Free drainage of catheters leading to the renal pelvis is of the utmost importance. Since the normal renal pelvis has only a 5 to 8 ml capacity, great pressure can be exerted on renal structures even when these catheters are obstructed for only a few minutes. Care must be taken to prevent kinking of the tubes while the patient is in the side-lying position in bed.

In some cases nephrostomy tubes may be left in place for several months, with the patient returning to the hospital later for their removal. Occasionally, the nephrostomy tube serves a form of urinary diversion for long-term use. The person at home with a catheter draining the kidney pelvis must know how to obtain medical assistance quickly should the catheter obstruct or become dislodged.

DRAINAGE OF THE BLADDER
CYSTOSTOMY TUBE

When obstruction occurs below the bladder, constant drainage must be provided to prevent renal damage, which may occur because of inadequate emptying of the lower urinary system. One means of providing drainage is by the use of a *cystostomy* tube (usually a Foley, Malecot, or Pezzar catheter), which is placed directly into the bladder through a suprapubic incision. This method is usually used when the urethra is completely obstructed or when the prolonged use of a urethral catheter is to be avoided in a male patient. During some operative procedures both a cystostomy tube and a small urethral catheter will be inserted to drain the bladder. Both catheters must be monitored for patency. If patency is assured, it is not necessary to record the output from each catheter separately, since both tubes drain the bladder. The catheters will not necessarily drain equal amounts of urine. As is true with nephrostomy and ureteral catheters, secure anchorage of these catheters is also necessary.

URETHRAL CATHETER

Urethral catheterization is the most common means of draining the bladder, and insertion of this type of catheter is a nursing responsibility in many settings. The Foley catheter is most frequently used for this purpose.

Catheterization is a major cause of urinary tract infections, and strict asepsis should be practiced by anyone carrying out this procedure or assembling the drainage equipment. The need for urethral catheterization must be carefully evaluated; use of urethral catheter drainage only for nursing convenience is not appropriate.

If the nurse finds it difficult to pass the catheter, the procedure is discontinued and the physician notified. Traumatic catheterization predisposes to urinary tract infection and formation of urethral strictures. In patients who have urethral disorders, resistance may be encountered with a standard catheter; special equipment such as catheter directors, filiform catheters, or sounds may be needed. The introduction of such equipment into the urinary tract is not a nursing procedure; neither is catheterization of a patient in the immediate postoperative period after surgery of the urethra or bladder.

The urethral catheter is anchored securely, not only for patient comfort, but also to prevent complications (Figure 49-2). For the female the catheter is taped to the inner thigh, allowing sufficient slack to prevent tension at the bladder neck. For the male the catheter

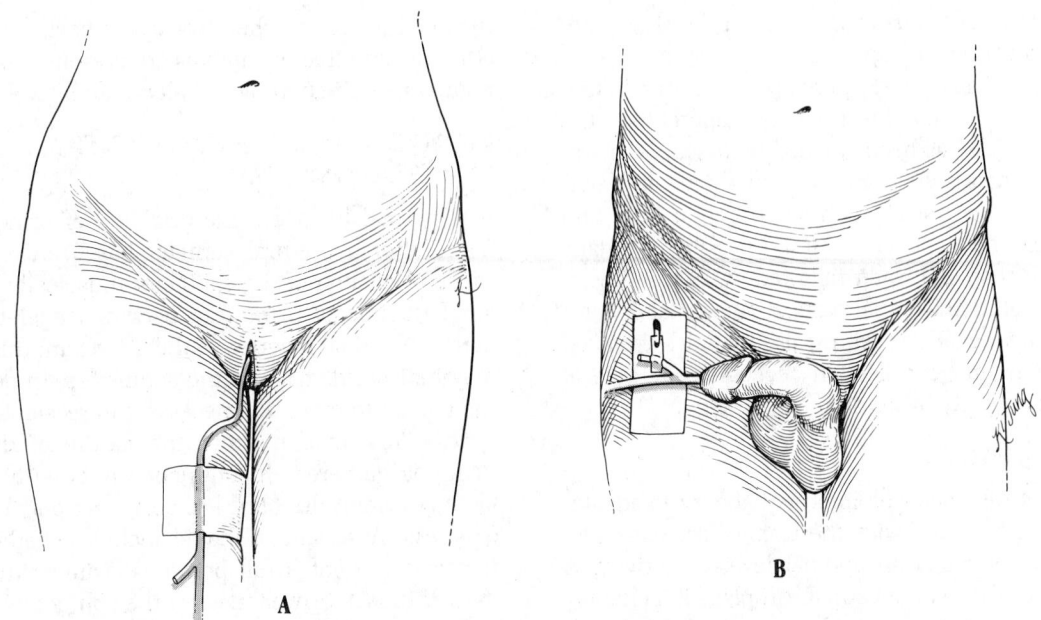

FIGURE 49-2 Anchoring of Foley catheter. **A,** In female patient. **B,** In male patient. Proper anchoring prevents accidental traction that could result in injury to bladder or urethra while at the same time keping catheter from moving in and out of urethra.

should be taped to upper thigh or lower abdomen. This avoids pressure and friction that can lead to necrosis of tissue and the formation of urethral ulceration and fistulas. In all patients the catheter should be securely anchored so that it does not move in and out of the urethra and track bacteria into the urethra.

The urethral catheter is changed when it is in danger of becoming obstructed by encrustations within its lumen. The person who will have an indwelling urethral catheter at home will need to learn to change the catheter or to have someone else do this.

HOME CARE FOR THE PERSON WITH URINARY CATHETER DRAINAGE

The person who requires catheter drainage at home on a temporary or permanent basis must be able to safely maintain the urinary drainage system. If the person is incapable of this because of physical or mental status, another person must be instructed in all necessary care. Written instructions are provided to supplement and reinforce the information. The services of a community health nurse may be indicated. The following areas must be included in home-going preparation of any person with indwelling catheter drainage: maintaining catheter patency, preventing urinary tract infection, maintaining activity, dealing with catheter problems, obtaining supplies, and continuing with urologic surveillance.

MAINTAINING PATENCY OF CATHETER

The person (or care provider) must know how to check for kinks in the tubing and should be aware of the most appropriate way to secure the catheter to prevent kinking. An adequate fluid intake of 2 to 3 L of fluid per day should be encouraged unless contraindicated by the person's condition. Persons who will be irrigating their own catheters at home should practice under supervision several times before discharge.

PREVENTING URINARY TRACT INFECTION

The person (or care provider) must be helped to understand the importance of cleanliness as a means of preventing complications. Instruction includes the necessity of good hand washing before and after working with the catheter. Instruction also includes cleansing the meatal-catheter junction with soap and water twice daily. The person should be reassured that cleansing the meatal-catheter junction will not dislodge or pull out the catheter. Ideally, frequent disconnection of the catheter and drainage tubing should be avoided. However, the person at home must disconnect the tubing at night to change from a leg bag to the overnight drainage bag and again in the morning to resume leg-bag drainage. To lessen the risk of contamination, the person is taught to wash the hands and then wipe the catheter and tubing with 70% alcohol before disconnection and reconnection. The disconnected ends of the drainage bags are protected with sterile gauze secured in place with a rubber band or a connector cap.

If equipment must be sterilized at home, instruction is given in how to do this properly. Before use, the equipment, which has been washed with soap and water, is boiled for a full 10 minutes in a pan of water. Other parts of the system such as collection bags and tubing should be kept as clean as possible by daily washing with soap and water followed by 15 minutes of soaking in a solution of equal parts of vinegar and water (half-strength vinegar). Teaching also includes the need to keep the drainage collection receptacle at a level lower than the cavity being drained.

PROMOTING ACTIVITY

The person needs to be well informed about the adaptations that can be made with the urinary drainage system to allow return to an optimal level of activity. A shower or tub bath with a catheter in place is generally permitted unless there is an unhealed surgical incision. The adhesive tape holding the catheter in place will need to be replaced after bathing. Leg bags are available in a variety of sizes and are concealed by clothing. There is no need for men or women to remove an indwelling catheter before intercourse—a question persons may be hesitant to ask. The male can fold the indwelling catheter over the penis to facilitate insertion during intercourse. Questions pertaining to resumption of usual lifestyle activities should be encouraged so that the person can be as well prepared as possible for self-care at home.

DEALING WITH CATHETER PROBLEMS

The patient (or care provider) is informed about how to handle problems such as obstruction of the catheter or displacement of the catheter. The person needs to know whether to contact the physician or to seek help through a clinic or emergency room. The amount of time that can safely elapse before obtaining help will depend on the type of catheter and its location.

OBTAINING SUPPLIES

At discharge the patient should be provided with adequate supplies for at least a few days. A list of names, addresses, and phone numbers of where additional supplies may be obtained and what resources are available to assist with payment if necessary should be given to the person before discharge. A written list of the specific supplies needed should be provided to aid the person, who is likely to be confused by the many products available.

PROVIDING ONGOING CARE

The person with a urinary catheter of any type will need continued urologic surveillance. Instruction includes the need to contact the physician if back pain, fever, or other urinary tract symptoms are present and to plan for regular examination by the physician as well.

INTERVENTION FOR PATIENT AFTER CATHETER REMOVAL

It is normal to note some dribbling of urine for a few hours after a urethral catheter has been removed because of dilation of the sphincter muscles by the catheter. Dribbling of urine that persists longer than a few hours should be reported to the physician; this symptom may indicate damage to the sphincters. In determining the type of intervention necessary to reestablish bladder control, information about the nature of the incontinency is gathered. Incontinence is described as complete (constant dribbling) or occurring only on urgency or stress. Assessment should include whether incontinence is present in all positions (lying, sitting, standing). If muscular weakness of the sphincters is the major problem, incontinence is least likely to occur when the person is in a prone position and most likely to be a problem when standing or walking. Perineal exercises (see Chapter 48) may help to regain control of voiding.

Another problem that may arise after removal of a catheter is inability to void. The patient is encouraged to drink fluids and then attempt to void. The nurse carefully assesses the patient's bladder for distention. Efforts are made to provide comfortable positioning and privacy to facilitate voiding. No patient with an adequate intake should go longer than 8 hours without voiding. It is not uncommon for a patient with edema of the bladder neck to require temporary reinsertion of a catheter to facilitate urinary output. The nurse's responsibility is to determine and record accurately all spontaneous voidings of the patient until adequacy of output has been well established.

Color and clarity of the urine are noted. *Cystitis* (inflammation of the bladder) may develop after catheter removal because of incomplete emptying of the bladder as muscle tone is being reestablished. Any abnormalities in color, odor, or sediment in the urine are reported.

Educating the patient about signs and symptoms of urinary retention, changes in the color and clarity of the urine, and incontinence and dysuria is undertaken when bladder drainage is discontinued. Often the first indicators of dysfunction are subjective judgments offered by the patient. This information enhances detection of early recurrence of urinary drainage problems.

INTERMITTENT CATHETER DRAINAGE
USE

Intermittent catheterization of the urinary bladder is being used with increasing frequency in the treatment of neurogenic bladder dysfunction secondary to spinal

RESEARCH

Williamson ML: Reducing postcatheterization bladder dysfunction by reconditioning, Nurs Res 31(1):28-30, 1982.

The purpose of this study was to determine the effect of reconditioning before catheter removal on bladder dysfunction following prolonged catheterization. Subjects were eight women with catheterization intervals of 36 to 106 hours. The four experimental subjects received a reconditioning program consisting of four episodes of 3-hour catheter clamping followed by 5 minutes of drainage before catheters were removed. The four control subjects did not receive any catheter clamping before removal. After catheter removal the reconditioned subjects resumed natural micturition significantly sooner than the control group. There was no significant difference in residual urine volumes (RUV) between the two groups, but the mean RUV of the reconditioned group stayed within normal limits (less than 25 ml), whereas the mean RUV of the control group increased to 42 ml. ∎

cord trauma, birth defects, urinary retention, and some chronic diseases. Because periodic complete emptying of the bladder eliminates residual urine (an excellent culture medium for multiplication of bacteria) and maintains a good blood supply to the bladder wall by avoiding high intrabladder pressures, infections are often decreased, even when only a clean technique is used.

The hospitalized patient with intermittent catheter drainage of the bladder may be one for whom the treatment is temporary (as in the early phases of spinal cord trauma), one who is learning the technique for home use, or one who has been using intermittent catheterization before admission.

ASSESSMENT

Individuals are evaluated for their appropriateness for this form of management by the urologist. Potential for success with this form of therapy should be further evaluated, using input from the nurse, psychologist, social worker, and other involved health care professionals. Teaching, however, is generally a nursing responsibility in either an inpatient or outpatient setting. Before a teaching plan can be made, the nurse must know whether a clean or sterile technique is to be taught and the frequency with which it is to be used. Knowledge of the person's physical, mental, and emotional status as well as usual lifestyle must also be used in planning a program suitable for each person.

The goals of intermittent catheterization may vary from patient to patient but are generally to prevent urinary retention and its sequelae (urinary tract infection

and renal damage) and to achieve continence. The patient should know exactly what is expected of the treatment plan in order to elicit full cooperation.

INTERVENTIONS

Method

Even though the clean technique is suitable for home use, sterile technique is necessary during hospitalization to decrease the possibility of hospital-acquired infection when the catheterization is performed by hospital personnel. When hospitalized, the patient who customarily performs self-catheterization may continue to use clean technique if this method is used at home, but preferably a sterile catheter will be used each time or special precautions are taken to store the reusable catheter in a closed container. Specimens for culture must be obtained by the usual sterile catheterization technique to avoid contamination of the specimen. The patient is informed about the reasons why sterile precautions are necessary in the hospital setting.

In the hospital, the size 14 Fr Robinson catheter is generally used for an adult. A special silicone catheter is used for intermittent catheterization. The volume of urine obtained with each catheterization is recorded to assure that schedule adjustments can be made if necessary. The adult bladder should not be permitted to hold more than 300 ml at any time, since greater amounts lead to overdistention of the bladder with greater susceptibility to infection. The frequency of catheterization is determined by the amount of residual urine. The person first attempts to void and then performs self-catheterization. A large amount of residual urine (more than 100 ml) means that more frequent catheterization is necessary. Usually such persons will need catheterization every 4 to 6 hours. A small amount of residual urine (less than 100 ml) after voiding means that the person will need to do self-catheterization only every 8 to 12 hours. Some persons eventually will be able to manage with once-a-day catheterization.[14] Some persons may also have a catheterize themselves at night if they have a large output of urine at night. The person who normally does not perform self-catheterization at night at home may need to do so when the fluid intake is greater than usual, as with intravenous fluid administration.

In some instances the physician will prescribe the frequency of catheterizations; in other instances, adjustment of the schedule may be a nursing judgment. If the nurse notes that excess volumes of urine are being obtained with a prescribed schedule, the physician is consulted about the need to alter the schedule.

Color, clarity, and odor of the urine are noted and any symptoms of urinary tract infection reported. Periodic urine specimens are obtained and sent for culture and sensitivity. Some individuals are given prophylactic long-term antibiotic therapy.

Patient Teaching

The person needs to understand the rationale for intermittent catheter drainage and for regularity of bladder emptying (see the box below). Basic anatomy of the genitalia and urinary tract is pointed out to aid the person's understanding where the catheter is inserted and to alleviate fears of causing damage by misplacement of the catheter.

Most persons require a great deal of support during the actual teaching but usually become comfortable with the procedure. Initially a mirror is used to teach women where to place the catheter. The woman should learn to catheterize while sitting on the commode, using palpation to locate the urethral meatus. Men may sit or stand to catheterize themselves. It is important that they use generous amounts of lubricant to avoid urethral irritation; women generally do not require lubrication of the catheter.

If the patient is unable to perform self-catheterization because of age or physical limitations, a care provider may be instructed in the technique. The person or care provider must know how to care for the catheters and where additional catheters may be obtained.

Home Care

In most cases, clean (not sterile) catheterization technique is prescribed for home use. Hand washing is advised before each catheterization, and the meatal area is cleansed with soap and water. After inserting the catheter and draining the bladder, the catheter is removed and washed with soap and water before being stored in a clean, closed container for the next use. The catheter is reused until it becomes either too soft or too hard to be directed properly.

If sterile catheterization technique is needed for home use, more time and practice will be required to learn good sterile technique. Careful explanation of sterilization of equipment must be provided, and planning for adapting sterile intermittent self-catheterization to the individual's usual lifestyle must be worked out with the person.

If teaching of self-catheterization is performed on an outpatient basis or if hospitalization is short, follow-up for adjustment of schedule and other concerns of adaptation to home routine should be provided. This may be done by the primary nurse, by the physician, or by referral to a visiting nurse. Ongoing urologic care is essential with periodic urine cultures.

PREVENTING FLUID IMBALANCE IN PERSONS WITH URINARY PROBLEMS

Management of fluid balance is a fundamental and common problem for persons requiring urologic procedures and nephrology care. Maintaining normal fluid balance helps to (1) preserve renal function in individuals having ongoing kidney insufficiency or failure, (2) prevent the development of acute renal failure caused by fluid depletion, (3) prevent inadequate tissue perfusion and shock from depletion of blood volume, (4) provide continuous urine formation to help alleviate stasis of urine and bacterial growth, and (5) prevent fluid overload, which would increase the work of the heart and lead to peripheral and cerebral edema. The potential for altered states of fluid balance in patients with urologic and renal problems commonly involves both abnormal losses and gains of fluid. Prevention of fluid imbalances in persons with urinary problems includes the following: (1) identification of persons at risk for fluid imbalances, (2) monitoring persons at high risk, and (3) teaching the patient management of fluid balance.

IDENTIFICATION OF PERSONS AT RISK

Individuals predisposed to developing *fluid overload* include (1) those with acute renal failure in which kidney shutdown and oliguria are the rule; (2) those with bilateral obstructive disease attributed to strictures, tumors, or calculi who present with anuria or severely decreased urinary output; and (3) those with chronic renal failure characterized by limited and fixed ability to excrete fluid through the kidneys. The common defect in the above situations is an inability to excrete more than a low and fixed volume of urine per day, regardless of fluid intake.

Individuals susceptible to *fluid depletion* or *dehydration* include (1) those recovering from acute renal failure and in a phase of the illness in which the kidneys do not appropriately conserve body fluid (diuretic phase); (2) those with chronic renal failure whose urinary output per day is fixed at a high volume (2000 ml/day or

---

TEACHING THE PATIENT WITH INTERMITTENT CATHETERIZATION

The patient or significant others can:
1. Explain the reason for the intermittent catheter drainage.
2. State the need for regular, periodic, complete emptying of the bladder.
3. Demonstrate self-catheterization using clean technique unless sterile technique is prescribed.
4. Describe how to adapt the catheterization routine to the individual lifestyle.
5. State how to obtain needed supplies.
6. Describe symptoms of urinary tract infection requiring medical care.
7. State plans for ongoing urologic care.

greater) and who are unable to obtain or retain fluids sufficient to replace those lost through the kidneys; and (3) persons on diuretic therapy whose oral intake does not keep up with renal and other body fluid losses. The kidneys of these persons are unable to conserve fluid when intake is low or when extrarenal losses are high. Such situations occur, for example, when there is vomiting or diarrhea over prolonged periods, when fluids are restricted for several diagnostic tests in succession, when there is sudden sodium restriction or loss that decreases thirst, or when individuals become weak and unable to replace fluid losses on their own.

In addition, certain urologic situations make it very difficult to measure fluid output accurately. These include copious wound drainage or continuous bladder irrigation after urologic surgery, ill-fitting urinary appliances, and incontinence.

MONITORING PERSONS AT RISK

A second consideration in preventing fluid imbalances involves collecting appropriate baseline data and continuing to monitor the patient who is at risk for developing fluid problems. Such data will assist both in diagnosing imbalances and in the ongoing management of these problems. For example, when the diagnosis is chronic renal failure, the nurse should obtain information about the ability to excrete fluid.

Data to identify possible fluid imbalances include the following:

1. Subjective data: weight gain, nausea, changes in mental status and voiding patterns
2. Objective data: intake and output, daily weights, condition of mucous membranes, skin turgor, neck vein distention, lung sounds, presence of edema, urine specific gravity

PATIENT TEACHING

Prevention of fluid imbalances is also achieved through efforts to educate individuals about potential problems they may have in handling fluids. Persons with chronic renal failure (see Chapter 50) and those on diuretic therapy in particular will need to be given guidelines about current goals for fluid management, potential problems with fluid balance, signs and symptoms indicating a problem, and mechanisms for correcting fluid problems or in receiving assistance when they cannot manage the problems on their own.

UROLOGIC SURGERY

GENERAL INTERVENTIONS

Before discussing in detail particular types of surgery of the urinary tract, general principles of care of the patient requiring urologic surgery will be described.

PREOPERATIVE CARE

The focus of preoperative care is preparation of the patient for the impending surgery and implementation of the medical regimen. Much of the patient's concern depends on the type of surgery and diagnosis. Since the surgery will temporarily or permanently alter urinary elimination, the person will be concerned about the degree of change that will occur.

Preoperative instructions may include a discussion of the type and length of surgery; type of anesthesia; and the need for an intravenous line, catheter, or other drains. Instructions in coughing and deep breathing are crucial since ventilation is a frequent problem postoperatively. The patient is informed of the pain medication routine—whether or not it will be offered or if it must be requested. A description of methods of decreasing pain, such as by splinting the incision, should be offered. Persons having a urinary diversion require bowel preparation (p. 1454).

POSTOPERATIVE CARE

The basic needs of the patient requiring urologic surgery are the same as those of any other surgical patient. Special emphasis must be placed on promotion of ventilation and adequate urinary output, prevention of distention and hemorrhage, and attention to drainage tubes and dressings (see the box below).

Ventilation

Surgery of the kidney or upper ureters usually involves a flank incision that can influence respiratory status. Because the incision is directly below the diaphragm, deep breathing is painful and the patient is reluctant to take deep breaths or to move about. Splinting of the chest is common; therefore, atelectasis or other respiratory complications must be guarded against. In addition,

---

GUIDELINES FOR CARE AFTER UROLOGIC SURGERY

1. Promote ventilation
   a. Encourage breathing exercises
   b. Encourage self-turning in bed frequently
   c. Encourage ambulation
2. Monitor patency and output of urinary catheters
3. Prevent complications
   a. Change wet dressings to protect skin
   b. Restrict food and oral fluids if paralytic ileus is present
   c. Encourage fluids to 3000 ml/day when permitted
   d. Monitor for bright red blood on dressings or in urine
4. Administer analgesics to control pain

because of the placement of the incision there is a greater incisional pull every time the person moves, as compared with an abdominal incision. The patient is often reluctant to turn in bed or to get up to ambulate. Most patients will be more comfortable turning themselves if they are given time, side rails to hold onto, and encouragement. Incisional pain usually requires a narcotic every 3 to 4 hours for 24 to 48 hours after surgery. Turning, ambulation, and deep breathing exercises should be planned so that these activities occur at the time the analgesic has the greatest effect. Patients may lie on the affected side unless a nephrostomy tube is in place. Even then they can be tilted to the affected side with pillows placed at the back for support. The nephrostomy tube must not be kinked and must be free of traction.

Monitoring Urinary Output

The urinary output is monitored carefully for several days postoperatively to ascertain adequate renal functioning and drainage. The output should be at least 50 ml/hr, preferably greater in order to prevent urinary stasis and subsequent infection. A urinary output of 20 to 30 ml/hr in a patient with satisfactory fluid intake (at least 1200 ml/day) and in the absence of signs of urinary retention is reported immediately to the physician. Urinary output includes drainage from nephrostomy or cystostomy tubes, urethral or ureteral catheters, and an estimate from urine-soaked dressings. Daily weights are compared with the preoperative weight and with previous days to identify fluid retention.

Preventing Distention

After kidney surgery most patients have some abdominal distention that may result in part from pressure on the stomach and intestinal tract during surgery. Patients who have had renal colic before surgery frequently develop paralytic ileus postoperatively. This condition may be related to the reflex gastrointestinal tract symptoms caused by postoperative pain. Because of the problem of abdominal distention after renal surgery, food and fluids by mouth are often restricted for 24 to 48 hours postoperatively. By the fourth postoperative day, most patients tolerate a regular diet. Fluids are usually encouraged to 3000 ml/day.

Preventing Hemorrhage

Hemorrhage may follow such operative procedures as prostatectomy, nephrolithotomy, or partial nephrectomy. It occurs most often when the highly vascular parenchyma of the kidney has been incised. The bleeding may occur on the day of surgery, or it may occur 8 to 12 days postoperatively, during the period when tissue sloughing normally occurs with healing. The presence of bright red blood on the dressing or in the urine is re-

ported immediately to the physician. The patient is observed for signs of shock. Since many patients with urologic disease have hypertension, the blood pressure may be relatively high but still represent a marked drop for the individual. Therefore, comparisons should be made with baseline data.

If hemorrhage occurs, a pressure dressing is applied over the incision while awaiting the physician's arrival. Measures to prevent shock are instituted (see Chapter 25). Several liters of sterile physiologic saline solution for irrigation should be available.

Care of Dressings

There may be large amounts of urinary drainage following urologic surgery except after nephrectomy. The drainage may be pink or dark red but should not be bright red. If the surgery involves a flank incision, drainage is usually the heaviest on the posterior edge of the dressing because of gravity flow. It is important, therefore, to turn the patient on the side opposite the surgery to examine the posterior edge of the dressing. When a suprapubic incision is present, drainage is heaviest on the side and in the inguinal region.

The dressings are usually held in place by Montgomery straps and must be changed frequently. Urinary drainage irritates the skin, has an unpleasant odor, and leads to discomfort. If a drain is present, the end of the drain should be placed over dressings, then covered with additional dressings to absorb the drainage. If a drainage tube is present, the presence of large amounts of drainage on the dressing with little drainage coming from the tube indicates blockage of the tube. If a large amount of drainage is present, a disposable drainage bag used for urinary stomas (p. 1456) may be applied over the drainage site.

Care of Drainage Tubes

A catheter is usually inserted during surgery to drain urine from the operative area and permit healing to occur. Different types of drainage tubes may be inserted, and each tube is connected to a separate drainage system. It is important to know the purpose of the catheter and the area to be drained.

SPECIFIC TYPES OF UROLOGIC SURGERY
SURGERY OF THE KIDNEY

Removal of a kidney (*nephrectomy*) may be indicated for some congenital anomalies or for irreparable damage to kidney tissue from trauma or diseases such as renal hypertension, tumor, multiple cysts, or kidney stones. Adequate waste removal can be maintained by the remaining kidney or by even less than half of one functional kidney. In some instances only a portion of a diseased kidney is removed (*partial nephrectomy*). If an entire kidney is removed, a drain may be placed to remove serous fluid from the space previously occupied by the kidney. In this situation there will be no urinary drainage. Urinary drainage will occur with partial nephrectomy.

The kidney may also be incised for removal of calculi, either through the pelvis of the kidney (*pyelolithotomy*) (see Chapter 48) or through the parenchyma (*nephrolithotomy*). There is usually a large amount of urinary drainage after these surgeries.

A kidney may become loosened and "float" or become displaced (*nephroptosis*). If symptoms of obstruction occur, the kidney may be sutured to its anatomic site (*nephropexy*). Postoperatively, the patient is positioned with the hips elevated to prevent tension on the sutures.

SURGERY OF THE URETERS AND BLADDER

Removal of stones (*calculi*) blocking a ureter is termed *ureterolithotomy*. The root word "lith" refers to stones. Obstruction at the ureteropelvic junction is corrected by means of a *pyeloplasty* (plastic repair of the renal pelvis).

The bladder may be incised (*cystotomy*) for removal of calculi or as part of one method of prostate removal (suprapubic prostatectomy) (see Chapter 48). A *cystostomy* (note the "s" in the middle of the word) is an opening made in the bladder for drainage, usually by means of a tube.

Partial removal of the bladder (*segmental resection*) is usually performed for tumors of the bladder. Bladder capacity will be small initially with a capacity of no more than 60 ml immediately postoperatively, but the elastic tissue of the bladder will regenerate so that the patient is able to retain from 200 to 400 ml of urine within several months.

The decreased bladder size, however, is of major importance in the postoperative period. The patient will return from surgery with catheters draining the bladder both from a cystostomy opening and from the urethra. This is to avoid the possibility of obstruction of drainage, since it would take only a very short time for the bladder to become distended and there would be danger of disrupting the suture line on the bladder. Because bladder capacity is limited, the catheters usually cause severe bladder spasm. The urethral catheter is usually removed 3 weeks after surgery, but it may be left in place longer if the cystotomy wound is not well healed.

As soon as the urethral catheter is removed, the patient becomes acutely aware of the small capacity of the bladder. Most patients will need to void at least every 20 minutes, and they need to be reassured that the bladder capacity will gradually increase. Meanwhile they should be urged to force fluids to 3000 ml but should be advised to space the fluids so that time spent in the bathroom is not an inconvenience. They also should not take large quantities of fluids at one time, should limit fluids

for several hours before planning to go out, and should take no fluids after 6 PM.

If the entire bladder is removed (*cystectomy*), diversion of the urinary tract is necessary. Immediately after the cystectomy, the patient is usually acutely ill, since not only the bladder but also large amounts of surrounding tissue will be removed if the diagnosis is a malignant tumor. These patients frequently need hemodynamic monitoring in an intensive care unit for 24 to 48 hours after surgery. A long vertical abdominal incision is present, along with one or more pelvic drains. A nasogastric tube is inserted in the operating room, and the patient is given nothing by mouth until gastrointestinal function returns. The nursing care is similar to that given any patient after major abdominal surgery, plus the care and monitoring of the diverted urinary tract.

URINARY DIVERSION PROCEDURES
PURPOSE AND TYPES

Urinary diversion procedures are required to treat malignancies of the urinary tract, birth defects, neurogenic bladder dysfunction, chronic progressive pyelonephritis, and irreparable trauma to the urinary tract. The most frequent urinary diversion procedures are ureterostomy, ileal conduit, and colonic or sigmoid conduit, all of which result in external stomas and the need for ostomy pouches. The *continent urostomy* is a surgical alternative that has an external stoma, but internally has a reservoir made from intestine that holds the urine. The stoma must be catheterized at regular intervals to drain the reservoir. The *Kock continent ileal reservoir* (Figure 49-3) is formed from loops of the small intestine. Other variations, such as the *Indiana pouch*, consist of portions of large intestine and ileum (cecoileal) (Figure 49-4). New surgical advances being studied consist of internal reservoirs anastomosed to the urethra.

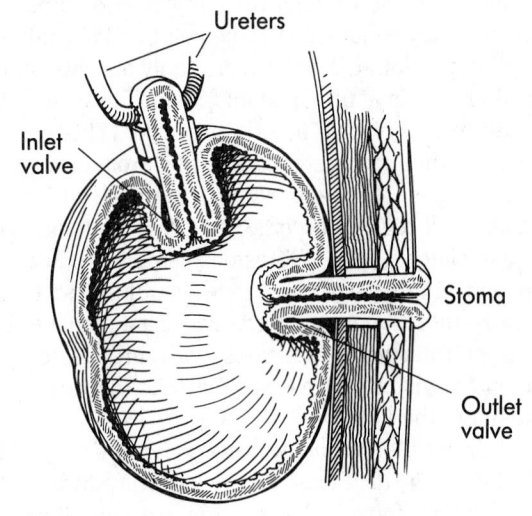

FIGURE 49-3 Kock continent ileal urinary reservoir.

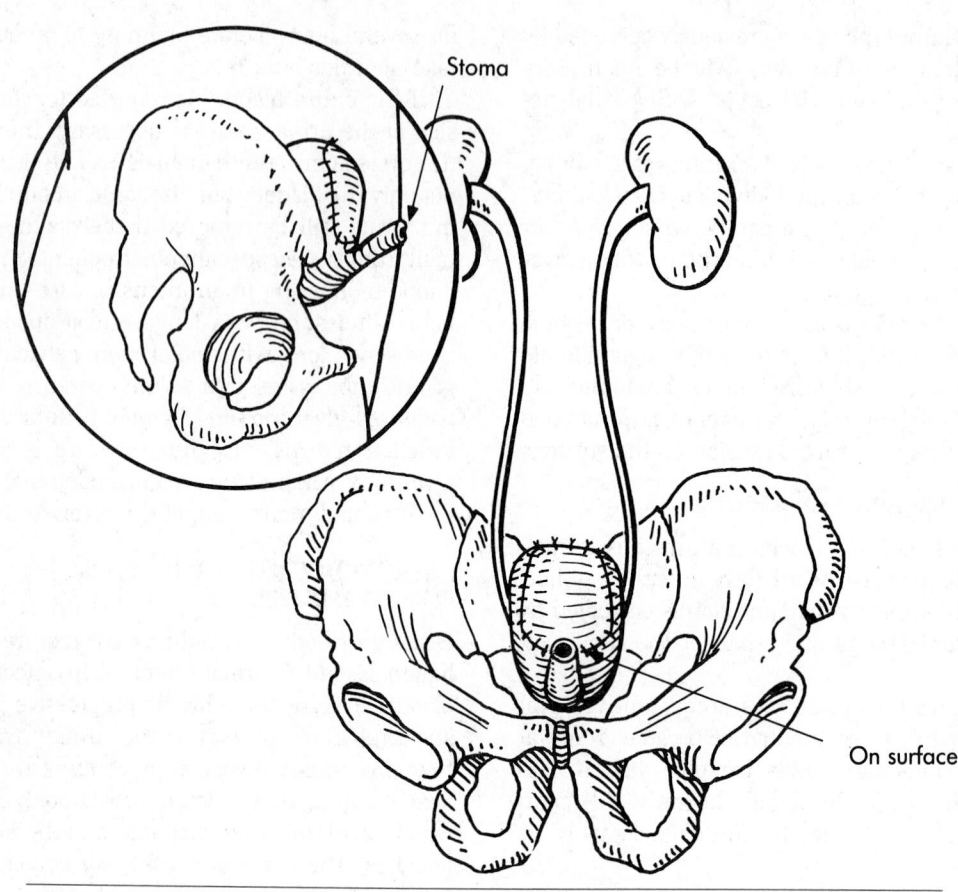

Stoma

On surface

FIGURE 49-4 Cecoileal continent urinary reservoir (Indiana pouch).

Cutaneous ureterostomy is used when the physical condition prohibits more extensive surgical procedures. One or both ureters are excised from the bladder and brought out through the skin, either on the flank or the anterior abdominal wall to create a small stoma. When both ureters are involved, each may be brought out to the skin surface separately, resulting in two stomas, or the ureters may be joined at some point and brought out through the abdominal wall to form only one stoma. Initially after surgery, ureterostomy stomas are pink, but they will turn very pale in several weeks. This surgery works best when the ureters are dilated from chronic reflux. Otherwise, the ureterostomy opening will be very small and will tend to become stenosed. The complications associated with ureterostomy stoma stenosis are inadequate drainage of the kidney resulting in hydronephrosis, infection, and progressive renal damage. Urinary tract infection in persons with ureterostomy is common because of the ease of reflux of the urine from the stoma to the kidney.

The *ureteroileocutaneous anastomosis* (also called an *ileal conduit, ileal loop,* or Bricker procedure) is the most common form of permanent urinary diversion. During the surgical procedure, the ureters are excised from the bladder and transplanted into one end of a 15 to 20 cm (6 or 8 inches) segment of ileum that has been resected from the intestinal tract with its mesentery, which contains the blood supply. The remaining intestinal segments are anastomosed, and gastrointestinal function is expected to return to its normal preoperative state after healing. The end of the resected ileum into which the ureters are connected is sutured closed and the other end is brought through the abdominal wall to the skin surface to create a stoma (Figure 49-5). The urinary bladder may be resected or left intact, depending on the reason for the diversion.

The ileal segment is intended to serve as a passageway for urinary flow rather than as a reservoir; therefore, in an ileal conduit urine flow is continuous. Electrolyte imbalance caused by reabsorption of waste products from the urine in the ileal segment is generally not a problem in a well-functioning ileal conduit.

The *colon conduit* (colonic loop) is basically performed like an ileal conduit except that a segment of colon (ascending, descending, transverse, or sigmoid colon) instead of ileum acts as the conduit for the urine. The colonic loop has reduced the incidence of urinary reflux for some persons. Preoperative and postoperative

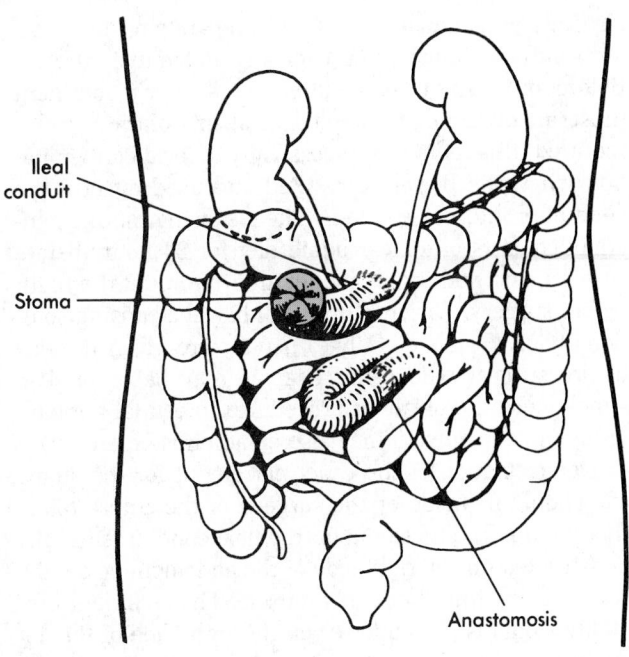

FIGURE 49-5 Ileal conduit or ileal loop.

nursing care and ongoing management are the same as those for ileal conduit surgery.

The *continent urostomy* (Kock pouch, Indiana pouch) consists of loops of intestine anastomosed together, separated from the rest of the intestine so that the gastrointestinal function occurs normally and then connected to the abdomen via the stomal segment. The ureters from the kidney are connected to the pouch above a valve. This valve prevents urine from refluxing to the kidney. The urine stays in the reservoir because a second valve is placed in the intestinal segment leading to the stoma. This valve prevents the leakage of urine, thus maintaining continence.[10] The end of the intestinal segment is brought out onto the skin surface, turned over on itself, and sutured to the skin to form the stoma. The stoma for the continent urostomy is usually flush to the skin and placed lower on the abdomen than the ileal conduit stoma.

The ileal conduit, colon conduit, and continent urostomy stomas should be a bright red color. Peristalsis of the stoma may be visualized when the pouch is removed. Early complications after surgery include breakdown of the anastomosis in the gastrointestinal tract, leakage from the ureteroileal or ureterosigmoid anastomosis, paralytic ileus, obstruction of the ureters, wound infection, mucocutaneous separation, and stomal necrosis. Complications that may occur after hospitalization include stomal problems (retraction, prolapse, hernia), urinary infections, crystal formation, and kidney stones.

Any procedure for diversion of urine that results in an external stoma leads to a significant change in the person's body image. Reactions may vary depending on the reason for the procedure, but virtually every person will require time and much nursing support while adapting to the altered means of urine elimination.

■ DATA ANALYSIS: NURSING DIAGNOSES

Nursing diagnoses are determined from assessment of patient data. Possible nursing diagnoses for the person with an urinary diversion may include, but are not limited to, the following:

Diagnostic Title	Possible Etiologies
Body image, disturbance	Loss of bladder, change in body appearance with the urinary stoma
Knowledge deficit	Lack of information about ileal or colon conduit, ureterostomy, or continent urostomy
Sexual dysfunction	Risk of impotence in male due to removal of bladder
Skin integrity, impaired potential	Potential for urine leakage, improper pouch fit

■ PLANNING: EXPECTED PATIENT OUTCOMES

Expected patient outcomes for the person with a urinary diversion may include, but are not limited to, the following:

1. The person or significant other can explain and describe the anatomic variation of own diversion.
2. The person can demonstrate care of the stoma and method for managing the urinary drainage (pouch for ileal or colon conduit or ureterostomy; catheterizations and irrigation of the continent urostomy).
3. The person can describe the signs and symptoms of a urinary tract infection and the need to notify the physician.
4. The person can recognize the normal appearance of the stoma and normal peristomal skin conditions and can state changes requiring medical assistance.
5. The person can describe any necessary activity restrictions and duration of limits (avoidance of heavy lifting for 6 weeks).
6. The person can describe potential for return to preoperative sexual performance and plans for adapting to body changes.
7. The person can state plans for follow-up care and continued urologic surveillance.

■ IMPLEMENTATION

Preoperative Care

Counseling and teaching. When the physician tells the person of the probable need for a urinary diversion, the first reaction is likely to be disappointment and disbelief. The reason for the surgery will influence a person's reactions. Time to go through the grieving process is essential whether it occurs before or during hospitalization. The nurse recognizes the need for the patient to grieve and can be a source of support during this time.

Much of the basis for successful adjustment can be provided in the preoperative period. Persons who have been well informed about the surgical procedure as well as the postoperative period and long-term management goals are generally better able to adjust to the entire experience than those who do not receive such preparation. As soon as a person learns that a urinary diversion is contemplated, many questions arise, and accurate answers must be given at this time.

The enterostomal therapy nurse specializes in the care and instruction of persons who have or will have an ostomy. If possible, a preoperative meeting with the patient and enterostomal therapy nurse should be arranged. In addition to providing information, the enterostomal therapy nurse can select and mark the site for the placement of the stoma. If time permits, a meeting with the patient and a visitor from the United Ostomy Association can be arranged. The visitor is a trained volunteer who has an ostomy and has adjusted well to it. The visitor can also arrange for a postoperative or home visit.

The nurse's goals for preoperative teaching must reflect the patient's needs. However, certain basic information must be included. An assessment of the patient will determine how much of the basic information is provided preoperatively. The patient should understand the surgical procedure and should know whether a pouch will have to be worn postoperatively.

Preoperative instruction also involves preparing the person for the appearance of the stoma. The patient should be told that the stoma will be red, that the tissue is similar to the mucosal lining in the mouth, and that it will not be painful. An anatomy chart or simple drawing supplements and clarifies explanations of the surgical procedure. The patient should be given definition of terms such as stoma, urostomy, and pouch.

Booklets designed for the person having a urinary diversion may be given to the patient preoperatively.[24,36] Some persons need this additional information to assist them in accepting the surgery. Others may be unable to review written materials until after surgery.

Finally, a brief description of the management of the urostomy is given. The person who will be having an ileal or colon conduit is informed of the need to wear the pouch, the frequency of changing and emptying the pouch, and the function of the urinary stoma. The person having a continent urostomy procedure is informed of the need to catheterize the stoma at regular intervals and to irrigate the internal reservoir to remove mucus. Assurance is given that the nurse will provide stoma care immediately after the surgery and that the patient will be assisted to master self-care before discharge.

Physical preparation. Physical preparation for ureterostomy is similar to that for any abdominal surgery. Before an ileal or colon conduit diversion or a continent urostomy diversion, a complete cleansing of the bowel is required; this reduces the possibility of fecal contamination when the bowel is resected and used to form the conduit or internal reservoir. The cleansing routine generally consists of a clear liquid diet for 24 hours before surgery, and nothing by mouth after midnight the night before surgery. Large volume oral bowel cleansing solutions (GoLYTELY or Colyte) usually are given the day before surgery. Cleansing enemas may be ordered to supplement the cleanout procedure. Intestinal antibiotics such as neomycin may also be administered orally.

Determination of the exact placement for the stoma site should be made by the surgeon or the enterostomal therapy nurse. The stoma for the ileal conduit is usually constructed on the right side of the abdomen, below the waist, and within the rectus muscle. The continent urostomy stoma is placed lower on the right side of the abdomen since a flat surface for a pouch is not needed. Selection of the site is ideally made before surgery and should include evaluation of the person's body when in the lying, sitting, and standing positions. Since a smooth, even skin surrounding the stoma is important for optimal adherence of the pouch, it is important that the site selected is free from scars, skin folds, and bony prominences.

Postoperative Care

After a cutaneous ureterostomy, the person generally returns from surgery with catheters or stents (tiny catheters) inserted through the ureters to drain the renal pelves. The stents are usually left in place for 7 to 14 days. Patency of the catheters must be maintained because hydronephrosis can rapidly ensue if obstruction occurs.

After an ileal or colon conduit procedure, stents are usually in place in the stoma for 1 week to 10 days. The stents promote urinary drainage. The person with a continent urostomy will usually have a catheter in the stoma sutured in place to allow drainage from the reservoir. Another drain tube may be placed into the pelvic area. The newly created internal reservoir must be protected from over distention to prevent leakage at the anastomoses.

A nasogastric tube with gastric suction will be used until effective intestinal peristalsis has returned. Adequate drainage through the nasogastric tube is maintained to prevent pressure on the intestinal anastomosis. Nothing by mouth is permitted until peristalsis has returned; then a normal diet is gradually resumed, beginning with small amounts of water. Intravenous fluids are continued until an adequate diet is possible.

Skin care. In any type of urinary diversion, care must be taken to prevent urine leakage onto the surrounding

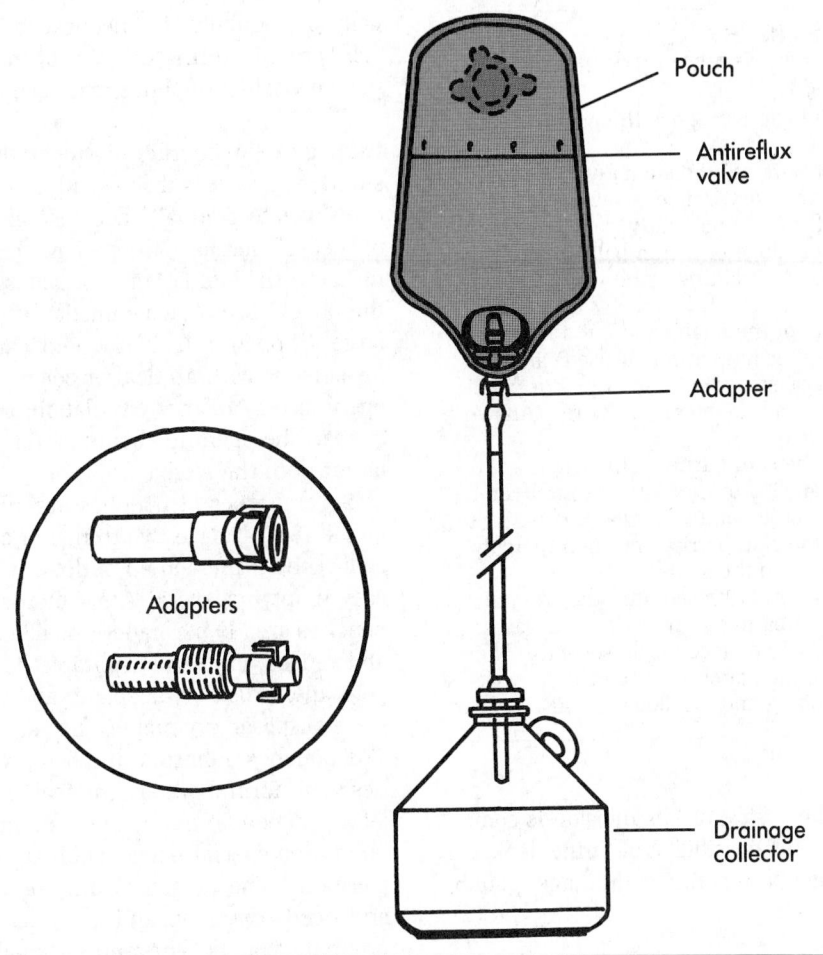

Pouch

Antireflux valve

Adapter

Adapters

Drainage collector

FIGURE 49-6 Urostomy pouch connected to continuous drainage.

skin and abdominal incision. For the ureterostomy and the ileal or colon conduit, a transparent pouch is placed around the stoma in the operating room. This allows visualization of the stoma, catheter or stents, and the stoma sutures. The stoma should be bright pink or red. Any evidence of gray or black discoloration is reported to the surgeon, since this may indicate necrosis of the stoma. Careful checking of the stoma that is in contact with a catheter is imperative because improper positioning of a catheter may exert pressure on the stoma mucosa, leading to necrosis. The pouch is changed within 24 to 48 hours after surgery to allow for better visualization and assessment of the stoma and the peristomal skin.

In the early postoperative period, the pouch is positioned so that it drains to the side of the bed, facilitating drainage and emptying of the pouch. The urostomy pouch has a valve at the bottom that permits emptying. Drainage tubing and a collection bag can be attached to the valve of the pouch to allow continuous drainage in the postoperative period (Figure 49-6). The procedure for changing the pouch is outlined in the box on p. 1456.

Monitoring urinary output. After any type of urinary diversion, urinary output must be carefully monitored in the postoperative phase. Edema of the stoma or of the ureteral anastomosis site may cause failure of adequate urine drainage that may lead to hydronephrosis or to a break in the anastomosis. Other complications that may first be detected by a decreased urinary output include dehydration, obstruction of the ureters, ileal loop ileus, or compromised renal function.

Decreased urinary output associated with symptoms of peritonitis (fever, abdominal distention, and pain) should alert the nurse to the possibility of intraperitoneal leakage caused by a leak at either the intestinal or ureterointestinal anastomosis. If this occurs, emergency surgery is required to repair the leak.

The color and nature of the urinary output are also noted. Blood in the urine is expected in the immediate postoperative period with gradual clearing. Mucus, a normal discharge from the intestinal segment, is normally secreted from an ileal or colon conduit, or continent urostomy.

The abdominal incision is observed *at least daily* for

CHANGING A URINARY POUCH

1. Assemble all supplies.
2. Empty the pouch and gently remove the pouch from the skin.
3. Cleanse the skin surrounding the stoma with mild soap and water. Rinse and pat dry. Mucous secretions should be washed off the stoma gently.
4. Place a rolled piece of gauze or cotton balls over the stomal opening to absorb draining urine while the skin is being cared for.
5. Measure the diameter of the stoma and cut a corresponding opening in the skin barrier (if used) and the pouch or select the corresponding size of precut pouch.
6. Apply skin sealant around the stoma if desired. Allow the area to dry completely.
7. Attach the pouch to the skin barrier. The pouch and skin barrier may be applied to the skin separately or together. In the early postoperative period it is easier to attach the pouch to the skin barrier and then to apply the system in one piece to the skin.
8. Apply the pouch and skin barrier around the stoma, keeping the adhesive area free of wrinkles or creases. Press gently but firmly into place for 30 seconds. The valve at the bottom of the pouch must be closed or attached to drainage tubing and a collection bag.

healing of the suture line. Care of this incision is sometimes complicated by the possibility of urine leakage onto it. An appropriate postoperative drainage pouch will minimize this problem.

Body image. A person having a urinary diversion will need time and assistance in adjusting to the change in body appearance, to the loss of the "normal" pattern of elimination, to the presence of an external pouch or an internal reservoir, and to the presence of a stoma. An opportunity should be provided for the patient to explore feelings and to begin to cope with all the changes. Competent nursing care is also important, because the person who experiences constant urine leakage and skin breakdown will most likely feel discouraged and depressed. The patient gains a sense of control and independence when management of the ostomy and its care is mastered.

Promoting self-care. Postoperative instruction is started as soon as a person feels able to participate in the urostomy care. Usually lessons begin after the nasogastric tube has been removed. This allows the patient to better visualize the stoma. During the active phases of teaching, the pouch is removed more often than is recommended after discharge. The patient (or caregiver) must learn how to manage the assembly, application, emptying, and changing of the selected pouch. A family member or friend is often included in the teaching to provide support at home, but the patient, unless limited physi-

cally or mentally, is encouraged to be responsible for self-care. Mastering the care of the stoma enhances the person's self-confidence and acceptance of the stoma.

Use and care of pouches. Postoperatively the edema of the stoma begins to subside within 7 days, but the stoma continues to gradually decrease in size for the next 6 to 8 weeks. Therefore, the patient should be taught how to measure the stoma before discharge and how to adjust the pouch size to accommodate the smaller stoma. Too large an opening is a frequent cause of skin problems for persons with an ileal or colon conduit. Too small an opening may restrict circulation or cause trauma to the stoma. The opening should be no more than 2 to 3 mm larger than the stoma.

Several types of pouches are available (Figures 49-7 and 49-8). All have two things in common—a pouch to collect the urine and an outlet or valve at the bottom for easy emptying every 3 to 4 hours. The basic types of pouches are (1) permanent pouches that can be washed and reused, (2) semidisposable pouches that fit onto a permanent disk or faceplate, and (3) one-piece or two-piece disposable pouches that are discarded after use. The pouches adhere to the body with some form of adhesive to form a watertight seal. The type of pouch selected depends upon the patient's preference, body build, and special needs, such as physical or visual impairment. The person is informed of choices available and needs direction and guidance in selecting the appropriate pouch. The enterostomal therapy nurse can assist the patient in the assessment and selection of the appropriate pouch.

Most persons can wear a pouch for 3 to 5 days between changes. An interval longer than 7 days should be discouraged because of potential odor, crystallization problems or risk of infection. An appropriate schedule that eliminates leakage and provides the best skin protection needs to be determined. For example, if the pouch tends to show signs of impending leakage or skin redness on the fifth day, then it should be changed every 3 or 4 days, before leakage and skin problems occur. This schedule must be individualized.

Proper cleaning of reusable equipment is essential for odor control, general hygiene, and prevention of stomal complications. Manufacturers include cleaning instructions with their equipment. Following are the principles for proper cleaning of reusable urinary appliances:

1. Clean equipment promptly.
2. Use adhesive remover as necessary to remove residue.
3. Avoid soaking equipment for prolonged periods of time (20 to 30 minutes in soap and water is sufficient). Longer soaking speeds deterioration of many appliances.

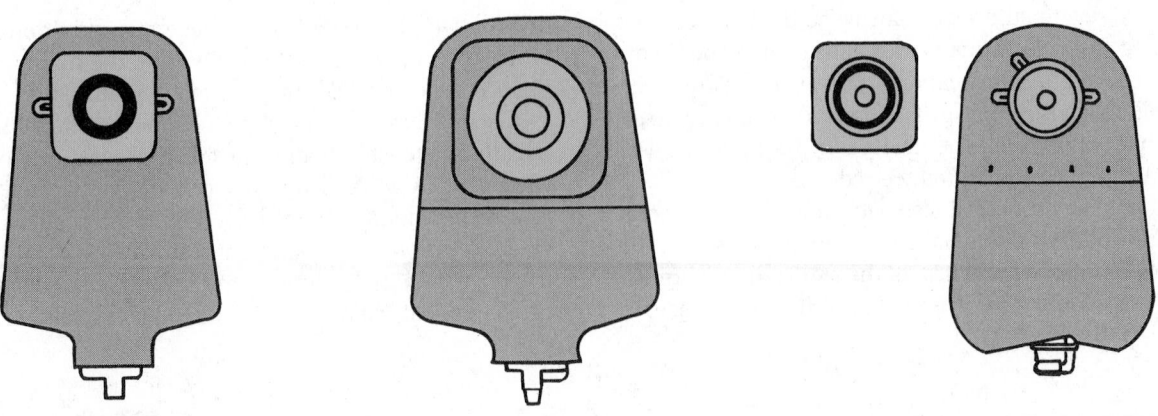

FIGURE 49-7 Disposable one- and two-piece pouches.

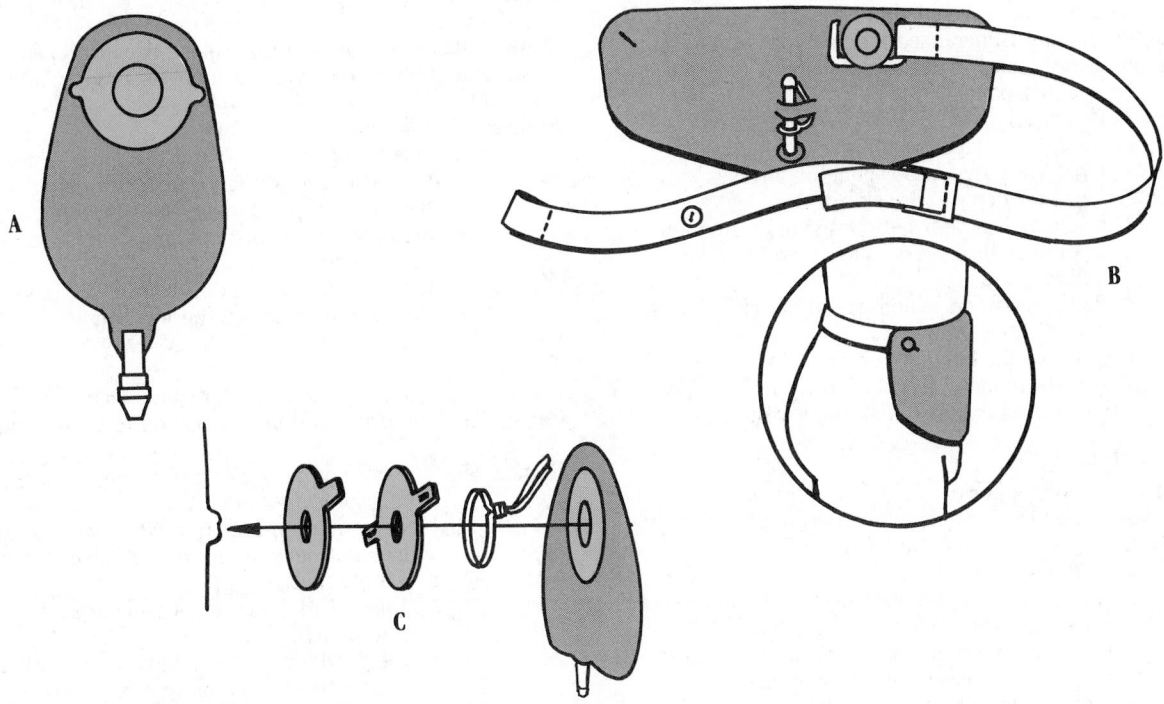

FIGURE 49-8 Reusable pouches. **A,** One-piece pouch. **B,** One-piece nonadhesive pouch. **C,** Two-piece reusable faceplate and reusable or disposable pouch.

4. For odor problems soak appliance in half-strength vinegar water for an additional 20 to 30 minutes.

POTENTIAL PROBLEMS OF URINARY DIVERSIONS

The person with a urinary diversion is at greater risk for *urinary tract infection* due to the shorter distance from the urinary diversion to the kidneys. The patient must be taught the signs and symptoms of urinary infection: cloudy urine, blood in the urine, strong odor to urine, flank pain, fever, and malaise. Urine cultures are correctly obtained by catheter from the ileal or colon con-duit stoma. A specimen taken from the pouch is likely to be contaminated. Catheterization of a ureterostomy stoma is generally performed by the physician unless nurses have been instructed in the procedure. A pouch with an antireflux valve is recommended to prevent infections from bacteria found in the pouch.

Problems with the stoma include bleeding, lacerations, crystal formation, stenosis, hernia, and prolapse. A small amount of bleeding from the stoma mucosa is not uncommon when the stoma is cleansed. This generally stops within a few seconds. If bleeding persists or is unusually severe, the physician is notified. Blood that originates from the urinary tract rather than the stoma may be related to complications such as infection or calculi. Patients also need to be forewarned about medicines that will discolor the urine. For example, doxorubicin (Adriamycin) will produce red urine.

A stoma laceration can also cause bleeding. A laceration can occur when the pouch opening is too small, the pouch is misapplied and lies on the stoma, or a belt misplaces the pouch. The laceration will heal if the source of irritation is removed. If the laceration is through the entire thickness of the stoma and into the lumen, creating a fistula, surgical intervention is required.

Crystal formation on the stoma or peristomal skin is usually related to alkaline urine. However, acidic crystals occur in a small number or patients. Crystals may also result in stomal bleeding. The urine pH should be checked before any treatment is initiated. A sample of the crystals may be sent to the laboratory to determine the chemical composition. Alkaline crystals may be

TREATMENT OF SKIN PROBLEMS

RASH OR IRRITATED HAIR FOLLICLES

Location: Rash can be located under tape, under pouch adhesive, and on any part of skin where pouch comes in contact with skin. Generalized reddish appearance that covers an entire area, similar to diaper rash will be seen.

Cause:
1. Leaking pouch
2. Perspiration
3. Allergies to tape or adhesive
4. Unshaven area under pouch adhesive

Remedy:
1. Use hair dryer to dry skin.*
2. Use a skin barrier between skin and pouch until skin clears. Try to leave on 24 to 28 hours.
3. Powder skin on which pouch lies (but not under adhesive area).
4. Make or buy a pouch cover.
5. If rash, redness do not clear up in 5 to 7 days, consult an enterostomal therapy nurse.

MONILIAL INFECTION

Location: On peristomal skin

Cause: Yeast infection is often seen when patient is on antibiotics, which alter normal bacterial flora.

Remedy:
1. Use hair dryer* for the area.
2. Apply nystatin (Mycostatin) powder to area, if prescribed, or other antifungal powder. Brush off excess powder, seal in with skin sealant, and apply pouch in usual manner.
3. Drink at least 2500 ml fluids.
4. If infection does not clear in 5 to 7 days, consult an enterostomal therapy nurse.

ULCERATED AREA ON STOMA

Location: Anywhere on stoma

Cause: Opening of pouch was too small, or activities were causing the pouch faceplate or wafer to rub or cut into the stoma.

Remedy:
1. Enlarge size of pouch opening, at least 1/8 inch larger than stoma.
2. Evaluate patient's activities; a different sized or shaped faceplate or wafer may be needed.
3. Loosen belt, if too tight. Belt may cause shifting of the pouch.
4. If ulcerated area does not clear up in 5 to 7 days, consult an enterostomal therapy nurse.

HYPERPLASIA

Location: Between opening of faceplate, wafer, or pouch and stoma

Cause: Maceration of skin from urine because opening in pouch system is too large. Skin is raised, gray, and painful to touch.

Remedy:
1. Use hair dryer* to dry.
2. Use Colly-Seel, Stomahesive, Durahesive, or Reliaseal under pouch, firmly hugging stoma.
3. If using faceplate, decrease size of opening. If using pouches with openings too large, decrease size.
4. If condition does not clear in 5 to 7 days, consult an enterostomal therapy nurse.

ALKALINE CRYSTALS

Location: On stoma and/or around stoma base

Cause: Alkaline urine and predisposition to stone formation

Remedy:
1. Vinegar compresses on the stoma when changing the pouch.
2. Insert vinegar into pouch while wearing it if it does not have an antireflux valve.
   a. Empty pouch.
   b. Instill 1 to 2 ounces of vinegar solution into pouch.
   c. Lie down so solution will bathe inside of pouch and stoma for approximately 20 minutes.
   d. Empty pouch and rinse with cool water.
3. Switch to vinyl or plastic pouches if using rubber pouches. Rubber pouches tend to precipitate crystals inside pouch, which may cause bleeding and irritation to stoma.
4. Use pouch with antireflux valve

From Broadwell DC and Sorrells SL: Summary of your urinary diversion care, unpublished material, 1976.
*A hair dryer should be set on a cool setting.

treated with vinegar soaks, disposable antireflux pouches, and treatment of any infection.

The combination of an improperly fitting pouch and alkaline urine can lead to the development of raised, painful, *wartlike areas* next to the stoma.[8] The exposed skin is covered by recalibrating the stomal opening and treating the affected skin area (see box on opposite page for treatment of skin problems.)

Peristomal hernias and *prolapse of the stoma* are other complications that may occur after hospitalization. The primary treatment is surgical intervention, however, some patients may elect not to have a hernia or prolapse repaired. The pouch opening may need to be adjusted or enlarged to accommodate the stoma.

Electrolyte imbalance may develop if the urine is retained in the conduit because of stomal or loop stenosis. The mucosa of the conduit reabsorbs chlorides from the urine, and the patient may develop a metabolic hyperchloremic acidosis. A person with optimal renal function has no difficulty excreting the reabsorbed chlorides. When the renal function is compromised, the patient is more likely to develop electrolyte problems. This reabsorption can also occur in those with internal reservoirs because the urine is retained within the internal pouch until the stoma is catheterized and the urine drained. Follow-up urologic visits and electrolyte studies are imperative.

DISCHARGE PLANNING

Before discharge from the hospital the nurse must be certain that the individual can manage the urinary drainage and can detect any deviations from normal. At least one return visit or an opportunity for telephone consultation with the primary nurse involved in the teaching or the enterostomal therapy nurse is extremely helpful so that questions that arise after returning home can be discussed. Visiting nurse assistance may be required for a period of time. Ongoing urologic care will be required, including urine cultures, which are correctly obtained by catheter from the ileal or sigmoid loop stoma. A specimen taken from the pouch is likely to be contaminated.

In summary, at the time of discharge the person should be able to explain the nature of the urinary diversion, expected appearance of the stoma, care of the stoma and pouch, and signs to be reported to the physician.

CHAPTER SUMMARY

✔ Under normal conditions, the person eating an adequate diet has a urinary output essentially equal to fluid input.

✔ Mechanical urinary obstruction refers to an anatomic blockage of urine flow at any level of the urinary tract and may be acquired or congenital.

✔ A cystostomy tube is placed directly into the bladder through a suprapubic incision to provide urinary drainage when an obstruction exists below the bladder.

✔ Clean technique, rather than sterile, is usually encouraged for home care intermittent catheterization.

✔ Fluid imbalances in persons with urinary problems can be prevented by identifying and monitoring high-risk persons and teaching patients management of fluid balance.

✔ Postoperative care for urologic surgery includes promoting ventilation, monitoring urinary output, monitoring for signs of distention and hemorrhage, protecting the skin from urinary drainage through the incision, and patient teaching.

✔ Four types of urinary drainage procedures include cutaneous ureterostomy, ileal conduit, colon conduit, and continent urostomy.

✔ Postoperative care after a urinary drainage procedure includes skin care, changing the pouch and teaching the patient self-care in pouch changing, monitoring urinary output, supporting the person adapting to the body image change, and teaching about care of potential problems.

QUESTIONS TO CONSIDER

- What are the major causes of urinary retention?

- Why is sterile technique used when caring for the hospitalized patient with intermittent catheterization, even when the patient was using clean technique at home?

- What are the major nursing considerations in managing nephrostomy drains?

- Compare and contrast the different types of urinary diversion procedures.

- What are potential remedies for skin irritations around urostomy stomas?

REFERENCES AND SELECTED READINGS

1. American Cancer Society Inc: Living with your urostomy (urinary diversion), New York, 1979, The Society.
2. American Cancer Society Inc: Colostomy, ileostomy and ureterostomy care: a guide of practical information for nurses, New York, 1977, The Society.
3. Anderson RU: Response of bladder and urethral mucosa to catheterization, JAMA 242:451-453, 1979.
4. *Bates P: A troubleshooter's guide to indwelling catheters, RN 44(3):62-68, 1981.

*References preceded by an asterisk are particularly well suited for student reading.

5. Bellinger MF: The history of diversion and undiversion, J Enterostom Ther 16:39-41, 1989.

6. Bielski M: Symposium on infection control: preventing infection in the catheterized patient, Nurs Clin North Am 15:703-713, 1980.

7. *Bristoll S et al: The mythical danger of rapid urinary drainage, Am J Nurs 89:344-345, 1989.

8. Broadwell DC and Jackson BS: Principles of ostomy care, St Louis, 1982, The CV Mosby Co.

9. Broadwell DC: Peristomal skin integrity, Nurs Clin N Am 22:321-332, 1987.

10. *Brogna L and Lakaszawski ML: Nursing management: the continent urostomy, J Enterostom Ther 13:139-147, 1986.

11. *Brogna L and Lakaszawski ML: The continent urostomy, Am J Nurs 86:160-163, 1986.

12. Brundage DJ: Nursing management of renal problems, ed 2, St Louis, 1980, The CV Mosby Co.

13. *Cain L and Bigongiari LR: The percutaneous nephrostomy tube, Am J Nur 82(2):296-298, 1982.

14. Campion V: Clean technique for intermittent self-catheterization, Nurs Res 25:13-18, 1976.

15. Chezem J: Urinary diversion: select aspects of nursing management, Nurs Clin North Am 11:445-456, 1976.

16. *Conti M and Eutropius L: Preventing UTI's: What works?, Am J Nurs 87:307-309, 1987.

17. Dowd JB: Urinary diversion: alternatives and techniques, Surg Clin North Am 60:687-702, 1980.

18. Glenn JF, editor: Urologic surgery, ed 3, Hagerstown, MD, 1983, Harper & Row, Publishers, Inc.

19. Gonzalez R, and DeWolf W: The artificial bladder sphincter AS-721 for treatment of incontinence in patients with neurogenic bladder, J Urol 121:71-72, 1979.

20. *Gray M: Treatment modalities for bladder cancer, Semins Oncol Nurs 2(4):260-264, 1986.

21. Greig, BJ: Interventions of the ET nurse with the continent urinary Kock pouch patient, J Enterstom Ther 13:226-231, 1986.

22. *Gurevich I: The new urine meters, Nursing '80 10:47-52, 1980.

23. *Hinkle MT and Bowditch RR: The great stent mystery: can you solve it? Nursing '81 11:94-95, April 1981.

24. *Hollister, Incorporated: Managing your ostomy: do more with your life than just cope with it, Libertyville, IL, 1985, Hollister, Inc.

25. Jete KF: Hyperplasia or what? J Enterostom Ther 10:181-184, 1983.

26. Kaplan J: Dilatation of a surgically ligated ureter through a percutaneous nephrostomy, AJR 139(1):188-189, 1982.

27. King AW: Nursing management of stomas of the genitourinary system. In Broadwell DC and Jackson BS, editors: Principles of ostomy care, St Louis, 1982, The CV Mosby Co.

28. *McCormack A, Itkin J, and Cloud C: Correcting acid-base imbalance, RN 48(5):39-40, 1985.

29. *Petillo MH: The patient with a urinary stoma, Nurs Clin North Am 22:263-279, 1987.

30. *Pickering L and Robbins D: Fluid, electrolyte, and acid-base balance in the renal patient, Nurs Clin North Am 15:577-592, 1980.

31. Rowland RG, Mitchell ME, and Bihrle R: Alternative techniques for a continent urinary reservoir, Urol Clin North Am 14(4):797-804, 1987.

32. Rowland RG et al: Indiana continent urinary reservoir, J Urol 137(6):1136-1139, 1987.

33. *Shipes E: Sexual function following ostomy surgery, Nurs Clin North Am 22:303-310, 1987.

34. Skinner DG, Boyd SD, and Lieskovsky G: An update on the Kock pouch for continent urinary diversion, Urol Clin North Am 14(4):789-795, 1987.

35. Smith DB: Clinical rounds: stomal complications, J Enterostom Ther 11(1):35-39, 1984.

36. *Squibb & Sons, Inc.: For a better way of living with a urostomy . . . every day, Princeton, NJ, 1987, Convatec.

37. Stables D: Percutaneous nephrostomy: techniques, indications and results, Urol Clin North Am 9(1):15-29, 1982.

38. Tebeau JL: Fluid, electrolyte, and acid-base balance: special considerations in gastrointestinal and urinary diversions. In Broadwell DC and Jackson BS, editors: Principles of ostomy care, St Louis, 1982, The CV Mosby Co.

39. *Toth JM: When your patient faces a urostomy, RN 48(11):50-56, 1985.

40. *Watt RC: Nursing management of a patient with a urinary diversion, Semins Oncol Nurs 2(4):265-269, 1986.

41. Wishnow KL et al: Ileal conduit in era of systemic chemotherapy, Urology 33(5):358-360, 1989.

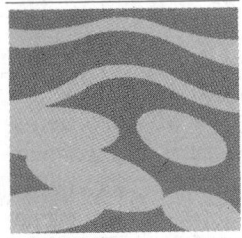

CHAPTER 50

Management of Persons with Renal Failure

H. FRED FARLEY, JR.

CHAPTER OBJECTIVES

After studying this chapter, the student should be able to:
1. Describe the pathophysiologic bases for the clinical manifestations of acute and chronic renal failure.
2. Describe the medical and nursing management of the patient during the oliguric and diuretic phases of acute renal failure.
3. Identify treatment goals for patients in chronic renal failure.
4. Describe the physiologic principles of dialysis.
5. Describe nursing assessment and management of the patient undergoing hemodialysis, peritoneal dialysis, and kidney transplantation.

Renal failure is the state of total or nearly total loss of kidney function. The kidneys have a tremendous ability to adapt to a decreasing number of functioning nephrons. With less than 25% of the original nephrons maintaining functional ability, the kidneys are able to excrete waste products and maintain fluid and electrolyte balance. As renal failure develops, laboratory tests reflect the changes in homeostasis, and the person appears clinically ill. The person in renal failure cannot independently sustain life.

Renal failure may be acute in onset or may develop slowly and progressively over a course of several years. When renal failure occurs suddenly, as within a few days, biochemical changes are often dramatic, and the person has little time to adjust to these changes. The person becomes very ill, and hospitalization is required, frequently involving placement in a critical care area.

When renal failure occurs as the end result of a chronic kidney illness in which kidney tissue is destroyed progressively over the course of several months or years, control of symptoms and preservation of functional abilities are achievable goals. Dietary adjustment, medications, and attention to preventing additional illnesses must compensate for loss of renal function in the early stages of progressing renal failure. As renal function continues to deteriorate, dialysis or transplantation becomes necessary to maintain life.

Renal insufficiency exists when significant loss of renal function has developed but with enough nephrons remaining functional to maintain an internal environment consistent with life. When renal insufficiency exists, any additional physiologic stressor, such as illness, nutritional overindulgence, or drugs, may lead to renal failure. The individual experiencing renal insufficiency may appear and feel well, even though laboratory data reflect deterioration in renal function. Renal insufficiency occurs as a phase in gradually and chronically progressive renal disease.

ACUTE RENAL FAILURE
EPIDEMIOLOGY/ETIOLOGY

Acute renal failure occurs as a sudden and frequently reversible decrease or cessation of kidney function related to prerenal, renal, or postrenal factors. It generally follows an identifiable trauma of either toxic or ischemic nature or a postrenal infection or obstruction.[29] The health of the individual before the insult is usually good.

Recovery from an episode of acute renal failure depends on the underlying illness, the condition of the patient, and the careful, supportive management given during the period of renal shutdown. Mortality associated with acute tubular necrosis approaches 40%; these statistics largely reflect the deaths of severely ill persons in whom renal failure is a sequela to extensive underlying illness. Owing to more widespread availability of dialysis, mortality directly attributable to decreased renal function from potassium intoxification, fluid overload, and acidosis has been reduced. The potential for recovery of renal function for those who survive the acute episode of tubular insufficiency is good. Although recovery statistics indicate that kidney tissue may regenerate more completely after toxic injury in comparison with ischemic injury, follow-up studies of persons several years after episodes of acute tubular insufficiency show normal or near-normal renal function.[37]

CONDITIONS AND SUBSTANCES THAT PRODUCE ISCHEMIC OR NEPHROTOXIC INJURY TO THE KIDNEYS

ISCHEMIC CAUSES* (prerenal)

Hypovolemia
Blood loss (surgery, trauma)
Plasma loss (burns, surgery, acute pancreatitis)
Sodium and water loss (prolonged diarrhea or vomiting, gastrointestinal tract drainage, sustained high fever)
Cardiac failure
Myocardial infarction
Cardiac dysrhythmias
Congestive heart failure
Septic shock

TOXIC SUBSTANCES† (renal)

Solvents (carbon tetrachloride, methanol, ethylene glycol)
Heavy metals (lead, arsenic, mercury)
Antibiotics (kanamycin, gentamicin, polymyxin B, amphotericin B, colistin, neomycin, phenazopyridine)
Pesticides
Mushrooms

———————————————————
*Inadequate perfusion of the kidney.
†Direct injury to functional component of kidney cells.

For those in whom acute renal failure has been caused by glomerular disease or severe infection of kidney tissue, the prognosis may not be as favorable. Return of renal function is determined by the extent of scarring and obliteration of functional renal tissue that has occurred during the acute episode of kidney failure. A significant number of adults who develop acute glomerulonephritis show some decrease in renal function, which may remain at a level not producing biochemical abnormalities or may progress to a chronic form of renal failure.

The major causes of ischemic and toxic injuries to the kidney that may lead to acute renal failure are listed in the box above. Additionally, other conditions can precipitate acute renal failure:

1. Acute glomerular disease
2. Acute severe infection of kidney tissue
3. Bilateral occlusion of renal arteries
4. Mechanical obstructions in the urinary tract
5. Hemoglobinemia and myoglobinemia

All of these conditions lead to massive and rapid destruction of kidney tissue.

PREVENTION

The incidence of acute renal failure can be reduced through two measures: (1) identification and observation of populations at risk and (2) identification and control of environmental risk factors. The greatest incidence of acute renal failure occurs in persons with the following:

1. Major trauma
2. Extensive burns
3. Aortic surgery
4. Massive blood loss
5. Severe myocardial infarction

Acute renal failure also frequently occurs in patients with sepsis and in those having abnormal intravascular coagulation, such as disseminated intravascular coagulation (DIC) because these acutely ill persons are prime candidates for inadequate kidney perfusion. Frequent monitoring of urinary output and detection of excessive losses of body fluid will help to identify instances of inadequate renal perfusion before renal failure develops.

Significant factors in preventive care for the general population include control of nephrotoxic drugs, increased medical supervision of persons with sore throats and upper respiratory tract infections, and increased case finding and treatment of individuals with bacteriuria and obstructive disease of the urinary system. Attempts to control the distribution and identification of nephrotoxic drugs and chemicals are primarily accomplished through the Food and Drug Administration (FDA). Identification of nephrotoxic drugs and chemicals, enforced labeling of these substances, and drug dispensing by prescription only are examples of the FDA's attempts to promote public health. Proper labeling and storage of potentially toxic drugs and chemicals in the home can further reduce the number of accidental ingestions of nephrotoxic substances.

PATHOPHYSIOLOGY AND CLINICAL MANIFESTATIONS

Renal ischemia occurs when blood flow to the kidneys is reduced. The response of the normal kidney is *vasoconstriction,* which compounds the problem of reduced renal blood flow and increases renal ischemia. Perfusion problems affect both kidneys. When ischemia is prolonged, renal tubular tissue dies and frank renal failure develops.

Substances that are toxic to the cells of the renal tubules affect the kidneys bilaterally. The kidney with its large blood flow and ability to concentrate fluid in the medullary portion (where the tubules are located) creates conditions in which exposure of tubular cells to toxins is maximized. Damage to the cells leads to decreased glomerular permeability and tubular obstruction.

The course of acute renal failure is usually characterized by an initial oliguric phase followed in a number of days (10 to 15) to a few weeks by a diuretic period. Major problems during the *oliguric* phase include inability to excrete fluid loads, regulate electrolytes, and excrete metabolic waste materials (Table 50-1). During the *diuretic* phase, large amounts of fluid (2 to 3 L/day) and electrolytes are lost.

TABLE 50-1 Symptoms caused by physiologic changes in acute renal failure

Physiologic Effect	Findings	Symptoms
OLIGURIC PHASE		
Inability to excrete metabolic wastes	Increased serum: Urea nitrogen Creatinine	Nausea Vomiting Drowsiness Confusion Coma Gastrointestinal bleeding Asterixis Pericarditis
Inability to regulate electrolytes	Hyperkalemia Hyponatremia Acidosis	Nausea Vomiting Cardiac dysrhythmias Kussmaul's breathing Drowsiness Confusion Coma
Inability to excrete fluid loads	Fluid overload Hypervolemia	Edema Congestive heart failure Pulmonary edema Hypertension
DIURETIC PHASE		
Increased production of urine (deficit in concentrating ability of tubules and osmotic diuretic effect of high BUN) Slowly increasing excretion of metabolic wastes	Hypovolemia Loss of sodium Loss of potassium High blood urea nitrogen (BUN) initially BUN gradually returns to baseline	Urinary output of up to 4-5 L/day Postural hypotension Tachycardia Improving mental alertness and activity

OLIGURIC PHASE

Inability to Excrete Fluid Loads

Because of the decreased kidney function, fluids are retained in the body, resulting in fluid overload and edema (see Chapter 23). When fluid overload is excessive, congestive heart failure and pulmonary edema may occur. Hypertension accompanies acute renal failure when the person is hypervolemic, although this is usually not a finding when fluid balance is controlled.

Inability to excrete fluid loads leads to decreased urinary output. Either *oliguria* (urinary output below 400 ml/day) or *anuria* (urinary output below 100 ml/day) may be present, although oliguria is more common. Classically, the patient in acute renal failure shows a fall in urinary output within 1 to 2 days to between 50 and 400 ml/day. The urine *specific gravity is low* (1.010), and the osmolality of the urine approaches that of the person's serum (280 to 320 mOsm). Specific gravity and urine osmolality remain within this fixed range and reflect tubular damage with loss of concentrating ability.

Electrolyte Imbalances

The three major electrolyte problems are retention of potassium, excretion of sodium, and metabolic acidosis.

Potassium imbalance. In the normal individual, the potassium ion is exchanged in the distal convoluted tubule of the nephron for either sodium or hydrogen ions; healthy person cannot conserve the potassium ion. However, in the individual with acute renal failure in whom a large number of tubular cells are no longer functional, no mechanism exists to remove potassium from the body. *Hyperkalemia* (the most sudden hazard in oliguric ARF) is said to exist when the serum concentration of this ion reaches a level of 5.5 mEq/L or higher. Serum concentrations of 7 to 10 mEq/L can be quickly reached in acute renal failure and are incompatible with normal cardiac function and life.

In monitoring for signs of potassium toxicity, electrocardiography and laboratory determinations of serum potassium are the most reliable indicators. Rarely does the patient become symptomatic, and pulse changes must not be relied on to indicate the degree of rise of potassium in the patient's system.

Sodium imbalance. *Hyponatremia* in acute renal failure most commonly develops with overhydration of the patient. The oliguric patient cannot excrete large volumes of urine; when the administration of sodium-free or low-sodium intravenous or oral fluids continues in such an individual, the serum is diluted and the serum concentration of sodium falls.

In this situation hyponatremia is accompanied or caused by hypervolemia. In the very acutely ill, the situation commonly occurs when the patient receives numerous drugs and fluids in an attempt to treat coexisting life-threatening problems. When the volume of drugs and fluids cannot be reduced to a safe level, dialysis is required to remove the excess fluid and restore sodium balance.

Signs and symptoms of hyponatremia include warm, moist, flushed skin; muscle weakness; muscle twitching; and behavioral changes involving confusion, delirium, coma, and convulsions. Serum sodium concentrations will be below 130 mEq/L. The hematocrit and hemoglobin values suddenly fall without evidence of bleeding, which is caused by hemodilution.

Increases in total body content of sodium also occur in acute renal failure. Commonly, this occurs when the patient is receiving medications high in sodium content and excess sodium in the diet. Edema and increasing blood pressure indicate retention of sodium and fluids even though the serum sodium concentration is normal or below normal.

Metabolic acidosis. Acidosis develops when hydrogen ion secretion and bicarbonate ion production diminish in the tubular cells. The pH of the blood decreases, the carbon dioxide content decreases, and central nervous system symptoms of drowsiness progressing to stupor and coma may appear. Although the lungs are unable to compensate totally for the increasing acid load, they help determine the rate at which acidosis develops and the frequency or need for dialysis. In compensating for increased metabolic acid loads, the lungs attempt to excrete more carbon dioxide. Kussmaul's breathing is noted.

Inability to Excrete Metabolic Wastes

Decreased kidney function alters the body's ability to get rid of metabolic waste materials, producing typical signs and symptoms referred to as *uremia*. BUN and serum creatinine values rise sharply. In the person who has already sustained illness and trauma, BUN values may increase at a rate of 30 mg/100 ml/day. Signs and symptoms include neurologic manifestations such as confusion, convulsions, coma, and asterixis. Gastrointestinal bleeding may result from uremic gastritis or colitis. Decreased cellular immunity causes an increased tendency for infections to develop. Bruising and bleeding result from changes in blood coagulation factors. Pericarditis (see Chapter 28) is thought to develop as a result of pericardial irritation from accumulated metabolic wastes.

DIURETIC PHASE

After a period of oliguria or anuria that may last a few days to several weeks, patients recovering renal function pass into another distinct phase of illness characterized by increased urinary output. Increased output indicates that the damaged nephrons are healing and are able to begin excreting urine. At first daily urine volume increases slowly, although within 1 to 2 days diuresis up to or exceeding 4 to 5 L/day may occur. Although fluid can be excreted, the kidneys are not yet healed. Often there is inability to excrete proportional amounts of waste materials, and BUN and creatinine may rise or remain elevated as urine volume increases. At times excessive excretion of sodium and potassium occurs during diuresis. Complete recovery of renal function is slow and requires anywhere from days to several months. Return of renal function to normal or near normal levels is evidenced when the kidney can both conserve and dilute urine and when serum electrolytes and nonprotein nitrogen levels become normal.

MEDICAL MANAGEMENT

Medical management of the patient in acute renal failure is specific to the cause and phase of the acute failure. During the *oliguric* phase, the goals are to control fluids, regulate electrolytes, control and promote excretion of metabolic waste buildup, and reduce tissue catabolism. This is accomplished by dialysis; fluid restrictions; low-protein, low-potassium, high-carbohydrate diet; exchange resins (such as Kayexalate) to increase potassium excretion if necessary; and prevention of infection with administration of antibiotics as needed. TPN, with a mixture of essential amino acids and glucose, may be given during dialysis to prevent excessive catabolism.

During the *diuretic* phase, medical management centers around maintaining adequate fluid balance while also regulating electrolytes. Even though the patient may be excreting large volumes of urine, dialysis may still be necessary to adequately control electrolyte balance. Protein restrictions are continued until BUN and serum creatinine levels decline.

■ ASSESSMENT
SUBJECTIVE DATA

Subjective data to obtain from the person with acute renal failure include the following:
1. Voiding patterns, including any recent changes
2. Weight gain (fluid retention)
3. Nausea and vomiting
4. Patient and family history of renal disease
5. Medication use (prescription and OTC)
6. Recent surgery, anesthesia, or trauma

OBJECTIVE DATA

Objective data include the following:

1. Amount of urine excreted in 24 hours
2. Blood pressure, particularly postural changes
3. Daily weights
4. Fluid status
   a. Peripheral edema, periorbital, sacral, or dependent edema
   b. Auscultated breath sounds
   c. Skin turgor
5. Halitosis as a result of acidosis and/or ammonia secretion
6. Changes in mental status
7. Pulse rate and rhythm

■ DATA ANALYSIS: NURSING DIAGNOSES

Nursing diagnoses are determined from assessment of patient data. Possible nursing diagnoses for the person with acute renal failure may include, but are not limited to, the following:

Diagnostic Title	Possible Etiologies
Fluid volume deficit (diuretic phase)	Abnormal fluid loss
Fluid volume excess (oliguric phase)	Compromised regulatory mechanism
Infection, potential for	Decreased nutrition, decreased immune response
Injury, potential for	Sensorimotor deficits, mental confusion
Knowledge deficit	Lack of exposure/recall, cognitive limitation
Nutrition, altered: less than body requirements	Anorexia, nausea, restricted diet
Urinary elimination, altered patterns	Decreased urine production

■ PLANNING: EXPECTED PATIENT OUTCOMES

Expected patient outcomes for the person with renal failure during the *oliguric* phase may include, but are not limited to, the following:

1. The patient will have:
   a. Absence of pulmonary edema
   b. Absence or control of peripheral edema
   c. Control of blood pressure (range between 170/100 and 100/60 mm Hg
   d. Restored or maintained mental alertness
   e. Control of electrolyte balance
      (1) Sodium range of 125 to 145 mEq/L
      (2) Potassium range of 3.0 to 6.0 mEq/L
      (3) Bicarbonate above 14 mEq/L
   f. Control of protein catabolism
      (1) Urea nitrogen below 100 mg/dl
      (2) Creatinine below 12 mg/dl
      (3) Absence of skin breakdown
   g. Absence of bleeding
   h. Resolution or control of intercurrent illness (congestive heart failure, shock)

2. The patient remains free of:
   a. Infection
   b. Injury resulting from decreased level of awareness and strength
   c. Toxicity from inadequately excreted medication

Expected patient outcomes for the person with renal failure during the *diuretic* phase may include, but are not limited to the following examples in which the patient will:

1. State extent of recovery of kidney function
2. Identify any preventable environmental or health factors involved in generating the illness
3. Plan a diet to maintain positive nitrogen balance and sufficient caloric intake
4. Identify signs and symptoms of dehydration and sodium and potassium loss
5. Describe plans for prevention of infection
6. State plans for follow-up health care

■ IMPLEMENTATION

OLIGURIC PHASE

During the oliguric phase of acute renal failure, the goals of nursing interventions are maintaining fluid and electrolyte balance and rest/activity balance, preventing infection and effects of altered bleeding and neurologic status, and promoting comfort and control of the environment (see the box on p. 1466).

Control of fluids is essential during the oliguric phase because of the decreased ability of the kidneys to excrete urine. Nursing care should have three broad objectives: (1) monitoring for signs of fluid overload, (2) maintaining the patient's energy expenditure at a level compatible with the individual's state of health, and (3) controlling or helping the patient to control fluid intake.

All observations about the patient's state of hydration need to be recorded so that hour-to-hour and day-to-day comparisons can be made. Any finding indicating retention of fluids is reported to the physician. Edema can first be noted in dependent areas such as the feet and legs, in the presacral area, and around the eyes. The person is observed carefully for signs of pulmonary edema and congestive heart failure (see Chapter 28). Central venous lines or arterial monitoring lines will help to provide data for short-term comparison in managing the fluid balance of the critically ill person. Positioning and activity are determined daily based on assessment of the energy level and ability to breathe adequately.

All fluid (parenteral and oral) must total only slightly more than daily output if severe overhydration is to be avoided. Devices that allow precise control of intravenous fluids are added safety measures when giving fluids parenterally to anuric or oliguric patients. Accuracy in fluid balance records is essential.

GUIDELINES FOR CARE DURING OLIGURIC PHASE OF ACUTE RENAL FAILURE

1. Fluid and electrolyte balance
   a. Assist in maintaining adequate nutrition
   b. Assist patient in remaining within limitations of diet (protein, sodium, potassium, phosphorus, and fluid limits)
   c. Maintain fluid restrictions
   d. Keep accurate records of intake and output
   e. Weigh patient daily
   f. Monitor vital signs frequently, including postural signs
   g. Frequently assess fluid status of patient
   h. Administer phosphate-binding medications as prescribed
2. Rest/activity balance
   a. Maintain strict bed rest in the acute phase
   b. Assist patient with activities of daily living (ADL) to conserve energy
   c. Promote early ambulation when renal status permits
   d. Maintain safe environment for patient
   e. Provide for planned rest periods
3. Prevention of infection
   a. Avoid patient contact by anyone with infection
   b. Assess patient for signs and symptoms of infection
   c. If catheterization is required, maintain asepsis during insertion (meticulous catheter care is essential)
   d. Maintain pulmonary hygiene while patient is on bed rest
   e. Turn patient frequently
   f. Administer antibiotics as prescribed
4. Altered bleeding tendency
   a. Protect patient from injury
   b. Administer stool softeners as prescribed
   c. Instruct patient to use soft toothbrush
   d. Assess patient for signs of bleeding
      (1) Bruising
      (2) Perform guaiac tests on stool, emesis, and nasogastric returns
      (3) Changes in vital signs
5. Altered neurologic status
   a. Assess orientation at least every 8 hours
   b. Assess level of consciousness at least every 8 hours
   c. Immediately report any changes in mental status to physician
   d. When patient is ambulatory, assess motor skills at least every 8 hours
6. Comfort and ADL
   a. Assist patient with ADL to conserve energy
   b. Instruct patient to breathe deeply when experiencing nausea
   c. Provide fluid in small amounts; ginger ale and other effervescent soft drinks are often tolerated better than other fluids
   d. Administer antiemetics as prescribed
   e. Provide patient with moist cloth to keep lips and mouth moist
   f. Provide meticulous mouth care
   g. Provide meticulous skin care
      (1) Assess skin for pruritus and rashes
      (2) Bathe patient every day or more often if necessary using superfatted soap
      (3) Administer antipruritics (Benedryl, Periactin) as prescribed
7. Control of environment
   a. Protect patient from chilling
   b. Maintain a calm, supportive environment
   c. Institute reverse isolation if necessary
   d. Use humidifier during dry months

Most patients in acute renal failure are too ill to tolerate oral feedings, either initially or for sustained periods of time. Some patients who are able to tolerate fluids orally find that eating food compounds the nausea they experience as a result of the altered biochemical environment and accompanying gastrointestinal tract irritation. If the patient is able to tolerate *oral feedings*, dietary protein and potassium are avoided unless dialysis has been initiated. In this case modest amounts of protein and potassium are allowed, thus increasing protein available for tissue building and increasing the palatability of the diet. Foods high in carbohydrate and fat content are encouraged.

The patient in acute renal failure is weak, may be confused, and may have visual changes. The amount of supervision required during daily care must be assessed continually and appropriate actions taken to prevent injury. During the acute phase of the illness, the bio-chemical alterations may affect not only the level of awareness but also the personality of the patient. The family members and occasionally the patient will be aware of these changes, such as faltering memory or an inability to think clearly. Simple conversations that attempt to structure the environment and the situation are useful in assisting the person to maintain orientation. Frequent repetition may be necessary. The person who perceives a decreased memory or ability to think clearly is assisted to express concerns and is given reassurance that mental capacities will return with recovery of physical health.

DIURETIC PHASE

During the diuretic phase, interventions to prevent infection, maintain rest/activity balance, and maintain control of the environment are continued. Of importance during the diuretic phase is the detection of fluid

GUIDELINES FOR CARE DURING THE DIURETIC PHASE OF ACUTE RENAL FAILURE

1. Fluid and electrolyte balance
   a. Frequently assess the patient for adequate hydration
   b. Assess for changes in mental status indicative of low serum levels
   c. Assess for presence of irregular apical pulse indicative of hypokalemia (from potassium lost in urine)
2. Activity
   a. Encourage independence in ADL as tolerated
   b. Encourage early ambulation as tolerated
3. Coping with illness
   a. Encourage the development of a nurse-patient relationship that will assist the patient in expressing perceptions of illness
   b. Promote patient independence
   c. Involve patient and significant others in patient care
4. Teaching
   a. Cause of renal failure
   b. Identification of preventable environmental or health factors contributing to the illness (for example, hypertension, nephrotoxic drugs)
   c. Prescribed medication regimen
   d. Prescribed dietary regimen
   e. Signs and symptoms of returning renal failure (decreased urinary output without decreased fluid input, signs of fluid retention)
   f. Signs and symptoms of infections
   g. Need for ongoing follow-up care

and electrolyte imbalances because of the large amount of fluid excreted by the kidneys (see the box above). During this phase, the patient is usually ready for the start of the education process that is necessary for patients with kidney disease. Items to include in the teaching plan are also listed in the box above. A nursing care plan is illustrated on pages 1468-1469.

CHRONIC RENAL FAILURE

EPIDEMIOLOGY/ETIOLOGY

Chronic renal failure exists when the kidneys are no longer capable of maintaining an internal environment that is consistent with life and when return of normal renal function is not anticipated. For the majority of individuals the transition from health to a state of chronic or permanent illness is a slow process that may occur over a number of years. Recurrent infections and exacerbations of nephritis, obstruction of the urinary tract, and destruction of blood vessels from diabetes and long-standing hypertension can lead to scarring of kidney tissue and progressive loss of renal function. Some individuals, however, develop total irreversible loss of renal

function acutely. Such loss of renal function usually develops in a matter of a few hours or days and follows a direct traumatic insult to the kidneys.

Chronic renal failure remains a significant health care problem in the United States. More than 60,000 deaths each year occur as a result of renal failure. In 1986, approximately 87,505 people were being treated with dialysis.[51]

PREVENTION

Obstruction and infection of the urinary tract and hypertensive disease are common and often asymptomatic causes of renal damage and renal failure. A significant reduction in the incidence of chronic renal failure can be effected through increasing attention to general health promotion. Yearly physical examinations in which blood pressure is determined, urinalysis is performed, and the person is questioned about dysuria or pain in the urinary tract assist in early detection of disease that may lead to chronic renal failure.

General health maintenance can reduce the number of individuals who progress from renal insufficiency into frank renal failure. The goals of care are adequately treating medical problems and closely supervising the person's health status in times of stress (for example, during infection or pregnancy).

PATHOPHYSIOLOGY AND CLINICAL MANIFESTATIONS

Chronic renal failure differs from acute renal failure in that it represents progressive and irreversible damage to the kidneys. Progression of the disorder is essentially through four stages: decreased renal reserve, renal insufficiency, renal failure, and end stage renal disease (ESRD) (Table 50-2). However, in practice no sharp division of these stages is apparent. Severe symptoms occur at the renal failure stage.

The specific pathophysiologic mechanisms depend on the underlying disease entity causing the tissue destruction. However, the following general pathophysiologic mechanism summarizes these changes. During chronic renal failure, some of the nephrons (including the glomerulus and tubules) are thought to remain intact while others are destroyed (intact nephron hypothesis). The intact nephrons hypertrophy and produce an increased volume of filtrate with increased tubular reabsorption despite a decreased glomerular filtration rate (GFR). This adaptive method permits the kidney to function until about three fourths of the nephrons become destroyed. The solute load then becomes greater than can be reabsorbed, producing an osmotic diuresis with polyuria and thirst. Eventually, as more nephrons are damaged, oliguria occurs with retention of waste products.

The clinical course of chronic renal failure varies

NURSING CARE PLAN

PERSON WITH ACUTE RENAL FAILURE

DATA: Mr. Woods is a 34-year-old factory worker who was involved in an industrial accident 2 weeks ago in which he sustained a leg fracture. He was admitted to the hospital for reduction of an open fracture of his left femur. After surgery, he was started on a course of antibiotic therapy. His recovery was uneventful until yesterday; however, in the last 24 hours, he experienced a weight gain of 4 kg and became short of breath with minimal exertion. The medical diagnosis is acute renal failure.

The nursing assessment identified the following:
- He appears short of breath when in a supine position; rales are present in all lobes on auscultation of lungs
- He states feeling nauseated and doesn't want to eat.
- He states that he tires easily.

- He is oriented to person but not to place and time; he becomes easily agitated on questioning.
- Blood pressure is 150/90; baseline is 120/70.
- In the past 24 hours, fluid intake was 4800 ml; fluid output was 1900 ml.

Collaborative nursing activities include those to assess Mr. Woods' response to the therapeutic regimen and the presence of any complications associated with that regimen. Nursing actions include monitoring the following: (1) daily weights, (2) intake and output, (3) response to exertion, especially cardiac (pulse rate and rhythm) and respiratory effort, (4) breath sounds, (5) blood pressure, and (6) serum electrolytes.

NURSING DIAGNOSIS

Tissue perfusion, altered, renal, related to renal ischemia (renal artery stenosis)

Expected Patient Outcomes	Nursing Interventions	Rationale
Mr. Woods' serum nitrogen, creatinine, sodium, potassium, and bicarbonate return to normal.	1. Monitor for signs of hyperkalemia, hyponatremia, or acidosis during oliguric phase and hypokalemia during diuretic phase. 2. Assess mental status for changes (confusion, convulsions, coma). 3. Assess for signs of GI bleeding or asterixis. 4. During oliguric phase, provide bed rest and assist with ADL. 5. During diuretic phase, encourage independence in ADL and early ambulation as tolerated. 6. Provide protein-sparing diet	Early identification of complications can be life-saving. Conservation of energy will promote recovery. Decreased protein intake will modify buildup of additional serum nitrogen (kidney cannot eliminate waste products).

NURSING DIAGNOSIS

Fluid volume excess (oliguric) or deficit (diuretic), related to compromised regulatory mechanism

Expected Patient Outcomes	Nursing Interventions	Rationale
Mr. Woods' breath sounds are clear. Mr. Woods does not show signs of tissue edema or weight gain. Mr. Woods' blood pressure is stabilized within normal range.	1. Monitor central venous pressure readings. 2. Monitor weight, intake and output, vital signs (including postural signs), breath sounds (use flow sheets). 3. Assess neck veins, skin turgor, and mucous membranes; note peripheral edema. 4. Use IV control devices during oliguric phase.	Excess fluid retention may cause pulmonary or tissue edema. Because of changes in body fluids during oliguric and diuretic phases, careful monitoring is essential. Blood pressure returns to normal as fluids are controlled.

NURSING DIAGNOSIS

Infection, potential for, related to decreased nutrition and decreased immune response.

Expected Patient Outcomes	Nursing Interventions	Rationale
Mr. Woods' skin remains intact. Mr. Woods' temperature remains in normal range. Mr. Woods' breath sounds are clear.	1. Assess for signs of infection; inspect skin daily. 2. Maintain strict asepsis of indwelling catheter. 3. Promote pulmonary hygiene. 4. Assist him to turn frequently. 5. Use measures to prevent skin breakdown. 6. Avoid exposure to persons with infections. 7. Administer prescribed antibiotics on a timely basis.	Primary sites for infection are pulmonary, urinary (from indwelling catheter), and skin (from immobility). Preventive measures are high priority during this high-risk period.

NURSING CARE PLAN

PERSON WITH ACUTE RENAL FAILURE—cont'd

NURSING DIAGNOSIS

Injury, potential for, related to sensorimotor deficit, fatigue, physiologic changes

Expected Patient Outcomes	Nursing Interventions	Rationale
Mr. Woods does not experience bleeding and trauma.	1. Assess for signs of bleeding from gums, guaiac-positive stools. 2. Instruct him to use soft toothbrush. 3. Give stool softeners as needed. 4. Provide assistance as needed because of his fatigue. 5. Provide a safe environment.	Ammonia produced by breakdown of urea in GI tract leads to GI mucosal bleeding. Bleeding is increased when the mucosa is irritated. Fatigue may lead to accidental injury.

NURSING DIAGNOSIS

Nutrition, altered: less than body requirements related to anorexia, nausea, and tissue catabolism

Expected Patient Outcomes	Nursing Interventions	Rationale
Mr. Woods' body weight becomes stabilized.	1. Assess nutrient intake. 2. Give good mouth care before oral feedings. 3. Use measures to encourage eating of prescribed diet (low protein, high carbohydrate, high fat).	Adequate caloric intake is necessary to reduce tissue catabolism. The calories must come from carbohydrate and fats; until renal function returns, the body cannot get rid of protein waste products.

NURSING DIAGNOSIS

Sensory perception, altered, related to decreased sensory reception

Expected Patient Outcomes	Nursing Interventions	Rationale
Mr. Woods identifies time and place.	1. Assess mental status. 2. Orient to place and time as necessary. 3. Provide simple explanations and repeat instruction as necessary. 4. Structure environment. 5. Reassure that mental capacities will return with recovery. 6. Explain rationale for patient's behavior to family/friends.	Providing structure in a situation of uncertainty or confusion allows the person to gain control.

NURSING DIAGNOSIS

Coping, ineffective, individual, related to situational crisis.

Expected Patient Outcomes	Nursing Interventions	Rationale
Mr. Woods participates in ongoing activities.	1. Give him opportunities to express feelings about condition. 2. Involve family/friends in his care. 3. Promote his independence when appropriate.	Providing patient with opportunity to express feelings and be independent will promote ability to cope.

NURSING DIAGNOSIS

Knowledge deficit related to lack of exposure.

Expected Patient Outcomes	Nursing Interventions	Rationale
Mr. Woods describes nature of disorder and therapeutic regimen.	Teach Mr. Woods: 1. Basis of symptoms and therapy. 2. Prescribed medication and dietary regimens. 3. Signs of returning problems or infection. 4. Need for follow-up care.	Understanding the rationale of therapy may ensure compliance. Providing information on signs of any returning problems helps the patient know when to seek care.

TABLE 50-2 Stages of chronic renal failure

Stage	Characteristics
Decreased renal reserve (renal impairment)	GFR 40%-50% of normal
	BUN and serum creatinine normal
	Patient asymptomatic
Renal insufficiency	GFR 20%-40% of normal
	BUN and serum creatinine begin to rise
	Mild anemia, mild azotemia except during stress
	Nocturia, polyuria
Renal failure	GFR 10%-20% of normal
	BUN and serum creatinine increase
	Anemia, azotemia, metabolic acidosis
	Urine specific gravity low
	Polyuria, nocturia
	Symptoms of renal failure
End-stage renal disease (ESRD)	GFR <10% of normal
	BUN and serum creatinine at high levels
	Anemia, azotemia, metabolic acidosis
	Urine specific gravity fixed at 1.010
	Oliguria
	Symptoms of renal failure

greatly from individual to individual; however, there are some common features to the disease process. Signs and symptoms result from disordered fluid and electrolyte balance, alterations in regulatory functions of the body, and retention of solutes. *Anemia* results from decreased red blood cell (RBC) production because of decreased secretion of erythropoietin by the kidney. RBC survival time is also decreased. *Azotemia* (excess nitrogenous products in the blood), and *acidosis* are always present. Potassium and hydrogen ion excretion is impaired. Fluid and sodium balance is abnormal and may involve either abnormal retention or secretion of sodium and water; thus urinary volume can be increased, normal, or decreased.

With end-stage renal disease, hyperuricemia is a common finding, although the varied serum levels of uric acid seem to have no definite relationship to the exact level of kidney function.[37] Increased levels of serum phosphate are characteristic, and calcium levels may be low or normal. These findings result from decreased renal excretions of phosphate and simultaneous reduction in ionized serum calcium. Through increased production of parathormone the body may reestablish a normal serum calcium level, although this is accomplished at the expense of the individual's bone matrix.

Hypertension may or may not be present. Often with the development of end-stage renal disease blood pressure is elevated as a result of increased total body water, a renally released vasopressor, and inadequately secreted vasodepressors.[29] Glucose intolerance may be

seen, although usually not of sufficient severity to warrant treatment. The rising blood sugar level appears to be the result of an altered biochemical environment produced by the failing kidneys and does not signify the development of diabetes mellitus. As renal failure progresses, the patient develops increased pigmentation of the skin; the skin becomes sallow or brownish in tone. With more advanced and insufficiently treated renal failure, the patient may develop muscular twitching, numbness in the feet and legs, pericarditis, and pleuritis. These signs usually resolve when the patient is treated by dietary modifications, medication, and/or dialysis.

The symptoms of uremia usually develop so slowly that the patient and family often do not recall the time of onset of the illness. Symptoms generally noted as *uremia* (more correctly called *azotemia*) develop, including lethargy, headaches, physical and mental fatigue, weight loss, irritability, and depression. Anorexia, persistent nausea and vomiting, shortness of breath on either mild or no exertion, and pitting edema are symptomatic of severe loss of renal function. Pruritus may be absent, mild, or severe. Table 50-3 provides a summary of the body systems affected by chronic renal failure.

As end-stage renal failure develops, most women note changes in their menstrual cycle. Bleeding may occur at more widely spaced intervals, may be heavier or lighter in flow than normal, or may cease all together. This obvious change in reproductive cycle is usually accompanied by changes in fertility. Ovulation may occur normally or may occur only a few times a year. Pregnancy in uremic women is of much lower incidence than in the normal population. In men impotence may occur as chronic renal failure progresses toward end stage disease. Dialysis or more vigorous treatment of uremia is indicated to return or maximize reproductive function. It should be stressed that sexual activity of some persons with chronic renal failure may remain quite normal even though changes in reproductive ability are present.

The point at which the patient becomes obviously symptomatic and displays signs typical of renal failure occurs when approximately 80% to 90% of renal function has been lost (Figure 50-1). At this level of renal function, creatinine clearance values will fall to 15 ml/min or less.

CONSERVATIVE MEDICAL MANAGEMENT

The medical management of patients with chronic (end-stage) renal disease can be categorized as follows:
1. Conservative management
2. Dialysis (p. 1481)
3. Renal transplantation (p. 1491)

Conservative medical management is primarily directed toward relief of symptoms. The focus is on fluid and

TABLE 50-3 Body system manifestations in chronic renal failure

Body System	Causes	Signs/Symptoms	Assessment Parameters
Hematopoetic	Suppression of RBC production Decreased survival time of RBCs Loss of blood through bleeding Loss of blood during dialysis Mild thrombocytopenia Decreased activity of platelets	Anemia Leukocytosis Defects in platelet function Thrombocytopenia	Hematocrit Hemoglobin Platelet count Observe for bruising, hatemate- sis, melana
Cardiovascular	Fluid overload Renin-angiotensin mechanism Fluid overload, anemia Chronic hypertension Calcification of soft tissues Uremic toxins in pericardial fluid Fibrin formation on epicardium	Hypervolemia Hypertension Tachycardia Arrhythmias Congestive heart failure Pericarditis	Vital signs Body weight ECG Heart sounds Monitor electrolytes Assess for pain
Gastrointestinal	Change in platelet activity Serum uremic toxins Electrolyte imbalances Urea converted to ammonia by saliva	Anorexia Nausea and vomiting Gastrointestinal bleeding Abdominal distention Diarrhea Constipation Uremic fetor (halitosis)	Monitor intake and output Hematocrit Hemoglobin Guaiac test all stools Assess quality of stools Assess for abdominal pain
Neurologic	Uremic toxins Electrolyte imbalances Cerebral swelling resulting from fluid shifting	Lethargy, confusion Convulsions Stupor, coma Sleep disturbances Unusual behavior Asterixis Muscle irritability	Level of orientation Level of consciousness Reflexes EEG Electrolyte levels
Skeletal	Decreased calcium absorption Decreased phosphate excretion	Osteodystrophy Renal rickets Joint pain Retarded growth	Serum phosphorus Serum calcium Assess for joint pain
Skin	Anemia Pigment retained Decreased size of sweat glands Decreased activity of oil glands Dry skin; phosphate deposits	Pallor Pigmentation Pruritus Ecchymosis Excoriation Uremic frost	Observe for bruising Assess color of skin Assess integrity of skin Observe for scratching
Genitourinary	Damaged nephrons	Decreased urine output Decreased urine specific gravity Proteinuria Casts and cells in urine Decreased urine sodium	Monitor intake and output Serum creatinine BUN Serum electrolytes Urine specific gravity Urine electrolytes
Reproductive	Hormonal abnormalities Anemia Hypertension Malnutrition Medications	Infertility Decreased libido Impotence Amenorrhea Delayed puberty	Monitor intake and output Monitor vital signs Hematocrit Hemoglobin

electrolyte regulation by control of fluids, electrolytes and diet, treatment of intercurrent disorders, and patient comfort. The major treatment goals are listed in the box on p. 1472.

FLUID AND ELECTROLYTE CONTROL

Fluid Control

Changes in the ability to regulate water and sodium are often the first clinical signs of renal failure. The ability to excrete sodium and water in the urine can vary considerably from one patient with chronic renal failure to the next. Although volume problems for most patients involve hypervolemia resulting from a marked inability to excrete sodium and water, some patients are unable to conserve these substances and hypovolemia results. With either marked inability to excrete or conserve body fluid, the patient can develop severe fluid imbalances in a relatively short time. Fluid imbalances are identified

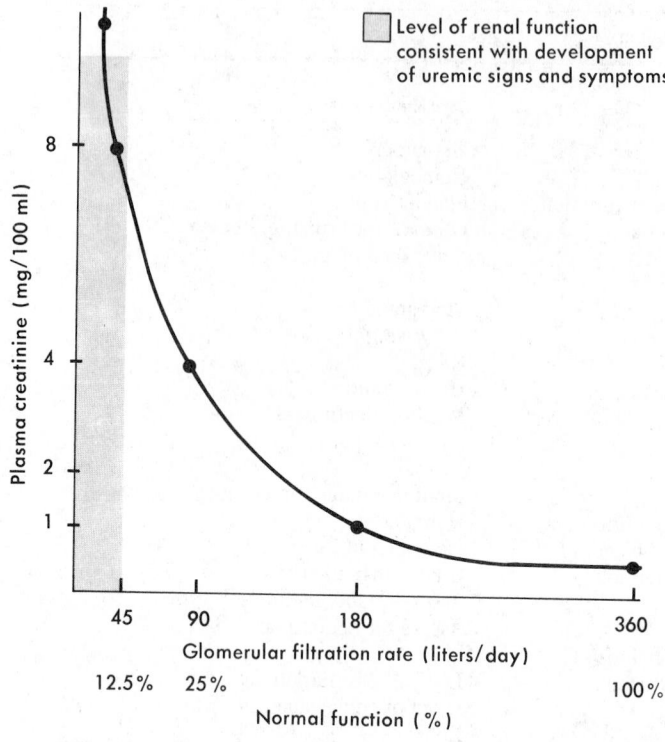

FIGURE 50-1 Glomerular filtration and plasma creatinine levels.

and an intake of sodium and water equivalent to the amount of these substances that are excreted is provided. The desired effect is to maintain the person in a normotensive, normovolemic state.

Electrolyte Control

Potassium and *phosphorus retention* occur in chronic renal failure. Serum potassium can be at least partially controlled by decreasing dietary and drug intake. Cation exchange resins may also be prescribed.

When the kidneys fail, the ability to excrete phosphorus decreases. This leads to a vicious cycle whereby Ca^{++} decreases, parathormone is stimulated, and bone demineralization occurs. Because the excess phosphorus is not excreted, calcium and phosphorus precipitate out in soft tissue. The serum phosphorus level rises again, the calcium level falls, and the cycle continues. Severe demineralization of bone may develop, and if the problem continues unabated, hyperparathyroidism can occur. Serum levels show elevated phosphorus with low to normal levels of Ca^{++}. Treatment is aimed at decreasing the serum phosphorus levels. Aluminum hydroxide preparations that bind phosphorus in the intestinal tract and allow it to be eliminated are administered in doses that range from 1 to 5 g daily. Cookies made with aluminum hydroxide may be more palatable. Aluminum hydroxide is constipating, and stool softeners or

TREATMENT GOALS FOR THE PERSON WITH CHRONIC RENAL FAILURE

1. Stabilization of the internal environment as demonstrated by:
   a. Mental alertness, attention span, and appropriate interactions
   b. Absence or control of peripheral and pulmonary edema
   c. Control of electrolyte balance within the following limits:

Sodium	125 to 145 mEq/L
Potassium	3 to 6 mEq/L
Bicarbonate	>15mEq/L
Calcium	9 to 11 mg/dl
Phosphate	3 to 5 mg/dl

   d. Serum albumin >2 g/dl
   e. Control of protein catabolism and protein metabolic wastes as indicated by the following parameters:

Urea nitrogen	<100 mg/dl
Creatinine	<10 mg/dl
Uric acid	<12 mg/dl

   f. Absence of joint inflammation and pain
2. Absence of infection
3. Absence of bleeding
4. Blood pressure is controlled at less than 160/100 mm Hg sitting, less than 30 mm Hg postural change on standing
5. Any intercurrent illness is controlled or resolved, including:
   a. Heart failure
   b. Anemia
   c. Dehydration
6. Absence of toxicity from inadequately excreted medications
7. Nutrient intake is sufficient to maintain positive nitrogen balance
8. Anorexia and nausea are controlled
9. Pruritus is controlled

laxatives may have to be given to patients receiving large doses of it.

Hypocalcemia may result not only from elevated levels of phosphorus but also from the inability of the diseased kidney to activate vitamin D. In the absence of vitamin D there is poor absorption of calcium from the intestinal tract. In some instances activated vitamin D or calcium supplements or both are prescribed.

In chronic renal failure the kidneys are unable to excrete hydrogen ions and to manufacture bicarbonate. *Metabolic acidosis* results. On the basis of laboratory data, acidosis may appear to be severe; however, persons with chronic renal failure adjust to lower serum bicarbonate levels and often do not become acutely symptomatic even when bicarbonate levels reach values of 15 to 16 mEq/L. Because of this adjustment, treatment with bicarbonate is not routine.

DIETARY CONTROL

Metabolic waste production can be significantly reduced by controlling dietary protein intake and by preventing catabolism of existing protein stores. The amount of protein allowed in the diet for the person with chronic renal failure can vary from 20 to 80 g/day. The specific level of protein intake prescribed depends on the presence of some means for clearing the products of protein breakdown from the patient's system. Dietary protein intake is more liberal for persons who have some ability to excrete wastes in the urine and for those being treated with dialysis. When restricting dietary protein, the quality of that allowed must be high.

When calories are provided in the form of carbohydrate and fat for immediate energy needs, smaller amounts of protein can suffice for cellular growth and repair. Catabolism of existing protein stores liberates nitrogenous wastes. For this reason sources of potential infection, such as indwelling catheters, are avoided, and when infection is noted, it is immediately treated.

TREATMENT OF INTERCURRENT DISORDERS

Anemia

Anemia universally accompanies chronic renal disease. Hematocrit values of 16% to 22% are not abnormal for these individuals. Dietary iron is of little value unless an iron deficiency exists. Iron is also not well absorbed by the gastrointestinal (GI) tract in chronic renal failure, and in some individuals it may cause nausea and vomiting. Since dietary sources of folate (folic acid) may be restricted in chronic renal failure, and food preparation may further decrease the amount of folate ingested by the patient, this vitamin may be given as a medication. A sufficient dose is 1 mg/day. Transfusions are not generally given unless the hematocrit level becomes extremely low and the patient is grossly symptomatic because when transfusions are given frequently, the patient's own stimulus to red cell production is decreased.

Gastrointestinal Disturbances

In patients with uremia, disturbances in fluid, electrolyte, and waste composition of body fluids produce changes in osmotic gradients in all cells. When these changes occur in the cells of the GI tract and the central nervous system, anorexia, nausea, and vomiting result. Persons with uremia are subject to *bleeding of the GI tract,* including the oral cavity. Urea is broken down to ammonia by the action of intestinal bacteria. Because ammonia is a mucosal irritant, ulceration and bleeding can occur. In addition to GI tract problems that lead to nausea and vomiting, there is a *decreased salivary flow* in persons with chronic renal disease. An ammonia smell and taste can quickly accumulate in the mouth and can further compound anorexia. Vinegar mouthwashes help neutralize the ammonia in the mouth and

promote comfort. Treatment includes administering antacids every 2 to 4 hours to decrease GI irritation. Dietary control of uremia, perhaps augmented by dialysis, helps to control disturbances in fluid, electrolyte, and water composition of body fluids and thus help to control nausea and vomiting.

Other Conditions

Hypertension is treated vigorously using a stepwise approach (see Chapter 29), starting with fluid and sodium restriction and diuretics. Other drugs are added, depending on the patient's response. Other conditions that are treated include *heart failure* and *infection.*

■ ASSESSMENT

The nursing assessment of the patient in chronic renal failure is extremely complex. The assessment must include physical, psychological, and social parameters. The basis of this assessment is the same as that described in Chapter 47 for the patient with suspected renal problems. The initial nursing history and physical assessment must elicit adequate information to generate the appropriate nursing diagnoses. An example of a comprehensive nursing history is found in Figure 50-2, and an example of a physical assessment in Figure 50-3.

The extent and nature of subsequent assessments are determined by the medical regimen and nursing diagnoses for the individual patient. The frequency of assessment is a function of the medical regimen and stability of the patient. For example, the patient being managed by conservative means may be able to go several months without follow-up assessments. On the other hand, the patient being treated with hemodialysis will require a thorough assessment at each treatment.

■ DATA ANALYSIS: NURSING DIAGNOSES

Nursing diagnoses are determined from assessment of patient data. Possible nursing diagnoses for the person with chronic renal failure may include, but are not limited to:

Diagnostic Title	Possible Etiologies
Fatigue	Anemia, decreased nutrition
Fluid volume excess	Compromised regulatory mechanism
Injury, potential for	Sensorimotor deficits, lack of awareness of environmental hazards, decreased level of consciousness
Knowledge deficit	Lack of exposure/recall, cognitive limitation
Noncompliance with medical prescription	Patient value systems, treatment side effects, cognitive/perceptual alterations

Text continued on p. 1478

HEMODIALYSIS NURSING NOTES
ADMISSION HISTORY

41   (Inpatient)/Patient Notes (Outpatient)

DATE	HOUR	
		I. Perception of Illness
		Why, initially, did you come to the hospital?
		What does the doctor plan for you while you are here?
		What do you expect to happen to you when you start dialysis?
		II. History of Past Illness (Include dates and hospitalizations).

MEDICATIONS	DOSE	FREQUENCY	LAST DOSE TAKEN	REASON FOR TAKING

Do you receive any special treatments or exercises?

III. Activity

Do you have difficulty walking or getting in and out of a chair?

Can you climb stairs?

Are you employed?

What are your usual daytime activities?

What are your recreational interests?

FIGURE 50-2 Hemodialysis nursing notes: admission history.

DATE	HOUR	IV.	Nutrition
			Are you on a special diet?
			Do you have difficutly following a diet?
			How many meals do you eat a day?
		V.	**Sleep Habits**
			Do you sleep through the night at home?
			What helps in getting to sleep at night?
			What are your usual sleeping habits?
		VI.	**Elimination**
			How often do you urinate?
			Do you have any difficulty with urination?
			Frequency Pain on urination
			Urgency Other
			Have you ever had urinary tract infections?
			24-hour urine output cc/24 hr
			Color of urine?
			What are your usual bowel habits?
			Do you have difficulty with diarrhea or constipation?
			How often do you use enemas or laxatives?
		VII.	**Reproductive System**
			When was your most recent menses?
			Have you recently had a change in menses?
			Have you had any changes in sexual function recently?
			Do you have any concerns about reproductive or sexual functions?
		VIII.	**Social**
			Do you live with anyone?
			Upon whom do you rely when you need help?
			What type of dwelling do you live in?
			Do you have to climb stairs?
			Financial resources/insurance

Admitting Nurse _____

FIGURE 50-2, cont'd. Hemodialysis nursing notes: admission history.

HEMODIALYSIS NURSING NOTES
ADMISSION ASSESSMENT

41   (Inpatient)/Patient Notes (Outpatient)

DATE	HOUR	A) Vital Signs			
		Temperature			
		Pulses	Apical		
			Radial		
			Rhythm		
		Weight			
		Height			
		B) Cardiopulmonary			
		Vascular Access			
		Peripheral Pulses:	Right		Left
		Radial			
		Femoral			
		Popliteal			
		Pedal			
		Peripheral Edema?			
		Periorbital Edema?			
		Friction Rub?			
		Neck Vein Distention?			
		Cough?	Sputum?		Smoking Habits?
		Adventitious Breath Sounds?			
		Shortness of Breath?			
		Orthopnea?			
		C) Neuromuscular			
		Orientation			
		Level of Alertness and Responsiveness?			
		Muscle Tone and Strength, Symmetry?			
		Weakness or Loss of Function of Extremities?			
		Balance			
		Numbness, Tingling or Tremors?			

FIGURE 50-3 Hemodialysis nursing notes: admission assessment.

DATE	HOUR	Patient Experiencing Difficulties with:
		Sight
		Speech
		Touch
		Taste/Smell
		D) Skin
		Color
		Turgor
		Temperature
		Lesions
		Condition of Nails
		E) General
		Presence of:
		Nausea
		Vomiting
		Headache
		Blurring of Vision
		Ability to perform ADL

Admitting Nurse _____

FIGURE 50-3, cont'd. Hemodialysis nursing notes: admission assessment.

Diagnostic Title	Possible Etiologies
Nutrition, altered: less than body requirements	Anorexia, nausea, decreased salivary flow, bad taste, pain
Pain: muscle cramping, pruritus, ocular irritation	Sodium depletion, uremia
Role performance, altered	Changes in social environment
Self-esteem, decreased	Changes in body appearance, change in social involvement
Sexual dysfunction	Physiologic limitations, stress
Skin integrity, impaired, potential	Immobility, edema, pressure points
Urinary elimination, altered patterns	Decreased urine production, motor impairment

■ PLANNING: EXPECTED PATIENT OUTCOMES

Expected patient outcomes for the person with chronic renal failure vary depending on the course of the disorder and the identified nursing diagnoses. Expected patient outcomes may include the following:

1. The patient will maintain fluid and electrolyte balance.
2. The patient does not experience injury and infection.
3. The patient does not become overly fatigued or short of breath.
4. The patient indicates plans to follow prescribed diet and fluid restrictions.
5. The patient states feeling more comfortable.
6. The patient can describe:
   a. The nature of the disorder
   b. Preventive health care measures
   c. Measures to monitor and control fluid balance
   d. Dietary regimen
   e. Medication regimen
   f. Plans for physical activity modified by rest
   g. Measures to promote comfort and minimize pruritus
   h. Plans for health care follow-up

■ IMPLEMENTATION

Because the condition of the person with chronic renal failure can vary to a considerable extent, nursing care focuses on the specific identified nursing diagnoses. Most persons, however, require some help or teaching to maintain fluid and electrolyte balance; prevent infection or injury; promote comfort, rest, and sleep; and cope with the effects of the disorder (see the box below.

MAINTAINING FLUID AND ELECTROLYTE BALANCE

The person with chronic renal failure must learn how to identify signs of imbalances, take fluids in the prescribed amounts, and eat within the prescribed limits.

Controlling sodium intake can be an extremely challenging problem for both the nurse and the patient. Any sudden increase in weight indicates accumulating fluid, and the source of this fluid must be sought with the patient. Often when the patient is not acutely ill and is responsible for diet restrictions, the problem can be traced to excess sodium ingestion, which produces thirst. In helping to avoid this cycle of sodium-driven thirst lead-

---

G UIDELINES FOR CARE OF THE PERSON WITH CHRONIC RENAL FAILURE

1. Maintain fluid and electrolyte balance
   a. Monitor for fluid and electrolyte excess
      (1) Assess intake and output every 8 hours
      (2) Weigh patient every day
      (3) Assess presence and extent of edema
      (4) Auscultate breath sounds
      (5) Monitor cardiac rhythm and blood pressure every 8 hours
      (6) Assess level of consciousness every 8 hours
   b. Encourage patient to remain within prescribed fluid restrictions
   c. Provide small quantities of fluid spaced over the day to stay within fluid restrictions
   d. Encourage a diet high in carbohydrates and within the prescribed sodium, potassium, phosphorus, and protein limits
   e. Administer phosphate binding agents (Basaljel, AlternaGEL, Amphojel) with meals as prescribed
2. Prevent infection and injury
   a. Promote meticulous skin care
   b. Encourage activity within prescribed limits but avoid fatigue
   c. Protect confused person from injury
   d. Protect person from exposure to infectious agents
   e. Maintain good medical/surgical asepsis during treatments and procedures
   f. Avoid aspirin products
   g. Encourage use of soft toothbrush
3. Promote comfort
   a. Medicate patient as needed for pain
   b. Medicate with prescribed antipruritics, use emollient baths, keep skin moist, and control environmental temperature to modify pruritus
   c. Encourage use of damp cloth to keep lips moist; give good oral hygiene
   d. Encourage rest for fatigue; however, encourage self-care as tolerated
   e. Provide calm, supportive atmosphere
4. Assist with coping in lifestyle and self-concept
   a. Promote hope
   b. Provide opportunity for patient to express feelings about self
   c. Identify available community resources

ing to increased fluid ingestion and overhydration, the patient is carefully taught about the amount of sodium and fluid allowed in the diet and what restrictions are to be observed in purchasing prepared foods. The words "sodium" and "salt" should be sought on all food labels when the person is on a severely sodium-restricted diet. Salt substitutes should be avoided by all patients with chronic renal failure because these substitutes contain large amounts of potassium.

At times the patient is unable to offer an explanation for increasing thirst and sodium ingestion. At this point the question of home self-medication is raised. The person may be taking over-the-counter antacids that are high in sodium. If the cause of the hypervolemia cannot be identified, the patient is asked to list all foods and fluids ingested over the period of 3 consecutive days. This list can be used to uncover dietary indiscretions as well as a teaching tool to reinforce the prescribed diet.

Persons usually need help in planning diets within the prescribed sodium, potassium, phosphorus, and protein limits. Modifying the diet as possible to the preferences of the individual can help to maintain intake of food. Dietary teaching and meal planning can be approached according to an exchange system similar to that used for persons with diabetes.

Actual eating of prepared food can be promoted through attempting to decrease emotional tension at the dinner table. Food that is attractively arranged and well flavored is also likely to encourage eating. Herbs and other flavorings can add variety to foods that are prepared without sodium. When the GI tract is ulcerated, bland foods may be tried in an attempt to increase ingestion of food.

PREVENTING INFECTION AND INJURY

Tissue breakdown leads to infection and significant rises in serum potassium, and thus must be avoided. Potassium is largely an intracellular cation, and extensive tissue damage can liberate a lethal amount of this ion into the system of the person with chronic renal failure. Edematous skin poses a high risk for skin breakdown; therefore, meticulous skin care is important. Patients with chronic renal failure should avoid others with infections; avoid fatigue, which lowers body resistance; and seek medical attention when symptoms of infections, GI bleeding, or other problems first appear.

Aluminum hydroxide, prescribed to bind phosphorus in the intestinal tract is best taken at mealtimes. It should not be taken with other medications because it can bind drugs in the intestinal tract. Because aluminum hydroxide is constipating, stool softeners or laxatives may be needed. The risk of constipation is also high in persons with chronic renal failure because of the fluid restrictions.

Other important nursing activities include helping the patient to control blood losses. A soft toothbrush is recommended for oral care. The patient is instructed to observe for melena and to report this without delay to the physician. Aspirin should be avoided because it is normally excreted by the kidneys and may rapidly build to toxic levels and prolong bleeding time. Anabolic steroids may be used, but the side effect of fluid retention may limit their usefulness.

The buildup of osmotically active particles and fluid in the body that occurs with azotemia produces changes in the cells of the brain that may lead to confusion and impairment in decision-making ability. Fluid accumulation and hypertension can produce visual changes. The person's environment is assessed for potential for injury. At times the person may need help in limiting activities to a level commensurate with mental processes and level of awareness. For example, blurred vision and delayed reaction time contraindicate driving an automobile.

PROMOTING COMFORT, REST, AND SLEEP

Rarely does the patient with chronic renal failure have acute, sharp pain; however, these persons are subject to a wide variety of chronic discomforts, including pruritus, muscle cramping, headaches, ocular irritation, and insomnia.

Most patients with end-stage renal disease develop *pruritus;* they describe a sensation of deep itching. Itching is largely symptomatic, and measures that are effective in controlling it vary from person to person. Reducing levels of serum phosphorus with aluminum hydroxide preparations decreases itching for most patients. Medications such as trimeprazine tartrate (Temaril) may prove effective for some patients. Keeping the skin moist and supple through use of lotions and bath oils, controlling the room temperature during sleep to prevent excessive warmth, and bathing with emollients or a vinegar solution are measures alone or in combination that may provide some relief from itching. (See Chapter 73 for a discussion of pruritus.) Since emotional stress seems to increase the itching, helping the patient verbalize feelings may provide for some resolution of conflict and help decrease itching. The urge to scratch the skin is acute in some patients. Because scratching is often vigorous, injury to the skin with subsequent infection can result. Fingernails are trimmed closely. In preference to fingernails, a soft cloth should be used to scratch the skin.

Muscle cramping in the lower extremities and the *hands* is common in renal failure. Often cramping can be correlated with sodium depletion. Primary treatment for muscle cramping involves controlling the state of uremia and fluid and electrolyte balance. Temporary measures of heat and massage are effective for some persons.

Ocular irritation in chronic renal failure is caused by calcium deposits in the conjunctiva that cause burning and watering of the eyes. Treatment involves controlling the plasma phosphate level through administration of oral aluminum hydroxide preparations. "Artificial tears" (methylcellulose) placed in the conjunctival sac every few hours also help to reduce irritation.

Insomnia and *chronic daytime fatigue* are common complaints of persons with chronic renal failure. This reversal of normal sleep patterns has been attributed to a variety of causes. These include (1) recurring occupation with thoughts concerning the disease state and resultant changes in lifestyle, (2) pruritus, and (3) the state of uremia itself. Reduction of high serum levels of urea nitrogen and creatinine through decreasing dietary intake of protein or dialysis may bring sleep patterns more toward normal. When control of uremia fails to cure insomnia, mild central nervous system depressants may be prescribed.

The severely anemic person complains of extreme fatigue and shortness of breath. Because of a lack of RBCs there is an inability to transport sufficient oxygen to cells for energy production. The anemic person may be unable to work or play without extended rest periods. Rest periods should be taken early enough in the day to prevent sleeplessness at night.

General comfort at bedtime is needed to induce sleep at any time and is especially important whenever sleeping problems arise. Comfort measures can include tepid baths, pursuing quiet activities an hour or two before bedtime, controlling itching, or anything the patient finds calming and soothing.

FACILITATING COPING WITH CHANGES IN LIFESTYLE AND FEELINGS REGARDING SELF

Numerous alterations in lifestyle, group membership, and feelings about the self occur for the patient with chronic renal failure. The numerous physical changes that occur often make it difficult to carry on activities that were once normally pursued. *Chronic fatigue* may make it impossible for the patient to continue to be used. Because the patient is often tired and not feeling well, it may be difficult to plan in advance for social events. The former roles of the sick member of the family must often be taken on by another. When roles cannot easily be changed or additionally assumed by other members of the family, serious threats to the organization of the family group occur. Physical appearance also changes and is of much concern to most patients. As uremia progresses, the individual often becomes thin and weaker and appears sallow. Thoughts concerning death and the quality of life are common.

Denial often becomes a chief defense mechanism for the patient. With it the individual can periodically forget the constant threat of life. The use of this mental mechanism for the person with chronic renal failure can be

quite appropriate as long as it is not manifested by maladaptive or harmful behavior. Inappropriate uses of denial involve continuous dietary indiscretion and failure to take prescribed medications.

Patients with chronic renal failure need encouragement and the hope that discomfort will be lessened with treatment, and they will be allowed to pursue what seems most productive and important to them. Hope should not be focused on cure, but on learning to manage a new lifestyle. In managing the changes that occur as a result of chronic renal failure, the patients are encouraged to be as independent and as active as possible. Patients should be taught to manage the treatment and should be given the responsibility of doing so. Nursing care should be provided as part of the team approach that assists patients in identifying problems and resources to meet them, and helps patients and their families adjust to the changes in lifestyle.

PATIENT TEACHING

The person with end-stage renal disease presents a unique opportunity for the nurse to promote optimal health through teaching and counseling. Important points to be included in patient teaching are listed in the box below. Education about medications is carried out in areas of both prescribed medications and over-

---

TEACHING THE PATIENT WITH CHRONIC RENAL FAILURE

1. Relationships between symptoms and their causes
2. Relationships among diet, fluid restriction, medication, and blood chemistries
3. Preventive health care measures: good oral hygiene, prevention of infection, avoidance of bleeding
4. Dietary regimen including fluid restrictions
   a. Prescribed sodium, potassium, phosphorus, and protein restrictions
   b. Means of identifying contents of foods
   c. Use of small frequent feedings to maintain nutrient intake when anorexic or nauseated
   d. Fluid prescription and sources of fluid in diet
   e. Avoidance of salt substitutes containing potassium
5. Monitoring for fluid excess
   a. Accurate measurement and recording of intake and output
   b. Monitoring for weight gain and edema
6. Medications
   a. Actions, doses, purpose, and side effects of prescribed medications
   b. Avoidance of over-the-counter drugs, especially aspirin and cold medications
7. Plan for gradual increase in physical activity including rest periods to conserve energy
8. Measures to control pruritus
9. Plans for follow-up health care
   a. Symptoms requiring immediate medical attention: changes in urine output, edema, weight gain, dyspnea, infection, increased symptoms of uremia
   b. Need for continual medical follow-up

the-counter or folk medicines. All medications taken by the person with chronic renal failure should be prescribed by the physician. Many cold preparations contain large amounts of sodium. Remembering to take prescribed medications can be a problem for the person who may have to take over two dozen pills each day. Thus "noncompliance" for medications may actually be simply difficulty in memory. Correlating pill-taking times with major activities of the day and use of aids to separate out the day's pills are helpful.

DIALYSIS

In 1960, a person with end-stage renal disease (ESRD) was treated for the first time with chronic intermittent hemodialysis by means of an artificial kidney.[19] That individual was successfully treated for more than 14 years. Before that time many patients were treated for acute renal failure with hemodialysis; however, once it was determined that the kidney disease was irreversible, the treatment was withdrawn. This practice continues today in many industrialized countries around the world.

In 1972, the United States Congress enacted legislation that provides for payment of health care costs for all U.S. citizens with ESRD.[20] Under this legislation, any person with documented chronic uremia is provided benefits under Medicare. As a result of this legislation, many persons are able to live extended lives. By December of 1986, almost 87,505 persons were on some form of dialysis.

Many technologic advances have been made in the treatment of persons with ESRD. Drastic changes in ar-

tificial kidneys allow for more efficient and comfortable hemodialysis treatments. Advances in the development of dialysis machines allow individuals the convenience of treatment in their own homes. Developments in peritoneal dialysis permit patients to treat themselves with continuous peritoneal and intermittent peritoneal dialysis. These advances provide persons with the opportunity to have more control over meeting their own health care needs.

Dialysis involves the movement of fluid and particles across a semipermeable membrane. It is a treatment that can help restore normal fluid and electrolyte balance, control acid-base balance, and remove waste and toxic material from the body. It is a treatment that can sustain life successfully in both acute and chronic situations where substitution for or augmentation of normal renal function is needed. Specifically, dialysis is used to remove excessive amounts of drugs and toxins in poisonings of both an intentional and accidental nature, to correct serious electrolyte and acid-base imbalances, to maintain kidney function when renal shutdown occurs as a result of transfusion reactions, to temporarily replace renal function in persons with acute renal failure of various origins, and to permanently substitute for loss of renal function in persons with chronic end-stage renal disease.

PHYSIOLOGIC PRINCIPLES OF DIALYSIS

Dialysis is based on three principles: diffusion, osmosis, and ultrafiltration (Figure 50-4). *Diffusion* involves the movement of particles from an area of greater to an area of lesser concentration. In the body this usually occurs across a semipermeable membrane. Diffusion is in-

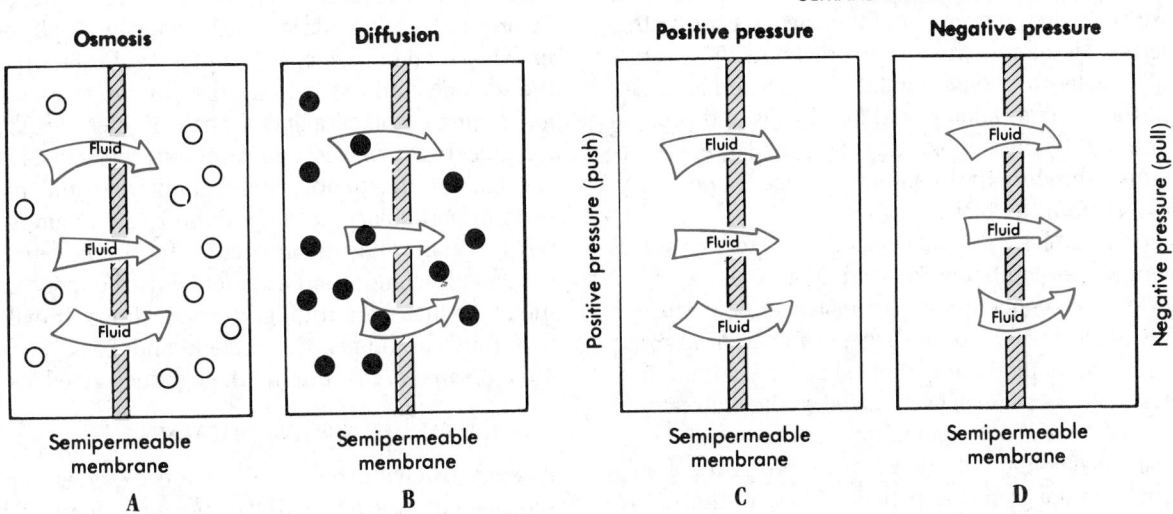

FIGURE 50-4 Dialysis is based on principles of osmosis: **A,** diffusion **B,** and ultrafiltration. Ultrafiltration occurs when either positive pressure **C,** or negative pressure **D,** is placed on system. Ultrafiltration can be maximized by exerting both positive and negative pressure on system simultaneously.

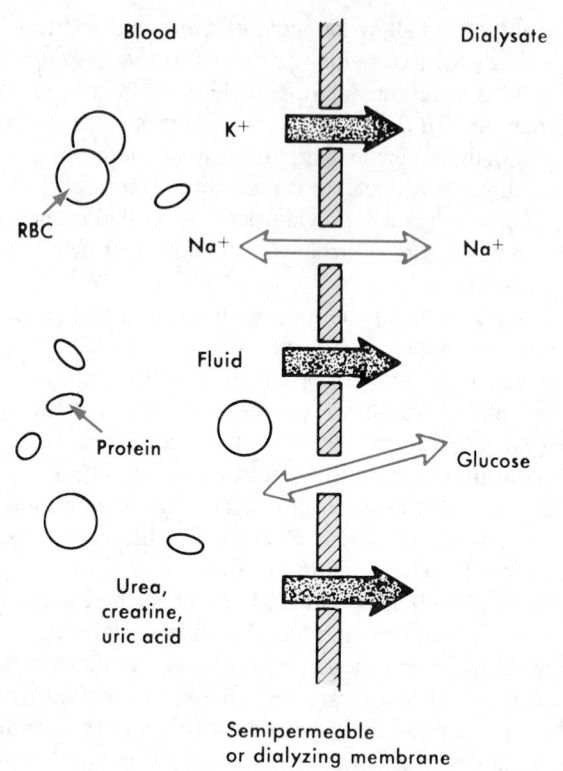

FIGURE 50-5 Osmosis and diffusion in dialysis. Net movement of major particles and fluid is illustrated.

volved in the clearance of solute from the patient's body in both hemodialysis and peritoneal dialysis. Diffusion results in the movement of urea, creatinine, and uric acid from the patient's blood into the dialysate solution. This solution contains fewer particles to be removed from the bloodstream and high concentrations of particles to be added to the blood (Figure 50-5). Since the dialysate contains no protein waste products, the concentration of these substances in the blood will decrease because of random movement of the particles across the semipermeable membrane into the dialysate. The same principle applies to the movement of potassium ions. Although the concentration of red blood cells and protein is high in blood, these molecules are quite large and do not diffuse through the membrane pores; hence they are not lost from the blood.

Osmosis involves the movement of water across a semipermeable membrane from an area of lesser to an area of greater concentration (osmolality) of particles. Osmosis is responsible for movement of extra fluid from the patient, particularly in peritoneal dialysis. Figure 50-5 shows that glucose has been added to the dialysate to make its particle concentration greater than that of the patient's blood. Fluid will then move through the pores of the membrane from the patient's blood to the dialysate.

Ultrafiltration involves the movement of fluid across a semipermeable membrane as a result of an artifically

created pressure gradient. Ultrafiltration is more efficient than osmosis for removal of fluid and is used in hemodialysis for this purpose. During dialysis, osmosis and diffusion or ultrafiltration and diffusion occur simultaneously.

HEMODIALYSIS
PROCEDURE

Hemodialysis involves shunting the patient's blood from the body through a dialyzer in which diffusion and ultrafiltration occur and back into the patient's circulation. To perform hemodialysis there must be access to the patient's blood, a mechanism to transport the blood to and from the dialyzer, and a dialyzer (area in which the exchange of fluid electrolytes and waste products occurs). Currently, there are five major means for gaining access to the patient's bloodstream. These include the following:

1. Arteriovenous fistula (Figure 50-6, *A*)
2. Arteriovenous graft (Figure 50-6, *B*)
3. External arteriovenous shunt (Figure 50-6, *C*)
4. Femoral vein catheterization (Figure 50-6, *D*)
5. Subclavian vein catheterization (Figure 50-6, *E*)

The indications and nursing implications for each access are summarized in Table 50-4.

Many patients expect to leave the dialysis treatment with a feeling of well-being. Few persons feel this way; most experience some minor discomfort that diminishes within several hours after dialysis. The greatest feeling of well-being seems to occur the day after dialysis.

Immediately before dialysis the patient is weighed, vital signs are taken, a sample of blood is drawn to determine the level of serum electrolytes and waste products, and the patient's physical status is assessed. Nursing care of the patient during hemodialysis centers around (1) monitoring the physical status of the patient before and during dialysis for evidence of physiologic imbalance and change, (2) comfort and safety needs of the patient, and (3) helping the patient to understand and adjust to the care and changes in lifestyle. This latter objective involves educating the person as to the specifics of the treatment program (diet and medications in particular) and how these relate to altered kidney function. The person is encouraged to express concerns and feelings, and attempts must be made to help the individual work through these feelings. If dialysis is performed at home, the patient and back-up person must be able to institute all the care described.

■ DATA ANALYSIS: NURSING DIAGNOSES

Patients receiving hemodialysis are experiencing endstage, renal disease (ESRD); therefore, it must be remembered that numerous nursing diagnoses are ongoing during hemodialysis that are not specific to hemodialysis. Additional nursing diagnoses pertinent to hemo-

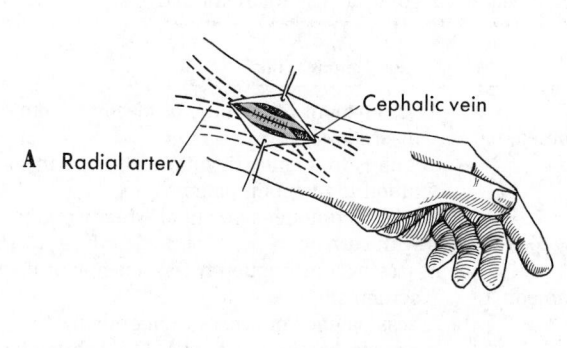

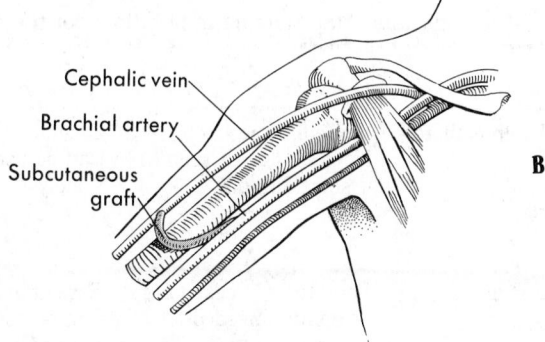

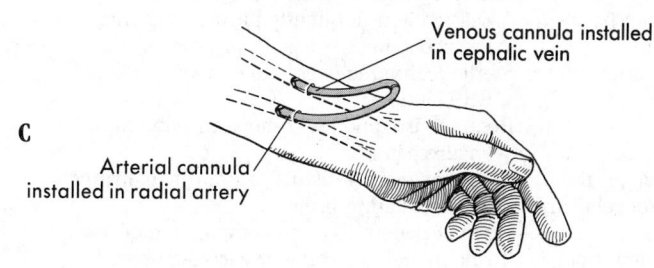

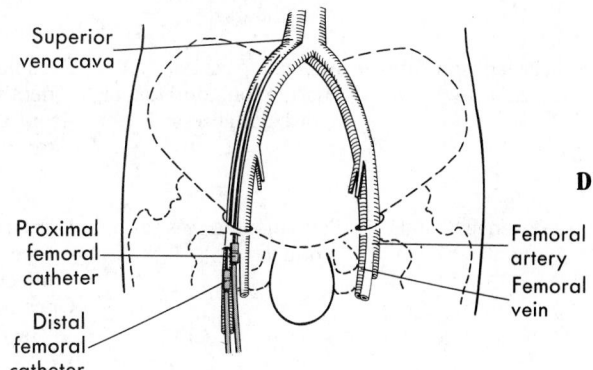

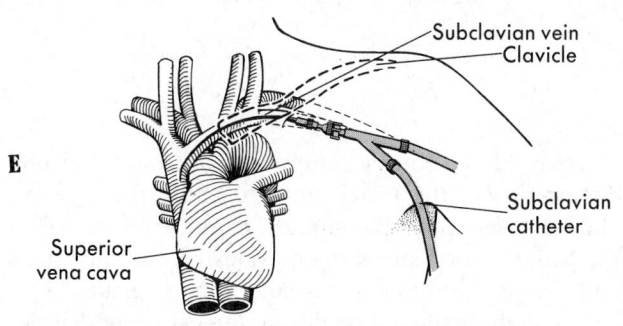

FIGURE 50-6 Frequently used means for gaining vascular access for hemodialysis include **A,** arteriovenous fistula, **B,** arteriovenous graft, **C,** external arteriovenous shunt, **D,** femoral vein catheterization, and **E,** subclavian vein catheterization.

dialysis may include, but are not limited to, the following:

Diagnostic Title	Possible Etiologies
Activity intolerance	Immobility, anemia
Anxiety	Effects of dialysis
Coping, ineffective, individual	Personal vulnerability
Diversional activities, deficit	Frequent lengthy treatments
Fluid volume deficit	Overvigorous dialysis
Hypothermia	Cooling of blood during dialysis
Infection, potential for	Vascular access, inadequate nutrition
Injury, potential for	Immobility, anticoagulants, mental confusion
Knowledge deficit	Lack of exposure/recall of hemodialysis effects
Nutrition, altered: less than body requirements	Effects of dialysis

Diagnostic Title	Possible Etiologies
Pain	Needle insertion for dialysis, headache and cramping during dialysis
Role performance, altered	Changes in social involvement
Sexual dysfunction	Physiologic limitations, stress, side effects of medications
Skin integrity, impaired potential	Immobility, edema, pressure points

■ **PLANNING: EXPECTED PATIENT OUTCOMES**

Expected patient outcomes for the person on hemodialysis include, but are not limited to, the following:

1. Patient achieves dry weight during dialysis.
2. Patient participates in a program to maintain activity levels.

TABLE 50-4 Indications and nursing implications for the major types of vascular access for hemodialysis

Type	Indications	Advantages	Nursing Implications
Femoral vein catheterization	Immediate access Need for access seen as short duration	Ease of access Can be used immediately	Assess patient frequently for bleeding from insertion sites Requires frequent irrigation with heparin solution to maintain patency Sterile technique is essential when working with catheters
External shunt	Long term (weeks to months) needed for vascular access Access required within a few hours	Ease of access Can be used immediately	Assess patient frequently for bleeding at insertion site Assess patency of access frequently by observing continuous flow of blood through shunt Shunt is potential source of infection
Subclavian vein catheterization	Immediate access Short or long duration of vascular access	Does not restrict patient's activity Requires only one catheter	Assess patient frequently for bleeding from insertion site Sterile technique is essential when working with catheter Requires irrigation with heparin solution to ensure patency
Arteriovenous fistula and graft	Permanent access required	Is least likely of all the accesses to develop an infection Once maintained it provides easy access	Assess patency of fistula or graft by palpating or auscultating bruit Instruct patient to avoid compression of fistula by tight clothing or carrying objects with arm bent Patient must be instructed to assess fistula for signs and symptoms of infection including pain, redness, swelling, or excessive warmth

3. Patient participates in diversional activities while on dialysis (such as art or music therapy programs).
4. Patient has no injury or infection.
5. Patient shows signs of decreased anxiety.
6. Patient states that discomfort decreases.
7. Patient describes the nature of dialysis, care of venous access routes, side effects, and work/activity schedule.

■ IMPLEMENTATION

Preventing Hypovolemia and Shock

Most physical problems that occur during dialysis are related to hypotension from removal of fluid and disequilibrium from a rapid reduction in extracellular electrolytes and wastes. *Hypovolemia* and *shock* can occur during dialysis as a result of rapid removal of fluid from the intravascular compartment. Because this can occur faster than reequilibration of intracellular and intravascular volume relationships, the person may appear edematous and yet exhibit signs of shock. Signs and symptoms that indicate that the intravascular volume is being rapidly depleted are anxiety, restlessness, dizziness, nausea and vomiting, diaphoresis, tachycardia, and hypotension.

To avoid depleting the intravascular space and producing shock, the blood pressure and pulse rate are checked every 30 to 60 minutes, more frequently when the patient shows any of the previously mentioned signs and symptoms. Blood pressure readings should show only a slight gradual drop during the course of dialysis. Because the rate and pressure at which blood flows through the dialyzer are proportional to the rate and amount of fluid removed, blood flow and dialyzer pressure settings are carefully monitored. (A flow rate of 200 to 250 ml of blood per minute is a reasonable rate for an adult.) Unless the individual is severely hypertensive, rapid-acting antihypertensive medications are usually withheld the morning of dialysis until after the treatment has been completed. Additionally, sedative drugs (analgesics, tranquilizers, hypnotics) and those primarily affecting the vasculature (nitroglycerin) predispose the patient to hypotensive episodes. Self-medication with these agents before and during dialysis must be carefully reviewed with each patient.

In treating a patient who shows signs of hypovolemia, initial nursing measures include determining the blood pressure and pulse, placing the head of the bed in a flat position, and raising the patient's feet. The ultrafiltration pressure is decreased and fluid replacement may be necessary to restore blood pressure. Throughout a hypotensive episode, vital signs, level of consciousness, and any complaints offered are closely monitored. It is important for the nurse to know that vomiting frequently accompanies severe hypotension. Because an upper extremity must be maintained fairly immobile during the dialysis, it may be awkward for the patient to clear the mouth if vomiting should occur. The patient is helped to a safe position so that aspiration is avoided.

The patient is weighed before and after dialysis to determine amount of fluid loss during treatment. When the weight losses of several dialysis treatments are correlated with the patient's blood pressure, pulse, and other indications of hypovolemia, an individual pattern of the patient's tolerance to fluid removal can be determined. This trend or pattern can be used to help adjust the rate and overall effect of the dialysis in keeping with the patient's physiologic tolerance.

Preventing Disequilibrium Phenomenon

A disequilibrium phenomenon occurs for many dialysis patients. This syndrome occurs toward the end of or after dialysis. Disequilibrium results when excess solutes (urea) are cleared from the blood more rapidly than they can diffuse from the body's cells (particularly those of the central nervous system) into the vascular compartment. Hence, disequilibrium exists in the concentration of solute inside and outside the cells. Since particle content is greater inside the cells, water is taken in and edema results. Intracellular pH changes are also present. To some degree, this process occurs with all patients with each dialysis procedure and helps to explain why patients do not feel their best immediately after treatment. *Severe disequilibrium* or *disequilibrium phenomenon* is most likely to be seen in the person whose blood chemistry values are exceptionally high before dialysis. Signs and symptoms of disequilibrium include *headache, hypertension, restlessness, mental confusion,* and *nausea* and *vomiting.* Severe disequilibrium may result in convulsions, especially in children, when blood urea nitrogen levels exceed the concentration of 100 mg/ml.

Treatment includes anticipation of severe disequilibrium. Often when a patient is beginning dialysis treatments, the procedures are kept short and may be spaced more frequently than normal during the first week. This allows solute to be cleared from the body without producing the extremely wide swings in body chemistry that would result in severe disequilibrium. Keeping the patient quiet, reducing environmental discomfort such as temperature extremes and bright lights, and closely supervising the patient to ensure physical safety are nursing care requirements. Mild analgesics may help to relieve headache. If disequilibrium becomes severe and the patient is still on dialysis, the therapy may be discontinued.

Preventing Blood Loss

Care of the patient on dialysis should also include preventing *blood loss.* To prevent the patient's blood from clotting as it flows through the dialyzer, heparin is administered. Protamine sulfate is not generally given to the patient to counteract the effect of heparin. The patient is watched for signs of bleeding anywhere in the body. At the end of the treatment when dialysis needles are removed from the fistula, pressure dressings are applied to the puncture sites. They are observed at frequent intervals to detect hemorrhage. During and shortly after dialysis, treatments that cause tissue trauma should not be performed. These commonly include venipuncture and intramuscular injections. The patient who has had recent surgery, dental extractions, or recent trauma to soft tissues will have clotting times monitored frequently during dialysis to prevent hemorrhage. These patterns need to be closely observed for signs of bleeding.

Providing Comfort

Lying relatively immobile for even a few hours can produce pressure over bony prominences and general restlessness. Changing the patient's position increases tolerance to limited movement. Mouth care is required if the patient is nauseated and vomiting. Because an upper extremity is generally kept immobile during dialysis, the patient may need help with activities requiring the use of both hands.

Before the procedure, patients should have an opportunity to become familiar with the dialysis unit. They should be given an explanation of what will happen and what will be expected of them during the treatment. Patients often want to know (1) what types of pain will be experienced during the treatment, (2) how long and how often the dialysis will be, (3) what they should feel like during and after the treatment, (4) what they will be allowed to do during dialysis, and (5) if family members may be present during the therapy.

When the patient has an external shunt, no pain should be experienced during initiation of dialysis. However, pain of a moderate degree may be present when venipuncture is performed in an arteriovenous fistula. A local anesthetic is used in most dialysis centers before insertion of the large bore needles.

Patients should be told that they may experience some headache and nausea during the treatment and for a few hours afterward. Headache and nausea result from change in fluid, acid-base, and waste balance during dialysis. The symptoms should never be extreme, and relief should be attained from rest and sleep, mild analgesics, or antiemetics. Postural hypotension may also occur after dialysis; it is transitory in nature and caused by a relative depletion of intravascular volume secondary to fluid removal. The hypotension may produce dizziness and faintness. Relief should be obtained within a few hours with rest. The patient is assured that all of these symptoms will abate and that frequent monitoring during the procedure will help to control the degree of change that occurs during dialysis and the development of these symptoms.

Maintaining Activity and Nutrition

A dialysis treatment lasts from 3 to 5 hours, depending on the type of dialyzer used and the time necessary to correct the fluid, electrolyte, acid-base, and waste problems that are present. Dialysis for an acute problem may be carried out daily or as often as the condition of the patient warrants. Hemodialysis for renal failure is usually performed two or three times a week. Activity during dialysis is largely a matter of individual preference. Some persons sleep throughout treatment; others read or carry on various activities.

Eating during dialysis is largely a matter of individual preference. Some individuals may become quite hungry, whereas for others the smell of food causes nausea. Patients may ask that they be allowed to eat foods not generally allowed during dialysis. Practice indicates that either allowing or discouraging eating freely during dialysis is a matter of individual unit philosophy. Because of the frequency of nausea, vomiting, and disequilibrium many patients experience during hemodialysis, it may be best to discourage eating to decrease the potential of aspiration.

Patient Teaching

The person or significant others can state, demonstrate, or plan the following:

1. The process of hemodialysis and relate to own body needs
2. Observations required of vascular access about infection and clotting as well as state means of obtaining care when these occur
3. Appropriate care of venous access
4. Common side effects of treatment, means for controlling mild symptoms, and means of obtaining medical attention for severe or persistent complications
5. Changes in medication schedule required before and after dialysis
6. A work and activity schedule as physical capabilities permit with minimal interference from scheduled dialysis time (see the research box above).

An example of a teaching care plan for the person on hemodialysis is illustrated in the box on pp. 1488-1489.

PERITONEAL DIALYSIS

In peritoneal dialysis the dialyzing fluid is instilled into the peritoneal cavity and the peritoneum becomes the dialyzing membrane (Figure 50-7). In comparison with

RESEARCH

Ferrans CE and Powers MJ: The employment potential of hemodialysis patients, Nurs Res 34:273-277, 1985.

The purpose of this study was to examine factors that may influence employment for persons experiencing dialysis. The subjects were 40 hemodialysis patients divided into two equal groups of those currently employed and those unemployed but rated by the physician to be able to work. All subjects had been employed before start of dialysis. The groups did not differ significantly in terms of biophysical status, perceptions of health, life satisfaction, dependence, or job satisfaction before dialysis. The family income of persons in both groups decreased 20% by the employed and 60% by the unemployed. In the employed group, 35% had changed jobs after dialysis without discrimination, whereas 25% of the unemployed stated being rejected for jobs and 10% were fired. A greater percentage of the employed were college educated, whereas a large number of the unemployed had held jobs requiring moderate or heavy physical labor.

Nursing implications consist of identifying persons who are receiving initial dialysis and who had physically taxing occupations and providing counseling about job changes and retraining. ■

---

hemodialysis treatments, which last 3 to 6 hours, peritoneal dialysis is maintained continuously for up to 36 hours. The procedure, once instituted, becomes largely a nursing responsibility. Peritoneal dialysis is used in treating acute and chronic renal failure. It can be performed in the hospital or at home (see p. 1430).

The major advantages of peritoneal dialysis include the following:

1. Provides a steady state of blood chemistries
2. Patient can dialyze alone in any location without need for machinery
3. Patient can readily be taught process
4. Patient has few dietary restrictions; because of loss of protein in dialysate the patient is usually placed on a high protein diet
5. Patient has much more control over daily life
6. Can be used for patients that are hemodynamically unstable

Procedure

Access to the peritoneum is gained through introduction of a catheter into the peritoneal space. For acutely ill patients and those who are chronically ill and require sporadic dialysis, a sterile catheter is inserted for each procedure. For the chronically ill person treated on a routine basis, a special catheter can be placed into the peritoneal space; the catheter remains until it malfunctions or another form of treatment is selected for the patient. These catheters present a continued potential en-

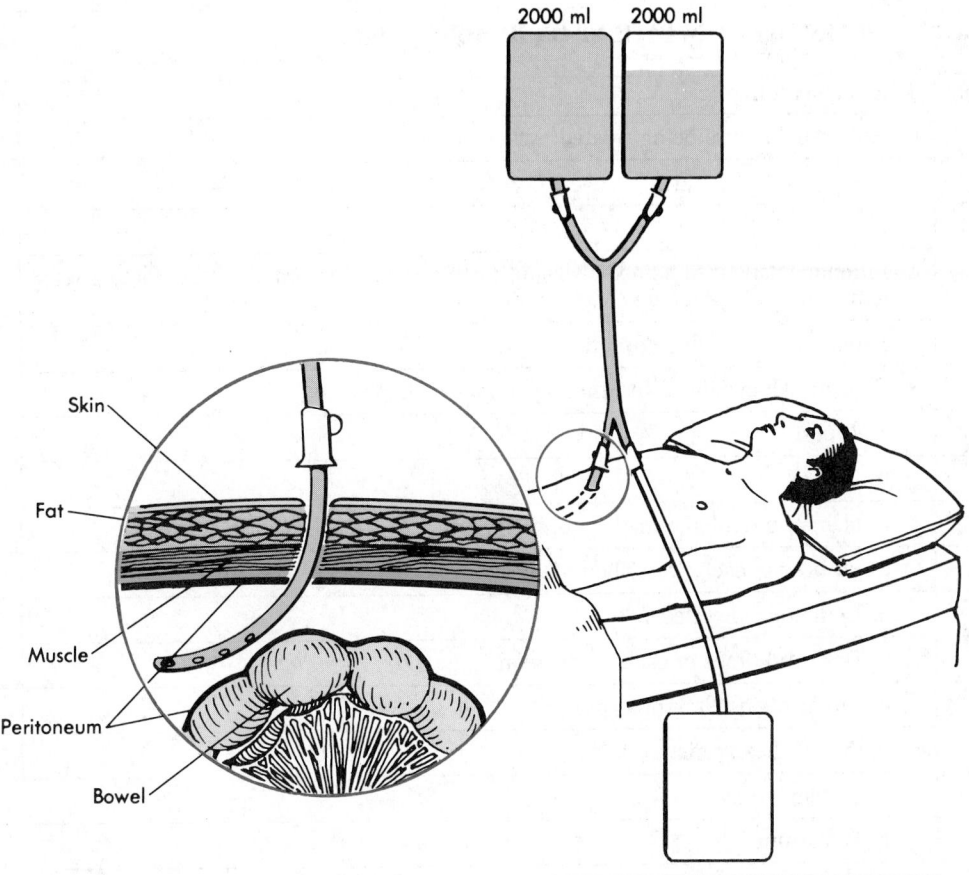

FIGURE 50-7 Patient receiving peritoneal dialysis. Dialysis fluid is being inserted into peritoneal cavity.

trance for organisms into the peritoneum. Each patient must be thoroughly instructed in the care of the catheter and the signs and symptoms indicative of local or peritoneal infection. These must be reported to the physician.

For all patients, weight, blood pressure, and pulse are recorded before initiating the procedure. These values serve as baseline information to assess changes in the patient's condition. For persons undergoing insertion of a peritoneal catheter before dialysis, assessment should be made of their knowledge of the procedure and their anxiety level. A mild sedative may help the severely anxious person to better tolerate the insertion of the catheter. It is important that these patients void just before catheter insertion; this decompresses the bladder and prevents accidental puncture during catheter placement.

To insert a peritoneal catheter, the physician cleanses the abdomen and anesthetizes a small area in the midline of the abdomen about 5 cm (2 inches) below the umbilicus. A small incision is made, and the many-eyed nylon catheter is inserted into the peritoneal cavity (Figure 50-7). A dressing is placed around the protruding catheter.

Approximately 2 L of sterile dialysate warmed to body temperature is attached by tubing to the catheter and allowed to run into the peritoneal cavity as rapidly as possible. This usually takes about 10 minutes. The tubing is then clamped, and 10 to 30 minutes are allowed for osmosis of fluid and diffusion of particles into the dialyzing solution. At the end of the dwell time, the tubing is unclamped and the fluid is allowed to flow by gravity from the abdomen. Fluid should drain in a steady stream. Drainage time should average about 10 to 15 minutes. The first drainage may be pink tinged as a result of the trauma of catheter insertion; however, this should clear with the second or third drainage. At no time should fluid draining from the abdomen appear grossly bloody. After fluid has drained from the abdomen, another cycle is started immediately. Dialysis is initiated for the person with a permanent catheter by carefully cleansing the catheter and surrounding skin with a bactericidal agent before the catheter is connected to the dialysate line. After the dialysis has been completed, the permanent catheter is again cleansed and a sterile cap is applied to the tip.

If the procedure is temporary, the catheter is removed, and the incision is covered with a dry sterile

EXAMPLE OF CARE FOR TEACHING THE PATIENT ON HEMODIALYSIS

Date	Hour	Teaching/learning	RN signature
		Chronic renal failure being treated by hemodialysis	
Start	Stop	Plan	
		1. Introduce patient to hemodialysis unit using available printed material and a visit to unit when appropriate	
		2. Explain normal kidney function	
		3. Explain kidney failure specific to patient's pathophysiology	
		a. Types	
		b. Causes	
		4. Explain and reinforce medication regimen	
		a. Purpose of each prescribed medication	
		b. Common side effects	
		c. Dose and times of each medication	
		d. Prescription filling procedure	
		5. Reinforce dietary instruction	
		a. Protein	
		b. Potassium	
		c. Sodium	
		d. Fluids	
		e. Calories	
		6. Instruct patient about need for and care of vascular access	
		a. Procedure for assessing presence of thrill and bruit; who to notify if thrill or bruit is absent	
		b. Guarding against constriction of fistula; that is, sleeping on arm or wearing tight clothing	
		c. Hygiene and removing dressing after dialysis	
		d. Signs and symptoms of infection; that is, redness, swelling, or tenderness	
		e. Measures to control hemorrhage should it develop while away from dialysis unit	

dressing. The small abdominal wound from the catheter should heal completely in 1 to 2 days.

Care During Peritoneal Dialysis

Problems most commonly associated with peritoneal dialysis include hypotension and hypovolemia, inadequate drainage of fluid from the peritoneal space, pain, atelectasis, respiratory distress, and peritonitis.

Regulating fluid volume and drainage. As with hemodialysis, *hypotension* is most likely to result from rapid removal of fluid from the intravascular space. In addition to checking vital signs and observing the patient's behavior, records of fluid balance are crucial in determining the amount of fluid that has been removed. The net gain or loss of fluid from the abdomen should be determined at the completion of each cycle. To decrease the

EXAMPLE OF CARE FOR TEACHING THE PATIENT ON HEMODIALYSIS—cont'd

		7. Instruct patient about process of hemodialysis	
		a. Explain principles of dialysis in sufficient detail for learning level of patient	
		b. Describe hemodialysis in full detail to patient	
		c. Explain common sights and sounds of dialysis unit to patient	
		d. Describe common complications of hemodialysis to patient as well as usual treatments	
		(1) Hypotension	
		(2) Nausea	
		(3) Vomiting	
		(4) Cramping	
		8. Instruct patient in interpretation of laboratory data and effects of hemodialysis, diet, and medications on these values	
		9. Introduce patient to alternative modes of treatment of end-stage renal disease	
		a. Free-standing hemodialysis centers	
		b. Self-dialysis (home)	
		c. Peritoneal dialysis	
		d. Transplantation	
Date		Status of problems at discharge	
Date		Patient knowledge	
Date		Follow-up plan	
		RN signature _____	

amount of fluid that is being removed from the vascular space, the physician may decrease the hypertonicity of the dialysate and may increase the rate at which fluid is administered through an intravenous line.

Drainage of fluid from the abdomen can be slow or impossible to start. Generally, this problem results when the tip of the catheter has become lodged against abdominal tissues. It may also result from plugging of the catheter with blood or fibrin that has accumulated as a result of tissue trauma. A small amount of heparin may be added to the dialysate to decrease the chance of a clot forming in the catheter. When the dialysate does not drain freely from the abdomen, the patient should be turned from side to side in an attempt to reposition the catheter in the peritoneal cavity. In addition, firm pressure may be applied to the abdomen with both hands and the head of the bed may be raised. If the flow of the dialysate does not increase, the physician is called to irrigate the catheter or reposition it.

Promoting comfort. Severe *pain* should not be experienced during peritoneal dialysis. Moderate levels of pain are often experienced as fluid is instilled and withdrawn from the peritoneal cavity. Procaine hydrochloride may be instilled with the dialysate in an attempt to control the patient's discomfort. Mild analgesics may be ordered for administration at 3- to 4-hour intervals during the procedure.

Although the patient is generally confined to a recumbent position for the length of the dialysis, comfort and diversion can be provided. The patient may turn from side to side and move about in bed as desired as long as the catheter remains undisturbed. The patient may be provided assistance with oral care and bathing as needed. Visiting and other diversional activities should be encouraged when the patient's physical condition permits. If peritoneal dialysis is carried out at home, the patient and a backup person need to be able to do all steps described above.

Preventing complications. When the patient is markedly overhydrated and shows evidence of congestive heart failure and pulmonary edema, *respiratory difficulty* may be encountered as the dialyzing fluid infuses. The quality and rate of respiration should be closely observed. The head of the bed can be raised to decrease the pressure of the dialysate on the diaphragm. The amount of dialyzing fluid used for each cycle may be decreased when respiratory distress becomes prolonged and severe. The patient, although encouraged to eat while being dialyzed, may find that this increases respiratory difficulty. To help overcome additional pressure created by a full stomach, frequent small meals may be provided.

Peritonitis is an ever present threat during peritoneal dialysis. Aseptic technique must be rigidly maintained during insertion of the catheter and throughout the procedure. Care should be taken to avoid contaminating the solution or the tubing when dialysate solution is hung. Cultures of the dialysate fluid are performed routinely to ensure continued attention to asepsis and to identify organisms if peritonitis should develop subsequently. The patient should be observed for signs of peritonitis. These include an elevated temperature, chills, tenderness or pain of the abdomen, nausea and vomiting, and cloudy outflow.

Other Approaches to Peritoneal Dialysis

Several advances in the management of patients with chronic end-stage renal disease have led to two variations of peritoneal dialysis. These technologies emphasize home and self-dialysis.[1,4,26]

Continuous ambulatory peritoneal dialysis (CAPD) is one method leading to safe self-dialysis that is practical, relatively inexpensive when compared to hemodialysis, and promotes patient independence. Basically, CAPD involves continuous contact of dialysate with the peritoneal membrane. Approximately 2 L of dialysate are maintained interperitoneally and exchanged by the patient through a permanent peritoneal catheter 4 to 5 times a day every week.[1] No special equipment is required for the exchanges and the patient, therefore, can lead a fairly normal lifestyle. Exchanges can take place at home or at work by connecting an empty bag to the catheter and opening a clamp to allow drainage. A full dialysate bag is then instilled and the patient has completed an exchange.

The second method is *continuous cyclic peritoneal dialysis* (CCPD). CCPD differs from CAPD in that a machine known as a cycler is used to instill and drain dialysate from the patient. The machine has a series of clamps that are controlled by timers. The timers open and close the clamps in sequence to allow for instillation and drainage of dialysate from the patient. The cycle times for patients with chronic renal failure generally allow for the patient to be dialyzed in 6 to 8 hours. A patient, therefore, can connect up to the cycler at bedtime, set the machine, and be dialyzed while sleeping. A number of alarms are built into the cycler to protect the patient from such malfunctions as dialysate that is too hot or cold, long or short dwell times, improper return of fluid, and changes in catheter pressures. The greatest advantage of CAPD and CCPD over other forms of dialysis is that both offer the patient unprecedented freedom in managing their own care.

Patient Teaching

The teaching requirements for the patient undergoing peritoneal dialysis is consistent with the teaching plan for hemodialysis. However, the patient will need to be instructed in the specifics of the process of peritoneal dialysis. If the patient will undergo CAPD, training should be accomplished in a home training center that is equipped to assist the patient in dealing with home care.

The person or significant others can explain, demonstrate, or plan the following:

1. The process of dialysis and relate work of dialysis to own body needs
2. Observation indicating infection of the peritoneal cavity or catheter and state means of obtaining care when these occur
3. Appropriate care of permanent peritoneal catheter
4. Common side effects of treatment, means for controlling mild symptoms, and means of obtaining medical attention for severe or persistent complications
5. Changes in medication schedule required before and after dialysis
6. A work and activity schedule as physical capabilities permit, with minimal interference from scheduled dialysis time

KIDNEY TRANSPLANTATION

Major advances have also been made in renal transplantation. In 1988 alone, more than 9000 victims of ESRD underwent transplantation since the first transplant was performed in the United States in 1954.[51] Developments in surgical technique, tissue typing, and antirejection drug therapy has made transplantation a reasonable therapy. However, the major block to further use of transplantation as a form of treatment for chronic uremia remains the availability of donor kidneys for transplantation. It has been estimated that of the 20,000 potential donors (clinically brain dead and of young to middle age), only 2500 will actually give organs.[51]

Kidney transplants are being performed with increasing frequency in an effort to prolong the lives of persons with end-stage renal disease. At present the ability to completely overcome the body's tendency to reject the grafted kidney has not been achieved. Persons undergoing kidney transplantation in essence exchange a program of chronic dialysis and its limitations for a new therapeutic program with new limitations and requirements. Unless the kidney has been donated by an identical twin, the body senses the graft as a foreign tissue and attempts to destroy it (rejection) (see Chapter 76).

DONOR SELECTION

Kidney allografts may be obtained from cadavers, matched family members, or an identical twin. Although more than half of the transplanted kidneys are from cadavers, better results are obtained from related donors. Currently, success rates 1 year after transplan-

tation are about 80% when a cadaveric kidney is used and greater than 90% when a living related organ is donated.[21]

The major requirement for the donated kidney is histocompatibility between the donor organ and the recipient. Rejection occurs from a cell-mediated (type IV hypersensitivity) response or from a humoral (type II cytotoxic hypersensitivity) response (see Chapter 76). The important antigens are the human leukocyte antigen (HLA) and the ABO blood groups. For the ABO groups the same rules apply as for blood transfusions.

One procedure currently being used that may significantly increase graft survival from living related donors is that of *donor-specific transfusions*.[45] In the last two months before transplantation the recipient receives three transfusions of the donor's blood, each about 2 weeks apart. After these transfusions, if the recipient and donor blood cross-match remains compatible, transplantation is performed. The purposes of donor-specific transfusion are (1) to identify those recipients who would respond unfavorably to the donated organ and (2) to desensitize the recipient to the donor's tissue.[48]

Living related donors must be in good general health, be highly motivated to be a donor, have good mental health, and not be receiving drugs such as barbiturates, which depress reflexes and electrical brain activity. The donor is given a complete medical evaluation and in some cases may be referred to a psychiatrist for further evaluation. Many transplant centers have a transplant team comprised of physicians, nurses, and social workers who all participate in the donor selection process. Normally, the living related donor organ is harvested and immediately transplanted to the donor. Both surgeries can occur simultaneously.

Cadavers should be free of renal disease, neoplasms (excluding those of the central nervous system and skin), and sepsis. Permission for cadaver donation is generally given by the next of kin or by the persons who plan in advance to donate their organs. Laws governing organ donation differ from state to state. Since 1986, many states have enacted "Required Request" legislation. Under required request, following the death of any hospitalized patient, the next-of-kin *must* be asked if they would consider donating organs or tissues of the deceased for transplantation. The goal of this legislation is to increase access to the much-needed organs and tissues. Hospital policy will often direct who will seek permission for organ donation. This responsibility is often left to the physician, but the nurse can play a very important part in this process.

Viability of the cadaveric donor kidney must be maintained until the time of transplantation surgery. Preservation times of 24 to 72 hours have been reported with proper technique. Methods of preservation include washing out the formed blood elements and perfusing a heparinized electrolyte solution at 2° to 4° C. Use of a pulsatile flow pump and oxygenator helps to preserve the kidney beyond 6 to 12 hours.

PREOPERATIVE CARE

Nursing care of the patient in the preoperative phase includes physical and emotional preparation for the surgery. The patient and family should understand the outcomes expected from the surgery and the follow-up care that will be required. They should be prepared for the possibility of the kidney not functioning after transplantation as well as the potential of rejection. The nature of the surgery and location of the transplant, possible need for postoperative dialysis, use of immunosuppressive drugs, and need for infection prevention after surgery must be explained to the patient and family.

Throughout the period from the patient's acceptance as a transplant candidate to the time of surgery, the concerns and anxieties of the patient and family regarding transplantation need to be identified. As appropriate, the nurse and other members of the health team are called on to help in dealing with these concerns and anxieties.

The patient must be in optimal physical condition for transplantation. Dialysis may be required before transplantation to ensure optimal fluid and electrolyte balance, acid-base balance, and removal of wastes. The integrity of the vascular access must be maintained. Before surgery the extremity containing the vascular access may be wrapped to draw attention to it and identify it as containing the patient's access for dialysis. This identification will help all individuals caring for the person to avoid using the affected extremity for blood pressure determinations, drawing of blood, or intravenous infusions.

SURGERY

During surgery the transplanted kidney is usually placed in the iliac fossa (Figure 50-8). Generally, the peritoneal cavity is not entered. The patient's own kidneys are not disturbed unless they are infected or are the cause of significant hypertension for which the recipient might undergo bilateral nephrectomy before the transplant surgery. The recipient's kidneys are left intact whenever possible to maintain erythropoietin production, blood pressure control, and prostaglandin synthesis and metabolism. The donor ureter is used to the extent that is possible. If long enough, it is connected to the bladder in such a way as to prevent reflux of urine. If the ureter is short, a ureteroureterostomy may be performed. A catheter is placed in the wound to promote drainage of any accumulating fluid.

POSTOPERATIVE CARE

Immediate postoperative care includes maintaining drainage of the urinary bladder and monitoring hourly output, assessing the adequacy of fluid and electrolyte balance, protecting the patient from infection, observing for signs and symptoms of rejection and other complications, and identifying the effects of medications that have been administered throughout the entire care cycle.[41] A free flow of communication must be maintained with the patient and significant others regarding the individual's progress.

In the operating room, a Foley catheter is inserted into the bladder to promote drainage of urine and to prevent bladder distention and pressure on the newly anastomosed ureter. If gross hematuria or clots are noted in the drainage system, the physician should be notified immediately.

As with any surgical patient, the possibility of hemorrhage and hypovolemia exists. Hemodynamic monitoring is instituted. Blood pressure and pulse are determined frequently. Because the patient may have little or no urinary output for a number of hours to days after transplantation, fluid and electrolyte balance must be monitored carefully. Parameters indicating disturbed fluid and electrolyte balance are listed in the discussion of care of the patient with chronic renal failure (p. 1472). Any drainage from dressings or tubes are carefully calculated into the patient's fluid balance record. The care of the patient following renal transplantation is summarized in the box on p. 1493, left.

REJECTION

Rejection, the leading cause of graft failure, may occur as a hyperacute event, as an accelerated event, as an acute event, or as a slow and progressive decline

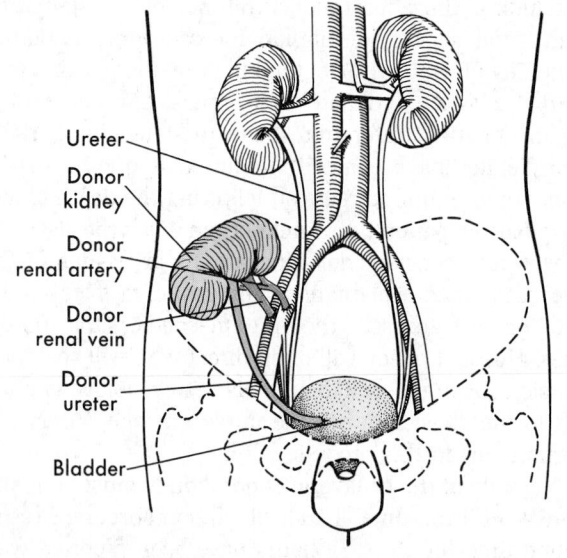

FIGURE 50-8 Location of transplanted kidney showing anastomosis of renal artery, renal vein, and ureter.

NURSING CARE OF THE PATIENT AFTER RENAL TRANSPLANTATION

1. Immediate postoperative period
   a. Maintain sterile technique in caring for wound and urinary drainage catheter
   b. Encourage early ambulation
   c. Administer medications as prescribed
   d. Assess patient for signs and symptoms of infection both at surgical incision and systemically
2. Fluid and electrolyte balance
   a. Maintain accurate intake and output
   b. Weigh patient daily at same time
   c. Monitor signs of fluid and electrolyte imbalance
   d. Monitor and regulate parenteral fluid replacement as prescribed by physician (usually 1 ml replacement for each 1 ml output)
   e. Encourage oral intake as tolerated
3. Assisting with comfort and ADL
   a. Promote rest periods when fatigue is present
   b. Administer pain medication as prescribed
   c. Assist with ADL as necessary but encourage independence
4. Control of environment
   a. Maintain calm reassuring environment
   b. Reverse isolation may be required while patient is immunosuppressed
   c. Restrict visitors with colds or other infections
   d. Provide diversional activities as tolerated

SIGNS AND SYMPTOMS OF ACUTE REJECTION OF A TRANSPLANTED KIDNEY

1. Decrease in urine output
   a. Oliguria
   b. Anuria
2. Fever greater than 37.7° C (100° F); this may be masked by steroid therapy
3. Pain or tenderness over grafted kidney
4. Edema
5. Sudden weight gain; 2 to 3 pounds in a 24-hour period
6. Hypertension
7. General malaise
8. Rise in serum creatinine BUN values
9. Decrease in creatinine clearance

(chronic rejection) in renal function. In a *hyperacute* event, rejection occurs immediately after surgical implantation. Instantly following arterial anastomosis, circulating cytotoxic antibodies infiltrate and infarct the foreign tissue. The kidney undergoing hyperacute rejection is usually removed immediately to prevent further complications. *Accelerated* rejection usually occurs 3 to 5 days after transplant. It is thought to be a secondary response resulting in antibody formation after contact with an antigen to which the patient has already been sensitized. It presents as a sudden severe episode of graft dysfunction, and it can sometimes be reversed with large doses of potent immunosuppressive-drug therapy. *Acute* rejection typically begins within the first 2 weeks but may be seen two or more years after transplantation. Most transplant patients undergo at least one episode of acute rejection. Rejection is caused by a cell-mediated immune response. The delay in occurrence of the first attack is related to the time it takes for T lymphocytes to become sensitized. Signs and symptoms indicative of acute rejection are listed in the box above, right.

Chronic rejection is a slow, progressive process. It occurs secondary to both cell-mediated and humoral immune responses. The signs and symptoms are similar to those that occur in acute rejection; however, they occur more slowly. In most instances the patient will eventu-

ally lose all renal function as chronic rejection progresses.

Treatment of acute rejection usually consists of large doses of SoluMedrol (methylprednisolone) administered intravenously. Local graft irradiation may be used to destroy infiltrating lymphocytes.

IMMUNOSUPPRESSION

Rejection of the grafted kidney is a function of the recipient's immune system; therefore, survival of such a graft depends on the suppression of the recipient's immune response. The major drugs used for immunosuppression in kidney transplants are azathioprine and cyclosporine (see below) in addition to adrenal corticosteroids and OKT3 (see Chapter 76). Total lymphoid irradiation may be performed to reduce dosage of the corticosteroids.

Azathioprine

Azathioprine (Imuran) is the most commonly used immunosuppressive drug. It functions by inhibiting DNA and RNA synthesis, thereby suppressing antibody synthesis. Cyclophosphamide (Cytoxan) and azathioprine have similar functions and are often used concomitantly. By using the two medications in combination, lower doses can be administered, thereby reducing the side effects of both drugs. Cyclophosphamide also functions by destroying circulating lymphocytes.

Cyclosporine

Cyclosporine (Sandimmune) has now become the immunosuppressive agent of choice for almost all cadaveric renal transplants.[47] The increase in 1-year survival rates of renal transplants is largely attributed to cyclosporine. Cyclosporine has also changed the picture for the elderly and diabetic patient with renal failure. Diabetic patients have proved to have increased risk of graft rejection when on regimens of other immunosuppressives. This increased risk of graft failure is eliminated with cyclosporine. The side effects of immunosuppression have also kept older patients from receiving transplants in the past. These side effects are not present with cyclosporine and 10% of all patients receiving the drug are over 55 years old.

The major immunologic advantage of cyclosporine is its specificity. Cyclosporine strongly inhibits antibody production that leads to graft rejection. However, this drug does not affect the antibody systems that provide protection against infection. The use of other types of immunosuppressive agents in renal transplantation has resulted in causing the patient to be almost defenseless against infection because of their broad action.[21]

Cyclosporine therapy usually begins several hours before the actual transplant surgery. A postsurgical dose of 14 to 18 mg/kg of body weight is then administered daily for 7 to 14 days. After this initial therapy, the daily dose is gradually tapered to a maintenance dose of 5 to 10 mg/kg of body weight. Once cyclosporine therapy is initiated, it must be continued as long as the graft survives or other immunosuppressive therapy is started.

Cyclosporine can be administered intravenously or orally. The intravenous route is used only when the patient is unable to take the oral form. The intravenous dose is usually about one third of the oral dose. An intravenous dose is administered as a slow drip over a period of 2 to 6 hours. Dosage is changed to the oral preparation as soon as possible.

Oral cyclosporine has a very unpleasant taste. Mixing the medication in milk or fruit juice makes it easier for the patient to drink. Many patients prefer using chocolate milk since it masks both the taste and oily texture. Cyclosporine should be mixed in a glass container since it is absorbed by Styrofoam and some plastics. After the patient takes the medication the glass should be partially refilled, stirred, and taken by the patient. This will ensure that the patient gets a complete dose. Doses of cyclosporine must be carefully monitored since there is often a narrow margin between drug toxicity and therapeutic value.

A major side effect of cyclosporine is *nephrotoxicity*. Because it is often difficult to differentiate between cyclosporine-induced nephrotoxicity and acute rejection, the patient must be closely monitored initially. Renal biopsy may be necessary to establish a definitive diagnosis. Other side effects include hypertension, tremor, excessive hair growth, hyperplasia of the gums, and hepatotoxicity. Stomach and liver carcinomas have also been associated with low-dose cyclosporine.

Side effects of therapy with immunosuppressive medications as well as nursing interventions are listed in Table 50-5.

PATIENT TEACHING

The person having had a renal transplant or the significant other can state or demonstrate the following:
1. The prescribed diet and how it will be achieved
2. The medication plan including:
   a. State name, dose, frequency, rationale, and side effects of prescribed medications (immunosuppressives, antacids, etc.)
   b. State method of obtaining medications

TABLE 50-5 Common side effects of immunosuppressive therapy and nursing interventions

Side Effect	Nursing Intervention
Leukopenia	1. Observe for signs of infection 2. Reverse isolation when necessary 3. Antibiotic therapy as prescribed
Gastrointestinal irritation and bleeding	1. Perform guaiac tests on stools, vomitus, and nasogastric aspirate 2. Administer antacids as prescribed 3. Provide calm, supportive environment 4. Assess postural vital signs
Increased appetite	1. Reinforce diet teaching 2. Encourage low-sodium diet
Alopecia	1. Suggest use of wig 2. Reassure patient that hair will grow back 3. Provide emotional support
Acne	1. Encourage frequent bathing 2. Instruct in use of appropriate soaps
Delayed wound healing	1. Maintain sterile technique for dressing changes 2. Assess wound each dressing change for signs of infection 3. Encourage adequate protein in diet
Change in mental status (mood swings)	1. Observe patient for changes in behavior and report to physician 2. Provide calm supportive environment 3. Provide diversional activities as tolerated

3. Accurate taking and recording of oral temperature, 24-hour urine specimens, weights, fluid intake, and urinary output
4. Recommended preventive health care measures
   a. State measures useful in preventing infection
   b. State plans for dental and gynecologic health care (if appropriate)
   c. State need to avoid immunization with live virus vaccines
5. A program for continued health supervision
   a. Explain concept of immunosuppression and relate this to health care needs
   b. Describe signs and symptoms requiring immediate medical attention
   c. Relate appropriate information regarding sexual functioning and family planning
   d. State need to preserve dialysis access
   e. State resources available for assistance with illness and rehabilitative concerns and means of contact with resources
   f. Explain specific plans for follow-up care

QUALITY OF LIFE

As a result of the development of new surgical techniques and immunosuppressive therapy, the success rates of renal transplantation as measured by graft survival at 1 year, has greatly improved. Attention is now being focused on other issues such as costs of care and the quality of life of patients on dialysis and following transplantation.[16,25] As a result of rising costs, concern has been raised as to whether all patients truly benefit from either transplantation or long-term dialysis.

One study suggests that patients who have undergone transplantation have a higher quality of life than patients on dialysis. Quality of life of transplant recipients compared favorably with that of the general population. Further, it was found that patients on home dialysis have a higher quality of life than patients being treated at dialysis centers. However, even though dialysis patients made favorable subjective assessments about their quality of life, these patients did not work or function at the same level as others in the general population.[16]

As costs to provide care to patients with end-stage renal disease continue to escalate, decisions will have to be made about treatment modalities and availability of those treatments. With the increasing success rates of transplantation, cost substantially lower than dialysis, and data to support that the quality of life is improved with transplantation, more efforts must be made to increase availability of kidneys for transplantation. The nurse can play an important role in these efforts by identifying potential donors and, when appropriate, discussing this issue with both patients and the lay public.

INTERVENTIONS FOR THE PERSON DYING OF RENAL FAILURE

At times nursing care must be provided for the patient dying from renal failure. Major objectives should be maintaining the comfort and safety of the patient and providing the opportunity for the patient and family to express their feelings and arrive at some degree of emotional comfort. In providing physical comfort to the patient, diets may be liberalized. Frequent turning and repositioning are necessary to prevent skin excoriation and breakdown. Oral care is extremely important, because sores in the mouth, once developed, are almost impossible to cure. Mineral oil is an acceptable protective lubricant for the alert patient. A water-soluble lubricant with a vegetable base (for example, K-Y Jelly) is preferable for the comatose patient. Hydrogen peroxide is helpful in removing blood from the mouth and the nose. Vinegar mouthwash neutralizes the ammonia.

As death approaches, the patient often becomes severely confused or comatose. As the patient's level of awareness and ability to control the environment decrease, it becomes the responsibility of the nursing staff to provide safety for the patient. The specific care required for the unconscious patient is described in Chapter 60.

Providing an opportunity for the patient and family to ventilate feelings is one of the more important aspects of nursing care for a patient with either acute or chronic onset of uremia. Thoughts concerning death and alarm over treatments can produce considerable anxiety. The wishes of the patient and family regarding spiritual counseling should be determined. Through demonstrating interest in the patient's needs and providing comfort measures the nurse can do a great deal to help the patient and family accept the patient's ultimate death.

CHAPTER SUMMARY

- Renal failure indicates a state of total or nearly total loss of the kidney's ability to excrete waste products and to maintain fluid and electrolyte balance.

- Signs and symptoms indicating the onset of acute renal failure appear rapidly and are a direct result of retention of fluids, metabolic wastes, and inability to regulate electrolytes.

- The oliguric phase of acute renal failure is characterized by inability to excrete fluid loads (oliguria), hyperkalemia, hyponatremia, metabolic acidosis, and uremia. The diuretic phase is characterized by excessive diuresis with loss of sodium and potassium; BUN remains elevated, then decreases slowly.

- Nursing care during the oliguric phase includes monitoring fluid and electrolyte imbalances, promoting rest/activity balance, preventing infection and bleeding, promoting comfort and ADL, and controlling the environment. During the diuretic phase, monitoring of fluid and electrolyte balance continues, activity is encouraged, coping is facilitated, and patient teaching is instituted.

✔ Chronic renal failure represents progressive and irreversible damage to the kidneys. It is characterized by altered fluid and electrolyte balance and regulatory functions of the body and by retention of solutes (uremia).

✔ Chronic renal failure can be treated by conservative medical management, hemodialysis, peritoneal dialysis or its variations (CAPD, CCPD), or kidney transplantation.

✔ Nursing interventions for chronic renal failure include maintaining fluid and electrolyte balance, preventing infection and injury, promoting comfort, assisting with coping in lifestyle and changes in self-concept, and teaching the patient.

✔ Dialysis involves movement of fluid and particles across a semipermeable membrane by diffusion, osmosis, and ultrafiltration. Hemodialysis involves shunting the patient's blood through a dialyzer to exchange fluids, electrolytes, and waste materials. With peritoneal dialysis, the peritoneum becomes the dialyzing membrane.

✔ Kidney transplantation should not be considered a cure for renal failure but rather an ongoing therapy with its own side effects and potential complications.

✔ Success with kidney transplantation has been greatly enhanced by pretransplantation donor-specific transfusions and by the use of cyclosporine to decrease rejection.

QUESTIONS TO CONSIDER

- How prevalent is renal failure in the United States and what are the major causes?
- How do fluid and electrolyte balance differ among the oliguric and diuretic phases of acute renal failure and chronic renal failure?
- How would the nursing care plan of a patient on hemodialysis differ from that of a patient on peritoneal dialysis?
- If you were assigned a patient who is to initiate continuous cyclic peritoneal dialysis (CCPD) at home, what information would you need?

REFERENCES AND SELECTED READINGS

1. *Arenz R: Do-it-yourself dialysis, RN 44:57-60, 1981.
2. Aroesty J and Reggig R: The cost effects of improved kidney transplantation, Contemp Dialysis and Nephrol, 5:32-36, 1984.
3. Bernbeck L: Conservative care of patients with renal failure. In Schlotter L, editor: Nursing and the nephrology patient, Flushing, NY, 1973, Medical Examination Publishing Co.
4. *Binkley L: Keeping up with peritoneal dialysis, Am J Nurs 84(6):729-733, 1984.
5. *Booth S and Dobberstein K: Living without kidneys, Am J Nurs 89(2):270, 1989.
6. Brundage D: Nursing management of renal problems, ed 2, St Louis, 1980, The CV Mosby Co.
7. Campbell JD and Campbell AR: The social and economic cost of end-stage renal disease: a patient's perspective, N Engl J Med 229:386-392, 1978.
8. *Chambers J: Bowel management in dialysis patients, Am J Nurs 83(7):1051-1052, 1983.
9. *Chambers J: Assessing the dialysis patient at home, Am J Nurs, 81(4):750-753, 1981.
10. *Cianci J et al: Renal transplantation, Am J Nurs 81:354-355, 1981.
11. *Cianci J and Lamb J: Organ transplantation: matching donors and recipients, Am J Nurs 81(3):544-545, 1981.
12. Clinical news: Dialysis on the double, Am J Nurs 85(8):864, 1985.
13. Clinical news: Transplanting islet cells along with kidneys, Am J Nurs 85(7):773, 1985.
14. Cohen D et al: Cyclosporine: a new immunosuppressive agent for organ transplantation, Ann Inter Med 101:667-682, 1984.
15. Denny D: Medicare mandated organ donor referrals, AKF Newsletter, 2(2):3-8, 1985.
16. *Evans R and others: The quality of life of patients with end-stage renal disease, N Engl J Med 312(9):553-559, 1985.
17. Flynn C: Subclavian vein catheter and clockwork pump, Dialysis Transplant, 9:556-557, 1980.
18. *Froberg J: The anemias: Causes and courses of action, RN 52(3):52-57, 1989.
19. Freeman R: Treatment of chronic renal failure: an update, N Engl J Med 312(9):577-579, 1985.
20. Gibson R: Dialysis. In Stone, W and Rabin, P, editors: Chronic end-stage renal disease: an integrated approach, New York, 1983, Academic Press.
21. *Golden D et al: Understanding the magic of cyclosporine, RN 48(6):53-54, 1985.
22. Gutch CF and Stoner MH: Review of hemodialysis for nurses and dialysis personnel, ed 4, St Louis, 1983, The CV Mosby Co.
23. Gutman R, Stead W, and Robinson R: Physical activity and employment staus of patients on maintenance dialysis, N Engl J Med, 304:309-313, 1985.
24. Irwin B: Now-peritoneal dialysis for chronic patients too, RN 44:49-52, 1981.
25. Johnson J, McCauley C, and Copley J: The quality of life of hemodialysis and transplant patients, Kidney Int, 22:286-291, 1982.
26. Johnson R: Home dialysis: the competition between CAPD and hemodialysis, JAMA 245(15):1511-1514, 1981.
27. Kappel D: The changing focus of state kidney programs, AKF Newsletter, 2(2):2, 1985.

*References preceded by an asterisk are particularly well suited for student reading.

28. Klahr S, Schreiner G, and Ichikawa I: The progression of renal disease, N Engl J Med 318(25):1657-1665, 1988.
29. Lancaster L: The patient with end stage renal disease, ed 2, New York, 1984, John Wiley & Co.
30. Latos DL: Chronic renal failure: an overview, Dialysis Transplant 9:435-440, 1980.
31. Levey A and Harrington J: Continuous peritoneal dialysis for chronic renal failure, Medicine 61:330-339, 1982.
32. *Luke B: Nutrition in renal disease: the adult patient on dialysis, Am J Nurs 79:1096-1099, 1979.
33. Nolph K, Lindblad A, and Novak J: Continuous ambulatory peritoneal dialysis, N Engl J Med 318(24):1595-1599, 1988.
34. Norris MK: Dialysis disequilibrium syndrome, Nursing 89, 19(4):33, 1989.
35. Norris MK: Management of acute conditions in chronic renal failure, Dimens Crit Care Nurs 2(6):328-337, 1983.
36. Overcast T et al: Problems in the identification of potential organ donors: misconceptions and fallacies associated with donor cards, JAMA 251:1559-1562, 1984.
37. Papper S: Clinical nephrology, ed 2, Boston, 1981, Little, Brown & Co.
38. *Perras S and Zappocosta A: The application of Orem's theory in promoting self-care in a peritoneal dialysis facility, AANNT J 9(3):37-39, 1982.
39. Popovitch RP, et al: Continuous ambulatory peritoneal dialysis, Ann Intern Med 88:449-456, 1978.
40. Porth C: Pathophysiology: Concepts of altered health states, ed 2, Philadelphia, 1986, JB Lippincott Co.
41. Prewit D: Postoperative complications: an overview, Nephrol Nurse 5:27-32, 1983.
42. Price SA and Wilson CM: Pathophysiology: Clinical concepts of disease processes, ed 3, New York, 1986, McGraw Hill Inc.
43. *Reckling J: Safeguarding the renal transplant patient, Nursing '82, 12(2):46-49, 1982.
44. *Reed S: Giving more than dialysis, Nursing '82, 12(4):58-63, 1982.
45. *Robbins K, Richard A, and Ronselli M: Donor specific transfusions as pre-treatment for living related donor transplants and nursing implications, Nephrol Nurs 5:4-8, 1983.
46. *Robson MD and Oroponlous DG: Continuous ambulatory peritoneal dialysis: an orientation in the treatment of chronic renal failure, Dialysis Transplant 7:999-1103, 1978.
47. *Rule R: Enthusiastic cyclosporine consensus, Am J Nurs 85(8):861-862, 1985.
48. Salvatiena O et al: Deliberate donor specific blood transfusions prior to living related renal transplantation, Ann Surg 192:543-552, 1980.
49. *Snyder T: An exercise program for dialysis patients, Am J Nurs 89(3):362-364, 1989.
50. Stark J and Hunt V: Helping your patient with chronic renal failure, Nursing 83, 13(9):56-63, 1983.
51. UNOS Releases, 1988 transplantation statistics, United Network for Organ Sharing Update 5(5):1-2, 1989.
52. Williams SR: Nutrition and diet therapy, ed 6, St Louis, 1989, The CV Mosby Co.
53. Younger S et al: Psychosocial and ethical implications of organ retrieval, N Engl J Med 313(5):321-323, 1985.

ALTERATIONS IN SEXUALITY AND REPRODUCTION

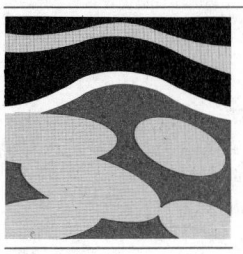

CHAPTER 51

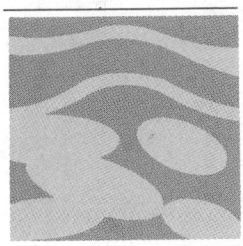

Assessment of Sexual Health

NANCY FUGATE WOODS

CHAPTER OBJECTIVES

After studying this chapter, the student should be able to:
1. Analyze the dimensions of sexual health in your personal life and professional practice.
2. Explore variations in sexual experience and expression and your personal responses to sexual variation.
3. Apply information about sexual development and human sexual response in nurse-client relationships.
4. Assess sexual health in specific client populations.

SEXUALITY AND HEALTH

DEFINITION OF SEXUALITY

Human sexuality is not merely a biologic phenomenon, but pervades the total person and involves a complex interplay of biologic, psychological, and sociocultural variables. Sexual health is an elusive concept, its definition involving a person's unique combination of feelings, attitudes, and values that shape what is "healthy" at a given moment and in specific social situations. The World Health Organization's "Report on Education and Treatment in Human Sexuality" asserts that: "Sexual health is the integration of the somatic, emotional, intellectual, and social aspects of sexual being, in ways that are positively enriching and that enhance personality, communication, and love.[11,17]

As with many definitions of health, sexual health is not restricted to a discrete state, but encompasses a range of behaviors, functions, and experiences. One way of thinking about sexual health involves consideration of sexual function, sexual self-concept, and sexual relationships. Sexual function implies the person's capacity to engage in and to experience pleasure from sexual activity. Although emphasis is frequently placed on ability to experience orgasm or to pleasure a partner, sexual function includes a wide variety of behaviors that make up the unique repertoire of that individual. Sexual self-concept pertains to the images we have of ourselves as men or women. It is evident in our feelings of adequacy, our masculinity, and our femininity. It is influenced by our body image, which is the mental image we have of our physical selves. Sexual relationships are those interpersonal relationships with others in which sexual activity is shared.

SEXUAL BEGINNINGS

We are sexual beings from the moment we are conceived. This event establishes chromosomal sex and is the first of a series of developmental influences on our sexuality. The paternal sperm contributes either an X or a Y chromosome, which combines with the maternal X chromosome; this results in the XX (female) or XY (male) combination. (There are, however, instances in which some other combinations occur.)[37] Indeed, the X or Y chromosome from the paternal sperm sets in motion a process analogous to a relay race; that is, each component has control of the process for a time, eventually yielding control to another.[37] (See Figure 51-1.)

After fertilization, there are probably two other critical points in the evolution of gender identity. The first is the induction of development of internal and external genitalia, and the second is the process by which the hypothalamus takes on a male or female pattern. At about 5 to 6 weeks of fetal life, the XX or XY chromosomal combination determines whether the undifferentiated fetal gonads will develop as ovaries or testes. Further differentiation occurs in response to the secretion of fetal androgen in the male fetus. If androgens are not present at critical periods and in appropriate amounts, male structures will not develop from the wolffian ducts; thus it is possible for a fetus with XY chromosomes to develop female genitalia. It is also believed that a müllerian-inhibiting substance is necessary in males to prevent development of the female (müllerian) duct system. Lack of Müllerian-inhibiting substance is thought to be responsible for some males being born with both male and female internal genitalia (for example, testes and ovaries, fallopian tubes, and uterus). In the absence of fetal gonadal hormones, female reproductive structures will begin to develop from the müllerian ducts, regardless of the chromosomal sex of the fe-

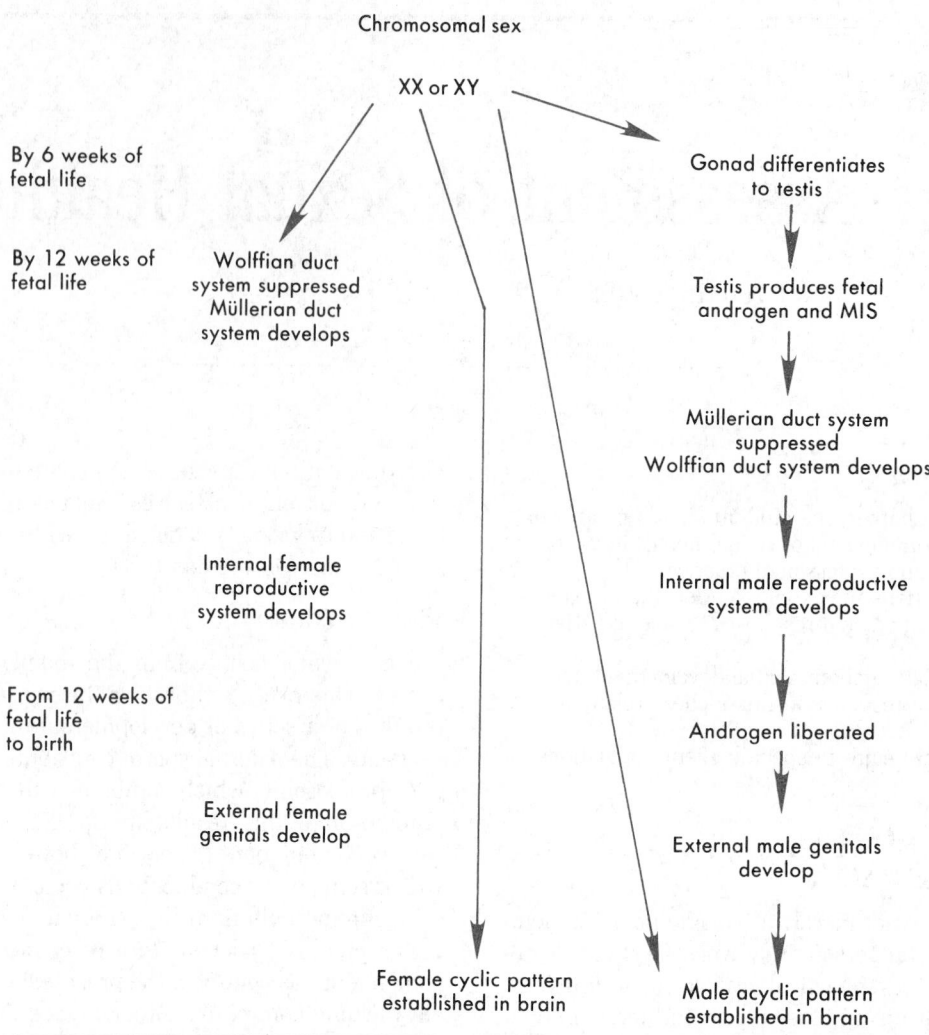

FIGURE 51-1 Fetal sexual development. (Modified from Money J and Ehrhardt AA: Man, woman, boy, girl: the differentiation and dimorphism of gender identity from conception to maturity, Baltimore, 1972, The Johns Hopkins University Press. In Woods NF: Human sexuality in health and illness, ed 3, St Louis, 1984, The CV Mosby Co.)

tus. By the twelfth week of fetal life, biologic sex is well established. Although there does not appear to be a hormone necessary for induction of the ovarian function in female fetuses, estrogen is necessary for full development of female genitalia.[37]

Another critical stage probably occurs just before or soon after birth, at which time another set of sexual controls is introduced. Testosterone is thought to influence the hypothalamus in such a way that the male hypothalamus develops a male acyclic pattern for the release of pituitary gonadotropins. In the female, a cyclic pattern of gonadotropin release is established. Although the infant is born with an established biologic sex (gender), gender identity and gender role are yet to be established. Gender identity is the feeling that one is male, female, or ambivalent. Typically, the child is labeled male or female by the parents or other caretakers

shortly after birth, and their subsequent behavior confirms and reinforces the child's sense of maleness or femaleness. Gender identity is probably solidified in children by the time they are 3 years of age.[37] Gender role is the outward expression of one's gender and is learned early in life. The distinctions between appropriate masculine and feminine behavior vary with the culture. In Western cultures, these distinctions are becoming less clear. Recently, Western societies have begun to appreciate the optimal characteristics of both sexes. Indeed, being androgynous (possessing characteristics once associated with both women and men) is now nearly synonymous with mentally healthy sex-role behavior.[9] If the processes described above proceed without interference, the person's biologic sex (female or male) will be congruent with gender identity (person sees herself or himself as a woman or a man) and gender role (outward manifestations of masculinity or femininity). (Consequences of lack of congruence between sex, gender identity, and gender role are explored briefly later in this chapter.)

This complex set of biologic and psychosocial variables set in motion by the event of conception has a pervasive influence on the remainder of our lives. The biologic component of sexuality, sexual function or expression, constantly interacts with gender identity, cognition, and affect as well as with social factors such as sanctioned roles and mores and folkways regulating sexual expression.

HUMAN SEXUAL RESPONSE

Throughout life, various components of sexual function develop and change. Many of the basic sexual functions are evident in infants and children (for example, the ability to have erections and orgasms) and persist well into the last decades of life. Human sexual response represents an opportunity for the integration of biologic aspects of sexuality with our thoughts, feelings, and interpersonal relationships.

Masters and Johnson,[32] pioneers in the scientific study of the physiologic aspects of sexual behavior, demonstrated that sexual response is a cyclic phenomenon consisting of four phases. The *excitement phase*, the initial component of the cycle, develops from sexually arousing stimuli such as touch; an increase in sexual tension is observed during this phase. Next, a consolidation period, the *plateau phase*, occurs, during which sexual tension becomes intensified. The involuntary climax of sexual tension, *orgasm*, follows and involves only a small portion of the sexual response cycle. During this period, changes attributable to muscular tension and congestion of blood vessels reach a peak and begin to dissipate. During the *resolution phase*, an involuntary period, the changes involving the blood vessels, sexual organs, and muscular tension are reversed. Women may at this time begin another sexual response cycle immediately; men cannot be restimulated to higher levels of sexual tension immediately.

The physiologic changes seen during human sexual response depend on two main principles: myotonia and vasocongestion. The congestion of pelvic blood vessels and involuntary muscular contractions in the pelvic organs and other parts of the body are responsible for arousal and orgasmic experience. Sexual response is a total body response, involving nearly every body system. Phase-specific descriptions of the sexual response cycle follow.

EXCITEMENT

The hallmark of sexual arousal in women is vaginal lubrication. Believed to result from transudation of a mucoidlike substance across the vaginal mucosa, lubrica-

tion appears within seconds of sexual stimulation. The vaginal barrel becomes longer and wider as the uterus begins to elevate in the pelvis. Vasocongestive changes are also seen in the external genitalia: the clitoris becomes longer and wider, and the labia minora flatten and separate from the vaginal opening. As the labia minora become vasocongested, they actually extend outward, lengthening the vaginal barrel. The man's penis rapidly becomes erect, tensing of the scrotal sac is noted, and the testes begin to rise toward the perineum.

Extragenital changes are also seen with sexual excitement: women's nipples become erect, the areolae become engorged, venous patterns in the breast become more evident, and breast size actually increases. The sex flush, which looks like a red, maculopapular rash, appears over the chest in some persons. Men's nipples may also become erect. An increase in both the heart rate and blood pressure is evident, paralleling the level of sexual excitement.[32]

PLATEAU

During the plateau phase, the clitoris retracts upward beneath the clitoral hood. Clitoral stimulation may still occur indirectly with traction on the labia. The orgasmic platform, the extremely vascular tissue at the outer portion of the vagina and the labia minora, becomes increasingly congested. The uterus continues to elevate in the pelvis, which creates a tenting effect in the innermost portion of the vagina. Externally, the labia majora become more congested, and the labia minora deepen in color as a result of vasocongestion. A few drops of mucoid-like material are secreted from Bartholin's glands, probably to assist with the lubrication of the outermost portion of the vagina. The diameter of the penis continues to increase, especially at the coronal ridge, and the testes increase in size to 50% over their unstimulated state as they elevate closer to the perineum. A few drops of mucoid material are secreted from Cowper's glands.

The woman's areolae may become so engorged that it is difficult to see the erect nipple. The sex flush continues to spread, sometimes involving the neck, face, and arms. Hyperventilation occurs along with heart rates of 100 to 175 beats/min. There is elevation of systolic blood pressure (20 to 60 mmHg for women, 20 to 80 mmHg for men) and diastolic blood pressure (10 to 20 mmHg for women, 10 to 40 mm Hg for men).[32]

ORGASM

Orgasm involves the climactic release of sexual tension and is evident in contractions throughout the body. The woman's orgasmic platform contracts rapidly, and expulsive contractions along the entire male urethra propel semen from the vas out through the penis. During orgasm, the internal bladder sphincter in men contracts, thus preventing semen from being propelled backward into the bladder. Uterine contractions are also noted in women with orgasm, much like those characteristic of labor. The rectal sphincter also contracts rapidly in both men and women during orgasm.

Recently investigators have explored orgasmic expulsion of fluid occurring in some women. Although earlier studies discussed ejaculation as the only physiologic phenomenon in sexual response that was not homologous in both sexes, there is a long history of literary and scientific reference to orgasmic expulsions, sometimes termed female ejaculation. Women who experience expulsions describe the experience as a gushing of fluid with orgasm. Often they have mistakenly been diagnosed as having stress incontinence.

Orgasmic expulsions seem to be triggered by stimulation of the Grafenberg spot, an area in the anterior vaginal wall corresponding to the site of Skene's glands. Stimulation of the Grafenberg spot produces first an urge to urinate, followed by intense pleasure. The site increases in size with sexual stimulation. Expulsions of fluids from the urethral meatus have been observed in response to stimulation of the Grafenberg spot, and chemical analysis of specimens in a single case study revealed the substance was not urine but a glandular secretion.[8]

Bullough and her colleagues found that 54% of the women she studied had experienced orgasmic expulsions. Most had experienced them with a male partner (88%) or with masturbation (82%), but others with a female partner (49%).[14]

RESOLUTION

During this phase, vasocongestion is lost gradually from the clitoris and breasts but rapidly from the orgasmic platform. The clitoris quickly returns to its usual position from under the clitoral hood. Vasocongestion of the labia dissipates, nipple erection recedes, and the uterus descends to its usual position in the pelvis. Cardiovascular and respiratory rates quickly return to normal. In men, there is initially a rapid loss of erection to 1 to 1.5 times the size of the penis in its unstimulated state. Later there is a slower resolution of vasocongestion until the penis returns to prestimulation size. The scrotum and testes lose their vasocongestive changes, and the testes rapidly descend into the scrotum. Occasionally, a thin film of perspiration may appear over the entire body.

TRIPHASIC CONCEPT OF HUMAN SEXUAL RESPONSE

Recently, Kaplan[25] has suggested a triphasic concept of human sexual response. She delineates three phases—desire, excitement, and orgasm—that are related components of sexual response but are governed by separate neurophysiologic systems. This notion is useful for understanding not only the functions of sexual response,

but also the consequences of pathology, the causes of sexual dysfunction, and appropriate therapies.

The *desire phase* refers to the experiences of sexual appetite or drive produced by the activation of a neural system in the brain. Sexual desire is experienced as sensations that move the person to seek sexual experiences. Although the precise neural circuitry involved in sexual desire is unknown, it is believed to involve the limbic system and the preoptic nuclei of the hypothalamus. It is likely that the sexual centers of the brain have either neural or chemical connections with the pleasure and pain centers of the brain. The pleasure centers are stimulated during a sexual experience, which accounts for the pleasurable quality of sexual behavior. On the other hand, the pain centers can inhibit the sexual system. Some persons suggest that the pleasure center is stimulated by release of endorphins in sexual behavior. If a sexual object or situation produces pain, then it will cease to evoke desire.

Testosterone is important in mediating sexual desire in both men and women. Luteinizing hormone also may be important in mediating sexual desire. Two neurotransmitters, serotonin (5HT) and dopamine, are also believed to be important in mediating sexual desire. Serotonin acts as an inhibitor, and dopamine acts as a stimulant to the sexual centers of the brain. Bonding to another person and love are powerful stimuli to sexual desire. There seem to be many stimuli capable of evoking sexual desire, such as sight, smell, and other sensory cues; and some of these are conditioned by the culture. Fear and pain, however, are potent inhibitors.

The connections between the sex center and other parts of the brain also make it possible for people to "turn off" sexual desire when other stimuli are more important or when it is not to the individual's advantage to pursue sexual activity. Hypoactive desire and inhibited sexual desire are common problems of the sexual desire phase.

The *excitement phase* of sexual response is similar to the excitement and plateau phases described by Masters and Johnson and is produced by reflex vasodilation of the genital blood vessels. Two centers in the spinal cord—S2 to S4 and T11 to L2—cause the arterioles to dilate. This vasodilation causes the genitalia to swell and changes their shape to adapt to their reproductive function. Vasocongestion is primarily a parasympathetically mediated response, and the intense sympathetic response such as that produced by fear and anxiety can instantly lead to loss of erection. It is believed that erection is governed by two spinal reflex centers. The thoracolumbar center (psychogenic) appears to respond more to psychic stimuli, whereas the sacral center is stimulated from tactile input to the genitalia. It is believed that the spinal reflex centers and the higher neural connections are analogous in men and women. Disorders of the excitement phase include difficulty in attaining or maintaining erection in men and difficulty with swelling and lubrication in women.

The *orgasm phase* of sexual response, which corresponds to orgasm as described by Masters and Johnson, is also a genital reflex governed by spinal neural centers, but it consists of reflex contractions of certain genital muscles. Sensory influences, which trigger orgasm, enter the cord in the pudendal nerve at the sacral level and the efferents are T11 to L2. Disorders of the orgasm phase include inadequate ejaculatory control (premature ejaculation) and retarded ejaculation in men and orgasmic dysfunction in women. Other disorders include painful intercourse and sexual phobias.

SUBJECTIVE EXPERIENCE OF SEXUAL RESPONSE

The persons in the sample studied by Masters and Johnson[32] were polled with regard to the subjective experience associated with orgasm. Women described three distinct stages of orgasmic experiences. The first stage of orgasm begins as a sensation of "stoppage" or "suspension." This instantaneous sensation is followed by an intense sensual awareness oriented to the clitoris. A loss of sensory acuity has been described during this period. Some women described a sense of bearing down occurring simultaneously with the clitoral-pelvic sensation. A feeling of receptive opening has also been expressed by parous women. This sensation has also been compared to sensations felt during the second stage of labor.

The second stage of the women's orgasmic response is described as a feeling of warmth that pervades the pelvis and then spreads throughout the body. The third stage of subjective experience is a feeling of involuntary contraction of the vagina followed by a sensation of pelvic throbbing; however, women's experience is highly individual and varied.

The Singers[47] have recently described three types of orgasmic experience for women—the vulval, uterine, and blended orgasms. The vulval orgasm involves involuntary contractions of the orgasmic platform, as described by Masters and Johnson. The uterine orgasm depends on deep stimulation of the cervix that displaces the uterus, thus stimulating the peritoneum; it is characterized by a gasping type of breathing, eventually culminating in an explosive type of exhalation. The blended orgasm combines features of both the vulval and uterine variety.

Men in Masters and Johnson's study reported two stages of the subjective orgasmic experience. The first stage is a feeling of ejaculatory inevitability that develops as seminal fluid collects in the prostatic urethra. Distention of the urethral bulb may also contribute to this sensation. The second stage of subjective experience involves two phases—the sensation of contractions of the urethral sphincter and the perception of the volume of seminal fluid as it is expelled through the penile urethra.[32]

VARIATIONS IN SEXUAL EXPRESSION

People experience sexual pleasure in a variety of ways. One's culture influences both the forms of sexual expression deemed acceptable and one's value system about sexual behavior. Indeed, what is considered normal varies widely among cultures. Comfort[15] suggests that health professionals should not use a personal concept of "normal" but rather should consider the meaning that a behavior has for any individual, whether it impoverishes or enriches the lives of that person and any others with whom the sexual relations are shared, and finally, whether the behavior is tolerable to the society.

Each culture provides for a variety of erotic behaviors, but nearly all are concerned with sexual modesty. Incest taboos are common to most societies, but the definition of incest varies among cultures. Each society has some form of legal system to regulate sexual behavior.

Ford and Beach[19] found that the approaches to sexual pleasuring were highly variable among and within cultures. Positions used for intercourse include the woman astride (on top), man astride, side-to-side, or squatting. Women are expected to initiate sexual activity in some cultures, but in other cultures only men are expected to do so. The duration of sexual acts is also regulated by the culture. In some cultures, men are encouraged to ejaculate rapidly, whereas in others the man's ability to prolong intromission is valued. Forms of sexual stimulation are also highly variable. Although kissing is nearly ubiquitous, some cultures deem it unsanitary. Stimulation of the breasts either manually or orally is common. Manipulation of women's genitalia by the men is a common prelude to intromission. Oral stimulation of women's genitalia (cunnilingus) is common to many cultures, and somewhat less common is oral stimulation of men's genitalia (fellatio). Painful stimulation is sometimes used to enhance arousal. Although the circumstances surrounding coitus vary among cultures, usually privacy is important. Sexual frequency is also often governed by cultural norms; for example, intercourse may be prohibited during menses, lactation, pregnancy, and in some cultures before hunts or wars.

Although heterosexuality is the most prevalent form of sexual expression in the cultures that have been studied, it is rarely the only type of sexual behavior in which people engage. Heterosexuals choose partners of the opposite sex, whereas homosexuals seek partners of the same sex. Bisexuals enjoy both same- and opposite-sexed partners at various points in time. The pedophile experiences sexual arousal with a child, whereas those who practice "swinging sex" have sexual relations as a couple with another person or persons. Incest implies having sexual relations with a close relative. In zoophilia, the sexual object is an animal; in fetishism, it is an inanimate object; and in necrophilia, it is a dead body. Transvestites experience sexual pleasure by dressing in clothes of the opposite sex. Some persons experience sexual pleasure from watching others (voyeurism), exposing their genitalia (exhibitionism), inflicting pain (sadism), or experiencing pain (masochism).

HOMOSEXUALITY

Homosexuality and heterosexuality are the most common sexual variations; yet homosexuality is poorly understood by health professionals. It has been regarded as an illness, a criminal offense, and a life-style in Western society. Nevertheless, Kinsey estimated that 13% of women and 37% of men had had at least one homosexual experience leading to orgasm. Because the extent to which people engaged in homosexual behavior varied greatly, Kinsey proposed a continuum, on which the two poles represented exclusive heterosexuality (0) and homosexuality (6) and the five remaining categories (1 through 5) represented a combination of the two. Individuals in categories 1 and 5 had predominant heterosexual or homosexual orientations, whereas those in categories 2 and 4 had a clear preference for heterosexual or homosexual relations, but retained an active interest in the other form. Category 3 represented persons who had equal heterosexual and homosexual interests.

Many explanations have been suggested for the origins of sexual orientation. Bell et al.[7] studied over 1400 homosexual and heterosexual men and women. Their data did not support psychological or social origins of homosexuality, except for an association between effeminate boys having a cold, rejecting father. Genetic or hormonal causes of homosexual sexual orientation have not been established.

The Institute for Sex Research studied 979 homosexual men and women and a comparison group of 477 heterosexuals from the San Francisco area. Through an extensive interview, these investigators determined that homosexuality involved more than just sexual practices. Homosexuals varied in the degree to which they were involved in homosexual and heterosexual experiences, ranging along a continuum from those with exclusively homosexual feelings and behaviors to those with more heterosexual than homosexual feelings and behaviors. They were predominantly covert about their homosexuality, although frequently their families were aware of their sexual preferences. Many common assumptions about homosexuality were not supported by this study. Homosexuals could not be typified as sexually hyperactive or hypoactive. The investigation made clear the uniqueness of homosexual life-styles and the differences in life-style for men and women. For example, cruising (purposefully searching for a partner) was common among men but less common among women. Men tended to have more partners than women, but both men and women preferred a relatively steady relationship with a lover.

The men and women in this study used a variety of sexual techniques. Men most frequently used fellatio, hand-genital contact, and anal intercourse; and women most frequently participated in masturbation and cunnilingus with their partners. Sexual problems were more commonly reported by men than by women and included difficulty meeting a partner and meeting the partner's sexual requests. Sexually transmitted disease was a common health problem for men, but this was not the case for women.

Bell and Weinberg[6] found that the homosexuals they interviewed were involved in a variety of relationships, ranging from a quasimarriage to having multiple short-term contacts. Some were not involved in a relationship, had little sexual interest, and regretted their homosexuality.

When psychologic adjustment of the homosexual group was compared with that of the heterosexual group, it was apparent that homosexuals who were in dysfunctional sexual relationships or situations and who were asexual were less well adjusted than heterosexuals. However, when the comparison was restricted to those who were functional (had little regret about homosexuality) or were in a coupled relationship, homosexuals were no more distressed than heterosexuals.

Masters and Johnson[31] compared the physiology of sexual response in homosexuals and heterosexuals in the laboratory setting. They found no significant difference in the homosexual and heterosexual subjects' facility for orgasm in response to masturbation, partner manipulation, fellatio, or cunnilingus; nor were there demonstrable physiologic differences in the sexual response cycles of homosexuals and heterosexuals.

Blumstein and Schwartz's study of American couples[12] revealed that physical contact still forms a major bond between members of a couple. They found that the frequency of sexual activity declines the longer the couple stays together, and sexual frequency declines with age. Sexual frequency also depends on whether a couple is married, gay, lesbian, or living together. Those with the highest frequency were gay men, followed by cohabitors, marrieds, and lesbians. The quality and quantity of sex seem to be important to the well-being of relationships for all types of couples, and when nonsexual parts of couples' lives were going badly, their sex life suffered.

Among contemporary couples, when having sex, many share initiation and refusal. When there is not sharing, men tend to initiate sexual activity and women tend to share. Cohabiting women initiate more frequently than do wives. Older cohabiting men resent women initiating sexual activity. Among heterosexual couples, a woman may hesitate to initiate sex when she believes her partner is feeling vulnerable. Equality of initiation of sexual activity is associated with a happier sex life than is role reversal in initiation. In gay, lesbian, married, and cohabiting couples, the more emotionally expressive partner initiates sex most often. The more powerful partner is more likely to refuse sex.[12]

Kissing occurs frequently when couples have sex. It is most consistent among lesbians and least consistent among gay men. Intercourse is a more essential part of having sex for heterosexual women than for heterosexual men. The less power a heterosexual woman has in her relationship, the more likely it is that the couple will have intercourse in the man astride (on top) position.[12]

Women, more than men, need to be in love to have sex; this has made them feel more possessive of their partners than is the case for men. Monogamy is still a strongly held moral ideal, even though not always observed. An occasional act of nonmonogamy does not assure a career of infidelity. A woman's nonmonogamy is more likely to be an affair than is the case for a man's nonmonogamy. Couples who live separate lives have more opportunity to be nonmonogamous, and they are.[12]

AGING AND SEXUALITY

It is commonly assumed that sexuality is not a concern for older people, and some consider that an elderly person's interest in sex is perverse. Research on sexuality and aging contradicts the stereotypes of the elderly as either disinterested in sex or abnormally obsessed with it. Instead, it appears that for many aging persons, sexuality is an important dimension of being alive. There is no single point in the life cycle at which sexual activity must cease, although there is a decline in reports of sexual interest and activity with increasing age. Even so, investigators have demonstrated that both sexual interest and activity persist well into the seventh, eighth, and ninth decades of life.[41,26,43] One study estimated that 40% to 65% of persons 60 to 71 years of age engaged in intercourse fairly frequently, and 10% to 20% of those over 78 years of age were sexually active. Indeed, 13% to 15% of the older persons in one study actually showed *increased* patterns of sexual activity and interest with age.[43]

If one were to compare sexual response in young men and women with their middle-aged and older counterparts, there would be more similarities than differences. The processes essential for sexual response occur more slowly with age, and the phase-specific changes may appear somewhat less intense. Neverthe-

less, the capacity for sexual pleasure exists in many elderly persons.

As women age, there is a gradual change in their genitalia and breasts, paralleling the change in estrogen levels associated with menopause. There is often a delay in the production of vaginal lubrication, although this appears to be much less a problem for women who have been consistently sexually active throughout their lives. As women age, the vagina becomes smaller in both length and diameter.

Also as women age, there is less marked elevation and tenting of the uterus during sexual excitement and less evidence of vasocongestive changes in the labia and breasts. Vasocongestion of the orgasmic platform is less apparent; and during orgasm, the frequency of contraction of the orgasmic platform is less than that for younger women. Indeed, some women report uncomfortable uterine contractions during orgasm. The resolution of sexual tension proceeds more slowly than in younger women.[32]

Age-related changes in sexual response in men parallel those changes in women. The time period necessary to experience an erection increases, and the erection is likely to be less full than earlier in life. There is usually less profound evidence of vasocongestion in the scrotum and testes. Because the plateau phase of the sexual response cycle is prolonged, the aging man attains better control of ejaculation. Orgasm encompasses a shorter time span. The intensity of the ejaculation decreases, and a man may feel satisfied ejaculating every second or third time he has intercourse.[32]

A gap between interest and sexual activity has been found for middle-aged persons. Usually the gap is much wider for men than women, with men exhibiting more interest in sexual activity than actual activity. An explanation for this gap was that men had impaired sexual function as a result of poor health. The absence of such a gap for women was attributed to their adaptively inhibiting sexual interest because of lack of opportunity— usually the result of the loss of a partner or the partner's sexual dysfunction.[41] An alternative explanation is the different sexual value systems held by men and women of the study cohort. In earlier generations, men were socialized to express their sexual desire and women were socialized to avoid discussing their desire.

SEXUAL HISTORY

Many health care providers may not be experienced in eliciting a sexual history and may initially be uneasy when doing so. No doubt this uneasiness is conditioned by social prohibitions about discussing intimate matters such as sexual experiences or behavior. However, clients expect health professionals to be informed, willing to discuss sexual matters openly with clients, and prepared to educate and counsel them appropriately.

Nurses who are hesitant to deal with sexual matters with clients will be helped by confronting their own feelings about sex and sexual matters. Seeking counsel from other nurses or health professionals who are comfortable with the topic is often helpful. Recently, special courses and workshops on sexuality for nurses have become available, and some nurses may find it helpful to attend one of these. During the past decade, the public has been exposed to explicit portrayals of sex and sexuality. Although sometimes criticized, this candor has had salutary effects: more people are willing and able to discuss their sexual concerns. As a result, health professionals are increasingly expected to be informed, willing to discuss these concerns, and able to educate and counsel clients.

Although there is no single approach to taking a sexual history, application of certain principles will facilitate both the client's and the practitioner's comfort. Absolute requirements for history taking include provision of privacy, such as a closed room; an atmosphere of trust between client and practitioner, such as assurance of confidentiality for the client; and comfort on the part of the practitioner with her or his own sexuality.

Some principles for promoting client-practitioner comfort follow. First, obtaining the sexual history early in the therapeutic relationship conveys to the client that sexuality is a legitimate component of health and that it is normal and usual for it to be examined in the context of a physical examination or health history. Next, the sexual history, itself, may be therapeutic. Within the context of obtaining the data, the practitioner can provide permission for the client to discuss her or his concerns, provide limited information or suggestions, or validate the normalcy and acceptability of the client's concerns and practices. Avoiding overreaction, such as shock and horror, to the information related by the client, as well as underreaction, such as boredom, facilitates accuracy on the part of the client. Using language that the client understands and with which the practitioner is comfortable will also facilitate obtaining an adequate picture of the client's concerns. It may be necessary for both the client and the practitioner to define their terms; "street' language may be unfamiliar to the nurse, and highly technical language may be confusing to the client. The technique of moving from less sensitive to more sensitive areas paves the way for both the client and the practitioner. For example, the nurse may explore a woman's sexual role before discussing her ability to have orgasm, her menstrual history before her experience with sexual variations, and her personal experiences with sex education before her actual sexual experiences.

"Unloading the question" is another technique useful in obtaining a sexual history. This consists of prefacing the question with a statement referring to the known variation in or prevalence of a specific behavior. For example, the question related to frequency of intercourse may be asked in the following fashion: "Some women have intercourse many times a week, some a few times a month, and still others not at all. On the average, how often do you have intercourse?" This approach conveys to the client that no matter what her practices, they fit into the framework of known behavioral patterns.

Referring to the ubiquity of sexual practices is another useful strategy. This consists of asking clients "how" or "when" they began certain sexual practices as opposed to the more threatening "did you ever?" approach. Prefacing an inquiry by a statement such as "Many people experience. . . ." conveys to the client that his or her practices or experiences are not too unusual to relate.

Following the life cycle chronology is another useful technique inasmuch as it provides for a logical unfolding of events. Finally, terminating the sexual history by inquiring whether the client has additional questions or issues to discuss conveys a willingness on the part of the practitioner to further explore sexual matters.

BRIEF SEXUAL ASSESSMENT

A brief assessment can be incorporated in the nursing history using three questions. The first of these deals with the person's role, the second with the affective-cognitional elements of sexuality, and the third with biologic aspects of sexual function. These questions may be modified to deal with illness, hospitalization, life events, or any other relevant entity that may influence or interfere with sexual health.

Has your (illness, pregnancy, hospitalization) affected your being a (husband, wife, father, mother)?

SAFETY OF SEXUAL PRACTICES

PROBABLY SAFE

Dry kissing, hugging
Mutual masturbation on healthy skin
Unshared sex toys
Massage, touching, fantasy

POSSIBLY SAFE

Deep kissing
Intercourse (vaginal or anal) with a condom
Oral sex with a condom
Urine-to-skin contact (external water sports)

UNSAFE

Intercourse without a condom (vaginal or anal)
Oral sex without condom
Oral-anal contact (rimming)
Hand in rectum (fisting)
Shared sex toys
Urinating into mouth, vagina, or rectum
Sharing a needle

Has your (abortion, heart attack) affected the way you see yourself as a (woman, man)? Has your (colostomy, hysterectomy) affected your ability to function sexually (or your sex life)? These questions may also be adapted to elicit the client's expectations of changes resulting from impending procedures or hospitalization. These brief items invite the client to explore sexual concerns. Often it is unnecessary for the practitioner to ask the second and third questions, because many clients proceed to discuss their concerns about masculinity, femininity, and sexual functioning.

Another dimension of sexual assessment focuses on safe sexual practices that prevent or limit transmission of sexually transmitted diseases, including AIDS. Direct questioning about safe, possibly safe, and unsafe sexual practices can be linked with teaching. Intercourse (vaginal or anal) without a condom and with multiple partners escalate risk for AIDS and other sexually transmitted diseases. (See box on opposite page).

SEXUAL PROBLEM HISTORY

The sexual problem history may be used in conjunction with the brief history described above or alone in the context of sexual counseling or therapy. Although the parameters explored in a sexual problem history will vary with the theoretical framework guiding the nurse's practice, there are commonalities to be explored regardless of the approach to therapy. The approach described below has been suggested by Annon.[3]

The first component of the sexual problem history is a description, in the client's terms, of the current problem or concern. Next, the onset and course of the problem are explored. The practitioner may wish to inquire about the age of the client when the problem began, whether it had an insidious onset or occurred suddenly, whether the client can identify any precipitating events, and whether there are other life events associated with the sexual problem. The course of the sexual problem can be described in terms of its fluctuations over time, such as with the changing intensity of a disease process, and whether the problem has any functional relationships to phenomena such as medication or alcohol use.

Of great importance is the client's conception of the cause and persistence of the problem. This data will enable the nurse to respond directly to the client's concerns rather than dealing with them indirectly.

Past attempts at treatment and their results may be explored, including evaluations by other health practitioners (for example, physicians), the use of other professional help (for example, counselors), and finally the attempts that the client has made to cope with the problem.

The last component of the sexual problem history includes an examination of the client's current expecta-

tions and the goals identified for treatment. A woman complaining of inability to have orgasm may have the expectations of having orgasm with intercourse rather than by self-stimulation. If her expectations are not stated precisely, the practitioner may inappropriately treat her with the latter goal in mind or refer her to a practitioner whose approach to therapy would not be congruent with her goals.

PHYSICAL ASSESSMENT*

An essential sequel to identification of sexual concerns or problems is a thorough physical examination. Because the genitals have special significance for sexuality, the following discussion will focus on the breast examination, pelvic examination for women, and genital examination for men. Treating both men and women with dignity and conveying respect for their sexuality is important in any aspect of the physical examination. It is particularly important for breast and genital examination because most people have been socialized to consider their genitals private and sometimes even unacceptable.

EXAMINATION OF WOMEN

Examination of women begins with inspection of the secondary sex characteristics, breast development, hair distribution, and the development of the external genitalia, including the mons, vulva, clitoris, labia minora and majora, and vaginal outlet. Women's breasts are inspected to determine size and symmetry, contour, and appearance of the skin. Although there is often some difference in breast size (for example, the left breast may be smaller than the right), the breasts usually are relatively symmetric. Variations in breast contour may include the presence of masses, dimpling, or flattening. The color of the skin of the breasts, presence of thickened areas, and abnormalities of the venous pattern may indicate pathologic processes. The nipples may be inverted, but this is usually not pathologic. However, the direction in which the nipples are pointing may provide clues to masses when there is asymmetry. Discharge from the nipples may indicate pathologic processes or may merely vary in certain women with the hormonal fluctuation of the menstrual cycle. Ulcerated areas and other nipple lesions require further exploration.

Making body contact with the woman, such as in palpation of the cervical nodes or auscultation of the chest, precedes the breast examination. Ideally, instruction in or a review of the breast self-examination can occur as the practitioner performs the breast examination. Women can be encouraged to examine their breasts on

---

*This section modified from Woods NF: Human sexuality in health and illness, ed 3, St Louis, 1984, The CV Mosby Co.

a monthly basis. The conclusion of their menstrual period or a few days thereafter is the best time for this, since premenstrual engorgement of the breasts may cause them to have a lumpy consistency or to be tender. Because of the cyclic changes in the consistency of breast tissue, it is recommended that the self-examination be performed at a consistent point in the menstrual cycle.

The practitioner inspects the external genitalia, including the labia majora, the mons, and the vulva, before the pelvic examination, noting inflammatory processes, ulcerations, congenital or surgical absence of structures, lesions, nodules, and discharge. It is customary to inspect the labia minora, clitoris, urethral opening, and vaginal introitus before the pelvic examination.

Examiners wear gloves on both hands during the genital examination. Although some women may safely practice self-examinations without gloves, practitioners commonly wear gloves to prevent the transmission of infection to their clients. The practitioner can explain the reason for wearing examination gloves to the woman so that she does not perceive the practice as an indication that she is abnormal or unclean.

Usually the examiner makes physical contact with the woman's knees before touching her thighs or genitals. The labia minora, clitoris, and urethral opening can be revealed by separating the labia majora. Evidences of pathologic processes cited earlier are noted. While the labia are separated with the examiner's middle and index fingers, the woman can be requested to bear down, allowing the examiner to note any bulging of the vaginal walls or gaping of the introitus. The former may be indicative of cystocele and rectocele, the latter of injury to the pubococcygeus muscle surrounding the vaginal outlet. Presence of surgical scarring, such as at an episiotomy site, may also be noted at this time. This part of the examination affords the practitioner the opportunity to teach the woman Kegel's exercises in the event that she does not already know how to do them. A set of instructions for exercises of the pubococcygeus muscle is given in the box above.

A pelvic examination is customarily performed as part of a total health assessment for women. It consists of two primary components: the speculum examination of the cervix and vagina and the manual palpation of the uterus and ovaries. Because this is described in detail in Chapter 53, only those aspects of the examination that are related to the woman's sexuality will be addressed here.

The pelvic examination can be an educational experience for the woman, as well as an experience that validates her sexuality. It is recommended that the practitioner avoid assumptions about whether the woman is sexually active and with whom, as well as assumptions about her desire for fertility control. The examination

---

EXERCISES FOR THE PUBOCOCCYGEUS MUSCLE

Sit on a toilet seat with your knees as far apart as possible. Start and stop the flow of urine. This will enable you to feel the pubococcygeus muscle.

Begin exercising this muscle gradually at intervals throughout the day. The following exercises can be done each day:

1. Contracting the pubococcygeus muscle and holding for 3 seconds (this feels the same as it did when you stopped the flow of urine)
2. Contracting the pubococcygeus muscle rapidly
3. Breathing deeply and tightening the pubococcygeus muscle as you inhale
4. Bearing down, then relaxing, and as you relax, tightening the pubococcygeus muscle

Ten to twenty-five contractions each day are usually sufficient to maintain good muscle tone.

---

should begin with the woman in a sitting position, rather than greeting the examiner from the lithotomy position (usually this produces poor, if any, eye contact and a feeling of being vulnerable). The examiner can offer the woman the choice of whether or not she would like a drape. Some women prefer to see what the examiner is doing. Some women prefer not to use a drape because this reinforces the idea that their bodies and the procedure are something shameful. Other women believe the drape adds to their dignity. Asking whether the woman would like a drape while offering it to show that it is available allows her to choose what is most comfortable. The examiner can also ask the woman whether she would like a mirror to enable her to see her cervix. The mirror may enable some women to see their genitals for the first time. Many examiners use a lighted speculum to facilitate the woman's viewing of her own anatomy.

By explaining what is happening, the examiner can validate the woman's sexuality and health. For example, the examiner might say "I'm going to look at your labia and clitoris now. They look very healthy." As the examiner gets ready to insert the speculum, she or he can advise the woman of any noise the speculum might make (plastic speculums are especially noisy) and also advise her of what will be done: for example, "Now I'm going to put two fingers in your vagina. I'm going to put the speculum into your vagina, and I'll open it up so you can see your cervix. Your vagina looks very healthy. Can you see your cervix?" Insertion of the speculum can be facilitated by using warm tap water as a lubricant. Some practitioners advocate inserting the speculum blades at only a slight oblique angle, whereas others advocate inserting the blades horizontally. The primary concern is avoiding pressure on the urethra, which causes pain. When removing the speculum, the blades are closed after the cervix is cleared, otherwise the cervix may become pinched between the speculum blades.

During the bimanual examination the woman can also be included. For example, she may wish to palpate her ovaries. This orientation to the pelvic examination affords many opportunities for teaching and modeling that sexuality is a wholesome, positive phenomenon.

EXAMINATION OF MEN

Inspection of the penis, scrotum, and testicles is usually integrated with the physical examination. As these structures are examined, the practitioner also notes the hair distribution pattern over the axillary and pelvic area, as in the examination of the woman. Abnormalities of the male breast may be noted, including the presence of gynecomastia, an enlargement of breast tissue that often occurs during normal puberty and at other times during the life cycle. The male breast may be inspected for deviations in contour, symmetry, abnormalities in the skin of the breast, and irregularities of the nipple. Men do develop breast cancers, so caution is in order if abnormal discharges or lesions are found.

Inspection of the penis includes observations of the skin for ulcers or lesions. The shaft is observed for deviations in shape and size or symmetry. The foreskin may be present in uncircumcised men, and the client may be asked to retract it to facilitate inspection of the glans area for the presence of lesions. Abnormalities of the glans and urethral meatus may also be noted, including deviations in the location of the urethra, ulcerations of the glans, and discharge from the urethral meatus.

The scrotal skin is usually inspected next for the presence of nodules or inflammation and to check contour. Usually the left testicle is somewhat lower in the scrotal sac than the right. Absence or atrophy of the testicles may also be identified by inspection. Palpation may be used to examine the penis, scrotal sac and contents, prostate gland, and rectum. Usually the genitalia are examined with a gloved hand. Inspection and palpation of the external genitalia can be accomplished with the client lying on the examination table. As with female clients, a drape may be offered. Inspection of the perineum and scrotum and palpation of the seminal vesicles and prostate can be easily accomplished by asking the client to turn on his left side with his legs flexed, a somewhat less vulnerable position than the spread-eagle position.

Approaches such as the explanations provided to women can be used when examining men. Some men may elect to use a mirror to see their own genitals. Instruction in testicular self-examination can be integrated with this portion of the physical examination (see Chapter 56).

OTHER USEFUL DATA

To fully evaluate clients' sexual difficulties, relevant historical and laboratory data are obtained. Clients are queried about their cardiovascular, respiratory, gastrointestinal, genitourinary, central nervous system, and endocrine functions, as well as the presence of intercurrent illnesses, their use of prescription and nonprescription drugs, and habits such as alcohol use. Problems in other body systems, use of medications affecting sexual performance, and habits interfering with sexual appreciation or function may be corrected with appropriate medical therapy, and, in turn, the sexual problems are often corrected.

Laboratory data useful in the determination of the cause of sexual dysfunction include blood work, such as complete blood counts, thyroid function tests, glucose tolerance tests, and chemistry determinations. Vaginal cytology, endocrine workups, electrocardiograms, and chest x-ray films may reveal underlying conditions responsible for sexual problems.

CHAPTER SUMMARY

- ✔ Sexual health is multidimensional, including sexual function, sexual self-concept, and sexual relationships.
- ✔ Human sexuality is the result of complex physiologic, psychosocial, and cultural influences.
- ✔ Sexual beginnings influence gender, gender identity, and gender role.
- ✔ Human sexual response is a total body response based on myotonia and vasocongestion. Desire, arousal, and orgasm result from different neurophysiologic systems in response to physical, interpersonal, and contextual stimuli.
- ✔ Variations in sexual experience and sexual expression reflect human development and individual differences. Homosexuality and heterosexuality represent common variations of sexual expression and experience and exist on a continuum.
- ✔ Although sexual interest and sexual activity may decline as people age, many continue an active sexual life well into their later years. Activity levels appear to be related to sexual activity during younger years.
- ✔ Sexual assessment includes history taking and a physical examination as the basis for a nursing diagnosis.
- ✔ Several formats are available for taking a sexual history. Inquiring directly about safe and unsafe sexual practices creates an opportunity for education about safe sex.

QUESTIONS TO CONSIDER

- Before taking a sexual history from a patient, think about your own sexual history. Try to respond to the following questions about your own sexual development as honestly as possible. If some of the questions do not apply to your experience, just skip to the next questions.
  a. How old were you when you discovered the differences between women's and men's anatomy?
  b. How did you find out about these differences?
  c. How did you feel about your discovery?
  d. What were your parents' attitudes about sex?
  e. How were these attitudes communicated to you?
  f. What were your peers' attitudes about sex?
  g. What was your response to your first menstruation? ejaculation? orgasm?
  h. How did you learn about it?
  i. Do you remember when you first stimulated yourself in a sexual way? How did you feel about it?
  j. Have you ever had sexual relations with another person? Do you remember the first time?
  k. What was it like?
  l. How do you feel about your body now?
  m. How do you feel about being a man? woman?
  n. How do you feel about your sexual relationship?
  o. Are you satisfied with your current sexual activities? How would you change them?
  p. If you have a partner, how does your partner feel?
  q. Can you describe a peak sexual experience?

- What behaviors by a nurse would enhance your comfort in discussing your sexual history? What behaviors would cause you to feel uncomfortable?

- Choose one portion of the life cycle that is most relevant to your clinical practice or your interests. Consider one client with whom you have been involved as a nurse. Describe the most significant aspects of sexuality for a person during this part of the life cycle. In what respects does your client differ from your expectations? What factors seem to contribute to these differences?

- List 10 different types of sexual behavior. Think about which of these are acceptable to you in relation to both yourself and others. For those behaviors that you find unacceptable, try to identify what specific aspect of the behavior "turns you off." What criteria do you seem to be using? For example, legal, religious, statistical, or social, cultural criteria may all be used as criteria for determining what sexual behaviors are acceptable in yourself and others.

Behavior	Acceptable in Me	Acceptable in Others	Unacceptable
1.			
2.			
3.			
4.			
5.			
6.			
7.			
8.			
9.			
10.			

REFERENCES AND SELECTED READINGS

1. Allen M: A holistic view of sexuality and the aged, Holistic Nurs Pract 1(4):76-83, 1987.
2. Andrist L: Taking a sexual history and educating clients about safe sex, Nurs Clin North Am 23(4):959-973, 1988.
3. Annon J: The behavioral treatment of sexual problems, Honolulu, 1974, Enabling Systems, Inc.
4. Assey J and Herbert J: Who is the seductive patient? Am J Nurs 83:530-532, 1983.
5. Beach F, editor: Human sexuality in four perspectives, Baltimore, 1977, The Johns Hopkins University Press.
6. Bell A and Weinberg M: Homosexualities, New York, 1978, Simon & Schuster, Inc.
7. Bell A, Weinberg M, and Keifer-Hammersmith S: Sexual preference: its development in men and women. Bloomington, 1981, Indiana University Press.
8. Belzer E: A review of female ejaculation and the Grafenberg spot, Women Health, 9(1):5-16, 1985.
9. Bem S: Probing the promise of androgyny. In Kaplan, A, and Bean, J: Beyond sex role stereotyping: readings toward a psychology of androgyny, Boston, 1976, Little, Brown & Co.
10. Bernhard L and Dan A: Redefining sexuality from women's own experiences, Nurs Clin North Am 21:125-136, 1986.
11. Bidwell R: The gay and lesbian teen: a case of denied adolescence, J Pediatr Health Care. 2(1):3-8, 1988.
12. Blumstein P and Schwartz P: American couples: Money, work, sex, New York, 1983, William Morrow.
13. Brink P: Cultural aspects of sexuality, Holistic Nursing Practice 1(4):12-20, 1987.
14. Bullough B et al: Subjective reports of female orgasmic expulsion of fluid, Nurse Pract 9:55-59, 1984.
15. Comfort A: The normal in sexual behavior: an ethological view, J Sex Educ Ther 2:1-7, 1975.

*References preceded by an asterisk are particularly well suited for student reading.

16. De Bow M: Safer sex, Imprint 35(1):33-34, 36, 1988.
17. Education and treatment in human sexuality: the training of health professionals: report of a WHO meeting, Geneva, 1975, World Health Organization.
18. Fogel C and Lauver D: Sexual health promotion, Philadelphia, 1989, WB Saunders Co.
19. Ford C and Beach F: Patterns of sexual behavior, New York, 1951, Harper & Row, Publishers, Inc.
20. Friend R: Sexual identity and human diversity: implications for nursing practice, Holistic Nurs Pract 1(4):21-41, 1987.
21. Green R: Taking a sexual history. In Green, R, editor: Human sexuality: a health practitioner's test, Baltimore, 1975, The Williams & Wilkins Co.
22. Hallstrom T: Sexuality of women in middle age: The Goteberg study, J Biosoc Sci., Suppl 6, 165-175, 1979.
23. *Hogan R: Human sexuality: a nursing perspective, ed 2, New York, 1985, Appleton-Century-Crofts.
24. Kaplan HS: The new sex therapy, New York, 1974, Brunner/Mazel, Inc.
25. Kaplan HS: Disorders of sexual desire and other new concepts and techniques in sex therapy, New York, 1979, Brunner/Mazel, Inc.
26. Kinsey AC et al: Sexual behavior in the human male, Philadelphia, 1948, WB Saunders Co.
27. Kus R: Sex, AIDS, and gay American men, Holistic Nurs Pract 1(4):42-51, 1987.
28. Lion E: Human sexuality in nursing process, New York, 1982, John Wiley & Sons, Inc.
29. LoPiccolo, J, and Steger, J: The sexual interaction inventory: a new instrument for assessment of sexual dysfunction, Arch Sex Behav 3:585-593, 1974.
30. Ludeman K: The sexuality of the older person: review of the literature, Gerontologist 21(2):203-208, 1981.
31. Masters W and Johnson V: Human sexual inadequacy, Boston, 1970, Little, Brown & Co.
32. Masters W and Johnson V: Human sexual response, Boston, 1966, Little, Brown & Co.
33. Masters W and Johnson V: Principles of the new sex therapy, Am J Psychol 133:548-584, 1976.
34. Mc Cracken A: Sexual practice by elders: the forgotten aspect of functional health, J Gerontolog Nurs 14(10):13-18, 1988.
35. Mims F: Sexual stress: coping and adaptation, Nurs Clin North Am 17:395-405, 1982.
36. *Mims F and Swenson M: Sexuality: a nursing perspective, New York, 1980, McGraw-Hill Book Co.
37. Money J and Erhardt A: Man, woman, boy, girl, Baltimore, 1972, The Johns Hopkins University Press.
38. Moses A and Hawkins R: Counseling lesbian women and gay men: a life issues approach, St Louis, 1982, The CV Mosby Co.
39. Parsons J: The psychology of sex difference, Washington, 1980, Hemisphere Publishing Co.
40. Paul W et al: Homosexuality: social, psychological and biological issues, Beverly Hills, 1982, Sage Publications.
41. Persson G: Sexuality in a seventy year old urban population. J Psychosom Res 24:335-342, 1980.
42. Pfeiffer E, Verwoerdt A, and Davis GC: Sexual behavior in middle life: Am J Psychiatry 128:1262-1267, 1972.
43. Pfeiffer E, Verwoerdt A, and Wang HS: The natural history of sexual behavior in a biologically advantaged group of aged individuals, J Gerontol 23:193-198, 1969.
44. Renhshaw D: Sex, intimacy, and the older woman, Women Health 8(4):43-54, 1983.
45. Saltzman S et al: Reliability of self reported sexual behavior risk factors for HIV infection in homosexual men, Public Health Rep 102(6):692-697, 1987.
46. Schecter M: Patterns of sexual behavior and condom use in a cohort of homosexual men, Am J Public Health 78(12):1535-1538.
47. Singer J and Singer J: Types of female orgasm, J Sex Res 8:255-267, 1972.
48. Starr B and Weiner M: The Starr-Weiner report on sex and sexuality in the mature years, New York, 1981, Stein & Day, Publishers.
49. Turner B and Adams C: The sexuality of older women. In Markson E: Older women, Lexington, Mass, 1983 Lexington Books.
50. *Watts R: Dimensions of sexual health, Am J Nurs 79:1568-1572, 1979.
51. Weg R, editor: Sexuality in the later years: roles and behaviors, New York, 1983, Academic Press Inc.
52. Whitley M and Willingham D: Adding a sexual assessment to the health interview, J Psychiatr Nurs Mental Health Serv 5(4):17-22, 1978.
53. Winter L: The role of sexual self concept in the use of contraceptives, Fam Plann Perspect 20(3):123-127, 1988.
54. *Woods NF: Human sexuality in health and illness, ed 3, St Louis, 1984, The CV Mosby Co.
55. Woods N: Toward a holistic perspective of human sexuality: alterations in sexual health and nursing diagnoses, Holistic Nurs Pract (4):1-11, 1987.

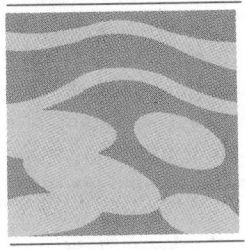

CHAPTER 52

Management of Persons with Sexual Problems

NANCY FUGATE WOODS

CHAPTER OBJECTIVES

After studying this chapter, the student should be able to:
1 Analyze data to identify diagnoses of sexual concerns, difficulties, and dysfunctions.
2 Analyze clinical data to identify risk factors for sexual concerns or problems.
3 Promote sexual health by providing permission and limited information to clients.
4 Refer clients to health professionals who can provide specific suggestions and intensive sexual therapy when needed.
5 Practice ways of promoting one's own sexual health and protecting one's own integrity.

This chapter examines common sexual concerns and problems people experience, risk factors that influence the experience of sexual concerns and problems, and nursing approaches to prevent or alleviate sexual concerns and problems. Outcome criteria for interventions for clients experiencing sexual problems will be specified.

DIAGNOSING SEXUAL CONCERNS, DIFFICULTIES, AND DYSFUNCTIONS

DEFINITIONS AND DIAGNOSES

People experience a variety of sexual problems ranging from concerns about sexual phenomena to sexual dysfunctions. Each type of problem has different antecedents, and each requires somewhat different therapeutic approaches. Sexual concerns include worry, dissatisfaction, or discomfort but do not produce difficulty in sexual function, profound problems in a sexual relationship, or a greatly altered sexual self-concept. These concerns often arise because of misinformation or lack of information, conflicting values, difficulty communicating about sexual issues, and anxiety or guilt about sexual phenomena. Such concerns are usually amenable to sex education strategies including permission giving, provision of limited information, values clarification ex-

ercises, rehearsal of communication, validation of normalcy, and provision of anticipatory guidance.

Sexual difficulties create discomfort in the sexual relationship, may occasionally interfere with sexual function, and sometimes may challenge the person's sexual self-image. Sexual difficulties include the inability to relax, disinterest in sexual activity, sexual dissatisfaction, inability to please or be pleased by a partner, and problems in the timing of sexual activities. These difficulties are amenable to counseling approaches, including relaxation training, exploration of alternatives in the sexual repertoire, provision of specific suggestions, and training in communication skills. Sexual dysfunction usually results not only in disruption of sexual function but also in severe strains on a sexual relationship and one's sexual self-image.

There are three categories of sexual dysfunction: (1) alterations in sexual desire, (2) alterations of arousal, and (3) alterations of orgasm. Each broad category of dysfunction includes several specific types of problems. Moreover, each problem can be described as lifelong versus time limited and global or situational. Qualifying information can also be included in the diagnostic statement.[116]

ALTERATIONS IN SEXUAL DESIRE

Alterations in sexual desire include low sexual desire and sexual aversion. Low desire is defined on the basis of frequency of self-pleasuring and partner activity as well as reports of desire for a partner and incidence of fantasy, erotic dreams, or seeking out erotic stimuli. Aversion is a clearly negative reaction to sex. Individuals with low sexual desire or sexual aversion may be able to experience lubrication or erection but do not experience much pleasure from their sexual activity.

Alterations in sexual desire, including low sexual desire and aversion, can be attributed to both physiologic and psychosocial factors. Depression, severe stress states, certain pharmacologic agents, low androgen levels, and certain illnesses can interfere with sexual desire. Low sexual desire is a frequent feature of depression and may occur with severe stress. Pharmacologic agents, including narcotics, sedatives, alcohol, centrally acting hypertensives such as reserpine and methyldopa, and testosterone antagonists, also are associated with low sexual desire, as are illnesses producing discomfort or malaise. Alterations in sexual desire may also occur in response to conscious or unconscious thought processes. Sexual desire can be turned off by physiologic responses associated with anger or fear, and these, in turn, may result from personal conflicts about success, intimacy, complex intrapsychic problems, or severe relationship problems. Anger may be directed at a partner. Anxieties linked to childhood experiences such as sexual abuse, pressure to have sex, repeated unpleasurable experiences, and guilt may also interfere with sexual desire.[69,116]

Some examples of nursing diagnoses related to low sexual desire are:

Diagnostic Title	Possible Etiologies
Sexuality patterns, altered, related to low sexual desire	Chronic pain— partner's inability to provide adequate stimulation Medication regimen— depression Sexual aversion related to rape

Therapies for low sexual desire and sexual aversion address underlying causes when they can be identified. When low sexual desire is related to chronic pain, some alternative therapies include positioning to avoid pain and using alternative stimulation to enhance sexual pleasure without producing pain.

ALTERATIONS IN SEXUAL AROUSAL

Alterations in sexual arousal, sometimes referred to as *excitement phase dysfunctions,* include decreased subjective arousal, difficulty attaining or maintaining an erection, difficulty in both attaining and maintaining an erection, decreased subjective arousal coupled with difficulty in attaining or maintaining an erection or in both attaining and maintaining an erection, decreased physiologic arousal in women, and decreased physiologic and subjective arousal in women. Feelings of subjective arousal and physiologic arousal can be distinguished. Some persons report diminished vasocongestion without a loss of erotic sensation. It is possible for men and women to experience problems in physiologic aspects of arousal without problems of subjective feelings of arousal or vice versa. Difficulty in attaining or maintaining arousal is common in both men and women, and short episodes are considered typical.

Problems related to sexual arousal originate in bodymind interaction. Pharmacologic agents, such as those given in Table 52-3, pp. 1524 can interfere with physiologic correlates of sexual arousal in men and women. Disorders that affect vascular function, such as diabetes or Leriche's syndrome, can impair erection and vasocongestion in women and men. The aging process is associated with less intense vasocongestive response to sexual stimuli. Problems with vaginal lubrication and swelling are associated with menopausal changes in estrogen levels in some women and in diabetic women. Performance anxiety and fear of failure are commonly associated with arousal phase dysfunctions.[70,116]

Alterations in sexual arousal become evident when individuals identify a history of sexual problems or during physical examination. For example, absence of alterations in sensation or reflex arousal may become apparent during physical examination.

Examples of diagnoses related to alteration in sexual arousal include:

Diagnostic Title	Possible Etiologies
Sexual dysfunction, related to decreased vasocongestion and vaginal lubrication	Diabetic neuropathy Anxiety about sexual activity
Sexual dysfunction, related to decreased vaginal swelling	Radiation therapy
Sexual dysfunction, related to difficulty attaining an erection	Medication regimen

Therapies for alterations in sexual arousal include decreasing anxiety about the problem and correcting or transcending the physiologic problems if possible. Anxiety can be reduced through desensitization exercises in which the person is instructed to use erotic imagery to approximate sexual situations evoking anxiety.

Structuring sexual encounters so that they are not demanding is another strategy. Exercises that emphasize pleasure rather than pressure to perform often begin by refocusing the person's attention on sensual aspects of touch without genital touching for a time. After the person has pleasure in sensual experiences without anxiety, sexual activity is gradually reintroduced.

Physiologic problems can sometimes be modified to restore sexual function. Drug regimens can be modified, and strategies can be introduced to amplify erotic sensations in parts of the body not affected by disease.

A penile prosthesis may be implanted in men as a method of treatment for organic erectile dysfunction. There are two types of penile prostheses. The older type consists of two sponge-filled silicone rods, which are implanted in the corpora cavernosa. This maintains the penis in a constant semierect position. The newer and more acceptable method for many men is the inflatable penile prosthesis (Figure 52-1). Both types of prostheses are implanted surgically and do not interfere with normal urinary elimination. The silicone implants are inserted through perineal or penile incisions and the in-

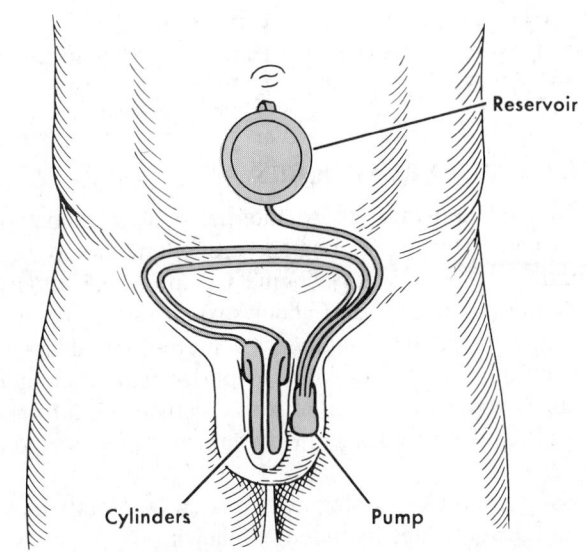

FIGURE 52-1 Inflatable penile prosthetic implant. Reservoir is implanted under abdominal muscles, inflatable cylinders in each corpus cavernosum, and pump inside scrotum. Man compresses pump to fill cylinders from reservoir, producing penile erection. Small release valve in lower portion of pump bulb releases fluid to return penis to flaccid state.

flatable prostheses through perineal and abdominal incisions. Penile edema is minimal, but scrotal edema may occur with the inflatable type. Pain may be severe during the first week, and mild pain may continue for several weeks after surgery.[57] As with any prosthetic device, there is a need to integrate it into one's self-image and the relationship.

ALTERATIONS IN ORGASM

Alterations in orgasm include problems with ejaculatory function and orgasm and with perception of pleasure associated with orgasm. *Ejaculatory dysfunctions* include premature ejaculation and inhibited ejaculation. Premature ejaculation occurs when men ejaculate too rapidly. Usually the definition is based on the individual's or couple's definition of what is too rapid. Premature ejaculation may occur before or shortly after intromission. Men who experience premature ejaculation often do not perceive erotic sensations that occur before orgasm, and instead progress rapidly from low to very high levels of arousal. Often an underlying problem is anxiety related to the experience of erotic sensations. A variety of mechanisms has been suggested including learning to ejaculate rapidly, fear, anger, and anxiety.[70,116]

Inhibited ejaculation, sometimes termed *retarded ejaculation,* implies inability to ejaculate at all during sexual activity or the requirement for an extended period of time to ejaculate, even in the presence of ade-

quate stimulation. Some men have never ejaculated even with masturbation; others have not ejaculated intravaginally. Inhibited ejaculation is often associated with lack of trust or with anger in a relationship. Neurophysiologic and other medical conditions, as well as medications, can interfere with ejaculation and stimulation and may be responsible for inhibited ejaculation.

Other problems men experience related to orgasm include anhedonic orgasm, which occurs when the person ejaculates with normal force but experiences no sensation; or inhibition of ejaculation, in which emission occurs as a seepage of semen rather than forceful ejaculation, and a lack of pleasurable sensation is experienced. Ejaculation sometimes occurs with a flaccid penis and in other instances anhedonic orgasms may occur with penile flaccidity. Rapid ejaculation with a flaccid penis may occur, with or without sensations of pleasure.[70,116]

Orgasmic dysfunctions in women include anorgasmia, a global incapacity to reach orgasm. Women may also be situationally inorgasmic, having orgasms with self-pleasuring or partner manipulation rather than during intercourse. Anorgasmia with intercourse is a common dysfunction. Diagnoses include inorgasmic except with masturbation; inorgasmic except with partner manipulation; inorgasmic except with masturbation or partner manipulation; infrequent coital orgasms; inorgasmic except for vibrator or mechanical stimulation. Mechanisms responsible for orgasmic phase dysfunctions include inadequate stimulation or obsessive self-observation. More remote mechanisms include fear of loss of control over sexual or aggressive impulses.[70,116]

Some examples of diagnoses related to alterations in orgasm include:

Diagnostic Title	Possible Etiologies
Sexual dysfunction, related to premature ejaculation	Anxiety
Sexual dysfunction, related to anorgasmia	Ineffective stimulation

Both physiologic and psychosocial factors influence orgasm phase alterations. The presence a physiologic problem does not justify attribution of the alteration to the disease; an emotional or cognitive process may be involved.

Therapeutic strategies for anorgasmia include structuring situations for sexual activity that reduce anxiety. Distraction from self-observation through the use of fantasy and imagery along with self-pleasuring exercises often reduce anxiety sufficiently to enhance awareness of erotic sensation and orgasm.

Strategies for premature ejaculation include use of the start-stop techniques in which stimulation is withdrawn intermittently, or the source of stimulation is stopped intermittently to increase awareness of erotic sensations and to increase tolerance of pleasure associated with arousal. Treatment of retarded ejaculation includes use of manual stimulation that gradually approximates intercourse. Relaxation and stimulation can be paired, or stimulation with distraction or with the use of fantasy can be helpful.

PAIN WITH COITUS

Vaginismus is a relatively rare sexual problem characterized by an involuntary, conditioned spasm of the vaginal outlet, causing it to shut tightly. This problem precludes sexual intercourse, but vaginismic women may be orgasmic with alternative methods of sexual stimulation. Vaginismus is often associated with sexual abuse and incest.

Dyspareunia, or painful intercourse, may be attributable to a number of factors ranging from full lower bowel to feelings of aversion toward sexual intercourse. It is sometimes experienced by women with steroid alterations, for example, the postpartum mother and the postmenopausal woman.

HOMOSEXUALITY AND SEXUAL DSYFUNCTION

Masters and Johnson[82] have conducted clinical studies with homosexual men and women who had a sexual dysfunction or were sexually dissatisfied. There appeared to be more similarity than difference in the kinds of sexual dysfunctions homosexuals and heterosexuals experienced.

ALTERATION IN SEXUAL SELF-CONCEPT

Sexual self-concept includes the notion we have of ourselves as men or women, masculine or feminine. It reflects body image and evaluation of one's adequacy as a man or woman. A person's sexual self-concept can be altered dramatically as a consequence of illness. Surgery or injuries may produce changes in body image affecting sexual self-concept. Sometimes a person who is ill takes on the identity of the illness, making it difficult to integrate sexuality with the role changes that accompany being ill. Embarrassment and shame associated with changes in one's body due to illness or disfiguring therapies may produce intense anxiety about sexual activity and a pervasive sense of inadequacy. Diagnoses associated with altered sexual self-concept include anxiety about sexual encounters related to altered body image, altered sexual self-concept related to illness role experiences, and altered sexual self-concept related to a partner's actual or potential response. Altered sexual self-concept exists independently of altered sexual function.

Some examples of diagnoses associated with alterations in sexual self-concept include the following:

Diagnostic Title	Possible Etiologies
Sexual dysfunction, related to anxiety about sexual activity	Body image changes after ostomy surgery
Sexual dysfunction, related to altered sexual self-concept	Partner's rejecting responses Low self-esteem related to unemployment

ALTERED SEXUAL RELATIONSHIPS

Sexual relationships, those interpersonal relationships in which sexuality is shared, are often altered profoundly by illness. Values conflicts about sexual activity, difficulty communicating about sexual issues, dissatisfaction with sexual frequency, a partner's inability to provide stimulation, inability to please a partner, and conflicts about the timing of sexual activity are a few of the difficulties couples can experience in their relationships.

Some examples of diagnoses related to alterations in sexual relationships include the following:

Diagnostic Title	Possible Etiology
Sexual dysfunction: value conflicts related to use of alternative forms of sexual expression	Alternate forms of expression required by partner's illness
Sexual dysfunction: value conflicts related to sexual frequency	Partner's inability to reconcile roles as caregiver and lover
Sexual dysfunction, related to sexual dissatisfaction	Related to partner's inability to provide sexual stimulation due to reduced mobility

Strategies for promoting healthy sexual relationships include facilitating involvement that is mutually acceptable to both partners. Communicating clearly and comfortably about concerns and problems, negotiating mutually acceptable solutions to conflicts, obtaining adequate information about the consequences of health problems for sexuality, and clarifying sexual values can enhance the quality of sexual relationships.

GENDER DISORDERS

Gender disorders, although numerous, are encountered less often in practice with ill adults than the problems discussed earlier. Recently, the media have focused on one gender identity problem, transsexualism, which nurses may encounter in adult health services. Transsexualism refers to the condition of people who are convinced that they are "trapped in the body of the wrong sex." These persons believe that they belong to the opposite sex and desire the body, appearance, and social status of the opposite sex. Many actually live in the role of the opposite sex before treatment. Male-to-female transsexuals are usually treated initially with hormonal therapy, and later surgical revision of their genitalia is performed. The surgery involves removal of the male genitalia and revision of the scrotal and neighboring tissue to resemble the female genitalia. Usually, the surgery is cosmetically successful, and an artificial but functional vagina can be created. These women, of course, are sterile, since they have neither ovaries nor uteri.

The female-to-male transsexual has a less cosmetically effective and functional surgical transformation. In a series of procedures, the breasts and vulva are revised and a phallus is created. Hormonal therapy is also used to effect the transformation. Often the creation of the penis requires extensive grafting and surgical revision, and the female-to-male transformation is consequently more difficult and usually less satisfactory. After the transformation these men are also sterile.

Both men and women electing transsexual surgery require considerable emotional support. Usually, they have careful psychological assessments before and after surgery. Because of their cultural conditioning, nurses sometimes find it difficult to relate appropriately to a transsexual. Often it is necessary to analyze one's attitudes and values carefully to be able to accept these patients.

Transsexualism should not be confused with tranvestism, the act of dressing in the clothing of the opposite sex. Additionally, transsexuals are not to be assumed to be homosexuals.

Hermaphroditism is a congenital condition in which the reproductive structures appear ambiguous. Early life experiences seem to have profound impact on our gender identities. Therefore, it is important that sexual assignment be correctly established very early in life to prevent gender confusion later on.[91]

OTHER PROBLEMS RELATED TO SEXUALITY

Rape and sexual abuse occur frequently. Nurses employed in emergency care facilities frequently are the first to provide care to victims of sexual abuse. These problems are discussed in detail in Chapter 79.

RISK FACTORS FOR SEXUAL CONCERNS OR PROBLEMS

Although many persons, themselves, will identify their sexual concerns and problems, in some instances nurses need to initiate discussion of issues of potential concern to the individual. In the context of clinical nursing practice, many persons are "at risk" for experiencing sexual concerns or problems. A framework for understanding the effects of altered health states on human sexuality will be described and examples given.

ALTERED HEALTH STATES AND SEXUAL HEALTH

Altered health states and their treatment can influence sexuality in several ways, some direct and some indirect. Some may have the ability to enhance sexuality, whereas others may interfere with sexual health. Some may affect the person's ability to engage in sexual activity, some may change the person's self-image as a sexual being, and others may induce changes in the sexual relationship. Some effects may pertain only to the client, whereas others affect the partner.

Although it may seem ironic, some illnesses and their therapies may improve sexual health. Confrontation with a critical illness or one that has a bad prognosis may lead couples to reassess the importance of their relationship and may be the prelude to a renewed closeness. Some therapies may lead to an enhanced feeling of general well-being and may even reverse sexual dysfunctions, such as problems getting an erection. This can occur when a debilitating disease is arrested or when the therapy, itself, improves the person's well-being, as is sometimes the case with the use of steroids. In both examples, the mechanisms are probably indirect, but one or more of the components of sexual health is enhanced.

Altered health states can interfere with the sexual health of the patient and the partner. Potential threats to sexual health include anatomic or physiologic changes, body image distortion, environmentally induced problems, and behavioral problems. Variations in life events and changes throughout the life cycle occur concomitantly. Even given optimal health, sexual response remains vulnerable to interference from behavioral and socioenvironmental factors. Kaplan[70] estimates that the number of sexually dysfunctional patients whose dysfunction is purely organic ranges from only 3% to 20%.

STRUCTURAL CHANGES INTERFERING WITH SEXUAL HEALTH

The person with a spinal cord injury best exemplifies the sexual consequences of structural alterations. Other conditions resulting in sexual problems or concerns as a result of structural changes are listed in Table 52-1. In general, structural changes that disrupt peripheral nerve transmission, spinal cord reflexes, blood supply to the genitalia, or removal of or structural changes in the genitalia threaten sexual function and in some cases threaten sexual self-concept and relationships.

After spinal cord injury, men and women alike are anxious to know about the future of their sexuality. Shortly after cord injury, it may be difficult to determine the extent to which sexual activity will return. However, after spinal shock subsides, many men regain their ability to have an erection.

One major difference between sexual response in spinal cord-injured persons and those who are not disabled in this manner is that genital sexual functioning and cerebral or cognitional eroticism become separated. In those persons who have complete transections of the cord, an erection or swelling may not be perceived unless the person can visualize it.

TABLE 52-1 Structural changes and their hypothesized interferences with sexual health

System	Hypothesized Mechanism of Interference
CENTRAL AND PERIPHERAL NERVOUS SYSTEMS	
Spinal cord injury	Disrupts integrity of peripheral nerves and spinal cord reflexes involved in sexual response (e.g., erection insensitivity or hypersensitivity to sexual stimuli)
Spinal cord tumors	
Herniated disk	
Multiple sclerosis	
Spina bifida	
Amyotrophic lateral sclerosis	
Tumors of frontal or temporal lobes	May interfere with function of centers controlling sexual drive
Cerebrovascular accident	
Trauma to frontal or temporal lobes	
CARDIOVASCULAR SYSTEM	
Thrombus formation in vessels of penis	May interfere with blood supply to penis, thus interfering with erection
Leriche's syndrome	
Sickle cell disorders	
Leukemia	
Trauma to vasculature supplying sexual organs	
REPRODUCTIVE/SEXUAL SYSTEM	
Prostatectomy, radical perineal	May destroy nerve supply, interfering with sensory and motor aspects of sexual response
Abdominal perineal resection	
Lumbar sympathectomy	May result in disturbed ejaculation
Rhizotomy	May result in impotence as well as disturbed ejaculation
Absence of penis or penile injury	Precludes or discourages intromission
Penectomy	
Imperforate hymen	
Congenital absence of vagina	
Pelvic exenteration	
Vaginectomy	
Obstetric trauma or poor episiotomy	Leaves gaping vaginal opening or painful scarring, thus discouraging intercourse
Damage to pubococcygeus muscle	

Often questions are raised about the likelihood of any form of sexual function among cord-injured persons. Most research investigating sexual function after spinal cord injury has focused on men. As a result, little information is available about women's experiences. In general, the higher the lesion, the more likely men will be able to experience an erection. Men with cervical lesions are able to achieve erections in a greater percentage of cases than those with lumbar or sacral lesions. In fact, if there is injury to the sacral cord, the nerves supplying the pelvis and involved in the reflex permitting erection are likely to be damaged, and thus reflexogenic erections often are not possible. When the lower motor neuron is damaged, there is sometimes the potential for psychogenically induced erections. In this case, feelings or thoughts perceived at higher levels of the cortex may trigger erections.

The major complication of cord injury is the decreased likelihood of experiencing ejaculation. Generally, ejaculation is infrequent and is much less frequent in men with complete transections than in those with partial lesions. Thus a person's sexual function after cord injury depends on two biologic variables: the number of fibers that were severed (complete versus incomplete lesions) and the level of the injury (cervical, thoracic, lumbar, or sacral). Erection can occur in response to local stimulation, which produces it reflexly, or in response to psychogenic stimuli. In the latter case, impulses from the brain can sometimes bypass the injured portion of the cord via the autonomic nervous system. Indeed, some men with complete denervation of the genitalia report experiencing erection and orgasm. Usually psychogenic erections are much less common than reflexogenic erections. Ejaculation usually cannot occur.[13]

Because of the sensory losses associated with cord injury, the experience of orgasm as it occurred before injury is usually impossible. However, many cord-injured persons report what is an orgasmlike experience in other parts of their bodies. This sensation is commonly referred to the breasts in women. Additionally, recent work with imagery or fantasy seems promising. In this technique, the person's thoughts and feelings are channeled to produce a psychic experience similar to orgasm.[25]

Sexual options available to cord-injured persons depend on numerous factors, including their sexual value systems, muscle strength in the upper extremities, presence of hip flexors and extensors, presence of appliances, and access to a partner. The first of these, the individual's sexual value system, in conjunction with a partner's, determines what range of behaviors is acceptable. For example, oral genital stimulation is a viable means for a cord-injured man to stimulate his partner, but this may not be acceptable within the couple's sexual value system. The muscle strength of the arms will determine to what extent the person can support the body weight, thus determining the variety of positions that can be used. The ability to flex and extend the hips may enable a man or woman to take a more active role in intercourse by thrusting the pelvis. Weakness in these muscles can be compensated by use of a water bed, which amplifies movement (and also decreases skin problems). The presence of a urinary appliance may not be a problem. Condom catheters and leg bags can be removed before intercourse, Foley catheters can be taped in place and left in the bladder, or the urinary collection system can be positioned in such a way that it is not likely to become clamped off or ruptured by the partner's weight. A man who has an indwelling catheter can leave it in during vaginal intercourse; most women are able to accommodate the catheter, providing they are sufficiently aroused and have vaginal lubrication.

With orgasmic release, some cord-injured persons experience severe muscle spasms. These can sometimes be managed with medication, but there is a trade-off involved—some antispasmodics precipitate sexual dysfunction.

For those cord-injured men who cannot obtain a full erection, the "stuffing" technique may be a useful approach. The penis is literally stuffed in the partner's vagina. By contracting her pubococcygeus muscle, a woman can experience sexual sensations similar to those previously associated with penile thrusting.[92]

Although not much has been written about adaptation of homosexuals to cord injury, probably similar concerns and options are appropriate. For those not currently involved in a relationship, opportunity is likely to be a problem just as it is for heterosexuals.

Perhaps one of the greatest assets of the cord-injured person is the presence of a caring partner. Those who are not involved in a caring relationship at the time of their injuries are faced with the problems of developing new relationships as well as experimenting with new sexual options.

Fertility is usually unimpaired in cord-injured women, but because of a number of factors, sperm may not be viable in cord-injured men. Use of artificial insemination (either with the man's own or a donor's semen) is an option for those who want children. Normal pregnancy is possible for women with cord injuries. Careful health monitoring is essential since the incidence of urinary tract infections may be greater in cord-injured women during pregnancy. Cord-injured women may fail to perceive the beginnings of labor because of loss of sensation, and in some instances cesarean section may be required.

Although in the past much emphasis has been placed on the cord-injured person's ability to help a partner achieve sexual gratification, new techniques, such as imagery, actively seek to help the person with a spinal cord injury adapt to the sexual changes experienced. Nurses as health professionals may be involved in long-term relationships with these persons and have an excellent opportunity to assess their sexual concerns and intervene by teaching or counseling.

Other structural changes that influence sexual health are those directly affecting the reproductive/sexual system. Penectomy and vaginectomy are obvious examples, but structural changes in the pelvis from obstetric trauma or abdominal-perineal resection for bowel malignancies also may impair sexual function.

Removal of the anus in gay men removes a source of sexual gratification. Injury to pelvic nerves or disruption of blood supply to the genitalia in both men and women can produce alterations in sexual arousal and orgasm, as well as changes in sexual self-concept and sexual relationships.

PHYSIOLOGIC CHANGES AND SEXUAL HEALTH

Many illnesses alter physiologic processes essential to the sexual response, including nervous transmission,

RESEARCH

Whitley M, and Berke P: Sexual response in diabetic women. In Woods, N: Human sexuality in health and illness, St Louis, 1984, The CV Mosby Co.

A study of 73 diabetic women and 55 women without diabetes revealed that among diabetics there was a greater prevalence of pain or discomfort with intercourse or foreplay and a greater prevalence of vaginal dryness. Moreover, the diabetic women reported vaginal dryness with self-pleasuring more frequently than the nondiabetic women. Difficulty with vaginal lubrication was seen more frequently among women who had diabetes for longer than 6 years and for those who had neuropathy. These results suggest that women with diabetes experience arousal-phase difficulties, not merely the difficulties with orgasm suggested by earlier studies. In addition, the progression of the disease seems to be related to arousal-phase difficulties. ▪

TABLE 52-2 Physiologic interferences with sexual health

Physiologic Interferences	Hypothesized Mechanism of Action	Physiologic Interferences	Hypothesized Mechanism of Action
SYSTEMIC DISEASES		**DISEASES OF THE GENITALIA**	
Pulmonary disease	Debility, pain, and depression probably interfere with sexual libido as well as expression	Priapism	Each of these problems involves damage to genital organs, which may result in painful intercourse
Renal disease		Peyronie's disease	
Malignancies		Balanitis	
Infections		Phimosis	
Degenerative diseases		Genital herpes	
Some cardiovascular diseases		Trauma to penis	
		Vaginal infections	
METABOLIC DISRUPTIONS		Senile vaginitis	
Cirrhosis	Hepatic problems in men result in estrogen buildup from inability of liver to conjugate estrogens; similar processes occur in women along with general debility	Vulvitis	
Mononucleosis		Leukoplakia	
Hepatitis		Bartholin's cyst	
		Allergic response to vaginal sprays and deodorants	
		Vaginitis after radiation therapy	
Hypothyroidism	By depression of CNS function, general debilitation, and depression, libido may be decreased, and impaired erectile abilities in men may result	Pelvic inflammatory disease	
Addison's disease		Fibroadenomas	
Hypogonadism		Endometriosis	
Hypopituitarism		Uterine prolapse	
Acromegaly		Anal fissures, hemorrhoids	
Feminizing tumors		Pelvis masses	
Cushing's disease		Ovarian cysts	
Diabetes mellitus		Prostatitis	Local irritability, damage to genitalia, and consequent interference with reflex mechanisms involved in erection and ejaculation
		Urethritis	
MEDICAL OR SURGICAL CASTRATION			
Orchiectomy	Lowered androgen levels depress libido and lead to impotence, retarded ejaculation, or impaired sexual responsiveness		
Radiation therapy			
Oophorectomy, adrenalectomy			

vasocongestion, hormonal metabolism, myotonia, and perception of pleasurable sensation. Pharmacologic agents that interfere with these basic physiologic activities have the potential to affect sexual drive as well as performance. Table 52-2 illustrates some illnesses and Table 52-3 some drugs that have the potential to interfere with sexual response and the hypothesized mechanism by which they limit sexual response.

In general, it appears that the *extent of a physiologic disorder* and its *chronicity* determine relative frequency of sexual problems. For example, frequency of sexual dysfunction among women with diabetes increases with the duration of the disease, although no correlation exists between sexual dysfunction and actual complications of the disease.[118] This relationship between chronicity and dysfunction is also observed in men with diabetes.[113] A high incidence of impotence is found among diabetic men during the first year after diagnosis. In this instance, the lack of diabetic control (physiologic derangement) may be responsible for the sexual dysfunction.

Other altered health states involve *endocrine* or *metabolic changes*. For example, both men and women experience a decrease in sexual desire when testosterone is absent. Erection and vaginal lubrication are diminished when the appropriate hormonal milieu is not present, for example after orchidectomy, orgasm and ejaculation may be impaired as well.

Painful conditions may make it difficult for the person to be physically close to a partner or may require special attention to positioning; for example, in arthritis the person's mobility may be limited, and he or she may require assistance with positioning or other preparations for lovemaking. *Depression* is an appropriate response to illness for some, and depression is often accompanied by decreased interest in sexual function and in some instances inability to function sexually.

The relationship between extent of physiologic change and degree of sexual dysfunction is also demonstrated by *pharmacologically induced changes*. For example, alcohol induces transiently positive changes; in small doses it initially promotes relaxation and release of

TABLE 52-3 Drug effects on human sexual behavior

Drug or Drug Category	Effect	Probable Mechanism of Action
Oral contraceptives	Positive	Permits separation of sexual activity from concern about conception
Antihypertensives Clonidine (Catapres) Guanethidine (Ismelin) Methyldopa (Aldomet) Propranolol (Inderal) Reserpine (Serpasil) Trimethaphan (Arfonad)	Negative	Peripheral blockade of nervous innervation of sex glands
Antidepressants Amitriptyline (Elavil) Desipramine (Norpramin, Pertofrane) Imipramine (Tofranil) Nortriptyline (Aventyl) Pargyline (Eutonyl) Phenelzine sulfate (Nardil) Protriptyline (Vivactil) Tranylcypromine sulfate (Parnate)	Negative	Central depression; peripheral blockade of nervous innervation of sex glands
Antihistamines Chlorpheniramine (Chlor-Trimeton) Diphenhydramine (Benadryl) Promethazine (Phenergan)	Negative	Blockade of parasympathetic nervous innervation of sex glands
Antispasmodics Glycopyrrolate methobromide (Robinul) Hexocyclium (Tral) Methantheline (Banthine) Poldine (Nacton)	Negative	Ganglionic blockade of nervous innervation of sex glands
Sedatives and tranquilizers Benperidol Chlordiazepoxide (Librium) Chlorpromazine (Thorazine, Megaphen) Chlorprothixene (Taractan) Diazepam (Valium) Mesoridazine (Serentil) Methaqualone (Quaalude) Phenoxybenzamine (Dibenzyline) Prochlorperazine (Compazine) Thioridazine (Mellaril)	Negative and positive	Central sedation; blockade of autonomic innervation of sex glands; suppression of hypothalamic and pituitary function Tranquilization and relaxation
Ethyl alcohol	Negative Transiently positive	Central depression; suppression of motor activity; diuresis Release of inhibitions; relaxation
Barbiturates	Negative	Central depression; suppression of motor activity; hypnosis
Diuretics Bendroflumethiazide (Naturetin) Chlorthiazide (Diuril) Spironolactone (Aldactone)	Negative	Diuresis
Sex hormone preparations Cyproterone acetate Methandrostenolone (Dianabol) Nandrolone phenpropionate (Durabolin) Norethandrolone (Nilevar)	Negative	Antiandrogenic effects on sexual function; loss of libido; decreased potency
Methadone	Negative	Suppresses secondary sex organ function in men
Potassium nitrate (saltpeter)	Questionable	Diuresis
Cantharis (Spanish fly)	Negative	Irritation and inflammation of genitourinary tract; systemic poisoning
Yohimbine	Questionable	Stimulation of lower spinal nerve centers
Strychnine	Questionable	Stimulation of neuraxis; priapism

Continued.

TABLE 52-3 Drug effects on human sexual behavior—cont'd

Drug or Drug Category	Effect	Probable Mechanism of Action
Narcotics and psychoactive drugs Amphetamines Cocaine	Negative	Central depression; decreased libido and impaired potency
Heroin LSD Marijuana Methadone Morphine	Transiently positive	Release of inhibitions; increased suggestibility; relaxation
L-Dopa and p-chlorophenylalanine (PCPA)	Questionable	Improvement of well-being
Amyl nitrite	Questionable	Vasodilation of genitourinary tract; smooth muscle relaxation
Caffeine	Questionable	Central nervous system stimulant
Vitamin E	Questionable	Supports fertility in laboratory animals
Selenium	Questionable	Supports fertility in laboratory animals
Lithium carbonate	Questionable	Produces broad endocrine changes; diuresis
Clomiphene citrate (Clomid)	Questionable	Stimulates gonadotropic hormones; enhances expectations of achieving pregnancy
Bromocriptine (Parlodel)	Questionable	Stimulates gonadotropic hormones
Cimetidine (Tagamet)	Negative	Unknown
Clofibrate (Atromid S)	Questionable	Unknown
Disulfram (Antabuse)	None by itself; negative with alcohol	Blocks alcohol metabolism; produces aldehyde syndrome

inhibitions as do other psychoactive drugs. However, in larger doses alcohol has negative effects on sexual function, leading to central nervous system depression and interference with motor activity.[113]

Several categories of drugs have negative effects on sexual function. These include antihypertensives, antidepressants, antihistamines, antispasmodics, sedatives and tranquilizers, ethyl alcohol, some sex hormone preparations, and some narcotics and psychoactive drugs. Examples of these drugs are listed in Table 52-3.

Although some medical-surgical conditions do not interfere directly with sexual function, their *perceived seriousness* or the *presence of symptoms* discourages persons from engaging in their usual sexual practices. One very common example is associated with cardiac disease, more specifically myocardial infarction. Although marital coitus probably does not demand a great energy expenditure, many persons are fearful of attempting intercourse after having a heart attack. One study of married men who had had myocardial infarctions demonstrated that heart rates with orgasm were much lower in this group (about 117 beats/min on the average) than among the younger group studied by Masters and Johnson.[64] An active physical conditioning program did produce significant improvements in the frequency and quality of sexual activity for men who had had a myocardial infarction. The energy expenditure associated with sex seemed to be better tolerated by those who exercised regularly.

In general, the person who has had a myocardial infarction may return to regular sexual activity provided that there are no symptoms of congestive heart failure. However, certain conditions that increase energy expenditure during coitus should be avoided. These include having intercourse shortly after a meal or soon after alcohol consumption, since both increase the heart rate and metabolic demands, and avoiding extremes in temperatures and anxiety-provoking or secretive situations. (Sample instructions to be given to cardiac patients appear in the boxed material on p. 1528.)

Often a change in health is accompanied by malaise or fatigue. As a consequence, the person experiences a decrease in sexual desire or difficulty becoming aroused. This effect may not be a direct function of the disease itself, but rather the consequence of an incompatibility between "feeling bad" and the stimulating thoughts and feelings an individual associates with sexual response.

BODY IMAGE CHANGES

The extent to which body image change influences sexuality often depends on the perceptions of at least two persons: oneself and a significant other. Multiple variables may influence the body image of a woman who has had a mastectomy. Among these are factors such as extent of the surgical procedure, the value she assigns to her breasts, her preoperative body image, and social factors such as the quality of her preoperative sexual re-

TABLE 52-4 Some health problems resulting in body image changes that may raise sexual concerns

Surgically Induced	Traumatically Induced	Others
Mastectomy	Burns	Dermatologic disorders
Ostomy	Lacerations, scarring	Obesity
Hysterectomy		Congenital anomalies of sexual organs (e.g., absence of penis, hypospadias)
Amputation of limb or limbs	Amputations	
		Unusual breast size, including immaturity or hypertrophy

lationship. A sexual partner's reaction may be similarly affected.[143]

The visibility of a change plays an important role in sexual adaptation. Goffman refers to individuals with "spoiled identities" whose interactions with others are marked by disgrace and rejection and who may elicit withdrawal on the part of others. Visibility of a change in one's body seems to be just as disruptive of marital and family relations as it is of other social relationships.[147]

The meaning and significance one attaches to a changed body part may interfere with sexual behavior. A male amputee who views his loss as castration, a woman who sees her hysterectomy as a neutering surgery, and a person who equates an ostomy with loss of adult control are likely to experience problems with self-image and, in turn, sexual adjustment. Some common health problems resulting in body image changes are listed in Table 52-4.

ENVIRONMENTAL FACTORS

Environmental factors, such as privacy, competing stimuli, and sexual segregation, interfere with sexual expression. Institutionalization rarely affords sufficient privacy for sexual expression. As indicated by Masters and Johnson's work, the presence of distracting stimuli can interfere with the progression of sexual arousal.[83] Finally, many institutions segregate persons on the basis of sex, which may elicit a range of adaptation including masturbation, homosexual activity, or withdrawal from human warmth. Often these adaptive behaviors are punished, and those who resort to them are stigmatized. In some institutions, staff members may adopt an in loco parentis stance, treating even aging persons as if they required protection from their sexual desires.

OTHER EFFECTS OF ILLNESS

Some individuals may not be able to integrate their sexuality with the role changes that accompany being ill. They may see their illnesses as precluding sexual expression.

The partner of a person with altered health can also experience changes in sexuality. For some, there may be no acceptable opportunity for sexual expression. When one partner is ill, the other partner may be forced to inhibit his or her sexual interest. This is often frequently the case for aging women. In some instances one partner may feel guilty about initiating sexual activity, particularly if he or she perceives the other partner as vulnerable to injury. Sometimes one partner may express guilt for being interested in sex when the other is not. In other instances a partner may experience role confusion when he or she is expected to be caregiver as well as lover. For example, a partner may not be able to integrate helping with a bowel program with being sexually involved.

PROMOTING SEXUAL HEALTH

PRINCIPLES FOR PROMOTING SEXUAL HEALTH

Mims and Swenson[89] cite basic principles involved in the promotion of sexual health. The first of these acknowledges that there is no single set of appropriate sexual values in our society; rather, the professional needs to accept that major conflicts of values exist. A second principle is that provision of accurate and adequate information is more helpful than indoctrination. Although it is often tempting to impose one's own solutions to sexual concerns or a values conflict on others, growth of the individual is more likely to be fostered by guidance rather than by indoctrination. Finally, individuals can be assisted to make their own informed choices rather than conform to guidelines established by a professional or an agency. It is the individuals, and not the health professional, who will have to cope with the consequences of their choices.

Examples of diagnoses related to alterations in sexual desire, arousal, orgasm, sexual self-concept, and relationships appeared earlier in this chapter. Risk factors for sexual concerns, difficulties, and dysfunctions include changes in structure, physiology, body image, and drug and environmental effects on sexual health. Diagnoses are based on collection of data from a sexual history coupled with findings from physical examination and laboratory tests.

PLANNING: EXPECTED PATIENT OUTCOMES

The first four criteria listed below apply to persons of all ages and health statuses. The last three are particularly relevant to those persons hospitalized for illness. The person can:

1. Express sexuality in a manner comfortable and rewarding to oneself and one's partner.
2. Express positive feelings about one's sexuality and oneself.
3. Maintain, with cooperation of the partner, a relationship conducive to sexual functioning.
4. Identify erotically pleasing stimuli that facilitate sexual arousal.
5. Express sexual feelings in a manner consistent with personal values and beliefs.
6. Relate knowledge of safe sexual practices to sexually transmitted disease prevention and family planning to personal sexual relationships.
7. Accurately describe how illness or treatment is likely or not likely to interfere with sexual functioning.
8. Explore with a partner any adaptations in sexual behavior necessitated by illness, hospitalization, or medication.

INTERVENTIONS

Annon[3] presents an extremely useful distinction between the various levels of intervention possible for persons with sexual concerns or problems. He terms these levels *permission, limited information, specific suggestions,* and *intensive therapy.* They are listed in order of increasing sophistication, with permission requiring the most basic preparation and intensive therapy requiring specific educational preparation in sex therapy theory and techniques. Annon contends that sexual problems may be resolved on a variety of levels and do not always require counseling or intensive therapy.

PERMISSION

Often individuals merely want to know that they are normal, acceptable, and not "perverted;" and they seek out the health professional for validation of their sexual normalcy. Permission is not merely a therapeutic measure but also a preventive one. It can be applied in a variety of community settings as well as in the hospital. Permission may be applied to thoughts, fantasies, dreams, and feelings as well as to overt sexual behaviors. At times nurses will be asked to provide individuals with permission *not* to engage in certain sexual behaviors if they choose. This may relieve them from feeling pressured to conform to someone else's standards for sexual behavior that are not necessarily their own.

Persons with diseases that interfere with their usual forms of sexual expression may seek permission to discuss alternative approaches to sexual pleasure. For example, spinal cord-injured persons may welcome the permission from staff members to discuss alternatives to penis-vagina intercourse. A male adolescent who is comparing his sexual prowess with that of peers may seek permission *not* to be sexually active. Female ado-

---

RESEARCH

Larson J et al: Heart rate and blood pressure: responses of coronary artery disease patients during sexual activity and a 2-flight stair climbing test, Heart Lung 9(6):1025-1030, 1980.

Effects of climbing two flights of stairs and of having intercourse were evaluated in eight men with coronary artery disease and nine men without coronary artery disease. For men with coronary artery disease (CAD), the mean maximal heart rate was 115 +/- 7/minute during sexual activity and 118 +/- 6/minute during stair climbing. Mean maximal heart rates were also similar for sexual activity and for stair climbing among the men without CAD. Mean maximal systolic blood pressure for the men with CAD was 144 +/- 6 mmHg at orgasm but 164 +/- 7 mmHg at the end of stair climbing. There were no significant differences in the pressure rate product across groups of men or between stair climbing and sexual intercourse. Four of the men with CAD did demonstrate electrocardiographic changes, ST segment changes, or premature atrial or ventricular contractions during sexual activity. ■

---

lescents may seek guidance about how and when to say "no." Permission to be assertive about safe sexual practices (see box in Chapter 51) can reduce the likelihood of transmission of sexually transmitted diseases (STDs) and AIDS.

In summary, permission-giving can help individuals break associations between behaviors, thoughts, fantasies, dreams, and labels. Usually, these labels bear negative connotations such as "dirty," "perverted," or "abnormal."[3] Even though most sexual acts could be considered normal in some sense (for example, statistically or phylogenetically), individuals do need to be aware of the consequences of their behavior. These consequences may include legal prosecution or social ostracism, and such concerns need to be explored with the individual before one gives blanket permission to engage in such practices.

LIMITED INFORMATION

The next level of intervention can also be therapeutic as well as preventive. It involves providing information to individuals that is directly relevant to their particular problems or concerns. Rather than condoning an individual's behavior, this approach may result in a change of behavior on the basis of an informed decision. Some common areas of sexual concern that may require only limited information include worry over breast and genital shape, and size, masturbation, sexual intercourse during menstruation, and oral-genital sex. The nurse familiar with famous myths associated with each of these topics can appreciate that providing individuals with basic factual information may resolve sexual worries.

A common concern among adolescent and young

RESEARCH

Gilliss C and Rankin S: Social and sexual activity after cardiac surgery. Prog Cardiovasc Nurs 3(3):93-97,1988.

Resuming social and sexual activities mark recovery from cardiac surgery. People who were having cardiac surgery were asked at hospitalization and at 3 and 6 months after surgery to compare the frequency of social and sexual activities with levels observed 6 months before their surgeries. Social activities increased significantly after 3 months. Sexual activities increased over the 6-month period, but patients were more likely to have reduced their sexual activities than to have increased them after surgery. Most reported no changes in sexual activities. Increased attention to discharge planning and follow-up seems warranted. ▪

RESEARCH

Hahn K: Sexuality and COPD. Rehabilitation Nursing 14(4):191-195, 1989.

A support group program designed to help persons with chronic obstructive pulmonary disease (COPD) become more knowledgeable and confident discussuing sexual matters was evaluated by participants. Group members wanted health professionals to ask matter-of-factly about their sexual concerns. They agreed unanimously that a simple, direct question would help them talk about their sexual needs. Dyspnea, coughing, energy management, sexual self-concept, and problems communicating about sex were addressed in the group. Participants were asked what had changed about their sex life since their breathing problems began. They indicated decreased mouth kissing, increased resting after position changes, and changed positions. They describe apprehension about sexual activity and fear of provoking dyspnea by both the patient and partner. The most frequently mentioned consequences of role changes were decreased sexual activity, frequency of intercourse, and threat to sexual self-concept. ▪

adult men is penis size. Giving the information that the smaller flaccid penis becomes about as large when erect as larger flaccid penises may be sufficient to relieve anxieties. A woman who is about to have a hysterectomy may be concerned that she will no longer be able to have intercourse or that she will no longer have sexual desire. Informing the woman before surgery that this is not true may remove unnecessary barriers from the resumption of sexual activity. Similar information would be helpful to a man about to undergo a transurethral prostatectomy. Even though the man having a transurethral resection is likely to experience retrograde ejaculation, he may still have an erection and enjoy intercourse. Having this information before surgery may avert dysfunctional sex later.

Currently many men and women share concerns about contracting AIDS or STDs during sexual activities. Providing limited information about unsafe sexual practices, such as having vaginal or anal intercourse without using a condom or oral-genital sex without using a condom, can be life-saving.

In sum, providing limited information can free the individual from anxieties connected with sexual performance or assumptions about negative effects of health-related conditions on sexual activity. Combating popular mythology with this approach is often a sufficient preventive or therapeutic measure.

SPECIFIC SUGGESTIONS

Before giving individuals specific suggestions about direct attempts to help them change their behavior to reach a designated goal, it is essential to obtain a sexual problem history (see Chapter 51). This approach presupposes a brief approach to counseling individuals with the understanding that if results are not achieved within a limited period, referral to someone prepared to

provide intensive sexual therapy will be made. Specific suggestions may be preventive as well as therapeutic. Some specific suggestions may relate to the conditions conducive to optimal sexual functioning, specific approaches to use in the presence of certain illnesses or surgeries, and directives for coping with some sexual dysfunctions.

One specific suggestion often incorporated in sexual counseling is that a couple having difficulties with intercourse abstain from it for a specified period. This reduces the "pressure to perform" perceived by a member of the dysfunctional couple.

The counseling approach applied to persons who have just had a myocardial infarction is outlined in the box below. These suggestions are designed to minimize the effects of cardiovascular problems during intercourse.* Similar specific suggestions can be given to cord-injured persons, including positions most likely to be comfortable, care of the catheter before and during intercourse, and techniques available to stimulate the noninjured partner. Use of imagery (fantasy) can also be incorporated as a specific suggestion.† Ostomy pa-

*Scheingold L and Wagner N: Sound sex and the aging heart, New York, 1974, Human Services Press.
†Bregman S: Sexuality and the spinal cord injured woman, 1975, Sister Kenny Institute, Office of Continuing Education, Dept 188, 1800 Chicago Ave, Minneapolis, MN 55404.
Mooney T, Cole T, and Chilgrin R: Sexual options for paraplegics and quadriplegics, Boston, 1975, Little, Brown & Co.
Toward intimacy: family planning and sexuality concerns of physically disabled women, Planned Parenthood of Snohomish County, 2730 Hoyt, Everett, WA 98201.

EXAMPLES OF SPECIFIC SUGGESTIONS FOR PERSONS RECOVERING FROM MYOCARDIAL INFARCTION

TO MINIMIZE CARDIAC WORKLOAD:

Avoid having intercourse in either very hot or very cold rooms.

Wait about 3 hours after eating a meal or drinking alcoholic beverages.

Allow plenty of time to rest afterwards.

Use comfortable positions.

CONSULT YOUR HEALTH CARE PROVIDER IF:

You have chest pain during or after intercourse.

You feel extremely tired after having intercourse.

You feel your heart beating very loudly for more than a few minutes after intercourse.

---

tients often have concerns about accidents involving their appliances during intercourse. Specific suggestions might include emptying the appliance before initiating sexual activity, using cosmetic covers for the stoma bag, and avoiding excess pressure over the stoma site until the ostomy incision is well healed.*

Finally, nurses can offer some rather simple directives for coping with specific sexual dysfunctions. The man with premature ejaculation can be taught to use the "squeeze technique," or the partner may learn to apply it. This technique consists of placing the thumb and second and third fingers at the coronal ridge of the glans, exerting enough pressure for 3 to 4 seconds to relieve the feeling of ejaculatory inevitability. Women who have inadequate lubrication and experience painful intercourse as a consequence of steroid changes during the postpartum period or menopause may benefit from the use of a water-soluble lubricant.

INTENSIVE SEXUAL THERAPY

Intensive sexual therapy combines techniques and concepts of psychotherapy with special approaches to intervention for individuals or couples having sexual problems. Usually the problems involved are one or more of the sexual dysfunctions discussed earlier. Since a discussion of the many approaches to intensive therapy is beyond the scope of this text, interested readers are referred to the references. These forms of therapy usually require intensive preparation beyond that provided in most schools of nursing. However, an awareness of the sexual dysfunctions discussed here will enable nurses

---

*Binder D: Sex, courtship, and the single ostomate, Los Angeles, 1973, United Ostomy Association.

Gambrell E: Sex and the male ostomate, Los Angeles, 1973, United Ostomy Association.

Norris C and Gambrell E: Sex, pregnancy, and the female ostomate, Los Angeles, 1972, United Ostomy Association.

---

to refer persons with complex problems to trained therapists.

PROMOTING SEXUAL HEALTH OF THE CLINICIAN

Nurses sometimes confront (1) patients whose actions are overtly and inappropriately sexual, (2) gender differences between nurse and patient that can lead to embarrassing situations, (3) their own sexual feelings as nurses for particular patients, and (4) sexual harassment in the work place.

Patients may expose their genitalia or make sexual overtures to nurses. Often these behaviors are manifestations of the patient's need for some validation of his or her sexuality, a need for feeling some control over a situation in which they feel dependent and out of control, or a need to attract attention. Some patients may simply be expressing sexual deprivation. Nurses can respond in a way that addresses these concerns, validating their patient's sexuality while simultaneously respecting their own integrity. It is important for nurses to assert their rights to have their own body boundaries respected as well as to empathize with the patient. It is also important for nurses to not automatically assume that they were responsible for eliciting the patient's sexual behavior.

Because of the intimate contact sanctioned by the nurse-patient relationship, many potentially embarrassing situations can occur, such as those in which nurses provide direct care to patients of the opposite gender. Maintaining privacy and preventing shaming experiences where possible can help protect the patient from unnecessary embarrassment. It is often useful to acknowledge uncomfortable feelings and discuss them.

It is not unusual for nurses to have sexual feelings for patients, and these feelings are often anxiety provoking. Professional ethics discourage sexual involvement with patients because they are in a vulnerable position. When sexual feelings interfere with one's practice, it is helpful to acknowledge this and request help for the patient from another professional. Nurses may feel sexually aroused, have physical manifestations of sexual arousal, or have a desire for and fantasies about a patient. It is important to recognize the difference between having these feelings and acting on them. Discussing these feelings with a peer often helps put them into perspective.

Sexual harassment occurs when one person is the recipient of unwanted sexual attention, and another person perpetrates the unwanted behavior. Although sexual harassment may occur between persons of the same sex, it occurs most commonly between women and men, and men are the most frequent perpetrators. Unwanted sexual attention may include a verbal remark, physical gesture, unwanted touch, sexually explicit pictures, or graffiti. Price-Spratlen[104] has developed an approach to sexual harassment counseling that allows the client to place details of an event in sequence and to gain skill as a participant observer of behaviors, thoughts, or feelings. Association between behavior and the consequences are made, thus reducing self-blame, loss of self-esteem, and self-confidence. Victims eventually confront their alleged harasser in a conciliatory conference. They are asked to identify the most personally damaging elements of sexual harassment and what actions will be most helpful in healing the interpersonal conflict.

CHAPTER SUMMARY

✔ Sexual concerns and difficulties generally do not produce profound problems in sexual response, although they may interfere temporarily with sexual functioning. Sexual concerns and difficulties are usually amenable to sex education and counseling.

✔ Alterations in sexual health include alterations in sexual function (desire, arousal, orgasm), in sexual self-concept, and in sexual relationships.

✔ Alterations in sexual desire include low sexual desire and sexual aversion. Therapy is directed toward underlying causes; intensive sex therapy or psychotherapy is often required for sexual aversion.

✔ Alterations in sexual arousal reflect body-mind-social interaction and may result from drugs, diseases affecting vascular function, age, and anxiety about sexual performance. Transient episodes of alteration in arousal are common. Therapies include anxiety-reducing approaches and exercises that emphasize pleasure rather than pressure to perform.

✔ Alterations in orgasm include ejaculatory problems in men and anorgasmy in women; both physiologic and psychological factors can produce orgasm-phase alterations. Therapies include anxiety-reducing strategies for anorgasmy and relaxation stimulation techniques for ejaculatory problems.

✔ Alterations in sexual self-concept may result from disease or injury. Therapies include strategies toward accepting and transcending body image changes, transcending the sick role, obtaining partner support, and enhancing a positive self-concept.

✔ Alterations in sexual relationships during illness result from value conflicts about sexual activity, problems with communication, or difficulties in sexual functioning. Therapies include promoting communication and providing education to resolve conflicts and promote sexuality.

✔ Illness may affect sexuality and sexual function through changes in body structure, changes in body functions, effects of pharmacologic agents, body image changes, or environmental restrictions (privacy, competing stimuli, partner segregation).

✔ Levels of intervention for persons with sexual problems include giving permission for engaging or not engaging in sexual behaviors (inner or overt), providing limited information directly related to the particular problems or concerns, giving specific suggestions, or providing intensive sexual therapy. The type of intervention depends on the nature of the problem and the level of expertise of the provider.

✔ Promoting the sexual health of the clinician involves obtaining support for dealing with patients whose actions are overtly and inappropriately sexual, gender differences between nurse and patient that can produce embarrassment, one's own sexual feelings for particular patients, and sexual harassment in the work place.

QUESTIONS TO CONSIDER

■ Review the health records and nursing histories for at least 10 clients for whom you have provided nursing care. Identify the following:
  a. What drugs are they receiving that are likely to interfere with their sexual functioning?

  b. How has their hospitalization affected their sexual health? self-concept? sexual function? sexual relationships?

  c. How has their primary and secondary medical diagnoses affected their sexual health? sexual function? sexual relationships? sexual self-concept?

■ Design a brief program to provide limited information to clients with cancer, diabetes, or heart disease. What information would you include? How will you present it? What adaptations will you make relating to individual clients?

REFERENCES AND SELECTED READINGS

1. Aletky P: Sexuality of the nursing home resident, Clin Nurs 1:53-60, 1980.
2. Anderson F and Bardach JL: Sexuality and neuromuscular disease: a pilot study, Int Rehabil Med 5:21-26, 1983.
3. Annon J: The behavioral treatment of sexual problems. Honolulu, 1974, Enabling Systems.

*References preceded by an asterisk are particularly well suited for student reading.

4. Bachers E: Sexual dysfunction after treatment for genitourinary cancers, Semin Oncol Nurs 1(1):18-24, 1985.

5. Baggs J et al: Sexual counseling of women with coronary heart disease, Heart Lung 15:154-159, 1987.

6. Benson C: Arthritis and sexuality, J Urol Nurs 7(1):370-372, 1988.

7. Bergman B et al: Sexual function in prostatic cancer patients treated with radiotherapy, orchiectomy or oestrogens. Br J Urol 56:64-69, 1984.

8. Berkman AH, Katz LH, and Weissman R: Sexuality and the lifestyle of home dialysis patients, Arch Phys Med Rehabil 63:272-275, 1982.

9. Berkum C: Changing appearance for women in the middle years of life: trauma? In Markson E, editor, Older women, Lexington, Mass, 1983, Lexington Books.

10. Bernhard L: Sexuality expectations and outcomes in women having hysterectomies, Chart 83(10):11-15, 1986.

11. Besterman EM: How disturbing are side effects of beta blockers? Eur Heart J, (Suppl) 4 D:143-134, 1983

12. Blackmore C: The impact of orchidectomy upon the sexuality of the man with testicular cancer, Cancer Nurs 11(1):33-40, 1988.

13. Bors E and Comarr AE: Neurological disturbances of sexual function with special reference to 529 patients with spinal cord injury, Urol Surv 10:191-222, 1960.

14. Boyer G and Boyer J: Sexuality and aging. Nurs Clin North Am 17:421-428, 1982.

15. Bransfield DD: Breast cancer and sexual functioning: a review of the literature and implications for future research, Int J Psychiatry Med 12:(3)197-211, 1982.

16. Brooks BN, and Chit M: Sexual problems related to the presence of a stoma, Sexual Disabil 3:154-155, 1980.

17. Brouillette JN, Pryor E, and Fox T: Evaluation of sexual dysfunction in the female following rectal resection and intestinal stoma, Dis Colon Rectum 24:96-102, 1981.

18. Burgener G: Sexuality concerns of the post-stroke patient, Rehabil Nurs 14(4):178-181, 1989.

19. Burnham WR, Lennard-Jones JE, and Brooke BN: Sexual problems among married ileostomists, Gut 18:673-677, 1977.

20. Bullard DG and Knight SE: Sexuality and physical disability: personal perspectives, St Louis, 1981, The CV Mosby Co.

21. Bush P: Drugs, alcohol and sex, New York, 1980, Richard Marek.

22. Campbell M: Sexual dysfunction in the COPD patient, DCCN Dimens Crit Care Nurs 6(2):70-74, 1987.

23. Coffman C et al: Sexual adaptation among single young adults with cystic fibrosis, Chest 86(3):412-418, 1984.

24. Cohen J: Sexual counseling of the patient following myocardial infarction, Crit Care Nurs 6(6):18-29, 1986.

25. Cole TM, Chilgren RA, and Rosenberg P: A new programme of sex education and counseling for spinal cord injured adults and health care professionals, Paraplegia 11:111-124, 1973.

26. Comarr A et al: Sleep dreams of sex among traumatic paraplegics and quadriplegics, Sexual. Disabil 6(1):25-29, 1983.

27. Cooley M et al: Sexual and reproductive issues for women with Hodgkin's disease: overview of issues, Cancer Nurs 9:188-193, 1986.

28. Cooper-Fraps C, et al: Denial: implications of a pilot study on activity level related to sexual competence in burned adults, Am J Occup Ther 38(8):529-534, 1984.

29. Csesko P: Sexuality and multiple sclerosis, J Neurosci Nurs 20(6):353-355, 1988.

30. Cummings V: Amputee and sexual dysfunction, Arch Phys Med Rehabil 56:12-13, 1975.

31. Cushman L: Sexual counseling in a rehabilitation program: a patient perspective, J Rehabil 54(2):65-69, 1988.

32. Davidson JM et al: Hormonal changes and sexual function in aging men, J Clin Endocrinol Metab 57:71-77, 1983.

33. deBaker E et al: Sexual behavior after prostatectomy, Eur Urol 3:295-298, 1977.

34. DeNour AK: Hemodialysis: sexual functioning, Psychosomatics 19(4):229-235, 1978.

35. Dewis M and Thornton N: Sexual dysfunction in multiple sclerosis, J Neurosci Nurs 21(3):175-179, 1989.

36. Donlou J et al: Psychosocial aspects of AIDS and AIDS related complex: a pilot study, J Psychosoc Oncol 3(2):39-55, 1985.

37. Dunn M: Sexual questions and comments on a spinal cord injury service, Sexual Disabil 6:126-134, 1983.

38. Eisenberg MG and Rustad LC: Sex and the spinal cord injured: some questions and answers, Cleveland Veterans Administration Hospital, 1975.

39. Ellenberg M: Sex and diabetes: a comparison between men and women, Diabetes Care 2(1):4-8, 1979.

40. Ellenberg M: Sexual aspects of the female diabetic, M Sinai J Med 44:495-500, 1977.

41. Ellis E, Calhoun K, and Atkeson B: Sexual dysfunction in victims of rape, Women Health 5(4):39-47, 1980.

42. Elst P: Sexual problems in rheumatoid arthritis and ankylosing spondylitis, Arthritis Rheum 27:217-220, 1984.

43. Fazio V, Fletcher J, and Montague D: Prospective study of the effect of resection of the rectum on male sexual function, World J Surg 4:149-152, 1980.

44. Fisher S: Psychosexual adjustment following total pelvic exenteration, Cancer Nurs, June 1979, pp 219-225.

45. Fitting MD et al: Self concept and the sexuality of spinal cord injured women, Arch Sex Behav 7:43-156, 1978.

46. Fletcher S: Learning needs related to sexual functioning of the neurologically impaired individual. In MJ Van Meter, editor, Neurological care: A guide to patient education New York, 1982, Appleton-Century-Crofts.

47. Florian V and Shurka E: Non-disabled opinions on sexual activities and family roles for disabled persons, and disabled persons' view of these opinions. Int Rehabil Med 5:17-20, 1983.

48. Foltz A: The influence of cancer on self concept and life quality, Semin Oncol Nurs 3(4):303-312, 1987.

49. Frank-Stromberg M: Sexuality and the elderly cancer patient, Semin Oncol Nurs 1(1):49-55, 1985.

50. Fuentes R et al: Sexual side effects: what to tell your patients, what not to say . . . commonly prescribed drugs, RN 46(2):34-41, 1983.

51. Garner W and Allen H: Sexual rehabilitation and heart disease, J Rehabil 55(1):69-73, 1989.

52. Gillis C and Rankin S: Social and sexual activity after cardiac surgery, Prog Cardiovasc Nurs 3(3):93-97, 1988.

53. Glasgow M, Halfin V, and Althausen A: Sexual response and cancer, CA 37(6):322-333.

54. Glass DD et al: Sexual adjustment in the handicapped, J Rehabil 44:43-47, 1978.

55. Gloeckner M: Perceptions of sexual attractiveness following ostomy surgery, Res Nurs Health 7(2):87-92, 1984.

56. Goddard L: Sexuality and spinal cord injury, J Neurosci Nurs 20(4):240-244, 1988.

57. Googe MCS and Mook TM: The inflatable penile prosthesis: new developments, Am J Nurs 83:1044-1047, 1983.

58. Greenberg DB: The measurement of sexual dysfunction in cancer patients, Cancer 15(10 Suppl):2281-2286, 1984.

59. Grunbert K: Sexual rehabilitation of the cancer patient un-

dergoing ostomy surgery, J Enterostomal Ther 13:148-152, 1986.

60. Hale J et al: Within reach: providing family planning services to physically disabled women, New York, 1978, Human Sciences Press.

61. Hallstrom T: Sexuality of women in middle age: the Goteborg study, J Biosoc Sci 6(suppl):165-175, 1979.

62. Halstead L et al: Disability SARs and the small group experience: a conceptual framework, Sexual Disabil 6:183-196, 1983.

63. Heinrich K: Effective response to sexual harassment, Nurs Outlook 35(2):70-72, 1987.

64. Hellerstein H and Friedman EG: Sexual activity and the postcoronary patient, Arch Intern Med 125:987-999, 1970.

65. Hogan R: Human sexuality: a nursing perspective, ed 2, New York, 1984, Appleton-Century-Crofts.

66. Humphrey M and Kinsella G: Sexual life after stroke. Sexual Disabil 3:150-153, 1980.

67. Jenkins B: Patients' reports of sexual changes after treatment for gynecological cancer, Oncol Nurs Forum 15(3):349-354, 1988.

68. Johnson C et al: Alcohol and sex: alcohol induced problems of sexual function, Heart Lung 12(1):93-97, 1983.

69. Kaplan HS: Disorders of sexual desire and other new concepts and techniques in sex therapy, New York, 1979, Simon & Schuster, Inc.

70. Kaplan HS: The new sex therapy, New York, 1974, Brunner/Mazel, Inc.

71. Kendall MJ and Beeley L: Beta-adrenoceptor blocking drugs: adverse reactions and drug interactions, Pharmacol Ther 21:351-369, 1983.

72. King BD et al: Impotence during therapy with verapamil, Arch Intern Med 143:1248-1249, 1983.

73. Kitzinger S: Woman's experience of sex, New York, 1983, Putnam.

74. Kolodny RC et al: Textbook of human sexuality for nurses, Boston, 1979, Little, Brown, & Co.

75. Kornfeld DS: Psychological and behavioral responses after coronary artery bypass surgery, Circulation 66:24-28, 1982.

76. Krueger JC et al: Relationship between nurse counseling and sexual adjustment after hysterectomy, Nurs Res 28:145-150, 1979.

77. Lamb M: Sexual dysfunction in the gynecologic oncology patient, Semin Oncol Nurs 1(1):9-17, 1985.

78. Lion E: Human sexuality in nursing process, New York, 1982, Wiley.

79. Lüedman K: The sexuality of the older person: review of the literature, Gerontologist 21(2):203-208, 1981.

80. Mac Elveen-Hoehn P: Understanding sexuality in progressive cancer, Semin Oncol Nurs 1(1):56-62, 1985.

81. Marks R: Sexual side effects: how drugs can change fertility, RN 46(3):61-63, 1983.

82. Masters W and Johnson V: Human sexual inadequacy, 1970, Boston, Little, Brown & Co.

83. Masters W and Johnson V: Human sexual response, Boston, 1966, Little, Brown & Co.

84. McCusker J, Zapka J, Stoddard A, and Mayer K: Responses to the AIDS epidemic among homosexually active men: factors associated with preventive behavior, Patient Education Counseling 13:15-30, 1989.

85. McKenzie F: Sexuality after total pelvic exenteration, Nurs Times 84(20):26-28, 1988.

86. Michal V: Arterial disease as a cause of impotence. Clin Endocrinol Metab 11:725-748, 1982.

87. Mims F: Sexual stress: coping and adaptation, Nurs Clin North Am 17:395-405, 1982.

88. Mims F, et al: Unwanted sexual experiences of young women, Psychosoc Nurs Mental Health Services 22(6):6-14, 1984.

89. Mims F and Swenson M: Sexuality: a nursing perspective, New York, 1980, Appleton-Century-Crofts.

90. Mitchell ME: Sexual counseling in cardiac rehabilitation, J Rehabil 48(4):15-18, 1982.

91. Money J and Ehrhardt A: Man and woman, boy and girl, Baltimore, 1972, The Johns Hopkins University Press.

92. Mooney T, Cole T, and Chilgren R: Sexual options for paraplegics and quadriplegics, Boston, 1975, Little, Brown & Co.

93. Morgan S: Sexuality after hysterectomy and castration, Women and Health 3(1):5-10, 1978.

94. Moses A and Hawkins R: Counseling lesbian women and gay men: a life issues approach, St Louis, 1982, The CV Mosby Co.

95. O'Brien KM et al: Sexual dysfunction in uremia, Proc Clin Dial Transplant Form 5:98-101, 1975.

96. Papadopoulos C et al: Sexual concerns and needs of the postcoronary patient's wife, Arch Intern Med 140:38-41, 1980.

97. Papadopoulos C: Myocardial infarction and sexual activity of the female patient, Arch Intern Med 143:1528-1530, 1983.

98. Papadoupolous C et al: Sexual activity after coronary bypass surgery, Chest 90:681-685, 1986.

99. Persaud D: Assessing sexual functions of the adult with traumatic quadriplegia, J Neurosurg Nurs 18(1):11-12, 1986.

100. Pfeiffer E, Verwoerdt A, and Wang HS: The natural history of sexual behavior in a biologically advantaged group of aged individuals, J Gerontol. 24:193-198, 1969.

101. Phelps G: Sexual experience and plasma testosterone levels in male veterans after spinal cord injury, Arch Phys Med Rehabil 64:47-52, 1983.

102. Pluchinotta A and Fabris G: Sexual function after abdominoperineal resection of the rectum, Am J Proctol Gastroenterol Colon Rect Surg 31(6):18-21, 1980.

103. Price J: Promoting sexual wellness in head injured patients, Rehabil Nurs 10(6):12-13, 1985.

104. Price-Spratlen L: Sexual harassment counseling, J Psychosoc Nurs Mental Health Services 26(2):28-33, 38,40, 1988.

105. Procci WR et al: Sexual functioning of renal transplant recipients, J Nerv Ment Dis 166:402-407, 1978.

106. Quinif NJ and Nasrallah PF: Sexuality after urinary diversion, J Urol 130:129-131, 1983.

107. Richards JS: Sex and arthritis, Sexual Disabil 3:96-104, 1980.

108. Roberts N: Advising patients on sex after surgery, AORN J 32:55-61, 1980.

109. Scalzi CC: Sexual counseling, In SL Underhill, et al: Cardiac nursing, Philadelphia, 1982, JB Lippincott.

110. Scalzi C et al: Sexual counseling of coronary patients, Heart Lung 7:840-845, 1978.

111. Schain W: Breast cancer surgeries and psychosexual sequelae: implications for remediation, Semin Oncol Nurs 1:200-205, 1985.

112. Schiavi R and Hogan B: Sexual problems in diabetes mellitus: psychological aspects, Diabetes Care 2(1):9-17, 1979.

113. Schöffling K et al: Disorders of sexual function in male diabetics, Diabetes 12:519-527, 1963.

114. Schover LR and von Eschenbach AC: Sexual and marital counseling with men treated for testicular cancer, J Sex Marital Ther 10:29-40, 1984.

115. Schover L et al: Multiaxial problem oriented systems for sexual dysfunctions, Arch Gen Psychiatry 39:614-619, 1982.

116. Schover LR et al: Sexual rehabilitation of urologic cancer patients: a practical approach, CA 34:66-73, 1984.

117. Schover L, Fife M, and Gershenson D: Sexual dysfunction and treatment for early stage cervical cancer, Cancer 63:204-212, 1989.
118. Schreiner-engel P: Diabetes mellitus and female sexuality, Sexual Disabil 6(2):83-92, 1983.
119. Schuler M: Sexual counseling for the spinal cord injured: a review of five programs, J Sex Marital Ther 8:241-252, 1982.
120. Seibel M: Hysterectomy for carcinoma in situ and sexual function, Gynecol Oncol 11:195-199, 1981.
121. Sex and Disability Project: Who cares? A handbook on sex education and counseling services for disabled people. Washington, DC, 1979, George Washington University.
122. Siegel K, Mesagno F, Chen J, and Christ G: Factors distinguishing homosexual males practicing risky and safer sex, Soc Sci Med 28(6):561-569, 1989.
123. Siewicki BJ and Mansfield LW: Determining readiness to resume sexual activity, Am J Nurs 77:604, 1977.
124. Sjogren K: Sexuality after stroke with hemiplegia. II: With special regard to partnership adjustment and to fulfillment. Scand J Rehabil Med 15:63-69, 1983.
125. Sjogren K, Damber JE, and Liliequist B: Sexuality after stroke with hemiplegia, I: Aspects of sexual function, Scand J Rehabil Med 15:55-61, 1983.
126. Sjorgren K and Fugl-Meyer AR: Some factors influencing quality of sexual life after myocardial infarction. Int Rehabil Med 5(4):197-201, 1983.
127. Smith D: Sexual rehabilitation of the cancer patient, Cancer Nurs 12(1):10-15, 1989.
128. Smith D: Sexuality and the homosexual person with a stoma, J Enterstomal Ther 15:118-120, 1988.
129. Solomon M and De Jong W: Preventing AIDS and other STD's through Condom promotion: a patient education intervention, Am J Public Health 79(4):453-458, 1989.
130. Spengler A: Radical prostatectomy and sexuality, Sexual Disabil 6:155-166, 1983.
131. Starr, B and Weiner M: The Starr-Weiner report on sex and sexuality in the mature years, New York, 1981, Stein & Day, Pub.

132. Stevenson J: Sexual dysfunction due to antihypertensive agents, Drug Intel Clin Pharmacol 18(2):113-121, 1984.
133. Taylor P: Understanding sexuality in the dying patient, Nursing 13(4)54-55, 1983.
134. Valentich M et al: Facilitating the sexual integration of the head injured person in the community, Sexual Disabil 7:28-42, 1984.
135. Valleroy M: Sexual dysfunction in multiple sclerosis, Arch Phys Med Rehabil. 65(3):125-128, 1984.
136. Wallace L: Sexual adjustment after radical genital surgery, Nurs Times 83(51):41-43, 1987.
137. Wasow M: Human sexuality and terminal illness, Health Soc Work 2(2):105-121, 1977.
138. Waterhouse J et al: Development of the sexual adjustment questionnaire: impact of cancer and surgery, Oncol Nurs Forum 13(3):53-59, 1986.
139. Weinberg JS: Human sexuality and spinal cord injury, Nurs Clin North Am 17:407-420, 1982.
140. Williams J and Slack W: A prospective study of sexual function after major colorectal surgery, Br J Surg 67:722-724, 1980.
141. Witkin MH: Sex therapy and mastectomy, J Sex Marital Ther 1:290-304, 1975.
142. Wood RY and Rose K: Penile implants for impotency, Am J Nurs 78:234-238, 1978.
143. Woods NF: Human sexuality in health and illness, ed 3, St Louis, 1984, The CV Mosby Co.
144. Woods NF: Influences on sexual adaptation to mastectomy, JOGN Nurs 4:33-37, 1975.
145. Woods NF, and Earp, JAL: Women with cured breast cancer: a study of mastectomy patients in North Carolina, Nurs Res 27:279-285, 1978.
146. Woods N: Toward a holistic perspective of human sexuality: alterations in sexual health and nursing diagnoses, Holistic Nurs Pract 1(4):1-11, 1987.
147. Zahn MA: Incapacity, impotence, and invisible impairment: their effects upon interpersonal relations, J Health Soc Behav 14:115-123, 1973.

CHAPTER 53

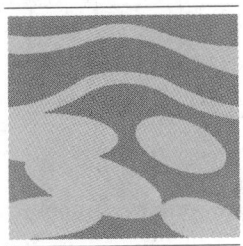

Assessment of Reproductive Health

GREER GLAZER

CHAPTER OBJECTIVES

After studying this chapter, the student should be able to:
1. Identify structures of the reproductive system and summarize the related endocrine functions.
2. Identify pertinent reproductive data to be collected by a nursing history.
3. Describe preparation of a woman for pelvic examination.
4. Recognize diagnostic tests used to diagnose problems of the reproductive system and nursing responsibilities associated with each.

Conditions affecting healthful functioning of the reproductive systems of men and women take a high toll in loss of life and acute and chronic physical and emotional stress. The nurse has a responsibility to assist in general health education, to refer patients to good health care, and to understand the treatment available and the nursing care needed when disease develops. A sound knowledge of the structure and functions of the reproductive system is essential to the assessment process.

ANATOMY AND PHYSIOLOGY
PELVIS

The bones of the pelvis are shown in Figure 53-1. The pelvis is the weight-bearing structure of the upper body and trunk. The pelvic bones consist of the innominate bones, the sacrum, and the coccyx. The two innominate bones are made up of the pubic bone, ilium, and ischium. Anteriorly, the pubic bones join at the symphysis pubis. The inferior borders of the pubic bones and symphysis form an inverted V, called the pubic arch. The sacrum and coccyx come together at the sacrococcygeal joint, which is movable. Caudal anesthetics are administered at the sacral hiatus.

The pelvis is divided into two parts (the true and the false pelvis) by a bony ridge called the pelvic brim. The false pelvis is the broad, expanded portion above the pelvic brim. The narrow part below the pelvic brim is the true pelvis. The true pelvis is further described as having an inlet and an outlet. The inlet is located at the pelvic brim, and the outlet is at the base of the pelvis. The iliac spines mark the midpoint between the inlet and the outlet. The distances between the bones of the true pelvis have special significance during childbirth, since it is through this bony canal that the baby must pass to be born.

Like other bones of the skeletal system, the pelvic bones undergo changes during periods of growth and development until maturity is reached. The major differences between the pelves of men and women are in the contour of the pelvis and thickness of the bones. Although variations are seen in both sexes, the female pelvis is more delicate because the bones are thinner and lighter in weight. The female pelvis is wider and more shallow because of the flaring of the iliac bones; the male pelvis tends to be narrow and deep. In women, the sacrum is shorter, wider, and less curved and the coccyx is more movable. The pubic arch is wider and more rounded in women, and the ischial spines are less prominent. Pelvic dimensions vary with age and race in addition to sex. The typical architecture of the female pelvis is especially suited for childbirth.

FEMALE GENITAL SYSTEM
EXTERNAL STRUCTURES

Figure 53-2 shows the external genitalia of a female. Collectively, the external genitalia are often referred to as the vulva and consist of the mons pubis (mons veneris), labia majora, labia minora, clitoris, prepuce, frenulum, vestibule, urethral meatus, Skene's (paraurethral) glands, vaginal orifice, hymen, fossa navicularis, Bartholin's (vulvovaginal) glands, fourchet, perineum, and escutcheon. The escutcheon is the triangular pubic hair

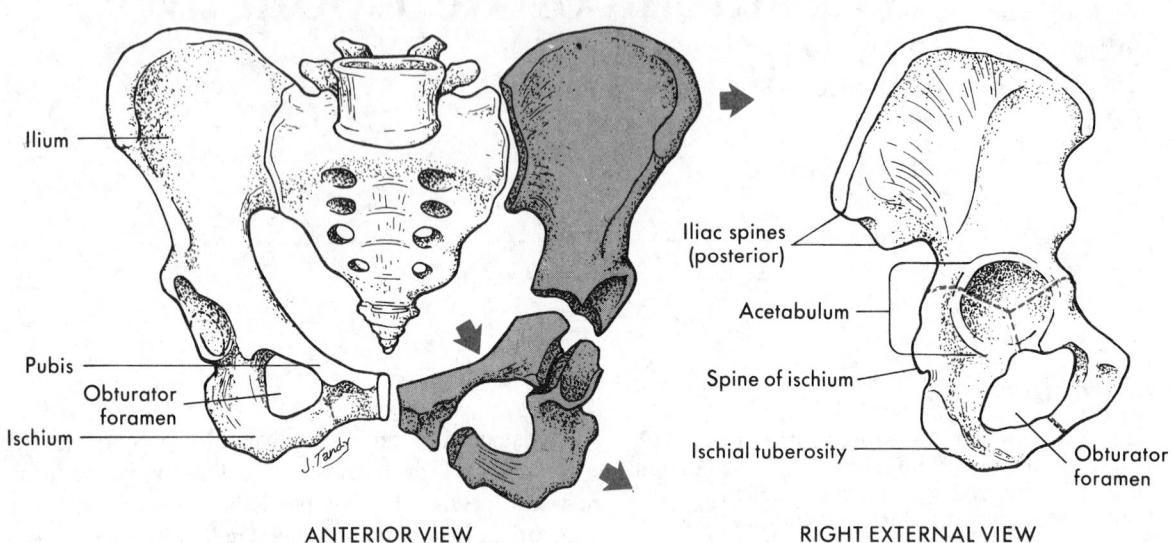

Ilium

Pubis

Obturator
foramen

Ischium

Iliac spines
(posterior)

Acetabulum

Spine of ischium

Ischial tuberosity

Obturator
foramen

ANTERIOR VIEW

RIGHT EXTERNAL VIEW

FIGURE 53-1 Adult female pelvis, showing origin of parts from separate embryonic bones. (From Jensen MD, Benson RC, and Bobak IM: Maternity care: the nurse and the family, ed 2, St Louis, 1981, The CV Mosby Co.)

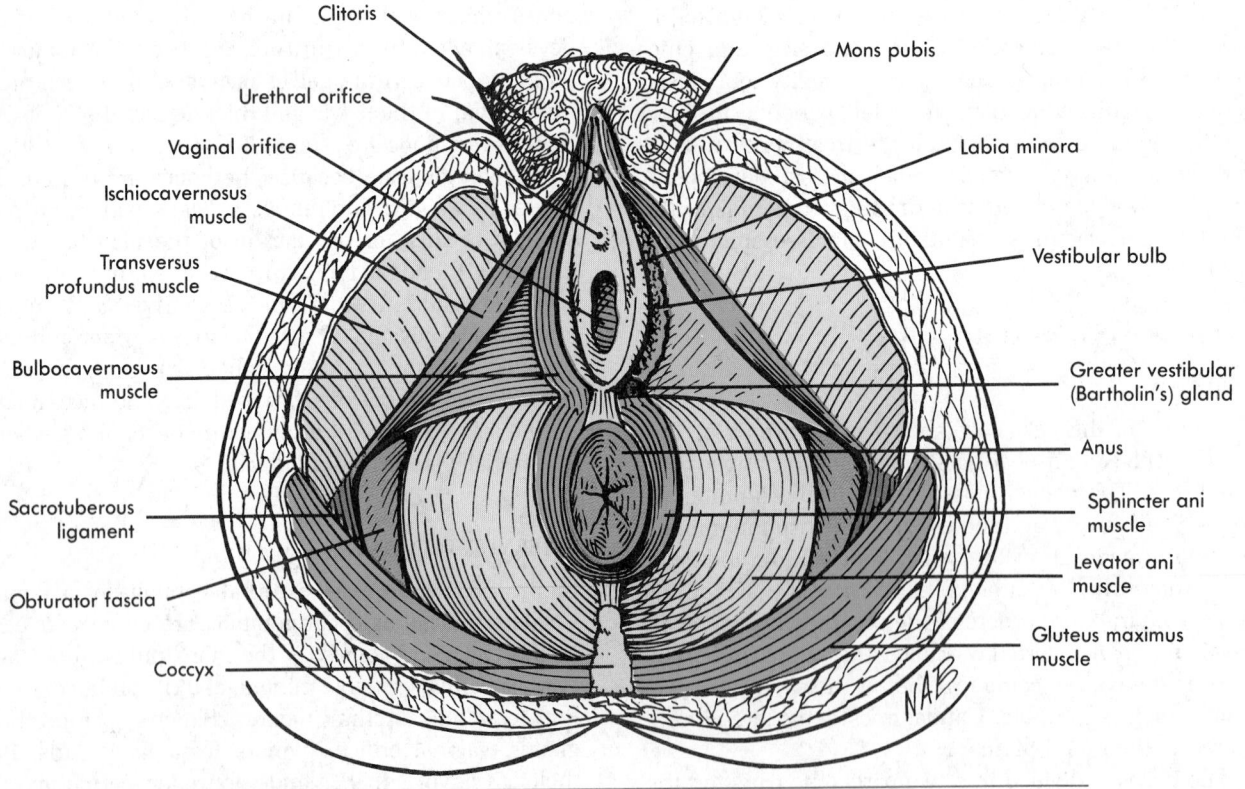

Clitoris

Urethral orifice

Vaginal orifice

Ischiocavernosus
muscle

Transversus
profundus muscle

Bulbocavernosus
muscle

Sacrotuberous
ligament

Obturator fascia

Coccyx

Mons pubis

Labia minora

Vestibular bulb

Greater vestibular
(Bartholin's) gland

Anus

Sphincter ani
muscle

Levator ani
muscle

Gluteus maximus
muscle

FIGURE 53-2 Female perineum.

pattern from the upper portion of the pubic bone to the lateral areas of the labia majora. The *mons pubis* is the rounded area in front of the symphysis pubis. It consists of a collection of fatty tissue beneath the skin and is covered with hair after puberty.

The *labia majora* are two prominent, longitudinal folds of tissue extending back from the mons pubis. These labia are thicker in front, gradually become thinner as they extend back, and appear to flatten out as they merge with the adjacent tissues in the area of the perineum. The labia majora have two surfaces. The outer surface is covered by a thin layer of skin containing hair follicles and sebaceous and sweat glands. The inner surfaces are smooth, lack hair, and are supplied with a large number of sebaceous follicles. The labia are homologous to the male scrotum.

The *labia minora* are two smaller folds of tissue parallel to the labia majora and sometimes concealed between the folds of the labia majora. In sexually active women and in women who have borne children, the labia minora may project beyond the labia majora. The labia minora join near the prepuce, which covers the clitoris, extend backward to enclose the urethral and vaginal openings, and merge with the labia majora in the perineum. The labia minora are made up of connective and elastic tissue and contain little fatty tissue. Sweat glands and hair follicles are absent from the labia minora, but sebaceous glands are present. Abnormal sexual differentiation is possible with maldevelopment or fusion of the labia. Vulvovaginitis affects the labia minora.

The *clitoris* is situated near the anterior folds of the labia minora. The glans of the clitoris is a small, rounded area consisting of erectile tissue enclosed in a layer of fibrous membrane. Although it is often compared with or said to be homologous to the penis in males because it consists of the glans, corpus, and crura, the clitoris is unique in that its sole physiologic functions are initiation and elevation of sexual tension levels. The clitoris serves as both receptor and transformer of sexual stimuli. Sexual stimulation initiates a process whereby the clitoris becomes enlarged, erect, and very sensitive to sexual stimuli. Female orgasm can occur from stimulation of the clitoris but also results from stimulation of other sites; in fact, female orgasm has been documented in instances where the clitoris had been surgically removed. Inflammation of the lower genital tract or cancer may develop on the clitoris.

The *vestibule* is a boat-shaped fossa formed between the labia minora, clitoris, and fourchet. The *fossa navicularis* is a small depression between the fourchet and hymen. On opening the labia minora, the vaginal and urethral orifices can be seen. These surfaces are thin, easily irritated, and especially subject to laceration during childbirth.

The *hymen* is an irregular membranous fold of con-nective tissue of varying thickness that partially covers the vaginal orifice. The hymen may be avulsed (broken) by coitus, digital examination, vigorous exercise, or surgery. Absence of the hymen does not denote lack of virginity. Remnants of the hymen usually persist after avulsion and form an irregular border around the vaginal opening.

The location of *Skene's* (paraurethral) glands and *Bartholin's* (vulvovaginal) glands should be noted, because they are common sites of infection. Skene's glands are located on each side of the urethral meatus. Bartholin's glands are situated at each side of the vaginal opening near the bases of the labia. Since both Skene's glands and Bartholin's glands are very small, their openings are just visible. They may not be palpable unless the woman is very thin or unless the glands are enlarged because of infection.

The *perineum* is the area between the vagina and anus. It is composed of muscles and subdermal and dermal tissue.

The appearance of the vulvar structures varies with age. Before puberty, the external genitalia are characterized by absence of pubic hair, and the labia minora are more prominent than the labia majora. With deposit of body fat and hormone effects during puberty, the labia majora increase in thickness and pubic hair appears. With the onset of the menopause and gradual withdrawal of hormones, the external genitalia again become less prominent and the pubic hair begins to thin. In elderly women, the vulva may appear wrinkled, shrunken, and almost flat. During the life span, congenital defects, childbirth, infection or other diseases, and surgery may alter the structure and appearance of the external genitalia.

INTERNAL ORGANS

The female internal reproductive organs are shown in Figure 53-3. In relation to the skeletal system, the internal reproductive organs are located in the true pelvis. Unless their size is increased by a disease process or by pregnancy, the internal organs of reproduction remain within the cavity of the true pelvis. An exception is noted during sexual response when the uterus elevates into the false pelvis.

Vagina

The vaginal orifice serves as the boundary between the external structures and the internal organs. The vagina is a musculofascial tube that connects the vulva with the cervix and uterus. The functions of the vagina are to receive the penis during intercourse, allow for childbirth, and permit discharge of the menstrual flow. The vagina is located between the rectum and urethra and is a soft, tubular structure that extends upward and back from the vaginal opening.

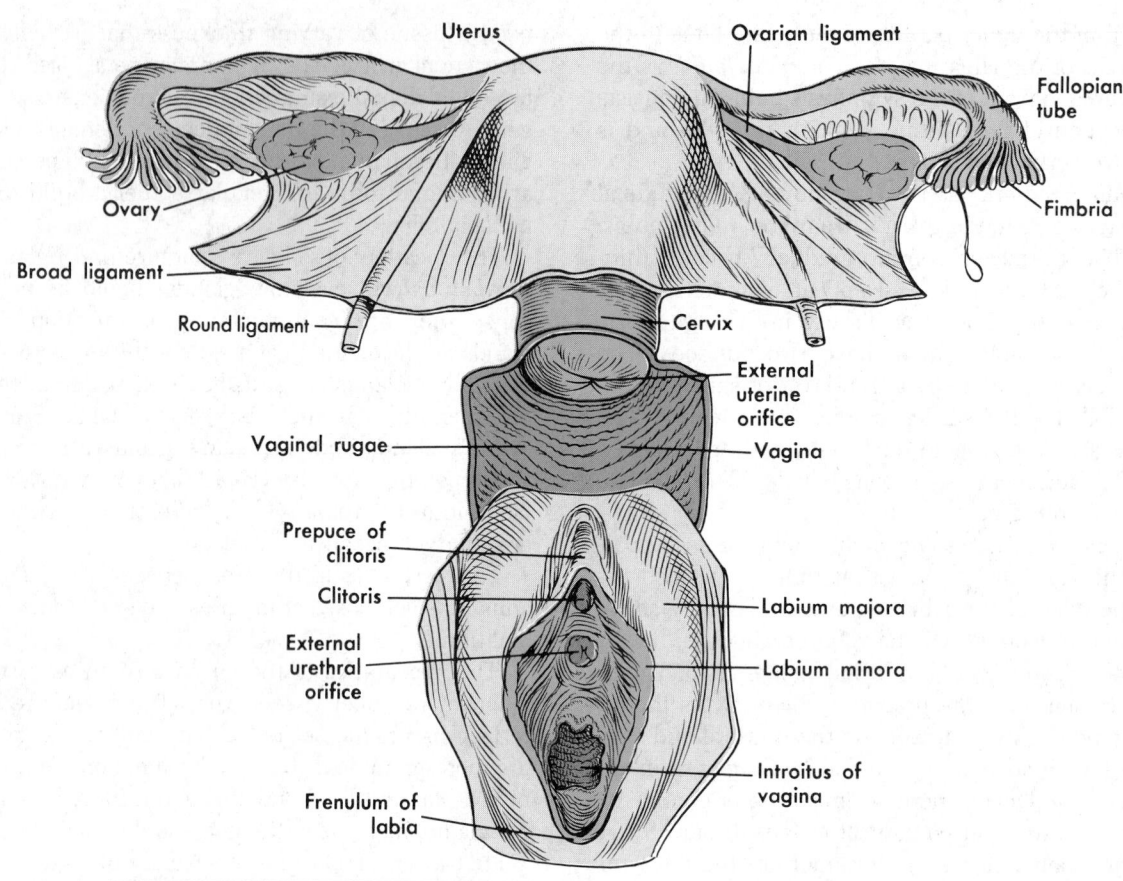

FIGURE 53-3 Female internal organs of reproduction. Major ligaments are shown.

The length of the vaginal canal varies, and the posterior wall is longer than the anterior wall. The anterior wall averages 6 to 8 cm long, whereas the posterior wall averages 8 to 9 cm.

The vagina is lined with pink mucous membrane arranged in folds called *rugae*. Physiologic events (for example, pregnancy) and pathologic conditions (for example, infections) often alter the color of the vaginal mucosa because of congestion with blood. The rugae make it possible for the vagina to distend and to stretch during coitus and childbirth. The rugated appearance of the vaginal canal is prominent during adolescence and tends to disappear with multiparity.

The vaginal walls end in a blind pouch *around* the cervix. Note that the vaginal epithelium is continuous with the epithelium of the cervix and that the cervix projects into the upper vagina. The groove formed by the termination of the vagina around the cervix is called the *vaginal vault*.

A cup-shaped *fornix* is formed by the protrusion of the cervix into the superior portion of the vagina. The fornix is divided into anterior, posterior, and lateral fornices.

The vagina is lubricated by secretions from its own cells and by secretions from the cervix and Bartholin's glands. The combined vaginal secretions are normally acid during the years of ovarian function. The presence of Döderlein bacilli and estrogen influences the acidity of the vagina. When adequate estrogen stimulation is present, the cells of the vagina and cervix contain glycogen. Lactic acid is produced by breakdown of glycogen, the degree of which is related to acidity of the vagina. Before puberty, the vaginal pH tends to be neutral. With the onset of puberty, the vaginal pH varies between 4.0 and 5.0, depending on the phase of the menstrual cycle and the level of estrogen. The pH is lowest at the time of ovulation and just before menstruation. During pregnancy, a pH of 4.0 or less is common. Neutral or alkaline values are normally found in postmenopausal women. The importance of vaginal acidity is demonstrated by the fact that most pathogenic bacteria produce signs of vaginal infection when the pH falls below 4.0 or rises above 5.0.

Until puberty, the vaginal epithelium is thin. The epithelium thickens at the time of puberty, and this state persists through the reproductive years until the menopause, when the epithelium again becomes thin. The thickness of the vaginal epithelium is closely related to estrogen levels.

The natural barriers to infection (thickness of the vaginal epithelium and acidity of the vagina) are minimal before puberty and after menopause, predisposing females in these age groups to vaginal infections and trauma of the vaginal mucosa.

Uterus

The uterus is a hollow, muscular organ located between the urinary bladder and rectum. It consists of two portions—the corpus (body) and the cervix. The body is composed of the fundus, which is the thick muscular region above insertion of the fallopian tubes; the body, which is the main portion of the uterus; and the isthmus, which is the lower region. The cervix is located between the isthmus and the vagina. The size of the uterus decreases from the fundus to the cervix, giving the contour of the uterus a triangular, pear-shaped appearance. The size of the uterus varies among women, ranging from 5.5 to 9 cm long, 3.5 to 6 cm wide, and 2 to 4 cm thick in nonparous women. All dimensions may be 2 to 3 cm larger in multiparas.

The position, shape, and size of the uterus vary at different periods of life and under different circumstances. Minor developmental abnormalities, probably the result of embryonic error, are relatively common. During infancy, the uterus is an abdominal organ, and the cervix is larger than the corpus. By puberty, the uterus has increased in size and has descended into the pelvic cavity. In women, the position of the uterus is subject to considerable variation (see Figure 55-2). The uterus is usually anteverted and slightly anteflexed, although it may be retroverted, retroflexed, or in mid-position. During pregnancy, the uterus changes remarkably in size, shape, structure, and position and returns to its prepregnancy state within 6 to 8 weeks after delivery. During menopause, the uterus begins to hypertrophy and decreases in size.

The body of the uterus is normally bent forward over the bladder so that the fundus is behind the symphysis pubis. The uterus is in direct contact with the bladder and may also touch the rectum, sigmoid colon, and small intestines.

The cervix curves forward. The relationship between the corpus and the cervix produces an angle of about 90 degrees. The angle is decreased as the urinary bladder fills and elevates the corpus.

The outer surfaces of the uterus are covered by peritoneum, which is reflected from the abdominal wall. The anterior and posterior reflections of the peritoneum join at the sides to enclose the fallopian tubes and ovaries. Reflection of the peritoneum over the top of the pelvic organs creates spaces between the uterus and

bladder anteriorly and the uterus and rectum posteriorly. The posterior space is known as the cul-de-sac of Douglas and is clinically important in that the peritoneal cavity can be entered through the posterior vaginal wall with little risk of damaging adjacent organs or structures. The cul-de-sac of Douglas is a common entry site for culdoscopy, culpotomy, and surgical drainage of the peritoneal cavity.

The uterus has three functional layers—the parametrium, which is the peritoneal and fascial outer layer; the myometrium, which is the middle muscular layer; and the endometrium, which is the mucous membrane-type tissue. The endometrial lining is thickest before the beginning of menstruation and thinnest after menstruation. The cavity of the uterus is continuous with the cervical canal and has an average capacity of 3 to 8 ml. Near the fundus, the uterus opens into the lumen of the fallopian tubes. Thus there is a direct route from the vagina through the cervix, uterus, and fallopian tubes to the peritoneum. This is important in prevention of infection and its spread by continuity of tissue.

The cervix is firm, smooth, and round. It is primarily made up of elastic and fibrous connective tissue and smooth muscle. Its color is usually lighter pink than that of the vagina. The lower portion of the cervix protrudes into the vagina, and in the center of the vaginal portion of the cervix is the external os. Extending upward from the external os is the cervical canal, which averages 2 to 3 cm long. The cervical canal terminates as it joins the corpus, and the junction of the cervical canal and the corpus is termed the internal cervical os. The functions of the cervix are to secrete mucus to facilitate transport of sperm, to dilate during labor, and to provide a channel for discharge of the menstrual flow. During childbirth, cervical lacerations are almost inevitable.

Changes in the physical properties and in the pH of the cervical mucus are significant in the treatment of infertility and in fertility control (see Chapter 54). At the time of ovulation, the cervical mucus becomes thinner and more elastic. These changes enhance penetration of the cervical mucus by sperm. The viscosity of the cervical mucus can be determined by studies of mucous flow and elasticity. The term *spinnbarkeit* is applied to describe the characteristic ability of the cervical mucus to stretch and recoil.

Fallopian Tubes

The fallopian tubes are two narrow, muscular canals ranging from 8 to 14 cm long. They extend outward from the corpus near the fundus at the cornua and are enclosed in the folds of the broad ligaments. The tubes are divided into three portions: The isthmus is the proximal portion of the tube nearest the cornu; the ampulla is the longer, middle portion where fertilization usually occurs; and the farthest, distal portion of the tube is fimbriated.

The walls of the fallopian tubes contain smooth muscles that possess peristaltic properties. The fallopian tubes are lined with a mucous membrane that contains cilia. At the time of ovulation, both the peristaltic action and the ciliary action increase, and it is likely that these combined actions provide the mechanism for ovum transport.

The functions of the fallopian tubes are to serve as a site for union of the sperm and ovum and to transport the ovum to the uterus. If a stricture of the fallopian tube exists in the proximal portion, the fertilized ovum may not be able to pass the point of obstruction and an ectopic (tubal) pregnancy may result.

Ovaries

The ovaries are endocrine glands as well as reproductive organs. There are normally two almond-shaped ovaries, ranging from 3 to 4 cm long, 2 cm wide, and 1 to 2 cm thick, each lying near the fimbriae of the fallopian tubes. They are partly enclosed by the broad ligaments. Each ovary contains an outer portion (cortex) and an inner portion (medulla). The term *adnexa* refers to the ovaries, fallopian tubes, and supporting tissues. The functions of the ovaries are to store primordial follicles; to produce mature ova; and to produce and secrete estrogen, progesterone, and androgens. Ovarian functions are readily disturbed by acute and chronic diseases. The functions can also be altered or interrupted by surgery, radiation, and the ingestion of drugs such as oral contraceptives.

The ovaries undergo histologic changes resulting from endocrine stimulation as well as physical changes in position, size, and shape during the life span. At birth, the ovaries are very small, round, smooth, and light pink and are located in the false pelvis. Between infancy and puberty the ovaries increase in size, become more flattened, assume a grayish color, and descend into the true pelvis. During the childbearing years, the ovaries appear long and flat, have a nodular surface caused by the presence of follicles, and lie close to the pelvic walls. During pregnancy, the ovaries are lifted out of the pelvis by the enlarging uterus, but they descend into the pelvis after childbirth. After menopause, the ovaries undergo rapid regressive changes. They decrease in size, their surfaces become wrinkled, and the color fades from gray to white. In most postmenopausal women, the ovaries are so small that they cannot be palpated during vaginal examination.

After puberty, the surfaces of the ovaries are covered by connective tissue fibers that form a layer called the *tunica albuginea*. Immediately below the connective tissue is the ovarian cortex containing a large number of minute vesicles, the primordial follicles. Each primor-

dial follicle contains an undeveloped ovum having the capacity to respond to stimulation by pituitary hormones. It is estimated that each ovary contains 500,000 primordial follicles at the time of birth. Many of the primordial follicles disintegrate before puberty, and the process of disintegration continues throughout the childbearing years. Consequently, few if any primordial follicles are found in the ovaries after menopause.

Unlike sperm, which are produced constantly by males, only one ovum matures at a time, and the process of ovum maturation requires an average of 28 days. When the ovum reaches maturity, it leaves the ovary by the process of ovulation.

MALE GENITAL SYSTEM

The male reproductive organs and associated structures are shown in Figure 53-4. The male reproductive organs produce sperm, suspend the sperm in a liquid, and deliver the sperm into the vagina to fertilize an ovum. Another important function is secretion of male hormones, the androgens. The male genitalia include the testes, vas deferens, seminal vesicles, ejaculatory ducts, and penis, along with the prostate and bulbourethral glands, which are accessory structures.

TESTES

The oval-shaped testes produce the sperm. During fetal life, the testes are located in the abdominal cavity behind the peritoneum. Before birth, the testes descend through the inguinal canals and inguinal rings into the scrotum and are suspended in position by the spermatic cords, which are attached to the posterior borders of the testes. At the lateral edge of each spermatic cord is the epididymis, which appears as a narrow, flattened structure.

The testes are composed of glandular tissue covered by fibrous tissue. The glandular tissue is composed of many lobules differing in size according to their location. The lobules consist of 600 to 1200 small convoluted structures, the seminiferous tubules. The seminiferous tubules produce the sperm, and spermatozoa in different stages of development can be seen along the cells of the tubules.

After puberty, the lining of the seminiferous tubules continually forms millions of sperm. Spermatogenesis follows a sequential pattern of maturation of germ cells from spermatogonium to the mature spermatozoa. The process involves mitosis, meiosis, and spermiogenesis. Approximately 74 days are required for conversion of immature sperm to mature sperm. Each mature sperm has a whiplike tail, making it possible for the sperm to move freely in the proper environment. Because of the environment of the testes, the sperm are passive. Some of the sperm are moved by peristaltic action in the epididymis and vas deferens to the prostate gland. The sem-

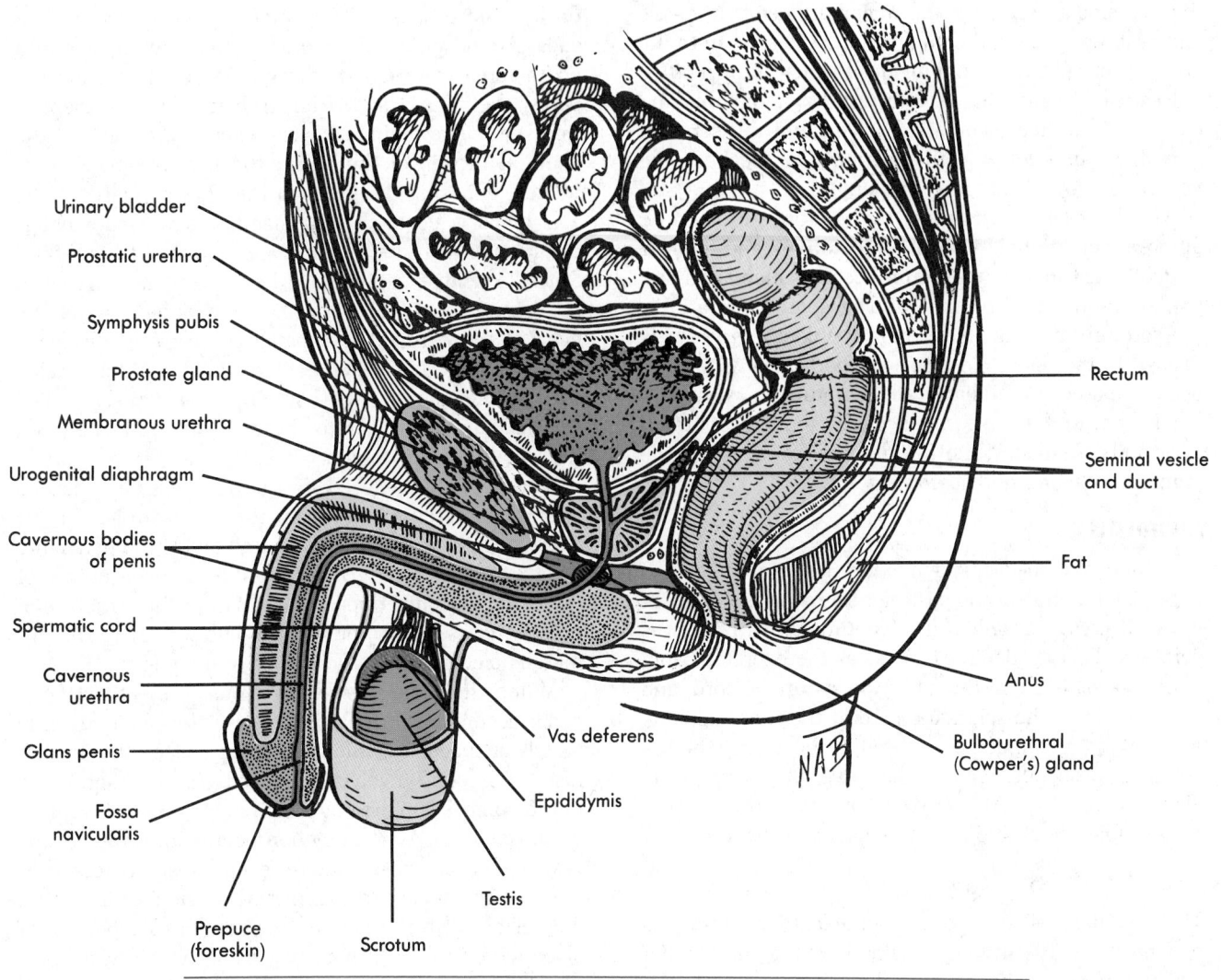

FIGURE 53-4 Male organs of reproduction.

inal vesicles and prostate gland produce most of the fluid in which the sperm can be suspended and made motile.

In addition to producing sperm, the testes function as an endocrine gland. The male hormone testosterone is produced by the interstitial cells of the testes and is responsible for development of the genitalia during puberty and for maintaining the genitalia in a functional state during life. Androgenic hormones are also responsible for the development of secondary sex characteristics, including growth of body hair and thickening of the vocal cords.

SPERMATIC CORDS

The spermatic cords extend from the deep inguinal rings and consist of arteries, veins, lymphatics, nerves, and the excretory duct of the testes held together by the spermatic fascia. At the deep inguinal rings, the structures of the spermatic cords converge with the struc-

tures of the testes. The spermatic cords then pass through the inguinal canals, emerge through the superficial inguinal rings, and pass downward into the scrotum.

SCROTUM

The scrotum is a cutaneous pouch that covers and protects the testes and spermatic cords. Because the testes are surrounded by serous membrane and are suspended in the cavity of the scrotum, the testes are capable of being moved about readily. The ease of movement of the testes within the scrotum protects them against injury.

The skin of the scrotum is thin, brownish, and very elastic because it contains rugae; and it contains sebaceous follicles. Thinly scattered hairs cover the skin. Because of the rugae, the skin of the scrotum is capable of great distention, and the scrotum may become greatly enlarged when edema is present. The surface of the scrotum is divided into two halves by a ridge (raphe) that extends anteriorly to the undersurface of the penis and posteriorly along the midline of the perineum to the anus. Internally, a septum divides the scrotum into two halves, each containing a testis and its epididymis and portion of spermatic cord. The left side of the scrotum normally hangs lower than the right side because the left spermatic cord is greater in length.

The external appearance of the scrotum varies under different conditions. In warm temperatures and in older or debilitated men, the scrotum becomes elongated and flat. In young, healthy men and in cool temperatures, the scrotum appears short, more wrinkled, and closely applied to the testes. In some newborn boys who have been exposed to chilling, the scrotum may appear empty, because the spermatic cords tend to contract. This pulls the testes into the inguinal canal when the inguinal rings are not closed.

EPIDIDYMIS

The comma-shaped epididymis can be visually located at the lateral edge of the posterior segment of the testes where it creates a bulge. It is continuous with the vas deferens. The vas deferens serves as the excretory duct of the testes, is a constituent of the spermatic cord, and separates from the spermatic cord at the inguinal ring. After taking a complex path through the pelvis, the vas deferens descends, enters the base of the prostate gland, becomes greatly narrowed, and joins the ducts of the seminal vesicles to form the ejaculatory duct.

SEMINAL VESICLES

The seminal vesicles are two lobulated, membranous pouches, 5 to 10 cm long, located between the bladder and the rectum. They secrete fluid to be added to the secretions of the testes. The lower end of each seminal vesicle becomes constricted into a straight duct and joins the vas deferens to form the ejaculatory duct. The ejaculatory duct begins at the base of the prostate gland, runs posteriorly and downward, and enters the prostate gland in the midline. In the prostate gland, the ejaculatory duct opens into the prostatic portion of the urethra.

PENIS

The penis is a conduit for elimination of ejaculate and urine through the urethral opening. It is attached to the front and sides of the pubic arch. When flaccid, the penis is cylindric in shape; when erect, it assumes a triangular shape with rounded angles. The penis consists of three masses of cavernous tissue held together by fibrous tissue. The three columns of erectile tissue are the two corpora cavernosa and the corpus spongiosum, which contains the urethra.

The skin covering the penis is dark in color, contains no fat, and is loosely connected to the underlying tissues. At the pubis, the skin is covered with hair in a characteristic triangular distribution. At the neck of the penis, the skin is folded on itself to form the prepuce (foreskin). The prepuce covers a variable amount of the glans at the tip of the penis; the prepuce may be retracted, exposing the glans in the uncircumcised male. The glans is covered by a membranous tissue that is continuous with the mucous membrane of the urethra. Small, sensitive papillae are located on the surface of the glans, the inner surface of the prepuce, and the neck of the penis. These papillae secrete a sebaceous substance and have a characteristic odor. When mixed with epithelial cells, the combined discharge is called *smegma* and is similar to the deposits found between the labial folds in women.

The penis is enclosed in a strong capsule of fascia. Numerous cords extend from the inner surface of the capsule, cross in all directions, and divide the penis into compartments. This gives the entire inner structure of the penis a spongy appearance. Within the structure of muscle fibers and fibrous and elastic tissue are the numerous blood vessels and nerves of the penis.

When the male is sexually aroused, erection of the penis occurs involuntarily. Because the penis consists largely of spaces in which blood can collect, the mechanism of erection involves the blood vessels. Each space in the penis is supplied by a vein having a small sphincter at its outlet. When erection begins, the walls of the vascular spaces relax, and the outlet sphincters contract. At the same time, the arteries bring an increased flow of blood to the penis. This results in collection of blood within the cavernous spaces of the penis, hardening of the penis, and erection. During erection, enough blood passes through the sphincters of the veins to maintain circulation but not enough to empty the spaces. The erection is normally maintained until repeated stimulation results in reflex, involuntary ejaculation.

Ejaculation, the male orgasm, involves contractions of the muscular walls of the epididymis and vas deferens. These contractions force the passive sperm upward to the prostate gland. The seminal vesicles, which also have muscular walls, contract and force their contents into the urethra with the sperm. The fluid secreted by the seminal vesicles makes up most of the volume of the ejaculate. In the seminal fluid, the sperm become motile and begin to move about actively. As the seminal fluid moves into the prostatic portion of the urethra, the urethral walls begin peristaltic movement. The semen is thus forced down the urethra and through the urinary meatus in a short series of spurts, called ejaculation. Shortly after ejaculation, erection of the penis begins to subside. The vascular spaces relax, causing the blood to flow freely from the spaces within the penis. The walls of the vascular spaces contract as they empty of blood, and the body of the penis returns to its flaccid state.

PROSTATE GLAND

The prostate gland is located below the internal urethral orifice, behind the symphysis pubis, and close to the rectal wall, extending around the beginning of the urethra. The prostate gland averages 4 cm wide at its base, 3 cm from top to bottom, 2 cm from front to back, and 20 weighs g.

The prostate gland, which grows to the size and shape of a walnut during puberty, is enveloped in a firm, adherent capsule. Internally, the prostate gland is partly muscular and partly glandular. The glandular substance of the prostate gland consists of numerous follicular pouches that open into long canals. These canals join to form 12 to 20 small excretory ducts. Prostatic ducts open into the prostatic portion of the urethra, thus adding the prostatic secretion to the seminal fluid.

Clinically, the prostate gland is important because of its affinity for congestive, inflammatory, hyperplastic, and malignant diseases. Since the prostate gland is close to the rectal wall, it is easily palpable by rectal examination, making early diagnosis of disease possible. Because of the anatomic relationship of the prostate gland to the urethra, most prostatic diseases present urinary tract symptoms.

COWPER'S GLANDS

Cowper's (bulbourethral) glands are two small, round bodies located at the sides and to the back of the membranous portion of the urethra. They are enclosed by the transverse fibers of the sphincter muscles of the urethra. Each gland has an excretory duct that opens into the urethra. The main excretory duct of a Cowper gland represents the joining of many ducts from the internal glandular tissue substance. Cowper's glands secrete an alkaline substance into the semen to counteract vaginal and urethral acidity.

PELVIC LIGAMENTS AND MUSCLES

The internal and external reproductive structures are maintained in their positions by groups of ligaments and muscles. In the female, the broad ligaments (consisting of peritoneum) extend from the surfaces of the uterus to the sides of the pelvis and support the uterus in a horizontal position. The free margins of the broad ligament enclose and support the fallopian tubes and ovaries. The ovaries are suspended from the broad ligament by the ovarian ligaments (Figure 53-3).

The round ligaments extend laterally from the anterior surface of the uterine fundus. They pass through the abdominal wall, inguinal canals, and inguinal rings and terminate by dissemination of their fibers in the labia majora and surrounding tissues, holding the corpus forward over the urinary bladder. These ligaments stretch to allow enlargement and alteration of position of the uterus during pregnancy. They appear to keep the uterus in an anteverted position.

The uterosacral ligaments originate from the posterior surface of the uterus at the level of the internal os. They arch posteriorly and are inserted into the sacrum at the level of the second and third sacral vertebrae. Because the uterosacral ligaments exert backward tension on the cervix, they maintain the cervix and vagina at right angles to each other. The uterosacral ligaments thus prevent prolapse of the uterus by preventing the corpus from taking a position in line with the vagina. It is likely that uterosacral ligaments contain sensory nerve fibers, which may contribute to dysmenorrhea.

The cardinal ligaments arise from the base of the broad ligaments. They integrate with the pelvic fascia and fan outward around the base of the uterus. The cardinal ligaments provide the chief support for the cervix and upper vagina, preventing descent of these structures.

The pubocervical ligaments extend from the posterior surface of the pubis to the anterolateral portion of the cervix. They provide some support to the bladder and cervix.

The muscles that actively and passively support the pelvic floor are shown in Figure 53-2. The pelvic diaphragm consists of the levator ani and coccygeus muscles together with the pelvic fascia and stretches across the bottom of the pelvic cavity. The anal cavity, the urethra, and in females the vagina pierce the pelvic diaphragm. The levator ani muscles contain striated muscle fibers that enable the vaginal and anal openings to be closed voluntarily. The pubococcygeus muscle (part of the levator ani muscle) is especially important to women in sexual functioning, in relaxation of the perineum, in expulsion of the fetus in birthing, and for bladder control.

The muscles of the perineum, commonly called the perineal body or perineal center, reinforce the support provided by the levator ani and coccygeus muscles. The perineal body consists of a mass of several muscles extending across the center of the pelvic outlet. It is located between the anus and bulb in males and between the anus and vagina in females. Together the pelvic diaphragm and perineum support the pelvic organs and external genitalia from below.

In females, the perineum is wider and thicker than it is in males. The muscles of the perineal body are the means of approach to the bladder and prostate gland in males, and they are the site of perineal incisions and lacerations during childbirth.

BLOOD, LYMPH, AND NERVE SUPPLY

In males and females the organs of reproduction are supplied with blood from the aorta as it branches downward and divides into the internal iliac (hypogastric) artery.

The ovarian and uterine arteries anastomose to furnish the ovaries with blood. The venous drainage is similar to the arterial supply to the reproductive organs, with the blood vessels emptying into the vena cava.

In males, blood is similarly supplied to and drained from the reproductive organs. The pudendal branches of the aorta divide into the testicular arteries, and arteries supplying the seminal vesicles are derived from the inferior vesical and middle rectal arteries. Most of the blood to the penis is furnished through the internal pudendal artery. Venous return is similar to the arterial supply. Blood from the penis, testes, and prostate gland is returned to the internal iliac vein and then to the vena cava.

In both males and females, lymphatic drainage of the external and internal organs of reproduction is extensive. Both superficial and deep lymphatics empty into the external iliac, internal iliac, and preaortic lymph nodes. Nerve supply is derived from sympathetic and parasympathetic fibers of the autonomic nervous system and by spinal nerve pathways.

ENDOCRINE FUNCTIONS

The major hormones produced by the ovaries are estrogen and progesterone. Estrogen is the hormone responsible for the development of secondary sex characteristics at the time of puberty. After puberty, the primary function of estrogen is to cause development of the endometrium in preparation for implantation of a fertilized ovum. Progesterone enhances the preceding action of estrogen on the endometrium.

MENSTRUAL CYCLE

Like production of a mature ovum, secretion of ovarian hormones occurs in a cyclic fashion, with each cycle requiring an average of 28 days. Unless stimulated by pituitary hormones, however, the ovaries do not fulfill their hormone-secreting and ovum-producing functions.

The menstrual cycle is divided into phases according to uterine or ovarian changes. The uterine cycle consists of the menstrual, proliferative, and secretory phases. The follicular phase in the ovarian cycle corresponds to the menstrual and proliferative phases of the uterine cycle. The luteal phase in the ovarian cycle corresponds to the uterine secretory phase.

The functioning of the menstrual cycle depends on the proper relationships between the central nervous system, anterior pituitary, ovaries, and uterus (Figure 53-5).

In describing the ovarian-pituitary-uterine cycles, it is common to relate the events occurring to phases of the menstrual cycle. The first day of the menstrual flow is the first day of the menstrual cycle.

Menstrual Phase

During the menstrual phase of the cycle (menstruation), the endometrium breaks down and is shed. Withdrawal of estrogen and progesterone before the onset of menstrual flow results in rupture of uterine capillaries and necrosis of endometrial tissue. The menstrual phase of the cycle lasts an average of 4 days.

Proliferative Phase

When menstruation ceases, the proliferative phase begins and extends over the next 14 days and ends with ovulation. During the proliferative (follicular) phase, the pituitary gland secretes increasing amounts of follicle stimulating hormone (FSH). Of the pituitary hormones, FSH is probably the most important for ovarian function because it stimulates a primordial follicle to develop into a mature graafian follicle containing a mature ovum. Because the graafian follicle produces estrogen, FSH is essential for estrogen production.

As the graafian follicle matures, it secretes increasing amounts of estrogen, resulting in proliferation of endometrial cells. The endometrium becomes thicker and softer as preparation for implantation of a fertilized ovum begins. While increasing in size, the graafian follicle moves toward the surface of the ovary, where it appears as a blisterlike structure. Finally, the graffian follicle ruptures (ovulation), allowing the ovum and follicular fluid to escape. The ovum enters the fallopian tube and is carried in the direction of the uterus.

Before ovulation, estrogen exerts still other effects. It influences the cervical epithelium in such a way that the cervical mucus increases in quantity and attains a clear, elastic state. This permits the sperm to more readily enter the cervix. The high level of estrogen before ovulation suppresses pituitary release of FSH and triggers release of luteinizing hormone (LH).

As the level of FSH is falling and the level of estrogen is rising in the proliferative phase, the pituitary gland secretes increasing amounts of LH. There is a sharp rise in LH levels 12 to 24 hours before ovulation, followed by a peak level about 8 hours after ovulation. This change in hormone levels is reflected in the basal body temperature, which drops just before and rises after ovulation.

On the day of ovulation, about 25% of women experience pain in the lower abdomen on the side of ovulation. This pain is referred to as *mittelschmerz* and is probably a result of peritoneal irritation from follicular fluid or blood released from the ovary with the ovum. This sign rarely occurs with every cycle and is thus an unreliable indicator of ovulation. If the pain is on the

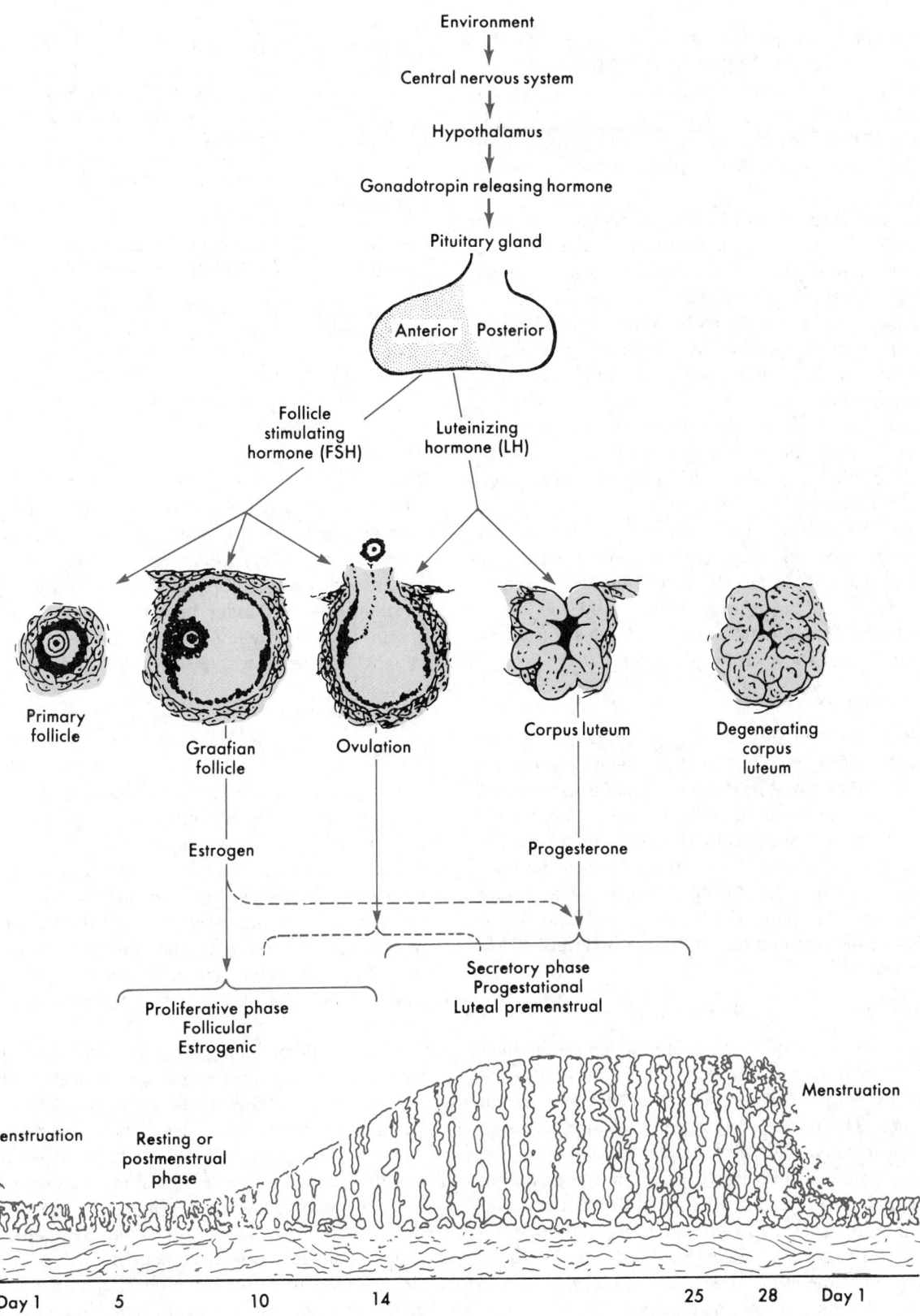

FIGURE 53-5 Hormone control of menstrual cycle.

right side and is severe, it may be mistaken for appendicitis.

Secretory Phase

With ovulation, the proliferative phase ends and the secretory phase begins. The secretory phase lasts for approximately 10 to 14 days. The secretory (luteal) phase is the least variable part of the menstrual cycle. Irregular menstrual cycles are most frequently related to longer or shorter menstrual or proliferative (follicular) phases.

Under the influence of LH, the corpus luteum forms in the ovary at the site of the ruptured graafian follicle. The hormone produced by the corpus luteum is progesterone. Progesterone further alters the endometrium by stimulating growth of cells and circulation of blood to the uterus. With these additional endometrial changes, the uterine environment is prepared for implantation of a fertilized ovum.

If pregnancy occurs, the corpus luteum remains secretory by the action of human chorionic gonadotropin (HGG), which is produced within a week of conception by the placenta. By 6 to 8 weeks after conception, the placenta is developed and assumes the function of secreting progesterone to maintain the endometrium. If pregnancy does not occur, the corpus luteum degenerates in about 10 days, progesterone secretion drops markedly, and the endometrium degenerates; menstruation results, and the cycle begins again.

MALE HORMONES

In males, secretion of the androgenic hormones increases at puberty, resulting in appearance of secondary sex characteristics and production of mature sperm. Of the androgens, testosterone is most closely related to reproduction, since it specifically stimulates maturation of sperm and is responsible for maintaining the reproductive organs in a functional state. Testosterone secretion is closely related to pituitary gland function. The rate of secretion of testosterone is determined by levels of LH in the blood.

PHYSIOLOGIC CHANGES WITH AGING

Changes in the reproductive tract in the female begin at middle age with menopause (Chapter 54). When ovulation ceases, no progesterone is produced and estrogen diminishes. The hormonal changes lead to changes in the uterus, ovaries, and vagina (see the box above). The physiologic changes may lead to discomfort or complications with sexual intercourse; vaginal dryness and narrowed introitus may cause dyspareunia (painful intercourse), and vaginal infections may occur more readily in the alkaline medium. Muscle weakness may lead to cystocele, rectocele, or uterine prolapse.

In the male, the production of testosterone decreases

PHYSIOLOGIC CHANGES IN REPRODUCTIVE TRACT WITH AGING

FEMALE

Uterus	Decreased size
Ovaries	Atrophy, with decreased size
Vagina	Decreased width and length
	Vaginal entrance (introitus) narrowed
	Vaginal secretions decrease and become more alkaline

MALE

Testes	Decreased size and firmness
Seminal fluid	Decreased amount and viscosity
Prostate gland	Hypertrophy (enlargement)
Penile erection	Slower, decreased frequency of involuntary morning erections

---

gradually until about age 60 and then levels off. Changes can be noted in the testes, seminal fluid, prostate, and in penile erections (see the box above). Contrary to the inability to procreate as seen in elderly females, males may still procreate but with less probability than when younger because of fewer, less viable sperm. Both elderly females and elderly males have the capacity for sexual response (see Chapter 51).

ASSESSMENT

SUBJECTIVE DATA

Men and women who present themselves for a checkup or with a complaint related to the genital tract should have a complete history taken. Some persons who at first appear to have no symptoms indicating involvement of the reproductive organs may be found to have a problem of the genital system. Careful eliciting of information will help define the problem or problems so that immediate attention can be directed to relieving the cause of the complaint or preventing problems from occurring.

Many of the problems that individuals bring to the attention of nurses and physicians concern subjects or body areas that they are hesitant to discuss. Careful, tactful questioning can assist them to feel more at ease, and often they are relieved that the topic has been raised by someone else. Establishing a trusting relationship between nurse and patient is imperative and should lead to open communication. Sympathy and understanding, along with respect for personal feelings, are essential in obtaining information that individuals might omit because of fear, tension, or embarrassment. Listening with attention and interest is reassuring to individuals and helps them to be more open and free in expression.

PERSONAL DATA

Sociocultural information is helpful to determine the patient's frame of reference. The data include the person's age, socioeconomic status, educational background, occupation, religion, ethnic group, living arrangements, family network, and support systems. Many superstitions related to the reproductive system are culture specific.

PAST MEDICAL HISTORY

The person's history of previous illnesses and surgery is carefully recorded and includes any previous treatment for conditions that might influence functioning of the reproductive organs.

Men are questioned about their past history concerning pain or swelling of the scrotum, testes, sores on the penis, discharges from the urethra, urinary tract problems, ability to achieve and maintain an erection, and previous surgery or treatments for problems of the genitourinary tract. Both men and women should be questioned about a history of discharge, syphilis, gonorrhea, or other venereal diseases.

FAMILY HISTORY

The incidence of diseases such as diabetes, hypertension, coronary occlusion, and cancer should be obtained and recorded. Some chronic diseases that tend to recur in families influence functioning of the reproductive organs. A history of the mother's past pregnancies is important especially if it involved use of diethylstilbestrol (DES), which leads to vaginal adenosis.

GYNECOLOGIC-OBSTETRIC HISTORY

In securing information about the gynecologic history, as with other aspects of the history, it is important to assess the person's level of understanding and to use words that are readily understood. Many persons are hesitant to give information because they are embarrassed that they lack knowledge of medical terms. Questions should be clearly stated to elicit accurate answers. For example, few women can answer questions about *menarche*, but most could answer the question, "How old were you when your periods began?"

When the nurse takes the history, it is usual to begin with previous illnesses or surgery related to the reproductive organs. The gynecologic-obstetric history is outlined in the box above.

Because countless women are using some form of contraception and because some of the contraceptives in use may affect the state of reproductive health, a complete contraceptive history should be taken if the woman has been determined to be heterosexually active

---

GYNECOLOGIC-OBSTETRIC HISTORY

1. Previous illness or surgery involving the reproductive organs
2. Menstrual history
   a. Age at menarche
   b. Interval and duration of menstrual periods
   c. Pain with menstruation, including days of cycle on which it occurs, duration, and factors that intensify or alleviate it
   d. Amount of flow (number of tampons or pads)
   e. Presence of clots, their size, and dates on which they appear
   f. Dates of onset of last two menstrual periods and duration of flow
3. Obstetric history
   a. Pregnancies (dates, length of gestation, type of delivery, birth weight, complications during or after pregnancy)
   b. Abortions, miscarriages (length of pregnancy, method of abortion, physical or psychological complications)

---

and of reproductive age. Information includes types of contraceptives used in the past and at present, how long each type was used, why a specific method was discontinued and another substituted, and any problems that occurred during the use of contraception.

URINARY AND GASTROINTESTINAL SYMPTOMS

Urinary and gastrointestinal symptoms are frequently reported by women and may be associated with various gynecologic disorders. Urinary symptoms that should be explored further are pain on urination, increased frequency of urination, hematuria, nocturia, and incontinence. Gastrointestinal symptoms that may relate to gynecologic disease are nausea and vomiting, constipation, bloating, discomfort after eating, and heartburn.

PATIENT'S COMPLAINT

The patient's complaint is recorded in the patient's own language to direct the questioning and to assess the urgency of any problem. The data should include location of the symptoms, duration, severity, treatment by a physician, and attempts made by the patient to relieve the problem.

Once a general statement or description of the patient's chief complaint is obtained, more specific questioning can follow. If pain is a complaint, the patient is asked to describe it in clear terms (for example, sharp, dull, cramping, steady, or intermittent). The site of the pain can usually be determined by asking the patient to show where it is. Identification of events or activities that increase or decrease the pain is important. Such facts as the use of heat or cold, self-medication, alterations in position, coughing, or having intercourse and their influence on the pain should be obtained.

When the patient complains of bleeding, as much specific information should be obtained as possible. If a woman complains of bleeding, vague statements such as "irregular periods" or "intermittent bleeding" are inadequate. Data about the last two menstrual periods are obtained. If the menstrual periods are irregular, the range of the cycles and duration of flow are recorded. Bleeding between menstrual periods is described in terms of number of days before or after a menstrual period and duration of bleeding at these times. In addition, characteristics of the blood lost are obtained and recorded.

In men, complaints of bleeding are often related to the presence of blood in the urine, and other symptoms such as pain on voiding may be present. Frank bleeding may be present in the form of bright or dark blood on the underwear, and the patient is questioned about this. Associated symptoms of other types of discharge, burning or itching or the genitalia, and ability to initiate urination are determined.

In a similar way, specific descriptions of complaints of a tumor, mass, swelling, sore on the genitalia, discharges other than bleeding, and symptoms related to the bladder and rectum are obtained by questioning the patient.

Because the reproductive tract is influenced by endocrine functioning, which is sensitive to medications, all patients are questioned about their use. In women, it is especially important to determine whether hormones or contraceptive pills are being taken.

OBJECTIVE DATA
PHYSICAL EXAMINATION

When patients present themselves for a checkup or because of a problem of the genital tract, a complete physical examination should be performed. Men should have a rectal examination, and woman should have a pelvic examination and thorough examination of the breasts. General items that are assessed include the patient's weight, height, body build, thyroid gland, heart, lungs, hair distribution, blood pressure, pulse, and urine for protein, glucose, and bacteria.

Both men and women may delay medical examinations of the reproductive tract because this type of examination may cause intense emotional reactions. Fear, embarrassment, and cultural mores play an important part in this emotional distress. In our culture, people frequently fear that their anxieties concerning carcinoma, venereal disease, sterility, or the climacteric will be verified. Many patients are embarrassed by the required exposure of the external genitalia during examination. Many patients also fear that some condition will be discovered that will require surgery resulting in ste-

rility or impotence. The nurse who is sensitive to the many thoughts and fears that may trouble patients will be better prepared to help them accept the necessary examination.

Men should be encouraged to have a yearly rectal examination to detect early prostatic disease. The positive aspects of such an examination should be pointed out.

Whether the physical examination is to be performed by a nurse or a physician, it is a function of the nurse to prepare the patient for the examination. Preparation includes informing the patient of what is to be done, by whom and why, what the patient needs to do to prepare for the examination and why, what the patient can do to feel more relaxed and comfortable during the examination, and when the patient will be informed of examination results.

ABDOMINAL EXAMINATION

Information related to the reproductive organs is obtained by inspection, palpation, percussion, and auscultation of the lower abdomen. *Inspection* is done first because pressure on the bowel by palpation and percussion alter bowel motility and heighten sounds. The abdomen is inspected for the presence of scars and for size and contour. If scars are noted, the patient is questioned about these, even though information may have been obtained during the history taking. Any localized areas of prominence are noted, as these may indicate enlargement of the reproductive organs or adjacent structures. The skin of the abdomen and pubic area is inspected for amount, distribution, and character of hair; abnormal pigmentation; and lesions. Abdominal muscle tone is assessed by having the patient cough or raise the head. Such actions reveal muscle weakness by producing bulging around the umbilicus, inguinal region, or in the midline between the rectus muscles. Women who have been pregnant are more likely to have diastasis recti.

Abdominal *palpation* follows inspection. Since the reproductive organs are normally situated in the pelvic cavity, they are usually not palpable through the abdominal wall. Therefore, abdominal palpation is performed to rule out or discover abnormalities. If an abdominal mass is felt, its position and relationship to any pelvic or abdominal organ, size, shape, consistency, contour, tenderness, and movability are described.

Enlargement of the uterus is detected by palpating in the midline of the lower abdomen. Palpation is started just below the umbilicus and continued in the direction of the symphysis pubis. In contrast to a full bladder, which feels soft, an enlarged uterus feels firm and may be round or asymmetric. During pregnancy, the uterus is not palpable as an abdominal organ until about the end of the third month. A firm, isolated area of enlargement may be caused by the presence of a tumor of the uterus.

Enlargement of the fallopian tubes and ovaries may be detected by palpation of the right and left lower quadrants. Even when enlarged, these organs are not always palpable through the abdominal wall. However, enlargement is often associated with pain or tenderness on palpation of the lower quadrants. The round ligaments are often palpable in the lower quadrants, stretching from the iliac crests to the pubic bones, and they should not be confused with the fallopian tubes.

Percussion of the lower abdomen is directed chiefly to the organs or masses that are palpable. A tumor, such as an ovarian cyst or fibroid tumor of the uterus, produces a flat note (dullness), over the area; whereas a uterus enlarged because of pregnancy usually produces a hollow note. The increased risk of benign liver tumors in women who use oral contraceptives necessitates palpation and percussion of the liver.

Auscultation is used to determine the presence and quality of peristaltic movement. During pregnancy, it is possible to hear the fetal heartbeat through the abdominal wall by the twentieth week if an ordinary stethoscope is used. If devices with Doppler signals and amplification are used, the fetal heartbeat may be heard at least 8 weeks earlier.

PELVIC EXAMINATION

Whereas some nurses perform pelvic examinations as part of their practices, in some instances the nurse's involvement includes encouraging the woman to relax and providing assistance as necessary. The nurse assisting with a pelvic examination has an ideal opportunity to create an educational atmosphere, encouraging the woman to learn more about her body and her sexuality and to explore concerns about her body and its functions (see research box). The nurse can also help women overcome negative aspects, such as pain, embarrassment, and anxiety. The higher the woman's level of concern before the examination, the higher the level of anxiety during and after the examination. After the examination, nurses can reinforce findings, discuss treatment plans, or provide necessary health education.

Preparation

Visual aids are useful when a pelvic examination is to be performed. Models of the pelvic organs and pamphlets assist with the presentation of information about the purpose of the examination, what is done, and what to expect. Three-dimensional, concrete visual aids should be used to teach adolescent girls because they may not have developed the ability to think abstractly.

To make the pelvic examination a positive experience, there must be open communication between the examiner and the patient. The examiner explains the procedure and answers questions before the patient is undressed and on the examination table. Some patients

RESEARCH

Latta W and Weismeier E: Effects of an educational gynecological exam on women's attitudes, J Obstet Gynecol Neonat Nurs 11:242-245, 1982.

Women between the ages of 18 and 25 who had had previous gynecologic examinations participated in a gynecologic educational examination or the traditional examination. The gynecologic educational experience included demonstration of the breast self-examination, explanation of each part of the external genitalia examination, demonstration of Kegel's exercises, discussion of dyspareunia and sexual satisfaction, description of the speculum and viewing of the cervix with a mirror, explanation of the findings of the speculum and internal examination, palpation of the woman's uterus with the help of the examiner, and explanation of the rectal-vaginal examination. The group receiving the educational examination demonstrated more positive attitudes toward the examination both before and after the examination, but there were no significant differences between the educational examination group and the traditional examination group 3 months after examination. ∎

may need to see and touch the speculum before it is inserted. The patient should have the option to use or not use drapes to cover her perineum. Some women feel that drapes prevent embarrassment and protect their modesty, whereas others feel that draping indicates something mysterious or shameful about the pelvic examination. During the examination, the examiner tells the patient what will be done next and informs her of the findings. The patient is told to relax *specific* tense body parts rather than generally to relax throughout the examination. The patient's face is monitored for responses.

Sharing information with the woman about sensory data has been found to be more important in reducing anxiety and pain than explanation of the procedure. The nurse should describe the pulling of the labia during inspection, the sensation of a finger in the vagina, the feeling of opening experienced when the speculum is inserted, and the pressure similar to having a bowel movement during the rectal examination.

After the pelvic examination, the examiner reviews findings and answers any patient questions. The pelvic examination is a unique opportunity to teach anatomy and physiology, as well as to discuss health practices.

Women who are scheduled ahead of time for pelvic examination should be advised to avoid douching and applying any vaginal preparations (medicinal or deodorant) for at least 24 hours before examination. Patients should void immediately before examination because an empty bladder makes palpation of the pelvic organs easier, decreases patient discomfort, eliminates possible distortion of the position of pelvic organs caused by a full bladder, and obviates the danger of incontinence during examination. The patient should be in the supine position with a small pillow under her head for comfort and under her knees to maintain slight leg flexion. Arms are at the side. Raising the head of the table to 30 degrees makes it easier for the examiner to make eye contact and for the woman to watch the examination if she chooses.[18]

A mirror used by the examiner enables the woman to visualize her genitalia, often correcting myths about the vagina and other structures. This educational approach to the pelvic examination may provide many women with their first opportunity to view and identify their genitalia.

Positions for Pelvic Examinations

Several positions may be used for the pelvic examination. Arthritis and other conditions that limit the woman's mobility may preclude some of these positions. Furthermore, some positions, such as the knee-chest position, are both uncomfortable and embarrassing for women of almost any age or physical condition. Nurses can interpret the necessity for such positions.

In *Sims' position* (used for rectal examination) (Figure 53-6, *A*) the woman is placed on her left side with her left arm and hand behind her. The left thigh is only slightly flexed, and the right knee is flexed sharply on the abdomen.

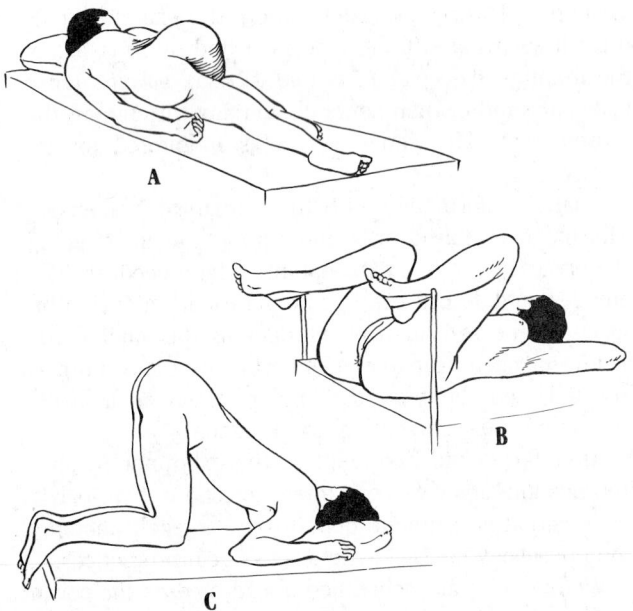

FIGURE 53-6 Various positions that can be assumed for examination of rectum and vagina. **A,** Sims's (lateral) position. Note position of left arm and right leg. **B,** Lithotomy position. Note position of buttocks on edge of examining table and support of feet. **C,** Knee-chest (genupectoral) position. Note placement of shoulders and head.

For the *dorsal recumbent position (lithotomy position)* (Figure 53-6, *B*) the lower leaf of the examining table is dropped before the woman gets onto the table, as dropping it may be frightening to her after her feet have been placed in the stirrups. There should be a footstool handy so that she can be guided to step on the stool, sit down on the edge of the table, and then lie back. Most women are able to place their own legs in the stirrups; they should be told to raise both legs and put them in the stirrups simultaneously. When a woman needs help, two persons may assist, with one on each side of the patient so that both can hold one leg and simultaneously place them in position without abruptly lifting the lower extremities. Gentleness and gradual positioning are essential to prevent strain or twisting of the hip joint. Metal stirrups are the most satisfactory; however, if they are used, the patient should wear her shoes because the heels help to hold the feet in the stirrups.

Care must be taken to see that there is no pressure on the legs when sling stirrups are used, since nerve damage and impairment of circulation can occur. The buttocks need to be moved down so that they are even with the end of the table. The pillow under the head is pulled down at the same time to assure comfort for the patient.

The pelvic examination can be performed with the woman in bed if it is inadvisable for her to be moved to an examining table. The woman can be helped to assume a position across the bed, and her feet can be supported on the seats of two straight chairs. Some practitioners find this a useful adaptation when the pelvic examination is performed at home.

For the *knee-chest position* (Figure 53-6, *C*), first the lower end of the examination table is dropped; then the woman is helped to get on her hands and knees on the table. Her buttocks will be uppermost, and her thighs will be sharply flexed on her trunk. The woman's head is turned to one side and rests on the table. Her arms are flexed and resting well forward (often above her head), and her knees are apart. Her feet extend over the lower edge of the table to prevent pressure on her toes. This examination can also be accomplished by positioning the woman crosswise on the bed.

Inspection and Palpation

This portion of the pelvic examination is performed before internal examination and includes external appearance of the genitalia, tissues and structures within labial folds, and the vaginal opening and perineum. Most often, irregularities of distortion of tissues at the vaginal opening are the result of scars from lacerations, an ulcer just inside the vagina, or infections and cysts in the location of Skene's or Bartholin's glands. These glands are common sites of infection, especially from the gonococ-

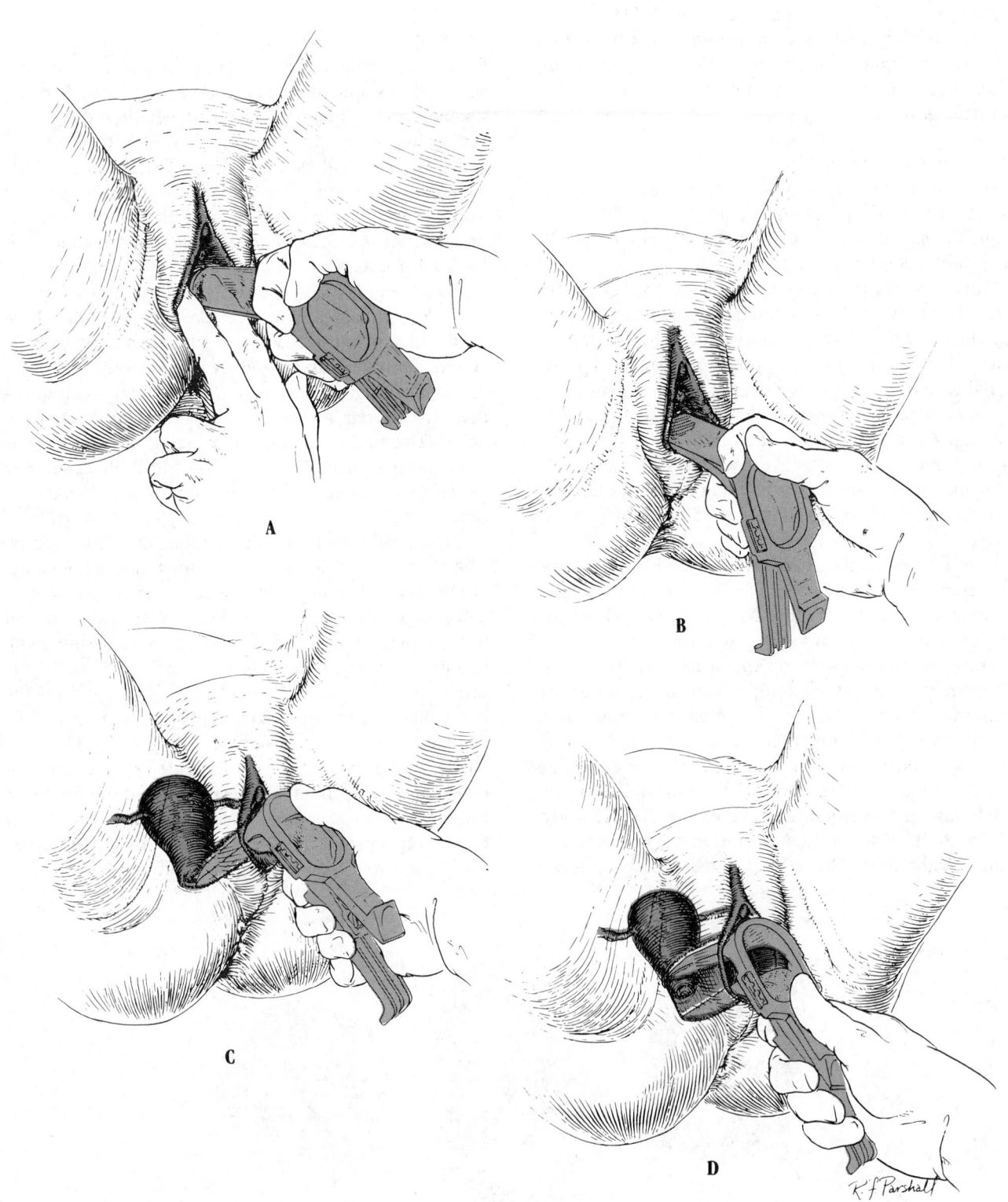

FIGURE 53-7 Procedure for speculum examination. **A,** Opening of introitus. **B,** Oblique insertion of speculum. **C,** Final insertion of speculum. **D,** Opening of speculum blades. (From Malasanos L et al: Health assessment, ed 3, St Louis, 1986, The CV Mosby Co.)

cus organisms. Clitoral enlargement or atrophy is abnormal. The clitoris is frequently a site for malignant lesions in older women and syphilitic chancres in younger women. Abnormalities of the urethral meatus include erythema, exudates, and masses. The labia are inspected for asymmetry, enlargement, atrophy before menopause, exudates, parasites, altered pigmentation, ulcerations, varicosities, and leukoplakia (white adherent patches).

Inspection of Vagina and Cervix

The vagina and cervix are inspected by means of insertion of a vaginal speculum (Figure 53-7). (The technique for speculum examination can be found in physical examination textbooks.)

The *cervix* is inspected for color, contour, position, size, symmetry, surface characteristics, discharge, projection into vaginal vault, consistency, shape, and patency of the external os. In nulliparous women the external os appears as a round depressed area (Figure 53-8). In multiparous women, the cervix os usually appears as a transverse slit in the center of the cervix. The color of the cervix varies but is usually pink. It becomes pale after menopause and cyanotic either during pregnancy or with any condition causing venous congestion or hypoxia.

The surface of the cervix is inspected to determine whether it is smooth, irregular, or raw and whether there is any purulent or other type of discharge from the os. It is not uncommon to see a red, somewhat raw appearing area (an erosion) on the surface of the cervix. Scars may appear as white or reddened slits radiating from the cervical os and are lacerations often present in women who have borne children (Figure 53-8). Occasionally, a stalked polyp may be seen extending through the cervical os as a bright or dark red mass. These polyps frequently cause bleeding and require further study.

The walls of the vagina are inspected as the speculum is withdrawn. The vaginal mucosa is observed for color, consistency, inflammation, ulcers, masses, presence of rugae, discharge, and odor. The vaginal wall is normally pink in color but is usually pallid after menopause.

Palpation

Palpation of the internal reproductive organs follows speculum examination. The cervix is palpated for consistency and contour. It is noted whether the cervix feels softer or harder than normal and whether the surface and shape feel regular or irregular. The cervix feels softer with pregnancy and harder with tumors. Areas of irregularity and abnormal tension should be carefully noted in terms of site. For example, abnormalities can be described as being in position 12, 6, or 9 o'clock.

An attempt is made to insert a finger into the cervical os to detect masses, but excessive force should not be used. In nulliparous women, the cervix is usually closed. In multiparous women, the cervix may admit one or two fingers. Movability of the cervix in all directions is checked, and any restrictions of movement are noted. The vaginal vault is palpated for areas of tenderness and presence of masses. Feces in the rectum may be palpated and can be verified later by rectal examination.

Bimanual palpation follows palpation of the cervix. The purpose of the bimanual examination is palpation of the internal reproductive organs and assessment of pelvic supports. The position of the uterus is determined first. It may be anteverted, midpositioned, retroverted, anteflexed, or retroflexed (see Chapter 54). Usually, the fundus can be felt anterior to the cervix between the two hands. If not, the uterus may lie posteriorly and be palpated through the posterior vaginal vault. The size, shape, and regularity of the uterine surface are palpated. Normally, the uterus feels firm and the fundus is round. The uterus is softer during pregnancy and firmer during menopause. Localized areas of enlargement are noted, and the approximate size and shape of masses

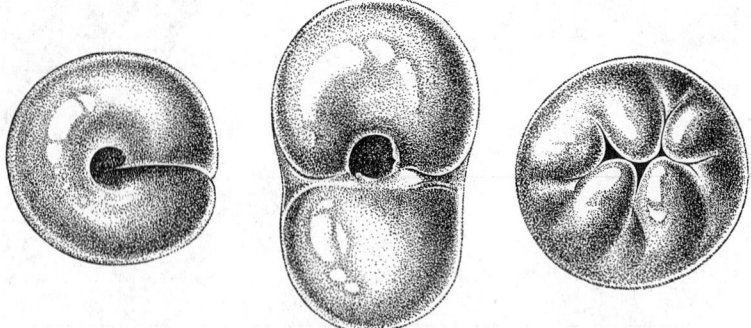

FIGURE 53-8 Nulliparous cervix and laceration of cervix. (From Malasanos L et al: Health assessment, ed 4, St Louis, 1989, The CV Mosby Co.)

are determined. Because the uterus is normally movable and easy to displace, loss of movability is readily detected. This, too, is noted and recorded.

The areas around the fallopian tubes and ovaries require deep palpation. Normally, the fallopian tubes are not palpable; therefore, any enlargement is significant. An enlarged fallopian tube resembles an enlarged ovary to a great extent, and it may not be possible to distinguish between the two.

On bimanual examination, the ovaries are normally slightly tender to palpation and are not always palpable, especially in obese women. When palpable, the ovaries feel smooth and oval in shape if no pathologic condition exists. Any readily palpable mass in the area of the fallopian tubes and ovaries that feels irregular, round, or very firm indicates a possible deviation from normal. Because the ovaries atrophy during the menopause, any mass felt in the areas of the ovaries in postmenopausal women is usually a sign of a problem.

The *rectovaginal examination* is performed to confirm uterine position, to reassess the adnexal areas, to follow up on complaints of pain or bleeding, and to determine rectal sphincter tone. The woman is told that it may be uncomfortable and she may feel as though she has to have a bowel movement. Hemorrhoids, fistulas, and fissures can be observed.

Rectal examination is usually performed to palpate masses in the rectum. If it is necessary for any reason to repeat any part of the examination requiring insertion of fingers into the vagina, the glove is changed after rectal examination to avoid contamination.

TERMINATING PELVIC EXAMINATION

After the pelvic examination, a woman may need assistance with removing lubricating jelly or discharge that may be on her genitalia, removing her legs from the stirrups, and getting down from the table. Elderly women merit careful assistance after pelvic examination because unnatural positions such as the knee-chest and lithotomy positions may alter the normal circulation of blood sufficiently to cause faintness.

EXAMINATION OF MALES

As with women, men should have an examination of the genital system during physical examination. Examination of the male genitourinary system includes inspection and palpation of the lower abdomen, inspection and palpation of the external genitalia, and palpation of the prostate gland by rectal examination.

Sometimes male patients are requested not to void until they are seen by the physician. This allows the physician to evaluate ability to start and maintain a stream and to assess characteristics of the urinary stream by observing the patient during voiding.

The *abdomen* is palpated above the symphysis pubis

to determine whether the bladder is distended; if so, as evidenced by a soft, palpable mass, the patient is questioned about the time of last voiding.

The *inguinal area* is inspected for areas of bulging caused by hernias. The man is requested to hold his breath and to bear down to make presence of herniation more evident. Straining is preferable to coughing because it produces more steady sustained pressure. The load test is used if a hernia is not palpated despite complaints of hernia symptoms. The man lifts something heavy, while the inguinal area is inspected.

The inguinal lymph nodes are palpated for enlargement, pain, or tenderness. The amount and distribution of pubic hair are noted.

The *penis* is inspected for abnormalities of prepuce, glans, and urethral meatus and for visible evidence of infection and masses. The prepuce is retracted to determine the presence and degree of phimosis, an elongation of the foreskin such that it constricts the urethral orifice and cannot be retracted. It is important to note whether the urethra is centrally located or whether it opens on the upper or lower surface of the glans. The urinary meatus is inspected for lesions, periurethral abscess, and purulent or bloody discharge. If a discharge is present, a specimen is obtained by milking the penis from the base to the urethra. The skin along the shaft of the penis is checked for lesions of any type and for general color.

The *scrotum* is observed for general appearance, color of the skin, tension of the skin surfaces, size, symmetry, and the presence of lesions on the skin surfaces.

The left testis is lower than the right testis, which causes the scrotum to appear asymmetric under normal conditions. Scrotal size is determined by the tone of the dartos muscle. The scrotum may look pendulous in older age as the dartos muscle becomes atonic and in warm temperatures with relaxation of the dartos muscle. Cold temperatures cause the dartos muscle to contract and the scrotum shrinks. The testes are inspected for shape, size, consistency, and response to pressure by simultaneous palpation between the thumb and first two fingers. The spermatic cords are palpated between the thumb and forefinger. Unilateral or bilateral enlargement usually indicates presence of a mass or edema.

Palpation of the scrotum is necessary to distinguish between enlargement caused by a mass and swelling caused by collection of fluid. The size, shape, location, tenderness, and consistency of any mass are carefully noted. Transillumination of the scrotum, by placing a flashlight behind the scrotal area in a dark room, is attempted to differentiate the cause of the scrotal mass. Serous fluid will transilluminate or produce a red glow; tissue and blood will not transilluminate.

The *prostate gland* is palpated by means of a rectal

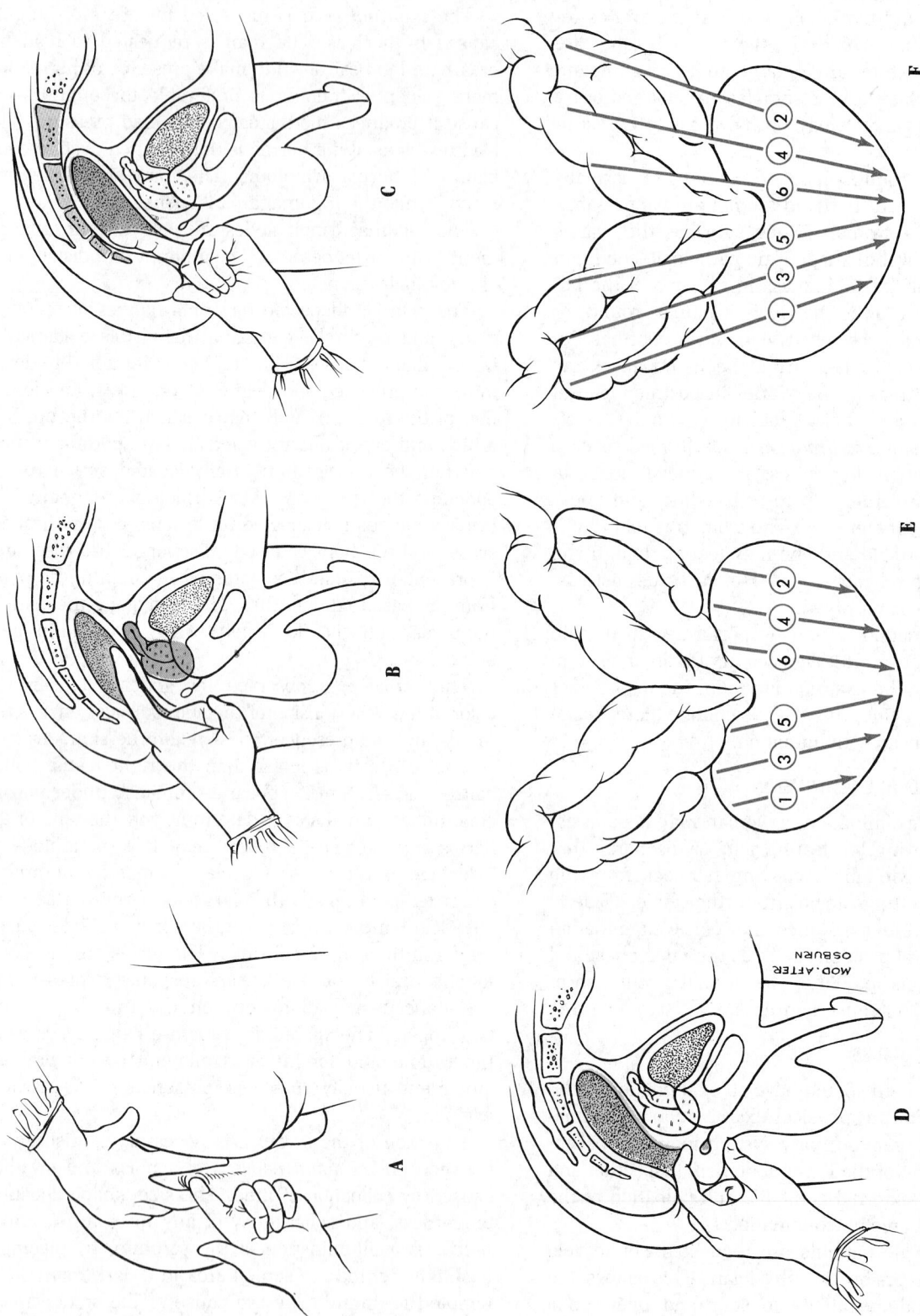

FIGURE 53-9 Rectal examination. **A,** Introduction of protected, well-lubricated finger. **B,** Palpation of prostate gland and seminal vesicles, lateral view. **C,** Palpation of anterior surface of sacrum and coccyx. **D,** Palpation of Cowper's glands. **E,** Massage of prostate gland for specimen collection or treatment; order of strokes is indicated by gradually working toward center (verumontanum). **F,** Massage of seminal vesicles and prostate gland. (From Campbell MF and Harrison JH: Urology, vol 1, ed 3, Philadelphia, 1970, WB Saunders Co.)

examination with the patient standing (Figure 53-9). Rectal examination on a regular basis is the most important step in the diagnosis of prostatic disease, especially carcinoma. Cancer of the prostate gland may start as a localized, hard nodule, palpable by rectal examination, before proceeding to an advanced, inoperable, or incurable stage. For this reason, it is recommended that all men, especially those over the age of 50 years, have a rectal examination at least once a year.[1]

DIAGNOSTIC TESTS

Laboratory data useful in the determination of the cause of reproductive or sexual dysfunction include blood work, such as complete blood counts, thyroid function tests, glucose tolerance tests, and chemistry determinations. Vaginal cytology, endocrine workups, electrocardiograms, and chest films may reveal underlying abnormalities responsible for reproductive or sexual problems. A number of conditions that affect the sexuality directly or indirectly are discussed in Chapter 52. In addition to routine urinalysis and blood count, some specific studies requiring samples of blood or urine may be performed.

LABORATORY TESTS
TESTS FOR SYPHILIS

Serologic testing is used for detecting syphilis. Two identifiable antibodies appear in the blood from 1 to 4 months after syphilis is contracted. The tests in common use require a sample of venous blood. Two types of tests, treponemal and nontreponemal, are presently available. The tests differ in the type of antibody measured and in the antigen used to detect antibodies.

The nontreponemal tests, commonly called serologic tests for syphilis (STS), measure an antibody-like substance called reagin. The Venereal Disease Research Laboratory (VDRL) test is the most frequently used serologic test for syphilis and is the test used most often for routine premarital and prenatal screening.

Syphilitic reagin is thought to form from tissue breakdown products resulting from the interaction of the organism and body tissues. STS are usually reported as nonreactive, weakly reactive, or reactive. If any degree of reactivity is found, a quantitative test is performed by diluting the serum progressively until an end point of reactivity is reached. Quantitative reactions are reported in rations and reflect the *highest dilution* at which the serum reacts. For example, a reaction reported as 1:16 means that the person's serum was diluted 16 times and still produced reaction, but no reaction occurred when the serum was diluted more than 16 times.

A reactive STS is confirmed by alternate serologic tests. For this purpose, the fluorescent treponemal antibody-absorption test (FTA-ABS) is most often used, as it is the most sensitive and specific test for syphilis available. A reactive STS, which occurs with no exposure to syphilis, frequently occurs in conjunction with a hypersensitivity reaction, acute bacterial or viral infection, recent vaccination, or chronic systemic illness such as tuberculosis, collagen disease, or malaria. It is important, therefore, not to tell patients they have syphilis based on the STS alone. A positive FTA-ABS must be established before the diagnosis of syphilis is made.

Because antibodies are not present in the serum of the infected person until the organism gains entry into the circulation, STS may be negative, and the individual may still be infected. A negative syphilis test may also occur when an individual is taking antibiotics. Once antibodies are present, they do not completely disappear from the serum. Although treated and noninfected, the person may have a positive serology test indefinitely. If successful therapy is given before antibodies develop, these tests may never be positive unless the person again becomes infected and develops antibodies. Therefore, serologic tests in use today do not always indicate an active syphilitic infection and only detect the presence of antibodies. There is presently an urgent need for a specific, rapid method of detecting infection caused by syphilis, and such methods are being studied. Until new tests are developed, the patient's history, clinical symptoms (if any), and serologic testing are the means most often used to make a diagnosis of syphilis. Patients infected with syphilis may be surprised, angry, anxious, and depressed. They may not know how they contacted the disease. The nurse needs to explore the patient's feelings and encourage the patient to bring in a partner or known contact for treatment.

TESTS FOR CHLAMYDIAL INFECTIONS

Chlamydial infections are approximately ten times more common than gonorrhea. Tests for *Chlamydia* using fluorescent tagging are very specific and sensitive. For these tests, the cervix is abraded to obtain cells rather than collecting cervical mucus. The material on the slide is fixed with ethyl acetate and fluorescently tagged monocolonal antibody is added. A diagnosis can be made in 20 to 30 minutes. The ELISA test (Chlamydiazyme) is another diagnostic test in which a diagnosis takes 4 hours.

Women who should be tested for chlamydial infections are those with mucopurulent cervicitis, sterile pyuria, a positive gonorrhea culture, pelvic inflammatory disease (PID), teenagers taking oral contraceptives, and pregnant women where the population has a high incidence of chlamydial infections.

PAPANICOLAOU (PAP) SMEAR

Women who are at high risk for developing cervical neoplasms (those with abnormal Pap smears or a history of intercourse at an early age or with multiple partners) should have Pap tests every year. The American Cancer Society recommends an annual Pap test and pelvic examination for 3 consecutive years for women who are or have been sexually active, or have reached age 18. After three consecutive normal annual examinations, the Pap test may be performed less frequently at the discretion of the physician.[1]

The Pap test makes it possible to detect abnormal cells, not all of which are malignant. However, the Pap test has made it possible through routine use to detect precancerous conditions and cancer of the cervix early enough to make treatment of these conditions almost 100% successful. For detection of atypical cells, the Pap test is 95% accurate. False-negative reports are most frequently the result of an inadequate sample or improperly fixed slide.

The Pap test is performed by microscopic examination of cells collected from the vaginal pool, exocervix, and endocervical canal. Secretions containing exfoliated cells are preferably obtained from the cervix or external os. Instructions for obtaining Pap smears include the following:

1. Obtain smear preferably 5 to 6 days after menstruation termination (menses makes interpretation difficult and may camouflage atypical cells).
2. Avoid taking a tub bath or douche of any type for at least 48 hours before the Pap test.
3. Delay obtaining a Pap test for a least 1 month after use of topical antibiotics (produce rapid, heavy shedding of cells).
4. Use a vaginal pipette with a rubber tip and a specially designed wooden spatula to collect the secretions.
5. Collect enough material to make a distinct blur on the slide.
6. Smear material on prelabeled glass slide.
7. Place the glass slides immediately in a wide-mouthed jar containing a fixative solution of 95% alcohol and ether (to prevent drying out and cell distortion).
8. Carefully label two specimens for site and place them in solution so that the unsmeared sides are back to back.

Many women experience some vaginal bleeding in the form of spotting after a Pap smear has been taken. They should be advised that this is expected and normal, but that any bleeding in excess of spotting is abnormal and should be reported to the health care provider.

When the Pap test is positive, additional tissue studies are indicated. The woman should understand that the Pap test is not necessarily conclusive and that biopsy or even surgery may be necessary to verify the diagnosis of premalignancy or malignancy. The false-positive rate is 5%. Any woman with a positive Pap smear will be anxious and upset. It is quite natural to worry about dying and to go through the grieving process. The nurse should give anticipatory guidance about future treatment and provide emotional support (see Chapter 17).

Many women are familiar with the Pap test because of the vast amount of publicity it has received. Securing the specimen does not cause pain. Since the procedure can be used to obtain cell samples for study in cases of infertility or when women are taking estrogen preparations, the woman may need to learn how to take the smear herself. It is imperative that the woman be taught how to insert the aspirator or spatula deeply enough to reach the cervix, how to prepare the slide, and how to place the slide in the fixative.

Do-it-yourself Pap tests are available. These can be used by women who are reluctant or unable to visit a physician for examination. The same instruction is required for an adequate specimen to be obtained. The Pap test alone is not a substitute for the more complete history and examination necessary for preventive care, and women should be encouraged to have a yearly pelvic examination.

OTHER SMEARS AND CULTURES

Smears or cultures are also taken from various sites when symptoms of infection are present. Most infectious diseases of the reproductive tract produce a purulent discharge. In men, the most common site of purulent discharge is the urinary meatus. The cervix, urethra, Skene's glands, and Bartholin's glands are the most common site of infection in women. Smears or cultures of the discharge are usually successful in identification of the organism responsible for the infection. The sexually transmitted diseases require a number of different diagnostic studies, which are discussed in Chapter 63.

ENDOCRINE STUDIES

Because the endocrine system is so closely related to reproductive function, almost any study for endocrine function may be ordered, such as thyroid function tests. In women having menstrual problems and in cases of infertility, ovarian function is often studied.

Endocrine studies may include determination of estrogen secretion and estrogen levels in women. Secretion of estrogen in the secretory phase of the menstrual cycle can be estimated by study of the elasticity of the cervical mucus. Quantitative determination of estradiol levels is accomplished by radioassay of serum. Twenty-four-hour urine estriol or serum estriol determinations can be obtained during pregnancy to measure the placental secretion of hormones indirectly. The 24-hour urine collection is kept cold until it is sent to the laboratory.

In addition to infertility, estrogen level determination

may be valuable in discovering whether amenorrhea is from pituitary, ovarian, or uterine failure of function. With pituitary or ovarian problems, the estrogen level is low; with uterine problems, the estrogen level is normal. A combination of urinary estriol levels with endometrial tissue studies helps to pinpoint failure of the uterus to respond to estrogen stimulation.

Determination of male hormone levels is sometimes helpful in treating fertility problems. The levels of 17-ketosteroids, pituitary gonadotropins, and corticosteroids may be determined. A 24-hour sample of urine is required, and the procedure for collection is the same as for urinary estriols.

Frequently, men and women show signs of anxiety and depression after diagnostic studies and procedures that require waiting for pathologic reports. Fear about the findings and about the possible ways in which sexuality and fertility might be affected is common. Many times, patients are poorly informed and worry needlessly. Nurses can reduce the distress associated with many of these procedures by providing factual information and by avoiding hedging. Collaboration with the physician may facilitate patients being informed as quickly as possible, thus avoiding unnecessary waiting and anxiety.

RADIOLOGIC TESTS
ULTRASONOGRAPHY

Ultrasonography (ultrasound) has become a useful diagnostic tool for gynecologic problems. It can be used to locate pelvic masses, intrauterine devices (IUDs), ec-

topic pregnancies, and prostatic neoplasms. Transvaginal sonography allows for improved ultrasonic picture clarity compared to transabdominal sonography in assessing gynecologic health.[13] Transvaginal sonography is currently being used to inspect and assess the uterus, ovaries, fallopian tubes, and extragenital structures (Table 53-1). Transvaginal probe use is increasingly common in guiding procedures involving needle puncture such as ova retrieval for in vitro fertilization.

SCANNING AND IMAGING

Computed tomography (CT) may be helpful in identifying very small lesions of the reproductive tract. *Magnetic resonance imaging* (MRI) is useful in visualizing normal pelvic and abdominal anatomy. Expected uses of MRI in the future include staging of uterine, ovarian, and cervical carcinoma; staging of endometriosis; determining the extent and rate of resolution of pelvic inflammatory disease; differentiating between uterine fibroids and ovarian cysts; and diagnosing tumors, inflammation, or secretions based on biochemical signatures or collections of pathologic cells.

SPECIAL TESTS
PREGNANCY TESTS

Pregnancy testing is commonly performed so that management can be started as soon as possible. This is true whether a woman intends to deliver her baby, whether she elects to have an abortion, or whether the physician suspects an ectopic pregnancy. Most of the commonly used pregnancy tests are based on two facts. First, human chorionic gonadotropin (HCG) is present in the serum of pregnant women within 10 to 14 days after the first missed menstrual period. Second, HCG produces antisera. Currently available methods of pregnancy testing fall into four groups: biologic, immunologic, radioreceptor assay, and immunoassay tests.

Biologic tests for pregnancy were first available in the mid-1920s. Among the better-known biologic tests are the *Ascheim-Zondek* test, the *Friedman* test, and the *Hogben* test. These tests require that an early morning voided urine specimen from the woman be injected into a laboratory animal. If HCG is present in the urine, the test is positive as indicated by rapid maturational changes in the ovaries of the laboratory animal. Biologic tests for pregnancy are 95% accurate 2 weeks after the first missed menstrual period. Because of their relative lack of sensitivity and difficulty doing them, biologic pregnancy tests are no longer used.

Since the early 1960s, a number of commercial *immunologic tests* for pregnancy have become available (*Ortho, Hyland,* and *Roche*). Depending on the specific test, blood or urine specimens are required from the woman. Results are obtained within 2 minutes to 2 hours depending on the test used. The short period for

TABLE 53-1 Uses of transvaginal sonography[13]

Organ	Uses
Uterus	Size, position
	Inspection of myometrium and endometrial lining
	Detection of malformations
	Identification of small fibroids
	Early pregnancy determination
	Early fetal heart beats
Ovaries	Size, texture, and location
	Monitoring follicular growth
	Evaluation of ovulation
	Identification of corpus luteum
	Identification of tumors and structural deformities
	Follicular aspiration
Fallopian tubes	Diagnosis of tubal pathology
	Detection of tubo-ovarian abscess
	Early recognition of tubal pregnancy
Extragenital structures	Evaluation of free pelvic fluid
	Detection of pelvic blood clots

obtaining results is an advantage of immunologic tests. However, these tests are not as sensitive in detecting pregnancy as are other tests. When used in women in whom menstruation is delayed for up to 2 weeks, they show positive results 50% of the time. Immunologic pregnancy tests are valuable in screening women who are possibly pregnant. It is generally believed that women with negative immunologic tests should have further examination for pregnancy.

The *radioreceptor assay* test for pregnancy is a rapid and reliable test for pregnancy. The test can be performed in 1 hour and is 90% to 95% accurate by 6 to 8 days after ovulation. A blood sample from the finger is taken. This test has proved to be very reliable clinically. *Ultrasensitive immunoassay* is accurate within 7 to 14 days after conception. It can be performed in a few hours and is commonly used for confirmation of normal pregnancy.

Do-it-yourself pregnancy tests are available to women through department and drug stores. These tests are sensitive and easy to perform.

Two conditions, *hydatidiform mole* and *choriocarcinoma*, produce false-positive pregnancy tests. In both of these conditions, trophoblastic tissue secretes chorionic gonadotropin in abundance.

CERVICAL TESTS

Schiller's Test

Schiller's test is a simple test that helps the physician decide whether other diagnostic procedures should be performed when cervical disease is suspected. For example, Schiller's test assists with identifying the area from which a cervical biopsy specimen should be taken. The test is currently being used less frequently because culposcopy is a more accurate method of obtaining the same information.

Schiller's test reveals the presence of atypical cervical cells. A solution of 3.5% iodine or Lugol's solution is applied to the cervix. Atypical cells, both malignant and benign, do not contain glycogen and will fail to stain. Early cancerous lesions and benign lesions, such as cervicitis, may appear as glistening areas of a lighter color than surrounding tissue. The tissue having lighter color indicates, for example, the site from which a biopsy specimen should be taken.

Cervical Biopsy

If the physician wishes to send a piece of cervical tissue to the laboratory for pathologic examination, a cervical biopsy is performed. Cervical biopsy is almost always performed with culposcopic direction. Bleeding is minimal and almost always maintained only by pressure and possibly a small amount of silver nitrate. The woman should know what is to be done and why. There may be momentary discomfort but an anesthetic is not required.

A cervical biopsy specimen can be secured by using a scalpel, but most often a special punch biopsy is used. A punch biopsy can be performed safely on an ambulatory surgery basis. A speculum is used to expose the cervix, and a small piece of the cervix is excised.

Instructions to the woman after cervical biopsy will vary but usually include the following:
1. Report to the physician or hospital if bleeding is excessive; usually more than occurs during normal menses is considered excessive.
2. Do not use an internal douche or have sexual relations until the next medical appointment, unless specific instructions have been given as to when intercourse can safely be resumed.
3. Leave the tampon or packing in place for the specified period (usually 8 to 24 hours).

Conization of Cervix

If the suspected cervical lesion is widespread or the location of abnormal cells found on the Pap smear cannot be located, conization of the cervix may be performed. This method of obtaining tissue from the cervix is also preferred when cancer of the cervix is suspected. Conization of the cervix is sometimes performed as a therapeutic measure in cases of chronic cervical infections in which the inflammatory process has involved the deep tissues of the cervix.

Women are sometimes hospitalized for conization, but most undergo the procedure as outpatients. A local or general anesthetic is administered. A cone-shaped portion of the cervix containing the suspected malignant or infected tissue is removed. Bleeding from the site of conization is greater than that occurring from punch biopsy. If the bleeding is excessive or if hemorrhage seems likely, the cervix is sutured to control loss of blood. Oozing is controlled by packing, which is kept in place for 24 to 48 hours. The nursing care is basically the same as that required after a dilation and curettage (D & C).

After the procedure, the woman needs to know that her next two or three menstrual periods may be heavy and prolonged. If conization was performed for carcinoma in situ, the woman will be observed by her physician more frequently, probably every 4 to 8 months. She will need support from the nurse to cope with the diagnosis, prognosis, and future implications of carcinoma.

ENDOMETRIAL TESTS

Screening for Endometrial Cancer

With the decline of mortality from cervical cancer, greater attention has been directed toward developing mass screening techniques to detect early cancer of the endometrium (uterus). An ideal method for mass screening has not yet been developed, but continued refinement of available methods and development of new methods will probably make it possible for screening for uterine cancer to become part of every woman's health care program. Since women over the age of 50 years are more likely to develop cancer of the uterus, screening of postmenopausal women assumes greater significance.

A variety of methods for screening and diagnosis of uterine cancer are now in use. It is generally agreed that the Pap test is not ideal for detecting uterine cancer. The best results are obtained when cervical aspiration is conscientiously performed as part of the Pap test. Variation in the reported rates of accuracy is probably caused by a combination of factors, including the site from which samples are taken, clinical grade of the uterine malignancy, and care exercised in obtaining specimens. Less than one half of women with uterine cancer have an abnormal Pap test at the time of routine screening. Probably the main reason the Pap test is inadequate is that cells rarely exfoliate from the endometrium in the early stages of uterine cancer.

Aspiration Smear

Endometrial cells obtained by aspiration smear show malignant changes between 75% and 90% of the time when uterine cancer exists. The aspiration method is popular because of its relative simplicity; however, it is not an acceptable method for the routine screening of symptomatic patients. In this method, a small cannula is inserted through the cervix into the uterine cavity, and suction is applied by means of a syringe attached to the cannula. The specimen obtained is prepared as for a Pap smear (p. 1553).

Endometrial Biopsy

Endometrial biopsy is performed by introducing a small curette into the uterus and obtaining several strips of endometrial tissue. The specimens are taken from several sites of the uterine cavity to increase the chances of obtaining malignant cells. For diagnosis of endometrial cancer, the biopsy method is considered to be about 90% accurate.

Vacuum Curettage

The procedure and apparatus used for vacuum curettage are similar to those used in suction curettage for performing an abortion except that the curette is much thinner. The cervix is dilated and the suction tip is inserted through the cervix into the uterus. Suction is applied and the entire uterine cavity is suctioned to secure specimens. Vacuum curettage is considered to be at least as good as conventional endometrial biopsy for diagnosing endometrial cancer.

Dilation and Curettage

The most prevalent and preferred method of obtaining endometrial cells for study is dilation and curettage (D & C). Because the entire uterine cavity is "scraped," a large tissue sample is obtained. This makes the likelihood of missing malignant cells minimal. In addition to suspected malignancy, endometrial tissue may be studied for influence of ovarian hormones on the endometrial cells and evaluation of other causes of infertility. D & C is sometimes used for the treatment of excessive or prolonged uterine bleeding. This procedure is often carried out to induce abortion and is frequently used after a spontaneous abortion to reduce the chances of hemorrhage. Occasionally, dilation alone is performed to treat dysmenorrhea or to correct a stricture or stenosis of the cervical canal. Most of the procedures used for screening and diagnosis of endometrial cancer require some dilation of the cervix to introduce instruments into the uterus.

For a D & C, metal dilators of graduated sizes are inserted into the cervical canal. Once the cervix is dilated, curettes having a sharp surface are used to remove endometrial tissue. The major complications of a D & C are hemorrhage and perforation of the uterus. Perforation is a greater risk during pregnancy because the uterus is much softer than in the nonpregnant state. Preoperative care includes informing the woman what will occur and why and preparing her for anesthesia. Most physicians now believe that preoperative shaving is not necessary and that the discomfort from regrowth of pubic hair can be avoided.

Following a D & C, the woman is monitored for excessive bleeding (see the box below). Most women are discharged on the day of surgery; some are discharged the next day. Normal daily activities can be resumed, increasing to normal activity in about 1 week. The degree of activity permitted depends partly on the reason for the D & C. Vigorous exercise is discouraged. Sexual intercourse may be resumed when the woman feels

---

POSTOPERATIVE CARE AFTER D & C

1. Place a perineal pad over perineum and anchor with a sanitary belt, to ensure all blood loss will be absorbed by the pad.
2. Take vital signs every 15 minutes until stable.
3. Monitor bleeding every 15 minutes for 2 hours; if active bleeding continues, monitor every hour for about 8 hours.
4. Record each pad change and amount of blood loss in estimated ml (60 ml saturates a perineal pad).
5. Monitor urinary output.
6. Give mild analgesics as prescribed: Report immediately any abdominal pain that is continuous, sharp, and not relieved by analgesics (may indicate perforation of uterus).
7. Encourage ambulation when patient is awake and vital signs are stable.

comfortable. The menstrual cycle usually is not upset by a D & C, and all vaginal bleeding should disappear in a week to 10 days. Women are advised to report recurrence of bright red blood or the development of a vaginal discharge with an unpleasant odor.

ENDOSCOPY

The pelvic organs and surrounding tissues can be visualized directly by endoscopy. The procedures by which this can be accomplished are colposcopy, culdoscopy, peritoneoscopy (laparoscopy), and hysteroscopy (see the box below). Depending on the organs and structures inspected, these methods are valuable for determining the cause of abnormal bleeding, in evaluating the stage of malignancies, and for inspecting organs for size, shape, and position.

Colposcopy is the technique in which a low-power microscope with a light source offers magnifications of 6 to 40 times the visible part of the cervix. The procedure is useful to evaluate women with abnormal Pap tests; to study neoplastic changes in the vulva, vagina, and cervix; and to follow patients after radiation therapy.

Culdoscopy is an examination in which a culdoscope is inserted through the posterior vaginal vault into the cul-de-sac of Douglas (Figure 53-10). The fallopian tubes and ovaries can be seen, as well as the presence of pus, blood, or other abnormal fluids in the cul-de-sac. If such fluids are observed, the physician may perform a *culdocentesis* by inserting a needle into the site and aspirating a specimen for laboratory study.

Laparoscopy, which has replaced culdoscopy, is a procedure by which the pelvic organs are studied by insertion of a laparoscope through the abdominal wall,

---

ENDOSCOPIC PROCEDURES FOR VISUALIZATION OF PELVIC ORGANS

Colposcopy	Visualization of vagina and cervix under low-power magnification
Culdoscopy	Insertion of a culdoscope through posterior vaginal vault into cul-de-sac of Douglas for visualization of fallopian tubes and ovaries
Hysteroscopy	Insertion of a hysteroscope through the cervix for visualization of inside of the uterus
Laparoscopy	Insertion of a laparoscope (under local anesthesia) through small incision in abdominal wall (inferior margin of umbilicus), which is insufflated with carbon dioxide; permits visualization of all pelvic organs).

---

which is insufflated with carbon dioxide (Figure 53-11). A local anesthetic is injected before insertion of the instrument. Laparoscopy is useful in inspecting the outer surfaces of the uterus, the fallopian tubes, and the ovaries for appearance. For example, a tubal pregnancy can be seen. In addition to inspection of the pelvic structures, the laparoscope is used for sterilization by tubal ligation.

Hysteroscopy is used to inspect the inside of the uterus and sometimes to treat adhesions. It is is indicated in abnormal uterine bleeding and localization and retrieval of lost IUDs, and it is becoming increasingly important in the evaluation of causes of infertility.[8] Hysteroscopy is performed before a D & C for diagnosis of uterine cancer, to decrease the chances of missing a lesion with a D & C. The hysteroscope is inserted through the cervix rather than through the abdomen. This procedure is contraindicated whenever a pregnancy is suspected.

Most of the procedures used for visualizing the pelvic organs can be performed on an ambulatory basis; this allows the physician to schedule at the patient's convenience and during the appropriate time of the menstrual cycle.

Maintaining asepsis throughout any of the endoscopic procedures is important in preventing infection. Air may enter the abdominal cavity during the procedures and cause discomfort; a prone position with a pillow under the abdomen may increase comfort. Douching and intercourse should be avoided for about 1 week after a culdoscopy. Complications such as hemorrhage and infection are rare, but women should be cautioned to report fever or pain in the lower abdomen.

SPECIAL TESTS FOR MALES
PROSTATIC TESTS

Prostatic Smear

For a prostatic smear, the physician first massages the prostate gland (see Figure 53-9). The next voided urine specimen is collected, and a smear is prepared in the laboratory. Some cases of cancer and tuberculosis of the prostate gland can be detected by this method.

Most often, biopsy specimens of the prostate gland are used for diagnosis. Various methods are used to obtain tissue specimens from the prostate gland.

Needle Biopsies

For a *perineal needle biopsy,* the patient is placed in the lithotomy position (Figure 53-6, *B*), and a finger is inserted into the rectum to identify the area from which the biopsy specimen is to be taken. The biopsy needle is inserted through the perineum into the prostate gland, and a core of tissue is removed. This technique is considered a minor procedure and can be accomplished on an outpatient basis.

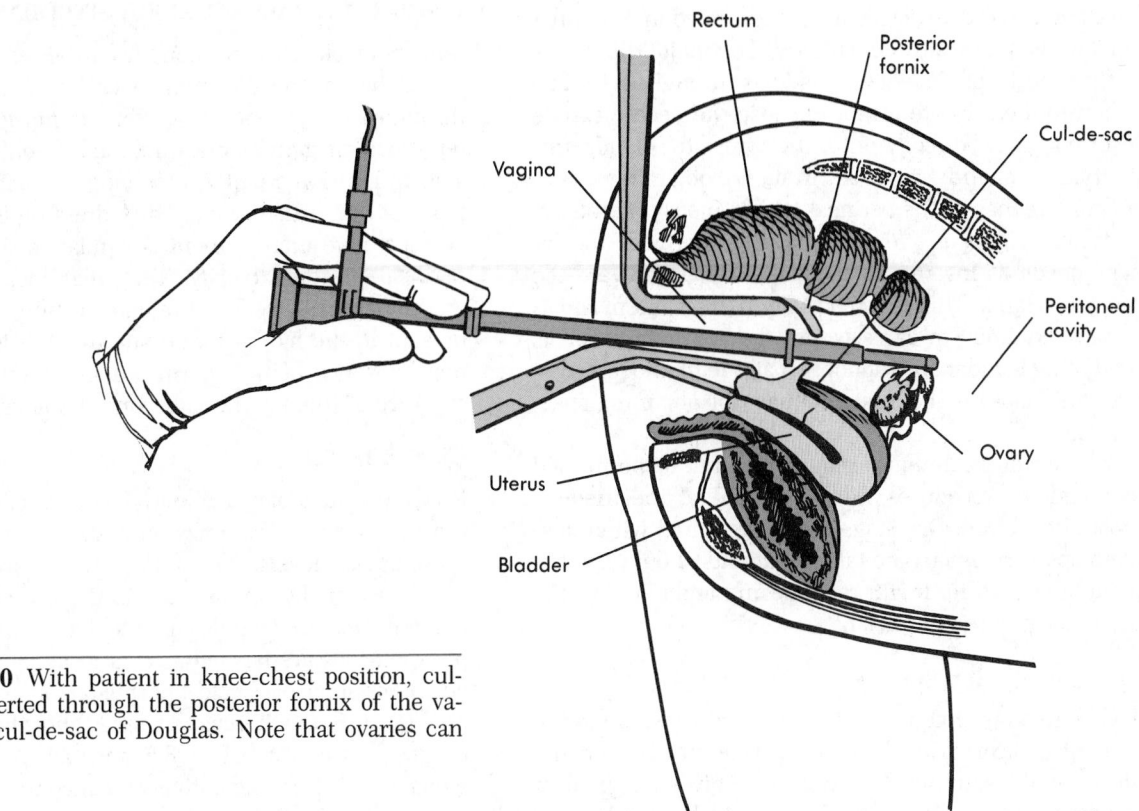

FIGURE 53-10 With patient in knee-chest position, culdoscope is inserted through the posterior fornix of the vagina into the cul-de-sac of Douglas. Note that ovaries can be seen.

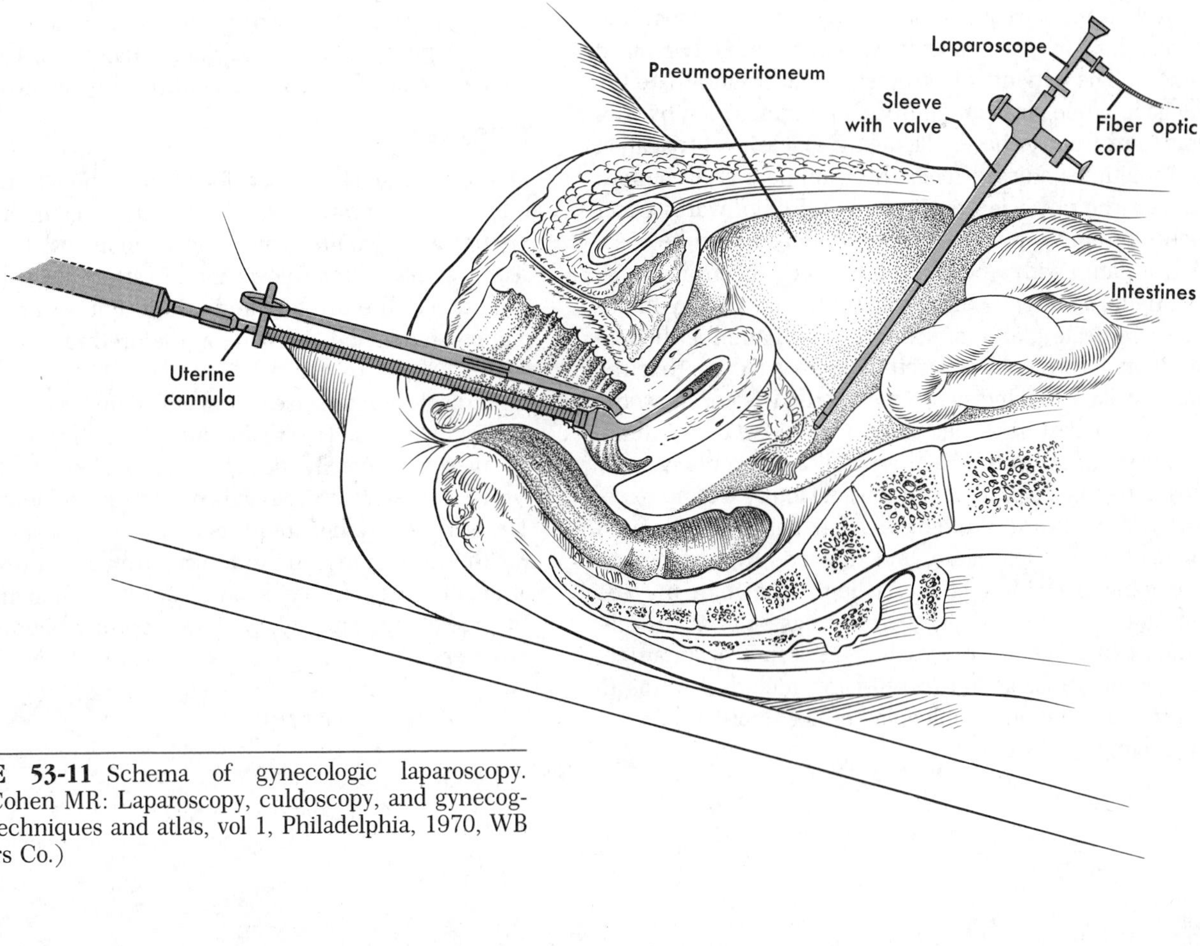

FIGURE 53-11 Schema of gynecologic laparoscopy. (From Cohen MR: Laparoscopy, culdoscopy, and gynecography: techniques and atlas, vol 1, Philadelphia, 1970, WB Saunders Co.)

A *transrectal needle biopsy* is performed in a manner similar to a perineal needle biopsy. The major difference is that the biopsy needle is inserted through the rectal wall into the prostate gland. Because the needle can be inserted more directly into the prostate gland, this method is slightly more accurate in obtaining tissue specimens than is the perineal needle biopsy method.

When a *transurethral biopsy* is performed, the biopsy needle is inserted through the urethra toward the prostate gland. This method is used least often and is usually confined to cases where the prostatic lesion is producing bladder obstruction. Of all the methods, transurethral biopsy is the least adequate for obtaining specimens.

The needle techniques may or may not be performed as inpatient procedures. A local or general anesthetic is most often given. Dressings are not required when needle biopsy specimens are taken. Patients should be cautioned to watch for bright red bleeding and to report the occurrence to the physician.

Open Perineal Biopsy

To obtain a specimen of tissue by *open perineal biopsy,* a small incision is made in the perineum between the anus and the scrotum. This technique gives the greatest accuracy because the suspect lesion can be clearly identified and multiple specimens can be taken from the prostate gland.

A dressing is required after open perineal biopsy and can be held in place for about 24 hours with a two-tailed binder. The patient is instructed not to contaminate the incision while cleansing himself after defecation by wiping from front to back. Cleansing by perineal irrigation is sometimes advised for both cleanliness and comfort. Unless the physician prescribes a solution, warm water poured from front to back over the incision can be used. A heat lamp with a 60-watt bulb placed 30 cm from the perineum is often used two or three times a day to encourage healing and for comfort. The man must be in a position in which the scrotum is elevated so that the heat strikes the incision. One method is to allow the scrotum to rest on a wide piece of adhesive tape extending from thigh to thigh. Alternately, exaggerated Sims' position (Figure 53-6, A) gives satisfactory wound exposure. After sutures are removed, sitz baths may be used instead of the heat lamp, and they add a great deal to the general comfort of the patient. The man may be hospitalized after an open perineal biopsy until the laboratory findings are reported. If he is not hospitalized, he requires instruction in self-care, including signs to report, prevention of infection of the incision, use of heat lamp, and sitz baths.

TESTICULAR SMEARS AND BIOPSY SPECIMENS

Smears or biopsy specimens from the testes can be obtained by the needle method or by an incision made through the scrotum. Most often an incision is used. After a local or general anesthetic has been administered, a small incision about 2.5 cm long is made, and a small piece of the testis is removed. A dressing is applied, and postoperative management is similar to that after open perineal prostatic biopsy. Testicular biopsy specimens are sometimes used to evaluate fertility. If sperm are present in the biopsy tissue but are absent from the semen, absence of the sperm is most often the result of stricture of tubal systems beyond the testes.

ENZYME VALUES

Enzyme values play a role in diagnosis of cancer of the prostate gland. The enzyme tests of most value are phosphatase levels. The phosphatases are secreted in the serum of the tumor mass in the prostate gland and are reflected in changes in the blood chemistry. The phosphatases are labeled as acid or alkaline, depending on the optimal pH. Acid phosphatase usually has a pH of 4.0 to 6.0, whereas alkaline phosphatase usually ranges between a pH of 8.5 and 9.5. A rise in phosphatase value is indicative of cancer of the prostate gland but is not conclusively diagnostic. Usually the phosphatase values are repeated for reliability because such events as rectal examination, prostate massage, or recent episodes of fever may cause either an elevation or drop in phosphatase level. Additional studies such as prostatic biopsy are done to confirm the diagnosis.

ENDOSCOPY

Methods most often used for visualization of the male reproductive organs and related structures include cystoscopy and visualization of the seminal vesicles. *Cystoscopic examination* allows the physician to inspect the condition of the urethral and bladder mucosa and to detect prostatic encroachment on the urethra (see Chapter 47).

Radiographs are used to diagnose obstruction of the seminal vesicles. Two techniques are in use. One method uses a specially designed panendoscope through which catheters are passed into the ejaculatory ducts. The second method requires surgical exposure of the vas through an incision in the scrotum and introduction of small plastic catheters into the vas. For both methods, radiographs are taken to inspect the positions of the catheters.

CHAPTER SUMMARY

- Major external structures of the female genital system include the mons pubis, labia majora, labia minora, clitoris, prepuce, frenulum, vestibule, urethral meatus, Skene's glands, vaginal orifice, hymen, fossa naviculares, Bartholin's glands, fourchet, perineum, and escutcheon.

- Major female internal reproductive organs are the vagina, uterus, fallopian tubes, and ovaries.

- The male genital system includes the testes, spermatic cords, vas deferens, seminal vesicles, ejaculatory ducts, penis, scrotum, prostate glands, and bulbourethral glands.

- The menstrual cycle is divided into phases according to uterine or ovarian changes. The ovarian cycle consists of the follicular and luteal phase, whereas the uterine cycle consists of the menstrual, proliferative, and secretory phases.

- Menstrual cycle function depends on the interrelationship of the central nervous system, anterior pituitary, ovaries, and uterus.

- The female and male reproductive system changes with aging.

- Preparation of the woman for a pelvic examination includes use of models, films, three-dimensional concrete visual aids, explanation of the procedure and answering questions, encouragement to see and touch equipment before its use, draping or nondraping per the patient's request, explanation of what is being done and findings during the examination, relaxation training, and sharing information about sensations she will feel.

- Laboratory tests used to assess reproductive health include tests for syphilis and chlamydia, the Pap smear, endocrine studies, and smears and cultures from various sites.

- Radiologic tests used to assess reproductive health include ultrasonography, CT scan, and MRI.

- Screening tests for endometrial cancer include aspiration smear, endometrial biopsy, vacuum curettage, and dilation & curettage.

- Endoscopy procedures to assess reproductive health include colposcopy, culdoscopy, laparoscopy, and hysteroscopy.

- Special tests for assessing reproductive health in males include prostatic smear, needle biopsies, open perineal biopsy, testicular smears and biopsy specimens, enzyme tests, and endoscopy.

QUESTIONS TO CONSIDER

- How would you provide anticipatory guidance to middle-aged men and women about changes to expect in their reproductive system with aging?

- What approach would you take to prepare a woman for a pelvic examination?

- What approach would you take to prepare a man for an examination of his reproductive system?

- What approaches might you consider for a sexually active person who tests positive for a sexually transmitted disease and doesn't want to tell his partner?

- How would you counsel a 21- or 70-year-old woman with a positive Pap smear?

REFERENCES AND SELECTED READINGS

1. American Cancer Society Inc: 1990 Cancer facts and figures, New York, 1990, The Society.
2. *Bates B: A guide to physical examination, ed 4, Philadelphia, 1987, JB Lippincott Co.
3. Dan A, Graham E, and Beecher C: The menstrual cycle: a synthesis of interdisciplinary research, vol 1, New York, 1981, Springer Publishing Co.
4. Droegemueller W et al: Comprehensive gynecology, St Louis, 1987, The CV Mosby Co.
5. *Ebersole P and Hess P: Toward healthy aging, ed 3, St Louis, 1989, The CV Mosby Co.
6. Komnenich R et al: The menstrual cycle: research and implications for women's health, vol 2, New York, 1981, Springer Publishing Co.
7. Koss LG: The Papanicolaou test for cervical cancer detection: a triumph and a tragedy, JAMA 261:737-743, 1989.
8. Lavy G: Hysteroscopy as a diagnostic aid, Obstet Gynecol Clin North Am 15:61-72, 1988.
9. Levinson JM: Laparoscopy in gynecology. In Pernoll ML, and Benson RC, editors: Current obstetrical and gynecologic diagnosis and treatment, ed 6, Norwalk, CT, 1987, Appleton & Lange.
10. *Malasanos L et al: Health assessment, ed 4, St Louis, 1989, The CV Mosby Co.
11. Mattison D, Kay H, and Heinrichs W: Widening window of magnetic resonance imaging, Contemp Obstet Gynecol 24:91-108, 1984.
12. Mead P and Sweet R: Looking for Chlamydia and finding it, Contemp Obstet Gynecol 25:50, 1985.
13. Modica MM and Timor-Tritsch IE: Transvaginal sonography provides a sharper view into the pelvis, J Obstet Gynecol Neonatal Nurs 17:89-95, 1988.
14. Pagana KD and Pagana TJ: Diagnostic testing and nursing implications, ed 2, St Louis, 1986, The CV Mosby Co.
15. Pernoll ML and Benson RC: Current obstetrical and gynecologic diagnosis and treatment, ed 6, Norwalk, CT, 1987, Appleton & Lange.
16. Pritchard JA, MacDonald PC, and Gant NF: Williams' obstetrics, ed 17, Norwalk, CT, 1989, Appleton-Century-Crofts.
17. Seidel HM et al: Mosby's guide to physical examination, St Louis, 1987, The CV Mosby Co.
18. Wawrznyniak MN: The painless pelvic, MCN 11:178-179, 1986.

*References preceded by an asterisk are particularly well suited for student reading.

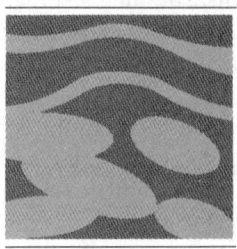

CHAPTER 54

Management of Persons with Alterations in Fertility

GREER GLAZER

CHAPTER OBJECTIVES

After studying this chapter, the student should be able to:

1 Describe factors affecting menstruation and menopause and interventions for related problems.
2 Describe and compare different approaches to family planning.
3 Describe factors affecting fertility and methods of assessment.
4 Identify nursing interventions for assisting women to cope with symptoms associated with alterations in the reproductive cycle.
5 Explain how nurses can assist couples experiencing infertility.

Health behaviors related to the reproductive tract are directed toward maintaining normal reproductive processes. As a woman develops, matures, and then ages, she must cope with menstruation, then fertility or infertility, and finally with menopause. Men are also involved with desiring or preventing conception. Various medical disorders can affect the menstrual cycle or the couple's ability to procreate. Health teaching related to these processes and conditions, therefore, is an integral part of medical-surgical nursing. The topics discussed in this chapter include menstruation, menopause, family planning and contraception, sterilization, and infertility.

MENSTRUATION

MENARCHE

The onset of menstruation in young girls is called *menarche*. Menarche is the external phenomenon used to identify the point of true puberty, the time when reproduction is first possible. The average age of the menarche, which has decreased over the past 100 years, is 12.5 to 12.8 years, with the normal range between 9.1 and 17.7 years.[46] The onset of menstruation occurs at an earlier age in the southern hemisphere. Other factors affecting the onset of menstruation are heredity, health,

The author acknowledges the assistance of Dr. James Goldfarb in the preparation of this chapter.

nutritional status, and weight. Approximately 97.5% of females in the United States begin normal menstrual cycles by 16 years of age.[39] The declining age at which menarche begins reflects improved nutritional status.[46]

It is not possible to predict the exact time at which the first menstrual period will occur. Menarche is caused by cyclic changes in estrogen levels. In general, most girls experience the following progression of somatic changes several months before the menarche: apocrine and other glandular development, increased diameter of the internal pelvis, growth of the ovaries and uterus, breast enlargement, appearance of pubic hair, and growth of the labia and vagina. It is believed that a critical body weight (47.8 kg/105 lbs.) and shift in body composition to a greater percent of fat (from 16.0% to 23.5%) must be attained by a girl to reach menarche.[13] This is supported by two occurrences: moderately obese girls have earlier menarches than girls of normal weight, and girls who are intense exercisers and anorectics may have delayed menarche or secondary amenorrhea.

Some irregularity in duration of menstrual cycles and in the amount of flow is normal for the first few years. Anovulatory cycles are common for the first 12 to 18 months after menarche and before the onset of menopause. The irregularity is probably caused by the lack of progesterone because progesterone is not produced until ovulation begins. By the age of 18 to 20 years, the menstrual cycle usually assumes a rhythmic pattern with minor variations. Theoretically, conception is possible with the menarche.

NORMAL MENSTRUATION
MENSTRUAL CYCLES

There is normal variation among women in the intervals between menstrual periods. Cycle length varies most during the perimenarchal and perimenopausal years (the years around the beginning and end of menstruation) when there is a higher incidence of both long and short cycles. A multinational study found a statistically significant variation in the number of days of menstrual bleeding in different countries and cultures.[58] Menstru-

RESEARCH

McKeever P and Galloway S: Effects of nongynecological surgery on the menstrual cycle, Nurs Res 33:42-46, 1984.

The purpose of this study was to analyze the nature and frequency of menstrual cycle alterations after nongynecologic surgery. The sample consisted of 77 women (46 women aged 19 to 45 and 31 adolescents ages 12 to 18) who had regular menstrual cycles. Data was collected by means of a stress rating scale and a questionnaire by interview 3 or more days after surgery and by telephone 6 weeks postoperatively. Menstrual cycle alterations were reported by two thirds of the subjects. An equal number of women reported delayed menses as did early menses, although adolescents reported more early menses. Women who experienced no menstrual alterations encountered relatively low levels of stress; delayed menses were associated with moderate stress and early menses with relatively high stress. ■

ation occurs on an average of every 28 days, but most cycles occur within a normal range of 26 to 36 days. A majority of women have cycles that normally vary in length by up to 5 days.

The pattern of the menstrual cycle may be upset by such things as changes in climate, changes in working hours, emotional trauma, fatigue, exercise, acute or chronic illness, or surgery (see the research box above). Any of these factors may alter the lifestyle temporarily and produce change in the menstrual cycle by way of the nerve centers of the hypothalamus that influence the rate and timing of pituitary stimulation of the ovaries. A period that is missed, earlier or later than expected, or shorter or longer than usual is not significant if it occurs for only 1 month. If any of these irregularities continue, a health professional should be consulted.

During pregnancy menstruation ceases and then usually returns within 6 to 8 weeks after delivery, although lactation suppresses the menses for varying periods of time. Unless disease occurs, the menstrual periods recur during adult life until menopause.

MENSTRUAL FLOW

The menstrual flow usually lasts for 3 to 7 days, with an average of 4 days. It can be divided into three phases: premenstrual discharge, major discharge, and postmenstrual discharge. Some women do not experience a premenstrual or postmenstrual flow. The premenstrual flow is initially light, lasting up to one or one and a half days and is pink mucoid to dark brown. The major discharge is the heaviest flow, lasts 3 to 5 days, and is bright red. The postmenstrual discharge gradually subsides in up to 2 days and may be pink mucoid, yellow-brown, red, or brown.

Some women have heavier flows than others. Normally, there is a loss of from 30 to 180 ml of menstrual fluid during the period, with an average blood loss of 45

ml. The woman's perception about the amount of blood loss often differs from objective measurements. Previous menstrual experience and preconceived ideas about what is normal blood loss greatly influence a woman's assessment of blood loss.

One half to three fourths of the fluid is blood; the remainder is mucus, fragments of endometrial cells, and desquamated vaginal epithelium. The average woman needs approximately one dozen pads or one dozen tampons for the entire period; however, this is highly variable in relation to both the amount of flow and esthetic concern. Normally, menstrual fluid does not clot unless it is retained in the uterus or vagina for a prolonged time. It is believed that the endometrium produces an anticoagulant that prevents clotting of blood in the uterus. An occasional very small "clot" may occur during the first 24 hours, and this is probably a particle of endometrial tissue. Large clots or pus is never normal in the menstrual flow.

PERIMENSTRUAL SYMPTOMS

A variety of symptoms that may be present before and during menstruation are considered normal. Research contradicts the notion that premenstrual and menstrual symptoms constitute mutually exclusive categories.[60] Daily stressors may influence the occurrence of perimenstrual symptoms (see the research box on p. 1565).

Fluid retention, with up to a 5 lb weight gain, is very common. The excess fluid is lost through increased urine production during the first few days after menstruation begins. Slight *aching in the lower back, legs, and pelvis,* especially on the day of onset of the flow, occurs frequently. A slight tendency toward *fatigue* during the menses is common, and many women experience a spurt of energy a few days before the period begins. *Breast changes,* consisting of tingling, fullness, tenderness, and increase in size, are usually noticed before the menses begin and last for 1 to 2 days after the flow starts. Some women note *mood changes* premenstrually.

Lower abdominal cramps caused by decreased uterine blood flow and increased contractility of the uterus may range from mild to severe. Dysmenorrhea (painful menstruation) is discussed on p. 1567. *Lower abdominal pain* may also be noticeable around the time of ovulation (mittelschmerz), resulting from minor bleeding from the follicle into the abdominal cavity. Most women report no symptoms or have very low severity symptoms.

PROMOTING POSITIVE ATTITUDES

Menstruation is a manifestation of normal body function and should be treated as such. The "period" and "monthly period" are sensible and accurate terms to use if the individual does not wish to say, "I am menstruating." Because of the negative connotations engendered

RESEARCH

Woods NF, Most A, and Longenecker AD: Major life events, daily stressors, and perimenstrual symptoms, Nurs Res 34:263-267, 1985.

The purpose of this study was to determine the relationship of major life events and daily stressors to perimenstrual symptoms (PS). The sample consisted of 74 women aged 18 to 35 who kept daily recordings of stressors and symptoms for 2 months and then completed the Schedule of Recent Events and the Moos Menstrual Distress Questionnaire. Daily stressors were more influential on PS reports than major life events. A generally stressful life context was more influential on PS than stressful episodes during a particular menstrual cycle phase. ■

---

by such terms as "being sick," or "having the curse," girls and women can be encouraged to avoid using them and to use appropriate terms instead. Some women consider the menstrual periods a time of great inconvenience, perhaps because of inadequate knowledge of the physiology of menstruation; inadequate information about how it is possible to maintain usual physical, mental, and social activities; sociocultural conditioning; or in some instances, because of symptoms. Menstruating women have been viewed as dangerous, vulnerable, sick, and contaminated throughout history.

HEALTH TEACHING

Before engaging in any discussion of menstruation, the nurse first assesses the individual's knowledge and level of understanding. Once this is accomplished, a teaching plan can be designed to meet the specific learning needs of the person. All information can be given in an open, factual manner, but latitude must be allowed for individuals to express their feelings, thoughts, beliefs, and concerns.

Girls and women often want and need information about menstruation. Their understanding may be limited or inaccurate because of word-of-mouth information passed along by peers, parents, and others who are poorly informed. On the other hand, nurses may find women who know about the entire menstrual cycle but have difficulty in accepting it as a normal process. Women need to know the physiology of menstruation. They also need to know what discomforts are normally associated with the menstrual period and what measures can be taken to relieve them. They need to know what signs indicate deviations from normal and what actions to take regarding possible problems (see the box above).

Nurses are often questioned about methods of sanitary protection during menstruation. Either pads or tampons can be used, depending on which is most com-

HEALTH TEACHING FOR MENSTRUATION

1. Knowledge of the physiologic process
2. Factors that may alter the menstrual cycle: stress, fatigue, exercise, acute and chronic illness, changes in climate or working hours, pregnancy
3. Personal hygiene
   a. Wear pads during early period of heavy flow
   b. Change tampons frequently to decrease risk of toxic shock syndrome
   c. Wear pads at night to decrease risk of TSS
   d. Consult a nurse practitioner or physician if tampons cause discomfort
   e. Take a daily bath for comfort (warm bath may relieve slight pelvic discomfort)
4. Exercise
   a. Exercise is not contraindicated and may help prevent discomfort
   b. Modify exercise if fatigue occurs
5. Diet
   a. Restrict salt intake if fluid retention is present
   b. Decrease foods that promote sodium retention such as caffeine, MSG.
   c. Consult nurse practitioner or physician if fluid retention persists after menstruation
6. Discomfort (dysmenorrhea)
   a. For mild discomfort take aspirin, acetaminophen, or antiprostaglandins, apply warmth, rest
   b. For prolonged severe discomfort, consult physician.

---

fortable and acceptable. Tampon use has been associated with an increased risk of developing toxic shock syndrome (see Chapter 55). Women should be encouraged to wear pads on their first menstrual day, to use regular tampons instead of super tampons, and to change tampons frequently during their menstrual period. Use of pads (not tampons) at night is also suggested to decrease the likelihood of toxic shock syndrome. If tampons are of the correct size and are properly inserted, there should be no discomfort when they are worn. If tampons are not easily inserted or produce pain when in place, a health professional should be consulted.

To increase knowledge and to reduce fear and anxiety, women can be informed of the events that may temporarily alter the menstrual cycle. However, they also need to be informed of symptoms indicating potential problems so that medical attention can be sought. To become knowledgeable about the patterns of their menstrual cycles, women can be encouraged to keep a written record. Establishing this habit makes it possible to predict the onset of the next menstrual period and to determine the range of cycles and duration of flow. Should it be necessary to seek the attention of a health professional for any reason, the date of onset of the last menstrual period (LMP) would be known.

Some women have marked discomfort during menstruation and take a variety of medications to relieve the symptoms. Women can be advised to treat minor discomforts with rest, warmth, acetylsalicylic acid, or antiprostaglandins. Women should be urged to seek medical evaluation if discomfort is incapacitating.

Daily bathing and frequent changing of sanitary devices add greatly to comfort and hygiene during menstruation. An unpleasant odor develops when the menstrual flow comes into contact with the air. A warm tub bath often relieves slight pelvic discomfort, although many women prefer to take showers during the menstrual period. Cold baths and showers may increase discomfort, but many women use tampons and go swimming during their periods with no ill effects.

Daily activities may be continued for both physical and mental health. If fatigue is associated with menstruation, exercise may need to be modified to provide for additional rest.

Most women experience some fluid retention preceding menstruation, and many notice weight gain that may be controlled to some extent by restricting the intake of salt and other foods high in sodium. Edema from other causes can be ruled out by having the woman observe her weight daily. If edema is present at times other than the premenstrual and menstrual periods, the woman should be advised to consult a physician.

INVESTIGATION OF MAJOR COMPLAINTS

Problems related to the menstrual cycle are common. They include a variety of symptoms directly or indirectly related to the pelvic organs and may result from any one or a combination of causes.

Women who seek care because of absence of menstruation (amenorrhea), irregular periods, excessive flow, or dysmenorrhea should have a complete history taken and undergo a physical examination. Close questioning about the menstrual periods and sexual activity is important (see Chapter 53). The history should include use of medication including tranquilizers and hormones, as well as daily exercise patterns as these often disrupt the menstrual cycle.

A pelvic examination to assess the state of the reproductive organs is essential. If a sexually active woman complains of amenorrhea, a pregnancy test is usually performed. Urinalysis, complete blood count, study of cervical and endometrial tissue, hormone assays, or visualization of the pelvic organs may be indicated to determine the cause of the problem.

Dilation and curettage (D & C) is often the method selected for obtaining endometrial tissue for study. In many cases, a D & C is temporarily therapeutic because it removes hypertrophied endometrium. Unless the direct cause of the menstrual problem is found, however, and unless treatment for the cause is instituted, symptoms tend to recur. Women having a D & C should understand the purpose of the procedure and should be urged to remain under medical care even though the D & C has helped the problem (see Chapter 53).

Endometrial biopsy is the best method to assess ovulation and the luteal phase of the menstrual cycle. The biopsy is done two to three days before the expected period. Endometrial tissue is obtained relatively painlessly using a plastic endometrial suction curette (3 mm diameter) inserted through the cervix and requiring no cervical dilatation.

PREMENSTRUAL SYNDROME

Premenstrual syndrome (PMS), which occurs in approximately 10% of all menstruating women, is the presence of symptoms in the premenstruum or early menstruation with the absence of postmenstrual symptoms. PMS is present if the symptoms interfere with activities of daily living and the woman seeks assistance from health care providers. Identical symptoms must occur in three consecutive cycles (during the last 7 to 10 days of each cycle) to confirm a diagnosis of PMS. Symptoms vary considerably among women and may include behavioral changes (tension, irritability, mood swings, anxiety, crying, depression, insomnia), fatigue, signs of water and sodium retention (edema, weight gain, breast enlargement and tenderness, abdominal bloating), acne, palpitations, increased appetite, migrainelike headache, joint pain, and backache.[20] In addition, some women have complained of a desire to be alone; a sensitivity to rejection; an intolerance of others; paranoia; panic attacks; decreased sexual desire; sensitivity to noise, light, and touch; a decreased ability to concentrate; and impaired judgment and memory.[20]

The etiology of PMS is unknown. However, investigators believe that it may result from a variety of factors, including an estrogen-progesterone imbalance, hypoglycemia, excess aldosterone, hyperprolactinemia, excess prostaglandin, psychogenic factors, low progesterone levels, high estrogen levels, falling estrogen levels, increased renin-angiotensin activity, increased adrenal activity, endogenous endorphin withdrawal, central changes in catecholamines, and vitamin deficiencies.[39,46]

Numerous treatments have been suggested to alleviate symptoms (Table 54-1). Although oral contraceptives may produce symptoms similar to those of PMS, symptoms may be relieved in some women with oral contraceptives. However, research has shown that oral contraceptives, vitamin B_6, bromocriptine, monoamine oxidase (MAO) inhibitors, and synthetic progestational agents have failed to demonstrate significant benefits over placebo.[46] No treatment has proven to be therapeutically effective for PMS.[4,43] Therefore, most clinicians treat specific symptoms with specific therapy (such as diuretics for edema). Four categories of PMS symptoms have been identified and treatment for each is indicated in table 54-1.).

There are three purposes of PMS treatment: to decrease the number and severity of symptoms, to restore

TABLE 54-1 Common symptoms and treatment of premenstrual tension symptoms[1,20]

Category	Symptoms	Traditional Therapy	Nontraditional Therapy
PMT-A	Anxiety, irritability, nervous tension	Progesterone, vitamin B$_6$, limit dairy products intake, increase outdoor exercise, lorazepam	Validation Education Exercise Family therapy Peer support groups Stress management Assertiveness training Sex and marital therapy
PMT-H	Water and sodium retention	Restrict intake of salt, coffee, tea, cola, chocolate; vitamin B$_6$, primrose oil, spironolactone, antiprostaglandins, oral contraceptives	
PMT-C	Increased appetite, especially for sweets, headache, fatigue, palpitations	Restrict free sugar, sodium, and animal fat intake; substitute complex carbohydrate for simple sugars	
PMT-D	Depression	Increase intake of foods high in B vitamins and magnesium (green leafy vegetables, legumes, whole-grain cereals)	

the woman's psychological health, and to deal with social and interpersonal problems resulting from PMS. The nurse can assist women with PMS by acknowledging the existence of the syndrome and its attendant fact, women commit violent crimes and suicide more frequently in the week before the onset of menstruation. Because some women have been made to feel that the symptoms are nonexistent or exaggerated, the nurse can encourage them to keep a menstrual symptom calendar to document the cyclic nature of the symptoms.[20]

Overall well-being and a reduction in symptoms can be achieved by simple measures such as alteration in diet, cessation of smoking and drinking, and exercise.[31] A diet high in complex carbohydrates, moderate in protein, and low in refined sugar and sodium should be eaten, especially during the premenstrual interval. Consumption of caffeine (in tea, coffee, caffeine-containing beverages), chocolate, and alcohol, and smoking should be reduced or eliminated. Regular exercise three to four times a week for 30 minutes is encouraged, especially

RESEARCH

Coyne C: Muscle tension and its relation to symptoms in the premenstruum, Res Nurs Health 6:199-206, 1983.

A study of 22 women who predicted they usually had premenstrual symptoms ranging from mild to severe revealed that electromyography levels (muscle tension) were elevated during the premenstruum relative to the follicular phase. Moreover, women who anticipated having symptoms had the highest levels of muscle tension during the premenstruum. The results suggest that training in muscle tension reduction may be beneficial for some women with premenstrual symptoms. ■

during the premenstrual interval. Other recommendations include 100 mg of vitamin B$_6$ daily, 1.5 g twice daily of evening primrose oil (contains linoleic acid, gamma linoleic acid, and vitamin E), 100 mg spironolactone daily, and prostaglandin inhibitors.

Women can also be encouraged to plan activities during the symptom-free part of their cycles. Because fatigue may exaggerate PMS symptoms, adequate rest, sleep, and relaxation are helpful. Information can be obtained from PMS Action, Inc.*

DYSMENORRHEA

Etiology/Epidemiology

Uterine pain with menstruation, commonly called "menstrual cramps" is properly termed *dysmenorrhea*. *Primary* dysmenorrhea, painful menstruation unassociated with pelvic pathology, usually develops when ovulatory function is established and occurs in the absence of organic disease. It often disappears or declines after pregnancy or by age 23 to 27. *Secondary* dysmenorrhea is painful menstruation caused by organic disease, usually pelvic inflammatory disease, endometriosis, or cervical stenosis, or rarely by a malpositioned uterus. *Membranous* dysmenorrhea (cast of endometrial cavity shed as a single entity) is extremely rare. The woman experiences extreme cramping pain resulting from the passage of the endometrial lining through an undilated cervix. Dysmenorrhea may also be caused by an intrauterine device (IUD).

Although estimates vary, it is generally believed that greater than 50% of menstruating women have some degree of dysmenorrhea, with 5% to 20% of women becoming incapacitated.[46] Studies in industry and schools

*PO Box 16292, Irvine, CA 92713.

SITUATIONS THAT PROVOKE HOT FLASHES

Exercise
Excitement
Eating
Alcohol beverages
Impairment of heat loss in hot weather
Excessive clothing

sult from a decline in estrogen that causes instability between the hypothalamus and the autonomic nervous system. Hot flashes may be so mild that they are hardly noticed or so severe that they produce distress. The hot flashes last seconds to minutes, ranging from 0.5 to 60 minutes, and can occur as frequently as one to two an hour to one to two a week. They are the most common symptom for which menopausal women seek treatment. At least 85% of postmenopausal women experience hot flashes.[46] Of these women, 82% will experience flushes for more than 1 year, and 25% to 85% will experience them for more than 5 years.[11a,39] Situations that may provoke hot flashes are listed in the box above. The hot flashes are usually most disturbing during sleep, perhaps because the hypothalamus is relatively inactive. Despite the commonality of hot flashes, they do not present a health hazard to women. However, many women go through the climacteric with little awareness of its occurrence.

Vaginal Changes

As a result of thinning of the vaginal mucosa because of decreased estrogen women may have pain during intercourse (dyspareunia), vaginal dryness, burning, itching, and occasional bleeding after menopause. The lack of estrogen also causes vaginal secretions to become more alkaline, leading to an increase in vaginal infections.

Urinary Tract Changes

Lower estrogen levels may cause atrophic changes in the bladder and urethra. Atrophic cystitis may be produced, resulting in urinary frequency and urgency, painful urination, and incontinence.

Breast Changes

Breast size may decrease. This may be distressing to some women or appreciated by others. The breast hangs more loosely because of tissue changes from glandular to fat.

Skeletal System Changes

Estrogen decrease causes a negative nitrogen balance and muscle is replaced by fibrous tissue. Women begin to lose bone at a rate of 0.75% to 1% per year between

RESEARCH

Carter L: Calcium intake in young adult women: implications for osteoporosis risk assessment, J Obstet Gynecol Neonatal Nurs 16:301-308, 1987.

This study of 41 women ages 25 to 35 revealed that daily calcium intake was insufficient for the majority of women. Thirty-one women consumed less than 1250 mg calcium daily, placing them at risk for osteoporosis after menopause. ■

the ages of 30 and 35. Because the rate of loss increases with age, the menopausal woman may lose from 2% to 3% yearly.[3] About 25% of postmenopausal women develop osteoporosis.[51]

Osteoporosis is characterized by a decrease in the quantity of bone, marked by reductions in the bone mineral content and bone calcium. Osteoporotic problems include back pain; reduced height and mobility; and fractures of the vertebral body, humerus, upper femur, distal forearm, and ribs. The increased bone loss in menopausal women has been related to the increased risk of hip fractures, and postmenopausal women account for approximately 250,000 hip fractures in the United States per year. The vertebral body is the most common site of fracture. Because the fractured femur is associated with appreciable mortality and morbidity, it is of particular concern. Women who are sedentary, thin, and white, and Asian women who smoke are at high risk for development of decreased bone density.[36]

An imbalance in the calcium/phosphorus ratio may be the most significant factor in the development of osteoporosis. The phosphorus excess may be related to eating foods high in phosphorus (for example, soft drinks, bread, cereal) and to the reduced ability of older adults to absorb calcium from the intestines. Increased calcium may be removed from the bones to buffer high nitrogen levels resulting from high protein diets. Women often obtain less than 500 mg of calcium from their food intake daily and less than 1250 mg from food and calcium supplements and may require 1200 mg of calcium daily to maintain a positive calcium balance. Women over age 50 may need up to 1500 mg of calcium daily[17] (see research box above). A daily calcium intake of 1000 mg to 1500 mg may retard bone loss and decrease the incidence of fractures in women with postmenopausal osteoporosis. For absorption of calcium, 400 IU of vitamin D/day is needed.

INTERVENTIONS

Counseling and Teaching

Most women have heard of the "change of life." The negative image of menopause is reinforced by the me-

HEALTH TEACHING FOR MENOPAUSE

1. Knowledge about menopause
   a. Cessation of ovarian function, with cessation of menstruation over 12 to 18 months
   b. Changes in reproductive ability
      (1) Conception still possible during the period of change
         (a) Contraception should be used for 1 year after last menstrual period
         (b) Rhythm method unreliable contraceptive method during this period
      (2) Ability to conceive ceases when menopause is completed
   c. Sexual ability still present
   d. Physical symptoms vary from mild to severe; estrogen therapy may be given to relieve severe symptoms
2. Promotion of health and physical appearance
   a. Moderate exercise to maintain muscle tone and help prevent osteoporosis
   b. Calcium supplement to prevent osteoporosis
   c. Dietary control to prevent weight gain
   d. Activities that encourage self-esteem and interest outside of self
   e. Peer support groups during menopause, if necessary
3. Prevention of discomfort
   a. Relief of vasomotor reactions (hot flashes)
      (1) Moderation of factors identified by patient as exacerbating hot flashes (excitement, alcoholic beverages, heavy eating, excessive clothing, impairment of heat loss in hot weather)
      (2) Vitamin E or B-complex vitamins
      (3) Estrogen, Bellergal
   b. Prevention of dyspareunia: local application of lubricant or vaginal cream
   c. Relief of vaginal itching: vitamin E or estrogen therapy

dia, books, health professionals, and the general public. Depending on the social attitudes in which they were reared and on their own changes in attitude toward normal functions of the reproductive organs, women may feel more or less free to discuss the menopause and their feelings and concerns during this period of life. Because many problems related to the reproductive organs occur in this age group, and because it is important for mental health that women be helped to make the menopause as comfortable as possible, it is important for nurses to identify women who can profit from interventions. It is especially important to discuss the patient's lifestyle during the climacteric because of its effect on symptoms.

Education about the menopause should precede its onset. Health teaching for menopause is summarized in the box above. Many women appreciate opportunities made by nurses to discuss the menopause. Women approaching the menopause, regardless of whether it is an event of normal aging or is artificially induced, need to know what the menopause is, why it occurs, the effects it has on reproductive and sexual ability, what can be done to make it more comfortable, and what symptoms require medical attention.

Some women feel that they are less attractive after menopause. Moderate exercise to maintain muscle tone is beneficial to both health and physical appearance. Feelings of depression and uselessness are common among women, particularly those who have been highly invested in the maternal role. Men also sometimes have feelings of depression and uselessness if they perceive a decline in sexual and other abilities. Peer support groups during menopause may be helpful.

Many women have heard of "change of life babies" and fear they may become pregnant during the menopause. During this time menstrual cycles and ovulation are irregular and if pregnancy is to be prevented, a highly reliable contraceptive method is necessary. The rhythm method is unreliable during the menopause because of the irregular cycles. Contraception should be used for 1 year after a woman's last menstrual period.

Because the incidence of cancer of the uterus is higher during this period, these patients should be urged to have physical examinations, including screening for cancer, at least once a year. All women are advised that bleeding after the menopause requires medical attention.

Estrogen Therapy

Over the years there has been much debate over the advantages and disadvantages of estrogen replacement therapy (ERT). There is evidence that appropriate ERT can have a major impact on the risk of fractures with a 50% to 60% decrease in fractures of the arm and hip.[11,22,54,57] Estrogen therapy combined with calcium supplementation has resulted in an 80% reduction in vertebral compression fractures.

Before initiation of ERT, menopause should be confirmed. Decreased serum estradiol levels below 40 pg/ml and increased FSH and LH above 100 mIU/ml indicate menopause. Estrogen therapy has been effective in treating hot flashes, vaginal atrophy, and osteoporosis; however, adverse effects have been found. Administration of estrogen by itself has been suggested as associated with a fourfold to eightfold increased risk of endometrial cancer. This risk can be avoided by taking progestin with estrogen for 12 days each. Because estrone, which has been linked to endometrial cancer, is made in adipose tissue of menopausal women, other types of synthetic estrogens, such as estriol or estradiol preparations, are preferred by some clinicians. Estrogens are likely to be taken for extended periods of time, but may be tapered and discontinued when women desire to stop taking them.

It is currently believed that estrogen is protective against osteoporosis only while women are maintained on the replacement therapy.[46] Present recommendations for estrogen-progestin replacement therapy are based on risk of fractures; it may be started as close to menopause as possible and maintained long term, if not life-long.

Literature generally supports reduced risk of cardiovascular disease in women taking estrogen replacement therapy.[46] The relationship between estrogen therapy and breast cancer is unproven; however, accumulating evidence suggests that exposure to progestational agents may offer protection against breast cancer.[15,58]

Women who take estrogen and progestin in combination after menopause have a lower risk for endometrial cancer and heart disease than untreated women.[17] However, adverse metabolic effects of a progestogen include alterations in lipoprotein fractions and the potential for carbohydrate intolerance and are a cause for concern.[27]

Because of these concerns and emerging data on ERT, the International Consensus Meeting convened in 1988 to consider the appropriate use of progestogens during menopause. A consensus statement was drafted that includes the following: (1) All postmenopausal women should be made aware of the consequences of untreated menopause and should be *offered* the opportunity to receive estrogen; (2) the routine use of progestogens in hysterectomized women is not indicated; (3) there is insufficient data to suggest a protective effect of progestogens against breast cancer; (4) with adequate estrogen therapy, the addition of progestogen to ERT affords no extra protection against bone loss or fracture incidence; and (5) because epidemiologic studies have linked the cardioprotective effects of ERT to increases in HDL-C, large amounts of progestogens (which decrease HDL-C) should be avoided.[27]

Guidelines for ERT are general because risks and benefits need to be judged on an individual basis. Since women assume risks whether or not estrogen is taken, they should receive enough information to make an informed choice. Standard hormone replacement therapy now includes a combination of estrogen with a progestational agent. Current standard hormone replacement includes 0.625 mg conjugated equine estrogens orally from days 1 to 25 and 10 mg of medroxyprogesterone acetate orally from days 16 to 25 for women with an intact uterus. Estrogen can also be administered intramuscularly. Subcutaneous implants (patches) provide continuous therapy that results in a high incidence of endometrial hyperplasia.

In general, it is desirable to use the lowest dose possible to relieve symptoms. Absolute contraindications to ERT include gallbladder, liver, cerebrovascular, and pancreatic disease; undiagnosed vaginal bleeding; sickle cell anemia; and a history of myocardial infarction, deep vein thrombosis of unknown cause, pulmonary embolism, estrogen-dependent tumors of the uterus and breasts, or hypertension.

During estrogen therapy, women should be seen at least every 6 months for examination and for review of menopausal symptoms. The examination should include the breasts and reproductive organs, Pap smear, and blood pressure. Women who are receiving estrogen need to be advised that they still would benefit from an exercise program three times a week, consumption of 1.5 g of calcium daily, and proper nutrition.

Relief of Symptoms

Research indicates that the more roles women assume, the less likely they are to experience climacteric symptoms. Adjustment to the marital role and an active recreational role were the best predictors of infrequent and mild climacteric symptoms (see research box below).

Medroxyprogesterone acetate has been associated with a 90% reduction in hot flashes.[39] Other natural methods reported to diminish or eliminate hot flashes are vitamins E and B-complex, and ginseng. Vitamins E and B complexes can be added to the diet or taken by supplementation. Dietary sources of vitamin E are vegetable oils, soybeans, spinach, peanuts, and wheat germ. Good dietary sources of vitamin B complexes are whole grains, brewer's yeast, wheat germ, yogurt, liver, and milk.

Pain during intercourse, resulting from thinning of the vaginal mucosa, is most often treated by local application of a vaginal cream. Vaginal estrogens are absorbed in much greater amounts than when given systemically; thus they must be used with caution. Vitamin E has been effective over time in alleviating dryness of vaginal tissue.

RESEARCH

Uphold C and Susman E: Child-rearing, marital, recreational and work role integration and climacteric symptoms in midlife women, Res Nurs Health 8:73-81, 1985.

An investigation of the relationship between the roles women enact during midlife and the frequency and severity of the symptoms they report at the climacteric revealed that for 185 healthy middle-aged women the more roles women assumed, the less likely they were to experience climacteric symptoms. Positive marital adjustment and an active recreational role were the best predictors of infrequent or mild symptoms. The child-rearing role was not related to symptoms, nor was the number of hours the woman worked. Successful marital adaptation and active role participation was associated with positive adaptation to the climacteric for women. ■

As with other menopausal symptoms, changes in the skeletal system are usually treated with estrogen therapy. As noted earlier, calcium intake should be increased by tablet and by diet. TUMS antacid tablets contain 250 mg calcium per tablet and have been advocated as an inexpensive, convenient source of calcium. Some rarely eaten foods that contain considerable calcium but no phosphorus are sesame seed and seaweed. Turnip greens, broccoli, nuts, and sardines are a good source of calcium in addition to dairy products. The addition of fluoride, which stimulates bone formation, may be beneficial; however, a significant proportion of women have encountered joint and tendon inflammation, gastrointestinal disturbances, and anemia.

Exercise, particularly when combined with calcium supplementation, can prevent or retard osteoporosis.[46] Weight-bearing exercise three times a week for at least 30 minutes per day will increase the bone mineral content of bone in older women.[8] The exercise program also improves vital capacity and minute volume, increases physical work capacity, decreases blood pressure, decreases percentage of body fat, and adds a sense of overall well-being. The best exercise programs include aerobic exercises for cardiopulmonary conditioning, flexibility, and relaxation, and muscle-strengthening exercises. Walking and ordinary calisthenics will also produce benefits.

FAMILY PLANNING AND CONTRACEPTION

Overpopulation and world hunger have become problems of such magnitude that they affect every living being. Ecologic insights force us to look at life and our environment. We now know that we have few choices left if we are to survive on this planet. Beyond the question of survival are questions of quality of life. Conclusions of the Project on Predicament of Mankind at the Massachusetts Institute of Technology include the prediction that "the quality of life will continue to decline if no curbs are placed on population, until pollution and other factors bring about their own curb on population."[39] Thus birth control and family planning not only become matters of personal concern but also take into consideration the rights of others.

For the first time in human history it is now possible to regulate conception with a high degree of reliability. During the past 20 to 30 years there has been a sharp decline in the birth rate in the United States and similarly developed nations. This drop is attributed to widespread use of highly effective fertility and birth control methods and new techniques for performing abortions and sterilizations.

Contraception remains a controversial issue. The incentives and imperatives for separating sexual and reproductive functions have been widely discussed from the standpoint of medical care, sociology, psychology, demography, economics, theology, and the law. Prevention of the birth of unwanted children and prevention of illness are two of the themes addressed pro and con in the literature.

Regardless of the personal and global issues involved, individuals and couples are required more than ever before to examine the consequences of their actions and to select from among the various alternatives the one most consistent with their beliefs, needs, and sense of responsibility. Bound into these issues and pressures for individual responsibility are controversies surrounding the use of particular methods of conception prevention, advantages and disadvantages of methods available for birth control, and the problems incurred by the use of individual methods of preventing pregnancy.

Mortality associated with the use of various methods of birth control has received much attention through the years. Reports continue that very low rates of mortality are associated with all *reversible* methods of fertility control as compared with mortality associated with pregnancy and childbirth. The view that any type of contraception is better than pregnancy needs to be qualified because maternal mortality is influenced by a woman's health and socioeconomic status before becoming pregnant. Mortality reported for tubal ligation for sterilization of women is higher than for any other form of birth control. However, these rates are still lower than rates for pregnancy and childbirth. No mortality from vasectomy is reported in the literature.

Family planning improves family health in the following ways as reflected in the mnemonic "FAMILY HEALTH"[17]:

1. Food is available in greater amounts
2. Anemia is diminished
3. Maternal mortality is decreased
4. Infertility may be prevented
5. Low birth weight is less likely
6. Young children and infants are less likely to die of infectious disease
7. Happier sexual relations
8. Educational opportunities are increased
9. Abortions are more safe and legal
10. Lactation can continue for longer
11. Teenage pregnancy rates are decreased
12. Health screening tests are done while providing family planning

COUNSELING OF INDIVIDUALS AND COUPLES
DECISION MAKING

Individuals choose a method of preventing pregnancy for reasons other than risk to health or life. These reasons include effectiveness, convenience, reversibility, ethical considerations, cost, lifestyle, and noninterference with enjoyment of sexual intercourse. Much of the literature is devoted to the concerns of risk to health and life and very little to other factors, including risks attended by reproduction.

For individuals to make a fully meaningful and responsible choice, they need to be informed of all advantages and disadvantages of all methods or combinations of methods available for preventing pregnancy. With the flood of publicity in the media, especially regarding congressional hearings and actions, considerable anxiety and confusion on the part of the public has resulted. Usually the publicity is directed toward one aspect of health risks associated with one method of conception control, and the risks are not presented in comparison with risks associated with pregnancy and childbirth. In addition, certain biases are inherent in the lay and professional literature about which forms of contraception are most desirable. Many family planners have biased their responses about contraceptive effectiveness largely in favor of oral contraceptives and the IUD. Family planners may bias their teaching in favor of methods clinicians provide more frequently.[17] Condoms, foam, and diaphragms get an underservedly low efficacy score despite their safety. This biased approach dissuades people from using diaphragms, foam, condoms, and fertility awareness methods of conception control. However, there seems to be a growing trend toward the lower risk methods. Thus health professionals are given the task of

fitting pieces of information together to form a whole picture with meaning and perspective and of presenting the total block of information to persons seeking information, advice, and help.

Individuals who use a reversible method of birth control and then decide to change have two alternatives: They can choose an alternate method or not use any method of birth control. When the second alternative is chosen, pregnancy is very likely. Pregnancy then may lead to either an abortion or continuation of the pregnancy resulting in the birth of an unplanned child. It is important, therefore, that information be fully given, including risks to health and life and risks of pregnancy. Only in this way can individuals make an intelligent judgment of the risks they are willing to take and assume responsibility for their actions. One of the greatest responsibilities of nurses is to assist sexually active individuals in making decisions about contraception, childbearing, and pregnancy spacing in a well-informed manner.

APPROACHES IN COUNSELING

Kurtzman and Block[24] present a family planning counseling model that assists nurses to counsel clients by values clarification (Figure 54-1). An evaluation of the family planning program 1 year after the model was introduced showed that 84% of the women who had given

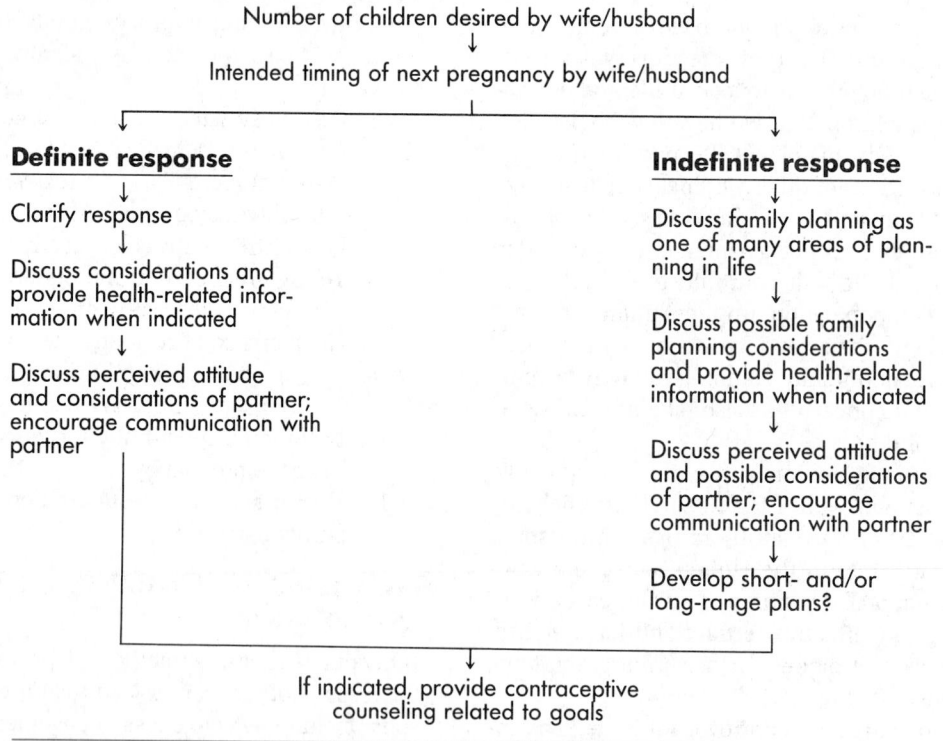

FIGURE 54-1 Family planning counseling model. (From Kurtzman C and Block DE: Family planning: beyond contraception. Matern Child Nurs J 11:341, 1986.)

TABLE 54-6 Lowest expected, typical, and lowest reported failure rates during the first year of use of a contraceptive method and first-year continuation rates, United States*

Method	Percent of Women Experiencing an Accidental Pregnancy in the First Year of Use			Percent of Women Continuing Use at One Year[d]	
	Lowest Expected[a] (1)	Typical[b] (2)	Lowest Reported[c] (3)	Excluding Pregnancy (4)	Including Pregnancy (5)
Chance[e]	85	85	43.1		
Spermicides[f]	3	21	0.0	55	43
Periodic abstinence		20		84	67
Calendar	9		14.4[g]		
Ovulation method	3		10.5[g]		
Symptothermal[h]	2		12.6		
Post-ovulation	1		2.0[g]		
Withdrawal	4	18	6.7[g]		
Cap[i]	6	18	8.0	77	63
Sponge					
Parous women	9	28	27.7	73	53
Nulliparous women	6	18	13.9	73	60
Diaphragm[i]	6	18	2.1	69	57
Condom[j]	2	12	4.2	73	64
IUD		3		75	73
Progestasert	2.0		1.9		
Copper T 380A	0.8		0.5		
Pill		3		75	73
Combined	0.1		0.0		
Progestogen only	0.5		1.1		
Injectable progestogen				70	70
DMPA	0.3	0.3	0.0		
NET	0.4	0.4	0.0		
Implants				90	90
NORPLANT (6 capsules)	0.04	0.04	0.0		
NORPLANT-2 (2 rods)	0.03	0.03	0.0		
Female sterilization	0.2	0.4	0.0		
Male sterilization	0.1	0.15	0.0		

*From Trussell et al.: Contraceptive failure in the United States: an update, Stud Fam Plan 21(1):52, Jan/Feb 1990.

[a]Among couples who initiate use of a method (not necessarily for the first time) and who use it *perfectly* (both consistently and correctly), the authors' best guess of the percentage expected to experience an accidental pregnancy during the first year if they do not stop use for any other reason.

[b]Among *typical* couples who initiate use of a method (not necessarily for the first time), the percentage who experience an accidental pregnancy during the first year if they do not stop use for any other reason.

[c]In the literature on contraceptive failure, the *lowest reported* percentage who experienced an accidental pregnancy during the first year following initiation of use (not necessarily for the first time) if they did not stop use for any other reason. However, see note h.

[d]Among couples attempting to avoid pregnancy, the percentage who continue to use a method for one year, under the alternative assumptions that no one becomes pregnant (column 4) and that the proportion becoming pregnant is given by column 1 (column 5).

[e]The lowest expected and typical percents are based on data from populations where contraception is not practiced and from women who cease practicing contraception in order to become pregnant. These represent our best guess of the percent who would conceive among women now relying on reversible methods of contraception if they abandoned contraception altogether. The lowest reported percent is based on US women who practice no contraception even though they do not wish to become pregnant. This group is selected for low fecundity or low coital frequency, and some fraction may use an unreported variant of periodic abstinence.

[f]Foams and vaginal suppositories.

[g]Too low, because rate is based on more than one year of exposure. See Trussell J. and Kost K.: Contraceptive failure in the United States: A critical review of the literature, Stud Fam Plan 18: 237-283, 1987.

[h]Cervical mucus (ovulation) method supplemented by calendar in the pre-ovulatory and basal body temperature in the post-ovulatory phases.

[i]With spermicidal cream or jelly.

[j]Without spermicides.

birth formulated definite family planning goals, compared to 69% of those who gave birth before the model was introduced.

Experience has shown that, on an individual basis, the best method of contraception is one that is acceptable and comfortable to both sexual partners, is readily available, is convenient and easy to use, is effective and safe, is inexpensive, does not interfere with the enjoyment of sex acts, and will be used consistently and correctly. These factors should be explored with persons seeking assistance with birth control.

Access to contraceptives for minors is a legal issue. Nurses need to be aware of federal and state laws about the constitutional right of adolescents to access to contraceptives. It is advisable when possible to involve a parent in the process.

It is essential to counsel people with more than one sexual partner to use condoms for all forms of penetration until the epidemiology of acquired immune deficiency syndrome (AIDS) and other sexually transmitted diseases is more completely known. However, no form of contraception provides complete protection from the risk of sexually transmitted disease.

CONTRACEPTIVE EFFECTIVENESS

Individuals are usually more concerned with effectiveness than any other factor when deciding among contraceptive methods. The most current way of understanding contraceptive effectiveness looks at lowest expected, typical, and lowest reported failure rate during the first year of use of a method, and first-year continuation rates (Table 54-6). The table applies to the first year a contraceptive is used and answers the question: "Of 100 women who start to use a method and continue use unless they fail, how many will become pregnant in the first year?" *Lowest effective failure rate* is the effectiveness of a method when used correctly, without error and according to instructions. *Typical failure rate* takes into consideration those who use the method correctly and incorrectly. All types of effectiveness rates must be presented when providing contraceptive counseling.

FACTORS AFFECTING TYPICAL CONTRACEPTIVE FAILURE RATE

Fear of method
Difficulty remembering to use method
Past unsuccessful attempts with method
Inability to use method as counseled
Unanswered questions or concerns
Cost
Side effects
Complications
Embarrassment
Inconsistency with personal beliefs

Changes in the technology of contraceptives will change lowest expected failure rates in the future. The typical failure rate of a specific contraceptive method may be lowered by numerous factors (see box below, left).

ROLE OF THE NURSE

In many settings, nurses take an active role in managing birth control programs. The nurse's role includes history taking, physical examination, counseling, and evaluating the effectiveness of various methods of birth control during follow-up visits. The nurse should include teaching efficacy concepts and numbers to patients:

1. Efficacy numbers must be understood in concept; for example, it would be unfair to tell a young teenager that oral contraceptives are 98% effective when they rarely are that effective in her age group.
2. Be consistent and neutral.
3. Explain that technology fails.
4. If two methods are used consistently, the risk of accidental pregnancy is significantly lowered.

In some settings nurses in extended roles prescribe the method of birth control. All nurses dealing with women of childbearing age in outpatient and inpatient settings need to assess and evaluate the use or nonuse of birth control by their clients. A 28-year-old woman admitted with kidney stones to a medical division has the same need for birth control information as a woman who just gave birth on a maternity division. Nurses cannot assume that a woman who has given birth is knowledgeable about birth control (see research box below).

Counseling of individuals or couples about birth control goes beyond teaching them how to use a method correctly. If couples are to accept the responsibility for conception control, nurses need to assess the extent to which misunderstanding, superstition, and fear may be factors and to take action by presenting facts about reproduction as well as facts about contraceptive meth-

RESEARCH

Panzarine S and Gould C: Knowledge about contraceptive use and conception among a group of urban, black, and adolescent mothers, J Obstet Gynecol Neonatal Nurs 17:279-282, 1988.

This study explored the knowledge that 62 urban, black, low-income adolescent mothers had about contraceptive use and conception. The majority had poor knowledge about conception and contraceptive use. Seventeen adolescents answered more than one half of six knowledge scale items incorrectly. Misinformation existed about methods of birth control other than oral contraceptives and about ineffective methods of pregnancy prevention. Increasing age was not related to greater knowledge. ■

ods. For example, lay people sometimes confuse contraception, which is temporary and reversible, with sterilization, and the differences need to be pointed out to them.

Individuals may have many questions about contraception, and the nurse can anticipate some of the following that are frequently asked:

1. What methods are most effective in preventing pregnancy?
2. How safe are the available methods? Will they harm the couple, the individual, or a future child?
3. Will contraception interfere with sexual intercourse in any way?
4. Do the methods hamper or prevent later desired pregnancies?
5. How convenient are the different methods?
6. What is the cost of different methods?

Often nurses must initiate the discussion about conception control, although this is now a commonly expressed concern of clients. In many instances women who are hesitant to pose questions about birth control are relieved when nurses indicate that this is an acceptable concern.

DATA FOR COUNSELING AND TEACHING

Direct or indirect questions may be used to initiate discussions. Questions may be more direct; that is, "Would you like help in planning your family?" "Do you want help in preventing pregnancy before you are ready for another child?" "Do you want information about birth control?" Questions can also be posed more indirectly and individualized for the patients' circumstances.

Pamphlets can be placed where patients have access to them, and this often gives the nurse a cue to the patient's interest. To verify this the nurse might say, "I noticed you looking at this pamphlet. What information or help can I give you?"

The records of hospitalized patients are a source of information about the patient's history, physical condition, and reason for current hospitalization. The medical and nursing records should be reviewed before the nurse offers assistance with birth control and family planning.

During the interview and physical examination, the patient's reliability is assessed. Ability to recall facts or to give information readily may give clues as to the most reliable method for the patient. For example, a woman who states she is taking vitamins but often forgets them, or a woman who, when questioned about self-medication, states she hates taking pills or does not believe in medicines may not be the best candidate for oral contraceptives. Although judgment about reliability needs to be reserved until follow-up visits reveal a repeated pattern of missed pills, the initial interview will alert the nurse to question the woman carefully during future visits.

Physical examination is directed toward discovering conditions that indicate which methods of contraception should not be used and why. During the examination, opportunities for health teaching arise, and nurses can take advantage of these. All women seeking assistance for conception prevention should have a Pap test and breast examination and should be encouraged to have an annual physical examination. In addition, serology and cervical smears and cultures are usually taken to detect infections, and individuals can be instructed at this time about how to prevent infection, how to recognize infection, and the need for medical care when infection occurs.

Finally, it is especially important that the woman's value system is respected even though it may not be congruent with that of the health care provider. The decisions about family size need to be made by the woman, not by the health professional.

METHODS OF CONTRACEPTION

When assisting patients to select a method of birth control, personal beliefs and biases must be avoided. The nurse's personal opinions about preferred methods may be dangerous to the patient's health and may force the patient to follow a practice not really desired; this in turn may result in the pregnancy the patient wishes to avoid. Information is given about each method, how the method works, the degree of protection against pregnancy provided by the method, self-care requirements, side effects of the method, contraindications to use, and the need for follow-up care (Tables 54-6 and 54-7). Information is repeated in the same way for each method. Once the patient has selected a method, information about that method is reviewed again. The patient should then demonstrate a complete understanding of the chosen contraceptive method.

HORMONAL CONTRACEPTIVES

Use

It has been estimated that 56 million women worldwide are using oral contraceptives ("the pill"), including 10 million women in the United States. Twenty percent to 40% of women of childbearing age in developed countries have used oral contraceptives to prevent conception. Twenty-five percent to 50% of women who begin taking birth control pills discontinue use of the pills within 1 year.[17] The majority of these women discontinue the pills for nonmedical reasons. Because of the high rate of discontinuation, every women receiving the pills is encouraged to think about an alternative method and receive instructions in the proper use of that method.

Many women using the pill are incorrectly or poorly informed about the correct use and side effects of the drug. According to a study of women using oral contra-

TABLE 54-7 Summary of major reversible methods of conception control

Method	Action	Effects

HORMONAL CONTRACEPTIVES
 	
Combination pill (estrogen and progestin
IM long-acting progestin
Low-dose oral progestin (minipill)
	ESTROGENIC EFFECTS
	
	Inhibit ovulation by suppression of pituitary FSH and LH
	Inhibit implantation by antiprogestational effect on uterus with high doses
	May accelerate ovum transport
	Prevent normal implantation and placental attachment by causing degeneration of corpus luteum and decreasing serum progesterone levels
	
	PROGESTIN EFFECTS
	
	Produce hostile cervical mucus, hampering transport of sperm and decreasing ability of sperm to penetrate cervical mucus
	May inhibit implantation by altering FSH and LH peaks
	May inhibit ovulation via subtle disturbance in hypothalamic-pituitary ovarian functioning
		BENEFICIAL EFFECTS
		
		Combination pill
		  Relief of premenstrual tension
		  Regulation of menstrual cycles
		  Relief of acne (80%-90%)
		  Increased sex drive
		  Improved feeling of well-being
		  ↓ Incidence of functional ovarian cysts
		  ↓ Fibrocystic breast disease and breast fibroadenomas
		  ↓ Endometrial and ovarian cancer
		  ↓ Pelvic inflammatory disease
		Pill and IM progestin
		  ↓ Incidence of iron deficiency anemia
		Pill, IM progestin, and minipill
		  Relief of dysmenorrhea (60%-90%)
		  ↓ Amount of blood and number of days of bleeding
		
		FAIRLY MINOR SIDE EFFECTS
		
		Pill
		  Breast tenderness, and increased breast size
		  Nausea
		  ↑ Incidence of yeast infection
		  Chloasma, cyclic weight gain
		Pill and IM progestin
		  Weight gain, mild headache
		  Mood changes, depression
		IM progestin
		  Decreased libido
		Pill, IM progestin, and minipill
		  Spotting, missed periods
		
		SERIOUS SIDE EFFECTS
		
		Pill
		  Hypertension
		  Gallbladder disease
		  Thromboembolic disorders

IUDS
 	
Lippes loop
Saf-T-Coil
Copper-7
Copper-T
Progestasert-T
	Unknown
	Suggested mechanisms
	  ↑ Motility of ovum in fallopian tube
	  Local foreign body inflammatory response preventing implantation and/or causing lysis of blastocyst
	  Immobilization of sperm
	  Mechanical dislodging of implanted blastocyst
	  Copper may interfere with estrogen uptake and its intracellular effects on endometrium
	  Progestin-induced thick mucus
	  Endometrial suppression and inhibition by disruption of proliferative-secretory maturation process with progestin
		Spotting
		↑ Amount of blood and length of bleeding: hemorrhage, irregular menstrual flow
		Anemia
		Cramping pain
		May expel IUD
		Uterine perforation or embedding
		Cervical perforation
		Pelvic inflammatory disease: endometritis, salpingitis, oophoritis, peritonitis, tubo-ovarian abscess, sepsis
		Ectopic pregnancy

Absolute Contraindications	Strong Relative Contraindications	Other Relative Contraindications
ALL HORMONAL CONTRACEPTIVES	**COMBINATION PILL**	**COMBINATION PILL**
History of cerebral vascular accident, coronary artery disease, hepatic adenoma, malignancy of breast or reproductive tract, thromboembolic disorder, estrogen-dependent neoplasia	Diabetes mellitus or strong family history of diabetes	History of cardiac or renal disease
Impaired liver function	Elective surgery within 4 wk	Unreliability to follow instructions (e.g., mental retardation)
Pregnancy	Fibrocystic breast disease or breast fibroadenomas	History of taking pills incorrectly
Undiagnosed abnormal vaginal bleeding	Gallbladder disease, active	Irregular menstrual cycle, infertility
	Hypertension with resting diastolic pressure >110 mm Hg or resting systolic pressure >140 mm Hg on three or more occasions	Lactation
	Long leg casts or major injury to lower leg	Use with caution if history of depression, hypertension with resting diastolic pressure 90-100 mm Hg, asthma, epilepsy, acne, uterine fibromyomata, varicose veins, hair loss related to pregnancy
	Mononucleosis, with acute phase over age 35	45+ years of age
	Severe vascular or migraine headaches	Term pregnancy terminated within past 10-14 days
	Sickle cell disease	Recent impaired liver function
	40+ years with a second risk factor for cardiovascular disease development	Strong family history of diabetes
	35+ years with heavy smoking	Previous cholestasis during pregnancy
	Weight gain of ≥10 lbs on pill	
Active pelvic infection	Pelvic infection (recent or recurrent)	Cervical stenosis, malignancy or premalignancy
Pregnancy	Acute cervicitis or vaginitis	Small or bicornuate uterus
Gonorrhea and chlamydia (known or suspected)	History of ectopic pregnancy	Endometriosis
	Concern for future fertility	Fibromyomata, leiomyomata
	Abnormal Pap test	Endometrial polyps or malignancy
	Diabetes mellitus	Severe dysmenorrhea or menorrhagia (Progestasert-T may be helpful)
	Steroid therapy	Anemia
	Blood coagulation disorders	Psychologic or intellectual inability to check for danger signals or string
	Abnormal bleeding (undiagnosed)	Valvular heart disease
	Multiple sex partners by woman or partner	Allergy to copper
	Postpartum endometriosis	Previous problems with IUD expulsion
		Past history of sexually transmitted disease
		Vaginal infection

Continued

TABLE 54-7 Summary of major reversible methods of conception control—cont'd

Method	Action	Effects
CONDOM		
Thin, comfortable plastic sheath worn over penis	Mechanical barrier to prevent transmission of semen into vagina	Reduced glans sensitivity Protection against sexually transmitted disease Possible prevention of cancer of cervix
DIAPHRAGM (WITH SPERMICIDE)		
Rubber dome attached to flexible metal ring; inserted into vagina to cover cervix	Mechanical barrier to ↓ contact between semen and cervix Spermicide kills sperm	Bladder pressure, pelvic discomfort, urethral irritation, urinary retention, uterine cramps Protects against sexually transmitted diseases and pelvic inflammatory disease May have some protective effect against development of cervical dysplasia Toxic shock syndrome Recurrent urinary tract infection Allergy to rubber and spermicide
CHEMICAL CONTRACEPTIVES: SPERMICIDES		
Foam, jelly, cream, suppository applied inside vagina by means of plunger-type applicator	Chemical immobilizes and kills sperm Contains medium to hold spermicide in vagina against cervix—mechanically blocks cervix and prevents entry of sperm	May irritate genitalia Unpleasant taste Foam decreases transmission of gonorrhea and trichomoniasis Provides vaginal lubrication
FERTILITY AWARENESS		
Calendar method Basal body temperature Cervical mucus	Sexual abstinence around time of ovulation	↑ Understanding/appreciation of own body Frustration May have lack of sexual gratification during abstinence if other lovemaking techniques not used

ceptives, most of them read the labeling and package insert and found the information useful, but after reading this information some women were still inadequately informed about correct use and side effects. When questioned, these women preferred getting information about oral contraceptives from health professionals. Merely handing printed information to clients and telling them to read it is inadequate. Such a procedure should be accompanied by verbal information and questioning to determine the accuracy and degree of knowledge about oral contraceptives. The printed information can then be used by the patient for future reference.

Types of Hormonal Contraceptives

Most hormonal contraceptives are taken orally. Birth control pills today most commonly contain 30 to 35 µg of an estrogen and 1 mg or less of a progestin (com-

paired to 100 to 150 µg of estrogen and 1 to 10 mg of a progestin used in the 1960s). Minipills, used by less than 5% of women taking oral contraceptives, do not contain estrogen and have less than 1 mg of a progestin. The *biphasic* pill was introduced in 1982. The estrogen content remains the same throughout the cycle and the progestin content differs from the first 10 days to the next 11 days. Ortho-Novum 10/11 provides 0.5 mg of norethindrone for the first 10 days of the cycle and 1.0 mg for the next 11 days.

Triphasic pills were introduced in the United States in 1983. The estrogen content of 0.035 mg remains the same throughout the cycle, but the progestin content differs. There are three triphasics available: Traphasil, Ortho-Novum 7/7/7, and Try-Norinyl. Advantages of triphasics are less progestin, fewer metabolic effects related to the progestin, and increased physician and pa-

Absolute Contraindications	Strong Relative Contraindications	Other Relative Contraindications
Allergy of either partner to rubber Inability of man to obtain an erection	None	Psychological inability to enjoy intercourse
History of toxic shock syndrome Allergy to rubber or spermicide Recurrent urinary tract infections Inability to obtain proper fitting as a result of uterine prolapse, cystocele, rectocele, extreme fixed uterine retroversion, vaginal fistula or septae Transient severe pelvic or introital pain Poor vaginal muscle tone Vaginal lesions or deep lacerations	None	Inability of either partner to learn proper insertion technique Lack of motivation to use method correctly Aversion to touching genitalia
Allergy to spermicide Inability to learn correct diaphragm insertion Full-term pregnancy delivered within last 6-12 weeks	None	Lack of motivation to use at time of intercourse Inability to properly insert spermicide
None	Irregular menstrual cycles History of anovulatory cycle Irregular temperature charts	Unwillingness to abstain from intercourse during fertile period Inability or unwillingness to keep proper records

tient interest because they are new and different. Disadvantages include increased patient confusion with three different-colored pills per cycle, increased breakthrough bleeding and spotting, less flexibility in doubling up on pills and starting on a day other than the day recommended on the package insert, and providing pills for more than 21 consecutive days.

The major synthetic estrogen steroid used in oral contraceptives is ethinyl estradiol. Six types of progestins, all 19-nortestosterone derivatives, are used. Major progestins are either norgestrel or norethindrone. The mechanism of action of the naturally occurring hormones compared to the synthetic hormones differs with respect to metabolism, binding properties, excretion, intracellular transport, and behavior in body fluids.[46]

Long-acting progestin injections (medroxyprogester-

one acetate [Depo-Provera] and norethindrone ethanate [Noristerat]) are used by approximately 5 million women in 130 countries. Women using this method receive an injection every 3 months. There is considerable controversy concerning the serious side effects of these drugs and the paternalism often involved in their prescription; as advocates, nurses cannot ignore these issues. *Subdermal* implants are approved in Sweden and Finland and could be approved by the FDA for use in the United States in 1990. Norplant implants are nonbiodegradable silastic capsules or rods that release levonorgestrel. Capsules are implanted under the skin of a woman's upper or lower arm through a 2 mm incision. Fifty to 80 μg of norgestrel are released daily during the first year, and 30 to 35 μg are released daily over the next 5 years.

Methods of Oral Contraceptive Administration

It was once thought that there was one right way to begin taking contraceptive pills, whereas it is now known that several approaches may be used. These approaches include:

1. Take the first pill from the first pack on the first day of bleeding during menstruation.
2. Take the first pill from the pack on the first Sunday after menstruation begins.
3. Take the first pill on the fifth day after menstruation begins.
4. Take the first pill *today* if there is no chance that pregnancy has occurred.

One pill is swallowed each day until the pack is finished. (Incidents have been reported of women inserting the pills in their vagina or giving them to their partner.) Women using the 21-day pack should stop taking pills for 1 week and start the new pack the first day of the next week. Women using the 28-day pack, with a placebo for the last 7 days, should begin the new pack when the old one is completed.

Pills work best if taken at the same time every day because this keeps estrogen and progestin at a constant level. Many women find it easier to remember taking pills if they associate taking pills with a daily activity such as bedtime or mealtime. A second birth control method should be used during the first month of taking the pill because the hormone levels may not be sufficient to suppress ovulation.

Most women will forget at some time to take one or more pills. Unfortunately "making up" pills can increase the risk of pregnancy. Low levels of estrogen and progestin resulting from missed pills may stimulate the pituitary gland to release FSH and LH, resulting in the development of a graafian follicle. If the woman takes two or three pills at one time, this causes a sharp rise in estrogen level and may trigger ovulation.

If one pill is missed, the woman should take the forgotten pill as soon as she remembers and then take the pill for the day at her regular time. If two pills are missed consecutively, two pills should be taken as soon as the woman remembers and two pills taken on the next day. Another method of contraception is necessary for the remainder of the cycle. If three or more pills are missed, ovulation will probably occur. The old pack of pills should be thrown away. A new pack of pills is started after three or more pills have been missed, and another method of birth control should be used until the new package of pills is used for 2 weeks. In this case the woman should seriously consider whether oral contraception is a good method of birth control for her. Women who have had several days of severe diarrhea, which may retard absorption of the contraceptives, should also use another method of birth control for the remainder of that cycle. There are anecdotal reports of women taking oral contraceptives conceiving while taking antibiotics. Rifampin decreases the efficacy of oral contraceptives by stimulating the liver's metabolic capacity.[46] It is recommended that women on medication that affect liver metabolism (rifampin, coumadin, phe-

TABLE 54-8 Laboratory tests affected by birth control pills

Type of Study	Increased (False-Positive) Results	Decreased (False-Negative) Results
Blood chemistry	Alkaline phosphate	
	Bilirubin, icteric index	
	Bromsulphalein (BSP) retention	
	Cholesterol	
	Glucose (fasting)	
	Glucose tolerance curve	
	^{131}I thyroid uptake (estrogen)	^{131}I thyroid uptake (progesterone)
	Iron, iron-binding capacity	
	Lipids, total	
	Lipoproteins	
	Protein-bound iodine (PBI)	Protein, total
	Serum glutamic-oxaloacetic transaminase (SGOT), serum glutamic-pyruvic transaminase (SGPT)	
	Sodium	
	Thyroxine-binding globulin	
	Thyroxine (T_4) uptake	Triiodothyronine (T_3) uptake
Hematology	Leukocyte count	Prothrombin time
	Platelet count and aggregation	
	Erythrocyte sedimentation rate (ESR)	
Urine	Porphyrins	17-Ketosteroids

nobarbital, phenytoin, carbamazepine, griseofulvin, and primidone) should use another method of contraception during treatment.

Women should also be advised about storing pills used for contraception. Appropriate places for strong pills are away from children's access and where temperature and humidity are not extremely high.

If women anticipate having multiple sexual partners, they should be encouraged to use condoms in addition to the pill because the pills do not offer a barrier to the transmission of sexually transmitted diseases (STD), including AIDS.

Follow-up Care

Women taking oral contraceptives require close supervision. Some laboratory tests, especially liver function and endocrine function tests, are altered by the use of birth control pills (Table 54-8). Birth control pills also interact with other drugs (see box at right) leading to possible decreased contraceptive effects or other side effects, and women must be monitored for adverse effects. To ensure that women will return for periodic examination, some are only given a prescription for only 1 to 3 months.

During interim care the woman is monitored for side effects and emerging problems. The most serious side effects and many of the fairly minor but annoying side effects likely to result in discontinuation of oral contraceptives are estrogen related (Table 54-9). This information can be used for instructing women about problems to report and as a guide for screening for problems during follow-up visits. Women are instructed to call their

DRUGS THAT INTERACT WITH BIRTH CONTROL PILLS[41]

Acetaminophen	Alcohol
Anticoagulants (oral)	Antidepressants
Barbiturates*	Benzodiazepine tranquilizers
Beta blockers	Carbamazepine*
Corticosteroids	Griseofulvin*
Guanethidine	Hypoglycemics
Methyldopa	Penicillin (Ampicillin*)
Phenytoin*	Primidone*
Rifampin*	Tetracycline*
Theophylline	Troleandomycin
Vitamin C	

*Decreased contraceptive effect.

health care provider if they develop one of the five symptoms (ACHES) that may signify serious trouble (Table 54-10). All women taking oral contraceptives should receive a copy of the symptoms.

The incidence of vaginal infections is higher among women using oral contraceptives because the pill alters the natural environment of the vagina. If infections occur and persist, a different oral contraceptive or an entirely different method of birth control may be needed.

Women who desire pregnancy should discontinue use of the pill and use another contraceptive until they have three spontaneous normal menstrual periods.

Women over 35 years who smoke are at highest risk for pill complications. Other predisposing risk factors are diabetes, obesity, elevated lipids and lipoproteins,

TABLE 54-9 Symptoms that may be associated with use of oral contraceptives

Due to Hormone Excess		Due to Hormone Deficiency	
Estrogen	**Progestogen**	**Estrogen**	**Progestogen**
Nausea, vomiting	Increased appetite, weight gain	Breakthrough bleeding early in cycle	Breakthrough bleeding late in cycle
Headache	Fatigue	Absence of withdrawal bleeding	Menorrhagia with clotting
Edema, weight gain	Decrease in libido	Hot flashes, nervousness	Delay of withdrawal bleeding
Vertigo	Depression	Candidal vaginitis	Weight loss
Uterine cramps	Absence of withdrawal bleeding	Dyspareunia	
Breast changes, mastalgia	Headache*		
Cervical erosion	Breast fullness*		
Cervical mucorrhea	Cholestatic jaundice		
Vein complications (e.g., thrombosis, phlebitis)	Increased tendency to thromboembolism		
Chloasma, acne, rashes	Hirsutism		
Increase in size of myoma (if present)	Loss of scalp hair		
Depression	Acneform rash		

From Effler SB: Postgrad. Med. 59:164-170, 1976.
*During medication-free period.

hypertension, and a strong family history of coronary artery disease. Women should be encouraged to limit and stop smoking because cigarette smoking has a synergistic effect with oral contraceptives and increases the woman's risk of myocardial infection, thromboembolic injury, and stroke. However, there is now considerable evidence that the pill protects against both ovarian and endometrial cancer.

INTRAUTERINE DEVICES

Intrauterine devices (IUDs) are used by approximately 85 million women worldwide and 1.4 million women in the United States.[17] IUDs that have been most widely used in the past are the Lippes loop (Figure 54-2), Saf-T-Coil, Copper-T, Copper-7, and Progestasert-T. Currently only two IUDs are being produced and distributed in the United States, the progestasert and Copper-T. The first-year failure rate in typical IUD users is 6%. The lowest expected/reported pregnancy rates in nonmedicated IUDs are 2% and 3%, respectively, and 1% and 5%, respectively, in medicated IUDs. The differences in rates of effectiveness are caused by IUD characteristics, such as form, size, amount of copper or progesterone, and to IUD-user characteristics, such as age,

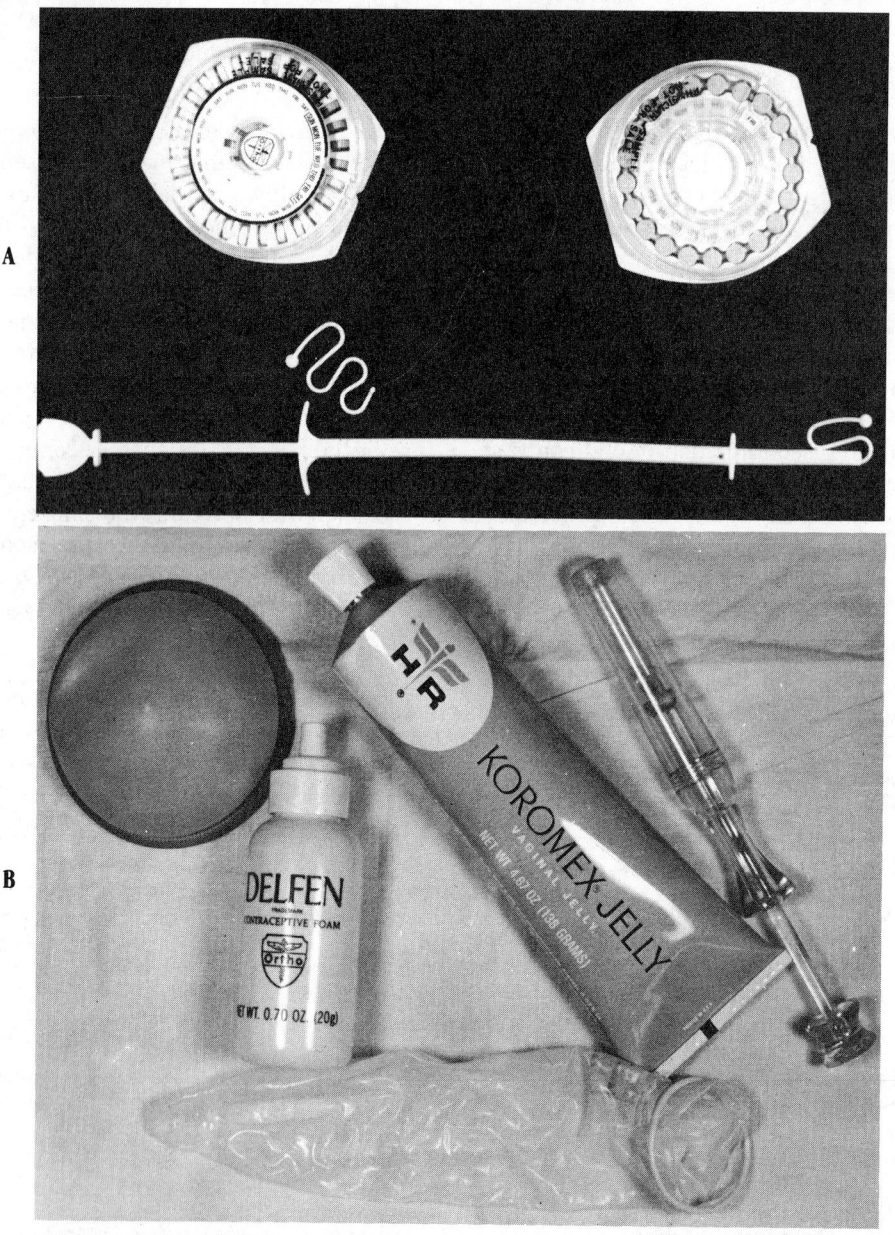

FIGURE 54-2 A, Two types of oral contraceptives and Lippes loop with applicator. **B,** (*left to right*), Diaphragm, contraceptive foam for vaginal application, contraceptive jelly and vaginal applicator, and condom.

TABLE 54-10 Symptoms that may indicate serious trouble when taking oral contraceptives

Symptom	Possible Problem
Abdominal pain, severe	Gallbladder disease, hepatic adenoma, blood clot, pancreatitis
Chest pain or shortness of breath, severe	Blood clot in lungs or myocardial infarction
Headaches, severe	Stroke, hypertension, or migraine headache
Eye problems: blurred vision, flashing lights, or blindness	Stroke, hypertension, or temporary vascular problems of many possible sites
Severe leg pain (calf or thigh)	Blood clot in legs

From Hatcher RA et al: Contraceptive technology, 1980-1981, ed 10, New York, 1980, Irvington Publishers, Inc.

parity, uterine shape and size, and frequency of intercourse. Effectiveness of IUDs is also determined by the expertise of the clinician inserting the IUD.

It is well known that women using IUDs have menstrual periods that are heavier and that they more often have intermenstrual spotting than do women using other methods of contraception. The bleeding experienced by women using IUDs may be due to spontaneous abortion. Some women using a copper-type IUD demonstrated human chorionic gonadotropin in their blood. This adds to the evidence that the IUD probably interferes with pregnancy by producing degeneration of a fertilized ovum, that fertilization of the ovum can and does occur, and that tubal pregnancy occurs more often in women using the IUD.

Women who decide to use an IUD for contraception are given a thorough explanation of the insertion procedure as well as of the side effects and potential complications. Women with a history of pelvic inflammatory disease (PID) or ectopic pregnancy and with multiple sexual partners should be discouraged from using an IUD, because of a high incidence of infertility. The IUD does not protect the woman against the virus that causes AIDS or against other sexually transmitted diseases. Some women experience cramping pain or nausea during and after insertion of the IUD. The discomforts can be relieved by bed rest, heat, and analgesics. Women using an IUD are required to feel for the string on the device before they leave the clinic or office to be sure it is still in place. The string is checked frequently (about once a week) in the first months and then after each period or if the woman is experiencing abdominal cramping.

Many women fear the device will get lost inside them, and occasionally this occurs. Showing them a model of the pelvis and how the device is situated when in place helps them overcome this fear. Informing the woman that the string becomes soft with body heat and that her sexual partner probably will not be aware of it during intercourse is usually reassuring. Use of tampons is permitted.

Pain, bleeding, or discharge in the days or weeks immediately after IUD insertion should be reported immediately, as they may be signs of infection of the uterus or fallopian tubes. Infection is most likely to develop during this period; however, it can occur at any time and usually requires IUD removal and antibiotics. IUD users also need to report inability to feel the string, if the string is shorter or longer, or if their period is late. Other symptoms to be reported include pain with intercourse, severe cramping, fever, chills, foul discharge, spotting, clots, or unusual vaginal bleeding, which may be signs of impending PID.

A Copper-T device must be replaced every 4 years because the copper loses its effectiveness. The Progestasert-T must be replaced every year because the progesterone also loses its effectiveness. The Dalkon Shield was taken off the market; any woman still wearing one should have it removed immediately.

DIAPHRAGM

The diaphragm is becoming increasingly popular because it protects the user from sexually transmitted infections. Protection against transmission of HIV is not known for the diaphragm and spermicide. There are four types of diaphragms: flat spring rim, coil spring rim, arching spring rim, and wide seal rim that comes in a variety of sizes.

Women choosing a diaphragm should receive written and verbal instruction, opportunity to practice insertion and removal, and assistance until placement is correct. Diaphragms must be used with contraceptive jelly or cream to provide maximal effectiveness. They must be inspected for holes or defects each time before use. Approximately 1 tablespoon of jelly or cream is placed into the dome and on the rim of the diaphragm up to 6 hours before intercourse. Petroleum products contained in Vaseline and some vaginal medication can damage the latex of the diaphragm. Placement of the diaphragm is checked to ascertain that the back rim of the diaphragm is below and behind the cervix and that the front edge is behind the pubic bone (Figure 54-3). Additional spermicide via an applicator is necessary after each act of intercourse. The diaphragm is not removed for 6 to 8 hours after intercourse. After removal, the diaphragm is washed in soapy water and dried before storage.

Women should see their health care providers if they experience one of the following signs indicating that the size of the diaphragm should possibly be changed: weight loss or gain greater than 5 kg (11 lb), birth, abor-

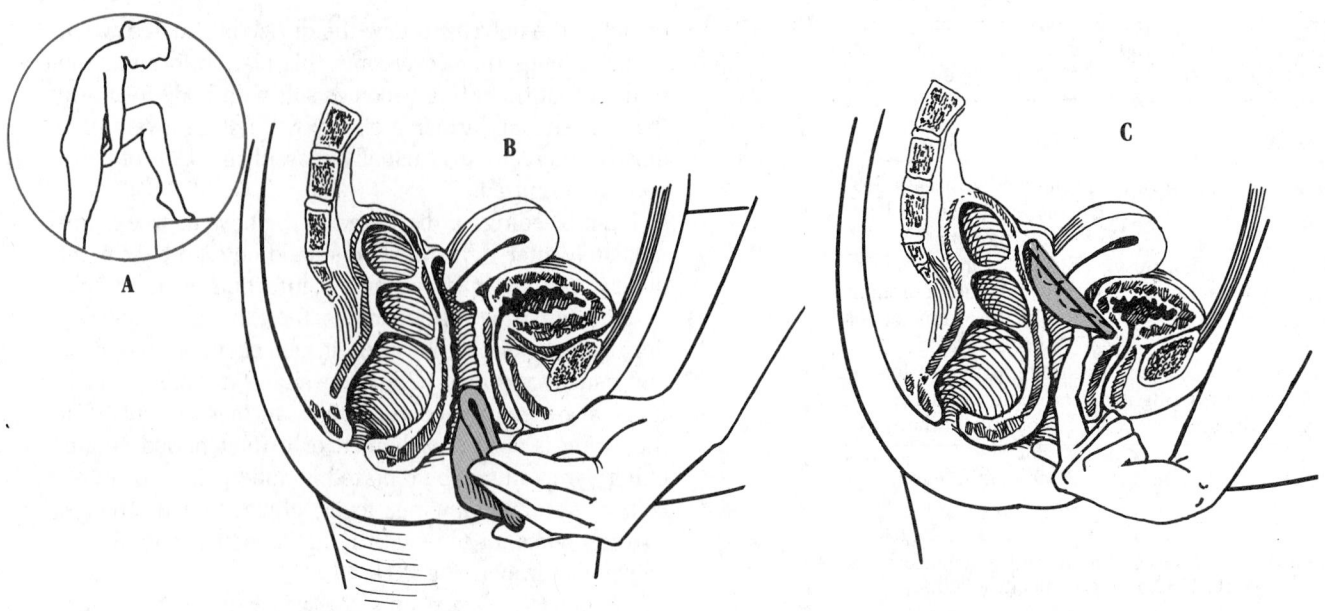

FIGURE 54-3 A, Diaphragm insertion in a standing position. **B,** Diaphragm is folded in half and inserted in vagina. **C,** The back rim is pushed behind the cervix; the front rim is slipped behind the pubic bone. The cervix is completely covered by the diaphragm.

tion, pelvic surgery, pain or discomfort caused by the diaphragm, or sensations of the diaphragm being too large or small.

To decrease the risk of developing toxic shock syndrome, women should not wear the diaphragm longer than 24 hours or during menstruation, vaginal bleeding, abnormal vaginal discharge, or the first 6 to 12 weeks after delivery. They should wash their hands with soap and water before insertion and removal of the diaphragm. If signs of toxic shock syndrome (fever greater than 101° F, diarrhea, vomiting, muscle aches, sunburnlike rash) occur, the woman should remove her diaphragm and call her health provider immediately.

The *cervical cap* is a miniature diaphragm with a dome that fits over the cervix and is held in place by suction. First-year failure rates range from 8 to 27 pregnancies per 100 women. Cervical caps have been granted FDA approval in the United States since 1988. The cervical cap can be left in place for as long as 24 hours, but should not be left in place longer because of the risk of toxic shock syndrome. The cap has great potential for use with women who want to use a diaphragm but cannot be fitted because of lax vaginal tone or marked cystocele or rectocele.

The vaginal contraceptive sponge is a small pillow-shaped polyurethane sponge containing spermicide. A concave dimple in one side fits over the cervix; the other side has a loop for removal. The sponge is moist-ened with water and then inserted into the vagina where it can provide contraception for up to 24 hours; it should be left in place for at least 6 hours. The sponge provides a barrier between sperm and the cervix, trapping the sperm in the sponge and destroying it via the spermicide. First-year failure rates range from 17 to 24.5 pregnancies/100 women. Parous sponge users are twice as likely to become pregnant as nulliparas.[32] There is only one size sponge and it is available without a prescription. The same precautions taken by diaphragm users to minimize the risk for toxic shock syndrome should be taken by women using the sponge.

CONDOM

Condoms are gaining increased acceptance due to their protection against the transmission of AIDS. Condoms are the best contraceptive available for AIDS prevention, although they do not eliminate the risk of HIV transmission. Forty-six million couples used condoms worldwide in 1987.[14] First-year failure rates among typical users is 12%.[17] Nevertheless, the health care provider should never assume that the person does not need instructions to use condoms correctly. The condom is placed on the penis before insertion in the vagina, and the rim of the condom is rolled to the base of the penis. One-half inch of empty space should be left at the tip unless the condom has a nipple tip to hold the semen. The condom is held as the penis is withdrawn. The penis should be withdrawn soon after ejaculation because loss of erection may cause the condom to slip off. If this occurs, contraceptive jelly or foam should be inserted immediately into the vagina.

Condoms may be stored away from heat for 2 years; those kept in wallets may deteriorate as a result of body heat. Petroleum jelly used as a lubricant will also cause the rubber to deteriorate. A new condom should be used each time a couple has intercourse. The spermicidal latex condom is the best condom to use to protect against transmission of the HIV virus because HIV is killed by spermicides in laboratory conditions.[17] The natural membrane or "skin" condoms do not provide as effective a barrier as latex condoms.

SPERMICIDAL FOAM AND SUPPOSITORY

There is a significant difference between lowest expected typical effectiveness and lowest reported effectiveness rates for both spermicidal foam and spermicidal suppositories (Table 54-6). First-year failures among typical users of vaginal spermicides is about 21% and contraceptive foam 0 to 36.9%.[17] The most common problem leading to accidental pregnancy is failure to use the method. It is important, therefore, for women to be taught how to use these methods correctly and consistently.

Foam

If the applicator is not preloaded, it is filled to the designated mark. When the can is shaken 20 times before using, the spermicide is mixed with the foam and there are enough bubbles to form a barrier. The applicator is inserted 3 to 4 inches into the vagina until it cannot go any farther and then withdrawn about ½ inch. The plunger is pushed to deposit the foam, and the applicator is then withdrawn. The foam is inserted no more than 30 minutes before intercourse, and additional foam must be added before each act of intercourse. The applicator is washed with soap and water.

Suppository

The spermicidal suppository is inserted high in the vagina at least 10 minutes but no longer than 1 hour before intercourse. An additional suppository must be used with each subsequent act of intercourse. The woman may feel warmth in the vagina as the suppository disintegrates. The major problem with this method of contraception is its actual use effectiveness rate of 18% to 20%.[17]

FERTILITY AWARENESS

Cyclic fertility can be evidenced by covert and overt signs that occur in fertile women. Many women can become aware of the following signs that relate to their own fertility: basal body temperature patterns, cervical mucus changes, a recorded history of menstrual dates, mittelschmerz (pain during ovulation), breast changes, placement and consistency of the cervix, mood, and sexual desire. The symptothermal method combines basal body temperature and mucus changes in the cervical os to detect ovulation (Figure 54-4).

Calendar Method

To be reliable, the calendar method (rhythm) requires that the woman be certain of the length of the menstrual cycles and the shortest and longest ranges of her cycles (Table 54-11). A woman records the length of her menstrual cycles over the preceding 8 months. The first day of bleeding is day one in each cycle. The earliest day that she is likely to be fertile is determined by subtracting 18 days from her shortest cycle. The last day she is likely to be fertile is computed by subtracting 11 days from the length of her longest cycle. The two numbers represent the beginning and end of the woman's fertile period. During the fertile period a woman may either avoid intercourse or use another method of birth control. Calculation of the fertile period is based on the following assumptions: ovulation occurs 14 days before the beginning of menstruation, sperm can survive for 2 to 3 days, and the ovum remains viable for 24 hours.

Basal Body Temperature

The basal body temperature (BBT) is the lowest body temperature of a healthy person during waking hours. A

Cycle day	Date	Basal body temperature 96 97 98 99	Vaginal discharge 0	Wet	Mucus	Blood	Premenstrual symptoms

FIGURE 54-4 Example of fertility awareness charting.

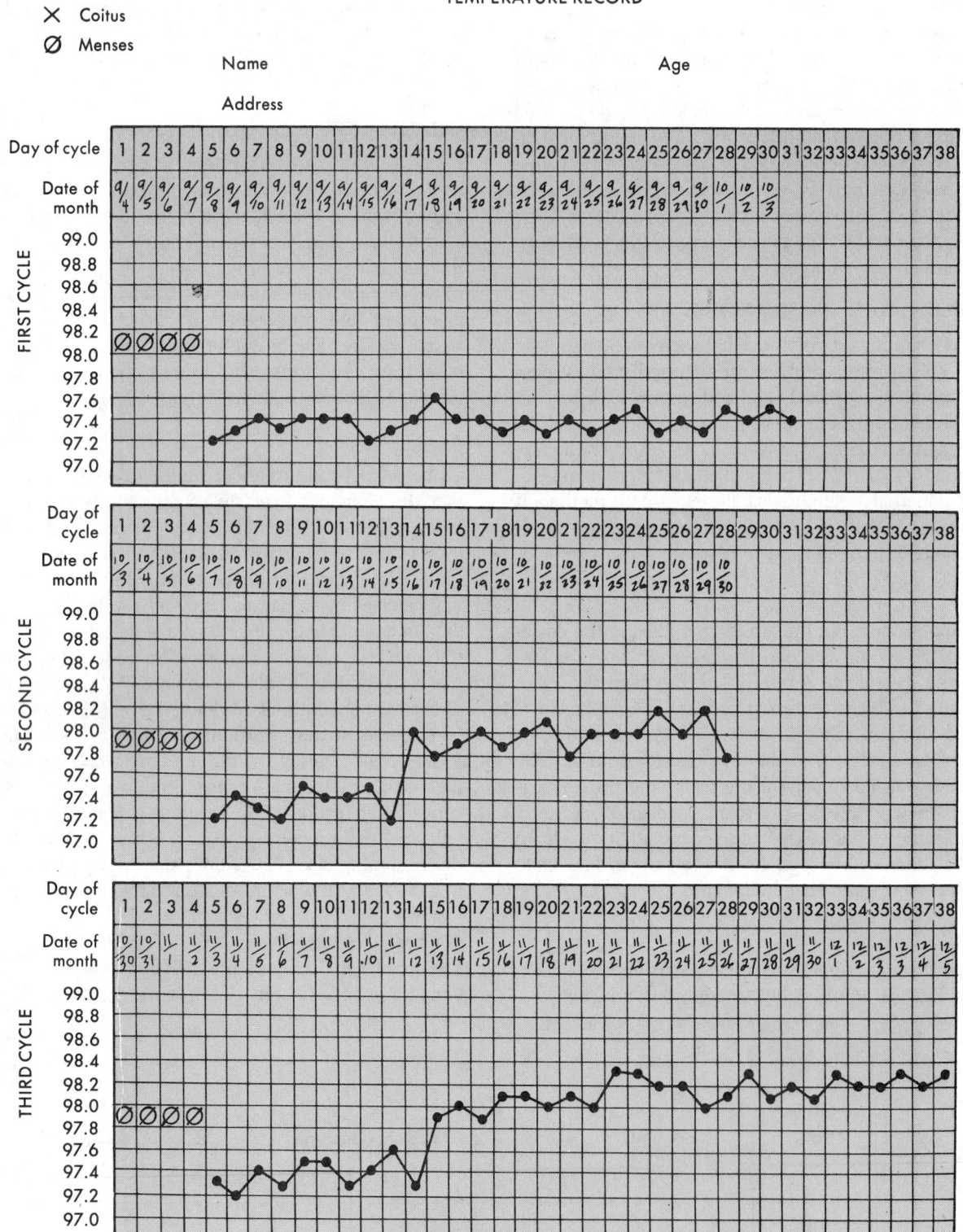

FIGURE 54-5 Basal body temperature (BBT) chart illustrating determination of ovulation. First cycle shows no midcycle rise in BBT. Second cycle shows a drop followed by a rise in BBT. Third cycle shows a BBT pattern consistent with pregnancy. (From Fogel CI and Woods NF: Health care of women: a nursing perspective St Louis, 1981, The CV Mosby Co.)

TABLE 54-11 Ovulation and the menstrual cycle

Shortest Cycle (in Days)	First Unsafe Day	Longest Cycle (in Days)	Last Unsafe Day
20	2nd	20	9th
21	3rd	21	10th
22	4th	22	11th
23	5th	23	12th
24	6th	24	13th
25	7th	25	14th
26	8th	26	15th
27	9th	27	16th
28*	10th*	28	17th
29	11th	29	18th
30	12th	30*	19th*
31	13th	31	20th
32	14th	32	21st
33	15th	33	22nd
34	16th	34	23rd
35	17th	35	24th
36	18th	36	25th

*Example: A woman whose cycles range from 28 to 30 days has her first "unsafe" day on the tenth day after the start of any period and her last "unsafe" day on the nineteenth day after the start of any period.

woman can determine when she ovulates by taking her temperature daily immediately after waking and before any activity, and recording it on a chart for 3 to 4 months (Figure 54-5). Some health care providers suggest using a special BBT thermometer, whereas others believe that a regular thermometer is adequate. This method is based on two temperature variations. Immediately preceding ovulation, some women's BBT drops slightly or remains the same. A noticeable rise in temperature occurs 24 to 72 hours after ovulation and remains elevated until menstruation.

A woman should avoid intercourse or use another contraceptive method until her temperature has remained elevated (a rise of 0.4° to 0.8° F above her normal BBT) for 3 consecutive days. Temperature elevations may not signify ovulation in cases of infections, irregular sleeping hours, or use of an electric blanket.

Cervical Mucus

Cervical mucus changes in amount, color, viscosity, spinnbarkeit (ability to stretch), and ferning pattern throughout the menstrual cycle (Table 54-12). A woman can observe these physical changes to determine when she is fertile. During ovulation the cervical mucus will be most abundant, clear, very thin and slippery, and very stretchable and will exhibit a well-developed ferning pattern (Figure 54-6). This is caused by a low saline content and high estrogen level.

The woman checks her vagina each day to notice wetness and if mucus is present. As soon as any mucus is present or wetness is noticed, she should consider herself fertile. The last fertile day should be the fourth day after the woman's peak day (last day of wetness and abundant, clear, slippery mucus). Intercourse should be avoided or another method of birth control used during the fertile period. The mucous pattern may be undetectable with vaginal infection, douching, use of contraceptive foams or jelly, or if semen is present in the vagina.

The fertile awareness methods of contraception can also be used to help women become pregnant. The BBT and mucous changes can be recorded to find the most fertile day of the woman's cycle.

FUTURE METHODS OF CONTRACEPTION

As research continues to provide insight into the control of female and male fertility, new methods of contraception will become available. In the *female,* it is known that the pituitary secretes LH and FSH in response to a signal from the hypothalamic releasing factors. Research is currently being conducted to produce hypothalamic releasing factors and compounds that could block the releasing factors.

Injectable progestin products using biodegradable copolymers are being developed that provide a daily release rate for 1, 3, or 6 months. Products being studied contain norethindrone, levonorgestrel, natural progesterone, and norgestimate. It is predicted that five new methods using a progestin will be available in the United States before the year 2000.[17] Other future technology includes biodegradable implants placed under the skin that dissolve over time, injectable microspheres

TABLE 54-12 Cervical mucus characteristics

Time of Cycle	Amount	Color	Viscosity	Spinnbarkeit	Ferning
Postmenstruation	Moderate	Cloudy, yellow or white	Thick	Small	None
Preovulation	Increasing	Clearing	Thinning	Increasing	Increasing
Ovulation	Greatest	Clear	Very thin and slippery	Greatest	Greatest
Postovulation	Decreasing	Becoming cloudy	Thickening	Decreasing	Decreasing or none
Premenstruation	Small	Cloudy	Thick	Small	None

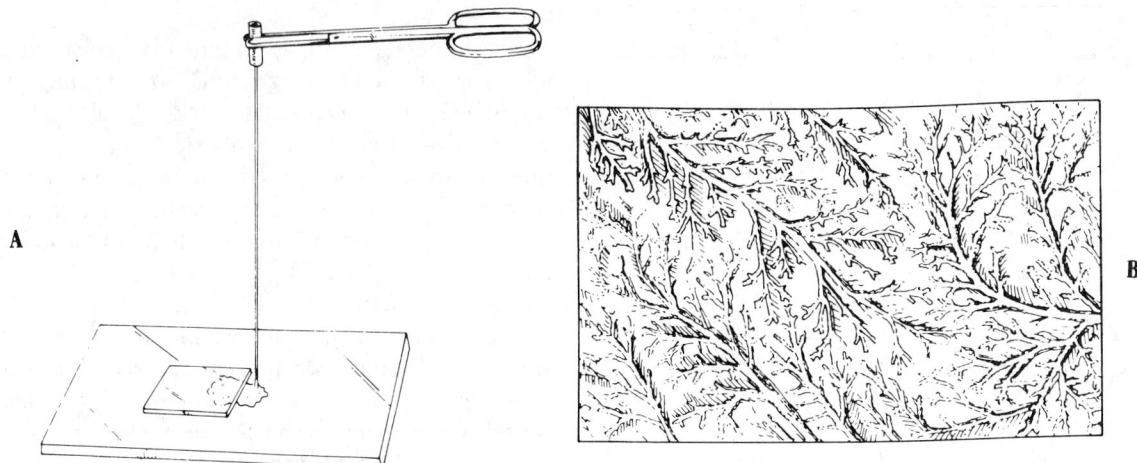

FIGURE 54-6 A, Spinnbarkeit. At midcycle the mucus resembles raw egg white, being clear, stretchy, and slippery. It will stretch without breaking or spin a thread. **B,** Ferning. When allowed to dry on a slide, the midcycle mucus gives a fern or palm-leaf pattern. (From Fogel CI and Woods NF: Health care of women, St Louis, 1981, The CV Mosby Co.)

and microcapsules containing hormones, monthly injectables containing hormones, vaginal rings containing hormones, postcoital contraceptives, an antifertility vaccine, and intracervical implant to neutralize sperm.

Most researchers believe that there will not be a *male* contraceptive in the United States in the next 5 years. This is in part a result of politics because some men equate fertility with potency. Significantly more money is spent doing research on female contraception than male contraception. Testosterone and progesterone, both inhibitors of spermatogenesis, have been used but have the following complications: slow acting, diminished return of fertility, and difficulty in the administration method. Gossypol, a phenolic compound derived from the seed, stem, or roots of cotton plants, has been used successfully since 1972 in China as an oral antifertility agent for men. Potential side effects are hypokalemia, cardiac arrhythmias, weakness, and, rarely, a decreased libido. Other future male methods of contraception include vas deferens blockade, and LH-RH analogs with androgens.

DISCONTINUING CONTRACEPTION

When a nurse counsels couples about birth control, it is important to make notations about their plans for having children and their desired family size. In this way couples can be advised about the appropriate time for discontinuing contraception. Removal of an IUD restores fertility immediately or within 1 to 2 months. After long-term use of oral contraceptives, about 75% of women are able to become pregnant within 1 year after discontinuing the pill. With all other temporary methods, fertility is restored immediately after the method is discontinued.

It is generally accepted that, for preservation of health, pregnancy and childbirth should be spaced to avoid the consequences of stress on the body. Most experts believe that an interval of at least 2 years between pregnancies is desirable. In the years between pregnancies, every effort needs to be made to improve and maintain health so that when pregnancy does occur the woman is more likely to face fewer risks and the fetus is more likely to have a better chance for growth and development in a healthful environment. To these ends, nurses can make a valuable contribution to the health of women and children.

STERILIZATION

In addition to the conception control methods mentioned above, voluntary sterilization has become increasingly acceptable to both men and women as a method of preventing pregnancy. It is the most commonly used method of fertility control for married couples over 30 years of age[17] and is the most widely used contraceptive method worldwide, protecting approximately 100 million couples. It has been estimated that greater than 13.7 million adults have been sterilized in the United States, and 100 million worldwide. Every year approximately 100,000 American women elect surgical sterilization. In addition, each year between 500,000 and 1,000,000 American men have vasectomies.

A profile of men and women seeking sterilization indicates they come from all strata of society, are between 25 and 50 years of age, are married, have large families, and are likely to be white and of the Protestant faith. The primary reason given by both men and women for wishing sterilization is a desire to limit family size. Other reasons include financial inability to support a large family, concern over population growth, problems with other methods of contraception, and age, with some couples preferring personal freedom over the risk of childbearing with advancing age. More frequently than women, men give as an important reason for sterilization their wish for an effective contraceptive that does not interfere with sexual pleasure. Also, men express concern over the health of their sex partners. Some men whose sexual partners (including wives) use oral contraceptives feel that the pill is actually or potentially harmful to the woman.

Medical indications for sterilization broadly include any condition or situation in which pregnancy would be attended by risks to health or life of the woman or her infant. Included in this category are severe heart disease and diabetes and probable genetic defects in the infant.

The laws governing sterilization vary from state to state and have undergone many changes. In general, if the surgery does not violate specific state provisions and if written, informed consent is given by a man or woman legally capable of giving permission, the surgery can be performed by a physician. Since sterilization is a permanent method of contraception, it is absolutely nec-

essary to obtain voluntary, informed consent. Patients using federal funds for sterilization must be at least 21 years old and mentally competent. There may be a prescribed waiting period for patients using Medicaid funds before the sterilization procedure can take place.

METHODS

Over 200 different techniques have been developed since the first tubal sterilization was performed in 1823.[39] Most methods of sterilization (Table 54-13) involve mechanical removal of a part of the male or female reproductive system so that the sperm and ovum cannot unite. The most common surgical procedure for elective sterilization of women is tubal sterilization. Hysterectomy is being performed for this purpose but should be done only when there are other indications for removal of the uterus. Bilateral salpingectomy, bilateral oophorectomy, and pelvic radiation in large doses also bring about cessation of childbearing, although the primary purposes of these procedures are not sterilization.

ABDOMINAL TUBAL STERILIZATION

Tubal sterilization can be accomplished by different surgical techniques. There are 100 variations of the abdominal approach, but the two primary methods are the minilaparotomy and the laparoscopic approach.[17] In the *minilaparotomy* a small (2 to 3 cm) transverse abdominal incision is made below the umbilicus in postpartum women or approximately 3 cm above the pubis in nonpregnant women. The peritoneal cavity is entered, and

TABLE 54-13 Methods of sterilization

Method	Description	Comments
FEMALE		
Tubal Sterilization		
Abdominal		
Minilaparotomy	Ligation or cutting of fallopian tubes under direct vision through small abdominal incision	Local or general anesthesia Complications: wound infection, hematoma, bladder injury Advantages: good chance for sterility reversal
Laparoscopy	Electrocoagulation of segment of fallopian tubes by laparoscopy through small abdominal incision	Local or general anesthesia Advantages: minimal discomfort, short procedure
Vaginal		
Culpotomy	Ligation or cutting of fallopian tube through small incision in cul-de-sac of Douglas	Local, spinal, or general anesthesia Higher complication rate than laparoscopy (infection, hemorrhage)
Culdoscopy	Electrocoagulation of segment of fallopian tubes by culdoscope through small incision in cul-de-sac of Douglas	Local anesthesia Higher complication rate than laparoscopy
MALE		
Vasectomy	Removal of a segment of vas deferens through small incision in scrotum	Local anesthesia Complications rare Bruising, mild edema, and mild discomfort common

the fallopian tubes are located. A loop of the midportion of the tube is elevated and the loop is ligated at the base. A small piece of each fallopian tube is excised. Cauterization can be performed, or the end of the tube may be tied off. This procedure may be performed as ambulatory surgery. A local or general anesthetic is given. Complications after minilaparotomy are wound infection, hematoma, medication reaction, and bladder injury. The major advantages are the relatively nondestructive nature of the procedure and relatively good chance for future reanastomosis if sterilization reversal is requested.

Laparoscopic tubal sterilization is more frequently performed than minilaparotomy and requires only a very small subumbilical incision for the purpose of introducing the laparoscope through the abdominal wall. A segment of each tube is grasped with forceps, and an electric current is passed through the forceps to bring about coagulation of the tissues, or clips or rings are applied to the tube. A local or general anesthetic may be used, and postoperative pain is minimal. Advantages of laparoscopy are its safety, minimal discomfort, small amount of time required to perform the procedure and for recovery, and inexpensiveness as compared to those procedures requiring hospitalization.

Tubal sterilization using one of the abdominal approaches is often performed in the early postpartum period or at the time of cesarean section, since the fallopian tubes have not descended into the pelvis and are more readily accessible at this time.

VAGINAL TUBAL STERILIZATION

Vaginal tubal sterilization is rarely performed today. Currently, culpotomy and culdoscopy are the two types of vaginal approaches in tubal ligation. *Culpotomy* is performed by way of a small incision in the cul-de-sac of Douglas with the woman in the lithotomy position. Each oviduct is brought into view, ligated, and cut. A general, conduction (caudal or spinal) or local anesthetic is used. No hospitalization is required. The complication rate of culpotomy is twice that of laparoscopy and has been attributed to increased rates of infection and hemorrhage.

The *culdoscopic* method is an endoscopic approach through the cul-de-sac of Douglas. The fallopian tubes are coagulated by means of an electric current under local anesthesia. The culdoscopic method results in little postoperative pain and a short period of hospitalization.

Successful sterilization (conception prevented) depends on the technique used, the health professional's experience in performing the procedure, other surgical factors, and the length of tube removed. The main causes of failure are recanalization of the fallopian tube, erroneous ligation, and pregnancy resulting from tubo-peritoneal fistula.

VASECTOMY

Bilateral vasectomy (Figure 54-7) is the surgical procedure for accomplishing sterilization of men. At least 11 techniques are described to accomplish what is generally considered to be a safe, simple procedure. Two reasons probably account for the variety of techniques developed. The first is the tendency of the vas deferens to rejoin spontaneously, a distressing long-term complication. The second reason centers around developing techniques having potential reversibility.

Bilateral partial vasectomy is the surgical method most often used. Because of its safety and simplicity, the procedure is most often performed on an outpatient basis in a clinic or a physician's office using a local anesthetic. A small incision is made in the scrotum to expose the sheath of the vas. The sheath is opened, the vas deferens is exposed, and a segment measuring 0.63 to 1.27 cm is removed. The segmented ends of the vas are then ligated. Some physicians prefer to coagulate the severed ends of the vas to ensure sterility. The incision is then closed by suturing.

Complications after vasectomy are rare and minor when they do occur. Most of the complications are preventable by using proper anesthetic doses, aseptic technique, and counseling against strenuous exercise for 1 to 2 days after the procedure. Bruising, mild edema, and mild discomfort are common and usually subside without treatment. Infection of the wound occurs in about 3% of patients. Hematoma, epididymitis, and granuloma formation may occur. The incidence of failure as a result of recanalization is reported to be between 0% and 6%.[40] The cause of spontaneous recanalization (reanastomosis) is unknown, but duplication of the vas has occasionally been noted. The literature does not report any occurrences of mortality from vasectomy.

After vasectomy, antibodies to sperm develop in about 50% to 66% of men.[17] There has not been any relationship found in humans between the presence of sperm antibodies and any systemic pathologic condition. In some studies with samples of 5 to 10 monkeys, atherosclerosis has developed more extensively in vasectomized monkeys. It is hypothesized that antisperm antibodies formed after vasectomy may result in circulating immune complexes that exacerbate atherosclerosis. A relationship between vasectomy and atherosclerotic changes in humans has been found.

PHYSIOLOGIC EFFECTS

Although tubal sterilization usually terminates a woman's ability to bear children, usually ovarian hormones and menstrual functioning are not altered and an artificial menopause is not induced. Ability to derive satisfaction from sexual intercourse should not be impaired, and some women may experience greater enjoyment from intercourse with the removal of fear of pregnancy.

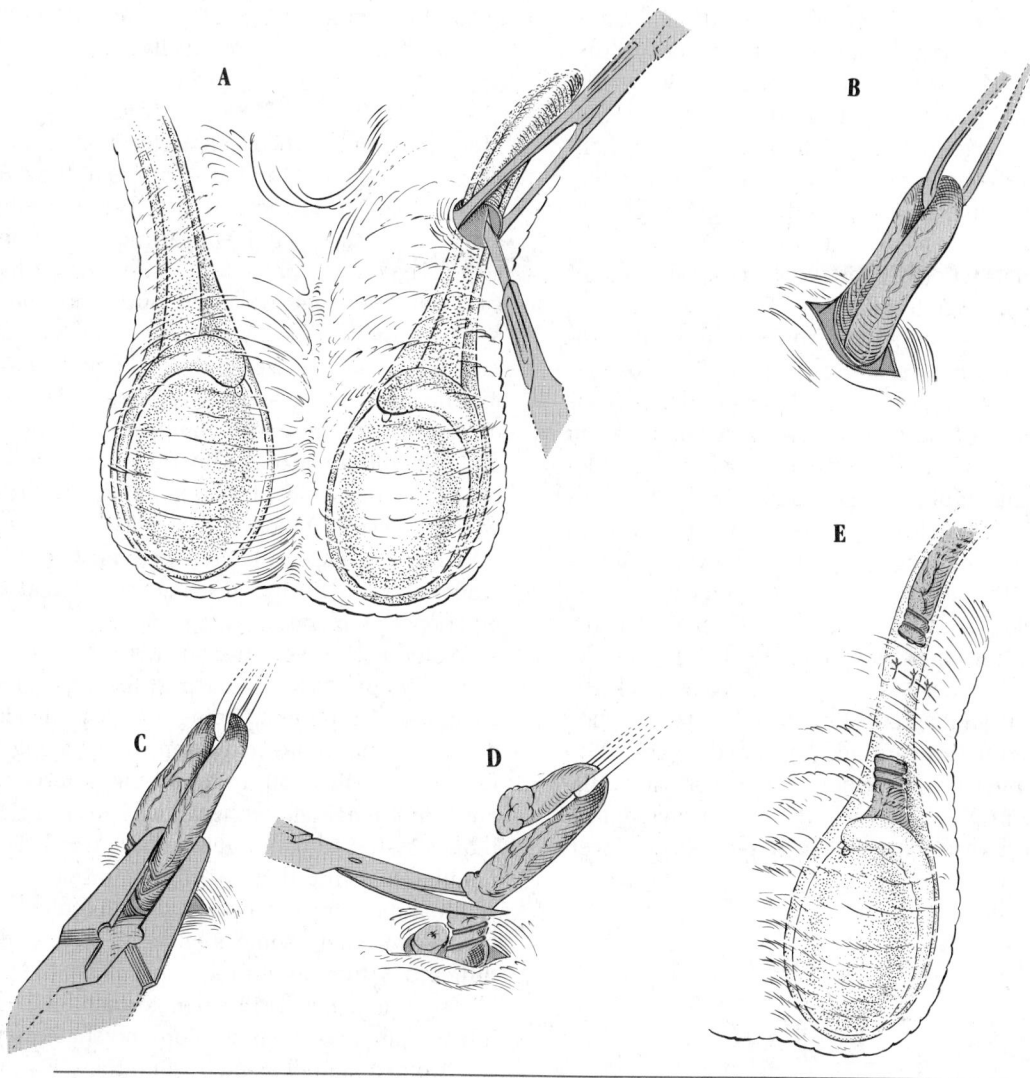

FIGURE 54-7 Vasectomy procedure. **A,** Bilateral incision used to expose sheath. **B** and **C,** Vas exposed and occluded. **D,** Segment is excised. **E,** Vas is replaced in sheath and skin sutured. (Modified from Davis JE: Vasectomy, Am J Nurs 72:509-513, 1972.)

Since vasectomy interrupts the continuity of the vas deferens, sperm are prevented from being ejaculated with other components of the semen. However, sperm are still produced, and the ejaculate is not noticeably diminished in amount. Residual fertility lasting for a variable period is present because of sperm in the semen beyond the point of occlusion of the vas. Sperm *gradually* disappears from the ejaculate; thus conception is possible in the immediate postoperative period. After a vasectomy it is important for the man to report for semen analysis as advised. Disappearance of the sperm from the semen and methods of determining this are described in Chapter 53.

STERILIZATION REVERSAL

Requests for reversal of previous sterilizations may be made because of divorce and remarriage, loss of chil-

dren through death, or change in economic status, as well as for other reasons. A profile of persons at high risk for requesting a reversal include those who were sterilized (1) before 30 years of age, (2) after therapeutic abortion, (3) after miscarriage or term delivery, and (4) for reasons of improving a marriage by preventing future pregnancies followed by a wish for a child during a subsequent marriage.[28]

Attempts at reconstruction of the fallopian tubes to restore fertility have been made for many years. Microsurgical procedures are the standard approach to reversal. The surgery performed primarily involves an end-to-end anastomosis of the ligated tubes. The success of restoring tubal function depends partly on the original surgery performed, especially regarding the amount of the tubal portion excised. Ligation of the tubes produces adhesions that must be dissected away to the point of tubal patency, and this reduces the amount of remaining tubal structure. Also, the length of the fallopian tube remaining after reconstruction may play a role in permitting adequate time for a fertilized ovum to undergo maturational changes in preparation for implantation. Some of these changes occur within the fallopian tube. Success in rendering the fallopian tubes functional after sterilization is usually measured in terms of pregnancy rate after reconstruction. Reports of success after microsurgical reversal range from 40% to 75% of women.[17]

A surgical attempt to restore male fertility after vasectomy is called a *vasovasostomy* (Figure 54-8). An attempt is made to rejoin the severed ends of the vas deferens. Success is measured by the presence of sperm in semen specimens after reconstruction. Reports of success in restoring fertility range from 29% to 85%.[17] A notable point is that although sperm may reappear in the semen, the pregnancy rate after vasovasostomy is not 100%, and the reason for this is unknown.

Considerable research is now in progress for the development of a reversible vasectomy device. Ideally, reversible vasectomy devices would effectively block the vas deferens, would permit simple and safe insertion and removal of the device, could be turned on and off to provide for timing of conception, would not cause discomfort when in place, and would not cause complications. The ideal vasectomy device has not been developed, and the incidence of pain and tissue reaction is high with the devices now available.

PSYCHOLOGIC ASPECTS

Men and women who elect sterilization seem to have little or no regret after the surgery if they understand what to expect during and after the procedure and are able to express their feelings and have questions answered before the procedure. Most women having tubal sterilization express no regret, but some women are disturbed emotionally by having been sterilized. The method of elective sterilization seems to have little effect on women's emotional responses. Depression, loss of self-esteem, physical complaints, feelings of guilt, and difficulty in sexual adjustment after surgery are reported to be some of the psychological responses of women to sterilization even when the surgery is elective. Psychological studies have suggested that women who regretted having been sterilized had preexisting emotional problems.

Women who were dissatisfied after sterilization describe themselves as having feelings of inferiority, weakness, emptiness, being torn up inside, being a damaged and changed person, and having less desire for and gratification from sexual intercourse. These emotional reactions are less likely to occur if a woman requests sterilization and it is performed for reasons of family size rather than for organic disease.

Most men are satisfied with the results of vasectomy but, like women, some men have increased emotional difficulties after sterilization.

There is a need to recognize that tubal sterilization affects men as well as women and that vasectomies affect women as well as men when there is mutual caring and concern between them. This concern may be best illustrated by a woman who described her feelings when she and her husband selected vasectomy as their method of contraception:

The worst part of the experience was that I had not anticipated the range of my reactions. Now it seems that these transitions may have been natural. Perhaps if I had known the experiences of others, I would have passed more easily through these feelings. We try to prepare husbands for childbirth; we should recognize the need to prepare wives for vasectomy.[19]

INTERVENTIONS
PREOPERATIVE COUNSELING AND CARE

The findings of studies about the psychological aspects of sterilization indicate a need to identify men and women before surgery who may later have strong regrets and emotional problems. One aim of counseling before surgery is to confirm that the decision for sterilization is made as objectively as possible. Asking hypothetical questions about the possibility of divorce, loss of

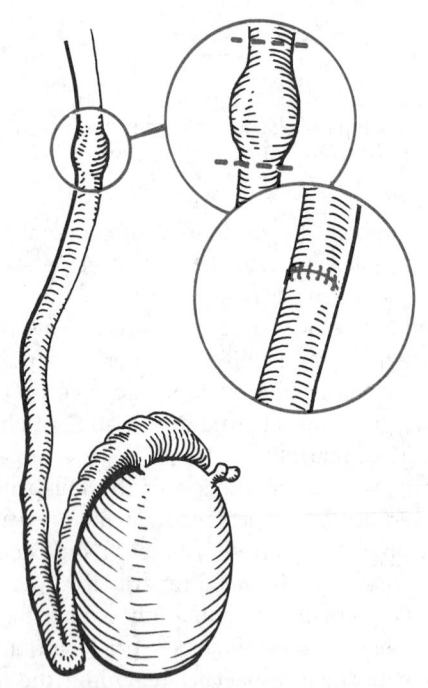

FIGURE 54-8 Vasovasostomy. Scar tissue is resected. Vas deferens is reanastomosed over a splint.

INFORMED CONSENT GUIDELINES (FEDERAL) RELATING TO STERILIZATION

1. Choice is made by patient. No pressures are placed on choice (for example, loss of welfare benefits, wrath of health care provider).
2. Benefits and risks of sterilization are described:
   a. Benefits: permanent, no further costs or decision making
   b. Risks: usual surgical risks, possibility of future pregnancy (that is, not 100% effective)
3. Alternative contraceptive methods are described.
4. Patient is encouraged to ask questions.
5. Patient may withdraw from using the method without penalty.
6. Explanations are given about the entire sterilization procedure, costs, and possible side effects (effects of hormones, weight changes, menstrual changes, sexual response).
7. Written instructions and risk factors are given to patient.
8. A written consent to the procedure is signed by patient and witnessed.

TEACHING FOR THE PATIENT WHO HAS HAD A STERILIZATION PROCEDURE

WOMAN

1. Rest for 24 to 48 hours after procedure
2. No heavy lifting or strenuous exercise for 1 week
3. Abstain from sexual intercourse
   a. Abdominal method: until wound is healed and no discomfort is present
   b. Vaginal method: 1 week
4. Report to physician signs of fever, persistent abdominal pain, or bleeding from incision

MAN

1. Apply ice to scrotum, take sitz baths for minor discomfort and swelling
2. Wear scrotal support for 48 hours
3. Rest for 48 hours after procedure
4. No heavy lifting or strenuous exercise for 1 week
5. Abstain from sexual intercourse for 3 days
6. Use an alternate method of contraception until physician reports semen no longer contains sperm
7. Report to physician signs of fever, persistent scrotal pain, or profuse incisional bleeding

the spouse, or loss of a child can assist in estimating whether the decision to be sterilized has been treated as a serious step.

Previous experience with other methods of contraception can be explored and reasons for dissatisfaction with the methods determined. It may be that an individual or couple lacks knowledge about contraceptive methods and with adequate information might choose something other than sterilization. Care must be taken, however, that persons who are knowledgeable and have made a firm, objective decision are not made to feel that their decision is a poor one or is unacceptable.

The discussion of sterilization methods should be based on the federal government's informed consent guidelines (see box above). The nature and consequences of the surgery must be explained to the patient. It is important to emphasize that the sterilization procedure does nothing to increase or decrease sexual performance or enjoyment but simply removes the chance of pregnancy. It is common for lay people to equate sterilization with castration and loss of femininity or masculinity. Even those patients who know the difference need reassurance.

Visual aids and models can be of great value in giving explanations about the surgery to patients. Films such as *Freedom from Pregnancy,** *Sterilization by Laparoscopy,†* and *Tubal Ligation†* and pamphlets

such as *Voluntary Sterilization for Men and Women** are useful in increasing patients' understanding.

The facts of reversibility, including current success rates, are discussed. In the case of vasectomy, the chance of recanalization and return of fertility should be pointed out. The man or couple also must be informed of progressive rather than immediate sterility after vasectomy, and alternate methods of protection until sterility results should be discussed.

For men having vasectomies, a preoperative specimen of semen is examined to serve as a baseline for interpreting sperm disappearance after surgery. The patient is instructed to shave the scrotal hair and to take a shower the night before surgery. He is advised to bring briefs-type underpants with him on the day of surgery to hold the postoperative dressing in place.

POSTOPERATIVE CARE

Most women having tubal sterilization can be discharged when effects of the general anesthetic have disappeared and when vital signs are stable. Exceptions are women who have recently delivered a baby and those having tubal sterilization by other than the laparoscopic abdominal method. Instructions for patients who have had sterilization procedures are described in the box above.

After vasectomy, men are advised to expect slight

---

*Allend'or Productions, Inc, 3449 Cahuenga West, Hollywood, CA 90068.
†Milner Fenwick, Inc, 3800 Liberty Heights Ave, Baltimore, MD 21215.

---

*Planned Parenthood World Population, 810 Seventh Ave, New York, NY 10019.

swelling of the scrotum, minor pain, and a small amount of bleeding. Ice to the scrotal area, sitz baths, time, and rest will ameliorate these discomforts (see the box, p. 1597). Different methods may be used to determine when sterility actually occurs. The standard procedure has been to take a sperm count 4 weeks after vasectomy. Two consecutive sperm-free specimens are usually considered necessary before the man can be considered sterile. Another method uses the number of ejaculations required to render the semen free of sperm. Most men require at least 24 to 36 ejaculations to become aspermatic (except those with spontaneous reanastomosis of the vas). Reanastomosis is suspected if sperm fail to disappear from the ejaculate despite an adequate number of ejaculations, if there is an increase in sperm in the semen after two successive sperm counts, if motile sperm are found in the semen beyond 3 months after vasectomy, and if, of course, pregnancy occurs.

In the postoperative period both men and women need opportunities to express their feelings about having been sterilized. Previously given information about sexual performance may need to be repeated. If the patient expresses feelings of regret or guilt, a review of the reasons for the sterilization may be of assistance in recognizing that the decision was made as objectively as possible.

INFERTILITY

Infertility is the inability to achieve a pregnancy within a stipulated period of time, usually within 1 year of regular unprotected sexual intercourse. Some authorities include the inability to carry pregnancies to a live birth. Infertility is classified as either primary or secondary. *Primary infertility* describes couples who have never conceived, whereas *secondary infertility* refers to couples who have previously conceived. *Sterility* is irreversible and refers to an individual who has an absolute factor preventing procreation.

EPIDEMIOLOGY

It has been estimated that 10% to 15% of all couples in the United States are infertile, and about 1% to 2% are sterile. This represents about 10 million Americans.[46] Approximately 50% of the couples who undergo assessment and treatment for infertility in major infertility settings are likely to conceive. Although infertility is most often attributed to women, about 40% of infertility results from infertility of men and 20% from a combination of partners. Some of the major factors that account for infertility are failure to ovulate (10% to 15%), tubal pathologic conditions (10% to 30%), cervical factors (5%), and STD (20% to 40%). There is no known cause in 10% to 20% of infertility problems.[46]

The risk of infertility is doubled for women 35 to 44 years of age as compared to those 30 to 34 years old. Approximately 33% of women who delay pregnancy until they are over 35 will have an infertility problem.[46] Infertility is becoming a more serious societal problem because of the increased prevalence of STD. In addition, because of the availability of abortion, fewer infertile couples are able to adopt.

EFFECTS OF INFERTILITY

Couples wishing to have children who find themselves unable to do so experience immeasurable emotional distress. The trauma of infertility affects every facet of an individual's and a couple's psychosocial functioning.[16] Feelings of inadequacy are common, as are anger and guilt.

The infertile couple must confront feelings about lack of control, self-image, self-esteem, and sexuality (see research box below). When the couple is faced with infertility, intercourse must be timed and goal-directed. A large proportion of couples experience sexual dysfunction at some point. Lack of sexual desire and interest, decreased lubrication, inability to achieve or sustain an erection, and painful intercourse are common complaints of these couples.

Couples who are informed that they will never be able to have children experience a life crisis with all of its ramifications and have a strong need to grieve. For those who are told they are a normal, fertile couple and for whom pregnancy does not result despite months or years or tests, studies, examinations, and advice, feelings of frustration alternating with hope are high. Couples undergo a stress response syndrome that typically includes four stages: denial and numbness, obsessional thoughts, working through, and completion.[42]

All of these couples require emotional support, including encouragement to grieve, to express their anger

RESEARCH

Hirsch AM and Hirsch SM: The effect of infertility on marriage and self-concept, J Obstet Gynecol Neonatal Nurs 18:13-20, 1989.

Questionnaires were completed by 92 subjects (58 seeking medical treatment for a perceived infertility problem and 34 who had not decided whether to have children) assessing the impact of infertility on their marriages and self-concept. Groups were compared as to self-esteem, marital satisfaction, sexual satisfaction, and general contentment. People experiencing infertility had greater dissatisfaction with themselves and their marriages. They experienced less sexual satisfaction and greater discontent than noninfertile persons. Infertile couples labeled noncommunicators had significantly higher levels of general discontent and marital dissatisfaction. ∎

and other feelings to regain objectivity, and to avoid premature decisions and actions about alternatives. The urgent need for such support is reflected in the emergence of support groups organized by infertile individuals and couples.*

It is important that couples who wish to have children and are unsuccessful after about a year of trying to achieve pregnancy seek medical advice. Infertility evaluation often requires a long time. Sometimes infertility cannot be treated successfully, and alternatives such as adoption, artificial insemination, or child-free living are considered.

ETIOLOGY AND PREVENTION

The fertility of a couple is affected by four factors: duration of pregnancy exposure, coital frequency, female's age, and male's age. In general, the likelihood of becoming pregnant is greater as the duration of exposure to pregnancy increases. Approximately 25% of women will become pregnant during the first month of noncontraceptive intercourse. Sixty-five percent become pregnant within 6 months, 75% within 9 months, 80% to 90% within 1 year, and 93% to 95% within 1½ years.[40]

Increased coital frequency enhances fertility to a point. In couples having intercourse four or five times a week, 83% become pregnant within 6 months, as compared to 16% of the couples having intercourse less than once a week.[40] Frequent ejaculation improves sperm motility unless ejaculation is excessive, resulting in depletion of available sperm.

Fertility in women is low during the early teenage years, peaks at 24 years of age, and declines after age 30. An infertility rate of 21.9% to 29.6% has been reported for married women 35 to 40 years old and 28.9% to 63.6% for women over age 40 to 44.[34] Fertility reaches its peak at 25 years of age in men and subsequently declines, although some 80- to 90-year-old men are fertile. The age of men younger than 60, per se, has little impact on reproduction; however, it has a significant effect on decreased coital frequency that results in decreased pregnancy rates.

There are many causes of infertility in men and women (see box at right). Some of these causes are preventable or treatable, whereas others are not. Individuals need to consider fertility consequences as part of birth control decision making.

One of the most common, preventable causes of infertility in women is infection of pelvic organs, especially as a result of gonorrhea and chlamydia that cause obstruction of fallopian tubes. An estimated 17% of women have symptoms of salpingitis as the first sign of

gonorrheal infection, and during the course of treatment about 5% are surgically sterilized. Such serious consequences are preventable through prophylactic use of penicillin for women exposed to gonorrhea and through early diagnosis and treatment of all vaginal and cervical infections. The prevention and treatment of STDs and PID can help prevent infertility. Gonococcal cultures should be obtained every 6 months for women with multiple partners. If infection is present and the woman has an IUD, it should be removed. Barrier contraceptives reduce the risk for infections and PID. Oral contraceptives decrease the incidence of acute gonococcal PID[45] but may increase the likelihood of *Chlamydia* infection.[2]

Many of the ovarian and hormonal problems that cause infertility produce symptoms such as menstrual irregularities and ill health before a problem with conception is ever recognized. Many of these problems can be managed with hormone therapy, provided women seek help for such problems at an early age or as soon as deviations are noticed. Birth control pills should be avoided by women who have not established normal menses, have irregular menstrual cycles, or have used birth control pills for over 2 years. Some authorities suggest a break from prolonged use of birth control pills to reactivate the hypothalamic controls.

Bilateral undescended testes (cryptorchism) in men should be corrected surgically before puberty. In later life cryptorchism may produce sterility because of fail-

---

CAUSES OF INFERTILITY

FEMALE

1. Developmental: uterine abnormalities
2. Endocrine: pituitary, thyroid, and adrenal dysfunctions, ovarian dysfunctions (inhibit release of ova)
3. Diseases: PID (especially from gonococcus, fallopian tube obstructions, diseases of cervix and uterus that inhibit passage of active sperm)
4. Other: malnutrition, severe anemia, anxiety

MALE

1. Developmental: undescended testes, other congenital anomalies (inhibit development of sperm)
2. Endocrine: hormonal deficiencies (pituitary, thyroid, adrenal) (inhibit development of sperm)
3. Diseases: testicular destruction from disease, orchitis from mumps, prostatitis
4. Other: excessive smoking, fatigue, alcohol

BOTH FEMALE AND MALE

1. Diseases: STDs, cancer-causing obstructions (inhibit transport of ovum or sperm)
2. Other: immunologic incompatibility (inhibit sperm penetration of ovum), marital problems
3. Diethylstilbesterol exposure in utero (suggested but not proven as a cause of male infertility)

---

*RESOLVE, Inc., 5 Water Street, Arlington, MA 02174; and for child-free living, National Organization for Non-Parents, 806 Reistertown Rd., Baltimore, MD 21208.

ure of the testes to develop their sperm-producing function, even if the condition is surgically corrected. Destruction of testicular tissue by infectious processes can be prevented through prompt treatment when symptoms first appear. Prepubescent boys should be immunized for mumps to prevent orchitis.

Abnormal quality and quantity of sperm can be caused by a small rise in scrotal temperature. Nurses should inform men and their partners about environmental sources of heat, such as excessively hot baths, hot tubs, use of jockey shorts instead of boxer shorts, or jobs requiring long hours of sitting, so that they can change their habits. Another preventable cause of infertility in men is heavy marijuana use, which depresses sperm counts and testosterone levels. Cigarette smoking has also been linked to decreased sperm motility. Other drugs that cause abnormal sperm development are chemotherapeutic agents, sulfasalazine, Furadantin, spironolactone, and cimetidine. Infertile men with ulcerative colitis should use mesalamine instead of sulfasalazine.[46]

ASSESSMENT OF INFERTILITY

The purposes of an infertility evaluation are to establish the cause of infertility and determine the diagnosis, to give a prognosis for future fertility, to provide a basis for medical or surgical treatment, and to plan for assisting the couple to accept their diagnosis, treatment, and future options. The assessment and intervention can be physically painful as well as emotionally and economically stressful.

Attempts to correct infertility are based on data obtained through a detailed history and physical examination as well as data obtained from laboratory tests and clinical studies. During the physical examination, close attention is given to the individual's general health; development of secondary sex characteristics; size, posi-

tion, and condition of the reproductive organs; and signs of metabolic diseases or infection. A sexual history is taken, and sexual practices are reviewed. Anyone considered at high risk for AIDS should be screened before proceeding with an infertility evaluation because women who have AIDS or who are HIV-positive are encouraged not to become pregnant due to the high incidence of transmission to the fetus.

The couple should attempt to be at the first interview together because they share responsibility for infertility. Information is needed by both partners, and this may be their first opportunity to confront their feelings about being infertile.

EXAMINATION OF THE MAN

Many physicians prefer to carry out examination of the man first, since it is more easily accomplished and less time consuming (Table 54-14). The first special test performed is multiple semen examinations to determine the presence, number, maturity, and motility of sperm. Normal findings indicate fertility. Abnormal findings on a single semen analysis does not necessarily mean that there is a significant male factor contributing to male infertility. Some experts believe that semen analysis needs to be performed four times to ascertain a man's mean sperm count because of extreme variability and sensitivity of the test. Follow-up to an abnormal semen analysis includes a repeat semen analysis, a postcoital test, a detailed history of exposure to heat, drugs, radiation or illness, and special studies with referral to a urologist if appropriate.

Absence of sperm in the semen may indicate a stricture along the vas deferens. A biopsy of the tests is performed, and if sperm are being produced, there is a stricture. The stricture can sometimes be successfully repaired by plastic surgery (vasovasostomy). Varicoceles (dilated veins of the spermatic cord) are also associated

---

TABLE 54-14 Examination for infertility

Sex	Tests	Data Obtained
Male	Multiple semen examination	Determine presence, number, and motility of sperm
	Testicular biopsy if sperm count low or absent	Presence of sperm indicates obstruction of vas deferens
Female	Basal body temperature chart	Determines that ovulation is occurring
	Postcoital test of cervical secretions	Measure ability of sperm to penetrate cervical mucus and remain active, and quality of the mucus
	Endometrial biopsy, serum progesterone and estradiol levels, laparoscopic inspection of ovaries	Determine whether ovulation is occurring (if in question)
	Laparoscopy	Determine patency of fallopian tubes
	Hysterosalpingography (x-ray after insertion of contrast media)	Determine patency of uterus and fallopian tubes
Male/Female	Hormonal tests	Determine whether the problem is hormonal

with decreased sperm counts. Approximately 25% of infertile males have a varicocele (see Chapter 56). Varicoceles probably reduce sperm count by raising testicular temperature.

If the sperm count and motility rate of sperm are low, thyroid extract and vitamins may be prescribed, along with a well-balanced diet, rest, and moderate exercise. A lack of vitamins A and E in the diet may cause some atrophy of the sperm-producing structures. The couple are advised to have intercourse every other day during the fertile period (usually 12 to 16 days before the beginning of the next menstrual period). When the man is completely aspermatic, conception is impossible, and the couple should be counseled about the alternatives open to them.

EXAMINATION OF THE WOMAN

If the man is found to be fertile, examination of the woman is carried out. A complete history and physical examination are performed. If there is an infection of the reproductive tract, it is treated. A systematic check is then made of each organ that might affect the woman's reproductive ability. Baseline laboratory tests should consist of a blood count, test for syphilis, sedimentation rate, urinalysis, TSH by radioimmunoassay to rule out hypothyroidism, and other specific tests to rule out suspected systemic disease.[39]

If menstruation occurs regularly, this usually indicates that the ovaries are producing estrogen and progesterone but does not indicate that amounts are sufficient for ovulation. To determine whether ovulation is occurring, the woman is instructed to keep a basal body temperature chart to help determine the presence and time of ovulation. In the interim, cervical secretions are examined for pH and spinnbarkeit. A postcoital test is usually performed. If sperm are being destroyed by vaginal and cervical secretions, smears from these sites are studied. If the secretions are too acid or too alkaline, medicated douches may be prescribed. A douche using sodium bicarbonate (15 ml to 1 L of water) taken just before intercourse has been found to increase the motility of sperm in many cases.

If a question remains about ovulation, endometrial biopsies and occasionally serum progesterone and estradiol levels may be obtained. Endometrial biopsy provides the most reliable assessment of ovulation and is performed 2 to 3 days before the expected period. Serum progesterone levels of 6.5 ng/ml or preferably 10 ng/ml or more at the midluteal phase (midpoint between ovulation and onset of menses) confirms ovulation. The woman can ascertain for herself whether ovulation has occurred with over-the-counter ovulation detection kits. Laparoscopic inspection of the ovaries may be carried out to determine if ovulation has, in fact, occurred.

If an obstruction of the fallopian tubes is suspected,

tubal patency studies by hysterosalpingography or laparoscopy are indicated.

Tubal strictures or obstructions are sometimes repaired by microsurgery. There is a significant correlation between the severity of the pathologic process affecting the fallopian tube and the cause. Fallopian tubes covered with peripheral adhesions caused by exosalpingitis are likely to have a greater success rate of repair than tubes with adhesions caused by endosalpingitis.[52] If ovulation is occurring, the couple may require advice about timing of intercourse and ovulation.

Metabolic disease processes can be detected by thyroid function tests, glucose tolerance tests, 17-ketosteroid assay or measures of circulating androgens, and prolactin assays to detect hyperprolactinemia. Usually, however, extensive laboratory evaluation is not necessary.

INFERTILITY STUDIES

Semen Analysis

Analysis of the semen is indicated in evaluation of male and female infertility. It is also used to follow-up male sterilization by vasectomy.

Multiple semen examinations are done to determine the presence, number, maturity, shape, and motility of sperm. The man may be instructed to secure a specimen of semen at home by masturbation or by coitus interruptus, but because of rapid deterioration of sperm, most physicians prefer a fresh sample collected in the physician's office or in the laboratory. If collected at home, the specimen of semen should be taken to the office or laboratory within 2 to 3 hours and protected from cold.

The semen is usually collected after a period of abstinence corresponding to the man's usual frequency of intercourse. An abstinence period of 2 to 5 days before semen collection is recommended.[46] The specimen is ejaculated into a clean, widemouthed jar supplied by the laboratory or physician. The dates of the last emission and of the current specimen are recorded.

A gross examination of the semen for its physical properties is first carried out. Semen is normally a highly viscous, opaque, grayish-white fluid that spontaneously liquefies by prostatic enzymes within 10 to 45 minutes after ejaculation. After this time, the semen appears translucent, turbid, and viscous. Semen is normally slightly alkaline, with a pH of about 7.7, which protects sperm from the acid environment in the vagina. The normal volume in an ejaculation of semen is 3 to 5 ml. Five to 10 white blood cells observed by higher power field on microscopic examination may be normal. Higher amounts of white blood cells are associated with decreased fertility.

After the semen liquefies, a sperm count is taken. A count repeatedly greater than 20 million/ml is considered to be associated with normal fertility if other parameters are normal. Twenty to 25% of men who are fertile have sperm counts less than 20 million/ml at some point in their lives.

The sperm are also examined for motility and for presence and number of abnormal forms. New methods currently available for objective measurement of sperm motility include time-exposure photomicrography, videotapes of semen, and motion analysis computers.[47] It is generally accepted that normal semen contains more than 70% motile sperm and fewer than 30% abnormal forms. Sperm motility under 40% and abnormal sperm forms over 25% are known to lower the chance of fertilization of an ovum. Also, men who are infertile may have an increased rather than a decreased volume of semen, and the increased volume is often associated with a significantly decreased sperm count.

The *zona-free hamster test* is being used occasionally in addition to routine semen analysis to assess the fertilizing capacity of spermatozoa (ability to capacitate, undergo the acrosome reaction, and to fuse with the oolemma).

Three tests to detect sperm-bound immunoglobulins are available:

1. Xenogenous antihuman antiserum and immunobinding: uses microsize polyacrylamide spheres covalently linked to rabbit antihuman antibodies[7]
2. Mixed agglutination reacter (MAR): Rh-positive human red blood cells previously exposed to a human anti-Rh antibody of the IgG class are mixed with the test semen
3. Radiolabeled antiglobulin assay: use of radioiodinated xenogenous antibodies raised against human immunoglobulins to detect antibodies bound to sperm

Postcoital Test

The postcoital test involves examination of the cervical mucus of women after intercourse to measure both the ability of sperm to penetrate the mucus and remain active and the quality of the cervical mucus. This test is valuable in evaluation of infertility. Similar tests are performed in cases of rape, where secretions from the vagina and cervix are examined for the presence of sperm.

For the postcoital test, mucus is aspirated from the cervical canal and examined for the presence and number of sperm. Characteristics of the cervical mucus (spinnbarkeit) (Figure 54-6) are also studied. At the time of ovulation under normal circumstances, the amount of cervical mucus is maximal, but the viscosity is decreased. This facilitates penetration of the cervical mucus by the sperm.

The prognostic value of the postcoital test has been questioned because of contradictory findings, such as

no difference in the pregnancy rate between groups having no sperm, no motile sperm, 1 to 5 motile sperm, 6 to 11 motile sperm, and 11 or more motile sperm.[9] Coital technique can be deemed adequate if the mucus is clear and plentiful with good spinnbarkeit and sperm are present in the mucus. The couple should be told that lubricants such as K-Y Jelly have a spermicidal effect and should not be used. Vegetable oil can be substituted.

A woman undergoing a postcoital test should see the physician within 12 hours after intercourse. She should be informed of the procedure for collection of the specimen, additional studies to be performed, and measures to be taken at home.

Hysterosalpingogram

A hysterosalpingogram is usually the initial screening procedure when investigation of ovulatory function, semen production, and sperm/mucus interacter yield no pathology. The uterus and fallopian tubes can be visualized when a contrast medium is used with x-ray. A sterile, opaque, aqueous contrast medium is injected through the cervix into the uterus for a hysterogram. For a hysterosalpingogram, the dye is also injected into the fallopian tubes. X-rays are then taken to observe the structure of the uterus and fallopian tubes. These studies are preferably performed 2 to 5 days after the end of a menstrual period to avoid interfering with ovum transport. In some institutions, hysterosalpingography for screening has been replaced by laparoscoy combined with hysteroscopy.[48]

The *Rubin test*, in which carbon dioxide is forced into the uterus and fallopian tubes, is now rarely performed because of numerous false-positive and false-negative results and patient discomfort. The Rubin test has been replaced by the hysterosalpingogram.

Hysteroscopy

Hysteroscopy (see Chapter 53) complements hysterosalpingography. Hysteroscopy should be used to follow up abnormalities identified on the hysterogram. Use as a screening tool is discouraged because of its higher cost.

Laparoscopy

Laparoscopy (see Chapter 53) is the final diagnostic procedure of an infertility workup. It is generally performed after 6 months have elapsed since the hysterosalpingogram because a fertility-enhancing effect has been related to the x-ray procedure.[46] A 6-month delay is not followed in women at high risk for pelvic infection or if the hysterosalpingogram shows major abnormalities. Laparoscopy has been able to detect pelvic adhesions and endometriosis that the hysterosalpingogram fails to detect. Manipulation through the laparoscope is attempted and many abnormalities can be treated.

■ **DATA ANALYSIS: NURSING DIAGNOSES**

Nursing diagnosis for individuals experiencing infertility may include, but are not limited to, the following:

Diagnostic Title	Possible Etiologies
Grieving, anticipatory	Loss of fertility, loss of imagined child
Knowledge deficit	Multiple treatment options
Self-esteem disturbance	Inability to become pregnant, inability to impregnate
Sexuality patterns, altered	Anxiety regarding ability to conceive; anxiety regarding sexual performance

■ **PLANNING: EXPECTED PATIENT OUTCOMES**

Expected patient outcomes for persons with infertility may include, but are not limited to, the following:

1. Patient demonstrates understanding of altered sexual desire, difficulty with sexual arousal related to anxiety.
2. Patient understands techniques for reducing sexual demands.
3. Patient demonstrates positive self concept.
4. Patient verbalizes understanding of diagnosis and prognosis.
5. Patient explains procedures necessary to diagnose and treat infertility and understands care that is expected of both professional and client.
6. Patient demonstrates understanding of options for parenthood and childfree living.
7. Patient verbalizes feelings regarding loss of pregnancy experience.

INTERVENTIONS FOR FERTILITY

FACILITATING SEXUAL RELATIONSHIPS

Sexual dysfunction resulting from the experience of infertility requires accurate diagnosis, education, and reassurance. Suggestions about sexual intercourse are given if this seems to be the problem. Behavioral techniques such as sensate-focus exercises may reduce performance anxiety. Couples can be reassured that most sexual dysfunction is temporary and can be corrected.

COPING WITH INFERTILITY

Couples found to be infertile are confronted with the need to make choices from among available alternatives. Remaining childless or adopting a child are the usual alternatives from which they must select. First the couple must deal with their feelings and accept their infertility. An excellent book for couples to read is *Infertility: A Guide for the Childless Couple* by Barbara Eck Menning.*

The couple needs objective guidance when making a decision, and they need help in making a sound decision to prevent regret stemming from premature and hastily made decisions. They need time to cope with the crisis of being told they are infertile, and they need to be permitted to handle their grief (see Chapter 14). They may grieve for their loss of fertility, loss of future children, or loss of the pregnancy experience. Once the initial crisis is dealt with, the couple is better prepared to discuss alternatives. Couples who elect to remain child-free need to be informed that with advancing age there is increased difficulty in adopting children, should they change their minds at a later time, but this must be done in such a way that they will not feel guilty about not wanting to adopt a child.

Those couples deciding on adoption need to be presented with the facts concerning their chances of success in locating the child of their choice and the need to undergo still another long process before obtaining a child. These couples need information about reliable adoption agencies and may need help in dealing with frustration during adoption procedures. Organizations to support persons seeking adoption are available.† Some couples will not be successful in their attempts to adopt a child and will need help in coping with still another crisis.

ARTIFICIAL INSEMINATION

Artificial insemination is an alternative in some cases of infertility. The major indication for artificial insemination is male infertility. Previous loss of children because of Rh or ABO incompatibility or severe hereditary defects transmitted by the man are other indications. Therefore, artificial insemination is not reserved only for infertile couples.

Medically, the procedure of artificial insemination is simple, safe, inexpensive, and highly successful. Accepted routes for insemination are intrauterine (which is painful and rarely necessary to use), cervical-vaginal, and intracervical. A few drops of semen are injected as close to the time of ovulation as possible. Having intercourse around the time of insemination or mixing the partner's semen with the donor's may be emotionally satisfying for the couple.

Artificial insemination is *homologous* (AIH) when the partner's semen is used and *heterologous* (AID) when donor semen is used. Homologous insemination may be used when there is a small volume of semen with normal density, oligospermia with normal sperm motility and morphology, impotence or refractory premature ejaculation, or congenital or acquired anomalies preventing adequate cervical insemination (procidentia, hy-

---

*Englewood Cliffs, NJ, 1977, Prentice-Hall, Inc.

†OURS (Organization for a United Response), 3418 Humboldt Ave, South Minneapolis, MN 55408.

pospadias, retrograde ejaculation, vaginismus, incompatible cervical mucus). Heterologous insemination is indicated in irreversible male infertility, a partner with a proven gene error, or an Rh incompatibility with a homozygous Rh-positive partner.

Donor selection in heterologous insemination is a very important part of the procedure. Criteria for donor selection is based on semen analysis as well as on a complete history and physical examination. AID couples are also concerned with intelligence. Attempts may be made to select donors who have similar physical characteristics to the partner. Donor candidates with venereal disease, diabetes, hepatitis, blood diseases, prostatic infection, and a family history of hereditary disorders are excluded.

Fertility of donors must be proved by semen analysis. Frozen sperm is typically used. The semen should show a sperm count of over 100 million/ml, have a predominance of normal sperm forms, and have a greater than 70% sperm motility. All sperm are now screened for AIDS. Karyotyping has been advocated by some authorities.

Artificial insemination is not well understood by the general public. Many people are poorly informed about it, and some people find the topic highly distressing or distasteful and refuse to discuss it. Others may not have considered artificial insemination, wish to have additional information, and welcome opportunities to discuss the subject.

OTHER INFERTILITY APPROACHES

In Vitro Fertilization

In vitro fertilization (IVF) was originally developed as a means of bypassing blocked or absent fallopian tubes. It involves recovering one or more of the woman's ova from her ovarian follicles through laparoscopy or her vagina via ultrasound and fertilizing the ova with the partner's sperm in a petri dish. If fertilization and cleavage occur, the resulting embryos are transferred into the woman's uterus about 48 hours after the ova retrieval has taken place. Although irreparable tubal damage or the absence of the fallopian tubes are the primary indications for in vitro fertilization, it is also indicated for male-factor infertility, endometriosis, unexplained infertility, and immunologic causes of infertility.[17] There are over 150 IVF programs in the United States. The infertile couple that enters an IVF program has already been through years of disappointment, anger, frustration, sadness, and intrusive physical procedures. They are vulnerable, desperate, anxious, and under physiologic and psychological stress. For these couples, in vitro fertilization represents the last hope of achieving a long-desired pregnancy. The couple must realize that the chance of a successful pregnancy is at best about 30% per IVF attempt, so the odds are very much against any one couple achieving a pregnancy.[39]

Surrogate Mothers

Surrogate mothers are women who contract to conceive by artificial insemination and give the baby to the semen donor after delivery. There are many social, moral, psychological, and legal implications surrounding this approach. The United States courts are currently trying cases of legitimacy and parents' rights to the child. In some states it is illegal.

Ovum Transfer

A donor provides the oocyte and site of fertilization and carries the embryo for a short period in this procedure. The donor is inseminated with the husband's sperm after synchronization of the donor's and recipient's expected times of ovulation. Five days later, the conceptus is transferred to the recipient's endometrial cavity via a small catheter. Primary indications for ovum transfer are uterine tube obstruction and women who are carriers of genetic disorders. Pregnancy rates are 12% per transfer and 6% per donor insemination.[39]

Gamete Intrafallopian Transfer

Gamete intrafallopian transfer (GIFT) occurs when oocytes that have been aspirated from follicles at laparoscopy are mixed with washed sperm and placed in the uterine tube via laparoscopy or minilaparotomy. Current data suggest that GIFT achieves a higher pregnancy rate than in vitro fertilization and embryo transfer.[38] GIFT is used when the woman has at least one working fallopian tube so that ovary and follicular aspiration can take place. The preembryo travels to the uterus for implantation 4 days after ovulation according to a natural timetable as compared to 44 hours after insemination in IVF.

CHAPTER SUMMARY

- The menstrual cycle is usually 26 to 36 days but may be altered by changes in climate, changes in working hours, emotional trauma, fatigue, exercise, illness, and surgery.

- Health teaching for menstruation includes information about the physiologic process, factors that may alter the menstrual cycle, personal hygiene, exercise, diet and dysmenorrhea.

- PMS occurs in about 10% of all menstruating women; and symptoms include behavioral changes, fatigue, signs of water and sodium retention, palpitations, headache, increased appetite, joint pain, and backache.

- Primary dysmenorrhea is caused by high levels of prostaglandin and can be treated with antiprostaglandins, some of which are now available without a prescription.

- Amenorrhea is classified as primary or secondary and results from a variety of causes.

- Abnormal types of vaginal bleeding include oligomenorrhea, menorrhagia, metrorrhagia, polymenorrhea, menometrorrhagia, cryptomenorrhea, and dysfunctional uterine bleeding.

- Approximately 10% of women have pronounced symptoms during menopause. Although many symptoms have been associated with menopause, the three major symptoms are osteoporosis, hot flashes, and vaginal dryness.

- Controversy surrounds the use of estrogen replacement therapy with many experts encouraging all women to take ERT to prevent or retard osteoporosis.

- Nonpharmacologic methods of menopause symptom relief include exercise, vitamins E and B-complex, ginseng, adequate nutrition and local application of a vaginal cream.

- It is essential to counsel people with more than one sexual partner to use condoms for all forms of penetration until the epidemiology of AIDS and other sexually transmitted diseases is more completely known.

- The most current way of understanding contraceptive effectiveness looks at lowest expected typical and lowest reported failure rate during the first year of a method, and first-year continuation rates.

- Major methods of contraception include hormonal contraceptives, IUDs, condom, diaphragm, chemical contraceptives, spermicides, and fertility awareness.

- Patient teaching about contraceptives includes information about each method, how the method works, the degree of protection against pregnancy provided by the method, self-care requirements, side effects of the method, contraindications to use, and the need for follow-up care.

- Blood chemistry, hematology, and urine tests are affected by birth control pills.

- Sterilization is the most widely used contraceptive method worldwide. Female methods of sterilization include abdominal tubal sterilization by minilaparotomy and laparoscopy and vaginal tubal sterilization (rarely performed) by culpotomy and culdoscopy. Male sterilization is by vasectomy.

- Sterilization reversal is performed via microsurgical procedures.

- Infertility affects 10% to 15% of all couples in the United States. Tests for males include multiple semen examination, hormonal tests, and testicular biopsy. Tests for females include the basal body temperature chart, postcoital test, endometrial biopsy, laparoscopy, hysterosalpingography, and hormonal tests.

- Nurses can assist couples experiencing infertility by providing emotional support, encouraging them to grieve and express their feelings, providing anticipatory guidance about testing, assisting the couple to consider their alternatives, and referring couples to support groups or other health care professionals.

QUESTIONS TO CONSIDER

- What would you include in health teaching about menstruation, and what age would be the best time to begin the teaching?

- How would you counsel a menopausal woman who asks you, "Should I take estrogen replacement therapy for my hot flashes?"

- How would your advice about contraception differ for a teenager compared to a 39-year-old woman who thinks that she doesn't want any more children?

- What approach would you consider for a couple experiencing infertility for 2 years without treatment if the woman wants to try anything available and the man wants nature to take its course?

REFERENCES AND SELECTED READINGS

1. Abraham G: Nutritional factors in the etiology of the premenstrual tension syndrome, J Reprod Med 28:446-464, 1983.
2. Aral S, Mosher W, and Cates W: Contraceptive use, pelvic inflammatory disease, and fertility problems among American women, Am J Obstet Gynecol 156:59-64, 1987.
3. Bachmann G: Optimizing the postmenopausal years, Contemp Obstet Gynecol 24:127-136, 1984.
4. Bancroft J, and Backstrom T: Premenstrual syndrome, Clin Endocrinol 22:313-324, 1985.
5. Blumenthal SJ and Nadelson CC: Late luteal phase dysphoric disorder (premenstrual syndrome): clinical implications, J Clin Psychiatry 49:469-473, 1988.
6. Boyd AS: Varicoceles and male infertility, Am Fam Physician 37:252-258, 1988.
7. Bronson R: Detecting autoimmunity to spermatozoa, Contemp Obstet Gynecol 25:205-216, 1985.
8. Chow R et al: Physical fitness effect on bone mass in postmenopausal women, Arch Phys Med Rehabil 67:231-234, 1986.
9. Collins J et al: The postcoital test as a predictor of pregnancy among 355 infertile couples, Fertil Steril 41:703-705, 1984.
10. *Dodek OI: The infertile couple, Am Fam Physician 38:101-112, 1988.
10a. Drage M, Woods N, and Mitchell E: Gender differences in the infertility experience, Health Care for Women Int 9:163-175, 1988.
11. Ettinger B, Genant H, and Cann C: Long-term estrogen replacement therapy prevents bone loss and fractures, Ann Intern Med 102:319-324, 1985.

*References preceded by an asterisk are particularly well suited for student reading.

11a. Feldman B, Voda A, and Gronseth E: The prevalence of hot flash and associated variables among premenopausal women, Research in Nursing and Health 8:261-268, 1985.

12. *Fogel CI and Woods NF: Health care of women: a nursing perspective, St Louis, 1981, The CV Mosby Co.

13. Frisch R et al: Body fat, menarche and reproductive ability, Semin Reprod Endocrinol 3:45-53, 1985.

14. *Gallen M, Liskin K, and Kak N: Men: new focus in family planning, Popul Rep 33:85-87, 1987.

15. Gambrell R, Maier R, and Sanders B: Decreased incidence of breast cancer in postmenopausal estrogen-progestogen users, Obstet Gynecol 62:435-44, 1983.

16. Goodman K, Goodman N, and Rothman B: Group work in infertility treatment (abstract), Fertil Steril 41:228, 1984.

17. Hatcher RA et al: Contraceptive technology 1988-1989, ed 14, New York, 1989, Irvington Publishers.

18. Havelock CM: The cervical smear test, Practitioner 231:74-80, 1987.

19. *Houghton B: Vasectomies affect women, too, Am J Nurs 81:821-825, 1981.

20. Keye WR: Premenstrual symptoms: evaluation and treatment, Compr Ther 14:19-26, 1988.

21. Khandwala SD: Laparoscopic sterilization: a comparison of current techniques, J Reprod Med 33:463-466, 1988.

22. Kiel D, et al: Hip fracture and use of estrogens in premenopausal women: the Framingham study, N Engl J Med 317:1169-1174, 1987.

23. Knopp RH: The effects of postmenopausal estrogen therapy on the incidence of arteriosclerotic vascular disease, Obstet Gynecol 72:23S-30S, 1988.

24. *Kurtzman C and Block DE: Family planning: beyond contraception, Matern Child Nurs J 11:340-343, 1986.

25. Lavy G: Hysteroscopy as a diagnostic aid, Obstet Gynecol Clin North Am 15:61-72, 1988.

26. Lindsay R: The menopause: sex, steroids, and osteoporosis, Clin Obstet Gynecol 95:963-972, 1987.

27. Lobo RA: Too much of a good thing? Use of progestens in the menopause: an international consensus statement, Fertil Steril 51:229-231, 1989.

28. Loffer F: Anticipating complications of laparoscopic sterilization, Contemp Obstet Gynecol 17:41-51, 1981.

29. *Loucks A: A comparison of satisfaction with types of diaphragms among women in a college population, J Obstet Gynecol Neonatal Nurs 18:194-200, 1989.

30. Mao C and Grimes DA: The sperm penetration assay: can it discriminate between fertile and infertile men? Am J Obstet Gynecol 159:279-286, 1988.

31. Massil H and O'Brien S: Approach to the management of premenstrual syndrome, Clin Obstet Gynecol 30:443-452, 1987.

32. McIntyre S and Higgins J: Parity and use-effectiveness with the contraceptive sponge, Am J Obstet Gynecol 153:796-801, 1986.

33. Meldrum D et al: Evolution of a highly successful in vitro fertilization-embryo transfer program, Fertil Steril 46:663-669, 1987.

34. *Menken J, Trussell J, and Larsen V: Age and infertility, Science 233:1389-1394, 1986.

35. *Milne BJ: Couples' experiences with in vitro fertilization, J Obstet Gynecol Neonatal Nurs 17:347-351, 1988.

36. *Nachtigall L, and Nachtigall R: Evaluating newly menopausal women, Contemp Obstet Gynecol 25:65-91, 1985.

37. Noakes TD and vanGend MV: Menstrual dysfunction in female athletes: a review for clinicians, South Afr Med J 73:350-355, 1987.

37a. Olshansky E: Infertility and its influence on women's career identities, Health Care for Women Int 8(2,3):185-196, 1987.

38. *Pace-Owens S: Gamete intrafallopian transfer (GIFT), J Obstet Gynecol Neonatal Nurs 18:93-97, 1989.

39. Pernoll ML and Benson RC, editors: Current obstetrical and gynecologic diagnosis and treatment, ed 6, Norwalk, CT: Appleton & Lange.

40. Pritchard JA, MacDonald PC, and Gant NF: Williams' obstetrics, ed 17, Norwalk, CT, Appleton-Century-Crofts, 1989.

41. Rizak MA, and Hillman CDM: The medical letter handbook of adverse drug interaction, New Rozelle, NY, 1985, The Medical Letter.

42. *Rosenthal M: Grappling with the emotional aspects of infertility, Contemp Obstet Gynecol 27:97-106, 1985.

43. Rubinow D et al: Changes in plasma hormones across the menstrual cycle in patients with menstrually related mood disorder and in control subjects, Am J Obstet Gynecol 158:5-11, 1988.

43a. Sandelowski M: The color gray: ambiguity and infertility, Image 19(2):70-74, 1987.

43b. Sandelowski M and Pollock C: Women's experiences of infertility, Image 18(4):140-144, 1986.

44. Siegler AM and Valle RF: Therapeutic hysteroscopic procedures, Fertil Steril 50:685-701, 1988.

45. Senanayake P and Kramer D: Contraception and etiology of pelvic inflammatory disease: new perspectives, Am J Obstet Gynecol 138:852-860, 1980.

46. Speroff L, Glass RH, and Kase N: Clinical gynecologic endocrinology infertility, ed 4, Baltimore, 1989, Williams & Wilkins.

47. Swerdloff RS, Wang C, and Kandeel FR: Evaluation of the infertile couple, Endocrinol Metab Clin North Am 17:301-337, 1988.

48. Taylor P: The case against HSG as a first time procedure, Contemp Obstet Gynecol 25:49-71, 1985.

49. Thatcher SS: Hysteroscopic sterilization, Obstet Gynecol Clin North Am 15:51-59, 1988.

50. Uphold C and Susman E: Child rearing, marital recreation and work role integration and climacteric symptoms in midlife women, Res Nurs Health 8:73-81, 1985.

51. Upton G: The perimenopause physiologic correlates and clinical management, J Reprod Med 27:1-8, 1982.

52. Utian W: Infertility microsurgery. In Proceedings of the Second Annual MacDonald Hospital Conference of Reproductive Endocrinology, University Hospitals of Cleveland, 1985, Case Western Reserve University.

53. Velduis JD: Management of amenorrhea, Hosp Pract 23(11A):40-56, 1988.

54. Weiss N et al: Estimated incidence of fractures of the lower forearm and hip in postmenopausal women, N Engl J Med 303:1195-1198, 1980.

55. Whitehead MI and Fraser D: Controversies concerning the safety of estrogen replacement therapy, Am J Obstet Gynecol 156:1313-1322, 1987.

56. *Wilson MA: Menstrual disorders: premenstrual syndrome: amenorrhea, J Obstet Gynecol Neonatal Nurs 11:167-179, 1982.

57. Wingate MB: Postmenopausal osteoporosis: concerns and costs in clinical management, J Medicine 15:323-332, 1984.

58. World Health Organization: Women's bleeding patterns: ability to recall and predict menstrual events, Stud Fam Plan 12:17-27, 1981.

59. World Health Organization: The WHO Collaborative Study of Neoplastic and Steroid Contraceptives: breast cancer, cervical cancer, and medroxyprogesterone acetate, Lancet 2:1207-1210, 1984.

60. Woods NF, Most A, and Dery GK: Prevalence of perimenstrual symptoms, Am J Public Health 72:1257-1264, 1982.

61. Yarbro ES and Howards SS: Vasovasostomy, Urol Clin North Am 14:515-526, 1987.

62. *Zion AB: Resources for infertile couples, J Obstet Gynecol Neonatal Nurs 17:255-258, 1988.

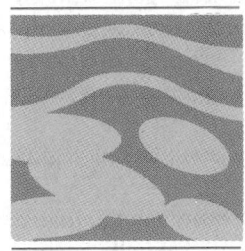

CHAPTER 55

Management of Women with Reproductive Problems

ELLEN F. OLSHANSKY
MARGARET LAMB

CHAPTER OBJECTIVES

After studying this chapter, the student should be able to:
1. Analyze the process of infectious diseases specific to women's reproductive health.
2. Analyze the process of development of structural problems specific to women's reproductive health.
3. Analyze the process of development of benign and malignant diseases specific to women's reproductive health.
4. Develop nursing diagnoses and nursing care plans related to the conditions discussed.

Since both professionals and lay persons have become more enlightened about prevention of problems of the reproductive system, there is heightened awareness of the importance of illness prevention and health promotion throughout the life span. This increased awareness has led many persons to initiate requests for information about or treatment of reproductive system problems.

Although men and women are better informed today about matters relating to reproductive health than they were previously, many neglect preventive measures and ignore signs or symptoms of illness because of embarrassment and the special significance they attach to the reproductive organs.

Despite advances in medicine, science, and technology, diseases and disorders of the genital system continue to threaten the lives and the physical and emotional health of women, sometimes needlessly. Many of these problems are preventable; many of them can be treated and cured. Nurses occupy a unique position because their daily contacts with women provide opportunities to (1) actively seek out persons in need of information and other forms of assistance, (2) help people find necessary information, (3) seek solutions to their problems, (4) increase their awareness of health-promoting measures, and (5) promote their comfort in discussing problems related to reproduction and their prevention and treatment.

INFECTIOUS PROCESSES

INFECTIONS OF THE VULVA AND VAGINA
EPIDEMIOLOGY AND ETIOLOGY

Although the vulva and vagina are considered to be relatively resistant to infections, these occur quite often. Many organisms play a causative role, including streptococci, staphylococci, *Pseudomonas*, *Escherichia coli*, *Candida albicans*, *Trichomonas vaginalis*, *Treponema pallidum*, *Neisseria gonorrhoeae*, chlamydiae, *Trachomatis*, bacteria that cause vaginosis, and the virus of herpes simplex. Parasites such as pinworms, mechanical irritants, and contact allergens can also be the cause of a vaginal discharge. However, women can harbor many of these organisms without developing an infection. Therefore one must consider the factors associated with increased risk of infection in some women. (See research box on p. 1608 for description of a study on *Chlamydia trichomatis* screening.)

PREVENTION

Recognition of predisposing factors is important in the prevention of vulvar and vaginal infections. Associated risk factors include pregnancy, premenarchal age, menopausal and postmenopausal status, allergies, diabetes, oral contraceptives, inadequate hygiene, excessive douching or use of vaginal inserts, treatment with broad-spectrum antibiotics, and intercourse with an infected partner. Women at greatest risk are those whose natural barriers to infection (low estrogen levels, thinness of the vaginal epithelium, reduced acidity of the vagina) are at a minimum.

Some women might require instruction in daily health and hygiene practices. Wearing cotton rather than nylon underwear helps provide ventilation, contributing to an environment less conducive to the growth of infectious organisms. In particular, it is important that women wipe from front to back after bowel movements to avoid fecal contamination of the vulva. Maintaining

RESEARCH

Woolard DB, Larson J, and Hudson L: Screening for *Chlamydia trachomatis* at a university health service, J Obstet Gynecol Neonatal Nurs 18(2):145-149, 1989.

A descriptive study based on retrospective data from a nonprobability sample of 419 female students at a small midwestern university was conducted to assess the usefulness of routine screening for *Chlamydia trachomatis*. The method involved routinely screening all family-planning patients for chlamydia regardless of history of symptoms or high-risk factors such as multiple sexual partners. Results indicated that 53 students (12.6%) were positive for *C. trachomatis;* of this group, 26% had clinical signs and 74% had no clinical signs. In addition, 85% of the 53 students had no symptoms. Thus no statistical significance was found between signs and symptoms and presence of *C. trachomatis* infection. A statistically significant difference was found between those infected with *C. trachomatis* and a higher mean number of sexual partners compared with those not infected, although reliability of subject reporting of number of sexual partners was questioned. Implications for nursing include the importance of routine screening for *C. trachomatis* regardless of presence or absence of signs and symptoms and education of nurses regarding current knowledge of *C. trachomatis*. ∎

cleanliness of the vulva and vagina without altering vaginal pH is essential. Frequent douching may alter vaginal pH, and using a high-pressure douche may irritate vaginal tissues and facilitate the spread of infection into the pelvis. In general, women should not douche unless advised to do so for treatment.

Women can also be advised to void shortly after having intercourse, thus removing organisms from the urethra and vulva. Women also may need to know the characteristics of normal vaginal discharges and how to distinguish between these and abnormal discharges. They must to be informed of the other signs of vulvar and vaginal infections and the particular significance of lesions on the vulva. Sexually active women may require information about how to recognize signs of infection in their partners and the importance of seeking medical attention when they suspect the partner is infected. Use of barrier methods of contraception (condoms, diaphragms) can decrease the risk of acquiring a sexually transmitted disease.[23] Pregnant and diabetic women need to know about their predisposition to infections and how to prevent infection from occurring. They must be urged to seek professional help as soon as signs of infection develop.

PATHOPHYSIOLOGY

Normally the vagina is protected from infection by its pH and the presence of *Döderlein's bacilli*. If the vaginal pH is altered, if the invading organisms are numerous, or if the woman's resistance is decreased by aging, malnutrition, stress, disease, or the use of drugs, the woman's risk of infection is increased. Yeast organisms grow best in an acid pH less than 4.7, whereas *Trichomonas* and organisms causing nonspecific vaginitis thrive in a pH greater than 5.

Organisms causing infection of the vulva and vagina are most often introduced from outside sources such as clothing, hands, douche nozzles, or other contaminated articles or during intercourse. In sexually active women, reinfection may occur following treatment unless their sexual partners are also successfully treated. Because vaginitis produced by *C. albicans*, *Trichomonas*, and bacterial vaginosis, is considered a sexually transmitted disease, it is discussed in greater detail later in Chapter 58.

Nonspecific vaginitis is a superficial vaginal infection that may be caused by bacterial vaginosis or unidentified organisms.

Bacterial vaginosis is a superficial vaginal infection that has undergone many changes in its label. It was first referred to as *corynebacterium vaginalis* and later as *Haemophilus* vaginitis, then called *Gardnerella vaginalis*. Recently its name has been changed to bacterial vaginosis, a more general term reflecting that this infection is caused by several organisms.[44]

Table 55-1 lists normal function, pathophysiology, and clinical picture of vulvar and vaginal infections.

Vaginitis in Mature Women

Women of menopausal and postmenopausal ages often develop vaginitis. (Some refer to this as atrophic or senile vaginitis; a less negative diagnostic label is preferable).

Many physiologic changes that occur secondary to decreased estrogen production during and after menopause predispose women to vaginitis. Pyogenic bacterial invasion of the thin vaginal mucosa produces symptoms of burning, pruritus, and leukorrhea. Vaginitis is usually treated with warm douches of a weak acid solution such as vinegar and water (15 ml [1 tbsp] vinegar to 1 L [1 qt] water). An estrogenic preparation, given orally or applied intravaginally as an ointment, may help to restore the vaginal epithelium to a normal state. Because of the link between estrogen use in menopausal women and endometrial cancer, this therapy should be used with caution.

Bartholinitis

Invasion of Bartholin's glands by streptococci, staphylococci, gonococci, *E. coli*, or anaerobes can result in infection. The infection is usually unilateral, but it can be bilateral. With infection, the duct from the gland becomes partially or completely obstructed, resulting in severe redness, enlargement of the gland, and edema of

TABLE 55-1 Normal function, primary pathophysiology, and clinical picture in infections of vulva and vagina

Normal Function	Pathophysiology	Clinical Picture
Vagina protected by Döderlein's bacilli	Vaginal pH altered; increased number of invading organisms; decreased resistance of woman (caused by aging, malnutrition, stress, drug use, or disease)	Inflammation of tissues, abnormal discharge, itching
Hormonal balance between estrogen and progesterone; during menopause, estrogen decreased	Pyogenic bacterial invasion of thin vaginal mucosa	Burning, pruritus, leukorrhea
Intact Bartholin's, urethral, and Skene's glands	Invasion of glands by organisms	Enlarged glands resulting from accumulation of pus; obstructed glands cause redness, edema of tissues, and pain

the surrounding tissues. The area becomes tender, and walking might become difficult because of the pain. Sometimes the abscess that forms ruptures and affords almost immediate relief of pain. Most often, however, this is followed by recurrence of symptoms. The usual course of the infectious process results in an abscess that does not rupture and requires surgical incision and drainage. A smear or culture is usually taken to identify the causative organism, and an appropriate antibiotic is prescribed. The cervix should be cultured for gonococci.

Occasionally, acute bartholinitis subsides, leaving fibrotic or scar tissue. When this occurs, Bartholin's cyst develops. The cyst may vary in size from a few centimeters in diameter to the size of a hen's egg; it is mobile, and not tender. If the cyst grows sufficiently to interfere with walking or intercourse, or if it shows signs of inflammation, it may be excised surgically.

Skene's glands are less often infected than are Bartholin's glands. When infection does occur, the local symptoms include redness, enlargement of the gland, tenderness, and accumulation of pus. These also may spontaneously rupture or require incision and drainage. Identification of the causative organism by smear or culture is important in determining the need for antibiotic therapy. Infections proved or strongly suspected to be sexually transmitted are discussed in Chapter 58.

In addition to cysts of Bartholin's and Skene's glands, cysts of epidermal origin and sebaceous and sweat gland cysts may arise in the vulva. These are usually asymptomatic but can become infected, sometimes requiring incision and drainage.[8]

CLINICAL MANIFESTATIONS

The common signs of infection of the vulva and vagina are inflammation of the tissues; abnormal discharge from the vagina, urethra, or Bartholin's glands; and itching (pruritus). The discharge may be purulent, white, and curdlike or grayish white. *Leukorrhea,* a white vaginal discharge, is a symptom of vaginal infec-

tions, but it is also associated with erosions of the cervix. This discharge differs from the normal vaginal discharge occurring just before menstruation in that it is more abundant and thicker and is associated with inflammation and pruritus.

Each of the organisms producing vaginitis is usually associated with a specific type of vaginal discharge. (Table 55-2). In addition, each organism might produce slightly different symptoms. Itching usually occurs with most, but *Trichomonas* infection is typically associated with intense itching of the vulva. *C. albicans* infection is also associated with itching. Severe itching may result from menopausal changes in the epithelium, vitamin A deficiency, irritation from chronic discharge, high urinary sugar content as in diabetes mellitus, pediculosis pubis, scabies, allergies, pinworms, and cancer of the vulva. With severe pruritus there are usually excoriations of the skin caused by scratching, and secondary infection may result. Dysuria may occur as a consequence of local irritation of the urinary meatus. Abdominal cramps and abdominal or pelvic fullness might also be associated with vaginal infections.

Lesions of various types may be seen on the vulva, between the labial folds, or inside the vagina. These might appear as macules, papules, boils, abscesses, vesicles, ulcers, or eroded areas. Skene's or Bartholin's glands might be enlarged because of accumulation of pus.

MEDICAL MANAGEMENT

Since most women having vulvar and vaginal infections are treated on an outpatient basis, it is imperative that they be actively involved in decisions and plans related to therapy. A variety of methods are available for management and treatment of vulvar and vaginal infections. The major goals are to (1) cure the infection, (2) prevent reinfection, (3) prevent complications associated with infections of the reproductive tract, and (4) prevent infection of the sexual partner or partners. In fact, with

TABLE 55-2 Common causes of vaginal discharge, symptoms, diagnostic measures, and treatment

Cause	Symptoms	Diagnostic Measures	Treatment
Infections			
Candida albicans (less than 50% of all vaginitis)	White, curdlike, cheesy discharge; characteristic patches on vaginal walls and cervix; itching; inflamed vagina and cervix	Potassium hydroxide (KOH) slide shows hyphae and/or spores; Nickerson culture	Miconazole (Monistat) cream used daily for 14 days Nystatin suppositories daily or bid for 14 days
Trichomonas vaginalis	Yellowish to greenish, frothy, copious discharge; "strawberry spots" on cervix; foul odor; severe burning, itching, and dyspareunia	Saline wet smears show *Trichomonas*	Metronidazole (Flagyl), 250 mg tid for 7 days or 2 g stat for both partners Symptomatic therapy
Bacterial vaginosis	Grayish white, homogenous discharge; scant amount; fishy or foul odor	Saline wet smear demonstrates typical "clue" cells	Oral antibiotics for both partners: ampicillin, 500 mg qid for 5 days; metronidazole (Flagyl), 250 mg tid for 7 days or 500 mg bid for 7 days
Foreign body	Blood-tinged, serosanguineous, or purulent discharge; usually foul odor; discharge may be thick or thin	Visualization of object	Removal of object; antibiotics specific to secondary infection
Allergens or irritants	Increase in usual type and amount of secretions; itching, burning, rash	By exclusion of other possible causes; identification of possible allergen or irritant	Removal of possible allergen or irritant; topical steroid ointment as needed
Cervicitis	Yellow, mucopurulent discharge; erosion seen on cervix; cervix appears inflamed and irritated with varying amounts of ulceration; nabothian cysts; mucosa around os everted	Pap smear; visualization of cervical lesions; gonorrhea or other culture to identify infecting organism	Cauterization; antibiotics; conization of cervix For *Chlamydia* infection: tetracycline, 250 mg qid for 14 days for both partners

From Fogel CI and Woods NF: Health care of women: a nursing perspective, St Louis, 1981, The CV Mosby Co.

TABLE 55-3 Alternative therapies for vaginitis

Infection	Intervention	Dosage	Administration
Candida (Monilia)	Gentian violet	Few drops/qt water 0.25%-2% (over-the-counter drug)	Douche or local application
	Vinegar (white)	1 tbsp/1 pt water	Douche every day for 5-7 days; twice daily for 2 days
	Acidophilus culture	2 tbsp/1 pt water	Douche twice daily
	Acidophilus yogurt Plain yogurt	1 application hourly and as needed to labia for symptom relief	
Trichomonas	1 handful chapparel chamomile	Steep in 1 qt water for 20 min	Douche 2-3 times/wk for 2 wk
Nonspecific vaginitis	Vinegar douche	5 tbsp/2 qt water	Every other day for 1 wk
	Salt (sea)	1 tbsp/1 qt water	Every other day for 1 wk
	1 tsp goldenseal and 1 clove minced garlic	Steep in 1 qt boiling water	Douche every day for 1 wk
	1 tsp goldenseal	Steep in 1 pt water; strain with cloth	Douche every day for 1 wk
	Povidone-iodine (Betadine) gel		Twice daily for 1 wk

From Fogel CI and Woods NF: Health care of women: a nursing perspective, St Louis, 1981, The CV Mosby Co.

Trichomonas infection or persistent nonspecific vaginitis, the partner is often treated as a contact, although he has no signs or symptoms. Usual methods for treating vaginal infections are given in Table 55-2. Some alternative therapies developed by women themselves are included in Table 55-3.

Abscesses require incision and drainage, and this is usually done at the time the woman first seeks medical attention. Some lesions may require biopsy. Antibiotics may be given if cervicitis or systemic effects of another infection are present. Relief from pain occurs almost immediately following incision and drainage. The woman may experience soreness or mild pain for about a day.

■ ASSESSMENT

The patient is asked to give a detailed account of her symptoms, including duration and what she has done to relieve them. The history should include sexual practices, including the last sexual exposure so that the incubation period can be calculated, and information about signs of infection in the partner. The history and physical examination may reveal predisposing factors, patterns of repeated infections, or evidence of concurrent problems. In such cases, further examination, laboratory tests, or clinical studies might be indicated.

The vulva and vagina are inspected and palpated (see Chapter 53). A smear or culture is taken from the vagina, and a Papanicolaou (Pap) smear might also be done. Palpation of the internal organs of reproduction helps to determine whether upward extension of infection has occurred.

■ DATA ANALYSIS: NURSING DIAGNOSES

Nursing diagnoses are determined from assessment of patient data. Possible nursing diagnoses for the woman with an infection of the vulva and/or vagina include but are not limited, to the following:

Diagnostic Title	Possible Etiologies
Infection	Lack of knowledge to avoid pathogens
Knowledge deficit	Unfamiliarity with information sources; lack of exposure and recall
Pain	Vaginal itching, irritation, and inflammation
Sexuality patterns, altered	Altered body structure/function; lack of knowledge; psychologic stress
Social isolation	Altered state of wellness; fear of passing infection to others

■ PLANNING: EXPECTED PATIENT OUTCOMES

Expected patient outcomes for the woman with infection of the vulva and/or vagina may include, but are not limited to, the following:

1. Demonstrate an increase in knowledge about her body and promoting her health.
2. Describe how infections occur and are spread.
3. Identify ways to prevent reinfection.
4. Practice habits that improve or promote her health.
5. State how changes in daily practices influence control of infection.
6. Follow therapies that assist in decreasing pain.
7. Demonstrate knowledge of relationship between sexual activity and infections.
8. Demonstrate improved communication with partner.

■ IMPLEMENTATION

Improving Knowledge

The woman and her partner should be given accurate information regarding how infections occur, spread, and recur, as well as ways to prevent infection and the spread of existing infection (see Chapter 58). In addition, women should be taught self-care techniques that promote healing.

When pruritus is present, the patient needs to know that any irritation, such as scratching, can aggravate the itching and predispose to secondary infection. Frequent bathing, sitz baths, and careful cleansing are essential for comfort as well as prevention of complications. Soothing lotions are sometimes prescribed to relieve itching. If the pruritus is severe enough to interfere with sleep, the physician might prescribe a mild sedative.

Decreasing Pain

Women can be advised to follow certain procedures to help them in decreasing the pain of infection. For example, heat increases circulation, promotes healing, and provides comfort. Applications of heat may be prescribed in the form of hot soaks, douches, perineal irrigations, or sitz baths. The patient may require instruction in these procedures. If both heat and local applications of medications are prescribed, the patient is instructed to use the medication after application of heat.

Improving Altered Sexuality Patterns

The woman and her partner should be encouraged to discuss their concerns regarding their sexuality patterns. Ideally, the partner should accompany the woman to her appointment with the health care provider so that the partner understands what changes, if any, are advised in their sexual relationship while the infection is being treated. In addition, misunderstandings regarding sexuality may be prevented or corrected. Discussing with one another the stresses that may have occurred in their relationship may also improve their sexual relationship.

Most women who have vaginal infections are advised to abstain from intercourse during the period of treatment. The extent to which abstinence is possible should be explored, and if this is not feasible for the woman, use of a condom by the male partner until symptoms of infection disappear can be suggested.

Women taking oral contraceptives should be carefully screened and examined during interim visits to the physician for signs of vaginal infection. If repeated episodes of infection occur, it might be necessary for the patient to try an alternate brand or different dosage of pill used as a contraceptive. If infections continue, it usually becomes necessary for the woman to use an entirely different method of birth control (see Chapter 54).

Decreasing Social Isolation

The fear of spreading the infection is often a cause of social isolation, many times because of misinformation and misunderstanding about how the infection is spread. This is interrelated with altered sexuality patterns. Thus, as with altered sexuality patterns, the woman and her partner should be encouraged to attend an appointment together with a health care provider.

Treating Infection

Douching is frequently prescribed for treatment of vaginal infections; for example, povidone-iodine (Betadine) douches are recommended for *Trichomonas* when metronidazole is contraindicated. Local applications in the form of vaginal suppositories, ointments, or creams are often used when vaginal infection occurs. A model of the pelvis is of value in showing women how to use these preparations. The woman is advised of the importance of handwashing before and after each application. Because the substances used to treat vaginitis melt with body heat, the patient is advised to lie down after insertion to facilitate distribution of the medication in the vaginal canal and to prevent loss of medication from the vagina. This medication is usually administered at bedtime for this reason. Women are advised not to douche but to wear a minipad.

Patient Teaching

Instructions for the woman with a vaginal infection include the following:
1. After incision and drainage:
   a. Expect a small amount of purulent drainage (may be blood tinged).
   b. Report signs of active, bright-red bleeding.
   c. Use warm water to cleanse involved area after each voiding or bowel movement.
2. Wash hands before and after medication applications or treatments.
3. Lie down after applying vaginal ointments or suppositories.
4. Use only prescribed douches during infective period; douche equipment should be washed and soaked in diluted bleach for 30 minutes.
5. Abstain from intercourse during period of treatment.
6. Report signs of unexplained fever and increased pain, discharge, or dysuria.
7. Return for follow-up care as instructed; avoid douching for 24 to 48 hours before an examination.

CERVICITIS

EPIDEMIOLOGY AND ETIOLOGY

Cervicitis, infection of the cervix, is the most common gynecologic disorder, affecting more than half of all women. Cervicitis can follow childbirth or abortion, or it can be caused by infection of a cervical laceration or erosion. In untreated cervicitis the tissues are constantly irritated, and some evidence suggests that this irritation predisposes to cancer.

PREVENTION

If the practice of a careful 6-week postpartum examination were adhered to and if women had yearly examinations, much acute and chronic cervicitis could be prevented. During childbirth the cervix is frequently lacerated as it stretches and thins to allow the baby to pass through the birth canal. These torn surfaces do not al-

TABLE 55-4 Normal function, primary pathophysiology, and clinical picture in cervicitis

Normal Function	Pathophysiology	Clinical Picture
Cervix is pink, nontender; no lesions; os is closed	Gonococcus, streptococcus, staphylococcus, herpesvirus, and chlamydia may invade cervix	Leukorrhea may be only sign; pain may occur if infection extends upward; grossly erythematous and edematous cervix Chronic: constant irritation; possible cervical laceration, purulent discharge, erythema, hypertrophy, hyperemia; potential infertility from thick cervical mucus

ways heal properly and thus serve as foci for infection. At the 6-week postpartum examination, improperly healed lacerations of the cervix and cervical erosions can be easily detected and treated.

Prompt detection and treatment of infections of the vulva and vagina can prevent upward spread of infection that results in cervicitis. The preventive aspects discussed under infection of the vulva and vagina are applicable to prevention of cervical infections. Opportunities similarly arise for teaching women about desirable health habits and prescribed therapy.

PATHOPHYSIOLOGY

The gonococcus, streptococcus, staphylococcus, a variety of other aerobic and anaerobic organisms, herpesvirus, and chlamydia may be responsible for the infection (see Table 55-4). There are two forms of cervicitis, acute and chronic. Chronic cervicitis is the most frequent of all the pathologic conditions of the cervix. Cervicitis usually progresses from the acute to the chronic form if not treated, and it can go undetected for a long period. The cervix might heal and appear quite healthy after the disease has spread upward. This condition presents few symptoms, and those symptoms that occur do not ordinarily lead women to seek medical attention. Leukorrhea may be the only sign, and if it is a small amount of discharge, the woman may not become concerned. Pain does not usually occur unless the infection extends upward and involves the uterus or adjacent pelvic structures. A long history of leukorrhea may lead the nurse or physician to suspect cervicitis.

CLINICAL MANIFESTATIONS

Acute cervicitis may be present without subjective symptoms. When inspected, however, the cervix is grossly erythematous and edematous, and the mucosa around the external os shows hypertrophic ectopy and looks everted. There is usually a mucoid, purulent discharge from the cervix, but the amount might be so small that it is not noticed by the patient. A smear or culture of the discharge is taken to determine the causative organism, as well as the number of white blood cells (WBCs).

Chronic cervicitis is a common cause of leukorrhea. On examination, a laceration or eversion of the cervix may be seen. Purulent discharge from the cervix often occurs, and erythema and hypertrophy of the cervix are usually present. Inclusion cysts, appearing as gray or white vesicles, may be seen on the surface of the cervix. A reddened, irritated area (an erosion) may or may not be present. Hyperemia of the infected cervix may produce intermenstrual or postcoital spotting. Some women may merely complain of infertility, as a result of the thick, viscid cervical mucus interrupting sperm

transport; pruritus; or vulvar burning. Others may experience lower abdominal pain or dyspareunia as a result of pelvic congestion.

A Pap smear or cervical biopsy specimen is frequently taken when patients have cervicitis. This is usually done as a precautionary measure to rule out malignancy. Often a Pap smear, indicating inflammatory changes, may be the first clue to cervicitis.

INTERVENTIONS

In acute cervicitis the associated vaginitis is usually treated first, and then the condition of the cervix is evaluated. Acute gonococcal cervicitis is usually treated with procaine penicillin G, 4.8 million units given intramuscularly. Women who are allergic to penicillin can be treated with tetracycline, 1.5 g, followed by 0.5 g four times daily for 3 days. Often chlamydial infection is present along with gonorrhea; therefore optimal treatment includes penicillin and tetracycline.[23] Usually the cervix is recultured in a week, and serologic tests for syphilis performed 6 to 9 weeks later.

Women with trichomoniasis are given metronidazole (Flagyl), 250 mg two times daily for 10 days. An alternative treatment is 2 g of metronidazole at once. Alcohol should not be ingested during treatment with Flagyl, since Flagyl contains Antabuse-like properties. For candidal infections, nystatin vaginal suppositories (100 mg) are used twice daily for 10 days, or miconazole (Monistat) cream may be used. Bacterial vaginosis are treated with metronidazole, 500 mg twice a day for 7 days, or with ampicillin, 500 mg four times daily for 7 days. Some physicians advocate treatment of acute cervicitis with tetracycline, 2 g daily for 7 days, because of the high prevalence of chlamydia as the causative organism in cervicitis, an organism that responds to tetracycline therapy.

When cervical lacerations or erosions are present, the area is usually cauterized. Silver nitrate sticks may be used to remove very small lesions. For larger areas requiring cauterization, an electric cautery unit is used. The woman is informed that a small, lubricated sheet of lead will be placed against the skin under the lumbar areas as a safety device for grounding electrical charges and that there will be slight bleeding, which will be controlled by a tampon or packing inserted by the physician. The odor of burning tissue when cautery is used is distressing to some patients. They should be told to expect an odor but that the odor is insignificant and that the procedure is over quickly.

Following cauterization, the nurse can ascertain that the patient understands instructions for follow-up care. Directions vary but usually include the following:

1. Leave the tampon or packing in place as long as the physician advises (usually 8 to 24 hours).

2. Report to the hospital or physician's office if bleeding is excessive (more than occurs during a normal menses is considered excessive).

3. Do not use a douche or have sexual relations until the next visit to the physician unless specific instructions have been given as to when intercourse can be safely resumed.

4. An unpleasant discharge caused by sloughing of destroyed cells may appear 4 to 5 days following cauterization; a warm bath several times a day will help this condition, which should not last more than a few days.

Additional opportunities for teaching and counseling may arise during the course of treatment of cervicitis.

PELVIC INFLAMMATORY DISEASE
EPIDEMIOLOGY AND ETIOLOGY

Pelvic inflammatory disease (PID) is an infectious process involving the fallopian tubes, ovaries, pelvic peritoneum, pelvic veins, or pelvic connective tissue. The infection may be confined to one structure, or it may be widespread and involve all of the pelvic structures. Inflammation of the fallopian tube is known as *salpingitis,* and inflammation of the ovary is known as *oophoritis.* (The routes of pelvic infection are shown in Figure 55-1.)

In addition to the gonococcus organisms, chlamydia, coliforms, *Haemophilus,* streptococcus, mycoplasma, and anaerobes have been implicated in severe or recurrent salpingitis. These pathogens may invade the pelvic organs during sexual intercourse, childbirth, the postpartum period, or when an abortion is done. The rupture of any adjacent structure may spill organisms into the pelvic cavity, thus producing secondary infection. For example, when the appendix perforates, pelvic peritonitis may follow. PID is reported to occur five times more often among women using intrauterine devices (IUDs) than among women using other birth control methods. These women must be urged to have regular checkups for signs of infection. Instruction in prevention and signs of infection is important.

PREVENTION

The potential destructive effects of PID on the reproductive organs, coupled with the prevalence of gonorrhea and other sexually transmitted diseases, should mobilize every nurse to engage in case finding for the purpose of education. To prevent PID and its serious consequences, it is important to prevent infections of the vulva, vagina, and cervix and to treat these infections promptly when they occur. Knowing the factors that predipose women to PID is important in identification of the population at risk.

Hospitalized women usually have decreased resistance and need protection against infection. Gynecologic disorders of long duration are especially debilitating. Surgery of the reproductive tract, childbearing, and abortion lower resistance and provide portals of entry for organisms. Cleanliness and asepsis are important in giving care to these women, and every attempt should be made to prevent introduction of organisms into the reproductive tract.

Every sexually active woman having a physical examination should have a routine cervical smear or culture taken to screen for gonorrhea. Women need to be informed of methods of preventing infection, how to recognize infection in their sexual partners, and what to do when they suspect infection has occurred.

PATHOPHYSIOLOGY

Pathogenic organisms are usually introduced from outside the body and pass up the cervical canal into the uterus. They seem to cause little trouble in the uterus but pass into the pelvis by way of the fallopian tubes through thrombosed uterine veins or through the lymphatics of the uterus. The invaded structures become involved in an acute or chronic inflammatory process. Many of the pathogens causing PID lodge in the fallopian tubes. Purulent material collects in the tubes, adhesions form, strictures may occur, and sterility is a frequent result. Infertility is one of the most serious consequences of PID. Although tubal surgery is available for correcting tubal adhesions, fertility after tubal surgery is not ensured. Obstruction of the fallopian tubes resulting from inflammation may be complete or partial. Complete obstruction of the tubes makes conception impossible. Partial tubal obstruction predisposes the woman to ectopic pregnancy, since the fertilized ovum cannot reach the uterus, although the sperm has been able to pass the stricture and produce conception. Adhesions resulting from inflammation may cause such distress that complete removal of the uterus, fallopian tubes, and ovaries may be necessary. Although generalized peritonitis can occur, the infection usually remains con-

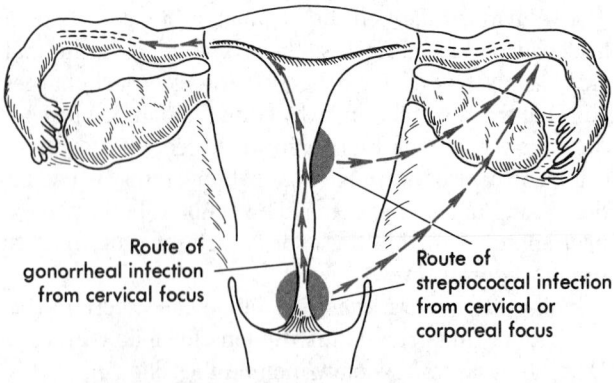

FIGURE 55-1 Two main routes of pelvic infection. (From Novak ER, Jones GJ, and Jones HW Jr: Novak's textbook of gynecology, ed 10, Baltimore, 1980, Williams & Wilkins.)

fined to the lower abdomen and pelvis. An abscess in Douglas' cul-de-sac often occurs.

CLINICAL MANIFESTATIONS

Signs and symptoms of *acute* PID include severe abdominal pain (or pressure and fullness), lower abdominal cramps, intermenstrual spotting, dyspareunia, fever and chills, malaise, nausea, and vomiting. There may be a foul-smelling purulent vaginal discharge. These symptoms last for a variable time. If they are mild and the woman ignores them, the symptoms may temporarily subside. Some cases of acute PID are never reported to a nurse or physician.

Chronic PID is generally considered to be a result of undiagnosed, inadequately treated, or neglected acute PID. This type of pelvic inflammation is characterized by chronic, dull, aching pain in the lower abdomen; backache; constipation; malaise; low-grade fever; and disturbances of menstruation. During periods of exacerbation, acute symptoms return. Occasionally a patient might be labeled neurotic because of the repeated, nonspecific nature of her complaints. The diagnosis of PID may be made when the patient seeks medical care for another problem, such as menstrual irregularity or infertility.

Abdominal palpation usually reveals the presence of pain and tenderness in the lower abdomen and lower quadrants. Most often, both lower quadrants are painful on palpation. On vaginal examination, the pain and tenderness increase with movement of the pelvic organs. Masses may be felt in either one or both quadrants, which indicates enlargement of the fallopian tubes or ovaries or an abscess. A mass may be palpated in Douglas' cul-de-sac when abscess formation occurs in this site. If adhesions are present, the pelvic organs may be less movable than normal.

Smears and cultures taken from the vagina, cervix, or Douglas' cul-de-sac may aid in identification of the causative organism and its sensitivity to antibiotics. Culdoscopy is usually done when an abscess in the cul-de-sac is suspected. If an abscess is seen, a specimen is secured by aspiration. Laparoscopy has gained popularity in the diagnosis of PID because it permits visualization of the reproductive organs and adjacent tissues.

INTERVENTIONS

Treatment for outpatients consists of cefoxitin, 2.0 g intramuscularly; or amoxicillin, 3.0 g orally; or ampicillin, 3.5 g orally; or aqueous procaine penicillin G, 4.8 million units at two sites. Each of these medications is administered with probenecid, 1.0 g orally twice a day for 10 to 14 days. Tetracycline, 500 mg four times a day for 10 days has been administered, but sources indicate that outpatient treatment of PID with either tetracyline alone or penicillin/ampicillin alone is less effective and not recommended.[23] Some patients with PID are hospi-

---

> ### PATIENT TEACHING FOR PELVIC INFLAMMATORY DISEASE
>
> 1. Effects of PID on general health and functioning of the reproductive organs
> 2. Method by which organisms gain entry to the reproductive organs and how infection can spread by continuity of tissue
> 3. Medication therapy and importance of taking medication for the prescribed period
> 4. Signs that should be reported to physician (return of symptoms, increased vaginal discharge)
> 5. Need to return for follow-up care as instructed

talized. They are usually placed on bed rest in mid-Fowler's position to provide dependent drainage so that abscesses will not form high in the abdomen, where they might rupture and cause generalized peritonitis. Intravenous fluids may be indicated. It is recommended that sexual partners of women with PID be treated as contacts.

Heat (a hot-water bottle or electric heating pad) applied to the abdomen may promote circulation and comfort. Analgesics may be necessary to alleviate pain. The woman is instructed to observe the amount, color, consistency, and odor of any vaginal discharge and changes in pain level. Her temperature is usually monitored every 4 hours until fever subsides. In some instances, women may need to be hospitalized for therapy. Patient teaching is described in the box above.

Salpingectomy may be necessary in the event of tubal abscess, and all the reproductive organs may require removal in severe cases of chronic inflammation.

TOXIC SHOCK SYNDROME
EPIDEMIOLOGY AND ETIOLOGY

Toxic shock syndrome (TSS) is a severe acute disease associated with strains of staphylococci of phage group I, which produce a unique epidermal toxin. The incidence of TSS is much greater among women during menstruation and among women using tampons, particularly superabsorbent tampons. Women at increased risk for developing TSS include those who insert tampons with their fingers rather than with inserters provided with many brands of tampons; those who have had a chronic vaginal infection; and those with herpes genitalis.

PREVENTION

The primary means for preventing TSS in women is through prevention of the introduction of organisms. Following hygienic principles for cleaning the perineum, caring for douche equipment, and handling tampons aseptically may help prevent vaginal colonization with *Staphylococcus aureus*. In addition, women can modify their use of tampons by avoiding superabsorbent brands, or they can use sanitary napkins instead of tampons. Tampon manufacturers now recommend that women use only the absorbency necessary, change tampons at least every 4 to 6 hours, and use sanitary napkins at night. More frequent changing of tampons may produce ulcerations, thus actually increasing the risk of infection. Recurrent TSS can be limited by use of the β-lactamase–resistant antibiotics. Women who carry *S. aureus* should be advised of this so they can make informed choices regarding menstrual hygiene. It is suggested that women who use the diaphragm for contraception limit its use to not more than 24 hours at one time.

PATHOPHYSIOLOGY

TSS recurs in some women during subsequent menstrual periods, although treatment of TSS with β-lactamase–resistant antibiotics (for example, cephalosporins and penicillinase-resistant penicillins) may decrease the likelihood of recurrence. It is suggested that the organism gains entry to the circulation through lesions in the vagina produced by tampons. Superabsorbent tampons maintain a milieu favorable to bacterial growth, since they can contain a large amount of menstrual blood and may be left in place several hours. TSS may also occur in men.

CLINICAL MANIFESTATIONS

The woman experiencing TSS exhibits a fever greater than 38.9° C (102° F), palmar or diffuse erythroderma followed by desquamation of the skin of the hands and feet, hypotension or orthostatic dizziness, hyperemia of the conjunctivae or mucous membranes, and multisystem dysfunction, including symptoms such as vomiting or diarrhea, alterations in consciousness, and impaired renal, hepatic, or cardiopulmonary function. TSS has caused death in some women. The diagnosis of TSS is usually confirmed by cultures for *S. aureus*.[17,46]

INTERVENTIONS

Women who are menstruating and develop a sudden high fever accompanied by vomiting or diarrhea should be counseled to seek immediate treatment. If the woman is wearing a tampon, she should remove it immediately. Treatment of TSS involves use of β-lactamase–resistant antibiotics. Women who are acutely ill with TSS require careful monitoring and supportive therapy similar to that given patients with septic shock (see Chapter 25).

STRUCTURAL PROBLEMS

UTERINE DISPLACEMENT
EPIDEMIOLOGY AND ETIOLOGY

Displacement of the uterus, bladder, and rectum can be congenital or acquired because of stretching of the liga-

ments supporting the uterus and stretching of the muscles of the perineal floor. Acquired displacement of these structures usually results from unrepaired lacerations during childbirth and ill-advised bearing down during labor. Repeated, close pregnancies especially predispose to loss of muscle tone and displacement of the uterus and other pelvic structures.

PREVENTION

With better obstetric care, use of episiotomies to prevent tearing of the pelvic muscles, immediate repair of all tears, and the trend toward fewer pregnancies and births per woman, fewer women should require vaginal wall repairs late in life. Perineal exercises practiced following delivery help to prevent relaxation. Apparently relaxation can also be caused by a congenital weakness of the muscles of the pelvis, because it occurs occasionally in women who have had no children.

PATHOPHYSIOLOGY

As the uterus begins to drop, the vaginal walls become relaxed, and a fold of vaginal mucosa may protrude outside the vaginal orifice. This is known as a *colpocele*. With the relaxation of the vaginal walls, the bladder may herniate into the vagina (a *cystocele*), or the rectal wall may herniate into the vagina (a *rectocele*) (Figure 55-2). Both conditions may occur simultaneously.

Older women may have suffered from these conditions for years and yet may not have sought medical attention. They may remember that their mothers had a similar condition and think that it is to be expected in women who have borne children. Since they are not incapacitated, some may decide not to have reparative surgery that they know is available. Some delay seeking treatment because they dread surgery or because of the expense. However, untreated displacements of the uterus can cause complications such as cervical ulceration and infection, cystitis, and hemorrhoids.

CLINICAL MANIFESTATIONS

A sign of relaxation of the pelvic musculature is a dragging pain in the back and in the pelvis. It worsens with standing or walking. The woman who has a cystocele may complain of urinary incontinence accompanying activity that increases intraabdominal pressure, such as coughing, laughing, walking, or lifting (*stress incontinence*). The cystocele may become so pronounced that, in order for the patient to void, the bladder must be pushed back into place by holding the finger against the anterior vaginal wall. The patient with a rectocele may complain of constipation and resultant hemorrhoids.

■ ASSESSMENT

Assessment of a woman with structural problems includes a careful history of symptoms such as pain, uri-

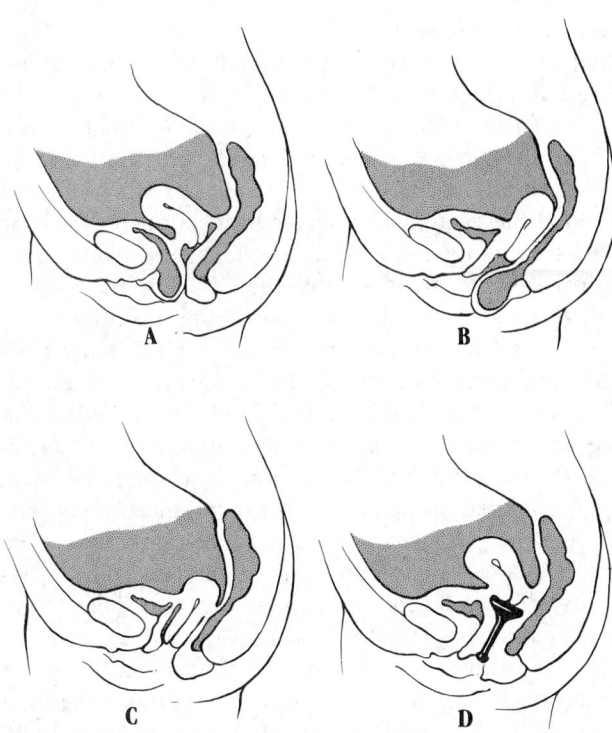

FIGURE 55-2 Abnormalities of vagina. **A,** Cystocele: downward displacement of bladder toward vaginal orifice. **B,** Rectocele: pouching of rectum into posterior wall of vagina. **C,** Prolapse of uterus into vaginal canal. **D,** Stem pessary in place to maintain normal anatomic position of uterus.

nary incontinence, or constipation. A physical examination includes a pelvic examination with careful inspection of the vaginal walls and adjacent organs.

■ DATA ANALYSIS: NURSING DIAGNOSES

Nursing diagnoses for a woman with structural problems of the reproductive system, including uterine displacement and fistulas, may include, but are not limited to, the following:

Diagnostic Title	Possible Etiologies
Body image disturbance	Drainage or changes in structure of reproductive organs
Constipation	Rectocele
Incontinence, stress	Cystocele
Knowledge deficit	Lack of information regarding the structural problem
Pain	Rectocele, fistulas, or postsurgical pain
Sexuality patterns, altered	Hygiene problems such as incontinence or drainage
Social isolation	Problem managing drainage or incontinence

■ PLANNING: EXPECTED PATIENT OUTCOMES

Expected patient outcomes for a woman with structural problems may include, but are not limited to, the following:

1. Patient demonstrates increased knowledge about structural problem and cause of condition such as uterine displacement or fistulas
2. Patient demonstrates understanding of surgical or medical plan of care
3. Patient describes therapies to enhance healing and decrease infection after surgery
4. Patient describes measures to relieve pain postoperatively
5. Patient describes safe sexual practices after surgery

INTERVENTIONS

Cystoceles and rectoceles are treated by surgical procedures designed to tighten the vaginal wall. The surgery is done through the vagina. The repair for a cystocele is called an *anterior colporrhaphy;* the repair for rectocele is called a *posterior colporrhaphy.* Previous tears of the pelvic floor, usually caused by childbearing, may also be repaired. Such repair is called a *perineorrhaphy.*

General Surgical Care

As part of the preoperative preparation, a cleansing douche is frequently ordered the morning of surgery. When surgery involving the vagina is performed, postoperative nursing care includes prevention of pressure on the vaginal suture line and prevention of wound infection (see box on p. 1618). Perineal dressings are seldom used.

Posterior Colporrhaphy

Women who are having a posterior colporrhaphy are given a cathartic approximately 24 hours before surgery, and several enemas usually are given preoperatively to help ensure an empty bowel at the time of surgery and immediately thereafter. Up to 24 hours preoperatively, she may be permitted only clear liquids orally to further reduce bowel contents. Postoperatively, the patient may be kept flat in bed or in a low Fowler's position to prevent increased intraabdominal pressure or strain on the wound. Special attention must be given to exercise for the patient's legs, to having her turn frequently, and to having her cough deeply. For 5 days only liquids are permitted orally, and camphorated tincture of opium (paregoric) is also given to inhibit bowel function. After this time, mineral oil is given each night, and an oil-retention enema is given the morning after the first laxative is given. Only a soft rectal tube and

GUIDELINES FOR CARE FOLLOWING VAGINAL OR PERINEAL SURGERY

1. Give perineal care after each voiding or defecation:
   a. Pour sterile normal saline over vulva and perineum.
   b. Cleanse perineum as needed with sterile cotton balls; cleanse away from vagina toward rectum.
   c. Dry perineum as needed with sterile cotton balls.
2. Use a heat lamp as needed to help dry the perineum and prevent tissue sloughing.
3. Encourage sitz baths after sutures are removed.
4. If douches are ordered during immediate postoperative period:
   a. Use sterile equipment and sterile solution.
   b. Insert douche nozzle very gently and rotate carefully.
5. Avoid pressure on suture line:
   a. Avoid a full bladder; keep urinary catheter patent.
   b. Use measures to prevent constipation.
   c. Teach patient to avoid Valsalva maneuver.
6. Provide an ice pack for perineal discomfort (covered, sealed plastic bags or gloves make an acceptable pack).
7. Teach patient to:
   a. Take daily douches and tub baths as prescribed.
   b. Take measures to avoid constipation; laxatives may be necessary until healing is complete.
   c. Avoid sexual intercourse until safe to do so.
   d. Avoid jarring activities and heavy lifting for 6 weeks postoperatively.

small amount of oil (200 ml) should be used. Straining to produce a bowel movement is discouraged. Enemas for relieving flatus and for cleansing the bowel usually are not given until at least a week postoperatively.

Anterior Colporrhaphy

After an anterior colporrhaphy, an indwelling catheter is usually left in the bladder for about 4 days. The catheter should keep the bladder completely empty. If the catheter is not used and if the patient is taking sufficient fluid, voiding should be checked at least every 4 hours. No more than 100 ml of urine should be allowed to accumulate in the bladder. It is usually very difficult to catheterize a patient following a vaginal repair, since the urethral orifice may be distorted and edematous. Having the patient take deep breaths may help in locating the orifice because it dilates slightly with each breath. A soft rubber catheter should be used. Ambulation is begun immediately after surgery. A regular diet is given, and mineral oil is taken each night to lessen the need to strain on defecation.

Urethral Suspension

Sometimes a vaginal plastic procedure does not relieve the stress incontinence caused by a cystocele and by general relaxation of the pelvic floor. When this happens, the ligaments about the bladder neck may be shortened in such a way that the bladder drops less easily into the vagina. The degree of incontinence may be tested by filling the bladder to various levels with sterile normal saline solution and then having the patient cough or strain while standing. If the incontinence is severe, the patient may be placed in a lithotomy position, and the physician fills the bladder with normal saline solution and supports the bladder neck with a finger or with a clamp in the vagina to test the effectiveness of the bladder with this support. If the patient can cough and strain down without being incontinent, she is considered a good candidate for the procedure. The surgery consists of a retropubic urethral suspension and is usually combined with further vaginal repair. A urethral catheter is inserted, and nursing care is similar to that following a vaginal repair. If the catheter does not drain freely or if the patient without a catheter does not void within 4 to 6 hours, the physician should be notified. Pressure from a full bladder may disrupt the repair.

PROLAPSE OF THE UTERUS
PATHOPHYSIOLOGY

Prolapse of the uterus, or procidentia uteri, is extreme downward displacement of the uterus. The severity of the displacement is designated as first, second, or third degree. In *first-degree* prolapse the cervix is still within the vagina. In *second-degree* prolapse the cervix protrudes from the vaginal orifice. In *third-degree* prolapse the entire uterus, which is suspended by its stretched ligaments, hangs below the vaginal orifice. In both second-degree and third-degree prolapses, the cervix becomes irritated from clothing, the circulation becomes impaired, and ulceration often follows.

CLINICAL MANIFESTATIONS

Displacement of the uterus may cause dysmenorrhea, although many women with known displacements have no pain. Some women with displacement complain of chronic backache, pelvic pressure, easy fatigue, and leukorrhea in addition to painful menstruation.

Common types of displacement are *anteflexion*, *retroflexion*, and *retroversion* of the uterus caused by congenitally weak uterine ligaments, adhesions following infections or surgery in the pelvic region, or the strain of pregnancy on the ligaments. A space-filling lesion in this region or even a full bladder or rectum may also displace the uterus enough to cause symptoms. Normally the body of the uterus flexes forward at a 45-degree angle at the cervix. In retroflexion, this angle is increased; in anteflexion, it is decreased; in retroversion, the whole uterus is tipped backward (Figure 55-3).

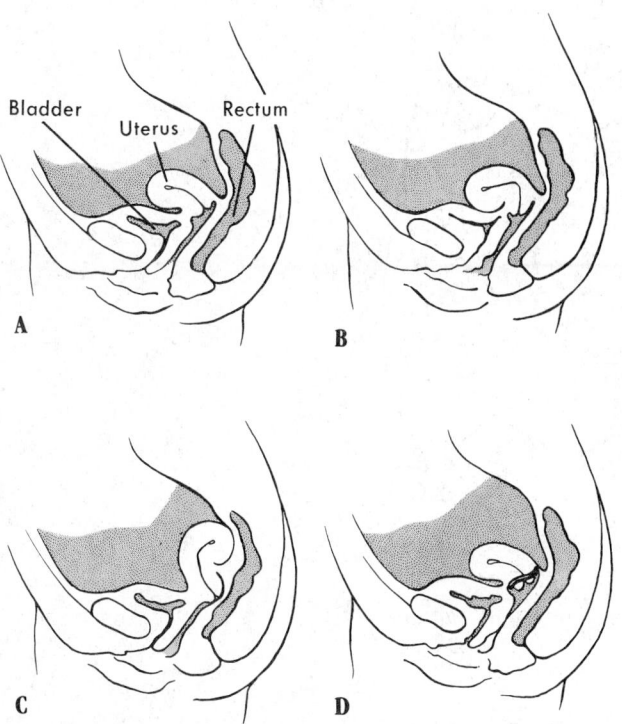

FIGURE 55-3 Normal and abnormal positions of uterus. **A,** Normal anatomic position of uterus in relation to adjacent structures. **B,** Anterior displacement of uterus. **C,** Retroversion or backward displacement of uterus. **D,** Normal anatomic position of uterus maintained by use of rubber S-shaped pessary.

INTERVENTIONS

If the displacement is not caused by some coexistent pelvic disease, various pelvic exercises may be recommended in an attempt to return the uterus to a normal position. These exercises, using the principles of gravity, stretch or strengthen the uterine ligaments. Some exercises used are knee-chest exercises, the "monkey trot," lying on the abdomen 2 hours a day, and premenstrual exercises. Corrective exercises for poor posture may also be prescribed.

In doing knee-chest exercises, the woman is instructed to assume a knee-chest position and to separate the labia to allow air to enter the vagina, since this helps to produce normal positioning of the uterus. This position should be maintained for 5 minutes two or three times a day.

In doing the monkey trot, the woman is instructed to walk about on her hands and feet, keeping the knees straight. This should be done for 5 minutes two or three times a day.

The usual treatment for a uterine prolapse is hysterectomy. This procedure may sometimes be done by the vaginal route. If any surgery is contraindicated because of the age or general condition of the patient, a pessary can be inserted to hold the uterus up in the pelvis (Fig-

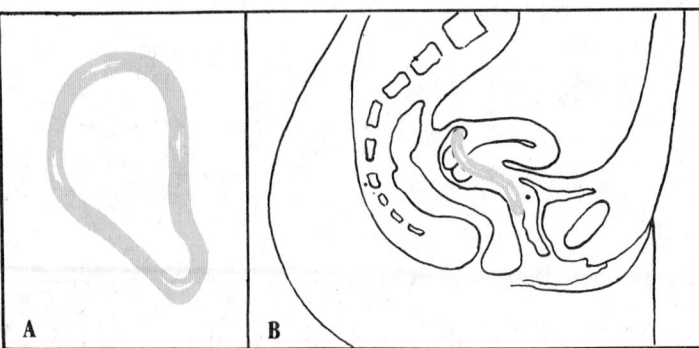

FIGURE 55-4 A, Albert Smith pessary. **B,** Pessary in place to hold posterior vaginal fornix, and with it attached cervix, well backward and upward in pelvis. (From Beacham DW and Beacham WD: Synopsis of gynecology, ed 10, St Louis, 1982, The CV Mosby Co.)

ure 55-4). A string should be attached to the pessary, and after its insertion the woman pins the string to her underclothing. This type of pessary occasionally becomes displaced and might cause the patient embarrassment.

FISTULAS

Fistulas can occur in several locations (Figure 55-5). They may develop when a malignant lesion has spread or when radiation treatment has been used for a malignancy, or they may be caused by trauma at surgery or delivery.

Women with vesicovaginal or rectovaginal fistulas may become withdrawn because of embarrassment about odors and soiling of their clothing. Sometimes women become immune to the odors associated with a fistula. Chlorine solution (for example, 5 ml [1 tsp] chlorine household bleach to 1 L [1 qt] water) makes a satisfactory deodorizing douche, and this solution is also excellent for external perineal irrigation. Sitz baths and thorough cleansing of the surrounding skin with mild soap and water are helpful. Deodorizing powders such as sodium borate can be used. Care is time consuming and must be repeated at regular intervals to ensure cleanliness. Protective pants can be worn.

The patient needs encouragement from the medical and nursing staff and needs assurance that they understand her problem. When fistulas persist, couples have special problems that require patience and understanding. Husband and wife should be encouraged to communicate with one another regarding interference with their sexual relationship.

URETEROVAGINAL FISTULAS

Ureterovaginal fistulas frequently complicate gynecologic treatment. In treating cancer of the uterus, either by radiation or by surgery or occasionally when a hyster-

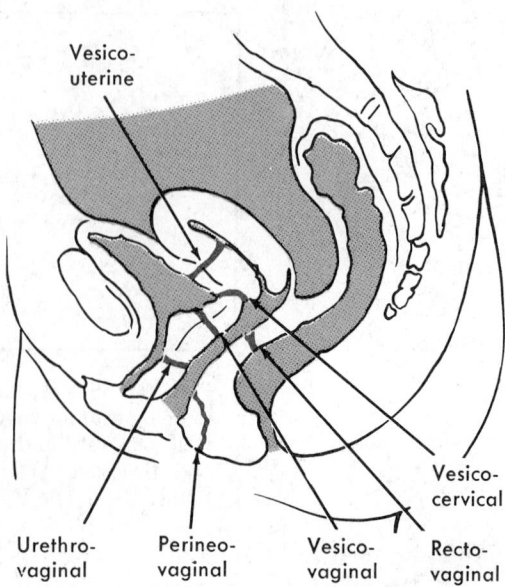

FIGURE 55-5 Types of fistulas that may develop in vagina and uterus.

ectomy is done, the blood supply to the ureter may be impaired, or other damage may occur. The ureteral wall sloughs, and a fistula opens from the ureter to the vagina. This causes a constant drip of urine through the vagina. A ureterovaginal fistula usually heals spontaneously after a time. If it does not, repair procedures may be attempted, and occasionally an ileobladder must be made (see Chapter 48).

VESICOVAGINAL AND URETHROVAGINAL FISTULAS

Vesicovaginal fistulas, or fistulas between the bladder and the vagina, and urethrovaginal fistulas, between the urethra and the vagina, may follow radiation of the cervix, gynecologic surgery, or trauma during delivery. It is impossible to perform surgery to repair the fistula until the inflammation and induration have subsided. This may take 3 to 4 months. A suprapubic incision is made into the bladder, the fistula tract is dissected out, and the defect is closed by primary closure or by using a graft from the bladder or adjacent mucosal wall.

Postoperatively, usually both a suprapubic tube and a urethral catheter are inserted to drain the bladder. These tubes are sometimes attached to a "bubble" suction drainage apparatus in order to ensure that the bladder is kept empty. Bladder drainage is maintained for about 1 week or until the wound is completely healed. The catheters should not be irrigated unless it is absolutely necessary, and only very gentle pressure should be used when irrigating them. Signs of urinary drainage from the vagina should be noted. Normally a small amount of serosanguineous drainage occurs from the vagina for a few days postoperatively. Vaginal douches

may be ordered and should be given gently and with little pressure from the fluid. Women may need to stay in bed for several days or may need to remain in their rooms if bubble suction is being used. Such confinement is tiring, and visitors, television, radio, reading materials, and a variety of occupational therapy activities may help to pass the time satisfactorily.

The results of repair surgery for fistulas are not always successful. The patient must sometimes have several procedures, and each successive hospitalization increases her anxiety about the outcome of surgery and lessens her ability to accept the discomforts and inconveniences entailed. All possible nursing measures should be taken to prevent infection and to be certain that free drainage of urine is ensured. Obstruction of drainage tubes may place pressure against the newly repaired vesicovaginal wall and cause healing tissue to break down, resulting in return of the fistula.

RECTOVAGINAL FISTULAS

Rectovaginal fistulas are less common than vesicovaginal fistulas. The constant escape of flatus and fecal material through the vagina is particularly distressing to the patient, especially because rectovaginal fistulas are quite resistant to satisfactory surgical treatment. They may be the result of the same causes as vesicovaginal fistulas. Surgical repair is usually done through the rectum. It may not be satisfactory, and procedures may have to be repeated. The nursing care is similar to that needed by patients following surgery for other types of rectal fistulas (see Chapter 44). In addition, the patient will need sympathetic understanding and encouragement because the emotional reactions are often severe.

If there is dribbling of fecal material into the vagina, it may be temporarily lessened by giving a high enema, and the woman at home is encouraged to do this before going out. After surgery, of course, enemas are never permitted until healing is complete. They may be given during the preoperative period. A soft rubber catheter should be used and should be directed carefully on the side of the rectum opposite the fistula. The catheter must go beyond the fistulous opening, or the fluid will return through the vagina and no benefit will be derived from the treatment. Although a constipating diet will temporarily prevent fecal material from going into the vagina, it eventually will cause pressure and may aggravate the condition and increase the size of the fistula. The woman therefore is advised against restricting diet and fluids in an effort to control bowel action.

BENIGN TUMORS OF THE FEMALE GENITAL TRACT

OVARIAN TUMORS AND CYSTS
EPIDEMIOLOGY AND PATHOPHYSIOLOGY

Many types of benign neoplasms affect the female reproductive tract. Neoplasms of the ovary alone account for several varieties. Almost a third of women have no symptoms of ovarian tumors at the time of diagnosis. Nearly 80% of these are discovered during routine pelvic examination. Women between the ages of 45 and 60 years are at greatest risk for developing ovarian tumors.

Benign neoplasms of the ovary include serous cystadenomas, mucinous adenomas, endometroid benign cysts, and benign mesonephric tumors. In addition, nonneoplastic cysts originating in the graafian follicle, cysts derived from the ruptured follicle (corpus luteum cyst), and simple cysts may occur. The follicle cysts are thin walled and translucent, arising during the evolution or involution of the graafian follicle, and do not grow autonomously. Corpus luteum cysts result from an abnormal persistence or exaggeration of the process of formation and resorption of the corpus luteum. After resorption, the cavity is normally distended with hemorrhagic or clear fluid. When exaggerated, the process results in the corpus luteum taking on a cystic structure. Simple cysts (that is, thin-walled structures containing serous fluid) occur frequently during menopause. Polycystic ovary (Stein-Leventhal) syndrome is characterized by enlargement of the ovaries, with numerous cystic follicles encased in a fibrotic capsule. Effects of these tumors are often not noted unless there is compression of a neighboring organ or blood supply, a menstrual disorder, or infertility.

CLINICAL MANIFESTATIONS

Symptoms are usually nonspecific. With rapidly growing cysts or tumors of the ovary, the first symptom may be an increase in abdominal size. Complaints of fatigue and sensations of weight, fullness, or pressure in the pelvis typically occur. Pain is an unusual symptom in the absence of acute complications such as twisting of an ovarian cyst on its pedicle. An increase in the size of the tumor may cause pressure symptoms such as urinary frequency and constipation, and backache may be present. Ovarian tumors and cysts are a frequent cause of menstrual irregularities.

Palpation of reproductive organs during pelvic examination usually reveals a mass or enlargement of the ovary. One or both ovaries normally atrophy and become nonpalpable after menopause; any mass palpated in the area of the ovaries requires further evaluation. Laparoscopy or exploratory laparotomy is usually done to confirm the diagnosis.

INTERVENTIONS

Ovarian tumors and cysts are treated surgically, and most often an oophorectomy is performed. If the woman is of childbearing age, however, reproductive goals must be weighed in determining the best course of treatment.

FIBROID TUMORS
EPIDEMIOLOGY AND ETIOLOGY

It has been estimated that 20% to 25% of women over 30 years of age develop uterine fibroid tumors (*myomas*). Uterine myomas occur more often in black women and in women who have never been pregnant. They rarely become malignant. Because their growth is stimulated by ovarian hormones, fibroid tumors of the uterus tend to disappear spontaneously with the advent of menopause.

PATHOPHYSIOLOGY

The cause of uterine myomas is unknown. They do not appear to be transmitted genetically. Because uterine myomas regress after menopause, it has been suggested that they are stimulated by estrogen. The sizes of myomas are variable. Most are found in the body of the uterus (corporeal), but some occur in the cervix or may involve the broad ligament. Subserous growths may extend outward into the folds of the broad ligament, cresting as intraligamentary tumors that burrow outward to form retroperitoneal masses. Intramural growths may cause no change in the contour of the uterus if they are small. When the growths are larger, they may produce an actual uterine enlargement. Submucous tumors may impinge on the blood vessels of the endometrium and produce bleeding. As they grow larger, they may impinge on the opposite uterine wall and distort the cavity of the uterus. In some instances, submucous tumors develop pedicles and may protrude through the vagina or cervix, resulting in infection or ulcerations.

CLINICAL MANIFESTATIONS

Menorrhagia is the most common symptom of myomas. If the tumor is very large, it may cause pelvic circulatory congestion and may press on surrounding viscera. The woman may complain of low abdominal pressure, backache, constipation, or dysmenorrhea. If a ureter is compressed by the tumor, signs and symptoms of ureteral obstruction may be present. Sometimes the pedicle on which a myoma is growing becomes twisted, causing severe pain. Large tumors growing into the opening of the fallopian tubes may cause sterility, those in the body of the uterus may cause spontaneous abortions, and those near the cervical opening may make the delivery of a baby difficult and may contribute to postpartum hemorrhage.

INTERVENTIONS

The treatment of fibroid tumors depends on the symptoms and the age of the patient, on whether more children are desired, and on how near she is to menopause. If the symptoms are not severe, the woman may simply need close health supervision. If the tumor is near the outer wall of the uterus, a *myomectomy* (surgical removal of the tumor) may be performed. This procedure leaves the muscle walls of the uterus relatively intact. If severe bleeding or obstruction occurs, a hysterectomy is usually necessary. Occasionally, if surgery is contraindicated or if the woman is approaching menopause, x-ray therapy or radiation is used to reduce the size of the tumor and to stop vaginal bleeding.

ENDOMETRIOSIS
EPIDEMIOLOGY

Endometriosis is a condition in which endometrial cells that normally line the uterus are seeded throughout the pelvis and occasionally extend to as distant a location as the umbilicus (Figure 55-6). The disease appears to be increasing, although the increased incidence may be a result of better diagnosis and recognition of the condition.

PREVENTION

Since theories on causes of endometriosis are merely speculation at present, it is difficult to know how to prevent this condition. However, it is believed that pregnancy may prevent the development of endometriosis. This is ironic, however, because infertility is often one of the first symptoms of the condition. It is not known how endometriosis first develops. Theories include congenital presence of endometrial cells out of their normal location, their transfer by means of blood vessels or the lymphatic system, and reflux of menstrual fluid containing endometrial cells up the fallopian tubes and into the pelvic cavity. None of these theories has been proved.

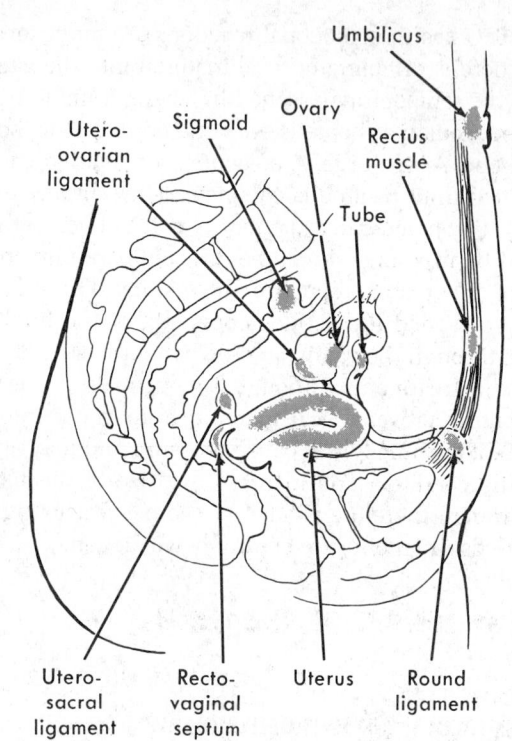

FIGURE 55-6 Sites of endometrial implants.

PATHOPHYSIOLOGY

With each menstrual period, the endometrial cells are stimulated by the ovarian hormones and bleed into the surrounding areas, causing an inflammation. Subsequent adhesions may be so severe that pelvic organs may become fused together, occasionally causing a stricture of the bowel or interference with bladder function. Encased blood may lead to palpable tumor masses, which often occur on the ovary and are known as *chocolate cysts*. Occasionally these cysts rupture and spread endometrial cells still farther throughout the pelvis. Some evidence suggests that women have a greater chance of developing endometriosis if a sibling or a parent has it. The highest incidence of endometriosis is among white women in higher socioeconomic classes who postpone childbearing until the later reproductive years. However, endometriosis does occur in other races and in earlier reproductive years.

CLINICAL MANIFESTATIONS

Usually endometriosis progresses gradually and does not produce symptoms until the ages of 30 to 40 years. Occasionally, however, symptoms appear when the woman is an adolescent. The characteristic symptom of endometriosis is pain and general discomfort accompanying menstruation that becomes progressively worse and that was not present at menarche. This one characteristic feature should alert the nurse to urge the woman to see a gynecologist at once. Many women with severe pain related to menstruation have been judged to be neurotic, when in reality they were suffering from endometriosis. Other symptoms of endometriosis are a feeling of fullness in the lower abdomen, dyspareunia, menorrhagia, irregular menstrual cycles, prostration, and general poor health. Sometimes the disease is far advanced and yet has caused no symptoms at all. Approximately 40% to 50% of women are infertile, and endometriosis is sometimes first detected when a woman complains of inability to conceive. On pelvic examination (done preferably during the first 24 hours of menses), tender, nodular uterosacral ligaments and sometimes fixed uterine retroversion are found. With endometriosis the uterus is enlarged, nodular, and tender, but Douglas' cul-de-sac is usually normal. The only definitive mode of diagnosing endometriosis is by laparoscopy.

INTERVENTIONS

Although extensive study of endometriosis is underway at present, its response to treatment is still variable and poorly understood. For this reason, treatment is highly individualized. If the woman is young and wants to have children, the treatment for endometriosis is usually as conservative as possible. Pregnancy is beneficial because menstruation ceases during this time. If a young women has endometriosis, she and her partner usually are advised to conceive early, if they want children, because the fertility rate is low, infertility caused by adhesions may occur, and a hysterectomy may have to be done within a reasonable time. Nursing the infant is also recommended because it delays the onset of menstruation following birth.

Because they imitate the state of pregnancy by inducing the ovaries to become anovulatory, antiovulatory drugs are frequently prescribed. Oral contraceptives with potent progestins and minimal amounts of estrogen are used for prolonged periods to produce endometrial atrophy and to lessen endometrial flow into the peritoneal cavity. The disadvantages of this treatment are that irregular bleeding may occur and that the symptoms of early pregnancy, including nausea, vomiting, depression, and fatigue, may be troublesome.

Drugs having reversible antigonadotropic action by suppressing ovarian activity, such as danazol, may be prescribed. These drugs are given in a dose of 200 mg twice a day for 3 to 6 months. Treatment can be extended up to 9 months if necessary, or it can be reinstituted if symptoms recur. Danazol is used to arrest proliferation of the endometrium, to prevent ovulation, and thus to produce atrophy of the ectopic endometrium. This therapy is expensive and may create hot flashes,

dry vagina, and depression and may foster weight gain. Antigonadotropic drugs are contraindicated if the woman has undiagnosed abnormal vaginal bleeding; has impaired hepatic, renal, or cardiac function; is pregnant; or is breast-feeding an infant.

Some women find their endometriosis disappears spontaneously, and some who become pregnant remain asymptomatic thereafter. For minimal symptoms, treatment with mild analgesics may be adequate. Regular pelvic examinations (every 6 months) are recommended to monitor the progress of endometriosis.

When the involvement is severe and does not respond to hormonal treatment, surgery may be necessary. A total hysterectomy, oophorectomy, and salpingectomy may be done. Removal of the ovaries prevents further bleeding of endometrial implants that cannot be removed. If the woman is premenopausal and the ovaries must be removed, she may be given very small amounts of estrogen. Menopause stops the progress of this condition.

Referral to endometriosis support groups is often beneficial for women and their partners. One such group is The Endometriosis Association,* which is a national organization that also includes Canada.

CERVICAL POLYPS

Cervical polyps form when an area of the cervical mucosa proliferates. These growths are usually visible at the cervical os as bright-red, vascular, fragile areas. They are most often pedunculated and appear to protrude from the cervical canal. Polyps may occur singly or in clusters.

Because of the vascularity of the polyp, bleeding is a common symptom. Generally, no other symptom is present. The characteristics of the bleeding associated with polyps closely resemble the signs of early cancer of the cervix. The bleeding is small in amount and occurs between menstrual periods. Especially characteristic is the contact bleeding produced by coitus, douching, or vaginal examination.

The pedicle by which the polyp is attached is usually quite small; thus that the polyp can easily be removed by twisting the pedicle at its base or by use of a biopsy forceps or sharp curette. Tissue examination of removed polyps is essential, since epidermoid cancer arises from cervical polyps in a small percentage of patients.

CANCER OF THE FEMALE GENITAL TRACT

Only three avenues are available to control and reduce the toll of gynecologic cancer morbidity and mortality:

---

*8585 N 76th Place, Milwaukee, WI 53223.

prevention, early detection, and improvements in treatment. Fortunately, many of the gynecologic malignancies have an associated high cure rate. This has been at least partly by a result of the development of diagnostic techniques that can identify precancerous conditions, the ability to apply highly effective treatments that are more restricted elsewhere in the body, better understanding of disease spread patterns, and more sophisticated and effective treatment in cancers that previously had poor prognoses.[18] Thus the patient with a gynecologic malignancy may look forward to earlier diagnosis, more effective treatment, and subsequently longer survival than was previously experienced. This optimism should be realistically transferred to the patient and significant others.

The nurse caring for the gynecologic oncology patient is responsible for coordination of patient care, which includes physical, psychosocial, and discharge planning needs. The nurse must understand that women with gynecologic cancers are faced with anxieties precipitated by threats to survival, body image, personal and cultural roles, and modesty. For many, genital cancer may symbolize cultural taboos or retribution for sexual transgressions and may cause embarrassment and reluctance to verbalize these concerns. Therefore the nurse must address these problems, placing emphasis on the patient's perception of femininity, the stigma associated with gynecologic cancer, and fears regarding future personal and sexual roles.[26]

CANCER OF THE CERVIX
EPIDEMIOLOGY AND ETIOLOGY

The annual mortality for cancer of the cervix has fallen steadily over the past 45 years. This decline has been attributed to early detection through annual examinations, including a Pap smear, and improved surgical and radiotherapeutic techniques. Nevertheless, despite these improved diagnostic and therapeutic techniques, the estimated mortality from cervical cancer in 1989 was 7000, with an estimated incidence of 13,000 new cases.[3]

The age of patients with carcinoma in situ is, on the average, 10 years less than the average patient with invasive cancer of the cervix. The average age of patients with invasive cancer of the cervix is 45 years. Many exceptions exist, however, and in the past 20 years an increasing number of young women (late teens and early 20s) have been diagnosed with invasive cancer of the cervix. The risk factors associated with cancer of the cervix include the following: first coitus at an early age, multiple sexual partners, low socioeconomic group, and exposure to herpesvirus type 2. There is no correlation with frequency of sexual intercourse.[58]

PREVENTION AND EARLY DETECTION

Dramatic decreases in deaths from cancer are associated with early detection and treatment. The decline in deaths from cervical cancer is primarily because of increased use of the Pap smear for mass screening combined with more frequent and more thorough gynecologic examinations.

To save more lives through diagnosis and treatment, it is important first to determine the population at risk and then to provide them with the means by which frequent, inexpensive screening can be accomplished. The risk factors associated with cervical cancer have been cited. Application of this knowledge in practice assists with identification of specific individuals at high risk for cancer.

Cervical cancer deaths could be greatly reduced if every adult woman had an annual physical examination, including a Pap smear. Many older women, especially those in rural areas, have not had a physical examination since their childbearing years. The American Cancer Society, in its report on *The Cancer-Related Health Checkup*, recommended the following:

. . . that all asymptomatic women age 20 and over, and those under 20 who are sexually active, have a Pap test annually for two negative examinations and then at least every three years until the age of 65. A pelvic examination should be done as part of a general physical examination every three years from age 20 to 40 and annually thereafter; women who are at a high risk of developing cervical cancer because of early age at first intercourse, multiple sexual partners, or other risk factors may need to be tested more frequently. Women who are relatively inactive sexually may prefer a less frequent interval.[1]

This report by the American Cancer Society has caused considerable concern about its possible adverse effect on the current successful cancer control in the United States. In response to this report, the American College of Obstetricians and Gynecologists recommended the continuation of annual cytologic screening for cervical neoplasia. A summation of this report states the following*:

The dramatic fall in cervical cancer incidence and death rates has been brought about largely as a result of annual cytologic screening. There is no existing clinical experience which can provide assurance that such reductions could be maintained with a program of less frequent screening. Any change in this pattern should take into account the following facts: the Papanicolaou smear is an inexpensive procedure, has no discernible morbidity, is easily obtained, and has the potential for a high degree of sensitivity.

The choice of a screening interval is arbitrary and is based on a subjective assessment of cost-effectiveness. Lengthening the screening interval inevitably detects the cancers or precan-

---

*From American College of Obstetricians and Gynecologists, Washington, DC, 1980, The College.

cerous states at a later stage and inevitably trades lives for dollars.

The Pap smear has an inherent false-negative rate of 15% to 40%. This problem has its greatest impact on the high-risk patient. Any screening interval that fails to recognize this fact introduces some increased risk to the individual woman's health and life.

The earlier that cervical neoplasia is detected, the more amenable it is to local, office-based treatment. Later stages, even of the cancer precursors, may require surgery (conization or hysterectomy) for diagnosis or therapy.

It has been recommended that high-risk women (those who have had early sexual intercourse, have had several sexual partners, or multiple marital events) should be screened annually.

Since a substantial proportion of women in the United States are at high risk for developing cervical neoplasia, they should be made aware of those factors that result in high-risk status.

Although the annual screening interval has been arrived at arbitrarily, it has served as a convenient benchmark. Abandoning this traditional interval may result in an increase in untreated cervical neoplasia. The annual interval may be too short for some populations and too long for others. Further attempts to codify this decision are potentially dangerous and may lead to an increase in cancer deaths.[4]

Nurses should take an active role in the prevention and detection of cervical cancer. Nurses can both educate and encourage their clients to assume responsibility for their health by routinely participating in screening programs. Emphasis should also be placed on identifying high-risk populations and participating in outreach programs.[49]

PATHOPHYSIOLOGY

Cervical carcinomas may arise in one of two cell types: squamous carcinomas (epidermal layer of the cervix) make up 95% of all cervical cancers; adenocarcinomas (cervical mucus-producing gland cells) primarily make up the remaining 5%.

The precursor lesions of cervical squamous cell carcinoma have been identified as dysplasia. *Cervical intraepithelial neoplasia* (CIN) is the term usually used to define the precursor state. CIN has been subdivided into the following three stages:

CIN I   Mild to moderate dysplasia
CIN II   Moderate to severe dysplasia
CIN III   Severe dysplasia to carcinoma in situ

It is generally agreed that patients with the earlier stages of CIN (the dysplasias) may have one of three courses: regression, persistence, or progression to carcinoma in situ or invasive carcinoma.[3]

Adenocarcinoma arises from the mucus-producing gland cells of the cervix. Unlike squamous cell carcinoma of the cervix, adenocarcinoma is not preceded by a well-recognized, prolonged precursor state. Also, be-

cause of its origin within the cervix, adenocarcinoma may be present for a considerable time before it can be clinically detected.[18]

CLINICAL MANIFESTATIONS

The 5-year survival rate for CIN is 100%; the 5-year survival rate for cervical cancer stage IV is 8%. In the early stages, cervical cancer is asymptomatic. With progression of disease, a slight watery vaginal discharge may appear, occasional bloody spotting following intercourse or between periods may occur, and as the disease progresses, a foul discharge or pain may develop.

■ ASSESSMENT

The diagnosis of cervical cancer can only be accomplished through biopsy-obtained tissue. The Pap smear is not a diagnostic tool. Rather, it is a screening measure used to pick up suspicious cells on the surface of the cervix. Once a Pap smear has been reported as "abnormal," biopsy-obtained tissue must be examined to confirm the diagnosis. Several techniques are used to obtain a cervical biopsy; a punch biopsy or a cervical conization are the two techniques employed most often.

Once the diagnosis has been confirmed pathologically, other diagnostic tests may be used to stage the disease. These tests include; chest roentgenogram, colposcopy, cystoscopy, proctosigmoidoscopy, intravenous pyelogram (IVP), and barium studies of the lower colon and rectum.[18]

Assessment also includes a careful history of symptoms that may be related to the diagnosis of a pelvic neoplasm such as vaginal discharge or spotting, abdominal pain, weight change, or change in abdominal girth. Symptoms may be specific to the type of neoplasm and its location, such as vaginal discharge, or may be common to several types of neoplasms, such as fatigue, or a woman may be asymptomatic at time of diagnosis.

■ DATA ANALYSIS: NURSING DIAGNOSES

Nursing diagnoses for a woman with a neoplasm of the reproductive system may include, but are not limited to, the following:

Diagnostic Title	Possible Etiologies
Anxiety	Related to cancer; diagnosis or fear of the unknown
Body image disturbance	Changed sexual and/or reproductive anatomy
Grieving, anticipatory	Loss of significant body part
Sexuality patterns, altered	Change in reproductive anatomy or change in energy level

■ PLANNING: EXPECTED PATIENT OUTCOMES

Expected patient outcomes for the patient with a neoplasm may include, but are not limited to, the following:
1. Patient demonstrates understanding of nature of diagnosis and prognosis
2. Patient demonstrates understanding of complete plan of care, including surgery, radiation therapy, or chemotherapy
3. Patient expresses less anxiety regarding treatment and the unknown
4. Patient verbalizes potential and actual loss
5. Patient participates actively in postoperative care
6. Patient experiences comfort
7. Patient discusses alterations in sexual pattern
8. Patient discusses alterations in sexual patterns and consequences of treatment for fertility
9. Patient demonstrates positive concept of self as a woman

INTERVENTIONS

Cervical cancer is treated according to the stage of the disease (Table 55-5), the woman's age and general health, and the presence of complications.

Treatment of carcinoma in situ may consist of an excisional conization of the cervix (or cryosurgery in some institutions) if the woman is young, she wishes to have more children, and invasive cancer has been ruled out. In other women, simple hysterectomy is preferred to radiotherapy, particularly for those in whom preservation of ovarian function is desirable.

Invasive cancer of the cervix can be treated by means of surgery or radiotherapy (Table 55-6). Usually the tumors beyond stages I and II are treated with radiotherapy. Surgery for stage I and early stage II disease may be reserved in some institutions for those women desiring preservation of ovarian function. Comparable cure rates are obtained with either surgery or radiother-

TABLE 55-5 Stages of cancer of the cervix

Stage	Involvement
0	Confined within epithelium of cervix
I	Completely confined to cervix
II	Extends outside cervix but does not involve pelvic wall or lower third of vagina
III	Involves pelvic wall and lower third of vagina
IV	Extends beyond stage III; involves bladder, rectum, or metastatic spread

apy; however, the morbidity associated with both approaches is considered in light of the individual and her problem.

Surgery

The surgery recommended for stage I and early stage II is a radical hysterectomy with pelvic lymph node dissection (Figure 55-7). The structures removed in this procedure are the uterus, nearby supporting tissues, uppermost part of the vagina, and pelvic lymph nodes. This surgery is more extensive than a simple hysterectomy, and the nursing care is more involved. (Figure 55-8 shows comparison with other types of hysterectomies.) A sample nursing care plan for the woman with sexual dysfunction following radical hysterectomy is described on pp 1627-1628.

Nursing management. If a radical hysterectomy is to be performed, the preoperative physical preparation is the same as that for any other abdominal surgery. A vaginal douche may be given. Postoperatively the patient has an abdominal dressing and wears a perineal pad. The dressings should be observed for any sign of bleeding every 15 minutes for 2 hours and then at least every

TABLE 55-6 Summary of treatment options for cervical cancer

Clinical Stage	Treatment Options	5-Year Survival (%)
Dysplasia	Cryosurgery/conization	100
CIN	Simple hysterectomy	100
Ia	Simple hysterectomy or radiation (cesium implant)	95-100
Microinvasive (3 mm below basement membrane)		
Microinvasive (3-5 mm depth)	Radical hysterectomy with nodes or radiotherapy (external and implant)	95-98
Ib and IIa	Radical hysterectomy with nodes or radiotherapy	75-90
IIb	Radiation	50-60
IIIa and IIIb	Radiation	30-40
IV	Radiation or chemotherapy	5-14
Recurrent	Pelvic exenteration, if operable	Varies according to site and extent of recurrence

DATA: Mrs. Conn, age 42, saw her gynecologist 2 weeks ago because of bleeding between periods and occasional postcoital bleeding. The result of her Pap smear 5 years previously had been negative. The Pap smear this time was positive, and a cervical biopsy confirmed cancer of the cervix, stage I. She was admitted yesterday for a total hysterectomy.

Admission notes indicate that Mrs. Conn is married and has two teenagers, a boy and a girl. Her husband accompanied her to the hospital and appeared to be supportive. Mrs. Conn is a bank teller and likes to read, knit, and watch TV. She has varicose veins but states these do not bother her. Her preoperative concerns centered mainly on the cancer: "I hope they get it all." She also stated, "Well, at least I hadn't planned any more children. My boy joked and said, 'You're going to be neutered like our cat was!' I wonder how it feels to be so-called neutered. I hope it won't affect my sex life." The nurse explored Mrs. Conn's knowledge of the surgery and explained that the surgery would not physically affect sexual relationships.

Mrs. Conn returned from the recovery room alert with an IV running and stable vital signs. The dressing was dry. She had an order for morphine sulfate (MS) q3h prn and received a half-dose in the recovery room.

Nursing activities include monitoring the following activities:
- Vital signs
- Breath sounds
- Urinary output
- Fluid intake
- Dressing checks

NURSING DIAGNOSIS
Pain, abdominal, related to abdominal incision

Expected Patient Outcomes	Nursing Interventions	Rationale
Mrs. Conn states she is feeling more comfortable	Give analgesic on a regular basis for first 24 h, then as necessary	Giving the analgesic regularly will prevent severe pain and thus be more effective; morphine sulfate (MS) also reduces anxiety
	Encourage frequent changes of position in bed and early ambulation	Activity decreases pain by increasing circulation and reducing muscle tension; ambulation will also encourage peristalsis, decreasing possibility of gas pains

NURSING DIAGNOSIS
Body image disturbance: potential, related to loss of uterus

Expected Patient Outcomes	Nursing Interventions	Rationale
·Mrs. Conn verbalizes concerns about loss of uterus	Provide patient opportunites to express feeling and concerns about loss of uterus	Patient may feel freer to talk about her feelings if opportunities are provided
	Be empathetic about patient's feelings, which may include grief, guilt, shame, or remorse	Feelings associated with grief may also be expressed when grieving over loss of a body part
	Encourage her to continue activities associated with femininity, such as fixing hair, makeup, wearing own apparel	Feelings of femininity will emphasize "feminine" rather than "neuter," and that she herself has not changed
Mrs. Conn makes plans for resuming her role	Help her make plans for resumption of former activities	If life pattern is not changed, her thoughts about her body changes may diminish

NURSING DIAGNOSIS
Constipation: potential, related to pelvic surgery

Expected Patient Outcomes	Nursing Interventions	Rationale
Stool is soft and formed	Monitor stool characteristics and frequency	Peristalsis may be decreased from handling of pelvic viscera
	Encourage oral fluids when permitted	Hydration will promote a soft stool
	Encourage ambulation	Ambulation promotes peristalsis

From Long BC and Phipps WJ: Medical-surgical nursing: a nursing process approach, ed 2, St. Louis, 1989, The CV Mosby Co.

Continued.

NURSING DIAGNOSIS
Urinary elimination, altered patterns: related to pelvic surgery

Expected Patient Outcomes	Nursing Interventions	Rationale
Patient voids in sufficient quantities	Monitor urinary output until she voids sufficiently Monitor for distention above symphysis pubis and for lower abdominal discomfort other than incisional pain	Handling of bladder during pelvic surgery may decrease bladder muscle tone, leading to urinary retention (Mrs. Conn did not have an indwelling catheter)

NURSING DIAGNOSIS
Tissue perfusion, altered peripheral: related to pelvic venous stasis from surgery

Expected Patient Outcomes	Nursing Interventions	Rationale
No leg or thigh pain occurs	Monitor for discomfort in legs/thighs or sudden dyspnea; assess for Homan's sign	Early detection will ensure early treatment of thrombophlebitis
	Encourage leg exercises and frequent turning in bed until ambulating well	Exercises promote venous return (muscle pumps)
	Avoid use of knee gatch or pillows under knees; encourage patient to keep knees flat when in bed	Pressure on popliteal veins or sharp knee flexion may increase venous stasis
	Encourage patient to lie completely flat in bed for short periods q2h for 24 h, then q4h until ambulating well	Lying flat for periods of time will help blood return from the pelvic veins
	Encourage ambulation	Ambulation promotes venous return (muscle pumps)
	Provide antiembolic stockings	Mrs. Conn is at higher risk for thrombophlebitis because of varicose veins (sluggish circulation) and sedentary life pattern

NURSING DIAGNOSIS
Knowledge deficit: related to surgery

Expected Patient Outcomes	Nursing Interventions	Rationale
Mrs. Conn describes self-care accurately	Teach patient: 1. When activities can be resumed (see text)	Activities are resumed gradually to permit healing; heavy activities are avoided for 6-8 weeks
	2. Signs of thrombophlebitis to be monitored and reported	Thrombophlebitis may occur 7-10 days postoperatively, after patient goes home
	3. Signs of vaginal bleeding to be reported; (excessive or persistent) possibility of slight vaginal discharge for 1-2 weeks	Bleeding could indicate impaired healing
	4. Bathing and light activity permitted after hospital discharge	
	5. Avoid driving car for 2-4 weeks, especially with standard shift	
	6. Avoid heavy activity and active sports for 4-6 weeks	
	7. Need for medical follow-up	To ensure that metastasis has not occurred
	Reinforce the preoperative explanations of the surgery and effect on sexual relationships	Preoperative anxiety may have decreased her awareness; hysterectomy does not interfere with satisfactory sexual relationships
	Find out what she has told her daughter about regular Pap smears	Regular Pap smears enhance early detection of cervical cancer
	Suggest she use support hose in her job as a bank teller	Preventive measure for thrombophlebitis because of her varicose veins

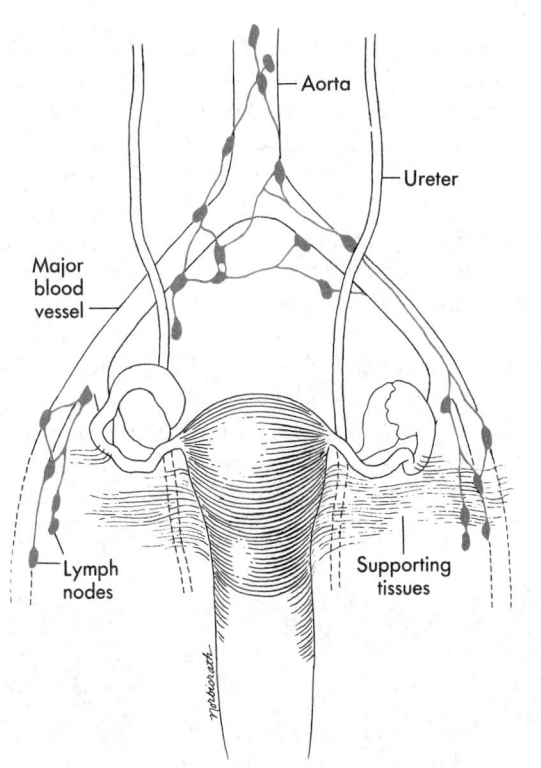

FIGURE 55-7 Radical hysterectomy includes removal of uterus, nearby supporting tissues, uppermost part of vagina, and pelvic lymph nodes.

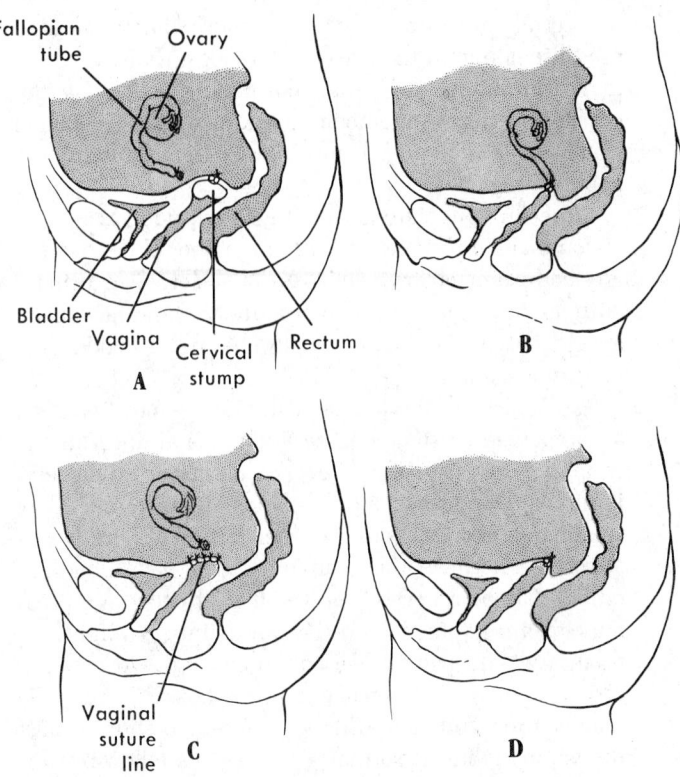

FIGURE 55-8 A, Cross section of subtotal hysterectomy. Note that cervical stump, fallopian tubes, and ovaries remain. **B,** Cross section of total hysterectomy. Note that fallopian tubes and ovaries remain. **C,** Cross section of vaginal hysterectomy. Note that fallopian tubes and ovaries remain. **D,** Total hysterectomy, salpingectomy, and oophorectomy. Note that uterus, fallopian tubes, and ovaries are completely removed.

hour for 8 hours. Normally a moderate amount of serosanguineous drainage occurs. Two catheters connected to hemovacs are placed below the incision to drain excess fluid from the surgical site. These drains are left in place until there is only a minimal amount of drainage from them (3 to 5 days).

Following a hysterectomy, especially one in which there has been extensive nodal and parametrial resection, the *bladder* may be temporarily *atonic* as a result of nerve trauma, and a Foley catheter is used to maintain constant drainage of the bladder. If no catheter is used and if the woman is unable to void within 8 hours, she is usually catheterized. The catheter is usually left in place for 2 to 3 weeks. After catheter removal, the woman is catheterized after voiding to check residual urine. If the residual urine is more than 100 ml, the catheter is left in place for an additional 1 to 2 weeks and is then rechecked.

Prevention of complications. Abdominal distention may complicate a hysterectomy. It is caused by nerve damage or by handling of the viscera during surgery. Some physicians insert a nasogastric tube prophylactically following surgery, and most physicians restrict food and fluids orally for 24 to 48 hours. Fleet's enema may be given on the second or third postoperative day.

When peristalsis returns, fluids and food are started gradually.

Interference with circulation may occur during hysterectomy, and thrombophlebitis of the vessels of the pelvis and upper thigh is a rather common complication. The patient should never rest with the knees bent or with the thighs sharply flexed. The knee gatch should not be used, and the bed should not be raised at the head to more than mid-Fowler's position. The woman should exercise her feet and legs every hour, and she should move about in bed, turning from her side to her back and to a partial face-lying position. A pillow can be used to support the abdominal wound. The head of the bed should be put completely flat for a short time every 2 hours during the first 24 hours postoperatively and then at least every 4 hours until the patient is ambulatory. These precautions help prevent stasis of blood in the pelvic vessels. If the woman has varicosities, the physician may order elevation of the legs for a few minutes every 2 to 3 hours to permit blood to drain from the legs. To lessen the possibility of thrombus formation, nurses need to ensure that no undue pressure is put on the calves of the legs, that the elevation is uniform, and that no flexing exists at the popliteal region. Antiembolic stockings may be applied from the toes to just below the knee, excluding the popliteal region.

Other nursing care is the same as that following any abdominal surgery. Special attention should be given to any complaint of low back pain or to lessened urinary output, since it is possible that a ureter could have been accidentally ligated. Occasionally the ureter, bladder, or rectum is traumatized.

Psychologic response. Radical hysterectomy is often accompanied by some degree of emotional upset. Some women worry about the effect it will have on their femininity and wonder about possible changes in secondary sex characteristics. Young women may feel bitterly disappointed because they can no longer have children; others may be relieved from the fear of becoming pregnant. Some women worry about gaining weight, although weight gain is most often caused by overeating rather than by hormonal changes. It is true that the childbearing function will be terminated, but usually the vagina is intact so that 4 to 6 weeks following surgery, women can resume normal sexual intercourse.

Older women may be less upset by the prospects of this surgery than are those who have not reached the menopause. Postoperatively, however, almost all patients feel depressed for several days. The patient often is unable to explain why she is depressed and crying. Grieflike responses to loss of a body part may appear as they do following surgery in other cases. The patient may have feelings of guilt, shame, and remorse. Encouraging the woman to continue activities associated with being feminine, such as using makeup, arranging her hair, and wearing her own clothing, often helps her to regain her feminine perspective. During this period, she needs understanding and sympathetic care. Families need to be helped to accept these responses calmly, and a partner may need help in understanding her need for reassurance of his continued love and affection.

Patient teaching. The woman should know what surgery has been done, what changes in herself she should expect, and what care she needs when she leaves the hospital. Most patients are more comfortable if they wear a girdle. Heavy lifting should be avoided for about 2 months. Activities such as riding over rough roads, walking swiftly, and dancing tend to cause congestion of blood in the pelvis and should be avoided for several months. Physical activity that does not cause strain, such as swimming, may be done because it is helpful for physical and mental well-being.

A comprehensive teaching booklet for the woman undergoing a radical hysterectomy has been published by Jusenius.[27]

Radiotherapy

The radiotherapy used in the treatment of cervical cancer usually consists of whole pelvic irradiation as well as two intracavitary implants (Figures 55-9 to 55-11). The amount of radioactive substance used and the number of hours it is left in place are determined by the amount of radiation needed to kill the less resistant cancer cells without damaging normal cells. (For a discussion of radiation treatment and the general nursing care and precautions involved, see Chapter 17.)

Nursing management. Premenopausal women who receive pelvic irradiation will lose their ovarian function. Counseling regarding use of hormones, vaginal lubricants, and other methods to prevent or alleviate menopausal symptoms is indicated (see research box on p. 1632).

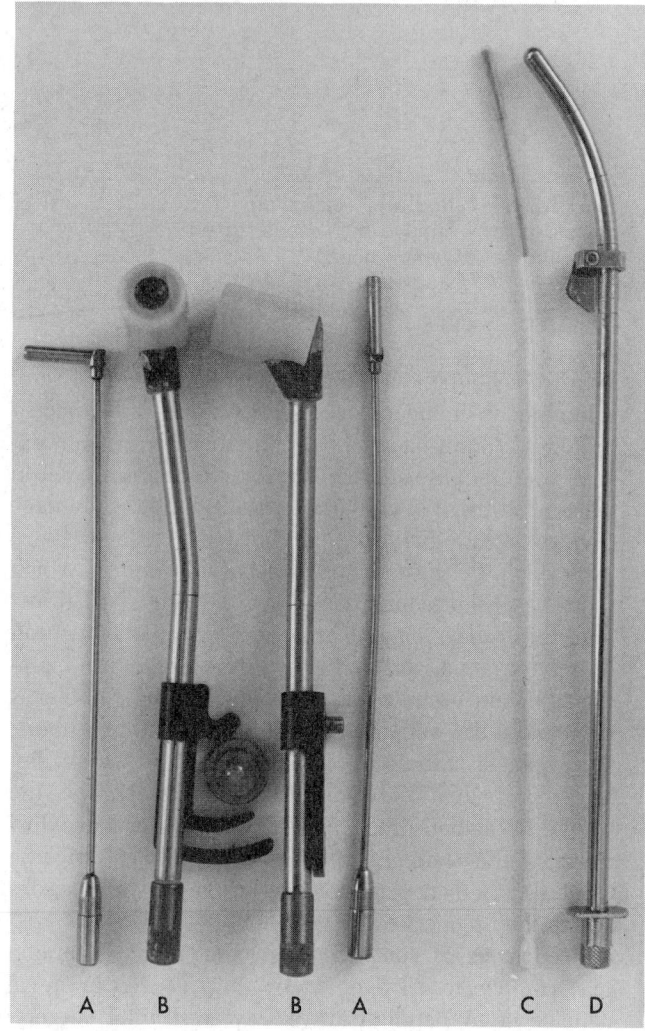

FIGURE 55-9 Intracavitary implant for treatment of cervical cancer. **A,** Inserts for colpostats to insert radium or cesium. **B,** Colpostats. **C,** Teflon tubing to insert radium or cesium into tandem. **D,** Tandem.

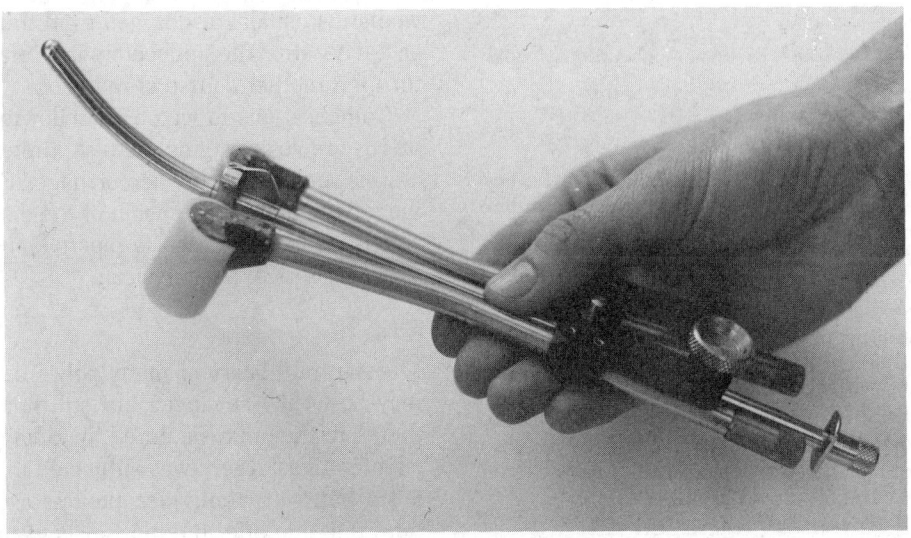

FIGURE 55-10 Assembled configuration of tandem and colpostat before displacement.

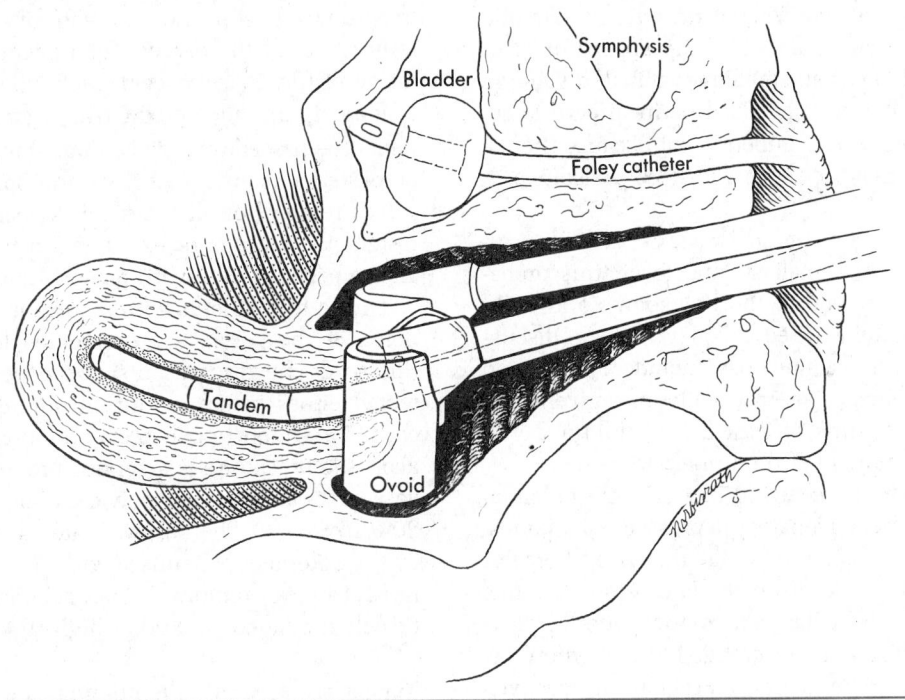

FIGURE 55-11 Placement of tandem and colpostats before vaginal packing.

During an intracavitary implant, it is important that all normal tissues remain in their natural position and do not come nearer to the radioactive substance than is anticipated and provided for by the protective materials used. Before treatment begins, a cleansing enema and a low-residue diet are given to prevent distention of the bowel. A catheter may be inserted to prevent distention of the bladder. Gauze packing is usually inserted into the vagina to push both the rectum and the bladder away from the area being irradiated. Cleansing enemas

are not given during the treatment. To prevent any displacement of the radioactive substance, the patient is kept flat in bed and is allowed to turn only from side to side. A roentgenogram is taken before the radioactive substance is inserted to determine the exact location of the tandem and colpostat (see Figures 55-10 and 55-11).

Since the presence of anything in the cervix stimulates *uterine contractions,* the woman who has a tandem or intrauterine applicator in place may have severe

RESEARCH

Jenkins B: Patients' reports of sexual changes after treatment for gynecological cancer, Oncol Nurs Forum 15(3):349-354, 1988.

Twenty sexually active women were studied for the occurrence of sexual changes following surgical and radiation treatments for endometrial and cervical cancer. In response to a mailed questionnaire, statistically significant negative changes were reported by 95% of the women in four indicators of sexual function: frequency of intercourse and orgasm and feelings of desire and enjoyment. Regarding the amount of sexual counseling received before and after treatment; 59% reported that they received no information. Most of the information was given to patients by radiotherapists. No sexual counseling was given by nurses. Eighty-eight percent of these women wanted sexual discussions initiated by the physician or nurse. ■

---

uterine contractions as a result of dilation of the cervix. She should know that they will occur. Often a narcotic is given at regular intervals while the applicator is in place. There will be foul-smelling vaginal discharge from the destruction of cells. Good perineal care is essential, and it must be remembered that because the patient must lie on her back, she will need assistance. A deodorizer is helpful.

Patients may develop *radiation sickness*, with nausea, vomiting, diarrhea, malaise, and fever; this probably is a systemic reaction to the breakdown and reabsorption of cell proteins. (See Chapter 17 for a discussion of care.) Local reaction may include cystitis and proctitis. Steroid enemas are also sometimes given. The woman is urged to drink at least 3 L of fluid a day to help relieve any irritation of the urinary system.

The woman who is receiving intracavitary radiation treatments often feels alienated, depressed, or anxious. Nurses can spend some time talking with her but should remain at a safe distance. The reason for this precaution should be explained to the patient. Close members of the family are encouraged to visit when it is considered safe for them to do so. Pregnant nurses, visitors, or any other personnel should avoid contact with the patient while the implant is in place.

Following removal of the radioactive agent, the catheter is removed, a cleansing enema is given, and the woman is allowed out of bed. Vaginal discharge will continue for some time, and the patient may need to take douches for as long as the odor and vaginal discharge persist. Usually douches are ordered twice a day. The woman who is returning home needs detailed instructions in how to give herself douches and what solutions to use. Some vaginal bleeding may occur for 1 to 3 months after irradiation of the cervix. Emollient enemas may be prescribed to be taken at home. The

woman is usually discharged from the hospital within 1 or 2 days after the applicators are removed but may return for another course of radiation.

Complications to watch for following radiation of the uterus are vesicovaginal fistulas, ureterovaginal fistulas, cystitis, phlebitis, and hemorrhage. Each is caused by the radiation or by extension of the disease process. The patient should be urged to report even minor symptoms or complaints to her physician.

Pelvic Exenteration

The natural history of many pelvic cancers is that they may be locally advanced but still limited to the pelvis; therefore they may be cured by radical resection. Pelvic exenterative surgery was subjected to severe initial criticism but is currently accepted as a worthwhile procedure that can offer life to a selected number of patients for whom no other possibility of cure exists.[18]

Although pelvic exenteration has been implemented for various pelvic malignancies, its greatest and most important role is in the treatment of advanced or recurrent cancer of the cervix. Total exenteration entails removal of the pelvic viscera, including the bladder, rectosigmoid, and all reproductive organs. In selected patients the procedure may be limited to either an anterior or posterior exenteration. An anterior exenteration involves removal of all the pelvic viscera except the rectosigmoid. A posterior exenteration involves removal of all the pelvic viscera with preservation of the bladder.

Only a few patients with recurrent or advanced carcinoma of the cervix are candidates for the procedure. Spread of the disease outside the pelvis, which is detected either before or during surgery, is an absolute contraindication to pelvic exenteration. The decision to abort the procedure is a serious prognostic sign. The 5-year survival rate after pelvic exenteration varies from 20% to 62%.[18] The survival rates are most influenced by the criteria of patient selection. For instance, survival rates can be improved by excluding elderly obese, heavily irradiated, and other high-risk patients.

Nursing management. The nursing care of the patient undergoing pelvic exenteration includes the care given the patient having a hysterectomy (pp. 1627-1628), the patient having an abdominal perineal resection of the bowel (see Chapter 44), and the patient having an ileobladder with transplantation of the ureters (see Chapter 49).

An essential aspect in the nursing care of the exenteration patient is teaching. It is essential that each patient be cognizant of the indications, goal, and scope of the surgical procedure. Explanations regarding female anatomy, alteration in body function, and impact on sexual function should be included in the preoperative teaching sessions. Also helpful are introductions to other members of the health care team who will be in-

NURSING CARE PLAN

WOMAN WITH SEXUAL DYSFUNCTION FOLLOWING RADICAL HYSTERECTOMY

DATA: Ms. Esther Barnes, a 49-year-old married woman, was recently diagnosed with uterine cancer. She has experienced a radical hysterectomy and will be leaving the hospital in a few days. As you discuss her future plans she tells you: "I'm really worried. My husband and I have always had a really active and enjoyable sex life. After this surgery I have to go to radiation therapy and have chemotherapy. I'm sure our relationship will never be the same."

NURSING DIAGNOSIS

Sexual dysfunction related to:

- Physiologic damage to pelvic organs, innervation, and/or vasculature as a result of disease process and/or therapy
- Emotional response to altered body image
- Hesitancy of partner to initiate sexual play as a result of patient's disease, altered anatomy, fear of contagion, or fear of injuring "sick" partner

Expected Patient Outcome	Nursing Interventions	Rationale
Resumption of optimal sexual relationship	Obtain sexual history (see Chapter 51) early in relationship with client.	History taking legitimizes sexual concerns.
	Perform physical assessment (see Chapter 51).	Assessment augments sexual history.
	Provide anticipatory guidance. Explain possible sexual changes that may result from disease and/or therapy; include sexual partner, if possible.	Providing structure in a situation of uncertainty allows persons to gain control and feel less anxious.
	Validate normalcy of sexual concerns; include partner, if possible.	Reassurance regarding sexual acceptability of concerns, thoughts, and activities can decrease anxiety
	Counsel regarding alternate sexual expressions; include sexual partner, if possible.	If clients are unable to continue customary modes of sexual expression, it may be necessary to explore alternate modes. Taking into consideration couple's values system is essential aspect of this intervention.
	Refer to sex therapist or other professional, if necessary.	If nurse is unable to address client's sexual problems adequately, referral to trained sexual counselor may be necessary. Ability to assess one's own abilities appropriately is essential component of nursing process. Identifying one's limitations is an asset, not an admission of failure.

volved in postoperative care (for example, enterostomal therapist, social worker, dietitian). Excellent teaching plans for patients undergoing pelvic exenteration are available.[15,53]

The psychosocial aspects of undergoing pelvic exenteration are understandably immense. The psychosexual adjustment to this radical surgery encompasses psychologic, social, and sexual factors (see nursing care plan above). Adaptation includes changes in body image, social life-style, and sexual relations. Nurses have the professional responsibility of nurturing these women so they redevelop and adjust their life to what they consider an acceptable and worthwhile level.

Chemotherapy

The control or cure of metastatic cancer of the cervix has not significantly improved with the progress of modern chemotherapy. This may be caused, in part by most cervical cancers (95%) being of the squamous cell variety, which are generally the least responsive to most chemotherapeutic agents. In addition to cell type, recurrent cancers often appear within a previously irradiated area that is fibrotic and avascular. The perfusion of this area is marginal, and therefore it is difficult to obtain a high tissue concentration of the drug in the recurrent neoplasm. The drugs most often used are mitomycin C, vincristine, bleomycin, doxorubicin (Adriamycin), cisplatin, 5-fluorouracil, cyclophosphamide, and methotrexate. These can be given alone or in various combinations at regular intervals. (For the nursing care of patients receiving these drugs, see Chapter 17).

CANCER OF THE ENDOMETRIUM
EPIDEMIOLOGY AND ETIOLOGY

Cancer of the endometrium (uterine corpus) affects mainly mature women; this diagnosis is most common in women between the ages of 50 and 64 years. The yearly estimated incidence of new cases in the United States is 34,000; the estimated mortality is 3000.[3] Seventy-five percent of all endometrial cancers occur in postmenopausal women.

Multiple risk factors for endometrial cancer have been identified. The most common risk factors are obesity, nulliparity, late menopause (after 52 years of age), diabetes mellitus, and hypertension. Use of exogenous estrogens has also been implicated as a risk factor.

PREVENTION AND EARLY DETECTION

Cancer of the endometrium is a slow-growing form of cancer and is very amenable to treatment if detected early. Women who are in the high-risk category (for example, obesity, late menopause, diabetes mellitus, hypertension) for developing endometrial cancer often have endometrial tissue samples taken periodically. This can be done in an ambulatory clinic, in a physician's office, or as an inpatient. The tissue samples can be obtained in a variety of ways (Table 55-7) with varying effectiveness.

PATHOPHYSIOLOGY

Uterine hyperplasia is somethat analogous to dysplasia of the cervix. Some of these lesions revert to normal, some persist as hyperplasia, and a few progress to endometrial adenocarcinoma. Unfortunately, unlike cervical dysplasia, no reliable, frequently used screening method for endometrial hyperplasia exists. Most women with this condition are diagnosed because they seek medical care with symptoms of abnormal uterine bleeding. The diagnosis of endometrial hypeplasia can be made only in pathologic examination of uterine tissue.

CLINICAL MANIFESTATIONS

The most common symptom associated with endometrial cancer is abnormal spotting and bleeding. Any postmenopausal woman with uterine bleeding should be evaluated for endometrial cancer. In the premenopausal woman or one who is currently going through

TABLE 55-7 Methods for detection of endometrial cancer

Method	Effectiveness (%)
Endometrial aspirations	70-80
Endometrial washings	80-90
Dilation and curettage (fractional)	85-90
Pap smear	45-50
Combination of above	90

menopause, these symptoms may be interpreted as normal menopausal symptoms. During this time in a woman's life, the menstrual periods should become lighter and further apart. Any other bleeding pattern should be evaluated.[18]

Other more vague symptoms include abdominal pain or pressure, nausea, and vomiting. These are late symptoms, however, and patients who have these symptoms and the subsequent diagnosis of uterine cancer usually have a history of abnormal bleeding.

INTERVENTIONS

Endometrial cancer is treated according to the stage of the disease (Table 55-8).

The treatment for cancer of the corpus is most often total abdominal hysterectomy and bilateral salpingo-oophorectomy (TAH/BSO). The nursing care for women who undergo a TAH/BSO is similar to that of any other patient receiving major abdominal surgery (see Chapter 44). If, on analysis of the tissue, the tumor has deeply invaded the uterus or spread to the pelvic lymph nodes, postoperative radiation will be given. In advanced stages, preoperative radiation is used (intrauterine radiation and external whole pelvic irradiation). This treatment can also be done preoperatively to shrink the tumor and decrease the amount of local infection so that the procedure will be safer and easier to perform. Since endometrial cancer often occurs in later life, some women who are poor operative risks will be given radiation therapy as opposed to being exposed to the risk of surgery. The nursing care of patients receiving radiation

TABLE 55-8 Stages of cancer of the endometrium

Stage	Involvement
I	Confined to corpus
II	Involves corpus and cervix
III	Extends outside corpus but not outside pelvis (vaginal wall but not bladder or rectum)
IV	Involves bladder, rectum, or outside pelvis

therapy for endometrial cancer is similar to the care given any patient receiving external radiation with a subsequent radium implant (see Chapter 17).

Treatment of patients with stage III or stage IV disease usually includes hormonal treatment and chemotherapy in addition to surgery and radiation. Progestins have been used for more than 20 years with good response, especially in patients with well-differentiated tumors. Progestin therapy may be administered in several different ways: medroxyprogesterone acetate (DepoProvera), 400 mg intramuscularly at weekly intervals; oral medroxyprogesterone in the range of 150 mg/day; or megestrol acetate (Megace), 160 mg/day. Side effects from these medications are rare. Most women tolerate this form of hormonal manipulation very well.

For patients who do not respond to progestins, doxorubicin, cyclophosphamide, and 5-fluorouracil have been used, either singularly or in combination. The effectiveness of these agents varies.

CANCER OF THE OVARY
EPIDEMIOLOGY AND ETIOLOGY

Ovarian cancer causes more deaths than any other female genital cancer. There are about 20,000 new cases diagnosed each year in the United States with about 12,000 deaths annually.[3] Malignant neoplasms of the ovaries occur at all ages, including infancy and childhood. The major histologic types occur in distinctive age ranges. Malignant germ cells are most common in women under age 20, whereas epithelial cancers of the ovary are primarily seen in women over 50 years. Most cases occur in the age group of 50 to 59 years.

No known specific risk factors exist for ovarian cancer. The nonspecific risk factors most frequently seen are familial history and environmental factors. The highest rates of ovarian cancer occur in highly industrialized countries, which suggests exposure to physical or chemical products of industry. The etiology of ovarian neoplasms is poorly understood. The mechanisms of development are virtually a mystery. Many retrospective studies are currently underway to determine preexisting gynecologic abnormalities.

PATHOPHYSIOLOGY

The pathophysiology of ovarian cancer is complex. Ovarian cancer is a broad term than can be divided into many categories depending on the cell type of origin. The four main types of ovarian neoplasms are shown in Table 55-9.

CLINICAL MANIFESTATIONS

The early diagnosis of an ovarian neoplasm is usually by chance rather than a result of frequent screening. No known method exists for detecting ovarian cancer at an early stage. The signs and symptoms of advancing dis-

TABLE 55-9 Classification of ovarian neoplasms

Source of Neoplasm	Examples
Epithelium	Serous, mucinous, endometroid
Germ cell	Teratoma (mature and immature), dysgerminoma
Gonadal stroma	Granulosa (theca, Sertoli's, Leydig's cells)
Mesenchyme	Fibroma, lymphoma, sarcoma

ease include abdominal girth enlargement, abdominal pain and pressure, nausea and vomiting, constipation, and urinary frequency. Any ovarian enlargement should be suspected of being an ovarian malignancy. Palpable ovaries in premenarchal or postmenopausal women are an abnormal physical finding.

INTERVENTIONS
Medical Management

Ovarian cancer is diagnosed and staged at the time of exploratory laparotomy. A TAH/BS0 is most often done in addition to the removal of as much of the tumor as possible. Any ascites encountered during the surgery are submitted for cytology and, if there is no ascitic fluid, "washings" are taken by lavaging the peritoneal cavity with normal saline and submitting this fluid for an analysis. Often the omentum is removed, as well as samples of the paraaortic and pelvic lymph nodes. All the remaining tissue in the pelvis and abdomen is carefully scrutinized, and a biopsy is done of any suspicious areas.

Ovarian cancer is *surgically* staged, unlike cervical and endometrial cancer, which are *clinically* staged. The staging of ovarian cancer is included in Table 55-10.

In addition to surgery, some form of adjuvant therapy is often recommended. The adjuvant therapy used is usually based on the stage of the disease. Long-term survival depends on the stage of the disease, the grade of differentiation of the tumor, the amount of tumor left after surgery, and the additional treatment used after surgery.

Additional or adjuvant therapy usually suggested for stage I disease is chemotherapy with an alkylating agent such as melphalan or intraperitoneal instillation of radioactive phosphorus (32-P). (For the nursing care of patients who have had 32-P instilled, see Chapter 17.)

Patients with stage II disease may be offered a variety of adjuvant therapies. The most common options include instillation of 32-P, external abdominal and pelvic irradiation, or systemic combined chemotherapy. Often,

TABLE 55-10 Stages of cancer of the ovary

Stage	Involvement
I	Limited to ovaries
II	Involving one or both ovaries with pelvic extension
III	Involving one or both ovaries with intraperitoneal metastasis outside pelvis or positive lymph nodes
IV	Involving one or both ovaries with distant metastasis (for example, liver, lungs)

after completion of systemic chemotherapy, "second-look" surgery is done to determine if any disease remains. This surgery is done only if the patient is clinically free of disease. If no disease is found during this procedure, no further therapy is given.

Patients with stage III or stage IV ovarian cancer have as much of the tumor removed as possible. It has been found that the survival rates of patients with stage III and stage IV disease are directly related to the amount of residual disease. Patients with minimal residual disease appear to have a better prognosis with adjuvant therapy.

The adjuvant therapy used in stage III and stage IV ovarian cancer is most often combined chemotherapy. Occasionally, in stage III disease, whole abdominal irradiation is implemented. For patients who cannot tolerate aggressive chemotherapy or radiation, a single alkylating agent such as melphalan is used.

Nursing Management

The nursing care for any patient with ovarian cancer includes management similar to that for patients undergoing major abdominal surgery (see Chapter 44). The nursing care for patients receiving external radiation therapy and chemotherapy is found in Chapter 17. Patients who receive the recommended number of courses of chemotherapy and who are clinically free of disease usually undergo a second-look procedure to determine if the disease has been completely eradicated.

Patient education regarding the diagnosis, surgery and adjuvant therapy for ovarian cancer is an integral aspect of patient care. Teaching should begin in the outpatient department, continue through hospitalization, and persist through the follow-up treatment and surveillance. A comprehensive teaching booklet for the woman with the diagnosis of ovarian cancer is available.[32]

CANCER OF THE VULVA
EPIDEMIOLOGY AND ETIOLOGY

Cancer of the vulva is the fourth most common malignant tumor of the female genital tract; cervical, uterine, and ovarian cancers occur more frequently. Cancer of the vulva accounts for 3% to 4% of all primary malignancies of the female genital tract.[18] It is most often a disease of elderly women; approximately 85% of the cases occur after menopause, particularly after 65 years of age.

Little is known of the cause of vulvar cancer. Parity, marital status, and racial differences have no causal relationship to this cancer.[47]

PREVENTION AND EARLY DETECTION

Since the etiology of vulvar cancer is vague, its prevention is difficult. Cancer of the vulva is usually (60% of the time) diagnosed in the localized stage.[18] Any mass, pigmented lesion, ulcer, or hypertrophic process of the vulva should be suspected of being vulvar cancer, and therefore a biopsy should be done. The 5-year survival rate for vulvar cancer diagnosed and treated in an early stage approaches 90%. This emphasizes the importance of early diagnosis and treatment. Many women delay seeking medical attention for vulvar problems. There are many reasons for these delays, including economic concerns, modesty, denial, and neglect. Occasionally, some patients are treated with topical creams or ointments without being initially examined.

PATHOPHYSIOLOGY

Most cancers of the vulva are squamous in origin. Approximately 86% of reported vulvar cancers are of the squamous cell type.[18] The vulva is covered with a layer of skin; therefore any malignancy that appears elsewhere on the skin can occur in this area. The initial lesion often arises from an area of intraepithelial neoplasia, which can eventually form a firm nodule that can ulcerate. The diagnosis of vulvar cancer can only be made by biopsy and histologic examination of the tissue.

CLINICAL MANIFESTATIONS

The lesion can develop anywhere on the vulva; 70% of vulvar cancers arise on the labia. The disease is usually localized and well demarcated. The most common complaints are vulvar itching (pruritus) and burning. On inspection, an ulcer may be noted; abnormal pigmentation or lack thereof (leukoplakia) and asymmetry may also be detected.

INTERVENTIONS
Medical Management

Surgery is the most common form of treatment used in vulvar cancer. More than 80% of patients are treated primarily by surgery.[18] A radical vulvectomy is often the treatment of choice for invasive disease. This involves dissection of bilateral inguinal lymph nodes, excision of the mons pubis and terminal portion of the urethra and vagina, and excision of portions of the round ligaments and saphenous veins. In some instances, much less radical surgery is performed. Patients with cancer of the vulva are often poor surgical risks because of concurrent physical disease.

Nursing Management

The woman requiring a vulvectomy has some special nursing needs in addition to routine preoperative and postoperative care. She is given enemas preoperatively and a low-residue diet postoperatively. Measures are taken to obviate the need for straining to defecate and help prevent contamination of the vulvar wound. A Foley catheter usually is used to provide urinary drainage. When the catheter is removed, the patient may be unable to void because of difficulty in relaxing the perineum; sitz baths may help. If the inguinal nodes have been dissected, a heat lamp can be directed to the groin. After all the sutures are removed, sitz baths may be substituted for the heat lamp. Large amounts of tissues are removed from the vulva and the groin during the procedure, and the sutures are usually taut, leading to severe discomfort. The patient will usually need analgesic medication at frequent intervals during the 2 or 3 weeks before sutures can be removed. Following an inguinal node dissection, pillows need to be arranged to prevent undue pulling on the taut inguinal sutures when the patient moves. If the patient is lying on her side, she will be more comfortable if her upper leg is supported by a pillow. If she is lying on her back, low Fowler's position puts less tension on the sutures. Wound breakdown is often a complication.

The vulvar wound is frequently left exposed, but if a dressing is used, it is held in place with a T binder. The wound is cleansed twice a day with solutions such as hydrogen peroxide, normal saline solution, benzalkonium chloride, or other antiseptic solutions. Following this, a heat lamp is used to dry the area. The heat also improves local circulation, thus stimulating healing.

The wounds following a vulvectomy or an inguinal node dissection heal slowly, and the woman may become quite discouraged. Diversional activities and socializing with other patients can help her to pass the time. Privacy should be ensured, and women should be encouraged to express their feelings concerning this disfiguring surgery. Some women feel that their femininity has been irreparably damaged or that the disfigurement may end their sexual life.[5] By the time of hospital discharge, however, the wounds are usually healed, and the convalescence will be similar to that following any surgical procedure. Sexual intercourse can usually be resumed after complete wound healing has been achieved, approximately 4 weeks.

Patient teaching before and during treatment, at discharge from the hospital, and through follow-up care and surveillance is an essential component of nursing care. A comprehensive teaching booklet for the woman undergoing a radical vulvectomy is available.[34]

GESTATIONAL TROPHOBLASTIC NEOPLASIA
EPIDEMIOLOGY AND ETIOLOGY

Gestational trophoblastic neoplasia (GTN) is the term now usually applied to hydatidiform mole, molar pregnancy, invasive mole, and choriocarcinoma.[27] GTN is recognized as one of the most curable gynecologic malignancies. This is mainly because this neoplasm is extremely sensitive to various chemotherapeutic agents. The reported incidence of GTN varies significantly in different regions of the world—in the Far East, it is about 1 in 120 pregnancies; in the United States, about 1 in 1200 pregnancies.

The cause of GTN is not thoroughly understood. Nutrition and socioeconomic factors have been correlated; however, no conclusive evidence has been found to directly relate these factors to the incidence of the disease.

PATHOPHYSIOLOGY

GTN is an abnormal pregnancy characterized by a degeneration, or an abnormal growth, of the trophoblastic tissue of the placenta. This anomaly of the placental tissue usually is associated with the absence of an intact fetus. One of the most important characteristics of GTN is the serum marker this tumor produces, human chorionic gonadotropin (HCG). The amount of this hormone present in the serum is directly related to the number of viable tumor cells.[18] Therefore, even in the absence of clinical disease, levels of serum HCG can determine the presence of disease recurrence in minute amounts.

CLINICAL MANIFESTATIONS

No known prevention exists for GTN, except to avoid conception. Early stages of GTN may be similar to normal pregnancy. As the disease progresses, most women have uterine bleeding. Uterine growth more rapid than gestational age, anemia, nausea, and vomiting are also common symptoms. The diagnosis of GTN is usually by pathologic examination of the products of conception. Before evaluation, amniography or ultrasonography can determine the presence of a molar pregnancy. Serum HCG titers are also routinely done before evacuation of the uterus.

INTERVENTIONS
Medical Management

Suction curettage is the most common method used for evacuation of a molar pregnancy. After a moderate amount of tissue has been removed, intravenous oxytocin (Pitocin) is begun. If the patient does not desire future pregnancies, a primary hysterectomy may be done as opposed to a suction dilation and curettage (D&C).

After the removal of the molar tissue, weekly serum HCG titers are drawn. This test is continued weekly until 2 consecutive weeks of normal values are reached. This indicates a spontaneous remission and should occur in 80% of patients.[18] The HCG titer should then be continued monthly for 6 months, then every month up to a year. After a full year without an elevated HCG titer, the woman may become pregnant. Pregnancy is not advised before this time because HCG is also secreted during normal pregnancy. If a patient becomes pregnant before 1 year has elapsed, it would be difficult to determine whether this hormone was being secreted by a normal pregnancy or by remaining molar tissue. Therefore it is essential to have patients use a reliable method of birth control.

Plateaus or rises of the HCG titer during the observation period indicates persistent or recurrent GTN, and the patient is evaluated and started on chemotherapy. The pretreatment evaluation includes a physical examination and a chest roentgenogram. Persistent disease can metastasize, and GTN usually disseminates widely by way of the bloodstream. The most common sites of metastasis are the lung, vagina, pelvis, brain, and liver.

Chemotherapy is used in the treatment of recurrent or persistent GTN. Methotrexate intravenously or intramuscularly for 5 days every 14 days, or actinomycin D intravenously for 5 days every 14 days, are the regimens most often used (see Chapter 17). Patients receive their courses of chemotherapy until the HCG titer returns to normal. Most institutions give one or two additional courses after a normal HCG titer is reached. Women who do not respond to single-agent chemotherapy may be given a multiple-drug regimen, have surgery (for example, hysterectomy or lobectomy), or receive radiation therapy.

Nursing Management

It is essential to address the social and emotional impact of the disease process on both the patient and her family. GTN is a unique neoplastic process because it is an aberration of pregnancy. Thus it cannot only raise concerns about malignancy and death, but also influence feelings about self-worth, self-image, future sexual relationships, and plans for future pregnancies. Patient and family teaching should include an understanding of the disease process compatible with the level of education and desire for knowledge, future pregnancies, change in body image, effect of chemotherapy (if given) on future children, chance of GTN developing with future pregnancy, and need for effective birth control.

CHAPTER SUMMARY

- Many organisms play a role in the development of infections of the vulva and vagina. In addition, women may be predisposed to developing such infections as a result of stress, malnutrition, aging, and decreased resistance.

- The clinical manifestations of such infections include inflammation of the tissues; abnormal discharge from the vaginal, urethra, or Bartholin's glands; and pruritus. Each specific organism that is the causative factor of the infection produces signs and symptoms specific to that organism.

- Medical management involves treatment of the infection, prevention of recurrence, and prevention of the spread of infection to others.

- Nursing management involves teaching regarding the prevention of infection. Such teaching includes self-care techniques, modifications of habits and activities of daily living, as well as correct adherence to therapeutic regimens.

- Specific conditions that require in-depth assessment, diagnosis, and management include cervicitis, pelvic inflammatory disease, toxic shock syndrome, structural problems of the uterus, ovarian tumors/cysts, fibroid tumors, endometriosis, and cervical polyps.

- Factors placing the woman at risk for developing cancer of the cervix include first coitus at an early age, multiple sexual partners, low socioeconomic group, and exposure to herpesvirus type 2.

- The incidence of and death rate associated with invasive cervical cancer can continue to be reduced through adequate screening using the Pap smear.

- Treatment for invasive cancer of the cervix depends on the stage of the disease. Surgery and radiation therapy are the most frequently used methods. Surgical techniques include radical hysterectomy for stages IB and IIA and pelvic exenteration for locally recurrent disease. Radiation therapy includes external beam irradiation followed by two implants.

- Teaching for the woman undergoing radical hysterectomy includes information about the disease and proposed surgery; diagnostic tests; diet, exercise recommendations, and bladder function following surgery; personal impact and sexuality; and follow-up care.

- Factors placing the woman at risk for developing cancer of the endometrium include obesity, nulliparity, late menopause, diabetes mellitus, hypertension, and the use of exogenous estrogens.

- Any postmenopausal woman with vaginal bleeding should be encouraged to seek medical advice.

- Treatment for endometrial cancer is most often abdominal hysterectomy. Radiation therapy, hormonal manipulation, and chemotherapy may also be used for patients with advanced disease or those who are not good surgical candidates.

- Teaching for the woman who has endometrial, ovarian, or vulvar cancer should include information about her specific treatment plan, the disease, diagnostic tests, diet and exercise recommendations during and after therapy, personal impact and sexuality, and follow-up recommendations.

- No known risk factors are associated with ovarian cancer; nonspecific risk factors include familial history and environmental factors.

- Treatment for ovarian caner usually includes extensive debulking surgery followed by chemotherapy.

- The usual treatment for invasive cancer of the vulva is a radical vulvectomy.

- Gestational trophoblastic neoplasia (GTN) results from degeneration of the placental tissue; therefore it can be considered an abnormal pregnancy. It is one of the most curable gynecologic malignancies.

- The treatment for GTN is evacuation of the uterine contents, close follow-up of human chorionic gonadotropin (HCG) levels, and possibly short-term chemotherapy.

- Teaching for the woman being treated for GTN or monitored for its occurrence includes information about the disease and proposed treatment, the need for frequent serum evaluations of HCG level, the contraindication of pregnancy until serum HCG titers return to normal levels, personal impact and sexuality, and follow-up recommendations.

QUESTIONS TO CONSIDER

- What are some of the factors that predispose a postmenopausal woman to infection of the vulva or vagina?

- What important factors must the nurse consider in caring for a patient complaining of altered patterns of sexuality related to vaginal or vulvar infection?

- How might a nurse approach a patient who is recently diagnosed with endometriosis, complains of chronic pelvic pain, and fears future infertility?

- Explain the important areas to cover in teaching patients about prevention and treatment of pelvic inflammatory disease.

- Describe the nursing care of women who have undergone perineal surgery for structural problems of the uterus.

- How would the diagnosis of a genital cancer affect the sexuality of a 35-year-old woman?

- Should a woman at risk for developing endometrial cancer take oral estrogens to allay the symptoms of menopause?

- How would the diagnosis of ovarian cancer affect the life plans of a 25-year-old single woman as opposed to those of a 55-year-old mother of three children?

- What methods of public education may encourage the population at risk for developing vulvar cancer to seek medical attention at the time symptoms first develop?

- How would immediate pregnancy affect the follow up of the woman recently treated for gestational trophoblastic neoplasia (GTN)?

REFERENCES AND SELECTED READINGS

1. American Cancer Society: Report on the cancer-related health check-up, New York, 1980, The Society.
2. American Cancer Society: Cancer facts and figures for minority Americans, New York, 1983, Springer Publishing Co.
3. American Cancer Society: 1989 cancer facts and figures, New York, 1989, The Society.
4. American College of Obstetricians and Gynecologists: Periodic cancer screening for women: statement of policy, Washington, DC, 1980, The College.
5. Anderson B and Hacker N: Psychosexual adjustment after vulvar surgery, Obstet Gynecol 62(4):457-462, 1983.
6. Ballon S: Gynecologic oncology: controversies in cancer treatment, Boston, 1981, GK Hall & Co.
7. Baluk U et al: Health professionals' perceptions of the psychological consequences of abortion, Am J Community Psychol 8(2):67-75, 1980.
8. Barclay DL: Disorders of the vulva and vagina. In Benson RC, editor: Current obstetric and gynecologic diagnosis and treatment, ed 4, Los Altos, Calif, 1982, Lange Medical Publications.
9. Berger M and Goldstein D: Impaired reproductive performance in DES-exposed women, Obstet Gynecol 55:25-27, 1980.
10. Berkowitz R et al: Psychological and social impact of gestational trophoblastic neoplasia, J Reprod Med 25:14-16, 1980.
11. Berkus M and Daly J: Cone biopsy: an outpatient procedure, Am J Obstet Gynecol 137:953-958, 1980.
12. Betts J and Buttram V: A plan for managing endometriosis, Contemp Obstet Gynecol 15:121-129, 1980.
13. Bouchard R and Owens NF: Nursing care of the cancer patient, ed 4, St Louis, 1980, The CV Mosby Co.
14. Brown L: Toxic shock syndrome, MCN 6:57-59, 1981.
15. Crosson K: A patient teaching aid for the pelvic exenteration patient, Oncol Nurs Forum 8:53-56, 1981.
16. Curran J: Economic consequences of pelvic inflammatory disease in the United States, Am J Obstet Gynecol 138:848-851, 1980.
17. Davis J et al: Toxic shock syndrome: epidemiologic features, recurrence, risk factors, and prevention, N Engl J Med 303:1429-1435, 1980.
18. DiSaia PJ and Creasman WT: Clinical gynecologic oncology, St Louis, ed 3, 1988, The CV Mosby Co.
19. Dodson MG and Faro S: The polymicrobial etiology of acute pelvic inflammatory disease and treatment regimens, Rev Infect Dis 4(suppl):696-702, 1985.
20. Fisher R and Goodpasture H: Toxic shock syndrome in menstruating women, Ann Intern Med 94:156-163, 1981.
21. *Fogel CI and Woods NF: Health care of women: a nursing perspective, St Louis, 1981, The CV Mosby Co.
22. Gorbach SL: Current experience with clindamycin in the treatment of abdominal and female pelvic infections, Scand J Infect Dis 43(suppl):82-88, 1984.
23. *Hatcher R: Contraceptive technology, ed 14, New York, 1988, Irvington Publishers.
24. Hill EC: Disorders of the uterine cervix. In Benson RC, editor: Current obstetrics and gynecology diagnosis and treatment, ed 4, Los Altos, Calif, 1982, Lange Medical Publications.
25. Ingram JM: Endometriosis. In Benson RC, editor: Current obstetric and gynecologic diagnosis and treatment, ed 4, Los Altos, Calif, 1982, Lange Medical Publications.
26. Jenkins B: Patients' report of sexual changes after treatment for gynecologic cancer, Oncol Nurs Forum 15(3):349-354, 1988.

27. Jusenius K: A teaching aid for the radical hysterectomy patient, Oncol Nurs Forum 10(2):71-75, 1983.
28. Kaufman D et al: Intrauterine contraceptive device use and pelvic inflammatory disease, Am J Obstet Gynecol 136:159-162, 1980.
29. Kaufman RH et al: Upper genital tract changes and pregnancy outcome in offspring exposed in utero to diethylstilbestrol, Am J Obstet Gynecol 137:299-308, 1980.
30. Keith LG et al: On the causation of pelvic inflammatory disease, Am J Obstet Gynecol 149(2):215-224, 1984.
31. *Kuczynski H: Pros and cons of douching: the nurse's role in counseling, J Obstet Gynecol Neonatal Nurs 9:90-93, 1980.
32. Lamb M: Ovarian cancer: patient information booklet, Oncol Nurs Forum 12(5):83-88, 1985.
33. Lamb M: Sexual dysfunction in the gynecologic oncology patient, Semin Oncol Nurs 1(1):9-17, 1985.
34. Lamb MA: Vulvar: patient information booklet, Oncol Nurs Forum 12(6):79-82, 1986.
35. Larsen B and Galask R: Vaginal microbial flora: practical and theoretic relevance, Obstet Gynecol 55(suppl):100-113, 1980.
36. Ledger WJ: Current problems in antibiotic treatment in obstetrics and gynecology, Rev Infect Dis 4(suppl):679-689, 1985.
37. Malkosian G, Annegers J, and Fountain K: Carcinoma of the endometrium: stage 1, Am J Obstet Gynecol 136:872-888, 1980.
38. Mardh P: An overview of infectious agents of salpingitis, their biology, and recent advances in methods of detection, Am J Obstet Gynecol 138:933-951, 1980.
39. McCarthy T, Roy AC, and Rotman SS: Intrauterine devices and pelvic inflammatory disease, Aust NZ J Obstet Gynecol 24(2):106-110, 1984.
40. Novak ER, Jones GS, and Jones HW Jr: Novak's textbook of gynecology, ed 10, Baltimore, 1980, Williams & Wilkins.
41. Rees E: The treatment of pelvic inflammatory disease, Am J Obstet Gynecol 138:1042-1047, 1980.
42. Rosenfeld D and Bronson R: Reproductive problems in the DES-exposed female, Obstet Gynecol 55:453-456, 1980.
43. Sargis N: Detecting ovarian cancer: a challenge for nursing assessment, Oncol Nurs Forum 10(2):48-53, 1983.
44. *Secor RMC: Bacterial vaginosis: a comprehensive review, Nurs Clin North Am 23:865-875, 1988.
45. Seibel M, Freeman M, and Graves W: Carcinoma of the cervix and sexual function, Obstet Gynecol 55:484-487, 1980.
46. Shands K et al: Toxic shock syndrome in menstruating women: association with tampon use and *Staphylococcus aureus* and clinical features in 52 cases, N Engl J Med 303:1436-1442, 1980.
47. Smith D: Gynecologic cancers: etiology and pathophysiology, Semin Oncol Nurs 2(4):270-274, 1986.
48. Sobel JD: Epidemiology and pathogenesis of recurrent vulvovaginal candidiasis, Am J Obstet Gynecol 157(7):924-935, 1985.
49. Studva K and White L: Cancer prevention and detection: cervical cancer, Cancer Nurs 7(4):335-345, 1984.
50. Toffe R and Williams D: Toxic shock syndrome: clinical and laboratory features in 15 patients, Ann Intern Med 94:149-155, 1981.
51. Walker A and Jick H: Declining rates of endometrial cancer, Obstet Gynecol 56:733-736, 1980.
52. Washington AE, Sweet RL, and Chafer MA: Pelvic inflammatory disease and its sequelae in adolescents, J Adolesc Health Care 6(4):298-310, 1985.
53. Yarborough B: Teaching plan for the patient undergoing total-pelvic exenteration, Oncol Nurs Forum 8:36-40, 1981.

*References preceded by an asterisk are particularly well suited for student reading.

CHAPTER 56

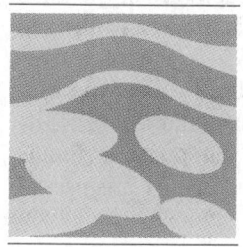

Management of Men with Reproductive Problems

MARGARET HEITKEMPER
DEBORAH POWER

CHAPTER OBJECTIVES

After studying this chapter, the student should be able to:
1. Analyze the process of infectious diseases specific to men's reproductive health.
2. Analyze the developmental process of structural problems specific to men's reproductive health.
3. Analyze the developmental process of benign and malignant neoplasms specific to men's reproductive health.
4. Develop nursing diagnoses related to the conditions discussed.
5. Develop nursing care plans related to the conditions discussed.

Men's reproductive health care is one dimension of an emerging specialty area of nursing practice, men's health. Currently a gap exists between expectations of male health care consumers and the health care options available to them. Like women, men have unique biological and social health care needs. Among these are a need for permission to have health concerns and discuss them; access to information about their bodies; instruction in self-care techniques; opportunities for physical examinations and history-taking, including the sexual-reproductive system; consideration of life-styles and male role influences on physical and mental health; concern for factors such as occupation, leisure, and personal relationships related to health; a health care system sensitive to their occupational demands that compete for time; and financial support to obtain health care.

This chapter includes a discussion of the most common health problems involving the reproductive system in men. Particular emphasis is on infectious processes, structural problems, and neoplasms of the reproductive tract. Table 56-1 summarizes the problems affecting men's reproductive health discussed in this chapter. Sexually transmitted diseases and methods of contraception are discussed in Chapters 58 and 54, respectively.

INFECTIOUS PROCESSES

EPIDEMIOLOGY AND ETIOLOGY

Both nonspecific pyogenic organisms and specific organisms such as the gonococci and tubercle bacilli may cause stubborn infections of men's reproductive systems. Urethritis, prostatitis, seminal vesiculitis, and epididymitis are the most common infections. The infecting organisms may reach the genital organs by spreading directly through the urethra, or they may be borne by blood or lymph.

ASSESSMENT

Assessment of men with reproductive system infections includes careful history regarding their likely exposure to infectious organisms and a careful physical examination and laboratory tests. Men are asked to give a careful account of their symptoms, including duration and what they have done to relieve them. The history includes sexual practices, such as the last sexual exposure so that the incubation period can be ascertained. Information about signs of infection in sexual partners is also

TABLE 56-1 Problems affecting the male reproductive organs

Organ	Infections	Structural Problems	Neoplasms
Penis		Phimosis Paraphimosis	Penile
Urethra	Nonspecific urethritis		
Scrotum		Hydrocele Varicocele Spermatocele	
Testes	Orchitis	Torsion of testicle	Seminomatous Nonseminomatous
Epididymis	Epididymitis		
Prostate	Prostatitis		Prostatic

obtained. The history may reveal information about predisposing factors, patterns of repeated infection, or evidence of concurrent problems.

The site of the infection will influence treatment. The physician may obtain segmented bacteriologic localization cultures to make the determination; four sterile culture tubes are used for collection. Men must be well hydrated, have a full bladder, and be able to cooperate. The first 5 to 10 ml of a voiding is collected and labeled VB1 (voided bladder 1). After approximately 200 ml, a 5-ml to 10-ml midstream specimen (VB2) is collected. The patient is asked to stop voiding, then the prostate is massaged rectally until the secretions (EPS [expressed prostatic secretions]) are collected. The next 5 to 10 ml of urine (VB3) is collected and the bladder emptied. The specimens must be refrigerated and taken to the laboratory for culture within 4 hours. If VB2 is profusely infected, the other specimens probably will be also. Antibiotics are given to sterilize the urine (eradicate cystitis, if present), and the segmented bacteriologic localization cultures are repeated.

■ DATA ANALYSIS: NURSING DIAGNOSES

Nursing diagnoses for men with an infection of the reproductive system may include, but are not limited to, the following:

Diagnostic Title	Possible Etiologies
Knowledge deficit	Lack of information about infection
Pain	Inflammation
Sexuality patterns, altered	Fear about infection, discomfort related to inflammation
Social isolation	Fear of infecting others

■ PLANNING: EXPECTED PATIENT OUTCOMES

Expected patient outcomes for men with infections of the reproductive system may include, but are not limited to, the following:

1. Demonstrates increased knowledge about their bodies
2. Describes how infections occur and are spread
3. Identifies ways of preventing reinfection
4. Practices habits that improve or promote health
5. Follows therapies that assist in decreasing pain
6. States how changes in daily practices influence control of infection
7. Demonstrates knowledge of relationship between sexual practices and infections
8. Demonstrates improved communication with sexual partners

PREVENTION

Because urethral infection spreads so readily to the genital organs, men should not be catheterized unless it is absolutely necessary. Every means should be used to help them void normally. They are often allowed to stand to void even when they are to be on bed rest otherwise. Because of the length and curvature of the male urethra, some trauma to the urethral mucosa is likely to accompany catheterization or the passage of instruments such as a cystoscope. The distal part of the urethra is not sterile, and trauma makes the urethra susceptible to attack from the bacteria present. Fluids should be given liberally after instruments are passed through the urethra.

NONSPECIFIC URETHRITIS

Nonspecific (nongonococcal) urethritis is an inflammation of the urethra caused by such organisms as *Chlamydia trachomatis, Ureaplasma urealyticum, Trichomonas vaginalis, Candida,* the herpes virus, or coliforms. The patient complains of urgency, frequency, and burning on urination, and there may be a purulent urethral discharge. Treatment of nonspecific urethritis is discussed in the chapter dealing with sexually transmitted diseases (Chapter 58). In approximately 25% of men with symptoms of acute dysuria and urethral discharge, no microbial cause is identified.[11]

PROSTATITIS
CLINICAL MANIFESTATIONS

Approximately 50% of all men will at some time during their adult lives experience symptoms suggesting prostate inflammation. However, only a small number of these cases will be due to bacterial infection.[11] The man with prostatitis usually has acute symptoms of urinary obstruction. He suddenly has difficulty in voiding, perineal tenderness and pain, and elevation of temperature. He may experience pain during or after ejaculation; hematuria may also be present.

Rotating specimens (also called *serial urine specimens* or *racking*) are collected to determine the change in the character of the urine (Figure 56-1). Three or more test tubes are used. Urine is voided into a container and mixed thoroughly; then a portion is poured into one of the test tubes and placed in a rack (hence its name). At the next voiding, the procedure is repeated; the first tube is moved toward the center of the rack, and the second specimen is placed at the end. The procedure is repeated a third time or until all test tubes and the rack are full. The first specimen is discarded at the subsequent voiding to make room for fresher specimens. Subtle changes in the degree of hematuria, cloudiness, sediment, and so on may be detected more easily without constant laboratory analysis, whereas if the specimens were discarded at the time of voiding, important signs might not be noticed. In addition, microscopic examination of the EPS is performed or a culture of the VB3 taken. Percutaneous cystotomy or computer tomography may be used to check for abscesses in the prostate gland.

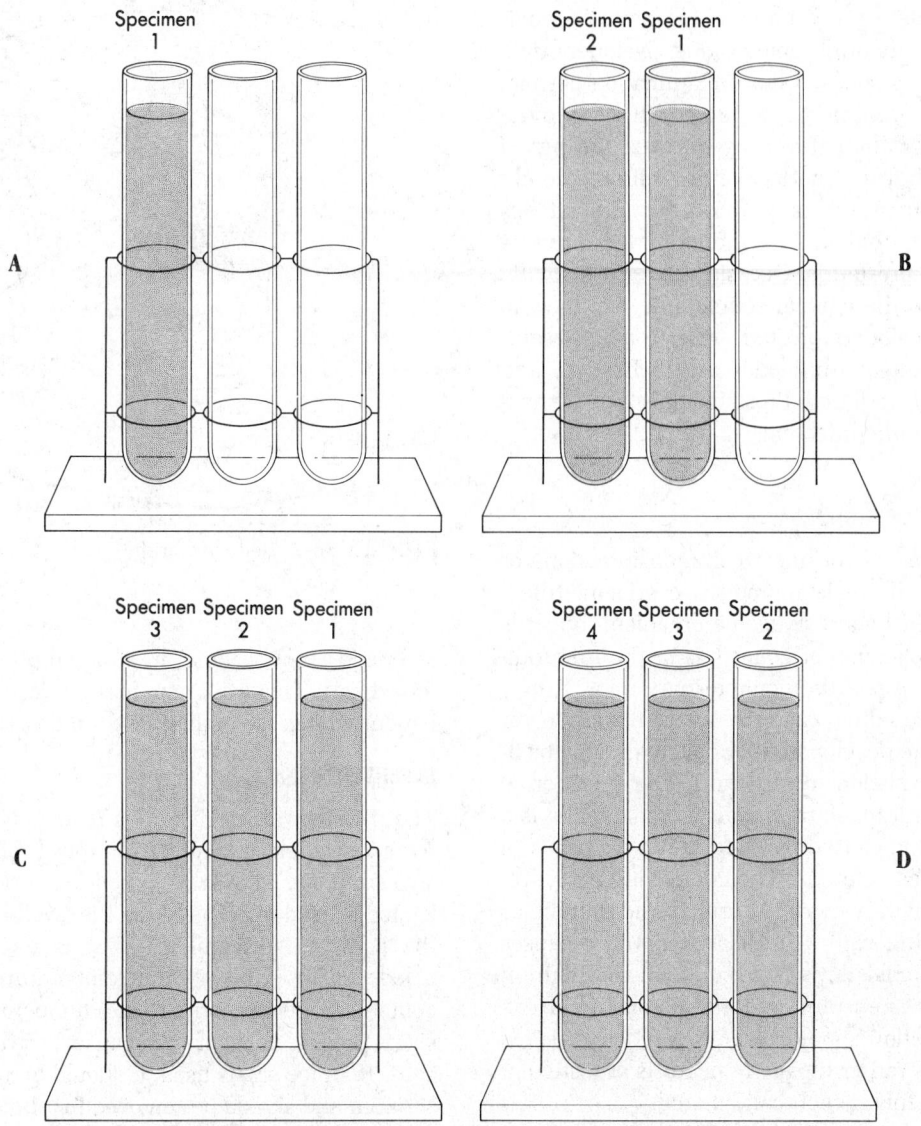

FIGURE 56-1 Rotating specimens. **A,** Specimen is obtained and placed in rack. **B,** Specimen 1 is moved to right when specimen 2 is obtained. **C,** Specimens 1 and 2 are moved to right when specimen 3 is obtained. **D,** Specimens 2 and 3 are moved to right and specimen 1 is discarded when specimen 4 is obtained.

INTERVENTIONS

Treatment is usually conservative, consisting of antibiotics for 30 days to prevent chronic infection, forcing fluids, physical rest, stool softeners to decrease rectal irritation of the prostate, and local application of heat by sitz baths.

Prompt treatment of prostatitis may prevent edema of the prostate with resultant obstruction of the urethra. If severe urinary retention occurs, suprapubic needle aspiration is safer than urethral straight or indwelling catheterization that would increase the risk of epididymitis. Prostatic massage to eliminate residual pus pockets is

contraindicated during the acute phase, since it may cause bacteremia; however, it may be used after the acute attack subsides.

Recurrent episodes of acute prostatitis may cause fibrotic tissue to form. The fibrosis causes a hardening of the prostate, which may initially be confused with carcinoma. In the granulomatous form of prostatitis, the enlargement may take 3 to 6 months to resolve.

Inadequate treatment of acute infection can result in chronic prostatitis. A subacute infection may also develop into a chronic prostatitis that remains asymptomatic. Therefore prostatic secretions should be examined routinely to detect infection and to prevent complications such as acute or chronic cystitis, pyelonephritis, or epididymitis. It is believed that inflammation permits entry of antibiotics that normally do not diffuse into the prostatic fluid. Although they may be used during an acute infection, they are ineffective in a chronic condition. Trimethoprim is the only antibiotic that diffuses into the prostatic fluid and is therefore the drug of choice in chronic prostatitis. Occasionally, *prostatic abscesses* complicate the clinical course and may have to be drained surgically. If prostatic calculi are present, they may be infected. Antibiotics are ineffective, and surgical excision is required. Prostatectomy may be necessary to eradicate the infection.

EPIDIDYMITIS

ETIOLOGY AND EPIDEMIOLOGY

Epididymitis is one of the most common infections or inflammations of the male reproductive system. Infection can be caused by any pyogenic organism, but it is frequently a complication of gonorrhea or the first indication of tuberculosis of the genitourinary tract. It may be caused by ascending bacteria, instrumentation, or prostatectomy. The development of epididymitis is facilitated by chronic bladder obstruction. The infection is rarely bilateral. Traumatic or chemical epididymitis is a sterile inflammation caused by direct injury or reflux of urine down the vas deferens. The chemical form is frequently seen in military recruits during basic training as a result of straining with a full bladder, which causes urinary reflux. Epididymitis is uncommon in children; therefore when it is encountered, the possibility of urinary tract obstruction should be considered. Untreated epididymitis leads rather rapidly to necrosis of testicular tissue and septicemia, which can be fatal.

PREVENTION

Since bilateral epididymitis usually causes sterility, special attention is given to the prevention of this infection. Frequently, epididymitis is a complication of prolonged indwelling catheterization. Therefore, when bladder drainage over a long period is necessary, a cystotomy is done so that a urethral catheter is avoided.

An older patient who must have surgery of the prostate such as transurethral resection that will require leaving a urethral catheter in place for a long time may be advised to have a *bilateral vasectomy* to prevent any infection from descending through the ductus deferens to the epididymis. The operation is done before any cystoscopic examination and only if the urine is sterile.

CLINICAL MANIFESTATIONS

The man with epididymitis complains of severe tenderness, pain, and swelling of the scrotum, which is hot to the touch. His temperature may be markedly elevated, and he has general malaise. He often walks with a char-

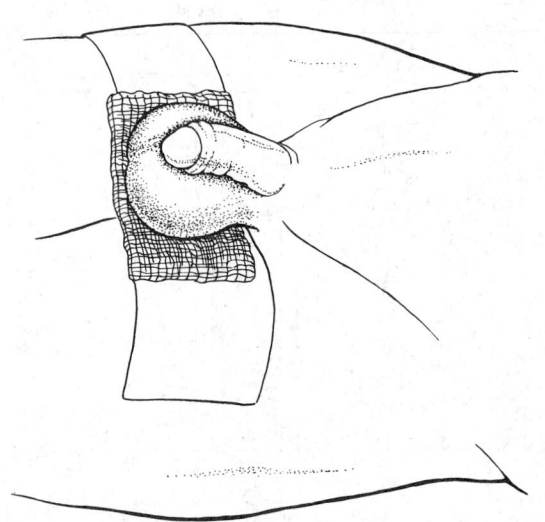

FIGURE 56-2 Bellevue bridge.

acteristic "duck waddle" in an attempt to protect the affected part. This walk may first disclose difficulty in the patient who is too embarrassed to describe his trouble.

INTERVENTIONS

The patient with epididymitis is usually put to bed and the scrotum elevated either on towel rolls or with adhesive strapping known as a Bellevue bridge (Figure 56-2). Ice is used to help reduce the swelling and to relieve the pain and discomfort. Heat is usually contraindicated, because the normal temperature of the scrotal contents is below normal body temperature and excessive exposure to heat can cause destruction of sperm cells. If an ice cap is used, it should be placed under the scrotum and should be removed for short intervals every hour to prevent ice burns. A plastic glove may also be filled with ice. With the palm of the glove placed under the scrotum, the fingers provide cold to the sides. Antibiotic therapy is given. Narcotic analgesics, antiinflammatory agents, and local anesthetics may also be used. Surgical excision (epididymectomy) may be required for severe or recurrent infection. If the testis is involved, an orchiectomy may be performed. The patient should drink at least 3 L of fluid daily. When the patient is pain free, he is allowed out of bed, at which time he should wear a scrotal support.

ORCHITIS

An inflammation or infection of the testicle is known as orchitis. It may be caused by pyogenic bacteria, virus (such as Paramyxovirus, the agent responsible for mumps), gonococci, or tubercle bacilli, or it may follow any septicemia. It rarely involves only the testis; usually the epididymis is also involved (epididymoorchitis). When mumps are contracted after puberty, approximately 20% of the cases are complicated by orchitis with symptom development 4 to 6 days after parotitis. If the case is mild, there may be no symptoms before the onset of orchitis.

The mumps virus is transmitted in respiratory secretions. Symptoms of low-grade fever, malaise, and headache occur 2 to 4 weeks after exposure. As a result of inflammation and fibrosis, some degree of testicular atrophy occurs in 50% of patients, but it does not appear to be related to the severity of the orchitis.

Unless both testes are severly involved, infertility is uncommon. Any postpubertal boy or man who is exposed to mumps usually is given gamma globulin immediately unless he has already had the disease. If there is any doubt, globulin usually is given. Although it may not prevent mumps, the disease is likely to be less severe with less likelihood of complications. Impotence and sterility are now rare sequelae. Traumatic orchitis may follow trauma, vasectomy, or surgical manipulation. There may be no prior history of inflammation or disease.

The signs and symptoms of orchitis are the same as those of epididymitis; there is also nausea, vomiting, pain radiating to the inguinal canal, and gonadal swelling. Parotid swelling and tenderness frequently precede testicular symptoms by 4 to 7 days. Treatment is the same for both conditions. Atrophy and sterility are caused by fibrosis that occurs during healing.

Hydrocele (a collection of fluid within the tunica vaginalis) is frequently associated with orchitis. The fluid may be aspirated to reduce pressure on the testis. If the hydrocele is surgically tapped within the first 2 days, it may decrease the atrophy; however, a tap should only be done in cases where edema is persistent, and there is a chance that surgical decompression may exacerbate inflammation.[11] Although effectiveness is questionable, stilbestrol (which inhibits normal testicular function), cortisone, and antibiotics may be given to reduce the severity of the disease. Abscesses of the testis require orchiectomy. A testicular prosthesis composed of Silastic gel is available for cosmetic purposes.[38] Possible complications of the prosthesis include infection and rejection. Unilateral orchiectomy may result in impotence and subfertility. Sexual counseling might be indicated.

PHIMOSIS

Phimosis is a condition in which the opening of the prepuce or foreskin is unable to be retracted behind the glans (Figure 56-3, A). It may be congenital or acquired as a result of inflammation or infection. Constriction may interfere with adequate hygiene. There may be a buildup of smegma, urine may be trapped in the preputial sac, and calculi may form, irritating the glans and predisposing to infection. Chronic irritation may be a cause of penile carcinoma. Healing is by fibrosis, which causes the acquired phimosis. If the constriction

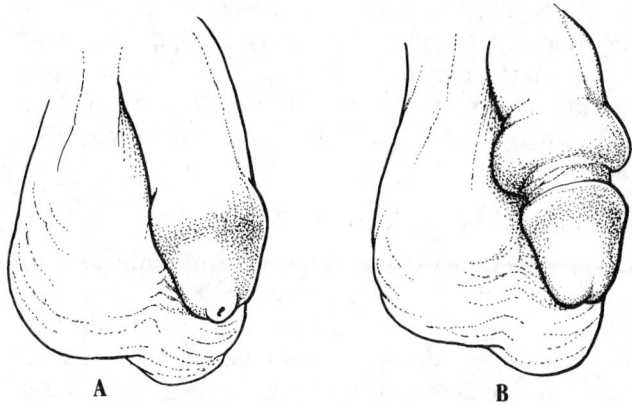

FIGURE 56-3 A, Phimosis. Note pinpoint opening of foreskin. **B,** Paraphimosis. Note foreskin is retracted but has become constricting band around penis.

is severe enough, it causes a urinary obstruction with straining and painful urination. This condition can be fatal in infants. Treatment for mild irritation and infection is hot soaks and antibiotics. If the case is severe, a dorsal slit or two lateral slits of the prepuce may be necessary. Circumcision, the surgical excision of the prepuce, should be performed when the tissue has returned to normal.

Treatment of congenital phimosis is stretching of the prepuce and repeated retraction behind the glans. If this does not permit adequate retraction, circumcision is the preferred treatment.

PARAPHIMOSIS

Paraphimosis is a condition in which the prepuce is retracted over the glans and forms a constriction that is sometimes impossible to reduce as edema develops in the glans (Figure 56-3, B). Cool compresses are applied to the penis, and it is elevated for a short time before a gentle attempt is made to reduce the prepuce. If this measure fails, emergency surgery must be done. A dorsal slit is made in the prepuce to prevent necrosis of the glans caused by impairment of its blood supply.

Circumcision is usually done later to prevent recurrences. The wound is covered with gauze generously impregnated with petrolatum. Bleeding usually is controlled by applying a pressure dressing that may be bulky and that sometimes must be removed before the patient can void. It should be removed cautiously and replaced after voiding with a petrolatum dressing. If the patient goes home on the same day as the surgery (or after the surgery), he (or his parent if the patient is a child) is taught to change the dressing at each voiding for a few days and to try to avoid fecal contamination of the area. An antibiotic ointment may be prescribed for the older child or adult. Instruction is also given to be alert for signs of bleeding. If severe bleeding occurs, a firm dressing should be applied to the penis, and the patient should be taken at once to the physician's office or the hospital emergency room. Very seldom, if bleeding persists, it is necessary to resuture the wound. An estrogen preparation may be prescribed for adult patients for several days after surgery to prevent painful penile erections.

LESIONS OF THE EXTERNAL GENITALIA

Any lesion of the external genitalia requires medical attention, and no ulcer of the genitalia should be treated by the patient before seeing a physician lest the diagnosis be obscured. Although lesions are present in a wide variety of conditions, they should always be considered infectious until proved otherwise, since many of the sexually transmitted diseases, with the exception of gonorrhea, produces a genital lesion or ulceration. These lesions will be discussed in the section that deals with the sexually transmitted diseases.

STRUCTURAL PROBLEMS

Immediate medical attention should be sought for any swelling of the scrotum or the testes within it. Any acute swelling of sudden onset must be considered twisting (torsion) of the testicles until proved otherwise. Torsion, as discussed below, leads to ischemia and necrosis of the affected testicle. Therefore scrotal enlargement should be diagnosed, not treated symptomatically with suspensories, which give relief and encourage procrastination about seeking appropriate medical care.

■ ASSESSMENT

Assessment of men with structural problems of the reproductive system includes a careful history of symptoms related to the structural problems such as pain or swelling. A physical examination focusing on the reproductive organs is usually accompanied with laboratory tests as discussed below.

■ DATA ANALYSIS: NURSING DIAGNOSES

Nursing diagnoses for men with structural prolems of the reproductive system may include, but are not limited to, the following:

Diagnostic Title	Possible etiologies
Altered sexuality patterns	Hygiene problems or pain
knowledge deficit	Lack of information about structural problems
Pain	Inflammation

■ PLANNING: EXPECTED PATIENT OUTCOMES

Expected patient outcomes for men with structural problems of the reproductive system may include, but are not limited to, the following:

1. Demonstrates increased knowledge about structural problems and their causes, for example varicocele
2. Demonstrates understanding of plan of care, including surgery or medical treatment
3. Describes therapy to enhance comfort and reduce pain
4. Describes safe sexual practices after therapy or surgery

HYDROCELE

Hydrocele, a common condition, is a benign, painless collection of clear, amber fluid within the tunica vaginalis that leads to swelling of the scrotum. It occurs fairly often in infant boys as well as in adult men. The cause of hydrocele is usually unknown, but it may be associated with trauma, acute nonspecific or tuberculous epididymitis, or orchitis. Hydrocele transilluminates when examined in a darkened room using a fiberoptic light.

If uncomplicated by other scrotal abnormalities, hydrocele is treated by aspirating the fluid and injecting a sclerosing drug such as urea hydrochloride into the scrotal sac. There is no pain, and only a Bandaid is required. Thirty percent of hydroceles recur and thus require repeated injections. Excision of the tunica vaginalis (hydrocelectomy) produces a permanent resolution. Postoperatively, a pressure dressing is applied on the scrotum, which is elevated. The patient should be observed carefully for any symptoms of hemorrhage, since bleeding may not be external. Hematoma formation occurs in up to 30% of cases. The patient needs a scrotal support when he is out of bed and may still require one after he is discharged from the hospital. He should have two scrotal suspensories, since the scrotal support should be washed each day. Immediately after surgery or after an infection, most patients require an extra large suspensory or perhaps an athletic support (jockstrap).

SPERMATOCELE

A spermatocele is a nontender cystic mass attached to the epididymis and containing a milky fluid and sperm. Since it also transilluminates, it should be distinguished from a hydrocele by the color of the fluid on aspiration. Because the lesion is benign and there are usually few symptoms, excision is rarely necessary. Occasionally, the patient is uncomfortable because of the size or heaviness of the cyst. Since excision of the cyst may affect fertility, if the patient desires children, he is usually advised to wear a scrotal support to prevent undue discomfort until after he has a family. Large masses may then be excised.

VARICOCELE

Approximately 15% of men in the United States have a varicocele. Varicocele is a dilation of the spermatic vein and is commonly seen on the left side only, probably because the left spermatic vein is much longer than the right. The venous valves are incompetent, resulting in pooling of blood. One third of men with subfertility or infertility have varicoceles.

Changes in blood flow through the testes is thought to cause a rise in intrascrotal temperature, which interferes with spermatogenesis. The ipsilateral testes may be atrophied. Ligation of the spermatic vein has been shown to improve semen quality with a pregnancy rate of 17% to 62%. Otherwise, unless severe, a scrotal support is usually all that is necessary to relieve any dragging sensation.

PRIAPISM

Priapism is a prolonged, sustained, nonsexual erection than can persist for hours or days. Its cause is unknown, but it is commonly seen in men with sickle cell anemia and leukemia. Men should be referred to an emergency room to have the erection surgically drained to prevent penile damage.

TORSION OF THE TESTES
ETIOLOGY AND PATHOPHYSIOLOGY

Torsion of the testes or kinking of the spermatic artery causes a sudden onset of severe pain, tenderness, and swelling of the testes. The affected testis will be elevated. Vascular obstruction and subsequent testicular infarction as a result of torsion have two peak periods of occurence: the perinatal period and puberty. As the testis becomes larger and heavier, the steadying action and support of the cremasteric muscle decrease and thus predispose the individual to torsion. Torsion often follows activity that puts a sudden pull on the cremasteric muscle such as may occur from jumping into cold water, blunt trauma during sporting events, or riding a bicycle. In severe trauma, rupture of the testis is the expected finding and torsion of the testis is often not considered, leading to misdiagnosis and inappropriate treatment. It may also occur spontaneously. In 40% of the cases, the individual is awakened at night by pain.

CLINICAL MANIFESTATIONS

Torsion interrupts the blood supply leading to ischemia and severe pain that is not relieved and may be aggravated by elevation. Absence of pain indicates infarction and necrosis. Gangrene may be a serious sequela. The patient experiences nausea and vomiting but is afebrile even if the testis is gangrenous. The scrotum may be red and swollen and look infected, but there are no urinary symptoms; that is, both urinalysis and blood tests are normal. An orchiogram, or testicular scan, which is performed in the nuclear medicine department, qualitatively measures the blood flow to the testis, and a Doppler examination differentiates between torsion and acute epididymitis.[30] If an orchiogram cannot be performed, surgical exploration is necessary.

INTERVENTIONS

Detorsion can be attempted manually. If detorsion is unsuccessful, surgical intervention is imperative within 6 to 12 hours to maintain viability of the testis. Even so, the testis may atrophy. Unless the testis is gangrenous, it is not excised, since it may still produce hormones, even if spermatogenesis is destroyed. The testis is fixed surgically to the scrotal wall (orchiopexy). The contralateral testis is usually fixed prophylactically at the same time. A small Penrose drain may be placed in the scrotum. Ice bags to reduce swelling and elevation of the scrotum may be ordered. Observation for signs of testicular necrosis and fever is continued. Body image disturbances may include fears of castration, loss of masculinity, sterility, and impotence. The possibility of these fears being justified depends on the degree of insult to the testis and the functioning of the remaining testicle.

After scrotal surgery, the patient should be instructed to limit stair climbing to two flights and not to lift or carry heavy objects for 4 weeks. He is to refrain from sexual activity for 6 weeks unless otherwise instructed by his physician. The use of a scrotal support for at least 3 weeks is recommended to control edema. Sitz baths may help relieve any discomfort.

NEOPLASMS OF THE MALE REPRODUCTIVE TRACT

CANCER OF THE TESTES
EPIDEMIOLOGY

Cancer of the testes is the second most common malignancy in men between the ages of 25 and 34 and is the second most common cause of death from cancer in this age group. On the whole, testicular neoplasms are relatively rare, affecting only two to three men per 100,000, but the frequency is increasing. Testicular cancer will most often be found in infancy, between 20 and 40 years of age, and over the age of 60. Testicular cancer is more common in white than in black men. If testicular cancer is untreated, death occurs in 2 to 3 years. If it is detected and treated early, there is a 90% to 100% chance of cure.

ETIOLOGY AND PATHOPHYSIOLOGY

The causes of testicular cancer are still unknown. Acquired causes being investigated are chemical carcinogens, trauma, and orchitis. Environmental factors are also being considered, since there is a greater incidence of testicular cancer in rural than in urban areas. Congenital causes implicated are familial predisposition, gonadal dysgenesis (developmental abnormality), and cryptorchidism.

Cryptorchidism is the failure of the testis to descend at birth. Most testes will descend within the first year. The incidence of true cryptorchidism (the undescended testes after 1 year of age) is 0.4%. However, the probability of developing testicular cancer is 30 to 50 times greater than in the normally descended testis. The increased occurrence of undescended testis in whites as compared with blacks matches the increased incidence of testicular cancer in these populations. A predisposing factor may be not the failure to descend but a developmental abnormality in the testis. In utero exposure to hormone preparations, such as to diethylstilbestrol (DES) and oral contraceptives, may also delay testicular descent.

Orchiopexy (a surgical procedure to bring the testis into the scrotum) is being recommended between the ages of 1 and 2 years. Hormonal therapy may also be used to cause the testes to descend. In some cases, descent is spontaneous. The effect of early treatment on the probability of cancer is not known at this time. Although the likelihood of cancer in the testis that descends after the age of 5 or 6 years is comparable to the likelihood of cancer in the testis that has always been outside the scrotum, regular examination of the descended testis does increase the chance of early cancer detection: the site of the testis makes no difference in the risk of developing cancer. Patients with current cryptorchidism or a history of cryptorchidism should be observed yearly; then after a 20-year latency period when testicular cancer is prone to develop, they should be examined every 6 months. Orchiectomy instead of orchiopexy is recommended in adults with cryptorchidism as a prophylaxis against cancer.

PREVENTION

Regular *testicular self-examination* (TSE) is recommended to detect cancer in its early stages when it is most likely to be localized and most curable. The best time to perform TSE is after a bath or shower when the scrotum is warm and most relaxed. Each testis is examined by holding and feeling it between the thumb and fingers of both hands (Figure 56-4). The testis should feel smooth, egg-shaped, and firm to the touch, without any lumps. The epididymis is found behind the testis and feels like a soft tube. The spermatic cord feels like rope. Each side should feel the same, except that the left testicle is lower than the right. By performing TSE routinely, each man can get to know what is normal for him and more readily identify any lumps or abnormali-

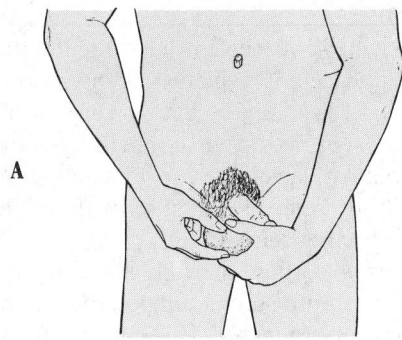

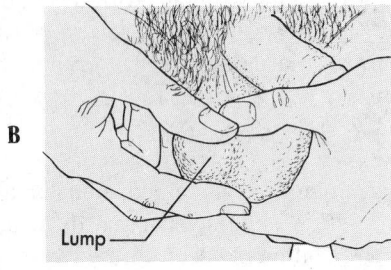

FIGURE 56-4 Testicular self-examination. **A,** Grasp testis with both hands; palpate gently between thumb and fingers. **B,** Abnormal lumps or irregularities are reported to physician. (Adapted from Fred Hutchinson Cancer Research Center, Cancer Control Program: Self breast and testicular exam (grant no. 2 R18-CA 16404), Seattle, 1980, Cancer Control Program).

ties. Anything that is not normal for that individual should be examined by a physician. Nine out of ten testicular cancers are detected by the patient or his sexual partner. Nurses should include knowledge about testicular cancer in assessment of all adolescent and adult male patients and include TSE in patient teaching.

CLINICAL MANIFESTATIONS

Frequently, a lump or swelling of the testis will be noted after bathing or trauma, although trauma is not usually the cause. Other symptoms include a heaviness or dragging sensation in the scrotum, a dull ache in the lower abdomen or inguinal area, and occasionally pain. A small or atrophied testis may grow to normal size. Pride (or embarrassment) may prevent the individual from seeking medical advice.

■ ASSESSMENT

Assessment of men with reproductive system malignancies includes a careful history of sypmtoms related to the diagnosis of a neoplasm such as a lump or pain. In addition to a physical examination focusing on the reproductive organs, diagnostic tests, some of which are specific to the organ involved are used.

■ DATA ANALYSIS: NURSING DIAGNOSES

Nursing diagnoses for a man with a neoplasm of the reproductive system may include, but are not limited to, the following:

Diagnostic Title	Possible Etiologies
Anxiety	Related to cancer diagnosis
Body image disturbance	Changed sexual or reproductive anatomy
Grieving, anticipatory	Loss of significant body part
Sexuality patterns, altered	Progression of disease process, medical or surgical treatment

■ PLANNING: EXPECTED PATIENT OUTCOMES

Expected patient outcomes for a man with neoplasms may include, but are not limited to, the following:

1. Demonstrates understanding of complete plan of care including surgery, radiation therapy and/or chemotherapy, and alternatives
2. Demonstrates understanding of the nature of the diagnossis and prognosis
3. Expresses less anxiety regarding diagnostic tests and therapies
4. Verbalizes losses related to surgery, treatments
5. Participates actively in postoperative care
6. Discusses possibility of changes in sexual patterns
7. Experiences comfort
8. Demonstrates a positive self concept as a man
9. Demonstrates TSE as appropriate
10. Performs TSE as appropriate

Testicular neoplasms are divided into two classifications: germinal and nongerminal. Germinal cancers make up 90% to 95% of all testicular neoplasms and are further divided into two groups: seminomatous (40%) and nonseminomatous (60%) tumors. In addition, tumors with mixed cell types can occur.

The determination of cell type, such as seminomatous versus nonseminomatous is crucial for treatment. Diagnostic workup includes chest x-ray films, computed tomograms, an intravenous pyelogram, skeletal surveys in the presence of an elevated alkaline phosphatase, and lymphangiography. Lymphangiography decreases pulmonary function by 10% because of oil embolism; therefore general anesthesia is contraindicated for 48 hours after the procedure. *Biopsy of the testis is contraindicated* because of the highly metastatic character of testicular carcinoma. Laboratory tests include evaluation of alphafetoprotein (AFP) and beta subunit of human chorionic gonadotropin (beta-HCG), AFP, and HCG are considered *markers* that indicate the presence of nonseminomatous disease, although a small number of men ($\approx$10%) with diagnosed seminoma will also have

elevations in some of these marker hormones. There is no one combination of elevated and normal markers to specifically indicate testicular neoplasm. These are monitored throughout the course of therapy to determine appropriate therapeutic regimens.

INTERVENTIONS

In any suspected testicular cancer, the testis is always removed immediately. *Orchiectomy* consists of en bloc excision of the spermatic cord, the contents of the inguinal canal, and the testis with the tunicae attached. The adjacent area is explored for metastases. The specimens are then examined to determine the cancer cell type (such as seminoma). Staging of the disease (see the box below), as well as pathologic findings, determines the course of treatment.

Seminoma is highly responsive to radiation therapy. For stage I seminoma, irradiation is started to the retroperitoneal nodes. In stage II, irradiation of the mediastinal and supraclavicular nodes is indicated. Chemotherapy is added for stage III. If markers are elevated after irradiation, nonseminomatous involvement must be suspected. Seminoma can metastasize into a different type of cancer. It is possible to develop a second primary lesion in the remaining testis. The prognosis in that case is the same as if it were the first lesion.

Nonseminomatous neoplasms are radioresistant. Therefore retroperitoneal lymphadenectomy or radical node dissection is performed immediately. If the nodes are free of metastases, careful follow-up every 2 months is mandatory. Chemotherapy is given for clinical, radiologic, or tumor marker evidence of metastasis. If the lymph node dissection is positive, the patient has stage II disease. Cyclic combination chemotherapy is started for 2 years with adjuvant surgery. In stage III, intensive cyclic combination chemotherapy is instituted for 10 to 12 months, followed by surgical excision of all metastatic sites. Drugs used in combination therapy include cisplatin, vinblastine, and bleomycin.

After a *radical node dissection*, there is danger of hemorrhage. Active movement may be contraindicated, since nodes may have been resected from around many large abdominal vessels, but gentle passive turning and leg and arm movement are essential to prevent postoperative development of pneumonia and thrombosis.

STAGING OF TESTICULAR NEOPLASIA

Stage I	No metastasis, confined to testis
Stage II	Metastasis to retroperitoneal lymph nodes or other subdiaphragmatic areas
Stage III	Metastasis to mediastinal and supraclavicular nodes or other areas above diaphragm

---

STAGING OF PROSTATIC NEOPLASIA

Stage I	Microscopic lesions found in the prostate removed because of benign hypertrophy	Stage III	Carcinoma involving prostatic capsule, seminal vesicles, urethra, bladder, and pelvic lymph nodes, or a malignant tumor of a lesser extent with an elevated serum acid phosphatase level
Stage II	Nodules confined to the prostate gland; no capsular adherence or urethral involvement; normal serum acid phosphatase level	Stage IV	Findings as in stage III plus evidence of extrapelvic lesions or osseous involvement

Deep breathing should be encouraged at hourly intervals. A turning sheet and a chest support are usually helpful. The patient is extremely uncomfortable and needs frequent and large doses of narcotics and sedative drugs.

Nongerminal testicular tumors are rare. Treatment consists of various combinations of the four modes of treatment (orchiectomy, radiation, lymphadenectomy, and chemotherapy) used in germinal neoplasms, depending on the specific type.

PROGNOSIS

Seminoma has the best prognosis of any of the germinal neoplasms. Five-year survival rates are as follows: for stage I, 95% to 100%; for stage II, 70% to 90%; for stage III, 50% to 70%. For those patients with advanced stage cancer, relapse is higher and thus chemotherapy with radiation will result in a higher percentage of persons with sustained remission.[31] For nonseminomatous neoplasms, 5-year survival rates are as follows: for stage I 90%; for stage II, 60% to 85%; and for stage III, 30% to 40%.

COMPLICATIONS OF TREATMENT

Radiation sickness and adverse reactions to chemotherapeutic agents have been addressed elsewhere (see Chapter 17). Although the normal testis is shielded during external radiation, it does receive radiation scattered from the abdomen and thighs. A period of 70 days is required to determine if spermatogenesis has been affected. Spermatogenesis may be decreased for 7 months to 5 years or more. Although genetic defects are possible after irradiation, there is currently no evidence to cause serious concern. Genetic counseling may be helpful for those couples desiring children. Orchiectomy alone does not result in impotence if the contralateral testis is normal. The remaining testis undergoes hyperplasia, producing sufficient testosterone to maintain sexual function, drive, and characteristics. Retroperitoneal lymphadenectomy results in decreased ejaculation in 90% of the patients as a result of disruption of the sympathetic nervous system pathways. Ejaculation is independent of other sexual functions; orgasm is still possible. The patient's perception of sexuality must be considered, as well as his physiologic capabilities.

CANCER OF THE PROSTATE GLAND
EPIDEMIOLOGY, ETIOLOGY, AND PATHOPHYSIOLOGY

The prostate gland is the second most common site of cancer among men, with 19% of all cancers in men occurring here; it is responsible for 10% of all deaths from cancer in men. Prostatic cancer rarely occurs before the age of 40, incidence increases with age, and there is an increased familial risk. Its incidence has increased by more than 20% since 1940. The increased incidence may reflect greater attention to the need for early diagnosis, improved diagnostic methods, and the fact that men are better informed about cancer than in the past.

Black Americans have the highest incidence of prostatic cancer in the world. Although white men in the United States have a lower incidence as compared to black men, they have a rate higher than men in other parts of the world.[24] There is a geographic distribution of prostatic cancer, so environmental factors may be causative. It may be caused by an oncogenic virus. Industrial exposure to cadmium has also been implicated. Another potential factor in the development of prostate cancer is hormonal stimulation by testosterone.

No classification system for the stages of prostatic cancer has been accepted. However, the information in the box above represents a sampling of classification systems most often used.

Cancer of the prostate may start as a discrete, localized, hard nodule, often in areas of senile atrophy. Although it can start anywhere and may be multifocal in origin, it usually arises in the peripheral lobes causing a palpable nodule before progressing to an advanced, inoperable, and incurable stage. For this reason, there is agreement that all men near and over the age of 40 should have an annual rectal examination.

Overall, 5-year survival rates of those with prostatic cancer are 70% for stages I and II, 61% for stage III, and 20% for stage IV.[1]

CLINICAL MANIFESTATIONS

Cancer of the prostate gland is most often diagnosed when the man seeks medical advice because of symptoms of urethral obstruction or because of sciatica (low back, hip, and leg pain). Urinary symptoms include dysuria, slow stream, urinary retention, dribbling, and hematuria. Pain is caused by metastasis of the cancer to the bones via the blood system. The pelvis, lumbar spine, and femur are the most common sites. This form of cancer frequently occurs concurrently with benign prostatic hypertrophy (Chapter 48). The relationship between the two is controversial. Benign prostatic hypertrophy causes urethral obstruction. However, the cancer itself may be so far advanced as to cause obstruction.

Most prostate gland cancers are adjacent to the rectal wall and can be detected by rectal examination before symptoms appear. Diagnosis is confirmed by histologic examination of a prostate biopsy. The majority of prostate tumors are adenocarcinomas.

Fine needle aspiration of prostate gland "tissue juice" is another technique used to gather a specimen for histologic evaluation. If the transrectal route is used, no bowel preparation is required. Prophylactic antibiotics are used only for high-risk patients. Vital signs should be monitored for possible hemorrhage because of the vascularity of the gland. Bleeding may be from the urethra or the bladder and may be internal. Rotating urine specimens should be used to monitor the amount of hematuria. Bacteremia is usually transient after transrectal biopsy,[24] but the patient should be observed for fever and septicemia. Other complications include acute urinary retention, rectal bleeding, and epididymoorchitis. If the biopsy is done on an outpatient basis, the patient should be informed of possible complications and instructed to notify his physician if any symptoms are persistent or severe.

Other routes for obtaining specimens include open biopsy, transperineal or transrectal biopsy, and transurethral biopsy. Diagnostic tests used to determine the extent of the disease include computerized tomography, lymphangiogram, serum alkaline phosphatase levels, and serum acid phosphatase levels.

INTERVENTIONS

In patients in whom a diagnosis is made before local extension of the cancer or distant metastasis, a radical resection of the prostate gland usually is curative. The entire prostate gland, including the capsule and the adjacent tissue, is removed. The remaining urethra is then anastomosed to the bladder neck.

Since the internal and external sphincters of the bladder lie in close approximation to the prostate gland, it is not unusual for the patient to have urinary incontinence after this type of surgery. The perineal approach is most used, but the procedure may be accomplished by the retropubic route.

Preoperative Care

If the patient is to have a perineal approach in surgery, he is given a bowel preparation, which includes enemas, cathartics, and phthalylsulfathiazole (Sulfathalidine) or neomycin preoperatively and only clear fluids the day before surgery to prevent fecal contamination of the operative site. Postoperatively, when food is permitted, a low-residue diet may be given until wound healing is well advanced. Camphorated tincture of opium may be prescribed to inhibit bowel action. If the retropubic approach is used, the preoperative care is similar to that of any patient having major surgery.

Postoperative Care

Regardless of the surgical approach, the patient returns from surgery with a urethral catheter inserted. A large amount of urinary drainage on the dressing for a number of hours is not unusual. This can be managed by use of an ostomy bag around the dressing. Urinary drainage should decrease rapidly, however. There should not be the amount of bleeding that follows other prostatic surgery. Since the catheter is not being used for hemostasis, the patient usually has little bladder spasm. The catheter is used both for urinary drainage and as a splint for the urethral anastomosis; therefore care should be taken that it does not become dislodged or blocked. Clinically, the risk of blockage from clots is greatest during the first hour. The catheter may be irrigated intermittently or continuously as ordered by the physician. The catheter is usually left in the bladder for 2 or 3 weeks.

The care of the perineal wound is the same as that after a perineal biopsy, except that healing is usually slower. If there has been a retropubic surgical approach, the wound and possible wound complications are the same as for a simple retropubic prostatectomy.

Since perineal surgery causes relaxation of the perineal musculature, the patient may suddenly have fecal incontinence. It is disturbing to the patient and sometimes can be avoided by starting perineal exercises (Chapter 49) within a day or two after surgery. Control of the rectal sphincter usually returns readily. Perineal exercises should be continued even after rectal sphincter control returns, since they also strengthen the bladder sphincters and, unless the bladder sphincters have been permanently damaged, the patient will retain urinary control more readily on removal of the catheter.

The patient with cancer of the prostate gland is often very depressed after radical prostatectomy, because he suddenly realizes the implications of being impotent and perhaps permanently incontinent (see research box on p. 1652). He usually has been told by the physician before the operation that these consequences are possible, but he may not have fully comprehended their meaning. A penile prosthesis may be considered to treat

RESEARCH

Scott D, Oberst M, and Bookbinder M: Stress-coping response to genitourinary carcinoma in men, Nurs Res 33(6):325-329, 1984.

Thirty men with chronic genitourinary cancer had minimal emotional distress in response to a periodic diagnostic procedure (cystoscopy). For men with negative biopsy results, stated anxiety levels and critical thinking ability before the procedure were not significantly different from the levels obtained 6 to 8 weeks after the procedure. Indeed, routine hospitalization for diagnostic monitoring was found to be less stressful than regular work or financial and family concerns. Men with higher current life stress had higher stated anxiety and had less resolution of their problems; 33% of the men had high anxiety on at least one testing occasion, and these men had more severe behavioral responses such as feelings of depression and helplessness and difficulty setting priorities. ■

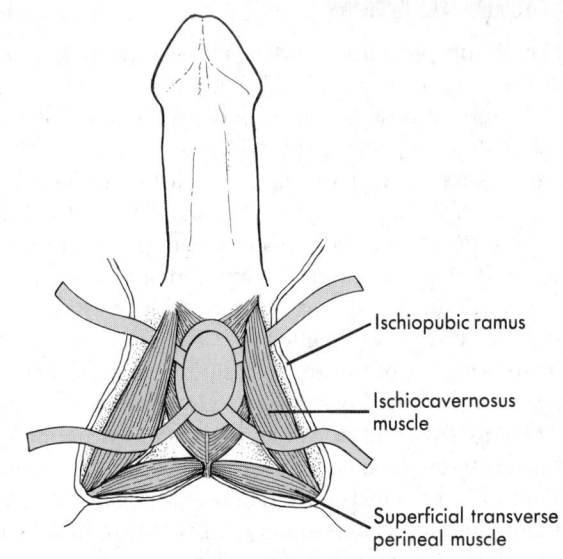

FIGURE 56-5 Placement of silicone gel prostatic prosthesis. Tapes are stapled to pubic rami or sutured to periosteum. (Adapted from Kauffman JJ: Urol Clin North Am 5:395, 1978.)

the impotence (erectile dysfunction) (Chapter 52). He needs to be encouraged, and provisions should be made to keep him dry so that he will feel able to be up and to socialize with others without fear of having obvious incontinence (see Chapter 49 for ways to manage incontinence). Until the physician has ascertained that return of urinary sphincter control is unlikely, a method that gives only partial protection, such as the use of a bathing cap, is preferable since the patient is more likely to attempt to regain voluntary control.

Prostatic Prosthesis

If voluntary urinary control has not been regained within 6 months to a year, a prostatic prosthesis is available to control urinary incontinence. This puts pressure on the urethra, and, if the pressure is too great, urethral erosion can occur. This will interfere with other forms of incontinence control such as artificial sphincters. Therefore intraurethral pressure is measured during surgery. The prosthesis consists of a silicone gel-filled sac placed at the base of the penis. Four tapes of polypropylene mesh are stapled to the pelvic rami or sutured to the periosteum to secure the prosthesis in place (Figure 56-5). If the pressure decreases within the prosthesis, injections may be used to increase it. There is a 60% success rate. Although it is better for the prosthesis to be applied loosely rather than too tight, if it is too loose it will fail. It may be repositioned surgically.

Because of their suppressed immune response, patients who have undergone radiation therapy have a greater risk of osteomyelitis, as well as wound complications; therefore they are not candidates for prostatic prosthesis. The prerequisite for surgery is a sterile urine culture. Preoperative antibiotics are given prophylactically and continued for 7 days postoperatively. An indwelling catheter is inserted during surgery and left for 48 hours. If difficulty with voiding persists, the patient can be discharged with the indwelling catheter or taught intermittent self-catheterization (Chapter 49). Residual urine of 50 to 100 ml may persist for a few weeks. A urinary antiseptic is given after the initial course of antibiotics and continued until the patient is voiding well.

Radiation Therapy

Irradiation is an alternate therapy for prostatic cancer. It may be delivered by external beam or by implant. The testes are shielded during external radiation. Iodine retropubic prostatic implantation may be used initially or after failure of external radiation therapy. The mortality and morbidity of internal irradiation when coupled with lymphadenectomy are less than for radical prostatectomy. Complications of ^{125}I implantation include blood loss from multiple needle punctures during implantation, deep vein thrombosis, pulmonary emboli, hematomas, and abscesses. Potency is retained. There is a greater risk of complications if radioactive implants are used after external beam radiation.[8] Irritability of the bladder caused by radioactive implants can produce urinary symptoms.

Hormone Therapy

When cancer of the prostate gland is inoperable, or when signs of metastasis occur after surgery, medical treatment is given. Relief from conservative treatment is quite dramatic in many patients and may last for 10 years or more in some instances. Usually, the response is quite good for about 1 year and then the patient's condition begins to deteriorate. Prostatic cancer has a slow growth rate; cytotoxic drugs are not indicated in prostatic cancer, because they are most effective against rapidly proliferating cells. Also, the elderly tolerate the side effects of these drugs poorly.

Huggins' treatment may be used for inoperable cancer of the prostate gland to cause atrophy of the local lesion, control metastases, and relieve pain. It is based on the elimination of androgens by removal of the testes or the administration of estrogenic hormones or both. The estrogen given is usually stilbestrol, 3 mg/day for 1 to 2 weeks. The dosage is then reduced to 1.5 to 3 mg/day. This measure frequently will relieve the pain. Stilbestrol causes engorgement and tenderness of the male breasts (gynecomastia). It may also cause nausea. Severe side effects should be reported to the physician so that the dosage or type of estrogenic preparation can be adjusted.

Estrogen preparations also result in fluid retention and dependent edema, which may be controlled with salt restriction and diuretics. Other problems include cardiovascular complications and increased blood coagulation. If a large tumor does not diminish in size with this treatment, some of the prostate gland may be resected to relieve obstruction. This procedure is most often done transurethrally (Chapter 48). The use of hormone therapy provides a longer symptom-free period but makes palliation more difficult when symptoms recur. If endocrine therapy is delayed, symptoms recur earlier, but longer palliation is possible.

When symptoms begin to recur, or if the patient is very uncomfortable and needs immediate relief when the diagnosis of cancer is first made, a bilateral orchiectomy (castration) may be performed. This operative procedure is technically minor and is often done under local anesthesia, but it may cause the patient considerable psychologic distress. The man's permission for sterilization must be obtained. If he is married, he is usually urged to discuss the operation with his wife. This surgery eliminates the testicular source of male hormones and seems to cause regression or at least slow the cancer growth. Very seldom, a hypophysectomy may be performed to further reduce hormonal stimulation.

SEXUAL DYSFUNCTION

As stated briefly above, sexual dysfunction can be an adverse effect of prostatic surgery. After transurethral resection of the prostate (TURP), erectile incompetence is usually the result of psychologic factors. Retrograde ejaculation is common after TURP. If the patient equates ejaculation with sexual competence, the de-

creased or absent fluid emission may be interpreted as impotence with concomitant dysfunction.

Total prostatectomy, which includes bilateral pelvic lymphadenectomy, results in physiologic sexual dysfunction as a result of disruption of genital innervation. Ninety percent of patients lose emission, ejaculation, and erectile potency. Ten percent do have satisfactory erections, possibly because some nerves escaped damage during surgery.

External radiation therapy causes erectile dysfunction more than does lymphadenectomy. Erectile impotence is not an automatic consequence of castration, since adult levels of testosterone are not required to maintain an erection. Erectile dysfunction during cytotoxic chemotherapy is felt to be caused more by the general ill health of the individual than by specific effects on sexual physiology. A test for nocturnal penile tumescence may be performed to help distinguish between psychologically and organically based erectile dysfunction. A penile implant (Chapter 52) might be a viable option.

Any time a procedure may result in loss of sexual function, the partner should be consulted. Recent court decisions have awarded compensation to wives who have lost conjugal relationships with their husbands as a result of medical therapy. In some cases, the partner is asked to sign a consent form for procedures that may result in sterility or impotence.[29]

CANCER OF THE PENIS
EPIDEMIOLOGY AND ETIOLOGY

In America, penile cancer accounts for 0.5% to 1.5% of all male malignancies. It is most common between the ages of 50 and 70, but it can occur in younger men and has been reported in children. There is a higher incidence in blacks than whites, possibly because of a lower incidence of circumcision. Penile cancer accounts for 10% to 20% of all male malignancies among African and Asian peoples.

The incidence of penile cancer is highly dependent on hygienic standards, as well as cultural and religious practices. It almost never occurs in a male who was circumcised at birth. Circumcision after puberty does not decrease the risk of cancer when compared with the incidence among uncircumcised males. Circumcision removes the prepuce, or foreskin, which provides a haven for bacteria. The bacteria act on desquamated cells producing smegma, which is irritating to the tissue of the glans penis and the prepuce. This chronic irritation is considered to be carcinogenic. Therefore adequate hygiene theoretically is sufficient prophylaxis against penile cancer, making circumcision unnecessary. In clinical practice this has not been substantiated and requires further study. Trauma and sexually transmitted diseases are felt to be coincidental to penile cancer rather

STAGES OF PENILE CANCER

Stage A   Lesions confined to glans or foreskin
Stage B   Shaft or corpora cavernosa invaded by tumors
Stage C   Shaft involvement; lymph nodes involved but operable
Stage D   Shaft involvement; lymph nodes inoperable; metastases to distant sites

than causative. The box above shows the stages of penile cancer.

PATHOPHYSIOLOGY

Penile cancer starts as a small lesion usually on or under the prepuce and extends until the entire glans and shaft are involved. It becomes autoamputative. If penile cancer is left untreated, death occurs in 2 to 3 years. The lesion may be papillary and exophytic (flowery). It may be a small bump or resemble a pimple or wart. It may also occur as a nonhealing ulcer with the edges rolled inward. The latter is associated with earlier metastases and a poorer 5-year survival.

The most common (95%) type of malignancy is squamous cell carcinoma. Phimosis (p. 1645), which occurs in 25% to 75% of penile cancer cases, may obscure the lesion. The lesion may then cause erosion through the prepuce with a foul odor and discharge. Bleeding may or may not be present. Urethral and bladder involvement is rare.

CLINICAL MANIFESTATIONS

Presenting complaints include weakness, fatigue, malaise, and weight loss. Men may complain of itching and burning under the prepuce and an occasional foul discharge. A delay of 1 year before seeking treatment is common in 15% to 50% of the cases. Biopsy is performed to establish the diagnosis; however, benign penile lesions are uncommon.

This delay in seeking health care may be related to denial or fear of a diagnosis of a sexually transmitted disease. Results of laboratory tests will indicate prolonged illness and chronic infection. Metastasis usually occurs at the regional femoral and iliac nodes and is associated with a significantly worse prognosis. Five-year survival with inguinal node involvement is 20% to 25%. If radiation therapy is instituted, the survival rate may approach 50%.

INTERVENTIONS

Treatment is usually surgical. Irradiation as the initial mode of treatment is indicated only in younger patients in whom sexual function is important and who have small superficial lesions.

If the lesion is confined to the prepuce, circumcision may be adequate. If the lesion is on the glans, partial penectomy or amputation of the penis is required. If the shaft of the penis is involved, total amputation may be necessary. The decision is based on the amount of penis remaining after excision with an adequate tumor-free margin. The remaining penis must be long enough for the patient to void standing, direct the stream, and not void on himself. If this is possible, the sexual function will probably be retained. If total amputation is required, a perineal urethrostomy is performed in which the urethra is redirected to an opening between the scrotum and the anus. With spread of the cancer to the scrotal contents, radical removal is required, either hemipelvectomy or hemicorporectomy.

Approximately one third of men with penile cancer have metastic nodal disease at the time of the initial diagnosis.[16] Radiation therapy is used as adjuvant therapy at all stages. Aside from common adverse reactions to irradiation, specific genitourinary reactions include penile necrosis (10%) and urethral strictures (30%).

Lymphadenectomy is indicated for lymph node involvement. Accurate detection of metastases is difficult, since enlarged lymph nodes may be free of cancerous tissue, whereas normal-sized lymph nodes may contain metastatic lesions. Either may contain undetectable lesions. Lymphedema of the lower extremities may be a debilitating complication of lymphadenectomy.

Chemotherapeutic agents have been used with some success, particularly in patients with stages A and B disease. Agents that have been used include high dose methotrexate, bleomycin, and cisplatin. Because of the rarity of the disease, large scale clinical studies to evaluate chemotherapeutic agents are lacking. Methotrexate given intravenously has been somewhat successful. Other chemotherapeutic agents have not been effective. If the disease is confined to the penis, 5-year survival is 80% to 85% with amputation. With metastasis to the lymph nodes, it is only 20%.

Sexual counseling is indicated for the patient with a total penectomy. Some patients with a urethrostomy have experienced orgasm and ejaculation after stimulation of the perineal, scrotal, and testicular regions.

CHAPTER SUMMARY

✔ The most common genital inflammations experienced by men are urethritis, prostatis, epididymitis, and orchitis. Bilateral epididymitis often causes sterility.

✔ Common structural disorders in men are hydrocele, spermatocele, varicocele, or torsion of the spermatic cord.

✔ Most genital cancers in men are prostatis cancers, occurring primarily in men over 60 years of age.

Young men have a higher incidence of cancer of the testes, which can be detected early by testicular self-examination (TSE).

QUESTIONS TO CONSIDER

- What factors predispose men to infections of the reproductive system? What can men do to decrease their risk of reproductive tract infection?

- What areas should nurses cover in explaining the consequences of structural changes in the reproductive system to men?

- How would the sexuality of a 35-year-old with penile cancer be affected? What sexual options exist for him?

- How would you recommend teaching testicular self-examination to adolescent men?

- What elements of nursing care are essential for men experiencing a prostatectomy?

REFERENCES AND SELECTED READINGS

1. American Cancer Society: 1989 cancer facts and figures, New York, 1989, The Society.
2. American Cancer Society: Report on the cancer-related health check-up, New York, 1980, The Society.
3. American Cancer Society: Cancer facts and figures for minority Americans, New York, 1983, Springer Publishing Co.
4. Babaryan R: When to refer: evaluation of scrotal masses, Hosp Pract 20(3)51-53, 1985.
5. Bozett F and Forrester D: A proposal for a men's health nurse practitioner, J Nurs Schol 21(3):158-161, 1989.
6. *Confer DJ and Beall ME: Evolved improvements in placement of the silicone gel prosthesis for post-prostatectomy incontinence, J Urol 126:605-608, 1981.
7. Crawford E: Diagnosis and treatment of prostatitis, Hosp Pract 20(9):77-80, 1985.
8. Cumes DM et al: Complications of ^{125}iodine implantation and pelvic lymphadenectomy for prostatic cancer with special reference to patients who had failed external beam therapy as their initial mode of therapy, J Urol 126:620-622, 1981.
9. Dosoretz DE et al: Megavoltage irradiation for pure testicular seminoma: results and patterns of failure, Cancer 48:2184-2190, 1981.
10. Ekman EP and Edsmyr F: Chemotherapy in nonseminomatous testicular tumors, stage I, Br J Urol 53:184-187, 1981.
11. Fowler J: Urinary tract infection and inflammation, Chicago, 1989, Year Book Medical Publishers, Inc.
12. Fred Hutchinson Cancer Research Center, Cancer Control Program: Self breast and testicular exam (grant no. 2 R18 CA 16404), Seattle, 1980, Cancer Control Program.
13. Fry R: Anorectal disorders, Clin Symp 37(6):2-32, 1985.
14. Galt P: Taking your part in the fight against testicular cancer, Nursing '81 11(5)45-50, 1981.
15. Glassburn J: Iodine 125 implantation for carcinoma of the prostate, Appl Radiol 14(3):49-52, 1985.
16. Grabstald H: Controversies concerning lymph node resection for cancer of the penis, Urol Clin North Am 7:793-799, 1980.
17. Kauffman JJ, editor: Current urologic therapy, ed 2, Philadelphia, 1980, WB Saunders Co.
18. Kursh ED: Traumatic torsion of testicle, Urology 1981 17:441-442, 1981.
19. Langemo D: Peyronie's disease, AUAA J 5(3):4-6, 1985.
20. Lawler P: Benign prostatic hyperplasia: knowing pathophysiology aids assessment, AORN J 40(5):745-8, 750, 1984.
21. Managing the patient with testicular cancer: nursing grand rounds, Nursing '86 16(8)42-45, 1985.
22. Martin DC: Testis (editorial), J Urol 124:388, 1980.
23. Payton T and Beilman AA: Caring for the urologic surgery patient. In West RS, Waring KS, and Lawson PK: Implementing urologic procedures, Horsham, Pa, 1981, Nursing '81 Books, Intermed Communications, Inc.
24. Ross R, Paganini-Hill A, and Henderson B: Epidemiology of prostatic cancer in diagnosis and management of genitourinary cancer, Philadelphia, 1988, WB Saunders Co.
25. Rothman CM, Newmark H, and Karson RA: The recurrent varicocele: a poorly recognized problem, Fertil Steril 35:552-556, 1981.
26. Scrinivas V et al: Penile carcinoma, Hosp Pract 20(1):154-5, 158-9, 1985.
27. Swanson J and Forrest K: Men's reproductive health, New York, 1984, Springer Publishing Co.
28. Tsuang MT, Weiss MA, and Evans AT: Transurethral resection of the prostate with partial resection of the seminal vesicle, J Urol 126:615-617, 1981.
29. Von Eschenbach AC and Rodriguez DB: Sexual rehabilitation of the urologic cancer patient, Boston, 1981, GK Hall & Co.
30. Vordermark JS et al: The testicular scan: use in diagnosis and management of acute epididymitis, JAMA 245:2512-2514, 1981.
31. Wheeler JE: Testicular tumors. In Hill GS: Uropathology, 1989, Churchill Livingstone Inc.

*References preceded by an asterisk are particularly well suited for student reading.

CHAPTER 57

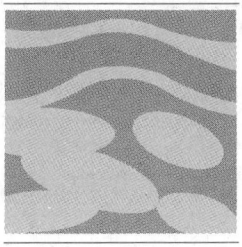

Management of Persons with Problems of the Breast

CAROL SUN REDFIELD
DORIS M. MOLBO

CHAPTER OBJECTIVES

After studying this chapter, the student should be able to:
1 Analyze clients' risk factor profile for developing breast cancer.
2 Develop a teaching plan to facilitate breast self-examination for the purpose of promoting breast health.
3 Explain early detection approaches to and diagnostic tests for breast evaluation.
4 Explain to clients the most frequently used approaches to treatment of breast cancer, including surgery, chemotherapy, and radiation therapy.
5 Develop a plan for caring for women who are receiving chemotherapy for breast cancer.
6 Develop a plan for caring for women who are receiving radiation therapy for breast cancer.
7 Develop a plan for caring for women who have a mastectomy, including the preoperative, postoperative, and rehabilitative phases of their experiences.
8 Explain to clients the differences between breast cancer and benign breast conditions.

The breasts are associated functionally with the reproductive system as an organ for milk production in the postpartum woman. The female sex hormones influence the development of the breasts and the production of milk (and the specific hormone prolactin). The breasts are also associated with feelings of sexuality and are an integral component of sexual behavior. The development of the breasts in the female adolescent indicates to her the approach of womanhood and emphasizes her femininity. The breasts, especially the nipples, which are erectile tissue, are erogenous areas in sexual activity. The advertising media emphasize the desirability of the female breast; femininity is typified by a fashion model's curved breasts, whereas masculinity is typified by a lifeguard's flat, expansive chest. Diseases of the breast therefore evoke varied feelings and cause fears and concerns that influence the practice of breast self-examination or the seeking of diagnostic and therapeutic care without delay.

The most common problems of the breast are dysplasia (fibrocystic condition), cancer, fibroadenoma, mammary duct ectasia, and infections. Although these conditions occur primarily in women, they can also occur in men. Cancer requires the most extensive nursing care and is discussed here in greater detail than the other diseases.

MALIGNANCIES OF THE BREAST

Nurses play a vital role in regard to cancer of the breast. Their responsibilities include (1) educating women so that cancer may be discovered and treated early, (2) caring for the patient receiving primary (first-line) therapy and possibly adjuvant (additional) therapy for the cancer, (3) assisting the patient with physical and emotional rehabilitation, and (4) caring for and assisting the patient when metastasis has occurred and second-line therapy or palliative therapy is needed.

Currently, major changes are being made in the modes of treatment and rehabilitation for the person with breast cancer. Nurses therefore have two additional important responsibilities:

1. Nurses must feel a real commitment to read and to keep current with the imminent controversies and actual changes taking place in the whole field of breast cancer so that the implications for women are understood.
2. Nurses are expected to be able to explain to the woman the many options she has heard about, differing detection methods, primary therapies, options for reconstructive surgery, and other rehabilitative resources.

This often also means assisting the woman to discuss most effectively these issues with her physician and to be able to ask those necessary questions so that wise choices for her future are made. Women today read current, accurate information about breast cancer in magazines and other publications. Nurses cannot be less informed. Since breast cancer is not one disease, the nurse can also assist a woman to accept the physician's professional advice that, considering her disease, all options may not be appropriate or adequate for her.

EPIDEMIOLOGY

The cancers of the breast are the most common malignancies in women, the second leading cause of cancer deaths in women, and the leading cause of death in women from ages 15 to 55 years. It is estimated that one of 10 women in the United States will develop cancer of the breast, and the probability increases with age. The chance of a 70-year-old woman developing breast cancer is six times greater than that of a 40-year-old woman. The American Cancer Society estimates that 150,900 new cases will be discovered in the United States during 1989 and that 44,000 women will die from the disease.[1] The incidence of breast cancer is increasing in almost all the populations considered, on the average approximately 2% each year. In one study the incidence rose impressively from an average annual rate of 53:100,000 population for 1935 to 1937 to 86.4: 100,000 for 1975 to 1979. Two thirds of all patients are over the age of 50 years.[27]

The mortality from breast cancer in the United States has remained about the same for the past 40 years. The present 5-year survival rate for all patients with breast cancer, whether treated or untreated, is approximately 65%.[3] This low survival rate is caused in part by the frequent failure to detect the early lesion and the delay in seeking medical treatment as soon as a lesion is discovered. Studies show that approximately 90% of all women treated when the lesion appears localized have a 5-year life expectancy, compared with 60% for those with obvious regional involvement at the time of treatment. As with any malignancy, however, survival at the end of 5 years cannot be considered synonymous with cure. Slightly fewer black than white women develop breast cancer. However, black women who develop this disease have a 5-year relative survival rate of 62%, compared to 75% for nonminority women. Low socioeconomic status and diagnosis at a later stage of disease have attributed to the lower survival rates for black women.[59] The average size of a breast tumor at diagnosis in black women is 5.5 cm. Tumors that are 1 cm or smaller are present at diagnosis in 21% of white women; only 8.3% of black women have such minimal-sized lesion.[35,42]

Breast cancer occurs in both premenopausal and postmenopausal women; peak incidence occurs between ages 45 and 49 and at age 65. It must be stressed, however, that when the comparison is made between the number of diagnosed breast cancer patients of a certain age and the total number of women in the population of that age, the resulting ratio will show

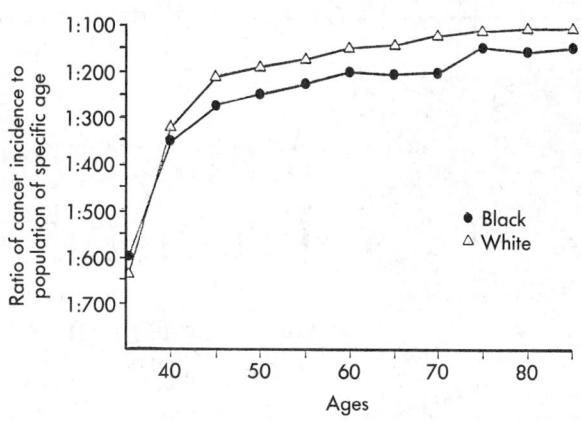

FIGURE 57-1 Ratio of breast cancer incidence to age-specific populations by 5-year cohorts. (Based on National Cancer institute data, 1986; from Carnevali D and Patrick M: Nursing management for the elderly, ed 2, Philadelphia, 1986, JB Lippincott Co.)

a steady rise in incidence as age increases (for example, one of every 420 women aged 45 years has breast cancer; one of every 110 women aged 70 years has breast cancer[38] (Figure 57-1). In addition, breast cancer is not one disease but many, depending on the tissue of the breast involved, its estrogen dependency, and the age at onset. Premenopausal breast malignancy is different from postmenopausal malignancy. Treatment response and prognosis differ with all malignancies.

Causes of breast cancer are not known but appear to include several factors rather than just one. High-risk factors are those that increase the possibility that breast cancer will occur. Whites have a slightly higher incidence of breast cancer than blacks, especially postmenopausal disease. Women with a family history and personal history of breast cancer have a higher risk. Obesity and alcohol consumption also appear to increase risk.[1] The person exposed to ionizing radiation with doses of 10 to 10,000 rad also appears to have an increased risk of breast cancer. When breast cancer occurs in the male, it is usually seen a decade later than in females, at an average age of about 60 years.[32]

Breast-feeding or injury to the breast does not influence the incidence of breast cancer. Frequently a neoplasm is discovered after a minor injury was already present, but the woman had not previously examined herself. However, a palpable hematoma could be caused by trauma.

Controversy still exists as to whether noncontraceptive preparations of estrogen increase the risk of breast cancer in postmenopausal women. Although some studies indicate no risk, other data are accumulating indicating that long-term treatment with preparations of estrogen for menopausal symptoms increases the risk of breast cancer. Among women with intact ovaries who were treated with a total estrogen accumulation in excess of 1500 mg, the risk is 2.5 times the risk of women not treated.[17]

Recently, some epidemiologic have suggested an increased risk of breast cancer in premenopausal women using oral contraceptives at an early age.[10,41,46] After reviewing these studies, the Fertility and Maternal Health Drugs Advisory Committee of the Food and Drug Administration (FDA) concluded no relationship exists between oral contraceptives and breast cancer.[2] However, further or continued epidemiologic studies are recommended.

PROGNOSIS

Favorable prognosis in cancer of the breast depends on early diagnosis, the type of cancer present, host factors, and complete therapeutic destruction or removal of all tissues containing malignant cells before metastasis occurs.

National statistics show breast cancer is discovered at a later stage with regional or distant spread in more than 50% of patients at initial diagnosis.[51] This is particularly true of black women; stage II disease is present at the time of diagnosis in 32% and stage III in 29% of these women.[35] Breast malignancy in men is often found and diagnosed at a later stage. Since the disease develops in a relatively accessible part of the body, it is unfortunate that early diagnosis is not made more often so that more lives might be saved.

At present, the American Cancer Society acknowledges several primary therapies, depending on the individual's preferences and medical situation—surgery of varying extent, radiation therapy, chemotherapy, or hormone manipulation. Often two or more methods may be used in combination.

PREVENTION AND EARLY DETECTION

Although measures to prevent breast cancer are not known, mortality from breast cancer can be prevented in many instances through early diagnosis and treatment. All women should have a complete medical examination that includes thorough palpation of the breasts at least once a year, and women over 30 years of age with a familial history of breast cancer should have an examination at least twice a year. A Gallup survey conducted for the American Cancer Society in late 1977 indicated that about 75% of the female population does have an annual breast examination by a physician. However, it was reported at the International Conference on Cancer in Black Populations that only 10% of black women have regular breast examinations by a physician.[42] The lack of examination is more prevalent among older women, poorly educated women, low-income women, and black women. For those in low-income levels, health-seeking services are on a crisis pri-

RESEARCH

Champion V: Use of the health belief model in determining frequency of breast self-examination, Res Nurs Health **8**:373-379, 1985.

Three hundred and one women responded to questionnaires about their perceived susceptibility and seriousness of breast cancer and the benefits and barriers related to breast self-examination (BSE), as well as general health motivation. Results indicated that benefits (BSE), barriers, and health motivation were important influences on the frequency of BSE. Those women who examined their breasts most frequently perceived fewer barriers, were motivated toward maintaining health, and perceived more benefits from BSE. ◼

ority. The elderly also refrain from annual checkups in the absence of symptoms. Further, the message to black women and to white and black elderly women has been inadequately delivered. Neither blacks nor the elderly population are aware of the rising incidence of breast cancer in their populations and the need for vigilance by each woman personally and by her health provider. The most accessible tool to detect early breast lesions is breast self-examination (BSE) (see box above).

Although 90% of all breast cancers are discovered by self-examination, many are not reported for several months. Fear of mutilation or of death are the two main reasons why some women delay seeking medical advice and treatment and hesitate to risk confirmation of their fears when a tumor is discovered. Publicized national statistics on death from breast cancer and knowing a relative or a friend who died from the disease increase the fear. Unfortunately, the average woman may tell only her closest friends when a breast cancer has been successfully treated. As a result, deaths from the disease are much better known than cures with no recurrence. A National Cancer Institute study has found that black women fear breast cancer more than any other disease and that both black and Hispanic women were more concerned about the changes in their lives that breast cancer would cause than were the white women studied.[42] Some women wish to avoid the expense or embarrassment of an examination, or they rationalize that their trouble would appear trivial to the busy physician. Therefore they sometimes seek the advice of nurses instead.

It then becomes the nurse's responsibility to stress the urgency of receiving medical advice at once. The publicized mastectomies of prominent women in recent years and their continued activity in life has encouraged other women to obtain breast examinations.

In an attempt to improve and assess the relative effectiveness of early detection of breast cancer, the National Cancer Institute and the American Cancer Society in 1973 jointly funded 27 screening centers in the United States to provide free diagnostic services to a population of presumed asymptomatic women. The objective of the program was to evaluate the ability of mammography, thermography, and palpation to find early breast cancers. A decision was made in 1977 to continue the nationwide screening project despite the controversy over the use of roentgenographic examinations used in the screening process. During the first 3 years of the project, the screening centers detected 1800 breast cancers in 280,000 women examined. The program did demonstrate that screening for early breast cancer is feasible and valuable.[5]

BREAST SELF-EXAMINATION

All women, beginning at high-school age, should know how to carry out BSE and should practice this monthly as a health habit. The 1973 Gallup survey reported that only 18% of the 1000 women sampled carried out monthly breast examinations. Other studies have also substantiated a low percentage of women who practice regularly.[6,30,52] This is attributed to lack of knowledge of the importance of and the method for doing BSE and fears concerning possible findings.[19] Other studies in compliance have revealed that, despite being taught BSE, women state they do not know what they are feeling.[6,30,52]

In response to the finding that women are confused by the lumpiness of their breasts, or that they cannot know whether they have a pathologic lump each month or not, a new teaching approach to BSE was begun in 1976. Called the Breast Health Program and initiated in Seattle and Washington state, it emphasizes a positive health approach and individually teaches each woman to distinguish her own healthy breast tissues from month to month. If she feels something that she knows is not her normal tissue, she confidently contacts her physician. A high rate of monthly BSE compliance (81%) had been achieved with this program. (Specific details may be obtained.*) Efforts are still being made to disseminate this approach of BSE, as seen in a local Seattle television station's 1988-1989 campaign to distribute their videotape "Getting in Touch with Yourself" to the public at low cost. This program has been very successful in its outreach and was given a National Emmy Award in 1989.[33]

Nurses working in the hospital or community settings have the responsibility of teaching women how to examine their breasts and of explaining why it is necessary. When working with groups of women, arrange-

ments can be made with the American Cancer Society or the local health department for showing movies developed for the general public describing the traditional method of self-examination. Specialized volunteers from the American Cancer Society, nurses, and other health care providers have been trained and certified in the traditional teaching of BSE to the public. The nurse follows through by teaching the women the actual BSE and by answering questions. The woman then practices palpation of the various breast tissue on herself or on models of the breast.

BSE should be done regularly each month. The best time is at the conclusion of or a few days following the menstrual period. Some women have engorgement of the breast premenstrually, and the breasts normally may have a lumpy consistency at this time. This condition usually disappears a few days after the onset of menstruation. Because of this possible change, it is important that the breasts be examined at the same time each month in relation to the menstrual cycle. Women who have passed menopause should examine their breasts at a set time each month.

Several approaches can be followed when carrying out BSE. All approaches follow these general guidelines: (1) the approach used is systematic; (2) the entire breast tissue is examined, including the tail (Figure 57-2) and the nipple; (3) examination is carried out in both

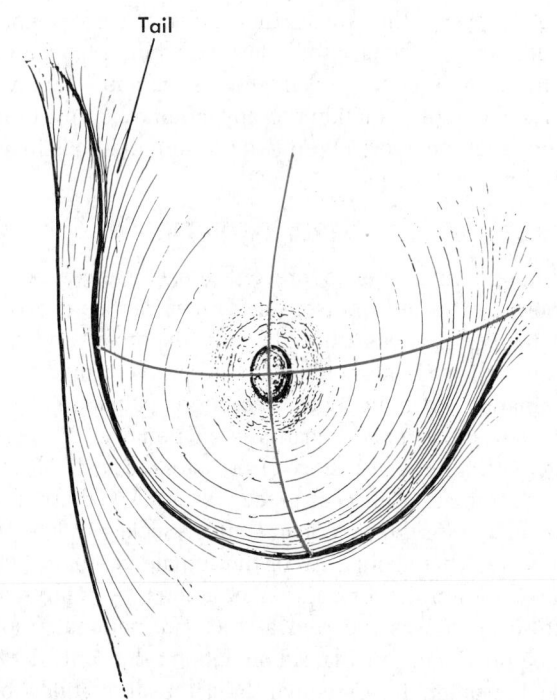

FIGURE 57-2 Breast mass includes "tail" that extends from upper, outer quadrant toward axilla. (From Malasanos L et al: Health assessment, ed 2, St Louis, 1981, The CV Mosby Co.)

*Doris Malbo, Breast Health Program, SM-28 School of Nursing, University of Washington, Seattle, WA 98195.

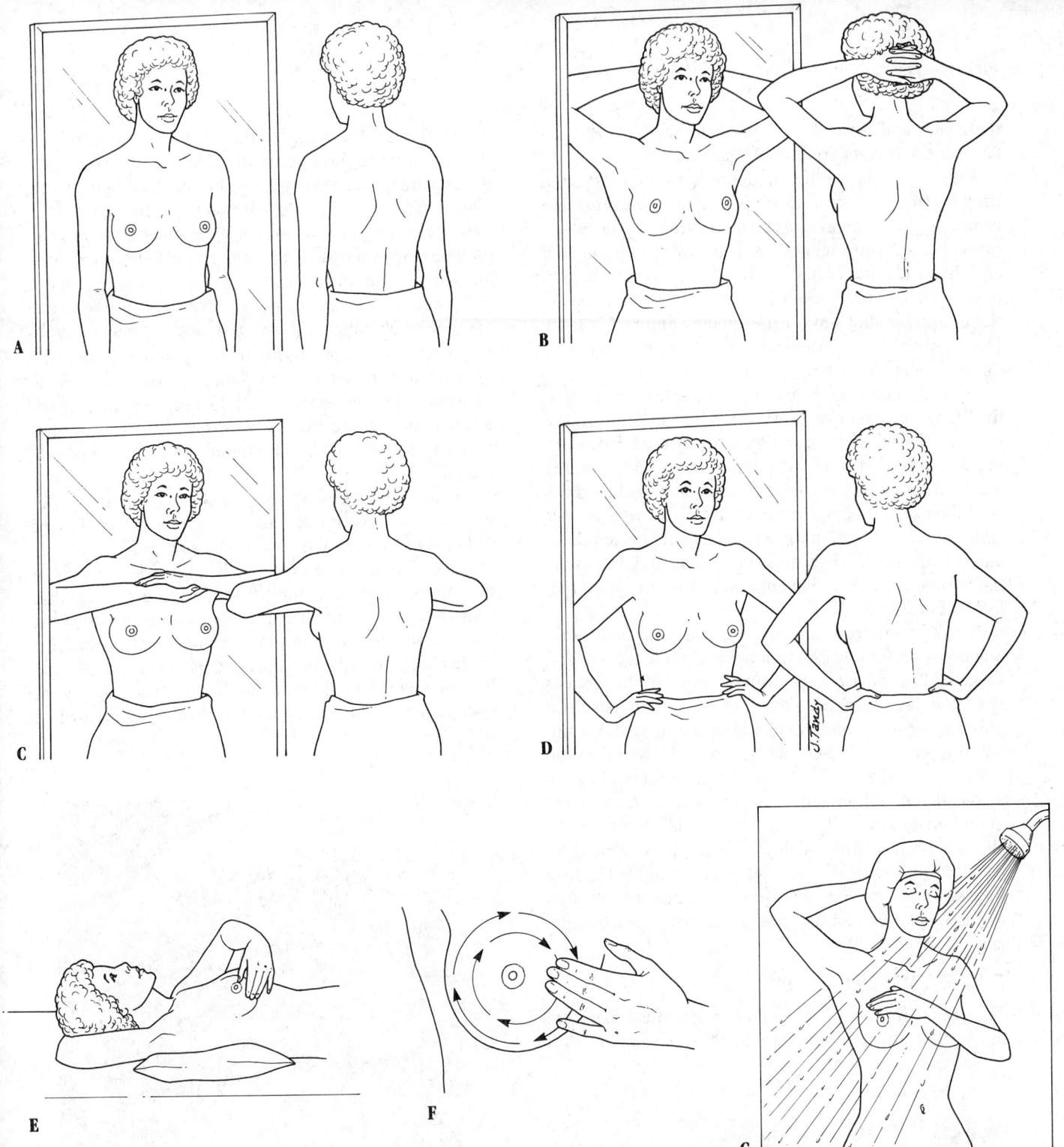

FIGURE 57-3 Breast examination (BSE). **A,** Stand in front of a mirror where you can see yourself from head to waist in good light. Observe your breasts from the front, then from the right and left sides, in each position described as follows. With arms at your side, notice the normal size, shape, color, contour, veins, nipple, and other characteristics of each breast. **B,** Raise your arms above your head; both breasts should rise when the arms are lifted. **C,** With your hands in front of you at shoulder height, press your palms firmly against each other to contract the chest wall muscles. Notice the manner in which your breasts move during position changes. **D,** Put your hands on your hips, squeeze your shoulders inward, and lean slightly forward and down. Look to see that the breasts appear normal for you. **E,** Lie down with one hand under your head and a pillow or folded towel under the scapula of the sides you will be examining. **F,** Bring your middle three fingers of the other hand together, and using the flat part of the fingers, move in small, concentric circles. It usually takes three circles to cover all breast tissue. Include the tail of the breast and axilla. Palpate areola; inspect and gently squeeze nipples to check for discharge. Move the nipples from side to side for mobility. Repeat for other breast. **G,** Repeat this technique during bath and shower, when soap and water allow fingers to glide easily over skin.

horizontal and vertical body positions; and (4) the flat parts of the fingers are used for palpation.

Essentially, three different approaches are most often used for BSE: (1) dividing the breast into quadrants and examining the area in each quadrant from the outer perimeter toward the nipple, (2) palpating the inner half and then the outer half of the breast, or (3) palpating in concentric circles beginning at the outer rim of breast tissue and moving toward the nipple (Figure 57-3, *F*). The method of approach suggested by the American Cancer Society is described in Figure 57-3.

Some women need help in learning self-examination; they may, for example, feel a rib when examining the medial half of the breast and become alarmed. However, most women learn the technique of palpation quite readily. If a lump of any kind is discovered, it should not be rubbed or touched excessively. It should be left alone, and the advice of a physician should be sought at once. Therefore women must be taught to differentiate the normal texture of glandular and fat tissues from that feels different.

It will be interesting to see if women will be less reluctant to perform self-examination of their breasts and seek medical advice concerning lumps in the breasts now that breast cancer has received such widespread publicity in the United States and now that the women's movement stresses self-health and awareness on one's body. Rosenstock[45] states that a person will take a medication or will practice a health procedure if (1) it is important to her to do it, (2) she can learn it, and (3) she is confident in her ability to do it. Many women report that they do BSE not at all or infrequently because they are not confident that they are competent enough to carry out this monthly responsibility.[57] (See box below.)

CLINICAL MANIFESTATIONS

The only early sign of breast cancer is a small, palpable mass. It is the primary sign in 90% of women with breast cancer. Dimpling of the skin, puckering of the skin, changes in the color of the skin over the lesion, alteration in the contour of the breast, distortion of the nipple, serous or bloody discharge from the nipple, and unusual scaling or inversion of the nipple are signs that the lesion is well established and has invaded surrounding tissues. An infrequent but very aggressive breast malignancy, inflammatory carcinoma, invades the mammary lymphatics early and appears as a totally edematous, red, hot breast. In the absence of mastitis associated with lactation, the woman should be quickly referred to her physician. In the advanced phases of neglected cases there may be ulceration of the skin and underlying tissue with subsequent infection of necrotic tissue.

Spread to the axillary lymph nodes occurs early. Because of the distribution of lymph vessels, malignant cells may spread rapidly, with metastasis to bone, lung, or brain. Discovery of enlarged lymph nodes or pain in the ribs or vertebrae may first alert the patient that something is wrong, particularly when the lesion is deep in the breast tissue or routine monthly BSE or medical palpation of the breast has not been carried out. It is now believed (1) that the finding of a subsequent malignancy in the contralateral or ipsilateral breast is a

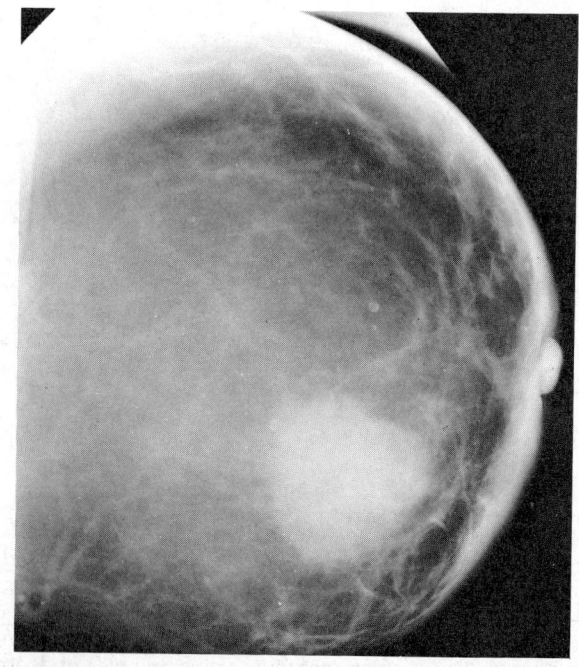

FIGURE 57-4 Mammogram of patient with area of density indicating carcinoma. (From Cramer LM and Lapayowker MS: Applied anatomy of the female breast: surgical, radiographic, and thermographic. In Masters FW and Lewis JR Jr, editors: Symposium on aesthetic surgery of the face, eyelid, and breast, vol 4, St Louis, 1972, The CV Mosby Co.)

RESEARCH

Benoliel JQ and Lierman LM: Adherence to breast examination study, 1987-1990, School of Nursing, Community Health Care Systems, University of Washington, Seattle.

The Fishbein model is currently being tested to predict adherence to breast self-examination. This model assumes that actions are under volitional control; that is, a person's intention to perform a behavior is the immediate determinant of action. Intention is a function of two basic determinants: attitude toward the behavior and the subjective norm (the person's perception of social pressure to perform or not perform the behavior). ■

primary tumor rather than a metastatic one and (2) that the subsequent malignancy was probably present at the time of the first malignancy but was undetectable because of size or location.[39]

DIAGNOSTIC TESTS

Mammography is an x-ray examination of the breast used to detect early lesions before they are palpable (Figure 57-4). Early cancers are often easily seen on the developed films as small densities with stippled calcifications within. Mammography is about 80% to 97% accurate in detecting early breast cancer. Mammography does have limitations, particularly in the penetration of dense breasts, as in adolescents, young nulliparous women, or women with large breasts.

Controversy still exists concerning the use of mammography as a screening device for women under 35 years of age. The routine screening of women under age 50 by mammography is questioned by some authorities because of the increased hazard of radiation carcinogenesis.

The American Cancer Society, however, has asserted that improved mammography techniques have decreased radiation dosage to low levels and that the positive potential for diagnosing breast cancer is considerably greater than the inherent risk. The society recommends mammography for women in whom breast cancer is suspected and for high-risk women regardless of age. Further, annual mammography is recommended for all women over age 50. *Guidelines for the Cancer-Related Checkup: Recommendations and Rationale* should be in the possession of all nurses. It can be obtained free from local American Cancer Society offices.

Xeroradiography (Figure 57-5) is a variation of mammography in which an aluminum plate with an electrically charged selenium layer is used in the place of the

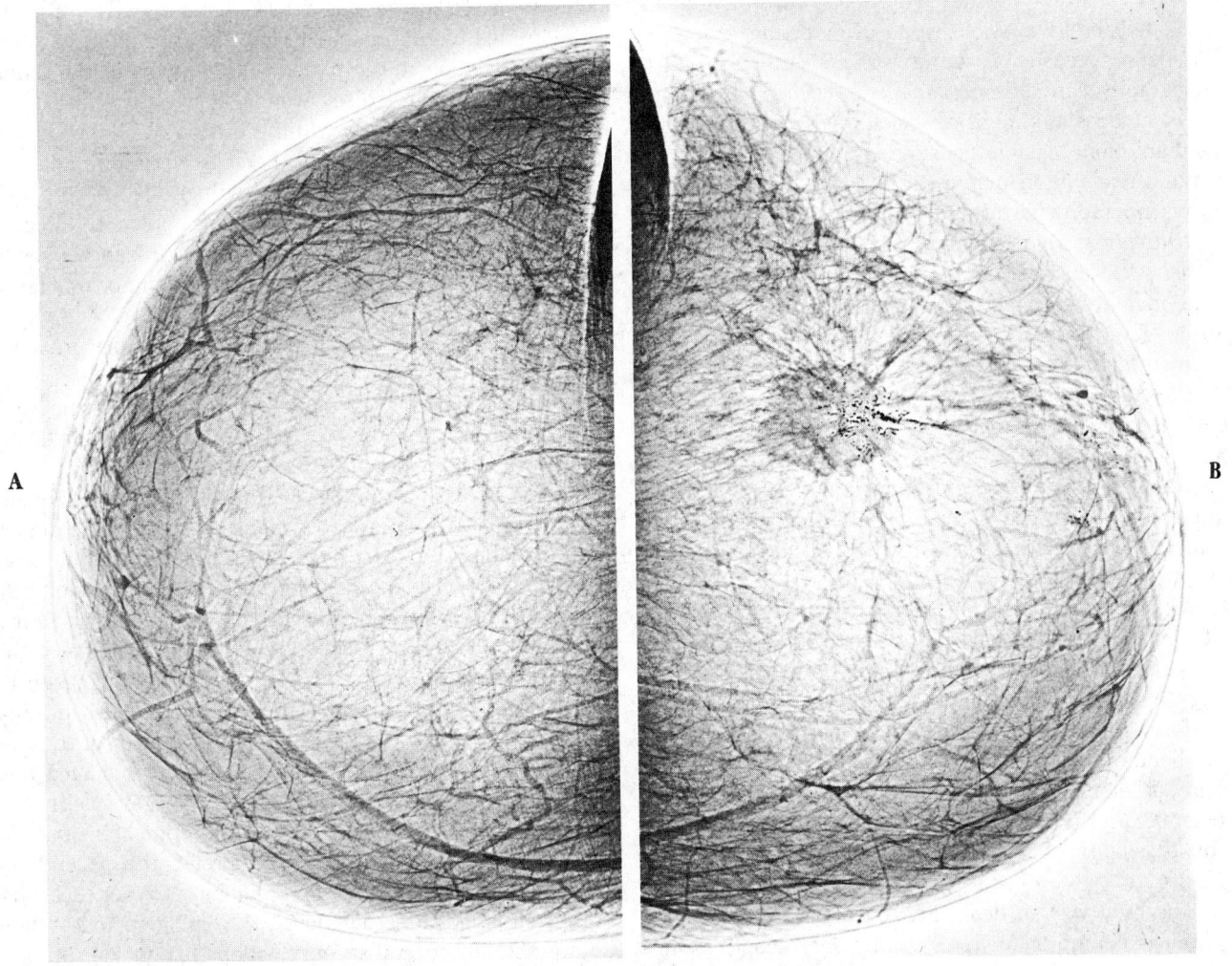

FIGURE 57-5 Xeroradiographs. **A,** Normal left breast. **B,** Right breast shows mass with spiculated margins characteristic of neoplasm. (Courtesy of University Hospitals of Cleveland.)

familiar black-and-white mammogram film. It is exposed in the usual manner with special mammoradiographic equipment. The resulting film is blue and white. Xeroradiography can detect some breast cancers in a preclinical stage, 1 or 2 years before the lesions reach a clinically palpable size of 1 cm.[53,61] Its ability to detect breast cancers at such an early stage (during which the prognosis for cure is excellent) without extensive procedures makes it a valuable tool for diagnosis.

Thermography is a less valuable screening device. In this procedure, an infrared scanner is used to measure the heat emissions coming from the breast. Abnormal variations in an area because of increased vascularization may indicate the presence of benign or malignant neoplasms. Also, some malignant lesions are not hot and some benign lesions are.[28] Thermography cannot diagnose a substantial number of tiny preclinical cancers.[7,13] In addition, it produces a high number of false-positive results and is therefore infrequently used.

Ultrasonography (ultrasound) is currently being evaluated for its possible value in detecting lesions in the dense breasts of young women. Although ultrasonography can differentiate the presence of a cystic mass, it does not indicate calcium deposits or tissue configurations, factors considered important in diagnosis and readable in mammograms. The future value of ultrasonography is yet undetermined.

Diaphanography (light scanning) has some limitations: poor sensitivity for carcinomas less than 1 cm in size, inability to detect microcalcifications, and inability to image a lesion located more than 2 cm beneath the skin surface.[28]

Computed tomography (CT) may be of use in diagnosis. Despite initial reports that breast cancer can cause increased uptake of iodinated contrast material, making identification of even small malignancies in dense breasts possible, use of CT in the screening of breast cancer clearly has not made any further impact on early diagnosis.[28]

Magnetic resonance imaging (MRI) may have more of a role in the area of diagnosis than in screening because of the high cost and increased time in interpreting the cross-sectional images. MRI has the potential to perform chemical analysis of breast tissue to differentiate benign from malignant leions. It also has the capability of identifying premalignant changes in the breast even before the cancer appears. Furthermore, MRI has the possibility of staging a breast cancer more accurately.[28]

The only way to determine conclusively whether a tumor is benign or malignant is by microscopic examination of a section of the tumor obtained by biopsy. Rarely, a palpable axillary node may be excised for microscopic study. Most surgeons believe that if the slight-

est possibility of cancer exists, it is safer to remove the entire tumor mass. Pieces of a tumor are seldom removed surgically because of the release of malignant cells into the blood and lymphatic systems at the time of surgery.

The success of mammography (and xeroradiography to detect early, nonpalpable lesions or areas of calcification) results in more and earlier biopsies. Sometimes the small size makes location of the lesion difficult or uncertain when biopsy is attempted. Therefore, to locate areas for surgical biopsy, a small methylene blue dye marker is injected within the area of the breast with a syringe and needle during mammographic monitoring. If mixed with iodinated contrast material, the position of the dye relative to the lesion can be located promptly, and the stained tissue containing the lesion can be excised.[29] This is called *needle localization* and is usually done in the diagnostic radiography department with the patient under local anesthesia. No color disfiguration is apparent on the breast surface because of this procedure, but it ensures that the biopsy tissue corresponds to the site identified by the mammogram. This procedure requires preinstruction to the patient and support in the radiology department. To the woman it is not routine, but a "tagging of the enemy within," during which she is consciously involved. Denial here is very difficult; the woman feels very helpless and vulnerable.

Until recently the most common approach has been to remove the tumor and examine a frozen section of the tissue under the microscope. If the tumor was found to be malignant, the surgical setup was completely changed, and the more extensive procedure was performed. In this approach to surgery, when the patient went for biopsy, she did not know in advance whether it was necessary for the breast to be removed or the extent of surgery that would be performed.

An increasing number of surgeons are now scheduling the patient for a biopsy alone. The patient then goes home and awaits the biopsy results. She thus has time to make decisions and prepare herself psychologically for the more extensive surgery if a malignancy is found. This is a two-step procedure. The disadvantage of this approach is the stress of waiting for the diagnostic results and then facing the prospect of a repeat hospital admission and a second surgical procedure. In the Gallup survey of 1973, 47% of the women indicated they would prefer to sign the consent for surgery along with the consent for biopsy (the first approach just described), whereas 48% would prefer the second approach in order to get other opinions (20%) or to discuss the situation after diagnosis (28%). Since today there are not only several surgery options to consider but also a therapy option that is nonsurgical, these figures may not reflect current thought. A National Cancer Institute study in 1980 reported 41% of white women would consent to a mastectomy at the time of biopsy, but 55% would want the two-step procedure, as would 52% of Hispanic women and 48% of black women.[38] It is believed that there is an understandable difference between a young woman's and an older woman's choice in this matter as well.

In either of these approaches, after excision of the tumor masses the pathologist sends tissue to a special laboratory for determination of hormone receptor by means of an estrogen receptor assay (ERA) and progesterone receptor assay (PRA) tests. Such studies reveal important prognostic factors and are helpful in future management of the patient. The hormone assay tests identify those breast cancers that are hormone dependent; that is, their growth is stimulated by estrogen and/or progesterone. Postmenopausal women have a higher incidence of hormone-dependent breast cancers. Treatment such as endocrine chemotherapy (hormonal therapy) and removal of the ovaries (oophorectomy) or adrenalectomy to remove the source of estrogen can retard growth and spread of the tumor. A negative ERA or PRA test indicates that a woman is less likely to benefit from hormonal therapy and even chemotherapy.

Another test that impacts treatment is the deoxyribonucleic acid (DNA) flow cytometry, which tests the nuclear grade of the tumor cell. It has significant predictive value for women with stage I disease.[36]

THERAPY PLANNING

The therapy proposed to the patient is planned and based on various factors: (1) the tissue involved and indications of its aggressiveness (histopathology of the biopsy specimen), (2) the hormonal milieu (that is, premenopausal, postmenopausal, estrogen or progesterone dependent), (3) identification of multifocal primary tumors in one breast or both (mammography), (4) the tumor's location, (5) the tumor's size, and (6) local containment or indications of extension to lymph nodes (as indicated by mammography, palpation, or biopsy) or to distant sites (as indicated by biopsy, bone scan, liver scan, or CT scan). Staging of the breast malignancy incorporates the TNM (tumor, node metastasis) classification, as shown in the box above.

When the diagnostic work is completed and classification of the tumor has been made, the physician, often with the consultative advantages of the hospital tumor board members (medical, surgical and radiation oncologists; pathologists; radiologists; surgeons; primary physicians), discusses and proposes the treatment protocol that would most successfully destroy the tumor and that offers the best prognosis for the patient.

The patient and family are often involved at some point in this treatment decision plan. If the patient is not involved, she should request to be informed of the findings of the diagnostic measures and of the determi-

---

STAGING AND TNM CLASSIFICATION

Stage 1 T_1 (Tumor 2 cm or less)
          N_0 (No palpable axillary nodes)
          M_0 (No evident mestastasis)

Stage 2 T_0 (No palpable tumor)
          T_1 (Tumor 2 cm or less)
          T_2 (Tumor less than 5 cm)
          N_1 (Palpable axillary nodes with histologic evidence of breast malignancy)
          M_0

Stage 3 T_3 (Tumor more than 5 cm; may be fixed to muscle or fascia)
          N_1 or N_2 (Fixed nodes)
          M_0

Stage 4 T_4 (Tumor any size with fixation to chest wall or skin; presence of edema, including peau d'orange; ulceration; skin nodules; inflammatory carcinoma)
          N_3 (supraclavicular or intraclavicular nodes or arm edema)
          M_1 (Distant metastasis present or suspected)

---

*International Union Against Cancer and the American Joint Committee for Cancer Staging and End-Result Reporting (UICC-AJC) clinical staging system.

---

nations considered in setting the therapy plan now being described to her. There are currently many treatments for breast malignancy. However, depending on the factors known about her tumor, only one treatment plan may exist, with no alternative plans and no options. (For example, when inflammatory carcinoma is present, immediate radiation therapy is the specific treatment for this serious type.) If the malignancy is small, nonaggressive, and present in a young woman, however, she may, for instance, have several options for therapy, offer a comparable prognosis with the knowledge available. Every woman should realize, that the latest therapy written up in magazines may or may not be best for her. If it is not best for her or does not have the same advantages as another therapy offers, it is then not an option for her decision making.

Nurses have the advantage of being able to assist a patient to understand these factors involved in the decision making from the expertise of the medical professional but still taking into consideration the subjective hesitations of the woman. The roles of teacher and advocate to both patient, family, and physician are important today, when both media and medical professionals voice controversial issues in the treatment of breast malignancy. Although decision making is always difficult during periods of stress and crisis, for the woman today with a breast malignancy, it has never been more so.

PRIMARY MEDICAL INTERVENTIONS

Several primary therapies for breast malignancies may be applied, depending on the individual woman's medical situation and preferences.

SURGERY

In the past, the treatment of choice for breast cancer has been surgery. However, within the last 2½ decades there has been a decline of cancer surgery on the basis of anatomic principles and conceptual changes that have resulted from new information concerning tumor biology. It is now clear that the primary goal of surgery is to effect local-regional disease control.[17,24]

Types of Surgery

Different types of surgeries can be performed:
1. Lumpectomy (tylectomy, tumorectomy): removal of the tumor mass without attention to margins
2. Partial mastectomy (segmental mastectomy, limited resection): excision of the tumor with grossly normal, clean margins
3. Quadrantectomy: en bloc excision of the tumor within a quadrant of breast tissue, along with excision the pectoralis major muscle fascia and overlying skin
4. Subcutaneous mastectomy (adenomammmectomy): removal of all underlying breast tissue, leaving skin, areola, and nipple intact
5. Simple mastectomy: removal of main breast structure, but not overlying skin, underlying chest muscles, or axillary lymph nodes
6. Modified radical mastectomy: complete removal of breast nipple, some of overlying skin, adjacent soft tissue, and axillary lymph nodes
7. Radical (Halsted) mastectomy: complete removal of breast, nipple, some of overlying skin, pectoralis muscles (minor and major), adjacent fat and fascia, and axillary lymph nodes
8. Extended radical mastectomy (supraradical): same as radical mastectomy plus removal of parasternal lymph nodes.

There has been considerable professional controversy in lay periodicals and medical journals about the surgical treatment of breast cancer.

Some suggest that a lumpectomy with irradiation is sufficient to treat small cancerous lesions up to 5 cm in size (stage II) and that a mastectomy is not necessary. At this time the 10- 20-year follow-up in retrospective series and prospective randomized trials with 8 or more years of follow-up have indicated (1) that local recurrence and survival rates are equal to those of mastectomy and (2) that incidence of contralateral breast cancer from radiation has not been substantiated.*

A modified radical mastectomy is often performed for early, well-localized, small lesions of the breast. It offers comparable therapy prognosis to the classic radical mastectomy. In the radical mastectomy the surgeon's judgment regarding the amount of overlying skin that can safely be left to cover the defect determines whether a skin graft will be necessary. Preoperatively the surgeon may order the skin of the anterior surface of one thigh shaved and prepared surgically in case the need for a graft should arise. If the lesion is located in the medial quadrant of the breast, particularly the upper medial quadrant, an extended radical mastectomy may be performed, since lesions of the medial quadrant tend to metastasize to the internal mammary chain of lymph nodes. A simple mastectomy sometimes is performed if cancer is believed to be limited to the breast or is done as a palliative measure to remove an ulcerated cancer of the breast in disease that is known to be advanced.

RADIATION THERAPY

Radiation therapy is the specific primary therapy of choice for inflammatory carcinoma and is also chosen as therapy for those whose physical condition could not tolerate anesthesia and surgery.

Some European surgeons have been doing a two-stage radiation therapy procedure for women with stage I or stage II disease. The therapy is done after biopsy of the lesion (and sometimes the axillary nodes) is performed. As an outpatient, the woman is given external beam therapy to the breast, lymph nodes, and the chest wall daily (Monday through Friday) for 5 weeks. This is then followed by a radiation "boost" to the biopsy site that can be divided in two different ways. One requires hospitalization for 3 or 4 days, when irridium needles are implanted in the breast under local anesthesia. They are then removed in 2 or 3 days and the therapy concluded. Another means of boost may be given with more external irradiation with electron beam.[12] The data collected and reported by these European oncologists seem to show similar therapy results for the modified radical surgery when comparable-sized lesions and aggressiveness of tissue are compared.[58] This treatment protocol is now being given in various parts of the United States, most often in connection with one of the cancer research centers. It seems to be gaining the attention and enthusiasm of many U.S. oncologists and their patients since 10 and 20 year results are encouraging for breast cancer patients threated by radical mastectomy and postoperative radiation without chemotherapy.[18a]

CHEMOTHERAPY (ADJUVANT)

The current emphasis is on treating women with breast malignancies as if they had metastatic disease or a high risk of recurrence. This type of treatment is called adjuvant chemotherapy, which supplements primary surgi-

---

*References 8, 12, 34, 37, 54, 58.

cal or radiation treatment. Today many combination therapy protocols are under study by regional cancer research groups, with varying timings for the therapies, use of specific cytotoxic agent or agents and dosage in chemotherapy, and possible hormonal therapy. Therefore the nurse must know what protocols are being used and keep current in this knowledge. The burgeoning field of oncology and especially the growing amount of information within the area of breast malignancy require professionals to assume responsibility for reliable and current reading sources. Thus, at present, chemotherapy generally may be given before, with, or after surgery or radiation therapy.

All three modes of therapy may be combined or may even integrate hormonal therapy. This complex therapeutic planning is rationally based on those factors cited on p. 1665 and on clinical indicators as the patient passes through the prescribed therapy or therapies.

■ ASSESSMENT

Subjective Data

If the woman is at high risk for breast cancer (see the box below), it is important to ascertain her knowledge of risk factors, BSE practices, and feelings concerning breast cancer. These data provide a base for health teaching and exploring of feelings. All women should be questioned concerning their knowledge and practices related to monthly BSE.

HIGH RISK FACTORS ASSOCIATED WITH BREAST CANCER

Sex	Female (99% in women)
Age	Over age 50 years (80% over age 35)
Familial history	Mother/sister with breast cancer, especially with premenopausal and bilateral condition
Parity	First live birth after age 30, or nullipara
Personal history	Primary breast cancer (seven times risk for a second primary cancer in breast)
	Other organ cancers, especially uterine or endometrium
	Benign breast disease
	Menarche before age 11
	Menopause after age 50
	Adverse hormonal milieu
	Lowered immunologic competence
	Other organ cancers, especially ovarian, uterine or endometrial
Environmental	Exposure to carcinogens
	High dietary intake of fat or alcohol
	Chronic psychologic stress
	Living in the western hemisphere or a cold climate. Belonging to upper socioeconomic group or being white

If the woman has been suspected of or diagnosed as having a breast tumor that is or may be malignant, the following additional data are obtained as a baseline for planning:

1. Identification of family relationships and the existence and availability of support persons
2. Usual coping mechanisms
3. Feelings and thoughts about her own sexuality and the relationship of the breast to these feelings
4. Thoughts about feelings of sex partner (if appropriate) concerning forthcoming diagnostic procedures or potential therapy options
5. Financial concerns over treatment and rehabilitation
6. Future goals, life expectancies, zest for living, and actual or perceived responsibilities to others

If possible, data are obtained from the sex partner (if appropriate) regarding his feelings about the forthcoming surgery. This identifies possible conflicts in perceptions, the degree of support that can be anticipated from the sex partner, and the potential effects of the partner's feelings on the woman's adaptation and relationships.

Objective Data

The woman's breasts are inspected to determine size and symmetry, contour, and appearance of the skin. Although there is often some difference in breast size, that is, the left breast may be smaller than the right, they usually are relatively symmetric. Variations in breast contour may include the presence of masses, dimpling, or flattening. The color of the skin, presence of thickened areas, or abnormalities of the venous pattern may be indicative of a pathologic condition. The nipple may be inverted; this is usually not pathologic unless it has not been previously present. The direction in which the nipples are pointing may provide clues to masses. Discharge from the nipple may be indicative of an abnormal condition; a clear fluid resembling colostrum may be present in certain women with monthly hormonal fluctuation. Nipple discharges unrelated to lactation should be evaluated by the physician without delay. Ulcerated areas and other lesions of the nipple require further exploration.

SURGERY

■ DATA ANALYSIS: NURSING DIAGNOSES

Nursing diagnoses are determined from assessment of patient data. Possible nursing diagnoses for the person requiring surgery for cancer of the breast include, but are not limited to, the following:

Diagnostic Title	Possible Etiologies
Preoperative	
Activity intolerance, potential	Mobility impairment and generalized weakness caused by surgery

Diagnostic Title	Possible Etiologies
Anxiety; fear	Surgery; threat of death; change in health status, socioeconomic status, and role functioning; situational crisis
Grieving, anticipatory	Loss of significant body part
Knowledge deficit	Lack of recall; cognitive limitation resulting from anxiety

Postoperative

Adjustment impaired	Inadequate support systems; assault to self-esteem; incomplete or dysfunctional grieving
Body image disturbance	Loss of body parts or functions; change in body appearance
Denial, ineffective	Threat to life
Disuse syndrome, potential for	Immobility; weakness
Family processes, altered	Situational crisis
Fatigue	Postsurgical period
Sleep pattern disturbance	Environmental changes; pain and discomfort; anxiety; medications
Fluid volume excess (lymphedema)	Compromised regulatory mechanism
Home maintenance management, impaired	Insufficient family resources; inadequate support systems
Infection, potential for	Compromised immune response
Mobility, impaired	Intolerance to activity, decreased strength and endurance; pain and discomfort; musculoskeletal impairment
Nutrition, altered: less than body requirement	Anorexia caused physiologic and psychologic changes
Pain	Trauma to tissue
Self-esteem disturbance	Change in body appearance
Sensory/perceptual alterations	Altered sensory reception or transmission integrity; psychologic stress
Sexual dysfunction	Altered body structure; physiologic limitations; psychologic stress
Skin integrity, impaired	Surgical procedure
Social isolation	Alteration in physical appearance; altered state of wellness; inadequate personal resources

■ PLANNING: EXPECTED PATIENT OUTCOMES

Expected patient outcomes for the person requiring surgery for cancer of the breast may include, but are not limited to, the following:

Preoperative

1. Patient will express less anxiety and fear about impending surgery and implications.
2. Patient will be able to verbalize loss of breast and its significance.
3. Patient will explain her disease, the surgical procedure and post-surgical care
4. Patient will understand importance of program of progressive activity for affected arm.

Postoperative

1. a. Patient learns and participates in wound care.
   b. Patient understands steps to take against infection.
2. a. Patient states she is feeling comfortable.
   b. Patient reports sensory alterations to health care provider.
   c. Patient participates in a program of progressive activity.
3. Patient ingests recommended dietary allowances (RDAs) of foods and fluids.
4. a. Patient is able to balance rest with activity.
   b. Patient takes rest frequently during the day.
5. Patient participates in postmastectomy arm exercise program.
6. a. Patient is able to: Verbalize loss of body parts/functions/appearance.
   b. Mobilize support systems.
   c. Work through grief of body loss.
   d. Accept altered body appearance and health status.
   e. Patient able to work through situational crisis
   f. Seek out community resources.
7. Patient talks about changes that impact sexual life with her partner.
8. Patient is able to focus on personal appearance as a woman.
9. Patient understands treatment to reduce lymphedema

■ IMPLEMENTATION

Preoperative Care

Relieving fear and anxiety: providing support and teaching. Since much emphasis is placed on the breast as a symbol of attractiveness, the thought of losing a breast becomes almost intolerable to many women. This is particularly true of those who depend largely on physical attractiveness for their work (for example, models), to hold the esteem of others and to secure gratification of their emotional needs. Psychologists have pointed out that a symbolic connection exists between the breasts and motherhood that is severely threatened when a breast must be removed. It is understandable that women may be seriously threatened emotionally by the loss of a part of the body that is so closely associated with sexual attractiveness and motherliness. Cancer of the breast often occurs at menopause or soon afterward when some women feel that they have lost much of their sexual attractiveness already. Surgical removal of the breast may save a woman's life, but it also may cause her to feel less feminine.

Although she may try to conceal fear, any woman who is hospitalized for removal of a breast tumor is always anxious, and some may be in a state of near panic.[20] Most of the fears are related to sexual acceptance, social isolation, disfigurement, recurrence, and death. Many of these women have been unable to discuss their worries and feelings with their significant others, including their partners. The nurse can help the patient to express feelings and to understand what breast surgery means to her as a person. The woman who is having breast surgery has a special need to feel understood and accepted by all persons who are giving preoperative care.

Simple explanations with repetition may decrease the patient's fear of the unknown. If it seems that the patient does not fully comprehend the surgeon's explanation, as the surgeon discusses the diagnosis and treatment with the patient and significant others, the nurse can repeat the explanation. The nurse then can report this to the surgeon, who in turn can talk with the patient again and clarify any misconceptions, alleviating needless anxiety. Since attention span, memory, and perception are limited when anxiety levels are high, it is helpful if the nurse can be present when information is given to the patient. The nurse can then repeat, reinforce, or clarify information given

The American Cancer Society sponsors a volunteer program, Reach to Recovery, in which the patient has an opportunity to visit with a woman who has had a mastectomy or lumpectomy. This encourages the patient, and she will receive practical help from someone who has made a satisfactory adjustment to the same procedure. Although most of the patient visits by the volunteer from Reach to Recovery occur during the postoperative period, preoperative visits may be very helpful to some women and can be requested.

Additional testing may be done. If a diagnosis of a malignancy is almost a certainty, roentgenographic examinations such as bone, lung, or liver scans or liver function studies may be ordered to rule out the possibility of metastases to these areas of the body or as baseline data for the future. Preparing the patient for procedures that will take place before and after surgery is of utmost importance in allaying her fears and in setting the stage for successful rehabilitation.

Preoperative teaching should include the following information if a mastectomy is planned. A dressing may be applied to the incision, and a catheter attached to suction may be used. The arm will be elevated. The woman should practice sitting up and turning to the nonoperative side by pushing up on the unaffected elbow. Postoperative exercises will be started early.

Teaching to prepare for postoperative activities and exercises. If the breast is removed, the shoulder will tend to droop on that side because of the inequality of weight; this can be prevented by close attention to posture and a properly weighted and fitted prosthesis. Exercises will be taught postoperatively to help maintain posture and to strengthen muscles. Telling the patient about the exercises helps to give her the feeling that there is something in the situation that she can control and contribute to, and thus she will begin to have a positive attitude toward rehabilitation. She will always need to be somewhat vigilant in protecting the arm on the side of the surgery. This will begin postoperatively as she too monitors that no blood pressure measurement, blood drawing, or injections are done on that arm. It is easier to prevent lymphedema than to treat it.

Arm measurements are taken by the nurse preoperatively, as baseline data; these measurements are also taken postoperatively, and the patient will continue to take them monthly. Measurements are made with a tape measure at the olecranon, at 6 inches above and at 6 inches below the olecranon. These measurements should be taken in both arms and the findings recorded in a permanent portion of the patient's record.

Postoperative Care

Promoting wound care. Following the completion of the mastectomy and closure, a stab wound may be made, and a catheter inserted and attached to a low constant suction such as that provided by a Hemovac or other low-suction system. The purpose of the catheter is to remove blood and serum that may collect under the skin flaps and that would prevent healing and predispose the woman to infection. The Hemovac must be checked frequently and emptied when half full to maintain constant suction through the catheter and prevent buildup of fluid under the skin flaps. There is usually no drainage from around the incision when a catheter is draining properly. The catheter may be clamped for short periods of ambulation and is usually removed within 3 to 5 days or when the amount of drainage is less than 5 to 10 ml in 24 hours.

At one time pressure dressings rather than a catheter were used to prevent the accumulation of fluid under the skin. Many surgeons now believe that the use of a catheter and a smaller dressing is preferable to the use of a large pressure dressing. This corresponds to the change from the radical procedure to the modified radical procedure.

The dressing is checked often for the first few hours to detect hemorrhage or excessive serous oozing. The bedclothes under the patient must be examined for

NURSING CARE PLAN

PERSON FOLLOWING MASTECTOMY FOR CANCER

DATA: Mrs. Litton, age 35, discovered a lump in her right breast quite accidentally while bathing. She is not familiar with breast self-examination. Mammography and a breast biopsy confirmed the diagnosis of cancer. In a conference with the surgeon and plastic surgeon, Mrs. Litton elected to have a modified radical mastectomy with consideration of breast reconstruction in 6 months.

Mrs. Litton was very quiet during the admission procedure. The primary nurse talked with her the evening before surgery, and Mrs. Litton stated that her major concern was "whether they would get it all." She is glad to know that breast reconstruction can be done in the near future because she doesn't think she wants to go through life with a deformed chest. She also said her husband had supported the surgery, and they both feel it will not affect their relationship. Mr. Litton accompanied his wife to the hospital for admission and spent the evening with her. Her mother is caring for their 3- and 6-year-old daughters while Mrs. Litton is hospitalized.

After surgery, Mrs. Litton returned to the division with intravenous fluids and a wound catheter attached to a Hemovac suction. Vital signs were stable.

Collaborative nursing actions included monitoring the dressing and catheter for wound drainage and observing the arm for signs of enlargement (lymphedema). Medical orders included keeping her right arm elevated on pillows to prevent lymphedema. A sign was placed on her door reminding others to avoid blood pressure readings and injections, or taking blood samples from Mrs. Litton's right arm.

NURSING DIAGNOSIS

Pain: related to surgical incision

Expected Patient Outcomes	Nursing Interventions	Rationale
Ms. Litton will report feeling more comfortable	Give prescribed narcotic on a regular basis for first 24 hr; then re-evaluate	Expected incisional pain is better controlled if not allowed to become severe; comfort will enhance participation in arm exercises
	Encourage deep breathing and coughing (DB & C) every 2-4 hr	Prevents lung problems that would increase her discomfort

NURSING DIAGNOSIS

Impaired physical mobility: related to shoulder immobility

Expected Patient Outcomes	Nursing Interventions	Rationale
Mrs. Litton participates early with arm exercises	Demonstrate early exercises (keep instructions simple) Visit her every 2 hours to provide encouragement Explain rationale of exercises to husband so he can encourage her	Because of discomfort and narcotic, she may have difficulty concentrating Exercises will help prevent stiffness and contractures of shoulder from disuse

NURSING CARE PLAN

PERSON FOLLOWING MASTECTOMY FOR CANCER—cont'd

NURSING DIAGNOSIS
Body image disturbance: related to loss of breast

Expected Patient Outcomes	Nursing Interventions	Rationale
Mrs. Litton begins to look at incision and to talk about loss of her breast	Spend planned time talking with her Give her opportunities to talk about her feelings without pushing her Observe for signs of touching her dressing and use this as an opening to discuss her thoughts about her surgery Check with her surgeon about a Reach to Recovery volunteer visitor and then explain the program Encourage her to put on makeup and wear her own clothes as soon as possible	As she begins to think about her surgery, she may need reassurance that the nurse is interested and willing to listen to her concerns Interacting with someone who has been through the experience is often helpful in adjustment She may need reassurance of her femininity

NURSING DIAGNOSIS
Knowledge deficit: related to lack of information

Expected Patient Outcomes	Nursing Interventions	Rationale
Mrs. Litton will: 1. Plan to do BSE regularly on other breast and teach her daughters when older	Teach BSE: demonstration with return demonstration Explain high risk of daughters for breast cancer and need for continued monitoring	Women who have a chance to practice BSE under supervision are more confident about doing BSE Mother's breast cancer is a high risk factor for daughter
2. Plan to continue exercises until full shoulder ROM returns	Demonstrate exercises to be done later; give her booklet from American Cancer Society with instructions	Seeing a demonstration and having written material for reference will promote follow-up of the activity
3. Plan for rest periods at home	Explain reason for expected fatigue after surgery and help her to plan her day to include rest periods	Care of young children is tiring and she still needs additional energy for healing; rest will give her additional energy for coping
4. Know where to obtain breast prostheses, if needed	Encourage visit by Reach to Recovery volunteer; if not, discuss types of prostheses and where to obtain them	She may postpone reconstructive surgery or may want to use a soft prosthesis before surgery
5. Report symptoms to her physician	Instruct her to report signs of arm edema, redness or infection of incision, or any mass in other breast	Lymphedema and incisional breakdown are better treated if identified early; she is at high risk for cancer in other breast

From Long BC and Phipps WJ: Medical-surgical nursing, a nursing process approach, ed 2, St. Louis, 1989, The CV Mosby Co.

blood that may flow down from the incision. Any evidence of bleeding is reported to the surgeon. If the wound is not covered with a dressing, a cradle may be used to protect it from the bed covers. Signs of circulatory obstruction, such as swelling and numbness of the lower arm or inability to move the fingers, must be reported at once. No dressings should be loosened without specific instruction from the surgeon.

Dressings may be removed in 24 hours, or they may not be changed for several days after the surgery. The skin sutures are often removed on the sixth to the eighth postoperative day. Usually this is after the patient's discharge from the hospital. If a graft has been taken from the thigh or back, this area may be covered with a firm pressure dressing or fine mesh gauze, and the wound exposed to the air. The patient may complain of severe discomfort in this donor site as soon as she recovers from anesthesia.

Promoting comfort. Pain in the surgical area also may be referred to the affected arm or shoulder. Sensations of numbness and tingling that is painful over the chest may cause the woman to take short, shallow breaths. She should be kept comfortable with analgesics, and a cough/deep breathing routine should be started. Each chest excursion may painfully discourage compliance. The nurse should be sympathetic and work with the patient.

When the patient recovers from the effects of anesthesia, she is usually only comfortable lying on her back with the head end of the bed elevated. If the affected arm is not incorporated in the dressing, the arm is elevated to enhance circulation and prevent edema. The pillows are arranged so that the hand is higher than the arm and the arm is above the level of the right atrium. No blood pressure readings, injections, or blood testing should be done on the affected arm because of potential circulatory impairment or infection (to prevent lymphedema). A sign or tape should be placed on this side of the bed with this message. The patient and family should be taught to be firm and aggressive in refusing procedures to the arm. The patient will be more comfortable sitting up straight during back care, since turning toward the affected side will be exceedingly painful and will place pressure on the area. To turn to the opposite side and to sit up, she should be taught to push up on the elbow of the unaffected side rather than pull up. She should lie down by using that arm in the same way.

Promoting nutrition. During the initial postoperative period of metabolic (adrenergic, mineralocorticoid) readjustment to the anesthesia and surgery, the patient probably will have little interest in food (1 to 1½ days). Relief that the surgery is over will collide with the impact of the nature of the surgery and its meaning to her.

For some women the assurance of removal of the malignancy will counterbalance the change in breast size and contour or total absence of the breast or breasts. For others, grieving focuses on these results of the surgery. Such depression becomes superimposed on the same period postoperatively (mineralocorticoid period), when normally the patient feels down and is tearful, introspective, and socially disinterested. Thirst would be assuaged; hunger, seldom thought about even if present; appetite, absent.

During this period the goals of nutrition for wound healing and esthetics for the feminine patient can be combined in small trays containing a very nourishing beverage, soup, or dessert, not all given at once but offered at short, unexpected intervals. The tray cover, a colorful napkin, a flower, or a note from the family not only restores to this patient protein nourishment but also reattaches her to the love of her family and friends and the realization that she still responds to gifts of beauty and surprise in a very feminine way.

In the wisdom of the body's conservation, wound healing has priority for all utilization of nutrients and energy. When the next postoperative metabolic (glucocorticoid) phase is reached (only in the absence of infection), the nurse can emphasize through teaching the importance of balanced nutrition, and she can assess and discuss with the patient her menu choice while she is hospitalized. Nutrition is very important to the cancer patient during and after treatment (no matter what modality), and it has been found that nutrition beneficially influences the success of the therapeutic outcome when optimal nutrition was present before therapy and maintained during therapy. For the woman who has surgical biopsies, to be followed by radiation therapy, wound healing and therefore good nutrition are imperative. Excellent cookbooks for cancer patients are available free from the National Cancer Institute and major cancer centers.[18] Nutrition introduced, learned, and reinforced during the initial therapy experience should be a patient care goal. Patients should be introduced at that time also to the literature available.[40]

Promoting rest. In the first few days after any surgery, energy reserve is accepted by patient, family, and staff to be limited and transitory. When the patient is also greatly grieving, lack of energy reserve is even more apparent. This must be acknowledged by staff and explained to family. One mastectomy patient cannot be compared to another.

During these 1 or 2 days of quick fatigue, more ambulation is required, and increasing exercise expected. At this time the nurse teaches the patient to plan for and anticipate those periods when energy will be needed. The nurse teaches the patient to conserve her energy for what is required, to recognize the early signs of tiredness that are uniquely hers, and to realize the importance of stopping activity before fatigue. When the patient becomes fatigued, she is depleted of energy and, closely following, emotionally distraught. Fatigue is unnecessary and detrimental. To be tired is to appreciate the support of a chair or the rest offered by a bed after the woman has achieved her realistic activity or exercise or social visiting goals for that period. After rest she is motivated to continue again.

A more difficult time to tolerate decreased energy reserves begins about the third postoperative day and extends for about a 5 to 6 weeks. During this glucocorticoid phase, the patient begins making and receiving more phone calls. She bathes and dresses and prepares her hair, face, and hands. This costs energy. She exercises, hears about prosthesis, and considers going home, more cost of energy. This time in the hospital and extending to 6 weeks postoperatively can be discouraging if the woman is not prepared to know that her energy now is more available. She feels better and better, but it is normal that her energy is capricious. Realistic plans, short tasks, and single interests and endeavors are necessary, all interspersed with planned rest periods. A pitfall at this time is for her to feel that she is not up to expectations, that something is wrong, and that she should not wilt so suddenly in the midst of activity. This is very important patient teaching for patient and family members alike. The priority of the body resources is for healing. She can initiate and partake in more and more energy-using activities, but this energy is limited until healing is fully completed.

Sleep at night should be facilitated in the hospital, with rest or sleep periods during the day. However, it is important that the patient establish a distinct day-night activity and sleep routine and that she gives this priority when she goes home as well. Sleeplessness or 3 AM awakening with insomnia is often symptomatic of grieving and can be a rewarding time for the night nurse to practice crisis intervention.

Promoting activity and exercise. Exercises are essential to prevent shortening of muscles, stiffness, and contracture of the shoulder girdle and to preserve muscle tone so that the affected arm can be used without limitations. To prevent additional deformities, exercises should be bilateral, with the patient using both arms simultaneously. When specific postoperative exercises should be started will depend on the extent of the surgery and whether skin grafting has been necessary.

Slings are to be avoided. Gentle exercises started early in the postoperative course help decrease muscle tension as well as regain muscle function more quickly. Usually the patient is encouraged to flex and extend her fingers immediately on return to her room. She should also be encouraged to pronate and supinate her fore-

POSTMASTECTOMY ARM EXERCISES

EXERCISE: BALL SQUEEZING

1. Lying in bed, hold a rubber ball in your hand.
2. Lift arm straight up and alternately squeeze and relax the ball.
3. Do this exercise as often as recommended by your physician.
4. If it is uncomfortable to hold arm straight up, support it using several pillows.

PULLEY MOTION

1. Toss the rope over the top of the door with unaffected arm.
2. Sit with legs hugging both sides of the door closely, and keep soles firmly planted on the floor.
3. Hold the ends of the rope in each hand with knots between third and fourth fingers.
4. Slowly raise affected arm as far as comfortable by pulling down on the rope with unaffected arm; the raised arm close to your head. Reverse the motion to raise unaffected arm by lowering affected arm. Rest and repeat.

HAND WALL CLIMBING

1. Start in standard position, with toes 6 to 12 inches from and facing wall.
2. Bend elbows and place palms against the wall at shoulder level.
3. Work both hands up the wall parallel to each other until incisional pulling or pain occurs. Mark spot so progress can be checked.
4. Work hands down to shoulder level. Move feet and body closer to wall as comfort allows and reach requires.
5. Return to standard position. Rest and repeat.

BACK SCRATCHER

1. Start in standard position.
2. Place hand of unoperated side on hip for balance.
3. Bend elbow of arm on operated side, placing back of hand on small of your back. Gradually work hand up your back until fingers reach the opposite shoulder blade.
4. Slowly lower arm and return to standard position. Rest and repeat.

ELBOW PULL-IN

1. Stand in standard position.
2. Extend arms sideways to shoulder level.
3. Bend elbows, clasping fingers at back of neck.
4. Pull elbows in toward each other until they touch.
5. Return to position 3, with elbows bent and fingers clasped at back of neck.
6. Unclasp fingers and extend arms sideways at shoulder level.
7. Return to standard position. Rest and repeat.

*From American Cancer Society: Reach to recovery, exercises after mastectomy, patient guide, New York, 1983, The Society.

arm; simply turning the palm up and down will do this. Squeezing a rubber ball is often started on the first postoperative day. Brushing the teeth and hair are encouraged later but as soon as they can be tolerated. Under close supervision, the patient is encouraged to exercise each day more and more to the limits of incisional pulling and discomfort. A specific exercise schedule planned by nurse and patient together is imperative.

Continuing exercises are shown in the box on p. 1673. With exercise, full range of motion will return; that is, both arms can be extended equally high above the head. This will not be achieved before the patient leaves the hospital; therefore the patient must learn and be motivated in the hospital so she will continue exercises at home on a regular basis. Following radical mastectomy, full muscle power for horizontal adduction may be decreased.

Participation in classes with others who have undergone the same surgery may stimulate the patient to learn the prescribed exercises. However, for most women this is best done individually while other teaching and grief work can be coordinated. As soon as possible, normal activities supplement the exercises; and the patient is taught how particular exercises can be accomplished by specific tasks. The patient must know what motion is intended in each exercise. For example, the patient may brush her hair with the arm on the affected side, but she may lower her head and hunch her shoulders in such a way that she does not achieve normal use of the shoulder girdle. The whole intent of the exercise may therefore be lost. A small handbook entitled *Reach to Recovery* is given to the patient by the American Cancer Society Reach to Recovery volunteers; the nurse uses this in teaching and reinforcing the exercising. In addition to the book of exercises, the Reach to Recovery volunteer, as a woman who has had surgical therapy for breast malignancy, gives a colorful gift bag to the patient containing a rubber ball, a rope for exercising, and in most states a temporary soft padded brassiere of her size for going home (to be used until it is time to be fitted for a weighted prosthesis). The Reach to Recovery volunteer holds the potential motivating the patient; extending hope; providing visible evidence that femininity, personality, and activity can be retained; and being a good resource person as the patient moves from hospital to community. All nurses should be familiar with the volunteers and should sponsor the program. Often, whether or not the patient has the opportunity to use this resource depends on a nurse's initiating the contact.

Later, after the patient returns to the community, swimming is excellent exercise. Bathing suits used with prostheses are available in retail stores. (Reach to Recovery volunteers also supply a current regional guide to such stores.) Some areas have swimming rehabilitation programs for women with mastectomies. The ENCORE program is sponsored by the YMCA or YWCA.

Providing emotional support. Loss of a breast involves two major concepts: change in body image and mourning over loss. This reflects a physical loss and a sexuality loss, as well as changes in goals, plans, and life span. The patient is trying to cope with the fear of cancer and its potential spread and death. Removal of a breast for cancer is therefore an extremely stressful situation. The initial response is usually shock. Denial may take the form of the woman speaking about "the cancer" and the "mastectomy" but never dealing with her loss or her fears on a feeling level. Denial here is a conservation of energy. If she is to express herself on a feeling level, she must have someone who is capable and responsible to support her according to her need. If she does not receive this professional assistance, the impact of her loss occurs at a later date, when support systems may not be available.

Phantom symptoms of the missing breast occur in women with painful breasts or nipples before surgery.

Avoidance of looking at the dressing or incision can be expected initially. The incision is large, and the feeling experienced by most women is that of mutilation. Postponing looking at the incision delays the impact that the breast is indeed gone. Preparing the woman in advance concerning the size of the incision is helpful,

RESEARCH

The impact of mastectomy on self-concept and social function: a combined cross-sectional and longitudinal study with comparison groups, Women Health 11:101-130, 1986.

Self-concept and social function following radical, modified radical or simple mastectomy for stage I or II breast cancer; breast biopsy for benign breast disease; cholecystectomy; or no surgical procedure were assessed across a 15-month period in a cross-sectional design and across a 12-month period in a repeated measure design. Women selected for study were without other preexisting mental or physical illness. The degree of disability observed following mastectomy was considerably less than previously reported in uncontrolled studies, with the incidence of actual disturbance extremely small. Women receiving adjuvant therapies following mastectomy, but not women treated by mastectomy alone, reported significantly more body image dissatisfaction and feminine self-image concerns than the comparison groups. The findings refute previously published impressions of severe psychologic maladjustments following mastectomy. The study suggests that postmastectomy women vulnerable to poorer outcomes are those with lower expectations of quality social support, other present life stressors, other preexisting chronic diseases, and a disposition to believe in life outcomes as being less under their own control. ■

but she still needs considerable support when viewing the incision and her new image. She is usually physically capable when she feels stronger and begins to respond to others socially (about the third day). She is encouraged to look at the incision several times before discharge from the hospital, while health professionals are available for support.

Feelings of anger and resentment may occur and, if present, frequently are projected on female staff or friends. Families may also express anger or anxiety and may complain without cause about the care the patient is receiving. Feelings of decreased self-worth and self-esteem on the part of the patient plus increased dependency often produce depression in the patient. The feeling of being isolated and alone during this experience can be helped by interaction with others who have had the same experience, such as a visitor from the Reach to Recovery program.

After the patient is discharged, she may experience periods of depression if she perceives her recovery as slow or if she tries to reenter her previous activities and responsibilities before her energy reserves return. She may have difficulty sleeping or concentrating if she is still acutely grieving, with little recognition or little support. Although she will be aware of this, she usually will not express her needs; significant others can be told of her continuing need for support and patience and can help to extend the support needed. Sometimes the nurse can assess how the newly discharged patient is coping when she makes a home discharge telephone call. Often, simple misunderstandings or forgotten discharge information can discourage, frighten, or depress a patient during the first days at home. Some patients remain at home, avoid their friends, and hesitate to engage in social activities. The reasons for withdrawal from social participation may include fatigue and fear of rejection by others because of loss of body intactness. Healing of the incision and the underlying area so that she is able to wear a fitted brassiere and prosthesis usually reassures the woman and encourages her to participate in home and social activities. Unfortunately, it must also be recognized that the woman's fear of rejection may be real.

Helping prepare for sexual adaptation. Woods has identified various factors that can influence sexual adaptation following mastectomy (Figure 57-6). Women with very small or very large breasts may have longstanding, unresolved feelings about breast size and may also experience more difficulty in obtaining a satisfactory breast prosthesis. The woman who perceives the surgery as mutilating may withdraw from the sexual relationship, fearing rejection from her partner. Women who felt sexually inadequate before surgery may find these feelings enhanced postoperatively and use the surgery as a rea-

son for withdrawing from sexual relationships. Sexual and marital counseling is helpful for couples who are unable to communicate their feelings openly with each other. The woman with a recent mastectomy (or following radiation therapy) has altered tactile perception over the operated site and over part of the upper arm, sometimes for 6 months or more. She needs to be touched. This should be discussed and begun by her spouse in the hospital and not left for the initial difficult period at home.

Providing information on breast prostheses and clothing. Information about breast prostheses is given to the patient whenever she asks about them or appears interested; this may occur preoperatively but usually occurs postoperatively. The volunteer from Reach to Recovery provides current information and suggestions concerning prostheses and clothing, where it can be purchased, and current prices. The volunteer is often of great assistance in accompanying the patient as she shops for her first prosthesis. It is often very difficult for her to request a prosthesis at a busy counter filled with two-breasted women. The volunteer supports her; she does not recommend types of prostheses. They are a very individual choice and require fitting. Breast prostheses are not fitted until at least 6 weeks postoperatively or until the incision is healed and is no longer tender.

Until the incision is well healed, the woman is advised to wear one of her own brassieres, which can be lightly padded with a soft, fluffy filling (Figure 57-7), or a temporary soft prosthesis, which will not shift and embarrass her and which is available from the Reach to Recovery volunteer. Knowing her brassiere size, a friend could also purchase one of these for her home trip if she desires that. Plain cotton can be covered with gauze and lightly tacked to the inside of the brassiere. Opaque, loose-hanging gowns are usually most acceptable to the patient. Both gown and robe should have wide armholes to prevent constriction of the underarm. When the woman goes home, loose-fitting clothes with wide armholes are suggested.[16,60]

Breast prostheses vary in price, type, and weight (Figure 57-8). All women will want the prosthesis to make them look bilaterally symmetric and feel bilaterally weighted. Even the small-breasted woman will change posture if weighting is not balanced. All women need the assurance that the prosthesis will not shift and, unknown to her, create some odd position beneath her clothing. Firm, molded prostheses have the disadvantage of remaining elevated when the woman is lying supine, whereas fluid types have a more natural look.

Treating lymphedema. Many patients develop a slight edema of the upper arm that disappears within a week. A few patients, however, develop a severe edema that

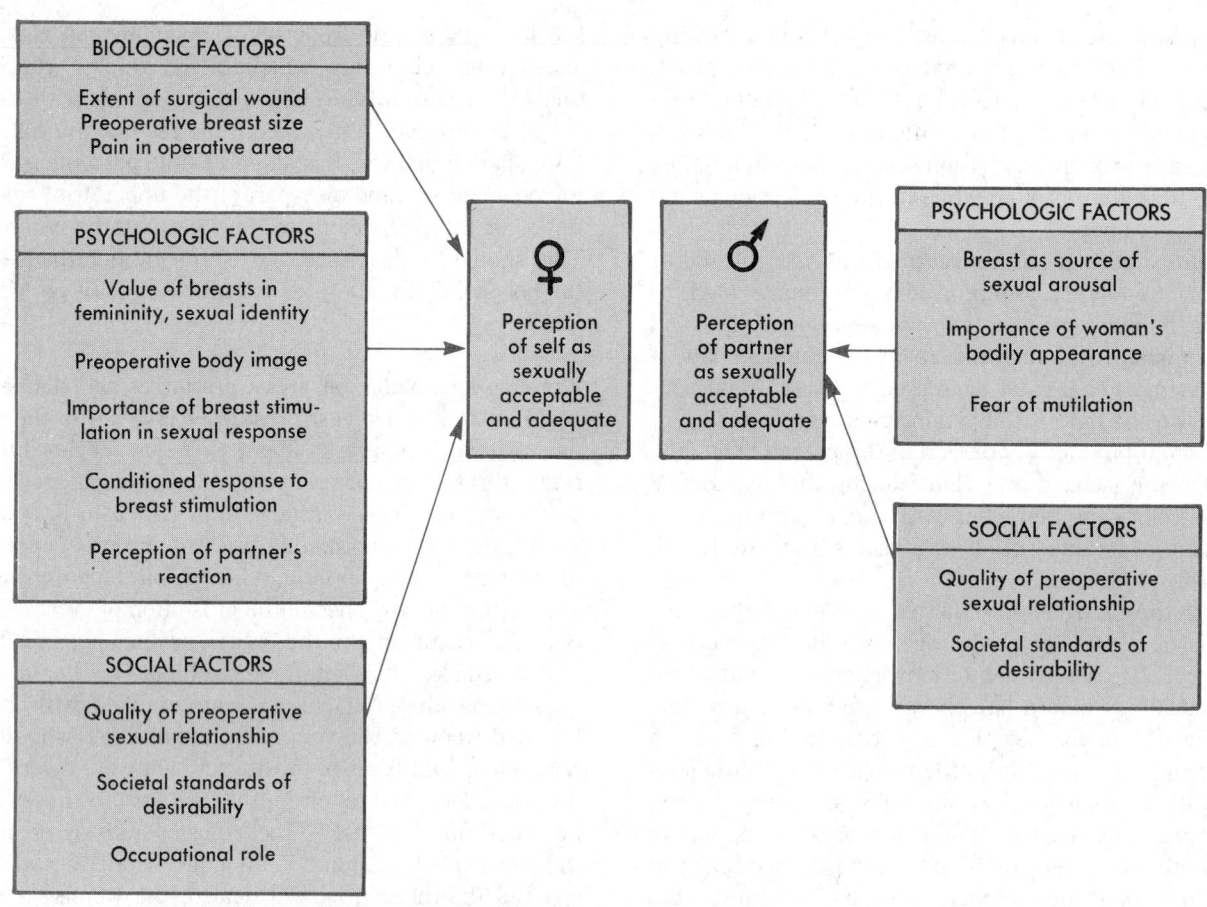

FIGURE 57-6 Factors influencing a couple's sexual adaptation to mastectomy. (From Woods NF: J Obstet Gynecol Neonatal Nurs 4:34, 1975.)

persists, that may become permanent, and that is caused by surgical interruption of lymph channels and nodes. The incidence is greater in women who are obese, develop infections, or are subjected to irradiation and chemotherapy. In some patients, lymphedema becomes more apparent after adjuvant chemotherapy. Some surgeons order an elastic sleeve that gives additional support to the vessels in the arm. This should extend from the wrist to the shoulder. It is similar to an elastic support stocking and usually may be removed when the patient is in bed. A diuretic such as chlorothiazide (Diuril) may be ordered to help relieve the edema.

Special care must be taken to prevent minor infections of the hands and arms in patients with lymphedema. If infections do occur, medical treatment should be sought at once, since the infection spreads quickly because of the improperly functioning lymph system. The patient is advised to use cuticle cream instead of cuticle scissors, to wear rubber gloves when using harsh household products, and to wear canvas gloves when gardening. The axillae should be kept clean with soap and water, deodorants used sparingly, and an elec-

tric razor used for shaving. Care is advised to prevent burns of the affected arm and hand. Injections, blood pressure measurements, and constricting clothing are to be avoided on the affected arm. These precautions should be taught to every women who has had a mastectomy (and radiation therapy), since they are also important to prevent lymphedema for the rest of her life.

Assisting with long-term adaptation. During the recovery period at home, many women experience varied symptoms that may last for several years. In a study of 49 women in North Carolina interviewed 4 years following a mastectomy, 53% reported one or more of the following symptoms still existing: swelling, weakness, stiffness, trouble moving and numbness of the arm, poor healing, and pain.[62] Approximately three fourths of the women experienced symptoms immediately following surgery, especially weakness and stiffness of the arm. The study also reported that women with many physical symptoms were more likely to have increased symptoms of depression. Measures that can be taken to prevent the symptoms from developing may assist the woman in

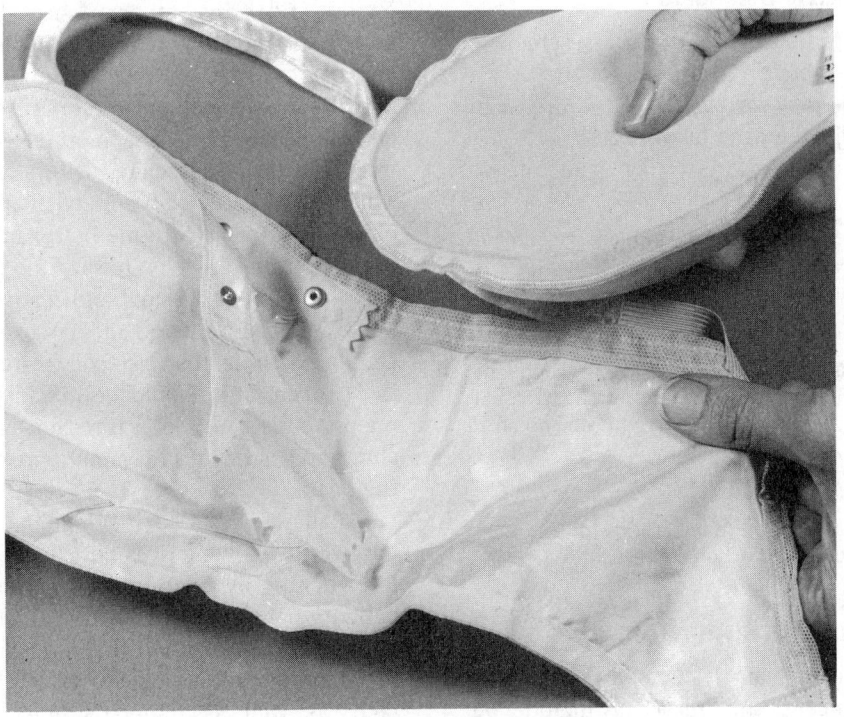

FIGURE 57-7 Inner pocket that will hold padding or breast prosthesis securely can be made in patient's own brassiere. Note snaps that simplify removal of padding.

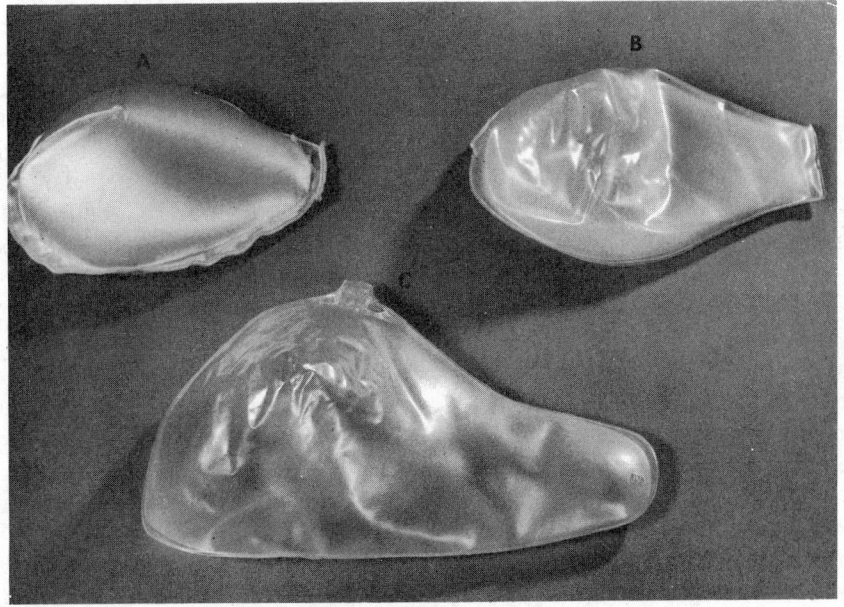

FIGURE 57-8 Three types of available breast prostheses. **A,** Foam rubber prosthesis. **B,** Prosthesis containing fluid. **C,** Prosthesis containing air.

her adaptation to the loss of the breast. She also needs to be prepared for potential occurrence of these symptoms.

RADIATION THERAPY

■ DATA ANALYSIS: NURSING DIAGNOSES

Nursing diagnoses are determined from assessment of patient data. Possible nursing diagnoses for the person receiving radiation therapy for cancer of the breast include, but are not limited to, the following:

Diagnostic Title	Possible Etiologies
External beam therapy	
Breathing pattern, ineffective	Therapy induced, pneumonitis cough
Fatigue	Therapy induced
Mobility, impaired physical	Difficulty obtaining transportation to treatment daily
Nutrition, altered: less than body requirements	Therapy induced, esophagitis, nausea, vomiting, dysphagia, altered taste and smell sensations
Skin integrity, impaired	Therapy induced
Interstitial therapy	
Knowledge deficit related to procedure and postanesthesia care	Unfamiliarity with information sources

■ PLANNING: EXPECTED PATIENT OUTCOMES

Expected patient outcomes for the person receiving radiation therapy for cancer of the breast may include, but are not limited to, the following:

External beam therapy

1. Patient is able to balance activities with frequent rest periods.
2. Patient lists ways to (a) minimize esophagitis, nausea, and vomiting and (b) increase adequate nutritional intake
3. Patient identifies and report symptoms to health care provider.
4. Patient mobilizes resources for daily treatment transportation.

Interstitial therapy

1. Patient identifies what to expect during procedure and postanesthesia period.

■ IMPLEMENTATION

External Beam Therapy

Intervention measures for the breast cancer patient receiving external beam radiation therapy include (1) promoting rest, (2) promoting nutrition, (3) preparing patient for possible side effects of therapy, and (4) assisting patient mobility.

Unless complicated by some other physical disability, the patient is an outpatient, traveling daily between her home and the hospital for therapy for a period of 5 weeks. Thus, although she may be surrounded by her usual support group at home, she may also try to carry full responsibilities at home. Often the outpatient is not recognized to be sick or to have as many needs as the person hospitalized. The woman receiving external beam therapy will have an extended period of waning energy and transient depression. Daily destruction of malignant and some normal tissue is taking place in her breast area; this controlled catabolic phase necessarily affects her. In addition to reduced energy, she may experience some nausea, sometimes some reflux discomfort (heartburn) associated with a transient esophagitis. This is especially pronounced if she also is receiving chemotherapy, as with methotrexate or 5-fluorouracil. A dry cough may develop toward the end of therapy. This may be frightening to her because she has probably heard and read enough media coverage on breast cancer to conclude that her cough indicates extension of the cancer. She should be quickly reassured that the pneumonitis cough is a transient result of minor exposure (unavoidable) of a small part of the lower lung to the beam.

To allay fears of such symptoms, since they may begin over a weekend, it is best to prepare the patient before therapy by relating some of the ways some other patients have experienced the treatment.[43] The patient requires assistance with handling nausea and fluctuating energies and an explanation of good nutrition intake, as well as understanding of the ever-present awareness that "I have cancer" and the attendant anxiety and grieving for her future.

The patient may also require assistance with transportation. Nurses should be aware of the American Cancer Society's Transportation Program and offer this resource before the patient becomes exhausted and considers dropping therapy. One of the greatest lessons of illness and convalescence is to be able to recognize that no one is independent or dependent; if we are mature individuals, we are interdependent. The nurse must help patients to be aware of the helping resources without feeling immature, inefficient, and afraid of losing face in their own eyes and others. The Washington Division of the American Cancer Society has started a Share-a-Ride Program through the offices of radiation oncologists. The Washington division also provides free housing at their Seattle headquarters for those who cannot make a daily trip involving 50 or more miles even with volunteer drivers. Details of these programs for patients may be obtained from the division office in Seattle.

The patient receiving external beam therapy for breast malignancy should receive the same considerations, emotional support, and teaching as she would have with surgery as primary therapy. A malignancy is present in her breast; it threatens her. Her breast may or may not ever look the same; it will not feel the same; she will mourn.

All the teaching, arm measurements, and precautions for lymphedema pertain to the patient receiving external beam therapy. Since few nurses usually work in the outpatient radiation therapy department, the patient may not receive this teaching. Emphasis on exercise is also lacking. All these measures should be started early for the patient's future benefit.

Interstitial Therapy

Preparing patient for procedure and postanesthesia period.
Interstitial therapy provides radiation "boost." It is the second part of the radiation therapy protocol for primary therapy of small lesions.

The patient may begin this phase immediately after completing the 5 weeks of external beam therapy. She will be hospitalized in a private room after iridium needles have been placed within the breast tissue under local anesthesia in the ambulatory surgery or special procedures room (Figure 57-9).

The woman's postanesthesia period should not be difficult, and she can move about her room with little discomfort. The needles are removed by a physician in her room after 3 days, and she is discharged. Unlike a patient with few needs, this woman requires support, teaching, sometimes crisis intervention, and always assistance with the isolating aspect that radiation safety policies impose on her, her visitors, and the staff.

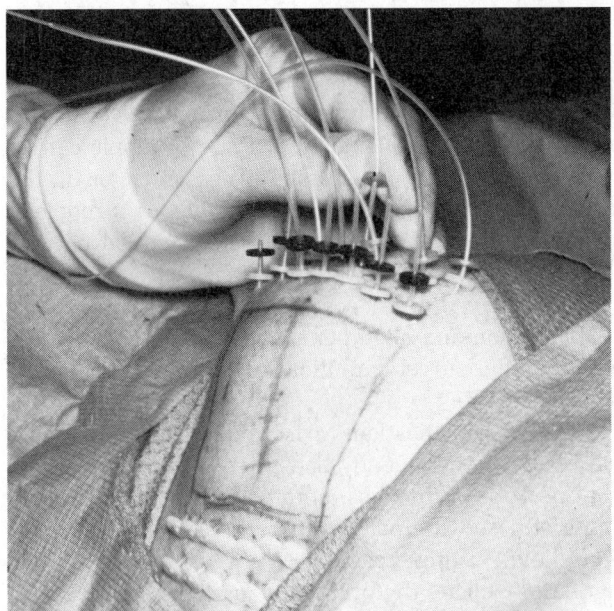

FIGURE 57-9 Interstitial therapy. Placement of iridium needles within breast tissue under local anesthesia.

CHEMOTHERAPY (ADJUVANT)

■ DATA ANALYSIS: NURSING DIAGNOSES

Nursing diagnoses are determined from assessment of patient data. Possible nursing diagnoses for the person receiving adjuvant chemotherapy for cancer of the breast include, but are not limited to, the following:

Diagnostic Title	Possible Etiologies
Coping, ineffective individual or family	Situational crisis over time
Knowledge deficit of medical information	Unfamiliar with information sources, information misinterpretation, cognitive limitation, lack of recall, anxiety

■ PLANNING: EXPECTED PATIENT OUTCOMES

Expected patient outcomes for the person receiving adjuvant chemotherapy for cancer of the breast may include, but are not limited to, the following:
1. Patient understands why side effects occur and will learn how to identify and report them appropriately and how to manage symptoms.
2. Patient mobilizes support systems.

■ IMPLEMENTATION

Intervention measures for the breast cancer patient receiving adjuvant chemotherapy include (1) preparing the patient for side effects of therapy and (2) providing support via teaching and continous monitoring of patient status.

Chemotherapy is usually administered on an outpatient basis. Depending on the therapy protocol, the woman with breast cancer may be traveling to the oncology clinic to receive her intravenous cytotoxic agents weekly to monthly for 6 to 12 months. Many of the outpatient issues that apply to the woman who receives radiation therapy also apply to the woman receiving chemotherapy. Teaching the patient about her drugs, possible side effects, and management is one of the major roles of the nurse. The cytotoxic agents most often used in adjuvant chemotherapy are cyclophosphamide, methotrexate, 5-fluorouracil, vincristine, prednisone, and doxorubicin (Adriamycin). Some side effects are minimal, whereas other drugs can cause discomfort (including nausea, which can lead to weight gain if improperly managed), temporary loss of hair, bone marrow depression, anemia, loss of appetite and fatigue, neurotoxicity, and rarely, cardiotoxicity. Some drugs may cause depressed reproductive function and change of life symptoms. If patients are irradiated concurrently, they may experience abnormally severe skin reactions, esophagitis, increase in other complications, and less satisfactory cosmetic effects.[57]

Since the patients often see the nurse more frequently than the physician, in addition to teaching and supporting, another important role for the nurse is continuous monitoring of patients' response to the multi-treatment modalities.

Many breast cancers are sensitive to hormones (estrogen, progesterone) and are partially controlled by them, depending on the hormone receptor assay results. In some breast cancers, beneficial effects can be received by adding hormones, removing glands that produce them, or administering antihormone drugs that counteract the hormones produced by the body.[55,56] Hormonal (endocrine) therapy often significantly increases the effectiveness of other cancer therapy. As with patients receiving cytotoxic agents, those receiving hormones need education, support, and close monitoring from the nurse.

BREAST RECONSTRUCTION

Mastectomy is the surgery women, especially black and Hispanic women, fear most; reconstructive surgery is the surgery women never thought possible.[49]

Reconstruction mammoplasty is a possibility for some women following a mastectomy. Both physical assessment and psychologic assessment are indicated before the procedure is considered. The patient must be realistic in what she thinks will be accomplished. The "you can be whole again" evangelism is detrimental. Preexisting psychosocial problems will not be solved by the surgery. Also, not all women think it is important or necessary to have a reconstruction. For some women, it is not essential to their positive self-image and esteem, femininity, or sexual experience. Many do not want the added surgery and attendant anesthesia, the costliness of time or money, or the pain. They are comfortable and active and successful without the added surgical procedure.

However, every woman should know about reconstructive surgery, whether it is appropriate for her stage of disease, and what it can and cannot do. She should have the opportunity to talk and read about breast reconstruction so she can determine its meaning for her. An excellent pamphlet, *Breast Reconstruction following Mastectomy for Cancer,* is available free from the American Cancer Society.[4] Attractive in format, it answers questions about such topics as insurance coverage, cost, how many procedures are necessary, and whether a nipple can be banked for later use or can be reconstructed. The pamphlet is designed for patient use but has been assessed for its readability at grade 13.[44] Since the woman contemplating breast surgery for a malignancy, whether educated or not, will have difficulty in concentrating on anything but the shortest words and sentences, this excellent pamphlet can be used to best advantage by nurses and patients speaking, reading, and interpreting the questions and answers in the bro-

chure together. It is recommended that all hospital units have a supply of this pamphlet and that professionals be familiar with it before discussion with patients.

In a study by Shain,[48] no difference was found in the degree of self-esteem, activity, or satisfaction with sex and "zest for living" between women who had reconstructive surgery and those who did not. The difference between these two groups of women lay in how the individual woman felt about her nude body. Reasons given by women who had reconstructive surgery were as follows: desire for a nipple; desire for greater freedom than an external prosthesis afforded in order to energetically play tennis, swim, and so on; desire for a feeling of normal contour when nude; desire to wear clothing that revealed breast cleavage; and desire to wear a wide range of clothes with no restrictions. Breast reconstruction is contraindicated when there is an aggressive tumor, a probability that metastasis has occurred, a concern about adequate healing being impaired, or unrealistic psychosocial expectation.

Reconstruction can be performed at the time of the mastectomy or, as is preferred by many plastic reconstruction surgeons, months later after some psychologic readjustment and physical strength and energy reserves have been achieved.

An early consultation with a plastic reconstruction surgeon is preferred; ideally the consultation should involve both the plastic surgeon and the oncologic surgeon working together. For the woman who makes her decision before her mastectomy, the plastic surgeon is often present at the mastectomy, when he can recommend incisional approaches, tissue salvage, or tissue banking, which is sometimes done for later use of the woman's nipple if it is free of disease. The surgery consists of a Silastic implant filled with silicone or saline placed under the subcutaneous tissue. A nipple can be reconstructed from labial tissue if necessary; or, in the absence of malignant cells, the patient's own nipple is sometimes banked on her inner thigh and salvaged at the appropriate time for reimplanting.

A brassiere is worn postoperatively to maintain implant position and alignment. Activity and exercise before and after surgery are individually prescribed by the plastic surgeon.

Possible complications exist: more anesthesia time for a person who recently had extensive surgery; infection; necrosis of the flaps, fibrotic contractures, or hardening of tissue around implant; and asymmetry in relation to the existing breast.

Shain[48] reports that women who have reconstruction surgery immediately after the mastectomy are less satisfied with reconstruction than those who have surgery after 6 months. This may result from not enough time to grieve for and see the loss. Grief cannot be hurried. A significant loss warrants significant grieving and an interval before a replacement is made.

The patient should have frequent medical checks by her physician and should know how to do a very thorough monthly BSE. She and her physician are somewhat handicapped, since tissue in back of the implants cannot be palpated or visualized by mammography. However, no current data seem to identify this as a risk to early detection of recurrent disease.

The American Cancer Society also has a program on breast reconstruction associated with their rehabilitation visitation program, Reach to Recovery. It includes volunteers who have had reconstruction because of cancer, who have been carefully screened as volunteers for the program, and who are carefully trained, supervised, and periodically evaluated. This is an additional resource for patients and professionals.

METASTATIC DISEASE

The progress of breast malignancy is from the primary mass foci (often more than one) through intramammary lymphatics to regional nodes and then to systemic dissemination, or it is from primary mass to extension of local structures (skin, rib) and then to systemic disseminated disease.

The most frequent metastasis of breast malignancy is to bone, lung, or brain. One of the most difficult concepts to live with when one has any cancer is the knowledge that it may metastasize. Cancer "cure" of 5, 10, or more years means cancer *control* for 5, 10, or more years. Thus all patients should be made knowledgeable about early symptoms that might signal disseminated disease and their responsibility to not delay further treatment, (often a different therapy protocol than before. This is difficult for a cancer patient and family because a cough along with coryza might cause spoken or unspoken anxiety: "Is it more than a cold?" Aching in a different area than the common arthritic pain may make an older patient wonder, "Is it more arthritis, or is it more than that?" Health providers must establish initial relationships with patients that make it comfortable and easy for them to recontact the professional for such anxious, nebulous, but often initial symptoms of disseminated disease. Guilt at treatment delay with initial disease need not be repeated again if relationships with the oncology team have been open and therapeutic.

Therapy for disseminated breast cancer is specific to the area involved. If the metastasis is found in the lung, surgical ablation, chemotherapy, and/or radiation may be used. The tumor board again becomes activated for the benefit of the patient's clinical management. Single and in-combination therapies are used. If the tumor was estrogen dependent, hormonal therapy and adrenalectomy may be performed. The sequelae of all these therapy interventions require further physiologic and psychologic adaptions. This is why strong coping mechanisms and supportive individuals and groups are necessary for the cancer patient and family. They live with cancer.

New battles must be fought by the patient's family with the occurrence of new therapies and their sequelae. For the first time the woman may have chemotherapy and meet a new adversary to her femininity; alopecia. The time to address this problem is when the chemotherapy protocol is planned; if alopecia is an expectation or possibility, she needs a wig prepared according to her hair and style. She should begin wearing it before she needs it, and she should wear it when she needs it. She may have new problems with eating because of stomatitis. Cookbooks especially written for cancer patients may be helpful. Bone metastasis will mean changes or cautions in ambulation and often pain. Adequate, round-the-clock, systematic administration of medication by patient or family is necessary for this deep, suffering pain. Radiation to the bone involved is also used to reduce pain.

The cancer patient is vulnerable to many infections, especially when metastatic disease has occurred. She must protect herself from others with infections and seek help from her physician at the early symptoms of infection.

Metastatic disease is a heavy burden. Patient and family may become overwhelmed with the disappointing hopes of successful therapy, a hiatus period of promise, and then recurrent symptoms. Hopelessness and giving up occur when coping is inappropriate or unsupported. These patients and families need help. Giving up and suicide ideation reflect perceived (and often real) inadequacy of help offered or given, often help by professionals themselves. Support groups offer one form of assistance to the patient and family. These may be held in the hospital setting or in the community by professional nurses or social workers. Helpful interventions by American Cancer Society volunteers, many of whom are physicians, nurses, and social workers, can also be obtained when the need is recognized and the helper alerted. Many communities have crisis clinics or crisis telephone hot lines. Use of the direct-dial Cancer Information Service through the American Cancer Society and the National Cancer Institute furnishes patients and families with immediate answers to their questions and their need of resources. Community resources for care, supplies, transportation, housing during treatment, assistance with insurance forms, and help seeking financial assistance are services offered to patients by the American Cancer Society in every state in the United States. Other programs also are needed by and available to the patient and family: (1) learning how to live with cancer, given in an 8-week group program called *I Can Cope;* (2) a support group of trained patients with cancer in a program called *Can Surmount;* and (3) local support groups facilitated by trained professionals. Information is available at all local offices of the American cancer Society as well as community hospitals.

Many facts about metastatic cancer are still unknown. Some involve the influences of the patient's interacting psychologies and spiritual and social aspects on the metastatic process, as well as the influence of the interfacing aspects of family, friends, and the helping-healing professionals on the patient and the metastatic process.

Cancer often kills. Sometimes, however, it seems that having cancer can become the beginning of living. The search for one's own being, the discovery of the life one needs to live, can be one of the strongest weapons.

Several years ago walking along a city street, I saw a familiar face in the crowd moving towards me. It was a woman patient I had not seen or heard from for over a year. She had had a terminal malignancy . . . . She was (now) walking so quickly with such a light but determined stride that she almost passed me by before she noticed me. She smiled happily, hugged me briefly, and then with a wave of her hand as she went her way, said she was in a hurry and shouted back to me, "I've been too busy living to get in touch with you." I watched her as she disappeared again. Going somewhere important; on her way. Alive. Living.*

NONMALIGNANT CONDITIONS OF THE BREAST
DYSPLASIA

Dysplasia (fibrocystic condition) constitutes the principal cause of benign breast problems, including lumps, breast pain (mastodynia), and nipple discharge. These changes are thought to be caused by hormonal imbalance or exaggerated response of breast tissue to ovarian hormones. Dysplasia is characterized by thickened nodular areas in the breast that usually become painful during or before menstruation. On palpation, cystic lesions are soft, well demarcated, and freely movable. The process is almost always bilateral. The most common site for the development of fibrocystic lesions in the upper outer quadrant of the breast. It occurs mainly in women between 30 years of age and menopause. In addition to palpable masses and mastodynia, fibrocystic changes may appear as clear, milky, straw-colored, or green nipple discharge.

The woman who discovers such a mass (or masses) in her breast should seek the advice of a physician, who will decide whether aspiration or biopsy should be con-

sidered. Little evidence suggests that dysplasia predisposes to the development of malignancy, but these women are considered more at risk than those who do not have fibrocystic disease. The presence of nodular tissue in the breast makes the early detection of malignant lesions more difficult. For this reason some physicians suggest periodic mammography or xeroradiography of the breast to detect any changes.

These women should be taught to recognize through touch their normal breast tissue and the location and size of areas of dysplasia. They should be encouraged to do monthly BSE. Other typically employed interventions include decaffeination, vitamin therapy, and hormonal therapy.

FIBROADENOMA

Fibroadenomas, or *adenofibromas,* comprise the second largest group of benign breast problems. These are tumors of fibroblastic and epithelial origin thought to be caused by hyperestrinism. Fibroadenomas are usually firm, rubbery, round, freely movable, nontender, and encapsulated; they are multiple and bilateral in about 14% to 25% of patients. They occur most often in women under 25 years of age. Fibroadenomas are usually slow growing and are often stimulated by pregnancy and lactation. Regression may occur following delivery. Fibroadenomas tend to appear more frequently in black women.[15] In general the association between fibroadenomas and breast cancer is very weak. However, it has been noted that women in their 40s are much more likely to have a malignancy within or adjacent to a fibroadenoma than are their younger counterparts.[14]

The woman who discovers such a mass should not delay in seeking medical consultation. Usually the tumor is removed with the woman under local anesthesia and is examined microscopically to ensure it is not malignant. The woman needs thoughtful nursing care, since she naturally is extremely fearful of cancer until the histology report reassures her otherwise.

MAMMARY DUCT ECTASIA

Mammary duct ectasia, also referred to as *comedomastitis* or *plasma cell mastitis,* ia a benign condition that involves inflammation of the ducts behind the nipple, duct enlargement, and a collection of cellular debris and fluid in the involved ducts. The primary risk factor for the development of duct ectasia is age, with a mean ranging from 45 to 55 years. Mammary duct ectasia apparently begins as periductal inflammation.[21] As the inflammatory response resolves, the involved ducts become fibrotic and dilated. Breast pain and a palpable mass are typical symptoms in premenopausal women; nipple discharge predominates in perimenopausal women; and nipple retractions secondary to periductal

---

*From LeShan L: You can fight for your life, New York, 1977, M Evans & Co, Inc. Reprinted by permission.

fibrosis are more often noted in postmenopausal women. Nipple itching may accompany transient pain in the subareolar and inner quadrant areas of the involved breast. Nipple discharge may be spontaneous and intermittent, ranging from serous to thick, sticky, or resembling toothpaste. The drainage may be green, greenish brown, or blood stained. On palpation, the areolar area may feel wormlike; the nipple may be red and swollen or may be flat or inverted.

Treatment plans vary depending on the severity of the problem. Most women with duct ectasia require nothing more than routine follow-up with physical examination. Nipples should be well cleansed to minimize the risk of infection. If an abscess develops, antibiotics and incision and drainage may be necessary. If a mass is present, surgical excision is performed.[15]

GYNECOMASTIA

Gynecomastia is a hyperplasia (overdevelopment) of the stroma and ducts in the mammary glands in the male. It usually appears as a firm, circular, disklike, circumscribed tender mass beneath the areola, usually unilateral at onset. It occurs most often during puberty and after 40 years of age. The cause is thought to be an abnormally large estrogen secretion. A gonadotropin (HCG-β) determination should be obtained, as well as chest and mediastinal roentgenograms and a careful testes examination, since germ cell testicular malignancy or lung cancer may show signs of gynecomastia and elevated HCG-β. Gynecomastia is also frequently seen following estrogen therapy for cancer of the prostate. It is a nonmalignant lesion, but physicians may suggest a biopsy specimen of the breast, because older men occasionally develop cancer of the breast.

The male is fraught with anxiety about the condition, which is little reduced by the information that it is a benign condition. This is the ultimate assault to the male self-image—enlarged breasts. The greater freedom of the male to be "topless" in the sun, at home, in construction work, and in recreation activities makes the developing and existent condition visible and joke provoking. Similarly, the infrequent male who develops breast cancer (unrelated to the dysplasia) and has primary surgical therapy has a publicly visible mastectomy, and the asymmetry is very apparent. The problems and needs of this patient still have not been fully recognized.

OTHER COMMON PROBLEMS OF THE BREAST
PERIODIC TENDER, PAINFUL, OR ENLARGED BREASTS

Although it is upsetting and uncomfortable to women, tender, painful, or enlarged breasts are normal functional changes in the breasts that respond to the monthly cyclic changes in estrogen and progesterone. Women who experience this "normal problem" require

reassurance, but above all they need health teaching about the normal changes that regularly occur in all women with functional ovaries or who have hormonal replacement. A reduction of dietary salt during the premenstrual period may be beneficial for some women.

BREAST PAIN

A small population of women experiences almost constant pain in one or both breasts. Careful assessment should be made to assure such a woman that infection, fibrocystic disease, or rarely a tumor mass is not present. This woman needs patient listening, understanding, and support from her physician and nurses. Breast pain is a problem unrelieved and unexplained to the woman who has it and is an idiopathic problem to the health professional, who currently can offer only symptomatic relief.

INFECTION
Skin

Women who wear no brassiere or who have large or pendulous breasts often have problems with yeast (*Candida albicans*) or *Staphylococcus aureus* infections, particularly during hot weather. This most frequently occurs under the breasts, where skin breakdown and maceration can occur quickly in the presence of heat, perspiration, and touching skin surfaces. It is accompanied by pruritus and bright, sharp pain and is often present for weeks before medical assistance is sought. Prevention could be taught to all women, in addition to teaching BSE. This would include encouraging frequent bathing of the breasts during hot weather, use of cornstarch to keep the areas under the breasts dry, and use of a supporting brassiere to reduce touching of skin surfaces.

Areolar Area

Some hair normally grows around the areola. If the hairs are plucked or if a depilatory is used, follicular infection by *S. aureus* or group A *Streptococcus* may occur. Women should be cautioned not to pluck hairs on their breast (rather, cut them close if unwanted) nor to squeeze any other pimple or skin lesion temporarily present on the breast. The local infection could progress to a breast cellulitis (mastitis).

Nipple

Infection usually results from cracks in the nipple during lactation. This condition occurs less often than previously because women are taught to "toughen" the nipple during pregnancy so that cracking during breastfeeding is less likely to occur. Since this infection often occurs when the new mother is at home, discharge teaching should involve care of the nipples, vigilance for problems that might develop, and encouragement for early treatment from her health provider. The most common organisms involved are *S. aureus,* group A *Streptococcus,* and *C. albicans* (rarely *Escherichia coli*); thus the untreated nursing mother can transmit the organisms to the feeding infant.

Breast

An infection can occur in the breast by direct spread from cracked or infected nipples, thus creating a cellulitis through the extensive breast lymphatic system. The pathogens may be transmitted to the mother's breast from the nasopharynx of the newborn infant who has been exposed to infected infants and hospital personnel or from the hands of the patient or hospital personnel. Staphylococcal and group A streptococcal infections develop most often.

Infections of the breast cause pain, redness, swelling, and elevated temperature. The woman's breasts feel "heavy" and "feverish," and the condition is not relieved by the baby's feeding; thus the symptoms are different from the engorged breast or "clogged ducts." The treatment is usually conservative. Antibiotics are typically given systemically. If the condition does not subside with conservative treatment and becomes localized to form an abscess, surgical drainage is necessary.

CHAPTER SUMMARY

✔ Factors placing the woman at high risk for breast cancer include age, personal or family history of breast cancer, parity, and environmental agents.

✔ Breast cancers can be detected early with regular breast self-examination (BSE), physical examination, and mammography.

✔ It appears that BSE skills are regularly practiced by women who are taught to look and feel for what is *normal* for them. This approach lessens their anxiety about finding "cancer" (pathology) each month, which discourages many from doing BSE regularly.

✔ Therapy for breast cancer depends on various factors, including histopathology, hormonal milieu, location and size of tumor, local or regional metastasis, and the woman's life-style.

✔ In the rehabilitation phase, women are working through the loss of a breast and its significance, learning to do wound care, initiating postmastectomy/lumpectomy exercises, mobilizing support systems, and pursuing prosthesis and clothing styles and possibly reconstruction options, if appropriate.

✔ Radiation therapy for women with breast cancer can last up to 6 weeks. Teaching includes mechanisms of radiation therapy's effect on cells, common side effects and management of side effects and symptoms. Interstitial therapy requires additional support and teaching on the isolating aspects imposed by radiation policies.

✔ Teaching the woman with breast cancer about chemotherapy includes information on medications and mechanisms for side effects and suggestions on managing and monitoring side effects and symptoms.

✔ Common benign breast conditions include dysplasia (fibrocystic condition), fibroadenoma (adenofibroma), mammary duct ectasia, and infections.

QUESTIONS TO CONSIDER

■ How would you help a woman who has a high risk for breast cancer, specifically in alleviating her anxiety and helping her understand the significance of a regular breast examination?

■ What approaches might you consider for a woman who has great difficulty accepting her diagnosis of cancer?

■ How would you respond when a woman tells you, "Most of our sex life has centered on my breasts. What am I going to do now that I will need a mastectomy?"?

■ When do you consult home care agencies to help a woman and her family live with her diagnosis of breast cancer?

■ How do you care for a woman who is so fatigued and weak from weekly chemotherapy treatments and ready to quit when therapy includes 6 more months of treatment?

REFERENCES AND SELECTED READINGS

1. American Cancer Society: 1990 Cancer facts and figures, New York, 1990.
2. American Cancer Society: oral contraceptives and breast cancer. FDA concludes no relationship—More Studies Recommended, Cancer Nurs 7:8, 1989.
3. American Cancer Society: Cancer statistics, New York, 1989, American Cancer Society Professional Education Publication.
4. American Cancer Society and American Society of Plastic and Reconstructive Surgeons: Breast reconstruction following mastectomy for cancer: questions and answers, New York, 1979, The Societies.
5. Baker LH: Breast Cancer Demonstration Project: 5-year summary report, New York, 1982, American Cancer Society Professional Education Publication.
6. *Bennett SE et al: Profile of women practicing breast self-examination. JAMA 249:488-491, 1983.
7. Byrne R: Utilization of thermography as a risk indicator in the detection of breast cancer, J Breast 2:43-47, 1976.
8. *Calle R et al: Local control and survival of breast cancer treated by limited surgery followed by irradiation, Int J Radiat Oncol Biol Phys 12:873-878, 1986.

---

*References preceded by an asterisk are particularly well suited for student reading.

9. *Chemotherapy and you: a guide to self-help during treatment, Pub No 88-1136, Washington, DC, 1985, National Institutes of Health.

10. Chilvers C et al: Oral contraceptive use and breast cancer risk in young women, UK National Case-Control Study Group, Lancet 1:973-982, 1989.

11. Cooper RG et al: Adjuvant chemotherapy of breast cancer, Cancer 44:793-798, 1979.

12. Danoff BF et al: Conservative surgery and irradiation in the treatment of early breast cancer, Ann Intern Med 102:634-642, 1985.

13. Dodd GD et al: Thermography and cancer of the breast. Cancer 23:797-802, 1969.

14. Duschenes L et al: Beware of breast fibroadenomas in middle-aged women, Can J Surg 28:372-374, 1985.

15. *Ellerhorst-Ryan JM et al: Evaluating benign breast disease, Nurse Pract 13:13-29, 1988.

16. Feather BL and Lanigan C: Looking good After your mastectomy, Am J Nurs 87:1048-1049, 1987.

17. Fisher B et al: The contribution of recent NSABP clinical trials of primary breast cancer: therapy to an understanding of tumor biopsy, Cancer 46:1009-1025, 1980.

18. Fishman J and Anrod B: Something's got to taste good: the cancer patient's cookbook, Farway, Kan, 1981, Andrews & McMeel, Inc.

18a. Fletcher GH et al: Long-range results for breast cancer patients treated by radical mastectomy and postoperative radiation without adjuvant chemotherapy: an update, Int J Rad Oncol Biol/Phys 17(1), 1989.

19. *Gallup polls: Women on attitudes on breast cancer, Am J Nurs 74:124, 1974.

20. *Gottschalk LA and Hoigaard-Martin J: The emotional impact of mastectomy, Psychiatry Res 17:153-167, 1986.

21. Haagensen CD: Mammary duct ectasta. In Diseases of the breast, Philadelphia, 1986, WB Saunders Co.

22. Harris JR et al: Breast disease, Philadelphia, 1987, JB Lippincott Co.

23. Hedley DW et al: Association of DNA index and S-phase fraction with prognosis of nodes positive early breast cancer, Cancer Res 47:4729-4735, 1987.

24. *Hellman S et al: Cancer of the breast. In DeVita V et al, editors: Cancer: principles and practice of oncology, ed 3, Philadelphia, 1989 JB Lippincott Co.

25. Henderson JC et al: Effects of adjuvant tamoxifen and of cytotoxic therapy on mortality in early breast cancer: an overview of 61 randomized trials among 28,896 women, N Engl J Med 319:1681-1692, 1988.

26. Hery M et al: Conservative treatment (chemotherapy/radiotherapy) of locally advanced breast cancer, Cancer 57:1744-1749, 1986.

27. Heston JF et al: Forty-five years of cancer incidence in Connecticut: 1935-1979, National Cancer Institute Monograph, (in press).

28. Homer M: Breast imaging: pitfalls, controversies and some practical thoughts, Radiol Clin North Am 23:459-472, 1985.

29. Horns JW and Arndt RD: Percutaneous spot localization of nonpalpable lesions, Am J Roentgenol 127:253-256, 1976.

30. Huguley CM Jr and Brown RL: The value of breast self-examination, Cancer 47:989-995, 1981.

31. Israel L et al: Two years of high-dose cyclophosphamide and S-fluorouracil followed by surgery after 3 months for acute inflammatory breast carcinomas, Cancer 57:24-28, 1986.

32. Jassak PF: Male Breast Cancer, Innovat Oncol Nurs 2:1, 1986.

33. *KOMO-TV 4: Getting in touch with yourself—a follow-along guide to breast self-examination (videotape), Seattle, 1988.

34. Kurtz JM et al: The second ten years: long-term risks of breast conservation in early breast cancer, Int J Radoat Oncol Biol Phys 9:1191-1194, 1983.

35. Leffall LD: Breast cancer in black women, Cancer 31:4, 1981.

36. McGuire WC and Dressler LG: Emerging impact of flow cytometry in practicing recurrence and survival in breast cancer patients, J Nat Cancer Inst 75:405-410, 1985.

37. Montague ED: Radiation therapy and breast cancer: past, present and the future, Am J Clin Oncol 8:455-462, 1985.

38. National Survey on Breast Cancer: A measure of progress in public understanding, Pub No 81-2306, Bethesda, Md, 1980, National Cancer Institute.

39. Nielsen M et al: Contralateral cancerous breast lesions in women with clinical invasive breast carcinoma, Cancer 57:897-903, 1986.

40. Nutrition and the cancer patient: an annotated bibliography of patient and professional information and education materials, Pub No 81-1511, ed 2, Bethesda, Md, 1981, National Institutes of Health.

41. Olsson H et al: Early oral contraceptive use and breast cancer among premenopausal women: final report from a study on southern Sweden, J Nat Cancer Inst 81:1000-1004, 1989.

42. Proceedings of the American Cancer Society National Conference: Meeting the challenge of cancer among black Americans, Washington, DC, 1979, The Society.

43. *Radiation therapy and you: a guide to self-help during treatment, Pub No 88-2227, Washington, DC, 1985, National Institutes of Health.

44. Readability testing in cancer communications, Pub No 81-1689, Washington, DC, 1981, National Institutes of Health.

45. Rosenstock I: The health belief model and personal health behavior, thorofare, NJ, 1974, Slack, Inc.

46. Rosner D et al: Influence of oral contraceptives on the prognosis of breast cancer in young women, Cancer 55:1556-1562, 1985.

47. Ross MB et al: Improved survival of patients with metastatic breast cancer receiving combination chemotherapy, Cancer 58:341-346, 1985.

48. Shain W: Facts every woman should know about breast reconstruction, New York, 1979, American Cancer Society.

49. Shain W: Reconstruction issues. In Proceedings of the Western States Conference on Cancer Rehabilitation, San Francisco, 1982.

50. *Schain WS: The sexual and intimate consequences of breast cancer treatment, Ca 38:154-161, 1988.

51. Silverberg E: Cancer statistics, Ca—A 35:19-35, 1985.

52. *Stillman MJ: Women's health belief about breast cancer and breast self-examination, Nurs Res 26:121-127, 1977.

53. Strax P: Results of mass screening for breast cancer in 50,000 examinations, Cancer 37:30-35, 1976.

54. Taylor EW: Results of limited surgery and irradiation for early stage breast cancer, Virginia Mason Clin Bull, 42:19-27, 1988.

55. Taylor SG: Adjuvant CMFVP versus CMFP plus tamoxifen versus observation alone in postmenopausal, node-positive breast cancer patients: three-year results of an eastern cooperative oncology group study, J Clin Oncol 3:144-154, 1985.

56. Tormey DC and Jordan VC: Long-term tamoxifen adjuvant therapy in node-positive breast cancer: a metabolic and pilot clinical study, Madison, Wis, 1984, Wisconsin Clinical Cancer Center.

57. Veronesi U et al: Comparing radical mastectomy with quadrantectomy, axillary dissection and radiotherapy in patients with small cancers of the breast, N Eng J M 305:6-11, 1981.

58. Veronesi U et al: Comparison of Halsted mastectomy with quadrantectomy, axillary dissection and radiotherapy in early

breast cancer: long-term results, Eur J C Clin Oncol 22:1085-1089, 1986.

59. Willis MA et al: Interagency collaboration: teaching breast self-examination to black women, Oncol Nurs Forum 16:171-177, 1989.

60. *Winkler WA: Choosing the prosthesis and clothing, Am J Nurs 77:1433-1436, 1977.

61. Wolfe JN: Risk of breast cancer development determined by mammographic parenchymal pattern, Cancer 37:2486-2492, 1976.

62. Woods NE and Earp JA: Women with cured breast cancer: a description of women's experiences four years after mastectomy, Unpublished manuscript.

63. *Zenmore R and Shepel LF: Effects of breast cancer and mastectomy on emotional support and adjustment, Soc Sci Med 28:19-27, 1989.

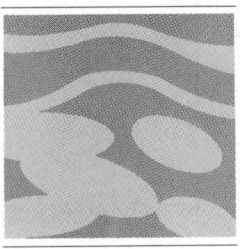

CHAPTER 58

Management of Persons with Sexually Transmitted Diseases

ELLEN FRANCES OLSHANSKY

CHAPTER OBJECTIVES

After studying this chapter, the student should be able to:
1. Analyze risk factors for development of sexually transmitted diseases (STDs).
2. Analyze the various organisms and associated clinical pictures for STDs.
3. Develop nursing diagnoses related to STDs.
4. Develop specific suggestions for persons with STDs and their partners.

SEXUALLY TRANSMITTED DISEASES

EPIDEMIOLOGY AND ETIOLOGY

Sexually transmitted diseases (STDs) are diseases that are *usually* or *can* be transmitted from one person to another with heterosexual or homosexual intercourse or intimate contact with the genitalia, mouth, or rectum. In addition to the five classic venereal diseases (syphilis, gonorrhea, chancroid, lymphogranuloma venereum, and granuloma inguinale), the STD category includes genital herpes infection, nonspecific urethritis, trichomoniasis, candidiasis, pediculosis pubic (crabs), scabies, genital or venereal warts, hepatitis B infections, molluscum contagiosum, and bacterial vaginosis (previously referred to as *Gardnerella vaginalis, Cornyebacterium vaginalis,* or *Haemophilus vaginalis* vagnitis).

These latter STDs might be considered the "new generation" of STDs, although they have probably existed since antiquity. Because of improved laboratory and epidemiologic methods, their prevalence, modes of transmission, and clinical consequences are better understood than in earlier decades. In addition, many of the newly recognized STDs have become epidemic or hyperendemic becauseof changing sexual behavioral patterns. Not only has the incidence of many STDs increased, but for agents with multiple modes of transmission (for example, hepatitis B virus, enteric pathogens), the proportion of infections transmitted sexually has also increased. In addition to the immediate consequences of STDs, there are newly recognized effects on

maternal and infant morbidity as well as on human reproduction and fertility.

AIDS (aquired immunodeficiency syndrome) is also considered a sexually transmitted disease but is addressed in Chapter 77.

All states require that each case of syphilis and gonorrhea be reported to the state or local health officer. Chancroid, granuloma inguinale, and lymphogranuloma venereum are reportable in most states. Herpes genitalis, trichomoniasis, and candidiasis are not reportable in any state. The true incidence of STDs is not known because of variable reporting requirements and also because many cases are not reported by the clinicians who treat them.

In explaining the trends of reported cases of STDs in the United States, *three changes* occurring in recent years are often referred to in the literature. The *first* of these concerns use of antibiotics and changes in the antibiotic susceptibility of pathogenic organisms. The widespread, perhaps indiscriminate, use of penicillin and other antibiotics between the late 1940s and early 1950s parallels the decline in both syphilis and gonorrhea. It is said that the organisms developed a greater resistance to antibiotics over time and that antibiotics have therefore become less effective than previously. No firm evidence indicates a decrease in effectiveness of penicillin against syphilis. However, the gonococcus tends to develop resistance to antibiotics.

A *second* explanation for the rise in incidence of STDs is that they are more likely to occur if a social system is permissive. During times of war and other catastrophes, it is easier for agencies to control interpersonal behavior, whereas in times of peace and absence of national crisis, civil liberties tend to flourish. The incidence curve of syphilis and gonorrhea (Figure 58-1) after the years of World War II seems to support this thesis.

The *third* explanation centers around sexual behavior patterns and includes permissiveness. Concern has

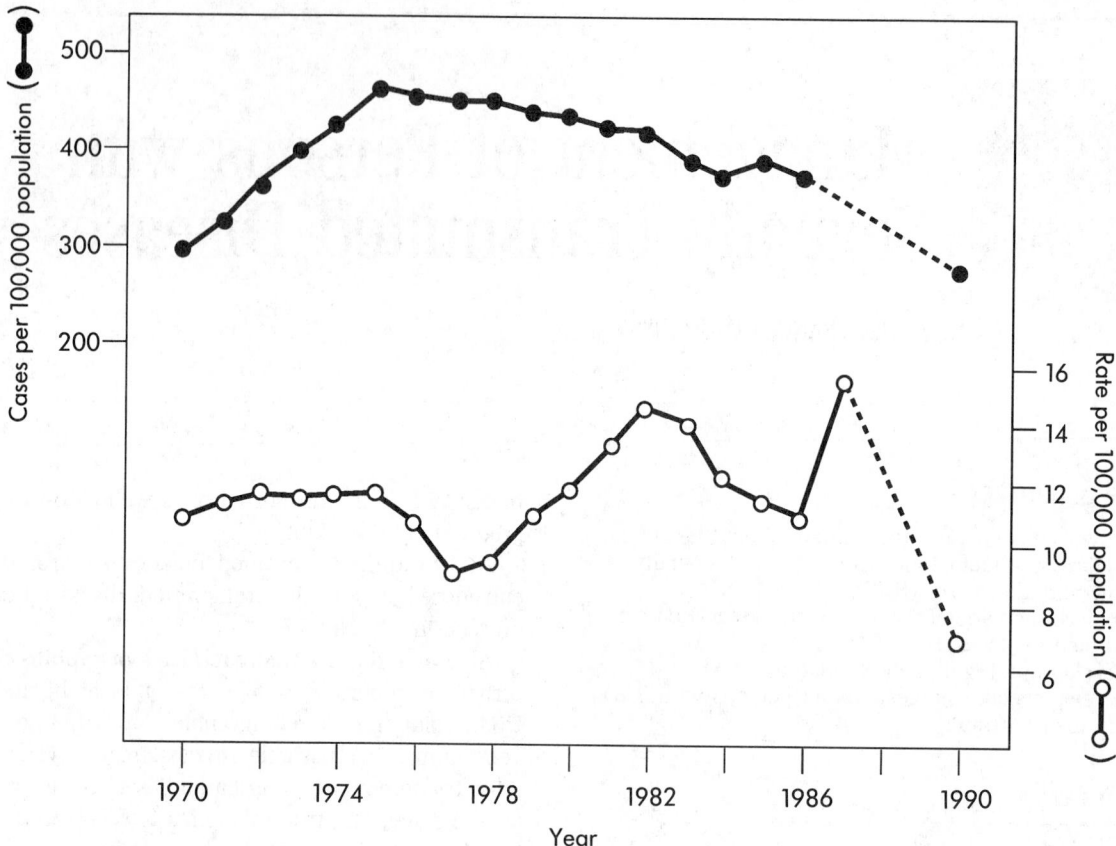

FIGURE 58-1 *(Top)* Incidence of gonorrhea in the United States by year, 1970 to 1990. The desired goal of 1990 is 280 cases per 100,000 population. *(Bottom)* Incidence of primary and secondary syphillis in the United States, 1970 to 1990. The desired goal of 1990 is 7 cases per 100,000 population. (From Centers for Disease Control: Progress toward achieving the national 1990 objectives for sexually transmitted diseases, MMWR 36(12):173-176, 1987; and 37(32):486-489, 1988.)

been expressed particularly about the prevalence of gonorrhea among adolescents and young adults who are considered to be promiscuous. Rates for gonorrhea show young adults 20 to 24 years of age accounted for 40% of reported cases of gonorrhea, whereas persons 15 to 19 years of age accounted for 25% of cases. The highest morbidity for males was in the 20- to 24-year age group; for females, the 15- to 19-year age group.[33]

The previous discussion makes an assumption of sexual promiscuity, and in doing so, requires acknowledgement of advances in contraceptive technology, especially "the pill." These social changes are often termed the three Ps (permissiveness, promiscuity, and the pill).[3] The underlying idea is that, with the advent of antibiotics and the pill, people began to lose fear of untreated venereal disease and pregnancy and that sexual promiscuity increased significantly, leading to increased exposure to infection.

If the definition of promiscuity is that sexual relations are not restricted to one partner, studies show that

patients diagnosed in clinics as having STD are not promiscuous. In one study, 66.4% of patients having an STD named only one sexual contact.[3] It must be realized, however, that persons may hesitate to admit to having more than one sex partner for various reasons.

In the past, prostitution has been considered a major force in the transmission of STDs. Before World War II it was estimated that approximately 75% of all STDs could be traced to prostitutes and that at least 10% of all prostitutes had contracted an STD at least once. Today less than 5% of patients with syphilis can be classed as prostitutes. Also, most persons with gonorrhea are single and under 25 years of age, and most clients of prostitutes are usually older, married men. *Chlamydia trachomatis* and herpes are two STDs that are very common in middle-class America.

Before 1960, homosexuals were rarely mentioned in the literature as carriers of STDs. Since the early 1970s, much more attention has been given to the risk of STDs among homosexual and bisexual men. Homosexual men carry pathogens in the rectum and colon, including gonococcus, *Giardia*, ameba, *Shigella*, and *Camphylobacter*. Although lesbians are at low risk for contracting STDs and gay males are at higher risk, it is important to note that sexual orientation does not prescribe individual forms of sexual behavior.

The condom was the main method of contraception used before the advent of antibiotics and oral contraceptives. The use of the condom may have prevented the spread of the STDs by providing a mechanical barrier to the organisms. The pill revolutionized contraception practices, and it is known that neutralization of the vaginal and cervical environment by estrogenic substances predisposes to infection. It would appear that individual characteristics of persons engaging in sexual activity need to be more closely studied before any conclusions about permissiveness, promiscuity, and use of oral contraceptives can be made.

The STDs are contagious diseases spread almost exclusively by contact during sexual intercourse; that is, when mucous membrane surfaces come in contact during genital, oral, or anal sexual activity. Since the causative organisms survive only very briefly outside a warm, moist environment, there is almost no way to contract STDs from toilet seats, towels, or bed linens. Although STDs are not usually transmitted in public restrooms, conditions caused by fungi, bacteria, and lice can be transmitted from water in unclean toilet bowls.

Women using a conventional toilet expose the vaginal and anal area to pathogens that can be introduced by the back splash of contaminated toilet water.

There are some notable exceptions to sexual transmission. During pregnancy the fetus may become infected in utero by placental transmission, and the infant may acquire congenital syphilis or be stillborn. Infants of mothers with gonorrhea may contract infections of the eyes (ophthalmia neonatorum) during birth, and unless treated, this can lead to permanent blindness.

PREVENTION AND CONTROL

Prevention and control measures for STDs include three levels of prevention. *Primary prevention* is directed at preventing the disease. This includes educating uninfected persons so that they can avoid contact with an infected person, identification and treatment of exposed persons who are asymptomatic, interviewing persons with infection for identification of contacts, examination and preventive treatment of contacts, educational programs for the public, and active involvement of professionals in programs of control. The goal of these efforts includes eradication of the reservoir of disease in the population. *Secondary prevention* is directed toward prevention of complications, and *tertiary prevention* focuses on decreasing the effects of complications.

The box below lists current guidelines regarding "safe sex."

SAFE SEX

One of the key elements of primary prevention of STDs is education regarding "safe (or safer) sex." The following guidelines are the current recommendations, based on updated information from Hatcher et al.[12]

1. A mutually monogamous relationship between two uninfected persons is considered the safest means of preventing STDs.
2. If a person is not in a mutually monogamous relationship, it is best for each partner to limit the number of other sexual partners.
3. When choosing a sexual partner, try not to engage in sexual relations with someone who has had many sexual partners in the past.
4. If one is not sure that his or her partner is free from any kind of infection, it is best always to use a condom made out of latex, with a spermicide (some condoms are made with spermicides; if not, spermicide can be used with the condom). Condoms should be used for vaginal and/or anal intercourse and for oral-penile contact.
5. If a couple is beginning a new sexual relationship, each partner should honestly tell the other about any known infections or risks for infection. If any symptoms are present or a question exists about possible infection, the person should be examined by a health care provider and treated when appropriate.

6. Oral-anal and finger-anal contact is considered unsafe. However, if this does occur, the hands should be washed well with soap and water before any other contact occurs.
7. Low-risk sexual activities (if no lesions present) include hugging, massage, body contact, dry kissing, and masturbation.
8. Probable low-risk sexual activities (if no lesions present) include vaginal or anal intercourse using a condom, oral-penile contact using a condom, oral-vulvar contact using a rubber barier, and mutual masturbation using a rubber glove.
9. Probably risky sexual activities include mutual masturbation without a glove and kissing with tongue contact.
10. Definitely risky sexual activities (unless each partner is certain that he or she is free from infection) include vaginal and anal intercourse without a condom, oral-penile contact, oral-vulvar contact, contact between a partner's semen or urine with a mucous membrane (vagina, rectum, urethra, mouth, eye), oral-anal contact, and blood contact (menstrual blood).

CONTACT INVESTIGATION

In the prevention and control of STDs, especially gonorrhea, emphasis was once placed on interviewing for information regarding sexual contacts. The named contacts were sought out for examination and treatment. Lay persons knowledgeable about the required reporting to the local health department of some of the diseases were very hesitant to name their sexual contacts. Young people often feared that their parents and the parents of the sexual partner would find out about their infection. Minors need to know that they can probably obtain treatment without parental consent. Presently most states permit physicians to treat minors for STD without obtaining parental consent, and several states are proposing changes in existing legislation restricting treatment of minors. People also may perceive reporting of STDs as a threat from an official agency and may hesitate to name their contacts out of a sense of protection if they do not know that no punishment is involved.

Interviewing the patient for contacts is done at the time of the initial visit in the event that the patient does not return for follow-up. This interview is probably best done after the patient is examined, the type of infection is determined, and treatment is prescribed. If assessment is accompanied by information giving, the person should be better informed about STDs and how they are treated, as well as more willing and able to give information about sexual contacts.

Interviewing for contacts involves two aspects. The patient is first asked to name sexual contacts. Second, the patient is interviewed for "cluster suspects," who are friends or acquaintances who may have been exposed to the same contacts or who have symptoms of an STD. Since one focus of STD control is on increasing self-referrals, the patient is asked to advise known contacts and cluster suspects to present themselves for examination and preventive treatment. Confidentiality is stressed. There is reason to believe that patients do not name all their contacts at the time of the first interview and that a reinterview will usually result in additional names of contacts. Because of the understandable reluctance of many people to name their sexual contacts, the patient may be given the responsibility of informing the contacts and advising them of their need for treatment. (The contacts are not named; instead, cards that permit both examination and treatment without identification are given to the contact by the patient.) The local health departments cooperate in locating, examining, and treating these contacts as necessary.

Whenever possible, the contacts of the infected person are located and advised to have an examination and tests as soon as possible. If the sexual contacts do not have symptoms of infection at the time of the first examination, treatment is instituted to halt infection. Giving preventive treatment to named contacts who have no clinical evidence of infection has gained popularity and acceptance in the United States, and indications are present that this same approach is being used more in management of patients having the "minor" STDs.

CURRENT AND FUTURE NEEDS

The epidemic nature of some STDs makes it evident that measures for control of spread need to be even more vigorously applied and that new measures may be necessary to check the spread of infection. Efforts to implement mass education and screening programs need to be continued. Program efforts are directed toward creating public awareness of the problem of STDs and their control methods and informing the public of the possible serious consequences of these diseases. There also is a need to expand screening, contact treatment, and diagnostic and treatment programs.

Little is known about some of the STDs. Surveillance over some of them is inadequate, so that even the true incidence of several sexually transmitted infections is not known. Treatment of several of these diseases is poorly understood because knowledge of the natural history of the causative organisms is inadequate. Such knowledge is necessary to understand the epidemiology of the spread of these diseases so that treatment and prevention can be better directed than is now possible. Diagnostic methods need to be improved so that they are more reliable and can be carried out inexpensively for large numbers of people. Alternative therapies for prophylaxis require the development of agents to be used specifically and with discretion for treatment of exposed individuals, for the treatment of persons sensitive to specific drugs, and for the management of pregnant women.

To better understand the modes of transmission and circumstances surrounding spread of the STDs, knowledge of human behavior is required. Considerable research has been done in recent years regarding sexual behavior patterns, contraceptive practices, and permissiveness. Although this has been helpful, little consensus exists about whether these variables influence the incidence and spread of STDs. Further study will add to the pool of knowledge, which can be applied in programs of detection, treatment, and prevention.

CLINICAL MANIFESTATIONS

Major STD syndromes include vaginitis, cervicitis, lower abdominal pain, urethritis, epididymitis, pharyngitis, proctitis, and skin or mucous membrane lesions. Some people may be asymptomatic. Please see discussion of specific STDs for detailed clinical manifestations.

MEDICAL MANAGEMENT

Treatment depends on the causative organisms identified through the history, physical examination, and laboratory tests and is discussed in detail in sections on the major STDs. It is not unusual for an individual to harbor two or more organisms simultaneously.

■ ASSESSMENT
SUBJECTIVE DATA

The following information is collected from the person suspected of having a STD:

1. Exposure to STD contact
2. Prior STD history, treatment
3. Sexual orientation: "Have you been having sex with men, women, or both?"
4. Timing of last sexual activity
5. Number of sexual partners in the past 2 months
6. Women are questioned about:
   a. Vaginal discharge
   b. Vulvar itching
   c. Dysuria
   d. Urinary urgency
   e. Lower abdominal pain
   f. Rectal symptoms
   g. Sore throat
   h. Genital lesians
   i. Skin rashes or itching
   j. Menstrual periods
7. Heterosexual men are questioned about:
   a. Urethral discharge
   b. Dysuria
   c. Genital lesions
   d. Skin rashes
   e. Itching
   f. Testicular pain
   g. Sore throat
8. Homosexual or bisexual men are asked the same questions as heterosexual men, plus about rectal symptoms such as pain, bleeding, discharge, and diarrhea
9. If hepatitis is also suspected, the person is questioned about:
   a. Dark-colored urine
   b. Clay-colored stools
   c. Fatigue
   d. Jaundice

OBJECTIVE DATA

Objective data include the following:

1. Inspection and palpation of the integumentary system, reproductive system, and anorectal area
2. Examination for women includes the following:
   a. Inspection of skin of lower abdomen, inguinal area, hands, palms, and forearms
   b. Inspection of pubic hair for lice and mites
   c. Inspection and palpation of external genitals, including perineum and anus
   d. Speculum examination of vagina and cervix

   e. Bimanual pelvic examination
   f. Palpation for inguinal and femoral lymphadenopathy
   g. Inspection of mouth and throat, including tonsils
3. Examination of heterosexual men includes:
   a. Inspection of the skin and pubic hair
   b. Inspection of the penis, including the meatus, with retraction of the foreskin and "milking" of the urethra
   c. Palpation of the scrotum
4. Examination of homosexual or bisexual men is the same as for heterosexual men plus the following:
   a. Inspection of the mouth, throat including the tonsils, and anorectal area
   b. Anoscopic examination if rectal symptoms present

■ DATA ANALYSIS: NURSING DIAGNOSES

Nursing diagnoses are determined from assessment of patient data. Possible nursing diagnoses for the person with an STD include, but are not limited to, the following:

Diagnostic Title	Possible Etiologies
Body image disturbance	Alteration of bodily function (sexuality) resulting from prevention of disease spread and prevention of reinfection
Knowledge deficit regarding cause of STDs	Lack of information regarding mode of infection transmission, ways of preventing infection
Sexual dysfunction	Alteration of bodily function (sexuality), lack of knowledge regarding "safer sex," psychologic stress caused by infection, and meaning of infection to sexual functioning

■ PLANNING: EXPECTED PATIENT OUTCOMES

Expected patient outcomes for the person with an STD may include, but are not limited to, the following:

1. Patients will state that they feel better about themselves and their body image.
2. Patient will demonstrate knowledge about cause, prevention, and treatment of infectious process.
3. Patient and partner will verbalize improvement in sexual functioning and satisfaction while engaging in "safer sex."

■ IMPLEMENTATION
PROMOTING BETTER BODY IMAGE

The nurse allows patients to verbalize their feelings of distress about body image and their sense of self related to the infection. The nurse validates these feelings and assist clients in putting them in perspective, encouraging ways of improving feelings about themselves, such as good hygiene, safer sex, and understanding the disease process and how to prevent and treat it.

IMPROVING KNOWLEDGE

The nurse teaches the patient about the etiology, mode of transmission, and spread of infection, as well as prevention of infection. The patient should understand self-care related to prevention and treatment. The nurse's first responsibility in STD control is to educate patients who may develop or have a sexually transmitted infection. Nurses must be knowledgeable about the diseases most prevalent, the signs and symptoms, methods used in diagnosis, treatments used, and where individuals can obtain help and information. Nurses also can influence the knowledge and attitudes of their colleagues and peers toward STD and its control. Nurses can exert influence in the community by taking an active role in programs of education. Perhaps the best way to reduce the risk of STD is for a person to know his or her sexual partner. Sexual activity with different partners increases the risk of infection.

Preventive measures such as washing or showering with soap and water and using condoms may also help but are no guarantee against STD. Good laundry and personal hygiene practices also may help reduce risk.

Before nurses can be effective in working with patients who have STDs, they must confront their own feelings and attitudes about STDs. The patient is often young, fearful of pain, and unaccustomed to surroundings in a clinic or physician's office. Young patients especially fear that their families and friends may learn they have an STD.

Once the diagnosis, tentative or conclusive, is made, focus should first be placed on obtaining a cure and preventing complications and reinfection. Many lay persons know that the treatment for syphilis and gonorrhea is penicillin, but they may not be fully informed about this and other aspects of treatment. Because some of the diseases respond to penicillin or other antibiotics, many people believe that all genital infections can be cured simply, and this is not so. Some people believe that antibiotics not only cure an infection but also produce immunity against reinfection as well. Persons receiving an antibiotic or other medications for STDs must be informed of the action of the drug, its duration of effectiveness, side effects, chances of cure, and the need for follow-up. They need to be advised that treatment failures do occur and that reinfection rates are high. Return visits should be encouraged whenever possible, since adequacy of treatment of all the STDs is evaluated best by laboratory analysis for the specific organism.

HELPING TO IMPROVE SEXUAL FUNCTIONING

The nurse encourages the person and his or her partner to attend a session to discuss their feelings and concerns related to sexuality. The nurse teaches them how to engage in "safer sex" while preserving their sexual satisfaction and desires.

PROVIDING SOCIAL AND EMOTIONAL SUPPORT

Many patients focus on how the diseases are spread rather than on the consequences of having an infection. For single persons, contracting an STD and securing help means they must admit to sexual activity, and some of them may feel guilty. Patients with an STD have not only a physical but a social, emotional, and perhaps economic problem as well. They need constructive and comprehensive help. The nurse who is successful in working with persons having an STD is one who can create an atmosphere of trust in which the person feels free to discuss all aspects of the problem.

Persons who seek help recognize they have a problem; they want to get better and stay well. Because of this, they are highly motivated to do what is necessary, are receptive to information and advice, and are attentive when advice is given. Nurses can take advantage of the patient's readiness to learn and motivation to improve and maintain health.

PROMOTING SELF-CARE

Persons treated for sexually transmitted infections need information about self-care. To understand their therapy and responsibly engage in self-care, they must be informed about the sexual nature of the infection, how it is transmitted, and the possibility of reinfection and infection of their sexual partner(s). The patient needs to know that it is important for sexual partners to be checked for signs of infection, to be advised of what the signs are, and have a culture done for asymptomatic infection. Patients should be advised to abstain from intercourse until cured. If sexual intercourse cannot be avoided, condoms should be used by men to prevent the possibility of infection or reinfection.

Teaching about hygiene and personal health practices is beneficial in reducing the chances of secondary infection, recurrence, and infections of various types in the future. Frequent bathing and handwashing are indicated. It is known that many of the organisms causing STDs are destroyed by soap and water. For women, douching is contraindicated unless it is prescribed for the purpose of applying heat or applying medication. All women should be informed that, for personal cleanliness, frequent douching at any time is not advisable, since this may disturb the vaginal and cervical environments and predispose the woman to infection. If douching is prescribed by the physician, the patient should be instructed in the procedure.

If the lesions are present on body surfaces, the patient should be instructed in their care. Unless contraindicated, a hot bath is taken two to three times a day, and lesions are kept as dry as possible between bathings. Both men and women should be advised to wear cotton underwear; women should be advised to avoid using pantyhose, since they tend to trap moisture and prevent circulation of air to the genitalia. Unless they are specifically prescribed as local medications, the patient should not apply any lotion, cream, or ointment to any of the lesions associated with STDs.

Self-examination is important for sexually active people, especially those with more than one partner. Inspecting skin, mouth, genitals, and perianal areas for lesions and discharges is recommended. In addition, people can learn to inspect their partners casually during the initial lovemaking to identify any signs of STDs. Urinating after sexual activity can be helpful in cleansing the urethra of organisms.

PROMOTING HEALTHY SEXUAL ATTITUDES

Opportunities for promoting healthy attitudes about sexual activity and STDs also frequently arise. These topics are approached tactfully and with consideration of the patient's feelings. Adolescents especially require an approach that indicates understanding balanced with the ability to help them set limits. Developmental tasks of adolescence require that young people find means of sexual gratification within the context of meaningful sexual relationships. In their search, adolescents need to be reassured that mutually rewarding relationships involving sexual gratification can be fulfilling. Within this context, however, adolescents need to recognize that consequences of their behavior may include unwanted pregnancy and STD.

Development of prophylactic vaccines, especially for gonorrhea and syphilis, needs to be given high priority. To accomplish this, techniques for growing the organisms must be developed, and this in turn requires knowledge of the natural history and evolution of specific organisms, including viruses.

History has revealed that treatment alone has never conquered any of the major communicable diseases. Rather, programs through which the public becomes better informed and demands services, as well as the development of protective vaccines, have almost always been universally successful in preventing disease.

GONORRHEA

EPIDEMIOLOGY, ETIOLOGY, AND PATHOPHYSIOLOGY

Almost 400 cases per 100,000 population were reported in the United States in 1986 (Figure 58-1), making it the most commonly reported communicable disease in the United States.[31] The Centers for Disease Control has estimated that, although only 1 million cases of gonorrhea are reported each year, it is likely that 3 million cases actually occur each year in the United States[8]

This is because only 25% to 50% of the patients with gonorrhea treated by private physicians are reported, and women have little or no signs or symptoms of infection, so underdiagnosis may occur. Young adults 20 to 24 years of age are at highest risk of acquiring gonorrhea, with the next highest rates found among adolescents 15 to 19 years of age. One of every 30 adolescents in this age group will acquire gonorrhea each year.[30]

Women and their offspring suffer the major physical, emotional, and economic burden of gonorrhea. Pelvic inflammatory diseases occur in 10% to 20% of women with gonorrhea; even when treated, these women are likely to suffer from recurrent salpingitis, ectopic pregnancy, infertility, and menstrual abnormalities and may face surgical removal of the pelvic organs as well as fetal loss.[30]

Asymptomatic persons or those with few symptoms are an important reservoir for infection, because they usually remain untreated. As many as 10% to 40% of gonorrheal infections in men are asymptomatic, and in women as many as 80% of infections are asymptomatic. Homosexual men can harbor reservoirs of anorectal and pharyngeal infections.[30]

Gonorrhea, often referred to as "GC" or "the clap" by lay persons, is caused by *Neisseria gonorrhoeae*. Gonorrhea is of great concern because of its epidemic rise, high reinfection rate, and seriousness of residual effects. The incubation period is 3 to 30 days in men and 3 days to an indefinite period in women.

PREVENTION

Prevention of gonorrhea and its complications can be achieved in three stages. The first and most crucial stage is prevention of the disease. The second stage involves prevention of complications of the disease, such as pelvic inflammatory disease. The third stage is reversal of the damage caused by the disease, such as by tubal reconstruction.

Early treatment of infected persons is currently the most effective measure to prevent new infection of sexual partners. Mechanical methods such as condoms appear effective when used. Education to acquaint people with the symptoms of gonorrhea, the efficacy of condoms, and the availability of diagnostic and treatment resources is also important. Early detection through contact tracing and screening can reduce the serious complications of gonorrhea. Experiments are currently in progress to develop and test an effective vaccine for gonorrhea.

CLINICAL MANIFESTATIONS
SIGNS AND SYMPTOMS

The most common signs and symptoms are listed in the box at right. In men the gonococcus is introduced into the anterior urethra during sexual activity. Because most men are diagnosed and treated early, complications and residual effects of gonorrhea are uncommon among men. Sterility from orchitis or epididymitis can occur as a residual effect, but this is rare.

The incidence of asymptomatic gonorrhea in men is believed to be low; however, there is an increasing awareness of the role men with asymptomatic infection have in the transmission of gonorrhea. Some men have been found to have no symptoms of infection despite positive tests for gonorrhea 2 weeks after exposure.

Gonorrhea in women most often begins as asymptomatic cervicitis, and the infection can be present for extended periods without causing noticeable signs. Thus there are many infected, asymptomatic women. These women do not receive treatment unless gonorrhea is diagnosed through screening or unless the woman is identified by the sexual partner and presents herself for treatment. Frequently, complications are the first indicators of gonorrhea in women. Salpingitis is the most common complication, with 10% to 20% of women presenting themselves with symptoms of salpingitis as the first sign of infection.[30] During the course of treatment for salpingitis, many women are surgically sterilized. In cases of untreated gonorrhea, the residual effects of chronic pelvic inflammatory disease, infertility, and ectopic pregnancy are well known.

Other complications of untreated gonorrhea in both men and women include dermatitis, carditis, meningitis, and arthritis. The incidence of these complications is higher among women because of the prolonged period of infection without symptoms.

DIAGNOSTIC TESTS

Gonorrheal infection may be suspected on the basis of history, symptoms, and clinical evidence obtained by physical examination. However, identification of the organism is necessary to confirm the diagnosis and to rule out other problems. In men the diagnosis is confirmed by Gram-stained smear of the discharge from the penis. Culture of the discharge from the penis is usually reserved for those whose smears are negative in the presence of strong clinical evidence.

Gram-stained cervical smears are inadequate for diagnosing gonorrhea in women. These smears are negative in about 50% of women having gonorrhea and are falsely positive in some cases. Therefore cultures from the cervix, urethra, throat, and anus are usually taken. Because of the long time required to obtain reports of cultures for gonorrhea, treatment is usually instituted on a presumptive basis.

SIGNS AND SYMPTOMS OF GONORRHEA

HETEROSEXUAL MEN

1. Urethritis—often first symptom
2. Severe dysuria—especially with first voiding in morning
3. Purulent discharge from urethra
4. Swelling of the penis and balanitis—rare symptoms

HOMOSEXUAL AND BISEXUAL MEN

5. Rectal gonorrhea common—usually asymptomatic and discovered by rectal culture
6. Pharyngeal gonorrhea—usually asymptomatic

WOMEN

Women rarely have early, distressing symptoms such as men have. When symptoms present, they include:
7. Slight purulent vaginal discharge
8. Vague feeling of fullness in pelvis
9. Discomfort or aching in abdomen
The above symptoms are so slight that they may be ignored.
If bladder involved—burning, frequency, and urgency, which usually cause the person to seek medical attention

INTERVENTIONS
MEDICAL MANAGEMENT

Therapy for gonorrhea presents a greater problem than for syphilis, because the gonococcus tends to develop resistance to antibiotics. It also is believed that inadequate therapy often occurs in the United States. Several drug regimens are in use, with emphasis on single-dose treatment to avoid problems with follow-up and patient cooperation. Recommended regimens include tetracycline, 500 mg four times daily for at least 7 days, or amoxicillin, 3 g (or ampicillin, 3.5 g) with probenicid; 1 g by mouth as a single-dose treatment for those who are unlikely to complete a multiple-dose schedule. Women and men with anorectal or pharyngeal infections are usually treated with 4.8 million units of aqueous procaine penicillin G injected intramuscularly in two sites, with 1 g of probenecid by mouth just before injection. The tetracycline regimen is effective against nongonococcal organisms such as chlamydiae, as well as gonococcus, but should not be given to pregnant women or children under 8 years of age.

Those who are allergic to penicillins or probenecid or who cannot tolerate tetracycline may be given spectinomycin, 2 g in one injection; ampicillin, 3.5 g; or amoxicillin, 3 g, all with 1 g of probenecid by mouth. Spectinomycin is the drug of choice for penicillinase-producing *N. gonorrhoeae*. The most common clinically significant reactions to penicillin are allergic reactions, of which urticaria is the most frequent. Before initiating treatment, it is important to screen for a history of previous reaction to penicillin.

NURSING MANAGEMENT

Nurses have a vital role in teaching patients about the mode of transmission and prevention of recurrence of gonorrhea. Nurses also assist patients and their partners to cope with the psychologic stresses and stigma of having an STD. Education regarding "safer sex" practices is essential. Encouraging proper adherence to the medical regimen is also an important nursing role.

SYPHILIS

EPIDEMIOLOGY, ETIOLOGY, AND

Syphilis is the third most frequently reported communicable disease in the United States, exceeded only by chickenpox and gonorrhea.[33]

Reported cases of syphilis reached an all-time high during World War II, with 575,593 cases being reported in 1943.

The number of cases dropped sharply in the 1950s and began to rise again in the 1960s. There was a steady yearly increase in the number of cases until 1977, when the total number of persons with infectious syphilis (both primary and secondary) decreased (Figure 58-1). This decrease has persisted each year since then. For example, the rate per 100,000 population decreased from 14.6 in 1982 to 14.1 in 1983.[33]

The trends for early congenital syphilis (CS) have parallelled the trends for primary and secondary syphilis among women. However, despite an increase of infectious syphilis in women between 1980 and 1983, the number of reported cases of early CS has stabilized. There were 259 reported cases of congenital syphilis in 1982. This number was reduced to 239 in 1983. However, an increase in congenital syphilis has been noted in 1985 and 1986.

Factors thought to contribute to the sustained level of early CS are (1) an increase in the incidence of early infectious syphilis among pregnant women, (2) lack of availability of prenatal care, and (3) failure of the prenatal system to provide timely serologic testing and prompt follow-up.

In addition, it is believed that the greatest percentage of cases of syphilis go unreported, and thus the incidence is much greater than the figures indicate.

Syphilis is caused by a spirochete, *Treponema pallidum,* that gains entry into the body through either the mucous membrane or the skin during intercourse. The organism is readily destroyed by physical and chemical agents, including heat, drying, and mild disinfectants such as soap and water.

The incubation period for syphilis is usually 3 weeks. However, symptoms can appear as early as 9 days or as long as 3 months after exposure; this is the case for rectal infections in homosexual men.

PREVENTION

As with gonorrhea, three levels of prevention are important. The first is prevention of the initial infection by finding and treating those with the disease. Secondary prevention is directed at early treatment of patients to prevent late syphilis or congenital syphilis. Finally, efforts can be made to treat the complications of syphilis when they occur.

CLINICAL MANIFESTATIONS
SIGNS AND SYMPTOMS

The signs and symptoms of the four stages of syphilis are listed in Table 58-1. If syphilis is adequately diagnosed and treated during the primary stage, the other stages can be prevented.

DIAGNOSTIC TESTS

Syphilis is most often diagnosed by standard serologic tests. Massive screening programs in the past made serologic diagnosis of syphilis very common. Mass screening with the Venereal Disease Research Laboratories (VDRL) test is no longer practiced except on high-risk populations, pregnant women, sexually active women, and couples who are applying for a marriage license. Dark-field microscopic examination of tissue scrapings from lesions or material obtained by aspiration of regional lymph nodes also reveals the presence of the spirochete, especially during the primary and secondary stages. A presumptive diagnosis is made on the basis of suspicious lesions, positive serologic tests, known exposure to infection, and involvement of regional lymph nodes. False-positive VDRL reactions are common among persons previously treated for syphilis, but fluorescent treponemal antibody (FTA) and absorption (ABS) tests are more specific (Table 58-2). Also, once a VDRL test is positive, it remains so and is not useful for identifying reinfection. Infectious mononucleosis, hepatitis, pregnancy, viral pneumonia, malaria, chickenpox, measles and smallpox vaccination, narcotic addiction, and terminal malignancy have also been associated with false-positive VDRL results.

INTERVENTIONS
MEDICAL MANAGEMENT

Syphilis can be successfully treated at any stage of the disease, although treatment may have to be more prolonged in latent and late syphilis. Although syphilis can be cured in late stages, the damage to the body is much less easily managed.

Because penicillin continues to be effective in the treatment of syphilis, it remains the drug of choice. All types of penicillin are effective, but penicillin G benzathine is preferred because it is long-acting and can be given in a limited number of injections.

Patients with primary, secondary, and latent syphilis

TABLE 58-1 Stages of syphilis

	Primary	Secondary	Latent	Late
Duration	2-8 wk	Appears 2-4 wk after chancre appears; extends over 2-4 yr	5-20 yr	Terminal if not treated
Signs and symptoms	Hard sore or pimple on vulva or penis that breaks and forms painless, draining chancre; may be a single chancre or groups of more than one; may be present also on lips, tongue, hands, rectum, or nipples; chancre heals leaving almost invisible scar	Depends on site; low-grade fever, headache, anorexia, weight loss, anemia, sore throat, hoarseness, reddened and sore eyes, jaundice with or without hepatitis, aching of joints, muscles, long bones; sores on body or generalized fine rash; condylomata lata (venereal warts) on rectum or genitalia	No clinical signs	Tumorlike mass, gumma, on any area of body; damage to heart valves and blood vessels; meningitis; paralysis, lack of coordination; paresis, insomnia, confusion, delusions, impaired judgment, slurred speech
Communicability	Exudates from lesions and chancre highly contagious	Exudates from lesions highly contagious; blood contains organisms	Contagious for about 2 yr; not contagious to others after that; blood contains organisms; may be transmitted placentally	Noncontagious; spinal fluid may contain organisms

TABLE 58-2 Serologic tests for syphilis (STSs)

Type	Description	Examples*	Comments
Flocculation	Antibody-antigen reaction produces a precipitation (flocculation)	VDRL RPR	Used primarily for screening; performed in standard laboratories
Complement fixation	Complement is used up in antigen-antibody reaction (fixed); hemolysis occurs	Reiter (Wasserman outdated)	Nonspecific; used less frequently; performed in standard laboratories
Fluorescent antibody	Antigen of killed *Treponema pallidum* is labeled with fluorescent dye	FTA FTA-ABS	More specific than flocculation or complement-fixation test; differentiates false-positive from true syphilis positive results; performed in special laboratories
T. pallidum immobilization (TPI)	Serum is mixed with live *T. pallidum;* paresence of antibody decreases organism mobility	TPI	Most sensitive test; performed at CDC laboratory in Atlanta

*VDRL, Venereal Disease Research Laboratories; RPR rapid plasma reagin;
FTA, fluorescent treponemal antibody; FTA-ABS, fluorescent treponemal antibody absorbed

(and their contacts) are usually given 2.4 million units of penicillin intramuscularly. Patients with late syphilis are generally given 2.4 million units intramuscularly at 7-day intervals until a total of 7.2 to 9.6 million units has been given. When the use of penicillin is contraindicated because of drug sensitivity, tetracycline in a total dose of 30 g over 15 days is effective (and over 30 days for late syphilis).

Pregnant women with penicillin sensitivity pose problems for treatment. In the large dosage required to treat syphilis, tetracycline produces mottling and staining of fetal teeth and possible abnormal bone formation may occur. If given the usual adult dose, inadequate placental transfer of tetracycline is likely, and congenital syphilis would probably develop. Erythromycin in a dose of 30 g over a 15 days seems to be the best alternative treatment for pregnant women with syphilis. Neurosyphilis is treated with intravenous penicillin. Contacts are treated with 2.4 million units of penicillin G benzathine.

NURSING MANAGEMENT

Nursing management of the patient with syphilis is similar to that for the patient with gonorrhea. Teaching is of prime importance, with emphasis on how the disease is transmitted and spread, as well as how it is prevented. Including both sexual partners in the teaching and counseling is ideal.

HERPES GENITALIS

EPIDEMIOLOGY, ETIOLOGY, AND PATHOPHYSIOLOGY

Herpes genitalis (genital herpes, HVH-2) is caused by infection with *Herpesvirus hominis* type 2 (HVH-2). Herpes genitalis is the most important STD of the past 15 years, though secondary to the more recent reports of AIDS. Its chronicity, frequent recurrences, and difficult treatment and prevention distinguish it from other STDs. It is estimated that about 400,000 to 600,000 new cases occur annually.[32] Conservative estimates are that 15% to 20% of Americans now suffer from genital herpes, and it is believed that because of poor control measures the number of cases is increasing dramatically.[30] Its peak incidence parallels the young age groups affected by other STDs. Once acquired, herpes genitalis is a lifelong disease and carries with it not only intense and recurrent discomfort, but also anxieties about future childbearing, malignancy, and sexual and marital function. In early pregnancy, women infected with herpes have an increased chance of miscarriage. Because genital herpetic lesions endanger the fetus during delivery, cesarean birth is often necessary. Genital herpes has also been associated with cervical cancer. It

is now generally accepted that HVH-2 is spread by sexual contact.

The incubation period is 3 to 7 days. The primary lesion appears as a vesicle on the external genitalia in men; often on the rectum in homosexual men; and on the vagina, cervix, or external genitalia in women. These lesions often ulcerate, especially when located on moist surfaces. Following primary herpes, the virus persists in a *latent* or *unrecognized* form in most patients. It is believed that latent infections are localized in the ganglia of sensory nerves to the genitalia. When the host factors favor it, the latent infection becomes clinically apparent as *recurrent herpes*.

PREVENTION

Primary prevention of herpes depends on limiting sexual contact between infected individuals and uninfected partners. Preliminary evidence indicates that the herpesvirus may survive on towels for up to 20 minutes; therefore it is important to use separate linens. Refraining from sexual intercourse while lesions are present and for 10 days after they heal is essential. Sexually active young persons should be taught to check themselves and prospective partners for such lesions. In some communities, groups of individuals with herpes have chosen to restrict themselves to sexual contact only with others who already have been exposed to herpes. Condoms may be helpful. Transmission to the fetus may be prevented by cesarean delivery. Infected neonates may develop subsequent mental retardation or die. If drug therapy for HVH-2 is effective, it will help limit new infections by eradicating at least some of the reservoir of infected individuals by preventing reactivation of HVH-2.

Secondary prevention is aimed at reducing or eliminating complications such as cervical cancer. A yearly Pap smear is recommended. Another important complication of the disease is its ability to create great psychologic pain and anxiety, disrupt normal social and sexual relationships, and stigmatize its victims. If secondary prevention is not possible, efforts are essential to detect and treat cervical cancer in its early stages.

CLINICAL MANIFESTATIONS
SIGNS AND SYMPTOMS

The common signs and symptoms of primary genital herpes infection are:
1. Local inflammation
2. Pain
3. Enlargement of inguinal lymph nodes
4. Generalized signs of infection, such as:
   a. Photophobia
   b. Headache
   c. Flulike symptoms

Primary infections are associated with local inflammation, pain, enlargement of the inguinal lymph nodes, and generalized signs of infection such as photophobia, headaches, and flulike symptoms. Although primary herpetic lesions begin as single or multiple reddish papules that then develop into clear, fluid-filled vesicles, once they rupture they form ulcerations that may fuse with other lesions to form large ulcerated areas. The disease tends to be more extensive in women than in men. In some women cervical infection accompanies the external lesions, and in certain cases it may be the only infected site. Cervical involvement may be mild or severe with extensive ulceration and pus. Genital lesions often worsen during the first 10 to 15 days but usually heal within 3 to 4 weeks. These symptoms usually lead the individual to seek medical attention.

Vaginal discharge is common among women, and discharge from the urethra is usual in men having primary infections. Urinary tract involvement may occur and is reflected in symptoms of dysuria or urinary retention. The lesions can cause severe pain, requiring hospitalization for parenteral analgesia. Subclinical infections, in which patients are unaware of any problem, occur in only about 10% of patients with genital herpes. Unfortunately, about 75% of all patients have at least one recurrence. Fortunately, recurrent infections are usually milder and of shorter duration than primary infections and usually produce local rather than systemic reaction. The patient experiencing a recurrent infection often has prodromal signs of paresthesia and burning at the site where the lesion will erupt. Factors known to predispose to recurrent infection include fever, emotional upsets, premenstrual states, and overexposure to heat and sunshine. Although the mode of recurrent infection is not clear, it has been theorized that during primary infection the virus ascends sensory nerve sheaths, localizing in corresponding nerve ganglia, and that when the environment becomes favorable, the virus is reactivated. Recurrent herpes usually begins with abnormal sensation or itching of a localized genital area. Lesions of recurrent infections usually occur in the site of primary infection. Herpes encephalitis may also occur.

DIAGNOSTIC TESTS

Diagnosis of herpes genitalis is made by isolation of the virus from specimens obtained from lesions. Pap smears or fluid from the vesicles collected in transport medium demonstrates cellular characteristics of viruses.

INTERVENTIONS
MEDICAL MANAGEMENT

Treatment for genital herpes has most often been symptomatic because no known cure exists for the disease. Acyclovir appears capable of inhibiting the replication of herpetic viruses in vitro, and in clinical trials with patients who had antibodies against herpes simplex viruses, acyclovir prevented active herpes infections.[24] Acyclovir ointment, 5%, is recommended for genital herpes. The ointment is applied to cover all lesions every 3 hours, six times a day for 7 days. The acyclovir treatment reduces viral shedding and the duration of the disease in patients with primary initial infections who are treated within 6 days of the onset of symptoms. *It does not prevent recurrences.* There is no effective treatment to prevent recurrences or to shorten their duration.

Persons with herpes should abstain from sexual contact while the lesions are present and for 10 days after the lesions heal. Risk of transmission during asymptomatic periods is unknown. Some advise using condoms to prevent transmission of the disease.

Symptomatic treatment consists of using Burow's solution of hydrogen peroxide and soap and water to cleanse the lesions. The involved areas are blown dry with a hair dryer, and the skin is then dusted with cornstarch. Women are advised to use a mirror to examine the vulva, vagina, and cervix for hidden lesions.

NURSING MANAGEMENT

Nursing management of the patient with herpes genitalis is similar to the management of patients with other STDs. However, one major difference is that herpes is an incurable disease. It is essential that nurses are sympathetic to the human response to this disease. Many patients are anxious and fearful that they will never be able to have a sexual relationship again because the partner is afraid of contracting the disease. Also, the patient may feel that he or she should not engage in sexual relations for fear of spreading the disease. Thus patient information and teaching are extremely important. With proper information, patients will be able to resume sexual relations and, with proper counseling of both partners, improve their communication with their partners.

CHLAMYDIAL INFECTION
EPIDEMIOLOGY, ETIOLOGY, AND PATHOPHYSIOLOGY

Chlamydia trachomatis infections are recognized as the most prevalent of the STDs in the United States. Because it is not a reportable disease, the actual number of cases is unknown. It is estimated, however, that each year 3 to 4 million Americans suffer from epidemic chlamydial infections. In Massachusetts, however, *Chlamydia* infection became a reportable disease; during 1986, 1200 cases were reported, whereas in 1987, 5470 cases were reported.[36] In England and Wales, where nongonococcal urethritis (about half the cases of

TABLE 58-3 *Chlamydia trachomatis* infections

Males	Females	Infants
TRANSMISSION		
Males ⟷	Females ⟶	Infants
INFECTIONS		
Urethritis	Cervicitis	Conjunctivitis
Postgonococcal urethritis	Urethritis	Pneumonia
Proctitis	Proctitis	Asymptomatic pharyngeal carriage
Conjunctivitis	Conjunctivitis	Asymptomatic gastrointestinal carriage
Pharyngitis	Pharyngitis	Otitis media
Subclinical lymphogranuloma venereum	Subclinical lymphogranuloma venereum	
COMPLICATIONS		
Epididymitis	Salpingitis	
Prostatitis	Endometritis	
Reiter's syndrome	Perihepatitis	
Sterility	Ectopic pregnancy	
Rectal strictures*	Infertility	
	Dysplasia	
	Postpartum endometritis	
	Prematurity	
	Stillbirth	
	Neonatal death	
	Vulvar/rectal carcinoma*	
	Rectal stricture*	

From Centers for Disease Control: MMWR Suppl 34(35):1, 1985.
*Associated with lymphogranuloma venereum.

which are caused by *C. trachomatis*) is a reportable disease, the incidence has nearly doubled in the 1970s and early 1980s.[28]

Chlamydial infections are responsible for about 20% of diagnosed pelvic inflammatory disease cases, and it is estimated that about 11,000 women each year become involuntarily sterilized and that 3600 have ectopic pregnancies as a result of this organism.[30] Chlamydial infections can be transmitted to infants during delivery, causing conjunctivitis and pneumonia in many. The ways in which chlamydia can be transmitted between males and females and children are shown in Table 58-3.

PREVENTION

Primary prevention of chlamydial infections consists of limiting sexual contact with infected partners. Secondary prevention requires early diagnosis and treatment.

CLINICAL MANIFESTATIONS

Chlamydial infections are usually diagnosed on the basis of history and pelvic examination. Women notice painful or difficult urination, abnormal vaginal discharge or bleeding, and possibly dyspareunia or other pelvic pain. Other women, however, are asymptomatic. Men usually have nonspecific urethritis or may seek treatment for epididymitis. Chlamydia can be diagnosed

by culture, but the test currently is expensive and inaccessible to many facilities.

INTERVENTIONS
MEDICAL MANAGEMENT

Urethritis is usually treated with tetracycline, 500 mg four times daily for at least 7 days, or doxycycline, 100 mg twice a day for at least 7 days. It is strongly recommended that partners of infected persons also be treated.

NURSING MANAGEMENT

As with other STDs, nurses play a key role in teaching patients about self-care and prevention of chlamydial infection, as well as about transmission and prevention of recurrence. In addition, *Chlamydia* specifically carries with it consequences for fertility; many women are infertile because of tubal damage secondary to untreated chlamydial infections. Much counseling is necessary in assisting patients to cope with this infertility.

LYMPHOGRANULOMA VENEREUM
EPIDEMIOLOGY AND ETIOLOGY

Lymphogranuloma venereum (LGV) is a systemic STD caused by *Chlamydia* organisms. Other species of

Chlamydia are the causative organisms of trachoma and psittacosis. The disease is contracted by vaginal, anal, or oral intercourse; and primary inoculation with the organism may occur at any site involved in close contact. The incubation period is 7 to 12 days. Lymphadenitis of regional lymph nodes draining the site of primary infection occurs, and the disease spreads by way of the lymphatic system.

LGV is most prevalent in the tropics. In the United States it is found most often in the southern states, but epidemiologic studies are needed to determine its true incidence. Reports of the incidence of LGV indicate less than 500 cases annually. The symptoms of LGV resemble those of other STDs, and its reported incidence may be influenced by this.

PATHOPHYSIOLOGY

There are three clinical phases of infection in LGV: (1) inoculation and appearance of the primary lesions, (2) lymphatic spread and generalized symptoms, and (3) late complications. In individual patients any one of the phases may be absent or go unnoticed.

The primary lesion, which is transient, appears as a papule, small erosion, or vesicle. The most common sites of the primary lesion are the prepuce and glans in men and the vagina and cervix in women. Since it is painless, the primary lesion may go unnoticed, especially in women. Localized edema may be present. If the rectum is infected, a bloody discharge is followed by a mucopurulent discharge, diarrhea, and cramping.

Involvement of the lymphatics follows appearance of the primary lesion in 1 to 4 weeks. If the primary lesion is on the penis, anal margin, clitoris, or upper vulva, the superficial inguinal lymph nodes are involved. Infection of the vagina or cervix as the primary site produces involvement of the deep iliac and anorectal lymph nodes. The large lymph nodes or buboes that appear are firm and lobular. The skin over the superficial nodes is bluish red and adheres to the nodes.

CLINICAL MANIFESTATIONS
SIGNS AND SYMPTOMS

The first indication of LGV infection in most patients is a feeling of stiffness and aching in the groin followed by swelling in the inguinal area. Symptoms of nongonococcal urethritis may be present. Constitutional symptoms of infection may or may not appear at this time. The involved lymph nodes may suppurate, causing extensive scarring. Obstruction of the lymphatics may result, leading to chronic edema and ulceration. Lymphatic spread of the infection is accompanied by generalized symptoms that vary. Mild to severe fever, malaise, nausea, and vomiting may occur. Abdominal pain, symptoms of cystitis, and urinary retention typically occur when pelvic lymph nodes are involved.

Acute proctocolitis is common in homosexual men.

Among the most severe complications of LGV are development of perianal abscesses, rectovaginal or rectovesical fistulas, and rectal strictures. In the final clinical phase, generalized infection is indicated by blood values showing anemia, leukocytosis, and elevated sedimentation rate.

DIAGNOSTIC TESTS

LGV is isolated from aspirate from an affected lymph node. The LGV complement-fixation test (LGV-CFT) is a test for antibodies. A positive LGV-CFT test along with a careful history and physical examination affords the best chances for diagnosing LGV.

INTERVENTIONS

Early antibiotic therapy is essential for controlling and reducing morbidity from LGV, and it is generally agreed that treatment should not be delayed until diagnostic test results are obtained. Tetracycline, 500 mg four times a day for at least 2 weeks, is the treatment of choice. If drug sensitivity or pregnancy precludes use of tetracycline, erythromycin, 500 mg four times daily for 2 to 6 weeks, is used. Flocculent lymph nodes may be aspirated to prevent scarring and destruction of lymphatic channels. This is usually done in conjunction with antibiotic therapy. Surgical removal of the lymph nodes is not advised, since this may increase lymphedema and elephantiasis.

If rectal stricture supervenes, rectal dilation at 2-week intervals may be attempted. Development of fistulas is especially distressing and requires that surgical repair be accomplished. LGV is a disease characterized by remissions and exacerbations, and thorough surveillance is important. Antibiotic therapy should be reinstituted as soon as symptoms of reactivation occur. Biopsy of lesions and lymph nodes is advised in chronic cases of LGV, because cancer may develop in the ulcerative lesions and may be overlooked as a result of similarity in appearance.

CHANCROID

EPIDEMIOLOGY, ETIOLOGY, AND PATHOPHYSIOLOGY

Chancroid is a sexually transmitted disease caused by a gram-negative bacillus, *Haemophilus ducreyi*. Although chancroid rarely occurs in the United States, with only about 1000 cases reported annually, a need exists for surveillance to determine an increase in incidence. Although it is found worldwide, chancroid is most prevalent in tropical and semitropical areas in the Orient, the West Indies, and North Africa. The disease occurs more often in men than in women and more often among nonwhite than white people. It is possible that returning military personnel may have introduced the disease into areas where it did not previously exist.

The incubation period varies from 1 to 14 days and averages 4 to 5 days. The primary lesion appears as an inflamed macule that rapidly progresses to vesicle and pustule stages. By the time the patient seeks medical care, the lesions have usually become ulcerated. Multiple lesions in various stages of progression may be seen and are caused by rupture of vesicles and pustules and autoinoculation. There may be single or multiple ulcers that are nonindurated and painful. Inguinal lymphadenopathy may or may not be present.

CLINICAL MANIFESTATIONS

In women the lesions of chancroid are most often found on the labia, anus, clitoris, vagina, and cervix. A few women do not have any lesions but may have signs of mild vaginitis. In men the lesions appear on the prepuce, glans, or shaft of the penis.

The ulcers found in chancroid are typically ragged and irregular. They are highly infectious and autoimmunity may occur, resulting in multiple lesions. The ulcers appear excavated, have a granulating, purulent surface, and are painful. Often, edema of the surrounding tissues is present. Involvement of the inguinal lymph nodes occurs in about 50% of all patients with chancroid within 2 weeks after appearance of the primary lesion. The buboes are most often unilateral, painful, and spheric in shape. The skin over the buboes is inflamed. The buboes tend to become softer as abscesses form. These abscesses in turn may suppurate and rupture, further spreading the infection. Generalized symptoms of infection usually appear when inguinal abscesses form.

Diagnosis of chancroid depends on demonstration of the organism. A specimen is collected by aspiration of a vesicle, pustule, or lymph node, or from the margin of an ulcer. A Gram-stained smear is prepared and visualized by microscopy.

INTERVENTIONS

Treatment consists of erythromycin by mouth 4 times a day for at least 10 days or an alternate regimen of sulfamethoxazole and trimethoprim twice daily for at least 10 days.

Local therapy for chancroid is beneficial for comfort and prevention of complications. Cleansing the lesions with a debriding solution three times a day aids in removing necrotic tissue and provides comfort as well. In men with ulcers of the glans or prepuce, the prepuce should be retracted during treatment unless there is edema of the prepuce. This site of ulceration may lead to phimosis, requiring circumcision once the lesions are healed. Cleanliness is essential for prevention of secondary infection.

DONOVANOSIS
EPIDEMIOLOGY AND ETIOLOGY

Donovanosis, usually called *granuloma inguinale* or *granuloma venereum*, is believed to be most often transmitted by sexual contact. The infection is caused by a gram-negative bacillus, *Calymmatobacterium (Donovania) granulomatis*, widely referred to as Donovan bacillus. The incubation period is unknown but is estimated to be 8 to 12 weeks.

Donovanosis occurs often in tropical and subtropical areas and rarely in the United States. It is very common in New Guinea, India, and the Caribbean. The disease is mildly contagious and probably requires repeated exposures for spread of infection. Predisposing factors are poorly understood. The disease more often affects men than women and is especially common among homosexual men.

CLINICAL MANIFESTATIONS

In donovanosis, lesions appear on the genitalia and in the perianal area. The most common sites of lesions are the prepuce and glans in men and the vagina and labia in women. The infection first appears with development of subcutaneous nodules. These elevated areas eventually ulcerate, producing sharply defined, painless lesions. The ulcers enlarge slowly and bleed on contact. With ulceration, the infection tends to spread along the pubic region. Involvement of the lymph nodes is uncommon but can occur and produce occlusion of the lymphatics, resulting in elephantiasis.

Smears of exudates taken from the lesions do not always demonstrate the causative organism, even when donovanosis is present. Therefore a sample of tissue is taken from the lesion, is crushed between two slides, and is stained. The specimen is examined for the presence of Donovan bodies, which represent the intracellular stage of the causative organism. Examination of a tissue sample also makes it possible to differentiate between donovanosis and cancer.

INTERVENTIONS

Tetracycline, streptomycin, and gentamycin are antibiotics used to treat the infection.

TRICHOMONIASIS
EPIDEMIOLOGY, ETIOLOGY, AND PATHOPHYSIOLOGY

A protozoan, *Trichomonas vaginalis*, is the causative organism of trichomoniasis. Evidence suggests that the incubation period ranges between 4 and 28 days.[21] Trichomoniasis may be the most frequently acquired STD in the United States, with an estimated incidence of 3 million cases occurring annually.[30] *T. vaginalis* organisms are found in 3% to 15% of women under the care of private physicians, 13% to 23% of women attending gynecologic clinics,[21] and 50% of women who have gonorrhea. There is no documentation of the rate at which asymptomatic carriers become symptomatic. Older women who experience changes in vaginal pH often exhibit the disease in the absence of new sexual contact.

Trichomoniasis is frequently viewed as an innocuous infection, but serious implications exist for health. During the postpartum period in women who have trichomoniasis, the rate of persistent fever, prolonged vaginal discharge, and endometritis is twice as high as in women who do not harbor the organism. About 90% of patients with trichomoniasis have cervical erosions and leukorrhea, and it has been suggested that chronic irritation may predispose to cervical cancer. Interpretation of cervical cytology, as in the Pap test, is unreliable in the presence of trichomoniasis, since the infection produces atypical cervical cells. Unless repeated cervical smears are taken, cancer of the cervix may be missed. Trichomoniasis results in urethritis; it also causes prostatitis in men 40% of the time; and finally, reversible sterility can occur as a result of inhibition of sperm motility by toxins produced by the organism.

CLINICAL MANIFESTATIONS

Only 25% of women harboring the organism are asymptomatic. Pruritus of the vulva and vagina is the predominant symptom among women. The itching may be so severe as to awaken the patient, and excoriation from scratching is common. Secondary infection of the broken skin may result.

Classically the symptoms of trichomoniasis in women are a copious, frothy, green or greenish yellow vaginal discharge, inflammation of the labia minora and lower vagina; and a red-speckled appearance of the vaginal canal and cervix. A small number of patients have this classic picture, which is usually described in texts. Most patients have a vaginal discharge, but it is small in amount and yellow, and some inflammation of the labia and vagina occurs. Itching is almost universally present, however, and dyspareunia, dysuria, and urinary frequency may also occur.

In men, urethritis and its symptoms of purulent discharge, itching, burning, and inflammation are the signs of trichomoniasis most often seen. Prostatitis, epididymitis, and urethral stricture may occur as complications among men. However, these consequences of trichomoniasis have not been extensively studied and are not well documented.

Diagnosis of trichomoniasis is most often made by preparing a hanging drop slide containing a specimen of the discharge and observing the motile organism under the microscope. Serologic and skin tests are currently being investigated but lack reliability so far. Because of the high incidence of coexisting gonorrhea, smears or cultures for gonococci should also be taken.

INTERVENTIONS

The treatment of choice for trichomoniasis is metronidazole (Flagyl) by mouth. Both partners should be treated simultaneously to prevent reinfection by the untreated partner at a later date. Vaginal inserts of metronidazole are less effective. The drug is known to cross the placental barrier. For this reason, it is not given to pregnant women until after the first trimester.

CANDIDIASIS

EPIDEMIOLOGY, ETIOLOGY, AND PATHOPHYSIOLOGY

Candidiasis, previously called monilial infection or monilial vaginitis, is an infection caused by a yeast form, *Candida albicans*. The overall incidence of candidiasis in the United States is unknown. Disagreement exists about whether yeast infections such as candidiasis should be classified as sexually transmitted. The organism is typically found on mucous membrane surfaces in women who have no symptoms of infection. The greatest incidence of candidiasis occurs during the ages of maximal sexual activity. The causative organism is frequently cultured from the urethra of regular male sexual partners, and urethritis and balanitis (inflammation of the glans penis) occur in up to 10% of men who engage in sexual activity with infected women. Women who respond to therapy and become reinfected are usually married women having one sex partner.

C. albicans is found in the mouth, gastrointestinal tract, and vagina of 25% to 50% of women. Differentiation between colonization and true infection may be difficult in some cases. Colonization rate and the chance of true infection increase in diabetic persons, during pregnancy, and with diseases or therapies that impair body defenses (use of broad-spectrum antibiotics, corticosteroids, oral contraceptives).

CLINICAL MANIFESTATIONS

Women having symptoms of candidiasis most often complain of pruritus of the vulva. A vaginal discharge that is thick, white, and curdlike is characteristic. The vulva appears inflamed and edematous, and excoriations from scratching are often present. White patches that appear to adhere to the mucosal surfaces are often seen in the vagina. Similar white, curdlike patches appear on the mucous membrane surfaces and tongue in newborn infants infected by the organism, causing a condition known as *thrush*.

Little is known about candidiasis among men. Symptoms of balanitis may be present, especially in uncircumcised men. Asymptomatic urethritis occurs in up to 10% of infected men.

Diagnosis may be suspected from the patient's history of predisposing factors and symptoms, but it is usually made by microscopic examination of a smear of the discharge.

INTERVENTIONS

Therapy for candidiasis consists of treatment with fungicidal creams, ointments, or tablets. The most frequently used fungicides are miconazole, nystatin, and candicidin. Relief from itching may be obtained from tepid sodium bicarbonate baths and clothing that allows adequate ventilation. Application of talcum powder or cornstarch is also helpful.

BACTERIAL VAGINOSIS

ETIOLOGY

Bacterial vaginosis, (previously known as *Gardnerella vaginalis, Cornyebacterium vaginalis* or *Haemophilus vaginalis*), can be cultured from 23% to 96% of women with vaginitis and is recovered from up to 50% of asymptomatic women.[25]

CLINICAL MANIFESTATIONS

Bacterial vaginosis is characterized by a small amount of homogeneous gray or grayish white discharge. The discharge usually has a disagreeable odor, and since it is less irritating than discharges caused by other organisms, pruritus is mild or absent. On inspection, the vaginal walls are slightly reddened, and the discharge appears to adhere to the mucosal lining. Some women are asymptomatic despite positive cultures. Diagnosis is confirmed by microscopic examination of a smear or culture of the vaginal discharge.

INTERVENTIONS

The treatment of choice for bacterial vaginosis is oral metronidazole (Flagyl), 500 mg twice a day for 5 to 7 days.[25] However, metronidazole is contraindicated during pregnancy. Other treatments are oral ampicillin given four times a day for 5 days; cephalosporin, 500 mg four times a day for 7 to 10 days; or tetracycline, 500 mg four times a day for 14 days. Many physicians recommend treating the patient's sexual partner at the same time.

HUMAN PAPILLOMAVIRUS

EPIDEMIOLOGY AND ETIOLOGY

Human *Papillomavirus* (HPV) has gained increasing attention because of its possible role in the development of cervical cancer. Forty-six HPV types have been identified related to a specific site of infection for each type.[16]

HPV was present 33% to 80% of women with invasive carcinoma of the cervix and in 22.6% to 93% of women with carcinoma in situ or severe cervical dysplasia.

The incidence of HPV has risen dramatically in the past decade. Estimates of 10% to 20% of American women of childbearing age having HPV are reported.[16] From 2% to 5% of pregnant American women are known to have HPV. This is significant in that infants born to women with HPV may develop laryngeal papilloma.

PREVENTION

Prevention of HPV consists of (1) avoiding sexual relations with persons in known high-risk groups; (2) using latex condoms if sexual intercourse is practiced; (3) avoiding any sexual behavior considered to be high risk, such as anal intercourse; (4) following up on persons who have a history of STDs, in utero exposure to diethylstilbesterol (DES), or immunodeficiency problems; and (5) encouraging cesarean birth for women with HPV.

PATHOPHYSIOLOGY

A hyperproliferative process occurs as warts develop; HPV causes warts known as *hyperproliferative benign epithelial neoplasms,* in which thickening of the squamous cell layer occurs. The transformation zone of the cervix is believed to be the area in which the infection occurs, and the anorectal region is thought to be similar to this cervical zone, a location susceptible to development of HPV.

CLINICAL MANIFESTATIONS

Keratinized, single or multiple painless growths develop, primarily around the anus, vulvovaginal region, penis, urethra, and perineum.[12]

INTERVENTIONS
MEDICAL MANAGEMENT

Medical management consists of accurate diagnosis based on visual appearance or with the assistance of culposcopy. Syphilis must be ruled out. Therapy usually consists of the application of podophyllin, 10% to 25% in tincture of benzoin. This is applied directly to the warts, avoiding contact with normal tissue by first applying K-Y jelly to the normal tissue. The podophyllin is washed off carefully within 4 hours of application. Several treatments with podophyllin may be necessary. Podophyllin is contraindicated during pregnancy. If this treatment is unsuccessful in removing the warts, alternative treatments are available, including cryotherapy, carbon dioxide laser surgery, electrosurgery, surgical removal, and 5-fluorouracil.[12]

NURSING CARE PLAN
PERSON WITH SEXUALLY TRANSMITTED DISEASE (STD)

DATA: Ms. Jones is a 24-year-old single woman who comes into the clinic with a chief complaint of vaginal discharge with an odor. On examination, not only is the discharge present, but herpetic lesions are noted as well. On wet mount, the discharge is found to contain trichomonads. The diagnosis is *Trichomonas* infection and primary herpes. Ms. Jones is treated with acyclovir and metronidazole.

The nursing history identified the following:
- Ms. Jones is currently sexually active with two men and has had sexual relations with five men during the past year.
- She has a history of *Trichomonas* infections and bacterial vaginosis.
- She uses oral contraceptives and has been for 2 years without problems.

- She is not taking any other medications. She drinks alcohol occasionally and does not smoke. She does not use street drugs.

Collaborative nursing activities include those to assess for:
- The presence of an STD
- Ms. Jones' response to a diagnosis of an STD
- Ms. Jones' ability to follow the prescribed therapeutic regimen

NURSING DIAGNOSIS

Body image disturbance related to alteration of bodily function (sexuality) resulting from prevention of disease spread and prevention of reinfection.

Expected Patient Outcomes	Nursing Interventions	Rationale
Patient states that she feels better about herself and her self-image.	Allow patient to verbalize and "ventilate" her feelings. Validate feelings where appropriate.	Expressing feelings may help gain perspective.

NURSING DIAGNOSIS

Knowledge deficit related to lack of information regarding mode of transmission of infection and ways of preventing reinfection

Expected Patient Outcomes	Nursing Interventions	Rationale
Patient demonstrates knowledge about causes, prevention, and treatment of infectious process.	Teach patient about etiology, mode of transmission, and spread of infection.	If patient understands situation, she may adhere to therapeutic regimen and understand how to engage in "safer sex."

NURSING DIAGNOSIS

Potential sexual dysfunction related to alteration of bodily function (sexuality), lack of knowledge regarding "safer sex," psychologic stress caused by infection, and meaning of infection to sexual functioning

Expected Patient Outcomes	Nursing Interventions	Rationale
Patient verbalizes improvement in sexual functioning, satisfaction in sexual relations, and understanding of "safer sex."	Discuss sexual relations and how they are related to infections; differentiate what is "safe" and what is "not safe."	Accurate information will give patient more confidence in having sex.
	Encourage sexual partner to attend counseling session (may be difficult in this case because she has two partners).	This improves communication between partners.

NURSING MANAGEMENT

Nursing management consists of teaching patients about the transmission, spread, recurrence, and prevention of HPV. In addition, teaching regarding the potential life-threatening consequences of untreated HPV and thus the need for careful follow-up after treatment is essential. Nurses also assist patients in dealing with the emotional sequelae of HPV, as with any STD.

OTHER SEXUALLY TRANSMITTED DISEASES

In addition to those diseases already enumerated, genital warts, hepatitis B infection, pediculosis pubis, and scabies are also considered to be STDs.

Genital warts (condylomata acuminata), caused by a papilloma virus, are the fourth most common STD in men and the third most common in women. Approximately 500,000 cases per year occur in the United States.[30] Genital warts occur in or around the vulva, vagina, cervix, perineum, anal canal, urethra, and glans penis. Their diagnosis is made by clinical appearance or histologic examination. Recommended treatment is podophyllin, 10% to 25% in tincture of benzoin applied weekly, or electrocautery. Recurrences are common. Genital warts enlarge during pregnancy and may cause hemorrhage or obstruction during delivery. They also sometimes undergo malignant change.

Viral hepatitis including A, B, and non-A, non-B, is more prevalent among homosexuals and prostitutes than the rest of the population, and is believed to transmitted by sexual contact.[30]

Pediculosis pubis, also known as "crabs," is caused by pubic lice. Although lice can be transmitted by bedding or clothing, they are often transmitted during sexual contact. They produce erythematous, itchy papules. The lice adhere to hair around the pubic area, anus, abdomen, and thighs. Diagnosis is made by observation of lice or microscopic observation of nits at the base of hair. Recommended treatment is 1% Kwell lotion or shampoo. One treatment per episode is necessary, but itching may persist.

Scabies, caused by mites known as *Sarcoptes scabiei,* is transmitted by close body contact, bedding, and clothing. Diagnosis is made from linear burrows, often characterized by a reddened papule containing the mite. Common sites are finger webs, wrists, elbows, ankles, and the penis. Nocturnal itching is common. A one-time use of 1% Kwell shampoo is recommended. Family, household, and sexual contacts should also be treated.

• • •

A sample nursing care plan for the person with an STD is found on p. 1704. The box above describes a study on condom promotion.

RESEARCH

Solomon MZ and DeJong W: Preventing AIDS and other STDs through condom promotion: a patient education intervention, Am J Public Health 79(4):453-458, 1989.

This article presents results of two studies that measured the effectiveness of showing a videotape to patients on knowledge and attitudes about condom use and patients' willingness to obtain condoms with free coupons. The videotape consisted of a story about a black woman who, after experiencing gonorrhea twice and pelvic inflammatory disease, learned to communicate with her partner about the use of condoms. The study used experimental design, with patients assigned to an experimental group who saw the videotape and a control group who did not. Results indicated that the experimental group demonstrated higher knowledge and more open attitudes regarding condoms, as well as greater redemption of free coupons for condoms. Implications of this study include the effectiveness of education and accessibility regarding condoms as a way of preventing STDs. ∎

CHAPTER SUMMARY

✔ Many organisms play a role in the development of sexually transmitted diseases (STDs). In addition, certain behaviors place persons at increased risk for contracting such diseases.

✔ The clinical manifestations of STDs vary with the particular causative organism. The sequelae of each also vary. Some may have consequences for future fertility, such as chlamydial infection, and others are incurable, such as herpes.

✔ Medical management involves treatment of the infection, prevention of recurrence, and prevention of the spread of infection to others. In addition, medical management involves prevention of adverse consequences from the infections.

✔ Nursing management involves teaching regarding the prevention of infection, as well as prevention of spread of existing infection and recurrence of infection. Such teaching includes self-care techniques, modifications of certain behaviors (for example, sexual behaviors), and correct adherence to therapeutic regimens.

✔ Counseling is a particularly important area for nurses as they assist persons in coping with the consequences of the particular diseases. Counseling regarding future fertility, infertility, and sexuality are key nursing roles.

✔ Including both partners in teaching and counseling is an ideal situation and should be encouraged.

QUESTIONS TO CONSIDER

- Describe the three levels of prevention for STDs and give examples of each.
- What important data must nurses obtain to make an accurate nursing assessment of a person with an STD?
- What are the goals of nursing care of persons with STDs?
- Describe some of the human responses to learning of the person with an STD.
- Describe the nurse's role in assisting patients who have learned that they have an STD.

REFERENCES AND SELECTED READINGS

1. Campbell C and Herten R: VD to STD: redefining veneral disease, Am J Nurs 81:1629-1634, 1981.
2. Chattopadhyay B: The role of *Gardnerella vaginalis* in "nonspecific" vaginitis, J Infec, 9(2):113-125, 1984.
3. Darrow WW: Changes in sexual behavior and venereal diseases, Clin Obstet Gynecol 18:255-267, 1975.
4. Darrow W: The gay report on sexually transmitted diseases, Am J Public Health 71:1004-1011, 1981.
5. DeMaria T: Sexually transmitted diseases. In Woods N, editor: Human sexuality in health and illness, ed 3 St Louis, 1984, The CV Mosby Co.
6. Eschenbach D: Recognizing chlamydial infections, Contemp Obstet Gynecol 16:15-30, 1980.
7. Felman J, and Nikitas J: Nongonococcal urethritis: a clinical review, JAMA 245:381-386, 1981.
8. *Fogel CI: Gonorrhea: not a new problem but a serious one, Nurs Clin of North Am 23:885-897, 1988.
9. Graduate education, gonorrhea: CDC recommended treatment schedules, 1979, Obstet Gynecol 55:255-258, 1980.
10. Grossman R et al: Management of genital herpes simplex infection during pregnancy, Obstet Gynecol 58:1-4, 1981.
11. Hacker S et al: Factors influencing the success of a community VD program held in a university facility, Public Health Rep 95:247-252, 1980.
12. *Hatcher RA et al: Contraceptive technology, ed 14, New York, 1988, Irvington Publishers, Inc.
13. Heller M: The gay bowel syndrome: a common problem of homosexual patients in the emergency department, Ann Emerg Med 9:487-493, 1980.
14. Herpes on delivery, Emerg Med 12:105-108, 1980.
15. Kramer M et al: Self-reported behavior patterns of patients attending a sexually transmitted disease clinic, Am J Public Health 70:997-1000, 1980.
16. *Lucas VA: Human papillomavirus infection: a potentially car-
cinogenic sexually transmitted disease (condylomata acuminata, genital warts), Nurs Clin of North Am 23:917-935, 1988.
17. Meheus A: Surveillance, prevention, and control of sexually transmitted disease, Am J Obstet Gynecol 138:1064-1070, 1980.
18. Meisels A: Is condyloma virus a potential human oncogen? Contemp Obstet Gynecol 16(3):100-106, 1980.
19. Miles P: Sexually transmissible diseases: fourteen sexually transmissible diseases currently recognized by the Center for Disease Control, Atlanta, Georgia, JEN 6(3):6-12, 1980.
20. Oill P: Herpesvirus type 2 infection of the genital tract, JEN 6(3):13-16, 1980.
21. Rein MF and Chapel TA: Trichomoniasis, candidiasis, and the other minor venereal diseases, Clin Obstet Gynecol 18:73-88, 1975.
22. *Ridenour N: Chlamydia, Nurse Pract 5(5):45-48, 1980.
23. *Romanowski B and Harris J: Sexually transmitted diseases, Clin Symp 36(1):2-32, 1985.
24. Saral R et al: Acyclovir prophylaxis of herpes-simplex virus infections: a randomized, double-blind, controlled trial in bone marrow transplant recipients, N Engl J Med 305:63-67, 1981.
25. *Secor RMC: Bacterial vaginosis: a comprehensive review, Nurs Clin of North Am 23:865-875, 1988.
26. Strauss R and Glimp T: Sexually transmitted diseases, Top Emerg Med 7(2):73-84, 1985.
27. Taylor-Robinson D: The bacteriology of gardnerella vaginitis, Scand J Urol Nephrol 86(suppl):41-55, 1984.
28. Thompson SE and Washington AE: Epidemiology of sexually transmitted *Chlamydia trachomatis* infections, Epidemiol Rev 5:96-123, 1983.
29. *Torrington J: Pelvic inflammatory disease, J Obstet Gynecol Neonatal Nurs 14(suppl):21-31, 1985.
30. US Department of Health, Education and Welfare, Public Health Service: Summary and recommendations of the National Institute of Allergy and Infectious Diseases study group on sexually transmitted diseases, Bethesda, Md 1980, National Institute of Allergy and Infectious Diseases.
31. US Department of Health and Human Services, Public Health Service: STD fact sheet, ed 35, HHS Pub No (CDC) 81-8195, Atlanta, 1981, Centers for Disease Control.
32. US Department of Health and Human Services: Sexually transmitted diseases: treatment guidelines, MMWR 31(2S), 1982.
33. US Department of Health and Human Services, Public Health Services: Annual summary 1983, reported morbidity and mortality in the United States, Atlanta, 1984, Centers for Disease Control.
34. US Department of Health and Human Services, Public Health Services: *Chlamydia trachomatis* infections: policy guidelines for prevention and control, MMWR 34(35), 1985.
35. Wasserheit JN and Holmen KK: Sexually transmitted diseases in women: approach to common syndromes in emergency medicine, Emerg Med Clin North Am 3(1):47-74, 1985.
36. *Whelan M: Nursing management of the patient with *Chlamydia trachomatis* infection, Nurs Clin of North Am 23:877-883, 1988.
37. Wilcox R: Sexual behavior and sexually transmitted disease patterns in male homosexuals, Br J Vener Dis 57:167-169, 1981.

---

*References preceded by an asterisk are particularly well suited for student reading.

ALTERATIONS IN COGNITION, SENSATION, AND MOTION

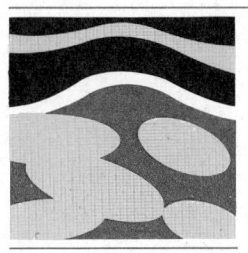

CHAPTER 59

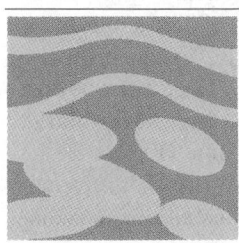

Assessment of the Nervous System

ELIZABETH A. SCHENK

CHAPTER OBJECTIVES

After studying this chapter, the student should be able to:

1 State the four general kinds of functions of the nervous system.
2 Name the three parts of the neuron and explain the function(s) of each part.
3 Define the following terms: *differential permeability, excitability, polarization, depolarization, action potential*, and *synapse*.
4 Name the two major divisions of the nervous system.
5 Name the three main areas of the brain and at least two functions of each part.
6 Name the four parts of the cerebral cortex and at least one function of each.
7 Explain what symptoms a patient may manifest with a tumor in the frontal lobe.
8 Name at least two special characteristics of circulation in the brain.
9 Name the three meningeal layers and the three potential spaces associated with the meninges.
10 Name at least four physiologic changes that occur in the nervous system with aging.
11 Describe the parts of the neurologic assessment that are assessed through the history.
12 Explain how aphasia is different from dysarthria.
13 Name the 12 cranial nerves and the function of each.
14 List and describe at least six diagnostic procedures used to evaluate neurologic disease.

Many systemic diseases have neurologic manifestations; thus, individuals may have their first neurologic assessments performed during a routine physical examination. Consequently, the physician generalist is often the first medical professional to document the neurologic problems. However, on referral to a physician specialist (neurologist), the individual will undergo a more detailed assessment to localize the particular lesion and to identify its pathophysiology. To enable the specialist to determine the specific diagnosis, the neurologist's examination will be more detailed, exact, and comprehensive than that of the generalist.

Persons with neurologic deficits require skilled as-

sessment by both physician and nurse. Neurologic assessment may be performed by generalists and specialists in both fields, and data collected will be used both collaboratively and independently to permit these professionals to provide their distinct services to the individual.

Professional nurses are involved in initial and ongoing assessments of a patient's neurologic status. The nurse's role is that of an independent professional as well as that of a collaborator.

The nurse generalist may become involved in baseline and continuing assessments early in the patient's course of therapy. Although data collected will also be useful to the physician, the primary purpose is to enable the nurse to identify the degree to which the patient is able to perform self-care activities and to assess how such activities are limited by the identified deficits in sensory, motor, affective, or intellectual capacities. With these problem areas identified, the nurse then is able to select appropriate strategies to maximize the patient's capabilities.

Because of additional experience and preparation in the speciality, the neurologic nurse specialist has developed skills beyond those of the generalist. Like the physician specialist, the neurologic nurse's assessments are more comprehensive and detailed in nature and, as such, they are more likely to overlap with those of the neurologist.

Again, although these data will be useful to the neurologist, the primary purpose is to enable the neurologic nurse specialist to formulate more comprehensive analyses of patient conditions. Problems identified may provide more thorough descriptions of deficits observed, patient responses to these deficits, and the effects of such deficits on the patient's family and lifestyle. This thorough analysis will lead to more comprehensive plans of care extending from the acute phase through rehabilitation. Also, the neurologic nurse specialist serves as a consultant to nurse generalists caring for patients with neurologic problems.

The purposes of this chapter are to review selected neuroanatomy and physiology, to discuss aspects of history taking, to present the components and methods of and the observations to be made during the neurologic examination, and to discuss selected tests and procedures used to assist in the diagnosis of neurologic problems.

ANATOMY AND PHYSIOLOGY

Neurologic assessment depends on the examiner's knowledge of normal neurophysiology and neuroanatomy and ability to interpret the degree of change in status from what is considered to be normal. The attainment of a logical diagnosis (nursing or medical) begins with a recognition of abnormality followed by grouping of the data, analysis of data, and conclusions about what the data mean in terms of a diagnosis.

The complexity of the nervous system limits what can be presented here. Only selected concepts relevant to neurologic assessment are included. The reader is referred to current texts for a more detailed and comprehensive coverage.[2,15,48] Emphasis is placed on key concepts including the *neuron, synapse, conduction, motor system pathways, sensory system pathways,* and *effector organs.*

FUNCTION

Functionally, the nervous system, like an electrical conductance system, coordinates and controls all activities of the body. Broadly, the nervous system carries out four general kinds of functions as related to informational processes:

1. Receives stimuli or information from the internal and external environments over varied afferent or *sensory pathways*
2. Communicates information between distant parts of the body (periphery) to the central nervous system
3. Computes or processes the information received at various *reflex* (spinal cord) and *conscious* (higher brain) levels to determine responses appropriate to existing situations
4. Transmits information rapidly over varied efferent or *motor pathways* to effector organs for body action control or modifications.

NEURON

The single *neuron* is the basic structural and functional unit of the nervous system. It shares all of the basic biologic and biochemical properties of other body cells. It is also a highly specialized and differentiated cell. The single neuron acts as a miniature nervous system and has properties specialized for its electrical function.

Microscopically, the neuron consists of a cell body, or *soma,* with two extensions that project from it: a *dendritic tree* and an elongated *cylindric axon.* A *cell membrane* encloses the outer boundary of the soma, dendrites, and axon, thus separating the inside from the outside of the cell. The presence of a large surface area of cell membrane makes it suitable to receive a large number of synaptic contacts at one time (Figure 59-1). The *axon* is specialized for the transmission of information along its extension *away from* the cell body to adjacent neurons; the *dendrite* or *dendrites* are specialized for receiving information from axon terminals at special sites called *synapses.* (It should be noted that the word *axon* is used in various ways. It may be used to describe the extension of one cell or the extension of several cells making up a nerve.)

CELL MEMBRANE

Many of the most important *functional* properties of the neuron lie within the *cell membrane* itself. Structurally, the membrane is made up of lipids and proteins and has the property of translocating materials across itself. The membrane exhibits *differential permeability* in that it is permeable to oxygen, carbon dioxide, and certain inorganic ions while it is impermeable to organic compounds (proteins) and other inorganic ions. This differential permeability results in a characteristic ionic distribution. The inside of the neuron contains a high concentration of proteins (which are impermeable) and potassium (K^+), whereas the outside of the cell is high in sodium (Na^+). This unequal distribution, or gradient, of K^+ and Na^+ across the membrane results in part from differential permeability and from the presence of an active *sodium-potassium pump* within the membrane. The pump requires metabolic energy for rapid movement of sodium and potassium across the membrane, and this produces an electrical potential difference, or charge, between the inside and the outside of the cell. The magnitude of the potential difference is a function of the ratio of charged particles on opposite sides of the membrane and is called the *resting membrane potential* (resting potential). All cells exhibit this property of resting potential, which essentially remains constant over time. Thus in the resting state all neurons possess a potential for action and are said to be *polarized* (a difference in voltage charge between inner and outer cell membrane or surface). This resting potential is quite small, -60 mV, with the inside of the cell being electronically negative compared with the outside of the cell.

EXCITABILITY

Additionally, the neuron exhibits the property of "*excitability*" as do muscles and certain glands. "*Excitability*" means that the resting potential of neurons is unstable under certain conditions; for example, as when a neu-

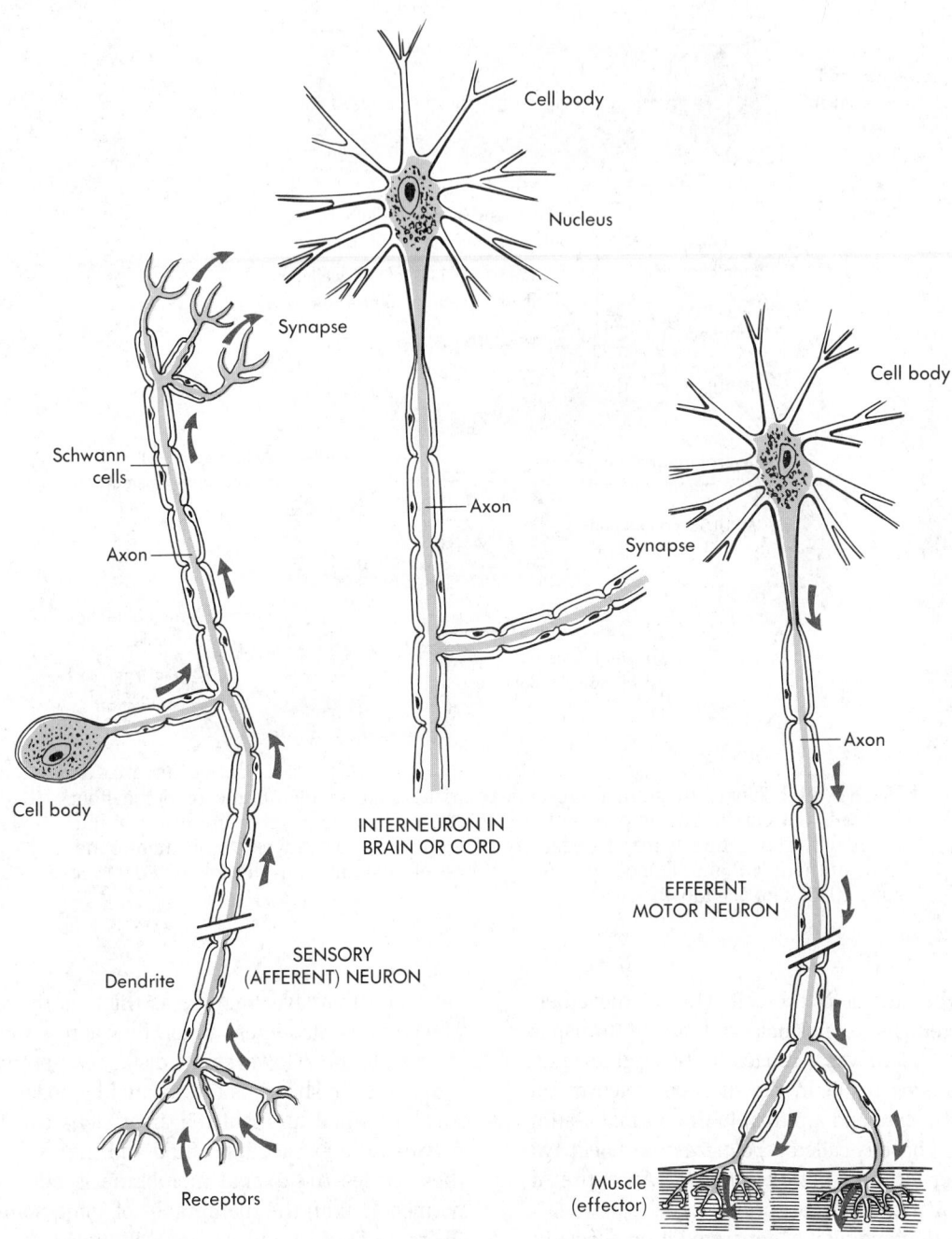

FIGURE 59-1 Diagram of neurons showing the cell body (soma), dendrites, and axon. Direction of impulse conduction indicated by arrows.

ronal membrane is subjected to stimulation, application of chemicals, or mechanical damage. This instability gives rise to the generation of *action potentials*. The generation of an action potential is a capacity unique to excitable cells, and it is the basic phenomenon underlying all nervous system functions. It is by means of action potentials that information is conducted within the nervous system.

An action potential occurs in the following manner:

When a neuron is stimulated, membrane permeability to Na^+ significantly increases, and there is a sudden movement of Na^+ to the inside of the membrane. These ions carry a sufficiently large positive charge, which causes the disappearance of the normal resting potential. In fact, a *positive state* develops within the cell and *depolarization* occurs.

Almost instantaneously the membrane pores return to the state of being virtually impermeable to Na^+ while

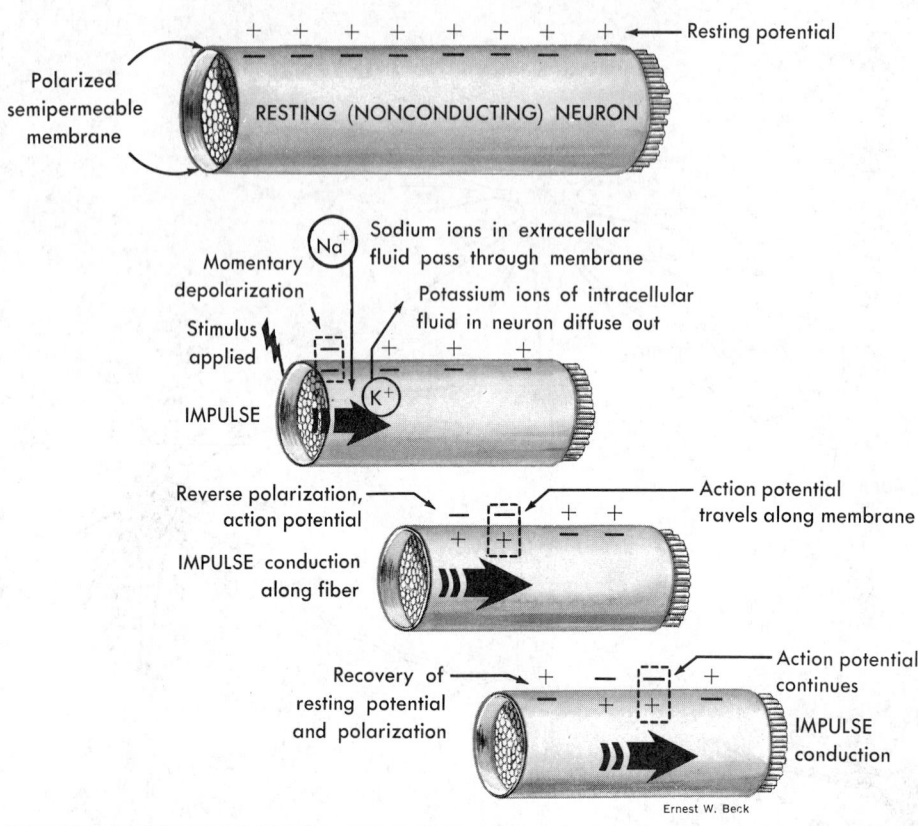

FIGURE 59-2 Upper diagram represents polarized state of membrane of nerve fiber when it is not conducting impulses. Lower diagrams represent nerve impulse conduction: A self-propagating wave of negativity or action potential travels along membrane. (From Anthony CP and Thibodeau GA: Textbook of anatomy and physiology, ed 11, St Louis, 1983, The CV Mosby Co.)

K^+ moves to the outside of the cell. The K^+ movement also quickly returns to normal, and active transport brings Na^+ and K^+ movement back to the original state. These mechanisms result in the disappearance of the internal positive state and a return to the normal resting potential. This phase is called *repolarization*. These two phases together form the *action potential*. An entire AP occurs within 1 to 2 msec (Figure 59-2).

When an action potential is generated it proceeds *automatically to completion*, independent of the property of the stimulus that initiated the depolarization; that is, a strong stimulus does not give rise to a larger action potential but does cause it to proceed to completion in an "all-or-none" fashion. The action potential is also spread, or propagated, over the entire membrane without a decrease in its velocity. The propagation velocity is related to the size of the axon (the larger the diameter, the higher the velocity) and to the presence or absence of myelin.

MYELIN

Myelin is an excellent insulator of axons. The myelin sheath is deposited around the axons by Schwann's cells, and this layer may be as thick as the axon itself. Myelin prevents almost all ion flow across the axon and its membrane. However, at distances approximately 1 mm apart the sheath is interrupted by nodes of Ranvier. At these small, uninsulated areas, ions can flow easily between the extracellular fluid and the axon. In fact, at these nodes the axonal membrane is 500 times more permeable than the membranes of some nonmyelinated fibers.[49] Thus impulses are conducted from node to node.

The presence of myelin causes such fibers to be called *large* fibers; those without myelin are called *small* fibers. Large fibers have a greater conduction velocity because (1) the jumping effect allows depolarization to proceed quickly and (2) energy is conserved since only the nodes depolarize. Large fibers appear white because of the myelin; the "white matter" of the nervous system is made up of myelinated fibers.

Many action potentials of neurons originate in a receptor neuron where internal and external stimuli are normally received. A receptor is like a transducer and can change one form of energy into another form. A receptor, however, responds or depolarizes to *only one* type of stimulus. For example, the retina of the eye responds only to the stimulus of light, which is converted to electrical energy and travels over the optic nerves to the visual cortices for perception. In this way the receptor neuron may initiate the depolarization. It does, however, limit what the neuron responds to, although the receptor neuron does obey the *all-or-none theory; a strong stimulus does make the receptor neuron fire* more action potentials *per unit of time* within its time limitations *than does a weak stimulus.*

SYNAPSE

Neurons make functional contact with one another at specialized sites called *synapses*. Whenever an action potential is generated in one neuron that invades a synapse site, a sequence of processes results in the action potential affecting the second neuron. Transmission across a synpase is essentially a *chemical process*. The end of the axon contains a chemical substance located within its vesicles. When an action potential reaches the vesicle, it releases a transmitter substance, which then diffuses across the synapse to the adjacent neuronal cell membrane. *Synaptic transmission* is both *excitatory* and *inhibitory* in nature. Inhibition means that the dendritic membrane becomes hyperpolarized because of the release of the specific neurotransmitter. The membrane potential shifts toward K^+ equilibrium, thus stabilizing the membrane and taking the potential further from threshold. Each neuron only acts when its membrane is *depolarized to threshold.* Thus, whether a neuron fires depends on the sum of excitatory and inhibitory inputs. *Chemicals* allowing *excitatory transmission* are *acetylcholine, norepinephrine, dopamine,* and *serotonin.* Those that *inhibit transmission* include *gamma aminobutyric acid (GABA) in brain tissue* and *glycine* in the *spinal cord.*

In summary, each single neuron contains all the structural and functional building elements of an electrical conductance system that also makes interconnections with adjacent neurons at synapses. Collectively, the neurons are in turn organized into larger and larger units of function that serve to coordinate all the activities of the body. All neurons function basically in the same manner. There is, however, a major difference in the functions carried out by sensory and motor neurons.

In neurologic assessment, the examiner should appreciate that any disruption in the conductance system results in dysfunction distal to the break. The degree of change in status of a particular function or functions depends on the location and nature of the stressor or lesion causing the disruption.

DIVISIONS OF THE NERVOUS SYSTEM

Macroscopically, the nervous system is divided into two major divisions: the central nervous system and the peripheral nervous system.

CENTRAL NERVOUS SYSTEM

The central nervous system (CNS) is made up of collections of neurons and their connections organized within the brain and spinal cord. All of the basic informational processes as summarized on p. 1710 occur within the CNS. Areas of the brain and spinal cord are distinguished where cell bodies are concentrated into *nuclei* and groups of axons running in *tracts* that interconnect the parts. Collections of neurons are connected in complex ways. The *connections* determine the capability of each collection of neurons. The neurons are organized into circuits, some of which are simple and made up of relatively few neurons and others that are very complex. A single neuron may be a component of a number of different neuronal circuits and thus play a role in different functions.

Structurally, the brain and spinal cord are continuous. They are protectively housed within the skull and vertebral column, respectively. When injured, centrally located neurons are unable to reproduce themselves because most cell bodies are located centrally and nerve cell bodies cannot reproduce. However, *nerve endings can regenerate because* of the presence of *neurilemma.* Neurilemma covers all peripheral nerves; it is theorized that the living neurilemma contains openings through which axonal growth occurs proximally to distally. This growth seems to occur at a rate of 1 to 4 mm/day. Rarely, however, is there 100% regrowth.

Brain

The brain (encephalon) is grossly divided rostrally to caudally into three main areas: the *cerebrum, brain stem* (diencephalon, midbrain, pons, and medulla), and *cerebellum.* Each circuit or area carries out unique functions.

Cerebrum. The cerebrum or cerebral cortex is comprised of two frontal lobes, two parietal lobes, two temporal lobes, and two occipital lobes. The cerebral cortex is separated into two hemispheres (left and right) by the *falx cerebri,* a tough dural tissue. Each of the hemispheres is further divided into the respective lobes by folds in the cerebral cortex called *fissures* or *sulci.* The frontal lobe is separated from the parietal lobe by the *fissure of Rolando* (also called the *central sulcus*) and from the temporal lobe by the *Sylvian fissure.* It is separated from the occipital lobe by the *parieto-occipital fissure.* The temporal lobe lies below the *Sylvian fissure.*

The *cortex* of the cerebrum is approximately ¼ inch thick. It controls over 14 billion neurons, receives and analyzes all impulses, controls voluntary movement, and stores knowledge of all impulses received.

Each cerebral lobe is named from overlying cranial bones (Figure 59-3) and carries out one or more functions as listed in Table 59-1.

TABLE 59-1 Specific functions of cerebral cortex

Lobe	Function
Frontal	Conceptualization
	Abstraction
	Motor ability
	Judgment formation
	Ability to write words
Parietal	Integrative and coordinating center for perception and interpretation of sensory information
	Ability to recognize body parts
	Left versus right
Temporal	Memory storage
	Integration of auditory stimuli
Occipital	Visual center
	Understanding of written material

Important to note is that speech is a function of the *dominant hemisphere* which for all right-handed people and most left-handed people is the left side. The two identified speech centers are *Broca's area* and *Wernicke's area*. Broca's area is located in the lateral inferior portion of the frontal lobe adjacent to the motor cortex and its projections. This area appears to control verbal, expressive speech. Wernicke's area is located in the posterior part of the superior temporal convolution and may extend to adjacent portions of the parietal lobe. This area is responsible for the reception and understanding of language. Other areas of the brain that are also involved in speech include an area in the frontal lobe, which governs the ability to write words, and an area in the occipital lobe, which governs the ability to understand written material (see Figure 59-4 for important cortical areas).

Finally, deep within the cerebrum are structures called the *basal ganglia*. These are masses of gray matter (cell bodies) and include such structures as the *caudate nucleus*, *putamen*, and *globus pallidus*. In general, the basal ganglia function as part of the *extrapyramidal* system and are responsible for postural adjustments and gross volitional movements.

Brain stem. The brain stem is placed deeply in the center of the hemispheres and is not visible when viewing the intact brain. It includes a series of parts making connections with the spinal cord at the level of the medulla (Figure 59-5), and it carries all nerve fibers passing between the hemispheres and the cord. All cranial nerves except the olfactory nerve (I) arise from it (Figure 59-6).

The brain stem is made up of several structures. The *diencephalon* surrounds the third ventricle and consists of the *thalamus, epithalamus, subthalamus*, and *hypothalamus*. Other structures include the *midbrain, pons*, and *medulla oblongata*. (See Table 59-2 for a more detailed explanation of the functions of the various structures and functions of the brain stem.)

Of special importance is the core of tissue extending throughout the entire brain stem. This is called the *reticular formation*. This interconnected network of cells has important integrating centers for respiration, cardiovascular function, afferent and motor systems, and

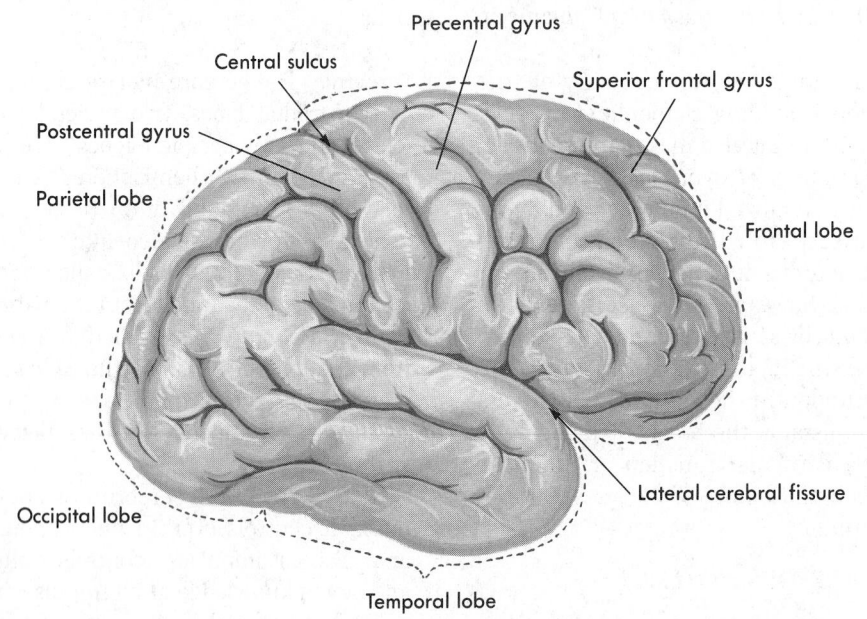

FIGURE 59-3 Lobes, sulci, and gyri of the brain.

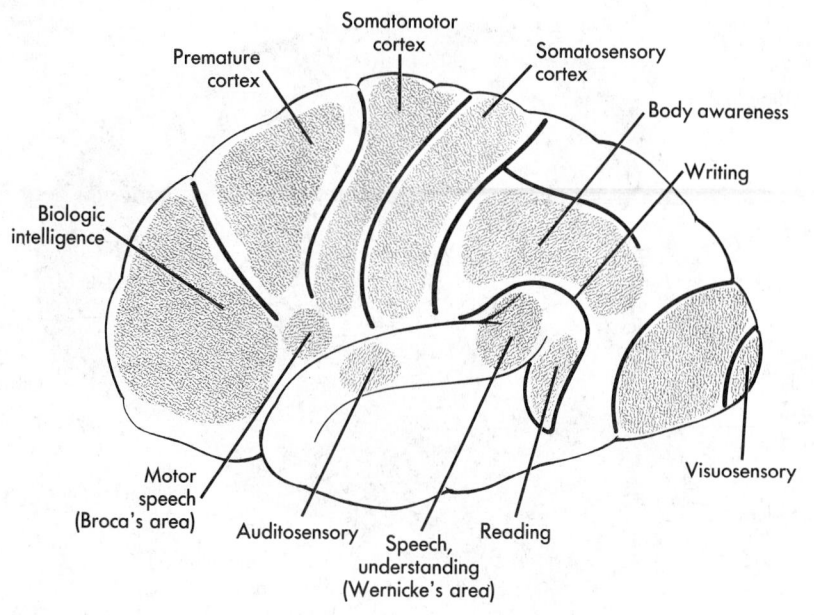

FIGURE 59-4 Lateral view of cerebral cortex with identification of major cortical areas.

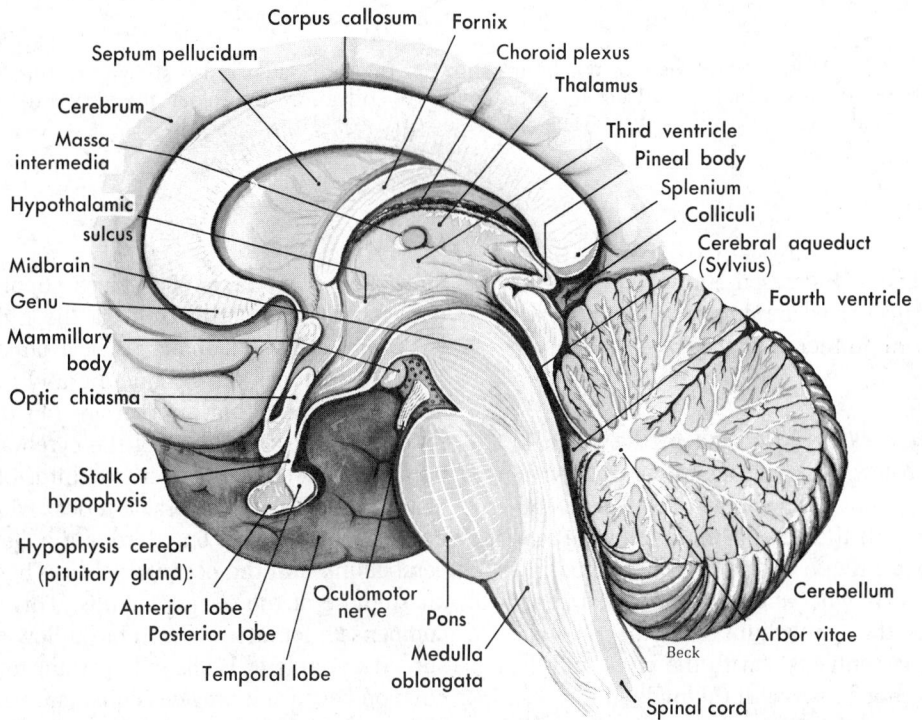

FIGURE 59-5 Sagittal section through midline of brain showing continuity of brain and spinal cord. (From Anthony CP and Thibodeau GA: Textbook of anatomy and physiology, ed 11, St Louis, 1983, The CV Mosby Co.)

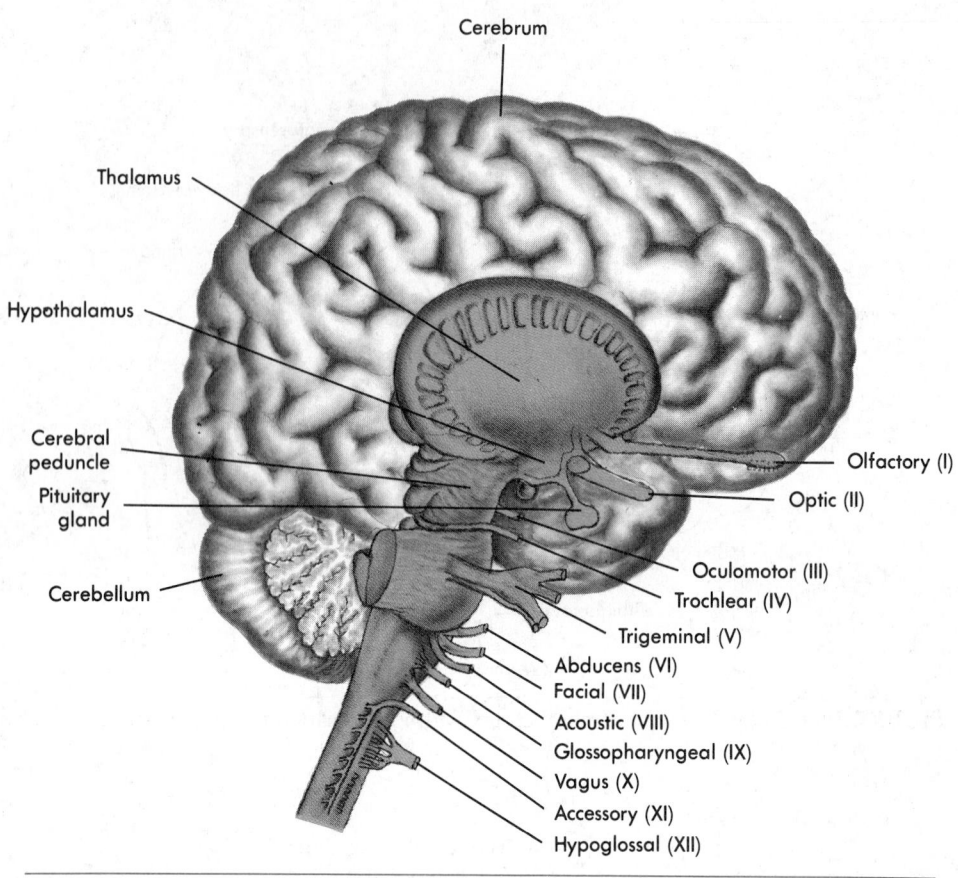

Cerebrum

Thalamus

Hypothalamus

Cerebral peduncle

Pituitary gland

Cerebellum

Olfactory (I)

Optic (II)

Oculomotor (III)

Trochlear (IV)

Trigeminal (V)

Abducens (VI)

Facial (VII)

Acoustic (VIII)

Glossopharyngeal (IX)

Vagus (X)

Accessory (XI)

Hypoglossal (XII)

FIGURE 59-6 Lateral view of the brain, showing the brain stem. Also shown are the cranial nerves, which arise from it. (From Rudy EB: Advanced neurological and neurosurgical nursing, St Louis, 1984, The CV Mosby Co.)

states of consciousness. Increased stimulation leads to wakefulness, and decreased stimulation (as in anoxia caused by increased intracranial pressure) results in sleepiness.

Cerebellum. The *cerebellum* is located in the posterior cranial fossa, just below the posterior cerebrum. It contains *short* and *long tracts*. The short tracts act as connections of nuclei with the cerebellum, while the long tracts enter and exit through *peduncles*. There are three peduncles—*inferior, middle,* and *superior*. The inferior peduncle connects the cerebellum with the medulla, the middle peduncle connects it with the pons, and the superior peduncle connects it with the midbrain.

The cerebellum has the following three main functions, all of which are related to monitoring and making corrective adjustments of body movements:

1. To keep persons oriented in space and to maintain truncal equilibrium
2. To control antigravity muscles
3. To check or halt volitional movements

Circulation of the brain. The blood supply for the brain derives from the aortic arch via the right innominate, left common carotid, and left subclavian arteries (Figure 59-7). It includes the conducting and penetrating vessels. The conducting arteries are (1) the internal carotids, which supply most of the cerebral hemispheres, basal ganglia, and the upper two thirds of the diencephalon, and (2) the vertebral arteries, which supply the brain stem, the lower one third of the diencephalon, the cerebellum, and the occipital lobes. These two systems anastomose at the *circle of Willis*. This allows them to compensate for alterations in blood flow and blood pressure. The circle of Willis is important to total brain circulation because it provides equal circulation bilaterally. If one side of the circle of Willis is unable to supply adequate blood, the other side provides blood to the area normally supplied by the damaged side (Figure 59-8).

The penetrating vessels are those that enter the brain substance at right angles after branching off from the conducting vessels; they supply nutrients to the neurons.

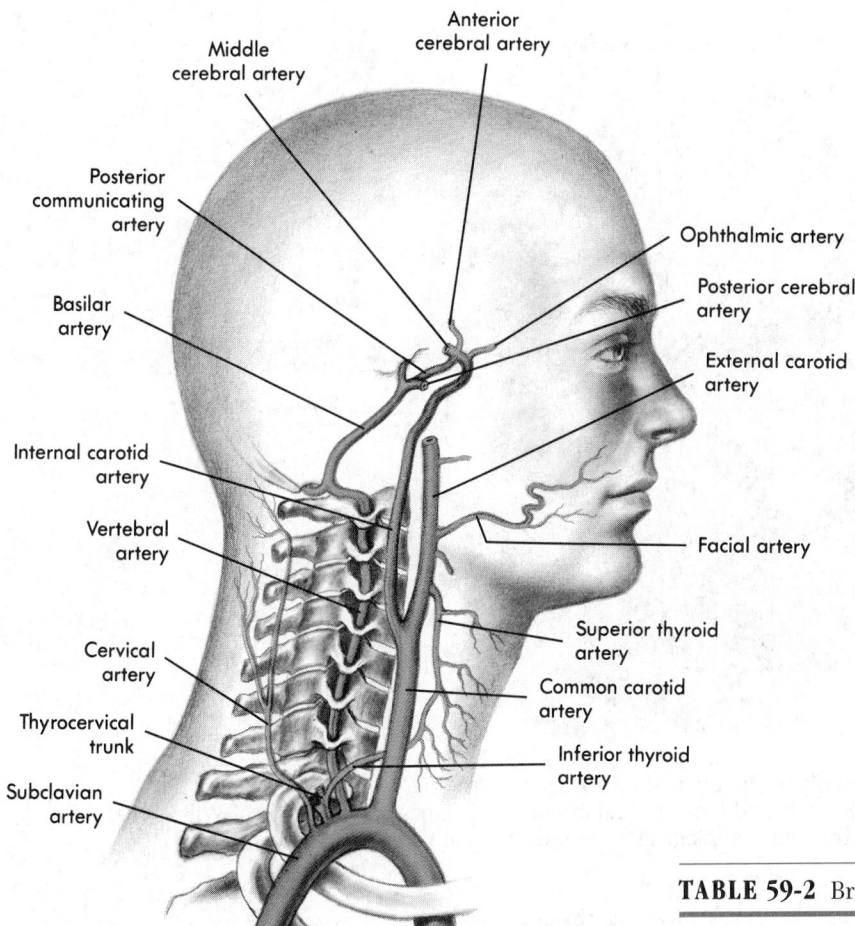

Middle cerebral artery

Anterior cerebral artery

Posterior communicating artery

Basilar artery

Internal carotid artery

Vertebral artery

Cervical artery

Thyrocervical trunk

Subclavian artery

Ophthalmic artery

Posterior cerebral artery

External carotid artery

Facial artery

Superior thyroid artery

Common carotid artery

Inferior thyroid artery

FIGURE 59-7 Conducting arteries of the brain, including the internal carotid arteries and the vertebral arteries. (From Rudy EB: Advanced neurological and neurosurgical nursing, St Louis, 1984, The CV Mosby Co.)

TABLE 59-2 Brain stem structures and functions

Structure	Function
Diencephalon	
Thalamus	Serves as end station for all sensory impulses
	All sensory fibers synapse for final relay to appropriate portion of sensory cortex
	General sensation perceived (meaning and locality imparted by cortex)
	Houses pain threshold
Epithalamus	Contains pineal body or epiphysis (thought to be endocrine gland whose secretion retards sexual development and growth)
Subthalamus	Receives fibers from globus pallidis, is part of afferent descending pathway
Hypothalamus	Contains cell bodies mediating most autonomic functions, endocrine functions, and emotional responses; contains stalk of pituitary
Midbrain	Relays impulses from cerebral cortex above and subcortical structures below
	Origin of righting and postural reflex located here
Pons	Connects medulla, midbrain, and cerebrum
	Contains pneumotaxic center—controls rhythmic quality of respirations
Medulla	Connects with central canal or spinal cord
	Vital centers of cardiac, respiration, vasomotor control, as well as swallowing and hiccoughing; gag and cough reflex

The venous system draining the brain is divided into vertebral veins that receive blood from the cerebrum and the cerebellar veins that receive blood from the cerebellum. The venous system of the brain is unique in that the cerebral veins have no valves. Also, all the veins of the brain terminate in dural sinuses, which eventually empty into the superior vena cava by means of the jugular veins.

Circulation in the brain possesses special characteristics. For example, systemic circulation favors the central nervous system over all other body parts. This helps provide a constant supply of nutrients (glucose and oxygen) to nervous tissue. The brain's vessels themselves also possess capabilities that allow them to assist in achieving a constant blood flow. The brain is able to autoregulate its blood flow to respond to changes in intraluminal pressure. In the presence of increased blood pressure, cerebral vessels constrict so as to decrease flow and possible tissue damage. Conversely, in the presence of decreased intraluminal pressure, cerebral vessels dilate to increase flow. Cerebral vessels also react to biochemical changes. For example, elevated carbon dioxide content causes notable vasodilation of cerebral vessels; hypoxia and elevated hydrogen ion concentration also causes vasodilation. However, these auto-

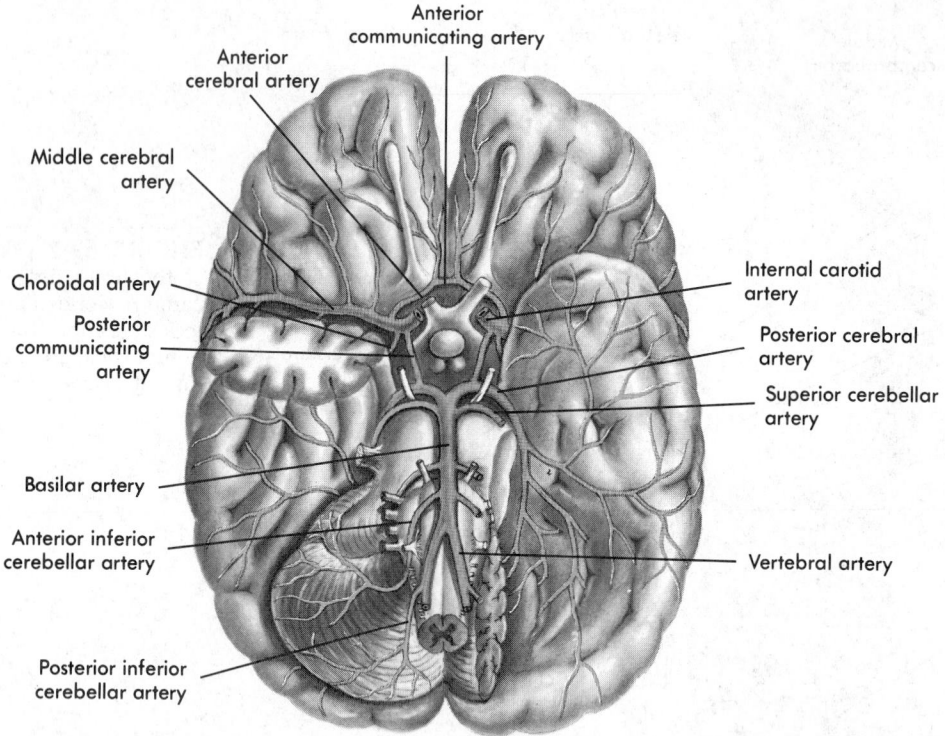

FIGURE 59-8 Blood supply of the brain showing the penetrating vessels and the circle of Willis. The internal carotids and the vertebral arteries anastamose at the circle of Willis. (From Rudy EB: Advanced neurological and neurosurgical nursing, St Louis, 1984, The CV Mosby Co.)

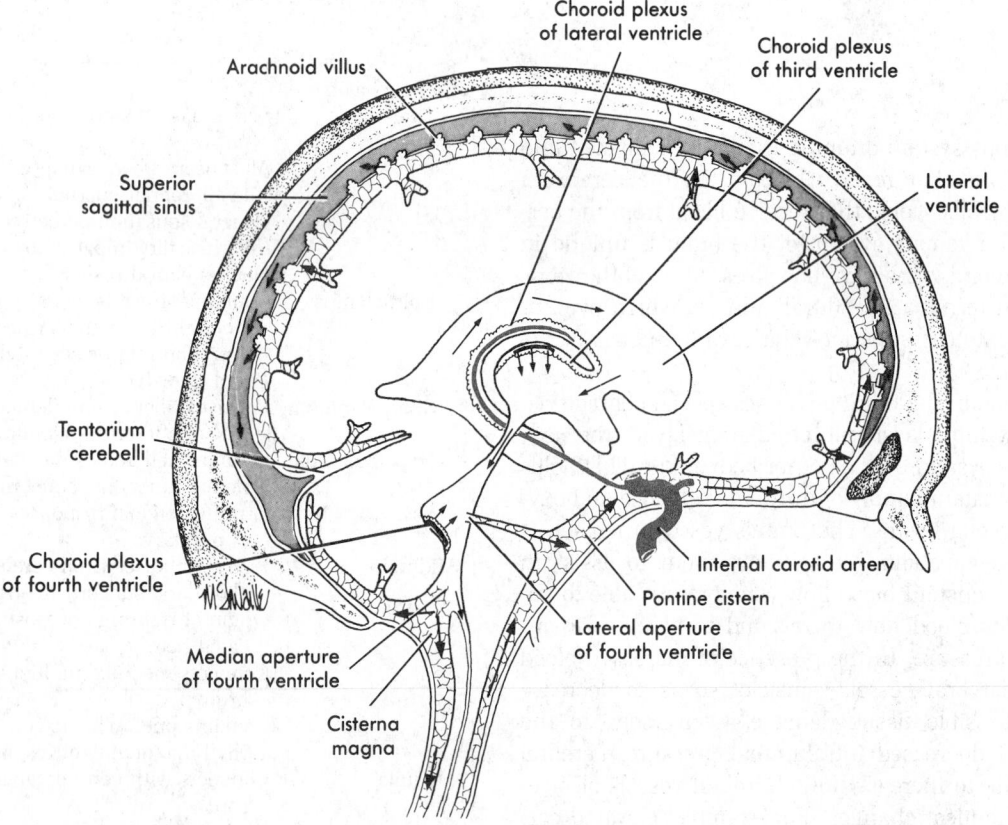

FIGURE 59-9 Path of circulation of cerebrospinal fluid from its formation in the ventricles to its absoprtion into the superior sagittal sinus. (From Notlte J: The human brain, St Louis, 1981, The CV Mosby Co.)

regulatory mechanisms become less responsive with increasing age and in the presence of arteriosclerosis.

Blood-brain barrier. In the nervous system a phenomenon exists that limits the free movement of substances from the blood to the brain tissue. Passage of substances into the brain is slower in comparison with passage into other body organs. The neurologic sheath, as well as capillaries that have thickened basement membranes, slows the process of diffusion in between the blood and the brain.

The barrier is selective, allowing entry of fluid, gases, and small molecular substances, while preventing the entry of toxic substances, plasma protein, and large molecules. The ability to overcome this barrier has proved instrumental in chemotherapy of brain lesions.

Cerebrospinal Fluid

Another fluid in the nervous system is *cerebrospinal fluid* (CSF). CSF is found in the ventricles of the brain, in the central canal of the spinal cord, and in the subarachnoid space. It serves as a fluid cushion for nervous tissue and helps to support the weight of the brain. It also carries nutrients to the brain and removes metabolites. CSF is continually formed by vessels of the *choroid plexus* at a rate of 18 ml/hr. In the adult there is 90 to 150 ml of CSF.

After circulating around the brain and spinal cord, CSF returns to the brain and is absorbed through the arachnoid villi. From here, CSF enters the venous system and follows its pathway through the jugular veins to the superior vena cava and into the systemic circulation (Figure 59-9).

Spinal Cord

The spinal cord weighs about 1 ounce and is approximately 1½ inches wide. It is elliptical in shape and appears wider from right to left than from anterior to posterior. Cervical and lumbar enlargements are areas of nerve origin to the upper and lower limbs.

The spinal cord forms a continuous structure with the medulla oblongata. It extends 42 to 45 cm from the foramen magnum through the spinal foramina of the vertebral column to the upper border of the second lumbar vertebra.

The spinal cord structurally includes H-shaped central gray matter (nerve cell bodies surrounded by white matter that is divided into three columns or *funiculi* according to their location (*anterior, ventral, lateral,* and *posterior* or *dorsal columns*). Each contains ascending and descending tracts that will be described in more detail later in the chapter (Figure 59-10). These tracts connect different segments of the spinal cord to each other and connect the spinal cord with the brain. The names of the tracts usually show the point of origin by

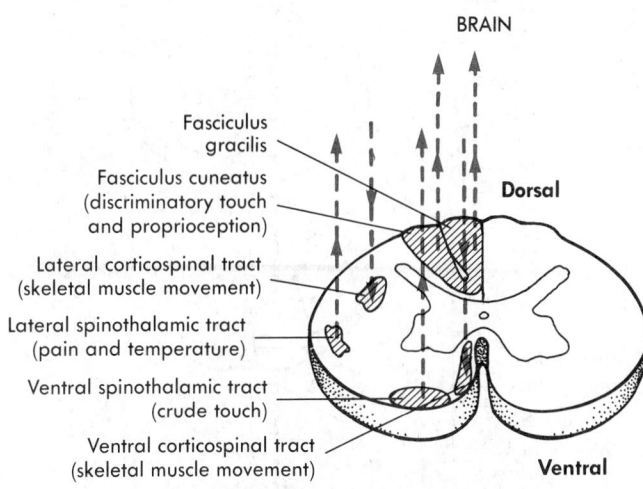

FIGURE 59-10 Nerve pathways arise from white matter of the spinal cord. Impulses travel to and from the spinal cord and brain along these pathways.

the first part of the name, and the end point by the last part of the name (see Table 59-3).

The spinal cord is also the site of reflex pathways. Reflexes are an example of the simplest neuronal circuit. They *do not* require relay to the brain level for action. A reflex action consists of a *specific stereotyped motor response to an adequate sensory stimulus.* The response may involve skeletal muscle movement or glandular secretion. It may involve only two neurons as in a simple monosynaptic reflex arch such as occurs with the myotactic knee jerk reflex. In the knee jerk reflex, a brisk tap over a partially stretched knee tendon stimulates sensory nerve endings within the tendons, and the stimulus travels over a sensory nerve fiber within a peripheral nerve toward the spinal cord where it synapses with a central motor neuron (anterior horn cell). Following this, the impulse is transmitted down the motor nerve (over the anterior nerve root of the spinal nerve or peripheral nerve) and across the neuromuscular junction to stimulate the muscle to contract. Figure 59-11 shows the reflex arc. In summary, a reflex arc depends on an intact sensory nerve, a functional synapse with a central neuron within the spinal cord, an intact motor nerve fiber and neuromuscular junction, and a competent muscle. A reflex may involve only one spinal cord level, as in the knee jerk reflex, or it may involve one or a few spinal cord levels (*segmental reflexes*), or it may involve structures in the brain that influence the spinal cord (*supraspinal* reflexes).

Meninges

Finally a word must be said about the *meninges*, the coverings of the nervous tissue in the brain and spinal cord. These fibrous coverings help support, protect, and

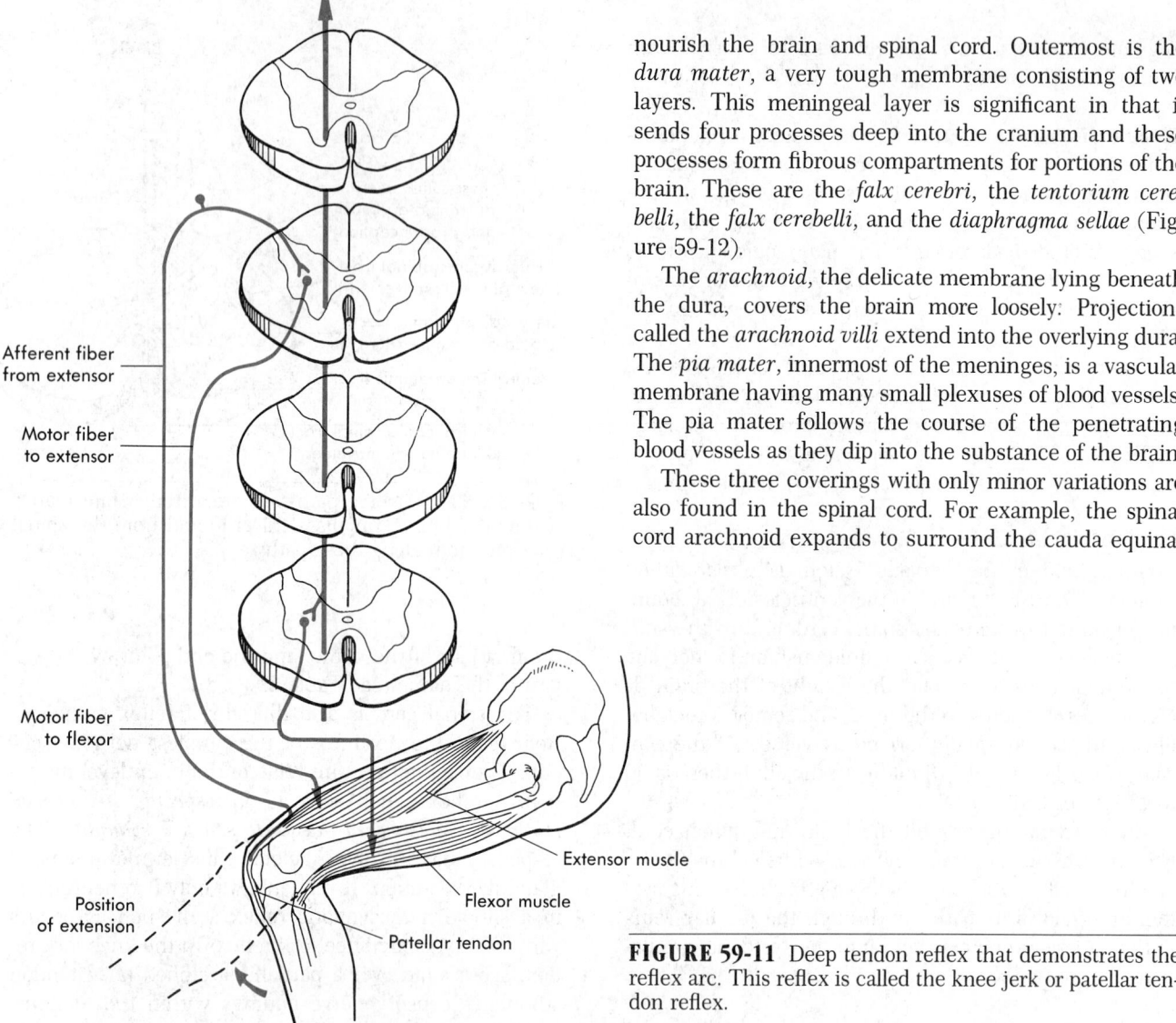

nourish the brain and spinal cord. Outermost is the *dura mater,* a very tough membrane consisting of two layers. This meningeal layer is significant in that it sends four processes deep into the cranium and these processes form fibrous compartments for portions of the brain. These are the *falx cerebri,* the *tentorium cerebelli,* the *falx cerebelli,* and the *diaphragma sellae* (Figure 59-12).

The *arachnoid,* the delicate membrane lying beneath the dura, covers the brain more loosely. Projections called the *arachnoid villi* extend into the overlying dura. The *pia mater,* innermost of the meninges, is a vascular membrane having many small plexuses of blood vessels. The pia mater follows the course of the penetrating blood vessels as they dip into the substance of the brain.

These three coverings with only minor variations are also found in the spinal cord. For example, the spinal cord arachnoid expands to surround the cauda equina;

FIGURE 59-11 Deep tendon reflex that demonstrates the reflex arc. This reflex is called the knee jerk or patellar tendon reflex.

TABLE 59-3 Tracts of the spinal cord

Tract	Column	Direction	Function
Ventral corticospinal	Anterior	Descending	Voluntary motion
Vestibulospinal	Anterior	Descending	Balance reflex
Tectospinal	Anterior	Descending	Sight and vision reflex
Reticulospinal	Anterior	Descending	Muscle tone
Ventral spinothalamic	Anterior	Ascending	Light touch
Spinoolivary	Anterior	Ascending	Proprioception reflex
Lateral corticospinal	Lateral	Descending	Voluntary movements
Rubrospinal	Lateral	Descending	Synergy and muscle tone
Olivospinal	Lateral	Descending	Reflex
Dorsal spinocerebellar	Lateral	Ascending	Reflex proprioception
Ventral spinocerebellar	Lateral	Ascending	Reflex proprioception
Lateral spinothalamic	Lateral	Ascending	Pain and temperature
Spinotectal	Lateral	Ascending	Reflex
Fasciculus interfascicularis	Posterior	Descending	Integration and association
Septomarginal fascicularis	Posterior	Descending	Integration and association
Fascicularis gracilis	Posterior	Ascending	Vibration, passive movement, joint, and two-point movement
Fascicularis cuneatus	Posterior	Ascending	Vibration, passive movement, joint, and two-point movement

thus the subarachnoid space ends at S2 in the adult and is most wide caudally. Also, the spinal cord pia mater is thicker and less vascular than that of the cranium.

It should be noted that three potential spaces are associated with the meninges: *epidural* (external to the dura); *subdural* (between dura and arachnoid); and *subarachnoid* (between arachnoid and pia mater).

PERIPHERAL NERVOUS SYSTEM

The peripheral nervous system (PNS) is basically a set of communication channels located outside the central nervous system. Peripheral nerves are *bundles of individual nerves* that are either *sensory, motor,* or *"mixed"* (having both sensory and motor fibers). Structurally, the PNS consists of 12 *pairs of cranial nerves and 31 pairs of spinal nerves.* The cranial nerves carry impulses to and from the brain. They originate mainly in the brain stem, except for the first nerve (olfactory) that arises in the olfactory bulb (see Table 59-7 for an explanation of the functions of each cranial nerve).

Spinal nerves are composed of a dorsal and ventral root. They correspond to the spinal cord segment from which they arise—8 cervical, 12 thoracic, 5 lumbar, 5 sacral, and 1 coccygeal (the first pair of cervical spinal nerves come off the cord *above* C_1). From L3 to S5, the spinal nerves branch out to form the *cauda equina.*

Peripheral nerves that transmit information toward the CNS are *afferent* or *sensory* in nature, whereas peripheral nerves that transmit information away from the CNS are *efferent,* or *motor,* in nature. Peripherally, the sensory and motor nerves usually travel together; however, they become separated centrally at the cord level into a *posterior* or *sensory root* and an *anterior* or *motor root,* respectively.

The peripheral nervous system is divided into the *somatic* and *autonomic* nervous systems. The somatic nervous system innervates skeletal (striated) muscles. Its neuronal cell bodies lie in groups within the CNS, and its axons exit the spinal cord at all levels. These fi-

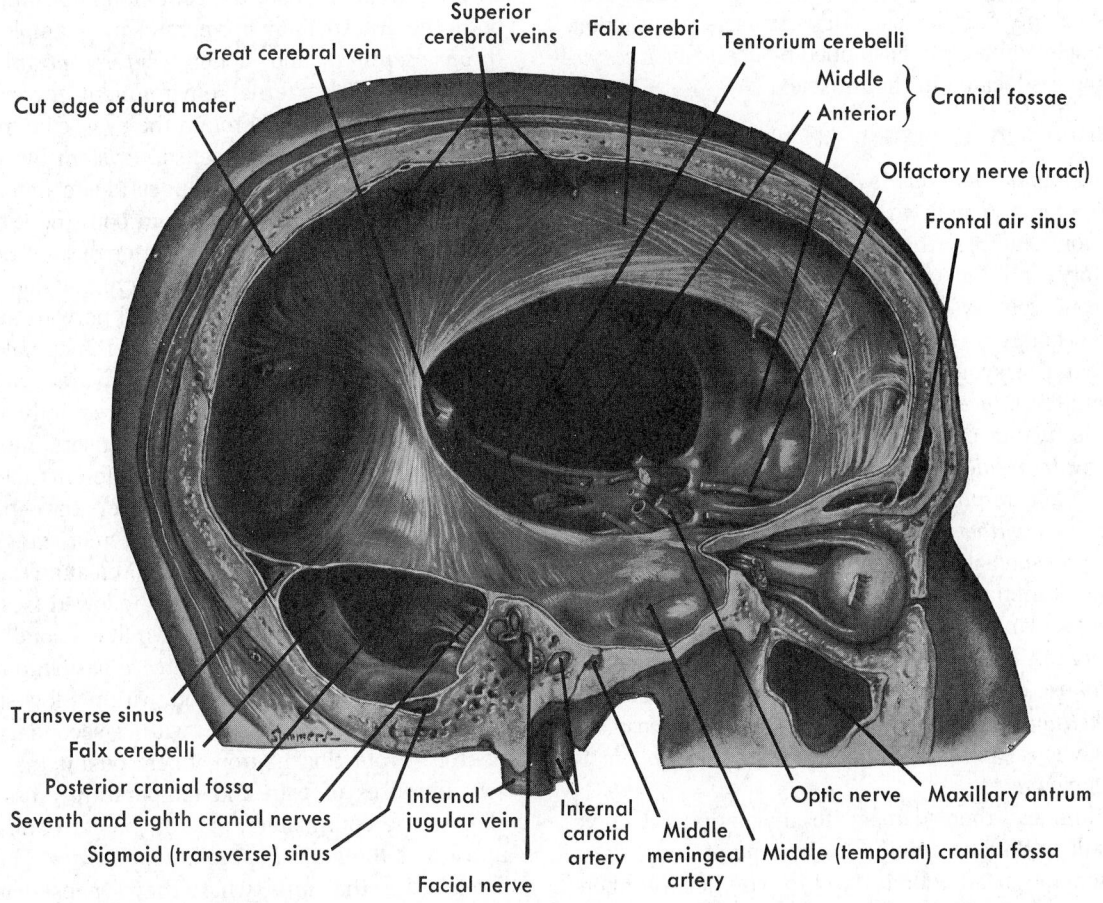

FIGURE 59-12 The brain and the meningeal layers. The subdural space and subarachnoid space are also shown. (From Mettler FA: Neuroanatomy, ed 2, St Louis, 1948, The CV Mosby Co.)

TABLE 59-4 Parasympathetic and sympathetic nervous system influence

Organ System	Parasympathetic Influence	Sympathetic Influence
Heart	Decreases rate	Increases rate
Blood vessels	Dilates visceral and brain vessels	Constricts
Lung	Constricts bronchi	Dilates bronchi
Gastrointestinal	Increases peristalsis	Decreases peristalsis
Anal sphincter	Opens	Closes
Urinary	Contracts bladder	Relaxes bladder
	Opens sphincter	Closes sphincter
Eye	Constricts pupil	Dilates pupil
	Accommodates for near vision	Accommodates for far vision
Skin	Not applicable	"Goose flesh"
Gastric and salivary secretions	Increases	Decreases
Liver	Not applicable	Stimulates glycogen
Adrenal medulla	Not applicable	Stimulates production of epinephrine

bers continue without synapse until they reach skeletal muscle cells. A small cleft exists between the nerve and the muscle. At the end of the nerve terminal are located *vesicles* containing *acetylcholine*. As the impulse moves down the nerve, the acetylcholine is released and crosses to the muscle, causing a muscle contraction. The muscle contraction is stopped by *acetyl cholinesterase,* which is located in the muscle.

AUTONOMIC NERVOUS SYSTEM

The *autonomic nervous system* regulates automatic body functions, usually in an effort to preserve homeostasis (for example, the regulation of cardiovascular, respiratory, and endocrine functions). Fibers of the autonomic nervous system synapse once after leaving the CNS and before arriving as the neuroeffector junction. The site of this synapse is called a *ganglion* and its neurotransmitter is *acetylcholine*. The autonomic nervous system is further divided into the *sympathetic nervous system (adrenergic)*, which functions to maintain homeostasis and to provide defense against stressors, and the *parasympathetic nervous system (cholinergic)*, which is responsible for conservative and restorative vegetative functions (see Table 59-4).

Fibers leaving the ganglia finally synapse at the effector organ. The neurotransmitter for the postganglionic synapse of the parasympathetic nervous system is *acetylcholine;* and the neurotransmitter for the postganglionic synapse of the sympathetic nervous system is *norepinephrine*.

In summary, then, damage to any peripheral nerve will result in deficits specific to the type of nerve damaged (somatic or autonomic) and to whether the fibers damaged are afferent, efferent, or mixed in nature. It is important to note that assessment of dysfunction will be directed to areas *distal* to the injury.

SENSORY SYSTEM PATHWAYS

Sensation as perceived by the individual is initiated by stimulation of *receptor neurons* located throughout the body. Receptor neurons function to provide the brain with information about the condition and composition of both the internal environment (for example, position [*proprioception*] and action [*enteroception*] of body parts) and the external environment [*exteroception*]. The latter is achieved through the eyes, ears, nose, skin, and tongue. The general sensory system by which this information is conveyed includes (1) receptor neurons responsive to special stimuli from both the internal and external environments, (2) posterior roots of the peripheral or afferent sensory nerves carrying action potentials (nerve impulses) toward the central nervous system, (3) ascending or sensory tracts within the spinal cord and upper brain centers, and (4) sensory areas of the cerebral cortex where stimuli are perceived and localized.

From the receptor neuron, the sensory impulse travels to the spinal cord along the afferent fibers of the nerve involved. These fibers enter the spinal cord through the posterior root (dorsal root ganglion) and may proceed along either the spinothalamic tracts or the posterior columns. The pathway followed is specific to the sensation. For example, nerve fibers conducting the sensations of *pain* and *temperature* pass into the posterior horn of the spinal cord and, within a few spinal segments from entry, synapse with a secondary sensory neuron. From this neuron, fibers conducting the sensory impulses of pain and temperature cross immediately to the contralateral side of the cord and continue upward as the *lateral spinothalamic tract*. These fibers arrive at the thalamus, where they synapse with a third sensory neuron. Fibers from this neuron terminate in the appropriate area of the sensory cortex.

Sensations for crude touch follow a very similar path-

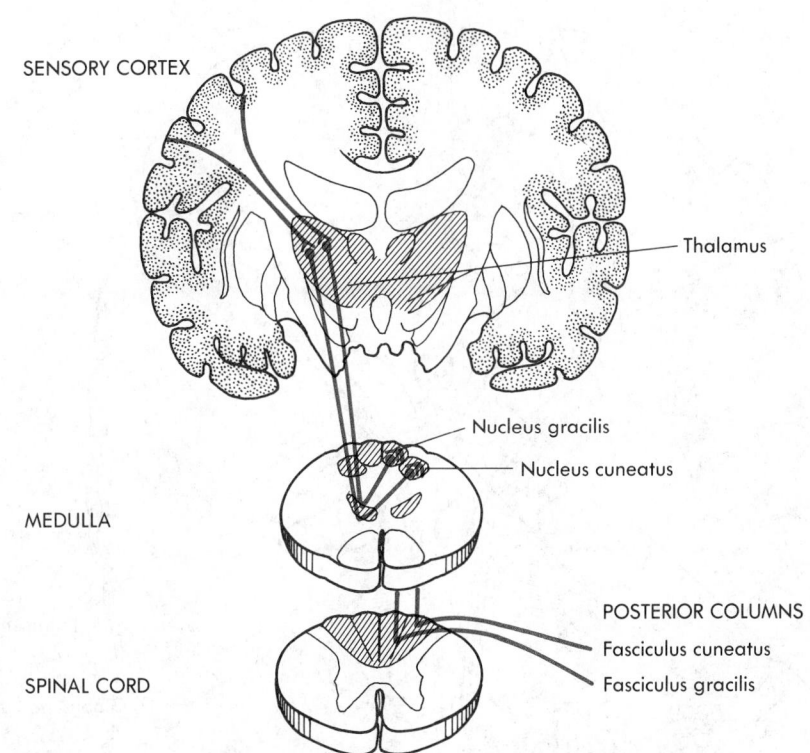

SENSORY CORTEX

Thalamus

Nucleus gracilis

Nucleus cuneatus

MEDULLA

POSTERIOR COLUMNS

Fasciculus cuneatus

Fasciculus gracilis

SPINAL CORD

FIGURE 59-13 Pathways for fine touch, deep touch and pressure, vibration, and proprioception. Note how stimuli entering through dorsal route (posterior) travel on the same side as posterior columns to medulla where they cross to the opposite side, ascend to the thalamus, and end in somasthetic area where perception occurs.

way to that for pain and temperature. Nerve fibers conducting the impulses pass into the posterior horn of the spinal cord and synapse with a secondary sensory neuron. The fibers from the secondary neuron cross to the contralateral side of the cord and continue upward as the *ventral spinothalamic* tract. These travel to the thalamus where they synapse with a third sensory neuron. Fibers from this neuron terminate in the appropriate area of the sensory cortex. Sensation of fine touch, deep touch/pressure, vibration, and proprioception, on the other hand, arriving at the spinal cord are conducted directly by the *posterior columns (fasciculus gracilis or fasciculus cuneatus)* to the level of the medulla before synapsing with a second neuron. These fibers then cross over to the contralateral side, where they continue to the thalamus. Here they also synapse with a third sensory neuron that terminates at the appropriate area of the sensory cortex (Figure 59-13).

MOTOR SYSTEM PATHWAYS

After the brain perceives the state of the body's internal and external environments, it may initiate corrective actions. These impulses are conveyed by the *descending motor pathways*—including the *corticospinal* (pyrami-

dal) tracts, the *extrapyramidal system,* and the *cerebellar system.* The corticospinal system is primarily concerned with skilled voluntary skeletal muscle movements of the distal extremities and, in particular, with the alpha (α) and gamma (γ) motor neurons. Fibers that combine to form the corticospinal *tracts* arise from the *upper motor neurons.* Their cell bodies are located in the primary motor area of the cerebral cortex in the precentral gyrus of the frontal lobe and in the premotor cortex in the frontal lobe.

After fibers leave the cerebral cortex, they descend through the posterior limb of the internal capsule, middle of the cerebral cerebri, break up into bundles in the basilar portion of the pons, and then collect into discrete bundles within the pyramids of the medulla. In the medulla, the majority of the fibers cross over, or *decussate,* to the opposite side of the medulla and become the *lateral corticospinal tract,* which then passes to all spinal cord levels in the lateral funiculus and terminally synapse in the lateral aspect of laminae IV through VIII (Figure 59-14). The remaining fibers descend directly from the medulla (do not decussate) and synapse directly with α- and γ-neurons in lamina IX of the spinal cord. The latter is known as the *anterior corticospinal*

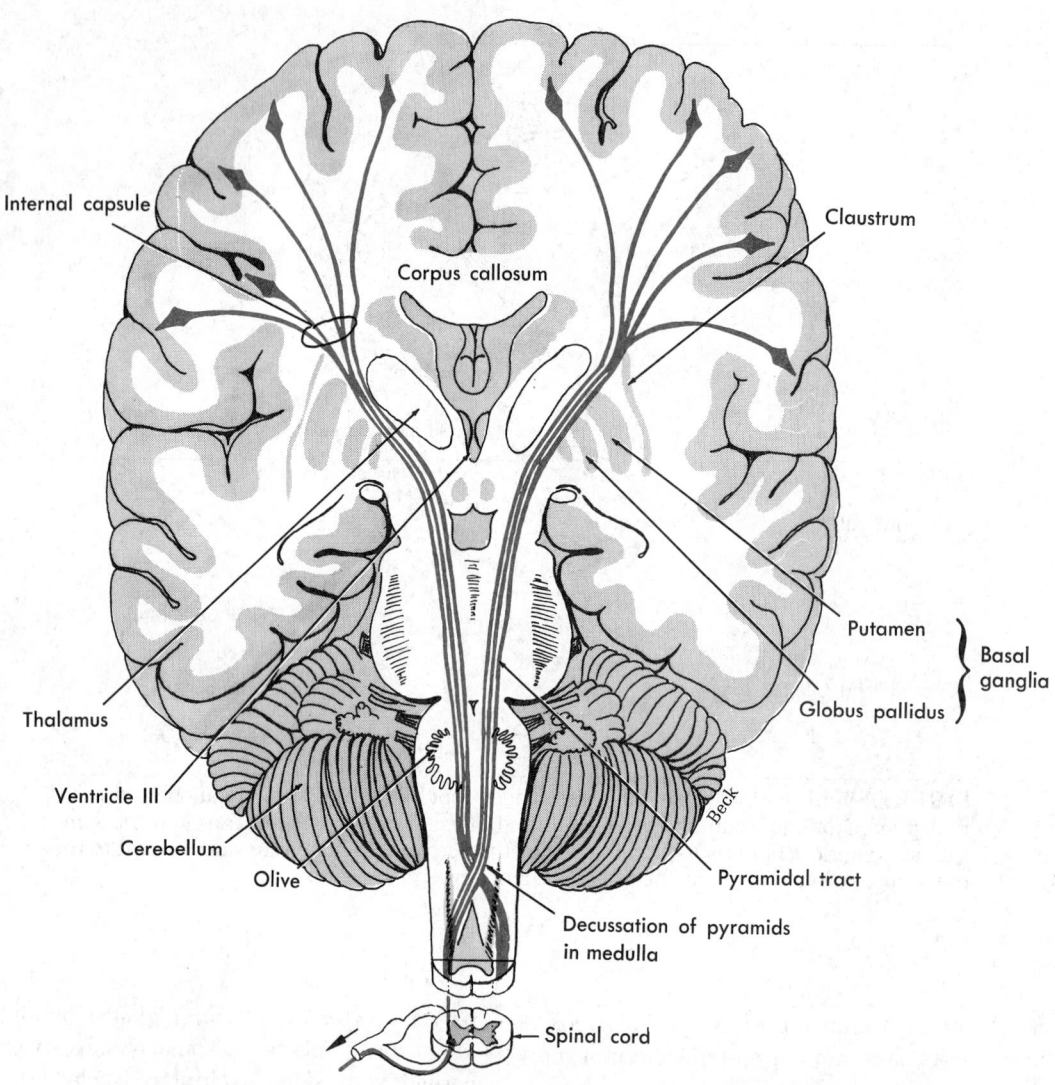

FIGURE 59-14 Crossed corticospinal (pyramidal) tracts. Axons that compose pyramidal tracts (corticospinal) come from neuron cell bodies in cerebral cortex. After they descend through the internal capsule of the cerebrum and white matter of the brain stem, about three fourths of fibers decussate (cross over from one side to the other) in the medulla, as shown. Then they continue downward in lateral corticospinal tract on opposite side of cord. Each crossed corticospinal tract, therefore, conducts motor impulses from one side of the brain to interneurons or anterior horn motoneurons on the opposite side of the cord. Therefore, impulses from one side of cerebrum cause movements of opposite side of the body. (From Anthony CP, and Thibodeau GA: Textbook of anatomy and physiology, ed 11, St Louis, 1983, The CV Mosby Co.)

tract. The *left* cerebral motor strip of the primary motor area controls the muscular movement of the right side of the body.

Eventually, these fibers synapse with large *anterior horn cells* located in the spinal cord as well as in the motor cranial nuclei in the brain stem. These cells are called the *lower motor neurons* and are responsible for providing the final direct link or *final common pathway* with muscles via the myoneural (neuromuscular) junction at the motor end plates. Thus skeletal muscle activ-

ity is the result of the net influence of upper motor neurons on the α- and γ-motor neurons through the anterior horn cells (lower motor neurons) in the spinal cord and motor cranial nuclei.

EXTRAPYRAMIDAL TRACTS

The *extrapyramidal tracts* are complex and provide separate pathways between the cortex, the basal ganglia, the brain stem, and the cord. In general, these include all descending motor pathways *other than* the corticospinal tract (indicating that they do not pass through the pyramids of the medulla). In general, these tracts are named from point of origin to termination. The extrapyramidal tracts collectively assist in maintaining muscle tonus and the control of gross automatic skeletal muscle movements. Some tracts tend to facilitate extensor activity and inhibit flexor activity (lateral vestibulospinal tract and pontine reticulospinal tract), whereas others facilitate flexor activity and inhibit extensor activity (lateral corticospinal tract and rubrospinal tract). It should be noted that some clinicians include as upper motor neurons the extrapyramidal descending fiber systems because such neurons also influence the lower motor neurons and help to modulate skeletal muscle tone and reflex activity.

CEREBELLAR SYSTEM

The *cerebellar system* is responsible for muscle synergy throughout the body. The cerebellum coordinates the action of muscle groups and controls their contractions so that movements are performed smoothly and accurately. Voluntary movements can proceed without the cerebellum, but movements would be clumsy and uncoordinated (*asynergia* and *cerebellar ataxia*). The cerebellum receives both *sensory* and *motor inputs*. There are feedback circuits with all the descending motor pathways. In addition, all sensory modalities, including tactile, auditory, and visual, also feed impulses to the cerebellum. The general scheme of cerebellar operation allows nerve impulses to be returned to or fed back to the same region from which they originated. These circuits can be compared with modern automatic control devices, or servomechanisms. The cerebellar cortex, similar to a computer, can detect any errors in muscle synergy and return the proper messages to adjust muscular control within the body.

Visceral efferent motor pathways from the spinal cord mediate the action of *involuntary*, or *smooth, muscles* located within walls of tubes, hollow organs, the heart, and the glands. *Most viscera are supplied by both excitatory* and *inhibitory fibers*.

EFFECTORS

Effectors may be thought of as the cells of the body that "do something." They in turn interact with the internal and external environments in some way and carry out the commands of the nervous system. The *two classes* of *effectors* are *muscles* and *glands*. They are both transducers and are capable of converting one form of energy into another. Effectors, like nerve tissue, are excitable tissues and are able to generate action potentials. The nervous system controls muscles and glands by directly turning them on or by altering their level of spontaneous activity through a neuron-to-effector chemical communication system.

PHYSIOLOGIC CHANGES WITH AGING

Changes in the nervous system occur with normal aging. It must be stressed, however, that normal aging cannot be equated with senility or Alzheimer's disease. The healthy older person continues to function mentally at a high level in most cases.

The changes in the nervous system associated with aging include the loss of brain cells with actual loss of brain weight. The nerve cell loss is frequently diffuse and gradual. The gyri of the brain surface also atrophy, causing widening and deepening of the spaces between the gyri. Other changes include a decrease in blood flow and increased reaction time and increased time required for decision making. Impairment in short-term memory may also be present. The ability of the brain to autoregulate its blood supply lessens with increased age.

The aged may also experience an altered sleep/wakefulness ratio and a decreased ability to regulate body temperature. These suggest changes in the function of the hypothalamus.

The control of the autonomic nervous system over various functions of the body is unpredictable and labile in the elderly, but some changes do occur. Additionally, sensory and motor conduction decreases in velocity of nerve impulses occur with aging, sensory conduction decreasing faster than motor. This occurs especially in peripheral nerves.

SUBJECTIVE DATA

Complete neurologic assessment is usually completed in phases and depends on the condition of the person and the urgency in collecting the data. The first phase is usually the *history*, where *subjective data* are obtained.

Several aspects of the neurologic examination contain largely subjective data. These are the assessment of *mental status, level of consciousness, language and speech, perceptual status*, and *sensory status*. Levels of consciousness will be discussed in Chapter 60. The others will be discussed in this chapter.

The reader is reminded that it is often difficult to separate subjective from objective data in the neurologic examination. One example of this is the testing of the cranial nerves. These will be discussed under objective data to prevent confusion, although many of these nerves have sensory components.

HISTORY

As in other specialties, a careful history precedes physical examination of the nervous system. In the course of history taking, the person's chief complaints are elicited through an interview. The person is asked to give a timewise account of the illness. The onset and progression of the condition, as well as the nature of symptoms, should be determined. As the person describes the onset of symptoms, note particularly the *speed of onset, frequency of remissions* (if any), and any *diurnal patterns or intensity changes in symptoms.* Symptoms often reported with vagueness and thus requiring sophisticated analyses are complaints of pain, headache, seizures, vertigo, numbness, visual changes, and weakness. Identification of specific patterns of these common neurologic manifestations may provide pertinent diagnostic information about the pathologic process and the person's perception of limitations. Ongoing collection of psychosociocultural data is of special importance. Information is collected about family members and their relationships and interactions, ethnic background, housing, recreational interests, occupation, education, coping mechanisms, dependence-independence characteristics, and how usual activities of daily living are correctly managed by the person. Particular *attention should be paid* to reports of any *recent changes in the person's usual behaviors;* for example, *increased irritability, memory loss,* or *complaints of increasing job-related pressure* or *tension.* A family health history and developmental history are also included. During the course of the neurologic or physical examination, some of the observations made during the history may be confirmed. A skillfully taken history with accurate analysis and interpretation of the collected data often holds the key to diagnosis. Some observations made during the history that are validated during the examination will require further study through special neurodiagnostic procedures.

MENTAL STATUS

Specific abnormalities to higher cerebral function are particularly significant in determining the presence of organic brain disease; therefore, clinical observation of mental function is important.

Along with level of consciousness, the patient is tested for *orientation* to time (day, month, week), place, and person. Disorientation to place and person indicates a more profound cerebral disorder. It is helpful to remember that orientation depends on the ongoing sensory impressions and involves the cerebral cortex. The nurse must be aware of the patient's access to sensory information before deciding the patient is disoriented.

The identification of *mood* and *behavior* is also included in a mental examination, because a particular mood may be associated with a specific disease. For example, *emotional lability is often seen in bilateral (diffuse) brain disease,* where the mood shifts easily and quickly from one extreme to the other. *Euphoria is a superficial elevation of mood* accompanied by unconcern even in the presence of threatening events. It needs to be determined if the person's mood is appropriate to the topic of conversation. *Personality changes* with the appearance of violent temper and aggressive

behavior may occur with destructive lesions of the inferior frontal parts of the limbic system. Such behaviors can be validated by family and friends.

The individual's *knowledge* and *vocabulary* are tested in reference to common knowledge of current events. The ability to think abstractly may be tested by asking the person to explain the meaning of a proverb. Calculation is tested by examining the ability to subtract serially 7 from 100. *Dyscalculia* is the inability to solve simple problems. *Recent memory loss* is more common in brain disease than is remote memory loss. The findings of these gross tests may indicate the need for more definitive tests of mental function. Thus, it can be seen that much data concerning mental status can be collected through a careful and thoughtful patient history.

LANGUAGE AND SPEECH

In assessing language and speech, one must first distinguish between *aphasia* and *dysarthria.* Aphasia is the general term for impairment of language function; it is a disorder of symbolic language. *Dyasrthria,* on the other hand, is an indistinctness in word articulation or enunciation resulting from *interference* with the *peripheral speech mechanisms* (for example, the muscles of the tongue, palate, pharynx, or lips).

Gross assessment of speech and language is made while the examinee's history is being taken. To further assess language, one must recall that language ability is concentrated in a cortical field that includes parts of the temporal lobe, the temporoparietal-occipital junction, the frontal lobe of the dominant (usually the left) hemisphere, and the occipital lobes. Lesions in any of the above areas will produce some impairment of language ability.

Aphasia

Several different types of aphasia have been identified: (1) fluent, (2) nonfluent, and (3) global. Although one type often predominates, often one or more of the other types will be detected to some degree. (See Table 59-5 for further information on the aphasias.)

Aphasic problems can be detected by assessing spontaneous speech and by asking the examinee to follow simple commands, written and oral, to read and interpret newspaper stories, or to write down thoughts. Once a problem is identified, referral may be made to a speech pathologist for a definitive diagnosis and suggestions for treatment.

Dysarthria

The ability to produce speech is tested through the detection of weakness or incoordination of muscles used in articulating speech. Limitations are observed during *cranial nerve testing* and particularly in reference to *cranial nerves V, VII, IX, X,* and XII. As previously dis-

TABLE 59-5 Types of aphasia

Type	Definition	Site of Lesion	Clinical Manifestations	Patient Awareness
Wernicke's	Type of fluent aphasia	Wernicke's area of left hemisphere	Fluent speech with normal and rapid rate; grammar and rhythm are intact, but with little content to speech. Paraphasias, neologisms, and verbal nonwords occur	Not aware of mistake
Anomic	Type of fluent aphasia	Area of angular gyrus	Speech is fluent but patient cannot name objects or places; may define or describe what he is trying to name	Is aware
Conduction	Type of fluent aphasia	Arcuate fasciculus	Speech characterized by literal paraphasia, but comprehension is intact	Is aware
Fluent	Impairment of ability to comprehend spoken language or written language			
Nonfluent	Loss of ability to express one's thoughts in speech and/or writing (motor, Broca's, expressive)	Motor cortex at Broca's area	Problems in selecting, organizing, and initiating motor speech patterns. Speech halting, with effort to produce each word. Limited vocabulary. Telegraphic speech—omission of small grammatic words	Knows what he or she wishes to say and comprehends disability. Often frustrated
Global	Occurs with extensive left damage and involves several speech areas. Few intact language skills	Several sites	Nonfluent speech, poor comprehension, limited ability to name objects or repeat words	Cannot comprehend world around him or her

cussed, involvement of the motor component of these nerves may produce alterations in phonation, resonance, and articulation. The examiner asks the individual to produce different speech sounds in order to localize the problem.

Dysarthrias are usually noticed during ordinary conversation or by having the examinee repeat a difficult phrase such as "Methodist Episcopal" or "third riding artillery brigade." Dysarthrias may be manifested by a single alteration or a variety of alterations. There are characteristic changes in particular diseases. For example, in cerebellar disease speech is often thick and explosive with a prolongation of speech sounds occurring at intervals (scanning). In parkinsonism, speech is referred to as being hyperkinetic and is characterized by a decrease in loudness and in vocal emphasis patterns that makes sounds seem monotonous to the listener.

Apractic speech is a rare, yet interesting, disorder in which there is difficulty in the production of speech volitionally in the absence of motor programming through cortical integration. (Apraxia is a general term that also relates to motor acts other than speech.)

PERCEPTION

All sensation is integrated and interpreted in the sensory cortex, especially in the parietal lobe. It is important for the nurse to recognize *perceptual problems*, for they can be more difficult to deal with than changes in the patient's ability to move or sense. Disorders of perception frequently involve *spatial-temporal relationships* or the *perception of self*.

The special ability to recognize objects through any of the special senses is known as *gnosia*. Lesions involving a specific association area of the cortex produce a specific type of gnosia (absence of this ability). One type of ability often tested is *stereogenesis*, the ability to perceive an object's nature and form by touch. This is assessed by asking the examinee to identify familiar objects placed in the hand one at a time.

Apraxia is an other perceptual problem often seen.

TABLE 59-6 Apraxia

Types	Impairment Produced	Lesion Site
Constructional	Impairment in producing designs in two or three dimensions Involves copying, drawing, or constructing	Occipitoparietal lobe of either hemisphere
Dressing	Inability to dress oneself accurately Makes mistakes, as putting clothes on backwards, upside-down, inside-out, or putting both legs in the same pant leg	Occipital or parietal lobe usually in nondominant hemisphere
Motor	Loss of kinesthetic memory patterns, which results in patient's inability to perform a purposeful motor task although it is understood	Frontal lobe of either hemisphere, precentral gyrus
Idiomotor	Inability to imitate gestures or perform a purposeful motor task on command May be able to do task spontaneously	Parietal lobe of dominant hemisphere, supramarginal gyrus
Ideational	Inability to carry out activities automatically or on command because of inability to understand the concept of the act	Parietal lobe of dominant hemisphere or diffuse brain damage as in arteriosclerosis

This is the inability to perform skilled, purposeful movements in the absence or loss of motor power, sensation, or coordination. (See Table 59-6 for examples of the different types of apraxia.)

SENSORY STATUS

Accurate assessment of sensory function depends on the person's cooperation, alertness, and responsiveness. The examinee should be relaxed and have the eyes closed during all portions of the sensory examination to avoid receiving visual clues. Also, sensation should be tested side to side and distally to proximally.

General sensory function of the trunk and extremities is tested for both superficial and deep sensations. Areas of sensory loss or abnormality are mapped out on a body diagram with a red pencil according to the distribution of the *spinal dermatomes* and peripheral nerves (see Figure 62-1). A dermatome, or skin segment, may be thought of as the area of skin supplied by one dorsal root of a cutaneous nerve. An area in which sensation is absent (*anesthesia*) is differentiated from areas in which a sensation is intensified (*hyperesthesia*) or lessened (*hypesthesia*). *Paresthesia* is an abnormal sensation that is perceived as burning, prickly, or itching.

Pain, Temperature, and Touch

Superficial pain perception is assessed by stimulating a suspected area by pinprick and asking the examinee to report discomfort. One can alternate sharp with dull objects for increased discrimination. *Deep pain* may be assessed by multiple means, some of which have the potential of causing tissue injury. It is only necessary to assess deep pain when the person being examined has a decreased level of consciousness. The method used

should be chosen carefully, and the reader is directed to use the expertise of a nurse specialist to learn the correct techniques.

Crude touch may be assessed by touching a suspected area with cotton and requesting that the examinee indicate when the touch is felt. *Temperature* is tested by touching particular areas with warm to hot and cool to cold objects and asking the person to state the sensations felt. Since *pain and temperature have the same nerve pathway, testing for temperature* can be *eliminated* in the routine examination *if the tests for pain perception are normal.*

Motion and Position

Proprioceptive fibers transmit sensory impulses from muscles, tendons, ligaments, and joints. This results in an awareness of the position of one's limbs in space (kinesthetic sense). *Proprioception* is tested by the examiner's grasping the sides of the examinee's distal phalanx and moving it up and down without assistance from the examinee. If proprioception is intact, the examinee will report correctly the direction in which the joint is being moved. (One can also assess proprioceptive abilities by the Romberg test.)

Vibration is tested by placing a low-frequency tuning fork on a bony prominence of each extremity and assessing the examinee's ability to feel it.

OBJECTIVE DATA

The sequence in performing the neurologic examination varies with the examiner, but it should be one that ensures completeness and thoroughness without exhausting the person being examined. Throughout the

EQUIPMENT NEEDED TO PERFORM A NEUROLOGIC EXAMINATION

1. Compass
2. Cotton applicators
3. Diagram of dermatomes
4. Dynamometer
5. Flashlight
6. Miscellaneous items of varied shapes and sizes (coin, key, marble)
7. Ophthalmoscope
8. Otoscope
9. Colored pencil
10. Pins with sharp and blunt ends
11. Printed page
12. Reflex hammer
13. Tape measure
14. Tongue depressors
15. Tuning fork
16. Snellen chart
17. Stoppered vials containing:
    a. Peppermint, oil of cloves, coffee, soap (smell)
    b. Sugar, salt, vinegar, quinine (taste)
    c. Cold and hot water (temperature)
18. Watch with second hand

examination the examiner attempts to localize the site of any abnormality. Using knowledge of normal neuroanatomy and neurophysiology, combined with a series of tests, the abnormal findings with reference to their *distribution* and *symmetry* of both sides of the body are noted.

The examination depends largely on inspection and palpation and only occasionally on percussion. Auscultation may be used to detect related vascular abnormalities. Varied instruments are used. Initially, functions may be tested grossly, followed by definitive testing should an abnormality be identified.

Equipment required to perform a neurologic examination (in addition to materials used for a general physical examination) is often assembled for convenience on a neurologic tray (see the box above).

CRANIAL NERVES

A general description of cranial nerve testing is included at this point. It is helpful to recall from anatomy the number of the nerve (the sequence of the nerve along the rostrocaudal axis of the brain) and the name (explains the function or distribution) and to be able to express in a few words the function or functions of each cranial nerve so that it has practical meaning. Knowledge of the brain stem anatomy assists in relating the cranial nerve locations (Figure 59-6).

The 12 cranial nerves may be tested in numbered sequence as presented on the following pages. Some nurses prefer to test at the same time those cranial nerves that have similarity of function, such as voluntary motor function and visceral motor function and special sensory and general sensory functions. It should be recalled, however, that some cranial nerves have both motor and sensory functions, whereas others are purely motor or sensory. It also should be recognized by the examiner that data collected from sensory testing are subjective. To counteract this, the person should be retested several times and in a random order to avoid memorization by the examinee (Table 59-7).

CRANIAL NERVE I (OLFACTORY)

The function of cranial nerve I is purely *sensory,* namely, smell. Special receptors located within the superior or uppermost part of each nasal chamber, when stimulated by odors, transmit neural impulses over the olfactory bulbs to the olfactory nerves terminating in the area of the central cortex concerned with olfaction. When testing this cranial nerve, it is first determined whether an odor is perceived. If so, then identification of the specific odor is requested by name. Data are collected in relation to the ability to perceive odor and identify substances by their odor. The ability to be aware of an odor must be differentiated from the ability to name a specific substance. *Anosmia* (absence of smell) or *hyposmia* (decreased sensitivity of the sense of smell) is often associated with complaints of lack of *taste,* even though tests may demonstrate that sense to be intact. Anosmia is caused by varied lesions involving any part of the olfactory pathways. Neoplasia at the base of the frontal lobe and trauma are the common causes of neurogenic anosmia. Intranasal disease affecting the epithelium containing the receptors should be excluded before a diagnosis is made.

CRANIAL NERVE II (OPTIC)

The function of cranial nerve II is purely *sensory,* namely, *sight or vision.* Rods and cones, the special receptors sensitive to light, are located within the retina of the eye. When the retina is stimulated, nerve impulses are transmitted over the optic nerves (extending from the optic disk to the chiasm), over the optic tracts with the radiations terminating in the visual cortex of the occipital lobes. It should be noted, as shown in Figure 59-15 *A* and *B,* that the medial (nasal) fibers of each optic nerve cross at the chiasm to the opposite side of the brain, while the lateral (temporal) fibers remain uncrossed. Thus fibers of the *left optic tract* contain only fibers from the left half of each retina and carry impulses to the left occipital lobe; fibers of the right optic tract contain only fibers from the right half of each retina and carry impulses to the right occipital lobe. Vision depends on the intactness of the visual pathways described previously. Optic nerve function is assessed in relation to visual acuity, visual fields, and the appear-

TABLE 59-7 Cranial nerves

Nerve	Origin	Function	Assessments
Olfactory (I)	Olfactory	Sensory—smell	Identification of odors
Optic (II)	Lateral geniculate body	Sensory—vision	Visual acuity; inspection of fundi; determination of visual fields
Oculomotor (III)	Midbrain	Motor—pupil constriction, elevation of upper eyelid, extraocular movements	Tested together for extraocular movements (Figure 34-15); also pupil reflex for CNIII
Trochlear (IV)	Midbrain	Motor—downward/inward eye movements	
Trigeminal (V)	Pons	Motor—jaw movement Sensory facial sensation	Jaw strength; facial sensation; corneal reflex
Abducens (VI)	Pons	Motor—lateral eye movements	
Facial (VII)	Pons	Motor—facial muscles Sensory taste on anterior two thirds of tongue	Facial movements; identification of tastes
Acoustic (VIII)	Pons	Hearing—cochlear division Balance—vestibular division	Whisper; caloric test
Glossopharyngeal (IX)	Medulla	Sensory—pharynx and posterior tongue, with taste	Identification of tastes
		Motor—pharynx Sensory—pharynx and larynx	Gag reflex; uvula motion; soft palate movement; hoarseness
Vagus (X)	Medulla	Motor—palate, pharynx and larynx	
Spinal accessory (XI)	Medulla	Motor—sternocleidomastoid, upper part of trapezius	Shoulder and neck motion
Hypoglossal (XII)	Medulla	Motor—tongue	Tongue motion

Adapted from Bates B: A guide to physical examination, ed 2, Philadelphia, 1979, JB Lippincott Co.

ance of the fundus (inner eye posterior to the lens). Each eye is tested separately.

Visual Acuity

Visual acuity is mediated by the *cones* of the retina. Central vision is grossly tested by reading fine newspaper print. Distant visual acuity is assessed through the use of the Snellen chart (see Chapter 64). Individuals with vision less than 20/20 are tested to determine light perception (LP), hand movement (HM), and finger count (FC).

Visual Fields

Field of vision is defined as that portion of space in which objects are visible during the fixation of vision in *one* direction. The field of vision thus relates to peripheral vision, or indirect vision. As in visual acuity, normality depends on the intactness of all parts of the visual pathway of the eye. The receptors for peripheral fields are the *rod* neurons of the retina. These are efficient for detection of form and movement but are poor for vision and color. Visual acuity and color are functions of the central field. The visual fields are tested grossly by *confrontation techniques.*

Visual fields may be altered in a variety of central nervous system diseases, such as neoplasia and vascular disease. Ocular disease such as glaucoma is a major

cause. Damage to one optic nerve anterior to the chiasm affects only the field of the involved eye. Lesions at the chiasm or posterior to it produce bilateral visual field defects of a wide variety. For example, a pituitary gland tumor compressing the optic chiasm damages the crossing fibers from the nasal retina and classically causes bitemporal hemianopia, or the loss of vision in the temporal halves of each eye. Loss of vision in the corresponding halves of both visual fields produces *homonymous hemianopia* and can be further designated as right or left. For example, patients with *right* cerebrovascular accidents often experience hemianopia with left visual field loss.

Ocular Fundus

The fundus is examined through the *ophthalmoscope*. The ocular fundus is defined as that portion of the interior of the eyeball that lies posterior to the lens. It includes the optic disk, blood vessels, retina, and macula. Examination, although painless in the normal eye, does require cooperation from the person being examined.

Examination and Interpretation of Ophthalmoscopic Findings

The optic disk (papilla) is normally the most prominent structure visible; *it is the center of observation from which the funduscopic* examination proceeds. The fu-

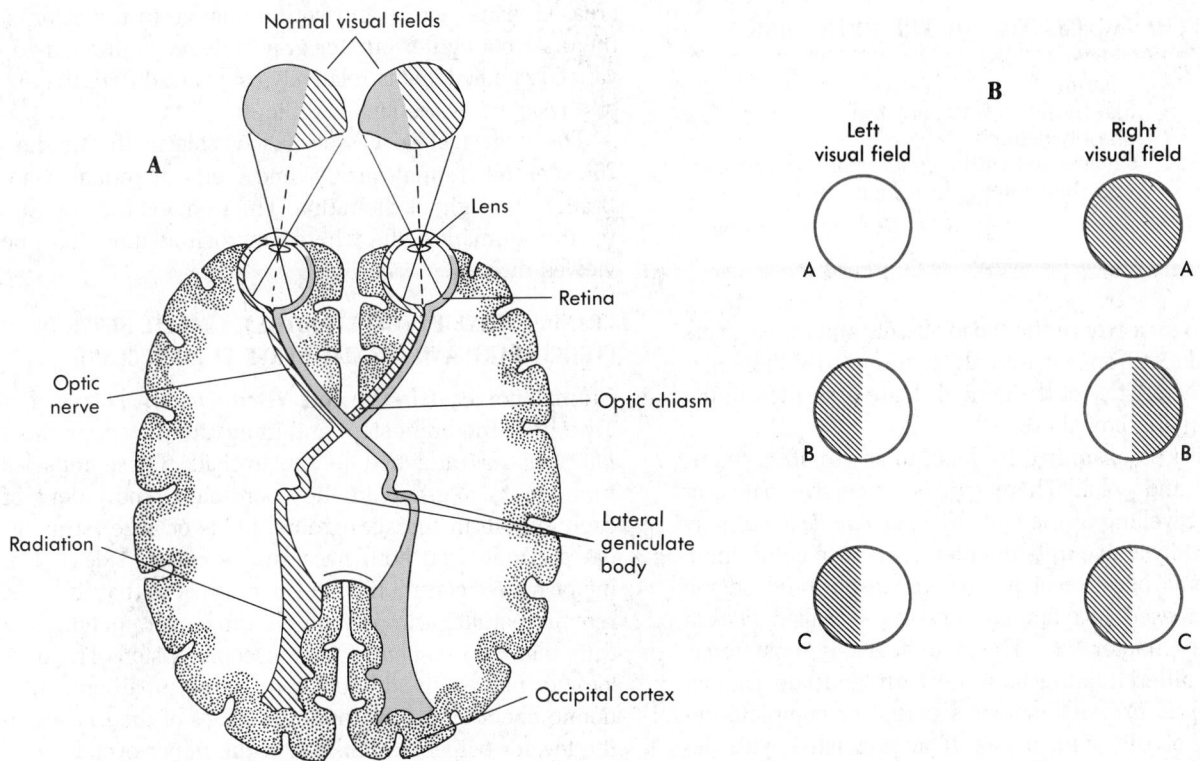

FIGURE 59-15 A, Visual pathways showing partial decussation at optic chiasm. Normal visual fields show reversal of light rays from the temporal and nasal sides to receptors in the retina. **B,** Abnormal visual fields. *A,* Normal left field of vision with loss of vision in right field as a result of complete lesion off right optic nerve. *B,* Loss of vision in temporal half of both fields as a result of lesion of optic chiasm (bitemporal hemianopia). *C,* Loss of vision in nasal field of right eye and temporal field of left eye caused by lesion of right optic tract (homonymous hemianopia).

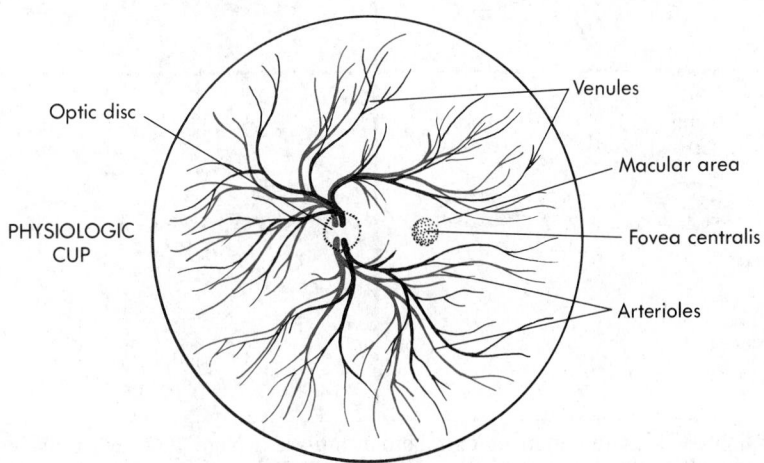

FIGURE 59-16 Structures of the left eye as visualized through the funduscope.

NORMAL CHARACTERISTICS OF THE OPTIC DISK

Size	1.5 mm
Shape	Flat round or vertically oval
Margins	Sharply defined
Color	Creamy red with a small whitish depression in the center (physiologic cup)

dus is the area where the blood vessels and nerve fibers enter and exit from the eyeball (Figure 59-16). The normal characteristics of the optic disk are presented in the accompanying box above.

The disk is examined in detail to assess size, shape, margins, and color. There can be excessive pallor or redness. Swelling of the optic disk, or *papilledema*, may be caused by active inflammation or passive congestion. Papilledema because of passive congestion and edema from increased intracranial pressure is called *choked disk* (see Chapter 62). The neurologist is most interested in differentiating between early and late papilledema. *Optic atrophy* indicates partial or complete destruction of the optic nerve. It is associated with de-

creased visual acuity and with a change in the color of the disk to a lighter pink or gray. The recognition of advanced papilledema is relatively easy, but differentiation of physiologic variations is difficult.

The largest blood vessels just visible in the fundus, the central retinal artery and central retinal vein, branch throughout the retina. The retina is the only site in the human body where microcirculation can be viewed directly.

CRANIAL NERVE III (OCULOMOTOR), CRANIAL NERVE IV (TROCHLEAR), AND CRANIAL NERVE VI (ABDUCENS)

Cranial nerves III, IV, and VI are *motor nerves* that arise from the brain stem and innervate the six *extraocular muscles* attached to the eyeball. These muscles function as a group in the coordinated movement of each eyeball in the six cardinal fields of gaze (straight, up, and down on both nasal and temporal sides). The motor nerves control the ocular muscles so that the eyes remain parallel throughout all ranges of motion and thus maintain *binocular* (stereoscopic) vision. The oculomotor nerves, in addition, send parasympathetic autonomic fibers to the constrictor muscles of the iris and to the levator palpebrae muscles of the upper eyelids.

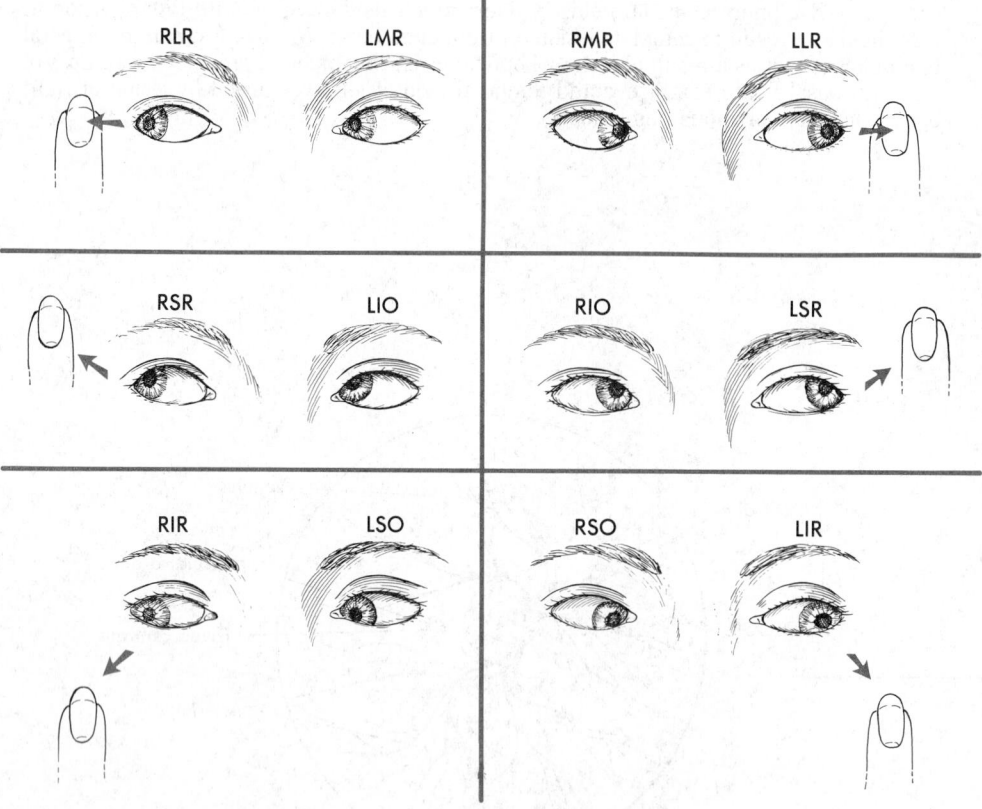

FIGURE 59-17 Examination of extraocular muscles. Note that two muscles are involved in each cardinal direction. R, right; L, left; LR, lateral rectus; MR, medial rectus; SR, superior rectus; IO, inferior oblique; IR, inferior rectus; SO, superior oblique.

Extraocular Movements

Individual eye movements are tested by covering one eye and following the examiner's finger in all fields of gaze with the uncovered eye while keeping the head stationary. Limitations of movement in all directions are observed as well as actual paralysis (*ophthalmoplegia*). If one of the extraocular muscles is paralyzed by damage to the nerve, the eye is unable to deviate fully into the corresponding field of gaze.

Conjugate movements of the eyes are also tested by asking the person to look with both eyes as far possible to either side then up and down. The examiner observes for parallel movements of the eyes in each direction or any deviation from normal (Figure 59-17).

Double vision (*diplopia*), squint (*strabismus*), and involuntary rhythmic movements of the eyeballs (*nystagmus*) may indicate weakness of some of the extraocular muscles because of deficits of the motor nerves. These nerves may be involved singly or in unison in some neurologic diseases. *Ptosis,* or dropping of the upper eyelid over the globe, may be caused by damage to the oculomotor nerve. Normally, the upper lid minimally overlaps the iris as the examinee moves the eyes downward. The person with ptosis is unable to raise the lid voluntarily.

Pupils

Each pupil should be inspected first as to size and then as to shape and equality. *Argyll Robertson* pupils, for example, are constricted and do not react to light, although they react to accommodation for near objects. Pupil inequality, or *anisocoria,* may assist in diagnosis of some neurologic diseases (Figure 59-18, *A, B*). The pupil is normally round, centrally placed, regular in outline, and equal in size to the other pupil. However, un-

equal pupils are found in approximately 25% of the normal population. Thus it is more significant to assess briskness of the pupillary response.

Pupillary Reflex

The examiner darkens the room before examination. A small beam of light is focused directly into each eye in turn. The examiner avoids shining the light into both eyes simultaneously and instructs the person not to focus on the light beam, thus producing an accommodation reaction. Normally, the pupil constricts quickly when a light is focused on the homolateral retina. Constriction is reported to be especially brisk in young people and those with blue eyes. After a head injury, for example, a *dilated, fixed* pupil may be observed on the side of the cranial injury (Fig. 59-18, *B*). A slow or sluggish pupil occurs as the pupil contracts slowly or imperfectly and relaxes immediately.

Consensual Light Reflex

Observations include inspection for constriction of the pupil *opposite* to the one directly stimulated. As a result of the decussation (crossing) of nerve fibers both in the optic chiasm and in the pretectal area, the homolateral pupil as well as the contralateral pupil normally reacts to light.

CRANIAL NERVE V (TRIGEMINAL)

Cranial nerve V is a *mixed* nerve with motor and sensory components. It is the largest cranial nerve. The motor part innervates the temporal and masseter muscles; the sensory part supplies the cornea, face, head, and mucous membrane.

In muscle weakness the opened jaw tends to deviate to the opposite side of the weakened muscles. The sensory components supplying the face are tested for touch, pain, and temperature and for any deficits noted as to distribution.

Next, bilateral *corneal reflexes* may be assessed if they are in question. Normally, the examinee will blink bilaterally. This is an especially important reflex to assess in persons with *decreased levels of consciousness* because corneal damage may result in its absence.

CRANIAL NERVE VII (FACIAL)

Cranial nerve VII is a *mixed nerve* that is concerned with facial movement and the sensation of taste. The inability to smile, close both eyes tightly, look upward and wrinkle the forehead, show the teeth, purse the lips, and blow out the cheeks constitutes weakness or paralysis of facial muscles innervated by this nerve. Distinction must be made between central and peripheral neurologic involvement. Special attention in examination is given to asymmetry. Peripheral involvement as in *Bell's palsy* is caused by compression of this cranial nerve and

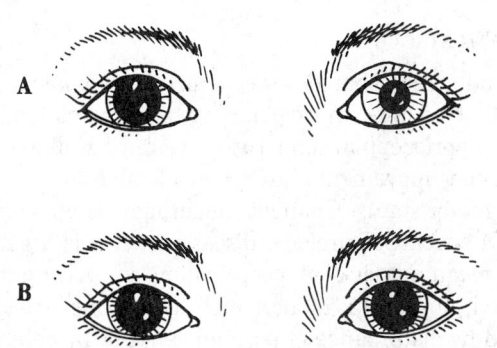

FIGURE 59-18 A, Unequal pupils, also called anisocoria. **B,** Dilated and fixed pupils, indicative of severe neurologic deficit.

is a common *lower motor neuron* type of facial paralysis. (This means the lesion affects the facial nerve or its nucleus). Lesions affecting the facial nerve produce paralysis of half of the entire face including the eyelids, forehead, and lips. Forehead function, by contrast, remains intact in *central or upper motor neuron* lesions. This suggests that the lesion lies somewhere on the path from the contralateral cerebral cortex to the nucleus of the facial nerve. The sensation of taste is tested by placing in turn, salty, sweet, bitter, and sour substances on the side of the protruded tongue for identification. A loss of taste over the anterior two-thirds of the tongue is present when the nerve is diseased, as in mastoid canal lesions.

CRANIAL NERVE VIII (ACOUSTIC)

Cranial nerve VIII is composed of a *cochlear* division related to hearing and a *vestibular* division related to equilibrium. The cochlear portion is tested grossly by having the examinee listen and identify whispered words. It is recommended that the ticking of a watch not be used routinely because it produces a high-pitched tone and such tones are not heard very well by the elderly. A more complete examination, including bone and air conduction of sound, involves testing with a tuning fork and audiometric testing (Chapter 64). The vestibular portion of the acoustic nerve may be tested in a variety of ways. In the *past-pointing test,* the examinee is asked to raise the arms and to bring the index finger down on the examiner's finger with the arm outstretched, first with the eyes open, then with eyes closed. Normally, the examinee's finger touches the examiner's without difficulty. In vestibular disease, the finger points to one side or the other consistently. The vestibular portion is also tested by looking for the presence of *nystagmus*, "to-and-fro" movements of the eyeballs on horizontal and vertical planes, as the examinee looks to one side and upward. True nystagmus is characterized by sustained movement of the eyeball including a fast jerk to the side of the deviation and a slow jerk back to the midline. Additional tests can include caloric tests and electronystagmography (see Chapter 64).

Disease of the *cochlea* is characterized by nerve deafness (perception deafness). There is loss or impairment of hearing. Nerve deafness is usually the result of disease of the peripheral nerve. It may also occur from central lesions involving *acoustic nerves* and *nerve pathways* in the brain stem and their *termination within the temporal lobe. The vestibular portion is frequently affected in diseases of the central nervous system, and the most prominent symptom is vertigo.*

CRANIAL NERVE IX (GLOSSOPHARYNGEAL) AND CRANIAL NERVE X (VAGUS)

Cranial nerves IX and X are tested together. The chief function of cranial nerve IX is *sensory* to the pharynx and taste to the posterior third of the tongue. Both nerves supply the posterior pharyngeal wall, and normally when the wall is touched there is prompt contraction of these muscles on both sides, with or without gagging. This test is thus unreliable in regard to either nerve alone. Since cranial nerve X is the chief *motor nerve* to the soft palatal, pharyngeal, and laryngeal muscles, the detection of abnormalities is made through testing of voice sounds and cough sounds. In unilateral involvement of the motor portion of the vagus nerve there is harshness and nasality of the voice. When the person says "ah" the soft palate does not stay in the midline but deviates to the intact side. Bilateral involvement produces more severe effects in speech; there is also difficulty in swallowing (*dysphagia*), and fluids regurgitate through the nose because of palatal and pharynge lainvolvement. Sensory function is not usually tested in the vagus nerve.

CRANIAL NERVE XI (SPINAL ACCESSORY)

Cranial nerve XI is a motor nerve that supplies the sternocleidomastoid muscle and upper part of the trapezius muscles. Weakness or paralysis of these muscles constitutes abnormality of this nerve.

CRANIAL NERVE XII (HYPOGLOSSAL)

Cranial nerve XII is a purely *motor* nerve. To begin, the examinee's tongue should first be inspected at rest in the mouth. Any asymmetry, unilaterality, decreased bulk, deviations, or fasciculations (fine twitching) should be noted. When this nerve is involved, there is deviation of the tongue toward the side of the lesion. Atrophy of the tongue is shown through wrinkling and loss of substance on the affected side. In an upper motor neuron lesion there is involvement of the tongue on the side opposite (contralateral) the lesion.

MOTOR STATUS

Function of the motor system is assessed as to gait and stance, muscle strength, muscle tonus, coordination, involuntary movements, and muscle stretch reflexes.

GAIT AND STANCE

Gait and stance should be recognized as complex activities that require muscle strength, coordination, balance, proprioception, and vision. Gait, or walking, and associated movements give considerable information about motor status. Changes in gait may be characteristic of a specific neurologic disease. *Ataxia* is a general term meaning lack of coordination in performing a planned, purposeful motion such as walking. It can be caused by disturbance of position sense or by cerebellar or other diseases. In evaluation of gait the person is asked to walk freely and naturally. A request may be made to walk *heel to toe* in a straight line, since this exaggerates any abnormalities. To evaluate stance, the person may perform the *Romberg test*. In this test the individual stands with feet close together, first with eyes open and then with eyes closed. Patients with problems of proprioception have difficulty maintaining balance with their eyes closed; patients with cerebellar disease have difficulty even with their eyes open.

The *hemiparetic gait* seen in upper motor neuron disease is characterized by circumduction of the affected leg and inversion of the foot. Persons with Parkinson's disease walk with a slow, shuffling gait, and as they start walking there is an increase in rapidity until they are almost running *(propulsive)*. They also have difficulty stopping, and deviation in the center of gravity causes retropulsion or lateropulsion. In addition, there is loss of associated movements of the arms in walking. Persons with cerebellar disease, on the other hand, walk with a wide-based, *staggering gait*.

Muscle strength, or power, is assessed systematically, including trunk and extremity muscles. During manual testing of each muscle group the examinee attempts to resist the examiner in moving his muscles when placed in fixed positions. Weakness of a specific muscle is identified by the examiner as to distribution and degree of muscle weaknesses. The examinee may also be tested for *drift*. This test is performed by asking the person to hold the arms straight out for 20 to 30 seconds with palms supine and eyes closed. *Hemiparesis* is suggested when there is pronation of one forearm or when there is a downward drift of the arm with elbow flexion. Evaluation may include all major muscles. *Hemiplegia* is complete paralysis of one half of the body (linear), whereas *hemiparesis* is weakness or incomplete paralysis in the same distribution. *Paraplegia* is paralysis of the lower extremities, and *quadriplegia* is paralysis of the four extremities. The reader should note the distribution of peripheral motor nerves to skeletal muscles. (The distribution varies from that of sensory nerve distributions.)

MUSCLE TONUS

Muscle tonus is tested by the examiner passively moving the examinee's limbs through a full range of motion. An increase *(hypertonia)* or a decrease *(hypotonia)* can be differentiated by the skilled examiner. In hypertonia extremities tend to stay in fixed positions and feel firm; in hypotonia the extremities assume a position governed by gravity. Overextension and overflexion are found in hypertonia; resistance to passive movement increases rapidly and then suddenly gives way to *pyramidal spasticity*, or *clasp-knife rigidity*. A steady, passive resistance throughout the full range of motion is characteristic of *parkinsonian rigidity;* the combination of passive resistance and parkinsonian tremor with small regular jerks is called *cogwheel rigidity*. In *decorticate rigidity*

the upper limbs are flexed and pronated and the lower limbs are extended. In *decerebrate rigidity*, on the other hand, the upper limbs are extended.

COORDINATION

Coordination of muscle movements, or the ability to perform skilled motor acts, may be impaired at any level of the motor system. However, the cerebellum is primarily responsible for control, so that movements take place in a smooth and precise manner. Disturbance in cerebellar function may result in ataxia (as discussed relative to gait), difficulty in controlling the range of muscular movement *(dysmetria), and an inability to alternate rapid opposite and successive movements (adiadochokinesia)*. Simple motor activities are evaluated on command of the examiner to perform rapid and rhythmic movements. For example, the nose-finger-nose test requires the individual to alternately touch the nose and the tip of the examiner's finger with variation in rate and level. Other tests include the knee pat (pronation-supination) and heel-knee or shin test, during which the examinee slides his heel over the shin toward the dorsum of the foot. There are many such tests, often modified by the examiner.

INVOLUNTARY MOVEMENTS

Involuntary movements also need to be observed and described during neurologic examination. Description of abnormal movements *(hyperkinesia)* is difficult but necessary. Observation of the following is helpful: location of muscles involved, amplitude of movement, speed of onset, duration of contraction and relaxation, and rhythm. The effects of posture, rest, sleep, diversion of attention, voluntary movements, and emotional stress on involuntary movement are determined. Involuntary movements are usually increased by emotional stress and may subside during sleep. They can be the result of organic disease, or they may be psychosomatic in origin. A few of the more common types of involuntary movements are considered next. *Tremor* consists of rhythmic to-and-fro movements that are usually of small amplitude. They are the result of alternate contractions of opposing groups of muscles; they are continuous while the patient is awake and may or may not be present during sleep. *Chorea* consists of short, sharp, rapid movements, usually of small excursion and irregular; movements occur in different parts of the body and persist during sleep. *Hemiballismus* is a variation of chorea in which movement is confined to one side of the body and affects the limbs to a great extent. *Athetosis* consists of slow, sinuous, and more sustained movements that may be of considerable amplitude; movements occur within the neck and trunk as well as the extremities and may be called *torsion spasms. Myoclonus* consists of irregular, abrupt, and arrhythmic contractions of a muscle or

TABLE 59-8 Grading of muscle stretch reflexes (MSR)

Scale	Interpretation
0	Areflexia
±	Hyporeflexia
1+ to 3+	Normal
3+ to 4+	Hyperreflexia

a group of muscles. Myoclonus may involve the extremities, the trunk, or the face and may be consistent in site.

REFLEXES

Although all muscles can be made to contract reflexly, only a few reflexes are tested clinically. The *muscle stretch reflexes* (MSRs) (also called myotactic and deep tendon reflexes) that are tested more routinely include the biceps, triceps, brachioradialis, quadriceps, and gastrocnemius and soleus muscles. (Superficial reflexes are omitted in this discussion.) Because the muscle reflexes are simply monosynaptic reflexes, they may be diminished in normal response *(hyporeflexia)* or lost completely *(areflexia)* because of interruption of afferent sensory fiber transmission or extensive destruction of efferent motor fibers of the anterior horn cells (lower motor neurons). On the other hand, release of the monosynaptic reflex from the influence of suprasegmental fibers (pyramidal and supplementary motor systems) (upper motor neuron influence) produces an increased muscular response *(hyperreflexia)*.

The degree of response of the reflex, above or below normal is noted and graded on a scale. The most important feature of any reflex pattern is not the absolute value on the scale but the difference between one side of the body and the other (asymmetry). Stick figures are commonly used to record the bilateral values (scale may range from 0 to 4+). See Table 59-8 for one example of how reflexes are graded on a scale. Because the threshold for muscle stretch reflexes has a normal range of variability, some individuals with generalized hyporeflexia or hyperreflexia will not have pathologic conditions but will rank at the end of the normal range. On the other hand, areflexia is usually a pathologic condition.

One *pathologic reflex* often referred to clinically is the *plantar reflex*. This reflex when present in adults results in extension of the great toe (moves toward dorsum) with fanning (abduction) of the other toes when pressure is applied to the plantar surface of the foot laterally from the heel toward the toes. This response is known as *Babinski's sign* and is associated with upper motor neuron disease (Table 59-9). Other reflexes may also be classified as pathologic. These are reflexes that are present in infancy for variable periods. They are thought to be released in adults by acquired diseases of the cerebrum. Examples include the sucking, pouting, and grasp reflexes.

A reflex when present may assist in localizing a lesion, as does the presence of a unilateral Babinski's sign. Reflex findings, however, are only used in relation to total assessment data and are not used alone. (Refer to neurology tests for techniques on eliciting specific reflexes.) Variations of grading-scale values used should be noted. It also should be recognized that grading is somewhat objective.

MENINGEAL IRRITATION

To test for meningeal irritation, or stiff neck, the head is passively flexed sharply toward the chest while the person is in a recumbent position. In the presence of meningeal irritation there is marked resistance to flexion, accompanied by rigidity of the neck (nuchal), spasm, and pain. There is also resistance to extension and rotary movements of the neck. *Brudzinski's sign*, indicating meningeal irritation, is also elicited by passive neck flexion. When the neck is flexed, the hips and legs flex involuntarily. *Kernig's sign* is a classic test used in the diagnosis of meningitis. In this test the examiner flexes one of the patient's thighs to a right angle and then attempts to extend the leg on the thigh (there are many variations of this test). A positive Kernig's sign is present when there is spasm of the hamstring muscles with resistance to extension of the leg and with neck and head pain.

TABLE 59-9 Clinical syndromes of upper motor neuron and lower motor neuron lesions

Motor Component	Upper Motor Neuron Characteristics	Lower Motor Neuron Characteristics
Reflex	Hyperreflexia, extensor toe sign (Babinski's sign)	Hyporeflexia or areflexia
Muscle tonus	Hypertonia, clasp-knife spasticity, clonus	Hypotonia, flaccidity
Muscle movement	Paralysis or paresis of movements in hemiplegic distribution	Paralysis or paresis of individual muscles in peripheral nerve distribution
Muscle wasting	Late atrophy from disuse	Early atrophy from denervation
Muscle fasciculations	Not present	Present

TABLE 59-10 Blood abnormalities

Element	Abnormality Seen	Possible Reason
Potassium	Decreased	Poor dietary intake
White blood cells	Increased	Infection such as meningitis
		Common steroid effect
Po_2	Decreased	Increased intracranial pressure
Red blood cells	Increased	Dehydration
	Decreased	Anemia
Hematocrit and hemoglobin	Increased	Dehydration
	Decreased	Anemia
Anticonvulsant drug	Increased	Toxicity or patient overdose
	Decreased	Patient not taking drug
Plasma cortisol	Increased	Acute head injury
Sodium	Decreased	Inappropriate antidiuretic hormone

TABLE 59-11 Urine abnormalities

Element	Abnormality Seen	Possible Reason
Urinary output	Decreased amount	Metabolic problem Kidney failure
	Increased amount	Diabetes insipidus
Specific gravity	Decreased	Diabetes insipidus
	Increased	Dehydration
Sugar and acetone	Present	Steroid effect—possible chemical diabetes
Sodium	Increased amount	Inappropriate antidiuretic hormone
		Diabetes insipidus

DIAGNOSTIC TESTS

Relevant diagnostic tests can be an important source of data in making a diagnosis of neurologic disease.

LABORATORY TESTS
BLOOD

A normal part of the neurologic assessment includes obtaining blood for screening. This usually includes electrolytes as well as a complete blood count. Serology screening is done to rule out syphilis which in the tertiary form of the disease may yield neurologic symptoms. Arterial blood gases may be obtained, especially if the patient is critically ill or comatose. One particular form of blood test that can be very helpful is the obtaining of drug levels, especially the level of anticonvulsants. The actual blood level can give the practitioner a sense not only of the way a person metabolizes the drug but also of how compliant the person is after following the prescribed medication regimen.

Abnormalities in any of the blood studies may be indicative of neurologic disease. (See Table 59-10 for some specific abnormalities that may be seen.)

URINE

Urinary output, as well as excretion of electrolytes, is easily influenced by cranial surgery and/or trauma. This is especially true if the pituitary gland has been traumatized from injury or surgery. See Table 59-11 for possible alterations in urinary results.

CEREBROSPINAL FLUID

Cerebrospinal fluid (CSF) is obtained either through a lumbar or cisternal puncture. These will be discussed later in this chapter. The cerebrospinal fluid is examined for an increase or decrease of its normal constituents; it is also examined for foreign substances such as pathogenic organisms and blood. Cerebrospinal fluid normally is a clear fluid that is formed in the lateral ventricles of the brain.

Spinal fluid normally is under slight positive pressure; 80 to 180 mm of water is considered normal. It is measured on a manometer when a spinal puncture is performed.

Normally each milliliter of spinal fluid contains up to eight lymphocytes. An increase in the number of cells may indicate an infection. Tuberculosis and viral infections may cause an increase in lymphocytes, whereas pyogenic infections may cause an increase in polymorphonuclear leukocytes, which may be in large enough numbers to make the fluid cloudy. Bacterial infections, such as tuberculosis meningitis, often lower the blood sugar levels. They may also reduce the chloride level. In the presence of degenerative diseases and when a brain tumor is present, the spinal fluid protein is usually increased. (See the box below for normal values of cerebrospinal fluid.)

Other tests of cerebrospinal fluid that may be helpful include the colloidal gold test that can be used to diagnose neurosyphilis or multiple sclerosis. CSF is abnormal in about 90% of patients with multiple sclerosis, in-

NORMAL VALUES OF CSF

Pressure	75 to 180 mm H_2O
Glucose	50 to 80 mg/100 ml
Chloride	118 to 132 mEq/L
Protein	20 to 50 mg/dl
Gamma globulin	3% to 9%
Lymphocytes	0 to 8/ml

cluding CSF pleocytosis and abnormal gamma globulins as demonstrated by electrophoresis. Cultures of CSF may indicate the actual organism causing disease. The spinal fluid serologic test for syphilis may be positive even when the blood serologic test is negative.

Blood in the spinal fluid indicates hemorrhage into the ventricular system. It may be caused by a fracture at the base of the skull that has torn blood vessels or it may be caused by the rupture of a blood vessel, which may occur, for example, with a congenital aneurysm. Occasionally, the first specimen of spinal fluid contains blood from slight bleeding at the point of puncture. For this reason, the specimens of fluid are numbered and the first one is not used to determine the cell count.

RADIOLOGIC TESTS

The multiple radiologic procedures of the brain and spinal cord are best carried out and interpreted by a neuroradiologist. These include plain radiographs, special contrast studies of the ventricular system (including the cisternal and subarachnoid space) and the cerebral vessels, and computed tomography.

ROUTINE OR PLAIN RADIOGRAPHS

Routine or plain radiographs of the brain and spinal cord are usually taken first, using varied projections to detect any developmental, traumatic, or degenerative

---

COMPUTED TOMOGRAPHY

Preparation of patient	No special physical preparation
	Patient teaching to include explanation of procedure
	Time is approximately 20 to 30 min for CT without contrast medium, 60 min if scan is performed with and without contrast medium
	Procedure is painless
	Intravenous fluid may be started
	Patient must lie still for duration of procedure
	Check for allergy to iodine if contrast medium is used
Procedure	Patient lies supine with head positioned in rubber head-holder
	Head is scanned
	If control study is desired, the patient receives the control medium and procedure is repeated
Postprocedure	No adverse effects except the risk of transient increased intracranial pressure in patients with masses or other brain pathology
	Patient may need rest

---

bone abnormalities. These films are still used frequently because of safety and availability.

COMPUTED TOMOGRAPHY (CT SCAN)

One of the most significant technologic advances in radiographic equipment is the electromagnetic imager (EMI) scanner, which is capable of providing up to 100% more information than conventional radiographic techniques. The EMI scanner is also referred to as CT scan and computerized assisted tomography. This technique offers increased versatility, efficiency, and enhanced image detail. The CT scanner is based on a technique of scanning the brain without isotopes in which series of images using the principles of tomography are x-rayed and each of the images is derived from a specific layer of brain tissue. The brain is thus scanned in successive layers by a very narrow beam of x-rays. The total system includes a scanning unit that houses the x-ray tube, two scintillation detectors, an x-ray control unit, a computer and magnetic disk unit, viewing unit, a line printer, and a teletyper. Data are thus collected in x-ray form and printout form, and information is also stored for future use. (See the box below for further information about this procedure.)

By comparing tissue densities found with the CT scan with norms, abnormalities can be detected. Tumor masses, infarctions, displacement of bone, and ventricles can be accurately detected. The CT scan is particularly efficient in detecting brain neoplasia and cerebrovascular lesions (Figure 59-19).

After the completion of the CT scan, the nurse should monitor the patient for any signs of increased in-

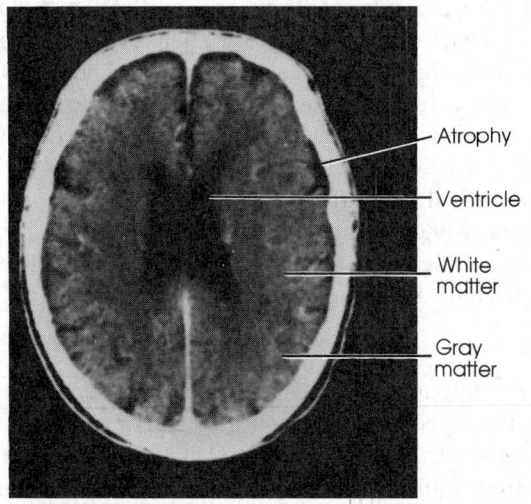

FIGURE 59-19 CT scan printouts. CT brain scan differentiates between gray and white brain matter. (From Ballinger PW: Merrill's atlas of radiographic positions and radiologic procedures, ed 5, St Louis, 1982, The CV Mosby Co.)

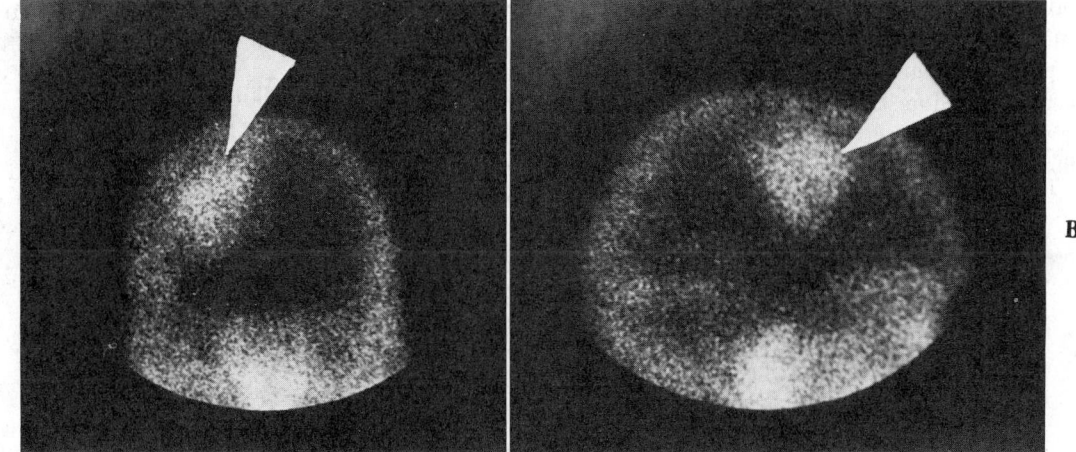

FIGURE 59-20 Brain scans. **A,** Anteroposterior view. **B,** Lateral view. White pointers indicate tumor seen in both views. (From Pagana K: Diagnostic testing and nursing implications: a case study approach, St Louis, 1982, The CV Mosby Co.)

tracranial pressure (if dye was used). If the patient has become disoriented as a result of the test, reassurance should be given and the patient protected from injury. The patient may need rest after the test.

BRAIN SCAN

Another radiologic test is the brain scan. The purpose of this test is to detect cerebral pathology using radioactive isotopes and a scanner (Figure 59-20). It is generally used as an adjunct to routine radiographs and CT. (See the box below for a description of the brain scan.) The

nurse may need to reassure and support the patient during the procedure. The injection site should be monitored for bleeding and the patient may need rest after the procedure.

MAGNETIC RESONANCE IMAGING

One of the newest methods of scanning the brain is magnetic resonance imaging (MRI). This procedure uses a very strong magnet combined with radiofrequency waves and a computer to produce x-ray-like images of body chemistry. No radiation is used. This pro-

---

BRAIN SCAN

Preparation of patient	No physical preparation of patient
	When mercury is used as the isotope indicator, a mercurial diuretic (mercuhydrin) is administered several hours before the procedure; this increases the uptake of radioactive mercury
	Patient teaching to include explanation of procedure: time is about 45 min; procedure is painless except for injection of radioactive isotope and need to lie still
Procedure	Patient is injected with radioisotope (mercury or sodium pertechnetate Tc^{99m})
	Patient lies still while scanner is passed over head
Postprocedure	No adverse effects
	Patient may need rest

MAGNETIC RESONANCE IMAGING SCAN

Preparation of patient	No physical preparation of patient
	Remove credit cards, watches, and other things that could be damaged by the magnet
	Check for presence of clips in brain, pacemakers, metal prostheses, or other implants that could be damaged by the magnet
	Patient teaching to include explanation of the procedure: time is about 60 min; procedure is painless except for need to lie still; procedure is noisy— machine makes several different sounds
Procedure	Patient lies supine with head positioned in holder
	Head is scanned
Postprocedure	No adverse effects
	Patient may need rest

cedure is often extremely helpful in visualizing areas of the brain not easily visualized, for instance the brain stem. (See the accompanying box on p. 1739 for a description of this procedure.) As with CT and brain scan, the patient who has undergone a MRI may need rest. The disoriented patient may have been frightened by the noises the machine makes during the scan and may need reassurance and monitoring for agitated behavior.

PNEUMOENCEPHALOGRAPHY

Pneumoencephalography (air encephalography) is a special contrast study of the ventricular and cisternal

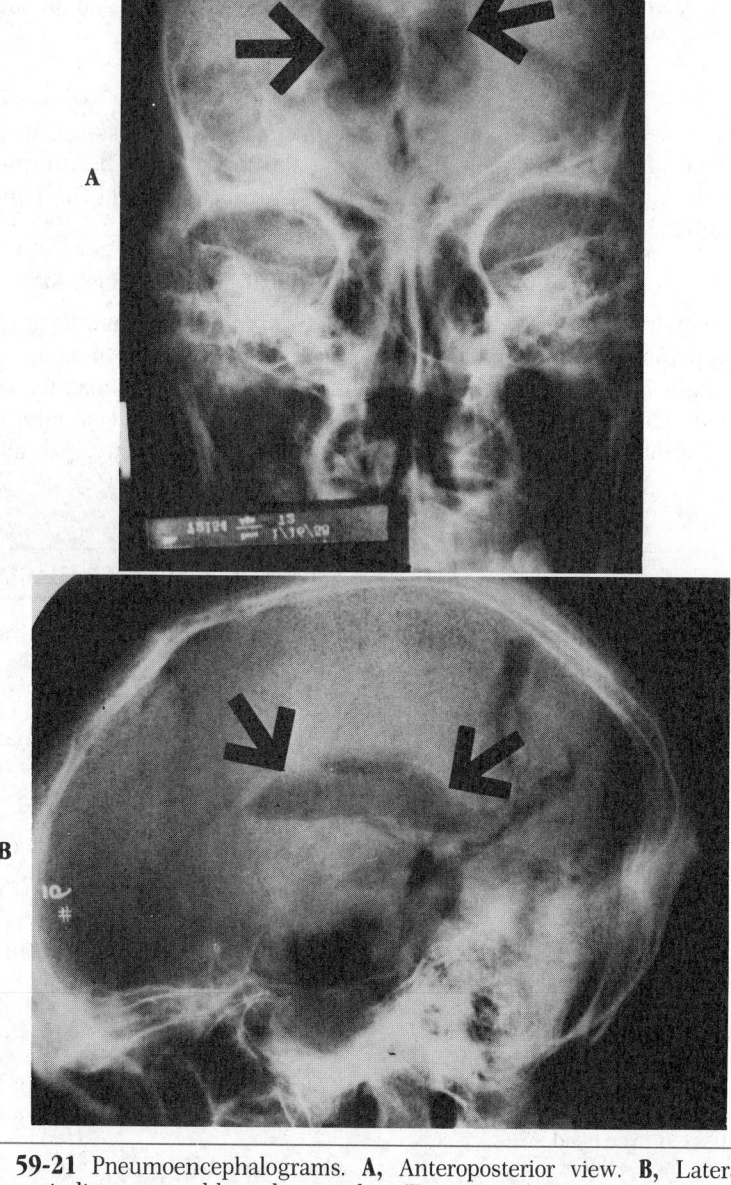

FIGURE 59-21 Pneumoencephalograms. **A,** Anteroposterior view. **B,** Lateral view. Black arrows indicate normal lateral ventricles. (From Pagana K: Diagnostic testing and nursing implications: a case study approach, St Louis, 1982, The CV Mosby Co.)

systems that permits accurate localization of brain lesions. It provides greater visualization of the posterior fossa than ventriculography. It combines a spinal or cisternal puncture with x-ray examination (Figure 59-21).

Pneumoencephalography is not used as frequently today because of the availability of other diagnostic measures, including CT and MRI. It is contraindicated when there is increased intracranial pressure because of the danger of herniation of the temporal uncus and the cerebellar tonsils, resulting in compression of the brain stem and possible death. Also, the procedure itself is extremely uncomfortable and may produce severe, life-threatening reactions. (See the box below for a description of this procedure.)

PNEUMOENCEPHALOGRAM

Preparation of patient	Prepare patient as if for surgery Make sure permit is signed Sedative may be given before procedure General anesthesia may be used Patient teaching to include explanation of procedure: time is about 2 hr; patient is usually very uncomfortable, with headache, nausea, or vomiting
Procedure	Patient is positioned as for lumbar puncture (p. 1744) or cisternal tap (p. 1746) After the tap is done and pressure is measured, the contrast medium (air or oxygen) is injected in amounts of 25 to 30 ml; patient is watched carefully for headache, nausea, vomiting, or any change in vital signs or color Head of the table is gradually raised and head may be rotated to assist air in filling ventricles
Postprocedure	Patient is placed flat in bed for 24 to 48 hr Constant attention to vital signs and neurologic checks is important until patient is awake and alert Severe headache is common and may last 48 hr (until air is absorbed) Seizure precautions should be maintained if patient has history of seizures Observe for respiratory difficulty Reactions to procedure may be severe and include vomiting, shock, respiratory difficulty, and increased intracranial pressure

VENTRICULOGRAPHY

Ventriculography is similar to pneumoencephalography except that air is introduced directly into the lateral ventricles through trepine openings (burr holes) into the skull. This procedure is always performed in the operating room. It may be used when the suspected diagnosis contraindicates performing a spinal or lumbar puncture because of the extreme pressure within the skull or because the spinal canal is blocked. (See the box below for additional information about the procedure.)

The nurse must closely monitor a patient who has had a ventriculogram or pneumoencephalogram for complications such as respiratory difficulty and seizures. Comfort measures, such as analgesics or a cold cloth to the forehead, may help relieve the headache that almost always occurs after the procedure. Because the patient will be on bed rest for a period of time after the test, the nurse will need to assist the patient with activities of daily living.

MYELOGRAPHY

In myelography, either gas or a radiopaque liquid is injected into the spinal subarachnoid space by way of a lumbar or cisternal puncture and radiographs are taken. It is useful in the identification of lesions in the intradu-

VENTRICULOGRAM

Preparation of patient	Procedure is performed in operating room Surgical permit must be signed Prepare patient as if for surgery Top or back of head is partially shaved—usually in operating room Intravenous or general anesthesia commonly used Patient teaching to include explanation of procedure: time is variable; often surgery may be performed immediately after test
Procedure	Patient positioned, usually supine Trephine openings (burr holes) are made into the lateral ventricles Air is introduced directly via the ventricle X-ray films of brain and ventricles are taken at intervals
Postprocedure	Same as for pneumoencephalogram Observe burr hole site for bleeding or drainage Observe for signs of neurologic deterioration that would indicate formation of intracerebral clot

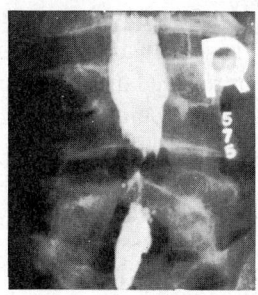

FIGURE 59-22 Myelogram showing almost complete block of interspace between fourth and fifth lumbar vertebrae. (From Moseley HF, editor: Textbook of surgery, ed 3, St Louis, 1959, The CV Mosby Co.)

ral or extradural compartments of the spinal canal. Observations of the flow of the radiopaque dye fluroscopically through the subarachnoid space provides valuable information. Lesions in the spinal cord in the subarachnoid space produce a blocking at some point (Figure 59-22).

The blockage may be complete or incomplete. The exact configuration of the defect causing the block may be helpful in determining whether the lesion is in-

tramedullary or extramedullary. Turning the patient in varied positions throughout the examination assists in securing a more complete visualization.

Another contrast medium, *metrizamide*, may be used in myelograms. However, it may precipitate seizure activity after the procedure, and special precautions must be taken. Side effects of metrizamide are nausea, vomiting, and seizures, and they are most likely to occur 4 to 8 hours after the procedure. However, the advantages of the metrizamide myelogram often outweigh the risks. Major advantages are that the metrizamide is water soluble, and thus the dye does not need to be removed. Also, metrizamide is less viscous than the iodine-based dye and, therefore, permits better visualization of small areas. (See the box below for a further description of the procedure.)

Patients who have undergone myelography should be assessed for leakage from the puncture site. Drinking fluids is encouraged after the procedure, and the patient is assessed for headache or loss of strength in the lower extremities. If metrizamide dye has been used, the patient may be nauseated and vomiting may occur. The patient should be medicated with a drug that does not increase the seizure threshhold.

MYELOGRAM (METRIZAMIDE AND PANTOPAQUE)

Preparation of patient	Permit must be signed If patient is to have metrizamide dye the following medications should be restricted for 24 to 48 hours before the test: phenothiazines, tricyclic antidepressants, and CNS stimulants, amphetamines With metrizamide dye fluids are encouraged Lower extremity strength and sensation should be assessed for baseline Patient teaching to include how procedure is performed: time is approximately 2 hours; slight pain and pressure may be felt as dura is entered; varied positions that must be assumed during procedure may be uncomfortable	Procedure—cont'd	Patient is turned to varied positions to visualize spinal cord while fluroscopic and radiologic films are taken After procedure, pantopaque dye is removed through another puncture; leaving it in will cause serious irritation to meninges With metrizamide dye, patient usually has CT scan of spinal cord 4 to 6 hours after the myelogram
Procedure	Patient is positioned on the side with both knees and head flexed at acute angle (as for lumbar puncture) Puncture is in lumbar region, or cisternally Dye is instilled and needle removed	Postprocedure	For pantopaque myelogram patient lies flat overnight For metrizamide myelogram head must be elevated 30 to 50 degrees for at least 8 hours and then elevated 30 degrees for 24 hours Fluids encouraged Strength and sensation of lower extremities must be assessed Site of puncture should be assessed for leakage of CSF Headache common with both types of myelogram With metrizamide dye, neausea and vomiting may occur For metrizamide procedure avoid previously listed drugs

CEREBRAL ANGIOGRAPHY (ANGIOGRAM)

Cerebral arteriography is a method of radiologic visualization of the cerebral arterial system during the injection of radiopaque material. The carotid or vertebral vessels or the femoral artery are the usual sources of entry for the catheter. Vessels are injected with dye as serial films are taken. The selection of needle puncture site is determined by the clinical problem under study. The large vessels of the *circle of Willis* and the large penetrating vessels can be visualized through arteriography (Figure 59-23). This test is effective in detecting arterial aneurysms, vessel anomalies, ruptured vessels, and displacement of vessels by mass lesions. (See box at the top of p. 1744 for a further description of this test.)

DIGITAL SUBTRACTION ANGIOGRAPHY

A digital subtraction angiogram (DSA) may be performed instead of the angiogram. The purpose is to identify abnormalities of the cerebrovascular system, using a process that removes overlying structures in an image so that the clinically significant details can be displayed with enhanced visibility. It is generally con-

sidered to be much safer than the angiogram, because it uses venous rather than arterial access. It can be done on an outpatient basis. (See the box on p. 1744 for a further description of this test.)

After the arteriogram or DSA, the patient should be monitored for any bleeding at the site of the puncture. A pressure dressing is usually left in place for at least 6 to 8 hours. With the femoral approach, the pulses in the lower extremities should be assessed; with the brachial approach, the radial pulse should be assessed. With the carotid approach the ability of the patient to breath and swallow without difficulty is important to assess. Because the dye used may raise intracranial pressure, the patient should be assessed for any change in level of consciousness.

POSITIVE EMISSION TOMOGRAPHY

One of the newest developments in the assessment of neurologic conditions is the positive emission tomography (PET). This scan involves use of radioactive substances that emit positive electrons (positrons) while CT scanning is done. It provides a metabolic profile by re-

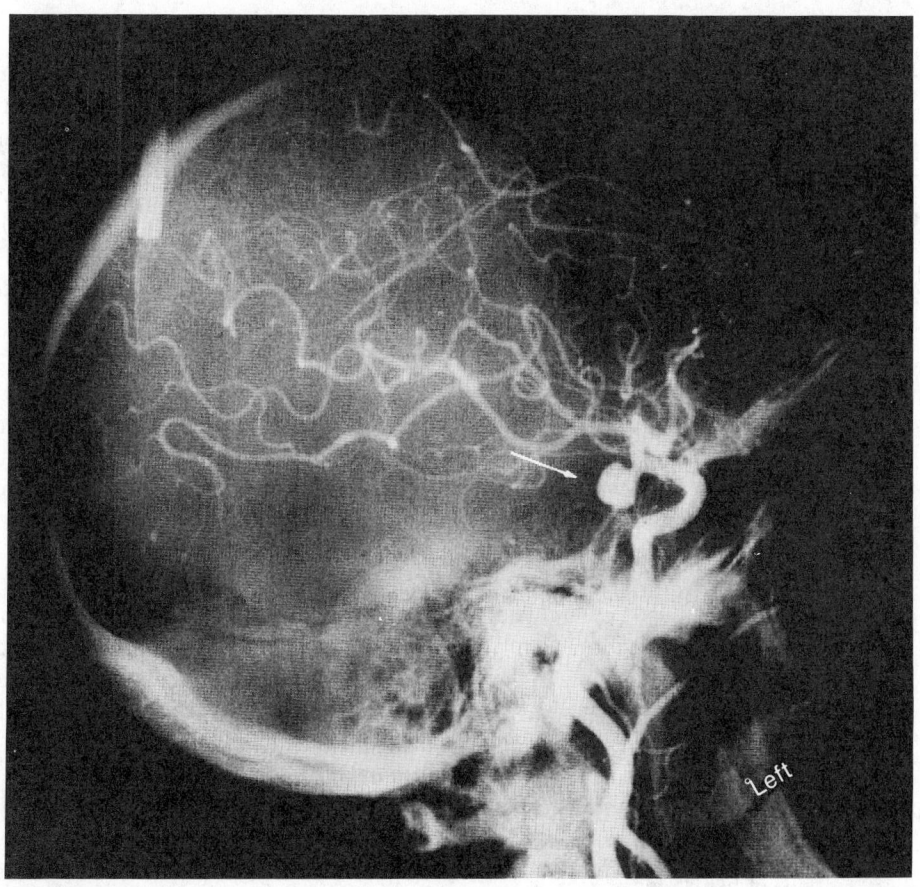

FIGURE 59-23 Cerebral angiography showing location of aneurysm at posterior communicating artery. (From Tortorici M: Fundamentals of angiography, St Louis, 1982, The CV Mosby Co.)

CEREBRAL ARTERIOGRAM (ANGIOGRAM)

Preparation of patient	Patient is given clear liquids the morning of procedure
	Assess patient for allergy to iodine
	If femoral approach is to be used, assess and mark locations of bilateral pedal pulses
	If carotid artery is used, assess neckline circumference
	Sedation may be given before procedure
	Check vital signs and baseline neurologic examination immediately before procedure
	Patient teaching to include explanation of test: time is 2 to 3 hours; lying still is uncomfortable; patients usually complain of hot feeling as dye is injected
Procedure	Patient is positioned supine on x-ray table
	Local anesthetic is used to anesthetize puncture site

Procedure—cont'd	Catheter is inserted percutaneously
	Each vessel is injected as films are taken
	Catheter is withdrawn and pressure applied to puncture site for at least 5 minutes
Postprocedure	Patient is kept on bed rest overnight
	Vital signs are checked frequently, along with neurologic checks
	Site of puncture is assessed frequently for presence of hematoma
	With carotid site check for difficulty in breathing or swallowing—check neck girth
	Dye used in angiogram may raise intracranial pressure and cause decreased extremity strength or change in level of consciousness

DIGITAL SUBTRACTION ANGIOGRAPHY (DSA)

Preparation of patient	Permit must be signed
	Food may be restricted
	Assess for allergy to iodine
	Patient teaching should include explanation of procedure: time is approximately 45 to 60 minutes; some patients may find injection of dye, along with need to lie still, uncomfortable
Procedure	Patient is positioned supine on x-ray table
	Local anesthetic may be used to anesthetize the are of puncture site
	Catheter is introduced into vein, usually in arm
	Dye is injected as films are taken
	Catheter is withdrawn
Postprocedure	Vital signs checked at completion of test
	Circulatory status of arm is assessed
	Injection site is checked for presence of hematoma
	Usually there are no activity restrictions

vealing the rate at which tissues metabolize glucose. The patient either inhales a radioactive gas or is injected with a radioactive substance. This material emits positrons, which combine with negatively charged electrons in body cells. Gamma rays are then given off, which can be seen by the scanning device. The computer translates the patterns of gamma ray emissions.

PET scanning is still not widely available because of the cost and lack of facilities to house the equipment.

SPECIAL TESTS

Other tests can be important in determining the nature of neurologic symptoms. These include the lumbar puncture, cisternal puncture, electroencephalogram, electromyogram, and evoked potentials.

LUMBAR PUNCTURE

The lumbar puncture is done to obtain CSF for examination (Figure 59-24). The importance of examining the constituents has already been described. A lumbar puncture may also be performed to relieve intracranial pressure in carefully selected cases. In most cases, a lumbar puncture is not performed in the presence of signs of increased intracranial pressure or when a brain tumor is suspected because the quick reduction in pressure produced by removal of spinal fluid causes the brain structures to herniate into the foramen magnum, which would put pressure on vital centers in the medulla and might cause sudden death.

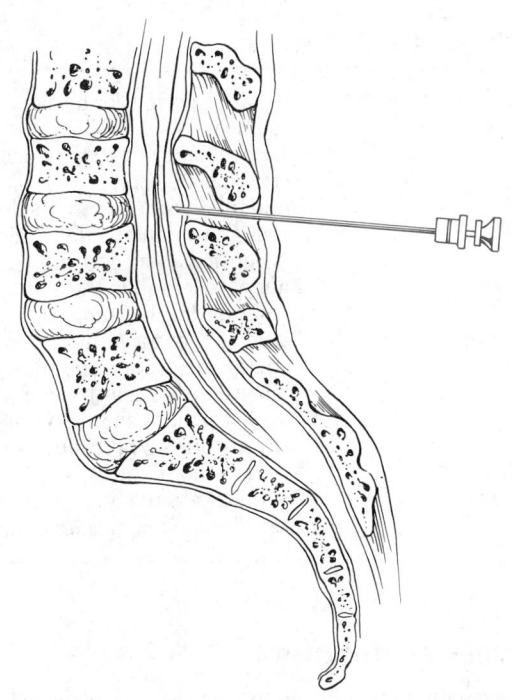

FIGURE 59-24 Position and angle of the needle when lumbar puncture is performed. Note that the needle is in the fourth lumbar interspace below the level of the spinal cord.

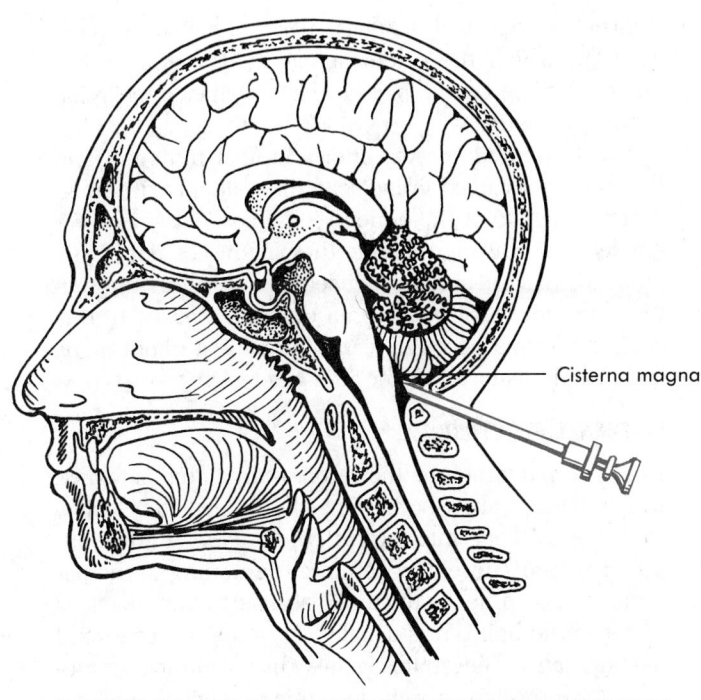

Cisterna magna

FIGURE 59-25 Position of needle when cisternal puncture is performed. Note needle length and short bevel.

LUMBAR PUNCTURE

Preparation of patient	A permit is usually signed Sedation may be given before the procedure Patient teaching should include an explanation of the test: time is approximately 10 to 15 minutes; a slight pain or pressure may be felt as the dura is entered; a sharp shooting pain down the leg may be felt if the needle comes to a nerve; patient must lie still during test	Procedure—cont'd	Level of fluid in manometer is read Fluid is collected as necessary *Queckenstedt's* test may be performed to test for subarachnoid block. The jugular veins are compressed for 10 seconds, first on one side then on the other side; any change in pressure of spinal fluid is noted Needle is withdrawn, dressing applied
Procedure	Patient is positioned on side with knees and head flexed at acute angle to allow lumbar flexion and separation of interspinous areas Local anesthetic is used to numb lumbar area Needle is inserted below level of spinal cord at the L4-L5 or L5-S1 interspace Inner needle is removed to allow drainage of fluid and measurement of pressure	Postprocedure	Patient lies flat for several hours Site of puncture is assessed for leakage of CSF Headache is fairly common and is thought to be caused by the leakage of fluid through the dura matter Headache is treated with bed rest, analgesics, and ice to head. The patient's emotional state may influence the development of a headache

Strict aseptic technique is mandatory in all procedures in which the cerebrospinal fluid system is entered. (See the box on p. 1745 for a further description of this procedure.)

Headache often occurs after a lumbar puncture and the nurse may need to medicate the patient with analgesics. The site of the puncture should be assessed for any leakage. During the time the patient lies flat, assistance with care may be needed. Some lumbar punctures are now performed on an outpatient basis. In this case, the nurse needs to teach the patient about signs and symptoms to watch for after the test.

CISTERNAL PUNCTURE

In a cisternal puncture, the cerebrospinal fluid is tapped by inserting a short-beveled needle immediately below the occipital bone into the *cisterna magna* (Figure 59-25). This procedure may be more frightening to the patient than a lumbar puncture because the approach is closer to the brain. It is usually very safe, however, and usually causes fewer headaches than a lumbar puncture. (See the box at right for a more detailed explanation of this procedure.) The nurse needs to observe the patient for any respiratory difficulties such as dyspnea, apnea, or cyanosis. The site of the puncture should be assessed for leakage.

CISTERNAL PUNCTURE

Preparation of patient	Usually a permit for surgery is signed
	The back of the patient's neck may be shaved
	Patient is positioned in a side-lying position at side of bed with head bent forward
	Patient teaching is the same as that for lumbar puncture
Procedure	Same as that for lumbar puncture, except for different site (between C1 and base of skull)
	Head of patient should be held firmly during procedure so that it does not rotate
Postprocedure	Patient is observed immediately for dyspnea, apnea, or cyanosis

ELECTROENCEPHALOGRAPHY

An electroencephalograph measures the electrical impulses of the brain. The electroencephalogram (EEG) is a pictured recording of the electrical activity of the brain amplified many times and recorded in a manner similar to that of the electrocardiogram (Figure 59-26). The re-

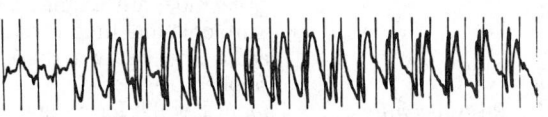

Frontal motor

Parietooccipital

Normal adult, 10/sec. activity in occipital area.

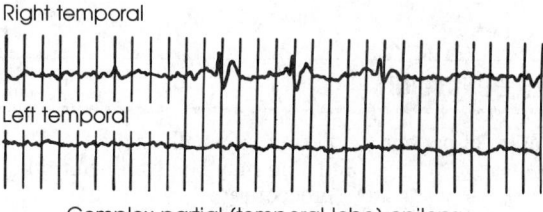

Right temporal

Left temporal

Complex-partial (temporal lobe) epilepsy. Right temporal spike focus.

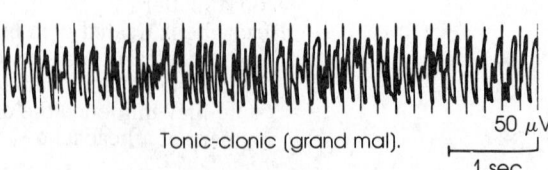

Absent attacks (petit mal seizures). Synchronous 3/sec. spikes and waves.

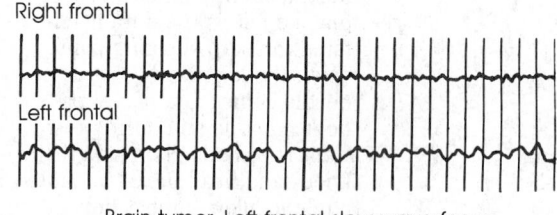

Right frontal

Left frontal

Brain tumor. Left frontal slow wave focus.

Tonic-clonic (grand mal). 50 μV 1 sec

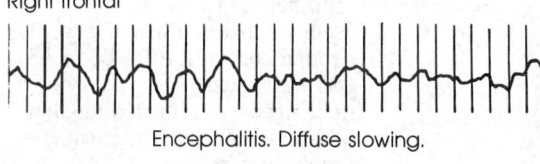

Right frontal

Encephalitis. Diffuse slowing.

FIGURE 59-26 Tracings of electroencephalogram. The normal tracing is demonstrated, as are several pathologic states.

ELECTROENCEPHALOGRAM (EEG)

Preparation of patient	No special preparation Patient is encouraged to rest and be quiet before procedure, except in the case of sleep-deprived EEG Scalp and hair should be clean Patient teaching to include explanation of test: time is 1 hour or more; the test is not painful—electrodes are attached to head with collodion	Procedure	Patient sits in a comfortable chair or lies on a cot with eyes closed Testing is conducted in room where electrical activity is eliminated Basic resting rhythm is affected by opening the eyes or altering attention Comparisons are made of different patterns of the recordings
		Postprocedure	Patient should be allowed to rest if tired Give assistance as needed to patient to wash hair and remove collodion

cording represents the synthesis of collective neurons. Certain characteristic patterns in the recordings are normal, and by study of the recordings of brain action, areas of abnormal action can be detected. This test is nonspecific and is only an adjunct to other diagnostic tests, but it may be helpful in locating the site of a lesion. (See the box above for further information about this procedure.) Most patients who return from an EEG require rest. The patient may need assistance in washing the hair to remove the collodion used to apply the electrodes. The EEG is often performed as an outpatient procedure.

ELECTROMYOGRAPHY

The electromyography measures the electrical activity of muscles; the electromyogram (EMG) is a recording of the variations of electric potentials (voltage) detected by a needle electrode inserted into skeletal muscles. The electrical activity can be heard over a loudspeaker and viewed on an oscilloscope and on a graph at the same time. No electrical activity can be detected in muscles at rest, but during volitional movement action potentials can be detected. However, in motor disease, electrical activity of various types of abnormal patterns appear in resting muscles. An EMG provides direct evidence of *motor dysfunction* and can be used to some extent to detect a dysfunction located in the motor neuron, the neuromuscular junction, or muscle fibers. This is particularly helpful in the detection of lower motor neuron disease, primary muscle disease, and defects in the transmission of electrical impulses at the neuromuscular junction. (See the accompanying box for an explanation of this procedure.) After the EMG the patient should be assessed for bleeding at the needle insertion sites. Medication may be needed for discomfort. The patient may also require rest, even if the procedure is performed on an outpatient basis.

ECHOENCEPHALOGRAPHY

Echoencephalography is a rapid and simple diagnostic procedure. Information provided is supplementary to an EEG and complementary to radiologic studies as to the nature and location of brain lesions.

Ultrasonic pulses (capable of reflection or refraction at cerebrospinal fluid and brain tissue surfaces) are delivered to the head in such a way that the beam intersects the site under study at a perpendicular angle, transverses the area, and is then reflected back. The returning echoes are then converted back to electrical impulses and recorded on a screen. This procedure pro-

ELECTROMYOGRAM (EMG)

Preparation of patient	No special preparation Patient teaching to include explanation of procedure: time is approximately 45 minutes for one muscle; some discomfort is experienced when electrodes are inserted; patients with sensory neuropathies may experience more intense pain; electrical current is uncomfortable; muscles may ache for a period of time after procedure
Procedure	Electrodes are inserted into skeletal muscles Electrical current is passed through electrodes Machine graphs the variations of muscle potentials (voltage)
Postprocedure	Observe for signs of bleeding at electrode insertion sites Patient may need rest period Medicate patient as needed for discomfort

vides a right, left, and lower trace or picture that gives reliable information as to the position of the midline of the brain. Shifts from midline, as caused by right or left hemispheric brain masses, can be inferred. Estimation of ventricular size can also be made from the traces.

EVOKED POTENTIALS

Evoked potentials are electrical measurements of physiologic maturation of the human nervous system. Used diagnostically, they can provide information about the maturational development of all the primary sensory areas of the cortex. Most commonly used are *auditory evoked potentials* and *visual evoked potentials*. Evoked potentials aid in the diagnosis of multiple sclerosis.

CHAPTER SUMMARY

- Neurologic assessment depends on the examiner's knowledge of normal neurophysiology and neuroanatomy and the ability to interpret the degree of change in status from normal.
- The nervous system coordinates and controls all activities of the body.
- The four general kinds of function carried out by the nervous system include receiving stimuli or information, communicating information, computing or processing the information, and transmitting information.
- The basic structural and functional unit of the nervous system is the neuron.
- The neuron is composed of a cell body (soma), a dendritic tree, a cylindric axon, and the cell membrane.
- The axon transmits information away from the cell body to adjacent neurons, whereas the dendrites communicate information to the cell body.
- The neuron cell membrane transmits information through properties called differential permeability and excitability.
- The myelin sheath is deposited around axons and assists in transmission of impulses.
- Synapses are specialized sites in the nervous system where neurons make functional contact with each other.
- The nervous system is divided into two major divisions: the central nervous system (CNS) and the peripheral nervous system (PNS).
- The CNS is made up of collections of neurons and their connections organized within the brain and spinal cord.
- The parts of the brain include the cerebrum, the brain stem (diencephalon, midbrain, pons and medulla), and the cerebellum, each of which carries out specific functions.

- Speech is a function of the dominant hemisphere, usually on the left side of the brain.
- The blood-brain barrier is a phenomenon that limits the free movement of substances from the blood to the brain tissue.
- Cerebrospinal fluid serves as a fluid cushion for nervous tissue, helps to support the weight of the brain, and carries nutrients to the brain and removes metabolites.
- The meninges are the coverings of the nervous tissue in the brain and spinal cord that help support, protect, and nourish the brain and spinal cord.
- Three potential spaces are associated with the meninges: epidural, subdural, and subarachnoid.
- The PNS is a set of communication channels located outside the CNS.
- The autonomic nervous system regulates autonomic body functions, usually in an effort to preserve homeostasis.
- The perceived sensation is initiated by stimulation of receptor neurons located throughout the body.
- Normal aging cannot be equated with senility or Alzheimer's disease.
- Subjective data collected during the neurologic examination includes mental status, level of consciousness, language and speech, perceptual status, and sensory status.
- The twelve cranial nerves carry out sensory, motor, or mixed functions.
- A lumbar puncture is not performed in the presence of signs of increased intracranial pressure or when a brain tumor is suspected because of the danger of brain herniation.
- Computed tomography (CT) has had significant impact on the diagnosis of neurologic abnormalities.

QUESTIONS TO CONSIDER

- How is the term *excitability* related to conduction of nervous impulses?
- Does nervous tissue ever regenerate? Please explain.
- Why is sensory and perceptual status difficult to measure in patients exhibiting neurologic disease?
- Why is doing a lumbar puncture contraindicated in the patient who is thought to have increased intracranial pressure?
- Coordination of muscle movements is a result of action of which part of the brain?

REFERENCES AND SELECTED READINGS

1. Anderson M: Assessment under pressure: when your patient says "my head hurts," Nursing 84, 149:34-42, 1984.
2. Anthony C and Thibodeau G: Textbook of anatomy and physiology, St Louis, 1983, The CV Mosby Co.
3. Bell T: Nurses' attitudes in caring for the comatose head-injured patient, J Neurosci Nurs 18:279-289, 1986.
4. Boss B: Dysphasia, dyspraxia, and dysarthria: distinguishing features, Part I, J Neurosurg Nurs 16:151-160, 194, 1984.
5. Boss B: Dysphasia, dyspraxia, and dysarthria: distinguishing features, Part II, J Neurosurg Nurs 16:211-216, 1984.
6. Boss B: Memory impairment: forgetfulness vs. amnesia, J Neurosci Nurs 20:151-158, 1988.
7. Boss B: The neuroanatomical and neurophysiological basis of learning, J Neurosci Nurs 18:256-264, 1986.
8. Boss B and Brewer L: Syncope: neuroscience assessment based on an understanding of underlying pathophysiological mechanisms, J Neurosci Nurs 20:245-252, 1988.
9. Burr L: Checking cranial nerve function, Patient Care, 17:86-89, 92-94, 1983.
10. Burr L: Evaluating sensory and motor systems, Patient Care, 17:121-123, 127, 1983.
11. Byers V and Gendell H: Using metrizamide for lumbar myelography: adverse reactions and nursing implications, J Neurosurg Nurs 14:315-317, 1982.
12. *Carlson C: Psychological aspects of neurologic disability, Nurs Clin North Am 15(2):309-320, 1980.
13. Chui L and Bhatt K: Autonomic dysreflexia, Rehabil Nurs 8:16-20, 1983.
14. Church M: Care of the elderly: clues to clarity, Neuropsychological deficits, Part 2, Nurs Times 81:35-37, 1985.
15. Chusid J: Correlative neuroanatomy and functional neurology, ed 19, Los Altos, Calif, 1985, Lange Medical Publications.
16. Clochesy J: Problems in interpreting abnormal auditory brainstem responses in comatose patients, J Neurosurg Nurs 17:253-255, 1985.
17. Condi J: Types and causes of nystagmus in the neurosurgical patient, J Neurosurg Nurs 15:56-64, 1983.
18. Dittmar S: Rehabilitation nursing: process and application, St Louis, 1989, The CV Mosby Co.
19. *Eliasson S et al: Neurological pathophysiology, New York, 1978, Oxford University Press.
20. Franges E: Assessment and management of carotid artery trauma associated with mild head injury, J Neurosci Nurs 18:272-274, 1986.
21. Gioiella E and Bevil C: Nursing care of the aging client: promoting healthy adaptation, Norwalk, Conn, 1985, Appleton-Century-Crofts.
22. Greenberg M: The neurological exam, Part 1, Emergency 15:22-26, 52-53, 1983.
23. Greenberg M: The neurological exam, Part 2, Emergency, 15:26-29, 1983.
24. Haberman B: Cognitive dysfunction and social rehabilitation in severely head-injured patients, J Neurosurg Nurs 14:220-224, 1982.
25. Jess L: Investigating impaired mental status: an assessment guide you can use. Nursing 88 18:42-50, 1988.
26. Johnson L: If your patient has increased intracranial pressure, your goal should be no surprises, Nursing 83 13:58-63, 1983.
27. *Jones S: Glasgow Coma Scale, Am J Nurs 79:1551-1554, 1979.
28. *Kolb D: Understanding aphasia and the aphasic, J Neurosurg Nurs 9:15-18, 1977.
29. Konikow N: Alterations in movement: nursing assessment and implications, J Neurosurg Nurs 17:61-65, 1985.
30. Long B and Phipps W: Medical-surgical nursing: a nursing process approach, ed 2, St Louis, 1989, The CV Mosby Co.
31. Lord-Feroli K and Maguire-McGinley M: Toward a more objective approach to pupil assessment, J Neurosurg Nurs 17:309-312, 1985.
32. Malasonas L et al: Health assessment, ed 3, St Louis, 1986, The CV Mosby Co.
33. March K: Look into my eyes: assessing the neurological patient, J Neurosurg Nurs 15:213-221, 1983.
34. McBride E, and DiStefano K: Explaining diagnostic tests for MS, Nursing 88 18:68-72, 1988.
35. *Mitchell P, and Irvin N: Neurological examination: nursing assessment for nursing purposes, J Neurosurg Nurs 9:23-38, 1977.
36. Nikas D: Neurological assessment of altered states of consciousness, Part 1, Focus Crit Care 10:10-13, 1983.
37. Nikas D: Neurological assessment of altered states of consciousness, Part 2, Focus Crit Care 10:20-23, 1983.
38. Nikas D: Neurological assessment of altered states of consciousness, Part 3, Focus Crit Care 11:54-58, 1984.
39. *Norman S: The pupil check, Am J Nurs 82:588-591, 1982.
40. *Olson E, et al: The hazards of immobility, Am J Nurs 67:779-797, 1967.
41. Olson E et al: An AJN classic: The hazards of immobility, Am J Nurs 90(3):43-48, 1990.
42. *Patient assessment: neurological examination, I, Am J Nurs 75:1511-1535, 1975.
43. *Patient assessment: neurological examination, II, Am J Nurs 75:2037-2057, 1975.
44. *Patient assessment: neurological examination, III, Am J Nurs 76:609-633, 1976.
45. Price M and DeVroom H: A quick and easy guide to neurological assessment, J Neurosurg Nurs 17:313-320, 1985.
46. Reinisch E: Quick assessment for hemiplegic's functioning, Am J Nurs 81:102-104, 1981.
47. *Ross A et al: Neuromuscular diagnostic procedures, Nurs Clin North Am 14:107-121, 1979.
48. Rudy E: Advanced neurological and neurosurgical nursing, St Louis, 1984, The CV Mosby Co.
49. Rudy E: Magnetic resonance imagery: new horizons in diagnostic testing, J Neurosurg Nurs 17:331-337, 1985.
50. *Seidel HM et al: Mosby's guide to physical examination, St. Louis, 1987, The C.V. Mosby, Co.
51. Spielman G: Metabolic complications associated with severe diffuse brain injury, J Neurosurg Nurs 17:83-88, 1985.
52. Stevens S and Becker K: A simple, step-by-step approach to neurologic assessment—Part 1. Nursing '88 18(9):53-61, 1988.
53. Stevens S and Becker K: A simple, step-by-step approach to neurologic assessment—Part 2. Nursing '88 18(10):51-58, 1988.
54. Turner H et al: Developing a brief neuropsychological mental status exam: a pilot study, J Neurosurg Nurs 16:257-261, 1984.
55. Walleck C: A neurologic assessment procedure that won't make you nervous, Nursing 82 12:50-57, 1982.
56. Young M: A bedside guide to understanding the signs of increased intracranial pressure, Nursing 81 11:59-62, 1981.

*References preceded by an asterisk are particularly well suited for student reading.

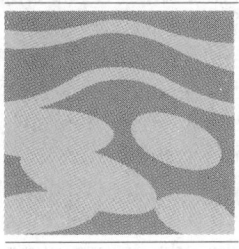

CHAPTER 60

Altered Levels
of Consciousness

ELIZABETH SCHENK

CHAPTER OBJECTIVES

After studying this chapter, the student should be able to:

1 Define the following terms: *arousal, delirium, illusion, hallucinations, agitation,* and *confusion.*
2 Name the five levels of consciousness and describe characteristics of each.
3 Name at least four diagnostic procedures that are helpful in determining the cause and nature of a decreased level of consciousness.
4 Define the term *brain death* and state two ways it is determined.
5 List at least four examples of subjective data and four examples of objective data that should be gathered from a patient with a decreased level of consciousness.
6 Describe the Glasgow Coma Scale and the Rancho Los Amigos Scale.
7 Explain three ways in which the comatose patient should be stimulated.
8 State at least five nursing interventions that are important for persons with a decreased level of consciousness.
9 Explain the importance of proper positioning of the patient with a decreased level of consciousness.
10 Describe at least two abnormal breathing patterns associated with a decreased level of consciousness and explain why they occur.

Consciousness is an ongoing process of awareness of the self and the environment; it is the mental ability to evoke feelings and provide meaning for that awareness based on previous experiences. One infers awareness in others on the basis of their observed behaviors.

Impaired consciousness may be the result of the following three general types of pathologic processes:

1. Conditions that widely and directly depress the function of the cerebral hemispheres
2. Conditions that depress or destroy the brain stem-activating mechanisms that lie in or near the central core of the gray matter of the diencephalon, midbrain, and rostral pons
3. Conditions that involve combined bilateral cortical

and brain stem failure (the latter are seen most commonly in cases of metabolic encephalopathy and intoxication in which the relative amount of the brain's impairment varies)

EPIDEMIOLOGY AND ETIOLOGY

The two aspects of consciousness that must be considered are arousal and awareness. *Arousal* is a physiologic function associated with wakefulness. It involves a primitive set of responses that are located entirely within the brain stem and are synchronized by a network of tracts and nuclei. The network is located in the core of the brain stem and extends from the medulla to the thalamus. *Awareness* (or content as it is differentiated by Plum and Posner[39]) is the sum of all cognitive and affective functions. It involves a higher level integration of multiple sensory inputs that allow meaningful understanding of self and environment.

There are multiple causes of impaired consciousness, many of which are not primarily neurologic. For this reason, a detailed history, extensive neurologic examination, and laboratory screening are often needed. These will be discussed later in the chapter. Generally, causes of impaired consciousness can be categorized into two broad categories. These are (1) primary brain injury or disease (usually a structured lesion) or (2) a systemic condition that secondarily affects the brain. (See the box on p. 1752 for a more complete listing of the possible causes of coma.)

PREVENTION

Primary prevention of decreased levels of consciousness involves avoidance of those factors that can contribute to it (such as carbon monoxide, drugs, or alcohol), as well as control of chronic diseases such as diabetes and chronic obstructive pulmonary disease (COPD). Avoidance of situations that can lead to head

POSSIBLE CAUSES OF DECREASED LEVELS OF CONSCIOUSNESS

1. Resulting from primary brain injury or disease
   a. Trauma (concussion, contusion, laceration, or traumatic intercerebral hemorrhage, subdural hematoma, epidural hematoma)
   b. Vascular disease (intracerebral hemorrhage, subarachnoid hemorrhage, infarction)
   c. Infections (meningitis, encephalitis, abscess)
   d. Neoplasms (primarily intracranial, metastatic, or nonmetastatic complication of malignancy)
   e. Seizures
2. Resulting from systemic conditions that secondarily affect the brain secondarily
   a. Metabolic encephalopathies (hypoglycemia, diabetic ketoacidosis, hyperglycemic nonketotic hyperosmolar states, uremia, hepatic encephalopathy, hyponatremia, myxedema, hypercalcemia, and hypocalcemia)
   b. Hypoxic encephalopathies (severe congestive heart failure, COPD with decompensation, severe anemia, and hypertensive encephalopathies)
   c. Toxicity (heavy metals, carbon monoxide, and drugs—especially opiates, barbiturates, and alcohol)
   d. Physical causes (heat stroke and hypothermia)
   e. Deficiency states (Wernicke's encephalopathy)

injury and subsequent trauma are important. With coma that results from vascular problems, it is important to avoid factors that can lead to decreased levels of consciousness. These include the following:

1. Cigarette smoking
2. Hypertension
3. Hypercholesterolemia
4. Obesity
5. Stress-related occupations and hectic pace of life

Secondary prevention, or early detection, is of the utmost importance in dealing with patients with a decreased level of consciousness. Many initial symptoms are so vague that it is easy to deny or minimize their importance. In addition, *tertiary prevention,* or prevention of complications, is vitally important in this type of patient. The dependence on nursing care that these patients usually exhibit makes it extremely important for the nurse to prevent *iatrogenic* problems. These will be discussed in more detail later in this chapter.

PATHOPHYSIOLOGY

Although it is not known precisely what the neural mechanisms are that make awareness possible, it is known that many different parts of the nervous system work together to determine the nature of a person's awareness. To date, our knowledge of brain mechanisms is insufficient to explain the functioning of the

mind as we experience it. No unified representation of one's environment exists in any single cortical area. The necessary conditions for consciousness, such as perception, memory, and language, depend on cortical functions. The presence of consciousness depends on a normally functioning interplay between certain neurons, the brain, and the reticular activating system (RAS).

The RAS, or deep central core of gray matter beginning in the brain stem, extends into the hypothalamus and thalamus either directly or indirectly, transmitting stimuli to the cerebral cortex and influencing arousal or wakefulness. Conscious behavior depends on an intact functioning cerebrum. The organization of the reticular network is vague; however, it does contain some distinct nuclei with long overlapping fibers and dendrites. Anatomic and physiologic details of brain stem nuclei are not yet fully understood. (For an indepth review of the anatomy and physiology of the consciousness system, the reader is referred to Plum and Posner.[39]) Impulses from the RAS keep us active and serve as an alerting system.

The RAS mediates responses such as eye opening to painful stimuli, as well as corneal reflexes, pupillary reaction, and ocular motility. The RAS acts as a relay to the cerebral cortex and functions like an on-off switch for the cortical awareness system. It is the cycling of this system that accounts for the sleep-wake cycle.

When the effects of an insult impinge on the RAS, the state of consciousness can be altered. As the severity of the insult or dysfunction increases, there is increasing impairment of responsiveness to events in the internal and external environment. If the dysfunction is great enough, unconsciousness or coma will result. Any impairment, reduction, or absence of consciousness indicates a serious dysfunction of the brain.

Cerebral function is most commonly affected by lack of oxygen or glucose. The brain is extremely sensitive to hypoxia, and only a few seconds of anoxia can lead to loss of consciousness. The amount of oxygen available to cells of the cerebral cortex depends on adequacy of blood flow, blood oxygen tension, hemoglobin concentration, and serum pH. *Delirium usually results with a PO_2 level below 55 mm Hg and coma* when the level falls below 25 mm Hg.

Cerebral cells are also affected by the same conditions that affect cellular metabolism elsewhere in the body. Thus, altered levels of consciousness can result from conditions such as fluid and electrolyte imbalances or toxins that interfere with metabolism of cerebral cells.

CLINICAL MANIFESTATIONS

The *conscious* person is able to respond to sensory stimuli, has subjective experiences, exercises will, and is capable of thought and reasoning. Consciousness may also be defined as self-awareness—ability to function mentally and physically in a manner appropriate to the level of one's normal ability and to experience life to the fullest degree. All body activities are controlled and coordinated by the nervous system. The cerebrum plays the central role in the higher functions. Rather than experiencing sensory inputs individually and discretely, they are integrated into a single consciousness, a perception; for example, one can identify items by touch that one has seen but not touched before.

In contrast, to be *unconscious* implies that there is no response to sensory stimuli—no thinking and no feelings or emotions. The conscious person is aware of what is going on in the environment. To differentiate between these two ends of the continuum are many levels of awareness and mental ability not so easily defined or precisely described.

Because consciousness is a complex expression of the mind and not just a single function, there is a wide spectrum of levels of consciousness between the two ends of the continuum: consciousness and coma. Although it is better to avoid labels, the nurse must have an understanding of them to have some idea of what is being said to communicate. The levels of consciousness can be divided into the following five levels of cerebral function:

1. Confusion
2. Drowsiness
3. Stupor
4. Light coma
5. Deep coma

(See Table 60-1 for further explanations of degrees of decreased levels of consciousness.)

Other terms have also been identified. These are *obtunded* and *locked-in states*. The term *obtunded* implies a reduction in alertness and a decreased interest in the surroundings. *Stupor* has been described as unresponsiveness from which the subject can be aroused only by vigorous and repeated stimuli; *coma* is unarousable responsiveness.[39] Different clinical pictures of coma have been described. The most common one is a *sleeplike condition* with *eyes closed;* the closed eyes are not seen in the chronic state. Second is a *hypersomnia* state very much like *normal sleep* because patients can be aroused, but they return to sleep immediately. The third state is one in which the individual's *eyes are open,* but *no movement or speech* can be elicited.

The chronically brain-damaged comatose patient may have periods when the eyes are open alternating with closed eye periods and may seem to be making some response to environmental stimuli. This is referred to as a *vegetative* state. Brain stem function may be intact and respirations remain normal, yet forebrain damage is too extensive to permit any awareness.

The *locked-in* state refers to the condition of persons who may be awake and alert, completely able to think and reason, yet who, because of a metabolic or structural disease in the nervous system, are unable to realize any motor expression of the cerebral function. Some

TABLE 60-1 Commonly used states of awareness and associated behaviors

	State					
	Conscious-Aware		**Semiconscious-Semicomatose**		**Unconscious-Comatose**	
Level	Alert	Confused	Obtunded, drowsy	Stupor	Light coma	Deep coma
Behaviors	Normal activity Aware, mentally functional	Poor coordination Delirium Hallucinations Restlessness Excitable May be combative Short attention span Inappropriate actions and judgments Decreased awareness Disorientation	Sleepy Very short attention span Ready arousal Responds appropriately when aroused Ability to respond verbally Fends off painful stimuli with purposeful movement	Apathetic Slow moving Blank expression Drooping head Staring Arousal only to vigorous stimuli Incomplete arousal to painful stimuli No verbal response or moaning Response to verbal communication is inconsistent and vague	Not oriented to time, place or person Response is only by grimace or withdrawing limb from pain Primitive and disorganized response to painful stimuli	Absence of response to even the most painful stimuli

of these patients have the ability to move their eyes in an up-and-down direction. Most commonly this state is caused by lesions in the brain stem.[12] There are three categories of events that may produce this state: (1) supratentorial masses or lesions that secondarily compress or damage both cerebral hemispheres; (2) subtentorial lesions or masses damaging the RAS, which normally activates the cerebral hemispheres; and (3) metabolic disorders that interrupt function of supratentorial and subtentorial brain structures.

PATHOLOGIC MOTOR RESPONSES

Damage to the central nervous system may be demonstrated by pathologic motor responses in the comatose

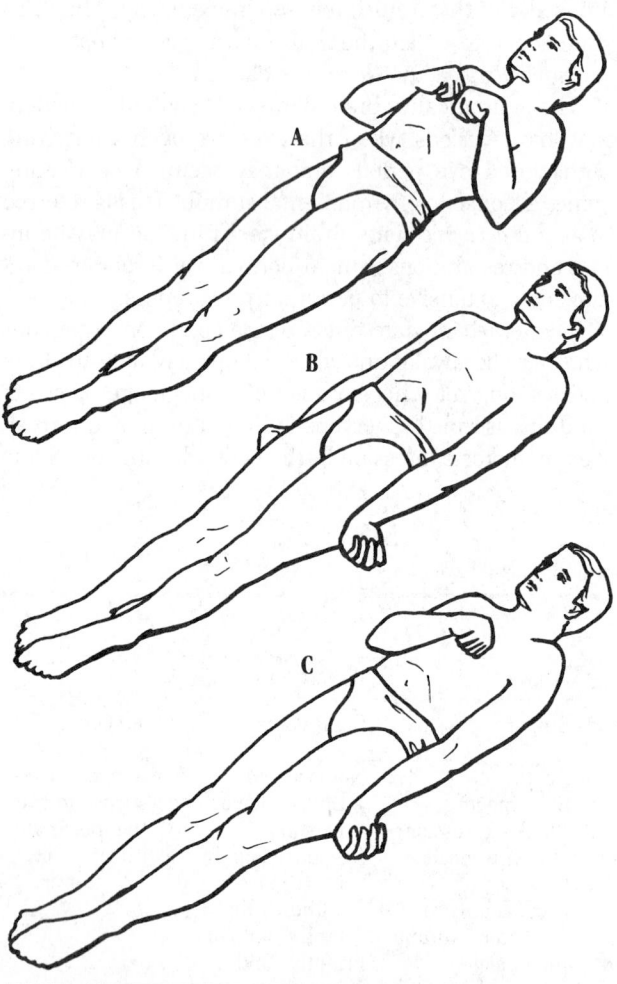

FIGURE 60-1 Decorticate and decerebrate responses. **A,** Decorticate response. Flexion of arms, wrists, and fingers with adduction in upper extremities. Extension, internal rotation, and plantar flexion in lower extremities. **B,** Decerebrate response. All four extremities in rigid extension, with hyperpronation of forearms and plantar extension of feet. **C,** Decorticate response on right side of body and decerebrate response on left side of body. (From Zschoche D: Mosby's comprehensive review of critical care, ed 2, St Louis, The CV Mosby Co.)

patient. These include decorticate and decerebrate posturing. *Decorticate posturing* includes flexion of the arms, wrists, and fingers, with adduction of the upper extremities. This indicates a lesion that involves large portions of the sensorimotor cortex, both anterior and posterior to the primary motor area. *Decerebrate posturing* is also called extensor spasm. In this pattern, all four extremities are rigid in extension, with hyperpronation of the forearm and extension of the feet. This response indicates a lesion at the level of the brain stem. With this response, the prognosis is grave. It is possible that a person may demonstrate both of these responses concurrently. These responses will often be accompanied by deep coma, rapid breathing, and dilation of both pupils (Figure 60-1).

BRAIN DEATH

With advanced means of prolonging life, the issue of when death occurs has arisen. From this has come debates about the nature of brain death. If a person is receiving artificial means of ventilation, it is possible to sustain breathing and circulation in the absence of brain activity. It is necessary in these cases to determine that all functions of the brain have ceased, including those of cerebrum and brain stem. Usually one or more electroencephalograms (EEG) are necessary to substantiate brain death. In addition, the following should be absent:

1. All cerebral responses to light, noise, motion, and pain
2. All reflex activity (except of spinal cord origin) and muscle activity
3. Spontaneous respirations
4. Cranial nerve reflexes and responses[42]

CONFUSED OR DISORIENTED PATIENT

When one has a disturbed consciousness, rather than a decrease in the level of consciousness, one is said to be experiencing a confused or disoriented state. It is the *content* of the consciousness that is altered. The disoriented person may experience hallucinations or have illusions or delusions or become agitated. With *disorientation* the patient is awake but perceives phenomena incorrectly. Thinking and reasoning are inappropriate, and remembering is difficult.

Delirium is a response often encountered in an intensive care unit. It is characterized by progressive disorientation first to time, then place, then person. *Illusions, hallucinations,* and *delusions* also commonly occur. Patients become agitated and combative or secretive and withdrawn. Sleep deprivation is implicated as a causative factor when it is impossible for the patient to get even one complete sleep cycle because of frequently interrupted sleep. Either too much stimulation (constant pain) or too little stimulation (eye patches) can initiate delirium. Microemboli in the postcardiotomy patient have been suggested as a possible cause. Analgesic and antipsychotic agents, metabolic imbalance, and shock are all contributory factors. High fevers, drug overdose, alcoholism, and strong fears can also lead to delirium.

An *illusion* is a sensory experience based on fact, but misinterpreted. This may happen when one of the senses is faulty or when environmental conditions prohibit a true interpretation of what is sensed. For example, the older person who has failing vision may think there is someone present in the room when a shadow moves.

A *hallucination* is an impression on any of the senses in the absence of a stimulus. The patient believes he or she sees, hears, tastes, feels, or smells something; but the source of this occurrence is within the patient's thinking rather than in reality. Confusion and hallucinations may be caused by injury, drugs, psychological problems, or organic problems. Organic causes may be acute infections with high fever, drug toxicity from alcohol or psychedelic drugs, withdrawal from drugs, brain tumor, senility, or exhaustion.

Agitation refers to a state of psychomotor excitement that is characterized by purposeless, restless activity. The person may pace, cry, and laugh without appropriate cause. Agitation may occur as a result of stress, fear, or anxiety.

DIAGNOSTIC TESTS

Diagnostic testing can be very important for the patient with a decreased level of consciousness (LOC). Routine laboratory tests should be performed and should include those tests found in the box below.

A toxicology screen should also be obtained on blood, urine, and gastric aspirate for opiates, barbiturates, sedatives, antidepressants, and alcohol. Other studies that are helpful to determine the cause and nature of decreased LOC include the following:

1. Skull roentgenogram
2. Brain scan
3. EEG
4. Computed tomography scan
5. Cerebral angiography

IMPORTANT LABORATORY TESTS FOR PATIENTS IN COMA

Complete blood count	Calcium
Urinalysis	PO_2
Electrolytes	Liver function studies
Blood urea nitrogen	Enzymes
Creatinine	Osmolality
Blood sugar	

---

6. Lumbar puncture (if there is a suspicion of intracranial infection such as meningitis or encephalitis)
7. Evoked potentials

(See Chapter 59 for a description of these tests.)

MEDICAL MANAGEMENT

Medical management of the patient with coma or decreased LOC depends to a great extent on the cause of the coma. The reader is referred to other sections of this text for appropriate treatments for the various disorders that can cause coma.

If there is some evidence that the decreased LOC is the result of an opiate overdose, naloxone should be given intravenously every 5 to 10 minutes until consciousness returns. The dose is 0.4 mg. Naloxone is a narcotic antagonist that reverses the effects of opioids. In patients with an opiate addiction, this might provoke an acute withdrawal state that will require treatment with narcotics.

In patients in coma who are found to have increased intracranial pressure (ICP), hyperosmolar agents, such as mannitol, and steroids, such as dexamethasone, are usually given. When other methods of controlling the increased ICP are ineffective, intravenous s barbiturates may be used to place the patient in a barbiturate coma. This requires both experienced personnel and a setting in which internal intracranial monitoring can take place.

■ ASSESSMENT

Both subjective and objective data about patients with decreased LOC should be collected.

SUBJECTIVE DATA

It may be impossible to obtain accurate information from the patient with a decreased level of consciousness. The history should always be obtained from the family or significant other, in addition to the patient. The following information should be gathered:

1. When the decreased LOC started
2. Concomitant symptoms
3. Patient's awareness of condition
4. Ability to think, calculate, and abstract
5. Presence of pain or discomfort, including stiff neck
6. Presence of visual symptoms
7. History of trauma

OBJECTIVE DATA

Objective data to be collected include the following:

1. Vital signs
2. Pupillary signs—size, equality, and reactivity

TABLE 60-2 Altered respiratory patterns in coma

Respiratory Pattern	Characteristics	Indications
Cheyne-Stokes	Periods of hyperventilation that gradually diminish to apnea of variable duration; respirations then resume and gradually build up to hyperventilation	Bilateral deep hemispheric and basal ganglionic dysfunction; the upper brain stem may be involved
Central neurogenic hyperventilation (CNHV)	Continuous rapid and deep respirations at a rate of 25/min	Systemic acidosis and hypoxemia should be excluded; has no segmental localizing influence; increasing regularity correlates with increasing depth of coma
Apneustic breathing	Prolonged inspiratory phase followed by apnea (inspiratory cramp)	Indicates lower pontine damage
Cluster breathing	Closely grouped respirations followed by apnea	Indicates lower pontine damage
Ataxic breathing	Chaotic respirations	Indicates damage to medullary centers; can precede respiratory arrest
Gasping breathing	Characterized by gasps followed by apnea of variable duration	Indicates damage to medullary centers; can precede respiratory arrest
Depressed breathing	Shallow, slow, and ineffective breathing	Usually caused by medullary depression

3. Focal motor or sensory signs—presence, symmetry, and character of movements, including eye movements
4. Presence of vomiting or hiccoughing
5. Eye changes including papilledema
6. Speech patterns
7. Odor of breath (a clue to diabetic ketoacidosis)
8. Abnormal reflexes

The respiratory rate is helpful in localizing and, in certain instances, determining the nature of the process. These patterns include the following:

1. Cheyne-Stokes respiration
2. Central neurogenic hyperventilation (CNHV)
3. Apneic breathing
4. Cluster breathing
5. Ataxic breathing
6. Gasping breathing
7. Depressed breathing

(See Table 60-2 for characteristics of each of these types of breathing.)

The reflex eye movements often used to evaluate brain stem functioning in the comatose patient include the oculocephalic reflex response (doll's eyes) and the oculovestibular reflex response. The *oculocephalic reflex* is demonstrated by holding the person's eyelids open and rotating the head from side to side. If the brain's pathways to the eye muscles are intact, the eyes will move to the left as the head is rotated to the right. This parallel or conjugate gaze is called positive or normal doll's eyes (Figure 60-2).

The *oculovestibular reflex* refers to reflex conjugate eye movements or *nystagmus* that is caused by stimulating the semicircular canals of the ear with ice water. This is an accurate method of assessing brain stem functioning. The reflex is evaluated by the caloric ice water test. What should be seen is horizontal nystagmus with slow eye movement toward the irrigated ear and rapid eye movement away. If warm water is used, the normal eye movements will be reversed (Figure 60-3).

Accuracy is best attained when a systematic approach is used by all persons involved in the continuing assessments. Although some efforts have been made to develop scales to measure LOC, there is a paucity of tools. What is vital is that all persons in a facility consistently use a single technique. The clues or evidence that might lead to the use of a descriptive term are recorded or reported as opposed to the descriptive term itself.

RANCHOS LOS AMIGOS SCALE

Another scale that has been developed is the Ranchos Los Amigos Levels of Cognitive Functioning. It was developed as a behavioral rating scale to aid in assessment and treatment of the head-injured person. It represents the progression of recovery of cognitive abilities as demonstrated through behavioral change. The tool is used to assess the patient and to give some structure to interventions. See the box on p. 1758 for the levels of cognitive functioning.

For purposes of management of the patient, eight levels of cognitive functioning are grouped in four basic recovery phases and intervention strategies. These include the following:

Level	Recovery Phase	Approach
II, III	Decreased response	Stimulation
IV	Agitated response	Structure
V, VI	Confused response	Structure
VII, VIII	Automatic response	Community

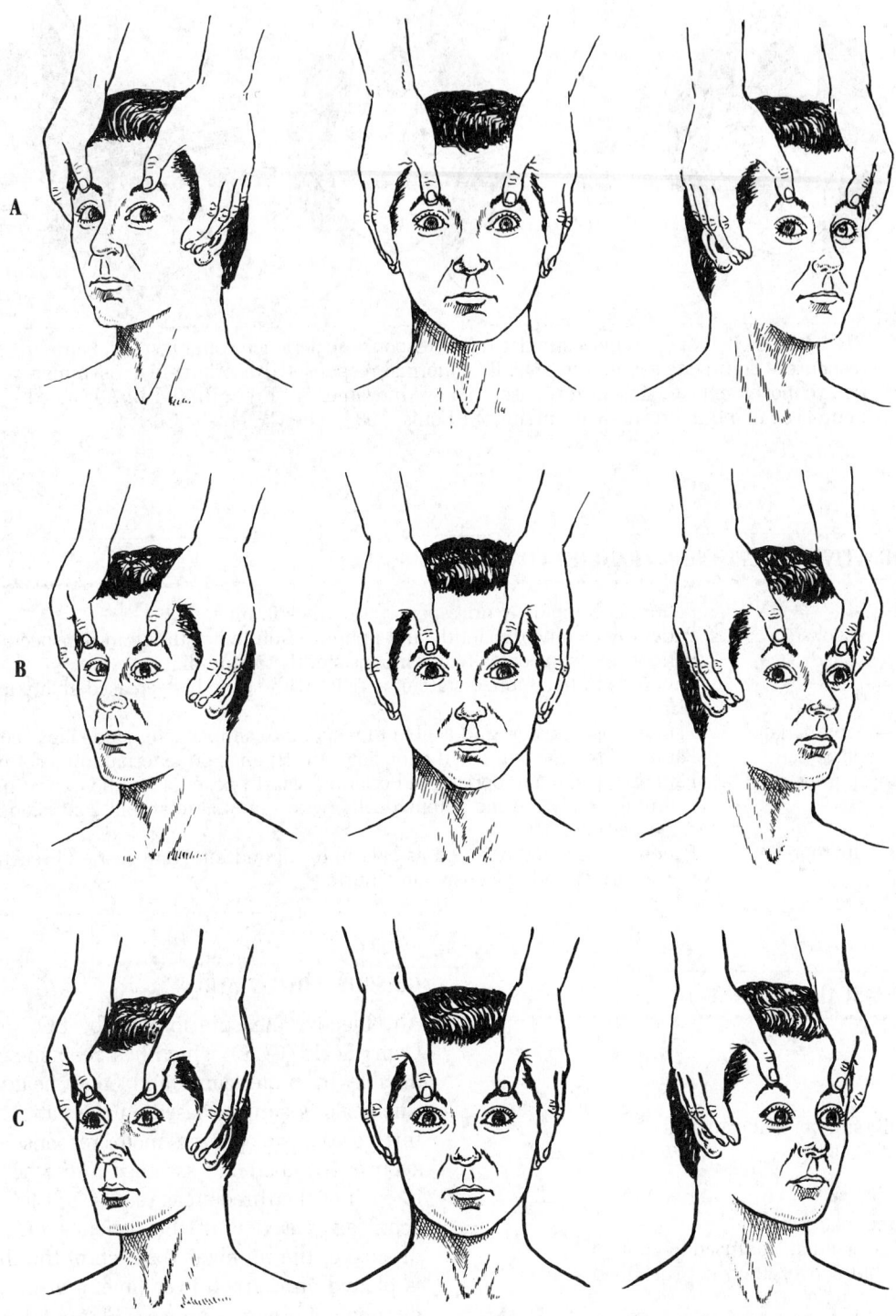

FIGURE 60-2 Test for oculocephalic reflex response (doll's eyes phenomenon). **A,** Normal response—eyes turn together to side opposite from turn of head. **B,** Abnormal response—eyes do not turn in conjugate manner. **C,** Absent response—eyes do not turn as head position is changed. (From Rudy EB: Advanced neurologic and neurosurgical nursing, St Louis, 1984, The CV Mosby Co.)

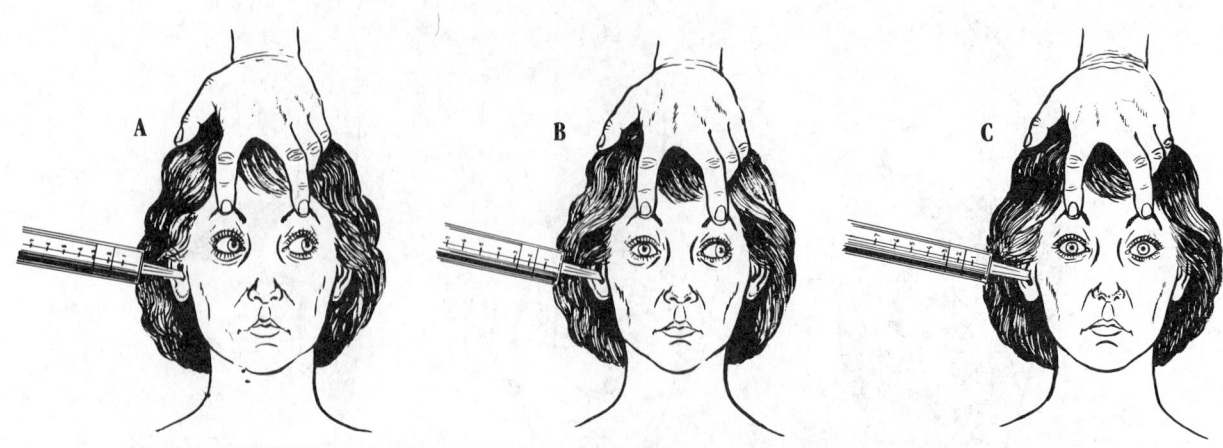

FIGURE 60-3 Test for oculovestibular reflex response (caloric ice water test). **A,** Normal response—conjugate eye movements. **B,** Abnormal response–dysconjugate or asymmetric eye movements. **C,** Absent response—no eye movements. (From Rudy EB: Advanced neurological and neurosurgical nursing, St Louis, 1984, The CV Mosby Co.)

LEVELS OF COGNITIVE FUNCTIONING (RANCHO LOS AMIGOS SCALE)

I. No response	Patient is completely unresponsive to any stimuli.
II. Generalized response	Patient reacts inconsistently and nonpurposefully to stimuli in nonspecific manner.
III. Localized response	Patient reacts specifically but inconsistently to stimuli.
IV. Confused—agitated	Patient is in heightened state of activity with severely decreased ability to process information.
V. Confused—inappropriate	Patient appears alert and is able to respond to simple commands fairly consistently.
VI. Confused—appropriate	Patient shows goal-directed behavior, but depends on external input for direction.
VII. Automatic—appropriate	Patient appears appropriate and oriented within hospital and home setting, goes through daily routine automatically, with minimal to absent confusion and has shallow recall of actions.
VII. Purposeful—appropriate	Patient is alert and oriented, is able to recall and integrate past and recent events, and is aware of and responsive to culture.[29]

GLASGOW COMA SCALE SCORING

EYES OPEN

4 Spontaneously
3 On request
2 To pain stimuli (supraorbital or digital)
1 No opening

BEST VERBAL RESPONSE

5 Oriented to time, place, person
4 Engages in conversation, confused in content
3 Words spoken but conversation not sustained
2 Groans evoked by pain
1 No response

BEST MOTOR RESPONSE

5 Obeys a command ("Hold out three fingers.")
4 Localizes a painful stimulus
3 Flexes either arm
2 Extends arm to painful stimulus
1 No response

Adapted from Teasdale G: Nurs Times 71(24):914-917, 1975.

GLASGOW COMA SCALE

An objective measure to describe LOC is the Glasgow Coma Scale (GCS), which has been shown to be reproducible by professional and other health personnel.[22] The scale is simple, based on the patient's response in three areas: eye opening, motor response, and verbal response. Numbers are assigned to the best performance in each of the three areas (see box at left) and the total score gives a view of the patient's LOC. When a sequence of the numbers for each of the three categories is plotted on a graph over time, a visual picture of the direction of progress evolves (Figure 60-4). It may show stability, or it may indicate deterioration or improvement in the condition. Although the GCS does not take the place of a comprehensive neurologic check, it is extremely useful in conjunction with motor and brain stem assessment in rapidly changing situations to detect deterioration in the patient's status. Scores of seven or less (but not scores of nine or more) represent coma.

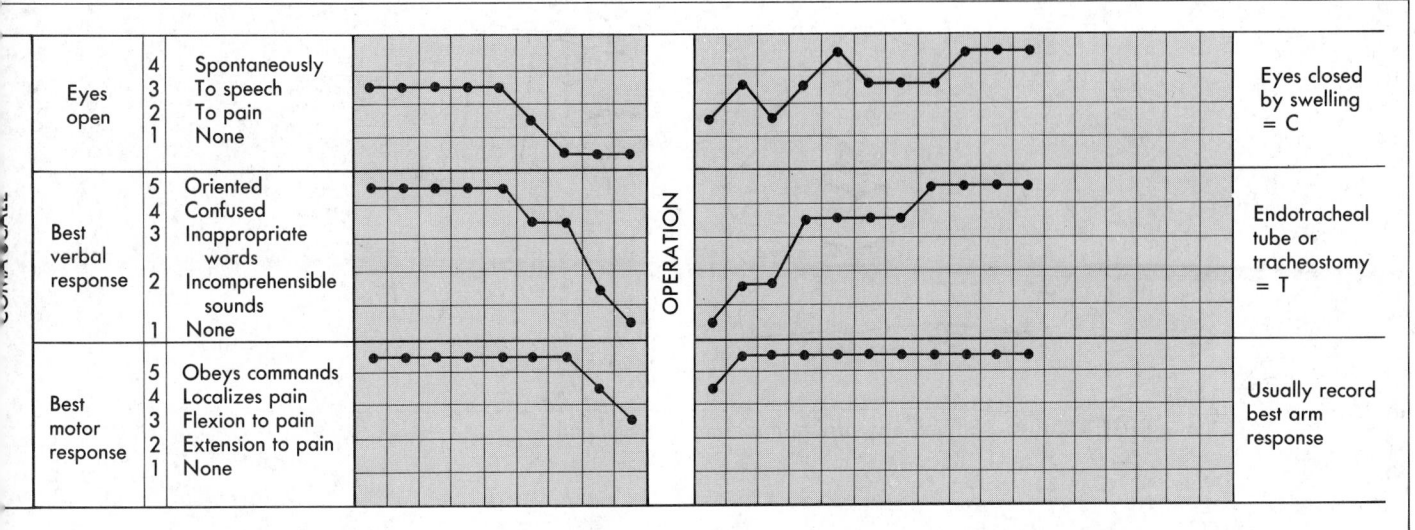

FIGURE 60-4 Glasgow Coma Scale, demonstrating measurement of level of consciousness. Notice change in patient's condition just before and after surgery.

When the onset of unconsciousness is *not* immediate, as it is with fainting or extreme shock or trauma, there is usually a consistent pattern of deterioration, although each patient is unique and may depart somewhat from the usual pattern. In the early stages of a deteriorating LOC the changes are so subtle they may not be noted. The behavior may appear to be a normal mood change. For instance, there may be less interest in the surroundings or in events taking place; the patient may seem bored or drowsy, inattentive or irritable, and restless. If these behaviors are noted and if there is any history that could lead one to suspect altered brain function, further exploration is necessary (see Chapter 59).

Another procedure for assessing level of consciousness is outlined in Figure 60-5. One begins by determining the patient's orientation by means of several questions about time, place, and person. The month and year are more readily recalled than days and dates. One can be satisfied if patients know they are in a hospital even if they cannot recall the name of the institution. Persons can be asked their name and occupation.

Next the person is requested to respond to simple commands such as blinking the eyes or touching the nose or ear with the fingers. Lack of symmetry can be noted by testing both sides of the body. This is important in localizing some lesions. The person can be asked

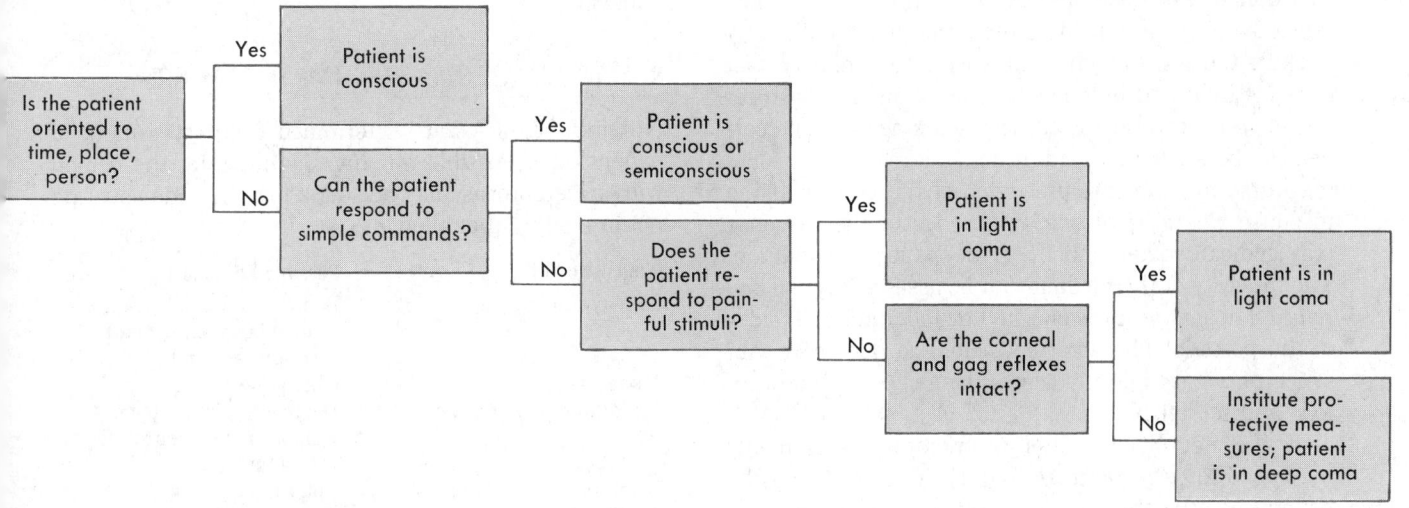

FIGURE 60-5 Procedure for assessing level of consciousness.

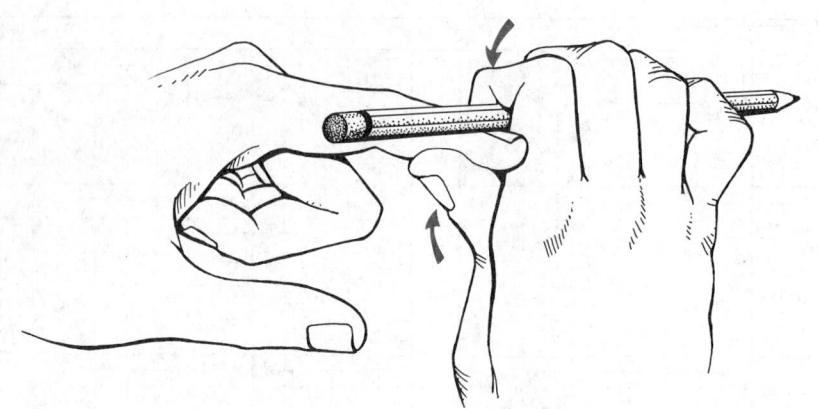

FIGURE 60-6 Nailbed pressure stimulation using pencil.

to squeeze your hand with first the right and then the left hand or to lift both feet simultaneously. If the person cannot perform in response to these commands, then proceed to assess the response to pain.

There are several techniques for checking response to pain that do not cause trauma to the patient. Pinching and pricking may damage tissues and are avoided when possible. The two preferred methods of delivering a pain stimulus are nail bed pressure and supraorbital pressure. Nail bed pressure is accomplished by placing a pen or similar object on the nail bed and squeezing it between the examiner's thumb and forefinger (Figure 60-6). If there is no response to nail bed pressure, supraorbital pressure is used.

To further assess brain stem function and to determine indications for nursing care, the integrity of the brainstem at the level of the pons can be assessed by checking the *lash reflex* or the *corneal reflex*. The lash reflex is checked by stroking the eyelashes with a finger. An intact reflex is indicated by immediate blinking (the eyes can be open or closed to do this). The corneal reflex is checked by holding the eyelid open and gently stroking the cornea with a thin wisp of cotton. An intact reflex is indicated by immediate blinking. The lash reflex is preferred over the corneal reflex because the cornea can be easily damaged. If no blink response is seen, the nurse must ensure protection of the cornea. If the response was present before, absence of the response may indicate deterioration of the patient's condition. The integrity of the medulla can be assessed by the *gag reflex*. The gag reflex is checked by touching both sides of the posterior pharynx with a tongue depressor. Absence of a gag reflex indicates danger of aspiration of food and secretions.

If the neurologic status deteriorates, assessments may need to be made more frequently. Likewise, if the patient's status improves, assessments may be made less frequently. The nurse independently institutes more frequent observations when the patient's status so indicates.

To perform the supraorbital pain maneuver, put the thumb on the upper edge of the bony groove of the eye socket about one third the distance from the inner aspect of the orbit and press. Probably the best check and the one with the least potential for harm is shown in Figure 60-6. One can apply pressure to the nail bed using a pencil held between the examiner's thumb and the patient's finger. One can also apply pressure to the trapezius by pinching it between the patient's neck and the shoulder. (Practice on yourself to see how much pressure is necessary.) The response showing the highest level of consciousness is for the patient to withdraw from the stimulus or try to push it away. If the response is by grimaces or by moving or thrashing around but in a nonpurposeful manner, the level of awareness is lower. Finally, with very deep coma there may be no response at all. Regardless of the response, be sure to record the type of stimulus and the patient's response behavior.

■ DATA ANALYSIS: NURSING DIAGNOSES

Nursing diagnoses are determined from assessment of patient data. Possible nursing diagnoses for the person with a cerebrovascular accident may include, but are not limited to, the following:

Diagnostic Title	Possible Etiologies
Activity intolerance	Bed rest, immobility, imbalance between oxygen supply/demand
Anxiety	Change in health status
Aspiration, potential for	Decreased consciousness, upper motor neuron lesion, dysphagia
Communication, impaired verbal	Aphasia
Constipation	Paralytic ileus

Diagnostic Title	Possible Etiologies
Coping, ineffective individual	Personal vulnerability
Disuse syndrome, potential for	Immobility, weakness
Fatigue	Muscle weakness, inadequate nutrition, inadequate rest
Home maintenance management	Individual injury/disease, impaired cognitive functioning
Incontinence, bowel	Neuromuscular impairment
Injury, potential for	Sensory/motor deficits
Knowledge deficit: cause of CVA and care required	Lack of exposure/recall, unfamiliarity with information sources
Mobility, impaired physical	Perceptual/cognitive impairment, neuromuscular impairment
Nutrition, altered: less than body requirements	Chewing or swallowing difficulties
Pain	Immobility
Self-care deficit: feeding, bathing/hygiene, dressing/grooming, feeding, toileting	Intolerance to activity, fatigue, perception/cognitive impairment, neuromuscular impairment
Sensory/perceptual alteration	Altered sensory reception/transmission, integration
Sexual dysfunction	Physiologic limitations
Skin integrity, impaired or potential	Mechanical forces (pressure, shearing forces, restraint), immobility
Social interaction, impaired	Poor communication skills, altered thought processes
Swallowing, impaired	Neuromuscular impairment, fatigue, limited awareness
Thought processes, altered	Neurologic disorders
Tissue perfusion, altered cerebral	Decreased blood flow (arterial)
Urinary elimination, altered patterns	Sensory-motor impairment

■ PLANNING: EXPECTED PATIENT OUTCOMES

Expected patient outcomes for the person with a cerebrovascular accident may include, but are not limited to, the following:

1. Patient makes progress toward independence in activities for daily living (ADL).
2. Patient can explain prescribed medication—side effects, desired effects, time, dose, route.
3. Patient demonstrates ability to communicate.
4. Patient can demonstrate exercises to maintain function.
5. Patient can explain importance of frequent position changes and demonstrate such positioning.
6. Patient can safely compensate for visual field cuts and perceptual, motor, and sensory losses.
7. Patient can explain plans for follow-up care.
8. Patient can demonstrate ability to check intactness of skin.
9. Skin remains intact.
10. Patient's anxiety is lessened.
11. Social interaction is maintained.
12. Disuse syndrome does not occur.
13. Sexual activity is maintained, if patient desires.
14. Swallowing is improved.
15. Nutritional status is improved.
16. Cerebral perfusion is maintained.
17. Mobility is improved.
18. Aspiration does not occur.
19. Patient remains free from injury.

■ IMPLEMENTATION

COMATOSE PATIENT
MAINTAINING STIMULATION

The nurse who cares for an already unconscious patient is always aware of the *patient's total dependency* on others. For the nurse the word *coma* is equated with helplessness. The unconscious patient cannot approve or disapprove of his or her care and cannot participate or select the person providing the care. Aside from involuntary motor activities such as cardiac, respiratory, and gastrointestinal actions, the patient is unresponsive. It then becomes paramount for others to provide for additional life-sustaining requirements, including nourishment, elimination, and protection of tissues.

Such a comatose state may lull the nurse into thinking that nothing is taking place in the patient's social world. We can only speculate about receptiveness. *Meaningful stimuli can be introduced* into the comatose patient's environment. To do this, the nurse must first learn as much of the patient's lifestyle as possible: social activities, work, friends, family. Key factors in the patient's former 24-hour routine are then selected, and the care should approximate previous habits. As an example, tube feedings should be scheduled about the same time of day as the patient was accustomed to eating, so that stomach distention is closely related to former habits. If the patient worked in a noisy factory, provide sound during the former working hours. Record familiar sounds and play them at appropriate times, for example, table talk when the family has dinner. For the long-term unconscious patient, this approach appears to have merit in keeping the focus of care from becoming too oriented to body functions to the exclusion of social factors.

Because *hearing is probably the last sense to be lost*, the monitoring of what is said in the presence of the unconscious person is vitally important. At present there is no sure device to assess when patients are no longer able to hear; therefore, even when patients appear incapable of receiving messages, they may still understand what is said. Grave prognoses or flippant comments are best kept outside a patient's range of hearing. In fact, positive and hopeful comments made in the patient's presence may give the patient motivation to struggle back to consciousness. Thus the nurse speaks to the patient and explains what is being done as if the patient were fully aware of what is going on.

The fourth factor to consider is the *therapeutic effect of touch*. The patient is spoken to before being touched and is handled with gentleness. Because there is no pain response to remind care providers when stress is increased, the tendency is to move the unconscious patient without consideration of soft tissue. Touch is one of the first sensations experienced by the human organism, and without proper touch, normal development would not take place. Touch is a medium for communication. Holding and cuddling infants seems to make them more tranquil and content. Research has shown positive results from the use of touch with disoriented and some mentally ill persons. It is highly possible that some of the same positive responses can be elicited in the unconscious patient. Using a firm hand grasp while talking to the patient about the day or the environment, smoothing the hair away from the face with the full palmar surface of the hand, or tucking the bed covers snuggly around the patient may stimulate the feeling of being cared for or encompassed.

A fifth factor relates to the patient's environment. The *environment should be low key*, with loud noises kept to a minimum. Soft music may be beneficial, but unnecessary sounds should be eliminated. The unconscious person with improving awareness often has an overly excitable nervous system response and is unable to attend to multiple stimuli. To facilitate the patient's ability to focus on any stimulus, eliminate all but necessary noises.

MAINTAINING NUTRITION

When a patient is experiencing rapidly decreasing awareness, nutrition is not a primary concern; however, if the patient becomes comatose and remains so for an extended period of time, nutritional support becomes a major concern. For the first few days of unconsciousness the patient will probably be maintained on intravenous fluids, as prescribed by the physician. Close observation of the needle site for inflammation or infiltration, as well as attention to flow rate to prevent excessive fluid intake, are essential. After 2 or 3 days a nasogastric tube, which will supply nourishment in liquid form, may be inserted into the stomach. Feedings are usually prescribed every 2 to 3 hours in small amounts to decrease the possibility of regurgitation and aspiration. The tube should be changed every 5 to 7 days unless it becomes clogged sooner, but the naris through which the tube is placed should be cleaned daily with warm water and lubricated with a water-soluble lubricant to decrease the formation of crusts.

The presence of a tube in the nostril is irritating and

RESEARCH

Ozuna J, and Friel P: Effect of internal tube feeding on serum phenytoin levels, J Neurosurg Nurs 16(6):289-291, 1984.

This study examined the relationship of timing of phenytoin (Dilantin) administration in relation to delivery of tube feedings and increasing the serum levels of phenytoin. Seven patients were studied. Tube feedings were stopped 2 hours before and 2 hours after administration of the phenytoin. No increase in levels were found. The study indicated that when increased phenytoin serum levels in patients receiving tube feedings are desired, the dose of phenytoin should be increased. ■

may cause tissue damage, so if coma lasts for an extended period of time, there may be a need for a gastrostomy tube to provide a means for feeding. The *gastrostomy tube* is inserted through the abdominal wall into the stomach. A catheter with an inflatable tip (to prevent the tube from slipping out of the stomach) is then sutured in place. This tube remains clamped or plugged except during feedings, and the area around the tube is cleaned daily and covered with a dry dressing. It has been found that patients receiving tube feedings often have decreased phenytoin levels (see the box above for relevant research about this topic).

MAINTAINING ELIMINATION
Bowel

Measures must be taken to assist in elimination and to maintain the tone of the bowel muscles. Without intervention, the tendency is for the comatose patient to become constipated and possibly impacted. Routinely palpate the abdomen to determine when a fecal mass is present. This palpation may also serve to stimulate peristalsis and induce a bowel movement. If possible, determine the patient's normal elimination schedule and place the patient on a bedpan at that hour. If a suppository is needed, administer it about 30 minutes before the regular elimination schedule. Bisacodyl (Dulcolax) is an effective suppository to use for bowel training. When laxatives are needed, a mild one such as milk of magnesia is often used and can be administered via the nasogastric tube.

Unconscious patients should be placed on a bowel program to ensure regular evacuation of stool (see Chapter 44).

Sometimes it becomes necessary to give a cleansing enema. Usual techniques for administering an enema are used; however, it may be necessary to hold the patient's buttocks together to prevent expulsion of the solution before the enema is ready to be expelled. The enema may also be administered through a Foley catheter placed in the rectum. The balloon is inflated before the fluid is introduced, thus preventing the expulsion of the fluid until the desired amount has been administered. The balloon is deflated (before removing the catheter) to allow expulsion of the enema. When placing the patient on the bedpan, care is taken to align the body correctly and to protect the skin. Gentle massage of the abdomen along the path of the transverse and descending colon will assist in the expulsion of the fecal mass. Stool softeners such as dioctyl sodium sulfosuccinate (Colace) administered via the nasogastric tube will also help facilitate elimination. Assuring an adequate liquid intake helps keep the fecal mass soft, and juices that have a laxative effect, such as prune juice, may be included in the diet. In the event that an impaction does occur, a retention enema is administered. If this is unsuccessful, the impaction may require manual removal; that is, using a gloved, lubricated finger to remove small pieces of the fecal material until the mass is eliminated.

The need for communication between health care providers is especially great with reference to bowel function. Only when bowel movements are carefully recorded as to time, amount, and consistency can the nurse make competent judgments about laxatives and enemas.

Bladder

A condom catheter connected to a urinary elimination bag may be placed on the male patient. The condom is unrolled on the penis and secured by an elasticized piece of tape around the penis. Care should be taken that the tape is not placed on the skin, but on the condom, and is wrapped around the penis snugly enough to prevent the condom from slipping, but not so tight as to interfere with circulation. Tactile stimulation may cause a temporary engorgement of the penis. When the size of the penis diminishes, the condom may slip off unless it has been securely attached. The condom is removed and the penis cleaned with soap and water daily.

An indwelling catheter with closed drainage may be needed for the female patient. While the catheter remains in, continual observation for signs of infection, chills, or fever is required. Accurate monitoring of intake in relation to output is essential. *Irrigation of the bladder through an indwelling catheter increases the possibility of introducing organisms; therefore, irrigate only when absolutely necessary.* Scrupulous sterile technique is indicated. Infections from prolonged use of an indwelling catheter cause the urine to become alkaline. This, in turn, causes inorganic materials such as phosphorus and calcium to settle out, and as a result bladder stones may form. A fluid intake of at least 3000 ml/day will keep the urine dilute enough to lessen the risk of bladder stones.

The catheter should be changed before mineral deposits plug the lumen or tip of the catheter. If no manufacturer's information is available about how frequently the catheter must be changed, a safe estimate is every 10 days.

MAINTAINING CIRCULATION

Circulation can be assisted in several ways. Conscientiously turning the patient from side to side at least every 2 hours will enhance circulation, because muscle movement stimulates circulation. Careful attention to positioning so that there are no constricted areas, as would be caused by twisted clothing, tight bedclothes, or a poorly positioned limb, will allow for maximum circulation. Joints bent at sharp angles slow circulation and should be avoided. Passive range of motion exercises planned into the nursing care regimen at least every 8 hours will increase blood flow. Padding of dependent bony prominences when they are being laid upon decreases pressure and helps to maintain good circulation. A commonly overlooked area is the ear. If it is folded over, circulation to the outer area is occluded and tissue necrosis occurs quickly. Always check the lower ear after turning the patient. Frequent monitoring of infusions to prevent overloading the circulatory system will also enhance circulation. The use of elastic stockings or wraps from toe to thigh on the lower extremities decreases the potential for stasis. These should be removed every 8 hours and the skin observed. They may be replaced after 30 minutes. When putting them on, raise the leg above the heart level.

MAINTAINING NORMAL BODY TEMPERATURE

A normal body temperature is generally considered to range from 36° C (97° F) to 37.2° C (99° F). Because the comatose patient is unable to express being too cold or too warm, it becomes the nurse's responsibility to monitor the body temperature at least every 4 hours and more frequently if a problem arises. If the heat center in the hypothalamus is disturbed, as it often is by trauma or by certain medical problems, the temperature may change rapidly. An excessively elevated temperature is called *hyperthermia*. An elevated temperature may also indicate an infection or dehydration. When a patient is experiencing hyperthermia, the nurse can assist in maintaining the temperature within a normal range by removing bedclothes and lowering the room temperature. If necessary, remove all of the patient's clothes except enough to protect modesty and the family's sense of propriety. Antipyretics may be given via the nasogastric or gastrostomy tube or by suppository. Ice bags covered with protective wraps to prevent tissue damage may be placed on the groin and axilla where there is a large blood supply. This helps to hasten body cooling. Sponging the body with a water and alcohol solution causes evaporation and subsequent cooling. The use of a fan to blow over the patient while the patient is being sponged further enhances cooling. Electrically controlled hypothermia blankets are often used to reduce fever when a patient suffers from hyperthermia. The patient should not be allowed to get chilled and shiver because shivering increases body metabolism and produces heat, thus raising the temperature. Continued hyperthermia will result in brain damage and ultimately death, so the temperature is kept as near normal as possible. On the other end of the continuum, a subnormal temperature (hypothermia) may be experienced. Additional clothing and covers and increased room temperature will help. Warmed blankets may help to elevate temperature in the hypothermic patient.

PROMOTING SAFETY

Numerous nursing activities are geared toward providing a safe environment for the comatose patient experiencing a changing level of consciousness. Side rails are kept up at all times for the unconscious patient unless the nurse is present. When the patient is restless and likely to be thrashing about, the railing should be padded. Equipment is placed far enough from the bed that a confused patient would be unlikely to interfere with its operation. Any prosthetic device such as false teeth, an artificial eye, or contact lenses should be removed and carefully stored in a safe place until the patient is lucid enough to use them appropriately. Restraint should be avoided unless the patient is agitated enough to do harm. When any type of restraint is used, caution should be taken to put it on properly and not too tightly. Periodic checks should be made for tissue damage.

When a person becomes unconscious, one of the first interventions is to remove contact lenses (Chapter 65). When properly done, there is little likelihood of causing damage. The cornea receives its oxygen supply primarily through exchange of gases in the atmosphere. When eyes are closed during sleep, the metabolic rate of the cornea decreases and the oxygen supply from the blood system is adequate to maintain health. When contact lenses are worn, however, the metabolic rate of the cornea increases. If the eyes are closed for a long time with the contact lenses in place, the cornea cannot remain healthy. The damage will be directly related to the time the lenses have been in place and the extent of interference with metabolic rate of the tissue. Contact lenses should be stored either in saline solution or distilled water, keeping the right and left lens separated and labeled.

Because the eyes are very precious and cannot be replaced, precautions should be taken to prevent their damage. Pull the lid back and check the eyes several times a day. Make sure they do not become dried out. Cleanse them with clear water or one of the commercial lubricants. Keep the eyelids closed. If there is any problem with keeping the eyelid closed, place a shield to cover the eye to prevent irritation from scratching or from dryness.

PROMOTING ACTIVITY

Positioning

Numerous interventions and aids are available to protect musculoskeletal integrity. Perhaps the most crucial is positioning. Improper positioning can lead to contractures, foot drop, wrist drop, and other deformities. The preferred position of the comatose patient is in the *side-lying position*. (Figure 60-7)

The comatose patient is at risk for pulmonary complications. Therefore, frequent changes of position are essential. Turning the patient from side to side at frequent intervals prevents pooling of pulmonary secretions. In some instances, tracheal suctioning may be necessary because of the patient's inability to cough. Unless neurologic complications contraindicate it, postural drainage may be initiated.

Comatose patients may be placed in a prone or supine position; however, care must be taken to ensure a patent airway. (Figures 62-7 and 62-8)

Patients who are comatose may be positioned without significant risk of increasing intracranial pressure. (See the box on p. 1765 for an example of relevant research.)

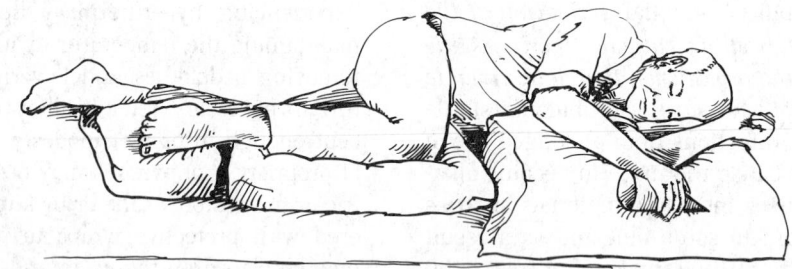

FIGURE 60-7 Lateral position with hand cone to prevent flexion contracture of hand. (From Dittmar S: Rehabilitation nursing, St Louis, 1989, The CV Mosby Co.)

RESEARCH

Parsons C and Wilson M: Cerebrovascular status of severe closed head injured patients following passive position changes, Nurs Res 33(2):68-75, 1984.

This study examined the effects of six body position changes, performed as part of routine nursing care on the cerebrovascular status of 18 head-injured patients. These changes included turning and positioning in bed, range of motion exercises, head rotation, and raising and lowering the head of the bed. All patients had baseline mean intracranial pressures of less than or equal to 15 mm Hg. All position changes except that of raising the head of the bed raised heart rate, blood pressure, intracranial pressure, and cerebral perfusion pressure. These elevations were transient and returned to baseline in 1 minute. This study indicates that passive position changes may safely be made in severely head-injured patients who have stable baseline mean intracranial pressures of 15 mm Hg or less, and cerebral perfusion pressures of about 50 mm Hg. ▪

Exercise

Passive range-of-motion (ROM) exercise is performed a minimum of twice daily and ideally several times a day. One way to accomplish this is to put the upper side of the body through complete range of motion each time the patient is turned. Doing it systematically helps assure that it is not postponed and subsequently overlooked. ROM will increase circulation and decrease the likelihood of thrombi.

When the physical condition is stable and consciousness returns, the patient should sit in a chair at least once and preferably twice a day. The upright posture fosters weight bearing on the long bones, thus limiting calcium loss, and enhances pulmonary expansion, circulation, and digestive motility. Unless the patient is small enough for two people to manage, use a mechanical lift. Position the patient so that he or she is seated squarely on the buttocks with the spine straight and feet flat on the floor or footrest. Support the arms and head with pillows. Use a chest harness support tied behind the chair or secure the patient's torso by wrapping a sheet around the torso and the chair.

MAINTAINING SKIN INTEGRITY

The integument of the comatose patient is prone to many assaults: being pulled across bed linens, lying too long on bony prominences, dryness or moisture, and increased bacteria from incontinence of urine and feces. A warm water bath daily is recommended. While tub baths are not always feasible, the patient can be placed in a tub or shower when consciousness returns if an adequate number of people are present to prevent injury.

Until such time, a daily bed bath should include a brisk rub (except when the skin is fragile) with sparing use of soap and a thorough rinse. Soap residue causes dryness and skin irritation, and moisture increases the potential for skin breakdown.

To prevent dryness, place a lotion (such as Alpha-Keri oil or Jeri-Bath) in the bath water. If this is not sufficient, rub the body with a lanolin preparation or other cream. The family may suggest a lotion the patient has used routinely.

The skin of the feet is especially prone to drying, and the nails harden with decreased circulation. Rub the feet daily with a lubricant such as Vaseline. Never use alcohol unless specially indicated, because it makes the skin extremely dry. Comatose patients perspire just as alert patients do. If talcum powder is used, it tends to hold perspiration. Because moist skin is more prone to necrosis, avoid using talcum.

Linens are kept dry. Keep them pulled taut so there will be no wrinkles underneath the patient that might cause decubitus ulcers. Protect the patient's skin from the shearing effect of sliding on the sheets by positioning the head of the bed at not more than a 10-degree angle unless otherwise ordered so that the patient will not constantly be sliding down in bed. The use of lamb's wool under pressure areas also helps prevent decubitus ulcers. A water or air mattress to equalize pressure can be used, although if the patient is turned carefully this is not necessary. Be sure never to use a doughnut or rubber ring, as they simply cause a circle of pressure and decrease the blood supply to the area within that circle, making skin breakdown more likely.

MAINTAINING GOOD HYGIENE

Hair

Shampoos are indicated every 1 or 2 weeks, unless contraindicated by the patient's underlying problems. The scalp of the comatose patient continues to secrete oils and perspiration, and the hair becomes sour-smelling, and difficult to manage when not properly cleansed. Comb hair daily, and braid or arrange long hair to prevent matting. Take care that there are no lumps of hair on the part of the head where the patient lies.

Hair care for black persons differs from that recommended for white persons. For the black person, cleansing the hair with a warm solution of one part alcohol with four parts of mineral oil is followed by an application of warm olive oil, baby oil, or Vaseline oil to the scalp and hair.[16] Excess oil may be removed with a towel. Long hair can be braided; very short hair can be left loose after combing. Afro combs or picks make combing less uncomfortable for the patient.

Hair care is important to the patient's sense of well-being and is comforting for the family because a well-groomed patient conveys that he or she is "cared about" as well as "cared for."

Mouth and Teeth

The unconscious patient is often a mouth breather and therefore has a dry mouth. Regardless of how he or she breathes, the patient experiencing a decreased level of consciousness will require mouth care. When not cleansed, the mouth becomes inflamed and more prone to infection. Mucus and bacteria form plaque. Plaque, tartar, and food debris collect in gingival crevices around the teeth and cause mechanical and bacterial irritation. The tissue becomes swollen and inflamed. In time, gingival tissue will separate from the teeth and form pockets where still more debris can accumulate. Teeth may be lost and bone may become involved. Elderly persons have thinner oral membranes and less flow of salivary juices to help wash the mouth, so their problem is compounded. Refer to Chapter 42 for oral care guidelines.

Nose

The nares are cleansed daily to help keep them patent. Inspect for secretions and note the type. If crusts are forming, gently remove with a moist applicator unless the patient's condition contraindicates. A thin application of a water-soluble lubricant helps decrease accumulation of debris. This is especially important when a nasogastric tube is in place because it causes some trauma to the tissues, and inflammation may ensue if the naris is not kept cleaned.

Ears

The folds of the ears are cleansed and dried carefully. The area behind the ear is easily overlooked when drying but is prone to skin irritation when soap or moisture is not removed. Check the ears for wax while bathing the patient. Over a period of time large amounts of wax may accumulate; this is easily removed with a small wire loop. When head trauma is the basis of coma, be very cautious about introducing anything into the ear

---

GUIDELINES FOR NURSING INTERVENTION FOR PERSONS WITH DECREASED LEVEL OF CONSCIOUSNESS OR COMA

1. Maintain stimulation
   a. Introduce meaningful stimuli
   b. Monitor what is said around patient
   c. Speak to patient before touching
   d. Use gentleness in handling patient
   e. Maintain low-key environment
2. Maintain nutrition
   a. Monitor intravenous fluids
   b. Administer tube feedings with patient in high Fowler's position
   c. Administer tube feedings at room temperature
   d. Change feeding tube every 5 to 7 days
   e. Cleanse and lubricate naris to prevent breakdown
   f. Begin oral feedings as soon as patient is able
3. Maintain elimination
   a. Institute suppository regimen, considering patient's normal routines
   b. Administer enemas only as last resort
   c. Stool softeners as ordered
   d. Give adequate fluids—use prune juice
   e. Regular toileting to institute regimen
   f. Use of condom catheter for male
   g. Adequately care for indwelling catheter
4. Maintain circulation
   a. Reposition frequently
   b. Avoid positioning joints at acute angles
   c. Use elastic stockings or Ace wraps to legs
5. Maintain normal body temperature
   a. Hyperthermia
      (1) Remove excess bedclothes and clothing
      (2) Lower room temperature
      (3) Ice bags to groin or axilla
      (4) Alcohol sponge baths

   (5) Use of hypothermia blankets
   (6) Use of antipyretics
   b. Hypothermia
      (1) Add additional clothing or blankets
      (2) Increase room temperature
      (3) Warmed blankets
6. Promote safety
   a. Side rails up at all times
   b. Pad rails as necessary
   c. Keep supplies and equipment out of reach of patient
   d. Use restraints only when absolutely necessary
   e. Remove contact lenses
   f. Cleanse eyes at least daily and check for redness or other signs of irritation or infection
7. Promote activity
   a. Position properly at least every 2 hours
   b. Use prone position if patient is able to tolerate
   c. Range of motion exercises at least twice a day
   d. Mobilize patient into chair as soon as possible
8. Maintain skin integrity
   a. Cleanse skin daily using warm water
   b. Judicious use of lotion to prevent dryness
   c. Keep linen pulled tight and free of crumbs or other residue
   d. Use air or water mattresses as necessary
   e. Inspect skin frequently
9. Maintain good hygiene
   a. Wash hair every 1 to 2 weeks, or more often if needed
   b. Braid or arrange long hair to prevent matting
   c. Give good mouth care at least three times a day

until it has been ascertained that there is no damage within the ear.

SUPPORTING SIGNIFICANT OTHERS

The unconscious patient has no awareness of the severity of the situation, but the alert family does. This awareness creates great anxiety and stress. During the initial phase of injury or onset of disease when consciousness is being affected, the family has many decisions to make about the patient's care. If the outcome of those decisions is not positive, family members may feel guilty for having made them. Additionally, they will experience feelings of loss and grief. As time passes, the family members remain in limbo, unable to complete the grieving process, yet equally unable to sustain the high pitch of grief initially experienced. Guilt feelings may be expressed as anger and hostility toward those who are providing care.[25] It is difficult for family members to understand what is going on, and it is very frightening to stand by feeling inadequate and unable to help. The family then becomes part of the responsibility of the nurse. From the beginning, they need special understanding and special consideration. For them, the patient's condition may precipitate a crisis. They can be helped to cope by being encouraged to participate in the patient's care.

A good way to involve the family in the care of the patient is by asking for help with positioning the patient. They are usually quite capable of doing an excellent job of monitoring and maintaining position and are often with the patient extended periods of time when the nurse cannot be. Their involvement not only ensures more consistent care for the patient, but it is very beneficial to the family, giving them a sense of accomplishment and purpose. The hours of waiting are lessened for significant others when they feel they are needed and involved. For this reason, carefully explain what is to be done and the principles underlying the actions; then allow them to help you, not only with positioning but in other aspects of care as they desire. Acknowledge the value of their contributions.

Family members often will wish to stay at the bedside. If they do, share with them that their talking is providing sensory stimulation to the patient. The assumption is made that some of this talking may be filtering through to the awareness of the patient even though the patient is unable to respond to it.

The nurse conveys to the family a willingness to listen, to be involved, and to help them explore their thoughts. Keeping the family informed of what is being done, what is planned, and changes in the patient's condition is very crucial. Provide the family with a comfortable environment. An expression of the nurse's willingness to help is frequently all that is required to comfort the family.

When a patient begins to recover, the first response often is to a familiar voice or face, and this may be in the form of a verbal comment. The patient will need the security of knowing that family, friends, and staff are concerned and will need much support and encouragement, as well as explanation. See box on p. 1766 for guidelines for care of a person in coma.

CONFUSED OR DISORIENTED PATIENT

The care of the *confused* patient begins with a thorough assessment to determine the cause of the confusion and the patient's needs (see box on p. 1768). Establish communication with the patient. A good way to get the patient's attention is through touch. Once the contact is made, use a calm, quiet, unhurried voice. To keep the patient oriented, explain in advance what you will do. Include the patient in planning and discussions. See that the room is well lighted. Keep a large calendar and clock in view. Introduce yourself each time you care for the patient. Talk slowly and distinctly and use short statements. Face the patient and stay within a conversational distance of 4 feet. When speaking to the patient, eliminate extra stimuli such as the radio and television, which would tend to clutter the sensory field and might prevent a clear communication between the nurse and patient. When it is possible, provide consistency by having the same staff members care for the patient every day. It is advisable to keep decision making at a minimum for the confused person. See box below and on p. 1768 for relevant research.

The nurse can minimize effects of confusion by recognizing environmental areas likely to precipitate delirium and teaching the patient what to expect before placement there. When emergency placement is required, discussion and explanation should take place as

---

RESEARCH

Williams M, et al: Predictors of acute confusional states in hospitalized elderly patients, Res Nurs Health 8:31-40, 1985.

One hundred seventy elderly (mean age = 78.8 years) patients from four hospitals with no prior history of mental impairment were studied during the first 5 postoperative days to determine the incidence of acute confusional state. Over half (51.5%) demonstrated some confusion postoperatively. Based on admission data, older people, those who made more errors on the mental status test given on admission, and those with lower levels of activity before injury were most likely to experience confusion. In addition, data were obtained during the hospitalization that were also used to predict confusion. Based on treatment and clinical progress data, the best set of predictors included age and performance on the mental status test, the previous day's confusion score, pain, narcotics, and mobility. ■

RESEARCH

Williams M, et al: Reducing acute confusional states in elderly patients with hip fractures, Res Nurs Health 8:329-337, 1985.

Interpersonal and environmental nursing interventions were carried out with 57 elderly (over 60 years) patients on orthopedic units in three hospitals to reduce the incidence of acute confusional state. Preventive approaches were related to strange environment, altered sensory input, loss of control and independence, disruption in life pattern, immobility and pain, and disruption in elimination patterns. Ameliorative approaches were related to mild behaviors suggestive of confusion, sundowning, unsafe behavior, hallucinations or illusions, and fright. The overall incidence of confusion was 51.5% for the nonintervention sample and 43.9% for the intervention sample. The difference was especially apparent for moderate to severe confusion, for which the incidence rates for the nonintervention and intervention groups were 16% and 8.8%, respectively. ∎

soon as possible after the crisis situation. Emphasize that physical and environmental factors are contributing to the confusion, fears, and memory loss; reassure the patient that the state will eventually pass. Other interventions include keeping the environment simplified and well organized. Place noisy machines as far from the patient's head as possible. Dim lighting to facilitate sleep. Organize care to provide the longest possible rest periods. Place familiar personal objects within view. Use touch judiciously. Treatment directed at known causes such as fever, shock, and drug overdose will result in decreasingly confused responses.

Regardless of the specific treatments, the nurse provides safety for the patient and protection from self-injury. This may include keeping the environment quiet and nonstimulating or using side rails if the patient is to be left alone. If the presence of side rails disturbs the patient, as they sometimes do, a judgment must be made whether to use them and risk increased agitation or not use them and risk a fall. Occasionally, it becomes necessary to restrain the patient.

One also monitors the physiologic processes, ensures the adequate intake of fluid and food, and monitors and supports elimination. Speak slowly and clearly. This facilitates communication with the person who experiences delirium. Recognizing that the patient cannot control behavior fosters acceptance and patience.

Help family members or significant others to understand what is happening and what such behavior might imply. Let them know that their presence provides a familiar stabilizing force. Let them make plans for the patient's care in the hospital and at home. Support them as much as possible in whatever they decide. (See the box above, right, for a summary of care for the confused or disoriented patient.)

GUIDELINES FOR NURSING INTERVENTIONS FOR PERSONS WITH CONFUSION OR DISORIENTATION

1. Promote communication
   a. Touch may be useful to establish communication
   b. Use calm, quiet, and unhurried voice to talk to patient
   c. Talk slowly and distinctly and use short sentences
   d. Face patient when talking and stay within conversational range
2. Promote orientation
   a. Explain procedures in advance
   b. Environment should be well lighted
   c. Keep large calendar and clock in view
   d. Introduce self when caring for patient
   e. Keep sensory stimulation to a minimum
   f. Provide consistency in staff caring for patient
   g. Keep decision making to a minimum
3. Support family

PATIENT TEACHING

Generally, the patient teaching that can be accomplished with a patient who is comatose or suffering from a decreased LOC is minimal. Family members, however, need a great deal of help and understanding, as well as teaching about the disease process and care involved.

CHAPTER SUMMARY

- ✔ Consciousness is the process of awareness of the self and the environment.
- ✔ Impaired consciousness may result from conditions that depress or destroy the brain stem or the cerebrum.
- ✔ Arousal is a physiologic function associated with wakefulness.
- ✔ Awareness is the sum of all cognitive and affective functions of the body.
- ✔ The presence of consciousness depends on a normally functioning interplay among certain neurons, the brain, and the reticular activating system (RAS).
- ✔ Five levels of cerebral function are confusion, drowsiness, stupor, light coma, and deep coma.
- ✔ In the comatose patient, damage to the central nervous system may be shown by pathologic motor responses that include decorticate and decerebrate posturing.
- ✔ If a patient is receiving artificial means of ventilation, it is possible to sustain breathing and circulation in the absence of brain activity.
- ✔ A confused or disoriented patient experiences a disturbance in the content of the consciousness.

✔ Medical management of the patient with coma or decreased LOC depends to a great extent on the cause of the coma.

✔ Abnormal respiratory patterns occur with decreased level of consciousness and may assist in determining the nature of the process.

✔ The Glasgow Coma Scale is an objective measure to describe levels of consciousness.

✔ It is important to maintain sensory stimulation of the unconscious patient.

✔ Because of the disabling nature of coma or other levels of decreased consciousness, patient outcomes are often the result of direct nursing and medical treatment.

✔ The nurse who cares for the unconscious patient should be aware of the patient's total dependency on others.

✔ It is important to speak to the unconscious patient before touching or giving care and to handle the patient with care.

✔ Important nursing measures for the patient with altered levels of consciousness include maintaining stimulation, nutrition, elimination, circulation, safety, activity, skin integrity, normal body temperature and good hygiene.

✔ Although the unconscious patient may not be aware of the severity of the situation, the family or significant others are aware and need support and education.

✔ The care of the confused patient begins with a thorough assessment to determine the cause and needs of the patient.

✔ With a confused or disoriented patient, it is essential for the nurse to provide safety for the patient and protection from self-injury.

QUESTIONS TO CONSIDER

- The mother of a comatose patient states, "Why worry about his skin and teeth. He's going to die anyway." What would your response be?

- Why are the Glasgow Coma Scale and the Rancho Los Amigos Scale important?

- Why is it important to consider hearing in the comatose patient?

- A patient is extremely agitated and has threatened staff. What should the nurse do?

- A patient is admitted with delirium. A toxicology drug screen indicates that she has ingested PCP. How should this alter her care?

REFERENCES AND SELECTED READINGS

1. Abelson N: Observations of the neurosurgical patient, Curationis 5:332-337, 1982.
2. *Adams M et al: The confused patient: psychological responses in critical care units, Am J Nurs 78:1505-1512, 1978.
3. *Adams N: Prolonged coma: your care makes all the difference, Nursing '77 7(8):21-27, 1977.
4. Adams R and Victor M: Principles of neurology, New York, 1985, McGraw-Hill Book Co.
5. *Allen N: Prognostic factors in coma, Heart Lung 8:1075-1082, 1979.
6. Ballenger M: The neurological system and level of consciousness, Emergency 16:52-55, 1984.
7. Boss B: Memory impairment: forgetfulness vs. amnesia, J Neurosci Nurs 20:151-158, 1988.
8. Clochesy J: Problems in interpreting abnormal auditory brainstem responses in comatose patient, J Neurosurg Nurs 17:253-255, 1984.
9. Crigger M et al: Selecting a nursing diagnosis for changes in consciousness, Digest of Crit Care Nurs 4:156-163, 1985.
10. Daily T: The diagnosis of brain death: an overview of neurosurgical nursing response, J Neurosurg Nurs 14:85-89, 1982.
10a. Duffey B: Demented, old, and alone, Amer J Nurs 89(2):212-218, 1989.
11. Findley L: Altered consciousness, Nursing '84 2:633-664, 666, 1984.
12. *Finklestein S and Ropper A: The diagnosis of coma: its pitfalls and limitation, Heart Lung 8:1059-1064, 1979.
13. *Gifford R and Plant M: Abnormal respiratory patterns in the comatose patient caused by intracranial dysfunction, J Neurosurg Nurs 7:57-61, 1975.
14. Giublilatom R: Evoked potentials, J Neurosurg Nurs 16:241-247, 1984.
15. *Gould H: How to remove contact lenses from comatose patients, Am J Nurs 76:1306-1311, 1976.
16. *Grier M: Hair care for the black patient, Am J Nurs 76:1781, 1976.
17. Haberman B: Cognitive dysfunction and social rehabilitation in severely head-injured patients, J Neurosurg Nurs 14:220-224, 1982.
18. Hummelgard AB et al: Prognostic value of brainstem auditory evoked potentials in head injury, J Neurosurg Nurs 16:181-187, 1984.
19. Jess L: Investigating impaired mental status: an assessment guide you can use, Nursing 88 18(6):42-50, 1988.
20. Johnson L: If your patient has increased intracranial pressure: your goal should be no surprises. Nursing 83 15:58-64, 1983.
21. Jones A et al: Side effects following metrizamide myelography and lumbar laminectomy, J Neurosci Nurs 19:90-94, 1987.
22. *Jones C: Glasgow Coma Scale, Am J Nurs 79:1551-1553, 1979.
23. Kirk E and Bradford L: Effects of alcohol on the CNS: implications for the neuroscience nurse, J Neurosci Nurs 19:326-335, 1987.
24. *Konikow N: Alterations in movement: nursing assessment and implications, J Neurosurg Nurs 17:61-65, 1985.
25. *Loen M and Snyder M: Psychosocial aspects of care of the long-term comatose patient, J Neurosurg Nurs 11:235-237, 1979.
26. Maher M and Strong S: Organ donation: a nursing perspective. J Neurosurg Nurs 21:357-361, 1989.
27. Mahon D and Elger C: Analysis of posttraumatic syndrome following head injury, J Neurosci Nurs 21:382-384, 1989.

*References preceded by an asterisk are particularly well suited for student readings.

28. Malasanos L et al: Health assessment, ed 3, St Louis, 1986, The CV Mosby Co.

29. *Malkmus D et al: Rehabilitation of the head injured adult-comprehensive cognitive management, Downey, Calif, 1980, Professional Staff Association of Ranchos Los Amigos Hospital, Inc.

30. Mauss-Clum N: Bringing the unconscious patient back safely: nursing makes all the critical difference, J Neurosurg Nurs 14:32-43, 1982.

31. Minnich A: Locked-in syndrome, J Neurosurg Nurs 15:77-79, 1983.

32. Mitchell P et al: Moving the patient in bed: effects on increased intracranial pressure, Nurs Res 30(4):212-218, 1981.

33. *Myco F and McGilloway F: Care of the unconscious patient: a complementary perspective, J Adv Nurs 5:273-283, 1980.

34. Nikas D: Neurological assessment of altered states of consciousness, Part 1, Focus Crit Care 10:10-14, 1983.

35. Nikas D: Neurological assessment of altered states of consciousness, Part 2, Focus Crit Care 10:20-23, 1983.

36. Nikas D: Neurological assessment of altered states of consciousness, Part 3, Focus Crit Care 11:54-58, 1984.

37. Ozuna J and Friez P: Effects of enteral tube feedings in serum phenytoin levels, J Neurosurg Nurs 16:289-290, 1984.

38. Parsons C and Wilson M: Cerebrovascular status of severe closed head injury following passive position changes, Nurs Res 33(2):68-75, 1984.

39. *Plum F and Posner J: The diagnosis of stupor and coma, ed 3, Philadelphia, 1980, FA Davis Co.

40. Plylar P: Management of the agitated and aggressive head injury patient in an acute hospital setting, J Neurosci Nurs 21:353-356, 1989.

41. Rainer J: Evaluation of the comatose patient, J Neurosurg Nurs 15:283-286, 1983.

42. Rudy E: Advanced neurological and neurosurgical nursing, St Louis, 1984, The CV Mosby Co.

43. Smith S: Continuous intracranial monitoring: implications and applications for critical care, Crit Care Nurs 3:42-51, 1983.

44. *Teasdale G and Jennett B: Assessment of coma and impaired consciousness: a practical scale, Lancet 2:81-84, 1974.

45. Tosch P: Patients recollections of their posttraumatic coma, J Neurosci Nurs 20:223-228, 1988.

46. Turner H et al: Comparison of nurse and computer recording of ICP in head injured patient, J Neurosci Nurs 20:236-239, 1988.

47. Vernberg K et al: The Glasgow Coma Scale, Nurse Education 8:33-37, 1983.

48. Warren J and Peck E: Factors which influence neuropsychological recovery from severe head injury, J Neurosurg Nurs 16:248-252, 1984.

CHAPTER 61

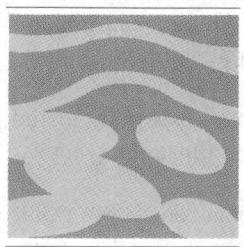

Sleep Disorders

DIANE BROADBENT FRIEDMAN

CHAPTER OBJECTIVES

After studying this chapter, the student should be able to:
1 Take a complete sleep history.
2 Describe the nature, pathophysiology, therapy, and teaching needs of persons with insomnia, narcolepsy, and sleep apnea.
3 Describe the relationship of sleep to chronobiology and the implications for nursing research.

We usually divide our lives into two parts, waking and sleeping. We also commonly believe that our important activity occurs while we are awake and that sleep is a passive state initiated by simply closing our eyes. This belief contains the two most basic *misunderstandings* about sleep: sleep is not active or very important to life, and sleep is something that simply comes "naturally." These misunderstandings contribute to health professionals and their patients overlooking sleep problems and the role sleep plays in healing and health maintenance.

INTRODUCTION TO SLEEP PROBLEMS

ASPECTS OF NORMAL SLEEP

Sleep is difficult to define because as yet it is incompletely understood by researchers. From the sleeper's point of view, sleep is experienced as (1) being the deliberate initiation of a change or reduction in consciousness lasting an average of 8 hours, (2) commencing about the same time each 24-hour period, and (3) usually resulting in a feeling of restored physical, emotional, and intellectual energy. This definition contains three important concepts about normal sleep: *changes in consciousness, deliberate initiation of sleep,* and *timing of sleep.*

Although the sleeping person or observers may believe the sleeper is unconscious, the sleeping brain alternates among several active states during sleep, producing a series of predictable 90-minute sleep cycles. Unlike the unconsciousness produced by anesthesia, the brain maintains all body systems during sleep, some

of which are more active in sleep (such as secretion of growth hormone), and allows for restoration of alertness if required. Also, unlike animals, only humans can deliberately postpone the initiation of sleep. The record for sleep postponement is about 10 days.

Sleep commences about the same time each 24-hour period. The study of biologic rhythms places the study of sleep into a larger context. The timing for sleep is regulated by many subtle external factors (see box below). Internal hormonal factors and neurologic activity maintain internal biologic clocks. These factors tend to occur at the same time every 24 hours; therefore they help to "anchor" the onset and termination of sleep. Sleep research at the cellular level indicates that changes in the neuronal cell membrane and in the cell nucleus in several brain areas alter the cell's excitability in different stages of sleep.

NORMAL SLEEP FUNCTION

Sleep usually is initiated in the late evening about 8 hours before arising for morning work or daily routine. Some people require more or less than 8 hours to feel refreshed. Some people are "larks," falling asleep within moments of lying down and awakening alert and ready to go, whereas others are "owls," taking up to 30 minutes to fall asleep and feeling their most alert in the afternoon or early evening.

Sleep usually is initiated within 30 minutes of lying down. Sleep cycles of 90 minutes occur, initiated by very light stage I/II, followed by deep stage III/IV, and

---

EXTERNAL FACTORS REGULATING SLEEP

Sunrise, sunset, and length of day
Ambient temperature
Physical activity and rest
Timing and composition of meals
Timing of social/environmental cues, such as increased
    morning traffic noise

---

ending with lighter rapid eye movement (REM)/dream sleep. If awakened from light stage I sleep, sleepers state that they were not asleep, whereas if awakened from other stages, they state that they were asleep or dreaming. Arousal can occur after each REM cycle. As the night progresses, the amount of time spent in stage III/IV shortens and the amount of REM lengthens. Thus more dreaming time occurs in the morning hours just before final awakening.

NATURE OF SLEEP PROBLEMS

It is estimated that more than one half of all adults cite difficulties with sleeping at some time in their lives. These problems result in suffering; risk of accident; worry about loss of emotional, intellectual, or neurologic functioning; embarrassment; and exacerbation of other health problems. In 1983 the National Institutes of Mental Health (NIMH) determined that 35% of a na-

tionally representative sample reported "trouble sleeping" in the previous year and that half this group reported this as a "serious" problem. This means that approximately one of every three patients a nurse encounters may describe a sleep problem. Sleep problems have been historically overlooked, however, especially in the hospitalized patient when other circumstances appear more compelling.

Nurses can have a primary impact on helping persons with sleep problems and preventing sleep problems. The following instances of sleep problems highlight the need to detect sleep concerns or to prevent sleep problems from developing.

1. A 50-year-old woman describes a 25-year history of inability to stay asleep beyond 5 AM, dating from the birth of her first child.
2. A 65-year-old man comes to the emergency room for contusions following a minor traffic accident.

CLASSIFICATION OF SLEEP AND AROUSAL DISORDERS*

DISORDERS OF INITIATING AND MAINTAINING SLEEP (DIMS)

1. Psychophysiologic: transient and situational, persistent
2. Associated with:
   a. Psychiatric disorders: symptom and personality disorders, affective disorders, other functional psychoses
   b. Use of drugs and alcohol: tolerance to or withdrawal from central nervous system (CNS) depressants, sustained use of CNS stimulants, sustained use or withdrawal from other drugs, chronic alcoholism
   c. Sleep-induced respiratory impairment: sleep apnea DIMS syndrome, alveolar hypoventilation DIMS syndrome
   d. Sleep-related (nocturnal) myoclonus DIMS syndrome and/or "restless legs"
   e. Other medical, toxic, and environmental conditions
   f. Child-onset DIMS
   g. Other DIMS conditions: repeated REM interruptions, atypical polysomnographic features
   h. No DIMS abnormality: "short sleeper," subjective DIMS complaints without objective findings

DISORDERS OF EXCESSIVE SOMNOLENCE (DOES)

1. Psychophysiologic: transient and situational, persistent
2. Associated with:
   a. Psychiatric disorders: symptom and personality disorders, affective disorders, other functional psychoses
   b. Use of drugs and alcohol: tolerance to or withdrawal from CNS stimulants, sustained use of CNS depressants
   c. Sleep-induced respiratory impairment: sleep apnea DOES syndrome, alveolar hypoventilation DOES syndrome
   d. Sleep-related (nocturnal) myoclonus DOES syndrome and/or "restless legs"

   e. Other medical, toxic, and environmental conditions
   f. Other DOES conditions
   g. Intermittent DOES (periodic) syndromes: Kleine-Levin syndrome, menstrual-associated syndrome
   h. Insufficient sleep
   i. Sleep drunkenness
3. Narcolepsy
4. Idiopathic CNS hypersomnolence
5. No DOES abnormality: "short sleeper," subjective DOES complaints without objective findings

DISORDERS OF THE SLEEP-WAKE SCHEDULE

1. Transient: time-zone (jet lag) syndrome, work shift change in conventional sleep-wake schedule
2. Persistent: frequently changing sleep-wake schedule, delayed sleep phase syndrome, advanced sleep phase syndrome, non-24-hour sleep-wake syndrome, irregular sleep-wake pattern

DYSFUNCTIONS ASSOCIATED WITH SLEEP, SLEEP STAGES, OR PARTIAL AROUSALS—PARASOMNIAS OR DISORDERS OF AROUSAL

1. Sleepwalking (somnambulism)
2. Sleep terror (pavor nocturnus, incubus)
3. Sleep-related enuresis
4. Other dysfunctions
   a. Dream anxiety attacks (nightmares)
   b. Familial sleep paralysis
   c. Impaired sleep-related penile tumescence
   d. Sleep-related epileptic seizures, bruxism, head banging (jactatio capitis nocturna), painful erections, cluster headaches and chronic paroxysmal hemicrania, abnormal swallowing syndrome, asthma, cardiovascular symptoms, gastroesophageal reflux, hemolysis (paroxysmal nocturnal hemoglobinuria)
   e. Asymptomatic polysomnographic findings

---

*Adapted from Association of Sleep Disorder Centers and the Association for the Psychophysiological Study of Sleep, the diagnostic classification of sleep and arousal disorders, Sleep 2(1):21, 1979.

He works the night shift, driving a newspaper delivery truck, and then stays awake during the day to care for his chronically ill wife.

3. A downcast young boy leaves the examining room after his mother describes how he must pass up summer camp because of bed-wetting.
4. An executive, whose head is immobilized in halo traction following a neck injury, describes sleeplessness at night, distorted conversations with physicians (probably related to medications), being awakened at night for procedures, and being disturbed by noises and vibrations amplified by the tongs.
5. A woman states that her husband falls asleep readily, even while sitting up in a chair, and that his skin color becomes bluish as he snorts and breathes irregularly.

Sleep problems can be categorized by the disruption in one or more of the aspects of normal sleep. The box on p. 1772 identifies different types of sleep problems. This chapter discusses only the most common types of sleep disorders:

parasomnias or **disorders of arousal** dysfunctions associated with sleep, sleep stages, or arousal
insomnia inability to initiate or maintain sleep
narcolepsy sleep intrusion into wakefulness
sleep apnea sleep problems involving other body systems

The last section of this chapter discusses research into sleep and circadian rhythms and its impact on nurses, both as researchers and as caregivers who must remain awake and alert at night.

PARASOMNIAS OR DISORDERS OF AROUSAL

Various types of parasomnias or disorders of arousal may occur (Table 61-1), especially in children who often outgrow the dysfunction.

SLEEPWALKING

Sleepwalking (*somnambulism*) usually occurs in children, although it may also be seen in adults. Children usually outgrow sleepwalking. It is characterized by sitting up or walking about during sleep. The sleepwalker's eyes are wide open, but the person appears in a daze, has purposeless movements, and may speak in short phrases, with no recollection in the morning. Twenty percent of sonambulists have a sleepwalking parent, and 5% to 15% of the population has sleepwalked at some time. Sleepwalking usually occurs in the first third of the night in stage III/IV sleep. Up to one half of all sleepwalkers either experience injury or narrowly avoid it.

Sleepwalkers should be led back to bed without awakening them. If the sleepwalker must be awakened, do not slap or shake the person or splash cold water on

---

TABLE 61-1 Parasomnias or disorders of arousal

Type of Dysfunction	Comments
Sleepwalking	Walking while asleep
Sleep terror	Panic attack while asleep
Sleep-related enuresis	Bed-wetting; event begins in stage III/IV sleep, and enuresis occurs as sleep lightens
Dream anxiety attacks	Nightmares; REM phenomenon
Sleep-related epileptic seizures	Seizures occur most often during sleep; explains why sleep encouraged during short routine electroencephalograms (EEGs)
Sleep-related bruxism	Teeth grinding; dental assistance may be needed to preserve teeth
Sleep-related head banging (jactatio capitis nocturna)	Rhythmic head rocking and banging common in young children under age 5 years; occurs in stage I/II sleep
Familial sleep paralysis	Inability to move muscles when first awakening
Sleep-related cluster headaches	Associated with REM and relieved by indomethacin
Sleep-related abnormal swallowing syndrome	Inadequate swallowing of saliva during sleep
Sleep-related asthma	Early morning increase in bronchoconstriction; 46% of asthmatic attacks occur during last third of night
Sleep-related cardiovascular symptoms	Include paroxysmal nocturnal dyspnea, myocardial infarction (peak incidence, 4 AM to 6 AM), nocturnal angina, and premature ventricular contractions (more common in REM sleep)
Sleep-related gastroesophageal reflux	Caused more by posture than sleep
Sleep-related hemolysis	Probably related to combination of respiratory acidosis, change in acid-base balance, and renal clearance of defective red blood cells
Morning headaches	May be related to sleeping longer on weekends and delaying usual morning dose of caffeine
Impairment in penile erections	Changes in normal incidence of erections; painful erections

the face, but do say the person's name over and over. If the sleepwalker lies down to sleep on the floor, simply let the person stay there covered until awakening.

Protect the sleepwalker from injury. Place a bell at the bedside that will ring if the bedside is moved, or use a two-way radio in a child's room to awaken the parent when the child stirs. A protective gate or screen door may be placed across the entrance to the bedroom, but note that this blocks escape if there is a fire. Lock windows and doors to balconies. Imipramine, a tricyclic antidepressant, is sometimes prescribed for adult sleepwalkers who walk frequently and have been injured.

SLEEP TERROR

Sleep terror (pavor nocturnus) usually occurs in children during the first part of the night in stage III/IV sleep. The child screams, arises from bed, wanders about in panic, and cannot be awakened or consoled. Autonomic changes (rapid pulse and respirations, sweating) can be noted. The child may be amnestic for the event. Sleep terror is often associated with sleepwalking.

Interventions include planning sleep on a regular schedule. Do not try to awaken the child because this may worsen the confusion. Usually the child will lie back on the pillow after several minutes, never having awakened. Benzodiazepines are sometimes given to patients with severe episodes, because these suppress stage III/IV sleep.

FAMILIAL SLEEP PARALYSIS

The person with familial sleep paralysis appears asleep but maintains consciousness. Occasionally, frighteningly vivid hallucinations may occur. The eyes may be open and can be moved, although the person is unable to move any other muscles. Although this is part of the tetrad of symptoms of narcolepsy, many normal people experience this. Intervention includes teaching family members to awaken the person by touch each day or allowing a pet dog or cat to awaken the person through touch.

PENILE ERECTIONS

Men experience erections during REM sleep regardless of sexual activity or dream content. If impairment of erections occurs during sleep, an underlying illness may be present, such as diabetes mellitus, or it may result from the effect of medications. *Painful erections* may occur during sleep, even though erections are not painful or difficult while awake. There may be a problem with the foreskin in uncircumcised men or a problem with the penile blood vessels. The man should be referred to a urologist for evaluation.

INSOMNIA

EPIDEMIOLOGY AND ETIOLOGY

Insomnia is the difficulty with initiating or maintaining sleep. Epidemiologic studies estimate the number of Americans experiencing insomnia to be in the millions. Insomnia is experienced by adults and children and affects males and females equally.

Insomnia can be caused by various factors:
1. Transient situations of emotional upset (such as loss of a job) or family needs (such as a child's illness)
2. Adoption of nonfunctional sleep habits
3. Psychiatric disorders, such as depression or psychoses
4. Use of drugs or alcohol
5. Respiratory impairment (see later section on sleep apnea)
6. Medical conditions associated with pain, anemia, fever, changes in nutritional status, or immobility
7. Attempting to sleep in nonconducive environmental conditions

It is important to remember that in many instances persons experience altered sleep patterns when the actual cause of the sleep changes may have been resolved long ago. For example, a woman may describe that she habitually arose at 5 AM to nurse her baby, and now several years later, she still awakens at that time and cannot go back to sleep. Another person may report inability to sleep following great anxiety associated with a job loss that has persisted, although the person has now been happily employed for several years.

PREVENTION

Prevention involves teaching persons and families about normal sleep and counseling them to be aware of events and activities that can enhance or detract from sleep. Often persons take steps to remedy a sleep problem, such as taking sleeping pills, taking naps, or drinking alcohol, which only exacerbate sleeping problems. Nurses must also teach persons that it is never too late to begin dealing with a sleep problem.

PATHOPHYSIOLOGY

Sleep onset can be delayed and arousal prolonged by active thought and worry, physical discomfort, or poor oxygenation. Worry and poor habits, such as sleeping with lights or a TV/radio on, prolong sleep onset and cause arousals during light stage I sleep. Staying in bed longer than 8 hours or napping during the day fragments sleep; the person still sleeps 8 hours, but the total sleep time lengthens to fill 10 hours spent in bed. The person then believes the sleep is "poor."

Normally there is a clear boundary between and regular timing of sleep time and awake time. Meals and social and physical activities occur at predictable times during awake hours, and sleep occurs at night in a dark, quiet, comfortable, secure place. Biologic clocks are anchored in time by the regular occurrence of these events. For the person with insomnia, the distinction between waking/sleeping time is blurred by spending a prolonged time in bed, by not initiating the day's activities at a prompt time, or by staying up too late at night. These events cause a distortion in sleep and lead to a continuing cycle of poor sleep at the wrong time.

CLINICAL MANIFESTATIONS

The person may describe insomnia in many ways, depending on which aspect of sleeplessness is most troubling. Typical comments include: "I cannot go to sleep," "I am awake all night," and "I awaken early and can't go back to sleep." Persons with insomnia often monitor sleep by watching the clock. They may turn on the TV, read, or eat while waiting to feel sleepy. They may try to go to sleep earlier, stay in bed longer, take naps, use sleeping pills or alcohol to initiate sleep, or use caffeine to increase alertness during the day. They may also change their pattern of daily activities to compensate for a distorted sleep pattern by declining or omitting activities from the daily routine, saying "I'm just too tired." Some persons may not recognize a sleep problem at first because they have adapted to a changed sleep schedule over many years.

DIAGNOSTIC TESTS

Routine blood work, such as a SMA 18 and complete blood count (CBC), is done to determine if any hematologic, metabolic, cardiac, or respiratory diseases are contributing to sleeplessness. A thorough assessment, including questions to elicit signs of underlying depression or psychosis, should be done.

A *polysomnogram* (PSG) consists of an all-night sleep study conducted in a certified sleep laboratory. Sleep technicians monitor the following:
1. Sleep time and quality
2. Brain EEG activity to determine stages of sleep
3. Respiratory activity: intercostal muscle movement, air passage from nose and mouth, oxygen saturation using an ear lobe oxymeter
4. Electrocardiogram (ECG) for monitoring cardiac rate
5. Electromyogram (EMG) monitoring of leg movement to detect abnormal movement of eye and face (to determine onset of REM sleep)
6. Occurrence of nightmares or "restless legs"

The PSG is performed when the person complains of insomnia and the physician is unable to make the diagnosis from a history and physical examination.

The *multiple sleep latency test* (MSLT) is a sleep study done in the sleep laboratory during the day to measure daytime sleepiness. At times it is needed to distinguish the sleepiness caused by poor nighttime sleep and sleepiness caused by narcolepsy.

MEDICAL MANAGEMENT

If the person has used sleeping pills or alcohol to help with sleep, supervised weaning from these substances is required. A schedule of reducing the dose of sleeping pills over a month or more, or a course of chlordiazepoxide hydrochloride (Librium) to assist with alcohol withdrawal, may be prescribed.

■ ASSESSMENT

A complete nursing assessment of sleep disorders is listed in the box on p. 1776. Never jump to a conclusion about a sleep problem without asking systematic questions about all sleep disorders, because one sleep problem can resemble another superficially. Keep in mind that many times insomnia begins as an understandable response to a stress, such as the loss of a spouse, illness of a family member, or after a difficult hospitalization. The person may come to terms with the stress or loss, but the new maladaptive sleep habits are now in place. The person may state that the sleep pattern began 5 years ago and that nothing is bothering him or her now to prevent sleep. This makes sense when one views insomnia as a series of decisions that *perpetuate* a certain sleep pattern, unfortunately a pattern that distresses instead of refreshes. The following data are important to highlight for a person with insomnia.

SUBJECTIVE DATA

1. Beliefs about the sleep problems and ability to sleep restfully. Some people believe that they have inherited or developed a permanent mental change or disorder that will prevent regaining normal sleep.
2. Knowledge about normal sleep.
3. Sources of pleasure and difficulty in the person's life and how the sleep problem has been affected by these.
4. Potential resources for life changes. For example, if a retired person has nothing to wake up for, can that person find transport to a senior citizens center, volunteer job, or activity group?

OBJECTIVE DATA

Objective data include results from diagnostic tests and reports from a bed partner. A person may be asked to keep a sleep diary, recording times of sleep initiation, arousals, naps, and time of awakening in morning.

SLEEP INTERVIEW

GENERAL DATA

1. Statement of the sleep problem by patient, bed partner, or family: obtain a quantifiable answer regarding sleep, such as never sleeps, dozes off for an hour several times a night, or has trouble sleeping five nights out of seven, every other night, or on weekends only
2. Initiation of sleep problem: when possible, elicit cause
3. Factors that make it worse or better
4. Previous occurrences to patient or to other family member or friend
5. Modifications that needed to be made for daytime activities or travel
6. Occurrences of frightening or upsetting incidences during sleep, such as sudden illness or death of a loved one or damage from storm, fire, or robbery
7. Occurrences of accidents or "near misses" as a result of sleep problems (*very important*)

INSOMNIA DATA

(Remember that a complaint of insomnia may be caused by sleep apnea or other difficulties with sleep.)
1. Time person gets into bed and time person falls asleep
2. Number and times of awakenings at night
3. Interval before returning to sleep after each awakening
4. Time of final awakening, time of arising from bed, and what wakes the person up, such as noises, alarm clock, or treatment
5. Daytime naps: number, when, and how long
6. Dozing off briefly (same question as napping, but some persons answer this question differently)
7. Lying down to rest on couch or "resting eyes for a moment" (this counts as napping because person may be falling asleep)
8. Practices used to assist with sleep: type and regularity of use
9. Changes in sleep patterns because of sleep deficit
10. Places where sleep occurs more readily, such as somewhere else in the house or on vacation
11. Concerns that delay getting into bed or falling asleep
12. Amount of and recent changes in caffeine intake (coffee, tea, colas, other caffeinated beverages, caffeinated gum) and alcohol
13. Types of weekly exercise and recreational activities
14. Measures of coping with concerns
15. Recent illness or loss of relatives, friends, or pets
16. Activities of others in house or neighborhood that affect sleep, such as child who returns home late, spouse who leaves home early in morning, noise from a neighbor or dog, and noise from a nearby highway or airport

SLEEP APNEA DATA

1. Description or reenactment by bed partner of the person's breathing pattern, including sound and volume of snoring, length of time that no air passes, and how the person starts to breathe again

2. Description by bed partner of differences in patient's breathing while on back, each side, and stomach and of changes in patient's skin color while asleep
3. Presence of morning headaches
4. Difficulty in awakening for the day
5. Number of pillows used; preference of sleeping in a certain chair
6. Degree of sleepiness during day; falling asleep at a movie, during a conversation, or while driving

NARCOLEPSY-RELATED DATA

1. Presence of sudden irresistible urges to sleep; falling asleep and then awakening a few minutes later feeling refreshed
2. Experiences of a sudden loss of muscle tone, leading to drooping of the head or slumping to the floor, that occur during episodes of strong emotions (surprise, laughter, anger)
3. Experiences on awakening of feeling paralyzed until touched by another
4. Presence of visual, auditory, or tactile hallucinations at time of sleep initiation or awakening
5. Family history of unusual experiences in sleep

SLEEP SCHEDULE DATA

1. Working hours
2. Experience of going to bed later each night
3. Daily scheduled activities, flexibility
4. Changes in sleep schedule as a result of changes in life schedule, such as retirement or hospitalization
5. Interruption of sleep because of family activities
6. Practice of sleeping through the day or staying up at night because of a specific purpose, such as fear that a calamity will befall during the night

OTHER SLEEP-RELATED EVENTS

1. Uncomfortable feelings in legs when ready to fall asleep: location, type of sensations, duration, actions that make it better or worse, attempted remedies, and effect on sleep
2. Reports from bed partner of patient kicking or moving legs in sleep
3. Bed-wetting: frequency, time of occurrence, actions that make it better or worse, and reports of any nights of dryness
4. Dreams: upsetting recurring dreams, frightening nightmares, or sleep terrors
5. Sleepwalking: initiation, frequency, ability to be awakened easily or guided back to bed, experience of injury while sleepwalking, actions that make it better or worse, and steps taken to keep the person safe
6. Teeth grinding during sleep
7. Dysfunctions associated with sleep, such as chest pain, shortness of breath, heartburn/ulcer pain, morning headache, asthmatic attacks, frequent awakenings to urinate, hot flashes in menopausal woman, coughing, choking and gagging, and arthritic or other neuromuscular pain

■ DATA ANALYSIS: NURSING DIAGNOSES

Nursing diagnoses are determined from assessment of patient data. Possible nursing diagnoses for the person with insomnia may include, but are not limited to, the following:

Diagnostic Title	Possible Etiologies
Coping, ineffective individual	Habit of seeking sleep to avoid facing problems or of reviewing problems at sleep initiation
Diversional activity deficit	Immobility, depressed feelings, perceived loss of usefulness or of need for activity
Fatigue	Reduced total sleep time
Fear	Personal concern about impossibility of ever sleeping well again
Injury, potential for	Sleepiness during the day
Knowledge deficit about insomnia	Incorrect self-monitoring and self-assessment of sleep
Sleep pattern disturbance	Adoption of counterproductive sleep habits

■ PLANNING: EXPECTED PATIENT OUTCOMES

Expected patient outcomes for the person with insomnia may include, but are not limited to, the following:

1. Patient/bed partner/family describe the basic aspects of normal sleep, with emphasis on factors that contribute to the person's problem.
2. Patient/family carry out measures to reduce the insomnia.
3. Patient has realistic expectations about the quality of sleep.
4. Patient identifies impediments to activity and develops and implements a plan for increasing diversional activity.
5. Patient participates in a plan to problem solve and cope with difficulties; patient does not think about problems at time of sleep.

■ IMPLEMENTATION

PROMOTING KNOWLEDGE OF NORMAL SLEEP

Teach aspects of normal sleep to patient and family. Persons typically monitor their own sleep. This can contribute to the sleep problem because the person may mistake a normal phenomenon for something abnormal or for a sign that the new sleep habits are not working.

PROMOTING SLEEP HYGIENE

A person with insomnia will benefit most from a reordering of sleep habits. Develop a plan for sleep hygiene with the patient and inform the physician of the plan, as appropriate. Physician advice may be required if intake patterns of alcohol, other drugs, or caffeine need to be changed. Patients must recognize that they must ad-

here to the plan faithfully every day, no matter what occurs. They are resetting their sleep-wake cycle, which takes several weeks to a month to accomplish. In developing the plan, choose from the elements listed here those that apply to the individual's sleep hygiene problem. Not all elements are appropriate for each person. The plan has three important parts: (1) what the person does during the day (use of time, naps, eating and drinking, exercise, diversion), (2) what the person does to prepare for sleep, and (3) how the person interprets his or her sleep experience.

The plan is to be followed faithfully for 1 month. If sleep is improved, adjustments can be made for one element at a time, such as resuming a reduced intake of alcohol or caffeine. Once the sleep pattern is established, however, only one element should be modified at a time. If the sleep pattern is weakened, the person can identify an element to which he or she is sensitive. Check with the person weekly to identify how the new plan is proceeding. Be generous with encouragement. Remember that a new way of sleeping is being taught to the person who is still partly convinced that he or she is one of the few persons in the world who never sleeps.

Time Spent in Bed, Sleep, and Wake-up Hours

The person, in collaboration with the health professional, selects a sleep time and a wake-up time for a total time spent in bed of 7 to 8 hours, depending on how much sleep the patient thinks is needed. Ask what constraints the person has, such as time to get up for work or time arriving home from evening work, and what time the person likes to go to bed, based on time spent with family members or favorite late-night TV shows. The bed time and wake-up time should be followed faithfully, without alteration, for 1 month, so planning ahead for life-style preferences is important. This means the person will follow this schedule even if he or she is out late on Saturday nights or wants to sleep in on Sunday mornings. If the person does not sleep well one night, the schedule must be kept because it is an investment in a better night's sleep the next night.

Napping

No naps should be taken. This means not lying down during the day and not closing the eyes while sitting in the chair after dinner. If the person gets sleepy reading the paper, the paper should be read while standing up at the counter. If the person is tired an hour before the agreed-on sleep time, he or she should walk around, engage in an activity, or stand up while watching TV. This gives the body a firm message that all sleep will take place in bed during the nighttime hours only. Taking naps at other times fragments nighttime sleep. If, in following the schedule, the person does not sleep much the night before, taking a nap only hinders the possibility that sleep will come more easily the next night, which perpetuates the problem.

Caffeine and Alcohol

The best and fastest change in sleep quality comes from the elimination of caffeine and alcohol from the diet during the start of this plan. However, persons who drink a lot of caffeine or even one alcoholic drink each day could experience withdrawal symptoms, so it is best to work with the physician on a safe plan for withdrawal. Also, the strength of this plan is to help the person experience improved sleep without experiencing uncomfortable symptoms that might lead the person to resume the previous, more comfortable patterns.

Nutrition

It is important to eat three meals a day comprised of balanced nutrition at about the same time each day. On awakening in the morning, the person should wash, dress, and have some breakfast to give the body yet another message that it is time for the day to start. Breakfast may be large or simply toast and juice; the point is to give a regular nutritional time cue.

Exercise

Increasing activity gives the body another biologic message that the day is here. Even if the person is confined to bed, exercises can be developed to enhance a feeling of well-being. For persons who experience tension, stress, or worry or who face difficult problems, exercise can bring a respite from troubling thoughts or can be a time for thinking through problems instead of at bedtime. Any exercise, from active sports to walking to stationary exercise, is encouraged.

Diversion

It is important for the person to do something each day that brings enjoyment. It is equally important to have both something in life a person can look forward to and something that requires a person's special participation, a feeling of being needed. A person facing a continuing illness often experiences a curtailing of usual outlets for diversion and participation. Remember that what a person does with time during the day influences sleep time as well. An important part of a plan for better sleep is life-participating activity. Even if the person is confined to bed, a telephone is a link with others who could use the person's support and good will.

Sleep Environment

Evening routines, such as checking door locks or letting the dog out, should be completed before the predetermined bedtime. By bedtime the person should be in night clothes and ready to get into bed. The bed covers should provide the proper comfort. Lights, TV, and radio should be off. The person should not read or eat in bed. Persons can be advised to turn the clock around so it cannot be checked during the night. The person needs to understand that awakening during the night is normal and sleep activity does not need to be monitored.

Relaxation

The final component of a sleep plan is the relearning of skills of relaxing when the person wants to go to sleep. A person can easily adopt the habit of postponing thoughts about troubling issues until in bed with the lights off. This is a habit and can be replaced by a more useful habit. A person cannot lie in bed "thinking about nothing" because the mind simply searches for something interesting to think about and usually selects some unfinished, compelling issues. Relaxation exercises can help persons regain and strengthen the ability to select something enjoyable to think about. If the person consciously selects something pleasant, the tendency to ruminate over troubles is weakened. Relaxation exercises must be practiced each night. If the person has difficulty mastering this task, a referral to a behavioral therapist may be appropriate.

PROMOTING REALISTIC EXPECTATIONS OF SLEEP

Reinforce that it is not realistic for the person to expect every night of sleep to be free of awakenings or disturbing thoughts and to be totally refreshing. The goal of the plan is to increase the number of nights that are restful. If sleep patterns unravel sometime in the future, the person now has the tools to get back on track.

NARCOLEPSY

Narcolepsy is a neurologic condition characterized by short, irresistible episodes of sleep intruding into wakefulness and recurring at frequent intervals. Five abnormal sleep features may be present: (1) irresistible sleep attacks with excessive daytime sleepiness, (2) hypnogogic hallucinations, (3) cataplexy, (4) sleep-onset REM periods, and (5) sleep paralysis. Any combination of the five features can be seen in narcolepsy, but at least two must be present to make a diagnosis.

EPIDEMIOLOGY

Narcolepsy is not a rare condition. Its prevalence has been estimated at 0.05% to 0.06%, which indicates that about one of every 2500 people have this disorder. Males are somewhat more affected than females. The age of onset varies from childhood to the 50s, with a peak incidence in the second decade of life, usually after puberty. Unrecognized and untreated, these irresistible, unwanted sleep attacks can be totally disabling.

They interfere with the concentration required in school or at work and can result in accidents, leading to injury and death.

ETIOLOGY

Two new research findings are fueling greater understanding of narcolepsy. First, several researchers have found a genetic link among persons with narcolepsy in which mild forms tend to cluster in some families, whereas more severe forms cluster in other families.[9] Some aspects of narcolepsy (cataplexy, excessive daytime sleepiness) are genetically transmitted in some breeds of dogs. Second, a genetic link has recently been discovered between narcolepsy and a class II antigen of the major histocompatibility complex known as DR2. Scientists theorize that narcolepsy may be a disease that links the involvement of the immune system and its response to severe psychologic stress with the development of disease in susceptible individuals.[9] This may help to explain the finding that in about one half of persons with narcolepsy, an abrupt change in the sleep/wake schedule and/or a major psychologic stress precede the first symptom.

PREVENTION

As yet, no clear evidence exists concerning the prevention of narcolepsy. More effort is being directed toward the early recognition of the disorder, particularly in relatives of affected family members. If a parent has narcolepsy, there is a 1 in 50 chance that each child will have it.

CHARACTERISTICS

Occasionally a person with normal sleep patterns may experience any one aspect of narcolepsy. The combination of symptoms, however, experienced consistently, sets narcolepsy apart.

IRRESISTIBLE SLEEP ATTACKS AND EXCESSIVE DAYTIME SLEEPINESS

The sleep attacks, unpredictable and lasting a few moments to an hour, occur not only during monotonous sedentary activity, but also during mental or physical stimulation. The person may also feel unpleasantly drowsy throughout the day, resulting in poor performance of tasks.

SLEEP-ONSET REM PERIODS

The normal sleeper passes through several stages of sleep and experiences REM sleep near the end of the 90-minute sleep cycle. In narcolepsy, when sleep occurs during the day in naps or during sleep attacks, the person goes into REM sleep within 5 minutes of going to sleep.

CATAPLEXY

Cataplexy is an abrupt, reversible loss of muscle tone usually brought on by strong emotions such as fright, laughter, anger, or sudden increased stress. Cataplexy can be experienced variously from a feeling of slight weakness to a loss of strength in skeletal muscles to a complete loss of posture. Typically, the jaw sags, the head nods, the arms droop, and the legs buckle. Because attacks can be precipitated by listening to a funny joke or reexperiencing in memory a strongly unpleasant experience, persons suffering from cataplexy often try to restrict their emotional responses to gain some control. *This atonia is similar to the atonia seen during REM sleep.*

HYPNOGOGIC HALLUCINATIONS

This is the experience of vivid, troubling hallucinations, usually on awakening. The hypnogogic hallucinations are usually visual but can be auditory or tactile.

SLEEP PARALYSIS

This frightening experience occurs just before falling asleep or on awakening. Sleepers find that, although they are completely awake, they cannot move the extremities, cannot speak, and may not even be able to breathe deeply. Sleep paralysis terminates spontaneously within several minutes but can be interrupted by being touched by someone. (One person plagued by sleep paralysis trained her dog to come and lick her hand each morning.) Often sleep paralysis is accompanied by hypnogogic hallucinations.

PATHOPHYSIOLOGY
LOSS OF ABILITY TO SUPPRESS SLEEP

Normally the thalamus and cortical gray matter are highly active in wakefulness, resulting in general enhanced excitability of neurons as well as selective inhibition of input. In drowsiness, reduction of synaptic transmissions occurs in the thalamus, despite an unchanged level of sensory input. It is unknown exactly what neurotransmitters and synaptic receptors relate to maintenance of alertness and initiation of sleep. Interestingly, the activity of the gray matter and thalamus in REM sleep closely resembles waking activity.

It is also unknown what neuronal changes occur with narcolepsy. Because this condition responds to stimulant drugs such as amphetamine, pemoline, and methylphenidate, however, it is hypothesized that some ratio of adrenergic/cholinergic neuronal activity is disrupted in sleep attacks and restored by these drugs.

EPISODIC ATONIA

Normally, muscle tone is maintained during wakefulness and during all sleep stages *except REM* by activity in the cerebellum. In REM sleep, centers in the pons activate, producing active inhibition of muscle tone in all muscle groups except those of the eye, respiration, and penis. Usually this atonia is briefly interrupted or overcome by powerful excitatory inputs to muscle groups, resulting in the muscle twitches and jerks seen in REM sleep.

In cataplexy, sudden time-limited atonia is experienced, although no change occurs in consciousness. Because this disorder responds to monoamine oxidase (MAO) inhibitors and other tricyclic antidepressants, it is theorized that cataplectic attacks (as well as sleep paralysis and hypnogogic hallucinations) result from some malfunction of norepinephrine, dopamine, and serotonin neurotransmitters or receptors in the brainstem.

ASPECTS OF DREAMING INTRUDING INTO WAKEFULNESS

Dreaming usually occurs in REM sleep. REM sleep occurs at the end of each 90-minute sleep cycle, and longer periods of REM sleep occur at the end of the night. On awakening, all features of REM sleep (atonia and resulting paralysis of all muscle groups except those for breathing and sight; dreaming) terminate. Less is known about the mechanisms of dreaming intruding into wakefulness. As just noted, however, because the person with narcolepsy responds to tricyclic antidepressants and MAO inhibitors, a disorder of neurotransmitters or receptors may exist somewhere in the brain.

CLINICAL MANIFESTATIONS

The person with narcolepsy feels chronically drowsy, exhibits memory lapses and poor work performance, and may experience *microsleeps*, sleep periods of a few seconds that may appear as daydreaming. Night sleep can be frequently interrupted by frightening dreams and awakenings. Cataplexy may develop as long as 20 years after the more common symptom of sleep attacks and excessive daytime drowsiness. The paralysis may last from a few seconds to a few minutes. No known measures can terminate an attack, except to remove the emotional trigger so that another attack will not immediately follow recovery from the first.

DIAGNOSTIC TESTS

The PSG and MSLT (see p. 1775) are the essential tests to distinguish narcolepsy from daytime sleepiness experienced by someone who simply sleeps poorly at night. The night sleep test (PSG) documents the night aspects of sleep. The MSLT, performed the following day, documents how readily the person falls asleep during a half-hour nap (four naps are observed during the next 8 hours after awakening from the PSG) and how quickly REM sleep occurs with each nap. A *normal* person may have one sleep-onset REM episode out of four naps and

may not be able to fall asleep for all the nap periods. A *sleepy* person may be able to fall asleep each time but does not have more than one sleep-onset REM period. A *narcoleptic* person falls asleep readily during each nap period and has more than one sleep-onset REM period. The physician may try to record a cataplectic attack if the patient reports a history of this with particular stressors.

MEDICAL MANAGEMENT

The person who has sleep attacks and excessive daytime sleepiness is given CNS stimulants such as amphetamine, pemoline (Cylert), or methylphenidate (Ritalin). Some side effects, such as irritability, tachycardia, and nocturnal sleep disturbances, as well as tolerance and drug dependence, may occur. Persons experiencing cataplexy, sleep paralysis, or hypnogogic hallucinations receive a tricyclic antidepressant. Doses are usually adjusted to achieve the best balance between improved daytime alertness and unwanted side effects. An experimental drug, gamma-hydroxybutyrate, shows some promise.

Daytime naps may also be prescribed to assist with daytime alertness. Three 15- to 20-minute naps spaced evenly throughout the day often help restore a feeling of alertness.

■ ASSESSMENT

A complete sleep history (see p. 1776) is obtained from the person suspected of having narcolepsy. Data of particular importance include the following:

1. Understanding of narcolepsy and factors that increase or decrease symptoms
2. Experience with antinarcoleptic drugs and side effects (Are the drugs taken on holidays? Are doses self-adjusted?)
3. Safety practices and accident history, especially if the person drives
4. Family understanding and support
5. Problems and adjustments in employment or school performance

■ DATA ANALYSIS: NURSING DIAGNOSES

Nursing diagnoses are determined from assessment of patient data. Possible nursing diagnoses for the person with narcolepsy may include, but are not limited to, the following:

Diagnostic Title	Possible Etiologies
Coping, ineffective individual	Purposeful emotional restriction and day-to-day difficulties
Fatigue	Excessive daytime sleepiness Difficulty with treatment regimen, misunderstanding by family and employer or teacher

Diagnostic Title	Possible Etiologies
Injury, potential for	Sleep attacks, cataplexy
Knowledge deficit about narcolepsy	Lack of information

■ PLANNING: EXPECTED PATIENT OUTCOMES

Expected patient outcomes for the person with narcolepsy may include, but are not limited to, the following:

1. Patient identifies purposeful avoidance of strong emotions to cope with cataleptic attacks.
2. Patient describes a level of participation that satisfies family and work responsibilities.
3. Patient reports feeling less fatigue.
4. Patient reports improved job or school performance.
5. Patient demonstrates effective strategies for reducing exposure to risk factors in the environment; avoidable accidents and injuries do not occur.
6. Patient describes the disorder and medication regimen and reports success with explaining narcolepsy to family or employer (or enlists the assistance of a person knowledgeable about narcolepsy).

■ IMPLEMENTATION

The major nursing strategies for the person with narcolepsy are teaching and support with effective ways of coping with the disorder. As control of sleepiness and cataleptic attacks is achieved, fatigue and job or school performance should improve and the potential for injury will decrease.

PROMOTING UNDERSTANDING OF NARCOLEPSY

Teach aspects of narcolepsy and rationale for the treatment plan. It is important that the person maintain close contact with the physician and nurse to monitor effectiveness of medications and treatment. Telephone follow-up may be used to maintain contact and support. Encourage the person and family to contact the American Narcolepsy Association,* which can provide information on local support networks. The association's newsletter contains up-to-date information on recent research findings and provides a forum for sharing ideas.

Assess and support the person's efforts to teach others about narcolepsy. Remind the person that it may take some practice before acquiring ease in teaching others.

PROMOTING SAFETY AND PERSONAL RISK ASSESSMENT

Teach the patient to consider carefully the risks of injury at home and at school or work. Rather than engage

_____

*PO Box 1187, San Carlos, CA 94070, 800-222-6085 (in California, 800-222-6086).

in denial or wishful thinking, the patient should consider problems caused by sleep attacks and cataleptic attacks. Some suggestions include the following:

1. Do not drive unless sleep attacks and cataleptic attacks are completely under control; then drive only for short distances.
2. Do food preparation or self-grooming activities (handling knives, curling or clothes iron; cooking on stove) during quiet times (such as before others in the house awaken) to avoid times of surprise or emotion that can trigger an attack.
3. Learn to use the microwave oven for cooking to avoid burns from the stove.
4. If possible, live in a dwelling that has either no stairs or an enclosed staircase to minimize injury during falls.
5. Ask family members/co-workers to use a gentle aural signal before approaching to prevent triggering a sleep attack.

PROMOTING PARTICIPATION IN FAMILY LIFE AND WORK

Encourage the person to meet with other persons with narcolepsy for mutual support or with the nurse in times of frustration as well as success. Suggest that family members join a local narcolepsy support group to help deal with their own concerns. Narcolepsy can be a very difficult disorder to live with, but personal isolation and withdrawal will only make life more difficult.

SLEEP APNEA

Sleep apnea is a sleep problem involving other body systems. A mutual relationship exists between sleep and other body systems; the sleep state affects the functioning of *all* body systems to some extent. In addition, the functioning of *any* body system affects the states of sleep. Many disease processes affect sleep or are affected by sleep, including asthma, gastroesophageal reflux, epilepsy, headache, fibrositis, myocardial instability, and chronic pain. This section focuses on sleep apnea and the mutual relationship between body systems and sleep.

ETIOLOGY

The gradual development of sleep apnea and its sequelae is incompletely understood. Although such factors as obesity and oropharyngeal architecture have been associated with this disorder, other neurologic and genetic factors may play a role even before any symptoms develop. Some researchers hypothesize that sleep apnea is a progressive illness resulting as a systemic response to years of decreased airway patency, reduced airflow, reduced ventilation,[9] stimulation of autonomic functioning, and disruption of reflexes required to maintain breathing during sleep. This produces a maladaptive response that results in a feedback loop of greater impairment.

Many unanswered questions remain concerning sleep apnea, including the following:

1. How much time does it take for sleep apnea syndrome to develop or for cardiac rhythm changes and hypertension to become severe?
2. How many sleepers who snore quietly and sporadically early in life will subsequently develop sleep apnea?
3. How can one predict who will develop milder or more severe forms of sleep apnea?

PREVENTION

Because sleep apnea is not yet fully understood, steps to prevent its development are not completely known. In addition to encouraging normal weight and good pulmonary habits, it is advisable not to overlook or discount any reported symptoms of sleep apnea.

PATHOPHYSIOLOGY

While reading the following discussion of normal and abnormal breathing during sleep, remember the following major points:

1. The understanding of breathing during sleep centers on the complex interrelationships and feedback loops between the neurologic and respiratory systems. These interrelationships have significant impact on the cardiovascular system and on sleep itself.
2. The two primary results of severely impaired breathing during sleep are (a) cardiac dysrhythmia, which can result in increased risk of cardiac fibrillation and death, and (b) excessive daytime sleepiness or reduction of daytime alertness, which can result in increased risk of accident, such as falling asleep while driving.

CONTROL OF BREATHING

Breathing is initiated by the respiratory center in the medulla. Breathing responds to body requirements through input from three sources: chemoreceptors in the carotid body, stretch/mechanical receptors located in the lung and chest wall, and input from other brain centers (see Chapter 31). In wakefulness, breathing is modified by conscious effort. In sleep, breathing patterns show clear differences between stage I, deeper, and REM (dreaming) sleep, indicating that brain centers controlling sleep have a direct impact on breathing centers as well. In persons with sleep apnea, chemoreceptor responsiveness is reduced, possibly as a result of years of decreased oxygen saturation and increased carbon dioxide levels during sleep. It is not known if ventilatory compensation for resistive loading (stretch receptor responsiveness) is maintained in sleep. During sleep

apnea, when many arousals occur in the night, the person becomes sleepier, leading to decreased arousability and longer apneas.

OPEN PASSAGEWAY TO LUNGS

The pharynx is the only nonrigid structure in the passageway to the lungs. The diameter is maintained by toned muscle in pharyngeal walls, allowing for closure only during swallowing, regurgitation, and speech. In non-REM sleep, this muscle tone is reduced; in REM sleep, it is greatly reduced. Only intercostal, diaphragmatic, and ocular muscles maintain tone in REM sleep. Some sleep experts theorize that the evidence of diminished upper airway tone with maintenance of diaphragmatic and intercostal muscle tone suggests separate neural control of these respiratory muscle groups.[9] The oropharynx of persons with sleep apnea may be anatomically small or may contain enlarged structures, or it may once have been large enough but now has a reduced diameter because of fat deposition in tissues.

RESPONSE TO INTERNAL/EXTERNAL STIMULI

Breathing also depends on responsiveness to changed internal and external stimuli. In sleep, responsiveness to the following factors is reduced:

1. *Bronchial irritation.* Cough is reduced in REM and non-REM sleep and resumes only on arousal.
2. *Isocapnic hypoxia.* Partial oxygen pressure (P_{O2}) may fall as low as 70% of normal before sleepers are aroused. In REM sleep, arousal threshold if further reduced.
3. *Hypercapnia.* Most sleepers awaken before partial carbon dioxide pressure (P_{CO2}) rises by 15 mm Hg above wakefulness level. In REM sleep, arousal is further reduced.
4. *Alcohol and CNS depressants.* During sleep, these substances suppress upper airway tone as well as arousal by medulla and higher cortical centers.

Responsiveness to all these factors is depressed further in a person whose sleep has been so fragmented as to lead to further depressed arousal thresholds. Moderate degrees of alcohol intoxication can decrease hypoxic and hypercapnic ventilatory responses to 50% of baseline values. Oxygen saturation less than 80% of normal is considered severe.

APNEAS/HYPOPNEAS

Different types of apneas occur (see box on p. 1783 for definitions). Normal sleepers experience a few apneas/hypopneas each night; the apneas may be obstructive, central, or mixed. These apneas are fewer and shorter in duration than those in sleep apnea syndrome. The normal sleeper has a transient drop in oxygen saturation, transient bradycardia or tachycardia, and a transient rise in blood pressure; all return to normal levels

DEFINITIONS OF APNEA/HYPOPNEA

Apnea	Cessation of breathing for more than 10 seconds.
Hypopnea	Reduction, rather than complete elimination, of breathing.
Obstructive apnea	Breathing effort occurs with diaphragmatic and intercostal muscles, but no air passes through the mouth and nose. The pharynx collapses, producing obstruction.
Central apnea	No breathing effort is expended by thoracic muscles (message to breathe not received by lungs from medulla).
Mixed apnea	Begins as an absence of respiratory effort; when effort begins, however, obstruction results.
Sleep apnea syndrome	More than five apneic events per hour of sleep.

when the apnea episode is over. The person with sleep apnea syndrome has decreased oxygen saturation (less than 80%) through the night that results in (1) maladaptive cardiovascular responses, (2) disrupted sleep, and (3) other difficulties, including morning headache, bed-wetting, and changes in mood, alertness, endurance, work performance, and intellectual and sexual functioning. The most serious life-threatening results are hypertension, cardiac dysrhythmias (bradycardia, tachycardia, premature ventricular contractions, second-degree atrioventricular block, prolonged sinus pauses, atrial fibrillation), and accidents from falling asleep while driving or doing other monotonous tasks.

CLINICAL MANIFESTATIONS

When sleep apnea is suspected, a sleeping partner is interviewed as well as the sleeper. The bed partner may report most or all of the following details:

He falls asleep very easily in the chair or when he goes to bed for the night. Sometimes he is restless and dozes on and off for a while. He may begin snoring as soon as he falls asleep, or it may not start until later in the night. He used to snore only when he fell asleep on his back, but now he snores in any position. He snores very loudly, and you can hear him from other rooms in the house. Sometimes he stops breathing; after several moments, he snorts loudly, shudders or kicks his legs, then takes a deep breath and goes back to sleep. He may answer me if I speak to him, but he doesn't recall it in the morning. He does this all night long, but I think it happens more often in the early morning. He may get up frequently to urinate in the night, and sometimes he perspires heavily from all the moving around in bed. I hate to admit it, but sometimes I have to sleep in another room because the noise and his restlessness keep me awake. Yet, I am worried that he needs me

there to wake him up if he goes too long without breathing. I think *I* am developing a sleep problem.

DIAGNOSTIC TESTS

The PSG (see p. 1775) is the primary test. It should be performed at night because apneic episodes may be more frequent during REM sleep, and a sleeper may not have any REM sleep during afternoon naps. The test may be repeated after the patient undergoes treatment for sleep apnea to determine the degree of response.

Almost routinely the patient is sent for a consulting examination with an otolaryngologist or maxillofacial specialist to determine the extent to which oropharyngeal architecture impacts on the obstructed airway. Pulmonary function tests may also be ordered to detect any underlying contributing factors. The physician may request that much of the pulmonary testing be done with the patient in a supine position.

MEDICAL MANAGEMENT

Medical management of the person with sleep apnea takes a graded approach to match the severity of the problem. For *mild* sleep apnea syndrome, the patient is advised to sleep on a side and to lose weight if obese. In addition, the patient should avoid all sleeping medication, CNS depressants, and alcohol. If these approaches do not provide improvement, drug therapy may be instituted. Medroxyprogesterone may be prescribed for those who also hypoventilate while awake. A trial of protriptyline is initiated for obese persons. Patients need to be followed closely because the side effects of the drugs may work against the patient taking them faithfully.

For *moderate* sleep apnea syndrome, an oral surgeon or ear, nose, and throat (ENT) specialist may suggest removal of tonsils or realignment of the bite, either through jaw surgery or use of an appliance during sleep, if specific upper airway obstruction is found. In the absence of obstruction, a nasal *continuous positive airway pressure* (CPAP) system may be recommended. A CPAP system consists of an air pump connected to a mask worn over the nose during sleep. This air pump (to which supplemental oxygen may be added) delivers air to the oropharynx at a pressure sufficient to prevent collapse of the pharynx during sleep. For the first several nights, the CPAP system is worn while the patient sleeps in the laboratory, where sleep technicians adjust the air pressure in the mask to the amount required. When the CPAP system reduces apneic events, the sleeper will experience deeper and longer periods of sleep for the next several nights; arousal to breathe is unnecessary. Because increased REM sleep also means increased time during which the sleeper does not arouse as easily, the person needs to be observed for any difficulties. Wearing the mask takes some personal adjustment; however, most patients experience quick relief from their problems of daytime sleepiness and nighttime symptoms.

When a patient demonstrates pronounced oxygen desaturation or frequent cardiac dysrhythmias (*severe sleep apnea syndrome*), more extreme therapy is recommended. A *uvulopalatopharyngoplasty* (UPPP) may be performed by an ENT surgeon experienced with the treatment of sleep apnea patients. This procedure removes almost all the soft tissue at the back of the mouth to widen the pharynx. The patient must be cautioned, however, that in some people snoring will disappear but apnea can still be present. In addition, during the first 3 days postoperatively, regional edema can occlude the airway. A tracheostomy may be required to prevent sudden death. It may take a week to 10 days for the patient to swallow comfortably again. Special attention must be given to the obese person so that the airway will not occlude with supine sleeping postures.

■ ASSESSMENT
SUBJECTIVE DATA

The following subjective data should be assessed:
1. The patient's and family's understanding of the cause of the sleep apnea and the possible risks to health and life
2. Understanding of the cardiac and respiratory system
3. Awareness of contributing factors of weight and alcohol intake
4. Sleep history, including use of sleeping pills; use of stimulants; and work, hobby, and accident history
5. Understanding of possible courses of action
6. Assessment of any emotional, social, or economic factors that may contribute to reluctance of patient and family to take part in treatment

OBJECTIVE DATA

The following data should be assessed:
1. Blood pressure, respiratory assessment (including breath sounds, chest movement, presence of any thoracic deformities), degree of obesity, oropharyngeal assessment, level of awareness, skin color
2. Results of CBC, pulmonary, cardiac, and sleep studies
3. Presence of any other health problems

■ DATA ANALYSIS: NURSING DIAGNOSES

Nursing diagnoses are determined from assessment of patient data. Possible nursing diagnoses for the person with sleep apnea include, but are not limited to, the following:

Diagnostic Title	Possible Etiologies
Breathing pattern, ineffective	Airway obstruction or episodic loss of neurologic stimulus to breathe at night
Fatigue	Altered sleep pattern; oxygen desaturation and frequent arousals at night
Injury, potential for	Increased daytime sleepiness, fatigue, reduced vigilance and response time
Knowledge deficit about sleep problem	Lack of information

■ PLANNING: EXPECTED PATIENT OUTCOMES

Expected patient outcomes for the person with sleep apnea may include, but are not limited to, the following:
1. Patient breathes easily at night.
2. Injuries do not occur as a result of daytime sleepiness, fatigue, or decreased awareness.
3. Patient/bed partner/family can describe the effects of sleep apnea.
4. Patient/family carry out a plan to remedy sleep apnea and will describe measures to take if sleep apnea does not respond to treatment.

■ IMPLEMENTATION
PATIENT TEACHING AND COUNSELING

Nursing intervention consists primarily of patient/family teaching and counseling. As sleep apnea decreases with treatment, fatigue and potential for injuries are decreased.

It is important that both patient and bed partner/family understand normal breathing in sleep, the effects of sleep apnea, measures to take to prevent injury, and treatment regimen. Teaching includes the following:
1. Relationship between the pulmonary and cardiac systems
2. How sleep affects breathing
3. How uninterrupted sleep contributes to daytime functioning
4. How sleep apnea contributes to cardiac problems and leads to increased accident risk
5. Restrictions on operating machinery, including appliances and equipment at home, until risk of fatigue-related accident subsides
6. Drug therapy regimen, side effects, expected time to determine efficacy, and who to contact if difficulties occur

The nurse may anticipate that the patient or someone in the family may minimize the seriousness of sleep apnea and may not be totally supportive of the means required to respond to the problem. It takes teaching and support to help a family come to the understanding that "plain old snoring" can indicate a serious health problem. In some sleep laboratories the sleeper is videotaped throughout a night (with consent). If patients or family members doubt the seriousness of the problem, it can be instructive to let them see parts of the tape or sleep record to illustrate how long breathing does not occur or how often during the night the sleeper arouses.

PROMOTING EFFECTIVE TEAM RESPONSE

Successful treatment involves members of separate disciplines providing several modalities of therapy. A satisfactory therapeutic response from the family's point of view often hinges on one team member, such as the nurse, being willing to handle questions and concerns from family and other team members.

Obese patients need to lose weight. Successful participation in weight loss programs requires knowledgeable referral and supportive follow-up by a member of the treatment team. Surgical treatment requires input from many specialists, and patients and families benefit from someone who can handle questions and respond to concerns. A patient placed on CPAP will need information for the insurance company, as well as a 24-hour telephone number to call should problems with equipment occur in the middle of the night.

CLINICAL CHRONOBIOLOGY: THE DEVELOPMENT OF A NEW AREA OF SCIENCE

The study of normal sleep and sleep problems falls within the broader area of inquiry known as *chronobiology,* or the study of biologic activities as they vary or oscillate predictably over time. Sleep is only one of many biologic events that occur at the same time every 24 hours. Other events that have predictable cyclic peaks and troughs every 24 hours include the following:

1. Core body temperature
2. Cell division
3. Production of red blood cells
4. Preferential migration of lymphocytes into spleen from the peripheral circulation
5. Production of hormones, such as cortisol and growth hormone
6. Muscle strength and alertness
7. Mental alertness[11]

Even more interestingly, some of these events are apparently controlled by the action of internal pacemakers that are somewhat insulated from the activity of the environment, whereas other biologic rhythms depend much more on and are driven by environmental cues. For example, some biologic events depend on the person turning out the lights and lapsing into sleep before they begin. Another compelling finding is that under circumstances of environmental change, such as changing time zones during airplane travel, working the night shift, or postponing sleep, some biologic rhythms are affected more than others and some take longer to readjust. Therefore, not only does an individual rhythm lose its pattern transiently, but all rhythms that act on this one rhythm can also become asynchronous.

These findings are pertinent at the clinical level because the biologic rhythms of both patients and caregivers are affected by the patient's hospitalization. Regarding the patient, the following is only a partial list of factors at work when someone is hospitalized:

1. Pain, fatigue, uncertainty, and anxiety
2. Different bed and bedclothes in an unusual sleeping environment
3. Being awakened for procedures, vital signs, or medications
4. Reduced opportunity for exercise
5. Nutrient timing changes or food withheld
6. Medications depressing or accelerating different biologic functions
7. Lights being turned on or off during the sleep time
8. Living in an environmental temperature (too hot or too cold) that is not under patient control

It is not yet known to what degree, if any, a change in environmental conditions affects healing, recovery time, feelings of well-being, or response to treatment. All these environmental factors and more are being studied as they impact sleep, response to treatment, and recovery time. What is most exciting for nursing research is that nurses make clinical decisions about many of these factors (see research box below). Nursing research in the future will contribute to the determination of optimal timing for assessments and treatments and the creation of the chronobiologically most synchronous or most supportive environments for the patient.

Nurses must also remember that their biologic rhythms are also responding to the environment. Ongoing research helps determine optimal designs for shift

RESEARCH

Clapin-French E: Sleep patterns of aged persons in long-term care facilities, J Adv Nurs 11:57-66, 1986.

In this study, 102 elderly residents of three long-term care facilities were interviewed to determine their current sleep patterns and problems and how they compared their current and preadmission patterns. In addition, the researchers compared this information with the quantity and quality of assessments documented by nursing staff at the three facilities. Residents reported that since their admission sleep was disturbed more by every factor except traffic noise. Many reported more napping, increased total sleep time, earlier bedtimes, and greater difficulty falling asleep. All these factors implied decreased satisfaction with sleep and were conceivably an explanation for increased sedative use after admission. The author cites the downward spiral of decreasing daytime alertness and vigor caused by patient's slower metabolism, a result of taking sedatives and hypnotics. This led to less active participation in daily activities and further sleep problems. Nursing assessment of sleep problems by all three staff groups was uneven. This study is a step toward a needed longitudinal study to determine what the nursing staff of a long-term facility can do to improve the sleep, rest, and daytime well-being of its residents. ■

hours and any effects on health or performance during the day, evening, or night shifts.

Florence Nightingale is often pictured with a lamp as she watches over wounded and sick soldiers through the night. No more apt picture could illustrate the growing body of knowledge concerning the interrelationships among biologic rhythms, especially sleep, as they are challenged in illness, modified because of professional commitment, and highlighted by new nursing contributions to this developing research area.

CHAPTER SUMMARY

✔ More than a half million adults have difficulty with sleeping at some time in their lives.

✔ Sleep disorders can be categorized by the type of disruption they cause including the following:
Parasomnia—disorders of arousal
Insomnia—inability to initiate or maintain sleep
Narcolepsy—sleep intrusion into wakefulness that can challenge the pattern of daily living
Sleep apnea—sleep problems that involve other body systems and can be life-threatening

✔ Persons with insomnia must be taught not to take naps, sleeping pills, caffeine, or alcohol because these may exacerbate insomnia.

✔ Nurses need to understand the importance of a sleep schedule in treating sleep disorders.

✔ Problems of initiating or maintaining sleep may continue over many years, even when the precipitating factor has been resolved.

✔ Helping a patient master a problem with insomnia requires education about normal sleep and careful initiation of new sleep practices.

✔ Loud snoring and breathing disturbances in sleep are symptoms of sleep apnea.

QUESTIONS TO CONSIDER

■ Taking into consideration the 90-minute sleep cycle, how could you best time the waking of a patient at night to take his or her vital signs?

■ If a man with newly diagnosed sleep attacks caused by narcolepsy calls and states that his medication is not helping at all, what factors would you consider as you assess the situation?

■ What conversation difficulties might you expect as you assess a 70-year-old man whose spouse of 45 years has just mentioned that his snoring is a little louder than before, "but it's probably nothing"?

■ What steps would you take to coordinate the care of a person having severe obstructive sleep apnea?

REFERENCES AND SELECTED READINGS

1. American Medical Association: Straight talk no-nonsense guide to better sleep, New York, 1984, Random House.
2. *Clapin-French E: Sleep patterns of aged persons in long-term care facilities, J Adv Nurs 11:57-66, 1986.
3. *Czeisler CA, Moore-Ede MC, and Coleman RM: Rotating shift work cycles that disrupt sleep are improved by applying circadian principles, Science 217:460-463, 1982.
4. Czeisler CA et al: Exposure to bright light and darkness to treat physiologic maladaptation to night work, N Eng J Med 322:18,253-1259.
5. Ferber R: Solve your child's sleep problems, New York, 1985, Simon and Schuster.
6. Guilleminault E, editor: Sleeping and waking disorders: indications and techniques, Menlo Park, Calif, 1982, Addison-Wesley Publishing Co, Inc.
7. Guilleminault E, editor: Sleep and its disorders in children, New York, 1987, Raven Press.
8. Kandel ER and Schwartz JH: Principles of neural science, New York, 1981, Elsevier Science Publishing Co Inc.
9. Kryger MH, Roth R, and Dement WB: Principles and practice of sleep medicine, Philadelphia, 1989, WB Saunders Co.
10. Metzler DJ and Finesilver CA: When to worry if your patient can't sleep, RN 53(3):52-57, 1990.
11. Moore-Ede MC, Sultzman FM, and Fuller CA: The clocks that time us: physiology of the circadian timing system, Cambridge, Mass, 1982, Harvard University Press.
12. Parkes JD: Sleep and its disorders, London, 1985, WB Saunders Co.
13. Saunders NA and Sullivan CE: Sleep and breathing. In Lung biology in health and disease, vol 21, New York, 1984, Marcel Dekker, Inc.

*References preceded by an asterisk are particularly well suited for student reading.

CHAPTER 62

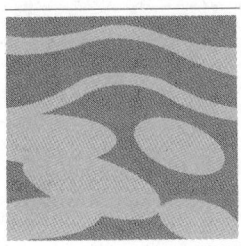

Management of Persons with Common Neurologic Manifestations

ELIZABETH SCHENK

CHAPTER OBJECTIVES

After studying this chapter, the student should be able to:

1 Name at least five causes of headache.
2 Differentiate between migraine, cluster, and tension headaches.
3 List at least six key points in assessing headache.
4 Name at least one nursing intervention for each type of headache discussed.
5 Define the following terms: paresthesia, hyperalgesia, hypoalgesia, analgesia, dysesthesia, referred pain, causalgia, and intractable pain.
6 State at least three nursing interventions to assist the patient with neurologic pain.
7 List at least five symptoms of increased intracranial pressure.
8 Explain the mechanism of increased intracranial pressure.
9 Explain how nursing interventions may decrease intracranial pressure, and give two examples of these interventions.
10 Define the terms *paralysis* and *paresis*.
11 Differentiate between upper motor neuron and lower motor neuron disease.
12 List at least five nursing diagnoses that may occur in the patient with a neurologic disease.
13 Define the term *aphasia,* and describe the difference between sensory, motor, and global aphasia.
14 Define the terms *proprioception, apraxia,* and *agnosia.*

This chapter discusses the care of persons with clinical manifestations resulting from (1) headache, (2) neurologic pain, (3) increased intracranial pressure, (4) alterations in muscle tone and motor function, (5) alterations in movement and posture, (6) alterations in communication, and (7) alterations in sensory and perceptual function.

HEADACHE

EPIDEMIOLOGY/ETIOLOGY

Headache, or head pain, is a common symptom experienced by many persons. As a symptom of an underlying disease, it varies in degree of severity from being relatively unimportant and transient to a very serious prognosis. This symptom clearly originates in many different pathologic processes. The source of recurring headache should be determined through careful physical examination and neurologic testing. Persons have been known to self-treat headache for months in the belief that it was not significant, only to learn later that it was caused by a more serious problem such as a brain tumor or hypertension. Because of the sites of some tumors in the brain, headache may be the only overt symptom for many months.

Headache from a neurologic perspective may have many causes, including:

1. Expanding masses, such as neoplasm
2. Intracranial bleeding
3. Inflammation of the meninges
4. Other infections of the brain and spinal cord
5. Dilation of cerebral vessels
6. Head trauma
7. Cerebral hypoxia
8. Psychologic factors, such as stress
9. Systemic disease of the eye, ear, or sinus

Generally, headaches can be divided into three categories: vascular, tension, and combinations of vascular and tension. This chapter discusses two types of vascular headaches, *migraine* and *cluster,* as well as tension headaches. See Table 62-1 for a comparison of these three types of headaches.

TABLE 62-1 Comparison of migraine, cluster, and tension headaches

Type	Onset	Frequency	Duration	Nature	Prodromal Symptoms/ Associated Symptoms	Treatment
Migraine headaches	Occur at any age Strongly hereditary More common in women than men	Episodic; tend to occur with stress or life crisis	Hours to days	Occur slowly; pain becomes severe, with one side of head affected more than other	Prodromal: vision field defects, confusion, paresthesias Associated: nausea, vomiting, chills, fatigue, irritability, sweating, edema	Ergotamine tartrate Propanolal Nonnarcotic analgesics Relaxation techniques
Cluster headaches	Early adulthood; precipitated by alcohol or nitrates More common in older men	Episodes clustered together in quick succession for few days or weeks with remissions that last for months	Few minutes to few hours	Intense, throbbing, deep, often unilateral pain; begin in infraorbital region and spread to head and neck	Prodromal: uncommon Associated: flushing, tearing of eyes, nasal stuffiness, sweating, swelling of temporal vessels	Narcotic analgesics during acute phase, often intramuscularly
Tension headaches (muscle contraction)	Often in adolescence; related to tension or anxiety No family history	Episodic; vary with stress	Variable; can be constant	Dull, constant, uncommon aggravating pain; vary in intensity; usually bilateral and involve neck and shoulders; pain may be poorly defined	Prodromal: uncommon Associated: sustained contraction of head and neck muscles	Nonnarcotic analgesics Relaxation techniques Amitriptyline (Elavil)

Each type of headache has certain characteristics. For instance, migraine headaches have a high hereditary influence, usually begin in persons between ages 16 and 30 years, and affect more women than men. Cluster headaches, on the other hand, usually begin in early adulthood and occur most often in middle-aged men.

PREVENTION

The key to prevention of headaches is the identification of triggering factors, if these can be found. An ongoing assessment of personality, habits, and activities of daily living (ADL) is helpful. The nurse should help the patient identify what purpose, if any, the headache serves. Internal conflicts and anxiety are frequent causes. Once identified, these causes can be decreased or eliminated. Clues to the source of headaches may be obtained by understanding the person's goals and aspirations, work habits, family relationships, coping mechanisms, and relaxation patterns. The person may be asked to keep a diary of ADL and the occurrence of the headaches, as well as their nature and treatment. Triggering factors that have been identified include fatigue, alcohol ingestion, stress, and hunger. Preventing these can prevent many headaches.

Prevention of migraine headaches may include the avoidance of certain foods, such as chocolate, nuts, and onions. Persons with cluster headaches may need to avoid the ingestion of alcohol.

PATHOPHYSIOLOGY

The pathophysiology of head pain is not fully known. The skull and brain tissues, from a neurophysiologic standpoint, are not capable of sensing pain. Rather, the pain arises from the scalp, its blood vessels, and muscles; from the dura mater and its venous sinuses; and from the blood vessels at the base of the brain. All these structures have pain receptors. Pain most often originates in muscles (face, neck, head), blood vessels, and the dura mater. The blood vessels dilate and become congested with blood extracranially and intracranially. The pain is thought to result from tension on or stretching of these tissues.

With migraine headaches, chemical changes in and around the cranial blood vessels seem to have a causative role.

CLINICAL MANIFESTATIONS
MIGRAINE HEADACHE

Prodromal signs and symptoms (aura) that occur before the acute attack may include the following:

1. Visual field defects
2. Confusion
3. Paresthesias
4. Paralysis in extreme cases

The usual signs and symptoms that occur at the attack are severe and vary in intensity and duration. The pain is usually severe and starts gradually. The headache is often present on awakening, and one side of the head is usually more affected than the other. Pain may be most severe over the temporal area but may occur anywhere in the head, including the face. Signs and symptoms that may occur at the attack, in addition to the pain, include the following:

1. Nausea and/or vomiting
2. Chilliness
3. Fatigue
4. Irritability
5. Diaphoresis
6. Edema
7. Associated autonomic signs
8. Temporary paralysis or paresis as well as aphasia

CLUSTER HEADACHE

In this type of headache, pain episodes are clustered or spaced together in quick succession for a few days or weeks and with relatively long remissions that may last for months. The frequency of the attacks is a unique characteristic. The duration of the pain is usually for a few minutes to a few hours. The pain is often described as very intense, throbbing, and deep. It is abrupt in onset and also stops abruptly. The pain, which is unilateral, most often starts in the face, usually in the infraorbital region, and spreads to the head and neck as it increases. The pain usually reaches its peak in 1 to 3 hours. Prodromal signs are uncommon, but associated signs may include the following:

1. Flushing
2. Lacrimation (tearing)
3. Nasal stuffiness
4. Diaphoresis
5. Swelling of temporal vessels

TENSION HEADACHE

Tension headaches vary in frequency and duration and are related to fatigue and stress. There is no aura. The pain is usually constant, bandlike, and bilateral and involves the occipital region, neck, and shoulders. The headache may be intermittent and transitory or may persist for days, weeks, and months. It may spread to all parts of the head and be poorly defined.

DIAGNOSTIC TESTS

It is important to evaluate severe and chronic headaches. Usual testing includes a neurologic examination, including a computed tomography (CT) scan (see Chapter 59 for description). A lumbar puncture may also be performed, but not if there is evidence of increased intracranial pressure (ICP) or if a brain tumor is suspected, since the quick reduction in pressure produced by removal of the spinal fluid may cause brain herniation.

MEDICAL MANAGEMENT

The medical management of headaches mainly involves prescribing medications appropriate to the particular type of headache (see following section on medications). Patients with chronic headaches may respond to psychotherapy. If the cause of the headache can be determined (for example, if sinus problems exist), appropriate medical care usually alleviates the headache.

■ ASSESSMENT

The collection of both subjective and objective data is important in the diagnosis of headache.

SUBJECTIVE DATA

Subjective data include the following:

1. Patient's understanding of headache and possible causes
2. Awareness of any precipitating factors, such as stress
3. Measures that relieve symptoms, including medications
4. Location, frequency, pattern, and character of head pain, including site of return, time of day, and intervals between headaches
5. Initial onset of headache
6. Presence of any prodromal symptoms
7. Presence of associated symptoms
8. Family history of headaches (especially important with migraine)
9. Situations that worsen headaches

OBJECTIVE DATA

Objective data include the following:

1. Behavior that indicates presence of stress, anxiety, or pain

1. Localized type of head pain is usually associated with migraine headaches or an organic disorder.
2. Generalized headache is usually related to psychologic causes or the presence of increased ICP.
3. Migraine headaches may change from one side of the head to the other.
4. Headaches that occur with increased ICP usually are present on awakening and may awaken the person from sleep.
5. Sinus headaches typically occur early in the morning and increase in intensity as the day progresses.
6. Pain described as dull, nagging, aggravating, and continuous often occurs with psychogenic headaches.
7. Organically caused pain tends to be constant and progressive.
8. Migraine headaches may be associated with menstruation.
9. Sleeping too long, fasting, or inhaling toxic fumes in work situations with inadequate ventilation may cause headaches.
10. Oral contraceptives may exacerbate migraine headaches.

2. Change in ability to carry on normal daily activities
3. Abnormalities found on neurologic examination
4. Elevated temperature or painful flexion of neck (may be present with meningitis)

Other key points to consider in assessing headache are listed in the box above.

■ DATA ANALYSIS: NURSING DIAGNOSES

Nursing diagnoses are determined from assessment of patient data. Possible nursing diagnoses for the person with headache include, but are not limited to, the following:

Diagnostic Title	Possible Etiologies
Coping, ineffective individual	Personal vulnerability
Fatigue	Inadequate rest
Knowledge deficit: cause of headache and needed treatment	Lack of exposure, unfamiliarity with information sources
Pain	Headache
Sleep pattern disturbance	Pain/discomfort

■ PLANNING: EXPECTED PATIENT OUTCOMES

Expected patient outcomes for the person with headache may include, but are not limited to, the following:
1. Headache pain will decrease.
2. Patient will explain prescribed medications.
   a. Dosage, action, side effects, and frequency
   b. Use of drugs as needed when headache recurs
   c. Reason for adequate and early treatment with prescribed drugs

3. Patient will describe the dangers of continuing use of unprescribed drugs for chronic recurring headache.
4. Patient will explain the importance of continued medical supervision for chronic recurring headache, whether the cause is known or unknown.
   a. Plan for follow-up care
   b. Dangers of undiagnosed headache
   c. Recognition of headache as a serious symptom
5. Patient will demonstrate prescribed relaxation techniques.
6. Patient will identify and discuss factors that trigger the headache and will state plans to avoid these factors.
7. Individual coping will be improved.
8. Patient will sleep at least 6 hours at night.

■ IMPLEMENTATION
MEDICATIONS

Treatment for headache often includes the use of selected medications. These are described in terms of their use for persons with migraine, cluster, and tension headaches.

Migraine Headaches

Acetylsalicylic acid (aspirin) may be helpful in the treatment of migraine headaches after the headache has developed. The drug of choice is ergotamine tartrate. If it is taken early in an attack, it may prevent the migraine from developing. The success of this drug in relieving the headache is often considered diagnostic of migraine. This medication acts by constricting cerebral blood vessel walls, thus reducing cerebral blood flow. It is usually administered orally, but it can be given rectally or sublingually in dosages of 2 to 4 mg or by injection in dosages of 0.25 to 0.5 mg. Ergot preparations are also available in combination with other drugs such as caffeine, phenobarbital, and belladonna. Side effects to watch for include nausea, vomiting, numbness and tingling, muscle pain, and changes in heart rate. This drug cannot be taken by pregnant women because it stimulates contraction of uterine smooth muscle.

Other medications that may be prescribed for migraine headaches include the following:
1. Phenacetin
2. Acetaminophen
3. Propoxyphene (Darvon)
4. Narcotics such as codeine
5. Propranolol (Inderal)

Cluster Headaches

Narcotic analgesics are often prescribed during the acute attack. Because the pain is so severe, it may be necessary to give these medications intramuscularly for optimal relief. Patients with cluster headaches usually feel no pain between attacks, so no analgesia is needed during these times.

Tension Headaches

Nonnarcotic analgesics are often prescribed for tension headaches. These include acetaminophen, propoxyphene, phenacetin, and acetylsalicylic acid. It is far better for the patient to learn to control the headaches with other means than to prescribe narcotics or sedatives to control tension and stress.

PROMOTING REST AND RELAXATION

Since tension and stress are triggering factors for headaches, nursing measures for persons with headache include those that facilitate relaxation and rest (see the box below for further details). Relaxation techniques, the use of biofeedback, regular sleeping patterns, and provisions for rest are all important. Regular physical exercise may help the patient relax.

Cold packs applied to the forehead or base of the brain may be helpful in decreasing pain. Some patients describe relief when pressure is applied to the temporal artery area. Patients with migraine headaches also find it more comfortable to be in a darkened room with minimal auditory stimulation.

PATIENT TEACHING

Patient teaching for the person with a headache should include the following:
1. Avoidance of factors found to increase the headache
2. Use of relaxation measures, including biofeedback when appropriate
3. Maintenance of regular sleep patterns
4. Importance of taking medication as prescribed and knowledge of expected action and side effects
5. Importance of follow-up medical care
6. Structuring of home and work environment to keep stressors at a reasonable level

---

GUIDELINES FOR NURSING INTERVENTIONS FOR PERSONS WITH HEADACHE

1. Promote rest and relaxation.
   a. Relaxation techniques, including biofeedback and meditation
   b. Regular sleeping patterns
   c. Provision for rest periods
2. Promote comfort.
   a. Cold packs to forehead or base of head
   b. Pressure applied to temporal artery area
   c. Rest in darkened room with minimal sensory stimulation
   d. Judicious use of medication

7. Importance of allowing others to assist with activities during headaches

NEUROLOGIC PAIN

EPIDEMIOLOGY/ETIOLOGY

Pain other than headache is one of the most common symptoms seen in neurology. It is sometimes difficult to distinguish between pain produced by lesions within the nervous system that cause objective sensory abnormalities and peripherally produced somatic pain in a distant organ. The nurse working with the patient in pain must appreciate the individuality of the pain experience and understand the multiple factors that influence the patient's perception and expression of pain.

The causes of pain are many and varied. Several sources of injury and disease that cause pain are discussed next.

PREVENTION

As with headache, little can be done to prevent neurologic pain unless the actual triggering factors are identified. With other types of pain, however, factors that make it worse can be addressed.

PATHOPHYSIOLOGY

Although in practice pain may be viewed from the standpoint of neural transmissions, the transmission of pain impulses is not fully understood. However, what is known about the neuroanatomy of pain transmission can serve to explain sources of neurologic pain and some of the interventions used (Table 62-2).

Receptors for temperature and touch are adaptable, whereas pain receptors are not. The pain impulses continue at the same rate as long as the stimulus is present. These receptors are considered specific for pain only and are present in layers of the skin, the periosteum, the adrenal walls, and the falx and tentorium of the dura. Factors that can activate pain receptors include the following:
1. Cellular damage
2. Certain chemicals, including histamine
3. Heat
4. Ischemia
5. Muscle spasms
6. Sensations of heat, cold, and itching that go beyond a specific level of intensity

CLINICAL MANIFESTATIONS

The quality of neurologic pain may vary from mild to excruciating. The sources of neurologic pain also vary, as described next.

The pain resulting from peripheral nerve lesions occurs as a direct result of stimulation of the pain receptors. The location and distribution of these pain recep-

TABLE 62-2 Site of problem and resulting neurologic pain

Site of Problem	Results	Characteristics of Pain
Peripheral cutaneous nerves	Pain usually limited to anatomic area supplied by affected nerve or nerves	Often described as burning sensation but may be sharp or dull and aching May be constant or permanent Often described as severe Also called local pain
Root pain	Limited to dermatomes supplied by affected sensory nerve roots (pain from lesion arising from deep somatic and visceral stimuli may radiate beyond dermatomes)	Aggravated by anything that causes direct or indirect movement of spinal cord (sneezing, coughing, or straining)
Central lesion within thalamus	Pain confined to contralateral side of body	Pain described as burning, pulling, and swelling Often aggravated by emotional stress and fatigue
Central spinothalamic tract	Pain sensation distributed to level of tract involved Hemisection of spinal cord produces loss of pain and temperature sensation on contralateral side at a level one or two segments below injury	May be similar to thalamic pain, but less disturbing

tors can be compared with charts showing the distribution of peripheral sensory fibers (Figure 62-1). Table 62-2 describes the site of the problem, the resulting neurologic pain, and the sensations accompanying the pain.

All peripheral nerves are mixed nerves (sensory and motor). Damage to a nerve at its periphery results in loss of both sensation and muscle function. An occasional sequela of peripheral injury is *causalgia*. An attack may arise spontaneously, in response to touch, or even as a result of emotions and stress. The quantity and quality of pain are disproportionate to sensory intake.

Root pain, or *radicular pain,* is limited to the dermatomes supplied by the affected sensory nerve roots (see Figure 62-1). However, pain from lesions arising from deep somatic and visceral structures may radiate beyond the dermatomes. It should be remembered that sensory (posterior) nerve roots are fixed directly to the spinal cord, and lesions in this area may extend to include the motor (anterior) nerve roots and may cause motor signs and symptoms.

Pain resulting from central lesions within the thalamus is confined to the contralateral side of the body, since the thalamus receives sensory pain impulses from the opposite side of the body. In massive thalamic lesions, only contiguous portions of the body may be affected. This type of pain is described as pulling, burning, and swelling.

Lesions that involve the central spinothalamic tract produce pain sensations distributed to the level of the tract involved. Hemisection of the spinal cord involving the spinothalamic tract usually produces loss of pain and temperature perception on the contralateral side at a level one or two segments below the injury. The pain is similar to thalamic pain.

Pain may also be called *referred;* that is, it occurs in a site other than its origin. This often occurs with visceral pain. Perhaps the most common example is chest pain that is referred to the left arm, shoulder, neck, or jaw.

DIAGNOSTIC TESTS

It is extremely difficult to evaluate pain objectively. Electrical stimulation may be used to define the pain to a greater extent. Psychologic testing also may be done as part of the workup. Other tests to rule out the cause of the pain may be helpful. One example is the myelogram, which is often done when the patient has back pain (see Chapter 59).

MEDICAL MANAGEMENT

The medical management for patients with neurologic pain is mainly symptomatic; medications are frequently given. If the source of the problem can be identified, medical or surgical intervention may be possible to cure the source. Psychotherapy may be used as a primary treatment or as an adjunct to palliative treatment.

Unbearable pain that does not respond to the definitive treatment of the causative lesion is classified as *intractable.* The pain is chronic and often disabling. It is usually possible to alleviate intractable pain surgically through deafferentation at varied sites by nerve block, neurectomy, rhizotomy, and cordotomy. Electrical stimulation may also be used. These techniques and the care required when instituted are described in Chapter 16.

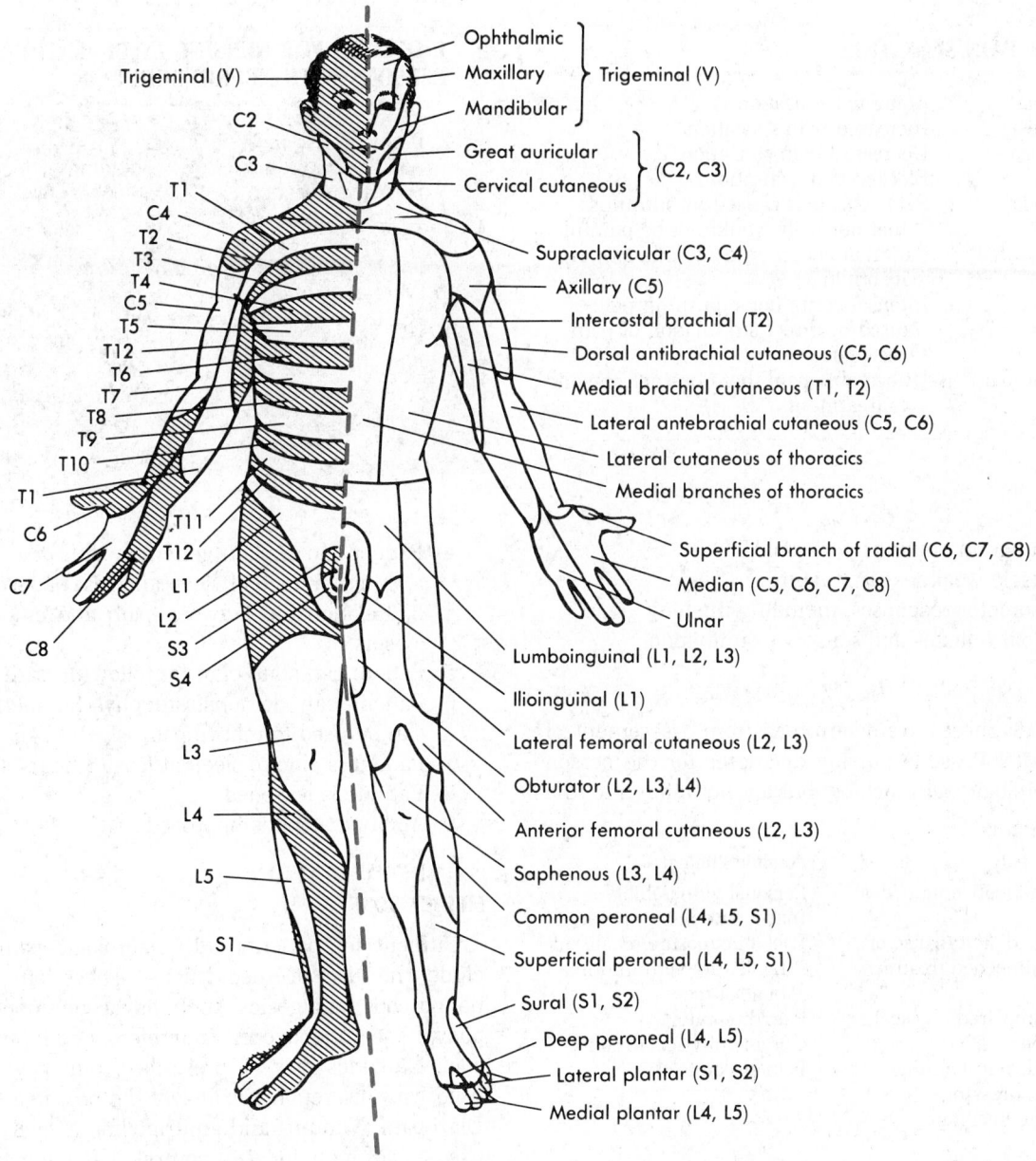

FIGURE 62-1 Peripheral distribution of sensory nerve fibers, anterior view. *Right,* Distribution of cutaneous nerves. *Left,* Dermatomes (*shaded areas*) and segmental distribution of cutaneous nerves.

■ ASSESSMENT

Both subjective and objective data are important to assess in the patient with neurologic pain. Since pain is a highly subjective experience, few objective data may accompany the subjective complaints.

SUBJECTIVE DATA

Subjective data include the following:
1. Patient's understanding of the pain
2. Any precipitating factors

3. Measures that relieve pain, including medication
4. Site, frequency, and nature of pain
5. Usual coping patterns when under stress
6. Presence of associated symptoms
7. Measures that worsen pain
8. Description of the pain (see the box on p. 1794)

OBJECTIVE DATA

Objective data include the following:
1. Behavior, including signs to indicate pain or stress

TYPES OF PAIN SENSATION

Paresthesia	Abnormal sensation
Hyperalgesia	Increased pain sensation
Hypoalgesia	Decreased pain sensation
Analgesia	Blocked pain sensation
Dysesthesia	Pain sensation caused by stimulus that normally would not be painful
Referred pain	Pain that occurs in a site other than its origin
Causalgia	Intense, continuous, burning pain
Local pain	Caused by direct stimulation of pain receptors
Intractable pain	Unbearable pain that does not respond to treatment

2. Change in ability to perform ADL
3. Muscle weakness or wasting
4. Vasomotor responses, including flushing
5. Spinal reflexes and sensory examination

■ DATA ANALYSIS: NURSING DIAGNOSES

Nursing diagnoses are determined from assessment of patient data. Possible nursing diagnoses for the person with neurologic pain include, but are not limited to, the following:

Diagnostic Title	Possible Etiology
Coping, ineffective individual	Personal vulnerability
Fatigue	Inadequate rest
Knowledge deficit: cause of pain and needed treatment	Lack of exposure/recall, unfamiliarity with information sources
Mobility, impaired physical	Pain/discomfort
Pain, chronic	Chronic physical disability
Self-care deficit: bathing/ hygiene, dressing/ grooming, feeding, toileting	Pain/discomfort
Sleep pattern disturbance	Pain/discomfort

■ PLANNING: EXPECTED PATIENT OUTCOMES

Expected patient outcomes for the person with neurologic pain may include, but are not limited to, the following:

1. Pain is decreased.
2. Patient can better carry on activities of daily living.
3. Patient can explain methods to control discomfort or pain.
   a. Prescribed analgesics or alternates as to action, side effects, and dosage schedules
   b. Positioning methods and relationships to occurrences of pain
   c. Advantages and disadvantages of surgical interventions to control pain

GUIDELINES FOR NURSING INTERVENTIONS FOR PERSONS WITH NEUROLOGIC PAIN

1. Promote rest and relaxation.
   a. Relaxation techniques, including biofeedback and meditation
   b. Regular periods of rest
   c. Regular sleeping patterns
   d. Structuring of environment to reduce stress
2. Promote comfort.
   a. Assume position of comfort
   b. Judicious use of medication
3. Promote ADL.
   a. Development of plan to handle ADL
   b. Frequent rest periods interspersed with periods of activity

4. Patient can explain general health practices.
   a. Maintenance of sleep and rest patterns
   b. Relationship between pain and emotional upsets
5. Patient can state plan for follow-up care.
6. Patient can demonstrate physical methods that can be used to relieve pain.
7. Patient is able to sleep at least 6 hours at night.
8. Fatigue is lessened.
9. Ability to cope is improved.

■ IMPLEMENTATION
MEDICATIONS

Treatment for patients with neurologic pain may include the use of medications. These often include nonnarcotic analgesics such as acetaminophen, propoxyphene, phenacetin, ibuprofen, and acetylsalicylic acid. Narcotics may be prescribed, but they should be used with discretion because of the potential for abuse. Diazepam (Valium) and amitriptyline (Elavil) are often used as adjuncts for pain control. The emphasis generally should be on helping the patient learn other measures to control pain.

PROMOTING COMFORT AND REST

It is important for the nurse to promote comfort, rest and relaxation, and the ability to carry out ADL in the patient with neurologic pain. See the box above for a summary of the nursing care.

Root pain is often aggravated by anything that causes direct or indirect movement of the spinal cord, leading to increased spinal pressure. Valsalva maneuvers such as sneezing, coughing, or straining at stool increase intrathoracic and intraabdominal pressure and indirectly produce distention of veins in the epidural space, thus affecting the dura mater surrounding the nerve roots. See the left box on p. 1795 for guidelines in caring for the patient with root pain.

GUIDELINES FOR NURSING INTERVENTIONS FOR PERSONS WITH ROOT PAIN

1. Avoid sharp flexion of the neck and extension of the leg.
2. Patient should not lie on horizontal plane for long periods.
3. Use stool softeners as indicated.
4. Sitting may relieve tension on nerve roots.

PATIENT TEACHING

Patient teaching for the person with neurologic pain is important and should include the following:
1. Avoid factors that increase pain.
2. Use relaxation measures when emotional tension is present.
3. Maintain regular rest and sleep pattern.
4. Take medication as prescribed.
5. Be aware of physical methods to control pain and use them appropriately.
6. Follow up with medical care as appropriate.
7. Structure home and work environment to keep stressors to a minimum.
8. Obtain help to complete ADL if needed.

INCREASED INTRACRANIAL PRESSURE

EPIDEMIOLOGY/ETIOLOGY

Increased intracranial pressure (ICP) is a complex manifestation that is caused by multiple neurologic conditions and often requires surgical intervention.

The cranial contents, including the brain tissues, vascular tissues, and cerebrospinal fluid (CSF), are contained within a bony vault for protection. Any increase in the volume of any of the cranial contents, singly or in combination, results in increased ICP because the cranial vault is rigid, closed, and nonexpandable. Several neurologic lesions, either by their nature or by causing cerebral edema, increase the volume of tissue within the cranium. Any lesion that increases tissue volume is known as a *space-occupying* lesion. Common examples are found in the box above, right.

Intracranial tumors arising from all types of brain tissue increase cell mass and thus increase ICP. An increase in the production of CSF, blockage of the ventricular system, or decreased absorption of CSF can likewise increase tissue fluid volume. Activities such as coughing, sneezing, or straining at stool or other Valsalva maneuvers also increase ICP for a short time. After activity ceases, the pressure then returns to its baseline.

It is also important to note that contrast dye used with cerebral angiography and CT scans may result in

SPACE-OCCUPYING LESIONS

1. Cerebral contusions
2. Hematomas
3. Infarctions
4. Abscesses
5. Intracranial tumors

irritation to cerebral blood vessels with resulting cerebral edema and increased ICP. Patients who have had either of these tests should be observed carefully for deterioration in neurologic status.

PREVENTION

Prevention of increased ICP involves the early detection of signs and symptoms so that corrective actions can be taken. This requires skill in nursing assessment (see assessment discussion).

Because many of the sources of increased ICP involve trauma, certain actions are important in prevention, including the following:
1. Use of seat belts
2. Use of helmets while riding motorcycles, snowmobiles, or bicycles
3. Safe use of firearms
4. Minimal use of drugs and alcohol
5. Not driving after taking drugs or drinking alcohol
6. Safe use of motor vehicles

PATHOPHYSIOLOGY

According to the *box theory* of the brain, an increase in any one of the contents of the cranium is usually accompanied by a reciprocal change in the volume of one of the others. Brain tissue cannot expand without serious effects on the flow and amount of CSF and cerebral circulation. Space-occupying lesions must displace and distort the brain and vascular tissues as pressure increases. Pressure may build up slowly over days or months or rapidly over minutes or hours. This usually depends on the cause. At first one hemisphere is more involved, depending on the lesion site, but eventually both hemispheres may become involved if the pressure continues to increase.

As pressure increases within the cranial cavity, it is initially compensated for by venous compression and CSF displacement. Although the brain has autoregulatory mechanisms to maintain a normal cerebral blood flow with some increase in ICP, as the pressure continues to rise, the cerebral blood flow decreases and *inadequate perfusion* occurs. The inadequate perfusion initiates a vicious cycle, causing the partial carbon dioxide pressure (PCO_2) to increase and the partial oxygen pressure (PO_2) and pH to decrease. These changes cause vasodilation and cerebral edema. The edema further increases ICP, causing increased compression of neural tissue and an even greater increase in ICP.

When the pressure within the cavity exceeds the compensatory mechanisms, the only escape for the brain hemisphere is to be displaced caudally or by downward herniation. The *falx cerebri* oppose medial shift of the hemispheres, and the *tentorium cerebelli* oppose downward shift to some extent. Structures that allow internal herniation are the cingulate gyrus, which permits medial subfacial herniation (under the falx); the uncus, which permits downward transtentorial herniation (across the free edge of the tentorium); and the cerebellar tonsil, which permits transforaminal herniation (through the foramen magnum). Because of the herniation, the brainstem is compressed at variable levels, which in turn compresses the vasomotor center, posterior cerebral artery, oculomotor nerve, corticospinal nerve pathways, and fibers of the ascending reticular activating system (RAS). Internal herniation in this way represents the critical state of decompensation. The life-sustaining mechanisms for consciousness, blood pressure, pulse, respirations, and temperature regulation fail.

CLINICAL MANIFESTATIONS

Increased ICP produces multiple signs and symptoms. One of the first is a decreasing level of consciousness (see Chapter 60).

PUPILLARY SIGNS

Pupillary responses are controlled by the oculomotor nerve (cranial nerve III), which carries sensory, motor, and parasympathetic fibers as well as sympathetic fibers. The oculomotor nerve is compressed by the herniating tissue and specifically by the downwardly displaced posterior cerebral artery. The pupilloconstrictor fibers of the oculomotor nerve run in a group in the top part of this nerve and are the first to be compressed. Consequently the ipsilateral pupil (when the lesion is in one hemisphere) remains dilated and is incapable of constricting. The pupil appears larger than in the other eye and does not react to light. Eventually, as cerebral pressure increases and both hemispheres are affected, bilateral pupil dilation and fixation occur. Inequality of the pupils may appear earlier than fixation when the nerve is only stretched. The pupil may respond to light slowly rather than with the usual brisk response. In examining the pupils, the nurse should note the size and equality first and then test the reaction of each pupil to light in a darkened room. Dilating pupils are a sign of impending tentorial herniation. When pupils dilate or change in their ability to react, the physician should be notified immediately. A pupil that is fixed and dilated is sometimes referred to as a "blown pupil" (see Figure 59-18, *B*).

BLOOD PRESSURE AND PULSE

The effect of cerebral pressure on blood pressure and pulse is variable. Compensatory changes occur in the cerebral vasculature relative to hypoxia or diminished blood flow. When the compensatory changes are no longer effective, however, compression of the brainstem occurs, and ischemia in the vasomotor center will be present. This excites the vasoconstrictor fibers, causing an increase in systolic blood pressure. If the ICP continues to increase, the ability of the vasomotor center to stimulate the vasoconstrictor fibers decreases and the blood pressure may fall. An increased systolic blood pressure with a widening pulse pressure followed by a sharp drop in blood pressure is often seen as the patient's condition deteriorates.

Pressure on the vasomotor center also increases the transmission of parasympathetic impulses via the vagus nerve to the heart, and the pulse rate is slowed. As the ICP continues to rise, however, the heart rate may sharply increase. *Slowing of the pulse rate in conjunction with a rising systolic blood pressure is a significant observation to be made and reported.* For consistency, blood pressure readings should be taken in the same arm, and the pulse should be taken for a full minute in the same location each time.

RESPIRATION

Herniation produces respiratory dysrhythmias that are variable and related to the level of brainstem compression or failure. The breathing pattern may be deep and stetorous or Cheyne-Stokes (periodic); fatal respiratory paralysis may follow. The beginning of periodic episodes of apnea is significant. The usual picture is slowing of respiration, a slow pulse, and a rising systolic blood pressure. The nurse should learn to look for variability in vital signs and detect trends as they occur. It is important to remember that the patient with a decreasing level of consciousness will require assistance in keeping the airway clear. Consequently, respiratory difficulty is further aggravated by this problem. Hypoxia also causes increased ICP. Persons who are experiencing increased ICP require supplemental oxygen.

TEMPERATURE REGULATION

Failure of the thermoregulatory center because of compression occurs later and gives rise to high uncontrolled temperatures. The nurse must understand that hyperthermia needs to be controlled, since it increases the metabolic needs of the brain tissues. Temperatures are taken rectally unless otherwise ordered.

FOCAL MOTOR AND SENSORY SIGNS

Compression of upper motor neuron pathways (corticospinal tract) interrupts the transmission of impulses to lower motor neurons, and progressive muscle weakness results. For example, a contralateral weakened hand grasp may progress to hemiparesis and hemiplegia; a weak hand, however, is not always a good indicator of motor weakness. More accurate is the observation and testing for *drift*, which requires the patient to close the eyes and extend the arms out straight in front for 30 seconds. If one arm is weakened, it will drift downward without the patient being aware of it. This can be tested in patients with increased ICP as long as they are capable of cooperating. Testing of the lower extremities includes the patient's ability to do straight leg raises as well as push and pull against the examiner. Ability to do plantar and dorsiflexion of the feet can also be evaluated.

When the patient is comatose, the response to tactile or painful stimuli is important. The nurse should note whether the person responds appropriately to pain or touch or whether the response is decorticate or decerebrate posturing.

The presence of Babinski's sign, hyperreflexia, and rigidity are additional motor signs that provide evidence of decreasing motor function from upper motor neuron involvement. Transtentorial herniation of the upper or rostral part of the brainstem produces decerebrate rigidity. The motor inhibitory fibers are blocked, and the person involuntarily assumes a fixed posture with arms, legs, and trunk extended and with flexion of the palmar and plantar joints; seizures may also be present. Decorticate rigidity may also occur (see Figure 60-1). This consists of a fixed posture with flexion of the arm, wrist, and fingers, with adduction of the arms and extension and internal rotation of the legs. Decorticate and decerebrate posturing may both be seen in the patient with herniation. The nurse should use gross tests or more definitive tests to determine motor changes. *The worsening of existing motor deficits is significant.*

VISUAL ACUITY AND PAPILLEDEMA

The blind spot of the retina measures the size and shape of the optic papilla, or optic disk. As venous congestion and ICP increase, the resulting pressure is transmitted to the eyes through the CSF and to the optic disk (choked disk). Since the meninges of the brain reflect out around the eyeball, they permit the direct transmission of pressure along the subarachnoid space through the CSF. As the optic disk swells, the retina adjacent to it is also compressed. The damaged retina cannot detect light rays. As the size of the blind spot enlarges, visual acuity decreases. The ability of the nurse to detect papilledema depends on skill in examination of the fundi (see Figure 59-16).

Many nurses will not have learned to observe for papilledema and must rely on other means to assess ICP. Decreasing visual acuity can be detected through the confrontation technique (see Chapter 59). Papille-

dema occurs most often when the increased ICP develops slowly. A rapid rise in ICP may not be reflected by papilledema.

HEADACHE

Headache may occur as an early symptom. It is thought to result from venous congestion and the tension on the intracranial blood vessels as the cerebral pressure rises. The onset of the headache should be noted along with its location and duration. It increases in intensity with cough, straining, and stooping.

VOMITING

The occurrence of projectile vomiting is often associated with increased ICP. Its frequency and character should be noted. The significance of vomiting and headache needs to be associated with other clinical signs, such as papilledema and vital signs.

DIAGNOSTIC TESTS

The diagnosis of increased ICP can be made with the CT scan, which can show the actual structural herniation as well as shifting of the brain. Most often, however, acute increased ICP is a medical emergency, and the diagnosis must be made on the basis of observation and neurologic testing alone.[2]

The frequency of "neurologic checks" of the patient is often ordered by the physician. However, with significant deteriorating changes in the aforementioned signs, the nurse should decide when more frequent assessments and recordings are indicated. On the basis of the results obtained from observations and the patient's medical history, the nurse must make a decision concerning the frequency of monitoring. Tools used for assessing the patient's neurologic condition may vary from institution to institution. The important point is that the patient's condition is regularly compared with an established baseline through continuous monitoring.

Various methods for measurement of ICP have been devised. One of the most frequent methods requires placement of a hollow screw through the skull into the subarachnoid space. The screw is attached to a Luer-Lok, which is connected to a transducer and oscilloscope for continued monitoring.[29] The transducer is fastened to the head of the bed and must be level with the screw for accurate monitoring. The screw may be attached to a manometer for intermittent readings. Directions for the use of this measurement device can be found in the literature[27] (Figure 62-2).

With more experience with the use of continuous internal intracranial monitoring, it has become evident that the traditional clinical signs of increased ICP do not always correlate with the actual pressure changes seen on the monitor. Studies have found that many of the classic signs of increased ICP do not appear until the pressure has reached extremely high levels and the opportunity to reverse the rising pressure and prevent permanent brain damage has already passed.[30]

It is important to note that ICP is not constant and unchanging. The nurse can significantly alter pressure depending on the interventions carried out. Intracranial monitoring of patients with increased ICP indicates that the pressure is in constant flux. When performing such monitoring, the nurse is responsible for reading the monitor and responding to significant changes as they occur.

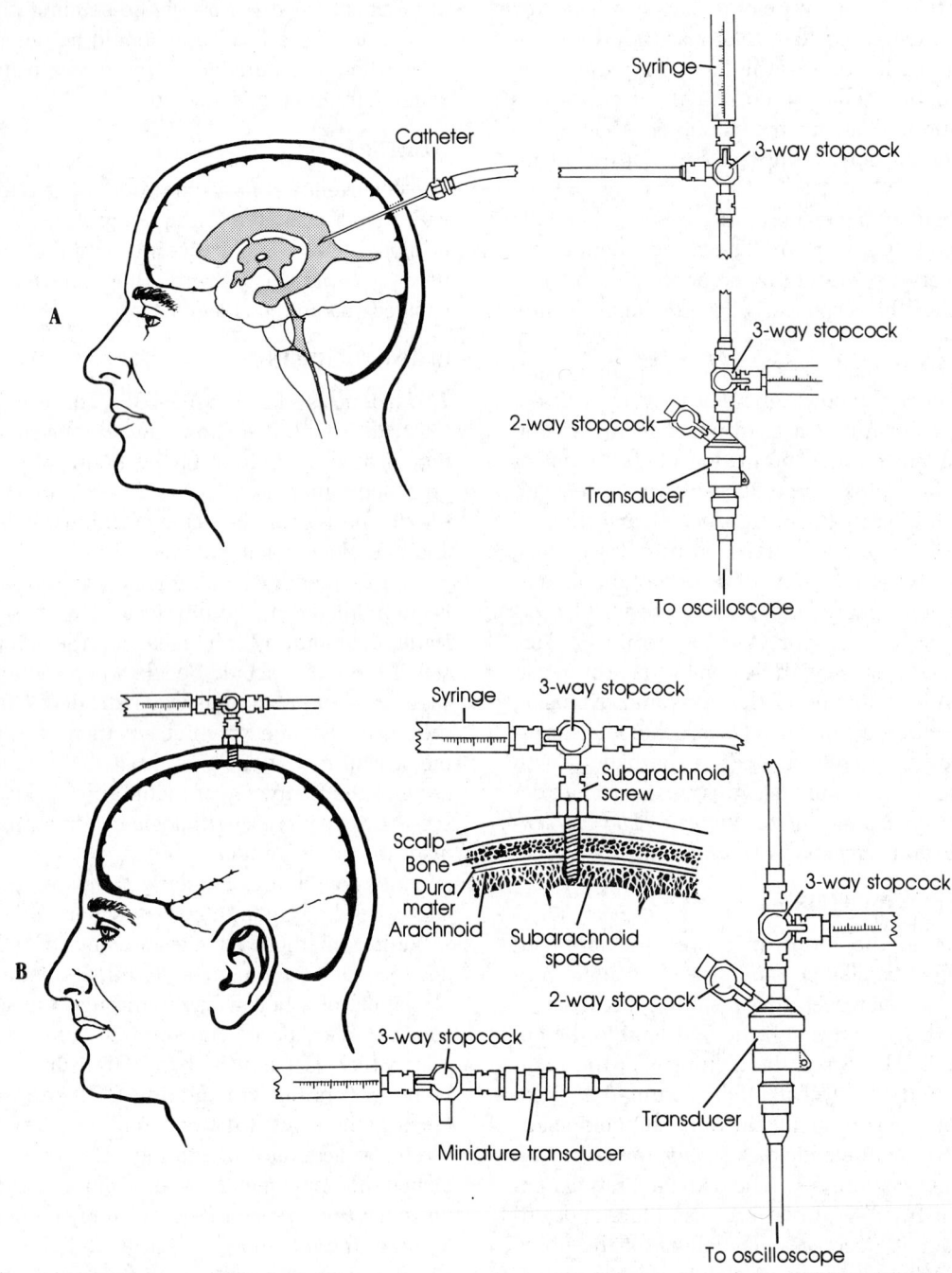

FIGURE 62-2 Equipment for ICP monitoring. **A,** Ventricular pressure monitoring. Catheter is inserted through a burr hole in the skull into the lateral ventricle and attached to a transducer and oscilloscope to monitor ICP. **B,** Subarachnoid screw pressure monitoring. Subarachnoid screw is inserted through a burr hole in the skull and attached to a transducer and oscilloscope for continuous monitoring. (From Rudy EB: Advanced neurological and neurosurgical nursing, St Louis, 1984, The CV Mosby Co.)

MEDICAL MANAGEMENT

The medical treatment of patients with increased ICP depends on the underlying cause. For example, if it is caused by an intracranial tumor, the tumor is removed surgically. When surgery is not possible (or indicated), efforts are made to reduce the pressure through the use of drug therapy or direct physical measures. The use of medications is discussed later.

Rapidly rising ICP must be relieved directly by mechanical decompression. This may be accomplished by a variety of procedures, including the following:

1. Ventricular puncture with withdrawal of CSF by needle or cannula
2. Continuous ventricular drainage via ventriculostomy tube
3. Removal of a piece of skull (craniotomy) to provide room for the cranial contents to expand
4. Burr holes made in the skull with or without evacuation of subdural hematoma
5. Continuous drainage of subdural hematoma via subdural drain

Each of these measures requires careful monitoring by the nurse for signs of increased ICP and the maintenance of asepsis at the entrance site into the skull.

■ ASSESSMENT

It is important to collect both subjective and objective data from the patient with increased ICP.

SUBJECTIVE DATA

Subjective data include the following:

1. Patient's understanding of condition
2. Presence of visual changes: diplopia or blurred vision
3. Ability to abstract, calculate, and reason
4. Presence of pain, especially headache

5. Ability to carry out ADL
6. Presence of nausea

The headache associated with increased ICP pressure usually increases in intensity with coughing, straining, or stooping. It is typically present in the early morning and may awaken the patient from sleep.

OBJECTIVE DATA

Objective data include the following:

1. Level of consciousness
2. Pupillary signs
3. Vital signs
4. Focal motor or sensory signs
5. Presence of vomiting or hiccoughing
6. Eye changes, including papilledema
7. Speech patterns
8. ICP

The detection of increased ICP must occur early, when it is reversible and before the stage of decompensation. The ability to make accurate observations, to interpret observations intelligently, and to record observations carefully is the most important part of nursing care of the patient experiencing increased ICP. (See boxes below for relevant research.)

■ DATA ANALYSIS: NURSING DIAGNOSES

Nursing diagnoses are determined from assessment of patient data. Possible nursing diagnoses for the person with increased ICP include, but are not limited to, the following:

Diagnostic Title	Possible Etiologies
Airway clearance, ineffective	Perceptual/cognitive impairment
Breathing pattern, ineffective	Neuromuscular impairment, perceptual/ cognitive impairment
Fluid volume excess	Compromised regulatory mechanism

RESEARCH

Stuart G et al: Head injury management without intracranial pressure monitoring, J Neurosurg Nurs 59:601-605, 1983.

This prospective study compared 100 patients with severe head injuries who were treated without benefit of intracranial monitoring with similar samples of patients who had intracranial monitoring that had been reported in the literature. Patients who were included in the study had a Glasgow Coma Scale score of eight or less for 6 hours within the first 48 hours after injury. The results of this study were very similar to those reported by other investigators of patients who were monitored with an intracranial monitoring device. The authors concluded that when proper assessment and early intervention have taken place, no difference exists in the quality of life in those patients who had intracranial monitoring and those who did not. ■

RESEARCH

Turner H et al: Comparison of nurse and computer recording of ICP in head injured patients, J Neurosci Nurs 20:236-239, 1988.

This study tested the ability of the nurse to describe the ICP course by a manual record and compared these results with an on-line computerized ICP monitoring system. The nurse recorded one value of ICP from the bedside monitor at the end of an hour, whereas the computer averaged 720 data samples of ICP during the hour. Data were collected from five patients who had suffered a head injury. Comparison of the two sets of scores showed that the nurse's "end-hour" value was a reasonable estimate of the patient's mean ICP for the entire hour as measured by the computer. ■

Diagnostic Title	Possible Etiologies
Knowledge deficit: symptoms of increased intracranial pressure	Cognitive limitation
Tissue perfusion, altered cerebral	Increased blood flow

■ PLANNING: EXPECTED PATIENT OUTCOMES

Because of the acute, emergent, and disabling nature of increased ICP, the outcomes are often the result of direct nursing and medical treatment. Expected patient outcomes for the person with increased ICP pressure may include, but are not limited to, the following:

1. Cerebral edema is reduced.
2. Cerebral hypoxia is prevented by the maintenance of a patent airway and reduction of cerebral pressure.
3. Activities that increase ICP are reduced.
4. Fluid intake is limited.
5. Intake and output are monitored.
6. Patient and family are supported, and explanations are given as appropriate.
7. Patient cooperates with the therapeutic plan as able.
8. Patient's airway remains patent.
9. Cerebral tissue perfusion is improved.
10. Effective breathing pattern is maintained.

If a person suffers from a more chronic form of increased ICP (for example the patient with a brain tumor), the following outcome criteria are important:

1. The patient can state the signs and symptoms that indicate the need for immediate medical assistance.
2. The patient can state the action, side effects, toxic effects, and dosage schedule of medications ordered to decrease ICP.
3. Patient can state plans for follow-up care.

■ IMPLEMENTATION

MEDICATIONS

Medications are usually ordered to promote rapid osmotic diuresis and to reduce ICP. Drugs often used include the following:

1. Intravenous urea (Urevert)
2. Intravenous mannitol
3. Hypertonic solutions of glucose (25% to 50%)
4. Corticosteroids such as dexamethasone (intravenous or intramuscular)

The corticosteroids act more slowly, but their effect is more sustained. All these drugs cause dehydration and promote the movement of excess fluid from the brain tissues into the blood so it can be eliminated. Narcotics and other drugs that cause respiratory depression are avoided. Phenytoin (Dilantin) may be prescribed to prevent seizures.

CONSERVATIVE MEASURES

Conservative measures to reduce venous volume may be implemented. See the box below left for more details.

PATIENT TEACHING

Teaching for the patient experiencing increased ICP will vary, depending on the patient's condition. In general the points that should be considered in teaching the patient or family include the following:

1. Use of medications, including actions, side effects, and schedule of use

---

GUIDELINES FOR NURSING INTERVENTION FOR PERSONS WITH INCREASED ICP

1. Decrease ICP.
   a. Elevate head of bed 15 to 30 degrees.
   b. Avoid flexion of hips, waist, and neck.
   c. Avoid rotation of head, especially to the right.
   d. Space out nursing activities to maintain lower pressure levels.
   e. Avoid Valsalva-type movements.
   f. Perform suctioning only as necessary.
2. Monitor fluid balance.
   a. Restrict fluids.
   b. Carefully monitor urinary output, often with indwelling catheter. Always use catheter if mannitol is being used.
   c. Use minidripper with intravenous fluids.
   d. Encourage use of normal saline as intravenous fluid.
3. Maintain oxygenation.
   a. Oxygenate patient before and after suctioning.
   b. Perform oxygen therapy via mask or cannula.
   c. Intubation may be necessary.
   d. Controlled respirations may be implemented to lower PCO_2, (thus causing a slightly alkaline pH and decreased vasodilation).

RESEARCH

Synder M: Relation of nursing activities to increases in intracranial pressure, J Adv Nurs 8:273-279, 1983.

This study examined the effects of nursing activities and environmental factors on ICP. All nine patients had an internal intracranial monitoring device in place. Activities were observed at the patient's bedside. Activities that increased ICP were tube manipulation, respiratory care, invasive procedures, neurologic assessment, movement, and conversation. The two activities that resulted in the greatest mean increase in ICP were respiratory care and repositioning. Invasive procedures were found to cause the longest periods of ICP elevation. ■

2. Signs and symptoms of increased ICP

3. How to obtain emergency or follow-up care
Research on the effects of nursing activities on ICP is discussed in the right box on p. 1800.

ALTERATIONS IN MUSCLE TONE AND MOTOR FUNCTION

EPIDEMIOLOGY/ETIOLOGY

Disturbances of motor function probably surpass all other clinical neurologic symptoms in frequency and importance. Since the nervous system is designed primarily for movement of the body in space and of the various parts in relation to each other, damages to the nervous system often cause serious problems in mobility.

PREVENTION

As with many neurologic diseases, often little can be done to prevent them. Much of the focus is on secondary prevention and tertiary prevention (prevention of complications). Some muscle injuries related to trauma, and the preventive aspects are discussed under the care of the comatose patient in Chapter 60.

PATHOPHYSIOLOGY

The term *paralysis* refers to a loss of function, either motor or sensory. When applied to motor function, it means loss of voluntary movement because of interruption of the descending efferent motor pathways. A lesser degree of paralysis is called *paresis*. Damage to sensory pathways that are intimately concerned with motor function may occur concomitantly with the loss of mo-

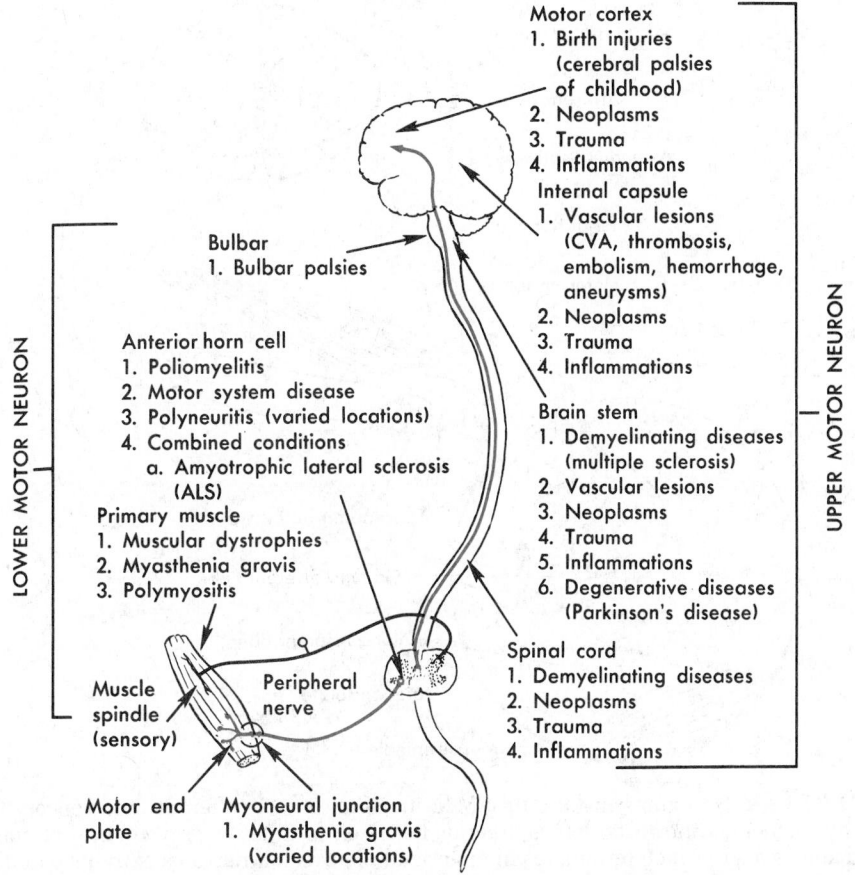

FIGURE 62-3 Disturbances in motor function are classified pathologically along upper motor neuron (UMN) and lower motor neuron (LMN) structures. It should be noted that the same pathologic condition occurs at more than one site in UMN area shown on right. A few pathologic conditions involve both UMN and LMN structures, as in amyotrophic lateral sclerosis. Other lesion sites include myoneural junctions and primary muscles, making it possible to classify conditions as neuromuscular and muscular, respectively. (Modified from Chusid JG: Correlative neuroanatomy and functional neurology, ed 15, Los Altos, Calif, 1970, Lange Medical Publications.)

tor function. Loss of sensory function is described later in this chapter.

Injury or disease of motor neurons and their extensions at any level results in alterations of muscle strength, tone, and reflex activity. The specific clinical manifestations differ according to whether the lesion involves an upper motor neuron or a lower motor neuron (Figure 62-3).

CLINICAL MANIFESTATIONS
LOWER MOTOR NEURON LESION

Recall that *lower motor neurons* (LMNs) consist of the large anterior horn cells located in the anterior gray matter of the spinal cord. They are also located in the motor cranial nuclei of the brainstem. Each anterior horn cell has a long axon that exits the cord via the an-

terior (ventral) spinal root and extends out the peripheral nerve, eventually synapsing at the motor end-plate of the neuromuscular junction. These structures together form a *motor unit* that controls skeletal muscle activity, both voluntary and reflex (Figures 62-4 and 62-5). When a lesion selectively involves some part (cell body, motor root, isolated peripheral nerve) of the LMN, it characteristically results in flaccid muscle weakness or paralysis, loss of reflex activity, loss of muscle tone, and atrophy confined to the involved muscle or muscles.

The *degree* of muscle weakness occurring in the involved muscle or muscles in a LMN lesion is directly related to the extent and severity of the lesion. Since each anterior horn cell innervates several separate muscle fibers and since several anterior horn cell columns exist at each spinal level, a lesion confined to *one* spinal seg-

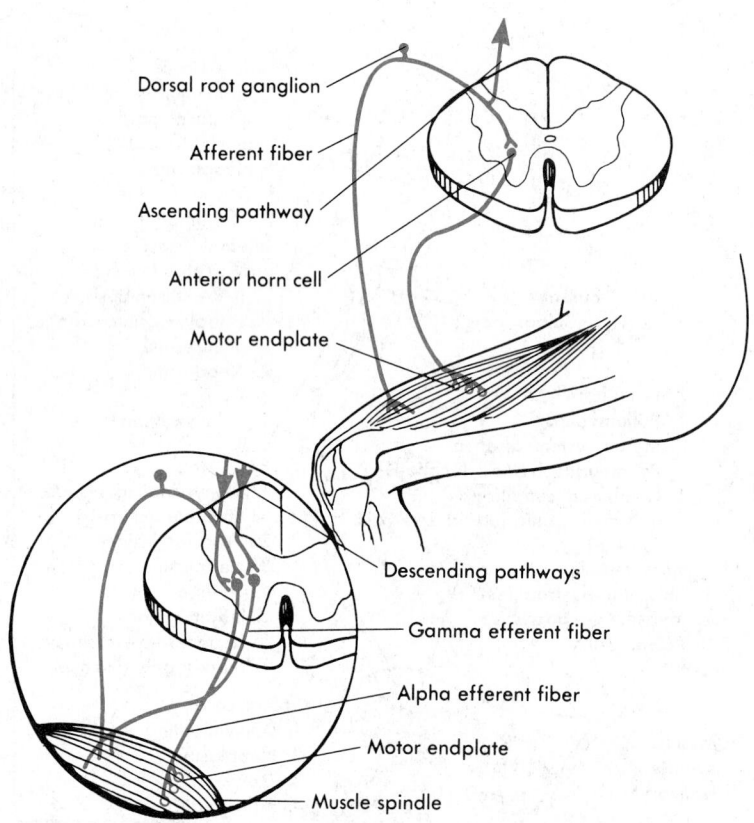

Dorsal root ganglion

Afferent fiber

Ascending pathway

Anterior horn cell

Motor endplate

Descending pathways

Gamma efferent fiber

Alpha efferent fiber

Motor endplate

Muscle spindle

FIGURE 62-4 Structures making up LMN, including motor (efferent) and sensory (afferent) elements. Shown on left is anterior horn cell in anterior gray column of spinal cord and its axon, which terminates in motor end-plate as it innervates extrafusal muscle fibers in the quadriceps muscle. Detailed in enlargement are sensory and motor elements of γ-loop system. γ-Efferent fiber is shown innervating polar or end region of muscle spindle (sensory receptor of skeletal muscle). Contraction of muscle spindle fibers stretch central portion of spindle and cause afferent spindle fiber to transmit impulse centrally to cord. Muscle spindle afferent fibers in turn synapse on anterior horn cell and are transmitted by way of α-efferent fibers to skeletal (extrafusal) muscle, causing it to contract. Muscle spindle discharge is interrupted by active contraction of extrafusal muscle fibers. (Modified from Truex RC and Carpenter MB: Human neuroanatomy, ed 6, Baltimore, 1969, Williams & Wilkins.)

ment may not damage all the anterior horn cells innervating an entire muscle. Thus such a lesion will cause muscle *weakness* (paresis) rather than paralysis of the entire muscle. Complete paralysis occurs in LMN lesions only when the lesion involves the column or anterior horn cells in several spinal segments that innervate an entire muscle or the ventral roots arising from these cells. A lesion in a single motor nerve root will cause varying degrees of muscle weakness in several muscles. If *all* or almost all the peripheral motor fibers supplying a muscle are destroyed, all voluntary postural and reflex movements are lost. The entire muscle becomes lax and soft, a condition known as *flaccidity*.

Muscle weakness itself cannot be classified as either lower or upper motor neuron, since it typically occurs to both. It is the *distribution* of the muscle weakness that is important to distinguish. In summary, a LMN lesion weakens individual muscles or sets of muscles in the spinal root or peripheral nerve distribution.

The involved muscle or muscles become flaccid because the motor unit has been damaged and normal reflex activity has been interrupted. This flaccidity is further evidenced by *hypotonia* and by reduced or absent muscle stretch reflexes (*hyporeflexia* and *areflexia*, respectively). This interruption of the primary motor unit results in localized muscle atrophy, or wasting, corresponding to the spinal segmental distribution of the anterior horn cells involved.

Atrophy also increases with nonuse of the muscle. In some LMN lesions the affected muscle bundle or unit exhibits small localized, spontaneous, and involuntary contractions known as *fasciculations*. These are visible through the skin and should not be confused with fibrillation. The fasciculations are thought to represent the discharge of isolated muscle fibers arising from a single-functioning LMN unit. They are coarse in large motor units but may be fine in smaller motor units, as in the hands.

The criteria for an LMN lesion site or disease include segmental or localized muscle weakness and atrophy in the same distribution, with absent or decreased muscle stretch reflexes in the affected muscles.

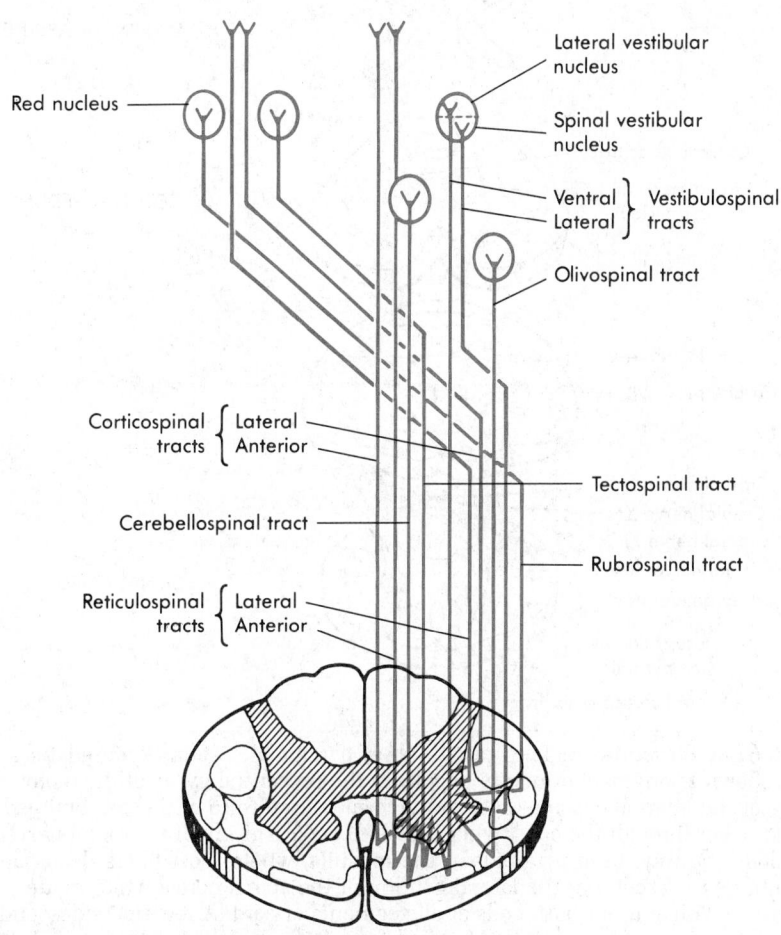

FIGURE 62-5 Nuclei and their respective pathways descend and terminate around the LMN in the ventral column of the spinal cord.

In summary, when a lesion involves the LMN, the following signs are present:
1. Flaccid muscle weakness or paralysis
2. Loss of reflex activity
3. Loss of muscle tone
4. Atrophy confined to the involved muscle or muscles

UPPER MOTOR NEURON LESION

Recall that *upper motor neurons* (UMNs) originate in the motor strip of the cerebral cortex and in multiple brainstem nuclei. From the cortex these axons pass through the internal capsule and brainstem, cross over (decussate) in the medulla, and continue descending in the spinal cord via the corticospinal tracts. These fibers

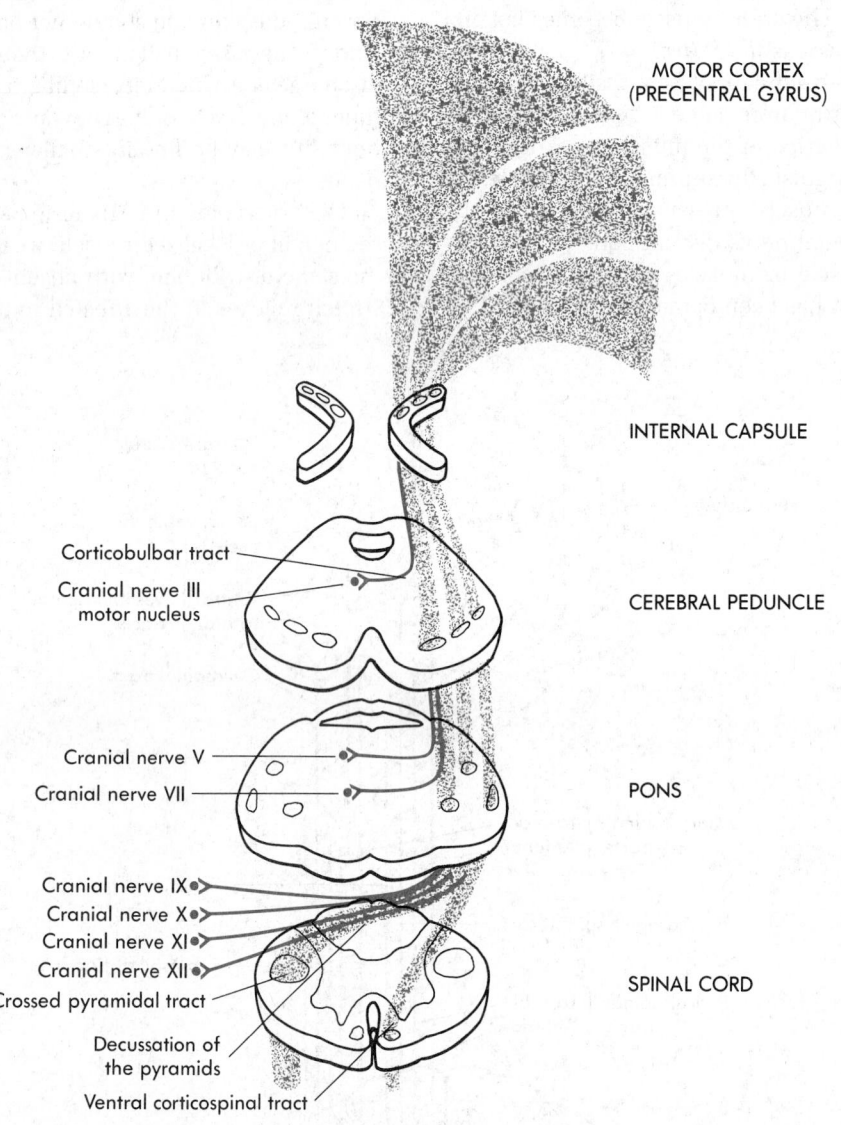

MOTOR CORTEX
(PRECENTRAL GYRUS)

INTERNAL CAPSULE

Corticobulbar tract
Cranial nerve III
motor nucleus

CEREBRAL PEDUNCLE

Cranial nerve V
Cranial nerve VII

PONS

Cranial nerve IX
Cranial nerve X
Cranial nerve XI
Cranial nerve XII
Crossed pyramidal tract

Decussation of
the pyramids

Ventral corticospinal tract

SPINAL CORD

FIGURE 62-6 Structures making up UMN, or pyramidal system. Pyramidal system fibers are shown to originate primarily in cells in the precentral gyrus of the motor cortex; converge at the internal capsule; descend to form central third of the cerebral peduncle; descend further through the pons, where small fibers are given off to cranial nerve motor nuclei along the way; form pyramids at the medulla, where most fibers decussate; and then continue to descend in the lateral column of the spinal cord's white matter, where they synapse with anterior horn cells at all segments of cord. A few fibers descend without crossing at the medulla level. (Modified from original painting by Frank H Netter. From the Ciba Collection of Medical Illustrations. Copyright by Ciba Pharmaceutical Co., division of Ciba-Geigy Corp. All rights reserved.)

eventually synapse with LMNs in the spinal cord (Figure 62-6).

The corticospinal tracts are thought to be primarily responsible for the execution of precise, fine, voluntary muscle movements. However, together with the extrapyramidal tracts descending to the LMNs, they assist in modulating muscle tone and reflex activity to some degree. Thus all descending systems collectively combine their influences on the LMNs so that efferent neural impulses are modified. This results in fine, orderly, and smooth muscle movements.

Any lesion that destroys UMNs or interferes with their influences over LMNs therefore is called a UMN lesion. When a UMN lesion is *rostral* to the medulla, as in a cerebrovascular accident (CVA), deficits will be contralateral to the lesion and will be demonstrated as a hemiplegia. The distribution or degree of paralysis is not always equal or the same within the hemiplegic distribution. For example, the face and arm may be weak or the weakness may involve the leg alone, depending on the part of the motor cortex involved. The following may be considered *UMN signs* following CVA: weakness of the mouth muscle associated with eye muscle weakness (forehead muscle is intact), weakness of forearm and wrist extensors, and weakness of the hip flexors and foot dorsiflexors. These muscle weaknesses result in the characteristic gait and appearance of the patient with a CVA. Circumduction of the affected leg occurs with inversion of the foot, which drags. The arm is held semiflexed at the elbow and wrist. The facial muscles around the eye and mouth droop.

Initially and for a variable period the muscles affected by the lesion are flaccid (hypotonic) and hyporeflexic. Gradually the flaccidity recedes, and the reflex arcs become increasingly hyperreactive in the absence of UMN modulation. Eventually, paresis or paralysis of voluntary muscle movement occurs with increased muscle tone and spasticity. The spasticity is characterized by increased resistance to passive movement, hyperreflexia, clasp-knife phenomenon, and *clonus*. Clonus is related to the hyperreflexia, in which the contraction of one muscle group is sufficient to stretch the antagonistic muscles and perpetuate the contractions. A unilateral Babinski's sign is present on the hemiparetic side. Atrophy of the muscle results from disuse and occurs late and to a lesser extent than in LMN disease.

UMN lesions within the brainstem also produce the characteristic motor manifestations just described and also cause involvement of the cranial nerve nuclei and sensory pathways near the midbrain lesion site. The problem of localizing the site of an UMN brainstem lesion is made more difficult by the proximity of the descending fiber systems and cranial motor nuclei in the brainstem area.

UMN lesions that are caudal to the medulla (as in spinal cord trauma) produce deficits ipsilateral to the lesion. If the cord is transected or the lesion extends into both halves of the spinal cord, deficits are demonstrated as a quadriplegia or paraplegia. A complete transection of the spinal cord immediately produces loss of motor function, muscle tone, and reflex activity as well as somatic and visceral sensations below the level of the injury. Usually, when examined after a year, voluntary motor losses remain, but there is increased spasticity of extensor muscles and hyperreflexia of *all* cord reflexes (muscle stretch, autonomic, nociceptive). Thus any stretch on the spastic muscles may result in extreme contraction. Likewise, contact with a noxious stimulus may cause flexion withdrawal of the limb along with variations of autonomic activity. Occasionally, all three types of reflex activity may occur simultaneously as a response to a single stimulus. For example, a full bladder or decubitus irritation may cause flexion of the lower extremities, reflex bladder or bowel emptying, and altered vasomotor response to that area. A bilateral, positive Babinski's sign is also present.

Table 62-3 summarizes and compares the characteristic clinical syndromes seen in UMN and LMN lesions.

In summary, when a lesion involves the UMN, the following signs are present:

1. Paresis or paralysis of voluntary muscle tone and spasticity
2. Hyperreflexia
3. Late atrophy from disuse
4. Increased muscle tone

DIAGNOSTIC TESTS

One of the most common diagnostic procedures used to evaluate muscle dysfunction is *electromyography*. In

TABLE 62-3 Clinical syndromes of UMN and LMN lesions

Motor Component	UMN Characteristics	LMN Characteristics
Reflex	Hyperreflexia, extensor toe sign (Babinski's sign)	Hyporeflexia or areflexia
Muscle tonus	Hypertonia, clasp-knife spasticity, clonus	Hypotonia, flaccidity
Muscle movement	Paralysis or paresis of movements in hemiplegic and other distributions	Paralysis or paresis of individual muscles in peripheral nerve distribution
Muscle wasting	Late atrophy from disuse	Early atrophy or denervation
Muscle fasciculations	Not present	Present

motor disease, electrical activity of various types and abnormal patterns appears in resting muscle. The electromyogram (EMG) provides direct evidence of motor dysfunction and can be used to detect a dysfunction located in the motor neuron, the neuromuscular junction, or muscle fibers. See Chapter 59 for a description of this procedure.

MEDICAL MANAGEMENT

Medical management for the patient with a neuromuscular disease is primarily supportive and palliative. Occasionally, surgery may help to alleviate the condition or its results, but this is usually not the case.

■ ASSESSMENT

Both subjective and objective data are important in determining more about abnormal muscle movements.[16]

SUBJECTIVE DATA

Subjective data include the following:
1. Patient's understanding of the problem and possible causes
2. Initial onset of problem
3. Measures that improve symptoms
4. Presence of clumsiness or incoordination
5. Presence of any abnormal sensation

Often, subjective symptoms occurring early in an illness involving muscle movements or sensations are ignored.

OBJECTIVE DATA

Objective data include the following:
1. Coordination
2. Muscle strength
3. Muscle tone
4. Any atrophy of muscles
5. Presence of clonus or fasciculations
6. Ability to move muscles; abnormal gait
7. Reflexes
8. Change in ability to carry out ADL

■ DATA ANALYSIS: NURSING DIAGNOSES

Nursing diagnoses are determined from patient data. Possible nursing diagnoses for the person with alterations in muscle tone and motor function include, but are not limited to, the following:

Diagnostic Title	Possible Etiologies
Activity intolerance	Generalized weakness
Disuse syndrome, potential for	Immobility, weakness
Home maintenance management, impaired	Individual disease/injury
Injury, potential for	Sensory/motor deficits
Knowledge deficit: required care	Lack of exposure/recall, unfamiliarity with information sources
Mobility, impaired physical	Neuromuscular impairment
Self-care deficit: bathing/hygiene, dressing/grooming, feeding, toileting	Neuromuscular impairment
Skin integrity, impaired, potential	Mechanical forces (pressure, shearing forces), immobility
Urinary elimination, altered patterns	Sensory/motor impairment

■ PLANNING: EXPECTED PATIENT OUTCOMES

Expected patient outcomes for the person with alterations in muscle tone and motor function may include, but are not limited to, the following:
1. Skin will remain intact and free of breakdown.
2. Joint deformities (contractures) will not develop.
3. Patient can describe medication dosage, function, side effects, and toxic effects.
4. Patient can demonstrate measures to prevent skin breakdown.
5. Patient can demonstrate measures to prevent muscle or joint deformities.
6. Patient can describe and demonstrate range of motion.
7. Patient can list signs of skin breakdown that require medical intervention.
8. Patient can describe bowel and bladder program.
9. Patient can demonstrate ADL that can be done alone and can describe methods of assistance for those functions that are dependent.
10. Patient can manage home management activities.

■ IMPLEMENTATION
MEDICATIONS

Patients experiencing ongoing problems with spasticity may be placed on one or more skeletal muscle relaxants to decrease tone and involuntary movements and to help relieve anxiety and tension. In general the centrally acting preparations specifically affect the spinal polysynaptic reflexes and, at the same time, depress the central nervous system. Common side effects include drowsiness and dizziness; these become intensified when combined with alcohol, barbiturates, sedatives, hypnotics, or tranquilizers. Some frequently prescribed drugs include the following:
1. Baclofen (Lioresal), a derivative of gamma aminobutyric acid (GABA) (an inhibitory neurotransmitter), acts on the spinal cord.
2. Dantrolene (Dantrium) acts directly on skeletal muscle. Effects from the drug become apparent about a week after it is started. It acts by impairing Ca^{++} release from the sarcoplasmic reticulum. Additional side effects include muscle weakness, slurred speech, drooling, and anuresis.

3. Diazepam (Valium) is a centrally acting muscle relaxant and antianxiety agent.

PROMOTING SAFETY

Patients who are paralyzed need to be protected from falling. The person with hemiplegia must have the side rail of the bed raised on the affected side when unattended. If permitted up in a chair, a chair restraint is used.

The *eye on the affected side* should be protected if the lid remains open and there is no blink reflex. Otherwise, damage to the cornea can lead to corneal ulcers and blindness. Irrigations with a physiologic solution of sodium chloride, followed by drops of sterile mineral oil, sterile castor oil, sterile petroleum jelly, or artificial tears solution (methylcellulose), are sometimes used. After the lid is gently closed, an eye pad may be taped over the affected eye. If a pad is used, it must be changed daily, and the eye cleansed and carefully examined for signs of inflammation or drying of the cornea. Eye shields are preferable to pads because they lessen the danger of lint entering the eye.

PROMOTING SKIN INTEGRITY

The skin of the paralyzed person needs to be inspected for signs of pressure. These patients are at risk for decubitus formation. The following factors account for this:

1. Muscles are not being used.
2. Interference with autonomic reflexes that monitor and maintain vasomotor tone may result in altered circulation in the paralyzed areas.
3. Sensory loss may prevent the patient from perceiving pain and pressure (the usual warning signs of tissue injury).

In monoplegic, hemiplegic, and quadriplegic distributions, successively larger areas of skin surface must be protected.

PROMOTING ACTIVITY

The limbs of a person with acute hemiplegia, as with those of the person with paraplegia, are often flaccid at first. Spasticity with a tendency to muscle contracture develops gradually. The joints then become flexed or extended and fixed in useless positions with deformity *unless preventive measures are taken by the nurse.* Shortening of joint capsules and ligaments occurs around the immobile joint, and the limb may be drawn into flexure or extensor contracture with or without muscle spasm.

Through assessment the nurse determines the specific joints that are vulnerable to contracture and deformity formation as related to the existing degree and type of paralysis. For example, greater contracture vulnerability will occur with quadriplegia than with paraplegia or hemiplegia, since the amount of muscle and joint involvement is greater. Assessment includes free range of motion (ROM) to determine the level of motion in all joints. On the basis of assessment, the nurse carefully positions the limbs in normal anatomic positions to prevent deformity. By having knowledge of the distribution patterns of paralysis in UMN or LMN lesions, *counterpositioning* can also be initiated. In hemiplegia, for example, the neglected upper limb is pulled inward at the shoulder joint and the wrist drops; in the lower limb the knee flexes and the foot drops. In counterpositioning the nurse plans for the shoulder and upper arm to be in abduction, the elbow slightly flexed, the wrist in dorsiflexion, the knee in neutral position, and the foot in dorsiflexion. If the person is supine, a pillow can be placed between the upper arm and body to hold the arm in abduction. A roll made of one or two washcloths or a styrofoam cup serves as a good support to prevent flexion of the fingers, and a splint made from a padded tongue blade may be used to ensure straightening of the thumb or other fingers for periods during the day. Dayhoff[10] questions the common use of soft devices to prevent hand deformity and believes that there should be experimentation with hard devices to improve hand functioning following an UMN lesion such as a CVA.

A firm box at the foot of the bed holds the feet at right angles and prevents contractures in the drop-foot position (Figure 62-7). Some physical therapists believe

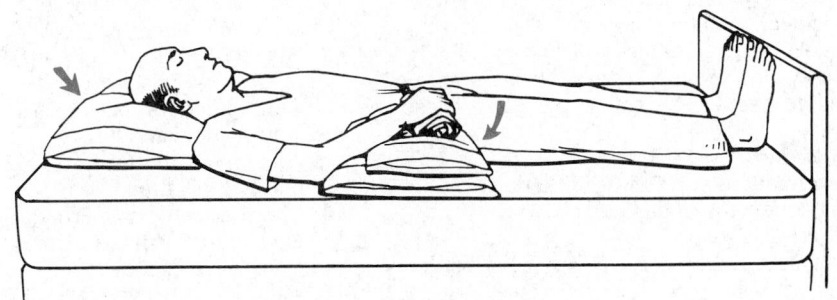

FIGURE 62-7 Patient lying supine with feet against foot board. Note that the lower arm is elevated on a small pillow and hand is flexed over a rolled towel.

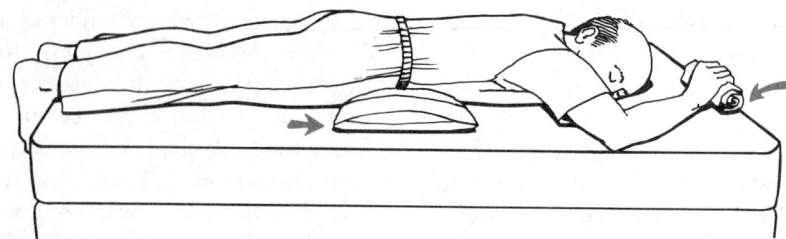

FIGURE 62-8 Patient lying prone with feet extending over end of mattress. Note that small pillow is positioned under patient's midsection and that hand is flexed around rolled towel.

that footboards used in the prevention of foot-drop contribute to increased spasticity and that their use should *not* be a routine practice for persons with UMN lesions.

Positioning is equally important as related to paraplegic and quadriplegic distributions. Knee flexion and foot-drop are severe complications that must be prevented. The development of a flexion contracture at the knee joint interferes with the ability of the person to bear weight later in an upright position and to transfer unaided from one place to another. As a consequence, the person's level of self-care and independence may be greatly diminished when a joint deformity occurs. Subluxation of a shoulder joint in a person with hemiplegia, related to inadequate support of the joint when in an upright position, causes pain and limits therapy of the limb. In addition, keeping the paralyzed person in a semiupright position for long periods, whether in or out of bed, results in hip deformities. Positioning in the prone position helps to counteract the formation of this type of deformity (Figure 62-8).

In summary, most joint deformities in a paralyzed person are *preventable* with early and continuing nursing interventions.

In addition to positioning, interventions for the person with paralysis include ROM exercises to all joints. Passive ROM exercises are indicated at least *twice daily* for all joints that the person cannot voluntarily move. Frequent active ROM of the unaffected joints must be carried out by the individual. The regularity of ROM is most important so that limitations do not develop.

PROMOTING NUTRITION

Patience and persistence are necessary in giving foods and fluid to the person with hemiplegia. So much difficulty may be encountered in swallowing food and fluids because of the paralysis that the patient may become easily frustrated. Important nursing measures are listed in the box below.

GUIDELINES FOR NURSING INTERVENTIONS FOR PERSONS WITH MOTOR DYSFUNCTION

1. Promote safety.
   a. Always keep side rail up on the affected side of hemiplegic patients.
   b. Use restraints judiciously as needed.
   c. Protect affected eye if there is no blink reflex.
      (1) Irrigate eye with normal saline solution as needed.
      (2) Use artificial tear solution if ordered.
      (3) Use eye shield to keep eye closed. Change daily and inspect eye for dryness, redness, or other sign of infection. (Eye shield is preferable to eye pad because of no lint).
2. Promote integrity of skin.
   a. Change position frequently; patient should do so if able.
   b. Shift weight for patients in chairs.
   c. Inspect skin at least daily.
   d. If sensory loss is present, avoid use of hot water bottles, heating pads, or hot water.

3. Promote activity.
   a. Position or counterposition as necessary.
   b. Use hand splints as needed.
   c. Use measures to protect from foot drop; that is, high-topped tennis shoes or footboards.
   d. Use sling for shoulder subluxation.
4. Promote nutrition.
   a. Give positive feedback to patient when progress is made.
   b. Turn patient on back or unaffected side to help swallowing.
   c. Avoid foods that cause choking such as mashed potatoes.
   d. Check affected side of mouth for accumulated food and poor mouth care.
   e. Encourage patient to feed self as soon as possible.
   f. Use dentures if patient has them.

PROMOTING ELIMINATION

The person with paralysis from a UMN or LMN lesion may experience problems with bowel and bladder control. This is discussed in Chapter 63.

PROMOTING ACTIVITIES OF DAILY LIVING

During the acute and rehabilitative phases, patients with paralysis are taught how to carry out ADL to the extent they are able. A variety of self-help devices are available that assist with dressing with one hand, for example. The occupational therapist becomes involved in many of these activities, including homemaking. It is important to stress the concept of the rehabilitative *team* in managing these patients.

PROMOTING PSYCHOLOGIC ADJUSTMENT

The person with paralysis will need assistance in adjusting to the change in the body. The loss of the ability to function independently when paralyzed is traumatic. The person may also have fears about the future and loss of self-esteem. A grief reaction similar to that described for the stages of death and dying may occur. At times, persons may relate to the paralyzed portion of the body as though it were not a part of them. Nursing interventions to help the patient cope with the loss of function and change in body image are essential.

PATIENT TEACHING

Teaching is an extremely important part of caring for the patient with motor problems. Relevant points include the following:
1. Safety needs
   a. Always lock wheelchair when transferring patient.
   b. Check condition of affected eye frequently.
   c. Be aware of placement of affected extremities before movement.
   d. Protect paralyzed limbs from injury.
   e. Stress the importance of wearing well-fitting shoes for ambulation.
2. Skin care
   a. Regular inspection of skin surfaces using mirror or other device as necessary
   b. Need to turn frequently
   c. Need to shift body weight from one position to another
   d. No use of heating pads, hot water bottles, or excessively hot water for bathing
3. Activity needs
   a. ROM exercises
   b. Proper positioning
   c. Frequent changes in position
4. Medications
   a. Use of medication, side effects, dosage, and timing
   b. Importance of reporting side effects to physician
   c. Importance of not combining medication with other mood-altering chemicals
5. Nutrition/diet
   a. Foods that can easily be tolerated
   b. Measures to decrease swallowing difficulty
   c. Use of special appliances to assist with eating
6. ADLs
   a. Teaching techniques of bathing, grooming, and dressing
   b. Importance of having meaningful recreational activities
   c. Bowel and bladder care
7. Other teaching
   a. Importance of good fluid intake
   b. Follow-up care such as where to procure equipment and supplies
   c. Methods of relieving or handling feelings of frustration

ALTERATIONS IN MOVEMENT AND POSTURE

EPIDEMIOLOGY/ETIOLOGY

Various neurologic lesions of the extrapyramidal motor system result in alterations of movement and posture. Clinically, this is seen most often in paralysis agitans, or *parkinsonism.* In this condition there is degeneration of various parts of the basal ganglia. This condition is discussed further in the next chapter. Other conditions that produce alterations in movement and posture include the following:
1. Drug-induced extrapyramidal syndromes
2. Idiopathic dyskinesias and dystonias
3. Huntington's chorea
4. Wilson's disease
5. Myoclonus
6. Tic
7. Cerebral palsy

The reader is referred to a neurologic text for a further description of these disorders.

PREVENTION

As with many of the neurologic diseases, the focus of prevention is on secondary and tertiary care. Because many of these diseases are genetically transmitted, appropriate genetic counseling may prevent their transmission.

CLINICAL MANIFESTATIONS

In contrast to UMN syndrome with the loss of volitional movement and spasticity, in extrapyramidal lesions there is characteristic muscle rigidity, involuntary movements, and bradykinesia without loss of voluntary movement. Muscle rigidity, or *hypertonus,* is present in all muscle groups, both flexor and extensor, but appears to be more prominent in those muscles that maintain a flexed posture. The smaller muscles of the face, tongue, and even the larynx become involved, with consequent difficulty in chewing, swallowing, and speech. The muscles remain continuously or intermittently firm and tense. Hypertonus is present even when the person is relaxed. There is an even or uniform quality to the hypertonus throughout the range of passive movement of a limb. The rigidity is often described as plastic. In addition, a superimposed rhythmic contraction of the muscle may be felt as the joint is moved through its range of motion. This is termed *cogwheel rigidity.*

Strength of muscle is not significantly decreased in bradykinesia. *Bradykinesia,* or *hypokinesia,* refers to slowness rather than lack of movement *(akinesia);* the actual time in carrying out a movement is longer than normal. There is also an extreme poverty of movement. The semiautomatic or habitual movements observed in the normal state, such as putting the hands to the face, folding the arms, or crossing the legs, are absent or greatly reduced. In looking to the side, the eyes move but not the head. In arising from a chair, the necessary adjustments such as putting the feet back and the hands on the arm of the chair are not made, although the person can do it with effort or will. The muscle is not paralyzed or apraxic. Various involuntary movements occur, such as static tremor or pill rolling of the fingers, as seen in parkinsonism; rest tremors that decrease when the limb is used; and chorea, athetosis, and dystonia. In all basal ganglia disorders, stress and nervous tension worsen motor performance; relaxation improves it.

MEDICAL MANAGEMENT

The medical management of motor problems is mainly pharmacologic and aimed at the relief of symptoms. No cures exist for most of the diseases that cause alterations in movement and posture.

NURSING ASSESSMENT

The nursing assessment (subjective and objective data) is the same as that for the patient with motor problems. The nurse should also ask about family members who may have the same symptoms. The reader is referred to the section on motor dysfunction for appropriate nursing diagnoses and patient outcomes.

■ IMPLEMENTATION

Muscle rigidity may be relieved by physical therapy. It is important that the person remain physically active in order to prevent the complications of immobility. It requires a great patience and understanding on the part of the family not to take over physical activities that the individual can perform, even though they will be per-

formed slowly and with much effort. Nursing interventions are planned to assist with feeding problems related to swallowing, with ambulation, and with speech. Often the person with parkinsonism is viewed as unintelligent because of the dysarthria produced by the rigid and bradykinesic muscles of articulation and phonation. Education of the patient and family is a nursing priority. They must understand the need to reduce stress and nervous tension to improve rigidity.

MEDICATIONS

Medications have been found to be very helpful in patients with spasticity. These include the following:
1. Dantrolene
2. Baclofen
3. Diazepam

It is possible to use combinations of drugs at doses low enough to prevent major side effects. With the use of these drugs, it is important to realize that spasticity may be necessary for gait training in the rehabilitation of the patient with a UMN lesion. The rigid legs are necessary for splinting.

OTHER TREATMENT MODALITIES

Other treatments that may be useful in patients with spasticity who do not respond to medications include intrathecal phenol (to alleviate painful spasm in lower extremities), individual peripheral nerve blocks, and physical therapy.

ALTERATIONS IN COMMUNICATION
EPIDEMIOLOGY/ETIOLOGY

Aphasia is a disorder of language caused by damage to the speech-controlling areas of the brain. It is a general term used to describe organic disturbances in language. It includes all areas of language, including speech, reading, writing, and understanding.

Cerebral hemorrhage and cerebral thrombosis are the most common causes of cortical damage, but tumors, multiple sclerosis, and trauma may also lead to aphasia. Aphasia caused by cerebral edema following trauma is usually temporary. Occasionally, a person cannot speak following a CVA because motor function of the vocal cords is affected, not because of damage to cortical speech centers. Defective innervation of the muscles of speech articulation, such as those in the vocal cords, tongue, cheeks, and palate, results in *dysarthria.*[6,7]

PREVENTION

Because many patients who suffer a CVA also experience aphasia or dysphasia, the elements concerning prevention of CVAs also apply here. The reader is referred to Chapter 63 for a discussion of these factors.

CLINICAL MANIFESTATIONS

A variety of abnormalities in communication can occur. The patient may be unable to comprehend the spoken word (*sensory aphasia*) or may comprehend and yet be unable to use the symbols of speech (*motor aphasia*). The patient may have both disorders at the same time (*global aphasia*). Writing may be possible even though speaking is not. Some patients may be able to speak, but the wrong words may be used. There may be a selective loss of words, or the patient may be able to read but be unable to speak or write.

DIAGNOSTIC TESTS

Many sophisticated tests are used to assess the degree and characteristics of a language problem. These are administered by the speech pathologist in most cases. The reader is referred to a more specific text on language and communication disorders for a description of these tests.

MEDICAL MANAGEMENT

The medical management of aphasia and dysphasia usually involves the referral of the person to a speech therapist, who can evaluate the disorder and institute necessary actions.

■ ASSESSMENT

Both objective and subjective information are important factors in assessment of the patient with a language disorder.

SUBJECTIVE DATA

Subjective data include the following:
1. Patient's understanding of problem
2. Other sensory deficits
3. Onset of problem
4. Ability to think clearly

OBJECTIVE DATA

Objective data include the following:
1. Change in level of consciousness
2. Ability to verbalize
3. Ability to write
4. Ability to name objects

Gross tests can be performed to determine what specific language abilities have been lost. These include the following:
1. Spread several familiar objects, such as keys, a pencil, and coins, before the patient.
2. Ask the patient to do the following:
   a. Name each object.
   b. As the nurse names each object, point to it.
   c. Write the name of each object as it is pointed to.
   d. Write the name of each object as it is stated aloud.
   e. When shown a card containing the printed name of each object, read the word aloud and point to the object.

■ DATA ANALYSIS: NURSING DIAGNOSES

Nursing diagnoses are determined from assessment of patient data. Possible nursing diagnoses for the person with alterations in communication include, but are not limited to, the following:

Diagnostic Title	Possible Etiologies
Communication, impaired verbal	Aphasia
Coping, ineffective individual	Personal vulnerability
Knowledge deficit: alternate ways to communicate	Lack of exposure, unfamiliarity with information sources

■ PLANNING: EXPECTED PATIENT OUTCOMES

Expected patient outcomes for the person with alterations in communication may include, but are not limited to, the following:
1. Patient demonstrates the ability to communicate within the constraints of the disease process.
2. Patient is able to communicate more effectively.
3. Compensatory techniques are used to aid communication.
4. Patient can state how to obtain assistance from community resources.
5. Patient can state plans for follow-up care.

■ IMPLEMENTATION

Each person reacts to language problems differently. Most persons with aphasia become tense and anxious. They may be irritable and emotionally upset because they are unable to evoke the words they need, and they become discouraged easily in their efforts to speak. Some may quickly refuse to attempt to communicate; others feel ashamed and withdraw from people, including their family and close friends. Yet desire to communicate and persistence in efforts to do so are the essential ingredients in speech rehabilitation.

Care is taken to reduce tension so that patients with aphasia can make satisfactory adjustments to their loss. The environment should be relatively free of excess stimuli. These patients are not deaf, and they should be spoken to in a normal voice. Procedures are explained to them in the same manner as that used with other patients. Recreational activities should be soothing and nonstimulating. Music is often relaxing, and some patients enjoy listening to the radio. If the patient is able to read and comprehend the written captions, watching television may be gratifying. Some patients do not enjoy listening to the radio or watching television when they cannot follow what is going on. Being alert to patients' facial expressions often gives clues to the activities that are most satisfying.

Specific interventions are based on whether the patient's aphasia is primarily one of *comprehension* or *expression*. Some approaches for patients with comprehension deficits are (1) to keep distractions to a minimum (that is, clear the patient's visual field of extraneous stimuli before initiating conversation), (2) to face the patient when speaking and speak simply and slowly, and (3) if the patient miscomprehends the message, to slow down the rate of speech and reword the message, using gestures to emphasize points. If the message is still not comprehended, go on to another topic after supplying the correct response.

Although the nurse does not initiate the formal speech therapy program with the patient, the nurse's cooperation is needed to reinforce the program. As the nurse cares for the patient, common objects should be named; the patient should be encouraged to handle them, to speak their names, and to write or copy their names. The family can supply these words and others that are particularly important for the patient. Speech retraining should be done for short periods because it is exceedingly trying, and fatigue tends to increase difficulty in speaking. Praising patients for each small improvement and encouraging them to take their mistakes good-naturedly helps to make this difficult problem more bearable. A patient's progress in language retraining will depend on the level of intelligence, the age (older patients have more difficulty), the severity of the damage, and whether the brain lesion is progressive. Complete language rehabilitation may require months of painstaking work on the part of skilled pathologists.* *A Guide to Clinical Services in Speech Pathology and Audiology*† lists clinics in the United States where speech and hearing services are available. Some of these clinics offer specialized help to persons with aphasia and dysphasia.

PATIENT TEACHING

The patient should be helped to understand that speech may be relearned. In the interim, gestures, pointing to objects, pointing to pictures or words on communication boards, or writing may be used to improve communication. After the most effective approach to communication is selected, it is shared with all who interact with the patient, including the family and other members of the health team.

---

*Some institutions that specialize in working with patients who have aphasia are ICD Rehabilitation and Research Center, New York, NY; The Institute of Logopedics, Wichita, Kan; and Vanderbilt University Hospital Clinic, Nashville, Tenn.
†American Speech-Language-Hearing Association, 10801 Rockville Pike, Rockville, MD 20852.

ALTERATIONS IN SENSORY AND PERCEPTUAL FUNCTION

ETIOLOGY/PATHOPHYSIOLOGY

The presence of a lesion anywhere within the sensory system pathways, from the receptor to the sensory cortex, alters the transmission or perception of sensory information. The parietal lobe cortex is of major importance for interpretation of sensation with the exception of sight, hearing, smell, taste, and thermoregulation. A loss, decrease, or increase in the sensation of pain, temperature, touch, and proprioception, singly or in combination, results in difficult problems in daily living for the person. Since these sensations normally help the person to be aware of alterations in the internal and external environments, any alteration in sensibility lessens the ability to be completely and accurately protected. As a consequence, there is a need to adapt to the alteration and plan for safety and comfort.

Some specific losses deserve to be mentioned. The loss of *proprioception,* or the ability to know the position of the body and its parts without looking directly at the part, is a serious loss that requires considerable adaptation. Lack of control of body temperature, or *hyperthermia,* occurs because of a malfunction in the thermoregulatory center in the brain, such as occurs following brain surgery near the hypothalamus or from head injury, brain tumors, and other cranial conditions. Hyperthermia is believed to occur as a result of hypoxia of the thermoregulatory center. Persons also often complain of *dysesthesia* or *paresthesia* (abnormalities of the sensation of touch). These are typically associated with peripheral neuropathies.

CLINICAL MANIFESTATIONS

SENSORY LOSSES

Figure 62-9 presents common patterns of sensory alteration. A cerebral lesion results in various alterations in sensation *contralateral* to the lesion. This distribution results from all sensory fibers having decussated before reaching the sensory cortex of the cerebrum. On the other hand, *transection* of the spinal cord results in total *bilateral* sensory loss distal to the lesion, since *all* pathways have been severed. Note, however, the characteristic distribution of deficits associated with hemisection of the cord (Brown-Séquard syndrome). In this situation the person experiences *ipsilateral* loss of proprioception and vibratory sense because the posterior columns decussate in the medulla. *Contralateral* loss of pain, temperature, and crude touch sensation results because the spinothalamic tracts decussate in the cord.

PERCEPTUAL PROBLEMS

Apraxia and agnosia are perceptual deficits that occur quite often in neurologic conditions (see Chapter 59 for

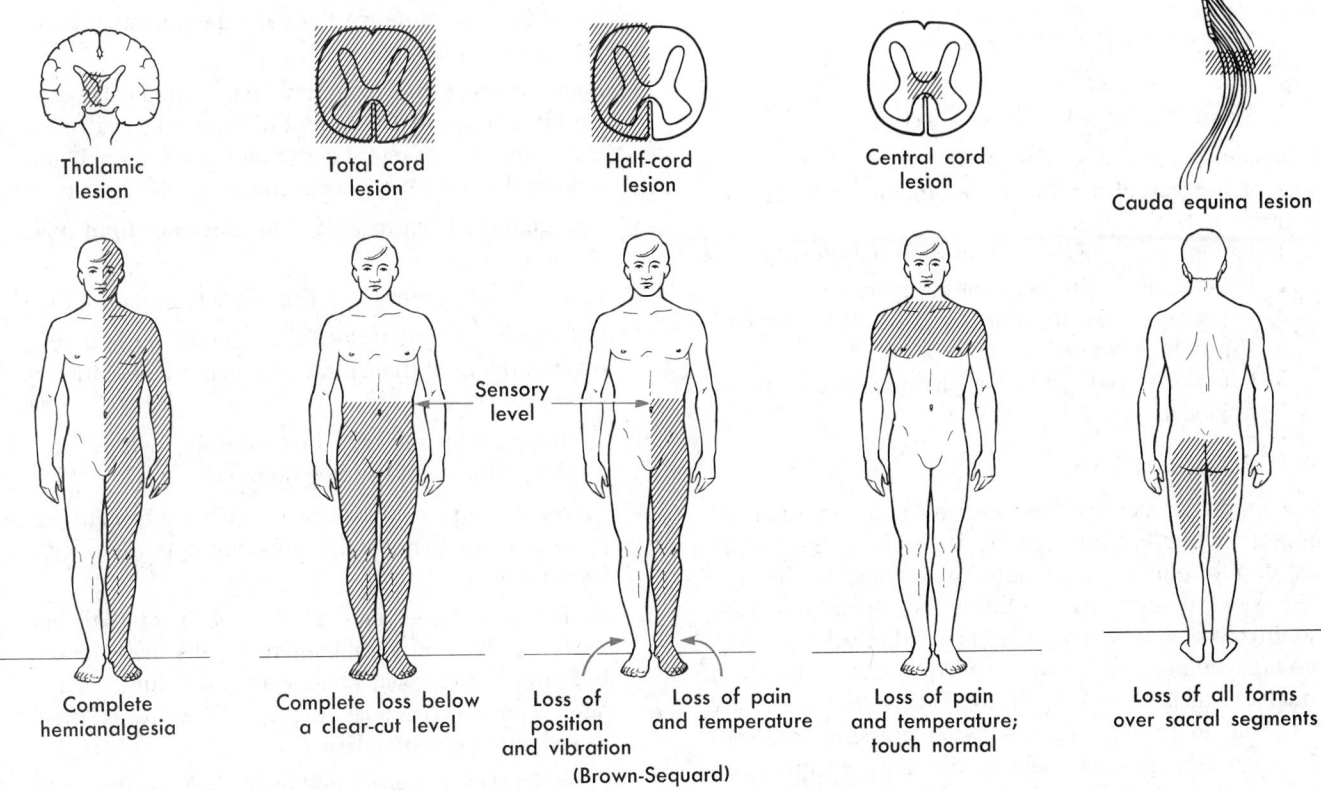

FIGURE 62-9 Common patterns of sensory abnormality. Upper diagrams show site of lesion; lower diagrams show distribution of corresponding sensory loss. (Modified from Bickerstaff ER: Neurology for nurses, ed 2, London, 1971, English Universities Press Ltd, and Hodder & Stoughton Ltd.)

details). They may occur in association with each other or separately. Research concerning perceptual problems is still in the early stages. Even though the perceptual deficits and their corresponding lesion sites have been described in the literature, the clinician is still concerned about to how to rehabilitate the person.

■ ASSESSMENT

The sensory and perceptual parts of the neurologic examination are the most difficult.

SUBJECTIVE DATA

Subjective data include the following:
1. Patient's understanding of the problem
2. Measures that relieve symptoms, including medications
3. Site of sensory abnormality
4. Onset of problem
5. Presence of associated symptoms
6. Alteration in sensation
   a. Pain
   b. Temperature
   c. Touch
   d. Proprioception
   e. Stereognosis

OBJECTIVE DATA

Objective data include the following:
1. Ability to perform purposeful movements in the absence of loss of motor power, sensation, or coordination
2. Ability to recognize familiar objects

■ DATA ANALYSIS: NURSING DIAGNOSES

Nursing diagnoses are determined from assessment of patient data. Possible nursing diagnoses for the person with a sensory or perceptual alteration include, but are not limited to, the following:

Diagnostic Title	Possible Etiologies
Injury, potential for	Sensory/motor deficits, lack of awareness of environmental hazards
Knowledge deficit: prevention of injury	Lack of exposure, unfamiliarity with information sources

Diagnostic Title	Possible Etiologies
Sensory/perceptual alterations: visual, tactile	Altered sensory reception/ integration

■ PLANNING: EXPECTED PATIENT OUTCOMES

Expected patient outcomes for the person with a sensory or perceptual alteration may include, but are not limited to, the following:

1. Patient can explain the nature of the disorder.
2. Patient can compensate for alterations.
3. Patient can explain safety factors to be observed.
4. Injury is prevented.
5. Patient can state plans for follow-up care with professionals.

■ IMPLEMENTATION

Once the alteration has been clearly identified, the most important nursing intervention is teaching the person and family protective measures in relation to the sensory deficit or alteration. Teaching the person to use the noninvolved senses more helps to avoid injuries. For example, teaching the person with hypoesthesia (lessened touch) to inspect visually involved body parts regularly will help to prevent injuries. Some nursing interventions, such as in hyperthermia, are more complex and require life-saving measures.

CHAPTER SUMMARY

✔ Headache is a typical symptom experienced by many persons that varies in degree of severity from relative unimportance to serious prognosis.

✔ Headache can be divided into three categories: vascular (includes migraine), tension, and a combination of vascular and tension.

✔ The influence of heredity is high with migraine headaches.

✔ Identification of triggering factors may help prevent headache.

✔ Prevention of migraine headaches may include the avoidance of certain foods, such as chocolate, nuts, and onions.

✔ Headache pain arises from the scalp, its blood vessels and muscles, from the dura mater and its venous sinuses, and from the blood vessels at the base of the brain.

✔ The aura that occurs before an acute migraine attack may include visual field defects, confusion, paresthesias, and in extreme cases paralysis.

✔ With cluster headaches the pain episodes are clustered or spaced together in quick succession for a few days or months with relatively long remissions that may last for months.

✔ The experience of pain is an individual matter, and many factors influence the patient's perception and expression of pain.

✔ Pain receptors may be activated by cellular damage, certain chemicals (including histamine), heat, ischemia, muscle spasm, or sensations of heat, cold, and itching that go beyond a specific level of intensity.

✔ The quality of neurogenic pain may vary from mild to excruciating.

✔ Referred pain occurs in a site other than its origin.

✔ Unbearable pain that does not respond to the definitive treatment of the causative lesion is called intractable.

✔ Techniques to relieve pain surgically include neurectomy, rhizotomy, and cordotomy.

✔ Increased intracranial pressure (ICP) is a complex manifestation that results from multiple neurologic conditions.

✔ An increase in the volume of any of the cranial contents, singly or in combination, results in increased ICP and a reciprocal change in the volume of the other contents because the cranial vault is rigid, closed, and nonexpandable.

✔ Prevention of increased ICP involves the early detection of signs and symptoms so that corrective actions can be instituted.

✔ One of the first symptoms of increased ICP is a decreasing level of consciousness.

✔ Slowing of the pulse rate in conjunction with a rising systolic blood pressure is a significant observation related to increased ICP.

✔ The medical treatment of increased ICP depends on the underlying cause.

✔ Rapidly rising ICP must be relieved by mechanical decompression.

✔ Damage to the nervous system often causes serious problems in mobility.

✔ Injury or disease of motor neurons and their extensions at any level results in alterations of muscle strength, tone, and reflex activity.

✔ Lower motor neurons (LMNs) consist of large anterior horn cells located in the anterior gray matter of the spinal cord, whereas upper motor neurons (UMNs) originate in the motor strip of the cerebral cortex and in multiple brainstem nuclei.

✔ Patients experiencing ongoing problems with spasticity may be treated with on one or more skeletal muscle relaxants to decrease muscle tone and involuntary movements.

✔ In persons with paralysis, the joints become flexed

and fixed in useless positions with resulting deformity unless the nurse takes preventive measures.

✔ Aphasia is a disorder of language (speech, reading, writing, understanding) caused by damage to the speech-controlling areas of the brain.

QUESTIONS TO CONSIDER

- What characteristics indicate that a headache is psychologic?

- What questions are important to ask a patient experiencing pain?

- What nursing measures increase intracranial pressure?

- How do you differentiate between an upper motor neuron lesion and a lower motor neuron lesion?

- How would you respond to another staff member who says, "Just leave him alone; after all, he's paralyzed and won't know if we turn him"?

REFERENCES AND SELECTED READINGS

1. Adams R and Victor M: Principles of neurology, New York, 1985, McGraw-Hill Book Co.
2. Anderson M: Assessment under pressure, when your patient says "my head hurts," Nursing '84 14:34-42, 1984.
3. Baggerly J: Epidural catheters for pain management: the nurse's role, J Neurosci Nurs 18:290-295, 1986.
4. *Belt L: Working with dysphasic patients, Am J Nurs 74:848-851, 1974.
5. Boortz-Marx R: Factors affecting intracranial pressure: a descriptive study, J Neurosurg Nurs 17:89-94, 1985.
6. *Boss B: Dysphasia, dyspraxia and dysarthria: distinguishing features. Part I, J Neurosurg Nurs 16:151-160, 1984.
7. *Boss B: Dysphasia, dyspraxia, and dysarthria: distinguishing factors. Part II, J Neurosurg Nurs 16:211-216, 1984.
8. *Carlson C: Psychological aspects of neurologic disability, Nurs Clin North Am 15:309-320, 1980.
9. Davenport-Fortune P and Dunnum L: Professional nursing care of the patient with increased intracranial pressure: planned or "hit or miss," J Neurosurg Nurs 17:367-370, 1985.
10. Dayhoff N: Rethinking stroke: soft or hard devices to position hands, Am J Nurs 75:1142-1144, 1975.
11. Haight K: What you should know about epidural analgesia, Nursing '87 17(9):58-59, 1987.
12. *Hendrickson S: Psychological care of the patient with neurological dysfunction, J Neurosurg Nurs 16:202-207, 1984.
13. *Hoskins L: Vascular and tension headaches, Am J Nurs 74:848-851, 1974.
14. Jones S: Glasgow Coma Scale, Am J Nurs 79:1551-1554, 1979.
15. Keller C et al: Psychological responses to aphasia: theoretical considerations and nursing implications, J Neurosci Nurs 21:290-294, 1989.
16. Konikow N: Alterations in movement: nursing assessment and implications, J Neurosurg Nurs 17:61-65, 1985.
17. Lamb S and Barbaro N: Neurosurgical approaches to the management of chronic pain syndromes, Orthop Nurs 6(1):23-29, 1987.
18. Leijon G and Boivie J: Central post-stroke pain—neurological symptoms and pain characteristics, Pain 36:13-25, 1989.
19. Long B and Phipps W: Medical-surgical nursing: a nursing process approach, St Louis, 1989, The CV Mosby Co.
20. McCaffery M and Beebe A: Giving narcotics for pain: a problem solver handbook, Nursing '89 19(10):161-168, 1989.
21. *Mitchell P: Intracranial hypertension: implication of research for nursing care, J Neurosurg Nurs 12:145-154, 1980.
22. *Mitchell P and Maus P: Relating of patients' nursing activities to intracranial pressure variation: a pilot study, Nurs Res 27:4-10, 1978.
23. *Mitchell P et al: Moving the patient in bed: effects on increased intracranial pressure, Nurs Res 30:212-218, 1981.
24. Muwaswes M: Increased intracranial pressure and its systemic effects, J Neurosurg Nurs 17:238-243, 1985.
25. *Olson E et al: The hazards of immobility, Am J Nurs 67:779-797, 1967.
26. Pettibone K: Management of spasticity in spinal cord injury: nursing concerns, J Neurosci Nurs 20:217-222, 1988.
27. Rudy E: Advanced neurological and neurosurgical nursing, St Louis, 1984, The CV Mosby Co.
28. Schaefer S: Relieving pain—an analgesic guide, Am J Nurs 88:815-827, 1988.
29. Shiminski-Maher T: Selective posterior rhizotomy in the pediatric cerebral palsy population: implications for nursing practice, J Neurosci Nurs 21:308-312, 1989.
30. *Smith S: Continuous intracranial monitoring: implications and applications for critical care, Crit Care Nurs 3:42-51, 1983.
31. *Snyder M: Relation of nursing activities to increases in intracranial pressure, J Adv Nurs 8:273-279, 1983.
32. *Stuart G et al: Head injury management without intracranial pressure monitoring, J Neurosurg Nurs 59:601-605, 1983.
33. *Terzian M: Neurosurgical intervention for the management of chronic intractable pain, Top Clin Nurs 1:75-88, 1980.
34. Turner H et al: Comparison of nurse and computer recording of ICP in head injured patients, J Neurosci Nurs 20:236-239, 1988.
35. *West B: Understanding endorphins: our natural pain relief system, Nursing '81 11:50-53, 1981.
36. Whitney C and Daroff R: An approach to migraines, J Neurosci Nurs 20:284-289, 1988.
37. Wilton L: Thalamic pain syndrome, J Neurosci Nurs 21:362-365, 1989.
38. *Young M: A bedside guide to understanding the signs of increased intracranial pressure, Nursing '81 11:59-62, 1981.

*References preceded by an asterisk are particularly well suited for student reading.

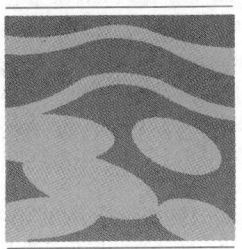

Management of Persons with Neurologic Problems

ELIZABETH A. SCHENK

CHAPTER OBJECTIVES

After studying this chapter, the student should be able to:

1 Define the term *epilepsy*.
2 List at least five causes of seizures.
3 Define the term *aura*.
4 Give examples of at least three different types of seizures.
5 Explain the observations that must be made about a person having a seizure.
6 Define the term *neurologic degenerative disease*.
7 Compare and contrast five neurologic degenerative diseases.
8 List at least six nursing diagnoses for the patient with multiple sclerosis, and describe at least three nursing interventions for each.
9 Describe the difference between myasthenia gravis and the Eaton-Lambert syndrome, and explain why it is important to make this differentiation.
10 Define the term *catastrophic reaction* as related to patients with Alzheimer's disease.
11 Describe the stages of Alzheimer's disease.
12 Differentiate between the causes of a cerebrovascular accident (CVA).
13 Explain the importance of rehabilitation for the patient who has had a CVA.
14 Explain how the nurse will know that function is beginning to return in a patient who has had a CVA.
15 List at least three infections that may occur in the nervous system.
16 Define the following terms in relation to craniocerebral trauma: contusion, coup, contrecoup, concussion, and laceration.
17 Explain why the extent of the original injury does not always indicate the degree of damage to the brain.
18 List at least three diagnostic tests that may be used to rule out head injury.
19 Explain the difference between an incomplete and complete spinal cord injury.
20 Explain the term *spinal shock*.
21 Describe the motor losses with cervical, thoracic, lumbar, and sacral levels of spinal cord injury.
22 List at least three symptoms of autonomic dysreflexia, and give examples of at least four nursing interventions in this emergency situation.
23 List at least three different types of intracranial tumors.

24 Discuss the preoperative and postoperative care of the patient undergoing a craniotomy.
25 List at least two complications that may occur as a result of brain surgery.
26 Explain why patients with AIDS often manifest neurologic symptoms, and list the possible causative agents.

The neurologic problems that have been selected for inclusion in this chapter are the ones most closely associated with the typical neurologic manifestations presented in Chapter 62.

CONVULSIVE DISORDERS: EPILEPSY

EPIDEMIOLOGY

Epilepsy (convulsive disorders) is one of the oldest diseases known to humans. It was described in detail by Hippocrates, as well as being described in the Bible. It has come to be defined as "seizure" or "cetate." For purposes of this chapter, the terms *epilepsy, seizure disorder,* and *convulsive disorder* are used interchangeably.

At one time epilepsy was thought to be of divine origin, and perhaps for this reason it has been linked in the public mind with the occult, the strange, and the unmentionable. No disease has been more carefully concealed within families, and many attitudes toward the disease have persisted from early times to the present. Attitudes may also be affected by the following:

1. The frightening experience of seeing a person during a severe seizure
2. The belief that mental deterioration occurs with epilepsy
3. The tendency to develop epilepsy possibly being inherited

The incidence of epilepsy is believed to be one in every 200 to 300 persons. This means that more than 1 million persons in the United States are subject to seizures. Seizures occur in all races and affect males and females equally. There seems to be no geographic distribution.

Epilepsy can begin at any age, but many persons have seizures before 20 years of age. The life expectancy of persons with seizures is somewhat less than that for the population as a whole, because these persons may die of an injury accidentally incurred during a seizure.

ETIOLOGY

Epilepsy may be defined as a transitory disturbance in consciousness or in motor, sensory, or autonomic function with or without loss of consciousness. Seizures are caused by uncontrolled electrical discharges in the brain. Seizures as a sign and symptom are of particular importance in neurologic diseases. Causes may include the following:

1. Cerebral anoxia
2. Hypoglycemia
3. Disturbance of calcium balance
4. Disturbance in hydration
5. Ingestion of drugs and poisons
6. Numerous metabolic disturbances and disorders
7. Infections that cause high temperature elevations
8. Electrolyte imbalances
9. Generalized inflammatory processes
10. Degenerative tissue disorders
11. Hysteria

In many patients with epilepsy, a localized organic lesion serves as the focus for the abnormal neuronal discharges from the damaged brain tissue. Often the lesion is microscopic in size. These organic lesions include the following:

1. Neoplasms
2. Inflamed areas or abscesses
3. Sclerosis
4. Vascular formations or hematomas
5. Congenital malformations
6. Trauma
7. Other space-occupying lesions

The role of heredity in the causation of epilepsy has not been completely clarified. The disease is not directly inherited, although abnormal brain waves, as shown on the electroencephalogram (EEG), are found in many relatives of persons who have seizures.

PATHOPHYSIOLOGY

Convulsions or seizures are brief cerebral storms. These are associated with sudden, excessive, and disorderly electrical discharges in the neurons of the brain. The patterns or forms of seizures vary and depend on the area of the brain from which the seizure arises. The pattern is stereotyped in the individual, although variations may occur with progression of the cerebral lesion. Seizures can involve essentially all parts of the brain at once, as in the generalized type, or only a minute focal spot.

In the generalized type, the excessive neuronal discharges are thought to originate in the brainstem portion of the reticular activating system (RAS); these then spread throughout the central nervous system (CNS) including the cortex and the deeper parts of the brain. The process may last from a few seconds to as long as 3 to 5 minutes, or it may stop immediately, as in a *petit mal seizure*. It is not known what stops the seizure at a given time, but it is believed to result from fatigue of the neurons involved in precipitating the seizure or by inhibition of certain structures within the brain. Focally, the excessive neuronal discharges may result in a *tonic convulsion,* with the contraction of all muscles at once, or a *clonic convulsion,* with alternate contraction and relaxation of opposing muscle groups and characteristic jerking movements of the body.

The seizure, regardless of origin or type, is always inappropriate to the immediate situation. It is followed by an inhibition of cerebral function, the length of which may last longer than the seizure itself. The inhibition of function is often incomplete and depends on the area of the brain from which the seizure arises.

CLINICAL MANIFESTATIONS

There are numerous ways to classify seizures. One frequently used method is the International Classification of Epileptic Seizures, which identifies them as partial, generalized, unilateral, or unclassified.

Most experts find it useful to classify seizures according to the clinical features. In this schema the following five groups can be identified:

1. Grand mal (major or generalized)
2. Petit mal
3. Psychomotor
4. Jacksonian, or focal
5. Miscellaneous

Table 63-1 shows the characteristics of each type of seizure.

TYPES OF SEIZURES

Grand Mal Seizures

The grand mal seizure is by far the most common and dramatic type. It is generalized and characterized by a loss of consciousness for several minutes and tonic and clonic convulsions. The seizures follow a typical course that includes the aura, cry, loss of consciousness, the fall, tonic and clonic convulsions, and incontinence.

Aura. The symptoms that occur during the prodrome are called an aura. Prodromal symptoms occur in about 50% of all patients and usually include a change in sensation or a change in affect. The exact character of the aura varies from person to person but may include any of the following:

1. Numbness

TABLE 63-1 Characteristics of seizures

Type of Seizure	Etiology	Characteristics	Clinical Signs	Aura	Postictal Period
Grand mal	Most common	Generalized, characterized by loss of consciousness for several minutes	Aura Cry Loss of consciousness Fall Tonic-clonic movements Incontinence	Present Flashing lights Smells Spots before eyes Dizziness	Present Need for sleep for 1 to 2 hours Headache common
Petit mal	Usually occurs during childhood and adolescence Frequency decreases as child gets older	Sudden impairment in or loss of consciousness with little or no tonic-clonic movement Occurs without warning Has tendency to appear a few hours after arising or when person is quiet	Sudden vacant facial expression with eyes focused straight ahead All motor activity ceases except perhaps for slight symmetric twitching about eyelids Possible loss of muscle tone Consciousness returns	Not present	Not present
Psychomotor	Occurs at any age	Sudden change in awareness associated with complex distortion of feeling and thinking and partially coordinated motor activity Longer than petit mal	Behaves as if partially conscious Often appears intoxicated May perform antisocial acts such as exposing self or carrying out violent acts Autonomic complaints may occur Chest pain Respiratory distress Tachycardia Gastrointestinal distress Urinary incontinence	Present Complex hallucinations or illusions	Present Confusion Amnesia Need for sleep
Jacksonian, or focal	Occurs almost entirely in patients with structural brain disease	Depends on site of focus May or may not be progressive	Typically begins in hand, foot, or face May end in grand mal seizure	Present Numbness Tingling Crawling feeling	Present
Myoclonic	May antedate grand mal by months or years	May be very mild or may cause rapid, forceful movements	Sudden involuntary contraction of muscle group, usually in extremities or trunk No loss of consciousness	Not present	Not present
Akinetic	Uncommon	Peculiar generalized tonelessness	Person falls in flaccid state Unconscious for 1 or 2 minutes	Rarely present	Not present

2. Flashing lights
3. Dizziness
4. Tingling of the arm
5. Smells
6. Spots before the eyes

The patient may find it difficult to describe the aura precisely, but it gives warning of the actual seizure activity. This serves a useful purpose in that it allows the person to seek safety and privacy before the onset of the seizure. Occasionally the aura occurs as much as a day before the actual seizure. The aura represents the local "signature" of the attack and is the result of an abnormal stimulation of the cortical area.

Almost at the same time that loss of consciousness occurs there is the so-called epileptic cry. It is caused by the spasm of the thoracic and abdominal muscles, which expels air through the glottis. Another type of cry results from an inspiratory effort. The loss of consciousness is sudden and variable in duration. It usually lasts several minutes.

The individual slumps or falls, depending on his or her position at the time. This is followed immediately by bilateral *tonic contraction* of all muscles: the legs are extended and the arms are flexed; the jaw is clenched and the tongue is frequently caught between the teeth; the eyes roll upward and pupils dilate and become fixed. Respiration ceases and cyanosis occurs. The tonic spasms may occasionally be so violent that a joint, such as the shoulder, hip, or temporomandibular, is dislocated. Fractures may also result. As the tonic phase ends, it is replaced by a series of *clonic contractions*. As the clonic movements continue, the contractions become stronger. Breathing returns and is shallow and irregular at first. There is often frothing at the mouth, which may be streaked with blood if the tongue and lips have been bitten during the convulsion. Fecal or urinary incontinence often occurs during the clonic phase or earlier. As the clonic phase subsides, within a few minutes the muscles relax, Partial consciousness is regained and color improves.

During the *postictal period* (postseizure) the individual appears groggy and confused. Complaints of headache or muscular pain are common. A deep sleep usually follows. During this phase the pupils may remain dilated and abnormal plantar reflexes may occur. After a variable period the patient awakens and is frequently unaware of the occurrence of the seizure. A dull headache and depression are common. The depression may be caused in part by knowledge that a seizure has occurred.

General fatigue may last 1 or 2 days. In addition to the injuries that may occur, the violent activity during a grand mal seizure may result in ruptures of blood vessels with the production of corneal and subconjunctival hemorrhages.

Seizures occur during sleep in some individuals. In such instances the occurrence of the seizure is recognized on awakening by the presence of blood on the pillow or by soiled linen resulting from fecal or urinary incontinence.

Petit Mal Seizures

Petit mal seizures are characterized by a sudden impairment in or loss of consciousness with little or no tonic-clonic movement. They usually occur without warning, and the arrest of voluntary activity is very brief, usually 10 to 20 seconds. The attacks have a tendency to appear a few hours after arising or when the person is quiet. In the classic petit mal seizure there is a sudden vacant facial expression with the eyes focused straight ahead. All motor activities cease except perhaps for a slight symmetric twitching about the eyelids or of the face and arms, or a loss of muscle tone. Consciousness returns as quickly as it left, and the individual may resume speaking at the point interrupted, unaware that the seizure occurred. The individual may learn to recognize when a few seconds of time have been lost. Petit mal seizures usually occur many times a day and have no aura, falling, or tonic and clonic phases.

This type of seizure usually occurs during childhood and adolescence, particularly at puberty. The frequency of the episodes usually diminishes as the child grows older. Although petit mal seizures do not have the dramatic and frightening aspects of grand mal seizures, they are disconcerting, and the momentary loss of consciousness presents safety problems.

Psychomotor Seizures

Psychomotor seizures are more complex and bizarre than either grand mal or petit mal seizures. They can occur at any age and are characterized by a sudden change in awareness or consciousness, associated with a complex distortion of feeling and thinking and partially coordinated motor activity. Any aura present is usually a complex hallucination or illusion. The length of the seizure is longer than that of petit mal. Persons with these seizures often behave as though they were partially conscious and perform antisocial acts such as exposing themselves or committing acts of violence. They often appear intoxicated. Talking with them during this type of seizure shows that they are out of contact with their environment. Smacking of the lips and chewing movements may take place. Visceral symptoms with autonomic complaints of chest pain, respiratory distress, tachycardia, urinary incontinence, and gastrointestinal distress may also occur. Abnormal smell and taste sensations are common.

These persons are likely to be confused and amnesic for a time and often fall asleep at the end of the seizure activity. A relationship has been found between psychomotor epilepsy and lesions in the temporal lobe of the brain. Because of the crimes that may occur during this type of seizure, the diagnosis is of interest not only to physicians but to law enforcement officials, lawyers, and judges as well.

Focal, or Jacksonian, Seizures

Focal, or jacksonian, seizures arise initially in the motor or sensory areas of the brain adjacent to the rolandic fissure or any localized part of the cerebral cortex. These seizures occur almost entirely in patients with structural brain disease and often occur as a symptom in persons with brain tumor, vascular malformations, scars, or infections. The clinical manifestations seen in this type of seizure thus depend on the site of the focus and differ from the generalized motor seizure (grand mal). If, for example, the abnormal neuronal discharge is initiated in the *precentral,* or *motor region* of the cortex for the thumb, the individual will experience a tonic contracture of the thumb muscles. If the abnormal neuronal discharge spreads to adjacent parts of the motor strip, there is progressive involvement of associated musculature with a progression (march) of movements from thumb to hand, arm, face, and so forth. The discharge may or may not progress. The localized seizure that does spread progressively to other muscles following initiation is known as a *jacksonian seizure.*

Focal motor seizures typically begin in the hand, face, and foot but may arise in any part of the motor strip. The seizure may end in a shower of clonic movements, or it may end in a generalized convulsion. Consciousness is retained unless the opposite half of the body is involved. When abnormal neuronal discharges arise in the lower part of the motor strip, which controls salivation and mastication, seizures are then manifested by chewing, smacking of the lips, and swallowing movements. Salivation may be profuse. Other seizures may begin with a forced turning of the head and eyes. Such attacks are termed *adversive* and originate in the eye-turning fields of the brain; the head turns away from the side of the lesion, or focus. When the abnormal neuronal discharges arise in the *postcentral,* or *sensory, strip* of the cortex, the seizure is initiated with complaints of disturbed sensations such as a numbness, tingling, prickling, or crawling feeling. As in a focal motor seizure, a march of sensations may or may not occur. The neuronal discharge may also spread from the sensory area to the motor area.

Miscellaneous Seizures

The category of miscellaneous seizures includes many different types, two of which are described here.

Myoclonic seizures. Myoclonic seizures are characterized by the sudden involuntary contraction of a muscle group, usually in the extremities or trunk. These contractions may be very mild, or they may result in rapid, forceful movement of the part. No loss of consciousness occurs. Some experts see myoclonus as a variant of petit mal seizures. The myoclonus may be found in some petit mal conditions. Myoclonus will sometimes antedate grand mal seizures by months or years.

Akinetic seizures. Akinetic seizures are characterized by a peculiar generalized tonelessness. An aura rarely occurs, but the person falls in a flaccid state and is unconscious for a moment or two. Recovery comes quickly, and the person is not postictal.

Status Epilepticus

When recurrent generalized seizure activity occurs with such frequency that full consciousness is not regained between seizures, it is referred to as status epilepticus. Although this condition is relatively rare, it can lead to death from brain damage secondary to prolonged hypoxia and exhaustion. *Status epilepticus is a medical emergency requiring intensive medical and nursing care.*

The person with status epilepticus is often in a coma for 12 to 24 hours or longer, during which time recurring seizures occur. The seizures may cease spontaneously with return of consciousness, or death may result from the repeated attacks. The attack usually is related to failure to take prescribed medication.

DIAGNOSTIC TESTS

By far the most common test used to evaluate seizure activity is the EEG. It is a safe and noninvasive test that allows for more specific diagnosis. It may be done with the patient in a sleep-deprived state. See Chapter 59 for a description of this test.

MEDICAL MANAGEMENT

Medical management of the patient with a seizure disorder is usually pharmocologic. Surgical treatment of seizures is done less frequently but may still be used in some cases when medical therapy is not effective.[17] *Cortical resection* is one surgical approach. It involves removal of the brain tissue where the focus of electrical discharge is located. The localization of tissue must occur in a part of the brain that is easily accessible to surgery or that can be removed without leaving the person with a serious disability. A *temporal lobectomy* is the most common resection. Data have shown a cure from seizure activity or a drastic reduction in the number of seizures in 60% to 90% of patients undergoing this procedure.[17]

A *corpus callostomy* is sometimes used. This procedure was first performed in the 1930s after it was observed that patients who suffered a CVA of the corpus callosum had fewer seizures. A *hemispherectomy* has been done in children with unilateral hemispheric disease and refractory epilepsy. Although often associated with significant morbidity, it has been found to improve the quality of life for some children.[17]

Another surgical approach involves *stereotactic* procedures with the use of electrical stimulation. This technique is used in an attempt to interrupt the pathways of seizure activity, to destroy the foci, or to alter the actions of the cortical nerve cells.

■ ASSESSMENT

Both subjective and objective data are important to assess with the patient with seizures.

SUBJECTIVE DATA

The following subjective data should be obtained from the patient with seizures:
1. Understanding of the seizure disorder and what may be causing it
2. Awareness of precipitating factors
3. Presence of aura
4. Postictal feelings

OBJECTIVE DATA

The following objective data should be ascertained:
1. Number of seizures occurring within a specific time
2. Behavior: signs of stress or fatigue

OBSERVATIONS TO BE MADE ABOUT A PERSON HAVING A SEIZURE

Aura	Presence or absence, nature of if present; ability of patient to describe it (somatic, visceral, psychic)
Cry	Presence or absence
Onset	Site of initial body movements, deviation of head and eyes, chewing and salivation, posture of body, sensory changes
Tonic and clonic phases	Movements of body as to progression, skin color and airway, pupillary changes, incontinence, duration of each phase
Relaxation (sleep)	Duration and behavior
Postictal phase	Duration, general behavior, ability to remember anything about the seizure, orientation, pupillary changes, headache, injuries present
Duration of entire seizure	
Level of consciousness	Length of unconsciousness if present

---

3. Results of EEG
4. Character of seizures (see the box below for observations to be made about a person having a seizure)

■ DATA ANALYSIS: NURSING DIAGNOSES

Nursing diagnoses are determined from assessment of patient data. Possible nursing diagnoses for the person with seizures include, but are not limited to, the following:

Diagnostic Title	Possible Etiologies
Adjustment, impaired	Disability requiring change in life-style
Aspiration, potential for	Decreased consciousness
Injury, potential for	Sensory/motor deficits
Knowledge deficit: cause of seizures and care needed	Lack of exposure to information

■ PLANNING: EXPECTED PATIENT OUTCOMES

Expected patient outcomes for the person with seizures may include, but are not limited to, the following:
1. Seizures are reduced or at least do not increase in severity or number.
2. Injury is prevented.
3. Aspiration does not occur.
4. Patient can explain any medications to be taken or treatment program to be carried out at home.
   a. Action, side effects, toxic effects, and dosage schedule for each anticonvulsant drug
   b. Importance of taking medication even though seizure free
   c. Need to seek medical assistance if side effects occur
   d. Incompatability of anticonvulsant drugs with alcohol and other drugs that counteract the anticonvulsants
5. Patient can explain schedule to carry out activities of daily living (ADLs) that includes a balance between rest and activity and avoidance of excesses in exercise, stress, or fatigue.
6. Patient can explain how to secure professional and community resources.
7. Patient will state plans for follow-up care.
8. Patient's significant others can demonstrate precautions to be followed during and after a seizure.

■ IMPLEMENTATION
PREVENTIVE CARE

Primary prevention of epilepsy is limited. Preventing problems such as electrolyte imbalances or other causes previously listed can prevent some seizures. Secondary prevention or early diagnosis is important, especially with the adult who experiences a first seizure after age 21 years. This almost always heralds an organic lesion that needs prompt attention.

ACUTE CARE

Status Epilepticus

With status epilepticus, vigorous therapy is directed toward arrest of the seizures. The first priority is ensuring an adequate airway, which may be compromised by the seizure and complications of certain drug therapy. The type of drugs used to stop status epilepticus may lead to pulmonary complications. Drug therapy is given intravenously. Medications used include sodium phenobarbital, diazepam (Valium), phenytoin (Dilantin), and paraldehyde. Optimal results appear to result from large or full (not divided) therapeutic dosages. At times it may be necessary to give a general anesthetic.

Constant monitoring of vital signs is necessary to assess for respiratory depression and cardiac changes. The responsibilities pertaining to the observation and recording of seizure activity are the same as those described in the box at right, top. It may not be possible to note the separate seizure phases because of the frequency of seizures. A safe environment is essential. See the box at right for guidelines for care of the person with status epilepticus.

Care During a Seizure: Potential for Injury

The primary goals of the nurse and the family caring for a patient having a seizure are to protect the person from injury and observe and record the seizure activity. Specific actions are listed in the box at right.

Accurate observation of the seizure from the beginning, when possible, is important because it provides needed information that may assist the physician in locating the site or focus of a cerebral lesion. It is more important to describe the seizure activity and sequence and determine where it started than to name or classify the seizure. See the bottom box at right for relevant research.

Maintaining the Airway

It is important to observe the patient for airway problems, which are sometimes caused by aspiration. If time is available, the nurse should insert an airway before the patient's mouth is clenched. The nurse should never attempt to insert anything into the clenched mouth because injury may result to both patient and nurse.

It may be helpful to position the person on the left side to encourage drainage of any secretions. A suction machine should be kept at the bedside or within easy access to the patient in the hospital. Oxygen may be administered. If the seizure is prolonged, it may be necessary to intubate or assist with ventilation.

Medications

Treatment of patients with a seizure disorder almost always includes the use of one or more of the anticonvulsant drugs (Table 63-2).[53] The choice of medications de-

---

GUIDELINES FOR NURSING INTERVENTIONS FOR PERSONS WITH STATUS EPILEPTICUS

1. Promote oxygenation.
   a. Ensure patent airway.
   b. Prepare for possible need to intubate or assist ventilation.
   c. Oxygenate.
2. Promote cessation of seizures.
   a. Provide quiet and nonstimulating environment.
   b. Give medications as ordered intravenously.
3. Promote safety.
   a. Lower head of bed.
   b. Turn patient to side-lying position.
   c. Put side rails up.
   d. Constantly observe vital signs and neurologic status.

CARE OF THE PERSON DURING A SEIZURE

1. Never leave person alone.
2. If person is standing, lower to floor or bed and move adjacent articles and equipment away to prevent injury.
3. Loosen constrictive clothing, especially around neck.
4. Turn head or body to one side to aid with airway.
5. Do not restrain, either manually or with restraints.
6. Do not pry jaw open to place padded tongue blade. Tongue blade may be inserted between the back teeth early in the seizure, if it can be accomplished before the tonic-clonic movements begin.
7. Pad side rails for patient who is confined to bed or has seizures during sleep. *Pillows should not be used* because of the danger of suffocation.
8. Observe seizure and make relevant recordings.

RESEARCH

Tucker C: Safety assessment for the postictal confusional phase following complex partial seizure, J Neurosurg Nurs 17(3):201-209, 1985.

This study examined the behavior of patients following a complex partial seizure (one in which consciousness is lost). All subjects who suffered seizures (20) were observed in a safe environment for at least 30 minutes following the seizure. They were asked a series of six questions that included orientation questions of name, year, month, day, place, and city. The results indicated that persons who responded to the six questions were safe to leave their rooms following the seizure. ■

TABLE 63-2 Anticonvulsants used to prevent seizures

Drug	Use Related to Seizure Type	Average Daily Dose	Toxic Effects
Phenytoin sodium (Dilantin)	Grand mal, focal, psychomotor	0.4-0.6 g (divided dose)	Ataxia, vomiting, nystagmus, drowsiness, rash, fever, gum hypertrophy, lymphadenopathy
Phenobarbital (Luminal)	Grand mal, focal, psychomotor (adjunctive)	0.1-0.4 g (divided dose)	Drowsiness, rash
Primidone (Mysoline)	Grand mal, focal, psychomotor	0.5-2.0 g	Drowsiness, ataxia
Mephenytoin (Mesantoin)	Grand mal, focal, psychomotor	0.3-0.5 g	Ataxia, nystagmus, pancytopenia, rash
Ethosuximide (Zarontin)	Petit mal, psychomotor, myoclonic, akinetic	750-1500 mg	Drowsiness, nausea, agranulocytosis
Trimethadione (Tridione)	Petit mal	0.3-2.0 g (divided dose)	Rash, photophobia, agranulocytosis, nephrosis
Diazepam (Valium)	Status epilepticus, mixed	8-30 mg	Drowsiness, ataxia
Carbamazepine (Tegretol)	Grand mal, psychomotor	0.3-2.0 g	Rash, drowsiness, ataxia
Valproic acid (Depakene)	Petit mal, absence of seizures	5-35 mg/kg body weight (at least tid dosage)	Nausea, vomiting, indigestion, sedation, emotional disturbance, weakness, altered blood coagulation
Clonazepam (Clonopin)	Petit mal, akinetic, myoclonic	5-20 g	Grand mal seizures, drowsiness, ataxia, hypotension, respiratory depression

pends on the type of seizure. Anticonvulsant medications act on the cerebral cortex generally and are not selective in acting on the part of the brain involved in abnormal neuronal discharges.

The dosages of anticonvulsant drugs are difficult to establish and regulate because of the high incidence of side effects and the toxicity of the drugs. The drug of choice is introduced in an average therapeutic dose and then increased until control of seizures is obtained. If toxicity is reached before control of the seizures, the dose is decreased to the previous nontoxic or tolerated dose. Additional secondary drugs may be introduced at this time to aid in control of the seizures.

Corticosteroids are used occasionally to treat myoclonus. Bromides are used less frequently than in the past and have been largely replaced by the anticonvulsant drugs. Occasionally a ketogenic diet may be prescribed for patients with petit mal seizures. The diet is not easy to follow, and the effectiveness of available medication has led to its decline in use.

Failure to take the prescribed medication or an adequate dose is often the cause of a failed treatment. Blood tests to determine the level of drugs in the blood are helpful to ensure compliance and prevent toxicity.

LONG-TERM CARE

Promoting Adjustment

Because most persons with seizures are without symptoms between attacks and most seizures can be controlled by medication, the person with seizures should be encouraged to lead as normal a life as possible. The person should not be made to feel that he or she is a chronic invalid. With treatment the person can live a useful, normal, and happy life. Until seizures are controlled, the person should avoid dangerous activities such as driving a car, working on or about machinery, or swimming. Once the seizures are controlled with medications and the person has learned the importance of taking the medication regularly and avoiding alcoholic beverages, these restrictions can be relaxed. Achieving adequate rest and maintaining nutritional intake are also important.

The issue of driving a car often poses a problem. Epilepsy is one condition that imposes driver limitations. Usually a waiting period of 1 seizure-free year should elapse before the person is eligible to drive and then *only* if seizures are completely controlled.

No special diet is needed for persons with a seizure disorder, unless mandated by the side effects of medications. The use of alcohol should be avoided, however. The person should be taught the importance of good mouth care if on long-term phenytoin (Dilantin) therapy because gingival hyperplasia is a common side effect.

The individual with seizures should use all resources to cope with feelings of self-consciousness and inferiority resulting from attacks. Adults should be encouraged to lead normal, productive lives. Children should be kept in school unless the frequency of attacks disturbs the activities of the classroom. Family members need to be assisted to discuss their attitudes and feelings about the individual's illness. Excessive attention to the overprotection of the person with seizures is to be avoided.

The family needs to understand the problems resulting from seizures and the prescribed therapy but should not make a chronic invalid of the person.

Public Attitudes

One of the most important aspects in epilepsy therapy is changing the public's attitude toward the disease. The individual subject to seizures and the public must view seizures not as bizarre catastrophies but as relatively normal events that can be dealt with rationally. Many persons with epilepsy lead normal, productive lives. Many outstanding figures in world history had seizures (Julius Caesar, Lord Byron, Napoleon). Studies do not bear out the popular assumption that mental deterioration occurs with epilepsy. Cognitive abilities vary among persons with epilepsy as with the population generally. Also, no evidence exists that personality changes are the result of pathologic processes; when they occur, they are probably the result of society's attitude toward the person with epilepsy. For example, some people who are found to have epilepsy are immediately suspended from their work even when they are not dangerous to themselves or others. Some employers refuse to hire a person with known epilepsy, but at least 80% of all persons with epilepsy are employable.

The Epilepsy Foundation of America has been active in trying to improve state laws regarding employment of persons with epilepsy. Children with epilepsy have been segregated to separate schools, and only recently have some major cities passed laws ensuring children with epilepsy the right to attend the public schools if they are under adequate medical care. In many schools children are barred from the classroom according to the inclination of the teacher. Limitation of environment and of education opportunity often limits the child's knowledge, but this does not mean that learning capacity is poor.

Interest in epilepsy and in the problems of the epileptic person has been increased by various organizations, such as the National Association to Control Epilepsy, Inc.,* National Epilepsy League, Inc.,† Epilepsy Foundation of America,‡ and United Epilepsy Association.§

The care of the person with a seizure disorder is summarized in the box below.

Patient Teaching

Teaching is an important part of the care of the person with seizures. This includes the individual as well as the members of the family who need to learn about care during and after a seizure. Teaching needs to include the following points:

1. Use of medication, including side effects, dose, timing, and reporting side effects to physician
2. Importance of avoiding use of alcohol if taking anticonvulsants
3. Safety measures to avoid injury in case of a seizure
4. Good oral hygiene for persons taking phenytoin (a side effect is gingival hyperplasia)
5. Importance of adequate rest
6. Importance of taking medication even when seizure free
7. Available community resources
8. Restrictions concerning driving
9. Importance of follow-up care

DEGENERATIVE DISEASES

The phrase *degenerative diseases* as used here refers to those neurologic diseases in which there is a premature senescence of nerve cells, is a known or suspected metabolic disturbance exists, or the cause is unknown. See Table 63-3 for a comparison of these degenerative neurologic diseases.

MULTIPLE SCLEROSIS
EPIDEMIOLOGY/ETIOLOGY

Multiple sclerosis is a common neurologic disease in northern climates. The exact prevalence of this disease is not known, because in many instances the diagnosis is not made, but probably at least 250,000 persons in the United States are known to have multiple sclerosis. The onset of symptoms usually occurs between 20 and 40 years of age. The course of the disease estimated to be 12 to 25 years. Multiple sclerosis has serious implications for family life, since it affects both men and

---

CARE OF THE PATIENT WITH A SEIZURE DISORDER

1. Prevent seizures.
   a. Take medication on regular basis.
   b. Avoid alcoholic beverages and other drugs that lower seizure threshold.
   c. Achieve adequate rest.
   d. Eat well-balanced diet.
2. Promote activity.
   a. Until seizures are controlled, avoid dangerous activities.
      (1) Driving car or other vehicle
      (2) Operating machinery
      (3) Swimming
   b. Once seizures are controlled, patient can lead normal life.
3. Promote mental health.
   a. Encourage to lead active life.
   b. Teach family not to overprotect patient.
   c. Patient and family should discuss concerns and feelings openly.

---

*Headquarters: 22 East 67th St, New York, NY 10021.
†Headquarters: 203 Wabash St, Chicago, IL 60604.
‡Headquarters: 1828 L St, NW, Washington, DC 20036.
§Headquarters: 113 West 57th St, New York, NY 10019.

TABLE 63-3 Comparison of neurologic degenerative diseases

Disease	Pathologic Signs	Effect
Multiple sclerosis	Multiple foci (patches) of nerve degeneration throughout brain and spinal cord	Demyelination causes nerve impulse to be interrupted (blocked) or distorted (slowed)
Myasthenia gravis	Decreased secretion of acetylcholine or an increase of cholinesterase enzyme at myoneural junction	Interference of nerve impulse across myoneural junction
Amyotrophic lateral sclerosis	Destruction of myelin sheath of motor neurons of lateral tracts in spinal cord and brain	Demyelination causes nerve impulse to be interrupted (blocked) or distorted (slowed)
Parkinsonism	Destruction of nerve cells of basal ganglia of brain	Decreased dopamine (neurotransmitter substance with anticholinergic effect)
Syringomyelia	Destruction of gray and then white matter of spinal cord by development of "syrinx" (cysts filled with cerebrospinal fluid)	Destruction of nerve pathways in spinal cord—interruption of nerve impulses
Muscular dystrophy	*Not a neurologic disease;* atrophy of voluntary muscles	Effect is a wasting away of the voluntary muscles; no nerve effect
Alzheimer's disease	Degeneration of neurofibrils and presence of plaques in brain	Destruction of neurons leading to impairment in intellectual functioning

women in the active productive years when their responsibilities are greatest. Women are affected twice as often as men. Several studies have demonstrated that an increased incidence of multiple sclerosis seems to occur among siblings and even distant relatives. No evidence has been found to suggest a conjugal relationship.

During the past 15 years, major advances have occurred concerning knowledge of the cause, pathology, diagnosis, and treatment of multiple sclerosis. The cause, however, remains unknown despite new findings and the numerous hypotheses that have been advanced as to cause. Mineral deficiency, toxic substances, disturbance of blood-clotting mechanism, viruses, and autoimmunity are a few of the causes studied. The latter two are currently the most favored. Experimental allergic encephalomyelitis has been produced in animals by the injection of the basic protein from a homologous neuron sheath. Despite the resemblance to multiple sclerosis, it is not yet clear to what extent this disease represents a human model for multiple sclerosis. The recent discovery of slow viruses (those with a long latent period) in association with the frequent findings of an increase of gamma (γ-) globulin and immunoglobulin (IgG) in the spinal fluid of patients with multiple sclerosis gives support to these theories. What constitutes an elevation of γ-globulin or of IgG is not clear. Whether the γ-globulin and IgG get into the spinal fluid by transudation or by increased permeability of the blood-brain barrier is still controversial.

PATHOPHYSIOLOGY

Multiple foci of demyelination are distributed randomly in the white matter of the brainstem, spinal cord, optic nerves, and cerebrum. During the demyelination process (primary degeneration) the myelin sheath and the sheath cells are destroyed, but early sparing of the axon cylinder occurs. The outer myelin sheath in the spinal cord neuronal pathways is often compared with the insulation of an electric wire. Its destruction causes interruption or distortion of the impulse so that it is *slowed* or *blocked*. This type of demyelination differs from that of *wallerian degeneration* in that damage is always primary to the myelin sheath or sheath cells. There is evidence of partial healing in areas of degeneration, which accounts for the transitory nature of early symptoms. In late stages the degeneration may extend to gray areas of the cord and limit healing.

Because of the wide distribution of areas of degeneration, *a greater variety of signs and symptoms in multiple sclerosis occurs than in other neurologic diseases.* The scarring that occurs at the degenerative lesions as well as the increasing number of lesions provides the name *disseminated sclerosis.*

Multiple sclerosis is a *chronic, remitting,* and *relapsing disease* although the clinical course may vary widely. Most people recover from their early episodes. Usually acute exacerbations and remissions may last for a year or more, although eventually exacerbations will recur. There is no record of any patients having recovered from the disease, although many have lived for 20 years or more and have died from other causes. Exacerbations may be aggravated or precipitated by fatigue, chilling, and emotional disturbances. In some cases the disease may terminate in death within a few months of onset. This so-called malignant multiple sclerosis is rare.

CLINICAL MANIFESTATIONS

Early symptoms are usually transitory and may include double vision (*diplopia*), spots before the eyes (*scotomas*), blindness, tremor, weakness or numbness of a body part such as the hand, fatigue, susceptibility to upper respiratory infections, emotional instability, or problems with the bowel or bladder. Many persons with early multiple sclerosis may be considered neurotic by their associates and sometimes by their physicians because of the wide variety and temporary nature of symptoms and because of the person's emotional instability. As the disease progresses, symptoms may include nystagmus, disorders of speech (*scanning*), urinary frequency and urgency, constipation, and changes in muscular coordination and gait. Other symptoms may include urinary incontinence, difficulty in swallowing, severe muscle spasm and contractures, and spastic ataxic gait.

A sense of optimism and well-being (*euphoria*) also seems to be characteristic of persons with multiple sclerosis, especially during remissions. It is suspected that this reaction is largely a result of patients' attempts to reassure themselves that their condition is not so serious. This response is helpful to patients in many ways, but sometimes it may lead them to overdo and thus increase symptoms. This euphoria may also be an indicator of involvement of selected areas of the brain.

Motor signs have upper motor neuron characteristics. Pain is not a common symptom of multiple sclerosis except when there is severe muscle spasm. Death generally is caused by infection, usually developing in the respiratory or genitourinary system.

Diagnostic Tests

Because multiple sclerosis involves multiple parts of the nervous system, is often characterized by exacerbactions and remissions, and frequently includes transient and bizarre signs and symptoms, it is difficult to diagnose with certainty. Because there is no specific diagnostic test, diagnosis is often a clinical judgment. The determination of cerebrospinal fluid (CSF) γ-globulin by chemical or electrophorectic methods or of CSF fluid IgG by electroimmunodiffusion appears to be the most valuable single laboratory test when used with the history and neurologic examination. Testing of *visual-evoked potentials* is now being performed to assess optic nerve integrity. Evidence of early damage has been closely linked with the diagnosis of multiple sclerosis.

MEDICAL MANAGEMENT

The medical management of patients with multiple sclerosis is mainly symptomatic. Use of various medications is helpful. In the patient with advanced disease who has developed contractures, surgical interventions may be necessary to facilitate mobility.

■ ASSESSMENT

Early symptoms of multiple sclerosis are usually transitory. As mentioned previously, persons with multiple

sclerosis may be considered neurotic because of the wide variety and temporary nature of symptoms and because of the emotional lability produced by the disease. Subjective and objective data are important in establishing the diagnosis.

Subjective Data

The following are subjective data obtained from the patient with multiple sclerosis:

1. Patient's understanding of disease
2. Presence of eye problems
   a. Diplopia
   b. Scotomas
   c. Blindness
3. Presence of weakness or numbness of part of the body such as the hand
4. Presence of unusual fatigue
5. Presence of tremor
6. Presence of emotional lability
7. Presence of bowel and bladder problems
8. Presence of impotence in males

Objective Data

The following are objective data obtained from the patient with multiple sclerosis:

1. Documented abnormalities of neurologic examination
   a. Nystagmus
   b. Scanning speech
   c. Muscle weakness and spasms
   d. Changes in coordination
   e. Spastic ataxic gait
2. Behavior: presence of euphoria
3. Urinary incontinence, frequency, or urgency
4. Difficulty in swallowing

■ DATA ANALYSIS: NURSING DIAGNOSES

Nursing diagnoses are determined from assessment of patient data. Possible nursing diagnoses for the person with multiple sclerosis include, but are not limited to, the following:

Diagnostic Title	Possible Etiologies
Activity intolerance	Generalized weakness
Anxiety	Change in health status
Communication, impaired verbal	Physical impairment
Constipation	Immobility
Disuse syndrome, potential for	Immobility, weakness
Fatigue	Muscle weakness
Incontinence, bowel	Neuromuscular impairment
Knowledge deficit: care required, cause of exacerbations	Lack of exposure/recall, unfamiliarity with information sources
Mobility, impaired physical	Intolerance to activity, decreased strength and endurance, neuromuscular impairment

Diagnostic Title	Possible Etiologies
Nutrition, altered: less than body requirements	Chewing or swallowing difficulties
Pain, chronic	Chronic physical disability
Self-care deficit, bathing/ hygiene, dressing/ grooming, feeding, toileting	Intolerance to activity, fatigue, pain/discomfort, perceptual/cognitive impairment
Skin integrity, impaired, potential	Mechanical forces (pressure, shearing forces), immobility
Social isolation	Altered state of wellness
Swallowing, impaired	Neuromuscular impairment
Urinary elimination, altered patterns	Sensory/motor impairment, urinary infection

■ PLANNING: EXPECTED PATIENT OUTCOMES

Expected patient outcomes for the person with multiple sclerosis may include, but are not limited to, the following:

1. Activity is maintained.
2. Anxiety is lessened.
3. Communication is enhanced.
4. Constipation and diarrhea are prevented.
5. Disuse syndrome does not occur.
6. Fatigue is minimized.
7. Bowel incontinence is minimized.
8. Patient can explain the action, desired effects, and side effects of medications to be taken at home.
9. Patient can explain plan for a balanced diet.
10. Patient can explain the importance of staying as active as possible.
11. Patient can explain the importance of skin care and demonstrate how to inspect the skin.
12. Patient can explain the importance of frequent changes of position.
13. Patient can state how to secure community help.
14. Patient can explain plan for follow-up care.
15. Adequate nutritional status is maintained.
16. Pain and discomfort are minimized.
17. Self-care deficit is minimized.
18. Social isolation is lessened.
19. Skin integrity is maintained.
20. Aspiration is prevented.
21. Urinary problems are minimized.

■ IMPLEMENTATION

Preventive Care

The cause of multiple sclerosis remains unclear; therefore no primary prevention for this disease is available. Again, the secondary and tertiary preventive aspects are important.

Acute Care

Medications. At present no specific treatment exists for multiple sclerosis.[5,87] Many physicians achieve favorable results from symptomatic treatments and the judicious use of adrenocorticotropic hormone (ACTH) or corticosteroids. Psychotherapy, social rehabilitation, physical therapy, patient education, and much compassion are also indicated. Although ACTH or the steroids are widely used, their efficacy remains controversial. These drugs have been shown to prevent experimental allergic encephalomyelitis. Currently, some clinicians prefer oral prednisone; others prefer intramuscular ACTH; still others prefer intravenous ACTH. Dexamethasone (Decadron), administered intramuscularly or orally, has become popular. Its demonstrated antiedema effect may explain the favorable results in acute attacks of multiple sclerosis. The effects of ACTH and the steroids on the demyelinating activity per se are not known. Testing has shown that (1) nothing is gained from long-term treatment with either steroids or ACTH and (2) some gain may result from taking high doses of steroids at the start of a fresh episode, since the episode tends to resolve itself more rapidly if patients are treated with intensive courses of these drugs. The mood-elevating drugs are used to relieve depression, which is often present in multiple sclerosis. Chemotherapy (low-dose cytoxan and interferon) is now being used to treat exacerbations of the disease (see research box below).

Persons with multiple sclerosis react similarly to others with a chronic illness. These reactions include fear, guilt, grief, denial, and depression.

Long-Term Care

Promoting activity/mobility. Persons with multiple sclerosis should have a daily routine for rest and activity. Rest must be balanced with adequate exercise. They are usually advised to exercise regularly but never to the point of extreme fatigue, Because persons with multiple sclerosis almost always feel tired, they must look for some special sign that tells them that they have exercised

---

RESEARCH

Jacobs L et al: Intrathecal interferon in multiple sclerosis, Arch Neurol 39:609-615, 1982.

This study examined the theories that a virus present in patients with multiple sclerosis causes exacerbations of the disease. Twenty patients with multiple sclerosis (15 females and 5 males) were studied over 2 years. Interferon was administered via lumbar puncture semiweekly for the first month, then once a month for the next 5 months. Ten control patients were also followed. The patients receiving interferon had a 80% decrease in exacerbations according to past disease behaviors. The results showed that intrathecal interferon could be tolerated and may change the course of multiple sclerosis. ■

enough. If they exercise more, they may suffer ill effects. For example, a tight feeling in the chest may indicate that the person must rest or else have severe discomfort. During the acute exacerbation, many physicians keep the patient as quiet as possible, limit all activities, and place the patient on bed rest. After an exacerbation, it may be difficult to resume exercises, but it is usually best that an established schedule be returned to as soon as possible. The person must conserve energy for priority activities.

One side of the body is usually affected more than the other, and the person may learn to stabilize gait by leaning toward the uninvolved side. The annoyance of having the foot slap forward in taking a step may sometimes be overcome by putting the heel down in a pronounced fashion and rolling the weight forward on the side of the foot.

Effort is made to maintain activity and work for as long as possible, and many persons have worked for 5 to 10 years and even longer after the onset of the first symptoms. Women at home can be helped to plan their shopping, housework, and other duties so that they may continue to function as wives and mothers even when the disease is advanced.[26] Many persons with multiple sclerosis remain mobile with only mild to moderate disability.

Promoting comfort. *Diplopia* can be relieved by an eye patch. Peripheral neurectomies, rhizotomies, and cordotomies are often used for the relief of *spasticity, pain,* and *parasthesias*. Relief from severe spasticity is often obtained from intrathecal injections of phenol. In more severe cases of spasticity when contractures have developed, surgical release of tendons may be necessary, followed by casting for a time.

Promoting skin integrity. Many persons with multiple sclerosis have motor involvement that prevents them from moving about and changing position easily. Also, they may experience sensory disturbances that affect how they sense pressure. As a result, these patients are especially prone to develop decubiti. They must be taught the importance of turning at least every 2 to 3 hours. Air mattresses or other devices may be used to help prevent pressure, but it is important to note that no substitute exists for regular turning.

Preventing bowel problems. The most common bowel problems are constipation and incontinence. Constipation may be minimized with the use of a fiber-rich diet and adequate fluid intake (at least eight glasses of water per day). If needed, prunes or prune juice may be helpful. The use of a stool softener may be necessary. Suppositories can be used to train the bowel and encourage evacuation of stool. Enemas may be used as a last resort, but the chronic use of them may lead to loss of bowel tone and dependency on them.

If incontinence of the bowel occurs, a bowel training program should be started. The use of suppositories as well as the other measures just mentioned can help the patient develop a regular pattern of evacuation and prevent incontinence. A good nursing assessment should include the time the patient usually had a bowel movement. This knowledge is incorporated into the bowel training program.

Preventing bladder problems. Urinary frequency and urgency, often the source of social disability, may respond to timed doses of propantheline bromide (Pro-Banthine). Prevention of urinary tract infection remains a problem, and such infections are a major cause of death. Cholinergic drugs such as bethanechol (Urecholine) may be of help in the patient with an atonic bladder. Oxybutynin chloride (Ditropan) is a newer drug used to treat neurogenic bladder. It acts by exerting a direct antispasmodic effect on smooth muscles. Some patients are placed on prophylactic doses of medications such as trimethoprim and sulfamethoxazole (Bactrim, Septra) or nitrofurantoin (Macrodantin) indefinitely. Cystometrographic study is important to detect the specific bladder problem.

Promoting adequate nutrition. A well-balanced diet with plenty of high-vitamin foods and fluids is important. Obesity must be avoided because it is more difficult for the obese person to maneuver, and this makes it more difficult to meet daily needs. High-fiber foods and prune juice may help to reduce constipation.

Controlling the environment. Persons with multiple sclerosis need a peaceful, relaxed environment. They should never be hurried and should not be expected to respond quickly either physically or mentally. They may be slow in speaking and being able to respond, and this difficulty should be ignored by persons around them. Family members and friends need help in understanding this problem and in meeting it calmly. The person may have sudden, explosive emotional outbursts of crying or laughing brought on by such simple acts as putting something hot into the mouth. Close family members must protect both patient and visitors from the embarrassment of prolonged emotional outbursts. Reminding the patient of something sad may stop the laughing, and holding the mouth open will sometimes stop the crying. The care of the patient with multiple sclerosis is summarized in the box on p. 1830.

Hot baths should be avoided because the heat can increase weakness in the person with multiple sclerosis. (In some centers, patients have been treated with ice water baths.) Traveling in hot weather should be care-

CARE OF THE PATIENT WITH MULTIPLE SCLEROSIS

1. Promote activity.
   a. Maintain daily routine for rest and activity.
   b. Avoid fatigue.
   c. Maintain work and activity as long as possible.
   d. Conserve energy for priority activities.
2. Provide comfort.
   a. Use eye patch for diplopia.
   b. Take prescribed medications to relieve spasticity.
3. Prevent bladder problems.
   a. Take medications as prescribed.
   b. Drink adequate fluids.
   c. Provide intermittent catheterization if needed.
4. Prevent bowel problems
   a. Eat fiber-rich diet.
   b. Drink adequate fluids
   c. Use stool softeners or suppositories if needed.
5. Promote adequate nutrition.
   a. Eat well-balanced meals.
   b. Encourage foods high in fiber.
   c. Avoid excessive fiber.
6. Control environment.
   a. Avoid hot baths and going out in hot weather.
   b. Avoid stressful situations.
7. Promote communication.
   a. Encourage patient to talk.
   b. Use compensatory measures if needed.

5. Need for balanced diet
6. Range of motion (ROM) exercises
7. Safety factors to prevent injury
8. Positioning to prevent contractures and decubiti
9. Importance of skin inspection and how to do it
10. Importance of avoiding temperature extremes
11. Community resources and how to obtain them
12. Education about the disease, what can bring on symptoms, and how to manage them.

The National Multiple Sclerosis Society* is a national voluntary, nonprofit organization founded in 1946. Its functions are to encourage and finance research, to gather statistics, and to act as an information center for patients and for the public. Some local chapters also supply equipment to patients. Membership is open to health and welfare workers and to patients and their families. Local organizations can be found in many large cities.

PARKINSON'S DISEASE (PARALYSIS AGITANS)
EPIDEMIOLOGY/ETIOLOGY

Parkinson's disease is one of the more common diseases of the nervous system. It was first described in 1817 by James Parkinson. It affects both men and women in their middle and late years (50 to 60 years old) and is seen in all races and classes of persons. It is estimated to affect 100 to 150 persons per 100,000 population.[112]

The cause is not known, but the cluster of symptoms was first observed in many patients following the 1916 to 1917 worldwide epidemic of encephalitis.

The characteristic symptoms of Parkinson's disease are sometimes found in patients with arteriosclerosis, leading some researchers to believe that arteriosclerosis may be a causative factor. Viral infections have also been suggested as a cause. Drug-induced parkinsonian syndromes have been linked with the phenothiazines, reserpine (Serpasil), and butyrophenones (for example, Haloperidol).

PATHOPHYSIOLOGY

The pathologic process that occurs with Parkinson's disease is basically a *depigmentation* of the *substantia nigra* of the basal ganglia. The loss of neurons in the substantia is severe. Also, selective depletion of dopamine occurs and can be correlated with the degree of striatal degeneration. Without dopamine, loss of inhibitory influence occurs and excitatory mechanisms are unopposed.

As mentioned, the cause of Parkinson's disease is not known. Its occurrence has been associated with arteriosclerosis, certain viruses, and the drugs listed under the epidemiology/etiology section.

fully planned to prevent travel during the warmest part of the day. It is essential that the person and the family understand the importance of checking the skin routinely and taking measures to relieve tissue pressure.

Promoting communication. The person with multiple sclerosis may develop problems in communicating verbally. They should be encouraged to express themselves through talking, even if this is difficult. The speech most often is described as scanning in nature. If the patient loses the ability to talk, compensatory measures should be instituted. These include the use of a communication board or a letter alphabet board. Sophisticated computers are available to patients who can afford them.

Patient teaching. Teaching is important for both patient and significant others. In the later stages of multiple sclerosis, all aspects of care may have to be assumed by someone other than the patient. The teaching needs include the following:

1. Use of medications, including side effects, dosage, timing, and desired effects
2. Importance of reporting side effects to the physician
3. Importance of good fluid intake
4. Importance of balancing activities to include relaxation and fun activities

*257 Park Ave South, New York, NY 10010.

CLINICAL MANIFESTATIONS

Parkinson's disease begins with a faint tremor and progresses so slowly that the person is seldom able to recall its onset. No true paralysis and no loss of sensation occur. Tremor (pill rolling of the fingers or resting tremor) is the outstanding sign of the disease. Two other frequent signs are muscular weakness (with rigidity) and loss of postural reflexes. Parkinson's disease has some characteristics of upper motor neuron involvement (see Chapter 62). It is essentially a problem with motion. Muscle rigidity prevents normal response in frequently performed acts and leads to characteristic changes that make the diagnosis almost unmistakable to persons who have observed patients with the disease.

There is a masklike appearance to the face and slowed, monotonous speech. Drooling may occur because of the difficulty of swallowing saliva. This may cause skin irritation, which is best prevented or treated by frequent sponging followed by protecting the skin with an emollient such as cold cream. There is a characteristic shuffling gait in which patients tend to walk on their toes. The trunk is bent forward, and the arms fall rigidly to the sides and do not swing in normal rhythmic gait. Neuromuscular control may be altered so that the patient is unable to stop this propulsive gait until an obstruction is met. The patient usually has moist, oily skin. Defects in judgment and emotional instability may occur, but intelligence is not impaired. The appetite may be increased, and there is heat intolerance. A decrease in blinking is seen. Fatigue is a common complaint, and pain in the arms or shoulder may be present. All signs and symptoms increase with fatigue, excitement, and frustration. As the disease progresses, the severity of symptoms increases. More and more symptoms develop. Patients with Parkinson's disease usually die from other causes, most often pulmonary or renal disease.

Diagnostic Tests

No test is diagnostic of Parkinson's disease. The clinical explanation and history, along with the patient's response to administration of medication used to treat the disease, confirm the diagnosis.

MEDICAL MANAGEMENT

In most cases, medical care of the patient with Parkinson's disease involves the use of medication. However, a surgical procedure has been used with some success in the treatment of selected patients. Descriptions of successful surgery in popular magazines have led some patients and their families to believe that a cure for all patients has been found. Many patients cannot be treated surgically. Results seem to be best in younger patients who have unilateral involvement following the disease

and who have severe tremor and rigidity. Treatment consists of destroying portions of the *globus pallidus* (relieves rigidity) or the *thalamus* (relieves tremor) in the brain by stereotactic methods through the use of cautery, removal, or injection of alcohol. Surgical techniques involving cooling or freezing with liquid nitrogen (cryogenic surgery) have been attempted with good results in selected patients and with fewer complications than when cautery or alcohol was used. Medications used to control rigidity and tremor are discontinued several days preoperatively so that patients' symptoms will be at their peak during surgery. Nursing care preoperatively includes seeing that nutrition is adequate, as well as other preoperative care.

Postoperative care includes the most careful attention to the vital signs; use of side rails to prevent accidents in the event of convulsions, disorientation, or temporary hemiplegia; and frequent turning and moving to prevent respiratory and circulatory complications. Excessive salivation and difficulty in blinking the eye on the surgically treated side may be problems requiring nursing attention.

■ ASSESSMENT

Subjective Data

The following are subjective data from the patient with Parkinson's disease:

1. Patient's understanding of disease
2. Complaints of fatigue
3. Presence of incoordination
4. Defects in judgment and emotional instability
5. Heat insensitivity

Objective Data

The following are objective data from the patient with Parkinson's disease:

1. Presence of tremor (pill-rolling motion of the fingers or resting tremor)
2. Muscular response to movement
3. Postural reflexes
4. Appearance of face, including skin
5. Presence of drooling
6. Gait disturbances
7. Sensory testing abnormalities
8. Inability to carry out daily activities

■ DATA ANALYSIS: NURSING DIAGNOSES

The nursing diagnoses for the patient with Parkinson's disease are the same as those for patients with multiple sclerosis, with the exception of sensory/perceptual alteration: visual.

■ PLANNING: EXPECTED PATIENT OUTCOMES

The reader is referred to the patient outcomes for the patient with multiple sclerosis on p. 1828. The following are additional outcomes for the person with Parkinson's disease:

1. Patient's tremor is controlled
2. Muscular rigidity is decreased.

■ IMPLEMENTATION

Preventive Care

Because the cause of Parkinson's disease is not known, primary prevention is difficult to achieve. With patients who have drug-induced symptoms, the judicious use of these drugs along with the use of anticholinergic drugs, such as benztropine mesylate (Cogentin) and trihexyphenidyl hydrochloride (Artane), may be helpful in preventing worsening symptomatology.

Early detection (secondary prevention) is important, as is prevention of complications (tertiary prevention).

Long-Term Care

Medications. Treatment for Parkinson's disease is palliative and symptomatic and depends on the pharmacologic manipulation of the pathophysiologic state. The severity of symptoms and presence of associated disease processes determine the drugs to be used. Anticholinergic alkaloids such as scopolamine hydrobromide and related drugs (hyoscyamine) have been used for more than a century. They act against cholinergic excitatory effects and are more effective in lessening muscle rigidity than in controlling tremor. Many synthetic anticholinergic drugs of varied chemical structure are also available. There is little to recommend one over the other, aside from personal preference, but each has some degree of central nervous system (CNS) anticholinergic action. However, they are incapable of restoring striatal balance. The preferred anticholinergic agents are trihexyphenidyl, benztropine, procyclidine (Kemadrin), and biperiden (Akineton). These drugs have some selectivity of action in that they have greater central than peripheral anticholinergic activity. Optimal results from these drugs depend on a dosage that provides a compromise between the limited symptomatic improvement given by these drugs and the disagreeable symptoms of central and peripheral cholinergic blockade (blurring of vision, dryness of mouth and throat, constipation, urinary urgency or retention, ataxia, dysarthria, mental disturbances). Antihistaminic drugs such as diphenhydramine (Benadryl), which are not primarily anticholinergic, exert mild central anticholinergic properties when used alone or in combination with other drugs.

Some patients with severe Parkinson's disease have experienced dramatic benefits from levodopa not experienced from anticholinergic drugs. Levodopa assists in restoring striatal dopamine deficiency because it is a precursor of dopamine. This drug does not affect the underlying process of parkinsonism. In this way, levodopa acts more as replacement drug than a cure.

Once benefits are obtained from levodopa, they are likely to be sustained. After prolonged periods of treatment, there may be an increase in side effects as well as a decrease in the effectiveness of the medication. The drug is usually increased gradually but cannot be increased indefinitely. It has been found helpful to admit some patients into the hospital for a "drug holiday" during which all medications are withdrawn for 7 to 10 days. The medications are then restarted, and often much smaller doses are able to produce favorable results. This drug holiday must take place within the hospital setting, however, because of the danger of aspiration pneumonia or other complications that can occur, since the immobility, rigidity, and other signs and symptoms will return when the drugs are withdrawn. Usually patients remain on anticholinergic drugs, or these may be added as an adjunct. Most individuals experience side effects from levodopa, such as nausea and vomiting, orthostatic hypotension, insomnia, agitation, and mental confusion, but these lessen with continued medication and dosage modification.

Kidney and liver damage have occurred in some patients taking levodopa. Candidates for levodopa should be selected carefully. Amantadine hydrochloride (Symmetrel), an antiviral agent, is known to have antiparkinsonian activity. It acts by blocking the reuptake and storage of catecholamines and allowing the accumulation of dopamine in extracellular or synaptic sites. This drug may not sustain its effectiveness for more than 3 months in some patients. Side effects, although infrequent, include mental confusion, visual disturbances, and seizures.

Carbidopa-levodopa (Sinemet) has recently been used more often in neurologic practice. It is a combination of levodopa with an inhibitor of the enzyme dopa decarboxylase, which limits the metabolism of levodopa peripherally and provides more levodopa for the brain. The reduction in peripheral metabolism and the reduction in dosage of levodopa that can occur reduce some of the side effects seen when levodopa is used alone.

Table 63-4 lists the drugs used to treat Parkinson's disease.

Surgery. A relatively new and still experimental treatment for Parkinson's disease is the adrenal medullary transplant. In this procedure tissue from the adrenal medulla is placed in contact with the substantia nigra with the hope of restoring the balance of dopamine and acetylcholine. The procedure is difficult because the patient undergoes three major surgeries at the same time: (1) stereotactic localization of the caudate nucleus, (2) craniotomy, and (3) laporotomy for the adrenalectomy. Results so far have been somewhat encouraging.[13]

Promoting activity/mobility. Special attention should be paid to *posture*. Lying on a firm bed without a pillow

TABLE 63-4 Medications used in Parkinson's disease

Medication	Action/Effects	Side Effects	Comments
Anticholinergic drugs Scopolamine hydrochloride Hyoscyamine	Act against cholinergic excitatory effects More effective in lessening muscle rigidity than in controlling tremor	Central and peripheral cholinergic actions Blurring of vision Dryness of mouth and throat Constipation Urinary retention or urgency Ataxia Dysarthria Mental disturbances	Optimal results depend on dosage that provides compromise between improvement and development of side effects
Synthetic anticholinergic drugs Trihexyphenidyl (Artane) Benztropine mesylate (Cogentin) Procyclidine ((Kemadrin) Biperiden (Akineton)	Some degree of CNS anticholinergic action, but incapable of restoring striatal balance	Same as for anticholinergic drugs	Same for anticholinergic drugs
Antihistaminic drugs Diphenhydramine (Benadryl)	Exert mild central anticholinergic properties	Sleepiness Dry mouth	Does not affect underlying process of Parkinson's disease
Levodopa	Assists in restoring striatal dopamine deficiency	Kidney, liver damage Nausea, vomiting Orthostatic hypotension Insomnia Agitation and mental confusion	Side effects common
Amantadine hydrochloride (Symmetrel)	Acts by blocking the reuptake and storage of catecholamines and allowing accumulation of dopamine in extracellular or synaptic sites	Mental confusion Visual disturbances Seizures	May not be effective for longer than 3 months
Carbidopa-levodopa (levodopa with inhibitor of the decarboxylase)	Inhibitor limits metabolism of levodopa peripherally and provides more levodopa to brain	Same as for levodopa	Fewer side effects than with levodopa used alone

during rest periods may help to prevent the spine from bending forward, and lying in the prone position also helps. Holding the hands folded behind the back when walking may help to keep the spine erect and prevent the annoyance of the arms falling stiffly at the sides. The tremor often is less apparent when persons are sitting in an armchair, since they can grip the arms of the chair and partially control the tremor in their hands and arms. The reader is referred to Chapter 62 for a discussion of alterations of movement and posture.

The patient with Parkinson's disease should continue to work as long as possible. Most physicians advise this unless the occupation is such that continued work is dangerous.

Promoting nutrition. *Feeding* the patient becomes a real problem when the disease is far advanced because of the *danger of choking* in attempts to swallow; eventually, aspiration pneumonia may terminate the patient's life. Unless the patient is well controlled by medication,

drooling can be a real problem and increases with general excitement. A bib can be used to protect the clothing during napping hours. When patients are dressed, garments with generous pockets well supplied with soft tissues will help them be less conspicuous and more comfortable.

Patient teaching. Teaching is important for both the caregiver and the patient. The teaching is the same as that for a person with multiple sclerosis on p. 1830.

MYASTHENIA GRAVIS
EPIDEMIOLOGY/ETIOLOGY

Myasthenia gravis is a relatively rare disease of unknown cause. It usually occurs in young adults and is thought to have a link with autoimmune reactions. It affects about one in 20,000 persons. In young persons, women are more often affected than men, but among older persons the distribution between the sexes is about equal. Occurrence within families is rare; however, infants of affected mothers may have symptoms at birth, but these symptoms usually disappear within several weeks.

PATHOPHYSIOLOGY

With myasthenia gravis, no observable structural change occurs in the muscle or nerve. Nerve impulses fail to pass to muscles at the *myoneural junction*. It is not known specifically why the motor nerve impulses fail to pass the muscle and cause it not to contract. Suggested causes include (1) the inability of the motor endplate to secrete adequate acetylcholine, (2) excessive quantities of the cholinesterase enzyme at the nerve ending, or a (3) nonresponse of the muscle fibers to acetylcholine. Relative to the third theory, myasthenia gravis may be considered a primary muscle disease; relative to the first two theories, it is a neuromuscular disease with lower motor neuron characteristics. About 25% of patients with myasthenia gravis have been found to have thymoma, and almost 80% have changes in the cellular structure of the thymus gland. Myasthenia gravis is considered a serious disorder because the respiratory muscles and the bulbar cranial nerves may be involved. During periods of exacerbation or lack of drug control, the patient may have to be cared for in a respiratory intensive care unit.[60]

CLINICAL MANIFESTATIONS

The outstanding symptoms of myasthenia gravis are muscle weakness and severe generalized fatigue that come on quickly, are usually more evident in the evening, and in the early stages of the disease, disappear quickly with rest. Weakness of arm and hand muscles may be first noticed when shaving or combing the hair. Facial muscles innervated by the cranial nerves are often affected, and it may not be possible for the person to hold the eyelids open (ptosis), to keep the mouth closed, or to chew or swallow. Diplopia (double vision) is also common. As the disease progresses, the trunk and lower limbs are affected, leading to difficulty with walking and sustained sitting. Usually the distal muscles are not as affected as the proximal muscles. Muscles weakness may become so severe that the person cannot

breathe without assistance. Exacerbations of the disease may be initiated by upper respiratory infections, emotional tension, and menstruation.

Eaton-Lambert Syndrome

The Eaton-Lambert syndrome is a condition associated with cancer that has many of the same symptoms as myasthenia gravis. It is important to differentiate between the two diseases. *The Eaton-Lambert syndrome is a special form of myasthenia that is found almost invariably in persons with oat cell carcinoma of the lung.* In this syndrome the muscles of the trunk as well as those of the pelvic and shoulder girdles are the ones most frequently involved by weakness, fatigue, and atrophy. Visual symptoms occur less frequently. Increasing weakness occurs after exertion, but muscle power may increase temporarily at first.

The onset of the Eaton-Lambert syndrome is usually insidious and the course progressive. Because the myasthenia may precede discovery of the lung tumor by months or years, it is important that a thorough check for malignancy be done at regular intervals. In addition to oat cell carcinoma of the lung, the syndrome has occurred with carcinoma of the rectum, stomach, prostate, and breast.

Table 63-5 compares myasthenia gravis and Eaton-Lambert syndrome.

Diagnostic Tests

Because of the slow, insidious onset and occurrence of symptoms with stress, myasthenia gravis is sometimes misdiagnosed as hysteria or neurosis. Actual diagnosis can be made partly on the basis of electromyography (EMG). A specific diagnostic test is the edrophonium chloride (Tensilon) test. In this test, Tensilon (a very short-acting anticholinesterase drug) is injected intravenously. When increased strength in a predetermined muscle group is seen, the test is considered positive. To obtain true results, it is important that the patient not know when the medication is being given.

The procedure for the test is as follows:

1. Edrophonium and normal saline are drawn up in separate syringes.

TABLE 63-5 Comparison of myasthenia gravis and Eaton-Lambert syndrome

	Myasthenia Gravis	Eaton-Lambert Syndrome
Onset	Slow and insidious	Slow and insidious
Vision	Diplopia common	Diplopia not as common
Muscle involvement	Cranial nerves, arms and hands, trunk and lower limbs affected (difficulty with walking and sitting); distal muscles not as affected as proximal muscles	Muscles of trunk as well as those of pelvic and shoulder girdle are most often involved
Weakness	Weakness and generalized fatigue that comes on quickly	Increased weakness with exertion, but temporary increase in muscle power may occur at first

2. Each is injected intravenously separately.
3. It is important that the patient not know which solution is being administered.
4. Increased strength in a predetermined muscle group with the administration of edrophonium is a positive test.

MEDICAL MANAGEMENT

Medical management involves the use of medication. In individuals who have thymomas, surgical removal of the thyoma often decreases the symptoms.

During acute exacerbations of the disease, and when the respiratory status is compromised, the patient may require intubation and mechanical ventilation. A tracheostomy may be necessary. See Chapter 34.

■ ASSESSMENT

Both subjective and objective data are important to collect in the patient with myasthenia gravis.

Subjective Data

The following subjective data should be obtained from the patient with myasthenia gravis:
1. Patient's understanding of disease
2. Fatigue—when it occurs and where it occurs
3. Profound muscle weakness
4. Presence of diplopia
5. Difficulty in keeping eyelids open and mouth closed or difficulty in chewing and swallowing
6. Effect of stress on symptoms
7. Patient's perception of muscle weakness

Objective Data

The following objective data should be obtained for the patient with myasthenia gravis:
1. Documented muscle weakness on neurologic testing
2. Presence of ptosis of eyelids
3. Documented weight loss
4. Breath sounds that are diminished
5. Muscle atrophy

■ DATA ANALYSIS: NURSING DIAGNOSES

Nursing diagnoses are determined from assessment of patient data. Possible nursing diagnoses for the person with myasthenia gravis include, but are not limited to, the following:[45]

Diagnostic Title	Possible Etiologies
Activity intolerance	Immobility, generalized weakness
Gas exchange, impaired	Ventilation/perfusion imbalance
Knowledge deficit; importance of preventing respiratory infections, taking medications	Lack of exposure/recall, unfamiliarity with information sources

Diagnostic Title	Possible Etiologies
Mobility, impaired physical	Intolerance to activity, decreased strength
Sensory/perceptual alterations: visual	Altered sensory reception

■ PLANNING: EXPECTED PATIENT OUTCOMES

Expected patient outcomes for the person with myasthenia gravis may include, but are not limited to, the following:
1. Mobility/activity is maintained.
2. Patient can explain each prescribed anticholinergic or cholinergic drug prescribed.
   a. Actions, side effects, and toxic effects
   b. Reason to take the drug at exact time prescribed
   c. Need to monitor effects of the medication, especially on respiration, swallowing, and general muscle strength
3. Patient can list the drugs that act on the neuromuscular junction and therefore must be avoided (see box below).
4. Patient can demonstrate the use of an airway and ventilatory equipment.
5. Patient can explain the need to avoid overexertion and emotional tension.
6. Patient can explain why it is better not to live alone.
7. Diplopia does not occur.

■ IMPLEMENTATION

Preventive Care

No known form of primary prevention exists for patients with myasthenia gravis. As noted, some patients have been found to have a thymoma. Surgical removal may decrease the symptoms of the disease or result in almost complete recovery.

As with all neurologic diseases, secondary and tertiary prevention is important.

Acute Care

Medications. No known cure exists for myasthenia gravis. However, great improvement follows the use of neostigmine (Prostigmin) or pyridostigmine (Mestinon). These drugs block the action of cholinesterase at the

---

DRUGS TO BE AVOIDED BY PERSONS WITH MYASTHENIA GRAVIS

1. Muscle relaxants
2. Barbiturates
3. Morphine sulfate
4. Tranquilizers
5. Neomycin (potentiates muscle weakness because of effect on myoneural junction)

---

myoneural junction and allow acetylcholine, a chemical necessary for transmission of impulses to the muscles, to act. Acetylcholine is the neurotransmitter between postganglionic parasympathetic fibers and receptor organs. Atropine or some other anticholinergic agent that blocks these *muscarinic effects* of acetylcholine may be used to treat the side effects of neostigmine and pyridostigmine. Treatment is planned so that the patient may continue to receive the amount of drug that can be tolerated without side effects and yet carry out activities essential for normal living. Usually the patient is permitted to adjust the dosage. *The nurse should teach the importance of taking medications at the time prescribed.* If the drug is delayed, dyspnea may result, followed by severe respiratory depression, which, if untreated, can cause death.

It is important also to teach that (1) dosage is individually determined and related to the person's activity, (2) dosage needs to be adjusted to maintain muscle strength, and (3) the effects of drugs need to be monitored. The nurse and family must understand that it is often difficult to distinguish between *myasthenic crisis* (too little drug) and *cholinergic crisis* (too much drug), since both conditions cause severe muscle weakness. Tensilon administered intravenously is used to differentiate between the two conditions. A positive test (increase in strength) usually indicates underdosage of medication. An increase in weakness when Tensilon is administered may be a sign of overdosage. Drugs to be avoided are muscle relaxants, morphine, barbiturates, tranquilizers, and neomycin. Because of their effects on the myoneural junction, they can potentiate the weakness associated with myasthenia gravis.

Promoting adequate ventilation. Respiratory problems typically occur in patients with myasthenia gravis. For this reason they are usually advised not to live alone. Upper respiratory infections occur because patients may not have the energy needed to cough effectively and may develop pneumonia or airway obstruction. Aspiration often occurs. Many patients keep airway equipment at their bedside at home.

During acute episodes of the disease, the patient will require hospitalization. The following are important measures to be taken:

1. Tracheostomy equipment at bedside because respiratory status may change suddenly
2. Serial determinations of vital capacity, minute volumes, and tidal volumes
3. Suction as necessary
4. Nasogastric tube if swallowing is too dangerous

Care must be taken that the nasogastric tube is in the stomach before fluid is introduced, because the patient cannot cough to indicate presence of fluid in the trachea.

Promoting mobility/activity. Persons with myasthenia gravis may have to change daily patterns of activity. The nurse can help the patient and family plan so that minimal energy is used in activities that are essential to remaining relatively self-sufficient and yet allow energy for activities in which the patient wishes to take part.

Patient teaching. The patient with myasthenia gravis is usually able to adjust the medication depending on his/her symptoms. Also, the patient can have much control over preventing respiratory complications. Therefore teaching is very important and should include:

1. Importance of taking medication at time prescribed
2. How to adjust dose to maintain muscle strength
3. Side effects and how to monitor
4. Medications to avoid
5. Importance of seeking medical attention at first sign of upper respiratory infections
6. Importance of eating only when sitting up
7. Avoiding crowds in flu and cold season
8. How to adjust to daily activities to allow for activities and rest periods
9. Plan to use minimal energy in activities that are essential, so that energy may be conserved for activities that patient enjoys

AMYOTROPHIC LATERAL SCLEROSIS

Amyotrophic lateral sclerosis (ALS) is a motor neuron disease that affects upper or lower motor neurons lying within the brain or spinal cord or a combination of the two.

EPIDEMIOLOGY/ETIOLOGY

ALS is sometimes called Lou Gehrig's disease because the famous New York Yankee ballplayer died of the disease. It affects men more than women. It usually occurs in middle age but may occur in younger persons. Some believe a familial or genetic component to ALS exists. The cause is unknown, but a slow viral infection has been suggested to be the causative agent.[15]

PATHOPHYSIOLOGY

Myelin sheaths are destroyed and are replaced by scar tissue in ALS. The lateral tracts of the spinal cord are directly involved, with possible eventual involvement of the medulla and the ventral tracts. The nerve impulses are distorted or blocked. Symptoms depend on which motor neurons are affected.

CLINICAL MANIFESTATIONS

Early symptoms of ALS include fatigue and awkwardness of fine finger movements and muscle wasting. Dysphagia may be the first symptoms in many persons.

Progressive muscle weakness, atrophy, and *fascicula-tions* occur. Spasticity of flexor muscles is typically present. With involvement of the brainstem and me-dulla, dysphagia, dysarthria, jaw clonus, tongue fascicu-lations, and respiratory difficulty are present. As the dis-eases progresses, disability is relative to both upper and lower limbs, and one side of the body becomes more in-volved than the other. The person remains alert. No sensory loss occurs with the disease. Death usually en-sues within 5 to 10 years, generally from respiratory or bulbar paralysis.

Diagnostic Tests

Initial testing for ALS may include an EMG (see Chap-ter 59) to rule out other muscle diseases. No definitive test exists for ALS.

MEDICAL MANAGEMENT

The medical management of ALS is mainly symptom-atic. As the disease progresses, surgical intervention to place a gastrostomy tube may be necessary.

■ ASSESSMENT

Subjective Data

The following subjective data should be obtained from the patient with ALS:

1. Patient's understanding of the disease
2. Presence of fatigue
3. Presence of dysphagia
4. Difficulty with tasks involving finger movement

Objective Data

The following objective data should be obtained for the patient with ALS:

1. Inability to carry out ADLs
2. Muscle abnormalities on testing
3. Evidence of involvement of brainstem and me-dulla
4. Weight loss

■ DATA ANALYSIS: NURSING DIAGNOSES

Nursing diagnoses are determined from assessment of patient data. Possible nursing diagnoses for the person with ALS include those for the patient with multiple sclerosis (p. 1827), as well as the following:

Diagnostic Title	Possible Etiologies
Airway clearance, ineffec-tive	Decreased energy/fatigue, tra-cheobronchial infection

■ PLANNING: EXPECTED PATIENT OUTCOMES

Expected patient outcomes for the patient with ALS are the same as those for the patient with multiple sclerosis (p. 1828), with the following addition:

Patient will maintain weight.

■ IMPLEMENTATION

Preventive Care

No cause for ALS is known; thus primary prevention cannot be implemented. However, prompt diagnosis (secondary prevention) and prevention of complications (tertiary prevention) remain extremely important.

Acute Care

Treatment is directed toward relieving the symptoms of the disease. Nursing interventions include assistance with ADLs as limb deficits increase. Protheses are often applied to support the weakened muscles. Providing ad-equate nutrition to the patient can be a real challenge. As swallowing becomes more difficult, a nasogastric or gastrostomy tube may be necessary.

Promoting effective airway clearance. As ALS progresses, the patient typically experiences increased difficulty in maintaining a clear airway. Aspiration often occurs. The patient should be taught to use a tucked chin position while eating or drinking to encourage more effective swallowing. Because the cough is weak, the person may not be able to clear the airway in this manner. A suction machine may be necessary. Many patients learn to suc-tion themselves using a tonsillar suction tip.

Providing emotional support. Emotional support is ex-tremely important. Patients with ALS and their families should be involved in making decisions about the types of interventions that will be used as the disease progresses. Some patients will decide to use ventilators at home as respiratory muscles become involved, whereas other patients will decide not to use any sup-portive devices. Patients and families need help and support in making decisions about how they are going to live their lives from the time the diagnosis is made until the disease causes the patient's complete depen-dency on others. Whatever decisions the patient and family make must be supported by the health team. Be-cause the patient remains alert until the end, nurses should not forget that they are caring for a person who is probably very afraid of what lies ahead. Patients should be helped to retain some control over their treat-ment as long as possible.

Patient teaching. Patient teaching is important for the pa-tient and caregiver. Significant points to consider in teaching are found in the section concerning teaching of the patient with multiple sclerosis on p. 1830.

ALZHEIMER'S DISEASE
EPIDEMIOLOGY/ETIOLOGY

Alzheimer's disease is a degenerative disorder that af-fects the cells of the brain and causes impairment of intellectual functioning. It affects 3 million American adults and is recognized as the most common cause of dementia in the older adult. It affects men and women equally. Most newly diagnosed persons are in late middle age, but the disease has been documented in some persons as young as 40 years old. By age 65, one person in 20 has been diagnosed with Alzheimer's disease; by age 75, one in 10; and over age 90, one in three persons.

The cause of Alzheimer's disease is not known. Some believe that perhaps it is an autoimmune disease. A slight hereditary disposition is suggested because family members of patients with Alzheimer's disease are slightly more likely to develop the disease.

PATHOPHYSIOLOGY

The changes in the brain of the patient with Alzheimer's disease are visible in the cerebral cortex. The first change is the presence of microscopic "plaques" found in brain tissue. These plaques consist of a core surrounded by strands of fiberlike material. In addition, there is degeneration of some of the small fibers (neurofibrils) that run through the body of the nerve cells. These changes were first discovered in 1907 by the German neurologist Alzheimer.

The diagnosis of Alzheimer's disease is usually made after other conditions in which memory loss occurs have been ruled out. Other conditions causing memory loss include the following:

1. Pernicious anemia
2. Drug reactions
3. Hormonal imbalances
4. Depression
5. Drug or alcohol abuse
6. Brain tumor
7. Chronic meningitis
8. Head trauma
9. Pick's disease
10. Parkinson's disease with dementia

CLINICAL MANIFESTATIONS

The patient with Alzheimer's disease goes through rather distinct clinical stages (see box above for details of a three-stage model).

One author cites *four* stages involved with Alzheimer's disease[46]:

Stage 1—mild memory lapses, difficulty with attention span, little interest in immediate surroundings or personal affairs

Stage 2—obvious short-term memory lapses, great hesitancy in verbal responses with confabulation to hide memory problems, disoriented to time, frequent losses of objects

Stage 3—disintegration of personality; disoriented to self, time, and place; apraxia; wandering behavior

---

CLINICAL STAGES OF ALZHEIMER'S DISEASE

STAGE ONE

Mild mental impairment
Forgetfulness
Impairment in judgment
Lessening of initiative
Lack of spontaneity

STAGE TWO

Confusion
Agitation
Irritability
Extreme restlessness
Incontinence of urine and stool
Need for constant supervision

STAGE THREE

Total inability to care for self
Inability to communicate
Total incontinence

Stage 4—terminal stage with severe physical and mental deterioration, incontinence, loss of ability to communicate, no recognition of family or self, swallowing problems

Although the signs and symptoms of Alzheimer's disease occur progressively, the rate at which they occur varies from person to person. A few patients have a very rapid decline, but usually many months pass with little change. As persons become more and more affected, they are more likely to develop pneumonia or other illnesses that may cause death.

Diagnostic Tests

No diagnostic test is specific for Alzheimer's disease. A computed tomography (CT) scan is often done to rule out other abnormalities. Often neuropsychologic testing can reveal characteristic changes in the ability to think.

MEDICAL MANAGEMENT

The care of the patient with Alzheimer's disease can be frustrating for the physician because the treatment options are so limited. Often, medication makes the problem worse. No medical treatment will improve the patient with Alzheimer's disease.

■ ASSESSMENT

Subjective Data

The following are the subjective data for the patient with Alzheimer's disease:

1. Patient's understanding of the disease
2. Change in mental status noticed by patient or family
3. Onset of symptoms

Objective Data

The following are the objective data for the patient with Alzheimer's disease:

1. Inability to carry out ADL
2. Behavior—evidence of agitation or restlessness
3. Presence of incontinence
4. Demonstrated change in mental status assessment

■ DATA ANALYSIS: NURSING DIAGNOSES

Nursing diagnoses are determined from assessment of patient data. Possible nursing diagnoses for the person with Alzheimer's disease include those for the patient with multiple sclerosis (p. 1827), as well as the following:

Diagnostic Title	Possible Etiologies
Injury, potential for	Sensory/motor deficits, lack of awareness of environmental hazards
Sleep pattern disturbance	Anxiety, environmental changes
Violence, potential for: self-directed or directed at others	Inability to control behavior, sensory/perceptual alterations

■ PLANNING: EXPECTED PATIENT OUTCOMES

The expected outcomes for the patient with Alzheimer's disease are the same as those for the patient with multiple sclerosis (p. 1828), with an additional outcome:
  "Safety is maintained."
Another difference is that in many cases the person with Alzheimer's disease is mentally incompetent; thus the caregiver must be closely involved in planning for the outcomes. The patient may not be able to have real input in the outcomes.

■ IMPLEMENTATION

Preventive Care

No known preventive measure or practice exists for Alzheimer's disease. Much of the focus of research includes finding a cause so that prevention can be implemented.

Acute Care

Preventing injury. It is important to protect the patient with Alzheimer's disease from injury. It may be necessary to install double locks on doors and windows to prevent the patient from leaving when there is no supervision. For example, this often occurs during the middle of the night. Controls on stoves may need to be removable to prevent the person from turning them on and possibly causing a fire. Matches should be stored in an inaccessible place, as should any poisonous fluids. The patient should be supervised at all times.[8]

Promoting activity. The patient with Alzheimer's disease may seem to have unlimited energy. They engage is many repetitive behaviors, such as walking for long periods or folding linens over and over. This activity should be somewhat encouraged because it keeps affected persons healthy for a longer time and tires them out, helping them sleep for longer periods at night. Walking can be an excellent activity for the patient, as well as for the caregiver.[8]

As the disease progresses, the person becomes more and more physically disabled. The nurse must then be aware of the need to turn the patient regularly to prevent skin breakdown and other complications of immobility. Range of motion should be done to prevent the development of contractures. Restraints used indiscriminately can hasten the person's physical decline.

At times patients are so active that, for example, it is difficult for them to sit long enough to eat. Finger foods that can be eaten while walking may be necessary. Patients should be encouraged to sit, and at times a soft waist restraint can help them do this at mealtime.

Promoting sleep. The tendency of patients with Alzheimer's disease to sleep for short periods can be very frustrating for caregivers.[43] It may be helpful to structure bedtime at same time each night. Caffeine should be restricted in the late afternoon and evening, and activities in the evening should be quiet if possible. Patients should be encouraged to exercise during the day to help tire them. At times the use of medications may be helpful in encouraging the patient to sleep, thus enabling the caregiver to rest as well.

Preventing agitation/violence. When persons are diagnosed with the disease, they face the beginning of many experiences, feelings, and fears. As the disease progresses, memory functions continue to deteriorate and patients become increasingly frustrated with their deficits. Significant depression, anxiety, and attempts at denial and rationalization occur as they observe their own brain failure. Patients are able to recognize that they are not reacting in a normal or predictable way. When asked, they can state that they are not thinking as well as they once did.[8]

Self-esteem is fostered by allowing and encouraging the patient to be as independent as possible. It is vital to avoid unnecessary frustrations so that complex tasks can be broken down into simpler components. Predictable routines are important. The caregiver must be aware of the patient's *stress threshold* and attempt to minimize stress to avoid angry, aggressive behavior.

Five basic groups of stressors that can produce dysfunctional behaviors include *fatigue, change of routine, excessive demands, overwhelming situations,* and *physical stressors* such as illness or pain. In the early stages of the disease, patients can be taught to structure their schedule and environment to maintain function. Memory aids can be helpful. As the disease becomes more disabling, the caregiver must assume more responsibility for monitoring and structuring the environment. Patients function best in predictable, known routines and environments.

When patients with Alzheimer's disease are put in situations where they cannot cope, overreaction to the stress may occur. This is described as a *catastrophic reaction*.

Patients are very aware of the feelings of those around them. Presenting care in a calm, unhurried manner helps reduce stress. It is important to treat the person with dignity and allow them to make whatever choices they are capable of making. Making decisions and choosing among the alternatives, however, requires higher-level cognitive processes and can be frustrating. If a decision or task precipitates a catastrophic reaction or if the patient becomes more agitated, decision making must be limited.

The patient should never be scolded or embarrassed. Arguing or reasoning with the patient increases patient resistance and escalates dysfunctional behavior. Reality-orientation techniques usually only increase confusion in these patients. If the patient is found to be depressed or distressed, counseling and possibly antidepressant medications may increase function.

Support groups for family members can be vital in supporting their care of the patient with Alzheimer's disease. Some areas also conduct groups for the patients themselves. The Alzheimer's Disease and Related Disorders Association,* which has chapters in many cities and may offer support groups for caregivers. Respite care services may assist the caregiver to cope (see Chapter 78).

VASCULAR DISEASES
CEREBROVASCULAR ACCIDENT
EPIDEMIOLOGY/ETIOLOGY

Cerebrovascular accident (CVA) is the most common disease of the nervous system and is the third highest cause of death in the United States. Five-hundred thousand Americans each year have an acute CVA.

In this chapter the term *cerebrovascular accident* is discussed as a general term. It should be recognized, however, that most neurologists and neurosurgeons more specifically refer to the disturbance in cerebral circulation as either a *thrombus, embolus, hemorrhage,* or *transient ischemic attack*. The nursing and medical care may differ depending on the specific cause. These

_____

*Alzheimer's Disease and Related Disorders Association, 360 N Michigan Ave, Suite 601, Chicago IL 60641.

CONDITIONS CAUSING CVA

THROMBUS

Atherosclerosis in intracranial and extracranial arteries
Adjacency to intracerebral hemorrhage
Arteritis caused by collagen (autoimmmune) disease or bacterial arteritis
Hypercoagulability such as in polycythemia
Cerebral venous thromboses

EMBOLI

Valves damaged by rheumatic heart disease (RHD)
Myocardial infarction
Atrial fibrillation (this dysrhythmia causes variable emptying of left ventricle; blood pools and small clots form; and then at times the ventricle is emptied completely with release of small emboli)
Bacterial endocarditis and nonbacterial endocarditis, causing clots to form on endocardium

HEMORRHAGE

Hypertensive intracerebral hemorrhage
Subarachnoid hemorrhage
Rupture of aneurysm
Arteriovenous (A-V) malformation
Hypocoagulation (as in patients with blood dyscrasias)

GENERALIZED HYPOXIA

Severe hypotension, cardiopulmonary arrest, or severe depression in cardiac output caused by dysrhythmias

LOCALIZED HYPOXIA

Cerebral artery spasms associated with subarachnoid hemorrhage
Cerebral artery vasoconstriction associated with migraine headaches

---

differences are discussed in each relevant section. *Hemiplegia* and *stroke* are also terms used when referring to CVA. Clinically, stroke refers to the sudden and dramatic development of focal neurologic deficits, and hemiplegia is one neurologic deficit that is typically seen.

The major causes of CVA are a thrombus, an embolus, or a hemorrhage, which can be precipitated by many underlying factors (see box above) frequently associated with other chronic diseases that cause vascular problems. These include heart disease, kidney disease, peripheral vascular disease, hypertension, and diabetes mellitus.

PATHOPHYSIOLOGY

The brain depends greatly on oxygen and has no reserve oxygen supply. Thus, when anoxia occurs, cerebral metabolism is promptly altered and cell death and permanent damage can occur within 3 to 10 minutes. Any condition that alters cerebral perfusion will cause hypoxia or anoxia. Hypoxia first leads to cerebral isch-

TABLE 63-6 Deficits resulting from disruption of blood flow in the brain

Artery	Areas of Brain Supplied*	Defects With Disruption of Flow
Internal carotid artery	Retina by its branch to retinal artery; lateral and medial surfaces of cerebral hemispheres by their branches to middle cerebral artery and anterior cerebral artery; portions of hypothalamus	Occasionally asymptomatic if good collateral circulation present Most frequently find the following: Intermittent ipsilateral visual impairment or blindness caused by retinal artery insufficiency Impairment similar to that seen with disruption of flow through middle cerebral artery Impairment caused by disruption of flow in anterior cerebral artery not frequently seen because both anterior cerebral arteries can be fed by one internal carotid artery Ipsilateral Horner's syndrome (ptosis, miosis, absence of sweating on same side of face) from hypothalamic damage
Anterior cerebral artery	Medial and superior surfaces of cerebral hemispheres; contains motor and sensory cortex for foot and leg and supplementary motor cortex; feeds large portion of frontal lobe	Contralateral hemiparesis or hemiplegia and contralateral sensory loss of lower extremities Upper extremities and face usually spared Confusion, dementia, and personality changes
Middle cerebral artery	Lateral portion of cerebral hemispheres, which contain motor and sensory areas for face and upper extremities and speech areas	Contralateral paralysis of paresis Contralateral sensory loss Sensory and motor loss are most noticeable in face, neck, and upper extremities Dysphasia or aphasia; may be global aphasia or only difficulty with expression without loss of comprehension; aphasia or dysphasia occurs if dominant hemisphere affected (left hemisphere in right-handed persons and most left-handed persons) Spatial perceptual problems (inability to judge distances, rate of movement, form and relationship of body parts); changes in judgment and behavior; neglect of paralyzed side; and inability to recognize paralyzed extremity as own (anosognosia) if nondominant hemisphere affected Contralateral homonymous hemianopia
Posterior cerebral artery	Posterior lateral and posterior medial surfaces of cerebral cortex, which contain primary visual receptive areas and internal structures; multiple branches that feed parts of optic pathway and diencephalic structure (thalamus and midbrain)	Paralysis usually absent Homonymous hemianopic field deficits If dominant side, difficulty with visual learning, visual recognition, and visual spatial orientation If branch to midbrain affected, can have ipsilateral oculomotor palsy and contralateral hemiparesis (Weber's syndrome) because of affect on cerebral peduncle; may have ataxia and choreoatherosis If bilateral occlusion to midbrain, will have quadriparesis (since all tracts pass through midbrain as they leave cortex); impaired consciousness; divergent gaze; and dilated, unresponsive pupils Patients in coma have unusual appearance in that they seem to be awake but do not communicate and do not respond; this has been termed *akinetic mutism* If thalamus affected, may have major sensory disturbances such as abnormal pain and dysesthesia, which are increased with emotional distress; the patient also may have emotional lability (crying, laughing without motivation); these symptoms are sometimes called *thalamic syndrome*

*Only major areas identified.

Continued.

TABLE 63-6 Deficits resulting from disruption of blood flow in the brain—cont'd

Artery	Areas of Brain Supplied	Defects With Disruption of Flow
Vertebral-basilar arteries	Multiple branches supply medulla oblongata, pans, midbrain, and cerebellum; no one structure receives all its blood supply from one branch; blood supply to ventral paramedian, ventrolateral, and dorsal brainstem structures all originate from different groups of arteries	Many different signs and symptoms depending on area of brainstem affected (pons, midbrain, or medulla) and what part of that area affected Because motor and sensory tracts pass through this area, paresis and sensory deficits affecting one to all four extremities may occur All cranial nerve nuclei are in this area, so disruption of their function may be present as visual impairment, focal paralysis, loss of sensory innervation to face, difficulty in swallowing, dysarthria, deafness, and so on Interference with cerebellar function can occur, causing ataxia, tremors, choreoatherosis, and so on Interference with reticular activating system causes alteration in consciousness Partial or complete Horner's syndrome caused by hypothalamic problem (ptosis of eyelid, constriction of pupil, absence of sweating on same side of face) Respiratory difficulty, syncope, nausea, and vomiting caused by dysfunction of major vital centers in brainstem

emia. Short-term ischemia (less than 10 to 15 minutes) causes temporary deficits but no permanent deficits. Long-term ischemia causes permanent cell death and results in a cerebral infarction. Cerebral edema accompanies the infarction and worsens the neurologic deficits seen in the patient.

The permanent focal deficits may be unknown when the patient is first seen because generalized cerebral dysfunction (coma) may be present. The generalized dysfunction may be a result of generalized ischemia affecting larger areas of the brain than the area of infarction and cerebral edema alone.

The type of permanent focal deficits will depend on the area of the brain that has been affected. The area of the brain affected depends on which cerebral vessels are involved. Table 63-6 lists the major vessels of the brain, the major areas of the brain perfused by each vessel, and the resultant deficits that occur when blood flow is disrupted.[33,50,51]

The *vessel most frequently affected is the middle cerebral artery*. The *second most frequently affected vessel is the internal carotid artery*. Other vessels are more rarely affected.

Because major differences exist in the clinical picture and care of the patient who suffers a CVA caused by hemorrhage, this is discussed in a separate section. The onset, pathologic process, and incidence of CVA from thombosis and embolism are different, and thus each is described before discussing care of the patient.

Cerebral Thrombosis

Thrombosis is the most frequent cause of a CVA; in one study of nonhemorrhagic causes of CVA it accounted for 92% of all CVAs. The most frequent cause of cerebral thrombosis is atherosclerosis. CVA secondary to thrombosis is seen most frequently in the 60-to-90-year age group, and many of these persons have a history of hypertension or diabetes mellitus.

It is important for nurses to be aware of the relationship between CVA and (1) atherosclerosis, (2) hypertension, and (3) diabetes mellitus so that they can be involved in appropriate preventive care.

The onset of symptoms of CVA secondary to thrombosis tends to occur during sleep or soon after arising. This may be related to elderly persons having decreased sympathetic activity and recumbency causing a lowering of blood pressure, which can lead to ischemia of the brain. In addition, these persons frequently have *postural hypotension and poor reflex response to changes in position*, which can cause hypotension on arising. Neurologic signs and symptoms very frequently deteriorate or worsen for the first 48 hours.

Cerebral arteriosclerosis may also lead to deterioration of brain tissue, even though CVAs do not occur. This condition, which usually is associated with high blood pressure, may occur in persons in their 50s, although it is usually considered a disease of old age.

Multiple small thrombi may occur in persons whose blood pressure is normal or even below normal if atheromatous changes have occurred in the lining of arteries. This condition causes frequent small, barely perceptible strokes. Both cerebral arteriosclerosis and multiple small strokes from thrombi may produce personality changes. The person who has arteriosclerosis is likely to have a more consistent downward course, whereas the one suffering from multiple small thrombi may have periods of apparently normal physical and mental episodes of confusion.

Both cerebral arteriosclerosis and multiple small thrombi cause slowly progressive changes that are particularly distressing to members of the person's family. Complete brain deterioration may occur. The person may feel irritable and unhappy with apparently little cause, and no amount of reassurance can make him or her feel better. The family must be prepared for gradual deterioration of the person's condition and should make provision for the person's safety and for the results of poor judgment. For example, the person may forget to dress appropriately, may give away family possessions, and may enter into unwise business dealings. The family needs help in learning how to treat the patient as an adult and yet deal with his or her limitations. The physician, the social workers, and the nurse can help family members care for the patient in such a way that their own lives are not completely disrupted and yet they are not plagued by guilt feelings when the patient dies. Institutional care is sometimes necessary, and the family needs encouragement and help in arriving at joint decisions that serve the best interests of all its members.

Cerebral Embolism

Embolism is the second most common cause of CVA. Patients who have CVAs secondary to embolism are usually younger, and most often the emboli originate from a thrombus in the heart. The myocardial thrombus is most frequently caused by rheumatic heart disease with mitral stenosis and atrial fibrillation. Therefore nurses can help to decrease the incidence of CVA from emboli by instituting the *preventive care measures* for persons with *rheumatic heart* disease described in Chapter 28. In addition, because cerebral embolism can originate from emboli in infarcted myocardium another set of preventive measures that nurses should be practicing are those described for the *prevention of myocardial infarctions* (see Chapter 28). Symptoms may occur at any time and progress rapidly. Emboli that originate from infected material can produce abscesses or other types of infections.

Transient Ischemic Attacks

CVA has just been discussed in relation to the causative agent or the vessel involved. CVA can also be described according to the temporal (time) character of the total clinical episode. Three profiles have been defined: transient ischemic attacks, stroke in evolution (progressive stroke), or completed stroke.

The term *transient ischemic attacks* (TIAs) refers to transient cerebral ischemia with temporary episodes of neurologic dysfunction. The neurologic dysfunction can be profound with complete loss of consciousness and loss of all sensory and motor function, or there may be only focal deficits of some sensory and motor functions. Focal deficits that occur depend on the area of the brain involved. The most *common deficit is contralateral weakness of the lower face, fingers, hands, arms and legs, transient dysphagia, and some sensory impairment.* Ischemic attacks may occur many times over days, weeks, months, or years. The neurologic deficit resolves, and between attacks the neurologic examination is normal.

TIAs may be caused by any of the conditions listed for CVA but most often precede cerebral thrombosis.

Stroke in evolution refers to development of a neurologic deficit over several hours to days. The clinical picture is the same as for a completed stroke; only the time course is different. *Completed stroke* refers to a permanent neurologic deficit.

The major importance of TIAs is that they warn the patient and health care provider of the existence of an underlying pathologic condition. At least one third of the patients who have TIAs will have a CVA within 2 to 5 years. Some patients will be treated with vasodilators, anticoagulant therapy, or drugs that inhibit platelet aggregation after they experience a TIA. The use of anticoagulants decreases the number of attacks. Aspirin (which prevents platelet aggregation) has also been shown to decrease subsequent attacks. The dose is 0.3 g four times per day. If an isolated, extracranial arterial lesion is found, surgical correction is possible.

CLINICAL MANIFESTATIONS

The exact clinical picture of CVA varies depending on the area of the brain affected. The most common focal neurologic signs and symptoms are those caused by disruption of flow through the midcerebral artery (see Table 63-6).

Frequently the patient is unconscious and may experience convulsions. Both unconsciousness and convulsions result from generalized ischemia and the brain's response to abrupt hypoxia.

Depending on the amount of cerebral edema present, the patient may have increased intracranial pressure (see Chapter 62 for a description of signs and symptoms of this condition).

Diagnostic Tests

A lumbar puncture is usually done and may reveal elevated spinal fluid pressure. If hemorrhage has occurred, there will be blood in the spinal fluid. In almost all instances a CT scan will be used to visualize the infarcted areas. If the patient is in a coma and it is uncertain how severe the increase in pressure is, CT may be used before the lumbar puncture. Lumbar puncture can precipitate tentorial or foraminal herniation when an expanding intracranial mass is present.

Following TIAs, a cerebral angiogram or digital subtraction angiogram may be done to discover blocked or occluded vessels.

MEDICAL MANAGEMENT

After the patient's condition is stable, or after the acute or rehabilitation phase, surgery may be used for selected patients. If the CVA is associated with a distinct atherosclerotic lesion in the extracranial system (internal carotid artery or common carotid artery), a carotid endarterectomy may be performed.

Surgical Intervention

A carotid endarterectomy involves the reaming out of the diseased vessel with the patient under either local or general anesthesia. Postoperative care includes the following:
1. Close attention to neurologic signs (changes in strength, mentation, speech, and level of consciousness)
2. Observation for bleeding in incisional area
3. Observation for swelling of the neck or complaints of dysphagia
4. Keep tracheostomy set in patient's room in case of severe respiratory distress

Revascularization procedures are now possible with the use of stereoscopic microscopes. Usually the superficial temporal artery is anastomosed to an artery within the brain such as the midcerebral artery. Other vessels can be used. The purpose is to provide for greater blood flow. The surgery usually does not resolve any permanent deficits but may prevent further problems. The care of the patient preoperatively and postoperatively is similar to that for any patient with cranial surgery but also includes the following:
1. Checking for pulse in anastomosed vessel
   a. Use of Doppler to detect pulse
   b. Gentle palpation
2. Keeping graft areas free of pressure
   a. Eyeglass frames bent out so as not to occlude vessel
   b. No other restricting bands around head

The patient will have a postoperative angiogram to assess the patency of the vessel.

■ ASSESSMENT

Subjective Data

The following list includes some subjective data for the patient who has had a CVA:
1. Patient's understanding of disease or symptoms

2. Characteristics of onset of symptoms
3. Presence of headache—nature and location
4. Any sensory deficits
5. Visual ability—presence of diplopia, blurred vision
6. Ability to think clearly
7. Any other concomitant symptom

Objective Data

The following objective data may be assessed in the patient who has had a CVA:
1. Motor strength—paresis or plegia common
2. Change in level of consciousness, including coma
3. Signs of increased intracranial pressure
4. Respiratory status
5. Ability to verbalize—presence of aphasia

■ DATA ANALYSIS: NURSING DIAGNOSES

Nursing diagnoses are determined from assessment of patient data. Possible nursing diagnoses for the person with a CVA include, but are not limited to, the following:

Diagnostic Title	Possible Etiologies
Airway clearance, ineffective	Perceptual/cognitive impairment
Anxiety	Threat/change in health status
Breathing pattern, ineffective	Neuromuscular impairment, perceptual/cognitive impairment
Communication, impaired verbal	Aphasia, physical impairment
Gas exchange, impaired	Ventilation/perfusion imbalance
Home maintenance management, impaired	Perceptual/cognitive impairment
Incontinence, total	Neurologic dysfunction/disease
Knowledge deficit: care required	Lack of exposure/recall, cognitive limitation
Mobility, impaired physical	Intolerance to activity, decreased strength and endurance, neuromuscular impairment
Nutrition, altered: less than body requirements	Anorexia, inability to obtain food
Self-care deficit: bathing/hygiene, dressing/grooming, feeding, toileting	Intolerance to activity, fatigue, perceptual/cognitive impairment, neuromuscular impairment
Sensory/perceptual alterations:	Altered sensory reception/transmission/integration
Skin integrity, impaired, potential	Mechanical forces, immobility
Thought processes, altered	Neurologic disorders
Tissue perfusion, altered cerebral	Decreased blood flow

■ PLANNING: EXPECTED PATIENT OUTCOMES

Expected patient outcomes for the person with a CVA may include, but are not limited to, the following:
1. Intracranial pressure is kept within safe limits.

2. Patent airway and adequate gas exchange are maintained.
3. Patient makes progress toward independence in ADLs.
4. Patient can safely compensate for visual field defects and perceptual, motor, and sensory losses.
5. Patient can explain prescribed therapy to follow at home.
6. Patient can demonstrate exercises to maintain function.
7. Patient can demonstrate the ability to communicate within disease process restrictions.
8. Patient can explain medication regimen at home and side effects, desired effects, time, dose, and route.
9. Patient can explain how to obtain assistance from community resources.
10. Patient can explain importance of frequent position changes and demonstrate such positioning.
11. Skin remains clear and intact.
12. Patient can state plans for follow-up care.
13. Continence is maintained to the extent possible.
14. Patient can manage home responsibilities.

■ IMPLEMENTATION

Preventive Care

Neurovascular disease can at times be prevented, or at least the results can be minimized. Many of the cerebrovascular diseases are thought to occur as a result of certain risk factors. These include the following:

1. Cigarette smoking
2. Hypertension
3. Hypercholesterolemia
4. Obesity
5. Stress-related occupations and a hectic-paced lifestyle

Secondary prevention is important with cerebrovascular disease because it is hoped the disease can be arrested before it causes irreversible results. The prevention of complications (tertiary prevention) is also important.

Acute Care

Emergency care. A CVA may occur when the person is at work or elsewhere outside the home and may be confused with convulsize seizures, diabetic coma, or drunkenness. Emergency care at the scene consists of turning the person carefully on to the affected side (determined by the puffiness of the cheek on this side) and elevating the head without tilting the neck forward, since tilting may constrict blood vessels and in turn cause congestion of blood within the cerebrum. Turning to the affected side permits saliva to drain out of the mouth and lessens the danger of aspiration into the lungs. Elevation of the head may help to prevent edema of the brain. Clothing should be loosened about the throat to aid further in preventing engorgement of blood vessels in the head, which may lead to cerebral edema. The person should be kept quiet, moved as little as possible, and protected from chilling. Medical assistance is sought at once.

Care in initial phase. Nursing intervention during the initial phase does not differ whether the person is in the hospital or at home, although oxygen is more likely to be given in the hospital. In an attempt to prevent further thrombosis or emboli, bishydroxycoumarin (Dicumarol) and heparin may be given in the hospital if it is certain that the cause is cerebral thrombosis or emboli and not cerebral hemorrhage. The use of anticoagulants is controversial. Some patients may be treated with various types of vasodilating agents, although the effectiveness of this type of therapy is not well established.

Goals are directed toward survival needs and preventing further brain damage. Care by the nurse is directed toward the unconscious state, if present (see Chapter 60). Neurologic assessment is done at regular intervals to detect changes in status and complications. The vital signs should be carefully checked, and the nurse should observe for such signs as a rise in temperature within the first day or two, slowing of pulse and respiration, and deepening of the coma, all of which indicate pressure on the vital centers and poor prognosis. Drugs to reduce intracranial pressure, such as dexamethasone (Decadron), may be given.

Care in acute phase. After the patient is stabilized physically, as just described, the nurse has the greatest influence of all health caregivers on the patient's recovery. Goals for care in the acute phase are directed toward preventing complications from the original CVA, from the immobility and dependency it causes, and from the loss of function caused by focal deficit.

Promoting nutrition. Fluids may be restricted for the first few days after a CVA in an effort to prevent edema of the brain. Patients are fed intravenous fluids, or the physician may insert a nasogastric tube and order tube feedings. When patients are no longer comatose, small amounts of fluid, 5 to 10 ml, can be given several times daily to determine patients' ability to swallow and to help them regain this function.[47] Returning as soon as possible to a regular diet and a normal fluid intake is desirable.

Promoting activity/mobility. Rest and quiet are important even if the CVA has not been serious enough to cause complete loss of consciousness. Some neurologists may prescribe that the head of the bed be kept flat for several days. This is believed to assist cerebral perfusion. No attempt should be made to rouse the patient from coma, although respiratory and circulatory stimulants may be prescribed by the physician if depression of these systems is present.

The time the patient remains in bed depends entirely on the type of CVA suffered and the judgment of the physician in regard to early mobilization. Some physicians prescribe fairly long periods of rest after CVAs, whereas others believe in *early mobilization of the patient with cerebral thrombosis.* Mobilization sometimes begins a day or two after the CVA has occurred.

Prevention of joint deformity is initiated during the acute stage. This includes positioning of affected limbs in anatomic position and ROM exercises. There should be a regular schedule for turning the patient to avoid the danger of circulatory stasis, hypostatic pneumonia, and decubitus ulcer.

Promoting bowel and bladder function. Urinary output should be noted carefully and recorded for several days after a CVA. Retention of urine may occur, but it is more likely that the patient will be incontinent. If urinary incontinence occurs, the patient who is not comatose may be told that control of excretory function probably will improve day by day. Offering a bedpan or a urinal immediately after meals and at other regular intervals helps to overcome incontinence. A retention catheter may be used for the first few days for female patients.

Fecal incontinence is fairly common following a CVA, and again the patient must be assured that as general improvement occurs, this condition will be overcome. Some patients develop constipation, and impactions develop readily. Elimination must be noted carefully, since diarrhea may develop in the presence of an impaction, causing the impaction to go unnoticed for several days. Suppositories such as bisacodyl (Dulcolax) are generally prescribed to be given daily or every other day. However, some physicians order stool softeners, laxatives, or enemas. Warm oil-retention enemas are sometimes given in an attempt to prevent impactions or to treat them when they occur. Milk of Magnesia by mouth is often given because straining during defecation increases ICP. The patient must be cautioned not to strain and must be assured that the suppositories can easily be repeated if no results are obtained. The patient usually needs assistance in getting on and off the bedpan. Side rails that can be held onto while turning or a trapeze that can be reached with the unaffected arm and hand help the patient to move independently and to get on and off the bedpan if this activity is allowed.

Providing emotional support. If the patient survives the first few days, consciousness may begin to return, and some of the paralysis may disappear. It is then that the greatest understanding is needed by persons attending the patient. The patient will become aware of the aphasia, drooling, paralysis, and unsteadiness and will be very upset by the awareness. It is at this point that the nurse's active part in rehabilitation begins. By quiet assurance a nurse can help the patient feel that progress toward recovery and self-sufficiency has begun and will continue.[21]

Promoting communication. The nurse can help by explaining what is going to be done even though the person may not be able to respond by speaking. If the patient has *aphasia* and also is unable to use the dominant *hand,* an additional problem of trying to write with the nondominant hand occurs. The nurse should try to anticipate patients' needs and should make every effort to understand indistinct speech, since repeated attempts to make themselves understood only augment misery and frustration.[65] Usually, if partial speech is present at the time of return to consciousness, speech probably will improve and the patient is heartened by this knowledge. Speech may also be affected because of involvement of the tongue, mouth, and throat muscles.

The patient who has sustained a CVA may be overly emotional. This reaction, combined with the fear and frustration on becoming aware of his or her condition, is upsetting to the family. Crying is common, and sometimes family members believe that they are responsible for this sadness when this is usually not true. Family, staff, and other patients need reassurance that they are not the cause of the reaction.

Compensating for perceptual difficulties. Following a stroke, persons may have difficulty relating to themselves and to their environment. After the acute stage a multibed environment is advocated because the sensory input from others is helpful. In the initial stage, bringing familiar articles into the patient's environment can be a very helpful stimulus. Examples are a clock, watch, family picture, or a Bible. *Hemianopsia,* or decreased visual field, occurs quite frequently. Approaching patients from the side of intact vision and teaching them to scan will not only make them more aware of stimuli but can help prevent injury. Diminished awareness or denial of the affected side (anosognosia) can occur and could be a safety hazard. This possibility should be considered when the patient runs into objects with the wheelchair or allows the affected arm or leg to drag behind when transferring from chair to bed.

The nurse's observations regarding the patient's mental status are important. The patient may be disoriented and have decreased judgment or poor memory. A constant environment and routine are helpful in improving orientation and the ability to function. Poor judgment and impulsiveness can be major safety hazards. Such behavior is brought to the attention of the physician. The family also must be aware of this if they are to care for the patient at home. See the left box on p. 1847 for summary of care.

CARE OF THE PATIENT WITH A CVA

1. Promote nutrition.
   a. Use intravenous or tube feeding until patient is able to eat.
   b. Begin attempts to feed as soon as patient is no longer comatose.
2. Promote activity.
   a. Position affected limbs to prevent contractures.
   b. Turn frequently.
   c. Perform ROM exercises.
   d. Begin mobilization as soon as medically possible.
3. Promote elimination.
   a. Monitor intake and output to check for urinary retention.
   b. Start bladder program early.
   c. Avoid urinary catheters.
   d. Start bowel program.
4. Provide emotional support.
   a. Reassure patient of progress.
   b. Explain what is being done.

RECOVERY STAGES FOLLOWING CVA

Flaccidity	No voluntary motion and no muscle tone are present.
Partial synergy	Muscle tone develops, and muscles contract either voluntarily or with spasticity. Patient can move extremities in part of synergy pattern.
Synergy	Spasticity is moderate to severe. Patient can move joints through all or most of synergy pattern.
Breaking out	Spasticity decreases. Patient can perform combinations of movements that are out of synergy.
Partially isolated	Spasticity has less influence. Movement combinations bear less resemblance to stereotyped patterns.
Isolated	Almost normal movement is present, with good control of voluntary movement and little spasticity.

PATIENT TEACHING

The teaching for a patient with a CVA is the same as that for the patient with a motor problem (see Chapter 62).

Rehabilitation Care

The greatest challenge for the nurse in care of the patient who has had a CVA comes after the patient is past the point of danger. Then the long, slow process of learning to use whatever abilities remain or can be relearned must be faced, and adjustments to limitations must be made if the patient and family are going to have fulfilling lives.

The nurse is an important member of the rehabilitation team. Three basic rehabilitation goals are:
1. Prevention of further impairment
2. Maintenance of existing abilities
3. Restoration of as much function as possible

Maximizing return of function. Return of motor impulses and subsequent return of function are evidenced by a tightening and spasticity of the affected part. The return occurs in stages. Theses stages can last from hours to months. Recovery may also halt at a specific stage and progress no further. Brunstrom[18] has defined these recovery stages in terms of degrees of synergy. *Synergy* has been defined as muscles acting together as a bound unit in stereotyped movement patterns. See the box above, right for these stages.

Return of motor impulses is significant for the future use of the affected part but presents new problems for the patient, nurse, and all others who may be involved in care. Muscles that draw the limbs toward the midline become very active, and the arm may be held tightly adducted against the body. The affected lower limb may be held inward and adducted to, or even beyond, the midline. Muscles that draw the limbs into flexion are also stimulated, with the result that the heel is lifted off the ground, the heel cord shortens, and the knee becomes bent. In the upper limb, flexor muscles draw the elbow into the bent position, the wrist is flexed, and fingers are curled in palmar flexion. This is often seen following a CVA because the adductor and flexor muscles are stronger than opposing muscles.

Persistent nursing efforts must be directed toward prevention of further impairment and keeping any part of the body from remaining in a position of flexion long enough for the occurrence of muscle shortening and joint changes that might interfere with free joint action. If a physical therapist is not available, the total responsibility for preventive measures may rest with the nurse. *Every minute counts in prevention, and the nurse must not miss one opportunity to move the patient's adducted or flexed limbs back to the correct position.*

Passive exercise stimulates circulation and may help to reestablish neuromuscular pathways. No difficulty is encountered with these procedures until tightening of the muscles begins to appear. Then other physical measures are needed, and at this point, if not earlier, a physical therapist should be involved in the patient's treatment. The occupational therapist may also be involved and may provide various kinds of splints (Figure 63-1).

Recently the Bobath technique has been found useful to assist in the functional recovery of the patient who has had a CVA. The Bobath technique is a treatment approach that attempts to make muscle tone more nor-

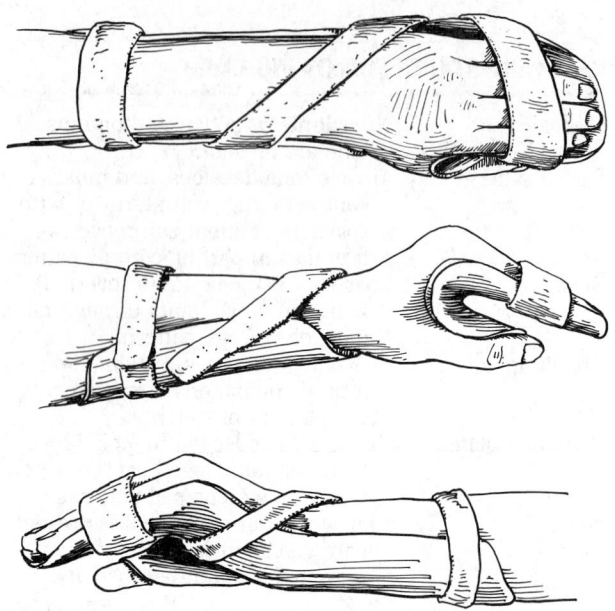

FIGURE 63-1 Volar resting splint provides support to wrist, thumb, and fingers of patient following CVA, maintaining them in position of extension. (From Dittmar SS: Rehabilitation nursing, St Louis, 1989, The CV Mosby Co.)

mal. This is done by providing as many sensations of normal muscle tone, posture, and movement as possible. The goal of treatment is to redirect short-term memory toward an appreciation of normal movement of the paralyzed side by using techniques of weight bearing, counterrotation, and protraction of the shoulder girdle and pelvis.[90] (The reader is referred to a rehabilitation nursing text for a further description of this technique.)

Promoting mobility/ambulation. *Active exercise* of the affected side also may be started early. In the hospital it may be directed by the physical therapist or nurse. In consultation with the physical therapist, the nurse plans the exercises while the patient is in the hospital, and the nurse or the physical therapist may teach the exercises to the family in preparation for the patient's return home.

Since the patient who has had a CVA will greatly depend on the unaffected arm and leg when moving about, the unaffected part of the body needs attention to prevent contractures and preserve muscle strength. Even while in bed, the patient should exercise the unaffected arm and use it in all normal positions. The unaffected leg should be in a position of slight *internal rotation* most of the time while the patient is in bed, and the knee should be bent several times each day. Exercises to strengthen the quadricep muscles should be done because the quadriceps is the most important muscle in

providing stability to the knee joint needed for walking (see Chapter 22).

Early *ambulation* facilitates vasomotor tone and has positive psychologic effects on the patient and family. Ambulation is usually started by the physical therapist by having the person walk between parallel bars. Transfer techniques are also taught to the patient and family (see following discussion).

When patients begin to move about and to try to help themselves, they may have several problems that can alter their ability to proceed. They may have loss of position sense, so that it is awkward for them to handle their bodies normally even when they have the muscular coordination to do so. They may have dizziness, spatial-perceptual deficits, diplopia, and alteration of skin sensation. They may also have to work harder than other persons to receive a normal amount of air on inhalation, because the involved side of the chest does not expand easily. This difficulty may lead to excessive fatigue unless those caring for the patient plan activities so that the patient's effort is not wasted.

Before standing or walking, patients may practice raising themselves up in bed and may sit on the side of the bed while holding firmly to an overbed table or to a strap with their good hand and pressing their feet on a chair or stool. The patient benefits from wearing shoes, because it is good for morale and keeps the paralyzed foot in good position.

If preparation for walking has been adequate, the patient usually needs only one crutch when walking begins; then a cane will be used as walking progresses. When walking first begins, the nurse must remain close to allay the fear of falling. Balancing may be practiced by standing between parallel bars or by leaning on the backs of two chairs (provided the chairs are heavy enough to support weight safely). Good walking patterns must be established early because incorrect patterns are difficult and sometimes impossible to change. A sideward shuffle should be watched for and avoided. The patient should begin by leaning rather heavily on the crutch or cane and lifting the body sufficiently to bring the leg and foot forward so that the toes point straight ahead and not inward. The cane or single crutch is held in the hand opposite the paralyzed or weakened side of the body. Pivot transfers may be the easiest way to transfer the patient from bed to chair, and vice versa. When a pivot transfer is used, the chair is always placed so that the unaffected side leads the transfer.

Promoting activities of daily living. The patient is evaluated on ability to carry out the usual ADL and is assisted by the occupational therapist or nurse in becoming independent in each activity to the extent possible. Assistive devices may be used (Figures 63-2 to 63-6). Reha-

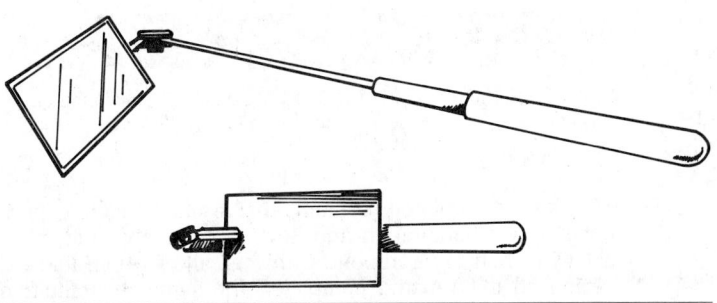

FIGURE 63-2 Long-handled skin inspection mirror. (From Dittmar SS: Rehabilitation nursing, St Louis, 1989, The CV Mosby Co.)

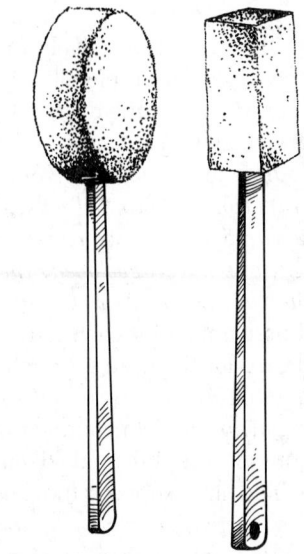

FIGURE 63-3 Long-handled bath sponge. (From Dittmar SS: Rehabilitation nursing, St Louis, 1989, The CV Mosby Co.)

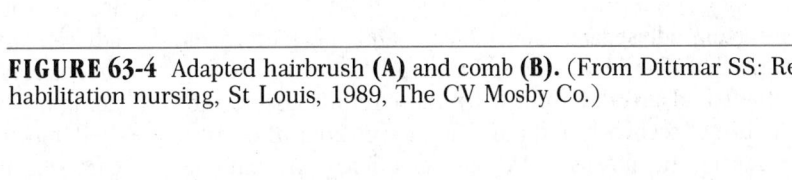

FIGURE 63-4 Adapted hairbrush **(A)** and comb **(B).** (From Dittmar SS: Rehabilitation nursing, St Louis, 1989, The CV Mosby Co.)

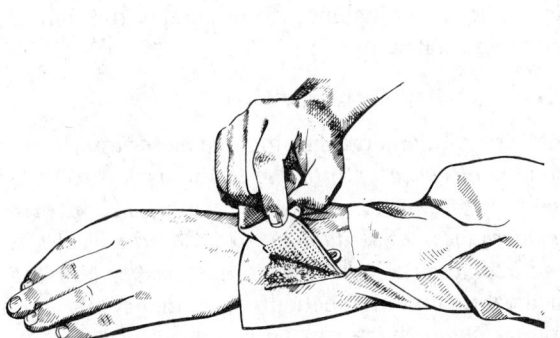

FIGURE 63-5 Velcro shirtsleeve to facilitate closure. (From Dittmar SS: Rehabilitation nursing, St Louis, 1989, The CV Mosby Co.)

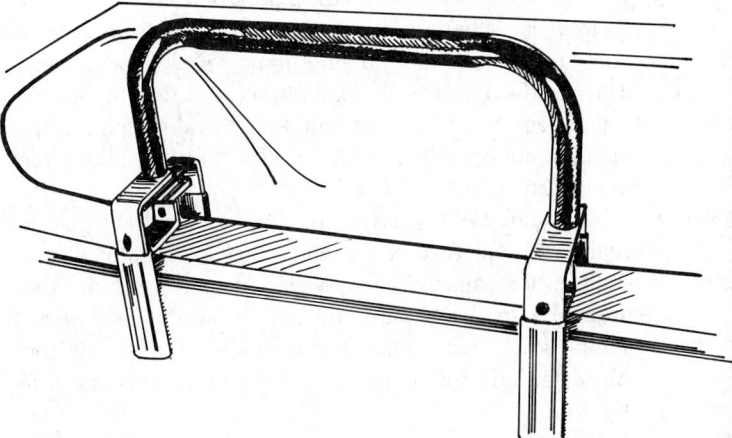

FIGURE 63-6 Bathtub with grab bars. (From Dittmar SS: Rehabilitation nursing, St Louis, 1989, The CV Mosby Co.)

bilitation in this way is essentially a teaching-learning process in which the patient is actively involved. Motivation is absolutely essential to rehabilitation but unfortunately is not found to the same degree in all patients. Some patients devote all their energies to their rehabilitation, whereas others just seem to "give up." *If there is return of hand function in 2 to 3 weeks, fecal incontinence has disappeared, and no contractures, decubiti, or other complications have developed, there is reason to believe that the patient can be independent in care.*

Patients need preparation for each new step in learning to move and care for themselves. Each new activity must be demonstrated by the nurse and then practiced by patients; supervision and encouragement must be given by the nurse. Careful and detailed instruction on how to hold and support the body will save patients much embarrassment, discomfort, and confusion. By using the unaffected hand, the patient may, for example, straighten out the flexed fingers on the affected side and move the affected arm to a position where, with the weight of gravity, the elbow will be straightened. Most patients can relearn to do ADL such as those pertaining to personal hygiene and dressing.

Promoting adjustment. General care and the pattern of living that should be followed after a CVA vary for each patient and are determined by the circumstances, the amount of recovery, and the guidance given in the early stages of the illness.[29] Despite all efforts, the patient may, for example, never be able to negotiate stairs. The social worker and the community health nurse are indispensable in helping to arrange the patient's home so that the greatest possible degree of self-sufficiency and independence is possible. Family members often need help in assisting the person to accept limitations, both physical and emotional. The family must also make adjustments to actual circumstances. Almost all persons who have CVAs need health supervision for the rest of their lives. Whether the patient will be able to return home or must go to a nursing home will depend a great deal on the family's understanding and acceptance of the patient and his or her limitations when maximal rehabilitation has been achieved. See the box above for relevant research.

Although CVAs may recur, the person may go for years with no further difficulty and eventually die of some other cause. The physician usually explains the prognosis to the person and to the family. The nurse should know what explanation has been given by the physician and sometimes must help in interpreting it to the family.

The person who has sustained a CVA and who has high blood pressure is usually advised to take prescribed antihypertensive medications as ordered, to get suffi-

RESEARCH

Davidson A and Young C: Repatterning of stroke rehabilitation clients following return to life in the community, J Neurosurg Nurs 17(2):123-128, 1985.

This study explored problems that stroke patients experience after rehabilitation and how they perceive and interact with their environment. Subjects, all of whom had experienced a CVA and completed the same rehabilitation program, were interviewed in their homes by means of a 16-question interview form developed and pretested by the investigators. The results indicated that although most subjects had gained some physical return of function, most energy was consumed with accomplishing ADL. To do pleasurable activities involved complex planning and timing. The study indicated that nurses need to consider individual life patterns, current patient goals, and the resources of the home and community in planning interventions. ∎

cient rest, and to avoid strain and excitement. Persons involved in strenuous work may be advised to reduce their work schedule and take more frequent vacations. Those who are overweight are advised to bring their weight within normal limits, and those who smoke are advised of the hazards of vasoconstriction caused by nicotine. ADL may be modified; sitting while shaving or doing other similar activities helps conserve energy.

Before discharge to the home or to another health care setting, certain outcomes should be achieved. The major emphasis is on maintaining structural and body integrity consistent with pathologic involvement. The parameters involved in achieving this are intact skin, normal range of joint motion with no contractures, loss of muscle tone confined to that which is consistent with pathologic condition, and maintenance of bladder and bowel function. When these outcomes are achieved at the highest degree possible, the person is ready for discharge. Obviously, some persons' conditions will limit their ability to become completely sufficient in ADL, and some persons will benefit from long-term rehabilitation either in a rehabilitation hospital or through regular outpatient follow-up care.

INTRACRANIAL HEMORRHAGE

Intracranial hemorrhages include *bleeding into the subarachnoid space or into the brain tissue itself.* Unlike cerebral thrombosis or cerebral embolism, *intracranial hemorrhages cause damage to the brain by destroying and replacing neighboring brain tissue.* Nursing and medical treatment of patients with aneurysms and intracranial hemorrhage can be significantly different from that of patients with CVAs caused by embolism or thrombosis. Because of this, intracranial hemorrhages are considered separately.

EPIDEMIOLOGY/ETIOLOGY

Intracranial hemorrhages are the third most frequent cause of CVAs. Bleeding may be from a vessel on the surface of the brain, and the bleeding may be limited to the subarachnoid space. This is called a *subarachnoid hemorrhage with intracerebral hemorrhage.*[23] Bleeding from a vessel in the brain substance is called an *intracerebral hemorrhage* and may form a cerebral hematoma. Intracerebral hemorrhages may extend through the brain tissue to the ventricles and the subarachnoid space.

The most common causes of cerebral hemorrhage are listed in Table 63-3. *Berry aneurysms* can result from congenital deficits. *Fusiform aneurysms* can develop from atherosclerosis. *Mycotic aneurysms* are caused by *necrotic vasculitis* occurring in the vessel at a site where septic emboli have lodged. The necrosis causes thinning of the vessel wall and aneurysm formation.

Hypertension causes thickening and degeneration of cerebral arterioles, making the small arteries vulnerable to rupture. Arteriovenous (A-V) anomalies are tangled, interconnected vessels that allow blood to pass directly from the artery to the vein without passing through the capillaries.[32] These vessels may be fed by one or several normal cerebral arteries and are usually malformed. Arterial pressure distends and eventually ruptures these vessels.

PATHOPHYSIOLOGY

Any of these problems (aneurysms, hypertensive vascular disease, A-V malformation) can result in a subarachnoid hemorrhage, intracerebral hemorrhage, or a combination of the two. The most common site for berry aneurysms is the anterior portion of the circle of Willis at the junction between the internal carotid and posterior communicating arteries. Other common sites are the middle cerebral artery or the anterior communicating artery. A small number of intracranial hemorrhages occur in the vertebral-basilar artery system. Multiple aneurysms are found in many persons. The rupture of a vessel causes disruption of the blood flow to a selected area, as well as focal ischemic changes and infarction of brain tissue. In addition, the sudden release of blood acts as a concussion and unconsciousness results. It also causes a rapid rise in cerebrospinal fluid (CSF) pressure with displacement of the brain. *Bleeding into brain tissue itself can cause brain damage by dissecting the brain along the fiber tracts.* The blood itself is a noxious agent, and as it is hemolyzed, it irritates the blood vessels, the meninges, and the brain. The blood and the release of vasoactive substances promote arterial spasms, which can further decrease cerebral perfusion.[38]

CLINICAL MANIFESTATIONS

Symptoms of an intracranial hemorrhage include sudden explosive headache, photophobia, and neck rigidity (if subarachnoid), nausea and vomiting, loss of consciousness (usually), convulsions, signs and symptoms of increased intracranial pressure, respiratory distress and shock.

The following system of grading has been developed to classify the clinical state of the patient with intracranial bleeding by level of consciousness and neurologic deficit.

grade I Minimal bleeding, alert, no neurologic deficit.
grade II Mild bleeding, alert, minimal neurologic deficit such as third nerve palsy and stiff neck.
grade III Moderate bleeding, drowsy or confused, stiff neck with or without neurologic deficit.
grade IV Moderate or severe bleeding, semicoma with or without neurologic deficit.
grade V Severe bleeding, coma, decerebrate movement.

Additional grades are also added for patients over 50 years of age and those with major heart, lung, kidney and liver conditions that increase risk for procedures.

Diagnostic Tests

The diagnostic tests used for intracranial hemorrhage are the same as those used for cerebrovascular accidents.

Laboratory findings include an abnormal CT scan, increased CSF pressure, and blood and white blood cells in the CSF. Lumbar puncture may not be performed if there is evidence of extensive brain damage for fear of precipitating *tentorial herniation.* An arteriogram is used to identify the exact cause of the problem.

MEDICAL MANAGEMENT

Surgery

The only satisfactory treatment for congenital aneurysm is surgery. If an intracerebral hematoma has formed, it may be evacuated after the patient's condition is stable. Before surgery can be performed, however, the location of the aneurysm must be determined by arteriography (angiography). The time after the acute rupture when arteriograms are taken and when surgery is performed varies with the person, age, the intensity and kind of symptoms present, and the surgeon's judgment. Because angiography may increase symptoms, it may be followed by immediate surgery.

Before surgical treatment of an aneurysm is attempted, the surgeon usually explains the hope for cure and the risks involved to the patient's family. The nurse must appreciate how distressing the situation is for the family and should realize that the time spent waiting to know whether the outcome will be favorable seems interminable to them. The nursing care the patient will receive postoperatively should be explained to the family if they are to be with the patient. For example, it is important that both the patient and the family know that blood pressure, pulse rate, respiratory rate, and other pertinent observations will be taken frequently, because these procedures can be most upsetting if their purpose and the need to check them so frequently is not understood. Some patients may spend the initial postoperative period in the intensive care unit. The family should be prepared for this possibility.

Surgery consists of a *craniotomy* and *location of the aneurysm*. When found, the aneurysm may be obliterated by ligation at its neck with the application of a silver clip. If the base of the aneurysm is too large for ligation to be practical, it may be wrapped or it may be coated with a liquid, adherent, plastic substance that hardens to form a firm support about the weakened vessel wall and thereby prevents rupture.[100] If the aneurysm has not ruptured but has produced symptoms, attempts may be made to produce thrombosis within the aneurysm by use of an electric current and other means. Both before and after surgery the nurse should observe for signs of increased intracranial pressure.

If the surgery is successful, patients will be cured, although usually they will be advised to avoid strenuous exercise and emotional stress for the remainder of their lives. Occasionally, they may have a severe physical or mental handicap resulting from damage to brain tissue during surgery. If so, they need the same type of care as discussed for patients with a CVA (see p. 1847).

Other Procedures

Not all aneurysms can be treated surgically at the site of the lesion. If surgery is not feasible, to reduce the chances of hemorrhage, the common carotid artery in the neck may be completely or partially obliterated to lessen the blood flow to the site of the aneurysm, *provided* enough blood can be supplied from collateral vessels to preserve vital brain function. The procedure usually is done in stages of several days.

A clamp (Silverstone or Salibi) that has a detachable screw stem and can be tightened gradually is used. Usually the surgeon adjusts it each day, and the nurse who attends the patient watches closely and is instructed to release the clamp at once if evidence of inadequate blood supply exists. Neurologic checks are done regularly by the nurse relative to placement of the clamp in the dominant or nondominant hemisphere. Any signs of muscle weakness in the face or in either extremity on the side opposite the incision or any changes in the level of consciousness, vital signs, or sensory or muscular coordination or control should be reported to the neurosurgeon at once. Immediate removal of the clamp may prevent irreversible complications such as hemiplegia, aphasia, and loss of consciousness.

If symptoms of inadequate blood supply appear, further surgical treatment cannot be done safely, although the clamp may be left indefinitely to partially obliterate the vessel. If complete occlusion can be tolerated, the vessel may be permanently ligated. Serial embolizations of blood vessels that "feed" the aneurysm may also be done via the femoral or axillary route.

The procedure is similar to a cerebral angiogram, and the postoperative care is the same. Thrombus formation with resultant cerebral embolism may complicate the patient's postoperative course following any surgery for a cerebral aneurysm. It is a feared and often fatal complication.

■ ASSESSMENT

The nursing assessment for the patient with intracranial hemorrhage includes the factors identified in the subjective and objective assessment for the patient who has had a CVA (see p. 1844).

■ DATA ANALYSIS: NURSING DIAGNOSES

Nursing diagnoses are determined from assessment of patient data. Possible nursing diagnoses include those found in the section on the patient who has had a CVA (p. 1844).

■ PLANNING: EXPECTED PATIENT OUTCOMES

In addition to those defined for the patient with a CVA (p. 1844), expected patient outcomes for the person with an intracranial hemorrhage also may include:
1. Does not develop signs of increased intracranial pressure.
2. Does not develop complications from immobility.
3. Patient can explain the need for surgery.
4. Patient can explain any restrictions in activity.

■ IMPLEMENTATION

Preventive Care

The prevention of intracranial hemorrhage is similar to prevention of CVA. Many same risk factors also apply.

Acute Care

The immediate treatment for intracranial hemorrhage is to keep the person absolutely quiet to prevent additional bleeding. Many of these patients are unconscious and require care as described in Chapter 60. In addition, because the bleeding causes an elevation in the intracranial pressure, they need care for this. An antifibrinolytic agent (Amicar) may be used to seal the clot. See the box on p. 1853 for further details of the nursing care of the patient with an intracranial hemorrhage.

Patient Teaching

If the patient with an intracranial hemorrhage has neurologic deficits consistent with a CVA, the patient teach-

NURSING CARE OF THE PATIENT WITH AN INTRACRANIAL HEMORRHAGE

1. Use gentleness in moving patient.
2. Keep room darkened.
3. Keep patient on bed rest; head of bed is usually elevated 30 degrees. Occasionally bathroom privileges are allowed.
4. Give patient no ice water.
5. Initiate a bowel program to prevent straining at stool.
6. Allow only a few visitors.
7. Decrease stimuli in room; no TV or radio in severe cases.
8. Take no rectal temperatures; give no enemas or suppositories.

ing is the same (see p. 1847). Also, several other points are important:

1. Importance of following activity restrictions
2. Importance of keeping as free of stress as possible
3. Very specific teaching about what activities are restricted
4. Use of medication and what it does
5. Information about preoperative and postoperative care

INFECTIONS/INFLAMMATIONS

The nervous system may be attacked by a variety of organisms and viruses and may suffer from toxic reactions to bacterial and viral disease. Sometimes the infection becomes walled off and causes an abscess; sometimes the meninges, or coverings of the brain and spinal cord, are involved; and sometimes the brain itself is affected most. Organisms and viruses may reach the nervous system by various routes. Untreated chronic otitis media and mastoiditis, chronic sinusitis, and fracture in any bone adjacent to the meninges may be the source of infection. Some organisms, such as the tubercle bacillus and probably the pneumococcus, reach the nervous system by means of the blood or the lymph system. Meningitis can also occur as a complication of invasive procedures such as lumbar puncture or procedures involving the use of contrast media. The exact route by which some infectious agents, such as the meningococcus in epidemic meningitis and the viruses that cause encephalitis, reach the central nervous system is not known.

Meningococcal meningitis (epidemic) and poliomyelitis are reportable communicable diseases. Because they are becoming less common and because they are discussed in specialized texts, they are mentioned only briefly here.

Several conditions that occur as a result of infection or inflammation of the nervous system are discussed in this section. These conditions include:

1. Meningitis
2. Encephalitis
3. Brain abscess
4. Poliomyelitis
5. Guillain-Barré syndrome
6. Neurosyphilis
7. Herpes zoster

Some aspects of these diseases are discussed together.

MENINGITIS
EPIDEMIOLOGY/ETIOLOGY

Meningitis is an acute infection of the meninges usually caused by pneumococci, meningococci (epidemic), staphylococci, streptococci, *Haemophilus influenzae*, or aseptic agents (usually viral). Any other pathogenic organism, such as the tubercle bacillus, that gains access to the subarachnoid spaces can also cause meningitis. Mild forms of the disease do occur and may be referred to as *meningism*. They may be caused by viruses. A common form of the disease is lymphocytic meningitis, believed in many instances to be associated with a virus.

The incidence of bacterial meningitis is higher in fall and winter when upper respiratory tract infections typically occur. Children are more often affected than adults because of frequent colds and ear infections. Disease caused by the enteroviruses is more common in the summer and early fall than in other seasons of the year.

PATHOPHYSIOLOGY

As previously stated, organisms and viruses reach the nervous system by many routes. Once organisms reach the brain, the CSF in the subarachnoid spaces and in the pia arachnoid membrane becomes infected. The infection then spreads rapidly throughout the meninges and eventually invades the ventricles. Pathologic alterations include hyperemia of the meningeal vessels, edema of brain tissue, increased intracranial pressure, and a generalized inflammatory reaction with exudation of white blood cells into the subarachnoid spaces. An associated hydrocephalus may be caused by exudate blocking the small passages between the ventricles.

CLINICAL MANIFESTATIONS

Meningitis can be a medical emergency. The onset (except when caused by tubercle bacilli) is usually sudden and characterized by severe headache, stiffness of the neck, irritability, malaise, and restlessness. Nausea, vomiting, delirium, and complete disorientation may develop quickly. *Kernig's sign* (the inability of the patient to extend the legs completely without extreme pain) is usually present with meningitis. When the neck of the patient with meningitis is flexed, the hip and knee also flex; this is known as *Brudzinski's sign*. Temperature, pulse rate, and respirations are increased. The diagnosis is usually confirmed by examination of spinal fluid obtained from a lumbar puncture. Usually the offending organism can be isolated from the spinal fluid; if a pyogenic organism is the cause, the fluid is cloudy. The CSF pressure is usually elevated, the protein level is elevated, and the sugar content is decreased.

Residual damage from meningitis includes deafness, blindness, paralysis, and mental retardation. These complications are usually the result of chronic arachnoiditis or subdural effusion. Hydrocephalus may also develop. These complications are now less common because the infection is effectively treated with antibiotics before permanent damage to the nervous system occurs.

Diagnostic Tests

Most of the infections involving the nervous system can be diagnosed by examining the CSF. A CT scan and an EEG may also be done. These procedures are discussed in Chapter 59.

MEDICAL MANAGEMENT

Medical management includes the use of antibiotics, as discussed under implementation. If the patient develops hydrocephalus as a result of the meningitis, medical management may include the insertion of a shunt to facilitate movement of the CSF.

■ ASSESSMENT

Subjective and objective data are important in any patient with an infection of the nervous system. This assessment includes common characteristics of all infections/inflammations discussed in this section.

Subjective Data

The following subjective data should be obtained from the patient with infection of the nervous system:
1. Patient's understanding of process and possible causes
2. Any history of infection, such as upper respiratory infections
3. Initial onset of symptoms
4. Measures that relieved symptoms
5. Presence of discomfort, including headache or stiff neck
6. Presence of difficulty in thinking
7. Presence of muscle weakness, soreness, or uncoordination

Objective Data

The following objective data for the patient with infection of the nervous system may be observed by the nurse:
1. Behavior—signs indicating discomfort or disorientation

2. Change in ability to carry out ADLs
3. Abnormalities on physical assessment part of neurologic examination
4. Temperature elevations
5. Presence of vomiting
6. Pulse and blood pressure
7. Respirations
8. Level of consciousness

■ DATA ANALYSIS: NURSING DIAGNOSES

Nursing diagnoses are determined from assessment of patient data. Possible nursing diagnoses for the person with a neurologic infection include, but are not limited to, the following:

Diagnostic Title	Possible Etiologies
Activity intolerance	Bed rest, immobility, generalized weakness
Breathing pattern, ineffective	Neuromuscular impairment
Communication, impaired verbal	Aphasia
Disuse syndrome, potential for	Immobility, weakness
Hyperthermia	Illness, trauma
Incontinence, total	Neurologic disease
Knowledge deficit: cause of infection and care required	Cognitive limitation, lack of exposure/recall
Mobility, impaired physical	Neuromuscular impairment
Self-care deficit: bathing/ hygiene, dressing/ grooming, feeding, toileting	Neuromuscular impairment
Skin integrity, impaired	Mechanical forces (pressure, shearing forces, restraint)
Thought processes, altered	Neurologic disorders

Not every diagnosis will apply to every infection. Much will depend on the severity of the deficit.

■ PLANNING: EXPECTED PATIENT OUTCOMES

Expected patient outcomes for the person with a neurologic infection may include, but are not limited to, the following:
1. Patient can state the nature of the infection, infectious agent, and method of transmission.
2. Patient can explain how to prevent further infection.
3. Patient can state and explain medications and side effects, action, route, and dosage.
4. Patient remains neurologically intact.
5. Patient can state plans for follow-up care.

■ IMPLEMENTATION

Preventive Care

Because meningitis is linked closely with upper respiratory and ear infections, prevention of these can help prevent meningitis. Prevention includes avoiding crowds during peak seasons for colds and other viral infections and receiving prompt treatment for ear or upper respiratory infections.

The prompt diagnosis and treatment of meningitis can prevent morbidity and mortality.

Acute Care

Medications. Treatment consists of massive doses of the antibiotic specific for the causative organism. Culture and sensitivity studies determine the most effective antibiotic. Usually a course of at least 10 days of parenteral administration is needed. The antibiotic may be given directly into the spinal canal (intrathecally). The use of hyperosmolar agents or steroids may also be necessary to decrease cerebral edema. Anticonvulsants may be administered to prevent seizures.

Preventing complications. Respiratory isolation is required until the pathogen can no longer be cultured from the nasopharynx. This is usually accomplished after 24 hours of effective antimicrobial therapy. Therapy is continued until the patient has been afebrile for 5 days or after 7 days of therapy (whichever is longer).

Supportive Nursing Care

Nursing care for the patient with meningitis includes the general care given a critically ill patient who may be irritable, confused, and unable to take fluids and yet is dehydrated because of elevation of temperature. The room is kept darkened, noise is kept at a minimum, and care is taken not to jar the bed because any increase in sensory stimulation can cause a seizure. The patient must be observed very carefully and must be constantly attended if disorientation is present. Padded side rails should be placed on the bed. The patient should be observed for symptoms of inappropriate secretion of antidiuretic hormone (see Chapter 23), which can occur readily in patients with meningitis.

ENCEPHALITIS
EPIDEMIOLOGY/ETIOLOGY

Encephalitis is inflammation of the brain tissues and its coverings. Occasionally the meninges of the spinal cord are also involved. Encephalitis can have a variety of causes. A generalized inflammation of the brain can be caused by syphilis, and encephalitis can follow exogenous poisoning, such as that following the ingestion of lead or arsenic or the inhalation of carbon monoxide. It can be caused by reaction to toxins produced by infections such as typhoid fever, measles, and chickenpox, and occasionally it follows vaccination.

Encephalitis caused by a virus and occurring in epidemic form was first described by von Economo in Austria, and the name Von Economo's disease is still used to identify the widespread epidemic in the United States

that followed the influenza epidemic in 1918. This form of the disease has not recurred since 1926. Von Economo's disease was also called encephalitis lethargica and sleeping sickness, a term still used by lay persons. The demonstration that viruses can affect the central nervous system after a prolonged incubation period has resulted in considerable search for viral agents in many chronic neurologic diseases.

The death rate from encephalitis varies with epidemics but is generally fairly high. The most common sequela for patients who do recover from the acute disease is *paralysis agitans,* which may come on suddenly or develop slowly. Other residual neurologic symptoms may also occur and occasionally incapacitate the patient completely.

ACUTE VIRAL ENCEPHALITIS
Epidemiology/Etiology

Viral encephalitis appears to be caused by several viruses, some of which may be interrelated. Acute viral encephalitis can be classified into epidemic and sporadic forms. The primary causes of acute epidemic encephalitis are members of the *arbovirus* (those transferred by a biting arthropod to humans) or *togavirus* group (named after properties of the virus). About 80 viruses of the arbovirus group cause disease in humans. Six of the viruses cause infections of the central nervous system (Table 63-7).

Clinical Manifestations

Clinical features of acute epidemic encephalitis, caused by the arboviruses that infect humans, are similar. The eastern equine form is more severe than the western form. The onset is abrupt, with a high fever, headache, meningeal signs, nuchal rigidity, and vomiting. Drowsiness or coma and focal or generalized convulsions develop within 24 to 48 hours after onset. Focal neurologic signs occur, such as hemiplegia and cranial nerve palsies. These are typical findings in the CSF. Fatality rates may be as high as 60%. Those who survive usually have no sequelae.

ACUTE ENCEPHALITIS (NONEPIDEMIC)

Acute encephalitis occurs sporadically and is caused by the herpes simplex virus (HSV). It occurs at any age, but more than half the persons are at least 15 years of age. Upper respiratory complaints often precede the onset of neurologic symptoms by at least 24 hours or longer. Headache and focal or major convulsions are the common early signs of cerebral involvement. A persistent high fever and coma typically occur. Spinal fluid proteins may be moderately elevated, and red blood cells are often present when spinal fluid is examined. Herpetic skin lesions do not usually occur.

TABLE 63-7 Arbovirus infections of the central nervous system occurring in the western hemisphere

Disease	Causal Agent	Location	Incubation Period (Days)	Clinical Manifestations
California encephalitis	Arbovirus of California virus (mosquitoborne)	United States, Canada, Alaska, Yukon, north-west territories	5-15	Aseptic meningitis, encephalitis
Eastern equine encephalitis	Eastern equine enceph-aencephalitis virus (mosquitoborne)	Eastern seaboard and Gulf states, Caribbean	5-15	Severe encephalitis (usually infants and children)
Powassan encephalitis	Powassan virus (tick-borne)	Canada, northeastern and north-central United States	4-8	Encephalitis
St. Louis encephalitis	St. Louis encephalitis virus (mosquitoborne)	Central, southern, northwestern, western, and central United States; southern Ontario; Caribbean	4-21	Encephalitis aseptic meningitis
Venezuelan equine encephalomyelitis	Venezuelan equine encephalomyelitis virus (mosquitoborne)	Texas, Florida, Mexico, Central and South America	2-5	Fever, headache, myalgia, malaise, cough, encephalitis
Western equine encephalomyelitis	Western equine encephalomyelitis virus (mosquitoborne)	Central and western United States and Canada, Central and South America	5-10	Encephalitis (infants), fever, aseptic meningitis

Adapted from Report of the Committee on Infectious Diseases, American Academy of Pediatrics, 1977.

MEDICAL MANAGEMENT

Medical management of acute encephalitis involves the use of antibiotics to eradicate the virus. Other measures to reduce increased intracranial pressure may be necessary.

■ ASSESSMENT/DIAGNOSES/OUTCOMES

The reader is referred to the section on meningitis for subjective and objective data, nursing diagnoses, and patient outcomes.

■ IMPLEMENTATION

Preventive Care

Prevention of arboviral infections consists of eradication of the mosquito or tick vector, including destruction of larvae and elimination of breeding places. Infection is controlled by avoiding mosquito or tick bites. Avoiding the substances that cause exogenous poisoning also helps decrease the occurrence of encephalitis. Proper, timely diagnosis is important with encephalitis.

Acute Viral Encephalitis

Nursing care consists mainly of symptomatic or supportive care and careful observation. Any change in appearance or behavior must be reported at once, since the progress of this disease sometimes is extremely rapid. The patient is kept in bed, and side rails are used if disorientation develops. The patient must be constantly attended to prevent injury. During the period when the temperature is high, sponging or other antipyretic measures may be ordered. Frequent changes of linen may be necessary if perspiration is excessive.

No specific medical treatment exists for acute viral encephalitis. No isolation is necessary because encephalitis is not transmitted from person to person.

Acute Encephalitis (Nonepidemic)

Treatment of acute nonepidemic encephalitis is supportive with anticonvulsant drugs and steroids to reduce cerebral edema. Adenine arabinoside (Ara-A) may be given parenterally.[113]

BRAIN ABSCESS
EPIDEMIOLOGY/ETIOLOGY

A brain abscess is almost always secondary to foci of infection somewhere else in the body. Common sites include the ear, sinus or mastoid, lung, heart, pelvic organs, teeth, or skin. The three most common organisms involved are streptococci, staphylococci, and pneumococci. Brain abscesses occur most often in older children and young adults but may be seen at any age. At times no organism is found, and the abscess is called a *sterile abscess*.

PATHOPHYSIOLOGY

In the first stage of brain abscess, a localized inflammation of the brain occurs with formation of exudate. Septic thrombosis of some vessels develops, and the surrounding brain tissue becomes edematous and necrotic. After days to weeks the inflammatory reaction decreases as the area is walled off. "Satellite" abscesses may occur, and the abscesses may rupture into the ventricles. Brain abscesses are most often found in the temporal lobe and the cerebellum.

CLINICAL MANIFESTATIONS

There may be a history of infection, although the person may not recall an infection. The most common symptom is a constant or intermittent headache that is not relieved by medication and that worsens with straining. There may be drowsiness, confusion, and mental slowness. Focal or generalized seizures may occur. Fever with bradycardia is often present. There may be signs and symptoms of increased intracranial pressure (see Chapter 62). The evolution of symptoms is variable. In some patients a rapid progression of symptoms may end in death, whereas in others the course is more benign. Generally, however, the mortality is high with brain abscess; residual disability often results. Brain abscess also may recur.

Diagnostic Tests

The diagnosis of brain abscess is made primarily on the basis of the history and examination of the CSF. EEG changes are present, and areas of increased uptake of dye are seen on the CT scan.

IMPLEMENTATION

Treatment consists of administering the appropriate antibiotics, often for extended periods. Because it may take some time to isolate the causative organism, broad-spectrum antibiotics or combined antibiotic therapy may be used. Appropriate agents to reduce intracranial pressure may be necessary.

Nursing care is supportive and directed toward ongoing assessment for signs and symptoms of increased intracranial pressure, seizures, and spread of the infection. Measures to prevent permanent damage from neurologic deficits that might be present should be instituted. The long hospitalization, length of treatment, neurologic deficits, and chance for recurrence all are major sources of stress. The nurse must be prepared to spend time with the patient and significant others to help them cope with these stressors.

POLIOMYELITIS
EPIDEMIOLOGY/ETIOLOGY

Poliomyelitis is an acute febrile disease caused by poliovirus types 1, 2, and 3; paralysis is more common with type 1. With discovery of the Salk vaccine, its wide use since 1956, and the availability of a safe "live virus" vaccine (Sabin vaccine), this disease, which had been a serious crippler of children and young adults, has become quite rare.

PATHOPHYSIOLOGY

The incubation period for poliomyelitis is 7 to 21 days. The virus attacks the anterior horn cells of the spinal cord where the motor pathways are located and may cause motor paralysis. Sensory perception is not affected since posterior horn cells are not attacked. Poliomyelitis sometimes takes a somewhat different form and attacks primarily the medulla and basal structures of the brain, including the cranial nerves; the term *bulbar poliomyelitis* is used for this form.

IMPLEMENTATION
Preventive Care

An essential part of the nurse's responsibility is to help prevent poliomyelitis by encouraging immunizations. It is important to have all children immunized.

Acute Care

Management of poliomyelitis usually includes bed rest, supportive therapy, and respiratory assistance if needed.

GUILLAIN-BARRE SYNDROME (POLYNEURITIS)
EPIDEMIOLOGY/ETIOLOGY

Guillain-Barré syndrome, known also as acute inflammatory polyradiculoneuropathy and postinfectious polyneuritis, is often serious because of the extent to which the nervous system may be affected. This condition has become better known to the public since it was identified as a sequela of swine flu immunization. The disease occurs most often in persons 30 to 50 years of age and is seen equally in men and women. The cause is unknown, but two theories are emerging: (1) that it is caused by a viral agent or (2) that it is an autoimmune reaction.

PATHOPHYSIOLOGY

Patchy demyelination occurs in the peripheral nerves, nerve roots, and root ganglia and spinal cord in Guillain-Barré syndrome. For this reason it may be classified as a neuritis. Axons are generally spared so that recovery may occur early; in severe forms, *wallerian degeneration* occurs with involvement of the axons, making recovery slow. In the severe form, protein in the CSF is elevated.

If the seventh, ninth, and tenth cranial nerves are involved, the patient may have varying degrees of difficulty in swallowing, speaking, and breathing. The vital centers in the medulla oblongata may be affected, and the patient may die of respiratory failure. Patients with

NURSING CARE PLAN

PERSON WITH GUILLAIN-BARRÉ SYNDROME

DATA: Mr. Doe is a 45-year-old married auto mechanic with a history of progressive weakness that began in his feet and legs. For the past day he has not been able to walk. He is also complaining of shortness of breath. He gives a history of an upper respiratory tract infection 2 weeks before admission. On admission he demonstrated weakness of all four extremities. His tidal volume was decreased and his respiratory rate was 32. He complained of discomfort in his lower extremities. The sensory examination was WNL. He was alert and oriented ×3. He was admitted to the neurologic unit for observation. He was started on corticosteroids, and his respiratory rate closely monitored. The day after admission the patient demonstrated paralysis of muscles below the waist.

The nursing history identified the following:
- He is unsure about what has happened to him and the reason for his weakness.
- He expresses anxiety about what to expect.
- He seems to have a close relationship with his wife.
- Leisure activities are mainly sports activities.

Collaborative nursing actions include those to prevent further complications caused by muscle weakness and respiratory weakness. Immediate reporting may prevent serious effects (respiratory arrest, clot formation). Nursing actions include monitoring for the following:
- Signs of respiratory compromise: decreased tidal volume, increased shortness of breath, tachnypnea, cyanosis, restlessness
- Signs of pulmonary embolism: chest pain, hemoptysis
- Signs of DVT (deep vein thrombosis): difference in leg girth, positive Homan's sign, leg pain, difference in temperature of legs

NURSING DIAGNOSIS
Anxiety related to change in health status

Expected Patient Outcomes	Nursing Interventions	Rationale
Patient verbalizes minimal anxiety.	Explain to patient procedures being done. Allow him time to verbalize feelings.	Explanations will help minimize anxiety. Expression of fears will lessen anxiety.
	Encourage his wife to spend time with him.	Family members are an important source of support.

NURSING DIAGNOSIS
Breathing pattern, ineffective, related to neuromuscular impairment

Expected Patient Outcomes	Nursing Interventions	Rationale
Patient will have adequate breathing pattern.	Assess respiratory rate, tidal volume, and color frequently. Notify physician of any changes immediately. Keep head of bed at 30 degrees. Give supplemental oxygen as ordered.	Ongoing assessment will detect critical changes. Changes in respiratory status can occur quickly. Position helps respiratory effort. Lowered oxygen levels in blood are common with impaired respiratory efforts.

NURSING DIAGNOSIS
Pain in legs related to Guillain-Barré syndrome

Expected Patient Outcomes	Nursing Interventions	Rationale
Patient states that leg pain is improved.	Position for comfort.	Positioning may relieve pain.
	Administer mild analgesic such as acetaminophen.	Pain relief is provided.
	Teach relaxation measures as appropriate.	This promotes rest and eases pain.

NURSING CARE PLAN

PERSON WITH GUILLAIN-BARRÉ SYNDROME—cont'd

NURSING DIAGNOSIS

Injury, potential for, related to possible trauma

Expected Patient Outcomes	Nursing Interventions	Rationale
Contractures do not develop.	Position patient with limbs in normal anatomic position.	Such positioning will prevent flexion contractures.
	Change position q2h.	
	Perform passive or active ROM to all extremities several times a day.	Activity stretches muscles and keeps joints movable.
	Assist out of bed at least daily.	Change in position helps prevent complications of immobility.
	Apply elastic stockings and keep legs elevated when up in chair.	This assists with venous return and helps prevent stasis.

NURSING DIAGNOSIS

Knowledge deficit related to lack of exposure to information

Expected Patient Outcomes	Nursing Interventions	Rationale
Patient can describe nature of disease and possible complications.	Review nature of disease with frequent reinforcement.	Teaching can raise patient's level of cooperation.
		Reinforcement of earlier teaching helps promote retention.

NURSING DIAGNOSIS

Mobility, impaired physical, related to neuromuscular impairment

Expected Patient Outcomes	Nursing Interventions	Rationale
Patient has minimal impairments in mobility.	Allow patient to do as much for self as possible.	Active exercise has positive effect on patient.
	See actions under "Injury, potential for."	

NURSING DIAGNOSIS

Self-care deficit: bathing/hygiene, dressing, toileting related to neuromuscular impairment

Expected Patient Outcomes	Nursing Interventions	Rationale
Patient carries out ADL at highest ability level.	Provide basic ADL needs as necessary but encourage patient to do what he can.	Self-care will promote positive self-concept.
	Provide sufficient time to do ADL.	Doing ADL when patient has deficits often takes more time.
	Work with therapists to optimize patient's learning needs.	Team work can accentuate care.

NURSING DIAGNOSIS

Body image disturbance; role performance, altered; related to loss of body functions and immobility

Expected Patient Outcomes	Nursing Interventions	Rationale
Patient verbalizes positive self-concept.	Provide information about disease and expected progress	Understanding of disease will improve self-concept.
	Provide privacy.	Patient may be embarrassed by need for physical care.
	Provide care but encourage patient to do as much for self as possible.	Ability to care for self will improve self-concept.
	Encourage family to visit.	Visitors will cheer patient.
	Give family chance to share their concerns.	If family concerns are met, they can be more supportive of patient.
	Encourage family to maintain previous role relationships, if possible.	There is comfort in knowing that role in family is intact.
	Identify patient's strengths and weaknesses.	This can assist nurse in planning care with patient.

Continued.

PERSON WITH GUILLAIN-BARRÉ SYNDROME—cont'd

NURSING DIAGNOSIS

Skin integrity, impaired; potential, related to mechanical forces and pressure

Expected Patient Outcomes	Nursing Interventions	Rationale
Skin remains intact.	Monitor pressure areas for signs of skin breakdown.	Early detection of pressure can allow time for measures to prevent breakdown.
	Use turning sheet when turning patient to prevent shearing effect.	Shearing forces lead to skin breakdown.
	Turn patient q2h.	Turning prevents pressure areas.
	Keep skin clean and dry.	Moisture leads to skin breakdown.
	Use air mattress or water mattress or special bed.	Can assist with relief of pressure areas.

less severe involvement may recover fully, although a year or more may transpire before the patient is completely well.

CLINICAL MANIFESTATIONS

The patient with Guillain-Barré syndrome has symmetric muscle weakness and lower motor paralysis characteristics (flaccidity). The paralysis usually starts in the lower extremities, and it ascends upward to include the thorax, upper extremities, and face. Selected cranial nerves may also be affected, as previously mentioned. Other symptoms that may be assessed clinically are paresthesias and sensory alteration as the sensory roots and nerves may also become involved. Respiratory failure may occur as intercostal muscles are affected, and without mechanical ventilation there is a 10% to 20% mortality. The bowel and bladder are rarely affected. Autonomic symptoms, such as a fluctuating blood pressure, may occur.

Variations may exist in the pattern of onset of weakness, as well as in the rate of progression of symptoms. The progression may stop at any point.

IMPLEMENTATION

A priority goal for the nurse and the patient with Guillain-Barré syndrome is the maintenance of respiratory function.[104] Close observation of respiratory function is necessary. This should include serial measurements of the patient's vital capacity, tidal volume, and minute volume. Urinary retention occurs in about 5% of patients. Patients who develop respiratory failure require mechanical ventilation and are usually placed in an intensive care unit. Nursing care of patients with respiratory failure is discussed in Chapter 33. Adrenocortical steroids are used empirically to treat symptoms. Conva-

lescence may require several months. Attention to the prevention of iatrogenic complications, such as contracture, decubitus ulcers, muscle atrophy, and loss of range of motion, is imperative. Recovery is usually complete.[14]

A nursing care plan for the person with Guillain-Barré syndrome can be found on p. 1858-1860.

NEUROSYPHILIS
PATHOPHYSIOLOGY

In the late or chronic stage of syphilis, infection may involve the brain and spinal cord. The oculomotor nerves may be involved, causing inability of the pupil to react to light (Argyll Robertson pupil). *Tabes dorsalis* is the name given to the involvement of the posterior columns of the spinal cord and the posterior nerve roots. Since the sensory nerves are primarily involved, sensory symptoms predominate. The patient may have severe paroxysmal pain anywhere in the body, although perhaps the most common location is in the stomach. This condition, known as *gastric crisis,* may be confused with ruptured peptic ulcer or other acute conditions of the stomach or gallbladder. Areas of severe paresthesia may be present. A common finding in tabes dorsalis is loss of position sense in the feet and legs. The patient is unable to sense where the feet are placed, and as a result there is a slapping gait that is highly characteristic of the disease. Increased difficulty walking in the dark occurs because the person relies on vision in placing the feet. Visual loss or even total blindness also occurs. Tabes dorsalis can cause trophic changes in the limbs and changes in the joints so that stability is lost (*Charcot's joint*).

General paresis is the term used to designate another late manifestation of syphilis in which degeneration of the brain, deterioration of mental function, and varying evidences of other neurologic disease occur. More specific information can be found in neurology texts.

With the success of penicillin in the treatment of syphilis, the incidence of neurosyphilis has decreased. However, the recent rise in the overall incidence of syphilis among young adults may indicate problems in the future.

HERPES ZOSTER
ETIOLOGY

Herpes zoster, also known as *shingles,* is a common disease that occurs at higher rates among the elderly and in patients with lymphomas, cancer, and Hodgkin's disease.

PATHOPHYSIOLOGY

The causative organism is the varicella virus, similar to the one that causes herpes simplex. It may occur as a result of reactivation of the viral infection that lies dormant in the ganglion following a primary case of chickenpox. It is not communicable, except in persons who have not had chickenpox. An acute inflammatory reaction develops in the spinal or cranial sensory ganglions, the posterior gray matter of the cord, and the meninges.

CLINICAL MANIFESTATIONS

The rash seen in herpes zoster consists of a vesicular, cutaneous eruption within a dermatome. It may be preceded by severe itching, pain in the area, fever, and malaise. There may be segmental weakness and atrophy in the same area as the sensory changes. A small percentage of patients are seen with ophthalmic herpes, with the rash and pain occurring along the distribution of the trigeminal nerve.

IMPLEMENTATION
Acute Care

Treatment for herpes zoster consists mainly of supportive care with medication for control of pain. The pain may persist for some time after the rash disappears. Phenytoin (Dilantin) and carbamazepine (Tegretol) may be helpful in control of persistent pain. Steroid therapy started early in the disease course is believed to shorten it. This is not recommended for patients who are immunosuppressed. Special emphasis on rest, nutrition, and hydration during the acute period is important.

Control of Environment

Isolation precautions may be necessary, especially to protect staff who have not had chickenpox and most especially to protect pregnant women. Also, patients with cancer, lymphomas, or Hodgkin's disease who have not had chickenpox should be protected from exposure to the patient.

ISOLATION MEASURES FOR HERPES ZOSTER

Private room with private toilet facilities
Gown, masks, and gloves required of care givers
Strict hand washing
Linen handled as isolation linens
Double-bagging of dressings
Disposable dishes if possible
Transport patients out of room only as necessary
Isolation procedure for all visitors

Because the virus is spread by direct contact and airborne routes, strict isolation is often necessary, at least until any drainage from the lesion stops. See the box above for isolation measures for herpes zoster.

TRAUMATIC LESIONS

Parts of the nervous system typically subjected to trauma include the craniocerebrum, the spinal cord, and the peripheral nerves. With the exception of the peripheral nerves, each is protected by a bony covering. The phrase *traumatic lesions,* as used here, includes lesions resulting from direct physical force and injuries that result from sustained compression. Attention is directed primarily to direct physical injuries in the following discussion.

CRANIOCEREBRAL TRAUMA
EPIDEMIOLOGY/ETIOLOGY

Craniocerebral trauma, or head injury, causes death and serious disability in people of all ages. In the United States, head injuries result in about 80,000 deaths yearly. Morbidity and mortality is higher in males. Primary traumatic lesions result from industrial, motor vehicle, and military accidents. Head injury is the second most common cause of major neurologic deficits, and the major cause of death between ages 1 and 35 years. It is estimated that 70% of motor accidents result in head injury. Brain injury causes more deaths than does injury to any other organ. In some states the repeal of laws requiring motorcyclists to wear helmets has resulted in an estimated threefold increase in death and injury resulting from damage to the brain sustained in motorcycle accidents.

PATHOPHYSIOLOGY

Craniocerebral trauma may result in injury to the scalp, skull, and brain tissues, either singly or collectively. Variables that may modify the extent of the injury to the head include the location and direction of the impact, rate of the energy transfer, the surface area of energy transfer, and the status of the head at the time of the impact. Injuries vary from minor scalp wounds to concussions and open fractures of the skull with severe damage to the brain. The amount of obvious damage is not indicative of the seriousness of the injury.

Contusions, abrasions, and lacerations of the scalp may occur. Lacerations of the scalp bleed profusely because of the scalp's large blood supply. Most bleeding is minor and controlled readily. An internal hematoma of the scalp may form as a result of the bleeding and resemble a depressed fracture. Infection of the scalp may result from the presence of foreign debris. It should be stressed that the absence of external scalp injury does not preclude serious craniocerebral damage.

The skull indents and deforms when a physical impact occurs. Fractures often result and are classified as in other parts of the body. Skull roentgenograms may detect the fractures; a negative x-ray film does not exclude the presence of a hairline fractures. Fractures can occur distal to the point of impact. A compound and depressed fracture causes serious complications. *The presence of a skull fracture does not necessarily indicate that brain injury has occurred.* A reverse correlation often exists between skull damage and brain damage. Complications of skull damage may include injury to cranial nerves, epidural hemorrhage, and brain contusion.

CLINICAL MANIFESTATIONS

Damage to the brain tissues per se may include concussion, contusion, or laceration. Each is discussed briefly here to differentiate them as to their degree of damage and significance. The dura may remain intact in brain damage (a *closed injury*), or the dura may be opened from a direct blow or from penetrating objects such as bone fragments or knives (an *open injury*).

A *concussion* is characterized by an immediate and transitory impairment of neurologic function caused by the mechanical force. No structural alteration is demonstrable. There may be loss of consciousness that is instant or delayed and is usually recovered. The effect of a blow on the cranium to the soft brain tissues contained within the closed cavity is one of sudden movement. This effect can be likened to what happens as one stops suddenly when moving quickly with an open dish of fluid—some of the fluid spills. The only difference is that instead of spilling in the closed cavity, the brain tissues strike the bony coverings forcibly. The damage sustained is variable in degree. Damage may occur to the brainstem centers and the cerebral hemispheres. There can be loss of consciousness, the cause of which is not clearly understood. Any person who exhibits an alteration in consciousness following a blow on the head should be under constant observation for a time, since damage is not always immediately apparent.

A *contusion* is a structural alteration characterized by extravasation of blood cells. It can be likened to

bruising without tearing of the tissues. The contusion may be at the site of the impact or on the opposite side. A concussion or contusion site may be classified as a *coup* (at the site), *contrecoup* (opposite the site), or *intermediate*. Contusions often damage the cortex.

Laceration of the brain tissues and blood vessels is a tearing of the tissues that may be caused by a sharp fragment or object or a shearing force. It is obvious that hemorrhage may be a serious complication.

In summary, when the head receives a direct blow or injury, the brain moves in the skull and suffers varying degrees of damage not always at the site of the injury. In addition, the brain swells to a great extent, and the capacity of the brain to swell may exceed the capacity of the closed cranial cavity to expand. Most deaths from head injury are from the brain swelling rather than from the actual primary destruction of vital centers. Brain edema is thus a major cause of increased intracranial pressure and its consequences (as previously discussed in Chapter 62). Along with the swelling, local and systemic disturbances in circulation occur with resulting anoxia. The brain damage may be minor or severe. A great disparity often exists between functional neurologic derangement and structural damage that can be demonstrated.

Table 63-8 compares the effects seen with the different types of head trauma.

Hemorrhage resulting from craniocerebral trauma may occur at the following sites: scalp, epidural, subdural, subarachnoid, intracerebral, and intraventricular. Epidural and subdural hematomas are discussed because of the need for careful and continuing observations by the nurse.

An *epidural hematoma* forms as blood collects between the dura and the skull. Since bleeding in this area is usually caused by laceration of the middle meningeal artery, it is capable of producing rapid clot formation. If *lethargy or unconsciousness develops after the patient regains consciousness,* an epidural hematoma may be suspected. Bleeding needs to be controlled promptly and the blood evacuated. Common sites for bleeding include basal and temporal skull fractures. The nurse should be alert for potential epidural hematomas when it is known that fractures exist in these sites.

A *subdural hematoma* forms as venous blood collects below the dural surface. Since the bleeding is under venous pressure, the hematoma formation is relatively slow. However, the clot formation will cause pressure on the brain surface and may eventually displace brain tissue. If this expanding clot is not evacuated, it can contribute to a rise in intracranial pressure and its sequelae. Thus a subdural hematoma can become serious because of its location and compression of vital areas. If a patient who has been conscious for several weeks or months after a head injury becomes unconscious and

TABLE 63-8 Damage of brain tissue caused by trauma

Trauma	Characteristics	Structural Alteration	Effects
Concussion	Characterized by immediate and transitory impairment of neurologic function caused by mechanical force	No	May be loss of consciousness that is instant or delayed; usually reversible
Contusion	Likened to bruising with extravasation of blood cells	Yes	Injury may be at site of impact or at opposite site; often damage is to cortex
Laceration	Tearing of tissues caused by sharp fragment or shearing force	Yes	Hemorrhage is serious complication

develops neurologic symptoms, a subdural hematoma should be suspected. *Nurses need to be aware of the delayed signs of head injury as well as the immediate and more obvious ones. The focal neurologic signs from clot formation can be related to the site of the clot.*

Fractures of the *base of the skull* are usually serious because of the site. When one is sustained, *vital centers, cranial nerves, and nerve pathways may be permanently damaged.* Trauma and the resulting edema may obstruct CSF flow directly or indirectly with resultant increased intracranial pressure. If the injury has caused a direct communication between the cranial cavity and the middle ear or the sinuses, meningitis or a brain abscess may develop. Bleeding from the nose and the ears suggests a basal fracture. Serosanguineous drainage from these orifices may contain CSF and should be noted. Intracranial bleeding as a result of trauma may cause the same signs and symptoms as nontraumatic hemorrhage.

Diagnostic Tests

Diagnostic procedures are performed as necessary and most often include CT scans, skull roentgenograms, and possibly cerebral angiography. When a hematoma is suspected, a trephine of the skull (burr holes) may be performed. It is important to remember that the contrast media used during the CT scan and angiography will increase intracranial pressure.

Many neurosurgeons believe that alert and intelligent nursing care is often the decisive factor in determining the outcome of the patient. Side rails should always be on the bed, and a padded tongue blade or an airway to protect the tongue should be kept at the bedside, since restlessness may come on suddenly and convulsions may occur. Usually the bed is kept flat, although some neurosurgeons believe that the danger of edema to the brain may be reduced by slight elevation of the head of the bed.

MEDICAL MANAGEMENT

If the head injury causes hematoma formation, the best medical approach may be surgery.

The surgical treatment for extradural hematoma consists of making a burr hole in the skull to relieve the pressure caused by the bleeding and to attempt to control the bleeding. Sometimes a craniotomy, removal of a large bony window, is necessary. Occasionally the patient has so much damage to the soft tissue of the brain that death occurs despite relief of pressure caused by the bleeding. Usually, such a patient is unconscious after the accident and is taken to the hospital at once.

■ **ASSESSMENT**

Subjective Data

Subjective data for a patient with a head injury who is conscious includes the following:
 1. Patient's understanding of injury and resulting pathology
 2. Patient's ability to understand
 3. Information about nature of injury—how it happened
 4. Presence of headache, nausea, or vomiting
 5. Presence of diplopia or other visual problems
 6. Unusual sensations (paresthesias, ringing in ears)
 7. History of bleeding from ear, nose, eye, or mouth
 8. History of loss of consciousness

Objective Data

Objective data for the patient with head injury includes the following:
 1. Respiratory status (presence of patient airway, need for suctioning, need for intubation and mechanical ventilation)
 2. Arterial blood gases
 3. Level of consciousness and alertness
 4. Pupils—size, equality, reactivity
 5. Orientation
 6. Motor status
 7. Vital signs
 8. Presence of bleeding
 9. Presence of vomiting
 10. Presence of discharge from ears or nose
 11. Speech pattern abnormalities

Because many persons with head injury, especially from motor vehicle accidents, have sustained other injuries, the intrathoracic and intraabdominal areas are checked carefully. The limbs are examined for fractures and injuries to nerves or arteries.

■ DATA ANALYSIS: NURSING DIAGNOSES

Nursing diagnoses are determined from assessment of patient data. Possible nursing diagnoses for the person with a head injury include, but are not limited to, the following:

Diagnostic Title	Possible Etiologies
Airway clearance, ineffective	Perceptual/cognitive impairment
Anxiety	Threat/change in health status
Breathing pattern, ineffective	Neuromuscular impairment, perceptual/cognitive impairment
Communication, impaired verbal	Aphasia, physical impairment
Gas exchange, impaired	Ventilation/perfusion imbalance
Incontinence, total	Neurologic dysfunction/disease
Knowledge deficit: care and monitoring required	Lack of exposure/recall, cognitive limitation
Mobility, impaired physical	Intolerance to activity, decreased strength and endurance, neuromuscular impairment
Nutrition, altered: less than body requirements	Anorexia, inability to obtain food
Pain	Trauma, immobility
Self-care deficit: bathing/hygiene, dressing/grooming, feeding, toileting	Intolerance to activity, fatigue, perceptual/cognitive impairment, neuromuscular impairment
Sensory/perceptual alterations: visual	Altered sensory reception/transmission/integration
Skin integrity, impaired, potential	Mechanical forces, immobility
Social interaction, impaired	Altered thought process
Thought processes, altered	Neurologic disorders
Tissue perfusion, altered cerebral	Decreased blood flow

■ PLANNING: EXPECTED PATIENT OUTCOMES

Expected patient outcomes for the person with a head injury may include, but are not limited to, the following:

1. Intracranial pressure is kept within safe limits.
2. Patent airway and adequate gas exchange are maintained.
3. Patient makes progress toward independence in ADLs.
4. Patient can safely compensate for visual field defects and perceptual, motor, and sensory losses.
5. Patient can explain prescribed therapy to follow at home.
6. Patient can demonstrate exercises to maintain function.
7. Patient can demonstrate the ability to communicate within disease process restrictions.
8. Patient can explain medications regimen at home and side effects, desired effects, time, dose, and route.
9. Patient can explain how to obtain assistance from community resources.
10. Patient can explain importance of frequent position changes and demonstrate such positioning.
11. Skin remains clear and intact.
12. Patient can state plans for follow-up care.
13. Continence is maintained to the extent possible.

With the patient who is severely injured and cannot respond, the caregiver should be taught to meet these outcomes.

■ IMPLEMENTATION

Preventive Care

Much can be done in terms of primary prevention of head injuries. Factors that can influence the outcome include the following:

1. Use of seat belts in automobiles
2. Use of helmets when riding motorcycles or snowmobiles
3. Practice of firearm safety
4. Minimal use of alcohol and drugs
5. Not driving after taking drugs or drinking alcohol
6. Use of precautions while swimming and especially not diving into shallow water

Acute Care

The patient who has a skull fracture or other serious head injury *must be attended constantly.* The major aims of medical and nursing management are as follows:

1. To be constantly alert for changes in the patient's condition, especially changes that indicate any increase in intracranial pressure
2. To sustain patient's vital functions until he/she has recovered sufficiently to resume own vital functions
3. To minimize complications that will be life threatening or interfere with full recovery

Promoting rest and control of convulsions. The patient should be kept as quiet as possible. No vigorous effort should be made to "clean the patient up" during the first few hours after an accident. Rest and constant observation are much more important. Sudden noises, flashes of light, and the clatter of equipment can increase the patient's restlessness and should be avoided. Portable equipment should be used to take roentgenograms. Nurses must remain in the room with patients to help them move and to protect them from exertion. Restlessness may be caused by the need for a slight change of position, the relaxation of a limb, or the need to empty the bladder. If nursing measures fail to allay extreme restlessness, the physician may order sodium amytal intramuscularly or paraldehyde. Morphine is not given to relieve pain because it will depress the patient's responsiveness and cause pupillary constriction, thus interfering with the necessary observation of pupillary change. Codeine or other mild analgesics may be necessary, however.

Twitching or convulsive movement of a body part is recorded in detail and reported at once. In some medical centers, anticonvulsants are given prophylactically when seizures are anticipated; they are always given once seizures occur.

Monitoring vital signs and maintaining temperature control.
Usually the blood pressure, pulse, and respiratory rate are taken and recorded every 15 minutes until they become stabilized and remain within safe limits. Leaving the deflated blood pressure cuff on the arm helps to prevent disturbing the patient unduly when the pressure must be taken often. Developing the habit of not forcing the mercury column much above the expected reading also sometimes enables the nurse to take the blood pressure and minimally disturb the patient. The eyes are observed for inequality of the pupils and the lips and fingernails for cyanosis. A sudden sharp rise in temperature, which may go to 42° C (106° F) or higher, and a sudden drop in blood pressure indicate that the regulatory mechanisms have lost control and the prognosis is poor. When temperature is elevated, measures need to be instituted to reduce it to normal. Although hypothermia has been used in the treatment of patients with severe brain contusions, it is being used less often because of some of the undesirable side effects. Instead, the nursing measures usually employed to reduce temperature, such as the administration of aspirin, tepid sponges, ice bags to the groin and axillae, and reduction of the temperature in the patient's room, are used. Electrically controlled cooling mattresses are also frequently used (Figure 63-7).

Promoting adequate respiration. One of the most common complications of severe head injury is respiratory failure. Cerebral anoxia, which is a sequela of respiratory failure, is a leading cause of death in these patients. The patient who has respiratory failure may have hypoxia, hypercarbia, hypotension, and dyspnea. Usually these patients are intubated and receive respiratory assistance with one of the mechanical respirators. Arterial blood gas levels and pH are checked frequently to determine whether respiratory exchange is adequate. The patient must be suctioned as necessary to maintain a patent air-

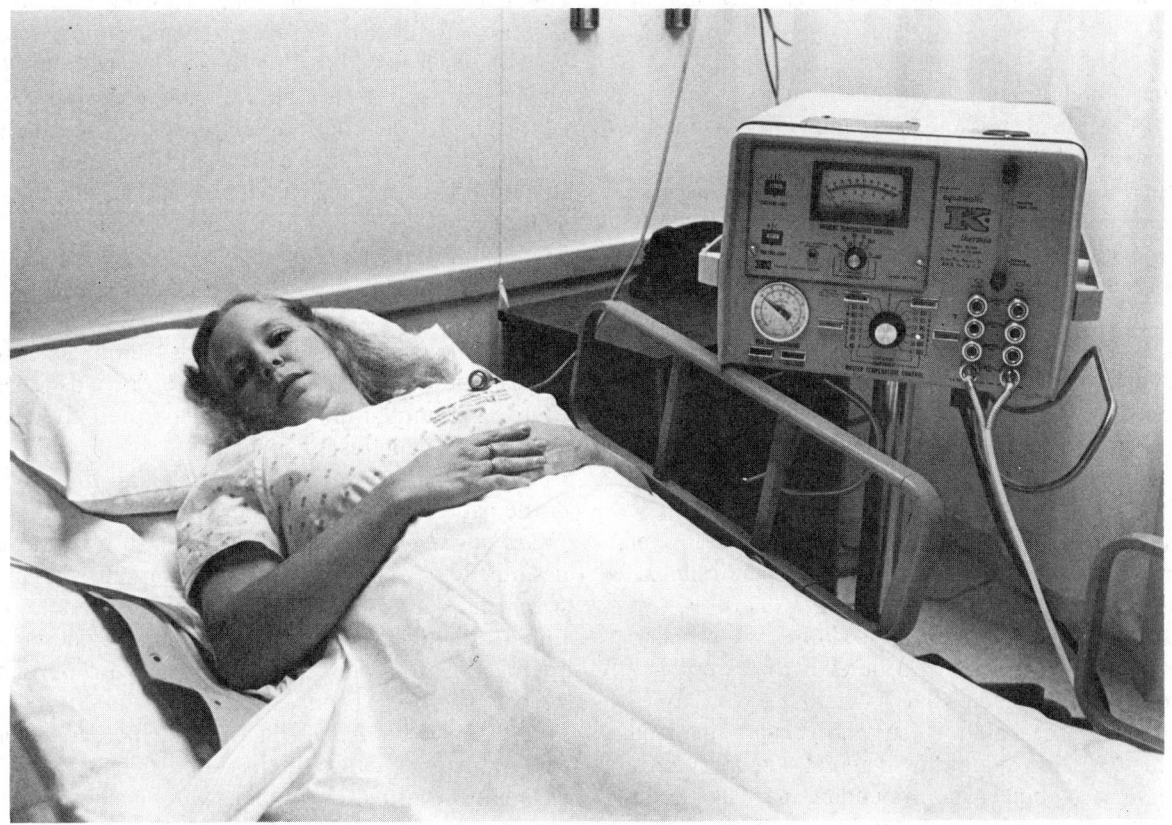

FIGURE 63-7 Patient lying on cooling mattress connected to hypothermia machine.

way. (See Chapter 34 for further nursing care of the intubated patient on a ventilator.)

Monitoring drainage from ears and nose. The patient's ears and nose are observed carefully for signs of blood and serous drainage, which may indicate that the meninges have been torn (common in basal skull fractures) and that spinal fluid is escaping. No attempt should be made to clean out these orifices. Loose, sterile cotton may be placed in the outer openings only. This procedure must be done with caution so that the cotton does not in any way act as a plug to interfere with free flow of fluid. The cotton should be changed as soon as it becomes moistened. Usually the flow of fluid subsides spontaneously. Antibiotics usually are given when a basal fracture has been sustained. Suction is never used to remove nasal secretions in any patient who has a head injury or who has undergone brain surgery because of the danger of causing further damage. *Meningitis is a possible complication when communication with the nose and ears occurs.* If evidence of drainage of spinal fluid from the nose exists, the patient should not cough, sneeze, or blow the nose. These activities may, in addition to contributing to the development of meningitis, enable air to enter the cranial cavity, where it may increase symptoms of intracranial pressure. Sometimes it is difficult to determine whether drainage from the nose is mucus or CSF. A Tes-Tape will give a positive sugar reaction to spinal fluid and a negative reaction to mucus.

Controlling cerebral edema. Cerebral edema and increased intracranial pressure are common problems in patients with head injuries. Osmotic diuretics that penetrate the brain slowly, such as 30% solution of urea in 10% invert sugar or 20% mannitol, may be given intravenously for several days. When the patient's condition is deteriorating because of cerebral edema, dexamethasone is usually administered intravenously. The usual dose is 10 mg initially, followed by 4 mg intramuscularly or intravenously every 4 hours thereafter. Steroids are also useful in combating shock associated with head injury. Usually they are employed only during the acute phase because of their side effects (see Chapter 62).

Maintaining electrolyte balance. Careful monitoring of electrolytes is necessary. Several types of sodium imbalance are known to occur in head injury. *Natriuresis,* or increased urinary excretion of sodium, is common. More recently this has been attributed to the inappropriate antidiuretic hormone (ADH) syndrome (with an increased plasma level of ADH, serum hyponatremia, and hypotonicity). This aggravates cerebral edema. *Hypernatremia,* or cerebral sodium retention, may also occur. No specific variations in potassium or chloride levels

have been noted. Plasma cortisol levels are also elevated in acute head injury. Plasma, blood urea nitrogen (BUN), pH, electrolytes, and urinary electrolyte levels are checked frequently.

Maintaining elimination. The patient's intake and output should be carefully measured and recorded. The specific gravity of the urine is also measured and recorded. These measures may be performed hourly when the patient's condition is acute.

Fluid intake may be restricted to 1500 to 2500 ml daily, and it is the nurse's responsibility to see that this is spread over the 24-hour period. Fluids may be given parenterally, by nasogastric tube, or by mouth, depending on the condition of the patient. The nurse must use caution in administering fluids orally, since the patient may have difficulty with vomiting and aspiration. The urinary output should be approximately 0.6 to 1 ml/kg of body weight/hour. This means that a person weighing 175 pounds (79 kg) should eliminate between 45 and 80 ml/hour, and if osmotic diuretics have been given, this amount may be greater. An indwelling catheter is essential when giving mannitol because of the large amounts of urine produced and the need to measure output exactly. The presence of an indwelling catheter increases the risk of urinary tract infection and should be removed as soon as possible.

Preventing complications. Patients with severe head injuries are candidates for several complications, some of which are discussed in this section. As with any other patient who is seriously ill, the patient may develop *atelectasis, pneumonia,* or a *urinary tract infection* (secondary to an indwelling catheter). These infections are treated with a suitable antibiotic. *Stress ulcers* of the stomach and duodenum also typically occur after a head injury and are apparently caused by autonomic imbalances associated with the injury. Cimetidine (Tagamet) can be given intravenously and acts to decrease the acid production of the stomach. Antacids can be given when the patient is able to take oral fluids. Antacids are especially important if the patient is on steroids such as prednisone, which is ulcerogenic.

See the box on opposite page for guidelines for care of the patient with a closed head injury.

Prolonged unconsciousness. General nursing care as described in Chapter 60 is necessary for the patient with a head injury who remains unconscious for some time. Patients may be unconscious for long periods and yet make a satisfactory recovery, provided good supportive care has been given.

Extradural hematoma. Because of the danger of extradural hematoma, as discussed previously, many physicians believe that any patient who has sustained any injury to the head with loss of consciousness should be

GUIDELINES FOR CARE OF THE PATIENT WITH A CLOSED HEAD INJURY

1. Promote rest and control convulsions.
   a. Provide quiet environment.
   b. Observe constantly.
   c. Give anticonvulsants.
   d. Medicate for pain as necessary.
2. Maintain temperature.
   a. Give tepid sponge baths.
   b. Administer aspirin as ordered.
   c. Use hypothermia blanket if ordered.
   d. Apply ice bags to groin and axilla.
   e. Reduce temperature in patient's room.
3. Promote adequate respiration.
   a. Suction only as necessary to provide adequate airway.
   b. Elevate head of bed to 30 degrees.
   c. Administer supplemental oxygen if ordered.
4. Observe for drainage from ears or nose.
   a. Make no attempt to clean out orifice.
   b. Use cotton in outer opening.
   c. Change cotton as soon as it is moistened.
   d. Do not suction nose if drainage is present.
   e. Use Tes-tape to verify presence of CSF.
   f. Have patient avoid coughing, sneezing, or blowing nose.
5. Control cerebral edema.
   a. Administer diuretics as ordered.
   b. Elevate head of bed to 30 degrees.
6. Maintain electrolyte balance.
   a. Observe for inappropriate ADH.
   b. Monitor electrolytes.
7. Maintain elimination.
   a. Keep accurate intake and output record.
   b. Restrict fluid if ordered.
   c. Monitor output.
   d. Remove catheter as soon as able.
8. Provide emotional support.
   a. Give firm but gentle care.
   b. Give specific guidelines for appropriate behaviors.
   c. Give positive feedback.
   d. Allow patient adequate time to complete tasks.

hospitalized for at least 24 hours. If patients are asleep during this time, they should be awakened hourly to determine the state of consciousness. Some physicians believe that fluids should be restricted to 1000 to 1500 ml for the first day or two and that an osmotic diuretic should be given. If patients remain at home, the families should be told to watch them closely for signs of increased intracranial pressure, to awaken them hourly during the night after injury, and to bring them to a hospital at once if drowsiness, stupor, paralysis, convulsions, or inequality of the pupil size should occur. A written handout with appropriate instructions about head injury can be extremely helpful to families of patients who are sent home instead of being hospitalized. It not only alerts them about signs to observe in the patient but may also help to allay their anxiety. (See the boxed material on p. 1868).

Providing emotional support. The patient with a head injury may manifest loss of memory and loss of initiative. Behavioral problems associated with lack of judgment and restlessness may also occur. These patients need firm but gentle care, with specific guidelines for what behavior is allowed. The patient and family need to have gains in functioning pointed out because it is easy to become frustrated and depressed when progress is slow.

Patient teaching. A patient with a head injury may be seen in the emergency room but not admitted to the hospital. These patients need teaching about observa-

tions for complications. A sample set of instructions is found in the box on p. 1868.

Teaching for the patient with a head injury who is left with deficits severe enough to require extended rehabilitation is similar to that for the patient with a motor problem. (See Chapter 62 for a description of this teaching.) In addition, the following points are important:
1. Causes of increased intracranial pressure
2. Factors that increase or decrease intracranial pressure
3. Signs and symptoms to report to the physician

Long-Term Care

Resumption of activities. The length of convalescence will depend entirely on how much damage has been done and how rapid recovery has been. Patients are usually urged to resume normal activity as soon as possible. Headache and occasional dizziness may be present for some time following a head injury. These difficulties should disappear within 3 to 4 months. Loss of memory and loss of initiative may also persist for a time.[57] Occasionally, convulsions develop because of the formation of scar tissue in injured brain substance or in its coverings. Such scar tissue may often be surgically removed to effect a complete cure. Loss of hearing and strabismus (cross-eye) sometimes complicate basal skull fractures and require a long period of rehabilitation. Sometimes corrective surgery can be performed for the strabismus.

Some persons require intensive rehabilitation in a re-

INSTRUCTIONS FOR PATIENTS WITH A HEAD INJURY

Patient should be awakened periodically through the first 24 hours to be sure he or she can wake up easily.

Also, for the first 24 to 48 hours, the family should watch carefully for the following warning signs:

1. Vomiting, often with force behind it
2. Unusual sleepiness, dizziness and loss of balance, or falling
3. Complaint of seeing two of everything or blurry objects; jerking movements of the eyes
4. Bleeding or discharge from nose or ears
5. A slight headache may be expected; however, if it worsens and the patient complains of feeling even worse when moving about, it should be reported
6. Convulsions (fits)—any twitching or movements of arms or legs that the patient is not able to stop
7. Any behavior or symptom that is not normal for the individual

Call a physician at once if any of these signs are observed by the family. Call either your personal physician or the emergency services.

Courtesy Department of Nursing, University Hospitals of Cleveland.

---

habilitation center. Recovery from head injury is most likely in those under age 20 years. Persons between the ages of 20 and 50 who remain in a coma longer than 2 weeks rarely recover.

SPINAL CORD TRAUMA
EPIDEMIOLOGY/ETIOLOGY

Spinal cord injury from accidents is a frequent and increasing cause of serious disability and death in the United States. It has been estimated that more than 100,000 individuals with serious spinal cord injury live in the United States today and approximately 6000 to 8000 new cases occur annually.[22]

Violent accidents are occurring more frequently, and because of medical advances the patients are living longer. Automobile accidents, diving and other athletic accidents, and gunshot wounds are major causes of spinal cord injuries.

PATHOPHYSIOLOGY

Important variations exist in the neuroanatomy of the vertebral column at the cervical, thoracic, and lumbar areas, and important segmental variations occur in the spinal cord itself. In the cervical area the vertebrae are unstable (to permit movement of the neck), and the cord at this level houses the most important neural structures in a copious dural tube. The anterior horn cells innervating the diaphragm (above C4) and the upper extremities are located in the cervical cord segments as well as in the long motor tracts to the remainder of the body. In the thoracic area, by contrast, a stable bony

column is supported by the rib structures. The thoracic spinal cord fills the subarachnoid space almost completely, and injuries in this area produce bony malalignments and are often associated with serious neurologic deficits. Finally, in the lumbar area the vertebrae are heavier and are supported by massive lumbar paraspinal muscles. The lumbar vertebrae thus have more stability than the cervical vertebrae but less than the thoracic vertebrae. The lumbar spine is more apt to be injured at the junction between the thoracic and lumbar area. The cauda equina, rather than the spinal cord, is housed below L1. The tip of the spinal cord, or the conus, houses the micturition center.

The spinal cord may be damaged by lesions arising outside the cord or by intramedullary lesions. The latter is a less common cause and is usually the result of intramedullary tumors (see Chapter 60). Various types of lesions arising *outside* the cord eventually cause damage within it. (The term *lesion* as used here includes both disease and injury.) For example, there may be direct extension of an extramedullary vertebral tumor to the cord, protrusion of a ruptured intervertebral disk into the spinal canal, or a fracture of the spine from direct trauma with resultant tearing of the spinal cord (Figure 63-8). All such lesions may produce compression of the cord. The anatomy and size of the spinal cord subject the cord to compression with even minimal inward encroachment by extramedullary lesions. Edema then forms and contributes even more to cord compression. With damage to any part of the vertebral column, the cord itself becomes more vulnerable to damage. Recognition of the function of the spinal cord as the only conducting system of nerve impulses to and from the brain makes one realize the seriousness of spinal cord damage from any cause.

Severe traumatic lesions of the spinal cord, as from accident, may result in total *transection* of the spinal cord or a tearing of the cord from side to side at a particular level. This represents the most serious damage to the cord, with a complete loss of spinal cord functions. This total transection injury is also referred to as a *complete cord injury*. With the complete injury there is a *loss of all voluntary movement below the level of the lesion and loss of all sensations below the level of the lesion.* A partial transection, or *incomplete injury,* involves a partial transection or injury of the cord. The symptoms of incomplete injuries can vary depending on the nature of the injury and the resultant syndrome. Possibilities include the anterior cord syndrome, central cord syndrome, Brown-Séquard's syndrome, conus medullaris syndrome, and cauda equina syndrome. (See a neurologic text for further descriptions of these syndromes and their respective symptoms.)

Initially in most spinal cord injuries, a period of flaccid paralysis and a complete (or almost complete) loss of

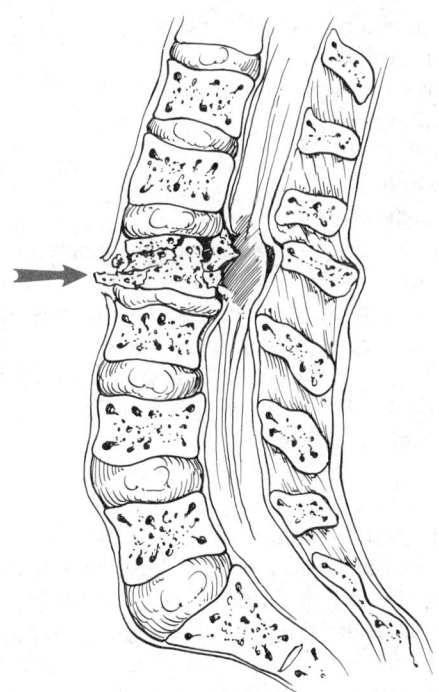

FIGURE 63-8 Damage to spinal cord and distortion of adjacent structures may occur in traumatic injuries to spine.

all reflexes occur. This is called *spinal* or *neural shock,* or *areflexia,* and is a transitory event. Following the injury, afferent impulses are unable to ascend from below the injured site to the brain, and efferent impulses are unable to descend to points below the site. Because transection represents an acute form of spinal cord damage, it is used as an example to relate and discuss the symptoms of spinal cord damage. *Considerable variability exists in the extent to which signs and symptoms are manifest in the individual patient.* The baseline assessment of the person with acute spinal cord injury should include the data listed in the box below.

BASELINE ASSESSMENT OF PERSON WITH ACUTE SPINAL CORD INJURY

1. Respiratory status
2. Level of alertness and consciousness
3. Orientation
4. Pupil size, equality, and reactivity
5. Proper alignment of body in neutral alignment
6. Motor strength
7. Absence of sensation-sensory level
8. Temperature, blood pressure, pulse
9. Bowel and bladder status; distention
10. Skin integrity
11. Pain control

CLINICAL MANIFESTATIONS

The signs and symptoms of cord transection and of lesser cord lesions depend on the level at which the lesion occurs and the degree of the damage (Table 63-9). In the *immediate stage of a transection* there is a complete loss or deficit of motor and sensory functions as well as somatic and visceral sensations below the level of the tear (areflexia). The individual has flaccid paralysis, areflexia, and hypotonia caused by the disruption of nerve impulses as related to the injured level. During this period persons may require temporary respiratory assistance until the body begins to recover.

Within hours, days, or weeks the involved muscles gradually become spastic and *hyperreflexic* with the characteristic signs of an upper motor neuron lesion.[94] These changes are thought to represent the release of the muscle stretch reflexes from the inhibitory influence of the damaged pyramidal tract, resulting in hyperactive responses. Another theory is that damage of the extrapyramidal descending fibers, in proximity to the pyramidal fibers, permits unmodified excitatory impulses to reach the lower motor neurons via the muscle spindles. Thus the lower motor neurons have increased sensitivity to afferent stimulation from the muscle spindles. Nurses need to be able to explain spinal cord damage to patients and their families so that involuntary movements are not confused with voluntary movements.

Damage at the cervical cord level is the most critical level for an injury to occur. It causes paralysis of all four extremities and the trunk (*quadriplegia*). The sparing of any one muscle movement of the shoulder, arms,

TABLE 63-9 Muscle function after spinal cord injury

Spinal Cord Injury	Muscle Function Remaining	Muscle Function Lost
Cervical		
Above C4	None	All including respiration
C5	Neck	Arms
	Scapular elevation	Chest
		All below chest
C6-C7	Neck	Some arm, fingers
	Some chest movement	Some chest
		All below chest
	Some arm movement	
Thoracic	Neck	Trunk
	Arms (full)	All below chest
	Some chest	
Lumbosacral	Neck	Legs
	Arms	
	Chest	
	Trunk	

and fingers depends on the specific cervical level of the injury. At the C5 level, for example, only scapular elevation movements would remain. All other muscle movements in the arms, chest, trunk, and legs are lost. In the immediate stage, muscles of internal organs such as the bladder and bowel are. atonic. Perspiration is diminished, as is touch sensation. Because the diaphragm and intercostal muscles are affected, respiratory failure and death may result unless the patient receives adequate respiratory assistance. Respiratory assistance is sometimes necessary during transportation of the patient to the hospital. Pain is not usually an early problem.

Injury at the thoracic level results in chest, trunk, bowel, bladder, and lower extremity muscle losses. The amount of remaining function varies in this area relative to the specific level. Fortunately, the individual has use of the upper extremities; the lower extremities are not functional (*paraplegia*).

Injury at the lumbar and sacral levels results in paralysis of the lower extremities. When injury occurs in the lower sacral area and the cauda equina nerve roots, away from the cord, the signs are variable and less severe. Paraparesis and scattered lower motor neuron signs often occur.

Voiding

The center for micturition is located in the conus medullaris (S2 to S4) and is linked to the detrusor muscle of the bladder by parasympathetic sensory and motor fibers that run in the pelvic nerves. Levels above the conus result in a bladder that is capable of emptying itself reflexly or involuntarily after the spinal shock phase. The bladder is hypertonic and is variously known as an *upper motor neuron bladder* and *reflex neurogenic bladder*. The emptying occurs spontaneously or automatically. The patient has no control over the act of micturition. Voiding may occur at intervals of 3 to 4 hours; there may be frequency, urgency, and incontinence. The reflex arc is intact in this type of bladder. When the cord lesion is at or below the micturition center, there is destruction of the center or the sacral nerve roots; the reflex arc is no longer intact. This type of bladder condition is known as a *lower motor neuron bladder* or *autonomous neurogenic bladder*. Contractions of the bladder muscle are the result of impulses transmitted through a mechanism within the bladder wall but are not of sufficient strength or duration to empty the bladder. Abdominal straining or manual compression is necessary for this to happen. Retention of urine and infection typically occur.

Autonomic Dysreflexia

One result of spinal cord injury that is extremely important to understand is *autonomic dysreflexia* (see Figure 63-9). It occurs in patients with cord lesions above T6 and most often in patients with cervical injuries.[10] The clinical signs include the following:

1. Bradycardia
2. Paroxysmal hypertension
3. Sweating
4. "Goose flesh"
5. Severe headache
6. Nasal stuffiness

Patients tend to develop individual symptoms of this condition and are soon able to recognize it.

The most common cause of autonomic dysreflexia is *visceral distention*, which may include a *distended bladder* or *impacted rectum. It is a medical emergency that requires immediate treatment because it can lead to CVA, blindness, or death*.[86,90]

Sexual Function

Most men with spinal cord injury experience impotence, decreased sensation, and difficulties with ejaculation. Impairment of fertility typically occurs. The act of erection is under the control of sensory and parasympathetic fibers, whereas ejaculation requires sympathetic and parasympathetic innervation. Lesions above S2 leave the parasympathetic reflex arc intact; patients may be able to have an erection, but ejaculation is usually not possible. Lesions in the S2 to S4 region usually prevent erection and ejaculation. The higher the level of injury, the more likely a man with complete cord injury is able to perform sexually. The experience of orgasm is described as different than before the injury.

Women with spinal cord injury are able to continue to perform sexually, although perception of sexual orgasm is usually altered. There usually is no decrease in fertility.[24,34,73]

Diagnostic Tests

It is most important to determine first if a cervical vertebra fracture or dislocation has occurred. Roentgenograms are usually taken to detect fracture-dislocation, which can occur when the patient is moved from the backboard or stretcher. Myelography may also be used to detect any blockage. It can be carried out without moving the patient if the dye is injected at the junction between C1 and the base of the skull. CT scanning may also be very helpful in ruling out spinal cord injury. (See Chapter 59 for details of these tests.) Further diagnostic measures are often delayed until any cervical fractures have been corrected. The presence of spinal compression in the thoracic, lumbar, and sacral spine areas must be determined, but the need for treatment is not as compelling as with a cervical injury. Both the lumbar and cervical spines are prone to flexion and extension movements that result from severe trauma.

MEDICAL MANAGEMENT

Immediate medical care after spinal cord injury with fracture is *directed toward realignment of the cervical column.* The following measures may be used to realign the cervical column:

1. Simple immobilization
2. Skeletal traction
   a. Crutchfield tongs
   b. Vinke tongs
   c. Virginia tongs
   d. Stryker or Foster frame
3. Surgery for spinal decompression[61]

Often surgical decompression is not performed until after a period of skeletal traction. This allows the patient's condition to stabilize and some initial swelling of the cord to subside. The beginning spontaneous healing of the fracture site provides more stability.

Sometimes, despite skeletal traction, extruded cervical disk materials produce continued compression of the cord. *With the introduction of the anterior surgical approach to the cervical spinal column, surgical intervention is safer and can be attempted earlier* in the hospitalization. The primary advantage of the anterior surgical approach (or anterior diskectomy or laminectomy) is that it provides immediate stabilization of the spinal column by techniques of interbody cervical fusion and the direct removal of any extruded disk materials. If evidence of spinal cord compression is demonstrated early, surgery may be warranted by the anterior approach.

Less immediate attention to *thoracic* fracture immobilization is necessary for the patient *with limited neurologic deficits.* The patient is often treated later with simple bed rest, hyperextension, and bracing (see Chapter 70). Diagnosis is necessary, however, to determine the presence or absence of spinal cord compression at this level. Patients who show subarachnoid blockage and have associated neurologic deficits are treated through early surgical decompression. The onset of instantaneous paraplegia following direct thoracic trauma is often reversible through spinal cord decompression.

An early to an intermediate laminectomy may be performed in the presence of even severe *lumbar* neurologic deficits. Stabilization of the spine is done at the time of the primary surgical intervention or delayed until later in the posttraumatic period. Long delays in lumbar laminectomies or explorations in patients who show early partial recovery are reported to be beneficial for recovery of some neurologic function.

■ ASSESSMENT

Assessment of the patient with a spinal cord injury includes both subjective and objective data.

Subjective Data

The following are subjective data for the patient with a spinal cord injury:

1. Patient's understanding of injury and the resulting deficit

2. Information about nature of injury—how it happened
3. Presence of shortness of breath
4. Unusual sensations (paresthesias and so on)
5. History of loss of consciousness
6. Presence of pain
7. Absence of sensation-sensory level

Objective Data

The following are objective data for the patient with a spinal cord injury:

1. Respiratory status
2. Level of alertness and consciousness
3. Orientation
4. Pupil size, equality, and reactivity
5. Proper alignment of body in neutral position
6. Motor strength
7. Temperature, blood pressure, and pulse
8. Skin integrity
9. Bowel and bladder status; distention
10. Presence or absence of anal wink reflex

The patient with a spinal cord injury should be assessed carefully for the presence of other injuries, especially head injuries or fractures.

■ DATA ANALYSIS: NURSING DIAGNOSES

Nursing diagnoses are determined from assessment of patient data. Possible nursing diagnoses for the person with a spinal cord injury include, but are not limited to, the following:

Diagnostic Title	Possible Etiologies
Anxiety	Threat to self-concept
Breathing pattern, ineffective	Neuromuscular impairment
Disuse syndrome, potential for	Immobility, weakness
Dysreflexia	Distended bladder, impacted rectum
Home maintenance management, impaired	Individual disease/injury, inadequate support systems
Incontinence, total	Neurologic dysfunction
Knowledge deficit: care required	Lack of exposure/recall, unfamiliarity with information sources
Mobility, impaired physical	Neuromuscular impairment
Pain	Spinal cord trauma
Self-care deficit: bathing/ hygiene, dressing/ grooming, feeding, toileting	Neuromuscular impairment
Sensory/perceptual alterations: tactile	Altered sensory transmission
Sexual dysfunction	Physiologic limitations
Skin integrity, impaired, potential	Mechanical forces

■ PLANNING: EXPECTED PATIENT OUTCOMES

The expected patient outcomes for a patient with spinal cord injury may include, but are not limited to, the following:

1. Function is preserved to the extent possible; no increase in level of injury.
2. Vital functions such as respirations compensated for until the spinal shock phase has passed.
3. Patient makes progress toward independence in ADLs.
4. Patient can explain prescribed therapy to follow at home.
5. Patient and/or caregiver can demonstrate exercises to maintain function.
6. Patient can explain medication regimen and side effects, desired effects, time, dose, and route.
7. Patient can explain importance of frequent position changes, including weight shifts.
8. Skin remain intact.
9. Patient can demonstrate inspection of skin.
10. Patient can explain need for assisted coughing and have caregiver demonstrate.
11. Patient remains free from respiratory complications.
12. Patient can explain bladder program and demonstrate intermittent catheterization if appropriate.
13. Patient can explain bowel program and demonstrate digital stimulation if able.
14. Patient can explain autonomic dysreflexia and actions to be taken when it occurs.
15. Patient can explain how to obtain community resources, including the Bureau of Vocational Rehabilitation.
16. Patient can state plans for follow-up care.
17. Disuse syndrome does not occur.

■ IMPLEMENTATION

Preventive Care

The reader is referred to the section on preventive care under head injury in this chapter on p. 1864.

Acute Care

Intubation. Intubation and respiratory assistance with a ventilator may be required in the immediate stage following upper cervical cord injury. In the conscious quadriplegic patient with a spinal cord lesion below C5, respiratory function generally is not compromised unless it is associated with acute blunt trauma to the chest. A lesion at the C5 level produces paralysis of the intercostal muscles, leaving only the diaphragm to function for respiration. The nerve roots C3, C4, and C5 innervate the diaphragm and make up the phrenic nerves. C4 supplies roots mainly to the phrenic nerves. Therefore any patient who has a cord lesion at the C4 level with quadriplegia probably will require *permanent ventilatory support.*

Medication. The use of adrenocorticosteroids for the prevention and alleviation of spinal cord edema has gained acceptance. The efficacy of steroids in the reestablishment of membrane stability and in the control of central nervous tissue edema has been documented clinically. Methylprednisolone (Solu-Medrol) at a dosage level of 60 to 80 mg/day (or equivalent dosage of other corticosteroids) may be used for the first week or longer following injury.

Spinal cord decompression. If the patient has surgery for spinal cord decompression, the nurse has an important role in making this a safe procedure. Guidelines for care are found in the box below.

G UIDELINES FOR CARE OF THE PATIENT UNDERGOING SPINAL CORD DECOMPRESSION

1. Provide preoperative care.
   a. Clarify patient's knowledge of surgery and expected changes.
   b. Explain expected postoperative measures (including positioning, bed rest).
   c. Encourage patient and family to verbalize fears.
   d. Assess and record baseline neurologic and physiologic data.
2. Provide postoperative care.
   a. Perform monitoring.
      (1) Assess ability to move legs, arms, and hands.
      (2) Assess degree and character of drainage on dressing (amount of drainage and bleeding should be minimal).
      (3) Assess ability of patient to swallow; observe neck for swelling (with anterior cervical fusions).
   b. Promote mobility.
      (1) Turn patient from side to side and onto back.
      (2) If decompression is in lumbar region, do not permit sitting.
      (3) If decompression is in thoracic area, patient should not use arms to pull or push; a trapeze *cannot* be used.
      (4) Assist with active ROM and quadriceps setting as well as other leg exercises.
   c. Promote psychologic comfort.
      (1) Encourage patient to verbalize fears and reactions.
      (2) Spend time with patient other than when giving direct care.
      (3) Share information about daily activities, tests, and procedures with patient.
      (4) Medicate as needed for pain.
   d. Prevent infections.
      (1) Keep area of incision clean and dry.
      (2) Check temperature frequently for several days.
      (3) Report any redness, drainage, or hardness of wound to physician.
      (4) Note that incision often left open to air after the first few days.

Throughout all stages of hospitalization of the spinal cord–injured person, nursing and medical interventions are directed toward restoration of structural or body integrity consistent with the pathologic condition present. This means that all efforts are taken to ensure (1) that the skin is intact, (2) that contractures do not develop, (3) that range of motion is maintained to the greatest degree possible, (4) that muscle tone is consistent with pathologic condition, and (5) that bladder and bowel functions are maintained. The following section discusses specific interventions to achieve these outcomes.

Maintaining mobility. Before moving a patient with acute spinal cord injury onto a bed from the stretcher, the physician should be consulted about the type of bed desired. The selection will depend on the physician's preference, the type of injury, the size of the patient, and the equipment available. If a regular bed is to be used, a full-length fracture board should be placed on top of the bedspring under the mattress. This board prevents sagging of the mattress and motion of the spine. If the bed is to be gatched, the board must be hinged, or two or more boards with correctly placed breaks can be used. Mattresses containing springs should not be used. Instead of springs and one mattress, some physicians prefer two air mattresses placed on top of the fracture board. Some use the knee gatch to provide hyperextension to the spine in selected thoracic and lumbar fractures; the bed must then be made up "head to foot." Sponge rubber mattresses are widely recommended and, when available, are often used when the patient may be moved very little and with extreme difficulty for some time. If available, an alternating air-pressure mattress often is used. Since the patient has loss of sensation and paralysis of part of the body, pressure areas develop easily. The mattress and entire bed foundation must be well protected with plastic sheeting so that incontinence will not cause damage.

To prevent injury when moving the patient, the bed foundation should be completely adjusted, with gatches raised as ordered, bolsters placed in the desired positions, and a turning sheet available so that minimal motion will be necessary. Three to five people are needed to move the patient from the stretcher to the bed, depending on the patient's size and the location of the spinal injury. The physician may supervise moving the patient and may support the head and neck during the transfer. The body should be supported in proper alignment, and if necessary, manual hyperextension should be applied to the spine as the patient is moved.

The nurse must carefully observe the patient with a spinal fracture, a cord tumor, or a ruptured intervertebral disk for signs of cord compression. The motion, strength, and sensation in the extremities should be tested at least every few hours for the first 24 to 36 hours and then at least four times a day. Any change in motion or sensation should be reported at once as related to level, since immediate surgery may be needed to relieve pressure on the cord. Some of the laminae may be removed to prevent pressure from edema.

Maintaining function. If cord damage has occurred, nursing care will depend on the level of the injury. Patients with cervical lesions, for instance, will be unable to do anything for themselves. Meticulous skin care, maintenance of correct body alignment, preservation of range of joint motion, and attempts to preserve muscle tone are imperative nursing measures as in the care of any paralyzed person. (See Chapter 62 for a discussion of the care of the person with paralysis.)

Maintaining elimination. The patient may have urinary retention because of injury to lumbar and sacral spinal nerves. Since there may be no sensation of needing to void, *the nurse should check carefully for voiding and for distention of the bladder.* A Foley catheter may be inserted into the bladder, or a cytostomy may be performed.

Most persons with spinal cord injuries have a reflex (autonomic or spastic) bladder, which occurs when the spinal cord reflexes are still present but the inhibiting influences from the higher cortical centers are lost. Reflex bladder is seen in persons with spinal cord injury or disease above the level of the sacral cord after the initial spinal shock phase. Because the pathways for motor and sensory impulses to the cord are still present, the reflex arc is intact. Any stimulation from the bladder wall leads to contraction of the detrusor muscle and relaxation of the internal and external sphincters, resulting in involuntary bladder emptying. The spastic bladder often responds to even minor stimulus such as touching or stroking the genitalia, thighs, or lower abdomen. Small, frequent voidings are common and demonstrate that the bladder empties long before it has reached normal capacity.

Some patients can be taught to recognize the stimulation for voiding and use it to induce voiding. Male patients often need to wear an external catheter for incontinence. Females unfortunately may have to wear pads and waterproof pants. One important measure that will help decrease the spasticity is the prevention of urinary tract infections.

Damage to the sacral cord or the peripheral nerves produces an atonic or areflexic bladder. Patients with spinal shock also have an atonic bladder. Any contraction from the bladder wall fails to stimulate the motor neurons in the cord. Because the reflex arc is disrupted, no sensations reach the brain. The person has no awareness of the need to void and no voluntary control.

Because the reflex arc and voluntary control are both absent, the bladder becomes increasingly distended. Overflow incontinence occurs, and if the bladder is not emptied, dribbling may occur almost continuously. The constant stretching of the bladder wall predisposes to infection and there may be reflux of urine. Depending on personal desire and residual functioning, the patient may be taught to use intermittent catheterization or Credé's maneuver or a combination of both. These procedures must routinely be used four times a day at intervals, at first by the nursing staff and then by the patient, if able. It may be necessary to continue intermittent catheterization for several months before the patient is able to stimulate voiding with Credé's maneuver alone.

The presence of an indwelling catheter makes the patient highly susceptible to urinary infection. The best means of preventing infection is maintenance of fluid intake (3 to 4 L daily) and meticulous aseptic technique in changing and irrigating catheters. The patient *must* know the signs of infection and *must* have a genitourinary checkup once a year or more frequently. Following an acute injury to the spinal cord, the patient often has abdominal distention. A rectal tube may be used, and neostigmine may be administered hypodermically to stimulate peristalsis. A nasogastric tube or a Miller-Abbott or Cantor tube attached to suction may be tried.

Stool softeners, adequate fluids, prune juice, and suppositories are recommended to obtain bowel function. Long-term use of laxatives and enemas is discouraged, although they may be necessary during spinal shock. If it is necessary to give an enema, 200 ml should be sufficient; no more than 500 ml should be used. Fecal incontinence may be caused by loss of sphincter control until the patient is regulated on a suppository regimen (see Chapter 62 for care of the incontinent person).

Alleviating pain. Patients with spinal injuries often have great pain at the level of the injury that radiates along the spinal nerves. A thoracic injury causes chest or back pain, whereas a lumbar injury causes pain in the legs. Analgesics such as acetylsalicylic acid (aspirin) or other nonnarcotic analgesics are ordered. Narcotics may be given for a short time but are contraindicated for long-term use because the patient's problem may be chronic and addiction is possible. Psychologic assistance is often recommended to help the patient learn to cope with pain. If the patient has a high cervical injury, no narcotics should be administered because respirations may be

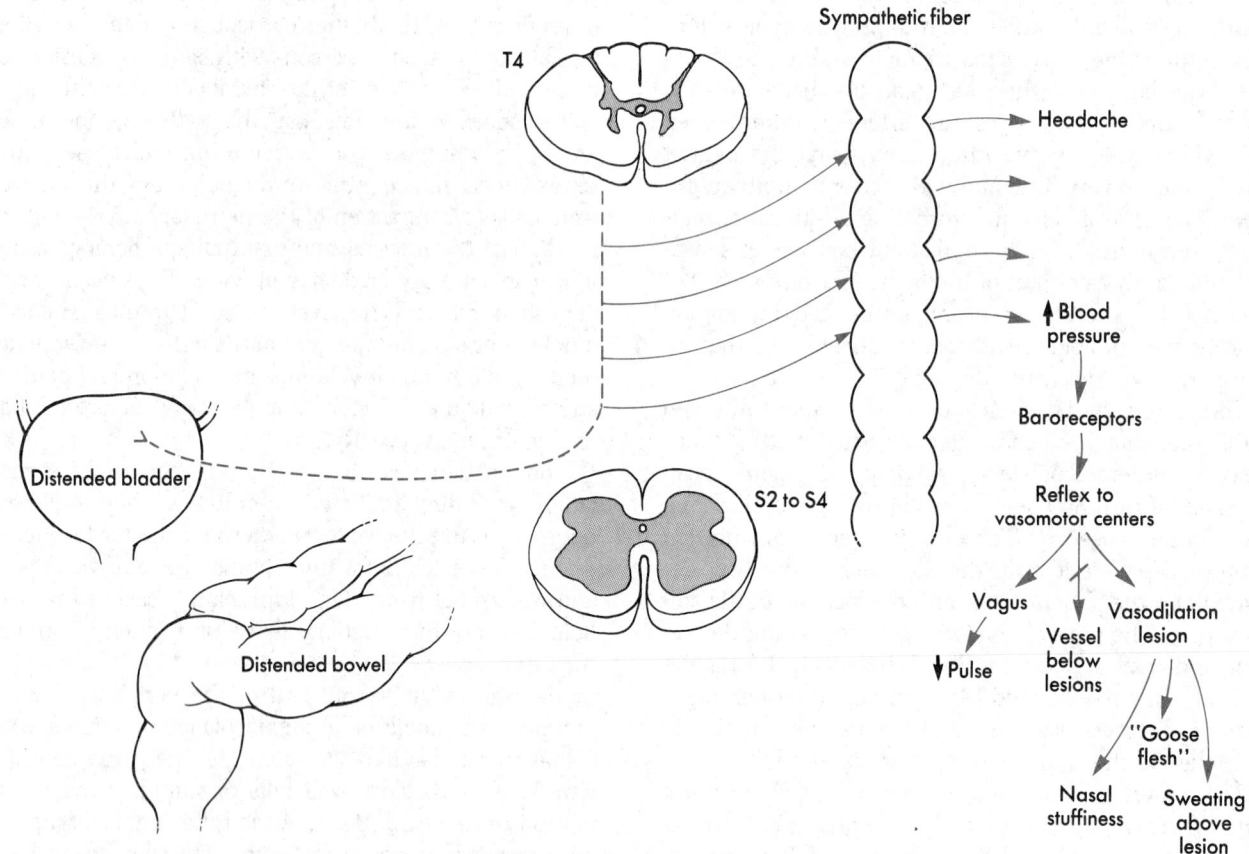

FIGURE 63-9 Pictorial diagram of cause of autonomic hyperreflexia and results.

further depressed. Sometimes the paravertebral nerves are injected with 95% alcohol to relieve thoracic pain. This measure may provide relief for several weeks or even months.

Preventing autonomic hyperreflexia. Autonomic hyperreflexia or autonomic dysreflexia (mass reflex) occurs in patients with cord lesions above the T6; most often it occurs in cervical injuries. The clinical signs are bradycardia, paroxysmal hypertension, sweating, "goose flesh," and severe headache (Figure 63-9). Patients tend to develop individual symptoms of this condition. They soon are able to recognize this complication when it occurs. For instance, some patients feel flushed but never develop a headache. The wise nurse learns to listen to what the patient says is happening to him or her.

The most common causes are visceral distention (distended bladder, impacted rectum). If the patient complains of these symptoms, the patency of the catheter should be checked for kinking and a new catheter inserted *immediately* if the catheter is plugged. The patient should be placed in a sitting position to decrease blood pressure. The rectum should be checked for impaction. If it is necessary to remove stool, dibucaine (Nupercaine ointment) should be instilled in the rectum for its anesthetic effect. At times urinary infections can lead to symptoms of autonomic dysreflexia. If no other obvious cause is found, a urine specimen is sent for culture.

Autonomic dysreflexia is a medical emergency (Figure 63-9). The hypertension can lead to CVA, blindness, or even death. If conservative measures are not effective, a ganglionic blocking agent such as hexamethonium chloride or a vasodilator such as nitroprusside (Nipride) is given intravenously. See the box above for details of care.

The major focus is to prevent such attacks. Before any bladder and bowel procedure such as cystoscopy or proctoscopy, the patient is given a local anesthetic. If autonomic dysreflexia is a continual problem, the patient may need long-term therapy to block sympathetic impulses.

Maintaining respiratory status. Respiratory complications are common following injury of the spinal cord. Any patient with a cord injury level at C4 or above can be expected to need assistance to maintain respiration, often on a long-term or permanent basis. In addition, patients with lower cervical fractures often have temporary respiratory difficulties until the spinal shock phase subsides.

Respiratory assistance may include intubation with ventilator assistance. Long-term ventilator assistance will require a tracheotomy. After the initial period these patients need continued respiratory support, including

CARE OF THE PATIENT WITH AUTONOMIC DYSREFLEXIA

1. Place patient in a sitting position to decrease blood pressure.
2. Check patency of catheter. Be sure it is not kinked. If catheter is plugged, insert new catheter immediately.
3. Check rectum for fecal impaction.
4. If it is necessary to remove an impaction, dibucaine (Nupercaine ointment) should be instilled in the rectum for anesthetic effect.
5. Send urine for culture if patient has elevated temperature and no other cause is found. A urinary tract infection may cause symptoms.
6. Administer ganglionic blocking agent such as hexamethonium chloride or a vasodilator such as nitroprusside (Nipride) if conservative measures are not effective.

postural drainage and clapping. Deep breathing and coughing, if medically approved, are essential. At times the rocking bed, a bed that rocks on a central axis, is employed by alternately elevating the head and foot. The bed assists in inspiration and expiration. Inspiration occurs as the diaphragm moves down as the head of the bed tilts up. With the reverse movement the patient exhales as the head is tilted down and the abdominal contents push upward against the diaphragm. If the patient is able to maintain respiration for a time, the bed may be turned off for eating and nursing care.

Persons who have injury at the cervical level may need respiratory assistance to prevent respiratory arrest. Those who have injury at the thoracic level tend to splint their chests and have shallow breathing; therefore measures to facilitate deep breathing and aeration of the alveoli are carried out (see Chapter 34). Because coughing can increase spinal pressure, the physician should be consulted before urging the patient to cough. Good nursing assessment of respiratory status in the patient with spinal cord injury is essential to prevent respiratory complications.

See the box on p. 1876 for guidelines for care of patients with a spinal cord injury.

Rehabilitative Care

Promoting rehabilitation. During the intermediate stage of treatment, rehabilitation and nursing care measures are focused on mobilization and patient-family education. Quadriplegics and paraplegics need to learn to live with the sequelae of paralysis. *The two goals of rehabilitation are to minimize the disability and to assist the patient toward independence to the extent possible.* Rehabilitation depends on the extent and level of the cord injury, the patient's emotional reactions, his or her age, and other factors.

Early mobilization of the patient is important regardless of the level of injury. At first, mobilization includes

GUIDELINES FOR CARE OF PATIENTS WITH A SPINAL CORD INJURY

1. Maintain mobility and function.
   a. Keep in neutral alignment when moving patient.
   b. Provide good skin care
   c. Assist with ROM exercises.
   d. Position in good body alignment at frequent intervals.
2. Maintain elimination.
   a. Reflex bladder
      (1) Provide stimulation of bladder.
      (2) Check for residual urine.
      (3) Use external catheters for males.
   b. Areflexic bladder
      (1) Use Credé's maneuver if effective.
      (2) Provide intermittent catheterization.
      (3) Check for residual urine.
   c. Encourage adequate fluids.
   d. Give cranberry juice to prevent medium conducive for infection.
   e. Place patient on bowel program.
3. Relieve pain.
   a. Use narcotics judiciously.
   b. Teach alternative methods of pain control, such as relaxation techniques or biofeedback.
4. Provide emotional support.
   a. Realize that patient probably will be very frustrated with limitations.
   b. Allow patient to vent feelings.
   c. Give patient positive feedback.

active or passive turning movements and ROM exercises to prevent pressure sores and contractures and to develop independence in bed activities. Later, mobilization is usually progressively effected through wheelchair activities. Most patients with spinal cord injury find it impractical to walk because of the energy required. Patients with very low cord injuries may be able to ambulate with braces. If ambulation is not possible, the patient may still use the braces to stand at intervals throughout the day. This helps to decrease Ca^{++} mobilization. Mat exercises and resistive exercises are initiated to increase muscle strength and endurance in remaining muscles.

When patients, especially quadriplegics, begin to sit up, it may be necessary to wrap their legs with Ace wraps to encourage venous return. Slowly increasing the angle of sitting is essential to prevent hypotension. For this reason the patient who has recently become a quadriplegic should use a recliner wheelchair until he or she is able to sit at 90 degrees for several hours.

The patient with paraplegia and the family are taught proper methods of transfer from bed to wheelchair or commode (Figures 63-10 and 63-11). Physical therapy activities facilitate learning to transfer. The patient also learns how to do weight shifts if able. Even patients who are not able physically to do weight shifts can take responsibility in getting others to help.

Before the patient is permitted to be up following a spinal injury, a brace may be prescribed. All braces and corsets must be custom made and are quite expensive. The cost of a back brace varies according to the materials used in construction. *The brace or corset should be applied before the patient gets out of bed.* Help is needed in getting into it. The patient should wear a thin, knitted undershirt next to the skin to keep the brace clean and to protect the skin. Correct use so that the brace fits contours of the buttocks and chest as designed makes a great difference in the patient's comfort. The patient's emotional reaction to wearing a brace or a corset is important because it vitally affects ultimate rehabilitation. Attention to small details that help in initial acceptance of this somewhat uncomfortable and unfamiliar piece of "clothing" is important. The patient should practice putting the brace on while in the hospital if it must be worn for some time after discharge. A close family member may visit the hospital and learn to assist the patient. Patients who live alone and are unable to care for their braces themselves may require a community health nurse to help them in the home or teach someone else to assist.

In addition to instruction about mobilization techniques, the patient is trained to be *functional in ADL,* with or without equipment and as related to his or her life-style. The patient needs to know how to obtain bowel and bladder automaticity and how to prevent bladder infection. One must understand how to prevent decubitus ulcers when one sits in a wheelchair most of the day and must know how to manage the wheelchair itself. *The patient's family or significant others are included in instruction, since many quadriplegic patients may require some supervision or assistance in ADL following discharge from the hospital.* The reaction of family members to spinal cord injury is often great. The family as well as the patient needs help in coping. In addition to medical and physical rehabilitation measures, psychologic, emotional, sociologic, and vocational rehabilitation is equally important. The trauma of spinal cord injury may result in numerous interpersonal problems and make adjustment to one's environment difficult. See the box on p. 1879 for relevant research.

Orthotics, or the application of external appliances to support a paralyzed muscle or to promote a specific motion required in ADLs, may require further follow-up care. Patients who have a ruptured cervical disk may need to use a neck brace. The brace extends well up under the chin and prevents flexion of the neck. Leg braces may be ordered for the paraplegic who is able to ambulate or stand.

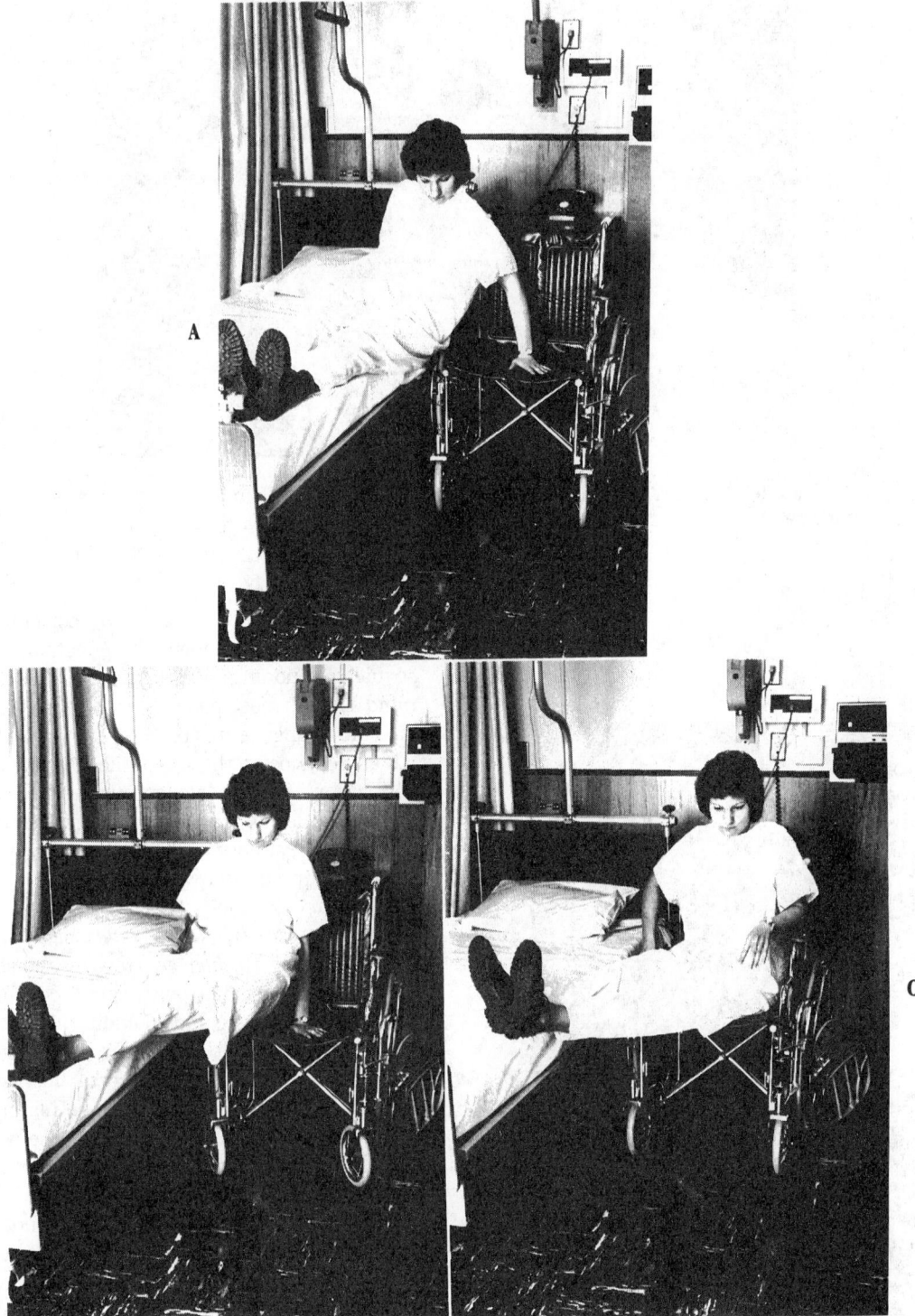

FIGURE 63-10 Two methods for patient with paraplegia and strong upper extremities to transfer from bed to chair. With one method: **A,** patient moves sideways (note wheelchair, with right armrest removed, placed next to bed); **B,** then patient uses her arms to lift trunk into chair seat; and **C,** patient settles her hips comfortabley into chair; she will then swing footrests into place and lift her legs from bed.

Continued.

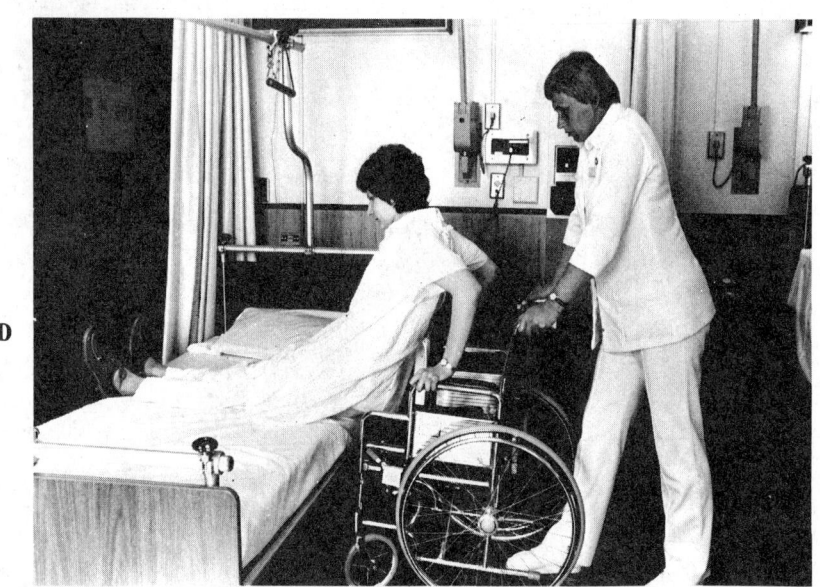

D

FIGURE 63-10, cont'd D, Second method involves patient pushing backward off bed into chair.

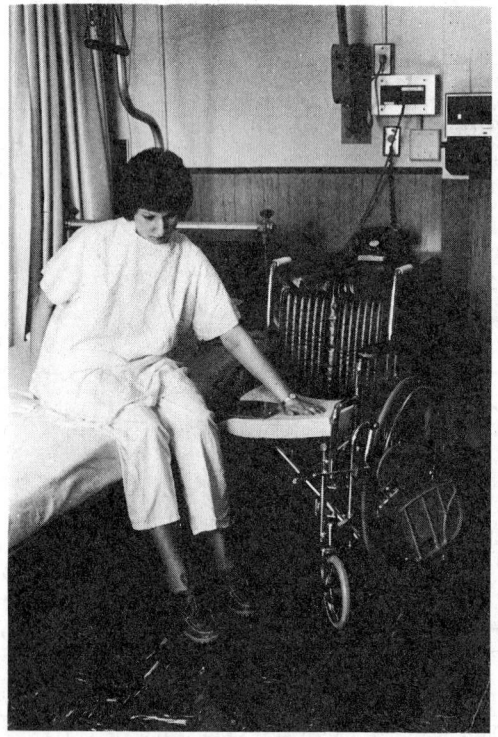

FIGURE 63-11 Paraplegic patient whose upper extremity strength is not yet developed can use a sliding board to transfer from bed to chair. Board provides a firm surface on which to move, and trunk is supported by board through the move.

Maintaining sexuality. Persons with cord injuries need assistance in learning about the effects of their injury on sexual functioning. The important thought to keep in mind is that most patients with a cooperative partner are able to engage in satisfying sexual activity. The limitation depends on the site of the lesion and whether the cord injury is complete or incomplete. Generally, the higher the lesion, the more normal sexual function is likely to be. Patients with sacral lesions are the only spinal cord injured men who are not able to have an erection and to ejaculate.

In men, erections are *reflexogenic* (secondary to stimulation) or *psychogenic* (response to sexual pictures and so on). Most men with spinal cord injury are not able to have psychogenic erections but are capable of reflexogenic erections. These occur not only as a result of direct stimulation of the genitalia but may also result from stroking the inner thigh, stimulating the rectum with a finger, or manipulating the catheter. The nursing staff can help point out these "trigger" points to the patient.

The ability to ejaculate usually is not present with complete injuries. With incomplete injuries, ejaculation may be possible. Even when patients have lost sensation, many report that there is increased intensity of feeling in other body parts, such as the breasts. Orgasms may be experienced, with release of tension.

Male patients with indwelling catheters can either remove the catheter just before sexual activity or turn it back on the penis, where it provides extra support. The bowels should be emptied before intercourse; otherwise, bowel incontinence typically occurs.

RESEARCH

DeJong G et al: Independent living outcomes in spinal cord injury: multivariate analysis, Arch Phys Med Rehabil 65:66-72, 1984.

This study examined what factors could best predict the ability of a person with spinal cord injury to live independently. Seventy-five patients were studied with the use of a variety of variables. The most important predictors of overall independent living were found to be marital status, transportation barriers, education, work disincentives, and severity of the disability. Being married and well educated positively correlated with independent living, whereas the other variables had a negative effect on independence. ■

RESEARCH

Borkowski C: A comparison of pulmonary complications in spinal cord–injured persons treated with two Modes of spinal immobilization, J of Neurosci Nurs 21:79-85, 1989.

This study investigated two modes of spinal immobilization, the Kinetic Treatment Table and the traditionally used wedge turning device and their relationship to the development of pulmonary complications in two groups of acutely injured patients with spinal cord injury. The following parameters were examined: incidence of pulmonary infection, length of need for mechanical ventilation, length of ICU stay, and length of hospitalization. Those clients turned with the Kinetic Treatment Table had a lower incidence of pulmonary infection and required less time on the ventilator. The length of ICU stay and the length of hospital stay did not differ. ■

Since many male patients who are able to ejaculate do so into the bladder (retrograde ejaculation), they are usually infertile. Without sperm counts, however, infertility cannot be guaranteed.

The spinal cord–injured woman is able to participate fully in sexual activity. She may not experience orgasm but can enjoy the sexual experience. Women who have a Foley catheter can keep it in place if desired.

Most spinal cord–injured women maintain their ability to conceive; for some reason many of these women do not realize this. All such sexually active women should have access to family planning information. If pregnancy is desired, the woman can usually have a normal vaginal delivery. However, she is at increased risk for autonomic dysreflexia and hydronephritis.

The nurse can be supportive and helpful to cord-injured patients by making it comfortable for them to discuss sexual matters. Nurses not prepared for sexual counseling need to be aware of resources available in the community to help the spinal cord–injured person. Some general suggestions that may be helpful include: (1) sex has many meanings, and for persons with no genital function, alternate ways of expression are available; (2) the partner will need time to adjust to the situation; openness in communication is helpful; and (3) it is sometimes difficult for a partner who routinely provides bladder and bowel care to view the person as sexually desirable; it may be helpful in this situation if this care can be provided by a community nurse or part-time attendant. See the box below for details of sexual functioning in spinal cord injury.

Patient Teaching

Teaching the patient with spinal cord injury encompasses all of the points covered under teaching the patient with a motor or sensory dysfunction. In addition, the patient needs to be taught about the effects of injury on sexual functioning, as just discussed.

RESEARCH

Research data on spinal cord injuries continue to be gathered (see research box above, right). Interestingly, electrostimulation of muscles of the bladder through remote control to regain micturition control in the paraplegic patient has been tested clinically. Success of this electronic spinal neuroprosthesis will assist in preventing urinary complications, which are often a cause of death. Functional intramuscular electrostimulation of paralyzed upper extremities muscles is also currently being tested. Since little or no external splinting is required in the latter orthosis, it will be cosmetically appealing to the quadriplegic person if successful.

In summary, although most complications of paralysis are now preventable, it is regrettable that complications do occur during and after hospitalization.

SEXUAL FUNCTIONING IN PATIENTS WITH SPINAL CORD INJURY

1. Reflexogenic erections occur not only as a result of stimulation of the genitalia, but also as a result of stimulation of the following "trigger points":
   a. Stroking the thigh
   b. Stimulating the rectum with a finger
   c. Manipulating the catheter
2. Males with catheters can either remove the catheter just before sexual activity or turn it back on the penis to provide extra support.
3. Bowels should be emptied before intercourse to prevent incontinence.
4. Women with a catheter can keep it in place during intercourse if desired.
5. Women maintain the ability to conceive; birth control should be used to avoid pregnancy

PERIPHERAL NERVE TRAUMA

EPIDEMIOLOGY/ETIOLOGY

The peripheral nerves that lie outside the brain and spinal cord include the cranial and spinal nerves and their branches and plexuses. The disorders involving the peripheral nerves are similar to those that affect the central nervous system and are the result of traumatic, degenerative, vascular, inflammatory, neoplastic, and metabolic causes. *Neuropathies,* noninflammatory disorders, may involve one peripheral nerve (mononeuropathy) or multiple nerves (polyneuropathies). *Neuritis* refers to an inflammatory disorder, whereas *neuralgia* means a painful nerve disorder. Although discussion in this section is limited to neuropathies caused by trauma, it should be clear that regardless of cause, the resulting nerve dysfunction will be similar and will be related to the site of the lesion. Some of the more common neuropathies (other than trauma) include nutritional, alcoholic, diabetic, lead, arsenic, hereditary, and infectious.

Traumatic causes of peripheral nerve injury typically include gunshot and knife wounds, fragmented fracture wounds, and surgical transections, as in denervation surgery and amputations. They variously result in stretching, laceration, and compression of the peripheral nerve; great variation also exists in the degree of injury. Fortunately, the axons of peripheral nerves are capable of regeneration under favorable conditions.

PATHOPHYSIOLOGY

Following trauma (or disease), the axon undergoes *secondary* or *wallerian degeneration* distal to the lesion (that is, distal to the cells of origin) and for several segments proximal. The axon and the myelin sheath (secondary) degenerate and immediately undergo fragmentation; the fragmented particles are completely ingested within several weeks; and the axis cylinder remains. Schwann's cells and fibroblasts begin to proliferate along the degenerated fibers. (Myelin in *peripheral fibers* is formed by Schwann's cells.) During the regenerative phase, new axoplasm forms at the proximal edge of the injury, and the regenerating fibers now grow distally and enter the empty neurolemmal sheath, which since has proliferated. Myelin then forms around the regenerated axon. When a nerve has been severely damaged and fibrous tissue is abundant, regeneration is interfered with by a tangled mass known as a *traumatic neuroma;* this may have to be removed surgically.

CLINICAL MANIFESTATIONS

The clinical signs and symptoms resulting from peripheral nerve lesions depend on the exact location of the lesion and the specific function of the involved nerve or nerves. Since peripheral nerves contain both sensory and motor components, deficits may exist in both components distal to the site. There will be alterations in pain, touch, temperature, proprioception, and stereognosis. Motor alterations include lower motor neuron signs such as flaccid paralysis and muscle wasting in those muscles innervated by the affected nerves.

Diagnostic Tests

The electromyogram (EMG) may be helpful in diagnosing peripheral nerve injuries. See Chapter 59 for a description of this test.

MEDICAL MANAGEMENT

Medical care of the patient with a peripheral nerve trauma depends on the nature of the individual nerve involved. Surgical intervention may be necessary.

■ ASSESSMENT

Assessment includes both subjective and objective data.

Subjective Data

The following are subjective data from a patient with peripheral nerve injury:

1. Patient's understanding of condition
2. Alteration in sensation
   a. Pain
   b. Touch
   c. Temperature
   d. Proprioception
3. Site of sensory problem
4. Onset of problem
5. Presence of associated symptoms

Objective Data

Motor alterations should be observed by the nurse caring for the patient with peripheral nerve injury.

■ NURSING DIAGNOSES/EXPECTED PATIENT OUTCOMES

The nursing diagnoses and expected patient outcomes for the patient with peripheral nerve trauma are the same as those for the patient who has a sensory or motor dysfunction (Chapter 62). See the box on p. 1881 for peripheral nerve trauma terminology.

■ IMPLEMENTATION

Preventive Care

The same measures taken to prevent head injury are applicable to peripheral nerve trauma (see p. 1864 in this chapter).

Acute Care

Nursing care is specific to the areas of the body affected by the sensory and motor deficits. Plans for care are based on the nurse's understanding of the distribution and function of the involved peripheral nerves. The flaccid muscles demand attention to prevent deformi-

COMMON TERMINOLOGY WITH PERIPHERAL NERVE TRAUMA

Neuropathies—noninflammatory disorders
Mononeuropathy—disorder affecting one peripheral nerve
Polyneuropathy—disorder involving multiple nerves
Neuritis—inflammatory disorder
Neuralgia—painful nerve disorder

ties. *Because of the atonia or hypotonia of the paralyzed muscles, they will be pulled excessively by the muscles that normally oppose them into abnormal or contracted positions.* When associated tendons shorten, the contracture is permanent. Positioning of extremities in neutral or counter positions will help in preventing joint deformities. Those areas of the body in which there is a loss of sensation need to be protected from injury. These patients need to be taught *protective measures* such as not staying in one position too long, since they cannot sense that damage is occurring in an area served by a damaged nerve. When positional sense is lost, patients must also be taught to protect themselves when walking and in other activities. Pain is usually localized, and more paresthesia may occur than pain. The painful areas need to be protected from external stimulation when present. Following surgical intervention, careful positioning of the operative area, as prescribed, is important. Finally, the promotion of good health measures assists in the creation of conditions favorable to nerve regeneration.

TRIGEMINAL NEURALGIA
EPIDEMIOLOGY/ETIOLOGY

Trigeminal neuralgia is one specific type of peripheral nerve problem. It is also called *tic douloureux.* More than 90% of cases of trigeminal neuralgia occur in persons over age 40 years. Women are affected somewhat more frequently than men. In most cases, no etiology for this disorder can be found. When it is associated with hypesthesia in the distribution of the fifth cranial nerve, with onset before age 40, or is associated with other cranial nerve palsies, a workup to rule out multiple sclerosis or a posterior fossa brain tumor is necessary.

Trigeminal neuralgia is characterized by *excruciating, burning pain* that radiates along one or more of the three divisions of the fifth cranial nerve (Figure 63-12). The pain typically extends only to the midline of the face and head, since this is the extent of the tissue supplied by the offending nerve. Areas along the course of the nerve are known as *trigger points,* and the slightest stimulation of these areas may initiate pain. Persons with trigeminal neuralgia try desperately to avoid "trig-

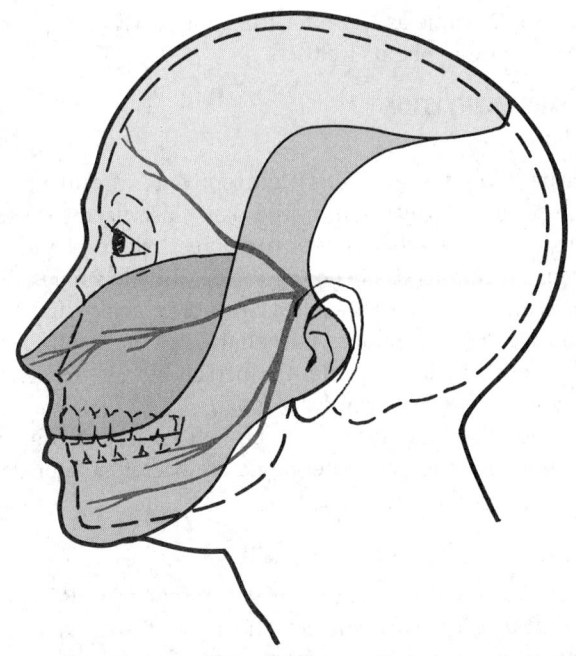

FIGURE 63-12 Pathway of trigeminal nerve and facial areas innervated by each of the three main divisions of this nerve.

gering" the pain. It is not unusual to see them lying in bed with the covers over their heads in an effort to avoid drafts. They frequently have been unable to eat properly for some time because chewing causes pain. They may therefore be undernourished and dehydrated. They may have slept poorly and have not washed, shaved, or combed their hair for some time. Oral hygiene may often be neglected because of pain.

MEDICAL MANAGEMENT

The peripheral branches of the trigeminal nerve may be injected with absolute alcohol. This provides relief for weeks or months, and the procedure may be repeated as necessary.[2] Permanent relief can be obtained only by surgery, which consists of dividing the sensory root of the trigeminal nerve, but this is not always successful.

An operating microscope is used during surgery on the trigeminal nerve. Microsurgery permits greater precision in selective cutting of fibers; also, the sensation of touch and the corneal reflex are preserved. A new method to sever the nerve inside the skull is presently being used. A thin electrode needle is inserted through the cheek and into the nerve. This avoids a surgical procedure and may provide permanent relief of pain.

■ ASSESSMENT/DIAGNOSES/OUTCOMES

The assessment, nursing diagnosis, and planning of expected outcomes for the patient with trigeminal neuralgia are the same as those for the patient with peripheral nerve trauma (see p. 1880).

■ IMPLEMENTATION

Medications

Carbamazepine (Tegretol) currently is the drug of choice for the treatment of the pain (also used for convulsions). The inhalation of trichloroethylene (10 to 15 drops on cotton) has been tried with variable success for relieving pain. Drugs such as nicotinic acid, thiamine chloride, cobra venom, and analgesics have all been tried, but usually they offer the person little if any relief. Sedatives may be given for sleep.

Two other drugs that may be helpful in treating the patient with trigeminal neuralgia are baclofen (Lioresal) and phenytoin (Dilantin).

Assisting with Comfort

In caring for the person with trigeminal neuralgia *preoperatively* or in caring for the patient who is being treated medically, it is important that members of the nursing staff be sympathetic toward the person's behavior. Comfort measures for the patient with trigeminal neuralgia are found in the box below, left.

Surgical Procedure

If the patient has had surgery to correct the pain, certain nursing measures are important. Postoperatively it is important to know which branches of the nerve have been cut or destroyed in the procedure so that necessary protection can be accomplished. If the *upper branch* is completely severed, the corneal reflex on that side will be lost. Usually an attempt is made to preserve a few of the fibers of the first division of the fifth nerve, because even a few intact fibers seem to preserve this vital function. Until the physician has tested the corneal reflex and verified its presence, an eye shield is used to prevent dust or lint from getting onto the cornea and causing injury.

When the *lower branch* of the fifth cranial nerve is interrupted, hot foods must be avoided because the per-

son will not be aware if the mucous membrane is burned. The patient may have difficulty chewing and swallowing at first.

Within 24 hours after a fifth nerve resection, many patients develop herpes simplex (cold sores) about the lips. Phenol and camphor (Campho-Phenique) applied frequently seems to give more relief than any other treatment. Usually the lesions heal in about 1 week. See the box below, right for postoperative care involved.

NEOPLASMS OF THE CENTRAL NERVOUS SYSTEM

Neoplasms of the central nervous system (CNS) include those arising from cells of structures within the cranium as well as those arising within or outside the spinal cord. In general, they occur in great variety; produce neurologic symptoms because of size, location, and invasive qualities; usually destroy the tissues in which they are situated and displace tissues around them; and are a frequent cause of increased intracranial pressure.

INTRACRANIAL TUMORS
EPIDEMIOLOGY/ETIOLOGY

Primary intracranial tumors, or *neoplasms,* arise from the intrinsic cells of brain tissues and from the pituitary and pineal glands. *Secondary* or *metastatic* tumors are also a frequent contributing type of intracranial tumor. Intracranial tumors are only one example of intracranial lesions. Variable intracranial lesions occur, such as hemorrhage, abscess, and trauma, and cause similar signs and symptoms as a neoplasm, depending on the site of the lesion.

COMFORT MEASURES FOR PATIENTS WITH TRIGEMINAL NEURALGIA

1. Keep room free of drafts.
2. Avoid walking briskly to bedside of patient.
3. Place bed out of traffic area to prevent jarring of bed.
4. Avoid touching the patient's face.
5. Advise patient *not* to wash or shave the affected area or to comb hair.
6. Avoid hot or cold liquids that trigger pain.
7. Food may have to be pureed and lukewarm and taken through a straw

---

POSTOPERATIVE CARE OF THE PATIENT WITH TRIGEMINAL NEURALGIA

1. Preserve eye function.
   a. If the upper branch of the nerve was cut, the corneal reflex is lost.
   b. Eye shield is used to prevent dust or lint from getting into cornea.
   c. Avoid contact with eye when washing face.
   d. Bathe eye with methylcellulose solution.
   e. Inspect eye several times a day.
2. Promote mouth function when lower branch of fifth cranial nerve is interrupted.
   a. Avoid hot food because of loss of sensation.
   b. Food should be placed on unaffected side of mouth because of difficulty in swallowing.
   c. Perform mouth care after each meal to remove retained food.
3. Promote safety (for example, electric razor should be used for shaving of face).

PREVENTION

No known primary prevention exists for intracranial tumors, except in cases in which the tumor results from metastatic disease. Cigarette smoking has a direct link to brain tumors because neoplasms of the lung often metastasize to the brain. In fact, a significant number of lung malignancies are discovered subsequent to signs and symptoms of brain metastasis.

PATHOPHYSIOLOGY

The symptoms of intracranial tumors result from both local and general effects of the tumor. Locally, the effects are from infiltration, invasion, and destruction of brain tissues at a particular site (see box below). There is also direct pressure on nerve structures, causing degeneration and interference with local circulation. Local edema develops, and if it is longstanding, it is often sufficient to interfere with the function of nerve tissues.

A brain tumor of any type situated anywhere in the cranial cavity may cause an increase in intracranial pressure. The increased intracranial pressure is then transmitted throughout the brain and the ventricular system. Eventually the ventricular system is distorted and displaced sufficiently to cause partial ventricular obstruction at some site, even though the tumor is some distance from the ventricular system. A tumor may directly obstruct a particular ventricle early when it grows adjacent to the ventricle. A tumor of the cerebrum can distort the lateral ventricles. A tumor that presses on the third ventricle, the aqueduct of Sylvius, or the fourth ventricle can result in obstruction of CSF flow into the central canal of the spinal cord. Cerebral edema forms even at some distance from the tumor and generally adds to the increasing pressure. As the edema increases, the blood supply to the brain is compromised and carbon dioxide is retained. The vessels dilate in an effort to increase blood oxygen supply. Unfortunately, this also increases edema, and the situation can deteriorate rapidly.

Papilledema results from the general effects of the increased intracranial pressure and is often a relatively late sign. Death is usually caused by brainstem compression resulting from herniation. The mechanism for the occasional acute focal symptoms that occur is thought to be caused by rapidly increasing cerebral edema or by functional decompensation of edematous tissues.

Common clinical circumstances in which intracranial tumors are present, or are likely to be found, include those persons with (1) general impairment of cerebral function or a seizure, (2) evidence of increased intracranial pressure, and (3) specific or focal intracranial tumor syndrome.

CLINICAL MANIFESTATIONS

Types of Tumors

Brain tumors are named for the tissues from which they arise. The more frequently encountered ones include gliomas, meningiomas, pituitary adenomas, and acoustic neuromas. In addition, the brain is a frequent site for secondary tumors from other organs.

Gliomas account for about one half of all brain tumors. They arise in any part of the brain connective tissue. As a rule, in adults they infiltrate primarily the cerebral hemisphere tissues and are not so well outlined that they can be completely excised surgically. They grow rapidly, and most persons do not live longer than a year after diagnosis.[1] The less malignant gliomas are the *astrocytomas* and the *oligodendrogliomas*. *Ependymomas* arise from the walls of the ventricular system. They cause death in about 3 years. The most malignant and rapidly growing forms are the *glioblastoma multiforme* and *medulloblastoma*. Gliomas sometimes start as one type and develop into more malignant forms if untreated.

The *meningiomas*, which account for 13% to 18% of all primary tumors in the intracranial cavity, arise from the meningeal coverings of the brain. They occur most frequently in the meninges over the cerebral hemispheres in the parasagittal region along the ridge of the sphenoid bone and in the anterior fossa in relation to the olfactory groove or the sella turcica. When located in the posterior fossa, they arise from the cerebellopontine angle, from the tentorium, or rarely in the region of the foramen magnum. Meningiomas vary widely as to size and histologic findings. They are usually benign but many undergo malignant changes. The neurologic signs and symptoms produced by meningiomas relative to these sites may include anosmia, optic atrophy, extraocular palsies, visual defects, papilledema, pituitary disturbances, and cerebellar dysfunction. Meningiomas

---

COMPARISON OF SYMPTOMS OF TUMORS FOUND IN SPECIFIC BRAIN LOBES

Frontal lobe	Personality disturbances (range from subtle personality changes to obvious psychotic behavior)
	Inappropriate affect
	Indifference of bodily functions
Precentral gyrus	Jacksonian seizures
Occipital lobe	Visual disturbances preceding convulsions
Temporal lobe	Olfactory, visual, or gustatory hallucinations
	Psychomotor seizures with automatic behavior
Parietal lobe	Inability to replicate pictures
	Loss of right-left discrimination

TABLE 63-10 Types of brain tumor

Type	Incidence	Pathology

Glioma
  Astrocytomas
  Oligodendrogliomas
  Ependymomas
  Medulloblastoma
  Glioblastoma multiforme—
  most malignant
	Accounts for one half of brain tumors	Arises in any part of brain connective tissue; infiltrates primarily cerebral hemisphere tissue; not so well outlined as to be incised completely; grows rapidly—most persons live months to years; tumors assigned grade from 1 to 4, with 4 the most malignant

Meningioma	13% to 18% of all primary tumors in intracranial cavity	Arises from meningeal coverings of brain; usually benign but may undergo malignant changes; usually encapsulated, and surgical cure possible; recurrence possible
Pituitary tumor	Occurs in all age groups, but more often in women	Arises from various tissues; surgical approach usually successful; recurrence possible
Neuroma (schwannoma, neurofibroma)	Acoustic neuroma is most common	Arises from Schwann's cells inside auditory meatus on vestibular portion of third cranial nerve; usually benign but may undergo cellular change and become malignant; will regrow if not completely excised; surgical resection often difficult because of location
Metastatic tumors	From 2% to 20% of all patients with cancer have metastasis to the brain	Cancer cells spread to brain via circulatory system; surgical resection very difficult; even with treatment, prognosis is very poor; survival beyond 1 or 2 years is uncommon

frequently cause seizures and involvement of the limbs as related to their presence in the convexity of a cerebral hemisphere.[12]

Acoustic neuromas constitute about 8% of all primary intracranial tumors. Neuromas may arise from any cranial nerve. The tumor affecting the acoustic nerve generally arises from its sheath but usually extends to affect the nerve fibers. The signs and symptoms resulting from these slowly growing tumors are related to compression of adjacent cranial nerves (trigeminal and facial), cerebellum, and the brainstem. Pituitary tumors are another intracranial tumor.

Metastatic tumors that arise primarily in the lung, kidney, breast, colon, and other organs account for about one fifth of all intracranial tumors. Primary brain tumors, conversely, rarely metastasize to other organs. See Table 63-10 for review of types of brain tumors.

Diagnostic Tests

No one procedure is entirely diagnostic for brain tumors, but the CT scan certainly has revolutionized the ease of diagnosis with minimal danger and discomfort to the patient. If the patient's condition is stable, an EEG, brain scan, or echoencephalogram may be used to help determine the exact site and nature of the tumor. Patients with increased intracranial pressure but with no evidence of specific neurologic deficits are evaluated as rapidly as possible. In emergency situations, arteriography or ventriculography may be used to locate the tumor.

A lumbar puncture may be helpful in assessment of patients with potential brain tumors. As mentioned previously, it is not carried out in patients with symptoms of increased intracranial pressure except in special circumstances because of the danger of herniation (see Chapter 62).

Brain scans are particularly useful in screening patients for suspected brain tumors by demonstrating the size and site of the tumor. A negative brain scan does not, however, exclude a tumor, since a small tumor may not be visualized. Conversely, a positive scan may be caused by a cranial lesion other than a tumor. An EEG is particularly useful in the detection of abnormal brain waves, generally or focally, within the cerebral hemispheres or their coverings. The echoencephalogram is helpful in identifying displacement of the ventricular system and the pineal gland from their normal midline positions. Displacement to the right of the midline or to the left may indicate a tumor within the respective hemisphere. This so-called displacement is also referred to as a *brain shift* and is a relatively late stage of increased intracranial pressure. Radiographic studies of the skull are carried out initially and may reveal increased intracranial pressure and abnormal calcifications.

Other tests that may be helpful in locating the tumor are arteriography or ventriculography. The ventriculogram is used when the suggested diagnosis is such that a spinal or lumbar puncture is contraindicated. Two newer procedures that can help with diagnosis of a brain tumor are the nuclear magnetic resonance (NMR) and positive emission tomography (PET) scans. These are described in Chapter 59.

MEDICAL MANAGEMENT

Intracranial surgery is typically used for all types of pathologic conditions of the brain, including tumor removal.

A surgical opening through the skull is known as a *craniotomy*. It is a basic preparatory procedure for intracranial surgery. A series of burr holes (trephine) is made first, and then the bone between the holes is cut with a special saw (Gigli's) to permit removal of the bone. Bone is then removed in such a way that it can be replaced if desired. The opening depends on the lesion site. Brain surgery may be performed under hypothermia to lessen bleeding during the procedure. Drugs such as levarterenol bitartrate (Levophed) may be used to maintain blood pressure. *Patients may also be placed in a barbiturate coma during the surgery and for several days following it to lessen brain activity, metabolism, and oxygen needs.* This may help to prevent worsening of deficits because of hypoxia.

When the brain lesion is in the *supratentorium* (above the tentorium or in the cerebrum), the incision is usually made behind the hairline. When the incision is into the *infratentorium* (below the tentorium or in the brainstem and cerebellum), it is made slightly above the nape of the neck. Neither of these incisions is apparent when the hair has regrown.

Tumors involving the pituitary gland that do not extend outside the sella turcica are usually removed by means of a transphenoidal approach. After the surgery, packing is placed inside the nose and remains for 3 to 4 days. A muscle graft from the thigh is used to close the defect in the dura. With this type of surgery, recovery is rapid and the patient has no loss of hair or external cranial incision.

Following craniotomy and removal of the bone, an incision is made into the meninges and the tumor is removed or other cranial surgery performed. The removed bone is carefully saved or preserved. Following brain surgery, *the bone may be replaced immediately (as in a bone flap with muscle attachment) when no evidence of infection or increased intracranial pressure exists.* At times the bone is left out for variable periods to prevent pressure from cerebral edema postoperatively or to permit expansion of an inoperable tumor. In this instance the preserved bone is used as a mold for a bone prosthesis, which is inserted with wire at a later date, or the preserved bone is reinserted. Sterile acrylic is the material presently used to make the bone prosthesis. The acrylic can be molded directly into the skull opening after covering the dura mater with a thin plastic sheet at surgery, or it can be molded from the preserved bone at

a later time. The removal of part of the skull without replacement is called *craniectomy*. When a tumor cannot be removed because of its location and nature, a subtemporal decompression is made by leaving an opening in the dura and skull. *Cranioplasty* is the repair of a cranial defect through use of substitute bone materials.

Limitation of some functions may necessarily follow the complete removal of brain tumors occurring in the cerebral hemispheres. Portions of the frontal lobe are removed in some instances with little residual damage. Patients with tumors located where they are rapidly accessible to removal, such as meningiomas and tumors of the outer cerebrum, have the best prognosis. Today, the decision to operate on persons with large tumors is weighed carefully by the neurosurgeon. If the surgery is likely to leave the patient with much permanent disability, the decision not to operate will often be made.

■ ASSESSMENT

It is important to assess both subjective and objective data in the patient with an intracranial tumor.

Subjective Data

The following are subjective data from the patient with intracranial tumor:

1. Patient's understanding of diagnosis
2. Changes in personality or judgment
3. Presence of abnormal sensation (paresthesia or anesthesia)
4. Visual problems—loss of visual acuity or diplopia
5. Complaints of unusual odors (especially with temporal lobe tumors)
6. Headache
7. Hearing loss
8. Inability to carry out ADL

Headache is an early symptom in about one third of patients with brain tumors and is variable in nature. The pain can be either slight or severe, dull or sharp, and transitory or intermittent. Possible characteristics of the headache is its nocturnal occurrence or its presence on first awaking and its deep nonpulsatile quality; however, these are not specific attributes because they occur in headaches from other causes. The mechanism for the headache is not known. In most patients the intracranial pressure is normal for the first weeks when headache is present. The headache may be caused by local swelling of tissues and distortion of blood vessels in and around the tumor. Later, headache seems to be related to increased intracranial pressure. Tumors above the tentorium cause headache on the side and in the vicinity of the tumor; those on the posterior fossae usually cause ipsilateral, retroauricular, or occipital headache. With elevated intracranial pressure, the headache becomes bilateral regardless of location.

Objective Data

The following are objective data from the patient with intracranial tumor:

1. Motor strength
2. Gait
3. Level of alertness and consciousness
4. Orientation
5. Pupils: size, equality, and reactivity
6. Vital signs
7. Funduscopic examination for evidence of papilledema
8. Seizures
9. Speech abnormalities
10. Cranial nerve abnormalities
11. Symptoms of increased intracranial pressure

■ DATA ANALYSIS: NURSING DIAGNOSES

Nursing diagnoses are determined from assessment of patient data. Possible nursing diagnoses for the person with an intracranial tumor include, but are not limited to, the following:

Diagnostic Title	Possible Etiologies
Anxiety	Threat of death
Body image disturbance	Change in body appearance
Disuse syndrome, potential for	Immobility, weakness
Fear	Surgery
Grieving, anticipatory	Actual or perceived loss
Incontinence, total	Neurologic dysfunction/ disease
Infection, potential for	Decreased nutrition, decreased immune response
Knowledge deficit: care and treatment required	Lack of exposure/recall, cognitive limitation, unfamiliarity with information sources
Mobility, impaired physical	Neuromuscular impairment, intolerance to activity
Nutrition, altered: less than body requirements	Chewing or swallowing difficulties, anorexia
Pain	Surgery
Self-care deficit: bathing/ hygiene, dressing/ grooming, feeding, toileting	Perceptual/cognitive impairment, neuromuscular impairment
Sensory/perceptual alterations: visual, tactile	Altered sensory reception/ transmission/integration
Thought processes, altered	Neurologic disorders
Tissue perfusion, altered cerebral	Decreased cerebral blood flow

■ PLANNING: EXPECTED PATIENT OUTCOMES

Expected patient outcomes for the person with an intracranial tumor may include, but are not limited to, the following:

1. Anxiety is lessened.
2. Body image is maintained.
3. Fear is minimized.
4. Disuse syndrome does not occur.
5. Appropriate grieving is facilitated.
6. Incontinence does not occur.
7. Patient remains infection free.
8. Patient verbalizes knowledge of necessary treatments and medications.
9. Mobility is maximized.
10. Optimal nutritional status is maintained.
11. Pain is minimized.
12. Patient maintains the ability to carry out ADL to the extent possible.
13. Patient compensates for any sensory/perceptual problems or impaired thought processes.
14. Patient remains mentally intact.
15. Cerebral perfusion is maintained.

■ IMPLEMENTATION

Acute Care

Prognosis. With the development of newer diagnostic techniques, modern surgical and radiologic methods, more effective chemotherapeutic agents, and an increased understanding of functional anatomy of the cerebrum, the prognosis for patients with intracranial tumors is more favorable today than in the past. The prognosis, however, depends on early diagnosis and treatment, since as the tumor grows within the cranial cavity, it exerts pressure on vital brain centers and causes irreparable brain damage and death. Although approximately one half of all brain tumors are benign, they also may cause death by exerting pressure on vital brain centers. It is important to remember that although cells of the CNS can regain function, even after cerebral edema, dead cells cannot regenerate. Early treatment is thus necessary to preserve cerebral functions. Early treatment also becomes important as newer techniques have been developed that improve surgical risks and postoperative prospects for patients with intracranial tumors. These techniques include *hypothermia*, the establishment of *controlled hypotensive states during surgery* by means of appropriate drugs, *hyperthermia to destroy tumor cells,*[117] and *dehydration of cerebral tissues* by administering osmotic diuretics such as urea compounds or mannitol before, during, and after surgery.

The nurse's attitude about the treatment of brain tumors cannot help but be communicated to the patient and family. The nurse should make an effort to communicate a positive attitude while stressing the importance of early diagnosis and treatment of intracranial tumors.

Preoperative Care

Baseline data of neurologic and physiologic status should be recorded by the nurse before surgery. Written permission for surgery on the brain must be given by the nearest relative unless the patient is able to sign.

Even when the patient has given consent, close relatives are usually consulted, and the neurosurgeon obtains their consent before surgery. The patient and family are usually very threatened by the prospect of brain surgery and should be encouraged to express their fears. Specific fears may be related to a permanent change in appearance, dependency, or death. Psychologic support of the patient and family is a priority intervention. The nursing staff should provide time for this as part of essential nursing care of the patient. The patient may also wish to see a spiritual advisor before surgery.

Treatments and procedures should be explained to the patient even though they *may not* seem to understand fully. Enemas may not be given before surgery because of the danger of increasing intracranial pressure further by exertion and by the absorption of fluid. Narcotics, except codeine, are rarely ordered preoperatively, since they may cause further depression of cerebral function. Any order for their use should be carefully verified by the nurse. If the head is to be shaved, the procedure may be delayed until the patient is in the operating room. Hair should not be discarded but should be returned to the patient unit because the patient may wish to have it made into a wig. Synthetic wigs are a good alternative for many patients. In many hospitals it is the practice to shave only the portion of the patient's head necessary to do the surgery. Hair along the front hairline can often be left so that after surgery it can be drawn backward to cover the scar. The hair is shampooed, and the condition of the scalp is noted.

Preparation of the family. The family of the patient needs to be prepared for what they will face when they see the patient after surgery. They need to know that the patient will have a head dressing and that edema may distort facial features. They also need to know that the patient may have discolored areas about the eyes (ecchymosis). If the patient is unconscious or has a limitation such as aphasia, this should be discussed with the family before they see the patient. If the patient is alert, the family will be advised to sit quietly at the bedside because talking will tire the patient.

The box above summarizes preoperative care.

Postoperative Care
Postanesthesia care. Whether in the patient unit or in the recovery room, the nurse should be certain that the following are readily available: side rails for the bed, suction machine or wall suction with disposable suction catheters, an airway, a padded tongue blade, a lumbar puncture set, and an emergency medication tray (cardiac and resporatory stimulants, amobarbital sodium [Amytal], anticonvulsive drugs), syringes, intravenous and hypodermic needles, and a tourniquet. An emer-

---

PREOPERATIVE CARE OF THE PATIENT HAVING INTRACRANIAL SURGERY

1. Baseline data of neurologic and physiologic status should be recorded.
2. Patient and family should be encouraged to verbalize fears.
3. Treatments and procedures are explained fully, even if unsure whether patient understands.
4. If head is shaved, it is usually done in the operating room.
5. Antiseptic shampoo may be ordered night before surgery and may be repeated in morning.
6. If hair is shaved, it is saved and given to patient or family.
7. Prepare family for appearance of patient following surgery.
   a. Head dressing
   b. Edema and ecchymosis of face common
   c. Temporary decreased mental status (possible)

---

gency tracheostomy tray should also be readily available on the unit.

The patient is observed regularly during the early postoperative period for signs of increased intracranial pressure (see Chapter 62). Frequency of making and recording specific observations depends on the patient's condition.

Any change in the patient's *vital signs, state of consciousness, pupillary response,* or *ability to use muscles* is reported at once. Restlessness, often secondary to tissue hypoxia, forewarnings of hemorrhage or irritation to the brain, or other symptoms of increased intracranial pressure should be watched for and reported immediately to the surgeon. These changes are described earlier in this chapter.

Maintaining proper position. Immediately after surgery the patient is placed on the side to ensure an adequate airway. To facilitate change of head dressings and other treatments following surgery, the patient may be placed in bed "head to foot." If a large brain tumor has been removed, the patient must not be turned on the affected side, since this position may cause displacement of brain structures by gravity. Otherwise, turning to either side is permitted. The primary objective is to eliminate pressure on the operative site. Handling of the brain tissues and surgical trauma causes cerebral edema, which contributes to increased intracranial pressure.

If there has been *supratentorial* surgery (above the cerebellum), *the head of the bed is elevated at least 45 degrees and a large pillow is placed under the patient's head and shoulders.* This position should lessen the possibility of hemorrhage, provide for better circulation of the CSF, and promote venous return. All these measures assist in decreasing cerebral edema and in preventing increased intracranial pressure. Internal bleeding would also contribute to a rise in intracranial pressure. If an *infratentorial* tumor has been removed, *the bed should be kept flat with only a small pillow under the nape of the neck and the patient turned to either side.* Any *flexion* of the neck should be avoided, either midline or laterally. Since infratentorial incisions are made adjacent to the medulla, vital centers, and ninth and tenth cranial nerves, there is more danger of respiratory complications and brainstem compression.

Coughing and *vomiting* are to be avoided because these increase intracranial pressure. Suctioning, if permitted, should be done gently and cautiously to avoid initiating coughing. Suctioning through the nose is also avoided. Deep breathing exercises should not be followed by coughing.

Preventing injury. Some patients must be protected from injuring themselves after surgery. Patients who pull at dressings or catheters or scratch or hit themselves must be attended constantly. Occasionally some type of hand restraint such as a large mitten made of dressings, bandages, and stockinette fastened at the wrist with adhesive tape may be used. Mittens usually upset patients less than arm restraints, since with mittens they can move their arms freely. The fingers should be separated with gauze to prevent skin irritation and should be curled around a large bandage roll in the palm to prevent hyperextension of the fingers. The hand is then well covered with dressings held in place with a bandage. A piece of stockinette is closed at one end and everted so that the tied end cannot cause injury to the eye. It is then slipped over the bandaged hand and fastened securely at the wrist with adhesive tape. The wrist should be shaved and the skin protected with tincture of benzoin before adhesive is used. At least every other day the mitten must be removed, the hand washed in warm water, and passive exercise given to the fingers before the mitten is reapplied.

Head dressing and care of wound. Usually the wound is covered with gauze dressings, and a special head dressing (neurosurgical roll) is then applied in a recurrent fashion from the back to the front of the head and anchored. The head *dressing* is inspected regularly for amount and type of drainage. Serosanguineous drainage on the dressings should be measured and marked, as is done with other dressings, so that it can be accurately checked for an increase in amount. Yellowish drainage should be reported immediately to the physician because it probably indicates loss of spinal fluid. If the head dressing appears to be soaked with drainage, the dressing should be reinforced. It may be necessary to apply a pressure dressing. Dressings that become wet should be removed by the neurosurgeon and replaced.

It is not unusual for dressings to be removed the day after surgery and the incision left open to the air.

When the final dressings are removed, the scalp can be gently cleansed with hydrogen peroxide to remove dried blood. Crusts can be loosened with mineral oil. Patients are usually advised to wait 7 to 10 days after the surgery before the head is shampooed. A head covering is usually worn to protect the wound, to help remind the patient not to scratch, and for cosmetic reasons until the hair has grown back. A cap can be made by tying one end of a 10-inch piece of tubular stockinette. Head scarves or wigs are usually preferred by women, and wigs can also be worn by men. Many patients prefer to wear disposable paper caps such as those worn by the operating room staff. The patient who has had a piece of bone left out will have a depression in the scalp and should be warned of the danger of bumping the head in this area.

Promoting nutrition. Fluid intake and output should be accurately recorded. Fluids can be resumed when the person has good bowel sounds, is awake enough to swallow, and has a stable neurologic status. If no orders exist to the contrary, 2500 to 3000 ml of fluid should be given each day. Some neurosurgeons routinely restrict fluids to 1500 ml/day for the first 3 days after a craniotomy.

Since the gag and swallowing reflexes may be depressed or absent after *infratentorial* brain surgery, fluids by mouth are usually withheld for at least a day and intravenous fluids are substituted. They should be run very slowly to prevent increased intracranial pressure. If reflexes are present, water is carefully given by mouth. The patient should be placed in a semisitting position. Fluid should never be forced on a patient who is still neurologically depressed because of the danger of aspiration. If after several days the gag and swallowing reflexes are still absent, a nasogastric tube may be inserted. A regular diet is given to all neurosurgical patients as soon as it can be tolerated.

Promoting elimination. Care must be taken to see that the patient voids sufficiently. Urinary output must be carefully recorded, and the specific gravity of most specimens should be measured. Sometimes an indwelling catheter may be used for a few days following surgery. A *decrease* in output must be reported because it may indicate the onset of a metabolic disorder of CNS origin. Correspondingly, an *increase* in urine output with low specific gravities should also be reported because it may herald the onset of *diabetes insipidus*. Although this condition occurs most frequently after hypophysectomy for pituitary tumor, it can also occur following trauma to the head or intracranial surgery (especially involving the area near the pituitary).

Because most patients who have intracranial surgery

will be on some type of steroids, it is important to test the urine for sugar and acetone. Patients who develop diabetes mellitus as a sequela of steroid treatment may require active treatment of the diabetes until the steroids are discontinued.

Laxatives or stool softeners should be used liberally to prevent constipation and straining while defecating. The patient should be instructed not to strain. Bowel function should be monitored by the nurse to prevent fecal impaction. If an impaction does develop, enemas or manual evacuation may be necessary. Suppositories may also be used after the initial postoperative period to promote bowel regularity.

Promoting comfort. Patients who are conscious after intracranial surgery may complain of a severe *headache* for 24 to 48 hours. CNS depressants, such as opiates and sedatives, are avoided. Codeine sulfate is often prescribed and is given parenterally. Acetylsalicylic acid (aspirin) or acetaminophen (Tylenol) may be given by rectum, or by mouth if fluids can be swallowed. An ice cap may be placed on the head, and sudden movement and jarring are avoided. The patient should be protected from loud noises and bright lights. The patient may need assistance with turning and other ADL.

Promoting early mobility. The patient who has had surgery for a *supratentorial* lesion usually is allowed out of bed on the second to third postoperative day. If the surgery was extensive or complications develop, bed rest

may be prescribed for longer periods. Activity is increased gradually, and the patient is watched carefully for signs of increased intracranial pressure. First the head of the bed should be elevated to high Fowler's position, and then the patient should sit on the edge of the bed with the feet dangling over the side. If this is tolerated, 4 to 6 hours later, with the help of two persons, the patient may be assisted to a chair and usually may sit up for a half hour. It is important to check the patient for postural hypotension while beginning progressive activity. Any drop in blood pressure of more than 20 points or complaints of dizziness by the patient should delay ambulation for several hours before another attempt is made. Patients then progress to normal activity as quickly as they desire and are able.

The patient who has had surgery for an *infratentorial* lesion usually is not permitted up for a much longer time. The trend is toward getting up earlier, depending on the patient's condition. Initial progress may be slower, since patients who have been kept flat in bed for some time may be dizzy and experience orthostatic hypotension when arising until the circulatory system readjusts to the change in position.

The box below contains a summary of postoperative care.

Preventing complications

Hydrocephalus. Occasionally, a catheter is placed in a ventricle of the brain to drain excess spinal fluid and prevent increased intracranial pressure. The catheter is

---

POSTOPERATIVE CARE OF THE PATIENT WITH INTRACRANIAL SURGERY

1. Perform monitoring.
   a. Assess neurologic status, including ability to move, level of orientation and alertness, and pupil checks.
   b. Assess degree and character of drainage.
      (1) Amount of drainage and bleeding should be minimal.
      (2) Initial head dressing can be reinforced as necessary.
      (3) Often incision is left open to air after first several days.
2. Promote mobility.
   a. Turning to either side is permitted except when large brain tumors have been removed. If this is the case, patient is not turned to affected side because gravity may cause displacement of brain structures.
   b. If supratentorial surgery was performed, the head of the bed is elevated at least 30 degrees.
   c. If infratentorial surgery was performed, the bed is flat or elevated only slightly and a small pillow is placed under the nape of the neck. Neck flexion is avoided.
   d. Early ambulation is encouraged to prevent complications of bed rest. Observe carefully for signs of postural hypotension and raise head of bed gradually; patient should always sit before standing.

3. Promote decreased intracranial pressure.
   a. Space nursing activities to allow patient to rest between them.
   b. Coughing and vomiting should be avoided.
   c. Suctioning should be done only as necessary, and then gently and cautiously.
4. Protect safety of patient.
   a. Use soft hand restraints if restraints are necessary.
   b. Use mittens as alternative to restraints; make sure fingers are separated and fingers are placed around large roll. Change mitt at least daily—give range of motion to hand at this time.
   c. Keep side rails up at all times.
5. Promote electrolyte balance.
   a. Perform accurate intake and output with measurement of specific gravity. Do frequent testing for sugar and acetone if patient is taking steroids.
   b. Have patient resume diet as soon as possible; assess for difficulty in swallowing or absence of gag reflex.
   c. Monitor electrolytes for evidence of abnormalities.
6. Promote comfort.
   a. Medicate for comfort with codeine sulfate or nonnarcotic analgesic.
   b. Ice cap to head for headache may be helpful.

usually attached to a drainage system. The collection bottle is frequently attached to the bed. The tubing and drainage receptacle should be sterile, and care must be taken to prevent kinking of the tubing. If drainage appears to stop, the neurosurgeon should be notified. The catheter is usually left in place for 24 to 48 hours and is then removed by the surgeon.[6]

Hydrocephalus of a more permanent nature also occurs in the presence of intracranial tumors and is manifested by symptoms of increased intracranial pressure. Treatment consists of a shunting procedure. The different types of shunting procedures are named for their point of origin and termination and include the following:

1. Cyst to peritoneal
2. Lumbar-peritoneal
3. Ventricular-jugular
4. Ventricular-peritoneal

In this type of surgery, excessive CSF is shunted away from the CNS and into either the peritoneal cavity (where it is absorbed) or into the jugular vein. At times, a Ryckham reservoir is placed through a burr hole into the ventricle. This device can easily be palpated through the skin. Some of the shunts have an on-off valve, as well as a part that may be pumped to facilitate drainage. Valves that are inserted can be set for a certain pressure, with some control over the amount of fluid drained.

See the box at right for key elements of the care of the patient having a shunt.

Meningitis. Meningitis is a relatively rare complication of brain surgery; it can follow infection intraoperatively or postoperatively. Following supratentorial surgery, the nurse should watch for any clear, watery drainage from the nose. This drainage may be present if there has been a tear in the meninges, which causes subsequent loss of CSF. The treatment consists of keeping the patient very quiet, avoiding suctioning the nose or blowing it, and administration of appropriate antibiotics. The leakage usually subsides spontaneously. Because of the danger of causing damage that might be followed by the drainage of CSF through the nose, many surgeons request that the nose never be suctioned when supratentorial surgery has been performed. A sign with this caution may be placed at the head of the bed.

Respiratory problems. _Respiratory collapse_ may follow infratentorial surgery. It is caused by edema of the brainstem or edema above the brainstem, which causes herniation of the brainstem into the foramen magnum and pressure on the respiratory center. Any irregularity of respiration, dyspnea, or cyanosis should be reported at once. Equipment should be ready for administering oxygen, doing a ventricular tap, and inserting an endotracheal tube if one is not already present. (For details

POSTOPERATIVE CARE OF THE PATIENT WITH A SHUNT

1. Perform monitoring.
   a. Assess neurologic status frequently for any decrease in mental status.
   b. Observe for symptoms of subdural hematoma, one of the possible side effects of the surgery.
   c. Monitor for symptoms of overdrainage, as evidenced by headache, especially when patient is sitting upright or standing.
   d. Assess degree and character of drainage.
      (1) Amount of drainage and bleeding should be minimal.
      (2) Reinforce dressing as needed.
      (3) Often incisional areas are left open to air after several days.
2. Maintain gastrointestinal status.
   a. Check frequently for signs of paralytic ileus; manipulation of the bowel that occurs with the placement of the shunt's peritoneal part can predispose the patient to this.
   b. Patient is usually given nothing by mouth for first day, and then clear liquids are started.
   c. Regular diet is resumed as soon as good bowel sounds are present and patient tolerates liquids.
3. Maintain comfort.
   a. Patient may need more frequent pain medication because of involvement of abdominal area.
   b. Keep pressure off incisional sites.
4. Promote mobility.
   a. Turning to either side is permitted.
   b. Raise head of bed gradually when mobilizing patient.
   c. Patient is encouraged to ambulate as much as possible to encourage adaption to decreased intracranial pressure.

of nursing care of the patient with an endotracheal tube, see Chapter 33). Occasionally a respirator is used.

Convulsions. Convulsions are not unusual after a craniotomy, and therefore side rails should be used even if the patient is unconscious and it is believed that movement is not possible. Phenytoin sodium (Dilantin) is often ordered prophylactically to prevent convulsions. It _should not_ be given intramuscularly because of its poor absorption via this route. If the patient has a history of seizures before surgery or if convulsions occurred in the postoperative period, this drug may be given for several months.

Corneal abrasions. _Loss of the corneal reflex_ may follow brain tumors of brain surgery. If the eye appears inflamed or if the patient does not seem to blink when objects approach the open eye, the neurosurgeon should be notified. Special eye care such as that given to patients who have had CVAs or who have had surgery for trigeminal neuralgia may be necessary (see earlier discussion on p. 1882).

The patient may complain of *diplopia* after brain surgery. This condition is often temporary, and the patient should know that it will probably improve. It can be relieved by placing an opaque eye shield over one eye. The eye covered usually is alternated each day to prevent atrophy of eye muscles through disuse.

Long-Term Care

Planning with patient's family. Few illnesses tax the entire physical and emotional resources of the patient's family as do the chronic neurologic diseases. It is imperative that the family participate in long-term plans for the patient. Family members may have severe emotional reactions and difficulties in adjustment that may require the assistance of a specially trained person such as a psychiatrist. Both patient and family need time to work through their feelings. Sometimes the enormity of the diagnosis cannot be grasped for weeks or even months by either patient or family members. Toxic polyneuritis in a young husband and father and multiple sclerosis in a young mother are examples of problems of such magnitude that long-term plans cannot be made quickly.

If the patient with neurologic disease has severe personality changes, aphasia, or convulsions, the family may even be afraid of the patient. Because the family is unaware that the patient may fully understand what is being said, they may make tactless remarks in front of the patient. When the patient is admitted to the hospital, it is often desirable to take the family aside to ascertain their insight into the situation. This interview provides an opportunity to help interpret the patient's actions and responses so that the family may better understand and be more supportive of the patient.

See Chapter 13 for more information about the general care of persons with prolonged illness.

Behavioral problems. Even the person who has suffered a mild head injury may experience long-term effects. These most often include cognitive problems such as difficulty with concentration and loss of memory. Recovery of intellectual functioning is often delayed, as frequently manifested in an inability to keep a job with increasing levels of unemployment.[57]

INTRAVERTEBRAL TUMORS
EPIDEMIOLOGY/ETIOLOGY

Primary intravertebral tumors, or neoplasms, occur either extramudullary (involving tissues outside the cord) or intramedullary (involving tissue cells within the cord). Secondary or metastatic tumors may also involve the spinal cord, its coverings, and the vertebrae.

CLINICAL MANIFESTATIONS

Extramedullary tumors of the intradural type may at first cause subjective nerve root pain. With tumor growth, this will include motor and sensory deficits relating to the level of the root and spinal cord involvement. As the tumor enlarges, it compresses the cord. Eventually the patient loses all motor and sensory function below the level of the tumor.

An intramedullary tumor, beginning within the spinal cord, often appears as a central cord syndrome, including segmental loss of pain and temperature function. In addition, loss of anterior horn cell function often occurs, especially in the hands. Most of the central long tracts of the nervous system become dysfunctional. There is gradual, progressive, and descending loss of pain and temperature sensations and motor weakness. Caudal motor and sensory functions are the last to be lost, including bowel and bladder function.

MEDICAL MANAGEMENT

The medical care of the patient with an intravertebral tumor may involve surgery. Radiation therapy may be used as an adjunct to surgery or as primary treatment when the tumor is considered to be inoperable. Chemotherapy also may be used.

A spinal decompression is typically done even when complete removal of the tumor is not considered possible. As much of the tumor as possible (and possibly bone) is removed to reduce the obstruction for a time. It can be performed at any level of the vertebral column and may include several vertebrae. The procedure is sometimes palliative.

IMPLEMENTATION

Convalescent care and rehabilitation of the patient depends on the type of tumor and whether it has been successfully removed. The decompression procedure may give relief of symptoms for years, if the tumor is a slow-growing one. The reader is referred to the previous section on spinal cord injury for further relevant care (see p. 1871).

ACQUIRED IMMUNODEFICIENCY SYNDROME (AIDS)
EPIDEMIOLOGY/ETIOLOGY

A significant number of patients with AIDS develop neurologic problems as the disease progresses.[3,9] At times subtle neurologic signs and symptoms may go unnoticed in patients with systemic illness. The incidence of patients with neurologic components to AIDS is increasing steadily. The reader is referred to Chapter 77 for a more complete discussion of AIDS.

PATHOPHYSIOLOGY

AIDS is associated with several abnormalities in the body's immune system, including decreased numbers of lymphocytes as well as impaired lymphocyte function.

The result is an immunosuppressed patient. In these patients the cellular response of the CNS is also decreased, enabling neurologic dysfunction to occur. Because the blood-brain barrier in some way protects the CNS from the systemic immune system, the CNS is relatively unable to resist organisms that do cross the blood-brain barrier, and they can increase rapidly.

The patient with AIDS can suffer neurologic disturbances as a result of three mechanisms. These include the following:

1. Frank infiltration of the CNS by specific organisms
2. Encephalopathy as a result of profound metabolic disturbances
3. Systemic peripheral neuropathy

The infiltration of the CNS may occur as a result of latent or inactive organisms in the CNS. Organisms that have been found to be particularly dangerous to the CNS include *Toxoplasma gondii*, cryptococcus, and cytomegalovirus.

Patients with AIDS also have been found to be at high risk for certain malignancies. Several of these have a high occurrence in the CNS. Primary CNS lymphoma or systemic lymphoma with CNS infiltration are common in patients with AIDS.

CLINICAL MANIFESTATIONS

The neurologic clinical manifestation seen most frequently is dementia. Other manifestations depend on the extent of cerebral involvement but include the following:

1. Neuropathies
2. Minor personality changes
3. Mild forgetfulness
4. Hemiparesis
5. Blindness
6. Seizures

DIAGNOSTIC TESTS

The diagnostic tests used to determine if a neurologic problem is related to AIDS include the following:

1. Serologic studies
2. Lumbar puncture
3. CT scan

At times, cerebral biopsy may be necessary to make the differential diagnosis.

MEDICAL MANAGEMENT

The treatment for patients with AIDS-related neurologic problems differs according to the actual pathologic process. Various methods used have included antiviral, antifungal, and antibacterial agents. Radiation used on the specific part of the brain affected has been used. Experimental therapies including interferon have been attempted. The mortality rate remains high despite aggressive therapy.

■ ASSESSMENT

The nursing assessment of the AIDS patient with neurologic manifestations varies depending on the specific pathology.

■ DATA ANALYSIS: NURSING DIAGNOSES

Nursing diagnoses are determined from assessment of patient data. Possible nursing diagnoses for the person with AIDS-related neurologic involvement include, but are not limited to, the following:

Diagnostic Title	Possible Etiologies
Activity intolerance	Generalized weakness
Adjustment, impaired	Disability requiring change in life-style
Body image disturbance	Change in body appearance
Coping, ineffective individual	Personal vulnerability
Grieving, anticipatory	Potential death
Hopelessness	Failing physical condition
Incontinence, total	Neurologic disease
Infection, potential for	Decreased immune response
Knowledge deficit: care required	Unfamiliarity with information sources
Nutrition, altered: less than body requirements	Chewing or swallowing difficulties, anorexia
Self-care deficit: bathing/ hygiene, dressing, toileting related to neuromuscular impairment	Intolerance to activity
Social isolation	Alteration in physical appearance, alteration in mental status
Thought processes, altered	Neurologic disorders

■ PLANNING: EXPECTED PATIENT OUTCOMES

Expected patient outcomes for the person with AIDS-related neurologic involvement may include, but are not limited to, the following:

1. Activity is maintained.
2. Coping and adjustment is facilitated.
3. Appropriate grieving is encouraged.
4. Patient has hope as long as possible.
5. Patient verbalizes knowledge of treatment options and use of medications.
6. Effects of incontinence is minimized.
7. Optimal nutritional status is maintained.
8. Infections are minimized.
9. Ability to care for self remains as long as possible.
10. Social isolation is minimized.
11. Compensatory mechanisms are used for altered thought processes.

■ IMPLEMENTATION

Care of the patient with AIDS will differ depending on the underlying problem causing the neurologic symptomatology. The reader is referred to other appropriate parts of this chapter for the necessary care of patients with neurologic involvement and to Chapter 77 for more information about care of the person with AIDS.

CHAPTER SUMMARY

- Epilepsy may be defined as a transitory disturbance in consciousness or in motor, sensory, or autonomic function with or without loss of consciousness and may be caused by neoplasms, abscesses, and trauma.

- Seizures or convulsions are associated with sudden, excessive, and disorderly electrical discharges in the neurons of the brain.

- The grand mal seizure is the most common and dramatic type of seizure and is characterized by a loss of consciousness for several minutes and tonic and clonic convulsions.

- An aura is a set of symptoms that occur before a seizure; the exact nature of the aura varies from person to person.

- The period following a seizure is called the postictal period.

- Status epilepticus is recurrent, generalized seizure activity that occurs at such frequency that full consciousness is not regained between seizures and can lead to death from hypoxia and exhaustion.

- Observations to be made about a person having a seizure include those associated with the aura, cry, onset, tonic and clonic phases, relaxation, postictal phase, duration of entire seizure, and level of consciousness.

- The primary goals of the care of the patient with a seizure disorder are to protect the person from injury, observe and record the seizure activity, and treat the seizure with one or more anticonvulsant drugs.

- The person with seizures should be encouraged to lead as normal a life as possible.

- Degenerative diseases are those neurologic diseases in which a premature senescence of nerve cells occurs and there is a known or suspected metabolic disturbance or the cause is unknown.

- Multiple sclerosis, the cause of which is unknown, is a common neurologic disease in northern climates that is chronic, remitting, and characterized by relapses.

- With multiple sclerosis, multiple foci of demyelination are distributed randomly in the white matter of the brainstem, spinal cord, optic nerves, and cerebrum. Because of the wide areas of distribution of degeneration, a greater variety of signs and symptoms is seen in multiple sclerosis than in other neurologic diseases. The treatment is symptomatic.

- The pathologic process that occurs with Parkinson's disease is basically a depigmentation of the substan-

tia nigra of the basal ganglia, which leads to multiple problems with motion.

- Treatment for Parkinson's disease is palliative and symptomatic and depends on the success of the drug used to treat it.

- Myasthenia gravis is a neurologic disease in which nerve impulses fail to pass to muscles at the myoneural junction.

- Respiratory problems are common in persons with myasthenia gravis.

- Alzheimer's disease, the most frequent cause of dementia in the older adult, is a degenerative disorder that affects the cells of the brain and causes impairment in intellectual functioning. No diagnostic test is specific for Alzheimer's disease.

- Nursing care of the patient with Alzheimer's disease is directed toward maintaining nutrition, continence, hydration, and safety.

- Cerebrovascular accident (CVA) is the most common disease of the nervous system and a major cause of death in the United States.

- The major causes of CVA are thrombus, embolus, or hemorrhage, all of which can be precipitated by many underlying factors. The blood vessel most frequently affected by a CVA is the middle cerebral artery.

- A transient ischemic attack (TIA) is a transient cerebral ischemia; temporary episodes of neurologic dysfunction serve to warn the patient of an underlying pathologic condition.

- Care of the patient with a CVA includes promoting nutrition, promoting activity, promoting elimination, providing emotional support, and beginning rehabilitation as soon as possible. Three goals of rehabilitation include prevention of further impairment, maintenance of existing abilities, and restoration of as much function as possible.

- Intracranial hemorrhages include bleeding into the subarachnoid space or into the brain tissue itself.

- The nervous system may be attacked by a variety of organisms and viruses and may be affected by toxic reactions to bacterial and viral disease.

- Infections that may affect the nervous system include meningitis, encephalitis, brain abscess, poliomyelitis, Guillain-Barré syndrome, herpes zoster, and neurosyphilis.

- Craniocerebral trauma, or head injury, causes death and serious disability in people of all ages.

- Damage to brain tissue by trauma can include concussion, contusion, and laceration.

- Automobile accidents, diving and other athletic accidents, and gunshot wounds are major causes of spinal cord injuries.

✔ A complete cord injury is one in which total transection of the spinal cord occurs with a complete loss of spinal cord functions, whereas an incomplete injury involves a partial transection or injury of the cord.

✔ Autonomic dysreflexia is a complication associated with spinal cord injury above the level of the sixth thoracic vertebra. It requires *immediate* nursing intervention.

✔ Primary intracranial tumors, or neoplasms, arise from the intrinsic cells of brain tissues and the pituitary and pineal glands and includes gliomas or astrocytomas, meningiomas, pituitary tumors, and neuromas.

✔ Hydrocephalus may occur in the presence of a brain tumor and is treated by a shunting procedure.

✔ Many patients with acquired immunodeficiency syndrome (AIDS) develop neurologic problems as the disease progresses.

✔ Neurologic problems in the patient with AIDS can occur because of infiltration of the central nervous system by specific organisms, encephalopathy, or systemic peripheral neuropathy.

✔ The outcomes and care of the patient with AIDS will differ depending on the underlying problem causing the neurologic symptoms.

QUESTIONS TO CONSIDER

■ Why is diagnosis of many of the neurologic diseases so difficult?

■ How would your care of the head-injured patient differ from that of the patient with a brain tumor?

■ Why is it important to do a workup for cancer in patients who have symptoms of myasthenia gravis?

■ Your patient with amyotrophic lateral sclerosis decides not to ever become ventilator dependent. What issues and nursing implications does this raise?

■ How would your care of a C5 quadriplegic differ from that of a L5 paraplegic person?

REFERENCES AND SELECTED READINGS

1. Adams R and Victor M: Principles of neurology, New York, 1985, McGraw-Hill Book Co.
2. Adler R: Trigeminal glycerol chemoneurolysis: nursing implications, J Neurosci Nurs 21:337-341, 1989.
3. Ake J and Perlstein L: AIDS: impact on neuroscience nursing practice, J Neurosci Nurs 19:300-304, 1987.
4. *Allan D: Treating subarachnoid hemorrhage using carotid ligation, Nurs Times 77:1383-1385, 1977.
5. Arnason B: Multiple sclerosis: current concepts and management, Hosp Pract 82:81-89, 1982.
6. Arsenault L: Selected postoperative complications of cranial surgery, J Neurosurg Nurs 17:155-163, 1985.
7. *Bartel M: Dialogue with dementia: nonverbal communication in patients with Alzheimer's disease, J Gerontol Nurs 5:21-31, 1979.
8. Beck C and Heacock P: Nursing interventions for patients with Alzheimer's disease, Nurs Clin North Am 23(1):95-124, 1988.
9. Beckham M and Rudy E: Acquired immunodeficiency syndrome: impact and implication for the neurological system, J Neurosci Nurs 10:5-10, 1986.
10. Bell J and Hannon J: Pathophysiology involved in autonomic hyperreflexia, J Neurosci Nurs 18:86-89, 1986.
11. Berger J and Sheremata W: Persistent neurological deficit precipitated by hot bath test in multiple sclerosis, JAMA 249:1751-1754, 1983.
12. Berkshire J and Watson-Evans H: Meningioma: a nursing perspective. J Neurosci Nurs 21:96-103, 1989.
13. Berry P and Ward-Smith P: Adrenal medullary transplant as a treatment for Parkinson's disease: perioperative considerations, J Neurosci Nurs 20:356-361, 1988.
14. Blanco K and Cuoma N: From the other side of the bedrail: a personal experience with Guillain-Barré syndrome, J Neurosurg Nurs 15:355-359, 1983.
15. *Blount M and Cluca R: Amyotrophic lateral sclerosis, Am J Nurs 76:66-68, 1976.
16. Borowski C: A comparison of pulmonmary complications in spinal cord—injured patients treated with two modes of spinal immobilization, J Neurosci Nurs 21:79-85, 1989.
17. Brewer K and Sperling M: Neurosurgical treatment of intractable epilepsy, J Neurosci Nurs 6:366-370, 1988.
18. *Brunstrom S: Movement therapy in hemiplegia, New York, 1970, Harper & Row, Publishers, Inc.
19. Burns E and Buckwalter K: Pathophysiology and etiology of Alzheimer's disease, Nurs Clin North Am 23(1):11-30, 1988.
20. *Burnside J: Alzheimer's disease: an overview, J Gerontol Nurs 5:14-20, 1979.
21. *Carlson C: Psychological aspects of neurologic disability, Nurs Clin North Am 15:309-320, 1980.
22. Chadwick A and Oesting H: Not for specialists only: caring for patients with spinal cord injuries, Nursing '89 19(11):52-56, 1989.
23. Chase M and Whelan-Decker E: Nursing management of a patient with a subarachnoid hemorrhage, J Neurosurg Nurs 16:23-29, 1984.
24. Chicano L: Humanistic aspects of sexuality as related to spinal cord injury, J Neurosci Nurs 21:366-369, 1989.
25. Connolly R et al: Update: head injury, J Neurosurg Nurs 13:195-201, 1981.
26. Csesko P: Sexuality and multiple sclerosis, J Neurosci Nurs 20:353-355, 1988.

*References preceded by an asterisk are particularly well suited for student reading.

27. Cyr L: Sequelae of SCI after discharge from initial rehabilitation program, Rehabil Nurs. 14:326-329, 337, 1989.

28. Daly B: Intensive care nursing, ed 2, Garden City, NY, 1985, Medical Exam Publishing Co.

29. Davidson A and Young C: Repatterning of stroke rehabilitation clients following return to life in the community, J Neurosurg Nurs 17:123-128, 1985.

30. DeJong G et al: Independent living outcomes in spinal cord injury: multivariant analysis, Arch Phys Med Rehabil 65:66-72, 1984.

31. *Donahue R: Symposium on care of the patient with neuromuscular disease: an overview of neuromuscular disease, Nurs Clin North Am 14:95-106, 1979.

32. Doolittle N: Arteriovenous malformation: the physiology, symptomatology and nursing care, J Neurosurg Nurs 11:222-226, 1979.

33. Doolittle N: Stroke recovery—review of the literature and suggestions for further research, J Neurosci Nurs 20:169-173, 1988.

34. *Eisenberg MG and Rustard LC: Sex and the spinal cord injured: some questions and answers, ed 2, Washington, DC, 1975, US Government Printing Office.

35. Elliott J and Smith D: Meeting family needs following severe head injury: a multidisciplinary approach, J Neurosurg Nurs 17:111-113, 1985.

36. *Fedun P: Postoperative evaluation of patients undergoing microanastomosis for brain ischemia, J Neurosurg Nurs 12:46-53, 1980.

37. *Felder L: Neurogenic bladder dysfunction, J Neurosurg Nurs 11:91-104, 1979.

38. Flynn E: Cerebral vasospasm following intracranial aneurysm rupture: a protocol for detection, J Neurosci Nurs 21:348-352, 1989.

39. Fode N: Subarachnoid hemorrhage from ruptured intracranial aneurysm, Am J Nurs 88:673-680, 1988.

40. Francabandera F: Multiple sclerosis rehabilitation: inpatient vs. outpatient, Rehabil Nurs 13:251-254, 1988.

41. Franco L: Cerebral contusions: a prototype for head injury, J Neurosurg Nurs 16:45-49, 1984.

42. Garrett E: Parkinsonism: forgotten considerations in medical treatment and nursing care, J Neurosurg Nurs 14:13-18, 1984.

43. Given C et al: Source of stress among families caring for relatives with Alzheimer's disease, Nurs Clin North Am 23(1):69-82, 1988.

44. Goddard L: Sexuality and spinal cord injury, J Neurosci Nurs 20:240-244, 1988.

45. Gould M: Nursing diagnoses concurrent with multiple sclerosis, J Neurosurg Nurs 15:339-345, 1983.

46. Gray-Vickrey P: Evaluating Alzheimer's patients: the importance of being thorough, Nursing '88 18(12):34-41, 1988.

47. Griffin C and Lockhart J: Learning to swallow again, Am J Nurs 87:314-318, 1987.

48. Guttman L: Spinal cord injuries: comprehensive management and research, ed 2, Oxford, 1976, Blackwell Scientific Publications, Ltd.

49. Haberman B: Cognitive dysfunction and social rehabilitation in severly head-injured patients, J Neurosurg Nurs 14:220-224, 1982.

50. Hahn K: Left vs. right: what a difference a side makes in stroke, Nursing '87 17(9):44-48, 1987.

51. Hart G: Strokes causing left versus right hemiplegia: different effects and nursing implications, Geriatr Nurs 4:39-43, 1983.

52. Hartshorn J: Immunosuppressive treatment of multiple sclerosis, J Neurosurg Nurs 16:275-278, 1984.

53. Hartshorn J and Hartshorn E: Nursing interventions for anticonvulsant drug interactions, J Neurosurg Nurs 18:250-255, 1986.

54. Hegeman K: A care plan for the family of a brain trauma client, Rehabil Nurs 13:254-258, 1988.

55. Hendrickson S: Psychological care of the patient with neurological dysfunction, J Neurosurg Nurs 16:202-207, 1984.

56. Hickey J: The clinical practice of neurological and neurosurgical nursing, New York, 1983, John Wiley & Sons, Inc.

57. Hinkle J et al: Restoring social competence in minor head-injury patients, J Neurosci Nurs 18:268-271, 1986.

58. Hodges K: Meningioma, astrocytoma, and germinoma: case presentations of three intracranial tumors, J Neurosci Nurs 21:113-121, 1989.

59. Hollans N et al: Overview of multiple sclerosis and nursing care of the multiple sclerosis patient, J Neurosurg Nurs 13:28-33, 1982.

60. Horvath M et al: Myasthenia gravis: a nursing approach, J Neurosurg Nurs 14:7-12, 1982.

61. Howard M et al: Psychological after effects of halo traction and review of acute care, Am J Nurs 12:1839-1843, 1982.

62. Hunt V and Walker F: Dysphagia in Huntington's disease, J Neurosci Nurs 21:92-95, 1989.

63. Ingersol G: Abdominal pathology in spinal cord injured patients, J Neurosurg Nurs 17:343-348, 1985.

64. Jacobs L et al: Intrathecal interferon in multiple sclerosis, Arch Neurol 39:609-615, 1982.

65. Keller C et al: Psychological responses in aphasia: theoretical considerations and nursing implications, J Neurosci Nurs 21:290-294, 1989.

66. Kelly B: Nursing care of the patient with multiple sclerosis, Rehabil Nurs 13:238-243, 1988.

67. Kim T: Hope as a mode of coping in amytrophic lateral sclerosis, J Neurosci Nurs 21:342-347, 1989.

68. *King R et al: Symposium on rehabilitation nursing: rehabilitation of the patient with spinal cord injury, Nurs Clin North Am 15:225-243, 1980.

69. Kirk E and Bradford L: Effects of alcohol on the CNS: implications for the neuroscience nurse, J Neurosci Nurs 19:326-335, 1987.

70. Kirkland J et al: Trigeminal neuralgia: approach to nursing care, J Neurosurg Nurs 15:149-153, 1983.

71. Leahy N: Intrarterial cisplatin infusion: nursing implications, J Neurosci Nurs 18:296-301, 1986.

72. Leopold N and Kage M: Swallowing, ingestion, and dysphagia: a reappraisal, Arch Phys Med Rehabil 64:372-375, 1983.

73. *Levitt R: Understanding sexuality and spinal cord injury, J Neurosurg Nurs 12:88-89, 1980.

74. Lipe H: Prevention of nervous system trauma from motor travel in motor vehicles, J Neurosurg Nurs 17:77-82, 1985.

75. Litchfield M and Noroian E: Changes in selected pulmonary functions in patients diagnosed with myasthenia gravis, J Neurosci Nurs 21:375-381, 1989.

76. Logemann J: Evaluation and treatment of swallowing disorders, San Diego, 1983, College Hill Press, Inc.

77. Long B and Phipps W: Medical-surgical nursing: a nursing process approach, ed 2, St Louis, 1989, The CV Mosby Co.

78. Maas M: Management of patients with Alzheimer's disease in long-term care facilities, Nurs Clin North Am 23(1):57-68, 1988.

79. MacDonald E: Aneurysmal subarachnoid hemorrhage, J NeuroSci Nurs 21:313-321, 1989.

80. Mahon D and Elger C: Analysis of posttraumatic syndrome following head injury, J Neurosci Nurs 21:382-384, 1989.

81. Markin D: Preoperative concerns of the patient undergoing craniotomy, J Neurosci Nurs 18:275-278, 1986.

82. Mauser G: Neuromuscular respiratory failure—what the nurse knows makes a difference, J Neurosci Nurs 20:110-117, 1988.

83. McArthur J and McArthur J: Neurological manifestations of acquired immunodeficiency syndrome, J Neurosci Nurs 18:242-249, 1986.

84. McClelland O: Behavioral problems after closed head injury, Top Emerg Med 4:42-50, 1983.

85. Mitchell S and Yates R: Extracranial-intracranial bypass surgery, J Neurosurg Nurs 17:288-292, 1985.

86. Monson R: Autonomic dysreflexia: a nursing challenge, Rehabil Nurs 6:18-19, 1981.

87. Morgante L et al: Research and treatment in multiple sclerosis: implications for nursing practice, J Neurosci Nurs 21:285-289, 1989.

88. Nemeroff D: Transphenoidal hypophysectomy, J Neurosurg Nurs 13:303-312, 1981.

89. Nicholsan C: Cranial bypass: a case study, J Neurosurg Nurs 15:165-168, 1983.

90. Niederpruem M: Autonomic dysreflexia, Rehabil Nurs 9:29-32, 1984.

91. *Olson E et al: The hazards of immobility, Am J Nurs 67:779-797, 1967.

92. Passarella P and Lewis N: Nursing application of Bobath principles in stroke care, J Neurosci Nurs 19:106-109, 1987.

93. Perlstein L and Ake J: AIDS: an overview for the neuroscience nurse, J Neurosci Nurs 19:296-299, 1987.

94. Pettibone K: Management of spasticity in spinal cord injury: nursing concerns, J Neurosci Nurs 20:217-222, 1988.

95. Pires M: Substance abuse: the silent saboteur in rehabilitation, Nurs Clin North Am 24(1):291-296, 1989.

96. *Plank N: Multiple sclerosis: an update and review, J Neurosurg Nurs 11:44-47, 1979.

97. Plylar P: Management of the agitated and aggressive head injury patient in an acute hospital setting, J Neurosci Nurs 21:353-356, 1989.

98. *Polhopek M: Stroke: an update on vascular disease, J Neurosurg Nurs 12:81-87, 1980.

99. Prendergast V: Bacterial meningitis update, J Neurosci Nurs 19:95-99, 1987.

100. Rhodes M et al: Complications of posterior fossa craniotomy, J Neurosurg Nurs 15:19-21, 1983.

101. *Ross A et al: Neuromuscular diagnostic procedures, Nurs Clin North Am 14:107-121, 1979.

102. Rudy E: Advanced neurological and neurosurgical nursing, St Louis, 1985, The CV Mosby Co.

103. Rutledge B: Aneurysm wrapping: principles applicable to the neuroscience nurse, J Neurosci Nurs 21:370-374, 1989.

104. *Samond R: Guillain-Barré syndrome: helping the patient in the acute state, Nursing '80 10:34-41, 1980.

104a. Scherer P: How AIDS attacks the brain, Am J Nurs 90(1):44-53, 1990.

104b. Sherman D: managing an acute head injury, Nurs '90 20(4):48-51, 1990.

105. Shpritz D: Craniocerebral trauma, Crit Care Nurs 3:49, 52, 55-56, 1983.

106. Smith S: Continuous intracranial monitoring: implications and applications for critical care, Crit Care Nurs 3:42-51, 1983.

107. Spielman G: Metabolic complications associated with severe diffuse brain injury, J Neurosurg Nurs 17:83-88, 1985.

108. *Stryker R: Rehabilitative aspects pf acute and chronic illness, ed 2, Philadelphia, 1977, WB Saunders Co.

109. *Terzian M: Neurosurgical intervention for the management of chronic intractable pain, Top Clin Nurs 1:75-88, 1980.

110. Tosch P: Patients' recollections of their posttraumatic coma, J Neurosci Nurs 20:223-228, 1988.

111. Tucker C: Safety assessment for the postictal confusional phase following complex partial seizure, J Neurosurg Nurs 17:201-209, 1985.

112. Vernon G: Parkinson's disease, J Neurosci Nurs 21:273-284, 1989.

113. Wahlquist G: A great nursing challenge: recover and effective management of the patient with herpes simplex encephalitis, J Neurosurg Nurs 13:220-225, 1982.

114. Wahlquist G: The family in rehabilitation, Rehabil Nurs 12:62, 1987.

115. Warren J and Peck E: Factors which influence neuropsychological recovery from severe head injury, J Neurosurg Nurs 16:248-252, 1984.

116. *Webb P: Neurological deficit after carotid endarderectomy, Am J Nurs 79:654-658, 1979.

117. Welsh D and Zumwalt C: Volumetric interstitial hyperthermia: nursing implications for brain tumor treatment, J Neurosci Nurs 20:229-235, 1988.

118. *Wheeler P: Care of the patient with a cerebellar tumor, Am J Nurs 77:263-266, 1977.

119. Whitney F: Relationship of laterality of stroke and emotional and functional outcome, J Neurosci Nurs 19:158-165, 1987.

120. *Wing S: Cervical spine injuries: treatment and related nursing care, J Neurosurg Nurs 9:138-140, 1977.

121. Woodward E: The total patient: implications for nursing care of the epileptic, J Neurosurg Nurs 14:166-169, 1982.

122. Zejdlik C: Management of spinal cord injury, Monterey, Calif, 1983, Wadsworth Health Services Division.

CHAPTER 64

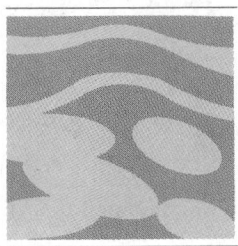

Assessment of the Eye

MARION ALLEN

CHAPTER OBJECTIVES

After studying this chapter, the student should be able to:
1   Describe the structure and function of the eye.
2   Identify the normal physiologic and anatomic changes that occur with aging.
3   Identify the subjective and objective data that should be obtained when assessing the eye.
4   Describe the purpose of the diagnostic studies used to assess the eye and its visual function.

Orientation to our world is primarily visual. We learn much about our environment and ourselves through our eyes. There is practically no behavior that is not affected by the visual sense. One hears a noise and looks in the direction from which it came. Something touches our body and we look to see what it was. Vision contributes meaning and pleasure to the human experience. Our eyes reflect the pleasure, sorrow, or pain that we feel in relation to human experiences. A world without the sight of children playing, the esthetic pleasure of the museum, or the beauty of the rainbow would be bleak indeed or, to some, almost unimaginable.

Although visual impairment is often not the initial problem or major diagnosis of persons for whom the nurse is providing care, it is often present. Nurses and other health workers need to be able to assess the person's visual abilities and plan care accordingly.

Nursing assessment is focused on the degree to which the vision loss affects the person's ability to carry out activities of daily living, the support systems available, and the coping skills that have been successfully used in the past. Nursing interventions are designed to help people meet their basic needs as they are affected by their disease, hospitalization, or illness; to strengthen existing support systems; and to encourage the use of successful coping mechanisms.

ANATOMY AND PHYSIOLOGY OF THE EYE

LAYERS OF THE EYE

The eyeball has three main coats or layers (Figure 64-1). The tough *outer layer* consists of the *opaque sclera*

(white); the *transparent cornea;* and their junction, the *corneoscleral sulcus* or *limbus.* The *middle vascular layer* or *uvea* is composed of the *choroid;* the *ciliary body;* and the *iris,* which contains the *pupil* in its center.

The *retina,* the *third* and *innermost layer* of the eye, is composed of *two parts, a sensory portion* and a layer of *pigmented epithelium. The sensory portion contains the photoreceptors (rods and cones).* These photoreceptors synapse in the retina with bipolar neurons and then with ganglion neurons, and these become the fibers of the optic nerve. The cones, which are less numerous than the rods, are concentrated near the center of the retina. They are considered to be the receptors for bright daylight and color vision and allow us to see sharp images. The rods, which are found mostly in the periphery of the retina, are receptors for dim or night vision. Rods contain rhodopsin, a photosensitive protein that rapidly becomes depleted in bright light. The slow regeneration of rhodopsin, which is dependent on the presence of vitamin A, explains the time needed to adjust from a bright to a dim light. Vitamin A deficiency affects night vision.

CHAMBERS OF THE EYE

The *interior* of the *eyeball* is divided into *two cavities,* the *anterior* and the *posterior.* The anterior cavity, which is in front of the lens, is further *subdivided* into an *anterior chamber* (between the cornea and the iris) and a *posterior chamber* (between the iris and the lens). The anterior cavity is filled with a clear liquid called *aqueous humor,* which is produced in the ciliary body, drains into the posterior chamber, and passes through the pupil into the anterior chamber. *Aqueous humor* leaves the eye through the filtration structures at the junction of the iris and cornea (anterior chamber angle). The filtration structures consist of a meshwork (trabeculum) and a tubular channel that encircles the anterior chamber (Schlemm's canal). Schlemm's canal has several exit channels that empty into the scleral and episcleral veins. Aqueous humor passes through these

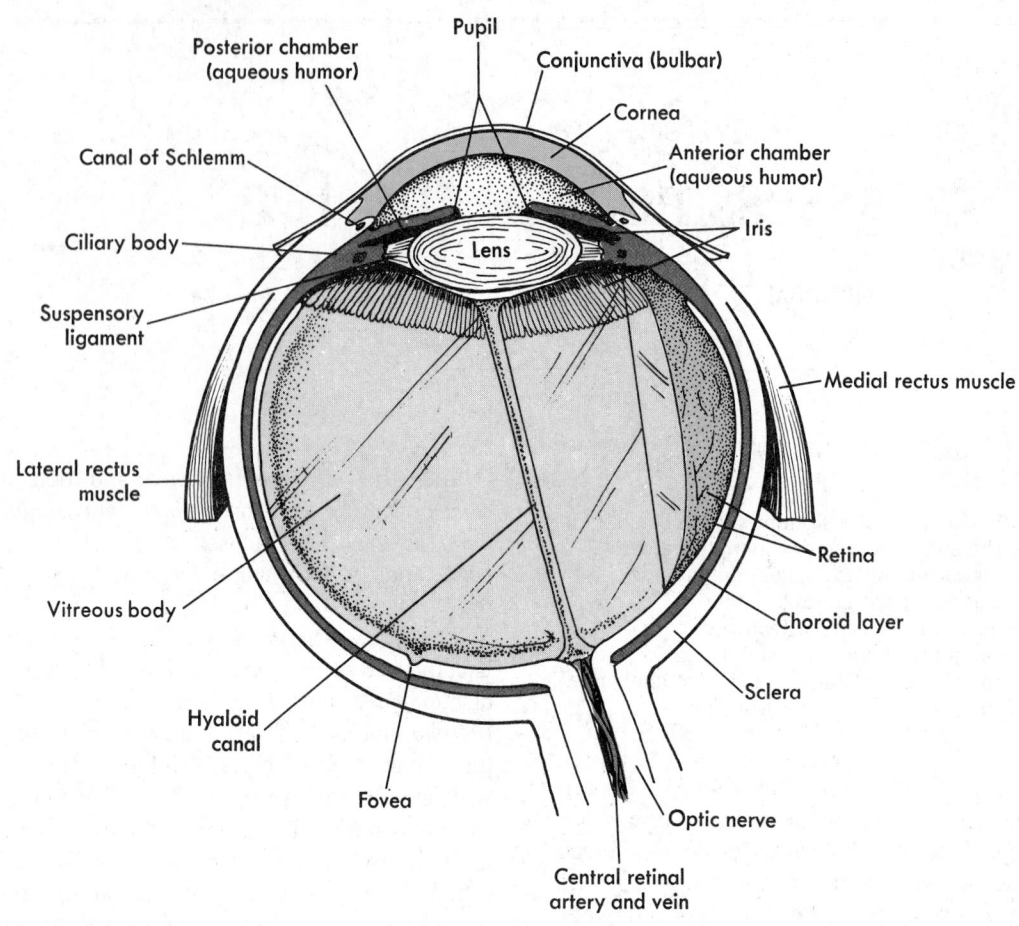

Pupil

Posterior chamber
(aqueous humor)

Conjunctiva (bulbar)

Cornea

Canal of Schlemm

Anterior chamber
(aqueous humor)

Ciliary body

Lens

Iris

Suspensory
ligament

Medial rectus muscle

Lateral rectus
muscle

Retina

Vitreous body

Choroid layer

Sclera

Hyaloid
canal

Fovea

Optic nerve

Central retinal
artery and vein

FIGURE 64-1 Horizontal section through left eyeball.

exit channels and eventually is absorbed into general circulation.

The *posterior or vitreous cavity* is the larger of the two cavities of the eye. It is filled with a clear gel-like substance called vitreous. The structure of the vitreous can be pictured as fine-collagen fibers crossing one another to form a scaffolding that helps to maintain the shape of the eyeball. This fibrous network becomes more dense toward the outermost portion of the vitreous, particularly in the areas of strong attachment between the vitreous and retina. These attachments occur at the anterior edge of the retina, the optic disc, the equator of the eye, and the macula.

LENS

The lens is a transparent biconvex structure located directly behind the iris and pupil. It is attached to the ciliary body by a suspensory ligament (zonule). The lens continues to form fibers throughout life. The old fibers are not removed but become compressed and form an increasingly larger and less elastic lens nucleus.

EYE MUSCLES

Eye muscles consist of *two types: extrinsic* and *intrinsic*. The extrinsic voluntary muscles outside the eyeball control extraocular movement (Table 64-1). The intrinsic involuntary muscles within the eye are the ciliary body, which controls the shape of the lens, and the iris, which controls pupil size and consequently the amount of light that enters the eye.

EYELIDS

The *eyelids* (palpebrae) are made up of *thin layers of skin, muscle, fibrous tissue, and mucous membrane.* The main purposes of the eyelids are to protect the eye from external irritation, spread tears over the front of the eye, and interrupt and restrict the amount of light entering the eye. The *conjunctiva,* the mucous membrane lining of the eyelid that extends over the anterior sclera, is of particular significance. This membrane and its blood vessels provide nutrients, antibodies, and leukocytes to the avascular cornea. The conjunctiva and glands within the eyelid secrete mucus and oil, which

TABLE 64-1 Extrinsic muscles

Name	Function
Superior rectus	Rotates eye upward and toward the nose
Inferior rectus	Rotates eye downward and toward the nose
Lateral rectus	Moves eye toward the temporal side
Medial rectus	Moves eye toward the nose
Inferior oblique	Rotates eye upward and toward the temporal side
Superior oblique	Rotates eye downward and toward the temporal side

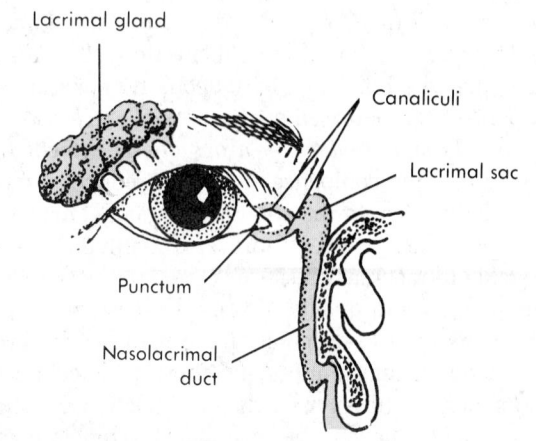

FIGURE 64-2 Lacrimal system.

help keep the cornea moist and clear and decrease friction when the lids blink over the cornea.

LACRIMAL SYSTEM

The lacrimal system consists of the *lacrimal gland* and a *tear drainage system* (Figure 64-2). The lacrimal gland produces the tears that flow nasally across the eye and enter into the drainage system. The tears flow through small holes in the eyelids (puncti) and ducts (canaliculi) to the lacrimal sac. They then drain into the nasolacrimal duct to the inferior meatus of the nasal cavity. Tears keep the surface of the eye and conjunctiva moistened and lubricated. Tears also contain an enzyme that functions as an antibacterial agent.

ORBIT

The eye rests within the confines of a bony orbit. This orbit is a *cone-shaped cavity* formed by the *union of cranial and facial bones*. The eyeball itself only occupies about one fifth of the space of the orbit. The remainder is filled with the lacrimal gland, muscles, blood vessels, nerves, and fatty tissue. This fatty tissue serves as a protective cushion for the eye.

PHYSIOLOGY OF VISION

Light rays entering the eye bend (*refraction*) as they pass over the curved surfaces of the cornea and through various structures of the eye (cornea, aqueous humor, lens, vitreous humor), which have different densities, to focus on the retina.

The eye can adjust (*accommodation*) to *seeing objects at various distances* by the *flattening or thickening of the lens*. Near vision requires contraction of the ciliary body, which decreases the distance between the edges of the ciliary body, thus relaxing the suspensory ligament attached to the lens. The lens then bulges to bend the light ray more acutely so that the rays will focus on the retina. Accommodation is also facilitated by changing the size of the pupil. With near vision the iris constricts the pupil to force light rays to pass through the shortened but thicker lens. The pupils also constrict with bright lights to protect the retina from intense stimulation.

Light rays are absorbed by the photoreceptors on the retina and are changed to electrical activity to transmit the image to the cortex. The fibers of the optic nerve (cranial nerve II, see Chapter 59) divide at the optic chiasm, the medial portion of each nerve crosses to the opposite side (see Figure 59-15), and the impulses are then transmitted to the visual cortex. *Bilateral vision provides depth perception.*

CHANGES WITH AGING

Aging affects many aspects of visual function, both physiologic and anatomic. Decreased flexibility and elasticity of the lens lead to one of the first noted signs of aging—the decreased ability of the eye to accommodate for near and detailed work (presbyopia).

The lens also yellows with age. This causes greater difficulty in distinguishing among colors at the blue end of the spectrum. A smaller sized pupil (senile miosis) aids in this distortion of color. It also affects the amount of light that reaches the retina and the ability of the person to adapt to dim light and darkness. Individuals over the age of 60 need about twice as much light to see things as they did when they were 20.[7]

This needed increase in light for close work can cause another aging problem—glare. Glare, a veil-like luminance super-imposed on the retinal image, masks and reduces the brightness of objects in the visual field.[17] Glare is related to increased light scatter in the eye caused by corneal, scleral, lens, and vitreal changes.

The field of vision also begins to decrease, affecting the breadth of vision that is possible. It is uncertain whether this decrease is caused by retinal changes, decreased pupil size, or loss of lens transparency.

The decrease in lens transparency, which begins to

appear in the fifth decade of life, is not fully understood. The compression of lens fibers, the yellowing of the lens, and the efficiency of aqueous humor may all play a part in the increased opaqueness of the lens.

Aqueous humor production drops off sharply in the sixth decade. This compensates for the reduced drainage and shallowness of the anterior chamber. This combination of events enables the eye to maintain a relatively stable intraocular pressure.[10]

The quantity and quality of tears decrease with age, and the tears tend to evaporate more readily. The eyes take on a duller appearance, and there is a feeling of tightness, scratchiness, or dryness. Instillation of artificial tears may relieve these symptoms. The drainage system for the tears also is less efficient. This may lead to a block in the system, with tearing as a result.

One of the more common eye changes from aging is *arcus senilis.* This *hazy gray ring around the periphery of the cornea is a result of fat deposits through the layers of the cornea.* Another important change in the cornea is its change in shape. It tends to flatten, resulting in an irregular curvature in the corneal surface. Light entering the eye tends to be refracted at varying angles leading to a distorted and blurred image (astigmatism).

ASSESSMENT OF EYES AND VISION

Examination of the eyes can be one of the most rewarding aspects of a physical examination. It is relatively easy to measure both the stimulus and the response of the entire visual system by the measurement of visual acuity. The tissues of the eye are for the most part transparent. Thus *abnormalities are easily detected* as opacities in a structure that should be transparent or as changes in the appearance of tissue. Ocular manifestations of systemic disease can be observed. Also, only the vascular system (retinal vascular system) and cranial nerve (optic nerve) of the eye can be visualized.

Assessment of the eye's structure and functioning is done by physicians, nurses, optometrists, and some paraprofessional health workers. Lay persons are often trained to conduct vision screening tests with preschool children. Assessment includes inspection of the external structures and gross measures of visual acuity. The more complex eye examinations such as electrophysiologic studies of the retina and other fundus examinations are performed by physicians or specially trained nurses or technicians.

The nurse's exact activities in assessment of the eye and vision depend on the place of employment, the nurse's preparation, and the patient's age and health. For instance, a nurse working in a community health agency may have the need and opportunity to do more extensive eye assessment than a nurse in a teaching hospital where physicians abound. Every nurse should

BASIC ASSESSMENT OF THE EYE AND VISION

Facial and ocular expression	Prominence of eyes, alert or dull expression
Eyelids	Symmetry, presence of edema, ptosis, itching, redness, discharges, blinking equality
Iris and pupils	Irregularities in color, shape, size
Pupillary reflex	Constriction of pupil in response to light in that eye (direct light reaction), equal amount of constriction in other eye (consensual light reaction)
Lens	Transparent or opaque
Peripheral vision	Ability to see movements and objects well on both sides of field of vision
Acuity with and without glasses	Ability to read newsprint, clocks on wall, and name pins, to recognize faces at bedside and at door
Supportive aids	Glasses, contact lenses, false eye

at least be able to carry out a basic assessment of the external eye structures and vision (see the box above).

A complete ocular assessment consists of subjective data elicited by means of an interview with the individual and objective data obtained by inspecting external structures and functions of the eye and some internal parts of the eye (see the box below).

SUBJECTIVE DATA: HISTORY

Because many eye disorders can be inherited, a family history is necessary. Questions are specifically directed to a family history of cataracts, glaucoma, diabetes, or to poor vision or blindness that could not be corrected by glasses. In addition to any current complaints, the person's previous eye problems, diagnoses, and treatment are recorded. It is important to note the presence of any systemic disease. The interviewer determines if the person perceives any of the following: changes in visual acuity; abnormal signs and symptoms such as burning, tearing, or blurred vision; and events surrounding onset of symptoms, duration of symptoms, and sources of relief.

OCULAR ASSESSMENT

Recording of history
Assessment of visual acuity
Assessment of ocular movement
Assessment of pupillary reflexes
Assessment of visual fields
Inspection of external structures
Inspection of internal structures
Estimation of intraocular pressure

OBJECTIVE DATA
ASSESSMENT OF VISUAL ACUITY

Visual acuity means acuteness or sharpness of vision and includes measurement of both distant and near vision.

Distant Vision

Distance vision is usually determined by the use of a *Snellen* chart (Figure 64-3, *A*), with the person standing 20 ft (6 m) from the chart. The chart consists of rows of letters, numbers, or other characters arranged with the larger ones at the top and the smaller ones at the bottom. The uppermost letter on the chart is scaled so that it can be read by the normal eye at 200 ft, and the successive rows are scaled so that they can be read at 100, 70, 50, 40, 30, 20, 15, and 10 ft, respectively. Visual acuity is expressed as a fraction, and a reading of 20/20 (6/6) is considered normal. The upper figure refers to the distance of the person from the chart, and the lower figure indicates the distance at which a normal eye can read the line. The distance from the chart to where the individual stands must be carefully measured. The examiner usually stands beside the chart and points to the line to be read so that no mistake occurs. Each eye is tested separately, and its performance is carefully recorded. The person is tested with and without distance lenses. When testing vision, a piece of stiff paper or a plastic occluder is placed over one eye while the other eye is tested.

For preschool children, illiterate adults, and others unable to read the English alphabet, a modified Snellen

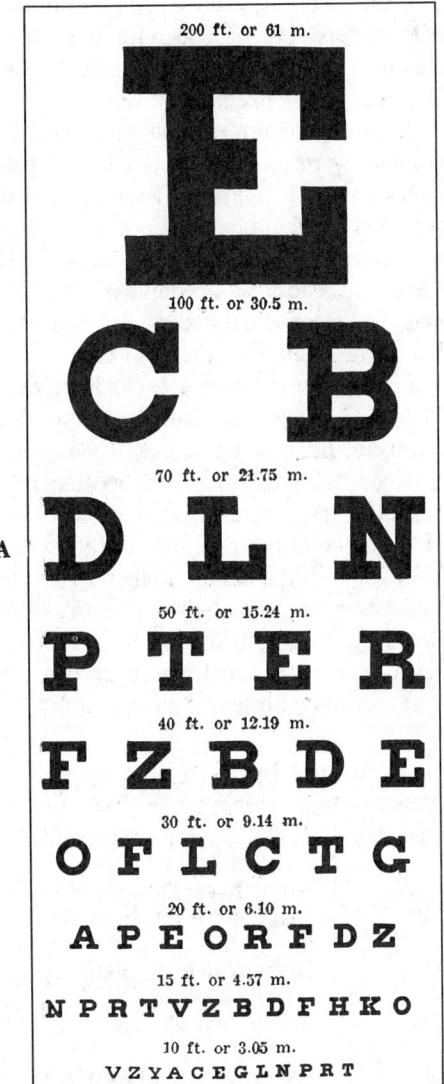

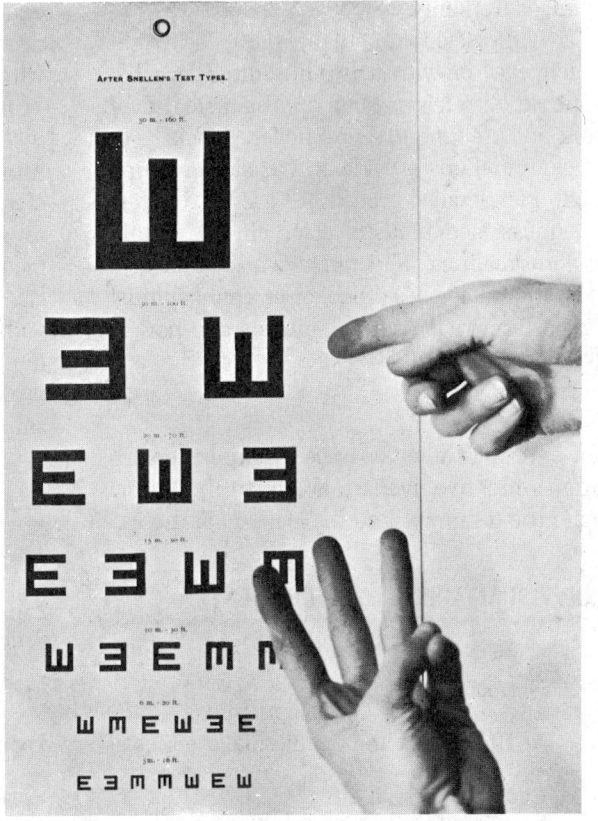

FIGURE 64-3 A, Snellen chart used in testing vision. **B,** Modified Snellen chart, called "E" game, for testing vision of small children, persons unfamiliar with English alphabet, and illiterate persons.

chart may be used (Figure 64-3, *B*). A block E is shown in varying positions and the individual is asked to indicate in which direction the "legs" or "fingers" of the E point. There now is a move away from using the E game with preschool children. It is believed that young children do not naturally understand that a symbol rotated in different directions has different meanings. Instead tests that use a limited number of letters and a matching card to which the child can point are being introduced.

Near Vision

Near vision can be tested with the use of a *Jaeger* chart or newsprint. The Jaegar chart is a card containing varying sizes of print and is held 35 cm (14 in) from the eye. The score obtained can be expressed in Snellen, metric, and percentage figures.

If persons are unable to read the letters on the charts, another method of assessing visual acuity is to hold fingers in front of the eyes and ask the person to count the number of fingers that they can see. Other persons may not be able to count fingers but can see hand movement. Still others may only be able to tell the direction from which light is coming (light projection) or just respond to light flashed in their eyes (light perception). The box below, left outlines some examples of visual acuity measurements.

Any person with vision less than 20/30 OD (right eye) or OS (left eye) or with a two-line difference between eyes should be referred to an ophthalmologist for further testing and treatment. The Snellen, block E, or Jaegar chart examinations provide only basic screening test data. Additional detailed procedures are used to test for nearsightedness, astigmatism, color blindness, and many other abnormalities. The nurse who works in a clinic, in an ophthalmologist's office, or in a school must know how to perform vision screening tests and how to teach others to do them.

Refraction

A ray of light entering the eye passes through the various transparent refractive media to focus on the retina. The bending of the light rays and the location of the image depend on the shape and condition of the eye. The eye has the ability to adjust to near or far objects (*accommodation*) by means of the ciliary muscles, which contract or relax, causing the lens to flatten or thicken as the need arises. If the anteroposterior dimension of the eye is abnormally long, the light rays will focus in front of the retina (*myopia*). Conversely, if the anteroposterior dimension is abnormally short, the rays will focus behind the retina (*hyperopia*). When the lens becomes less elastic and responds less to the need for accommodation, as occurs in persons past the age of 40, blurring of near objects (*presbyopia*) results. The curvature of the cornea may also be asymmetric or irregular so that rays in the horizontal and vertical planes do not focus at the same point (*astigmatism*).

When the image is not clearly focused on the retina, *refractive error* is present (see the box below, right). Refractive errors account for the largest number of impairments of good vision. The refractive error is tested by means of trial lenses and the Snellen chart. (Figure 64-3, *A*). Suitable corrective lenses are prescribed if needed. If refractive errors involving both distant and close vision are present, bifocal or trifocal lenses or separate glasses will be required. In situations where formal acuity testing equipment is not available, estimates of refractive error can be made. For instance, the person can be asked to read print or identify pictures at varying distances. The person's visual acuity can be compared with that of the examiner's.

Before refraction is done, a cycloplegic drug may be instilled into the eyes to dilate the pupils and temporarily paralyze the ciliary muscles. Cyclopentolate (Cyclogyl), 1% or 2%, is usually used, because it is effective in 30 minutes and the effect generally wears off completely by the end of 6 hours. The duration of effect will vary, however, lasting longer than 6 hours in persons with a light blue iris. A blue-eyed person's iris will dilate more rapidly and remain dilated longer than that of a brown-eyed person because more of the drug is absorbed into an iris with less pigmentation.

EXAMPLES OF VISUAL ACUITY MEASUREMENT

MEASUREMENT	MEANING
20/20	Normal
20/40-2	Missed two letters of the 20/40 line
10/400	At 10 ft, reads line that normal eye sees at 400 ft
CF/2 ft	Counts fingers at 2 ft
HM/3 ft	Sees hand movement at 3 ft
LP/Proj.	Light perception with projection
NLP	No light perception

TERMS DESCRIBING REFRACTIVE ERRORS

Accommodation	Ability to adjust between far and near objects
Emmetropia	Normal eye; light rays focus on retina
Ametropia	Refractive error; light rays do not focus on retina
Myopia	Nearsightedness; light rays focus in front of retina
Hyperopia	Farsightedness; light rays focus behind retina
Presbyopia	Hyperopia from loss of lens elasticity because of age
Astigmatism	Irregular curvature of cornea; light rays do not focus at same point

When the appointment is made for an eye examination with the use of a cycloplegic drug, the person is told that blurred vision will be present after the examination. It should be explained that driving or reading will not be possible until the effect of the drug subsides. In some cases a miotic drug, pilocarpine, is instilled after the examination to constrict the pupil and reduce the uncomfortable glare from lights. Homatropine occasionally is used for adults and school-age children and atropine for younger children to dilate the pupils for refraction; but both of these drugs require longer to take effect, and their effects persist longer. Atropine must be instilled at intervals for 3 days before examination and persists in its action for at least 10 days with some residual effect for up to 3 to 4 weeks.

ASSESSMENT OF OCULAR MOVEMENTS

Ocular movements are evaluated to determine whether the eyes are moving in a synchronous manner. Muscle imbalances and cranial nerve damage also can be detected.

To test ocular muscles the examiner and person being tested are seated facing each other. While the person looks straight ahead at a target, a penlight is shined on the cornea. The corneal light reflex should be in exactly the same position on each pupil. The examiner then covers one of the person's eyes while the person looks at the light. When the cover is quickly removed, the examiner notes whether that eye moves to regain fixation on the light. Movement may indicate a drift of the eye behind the cover, which can indicate muscle imbalances.

To evaluate possible weaknesses of individual extraocular muscles, muscle balance testing can be done in six cardinal fields of gaze, as well as straight ahead. The reader is referred to Chapter 59 (Neurological Assessment) for more detailed information about assessment of ocular movements.

INSPECTION OF EXTERNAL STRUCTURES

The general appearance of the face and eyes is observed for the type of expression (dull or alert) and prominence of the eyes. When there is an abnormal protrusion or bulging of an eye, the condition is called *exophthalmia* or *exophthalmos*. In elderly persons the eyes tend to sink into the orbit (*enophthalmos*). This is primarily caused by the loss of orbital fat.

The appearance of the *eyelids* is noted in relation to color, texture, mobility, and position. The lids should be able to close completely to prevent drying of the conjunctiva and cornea. Any swelling, redness, or discharge is noted. If one upper lid seems to be in a position lower than the other, or "droops," the condition may be *ptosis* of the eyelid. When there is ptosis in both eyes, the upper lid will be observed to be in an abnor-

mally low position covering the upper portion or more of the iris. Ptosis of the upper lids may be the result of extreme debility or neuromuscular disease. Extreme ptosis can interfere with vision by covering the pupil.

As the person ages, the eyelids become thinner and less elastic and positional defects may occur. Besides ptosis, ectropion, entropion, and dermatochalasis may be present. *Ectropion* is eversion of the lower lid. It is usually bilateral, and symptoms include tearing and irritation. *Entropion* is the turning in of the eyelids. The person experiences a foreign body sensation caused by the eyelashes rubbing against the cornea. *Dermatochalasis* is a redundancy of upper or lower lid tissues. This usually occurs from loss of elasticity and results in wrinkles and drooping folds.

The *conjunctiva* of the lower lid is examined by pulling downward on the lid as the individual looks upward (Figure 64-4). In order to examine the conjunctiva of the upper lid, the lid must be everted (Figure 64-5).

Small blood vessels are normally visible in the conjunctiva. The *sclera* shows through the conjunctiva and has a shiny porcelain-like appearance. Dilation of blood vessels of the conjunctiva may indicate disease of the cornea or disease within the eye. Spontaneous small hemorrhages may occur beneath the conjunctiva in the normal eye. A yellow discoloration of the sclera indicates jaundice.

The lacrimal gland is not normally observable. Enlargement of the gland may occur in certain disorders such as inflammation. This may be most evident when the upper lid is everted. The lacrimal sac may be palpated on the temporal side of the nasal bone for patency of the lacrimal puncta.

The *cornea*, which is normally visible except for surface reflections, must be smooth and transparent for good vision. It should look shiny and bright when exam-

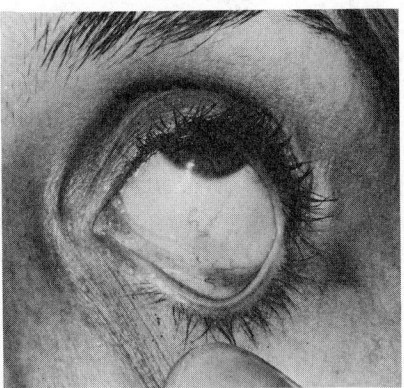

FIGURE 64-4 Eversion of lower eyelid by drawing the margin downward as subject looks upward. (From Newell F: Ophthalmology: principles and concepts, ed 6, St Louis, 1986, The CV Mosby Co.)

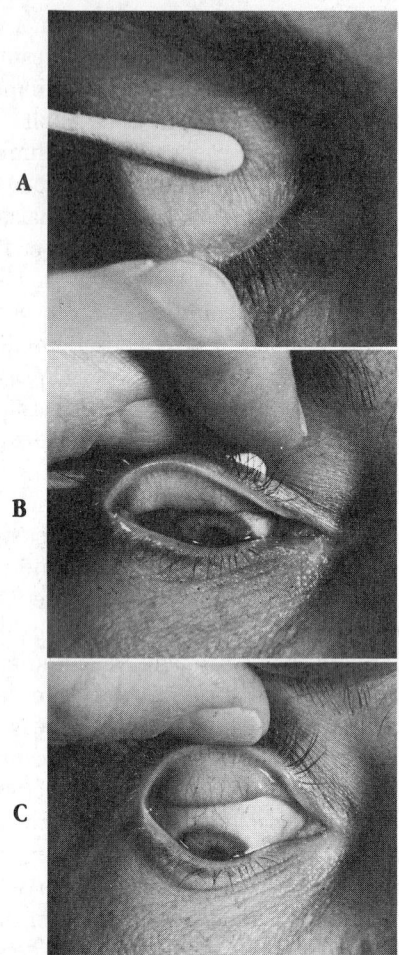

FIGURE 64-5 Eversion of upper eyelid. Patient is instructed to look downward, and lashes of upper eyelid are grasped between thumb and index finger. **A,** Cotton-tipped applicator is placed at level of tarsal fold. **B,** Eyelid is folded back on applicator while patient continues to look downward. **C,** Applicator is removed. (From Newell F: Ophthalmology: principles and concepts, ed 6, St. Louis, 1986, The CV Mosby Co.)

ined with a penlight. Moving the light and directing it from the side, the examiner looks for abrasions and opacities.

The *iris* of each eye is compared for color, pattern, and shape. When looking through the pupillary opening, the examiner is also inspecting the *lens,* which is normally transparent. An opaque lens is termed a *cataract.*

PUPILLARY REFLEXES

While approaching from the side, the examiner quickly shines a light into one eye causing constriction of the pupil in that eye (direct light reaction). The pupil of the other eye should also constrict the same amount (con-

sensual light reaction) (see Chapter 59). The other eye is then tested in the same manner.

A light shining into a blind eye will not produce a pupillary response; however, a light shining into a normal eye will produce a pupillary response in the blind eye by consensual reaction if the oculomotor nerve is intact.[1]

Another test of the pupillary reflex is to have the person focus on an object that is moved directly toward the nose. When focusing on the near object, the pupils of both eyes should constrict (near reaction, reaction in accommodation). The examiner looks for the presence of a response and whether the response is equal in both eyes. Loss of pupillary reflexes when sight is present is caused by neurologic disease.

VISUAL FIELDS

The visual field for an individual is that portion of the world that the eye can perceive. Lesions of the retina, optic pathways, and the central nervous system affect sections of the field of vision. The location of visual field loss indicates the location of the lesion. For instance, glaucoma decreases peripheral vision, indicating damage to the optic nerve at its head or the optic disk. A rough measurement of the visual fields can be made with the confrontation test (see Chapter 59). If there appears to be any abnormality in the field of vision, more precise testing should be done with precision instruments by an ophthalmologist or a specially trained technician. One precise method by which the person's peripheral vision can be plotted is the perimeter, an instrument that measures the visual fields in degrees of arc. The tangent screen is the simplest perimeter, in which peripheral vision is plotted as a test object is moved against a black screen. Also, several automated and computer-assisted perimeters, such as the Octopus, are now available.

EVALUATION OF THE OCULAR FUNDUS

The fundus of the eye is examined with an ophthalmoscope that magnifies the view of the back of the eye so that the optic nerve, retina, blood vessels, and macula can be seen through the pupil. The examiner may use either the *direct* (Figure 64-6) or the *indirect* (Figure 64-7) *method of ophthalmoscopic examination.* The indirect ophthalmoscope offers not only stereoscopic observation but also binocular vision. This method provides visualization of the ocular fundus as far as the ora serrata (anterior margin of the retina). The indirect method requires a great degree of skill to use and is not as readily available as the direct method. Thus the direct method is the more commonly used approach. The entire retina is not visualized at one time, so the examiner moves the ophthalmoscope until the entire fundus is visualized. (For further discussion on the use of the ophthalmoscope, see Chapter 59.)

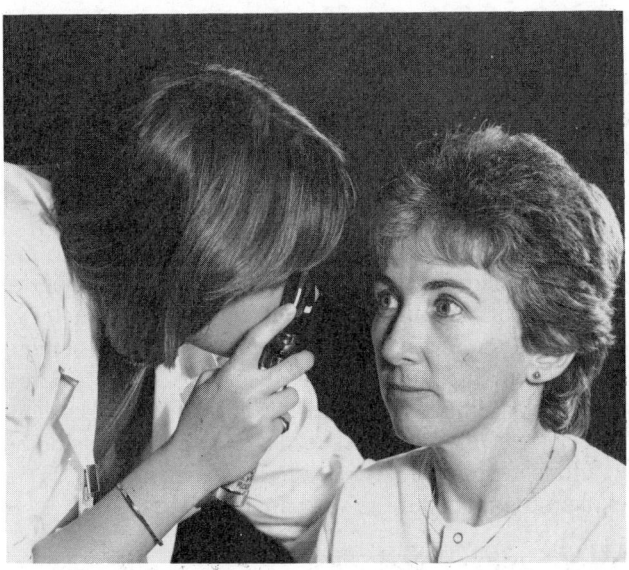

FIGURE 64-6 Direct method of ophthalmoscopic examination.

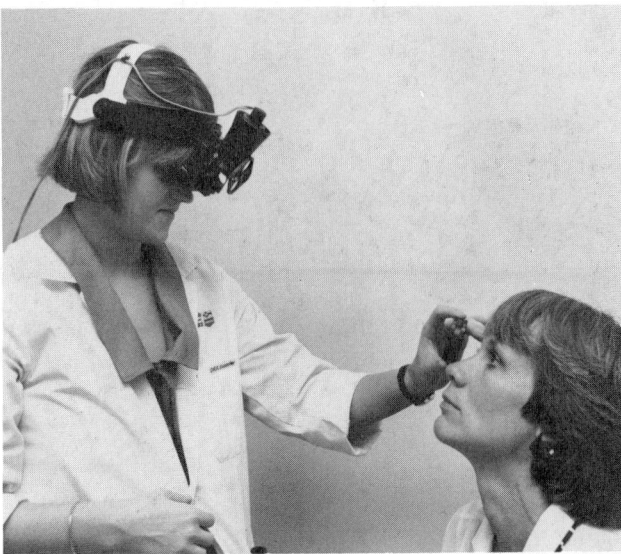

FIGURE 64-7 Indirect method of ophthalmoscopic examination.

Difficulty in perceiving the fundus may be caused by interference with the light penetrating the eye as a result of intraocular inflammation, corneal scarring, or cataract. Data obtained from visualization of the fundus may indicate eye disease (cupping of the disk in glaucoma) or systemic disease (arteriosclerosis or hypertension). Hemorrhages in deep retinal layers occur in advanced hypertension, severe renal disease, certain collagen diseases, advanced diabetes, and blood dyscrasias.

The interior of the eye can also be examined by the ophthalmologist using a slit-lamp microscope in a darkened room. The slit-lamp is an instrument that combines a microscope and a light source and is used to examine the anterior segment of the eye. By adjusting the lens, the examiner can test the person's eye for such changes as corneal ulcerations, lens changes, foreign bodies in the vitreous, or retinal changes. With the use of a contact lens on the surface of the cornea, the slit-lamp can also be used to examine the retina.

ESTIMATION OF INTRAOCULAR PRESSURE

An instrument known as a *tonometer* is used to measure ocular tension and is helpful in detecting early glaucoma. Some ophthalmologists suggest that tonometric readings be taken by the medical internist or the family physician as part of a regular annual physical examination. The most common indentation tonometer in clinical use is that of Schiøtz. The procedure is performed with the individual lying down or in the chair with the head back and looking upward at some fixed point. The eye may be anesthetized with one or two drops of proparacaine hydrochloride (Ophthaine), 0.5%,

after which the tonometer is placed on the cornea (Figure 64-8). While the weight of the tonometer is supported by the cornea, the amount of indentation that the plunger of the instrument makes in the cornea is measured on the attached scale. This reading is used to determine the pressure within the eye. Readings over 24 torr (Schiøtz) may suggest glaucoma, but tests usually are repeated because temporary increases sometimes may be caused by such things as emotional stress. The applanation tonometer (Goldmann) is more accurate in

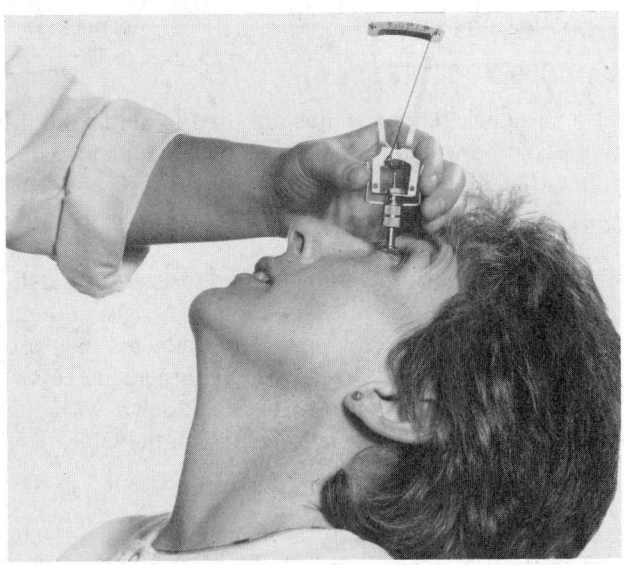

FIGURE 64-8 Measurement of intraocular pressure with Schiøtz tonometer.

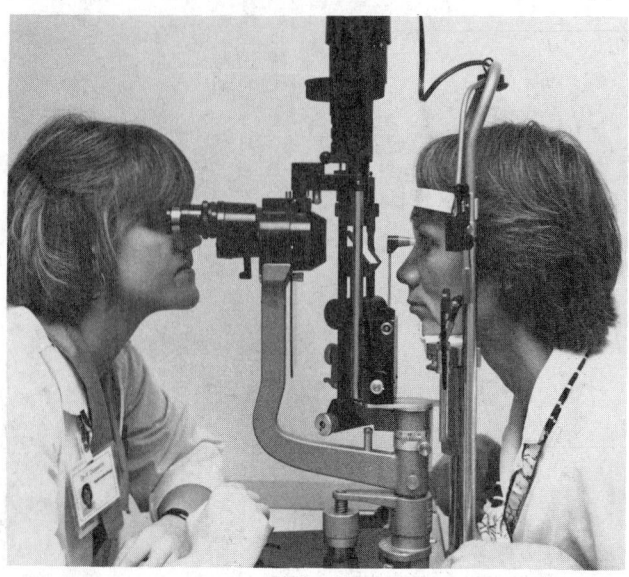

FIGURE 64-9 Measurement of ocular tension with applanation tonometer.

estimating intraocular pressure (Figure 64-9). The commonly used *applanation tonometer* is attached to the slit lamp, although handheld models are available. Instead of indenting the eye, a small area of the cornea is flattened to counterbalance a spring-loaded measuring device, and the pressure is measured directly. The noncontact tonometer has gained considerable popularity in the last few years. This applanation instrument uses a puff of air to flatten a circular area of the cornea, thus bypassing the necessity for physical contact between the tonometer and the eye.

DIAGNOSTIC TESTS

RADIOLOGIC TESTS

Several radiologic procedures are used to aid in the diagnosis of eye problems. These include plain x-ray films, CAT scans, and ultrasonography.

PLAIN X-RAY FILMS

Plain x-ray films of the orbit are used to assist in the diagnosis of orbital fractures and tumors. A right and left oblique view and lateral view of the affected side are usually able to provide the needed information. To obtain these views, the person lies face down with the forehead and nose or the chin resting on the table.

CAT SCAN

The CAT scan is a rapid, safe, and noninvasive technique for the investigation of the orbit and eye. The globe, lens, vitreous, optic nerve, and extraocular muscles can be evaluated. The CAT scan is of value, then,

in the diagnosis of orbital disease, retrobulbar tumors, and intraocular eye masses. The examination can be augmented by the intravenous injection of contrast material that increases the density of inflammatory or vascularized orbital lesions.[14]

ULTRASONOGRAPHY

Ultrasonography is used to detect and characterize intraocular and orbital tumors. Two types of ultrasonography, A-scan and B-scan, are used in ophthalmology. The A-scan is useful in differentiating between benign and malignant tumors. The B-scan provides a two-dimensional image that helps visualize tumors, swollen muscles, or inflamed tissue. The nurse's responsibility in ultrasonography, as it is in all radiologic tests, is to explain the procedure to the patient.

ELECTRODIAGNOSTIC EXAMINATION

Two of the electrodiagnostic examinations performed in ophthalmology are electroretinography (ERG) and visual-evoked potentials.

ELECTRORETINOGRAPHY

Electroretinography is a process of graphing the electrical response from the retina that occurs as a consequence of light stimulation. When undergoing this test, the person's pupil is dilated, a topical anesthetic is applied, and a corneal electrode is placed on the cornea. A grounding electrode is placed on the ear. Lights at various intensities and intervals are then flashed, and the nervous response graphed.

ERGs are helpful in evaluating widespread retinal disease such as retinitis pigmentosa. The visual potential of an eye that has a dense cataract or other opacification can also be assessed with ERGs. However, normal results do not rule out the presence of macular or optic nerve disease.

VISUAL-EVOKED POTENTIALS

The visual-evoked potential (VEP) is the measurement of visual function that is monitored at the level of the occipital cortex with scalp electrodes. Stimulation of the retina with light will change the electrical activity of the cortex. Through various computer activities, the electrical activity that is synchronized with this stimulation of the retina is summed and shown as a measurable electrical wave. This wave is altered in persons with *optic neuritis and demyelinating disease.*

SPECIAL DIAGNOSTIC TESTS AND PROCEDURES
CORNEAL STAINING

Defects in the epithelium of the cornea may be demonstrated with the use of topical dyes. The dye is put in the conjunctiva by drops or by touching the conjunctiva with a moistened strip of filter paper that has been impregnated with the dye. The injured tissue remains stained; and, as a consequence, visualization of foreign bodies, abrasions, and inflammation of the cornea is possible.

Fluorescein is the most common dye used, although rose bengal and methylene blue are also available. The latter two dyes stain more deeply than fluorescein does but are more irritating. The dyes should not be used while contact lenses are worn, because they tend to stain soft contact lenses.

TEAR TEST (SCHIRMER)

The quantity of tears is measured with a strip of filter paper 5 mm × 35 mm that is folded 5 mm from the end. The folded end is hooked over the lower lid and is left in place for approximately 5 minutes. The extent to which the filter paper is soaked with tears beyond the fold is then measured. Tear formation is generally considered normal if 10 to 15 mm or more of the filter paper is moistened. More than 25 mm of moistened paper is indicative of excessive tear formation. Patients need to be informed by the nurse that the test may be annoying, but is not painful.

COLOR VISION TESTING

Color vision testing is not always part of the normal eye examination. It is used most frequently to test for color blindness in those persons seeking motor vehicle licenses or jobs in which color discrimination is important.

There are both gross and sensitive measures of color vision. A common test consists of color plates on which numbers are outlined in primary colors and surrounded by confusion colors. The person with a color vision problem is unable to recognize the figure. The more sensitive tests involve hue discrimination. One such test consists of 84 chips of color that are matched in terms of increasing hue.

Color vision deficiencies occur as a hereditary defect in both men (7%) and women (0.5%). Nutritional deficiencies and various disorders of the optic nerve and fovea centralis can also alter color perception.

AMSLER GRID

The Amsler grid is a 20 cm square that is divided into 5 mm squares with a dot in the center (Figure 64-10). The grid is employed to detect and follow a *central area of blindness (scotoma)*. It most commonly is used at home by the patient to detect progression of a macular disease.

With glasses on and one eye closed, the person holds the grid at the customary reading distance (12 in). While he or she is fixating at the central dot, the person is asked to describe and outline any area of distortion or

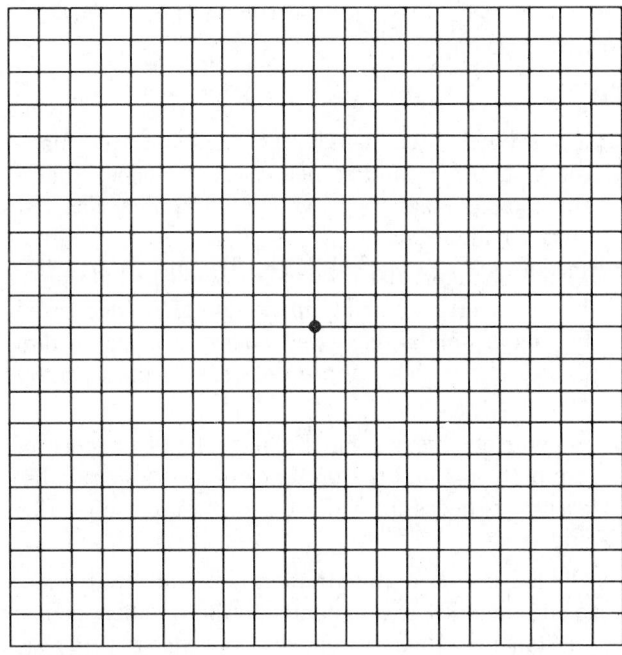

FIGURE 64-10 The Amsler grid.

absence of the grid. Abnormalities include all areas of blindness or distortion.

FLUORESCEIN ANGIOGRAPHY

Fluorescein angiography plays an important role in the diagnosis and monitoring of the progression of eye diseases. Following dilation of the pupil, fluorescein dye is injected into the antecubital vein. The retinal and ciliary arteries transmit the dye into the eyes, and the *retinal arteriovenous circulation* is visualized. To provide a permanent record of this circulation, photographs are taken with a specially designed camera, appropriate filters, and film. A rapid sequence of photographs is taken at approximately 1-second intervals from about 9 until 30 seconds after injection. Photographs are also taken at 1 to 5 minutes, and occasionally 1 hour, after injection. The frequent photographs are needed to capture the movement of the dye through the circulation. The dye reaches the retinal arteries 10 to 16 seconds following injection, and the veins are filled within 25 seconds. When the photographs are assessed, they provide much information about any vascular obstruction, the growth of new vessels (neovascularization), microaneurysms, abnormal capillary permeability, and defects in the pigmented layer of the retina.

Fluorescein angiography is a relatively safe procedure with few untoward effects. The dye can cause intense burning at the injection site if leakage into subcutaneous tissue occurs. Patients should be forewarned that yellowing of the skin and discoloration of the urine are to be expected. Allergic reactions and transient nausea may also occur.

CHAPTER SUMMARY

↙ The eye has three main layers: the outer layer, made up of the sclera and cornea; the uvea, consisting of the choroid, ciliary body, and iris; and the innermost layer, or the retina.

↙ Visual changes that occur with aging include presbyopia, decreased ability to tolerate glare, decreased peripheral fields, decreased ability to adapt to dim light and darkness, and a decrease in the quantity and quality of tears.

↙ A complete history—including a family history of eye problems and the presence of any systemic diseases—is necessary when assessing a person's eyes and vision.

↙ Objective data required when doing an eye assessment includes assessment of visual acuity, ocular movement, pupillary reflexes, and visual fields, as well as inspection of internal and external structures and an estimation of intraocular pressure.

↙ Radiologic tests used to aid diagnosis of eye problems include x-ray films, CAT scans, and ultrasonography.

↙ Electrodiagnostic examinations are used mainly to evaluate retinal and optic nerve diseases.

↙ The main nursing responsibility is to explain diagnostic tests, including any discomfort or alteration in vision that they may be experienced.

QUESTIONS TO CONSIDER

- What would you tell your 65 year old neighbor if she told you that she can't see to drive at night as well as she used to?

- What questions would you ask a person who stated that he or she did not see very well?

- Your patient has a sudden loss of vision and the ophthalmologist has scheduled her for fluorescein angiography. She asks you many questions about the test—how it works and what it might show. What information would you give to prepare her for the test and to help her better understand the possible results?

REFERENCES AND SELECTED READINGS

1. Bates B: A guide to physical examination and history taking, ed 4, Philadelphia, 1987, JB Lippincott Co.
2. *Boyd-Monk H: Examining the external eye. I, Nursing '80 10(5):58-63, 1980.
3. *Boyd-Monk H: Examining the external eye. II, Nursing '80 10(6):58-63, 1980.
4. Boyd-Monk H: How to use a direct ophthalmoscope, Occup Health Nurs 8:13-16, 1983.
5. Boyd-Monk H: The structure and function of the eye and its adnexa, J Ophthalmic Nurs Techol 6:176-183, 1987.
6. Boyd-Monk H and Steinmetz CG: Nursing care of the eye, Norwalk, CT, 1987, Appleton & Lange.
7. Ebersole P and Hess P: Toward healthy aging, ed 3 St Louis, 1989, The CV Mosby Co.
8. *Important clues in the external eye examination, Hosp Med 24(4):94-98, 1988.
9. Leitman MW: Manual for eye examination and diagnosis, ed 3, Oradell, NJ, 1988, Medical Economics Books.
10. Kapperud MJ: The aging eye: a guide for nurses, St Paul, 1983, The Minnesota Society for the Prevention of Blindness and Preservation of Hearing.
11. *Kopac CA: Sensory loss in the aged: the role of the nurse and family, Nurs Clin North Am 18:373-84, 1983.
12. Malasanos L et al: Health assessment, ed 3, St. Louis, 1986, The CV Mosby Co.
13. Meltzer MA: Diagnosis of eyelid and periorbital abnormalities, Hosp Pract 19(19):67-9, 72, 74-76, 1984.
14. Newell F: Ophthalmology; principles and concepts, ed 6, St. Louis, 1986, The CV Mosby Co.
15. Rosenbloom AA and Morgan MW, editors: Vision and aging: general and clinical perspectives, New York, 1986, Professional Press Books.
16. Sekuler R, Kline D, and Dismukes K, editors: Aging and human visual function, New York, 1982, Alan R Liss, Inc.
17. *Sullivan N: Vision in the elderly, J Gerontol Nurs 9:228-235, 1983.
18. Vaughan D and Asbury T: General ophthalmology, ed 11, Los Altos, CA, 1986, Lange Medical Publications.

*References preceded by an asterisk are particularly well suited for student reading

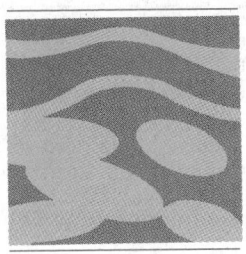

CHAPTER 65

Management of Persons with Problems of the Eye

MARION ALLEN

CHAPTER OBJECTIVES

After studying this chapter, the student should be able to:
1. Describe the care of healthy eyes, including safety and first aid measures.
2. State the common types of eye medications and their role in diagnosing and treating eye diseases.
3. Outline three common systemic diseases that have eye manifestations.
4. State the correct methods for carrying out nursing procedures related to eye care including instillation of eye medications, eye irrigations, eye compresses, insertion and removal of contact lenses and an artificial eye.
5. Discuss the epidemiology/etiology, pathophysiology, clinical manifestations, and medical and nursing management of cataracts and glaucoma.
6. Describe the nursing assessment, nursing diagnoses, expected patient outcomes, and the preventative, acute, and long-term care for persons with diabetic retinopathy.
7. Discuss the demands and the factors that facilitate or hinder adjustment to a visual impairment.
8. Describe the nurse's role in assisting a person to learn to live with visual impairment.

Eye disease and blindness cause suffering, disability, and loss of productivity for millions of people throughout the world. In the United States alone nearly 11.5 million people have some degree of impairment. Of these 11.5 million approximately 1.5 million either cannot read the newspaper with corrective lenses or do not have useful vision in one or both eyes.[14]

The major causes of severe impairment in the adult in decreasing order of frequency are retinal and choroidal disease, cataract, glaucoma, optic nerve atrophy, and corneal disease. In addition, trauma to the eye and inflammatory disorders of the eyelids, conjunctiva, cornea, and uveal tract are frequently seen.

PREVENTION

To decrease the problem of visual impairment, health workers need to focus on prevention and early detection of eye disease and injury, as well as on adequate treatment. Because of the involvement with persons of all age groups, nurses have a unique opportunity to be active in the promotion of health care of the eyes. Health care includes health education, care of the healthy eye, including eye examination and eye safety.

HEALTH EDUCATION IN THE CARE OF THE EYES

The education of individuals, families, and the public about the care of healthy eyes, prevention of eye disease, and impairment is an important nursing function. Nurses can carry out this function by:
1. Teaching and providing safety measures and first aid
2. Promoting regular eye examinations by an eye specialist
3. Detecting evidence of disease or impaired acuity
4. Explaining and administering treatments used to improve sight or prevent further loss (for example, medications)

To implement these actions, nurses should have knowledge about common eye diseases and their treatment, ophthalmic drugs, corrective lenses, methods of assessment, and first aid for eye trauma. In addition the nurse should recognize signs suggestive of eye disease and teach them to others (Table 65-1).

CARE OF HEALTHY EYES

Normal healthy eyes do not need special local treatment. The secretions of the conjunctiva are protective and should not be removed by frequent bathing with unprescribed solutions. Boric acid solution and numerous over-the-counter (OTC) preparations recommended to cleanse the eyes are usually unnecessary. Although these preparations are generally harmless, some proprietary solutions contain substances that may cause allergic reactions in sensitive persons.

People frequently treat eye ailments with OTC remedies or with eyedrops and other medication that they

TABLE 65-1 Symptoms suggestive of eye disease

Symptom	Eye Disease
Conjunctival redness	Conjunctivitis, blepharitis, sty
Crusting discharge	Conjunctivitis, blepharitis, sty
Ocular pain	Foreign body, sty, acute lid infection, glaucoma, keratitis, uveitis
Foreign body sensation	Foreign body, corneal erosion, blepharitis, chronic conjunctivitis
Blepharospasm	Keratitis, corneal ulcer
Multiple spots ("floaters")	Retinal detachment, intraocular hemorrhage, diabetic retinopathy
Photophobia	Uveitis, keratitis, glaucoma, corneal abrasions
Vision Changes	
Blurred vision	Refractive error, cataract, glaucoma, uveitis, retinal detachment
Double vision	Strabismus
Halos around lights	Glaucoma
Blind spots	Hemorrhage, choroiditis
Sudden vision loss	Central retinal artery or vein occlusion

COMMON EYE MYTHS

Children will outgrow crossed eyes
Night vision will improve by eating more carrots
Reading in dim light for long periods can harm the eyes
Watching TV is bad for the eyes
Older people who may have trouble seeing should not use their eyes too much, because they will wear out sooner
Wearing glasses makes you dependent on them
People with weak eyes should rest their eyes often to strengthen them

---

or others have used at some time in the past. Self-treatment of the eyes is not only dangerous but may also lead to loss of much valuable time for more helpful treatment. There are many disorders that can affect the eyes for which many different drugs are used, each of which has a specific purpose. Two drugs may have completely opposite effects. Because liquids evaporate and drugs deteriorate or become contaminated with bacteria or fungi, use of preparations that a person or friend has on hand can contribute to actual damage.

Boric acid solution, like other ophthalmic solutions, may present the problem of drug crystals precipitating on the tip of the dropper and irritating the eye. Preparations having mydriatic properties such as phenylephrine hydrochloride 0.8%, have the potential to produce sufficient dilation of the pupil to cause an attack of narrow-angle glaucoma in susceptible persons. Contamination of ophthalmic solutions may also be a problem. It is best to *discard* any ophthalmic solution that is cloudy, is discolored, has been opened for 3 months, or contains particles.

Many people believe erroneously that eyestrain causes permanent eye damage. Eyestrain actually refers to strain of the ciliary muscles when there is difficulty in accommodation. It causes a sense of fatigue but does not produce serious damage to the eyes. To avoid eyestrain, a good light should be used when reading and doing work that requires careful visual focus, and ex-

tremely fine work should not be done for long periods of time without giving the eye muscles periodic rest. Looking at distant objects for a few minutes helps to rest the eyes after close work. Besides the belief about eyestrain, many other myths are held about the eye. Some of these are outlined in the box above.

Care should be taken not to irritate the eyes or introduce bacteria into the eyes by rubbing them. Rubbing the eyes may be a natural response of many persons who are nervous, are fatigued, or wear contact lenses. It also may be the result of eczematous scaling, infection of the lids from contaminated eye makeup, or occasionally louse attachment on the lashes. The cause of severe or chronic irritation should be investigated.

Adequate nutrition is as important for eye health as it is for maintaining other body functions. Although many persons eat a diet that does not supply adequate amounts of needed nutrients, persons with nutritionally caused eye disorders are rarely found in the United States. Vitamin deficiencies can cause night blindness (vitamin A), corneal damage (vitamin A), optic neuritis (vitamin B) and other disorders. Although a sufficient vitamin intake is necessary, an excessive amount is wasted and may actually do more harm than good. For example, too much vitamin A can damage the optic nerve.

SAFETY MEASURES

Prevention of accidental injury to the eyes should be stressed in child and adult education. Slingshots, BB guns, and even seemingly harmless rubber bands and paper wads can be dangerous.

Protective goggles and break-resistant corrective lenses are available for persons engaging in active sports and selected occupations. The eyes should be protected by goggles or special dark glasses from prolonged exposure to very bright light such as sunlight on snow. They also need special protection from sudden flashes of light and heat that occur in some industrial occupations. Contact lenses may be prohibited for some industrial occupations because of concern for corneal irritation from particles or chemicals trapped under the lens.

EYE IRRIGATIONS

PURPOSE

1. Remove chemical irritants, foreign bodies, and secretions.
2. Cleanse the eye postoperatively (may be done preoperatively).

PROCEDURE

1. Prepare solution. Physiologic solutions of sodium chloride or lactated Ringer's solution are most commonly used.
2. Position person comfortably toward one side so that fluid cannot flow into the other eye.
3. Use appropriate means (for example, kidney basin) to catch irrigating fluid.
4. Use appropriate amounts of solution.
   a. If small amounts are needed (to cleanse eye postoperatively) sterile cotton balls moistened with solution can be used.
   b. If moderate amounts of fluid are needed (removing secretions) a plastic squeeze bottle is used to direct irrigating fluid along the conjunctiva and over the eyeball from inner to outer canthus(Figure 65-1).
   c. If copious amounts of fluid are needed (that is, for removing chemical irritants), bags of solution such as intravenous bags along with the tubing to direct the flow onto the eye can be used (Figure 65-2).
5. Avoid directing a forceful stream onto the eye.
6. Avoid touching any eye structures with the irrigating equipment.
7. If there is drainage, wrap a piece of gauze around the index finger to raise the lid and ensure thorough cleansing.

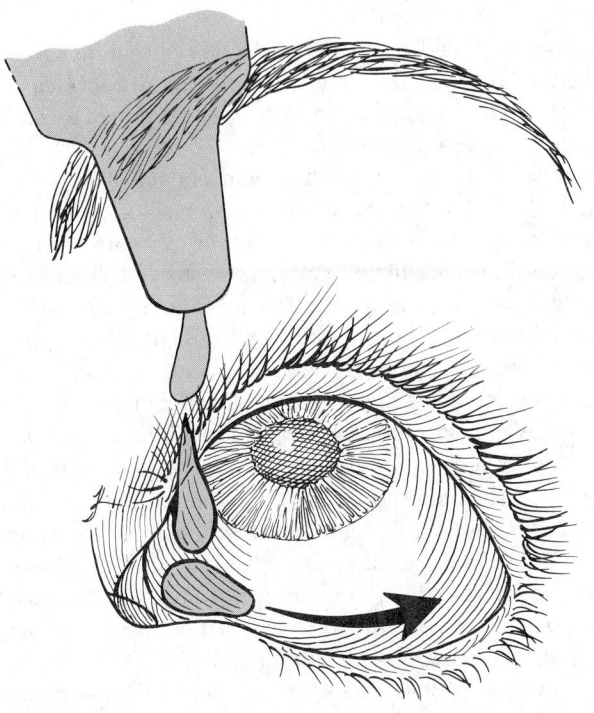

FIGURE 65-1 Irrigating the eye. Fluid is directed along conjunctiva and over eyeball from inner to outer canthus. (From Long BL and Phipps WJ: Medical-Surgical nursing: a nursing process approach, ed 2, St Louis, 1989, The CV Mosby Co.)

First aid measures necessary in the event of eye injury should be known by everyone; these measures can be taught in schools and industry (Table 65-5). The sight of many persons could be saved each year if everyone understood the need for immediate copious flushing of the eye with water when an acid, alkali, or other irritating substance has been accidentally introduced (see the box above). Much damage is done by the layperson's well-intentioned efforts to remove foreign bodies from the eye and by not obeying the important rule of always washing the hands before attempting to examine the eye or to remove a foreign object.

It is essential to know that a person who has a foreign object lodged on the cornea must be referred to a physician; the layperson should never attempt to remove it. The eye should be closed to prevent further irritation and the lids loosely covered with a dressing or patch anchored with a piece of transparent or adhesive tape. The person should be advised not to squeeze the eye and should be taken to an ophthalmologist at once.

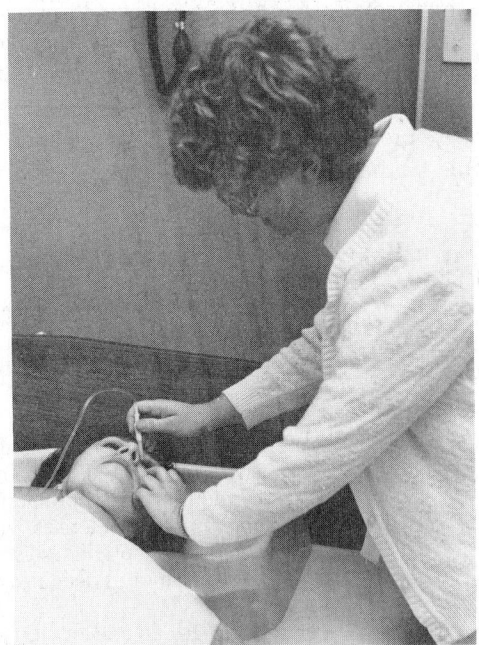

FIGURE 65-2 Eye irrigation using an intravenous bag and tubing.

REGULAR EYE EXAMINATIONS

The eyes should be examined by an ophthalmologist at regular intervals throughout life. Many authorities believe children should have their eyes examined at birth, at age 3 or 4, at approximately age 10, and in early adolescence. The young adult should consult an ophthalmologist at least every 3 to 5 years. Medical specialists recommend an eye examination every 2 years after the age of 35, especially with a family history of glaucoma.

Because the eyes are often profoundly affected by conditions within other areas of the body, they cannot be considered alone. In fact, nearly all diseases cause some eye changes that are diagnostically important. The nurse who is teaching eye health must be aware of *total health*. When apparently minor disease or abnormality of the eyes occurs, the nurse must be particularly alert for other signs of disease. Many serious medical conditions such as diabetes, renal disease, neurologic disease, and generalized arteriosclerosis may be diagnosed through early recognition of eye symptoms and examination of the eyes by an ophthalmologist.

There is widespread confusion and misunderstanding on the part of the public as to the proper specialist to consult about visual problems (see the box below). People who demand the best care when other medical and surgical problems arise may fail to seek help from an ophthalmologist when they have eye problems. The ophthalmologist is a physician and surgeon who can diagnose and treat diseases of the eye. The optometrist does not treat eye diseases but assesses vision and prescribes corrective lenses or exercises.

In their search for help, some people may purchase glasses from stores or use glasses originally prescribed for friends or relatives. Nurses can explain that eye conditions cannot always be remedied simply by the purchase of a pair of glasses or a change of lenses. A serious disease process such as glaucoma or cataract formation could be the cause of the problem.

PERSONS WHO SPECIALIZE IN EYE PROBLEMS OR IN VISUAL PROSTHESES

Ophthalmologist	Physician who specializes in the diagnosis and treatment of eye diseases; may also prescribe lenses
Oculist	Same as ophthalmologist
Optometrist	Professional person with special preparation in assessment of vision and in treatment of visual problems (for example, prescribes lenses, visual training, or orthoptic exercises); is not a physician and does not treat eye diseases
Optician	Person who grinds and fits lenses according to prescriptions written by ophthalmologist or optometrist

LENSES
EYEGLASSES

Acceptance of glasses seems to be influenced by the improvement in vision that they afford, the personality of the wearer, and current fashion trends. To some persons, however, glasses may appear as a cosmetic blemish. Because some stigma may be attached to wearing glasses, the young child will have a period of adjustment after receiving glasses. Acceptance of glasses may increase when children start school and realize that the glasses are needed to see the blackboard. The vogue for attractive frames makes the wearing of glasses more acceptable to teenagers and adults. All persons should be encouraged to wear their glasses as prescribed and to have periodic examinations of their eyes by an ophthalmologist or an optometrist. Instructions for persons who wear glasses include how to clean their glasses, how to protect them from being scratched or broken, and how to care for them when they are removed.

Federal law now requires that all prescription glasses be made with impact-resistant lenses. Each finished lens must pass an impact test before it is dispensed. *Plastic* lenses weigh less than half of equivalent glass lenses but cost more and scratch more easily. They are useful for persons who wear thick lenses that are heavy when made of glass and for those who are active in sports. *Hardened* lenses have been exposed to a tempering process that makes them extremely hard and resistant to impact and breakage. *Safety* lenses are similar to hardened lenses but are 1 mm thicker. They are used in goggles worn by workers whose eyes may be injured by such articles as chips of metal or glass.

Bifocal lenses consist of an upper portion of one focus used for distance and a lower part of another focus used for reading and close work. They make constant changing from distance to reading glasses unnecessary. *Trifocal* lenses are divided into three focuses to give correction for distance, intermediate, and near vision. *Sunglasses* should be carefully ground, large enough to exclude bright light around their edges, and dark enough to exclude about 30% of the light. The amount of light filtered can be varied according to the needs of the person.

CONTACT LENSES

Over the last several years there has been a great interest in and a desire for contact lenses by the public. The lenses are used mainly for cosmetic reasons or by persons who engage in sports, because the lenses do not fog or break easily. In some cases they provide better vision than can be achieved by glasses. This may be seen in *keratoconus*, a cone-shaped deformity of the cornea, which can prevent satisfactory fitting with conventional glasses. Also, persons who have had a cataract extraction, who are not candidates for intraocular lenses, achieve better vision wearing contact lenses than with the use of conventional glasses.

Contact lenses are small corrective lenses made of different types of ground plastic worn over the cornea of the eye or over the cornea and sclera (scleral lens). The lenses are held in place by capillary attraction and the upper lid. Conjunctival secretions provide the lubrication needed for the lenses to be worn in comfort. Contact lenses may be rigid, soft, gas permeable (rigid), or extended wear (soft). At present *rigid* lenses give better vision than the soft lenses but are generally more uncomfortable. Also, they require adaptation by progressive increase in wearing time, which does not usually exceed 12 to 14 hours.

Soft lenses are very flexible and have been used successfully by many persons who cannot tolerate hard lenses. The disadvantages of soft lenses may include a higher initial cost and more frequent replacement. They are also more difficult to clean and maintain. *Extended-wear* (soft) *contact lenses* have increased in use in the United States. Although some of these lenses can be left in place for as long as a month, the current trend is to limit wear to 1 week before removal for cleaning and disinfection. Those persons who use extended wear lenses must be educated in and prepared for the extra care required for these lenses. Scleral lenses are harder to wear than the corneal lenses and are less frequently used.

Gas permeable contact lenses with the optical qualities of the hard lenses and the comfort of the soft lenses are now more readily available. Because they are permeable to oxygen and other gases, some of the complications associated with both the hard and soft lenses are being avoided. Gas permeable lenses are also better candidates for safe extended wear than the currently available soft lenses.

Successful wearing of contact lenses requires careful personal hygiene and cleansing of the lenses. Instructions for cleansing and storage must be followed. Hands should be washed before insertion and removal of the lenses. Lenses should also not be worn longer than the prescribed length of time. Overwearing can cause edema and abrasion of the cornea. All contact lenses can cause problems. Most are minor and can be handled by changes in routine or lenses. However, problems should not be ignored, because they may lead to or be indicative of more serious difficulties.

Persons interested in wearing contact lenses are encouraged to consult an ophthalmologist who will make recommendations regarding their use. The person who dispenses the contact lenses may be an ophthalmologist, optometrist or technician supervised by the ophthalmologist. Persons with astigmatism are not candidates for contact lenses. Other persons may never be able to physiologically or psychologically tolerate the

REMOVAL OF CONTACT LENSES

RIGID LENS

Method 1:
a. Place finger at outer canthus of eye.
b. Pull skin obliquely upward, then straight down.
c. Lens will appear on lower lashes as the upper lid moves downward.
d. If lens moves off center, reposition it by gentle pressure on lid or lens itself and repeat steps a, b, and c.
Method 2:
a. Place finger or thumb of each hand at base of eyelashes (upper and lower).
b. Bring eyelids together, trapping the lens (the lens will eject).
c. If lens moves off center, reposition it by gentle pressure on lid or lens itself and repeat steps a, b, and c.
Method 3:
a. Using eye irrigation set, gently flush eye with sterile normal saline.
b. Retrieve lens in curved basin.
Method 4:
a. Use small suction device shaped like a miniature "plumber's helper."
b. Place over center of lens and pull lens off gently.

SOFT LENS

a. Ensure that lens is in place before attempting removal.
b. Pull up upper lid with one thumb.
c. Move lens over conjunctiva before grasping it, if possible. If lens does not move freely, put several drops of sterile saline in eye, close lid, and wait 1 min before trying again.
d. Grasp lens with thumb and forefinger of other hand and pinch the soft lens (it will pop off the cornea).

SCLERAL LENS

a. Spread eyelids with both thumbs.
b. Exert slight downward pressure on upper lid (the lower edge of the lens will lift above the lid margin).
c. Slide thumbs to outer canthus to eject lens.

---

presence of a foreign object in the eye, even for a short time.

Badly injured or unconscious persons should be checked for the presence of contact lenses, which must be removed (see the box above). The lenses are stored separately in suitable containers such as capped test tubes filled with sterile normal saline. It is important to note that the risk of HIV and HBV from tears is extremely low or nonexistent. Universal precautions apply to tears when they contain visible blood.

Soft contact lenses must be kept wet at all times; drying causes the soft lens to deteriorate. If a soft lens does dry, add sterile saline to soften it before handling. Label the lens storage containers with the patient's name and whether it is the right or left lens. Place the containers in a safe location and record this in the appropriate record.

ADMINISTERING MEDICATIONS

Accuracy in the administration of medications and treatments is essential. Irreparable damage can follow instillation of unprescribed or deteriorated preparations into the eyes. All medication bottles must be checked frequently for smearing or obliteration of labels. Solutions that have changed in color, that are cloudy, that contain sediment, or whose expiration date has passed should not be used. Eye medications in the home are discarded when the course of the treatment is completed. The nurse must know the usual dosage and strength, desired action, and side effects of medications being used, as well as signs of toxicity. For example, osmotic agents that reduce intraocular pressure by increasing plasma osmolarity are contraindicated in patients with poor kidney function. Steroids may cause an exacerbation of an already existing herpes corneal ulcer or increase the intraocular pressure.[14] Children and elderly persons are particularly susceptible to side effects of medications.

OPHTHALMIC DRUGS

A large variety of drugs are used for treatment of eye diseases (Tables 65-2 and 65-3). Most of the drugs are applied as drops, irrigations, or ointments.

Mydriatics are drugs that *dilate the pupil*. Mydriasis is necessary for thorough examination of the back of the interior of the eye (fundus). An example is phenylephrine (Neo-Synephrine).

Cycloplegics are drugs that not only *dilate the pupil* but also *block accommodation* by paralyzing the ciliary muscles. These drugs are used to keep the pupil dilated as part of the treatment for diseases of the cornea and for inflammatory diseases of the iris and ciliary body, after certain operations, and for eye examination. Commonly used cycloplegics are cyclopentolate (Cyclogyl), tropicamide (Mydriacyl), and atropine. Cycloplegic and mydriatric drugs should not be instilled in the eyes of a person with glaucoma, because they prevent drainage of the aqueous humor, thus increasing intraocular pressure to levels where eye damage can occur.

Miotics are drugs that constrict the pupil, permitting the aqueous humor to flow out more readily and thus reduce intraocular pressure. Miotics such as pilocarpine are the drugs most often used in the *treatment of glaucoma*. *Osmotic agents* may also be used to reduce intraocular pressure. These drugs—for example, urea and mannitol—are given intravenously in the treatment of accute glaucoma or to reduce intraocular pressure during eye surgery. β-Blockers may be prescribed to help control intraocular pressure (IOP). Timolol maleate (Timoptic), the prototype drug in this class, is used widely in the treatment of glaucoma.

Secretory inhibitors decrease intraocular pressure by reducing aqueous humor production. Drugs in this classification inhibit the enzyme carbonic anhydrase, which is necessary for the production of aqueous humor. These drugs are given orally and include acetazolamide (Diamox).

Local topical anesthetics such as proparacaine and tetracaine are used frequently for diagnostic and therapeutic purposes. Local injectable anesthetics (lidocaine, procaine) are used frequently for eye surgery and treatments. Epinephrine (Adrenalin), 1:50,000 or 1:100,000, may be used in combination with local anesthetics to prolong the duration of anesthetics by constricting blood vessels so that the anesthetic remains longer in the injected area and its absorption is delayed. Hyaluronidase (Wydase), which makes cell membranes more permeable, often is mixed with local anesthetic solutions to increase the diffusion of the anesthetic through the tissues.

Antibiotics such as bacitracin, polymyxin B, gentamicin, and neomycin may be prescribed for ocular instillation, because bacteria are less likely to be resistant to them. Because penicillin causes ocular allergy in about 5% of adult patients, it is not often prescribed.

TABLE 65-2 Mydriatic and cycloplegic drugs

Drug	Form and Concentrations	Duration of Effect
MYDRIATIC ACTION		
Phenylephrine (Neo-Synephrine), Myafrin	Eyedrops, 2.5%-10%	2-3 hr
Hydroxyamphetamine HBr (Paredine)	Eyedrops 1%	2 hr
CYCLOPLEGIC AND MYDRIATIC ACTION		
Atropine sulfate (Atropisol, Isopto-Atropine)	Eyedrops, 0.5%-1% Ointment 0.5%-1%	Up to 2 wk
Cyclopenetolate (Cyclogyl)	Eyedrops, 0.5%-2%	24 hr
Homatropine (Isopto-Homatropine)	Eyedrops, 0.5%-5%	1-2 days
Scopolamine hydrobromide	Eyedrops, 0.25%-0.5%	1-2 days
Tropicamide (Mydriacyl)	Eyedrops, 0.5%-1%	4-6 hr

TABLE 65-3 Other ophthalmic drugs

Drug	Form	Dose
ANTIBIOTICS AND ANTIVIRAL DRUGS		
Polymyxin B, bacitracin (Polysporin)	Ointment or eyedrops, 0.1%-0.5%	As directed
Polymyxin B, neomycin, bacitracin (Neosporin)	Ointment	As directed
Bacitracin	Ointment, 500-1000 Ug	As directed
Idoxuridine (IDU)	Eyedrops, 0.1% solution	As directed
	Ointment, 0.5%	
Gentamicin sulfate (Garamycin)	Eyedrops, 3% solution	2-4 drops q 6 hr
	Ointment	2-3 times daily
Chloramphenicol (Chloromycetin, Chloroptic)	Oral, IV, subconjunctival	50 mg/kg/day
	Eyedrops, ointment	As directed
STEROIDS		
Prednisone	Topical, 0.25%-0.5% suspension	As directed
	Oral, 5-15 mg	1 tablet q 6 hr
Prednisolone acetate (predFoi-te)	Eyedrops, 0.12-1% solution	1-2 drops q 6-12 hr
Methylprednisolone (Depo-Medrol)	Subconjunctival, 0.5 mg	q 2-4 wk
Triamcinolone (Aristocort)	Solution or ointment, 1%, subconjunctival	As directed
Dexamethasone (Decadron, Maxidex)	Solution, 0.1%, ointment,	As directed
	Injection, 4 mg	
Fluorometholone (FML)	Eyedrops, 0.1% suspension	As directed
	Ointment, 0.1%	
ANESTHETICS		
Proparacaine (Ophthaine, Ophthetic, Alcaine)	Eyedrops, 0.5% solution	1-2 drops
Lidocaine (Xylocaine)	Local infiltration, 1%-2% solution	4 ml
LUBRICANTS AND TEAR SUBSTITUTES		
Methylcellulose, gonioscopic	Eyedrops, 1% solution	As needed
Methylcellulose	Eyedrops, 0.1% solution	As needed

If the patient is being treated for an active infection, individual medicine bottles, droppers, tubes of ointment, and other equipment are mandatory. This precaution is also necessary when an infected eye is being treated with an antibacterial drug such as bacitracin and the same medication is ordered prophylactically for the other eye. In this situation, the unaffected eye is treated first.

A *lubricant* such as methylcellulose (artificial tears) may be used for dryness of the cornea and conjunctiva caused by deficiency in production of tears or faulty lid closure as a result of nerve involvement or unconsciousness.

Antiinflammatory drugs such as prednisolone, dexamethasone, and hydrocortisone as drops or ointment are used to control inflammatory and allergic reactions postoperatively, as well as for a variety of conditions involving the eyelids, the conjunctiva, and the cornea. Steroids also may be given systemically for the treatment of acute or subacute infections such as those of the iris and choroid.

Astringents such as zinc sulfate preparations are often useful in treating chronic conjunctivitis. The *dye* fluorescein is used for applanation tonometry and to stain and thereby outline superficial injuries and infections of the external globe of the eye. Strips of filter paper impregnated with the dry dye are used in place of prepared solutions, because the solution is easily contaminated by *Pseudomonas aeruginosa*.[40]

SYSTEMIC EFFECTS

Drugs applied topically to the eye can be absorbed and may cause systemic side effects. Systemic reactions may occur when anticholinergic drugs are instilled into the eye to produce mydriasis. Atropine is the anticholinergic drug that most frequently causes systemic reactions. Signs and symptoms of systemic atropine toxicity include flushing, dryness of mouth and skin, fever, rash, tachycardia, and confusion, but rarely progression to coma and death.

Topically instilled miotic drugs can also cause unwanted systemic effects, most frequently with the long-acting anticholinesterase drugs such as echothiophate. Signs and symptoms include hypersalivation, sweating, gastrointestinal tract disturbances, decrease in heart rate and blood pressure, and bronchoconstriction. These drugs should be used with caution in patients with intestinal obstruction or bronchial asthma.

Brown MM, Brown GC, and Spareth GL: Improper topical self-administration of ocular medications among patients with glaucoma, Can J Ophthalmol 19:(1):2-5, 1984.

RESEARCH

One hundred fifty patients with glaucoma were studied to determine the extent of improper topical self-administration of ocular medications. Using their customary methods of administration, 13% of the patients were unable to place drops in both eyes after one or more attempts, and 80% failed to maintain the bottle's sterility during application. No significant relationship was found between performance and age, sex, educational level, visual field or acuity, intraocular pressure, and length of time the patient had been using eyedrops. There was a difference between the performance of clinic patients (N = 100) and private-practice patients (N = 50). Significantly more (p 0.05) of the clinic patients failed to wash their hands before instilling the drops (97% versus 78%) and were unable to properly instill the drops in both eyes after one or more attempts (18% versus 2%). The researchers noted that the private-practice patients all had received prior instruction by one physician, whereas only 62% of the clinic patients had. They noted that there had been several instructors present in the clinic. Also there was no significant difference between clinic patients who had received instructions and those who had not. The researchers suggest that uniform teaching probably improves the ability of patients to topically administer ocular medications. ∎

To avoid undesired systemic reactions, care should be taken with topically applied medications to give exactly what is ordered and no more. Pressure applied at the inner canthus after instillation will minimize drainage into the nose and throat, thereby decreasing systematic absorption.

INSTILLATION OF MEDICATIONS

Solutions such as eyedrops are the most commonly used preparations in the local treatment of eye disease. Advantages of solutions are that they (1) are easily instilled, (2) do not interfere with vision, (3) cause few skin reactions, and (4) do not interfere with the mitosis of the corneal epithelium.

The major disadvantage of eyedrops is that they do not remain in contact with the eye very long (see the research box at left). Approximately 90% of aqueous solutions are eliminated from the eye within the first minute of application. It is sometimes necessary to instill the solution at frequent intervals to achieve therapeutic results.

Eyedrops and eyedroppers must be sterile. Each patient should have his or her own bottle of medication. If the bottle is small, it may be warmed slightly by holding it in the hands for a few moments. Blunt-edged eyedroppers are available and may be used for children. The dropper is held downward so that medication does not flow into the rubber bulb, because foreign material from the bulb can contaminate the solution. Most eyedrops are packaged in small plastic bottles with an attached dropper (Figure 65-3, *A*).

If crusting or discharge is present, the eye is cleaned before instillation of medication. When eyedrops are in-

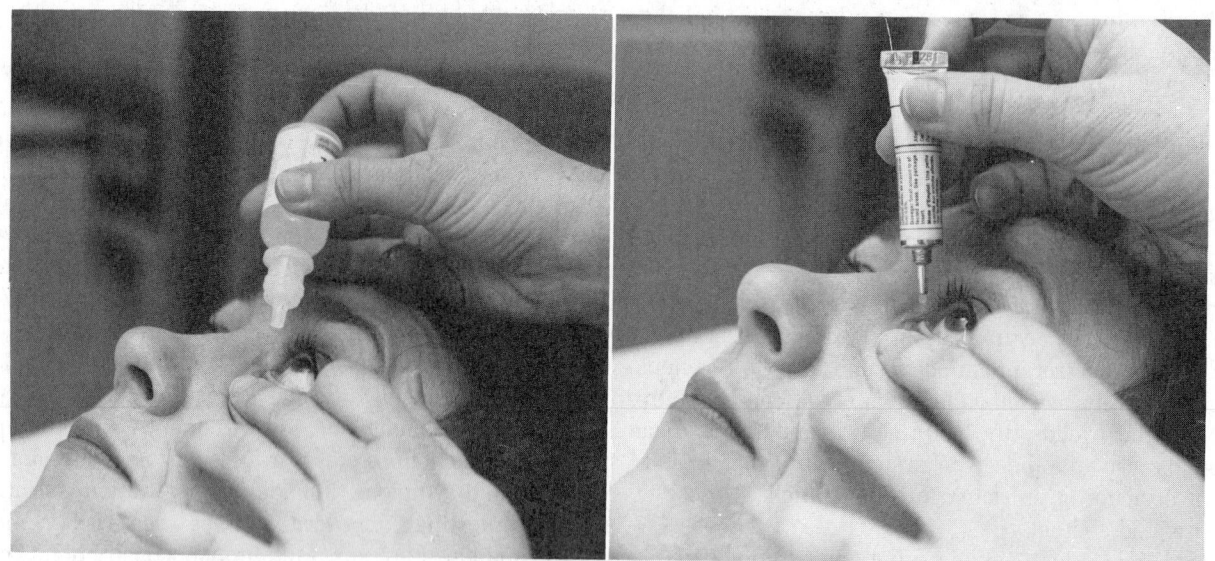

FIGURE 65-3 A, Ophthalmic solution is dropped onto conjunctiva of lower lid. **B,** Ophthalmic ointment is squeezed onto conjunctiva of lower lid.

stilled, the patient is asked to tilt the head back and look toward the ceiling. The lower lid is pulled gently outward, and the dropper should approach the patient's eye from the side and not directly from the front (Figure 65-3, *A*). Drops are placed on the lower conjunctiva. Care must be taken not to touch the eyelids, the conjunctiva, or the eyeball with the dropper. The eyelids should then be closed. The person is reminded not to squeeze the eye shut because this causes the medication to escape. Absorbent tissue or cotton held against the cheek will prevent the drops from running down the cheek. If two types of drops are to be administered, wait approximately 5 minutes before instilling the second drop. Two drops stimulate tear formation, dilute the drug, and may cause overflow of the conjunctival sac.

Ointments remain in contact with the eye much longer, providing a prolonged effect. They usually do not cause discomfort when instilled. There is less absorption into lacrimal passages than with eyedrops. Ointments, particularly those containing antibiotics, are more stable than solutions. Disadvantages of ointments are that they (1) produce a film in front of the eye that may blur vision, (2) cause contact dermatitis reaction more frequently, and (3) may inhibit mitosis of the corneal epithelial cells.

To instill ointment, the person tilts the head back and looks toward the ceiling. The lower lid is gently pulled down and the ointment is expressed directly onto the exposed conjunctiva from inner to outer canthus with a small individual tube (Figure 65-3, *B*). Care is taken not to touch the eye tissues with the tube.

EYE MANIFESTATIONS OF SYSTEMIC DISEASES

Diseases and infections that affect other parts of the body also affect the eye. The eye has been described as the most important square inch of body surface, both diagnostically and functionally. By examining the back portion of the interior of the eyeball (fundus) with an ophthalmoscope, many major diseases can be recognized. Some of the diseases and pathologic states that can be identified through their typical fundus picture and other eye assessment include metabolic diseases, vascular and hematologic disorders, neurologic problems, connective tissue disease, and nutritional deficiencies. Assessment of the eye often will indicate the severity of the disease.

METABOLIC DISEASE

Of the metabolic diseases affecting the eye, *diabetes* is the most common. Diabetes may affect any of the structures of the eye. *Senile cataracts* occur *earlier* in *persons* who have *diabetes* and progress more rapidly than in most elderly people. *Diabetic retinopathy* produces characteristic changes in the retina that can cause se-

vere visual damage and eventually result in blindness. Diabetes also causes the growth of new blood vessels on the surface of the retina and optic disc that later extend into the vitreous humor (*retinitis proliferans*). This condition often causes *blindness* because of recurrent *vitreous hemorrhages* and *retinal detachment*.

VASCULAR AND HEMATOLOGIC DISORDERS

Vascular disorders such as persistent systemic hypertension will eventually produce changes in the retina (hemorrhage, edema, and exudates) that may result in the loss of sight. If the cause of the elevated blood pressure is pregnancy induced hypertension and is of short duration, the *retinopathy* (any disorder of the retina) usually subsides when the pregnancy is terminated. Retinopathy caused by hypertension resulting from renal arteriosclerosis or diffuse glomerulonephritis is usually progressive and irreversible. Severe hypertension causes narrowing of the retinal arteries; and the blood flow through the retina and choroid is diminished, resulting in degenerative changes in the retina and loss of vision.

Visual loss may follow vascular accidents to vessels anywhere in the eye or in the main blood vessels outside the eye. A *cerebrovascular accident* may cause hemianopia (blindness for one half of the field of vision in one or both eyes) or total blindness, depending on its location. Arteriosclerosis and atheromatosis, particularly involving the carotid and cranial arteries, may release emboli that lead to occlusion of the retinal vessels.

Hematologic disorders cause characteristic retinal hemorrhages or neovascularization, as in the case of sickle cell disease.

NEUROLOGIC PROBLEMS

Neurologic disorders include a wide range of problems. Eye examination aids in evaluation of seven of the twelve cranial nerves (II through VIII) and provides information about the sympathetic and parasympathetic pathways (see Chapter 59). Demyelinating disorders (for example, multiple sclerosis) and infections (for example, syphilis) cause typical nerve damage to the eye. Increased intracranial pressure causes swelling of the optic disc (papilledema). Through eye examination (such as perimetry studies), lesions of the brain can be attributed to a specific lobe in the brain (temporal, parietal, or occipital). Unilateral dilation of the pupil helps diagnose severity and location of head injury.

CONNECTIVE TISSUE DISEASE

Persons with connective tissue disease commonly have eye involvement. One of the more frequent eye manifestations is dry eyes. Patients complain of a scratchy burning sensation with possible redness of the eye and photophobia (sensitivity to light). Any eye structure can be involved; the tissues of the eye that are affected are, in general, of the same type as the tissue involved in the primary manifestation of the disease. For example, rheumatoid diseases most commonly affect the cornea, sclera, and uveal tract, whereas systemic lupus erythematosus usually involves the vasculature of the eye.

NUTRITIONAL DEFICIENCIES

Nutritional deficiencies can cause pathologic changes in the eye. There seems to be a direct relationship between good nutrition and eye health. *A lack of vitamins A and B* in the diet can cause *changes* in the *conjunctiva, corneal epithelium, and retina.* The lack of vitamins available for body use may also be caused by interference with absorptive, storage, or transport capacities. Tears are reduced, and eyes and lid margins become reddened and inflamed. Sensitivity to light is often present, and some loss of visual acuity is noticed at night. Significant difficulty is called night blindness (*nyctalopia*). If night blindness is nutritionally caused, it may respond favorably to ingestion of a nutritious diet and vitamin A. On the other hand, *excessive* amounts of vitamin A can damage the retina. Vitamin B deficiency may cause *bilateral optic neuritis,* especially in individuals who drink large quantities of alcohol. When damage to the optic nerve has been severe and prolonged, a diet high in vitamin B and other essential nutrients can accomplish only partial recovery. Fortunately, eye problems from nutritional deficiency are rarely found in the developed countries.

TRAUMA

PREVENTION

Although the eye is vulnerable to trauma, natural protective mechanisms can prevent or minimize injury (Table 65-4).

In addition to the body's natural defenses against injury, *protective equipment* such as goggles, shields, and

shatterproof safety lenses are advised for certain occupations and sports activities. Knowledge of safety precautions and first-aid techniques are valuable in preventing serious damage from trauma.

Prompt and appropriate care of the injured eye may prevent serious vision impairment or loss of the eye. (Table 65-5). The two major categories of trauma are *burns* and *contact* (mechanical) *trauma.*

BURNS

Chemical burns such as those caused by acid or alkali must be treated immediately to prevent the possibility of permanent visual impairment from damage to the cornea. For chemical trauma of any nature, prompt immediate irrigation is the essential action that may result in salvaging an otherwise irrevocably lost eye. Irrigation after chemical trauma should be performed immediately after the injury and continued for a prolonged period of time, a minimum of 15 minutes. Although cool tap water is excellent for irrigation, any nontoxic solution can be used. After irrigation, and *only* after irrigation, is the patient transported to a physician.

Ultraviolet burns of the cornea may occur from exposure under a sunlamp or from exposure to the sun (outdoor workers, fishermen, sunbathers). The individual becomes aware of painful eyes several hours after exposure. Treatment consists of cold compresses, analgesics (for example, aspirin or codeine), and topical ophthalmic anesthetics. Topical antibiotics may also be used to prevent infection. Most patients are comfortable within 24 hours after treatment begins. Rarely is the cornea scarred permanently. Ultraviolet burns may also

TABLE 65-4 Protective mechanisms of the eye

Protective Feature	Function
Bony orbital rim	Prevents many mechanical injuries
Orbital fluids and tissues	Cushion direct blows
Eyelashes and eyelids	Quickly close reflexly (blink) from visual or mechanical stimuli
Bell phenomenon	Eyes reflexly rotate upward with lid closing to protect cornea
Lacrimal secretions	Can flush away chemicals or foreign bodies

TABLE 65-5 First aid for eye injuries

Injury	Interventions
Burns: chemical, flame	Flush eye immediately for 15 min with cool water or any available nontoxic liquid; seek medical assistance
Loose substance on conjunctiva: dirt, insects	Lift upper lid over lower lid to dislodge substance, produce tearing; irrigate eye with water if necessary; do not rub eye; obtain medical assistance if above interventions fail
Contact injury: contusion, ecchymosis, laceration	Apply cold compresses if no laceration present; cover eye if laceration present; seek medical assistance
Penetrating objects	Do not remove object; place protective shield over eye (for example, paper cup); cover uninjured eye to prevent excess movement of injured eye; seek medical assistance

occur from the use of germicidal lamps, electric flashes, and arc welding.

Thermal burns of the eyelids can cause lid contracture. Skin grafting may be necessary to prevent severe contractures and exposure of the eye. Full-thickness grafts can be taken from the uninjured eyelid, the inner aspect of the forearm, or behind the ear.

CONTACT TRAUMA
LACERATIONS OF EYELID

Lacerations of the eyelid require treatment by an eye specialist, because there is danger of scar formation as healing occurs. Although lid lacerations may bleed freely, pressure against the lid to stop bleeding can cause damage to the eye beneath. Cuts or tears in the eyelid may need to be sutured after bleeding is controlled and any foreign material is removed. Antitetanus serum usually is given to all patients who sustain eye wounds.

INJURIES TO CILIARY BODY, SCLERA, AND ORBIT

Injuries to the ciliary body and sclera and injuries involving the orbit are critical, because adjacent tissues usually are injured also and contents of the eyeball may escape and possible infection of the interior of the eye may occur. If these injuries result in wounds that are small and clean, treatment consists of bed rest, antibiotics given systemically and topically, suturing the wound, instilling atropine to put the iris and the ciliary body at rest, and a firm dressing. If the injury is extensive and if sight is lost, *enucleation* (removal of the eyeball) may be necessary.

ECCHYMOSIS

Persons with ecchymosis of the eyelid and surrounding tissues (black eye) should be examined to rule out coexisting skull fractures and intraocular bleeding or other eye damage. Initially, cold compresses will help to control the bleeding. Subsequent warm compresses after 48 hours will speed up the reabsorption of blood from the tissues. The discoloration, which lasts about 2 weeks, can be covered to some extent with cosmetics.

PENETRATING INJURY

Penetrating injury of the eye requires medical care as soon as possible. The most important goal is to prevent further damage before reaching the ophthalmologist. It is easy to convert a minor corneal laceration without iris prolapse into the loss of an eye when applying even gentle pressure on the eye during transportation of the patient. To protect the eye against pressure, a shield can be used. A cardboard cone or a paper cup can be taped securely over the patient's eye to prevent anyone or anything from touching it. Tears, blood, and other discharges cannot be wiped away without risking danger-

ous pressure changes. Also, covering the *uninjured* eye prevents excessive movement of the *injured* eye. Although the patient may walk or be transported sitting up in an automobile, *unnecessary exertion such as bending over or carrying heavy objects should be avoided.* These activities could *increase the intraocular pressure* and cause more *damage to the eye.*

CORNEAL INJURIES

Corneal injuries are serious, because resistance to infection is low in the cornea and scarring can impair vision. It has been estimated that foreign bodies on the surface of the cornea constitute about 25% of ocular injuries.[40] Tearing, photophobia, and a sensation of "something in the eye" warn a person that a foreign body is present if neuromuscular networks are functioning properly. If an abrasion of the cornea occurs, there may be considerable pain. For those persons with impaired sensorimotor function, the nurse must assess for corneal damage.

SYMPATHETIC OPHTHALMIA

Sympathetic ophthalmia is a serious inflammation of the uveal tract (ciliary body, iris, and choroid) in the *uninjured* eye that follows a penetrating injury or retained foreign body to the other eye. Although the cause of this condition is unknown, it may be the result of an *autoimmune inflammatory response* to *uveal pigment.* This inflammation spreads from the uvea to the optic nerve. Children are especially susceptible to sympathetic ophthalmia; however, it may occur at any age. The uninjured eye becomes inflamed; photophobia, lacrimation, dimness of vision, and pain in the eye may be experienced. *Sympathetic ophthalmia may appear 3 to 8 weeks after the eye injury or months or years later.* A severely injured blind eye may be removed soon after the injury in an attempt to prevent the development of sympathetic ophthalmia. Because of increased medical skill in treating perforating wounds and the administration of cortisone at the earliest suggestion of inflammation, sympathetic ophthalmia has become a rare disease in recent years.

INFECTIONS AND INFLAMMATION

Infections and inflammation can occur in any of the eye structures and may be caused by microorganisms, mechanical irritation, or sensitivity to some substance. Inflammation of the eye accounts for more than one half of the total incidence of acute disease conditions, with more than 1 million cases per year. Conjunctivitis represents about two thirds of the total.

STYES

Styes (hordeola) are relatively mild but extremely common infections of the small glands of the lid margins.

Guidelines for Application of Warm Moist Compresses

1. Use sterile technique when infection or ulceration are present; clean technique may be used for allergic reactions.
2. Use separate equipment for bilateral eye infections.
3. Wash hands before treating each eye.
4. Temperature of compress should not exceed 49° C (120° F).
5. Change compresses frequently every 10 to 20 minutes. Always wash hands first.
6. Do not exert pressure on the eyeball.
7. Sterile petrolatum may be used on skin around eyes, if desired, to protect the skin.
8. If sterility is not required, moist heat may be applied by means of a clean face cloth.

Staphylococci are often the infecting organisms. Poor hygiene and excessive use of cosmetics may be contributing causes. Patients should be taught not to squeeze styes, because the infection may spread and cause cellulitis of the lids. Warm moist compresses (see the box above) are used, and styes usually open and drain without surgery. A topical ophthalmic antibiotic may hasten healing.

CHALAZION

A chalazion is a sterile granulomatous inflammation of the sebaceous glands (meibomian glands) located in the connective tissue in the free edges of the eyelids. The cysts present a hard, shiny, lumpy appearance as viewed from the inner side of the lid. They may cause pressure on the cornea. Small chalazions may disappear after massage, hot compresses, and topical antibiotics. If they are large or become infected, they usually require surgical incision and curettage. Chalazions usually are removed in the physician's office or in the clinic with the patient under local anesthesia. An antibacterial ointment (for example, neomycin sulfate) may be applied to the conjunctiva; and an eyepad is worn for a few hours.

CONJUNCTIVITIS AND BLEPHARITIS
ETIOLOGY

Conjunctivitis (inflammation of conjunctiva) and blepharitis (inflammation of the eyelids) are common infections that can occur from a variety of causes. They may result from mechanical trauma such as that caused by sunburn or from infection with organisms such as staphylococci, viruses, streptococci, or gonococci. Inflammation is often caused by allergic reactions within the body or by external irritants (for example, poison ivy or cosmetics). Two of the viral agents that cause conjunctivitis are *trachoma* and *herpes simplex*.

ACUTE BACTERIAL CONJUNCTIVITIS

Acute bacterial conjunctivitis is often called "pinkeye." Common in school children, pinkeye is highly infectious. Conjunctival redness and crusting discharge deposited on the lashes and corners of the eye are the characteristic findings. Treatment includes cleansing of the lids and lashes, use of topical antibiotics, and precautions to prevent the spread to others. Firm adherent crusts may be softened by use of warm moist compresses. Because the material is infectious it should be disposed of in a sanitary way. Fortunately, acute bacterial conjunctivitis is usually self-limited, and leaves no permanent scars.

SEBORRHEIC BLEPHARITIS

Seborrheic blepharitis often begins in childhood and continues frequently throughout life. The lid margins of upper and lower lids are reddened with scales attached to the base of the lashes. The eyebrows and lid margins must be kept clean with water and a mild shampoo. Scales can be removed daily with a moistened cotton applicator. Frequently, some degree of conjunctivitis is present. Application of local antibiotics is helpful if infection is present. The condition can be kept under control if treated effectively before any serious eye involvement (for example, keratitis) develops.

TRACHOMA

Trachoma (a form of conjunctivitis), although rare in the United States, is endemic in low-income persons living in the dry, hot Mediterranean countries and the Far East and is a major cause of blindness in these areas. It is caused by a strain of the virus *Chlamydia trachomatis*. It is highly contagious in the early conjunctivitis stage and is spread by direct contact with the ocular discharge. Following the acute conjunctivitis stage, the eyelids become scarred, and granulations form on the inner surface of the lids and invade the cornea. The entire cornea may eventually become involved with subsequent loss of vision. Secondary bacterial infection is common.

Trachoma can be arrested in the early stages with topical and oral tetracycline. Eyelid granules may be removed surgically.

KERATITIS
ETIOLOGY

Inflammation of the cornea is called keratitis. It may be acute, chronic and superficial, or deep (interstitial). Acute epithelial keratitis commonly occurs in association with bacterial conjunctivitis caused by *Staphylococcus aureus*, *Streptococcus pneumoniae*, *Moraxella*, organisms, and *Pseudomonas aeruginosa*. Viruses such as herpes simplex may also cause a type of keratitis. Keratitis may be associated with a corneal ulcer or be caused by diseases such as tuberculosis and syphilis. Allergic reactions, vitamin A deficiency, or viral diseases (for example, mumps, measles, and herpes simplex) may contribute to its development in children.

CLINICAL MANIFESTATIONS

Keratitis causes severe pain in the eye, photophobia (sensitivity to light), tearing, and blepharospasm (spasm of the eyelids). Uncontrolled keratitis can result in loss of vision caused by impairment of corneal transparency or destruction of the eye by corneal perforation.

INTERVENTIONS

Medical Management

If possible, the systemic cause is found and treated. Cortisone may be used cautiously to control the inflammation. Except for herpes simplex, topical antibiotics are given to treat the infection. Cycloplegic agents, which will keep the iris and ciliary body at rest; hot compresses will help promote healing. Medications such as idoxuridine (IDU) applied locally are effective in helping to clear keratitis caused by herpes simplex in 80% of cases. The eyes may be covered to limit eye movements, and bed rest may be prescribed.

Corneal Transplantation

When the cornea is so damaged that severe vision impairment occurs, *corneal grafting (keratoplasty)* may be necessary. Loss of vision caused by an opaque or destroyed cornea may be restored by replacing the damaged layers with a corneal graft obtained from a new cadaver or from an eye freshly removed by operation. For best results the donor cornea must be removed within 6 hours of death and should be grafted within 24 to 48 hours. Transplants preserved for longer periods may be used for lamellar grafts and are discussed below. The present practice is to keep a waiting list of persons who need grafts, because eye banks are not able to keep up with the demand. Eye Bank for Sight Restoration, Inc.,* is a nonprofit organization that collects and distributes donated eyes throughout the country. Donors or their relatives usually make arrangements before death for donating the eyes.

Corneal transplantation cannot be performed if there is any infection. The kind of corneal graft used depends on the depth and size of the damaged part that must be replaced (Figure 65-4). Corneal transplants or grafts may involve the entire thickness of the cornea (total penetrating), only part of the depth of the cornea (lamellar), or a combination of these, in which a small part of the graft involves the entire thickness of the cornea (partial penetrating). Obviously, the more penetrating graft is more difficult to establish and requires more

*210 E. 64th St., New York, NY 10021.

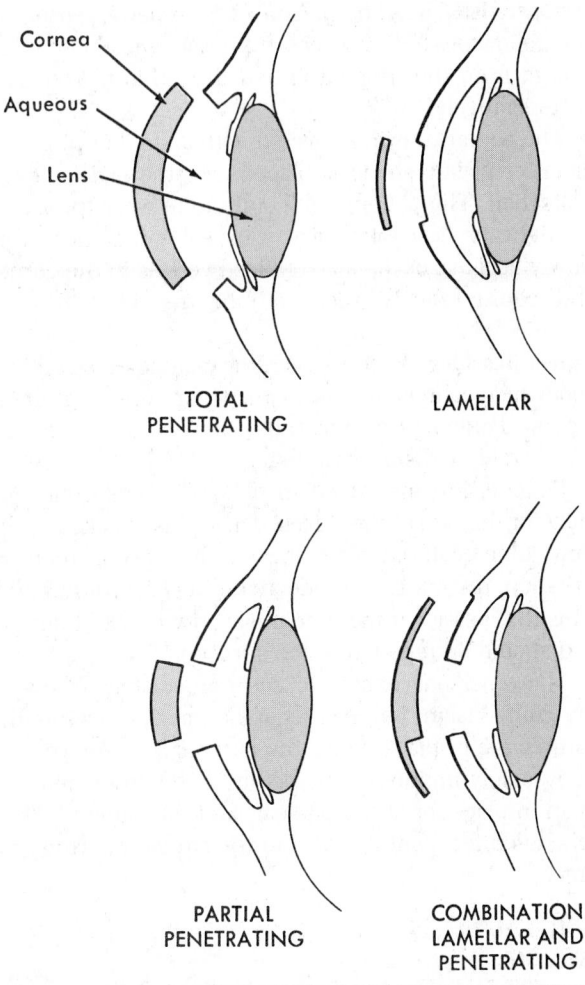

FIGURE 65-4 Types of corneal grafts currently in use. Note that in lamellar graft defect does not penetrate entire thickness of cornea.

definitive care postoperatively. For the penetrating graft, the eye surgeon seldom uses a donor eye that is over 48 hours old.

Nursing Management

Specific nursing interventions for persons undergoing a corneal transplant involve preparation for surgery, postoperative management, and patient education.

Preoperative Care. Persons usually have only a short notice that they are to be admitted to the hospital for surgery. Although they have been waiting for a donor cornea, this short period for actual preparation may find them feeling hurried and uneasy. They may be anxious about the surgical procedure itself and more specifically about its chances of success. A calm efficient manner on part of the nurse, along with explanation of the routine preoperative preparation, will help ease this anxiety.

Postoperative Care. The person may be permitted out of bed following full recovery from the anesthetic. Discharge from the hospital is usually within 2 to 4 days postoperatively.

The operative eye is covered with a sterile eye pad. A metal or plastic shield is placed over the pad for extra protection. The patient will continue to wear the shield at night for several weeks. Corneal grafts heal very slowly because of the lack of blood vessels in the cornea and require from 12 weeks to 6 months to heal firmly.

Patient Teaching. Patient teaching includes instructions about medications and assessment for corneal graft rejection. Patients are frequently sent home on cycloplegic, steroid, and sulfa eye drops.

Patients are instructed to check for graft rejection daily for the rest of their lives. The eye is checked at the same time each day for redness or increase in redness, irritation, discomfort, or a decrease in vision. Any symptoms that persist or increase in severity in a 24-hour period should be reported to the surgeon.

Many persons expect to see immediately following the graft. Vision, however, is sometimes poor while the sutures are in place. Once the sutures are removed, vision usually improves remarkably. The sutures may remain in place for at least a year, and the patient will be scheduled for monthly visits to the surgeon during that time.

CORNEAL ULCER
ETIOLOGY

Because of its location, the cornea is vulnerable to trauma and contamination with microorganisms. Infections of the cornea are not common occurrences. When present, however, they *can lead to scarring, perforation, extensive intraocular infection, and loss of the eye*. The ulcer may be caused by trauma, by contact lenses, or by infections of the conjunctiva that have spread to the cornea. Prompt treatment of ocular injuries can usually prevent the complication of infection. Persons at risk for infection may develop ulcers from little apparent cause (for example, the individual whose immune system is compromised).

CLINICAL MANIFESTATIONS

Persons with a corneal ulcer may complain of pain, photophobia, tearing, and spasms of the eyelid (blepharospasm). Reduced vision may also occur.

Assessment of the corneal ulcer is accomplished with the use of the slit lamp or with a bright movable light such as a small flashlight. With oblique illumination from a flashlight, directed from the side rather than straight on, details are seen more clearly. A greyish-white to yellowish-white opacity on the cornea may be

seen. The shape, size, and depth of the ulcer can be outlined by instilling sterile fluorescein. A *hypopyon* (pus in the anterior chamber) may also be noted. If pain and blepharospasm interfere with examination, a drop of an anesthetic such as 0.5% proparacaine may be used.

INTERVENTIONS
Medical Management

1. Culture and sensitivity, as required
2. Antibiotics, antiviral, or antifungal agents (depending on the causative agent) (Some given topically or subconjunctivally)
3. Cycloplegic agent
4. Steroid therapy, with caution
5. Cleansing of deep ulcers with an antiseptic solution, cauterization, and covering with a firm patch
6. Corneal transplant, if the ulcer causes permanent impaired vision

Nursing Management

The expected patient outcomes and nursing interventions are similar to those for persons with eye inflammations (see the box below).

UVEITIS
ETIOLOGY

Inflammation of the uvea is referred to as uveitis. Uveitis is caused by a wide variety of factors and infectious agents that may involve the choroid, the ciliary body, the iris, or all three simultaneously. Classification by cause includes *infection, allergy, trauma, toxic agents, noninfective systemic diseases such as diabetes, and unknown factors*. The specific cause of most cases of uveitis cannot be determined.

NURSING INTERVENTIONS FOR A PERSON WITH AN EYE INFLAMMATION

1. Promoting comfort
   a. Applying compresses as prescribed to decrease pain and promote healing
   b. Dimming lights and encouraging use of dark glasses if photophobic
   c. Administering analgesics, as prescribed
   d. Applying eye patch, as recommended
2. Teaching, as appropriate
   a. Self-care techniques
      (1) Instillation of eyedrops or ointment
      (2) Application of compresses, eye patch
   b. Prevention of spread of infection
      (1) Washing of hands before and after treatment of eye
      (2) Using separate medicine bottles or tubes for each eye
      (3) Using compresses one time only if infection present

---

CLINICAL MANIFESTATIONS

Uveitis produces pain in the eyeball radiating to the forehead and temple, photophobia (sensitivity to light), lacrimation, and interference with vision. There is edema of the upper lid, the iris is swollen because of congestion and exudation of cells and fibrin, and the pupil is contracted and irregular as a result of the formation of adhesions. The clinical picture may vary somewhat depending on the portion of the uveal tract involved.

INTERVENTIONS

Medical and Nursing Management

In self-limited acute inflammations, the cause is frequently not actively sought. In chronic uveitis, attempts are made to discover the possible cause such as sarcoid, histoplasmosis, toxoplasmosis, and connective tissue disease.

The instillation of scopolamine or atropine in the eye puts the iris and ciliary body at rest, relieves pain and photophobia, and diminishes congestion. By keeping the pupil dilated, the cycloplegic drug prevents adhesions from forming between the anterior capsule of the lens and the iris and tends to cause those already formed to regress. Moist, warm compresses may be applied several times each day to help diminish pain and inflammation. The eyes usually are covered, and in the convalescent period dark glasses are prescribed. Systemic analgesics are given as necessary for pain. Cortisone preparations are of great value in controlling the inflammation in many persons, but the inflammation in others resists almost all forms of treatment. Complications of uveitis include the formation of adhesions, keratitis, secondary glaucoma, and the loss of vision.

CATARACT

A cataract is a clouding or opacity of the lens that leads to gradual painless blurring of vision and eventual loss of sight (Figure 65-5). See Table 65-6 for a comparison of normal function, pathophysiology and clinical picture found with a cataract.

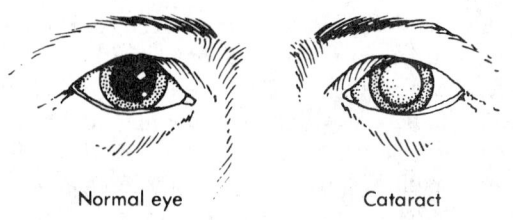

FIGURE 65-5 Cataract, visible in left eye as white opacity of lens, is seen through pupil.

Normal eye   Cataract

ETIOLOGY

In general, cataracts are classified as *senile,* those associated with aging; *traumatic,* those associated with injury; *congenital,* those that occur at birth; or *secondary,* those that occur following other eye diseases.

Cataracts occur so often in the elderly that the term *senile cataract* is used. At 80 years of age, about 85% of all persons have some clouding of the lens. Senile cataracts are listed as the most common cause of blindness in older persons, yet the response of the condition to surgery often is excellent.

After aging, the next most common cause of cataract is injury to the eye. The transparency of the lens may be destroyed by either a penetrating wound or a contusion. Cataracts may result from the ingestion of injurious substances such as dinitrophenol or naphthalene. Some researchers report that cataracts may result from systemic absorption of hair dyes.

Cataracts may also occur secondary to eye diseases, such as uveitis or eye trauma; or with systemic diseases, such as diabetes mellitus, galactosemia, or sarcoidosis.

CLINICAL MANIFESTATIONS

Cataracts resulting from aging or disease usually develop gradually. Both eyes may develop cataracts, but they usually develop at different rates. Blurring of vision may occur immediately following trauma. The predominant symptom is progressive loss of vision; the degree of

TABLE 65-6 Normal function, pathophysiology and clinical picture in cataract formation

Normal Function	Pathophysiology	Clinical Picture
Lens fibers continuously produced, with older fibers being compressed toward center of lens	With aging, nuclear portion of lens becomes increasingly dense; normal transparency of lens decreases	Gradual decrease in vision
Focuses light on retina	Light rays that strike opacity scatter	Glare, halos around lights
	Opacity filters out blue end of visible light spectrum	Ability to discriminate hues decreases; vision "rosier"
	Trauma to lens leads to rupture or break in lens capsule causing rapid swelling and opacification of lens	Sudden decrease in vision

loss depends on the location and extent of the opacity. Persons with an opacity in the center portion of the lens can generally see better in dim light when the pupil is dilated. The person with presbyopia may find that reading without glasses is possible in the early stages because of resulting myopia. To diagnose cataract(s) the pupil is dilated and the lens of the eye is examined with the ophthalmoscope and the slit lamp.

MEDICAL MANAGEMENT

Surgery

Operative treatment is the only method for treating cataracts. Unlike most other damaging diseases of the eye, vision loss from cataract can be restored by surgical removal of the cataract. Even patients who are in their 90s can often be operated on with good results. Between 90% to 95% of all cataract operations are successful. The decision as to when to remove the cataract depends on the general health of the patient and how much the cataract interferes with the person's activities.

It was previously thought that a cataract had to become mature or "ripe" before it could be extracted, that is, separated easily from the lens capsule. Now cataracts are removed whenever the decreased vision interferes with the person's activities of daily living or when the cataract may lead to other eye complications such as glaucoma.

Cataracts are usually removed with the patient under a local anesthetic. The most popular method of cataract removal is the extracapsular cataract extraction (ECCE). In this method, only the anterior portion of the lens capsule plus the capsule contents are removed, using techniques such as irrigation and aspiration or phacoemulsification (ultrasonic vibration to break up lens). Cataracts can also be removed within their capsule (intracapsular cataract extraction) using a freezing (cryo) probe that adheres to the surface of the lens.

Corrective Lenses

Because the lens or lens content has been removed, something is needed to replace the lost focusing power. The *intraocular lens* is most commonly used. When this is not possible, cataract glasses or contact lenses are necessary.

Intraocular lens. The intraocular lens, made of polymethylmethacrylate, is implanted within the eye at the time of surgery. It can also be secondarily implanted months or years after cataract extraction. The intraocular lens is the primary form of lens replacement today because it restores vision to near 20/20 (Figure 65-6)..

There are two types of intraocular lens implants being used. The *anterior chamber lens* is placed in front of the iris and is supported by it. This type of implant is used following an intracapsular cataract extraction or when the lens capsule cannot support a lens. The *poste-*

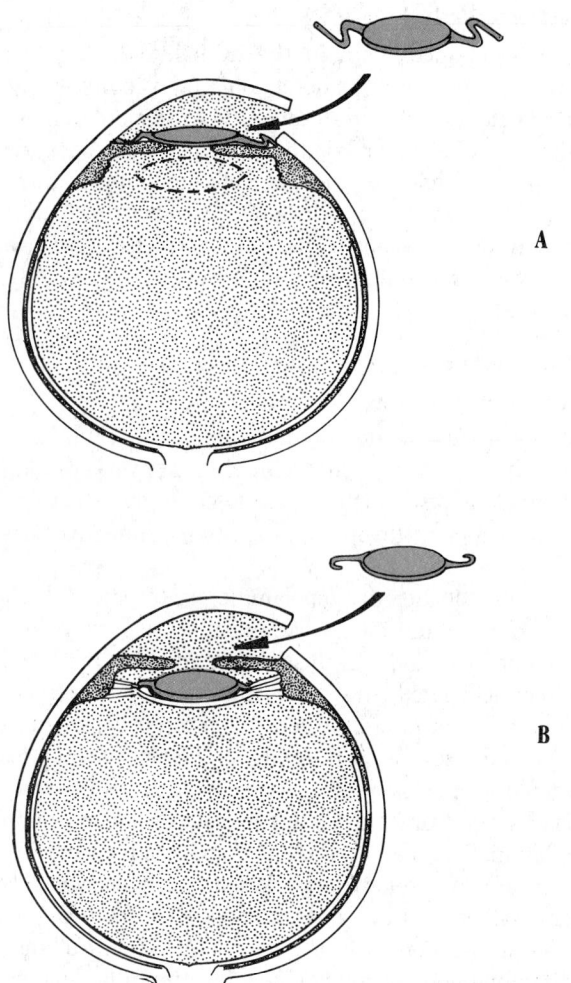

FIGURE FIG 65-6 Intraocular lens. **A,** Anterior lens implant in front of iris.**B,** Posterior lens implant behind iris. (From Lang BL and Phipps WJ: Medical-Surgical Nursing: a nursing process approach, ed 2, St Louis, 1989, The CV Mosby Co.)

rior chamber lens is placed behind the iris and is supported by the posterior portion of the lens capsule that was left in place (extracapsular technique). This type of implant is not dependent on the pupil or iris for support and rarely moves out of position. It is the most frequently used type of lens implant, because it is believed that the lens position most closely approximates the natural lens and magnification is minimized.

External lenses, cataract glasses, or contact lenses. If an intraocular lens is not inserted during surgery, the person must wear an external lens. Cataract glasses are the least desirable but are used for the person who cannot use contact lenses. Loss of depth perception and some peripheral vision make walking difficult. The final pair of glasses is not prescribed until vision has stabilized several months after surgery.

Contact lenses correct some of the problems encountered with cataract glasses but not entirely. The extended-wear soft contact lens is commonly used. Interruption of the nerve supply to the cornea from surgery usually facilitates the wearing of a contact lens. Persons with rheumatoid arthritis, hemiplegia, parkinsonism or Alzheimer's disease may have difficulty inserting and maintaining contact lenses.

NURSING MANAGEMENT

Preoperative Care

Most cataract surgery is now performed in ambulatory surgery centers; few patients require hospitalization. Routines for preoperative care vary with the setting and the eye surgeon. Eyelashes may be cut; this is done with curved sharp scissors with fairly short blades that have been lubricated with petrolatum to help prevent the cut lashes from entering the eye. Face scrubs may also be prescribed.

Before surgery the pupil of the operative eye is well dilated. The medications must be given at the prescribed times so that the eye is prepared at the time of surgery. Sedation may also be given, particularly for persons who are apprehensive.

Surgery is usually performed under a local anesthetic injected behind the eyeball and in and around the eyelids. The patient usually can go home within 1 to 3 hours after surgery. General anesthesia may be necessary for patients who cannot hold still during surgery.

Postoperative Care

The general goals of postoperative care are to prevent increased IOP, stress on the suture line, hemorrhage into the anterior chamber, and infection. Immediate postoperative care includes the following:

1. Position patient on *unoperative* side to prevent pressure on operated eye.
2. Keep side rails up as necessary for protection.
3. Place bedside table on side of unoperated eye (patient then turns toward unoperated side).
4. Place call light within reach.
5. Stress avoidance of actions that increase IOP (for example, sneezing, coughing, vomiting, straining, or sudden bending over with the head below the waist).

Following any cataract operation a dressing is applied to the eye and covered with a metal shield to protect the eye from injury. The dressing is usually removed the day of or a day after surgery, but an eye shield is worn at night for a few weeks until the eye is healed to avoid accidental bumping.

Currently, resumption of normal activities is much more rapid than before because of advancement in techniques of lens extraction. As mentioned above, most pa-

RESEARCH

Smith SJ and Drance SM: Difficulties patients have at home after cataract surgery, Can J Ophthalmol 19(1):6-9, 1984.

Twenty patients were interviewed to investigate their ability to manage eye care and daily living routines at home following uncomplicated unilateral cataract extraction without implantation of an artificial lens. Although there was a high degree of compliance to the medical regimen, difficulties were incurred in obtaining medications, reading labels, instilling eye drops, applying the eye shield, and providing a safe environment. Daily living routines were no problem if help was available with shopping and heavy household tasks. Knowledge about cataracts, treatment, and the home care required facilitated care at home. Also of importance was time to practice necessary eye care procedures and discuss concerns with the doctor. Support from relatives, friends, and home care nurses was also identified as a factor that aided self-care and reduced anxiety. ∎

tients have their cataracts removed in day surgical units and are discharged following recovery from the surgery. Normal activities of daily living are resumed as the patient feels able. The patient is cautioned not to sleep on the operative side for 3 to 4 weeks to prevent pressure on the operative eye. They are also taught not to bend the head lower than the waist for about 2 weeks.

Care should be taken in washing the face and hair to prevent any soap or water from entering the operated eye. Restrictions on activities such as heavy lifting may continue until complete healing has occurred (6 to 8 weeks). Patient teaching about follow-up care includes activity restrictions, the use of eye medications, and the eye shield. Patients should be given written instructions and a phone number to call if they have any questions. A research study describes the problems of persons who have undergone cataract surgery (see the research box above and the nursing care plan on pp. 1926-1927).

GLAUCOMA

EPIDEMIOLOGY

The term *glaucoma* designates eye disease characterized by increased intraocular pressure associated with progressive loss of peripheral visual fields. Glaucoma is responsible for 12% to 15% of all blindness in the United States today.[40] About 2% of persons over the age of 40 years have glaucoma. In black persons between 45 and 65 years of age, the prevalence of glaucoma is 15 times that of whites in the same age group. It has been estimated that nearly 1 million persons in the United States have glaucoma that has not been diagnosed. The

NURSING CARE PLAN

PERSON WITH A CATARACT

DATA: Mrs. Wilson is a 75-year-old woman who has had gradually decreasing vision in her right eye from a cataract. She states that it hasn't interfered too much with her activities until the last year. She remarks that now she can no longer drive at night because the car lights bother her and she has found it increasingly difficult to read large print books. She comments that she is still able to look after herself and her home, although she occasionally misses some of the dust. Mrs. Wilson has been admitted to the day surgery unit for an extracapsular cataract extraction with intraocular lens implant.

The nursing history identified the following:
- Mrs. Wilson is widowed and lives alone.
- She defines her cataract as a "growth on my eye" and thinks the physician needs to take "my eye out to fix it and then put it back in."
- Mrs. Wilson perceives herself as healthy except for some osteoarthritis in her hip.
- She states that she is anxious about the surgery because she depends on her eyes for everything.

NURSING DIAGNOSIS

Anxiety related to surgical procedure and possible loss of vision

Expected Patient Outcomes	Nursing Interventions	Rationale
Patient shows decreased signs of anxiety. Patient verbalizes feelings of anxiety.	Give patient an opportunity to explore concerns about possible loss of vision. Explore knowledge of cataracts and pre- and postoperative events; correct any misunderstandings, answer questions honestly.	Talking may help decrease anxiety and identify specific fears. Information decreases uncertainty and helps patient to gain control and feel less anxious.

NURSING DIAGNOSIS

Infection, potential for related to invasive procedure (cataract extraction)

Expected Patient Outcomes	Nursing Interventions	Rationale
Absence of signs or symptoms of infection.	Observe patient for signs and symptoms of infection. Use sterile technique when performing eye care and changing dressings. Administer antibiotic/steroid drops. Stress importance of not touching or rubbing operated eye.	Allows for early detection. Decreases possibility of introducing pathogens. Helps prevent infection. Prevents contamination and disruption of operative site.

NURSING DIAGNOSIS

Injury, potential for related to increased intraocular pressure, vitreous humar loss, hemorrhage

Expected Patient Outcomes	Nursing Interventions	Rationale
Patient describes factors that increase risk of injury. Patient demonstrates behaviors to protect self from injury.	Discuss postoperative course: pain, activity restrictions, and use of shield. Keep bed at lowest position and side rail up on right side. Assist patient when first getting up after surgery. Instruct patient to avoid sneezing, coughing, straining, and vomiting. Administer cough medicine, antiemetics as required. Instruct patient to wear eye shield at night or when taking a nap for 6 weeks following surgery. Instruct patient not to put pressure on eye when administering eye medications. Observe for flat anterior chamber, pear shaped pupil or bulging of wound.	Information enhances cooperation with necessary restrictions. Ensures safety. Ensures safety (strange environment). Helps avoid increasing intraocular pressure (IOP). To control cough and vomiting as they occur Prevents accidental bumping of the eye. External pressure can increase IOP causing rupture of the sutures. Indicates wound rupture, prolapse of iris related to loose sutures or pressure on eye.

NURSING DIAGNOSIS

Knowledge deficit regarding condition, surgery, pre- and post-operative care, self-care at home, related to lack of exposure to information

NURSING CARE PLAN

PERSON WITH A CATARACT—cont'd

Expected Patient Outcomes	Nursing Intervention	Rationale
Patient can describe a cataract and explain the basis for the symptoms experienced. Patient verbalizes or demonstrates knowledge of surgery, pre- and postoperative care, and self-care at home.	Teach about the eye and the role of the lens in vision. Explain why patient experienced decreased vision and difficulty driving at night. Teach about preoperative routine, surgery. Instruct patient in permitted activities postoperatively: 1. may climb stairs, watch TV, read, carry out ADL as long as eye is comfortable 2. avoid heavy physical activity for 6 weeks (lifting heavy objects, heavy house or yardwork, sports, shovelling) 3. do not lift any object over 10 lbs 4. may bathe in tub or take shower, avoid splashing eyes when washing face 5. protect eye with patch and shield when washing hair; tilt head backwards 6. do not bend head below waist; avoid sudden movements Demonstrate proper technique in cleaning eye from inner to outer canthus using clean cotton ball for each wipe. Stress handwashing. Demonstrate proper technique to put in drops and ointment, apply shield. Stress handwashing. Instruct patient to call doctor if: 1. eye pain is severe or persistent 2. redness of eye or lid increases 3. quantity of discharge from eye increases or drainage changes to greenish color 4. vision decreases	Increases understanding and promotes cooperation with post operative routine. Increases understanding and promotes cooperation with postoperative routine. Activities that cause eyestrain or increase IOP may compromise surgery. Prevents increasing IOP Good technique reduces risk of spread of bacteria within eye. Good technique reduces risk of introducing infection. These are early signs of infection and require immediate attention.

NURSING DIAGNOSIS

Pain related to inflammation, increased intraocular pressure

Expected Patient Outcomes	Nursing Interventions	Rationale
Patient states eye feels comfortable.	Assess the level of discomfort. Administer analgesics as required. Instruct patient to avoid rapid head movements and not to bend head below waist. To put on shoes, pick things up from floor, feed pet and so on. A long handled reacher may be helpful in reaching things on floor. Stooping with knees bent is acceptable.	Mild discomfort is expected postoperatively; acute pain suggests increased IOP or hemorrhage. Promotes comfort, Avoids increasing intraocular pressure (IOP) and pain.

NURSING DIAGNOSIS

Sensory alteration: visual, related to altered sensory reception/transmission

Expected Patient Outcomes	Nursing Intervention	Rationale
Patient understands that minimal alteration in normal sensory perception will be experienced.	Orient patient to physical surroundings and prepare her for the sensations and sounds she will feel and hear during surgery. Approach patient from unoperated side. Explain that vision will not be "normal" until the eye heals and glasses may be necessary in some cases (astigmatism).	Provides for increased comfort and familiarity. Aids orientation. Increases awareness of expected sensory alterations.

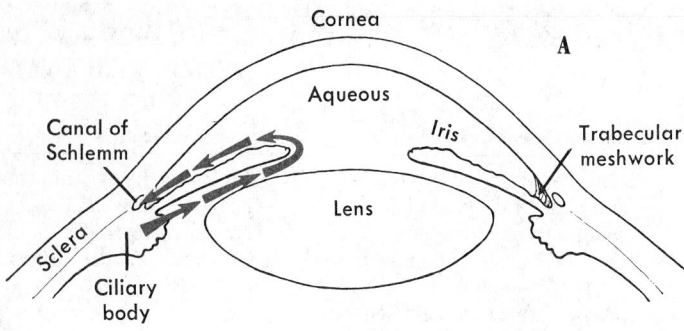

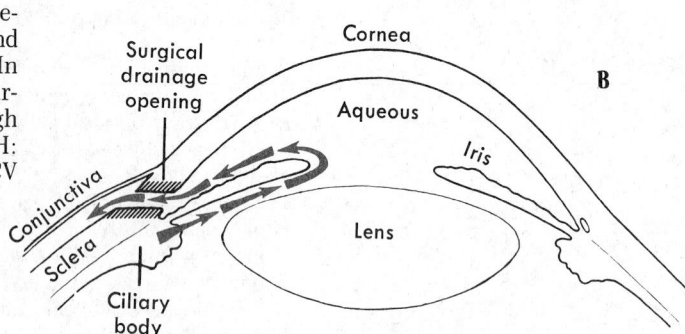

FIGURE 65-7 A, Originating from ciliary processes, aqueous humor flows through pupil into anterior chamber and normally leaves eye by way of canal of Schlemm. **B,** In glaucoma, normal aqueous humor outflow is blocked. Purpose of glaucoma surgery is to create new channel through which aqueous humor can leave eye. (From Havener WH: Synopsis of ophthalmology, ed 5, St Louis, 1979, The CV Mosby Co.)

TABLE 65-7 Types of glaucoma

Type	Characteristic	Manifestations	Treatment
Open-angle (chronic, simple)	Most common type (90%) Usually caused by obstruction in trabecular meshwork	Frequently no signs or symptoms in early stages Slow loss of vision Peripheral vision lost before central (Figure 65-8) Tunnel vision Persistent dull eye pain Difficulty adjusting to darkness Failure to detect color changes Later: headache, pain, blurred vision, halos around lights	Medical: miotics, carbonic anhydrase inhibitors, β-blockers Surgical: trabeculectomy, trabeculoplasty
Angle closure (narrow angle, acute)	Outflow impaired as result of narrowing or closing of angle between iris and cornea Intermittent attacks-pressure normal when angle open; if persistent, acute ocular emergency	Acute: severe prostrating pain, decreased vision, pupil enlarged and fixed, colored halos around lights, eye red, steamy cornea Permanent blindness if marked increase in IOP for 24-48 hours	Medical: osmotic diuretics, carbonic anhydrase inhibitors, miotics Surgical: peripheral iridectomy, iridotomy
Congenital	Abnormal development of filtration angle; can occur secondary to other systemic eye disorders Rare (0.05%)	Enlargement of eye, lacrimation, photophobia, blepharospasm	Goniotomy (incision into region of trabecular meshwork) Trabeculotomy
Secondary	Can result from ocular inflammation, blood vessel changes, trauma	May be similar to open angle and angle closure, depending on cause	Directed at cause as well as at decreasing the IOP

incidence of glaucoma is increasing as the number of older persons in our population increases. Glaucoma is the greatest threat to vision in older persons. Although it is seldom seen in persons under 35 years of age, it does occur in infancy.

In either chronic or acute glaucoma, early diagnosis and treatment are mandatory to prevent destruction of nerve fibers on the optic disk from increased IOP. Mass screening programs are important in detecting possible glaucoma in persons who do not have periodic medical eye examinations. It is important to detect and treat this disease, because the *permanent vision loss* it causes is *preventable*.

PATHOPHYSIOLOGY

Glaucoma results when the IOP is increased sufficiently to produce damage to the optic nerve. Normally there is a balance between the production and drainage of aqueous humor permitting the IOP to remain relatively constant (Figure 65-7). The normal range of IOP is 10 to 21 mmHg, with a mean of 16 mmHg. The pressure may vary up to 5 mmHg as a result of diurnal changes. Obstruction in any part of the outflow channels results in backup of fluid and increased pressure. This may occur as a primary condition or it may be secondary to infection or trauma. Most rarely, glaucoma results from abnormal placement of the iris against the angle of the anterior chamber, thus blocking the outflow of aqueous humor (acute angle closure glaucoma). Table 65-7 outlines the different types of glaucoma along with their characteristics and treatment.

■ ASSESSMENT

Assessment in glaucoma includes monitoring the patient's IOP, visual fields, and optic disc. Tonometry will reveal an elevated IOP, and visual field testing (perimetry) may show decreased peripheral vision. Ophthalmoscopy will reveal cupping of the optic disc, **if** the IOP is beyond the tolerance level of the patient. The nurse can also identify any change in vision, as well as any discomfort described by the patient.

■ DATA ANALYSIS: NURSING DIAGNOSES

Nursing diagnoses are determined from assessment of patient data. Possible nursing diagnoses for the person with glaucoma may include, but are not limited to, the following:

Diagnostic Title	Possible Etiologies
Health maintenance, altered	Impairment in vision
Knowledge deficit about glaucoma	Lack of exposure/recall of information or misinterpretation of information
Pain	Increased tension within the eye
Sensory alteration: visual	Altered sensory reception/ transmission

■ PLANNING: EXPECTED PATIENT OUTCOMES

For the patient with glaucoma, patient outcomes may include, but are not limited to, the following:
1. Vision not decreased further
2. Patient states discomfort is decreased
3. Patient can describe the following:
   a. Need for lifetime use of eye medications
   b. Prescribed medication therapy
   c. Preventive measures
   d. Signs and symptoms requiring immediate medical attention
4. Patient can maintain health despite alteration in vision.

■ IMPLEMENTATION
MEDICATIONS

Persons with glaucoma may be on medication for the rest of their lives. The goals of medication therapy are to provide better drainage of aqueous humor and to decrease the amount of aqueous humor produced. It is important that patients understand the necessity of taking the medication when prescribed to control the IOP and thus help prevent vision loss. The patient and family should know specifically what to do if essential eyedrops are accidentally spilled; for example, they should know which local drugstore is open at night and on holidays. The person often is advised to have an extra bottle of medication in the home and to carry one if working away from the home. It is advisable for the person to carry a card or other information that identifies him or her as having glaucoma in case an accident occurs. Drugs used in glaucoma are outlined in Table 65-8. Pilocarpine, a miotic, and timolol maleate, a β-blocker, are two of the most common drugs used.

SURGERY

Surgical intervention is indicated when conservative treatment fails to control the IOP. Two common procedures are trabeculoplasty and trabeculectomy. *Trabeculoplasty* is the application of a laser beam (argon) on the trabecular meshwork. This produces a nonpenetrating thermal burn that changes the configuration of the meshwork and leads to increased outflow of aqueous humor. *Trabeculectomy* is a filtering procedure in which an opening or fistula is made at the limbus under a partial-thickness scleral flap. The new opening circumvents the obstruction, and aqueous humor flows into the subconjunctival spaces.

Trabeculectomy usually requires overnight hospitalization. Trabeculoplasty, however, is frequently performed on an ambulatory basis, and the person usually remains for 3 to 4 hours following the procedure so that IOP can be checked. A complication of the procedure is a sudden rise of IOP immediately after surgery. It takes 4 to 8 weeks to see if the procedure is effective. How-

TABLE 65-8 Drugs used in treatment of glaucoma

Drug	Form	Dose
CHOLINERGIC DRUGS (MIOTICS)		
Pilocarpine	0.5%-10% solution	1 drop q 4-6 hr
	Ocusert continuous release	Replace weekly; ½ strip at bedtime
Carbachol (Carbacel)	0.75%-3% solution	1 drop q 6-8 hr
CHOLINESTERASE INHIBITORS (MIOTICS)		
Physostigmine (Eserine)	0.25%-1% solution or ointment	1 drop q 6-8 hr
Isoflurophate (DFP) (Floropryl)	0.01%-0.1% solution; 0.25% ointment	1 drop q 24-48 hr
Demecarium bromide (Humorsol)	0.125%-0.25% solution	1 drop q 12-24 hr
Echothiophate iodide (Phospholine iodide)	0.03%-0.25% solution	1 drop q 12-24 hr
ADRENERGIC AGENTS		
Epinephryl borate (Eppy)	0.25%-1% solution	1 drop q 12 hr, often used with miotic such as cholinesterase inhibitor
Epinephrine hydrochloride (Glaucon)	0.5%-2% solution	
Epinephrine bitartrate (Epitrate)	2% solution	
Dipivefrin (Propine)	0.1% solution	1 drop q 12 hr
CARBONIC ANHYDRASE INHIBITORS		
Acetazolamide (Diamox)	125-250 mg tablets	1 tablet q 6 hr
	500 mg capsules, sequential	1 capsule q 12 hr
	500 mg vials for IM or IV use	IM or IV if patient vomiting
Ethoxzolamide (Cardrase)	125-250 mg tablets	1 tablet q 6-12 hr
Dichlorphenamide (Daranide)	50 mg tablets	1 tablet q 6-12 hr
Methazolamide (Neptazone)	50 mg tablets	1 tablet q 4-6 hr
OSMOTIC AGENTS		
Glycerin (glycerol, Osmoglyn)	50%-75% solution: mix with equal amount of orange juice (oral)	1-1.5 g/kg body wt
Mannitol (Osmitrol)	5%-20% solution for IV use	0.5-2 g/kg body wt
Urea (Ureaphil, Urevert)	30% solution for IV use	0.5-2 g/kg body wt
β-ADRENERGIC BLOCKER		
Timolol maleate (Timoptic)	0.25%-0.5% solution	1 drop q 12 hr

NURSING CARE FOLLOWING TRABECULECTOMY

Nursing care for the patient following trabeculectomy includes:
1. Routine postanesthesia care
2. Protection of operative eye with patch, shield, positioning, patient on back or unoperative side, and safety measures
3. Maintaining comfort in the operative eye
4. Assessment, as appropriate, of the IOP, appearance of the bleb, and anterior chamber depth
5. Administration of medications such as a cycloplegic, a mydriatic and a combination antibiotic and steroid

TEACHING THE PATIENT WITH GLAUCOMA

1. Lifetime eye medication required
2. Preventive measures
   a. Have reserve bottle of eyedrops at home.
   b. Carry eyedrops when away from home.
   c. Carry identification for glaucoma and the prescribed eyedrop solution.
   d. Be aware of location of local drugstore open nights, weekends, and holidays.
3. Name, dosage, frequency, and side effects of prescribed eye medications
4. Signs and symptoms requiring immediate reporting to physician (for example, eye pain, sudden change in vision, halos around light)

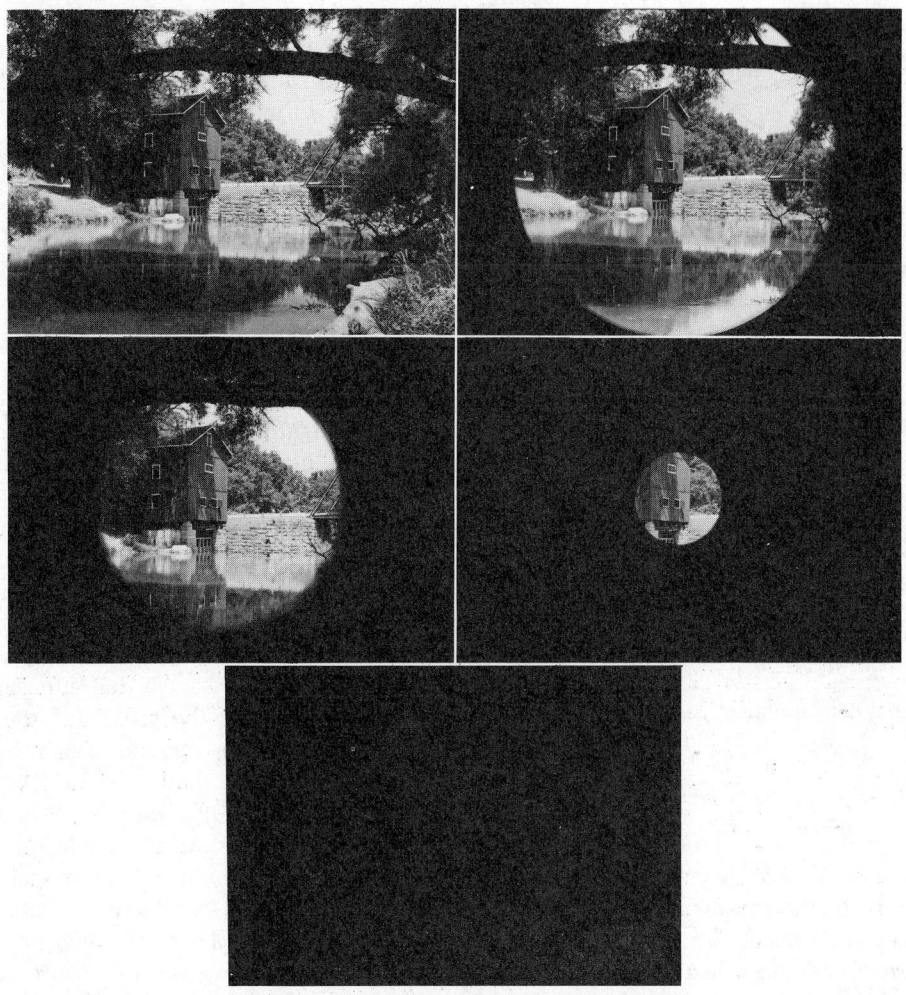

FIGURE 65-8 Gradual loss of sight from glaucoma so insidiously destroys vision that person is unaware of impending blindness until extensive and irreversible damage is present. Note loss of peripheral vision. (From Saunders WH et al: Nursing care in eye, ear, nose, and throat disorders, ed 4, St Louis, 1979, The CV Mosby Co.)

ever, glaucoma medications usually must be continued. Nursing care for the person following trabeculectomy is summarized in the box on p. 1930.

PROMOTING COMFORT

The eye usually becomes more comfortable when the IOP decreases. Analgesics may be prescribed. Cold eye compresses may also increase comfort.

PATIENT TEACHING

Glaucoma is a chronic disease, and the person with glaucoma needs help in understanding and learning to live with the disease. Despite explanations from the physician, the person frequently hopes that an operation will cure the condition, that no further treatment will be necessary, and perhaps that lost sight will be restored. It should be explained that the lost vision cannot be re-

stored, but that further loss can usually be prevented and life can be quite normal if the person continues under medical care. Usually no restrictions are placed on the use of the eyes. Fluid intake generally is not curtailed, and exercise is permitted. Bright lights or darkness are not harmful to the eyes of the person with glaucoma. Patient teaching is summarized in the box on p. 1930.

DETACHMENT OF THE RETINA

ETIOLOGY AND PATHOPHYSIOLOGY

Retinal detachment occurs when the two retinal layers (outer pigmented epithelium and inner sensory layer) separate as a result of accumulation of fluid or traction produced by contraction of the vitreous body (Figure 65-9). As the detachment extends and becomes com-

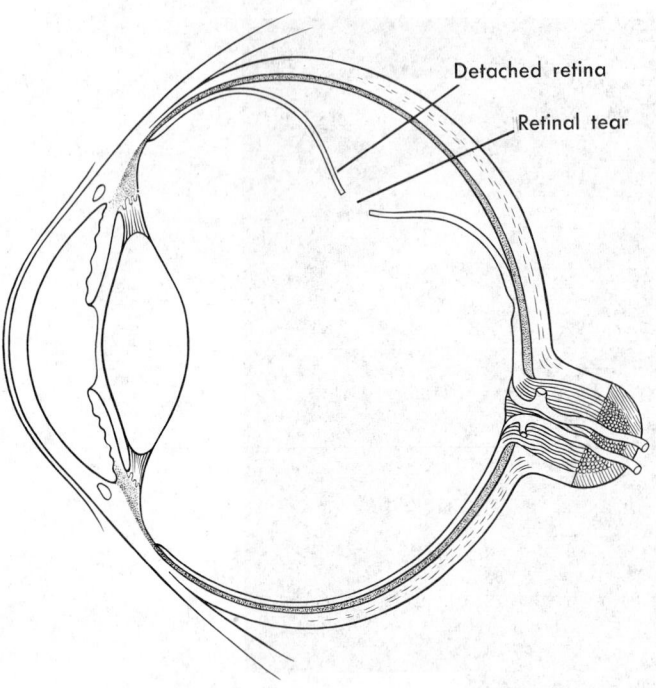

FIGURE 65-9 Retinal detachment.

plete, blindness results. Myopic degeneration, trauma, and aphakia (absence of the crystalline lens) are the most frequent causes of retinal detachment. It may also result from hemorrhage, tumor, or exudates that occur in front of or behind the retina. Detachment of the retina may follow sudden severe physical exertion, especially in persons who are debilitated. Most often, however, no apparent cause is identified.

CLINICAL MANIFESTATIONS

Retinal detachment may occur suddenly or may develop slowly. Symptoms include floating spots or opacities before the eyes, flashes of light, and progressive loss of vision in one area. The floating spots are blood and retinal cells that are freed at the time of the tear and cast shadows on the retina as they seem to drift about the eye. The flashes of light are caused by vitreous traction on the retina. The area of visual loss depends entirely on the location of the detachment. When the detachment is extensive and occurs quickly, the patient may have the sensation that a curtain has been drawn before the eyes. The diagnosis of retinal separation is based on the ophthalmoscopic appearance of the retina.

INTERVENTIONS
MEDICAL MANAGEMENT

Immediate care for the detachment is dependent on its degree and site. There may be moderate to little restric-

tion on activity, as well as bilateral to no patching of the eyes. If the macular region is threatened or a large detachment has occurred, care may include keeping the patient quiet in bed with the eyes covered to try to prevent further detachment and aid absorption of subretinal fluid. The head is positioned so that the retinal hole is in the lowest part of the eye. Activity may also be restricted (see nursing care plan on p. 1933).

Surgical Procedure

Surgery may be performed under either local or general anesthesia. Cyclopentolate or phenylephrine is used to keep the pupils widely dilated so that tears in the retina may be identified during the operation. The surgical procedure may include draining the fluid from the subretinal space so that the retina returns to its normal position, thereby closing the opening in the retina. To drain the fluid from the subretinal space, the sclera and choroid are perforated at the time of the operation.

The retinal breaks are sealed off by various methods that produce an inflammatory reaction (*chorioretinitis*) in the area of the tear so that adhesions will form between the edges of the break and the underlying choroid to obliterate the opening. When the tears are small or of recent origin, diathermy may be applied through the sclera with needlepoint electrodes to produce the inflammatory process. An intense beam of visible light directed to the area by means of an elaborate ophthalmoscope may be used to close a retinal tear when the retina is not elevated (*photocoagulation*). The *laser beam* is used by some surgeons as a source of intense energy to produce chorioretinitis. Subfreezing temperatures ($-40°$ to $-60°$ C) may be applied to the surface of the sclera in the area of the hole to produce the inflammatory reaction (cryotherapy). Nitrous oxide or carbon dioxide under pressure, flowing through a tube attached to a delicate instrument, is used to produce these low temperatures.

For most retinal detachments, *scleral buckling* procedures are used. In this procedure, the sclera and choroid are indented (buckled) toward the retinal break. Buckling is accomplished by placing silicone of various shapes and sizes in the region of the break (Figure 65-9). In addition an encircling tape of silicone can be placed around the entire eye. By these procedures, the choroid is pushed into contact with the retinal tear during healing, and vitreous adhesions that have exerted traction, or pull, on the retinal break are relaxed as the size of the scleral shell is decreased.

NURSING MANAGEMENT
Postoperative Care

The postoperative care for the person with retinal detachment includes the following:
1. Position and ambulate the patient as ordered.

NURSING CARE PLAN

PATIENT WITH RETINAL DETACHMENT

DATA: Mr. Arthurs is a 56-year-old warehouse clerk who complains of decreasing vision in his left eye over the last few days, like "a curtain coming over my eye." He comments that he began to notice spots floating in front of his eye about 2 weeks ago and flashes of light out of the corner of his eye a week ago. He states that he did not get concerned about these, because he thought they were just normal aging changes. He remarks, "I began to get scared when I started to go blind in that eye, and it didn't take me long to get to my eye doctor." He continues, "I got more scared when the doctor sent me straight to the hospital." Mr. Arthur states that, except for nearsightedness, he has had no trouble with his eyes. He is generally healthy except for high blood pressure, which is well controlled with medication and diet. Examination of his left eye revealed a superior retinal detachment with inferior visual loss. His visual acuity is 20/80. He is scheduled for retinal detachment surgery (scleral buckling). His left eye is patched, and his orders are for bed rest with bathroom privileges.

The nursing history identified the following:
- He and his wife have little understanding of what has happened to his eye or what the physician is going to do to his eye in the hospital.
- The loss of vision is very frightening to Mr. and Mrs. Arthur. They are also concerned about whether Mr. Arthur will get any vision back in the eye and whether it will spread to the other eye.
- Mr. Arthur has not had any accidents or injuries to his eyes that he can remember.
- Mr. Arthur is a very active man, swimming and jogging regularly. He comments that he has to do some "good" activity every day so he can feel his best.

NURSING DIAGNOSIS

Anxiety/fear related to surgical procedure and possible loss of vision

Expected Patient Outcomes	Nursing Interventions	Rationale
Patient shows decreased signs of anxiety Patient verbalizes fears and feelings of anxiety.	Give patient and spouse an opportunity to explore concerns about possible loss of vision. Answer questions honestly.	Talking may help decrease anxiety and identify specific fears. Information decreases uncertainty and helps person to gain control and feel less anxious.
	Encourage realistic hope about maintaining vision.	Helps relieve their anxiety.
	Explore knowledge of disorder and planned therapy, and correct misunderstandings.	Clarification assists in understanding.

NURSING DIAGNOSIS

Diversional activity deficit related to inability to participate in routine recreational activities (jogging, swimming)

Expected Patient Outcomes	Nursing Interventions	Rationale
Mr. A. will participate in activities to decrease boredom and maintain sense of fitness.	Encourage patient to perform leg exercises.	Decreases monotony and hazards of immobility.
	Vary patient's daily routine; provide tapes, and radio. Allow Mr. A. to make as many decisions as possible.	Decreases boredom and increases sense of control.
	Encourage postoperative resumption of normal activities, as permitted.	Increases feelings of normalcy.

NURSING DIAGNOSIS

Infection, potential for related to surgical repair of detached retina

Expected Patient Outcomes	Nursing Interventions	Rationale
Absence of signs or symptoms of infection.	Assess for signs and symptoms of infection.	Allows for early detection.
	Use sterile technique when performing eye care and changing dressings. Administer antibiotic drops.	Decreases possibility of introducing pathogens. Helps prevent infection.

Continued.

NURSING CARE PLAN

PATIENT WITH RETINAL DETACHMENT—cont'd

NURSING DIAGNOSIS

Injury, potential for related to sensory deficit, lack of awareness of environmental hazards

Expected Patient Outcomes	Nursing Interventions	Rationale
No injury occurs.	Orient patient to physical surroundings.	Increases awareness of potential hazards.
Vision is not decreased.	Keep bed at lowest position and side rail up on left side.	Ensures safety when patient has eyes patched and is in strange environment.
	Assist patient when first getting up after surgery.	Ensures safety.
	Instruct patient to avoid sneezing, coughing, and vomiting. Administer cough medicine, anti-emetics, if required.	Helps avoid increasing intraocular pressure (IOP).
	Instruct patient to wear eye shield at night or when taking a nap for 2 weeks following surgery.	Prevents accidental bumping of the eye.

NURSING DIAGNOSIS

Knowledge deficit regarding condition, surgery, pre- and postoperative care, and self care at home related to lack of exposure

Expected Patient Outcomes	Nursing Intervention	Rationale
Patient and his wife can describe retinal detachment and explain the basis for the symptoms experienced.	Teach about the eye and the role of the retina in vision. Explain why flashing lights, spots before the eyes, and decreased vision occur.	Increases understanding and promotes cooperation with post operative routine.
Patient and wife can verbalize or demonstrate knowledge of surgery, pre- and postoperative care, and self-care at home.	Teach about preoperative routine and surgery. Instruct patient in permitted postoperative activities: 1. ask physician when a return to work can be made 2. may climb stairs, watch TV, read, carry out ADL as long as eye is comfortable 3. avoid driving, heavy house or yardwork, or sporting activities before checking with physician 4. may bathe in tub; avoid splashing eyes when washing face 5. do not bend head below waist; avoid sudden movements	Activities that cause eye strain, or increase IOP, may compromise surgery.
	Demonstrate proper technique in cleaning eye from inner to to outer canthus using clean cotton ball for each wipe. Stress handwashing.	Good technique reduces risk of spread of bacteria.
	Demonstrate proper technique to administer drops and ointment and apply shield. Stress handwashing.	
	Instruct patient and spouse to call doctor if: 1. new flashing lights, floaters, or shadows appear 2. eye pain is severe or persistent 3. redness of eye or lid increases 4. quantity of discharge from eye increases or changes to greenish color	Early intervention can prevent development of complications.

NURSING CARE PLAN

PATIENT WITH RETINAL DETACHMENT—cont'd

NURSING DIAGNOSIS

Pain related to inflammation, increased intraocular pressure

Expected Patient Outcomes	Nursing Interventions	Rationale
Patient states eye feels comfortable.	Assess the level of discomfort.	Postoperative discomfort is expected, but acute pain suggests increased IOP or hemorrhage.
	Apply cool, moist compresses.	Reduces swelling and promotes comfort.
	Administer analgesics as required.	Promotes comfort.
	Instruct patient to avoid rapid head movements and not to bend head below waist.	Avoids increasing intraocular pressure (IOP) and pain.

NURSING DIAGNOSIS

Sensory alteration: visual related to altered sensory reception/transmission

Expected Patient Outcomes	Nursing Interventions	Rationale
Vision is not decreased further.	Maintain prescribed activity and position restrictions.	Restricted eye movement helps decrease risk of further detachment.
	Place bedside table within patient's reach without need to turn head.	Gravity is used to help keep the retina in its proper position.
ADL are met.	Assist with ADL as necessary.	Decreased vision and restrictions in activity alter or interfere with familiar ways of doing things.
Patient can describe physical surroundings.	Orient patient to physical surroundings.	Provides for increased comfort and familiarity.
	Place bed so patient is not facing wall and can see others approaching. Approach patient from unaffected side.	Offsets isolation and aids orientation to surrounding environment.
	Encourage diversional activities such as radio and conversation.	Provides sensory input and feelings of normalcy.

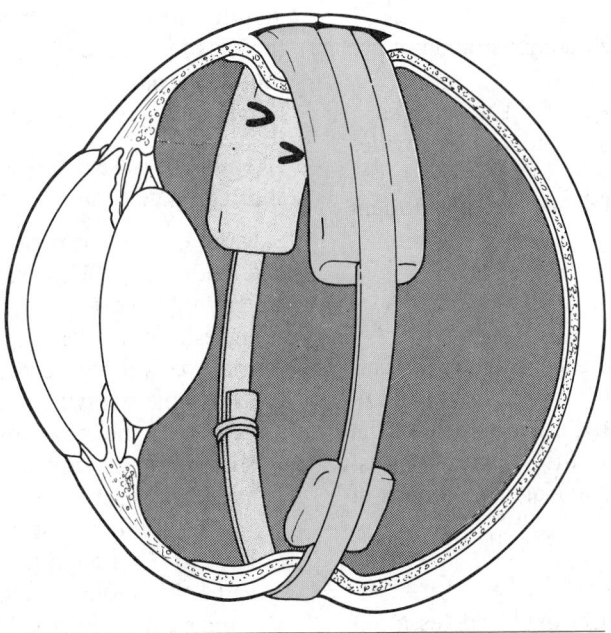

FIGURE 65-10 Scleral buckle.

2. Assist with activities of daily living, as required.
3. Administer eye medications as ordered (mydriatics, cycloplegics, and combination steroid/antibiotic).
4. Apply cold compresses as ordered to reduce swelling and promote comfort.
5. Implement safety measures such as side rails.
6. Instruct the patient to avoid jerking motions of the head (sneezing, coughing, vomiting).
   a. Administer antiemetics, as required.
   b. Administer cough medication, as required.

Promoting Safety

Although most surgeons do not patch both eyes (binocular) some do patch both eyes preoperatively and for 2 or 3 days postoperatively. Safety precautions such as side rails are essential if binocular patching is used. Call signals need to be kept within reach. Explanation of the immediate environment is also indicated.

Counseling

Patients are usually anxious and apprehensive when admitted to the hospital. Generally there has been a rapid loss of vision, and patients fear losing more vision. Restoration of sight will depend on the extent and duration of the detachment and the success of the surgery. Opportunity to discuss concerns needs to be provided. Nurses can do much to allay apprehension by answering questions honestly and instilling realistic hope.

Patient Teaching

Patient teaching for persons with retinal detachment includes:
1. Report to ophthalmologist any signs of redetachment (increase in floaters, flashes of light, decreased vision).
2. Use appropriate techniques for administration of eye medications.
3. Limit activities to sedentary work for 1 to 2 weeks
4. Check with physician about resumption of activities such as sports or heavy lifting.
5. Discuss plan for medical follow-up (appointment with doctor and so on).

DIABETIC RETINOPATHY

The quality of health and the life expectancy of the person with diabetes have improved as a result of the use of insulin and regulated exercise and diet. Because of the longer life span, however, some of the complications associated with diabetes such as pathologic conditions of the retina have increased.

ETIOLOGY/EPIDEMIOLOGY

Diabetic retinopathy is a disorder of the blood vessels of the retina, which usually appears about 10 years after onset of diabetes mellitus. The incidence seems to depend mainly on the duration of the diabetes. Retinopathy can be detected in approximatley 65% of persons who have had diabetes for 15 years and in about 90% of persons who have had diabetes for 30 to 40 years.[48] Diabetic retinopathy is responsible for at least 10% of cases of newly reported blindness each year and 20% of cases in persons 45 to 75 years of age.[14,38]

PATHOPHYSIOLOGY

In the initial phase of diabetic retinopathy, which usually lasts several years, the retinal capillary walls thicken and develop tiny pouchings (microaneurysms), and the retinal veins widen and become tortuous. Small hemorrhages develop, which may eventually disappear, leaving small scars that decrease vision in those areas. Protein leaks from the vessels as a result of increased capillary permeability causing retinal edema, especially in the area of the macula.

In advanced disease, small blood vessels develop on the retina and grow out into the vitreous. These vessels frequently rupture, causing decreased vision. Some of the blood may reabsorb and vision will increase until the next hemorrhage, but the continuing hemorrhagic process eventually leads to marked visual loss. Resolving of the hemorrhagic products may create a pull on the retina leading to tearing and detachment of the retina.

CLINICAL MANIFESTATIONS

The signs of diabetic retinopathy—tortuous vessels, small dots (microaneurysms), "fluffy wool" exudates on the retina, and new vessel formation—can only be identified by examining the retina through ophthalmoscopy and fluorescein angiography. As the disease progresses, the person describes increasing loss of vision and sees multiple spots (floaters). The floaters are minute hemorrhagic products in the vitreous humor.

INTERVENTIONS
MEDICAL MANAGEMENT

Several methods of treatment are currently being used and studied for effectiveness. These include:
1. *Photocoagulation.* In this therapy an intense beam of light from a laser (argon or zenon) is directed into the eye and focused on a small spot on the retina. The light energy is transformed into heat energy, coagulating the new vessels and preventing hemorrhage into the vitreous. At present, the *panretinal* or *scatter type* of treatment is the preferred approach. In this approach the physician scatters 200 to 2000 laser burns around the retina. Recent research indicates that retinal photocoagulation reduced, at least temporarily, the risk of blindness by about 60% in

those persons with moderate to severe retinopathy.[48]

2. *Vitrectomy.* Eyes that cannot be treated by photocoagulation can sometimes be treated surgically by a *vitrectomy.* Although the effectiveness of this procedure has steadily improved, it still is a difficult procedure, and complications occur. In this procedure the surgeon removes (a), the opaque bloody fluid (from hemorrhage) in the vitreous and replaces it with a saline solution, (b) the fibrous or scar tissue that could pull on the retina causing it to detach, and (c) the tissue that could serve as a scaffold for the growth of new vessels between the retina and vitreous. Retinal reattachment procedures, such as scleral buckling and injection of air/gases into the eye may be performed at the same time.

3. *Methods Under Investigation.* Because of the limitations of surgical methods to preserve vision in diabetic retinopathy, efforts are continually being made to find medical means of preventing development of the condition. Methods being investigated include (a) metabolic control such as blood sugar control, (b) aldase reductase inhibitors, and (c) laser and aspirin therapy.

NURSING MANAGEMENT

Nursing management of the person with diabetic retinopathy includes the following:

1. Teaching the patient about the importance of regular eye examinations.
   a. All diabetics should have their visual acuity and fundi checked yearly.
   b. Children should be examined 3 to 5 years after the onset of diabetes or at puberty.
   c. Those persons with mild forms of retinopathy are urged to have three to four examinations a year.
2. Teaching the patient about photocoagulation, as appropriate.
   a. Procedure usually is done on outpatient basis.
   b. There may be mild to moderate discomfort.
   c. Analgesia will be prescribed as necessary.
   d. Vision may be blurred following the procedure.
3. Assessing knowledge of diabetes, and implement teaching as required.
4. When vision is impaired, assess ability to administer own insulin and test own blood sugar.
5. Altering patient's self-management techniques as required (see discussion on diabetes in Chapter 37).
6. Providing opportunity for patients to discuss concerns and fears about disease and visual impairment.
7. If admitted for vitrectomy, carry out routine preoperative and postoperative nursing care for persons having eye surgery (p. 1932). Remember that many of these patients have poor vision.

MACULAR DEGENERATION

Macular degeneration is a disease of the aging retina caused by degenerative changes in the *choriocapillaris, Bruch's membrane,* or the *retinal pigment epithelium.* The choriocapillaris is a thin layer of blood vessels originating in the retina and extending into the choroid. Bruch's membrane separates the choriocapillaris from the retinal pigment epithelium.

ETIOLOGY/EPIDEMIOLOGY

The two types of macular degeneration generally seen are the wet and dry types. The *wet type* is characterized by a sudden growth of new vessels in the macular region. These vessels are fragile and tend to leak blood and fluid that displaces and damages the macula by interfering with its blood supply. Scarring occurs, and the function of the macula is destroyed, frequently very quickly. The *dry type* is the most common and is caused by degenerative processes other than neovascularization. Scattered round spots (drusen) begin to appear in the macular region of the retina. Drusen are discrete deposits that may in fact be waste products that could not be properly eliminated from the pigment epithelium. Sometimes following the appearance of drusen, there is a slow atrophy of the choroid, pigment epithelium, and retina in the macular region.

The most common form of macular degeneration is called *involutional macular degeneration,* which is associated with aging. This form of macular degeneration accounts for 70% of all cases.

CLINICAL MANIFESTATIONS

The main manifestations of macular degeneration are:
1. Varying degree of central vision loss in one or both eyes
2. Decreased ability to distinguish colors

INTERVENTIONS
MEDICAL MANAGEMENT

No treatment is available for the dry type of macular degeneration. Laser therapy is used in a small percentage of those with the wet type. This is only possible if the person is treated before the abnormal blood vessels have begun to grow into the center of the macula. Treatment *must* begin as soon as possible following the onset of symptoms. Each day that elapses before treatment is sought significantly decreases the chance of preserving vision.

NURSING MANAGEMENT
Counseling

Fear of blindness is a frequent concern. Opportunity to discuss this fear along with the frustration of changing vision must be provided. Support and help are also needed as the person learns new and different ways to carry out normal routines.

Patient Teaching

It is difficult to predict the degree of vision loss for each person. However, the disease, type of vision loss, and prognosis can be discussed. Optical aids such as magnification spectacles, magnifying glasses, and special lights may be helpful. The fact that peripheral vision will be maintained needs to be emphasized. Preparation for diagnostic testing (fluorescein angiography and retinal photographs) also needs to be done.

Prevention

Although there is no primary prevention for macular degeneration, early signs or changes in existing disease can be detected. This is done with the Amsler grid (see Figure 64-10). Distorted lines, dark spots, or areas that are completely missing will be noted by persons with macular degeneration. This test should be done two to three times a week by those at risk and may be done daily by those with existing disease. Any changes should be reported immediately to the ophthalmologist.

TUMORS

Both *benign* and *malignant* tumors may occur in the eye or related structures such as the eyelid. Neoplasms may originate in the retina or the uveal tract or metastasize to the eye from a primary site. Orbital neoplasms include *benign hemangiomas, pseudotumors, lymphomas, mucoceles* from the sinuses, *malignant melanomas, retinoblastomas,* and others. If tumors are malignant, both vision and life are endangered. Tumors within the eyeball are often silent except for a bloodshot appearance of the eye. As in all malignant tumors, the prognosis depends on early diagnosis and prompt treatment.

TYPES OF TUMORS
TUMORS OF THE EYELIDS

The eyelids are subject to the usual tumors of the skin such as *nevi xanthelasma* and *verrucae* (warts). Carcinoma of the lids is a common type of ocular malignancy. Any warty growth in the eyelids should be removed for histologic examination. Treatment consists of surgical excision of the growth.

RETINOBLASTOMA

Retinoblastoma is a *highly malignant intraocular neoplasm.* The neoplasm arises from mutations in the retinal cells (noninheritable form) or in the germinal cells (inheritable form). It is the most frequent ocular malignancy in childhood, occurring in one of every 23,000 to 34,000 births.[40] The diagnosis is made in 90% of patients by the age of 4 years. Signs and symptoms may include decreased vision, strabismus, retinal detachment, white pupillary reflex, and secondary glaucoma. In about one third of patients, the tumors invade both eyes. Retinoblastomas grow rapidly and spread backward along the optic nerve and invade the brain. Retinoblastomas can also metastasize to distant sites by way of the bloodstream and lymphatics.

Treatment of large retinoblastomas consists of enucleation, with removal of as much of the optic nerve as possible. Treatment modalities such as cobalt,[60] plaque irradiation, photocoagulation, and cryotherapy may be used for selected small retinoblastomas. Frequent examination of the remaining eye is recommended. When the tumor is bilateral, the more involved eye is removed. An attempt is made to save the other eye by using radiation, chemotherapy, or both. If the tumor is very advanced, removal of both eyes may be necessary to save the child's life. When the tumor is unilateral and diagnosed and treated early, there is a 90% survival rate.

When normal parents have one child with retinoblastoma, there is a likelihood of less than 4% that a subsequent child will have such a tumor. There is a 50% chance that children of the individual who has survived a proved hereditary retinoblastoma will also be so affected. Persons who survive the tumors should receive *genetic counseling* to alert them to the danger of transmission to their offspring.

MALIGNANT MELANOMAS

Malignant melanomas are neoplasms that occur in the choroid, ciliary body, and iris of adults. They grow slowly, but because of the vascularity of the choroid, they metastasize early to the liver and lungs.

INTERVENTIONS

Medical treatment of tumors of the eye may include cryotherapy, enucleation, radiation treatment, chemotherapeutic agents, and photocoagulation.

The emotional response to a tumor of the eye is perhaps even greater than to malignancies elsewhere. The surgeon may advise immediate enucleation of the eye in the hope of saving life. Both the patient and family need to be encouraged to talk about their feelings and concerns and to be helped to readjust their lives when confronted by this serious situation.

REMOVAL OF AN EYE
Medical and Nursing Management

An eye, with or without its supportive structures, may be removed surgically for four reasons: (1) in an attempt to save a life when a malignant tumor has developed, (2) to save sight in the other eye when *sympathetic ophthalmia* is feared or threatens, (3) to control pain in an eye blinded by disease such as chronic glaucoma or chronic infection, or (4) for cosmetic reasons following blindness from trauma or disease.

Three types of surgery may be performed. *Enucleation* is surgical removal of the entire eye including the sclera. *Evisceration* is removal of the contents of the eye with retention of the sclera. *Exenteration* involves removal of the entire eye and all other soft tissues in the bony orbit.

If feasible, the eyeball alone is removed, leaving the surrounding layers of fascia (Tenon's capsule) and the muscle attachments. A *silicone, plastic,* or *tantalum implant* is inserted into the eye socket, the cut ends of the muscle attachment are overlapped and sutured around it, and the Tenon's capsule and the conjunctiva are closed. This procedure provides a stump that supplies both support and motion for an artificial eye and therefore gives the patient whose eye has been removed a more normal appearance. The ball-shaped implant is left in place permanently. A plastic conformer is placed in the socket until edema subsides and an artificial eye can be inserted.

Postoperative Care

Hemorrhage, thrombosis of blood vessels, and *infection* are possible complications following enucleation, exenteration, or evisceration of an eye. Pressure dressings are used for 1 or 2 days to help control possible hemorrhage. Headaches or pain in the side of the head operated on should be reported at once, because meningitis occasionally occurs as a complication following thrombosis of adjacent veins. The patient is usually allowed out of bed the day following surgery. Antibiotic or steroid ointment or both may be prescribed until the patient receives the ocular prosthesis.

When a person has lost one eye, the preservation of sight in the other eye becomes crucial. Wearing impact-resistant glasses provides some protection from injury. Because binocular vision is gone when there is only one functioning eye, depth perception is affected. The individual needs to be taught about the adjustments necessary in learning to carry out normal activities with one eye and about the potential safety hazards. Driving a car, for example, is dangerous for the person who suddenly must use only one eye and is not accustomed to the alteration in depth perception. With patience and practice, however, almost all normal activities are possible; for instance, surgeons who have had an eye removed have been able to operate successfully.

Artificial Eye

An artificial eye can be used as soon as healing is complete and edema has disappeared, usually 4 to 8 weeks after surgery, although many patients begin to wear an artificial eye after only 2 to 3 weeks.

REMOVAL AND CLEANING OF ARTIFICIAL EYE

1. Remove prosthesis: gently depress the lower lid and exert a small amount of pressure under lower edge of prosthesis.
2. Wash prosthesis with soap (for example, Ivory) and water. Soap is less irritating than detergents. Rinse thoroughly.
3. Irrigate socket with water, if necessary.
4. Reinsert prosthesis: place upper portion under upper lid, pull down lower lid and slip lower edge behind lower lid. With finger or thumb, gently pull down on lower lid and slide prosthesis in place.

Today artificial eyes are made of plastic instead of glass. They can be bought in shades that closely match the normal eye or they can be specifically made by the ocularist. The ocularist will take an impression of the socket and paint the prosthesis to match the persons own eye. The majority of patients have custom made eyes, with stock eyes used for temporary fitting following surgery.

Follow up care is provided by the ocularist who polishes the eye to remove build up of salt and protein and assesses fit and appearance. At one time it was recommended that the artificial eye be removed and cleaned on a regular basis. It was discovered that this frequent removal kept the eye socket mildly irritated. Because of improved fitting and polishing techniques, some patients do not need to remove their artificial eye between yearly visits to the ocularist. For those who clean the eye more frequently, removal and cleansing is an easy process (see box above).

General tips on care of the artificial eye are outlined in the box on p. 1940.

Instead of a regular artificial eye, a scleral cover shell may be prescribed. In general, scleral cover shells are indicated for blind and disfigured eyes. The cover shell is made of the same material as hard contact lenses and is customarily made to match the color of the other eye. Wearing time of the shell is increased until it can be worn all day. It is usually removed at night to rest the eye. The shell is stored in water, hard contact lens solution or saline. Cleansing is the same as for a plastic artificial eye (see box).

VISUAL IMPAIRMENT

A person is considered legally blind when either of the following conditions exist: (1) the person's visual field is no greater than 20 degrees or (2) central distance vision in the better eye is 20/200 or worse with use of corrective lenses. In the United States there are an estimated 1 million legally blind persons. Annually, more than 46,000 persons become blind. Most blind people are 65

CARE OF ARTIFICIAL EYES

1. If the eye is left out of the socket, store it in water or contact lens solution.
2. Do not expose the plastic eye to alcohol, ether, chloroform, or any other solvent because they can damage the eye beyond repair.
3. If rubbing the eye, rub toward the nose. Wiping away from the nose may cause the eye to fall out.
4. Wear a protective patch or goggles when swimming, diving, or water skiing—or remove the eye and store safely.

years or older and in this older population more women than men are blind.

There is a broad diversity of characteristics in persons classified as legally blind. Loss of visual acuity may range from profound to slight; visual field loss may be peripheral or central; or there may be other visual functions affected such as "dark adaptation." Thus many persons classified as legally blind do have useful vision. Of the total blind population, only 25% have no useful vision, that is, they are totally blind or have light perception or light projection only.[38]

The visually impaired population does not only include those who are legally blind. There are well over a million people who, although unable to see well enough to read a newspaper, have vision better than 20/200. Also, over 3 million are monocularly blind, with a small proportion having a defective but not blind second eye.[38] Most persons in this visually impaired but not legally blind population are between the ages of 25 to 64.

CONSEQUENCES OF VISUAL IMPAIRMENT

Blindness imposes limitations in the range and variety of experiences, in mobility, and in the interaction with the environment. Limitations in the range and variety of experiences are related to the fact that a person who cannot see must use touch and kinesthetic experience to gain knowledge of the world. Objects too large or too small to handle are not perceivable.

Many blind persons feel that the restriction in mobility resulting from blindness is its most serious effect. Blind persons cannot move about as quickly, as securely, or as easily as sighted peers. They need to rely on aids or other persons, particularly in unfamiliar areas.

Vision is the sense that permits persons to control their environment and themselves in relation to that environment. Loss of vision can limit the interaction between persons and their environment. It may be that blind persons withdraw from others or that others pull away from the blind. Limitations in social interaction may also be related to difficulties in nonverbal commu-

nication. Glances, smiles, and frowns, for example, are missed.

Not only are blind persons restricted in nonverbal communication, they are also limited in the ways they can process information. Decreased ability to read and communicate in conventional ways can lead to decreased opportunities for learning experiences and may alter established careers.

Visual impairment can cause more than just difficulty in mobility and communication. Difficulties also arise in carrying out personal care, housework, cooking, and home maintenance. These limitations in activities may even be greater in older persons who tend to have more severe impairments.

ADJUSTMENT TO VISUAL IMPAIRMENT

Visual impairment requires a major life adjustment. Persons need to adjust to both the initial impact of the loss and the subsequent changes that will occur in their life because of the loss of vision. The initial reaction is often characterized by disbelief and then depression, withdrawal, self-pity, and, at times, embarrassment over changed abilities. In time, most persons make a decision, consciously or unconsciously, to live with their impairment. They learn new ways or adapt their present ways of doing things to carry out their normal activities. Most recognize that there are some things that they will never be able to do again on their own or that they can only do with help.

Adjustment is an ongoing process. New situations occur to which the blind person must adjust. These new situations can cause frustration and annoyance. However, these feelings do not occur as frequently nor do they last as long as they did initially.

The key variable in this process of adjustment is time. Time is needed to grieve for the lost sight and to recognize and come to terms with the implications of the loss. Time is also needed to master many of the difficult tasks and work associated with adjustment to a visual impairment.

DIFFICULT AREAS IN ADJUSTING

For many blind persons the dependence on others for help in carrying out normal routines and the necessity to ask for help are two of the most difficult things to which they must adjust. The inability to carry out tasks or role obligations in the usual way and the inability to recognize friends and acquaintances are also difficult areas. Fluctuating vision, a common occurrence for many visually impaired persons, leads to frustration and difficulties in planning or implementing tasks. Fears and uncertainties about the progression of visual impairment can lead to concern about the ability to cope with further deterioration of vision or the necessity of preparing for the future.

GUIDELINES FOR COMMUNICATING WITH BLIND PERSONS

1. Talk in a normal tone of voice.
2. Do *not* try to avoid common phrases in speech, such as "See what I mean."
3. Introduce yourself with each contact (unless well known to the person). If in hospital, knock on the door before entering.
4. Explain any activity occurring in the room or what you will be doing.
5. Announce when you are leaving the room so the person is not put in the position of talking to someone who is no longer there.

FACTORS ASSOCIATED WITH ADJUSTMENT

Many factors are associated with adjusting to a visual impairment. The ability to maintain the give and take in a relationship, especially with those who provide some form of service, helps to counteract some of the feelings of dependence on that person. Other factors that are associated with adjustment include age, amount of residual vision, gradual loss of vision, self-concept, previous coping patterns, and social support.

FACTORS HINDERING ADJUSTMENT

There are factors that do not help in the adjustment process. Other health problems, especially if they also limit or alter normal functioning, make learning to live with the visual impairment more difficult. Lack of social support can lead to a sense of isolation and loneliness. Insufficient information about the impairment in terms of diagnosis, prognosis, and aids and strategies to help live with the impairment may affect their ability to cope. Blind persons relate experiences of being ignored, "yelled at" as if deaf, and not addressed directly when with companions (see the box above for guidelines in communicating). These unhelpful or negative behaviors of others do not help adjustment. Blind persons are sensitive to being treated differently at the onset of their blindness. Helen Keller observed that the attitudes of the seeing toward the blind rather than blindness itself was the hardest burden for her to bear. See the research box above right, for a research study that examined blind persons' perceptions of behaviors of others.

NURSING MANAGEMENT
SUPPORT AND COUNSELING

The newly blind person and those with deteriorating vision need an opportunity to talk about their feelings and their fears and concerns about the future and their ability to cope. Nurses can provide this opportunity along with the support that persons need as they reorganize

RESEARCH

Rickelman BL, and Blaylock JN: Behaviors of sighted individuals perceived by blind persons as hindrances to self-reliance in blind persons, J Vision Imp Blindness 77:8-11, 1983.

The purpose of this descriptive study was to determine which behaviors of sighted persons are perceived by blind persons as hindering self-reliance in blind persons. Subjective reactions of the 60 blind men and women who took part in the study to the various behaviors of the sighted along with any actions taken were determined. Following a content analysis, 10 categories of situations evolved that described the behaviors of sighted persons that made the blind person feel less self-reliant. These included the following: (1) patronizing or derogatory statements were made or actions taken that caused anger, hurt, frustration; (2) equal opportunity or treatment was not accorded, and discrimination or prejudice was real or suspected; (3) assumptions were made that the blind were not responsible capable adults; (4) dependency was automatically assumed, and help was given when it was not needed or desired; (5) information regarding needs or desires was solicited from sighted companions; (6) sighted persons responded with embarrassment or avoidance of the blind; (7) help was needed, but the manner in which it was given was demeaning; (8) helpful acts were omitted although they would have been appropriate and were desired; and (9) assumptions were made that, if the person was blind, he or she also had other disabilities. The visually impaired person's principal response to these situations reflected mainly a passive or withdrawn response (57%). This was followed by an assertive response (34%) and an aggressive one (9%). The study findings indicated a significant lack of knowledge and understanding by sighted persons of the skills, abilities, and feelings of individuals with significant visual impairment. Negative incidents occurred not only with the general public but also with nurses, doctors, assistants in the doctor's office, family, and friends. ∎

their lives or come to terms with the need to change life goals or priorities. Social support is a key factor in adjusting to visual impairment. Assistance may be needed from nurses to help in the establishment and maintenance of social networks that include both sighted and visually impaired persons.

Integration of blindness and decreasing vision into one's self-concept can take a long time. It may be difficult to accept such things as the white cane; or being labeled as "blind" and are consequently different. Patience and understanding are required.

Fear of many of the aspects and consequences of visual impairment frequently occurs within the process of adjustment. The specific fears and the context in which they occur need to be elicited by the nurse. This can lead to development of appropriate interventions to alleviate or decrease these fears.

ASSISTANCE WITH ACTIVITIES OF DAILY LIVING

Although most visually impaired persons develop ways of coping with their activities of daily living, they do need ongoing assistance in learning techniques that can help them to maintain or regain this ability. Nurses can provide specific guidance to aid patients in this process of relearning (see the box below, right).

PATIENT TEACHING

Information is needed by blind persons, not only about their particular disease and prognosis, but also on aids and strategies to help them live with a visual impairment. Nurses, working in collaboration with other health team members and rehabilitation centers for the blind, can help provide this needed information.

COMMUNITY SERVICES

Many federal, state, and local agencies provide services to persons with severe visual impairment. The health professional can refer these persons and their families to a social worker who is familiar with services and facilities available in their home area. Community health nurses often have this information readily available. Services to visually impaired persons include mobility training, personal counseling, vocational rehabilitation, relearning independent self-care, special education, and financial compensation in some instances.

NATIONAL VOLUNTARY ORGANIZATIONS

Two national voluntary health agencies concerned with blindness and the prevention of blindness are the American Foundation for the Blind* and the National Society for the Prevention of Blindness, Inc.† Both organizations have literature that is available to nurses and patients on request. The American Foundation for the Blind distributes a free catalog, *Aids and Appliances* (also available in braille, free of charge to blind persons), which contains a list of devices for the visually handicapped. The catalog includes sewing and kitchen utensils as well as various kinds of tools and instruments (Figure 65-12). Medical appliances such as special syringes and aids for persons who must give themselves insulin or other parenteral medication can also be obtained. The National Society for the Prevention of Blindness, Inc., is engaged in the prevention of blindness through a comprehensive program of community services, public and professional education, and research. Publications, films, lecture, charts, and advisory service are available on request.

Recording for the Blind, Inc.* is a national, nonprofit voluntary organization that provides audio-tapes or records free on loan to anyone who cannot read normal printed material because of visual or physical handicaps. "Talking" books produced by this organization are fundamental aids to high school and college students and persons who require educational or specialized material in the pursuit of their occupations. These recordings also may be obtained from many local and state libraries. Tape players or record players are loaned free to persons who are legally blind. Information can be obtained from public libraries or organizations for blind persons.

FACILITATING INDEPENDENCE IN ADL FOR BLIND PERSONS

1. Place clothing in specific locations in drawers and closets.
2. Place food and cooking utensils in specific locations in cupboards and/or refrigerator.
3. Encourage use of cane when walking.
4. Keep furniture and household objects in specific places.
5. When assisting a blind person in walking, let the person take your arm (Figure 65-11).
6. Provide descriptions of food on the plate using clock placement of food; for example, put the peas at "7 o'clock." Cut food as appropriate.
7. Always permit blind persons to pull out their own chairs and seat themselves.

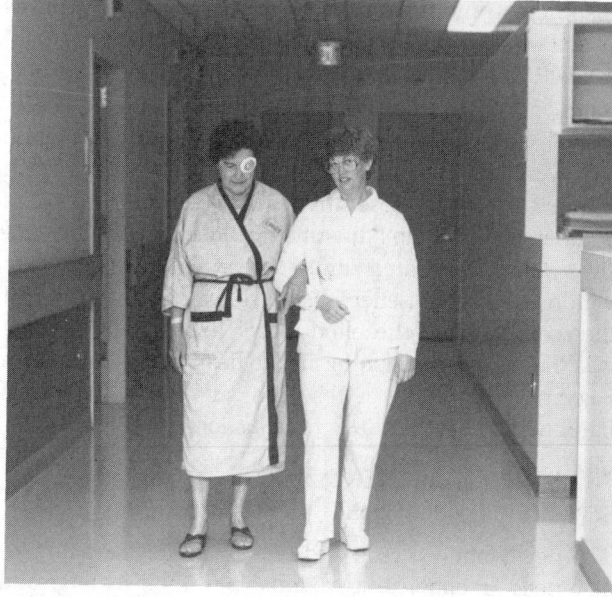

FIGURE 65-11 Ambulation of peson who cannot see. Note that patient is holding nurse's arm and is led without being held.

*15 W. 16th St., New York, NY 10011.
†79 Madison Ave, New York, NY 10016.
*20 Roszell Rd, Princeton, NJ 08540.

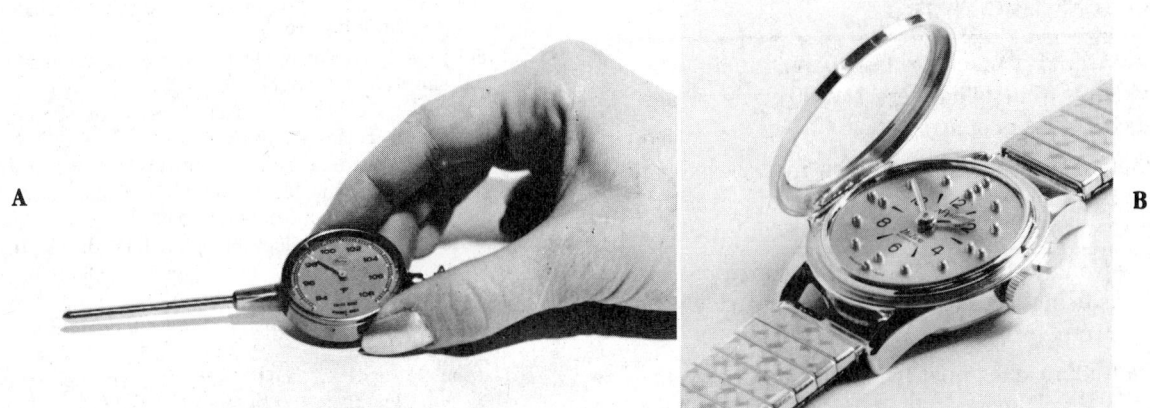

FIGURE 65-12 A, Dial-type clinical thermometer with unbreakable stem. Braille (raised) dots mark scale, one dot at odd numbers and two at even numbers. Raised line is at 98°6 F. Button is pushed to register temperature, which remains set until button is released. Needle then returns to zero. **B,** One of many models of watches available in both braille and ink print. (Courtesy American Foundation for the Blind, New York.)

GOVERNMENT ASSISTANCE

Legal blindness entitles a person to certain federal assistance. An amendment to the Social Security Act made provision for assistance to blind persons, and now all 50 states and all territories have approved plans for such aid. Assistance through this program is based on need. The Internal Revenue Act of 1948 permits blind persons an extra personal deduction in reporting income. In 1943 the federal government established a counseling and placement service for the blind in the Vocational Rehabilitation Administration. This agency, now called the Social and Rehabilitation Service (SRS), shares rehabilitation costs with the states. The Veterans Administration provides a substantial pension for the veteran who has had an enucleation of both eyes.

CHAPTER SUMMARY

- Normal healthy eyes do not need special treatment.
- The eyes should be examined by an ophthalmologist or optometrist at regular intervals throughout life.
- When administering more than one eye drop at a time, wait 5 minutes between installations.
- Many systemic diseases have eye manifestations.
- Following any chemical burn, the eye must be irrigated immediately before transportation to a physician.
- Acute bacterial conjunctivitis (pinkeye) is highly contagious.
- Teaching the person who has a corneal transplant includes instruction about medications and assessment for corneal graft rejection.
- Cataracts most commonly occur as a result of the aging process.
- The person with glaucoma may need help to adhere to a lifetime of medication therapy.
- Common factors placing the person at risk for a retinal detachment include myopia, trauma, and aphakia.
- Diabetic retinopathy occurs in about 90% of persons who have had diabetes for 30 years.
- Macular degeneration causes loss of central vision and decreased ability to distinguish colors.
- Blindness imposes limitations on mobility, interaction with the environment, and the range of experiences readily available to the sighted person.
- Loss of social supports is a major factor hindering adjustment to a visual impairment.
- Nursing care of the person with a visual impairment includes support and counseling, instruction about the aids and strategies that facilitate living with a visual impairment, and referral to appropriate community agencies.

QUESTIONS TO CONSIDER

- How would your care differ if the patient who suddenly went blind were age 20 years of age versus 70 years of age?

- What areas would you include in a class that you are teaching on the care of the eyes for nurses working in occupational health?

- How would you teach a visually impaired person who is using three different eye drops to identify the correct drops?

- What approaches might you consider for a person with glaucoma who refuses to administer eye drops four times a day as prescribed by the physician?

REFERENCES AND SELECTED READINGS

1. American Foundation for the Blind: Directory of Services for the blind and visually impaired in the US, ed 23, New York, 1988, The Foundation.
2. Arentsen JJ: The dry eye, J Ophthalmic Nurs Technol 6:134-137, 1987.
3. *Barker-Stotts K: Action STAT! hyphema, Nursing 18(12):33, 1988.
4. Bentz LN: Caring for and communicating with blind and visually impaired persons, J Visual Impair Blindness 81:472-481, 1987.
5. Bishop VE: Visually handicapped people and the law, J Visual Impair Blindness 81:53-58, 1987.
6. Boyd-Monk H and Steinmetz CG: Nursing care of the eye, Norwalk, CT, 1987, Appleton & Lange.
7. Brown MM and Spaeth GL: Improper topical self-administration of ocular medication among patients with glaucoma, Can J Ophthalmol 19(1):2-5, 1984.
8. Capino DG and Leibowitz HM: The elderly patient with cataract, Hosp Pract 22(3A):19-20, 23-24, 26, 33-37, 1987.
9. Capino DG and Leibowitz HM: Age-related macular degeneration, Hosp Pract 23(3):23-25, 29-30, 36,38+, 1988.
10. Carver JA: Cataract care made plain, Am J Nurs 87:626-630, 1987.
11. Centers for Disease Control: Recommendations for prevention of HIV transmission in health care settings, MMWR 36 (suppl 2:1S-18S, 1987.
12. Conant S and Budoff M: The development of sighted peoples' understanding of blindness, J Visual Impair Blindness 76(3):86-90, 1982.
13. *DeBase R et al: Postintraocular lens implants, Geriatr Nurs 9(6):342-343, 1988.
14. Department of Health and Human Services: Vision research: a national plan 1983-1987—the 1983 report of the National Advisory Eye Counsil, NIH Pub. No. 83-2469, 1983, Washington, DC, The Department.
15. Emerson DL: Facing loss of vision: the response of adults to visual impairment, J Visual Impair Blindness 75(2):41-45, 1981.

16. Folley FM et al: Alkaline injury to the eye, Ophthalmic Nurs Forum 5(1):1-4, 6-8, 1989.
17. Frank A and Werfel N: ECCE with phacoemulsification, J Ophthalmic Nurs Technol 7:62-67.
18. Goldstein J: Ocular side effects of systemic drugs, J Ophthalmic Nurs Technol 5:103-105, 1986.
19. Goldstein J: Pharmacology of ophthalmic drugs. I. Anesthetics, mydriatics, cycloplegics and ocular hypotensives, J Ophthalmic Nurs Technol 6:146-150, 1987.
20. Goldstein J: Pharmacology of ophthalmic drugs. II. Antiinflammatory and antiinfective agents, J Ophthalmic Nurs Technol 6:193-197, 1987.
21. Hamrick S et al: Therapeutic ultrasound, AORN-J 47:950-960, 1988.
22. Hanson CM et al: Glaucoma screening: an important role for NP's, Nurs Practi 12(12):14, 18, 21+, 1987.
23. Harrell RL and Strauss MA: Approaches to increasing assertive behavior and communication skills in blind and visually impaired persons. J Visual Impair Blindness 80:794-798, 1986.
24. Hill MM and Harley RK: Orientation and mobility for aged visually impaired people, J Visual Impair Blindness 78(2):49-53, 1984.
25. Hosein AM: The use of silicone oil in vitreoretinal surgery, J Ophthalmic Nurs Technol 7:126-129, 1988.
25a. Karb VK, Queener SF, and Freeman JB: Handbook of drugs for nursing practice, St. Louis, The CV Mosby Co, 1989.
26. Keller H: Out of the dark, Garden City, NY, 1913, Doubleday, Page & Co.
27. Kirchner C: Data on blindness and visual impairment in the US: a resource manual on social demographic characteristics, education, employment, income, and service delivery, ed 2, New York, 1989, American Foundation for the Blind.
28. Kohrman BD et al: Eye pain: ocular and nonocular causes, Hosp Pract 22(12):33-35, 38, 40+, 1987.
29. Lambert RM, West M, and Carlin K: Psychology of adjustment to visual deficiency: a conceptual model, J Visual Impair Blindness 75:193-196, 1981.
30. Large T: The effects of attitudes upon the blind: a reexamination, J Rehabil 48(2):33-34,45, 1982.
31. Lawlor MC: Common ocular injuries and disorders, J Emer Nurs 15(1):36-43, 1989.
32. MacInnis B: Lasers and the eye, Med Clin N Am 33:6045-47,6051, 1989.
33. Maerov PH: Ocular emergencies, Med Clin N Am 33:6004-6013, 1989.
34. Maise AR, Silberman R, and Trief E: Aging and visual impairment, J Visual Impair Blindness 81:323-325, 1987.
35. Melamed M: The injured eye at first sight, Emerg Med 20(17):89-9, 92, 97-8, 1988.
36. Mettler R: Blindness and managing the environment, J Visual Impair Blindness 81:472-481, 1987.
37. Moore JE: Impact of family attitudes toward blindness/visual impairment on the rehabilitation process, J Visual Impair Blindness 78:100-105, 1984.
38. National Society to Prevent Blindness, Operational Research Department: Vision problems in the United States: a statistical analysis, New York, 1980, The Society.
39. Nemshick LA, McCay V, and Ludman F: The impact of retinitis pigmentosa on young adults: psychological, educational, vocational, and social considerations, J Visual Impair Blindness 80:859-862, 1986.
40. Newell F: Ophthalmology: principles and practices, ed 6, St Louis, 1986, The CV Mosby Co.
40a. Nowell P: Lasers in ophthamology, Nurs Clin N Am 25(3):635-643, 1990.

*References preceded by an asterisk are particularly well suited for student reading.

41. *OTC eye drops and blindness, Nurses Drug Alert 12(7):56, 1988.

42. *Pashby T: Eye injuries in sports, J Ophthalmic Nurs Technol 8:99-101, 1989.

43. Peck AF and Uslan MM: Beliefs about public attitudes toward the blind. J Rehabil 46(2):36-39, 1980.

44. Ponchillia SV and LaGrow S: Independent glucose monitoring by functionally blind diabetics, J Visual Impair Blindness 82:50-53, 1988.

45. Rakes SM and Reed WH: Psychological management of loss of vision, Am J Ophthalmol 17(4):178-180, 1982.

46. Resnick R: An exploratory study of the lifestyles of congenitally blind adults, J Visual Impair Blindness 77:476-481, 1983.

47. Rickelman BL and Blaylock JN: Behaviors of sighted individuals perceived by blind persons as hindrances to self-reliance in blind persons, J Visual Impair Blindness 778:11, 1983.

48. Roach VG: What you should know about diabetic retinopathy, J Ophthalmic Nurs Technol 7:166-169, 1988.

49. Schein JD: Acquired monocular disability, J Visual Impair Blindness 82:279-281, 1988.

50. Smith S: Day care cataract surgery. The patient's perspective, J Ophthalmic Nurs Technol 6:50-55, 1987.

51. Smith S: Diabetic Retinopathy, Insight XIV(4):22-26, 1989.

52. Smith SJ: Sensory deprivation and the ophthalmic patient, J Ophthalmic Nurs Technol 8:148-154, 1989.

53. Smith SJ and Drance SM: Difficulties patients have at home after cataract surgery, Can J Ophthalmol 19(1):6-9, 1984.

54. Spencer RE: Transitions: being blind in a sighted world, J Ophthalmic Nurs Technol 7:220-222, 1988.

55. Stetten D: Sounding Board: Coping with blindness, N Engl J Med 305:458-460, 1981.

56. Stout JP: Psychological problems of visually impaired diabetic patients, Semin Ophth 2:62-67, 1987.

57. Vaughan D and Asbury T: General ophthalmology, ed 11, Los Altos, 1986, Lange Publications.

58. Vader L: End stage glaucoma and enucleation: an ophthalmic nursing challenge, Ophthalmic Nurs Forum 3(4):1-8, 1987.

59. Vickers R: A psychological approach to attitudes toward blind persons, J Visual Impair Blindness 81:326-327, 1987.

60. Wagner-Lampl A and Oliver GW: Bringing imagery into the world of visual impairment, J Visual Impair Blindness 82:373-377, 1988.

61. Whitton S: Managing detachment with retinal tacks, J Ophthalmic Nurs Technol 5:91-93, 1986.

62. Yanuzzi LA, Gitter K, and Judson PH: Lasers in ophthalmology, J Ophthalmic Nurs Technol 7:199-203, 1988.

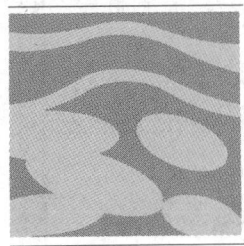

CHAPTER 66

Assessment of the Ear

LINDA T. SCHURING

CHAPTER OBJECTIVES

After studying this chapter, the student should be able to:
1 Describe the basic structure and function of the temporal bone and ear.
2 Describe behavioral clues suggesting loss of hearing.
3 Perform a nursing assessment of the ear for hearing and balance.
4 Recognize normal findings in the ears.
5 Identify specific diagnostic tests for hearing and balance.
6 Describe the role of the nurse in the detection of hearing and balance problems.

Nurses are involved in every aspect of the care of the patient with ear problems, including prevention, detection, and treatment of hearing and vestibular disorders. Ear problems are very common, can occur at any age, and often require immediate attention.

The ear and hearing are recognized together as one of the five senses of the human body. Hearing and balance are very important in our activities of daily living. Sound helps us to be in touch with our environment, adding aesthetic pleasure, as well as warnings of danger. The sense of hearing is essential for normal development and maintenance of speech. The ability to communicate with others depends on the ability to hear. The ear also contains the organs of balance that relay information about the body's position and direction of body motions to the brain.

ROLE OF NURSE

The nurse must be able to look at the patient with ear problems holistically. In other words, does the ear problem interfere with the patient's activities of daily living such as working, talking on the telephone, or walking? How does the patient cope with the temporary or permanent loss of hearing or balance?

A nurse might choose to specialize in the field of otolaryngology. Otolaryngology is the sum of the knowledge concerning the ears, nose, and throat or the head and neck. An otolaryngologist is a physician who treats diseases of the ear, nose, and throat. The subspecialty of otolaryngology is otology, the branch of medicine dealing only with the ear and its diseases. An otologist is a physician who has specialized in studying and treating the ear and its diseases. A nurse may choose to focus the practice of nursing on patients with ear problems. The Society of Otorhinolaryngology and Head-Neck Nurses, Inc., a specialty organization, provides education and growth opportunities.

However, every nurse, regardless of education or focus of care, should be prepared to both examine the outer ear and grossly assess the patient's hearing and equilibrium. Very often nurses participate in case findings of persons with hearing and balance disorders, as well as in the rehabilitation of these individuals.

The nurse can help find and direct the person with a hearing loss or balance problem and the family to the appropriate agencies for assistance. There might be ways of improving hearing through medical or surgical therapy. If the loss is irreversible, aural rehabilitation might make it possible for the person with a hearing loss to understand and communicate with others. The detection of patients with some degree of hearing impairment is an important nursing responsibility. Often the nurse is the first member of the health team to be approached by the patient regarding problems with the ear.

THE EAR AND COMMUNICATION

Personal communication involves two aspects of hearing. Hearing is used not only to receive information but also to monitor one's own voice. Therefore a person who is deaf from birth will have difficulty in learning to speak and difficulty in speaking normally. In addition, any level of hearing impairment will alter both aspects of communication.

Behavioral clues are useful in the assessment of hearing difficulties as seen in the box on p. 1948. Per-

BEHAVIORAL CLUES SUGGESTING LOSS OF HEARING

Any adult who exhibits one or more of the following traits:

Is irritable, hostile, hypersensitive in interpersonal relations

Has difficulty in hearing upper frequency consonants

Complains about people mumbling

Turns up volume on television

Asks for frequent repetition and answers questions inappropriately

Loses sense of humor, becomes grim

Leans forward to hear better, face serious and strained

Shuns large- and small-group audience situations

Might appear aloof and "stuck up"

Complains of ringing in the ears

Has an unusually soft or loud voice

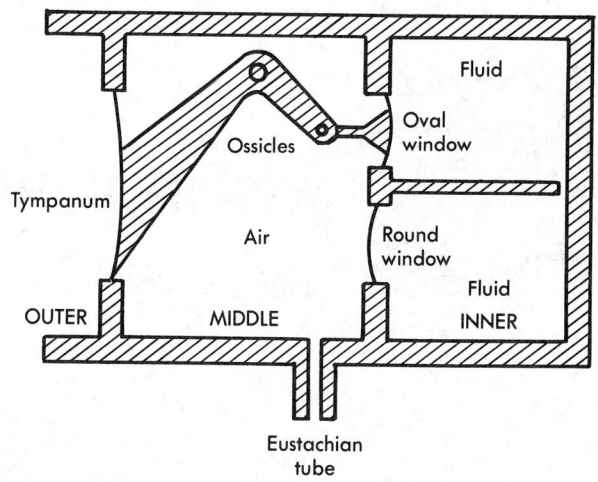

FIGURE 66-1 Diagrammatic representation of transmission of sound impulses from outer to inner ear.

sons who exhibit any of these behavioral clues should have their ears examined by an otolaryngologist who will obtain a hearing test. In this way a complete evaluation of the hearing problem can be made to determine the extent of the loss and its possible correction and the cause of the hearing loss.

The ears are a pair of complex sensory organs located midway on either side of the head. The position of the ears is important, because the use of both ears simultaneously produces binaural hearing and allows us to detect the direction of sound. A person detects the direction from which a sound comes in two ways: (1) by the time lag between the sound entry into one ear compared to the sound entry into the other ear, and (2) by the intensities of sounds in both ears. Each ear is also responsible for sending signals to the brain for the maintenance of equilibrium. Therefore the two *major functions* of the ears are *hearing* and *balance*.

Nerve impulses are transmitted between the ear and the brain by way of the eighth cranial nerve, called the acoustic or vestibulocochlear nerve. The acoustic portion of the ear responsible for hearing is innervated by the cochlear branch, and the vestibular portion responsible for equilibrium and posture is innervated by the vestibular branch.

Sound is transmitted from the external ear to the inner ear by two routes, *air conduction* and *bone conduction*. Air conduction is the transmission of sound vibration through the middle ear, involving the tympanic membrane and the ossicles (Figure 66-1). Bone conduction is the transmission of sound vibration through the skull to the inner ear. A comparison between the air conduction measurement and the bone conduction measurement gives valuable information for diagnosis.

Sound energy (mechanical energy) is first transformed into neural energy (electrical energy) and is

then decoded by the brain for hearing. In a similar way, the inner ears send impulses to the brain that are decoded to maintain normal balance.

EAR STRUCTURE, FUNCTION, AND ASSESSMENT

The ears are housed in the temporal bones of the skull. Each ear is divided into three parts. The first part is the *external ear,* which contains a sound-collecting portion (a short conducting tube with a membrane at its deepest end) (Figure 66-2). The second part is the *middle ear,* which is an air-containing cavity in the petrous portion of the temporal bone. Three small bones traverse this cavity, and a small (eustachian) tube connects the middle ear to the pharynx. The third part is the *internal ear,* which consists of membranous sacs and ducts encased in bony canals. The cochlea, which is specific for hearing, and the vestibular canals, which help to maintain equilibrium, are found in the internal ear.

THE TEMPORAL BONE

Understanding the structure and function of the temporal bone is necessary not only for physical assessment, but also as a basis for understanding the hearing and balance tests and the normal hearing and balance process.

The human skull is composed of 22 bones: 13 facial bones, eight cranial bones, and the mandible. Two of the eight cranial bones are the temporal bones that house the ears. The paired temporal bones are part of both the base and the lateral wall of the skull. Each of the *temporal bones* can be *divided* into *four parts: squamous, mastoid, petrous,* and *tympanic.* If the external opening of the ear canal is used as a reference point, the squamous part is upward, the mastoid part is backward, the tympanic part is forward and downward,

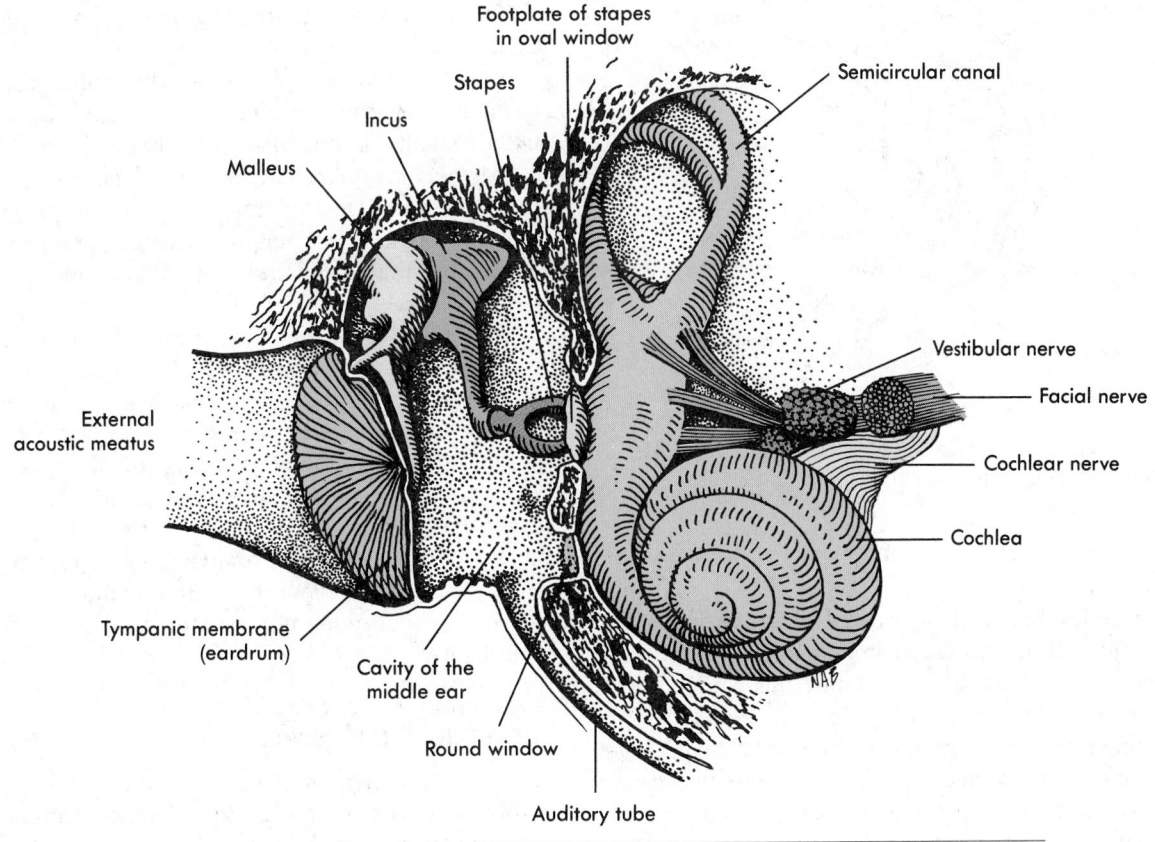

FIGURE 66-2 Structures of the ear.

and the petrous portion is forward toward the face. The temporal bone interfaces with the sphenoid, parietal, and occipital bones.

The temporal bone is the hardest bone in the human body and provides adequate protection for the organs of hearing and balance. The function of the temporal bone is to house the external and internal auditory canals, the mastoid air cells, the blood vessels and nerves, the labyrinth, and the cochlea.

THE EXTERNAL EAR
STRUCTURE AND FUNCTION

The external ear or auricle consists of the *pinna* and the *external auditory canal,* or the ear canal. The ears are located on each side of the head at approximately eye level. An imaginary line drawn from the outer canthus of the eye to the top of the ear should be straight and almost parallel to the floor. The pinna is attached to the side of the head at approximately a 10-degree angle.

The pinna is composed of cartilage covered by skin. There is little fat except in the lobule. Hair covers most of the ear but is usually rudimentary except in the region of the tragus and the antitragus. Sebaceous glands also are found on the surface.

The pinna is attached to the side of the head by skin,

ligaments, and muscles. Muscles of the pinna are innervated by a branch of the facial nerve.

The parts of the pinna are illustrated in Figure 66-3. The *concha* is the deepest part and leads to the ear canal. The *helix* is the outmost rim of the ear and leads inferiorly into the lobule. The concha is bounded anteriorly by a prominent process called the tragus, which projects posteriorly over the entrance to the ear canal.

In human embryology, the ears are formed at the same time as the renal system. Therefore abnormalities in the shape and form of the pinna might be found in conjunction with renal abnormalities. In addition, in the sixth month of fetal life, the human ear possesses a small tubercle, a downward protrusion of the helix (close to the resemblance of the ears of some adult monkeys) named Darwin's tubercle. If present, Darwin's tubercle is a normal finding.

The ear canal extends from the concha of the pinna at one end to the eardrum at the other end, in a path inward, forward, and downward in an adult. It is an S-shaped curve through the temporal bone, approximately 2.5 cm (1 in.) in length. The lumen is irregular in outline and constricts about midway in its course and again near the eardrum. Skin lines the ear canal and furnishes an external covering for the eardrum. Approxi-

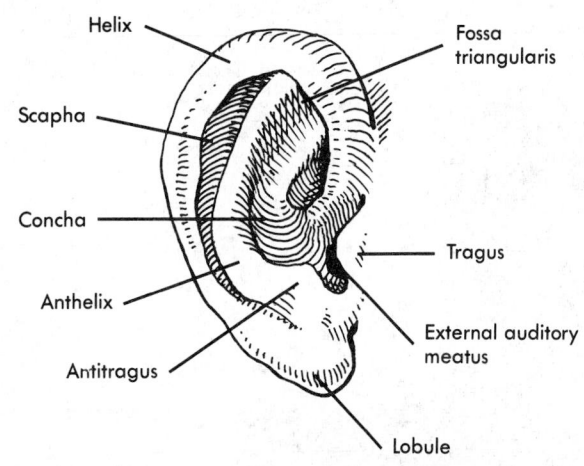

FIGURE 66-3 Pinna of the ear.

mately the first half of the ear canal is *cartilaginous*. In the second half, the cartilage stops and the supporting wall becomes *osseous*. The skin lining this bony portion of the canal is thin and highly sensitive. The skin contains numerous fine hairs and sebaceous glands. *Ceruminous glands* (modified sweat glands) produce *cerumen* or *ear wax*. The openings of these ducts appear as dark points to the unaided eye.

The funnel shape of the external ear provides for collection and direction of sound. Together with the head, the pinna and ear canal act as an integrated system that transforms sound on its way to the eardrum. For example, the external ear actually amplifies certain frequencies.

The secretion of wax functions as a protective mechanism. Wax is to the ears as tears are to the eyes. The sticky consistency of wax, along with the fine hairs of the ears, help to cleanse the ear canal of foreign matter. At times the wax must be mechanically removed from the ear.

ASSESSMENT OF THE EXTERNAL EAR

Inspection and *palpation* are the two methods used to assess the external ear. The external ear should be inspected for size, configuration, and angle of attachment to head. An imaginary line is drawn from the greatest protruberance on the occiput to the outside corner (lateral canthus) of the eye. When the top of the pinna falls below the eye-occipital line, the angle of attachment is significantly more than 10 degrees. The configuration of the pinna is observed for gross deformity. Whether the ears protrude and the degree of protrusion, the color of the skin of the ear, and whether any additional skin tags are present is noted. The skin of the ear should be smooth and without breaks or inflammation, especially behind the ear in the crevice. Note any lumps, skin le-

sions, or cysts by charting approximate size and location.

Palpation and manipulation of the pinna produce information regarding tenderness, nodules, or tophi. *Tophi* are small, hard nodules in the helix that are deposits of uric acid crystals characteristic of gout. In palpation, move the pinna, feel the mastoid area, and press on the tragus. Note if any of the manipulations produce pain or discomfort that could indicate inflammation or infection.

Inspection of the ear canal is carried out by direct observation, otoscopy, or microscopic examination. For direct observation, the *adult* is asked to tip the head slightly to the opposite side while the nurse pulls the pinna, up, back, and out. A penlight is then used to inspect the ear canal for any abnormalities such as extreme narrowing of the ear canal, excessive wax, redness, scaliness, swelling, drainage, cysts, or foreign objects. Normally, none of these aforementioned signs are present. Visualization of the eardrum with this method is unlikely.

THE TYMPANIC MEMBRANE
STRUCTURE AND FUNCTION

The tympanic membrane separates the middle ear (tympanic cavity) from the ear canal. The eardrum is a thin, semitransparent membrane, obliquely directed downward and inward. Nearly oval in shape, this membrane is approximately 9 mm in diameter and pearly gray in color.

A few distinguishing landmarks of the normal eardrum are the *annulus,* which is the thickened border that attaches the eardrum to the temporal bone; the *umbo,* the most depressed point where the first ossicle attaches to the eardrum, almost in the center; the *pars flaccida,* a small triangular area above the short process of the malleus; and the largest portion of the tympanic membrane, the *pars tensa* (Figure 66-4).

The *tympanic membrane* is formed by three layers: an outer skin layer continuous with the skin of the external ear canal, a fibrous supporting middle layer, and an inner mucosal layer continuous with the mucosal lining of the middle ear cavity. The pars tensa (about four fifths of the eardrum) contains all three layers, whereas the pars flaccida is composed of only two layers. The fibrous middle layer is missing and allows the pars flaccida to be more vulnerable to negative pressure.

The tympanic membrane serves as a common membrane between the external ear canal and the middle ear cleft. The tympanic membrane protects the middle ear and conducts sound vibrations from the external ear to the ossicles. The sound pressure applied to the *stapes* in the oval window connecting to the inner ear is 22 times greater than the pressure exerted by the sound pressure on the eardrum. The force of the sound vibra-

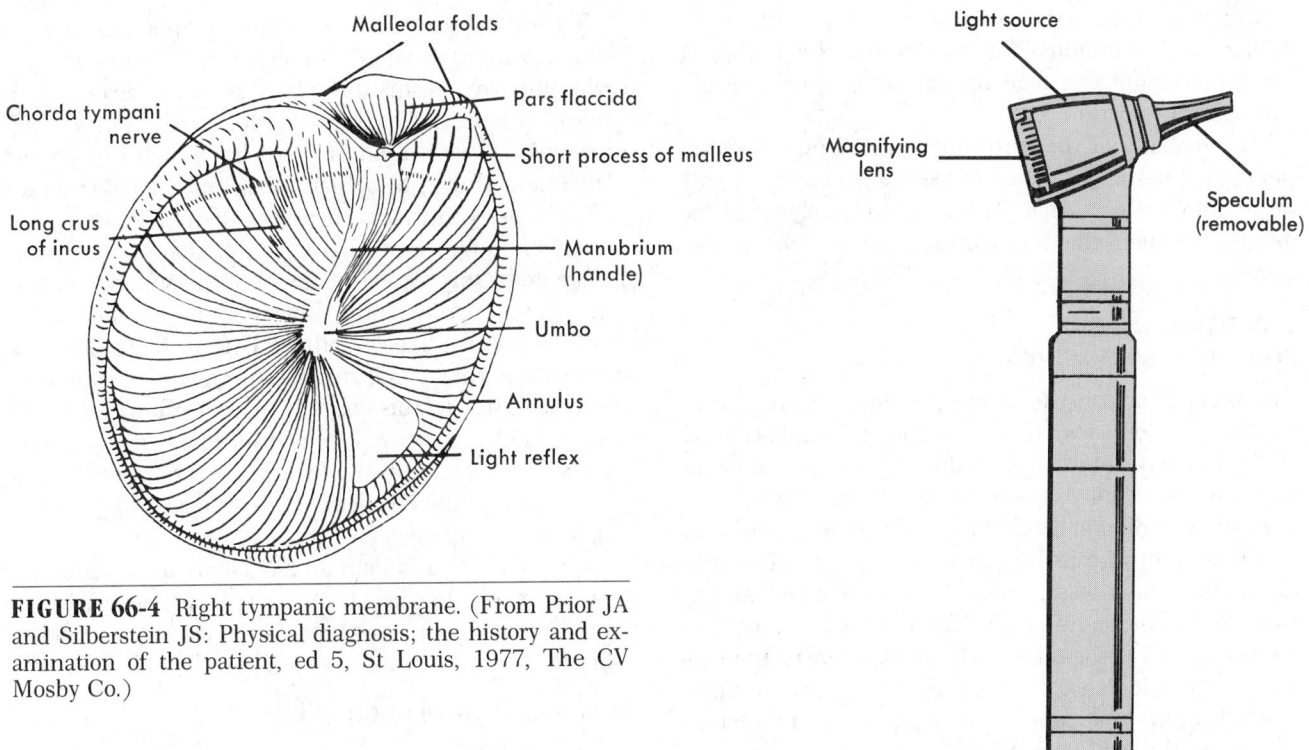

FIGURE 66-4 Right tympanic membrane. (From Prior JA and Silberstein JS: Physical diagnosis; the history and examination of the patient, ed 5, St Louis, 1977, The CV Mosby Co.)

FIGURE 66-5 Otoscope.

tions increases after transmission from a larger area to a smaller area.

ASSESSMENT OF THE EARDRUM

The eardrum is located within the head at the end of the only skin-lined canal in the body, the ear canal. Therefore visualization is difficult and requires illumination. The addition of magnification also allows a more accurate assessment of the ear. Portable otoscopes are the most common instrumentation used; therefore nurses should know how to use an otoscope. An otoscope is a device consisting of a handle, a light source, a magnifying lens, and an attachment for visualizing the ear canal and eardrum (Figure 66-5). Some otoscopes have a pneumatic device for injecting air into the ear canal to test the mobility and integrity of the eardrum.

Specula for the otoscope come in a variety of sizes. The diameter of the meatus and the length of the ear canal vary; thus the one with the largest diameter that fits comfortably into the ear canal should be chosen. The light source must be checked for brightness. If the light appears yellowish or dim (like a flashlight with weak batteries), the batteries must be recharged or replaced.

The otoscope is held with the dominant hand, with the hand resting against the patient's head. In this manner, should the patient move suddenly, the otoscope will move also, so that the nurse will be less likely to damage the external canal. With the nondominant hand, the pinna is pulled up, back, and out, thus straightening the

ear canal. While doing this, the patient's head should be gently tilted away from the nurse and the speculum inserted slowly and carefully into the ear canal. The nurse's eye is brought close to the magnifying lens to view the ear canal and eardrum. The otoscope should be advanced far enough to make a good seal to facilitate the use of the pneumatic bulb.

The ear canal is observed while the speculum is entering and leaving. The otoscope is moved in a circular fashion to allow for visualization of the entire ear canal. Any abnormalities such as extreme narrowing of the ear canal, nodules, redness, scaliness, swelling, drainage, cysts, foreign objects, or excessive wax should be noted. Visualization of the eardrum will be impaired by most of these abnormalities. Sometimes the ear canal must be cleaned of wax, dead skin, and other debris. Wax and debris can be removed with a cerumen spoon, suction aspirator, and irrigation (see Chapter 67).

The normal eardrum is slightly conical, quite shiny and smooth, and pearly gray in color. The position of the drumhead is oblique with respect to the ear canal. In the presence of disease, not only does the color of the eardrum change but also other abnormalities such as retraction of the eardrum, bulging of the eardrum, perforation of the eardrum, or a white plaque in the eardrum may exist.

Carefully inspect the entire eardrum, including the border or the annulus. The umbo and the long and short process of the malleus should be easily visible through the eardrum.

The mobility of the eardrum is tested by using the pneumatic device on the otoscope to inject a small puff of air into the ear canal. The eardrum is observed for gentle movement that normally accompanies this procedure.

THE MIDDLE EAR
STRUCTURE AND FUNCTION

The middle ear consists of the middle ear cleft and its contents, the ossicles, the oval and round windows, and the eustachian tube. The middle ear cleft or tympanic cavity is an air-filled space located within the petrous bone of the temporal bone. If the middle ear is viewed in relationship to surrounding structures, the middle ear is above the jugular fossa, behind the carotid canal, and in front of the mastoid air cells. The external auditory canal is external to the middle ear, and the labyrinth is internal. The middle ear is transversed by a chain of three movable bones that connect the tympanic membrane to the labyrinth (see Figure 66-2).

The three smallest bones in the body are called the *malleus* (hammer), the *incus* (anvil), and the *stapes* (stirrup). The ossicles have been given these common names because of their appearance. The outermost ossicle is the malleus, which is firmly attached to the tympanic membrane and is the largest of the auditory ossicles. The innermost ossicle is the stapes, which is fixed in the oval window, in direct contact with the perilymph of the inner ear, and the smallest of the auditory ossicles. The incus lies between the other two and has the same shape as a tooth with two roots.

The function of these *ossicles* is to *mechanically transmit sound* vibrations. The ossicles are held in place by muscles, ligaments, and joints and offer protective mechanisms from loud sounds. The light weight of these ossicles allows for ease of transmission, particularly of high-frequency sounds. The ossicles provide an efficient means by which the movement of air molecules can be transferred as movement to the fluid molecules that circulate in the inner ear. Liquids offer more resistance than air and need more force to produce movement; the ossicular chain produces this force against the inner ear fluids.

There are two windows in the middle ear, the oval window and the round window, so named because of their shape. The *oval window* is not a true window, since the footplate of the stapes covers it. The oval window is the opening into the inner ear where sound vibrations enter. The *round window* is a true window and provides an exit for sound vibrations from the inner ear. The windows are discussed more fully in a later section.

The *eustachian tube* is a channel approximately 35 mm (1½ inch) in length through which the middle ear communicates with the pharynx. The structure is mostly bone, cartilage, and fibrous tissue and extends downward, forward, and inward from each middle ear. The lining of the eustachian tube is mucous membrane continuous with that which lines the middle ear cavity at one end and that which lines the pharynx at the opposite end. Only a small segment at the superior end remains open permanently; otherwise the walls are in direct contact with each other. This is to prevent the sound of normal nasal respiration and one's own voice from passing up the eustachian tube into the middle ear. A failure of normal function leads to many middle ear disorders. However, during yawning, swallowing, and sneezing, the eustachian tube is opened by the tensor veli palatine muscle.

The eustachian tube normally allows air to enter and leave the middle ear. This tube is responsible for both ventilation and pressure regulation, which are necessary for normal hearing.

ASSESSMENT OF THE MIDDLE EAR
Objective Data

Assessment of the middle ear involves both measuring hearing and inspecting the middle ear through the tympanic membrane with the otoscope or other ear microscopes. Gross assessment of hearing can be accomplished by the presentation of a sound (whisper or watch tick) and the comparison of one ear to the other, as well as the comparison of the nurse's hearing and responses (provided the nurse has normal hearing) to the patient's responses. Tuning forks are also used to assess hearing. Typical tuning fork tests are the *Weber* and *Rinne* tests (p. 1948). *Behavior clues* (p. 1954) may indicate a hearing loss. Table 66-1 lists *subjective data* to be collected.

TABLE 66-1 Subjective data to be collected

Symptoms	Characteristics
Pain (earache)	Onset, severity, radiation
Itching	Site, intensity duration
Drainage	Onset, occurrence, consistency, type
Fullness (pressure)	Duration, association with other symptoms
Loss of hearing	Onset, location, duration
Ringing in the ear (tinnitus)	Onset, frequency, loudness, location, duration
Dizziness (vertigo)	Onset, frequency, sensation, duration
Facial weakness	Onset, extent, pain

THE MASTOID
STRUCTURE AND FUNCTION

The term *mastoid* (which means breastlike) pertains to the mastoid bone, part of the temporal bone; the mastoid process, which is conical-shaped and part of the mastoid bone; the mastoid antrum, a cavity that is a large cavity continuous with the middle ear; and the mastoid air cells that branch off of the mastoid cavity. The mastoid cavity and cells are within the mastoid bone, which is located directly posterior to the pinna or external ear. The mastoid process can be felt as a bony protuberance behind the lower portion of the pinna.

The system of air-filled cells and cavity of the mastoid bone aids the middle ear in adjusting to changes in pressure. Therefore the mastoid system is a buffer to the middle ear. Equally important, this system of cavities and air cells lightens the mastoid bone. Because humans stand erect and have a slender neck, the weight of the skull becomes important. The denseness of the temporal bone is necessary for inner ear protection, and the mastoid air system lightens the weight of this protective bony structure.

ASSESSMENT OF THE MASTOID

The assessment of the mastoid bone and process is performed by palpating the bone behind the pinna. A normal mastoid bone is smooth, hard, and not tender. In comparing the mastoid bones on either side, the mas-

toid process is not always equal in size. This fact is sometimes mentioned by a patient but is not pathologic. Inspection of the mastoid area should show normal skin.

THE INNER EAR
STRUCTURE AND FUNCTION

The *inner ear* is located deep in the petrous part of the temporal bone and is the *organ for hearing* and *equilibrium.* The inner ear is a complex system of intercommunicating chambers and connecting tubes composed of two major structures: the *bony labyrinth* and the *membranous labyrinth,* which lies within but does not completely fill the bony labyrinth. The bony labyrinth is the rigid capsule in which the membranous labyrinth lies and consists of the vestibule, the three semicircular canals, and the cochlea (Figure 66-6). The *vestibule* is the connecting chamber between the semicircular canals posteriorly and the cochlea anteriorly. The *cochlea* looks like a snail shell and has two compartments. In cross section, the upper compartment is called the *scala vestibuli* and leads from the oval window to the apex of the spiral. The lower compartment is called the *scala tympani* and continues from the apex of the cochlea to the round window. Thus this system allows sound vibrations to enter at the oval window and exit at the round window. The main function of the cochlea is hearing. There are three semicircular canals: the supe-

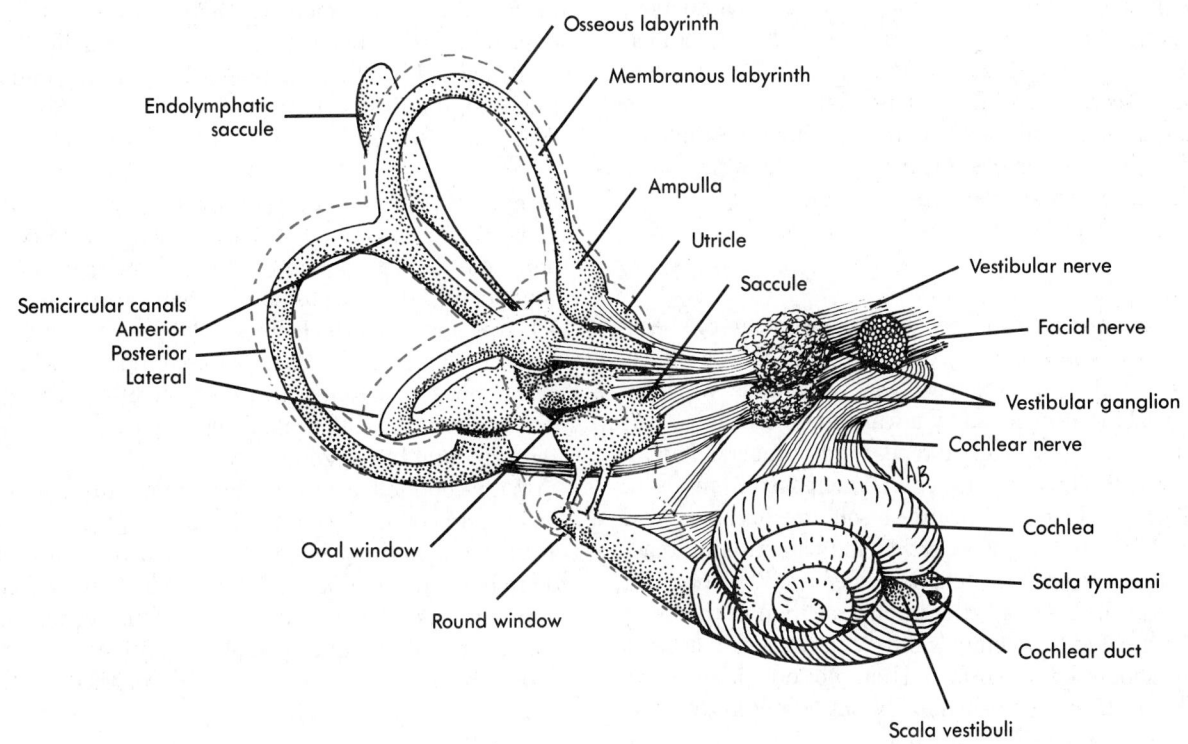

FIGURE 66-6 Structures of inner the ear.

rior, the lateral (horizontal), and the posterior. These canals provide the sense of balance.

The membranous labyrinth within the bony labyrinth is bathed in a fluid called *perilymph*. The membranous labyrinth consists of the utricle, saccule, three semicircular ducts, the cochlear duct, and the end organ for hearing called the organ of Corti. The membranous labyrinth contains a fluid called *endolymph*. The utricle, saccule, and the three semicircular canals are the sense organs responsible for position and balance. The semicircular canals are arranged to sense rotational movement, whereas the utricle and saccule are involved with linear movements. The cochlear duct is located in the cochlea between the scala vestibuli and the scala tympani. Membranes separate the cochlear duct from the scala vestibuli, and the scala tympani (called the vestibular membrane) from the basilar membranes. As sound vibrations enter the perilymph at the oval window and travel along the scala vestibuli, they pass through the vestibular membrane, enter the cochlear duct, and cause movement of the basilar membrane.

The organ of Corti is located on the basilar membrane and stretches from the base to the apex of the cochlea. This structure transforms mechanical sound vibrations into neural activity and separates sound into different frequencies. This electrochemical impulse travels via the acoustic nerve to the temporal cortex of the brain and is interpreted as meaningful sound.

ASSESSMENT OF THE INNER EAR

The inner ears are inaccessible to direct examination. However, some inferences concerning their condition can be made by testing auditory and vestibular function. A gross assessment of the patient's hearing can be made simply through conversation and by evaluating the logical sequences of replies. Assessment of the inner ear is divided into two sections: tests for auditory acuity and tests for balance.

Auditory Acuity

Each ear must be tested separately to estimate the hearing. One of the patient's ears is occluded with a finger. While standing 1 to 2 feet away, the nurse whispers two-syllable numbers softly toward the unoccluded ear, and the patient is asked to repeat the numbers. The intensity of the nurses voice can be increased from a soft, medium, or loud whisper to a soft, medium, or loud voice. If the nurse suspects that the patient is lip reading, the nurse's face should be turned away. The patient is asked if hearing is better in one ear than in the other ear. If the auditory acuity is different, the ear that hears better should be tested first. Then, noise is produced in the better-hearing ear by rapidly but gently moving the finger in the patient's ear canal while testing the other ear.

TABLE 66-2 Tuning fork tests for auditory acuity

Site of Problem	Weber Test	Rinne Test
NORMAL HEARING		
No problem	Tone heard in center of head	Air conduction lasts longer than bone conduction
CONDUCTIVE LOSS		
External or middle ear	Tone heard in poorer ear because ear not distracted by room noise	Bone conduction lasts longer than air conduction
SENSORINEURAL LOSS		
Inner ear	Tone heard in better ear because inner ear less able to receive vibrations[1]	Air conduction lasts longer than bone conduction

A watch tick can also be used to test hearing. However, a watch tick is a higher-pitched sound and less relevant to functional hearing than the voice test.

The tuning fork also provides a general estimate of hearing loss. The three major tuning fork tests date from the nineteenth century and are named after their originators: Weber, Rinne, and Schwabach.

Weber test. The tuning fork is set into vibration by striking the tines on the examiner's knuckles or knee. The rounded tip of the handle is placed on the patient's forehead or teeth. Placement on the teeth (even if the patient has false teeth) is generally more reliable. The patient is asked whether the tone is heard in the middle of the head, the right ear, or the left ear (Table 66-2). The Weber test is useful in cases of *unilateral loss*.

Rinne test. The vibrating tuning fork is shifted between two positions: against the mastoid bone (bone conduction) and 2 in. from the opening of the ear canal (air conduction). As the position is changed, the patient is asked to indicate which tone is louder (in front of the ear or behind the ear) or is asked to indicate when one of the tones is no longer heard (Table 66-2). The Rinne test is useful to differentiate between conductive and sensorineural hearing losses.

With conductive hearing loss, the pathways of normal sound conduction are blocked. However, vibrations against the mastoid bone can bypass the obstruction; therefore bone conduction lasts longer than air conduction. With sensorineural hearing loss, the acoustic nerve has decreased ability to perceive vibrations from either route; therefore normal patterns are reported by the patient.[3]

Schwabach test. This test is also used to differentiate between a conductive and sensorineural hearing loss. The Schwabach test compares the hearing of the examiner (who must have normal hearing) with the patient. However, the Rinne test has replaced this test.

These aforementioned tests can be performed at the bedside by the nurse to give some indication of the amount of hearing. More elaborate and specific hearing tests are performed in a soundproofed room.

Balance

Balance and equilibrium depend on *four systems* being intact: the *vestibular* (the labyrinth or inner ear), the *proprioceptive* (somatosensors) of joints and muscles, the *visual* (the eye), and the *cerebellar* (coordination). The sensations transmitted from the ears (that is, the somatosensors) and the inner ears are integrated in the brainstem and cerebellum and perceived in the cerebral cortex. *Dizziness* is most likely to occur when *two or more systems* are *impaired simultaneously* or when they transmit sensory information that is contradictory.

Assessment of the inner ear for balance should be accomplished by a thorough *history, observation of gait, gaze test for nystagmus,* and the *Romberg test.* The importance of the history and interview cannot be overemphasized. All patients bring some degree of anxiety regarding the illness to the interview and examination. Dizziness can have devastating effects on the patient's behavior. The disruption of the patient's routine, the severity of the attacks, and the fear of the unknown, can make the patient agitated, anxious, and depressed. The nurse must be aware of these feelings and demonstrate self-confidence, patience, courtesy, consideration, and gentleness.

The patient is asked to walk in one direction away from the examiner and then to turn and walk back. Posture, balance, swinging of the arms and movement of the legs should be observed. Normally, balance is easy; the arms swing at the sides, and when the patient turns, the face and head lead the rest of the body.

Nystagmus is the involuntary, rhythmic oscillation of the eyes. It is essentially a disorder of ocular posture but is associated with vestibular dysfunction. Nystagmus occurs normally when a person watches a rapidly moving object. To check for *gaze nystagmus*, the finger of the examiner is placed directly in front of the patient at eye level. The patient is asked to follow the finger without moving the head. The finger is moved slowly from the midline toward the ear in each direction. The eyes should be observed for any jerking movements. For example, if the eyes jerk quickly to the left and drift slowly back to the right, the patient has a left nystagmus. Nystagmus can be horizontal, vertical, or rotary.

For a *Romberg test*, the patient stands with feet together, without arm support, and with eyes open. Note ability to maintain an upright posture. Perform the same test with the eyes closed. Normally only a minimal amount of swaying exists. If the patient loses balance, this might indicate an inner ear problem (vestibular problem) or cerebellar ataxia. Dysfunction will be unbalance or positive Romberg test results.

Other noninvasive tests include hyperventilation, Valsalva maneuver, neck twist, and fistula test. Because these tests may simulate dizziness comparable to that which the patient is experiencing, more knowledge and special training is necessary to perform and interpret them.

DIAGNOSTIC OTOLOGIC TESTS

LABORATORY TESTS

Four laboratory tests are useful for assessment of ear problems: (1) blood tests, (2) ear cultures, (3) cerebral spinal fluid identification, and (4) pathologic tissue examination.

Blood tests that are diagnostic for systemic abnormalities are only secondarily significant for ear disease. For example, an elevated white blood count points to an infection, but is not diagnostic of ear disease. However, in the face of ear infection and in the absence of other infection, blood tests for infection are necessary for assessing ear infection.

Drainage from the ear canal or a surgical incision is usually *cultured* to identify the organism. This is especially necessary in acute infections to choose the appropriate antibiotic. When long-term drainage is present, such as in chronic otitis media, cultures are less helpful because gram negative bacillus cover up the original pathogen. In these cases many surgeons do not culture the drainage, but begin treatment with broad spectrum antibiotics.

When drainage is found in the ear, a dilemma is presented. Is this clear fluid *cerebral spinal fluid*? A fistula from the inner ear to the middle ear and external ear can produce cerebral spinal fluid. This pathway also can lead to meningitis by retrograde contamination. Therefore an analysis of clear fluid is often helpful in diagnosing the problem.

Pathologic examination of abnormal tissue from the ear canal or from other tissue harvested during surgery is necessary to both rule out a malignancy and identify unusual problems. In an infected ear, affected tissue is readily identified with pathologic assessment. If the surgeon is in doubt as to the findings, then a tissue sample (biopsy) is taken for examination. The surgical finding of *cholesteatoma* is usually documented by a pathologic examination.

RADIOLOGIC TESTS

The temporal bone and its structures are easily examined by diagnostic radiography because of the propensity of x-ray films to show bony structures. The oldest but not necessarily most useful tests are plane film radiography of the mastoid bone. To bypass certain bony structures and enhance other structures, specific views have been standardized. A standard mastoid series might include the Stenver, Owen, and Towne views. More recent x-ray film techniques, which are outlined in the following discussion, have largely replaced plane film radiography.

Polytomography, with its advantage of being able to focus on one plane, revealed the temporal bone for the first time. With frontal or lateral views, very small structures within the temporal bone (such as the ossicles) could be identified. In addition, the surgeon could assess the problems before surgery and anticipate the surgical treatment more closely.

The advantages of polytomography were further enhanced by *computed tomography (CAT) scanning.* The computer in a CAT scan mathematically reconstructs a cross section of the temporal bone from measurement of the x-ray film transmission. To show better soft tissue detail in the temporal bone, iodine enhancement is generally used. Thus an *enhanced CAT scan is the most commonly ordered CAT scan for the ear.*

Magnetic resonance imaging (MRI) is a totally different process. The advantage of MRI is that soft tissue details rather than bony structures are enhanced. Therefore, for the first time, the membranous organs, nerves, and blood vessels of the temporal bone can be examined.

An adjunct to radiography is *arteriography* and *venography* in which contrast dye is injected into blood vessels. These studies are specially useful for diagnosing vascular abnormalities in the temporal bone. Compression of the vessels can be recognized, and tumors of the temporal bone and related structures can be recognized in greater detail.

AUDIOMETRIC TESTS

Audiology is the study of hearing and hearing testing. A certified audiologist has a master's or Ph.D. degree and has a private practice associated with a hospital, with a speech and hearing clinic, or in an academic setting.

Hearing tests are conducted in soundproofed booths by an *audiologist.* *Hearing* is *measured* in a special unit named the *decibel,* a logarithmic function of sound intensity. The basic test of hearing is recorded on an audiogram, which records each ear according to air conduction of sound, bone conduction, and speech testing. The sound, in puretones or as speech, is presented through an audiometer. By varying the loudness of the puretones or speech, a hearing level is established. The use of earphones results in a puretone level or air conduction. The earphones are also used to measure the *level* of speech hearing (speech reception threshold) and the *understanding* of speech (discrimination). By pre-

senting the sound through a bone conduction oscillator placed on the mastoid bone, the middle ear structures are bypassed, and a bone conduction level is established. The bone conduction level is a level at which the cochlea can hear and is commonly referred to as the nerve hearing level.

A person with *normal* hearing would have the same air conduction as bone conduction hearing levels. Normal hearing is a range that was established nationally by measuring the hearing levels of the population, including all ages. Figure 66-7 relates normal hearing to other common noises.

Because the middle ear structures serve as a transformer that enhances sound and transfers sound to the inner ear (cochlea), a difference in hearing levels between air conduction and bone conduction results in a *conductive hearing loss.* A patient with a conductive hearing loss has a problem with the tympanic membrane, middle ear, or mastoid. Fortunately, most disorders causing a conductive hearing loss can be corrected

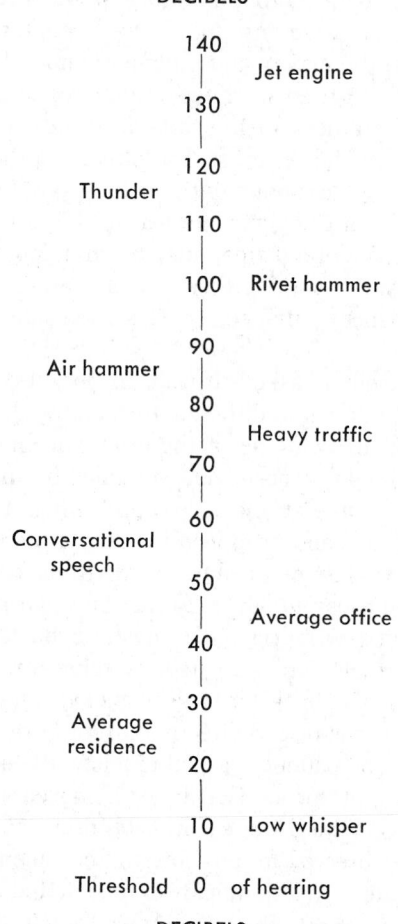

FIGURE 66-7 Intensity range of human hearing. Intensity levels of various environmental sounds and situations. (From Saunders WH et al: Nursing care in eye, nose, and throat disorders, ed 4, St Louis, 1979, The CV Mosby Co.)

by microsurgery. If the air and bone conduction levels are equal but not normal, a sensorineural nerve hearing loss occurs. Surgery cannot correct the problems that cause a *sensorineural hearing loss,* although a hearing aid is very useful if the discrimination of speech is adequate. A distinction is now being made between the sensory (cochlea) and neural (acoustic nerve) portions of a sensorineural hearing loss. It is quite common to find a patient with both a conductive and sensorineural hearing loss; this combination is called a *mixed hearing loss* (see Chapter 67).

Like any science, special testing of hearing is a large field in itself. Some of these tests are performed by the audiometer, whereas others are accomplished through computer-assisted instruments. The object of these special tests is to determine whether a lesion of the hearing system is located in the cochlea, in the acoustic nerve, or in the brain stem. The most common special tests performed by the audiometer are automatic audiometry or *Bekesy audiometry, tone decay* tests that measure the adaptation of sound, and the *short increment sensitivity index* (Sisi), useful to distinguish between cochlea or acoustic nerve lesions.

The most common test that uses other instruments is *brainstem audiology.* This test can be compared to an electroencephalogram (EEG) for hearing. By presenting a sound to the ear and measuring the response (computer averaging) in the brainstem, accurate diagnostic information can be obtained. Abnormal test results point to a lesion of the acoustic nerve or brainstem. Although there are other aspects of electrophysiologic assessments, *electrocochleography* is the only one clinically useful as of yet. In this test, the measurement of sound is taken from an electrode on the promontory passed through the tympanic membrane. In addition, the advent of the cochlear implant for patients with no usable hearing has generated new batteries of special tests.

A popular test used for differentiating problems in the middle ear is *tympanometry* or *impedance audiometry.* This automatic test of applying pressure to the tympanic membrane and measuring the result creates a distinctive tracing on a graft called a *tympanogram.* Abnormalities of the tympanogram point to the status of the middle ear, eustachian tube, and the ossicles. Tympanometry can also be used to measure the stapedial muscle reflex and its decay. This test measures the status of the acoustic nerve.

A series of tests for the vestibular system that assess balance by electrophysiologic means is also available. In some settings the tests are performed by audiologists, because audiometry is also used secondarily to assess balance problems. The physical proximity of the vestibular and cochlear systems in the labyrinth mirrors the juxtaposition of the clinical tests. Although the physical assessment of balance is important, the most common objective measurement of balance is accomplished by *electronystagmography* (ENG). The ENG instrument was developed to measure nystagmus in response to stimulation of the vestibular system. This stimulation includes testing the patient at rest in different positions for both the eyes and the head and with different temperatures in the ear canals, thus stimulating the semicircular canals. The different test results give an *electronystagmogram* that reflects the status of each labyrinth and can point to central nervous system disorders. Other means of testing the balance system, mostly research tools, include stimulation by rotary chair, pendulum swings, and postural changes. *Platform posturography* is a computerized test performed while the person is standing. This test can separate the balance problem into inner ear, visual and muscle stretch origins. The platform test helps to identify, quantify, and localize the source of vestibular disorders.

In addition to the tests of the eighth cranial nerve discussed above, mention of seventh facial nerve testing is necessary. Tests of the seventh cranial nerve are related to audiometric tests because the facial and acoustic nerves share the internal acoustic canal. The facial nerve is tested in the same way as other motor nerves with nerve conduction tests and muscle excitability tests. Also, the axillary functions of the facial nerve (taste and tearing) can also be measured. The facial and acoustic nerves are usually both involved in lesions of the temporal bone.

CHAPTER SUMMARY

✔ Detection of patients with a hearing impairment or a balance problem is an important nursing responsibility.

✔ Behavior can alert the nurse to the possibility of hearing impairment.

✔ The ear is housed in the temporal bone and divided into the external, middle, and inner ear.

✔ Sound vibrations reach the inner ear by mechanical energy through air conduction and bone conduction.

✔ The tympanic membrane is a common membrane between the external ear canal and the middle ear cleft.

✔ The otoscope is the most common instrument used to examine the ear.

✔ The functions of the eustachian tube are ventilation and pressure regulation, both of which are essential for normal hearing.

✔ The functions of the mastoid bone include helping the middle ear to adjust to pressure changes and lightening the weight of the skull.

✔ The inner ear transforms mechanical energy into electrochemical impulses that travel via the acoustic nerve to the temporal cortex of the brain. The brain interprets these impulses as meaningful sound and as balance.

✔ Nystagmus can be an objective sign of a vestibular problem.

✔ Electronystagmography is the test used to measure nystagmus.

✔ Audiometric tests, usually performed by audiologists, are used to evaluate the ear for hearing.

QUESTIONS TO CONSIDER

- Why does a comparison between air conduction and bone conduction give valuable information for a diagnosis?

- The vestibular system (inner ear) is only one of three systems responsible for balance. What are the other two systems?

- How would you help a person with a permanent loss of hearing or balance to cope?

REFERENCES AND SELECTED READINGS

1. Alberti PW and Ruben RJ, editors: Otologic medicine and surgery, vol 1, New York, 1988, Churchill Livingstone Inc.
2. Alberti PW and Ruben, RJ, editors: Otologic medicine and surgery, vol 2, New York, 1988, Churchill Livingstone Inc.
3. Bates B: A guide to physical examination, ed 4, Philadelphia, 1987, JB Lippincott Co.
4. Buckingham RA et al: Correlation between micro-otoscopy, micropneumatoscopy and otoadmittance tympanometry, Laryngoscope 90:127-1304, 1980.
5. Counter RT: Color atlas of temporal bone surgical anatomy, England, 1980, Year Book Medical Publishers Inc.
6. Hawke M, Keene M, and Albertin PW: Clinical otoscopy, New York, 1990, Churchill Livingstone Inc.
7. How to test your patient's hearing, Nursing 10(7):60-61, 1980.
8. Hughes GB:Textbook of clinical otology, New York, 1985, Thieme-Stratton Inc.
8a. Karb VK, Queener SF, and Freeman JB: Handbook of drugs for nursing practice, St. Louis, 1989, The C.V. Mosby Co.
9. Lee KF, editor: Comprehensive surgical atlas in otolaryngology and head and neck surgery, New York, 1983, Grune & Stratton Inc.
10. Northern JL: Impedance screening, an integral part of hearing screening, Ann Otol Rhinol Laryngol 89:233-235, 1980.
11. *Paparella MM and Schumrick DA: Otolaryngology, vol 2, Philadephia, 1973, WB Saunders Co.
12. *Portman M: The ear and temporal bone, New York, 1979, Masson Publishing USA.
13. *Programmed instruction: patient assessment of the ear, Am J Nurs 75(3):457-476, 1975.
14. Report of the task force on the National Strategic Research Plan of the National Institute on Deafness and Other Communication Disorders, Bethesda, Maryland, 1989, National Institute of Health.
15. Riley MAK: Nursing care of the client with ear, nose and throat disorders, New York, 1987, Springer Publishing Co Inc.
16. *Saunders WH, et al: Nursing care in the eye, ear, nose and throat disorders, ed 4, St Louis, 1979, The CV Mosby Co.
17. Serra AM, Bailey CM, and Jackson P: Ear, nose and throat nursing, Oxford, England, 1986, Blackwell Scientific Publications Inc.
18. Voke J: Aspects of hearing, physiology, of the ear, Part I, Nurs Time 80(33):28-30, Aug 15-21, 1984.
19. Voke J: Aspects of hearing, functions of the cochlea, Nurs Time 80(34):60-64, Aug 22-28, 1984.

*References preceded by an asterisk are particularly well suited for student reading.

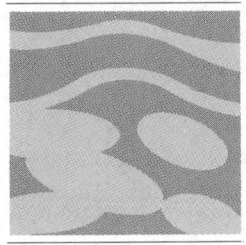

CHAPTER 67

Management of Persons with Problems of the Ear

LINDA T. SCHURING

CHAPTER OBJECTIVES

After studying this chapter, the student should be able to:

1. Discuss three measures that are important in preventing hearing loss.
2. Differentiate between conductive and sensorineural hearing loss and describe methods for assessing each.
3. Describe the pathophysiology and nursing requirements of the patient wth otitis media.
4. Describe the preoperative and postoperative care of the patient undergoing ear surgery. Explain the rationale for each measure.
5. Discuss the signs and symptoms and nursing care of the person with Ménière's disease.
6. Describe methods of aural rehabitation and communication with hearing impaired persons.
7. Describe the pathophysiology and nursing care of the person with a balance disorder.

HEARING LOSS

Hearing loss has become the nation's number one disability, affecting 1 of 15 Americans. More than 13 million people in the United States, 10 million of whom are age 65 or older, have some kind of hearing impairment. By the year 2050, approximately 1 out of every 5 persons in this country will be 55 years of age or older. Of these estimated 58 million persons, 26 million are expected to have a hearing impairment. Hearing impairment ranges from difficulty in understanding words or hearing certain sounds, such as ringing or buzzing, to total deafness.

Nurses have a responsibility not only to communicate with those with hearing loss and provide them with necessary information regarding health care but also to develop ways in which to relate to persons with hearing impairments. Very often, persons with ear problems must be motivated to seek professional help. Although some diseases of the ear canal can be helped with medicine or surgery, the vast majority of persons with a hearing impairment cannot be treated effectively. Of all hearing impairments, 80% are caused by nerve deafness for which there is no presently known cure.

Hearing impairment and dizziness (a major symptom

of inner ear problems) can hinder communication with others, limit social activities, and reduce constructive use of leisure time. Career options, job opportunities, and financial security may be affected negatively. These problems may influence the person's ability to remain independent or to feel that he or she is a contributing member of society. Last, the esthetic enjoyment of that which is pleasurable or beautiful may be decreased, and the ability to share the human experience is temporarily or permanently diminished. All of these variables could ultimately affect the person's quality of life. Hearing impairment diminishes the quality of life for one-third of U.S. adults who are between 65 and 75 years of age.

CLASSIFICATION OF HEARING LOSS
CONDUCTIVE HEARING LOSS

Any interference with the conduction of sound impulses through the external auditory canal, the eardrum, or the middle ear results in a *conductive hearing loss* or transmission deafness. The inner ear is not involved in a pure conductive loss, and sound amplification will reach the inner ear (Figure 67-1).

Conductive hearing loss may be caused by anything that blocks the external ear such as wax, infection, or a foreign body; a thickening, retraction, scarring, or perforation of the tympanic membrane; or any pathophysiologic changes in the middle ear affecting or fixing one or more of the ossicles.

SENSORINEURAL HEARING LOSS

Sensorineural hearing loss results from disease or trauma to the *inner ear*, neural structures, or nerve pathways leading to the brainstem. Some of the causes of "nerve" deafness include infectious diseases (measles, mumps, and meningitis), arteriosclerosis, ototoxic drugs (see the box on p. 2128), neuromas of cranial nerve VIII, otospongiosis (form of progressive deafness caused by the formation of new, abnormal spongy bone, in labyrinth), trauma to the head or ear, or degeneration of the organ of Corti occurring most commonly from advancing age (presbycusis).

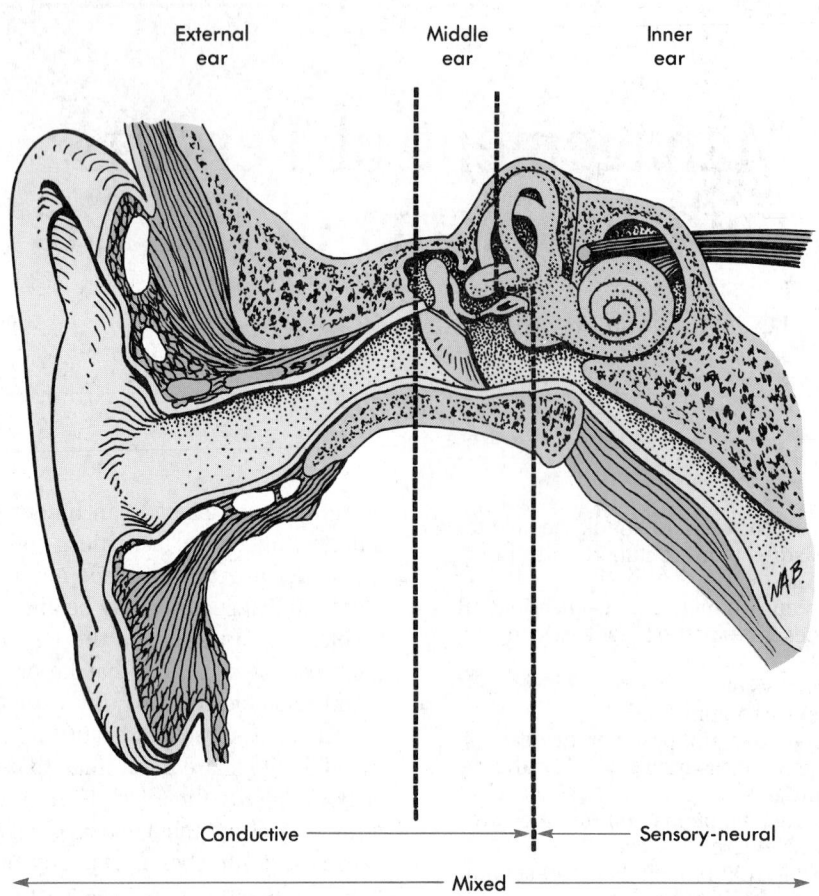

FIGURE 67-1 Three types of hearing loss. Conductive loss results from interference with conduction in external and middle ears; sensorineural loss from interference with conduction in inner ear; and mixed hearing loss results from interference with conduction in all three areas.

CENTRAL DEAFNESS

Central deafness is also known as central auditory dysfunction. With this phenomenon, the central nervous system cannot interpret normal auditory signals. Therefore the ability to hear tests as normal, although the patient is "deaf." Diseases that alter the central nervous system, such as cerebrovascular accidents and tumors, are the cause of this rare form of sensorineural hearing loss.

OTHER TYPES OF HEARING LOSS

Different types of hearing loss are listed in the box on p. 1961. A person is considered to have a *mixed* loss when both a conductive and a sensorineural hearing loss are present simultaneously (Figure 67-1). A *functional* loss is a hearing loss for which no organic lesion can be found. A hearing loss may also be congenital or acquired. *The majority of persons with ear problems have some degree of hearing loss.*

HEARING RESEARCH

Hearing and balance research is now conducted at the National Institute of Deafness and Other Communication Disorders (NIDCD). This newly formed division of the National Institutes of Health will vastly improve the care of patients with hearing impairments. Research grants are available to nurses as well as to other health care providers.

PREVENTION AND HEALTH EDUCATION

To maintain normal ear function, adequate protection of the ears is important and involves several activities:
1. Proper care of the healthy ear
2. Early, adequate treatment of ear diseases
3. Prevention of trauma to the ear
4. Early detection of hearing losses
5. Monitoring side effects of ototoxic drugs
6. Monitoring noise pollution
7. Periodic ear examinations

TYPES OF HEARING LOSS

Air conduction hearing loss: loss of hearing through the external and middle ears

Bone conduction hearing loss: loss of hearing through the inner ear

Central hearing loss: loss of hearing from damage to the brain's auditory pathways or auditory center

Conductive hearing loss: loss of hearing in which air conduction is worse than bone conduction

Fluctuating hearing loss: a sensorineural hearing loss that varies with time

Functional hearing loss: loss of hearing for which no organic lesion can be found

Mixed hearing loss: both elements of air and bone conduction hearing loss occur

Neural hearing loss: a sensorineural hearing loss originating in the nerve or brainstem

Sensorineural hearing loss: loss of hearing involving the cochlea and hearing nerve; bone and air conduction are equal but diminished

Sensory hearing loss: a sensorineural hearing loss originating in the cochlea and involving the hair cells and nerve endings

Sudden hearing loss: a sensorineural hearing loss with a sudden onset

PROPER CARE OF HEALTHY EARS

The external ear may be washed with soap and water daily while bathing or showering. The ear canal is generally "self cleaning." Wax is to the ears as tears are to the eyes and serves as a protective mechanism. Earwax lubricates the skin and traps foreign material that enters the canal. Therefore wax should not be cleaned out of the ear routinely. Although recommendations have been made that the ear should be cleaned only with a wet washcloth over the tip of a finger, cotton-tipped applicators may be used. The applicator should be moistened with alcohol and inserted into the canal only the length of the cotton tip. The ear canal is approximately 1 to 1½ in. long in an adult from the external opening to the eardrum, more than enough area to clean with a cotton-tipped applicator.

EARLY, ADEQUATE TREATMENT OF EAR DISEASES

Any disease that causes prolonged symptoms of the ear such as pain, swelling, drainage, "plugged" feeling, or decreased hearing should be promptly assessed and treated by a physician. The nurse must encourage persons with these symptoms to seek professional help. Many chronic problems such as perforations and necrotic ossicles could be prevented with prompt and adequate medical attention.

During upper respiratory infections (colds), the nose should be blown with both nostrils open. Excessive pressure occurs when one nostril is closed and can force infected secretions up the eustachian tube into the middle ear.

PREVENTION OF TRAUMA TO THE EAR

People should be taught to avoid inserting hard articles into the ear canal, obstructing the ear canal with any object, inserting unclean articles or solutions into the ear, or swimming in water identified as being polluted. These practices can lead to damage to the tympanic membrane or to ear infections. Adults often traumatize the ear by inserting hard articles into the outer ear in an attempt to remove cerumen or to scratch the ear canal.

EARLY DETECTION OF HEARING LOSS

Because the hearing (auditory) nerve does not regain function; early detection of hearing loss is important so that the cause of the loss can be diagnosed and, hopefully, the problem can be corrected or arrested. However, the signs of a small loss of hearing are illusive and are often ignored.

A hearing loss in both ears may first be detected by a family member rather than the person affected. The earliest sign is not hearing what once you heard. Another common sign is asking for a repetition of what was said. Usually the request is in the form of a question such as "What did you say?" Sometimes the hard of hearing person may repeat the information, even incorrectly, to provoke a response and thus a repetition of the information.

A hearing loss in one ear is more difficult to detect. The person may notice the loss only when using a telephone or when having difficulty determining the direction of sounds.

MONITORING SIDE EFFECTS OF OTOTOXIC DRUGS

Some drugs may affect the cochlea, the vestibule of the ear, or the eighth cranial nerve (see the box, p. 1962). Persons taking ototoxic drugs need to know the signs and symptoms of side effects of these drugs to prevent loss of hearing from developing. If these symptoms (dizziness, decreased hearing acuity, tinnitus) occur, the next dose of the drug is omitted, and the physician is consulted. Audiometric testing (see Chapter 66) may be necessary.

MONITORING NOISE POLLUTION

Industrial noise and occupational or noise-induced hearing loss are primary causes of hearing loss in our society. The most common type of occupational hearing loss is caused by loud noise. In the United States, the Occu-

SELECTED OTOTOXIC DRUGS

AMINOGLYCOSIDE ANTIBIOTICS
Streptomycin
Neomycin
Kanamycin
Gentamycin
Tobramycin
Netromycin
Amikacin

OTHER ANTIBIOTICS
Vancomycin
Viomycin
Polymyxin B (Aerosporin)
Polymyxin E (Colistin/Coly-Mycin)
Erythromycin
Minocycline
Capreomycin

DIURETICS
Ethacrynic acid (Edecrin)
Furosemide (Lasix)
Acetazolamide (Diamox)

OTHER DRUGS
Quinine
Chloroquine
Nitrogen mustard
Bleomycin
Quinidine
Cisplastin
Salicylates

pational Safety and Health Administration (OSHA) has established acceptable levels of noise in work environments. The provisions regarding noise protection are complex; but, in general, exposure to noise levels in excess of 90 dB over an 8-hour day are considered excessive and should be avoided. Sound intensity is measured in decibles (dB). Ordinary speech level is about 50 dB; heavy traffic is about 70 dB; and above 80 dB noise becomes uncomfortable to the human ear. Exposure to levels greater than 85 to 90 dB for months or years can cause cochlear damage. The nurse must participate in teaching the proper use of protective ear devices or earplugs for persons working in areas of high decibel-noise. Courses are available to educate nurses about industrial hearing conservation requirements.

Other causes of noise-induced hearing loss include the use of firearms and high-intensity music. A person firing guns who notices tinnitus, sensation of fullness in the ear, or a temporary hearing loss should stop firing the guns or wear suitable ear protection. Sound in front of a rock band can reach up to 120 dB, and hearing losses have been measured in some members of rock

bands. If proximity to the high noise level cannot be avoided, earplugs should be worn during exposure.

The earplugs are inserted into the external auditory canal and are capable of reducing the noise that reaches the middle ear by 10 to 30 dB. Usually standardized plugs are effective, but custom-made plugs molded to the individual's ear canal may be purchased. For noise levels reaching 140 dB and above, such as around jet airplanes, individuals must wear earmuffs.

PERIODIC EAR EXAMINATIONS

Periodic (every 2 to 3 years) ear examinations for evaluation of hearing are important in the adult, because aging frequently causes degenerative changes in the ear, as well as in other body tissues.

TYPES OF EAR DISORDERS

The same types of disorders that occur in other parts of the body also occur in the ear and include: *obstructions* or *blockage; trauma; inflammation, infection,* and *scarring;* and *skin disorders.* Some disorders that only affect the ear include hearing loss, dizziness and balance (disorders of the inner ear), and tinnitus (ringing in the ears).

In this chapter, the discussion of ear problems is divided into three parts: (1) problems of the external ear; (2) problems of the tympanic membrane, middle ear, and mastoid; and (3) problems of the inner ear.

PROBLEMS OF THE EXTERNAL EAR

ETIOLOGY AND PATHOPHYSIOLOGY
CONGENITAL EAR PROBLEMS

The auricle and external ear canal develop separately embryologically, resulting in two types of congenital disorders of the external ear. The pinna can be deformed or absent with a normal external ear canal, or the pinna and ear canal together can show congenital changes. External ear canal abnormalities result in different degrees of incomplete development or *canal atresia.* Congenital findings of the external ear do not necessarily mean that the middle or inner ears are involved. A minor congenital finding is protruding ears in which the auricle has a greater than normal angle to the head. Also, cysts and skin tracts that develop from incomplete formation of the pinna are quite common.

INFECTIONS

The most common problems found in the external ear are infections, primarily bacterial or fungal. The most frequent infection, called *external otitis,* involves the external ear canal (Table 67-1). This infection begins in the skin lining of the ear canal and can occlude the canal. External otitis occurs more frequently in the sum-

TABLE 67-1 Normal function, pathophysiology, and clinical picture in external otitis

Normal Function	Pathophysiology	Clinical Picture
The pinna of the external ear channels act like a funnel into the ear canal. The ear canal is 1-1½ in in length and lined with epithelium that contains modified sweat glands, cerumen glands, and hair.	Exposure to moisture, contamination or local trauma produces an environment conducive to the growth of normal flora.	Tenderness on pulling the pinna, whitish drainage, inflammation of the ear canal including redness, swelling, itching, decreased hearing because of debris, and narrowing of the ear canal.

mer than in the winter. A localized form of this infection is seen as an *ear canal furuncle* or *abscess*. When a systemic disease such as diabetes is present, the external otitis can spread wildly through cartilage and bone and is then named *malignant external otitis*. The most common form of external otitis is also called *swimmer's ear,* because it is prevalent when water remains in the ear canal. In addition, opportunistic fungal infections are common. Occasionally, infection can involve only the cartilage of the auricle *(perichondritis),* resulting in necrosis of the cartilage and loss of the distinctive shape of the auricle if not treated quickly.

MASSES

Benign masses of the external ear canal are usually cysts arising from a sebaceous gland, rarely from the cerumen (earwax) glands. Cysts can also be congenital in nature. Bony protrusions seen in the lower bony portion of the ear canal are called *exostosis*. The skin covering the exostosis is normal. If the skin is red, the mass is usually an abscess. *Infectious polyps* found in the ear canal arise from either the tympanic membrane or, more commonly, the middle ear through a hole in the tympanic membrane. Malignant tumors are also found in the external ear. The *cutaneous carcinomas* are most often *basal cell carcinoma* on the pinna and *squamous cell carcinoma* in the ear canal. These carcinomas can invade the underlying tissue if not treated, and squamous cell carcinoma may spread throughout the temporal bone. Rare tumors of the cerumen glands are of the *adenoma* cell type.

MISCELLANEOUS PROBLEMS

On inspection of the external canal, the most frequent problematic finding is *impacted cerumen* (wax). Although the ear canal is self-cleaning, cerumen may become impacted from a disorder or from improper cleaning. Removal of cerumen must be performed carefully and may be necessary before the tympanic membrane can be examined.

Trauma, either sharp or blunt, is becoming a more common finding. A residual finding of repeated blunt

trauma is a hypertrophic scar formation known as *cauliflower ears,* an occupational hazard for boxers. With prompt treatment, traumatic injuries can be corrected successfully.

Surprisingly, a wide array of *foreign bodies* fit into the ear canal. The most common foreign body found in adults is either a piece of cotton or, most annoying, an insect. In children, it is a small toy. Equally surprising is the difficulty that can be encountered in removing a foreign body. The least traumatic method of removing a foreign body is with the aid of an *operating microscope.* For removal of a live insect, the ear canal is filled with mineral oil, *NOT WATER.* Water causes the insect to swell and it becomes difficult to remove.

Finally, an allergic reaction involving the pinna can occur. This reaction is usually generalized and does not involve the ear canal.

CLINICAL MANIFESTATIONS

Pain in the external ear is the most *common symptom* of infection. Painful sites are also tender because of the close proximity of bone (a hard surface) when palpating the ear. A clue to early external otitis is tenderness when gently pulling on the pinna. *A forerunner of pain* in external otitis is *itching in the ear canal. Inflammation (redness)* is easily identified with an otoscope. At different stages of infection, *drainage* is found exiting the ear canal. In early infectious disorders, the drainage may be clear and not discolored by pus.

A common complaint of patients with occlusion of the ear canal is a *loss of hearing.* Both infection and cerumen can cause a sudden hearing loss. Accompanying the loss of hearing may be the complaint of a *blocked* ear.

MEDICAL MANAGEMENT

The most common external ear problems are infections and are treated with antibiotics in the form of drops and ointments, as well as systemically. However, the first rule of treating infection is meticulous cleaning of the site so that the local antibiotic can reach the infected area. Then external otitis must be treated by microscopic cleaning before applying antibiotic drops or ointments. If the ear canal is swollen shut, a *wick* must be inserted to allow the drops to penetrate the canal. If the infection is not localized, systemic antibiotics are standard. And if debris that cannot be removed accumulates in the ear canal, irrigations (with an ear syringe) can be used. Because external otitis is one of the most painful disorders of the ear, appropriate analgesics are in order.

The removal of cerumen by medicinal means often leads to minor complications caused by irritation resulting from mild caustic commercial products. An infection that involves cartilage has to be treated aggressively and quickly with systemic antibiotics to avoid complications.

SURGICAL MANAGEMENT

The surgical treatment of infections involves *incision and drainage* in the acute phase for abscesses and, at times, for perichondritis. Chronic infection can also require surgical treatment. The most common surgical treatment is *excision of cysts* and *cutaneous carcinomas*. For the most part, the surgery involved is minimal. For conditions that occlude the ear canal, more extensive surgery involving skin grafting (*canalplasty*) is performed. Extensive surgery of the external ear is usually necessary to repair congenital defects. The correction of protruding ears is called *otoplasty*.

■ ASSESSMENT
SUBJECTIVE DATA

The most frequent problems of the external ear seen by the nurse are *inflammation* and *infection*. *Pain* is the *chief symptom*, followed by a *sense of fullness* in the ear, *hearing loss,* and *itching.* Data to collect include onset, duration, and degree of severity of symptoms.

OBJECTIVE DATA

When assessing the external ear, manipulation of the ear is important. If the patient complains of pain when any part of the ear is palpated, a *furuncle, lesion,* or some kind of inflammatory process *of the ear canal* is *suspected.* If an otoscopic examination is performed, care must be taken not to cause the person unnecessary pain. A furuncle may be close to the opening of the canal, causing increased pain from the pressure of the speculum. Water in the ear canal from showering or swimming may aggravate the symptoms.

The external ear is inspected for signs of drainage, either serous or purulent. The auricle is also inspected for signs of redness, scaliness, and crusting.

The Operating Microscope

The binocular-operating microscope is found in the offices and clinics of most otologists. With specialized instruction the nurse may learn to use the microscope and manipulate instruments inserted through a speculum into the external ear. The speculum holds open the outermost portion of the external ear canal and allows the passage of both light and instruments. The appropriate speculum size for adults is from 4 to 7 mm in diameter. The microscope provides the examiner with excellent illumination, increased depth perception, and three-dimensional vision. Most operating microscopes allow changes in magnification to be made. The nurse can use the microscope to assess normal from abnormal, remove cerumen, and suction out drainage.

■ DATA ANALYSIS:NURSING DIAGNOSES

Nursing diagnoses are determined from assessment of patient data. Possible nursing diagnoses for the person with an external ear problem may include but are not limited to, the following:

Diagnostic Title	Possible Etiologies
Knowledge deficit about problem	Lack of exposure to information; unfamiliarity with information sources
Pain	Pathophysiologic ear pain caused by infection, inflammation, and swelling
Sensory/perceptual alteration auditory	Decreased hearing caused by debris and infection in ear canal

■ PLANNING: EXPECTED PATIENT OUTCOMES

Expected patient outcomes for the person with an external ear problem may include but are not limited to, the following:
1. The patient can describe preventive measures for external ear problems.
2. The patient can describe symptoms requiring medical attention.
3. Discomfort in the ear is decreased.
4. The patient demonstrates correct technique in application of eardrops and ear ointment.
5. The patient is prepared for the possibility of minor surgery.

■ IMPLEMENTATION

The box on p. 1965 lists the general guidelines for ear care.

PATIENT TEACHING

Patients with inflammations or infections of the external ear may be diagnosed and treated on an ambulatory basis. These problems are not life-threatening or life-shortening and are usually easily treated with topical antibiotic solutions. During the infection, patients should avoid getting water in the ear by using earplugs or cotton with vaseline on it. If earplugs are used, thorough cleansing with alcohol or a mild detergent between uses is recommended to prevent reinfection. No swimming is permitted during this time.

GUIDELINES FOR EAR CARE

The following guidelines are imperative when caring for a patient with a problem of the ear:
1. Teach patients how to care for their ears, whether lessons are preventive, therapeutic, or rehabilitative in nature.
2. Wash hands before and after caring for the patient's ear and between procedures for both ears to prevent cross-contamination.
3. Observe sterile technique when the middle ear or inner ear has been opened traumatically or surgically.
4. Be aware that certain conditions make the ear extremely sensitive. Be gentle when manipulating the external ear.
5. Have an adjustable light source for good visualization.
6. Place nothing in the ear canal without a physician's order, not even water.
7. Solutions for instillation or irrigation should be at body temperature.

PROMOTING COMFORT

Analgesics such as codeine 30 mg q4h are often helpful. After the physician has prescribed the analgesic, instruct the patient as to amount, frequency, and duration. Ear pain usually results from the buildup of fluid in the small bony spaces of the ear, leading to pressure and pain. Once the swelling and drainage are reduced by treatment, the pain subsides.

ADMINISTERING MEDICATIONS AND TREATMENTS

Eardrops

Antibiotics and antiinflammatory agents are usually administered locally rather than systemically in problems involving the external ear. The procedure and directions for administration of eardrops are as follows:
1. Wash hands before and after the procedure.
2. Warm the eardrops to body temperature by holding vial in the hand for a few minutes or by placing it in a dish of warm water. (Dizziness may occur from insertion of drops that are too warm or too cold.)
3. Patient should tilt the head so that the ear to be treated is up.
4. Straighten the ear canal by pulling up and back.
5. Instill prescribed number of drops to run along ear canal.
6. Press gently several times on the tragus of the ear to ensure proper instillation, or hold the head in position for 2 to 3 minutes.
7. Wipe the external ear with cotton ball or tissue to prevent skin irritation.
8. A cotton ball may be placed in the ear but is not necessary.

A wick may have been inserted by the physician to allow the drops to penetrate if the canal is swollen shut. In this case, the prescribed number of eardrops are placed directly on the wick. The wick serves not only as a bandage but also as an excellent vehicle to medicate the ear canal.

Ear Ointment

To apply ointment to the ear canal, use a Q-tip or an applicator with a tufted end. Care must be taken not to damage the ear canal or eardrum. Insert the cotton applicator no farther than the cotton end, remembering that the adult ear canal is approximately 1 inch in length. Instruct the patient not to move the head during the procedure and to use a new applicator each time the ointment is applied.

Removal of Cerumen

Wax that is visible in the ear canal can be removed with a Q-tip. *Do not put more than the cotton portion in the ear.* Impacted accumulations of earwax may be softened and loosened for removal by alternate instillation of glycerine and hydrogen peroxide. Three drops of glycerine are used at bedtime to soften the wax, and three drops of hydrogen peroxide are used twice a day to loosen the wax. The eardrops are warmed to body temperature and used daily as directed for 1 to 2 weeks. The ear is then irrigated with warm water to remove the softened wax or cleaned under magnification with a cerumen spoon. Wax that is on the tympanic membrane must be removed by a physician or a clinical nurse specialist in otology.

Ear Irrigation

The ear is commonly irrigated either to cleanse the external auditory canal or to remove impacted wax. Irrigations are not used for persons with a previous history of a perforated eardrum. The irrigating solution (usually water) is warmed to body temperature and placed in the irrigating syringe. The patients' clothes are protected with a plastic drape, and a kidney-shaped basin is placed below the ear to catch the irrigating solution. The patient sits with the ear to be syringed toward the nurse and with the head tilted toward the opposite ear. The external ear is pulled upward and backward for the adult, and the tip of the syringe is directed along the upper wall of the ear canal (Figure 67-2). The canal should not be completely obstructed by the syringe to allow for the backflow of solution. When charting the ear irrigation, record the nature of returned solution including amount, texture, and color of cerumen.

Insertion and Removal of Earwicks

Commercially prepared wicks or single pieces of ¼-inch gauze are used in the ear to promote drainage or to pro-

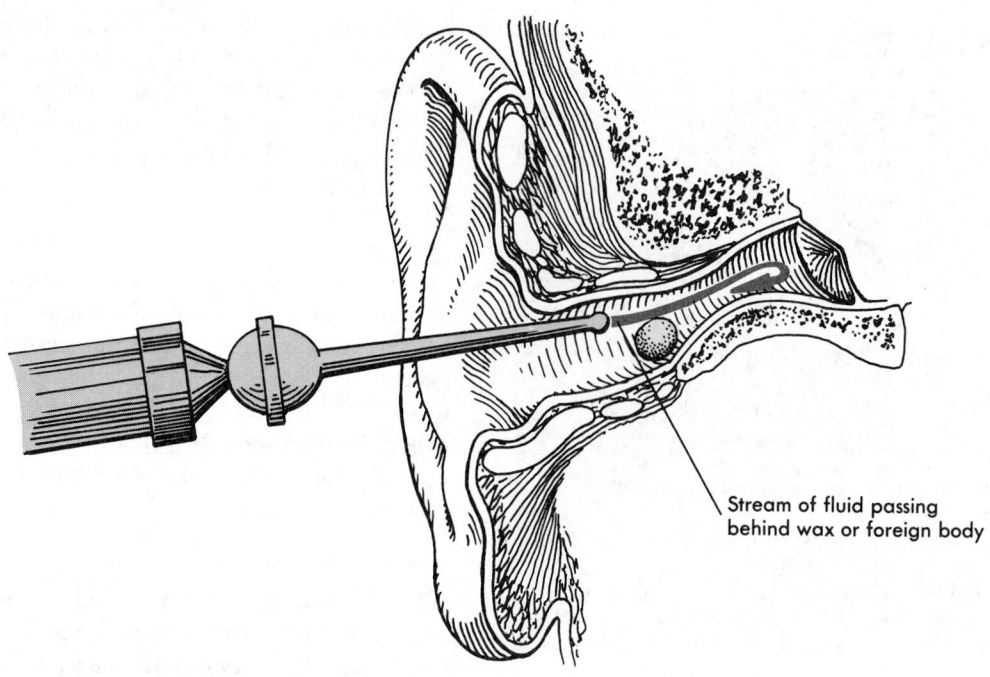

Stream of fluid passing
behind wax or foreign body

FIGURE 67-2 Ear irrigation. Note that fluid is directed toward upper canal wall so that stream will pass behind wax or object.

vide a pathway for the instillation of eardrops. The wick is gently inserted into the ear canal by means of bayonet forceps while gently pulling upward and backward on the external ear. The wick is usually slightly less than 1 inch in length. Frequently, a wick is inserted for swollen ear canals, commonly seen in acute external otitis.

PROBLEMS OF THE TYMPANIC MEMBRANE, MIDDLE EAR, AND MASTOID

PROBLEMS OF THE TYMPANIC MEMBRANE
ETIOLOGY AND PATHOPHYSIOLOGY

Congenital Disorders
The tympanic membrane is the end of the external ear canal and the beginning of the middle ear and thus is involved with problems of both structures. Therefore congenital problems of the tympanic membrane are also problems of the adjacent structures.

Infection
Likewise, infections of the external ear canal can involve the surface of the tympanic membrane, and the tympanic membrane will be a "window" for infection of the middle ear. Infection can cause hard deposits in the tympanic membrane known as *tympanosclerosis*, which is discussed in the section on the middle ear. A specific viral infection of the tympanic membrane is *bullous myringitis*. In this inflammatory disease blisters or bullae form on the tympanic membrane. Holes or *perforations*

of the tympanic membrane can be caused by infection or trauma.

Tumors
Both benign and malignant tumors can involve the tympanic membrane but seldom arise from it. However, an infectious glandular polyp can be isolated to the tympanic membrane.

CLINICAL MANIFESTATIONS
Because the tympanic membrane is a semitransparent membrane, it can reflect what lies underneath it, as well as discoloration and displacement of the membrane. Therefore both *fluid* in the *middle ear* and *infection can be seen*. The tympanic membrane may be dull or red in addition to the normal pearl grey coloration. The membrane may be bulging as a result of positive pressure in the middle ear that results from infection. This pressure is strong enough in some cases to "burst" the eardrum and cause drainage. A ruptured eardrum is more common in children than adults and usually heals spontaneously. *Disorders* involving the tympanic membrane are painful, *perhaps the most painful of all ear disorders*. A negative pressure in the ear causes a retraction of the tympanic membrane, outlying the ossicles. In these cases fluid is also found. Finally, any alteration of the tympanic membrane can cause a hearing loss.

Perforation

The major finding in tympanic membrane disorders is a perforation. A *perforation* may be either *acute,* as seen in trauma and acute infection, or *chronic,* as seen in repeated infection. *An acute perforation has a better chance of healing spontaneously than a chronic perforation.* A perforation that is located away from the annulus of the tympanic membrane is a *central perforation.* A perforation involving the annulus is a *marginal perforation.* A marginal perforation has less chance of spontaneous closure and a greater chance of invasion of skin from the external ear, thus causing a cholesteatoma (see p. 1970). A perforation causes a hearing loss, depending on its size and location. The largest hearing loss found with a perforation is approximately 35 dB (one third of the hearing). If a perforation is present, damage to the ossicles should be suspected, which will cause an even greater hearing loss.

INTERVENTIONS

Medical and Surgical Management

The medical management of tympanic membrane disorders involves both systemic and local antibiotics. Local antibiotics are used in the form of eardrops.

Surgical treatment involves using a surgical microscope to enlarge the tympanic membrane; the power of magnification most commonly used is 6 to 25 times normal. The major surgical procedure performed is closure of a perforation. This procedure is called a *myringoplasty* if only the perforation is in the surgical field or a *tympanoplasty* if more of the middle ear is involved. Sometimes the ossicles must also be reconstructed, altering the type of tympanoplasty performed (types I through IV). A tympanoplasty may also be performed in conjunction with surgery involving the mastoid. The most common material that is used as a free graft to close the perforation is fascia taken from the temporalis muscle. Less commonly used tissue is perichondrium or vein. At the present time, *tympanoplasty is a common surgical procedure of the ear with a high rate of success.*

PROBLEMS OF THE MIDDLE EAR
ETIOLOGY AND PATHOPHYSIOLOGY

Congenital Disorders

Congenital malformations of the ear include incomplete development of the ossicles, causing the absence or deformity of the ossicles. Another common congenital finding is the absence of the bony canal covering the facial (seventh) nerve or, very rarely, an abnormal course throughout the middle ear. Congenital disorders of the middle ear usually involve the tympanic membrane and, more often than not, the external ear canal and the auricle.

Infection

The most prevalent diseases of the middle ear are infections and are known as *otitis media.* Otitis media is caused by various types of bacteria, depending on the age of the patient and type of infection. When the infection is sudden in onset and short in duration, the diagnosis is *acute otitis media* (See Table 67-2). When the infection recurs, usually causing drainage and perforation, the problem is called *chronic otitis media.* In between bouts of otitis media, fluid may form in the middle ear *(serous otitis media).* This fluid is formed by a vacuum in the middle ear caused by a blocked eustachian tube. Infection causes swelling of the mucosa throughout the middle ear and eustachian tube. When the swelling subsides, the remaining fluid can be too thick to drain. At times, serous otitis media is found in conjunction with upper respiratory infections or allergies. If the fluid remains over a period of years, causing tympanic membrane retraction, *adhesive otitis media* becomes the diagnosis. Infection present over a long period of time can cause necrosis of the tympanic membrane (perforations) or of the ossicles. Both problems create a conductive hearing loss. Necrosis of the bony covering of the facial nerve may cause facial paralysis. *Because of the extraordinary anatomy of the temporal bone, middle ear infection can also lead to a brain abscess that is life-threatening if not treated properly.*

TABLE 67-2 Normal function, pathophysiology, and clinical picture in otitis media

Normal Function	Pathophysiology	Clinical Picture
The middle ear is separated from the external ear by the tympanic membrane. The middle ear is transversed by ossicles that transmit sound from the ear drum to the inner ear. The middle ear is aerated by the eustachian tube, which connects the nasopharynx to and equalizes pressure in the middle ear.	Blockage of the eustachian tube from allergic swelling, throat infection, or adenoiditis produces negative pressure and fluid in the middle ear. This fluid can become infected.	Throbbing pain, drainage, fever, decreased hearing, inflammation, and bulging of the eardrum with a possible perforation.

TABLE 67-3 Normal function, pathophysiology, and clinical picture in otosclerosis

Normal Function	Pathophysiology	Clinical Picture
The stapes articulates with the incus and oval window and transmits sound from the other ossicles to the inner ear.	Progressive loss of stapes movement caused by the formation of sclerotic bone, which fixes the stapes footplate. The stapes becomes immobile, causing a conductive hearing loss.	Normal ear canal, normal ear drum, progressive conductive hearing loss, or mixed hearing loss.

Tympanosclerosis is a result of repeated infection and deserves special emphasis. Tympanosclerosis is a deposit of collagen and calcium within the middle ear that can harden around the ossicles, causing a conductive hearing loss. Tympanosclerosis can also be found mounded up in the middle ear or as plaque on the tympanic membrane.

Cholesteatoma is a complication from otitis media but is primarily a problem of the mastoid (see p. 1970).

Otosclerosis

Otosclerosis or "hardening of the ear," which involves the stapes, is important in middle ear disorders. (See Table 67-3). This bony disease of the otic capsule causes excess bone to form, impeding normal movement of the stapes. *The conductive hearing loss that results is the second most common correctable middle ear disorder following an infection of the ear.* Another form of otosclerosis that does not involve the stapes is *cochlear otospongiosis*, which can cause a toxic sensorineural hearing loss.

Tumors

The *most common benign* growth in the middle ear is an *infectious polyp*. Next in frequency is a *cholesteatoma*. The rarest forms of benign middle ear tumors involve either the blood vessels or the facial nerve. Arising from the jugular vein is a *glomus jugulare*, known as a *glomus tympanicum* when limited to the middle ear. A *facial nerve neuroma* is found along the course of the facial nerve. Malignant tumors involving the middle ear can be primary or secondary in nature.

Trauma

Trauma to the tympanic membrane from a blast or blunt injury can involve the middle ear, causing a fracture or dislocation of the ossicles and tearing the tympanic membrane. The facial nerve is also vulnerable to trauma. A *basal skull fracture* involves the temporal bone and, depending on the fracture site, causes ossicular damage as well as facial nerve paralysis.

Eustachian Tube Disorders

The eustachian tube is part of the middle ear but presents separate problems. Because the eustachian tube connects the middle ear to the nasopharynx, pharyngeal disorders cause eustachian tube dysfunction and thus secondary middle ear problems. For example, the most common disorder is blockage of the eustachian tube by enlarged adenoid tissue in children. The most common blockage in adults is swelling of the mucosa in the eustachian tube during an upper respiratory infection that can lead to serous otitis media. In a unilateral blocked eustachian tube, a malignant tumor must be ruled out as the cause. Acute blockage from *barotrauma* (altitude changes) caused by flying or underwater diving also cause middle ear problems. *Any long-term blockage of the eustachian tube leads to a serous otitis media and a hearing loss.*

CLINICAL MANIFESTATIONS

Because the middle ear is the transformer for hearing (that is, it transmits the sound vibrations from the tympanic membrane to the inner ear), a *hearing loss is the most frequent middle ear finding.* Fortunately, a conductive hearing loss is found in 95% of problems and is correctable by either medical or surgical treatment. *Pain is also quite common because of pressure from infection or fluid behind the tympanic membrane.* Once a perforation is caused by infection, drainage of pus, blood, and other material is often found. In chronic middle ear and mastoid problems, a thick yellow pus discharge is common. *With an acute otitis media, all three findings (hearing loss, pain, and discharge) can be present.*

INTERVENTIONS

Medical Management

With any form of otitis media, appropriate antibiotic therapy may be necessary. If drainage is present, a culture and sensitivity should be performed. However, most episodes of acute otitis media do not produce a drainage, and the most probable bacterial cause must be identified. In chronic ear discharge, the normal contaminants of the ear abound and unfortunately do not respond to the common antibiotics. Thus local treatment such as ear irrigations, drops, and powders are used.

Blood in the ear canal usually points to a minor problem such as a scratch and not a major disease. Persistent hemorrhage must be checked by an otologist.

Because the eustachian tube is an integral part of

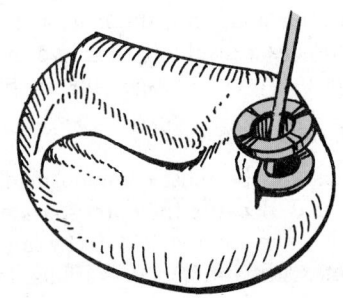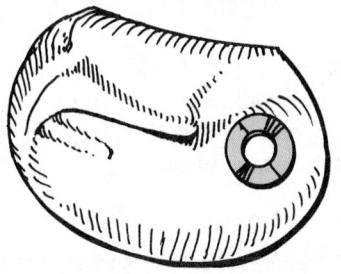

FIGURE 67-3 Insertion of Sheehy button through the eardrum to permit drainage of secretions (myringotomy) for chronic serous otitis media.

middle ear disorders, decongestants and antihistamines are used to decrease the swelling and open the eustachian tube. Pain medication is used appropriately when necessary.

Surgical Management

Repairing the damage from middle ear infection is the most challenging microscopic surgical procedure facing the surgeon. But removing fluid from the middle ear is the easiest and most common procedure. A simple incision in the tympanic membrane is a *myringotomy* through which fluid is removed by suction. To keep the incision open and prevent a recurrence of fluid, various types of *transtympanic tubes* can be inserted into the incision (Figure 67-3). These tubes extrude in 3 to 12 months by themselves and rarely have to be removed.

Reconstruction of the necrotic ossicles is not yet an exact science. Various methods of repositioning these tiny ear bones are now in use, although the surgery is difficult to perform and unfortunately is not always suc-

cessful over the long term. Therefore various prostheses have been used to reconnect the ossicles to carry sound. Extrusion of prostheses through the eardrum has also plagued the surgeon during the past few decades. In an attempt to solve this problem, the tissue is combined with a prostheses to connect the ossicles and prevent extrusion. This method is now used in different forms by the majority of otologic surgeons.

The surgical procedure of ossicular reconstruction is called *ossiculoplasty* (Figure 67-4). But many surgeons use the term tympanoplasty, meaning to make a new eardrum, to include ossiculoplasty.

Surgery on the facial nerve in the middle ear is limited. In the past, facial nerve decompression for idiopathic facial paralysis (Bell's palsy) was routine, but not today. *A controversy is raging, with physician's who advocate no surgery for Bell's palsy in the forefront.* Other middle ear lesions are excised often in combination with other recognized middle ear procedures. For example, tympanosclerosis is removed routinely during tympano-

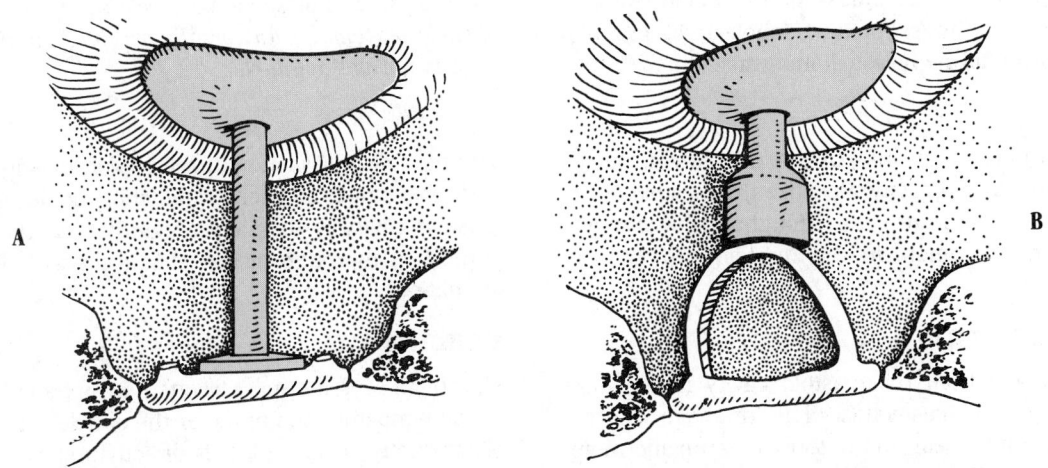

FIGURE 67-4 Middle ear prostheses. **A,** Schuring ossicle columnella prosthesis for total ossicular replacement surgery. **B,** Schuring ossicle cup prosthesis for incus replacement surgery.

plasty or ossiculoplasty without recognition in the procedures' names.

Stapedectomy, removing and replacing the stapes, was once a common middle ear procedure. The fixed stapes is replaced by an artificial stapes constructed of stainless steel or other exotic plastics.

PROBLEMS OF THE MASTOID
ETIOLOGY AND PATHOPHYSIOLOGY
Congenital Disorders

Because the mastoid cavity is irregular in dimensions and is often influenced by infection early in life, congenital irregularities are less significant. Of more significance are the structures directly surrounding the mastoid cavity. For the surgeon, the congenital abnormality of the course of the facial nerve is of primary concern in avoiding injury. Likewise, knowledge of a congenital change in the brain or sigmoid sinus is surgically very important. Therefore the surgeon obtains mastoid x-ray films before surgery.

Infection

Before the discovery of antibiotics, a mastoid infection was a life-threatening event. Now with the use of antibiotics, *acute mastoiditis* is indeed rare. On the other hand, *chronic mastoiditis* is still present. With repeated middle ear infections, the mastoid cavity becomes part of the problem, increasing the amount of drainage. A chronic infection also leads to the development of *cholesteatoma*. Although a benign growth, a cholesteatoma tends to erode the surrounding structures, causing other secondary problems. In the past, cholesteatoma has given rise to the "stories" of brain abscesses, dizziness, and facial paralysis. These conditions are still seen today but, like acute mastoiditis, are becoming less frequent. *A cholesteatoma is a skin-lined sac that sheds debris into its center, thus enlarging the sac.* Often infection is present in the mass of the cholesteatoma. These chronic changes produce cholesterol granules from which the term cholesteatoma was coined.

Tumors

The same tumors that arise in the middle ear can be found in the mastoid cavity. Because the mastoid cavity is connected to other air cells throughout the temporal bone, malignant tumors in the mastoid carry a poor prognosis.

CLINICAL MANIFESTATIONS

Today, drainage from the mastoid cavity is the most common sign of mastoiditis. The drainage courses through the middle ear and out of the tympanic membrane through a perforation. Tenderness over the mastoid cavity behind the ear points to an infection but usually is caused by an acute exacerbation of chronic mas-

toiditis rather than an acute mastoiditis. The protrusion of the pinna as a result of swelling over the mastoid may be part of this process, especially in children.

MEDICAL MANAGEMENT

Antibiotics are the most common medical therapy currently in use. Because infection starts in the middle ear, the problems in the mastoid cavity are avoided by early treatment with antibiotics. Various irrigations of the mastoid and middle ear are used in chronic infections, along with antibiotic eardrops or powders.

SURGICAL MANAGEMENT

At the turn of the century, a mastoidectomy was used as an incision and drainage of a mastoid infection, thus saving the life of the patient. Also around this time, the radical removal of the mastoid bone was first advocated and is even used today for both infection and cholesteatoma. Since the *radical mastoidectomy* sacrificed hearing, a *modified radical mastoidectomy* was advocated that saved the remaining middle ear structures. At the onset of the period of antibiotics, a *simple mastoidectomy* was performed, maintaining a normal appearing ear. Because the radical and modified mastoidectomy exteriorize the mastoid cavity to the external ear canal, they are known as *open mastoidectomies*. Closed mastoidectomies are simple mastoidectomies with modifications in conjunction with tympanoplasty and ossiculoplasty. Today, even the open mastoidectomy is performed with various tympanoplasties.

The excision of cholesteatoma by mastoidectomy is still in controversy. The historic and safe procedure is to perform an open mastoidectomy and to ignore the hearing. The advocates of the closed mastoidectomy point out that the cholesteatoma can be removed safely and better hearing can be achieved if a *staged mastoidectomy* is performed after the original procedure to check for reforming cholesteatoma. *Because of the recurrence of cholesteatoma, a universally accepted surgical procedure is not yet available.*

◾ ASSESSMENT

The nursing assessment of the person having problems with the tympanic membrane, the middle ear, or the mastoid cavity is the same, regardless of the need for surgery. A thorough history should precede the ear examination.

SUBJECTIVE DATA

Hearing loss is the most frequent symptom of blockage of the tympanic membrane or the ossicles. The amount of conductive hearing loss is directly proportional to the amount of damage to the eardrum, the middle ear, or the mastoid cavity. *Pain* may also be present because of pressure from infection or fluid behind or in the tympanic membrane. Data are collected about the onset, duration, and severity of these symptoms.

OBJECTIVE DATA

The tympanic membrane is the only structure that can be visualized directly; the middle ear and mastoid cavity must be evaluated by indirect means. The eardrum may be normal, perforated, infected, retracted, or bulging according to the disease process involved. Pain is not usually elicited on palpation of the external ear; this phenomenon usually provides a differential diagnosis between problems of the external ear and middle ear structures. The mastoid prominences postauricularly may be tender or enlarged in acute mastoiditis (usually in children). Serous, purulent, or bloody drainage may be present.

The ear is examined in the following manner:

1. Inspect the external ear for shape, color, and skin condition.
2. Palpate the external ear for pain, unusual movement, or nodules.
3. Palpate the mastoid prominences for tenderness and enlargement.
4. Examine the ear with an otoscope, noting the following conditions:
   a. Condition of external ear canal
   b. Presence of wax or drainage in external ear canal
   c. Appearance of tympanic membrane
      (1) Bony landmarks, color, and appearance of the light reflex
      (2) Signs of scarring or perforation
      (3) Signs of bulging or retraction
5. Test gross hearing in each ear (see Chapter 66).
6. Perform the Weber and Rinne tests (see Chapter 66).

■ DATA ANALYSIS: NURSING DIAGNOSES

Nursing diagnoses are determined from assessment of patient data. Possible nursing diagnoses for patients with problems of the middle ear may include, but are not limited to, the following:

Diagnostic Title	Possible Etiologies
Knowledge deficit about ear infection	Lack of exposure to information
	Unfamiliarity with information sources
Pain	Pathopsychiologic ear pain caused by infection, inflammation, and swelling
Fear	Possibility of hearing loss and/or chronic hearing problem
Injury, potential for	Chance of permanent damage to hearing caused by middle ear problems
Sensory perceptual alteration: auditory	Decreased hearing caused by infection, drainage, or fixation of ear bones in the middle ear

■ PLANNING: EXPECTED PATIENT OUTCOMES

For problems requiring medical intervention for the middle ear, expected patient outcomes may include, but are not limited to, the following:

1. The patient can describe the following:
   a. Measures to be taken to prevent further problems of the tympanic membrane, middle ear, or mastoid cavity
   b. Symptoms requiring medical attention (decreased hearing, pain, drainage from ear canal)
2. Discomfort in the ear is decreased.
3. The patient demonstrates correct technique for application of eardrops, ear ointment, or ear wash, if appropriate.
4. Hearing is improved.

There are additional patient outcomes for persons requiring *surgery* of the middle ear structures. The patient can describe the following:

1. Operative regimen including preoperative preparation, postoperative positioning and movement, prevention of infection, and temporary decrease in hearing
2. The rationale for and desired outcome of the surgical procedure
3. The rationale for and types of safety precautions to be followed
   a. Change dressing as instructed
   b. Prevent water from entering ear by not shampooing for 10 to 14 days and not showering or swimming for 6 weeks
   c. Avoid persons with colds
4. Required ear care
   a. Avoid blowing nose or sneezing to prevent sudden pressure changes
   b. Avoid sudden rapid movements for at least one month
   c. Do not bend from waist, strain at defecation, or lift heavy objects
5. Symptoms requiring medical attention and need for follow-up care (pain, dizziness, or any unusual sign or symptom)

■ IMPLEMENTATION

Hospitalization is rarely necessary for the nonsurgical ear patient and usually does not exceed 2 to 3 days for surgical ear patients. Surgical intervention normally follows unsuccessful attempts to treat the patient medically.

Eardrops and ear ointment may be prescribed for the patient with problems of the tympanic membrane, middle ear, or mastoid cavity. In addition, oral antibiotics and analgesics may be required. The patient is instructed as to the amount, frequency, and duration of medications.

EAR WASH

In addition to other treatment, the patient may be asked to use ear wash. The most common solution for ear

Guidelines for an Ear Wash

1. Wash hands before and after procedure.
2. Warm solution to body temperature by placing bottle in a pan of hot water. Do *not* warm solution on the stove. Solution that is too warm or too cold may cause dizziness.
3. Fill ear syringe with warmed solution.
4. Have patient lie down with affected ear uppermost.
5. Pull external ear up and out, and place tip of ear syringe in ear canal. Do not be afraid to put it down into the ear, but a return flow should occur; if not, pull syringe out slightly.
6. Pump warmed solution vigorously and repeatedly from syringe back and forth into ear by squeezing and releasing bulb of syringe. The ear wash must be forced back and forth, in and out of ear canal.
7. Have patient lean over and let solution run out of ear into a basin.
8. If solution burns too much at first, dilute solution (mix 2 ounces of water with 2 ounces of solution).
9. Use the wash twice a day for 2 weeks and then until the ear stops running or becomes dry. Dryness can be checked by putting a Q-tip down into ear canal. If Q-tip is wet or if there is an odor, continue using the wash until ear is dry.

wash is boric acid and alcohol, which is obtained by prescription at the drugstore. This solution cleanses the ear of debris and infection and provides a drying agent. A 2- or 3-ounce ear syringe, which also can be purchased at the drugstore, will be needed for the ear wash. A family member performs the ear wash for the patient (see the box above for guidelines). Usually the ear wash is followed by the use of eardrops.

PATIENT TEACHING

Teaching for persons with an infection of the tympanic membrane, middle ear, or mastoid cavity includes the following information:

1. Prevent further infections.
   a. Provide adequate treatment of allergic or persistent upper respiratory infections by seeking medical attention and taking medications as prescribed.
   b. Persons with a tympanic perforation should avoid water in the ear (such as while showering, shampooing the hair, or swimming).
2. During treatment for infection, avoid getting water in the ear. If the possibility exists, place two pieces of cotton in the ear, the first piece dry and the second piece saturated with petrolatum.
3. Seek medical attention for signs of decreased hearing, pain in the ear, or drainage from the ear.

CARE OF THE PATIENT UNDERGOING EAR SURGERY

Preoperative Care

The responsibilities of the nurse begin in the preoperative phase when the decision for surgical intervention is made. The scope of nursing activities for the patient having ear surgery can be as broad as a preoperative assessment performed in an office or clinic or as limited as an assessment performed in the holding area of the surgical suite. Data are collected to assess the following about the patient: (1) knowledge of events that are going to occur, (2) mental readiness for surgery, and (3) physiologic status.

The person undergoing ear surgery should be told what to expect in surgery because frequently the patient is given only local anesthesia. The patient is awake but sedated during surgery. The patient is instructed about the length of the procedure and the estimated length of hospital stay. Immediate postoperative instructions should also be discussed. Very often, fear of the unknown can be decreased by an understanding of events that will occur.

Postoperative Care

Immediate postoperative instructions include the following:

1. Lie with the operative ear up for 4 hours after surgery.
2. If necessary, blow nose gently one side at a time.
3. Sneeze or cough with mouth open.
4. Normal occurrences in the initial period may include the following:
   a. Decreased hearing in the operated ear from the packing (possibly, like the sound of talking in a barrel)
   b. Noises in the ear such as cracking or popping
   c. Minor earache and discomfort in the cheek and jaw
   d. Swelling of the ear

Most persons having ear surgery have a short hospitalization. Pain is not usually a major problem. Dizziness or light-headedness may occur when ambulating for the first time. Patients require supervision when ambulating on the day of surgery to protect them from falling. Some persons who are quite dizzy exhibit nystagmus from stimulation of the inner ear. The dizziness usually passes very quickly and seldom requires medication.

The ear rarely bleeds after surgery. Small amounts of serosanguineous drainage on a cotton ball is expected. Most ear surgeries require only a cotton ball in the ear postoperatively, although a dressing over the ear may be necessary following a *tympanomastoidectomy*. Postoperative patient teaching is listed in the box on p. 1973.

PATIENT TEACHING FOLLOWING EAR SURGERY

1. Continue to blow the nose gently one side at a time and to sneeze or cough with mouth open for 1 week after surgery.
2. Avoid physical activity for 1 week and exercises or sports for 3 weeks after surgery.
3. Return to work 1 week after surgery (3 weeks if work is strenuous).
4. Change cotton ball in ear daily as prescribed.
5. Keep ear dry for 6 weeks after surgery.
   a. Do not shampoo hair for 1 week after surgery.
   b. Protect ear when necessary with two pieces of cotton (outer piece saturated with petrolatum).
6. Avoid airplane flights for first week after surgery. For sensation of ear pressure, hold nose, close mouth, and swallow to equalize pressure.
7. Wear noise defenders such as ear muffs for loud noise environments.
8. Report any drainage other than a slight amount of bleeding to the physician.

PROBLEMS OF THE INNER EAR

ETIOLOGY AND PATHOPHYSIOLOGY

CONGENITAL DISORDERS

Incomplete development of the cochlea is the most frequent congenital disorder of the inner ear and results in a sensorineural hearing loss. In contrast, congenital disorders of the vestibular system do not usually cause dizziness or equilibrium problems.

INFECTION

An infection of the inner ear called *labyrinthitis* can be either viral or bacterial in origin. Viral labyrinthitis is usually isolated to the inner ear, whereas the rarer bacterial labyrinthitis is associated with infection in the middle ear and mastoid.

TUMORS

Both benign and malignant tumors of the temporal bone can involve the inner ear. The most common *benign tumor* is an *acoustic neuroma* of the eighth nerve arising in the internal ear canal. Spread of this tumor out of the internal ear canal toward the brain stem causes other neurologic problems and can be life-threatening. Other tumors in the *cerebellar-pontine angle* likewise involve the seventh (facial) and eighth (acoustic) cranial nerves as they enter the internal acoustic meatus.

BALANCE DISORDERS

Disorders of the vestibular structures are lumped under the term *dizziness*. In the true sense, dizziness is only a symptom but is commonly used to describe an illness. The most common balance disorder is a *viral labyrinthitis;* other problems include toxic reactions from drugs, trauma causing fractures of bones of the ear, and tumors such as an acoustic neuroma. A specific balance disorder called *Ménière's disease* is characterized by a triad of symptoms, including *dizziness, hearing loss,* and *tinnitus* (See Table 67-4). The cause is unknown but is thought to be from a virus. Recurring episodic incapacitating bouts of dizziness and hearing loss characterize this disorder. Because of the violent nature of Ménière's disease, the diagnosis is usually dreaded. However, control of the episodes is possible in about 80 to 90 percent of patients. A variety of tretments are used, which include tranquilizers, vagal blockers (such as atropine), antihistamines, vasodilators, diuretics, and avoidance of alcohol, caffeine, and tobacco.[16]

HEARING DISORDERS

A *sensorineural hearing loss* is the most common inner ear disorder. This hearing loss may occur in conjunction with a known disorder but is usually an isolated finding. Factors that influence the type and amount of hearing loss include hereditary disease, toxic substances, and noise-induced hearing loss. At times, the hearing loss may fluctuate, usually ending in progressive hearing loss.

Noise-induced hearing loss can be traumatic; for example, a sudden loud noise such as a blast injury. More commonly, a hearing loss occurs over time from repeated injury from noise. The major cause is industrial noise; the use of firearms is a distant second cause. Whatever the cause, this type of hearing loss is charac-

---

TABLE 67-4 Normal function, pathophysiology, and clinical picture in Ménière's disease

Normal Function	Pathophysiology	Clinical Picture
The vestibular labyrinth contains fluid and hair cells that convert mechanical energy into neural impulses to maintain balance. The fluids of the inner ear are perilymph and endolymph, which are separated by a thin membrane.	Tissue changes in the labyrinth cause an excess of endolymph, which distorts the membranous labyrinth. The cause is thought to be a virus, but this has not been definitely established.	Episodic attacks of incapacitating vertigo, fluctuating hearing loss, tinnitus, and ear fullness occur, often accompanied by nausea and vomiting. Symptoms relieved by rest and medications (see text above.

NURSING CARE PLAN

PERSON WITH MÉNIÈRE'S DISEASE

DATA: Mrs. Bell is a 59-year-old schoolteacher. During the past 6 months, she has had three attacks of "whirling in space" or vertigo, fluctuating hearing in the left ear, noise in the left ear or tinnitus, nausea and vomiting, and a sense of fullness or pressure in the left ear. Two attacks have occurred during class, and one attack occurred at home where she lives alone. Embarrassment, fear, anxiety, and uncertainty are some of her feelings. Mrs. Bell made an appointment at an otology office where diagnostic tests were performed.

These tests included an audiogram, tympanometry, electronystagmography, electrocochleography, a nursing assessment, and physical examination. A diagnosis of Ménière's disease was made. A 1500 mg sodium restricted diet, Dyazide po qd, labyrinthine compensatory exercises, and Niacin 100 mg t.i.d. were prescribed to control the incapacitating attacks of vertigo.

NURSING DIAGNOSIS

Anxiety related to effects of disorder

Expected Patient Outcomes	Nursing Interventions	Rationale
Signs of anxiety are decreased.	Encourage patient to explore concerns about decreased hearing and effects of dizziness attacks and to take action in relation to the concerns. Explore patient's knowledge of the disorder and correct misunderstandings. Encourage realistic hope about expected hearing ability as described by physician. Refer patient to necessary support services, such as social worker or audiologist.	Expressing concerns and receiving realistic counseling and support reduces helplessness and apprehension.

NURSING DIAGNOSIS

Sensory perception, alteration in vestibular, auditory

Expected Patient Outcomes	Nursing Interventions	Rationale
Patient describes actions to avoid dizziness. Patient interacts with others accurately.	Help patient identify avoidable actions that precipitate dizziness attacks. Encourage patient to move slowly and not turn head suddenly when dizziness is present. If tinnitus is distressing, increase background noises such as music. If hearing is decreased: 1. Use measures to facilitate communication with hearing impaired (see text). 2. Refer patient to audiologist, if appropriate.	Understanding cause of dizziness and measures to reduce it may lessen occurrence.

NURSING DIAGNOSIS

Injury, potential for trauma related to dizziness

Expected Patient Outcomes	Nursing Interventions	Rationale
Injury does not occur.	Keep side rails up when patient with dizziness is in bed. Assist with ambulation as needed. Encourage patient to sit or lie down and to remain immobile if signs of dizziness occur. Teach patient to stop car at side of road and turn ignition off immediately at first signs of dizziness while driving.	Knowledge of safety measures reduces possibility of injuries.

NURSING CARE PLAN

PERSON WITH MÉNIÈRE'S DISEASE—CONT'D

NURSING DIAGNOSIS
Self-care deficit, potential

Expected Patient Outcome	Nursing Intervention	Rationale
ADL needs are met. Patient functions as independently as condition permits.	Provide desired foods and fluids if nausea is present. Assist with hygiene as needed while encouraging independence; place hygiene supplies so that patient does not have to turn head. Provide sufficient time for ADL so patient can move slowly.	Assistance with ADL makes it possible for patient to function independently and feel in control of situation.

NURSING DIAGNOSIS
Coping inneffective, individual

Expected Patient Outcomes	Nursing Intervention	Rationale
Patient identifies coping pattern and resultant effects. Patient describes alternative coping behaviors.	Make decisions regarding safety of patient and others when patient is unable to do so. Assist patient to identify usual coping behaviors and the consequences of the behaviors. Assist patient to identify personal strengths. Teach patient alternative coping behaviors (see Chapter 10).	Support and understanding by caregivers improves coping. Discussing possible coping behaviors assists the patient to choose behaviors that are most functional for her.

NURSING DIAGNOSIS
Knowledge deficit about pathophysiology of Méniére's disease related to lack of exposure to information

Expected Patient Outcomes	Nursing Intervention	Rationale
Patient describes nature of disorder, therapy, and safety measures.	Teach patient about the disorder, therapy, and need for medical follow-up (see text). Teach patient ways to protect self from injury and to prevent dizziness attacks when possible.	Need for information regarding disease increases learning that assists the patient to care for self and to live as independently as, possible.

terized by a greater loss in the higher frequencies. The only treatment for noise-induced hearing loss is to prevent the injury by avoiding noise or by wearing ear protection.

Sudden or fluctuating hearing loss is recognized as a separate hearing disorder because of the isolated findings and dramatic outcome. Although the exact cause of the disorder is not known, it is thought to be vascular in nature. Therefore attempted treatments are made to alter the vascular system in some way. Occasionally, the hearing may return to normal without apparent reason. Unfortunately, most patients do not regain normal hearing. One cause that is becoming better recognized is a fistula from the inner ear to the middle ear via the oval or round windows. If this is suspected, the fistulas are closed by a tissue graft.

Presbycusis is a hearing loss found in the elderly. Changes in the delicate labyrinthine structures over the decades causes a *hearing loss predominantly in the higher frequencies.* The amount of the hearing loss will have familial differences and can start in middle age. Tinnitus usually accompanies presbycusis. The vast majority of people eventually suffer from presbycusis during the aging process. In some of these people, the amount of hearing loss warrants the use of a hearing aid. Presbycusis cannot be cured.

CLINICAL MANIFESTATIONS

HEARING LOSS

A sensorineural hearing loss is found with almost any inner ear disorder. The hearing loss is usually incomplete but can be progressive in some illnesses. A characteristic of a severe hearing loss is the loss of discrimination (understanding of words).

TINNITUS

Ringing, or any other noises, in the ear are called tinnitus. Tinnitus accompanies most sensorineural hearing losses and is very annoying. In some patients, the tinnitus becomes the problem, and the underlying cause may be forgotten. Unfortunately, the only cure for tinnitus is correction of the underlying cause; however, new and unproven cures are still advertised for this chronic ailment. The best treatment is to mask the tinnitus with background sounds such as music, which may help the patient adjust to the ear noise.

DIZZINESS

Dizziness also is associated with inner ear problems. The close anatomic relationship between the balance and hearing systems sometimes, but not always, causes the sensation of dizziness in conjunction with a hearing loss. However, in most instances, dizziness is present without a hearing loss.

Vertigo, or spinning, is the medical term for dizziness, but specific descriptions of vertigo are not helpful in diagnosing the vestibular abnormality. Dizziness is described in such varied terms that it is almost impossible to define the symptom. All descriptions should be accepted as the symptom caused by a disorder of the balance system. Because the balance system can compensate, *dizziness is usually* not present consistently but is *episodic in nature.* Dizziness, like pain, is subject to psychologic influences. *Dizziness is second only to headache as the most common symptom currently found in America.*

For the patient with dizziness, the differential diagnosis may be accomplished by a thorough medical as-sessment, including audiometry, vestibular tests, radiologic evaluation, and laboratory studies (see Chapter 66). The nurse may be involved in any or all of these procedures, according to the setting, and must be able to explain the procedures to the patient to promote understanding and to gain the patient's trust.

MEDICAL MANAGEMENT

Other than antibiotics for infections, the medical treatment of hearing loss is dismal. General modalities include steroids and vasodilators, but specific therapy is still lacking. Dizziness can be helped by labyrinthine suppressants and other medicines, but a specific medicinal cure for dizziness does not exist. Likewise, treatment for Menière's disease consists of over fifty different medicines. Usually a combination of medical therapy will control the dizziness, but no cure has been found.

HEARING AIDS

Because most hearing losses are permanent, the use of a hearing aid should always be considered. A patient should undergo a trial period to establish its benefit before purchasing the aid. Bilateral or binaural aids are desirable.

The technology of aided hearing is part of the current electronic explosion (see Aural Rehabilitation, p. 1980). The evolution in hearing aid development has led to

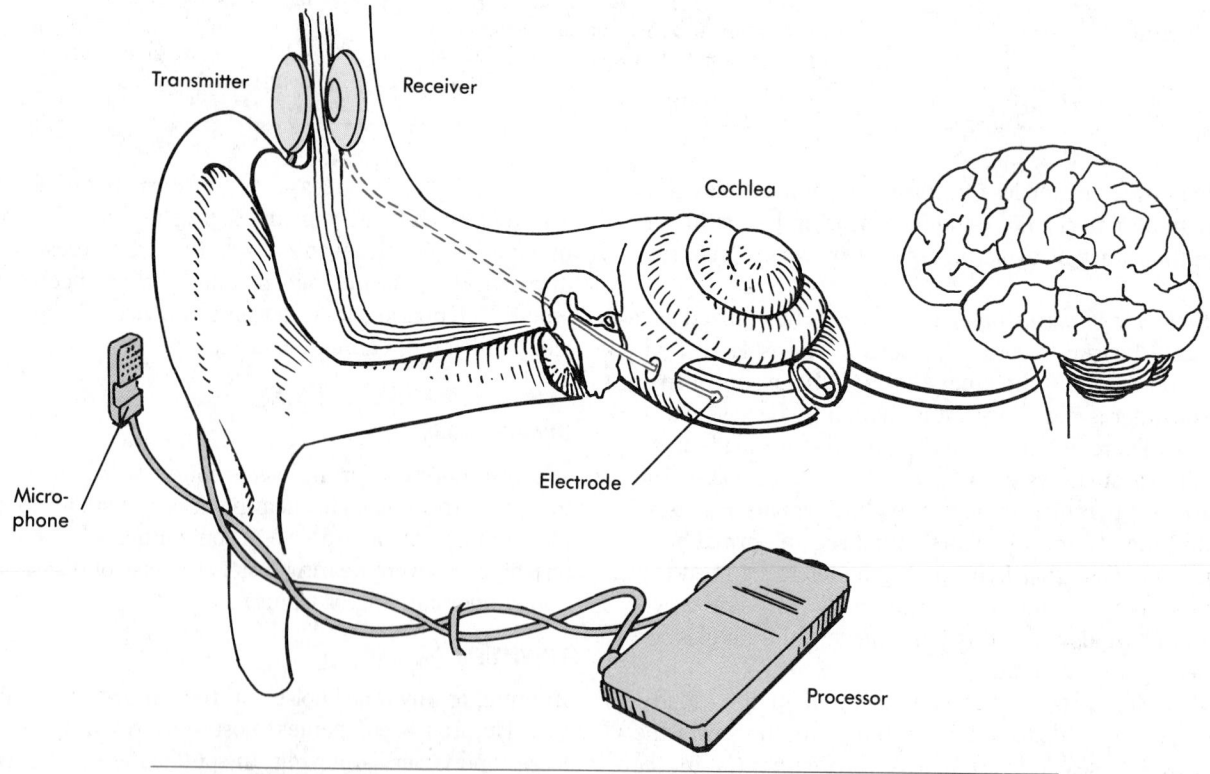

FIGURE 67-5 Cochlear implant.

smaller and more effective aids. Small hearing aids currently are available that fit into the ear canal; however, the greater the hearing loss is, the larger the hearing aid. Hearing aids also are available for placement within the ear concha or behind the ear. Special hearing aids can transmit sound by radio waves to the opposite ear or by vibration to the inner ear through the skull. In the future, hearing aids will be semi-implantable and finally totally implantable within the middle ear and mastoid.

IMPLANTABLE HEARING DEVICES

Three types of implanted hearing devices are either available for use or in the investigation stage. They are *cochlear implants, bone hearing devices,* and *semi-implantable hearing devices.*

Cochlear implants for those patients with no hearing at all are currently available (Figure 67-5). This device incorporates a small computer that changes the spoken word to electrical impulses. The impulses are transmitted across the skin to an implanted coil that carries the impulse to the hearing nerve endings in the cochlea by an electrode introduced through the round windows. The best of the cochlear implants use multichannels and are able to return about half of the patient's hearing and understanding. Cochlear implants are available for both children and adults.

In some cases of hearing loss, sound can be transmitted through the skull to the inner ear. Patients with a conductive hearing loss can use a device in which the receiver is implanted under the skin into the skull. The external device transmits the sound through the skin. This device is worn above the ear and not in the ear canal.

Patients who already use a hearing aid will gain the most from the implantable device. Clinical research has shown that a magnet implanted in the middle ear can be stimulated by an ear canal driver which changes sound to a magnetic force. This system eliminates several bothersome problems of hearing aids, such as feedback and difficulties with hearing in noisy environments. A semi-implantable hearing device is the first step to a totally implantable device that would eliminate any external device. However, many challenges have yet to be met before a workable device is available.

SURGICAL MANAGEMENT

The delicate inner ear does not lend itself to surgical treatment, except for destructive procedures. Nonetheless, surgeons have gingerly approached surgical methods involving the inner ear in an attempt to alleviate dizziness. The *endolymphatic sac procedures* include decompression and various forms of shunts. The intent of these procedures is to lessen the fluid pressure within the labyrinth and control dizziness. Other attempts to do the same are performed through the oval or round windows. A destructive procedure to remove the membranous labyrinth, either subtotally through the oval window or totally through the mastoid bone, is called *labyrinthectomy.* Also, *vestibular nerve section* alone can be performed to alleviate dizziness. Alleviation of the patient's dizziness is usually immediate. Because of the compensation by all of the other structures related to maintaining balance, a person can function with only one labyrinth.

The necessity of removing tumors of the inner ear and internal auditory canal has led to various approaches through and around the temporal bone. These procedures are sometimes performed in conjunction with a neurosurgeon. As time passes, a greater number of patients will undergo this surgery and thus retain facial nerve function and, rarely, hearing function. Because of the limited exposure of the central nervous system by the new techniques, the mortality and morbidity of the surgery is lessened. Facial nerve disorders are also treated by the same surgical approaches. Malignant tumors in this area can be excised by a *temporal bone resection.* However, surgery of the inner ear is still in a pioneering stage.

■ MANAGEMENT OF THE PERSON WITH DIZZINESS

Because dizziness is only a symptom, the diagnosis and treatment of the underlying disease is frustrating to both the patient and the health care providers. The nurse's role becomes even more important as psychologic factors, such as social isolation or fear of participating in activities because of the possibility of dizziness, complicate the illness. The nurse's ability to understand and to assess the person with dizziness will aid in providing care that will contribute toward the patient's recovery.

Balance and equilibrium depend on four systems being intact: the *vestibular* (labyrinth of the inner ear), the *proprioceptive* (somatosensors of joints and muscles), the *visual* (eye), and the *cerebellar systems.* The sensations transmitted from the eyes, the somatosensors, and the inner ears are integrated in the brain stem and cerebellum and perceived in the cerebral cortex. Dizziness is most likely to occur when two or more systems are impaired simultaneously or when they transmit sensory information that is contradictory.

■ ASSESSMENT

Dizziness is a common vague symptom with a wide variety of unpleasant meanings and with multiple individual interpretations. Spinning may be the most common form of dizziness. Other "feelings" include light-headedness, giddiness, imbalance, veering in one direction while walking, unsteadiness, or a vague feeling of uncertainty during changes in body position.

Nursing assessment of dizziness may include the following:

1. A patient interview obtaining a health history and specific data about the onset and characteristics of the dizziness
2. An interview with the family to identify the effect of the person's dizziness on others
3. Physical examination—with specific emphasis on eyes, ears, thyroid, heart, and lungs—and a neurologic examination
4. Review of laboratory tests

The importance of the history and interview cannot be overemphasized. All patients experience some degree of anxiety regarding the illness, and dizziness can have devastating effects on the person's behavior. The disruption of the person's routine, the severity of the "attacks," and the fear of the unknown may make the patient agitated, anxious, and depressed. The nurse must be aware of these feelings and demonstrate self-confidence, patience, courtesy, consideration, and gentleness.

■ DATA ANALYSIS: NURSING DIAGNOSES

Nursing diagnoses are determined from assessment of patient data. Possible nursing diagnoses for the person with inner ear problems may include, but are not limited to, the following:

Diagnostic Title	Possible Etiologies
Injury: potential for	Dizziness can cause person to fall
Knowledge deficit about condition	Lack of exposure to information about causes of dizziness
	Unfamiliarity with information sources
Anxiety	Vertigo is threat to self-concept and to successful role functioning
Coping ineffective, individual	Personal vulnerability because unable to control attacks of dizziness
Self-care deficit: activities of daily living	Perception/cognition impairment caused by vertigo
Sensory/perceptual alteration: auditory, vestibular	Decreased hearing caused by damage to the inner ear
	Altered vestibular function caused by damage to the inner ear

■ PLANNING: EXPECTED PATIENT OUTCOMES

Expected patient outcomes for the person with inner ear problems may include, but are not limited to, the following:

1. The patient can describe:
   a. The reason for the dizziness
   b. Circumstances that may precipitate an attack of dizziness and what to do when one occurs
   c. Safety precautions during episodes of dizziness
   d. Symptoms requiring medical intervention
   e. Dosage and side effects of medications

2. No injury from complications of dizziness
3. The patient is prepared for surgery, if indicated
4. Anxiety decreases after providing explanation for symptoms
5. Appropriate coping mechanisms to deal with the uncertainty of dizziness

■ IMPLEMENTATION

Although patients have been hospitalized for medical treatment of dizziness in the past, this trend is decreasing for three reasons: (1) increased use of prophylactic treatment, (2) increased specialization in the care of the person with dizziness by physicians and nurses, and (3) economic pressures such as diagnostic related groups [DRGs] which are discussed in Chapter 1.

At present, approximately 5% of all patients with dizziness undergo surgical intervention. However, an increasing number of patients will undergo surgical procedures in the future because of new surgical developments and advanced technology. The care of the person experiencing surgery of the inner ear is the same as that described on p. 1972.

Responsibilities of the nurse caring for a patient with dizziness include the promotion of comfort and safety. Patients who are experiencing dizziness are sometimes reluctant to move because movement aggravates the symptoms. Specific nursing care activities include the following:

1. Encourage patient to move slowly.
2. Encourage and facilitate eating by providing patient with desired foods and fluids (dizziness may cause nausea and vomiting).
3. Assist patient with hygiene as needed while encouraging independence.
4. Keep side rails up when patient is in bed.
5. Assist patient as needed in ambulation.
6. Encourage patient to verbalize specific problems created by the dizziness.
7. Teach the patient:
   a. Nature of the disorder
   b. Diagnostic tests and planned medical or surgical therapy for the dizziness
   c. Ways to protect self from injury when dizzy, such as lying down and remaining immobile or using an aid such as a cane for walking
   d. Information about prescribed medications
   e. Symptoms requiring medical attention

MANAGEMENT OF THE PERSON WITH SENSORINEURAL HEARING LOSS
■ ASSESSMENT

Of the 10 million people in the United States with a hearing loss who are over 65 years of age or older, over 90% have a sensorineural hearing loss. Because of fear, misinformation, lack of information, or vanity, many people do not admit that they have a hearing problem.

The nurse can identify persons with impaired hearing and encourage them to seek professional diagnosis and treatment. Indications of a hearing loss may include the following:

1. Failure to respond to oral communication
2. Inappropriate response to oral communication
3. Excessively loud speech
4. Abnormal awareness of sounds
5. Strained facial expressions
6. Tilted head when listening
7. Constant need for clarification of conversation
8. Faulty speech articulation
9. Behavioral clues (see Chapter 66)

The impact of not hearing others may make some people withdraw from social situations and become anxious and insecure. People with hearing losses may experience fears of inadequacy, feelings of inferiority, depression, and varying degrees of stress and isolation. Important nursing assessments include the extent and duration of the hearing loss, how the person has coped with stress previously, and what support systems are available to the person.

The sensorineural hearing loss is assessed by history, physical examination, and audiometry. The diagnosis is usually reached quickly and inexpensively in the physician's office or in a clinic. Occasionally, laboratory, radiologic, and vestibular examinations are used. In an otology office, the nurse may have the responsibility for performing the history, otologic examination, and screening audiometry. The history is often the most important part of the clinical assessment. The following questions are included in the history for a person with a sensorineural hearing loss:

1. When was the age of onset of the hearing loss?
2. Was the hearing loss progressive?
3. Is there a fluctuation in hearing loss?
4. Is the hearing loss in one ear or both?
5. Is there a family history of hearing loss?
6. Is there pressure in the ears?
7. Is there ringing in the ears?
8. Is there any dizziness?
9. What medications are currently being taken? (Determine whether a possibility of ototoxicity from medication exists.)
10. Has there been any head trauma?
11. What is the person's exposure to noise (present and past)?
12. Has the person experienced any other neurologic disturbances?
13. Has the person experienced any speech or visual disturbances?
14. Is there any ear pain or drainage?

The extent of the assessment of the sensorineural hearing loss by the nurse depends on the setting and the nurse's educational preparation and experience. All nurses, however, should be able to inspect the outer ear and grossly assess the auditory acuity (see Chapter 66).

■ **DATA ANALYSIS: NURSING DIAGNOSES**

Nursing diagnoses are determined from assessment of patient data. Possible nursing diagnoses for the person with sensorineural hearing loss may include, but are not limited to, the following:

Diagnostic Title	Possible Etiologies
Anxiety	Hearing loss is a threat to self-concept and to successful role functioning
Coping, ineffective, individual	Personal vulnerability and communication process threatened by hearing loss
Knowledge deficit about hearing	Lack of exposure to information Unfamiliarity with information sources
Sensory/perceptual alteration:auditory	Permanent or temprorary (surgical) loss of hearing

■ **PLANNING: EXPECTED PATIENT OUTCOMES**

Expected patient outcomes for the person with sensorineural hearing loss may include, but are not limited to, the following:

1. Patient can describe:
   a. The basis of the sensorineural hearing loss and the treatment plan
   b. The dosage and side effects of any prescribed medications
   c. Care of hearing aid, if one is prescribed
   d. Available community resources for the hearing-impaired person
2. Patient copes with the loss of hearing as evidenced by appropriate aural rehabilitation, wearing hearing aid, appropriate behavior, and effective communication with others

■ **IMPLEMENTATION**

Communicating with the Hearing-Impaired

Less than 1% of all persons with a sensorineural hearing loss require surgery of the inner ear. However, the hearing loss may be the secondary diagnosis of many hospitalized patients. The nurse must therefore understand the nursing interventions for this common health problem and facilitate communication for persons with hearing loss. The suggestions listed below can apply to communicating with all persons, regardless of the type or severity of hearing loss.

1. Get the person's attention by raising an arm or hand.
2. Stand with the light on your face; this will help the person speech (lip) read.
3. Talk directly to the person, facing him or her.
4. Speak clearly, but do not overaccentuate words.
5. Speak in a normal tone; do not shout. Shouting overuses normal speaking movements and may

cause distortion and be too loud for the person with sensorineural damage. If the person has conductive loss only, sometimes making the voice louder without shouting is helpful.

6. If the person does not seem to understand what is said, express it differently. Some words are difficult to "see" in speech reading, such as white and red.

7. Move closer to the person and toward the better ear if he or she does not hear you.

8. Write out proper names or any statement that you are not sure was understood.

9. Do not smile, chew gum, or cover the mouth when talking to a person with limited hearing.

10. Inattention may indicate tiredness or lack of understanding.

11. Use phrases to convey meaning rather than one-word answers. State the major topic of the discussion first and then give details.

12. Do not show annoyance by careless facial expression. Persons who are hard of hearing depend more on visual clues for acceptance.

13. Encourage the use of a hearing aid if the person has one; allow him or her to adjust it before speaking.

14. If in a group, repeat important statements and avoid asides to others in the group.

15. Avoid the use of the intercom when communicating with patient. The intercom may distort sound and cause poor communication.

16. Do not avoid conversation with a person who has hearing loss. It has been said that to live in a silent world is much more devastating than to live in darkness, and persons with hearing loss appear, by and large, to have more emotional difficulties than those who are blind.*

AURAL REHABILITATION

If hearing loss is irreversible or not amenable to surgical intervention or if the person elects not to have surgery, aural rehabilitation may increase communication. The purpose of aural rehabilitation is to maximize the hearing-impaired person's communication skills.

The auditory sense is our primary mode of communication, and rehabilitation is directed toward teaching the person more effective use of the senses of vision, touch, and vibration plus maximizing the use of any remaining hearing ability. Rehabilitation is affected by the person's background and by the severity of impairment. As with other forms of rehabilitation, success depends on the degree of the patient's motivation.

*Adapted from Conover M and Cober J: Nurs Clin North Am 5:497, 1970.

Types of Aural Rehabilitation

Aural rehabilitation includes *auditory training, speech reading, speech training,* and the *use of hearing aids.* The use of instruments and training are involved. *Auditory training* is an approach to enhance listening skills. The hearing-impaired person is initially exposed to gross differences in sound and then gradually "fine tuned" so that subtle differences in discrimination of two similar sounds can be made. The primary purpose of auditory training exercises is to help the person concentrate on the speaker. For some persons, only gross differences between sounds may be recognized.

Speech reading is the current term used for lip reading and is an important means of communication. Speech training is the process of understanding vocal communication by the integration of lip movements with facial expressions, gestures, environmental clues, and conversation contexts. Speech reading is very difficult, however, without auditory cues. Many movements for speech are very rapid, many sounds are very similar (b, m, p), and certain sounds of any language are invisible (the h in English). A high percentage of the words have to be guessed at by the hearing-impaired person. Knowledge of this fact alone will help the nurse be more understanding of the person who is speech (lip) reading.

Because of reduced auditory feedback (the inability of hearing-impaired persons to monitor their own speech), the clearness, pitch quality, or rate of their speech may deteriorate. These abnormal effects alter the efficiency of communication and reduce the intelligibility of speech. The goal of *speech training* is to conserve, develop, or prevent deterioration of speech skills.

Hearing Aids

Hearing aids are instruments made up of miniature parts working together as a system to amplify sound in a controlled manner. They are used by both hard-of-hearing persons (slight or moderate hearing loss) and deaf persons (severe or profound hearing loss). Hearing aids make sound louder but *do not improve the ability to hear.* Therefore persons with decreased discrimination (the ability to understand what is spoken) benefit less from a hearing aid. Appropriate aural rehabilitation will ensure successful adjustment of most problems. The hearing aid amplifies all background noises such as hospital machinery, footsteps, and department store noises, as well as speech. These noises may mask conversation or confuse the hearing-impaired person, especially the elderly.

Several types of hearing aids exist according to size and location to be worn (see the box top left on p. 1981). Regardless of the type of aid, the hearing aid consists of the following parts:

1. Microphone to receive sound waves from the air and change sounds into electrical signals

TYPES OF HEARING AIDS

Body-worn aid for hearing loss of 40-110 dB: usually worn on middle of chest

Eyeglass aid for hearing loss of 25-70 dB: worn in temple of eyeglasses

Postauricular aid for hearing loss of 25-80 dB: worn behind the ear

In-the-ear aid for hearing loss of 25-55 dB: worn in ear canal

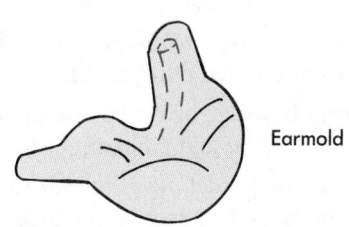

Earmold

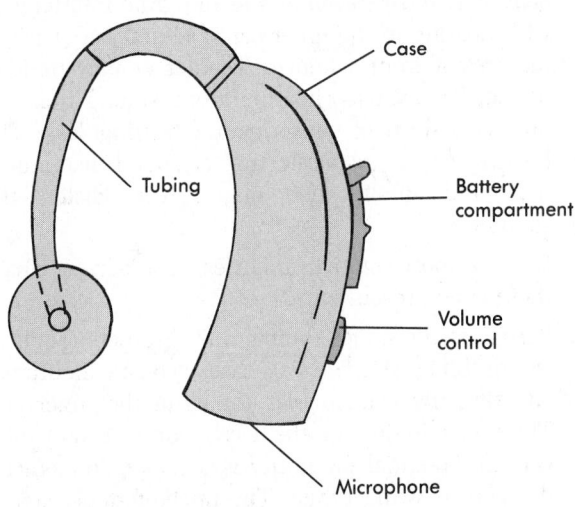

Case

Tubing

Battery compartment

Volume control

Microphone

FIGURE 67-6 Parts of hearing aid.

CARE OF A HEARING AID

1. Turn the hearing aid off when not in use.
2. Open the battery compartment at night to avoid accidental drainage of the battery.
3. Keep an extra battery available at all times.
4. Wash the earmold frequently (daily if necessary) with mild soap and warm water with the use of a pipe cleaner to cleanse the cannula.
5. Dry the earmold completely before reconnecting it to the receiver.
6. Do not wear the hearing aid during an ear infection.

WHAT TO DO IF HEARING AID FAILS TO WORK

1. Check the on-off switch.
2. Inspect the earmold for cleanliness.
3. Examine the battery for correct insertion.
4. Examine cord plug for correct insertion.
5. Examine cord for breaks.
6. Replace battery, cord, or both, if necessary. The life of batteries varies according to amount of use and power requirements of the aid. Batteries last from 2 to 14 days.
7. Check the position of the earmold in the ear. If the hearing aid "whistles," the earmold is probably not inserted properly into the ear canal, or the person needs to have a new earmold made.

2. Amplifier to increase the strength of electrical signals
3. Battery to provide the electrical energy needed to operate the hearing aid
4. Receiver (loudspeaker) to change the electrical signals back into sound waves

On all types of hearing aids but the body-worn type, all four components are housed in one small case. The louder sounds are then directed into the ear through a custom-fitted earmold (Figure 67-6).

The person with a hearing aid should know how to care for the aid (see the box below, left) and what to do if the aid does not work (see the box above). The nurse must also have a basic knowledge of the hearing aid to assist the person unable or unwilling to do this when ill. The person is encouraged to use the hearing aid and to store it safely in its case when it is not in use.

Community Services

Many agencies and associations exist for the hearing-impaired person. Services are offered by audiology clinics sponsored by universities, hospitals, community programs, state or local departments of health, or the Veteran's Administration. National organizations are available to give information and counseling and include the following:

1. American Academy of Otolaryngology—Head and Neck Surgeons, 1 Prince St, Alexandria, VA, a professional society for physicians specializing in diseases of the ear and related areas; it can provide information on hearing and balance disorders.
2. American Annals of the Deaf, 5034 Wisconsin Ave., NW, Washington, DC 20016. The April issue every year lists a directory of programs and services for the deaf available by state and includes information about the type of facilities.
3. American Federation of the Physically Handicapped, Inc., 1370 National Press Building, Washington, DC 20004; provides counseling and information.

4. American Speech-Language-Hearing Association, 10801 Rockville Pike, Dept AP, Rockville, MD 20852. This association can answer questions or mail information on hearing aids or hearing loss and communication problems in the elderly and provide a list of certified audiologists in each state.

5. Gallaudet College, 7th and Florida Ave, Washington, DC 20002; the only liberal arts college for the deaf in the world.

6. National Association of Hearing and Speech Agencies, 919 18th St NW, Washington, DC 20006; provides counseling and information.

7. Office of Scientific and Health Reports, National Institute of Neurological and Communicative Disorders and Stroke Bldg 31, Rm 8A06, Bethesda, MD 20205; a focal point for research on hearing loss and other communication disorders. (Pamphlet: Hearing loss: hope through research.)

8. Self-Help for Hard-of-Hearing People (Shhh), 4848 Battery Lane, Dept E, Bethesda, MD 20814; a nationwide organization for the hard-of-hearing; publishes a bimonthly magazine that includes experiences of the hard-of-hearing and new developments in the field of hearing loss; publications and reprints available.

9. Society of Otorhinolaryngology and Head–Neck Nurses, Inc., 439 N Causeway, New Smyrna Beach, FL 32069; a professional nursing society for nurses specializing in caring for patients with problems of the ear, nose, or throat; information on hearing and balance disorders.

10. State Office of Vocational Rehabilitation (in each state); provides vocational training and placement services.

11. Veterans Administration; provides audiology clinics and rehabilitation services for veterans.

CHAPTER SUMMARY

- Disorders that plug the outer ear, add fluid to the middle ear, make the ossicles unmovable, destroy the hair cells of the organ of Corti, or interfere with nerve stimulus transmission over the acoustic nerve will lead to decreased hearing.

- Hearing can be preserved by preventing infection or trauma of the ear, by using ototoxic drugs with caution and seeking medical attention if symptoms occur, and by preventing frequent exposure to loud noises (or using ear protection for constant loud noises).

- Ear infections are the most common disorders of the external and middle ears; pain results from pressure by fluid buildup within the enclosed spaces.

- Serous otitis media develops from collection of serous fluid in the middle ear when the eustachian tube becomes blocked. Purulent otitis media develops from bacteria entering the middle ear through the eustachian tube; pus collects in the middle ear.

- Ear infections are treated with antibiotics, given by eardrops, ear ointments, or systemically. Treatments to remove drainage may include ear wash, ear irrigation, or surgery of the eardrum.

- The person with an ear infection should avoid getting water in the ear (care during showering and shampooing and avoiding swimming).

- *Tympanosclerosis* and *cholesteatoma* are both complications from repeated otitis media.

- Any long-term blockage of the eustachian tube leads to *serous otitis media* and a hearing loss.

- Otosclerosis is the *hardening of the ear* that involves the stapes bone and causes a conductive hearing loss. *Stapedectomy* is the surgical procedure that removes and replaces the stapes.

- *Cochlear implants* are used for patients with no usable hearing at all in either ear.

- *Sensorineural hearing loss* results from interference with hearing in the inner ear or neural pathways; it may result from a known disorder or may be idiopathic. Presbycusis (hearing loss resulting from aging) is a form of sensorineural hearing loss. The hearing loss is primarily that of sound discrimination, and amplification may further distort the sound.

- It is the most common inner ear disorder for which there is no present cure.

- Vertigo is the major symptom of disorders (such as labyrinthitis, Ménière's disease, acoustic neuroma) affecting the semicircular canals of the inner ear. Tinnitus (ringing in the ears) often accompanies vertigo. Potential for injury is a major problem for the person with vertigo. The uncomfortable sensation of vertigo can be minimized by lying down and holding the head still.

- Dizziness, like pain, is subject to psychological influences and is second to headache as the most common symptom currently found in the United States.

- The nurse's ability to understand and assess the person with dizziness will aid in providing care contributing toward the person's recovery.

- The purpose of aural rehabilitation is to maximize the hearing-impaired person's communication skills.

- Aural rehabilitation includes auditory training, speech-reading (lip-reading), speech training, (improving speech clarity) and the use of hearing aids.

QUESTIONS TO CONSIDER

- Walk around for a day with earplugs in your ears. Describe your reactions. How do you think you would feel if you were told you would never hear well again?

- What are the predisposing factors for a conductive hearing loss? For a sensorineural loss?

- Which agencies are available in your community to aid in the rehabilitation of the hearing impaired?

- What are the major causes of dizziness?

REFERENCES AND SELECTED READINGS

1. Adams R and Victor M: Principles of neurology, ed 3, New York, 1985, McGraw-Hill Book Co.
2. Alberti PM and Ruben RJ editors: Otologic medicine and surgery, vol 1, New York, 1988, Churchill Livingstone Inc.
3. Alberti PM and Ruben RJ editors: Otologic medicine and surgery, vol 2, New York, 1988, Churchill Livingstone Inc.
4. Antibiotic treatment of ototis media, J Nurs Care 13:26-27, 1980.
5. Bates B: A guide to physical examination, ed 4, Philadelphia, 1986, JB Lippincott Co.
6. Becker G and Nadler G: The aged deaf: integration of a disabled group into an agency serving elderly people, Gerontologist 20:214-221, 1980.
7. Berger KW: The hearing aid: its operation and development, ed 3, Livonia, Mich, 1984, The National Hearing Aid Society.
8. Brackman D and Anderson RG: Meniere's disease, treatment with the endolymphatic shunt, Otolaryngol Head Neck Surg 88:174-182, 1980.
9. Bulechek GM and McCloskey JC: Nursing interventions, treatments for nursing diagnosis, Philadelphia, 1985, WB Saunders Co.
10. Chusid JG: Correlative neuroanatomy and functional neurology, Los Altos, Calif, 1982, Lange Medical Publications.
11. *Conover M and Cober J: Understanding and caring for the hearing impaired, Nurs Clin North Am 5:497-506, 1970.
12. The American Association of Neuroscience Nurses: Core curriculum for neurosurgical nursing, 1984, The Association.
13. Counter RT: Color atlas of temporal bone surgical anatomy, London England, 1980, Year Book Publishers Inc.
14. DeWeese DD and Suanders WH: Textbook of otolaryngology, ed 6, St Louis, 1982, The CV Mosby Co.
15. *Edsall J.: Relationship between loss of auditory and visual acuity and social disengagement in an aged population, Nurs Res 27(5):296-298, 1978.
16. Gardner G: Ménière's disease, in Rukel RE, ed. Conn's current therapy 1990, Philadelphia, 1990, WB Saunders Co.
17. Hawke M, Keene M, and Alberti PW: Clinical otoscopy, New York, 1984, Churchill Livingstone.
18. Healy GB: Hearing loss and vertigo secondary to head injury, N Engl J Med 306(17):1029-1031, 1982.
19. Heller BR and Gaynor EB: Hearing loss and aural rehabilitation of the elderly, Top Clin Nurs 31(1):21-29, 1981.
20. Holder L: Hearing aids: handle with care, Nurs '82 12(4):64-67, 1982.
21. *Holm C: Deafness: common misunderstandings, Am J Nurs 78:1910-1912, 1978.
22. Holm C: How to test your patient's hearing acuity, Nurs '80 10(7):60-61, 1980.
23. Hughes GB: Textbook of clinical otology, New York, 1985, Thieme-Stratton, Inc.
24. Kamenir S and Fothersill R: Hands-on-skill for dealing with hearing aids, Cancer Nurs 78(11):44-45, 1982.
25. Karb VK, Queener SF, and Freeman JB: Handbook of drugs for nursing practice, St. Louis, 1989, The CV Mosby Co.
26. Malkiewicz J: The fine art of giving a physical: how to assess the ears and test hearing acuity, RN 45(3):56-63, 1982.
27. * Mamaril AP: Sudden deafness, AM J Nurs 76:1992-1994, 1976.
28. McCormick GP, et al: Artificial speech devices, Am J Nurs 82:121-122, 1982.
29. Moore JC: Establishment of an outpatient ENT clinic, AORN J 31:620-626, 1980.
30. *Programmed instruction: patient assessment: examination of the ear, Am J Nurs 75:457-476, 1975.
31. Reiner A: Manual of patient care standards, Rockville, Md 1988, Aspen Publishers, Inc.
32. Report of the task force on the National Strategic Research Plan of the National Institute on Deafness and Other Communication Disorders, Bethesda, Md, 1989, Institute of Health.
33. Riley MAK: Nursing care of the client with ear, nose and throat disorders, New York, 1987, Springer Publishing Co, Inc.
34. *Saunders WH et al: Nursing care in the eye, ear, nose and throat disorders, ed 4, St Louis, 1979, The CV Mosby Co.
35. Serra AM, Bailey CM, and Jackson P: Ear, nose and throat nursing, England, 1986, Blackwell Scientific Publications.
36. Tortorelli B: Acoustic neuroma: an overview of the disorder and nursing care for these patients, J Neurosurg Nurs :170-171, August 1981.
37. Voke J: Aspects of hearing, physiology of the ear, part I, Nurs Time 80(33):28-30, Aug 15-21, 1984.
38. Voke J: Aspects of hearing, functions of the cochlea, Nurs Time 80(34):60-62, Aug 22-28, 1984.
39. Wilson WR and Nadol JR: Quick reference to ear, nose and throat disorders, Philadelphia, 1983, JB Lippincott Co.

*References preceded by an asterisk are particularly well suited for student reading.

CHAPTER 68

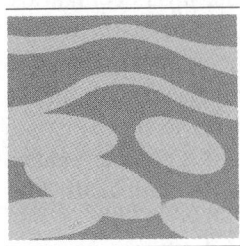

Assessment of the Musculoskeletal System

PATRICIA S. BUERGIN
KYLE M. PASKERT

CHAPTER OBJECTIVES

After studying this chapter, the student should be able to:
1   Describe the structure and function of the tissues that compose the musculoskeletal system.
2   Explain the interrelationship of the tissues of the musculoskeletal system to the overall functioning of the system.
3   Describe the physiologic changes that occur in the musculoskeletal system with aging.
4   Explain the nature of pathologic conditions that can occur within the musculoskeletal system.
5   Describe the subjective data that should be obtained during initial nursing assessment of the person who has a musculoskeletal problem.
6   Describe the components of objective assessment to be carried out with the person who has a musculoskeletal problem.
7   Describe the diagnostic tests that could be performed for the patient with a musculoskeletal problem, and explain the rationale for each test.
8   Identify the relevance of subjective and objective data and diagnostic tests in planning care for persons with musculoskeletal problems.

The eagle that cannot fly will starve to death. The deer that cannot run becomes the easy prey of its enemies. And if humans could not move, they too would surely die. The musculoskeletal system enables humans to move about freely. Thus illnesses and disorders that deprive persons of this ability can be very serious.

Planning appropriate interventions for individuals who have locomotor disabilities requires that the disabilities and the individual's reaction to them are carefully assessed. Such assessment is made on the basis of knowledge and understanding of the anatomy and physiology of the musculoskeletal system, as well as of the diagnostic studies involved and what the results of these studies mean. In this chapter the anatomy and physiology of the musculoskeletal system, methods and rationale for obtaining subjective and objective data about patients and their disabilities, and the pertinence of selected diagnostic studies are discussed.

ANATOMY AND PHYSIOLOGY

BONE

FUNCTION

Bones have three *mechanical* functions:
1. *Support* of body tissues as provided by the skeletal framework
2. *Protection* of body organs (for example, the bony casing of the skull that protects the brain)
3. *Movement,* affected by contraction of muscles pulling on bones that provide leverage for motion

Bones have two additional functions. They are a storehouse for calcium, and their marrow produces red blood cells (RBCs) (*hematopoiesis*).

COMPOSITION AND DEVELOPMENT

Bones are composed of both living cells and nonliving intracellular material. The living cells are the *osteoblasts, osteoclasts,* and *osteocytes.* Nonliving intracellular material, or *bone matrix,* consists of mucopolysaccharides and collagen. Bones are derived from embryonic hyaline cartilage that undergoes a process known as *osteogenesis,* or *endochondral ossification.* This process is accomplished through the synthesis of mucopolysaccharides and collagen by the *osteoblasts* (bone building cells). Calcium salts are deposited in the bone matrix, giving bone the "hard" quality that characterizes it.

TYPES, STRUCTURE, AND GROWTH OF BONE

Bones are divided into four types, according to their shape:
1. Long (femur, humerus)
2. Short (carpals)

3. Flat (skull)

4. Irregular (vertebrae)

Each bone is composed of *cancellous* (spongy) and *compact* (dense) bone. In the long bones the cancellous portions are found in the ends of the bones, and compact bone is located in the shaft. The short and irregular bones have an inner core of cancellous bone with an outer layer of compact bone. Flat bones have two outer plates of compact bone with an inner layer of cancellous bone.

Cancellous bone and compact bone are differentiated from one another by the arrangement of the *lamellae* within them. Lamellae are concentric cylindric layers of calcified matrix. At the center of this arrangement of concentric rings is a canal, called the *haversian canal*. This canal contains a capillary. Some canals also contain a small arteriole, venule, and lymphatics. Small spaces between the rings of the lamellae, called *lacunae,* are occupied by bone cells (*osteocytes*). Lacunae are connected with the haversian canal and therefore with the nutrient supply by very small canals called *canaliculi.* The lamella with its haversian canal, lacunae, and canaliculi is called a *haversian unit* (Figure 68-1). Haversian units fit closely together in compact bone. In cancellous bone, however, many open spaces exist between thin interconnecting processes of bone called *trabeculae.* The fine, thready structure of trabecular bone not only provides strength to the bone but reduces its weight.

A typical long bone is covered, except on its articular surfaces, by a white, fibrous membrane called the *periosteum.* The articular surfaces are covered with resilient *hyaline cartilage.* The periosteum provides a place for muscle fibers to attach, and its inner layers contain osteoblasts. Because of the presence of osteoblasts, the periosteum is considered an organ of growth and repair. The membranous *endosteum,* which also contains some osteoblasts, lines the marrow-filled medullary cavity and the haversian canals. The ends of the bone are called *epiphyses,* and the shaft is known as the *diaphysis* (Figure 68-2).

Longitudinal growth of the long bones emanates from the epiphyseal cartilage, located between the diaphyseal and epiphyseal centers of ossification. The epiphyseal cartilage thickens because of rapid proliferation of the cartilage cells, and this additional cartilage undergoes ossification. Growth in the diameter of the bone is accomplished as *osteoclasts* (bone-destroying cells) enlarge the medullary cavity while *osteoblasts* in the periosteum produce new bone at the outside of the bone (*membranous ossification*). In older people or in people who are quite inactive, degeneration and reabsorption of bone occur more rapidly than growth of new bone. This leads to *osteoporosis*, a condition in which bone is porous and fragile.

Bone has the capacity to remodel or reshape itself in response to alterations of its mechanical function. This response is in accordance with Wolff's law: "Every change in the form and function of bones or their function alone is followed by certain definite changes in their external configuration in accordance with mathematical laws." Trabeculae within the bone develop and align themselves along lines of stress, and osteogenesis occurs along those lines. If the bone is not stressed,

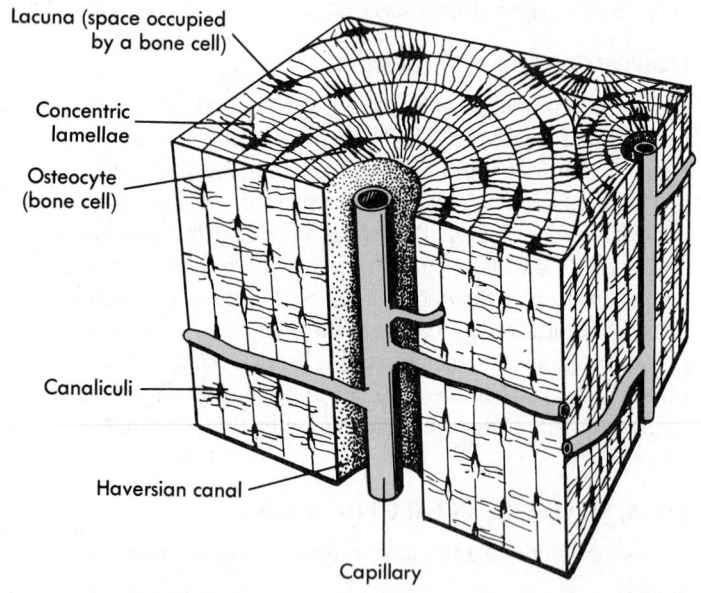

Lacuna (space occupied by a bone cell)

Concentric lamellae

Osteocyte (bone cell)

Canaliculi

Haversian canal

Capillary

FIGURE 68-1 Section of compact bone showing details of haversian system.

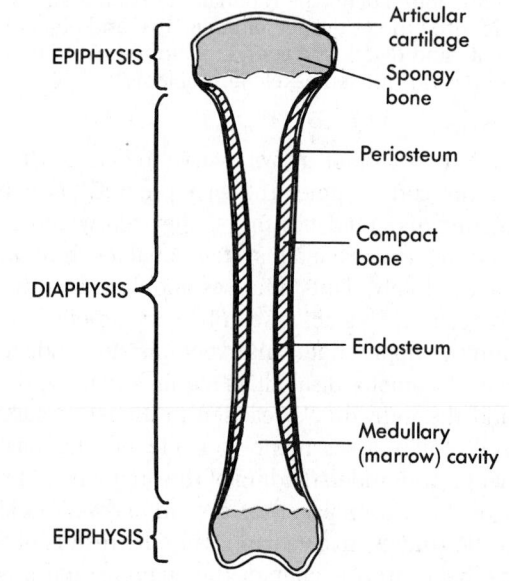

EPIPHYSIS

Articular cartilage

Spongy bone

Periosteum

Compact bone

DIAPHYSIS

Endosteum

Medullary (marrow) cavity

EPIPHYSIS

FIGURE 68-2 Structure of long bone as seen in longitudinal section.

bone resorption occurs. Thus the individual who begins a program of running can expect to have some hypertrophy (increase in bone mass) in the bones of the lower extremities, whereas the individual who is sedentary will experience bone atrophy (loss of bone substance).

CIRCULATORY SUPPLY AND INNERVATION

Adequate circulation of blood to bone is necessary to supply oxygen and nutrients. Blood is supplied to the bone through three routes:

1. The arterioles in the haversian canals
2. Vessels located in the periosteum that penetrate the bone through structures known as *Volkmann's canals*
3. Vessels in the marrow and the ends of the bone

Therefore if there is damage to a nutrient artery, the periosteum, or the bone itself, resulting in separation of the broken ends of the bone, blood supply to the bone will be interrupted.

Furthermore, bones are supplied with sensory nerve endings in the periosteum that connect with the central nervous system. Consequently, pain will result if bone is damaged, for instance, by fracture, infection, or other lesion.

PHYSIOLOGY OF BONE HEALING

Bone heals by a process known as *callus formation*. New growth of bone is called a *callus*. Callus formation proceeds in five general stages (Figure 68-3):

1. *Hematoma formation:* Because bone is highly vascular, bleeding occurs at both ends of the fractured bone. Increased capillary permeability permits further extravasation of blood into the injured area. Blood collects in the periosteal sheath or adjacent tissues and fastens the broken ends together.
2. *Fibrin meshwork formation:* Fibroblasts invade the hematoma, causing it to become organized into a fibrin meshwork. White blood cells (WBCs) wall off the area, localizing the inflammation.
3. *Invasion by osteoblasts:* As osteoblasts invade the fibrous union to make it firm, blood vessels develop from capillary buds, thereby establishing a source of supply for nutrients to build collagen. Collagen strands become longer and begin to incorporate calcium deposits.
4. *Callus formation:* Osteoblasts continue to lay the network for bone build-up as osteoclasts destroy dead bone and help synthesize new bone. Collagen strengthens and becomes further impregnated with calcium.
5. *Remodeling:* Excess callus is reabsorbed, and trabecular bone is laid down along lines of stress in accordance with Wolff's law.

Factors impeding good callus formation are (1) inadequate reduction of the fracture (see Chapter 69), (2) excessive edema at the fracture site impeding the supply of nutrients to the area, (3) too much bone lost at the time of injury to permit sufficient bridging of the broken ends, (4) inefficient immobilization, (5) infection at the site of injury, (6) bone necrosis, (7) anemia or other systemic conditions, (8) endocrine imbalance, and (9) poor dietary intake. If callus formation does not occur normally and efficiently, the resulting lack of repair is termed *nonunion*, or an *ununited fracture*.

MUSCLE

MUSCLE TYPES

Muscles are divided into three major groups:

1. Skeletal (striated, voluntary)
2. Visceral (smooth, involuntary)
3. Cardiac

Visceral muscle, such as that in the stomach and intestines, is innervated by the autonomic nervous system and therefore cannot be controlled at will. Skeletal muscle, however, is innervated by nerve fibers from the

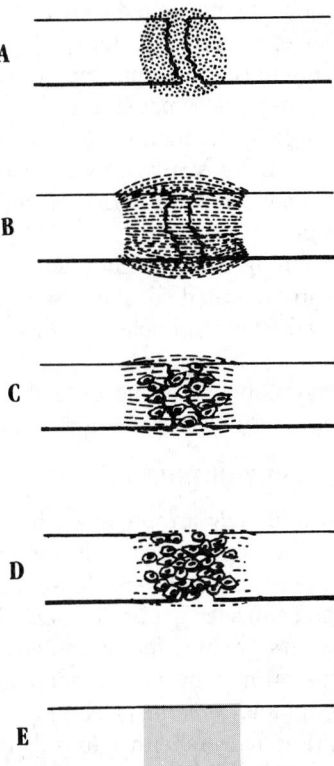

FIGURE 68-3 Bone healing (schematic representation). **A,** Bleeding at broken ends of the bone with subsequent hematoma formation. **B,** Organization of hematoma into fibrous network. **C,** Invasion of osteoblasts, lengthening of collagen strands, and deposition of calcium. **D,** Callus formation: new bone is built up as osteoclasts destroy dead bone. **E,** Remodeling is accomplished as excess callus is reabsorbed and trabecular bone is laid down.

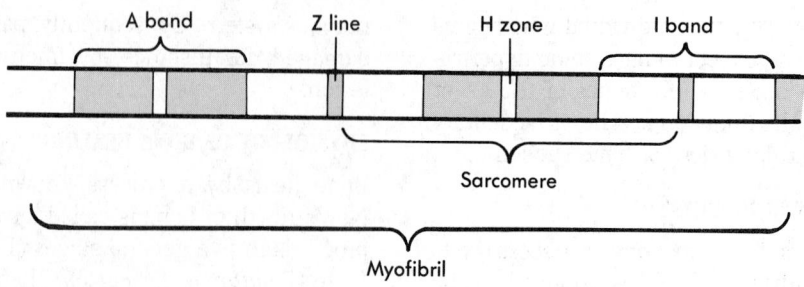

FIGURE 68-4 Schematic drawing of structure of myofibril.

cerebrospinal system and can be controlled by will. Skeletal muscle provides controlled movement, maintains posture, and produces heat.

SKELETAL MUSCLE STRUCTURE

Skeletal, or striated, muscle cells are long and narrow. Their structure causes them to be classified as fibers rather than cells. They are composed of a *sarcolemma*, or cell membrane, and *sarcoplasm*, or cytoplasm. Small, closely packed fibers within the sarcoplasm, called *myofibrils*, that alternate light and dark horizontal stripes, produce the striated appearance that lends this type of muscle its name. The dark stripes are *A bands*, and the light stripes are *I bands*. Light bands crossing the middle of the dark stripes are called the *H zone*, and dark lines crossing the middle of the light, stripes are called *Z lines*. Myofibrils consist of several sections called *sarcomeres*. Each sarcomere is a section that extends from one Z line of a myofibril to the next (Figure 68-4).[1] Bundles of muscle fibers (cells) make up the muscle itself.

PHYSIOLOGY OF MUSCLE CONTRACTION

It is the function of muscles to contract. This is accomplished by a complex process triggered by nerve impulses arriving at the muscle fiber. Calcium ions, released when the impulse is received, bind to troponin (an inhibitor of the molecular myosin-actin interaction). Once troponin is bound, the myosin-actin interaction takes place, and the sarcomeres of the myofibrils contract. The energy for muscle contraction is supplied by the breakdown of adenosinetriphosphate (ATP), a substance muscle cells produce by combining adenosine diphosphate (ADP) with creatine phosphate. Relaxation of the muscle occurs when the calcium separates from the troponin[1] (Figure 68-5).

Muscle cells obey the *"all or none" law;* that is, they contract fully or not at all. This does not mean that the entire muscle contracts fully. Only those individual cells that receive the nerve impulse contract. Muscle fibers that are adequately oxygenated contract more forcefully than those not adequately oxygenated.

TYPES OF CONTRACTIONS

Skeletal muscles vary in size and shape, from long and thin to broad and flat, or they may form bulky masses. The arrangement of the fibers within the muscle determines the capacity of the forceful contraction of the muscle. Skeletal muscles contract only if they are stimulated. There are many types of contractions[1]:

1. *Tonic:* a continual partial contraction that is vital in maintenance of posture
2. *Isotonic:* a contraction in which tension within the muscle is unchanged, but the length of the muscle does change (shortens)
3. *Isometric:* tension within the muscle increases but the muscle does not shorten
4. *Twitch:* a jerky reaction to a single stimulus
5. *Tetanic:* a more sustained contraction than the twitch, produced by a series of stimuli in rapid succession
6. *Treppe:* stronger twitch contractions in response to regularly repeated constant strength stimuli
7. *Fibrillation:* asynchronous contraction of individual fibers
8. *Convulsion:* abnormal uncoordinated tetanic contractions occurring in varying groups of muscles

MECHANISM OF BODY MOVEMENT

Movements of the body are produced by muscles pulling on bones; the bones serve as levers and the joints serve as fulcrums for the levers. Most movements depend on several muscles acting in a coordinated manner. *Prime movers* produce the movement; *antagonists* relax when the prime movers contract, thereby permitting movement; and *synergists* contract at the same time as the prime movers, either to produce the movement or to stabilize a body part so contraction of the prime movers is more efficient.[1]

CIRCULATION TO MUSCLE

Efficient muscle contraction is dependent on an adequate blood supply to and from the muscle fibers. Therefore skeletal muscle is highly vascular. Waste products resulting from the chemical changes that oc-

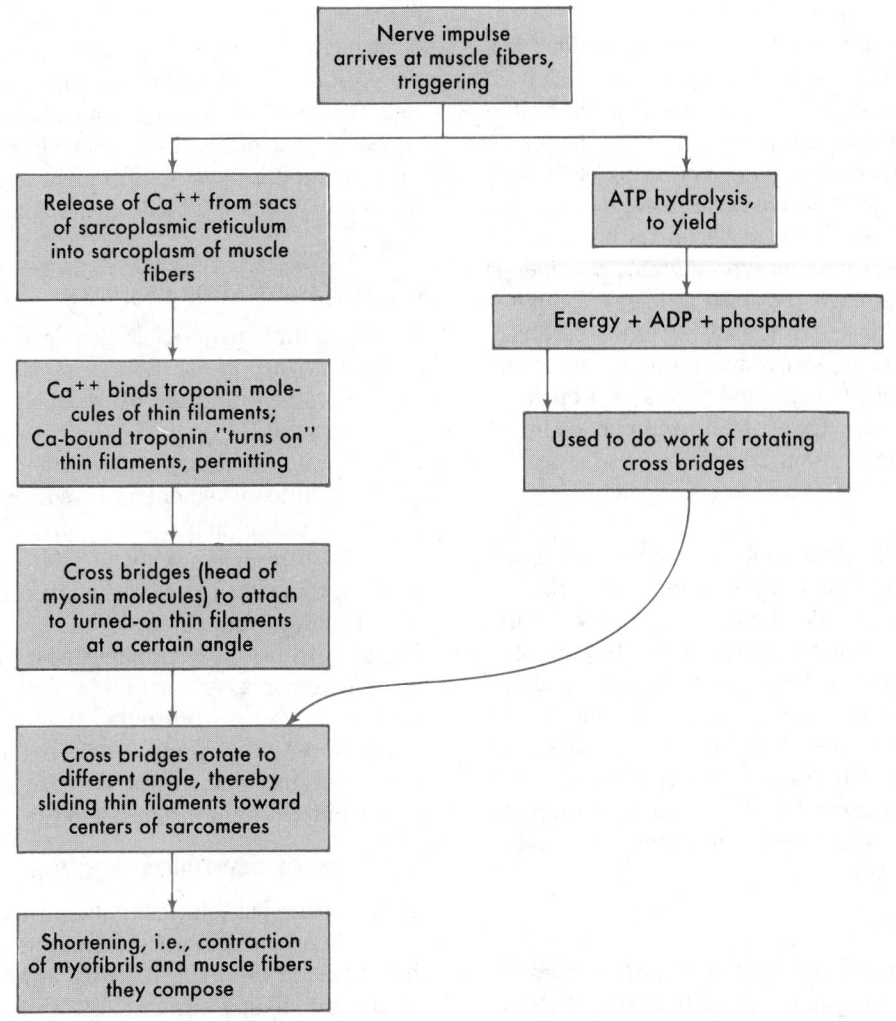

FIGURE 68-5 Mechanism of skeletal muscle contraction. (From Anthony CP and Thibodeau GA: Textbook of anatomy and physiology, ed 11, St Louis, 1983, The CV Mosby Co.)

cur during muscle contraction must be transported to the liver to be resynthesized. When waste products are not adequately carried off, muscle fatigue and pain result. Conversely, oxygen must be transported to the muscle fibers to support the work of muscle contraction. Poor muscle work occurs when the oxygen supply is inadequate, for example, in conditions such as anemia in which the amount of oxygen-carrying hemoglobin is reduced or trauma in which circulation to the muscle fibers is interrupted.

INNERVATION OF MUSCLE

Adequate muscle contraction also depends on effective innervation. The cerebellum is primarily responsible for control of muscle movement (see Chapter 59). Every muscle cell is supplied with the axon of a nerve cell. Nerve cells that transmit impulses to skeletal muscles are known as *somatic motor neurons*. The neuron and the muscle cell it activates are called a *motor unit*. The axon of one somatic motor neuron may be divided into any number of branches and therefore innervates a like number of muscle cells. The fewer muscle cells innervated, the more precise (or fine) are the resultant movements. The actual contraction of the muscle is set off by the release of *acetylcholine*, a chemical contained in small vesicles in the axon terminal. When acetylcholine contacts the sarcolemma, it stimulates the contraction. This reaction takes place across a structure known as the *motor end-plate*, or *neuromuscular junction*, where the muscle and the nerve are in contact. Damage to the nervous system at the cerebrospinal level or at any point in the nerve's course through the local motor neuron level will result in muscular dysfunction.

CARTILAGE

Cartilage is a material composed of fibers embedded in a firm gel. It is a strong but flexible material and is avascular. Nutrients must reach the cartilage cells by the process of diffusion through the gel from capillaries located in the *perichondrium* (fibrous covering of the cartilage), or in the case of articular cartilage, through the synovial fluid. The number of collagenous fibers found in the cartilage determine its type: *fibrous, hyaline,* or *elastic.* Fibrous cartilage (or fibrocartilage) composes the intervertebral disks. Articular (hyaline) cartilage, which is smooth, white, shiny, and resilient, covers the articular surfaces of the bone and serves as a cushion. Elastic cartilage has the fewest fibers and may be found in areas such as the external ear.

LIGAMENTS

Ligaments are bands of dense fibrous connective tissue that are flexible and tough. They connect the articular ends of bones and provide stability. Examples are the medial and lateral collateral ligaments of the knee that provide mediolateral stability to the knee joint, and the anterior and posterior cruciate ligaments within the joint capsule of the knee that provide anteroposterior stability. Ligaments may also attach to soft tissue to suspend structures. An example of this is the suspensory ligament of the ovary that passes from the tubal end of the ovary to the peritoneum.

TENDONS

Tendons are bands of dense fibrous tissue that form the termination of a muscle and attach it to a bone. The tendon is an extension of the fibrous sheath that envelops each muscle and is continuous with the periosteum at its other end. *Tendon sheaths* are tubular structures of connective tissue that enclose certain tendons, especially in the wrist and ankle. These sheaths are lined with a synovial membrane that provides lubrication (synovial fluid) for easy movement of the tendon.

FASCIA

Fascia is a sheet of loose connective tissue that may be found directly under the skin as *superficial fascia,* or as a sheet of dense, fibrous connective tissue making up the sheath of muscles, nerves, and blood vessels. The latter is known as *deep fascia.*

BURSAE

Bursae are small sacs of connective tissue located wherever pressure is exerted over moving parts. They may, for example, occur between skin and bone, between tendons and bone, or between muscles. Bursae are lined with synovial membrane and contain synovial fluid. They serve as cushions between moving parts. One such bursa, the olecranon bursa, is located between the olecranon process and the skin.

JOINTS

Movement would not be possible unless some flexibility were provided within the skeletal framework. This flexibility is provided by the joints, or places where the bones come together. The shape of the joint determines the amount and type of movement possible. The classification of joints is based on the amount of movement they allow.

MAJOR CLASSIFICATION OF JOINTS

There are three major classifications of joints:
1. *Synarthroses,* or *fibrous joints,* which allow no movement and are exemplified by the sutures of the skull
2. *Amphiarthroses,* or *cartilaginous joints,* which allow little movement and are exemplified by the intervertebral joints
3. *Diarthroses,* or *synovial joints,* which allow free movement and are exemplified by the hip, knee, shoulder, and elbow

The synarthroses and amphiarthroses may also be classified together as synarthroses, designating that both have no joint cavity but rather tissue (fibrous, cartilaginous, or osseous) grows between their articular surfaces. Because diarthroses are the joints that permit movement, they are discussed in the most detail.

STRUCTURE OF DIARTHRODIAL JOINTS

Each diarthrodial joint contains a small space, or *joint cavity,* between the articulating surfaces of the bones that make up the joint. Articular hyaline cartilage covers the articulating surfaces of both bones, allowing for the smooth, gliding motion of the joint. A *joint capsule,* or sleeve of fibrous tissue, encases the joint. The capsule is lined with tissue called *synovial membrane.* Synovial membrane secretes *synovial fluid* into the joint capsule. Synovial fluid lubricates the joint (Figure 68-6). In addition, ligaments may be present between the bones (as with the cruciate ligaments of the knee) to provide internal stability to the joint. Small pieces of

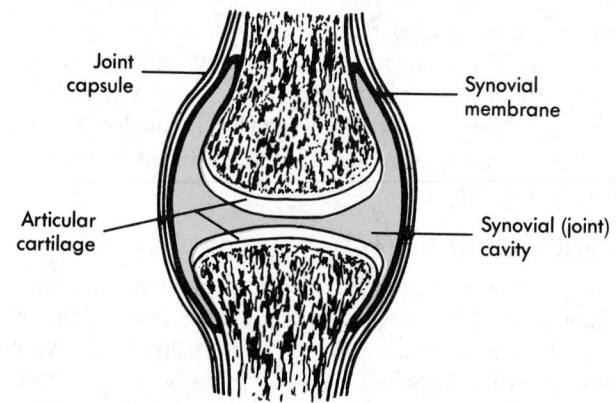

FIGURE 68-6 Structure of diarthrodial joint.

dense cartilage may also be interposed between the articulating surfaces. These are crescent shaped or half moon-shaped structures (*menisci*) that provide additional cushioning for the joint. Examples are the medial meniscus and lateral meniscus of the knee joint.

CLASSIFICATION OF DIARHRODIAL JOINTS

Diarthrodial joints are further classified by the shape of their surfaces and the type of movement they permit. Specialized texts should be consulted for discussion of these subtypes.[23] However, it may be generally stated that the diarthrodial joints permit one or more of the following movements: flexion, extension, adduction, abduction, rotation, circumduction, supination, pronation, inversion, eversion, protraction, or retraction. The latter six are considered special movements (Figures 68-12, 68-13, and 68-14).

PHYSIOLOGIC CHANGES WITH AGING

Physiologic changes occur in the musculoskeletal system throughout a person's lifespan. Childhood and adolescence are a time of rapid growth and development of the structures of the system. However, at maturity and into older age, tissue strength and integrity begins to decline as the total number of body cells decreases. Connective tissues lose some of their elasticity and resilience, particularly the articular cartilage of the joints and the intervertebral discs of the spine. As the amount of vigorous activity an individual engages in decreases, muscles lose bulk, tone, and strength. Bone reabsorption takes place more rapidly than bone growth; and particularly in postmenopausal women, calcium is lost from bone, rendering it softer and less resistant to fracture. The shoulders may become stooped and narrower. The knees and hips may be slightly flexed when standing or walking, often because of pain associated with joint degeneration. Posture becomes stooped as the body attempts to compensate for changes in the center of gravity caused by lower extremity joint flexion and forward thrusting of the head, neck, and shoulders. With these changes, height decreases from 6 to 10 cm. Gait may become unsteady because of loss of muscle strength and coordination, and the individual is more subject to falls.

NATURE OF PATHOLOGIC CONDITIONS IN THE MUSCULOSKELETAL SYSTEM

As discussed in the section on the anatomy and physiology of the musculoskeletal system, the musculoskeletal and nervous systems are interrelated. The muscles, bones, joints, supportive structures, and sensory and motor nerves all work together to provide controlled movement and to maintain posture. However, any problem that causes interference or disturbance at any level—innervation, contractility, articulation, or support—of this well integrated system results in muscu-loskeletal dysfunction. Problems can occur as a result of the interruption of blood supply to the involved structures; disease affecting the contour of bones or joints; disease affecting the nerves that innervate the musculoskeletal system; or trauma, of whatever origin, that interrupts the integrity of any of the involved structures.

SUBJECTIVE DATA

Plans for the care of any person with a musculoskeletal problem are based on a systematic assessment of needs, capabilities, and resources. A thorough assessment must include subjective data gathered from interviews with the person and his or her family.

DESCRIPTION OF PRESENT PROBLEM OR DYSFUNCTION
ONSET AND DURATION OF THE PROBLEM

Questions related to the history of the problem should help the patient explain the following:
1. Onset of the problem
2. Circumstances surrounding the onset of the problem
3. Duration of problem
4. Patient's perception of what the problem is

PAIN OR DISCOMFORT ASSOCIATED WITH THE PROBLEM

Because many musculoskeletal problems are marked by pain or discomfort, questions should elicit the following information about that pain or discomfort:
1. Nature
2. Location
3. Duration
4. Measures the person has taken to alleviate pain or discomfort
5. Effectiveness of measures taken

CURRENT MEDICATIONS

Many persons who have musculoskeletal problems are taking medications, either for the musculoskeletal problem or for additional problems. Interviewers should try to elicit the following information:
1. A complete listing of the person's current medications
2. Medications that have been used in the past and their effectiveness
3. Drug allergies the person has experienced and nature of the allergy

EFFECT OF PROBLEM/DYSFUNCTION ON PERFORMANCE OF ACTIVITIES OF DAILY LIVING

Because dysfunction of the musculoskeletal system often leads to impairment or loss of independence in activities of daily living (ADL), information relating to ADL performance is helpful in determining the extent and nature of nursing interventions that will be required. Questions should elicit information related to both personal ADL (feeding, bathing, dressing, transfer, ambulation, and sleep), as well as social ADL (household, work, recreational, and sexual activities). Interviewers should try to elicit the following information:

1. The amount and type of assistance needed to perform any ADL
2. Special techniques developed to assist in performance
3. Assistive or adaptive devices used
4. Availability of other persons to provide assistance
5. Adequacy of assistance provided by others
6. Modifications made in the home or work environment
7. Effectiveness of modifications

PERSON'S PERCEPTION OF THE PROBLEM/DYSFUNCTION

As part of the nursing interview, some specific questions may be helpful in determining the individual's perception of the problem. These questions include the following:

1. What effect has your problem had on the way you live?
2. Have you had to modify your ADL?
3. How do you feel about the changes that you have had to make in the way you live?
4. What have you found helpful in adapting to these changes?
5. How do you carry out the treatment program prescribed by your physician?
6. Has your treatment plan been effective for you?

Sometimes no direct questions will be necessary because the person may readily offer comments about each of the above areas. Persons who are dissatisfied with their current therapy may either perceive no need for further therapy or may be overly confident in their expectations about new therapy. Persons who believe they know all there is to know about their problem and its treatment may be less open to teaching by those involved in their care. Others may be confronting a problem for the first time and may be overwhelmed by it. The more information the nurse can gain from the person about perceptions, coping skills, and adaptive abilities, the better the plans developed for that person's care will be.

FAMILY'S PERCEPTION OF THE PERSON'S PROBLEM

An individual's problem or dysfunction generally has some effect on the other people who are intimately associated with that individual. Therefore it is important to determine the effects of the person's problem on the family or significant others. The degree to which the problem affects the lives of significant others, and the degree to which they can be supportive to the person and the role changes the problem may necessitate, can significantly affect the outcome of any proposed plan of care. It is important to determine the following from the family:

1. How do they feel they are able to support the patient?
2. How do they perceive their own and the patient's roles changing?
3. How do they perceive the patient feels about himself or herself, the problem, and his or her relationships with others?
4. How is the person's problem/dysfunction affecting their lives?
5. Are they aware of supportive resources in the community?

Frequently, when a person has a disabling temporary or chronic musculoskeletal illness or injury, family roles are changed. Not infrequently, these changes in roles and status are resented, not only by the family, but by the patient, who may feel worthless or inadequate. When these conditions prevail, some intervention by health personnel (physician, nurse, social worker, psychologist, or psychiatrist) may be necessary to assist the person and family to work through these feelings and to provide support. Listening to what the person and family have to say about the illness, the treatment, the short- or long-term outcomes of the problem or illness, and their feelings about the changes it has necessitated in their lives will give clues for interventions that might be tried to alleviate existing problems.

OBJECTIVE DATA

The second area of data collection of a thorough assessment concerns observations about the person. General observations are made regarding behavior, general appearance, skin, nails, and hair (see the box on p. 1993). In addition, data are collected regarding deformities, strength and range of motion, ability to transfer and ambulate, and ability to perform other ADL.

DEFORMITY

Many musculoskeletal problems are marked by deformity of one or more extremities or joints or the spine. Deformities should be specifically noted and described, and some evaluation should be made of the extent to which they curtail normal function. Deformity can be thought of as a change in size, shape, or position of a body part. Some common deformities are described in the box.

STRENGTH AND RANGE OF MOTION

Assessments of strength and range of motion are, in effect, measurements of the person's functional capacity. Before discussing this area, the following terms must first be defined:

OBJECTIVE DATA (BEHAVIOR, APPEARANCE, SKIN)

OBSERVATIONS	RATIONALE
Behavior	
Mental status	Interventions must be based on the person's:
Orientation to time, place, person	Ability to relate to reality
Ability to understand directions	Ability to act on and retain instruction
Capacity to retain information	
Span of attention	
Ability to relate to others	Ability to relate to instruction/intervention in a positive way
Is the person's attitude: quiet, talkative, tense, guarded, negative, appropriate, inappropriate	
General Appearance	
Age, sex	May relate to a specific disorder or attitude toward the disorder
Posture	May be characteristic of a specific problem, e.g., kyphotic posture in ankylosing spondylitis (Figure 68-7); guarding of head, neck, and shoulders following whiplash
Nutritional status	
Overweight	May be indicative of diminished ability to perform regular exercise or activity
Underweight	May be indicative of inability to secure or prepare nutritional meals or to carry out feeding activities adequately
	May relate to specific systemic condition causing anorexia, nausea, vomiting, or malabsorption of food
Skin	
Turgor (fullness)	Thin papery skin may indicate systemic connective tissue disease or long-term steroid use; skin is easily broken
Texture (feel)	Thick leathery patches over forearms, hands, chest, and face indicative of scleroderma; ulcerates easily, especially over joints
Integrity	
Breaks in skin, ulcerations, reddened areas	Individuals with limited mobility are subject to skin breakdown from pressure over skin areas, which interferes with circulation; consequent breakdown is known as *decubitus ulcer;* possibility of shearing forces against sheets, chair surfaces, bedpans, or other surfaces tearing or abrading skin; accurate assessment of potential for skin breakdown is vital in planning for prevention
Impaired circulation to extremities	Increased risk of skin breakdown in distal extremities
Temperature	Warmth, especially over painful joints, indicative of presence and degree of inflammatory or infectious process within joint
Erythema over joints	Indicative of inflammation and the need to keep joint at rest
Rash	May be present in systemic connective tissue disorders (psoriasis, scleroderma, dermatomyositis); initial observations provide useful baseline to determine effectiveness of treatment
Color change on exposure to cold	Change from *white* (resulting from arteriolar spasm) to *blue* (cyanosis caused by stagnation of blood) to *red* (warming and reactive vasodilation) present in some connective tissue disorders (*Raynaud's phenomenon*)[20]; requires specific interventions
Bruising	Often present following trauma and consequent to long-term treatment of connective tissue disease with corticosteroids; areas may slough easily and become infected (Figure 68-8)

Continued.

OBJECTIVE DATA (BEHAVIOR, APPEARANCE, SKIN)—cont'd

OBSERVATIONS	RATIONALE
Swelling of extremities or joints	In extremities, may denote prolonged dependent position, lack of activity, circulatory or renal impairment
	In joints, may indicate presence of *effusion* (serous, purulent, or bloody fluid in the joint capsule); inflamed synovium (feels boggy): indication of need to rest joints involved
Bony enlargements	Indicative of disease process, for example, *Heberden's nodes* in osteoarthritis (hard, irregular swellings over the distal interphalangeal joints of the fingers)
Subcutaneous nodules	Indicative of rheumatoid arthritis: hard, mobile swellings commonly found in the subolecranon area
Bursal swelling	Indicative of bursal inflammation: felt as soft swelling over the bursa
Synovial cyst	Indicative of hypertrophy of synovial tissue, for example, *Baker's cyst* (swelling in the popliteal area, often extending into the calf)
Tophaceous deposits	Indicative of gout: hard translucent swellings over joints or in cartilage such as that of the ear
Tenderness	
May be elicited by direct pressure, and graded by the amount of pressure required to produce discomfort	Degree of tenderness is usually in direct proportion to severity of inflammation or trauma, e.g., in joint inflammation or injured soft tissue or overlying fracture
General hygiene	
Evidence of uncleanliness of body, clothing	May indicate inability to adequately carry out hygienic requirements (because this may be embarrassing for the individual, plans must be made to introduce self-help devices or to provide assistance in ways that will not be demeaning)
Nails and Hair	
Poorly kept or diseased nails	May indicate lack of strength or inability to reach nails to care for them
	Change in nail structure may indicate presence of connective tissue disease
Poorly kept hair	May indicate inability to lift arms to comb hair
Alopecia, scaling of scalp	May indicate connective tissue disease

1. *Strength:* the capacity to perform work
2. *Range of motion:* the normal arc of movement provided for by the structure of a joint
3. *Active range of motion:* the movement of a joint that can be accomplished without assistance
4. *Passive range of motion:* movement of a joint through its normal range by someone else or some mechanical device
5. *Active assisted range of motion:* active movement of a joint by the person, but with assistance from someone else or a mechanical device to complete the motion
6. *Dexterity:* the coordination and agility with which movements are performed

Additionally, the following terms are applied to the extremities to accurately describe their capacity for strength and motion:

1. *Flaccid:* having defective or absent muscle tone
2. *Paralyzed:* having loss of function, especially loss of sensation or voluntary motion
3. *-plegia:* suffix to describe paralysis
4. *-paresis:* suffix to describe incomplete loss of muscle power or partial paralysis
5. *Mono-:* prefix to describe involvement of one extremity (for example, monoplegia)
6. *Hemi-:* prefix to describe involvement of both extremities on the same side of the body
7. *Para-:* prefix to describe involvement of both lower extremities
8. *Quadri-:* prefix to describe involvement of all four extremities

Before testing the muscle strength or range of motion of a joint, some assessment of the position of the person's extremities must be made. Positions that vary from the normal and that have had an acute onset may indicate the presence of fractures, dislocations, or ruptures of supporting structures. Typical of this kind of sudden change is the marked external rotation and shortening of the leg following a hip fracture; the inability to extend a "dropped" finger following rupture of an extensor tendon in the hand; or postoperative "drop foot," a complication that may occur following surgical procedures to the back, hip, or knee because of pressure on or stretching of the sciatic or peroneal nerve.

Subluxation, or partial dislocation of a joint, should also be noted. This is often a chronic problem, as in the shoulder of the hemiplegic or in the wrist of the arthritic. Its presence is usually accompanied by some loss of function or need for support. Subluxation of the shoulder may be detected by examination—a space can be felt between the head of the humerus and the glenoid cavity of the scapula.

Loss of strength or limitation of joint motion will result in some degree of loss of function. Loss of strength or joint range may be the result of a neurologic, skeletal, muscular, or traumatic disorder. Detailed tests of strength and joint range of motion require instruments such as the *dynamometer,* which measures grip strength in the hand, and the *goniometer* (an instrument resembling a protractor), which measures joint motion (Figure 68-11).

Gross testing of strength, however, may be accomplished very simply. To test the upper extremities, apply moderate pressure with your hand against the person's

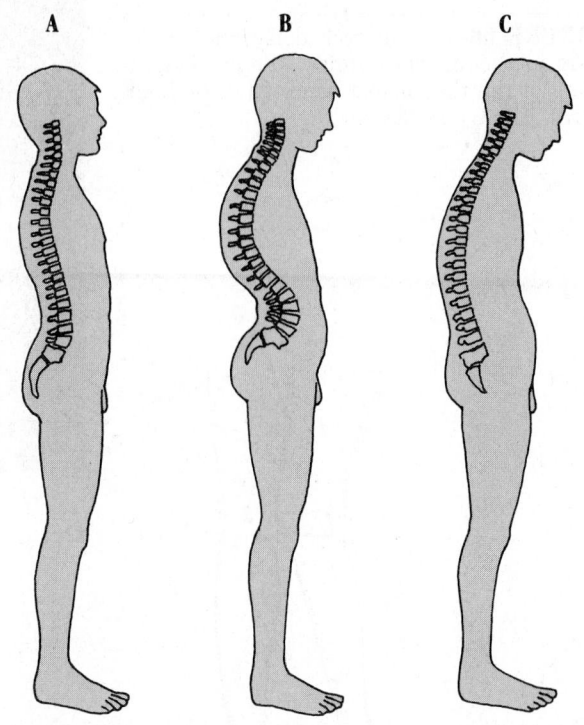

FIGURE 68-7 A, Curves of spine in good posture. **B,** Curves of spine in slumping posture. **C,** Obliteration of apinal curves such as in early spondylitis.

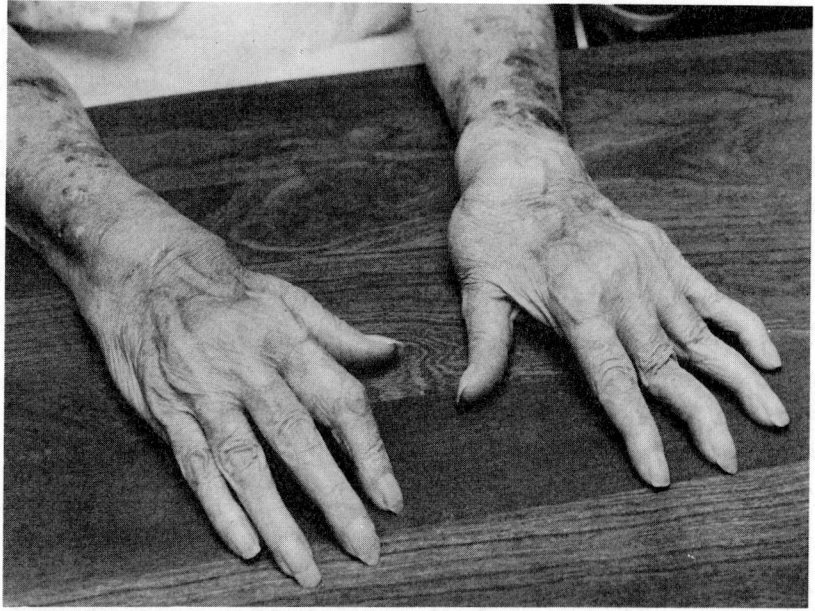

FIGURE 68-8 Hands and forearms of woman with advanced rheumatoid arthritis. Note areas of bruising on forearms. Such ecchymoses are common in individuals who have rheumatoid arthritis and who take steroids for treatment. Handling of such individuals must be extremely gentle, to avoid both bruising and potential sloughing of these areas.

FIGURE 68-9 Swan-neck deformities of fingers in rheumatoid arthritis. (From Flatt AE: Care of the rheumatoid hand, ed 3, St Louis, 1974, The CV Mosby Co.)

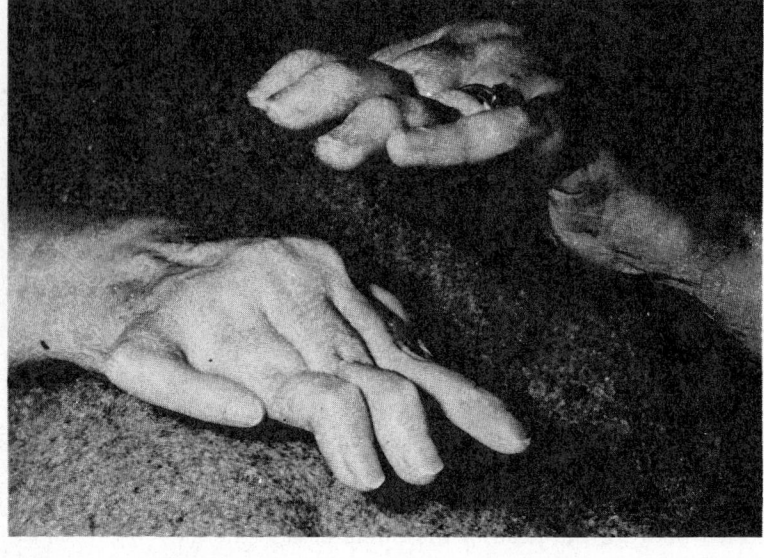

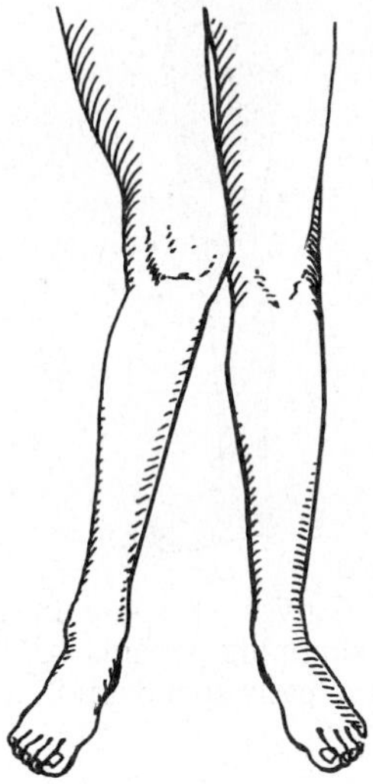

FIGURE 68-10 Valgus deformity of knee.

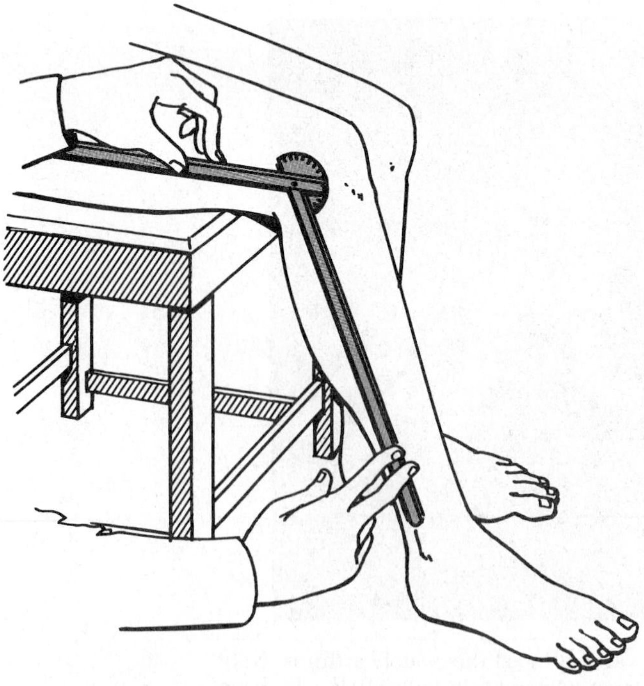

FIGURE 68-11 Use of goniometer in measuring joint range of motion.

COMMON MUSCULOSKELETAL DEFORMITIES

DEFORMITY	DESCRIPTION
Swan neck deformity	Flexion contracture of the metacarpophalangeal joint, hyperextension of the proximal interphalangeal joint, and flexion of the distal interphalangeal joints of the fingers (Figure 68-9); found in advanced rheumatoid arthritis
Ulnar deviation or drift	Fingers deviate at the metacarpophalangeal joints toward the ulnar aspect of the hand
Valgus deformities	Distal arm of the angle of the joint points away from the midline of the body
Hallux valgus	Great toe turns toward the other toes
Genu valgum	"Knock-knees" (Figure 68-10)
Talipes valgus	Eversion of the foot
Varus deformities	Distal arm of the angle of the joint points toward the midline of the body
Genu varum	Bowing of the knees (see Figure 70-20)
Talipes varus	Inversion of the foot
Scoliosis	Lateral curvature of the spine
Kyphosis	Thoracic spinal curvature, the convexity of the curve being posterior
Atrophy	Reduction in size of an extremity or body part, for example, wasting of muscles so that they appear to lack the bulk of normal muscle; can result from lack of use or disease process, for example, polymyositis
Hypertrophy	Abnormal enlargement of an organ or body part; limitation of function may be associated with enlargement

upper arm to resist movement; have the person flex, extend, and abduct the shoulder. Next, resist the patient's forearm movement with your hand, while he or she flexes and extends the elbow. Applying pressure to resist motion of the patient's hand, have the patient flex and extend the wrist. Hand grip strength may be tested by having the person squeeze your hand. The same maneuvers can be performed with the lower extremities. In all these instances the area proximal to the joint being moved is stabilized by one of the examiner's hands, while moderate resistance to movement distal to the joint being moved is provided by the other hand. Trunk strength may be tested by having the person attempt to sit up from the supine position. Gross muscle testing

provides very useful data for determining the amount of assistance the patient needs. More specific testing done by a physical therapist is useful to the physician in diagnosis and to the therapist in planning a program of muscle strengthening exercises.

Coordination of the upper extremities can be tested by having the person extend an arm and, with one finger, touch one of the examiner's fingers, then his or her own nose, then the examiner's finger again, and so on. The ability to pick up small objects such as a coin or a pen from a smooth, hard surface provides some indication of the person's manual *dexterity*.

Range of motion is tested by having the person actively perform with each joint those motions that partic-

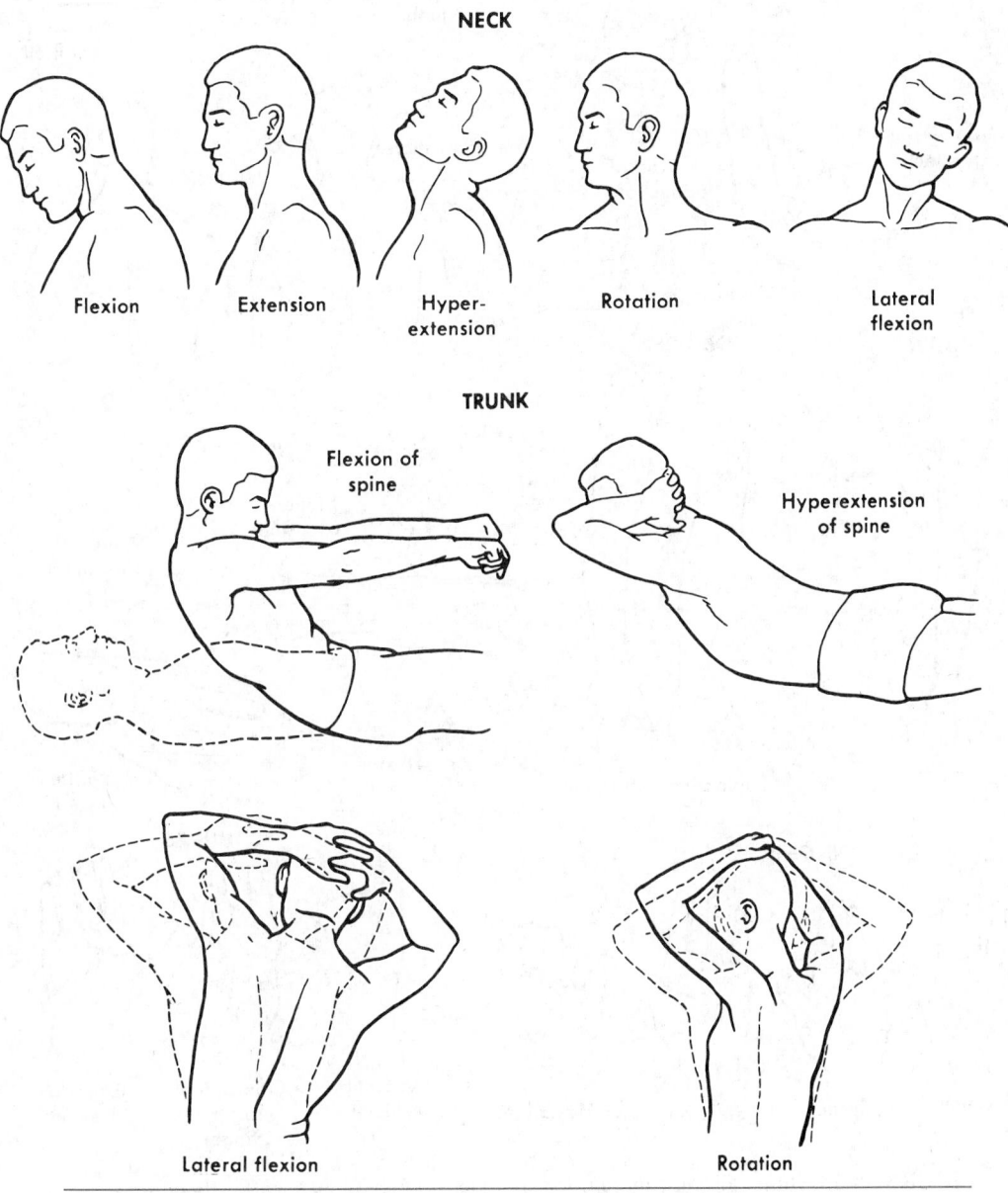

FIGURE 68-12 Range of motion for neck and trunk.

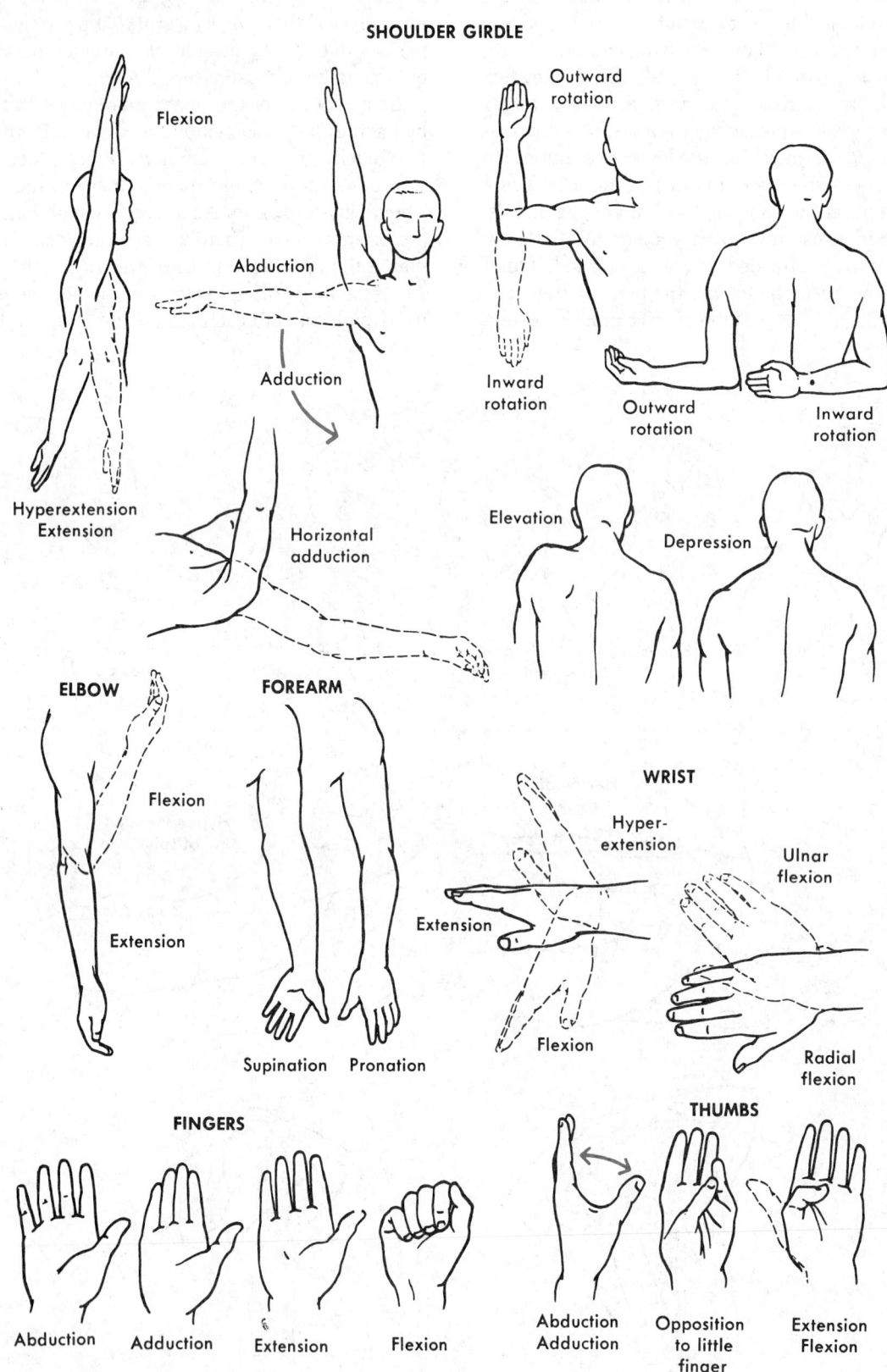

FIGURE 68-13 Range of joint motion for shoulder and shoulder girdle, elbow, forearm, and wrist.

ular joint is capable of performing (Figures 68-12, 68-13, and 68-14). In some instances when the person cannot actively move a joint, as with the person who has some form of paralysis, the joint may be passively moved. (Refer to Chapter 70 for discussion of passive range of motion and joint instability.) When passive

range of motion is performed, support must be given proximal to the joint being moved (Figure 68-15). Comparing the limitation of movement or instability present in one joint with its contralateral joint is helpful in differentiating normal from abnormal findings.

If a joint cannot be moved beyond a certain point in

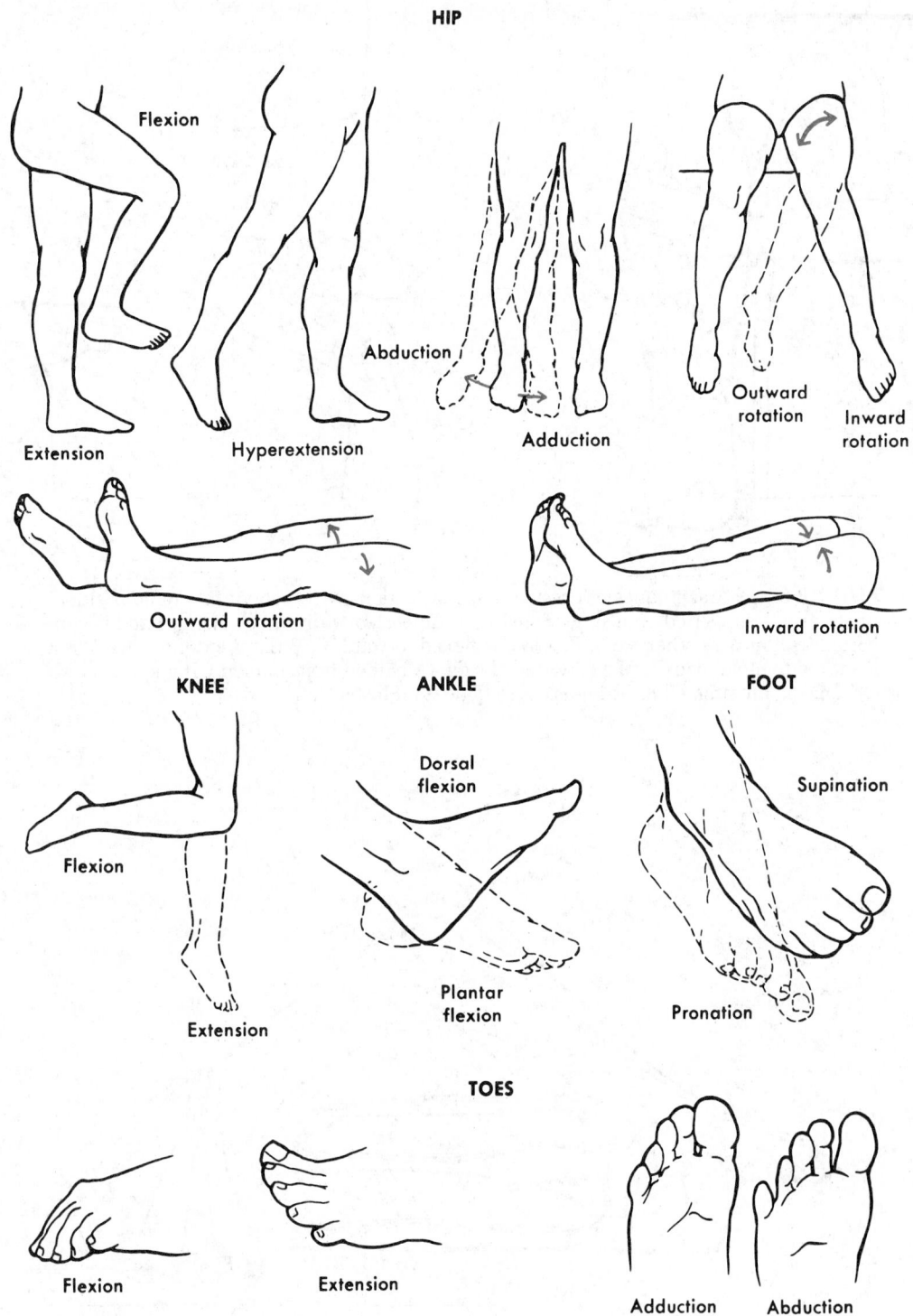

FIGURE 68-14 Range of joint motion for hip, knee, ankle, foot, and toes.

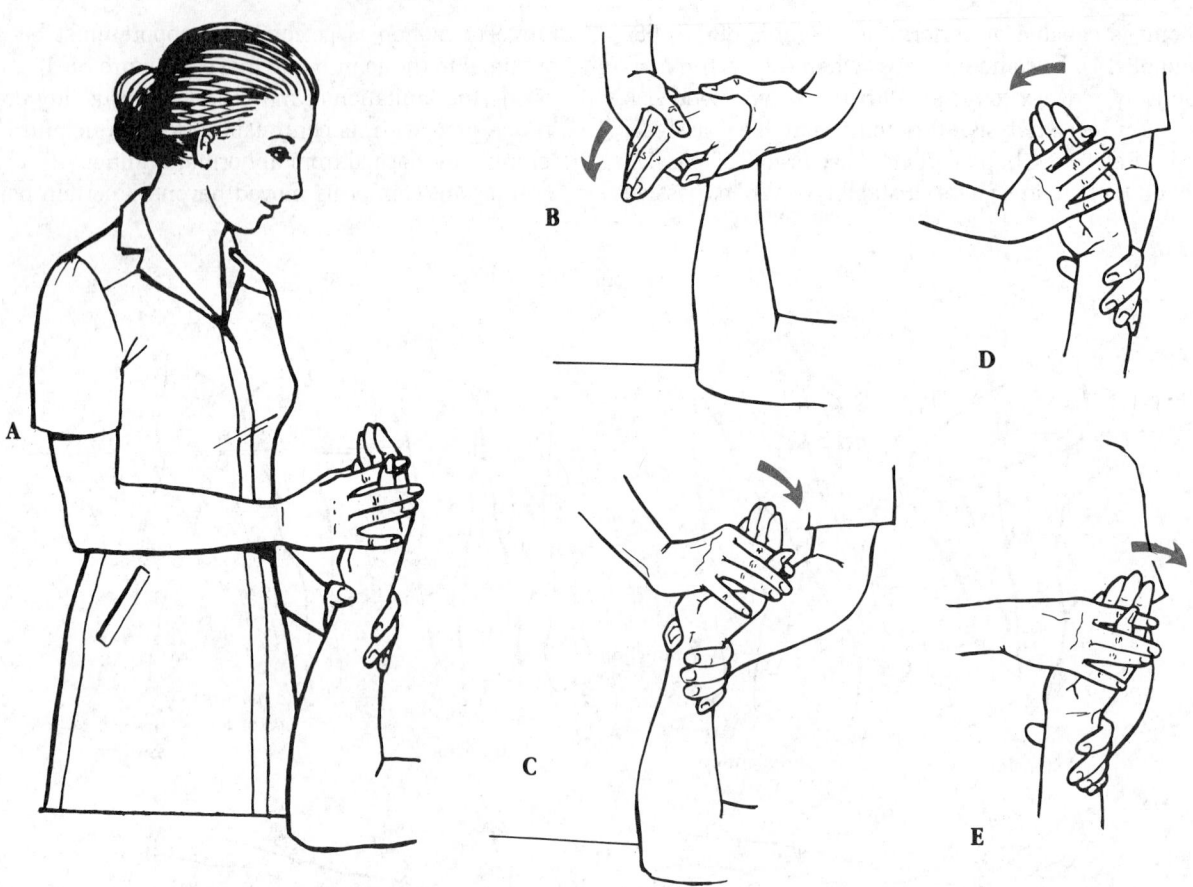

FIGURE 68-15 Techniques of passive range of motion. With patient in supine position, upper arm is supported on bed. **A,** Forearm is supported with nurse's hand; hand is supported with nurse's other hand. **B,** Wrist is flexed forward. **C,** Wrist is extended. **D,** Wrist is moved to ulnar side. **E,** Moved to radial side. (Modified from Larson CB and Gould M: Orthopedic nursing, ed 8, St Louis, 1974, The CV Mosby Co.)

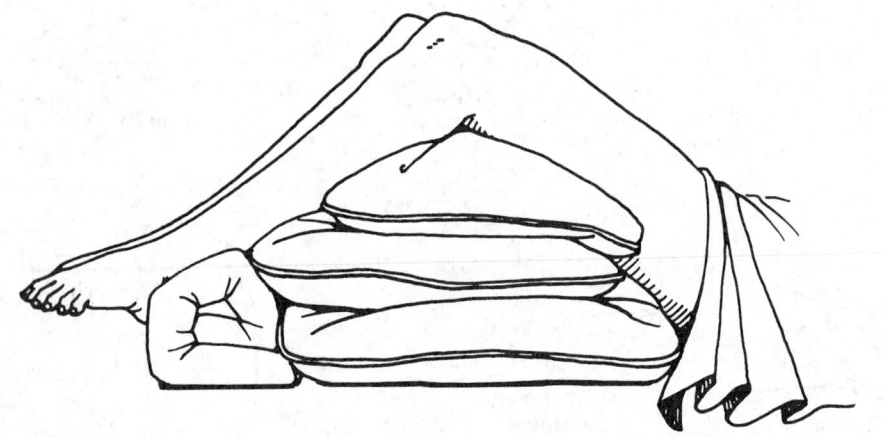

FIGURE 68-16 Contractures of hips and knees in patient with rheumatoid arthritis caused by continuous use of pillows to support knees in flexed position.

its range (for example, a knee that does not extend beyond 30 degrees of flexion), it is said that the joint is contracted, or that a *contracture* is present. Contractures may exist because of soft tissue limitation (following immobilization for treatment of a fracture) or because of bony limitation (Figure 68-16). The location and nature of contractures can significantly limit function. For example, a person who can flex one knee only 15 degrees must climb stairs one at a time.

Crepitus, or a crunching or grating sound when the joint is actively or passively moved, is a significant indicator of the presence of a pathologic condition within the joint. This sound will also be heard if the two broken ends of a bone move against one another. *In the presence of a possible fracture, no attempt should be made to elicit crepitus.* At times, grating within a joint may be felt, rather than heard, by placing a hand over the joint as it moves.

The preceding tests of strength, dexterity, and range of motion are simple to perform; however, it must be noted that the person's ability to perform the movements described may be limited by pain rather than by weakness, lack of coordination, or joint limitation. It is often difficult to differentiate these factors. Although the effect of the pain is quantitatively the same as the effect of the weakness or limitation (that is, diminished function), it is qualitatively different because treatment measures will be geared to relief of pain rather than to muscle strengthening. To further confuse the situation, the person with pain may have actual muscle weakness because of long-standing pain and consequent lack of use of muscles. It must be remembered that in performing these kinds of tests the person *must not be moved beyond the point of pain.* Pain is an indication that something is wrong. Injudicious testing techniques can produce untoward results, for example, the fracture of an osteoporotic bone. The desired result of such testing is the establishment of a baseline of strength, motion, and dexterity from which interventions to assist the person to gain strength, regain lost motion, and increase functional capacity may be planned and evaluated.

TRANSFER

An assessment should also be made of the patient's ability to transfer or move from one surface to another—from bed to chair, chair to toilet, and toilet to bed again (Figure 68-17). The person may have no difficulty with such movements, may have made some environmental modification to accomplish the transfer without help, or may need assistance.

A basic understanding of the principles of transfer techniques is required to assess the person's transfer ability (see Chapter 70). The nurse must follow certain steps in this assessment (see the box on p. 2003). Obviously, transfer is not evaluated in those persons who are not permitted to be out of bed, such as patients who are in traction.

The results of transfer assessment should reflect how much if any assistance will be required, what modifications need to be made in the environment, and whether the transfer can be performed safely.

AMBULATION

Assessment of ambulatory ability follows assessment of transfer ability. Some individuals are not able to ambulate because of pain, contractures, immobilization, frac-

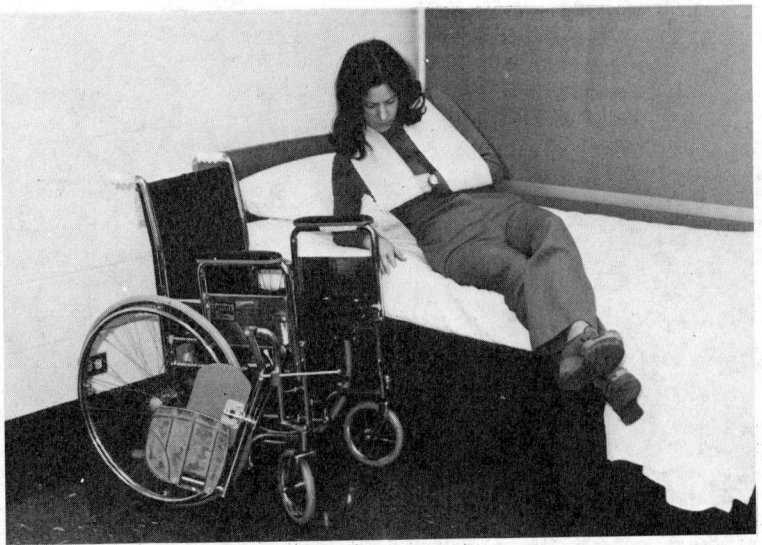

FIGURE 68-17 Independent transfer from bed to chair. Chair is placed within reach of patient's uninvolved side. Movements are made leading with uninvolved or stronger side. Position of chair is reversed for return to bed. *Continued.*

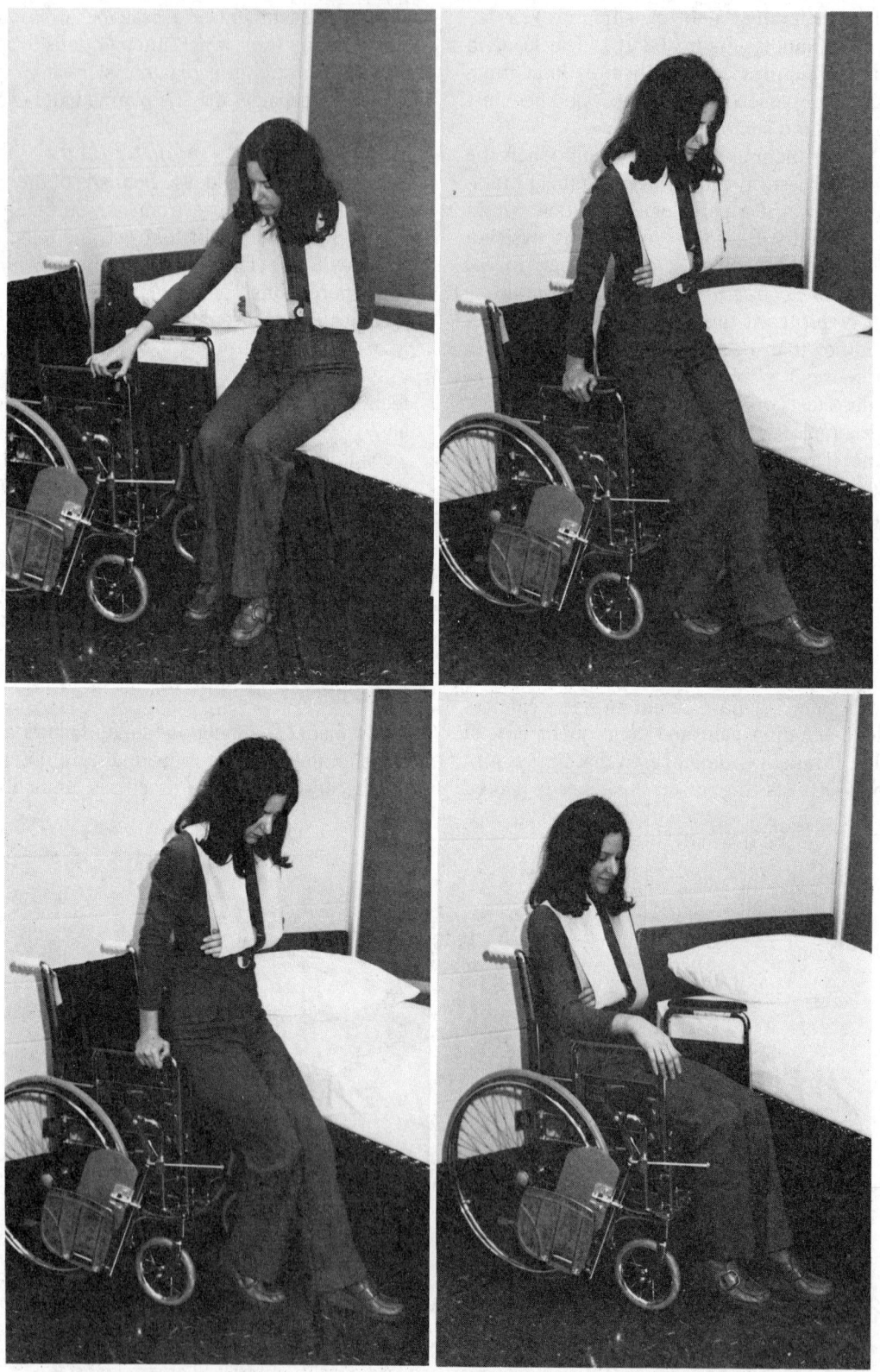

FIGURE 68-17, cont'd Independent transfer from bed to chair.

STEPS IN ASSESSING TRANSFER ABILITY

STEPS	EXAMPLES
1. Correlate data already obtained in interview to anticipate problems.	If person is a bilateral amputee or paraparetic, a transfer board may be necessary instead of employing a standing technique.
2. Solicit data from the person regarding modifications made in the home environment to effect safe transfer, and try to simulate those conditions in present situation.	Person may use grab bar on bathroom wall, have raised bed or chair surfaces, or use arms of chair for leverage.
3. Assess balance by having the person sit on the side of the bed without using hands for support, after attaining sitting position.	Persons who cannot sit unaided will probably not be able to stand safely.
4. Consider the person's ability to follow instructions, attention span, and fear of pain on movement.	Persons unable to follow instructions, retain instructions or fearful of pain will resist transfer or will follow through motions unsafely.

ture, weakness, or balance problems. Others are able to walk only with assistive devices such as a cane, crutches, or walker. These devices are sometimes used improperly. For example, a patient may use a cane on the wrong side of the body or support the weight of the body on the axillae when using axillary crutches. Note should be taken of this kind of problem, and interventions that will correct it should be planned.

Nursing assessment of ambulatory ability can usually be accomplished with the patient walking only a short distance (20 to 25 feet). Observations should be made regarding the use of assistive devices, balance, and gait pattern. If unsupported sitting balance is very poor, no attempt should be made to ambulate the patient without the assistance of another person.

Gait (see the box, upper right) is the manner or style of walking. An altered gait pattern is indicative of the presence of a pathologic process. While ambulation is being observed, note should be taken of the presence and type of limp displayed, the joints in which there is complaint or evidence of pain (for example, guarding), the degree to which there is reliance on assistance for weight bearing (either on devices or on a person), the person's balance, and the degree of deformity in the lower extremities. Deformity of the lower extremities

NORMAL GAIT CYCLE

Stance phase	Begins with heel strike and ends with toe-off
Swing phase	Begins with toe-off and continues through heel strike
Double support	Brief period when both feet are on ground

NOTE: Stance and swing phase are usually rhythmic and symmetric. When they are markedly asymmetric, alteration in gait is called a limp.

(genu varum, talipes varus, and so on) may not be as apparent when the joint is examined at rest as when weight-bearing forces are exerted across the joint. Furthermore, in persons with significant upper extremity involvement, some consideration must be given both to the amount of weight bearing that might be expected from the arms and hands and to the type of assistive device that would be appropriate. For example, an individ-

ASSESSMENT OF ACTIVITIES OF DAILY LIVING (ADL)

ADL FUNCTION	PERFORMANCE OF FUNCTION
Bathing	Independent
	Uses assistive devices
	Possesses ability, but function is performed by someone else
	Lacks ability
	Style of bathing—tub, shower, sponge, bed
Dressing	Independent
	Uses assistive devices (for example, buttonhook)
	Possesses ability, but function is performed by someone else
	Lacks ability
	Type of clothing or modifications (for example, Velcro fasteners, front opening, split seam to accommodate cast, elastic shoelaces)
Toileting	Independent
	Special equipment (for example, bedside commode, raised toilet seat)
	Functional problems (for example, constipation, diarrhea, urinary frequency, bowel or bladder incontinence)
	Recurrent bladder infections
	Special bowel maintenance programs
Sleep	No problem, usual sleep schedule
	Medications used to enhance sleep and their effect
	Interfered with by pain or inability to move freely
Relating with others	Note both positive and negative interactions with hospital staff, family, friends

ual with severe rheumatoid involvement of the hands might need a device that permits weight bearing on the forearms.

Other problems such as cardiovascular disease, respiratory impairment, or anemia may also affect ambulatory ability and must be taken into consideration during the assessment of ambulation. Assessment of transfer ability and ambulatory ability will help to determine a suitable level of activity for the patient.

OTHER ADL ASSESSMENT

Nurses should also assess other ADLs both to determine what functions the person may need assistance with and to plan for interventions that might restore a degree of independence to performance of those functions (see the box on p. 2003, lower right).

If a physical problem is long standing, the individual may have devised ways of managing ADL despite physical limitations that appear prohibitive. On the other

hand, if the problem had an acute onset, methods of handling ADL may need to be taught. Because abilities may change on a day-to-day basis, assessment of ADL abilities is an ongoing process throughout the period of time the nurse has contact with the individual. Data gathered and interventions based on that data are helpful in devising teaching approaches for both the patient and family, as well as in planning with the patient and family for the patient's eventual discharge.

DIAGNOSTIC TESTS

As with other illnesses, diagnostic tests are employed to provide information to assist in diagnosing a patient's musculoskeletal illness and to aid in devising a treatment program for the patient. Elements of the patient's care may be dependent on the outcome of diagnostic studies. Some of the principal studies that may be per-

SEROLOGIC TESTS

TEST	REASON FOR PERFORMING TEST
Serum muscle enzymes SGOT (serum glutamic-oxaloacetic transaminase) Aldolase CPK (creatine phosphokinase)	Enzymes can be elevated in the presence of primary myopathic (muscle) diseases. Elevated levels may result from degeneration of muscle fibers or from diffusion through a muscle membrane that has increased permeability. Enzyme levels are an index of both progress of the myopathic disorder and effectiveness of treatment. NURSING PRECAUTION: Intramuscular injections should be avoided when these enzymes are being monitored.
STS (serologic test for syphilis) FTA-ABS (fluorescent treponemal antibody absorption)	False positive STS results occur in 10% to 15% of persons with connective tissue diseases, so test may aid diagnosis. FTA-ABS excludes the presence of syphilis.
Rheumatoid factor or latex fixation (reaction of rheumatoid factor antibodies with IgG (7S) gamma globulin	Rheumatoid factor antibodies are found in the sera of individuals with rheumatoid arthritis. Test considered positive if rheumatoid factor is found in titrations of 1:40 or greater. CAUTION: Rheumatoid factor may be found in other conditions, that is, in aging, scleroderma, acute pulmonary tuberculosis, and parenteral narcotic addiction.
Antinuclear antibodies (ANA)	Circulating antibodies, which are composed of protein material and called *antinuclear antibodies* and which react with cellular nuclei and various individual constituents of cellular nuclei, can be identified by fluorescent techniques utilizing antihuman gamma globulin labeled with fluorescein. Positive tests are helpful in diagnosing Sjögren's syndrome, scleroderma, and systemic lupus erythematosus (SLE). Pattern of nuclear staining varies with different diseases.
Serum complement	Protein substances that are found in serum and synovial fluid and are associated with immune and inflammatory mechanisms; low levels often occur in SLE and rheumatoid arthritis.
Erythrocyte sedimentation rate (ESR) Hematocrit	Increased rate of settling of erythrocytes is an important index of the presence of inflammation. *Normal values:* Men, 1 to 3 mm/hr; women, 4 to 7 mm/hr Individuals with systemic connective tissue disease often have normocytic (normal RBCs), normochromic (normal amount of iron carried by RBCs) anemia, in the absence of any abnormal bleeding. Individuals who suffer trauma or undergo major surgery to the musculoskeletal system sustain significant blood loss. Symptoms of anemia (that is, extreme tiredness, fatigue, weakness) are experienced when hematocrit drops quickly; acute symptoms may be absent if anemia develops gradually or is chronic. Individuals with acute anemia should not be physically stressed. *Normal values:* Men, 45-50 vol/dl; women, 40-45 vol/dl

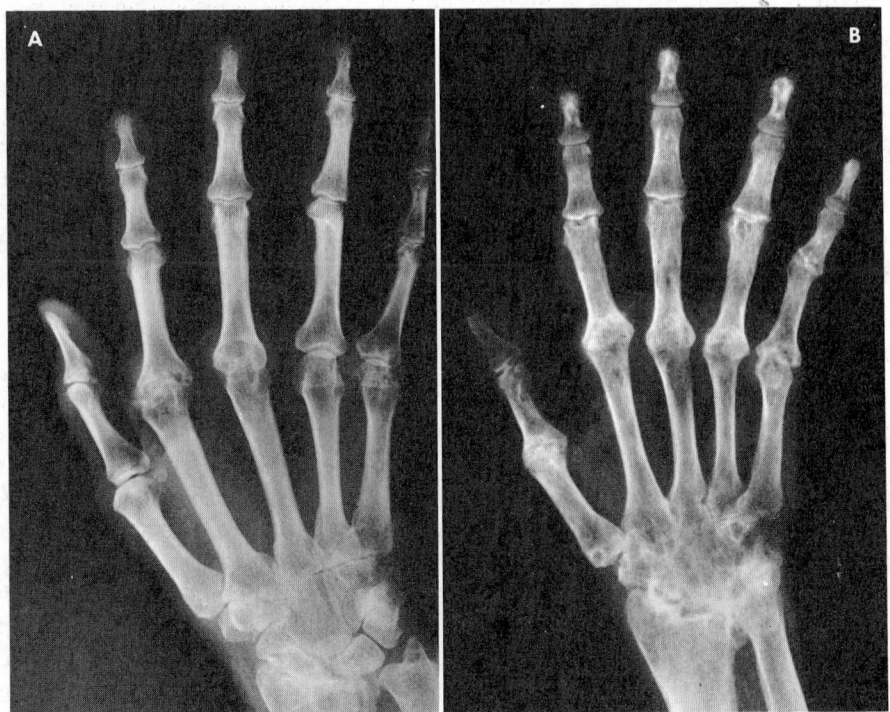

FIGURE 68-18 X-ray films of rheumatoid arthritis in hand and wrist. **A,** Moderate changes ranging from atrophic bone areas and narrowed cartilage spaces to subluxation of second and third metacarpophalangeal joints. **B,** More advanced case with severe destructive changes including multiple subluxations in digits and ankyloses in carpus. (From Raney R and Brashear H: Shand's handbook of orthopaedic surgery, ed 8, St Louis, 1971, The CV Mosby Co.)

formed on the person who has a musculoskeletal problem are described in the following sections.

LABORATORY EXAMINATIONS

Laboratory examinations consist of two major categories of study, serologic and urinary, as described in the box on p. 2004 and in the box at right.

RADIOLOGIC EXAMINATIONS
BONES AND JOINTS

Radiologic examination of bones and joints is imperative for the identification and treatment of fractures. It is also most helpful in determining the presence of disease (such as rheumatoid arthritis, spondylitis, avascular necrosis, and tumor), as well as the progress of and effects of treatment on these disorders (Figure 68-18). Specialized texts should be consulted for reference to the variety of views that are obtained in such examinations and for the specific findings that are present in the various disorders.[15]

It is important for nurses to remember that many patients are not able to lie on x-ray examination tables for long periods of time. In particular, persons with arthritis develop joint stiffness and pain if their ability to move

URINARY TESTS

DIAGNOSTIC TEST	RATIONALE FOR TEST
24-hour urine for creatine-creatinine ratio	In the presence of muscle disease, the ability of muscle to convert creatine is decreased, the amount of creatine excreted by the kidneys increases, and the ratio of urinary creatine to creatinine increases. Periodic studies are helpful in diagnosis and evaluation of progress of treatment of primary myopathies.
Urinary uric acid levels (24-hour collection)*	Helpful in diagnosis and decisions regarding treatment modalities for gout. *Normal value:* should not exceed 900 mg uric acid excretion per day

*NOTE: 24-hour urine collections must be accurate to facilitate proper diagnosis and treatment.

about is restricted. Because radiologic examinations for individuals with rheumatic diseases are often quite extensive, careful thought should be given to the scheduling of these examinations. Very few of these patients can tolerate a single session in which all the required views of all the involved joints are taken. Instead, 1 or 2 days of rest between shorter sessions may be required. Analgesics or local heat applications for relief of joint pain following x-ray examinations may be necessary for some patients.

SYSTEMIC RADIOLOGIC STUDIES

Systemic radiologic studies such as the barium enema, upper gastrointestinal series, esophogram, and intravenous pyelogram are helpful in determining the extent of involvement of various internal organs (bowel, kidneys) in systemic rheumatic diseases. Discussion of these examinations can be found in Chapters 41 and 47.

MYELOGRAPHY

Myelography is useful in identifying lesions such as a herniated nucleus pulposus that are blocking the subarachnoid space. Discussion of this procedure and the precautions that must be exercised in caring for the patient after the procedure are discussed in Chapter 70.

ARTHROGRAPHY

Arthrography permits visualization of structures within the joint that are not normally seen on routine radiographic films. The joint cavity is injected with radiopaque dye, air, or both. The latter is called a *double-contrast* arthrogram. The dye or air serves as a contrast medium against which the outlines of soft tissue components of the joint may be seen. Tears of the menisci, internal derangements of the joint, and synovial cysts can be diagnosed with the aid of arthrograms. Patients may experience pain while the joint is expanded by the dye or air, and some patients may be allergic to radiopaque dye. The procedure should be explained to the patient and the possibility of allergy to the dye should be excluded before an arthrographic examination.

RADIOISOTOPE BONE SCANS

Radioisotope *bone scans* are performed primarily to demonstrate the presence of metastatic disease. Intravenously injected sodium pertechnetate ^{99m}Tc (Technetium) is the isotope most frequently used in this study. The ^{99m}Tc concentrates in areas of osteoblastic activity involved in the exchange of calcium. In malignancies, this activity is accelerated. Lesions may be visualized on bone scans as early as 6 months before there is evidence of the lesions on routine X-ray films.[12] Sometimes, scans are performed to detect healing activity in bone following a complicated fracture.

Technetium scans are also of some use in determin-ing the degree of parotid gland involvement in Sjögren's syndrome. The uptake, concentration, and excretion of the isotope by the major salivary glands are measured by a technique called sequential scintiphotography.[20]

Persons being prepared for these procedures should know that the procedures will not cause them pain and that the isotopes will not harm them, but that they may have to remain quietly in one position for an hour or more.

COMPUTERIZED AXIAL TOMOGRAPHY

Tomography is an X-ray technique by which detailed images of "slices" of tissue are obtained by focusing X-ray beams at predetermined planes or depths of the tissue being studied. Detailed images of the stuctures at that level are produced, while details of structures surrounding that level are blurred or eliminated. *Computerized axial tomography (CAT scanning)* is tomography employing a computer to compose a picture of the tissue being studied. A series of X-ray beams are rotated, one degree at a time, around the specific area being examined. With each rotation, a picture is generated that depicts the difference in tissue density. These pictures are very clear and detailed. The procedure is noninvasive and does not require repositioning of the patient as does conventional tomography. Patients who are claustrophobic may have some difficulty tolerating the procedure as it does require lying in a cylindrical metal scanner for up to an hour.

MAGNETIC RESONANCE IMAGING

Magnetic resonance imaging (MRI) is a scanning technique that produces tomographic images by using magnetic forces rather than X-ray beams. The patient lies on a nonmagnetic scanning table that slides, head first, into a giant cylindrical magnet. The magnet causes the body's atomic protons to line up and spin in the same direction. A radio frequency signal is beamed into the magnetic field causing the protons to move out of alignment. When the signal stops, the protons move back into alignment and release energy. A receiver coil measures the energy released by the movement of the protons and the time it takes for the protons to return to their aligned position. These measurements provide information regarding the type of tissue in which the protons lie, as well as the condition of the tissue. A computer uses this information to construct an image on a television screen, showing the distribution of protons of certain atoms (usually hydrogen); and the television image can be recorded on film or magnetic tape. The images obtained by MRI are exquisitely clear, more so than CAT images (Figure 68-19). MRI is frequently performed following myelography to delineate the pathology grossly identified by the myelogram.

Patients being prepared for MRI should know that

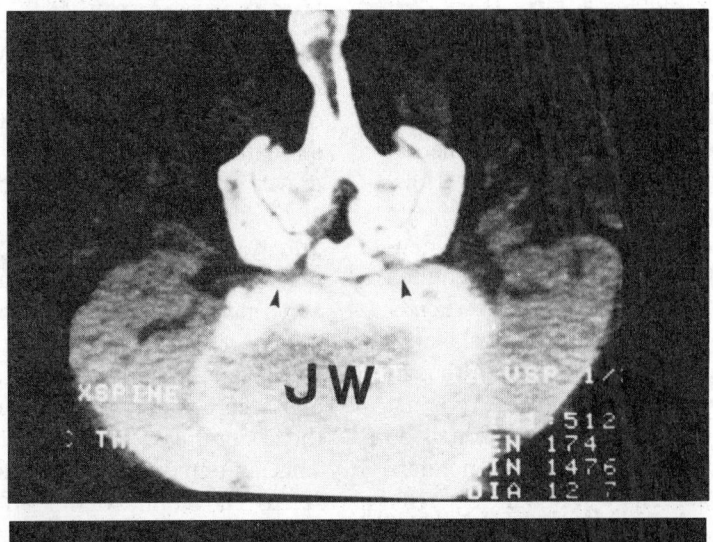
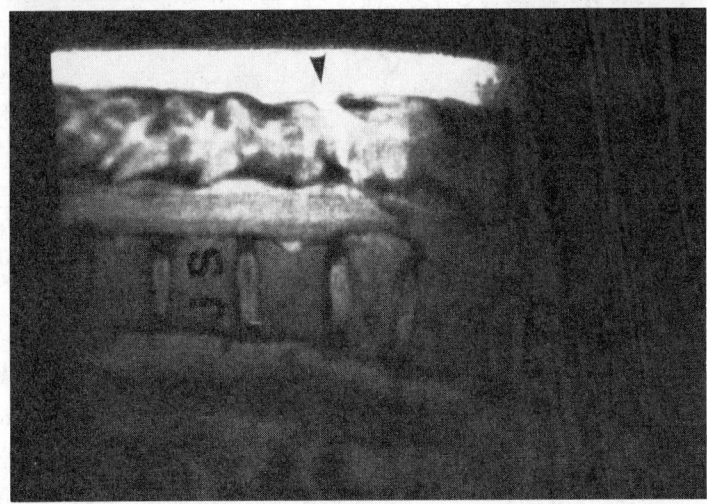

FIGURE 68-19 MRI scan showing sagittal and longitudinal views of the spine. Note the clarity of both the bony and soft tissue structures. This clarity cannot be achieved with routine x-ray studies. (Courtesy Sanford Emery, M.D., University Hospitals of Cleveland, Cleveland, Ohio.)

the procedure is painless and that there is no special preparation for the test. However, because a magnetic field is used, the patient will be asked to remove any metallic objects, such as jewelry or hairpins, and non-permanent dentures. Patients who have cardiac pace-makers or intracranial vascular aneurysm clips are excluded from MRI. As with CAT scanning, patients who are claustrophobic may have difficulty being placed in the scanner. Sometimes medication such as diazepam (Valium) is prescribed to help the patient relax. During the scan, the patient will hear the hum of the machine, a loud thump when the radio waves are turned on and off, and other machine-like noises. The thumping can be particularly annoying to patients, and many are frightened by it if they are not told it will happen. Scanning time is usually 30 to 90 minutes.

SPECIAL TESTS
ELECTROMYOGRAPHY

Electromyography measures the electrical activity of muscles; and an *electromyogram* (EMG) is a recording of the variations of electrical potentials (voltage) detected by a needle electrode inserted into skeletal muscle. The electrical activity can be heard over a loud speaker and viewed on an oscilloscope and on a graph at the same time. No electrical activity can be detected in normal muscles at rest, but during volitional movement, action potentials can be detected. In both primary myopathic and neuropathic disorders, specific variations exist in the size of individual motor unit potentials. In neurogenic atrophy, fibrillations may be present in the resting muscle. An EMG provides direct evidence of motor dysfunction and can be used to some extent to detect a dysfunction located in the motor neuron, the neuromuscular junction, or the muscle fibers. Thus it is particularly helpful in the diagnosis of lower motor neuron (LMN) disease, primary muscle disease, and defects in the transmission of electrical impulses at the neuromuscular junction, such as myasthenia gravis. However, electromyography *cannot* be used to differentiate *specific* disease entities in either the myopathic or neuropathic categories. No special preparation is required for this procedure. The patient may fear that insertion of electrode needles will be painful or that electrical stimulation of the needles will cause severe shock. Although the patient may be reassured that the procedure is not dangerous, it should be noted that some individuals do experience mild to moderate discomfort. Therefore nurses preparing patients for this test should not refer to the test as "painless."

MANUAL MUSCLE TEST

The manual muscle test (MMT) is performed to determine the degree of muscular weakness resulting from disease, injury, or lack of use. The MMT rates the strength of muscles by their performance in relation to gravity and manually applied resistance. The test is usually performed by a physical therapist. Factors such as gravity, stabilization of the tested part, proper positioning, amounts of resistance, range of the joint, pain, and abnormal muscle tone must be considered in the performance of the test and can influence the test's objectivity. Several grading systems are used, such as a 0 to 5 and a percentage system. The Lovett scale is probably the system most frequently used by physical therapists. This system rates muscle strength on a scale from "zero" (no contraction seen or felt) through "trace," "poor," "fair," "good," and "normal" (the muscle con-

TABLE 68-1 Types of biopsies

Organ	Test(s) Performed	Positive Results	Nursing Considerations
Skin (punch biopsy)	Immunofluorescent staining—tissue is washed with solution of fluorescein-labeled anti-human gamma globulin antibody	Band of immunofluorescence at epidermal-dermal junction, indicating presence of rheumatic disease (that is, scleroderma, SLE, psoriatic arthritis)	Biopsy site kept clean and dry with small adhesive bandage until scab develops; hydrogen peroxide (3%) used to cleanse open area p.r.n; only very mild discomfort experienced by patient
Muscle (operative procedure)	Histochemical staining	Tissue reveals features of lower motor neuron disease, degeneration, inflammatory reaction as in polymyositis, or involvement of specific fibers indicating primary myopathic disease	Patient instructed and prepared for surgery; patient monitored per post-anesthesia routine (local or general); mild to moderate pain and stiffness in biopsy area; routine activity encouraged within 24 hours to avoid undue stiffness; dressings changed as necessary
Synovium (closed—performed with needle; open—performed in surgery)	Histologic examination—synovial fluid obtained at the same time; may be cultured to determine presence of infection	Differentiates various forms of arthritis	Patient instructed about procedure; patient may require post-anesthesia monitoring; strict asepsis observed throughout procedure and in caring for the wound; small compression dressing applied to joint, and joint rested for 24 hours to prevent hemorrhage or effusion
Buccal mucosa (punch biopsy)	Histologic examination of tissue from inside lower lip	Helpful in diagnosing Sjögren's syndrome	Patient instructed about procedure; generally minor discomfort experienced; diet altered to avoid rough and very hot foods (they will irritate the site)
Bone (operative procedure)	Microscopic analysis	Can confirm presence of infection or neoplasm	Patient instructed and prepared for surgery; patient monitored per post-anesthesia routine; mild to severe discomfort may be experienced; activity restricted dependent on location and extent of surgical procedure; dressings changed as necessary

tracts to overcome greater resistance than a "good" muscle).

Muscle testing is particularly helpful in determining on which muscle a biopsy should be performed when confirmation of the diagnosis of myopathic disorders is required. Furthermore, the initial test is used as a baseline examination against which later test results can be compared to demonstrate progress or lack of progress in the treatment of myopathic and other musculoskeletal diseases. When muscle-strengthening exercises are indicated, the test will indicate the group of muscles that requires the most therapy.

BIOPSY

Biopsies of tissue from a variety of organs are helpful in the diagnoses of diseases or disorders affecting the musculoskeletal system. Table 68-1 lists the organs that may be biopsied, the test(s) performed on the biopsied tissue, what a positive result of testing indicates, and general nursing considerations in caring for the patient on whom the biopsy is performed.

JOINT ASPIRATION

Joint aspiration is performed to obtain a sample of synovial fluid from within the joint cavity. This procedure (performed by introducing a needle into the joint cavity and withdrawing fluid) aids in determining the presence of an aseptic inflammatory process such as rheumatoid arthritis or a septic process such as bacterial arthritis. Samples of synovial fluid are cultured and examined both microscopically and chemically.

The synovial fluid is normally straw colored and clear. Its viscosity resembles that of motor oil. In the presence of inflammation it becomes turbid and watery. The *mucin clot test* is performed by mixing synovial fluid with glacial acetic acid. Normal synovial fluid will form a white, ropey mucin clot. When inflammation is present, the clot breaks apart easily and becomes flaky (flocculent). The degree of flocculence increases with the degree of inflammation. Also, when inflammation is present, the number of WBCs, the protein content, and the number of polymorphonuclear cells in the synovial fluid are increased; glucose content is decreased.[14]

A local anesthetic is usually administered before the procedure. Strict asepsis is observed during the procedure. After the procedure the joint is often wrapped in a small compression (Ace) dressing. The joint may be rested for 8 to 24 hours. Drainage should be managed in accordance with universal body substance isolation techniques.

SCOLIOSIS SCREENING

Scoliosis screening programs, particularly for school-age children, are effective in identifying early indications of scoliosis. Such indications include "wing" (or protrusion) deformity of one scapula, uneven shoulder height, one arm hanging closer to the body than the other when standing erect, demonstrable curve of the spine, and rib hump (elevation of the rib cage posteriorly and laterally in the thoracic area) on forward bending. If scoliosis is detected early, nonsurgical treatment may be effective in arresting the progression of the curvature.

ENDOSCOPY
ARTHROSCOPY

Arthroscopy (visualization of a joint) is a procedure performed in the operating room. A specially designed endoscope (arthroscope) is inserted through a small incision into the joint cavity, enabling the physician to visualize the structure and contents of the joint. The majority of arthroscopic procedures are performed on the knee, although other joints, notably the shoulder, are also examined and treated with this technique. The procedure permits biopsy of the synovium or cartilage, is useful in the diagnosis and often repair of torn meniscus and ligament damage, and permits the removal of loose bodies from the joint space. The patient is treated in much the same manner as following a synovial biopsy; however, the period of time the joint is rested and the use of any immobilizing device is determined by the extent of the procedure. The surgeon should be consulted regarding the activity the patient is permitted following the procedure so that damage to the joint may be avoided.

CHAPTER SUMMARY

- ✔ Support, protection, and movement are the three mechanical functions of bone. Bones also store calcium and produce RBCs.

- ✔ Bone is produced by the process of osteogenesis or endochondral ossification. The bone building cells are known as osteoblasts; bone cells are osteocytes. Calcium salts in the matrix give bone its characteristic "hard" quality.

- ✔ Bones are classified into four groups based on shape: long, short, flat, and irregular.

- ✔ Bone is composed of cancellous (spongy) and compact (dense) bone. Lamellae are concentric cylindric layers of calcified matrix. The arrangement of lamellae within bone differentiates cancellous and compact bone. The haversian canal is at the center of the lamella.

- ✔ Periosteum is a white, fibrous membrane that covers bone except on the articular surface, which is covered with hyaline cartilage. The inner layers of the periosteum contain osteoblasts, thus the periosteum is considered a growth organ.

- ✔ Epiphyses are the ends of bone; the diaphysis is the shaft. Longitudinal bone growth begins in the epiphyseal cartilage between the diaphyseal and epiphyseal centers of ossification. Cartilage cells rapidly proliferate and the cartilage undergoes ossification.

Growth in the diameter of bone is accomplished through the simultaneous processes of bone destruction, by osteoclasts enlarging the medullary cavity, and bone production, by osteoblasts in the periosteum.

⮱ Bone reshapes itself in response to alterations of its mechanical function. Osteogenesis occurs along lines of stress. This explains why a person who regularly exercises may have some increase in bone mass (hypertrophy), whereas a sedentary person may experience loss of bone substance (atrophy).

⮱ Circulation of blood to bone is supplied by three routes: through arterioles in the haversian canals, through Volkmann's canals (located in the periosteum), and through vessels in the marrow and the ends of bone. Blood supply to the bone can be interrupted by injury to an artery, the periosteum, or the bone itself. Because bones are supplied with sensory nerve endings, pain will result if bone is damaged.

⮱ Callus formation is the process of bone healing and proceeds in five general stages: hematoma formation, fibrin meshwork formation, invasion by osteoblasts, callus formation, and remodeling. Good callus formation can be impeded by inadequate reduction of a fracture, excessive edema at a fracture site, too much bone loss at the time of injury, inefficient immobilization, infection, bone necrosis, anemia or other systemic conditions, endocrine imbalance, and poor dietary intake. Nonunion, or an ununited fracture, is the resulting lack of repair or of abnormal or inefficient callus formation.

⮱ The three major types of muscle are skeletal, visceral, and cardiac. Skeletal muscle is innervated by nerve fibers from the cerebrospinal system and can be controlled at will. It provides controlled movement, maintains posture, and produces heat.

⮱ Skeletal muscle cells are long and narrow and are made up of bundles of muscle fibers. Myofibrils are small, closely packed fibers within the sarcoplasm. They consist of several sections called sarcomeres.

⮱ The function of muscles is to contract. The triggering of nerve impulses at the muscle fiber accomplishes this complex process. Calcium ions released when the impulse is received bind to troponin. Once calcium ions are bound, the sarcomeres contract. Energy is supplied by the breakdown of ATP. Relaxation occurs when calcium ions separate from troponin.

⮱ Body movement is produced by muscles pulling on bones, with bones serving as levers and joints serving as fulcrums for the levers. Muscles act in a coordinated manner, involving prime movers, antagonists, and synergists.

⮱ Skeletal muscle is highly vascular because efficient muscle contraction is dependent on an adequate blood supply _to and from_ the muscle fibers.

⮱ Effective innervation is necessary for adequate muscle contraction. Somatic motor neurons transmit impulses to skeletal muscles. Contraction of the muscle is set off by the release of acetylcholine across the motor end-plate or neuromuscular junction.

⮱ Cartilage is a material composed of fibers embedded in a firm gel. It is strong, flexible, and avascular. The type of cartilage (fibrous, hyaline, or elastic) is determined by the number of collagenous fibers.

⮱ Ligaments connect the articular ends of bones and provide stability. They also may attach to soft tissue to suspend structures. Ligaments consist of dense fibrous bands of connective tissue.

⮱ Tendons are dense fibrous tissue bands that form the termination of a muscle and attach it to a bone. They are extensions of the fibrous sheaths that cover each muscle and are continuous with the periosteum at the other end. Tendon sheaths are tubular structures that enclose certain tendons, especially at the wrist and ankle.

⮱ Small sacs of connective tissue are called bursae. They are located wherever pressure is exerted over moving parts.

⮱ Joints, or the places where bones come together, provide flexibility within the skeletal framework. The type and amount of movement possible is determined by the shape of the joint. There are three major classifications of joints: Synarthroses, or fibrous, joints provide no movement; amphiarthroses, or cartilaginous, joints allow little movement; diarthroses, or synovial, joints allow free movement.

⮱ Diarthroidal joints contain a joint cavity between the articulating surfaces of the bones that compose the joint. The articulating surfaces of both bones are covered by articular hyaline cartilage, allowing smooth motion. The joint is encased in a joint capsule, and the capsule is lined with a synovial membrane. Lubrication is provided by synovial fluid secreted by the synovial membrane. Ligaments may be present to provide internal stability to the joint. Menisci (small pieces of dense cartilage) may also be present to provide additional cushioning.

⮱ Physiologic changes with aging occur as the total number of body cells decrease, resulting in the decline of tissue strength and integrity. Connective tissues lose elasticity; muscles lose bulk, tone and strength; bone reabsorption is more rapid than bone growth; and, particularly in postmenopausal women, calcium is lost from bone, making it softer and more prone to fracture.

- The musculoskeletal, circulatory, and nervous systems are interrelated. Any problem that causes interruption of innervation, contractility, articulation, circulation, or support results in musculoskeletal dysfunction.

- Assessment of any person with a musculoskeletal problem must include subjective data elicited from the person and his or her family. This includes a description of the present problem, such as onset and duration, associated pain or discomfort, current medications, and effect on performance of ADL; the person's perception of the problem or dysfunction; and the family's perception of the person's problem.

- Objective data involves observations of the person. Observations are made regarding behavior, general appearance, and the condition of skin, nails, and hair. Data also is collected about deformities, strength and range of motion, ability to transfer and ambulate, and ability to perform ADL. (Refer to the text and boxes for specifics.)

- Some of the principal diagnostic studies that may be performed on a person with a musculoskeletal problem include laboratory examinations (such as serologic and urinary tests); radiologic examinations (such as radiographs of bones and joints, systemic radiologic studies [to determine the extent of internal organ involvement], myelography, arthrography, radioisotope scans, CAT scans, and MRI); and special tests (such as EMG, MMT, biopsies, and joint aspiration).

- Arthroscopy is a surgical procedure that provides visualization of a joint via a specially designed endoscope. Biopsy, diagnosis, repair of torn meniscus or ligament, and removal of loose bodies from the joint space can be accomplished with this approach.

QUESTIONS TO CONSIDER

- Name the tissues that compose the musculoskeletal system, and discuss the function of this system.

- Describe the functions of bone.

- What is the process of osteogenesis, and how does it occur?

- What are the four types of bone, and how are they classified? Describe the anatomic structure of bones.

- Describe the physiology of bone healing.

- What are the three major groups of muscles, and how do they differ?

- Outline the physiology of muscle contraction.

- How is movement of the body produced?

- Define cartilage, ligament, tendon, fascia, and bursa.

- List the three major classifications of joints. How do they differ?

- Summarize the physiologic changes of the musculoskeletal system that occur with aging.

- Describe the most common laboratory, radiologic, and special tests that may be performed on a person with a musculoskeletal problem.

REFERENCES AND SELECTED READINGS

1. Anthony CP and Thibodeau GA: Textbook of anatomy and physiology, ed 11, St Louis, 1983, The CV Mosby Co.
2. Bates B: A guide to physical examination, ed 4, Philadelphia, 1987, JB Lippincott Co.
3. Beetham WP et al.: Physical examination of the joints, Philadelphia, 1965, WB Saunders Co.
4. Blauvelt C and Nelson F: A manual of orthopaedic terminology, ed 3, St. Louis, 1985, The CV Mosby Co.
5. Bluestone R, editor: Rheumatology, Boston, 1980, Houghton Mifflin Professional Publishers.
6. *Brunner NA: Orthopedic nursing: a programmed approach, ed 4, St Louis, 1983, The CV Mosby Co.
7. *Collier IC: Assessing functional status of the elderly, Arthritis Care Res 1(1):45-52, 1988.
8. *Cohen S and Viellion G: Patient assessment: examining joints of the upper and lower extremities, Am J Nurs 81(4):763-786, 1981.
9. *Farrell J: Orthopedic pain: what does it mean? Am J Nurs 84(4):466-469, 1984.
10. Farrell J: Illustrated guide to orthopedic nursing, ed 3, Philadelphia, 1986, JB Lippincott Co.
11. Flatt AE: Care of the arthritic hand, ed 4, St Louis, 1982, The CV Mosby Co.
12. French RM: Guide to diagnostic procedures, ed 5, New York, 1980, McGraw-Hill Book Co.
13. Fritzler MJ: Antinuclear antibodies in the investigation of rheumatic diseases, Bulletin on the Rheumatic Diseases 35(6):1-10, 1985.
14. Hilt NE, editor: Arthroscopy of the knee, Monograph Library National Association of Orthopaedic Nurses, Feb 1983, Anthony J Jannetti, Inc
15. Hilt NE and Cogburn SB: Manual of orthopedics, St Louis, 1980, The CV Mosby Co.
16. *Johnson C, editor: Symposium on orthopedic nursing, Nurs Clin North Am 16(4):707-766, 1981.
17. Magnetic resonance imaging, South Deerfield, Mass, 1986, Channing L Bete Co Inc.
18. Malasanos L et al: Health assessment, ed 3, St Louis, 1986, The CV Mosby Co.
19. McCarty DJ, editor: Arthritis and allied conditions: a textbook of rheumatology, ed 11, Philadelphia, 1989, Lea & Febiger.
20. Moskowitz RW: Clinical rheumatology: a problem oriented approach to diagnosis and management, ed 2, Philadelphia, 1982, Lea & Febiger.
21. Moskowitz RW et al.: Osteoarthritis: diagnosis and management, Philadelphia, 1984, WB Saunders Co.
22. *Mourad L and Droste M: The nursing process in the care of adults with orthopaedic conditions, ed 2, New York, 1988, John Wiley & Sons.
23. Norkin C and Levangie P: Joint structure & function: a comprehensive analysis, Philadelphia, 1983, FA Davis Company.
24. Perricone N: Overview of joint anatomy and physiology: a basis for understanding and assessing rheumatic conditions, Occup Health Nurs 32(7):352-355, 1984.
25. Pigg J, Driscoll P, and Caniff R: Rheumatology nursing: a problem-oriented approach, New York, 1985, John Wiley & Sons Inc.
26. *Ross D: Musculoskeletal assessment: ROM of fingers and hand, Orthopaedic Nursing 1(5):11-17, 1982.
27. Salter RB: Textbook of disorders and injuries of musculoskeletal structure, ed. 2, Baltimore, 1983, The Williams & Wilkins Co.
28. Schumacher HR: Primer on the rheumatic diseases, ed 9, Atlanta, 1988, Arthritis Foundation.
29. Turek SL: Orthopaedics: principles and their application, ed. 4, Philadelphia, 1984, JB Lippincott Company.
30. *Vanderbeck KA: Getting the facts: a guide to orthopaedic assessment, Orthop Nurs 3(5):31-34, 1984.
31. *Zubay RL: Understanding magnetic resonance imaging from a nursing perspective, Orthop Nurs 7(6):17-23, 1988.

*References preceded by an asterisk are particularly well suited for student reading.

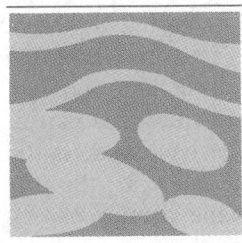

Management of Persons with Trauma to the Musculoskeletal System

PATRICIA S. BUERGIN

KYLE M. PASKERT

CHAPTER OBJECTIVES

After studying this chapter, the student should be able to:

1. Describe three causes of bone fracture and four measures that can be taken to prevent fracture.
2. Define the three mechanisms of immobilization by which fractured bone can heal.
3. Discuss the medical management of fractures, including definitions of the terms "closed reduction" and "open reduction."
4. List three major complications of bone fracture and explain how they are treated.
5. Describe what subjective and objective data the nurse should collect when assessing the person who has a fracture.
6. Describe the nursing measures that can be used in relation to the following:
   a Patient teaching
   b Pain management
   c Positioning
   d Neurocirculatory monitoring
   e Preservation of strength and mobility
   f Maintenance of skin integrity
7. Discuss four systemic complications that might occur after a fracture and the nursing measures that can be used to help prevent them.
8. Discuss the special nursing care measures required for the patient who has (1) a cast, (2), traction, and (3) an internal fixation device.
9. Describe the special nursing care measures required for the person whose hip fracture has been treated with a prosthetic implant.
10. Discuss the special nursing considerations in caring for the patient with a spine fracture.
11. Discuss the various types of trauma that can occur to ligaments, tendons, and muscles and the nursing care associated with each of these.
12. Discuss the various types of injuries that can occur to joints and the nursing care that is required.
13. Discuss the special care considerations required by the patient who has sustained multiple trauma.

The person who has had trauma to the musculoskeletal system has sustained an interruption in the integrity of one or more components of the system. Musculoskeletal trauma is most frequently manifested as bone fracture, but it may also include injury to soft tissue, muscle, ligament, meniscus, tendon, or joint.

TRAUMA TO BONE

FRACTURE OF BONE
EPIDEMIOLOGY/ETIOLOGY

Fracture of bone usually occurs as a result of a blow to the body, a fall, or another accident. However, fracture may occur during normal activity or after a minimal injury, if the bone has been weakened by a disease such as primary or metastatic cancer or osteoporosis. This is called a *pathologic fracture*, or collapse of the bone. Bone may also fracture when the muscles associated with it are unable to absorb energy as they usually do. This type of fracture is called a *fatigue* or *stress fracture*. *Avulsion* fractures occur when a strong ligamentous or tendinous attachment pulls a fragment of bone away from the rest of the bone. Fracture can occur at any age, although older persons, persons with balance or mobility problems, persons who work at high-risk occupations (for example, steelworkers and race car drivers), and persons with chronic degenerative or neoplastic diseases are at higher risk for injury.

PREVENTION

One approach to preventing fracture is to make the environment safer. Examples of measures that can be taken include the following:

1. Mounting grab bars on the wall next to a tub or toilet

2. Attaching safety arms around a toilet
3. Removing throw rugs and obstacles from areas used by individuals with locomotor difficulties
4. Ensuring that wheelchairs have adequate locking devices
5. Teaching individuals who must use ambulatory devices and wheelchairs how to use them properly

A second approach is to continue to educate the public regarding the following:

1. The dangers of drinking and driving
2. The advisability of using seat belts while driving
3. Attending to safety precautions when climbing ladders and using power tools or heavy equipment
4. Wearing recommended protective clothing (for example, steel-toed shoes and hard hats for hazardous work at home or on the job)
5. Wearing proper protective clothing while engaging in sports (for example, protective padding and well-fitting running shoes)

A third approach is to continue to educate women about the problem of *osteoporosis*. Individuals most at risk to develop osteoporosis are small-framed, nonobese, menopausal White females. Contributing factors are diets low in calcium, smoking, excessive coffee intake, too much protein in the diet, and a sedentary life-style. Measures that can be taken to retard osteoporosis include the following:

1. Increasing calcium intake
2. Refraining from smoking
3. Decreasing coffee intake
4. Decreasing excess protein in the diet
5. Engaging in some regular moderate activity such as walking
6. Exploring with a physician the advisability of estrogen replacement at menopause

PATHOPHYSIOLOGY

Definition and Types of Fractures

A bone is fractured when there is a complete or partial interruption of the osseous tissue. A fracture is *complete* when there is complete separation of the bone, producing two fragments; it is *incomplete* when only part of the bone is broken. The part of the bone nearest the body is referred to as the *proximal fragment;* the part more distant from the body is called the *distal fragment.* The proximal fragment is also called the *uncontrollable fragment,* because its location and muscle attachments prevent it from being moved or manipulated when attempting to bring the separate fragments into alignment. The distal fragment is called the *controllable fragment,* because it can usually be moved to bring it into correct relationship to the proximal fragment. Fractures in long bones are designated as being in the proximal, middle, or distal third of the bone.

If the skin over the fracture is intact, the fracture is classified as *simple* or *closed.* A fracture is classified as *compound* or *open* when there is a direct communication between a skin wound and the fracture site. An open or compound fracture has a high risk of contamination, and this is an important factor in its treatment. When the two bone fragments are in good alignment with no change from normal position despite the break in continuity of bone, the fracture is referred to as a *fracture without displacement.* If the bone fragments have separated at the point of fracture, it is referred to as a *fracture with displacement.* Displacement may be slight, moderate, or marked.

The *line of fracture* as revealed by x-ray film or fluoroscopy is usually classified according to type. It may be *greenstick,* with splintering on one side of the bone (this occurs most often in young children); *transverse,* with

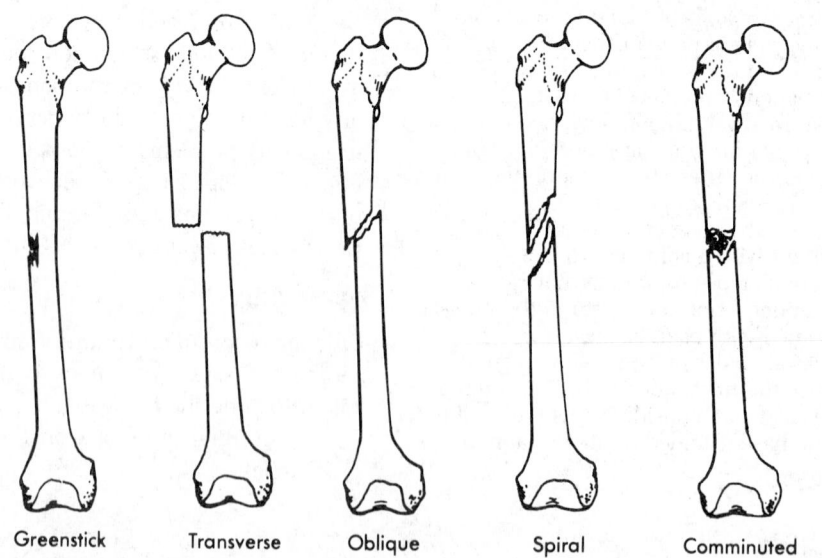

Greenstick   Transverse   Oblique   Spiral   Comminuted

FIGURE 69-1 Types of fractures.

the break being straight across the bone; *oblique,* with the line of the fracture being at an oblique angle to the bone shaft; or *spiral,* with the fracture lines partially encircling the bone. The fracture may be referred to as *telescoped* or *impacted* if the distal fragment is forcibly pushed against and into the proximal fragment. If there are several bone fragments, the fracture is called *comminuted.* (see Figure 69-1 for examples of fractures.)

Because bones are firmer than their surrounding structures, any injury severe enough to cause bone fracture may also cause injury to adjacent muscles, nerves, connective tissue, and blood vessels. The force that causes the fracture is dissipated through the surrounding soft tissue, and small fragments of bone may become embedded in muscle, blood vessels, or nerves.

Healing of Fractures

Immobilization of a fractured bone is necessary for healing to take place. Immobilization may be effected in any of the following three ways:

1. *Physiologic splintage,* a naturally occurring phenomenon related to pain in the affected area that causes guarding, muscle spasm, and avoidance of use; further, there will be a desire to rest the whole body until some repair has occurred
2. *External orthopaedic splinting* with devices such as casts

---

MAJOR FACTORS THAT IMPEDE BONE HEALING

PROBLEM	CAUSE
Poor approximation of fracture fragments	Inaccurate reduction or malalignment of fracture fragments
	Inadequate immobilization, resulting in movement of fragments
	Excessive bone loss at time of fracture, preventing sufficient bridging of broken ends
	Excessive fragmentation of bone, allowing soft tissue to be interposed between bone ends
	Inability of patient to comply with restrictions imposed by immobilizing/fixation device(s), resulting in movement of fragments
Excessive edema at fracture site	Tissue swelling impedes supply of nutrients to the area of fracture
Bone necrosis	Injury to blood vessels impedes supply of nutrients to involved bone
Infection at fracture site	Infection disrupts normal callus formation

3. *Internal fixation* with screws, plates, or rods to hold the opposing ends of the fracture in place

Once immobilization is accomplished, the bone heals by the process of *callus formation* (see Chapter 68). Factors that impede healing are described in the box below. Failure of a fracture to consolidate in the time usually required is called *delayed union,* failure to form a stable union after 6 to 9 months is called *nonunion,* and healing with angulation or deformity is called *malunion.* If a fracture is nonunited, there will be excessive mobility at the fracture site, creating a false joint. This is called a *pseudarthrosis.*

CLINICAL MANIFESTATIONS

The signs and symptoms of fracture vary according to the location and function of the involved bone, the strength of its muscle attachments, the type of fracture sustained, and the amount of related soft tissue damage; the following are possible signs and symptoms:

1. Pain (caused by swelling at the site, muscle spasm, damage to periosteum)
   a. Immediate
   b. Severe.
   c. Aggravated by pressure at the site of injury
   d. Aggravated by attempted motion
2. Loss of normal function (the injured part incapable of voluntary movement)
3. Obvious deformity resulting from loss of bone continuity
4. Excessive motion at site (that is, motion where motion does not usually occur)
5. *Crepitus** or grating sound if limb is moved gently
6. Soft tissue edema in area of injury resulting from extravasation of blood and tissue fluid
7. Warmth over injured area resulting from increased blood flow to the area
8. Ecchymosis of skin surrounding injured area (may not be apparent for several days)
9. Loss of sensation or paralysis distal to injury resulting from nerve entrapment
10. Signs of shock related to severe tissue injury, blood loss, or intense pain
11. Evidence of fracture on x-ray film

INTERVENTIONS

Medical Management

Management objectives include the following:

1. Reduction of fracture by approximating the fracture fragments
2. Maintenance of fragments in correct alignment through immobilization

---

*No attempt should be made to elicit this sign when fracture is suspected, because it may cause further damage and increase pain.

3. Prevention of excessive loss of joint mobility and muscle tone

Immediate management. Immediate management objectives include the following:

1. Splinting of fracture to prevent movement of the injured part
2. Preservation of body alignment
3. Elevation of body part to limit edema
4. Application of cold packs (during first 24 hours) to reduce hemorrhage, edema, and pain

5. Administration of analgesics
6. Observation for changes in color, sensation, or temperature of injured part
7. Observation for signs of shock

Secondary management. Secondary management goals include the following:

1. For simple fracture
   a. Optimal reduction (replacing bone fragments in their correct anatomic position)
      (1) Manual manipulation, or *closed reduction* (moving bone fragments into position by

TABLE 69-1 Complications of fracture

Complication	Mechanism	Signs	Onset	Treatment
Fat embolism	Pressure changes in interior of fractured bones force molecules of fat from marrow into systemic circulation, resulting in occlusion of vessels in the lungs and brain	Chest pain, pallor, dyspnea, prostration, confusion, petechial hemorrhage of skin and conjunctivae	2-3 days after injury	Supportive measures: high Fowler's position, oxygen therapy, blood transfusion to relieve hypovolemic shock, digitalization for heart failure Diuretics, bronchodilators, corticosteroids Proper immobilization of fracture and careful handling of fracture area may be helpful in preventing fat embolism
Ischemic paralysis (contracture)	Arterial flow is interrupted to injured part by trauma or pressure	Coldness, pallor, cyanosis, pain, swelling distal to injury or cast	At time of injury or after cast application	Treatment of fracture Release of cast or constricting bandages
Osteomyelitis	Infection occurs in marrow spaces, haversian canals, and subperiosteal space with subsequent destruction of bone by proteolytic enzymes	Hyperemia, edema, pain, pus		Culture and sensitivity testing, antibiotics, surgical drainage, and debridement Prevention: use of aseptic technique when caring for open wound
Acute	Bacteria are introduced through a wound	At time of fracture (compound) or at surgery	Intravenous antibiotic therapy	
Hematogenous	Bacteria spread from a preexisting focus; for example, a boil		Intravenous antibiotic therapy; treatment of primary focus	
Chronic	Inadequate treatment of acute infection; infected dead bone separates from living bone and becomes a sequestrum		Removal of sequestrum by natural processes or surgery.	
Nonunion	There is inefficient callus formation (Chapter 68)	Callus not visible on x-ray film	6 wk to 2 mo after reduction	Bracing, surgery (bone grafting)
Compartment syndrome	Pressure from accumulating blood and tissue fluid builds up in tissue confined by fascia or immobilizing devices	Extreme pain, unrelieved by medication, and elevation of part	Usually within 48 hr of fracture or reduction	Release of constricting bandages, casts; release of fascia (fasciotomy)

applying traction and pressure to distal fragment)

    (2) Traction

    (3) *Open reduction* (surgical intervention that may incorporate use of an internal fixation device)

  b. Immobilization

    (1) External fixation—cast or splint

    (2) Traction

    (3) Internal fixation such as pins, plates, screws, wires, and prostheses

    (4) Combinations of the above

2. For compound fracture

  a. Surgical debridement of wound to remove dirt, foreign material, devitalized tissue, and necrotic bone

  b. Administration of tetanus toxoid

  c. Culture of wound

  d. Packing of wound

  e. Treatment with antibiotics

  f. Observation for signs of osteomyelitis, tetanus, and gas gangrene

  g. Closure of wound when there is no sign of infection

  h. Reduction of fracture

  i. Immobilization of fracture

3. Treatment of complications (Table 69-1)

■ ASSESSMENT

Subjective and Objective Data

Subjective data to be collected include patient's complaint concerning, or description of, the following:

1. Pain at site of injury
2. Loss of sensation or movement of affected part
3. How trauma occurred
4. Understanding of injury sustained (may report having heard bone snap)

Objective data to be collected include the following:

1. Warmth, edema, and/or ecchymosis over and surrounding the injured part
2. Obvious deformity
3. Loss of normal function in the injured part
4. Immobilization device(s) applied to the injured part
5. Signs of systemic shock
6. Signs of circulatory, motor, or sensory impairment to the injured part (Table 69-2)
7. Indicators of apprehension or fear

■ DATA ANALYSIS: NURSING DIAGNOSES

Nursing diagnoses are determined from assessment data. Possible nursing diagnoses for the person with a fracture may include, but are not limited to, the following:

Nursing Diagnoses	Possible Etiologies
Infection, potential for	Tissue trauma, surgical intervention
Injury, potential for	Sensory/motor deficits
Knowledge deficit: fracture	Lack of experience with fracture
Mobility, impaired physical	Musculoskeletal impairment, decreased strength and endurance, pain
Nutrition, altered: less than body requirements	Fatigue, pain, chewing or swallowing difficulties
Pain	Injury to bone, injury to soft tissue at fracture site, muscle spasm, immobility, improper positioning, pressure points
Powerlessness	Health care environment, decreased mobility
Self-care deficit	Musculoskeletal impairment, pain/discomfort, intolerance to activity
Skin integrity, impaired, actual or potential	Decreased mobility, pressure, shearing forces
Tissue perfusion, altered: peripheral	Decreased mobility, pressure, trauma

TABLE 69-2 Observations* for signs and symptoms of neurocirculatory impairment

Observation	Interpretation
Tissue color white	Decreased arterial blood supply
Tissue color blue	Venous stasis and poorly oxygenated tissue
Color slow to return to nail bed after application of moderate pressure	Decreased arterial blood supply
Edema	Fluid accumulating in tissues; poor venous return
Tissue cold or cool to touch	Decreased arterial blood supply
Patient unable to move parts distal to injury or external fixation device	Pressure on nerves innervating parts distal to injury or underlying external fixation device
Patient complaint of extreme pain unrelieved by elevation, analgesic, or repositioning	Pressure on nerves innervating parts distal to injury or underlying external fixation device
Patient complaint of heightened or decreased sensation or paresthesia in part distal to injury or underlying external fixation device	Pressure on nerves innervating parts distal to injury or underlying external fixation device

*Comparison of tissue should be made with uninvolved limb to determine extent of deviation from normal.

■ **PLANNING: EXPECTED PATIENT OUTCOMES**

Expected patient outcomes for the person with a fracture may include, but are not limited to, the following:

1. Patient participates in a program of progressive activity.
2. Patient states feeling more comfortable.
3. Patient and/or significant others can explain the following:
   a. Nature of injury and course of treatment that must be followed to prevent injury or infection and to achieve desired result
   b. Limitations of motion and restrictions of activity to be observed and for how long
   c. How to perform or modify ADL within the limitations of activity and motion that must be observed
   d. How to care for cast, pins, or other immobilization devices, if applicable
   e. Safe use of an ambulatory or other ADL assistive device, if necessary
   f. Safe technique in carrying out wound care, if necessary
   g. Techniques appropriate to prevent skin breakdown, swelling, and neurocirculatory impairment
   h. Measures that can be taken for relief of pain or discomfort
   i. How to use prescribed medications
   j. Plans for follow-up care

■ **IMPLEMENTATION**

Promoting Knowledge

Treatment of the acute fracture is usually carried out in the hospital's emergency room or in the operating room before the patient is admitted to the general hospital unit. Patients will have had little or no opportunity to become oriented to the hospital or to the care they will be receiving. In addition, they will probably be frightened or overwhelmed by what has happened to them, be experiencing pain, and possibly be groggy from pain medication or anesthesia. Careful and often repeated explanation and direction regarding the following will be necessary:

1. Nature of injury and course of treatment
2. Positioning
3. Skin care routines
4. Deep breathing and coughing
5. Pain relief measures
6. Exercises to be performed to prevent complications

Direction, explanation, and physical handling must be accomplished gently but efficiently during the initial stages of hospitalization. Patients must be given time to adjust to their situation before they can begin to understand how they can cooperate in their care.

As healing progresses and pain diminishes, patients will be more receptive to learning what will be necessary for safe return home. The following instructions should include:

1. How to move comfortably in bed
2. How to transfer safely in and out of bed
3. What weight-bearing restrictions to observe and for how long
4. What activity limitations to observe and for how long
5. How to properly use ambulatory or other ADL assistive devices
6. What assistance will be needed to perform ADL
7. What equipment will be needed and how it can be obtained
8. How to use and/or care for immobilization devices (slings, casts, and pins)
9. How to avoid swelling in the affected part by proper elevation
10. How to control pain or discomfort in the affected part
11. What exercises to perform to maintain strength and enhance circulation

The easiest and most effective way to teach patients how to manage themselves is to have them function as independently as possible within their prescribed limitations and with whatever assistive aids they need while they are in the hospital.

Relieving Pain

The person with a fracture will most often have severe pain at the fracture site, pressure from edema in the damaged soft tissues adjacent to the fracture, and spasm of the muscles in the fracture area. Continued pain and the muscle spasm accompanying it can put undue stress on the fracture fragments and retard efforts both to reduce and to maintain reduction of the fracture. Patients who are in severe pain will resist efforts to help them carry out measures designed to prevent complications. If the fracture is repaired by *open reduction* and *internal fixation*, the patient will have operative pain.

Measures the nurse can take to help reduce pain include the following:

1. During initial stages of treatment, administer prescribed narcotic and nonnarcotic analgesics in appropriate doses at timely intervals.
2. Administer prescribed agents such as diazepam (Valium) to reduce muscle spasm.
3. Apply ice compresses, as ordered, to the affected part to reduce swelling.
4. Reposition patient frequently within prescribed position or activity limitations to avoid prolonged pressure over bony prominences and to prevent stiffness.

5. Instruct patient how to use relaxation techniques (deep breathing, imagery) to reduce tension.
6. As pain subsides, negotiate with the patient a reduction in the strength and/or frequency of analgesic administration.

With the use of analgesics, it is important to try to maintain a balance of having the patient comfortable enough to perform required exercises and other activities but not so overly medicated as to risk potential damage through overextending activity or heavy sedation. Devices that allow patients to self-administer intravenous narcotics (*patient-controlled analgesia* [PCA] pumps) are extremely effective in managing posttraumatic and postoperative pain, because they eliminate the highs and lows of drug concentrations characteristic of intermittent parenteral dosing.[35]

Positioning is a measure that promotes comfort, provides for adequate ventilation and mobilization of pulmonary secretions, enhances circulation, and relieves pressure on skin areas. However, there is certain knowledge the nurse must have before positioning a patient with a fracture:

1. Where is the fracture?
2. What is the nature of the fracture?
3. Has the fracture been reduced?
4. What method was used to reduce the fracture?
5. What are the tolerances of the method used to reduce the fracture?
6. Is the fracture stable?
7. Has the orthopaedist requested special precautions?

After this information is obtained, positioning should be done with careful attention to avoid the following:

1. Altering the alignment of the fracture
2. Changing the direction of the pull of traction (if used)
3. Compromising the integrity of the cast (if used)
4. Placing undue stress on the internal fixation device (if used)

Generally, nurses should avoid changing the position of patients with unreduced, unsplinted fractures.

Once the parameters for safe positioning are defined, the nurse should assist the patient to change position at least every 2 hours until the patient can independently perform this function. Providing an overhead frame with a trapeze will assist the patient to move about in bed.

Promoting Safety

Monitoring for neurocirculatory compromise must be carried out every hour in the initial stages of fracture. Damage to blood vessels and/or nerves may occur at the time of the fracture or subsequent to the fracture or its reduction. Some swelling of a fractured extremity may be expected and is often well controlled by elevating the extremity. However, unrelieved swelling of an extremity that is confined in a cast or compression dressing causes undue pressure on vessel and nerves and can result in circulatory and/or neurologic impairment. *Evidence of impaired circulation or sensation must be reported to the physician immediately.* Frequency of neurocirculatory checks can usually be reduced if there is no evidence of compromise within 48 hours of the fracture or reduction (see Table 69-2). Observations of the involved extremity should be compared with observations of the uninvolved, or normal, extremity to validate deviations from "normal."

Monitoring neurocirculatory status of the injured part includes the following:

1. Palpating for warmth
2. Observing color
3. Applying moderate pressure to nail bed and observing speed of capillary refill
4. Questioning patient about pain and paresthesias in injured part
5. Touching injured part to test patient's ability to discriminate sensation
6. Observing patient's ability to voluntarily move body part distal to fracture

Maintaining Strength and Mobility

One objective in the care of the patient who has sustained a fracture is to prevent loss of mobility and muscle tone. This is true for the fractured part, as well as for the rest of the body. The nurse can use the following interventions to maintain mobility, muscle tone, and strength:

1. Allow and encourage the patient to move about to the greatest extent possible within the restrictions of the fracture reduction and the immobilizing devices.
2. Allow and encourage the patient to accomplish as much of his or her own self-care as possible.
3. Encourage the patient to perform muscle toning (isometric) exercises on a regular basis, for example, quadriceps setting, gluteal setting (see Chapter 20).
4. Encourage and assist the patient to follow through with exercise programs (including ambulation) prescribed by the physician and taught by the physical therapist.
5. Encourage and assist patient to resume normal functioning for all ADL (within limits of immobilization or fixation device) as soon as possible, for example, using bedside commode or toilet instead of bedpan.

Maintaining Skin Integrity

When determining interventions to maintain skin integrity, the nurse must consider ways to prevent skin breakdown, as well as ways to promote wound healing. Measures to prevent skin breakdown include the following:

1. Identifying skin areas at risk, particularly areas over bony prominences (for example, heels, sacrum, elbows, and ischial tuberosities)
2. Applying a skin-toughening agent such as tincture of benzoin two to three times a day to areas identified as being at risk
3. Inspecting skin (at least every 8 hours) for signs of pressure, for example, erythema or induration
4. Turning (at least every 2 hours) within limits of system of fracture immobilization using a turning sheet (see Figure 70-12)
5. Moving patient from one surface to another with a pull sheet or roller board (see Figure 70-13)
6. Rolling patient onto side or lifting patient to place him or her on a bedpan rather than sliding pan under patient
7. For patient who cannot be fully turned because of traction apparatus or other limiting factors, possibly using one or more of the following pressure relieving devices:
   a. Sheepskin pads
   b. Flotation pads
   c. Alternating air pressure mattress, or alternating air pressure system such as Lapidus system
   d. Foam mattress
   e. Foam heel and/or elbow pads
   f. Special bed such as the Clinitron, Mediscus, or Biodyne
   g. Turning frames such as the Foster or Stryker frames
8. Regularly inspecting skin areas in contact with cast edges or traction apparatus and taking appropriate measures to eliminate chafing or rubbing in those areas (see p. 2022 and 2023)
9. Assisting patient to keep skin clean and dry, especially under casts, slings, and traction apparatus

Interventions to promote wound healing include the following:

1. Carefully attending to aseptic technique during dressing changes to prevent infection
2. Attending to drains to maintain their placement and patency to prevent the development of hematoma
3. Observing pin sites regularly and caring for them as ordered to prevent infection (see box on p. 2017)
4. Providing and encouraging patient to eat a well-balanced diet to provide the essential nutritional elements necessary for tissue healing

Preventing Systemic Complications

Preventing circulatory complications. Individuals who have sustained trauma and are wholly or partially immobilized are at risk to develop circulatory complications because of the following:

1. Vessels in the legs fail to assume or maintain a state of vasoconstriction.
2. Pooling of venous blood and decreased venous return.
3. Decreased cardiac output.
4. Increased prothrombin time and platelet adhesiveness.

These factors contribute to decreased ability to adapt to an erect posture, increased incidence of deep-vein thrombosis and pulmonary embolus, increased workload on the heart, and decreased tolerance to exercise or activity.

Interventions the nurse can use to help offset or prevent these complications are as follows:

1. Encourage and assist the patient to perform routine active or active-assisted range-of-motion exercises (at least 4 times a day).
2. Teach and encourage the patient to perform active dorsiplantar flexion and quadriceps setting exercises every 1 to 2 hours.
3. Position the patient so that pressure is not exerted over major vessels.
4. Mobilize the patient slowly and increase activity gradually.
5. Elevate the affected extremity for the first 48 hours; thereafter, elevate the extremity when the patient is at rest (see Figure 70-24).

The sequential compression device (SCD) promises to be an important adjunct to routine nursing measures in the prevention of deep vein thrombosis (DVT) and pulmonary embolus (PE). The SCD consists of an electric motor, plastic tubing, and two plastic leg sleeves containing chambers for air. One sleeve is wrapped around each of the patient's legs, and each is secured with a Velcro closure. The motor pumps air through the tubing and into the chambers in the sleeves. The chambers fill with air at controlled pressure gradients, the pressure being greater at the ankle and decreasing at the top of the thigh. The SCD promotes venous return by filling and then decompressing, thus "pumping" blood through the veins and substituting for the pumping effect of the muscles in the person who is ambulatory. This device can be applied before a fracture is reduced and should be continued for 72 hours after reduction or until the patient is ambulatory.

Preventing respiratory complications. Factors that contribute to pooling of secretions in the bronchi and bronchioles are pain on movement or deep breathing, decreased movement, decreased stimulus to cough, and decreased depth of respiration.

Unless interventions are used to facilitate movement and removal of secretions, hypostatic pneumonia can result. Nursing interventions include the following:

1. Turning patient frequently to mobilize secretions
2. Encouraging patient to perform active or active-assisted range-of-motion exercises to increase depth of respiration
3. Using appropriate pain control measures to improve respiratory effort
4. Teaching and encouraging patient to take maximal sustained inhalations and to cough to mobilize and clear secretions every two hours
5. Encouraging patient to move independently as much as possible to solicit improved respiratory effort

Preventing gastrointestinal complications. Individuals who sustain trauma to the spine, fracture one or more of the lower extremities, or undergo surgery for spine or lower extremity fracture fixation, will frequently experience a slowing or temporary cessation of bowel function. If these persons eat or drink, they are at risk to develop paralytic ileus (Chapter 44). Therefore nurses must withhold food and fluid until the presence of bowel sounds is established, or preferably, until the patient is passing flatus.

Additionally, individuals with fractures who are wholly or partially immobilized are frequently constipated. Contributing factors are changes in normal dietary habits and fluid intake, lack of activity, and use of a bedpan. Interventions the nurse can use to promote gastric motility and prevent constipation include the following:

1. Turning the patient frequently
2. Elevating the head of the bed (as permitted)
3. Administering stool-softening agents, laxatives, or suppositories
4. Encouraging the patient to incorporate in the diet bulk-building foods such as bran
5. Encouraging a fluid intake of 2000 to 3000 ml per day
6. Assisting the patient to use a bedside commode or toilet instead of a bedpan, when possible

Preventing urinary complications. Patients with fractures, particularly if immobilized, are at risk to develop bladder infections and renal stones for the following reasons:

1. Increased serum calcium, because of bone destruction
2. Increased urinary pH (alkaline)
3. Increased citric acid (which precipitates calcium salts)

4. Stasis of urine in bladder, because of difficulty emptying bladder when using a urinal or bedpan in bed

Nursing interventions to decrease risk of these problems include the following:

1. Encouraging a fluid intake of 2000 to 3000 ml per day
2. Encouraging patient to decrease calcium intake
3. Encouraging patient to limit intake of citrus fruits and juices
4. Assisting patient to use a bedside commode or toilet when possible to facilitate emptying bladder

Promoting Nutrition

The essentials of a nutritious diet, which includes fruits, vegetables, proteins, and vitamins, are as important for the individual after a fracture as for anyone else. *If mobility is restricted, catabolic activity is accelerated,* producing a rapid breakdown of cellular materials, leading to *protein deficiency* and *negative nitrogen balance.* Decalcification and demineralization of bone take place during immobility, regardless of the quantity of calcium intake. Therefore increasing calcium in the diet above normal requirements is not recommended, because the excess calcium cannot be used. However, a diet high in protein is indicated to overcome protein deficiency and to return the body to a state of positive nitrogen balance. Patients who have had fractures have increased needs for iron, protein, and vitamins if bone repair is to progress normally. Weight gain is to be avoided, especially if the patient is in a cast or molded brace.

Interventions the nurse can use to ensure adequate nutrition for the patient include the following:

1. Encourage the patient to eat regular meals.
2. Allow the patient adequate time to eat.
3. Encourage self-feeding, but help the patient or provide special assistive utensils as necessary.
4. Attend to the patient's need for roughage and fluid as noted and encourage protein intake of 150 to 300 g per day.
5. Position the patient to facilitate comfortable intake of food and fluid (Figure 69-2).

Maintaining Immobilization of the Reduced Fracture

The purpose of immobilization is to hold the broken bone fragments in contact with each other (or in very close approximation) until healing takes place. *Immobilization can be accomplished externally with a cast, splint, brace, cast brace, or traction or internally with metal plates, pins, screws, and nails; bone grafts* with addition of such devices as *metal plates and pins;* or prosthetic implants. Both external and internal methods can be used, with combinations of the above.

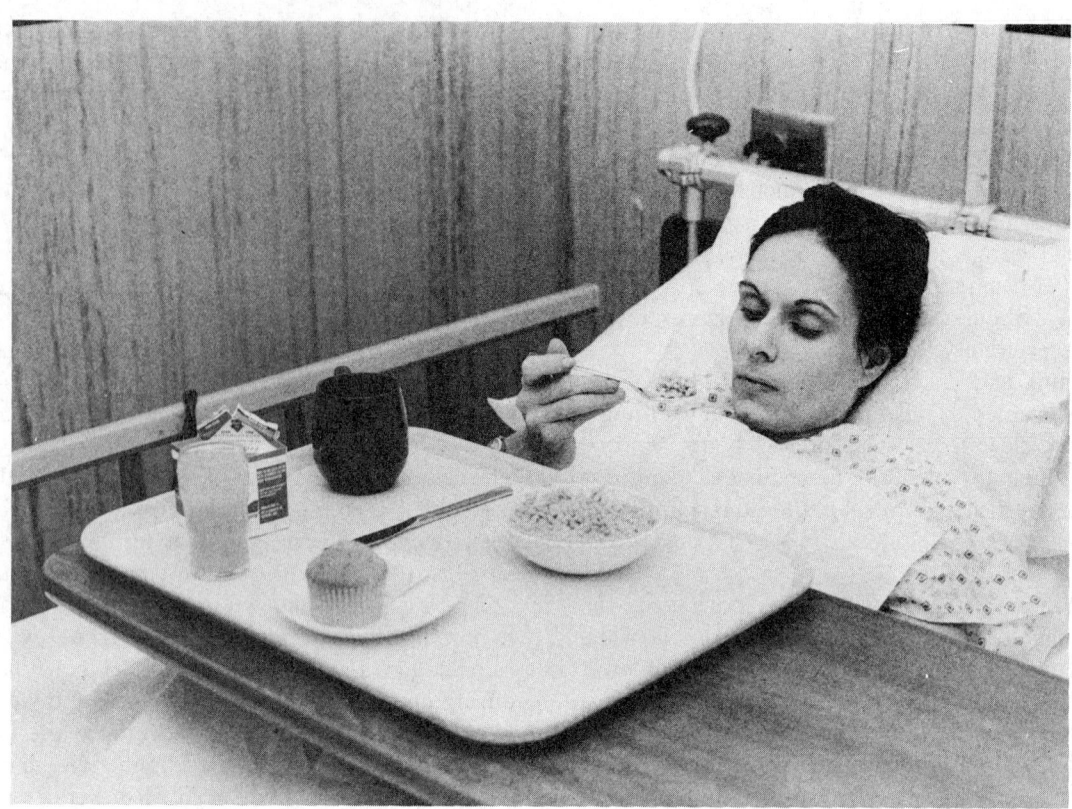

FIGURE 69-2 Patient who can neither sit up nor lie on one side to eat meals can still be made comfortable with some elevation of the head and shoulders on pillows. Additional means of elevating patient to a more upright position is to put frame of bed in reverse Trendelenburg's position.

Management of patients with external fixation devices

Casts. Probably the most common external fixation device is the cast. Materials used for casts include plaster of paris, fiberglass, and plastic. All three of these materials are available in the form of rolled bandages and are applied over the body part to be immobilized in much the same manner as an Ace bandage is wrapped. *Plaster,* which has to be moistened before application, dries very slowly, is heavy, and will lose its strength and integrity if it becomes wet after initial drying. If a plaster cast requires revision, it usually must be removed and a new one applied. However, plaster is less expensive than fiberglass or plastic. *Fiberglass* and *plastic* dry quickly, are lightweight, and may be immersed in water without losing their strength. Plastic casts may be reheated and remolded if revision is necessary. Disadvantages include the fact that some types of fiberglass require drying under special ultraviolet lights, and persons wearing fiberglass or plastic casts may suffer maceration of the skin unless they dry the skin thoroughly with a warm-air dryer after bathing or showering. Specific advantages and disadvantages of various cast materials are discussed in orthopaedic texts.[28]

A cast may incorporate (1) all or a portion of an extremity (Figure 69-3), (2) all or a portion of the trunk and cervical area, or (3) all or a portion of the trunk with all or a portion of one or more extremities. The latter type of cast is called a *spica* cast (Figure 69-4). *Splints* are made from cast material, but they may be thought of as half-casts because they do not encompass a body part. They are applied anteriorly, posteriorly, medially, and/or laterally and are wrapped in place with bandages, usually Ace bandages. *Cast braces* are made of two separate casts, one applied above a joint and the other below the joint. The two casts are joined by metal or heavy polyethylene hinges that are incorporated into the cast material. Cast braces are applied to permit the patient joint mobility below the fracture while still providing immobilization for the fracture fragments.

Casts are applied over skin that has been cleansed and inspected for cuts or abrasions that may become infected. Skin lesions are treated with disinfectant before cast application. Also, before the cast is applied, the skin may be treated with tincture of benzoin and wrapped with cotton padding or stockinette. Bony prominences are padded with material—sheet wadding or felt—to protect them from pressure. For specific techniques of cast application, consult specialized texts.[28]

Cast removal is accomplished by splitting the cast with an electric cast saw. The saw is very noisy, but if used properly, it will not damage the skin beneath the cast. Skin enclosed in a cast for a time will be covered with an exudate of built-up secretions and dead skin. To remove this exudate, mineral oil is applied, followed by numerous soaks with warm water. This process may take several days, but attempts to remove the exudate more rapidly may result in uncomfortable skin irritation. Special considerations in caring for the patient in a cast are described in the box on p. 2024.

Traction. *Traction* is the mechanism by which a steady pull is placed on a part or parts of the body. Traction may be used to perform the following:

1. Reduce a fracture
2. Maintain correct position of bone fragments during healing
3. Immobilize a limb while soft tissue healing takes place
4. Overcome muscle spasm
5. Stretch adhesions
6. Correct deformities

Countertraction is a force that counteracts the pull of traction.

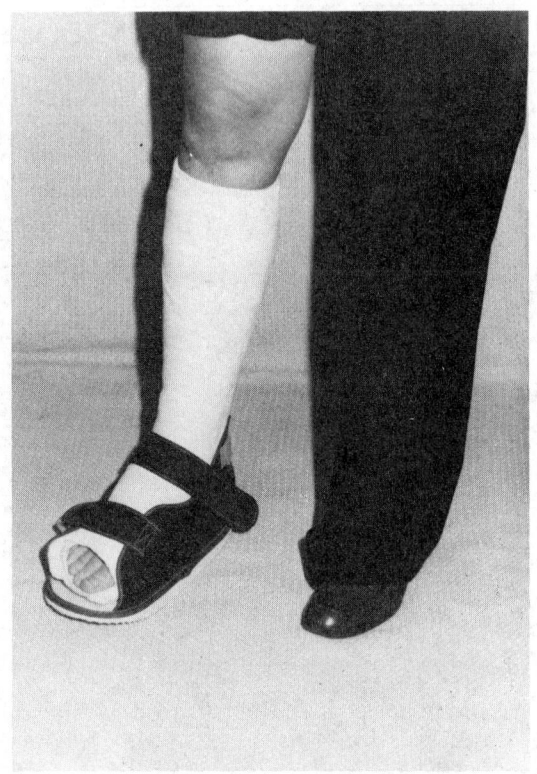

FIGURE 69-3 Short leg walking cast with cast shoe.

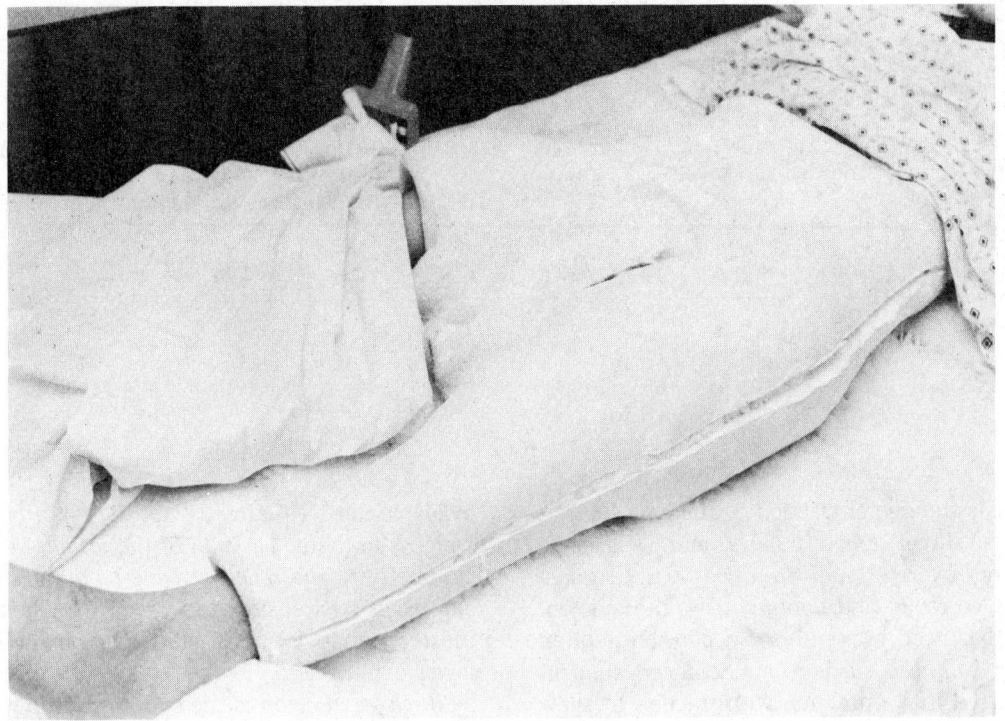

FIGURE 69-4 Hip spica cast, applied to provide immobilization of left femoral fracture, was bivalved when patient developed severe pain and swelling of left leg several hours after cast was applied. Ace bandages wrapped over cast to provide support have been removed for purposes of this picture.

GUIDELINES FOR CARE OF THE PERSON IN A CAST

1. Patient education
   a. Before cast application, explain why and how the cast will be applied.
   b. Advise the patient that the plaster cast will feel warm as it dries.
   c. Explain the extent to which the patient will be immobilized.
   d. Following cast application, explain care of the cast and expectations after discharge.
   e. Instruct patient not to insert sharp objects (coat hangers or pencils) under the cast, because these may abrade the skin and lead to infection.
2. Handling the new cast
   a. Support wet cast with the flat of the hands or on pillows to avoid indentations that will cause pressure on underlying skin.
   b. Place cotton blankets or other absorbent material under the cast to aid the drying process.
   c. Expose the cast to air as much as possible to aid the drying process.
   d. Turn the patient frequently to aid the drying process.
   e. Use a fan to circulate air over the cast.
   f. *Do not apply paint, varnish, or shellac to the cast; plaster is a porous material that allows air to circulate to the skin.*
3. Skin care
   a. Inspect skin at edges of cast and underlying the cast for redness or irritation; apply petal-shaped strips of adhesive tape or moleskin around rough edges of cast.
   b. Remove plaster crumbs from skin with a washcloth moistened with warm water.
   c. Use creams and lotions sparingly, since they may soften the skin and cause the cast to stick to the skin.
   d. Apply waterproof material around perineal area to prevent soiling of and damage to cast and irritation of the skin.
   e. Attend to patient's complaint of pain under the cast, particularly over bony prominences, since

this may indicate pressure on the skin. If discomfort is not relieved by repositioning, report to physician. Cast pressure may need to be relieved by windowing or bivalving (cutting cast into two halves).

4. Turning
   a. Turning to any position is generally permitted, as long as the integrity of the cast is not compromised and the patient is comfortable.
5. Toileting (for a long leg or hip spica cast)
   a. Use a fracture pan with blanket roll or padding as support under the small of the back.
   b. Elevate the head of the bed, if permitted; or place the bed in reverse Trendelenburg's position.
6. Abdominal discomfort
   a. Cast may be "windowed" (an opening cut into it) to provide relief of abdominal distention or a port for checking bladder distention.
7. Mobilization
   a. Weight bearing is at the discretion of the physician, and the amount of weight bearing will be prescribed.
   b. A cast shoe or a walking heel incorporated into a lower extremity cast will permit weight bearing without damaging the cast.
8. Prevention of neurocirculatory problems
   a. Perform neurocirculatory checks every hour for at least 24 hours after cast application to detect difficulty from swelling or pressure of cast on nerves or vessels. Notify physician of color changes, alterations in sensation, or motion unrelieved by position change; cast may need to be bivalved (cut in two) to relieve pressure.
   b. Elevate affected extremity on pillows until danger of swelling is over (usually 24 to 48 hours).
   c. After mobilization of patient with lower extremity or upper extremity cast, avoid keeping extremity in dependent position for prolonged periods.
   d. After lower extremity cast is removed, encourage patient to wear elastic stocking and elevate affected leg at rest until full mobility is regained.

Suspension is the use of traction equipment such as frames, splints, slings, ropes, pulleys, and weights to suspend but not exert a "pull" on a body part. To suspend the part correctly and continuously, the suspension must be balanced by weights. Suspension is often referred to as *balanced suspension*. Balanced suspension is often used in conjunction with traction to allow the patient to move about more freely and easily in bed.

Two types of traction are used: skin traction and skeletal traction. *Skin traction* is achieved by applying wide bands of moleskin, adhesive, or commercially

available devices directly to the skin and attaching weights to them. *The pull of the weights is transmitted indirectly to the involved bone or other connective tissue.* Buck's extension and Russell traction are the two most common forms of skin traction for injury to the lower extremities.

Buck's extension is the simplest form of skin traction and provides for straight pull on the affected extremity (Figure 69-5). It is often used to relieve muscle spasm and to immobilize a limb temporarily, for example, for a hip fracture before open reduction and internal fixation.

If adhesive substances are to be used, the skin of the leg is shaved and tincture of benzoin is applied to protect the skin. Adhesive tape or moleskin is then placed on the lateral and medial aspects of the leg and secured with a circular gauze or elastic bandage. The adhesive material should not cover the malleoli, because the skin would break down over these bony prominences. The tapes are attached to a spreader bar wide enough to pull the tapes away from the malleoli. Rope is attached to the spreader, passed through a pulley on a crossbar at the foot of the bed, and suspended with weights. The maximal weight that should be applied by skin traction is 3.6 kg (8 pounds). Greater amounts of weight can cause skin damage. Commercial foam rubber Buck's extension splints are widely used and are applied simply with Velcro straps. Contraindications to placing a patient in Buck's extension are stasis dermatitis, arteriosclerosis, allergy to adhesive tape, severe varicosities or varicose ulcers, diabetic gangrene, or marked overriding of bone fragments that would require more than 3.6 kg of weight to reduce the fracture.

Russell traction is sometimes used, because it permits the patient to move somewhat freely in the bed and permits flexion of the knee joint (Figure 69-6). It requires an overhead frame attached to the bed and preparation of the leg as for Buck's extension. A foot plate with pulley attachments is used instead of a spreader

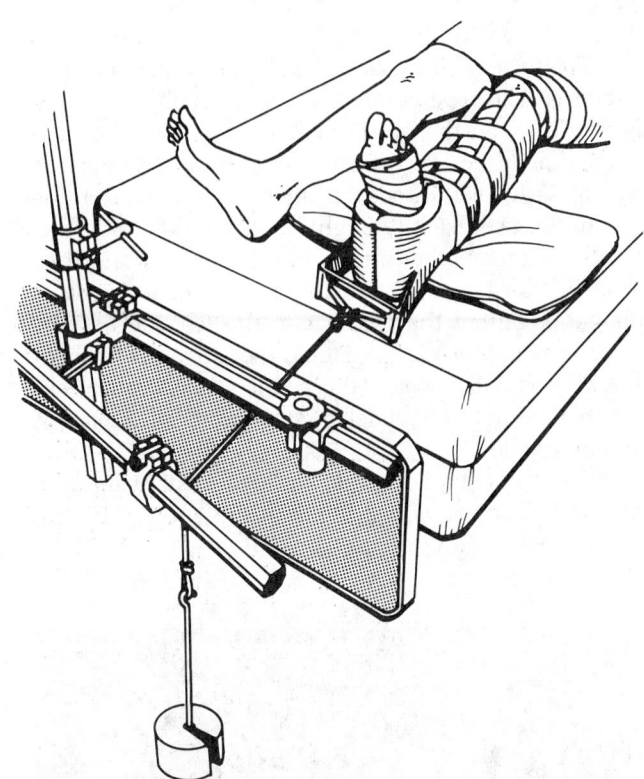

FIGURE 69-5 Buck's extension. Heel is supported off bed to prevent pressure on heel, weight hangs free of the bed, and foot is well away from footboard of bed. The limb should lie parallel to the bed unless prevented, as in this case, by a slight knee flexion contracture.

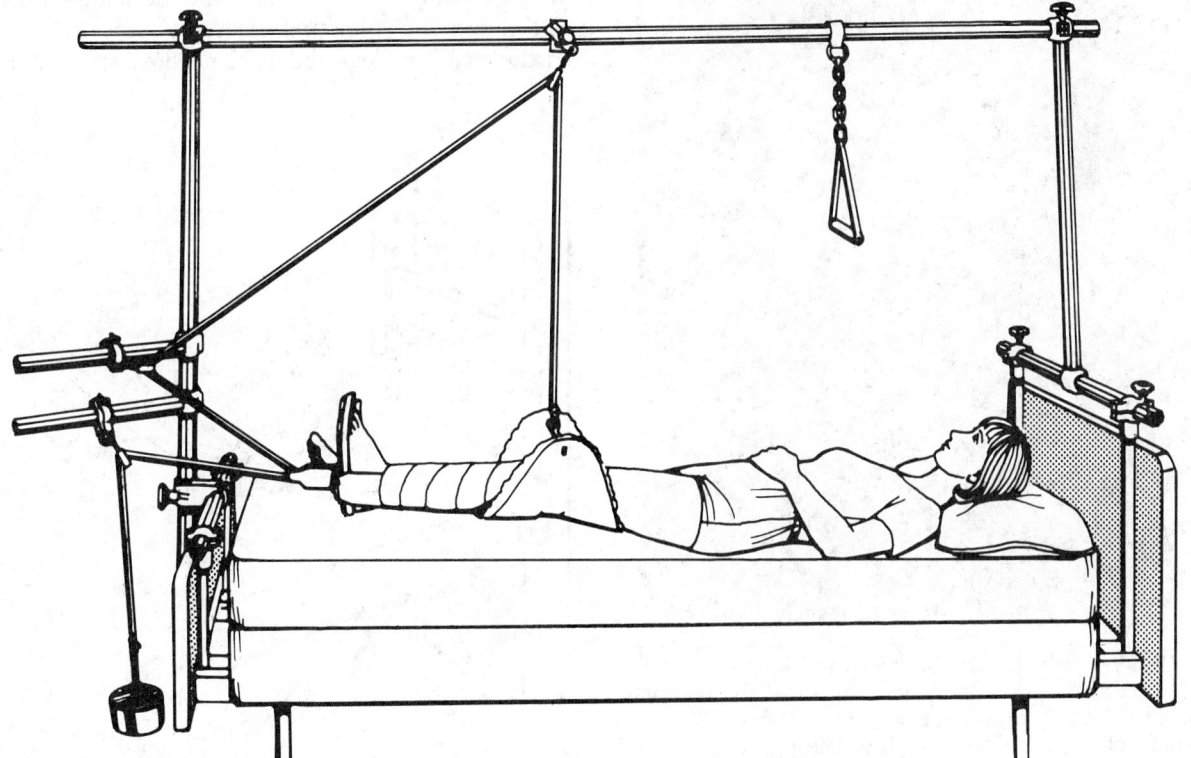

FIGURE 69-6 Russell traction. Hip is slightly flexed. Pillows may be used under lower leg to provide support and keep the heel free of the bed.

bar. The knee is suspended in a sling to which a rope is attached. The rope is directed up to a pulley that has been placed on the overhead frame directly above the tibial tubercle of the affected extremity. The rope is then passed down through a pulley on a crossbar at the foot of the bed, back through a pulley on the footplate, back again to another pulley on the crossbar, and then suspended with weights. This arrangement effects a double pull from the crossbar to the footplate, so the traction is approximately double the amount of weight used. Usually the foot of the bed is elevated on blocks (or the bed put in Trendelenburg's position) to provide countertraction.

Russell traction is used in the treatment of intertrochanteric fracture of the femur when surgery is con-

traindicated. Either bilateral Russell traction or Buck's extension may be used to treat back pain, because both partially immobilize the patient and reduce muscle spasm.

Skeletal traction is traction applied directly to bone. Under local or general anesthesia, a Kirschner's wire or Steinmann pin is inserted through bone distal to the fracture; the site of insertion varies with the type of fracture (Figure 69-7). The pin protrudes through the skin on both sides of the extremity, and the ends of the pin are covered with cork or metal protectors. Small sterile dressings are usually placed over the entry and exit sites of the pin or pin sites may be left uncovered for easier observation. A metal U-shaped spreader or bow is attached to the pin, and the rope on which the traction weights are hung is tied onto the spreader. Skeletal traction can be used for fractures of the tibia, femur, humerus, and cervical spine. Skeletal traction applied to the cervical spine is achieved through use of tongs applied to the skull (Figure 69-8).

When a balanced suspension apparatus is used in conjunction with skin or skeletal traction, the patient is able to move about in bed more freely without disturbing the line of pull of the traction. The use of a balancing apparatus facilitates nursing measures such as bathing, skin care, and positioning the bedpan. A full or half-ring Thomas or Hodgen splint (Figure 69-9) is frequently used for suspension of the lower extremity. Straps of canvas, muslin, or synthetic lamb's wool are placed over the splint and secured to provide a support for the leg. The areas under the popliteal space and heel

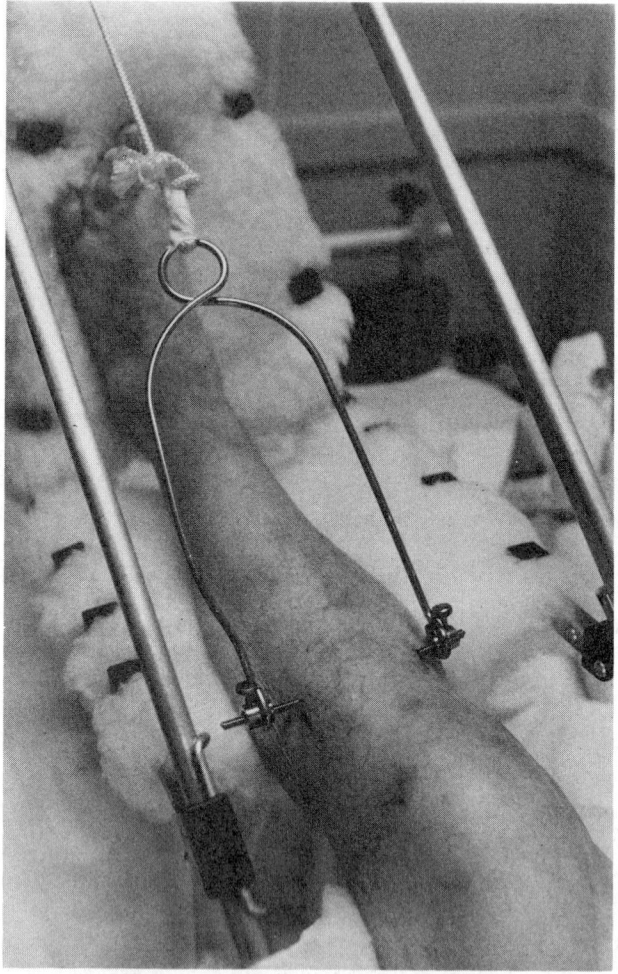

FIGURE 69-7 Tibial pin traction with Steinmann pin used in treatment of a distal femoral fracture. The bow attached to the pin provides a place of attachment for the rope that holds the traction weights. The pull exerted by the weight keeps the fracture fragments aligned. Pin sites must be inspected at least daily to detect signs of pin reaction or infection.

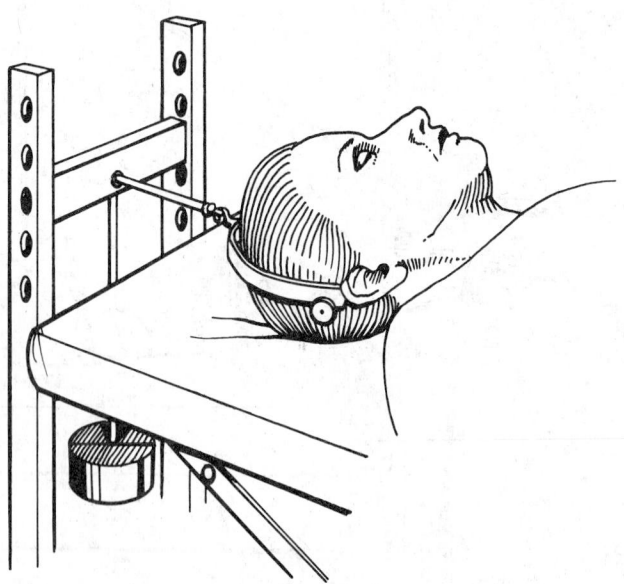

FIGURE 69-8 Traction to the cervical spine can be maintained through the use of Crutchfield tongs inserted into the skull.

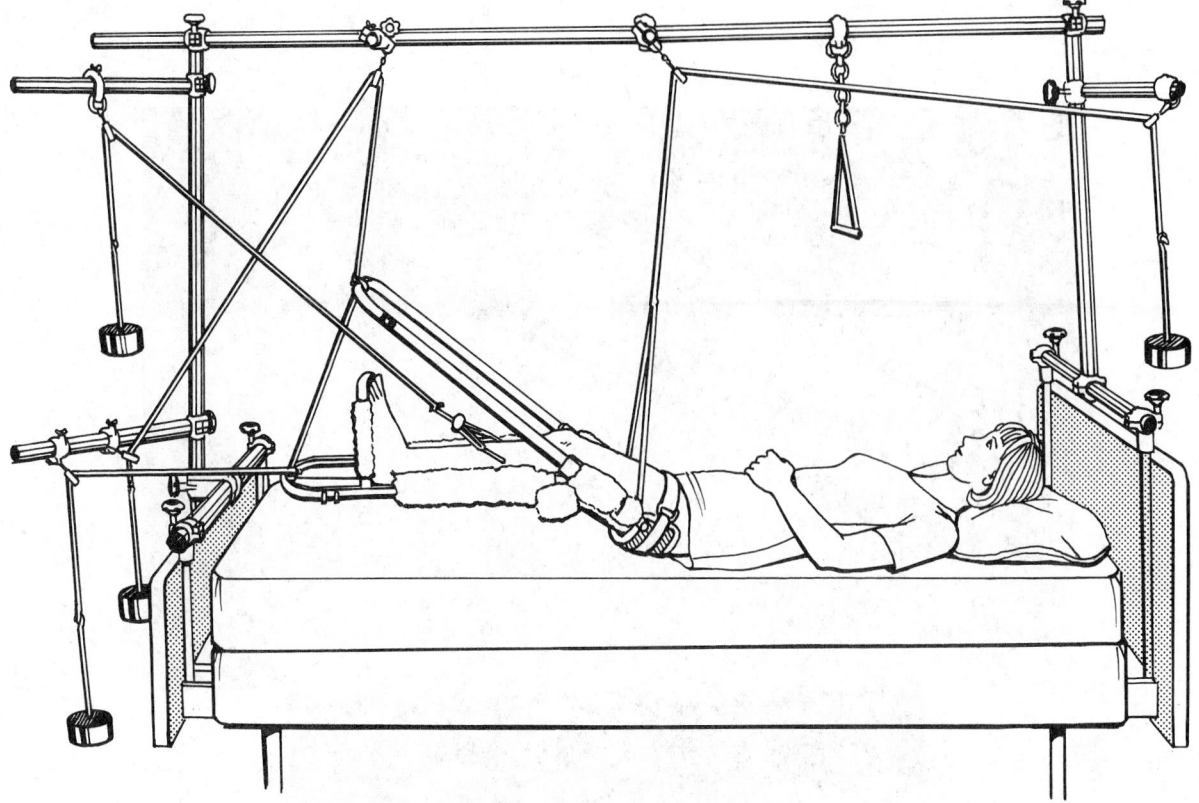

FIGURE 69-9 Balanced suspension with Thomas splint and Pearson attachment. This apparatus can be used alone or, as in this case, with skeletal traction.

GUIDELINES FOR CARE OF THE PERSON IN TRACTION

1. Patient education
   a. Explain traction in relation to fracture and physician's plan of treatment.
   b. Explain amount of movement permitted and how to achieve it (for example, how trapeze can be used to assist with movement).
   c. Explain correct body positioning.
2. Maintaining the traction
   a. Inspect traction apparatus frequently to ensure that ropes are running straight and through the middle of the pulleys; that weights are hanging free; that bedclothes, the bed, or the frame and bars on the bed are not impinging on any part of the traction apparatus.
   b. Check ropes frequently to be sure they are not frayed.
   c. Avoid releasing weights from or altering the line of pull of the traction.
   d. Avoid adding weight to the traction.
   e. Check the position of the Thomas splint frequently; if the ring has slid away from the groin, readjust the splint to its proper position without releasing traction.
   f. Avoid bumping into or jarring the bed or traction equipment.
   g. Be sure weights are securely fastened to their ropes.
   h. Avoid manipulation of pins.
3. Skin care
   a. Encourage the patient to turn slightly from side to side and to lift up on the trapeze to relieve pressure on the skin of the sacrum and scapulae; have the patient lift up for routine skin care.
   b. Avoid padding the ring of the Thomas splint, since this will create dampness next to the skin. Bathe the skin beneath the ring, dry it thoroughly, and powder the skin lightly.
   c. Inspect skin frequently to be sure it is not being rubbed, contused, or macerated by traction equipment; readjust splints or the extremity in the splint to free the skin from pressure.
   d. Keep skin areas around pin sites clean and dry; direct care to pin sites (for example, cleansing with cotton applicators and hydrogen peroxide or alcohol) is controversial, so check with patient's physician to determine if pin care is to be done routinely and what method the physician prefers. (See the research box on p. 2029.)
4. Toileting
   a. Use a fracture pan with blanket roll or padding as support under the small of the back.
   b. Protect the ring of the Thomas splint with waterproof material when female patients are using the bedpan.

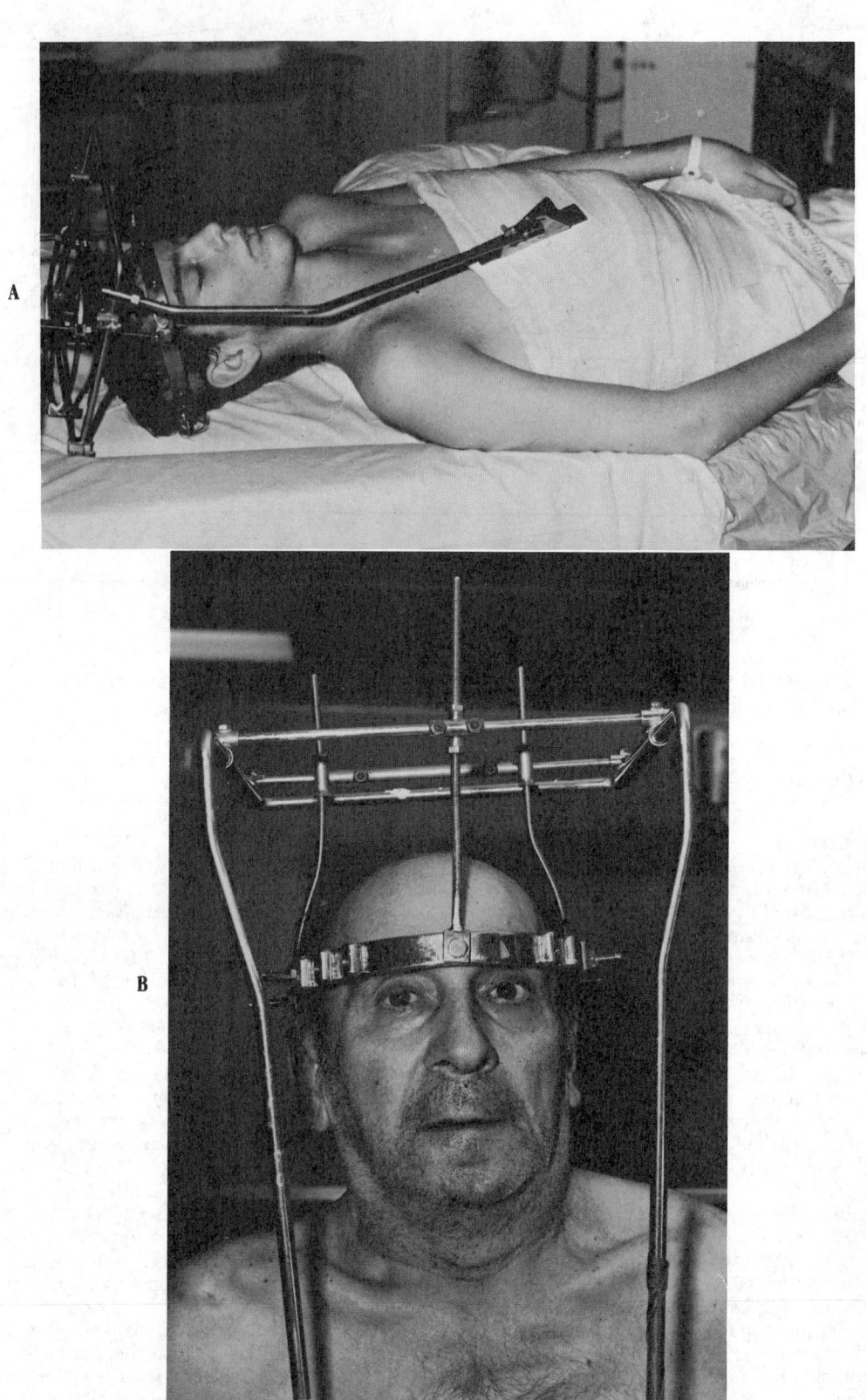

FIGURE 69-10 A, Halo attached to body cast. Metal strut will be anchored firmly into body cast with additional plaster. **B,** Metal ring, or halo, that attaches to skull. (Courtesy Dr. Henry Bohlman, Cleveland, Ohio.)

RESEARCH

Jones-Walton P: Effects of pin care on pin reactions in adults with extremity fracture treated with skeletal traction and external fixation, Orthop Nurs 7(4):29-33, 1988.

This retrospective, descriptive study examined 12 case records relative to fracture injury characteristics, pin site appearance and reaction incidence, pin care treatments, health deviation history, and routine medication therapy. The investigation was conducted in an attempt to contribute information to the very limited body of scientific knowledge available for making pin care treatment decisions. The following research questions were posed: (1) What are the clinical manifestations of pin reactions in adult fracture patients treated with skeletal traction and consistent pin care treatments? and (2) What is the incidence of pin reactions in adult fracture patients with skeletal traction? Pin care, pin reaction, host factors, and five criteria for case selection were defined; each of the 12 cases meeting the selection criteria were reviewed with regard to patient demographics, fracture injury characteristics, pin reaction manifestations, pin care implementation, health deviation history, and routine medication therapy. Results of the study indicated that pin care in and of itself did not prevent the development of pin reaction but supported findings from an earlier study by Sproles[38] indicating that pin reaction may be related more to host variables (alcoholism, oral infection) than to pins or pin care. The study indicates that further intensive study of the current methods of treating skeletal traction pin sites must be conducted if patients at risk to develop pin site reaction are to be identified and if care is to be delivered on a scientific rather than a traditional or ritualistic basis. ■

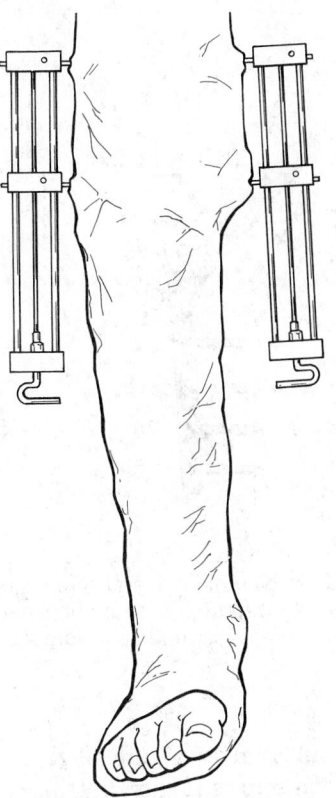

FIGURE 69-11 Example of an external fixator, in this case a Charnley compression apparatus. Skeletal pins through bone above and below the area of fracture or repair attach to the external metal supports to maintain rigid fixation. This particular device is equipped with hand screws that allow the pins to be brought closer together, thus providing increased compression.

are left open to prevent pressure on these parts. If it is desirable to have the knee flexed or to permit movement of the lower leg, a Pearson attachment is clamped or fixed to the Thomas splint at the level of the knee. Special considerations in caring for the patient in traction are described in the box on p. 2027.

Other types of external immobilization. Other devices for external immobilization of fractures include the following:

1. Braces made of rigid plastic material
2. Plaster or plastic braces that incorporate metal struts attached to pins inserted into bone, such as a halo brace (Figure 69-10)
3. Metal struts attached to pins inserted into bone (for example, the various types of Hoffman or Charnley external fixation devices) (Figure 69-11)

Devices such as the Hoffman or Charnley devices may be used in conjunction with plaster or alone. All of these devices provide extremely rigid fixation while allowing the patient some degree of mobility. It is quite possible for the patient in a halo brace to ambulate. The patient with an external fixator on the lower leg can be out of bed in a wheelchair or even ambulate without bearing weight on the affected leg.

Nursing care for patients in these devices is essentially the same as for patients in casts and/or skeletal traction, with the exception that patients in these devices may be mobile earlier.

Management of patients with internal fixation devices. Open surgical reduction of fractures has the advantage of allowing visualization of the fracture and surrounding tissues. It is particularly indicated when soft tissue is caught between bone fragments or when nerves or blood vessels are damaged. The disadvantages of internal fixation are that it requires anesthesia and carries the risk of infection at the time of surgery. *Internal fixation is carried out under the most vigorous aseptic conditions, and patients may receive a short course of prophylactic intravenous antibiotics postoperatively.*

A variety of internal fixation devices are available:

1. Plates and nails (Figure 69-12, *A*)

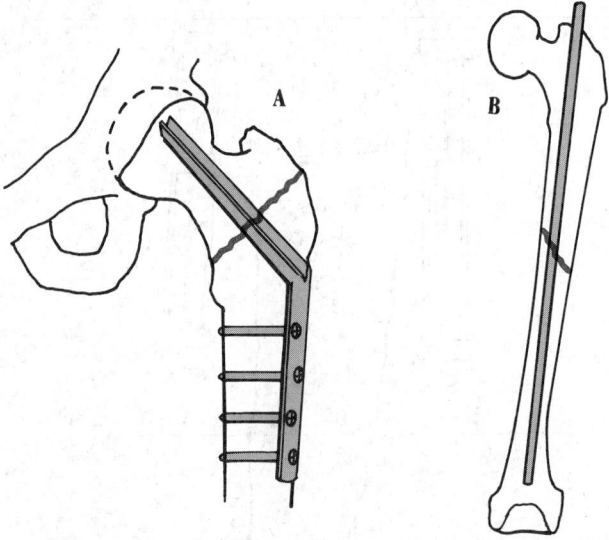

FIGURE 69-12 A, Neufeld nail and screws, used in repair of intertrochanteric fracture. **B,** Kuntchner nail (intramedullary rod) used in repair of mid-shaft femoral fracture

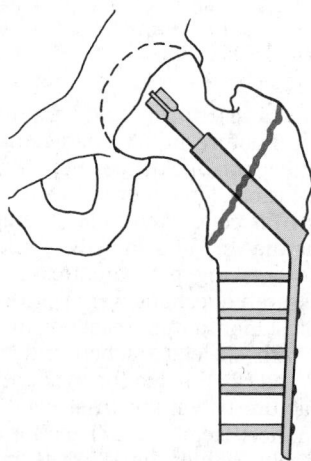

FIGURE 69-13 Ken sliding nail used in repair of intertrochanteric fracture. Sliding nails will usually permit the patient to bear weight to some degree, because they will "give" slightly when subjected to weight-bearing forces without shifting their placement or "cutting out" (penetrating) through the femur.

2. Intramedullary rods (Figure 69-12, *B*)
3. Transfixion screws (Figure 69-13)
4. Prosthetic implants (Figure 69-14)—used particularly when survival of the proximal fragment of the fracture is jeopardized, for example, a fracture through or immediately below the femoral head

Bone grafts, either *autograft* (the patient's own bone) or *allograft* (cadaver bone), may be used either in conjunction with internal fixation devices when excessive bone is lost at the fracture site, or alone, as in spine surgery. Fixation with internal devices does not preclude additional fixation with external devices (casts, braces, or traction), particularly in cases of very complicated fracture or multiple trauma.

In general, the major objective of care is to protect the fixation until healing takes place. Metal that can fatigue and break cannot be expected to substitute for intact bone. If the fixation device breaks, healing of the fracture will be disrupted. However, *mobilization of patients who have had internal fixation is usually much faster than for those who have had external fixation.* Nursing care of patients with internal fixation includes the following:

1. Patient education
   a. Prepare the patient for general anesthesia
   b. Explain the surgical procedure and general nursing care after surgery
   c. Postoperatively, explain the limits of motion and weight bearing to the affected part
2. Promoting mobility
   a. Determine, in consultation with the physician, the limits of motion and weight bearing permitted

   b. Instruct and assist the patient to turn within the prescribed limits
   c. Assist the patient to transfer and ambulate within the prescribed limits (mobilization may begin as early as the first postoperative day)
   d. Instruct and assist patient to use appropriate ambulatory aid if the fracture is of a lower extremity
3. Prevention of neurocirculatory problems
   a. Perform neurocirculatory checks every hour for the first 24 to 48 hours; notify the physician of any change from preoperative status, since this may indicate pressure from swelling, constricting bandages, or damage to nerves or vessels at surgery
   b. Maintain elevation of the affected extremity in bed
4. Maintenance of immobilization of fracture; considerations for care would be the same as for patients in cast/traction if those devices are used (see p. 2022 and 2023)

FRACTURE OF THE HIP
EPIDEMIOLOGY/ETIOLOGY

Fractures of the hip are perhaps the most common fracture seen in the hospital. They occur more frequently in women than in men, because women have a wider pelvis with a tendency to coxa vara; women experience postmenopausal hormonal changes, which are associ-

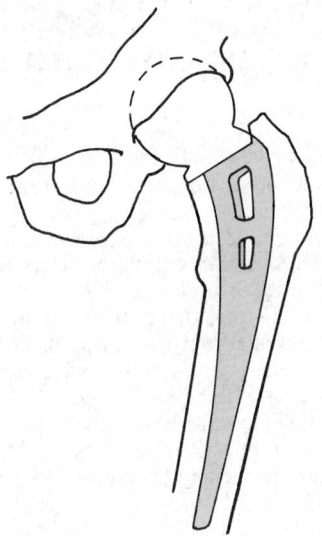

FIGURE 69-14 Regular stem Austin Moore prosthesis, commonly used to replace the femoral head and neck in hip fractures when the vascular supply to the femoral head may eventually be compromised.

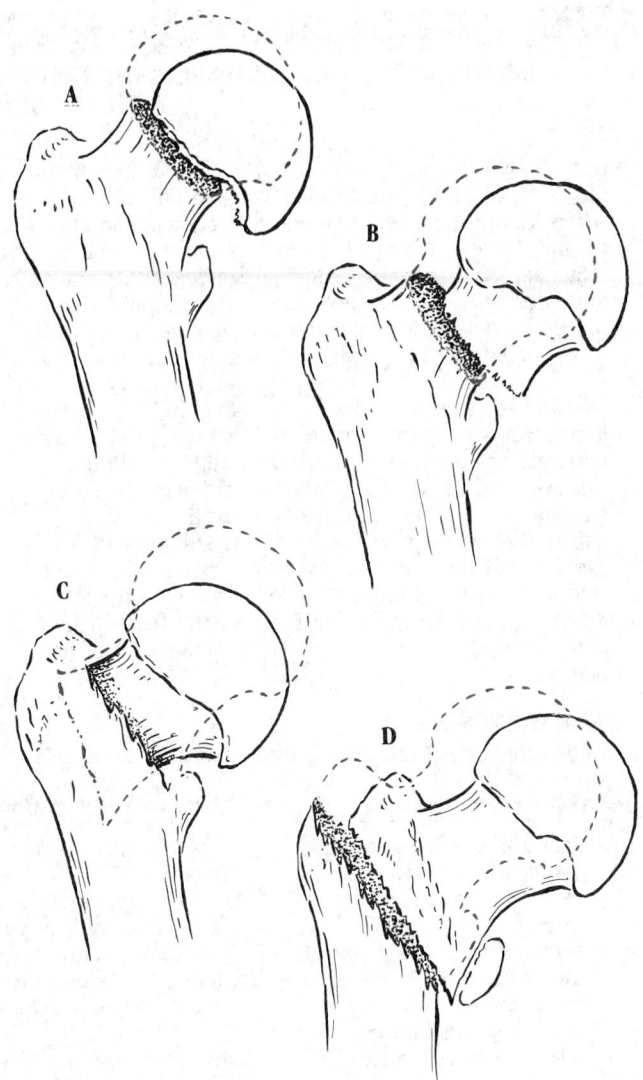

FIGURE 69-15 Fractures of the hip. **A,** Subcapital fracture. **B,** Transcervical fracture. **C,** Impacted fracture of base of neck. **D,** Intertrochanteric fracture.

ated with an increased incidence of osteoporosis; and women's life expectancy is greater than that of men.

PATHOPHYSIOLOGY

Fractures of the hip may be the classified in the two following general categories (Figure 69-15):

1. *Intracapsular*—occurring within the hip joint and capsule; these include the following types:
   a. Subcapital fracture
   b. Transcervical fracture
   c. Basal neck fracture
2. *Extracapsular*—occurring outside the hip joint and capsule to an area 5 cm (2 inches) below the lesser trochanter; called *intertrochanteric* fractures

Blood supply to the head of the femur comes up through the neck of the femur and is often disrupted in an intracapsular fracture (Figure 69-16). When blood supply is interrupted, there may be eventual death (*avascular necrosis*) of the femoral head.

CLINICAL MANIFESTATIONS

Signs and symptoms of hip fracture are severe pain at the fracture site, inability to move the leg voluntarily, shortening and external rotation of the leg, and other signs and symptoms consistent with those of any fracture (see nursing care plan, pp. 2032-2034).

Medical Management

Choice of fixation device depends on the location of the fracture, potential for avascular necrosis of the femoral

head, and the personal preference of the surgeon. An *impacted intracapsular fracture without displacement* may be treated with bed rest alone. The following treatments are often chosen for other fractures:

1. Stable plate and screw fixation; implies non–weight-bearing status for 6 weeks to 3 months
2. Telescoping nail fixation; implies minimal to partial weight-bearing status for 6 weeks to 3 months
3. Prosthetic implant, usually Austin Moore prosthesis or Bi-Polar prosthesis, to replace femoral head and neck; implies some *position restrictions* for 2 weeks to 2 months and *partial weight-bearing restrictions* for up to 2 months
4. Closed reduction and external fixation, if general medical condition precludes surgery

NURSING CARE PLAN

PERSON WITH AN INTRACAPSULAR HIP FRACTURE, OPEN REDUCTION, AND INTERNAL FIXATION WITH A PROSTHETIC IMPLANT

DATA: Mrs. W. is an 81-year-old widowed, retired secretary. This evening she tripped and fell on an icy step when leaving her niece's home. She complained of immediate, severe pain in her left hip and was unable to move her leg. Emergency Medical Services was phoned, and Mrs. W. was accompanied to the hospital by her niece and her niece's husband. In the emergency room it was noted that her left leg was shorter than her right, and it was externally rotated. Her vital signs were stable, and the neurocirculatory status of the left leg was intact. An x-ray examination revealed an intracapsular femoral neck fracture. Intravenous fluids were initiated. An ECG, urinalysis, CBC, and serum electrolyte study were obtained. She was transferred to the nursing unit with physician's orders for morphine sulfate 4 to 6 mg every 3 to 4 hours as necessary for pain. Buck's extension was applied. Consent was obtained for surgical repair in the morning. Replacement of the femoral head and neck with a regular stem Austin Moore prosthesis is planned.

The nursing history identified the following:
- Mrs. W. lives alone in her own apartment in a senior citizen complex.
- Mrs. W. has no children but has nieces and nephews in the area who see her regularly. They assist with shopping and other errands.
- Mrs. W. would like to return to her own apartment after being discharged from the hospital, but she worries that she might need help at home. Her family is considering hiring a home health aide.
- She takes no medications other than aspirin for occasional "stiffness" on awakening.
- She has never been hospitalized and last saw a physician 2 years ago for "the flu."

NURSING DIAGNOSIS

Knowledge deficit related to lack of exposure to surgery

Expected Patient Outcomes	Nursing Interventions (Preoperative)	Rationale
Patient can explain the teaching provided by the nurse about preoperative and general postoperative care.	Assess need for instruction and provide as necessary.	Understanding the surgical procedure and postoperative care should lessen anxiety and promote desired behaviors for recovery from surgery.
Patient states that she is experiencing less anxiety related to fear of the unknown and/or misconceptions about surgery and the recovery period.	Provide written materials pertaining to the surgery, if available in the institution. Review preoperative instruction with patient and family before the surgery. Evaluate patient's understanding of the information taught.	

Nursing Interventions (Postoperative)

Collaborative nursing actions include those to identify possible complications of surgery. Immediate reporting of and treatment of early signs may prevent serious effects. Nursing actions include monitoring for the following:

1. Neurocirculatory compromise: Perform neurocirculatory checks q2h for the first 24-48 hr. Notify physician of any changes from preoperative status.
2. Dislocation of the prosthesis: Notify physician if patient complains of sudden onset of increased pain, especially groin pain, particularly if accompanied by deformity or external rotation.
3. Impaired skin integrity and/or impaired wound healing: Monitor pressure areas for signs of redness, monitor temperature, and assess incision for signs or symptoms of infection or excessive drainage.
4. Atelectasis/respiratory infection: Monitor breath sounds until patient is ambulatory.
5. Urinary retention: Assess for urinary retention or stasis.

NURSING CARE PLAN

PERSON WITH AN INTRACAPSULAR HIP FRACTURE, OPEN REDUCTION, AND INTERNAL FIXATION WITH A PROSTHETIC IMPLANT—cont'd

Expected Patient Outcomes	Nursing Interventions	Rationale
	6. Constipation: Assess bowel status each day until patient is able to have a bowel movement. 7. Fluid and electrolyte imbalance: Monitor intake and output until patient is taking oral fluids without difficulty, monitor IV fluid rates, and assess patient for fluid volume excess or deficit. By discharge the patient should be instructed in and be able to explain or demonstrate the following: 1. Independent ambulation on level surfaces with appropriate ambulatory aid and independent stair climbing 2. Activity restrictions to be observed for approximately 2 months or until follow-up with physician, for example, limiting flexion of the affected hip to 90 degrees, avoiding adduction of the affected leg beyond midline, avoiding extreme internal and external rotation of the affected hip, and maintaining partial weight-bearing status with the walker or crutches 3. Independent ADL with assistive devices	

NURSING DIAGNOSIS

Pain related to surgical procedure

Expected Patient Outcomes	Nursing Interventions	Rationale
Patient states feeling comfortable. Patient is able to perform necessary postoperative routines/exercises.	Assess patient's pain and evaluate response to comfort measures provided. Administer prescribed analgesics (usually narcotic) at timely intervals during initial postoperative period. Teach relaxation techniques as appropriate. Use other pain relieving techniques as appropriate, for example, back rubs, repositioning. As pain decreases, use milder analgesics as prescribed.	Subjective and objective data are important in ascertaining the nature of the patient's postoperative pain and determining its management. It is usually necessary to administer narcotics in the first 48-72 hr after surgery. Analgesics have a greater effect if they are administered before pain becomes severe. Relaxation facilitates rest and may modify the response to pain. A change in type of cutaneous stimulation may result in pain relief. Pain may be controlled by less potent analgesics (with fewer untoward side effects) as pain lessens in severity.

Continued.

PERSON WITH AN INTRACAPSULAR HIP FRACTURE, OPEN REDUCTION, AND INTERNAL FIXATION WITH A PROSTHETIC IMPLANT—cont'd

NURSING DIAGNOSIS

Mobility, impaired physical related to alteration in lower limb status after surgical repair of hip fracture

Expected Patient Outcomes	Nursing Interventions	Rationale
Patient will demonstrate optimal level of mobility with adaptive devices within prescribed limitations of activity by time of discharge.	Have patient deep breathe and cough every 1-2 hr until fully ambulatory.	If carried out correctly and at appropriate intervals, pulmonary exercises can effectively prevent atelectasis and pneumonia.
No injury will have occurred during patient's hospitalization.	Encourage patient to perform active dorsiflexion, plantar flexion, isometric quadriceps setting and gluteal setting, and active range of motion of unaffected limbs q2h until ambulatory.	Exercising promotes venous return, prevents thrombus formation, and helps to maintain muscle tone.
	Determine from surgeon the limits of motion and weight bearing permitted, keeping in mind the following guidelines: 1. Hip flexion is usually limited to 90 degrees for 2-3 mo. 2. Adduction beyond midline is prohibited for 2-3 mo. 3. Extreme internal or external rotation is prohibited for 2-3 mo. 4. Partial weight bearing on affected body part with the aid of a walker or crutches is usually observed for 2-3 mo.	Restrictions on positioning are designed to avoid dislocation of the prosthesis.
	Turn patient from back to unoperated side q2h and prn. Avoid positioning patient on operative side, and observe flexion restrictions when elevating the head of the bed.	Turning and repositioning frequently promotes circulation, respiratory effort, and muscle activity.
	When turning the patient, hold the operative leg in abduction; use pillows to maintain 30-degree abduction when turning is accomplished.	Prevents adduction of leg.
	Assist patient to walk using the appropriate ambulatory aid. Begin walking the first or second postoperative day and increase the frequency and distance of ambulation as tolerated.	Early postoperative activity, including walking, can hasten recovery and prevent postoperative complications.
	Begin sitting when patient demonstrates sufficient control of the affected leg to sit within flexion restrictions.	Prepare patient for discharge while assuring that patient can sit safely within prescribed limits on flexion.
	Elevate sitting surface with pillows to keep angle of hip within prescribed limits.	Limits hip flexion to 90 degrees.

NURSING DIAGNOSIS

Potential for impaired home maintenance management related to independent living situation

Expected Patient Outcomes	Nursing Interventions	Rationale
Patient and family will express satisfaction with arrangements made to facilitate self-care at home.	Discuss with the patient and family their plans for the patient's care after discharge from the hospital.	Adequate discharge planning will foster successful completion of rehabilitation at home or will help to identify areas in the patient's performance of required functional abilities indicating a need for a skilled nursing facility, rehabilitation hospital, or other form of intermediate care.
	Determine with the patient what she must do for herself to return to her own home.	
	Determine with the patient the type of equipment and services needed for return home (for example, crutches, walker, elevated toilet seat, homemaker, companion, physical therapy, Meals on Wheels, and shopping services).	
	Assess patient's progress at regular intervals to determine whether her functional ability will permit carrying out of the above plans.	
	Involve appropriate department (for example, social service department) for assistance in planning, if patient is unable to achieve functional levels consistent with the initial plan.	

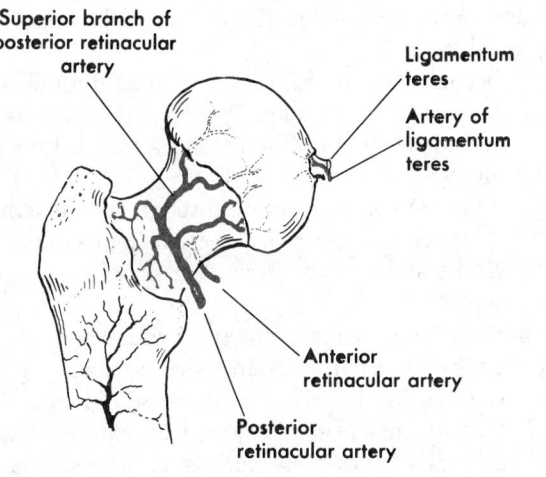

FIGURE 69-16 Posterior view of blood supply to head of femur.

Nursing Management

Nursing management should include those interventions already noted for general care of patients with fractures, with specific attention to interventions for persons with internal fixation. *Special consideration should be given to persons who have had a prosthetic implant, because there will be specific position restrictions, unless they have external fixation as well.* These include the following:

1. Avoidance of hip flexion beyond 60 degrees for up to 10 days
2. Avoidance of hip flexion beyond 90 degrees from day 10 to 2 months
3. Avoidance of adduction of the affected leg beyond midline for 2 months
4. Maintenance of partial weight-bearing status for approximately 2 months

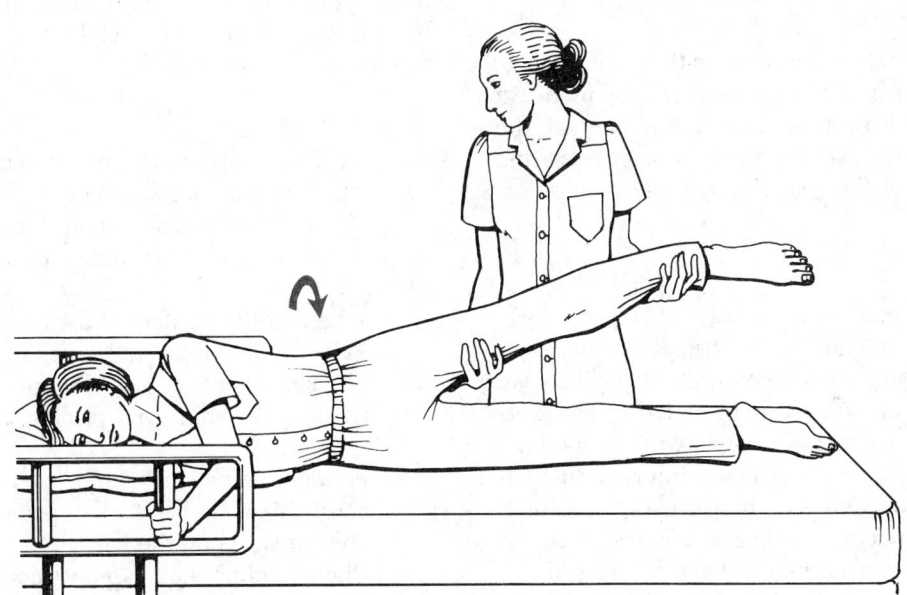

FIGURE 69-17 Assisting patient to turn while maintaining *abduction of the hip*. Leg is supported at the thigh and just above the ankle to avoid putting undue stress on the hip.

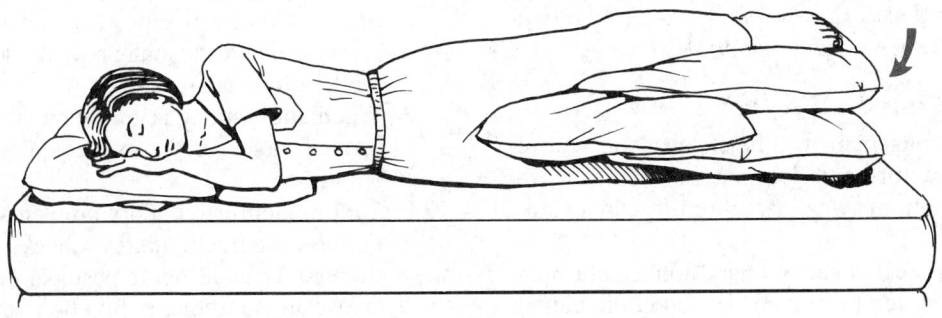

FIGURE 69-18 Pillows are staggered in a wedge-shaped arrangement to maintain *abduction of the hip*.

Suggestions for nursing management are the following:

1. Instruct the patient on the limits of motion to be observed.
2. Avoid positioning the patient on the operative side in bed.
3. Assist patient to maintain abduction of hip (Figures 69-17 and 69-18).
4. Carefully monitor the patient's position through transfer (while patient is standing and sitting).
5. Provide a chair with a firm, nonreclining seat and arms; elevate the sitting surface as necessary with pillows or foam cushions to keep the angle of the hip within the prescribed limits when the patient is sitting.

In general, patients who have had *any* kind of internal fixation for fractured hip should avoid elevation of the operated leg when sitting in a chair, because this puts excessive strain on the fixation device.

FRACTURE OF THE SPINE
EPIDEMIOLOGY/ETIOLOGY

Spinal, or vertebral, fractures occur as the result of falls, diving accidents, or blows to the head or body by heavy objects. With increasing frequency, fractures of the spine are also occurring as the result of osteoporosis and metastatic lesions of the spine. Spinal fracture can occur at any age.

PATHOPHYSIOLOGY

Vertebral fracture may occur with or without displacement. If fracture fragments are displaced, they may place pressure on spinal nerves or injure the spinal cord itself. Such pressure will result in partial or complete dysfunction of the body parts innervated from the level of injury. Depending on the extent of injury to the nervous system, dysfunction may be permanent, partially permanent, or temporary. Fracture can occur at any level of the spine, from occiput through the sacrum.

CLINICAL MANIFESTATIONS

Signs and symptoms of vertebral fracture include *pain at the site of injury, partial or complete loss of mobility or sensation below the level of injury, and evidence of fracture/fracture dislocation on routine x-ray examination, myelography, CAT scan, and/or MR scan.*

Medical Management

Objectives in management will be stabilization and reduction of the fracture and decompression (that is, removal of pressure from spinal nerves or the spinal cord).

Emergency management at site of injury. Immediate management objectives are (1) immobilization of the patient with backboard and cervical collar and (2) immediate transport to a hospital.

Surgical management. Objectives of surgical management are as follows:

1. Decompression of nerve structures through laminectomy (see Chapter 70) or appropriate reduction of the fracture and removal of fracture fragments
2. Reduction of the fracture through operative procedures, or in some cases, traction (for example, cervical traction through application of tongs to the skull)
3. Stabilization of the fracture with bone grafting and/or internal fixation devices such as Harrington, Jacobs, or Luque rods (see Chapter 70)
4. Maintenance of stabilization with external fixation devices such as casts, corsets, or braces, as necessary

If there is no displacement of fracture fragments and no pressure on spinal nerves or the spinal cord, *compression fractures may be treated with bed rest until the patient's pain subsides.* Then the patient is gradually mobilized, sometimes with stabilization by a corset or brace.

Nursing Management

Many of the nursing interventions required by the patient with spinal fracture are identical to those outlined for the patient with spinal cord injury in Chapter 63. Of special concern are interventions designed for the following:

1. Maintaining the stability of the fracture fixation
   a. Pay strict attention to "logrolling" the patient for position changes (see Figure 70-27) to avoid twisting the spine and placing stress at the fracture site.
   b. Position the patient with pillows between the legs and behind the back when patient is sidelying to prevent strain on the back.
   c. Changes of position can be accomplished with the use of special beds that rotate 45 degrees from side to side. *Recent literature indicates that when the spine is unstable, logrolling and/or the use of turning frames are contraindicated because they can stress the fracture site.*
   c. Avoid elevating the head of the bed beyond the prescribed level (usually only 30 degrees and only on the physician's order).
   d. When the patient is to be mobilized, apply prescribed corsets or braces *before* getting the patient out of bed.
2. Preventing neurocirculatory problems
   a. Perform neurocirculatory checks every hour in the first 24 to 48 hours postoperatively; report decrease in neuromotor function to the physician, because this may indicate displacement or pressure at the fracture site.

b. Perform passive range of motion to involved extremities at least four times daily to maintain joint motion.

c. Encourage patient to actively move noninvolved extremities to the extent possible as frequently as possible to maintain joint motion and promote circulation.

3. Promoting comfort—in addition to usual comfort measures
   a. Reposition the patient frequently.
   b. Wait a few minutes to ascertain the patient's comfort, because small adjustments may be necessary and may not be immediately recognized.

4. Promoting psychologic comfort
   a. Recognize that the patient may have feelings of powerlessness, anger, and/or fear about the situation, particularly if there is neuromotor deficit.
   b. Encourage the patient to express his or her feelings.
   c. Encourage the patient to take advantage of psychologic and/or social counseling, when it is available.
   d. If long-term rehabilitation is indicated, prepare the patient for care in a rehabilitation setting.

Other nursing interventions are similar to those for any patient who has a fracture, including interventions for individuals in casts or traction, which are discussed earlier in this chapter.

TRAUMA TO SOFT TISSUE STRUCTURES

TRAUMA TO LIGAMENTS AND TENDONS
EPIDEMIOLOGY/ETIOLOGY

Trauma to ligaments and tendons is usually seen in connection with injury to a joint caused by a blow, twisting, or severe stretching. The most common site of ligament damage is the knee, often resulting from a sports injury. A common tendon injury is *rupture of the Achilles tendon.*

PATHOPHYSIOLOGY

The most common ligamentous or tendon injuries are partial or complete tears. In the knee there may be damage to the medial, lateral, and posterior ligaments and to the anterior and posterior cruciate ligaments. Injuries may be classified as mild, moderate, or severe.

CLINICAL MANIFESTATIONS

Signs and symptoms may include tenderness, swelling, pain, effusion, hematoma, disability (for example, the knee "gives away"), and abnormal motion at the joint. These may or may not be present or may vary in intensity, depending on the extent of the injury.

Medical Management
Medical management includes the following:

1. Mild injuries
   a. Rest
   b. Compression
2. Moderate injuries
   a. Rest
   b. Possible aspiration of excess fluid
   c. Compression to control swelling and further effusion
   d. Support—splint or brace
   e. Strengthening exercises
3. Severe injuries
   a. Surgical repair to prevent disability and instability; possible knee surgery performed through an *arthroscope*
   b. Modified compression dressing to prevent effusion
   c. Immobilization of the joint for a prescribed time
   d. Remobilization of the joint, sometimes with the aid of a continuous passive motion machine, appropriate strengthening exercises through a program of physical therapy

Nursing Management

Postoperative nursing interventions for the patient with a ligamentous or tendon tear include the same considerations as for the partially immobilized patient after fracture reduction and application of an external fixation device. Of particular importance is patient teaching. The following information should be included:

1. Information about the nature of the injury and the general nursing care after surgery
2. Use of the brace/cast postoperatively (see p. 2022)
3. Limitations of motion and weight bearing
4. Use of appropriate ambulatory aids
5. Exercises to perform and frequency of exercising
6. Plans for follow-up with the physician

TRAUMA TO MUSCLE
EPIDEMIOLOGY/ETIOLOGY

Muscle strains result from using muscles beyond their intended or functional ability. *Strain may result from a one-time occurrence or as a cumulative effect of overuse.* Common strains are back strains. Muscle may rupture as the result of severe overuse.

PATHOPHYSIOLOGY

Acute strain may disrupt tissue surrounding the involved muscle, and there may be localized hemorrhage. Chronic strain may produce the same symptoms but with a more gradual onset.

CLINICAL MANIFESTATIONS

The following signs and symptoms of muscle strain may include: *mild aching to severe pain, depending on sever-*

ity of the injury, disability, swelling, and tenderness.

INTERVENTIONS

Medical Management

Medical management includes immediate *application of ice to control swelling, rest, application of heat after 24 to 48 hours to control pain, and surgical intervention and immobilization of the part to repair ruptured muscle.*

Nursing Management

Individuals who sustain only mild to moderate strain of a muscle seldom require hospitalization. Those who require surgical intervention (for example, a person with a ruptured quadriceps muscle) will need such nursing interventions as pain management and preservation of strength and mobility, similar to those for the patient who has sustained a fracture that requires surgical repair and external immobilization. Additionally, the nurse should explain the following:

1. The nature of the injury and what nursing care to expect postoperatively
2. How to modify ADL within the limitations of activity and motion that must be observed
3. How to keep the involved muscle at rest until the physician permits activity of the muscle; for example, no active movement of the involved part, no isometric exercise of the involved muscle
4. How to use and care for the immobilizing device being used

TRAUMA TO JOINTS AND JOINT STRUCTURES

Injuries to joints and joint structures may occur as a *sprain* (tearing of the capsule or ligaments surrounding a joint, including disruption of the synovial membrane), meniscus tears, joint dislocation, or joint subluxation.

EPIDEMIOLOGY/ETIOLOGY

Sprains are almost always the result of twisting injuries, as are meniscus tears. Dislocation and subluxation (partial dislocation) of a joint occur as the result of excessive stress being applied to the joint, forcing it in an abnormal direction. Many of these injuries are incurred in running or contact sports such as football. Cervical sprains (whiplash) may result from rear-end automobile collisions.

PATHOPHYSIOLOGY

When a sprain occurs, the ligaments and capsule surrounding the joint are partially torn, producing *hemorrhage and swelling*. Function may not be limited. A meniscus tear results in decreased ability of the meniscus to absorb shock and stabilize the joint. With a *dislocation, contact is lost between the articulating bones of*

the involved joint, whereas a subluxation causes a partial loss of contact between the articulating bones of the involved joint.

CLINICAL MANIFESTATIONS

Signs and symptoms of trauma to joints and joint structures include the following:

1. *Sprain*
   a. Pain
   b. Limitation of motion
   c. Edema
   d. Superficial bruising
   e. Tenderness over the involved joint
   f. Cervical sprain, possibly accompanied by dizziness, visual disturbance, headache, and nausea
2. *Meniscus tears*
   a. Pain
   b. Swelling
   c. Limited motion, especially flexion/extension
   d. "Locking" or "slipping" of the joint
   e. Evidence of tissue tear on arthrography or arthroscopy
3. *Tear of ligaments within the joint*
   a. Pain
   b. Swelling
   c. Instability of the joint
   d. Evidence of tissue tear on arthrography or arthroscopy
4. *Dislocation*
   a. Pain
   b. Loss of function
   c. Obvious deformity
   d. Possible impairment of neurovascular status
   e. Evidence of loss of articulation on x-ray film examination
5. *Subluxation*: signs and symptoms are similar to dislocation, but less severe

Medical Management

Medical management includes the following:

1. *Sprain*
   a. Application of ice to retard swelling and relieve pain
   b. Possible immobilization of joint with cast or splint
   c. Isometric exercises for involved joint
   d. Cervical collar for whiplash
2. *Meniscus tears*
   a. Strengthening exercises; for example, quadriceps setting, straight leg raising, progressive resistive exercises
   b. Surgical repair as necessary, often through arthroscope
3. *Tears of ligaments within the joint*
   a. Strengthening exercises

b. Surgical repair or reconstruction of the ligament, often through arthroscope
4. *Dislocation*
   a. Reduction, either closed (by manipulation) or open (surgical)
   b. Immobilization for a specified period of time
5. *Subluxation*
   a. Reduction
   b. Immobilization for a specified period of time

Nursing Management

Individuals who require surgical intervention for repair of joint injury may require short-term hospitalization or may be managed on an ambulatory surgery basis. Nursing interventions are essentially the same as for the person with severe strain, except that the emphasis will be on maintaining and improving muscle strength around the involved joint instead of resting the muscles. The joint may be immobilized for a relatively short period (1 to 5 days depending on the nature and extent of the injury) and gradually mobilized, either with a continuous passive motion machine in combination with a program of physical therapy exercises or with a program of physical therapy exercises alone. Programs of physical therapy may be extensive and rigorous; for example, *programs for anterior cruciate ligament reconstruction may last up to 6 months*. The nurse will want to concentrate on patient teaching, with special emphasis on prescribed exercises and following through with the prescribed program of physical therapy.

MULTIPLE TRAUMA

EPIDEMIOLOGY/ETIOLOGY

The leading cause of death in the United States for persons under the age of 45 is trauma. Causes of trauma include falls, crushing, vehicular (including airplane) accidents, and gunshot wounds. The nature of the injuries sustained in trauma are often extensive, involving multiple organ systems and multiple sites of injury. The fact that many individuals who sustain such extensive injuries are able to survive and reach treatment facilities is related to improvements in scene of the accident treatment and methods of transport to hospitals (including airlift by helicopter), as well as to increasing knowledge and skill in the field of emergency medicine. Regional trauma centers have been established across the country and, when possible, patients are transproted there. However, personnel in any hospital may be confronted with a multiply injured patient and should be prepared to treat the patient. Often the patient is stabilized and then airlifted to a trauma center.

MEDICAL AND NURSING MANAGEMENT

The goals of medical management are to correct or stabilize any life-threatening problems (for example, ob-

structed airway, pneumothorax, bleeding) and then to reestablish the continuity of injured tissues. Musculoskeletal injury may require reduction of fractures and repair of related soft tissue injury. *Because life-threatening problems must be addressed first, musculoskeletal injuries are usually not repaired until the patient has been stabilized*. However, sites of fracture or potential fracture must be splinted or otherwise protected until reduction can be effected.

The principles of nursing management are as follows:

1. *Before reduction*, protection of all actual or potential sites of fracture through maintaining splints, traction, and/or positioning precautions
2. *After reduction*, observation of all the previously discussed principles of nursing management of the patient with a fracture

The challenge for the nurse is to devise a plan of care that will take into account the demands of the variety of fixation techniques, fracture sites, and mobilization/immobilization requirements for that patient. It should also be noted that the rehabilitation requirements for individuals who have sustained multiple trauma are often long-term and very extensive. Consideration of rehabilitation requirements must occur early in the patient's hospital course and be reviewed frequently (see Chapter 13).

CHAPTER SUMMARY

✔ Musculoskeletal trauma is most frequently manifested as bone fracture but may include injury to other structures of the system.

a. Fracture of bone is usually the result of a blow to the body, a fall, or accident, but it may occur during normal activity if the bone is weakened by disease (pathologic fracture). A fatigue or stress fracture results when muscles associated with the fractured bone are unable to absorb energy as they usually do.

b. Making the home and work environment safer, educating the public about safety hazards, and teaching women about the problem of osteoporosis are all measures to prevent fracture.

c. A bone is fractured when there is a complete or partial (incomplete) interruption of the osseous tissue. Fractures may be further classified as simple (closed) or compound (open), depending on whether the skin over the fracture remains intact. If fracture fragments are moved away from the normal alignment of the bone, the fracture is "displaced;" if the fragments are not moved out of alignment, the fracture is "nondisplaced."

d. Greenstick, transverse, oblique, spiral, telescoped (impacted), and comminuted are terms that describe the line of the fracture.

e. Immobilization of fractured bone is necessary for healing to take place. This can be accomplished through physiologic splintage, external orthopaedic splinting, or internal fixation. Bone heals by the process of callus formation. Complications of bone healing, such as delayed union, nonunion, malunion, and pseudoarthrosis can occur.

f. The most pronounced signs and symptoms of fracture usually include pain, loss of normal function, obvious deformity, edema, and ecchymosis.

g. Medical management of the patient with a fracture focuses on reduction of the fracture, maintenance of correct alignment of the bone fragments, and prevention of excessive loss of joint mobility and muscle tone.

h. Nursing management is planned in collaboration with the medical plan. Nursing interventions emphasize promoting knowledge, controlling pain, maintaining safety; preserving strength and mobility; maintaining skin integrity; preventing systemic complications (circulatory, respiratory, gastrointestinal, and urinary); promoting nutrition; and maintaining immobilization of the reduced fracture. A major objective of nursing care is to protect external or internal fixation devices until healing takes place.

i. Internal fixation is carried out under anesthesia in the operating room. The result is open surgical reduction of the fracture. Fixation with external devices may be used in conjunction with internal devices.

j. Nursing care of the patient with internal fixation will be similar to that for patients with external fixation, except that mobilization is usually much faster.

✔ Fractures of the hip are common; they occur more frequently in women than in men.

✔ *Intracapsular fractures* occur within the hip joint and capsule. *Extracapsular fractures* occur outside the hip joint and capsule. *Avascular necrosis* may result if blood supply to the head of the femur is disrupted as a result of the fracture.

a. The signs and symptoms of hip fracture include severe pain, inability to move the leg, and shortening and external rotation of the leg.

b. Medical management of the patient with a hip fracture focuses on reduction and fixation of the fracture. Choice of fixation device depends on the location of the fracture, potential for avascular necrosis of the femoral head, and personal preference of the surgeon.

c. Nursing management of the patient with a hip fracture includes the same considerations and interventions as for any patient with a fracture. Spe-

cial considerations relate to specific position restrictions for persons who have had a prosthetic implant. Patients who have had any kind of internal fixation for fractured hip should avoid elevation of the operative leg when seated in a chair, because this puts excessive strain on the fixation device.

✔ Spinal fracture can occur at any age, usually as a result of trauma or, with increasing frequency, as the result of osteoporosis and metastatic lesions.

a. Fracture can occur at any level of the spine. If fracture fragments are displaced, they may injure the spinal nerves or spinal cord, resulting in partial or complete dysfunction of the body parts innervated from the level of injury. Dysfunction may be permanent, partially permanent, or temporary, depending on the extent of the injury.

b. The signs and symptoms of vertebral fracture include pain, loss of sensation or mobility below the level of injury, and evidence of fracture/dislocation on x-ray film or other radiologic studies.

c. Immediate medical management of the patient with suspected spinal fracture includes immobilization with backboard and cervical collar and transport to a hospital. The general medical management objectives are stabilization and reduction of the fracture, and decompression (that is, removal of pressure from spinal nerves or the spinal cord). This may be accomplished surgically or with traction. Surgical intervention often requires bone grafting and/or internal fixation devices.

d. Nursing management of the patient with spinal fracture may include both interventions required by any patient who has a fracture and those for a patient with a spinal cord injury.

✔ Trauma to ligaments and tendons is usually seen with injury to a joint. The most common site of ligament damage is the knee. A common tendon injury is a ruptured Achilles tendon. Ligament and tendon injuries may be classified as mild, moderate, or severe depending on the extent of the tear.

a. The signs and symptoms of ligament and tendon injury may include tenderness, swelling, pain, effusion, hematoma, disability, and abnormal joint motion. These are not always present and may vary in intensity.

b. Medical management of trauma to ligaments and tendons is determined by the extent of the damage and may range from rest and immobilization for mild injuries to surgical repair for severe injuries.

c. Specific nursing management takes into consideration all of the principles that are observed in the care of the patient who has a fracture.

✔ *Trauma* to muscle is manifested as *muscle strain,* which results from using muscles beyond their capacity. The signs and symptoms of muscle strain include pain, disability, swelling, and tenderness.

   a. Medical management of strains includes control of swelling and pain and rest. Surgery and immobilization are warranted if muscle is ruptured.

   b. Nursing management of patients with muscle strain is similar to that for patients who have sustained a fracture and require surgical repair and/or external immobilization.

✔ *Injuries to joints* and their structures may occur as *sprains, tears of the capsule surrounding the joint, meniscus tears, joint dislocations, or subluxation.* Joint sprains and meniscus tears are almost always the result of twisting injuries. Dislocation and subluxation occur as the result of extreme stress applied to the joint, forcing it in an abnormal direction.

   a. The signs and symptoms of trauma to the joints and their structures are specific to the type of injury and include pain, swelling, limitation of motion, instability of the joint, and possible impairment of neurovascular status.

   b. Medical management for sprains includes treatment of swelling, possible immobilization, and isometric exercise. Joint dislocation and subluxation require reduction and immobilization.

   c. Nursing management of the patient with trauma to joints and joint structures is the same as for the person with severe strain, except there will be emphasis on maintaining and improving muscle strength around the injured joint. Patient teaching is a priority and emphasizes performing the prescribed exercises and following through with physical therapy regimens.

✔ *Trauma is the leading cause of death in the United States for persons under age 45.*

   a. Causes of trauma include falls, crushing injuries, vehicular accidents, and gunshot wounds. These injuries are often extensive and involve multiple organ systems and multiple sites of injury.

   b. The goals of medical management in multiple trauma are to *correct or stabilize any life-threatening problems and to repair injured tissues.* This would include reduction of fractures and repair of related soft tissue injury. Because attention to life-threatening problems is the priority of immediate care, musculoskeletal injuries may not be repaired until after the patient has been stabilized. Fracture sites must be splinted until this can be accomplished.

   c. Immediate nursing management of the patient with musculoskeletal trauma focuses on protection of actual and potential sites of injury until they can be repaired. After repair, nursing interventions are similar to those carried out for the patient with a fracture.

   d. Nursing care takes into account a variety of challenging considerations, for example, fracture sites, fixation devices, and mobilization/immobilization requirements. Planning for long-term and extensive rehabilitation begins early in the patient's hospitalization.

QUESTIONS TO CONSIDER

- Name three causes of bone fracture and describe some measures that can be taken to prevent fracture.

- Define bone fracture. Include an explanation of the terms "complete," "incomplete," "simple," "closed," "compound," and "open." Name several of the various classifications of bone fracture.

- List three ways a fractured bone can be immobilized.

- Discuss the process by which bone heals and list some factors that might impede bone healing.

- Describe the five most common signs and symptoms of fracture and explain why they occur.

- Discuss immediate and secondary medical management of the patient with a fracture. Define the terms "closed reduction" and "open reduction". What additional special treatment is required in the treatment of a compound fracture?

- Identify three major complications of fracture and discuss how those complications are treated.

- Identify what subjective and objective data the nurse should collect about the person with a fracture. List four possible nursing diagnoses that can be identified for the patient, based on this assessment.

- Identify four potential *systemic* complications of fracture and the nursing measures carried out to help prevent them.

- Describe the nursing measures for the patient who has the following: (1) a cast, (2) traction, (3) internal fixation device.

- Explain why hip fractures are more common in women than men. Define the two general categories of hip fracture, explain the pathophysiology of each, and describe the signs and symptoms of hip fracture.

- List three methods for reducing a hip fracture and identify factors that the surgeon considers in choosing a fixation device.

- Describe the specific position restrictions and nursing care requirements for the patient with a prosthetic hip implant.

- What are some of the common causes of spinal fractures?

- Discuss the clinical significance of vertebral fractures without displacement versus fracture with displacement.

- Describe the signs and symptoms of vertebral fracture.

- What are the primary objectives of medical management for the patient with vertebral fracture? Discuss immediate versus surgical management.

- Discuss the nursing interventions of special concern for the patient with spinal fracture.

- Describe the types of injuries that can occur to joints and joint structures and how they are usually incurred. What are the signs and symptoms?

- What are the primary goals of both medical and nursing management for the person who has sustained multiple trauma?

- Discuss the special challenges the nurse encounters when caring for the multiple trauma patient. Include consideration of acute and long-term care needs.

REFERENCES AND SELECTED READINGS

1. *American Nurses' Association and National Association of Orthopaedic Nurses: Orthopaedic nursing practice: process and outcome criteria for selected diagnoses, Orthop Nurs 6(2):11-16, 1987.

2. Blauvelt C and Nelson F: A manual of orthopaedic terminology, ed 3, St Louis, 1985, The CV Mosby Co.

3. Brunner NA: Orthopedic nursing: a programmed approach, ed 4, St Louis, 1983, The CV Mosby Co.

4. Callahan J: Compartment syndrome, Orthop Nurs 4(4):11-18, 1985.

5. *Cochran S: Action stat! Open fracture, Nursing 87 17(5):33, 1987.

6. *Crocker C: Acute postoperative pain: cause and control, Orthop Nurs 5(2):11-16, 1986.

7. Duckworth T: Lecture notes on orthopaedics and fractures, ed 2, Oxford, 1984, Blackwell Scientific Publications.

8. Duthie RB and Bentley G: Mercer's orthopaedic surgery, ed 8, 1983, Baltimore, University Park Press.

9. Dwyer AP, editor: Symposium on spinal column fractures, Clin Orthop 189:3-208, 1984.

10. Edmonson AS and Crenshaw AH, editors: Campbell's operative orthopaedics, ed 6, St Louis, 1980, The CV Mosby Co.

11. Farrell J: Illustrated guide to orthopedic nursing, ed 3, Philadelphia, 1986, JB Lippincott Co.

12. Friedlaender GE, Mankin HJ, and Sell KW, editors: Osteochondral allografts: biology, banking, and clinical applications, Boston, 1983, Little, Brown & Co.

13. *Gamron R: Taking the pressure out of compartment syndrome, Am J Nurs 88(8):1076-1080, 1988.

14. *Hansell M: Fractures and the healing process, Orthop Nurs 7(1):43-50, 1988.

15. Hilt NE and Cogburn SB: Manual of orthopedics, St Louis, 1980, The CV Mosby Co.

16. Hilt NE, editor: Assessment and fracture management of the lower extremities, United States, 1984, Anthony J Jannetti, Inc.

17. *Hines N and Bates M: Discharging the patient in skeletal traction, Orthop Nurs 6(4):21-24, 1987.

18. *Hoyt N: Infections following orthopaedic injury, Orthop Nurs 5(5):15-24, 1986.

19. *Johnson C, editor: Symposium on orthopedic nursing, Nurs Clin North Am 16(4):707-766, 1981.

20. *Johnson J: Respiratory complications of orthopaedic injuries, Orthop Nurs 5(1):24-28, 1986.

21. *Johnson L: Operative management of unstable pelvic fractures, Orthop Nurs 8(4):21-25, 1989.

22. Jones-Walton P: Effects of pin care on pin reactions in adults with extremity fracture treated with skeletal traction and external fixation, Orthop Nurs 7(4):29-33, 1988.

23. *Lamb K, Miller J, and Hernandez M: Falls in the elderly: causes and prevention, Orthop Nurs 6(2):45-49, 1987.

24. Leach RE, editor: Progress in sports medicine, Philadelphia, 1985, JB Lippincott Co.

25. Maher AB: After the emergency is over: delayed and occult injuries in the trauma patient, Orthop Nurs 4(2):25-27, 1985.

26. *Maher AB: Early assessment and management of musculoskeletal injuries, Nurs Clin North Am 21:717-727, 1986.

27. *McFarland MB: Encircling cast drainage: is it valuable?, Orthop Nurs 3(2):41-43, 1984.

28. Mourad L and Droste M: The nursing process in the care of adults with orthopedic conditions, ed 2, New York, 1988, John Wiley & Sons, Inc.

*References preceded by an asterisk are particularly well suited for student reading.

29. National Institute of Arthritis and Musculoskeletal and Skin Diseases, NIH: Osteoporosis: cause, treatment, prevention, Orthop Nurs 5(6):29-38, 1986.
30. Omer G: Assessment of hand trauma, Orthop Nurs 4(2):29-33, 1985.
31. *Osborne L and DiGiacomo I: Traction: a review with nursing diagnoses and interventions, Orthop Nurs 6(4):13-19, 1987.
32. Robinson JE and Marx LO: A nail-safe method, Am J Nurs 85(2):158-161, 1985.
33. *Salmond SW: Trauma and fractures: meeting your patient's nutritional needs, Orthop Nurs 3(4):27-33, 1984.
34. Salter RB: Textbook of disorders and injuries of musculoskeletal structure, ed 2, Baltimore, 1983, The Williams & Wilkins Co.
35. *Sheidler V: Patient-controlled analgesia, Curr Concepts Nurs 1(1):13-16, 1987.
36. Spickler LL: Knee injuries of the athlete, Orthop Nurs 2(5):11-19, 1983.
37. Spiegel PG and Mast JW, editors: Complex fractures of the ankle and hindfoot, Clin Orthop 199:3-144, 1985.
38. *Sproles KJ: Nursing care of skeletal pins: a closer look, Orthop Nurs 4(1):11-20, 1985.
39. Turek SL: Orthopaedics: principles and their application, Philadelphia, 1984, JB Lippincott Co.
40. Unkle D and DeLong W: Abdominal trauma associated with pelvic fractures, Orthop Nurs 8(4):27-29, 1989.
41. *Wagner MM: Assessment of patients with multiple injuries, Am J Nurs 72(10):1822-1827, 1972.
42. Wittert D and Barden R: Deep vein thrombosis, pulmonary embolism, and prophylaxis in the orthopaedic patient, Orthop Nurs 4(4):27-37, 1985.

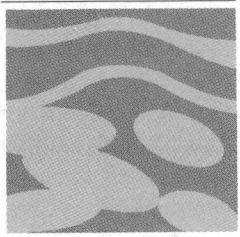

CHAPTER 70

Management of Persons with Degenerative Disorders of the Musculoskeletal System

PATRICIA S. BUERGIN

KYLE M. PASKERT

CHAPTER OBJECTIVES

After studying this chapter, the student should be able to:

1 Explain the five physiologic problems commonly experienced by persons who have disorders of the musculoskeletal system.
2 Discuss at least five interventions used in the management of physiologic problems experienced by persons with musculoskeletal disorders and give rationales for each.
3 Discuss the five psychosocial problems commonly experienced by persons with musculoskeletal disorders and explain the interventions that can be used in managing those problems.
4 Discuss both nonpreventable and preventable factors related to musculoskeletal disorders.
5 Explain the epidemiology/etiology, pathophysiology, and clinical manifestations of rheumatoid arthritis.
6 Explain the medical management and nursing management of persons who have rheumatoid arthritis.
7 Discuss the orthopaedic surgeries commonly employed to treat persons with rheumatoid arthritis and the nursing care associated with each of the surgeries.
8 Discuss the epidemiology/etiology, pathophysiology, and clinical manifestations of systemic lupus erythematosus (SLE).
9 Explain the medical and nursing interventions used in the care of persons with SLE.
10 Discuss the epidemiology/etiology, pathophysiology, and clinical manifestations of polymyositis, and explain the medical and nursing interventions used in the care of persons who have polymyositis.
11 Discuss the epidemiology/etiology, pathophysiology, and clinical manifestations of ankylosing spondylitis and explain the medical and nursing interventions used in the care of persons who have the disease.
12 Describe three forms of nonarticular rheumatism and describe the medical and nursing interventions used in the care of each.
13 Explain the epidemiology/etiology, pathophysiology, and clinical manifestations of degenerative joint disease (DJD) and discuss its preventable aspects.
14 Describe the medical and nursing management of persons who have DJD, including surgical intervention and postoperative nursing interventions.
15 Explain the pathophysiology and clinical manifestations of degenerative disease of the spine.
16 Discuss the medical management of persons who have DJD of the spine and explain the nursing care required for individuals being treated (a) conservatively and (b) surgically.
17 Explain the pathophysiology and clinical manifestations of scoliosis.
18 Describe the medical management of persons who have scoliosis and explain the nursing care required for individuals being treated (a) conservatively and (b) surgically.
19 Give three examples of other disorders that can affect the musculoskeletal system, describe how they differ from disorders previously discussed, and explain the essential medical and nursing nursing management required for persons affected by them.

The essence of nursing individuals with musculoskeletal problems lies in helping them to make the physiologic and psychosocial adaptations necessary to minimize their temporary or permanent disability. It is the purpose of this chapter to define some of the common problems (both physiologic and psychosocial) experienced by individuals with motor disabilities and to discuss specific methods that may be used in managing these problems.

PHYSIOLOGIC DISABILITIES

COMMON PROBLEMS

Five major problems must be considered in the area of physiologic disability. Most patients with a motor disability will have one or more of them.

PAIN

Pain is the priority problem that must be dealt with in planning care. Regardless of its intensity, unrelieved pain can become so all consuming a concern that the individual's entire attention is focused on relieving it. *Pain prevents activity, predisposes the patient to the complications of immobility, and dulls receptiveness to care and teaching.* In the extreme, it can affect the individual's attitude toward life. Therefore pain must be relieved to the greatest extent possible before other needed interventions can be implemented.

STIFFNESS

Stiffness (decreased flexibility) can be a result of pain or of disuse (as in the case of persons who are immobilized), or it can be a result of pathophysiologic changes (as in degenerative joint disease.) Stiffness cannot be defined as pain; however, an attempt to use an extremity that is stiff may cause pain. Stiffness may discourage activity, thereby affecting the person in much the same manner as pain.

Decrease in Muscle Strength

Decrease in muscle strength is sometimes a primary problem, as with some *myopathic and neuropathic disorders, or it can result from prolonged bed rest or immobility.* Interventions designed to improve strength (such as increasing mobility or exercising) can be implemented when some progress is made with treatment of the primary problem. When it is not possible for the person to regain muscle strength, some means of modifying activity to maintain function must be provided.

Loss of Dexterity

Loss of dexterity (skillful use of the hands or body) is another problem encountered either as a result of a primary pathophysiologic process (such as rheumatoid arthritis or ataxic neurologic disorders) or as a result of pain, stiffness, or enforced immobility. Again, the primary problem must be treated before measures to improve dexterity can be implemented. If the primary problem cannot be controlled, measures can be taken to provide alternative methods of performing activities so that function can be maintained.

Loss of Locomotor Ability

Perhaps the most threatening component of many musculoskeletal disorders is the temporary or complete loss (or potential for loss) of the ability to move freely from one place to another or care for one's self. While some problems present only short-term immobility, others, such as spinal cord damage, can cause lifelong disability.

Various groups of handicapped persons throughout the United States have been active socially and politically to inform the general public of the architectural barriers encountered by individuals with limited mobility. As a result, federally funded building projects must now be equipped with facilities to accommodate the handicapped individual. All new public buildings must have wheelchair ramps, special toilet facilities, and easy-access parking spaces.

The concern of those caring for hospitalized persons with activity or motor restrictions must be directed toward preventing complications (contractures), helping them work through their feelings about and adapt to restricted mobility, providing them with alternative means for moving about or performing activities of daily living (ADL), and helping them plan for adaptations they will have to make in their home environments and lifestyles.

Complications of immobility. Immobility may be accompanied by a number of potential or actual complications that can involve any or all of the major systems of the body (see Table 70-1).

COMMON INTERVENTIONS

Some interventions are common to a number of musculoskeletal disorders. They will be discussed generally here and will be referred to under specific interventions later in this chapter.

REST, ACTIVITY, JOINT PROTECTION, AND ENERGY CONSERVATION

Rest

Rest is a therapeutic measure used in many inflammatory and traumatic conditions of the musculoskeletal system. However, too much rest can at times be as detrimental as too much activity. There are two forms of rest:
1. *Absolute rest or no activity*
   a. May be required for the whole body or for a specific part of the body
   b. Is accomplished through avoidance of use of the part
   c. Is possibly enhanced by some method of external immobilization (splint, cast, traction) to ensure inactivity
2. *Partial rest or limited activity*
   a. Some activity is permitted, but other activities (for example, weight bearing, certain movements) are limited

The nurse's responsibility in helping the patient rest is as follows:
1. Help patient understand the meaning of "rest" as it applies to him or her
2. Take over functions for the patient that would require use of body part beyond limits prescribed
3. Teach the patient how to effectively use body parts not required to rest

TABLE 70-1 Complications of immobility

System Involved	Mechanism	Potential Complication	Intervention
CARDIOVASCULAR	Failure of vessels in legs to assume or maintain a state of vasoconstriction, resulting in pooling of venous blood	Deep vein thrombosis (DVT) Pulmonary embolism (PE) Increased work load on heart Diminished cardiac output Decreased ability to adapt to erect posture	Active and passive range of motion (ROM) Frequent turning Slow mobilization Positioning to avoid pressure over major vessels
RESPIRATORY	Decreased movement Decreased stimulus to cough Decreased depth of ventilation	Pooling of secretions in bronchi, bronchioles Hypostatic pneumonia	Active and passive ROM Stimulation to take maximal sustained inhalations and cough Frequent turning
SKIN	Pressure or shearing forces (two or more tissue layers sliding on each other or tissue sliding on another surface) disrupting or decreasing circulation to an area	Skin breakdown (abrasion or decubitus ulcer)	Early identification of areas at risk Turning on regular schedule Pressure-relieving pads, mattresses, flotation devices, special beds
GASTROINTESTINAL	Decreased bowel motility Change in dietary habits Disadvantageous positioning for defecation	Constipation Impaction	Increase fluid intake Add roughage to diet Encourage use of bedside commode or toilet when possible
MUSCULOSKELETAL MUSCLES	Disuse	Atrophy Weakness	Active ROM Exercise
JOINTS	Limited motion leads to muscle, tendon shortening	Contracture Fibrosis or bony ankylosis around joints	Active and passive ROM Exercise Encourage to perform own ADL as possible
BONES	Disruption of balance of osteoblastic/osteoclastic activity with destruction of bone matrix and release of calcium	Osteoporosis	Isometric and active exercise to tolerance
URINARY	Increased urinary pH, increased citric acid	Renal stones	Increase fluid intake Decrease calcium intake
	Poor bladder emptying	Urinary stasis	Improve position for bladder emptying (i.e., bedside commode or toilet when possible)
NEUROLOGIC	Loss of normal stimuli	Confusion, restlessness, forgetfulness	Provide stimulation and diversionary material

4. Gradually return functions to the patient when rest is no longer required

Activity

Activity, particularly in chronic conditions, must be balanced with adequate rest. Individuals who have pain with certain activities or increased pain and stiffness following certain activities must learn to recognize their tolerances and adapt their ADL accordingly. This does not mean stopping all activity; it means *modifying* activity. For the individual with degenerative arthritis of the hips, for example, it may mean walking 1 mile a day instead of 2.

Nurses can help patients determine their activity needs in the following ways:

1. Teach the patient the advantages of continuing, but modifying, activity

2. Help the patient identify his or her own activity tolerances
3. Help the patient work out an activity schedule approximating rest/activity requirements at home
4. Help the patient work through concerns about not being able to perform all activities he or she believes are necessary or desired.

Joint Protection and Energy Conservation

Individuals with joint involvement and/or activity intolerances can learn to protect their joints and themselves from overuse, misuse, and stress by becoming aware of and practicing joint protection and energy conservation techniques (see the box below). External pressures that put stress on joints in the wrong direction and internal pressures from muscles can produce deformities in joints that have been affected by chronic inflammatory processes. Fatigue and an increase in pain are symptoms of overactivity and overuse or misuse of joints. Nursing interventions are as follows:

JOINT PROTECTION AND ENERGY CONSERVATION TECHNIQUES

TECHNIQUE	EXAMPLES
Avoid positions of possible joint deformity	Avoid keeping joints in positions of flexion for prolonged periods of time
	Avoid twisting motions such as turning a jar lid with small joints
Avoid holding muscles or joints in one position for a long time	When working at a desk, stand up and walk about for a few minutes every half hour
Use the strongest joints for all activities	Use the knees, not the back, when lifting heavy objects
	Push a door open with the shoulder, not the wrist
	Use a shoulder strap, not a hand-held strap, to carry a heavy purse
Use joints in their best position, maintaining good standing and sitting posture	Avoid reaching or bending when another approach would work as well
	Work at a comfortable height
Conserve energy	Avoid trying to accomplish difficult tasks in a single time period
	Take breaks during work periods
	Slide, rather than lift objects
	Use a wheeled cart to move objects from one place to another

---

SOME ASSISTIVE DEVICES FOR PERSONS WITH MOTOR IMPAIRMENTS

ASSISTIVE DEVICE	PATIENT LIMITATION
Utensil with built up handle (Figure 70-1)	Cannot adequately close hand
Utensil with cuffed handle	Loss of opposition of thumb
Combination knife-fork (Figure 70-2)	Use of only one hand
Mug with special handle (Figure 70-3)	Unable to grasp regular cup handle
Long-handled shoehorn (Figure 70-4)	Unable to bend to reach feet
Long-handled reacher (to reach for or pick up objects) (Figure 70-5)	Unable to stoop or reach
Stocking guide (Figure 70-6)	Inability to reach feet

---

1. Teach the patient to recognize the symptoms of overactivity.
2. Teach the patient appropriate energy conservation and joint protection techniques.
3. Encourage the patient to use those techniques in ADL.

ASSISTIVE, SUPPORTIVE, AND SAFETY DEVICES

Many *assistive devices* are available for individuals who have impairment of upper and/or lower extremity function (see the box above). Although the occupational therapist is generally the person who evaluates the patient's disability, recommends specific assistive devices, and teaches the patient how to use them, the nurse is often the person who recognizes the need for referral to the occupational therapist and encourages the patient to use devices appropriately in the hospital or at home. For

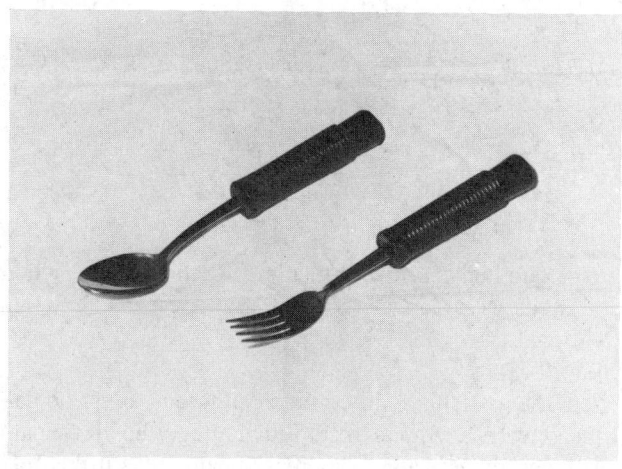

FIGURE 70-1 Utensils with built-up handles.

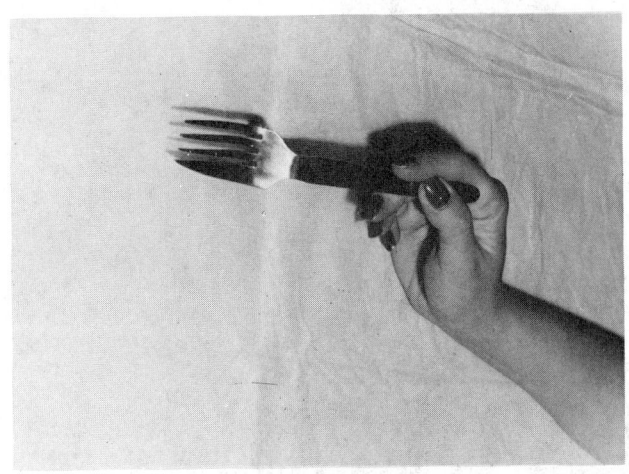

FIGURE 70-2 Combination knife-fork.

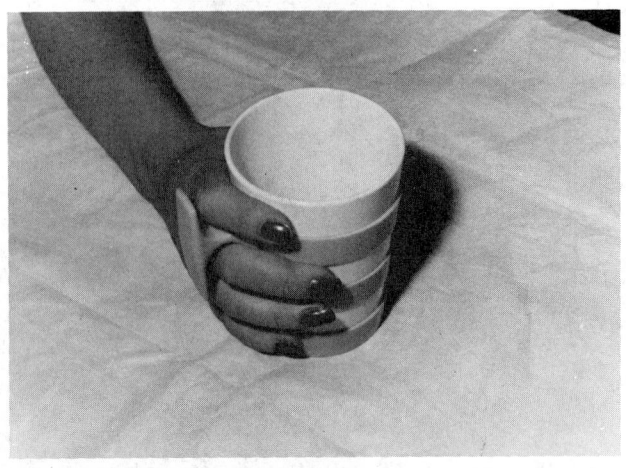

FIGURE 70-3 Mug with special handle.

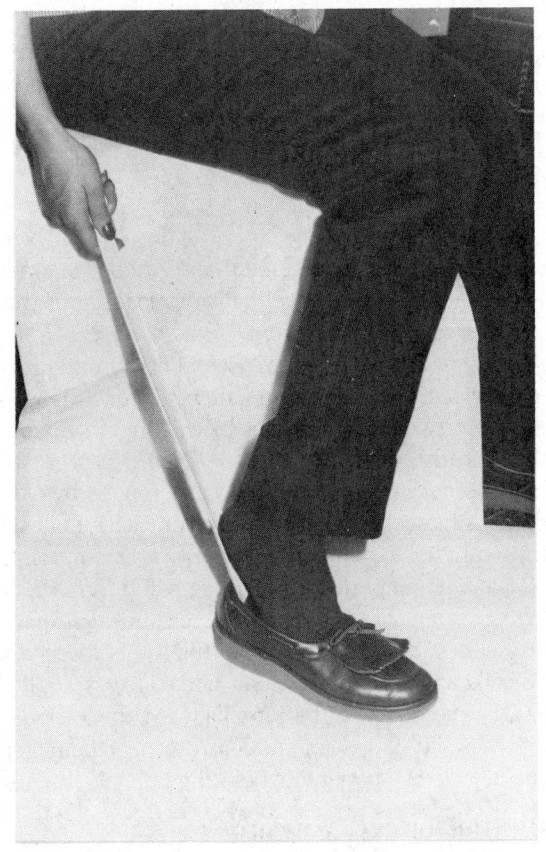

FIGURE 70-4 Long-handled shoehorn.

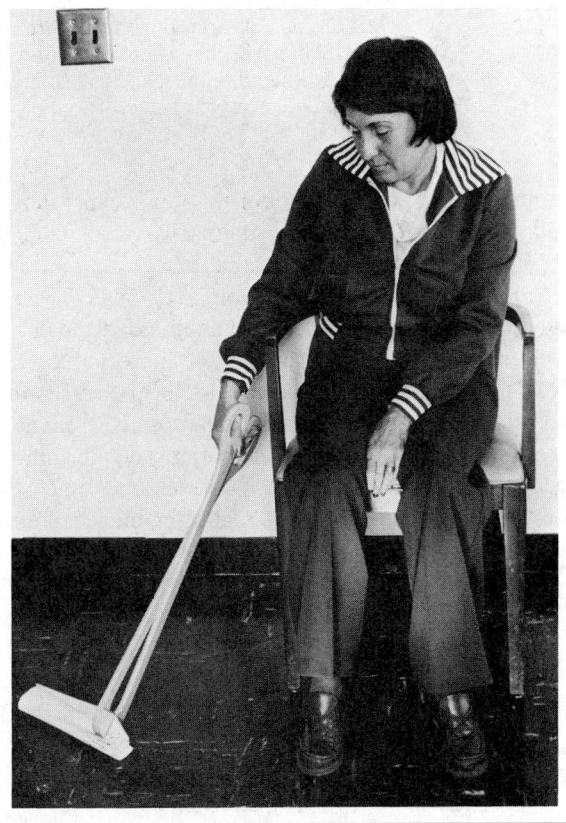

FIGURE 70-5 Long-handled reachers are handy for picking things up off floor if person is not to bend or stoop.

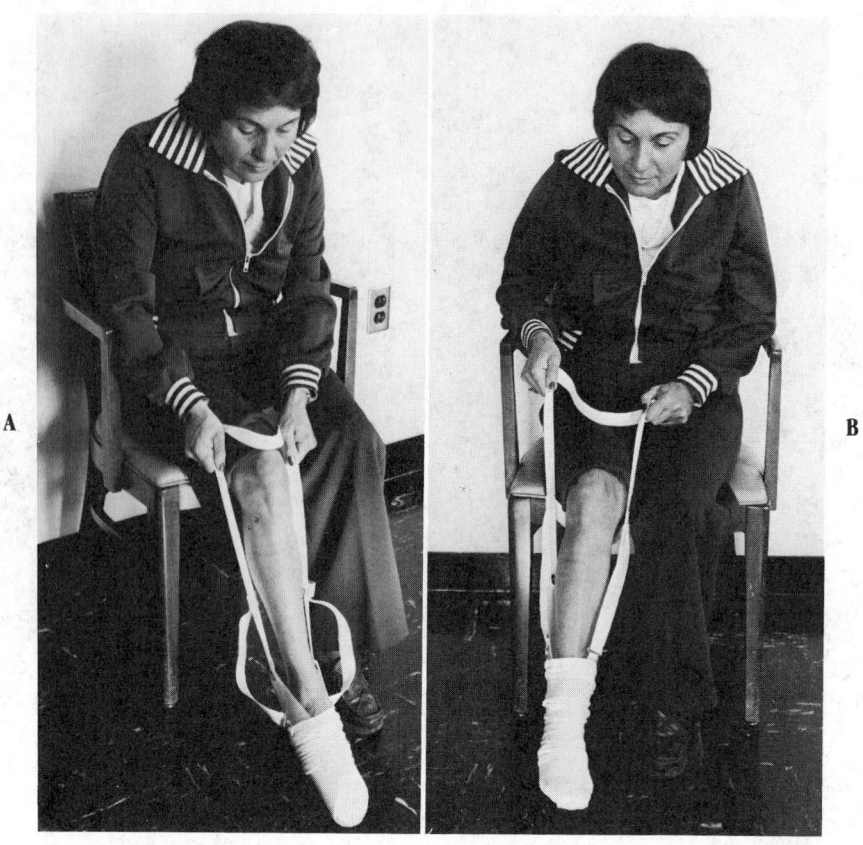

FIGURE 70-6 A, Using stocking aid. Stocking has been placed over plastic guide; garter clips at ends of strap have been attached to top of stocking. Woman then places her foot into stocking. **B,** Straps are used to pull stocking over foot and up leg; when top of stocking is at knee, patient can release garters. This apparatus is useful for persons who cannot bend over to reach feet.

example, it is nontherapeutic and time consuming to feed persons who can feed themselves independently with aids that have been provided.

Supportive devices or ambulatory aids (walkers, canes, crutches) are usually recommended for persons who cannot bear weight on one or more joints of the lower extremities. Other indications for their use are instability, poor balance, or pain on weight bearing. The physical therapist evaluates the patient to determine the specific device that will match the patient's needs and abilities. Some considerations regarding choice of device include the following:

1. Axillary crutches
   a. Require dexterity and a good sense of balance
   b. Permit faster ambulation than walkers
   c. Can be used on stairs
2. Walkers
   a. Provide solid support
   b. Can be used by individuals with balance problems
   c. Limit speed of ambulation
   d. Are hazardous on stairs or uneven ground

3. Canes
   a. Are less cumbersome than crutches or walkers
   b. Do not permit as effective unloading of weight as a double support

Nurses are expected to supervise patients in their use of these devices and encourage patients to use their walking aids correctly. Techniques of walking with aids are outlined in the box on p. 2051.

Safety devices are items that can be used by the patient to enhance function and prevent accidents when normal function, balance, or dexterity are compromised. Examples of safety devices include safety arms around toilets, grab bars mounted at tubs or showers, elevated toilet seats, adhesive strips on tub or shower floors, hand rails along staircases, and nonskid wax applied to floors. Nurses need to be familiar with the various devices available, help patients learn to use them, and if necessary, advise patients where they may be obtained.

APPLICATION OF HEAT AND COLD

Heat and cold have a variety of uses for individuals with musculoskeletal problems. *Heat,* particularly moist

TECHNIQUES OF WALKING WITH AMBULATORY AIDS

DEVICE	GAIT
Single-support device (cane, quad cane, single crutch)	Device is held in the hand opposite the involved leg Device and involved leg are advanced first, followed by the uninvolved leg
Double-support device Walker	Walker is advanced first, then the involved extremity, then the noninvolved extremity
Crutches	3-point gait—the same as walker gait 4-point gait—crutch, opposite leg, opposite crutch, other leg 2-point gait—both crutches, both legs (one leg may be non-weight bearing)

Special Note: Climbing up stairs is accomplished by moving the uninvolved leg first, then the device and the involved leg; to descend stairs, the involved leg and the device are moved first, then the uninvolved leg. The device and the involved leg always move together.

heat, is used for relieving stiffness and relaxing muscles and for analgesic effect and sedative effect. Heat may be applied in a variety of ways:

1. Dry heat
   a. Electric heating pad
   b. Warm towels
   c. Aqua-K pads
2. Moist heat
   a. Hydrocollator packs (packs containing chemical filler that expands in water and retains heat; may be heated in pot of water or special machines that have constant heat of 80° C [174° F])
   b. Paraffin baths
   c. Electric heating pads that are approved for use with moist towels
   d. Warm soaks, tub soaks, or showers

Application of *cold* or ice packs is helpful in reducing or preventing swelling (especially after trauma), reducing pain, and relieving stiffness. Cold packs may take the form of plastic bags containing ice, commercially available gel packs that can be refrozen and reused, or large bags of frozen vegetables (especially for home use).

Whenever heat or cold is applied, it should be left on for 15 to 20 minutes to achieve maximum effect. Cold packs and moist heat packs should be wrapped in protective towels to prevent burns to the skin, and the skin should be checked 5 minutes after application for any evidence of tissue damage. *Heat or cold should be ap-*

plied with caution to any individual with decreased sensation, because that person will not be able to determine if damage is occurring.

Nursing interventions with heat or cold therapy include:

1. Helping patient determine which type of application works best
2. Instructing patient about safety precautions to be observed with that method
3. Instructing patient about timely application of heat or cold (for example, before activity or exercise, or before going to bed at night) depending on patient's particular needs
4. Assisting the patient with application

TRACTION

Traction can be used to help reduce contractures or to relieve pain in the presence of muscle spasm. It can be applied intermittently or constantly and usually in the form of skin traction, that is, *Buck's* extension, *Russell* traction, or pelvic traction. Patients who are receiving this form of therapy can usually be taken out of traction if the traction itself is causing discomfort, and the traction can be reapplied when the patient believes it can be tolerated. The principles of maintaining the patient's comfort and safety while in traction are discussed in Chapter 69.

SPLINTING AND BRACING

Splints and braces (orthoses) are used for the following purposes:

1. Stabilize or support a joint
2. Protect a joint or body part from external trauma
3. Mechanically correct dysfunction such as footdrop by supporting the joint in its functional position
4. Assist patients to exercise specific joints

Splints and braces (see the box on p. 2052) are designed to be as lightweight and cosmetically acceptable as possible. Advances have been made in this area by orthotists (brace makers) who have developed plastic molded braces made out of lightweight materials; these braces are custom fitted to the patient (Figure 70-7). In many instances these have replaced the cumbersome metal and leather braces that are often obvious, even though worn under loose-fitting clothing. *Shoes* may be modified, or corrective shoes may be prescribed, to provide special support for the feet.

When patients need to use braces or splints, nurses need to:

1. Inspect patient's skin after the orthosis has been applied for a short time to be certain it has caused no skin irritation
2. Notify the orthotist if adjustments in the orthosis need to be made to make it more comfortable or relieve chafing

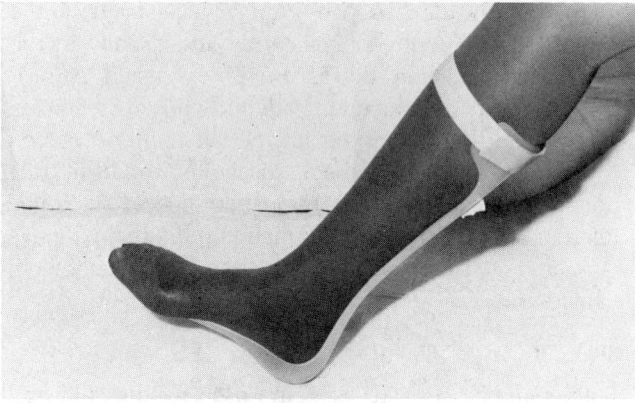

FIGURE 70-7 A, Molded footdrop brace. **B,** Brace in place on foot.

TYPES OF SPLINTS AND BRACES AND THEIR FUNCTION

TYPE	FUNCTION
Spring-loaded braces	Oppose the action of unparalyzed muscles and act as partial functional substitutes for paralyzed muscles (Figure 70-8)
Resting splints	Maintain a limb or joint in a functional position while permitting the muscles around the joint to relax (Figure 70-9)
Functional splints	Maintain the joint or limb in a usable position to enable the body part to be used correctly
Dynamic splints	Permit assisted exercise to joints, particularly following surgery to finger joints (Figure 70-10)

3. Instruct the patient in the proper application and care of the orthosis
   a. Metal braces should be stored upright
   b. Leather materials should be treated occasionally with Neatsfoot Compound or other leather preservative to prevent cracking and drying
   c. Orthoses fabricated of molded materials should be stored away from sources of heat
   d. Patients fitted with molded orthoses should avoid gaining or losing weight as the brace would have to be adjusted or refabricated
4. Assist the patient to make the psychologic adjustment to wearing the orthosis

POSITIONING AND TRANSFER

Principles of positioning (Figure 70-11) can be found in most fundamentals of nursing texts. However, because pain accompanies nearly all musculoskeletal problems, preventing or minimizing pain must be taken into consideration when positioning the patient. Nurses should be aware that patients in the acute stages of their disorders require the greatest care and gentleness when they must be moved. *Fear of pain often causes irritability and can lead to muscular resistance, which increases pain.* Care must be taken not to jar the bed. Heavy bedclothes over painful extremities may cause added pain. If bed cradles are used to support linen, caution must be taken not to accidentally bump an involved part of the body when adjusting or removing the cradle. Placing a very painful joint or extremity on a pillow or pillows to move it can reduce pain. Moving patients off the bed using a pull sheet (Figure 70-12) or a roller board (Figure 70-13) also facilitates comfort through the move. Frequently, patients would prefer to move themselves rather than risk pain from having someone else move them; when it is safe for the patient to do so, the nurse should permit it.

If the patient must use a wheelchair, it should be adjusted to fit that individual. No wheelchair should be purchased for permanent use by a patient unless someone knowledgeable about wheelchairs, preferably a physical therapist, has evaluated the patient and determined what special equipment is needed. Chairs poorly fitted to the patient's needs can be unsafe and encourage poor posture. Principles of transfer are summarized in the box on p. 2055.

EXERCISE

Exercise is a prescribed form of activity designed to accomplish the following:
1. Preserve joint mobility (active and passive range of motion)
2. Maintain muscle tone (active range of motion and isometrics)
3. Strengthen selected muscle groups (resistive ex-

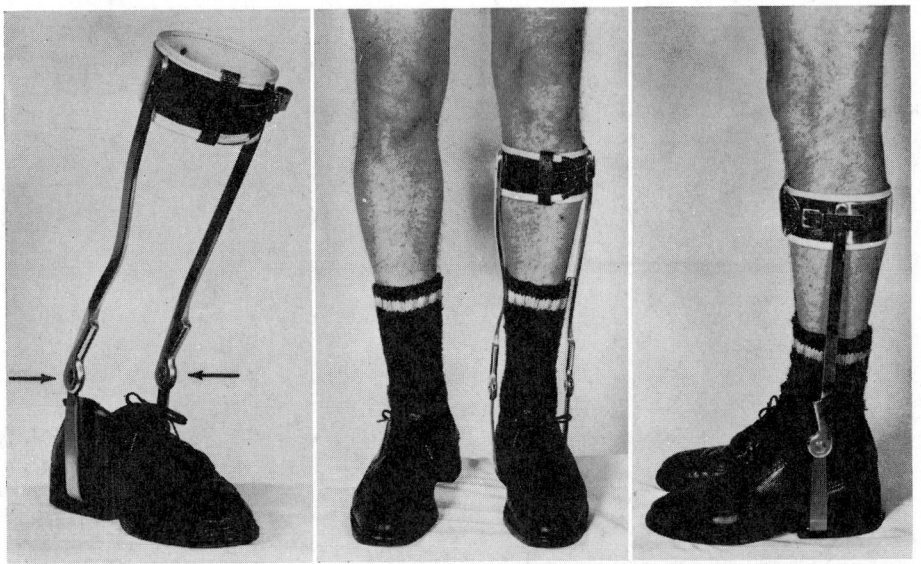

FIGURE 70-8 Spring footdrop brace. When weak dorsiflexor muscles are overbalanced by stronger plantar flexors, adjustable spring at ankle hinge of each upright (Klenzak joint, Pope Foundation, Inc.) is used to supply passive dorsiflexion and thus prevent footdrop and an equinus limp. (From Brashear H and Raney R: Shand's handbook of orthopaedic surgery, ed 9, St Louis, 1978, The CV Mosby Co.)

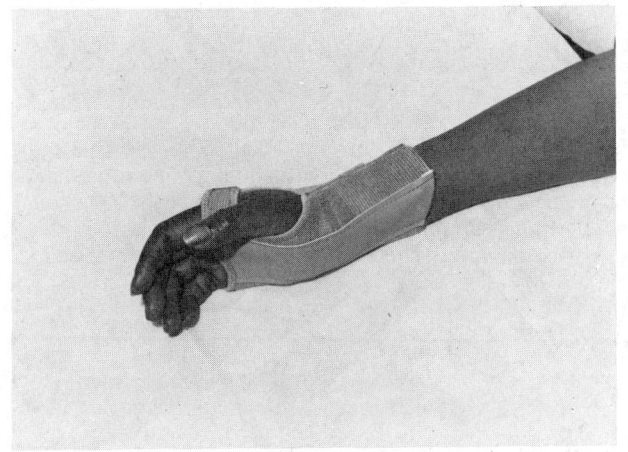

FIGURE 70-9 Commercially available resting splint for wrist.

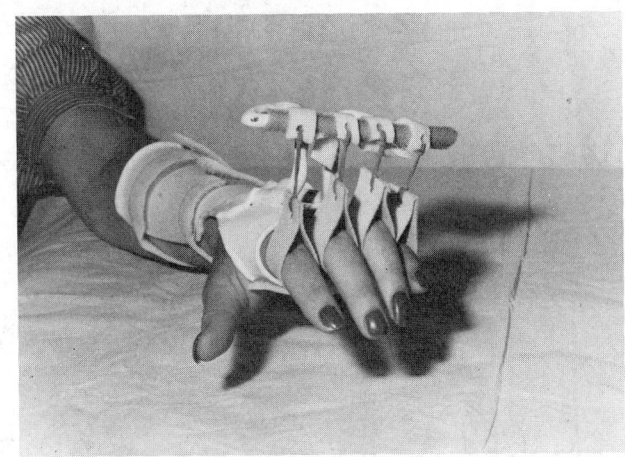

FIGURE 70-10 Dynamic hand splint.

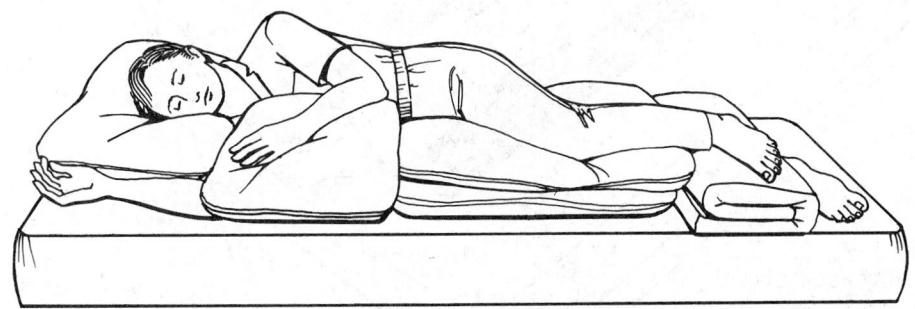

FIGURE 70-11 Side-lying position with extremities properly supported with pillows and rolled blankets.

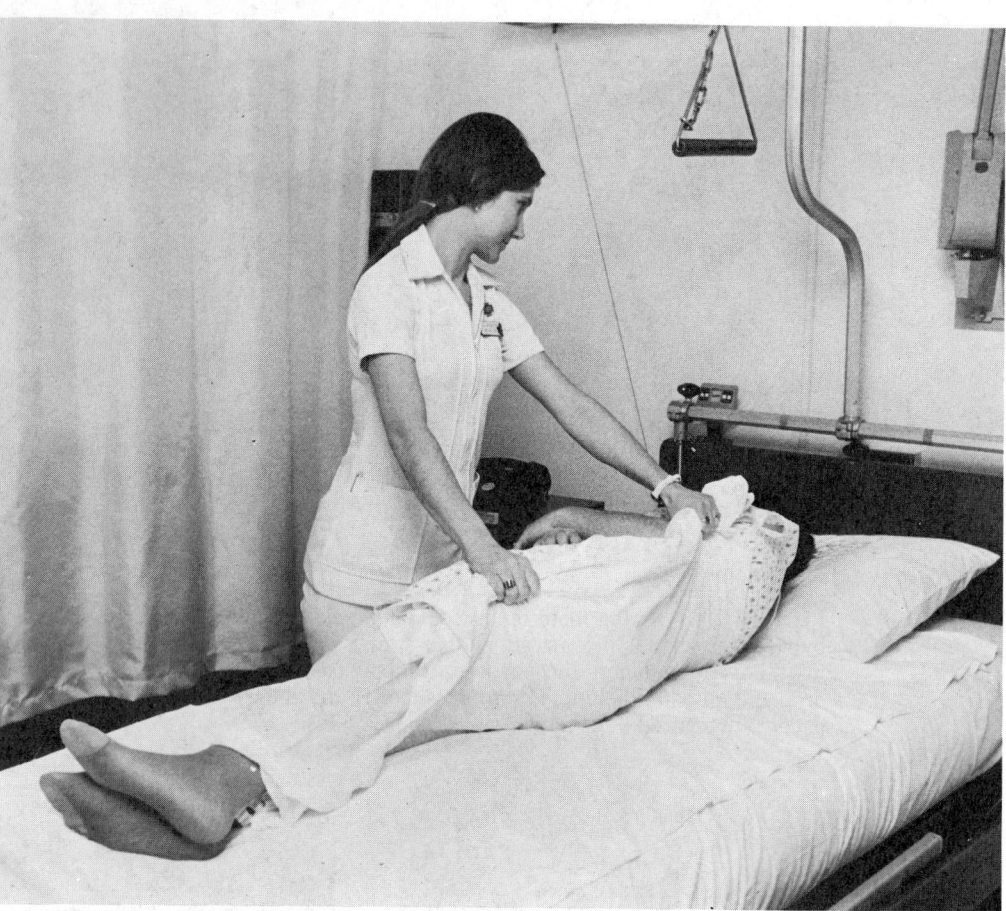

FIGURE 70-12 Use of turning sheet. Sheet is held taut with one hand at level of patient's shoulder and other hand below patient's buttocks, providing patient with a sense of support and control. A sheet so placed may also be effectively used as a pull sheet when moving patient from bed to cart.

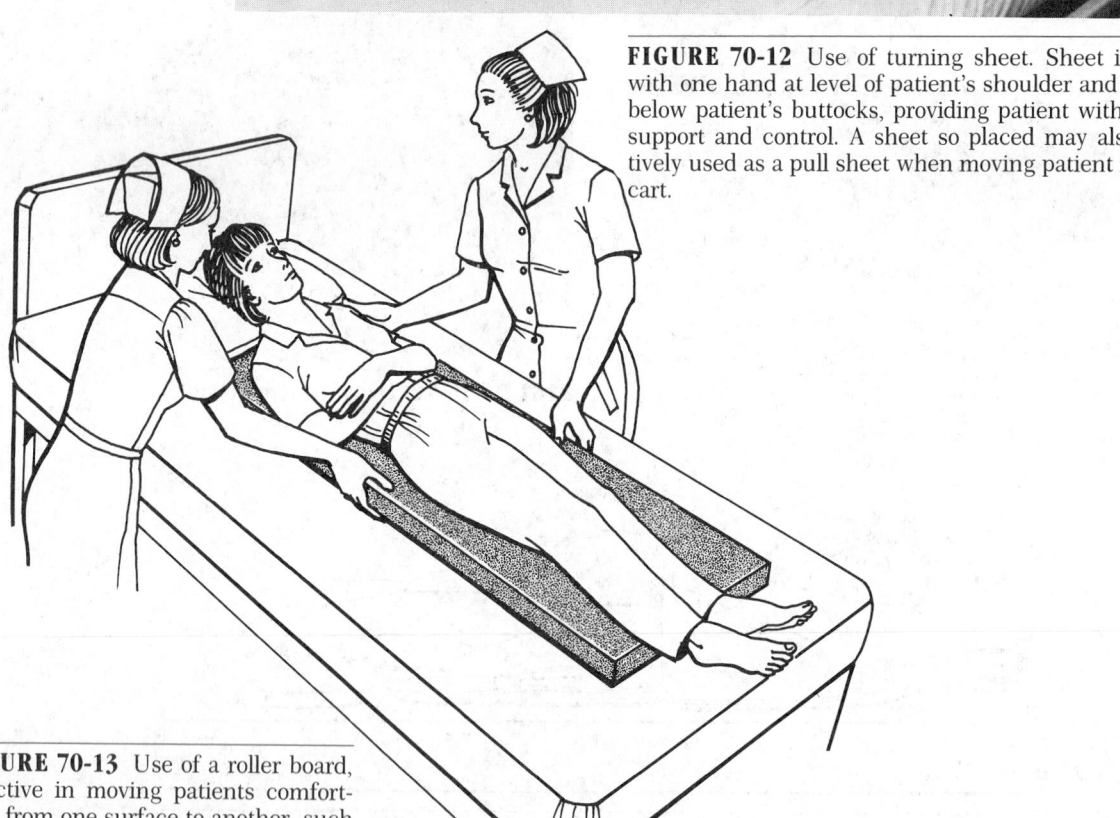

FIGURE 70-13 Use of a roller board, effective in moving patients comfortably from one surface to another, such as from bed to stretcher and stretcher to bed.

PRINCIPLES OF TRANSFER

The patient should always be moved toward his or her strong side.

The person assisting supports the *strong* side.

If there is any question regarding the patient's ability to cooperate with the transfer, a second person should be standing by for assistance.

If the person assisting with the transfer has any doubt about his or her ability to do so safely, a second person should be asked to help.

The transfer should be accomplished using the strong muscles of the legs rather than the weak muscles of the back.

If lifting is required, adequate help should be available. If help is not available, the transfer should not be attempted at that time.

ercises performed against resistance provided by another person or by weights)

Exercise may be facilitated by the application of heat or cold or the administration of an analgesic before the exercise period. *Exercise is contraindicated in the presence of acute joint or muscle inflammation* until the inflammatory process subsides.

Exercise programs should be tailored to the patient's specific needs and capabilities. Nurses need to be aware of the specific exercise program the patient is following and be prepared to provide support and assistance to perform the exercises as needed and reinforce with the patient the purpose, technique, frequency, and duration for performing the exercises. (See the Research Box above right.)

MEDICATIONS

Many of the medications used in the treatment of musculoskeletal problems are antiinflammatory analgesics. Specific drugs are addressed in Table 70-6 and in conjunction with discussion of specific disorders. Nurses caring for patients taking these drugs should be prepared to teach patients the expected effects of the drugs, how to use them appropriately, and how to recognize side effects or toxic effects. Additionally, nurses should be aware that *use of narcotic analgesics in chronic inflammatory musculoskeletal conditions is generally contraindicated,* because they are not antiinflammatory and the patient will develop a tolerance to them. Narcotic analgesics do have their place in the treatment of acute injuries and postoperative pain.

PROMOTING NUTRITION

The essentials of good nutrition are as important for individuals with musculoskeletal problems as for anyone else. Special diets, however, are usually not recom-

RESEARCH

Byers PH: Effect of exercise on morning stiffness and mobility in patients with rheumatoid arthritis, Res Nurs Health 8(3):275-281, 1985.

The purpose of this study was to evaluate the hypothesis that exercise before bedtime by the person with rheumatoid arthritis reduces morning stiffness and increases joint mobility. Graphic goniometric measures of finger mobility, arthrographic measures of finger stiffness, and subjective ratings of stiffness were obtained from 30 persons with rheumatoid arthritis who had stiffness of the right hand. All subjects performed nonweight-bearing, active range-of-motion exercise on one of two consecutive evenings (randomly selected). Exercises were repeated on both mornings. Measurements of stiffness and mobility were obtained before and after each morning exercise period. Performance of evening exercises resulted in less elastic stiffness and greater finger mobility the following morning than when evening exercises were not performed. Effects of evening exercise were subjectively reported as greater when elastic stiffness was greater. ■

mended except where other medical conditions require them. Patients should pay particular attention to avoiding weight gain. Added weight increases the patient's energy consumption and causes weight-bearing joints to be abnormally stressed. For many individuals with mobility problems, however, the problem of weight and mobility becomes a vicious circle. Mobility is impaired, therefore activity is limited, calories are not used in activity, more weight is added, and further immobility results as the individual finds it harder to move the weight. This cycle can be broken only by weight loss through a properly supervised reduction diet.

Nurses can help in the following ways:

1. Teach patients the importance of a well-balanced diet
2. Teach patients the importance of restricting weight gain
3. Encourage patients to select food wisely
4. Encourage the patient's family to bring home cooked food if the patient is not eating hospital food particularly following surgery when the patient needs to maintain a positive nitrogen balance

SURGICAL INTERVENTIONS
Indications for Surgery

Individuals who have surgery to the musculoskeletal system usually fall into one of two categories: those who have suffered trauma such as a fracture (Chapter 69) or those who require an elective orthopaedic procedure for correction of deformity, relief of pain, or restoration of

TABLE 70-2 Surgical procedures to the musculoskeletal system (except spine surgery)

Surgical Procedure	Definition of Procedure	Reason for Performing
Arthrotomy	Opening of a joint	Exploration of joint Drainage of joint Removal of damaged tissue or foreign body
Arthroplasty	Reconstruction of a joint	Restore motion Relieve pain Correct deformity
Interposition	Replacement of part of a joint with a prosthesis or with soft tissue	
Replacement	Replacement of both sides of a joint with prosthetic implants	
Synovectomy	Removal of part or all of the synovial membrane	Delay the progress of rheumatoid arthritis
Osteotomy	Cutting a bone to change its alignment	Correct deformity Alter the weight-bearing surface of diseased joint to relieve pain
Arthrodesis	Causing the bones of a joint to grow together by removing articular hyaline cartilage, introducing bone grafts, and stabilizing with external fixation	Stabilize a joint Relieve pain
Tendon transplants	Moving a tendon from its usual position	Substitute one tendon for another that is not working Realign tendon function; for example, for stability

musculoskeletal function. The four major objectives of orthopaedic treatment are as follows:

1. Restoration or maintenance of function of a body part
2. Prevention of deformity
3. Correction of deformity if it already exists
4. Development of the patient's powers of compensation and adaptation if loss of function or permanent deformity is not preventable

Before performing surgery, the orthopaedist considers what procedure is best suited to achieve the desired objectives for the individual patient. It is important that those caring for the patient know and understand what the expected outcomes are so that care may be adapted to achieving them. *Orthopaedic care is highly individualized to the patient being treated, and those who work with orthopaedic patients must not lose sight of the practical aspects of the treatment rationale.*

Types of Surgery

Table 70-2 defines the common types of surgery that are performed on the musculoskeletal system and the reasons they are performed. Specific interventions for these surgeries will be discussed under the appropriate disorder.

PSYCHOSOCIAL PROBLEMS

COMMON PROBLEMS
REACTION TO DISFIGUREMENT OR DISABILITY

A major problem faced by many individuals who have musculoskeletal problems is that the disorder may dis-

figure them as well as impair their motor function. Not only must they adapt to functional disability, but they also may have to adapt to "looking different" from other people. (For further information on body image, see Chapter 18.) Loss or alteration of function or the need to use an assistive device or prosthesis can also cause them to view themselves as different from others. Depending on the nature and strength of pressures from family, social, or work situations, or the *individual's degree of self-esteem,* the individual may attempt to cover up the disability so as not to lose support, esteem, or a livelihood. If the disability cannot be covered up, some persons may withdraw or limit their contact with others.

DEPENDENCE, INDEPENDENCE, AND INTERDEPENDENCE

Most people want to be able to live their lives independently. In the sense of this discussion, *independence* would mean freedom from having to make demands on others for personal and social ADL. However, persons with musculoskeletal problems may be unable to manage one or more activities for themselves. If help from another person is needed to perform a certain function, such as buttoning buttons, the individual is *dependent* in that area. If an assistive device (for example, button hook, Velcro closures) can be made available and the use of it can be mastered, the individual can again be independent in that function.

Very few people live truly independent lives. As a society, we depend on the farmer to grow our food, the lawyer to attend to our legal affairs, the mechanic to repair our automobile. We are *interdependent.* Families are also structured around interdependent functions. Persons with motor disability may at some time be faced with losing their interdependent role; that is, they may no longer believe they are useful or needed by anyone else.

ADAPTATION TO ASSISTIVE, SUPPORTIVE, AND CORRECTIVE DEVICES

Walkers, canes, crutches, splints, braces, and feeding aids often have negative connotations in our society. Individuals may have great difficulty overcoming their aversion to such devices and accepting them as a means of maintaining their independence and safety.

SOCIOECONOMIC IMPACT

Many disorders that affect motor function occur at an age when wage earning, child rearing, and other functions can be seriously impaired. Loss of income and self-esteem, the inability to maintain one's standard of living, and increased stress on the family can all result. By no means, however, is motor impairment less of a problem for the older person. Living alone or on a fixed income and faced with the possibility of not being able to maintain independence, the person can become very frightened, depressed, or withdrawn. Nursing homes are costly, as are persons who are hired to help in the home, if they are even available in a community. The idea of giving up one's home and way of life can be very threatening and demoralizing.

FAMILY RELATIONSHIPS

Reference has already been made to the fact that family roles and relationships (social and economic) may be changed owing to a patient's restricted motor function and areas of dependency. It is important that those caring for the patient recognize when those relationships are destructive and help the patient and family obtain appropriate guidance. Whenever it is possible, support should be given to "healthy," caring relationships that are identified.

COMMON INTERVENTIONS

Interventions for psychosocial problems should relate to the following outcomes:

1. Patients can maintain or achieve a state of independence consistent with their physical abilities.
2. Patients can define and share with their families or significant others the areas in *which they are dependent.*
3. Patients can return to their living situations able to resume interdependent roles with their families.
4. Patients will be able to name/utilize resources within their communities to assist them in maintaining their optimum level of function.

These outcomes may be achieved through support, teaching, and guidance.

SUPPORT

The nurse can provide support in the following ways:

1. Recognizing that the patient does have a problem
2. Defining with the patient what the problem is
3. Allowing the patient to do what he or she can do independently
4. Devising methods to help the patient achieve independent function in impaired areas
5. Assisting the patient, to the extent necessary, in areas where independent function cannot be achieved
6. Involving family or significant others in care so they know what the patient can and cannot do and so thus can provide positive encouragement.

If individuals are not allowed to perform functions that they can perform, they can quickly become angry and discouraged and lose motivation. *Loss of the desire to be independent, subjecting oneself to a state of dependence, can be the most destructive element of a musculoskeletal disorder.*

COUNSELING

Counseling by members of the health team concerning the nature of the patient's disability and areas of independence and dependence may be helpful in assisting patients and their families to define new roles for themselves, that is, roles in which patients can have an active part in their families' lives and concerns. Individuals with severe difficulties in adaptation may benefit from psychiatric counseling or spiritual support. Recognition of the need for counseling and the type of counseling the patient is most likely to respond to are important assessment factors in determining the correct intervention.

TEACHING

Teaching may take the form of demonstrating the positive advantages of physical interventions. The individual who resists taking medication or using a walking device may be positively influenced to continue therapy once the effectiveness of therapy in relieving pain or eliminating dependence in an area of functioning is demonstrated. Teaching may also include making the patient or family aware of community resources, for example, Visiting Nurse Association, Meals on Wheels, job retraining programs, community housing programs, or community responsive transport systems for the handicapped. For individuals with economic limitations, suggestions for inexpensive modifications in their living environment may influence their ability to continue living in their present circumstances. An example would be teaching the patient how to bathe while sitting on a chair in the bath tub and using a shower hose extension on the faucet. This is much less expensive than purchasing a hydraulic tub lift and is more satisfying than a sponge bath. Such teaching requires that nurses be inventive and innovative and possess a working knowledge of community resources available to help patients to continue to function satisfactorily in settings that they can afford.

PREVENTION

Whatever the nature of the musculoskeletal disability, certain factors of prevention and teaching must be considered.

NONPREVENTABLE FACTORS

Many of the diseases that affect the musculoskeletal system have at this time an unknown cause. Rheumatoid arthritis and the systemic connective tissue diseases are but a few examples. While these diseases are not now preventable, some complications of the diseases are preventable (for example, contractures, atrophy, skin breakdown, and others). In these instances, prevention depends on teaching the patient to understand the disease process and to use preventive measures.

PREVENTABLE FACTORS

Polio vaccine, screening of school-aged children for scoliosis, community programs for education of women in the prevention of osteoporosis, and screening tests for streptococcal infections with early treatment of the infection to prevent rheumatic fever are examples of preventive measures that can be employed on a community-wide basis to combat illnesses that cause musculoskeletal disability. Early attention to posture; good dietary habits; genetic counseling for individuals with sickle cell anemia and hemophilia; teaching of good body mechanics for individuals whose jobs entail lifting or carrying heavy objects; and concern and attention to the recommendations of the governmental agencies and community action groups to help avoid accidents at home, on the job, and on the road are all examples of preventive measures that may be used to decrease musculoskeletal disability within the general population.

PROMOTION OF SAFETY

For those individuals who have limitations of motion or mobility, a variety of precautions and protective or safety devices can be employed in the hospital or the home. Examples would include the following:

1. Grab bars mounted on a wall near a tub or toilet
2. Safety arms fitted around a toilet
3. Elevated toilet seats
4. Removal of throw rugs and obstacles from areas used by individuals with ambulatory difficulties
5. Adequate, easy to operate locking devices on wheelchairs
6. Hand rails on staircases

While some of these measures may seem to be common knowledge, patients are frequently not aware of them or their need for them. One of the most important functions nurses can perform is to assess the safety requirements of their patients and then teach the patient or family what steps are necessary to ensure safety. It is helpful if nurses know where in the community needed equipment can be obtained. Often the hospital social worker or physical therapist provides this information and assists the patient or family in obtaining the equipment. By the time of discharge from the hospital, arrangements should be made for the patient to have the equipment and instruction required for safe functioning at home.

MAINTENANCE OF POSTURE

Although maintenance of good posture (see the box below) is important for all persons, it is especially important for individuals with chronic musculoskeletal disease. Poor posture exerts further strain on already damaged joints and supportive structures, and it not only may cause pain and fatigue, but it also predisposes to increased deformity.

PRINCIPLES TO BE OBSERVED IN MAINTAINING CORRECT POSTURE

FOR THE GENERAL PUBLIC

Standing erect decreases strain on the back, hips, and knees.

Sitting erect decreases strain on the back and hips.

Holding the head erect with the chin in relieves strain from the joints of the upper spine.

Stooping with the knees and hips flexed (Figure 70-14) prevents strain on the back.

Using the strong muscles of the legs instead of the weak muscles of the back when lifting heavy objects prevents injury to the back.

FOR THE HOSPITALIZED PATIENT

Using a firm mattress and bedboard for the individual for whom prolonged bed rest has been ordered lessens pull on painful joints and helps keep the spine in good alignment.

Lying prone (when possible) relieves supine pressure areas (inferior scapular areas and ischial tuberosities) (Figure 70-15).

Using pillows to support extremities: pillows should not be placed in such fashion or for such periods of time that they promote flexion contractures of joints.

Bracing or supporting extremities or the trunk with pillows, trochanter rolls, and bath blankets: they must be placed with care to avoid compression of nerves or arteries.

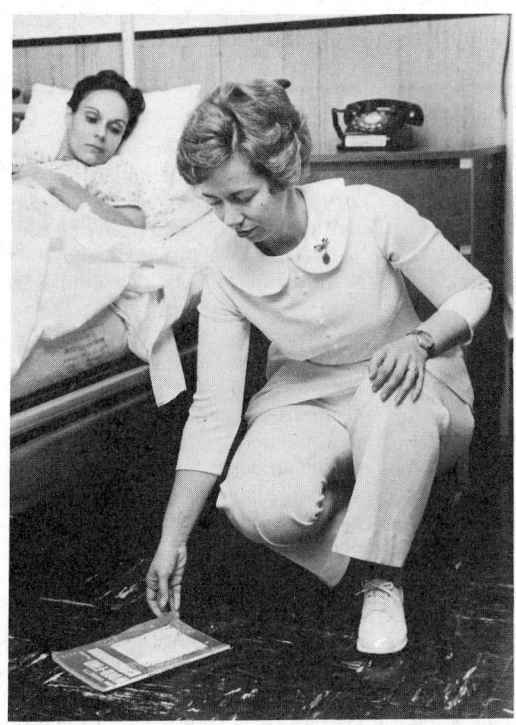

FIGURE 70-14 Good body mechanics being used to pick up object from floor. Note that nurse's back is straight while her knees and hips are flexed sharply.

INFLAMMATORY DISORDERS OF THE MUSCULOSKELETAL SYSTEM

The disorders and injuries of the musculoskeletal system are vast in scope. They range from those that cause the patient minor discomfort and inconvenience to those that are life threatening. Among the more troublesome are the inflammatory or rheumatic diseases. These diseases, though they may involve many systems, very often have an arthritic component. There are more than 100 arthritic diseases. One in every seven people in the United States has some form of arthritis. One in every three families in the United States is somehow affected by arthritis. The total economic cost of arthritis in the United States in 1980s, including both direct (med-

ical care) and indirect cost (lost wages), was estimated to be more than 13 million dollars.

RHEUMATOID ARTHRITIS
EPIDEMIOLOGY/ETIOLOGY

Rheumatoid arthritis is a chronic *systemic* disease. The disease process, while most prominent as a nonsuppurative inflammation in the diarthrodial joints, may also be manifested by lesions of the vasculature, lungs, nervous system, and other major organs of the body.

Rheumatoid arthritis is more prevalent in women than men by a ratio of 2:1 or 3:1. Usually it appears during the productive years of life when career and family responsibilities are greatest. While the cause of this disease is unknown, several theories of causation are under investigation. Areas of study include (1) immune mechanisms, such as the interaction of the IgG class of immunoglobins with the rheumatoid factor that appears to play a role in perpetuating rheumatoid inflammation; (2) metabolic factors; and (3) infection, with particular attention to viruses.

PATHOPHYSIOLOGY

The disease process within the joints (intraarticular) begins as an inflammation of the synovium with edema, vascular congestion, fibrin exudate, and cellular infiltrate. The inflammatory process is set off by some sort of irritation or damage to joint tissue. This is called a "triggering" event. White blood cells rush into the area, releasing chemicals (including superoxide radicals and hydrogen peroxide) useful in destroying bacteria, but also harmful to tissue cells. Also released are prostaglandins (chemicals that mediate inflammation), leukotrienes (producers of inflammation), and digestive enzymes. Particularly damaging to joint tissue is the *enzyme collagenase* because it breaks down collagen, the main structural protein of connective tissue. The presence of these substances within the joint attracts still more white blood cells, and in rheumatoid arthritis, the process becomes chronic. Continued inflammation leads to thickening of the synovium, particularly where it joins the articular cartilage. At these junctures, granulation tissue forms a *pannus*, or mantle, that covers

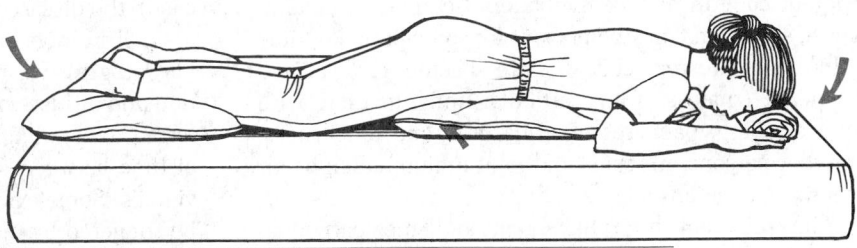

FIGURE 70-15 Good prone lying posture, with head, abdomen, and lower legs supported on pillows to keep body in good alignment.

TABLE 70-3 Normal function, primary pathophysiology, and the clinical picture in joint manifestations of rheumatoid arthritis

Normal Function	Pathophysiology	Clinical Picture
Synovial tissue secretes synovial fluid that both lubricates the joint and is the medium through which nutrients are supplied to the articular cartilage.	Inflammation causes edema, vascular congestion, fibrin exudate, and cellular infiltrate to build up around synovium. WBCs move into the synovium releasing superoxide radicals, H_2O_2, prostaglandins, leukotrienes, and collagenase.	Synovium thickens, particularly at articular junctions. Symptoms of inflammation occur within and overlying the joint (pain, swelling, erythema, warmth). Joint mobility is limited by pain.
Articular cartilage covers the ends of articulating bones to provide a smooth surface for movement.	Granulation tissue (pannus) forms at junctions of synovial tissue and articular cartilage, interfering with nutrition of cartilage. Articular cartilage becomes necrotic. Pannus invades *subchondral bone* (underlying cartilage) and supporting soft tissue structures (ligaments, tendons), destroying them.	Joint pain increases at rest and with movement. Destruction of soft tissue structures (ligaments, tendons) causes joint to sublux or dislocate. Depending on the amount of articular cartilage destroyed, adhesions can develop and the joints can fuse, prohibiting joint motion.

the surface of the cartilage. The pannus also invades subchondral bone (bone underlying the cartilage). As the amount of granulation tissue from inflammation increases, it interferes with normal nutrition of the articular cartilage and the cartilage becomes necrotic. The degree of erosion of the articular cartilage will determine the amount of articular disability. If large areas of cartilage are destroyed, adhesions form between the joint surfaces, and fibrous or bony union (ankylosis) develops between what were previously free-moving surfaces. Destruction of cartilage and bone, in addition to some weakening of tendons and ligaments, may lead to subluxation or dislocation of joints. Invasion of the subchondral bone may cause eventual regional osteoporosis (Table 70-3).

CLINICAL MANIFESTATIONS

The early manifestations of the disease may include fever, weight loss, fatigue, and generalized aching. *Early morning stiffness* lasting a few minutes to an hour or more is characteristic. The person may describe the location of aching and stiffness in general terms as opposed to naming specific joints. This kind of *discomfort, commonly referred to as fibrositis, is poorly localized.* Such discomfort may be the patient's earliest complaint. These symptoms may be present for some period of time before they are replaced by more specific, or localized, problems (that is, frank articular inflammation with joint swelling, pain, redness, warmth, and tenderness. In other persons, fibrositis and joint inflammation occur together at the onset.

The proximal interphalangeal and metacarpophalangeal joints of the hands and the metatarsophalangeal joints of the feet are often affected early. As the disease

progresses, the fingers develop a characteristic tapering (fusiform) appearance with a classic ulnar deviation of the hand (Figures 70-16, *A* and *B*). Virtually all joints can become involved but most common are the joints of the hands, wrists, feet, ankles, elbows, and knees. Shoulder and hip involvement are later phenomena. Joint involvement most often occurs in a *bilaterally symmetric* pattern with involvement of the same joints on both sides of the body.

Inflammation of the tendon sheaths, particularly in the wrist, may occur. There is spasm of the muscles attached to the involved joints. Such spasm is believed to contribute to deformity of the involved joints, and because the patient will tend to guard painful joints, some atrophy of muscles from disuse may occur (Figure 70-16, *C*). Painless subcutaneous nodules may develop near joints, over bony prominences, or along extensor surfaces.

The course of rheumatoid arthritis varies greatly from patient to patient. It is marked by periods of exacerbation and remission. Some individuals have been known to recover from a first attack and never suffer a recurrence. For others, particularly those in whom the rheumatoid factor is found (seropositive rheumatoid disease), the disease tends to be chronically progressive. In a small number of individuals the disease may be rapidly progressive, marked by unremitting joint destruction and diffuse vasculitis. This form of the disease is referred to as *malignant rheumatoid disease.* The length of time between exacerbations varies greatly with individuals. Some evidence suggests that exacerbations can be triggered by mental stress such as worry or grief, by overexertion, and at times by physical trauma such as surgery. The likelihood that the patient will enter a

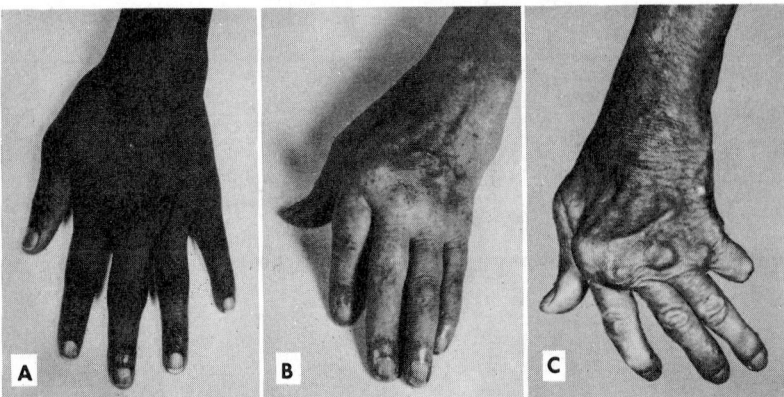

FIGURE 70-16 Rheumatoid arthritis of hand. **A,** Early stage. Note fusiform swelling of proximal interphalangeal joints, especially that of middle finger. **B,** Moderate involvement. Note swelling from chronic synovitis of metacarpophalangeal joints and early ulnar drift. **C,** Advanced stage. Note marked ulnar drift and subluxation of metacarpophalangeal joints with extension of proximal interphalangeal joints and flexion of distal joints. Note also deformed position of thumb. Hand has wasted appearance. (From Raney R and Brashear H: Shand's handbook of orthopaedic surgery, ed 8, St Louis, 1971, The CV Mosby Co.)

complete remission after 3 years of sustained disease activity is very slight.

If it is not treated, rheumatoid arthritis has a tendency to relapse and to recur in more severe form. Continued competent medical care is of the utmost importance for anyone who has rheumatoid arthritis. Some individuals, when having a remission of their symptoms, believe they are cured and discontinue their therapy, only to have a later and more severe exacerbation of the disease. Even with careful management, approximately 10% of patients with rheumatoid arthritis progress to a crippling state of complete incapacity.[53]

Laboratory findings usually include the following:

1. An elevated erythrocyte sedimentation rate
2. Mild leukocytosis
3. Positive rheumatoid factor or latex fixation test (present in 50% to 90% of patients, depending on disease duration and severity)
4. Narrowing of the joint spaces and erosion of articular surfaces on roentgenographic examination
5. Inflammatory changes in synovial tissue obtained by biopsy
6. Increased turbidity and decreased viscosity of synovial fluid obtained by needle aspiration

MEDICAL MANAGEMENT

Medical management is generally described as a pyramid of therapy. The pyramid is usually represented as having its foundation in a good history and physical ex-

Corticosteroids

or

Cytotoxic agents

or

Experimental agents

_____

Penicillamine

_____

Antimalarials   Gold salts

_____

Nonsteroidal antiinflammatory drugs

_____

Salicylates

_____

History	Rest	Patient	Measurement
Physical	and	and	of response
Lab and X-ray	exercise	family	to therapy
examination		education	

FIGURE 70-17 Pyramid of therapy used to treat rheumatoid arthritis..

TABLE 70-4 Medications prescribed in the treatment of rheumatoid arthritis*

Medication	Action	Side Effects/Toxic Effects	Precautions
SALICYLATES			
Examples: acetylsalicylic acid, choline salicylates	Analgesic, antipyretic, antiinflammatory	Gastric irritation; dose-related salicylism; skin rash; hypersensitivity	Take with food, milk, or antacid; space q 4-6 hr to maintain antiinflammatory effect
NONSTEROIDAL ANTIINFLAMMATORY AGENTS (NSAIAS)†			
Indomethacin (Indocin)	Analgesic, antiinflammatory	Headache; dizziness; insomnia; confusion; GI irritation	Take with food, milk, or antacid; discontinue if CNS symptoms develop and notify physician
Ibuprofen (Motrin)	Same as indomethacin	Same as indomethacin but believed less irritating to GI tract; fluid retention	Absorption is delayed if taken with food
Tolmetin sodium (Tolectin)	Same as ibuprofen	Same as ibuprofen	Take with food or milk
Naproxen (Naprosyn)	Same as ibuprofen	Same as ibuprofen; also drowsiness	Take with food, milk, or antacid; avoid driving until dosage effect is established
Fenoprofen (Nalfon)	Same as ibuprofen	Same as naproxen	Delayed absorption if taken with food; avoid driving until dosage effect established
Sulindac (Clinoril)	Same as ibuprofen	Same as ibuprofen; also skin rash	Take with food, milk, or antacid; do not use with acetylsalicylic acid
Diflunisal (Dolobid)	Analgesic, antiinflammatory	Gastric irritation; headache; dizziness; skin rash; tinnitus; fluid retention	Take with food or milk; do not use with salicylates or other antiinflammatory medications
Piroxicam (Feldene)	Analgesic, antiinflammatory	Gastric irritation; anemia; skin rash; fluid retention; dizziness; headache	Take with food or antacid
Diclofenac sodium (Volteran)	Analgesic, antiinflammatory	Possible intestinal irritation, headache, drowsiness, fatigue	Enteric coated; may be taken with food or milk
POTENT ANTIINFLAMMATORY AGENTS			
Adrenocorticosteroids (for example, Prednisone)	Interfere with body's normal inflammatory response	Fluid retention, sodium retention, potassium depletion; hypertension; decreased healing potential; increased susceptibility to infection; gastrointestinal irritation; hirsutism; osteoporosis; fat deposits; diabetes mellitus; myopathy; adrenal insufficiency or adrenal crisis if abruptly withdrawn	Take with food, milk, or antacid; dosage not to be increased or decreased without physician supervision; take in morning if taken once a day
Phenylbutazone (Butazolidin)	Antiinflammatory; analgesic at subcortical site in brain	Gastrointestinal irritation; hematologic toxicity; hypertension; impaired renal function	Used for a short term (7-10 days); take with food or milk

*NOTE: Adjunctive therapy, at any level of the pyramid of management, may include the use of intraarticular steroids, therapy with analgesic agents that do not have antiinflammatory effects (for example, acetomenophen [Tylenol], propoxyphene [Darvon], surgery, and/or antidepressant drugs.
†Acetylsalicylic acid (aspirin) is the drug of choice in the initial treatment of rheumatoid arthritis. Nonsteroidal antiinflammatory drugs are aspirin-like drugs. Many patients prefer the NSAIAs over aspirin because they tend to produce less gastric irritation and some of them need be taken only once or twice a day.
‡It should also be noted that the immunosuppressive agents azathioprine (Imuran), cyclophosphamide (Cytoxan), and chlorambucil (Leukeran) have been used on an investigational basis in patients with severe disease that has not responded to the conventional medications. These are used with great care because of their severe side effects and the attendant risks of the development of neoplasms. The drug methotrexate has recently received F.D.A. approval for use in rheumatoid arthritis.

TABLE 70-4   Medications prescribed in the treatment of rheumatoid arthritis*—cont'd

Medication	Action	Side Effects/Toxic Effects	Precautions
SLOW-ACTING ANTIINFLAMMATORY AGENTS‡			
Antimalarials			
Hydroxychloroquine (Plaquenil)	Antiinflammatory (mechanism unknown); effect not expected to be noted for 6-12 mo after beginning therapy	Gastrointestinal disturbances; retinal edema that may result in blindness	Eye examination before beginning therapy and every 6 mo thereafter
Chloroquine (Aralen)	Same as hydroxychloroquine	Same as hydroxychloroquine	Same as hydroxychloroquine
Quinacrine (Atabrine)	Same as hydroxychloroquine	Same as hydroxychloroquine but may be better tolerated; yellow discoloration of skin	May be stopped periodically to prevent deepening of skin discoloration
Gold salts - I.M. Gold Sodium Thiomalate (Myochrysine) Gold Thioglucose (Solganol) Gold, - oral Auranofin (Ridaura)	Antiinflammatory; effect not noted for 3-6 mo after beginning therapy	Renal and hepatic damage; corneal deposits; dermatitis; ulcerations in mouth; hematologic changes	Urinalysis and CBC before each injection; report dermatitis, metallic taste in mouth, or lesions in mouth to physician Oral gold may produce fewer side effects than injectable, but periodic laboratory tests are required
Penicillamine (Cuprimine)	Antiinflammatory (mechanism unclear); effect not expected to be noted until several months after beginning treatment	Fever; skin rash; nephrotic syndrome; hematologic changes; gastrointestinal irritation; lupus-like syndromes; allergic reactions (33% probability if allergic to penicillin); retarded wound healing	Urinalysis, CBC, differential, hemoglobin and platelet count at least weekly for 3 mo, then monthly; report skin rash, fever to physician; food interferes with absorption—take on empty stomach between meals

amination, prescription of rest and appropriate exercise, education of patient and family, and control of inflammation with salicylates. Medications are progressively added based on the patient's response to basic therapy and with regard to the toxicity of the medications. Goals of therapy include the following:

1. Relief of pain
2. Maintenance of joint function
3. Prevention and correction of deformity by application of orthopaedic principles
4. Correction of other health factors

The pyramid of therapy is usually represented as illustrated in Figure 70-17. It should be noted that adjunctive therapy, at any level of the pyramid of management, may include the use of intraarticular steroids, therapy with analgesic agents that do not have antiinflammatory effects (for example, acetomenophen [Tylenol], propoxyphene [Darvon]), surgery, and/or antidepressant drugs. Specific drugs are listed in Table 70-4.

■ ASSESSMENT

Subjective and Objective Data

Early in the course of the disease, the patient may complain of chronic "tiredness," "aching and stiffness in my arms" or "in my legs," and loss of weight. As the disease progresses, the patient will be able to identify particular joints that are painful, will complain of loss of strength and ability to move joints freely, early morning stiffness lasting up to 2 hours (see research box on p 2055), and will express concern that pain interferes with normal ADL. The patient will also note that affected joints are changing in appearance. Many patients will express fear or despair over what is happening to them. (For a comprehensive assessment, see Chapter 68.)

Specific objective data to be gathered by the nurse include:

1. Inspection and palpation of the same joints on both sides of the body for symmetry, skin color, size, shape, tenderness, heat, and swelling
2. Limitation of active joint range of motion
3. Evidence of pain with active range of motion
4. Evidence of atrophy, loss of tone or tenderness in muscles associated with involved joints

■ DATA ANALYSIS: NURSING DIAGNOSES

Nursing diagnoses for the person with rheumatoid arthritis may include, but are not limited to, the following:

Diagnostic Title	Possible Etiologies
Knowledge deficit regarding arthritis	Lack of exposure

RESEARCH

Lambert Vickie A, RN, DNSc: Study of factors associated with psychological well-being in rheumatoid arthritic women, Image: The Journal of Nursing Scholarship 17(2):50-53, Spring 1985.

The author designed a study to identify and describe factors associated with psychological well-being in women afflicted with rheumatoid arthritis. Review of the literature had indicated that arthritic women not severely impaired by their illness were not necessarily capable of coping with the demands of the disease while in a work situation. The study examined social support, severity of illness, and demographic characteristics in relationship to each other and to the level of psychological well-being. The research questions sought correlations between social support, severity of illness, and demographic characteristics; correlations between these independent variables and the dependent variable of psychological well-being; and what combination of independent variables is the best predictor of the dependent variable. A sample of 92 women was selected by defined criteria and interviewed using the Bradburn Morale Scale, the Social Support Questionnaire, and the Functional Status Index. Results of the study indicated significant correlations between the variables of dependence on others, difficulty in performing tasks, and pain and the variable severity of illness. Negative correlation was identified between the variables of difficulty performing tasks and pain and the variable of psychological well-being. Pain emerged as the primary predictor of psychological well-being.

Implications for nurses are the need to identify pain, introduce pain management methods, teach preventive measures (for example, joint protection measures, exercise), and identify alternative support systems for the older arthritic woman in order to enhance psychological well-being. ■

Diagnostic Title	Possible Etiologies
Pain	Inflammation and swelling in joints
Injury, potential for	Loss of muscle strength and joint motion
Self-esteem, disturbance in	Change in body appearance
Self-care deficit: bathing/ hygiene, dressing/ grooming, feeding, toileting	Pain and musculoskeletal impairment

■ PLANNING: EXPECTED PATIENT OUTCOMES

Expected patient outcomes for the person with rheumatoid arthritis may include but are not limited to, the following:

1. The patient can explain the disease process, the applicability of treatment measures, and plans for follow-up with the physician.
2. The patient states he or she is feeling more comfortable.

RESEARCH

Crosby LJ: Stress factors, emotional stress and rheumatoid arthritis disease activity, J Adv Nurs 13(4):452-461, 1988.

The purpose of the study was to "determine the relationship between stress factors, emotional stress and rheumatoid arthritis disease activity." A correlation research design utilizing several instruments for measurement (including the Daily Hassles Scale, the State Trait Anxiety Inventory, Visual Analogue, a Rheumatoid Arthritis Disease Activity scale, and the serologic test erythrocyte sedimentation rate) permitted assessment "of the extent to which variation in RA disease activity corresponded with variation in other investigated variables." There were 101 subjects included in the study, 68 females and 33 males. Findings demonstrated a significant relationship between emotional stress experienced by the subjects and the level of their rheumatoid disease activity. It was also found that subjects were most concerned about health-related issues and that many of those health issues could be addressed by nursing interventions including instruction about energy conservation, rest therapy, and progressive relaxation. The author concludes that nurses must acknowledge the "powerful interaction between the mind and the body" and continue to incorporate a holistic approach in providing care. ■

3. The patient demonstrates improved active joint range of motion.
4. The patient describes a more positive self-concept.
5. The patient demonstrates improved ability to perform self-care activities.

■ IMPLEMENTATION

Patient Teaching

As for any chronic illness, patient teaching is perhaps the most important aspect of nursing care of patients with rheumatoid arthritis. It is, after all, the patient who will have to recognize response to prescribed therapy, who will have to follow the prescribed therapy correctly, and who will have to report the effectiveness of therapy to the physician. It is estimated that hundreds of millions of dollars are spent each year on gadgets, programs, and "medicines" allegedly able to "cure" arthritis. This money is spent by arthritics who often can ill afford the expense. It should be recognized that in some instances, the disease and disability associated with it may increase in spite of all legitimate efforts to control it; this is extremely discouraging for both patient and family and members of the health team. But many more persons are able to live reasonably normal, productive lives while managing their arthritis. To large extent, their ability to do so depends on their knowledge of the disease and its treatment.

Nurses teaching persons about rheumatoid arthritis (and other rheumatic diseases) may find it helpful to use some of the patient teaching material that has been prepared by the Arthritis Foundation. Booklets, such as *Arthritis: the basic facts,* are written in such a way that most patients can understand and learn from them. (See the research boxes on p. 2064.)

Patient teaching should include information about the following:

1. Proper balance of rest and activity
2. Joint protection and energy conservation techniques
3. Proper use of medications (that is, names of drugs, dosages, precautions in administration, and side effects or toxic effects)
4. Plans for implementation of the exercise program prescribed by the physician or physical therapist
5. Proper application of heat and/or cold packs
6. Proper use of walking aids and other assistive devices
7. Safety measures to prevent injury
8. Application of, appropriate use of, and care of splints, braces
9. Basics of good nutrition and the importance of avoiding weight gain
10. Importance of regular follow-up with the physician
11. Risks of following programs that promise a "cure"
12. Information about local arthritis support groups and programs, services of the Arthritis Foundation

Other Interventions

In addition to patient teaching, nursing interventions for the person with rheumatoid arthritis include measures to promote comfort, promote mobility, encourage good nutrition, and promote improved self-esteem. The guidelines for care of persons with rheumatoid arthritis can be found in the box at right.

Special Postoperative Care

When rheumatoid arthritis is relentless in its progression or has caused severe joint destruction, patients may achieve relief of pain and improved function through selected surgical intervention. Common procedures and postoperative care are outlined in Table 70-5.

SYSTEMIC LUPUS ERYTHEMATOSUS
EPIDEMIOLOGY/ETIOLOGY

Systemic lupus erythematosus (SLE) is a chronic inflammatory disease of unknown cause. It affects women, particularly adolescents and young adults, 8 to 10 times more often than men. The disease was named after its characteristic rash, the erosive nature of the rash being "likened to the damage wrought by a hungry

---

GUIDELINES FOR CARE OF PERSONS WITH RHEUMATOID ARTHRITIS

PROMOTE COMFORT

Provide prescribed medications on time and in prescribed doses (Table 70-4).
Provide heat or cold treatments as appropriate.
Promote frequent changes of position (patients are often more comfortable changing position themselves rather than having someone handle their sore joints).
Provide for adequate periods of rest.
Encourage use of resting splints.

PROMOTE MOBILITY

Avoid positioning joints in such a way as to encourage contracture (for example, pillows under knees when supine, pillows forcing neck into forward flexion).
Encourage regular active range of motion of joints to greatest degree possible.
Encourage patient to assist with own ADL to greatest degree possible, with assistive aids if necessary.
Encourage patient to perform prescribed exercises on a regular basis.
Provide appropriate ambulatory devices.
Encourage patient to wear *shoes,* not slippers, for ambulation.

PROMOTE NUTRITION

Encourage patient to eat well-balanced diet.
Encourage patient not to exceed ideal body weight.

PROMOTE IMPROVED SELF ESTEEM

Listen to patient
Reinforce patient's progress
Support patient's efforts
Refer for counseling if indicated (see p. 2057)

PROVIDE PATIENT TEACHING, SEE P. 2064.

---

wolf."[53] Once thought to be relatively rare and always fatal, better techniques for recognition of the disease have demonstrated it to be fairly common, and its course can be controlled by corticosteroids. Some patients do, however, die as a result of lesions affecting major organs or from secondary infections.

The cause of the disease is unknown, though two major areas are being investigated as possible causes. One possibility is that an aberration of the immune system causes immune complexes containing antibodies to be deposited in tissue, thereby causing tissue damage; the second possibility is the presence of a viral infection caused by or resulting from some immunologic abnormality. A third possibility is that both of these factors combine to produce the disease. Some drugs, notably procainamide (Pronestyl), isonicotinic acid hydrazide

TABLE 70-5 Surgical procedures and postoperative care for the patient with rheumatoid arthritis

Surgical Procedure	Purpose	Postoperative Care
Synovectomy	Commonly performed on the wrist or knee to arrest the course of rheumatoid arthritis in that joint, to maintain joint function, and to prevent episodic inflammation. (Synovium does grow back, so the disease process may recur; however, relief from discomfort will persist for a prolonged period.)	Joint is maintained at rest for 3-5 days or is passively exercised in continuous passive motion machine to ensure even healing of tissue. Active motion of joint is permitted 3-5 days after surgery. For the knee: 　Patient is instructed to perform quadriceps setting exercises in repetitions of 10 every 1-2 hr from the time of surgery. 　Patient is assisted to perform straight leg raising exercises four times a day until able to perform them independently. 　Patient begins partial weight-bearing ambulation with appropriate assistive devices when able to demonstrate independent straight leg raising and active flexion to at least 45 degrees.
Arthrotomy	Performed to explore or drain a joint or remove damaged tissue or foreign bodies (most often performed on the knee).	Care is essentially the same as for synovectomy, but motion and weight-bearing restrictions may not be observed for as long. (*Continuous passive motion machine is not likely to be used.*)
Arthrodesis	Surgical fusion of joint performed to eliminate painful motion and provide stability; commonly performed on knee, wrist, and ankle.	Joint is immobilized in cast and/or with external fixation device until healing (fusion) is accomplished. If joint is the knee, quadriceps setting and straight leg raising are taught as for synovectomy; partial weight bearing may be permitted after 10-14 days. If joint is the ankle, weight bearing will not be permitted for 1-3 mo.
Arthroplasty	Resurfacing of one or both sides of diseased joint to eliminate pain and improve motion.	Refer to page 2076 for special postoperative care.

(INH, Isoniazid), and penicillin are known to induce lupus-like syndromes.[43]

PATHOPHYSIOLOGY

Pathologic manifestations of the disease include the following:

1. Synovial involvement as a fibrous villous synovitis
2. Severe vasculitis with necrosis of the walls of the small arteries
3. Renal involvement with thickening of the basement membrane of the glomerular tufts and necrosis of the glomerular capillaries
4. Lymph node necrosis
5. Development of small white spots in the retina called *cytoid bodies*
6. Lesions of the nervous system

CLINICAL MANIFESTATIONS

The initial manifestation of SLE is often arthritis. In many instances the joint symptoms are transient and respond to treatment. Weakness, fatigue, and weight loss may be present. The patient may complain of sensi-

tivity to the sun, and developing a rash, and at times fever or arthritis on exposure to sunlight. *Erythema*, usually in a *butterfly pattern*, appears over the *cheeks and bridge of the nose.* The margins of these lesions are bright red, and the lesions may extend beyond the hairline with partial alopecia (loss of hair) above the ears. Lesions may also occur on the exposed part of the neck. Lesions spread slowly to the mucous membranes and other tissues of the body, or they may originate there. These lesions do not ulcerate, but cause degeneration and atrophy of tissues.

Depending on the organs involved, the patient may have findings of *glomerulonephritis, pleuritis, pericarditis, peritonitis, neuritis, or anemia. Renal and neurologic manifestations are among the more serious manifestations of the disease.*

Laboratory findings may be specific to the organs involved, as with proteinuria, abnormal cerebrospinal fluid, or x-ray film evidence of pleural reactions. *Positive antinuclear antigen* and *immunofluorescent studies are helpful in making the diagnosis of the disease.*

INTERVENTIONS
Medical Management

1. Rest when the disease is active
2. Exercise to maintain mobility
3. Avoidance of exposure to the sun
4. Medications
   a. Antiinflammatory analgesics to control arthritic pain
   b. Antimalarial drugs, particularly if rash is extensive
   c. Corticosteroids for severe neurologic and renal involvement
   d. Cytotoxic agents if other drugs fail
   e. Ointments or skin creams for rash
5. Kidney dialysis or transplant for uncontrolled lupus nephritis
6. Total hip replacement for avascular necrosis consequent to high-dose steroid therapy

Nursing Management

Patient teaching. Guiding and teaching the patient and family to understand and manage the disease is perhaps the most important function the nurse performs in relation to SLE. Teaching should include the following:

1. Nature, course and treatment of disease
2. Appropriate balance of rest and activity
3. Appropriate exercise
4. How to avoid exposing skin to sunlight; for example, wearing long-sleeved blouses or dresses, slacks, broad-brimmed hats, and cotton gloves
5. Appropriate use of prescribed medications (that is, dosage, frequency, precautions in administration, potential side effects)
6. Application of cosmetics (for example, hypoallergenic, approved by physician) to mask skin lesions, and/or wigs to mask hair loss
7. Information about lupus support groups (if available in patient's area)

Promoting comfort and ADL. The nurse can promote comfort by the following:

1. Administering prescribed medications for control of joint pain
2. Providing appropriate periods of rest
3. Assisting patient to gradually resume independence in ADL
4. Provide appropriate nursing care following renal transplant (Chapter 50) or total hip replacement (p. 2076), or during kidney dialysis (see Chapter 50)

POLYMYOSITIS (DERMATOMYOSITIS)
EPIDEMIOLOGY/ETIOLOGY

Polymyositis (dermatomyositis), an inflammatory disease involving striated (voluntary) muscle occurs two times more frequently in women than men. It may occur at any age, and is believed to affect 5 in every 1 million people in the United States. The cause of the disease is unknown; however, it is thought that some reaction of the autoimmune system is involved, perhaps triggered by a virus.

PATHOPHYSIOLOGY

Pathologic findings on histologic studies of biopsied muscle are variable, but the alterations found, in order of their frequency, are the following:

1. Primary degeneration of muscle fibers, either focal or extensive
2. Basophilia of some fibers with central migration of the sarcolemmal nuclei
3. Necrosis of parts or entire groups of muscle fibers
4. Inflammation of blood vessels supplying the muscles
5. Interstitial fibrosis varying in severity with the duration and, to some extent, the type of the disease
6. Variation in the cross-sectional diameter of fibers[55]

CLINICAL MANIFESTATIONS

The disease, which usually runs a *course of exacerbations and remissions*, is usually *first noted in proximal muscles, in particular the pelvic and shoulder girdles*. Climbing stairs, arising from a chair, and other activities that involve lifting the body become increasingly difficult or impossible. Lifting the arms becomes progressively more difficult, and hair combing may be impossible. Other muscles such as the neck flexors and the muscles of swallowing may also become involved. Muscle pain or tenderness is present in some instances in the early stages but not necessarily. Involvement of the skin in the form of a rash marks the disease as *dermatomyositis*. A *dusky red lesion* may be found in *the periorbital region*, along *with periorbital edema*. This dusky red rash may extend over the face, forehead, neck, upper shoulders, chest, and upper back. Lesions on the arms and legs commonly affect the extensor surfaces. These patches are sometimes scaly.

The *weakness of myositis, if it persists, can lead to contractures and atrophy. Individuals with the dermatomyositis form of the disease, particularly if they are over 40 years of age, have a 40% to 50% greater chance of having evidence of a malignant neoplasm found during the first 5 years of illness than the population at large.* Some physicians believe that routine yearly examinations should be performed to define or exclude the presence of neoplasms in these patients during that 5-year period.

Diagnostic tests include:

1. Manual muscle test to delineate weakness in specific muscles
2. Electromyogram to delineate a specific pattern of

findings to differentiate polymyositis from other types of muscle disease

3. Muscle biopsy to define specific pathologic changes in muscle

4. Serum enzymes (SGOT, CPK, aldolase) (elevated in presence of active disease)

5. 24-hour urine tests to determine abnormal creatine/creatinine ratio

INTERVENTIONS

Medical Management

Medical management for the person with polymyositis includes:

1. Rest

2. Corticosteroids in sufficient doses to effect remission of symptoms and reversal of abnormal laboratory values

Nursing Management

Nursing management is as follows:

1. Teaching
   a. Instruct patient and family in nature and course of disease
   b. Instruct patient in appropriate balance of rest and activity
   c. Instruct patient in use of selected ADL devices to enhance function (for example, long-handled comb)
   d. Instruct patient in appropriate use of prescribed steroids (how to take them, dosage, side effects, precautions

2. Promote comfort
   a. During acute episodes, assist with frequent changes of position
   b. Administer prescribed analgesics
   c. Assist with ADL
   d. Provide adequate rest

3. Promote mobility
   a. Elevate sitting surfaces to facilitate transfer
   b. Provide appropriate ambulatory device to facilitate comfortable walking
   c. Provide for frequent changes of position and range of motion to prevent contractures
   d. Encourage patient to gradually resume independent ADL as symptoms subside

4. Prevent skin breakdown
   a. Reposition patient frequently
   b. Avoid pressure over bony prominences with appropriate protective devices (see Chapter 69)

ANKYLOSING SPONDYLITIS

EPIDEMIOLOGY/ETIOLOGY

Ankylosing spondylitis is a *chronic progressive disorder affecting the joints of the hips and spine that occurs 9 times more frequently in men than women, usually be-* tween the ages of 10 and 30. The cause of the disease is unknown and its progression cannot be stopped by any treatment now known. There is a strong genetic link with the genetic marker HLA-B27, and it is thought that a link between the marker and some form of trigger (perhaps an infection) sets off a reaction in the immune system that leads to the inflammatory process. Approximately 400,000 people in the United States have the disease.[55]

PATHOPHYSIOLOGY

Spondylitis means inflammation of the spine. As a result of inflammation, the bones of the spine grow together, or ankylose (fuse). Inflammation usually begins around the sacroiliac joints, eventually obliterating articular cartilage of the affected bones. The cartilage is replaced by new bony growth. The inflammatory process progresses up the spine, eventually resulting in fusion of the entire spine.

CLINICAL MANIFESTATIONS

Initial symptoms may include *low back pain or aching; pain and swelling of the hips, knees, or shoulders; mild fever; loss of appetite; and fatigue.* Low back pain flares and subsides intermittently. Over a period of time, pain subsides and motion of the back becomes restricted. *Fusion of the sacroiliac joints and spine up through the cervical vertebrae may occur over a period of 10 to 20 years;* as a result, *the patient may have either a "poker-back" deformity or a kyphosis at the cervicodorsal junc-*

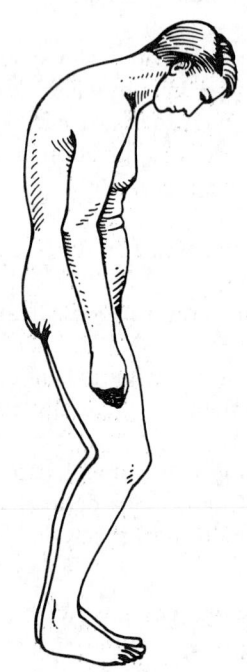

FIGURE 70-18 Characteristic posture in advanced ankylosing spondylitis.

tion (Figure 70-18). Knees are flexed as the person attempts to move the head into an upright position.

Diagnostic tests helpful in defining this disease are:

1. Presence in the serum of HLA-B27
2. X-ray films showing bony growths, called *syndesmophytes*, that bridge adjacent vertebrae to give the spine a "bamboo" appearance

INTERVENTIONS

Medical Management

Goals of treatment are to relieve pain, achieve and maintain the best possible alignment of the spine, strengthen the paraspinal muscles, and prevent interference with breathing capacity. Following are the most common interventions.

1. Prescription of postural exercises; for example, prone lying (extension) 3 to 4 times a day for 15 to 30 minutes
2. Rest
3. Heat
4. Antiinflammatory analgesics
   a. Salicylates
   b. NSAIA
   c. Potent antiinflammatory agents on short-term basis (phenylbutazone)
5. Spinal osteotomy or hip arthroplasty for persons with severe symptoms

Nursing Management

Nursing management focuses on the following:

1. Patient teaching
   a. Nature and course of disease
   b. Prescribed postural exercises
   c. Appropriate use of prescribed medications
   d. Methods of applying heat to back and hips
2. Promote correct posture and prevent complications
   a. Provide firm mattress and bedboard
   b. Encourage patient to sleep without pillow under the head
   c. Supervise and encourage regular postural exercises
   d. Encourage respiratory exercises
3. Promote comfort and relieve pain
   a. Provide heat applications/hydrotherapy, especially before exercises
   b. Administer prescribed medications on time

NONARTICULAR RHEUMATISM

Nonarticular rheumatic diseases include those disorders in which the supportive structures and structures located near the joints are inflamed, but the joints themselves are not involved except by the limitations imposed by the supportive structures. *Some of these disorders are fibrositis, tenosynovitis, bursitis, and carpal tunnel syndrome.*

BURSITIS

EPIDEMIOLOGY/ETIOLOGY

Bursitis, or inflammation of the bursa, may be acute or chronic. It is usually caused by trauma, strain, and overuse of the joint with which the bursa is associated. The shoulder bursa is most often affected.

PATHOPHYSIOLOGY/CLINICAL MANIFESTATIONS

The synovial lining of the bursal sac becomes inflamed, more fluid is secreted, and the bursa swells. Occasionally, large calcium deposits are present. The swelling is accompanied by pain and limited ability to move the associated joint or the entire extremity.

INTERVENTIONS

Medical Management

Medical management includes the following:

1. Rest for the involved area
2. Antiinflammatory agents
   a. Salicylates
   b. Phenylbutazone
   c. Indomethacin
   d. Injection of adrenocorticosteroids into bursa
3. Application of cold during early acute phase (heat is avoided because it increases fluid exudate in the bursa during early inflammatory period)
4. Surgical removal of calcium deposits

Nursing Management

Nursing management includes the following:

1. Patient teaching regarding rest, appropriate use of cold applications and prescribed medications
2. Promoting comfort through provision of rest, cold applications, and assistance with ADL

CARPAL TUNNEL SYNDROME

EPIDEMIOLOGY/ETIOLOGY

Carpal tunnel syndrome is caused by pressure being exerted on the median nerve of the wrist. The condition is *most common in middle-aged women and may occur as a result of trauma or of swelling of tendon sheaths caused by processes like rheumatoid arthritis.*

PATHOPHYSIOLOGY

The median nerve passes through a tunnel bounded by the carpal bones dorsally and the transverse carpal ligament volarly (Figure 70-19). Flexor tendons run through the tunnel parallel to the median nerve. Inflammation and swelling of the synovial lining of tendon sheaths narrow the space available and cause compression of the median nerve.

CLINICAL MANIFESTATIONS

The patient will complain of *dysesthesia, paresthesia, and hypesthesia of the thumb, index, and middle fin-*

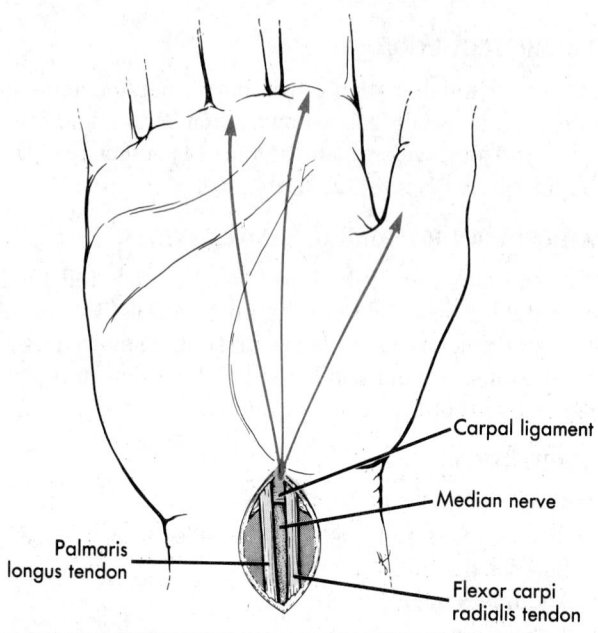

Palmaris
longus tendon

Carpal ligament

Median nerve

Flexor carpi
radialis tendon

FIGURE 70-19 Carpal tunnel syndrome. Volar aspect of wrist retracted to demonstrate position of median nerve. Distribution of median nerve is to thumb and first two fingers. (Adapted from Compere EL: Orthopaedic surgery, Chicago, 1974, Year Book Medical Publishers, Inc.)

gers. Complaints will usually increase when there has been forced flexion of the hand for long periods, such as when knitting. The symptoms can be elicited by tapping the median nerve at the wrist (Tinel's sign). The patient may feel that the hand is "swollen" and may complain of clumsiness when using the hand, especially when grasping or holding on to small objects. Referred pain to the upper extremity is common. Atrophy of the thenar eminence (the padded area of the palm below the base of the thumb) may be present in late disease.

INTERVENTIONS

Medical Management

Medical management of carpal tunnel syndrome includes the following:
1. Rest
2. Splinting of the wrist
3. Local steroid injections
4. Surgical release of the transverse carpal ligament to decompress the median nerve (usually an ambulatory procedure)

Nursing Management

Nursing management includes the following:
1. Patient teaching
   a. Instruct patient regarding rest, splinting
   b. Provide preoperative instruction if surgery is planned

2. Postoperative care and instruction
   a. Promoting comfort and circulation
      (1) Elevating hand and arm for 24 hours
      (2) Encouraging active thumb and finger motion within limits imposed by dressing
      (3) Administering prescribed analgesic as necessary
   b. Promoting safety
      (1) Check fingers for circulation, sensation, and movement every 1 to 2 hours for 24 hours
   c. Promoting self care
      (1) Encourage patient to use hand in normal ADL 2 to 3 days following surgery

DUPUYTREN'S CONTRACTURE
PATHOPHYSIOLOGY AND CLINICAL MANIFESTATIONS

Dupuytren's contracture is a *common problem, particularly in men past middle age. It often occurs bilaterally. Hyperplasia and progressive fibrosis of the palmar fascia on the ulnar side of the hand cause progressive shortening of the pretendinous bands to the ring and sometimes the small fingers.* The bands shorten, and the fingers are pulled into fixed flexion. The skin of the palm is drawn down, forming tight puckers and nodules.

INTERVENTIONS

Medical Management

Medical management includes the following:
1. Avoidance of activities that require grasping an object, for example, a hammer
2. Soaking hand in warm water while actively performing finger extension exercise
3. Surgical removal of involved palmar fascia (usually an ambulatory procedure)

Nursing Management/Postoperative Care

Nursing management includes the following:
1. Elevate hand to control swelling for at least 24 hours.
2. Check fingers for circulation, sensation, movement every 1 to 2 hours for 24 hours.
3. Administer prescribed analgesics as necessary to maintain comfort.
4. Encourage active extension of fingers.
5. Avoid passive extension of fingers.
6. Encourage patient to begin using hand in self-care activities after 2 to 3 days.

DEGENERATIVE DISORDERS

DEGENERATIVE JOINT DISEASE
EPIDEMIOLOGY/ETIOLOGY

Degenerative joint disease, also known as *osteoarthritis, hypertrophic arthritis, osteoarthrosis,* or *sene-*

scent arthritis, is an *extremely common disease that is probably as old as civilization*. Almost everyone past 40 years of age has hypertrophic changes in the joints. Although symptomatic degenerative joint disease is usually noted in the 50- to 70-year age group, it has been observed as early as age 20. *It is estimated that 17 million people in the United States have osteoarthritis serious enough to cause pain*. There are two forms of osteoarthritis: *primary*, for which the cause is unknown; and *secondary*, a result of trauma, infections, previous fractures, another type of arthritis (such as rheumatoid arthritis), the stress put on weight-bearing joints from long-term obesity, or the wear and tear on joints associated with some occupations (for example, coal mining and boxing). There may also be a genetic predisposition to the development of osteoarthritis.[55]

PREVENTION

Factors to be considered in the prevention of osteoarthritis are the following:
1. Avoidance of obesity
2. Avoidance of repeated trauma to joints
3. Practice of joint protection techniques in occupations that put joints at risk

PATHOPHYSIOLOGY

Degenerative joint disease (DJD) is a disease of the articular cartilage. Normally this cartilage is white, translucent, and smooth. When affected by the disease, it becomes yellow and opaque. Areas of cartilage soften and the surface becomes rough, frayed, and cracked. This process is thought to occur as a result of digestion of the cartilage by enzymes and alteration of the nutrition of the cartilage. Eventually the cartilage is destroyed, and the underlying subchondral bone goes through a remodeling process. *Osteophytes*, or spurs of new bone, appear at the joint margins and at the sites of attachment of supporting structures. These may break off and appear in the joint cavity as "joint mice." Unlike rheumatoid arthritis, *DJD affects only the joints and their surrounding tissue. It is not a systemic disease.*

CLINICAL MANIFESTATIONS

Individuals with DJD have pain in the movable joints, particularly the large weight-bearing joints (hips and knees) and the joints of the hand. Inflammation is usually not present, and tenderness is mild; however, the joints may become enlarged. Crepitation may be present on movement, and changes may occur in the alignment of the extremity. The patient's joints are usually stiff after periods of rest.

The following characteristic changes or symptoms occur in certain joints:
1. *Heberden's nodes*—bony protuberances occurring on the dorsal surface of the distal interphalangeal joints of the fingers (Figure 70-20)
2. *Bouchard's nodes*—bony protuberances occurring on the proximal interphalangeal joints of the fingers
3. *Coxarthrosis* (DJD of the hip)—pain in the hip on weight bearing, with pain progressing to include groin and medial knee pain and limited range of motion

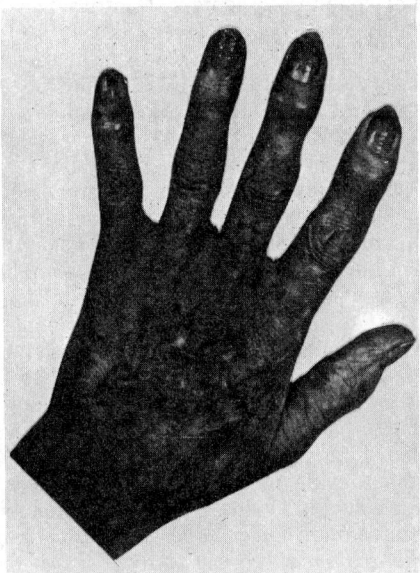

FIGURE 70-20 Osteoarthritis of hand. Note enlargement of distal joints of index, middle, and little finger (Heberden's nodes). (From Brashear H and Raney R: Shand's handbook of orthopaedic surgery, ed 9, St Louis, 1978, The CV Mosby Co.)

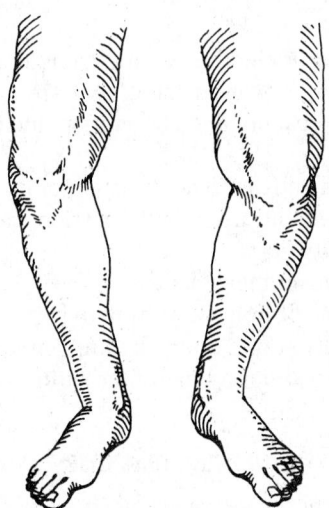

FIGURE 70-21 Characteristic bowing deformity of knees in degenerative arthritis. This deformity can be corrected by tibial osteotomy or total knee replacement.

4. Knee involvement—varus (Figure 70-21), valgus, or flexion deformity, crepitus, and limited range of motion

Serologic and synovial fluid examinations will be essentially normal. However, X-ray films will reveal narrowing of the joint space, osteophyte formation, and *eburnation* (sclerosis) of subchondral bone.

Medical Management

Objectives in management include relief of pain, restoration of joint function, and prevention of disability or further progression of the disease. Management methods include the following:

1. Medication
   a. Salicylates, NSAIAs
   b. Intraarticular injection of steroids for severe discomfort
   c. Adjunctive analgesics (Tylenol, Darvon)
2. Unloading painful weight-bearing joints through use of canes, walkers, crutches
3. Rest
4. Exercise
5. Joint protection
6. Surgery
   a. Removal of bits of broken cartilage or bone (débridement, usually by arthroscopic surgery)
   b. Realignment (osteotomy)
   c. Fusion (arthrodesis)
   d. Joint replacement (replacement arthroplasty)

■ ASSESSMENT

Subjective data include the following:

1. Where does pain occur?
2. When does pain occur?
3. What measures give relief?
4. What modifications in ADL have been made necessary by pain?

Objective data include assessing signs that are usually localized to the involved joints and are determined by inspection, palpation, and observation, including the following:

1. Limited active range of motion of involved joints
2. Enlargement; irregularity; flexion, varus or valgus deformity
3. Crepitus on movement
4. Presence of limp when walking
5. Difficulty sitting after standing for a period of time or arising from a chair after sitting for a period of time

■ DATA ANALYSIS: NURSING DIAGNOSES

Nursing diagnoses are determined from assessment of patient data. Possible nursing diagnoses for the person with DJD may include, but are not limited to the following:

Diagnostic Title	Possible Etiologies
Knowledge deficit: regarding DJD	Lack of exposure, unfamiliarity with information resources
Pain	Pathologic changes in articular cartilage and stiffness in affected joints
Mobility, impaired physical	Pain/discomfort
Activity intolerance	Pain/discomfort
Self-care deficit: bathing/ hygiene, dressing/ grooming, toileting	Pain and limited joint movement
Nutrition, altered: more than body requirements	Excessive intake in relation to ability to exercise

RESEARCH

Laborde JM and Powers MJ: Life satisfaction, health control orientation, and illness-related factors in persons with osteoarthritis, Res Nurs Health 8(1):183-190, 1985.

This study was based on the hypothesis that as a result of living with chronic pain, osteoarthritics' satisfaction with life may decrease. An earlier study by the same authors (1980) indicated that activities associated with a productive life were more compromised for arthritics with pain than for patients undergoing hemodialysis. The aim of this study was to explore "changes over time in levels of life satisfaction in a group of osteoarthritics and to examine the relative impact of illness-related and health belief factors on present life situation." A convenience sample of 160 osteoarthritic subjects was obtained at 4 different settings: an urban senior center, an outpatient clinic at a university hospital, an outpatient clinic at an urban private hospital, and 2 rural community centers. Cantril's Self-Anchoring Striving scale was used to assess the subjects' general sense of well-being, or life satisfaction, at three points in time: past, present, and future. The Health Locus of Control measure was administered to determine whether the subjects perceived their health-related expectations in terms of external or internal control. Additionally, subjects were interviewed for demographic and arthritis-related information. Measurements of past, present, and anticipated life satisfaction were obtained. Results indicated that past and present life satisfaction were viewed favorably by subjects, but "aspirations for future life satisfaction declined appreciably." The mean score for the total sample indicated "an external orientation in health beliefs for the entire group." Present life satisfaction was "found to be significantly associated with better health perception, internal health locus of control, and less joint pain." The authors suggest that "internally oriented individuals . . . engage in lifestyles that provide more satisfying experiences" than externally controlled individuals, and they conclude that osteoarthritics who are *given educational programs adjunctive to therapy may become more positive about their present satisfaction with life.* These conclusions were supported by a study by Bradbury and Catanzaro (Bradbury VL and Catanzaro M-L: The quality of life in a male population suffering from arthritis, Rehabil Nurs 14(4):187-190, 1989.) ■

■ PLANNING: EXPECTED PATIENT OUTCOMES

Expected patient outcomes for the person with DJD may include, but are not limited to, the following:

1. Patient can explain the disease process, the applicability of treatment measures, and plans for follow-up with the physician.
2. Patient states he or she is feeling more comfortable.
3. Patient is able to be more physically active.
4. Patient balances rest and activity appropriately.
5. Patient demonstrates improved ability to perform self-care activities.
6. Patient can state rationale for not exceeding ideal weight.

■ IMPLEMENTATION

As with rheumatoid arthritis, teaching the person with DJD about the disease process and the steps to take to control that process is the most important aspect of nursing care. (See the research box on p. 2072.) Patient teaching should include the same types of information outlined on p. 2064. Other interventions are the same as those outlined in guidelines for care of persons with rheumatoid arthritis, p. 2065.

Special Postoperative Care

As noted above, surgical intervention may be necessary to remove damaged bone or cartilage from the joint, realign or change the weight-bearing surfaces of the joint,

or resurface the joint. The objectives of surgery are to relieve pain, restore joint function (if possible), and prevent disability or further progression of the disease.

Surgery to the knee and hip are most common, but shoulder surgery is becoming more practical and effective. The following specific surgeries are performed:

1. Debridement (usually by arthroscopic surgery or arthrotomy).
   a. See Table 70-5 on p. 2066 for postoperative nursing care
2. Arthrodesis
   a. Through fusion of the joint, pain is relieved; joint motion is lost, but weight-bearing function is maintained. See Table 70-5 on p. 2066 for postoperative care.
3. Osteotomy
   a. Bone is cut to change alignment, thereby correcting deformity in the bone or adjacent joint. The procedure corrects angulation or rotational deformities or alters the weight-bearing surface in a diseased joint (Figure 70-22). Osteotomy may be thought of as a surgical or intentional fracture, and the extremity is treated as following a fracture with the exception that weight bearing may be started earlier to promote healing. Immobilization of the extremity and nursing interventions are similar to those used following a fracture (see Chapter 69).

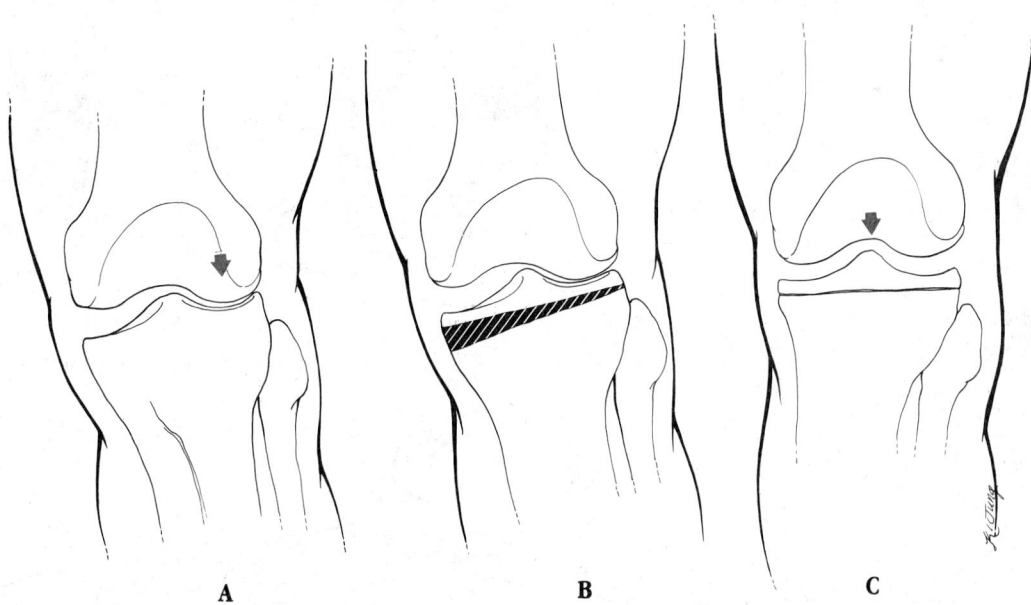

FIGURE 70-22 Osteotomy of tibia. Genu valgum (anterior view of left knee). **A,** Weight-bearing force is concentrated on one compartment of knee. **B,** Wedge of bone is removed from tibia. Amount of bone removed is determined by how much correction in angulation is necessary. **C,** Distal portion of tibia is swung to proximal portion. Correction of angulation obtained allows weight-bearing forces to be more evenly distributed through both compartments of knee. (Adapted from Hollander JL and McCarty DR Jr: Arthritis and allied conditions, ed 8, Philadelphia, 1972, Lea & Febiger.)

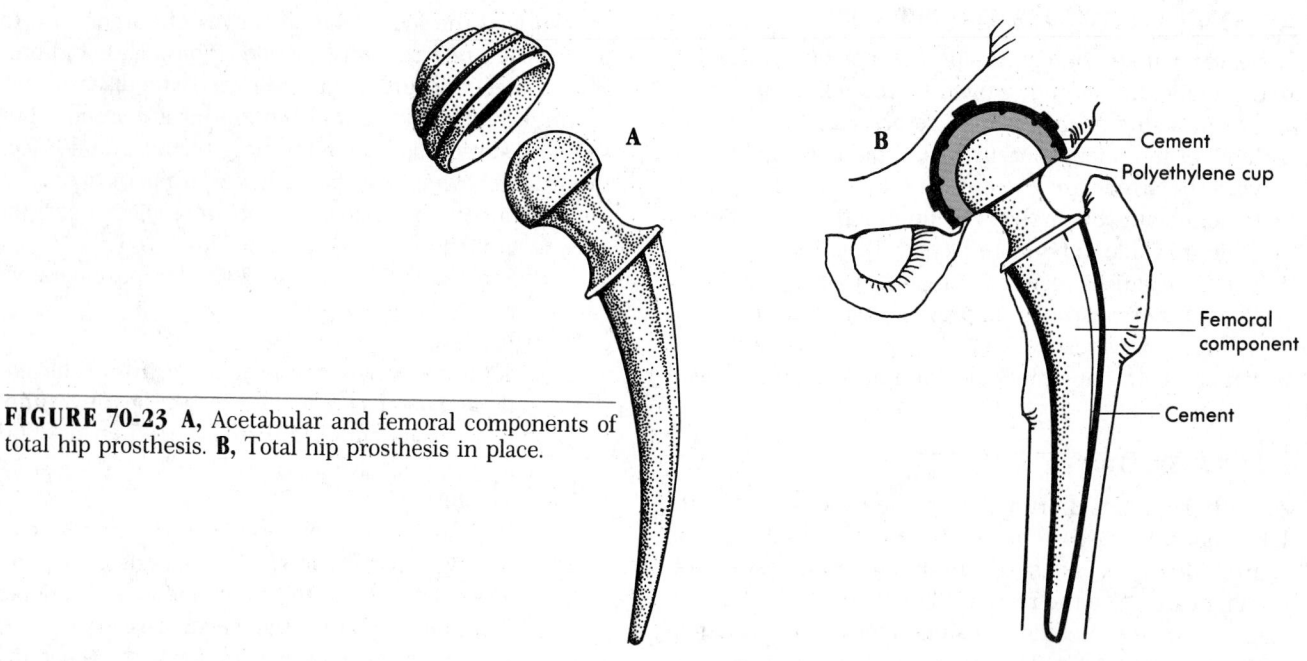

FIGURE 70-23 A, Acetabular and femoral components of total hip prosthesis. **B,** Total hip prosthesis in place.

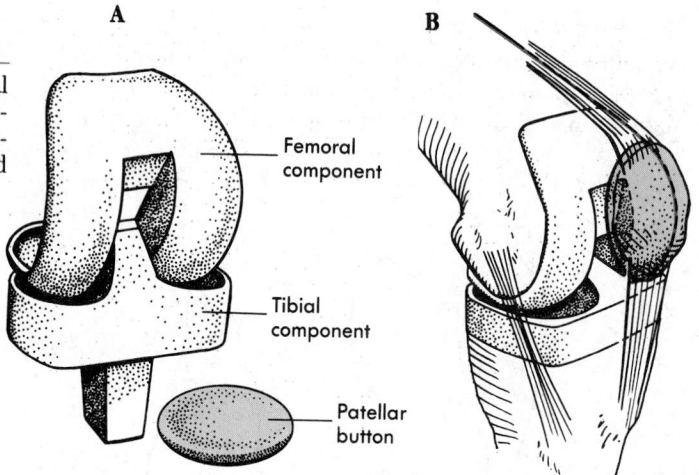

FIGURE 70-24 A, Tibial and femoral components of total knee prosthesis. Patellar button, made of polyethylene, protects posterior surface of patella from friction against femoral component when knee is moved through flexion and extension. **B,** Total knee prosthesis in place.

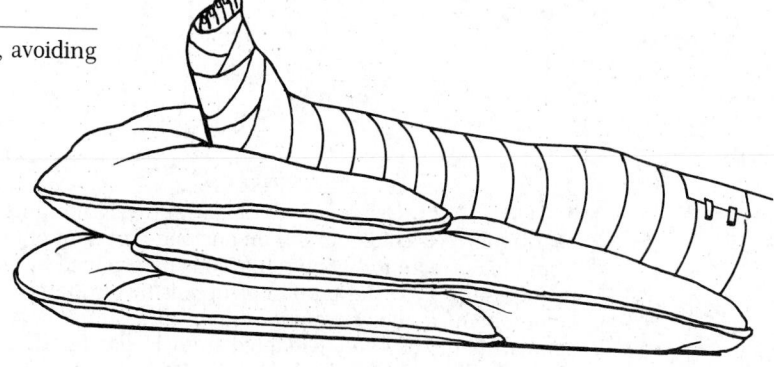

FIGURE 70-25 Leg properly elevated on pillows, avoiding knee flexion.

4. Two types of arthroplasty
   a. Interposition involves resurfacing of one side of the joint with metal or other inert material or soft tissue such as fascia.
   b. Replacement involves resurfacing of both sides of the joint with metal or polyethelyene implants. Replacement implants are available for the hip (Figure 70-23), knee (Figure 70-24), shoulder, ankle, elbow, wrist, and interphalangeal joints of the fingers. Replacement prostheses may be either *cemented* (held into bone with polymethylmethacrylate) or *uncemented* (treated with a special porous coating that promotes ingrowth of bone).

The care of persons experiencing total hip or knee replacement are described in the box below and in the box on p. 2076. Understanding the mobility restrictions is of utmost importance when providing patient care (see nursing care plan on p. 2077). Of equal importance is the prevention of infection. The area of the operation must be kept free of contamination. Infection of bone implanted with prosthetic materials will require removal of the prostheses. *Prevention of infection continues after the wound has healed; antibiotic prophylaxis must be given for future surgeries, dental work involving scraping or extraction, severe trauma or contaminated skin wounds, or systemic bacterial infection (respiratory or urinary).*

GUIDELINES FOR NURSING INTERVENTIONS FOR THE PERSON WITH TOTAL KNEE REPLACEMENT

PREOPERATIVE CARE
Same as for total hip replacement

POSTOPERATIVE CARE
1. Positioning
   a. The operative leg(s) is elevated on pillows to enhance venous return for the first 48 hours. Pillows are placed with caution not to flex the knee(s) (Figure 70-25). It is becoming more common for patients to have bilateral total knee replacements at one surgery.
   b. The patient may be turned from side to back to side.
2. Wound care
   a. Care of drains as for total hip replacement.
   b. Patient is assessed for systemic evidence of loss of blood (hypotension, tachycardia) if bulky compression dressing is used, since it may hold large quantities of drainage before drainage is visible.
   c. Bulky dressings are removed before the patient begins active flexion.
3. Activity
   a. Passive flexion in a continuous passive motion machine (CPM) within prescribed flexion-extension limits may be started in the recovery room. Patient's leg may remain in machine as much as tolerated (up to 22 hours per day) to facilitate even healing of tissue.
   b. Patient is encouraged to perform active dorsiplantar flexion of the ankles, quadriceps setting, and, after the drain is removed, straight leg-raising exercises.
   c. Patient begins active flexion exercises three to four times a day about the third to fifth postoperative day.
   d. Light weight bearing with an assistive device may be started as early as the first postoperative day and increased as the patient tolerates.
   e. Sitting in a chair with the leg(s) elevated may be started on the first postoperative day.
   f. Patient may be encouraged to wear a resting knee extension splint (immobilizer) on the operated leg(s) until able to demonstrate quadriceps control (independent straight leg raising).
4. Pain control
   a. Initial control of pain is with narcotics, positioning; medication is gradually decreased to nonnarcotic analgesics as patient tolerates.
   b. Patient is encouraged to apply ice to knee(s) for 20 to 30 minutes before and following active flexion exercise.
   c. Ice may be prescribed more frequently to reduce pain in some patients
5. Discharge instructions
   a. Patient must observe partial weight-bearing restriction and use ambulatory aid for approximately 2 months following discharge.
   b. Patient should continue active flexion and straight leg raising exercises at home.
   c. Patient must be made aware of the lifelong need for antibiotic prophylaxis before surgery or dental work.

GUIDELINES FOR NURSING INTERVENTIONS FOR THE PERSON WITH TOTAL HIP REPLACEMENT

PREOPERATIVE CARE

1. Skin care
   a. Preparation of the skin will follow the hospital's written procedure or the physician's written orders.
   b. Patient's environment must be as free as possible from potential sources of infection.
2. Reassurance and education
   a. Patient needs to understand about the surgical procedure, postoperative care, and limitations after discharge.
   b. Both hips may be replaced at one surgery.

POSTOPERATIVE CARE

1. Positioning
   a. Positioning will depend on the design of the prosthesis and the method of insertion. Restrictions designed to avoid dislocation of the prosthesis usually include these:
      (1) Flexion is limited to 60 degrees for 6 to 7 days, then 90 degrees for 2 to 3 months.
      (2) No adduction is permitted beyond midline for 2 to 3 months, therefore no sidelying on operative side unless ordered by the surgeon. Leg is maintained in abduction when lying supine or on nonoperative side.
      (3) No extreme internal or external rotation is permitted.
2. Wound care
   a. Drains are placed in wound to prevent formation of hematoma.
   b. Maintain constant suction through self-contained suction device (for example, Porto-Vac).
   c. Note amount and types of drainage.
   d. Keep area free from contamination.
3. Activity
   a. Observe flexion restrictions when elevating head of bed.
   b. Encourage periodic elevation and lowering of head of bed to provide motion at hip.
   c. Instruct patient in use of overhead trapeze to shift weight and lift for bedpan, change of linen.
   d. Encourage active dorsiplantar flexion exercise of ankles and quadriceps and gluteal setting exercises to promote venous return, prevent thrombus formation, and maintain muscle tone (see Chapter 24).
   e. Patient may be turned to unoperative side with operative leg maintained in abduction and extension.
   f. Begin ambulation as early as the first postoperative day, if tolerated.
      (1) Observe flexion and adduction restrictions.
      (2) Observe weight-bearing restrictions prescribed by surgeon (usually partial weight bearing assisted with walker or crutches).
      (3) Increase amount of walking each day according to patient's tolerance.
   g. Begin sitting when patient demonstrates sufficient control of leg to sit within flexion restrictions (usually requires elevation of sitting surfaces, including use of raised toilet seat).
4. Medications
   a. Prophylactic anticoagulant drugs (acetylsalicylic acid, low-dose heparin, or coumadin) may be prescribed to decrease risk of thrombus formation.
   b. Initially, control pain with positioning; use narcotics, gradually tapered to nonnarcotic analgesics according to patient's tolerance.
5. Discharge instructions
   a. Patient must use ambulatory aid, avoid adduction, and limit hip flexion to 90 degrees for about 2 to 3 months.
   b. A raised toilet seat is to be obtained and used at home until flexion restrictions are removed.
   c. Patient may need a long-handled shoe horn and reacher to facilitate ADL within flexion restriction.
   d. Patient must be made aware of the lifelong need for antibiotic prophylaxis to protect the prosthesis from bacteremic infection (see p. 2075).

DEGENERATIVE DISEASE OF THE SPINE
PATHOPHYSIOLOGY

Degenerative disease of the spine is a common but difficult problem that merits special consideration. The spine has 23 intervertebral disk joints and 46 posterior facet joints (Figure 70-26), all of which are subjected to stresses and strains in holding the human body upright and moving it about. The vertebrae in the spinal column are articulated in a series of "couplets" that are able to move through an intervertebral disk joint and two poste-

rior facet joints. The intervertebral disks are composed of an outer layer of cartilage called the *anulus fibrosus* and an inner layer of cartilage called the *nucleus pulposus*. Several common problems arise with these structures in degenerative disease of the spine.

1. *Herniated nucleus pulposus* (HNP), degeneration and dehydration of the cartilage composing the anulus and the nucleus, results in a loss of elasticity. As the disk loses its resiliency, a strong force exerted across it can result in herniation of the nucleus through the an-

NURSING CARE PLAN

PERSON WITH TOTAL KNEE REPLACEMENT

DATA: Mr. K. is a 59-year-old married office manager with osteoarthritis of the right knee. Over the past 8 months, he has had increased pain in his knee with only minimal relief from nonsteroidal antiinflammatory medications prescribed by his internist. He reports that he must now ambulate with a cane when his pain is severe. He can no longer participate in many activities he used to enjoy because of his discomfort and limited mobility. After consulting his internist and an orthopaedic surgeon, he has decided to undergo elective total knee replacement. Mr. K. is admitted to the nursing division on the morning of the day he is scheduled for surgery. Collaborative nursing actions include those to identify possible complications of the surgery.

The nursing history identified the following:
- Mr. and Mrs. K. reside in a two-story colonial house with the bedroom upstairs.
- Mr. K. plans to return home after this hospitalization and has received a 6 weeks' leave of absence from his job.
- He is not prescribed any medications other than his "arthritis pills," and has no other preexisting medical problems.
- Mr. K. was last hospitalized 18 years ago for a cholecystectomy.
- He attended a total knee replacement class 2 weeks ago as part of his preadmission screening.

Immediate reporting of and treatment of early signs and symptoms may prevent serious effects. Nursing actions include monitoring for the following:
- Neurocirculatory compromise: Perform neurocirculatory checks every 2 hours for the first 24 to 48 hours; notify physician of any changes from preoperative status.
- Impaired skin integrity and/or wound healing: Monitor pressure areas for signs of redness, monitor temperature, assess incision for signs or symptoms or infection or excessive drainage.
- Atelectasis/respiratory infection: Monitor breath sounds until ambulatory, encourage deep breathing and coughing until ambulatory.
- Problems with elimination: Assess for urinary stasis and constipation.
- Fluid and electrolyte imbalance: Monitor intake and output until patient is taking oral fluids comfortably, monitor IV fluid flow, assess patient for fluid volume excess or deficit.

NURSING DIAGNOSIS

Knowledge deficit related to lack of exposure to total knee replacement surgery

Expected Patient Outcomes	Nursing Interventions	Rationale

Patient states he understands the teaching provided. Patient will have less anxiety related to fear of the unknown and/or misconceptions regarding the surgery and recovery period.	Preoperatively:
	 1. Assess need for further instruction and provide as necessary.
	 2. Review preoperative instruction with patient and family before surgery. Use written materials if they are available.
	 3. Evaluate patient's understanding of the information taught.
	
	 Postoperatively:
	 1. Assure that patient can explain or demonstrate the following:
	   a. Independent transfer and ambulation with appropriate ambulatory aid.
	   b. Exercises to be performed at home (straight leg raising and active flexion) and with what frequency.
	   c. Activity restrictions, including avoidance of kneeling and jarring activities, that are to be observed for 2 mo or until follow-up with the surgeon.
	 2. Evaluate patient's understanding of the need for antibiotic prophylaxis in the future, and reinforce as necessary.
		Understanding the surgical procedure and postoperative recovery should lessen anxiety and promote behaviors that will enhance recovery from surgery.

Continued.

NURSING CARE PLAN

PERSON WITH TOTAL KNEE REPLACEMENT—cont'd

NURSING DIAGNOSIS

Pain, related to knee replacement surgery

Expected Patient Outcomes	Nursing Interventions	Rationale
Patient states feeling comfortable.	Assess patient's pain and evaluate response to comfort measures provided.	Subjective and objective data are important to ascertain the nature of the patient's postoperative pain and how to manage it.
Patient is able to perform necessary postoperative routines/exercises because pain is adequately managed.	Administer prescribed narcotic analgesics at timely intervals throughout postoperative course, particularly before exercise periods. Patient may be taking patient-controlled analgesia (PCA)	It is usually necessary to administer narcotic analgesics the first 48-72 hr after surgery. Analgesics have a greater effect if they are administered before pain becomes severe.
	Teach relaxation techniques as appropriate.	Relaxation facilitates rest and may modify the patient's response to pain.
	Use other pain-relieving measures as pertinent (for example, back rubs, repositioning, ice to knee for 30 min before and after active flexion exercises).	A change in type of cutaneous stimulation may result in pain relief. Ice is analgesic and retards swelling.
	As pain decreases, use milder analgesics.	Pain, as it lessens in severity, can be controlled by less potent analgesics that have fewer side effects.

NURSING DIAGNOSIS

Mobility, impaired physical: related to alterations in lower limb following total knee replacement surgery

Expected Patient Outcomes	Nursing Interventions	Rationale
Patient will demonstrate optimal level of mobility with adaptive devices by time of discharge from hospital.	Turn patient side to back to side every 2 hr and as necessary while bed rest is ordered.	Turning and repositioning frequently provides for better ventilation of the lungs.
No injury will occur during hospitalization.	Encourage patient to perform active dorsiplantar flexion, isometric quadriceps setting exercises, and, after drain is removed, straight let raises every 2 hr until fully ambulatory, then 4 times/day.	Exercises of the lower extremities will prevent venous stasis and promote muscle strengthening.
	Elevate operative leg on pillows in bed and when patient is up in chair for the first 24-48 hours. Place pillows so that passive flexion of the knee is avoided.	Elevation of the operative leg on pillows enhances venous return. Flexion contracture is to be avoided.
	Assist patient to transfer out of bed on first postoperative day. Light weight bearing on the operated leg is generally permitted using an assistive device.	The exercise of getting in and out of bed is one means of increasing activity in the early postoperative period. The patient accrues numerous physiologic benefits from such activity.
	Assist patient to walk as tolerated, increasing the frequency and the distance walked each day.	Early ambulation is a significant factor in hastening recovery and preventing postoperative complications.

NURSING CARE PLAN

PERSON WITH TOTAL KNEE REPLACEMENT—cont'd

Encourage patient to sit up in a chair as tolerated, especially for meals.	
If continuous passive motion machine is used, patient's leg should be in the machine a minimum of 8-12 hr/day and can be in the machine up to 22 hr/day if tolerated. Advance the degrees of flexion being obtained in the machine according to the surgeon's prescription.	Passive flexion of the knee may prevent excessive swelling and bruising at the site of the surgery, and it may promote more even healing of the involved joint tissues.
Begin active flexion exercise of the knee on the second postoperative day, and encourage flexion 4 times/day.	Active flexion of the knee is necessary to promote return of function. It is desired that the patient achieve approximately 90 degrees of active flexion before discharge from the hospital.
A knee immobilizer may be worn at night as a night resting splint.	The knee immobilizer splints the resting knee, helping to prevent painful muscle spasm.

NURSING DIAGNOSIS

Home maintenance management, impaired, related to discharge needs

Expected Patient Outcomes	Nursing Interventions	Rationale
Patient and family will express satisfaction with arrangements made to manage self-care at home.	Discuss with patient and family any problems they anticipate with management of self-care at home. Determine the type of equipment needed, for example, crutches, walker, elevated toilet seat; consult appropriate department or agency for assistance in procuring these supplies. Assure that the patient can climb stairs. If not, help the patient to arrange for first floor sleeping arrangements.	Adequate discharge planning will foster safe, successful completion of rehabilitation at home.

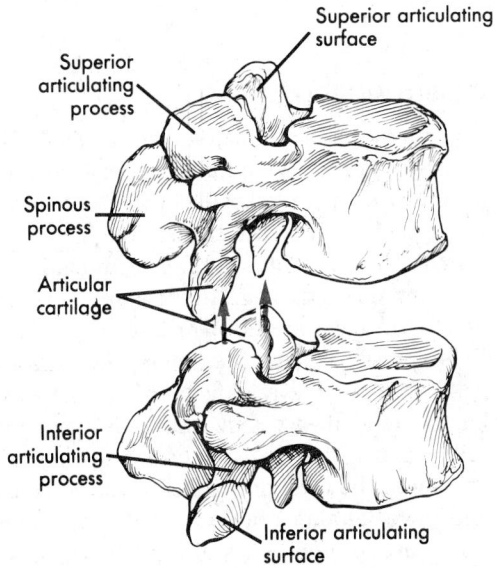

FIGURE 70-26 Posterior facet joints of lumbar vertebrae. Each vertebra has four surfaces by which it articulates with its adjacent vertebrae: two on its superior aspect and two on the inferior. Superior articulating surfaces are medially located; the inferior, laterally. These joints are diarthrotic, having a joint capsule with a synovial lining.

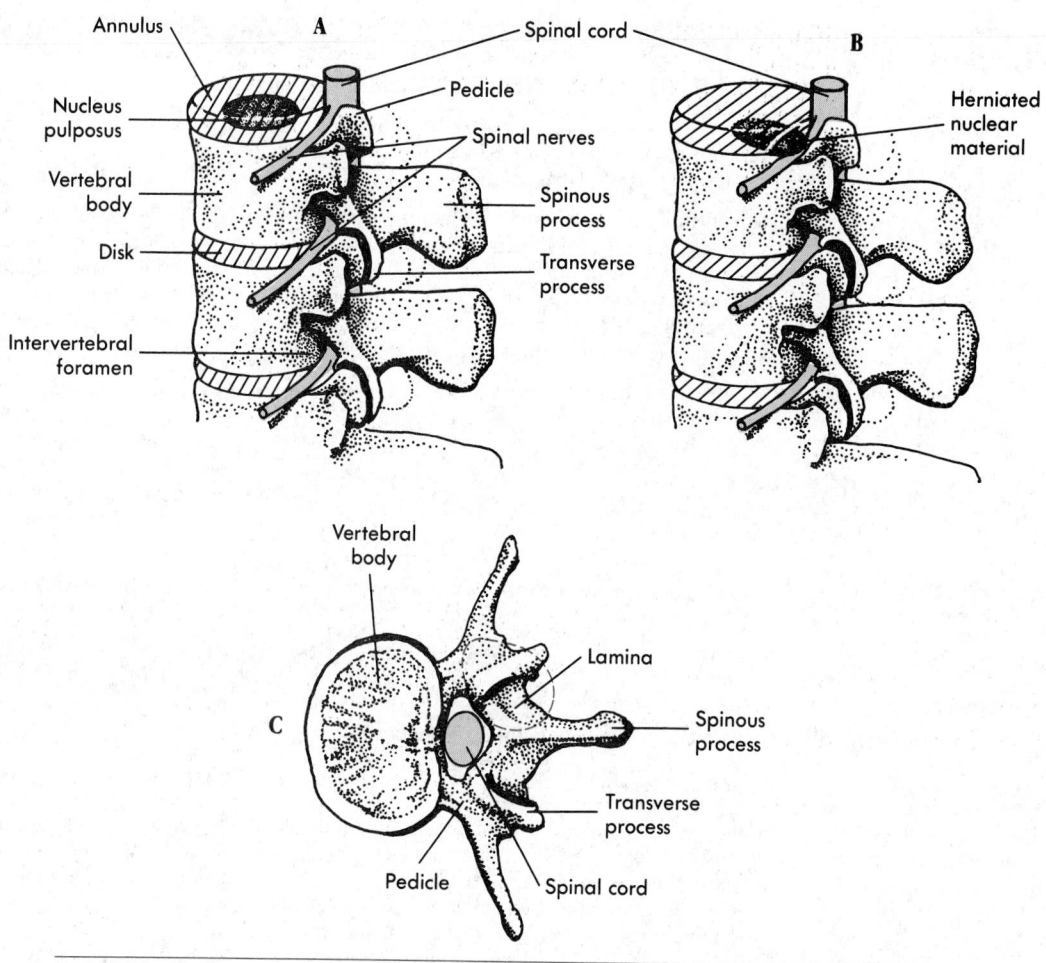

FIGURE 70-27 Compression of spinal cord and nerve root. **A,** Disks, composed of cartilaginous outer layer (anulus fibrosus) and gel-like inner layer (nucleus pulposus), lie between vertebral bodies. Spinal nerves exit the spinal cord laterally just above the pedicle. **B,** Laminae compose posterior portion of vertebrae. Each pedicle joins with a lamina *(dotted line);* the transverse and spinous processes project from laminae. **C,** When nucleus pulposus herniates posteriorly through its fibrous covering and the posterior longitudinal ligament, it may compress the spinal cord and trap the nerve root. Surgical approach to relieve this compresion is through lamina, posterior to transverse process.

ulus, either posteriorly or laterally. This results in compression of a spinal nerve root and subsequent pain (Figure 70-27).

2. *Osteophyte* formation along the vertebral column can cause fusion of vertebrae with consequent limitation of motion, usually in the lumbodorsal region.

3. *Spinal stenosis,* or narrowing of the intervertebral foramina at any level of the spine, creates pressure on nerve roots in the involved area, resulting in neurologic symptoms including pain.

4. *Degenerative and/or rheumatoid involvement of the hyaline articular surfaces of the facet joints* results in pain and limited motion. Rheumatoid involvement with consequent loss of vertebral stability is particularly troublesome in the cervical spine.

CLINICAL MANIFESTATIONS

The diagnosis of herniated disk is usually made on the basis of the history and physical examination. A history of low back pain relieved by recumbency and aggravated by flexion of the trunk, coughing, or sneezing is typical. The patient will often complain of sciatic pain radiating down the leg. After the initial injury, some patients will have sciatic pain but no pain in their back. Deep pressure over the interspace will usually elicit pain. Straight leg raising with the hip flexed and the knee extended (a positive Lasegue's sign) will produce sciatic pain. Neurologic signs and symptoms help in determining the level of the disk involved because sensory and motor changes depend on the nerve root involved. The most common sites of lumbar herniation are L3-4, L4-5, and L5-S1.

Compression of nerve roots from other causes—stenosis, vertebral instability, osteophyte formation—will also cause neurologic signs and symptoms relative to the level of the nerve root(s) involved. Signs and symptoms may include:

1. Numbness, tingling, and/or decreased motion in one or more extremities
2. Pain
3. Weakness of one or more extremities
4. Muscle wasting in one or more extremities
5. Partial or complete loss of bowel and bladder control

Diagnostic tests to determine defects in the spine include X-ray films, myelography, CAT scanning, and magnetic resonance imaging (MRI).

INTERVENTIONS

Medical Management

Interventions for degenerative problems of the spine may be conservative or surgical. *Conservative* management includes the following:

1. Rest (complete or modified depending on the severity of symptoms)
2. Heat
3. Medications
   a. Analgesics and/or antiinflammatory agents
   b. Muscle relaxants (for example, diazepam)
4. Traction to relieve muscle spasm
   a. Bilateral Buck's traction (see Chapter 69 for discussion of types of traction)
   b. Pelvic traction
5. If treatment is effective, a corset may be prescribed to provide external support to the spine when activity is resumed

Surgical Management

Surgical interventions are designed to relieve pressure on (decompress) nerve roots and to stabilize the spine. They may consist of removal of lamina or intervetebral disk, widening of the foramen, or fusion of two or more vertebrae (see the box for a description of spine surgery).

Nursing Management

Management of patients being treated conservatively. Nursing management includes the following:

1. Patient teaching
   a. Instruct patient in nature of and goals of management.
   b. Instruct patient in logrolling (Figure 70-28)
   c. Instruct patient in proper positioning.
   d. Instruct patient in good body mechanics (Figure 70-14).
2. Promoting comfort
   a. Encourage slight elevation of head of bed and

TYPES OF SPINE SURGERY

PROCEDURE	DESCRIPTION
Laminectomy	Removal of a portion of the lamina (Figure 70-27, *C*)
Diskectomy	Removal of all or part of a herniated intervertebral disk
Foraminotomy	Widening of the intervertebral foramen to allow free passage of the spinal nerve
Spinal fusion	Fusion of two or more vertebrae by insertion of bone grafts with or without the addition of metal rods or wires to achieve vertebral stability; fusion is required when thoracic and cervical vertebrae are involved because of mobility of the spine in these areas

flexion of the knees when supine (Figure 70-29).
   b. Roll patient onto bedpan rather than lifting onto bedpan.
   c. Use fracture bedpan or small bedpan.
   d. Apply heat as patient desires and tolerates it.
   e. Remove skin traction for periods of time if it causes patient discomfort.
   f. Provide analgesics and/or antispasmodics at regular intervals as necessary.
3. Promoting circulation
   a. Encourage patient to perform active dorsiplantar flexion of the ankles at regular intervals.

Nursing management of patients being treated surgically. Care following spinal surgery (lumbar, thoracic, or cervical) focuses on positioning and mobility, wound care, and patient comfort (see the appropriate boxes on pp. 2083 and 2084 for guidelines about nursing interventions after surgery). Changing position in bed following spinal surgery must be performed by logrolling; assistance is given as necessary, but patients can learn to do this for themselves. Because patients tolerate sitting less well than walking or lying, sitting is avoided until the person can tolerate it.

Thoracic spinal surgery may involve entering the chest cavity, and if so, nursing care will include postoperative measures required following chest surgery (see Chapter 34). Mobility restrictions are more prolonged than with lumbar surgery, because the thoracic spine is more mobile; consequently, there is greater risk of dislodging grafts through improper motion.

Persons with *cervical* spinal surgery may require tong or halo traction (see Chapter 69) or a halo brace. The person has edema of the throat in the early postop-

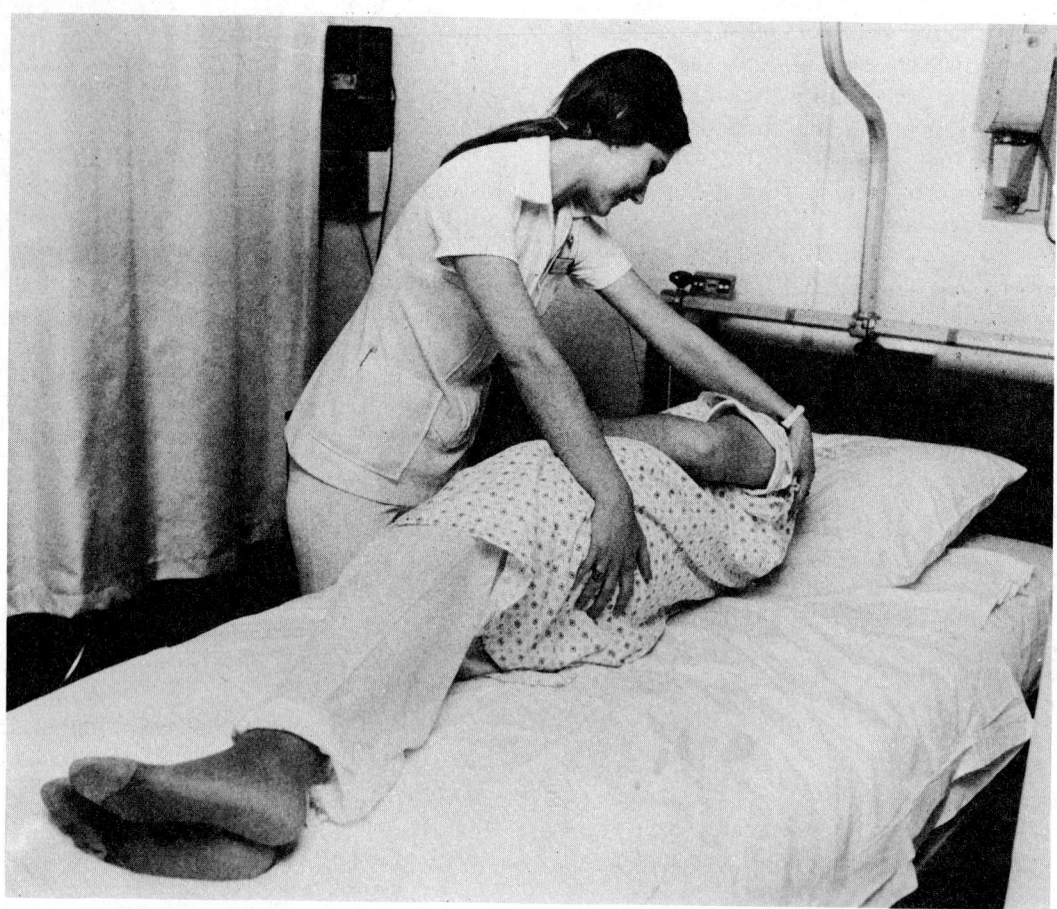

FIGURE 70-28 Logrolling patient. Patient crosses arms over chest, holds legs in extension and feet together. Nurse supports patient at level of shoulders and buttocks.

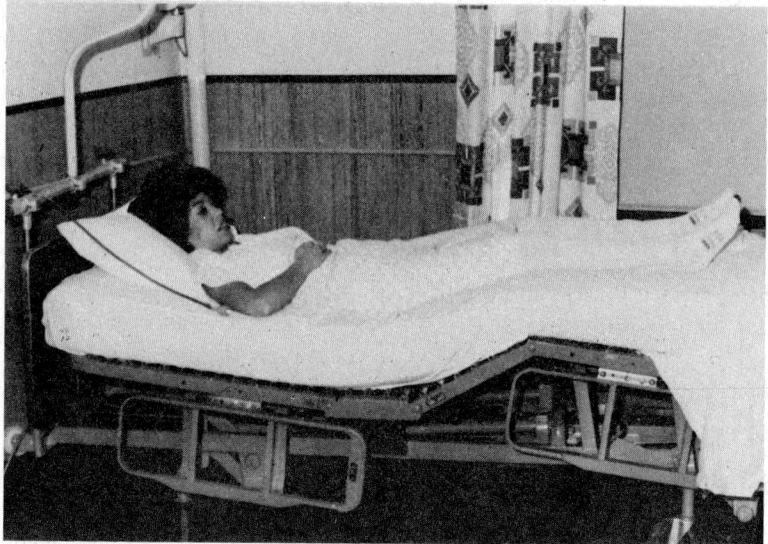

FIGURE 70-29 Elevating head of bed 20 to 30 degrees and flexing knees provides comfortable position for patients with acute back pain.

GUIDELINES FOR NURSING INTERVENTIONS FOR PERSONS WITH LUMBAR SURGERY

PREOPERATIVE CARE

1. Instruct patient in logrolling and performance of dorsiplantar flexion exercises.
2. Instruct patient about the surgical procedure, postoperative care, and expectations at discharge.

POSTOPERATIVE CARE

1. Positioning
   a. Head of bed is kept flat.
   b. Patient is encouraged to logroll to change position from side, back, side.
   c. Use of a turning sheet is advised until patient can assist with turning.
2. Wound care (drains placed in wound to prevent hematoma formation, if necessary)
   a. Maintain constant suction through drain as required.
   b. Maintain drain free of contamination.
   c. Inspect surgical area frequently for evidence of excess drainage or formation of hematoma (bulging of tissues surrounding surgical site).
   d. If a spinal fusion, inspect donor sites (usually iliac crest) for drainage, hematoma.
3. Promoting comfort
   a. Reposition patient frequently.
   b. Administer narcotic medications as needed; gradually reduce to nonnarcotic analgesics as patient tolerates.
   c. Use fracture bedpan or small bedpan.
4. Promoting mobility
   a. Activity out of bed may begin as early as 1 day after surgery (laminectomy) or 3 to 5 days after surgery (laminectomy and fusion).
   b. Transfer patient out of bed with as little time spent in the sitting position as possible.
      (1) Start transfer with patient in a side-lying position at the edge of the bed.
      (2) Have patient push off the bed with the uppermost hand and the lowermost elbow.
      (3) One person assists by guiding the patient's trunk, another assists the patient's legs over the side of the bed.
      (4) Reverse process for return to bed.
   c. The patient may be permitted to walk as much as tolerated, with assistive aid if necessary.
   d. Braces or corsets, if prescribed, are applied *before* the patient gets out of bed.
   e. Encourage patient to participate in ADL within prescribed limits of mobility.
5. Discharge instruction
   a. Do not lift or carry anything heavier than 2.25 kg (5 lb).
   b. Do not drive a car until permitted by surgeon.
   c. Avoid twisting motions of the trunk.

GUIDELINES FOR NURSING INTERVENTIONS FOR PATIENT WITH THORACIC SPINE SURGERY

PREOPERATIVE CARE

Same as for lumbar surgery

POSTOPERATIVE CARE

Same as for lumbar surgery *with the following additions and exceptions*

1. Positioning
   a. Head of bed may often be elevated to 30 degrees.
2. Wound care
   a. If pleural cavity is entered, a chest tube will be inserted and must be managed postoperatively (see Chapter 34).
3. Promoting comfort
   a. Assist patient to splint chest while coughing.
4. Promoting mobility
   a. Encourage and assist patient in vigorous pulmonary toileting.
   b. Assist patient to maintain bedrest for 1 week or longer with strict attention to avoidance of twisting or bending motions to prevent dislodging grafts.
   c. Discourage patient from vigorous pulling or pushing with the arms because weight bearing through the arms poses a threat to the integrity of the graft.
   d. Brace is routinely prescribed and must be applied before patient is allowed out of bed.
   e. Permit patient to perform whatever activities are comfortable within the limitations of the brace.
   f. Encourage patient to participate in ADL within prescribed limits of mobility.
5. Discharge instruction
   a. Apply and remove the brace before getting out of bed.
   b. Wear the brace whenever out of bed.

GUIDELINES FOR NURSING INTERVENTIONS FOR PERSONS WITH CERVICAL SPINE SURGERY

PREOPERATIVE CARE

1. Follow general instruction as for any spine surgery.
2. If tong or halo traction or halo brace is to be used postoperatively, familiarize patient with the apparatus before surgery.

POSTOPERATIVE CARE

1. Positioning
   a. Keep head of bed elevated 30 to 45 degrees, particularly if anterior surgical approach was used, to decrease swelling in throat.
   b. If patient is in cervical brace, position is not restricted except by patient's tolerance.
   c. If patient is in cervical traction, patient may be turned side to back to side to patient's tolerance.
2. Wound care
   a. Inspect surgical area, including iliac crest donor site, frequently for evidence of excess drainage or formation of hematoma.
   b. If *tong* or *halo traction* is being used, pin care may be required (See Chapter 69).
3. Promoting comfort and relieving pain
   a. Provide ice chips to soothe sore throat.
   b. Make progressive diet changes slowly; patient will have difficulty swallowing and will be afraid of choking. Full liquids (ice cream, custards, jello, nectars) are often better tolerated than clear juice or broth; however, milk products may increase mucus production.
   c. Administer analgesics as for any spine surgery. Donor sites often cause more discomfort than does neck incision.

d. Patient may require aerosol treatments or humidification of air to loosen mucus secretions or make breathing more comfortable.
4. Promoting mobility
   a. If patient is in traction, encourage patient to perform ankle dorsiplantar flexion exercises and quadriceps setting on a regular basis to promote circulation and maintain leg strength.
   b. If patient is in brace, out-of-bed activity, including walking may begin as soon as patient tolerates.
   c. Provide for temporary use of walker if donor site pain restricts mobility.
   d. Encourage patient to participate in ADL to greatest extent possible.
5. Promoting safety
   a. Provide suction equipment and tracheotomy set in patient's room until swelling in throat subsides and patient is swallowing and breathing normally.
   b. Check adjustment screws and straps frequently to ensure there is no loosening of the brace.
   c. Advise physician or orthotist of loosening of brace consequent to decrease in edema so brace can be readjusted.
6. Discharge instruction
   a. Wear brace at all times.
   b. Report any difficulty with brace to physician immediately.
   c. Do not drive a car during period that brace must be worn.

---

erative period, requiring attention to the person's ability to breathe and swallow.

RESTRICTIVE DISORDERS

SCOLIOSIS
EPIDEMIOLOGY/ETIOLOGY

Lateral deviation of the spine from the midline is known as scoliosis. The classifications of scoliosis are:

1. Congenital—present at birth
2. Acquired—not present at birth but develops at a later time
3. Idiopathic—most common type, usually develops in adolescence
4. Functional (postural or nonstructural)—develops from temporary postural influences; easily correctable
5. Structural—changes in structure of spine from various causes

6. Paralytic—develops following neurologic disease such as poliomyelitis

Scoliosis may be present in both children and adults.

PREVENTION

Screening programs for school age children are effective in identifying early indications of scoliosis. Attention to good posture may be effective in preventing the disorder in both children and adults.

PATHOPHYSIOLOGY

Scoliosis may develop in localized areas of the spinal column or involve the whole spinal column. Curves may be S-shaped or C-shaped. The degree of rotation of the curve is important as it determines the amount of impingement on the rib cage. Significant cardiac and pulmonary restrictions may be imposed by curves with a large degree of rotation. The balance of the curve is also important as it affects the stability of the spine and mobility of the trunk. Significant deviations in balance of the curve affect gait patterns.

CLINICAL MANIFESTATIONS

The individual can initially have slight, mild, or severe deformity. Early deformity may not be obvious except on specific examination. Deformity will increase with growth and age. In the early stages, individuals may note that clothing does not fit correctly or hang evenly. The height of the shoulders is uneven. Pain is not usually an accompanying factor. In advanced scoliosis, when there is impairment of the cardiorespiratory system, respiration is restricted and cardiac output is compromised.

MEDICAL MANAGEMENT

Medical management includes the following:
1. Early or postural scoliosis may be amenable to postural exercise or exercise combined with traction (for example, Cotrel's traction)
2. In scoliosis where the curve is flexible, less than 40 degrees, and the patient is cooperative, bracing, in combination with exercise, may be sufficient to correct the deformity (for example, Milwaukee brace, Risser cast, or halofemoral or halopelvic traction)
3. Corrective surgery (realignment of vertebrae and fusion) when curve exceeds 40 degrees and/or bracing has failed; it is usually accomplished with bone grafting and instrumentation
   a. Harrington rod instrumentation—a series of rods and hooks that apply compression to the posterior spinal elements

b. Dwyer instrumentation—titanium cables passed through heads of titanium screws imbedded in the vertebral bodies (Figure 70-30)
c. Luque instrumentation—two L-shaped rods and a series of sublaminar wires that apply transverse traction to the vertebral bodies
d. A combination of Harrington and Luque instrumentation
e. Cotrel-Dubosset instrumentation that derotates the spine

■ ASSESSMENT

Subjective data include the following:
1. Patient describes that clothes do not fit or hang well
2. Patient may describe not being able to breath comfortably
3. Patient complains of progressive difficulty with ambulation
4. Patient states negative feelings about appearance

Objective data includes the following:
1. Visible curvature in spine and/or a pronounced rib hump when patient bends forward from the waist
2. Palpation of spinal curve with patient in upright position
3. Notable limp
4. Shoulders are uneven in height
5. One arm hangs closer to the body than the other

■ DATA ANALYSIS: NURSING DIAGNOSES

Nursing diagnoses are determined from assessment of patient data. Possible nursing diagnoses for the person

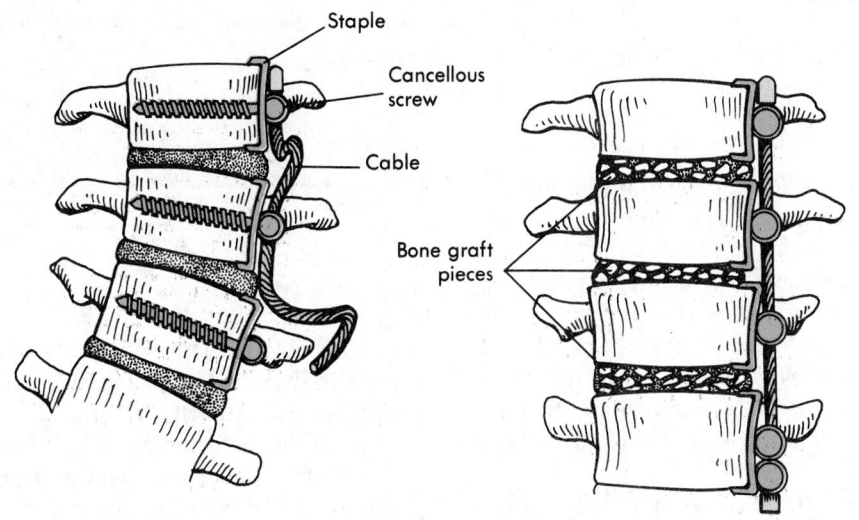

FIGURE 70-30 Scoliosis fusion with Dwyer instrumentation. Cable is passed through openings in heads of screws that are imbedded in vertebral bodies. Spaces between vertebrae are filled with bone chips as grafting material. Cable is pulled taut to secure and maintain correct alignment of vertebrae.

with scoliosis may include, but are not limited to, the following:

Diagnostic Title	Possible Etiologies
Knowledge deficit about scoliosis	Lack of exposure
Mobility, impaired physical	Musculoskeletal impairment
Activity intolerance	Imbalance between oxygen supply/demand
Self-esteem, disturbance in	Change in body appearance
Breathing patterns, ineffective	Musculoskeletal impairment
Pain, postoperative	Surgical intervention to correct deformity

■ PLANNING: EXPECTED PATIENT OUTCOMES

Expected patient outcomes for the person with scoliosis may include, but are not limited to, the following:
1. Potential complications are avoided.
2. Maximal functioning and independence are maintained.
3. Patient can explain applicability of treatment measures and plans for follow-up with the physician.

■ IMPLEMENTATION

Patient Teaching

For individuals with whom conservative interventions are being employed, patient instruction is most important for achieving the desired outcomes.
1. Instruct patient how to apply, remove, and care for brace.
2. Instruct and supervise patient in performance of prescribed exercises and use of traction equipment.
3. Advise patient regarding the selection of loose fitting, but attractive, clothing that conceals brace (particularly important for women and adolescents).
4. Advise patient that wearing brace need not restrict normal or desired activities.

Postoperative Care

The care of the person following spinal fusion for scoliosis is described in the box at right. There is a high risk of postoperative pulmonary complications as a result of postoperative immobilization; therefore preventive measures are important. *Paralytic ileus is a common complication and a nasogastric suction may be used in the first 24 to 72 hours postoperatively.* Patients with major spinal procedures also tend to retain fluid; therefore *they are at risk for fluid overload in the early postoperative period.*

Following surgery, a brace or cast is usually required for a period of time, and instructions are given to the person for the care of the brace or cast. A bed board is suggested for use at home to provide firm support for sleeping.

GUIDELINES FOR NURSING INTERVENTIONS FOR THE PATIENT WITH SCOLIOSIS FUSION

PREOPERATIVE CARE
1. Instruct the patient regarding the surgery, postoperative care, expectations after discharge.

POSTOPERATIVE CARE
1. Promoting comfort
   a. Administer narcotic analgesics as necessary; gradually decrease to nonnarcotic analgesics as patient tolerates.
   b. Turn and position frequently.
   c. Use a small bedpan or a fracture bedpan.
2. Positioning
   a. Bed is kept flat from 1 to 14 days, depending on the surgical technique used.
   b. Position patient side to back to side with use of a turning sheet and pillows between the legs to maintain alignment.
3. Promoting safety
   a. Monitor vital signs, motor function, and sensation in the lower extremities frequently.
   b. Monitor closely for respiratory impairment.
4. Promoting mobility
   a. Encourage leg exercise as for other spinal surgery.
   b. Encourage participation in ADL to extent possible within restrictions imposed by surgery and/or brace or cast.
   c. Begin activity out of bed, in brace or cast if prescribed, as soon as surgeon permits. (Commencement of activity depends on surgical technique.)
5. Preventing complications
   a. Encourage breathing exercises.
   b. Delay administration of oral food and fluid until patient is actively passing flatus.
   c. Monitor intravenous intake and urine output closely to prevent fluid overload until patient experiences postoperative diuresis (usually 3 to 4 days).
6. Wound care (as for any spine surgery)
7. Discharge instruction
   a. Care of brace or cast if required.
   b. Use of bed board at home.
   c. Plans for follow-up with physician.

OTHER DISORDERS

Some other disorders of the musculoskeletal system involve malposition of supportive structures, metabolic disorders, or problems arising as a result of infection. Three of the more common disorders (recurrent dislocation of the patella, gout, and bacterial arthritis) are examined in the following discussion.

RECURRENT DISLOCATION OF THE PATELLA
PATHOPHYSIOLOGY AND CLINICAL MANIFESTATIONS

Recurrent dislocation of the patella is representative of those problems in which a tendon or other supportive

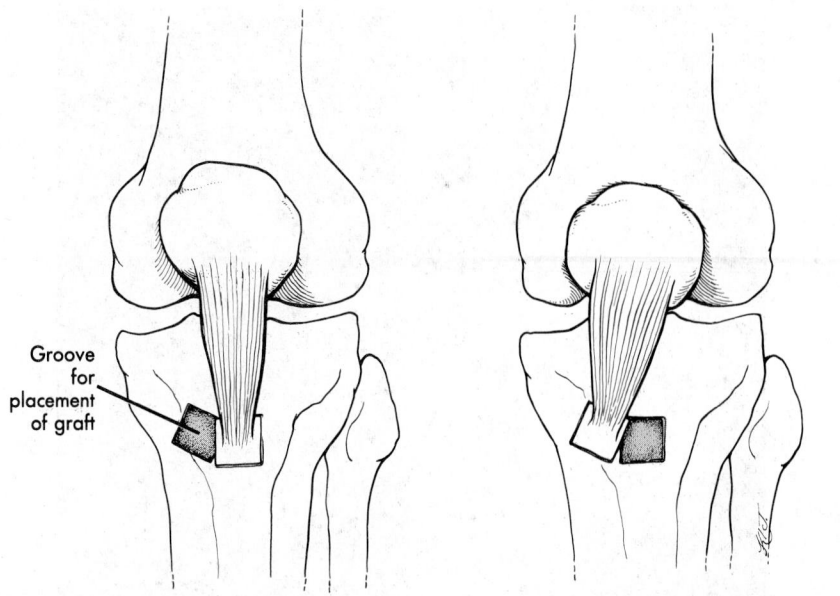

FIGURE 70-31 Tendon transplant. Movement of patellar tendon medially by detaching it and bone it is attached to in order to correct recurrent dislocation of patella. (Adapted from Helfet AJ: Disorders of the knee, Philadelphia, 1974, JB Lippincott Co.)

structure is malplaced or not functioning in a normal fashion. In this disorder, the patellar tendon is more laterally placed in its distal attachment than normal. Consequently, the patella is pulled laterally when the quadriceps contracts and it dislocates to the lateral side of the knee. *The disorder is painful and can restrict knee function.*

INTERVENTIONS

Medical Management

This condition is usually treated surgically.

1. The distal end of the tendon is transplanted from its insertion on the tibial tubercle to a point more medial and distal to the preoperative insertion (Figure 70-31).
2. Leg is protected postoperatively with splints and a compression dressing for 3 to 5 days.
3. Cylinder cast is applied after dressing is removed.
4. Active flexion exercises are begun in about 6 weeks.

Nursing Management

Major nursing interventions include the following:

1. Instructing the patient about the surgery, postoperative care, and expectations after discharge
2. Encouraging the patient to perform prescribed exercises
3. Promoting mobility while observing restrictions on active flexion
4. Promoting involvement in self-care
5. Instructing the patient how to care for self after leaving hospital

   a. Care of cast
   b. Performance of exercises
   c. Use of ambulatory aid
   d. Follow-up plans with the physician and physical therapist

GOUT

EPIDEMIOLOGY/ETIOLOGY

Gout or gouty arthritis is a metabolic disorder that affects men eight to nine times more frequently than women. It can occur at any age, the peak age of onset occurring in the fifth decade. Eighty-five percent of all persons with gout have a genetic or familial tendency to develop the disease. *Gout develops as a result of prolonged hyperuricemia (elevated serum uric acid) caused by problems either in synthesizing purines or by poor renal excretion of uric acid.*

PATHOPHYSIOLOGY/CLINICAL MANIFESTATIONS

Urate crystals form in the synovial tissue, causing severe inflammation. The inflammatory process is extremely rapid, occurring over a few hours. *Acute symptoms are extreme pain, swelling, and erythema of the involved joints.* Typically the first metatarsophalangeal joint of the great toe is involved (podagra), but other joints, such as the ankle, heel, or knee, may also be affected. Pain is so severe that the patient may not tolerate even the weight of a sheet over the joint. Renal damage may occur, especially if recurrent uric acid stones have been present. Between attacks of gout, the patient may be asymptomatic, but repeated attacks can occur with gradually increasing frequency if the disease

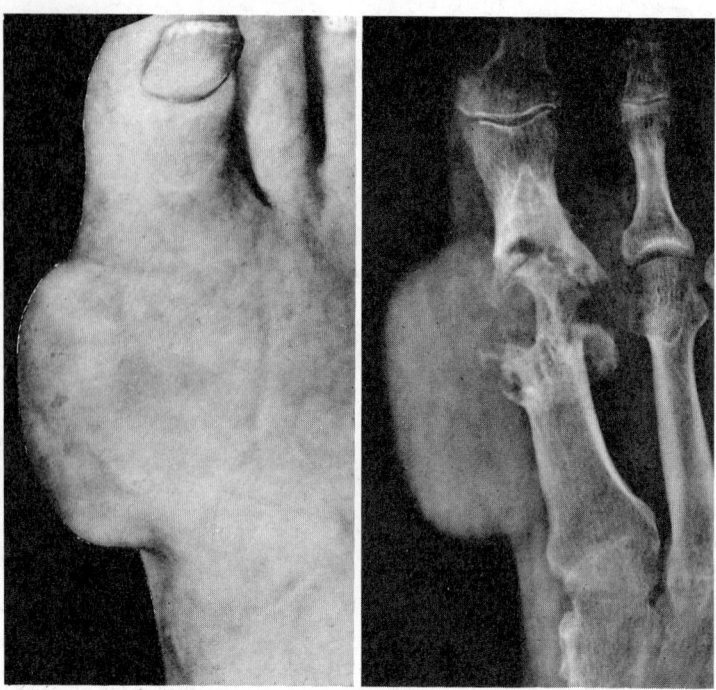

FIGURE 70-32 Gout of long duration. Tophaceous mass at base of great toe, as well as destructive bone and joint changes shown in roentgenogram, are associated with extensive urate deposits. (From Brashear H and Raney R: Shand's handbook of orthopaedic surgery, ed 9, St Louis, 1978, The CV Mosby Co.)

is untreated. Patients with gouty symptoms may develop *tophi,* or deposits of monosodium urate in their tissues. These consist of a core of monosodium urate with a surrounding inflammatory reaction. *Patients with tophaceous deposits* (Figure 70-32) *tend to have more frequent and more severe episodes of gouty arthritis.*

Laboratory studies will indicate an *elevated serum uric acid, normal or increased urinary uric acid* over a 24-hour period, and the presence of *monosodium urate* monohydrate crystals in the synovial fluid and in the tophi.

INTERVENTIONS

Medical Management

Management is directed toward control of acute attacks and prevention of recurrent attacks. Treatment of *acute* attacks includes the following:
1. Medications
   a. Colchicine (0.6 mg), oral administration of 2 tablets initially, then 1 tablet each hour until nausea, vomiting or diarrhea develop, or joint symptoms subside. Limit is 6.0 to 8.0 mg
   b. Colchicine 1.0 to 3.0 mg in saline intravenously over a 10-minute period
   c. Phenylbutazone (Butazolidin)
   d. Indomethacin (Indocin)
2. Absolute rest of the joint

Preventive therapy (interval therapy) consists of reduction of the body pool of urates by one of two methods:
1. *Enhancing uric acid excretion*
   a. Probenecid (Benemid), 0.5 g daily for 1 week, then increased by 0.5 g weekly until serum uric acid is in normal range
   b. Sulfinpyrazone (Anturane), used for patients who do not tolerate Benemid
   c. Daily prophylactic therapy for life
2. *Decreasing uric acid formation*
   a. Allopurinol (Zyloprim), 100 mg twice a day initially, increased by 100 mg every 2 to 4 weeks until serum uric acid level is normal
   b. Daily prophylactic therapy for life

Nursing Management

Nursing management includes the following:
1. Patient teaching
   a. Instruct patient in nature of disease.
   b. Instruct patient in proper use of prescribed medications.
   c. Encourage patient to lose weight if overweight.
   d. Encourage patient to take in sufficient fluid to assure daily *output* of 2000 to 3000 ml.
2. Promoting comfort
   a. Provide absolute rest until pain of acute attack subsides.

b. Avoid touching joint or moving affected extremity until acute pain subsides.

BACTERIAL ARTHRITIS
EPIDEMIOLOGY/ETIOLOGY

Bacterial arthritis is the result of invasion of the synovial membrane by microorganisms, most often *gonococci, meningococci, staphylococci, coliforms, salmonellae,* and *haemophilus influenzae.* Factors that predispose to such infections are a high degree of susceptibility on the part of the patient, recent joint surgery or trauma, intraarticular injections, and rheumatoid arthritis.

PATHOPHYSIOLOGY AND CLINICAL MANIFESTATIONS

Synovial tissues respond to bacterial invasion by becoming inflamed. The joint cavity may become involved, and pus will be present in the synovial membrane and the synovial fluid. If allowed to progress, the infection will cause abscesses in the synovium and subchondral bone, eventually destroying cartilage. *Ankylosis* of the *joint* may result. The patient will complain of pain, swelling, and tenderness of the joint.

Joint aspiration is helpful in making the diagnosis if the presence of organisms can be demonstrated in the synovial fluid. White cell counts will be high, and glucose content of synovial fluid may be reduced. X-ray films taken days to weeks after onset of the infection may reveal loss of joint space and lytic changes in bone.

INTERVENTIONS
Medical Management

Medical management includes the following:
1. Appropriate antibiotic therapy
2. Rest or immobilization of the joint
3. Surgical drainage or a system of irrigation and drainage if infection does not respond to antibiotic therapy or if osteomyelitis is present
4. Resumption of active range of motion when infection subsides and motion can be tolerated

Nursing Management

Nursing management includes the following:
1. Promoting rest of the affected joint
2. Administering antibiotics on time and as prescribed
3. Administering prescribed pain medication as necessary
4. Encourage patient to participate in self-care to extent possible within restrictions of prescribed rest for joint
5. Patient teaching
   a. Instructing in care of cast or other immobilizing device
   b. Encouraging active joint motion when motion is permitted
   c. Instructing in proper administration of antibiotics if therapy is to be continued after discharge
   d. Assuring that patient is aware of plans for follow-up with physician

CHAPTER SUMMARY

✔ Most persons with a musculoskeletal disorder have one or more of five common problems. These include pain, stiffness, decrease in muscle strength, loss of dexterity, and loss of locomotor ability.

✔ A number of potential or actual complications may accompany immobility. Any or all of the major body systems may be involved.

✔ Rest, activity, joint protection, and energy conservation are some interventions common to a number of musculoskeletal disorders. The nurse's responsibility is to help the patient understand the meaning of these interventions and to teach the patient how to carry out these activities.

✔ Assistive, supportive, and safety devices are available for persons with musculoskeletal disorders. These include ambulatory, feeding, bathing, and dressing aids. Safety devices such as arms mounted around toilets are designed to help prevent falls and accidents.

✔ The application of heat and cold can be used for persons with musculoskeletal disorders to relieve stiffness and pain. Heat may also have a sedative or relaxing effect. Cold is helpful in reducing or preventing swelling. Caution must be used whenever heat or cold is applied to prevent tissue damage.

✔ Intermittent or constant traction can be used to help reduce contractures or to relieve pain. It is usually applied in the form of skin traction, such as Buck's extension, Russell traction, or pelvic traction.

✔ Splints and braces (orthoses) can be used to stabilize or support a joint, protect a joint or body part from external trauma, mechanically correct dysfunction by supporting the joint in its functional position, and to assist patients in exercising specific joints. When patients must wear orthoses, nurses need to inspect the patient's skin for irritation, notify the orthotist when adjustments need to be made, instruct the patient in the proper application and care of the orthosis, and assist the patient in making the psychologic adjustment to wearing the orthosis.

✔ Principles of positioning and transfer are fundamental to most nursing care, but nurses must consider the special need for prevention or minimization of pain when moving patients with musculoskeletal problems.

✔ Exercise is a prescribed form of activity to preserve joint mobility, maintain muscle tone, and strengthen certain muscle groups. The ability to exercise may be enhanced by the application of heat or cold and the administration of analgesics before the exercise session. Patients should not exercise when joints or muscles are acutely inflamed. The nurse should be aware of the patient's specific exercise program and provide support and assistance to perform the exercises.

✔ Many of the medications used for the treatment of musculoskeletal problems are antiinflammatory analgesics. The use of narcotic analgesics in chronic inflammatory musculoskeletal conditions is generally contraindicated, although narcotics are used in the treatment of acute injuries and postoperative pain. The nurse's role when caring for patients taking antiinflammatory medications includes teaching about the action of the medication, correct dose and method of administration, and how to recognize untoward side effects.

✔ Special diets are usually not recommended for persons with musculoskeletal disorders, but patients should be careful about not gaining weight. Added weight increases the patient's energy consumption and causes weight-bearing joints to be overly stressed. Nurses can help promote weight loss by teaching the patient about a properly supervised reduction diet.

✔ Persons with a musculoskeletal problem may require elective surgery for correction of deformity, relief of pain, or restoration of musculoskeletal function. The major objectives of orthopaedic treatment are restoration or maintenance of function of a body part, prevention of deformity, correction of deformity if it already exists, and development of the patient's powers of compensation and adaptation if loss of function or permanent deformity is not preventable. The orthopaedist considers what procedure is best suited to achieve the desired objective for the patient. Orthopaedic care is highly individualized to the patient being treated. Refer to Table 70-4 for a summary of the surgical procedures to the musculoskeletal system.

✔ Persons with musculoskeletal disorders may have some common psychosocial problems. These can include difficulty with their reaction to disfigurement or disability; difficulty with dependence, independence, or interdependence; adaptation to assistive, supportive, or corrective devices; the socioeconomic impact of their disorder; and their family relationships.

✔ Support, teaching, and guidance (counseling) are the nursing interventions employed to achieve therapeutic outcomes for psychosocial problems.

✔ Factors of prevention and teaching must be consid-

ered for persons with musculoskeletal disability. Preventive measures to combat illnesses that cause musculoskeletal disorders can be used on a community-wide basis. For those conditions in which the cause is unknown, attention is focused on preventing complications. General teaching on an individual basis can include early attention to good posture, body mechanics, dietary habits, and promotion of safety.

✔ Rheumatoid arthritis is a chronic systemic disease most prominently manifested as an inflammation in the synovium of the diarthrodial joints. It is more prevalent in women than men. The cause of this disease is unknown.

✔ The disease process begins as an inflammation of the synovium. The inflammatory process is set off by a "triggering" event such as some sort of irritation or damage. WBCs rush into the area releasing chemicals, prostaglandins, leukotrienes, and digestive enzymes. Collagen (the main structural protein of connective tissue) is broken down. The process becomes chronic and leads to thickening of the synovium and formation of granulation tissue. The cartilage becomes necrotic. Destruction of cartilage and bone may lead to dislocation of the joints.

✔ Early manifestations of the disease may include complaints of fever, weight loss, fatigue, generalized discomfort that is poorly localized (fibrositis), and morning stiffness. These symptoms may later be replaced by more specific (localized) pain and articular inflammation with swelling, redness, warmth, and tenderness.

✔ The joints of the hands and the feet are often affected early. The joints of the hands, wrists, feet, ankles, elbows, and knees are most commonly involved, usually in a bilaterally symmetric pattern. Shoulder and hip involvement are later phenomena.

✔ The course of rheumatoid arthritis varies greatly from patient to patient and is marked by periods of exacerbation and remission. Some evidence suggests that exacerbations can be triggered by mental stress or physical trauma.

✔ Laboratory findings usually indicative of rheumatoid arthritis include an elevated erythrocyte sedimentation rate, mild leukocytosis, positive rheumatoid factor, narrowing of the joint spaces and erosion of articular surfaces on X-ray films, inflammatory changes in synovial tissue (biopsy), and increased turbidity and decreased viscosity of synovial fluid (needle aspiration).

✔ Medical management of rheumatoid arthritis is generally described as a pyramid of therapy. The foundation is a good history and physical examination, prescription of rest and appropriate exercise, education of patient and family, and control of inflammation with salicylates. Medications are added based on the patients's response to conservative therapy. The goals of therapy are relief of pain, maintenance of joint function, prevention and correction of deformity, and correction of other health factors.

✔ Nursing management consists of measures to promote comfort, promote mobility, encourage good nutrition, and promote improved self-esteem. Patient teaching is stressed.

✔ Surgical intervention may be warranted when rheumatoid arthritis has caused severe joint destruction. Common procedures are synovectomy, arthrotomy, arthrodesis, and arthroplasty.

✔ Systemic lupus erythematosus (SLE) is a chronic inflammatory disease of unknown cause. It affects women more often than men. Its course can be controlled by corticosteroids, but some patients do die as a result of lesions affecting major organs or from secondary infections.

✔ Pathologic manifestations of SLE include synovial involvement, severe vasculitis, renal involvement, lymph node necrosis, development of small white spots in the retina (cytoid bodies), and lesions of the nervous system.

✔ The initial manifestation of SLE is often arthritis, but the joint symptoms may be transient. The patient may complain of sensitivity to the sun. Erythema, usually in a butterfly pattern, can appear over the cheeks and bridge of the nose. The patient may also have findings of glomerulonephritis, pleuritis, pericarditis, peritonitis, neuritis, or anemia. Laboratory findings are specific to the organs involved.

✔ Medical management begins conservatively with rest, exercise, and medications. Kidney dialysis or transplant may be necessary for uncontrolled lupus nephritis, or total hip replacement may be necessary for avascular necrosis resulting from high-dose steroid therapy.

✔ Nursing management centers on patient teaching and promoting comfort and ADL.

✔ Polymyositis (dermatomyositis) is an inflammatory disease of striated (voluntary) muscle. It occurs more frequently in women than men. The cause is unknown.

✔ Diagnostic tests for polymyositis include manual muscle test, electromyogram, muscle biopsy, serum enzymes, and 24-hour urine tests.

✔ Medical management consists of rest and treatment with corticosteroids, and nursing management addresses teaching, prevention of skin breakdown, and promotion of comfort and mobility.

✔ Ankylosing spondylitis is a chronic, progressive disorder affecting the joints of the hips and spine. It occurs more frequently in men than women. The cause is unknown, although there may be a genetic link. Progression of the disease cannot be stopped by any known treatment at present.

✔ As a result of the inflammatory process within the spine, the bones of the spine fuse (ankylose). Inflammation usually begins at the sacroiliac joints and progresses up the spine, resulting in fusion of the entire spine.

✔ Early symptoms may include low back pain and pain and swelling of the hips, knees, or shoulders. Mild fever, anorexia, and fatigue may also be present. Symptoms flare and subside. Eventually pain may decrease and motion of the back becomes restricted. Fusion of the sacroiliac joints and spine may occur, resulting in a kyphosis at the cervicodorsal junction.

✔ Presence in the serum of the HLA-B27 genetic marker and X-ray films showing bony growths (syndesmophytes) can be indicative of ankylosing spondylitis.

✔ Medical management consists of exercise, rest, heat, and antiinflammatory analgesics. Spinal osteotomy or hip arthroplasty may be necessary for persons with severe symptoms.

✔ Nursing management centers on patient teaching, promotion of comfort and correct posture, and prevention of complications.

✔ Inflammation of the supportive structures and structures located near the joints is referred to as nonarticular rheumatism. Disorders in this category include fibrositis, tenosynovitis, bursitis, and carpal tunnel syndrome.

✔ Most nonarticular rheumatic diseases are caused by trauma, strain, and overuse of the related joint. The patient will complain of swelling, pain, and limited ability to move the associated joint. With carpal tunnel syndrome, the patient will complain of dysesthesia, paresthesia, or hypesthesia of the thumb, index, and middle fingers related to pressure on the median nerve of the wrist.

✔ Medical management of nonarticular rheumatic diseases consists primarily of rest of the involved area, splinting, antiinflammatory agents, or local steroid injections. Surgery may be required for removal of calcium deposits (for example, in bursitis) or release of inflamed ligaments (for example, the carpal ligament in carpal tunnel syndrome). Nursing management focuses on patient teaching and promoting comfort. Postoperative care measures are provided for patients treated with surgical interventions.

✔ Dupuytren's contracture is contracture of the palmar fascia causing the ring and sometimes the little finger to flex into the palm and lose the capacity to be extended. Surgical removal of the involved palmar fascia may be required if conservative measures to relieve symptoms are ineffective. Nursing management then addresses postoperative care.

✔ Degenerative joint disease (DJD) is the result of degeneration of the articular cartilage of the synovial joints. Unlike rheumatoid arthritis, it is not systemic. DJD is also known as osteoarthritis, hypertrophic arthritis, osteoarthrosis, or senescent arthritis. It is an extremely common disease. Symptomatic DJD is usually noted in the 50 to 70 year age group, although most persons past age 40 have hypertrophic changes of the joints.

✔ Two forms of osteoarthritis exist: primary, for which the cause is unknown; and secondary, which can be the result of trauma, infection, fracture, another type of arthritis, stress on weight-bearing joints from obesity, unusual wear and tear on joints associated with certain occupations, or a genetic disposition.

✔ The target organ of DJD is the articular cartilage. This normally white, translucent, smooth cartilage becomes yellow and opaque with softened areas and a rough or frayed surface. The cartilage is digested by enzymes and is eventually destroyed. The underlying bone develops osteophytes (spurs of new bone) that may break off into the joint cavity.

✔ Persons with DJD have pain, stiffness, and limited range of motion, particularly in the large weight-bearing joints and in the joints of the hand. Inflammation is usually not present, and tenderness is mild. The joints may become enlarged (deformed). Crepitation and changes in the alignment of the extremity may be present.

✔ Medical management objectives include relief of pain, restoration of joint function, and prevention of disability or further disease progression. Treatment includes medications, rest, exercise, joint protection, and the use of walking aids to decrease weight bearing on painful joints. Surgery may be indicated. Common surgical procedures include arthroscopic surgery for débridement, osteotomy for realignment, arthrodesis, and replacement arthroplasty.

✔ Nursing management of persons with DJD focuses on teaching persons about the disease process and measures to exert control over their situation. Patients who undergo surgery require special postoperative care. Of particular importance are the mobility restrictions following total hip replacement, and the exercise program following total knee replacement, and prevention of infection following any total joint replacement.

✔ Degenerative disease of the spine is a common but difficult problem. The intervertebral disks and facet joints of the spine are subjected to a great deal of stress in maintaining upright posture and providing mobility. Herniated nucleus pulposus (HNP), osteophyte formation, and spinal stenosis are several conditions that result from degenerative changes in the spine.

✔ Degenerative diseases of the spine are clinically manifested as low back pain, sciatic pain radiating down the leg (for example, with HNP), and neurologic signs and symptoms (for example, with HNP, stenosis, and osteophyte formation). Conservative medical management consists of rest, heat, medications, and traction to relieve muscle spasm. Surgical interventions are carried out to decompress nerve roots and to stabilize the spine. Spine surgery procedures include laminectomy, diskectomy, foraminotomy, and spinal fusion.

✔ Conservative nursing management consists of patient teaching, promoting comfort, and promoting lower extremity circulation.

✔ Nursing care following spinal surgery focuses on positioning (logrolling) and mobility, wound care, and patient comfort. Postoperative nursing interventions will differ depending on the level at which the spinal surgery was performed (for example, lumbar, thoracic, or cervical).

✔ Scoliosis is a restrictive disorder of the spine in which there is a lateral deviation of the spine from the midline. There are six classifications of scoliosis. Scoliosis may be present in both children and adults. Scoliosis may develop in localized areas of the spine or involve the whole spinal column. Curves may be S-shaped or C-shaped. The amount of impingement on the rib cage is determined by the degree of rotation of the curve. Stability of the spine and mobility of the trunk are affected by the balance of the curve.

✔ Scoliosis deformity can be slight, mild, or severe. Early deformity may not be easily detected but will increase with growth and age. Pain does not usually accompany scoliosis. The cardiopulmonary system can be impaired in advanced scoliosis. Medical management for early scoliosis includes exercise with or without traction, bracing in combination with exercise for curves less than 40 degrees, and corrective surgery if the curve exceeds 40 degrees and other measures have failed. Bone grafting and instrumentation is usually done to fuse the spine.

✔ Nursing management of persons with scoliosis consists of patient instruction for persons who are being treated conservatively. Patients who undergo surgery require special postoperative care. There is a high risk for pulmonary, gastrointestinal, and fluid balance complications following spinal fusion for scoliosis. Preventing such problems is a primary objective of the nurse. Instructing the patient about the brace he or she will be required to wear is another nursing responsibility.

✔ Other disorders of the musculoskeletal system include recurrent dislocation of the patella, gout, and bacterial arthritis. Recurrent dislocation of the patella involves malposition of the patellar tendon of the knee. Gout is a metabolic disorder that results from prolonged hyperuricemia. Urates are deposited in and around joints, usually in the knee or foot. Bacterial arthritis is a result of infection in which the synovial membrane is invaded by microorganisms.

✔ Recurrent dislocation of the patella is usually treated surgically. Management of gout is directed toward control of acute attacks and prevention of recurrent attacks. Medications and rest are prescribed to control joint symptoms. Medications are also used to enhance uric acid excretion or to decrease uric acid formation. Bacterial arthritis is treated with appropriate antibiotic therapy and rest (immobilization) of the joint. Irrigation and drainage may be necessary if antibiotic therapy is ineffective or if osteomyelitis is present.

✔ Nursing management of the above disorders is in collaboration with the medical plan of care. Patient teaching, promotion of rest or exercise as appropriate, promotion of comfort, and encouragement of participation in self care are emphasized.

QUESTIONS TO CONSIDER

- Describe five psychosocial problems persons with musculoskeletal disorders may have. What interventions could you use to help the patient manage these problems? How would you provide support to the patient?

- What is the nurse's role when considering preventable factors of musculoskeletal disorders?

- What are some of the current theories of causation of rheumatoid arthritis?

- What are the early clinical manifestations of rheumatoid arthritis, and how do they change as the disease progresses?

- What laboratory findings are usually indicative of rheumatoid arthritis?

- What is meant by the pyramid of therapy of rheumatoid arthritis? Describe some forms of adjunctive therapy.

- What are some nursing diagnoses commonly identified for persons with rheumatoid arthritis? List their related interventions.

- List the name and purpose of some of the surgeries performed to treat persons with rheumatoid arthritis. Describe the postoperative nursing care associated with each.

- What types of treatment or surgery may be necessary for uncontrolled SLE or secondary to complications of therapy?

- Describe the epidemiology/etiology, pathophysiology, and clinical manifestations of polymyositis. What marks the disease as dermatomyositis?

- Discuss the medical and nursing management of persons with polymyositis.

- What type of deformity may develop as a result of progression of ankylosing spondylitis?

- What are the goals of treatment for persons with ankylosing spondylitis?

- What are some of the other names for DJD? How are DJD and rheumatoid arthritis differentiated?

- What are some of the characteristic changes or symptoms that occur in certain joints as a result of DJD.

- Name two of the surgical procedures that may be performed for persons with DJD?

- What are some nursing diagnoses commonly identified for persons with DJD? List the related nursing interventions.

- What two postoperative considerations are of utmost importance when caring for a patient who has had a total joint replacement?

- Name some of the disorders that can result from degenerative changes in the spine.

- Describe the conservative treatment of DJD of the spine. List some of the surgical procedures that may be performed on the spine. What special positioning technique will the nurse assist the patient with postoperatively?

- Explain the signs and symptoms of slight, mild, and severe deformity in scoliosis.

- Outline both conservative and surgical treatment for scoliosis. What is the importance of the degree of the curve?

- What are some nursing diagnoses commonly identified for persons with scoliosis? List their related nursing interventions.

REFERENCES AND SELECTED READINGS

1. Allard JL and Dibble SL: Scoliosis surgery: a look at Luque rods, Am J Nurs 84:(5) 609-611, May 1984.
2. *Anderson LP: Carpal tunnel syndrome, Orthopaedic Nurs 5(4):40-42, 1986.
3. Bailey RW et al, editors: The cervical spine, Philadelphia, 1983, The JB Lippincott Co.
4. Barden RM: Osteonecrosis of the femoral head, Orthopaedic Nurs 4:(4) 45-51, July/Aug 1985.
5. *Blaha JD and Pickett JC, editors: Controversy on total knee arthroplasty, Clin Orthop 192S:2-112, 1985.
6. Blake SA: Non-cemented femoral prostheses: intraoperative focus, Orthop Nurs 4(1):40-42, Jan-Feb 1985.
7. Bluestone R, editor: Rheumatology, Boston, 1980, Houghton Mifflin Professional Publishers.
8. Brunner NA: Orthopedic nursing: a programmed approach, ed 4, St Louis, 1983, The CV Mosby Co.
9. *Cave L: Lowering the uncertainties of arthritis with a nurse-led support group, Orthop Nurs 3(5):39-42, Sept-Oct 1984.
10. *Ceccio CM: Postoperative pain relief through relaxation in elderly patients with fractured hips, Orthop Nurs 3(3):11-19, 1984.
11. Doheny MO: Porous coated femoral prosthesis: concepts and care considerations, Orthop Nurs 4(1):43-45, Jan-Feb 1985.
12. *Doheny MO and Ceccio CM: Total shoulder replacement: preparing patients for discharge, Orthop Nurs 7(3):13-21, 1988.
13. Edmonson AS and Crenshaw AH, editors: Campbell's operative orthopaedics, ed 6, St Louis, 1980, The CV Mosby Co.
14. Falkenburg SA: Choosing hand splints to aid carpal tunnel syndrome recovery, Occup Health Saf 56(5):60-64, 1987.
15. Flatt AE: Care of the arthritic hand, ed 4, St Louis, 1983, The CV Mosby Co.
16. Ghosh P: Articular cartilage: what it is, why it fails in osteoarthritis, and what can be done about it, Arthritis Care Res 1(4):211-221, 1988.
17. Hausman KL et al: Percutaneous lateral discectomy: another approach for the treatment of a herniated nucleus pulposus, Orthop Nurs 3(6):9-17, Nov-Dec 1984.
18. *Hennig LM et al: Keeping up on arthritis meds, RN 49(2):32-38, 1986.
19. Hilt NE and Cogburn SB: Manual of orthopedics, St Louis, 1980, The CV Mosby Co.
20. Hoyt NJ: Infections following orthopaedic surgery, Orthop Nurs 5(5):15-24, 1986.
21. *Ignatavicius DO: Meeting the psychosocial needs of patients with rheumatoid arthritis, Orthop Nurs 6(3):16-21, 1987.
22. Ivey M and Clark R: Arthroscopic debridement of the knee for septic arthritis, Clin Orthop 199:201-206, 1985.
23. *Joseph N: Arthritis medications from A to Z, Caring 8(1):14-16, 1989.

---

*References preceded by an asterisk are particularly well suited for student reading.

24. *Karn MA and Crawford AH: Postoperative nursing management of the patient following posterior spinal fusion, Orthop Nurs 3(2):21-25, 1984.

25. Keim HA and Hensinger RN: Spinal deformities: scoliosis and kyphosis, Clin Symp 41(4):3-32, 1989.

25a. Klippel JH: Systemic lupus erythematosus, treatment related complications superimposed on chronic disease, JAMA 263(13):1812-1815, 1990.

26. *Klippel JH, Strober S, and Wofsy D: New therapies for the rheumatic diseases, Bull Rheum Dis 38(4):1-7, 1989.

27. Koerner ME and Dickinson GR: Adult arthritis, Am J Nurs 83(2):253-278, Feb 1983.

28. Koffler D: Immunology of systemic lupus erythematosus and related rheumatic diseases, Clin Symp 39(2):2-36, 1987.

29. Kushner I et al, editors: Understanding arthritis, New York, 1984, Arthritis Foundation, Charles Scribner's Sons.

30. *Laborde JM and Powers MJ: Life satisfaction, health control orientation, and illness-related factors in persons with osteoarthritis, Res Nurs Health 8:183-190, 1985.

31. *Lambert VA et al: Coping with rheumatoid arthritis, Nurs Clin North Am 22:551-558, 1987.

32. Lamphier PC: Primary bone tumors, Orthop Nurs 4(5):17-23, 1985.

33. Ledo KM: Diagnostic overview: ankylosing spondylitis, Orthop Nurs 2(6):39-40, Nov-Dec 1983.

34. Levy RN et al: Progress in arthritis surgery: with special reference to current status of total joint arthroplasty, Clin Orthop 200:299-321, 1985.

35. Liang MH: Living with arthritis, HMS Health Letter, pp 5-8, Dec 1988.

36. Lin P, editor: Posterior lumbar interbody fusion, Clin Orthop 193:2-132, 1985.

37. Lorish C, Richards B, and Brown S: Missed medication doses in rheumatic arthritis patients: intentional and unintentional reasons, Arthritis Care Res 2(1):3-9, 1989.

38. *Mankin HJ and Treadwell BV: Osteoarthritis: a 1987 update, Bull Rheum Dis 36(5):1-10, 1986.

39. *Marchette L and Marchette B: Back injury: a preventable occupational hazard, Orthop Nurs 4(6):25-29, Nov-Dec 1985.

40. McCarty DJ, editor: Arthritis and allied conditions: a textbook of rheumatology, ed 11, Philadelphia, 1989, Lea & Febiger.

41. *Miller B: Osteoarthritis in the primary health care setting, Orthop Nurs 6(5):42-46, 1987.

42. Morrey BF and Kavanagh BF: Cementless joint replacement: current status and future, Bull Rheum Dis 37(4):1-7, 1987.

43. Moskowitz RW: Clinical rheumatology: a problem oriented approach to diagnosis and management, ed 2, Philadelphia, 1982, Lea & Febiger.

44. Moskowitz RW et al: Osteoarthritis: diagnosis and management, Philadelphia, 1984, WB Saunders Co.

45. Mourad L and Droste M: The nursing process in the care of adults with orthopedic conditions, ed 2, New York, 1988, John Wiley & Sons Inc.

46. Newschwander GE and Dunst RM: Limb lengthening with the Ilizarov external fixator, Orthop Nurs 8(3):15-21, 1989.

47. Nordby EJ: A comparison of discectomy and chemonucleolysis, Clin Orthop 200:279-283, 1985.

48. *Olson EV, editor: The hazards of immobility, Am J Nurs 67:780-797, 1967.

49. Panush RS: Controversial arthritis remedies, Bull Rheum Dis 34(5):1-10, 1984.

50. Pfeiffer CA and Wetstone SL: Health locus on control and well-being in systemic lupus erythematosus, Arthritis Care Res 1(3):131-138, 1988.

51. Phillips KF: The use of gold therapy with rheumatoid arthritis, Orthop Nurs 2(4):31-34, July-Aug 1983.

52. Pigg J, Driscoll P, and Caniff R: Rheumatology nursing: a problem-oriented approach, New York, 1985, John Wiley & Sons Inc.

53. *Rodts MF: Surgical intervention for adult scoliosis, Orthop Nurs 6(6):11-17, 1987.

54. *Schumacher HR: Primer on the rheumatic diseases, ed 9, Atlanta, 1988, Arthritis Foundation.

55. *Schlegel SI and Paulus HE: Update on NSAID use in rheumatic diseases, Bull Rheum Dis 36(6):1-8, 1986.

56. *Spindler CE: Audiovisual preoperative teaching for the total hip patient, Orthop Nurs 3(1):30-40, Jan-Feb 1984.

57. *Strang EL and Johns JL: Nursing care of the patient treated with continuous passive motion following total knee arthroplasty, Orthop Nurs 3(6):27-32, Nov-Dec 1984.

58. Swezey RL, editor: Straight talk on ankylosing spondylitis, Sherman Oaks, Calif, 1985, Ankylosing Spondylitis Association, Inc.

59. Swinson DR and Swinburn WR: Rheumatology, New York, 1980, John Wiley & Sons, Inc.

60. *Walsh CR and Wirth CR: Total knee arthroplasty: biomechanical and nursing considerations, Orthop Nurs 4(1):29-34, Jan-Feb 1985.

61. Wick JL: The role of ergonomics in the elimination and prevention of work-related musculoskeletal problems, Orthop Nurs 8(1):41-42, 1989.

62. *Willey T: High-tech beds and mattress overlays: a decision guide, Am J Nurs 89(9):1142-1145, 1989.

63. Wittert D: Rotator cuff tears, Orthop Nurs 5(4):17-25, 1986.

ALTERATIONS IN DEFENSE AND PROTECTION

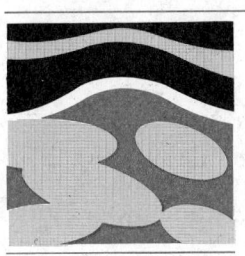

CHAPTER 71

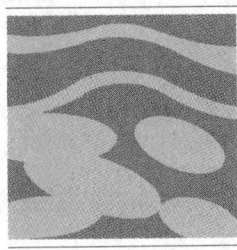

Assessment of the Skin

BARBARA C. LONG

CHAPTER OBJECTIVES

After studying this chapter, the student should be able to:
1   Identify the structures and functions of the skin.
2   Explain physiologic skin changes in the elderly.
3   Describe guidelines and parameters for assessment of the skin and accessory structures.
4   Differentiate among various skin lesions.

The integument, or skin, is the largest organ of the body. It is exposed to the external environment and provides the first line of defense of the body; yet at the same time it is affected by changes in the internal environment. (See Chapter 8 for a review of biologic defense mechanisms.) Assessment of the integument provides data about how the person is affected by and is coping with both external and internal environments. Data obtained in the assessment provide the bases for identification of nursing problems related to the skin, potential for infection, fluid and electrolyte imbalances, nutritional imbalances, or inadequate oxygenation of tissues. Baseline observations are useful for identifying changes that may occur.

ANATOMY AND PHYSIOLOGY OF THE SKIN

STRUCTURE OF THE SKIN

The skin is composed of two main layers, the epidermis and the dermis (Figure 71-1). The *epidermis* is composed of two parts: a thin layer of closely packed, dead squamous cells covering a second layer of cells containing melanin, which gives skin its color. The dead cells are constantly being shed and replaced by deeper cells. Blood vessels do not reach into the epidermis.

The second main layer, the *dermis* or corium, is connected to the epidermis by a convoluted layer of cells that produces new cells for the epidermis. The dermis is composed of bundles of collagen fibers that act to support the epidermis. It is well supplied with nerves and blood vessels and contains the sweat glands, sebaceous glands, and hair follicles.

Thickness of the skin varies over different areas of the body. Exposed areas such as hands and face are usually thicker. The skin on the inner aspect of the arms is thinner and therefore more sensitive to heat.

Sweat glands excrete directly to the surface of the skin and are under control of the sympathetic nervous system. There are two types of sweat glands, *eccrine* and *apocrine*. The eccrine glands are distributed throughout the body and are more abundant in the forehead, palms, and soles of the feet. Eccrine glands assist in the heat-regulating mechanisms of the body. The apocrine glands are found mainly in the axillary and genital regions. Some of the protoplasm of these secretory cells is secreted with the fluid, and it is bacterial decomposition of the sweat from these glands that is responsible for body odor.[1] Sweat glands of the axilla, palms, and soles are mostly under psychic control.

Sebaceous glands secrete an oily, odorless fluid (*sebum*) into the hair follicles. Ear wax is sebum from glands in the external ear canal. Sebum protects the hair follicle from infection and lubricates the skin.

Beneath the skin is the subcutaneous tissue composed of loose connective tissue filled with fat cells. Fat conducts heat only one fourth as rapidly as do other tissues and thus serves as the heat insulator of the body.

FUNCTIONS OF THE SKIN
PROTECTION

The outermost layer of the epidermis, the stratum corneum, is a relatively impermeable layer of tightly packed flat cells that provide protection of the underlying tissue from the outer environment. There are numerous nonpathogenic bacteria on the outer surface of the skin, but the dryness of the surface keeps the number small because microorganisms require moisture for growth. Bacteria that penetrate hair follicles are usually removed by the sebum. Fat-soluble substances can penetrate the skin by passing through the hair follicles and sebaceous glands. Atrophic or senile skin contains fewer hair follicles; thus permeability of fat-soluble substances through the skin is decreased in the elderly.

An intact skin is the first line of defense against bac-

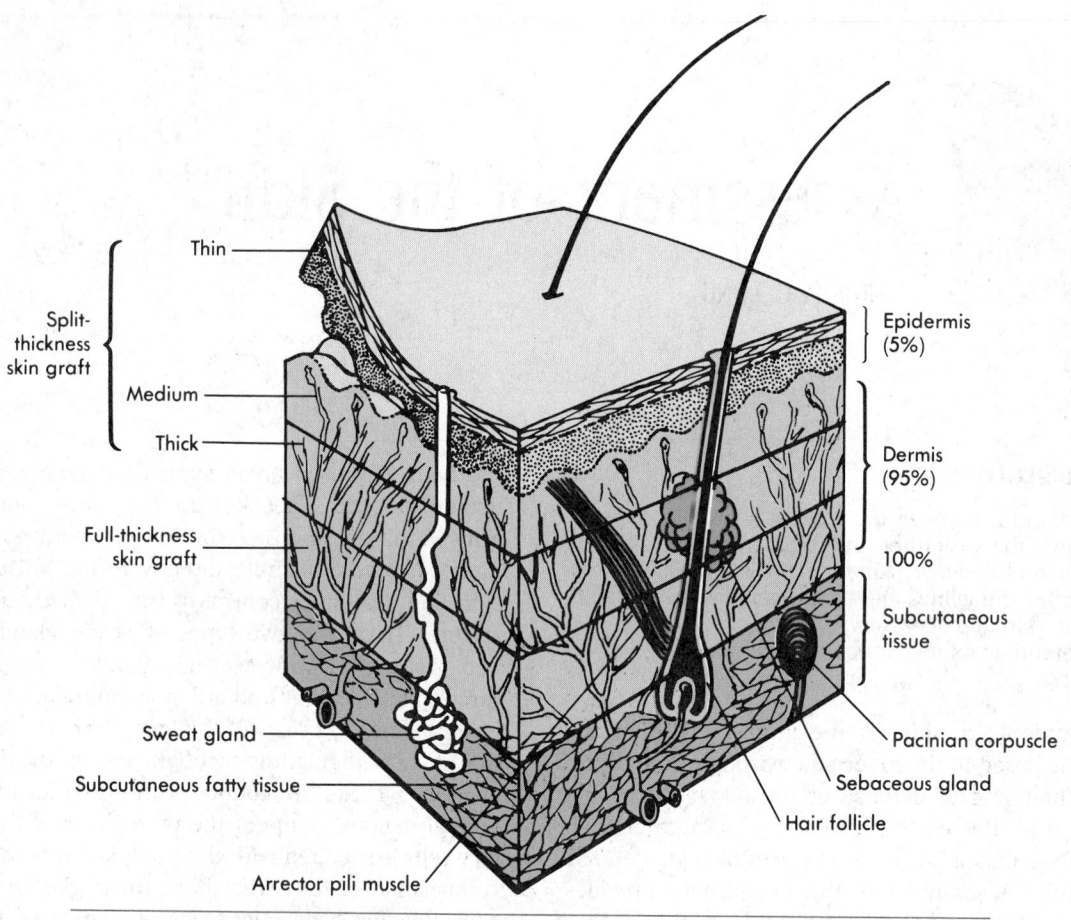

FIGURE 71-1 Structures of the skin and skin layers.

terial and foreign substance invasion, slight physical trauma, heat, or rays. The epidermis can be weakened by scraping or stripping the surface, such as by dry razors or by removal of tape. Once the barrier has weakened, permeability to bacteria, drugs, and so forth is increased. Large amounts of drugs can be absorbed by extensive denuded skin areas. Epidermis that becomes overdry may crack and lead to breaks in the surface. If it remains wet for long periods of time, it becomes macerated and the moisture provides a medium for bacterial growth.

The stratum corneum is not found in mucous membranes since these areas are somewhat protected from the external environment. Fluids and other substances such as certain drugs can be absorbed through the mucous membranes.

HEAT REGULATION

Body temperature is controlled by *radiation* of heat from the surface of the skin, *conduction* of heat from skin to other objects or air, removal of heat by air currents on the skin (*convection*), or *evaporation* of water from skin surfaces. Insensible water evaporation from the skin and lungs occurs at a rate of 600 to 1000 ml/

day. On a hot day the only way the body can lose heat is by evaporation, and anything that restricts evaporation under these conditions will increase body temperature. Blood vessels of the skin assist in control of body temperature by constriction in cold environments to promote conservation of heat, and dilation in warm environments to promote loss of heat by radiation. These mechanisms help maintain a constant internal body temperature.

SENSORY PERCEPTION

Receptors for pain, touch, heat, and cold are present in the skin.

EXCRETION

Water lost through the skin is a factor in maintaining water balance in the body. Salt is lost through excessive sweating in addition to water loss. A person can become acclimatized to a continually hot environment, however, and the amount of salt lost decreases over time.

VITAMIN D PRODUCTION

Synthesis of vitamin D takes place in the skin by the effect of sunlight (ultraviolet rays). Vitamin D is neces-

TABLE 71-1 Changes from aging in skin, hair, and nails

Parameters	Observable Changes	Cause
SKIN		
Color	Paleness in white skin	Decreased vascularity of dermis; loss of melanocytes
	Brown spots (senile lentigenes)	Hyperpigmentation
	Purple patches (senile purpura)	Blood leaking from poorly supported fragile capillaries
Moisture	Dry skin, decreased perspiration	Decreased sebaceous and sweat gland activity
Elasticity, turgor	Decreased elasticity	Loss of collagen and elastic fibers
	Loose folds and wrinkles	
	Decreased turgor	
Texture	Some rough areas	Environmental effects over time and less moisture
	Thin, more transparent skin	Thinning of epidermis from decreased vascularity of dermis; loss of underlying tissue
HAIR		
Color	Grayness	Decreased number of melanocytes in hair
Consistency	Thinner on head and body	Decreased density and rate of hair growth
	Coarser in nose of men	Increased density of nasal hair
Distribution	Loss of hair on head and body	Decreased rate of hair growth; decreased hormones; decreased peripheral circulation
	Increased hair on face of women	Higher androgen to estrogen ratio
NAILS		
	More brittle	Slowing of nail growth; decreased peripheral circulation
	Longitudinal ridges	
	Thickening and yellowing of toenails	

sary in the metabolism of calcium and phosphorus (Chapter 23).

EXPRESSION

Because the skin is the part of the body that is visible to others, it is a means of communicating feelings. Also, because of its visibility, skin is largely involved in a person's feelings of *body image*. Individuals become concerned when there is fear of or presence of disfigurement. (See Chapter 18 for a discussion of body image.)

PHYSIOLOGIC CHANGES WITH AGING

Many skin changes may be observed as the person ages (Table 71-1). These changes result primarily from loss of subcutaneous tissue, degeneration of collagen and elastic fibers, loss of melanocytes, increased capillary fragility, decreased secretion of sweat glands, hormonal changes, and overexposure to environmental elements.

The skin loses its elasticity and becomes loose and wrinkled. Exposed areas may be thickened, but in general the skin becomes thinner, drier, and more fragile. Lesions appear, the most common of which are *senile lentigines* (brown spots, Figure 71-2) or *senile purpura* (red to purple ecchymoses seen on exposed areas). Seborrheic keratoses (Chapter 72) are more common than actinic keratoses. Changes in appearance of the hair and nails also occur.

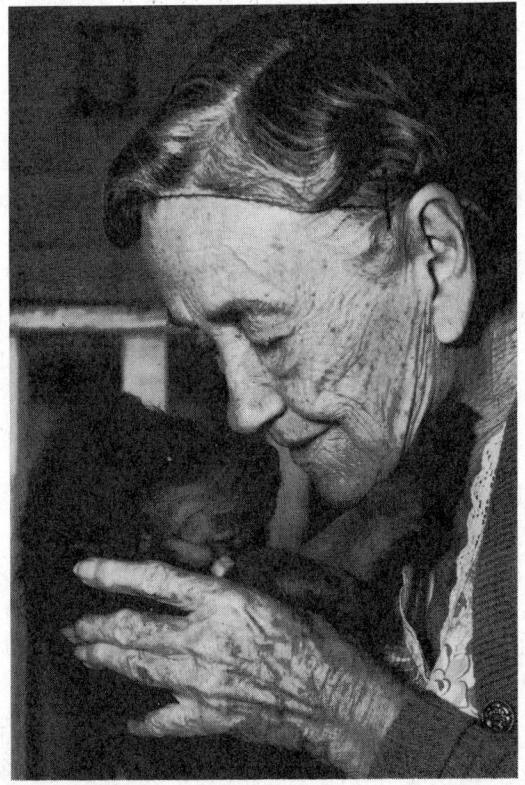

FIGURE 71-2 Elderly patients have skin changes. Note discolored spots on skin and tiny raised area on this woman's eyelid. (VanDerMeid from Monkmeyer Press Photo Service.)

The elderly person is also more likely to have one or more chronic diseases and to be taking medications that can cause skin changes. Dry skin may cause itching and may lead to skin breakdown if scratched. Stasis dermatitis may occur if there is marked decrease of circulation to the legs. Skin infections occur more readily because of increased epidermal permeability.

SUBJECTIVE DATA

The patient history is of less importance in skin disorders than is the physical assessment. If during a general history the patient describes a skin problem or skin discomfort (itching, superficial pain), then further data are obtained, including the following information:

1. *Onset of the problem:* initial sites: when were changes first noticed; skin appearance at onset; any other symptoms noted at time of onset, such as pain, itching
2. *Changes since onset:* changes in location of lesions; changes in appearance; new symptoms such as pain or itching
3. *Specific known cause:* for example, contact with poison ivy, exposure to a known allergen, stress
4. *If cause is unknown:*
   a. Recent exposure to sensitizing substances, such as metals, chemicals, detergents, poisonous plants
   b. New drug prescriptions such as penicillin
   c. Occupation: contact with potential skin irritants, hands constantly in water
   d. Recreational activities: for example, painting, camping, gardening
   e. Exposure to sun (burn, photosensitivity, skin cancer) or cold (frostbite)
5. *Alleviating factors:* physician-prescribed or self-prescribed
6. *Psychologic reaction to problem:* withdrawal from social activities; cosmetics for cover up; feelings concerning self in view of the problem (body image)

OBJECTIVE DATA
METHODS OF ASSESSMENT

The skin is an organ that can be examined by *direct inspection* and *observation* with no tools but a good light. *Palpation* is also used in gathering data related to certain types of lesions.

Considerable data can be obtained from physical assessment of the skin, not only concerning dermatologic problems, but also concerning the health status of the individual. A systematic head-to-toe skin assessment is usually carried out while gathering other significant data in the initial interview and physical assessment of the person. Specific areas of the skin are reassessed as potential or existing problems are identified.

GUIDELINES FOR SKIN ASSESSMENT

1. Be prepared; have a good light available. If the lighting is inadequate, lesions may be missed or described inaccurately.
2. Be systematic: if only some parts of the skin are inspected, an important parameter may be omitted or a lesion missed.
3. Be thorough: look at all areas carefully. If the person is lying down, be sure to examine the back, especially the sacral area. Lift folds of tissue, such as under the breasts or gluteal folds. Embarrassment by the examiner or anticipated embarrassment of the examinee may result in inadequate data.
4. Be specific: when lesions are identified, describe the lesions using the metric system and established parameters (for example, color, size, shape).
5. Compare right side with left side: when observing changes in skin color or tissue shape, always compare one side of the body with the other to differentiate structural from pathologic changes.
6. Record the data: unrecorded data is lost data. Baseline observations indicating normality or abnormality are needed for comparison with subsequent findings. Changes need to be recorded to determine progress toward achieving desired outcomes.

PARAMETERS OF GENERAL SKIN ASSESSMENT

The objective data to be collected when examining the skin for general health status include skin color, temperature, moisture, elasticity, turgor, texture, and odor.

COLOR

Changes in skin color are best observed in the lips, mucous membranes of the mouth, earlobes, fingernails and toenails, and the extremities. The lips show rapid color changes. Color of the skin varies with the amount of *melanin* in the cells and with the *blood supply* (Table 71-2). Skin color may be masked by cosmetics or tanning.

Pigmentation

Melanin formation requires the amino acid tyrosine, the enzyme tyrosinase, and molecular oxygen. Variations of general pigmentation are seen within one individual; an increase in pigmentation is usually seen on exposed surfaces and in the areola of the nipples. Conversely, decreased pigmentation is seen on unexposed surfaces and on the palms and soles of dark-skinned persons.

Hyperpigmentation occurs normally in some persons as a genetic factor (dark skin). Light-skinned persons may have increased pigmentation from the effects of sunlight (tanning). Melanin is formed in the basal cells

TABLE 71-2 Skin color changes

Color	Physiology	Conditions
Redness	Vasodilation: more rapid blood flow, more oxygenated blood giving a reddish hue (erythema)	Blushing heat, inflammation, fever, alcohol ingestion, extreme cold (below 15° C), hot flushes, polycythemia
Whiteness (pallor)	Vasoconstriction: slower blood flow, less blood in capillaries	Cold, fear, shock
	Partially obstructed blood flow: less blood in capillaries	Vasospasm, thrombus, narrowed vessels
	Fluid between blood vessels and skin surface	Edema
	Decreased oxygenation of blood from decreased hemoglobin	Anemia
	Loss of melanin	Vitiligo
Bluish	Deoxygenated hemoglobin (cyanosis) seen in earlobes, lips, mucous membranes of mouth, nail beds	Heart or lung disease, inadequate respiration, peripheral blood vessel obstruction
Yellow	Increased bile pigment in blood eventually distributed to skin and mucous membranes and to sclera of eye	Liver disease, obstruction of bile ducts, chronic uremia, rapid hemolysis
Brown	Increased melanin deposits: normal in brown-black races	Aging, sunburn, pituitary, adrenal or liver disease
Dullness	Vasoconstriction in dark skin	Cold, fear, shock

of the stratum basale and then gradually moves to the surface, where it is cast off and the tan fades. Elderly light-skinned persons may normally develop irregular brown patches. Hyperpigmentation may be seen with x-ray therapy as a result of activation of tyrosinase. This type of hyperpigmentation fades slowly but may be long lasting. Hydroquinone with salicylic acid or with retinoic acid (Atra) inhibits the tyrosinase reaction. Hyperpigmentation also occurs with inflammations, acne vulgaris, drug eruptions, neurodermatitis, and pityriasis rosea.

Hypopigmentation occurs normally in some persons as a genetic factor (light skin). Albinos have a congenital inability to produce melanin. Severe trauma can destroy cells producing melanin and result in hypopigmentation (scar tissue). Some healthy persons develop a condition called *vitiligo* in which there is a failure of melanin formation in certain areas, primarily around orifices and hairy areas, producing sharply demarcated white patches. Vitiligo can also occur with hyperthyroidism, pernicious anemia, and adrenocortical insufficiency. One treatment for small patches of vitiligo is methoxypsoralen orally plus exposure to sunlight or longwave ultraviolet light.

Blood Supply

The degree of blood supplied to the skin produces color changes. The rate of blood flow through the skin is highly variable because of its function in heat control. The blood vessels are innervated by the sympathetic nervous system; thus vasoconstriction occurs with the stress response. With *vasoconstriction*, smaller amounts of blood pass through the vessels, producing decreased redness; a dark skin becomes duller and a light skin whiter (pallor). *Vasodilation* increases the amount of oxygenated blood flow, and the skin acquires a reddish color (erythema). Vascular flush areas of the body are the "butterfly" band from cheek to cheek across the nose, the neck, upper chest, flexor surfaces of the extremities, and genital areas.

Changes in blood composition can also alter skin color. Excess deoxygenated hemoglobin gives a bluish tint *(cyanosis)* to the skin and mucous membranes. An excess of bile pigment results in a yellowish tint to the skin and sclera of the eyes. Increased RBCs (seen in polycythemia) give a reddish tint to the skin.

TEMPERATURE

The temperature of the skin is regulated by vasoconstriction or vasodilation. If an excess amount of heat is being produced within the body such as with fever or exercise, or if heat from the external environment increases, the sympathetic centers in the hypothalamus are inhibited and vasodilation occurs. An increase in the amount of blood flow creates a sensation of warmth on the skin. A local inflammation of the skin or underlying tissue also produces vasodilation; this is part of the inflammatory response. Cold skin is caused by vasoconstriction as a result of sympathetic stimulation. To assess the temperature of the skin, the backs of the fingers, which are more sensitive than the finger tips, should be used.

MOISTURE

Skin is assessed as being dry, moist, or oily. *Dry skin* is frequently seen in the elderly person because of decreased activity of the sebaceous glands. Dry skin and mucous membranes are also seen in persons who are dehydrated as water moves from the cells into the intravascular compartments. Persons with hypothyrodism have thick, dry, leathery skin.

Moist skin is caused by the presence of water or sweat on the surface. Overheating produces sweating. Persons with hyperthyroidism have moist, smooth skin. Some persons have more effective sweat mechanisms than others. Stress, shock, or any situation that stimulates the sympathetic nervous system will cause increased fluid loss through the sweat glands. Since vasoconstriction is also occurring with stimulation of the sympathetic nervous system, the skin is cold and wet (clammy).

Oily skin is frequently seen in the adolescent. Excess sebum formation by the sebaceous glands may lead to blocking of the follicular orifices, resulting in blackheads (*comedo*), acne, or sebaceous cysts.

ELASTICITY, MOBILITY, AND TURGOR

The skin is very elastic and moves freely over most areas. It loses its mobility when it becomes stretched; this occurs with edema when the interstitial spaces become filled with fluid and swelling occurs. Skin becomes rigid in the person with scleroderma, a collagen disease, as a result of collagenous fibrosis of the tissue. *Turgor* is tissue tension and is measured by the speed of skin return to normal position of fullness after it has been stretched. Decreased turgor indicates dehydration of the tissue. To assess elasticity and turgor, a portion of skin over the sternum is picked up (elasticity) and the speed of return to normal is assessed (turgor). Skin that has decreased turgor will remain for a few seconds in a fold before returning slowly to normal (Figure 71-3).

TEXTURE

Roughness may occur normally on exposed areas, especially elbows and the soles of the feet. The skin of an infant is usually soft and smooth, whereas that of an elderly person may be rough and lack underlying tissue substance (atrophy). Roughness may occur with hypothyroidism.

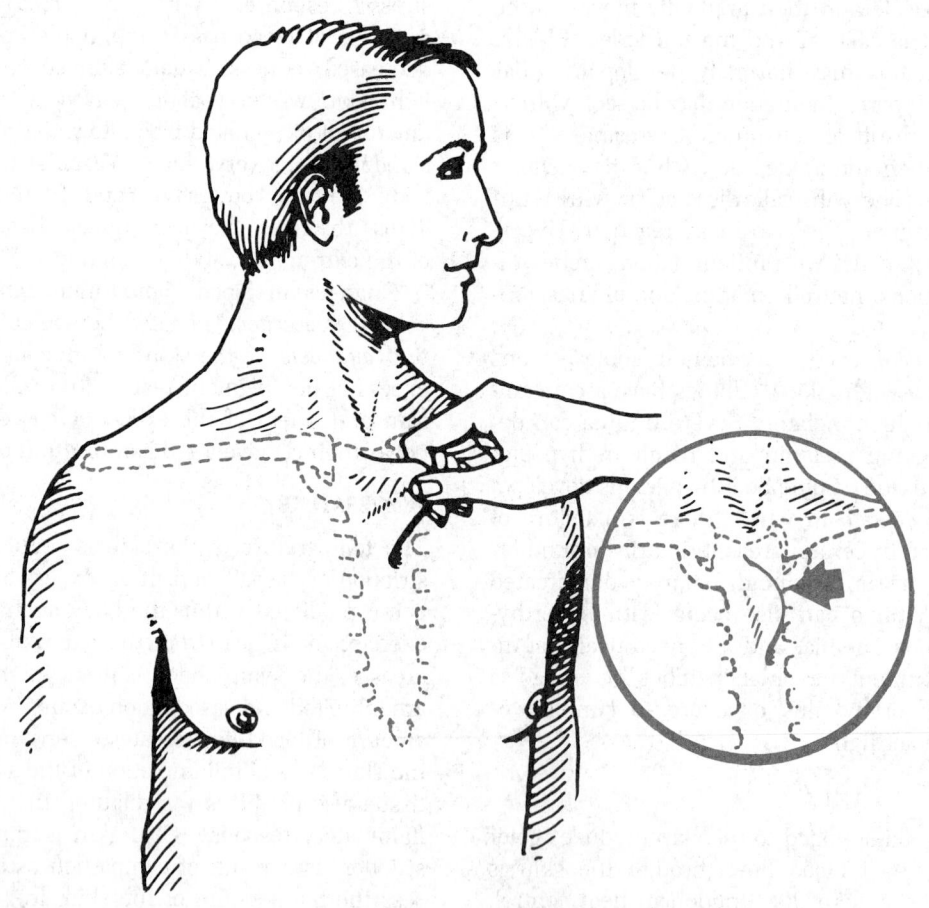

FIGURE 71-3 Examination of skin turgor. When skin over sternum is picked up, a fold of skin remains for a few seconds when poor turgor is present.

ODOR

Normal clean skin is usually free of odor except for areas containing apocrine sweat glands. Odor occurs because of bacterial composition of protein matter. Some draining skin lesions may produce an odor.

ACCESSORY STRUCTURES
HAIR

If the patient is wearing a wig or other hairpiece, this should be removed temporarily for inspection of the hair and scalp. It is easy to miss lesions on the scalp, and the patient can assist by indicating areas of itching, pain, or roughness.

Hair growth, pattern and distribution are indicators of the general state of health of an individual.[3] Excessive hair growth (*hirsutism*) is usually related to hormonal changes. Hair loss (*alopecia*) occurs normally with age, especially in some men. Abnormal hair loss may be caused by hormonal imbalance, general ill health, infections of the scalp, typhoid fever, chronic liver disease, stress, or drugs (antimetabolites, heparin). Changes in hair distribution on the body may be caused by hormonal changes. Hair loss on the dorsum of the toes may be indicative of decreased arterial circulation. Contrary to popular belief, shaving does not promote the growth of dark coarse hairs, singeing hair does not alter growth, brushing and massaging do not increase hair growth, nor does hair "turn gray overnight."[7] The hair shaft is an inert structure, and changes occur over time as a result of hormonal activity and the availability of nutrients to the bulb at the base of the hair root.

Hair should also be free of lice or nits. Nits are the eggs of the lice and are usually found embedded on hair strands behind the ears. They are observed as small, glistening, grayish specks along the hair shaft near the scalp.

NAILS

The appearance of the nails changes with age and with ill health. Changes in hardness, brittleness, roughness, or shape may be indicative of some metabolic diseases, nutritional imbalances including vitamin deficiencies, or digestive disturbances. Pale nail beds and poor capillary return (slow return to normal color after the nail is pinched) may indicate hypoxia or anemia. Clubbing of the nails refers to the elimination of the small concave portion at the base of the nail by soft tissue growth; this occurs with certain pulmonary diseases (Figure 71-4).

The epithelial lining of the nail bed is usually inert. The nail is affixed to the nail bed, and both move outward as the nail grows. The epithelial lining of the nail bed loses its inert quality in the presence of inflammatory lesions of the nail bed, such as occur with psoriasis or ringworm, and the nail bed begins to keratinize. Horny masses collect under the nail, resulting in a

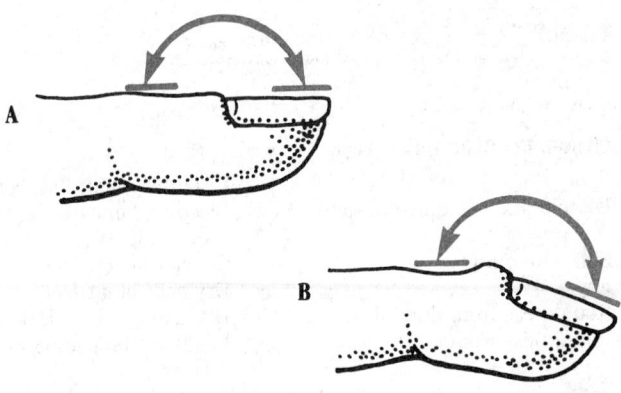

FIGURE 71-4 A, Normal nail angle. **B,** Abnormal nail angle seen in clubbing.

thickening deformity of the nail and possible separation from the nail bed.[7]

Infections of the tissue around the nail may occur (*paronychia*) characterized by red, shiny skin and painful swelling around the edge of the nail. The infection may result from trauma or from certain diseases such as psoriasis or dermatitis. If the nail is lost, it will usually grow back unless the nail bed has been injured.

LESIONS

When lesions are observed, the following parameters are used for description: type, color, size, shape and configuration, texture, effect of pressure, distribution, arrangement, and variety.

TYPE

Use of medical terminology facilitates communication (Table 71-3). For example, use of the term *vesicle* will immediately establish the lesion as a clear, fluid-filled lesion smaller than 1 cm (Figure 71-5).

SIZE

The metric system is used for descriptions. A helpful hint is to measure a portion of one's own fingers, such as the distance from the tip of the right thumb to the first joint, or the width of the nail on the right little finger. This can then be used as a gauge for estimating the size of a lesion.

SHAPE AND CONFIGURATION

Shape can be described as round, oval, and so on. *Configuration* refers to the sharpness of demarcation of the lesion, that is, if it is discrete or diffuse.

TEXTURE

The lesion is described as being rough or smooth, dry or moist, and on the surface or deeply penetrating into the tissue.

TABLE 71-3 Types of skin lesions

Observed Skin Changes	Differentiation	Term	Example
CHANGE IN COLOR OR TEXTURE			
Spot	Circumscribed; flat; color change	Macule	Freckle
Discoloration (reddish purple)	Bleeding beneath the surface; injury to tissue	Contusion	Bruise
Soft whitening	Caused by repeated wetting of skin	Maceration	Between toes after soaking
Flake	Dry cells of surface	Scale	Dandruff; psoriasis
Roughness from dried fluid	Dry exudate over lesions	Crust	Eczema, impetigo
Roughness from cells	Leathery thickening of outer skin layer	Lichenification	Callus on foot
CHANGE IN SHAPE			
Fluid-filled lesions	Less than 1 cm; clear fluid	Vesicle	Blister; chickenpox
	Greater than 1 cm; clear fluid	Bulla	Large blister, pemphigus
	Small, thick yellowish fluid (pus)	Pustule	Acne
Solid mass, *cellular* growth	Less than 5 mm	Papule	Small mole; raised rash
	5 mm to 2 cm	Nodule	Enlarged lymph node
	Greater than 2 cm	Tumor	Benign or malignant tumor
	Excess connective tissue over scar	Keloid	Overgrown scar
Swelling of tissue	Generalized swelling; fluid between cells	Edema	Inflammation; swelling of feet
	Circumscribed surface edema; transient; some itching	Wheal	Allergic reaction
BREAKS IN SKIN SURFACES			
Oozing, scraped surface	Loss of superficial structure of skin	Abrasion	"Floor burn"; scrape
Scooped-out depression	Loss of deeper layers of skin	Ulcer	Decubitus or stasis ulcer
Superficial linear skin breaks	Scratch marks, frequently by finger nails	Excoriations	Scratching
Linear cracks or cleft	Slit or splitting of skin layers	Fissure	Athlete's foot
Jagged cut	Tearing of skin surface	Laceration	Accidental cut by blunt object
Linear cut, edges approximated	Cutting by sharp instrument	Incision	Knife cut
VASCULAR LESIONS			
Small, flat, round, purplish, red spot	Intradermal or submucous hemorrhage	Petechia	Bleeding tendency; vitamin C deficiency
Spiderlike, red, small	Dilation of capillaries, arterioles, or venules	Telangiectasis	Liver disease, vitamin B deficiency
Discoloration, reddish purple	Escape of blood into tissue	Ecchymosis	Trauma to blood vessels

EFFECT OF PRESSURE

Some vascular lesions blanch when pressure is applied and then return to their original color. Other lesions remain the same with pressure.

ARRANGEMENT

Some lesions occur in patches, whereas others occur diffusely over the body. This is an important parameter when describing rashes.

DISTRIBUTION

Some lesions occur in certain parts of the body, such as on exposed areas as with contact dermatitis, or on main body areas as in chickenpox. The lesions may follow the area of distribution of one of the spinal nerves as in herpes zoster.

VARIETY

In some diseases, such as smallpox, the lesions may all occur at the same time, whereas in chickenpox the lesions occur in crops so that there may be lesions at different stages of development occurring at the same time.

ASSESSMENT OF DARK SKIN

Assessment of dark-skinned persons is more difficult than that of light-skinned persons because color changes are less obvious. Often other signs and symp-

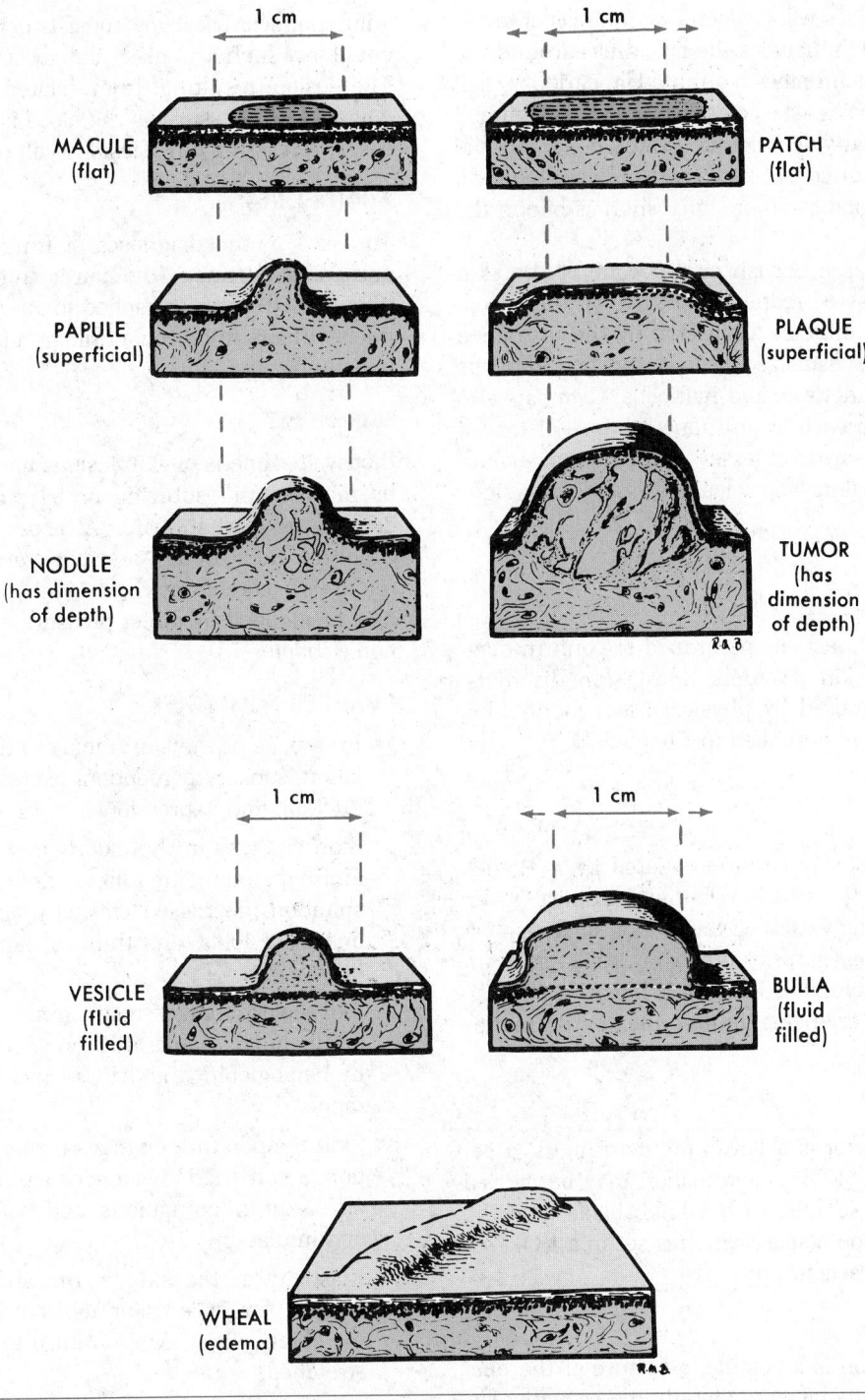

FIGURE 71-5 Skin lesions. (From Stewart WD, Danto JL, and Madden S: Dermatology: diagnosis and treatment of cutaneous disorders, ed 4, St Louis, 1978, The CV Mosby Co.)

toms must be used to reach a conclusion. For example, when a skin area is inflamed, the erythema may not be noticeable and the involved area must be palpated for warmth and edema. Rashes may not be visible and must be determined by palpation if the rash is papular or by patient reports of pruritus.

Melanin, which gives skin its general color, is produced by melanocytes. The skin of darkly pigmented persons does not contain more melanocytes, but the melanocytes are larger and produce more melanin.[7] Pigmented skin offers more protection from ultraviolet radiation; hence dark skin reacts less to sunlight and skin cancers occur less frequently.

Skin color changes will be seen best in areas of lesser pigmentation, which includes the lips, areas around the mouth, mucous membranes, conjunctiva, earlobes, nail beds, palms, and soles. The sclera of many dark-skinned persons contains fatty deposits with carotene, giving the sclera a yellowish tinge.[9] In these persons, jaundice will have to be concluded by other signs, such as bile in the urine or feces.

Pallor is seen as a grayish or dull tone of the skin caused by the loss of redness provided by the blood. This sign may be difficult to observe by the untrained eye. Pallor can be visualized best in the lips, mucous membranes, conjunctivae, and nail beds. *Cyanosis* also gives the skin a grayish or dull tone because of loss of redness. All of the areas of lesser pigmentation, including the earlobes, palms, and soles, are assessed for signs of cyanosis.

DIAGNOSTIC TESTS

Diagnostic tests are usually performed to confirm diagnoses of certain skin disorders. Most skin disorders, however, are diagnosed by physical assessment. Skin tests for allergies are described in Chapter 75.

LABORATORY TESTS
TZANCK SMEAR

Vesicular disorders may be differentiated by a Tzanck smear. The top of the vesicle is cut and a smear taken from the base of the vesicle. Examination of the smear may identify a virus (herpes simplex or zoster) or acantholytic cells (pemphigus). The test is negative for vesicles from burns, erythema multiforme, or dermatitis herpetiforme.

KOH TEST

If the causative factor is believed to be a fungus, a potassium hydroxide (KOH) examination may be carried out. The lesion is scraped with a knife blade, and the scraping is placed on a slide, which is set in a KOH solution before microscopic study.

CULTURE

If the primary lesion is a pustule, a culture of the pustule contents may be taken to identify the causative organism. Streptococci and staphylococci are commonly seen.

SPECIAL TESTS
DIASCOPY

Pigmented lesions resulting from increased blood in dilated vessels (such as erythema, spider angiomas, telangiectasis) can be differentiated from other lesions resulting from blood that has escaped into the tissue (such as petechiae, ecchymoses) or resulting from melanin changes. Diascopy consists of pressing a transparent object such as a glass slide over a pigmented lesion. The lesion resulting from dilated blood vessels will whiten with pressure as the blood is pushed to other areas, whereas the other lesions will not change color.

WOOD'S LIGHT

To assist in the diagnoses of fungal infections of the hair and skin (tinea), the hair is illuminated by a special filter (Wood's filter) attached to an ultraviolet lamp. The infected hairs fluoresce a brilliant green or appear luminous under the light.

SKIN BIOPSY

Biopsy specimens of skin lesions may be obtained either by incision and suturing or by punch biopsy, which does not require suturing. A biopsy punch has a sharp edge that cuts through previously anesthetized skin and removes a core from the lesion for analysis. Bleeding may be stopped by direct pressure or by electrodesiccation (Chapter 73).

CHAPTER SUMMARY

- Functions of the skin include protection, heat regulation, sensory perception, excretion, vitamin D production, and expression.

- Skin changes in the elderly include hypopigmented and hyperpigmented areas, dry skin, decreased perspiration, decreased elasticity and turgor, wrinkles and loose folds, and thinner skin with some roughened areas.

- Skin color changes result from changes in melanin production, vascular dilation or constriction, changes in hemoglobin and RBCs, and increased bile pigment.

- Skin temperature changes result from vascular dilation or constriction; some causes include fever, exercise, skin inflammations, and sympathetic inhibition or stimulation.

- Elasticity of the skin is the ability of the skin to stretch; turgor is tissue tension and is measured by the ability of the skin to return to normal after being stretched.

- Hair loss results normally from aging; hair may also be lost by decreased oxygenation, general ill health, stress, drugs, or chronic liver disease.

- Nail changes may occur from aging, metabolic diseases, nutritional deficiencies, or decreased oxygenation.

- Solid tissue growths, according to size, include papules, nodules, and tumors. Fluid-filled lesions by size include vesicle and bulla; if the fluid is pus, it forms a pustule.

✔ Breaks in skin surfaces include abrasions, ulcers, excoriations, fissures, lacerations, and incisions.

✔ Vascular lesions include petechia (intradermal or submucous bleeding), telangiectasis (dilated capillaries), or ecchymosis (bruise).

✔ Skin diseases are primarily diagnosed by direct observation; diagnostic tests include the Tzanck smear, KOH test, culture of a pustule, diascopy, Wood's light test, or skin biopsy.

QUESTIONS TO CONSIDER

■ Get together with several classmates and do a skin assessment on the face and arms of each other. Write down your observations using the parameters listed in the text. Describe any observed lesion in terms of its characteristics and label it using the terms in Table 71-3. Compare notes with each other. Why were all the descriptions probably not identical?

■ What could you do to improve your skills in skin assessment?

REFERENCES AND SELECTED READINGS

1. Bates B: A guide to physical examination, ed 4, Philadelphia, 1987, JB Lippincott Co.
2. *Brown ME: Introduction to assessment of the skin, Occup Health Nurs 28(8):13-16, 1980.
3. Guyton A: Textbook of medical physiology, ed 7, Philadelphia, 1986, WB Saunders Co.
4. Kaye D and Rose LF: Fundamentals of internal medicine, St Louis, 1983, The CV Mosby Co.
5. *Malasanos L et al: Health assessment, ed 4, St Louis, 1989, The CV Mosby Co.
6. *Mangieri D: Saving your elderly patient's skin, Nursing '82 12(10):44-45, 1982.
7. Pillsbury DM: A manual of dermatology, ed 2, Philadelphia, 1980, WB Saunders Co.
8. *Roach LB: Color changes in dark skin, Nursing '77 7(1):48-51, 1977.
9. Schroeder SA et al: Current medical diagnosis and treatment, Norwalk, Conn, 1989, Appleton & Lange.
10. Seidel HM et al: Mosby's guide to physical examination, St Louis, 1987, The CV Mosby Co.
11. *Uhler DM: Common skin changes in the elderly, Am J Nurs 78:1342-1344, 1978.
12. Wyngaarden JB and Smith LH: Cecil textbook of medicine, ed 18, Philadelphia, 1988, WB Saunders Co.

*References preceded by an asterisk are particularly well suited for student reading.

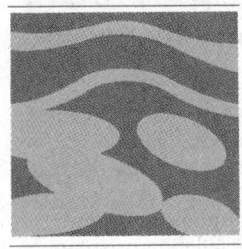

CHAPTER 72

Management of Persons with Problems of the Skin

BARBARA C. LONG

CHAPTER OBJECTIVES

After studying this chapter, the student should be able to:
1 Identify the etiology, clinical manifestations, and interventions for parasitic infestations, fungal and bacterial infections, and viral diseases of the skin.
2 Describe the nature, preventive measures, and therapy for acne.
3 Compare and contrast the different types of dermatitis, preventive measures, and interventions, especially patient teaching.
4 Identify different skin reactions that may result from systemic factors.
5 Describe the nature and management of psoriasis.
6 Describe the different benign and malignant skin tumors and their management.

Skin problems may result from various causes, such as parasitic infestations, fungal, bacterial or viral infections, reactions to substances encountered externally or taken internally, and new growths. Many skin manifestations have no known cause, whereas others are hereditary. This chapter provides an overview of the more common dermatologic disorders.

PARASITIC INFESTATIONS

The major parasitic infestations are pediculosis and scabies.

PEDICULOSIS
ETIOLOGY

Pediculi (lice) are most often found among people who live in overcrowded dwellings with inadequate hygiene facilities.[43] Many children get head lice from their classmates or from people on crowded buses. Control and treatment of pediculosis (lice infestation) in middle- or upper-income populations can be hampered by refusal of parents to admit that their children have pediculosis. Pediculosis is rare among blacks and occurs mostly among children.

Lice obtain their nutrition by sucking blood from the skin. They leave their eggs on the skin surface attached to hair shafts, and this results in the transfer from person to person.

Three types of lice infest humans: the head louse, the body louse, and the pubic louse. The head louse (*Pediculus capitis*) attaches itself to the hair shaft, laying about eight eggs a day. The eggs, or *nits,* are firmly attached to the hair or threads of clothing. They may be viewed with a hand lens and appear as grayish, glistening oval bodies. The head louse is usually confined to the scalp and beard.

The body louse (*Pediculus corporis*) resides chiefly in the seams of clothing around the neck, waist, and thighs. The bite causes minute hemorrhagic points and severe itching. Transmission is by direct contact or by way of clothing, bedding, and towels.

The pubic louse (*Phthirus pubis*) differs slightly from the head and body louse. It resembles a tiny crab, having clawlike pincers that attach firmly to the pubic hair. Nits are visible in the pubic hair. *P. pubis* is transmitted by sexual contact, bed clothing, towels, and occasionally toilet seats.

CLINICAL MANIFESTATIONS

Diagnosis is made by finding nits or lice on a person who also has pinpoint erythema; raised macules, and a complaint of pruritus. The bite of the insect, with contamination from saliva, head parts, and feces, causes intense itching. Scratching may lead to further trauma with the possibility of secondary infection and enlarged cervical lymph nodes.

INTERVENTIONS
Medical Management

Treatment of pediculosis consists of topical application of a pediculicide, such as lindane (Kwell, Scabene), permethrin (Nix), pyrethrin (RID, A-200 Pyrinate), or malathion 0.5% (Prioderm). Directions for applications differ according to the product and body location (see

APPLICATION OF PEDICULICIDES

HAIR

1. Apply to dry hair until hair is thoroughly saturated; a pediculicide shampoo is worked into a lather
2. Allow product to remain on hair for stated period of time (varies with product)
3. Rinse hair and allow to dry
4. Use a fine-toothed comb to remove dead lice and nits; rinse comb in vinegar after treatment; comb should not be shared by other family members
5. Repeat treatment in 8 to 10 days to remove any hatched nits

BODY

1. Apply pediculicide lotion or cream to affected areas
2. Bathe after 12 hours and put on clean clothes

TEACHING THE PATIENT WITH PEDICULOSIS

1. Use only the prescribed amount of pediculicide, to prevent toxicity.
2. If pediculicide accidently contacts the eyes, flush eyes immediately with water.
3. Wash brushes and combs with pediculicide.
4. Wash or dry-clean clothing and linens (garments can be stored for 1 month and will no longer be infested).
5. Vacuum carpets, mattresses, and upholstery.
6. All persons in household should use lotion or shampoo and use separate combs or brushes to decrease spread of infection.
7. Itching may continue for 4 to 6 weeks; use a menthol or phenol lotion for comfort.

box above, left). Pediculicides are not used on eyebrows or eyelashes because of potential eye irritation or sensitization. If eyelashes are infested, nits are removed and petrolatum jelly is applied to smother the lice.

Nursing Management

Patients are usually able to carry out their own treatment. The focus of nursing care is to identify infected persons and to teach about the nature of pediculosis and prevention of its spread (see box above, right).

SCABIES
EPIDEMIOLOGY

Scabies is highly prevalent during periods of overcrowding, such as occurs during wars. Since the 1960s, however, there has been a rise in the incidence of scabies worldwide. The reason for the pandemic is unknown and is thought to be multifactorial, including sexual promiscuity, increased worldwide travel, and ecologic changes.[37]

ETIOLOGY AND PATHOPHYSIOLOGY

Scabies is caused by the female itch mite (*Sarcoptes scabiei*), which penetrates the stratum corneum and burrows into the skin. Within several hours after skin penetration, the itch mite lays enormous eggs and deposits fecal material. The larvae mature in 10 days and move to the skin surface where the female is impregnated; then the cycle repeats itself. The incubation period varies, but there is often a long period of time before symptoms are noted. Delayed hypersensitivity is thought to be a major factor. Scabies is usually transmitted by prolonged contact, so that it is frequently observed among several members of a family. Young adults may transmit it by sleeping together as opposed to a brief sexual contact. Scabies occurs among all age groups and socioeconomic levels.

CLINICAL MANIFESTATIONS

The *classic* symptoms of scabies include lesions that resemble wavy, brownish, threadlike lines occurring most frequently on the hands (especially the interdigital webs), flexor surface of the wrists, posterior inner surface of the elbows, anterior axillary folds, nipples in the female, belt line, gluteal creases, and male genitalia. The head and neck are rarely involved. Pruritus may be severe, especially at night. Secondary infections with excoriations and pustules may result from scratching.

In the recent pandemic, the classic symptoms have been less frequently seen and the lesions may imitate different dermatoses. Distribution of lesions has also been atypical.[37] Scabies can be suspected if several family members have similar symptoms.

Diagnosis is made by identifying the itch mite. The mite is removed from the end of a burrow with a pointed scalpel blade, or the entire burrow is sliced off, placed on a slide with glycerol or mineral oil, and examined under a microscope.

INTERVENTIONS
Medical Management

Medical therapy is directed to elimination of the itch mite and treatment of complications.

1. Scabies treatment (patient, all family members)
   a. Lindane (Kwell, Scabene)
      (1) Apply at bedtime in a thin layer over the *entire* body from *neck down*
      (2) Wash off in 8 to 12 hours
      (3) Give a second treatment in 24 hours if prescribed
   b. Crotamiton 10% (Eurax)
      (1) Less effective than lindane
      (2) Bathe before initial application and after each treatment
      (3) Repeat treatment as prescribed

c. Benzyl benzoate
   (1) Give two overnight treatments 1 week apart as prescribed
   (2) Not widely available; apply as directed by physician
2. Treatment for complications from scabies
   a. Postscabies dermatitis with pruritus: topical or oral corticosteroids
   b. Secondary infections: systemic antibiotics
   c. Postscabies papules or nodules: coal tar gels

Nursing Management

As with pediculosis, nursing management is primarily teaching. Because scabies spreads within families, the patient and family members need to know the nature of the disease and the need for all family members to receive treatment, even if they are asymptomatic. Some patients experience shame and guilt feelings when they learn the diagnosis; a nonjudgmental attitude with explanations of methods of control may help these patients cope with their feelings.

Despite controversy about the potential for spread of the disease by clothing or linens, preventive measures are still being recommended. *Teaching* the patient with scabies includes the following:

1. All family members should be treated simultaneously, whether or not symptoms are present.
2. Be sure that *all* external body areas below the neck are covered by the prescribed scabicide.
3. Wash underclothing and bed and bath linens in hot water on the day of treatment; dry in dryer or iron after dry, change linens daily.
4. Signs and symptoms may not disappear until 1 or 2 weeks after treatment; pruritus of hands and feet may persist for up to 3 months.[15]

FUNGAL INFECTIONS

Fungi are larger and more complex than bacteria. They may be unicellular, such as yeasts, or multicellular, such as molds. Many types are pathogenic to humans, causing common skin disorders or serious systemic diseases such as blastomycosis. Certain types of fungi cause few symptoms, whereas others produce inflammatory or hypersensitivity reactions.

CANDIDIASIS
ETIOLOGY

Candida albicans, a yeastlike fungus, normally inhabits the gastrointestinal tract, mouth, and vagina but not usually the skin. Candidiasis (moniliasis), the inflammation associated with the organism's overgrowth on the skin, is caused by the toxins that are released. Some predisposing factors causing an overgrowth of *C. albicans* are pregnancy, use of birth control pills, poor nutri-

tion, antibiotic therapy, diabetes mellitus, other endocrine diseases, inhalational corticosteroids, and immunosuppressed conditions. Yeast thrives in a warm, moist environment such as the perineum and intertriginous areas.

CLINICAL MANIFESTATIONS

Thrush is candidiasis of the mucous membrane. The lesions are white spots that look like milk curd on the buccal mucosa and may extend down the esophagus. Vaginal thrush causes intense itching with a cheesy vaginal discharge. Skin lesions appear as pruritic, eroded, moist, inflamed areas with vesicles and pustules, and occur mostly in body folds, such as beneath the breasts, in the intergluteal fold, or in the groin. Diagnosis of candidiasis at any site is made by clinical appearance and microscopic examination.

INTERVENTIONS

Treatment is aimed at the precipitating factors. Other measures include keeping the skin dry to avoid maceration, wearing loose, absorbent clothing, and using topical medications such as powders that help to keep the skin dry. Nystatin (Mycostatin), an antibiotic available in tablets, powder, or vaginal suppositories; amphotericin, clotrimazole (Mycelex), ciclopirox (Loprox), and ketoconazole (Nixoral) are effective against yeast infections.

DERMATOPHYTOSES

There are several different types of dermatophytoses (tinea) or superficial fungal infections of the skin and its appendages. The most common types are tinea capitis, tinea corporis, tinea cruris, and tinea pedis.

TINEA CAPITIS

Tinea capitis, inappropriately called ringworm of the scalp, has a worldwide distribution, primarily among prepubertal children. It can be caused either by a species of *Microsporum* or by *Trichophyton* fungi. The most common causative agent in the United States is *Microsporum audouini*. The infection is transmitted readily, especially in crowded conditions where poor hygiene exists, although many children show a high resistance. Minor scalp trauma facilitates implantation of the spores; therefore, the infection can be spread by contaminated barber's instruments, combs, or sharp brushes.

The characteristic lesion is round, with erythema, a slight scaling, and some pustules appearing at the edge of the lesion (Figure 72-1, *A*). Hair loss occurs, with the hair shaft broken off at skin level. The hair loss is only temporary, since the lesions usually heal without scarring. Although tinea capitis is usually noninflammatory, a painful inflammatory condition called a *kerion* may

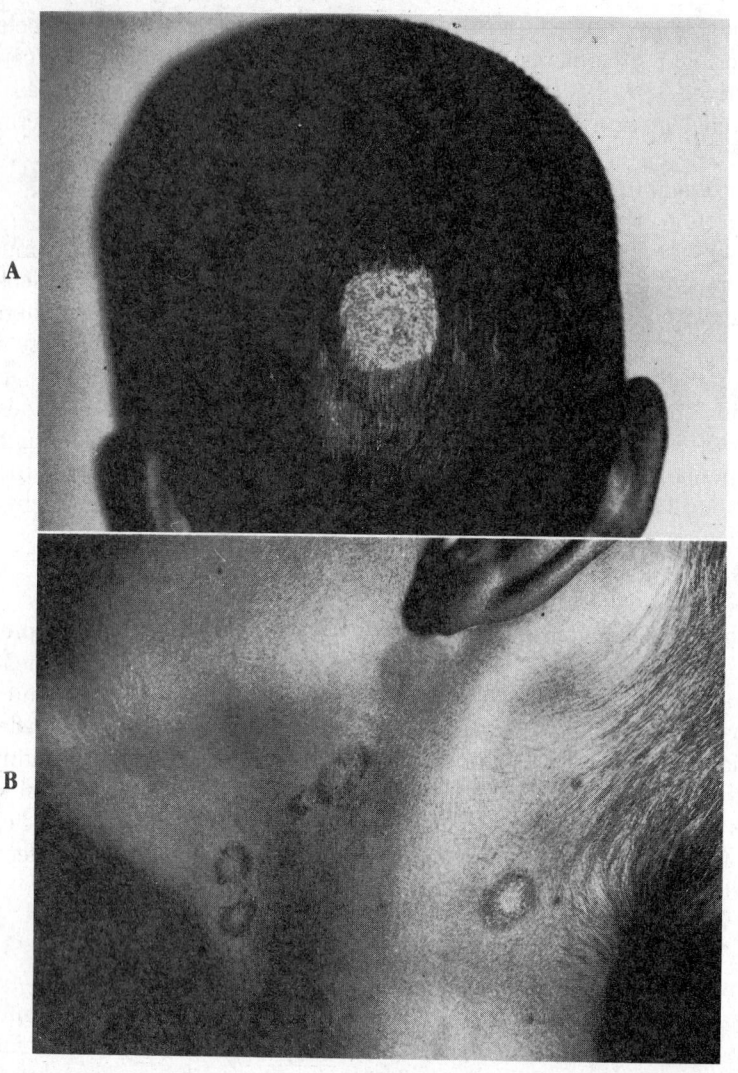

FIGURE 72-1 A, Tinea capitis. **B,** Tinea corporis. (From Stewart WD, Danto JL, and Maddin S: Dermatology: diagnosis and treatment of cutaneous disorders, ed 4, St Louis, 1978, The CV Mosby Co.)

develop. Infected hairs placed under Wood's light will fluoresce a blue-green color.

Interventions

Griseofulvin is an effective antifungal agent in the treatment of all the dermatophytoses. The adult dose for tinea capitis is 500 mg orally, and absorption is enhanced when the medication is administered after a high-fat meal. Four to 6 weeks are usually necessary before the infection is resolved.

The scalp should be shampooed at least twice a week. Cutting the hair short facilitates shampooing, but may pose psychological trauma for some children and is best left at an acceptable length. A mild antifungal agent, such as tolnaftate (1%) or haloprogin, may be ap-

plied topically twice daily. If inflammation occurs, the scalp is shampooed daily.

TINEA CORPORIS AND TINEA CRURIS

Tinea corporis is a dermatophytic infection of nonhairy parts of the body, commonly seen in children living in hot, humid climates. Typical lesions appear flat with an erythematous scaling border and clearing center (Figure 72-1, *B*). Tinea cruris, commonly referred to as "jock itch," occurs in warm, moist, intertriginous areas of the groin. It occurs frequently in men, especially those who have tinea pedis and those who frequently wear athletic supporters or tight shorts, and in women who wear tight pantyhose or slacks. The lesions are bilateral and extend outward from the groin along the in-

TOPICAL ANTIFUNGAL DRUGS

Miconazole (Micatin, Monistat)
Clotrimazole (Mycelex)
Econazole (Ecostatin, Spectazole)
Oxiconazole (Glaxo, Oxistat)
Ciclopirox (Loprox)
Haloprogin (Halotex)
Tolnaftate (Aftate, Pitrex, Tinactin)

ner thigh. The color ranges from brown to red, scaling is absent, and pruritus is usually present.

Interventions

Because the dermatophytes thrive in moist warm environments, the affected areas should be kept clean and dry, and overbathing should be avoided. A bland dusting powder can be used to promote dryness. Loose underclothing should be worn. Mild infections are treated with topical fungicides (see box above). Oral griseofulvin is given for severe infections.

TINEA PEDIS

The most common dermatophytosis is tinea pedis, or athlete's foot. There are many misconceptions about prevention and treatment of athlete's foot. It is rarely seen in children or women but is widespread among young men, especially those wearing shoes in hot climates. It is often confused with other foot eruptions such as simple intertrigo (chronic bacterial infection of the intertriginous areas of the toes), contact dermatitis, or psoriasis. Walking barefoot in gymnasiums or around swimming pools will not necessarily lead to a tinea infection, but susceptible persons will acquire it regardless of their activities. Preventive actions commonly taken, such as prophylactic foot baths in public places, are ineffective. Wearing white socks does not affect the course of the infection.[34] Factors that may lessen infection include wearing sandal-type shoes or going barefoot (to decrease tissue moisture), and using good foot hygiene, which includes washing the feet frequently and drying well between the toes.

There are several forms of tinea pedis, the most common being the intertriginous form. The fungus involvement usually begins in the toe webs, especially in the fourth interspace, and may extend to the undersurface of the toes or onto the plantar surface. The person may be asymptomatic or may experience itching and burning in the affected area. The nails may become discolored, thickened, or distorted (onychomycosis).

Interventions

Treatment depends on the stage of infection. Most persons have a chronic low-grade infection that is control-

lable with topical antifungal drugs (see box at left). When thick chronic scaling lesions are present, the topical antifungal drugs cannot penetrate the lesion; therefore, a strong peeling ointment, such as Whitfield's ointment, can be applied thinly to the lesions at bedtime, followed by an antifungal cream in the morning.[14] If the lesions become acutely inflamed, they are treated with foot soaks with a bland solution, such as Burow's solution (Chapter 73), followed by a topical antimicrobial agent. A systemic antibacterial agent, such as penicillin or erythromycin, may be prescribed. Oral griseofulvin is only prescribed for severe infections that do not respond to local treatment.[43]

The person with tinea pedis needs to carry out meticulous foot hygiene. After drying the toes thoroughly, a light dusting of antifungal powder is applied to promote dryness. Caking of the powder should be avoided. Socks should be of an absorbent material such as cotton and may need to be changed more than once daily to promote dryness.

Tinea Versicolor

Tinea versicolor is a mild, superficial fungal infection seen mostly in persons who perspire heavily, such as athletes or people living in warm climates. It is frequently noted during migrant health screening. Patches of variable coloring and mild scaling can be observed, primarily on the trunk. The involved areas do not tan. Pruritus is mild. Treatment includes application of selenium sulfide lotion (Selsun, Exsel) daily for 10 minutes before showering. Other topical antifungal drugs (see box above) may be used if selenium sulfide is ineffective. Encourage good hygiene and daily linen changes.

BACTERIAL INFECTIONS

Skin infections may result from loss of skin integrity or from altered host resistance. Most bacteria that normally inhabit the skin are nonpathogenic. Pathogenic bacteria that penetrate the outer skin layer may cause a superficial skin infection such as impetigo or superficial folliculitis, or they may penetrate deeper causing a deep folliculitis or a furuncle.

General principles of treatment for bacterial skin infections include cleansing the skin well and applying a topical antibiotic. The skin is cleansed with soap and water or with hexachlorophene. Water or saline compresses may be used to dry the horny layer of the skin or heat may be applied. Topical antibiotics commonly used include the hydroxyquinilones such as Vioform; neomycin, bacitracin, or polymyxin (Polysporin) either alone or in combination; and gentamicin or erythromycin. Systemic antibiotics are used only when systemic signs such as fever and malaise are present, when the infection is widespread, or when there is an epidemic.

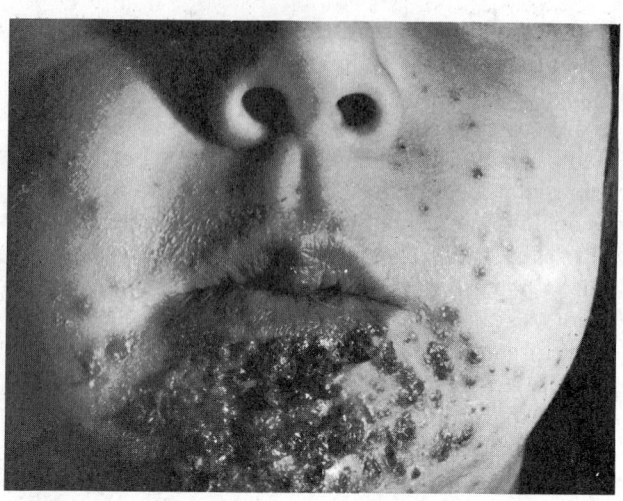

FIGURE 72-2 Impetigo contagiosa. (From Stewart WD, Danto JL, and Maddin S: Dermatology: diagnosis and treatment of cutaneous disorders ed 4, St Louis, 1978, The CV Mosby Co.)

IMPETIGO
ETIOLOGY

Impetigo is a common skin infection caused by staphylococci or β-hemolytic streptococci. Although impetigo may occur at any age, children are most often affected. It occurs more commonly in the summer or early fall. Factors that promote development of impetigo include tropical climates, uncleanliness, poor hygiene, poor nutrition, and poor health.

CLINICAL MANIFESTATIONS

Impetigo begins as a small thin-walled vesicle that ruptures easily and leaves a weeping denuded spot. It becomes pustular and dries to form a honey-colored crust that appears stuck on the skin (Figure 72-2). The process, which is superficial, may extend below the crust. Impetigo is usually confined to the face but may occur elsewhere. If untreated, impetigo may last for several weeks with new lesions forming.

INTERVENTIONS

Treatment consists of maintaining cleanliness and applying topical antibiotics. The crusts must be removed and the lesions washed gently two to three times daily to prevent further crust formation. Warm soaks or saline compresses may be necessary to soften crusts that adhere firmly. Topical antibiotics are applied at least three times daily. Systemic antibiotics may be prescribed.

Family or health care providers should wash their hands thoroughly with a bacteriostatic soap after contact. Patients should use personal towels. Linens should be laundered after the first day of treatment.

FOLLICULITIS

Bacterial infections of the hair follicle may be superficial in the epidermis around the hair follicle or deep in the tissue surrounding both the lower and upper portions of the hair follicle. *Superficial folliculitis* is usually caused by a staphylococcus organism, but occasionally it is caused by other bacteria, both gram negative and gram positive. The infection may occur secondary to drainage from other infected lesions. Predisposing factors include uncleanliness, maceration, exposure to oils and solvents, traction of hair by tar therapy, or occlusion therapy. Treatment of superficial folliculitis includes cleansing with soap and water and applying topical antibiotics.

Deep folliculitis produces a more severe inflammatory response. *Sycosis barbae* (barber's itch) is a deep folliculitis of the beard. The hairs do not fall out or break, such as occurs with tinea barbae. *Hordeolum* (stye) is a deep folliculitis of the cilia of the eyelids. There is usually swelling of the surrounding eyelid with crusting along the edge of the eyelid. Warm compresses are applied to encourage resolution. Topical antibiotics such as Neosporin hasten healing.

FURUNCLES AND CARBUNCLES
ETIOLOGY AND PATHOPHYSIOLOGY

Furuncles (boils) are a deep folliculitis that originates either from a superficial folliculitis or as a deep nodule around the hair follicle. *Furunculosis* is the appearance of several furuncles. An infection that involves several surrounding hair follicles is termed a *carbuncle*.

Furuncles are likely to occur on the face, neck, forearms, groin, and legs, whereas carbuncles are usually limited to the nape of the neck and the back. Both occur most often in obese, poorly nourished, fatigued, or otherwise susceptible persons whose hygiene may be poor, in debilitated elderly people, and in persons who have inadequately treated diabetes mellitus.

CLINICAL MANIFESTATIONS

Local swelling and redness occur, and there is severe local pain, which is decreased by moving the involved part as little as possible. Within 3 to 5 days the lesion becomes elevated or "points up," the surrounding skin becomes shiny, and the center or "core" turns yellow. A carbuncle has several cores. The boil will usually rupture spontaneously, but it may be surgically incised and drained. As drainage occurs, the pain is immediately relieved. The drainage soon changes from a yellow purulent material to a serosanguineous discharge. All drainage usually subsides within a few hours to a few days; the redness and swelling subside gradually.

INTERVENTIONS

Hot, wet dressings are used to help bring the boil to a head, but these dressings are discontinued as soon as drainage occurs to prevent skin maceration and spread of infection. As the boil drains, care must be taken to keep the infected discharge off the surrounding skin because organisms may be harbored in hair follicles and furunculosis may recur. Patients are cautioned to keep their hands away from the discharge to prevent spread of infection. Systemic antibiotics may be prescribed.

If the patient is hospitalized, wound isolation procedures are followed until the discharge subsides lest the organism be carried to others. Health personnel should wash their hands thoroughly after caring for the patient and should avoid getting the discharge on their own skin.

The patient who is at home must be taught to be scrupulously careful in hygiene practices to prevent accidentally passing the organisms to others in the family or to persons at work. It is not uncommon for entire families to have some type of staphylococcal infection after one member has had a boil. Both the patient and the family should *bathe and shampoo daily* with bacteriostatic soap for as long as infection is present. Razor blades should be discarded after each use. Each family member needs *separate bath linens* that are changed daily to prevent the spread of infection.

Furuncles and carbuncles tend to recur in susceptible individuals, and the staphylococci causing them often are resistant to local treatment and to antibiotics.

ERYSIPELAS

Erysipelas is an acute febrile disease caused by the hemolytic streptococcus and characterized by localized inflammation and swelling of the skin and subcutaneous tissues, usually of the face. A bright, sharp line separates the diseased skin from the normal skin. Elderly people with poor resistance are most often affected. Erysipelas was a serious disease before the advent of antibiotics. Penicillin is the drug of choice.

VIRAL DISEASES

WARTS

ETIOLOGY AND PATHOPHYSIOLOGY

Warts are benign skin growths that develop from hypertrophy of epidermal cells as a result of a viral infection. The infection is not highly contagious but does spread along the dermis through autoinfection. It is seen most commonly in older children and young adults.

Warts grow in a variety of shapes. The common wart is a small, circumscribed, painless, hyperkeratotic papule usually seen on the extremities, especially the hands. *Filiform warts* are slender fingerlike projections occurring mostly on the face and neck. *Plantar warts* grow inward from the pressure on the soles of the feet and are frequently painful. They are differentiated from calluses by lack of skin lines over the surface. Warts

that develop in the anogenital region have a lighter-colored surface and a cauliflower-like appearance, and they may cause itching. Anogenital warts may be spread either by sexual activity or by other means. Some genital warts in women may predispose cancer of the cervix.

INTERVENTIONS

There are numerous treatments for warts but no one major effective method. Warts sometimes disappear spontaneously or under psychological suggestion, thus creating a basis for numerous folktales concerning how to get rid of warts. If only a few painless warts are present, no treatment is necessary and the warts will probably disappear in time.

The most commonly used therapeutic measures for common warts are electrodesiccation and cryosurgery (see Chapter 73). In electrodesiccation the top of the wart is seared gently to soften the keratinized surface, curetted off, and the bleeding points cauterized. This method is not used for plantar warts. Cryosurgery consists of freezing the lesion with a substance such as liquid nitrogen. Cauterant chemicals such as formalin, phenol, nitric acid, cantharidin, salicylic acid, or podophyllum may be used. Recalcitrant warts may respond to radiation therapy. Surgical excision is seldom used because painful scarring may result.

HERPES SIMPLEX

ETIOLOGY AND PATHOPHYSIOLOGY

One of the most common viruses found in humans is the herpes simplex virus (HSV). It occurs as two similar yet serologically different strains, type 1 and type 2. The type 1 virus is found primarily in lesions of the face and mouth (fever blister, cold sore), eye (keratitis), and brain (encephalitis). Type 2 is associated with a lesion of the genitalia that can be transmitted by sexual contact (see Chapter 58). HSV has a DNA-containing core surrounded by a phospholipid covering. Factors that may precipitate recurrence of herpes simplex lesions include fever, upper respiratory tract infection, exhaustion, and nervous tension. Lesions also are more common during the menses or after direct exposure to the sun's rays.

CLINICAL MANIFESTATIONS

Most persons experience the initial contact with HSV (type 1) as young children. The HSV remains in the cells of the sensory nerves that supply the affected areas and causes recurrent lesions when the person is subjected to stress. The appearance of vesicles is preceded by several hours by a sensation of burning or itching. A cluster of vesicles on an erythematous base appears at the mucocutaneous junctions of the lips or nose or as an inflammation of the cornea of one eye with photophobia and tearing. The type 2 virus lesions occur in the vagina or cervix of the woman or on the penile skin of the man. The lesions are painful and frequently crack open. A crust gradually forms, and the lesions heal in about 10 days. HSV can be identified by a Tzanck smear (see Chapter 71).

INTERVENTIONS

No effective treatment of recurrent HSV infections is available at this time. Acyclovir (Zovirax) may be prescribed orally or given intravenously for severe infections.

Local treatments of herpes simplex lesions do not cure the lesions but may alleviate discomfort and prevent development of more extensive lesions. Astringent or drying agents include a moistened styptic pencil, epinephrine 1:100, 37.5% alcohol in gel base (Blister-Klear), or zinc sulfate 0.025-0.05%.[43]

HERPETIC WHITLOW

Herpetic whitlow is an HSV infection of the finger, occurring most commonly among nurses, physicians, and dentists. The source of infection may be direct contact with vesicular fluid of oral herpetic lesions or from viruses present in oral secretions of asymptomatic persons.[32] The lesion is preceded by itching and intense pain and sometimes by fever, chills, and malaise. Vesicles form as with other HSV infections. Healing occurs within 3 to 4 weeks but lesions will reappear. Treatment is essentially symptomatic with elevation and immobilization of the finger and analgesics. Personal linens and utensils should be used to avoid infecting others.[32] Contact with oral secretions of persons with known HSV lesions can be prevented by using gloves when providing oral care.

HERPES ZOSTER
ETIOLOGY AND PATHOPHYSIOLOGY

Herpes zoster, or shingles, is caused by the same virus (V-Z) that causes varicella (chickenpox). Varicella is believed to be the primary infection in a nonimmune host, whereas herpes zoster is thought to be the response in a partially immune host. Although herpes zoster is far less communicable than chickenpox, persons who have not had chickenpox may develop it after exposure to the vesicular lesions of persons with herpes zoster. For this reason, susceptible persons should not care for patients with herpes zoster. It is one of the most drawn out and exasperating conditions found in elderly patients and leads to discouragement and demoralization. Herpes zoster may recur in rare circumstances. Herpes zoster often occurs in persons with AIDS, Hodgkin's disease, and in individuals with lymphoid and some bone cancers because of reduced cell-mediated immunity.

CLINICAL MANIFESTATIONS

In herpes zoster, clusters of small vesicles usually form in a line. They follow the course of the peripheral sensory nerves and often are unilateral (Figure 72-3). Because they follow nerve pathways, the lesions never cross the midline of the body. However, nerves on both

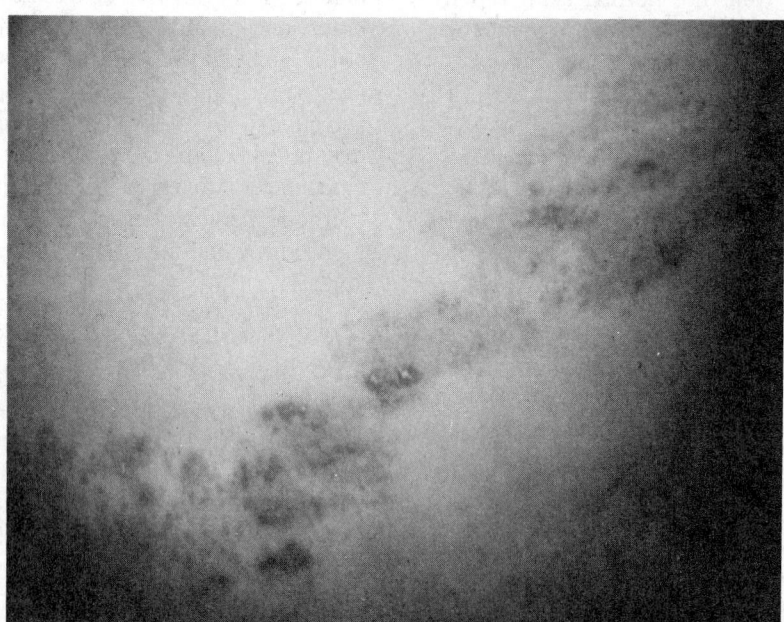

FIGURE 72-3 Herpes zoster. (Courtesy David Bickers, MD, Cleveland Ohio.)

sides of the body can be involved. Two thirds of persons with herpes zoster develop lesions over thoracic dermatomes, and the remainder show involvement of the trigeminal nerve with lesions on the face, eye, and scalp. The rash develops first as macules but progresses rapidly to vesicles. The fluid becomes turbid, and crusts develop and drop off in about 10 days.

Malaise, fever, itching, and pain over the involved area may precede the eruption of the lesions. If vesicles develop within 1 to 2 days after the initial pain symptoms, the lesions usually clear in 2 to 3 weeks, but if the vesicles develop over the period of a week, a prolonged course can be expected.[34]

Discomfort from pain and itching is the major problem with herpes zoster. The pain may vary from a light burning sensation to a deep visceral-type pain, and it may be intermittent or constant. It usually persists for up to 4 weeks. In approximately 50% of persons over age 60, the pain may last for months or years.[50] Enlargement of the lymph nodes may also occur with the rash.

INTERVENTIONS

Acyclovir (Zovirax) accelerates healing and reduces acute pain and is given orally in high doses (400 mg to 800 mg, every 4 hours, five times a day for 5 to 6 days). In severe infections, acyclovir may be given intravenously; lower doses are effective intravenously. Because acyclovir may precipitate in renal tubules, drinking fluids should be encouraged. Acyclovir has no effect in preventing postherpetic neuralgia.

Analgesics are prescribed for pain relief. Aspirin, with or without codeine, is often effective; meperidine hydrochloride (Demerol) may be needed for severe pain. Herpetic pain may be decreased by systemic steroids, such as prednisone; steroid therapy may decrease the incidence of postherpetic neuralgia. Sedatives may also be helpful, especially at bedtime. Local discomfort may be relieved by calamine lotion or by application of a vinegar solution (one-fourth cup white vinegar in 2 quarts lukewarm water.)[14] Loose clothing helps to minimize contact with the affected area. Patients should avoid exposure to highly susceptible persons (those who have not had chickenpox or who are immunocompromised.)

Postherpetic neuralgia (PHN) occurs in about 10% of persons following herpes zoster infection, mostly in elderly persons.[30] The pain usually lasts less than 1 year but may persist for many years. The pain is always present with superimposed sharp pain episodes. Because the pain results from nervous system damage, it does not respond well to usual pain therapies, and thus a multimodal approach is more effective.[29] A tricyclic antidepressant is commonly prescribed. Transcutaneous electrical nerve stimulation (TENS) may be tried initially, although it usually is not effective on a long-term

basis. Narcotics are avoided because of the persistence of the pain and potential for addiction. Neurosurgical procedures are usually ineffective. Because the pain becomes an all-consuming part of the patient's life, ongoing evaluation of the impact on the patient functionally and socially and ongoing supportive counseling are helpful. (For further interventions for chronic pain, see Chapter 16.)

ACNE

ACNE VULGARIS
ETIOLOGY

Acne vulgaris is a very common skin disease seen in 80% of adolescents. It may also occur in adults. The cause of acne is still unknown but is thought to be multifactorial. Some of the common causes that have been postulated are free fatty acids, endocrine effects, stress, diet, heredity, and infection. Diet has been essentially ruled out as a causative factor, but none of the other factors have been demonstrated conclusively. Acne occurs at puberty when the sebaceous glands are stimulated by androgens, and it is often found to be common within families. Acne is more quiescent in summer months.

PREVENTION

The lesions in acne develop when the pilosebaceous follicles become plugged; therefore, activities that contribute to occlusion of the follicles are to be avoided. Hair and hands should be kept away from the face. Loose clothing prevents pressure over the follicles, and tight collars should not be worn. The skin should be kept clean. Greasy, oil-based cosmetics may be occlusive and plug up the follicles. Any food that appears to cause acne flare-ups in a given individual is best avoided.

PATHOPHYSIOLOGY

At puberty, sebaceous glands undergo enlargement from androgen stimulation. When sebum is released it passes through the follicular canal, where it is combined with sebaceous gland cell fragments, epidermal cells (keratin), and bacteria. At this time the triglycerides in the sebum are hydrolyzed to glycerol and free fatty acids. The sebum and debris may become plugged in the hair follicle (Figure 72-4) to form an open comedo (blackhead) if it is at the surface or a closed comedo (whitehead) if it is below the surface. The dark color of the blackhead is melanin, not dirt, and results from passage of melanin from the adjoining epidermal cells.

Inflammatory lesions apparently develop from escape of sebum into the dermis, which then serves as an irritant causing an inflammatory reaction. Free fatty acids may also be an irritant in the follicle itself.

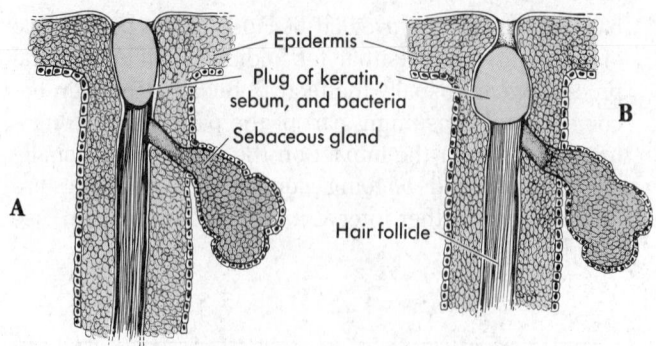

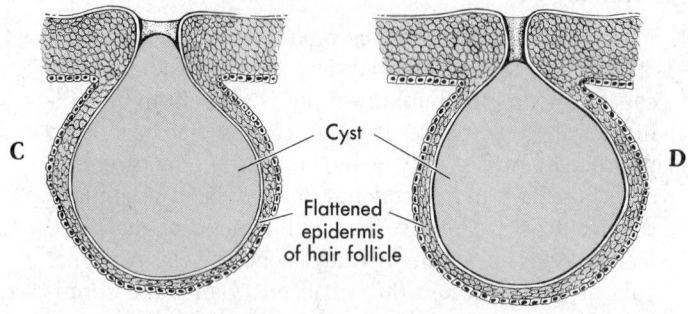

FIGURE 72-4 Formation of lesions in acne vulgaris. **A,** Open comedo (blackhead), early stage. **B,** Closed comedo (whitehead), early stage. **C,** Cyst formation in open comedo, advanced stage. **D,** Cyst formation in closed comedo, advanced stage. (From Parrish JH: Dermatology and skin care, New York 1975, McGraw-Hill Book Co. Used with the permission of McGraw-Hill Book Co.)

CLINICAL MANIFESTATIONS

Acne occurs mostly on the face and neck, upper chest, and back, although the upper arms, buttocks, and thighs may also be involved. Comedones are the first visible signs, and the skin is characteristically oily. The inflammatory lesions include papules, pustules, nodules, and cysts. Superficial lesions may resolve in 5 to 10 days without scarring, but large lesions last for several weeks and often result in scarring. The typical scar resembles an old volcano (ice-pick scar); however, many other sizes and shapes may result, depending on the depth and extent of the inflammatory lesions.

There is great variability in the extent of the lesions. Some persons have only a few small lesions. Many adolescents have several lesions that peak at ages 16 to 18 years of age and then slowly resolve. A few persons develop severe nodular acne that may not resolve for 10 to 15 years.

INTERVENTIONS
Medical Management

Medical therapy may be topical, systemic, intralesional, or surgical and includes the following:

1. Topical therapy
   a. Basic method of therapy
   b. Agents: benzoyl peroxide, vitamin A acid (tretinoin), antibiotics (topical erythromycin), sulfur-zinc lotion
2. Removal of comedones with a comedo extractor
3. Systemic therapy
   a. Used with topical therapy for *severe* nodular or cystic acne
   b. Isoretinoic acid (Accutane)
      (1) A vitamin A acid analog
      (2) Side effects: dry lips and conjunctiva, brittle hair, tenderness of fingertips and toetips, hypertriglyceridemia, birth defects
   c. Systemic antibiotics
   d. Estrogens for females who have not responded to other therapies
4. Intralesional corticosteroid therapy for cysts of severe acne
5. Surgery: dermabrasion (see Chapter 73) to remove scars

Nursing Management

Counseling and teaching are the major nursing strategies. Stress appears to be one of the causative factors; therefore, attempts to identify and cope with stressors (see Chapter 10) may be helpful. Acne, per se, can be a stressor, producing facial disfigurements and sometimes leading to behavior that is hostile, aggressive, and anxious, as well as shy and withdrawn. Psychological counseling is often desirable.

Knowledge of the nature of acne helps the person to understand the necessary care. Teaching is directed toward general health care of the skin and guidelines for therapy (see the box on the opposite page).

ACNE ROSACEA

Acne rosacea is a skin condition that usually affects persons over 25 years of age. The actual cause is unknown. Over the years many causative factors have been suggested, including bacteria, vitamin deficiency, hormonal imbalance, alcohol, caffeine, psychological factors, and heredity. Acne rosacea begins with redness over the cheeks and nose, followed by papules, pustules, and enlargement of superficial blood vessels. Years of acne rosacea lead to an irregular, bulbous thickening of the skin of the distal part of the nose (rhinophyma), with a red-purple discoloration and dilated follicles.

There is no specific treatment for acne rosacea. Some persons respond to tetracycline and topical peeling agents, but there is no specific treatment for the vascular component. Avoiding stimuli that cause vasodilation seems appropriate. Rhinophyma may be treated by plastic surgery.

TEACHING THE PERSON WITH ACNE

1. Preventive measures
   a. Keep hands and hair away from the face
   b. Avoid constricting clothing over lesions
   c. Shampoo hair and scalp frequently
   d. Avoid exposure to oils and greases
   e. Eat a well-balanced diet and avoid any foods that appear to cause skin flare-ups
2. General skin care
   a. Keep skin clean; wash face 2 to 3 times daily
   b. Use a medicated soap or agent prescribed by physician
   c. Avoid vigorous rubbing of the skin
   d. Use cosmetics that are water-based rather than cream-based and avoid those that contain wax esters (myristates, palmitates, stearates)
   e. Never leave cosmetics on face at night
3. During therapy
   a. Follow the prescribed therapy even when immediate improvement is not noted for 2 to 3 weeks
   b. Expect skin desquamation during therapy
   c. Avoid using self-remedies during therapy
   d. Remove cosmetics before applying topical medications
   e. Avoid exposure to direct sunlight if using tretinoin or taking tetracycline (photosensitivity)
   f. Avoid pregnancy if taking Accutane (possibility of birth defects)

TABLE 72-1 Types of dermatitis

Type	Cause	Characteristics
Contact	External agents	Site and pattern of lesions depend on exposure pattern (linear, angular, etc.)
		Itching a major symptom
Atopic	Hypersensitivity reaction, hereditary	Itching a major symptom
		Lesions caused by scratching
Lichen simplex chronicus	Stasis, irritants, psychic factors	Itching a major symptom
		Lesions caused by scratching
Seborrheic	Unknown	Erythematous, scaly (e.g., dandruff)
Nummular	Unknown	Coin-shaped lesions
		Severe itching
Stasis	Decreased circulation	Erythema, edema
		Lesions may develop from trauma
		Itching may be severe

DERMATITIS

Dermatitis, a superficial inflammation of the skin, refers to several different conditions resulting in the same type of lesions. Dermatitis is often classified arbitrarily according to specific features such as cause, pattern, age, or type of treatment required. Some of the common types of dermatitis are listed in Table 72-1 and are discussed in more detail in succeeding paragraphs. The term *eczema* is often used synonymously with dermatitis but frequently refers to the chronic type.

Regardless of the cause, the lesions in any dermatitis follow a characteristic pattern. Initially, there is erythema and local edema, followed by vesicle formation with oozing and then crusting and scaling. If the dermatitis persists, there will be evidence of excoriation from scratching and thickening of the skin, and the color becomes more brownish. Secondary infection may result.

CONTACT DERMATITIS
ETIOLOGY AND PATHOPHYSIOLOGY

Contact dermatitis is caused by external agents and may affect various parts of the body (Table 72-2). There are two types of contact dermatitis, irritant and allergic. *Irritant contact dermatitis* can occur in any person on

TABLE 72-2 Common causes of contact dermatitis of different areas*

Area	Cause
Face	Cosmetics, hair sprays, hair dyes, airborne contactants
Earlobes	Nickel
Ears	
Pinnae	Photosensitizers
Canals	Medications
Eyelids	Cosmetics, airborne sensitizers, transfer by hands
Nose (bridge)	Metal or plastic spectacle supports
Lips and perioral area	Toothpaste, lipstick
Neck	Perfumes, clothing (especially wool)
Axillae	Deodorants, clothing, perfumes
Scapular area	Nickel in clasps on straps
Breasts	Elastic and other brassiere material
Waist	Elastic
Perianal area	Dibucaine (Nupercaine) and other medications, excessive use of cleansers
Arms and legs	Poison ivy and other plants
Wrists	Nickel, etc., in watchbands
Hands	Detergents and other cleansers, gloves
Feet	Medication for "athlete's foot," shoes

*From Moschella, SL, and Hurley, HJ: Dermatology, ed 2, Philadelphia, 1985, WB Saunders Co.

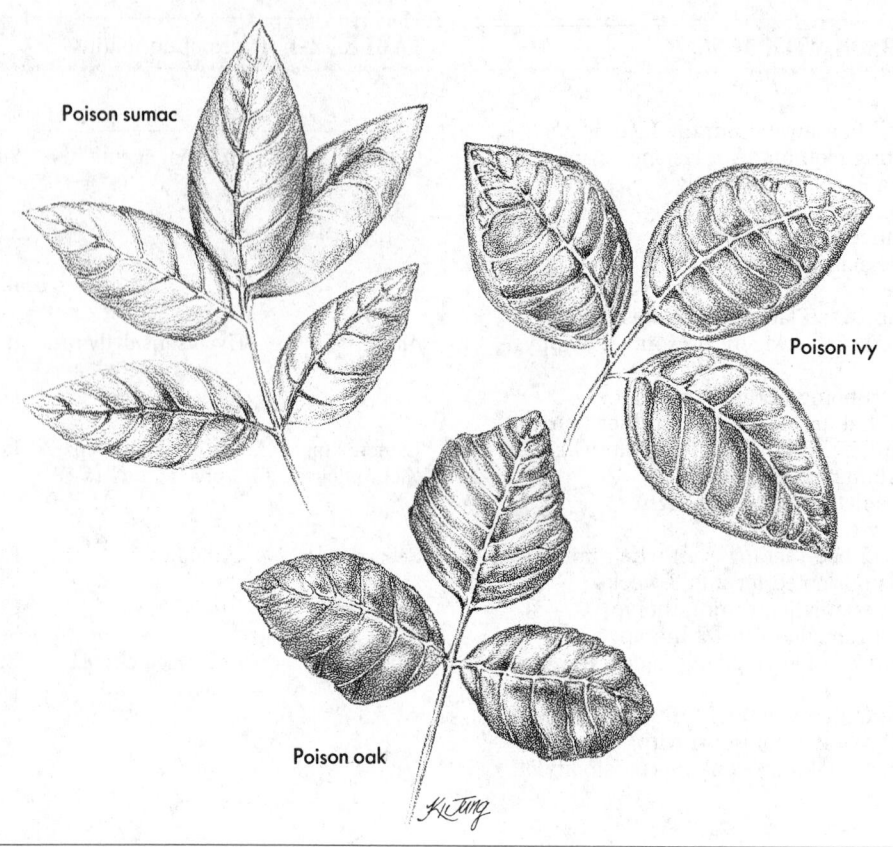

FIGURE 72-5 Typical leaves of poison sumac, poison ivy, and poison oak.

contact with a sufficient concentration of an irritant. Mechanical irritation may result from wool or glass fibers. Chemical irritants include acids, alkalies, solvents, detergents, or oils commonly found in cleaning compounds, insecticides, or industrial compounds. Biologic irritants include urine, fecal drainage, and toxins from insects or aquatic plants. People who are exposed to constant wetting of the hands or feet often develop irritant contact dermatitis.

Allergic contact dermatitis is a cell-mediated hypersensitivity immune reaction from contact with a specific antigen (see Chapter 76). Many compounds are capable of causing sensitization under specified conditions. Typical antigens include poison ivy, synthetics, industrial chemicals, drugs (for example, sulfanilamide or penicillin), and metals (especially nickel and chromate). Once the skin has been sensitized, further contact with the sensitizing substance will produce an eczematous reaction. The sensitizing allergen may reach the site by direct contact; by indirect contact such as transmission by animals, from one part of the body to the other by the hands, or on clothing; or by the air as in smoke.

PREVENTION

Contact dermatitis may be prevented by avoiding the irritating or sensitizing substance whenever possible. A person should know how to recognize the leaves of poisonous plants such as poison ivy, poison oak, or poison sumac that grow where they live (Figure 72-5). Persons walking in areas where poison ivy grows need to protect the skin by clothing. If contact with poison ivy is suspected, symptoms may be averted by immediately rinsing the skin for 15 minutes with running water to remove the resin before skin penetration occurs.

The person who develops a sensitivity to material encountered in the living or working environment may need to consider a permanent change of environment if other measures are unsuccessful. Gloves may be used if the person is handling irritant or allergenic substances. Persons sensitive to detergents may need to wash their clothes and to bathe with a mild soap such as Ivory.

CLINICAL MANIFESTATIONS

Characteristic dermatitis lesions appear sooner in irritant contact dermatitis than in the allergic type; however, the onset and appearance vary depending on the type and concentration of the irritant. The lesions develop on the exposed areas, particularly the more sensitive areas such as the dorsal rather than the palmar surface of the hands. If the irritant can be spread by the hands, as in poison ivy, lesions may involve other nonexposed areas.

When contact dermatitis is suspected but the agent is unknown, patch testing (see Chapter 75) may be carried out or the environment may be manipulated to exclude suspected agents.

INTERVENTIONS

Weeping uninfected lesions respond rapidly to wet dressings with water or Burow's solution (1:40 dilution of aluminum acetate) for 20 minutes four times daily (see Chapter 73). Crusts and scales are not removed but are allowed to drop off naturally as the skin heals. Topical corticosteroids are applied to dry lesions. Systemic corticosteroids may be given in acute extensive exacerbations but are not used to treat a mild contact dermatitis. Systemic antibiotics are prescribed when infection is present. Severe pruritus may be eased by antihistamines; *plain* calamine lotion may be applied for pruritus from poison ivy.

ATOPIC DERMATITIS (ECZEMA)
ETIOLOGY

Atopy refers to a type I hypersensitivity that is hereditary (see Chapter 76) and includes asthma, hay fever, and eczema. About 50% of persons with atopic dermatitis develop asthma or hay fever. The person who has inherited the tendency to eczema may not necessarily demonstrate symptoms. Exacerbating factors include sudden changes in temperature or humidity; exercise; psychologic stress; fibers such as wool, fur, or nylon; detergents; and perfumes.

PATHOPHYSIOLOGY

Persons with atopic dermatitis have a dry, highly sensitive skin with a lowered threshold to pruritus so that minor stimuli cause intense itching. There is a marked tendency toward vasoconstriction of superficial blood vessels and the skin blanches readily.[38] Cold and low humidity are poorly tolerated because of drying effects. Heat and high humidity are also poorly tolerated because vasodilation increases the inflammatory reaction, thus aggravating the dermatitis and causing increased itching and discomfort.

CLINICAL MANIFESTATIONS

The major symptom of atopic dermatitis is *pruritus*. Chronic scratching leads to eczematous lesions and subsequent lichenification. Healing usually occurs without scarring, but hypopigmentation or hyperpigmentation may result.

Atopic dermatitis in the infant is usually first noted about the third month. It usually disappear or becomes less severe about the age of 2 to 3 years, but recurs in late childhood or adolescence in a large number of persons. The lesions become localized to the flexor surfaces of the neck, to the eyelids, behind the ears, in the antecubital and popliteal areas (Figure 72-6), and at the

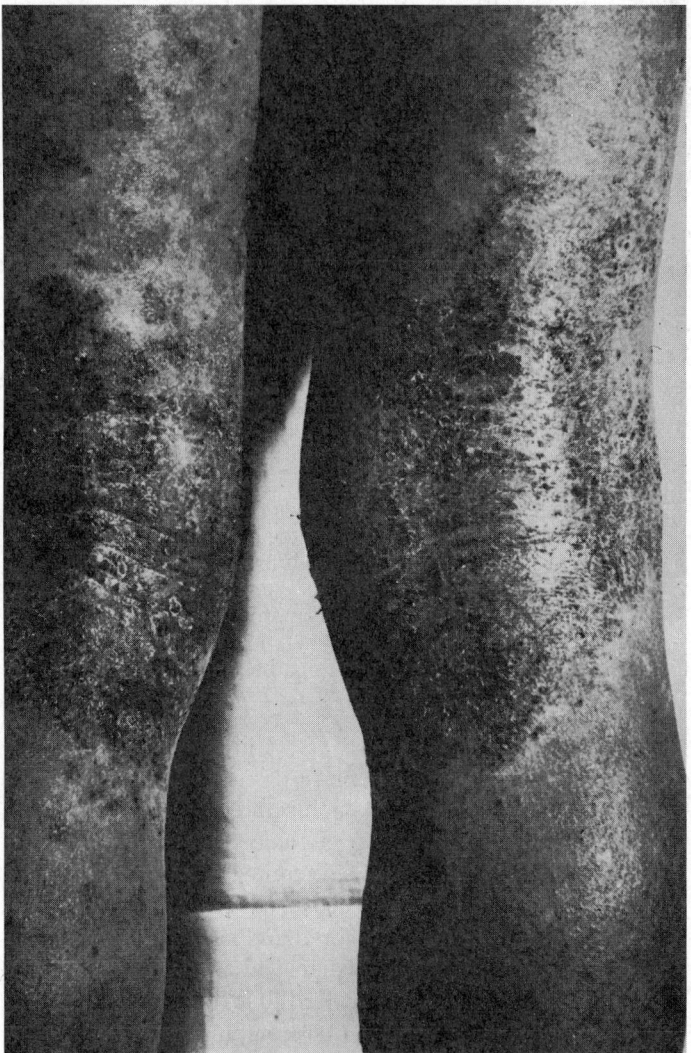

FIGURE 72-6 Atopic dermatitis with characteristic flexural involvement and crusting. (From Stewart WD, Danto JL, and Maddin S: Dermatology: diagnosis and treatment of cutaneous disorders, ed 4, St Louis, 1978, The CV Mosby Co.)

wrists. The erythema is now dusky in color, and excoriations may become secondarily infected. By the late twenties or early thirties the lesions usually disappear, but they may recur at a later date as chronic hand or foot eczema.[34]

Persons with atopic dermatitis are highly susceptible to viral infections, especially herpes, and to bacterial infections such as those caused by staphylococcus or β-hemolytic streptococcus. There is also an increased incidence of fungal infections such as tinea. Lymph nodes draining affected areas may be enlarged.

INTERVENTIONS

There is no cure for atopic dermatitis, but symptoms can be controlled. The focus of therapy is relief of pruri-

TEACHING THE PATIENT WITH ATOPIC DERMATITIS

1. Avoid soap over lesions (soap is an irritant); use soap minimally over nonaffected areas.
2. Soak affected areas for 15 to 20 minutes in warm water for hydration; pat skin dry, then *immediately* apply recommended lotion or cream to seal in moisture.
3. Wet wraps may be used in place of soaking; wraps permit evaporation that cools the skin, thus decreasing pruritus.
4. Apply corticosteroids in a thin layer and rub in well; do not use fluorinated corticosteroid on the face.
5. Avoid wool, fur, or rough fibers against the skin; they act as irritants and cause itching.
6. Avoid overheating that increases sweating, leading to itching. Wear loose, light clothing in hot weather. Air conditioning promotes comfort. Sunlight is beneficial to the skin.
7. Avoid excessive cold that dries the skin.
8. Avoid anything that aggravates the eczema.
9. Rinse all garments and bed linens twice to avoid residue of cleansing agents.
10. Consult dermatologist for appropriate laundry agents to prevent irritations from clothing.
11. Seek medical care if eczema becomes worse.

tus in order to break the itch-scratch cycle that leads to lesions. The major form of *topical* therapy consists of corticosteroid cream or ointment. Fluorinated corticosteroids may be used for localized lesions in adults but are used less often in children and *never on the face*. An occlusion wrap over the steroid in adults may enhance the steroid effect but may lead to folliculitis. Topical antibiotics are rarely used. Cool compresses with water or Burow's solution are helpful for acute phases when weeping lesions are present.

Systemic therapy includes antihistamines especially at night when itching is more intense. Antibiotics such as penicillin or erythromycin may be given systemically for bacterial infections. Systemic corticosteroids may be given for a limited period with severe atopic eczema. Patients should keep the skin hydrated, and avoid temperature extremes and irritating substances (see box above for patient teaching).

OTHER TYPES OF DERMATITIS
LICHEN SIMPLEX CHRONICUS

Lichen simplex chronicus (LSC) is a chronic skin condition that results from repeated scratching. Although it is more common in females and Orientals, it may occur in both sexes and all races. Itching initiates the condition in normal skin and may occur as a result of stasis or an irritant, or it may occur without any known cause. Psychological factors are thought to be involved. LSC is more commonly found in the occipital region of the scalp, hands, perineum, and legs.

Once itching starts, the itch-scratch cycle is initiated and scratching becomes a habit. The skin becomes excoriated, and lichenified plaques result. Lesions disappear if scratching ceases, but it is difficult for the person to stop scratching. Itching is often worse at night. Topical corticosteroids are the treatment of choice. In non-hairy areas, corticosteroid tape (Cordran tape) is effective if the medicated tape covers the area so that further excoriation is reduced.

SEBORRHEIC DERMATITIS

Dermatitis may occur primarily in areas of increased sebaceous gland activity on the face, ears, scalp, chest, and back. The cause is unknown. Mild seborrheic dermatitis is often seen in the scalp in the form of erythema and dandruff and can be controlled easily by shampooing with selenium sulfide (Selsun Blue) shampoo. More extensive seborrheic dermatitis leads to red scaly plaques and is treated with topical hydrocortisone.

NUMMULAR DERMATITIS

The lesions of nummular dermatitis are coin shaped and are found on the dorsum of the hand, the extensor surfaces of the extremities, and the the buttocks. It occurs most frequently in middle-aged or older men. The cause is uncertain, and the condition is chronic. Itching is often severe. The skin is usually dry; therefore, frequent bathing is inadvisable. Exposure to sunlight may be helpful. Treatment consists of topical corticosteroids and antibiotic therapy if bacteria are isolated by culture.

STASIS DERMATITIS

Stasis dermatitis is a common skin condition of the lower extremities in older persons. It is usually preceded by varicosities and poor circulation. With the reduction in venous return from the legs, substances normally carried away by the circulation remain in the tissues and irritate them. The skin is often reddened and edematous. Pruritus may be quite severe. Breaks in the skin are often caused by scratching, and infection then is introduced by the hands, clothing, and other sources.

The most important treatment for stasis dermatitis is prevention by careful attention to the treatment of peripheral vascular conditions and preventing the constriction of the circulation to the extremities. When acute weeping lesions are present, wet compresses and elevation of the legs are advised.

SKIN REACTIONS FROM SYSTEMIC FACTORS
DERMATITIS MEDICAMENTOSA

Skin manifestations resulting from drugs may have a nonallergic or an allergic basis. Commonly seen skin reactions include erythematous rashes, purpura, vesicles, bullae, ulcers, and urticaria (Table 72-3). The

TABLE 72-3 Skin reactions to common medications

Reaction	Medication
Erythematous rash	Antibiotics, sulfonamides, thiazide diuretics, barbiturates, phenylbutazone
Purpura (ecchymosis, petechiae)	Thiazides, sulfonamides, barbiturates, anticoagulants
Mucocutaneous lesions (vesicles, bullae, ulcers)	Sulfonamides, penicillin, barbiturates, phenylbutazone
Urticaria	Penicillin, streptomycin, tetracycline, insulin, aspirin, dyes, ACTH, antiserum

TABLE 72-4 Drug photosensitivity

Reaction	Symptoms	Drugs
Phototoxicity	Resembles sunburn (erythema, edema, vesicles)	Coal tar derivatives Psoralens Tetracycline Nalidixic acid Sulfanilamide Declomycin Chlorpromazine Certain dyes
Photoallergy	Resembles eczema (exudative papules, and vesicles, urticaria, lichenification)	Diuretics (thiazides) Phenothiazines Oral hypoglycemics Griseofulvin

reactions can appear at any time but the onset is usually sudden.

Hypersensitivity reactions (see Chapter 76) are the most common and may be either type I anaphylactic (urticaria, angioedema), type II cytotoxic (cellular injury), type III immune complexes (serum sickness), or type IV cell mediated (allergic contact dermatitis, allergic photosensitivity).[33] Some drugs may have combined reactions; for example, penicillin may produce both type I and type III reactions. Allergic contact dermatitis is commonly seen with drugs used topically. The rash is often bright red, semiconfluent, macular and papular, generalized, and bilateral. Hypersensitivity occurs early when previous sensitization has taken place.

Photosensitivity may also occur with certain drugs and may take one of two forms, phototoxicity or photoallergy (Table 72-4). *Phototoxicity* may occur with any person taking a photosensitive drug, and results from the reaction of the drug (chemical) with radiant energy, particularly ultraviolet light. Sunscreens are not effective in preventing photosensitivity reactions.[3] *Photoallergic* reactions are cell-mediated (type IV) hypersensitivity reactions; therefore, they affect only a small group of persons after several sensitizing exposures of drug and sunlight.

Treatment of dermatitis medicamentosa consists of stopping the drug and treating the symptoms with cool moist compresses, antihistamines (for pruritus), and topical and systemic corticosteroids. Photosensitivity can be prevented by avoiding direct sunlight on the skin when taking a drug with photosensitivity effects.

EXFOLIATIVE DERMATITIS

Exfoliative dermatitis is a rare, generalized dermatitis characterized by erythema and marked scaling. In most cases, the cause is unknown, but the disease may be associated with other types of dermatitis or with a lymphoma, or it may be the result of a drug reaction.

The onset may be rapid or insidious and consists of an elevated temperature and a generalized erythema followed by extensive scaling (exfoliation). Pruritus may be present, and the lesions often become infected. Loss of large amounts of water and protein from the skin leads to hypoproteinemia, weight loss, and difficulty with temperature control. Heart failure may occur in elderly patients. Death may result from overwhelming infection or circulatory collapse.

Therapy consists of maintaining fluid balance and preventing infection. Methods used to prevent infection in patients with burns are applicable (see Chapter 74). All drugs are discontinued as potential causative factors, although antibiotics may be started after culture and sensitivity tests of infected lesions. Oral corticosteroids are given for severe cases. Daily baths followed by application of petrolatum to the skin promote comfort.

ERYTHEMA MULTIFORME

Erythema multiforme is a skin condition believed to occur secondary to an underlying systemic disease such as an infection or to drugs. The skin eruption is characterized by red to purple macules, papules, and vesicles. Most often lesions occur on the wrists, back of the hands, ankles, tops of the feet, knees, elbows, face, palms, and soles of the feet; the entire body may be involved. The skin eruption may be preceded by fever, chest pain, and arthralgia. Treatment is to seek out the underlying cause and eliminate it if possible. Other treatment is supportive, and corticosteroids are often used. Local treatment includes baths, soaks, and dressings. If lesions appear in the mouth, special mouth care is indicated, including irrigations with warm salt solution.

INFECTIOUS DISEASES

Communicable diseases such as measles, chickenpox, smallpox, scarlet fever, and typhoid fever produce skin

TABLE 72-5 Skin reactions of some communicable diseases

Disease	Cause	Incubation Period (Days)	Place of Rash Origin	Skin Lesions
Measles (rubeola)	Rubeola virus	11 (8-14)	Face	Pink macular-papular rash; lesions coalesce
German measles; 3-day measles (rubella)	Rubella virus	14-21	Face	Pink macular-papular rash; lesions usually discrete; may coalesce
Scarlet fever (scarlatina)	Hemolytic streptococcus	1-3	Neck, chest	Bright red (scarlet) macules (pinpoint)
Chickenpox (varicella)	V-Z virus	14-21	Back, chest	Macule, papule, vesicle, crust, lesions at different stages
Smallpox (variola)	Variola virus	12 (7-21)	Face	Macule, papule, vesicle, crust, lesions all at same stage
Typhoid fever	*Salmonella typhosa*	14 (7-21)	Abdomen	Macular rash

reactions (Table 72-5). Nodes and hemorrhagic spots in the skin also accompany severe acute rheumatic fever.

LUPUS ERYTHEMATOSUS

One of the more common tissue diseases that may result in skin conditions is lupus erythematosus (LE), which occurs in two forms, systemic (SLE) (see Chapter 70) and discoid (DLE). *Discoid lupus erythematosus* is a chronic, relatively benign skin condition that has worldwide distribution among all races and that occurs most often in the fourth decade of life. It is rarely seen in children or the elderly. Precipitating factors include physical trauma and stress.

The lesions of DLE are well demarcated and erythematous, have a characteristic scaly border with an atrophied center, and vary in size. The most common sites are the cheeks (butterfly pattern), nose, ears, scalp, and chest, although other parts of the body, including mucous membranes, may also be involved. In addition to the skin lesions, the person may have leukopenia, an increased sedimentation rate, a positive rheumatoid factor test, a positive serologic test for syphilis (STS), and a low titer of antinuclear factors.

Preventive measures include avoiding physical trauma, such as by using protective lotions to prevent sunburn, and wearing warm clothing to protect against cold and wind. If stress is a precipitating factor, measures to reduce stress (see Chapter 10) can be instituted. There is no cure for DLE. Palliative measures include topical steroid therapy under occlusive wraps, intralesional steroid therapy, or antimalarial therapy with chloroquine (Aralen), hydroxychloroquine sulfate (Plaquenil), or quinacrine hydrochloride (Atabrine).

PAPULOSQUAMOUS DISEASES

Papulosquamous diseases are characterized by papular, scaly lesions. Common disorders are psoriasis, pityriasis rosea, and lichen planus.

PSORIASIS
EPIDEMIOLOGY AND ETIOLOGY

Psoriasis is a genetically determined, chronic, epidermal proliferative disease. It is not infectious or contagious and is not a nervous disorder. Approximately 1% to 2% of the population of the United States have psoriasis; 5% of this group have associated inflammatory arthritis. There is a higher incidence of psoriasis among whites and a lower incidence among the Japanese, American Indians, and blacks of West African origin. Men and women are equally affected. Psoriasis occurs in all ages but is less common among children and the elderly. There are no specific precipitating factors for the majority of persons; however, some people may develop exacerbations after climatic changes, stress, trauma, infections or drugs (propranolol, lithium). Pregnant women often see a remission of symptoms.

CLINICAL MANIFESTATIONS

The turnover time for normal skin is 28 days. After the basal cell divides, it normally takes 14 days to reach the stratum corneum and an additional 14 days for this cell to be sloughed off. In psoriasis the time is accelerated to 4 to 7 days.

The lesions of psoriasis are elevated, erythematous, sharply circumscribed, scaling plaques (Figure 72-7). The primary lesion is a papule; these papules then join to form plaques. In the black person the plaques may appear purple. Lesions may occur over the entire body but are found more commonly on the scalp, elbows, shins, and trunk. Beefy red lesions may be observed in an acute flare-up. The nails of persons with psoriasis have characteristic involvement; there may be pitting of the nails, yellowish discoloration, and onycholysis (separation of the nail from the nail bed).

Psoriasis takes many forms. *Arthropathic psoriasis* is one of the cruelest forms and may produce crippling. The nails are always involved and show denting and pit-

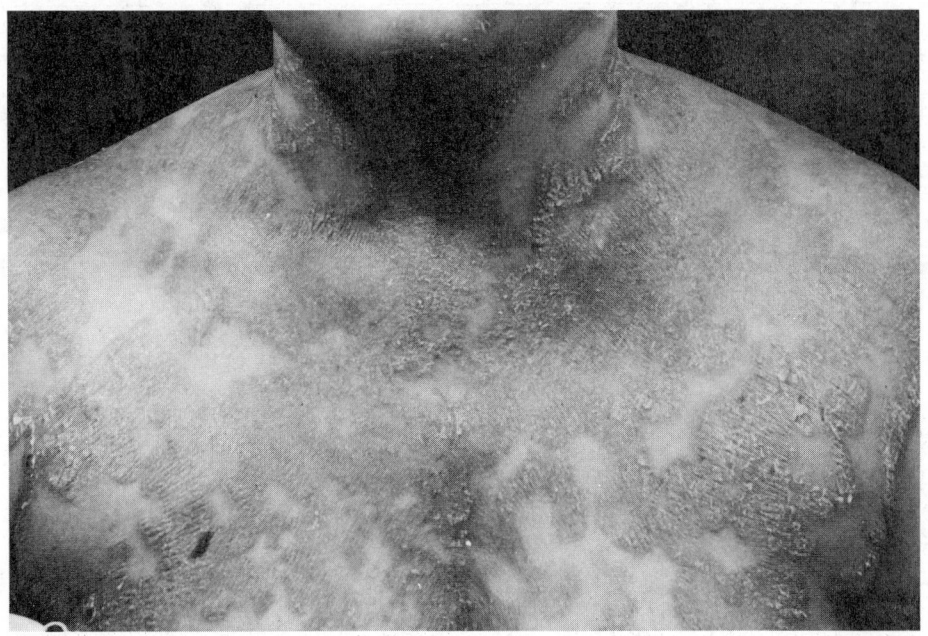

FIGURE 72-7 Generalized psoriasis. (From Rosai J: Ackerman's surgical pathology, ed 6, St Louis, 1981, The CV Mosby Co.)

ting. *Pustular psoriasis* (von Zumbusch) may present with fever, tenderness of the skin, and sterile pustules. Fortunately, only a small percentage of persons with psoriasis have eruptions that require adaptations in lifestyles.

INTERVENTIONS

Medical Management

Because of the overproduction of skin in psoriasis, treatment is based on slowing mitotic activity. Initially the lesions may be treated with topical keratolytic agents or topical steroids with occlusive wraps and wet dressings to decrease inflammation (Table 72-6). Use of topical medications and wet dressings is discussed in Chapter 73. If the psoriasis becomes resistant to these treatments, coal tar or anthralin therapy is used.

Ultraviolet light inhibits DNA synthesis, thus slowing the rapid skin cell growth. Ultraviolet light is divided into different waves: UVA (short), UVB (middle), and UVC (long). UVC is a potent carcinogen and can cause severe burns, so it is not used in treatment of psoriasis. Exposure to sunlamps or blacklight lamps without other therapy may benefit psoriasis. The combination of tar and ultraviolet (UVB) light known as the Goeckerman regimen (see the box at right) is one of the oldest forms of therapy for psoriasis but is still effective and widely used.

Photochemotherapy (Psoralen with ultraviolet (UVA) light [PUVA]) is used for severe psoriasis when other therapies have not been effective. Etretinate (Tegison), a vitamin A derivative, and methoxsalen (Psoralen) are photosensitizing agents that react with the ultraviolet energy. The drugs are taken 2 hours before exposure to the ultraviolet light; dose is based on body weight. Moderate flare-up of psoriasis (Koebner's phenomenon) may occur after treatment. Methotrexate is also reserved for persons with severe psoriasis who are recalcitrant to other treatments.

Nursing Management

Most patients with psoriasis are treated on an ambulatory basis. A new approach to therapy has been the establishment of psoriasis day care centers where patients come daily for treatments, rest, and counseling. Because the lesions are commonly found in visible skin areas, persons with psoriasis are faced with a socially disabling disease. They may need help in identifying and coping with their feelings and with changes that may occur in their lifestyle (see Chapter 18).

GOECKERMAN REGIMEN FOR PSORIASIS

1. Apply crude coal tar two to three times a day over all affected areas.
2. Remove tar with corn oil before ultraviolet therapy, leaving a thin film on skin.
3. Give ultraviolet light therapy.
4. Give tub bath with soap and oil. Shampoo scalp.
5. Reapply tar to skin and lotion to scalp.
6. Have person wear pajamas for 3 days to act as a dressing.

TABLE 72-6 Psoriasis therapy

Type	Action	Comments
Bland emollients (petrolatum, mineral oil)	Hydration of skin	Use for mild lesions Facilitates scale removal
Keratolytics (salicylic acid, ammoniated mercury)	Hydration and softening of skin Antimitotic	Avoid using on face Cover with occlusive wraps May cause skin maceration and folliculitis Not applied to irritated skin
Corticosteroids	Antimitotic Antiinflammatory	Topical use for most lesions; cover with occlusive wraps; may cause folliculitis Intralesional use for plaques Rarely given systemically May produce rebound psoriasis when withdrawn
Coal tar preparations	Action unknown Have keratolytic, antipruritic, and photosensitizing effects	May develop folliculitis with long-term use Avoid direct sunlight for 24 hours after use Avoid use on face Stains skin, hair, and clothing Available as cream, lotion, gel, solution, and shampoo May be used with ultraviolet light therapy (Goeckerman regimen)
Anthralin products	Antimitotic Inhibits enzyme metabolism	May cause skin irritation Not applied to open skin areas Petrolatum is used to protect normal skin during therapy Wear gloves during application; stains skin, hair, and clothing Avoid using on face
Photochemotherapy with ultraviolet light	Inhibition of DNA synthesis	May cause pruritus, erythema, vesicles, flare-up of lesions, transient nausea May be carcinogenic for light-skinned persons or those previously exposed to x-ray therapy Avoid direct sunlight for 12 to 24 hours after ingestion of Psoralen
Methotrexate	Antimitotic Inhibition of DNA synthesis	For severe lesions not amenable to other treatment Given orally unless nausea is present Requires close monitoring of hematologic, renal, and liver functioning
Synthetic retinoids	Corrects abnormal cell differentiation	Experimental Side effects: pruritus, lip edema, sore mouth, thirst, fragile skin, peeling of palms and soles May be used with anthralin or ultraviolet therapies

TEACHING THE PATIENT WITH PSORIASIS

1. Nature of psoriasis: noncurable, recurrence of symptoms
2. Reduce episodes of rapid-spreading psoriasis (flare-ups) by avoiding skin trauma (injuries, sunburn, infections), extremes of temperature, and stress.
3. Shampoo hair frequently to remove scales. If scalp has plaques, use a tar shampoo (Polytar, Sebutone) for 10 minutes before rinsing. Presoften thick plaques with mineral oil the night before a morning shampoo; use a fine-toothed comb to remove loose scales.[12]
4. Avoid self-medication, particularly when receiving prescribed therapy.
5. Apply topical medications in a thin layer for most lesions; use a thick layer over plaques.
6. Monitor for side effects of medications (Table 72-6).
7. Seek medical follow-up during periods of exacerbation.

The disease is not curable and may wax and wane continuously. Lesions may fade with treatment only to recur eventually in the same area or elsewhere. Patients who are not aware of this may lose confidence in the physician and may seek a quick cure elsewhere. Because psoriasis is so common and so stubborn in response to treatment, manufacturers of patent remedies find a lucrative field for their products among persons with the disease.

Teaching for individuals who have psoriasis is summarized in the box at left. A sample nursing care plan can be found on p. 2129.

PITYRIASIS ROSEA

Pityriasis rosea is a common skin condition with worldwide distribution affecting all races. It occurs more commonly in women and in adolescents and young adults. The cause is unknown but thought to be viral; the disease is not contagious.

NURSING CARE PLAN

PERSON WITH PSORIASIS

DATA: Mrs. Lee, aged 35, was referred to a psoriasis day care center for a 6-day Goeckerman regimen therapy (crude tar with exposure to ultraviolet light). Mrs. Lee told the nurse that she recently sent away for a new ointment that was supposed to cure her psoriasis, but the lesions began to flare up and itching increased.

She also said that her husband has been urging her to go out with him more to social events, but her arms and legs have "looked so bad," that she hasn't wanted others to see her until she's better.

NURSING DIAGNOSIS:

Body image disturbance related to lesions on arms and legs

Expected Patient Outcomes	Nursing Interventions	Rationale
Mrs. Lee states plans to go out socially with husband.	Help Mrs. Lee identify her positive attributes.	Awareness of positive attributes helps to increase self-esteem.
	Discuss with Mrs. Lee types of clothing that could hide the more obvious lesions.	Hiding the lesions may help her feel better about herself and desire to interact with others.

NURSING DIAGNOSIS:

Knowledge deficit related to information misinterpretation

Expected Patient Outcomes	Nursing Interventions	Rationale
Mrs. Lee describes chronicity of psoriasis and plans to follow only prescribed treatment.	Review her understanding of the nature of psoriasis.	Psoriasis is a chronic condition; understanding facilitates compliance with therapy.
	Explain the lack of cure for psoriasis and problems with self-treatment.	Lesions may fade with treatment only to recur.
	Suggest she discuss with physician lotions or ointments to use after her present treatment when lesions itch or flare up.	Self-treatment products are often ineffective and costly.
	Review with her how to apply ointments.	Ointment is more effective if spread in thin layer over plaques.

The initial symptom is usually a single oval lesion with a thin scaly border and yellowish center appearing most often on the trunk, upper arm, or thigh. This lesion is followed within a few hours, days, or weeks by similar smaller erythematous lesions with the long axis of the oval lesion along lines of skin cleavage and by scaling of the peripheral borders. The skin usually clears in 6 to 8 weeks, and the condition does not recur.

Treatment is essentially symptomatic and includes topical steroids and colloid baths if itching is present. Ultraviolet light therapy may be used.

LICHEN PLANUS

Lichen planus is a relatively common papulosquamous eruption of unknown origin. Lesions occur initially as shiny flat-topped papules on the flexor surfaces of the wrist, ankles, trunk, mucous membranes, and genitalia. The mouth is frequently involved. Bullous or hypertrophic lesions may also occur. Itching is severe, and new lesions may occur at the scratched sites. Nails may become distorted. Oral or hypertrophic lesions may be-

come chronic. A number of drugs (streptomycin, paraaminosalicylic acid, methyldopa, thiazides, antimalarials) may also cause lichen planuslike eruptions.

Colloid baths and antipruritic lotions are prescribed for itching. Benadryl or sedatives may be given at bedtime. Corticosteroids may be prescribed as topical therapy under occlusive wraps or as intralesional or systemic therapy. Psoralen with ultraviolet light (PUVA) therapy is effective. Persons with oral lesions should avoid smoking or ingesting hot or irritating foods or liquids. Acute lichen planus usually resolves in 6 to 18 months, but the chronic types frequently last for many years.

BULLOUS DISEASES

Bullous diseases are characterized by the formation of bullae (blisters). Bullous diseases include pemphigous vulgaris, bullous pemphigoid, and dermatitis hepetiformis.

PEMPHIGUS VULGARIS

Pemphigus vulgaris is a rare skin condition characterized by enormous bullae that appear all over the body and on the mucous membranes. The lesions break and are followed by crusts and scarring. The disease is characterized by *acantholysis* (cells slip past one another and fluid accumulates between the cells). By placing the thumb firmly on the skin and exerting lateral sliding pressure, the upper epidermis can be dislodged, resulting in erosion or blister (Nikolsky's sign). A Tzanck test (see Chapter 71) will identify acantholytic cells. Infection of the crust produces a mousy odor, and toxemia occurs.

The cause of pemphigus is unknown, but it is thought to have an autoimmune basis. It occurs worldwide, primarily in persons between the ages of 40 and 60, and has a higher incidence among Jews. If untreated, death usually ensues in about 1 year.

Hospitalization is usually required for skin care and monitoring of drug effects. The treatment of choice for severe pemphigus is systemic corticosteroids in large doses; the dose is gradually reduced as improvement is noted. Immunosuppressants, such as methotrexate, cyclophosphamide, and azathioprine may be given to reduce the corticosteroid dose. Gold therapy (gold sodium thiomalate) may be given alone or in combination with corticosteroids for chronic therapy.[43]

Nursing care of the person with severe pemphigus can be a challenge. Stryker frames may be used to help the person change position more painlessly and to prevent weight bearing on raw surfaces. Air mattress or flotation systems may be used. Dakin's solution compresses may be applied to oozing lesions to help control odor and infection. Infection is a major concern because of the immunosuppressive effects of drug therapy. Special mouth care is required for mouth lesions, and bland diets are more easily tolerated.

Emotional support and encouragement of both patient and family are extremely important. Patients may fear rejection by others because of their appearance, and they need evidence of continued interest and attention by family and staff. The potential for altered body image and social isolation is high.

BULLOUS PEMPHIGOID

Pemphigoid differs from pemphigus; it occurs more frequently and is a benign, chronic bullous disorder. The blisters are subepidermal rather than intraepidermal and acantholysis does not occur. It occurs primarily in persons 60 years of age or older and is thought to have an autoimmune basis.

The lesions of pemphigoid are usually preceded by a pruritic or eczematous eruption. The bullae may appear anywhere but are seen mostly on the abdomen and flexor surfaces of the extremities. Lower doses of corticosteroids are required for pemphigoid than for pemphigus. Immunosuppressive drugs are combined with steroids if treatment must be long term.

DERMATITIS HERPETIFORMIS

Dermatitis herpetiformis is a chronic skin condition seen mostly in men. The lesion is a vesicular, papular, pruritic eruption of unknown cause. The characteristic distribution of lesions, is usually symmetric; bilateral; and over the surfaces of the limbs, buttocks, and scalp. Scarring and hyperpigmentation may occur after the lesions heal. Many persons have an associated gluten-sensitive enteropathy.

Treatment consists of systemic sulfones, and the response is often diagnostic because of the improvement. Antipruritic drugs may or may not relieve the intense pruritus. A gluten-free diet helps to control the skin symptoms.

TUMORS OF THE SKIN

Growths of skin cells may develop from the epidermis, from sebaceous or sweat glands, from the melanocyte system, or from mesodermal tissue (for example, connective or vascular tissue). Most skin tumors are benign, and even those that are malignant, with the exception of some tumors such as malignant melanoma, are often of less serious consequence than tumors elsewhere in the body.

KERATOSES (BENIGN LESIONS)

The term *keratosis* refers to any cornification or growth of the horny layer of the skin. There are several different types of keratoses, including corns and calluses, warts (p. 2117), and seborrheic and actinic (senile) keratoses.

CORNS AND CALLUSES

Corns are thickened skin lesions with a center core that thickens inwardly and causes acute pain on pressure. They are often caused by the pressure of ill-fitting shoes and occur on the toes. A corn is best treated by placing over it a small felt pad with a hole in the center to relieve pressure and by correction of shoes. Popular corn remedies seldom produce a cure because their active ingredient is usually salicylic acid, which only dissolves the outer layer of skin. As soon as the medicated pad is removed, a new layer of skin forms unless pressure is relieved.

Calluses, or thickening of circumscribed areas of the horny layer of the skin, often appear on the plantar surface of the foot when the metatarsal arch has fallen and there is constant pressure against the sole of the shoe. They are often successfully treated by relief of the pressure and by regular massage with softening lotions and creams.

SEBORRHEIC KERATOSES

The most common benign keratotic tumors seen in older persons are the seborrheic keratoses. The lesions, which resemble large, darkened, greasy warts, are usually seen on the trunk but may also occur on the face, scalp, and proximal extremities (Figure 72-8, *A*). Development of malignancy from seborrheic keratoses is rare, but a sudden increase in the number and size of the lesions may indicate an internal gastrointestinal malignancy. Blacks at an earlier age develop a type of seborrheic keratosis called *dermatosis papulosa nigra* with lesions that are small, pedunculated, and heavily pigmented.

Most seborrheic keratoses do not require treatment except for cosmetic reasons or at areas of frequent irritation. They may be removed with a curette followed by light electrodesiccation or by application of liquid nitrogen (see Chapter 73).

ACTINIC KERATOSES

Actinic (senile, solar) keratoses result from exposure of the skin to irradiation, primarily solar. They are noted most often on exposed skin areas of persons who work outdoors and on older persons. Light-skinned persons are more vulnerable to skin changes from irradiation. The number of lesions can be restricted by the use of clothing and sunscreen lotions over skin areas frequently exposed to the sun. The skin lesions are round or irregular, red-brown to gray in color, and have a dry, scaly appearance. The surrounding skin is usually dry and wrinkled from overexposure to the sun (Figure 72-8, *B*).

About 25% of the lesions become malignant (squamous cell carcinoma), evidenced by inflammation and a rapid increase in size of the lesion. The lesions of actinic keratoses are removed by curettage and light electrodesiccation. Large lesions or lesions suspected of possible malignancy are removed by excision. Multiple lesions may be treated with a topical application of a 1% to 5% 5-fluorouracil cream.

PREMALIGNANT LESIONS

Skin lesions that may lead to malignancy include actinic keratoses (as previously described), leukoplakia, Bowen's disease, and pigmented moles. The term *premalignant* does not infer that all of the lesions become malignant but that the tendency to become malignant exists.

LEUKOPLAKIA

The mucous membranes of the mouth or vagina may develop a thickened white patch of keratinized cells,

A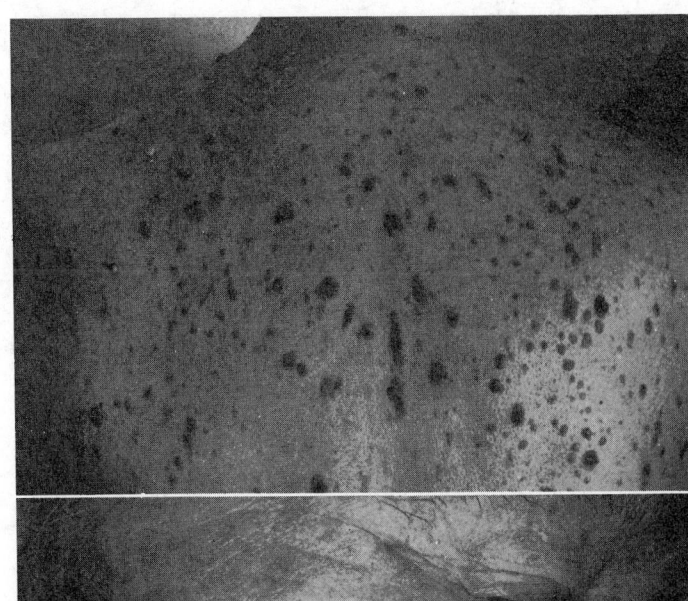

B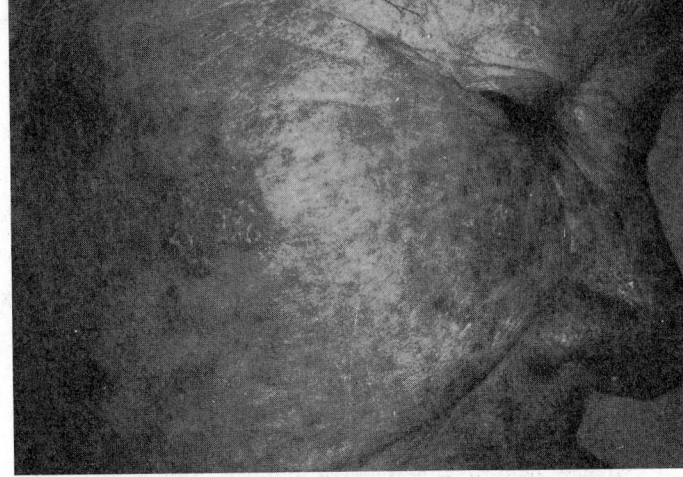

FIGURE 72-8 A, Seborrheic keratosis. **B,** Actinic (senile) keratoses. (From Stewart WD, Danto JL, and Maddin S: Dermatology: diagnosis and treatment of cutaneous disorders, ed 4, St Louis, 1978, The CV Mosby Co.)

which may eventually develop into invasive squamous cell carcinoma. Red or red and white patches of the mouth (erythroleukoplakia) may also occur and have a higher malignancy potential than the white patches. External irritants that appear to have an etiologic relationship to oral leukoplakia include poorly fitting dentures, cheek biting, and pipe or cigarette smoking. Chronic maceration, friction, and senile atrophy may lead to leukoplakia of the vagina.

Preventive measures include removal of potentially causative factors. Persons who continue to smoke need to inspect their mouths for signs of changes. Dental care should be sought for rough-edged teeth. Large lesions are usually surgically excised and a biopsy is performed. Benign lesions may be removed by electrodessication.

DIFFERENTIATION OF BENIGN AND MALIGNANT MOLES

BENIGN MOLES	MALIGNANT MELANOMAS
Symmetric	**A**symetric
Borders: even	**B**orders: uneven
Color: uniform	**C**olor: multiple shades
Diameter: <6 mm	**D**iameter: >6 mm

BOWEN'S DISEASE

Bowen's disease is a chronic skin disease that can be considered as squamous cell carcinoma *in situ*. It occurs mostly in older light-skinned men and is thought to be related to chemical carcinogens.[38] The lesions are sharply demarcated brown plaques that are widely distributed, although a single lesion may be present. Persons with Bowen's disease are at high risk for developing other malignant diseases. Treatment is by surgical excision.

PIGMENTED NEVI

Almost all persons have some pigmented nevi (moles), which usually develop during childhood, becoming more raised and prominent, and often containing hair. Moles, per se, are not generally significant except for cosmetic reasons or for their potential to develop into malignant melanomas. To facilitate differentiation between benign and malignant moles, the Skin Cancer Foundation has developed the mnemonic ABCD (see box above).

Small, evenly colored brown moles with hair are benign. A blue or greenish-black color does not usually indicate malignancy if the color is even. Changes in moles that should be reported immediately to the physician for further diagnosis include (1) development of a ring of new pigment around the base, (2) development of uneven pigmentation, (3) sudden growth, (4) loss of hair in a mole, or (5) bleeding in a mole.[43]

MALIGNANT LESIONS
SQUAMOUS CELL CARCINOMA

Squamous cell carcinoma is a malignant tumor of the surface epidermis that may appear on the exposed skin surface of older persons or at areas of chronic irritation or skin damaged from irradiation or burns. If the growth developed from actinic keratosis, Bowen's disease, or leukoplakia, the lesion will be indurated and surrounded by an inflammatory base. A new lesion appears as a firm keratotic nodule with an indurated base (Figure 72-9). Lesions that develop on hair-bearing skin rarely metastasize, but lesions of the lip or ear frequently metastasize to regional lymph nodes.

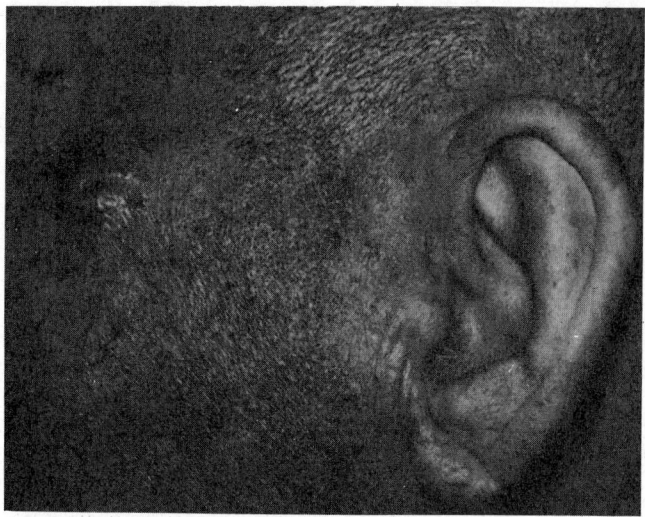

FIGURE 72-9 Squamous cell carcinoma in infratemporal area, one of the most common sites for this tumor. (From Stewart WD, Danto JL, and Maddin S: Dermatology: diagnosis and treatment of cutaneous disorders, ed 4, St Louis, 1978, The CV Mosby Co.)

Protection of the skin from excessive solar radiation and early detection of lesions are important preventive measures. Lesions may be removed by surgical excision, curettage with electrodesiccation, irradiation, or chemosurgery. *Chemosurgery* involves application of a dressing with a fixative paste such as zinc chloride and then removal of the dressing with some tissue fixed to it. Reapplication is often necessary until all malignant tissue has been removed. Chemosurgery is used for tumors without well-defined borders.

KERATOACANTHOMA

Keratoacanthoma is a skin tumor that has microscopic characteristics similar to squamous cell carcinoma but that is relatively noninvasive and does not metastasize. The lesions occur mostly on normal skin areas exposed to sun, tar, and oils. The tumor grows rapidly to a 1- to 2-cm size, remains quiescent for 2 to 8 weeks, and then begins to regress spontaneously.[34] The dome-shaped, shiny, pink lesion is filled with a keratinous plug that is expelled as the nodule shrinks. The lesion is usually excised and a biopsy performed because of its similarity to squamous cell carcinoma.

BASAL CELL EPITHELIOMA

Basal cell epithelioma or carcinoma is the most common malignant tumor affecting light-skinned people over 40 years of age. It is uncommon among blacks and Orientals. It occurs primarily over hairy areas, those containing pilosebaceous follicles. The growths initially have a characteristic translucent appearance, ranging from

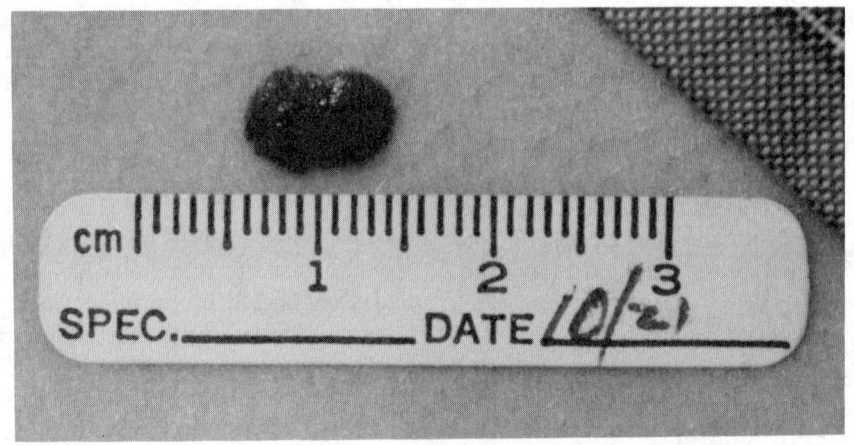

FIGURE 72-10 Malignant melanoma. (Courtesy David Bickers, MD, Cleveland, Ohio.)

flesh color to a pale pink with a few telangiectatic vessels across the surface. Because the lesion grows slowly, the center becomes indurated. Basal cell epitheliomas rarely metastasize, but untreated tumors can become locally invasive with severe tissue destruction, infection, and hemorrhage.

Treatment of basal cell epitheliomas depends on the site and extent of the tumor. The four treatment modalities include curettage with electrodessication, surgical excision, irradiation, and chemosurgery (see Chapter 73).

MALIGNANT MELANOMA

Malignant melanoma is one of the most serious of malignant tumors, affecting over 27,000 persons in the United States each year; it has been increasing at the rate of 3.4% per year.[1] Of the estimated 7800 deaths from skin cancers each year, 5800 are from melanoma.[1] It is seen more often in whites than blacks, especially in those who have had frequent exposure to the sun. It may develop from a pigmented nevus or arise from healthy skin and occurs mostly on the head, neck, and lower extremities. The lesions vary considerably in appearance, some with deep pigmentation, irregular borders, and surrounding erythema, and others with irregular pigmentation (yellow, blue, black) and irregular surfaces (Figure 72-10). The rate of growth is variable. Late changes include bleeding and ulceration. The incidence of metastasis from malignant melanoma is high and depends on the depth of invasion. Metastasis occurs first to the regional lymph nodes and then by hematogenous spread to the lungs and liver and to other areas.

Early diagnosis leads to a more favorable prognosis. Treatment consists of total wide excision, and skin grafts may be needed to cover the defect. Chemotherapy by regional perfusion or systemic therapy, or immunotherapy may be given when metastasis has occurred.

KAPOSI'S SARCOMA

Kaposi's sarcoma was a rare malignant disorder in older men in the United States until recently, although it was endemic in young black men of equatorial Africa. The disorder is now commonly seen as one of the opportunistic disorders occurring in conjunction with acquired immunodeficiency syndrome (AIDS), especially in homosexual men.

Persons with Kaposi's sarcoma develop discrete, red, purple, or dark plaques or nodules scattered widely over the body on the skin and mucous membranes, especially the mouth. Single lesions may occur. Some lesions may regress spontaneously. The disorder is slowly progressive, and successful treatment of the sarcoma does not affect survival. Many persons die of an associated opportunistic infection (see Chapter 74).

Treatment is primarily for cosmetic and psychological reasons. Individual lesions may be excised, but because lesions are usually numerous, therapy consists mainly of phototherapy, radiation for accessible tumors, or chemotherapy (vinblastine) given intralesionally or intravenously.[43]

SKIN DISORDERS IN BLACKS

The reported incidence of dermatologic disorders varies among different races, and some disorders are reported to be higher among blacks. Socioeconomic conditions must be considered when interpreting the data, and the reported incidence may actually reflect poor diet or poor health care rather than a racial difference.[38] Disorders commonly seen among blacks include lichen planus, follicular syphilis, acne, and follicular eczema. Because the pigment of black skin screens out the sun's rays, those disorders that are affected by solar irradiation, such as squamous cell carcinoma, keratoacanthoma, and basal cell epithelioma, rarely occur.

Pigmentary changes more commonly result from dermatologic disorders in blacks than whites because of the greater amount of melanin present. *Hyperpigmentation* is commonly seen after acne vulgaris, drug eruptions, lichen simplex chronicus, and pityriasis rosea. *Hypopigmentation* may result from atopic dermatitis, tinea, and pityriasis alba. Some dermatologic disorders that are unique to blacks include traumatic alopecia, pseudofolliculitis barbae, keloids, dermatosis papulosa nigra, and perifolliculitis abscedens.

TRAUMATIC ALOPECIA

Black hair shafts are highly susceptible to breakage, and hair loss may result from hair care practices sometimes used by blacks, such as tight hair curlers, cornrow braiding, hot combing, or the use of picks. Wetting or "softening" the hair before the use of a pick may help prevent trauma to the hair. The hair usually grows back when the specific hair practice is discontinued.

PSEUDOFOLLICULITIS BARBAE

Hair follicles in blacks are curved rather than straight; therefore, the hair curls back as it grows. After shaving, the sharpened point of the hair shaft (especially if a straight razor has been used) acts like a hook and reenters the skin, causing an inflammatory response. The most commonly affected areas include the chin and upper anterior neck. The legs and axilla may also develop pseudofolliculitis from shaving.

The lesions consist of papules and pustules, with some postinflammatory hyperpigmentation. Treatment consists of growing a beard or shaving with a foil-guarded shaver. As the beard is growing, a brush or rough washcloth may be used to dislodge ingrowing hairs. A mild depilatory may be used in place of shaving. Lesions may be treated with topical steroids or antibiotics.

KELOIDS

Although keloids are seen in all races, they are much more prevalent in blacks than whites. Keloids are hard, raised, shiny growths of collagen tissue that usually originate from a scar and then grow beyond the wound, often with clawlike projections. Keloids occur most often in young adults but may require many years to reach full growth. Highly susceptible areas for keloid growth include the sternum, mandible, ear, and neck. Keloids may recur after simple excision; therefore, surgery is followed by intralesional steroid therapy, radiation therapy, electron beam therapy, or pressure garments.

DERMATOSIS PAPULOSA NIGRA

Almost 35% of blacks develop a seborrheic keratosis consisting of small (5 mm) brown or black papules appearing in varying numbers primarily on the face but also on the neck, chest, and upper back. Pruritus may occur but is usually absent. Treatment consists of light electrodesiccation or cryotherapy.

PERIFOLLICULITIS ABSCEDENS

Perifolliculitis abscedens is a rare, chronic skin disorder seen in black males. It occurs on the scalp, and the lesions consist of numerous firm or fluctuant small nodules connected by purulent sinus tracts. Alopecia and scarring occur in the affected areas. Treatment is difficult. Antibiotics are ineffective, and intralesional steroid therapy provides only temporary relief. X-ray therapy is more effective, but in severe cases scalp excision with split-thickness grafting may be necessary.[34]

CHAPTER SUMMARY

- Parasitic infestations include pediculosis and scabies; treatment includes applications of pediculicides and scabicides; patient and family members need to learn measures to prevent spread of infection.

- Fungal skin infections include candidiasis and the dermatophytoses (tinea). Treatment includes applying topical fungicides, keeping the skin dry, and wearing loose clothing or shoes, as appropriate.

- Bacterial skin infections include impetigo, folliculitis, furuncles and carbuncles, and erysipelas. Management includes cleansing the skin well and applying topical antibiotics; soaks are used to remove crusts. Heat is applied to furuncles until drainage occurs; incision and drainage may be necessary. Care must be taken to prevent spread of infection to other skin areas or to other persons.

- Viral skin infections include warts, herpes simplex (fever blister), and herpes zoster (shingles). Acyclovir may be prescribed for herpes infections. Pain is a problem with herpes infections and may persist after the lesions have healed.

- Acne results from multiple factors and is seen mostly in adolescents. The lesions result from blockage of hair follicles by sebum, leading to inflammations. Treatment may be with topical drying agents; removal of comedones; and systemic therapy with isoretinoic acid, antibiotics, estrogens, or intralesional corticosteroids for severe acne.

- Types of dermatitis include contact (from external agents), atopic (hypersensitivity reaction), seborrheic, nummular, and stasis dermatitis and lichen simplex chronicus. Typical lesions include erythema, followed by vesicle formation with oozing followed by crusting and scaling; itching is common. Treatment commonly includes wet dressings with water or Burow's solution and corticosteroid therapy. Antibiotics are given for superimposed infections.

✔ Skin reactions from systemic factors include dermatitis medicamentosa (drugs), exfoliative dermatitis, erythema multiforme, lesions of communicable diseases, and lupus erythematosus.

✔ Psoriasis is a genetically determined, papulosquamous disease; no cure exists. The lesions are scaling plaques. Treatment consists of bland emollients and keratolytics to hydrate and soften the skin, corticosteroids, coal tar preparations, anthralin products (antimitotic), and photochemotherapy.

✔ Benign skin growths are keratoses (corns, calluses, seborrheic, actinic); premalignant growths include leukoplakia, Bowen's disease, and pigmented nevi.

✔ Benign nevi (moles) are symmetric with even borders, uniform color, and usually less than 6 mm in size; malignant melanomas are asymetric with uneven borders, multiple colors, and usually larger than 6 mm.

✔ A major contributing factor to the incidence of some skin growths (actinic keratoses, squamous cell carcinomas, keratocanthomas, malignant melanomas) is unprotected exposure to the sun. Most skin cancers, with the *exception* of malignant melanomas and some squamous cell carcinomas (on lips or ears), do not metastasize.

✔ Changes in moles that should be reported to the physician include change in pigmentation, sudden growth in size, loss of hair in the mole, and bleeding.

✔ Kaposi's sarcoma is widely scattered red, purple, or dark plaques, occurring mostly in persons with AIDS. The disorder is slowly progressive and treatment is primarily cosmetic; the person usually dies of another opportunistic infection.

✔ Skin disorders commonly seen in blacks include traumatic alopecia, pseudofolliculitis barbae, keloids, dermatosis papulosa nigra, and perifolliculitis abscedens.

QUESTIONS TO CONSIDER

■ Make a chart comparing the lesions and treatment of the four types of skin infections or infestations. How do they differ? What are nursing implications for each type?

■ Why are there several different treatments for psoriasis? What would you say to a person with psoriasis who complains that no one has been able to help her?

■ What teaching is important in prevention of skin tumors?

REFERENCES AND SELECTED READINGS

1. American Cancer Society: Cancer Facts and Figures, New York, 1989, The Society.
2. Anderson TF: Psoriasis, Med Clin North Am 66:769-793, 1982.
3. Bickers DR: Treatment of selected photosensitivity diseases, Med Clin North Am 66:927-937, 1982.
4. Black skin problems, Am J Nurs 79:1092-1094, 1979.
5. Bodey GP: Topical and systemic antifungal agents, Med Clin North Am 72:637-659, 1988.
6. Buxton PK: ABC of dermatology: eczema and inflammatory dermatoses, Br Med J 295:1112-1114, 1987.
7. Buxton PK: ABC of dermatology: acne and rosacea, Br Med J (Clin Res): 296:41-45, 1988.
8. Callen JP: Therapy of cutaneous lupus erythematosus, Med Clin North Am 66:795-805, 1982.
9. Chak LY et al: Radiation therapy for acquired immunodeficiency syndrome-related Kaposi's sarcoma, J Clin Oncol 6:863-867, 1988.
10. Cunha BA et al: Clinical clues to AIDS: recognizing the dermatologic and nondermatologic manifestations, Postgrad Med 83:165-174, 1988.
11. Douglas RG Jr: Antiviral drugs, Med Clin North Am 67:1163-1171, 1983.
12. *Dunn ML, Cockerline EB, and Rice MR: Treatment options for psoriasis, Am J Nurs 88:1082-1087, 1988.
13. Edwards KS: Diagnosing and treating AIDS-related Kaposi's sarcoma and carcinoma, Ohio Med 84:525-526, 1988.
14. Epstein E: Common skin disorders, ed 3, Oradell, NJ, 1988, Medical Economics Books.
15. Estes SA: Diagnosis and management of scabies, Med Clin North Am 66:955-963, 1982.
16. *Fraser MC and McGuire DB: Skin cancer's early warning system, Am J Nurs 84:1232-1236, 1984.
17. Greany D and Goldsmith HS: Cutaneous melanoma: diagnosis and surgical intervention, AORN J 42:43-49, 1985.
18. Habif TP: Clinical dermatology: a color guide to diagnosis and treatment, ed 2, St Louis, 1989, The CV Mosby Co.
19. Hanifin JM: Atopic dermatitis, J Allergy Clin Immunol 73:211-226, 1984.
20. Harber LC and Whitman GB: Photosensitivity: classification, Dermatol Clin 4:167-170, 1986.
21. *Heckel P: Teaching patients to cope with psoriasis: the unshared disease, Nursing '81 11(6):49-51, 1981.
22. *Hetland JR: Scabies: managing an outbreak, Geriatr Nurs 8:319-321, 1987.
23. *Hood LM: Scabies: are your patients at risk? Geriatr Nurs 8:312-315, 1987.
24. Jones HE: Therapy of superficial fungal infections, Med Clin North Am 66:851-871, 1982.
25. Kaplan AP: Drug-induced skin disease, J Allergy Clin Immunol 74:573-579, 1984.
26. Kaplan AP et al: Allergic skin disorders, JAMA 258:2900-2909, 1987.
27. *Kleinsmith D and Perricone NV: Common skin problems in the elderly, Dermatol Clin 4:485-499, 1986.
28. Kopf AW: Prevention and early detection of skin cancer/melanoma, Cancer 62(8 Suppl):1791-1795, 1988.
29. *LeFort SM: Herpes zoster and postherpetic neuralgia: the need for early intervention in the elderly, Nurse Practitioner 14(3):30-41, 1989.

*References preceded by an asterisk are particularly well suited for student reading.

30. Loeser JD: Herpes zoster and postherpetic neuralgia, Pain 25:149-164, 1986.

31. *Lombardo BL et al: Group support for derm patients, Am J Nurs 88:1088-1090, 1988.

32. *Lucey J and Baroni M: Herpetic whitlow, Am J Nurs 84:60-61, 1984.

33. Matthews KP: Clinical spectrum of allergic and pseudoallergic drug reactions, J Allergy Clin Immunol 74:558-566, 1984.

34. Moschella SL and Hurley HA: Dermatology, ed 2, Philadelphia, 1985, WB Saunders Co.

35. *Nicol NH: Atopic dermatitis, the (wet) wrap up, Am J Nurs 87:560-1563, 1987.

36. Olsen TG: Therapy of acne, Med Clin North Am 66:851-871, 1982.

37. *Orkin M and Maibach HI: Scabies, a current pandemic, Postgrad Med 66:53-62, 1979.

38. Pillsbury DM, and Heaton CL: A manual of dermatology, ed 2, Philadelphia, 1980, WB Saunders Co.

39. *Prigel CL: How to spot melanoma, Nursing '87 17(6):60-62, 1987.

40. Quan M et al: Management of acne vulgaris, Am Fam Physician 38:207-218, 1988.

41. Sauer GC: Manual of skin diseases, ed 5, Philadelphia, 1986, JB Lippincott Co.

42. Schaefer DG and Wolf JE: Common dermatologic disorders, Clin Plast Surg 14:201-208, 1987.

43. Schroeder SA et al: Current medical diagnosis and treatment, Norwalk, Conn, 1989, Appleton & Lange.

44. *Sheahan SL and Seabolt JP: Management of common parasitic infections encountered in primary care, Nurse Practitioner 12(8):19-33, 1987.

45. *Stern C: Melanoma, the most lethal skin cancer, RN 50(7):12-14, 1987.

46. Strommen GL et al: Human infection with herpes zoster: etiology, pathophysiology, diagnosis, clinical course, and treatment, Pharmacotherapy 8(1):52-68, 1988.

47. Toback AC and Anders H: Phototoxicity from systemic agents, Dermatol Clin 4:223-229, 1986.

48. *Todaro W: Scabies: treating the symptoms and masking the cause, Geriat Nurs 8:316-318, 1987.

49. Weinstein GD and Voorhees JJ, editors: Symposium on psoriasis, Dermatol Clin 2:355-516, 1984.

50. Wyngaarden JB and Smith LH: Textbook of medicine, ed 18, Philadelphia, 1988, WB Saunders Co.

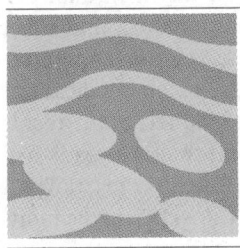

CHAPTER 73

Common Interventions for Skin Problems

BARBARA C. LONG

CHAPTER OBJECTIVES

After studying this chapter, the student should be able to:
1 Identify preventive measures for dermatologic disorders.
2 Describe psychological effects of dermatologic problems.
3 Describe general nursing interventions for dermatologic problems.
4 Identify types of dermatologic and plastic surgery and describe appropriate patient care.

The specific management of persons with dermatologic problems varies with each disease entity. There are general principles, however, that the nurse should follow in the care of these individuals.

Prevention of dermatologic conditions not only relieves the patient of discomfort but is cost effective, since many skin conditions are chronic. This chapter discusses methods of prevention, measures to alleviate common patient discomforts, care of skin lesions, and care of persons experiencing dermatologic or plastic surgery. Interventions for persons with specific dermatologic problems are discussed in Chapter 72.

PREVENTION OF DERMATOLOGIC DISORDERS

AVOIDANCE OF CAUSATIVE AGENTS

The first step in prevention of dermatologic conditions may be directed to avoiding the causative agent. This may be a specific antigen, contact irritant, microorganism, trauma, direct sunlight, or insect. Instructing the person to avoid a known causative agent is preventive medicine; however, it may not be that simple. Many dermatologic diseases have no known cause or are hereditary; or once the mechanism of the disease is known, it is not always possible to remove the trigger factors. Finally, symptoms may persist long after the agent is removed. Therefore the nurse's responsibility is one of educating the patient about good skin care, the importance of rest and avoidance of emotional stress,

good nutrition, and, lastly, close observation to determine changes in skin conditions.

SUNLIGHT

Sunlight, particularly ultraviolet (UV) rays, are damaging to the skin. These rays are termed *actinic,* meaning photochemically active radiation. UV-A waves contribute to aging and carcinogenesis of the skin.[41] UV-B waves lead to burning and activation of melanin that produces tanning. Suntans eventually lead to permanent roughening and wrinkling of the skin; therefore, there is no such thing as a "safe tan." *Tanning parlors should be avoided* because they use UV waves to produce the tan. Sun damage is the major cause of skin cancer (see Chapter 72).

There are two ways to protect against UV rays, by blocking or by absorbing the rays. The rays may be *blocked* by opaque clothing or by selected sunscreens containing titanium dioxide, zinc oxide, kaolin, or iron oxide.[41] UV-B rays may be *absorbed* by the use of sunscreens containing PABA (para-aminobenzoic acid), a PABA derivative, or a benzophenone compound. The best sunscreens have a sun-protection factor (SPF) of 15 or more. Sunscreens are removed easily with water and must be reapplied after swimming or heavy sweating. Lips must also be protected with sunscreens or dark lipstick. UV rays have stronger effects at high altitudes (where there is less atmosphere to absorb the rays) and at the equator (where the sun is closer to the earth); therefore, additional protection is required in these places. People who have been diagnosed as having a skin condition that is aggravated by UV light, or who are taking photosensitive drugs (see Chapter 72) should avoid the sun, if possible, or take adequate protection.

CLEANSING

The outer layer of skin cells and the perspiration are acid in reaction, and their presence inhibits the life and growth of bacteria. Strong soaps that are alkaline in reaction may neutralize this protective acid condition of the skin. They may also remove the oily secretion of the sebaceous glands, which lubricate the outer skin layers and contribute to their health. It is sometimes necessary to remove excess oil and scale or debris to facilitate the absorption of medication, promote healing, and enhance the appearance of the skin. In psoriasis, for example, removal of scale by mechanical means and slowing of skin metabolism are prime objectives.

Normal skin should be washed often enough to remove excess oils and excretions and to prevent odor. Care must be taken not to cause drying or irritation. Maintaining a proper degree of hydration in the skin will prevent dryness and itching, which may lead to scratching, excoriation, and further trauma. Hydrating the stratum corneum, or outer layer of skin, may be accomplished by soaking in a tub of water for 20 to 30 minutes and then immediately applying a lubricating lotion or cream. This application of a cream prevents the rapid loss of water from the skin surface.

NUTRITION

Good diet and nutrition play an important role in preventing the occurrence of skin lesions. Some skin lesions may be directly associated with dietary intake. Excessive dryness of the skin and thickening of the stratum corneum at the hair follicle openings may be caused by nutritional deficiencies. Elevated blood lipids secondary to hyperlipoproteinemia may take the form of xanthomas on the skin surface. Restriction of sodium in patients who are on steroids may lessen or prevent edema as a side effect.

Hypersensitive individuals may be placed on restrictive diets to exclude intake of known causative agents or as a diagnostic tool to identify causative agents. Food labels should be read carefully to determine whether the product or food additive contains the agent the hypersensitive person is to avoid. It also may be necessary to request information from the manufacturer if questions about food additives arise. The patient should know the type of diet to be followed. This includes knowledge of any restrictions, methods of preparing these foods, if necessary, and the duration of the prescribed diet.

OBSERVATIONS OF CHANGES

Care of normal skin includes regular observation of pigmented skin areas, moles, or other apparently minor skin lesions. Any change in size, color, or general appearance should be reported to a physician at once, since a change in moles or new skin growths is one of the danger signals of cancer.

DANGERS OF SELF-TREATMENT

People should be urged to seek competent medical help when skin conditions develop. Although skin diseases rarely cause death, they may be reflections of serious systemic illness and can account for much human discomfort and for serious interruption of work and other activities. Many persons are inclined to rely on the advice of friends or the local druggist or on medications they may have on hand. Each individual's skin reacts differently to treatment, and the skin that is already irritated or diseased may respond violently to inexpert treatment. Because of changes in the skin, medications prescribed even for a similar skin ailment in the same patient some time previously may not produce a favorable response. Medications may deteriorate, and for this reason old medications are not safe. The person may be spared much discomfort and expense by consulting a specialist when symptoms first develop and before a mild skin condition becomes a real problem.

PSYCHOLOGIC EFFECTS OF DERMATOLOGIC PROBLEMS

There is a certain degree of "beauty orientation" in Western culture. Beauty pageants are popular, advertisements in the media use beautiful models to attract the reader, and in public groups heads turn as a good-looking person walks by. Cosmetics to enhance good looks are extensively used by men as well as women. It is no wonder, therefore, that skin diseases or physical defects that detract from "good looks" produce psychological reactions.

A person's emotional reaction to a deformity or defect must not be underestimated. One's pride in oneself and the ability to think well of oneself and to regard oneself favorably in comparison with others are essential to the development and maintenance of a well-integrated personality. Every person who has a defect or a handicap, particularly if it is conspicuous to others, suffers from some threat to emotional security. The extent of the emotional reaction and the amount of maladjustment that follows depend on the individual's makeup and ability to cope with emotional insults. Disfigurements almost invariably lead to disturbing experiences. The child who has webbed fingers may be ridiculed at school; the adolescent girl who has acne scars may be self-conscious and avoid social situations; and the young man with a posttraumatic scar on his face may be refused a salesman's job. Under any of these circumstances it is not unusual for the individual to withdraw from a society that is unkind. The defect may be used to justify failure, to assume responsibility, or to justify striking out against an unkind society.

Skin diseases that produce marked disfigurement of visible body surfaces, therefore, can effect alterations in the person's body image, as described in Chapter 18. Feelings of decreased worth by persons with large draining lesions or with severe disfigurement are reinforced during interactions with others. Some people are repelled when viewing persons with severe skin diseases, or they may experience a threat to their own body integrity and physically withdraw to avoid interaction. Persons may also frequently experience nonverbal messages of disgust when others view them for the first time. This is markedly poignant when those nonverbal messages are sent by significant others or by health professionals.

The person with severe facial disfigurement may also experience job discrimination. One woman was moved sequentially from a large office to a smaller office to a single office and finally to the evening hours in a lonely room so that co-workers could avoid looking at her. She lived alone and was increasingly deprived of social contacts with others. It was only after her eyesight failed and she was encouraged to attend groups for the blind that she was able to develop meaningful relationships again.

In working with the person with severe skin disease, the nurse first examines his or her own feelings that could be expressed nonverbally in a negative manner. Measures to assist the patient and family to deal with and cope with their feelings are described in Chapter 10.

GENERAL INTERVENTIONS

RELIEF OF PRURITUS

ETIOLOGY AND PATHOPHYSIOLOGY

Pruritus or itching is a cutaneous symptom that provokes the desire to scratch. It is caused by repetitive low-frequency stimulation of C fibers that are similar to but different from C fibers that transmit pain stimuli. Itching can be produced by mechanical stimulation of the skin or by chemical mediators, primarily the kinins.[16] Itching occurs only in the skin, certain mucous membranes, and the eyes. The areas most sensitive to itching are the nostrils, mucocutaneous junctions, external ear canals, and perineum.

Pruritus can be caused by any irritating substance that interrupts the stratum corneum layer of the skin, or it can be a result of certain systemic diseases (see the box above). Not all infectious diseases producing rashes cause itching. One of the most common causes is dry skin, sometimes occurring as a result of excessive bathing, particularly with "bubble bath," which has a drying effect. Factors that can intensify itching include vasodilation, tissue anoxia, and stasis of circulation. Whatever the cause, pruritus ranges from an annoyance to a severe, distressing, or exhausting system.

CLINICAL MANIFESTATIONS

Pruritus leads to the motor response of scratching. Persons with very intense itching may excoriate the skin

COMMON CAUSES OF ITCHING

Dry skin
Skin irritants: plastic or glass fibers, wool, plant products, insects
Drug reactions
Psychogenic reactions
Infectious diseases
Infestation: hookworm
Systemic diseases: obstructive biliary disease, uremia, diabetes mellitus
Neoplasia: Hodgkin's disease, leukemia, lymphoma

severely by digging deeply into the skin with their fingernails when trying to alleviate the itch. Persons with generalized itching may be observed to be in almost constant motion—twisting, rubbing, and scratching.

INTERVENTIONS

A major step in treating pruritus is to attempt to remove the itch stimuli and break the itch-scratch cycle. Cold causes vasoconstriction and will provide some relief. Hydration in a tepid bath followed by the application of an emollient lotion is helpful. Cornstarch or oatmeal preparations (p. 2140) may be added to the bath. Topical corticosteroids decrease inflammation leading to vasoconstriction. In some persons antihistamines or tranquilizers are of some value.

The awareness of pruritus may be more acute during the night because of a decrease in diverting stimuli. Cool, light, nonrestrictive bed clothing may help allay itching. Excessive drying of the skin caused by high room temperature and low humidity can also increase pruritus. It occurs readily in an elderly person who already has dry skin. Usually a room temperature of 20° C (68° to 70° F) and humidity of 30% to 40% are best for the person with pruritus.

TEMPERATURE CONTROL

The individual who has a generalized flush, or erythema, and the one who has an extensive exfoliative dermatitis may be losing body heat at an abnormally increased rate and may need a room temperature of 32.2° C (90° F) or more to maintain normal body temperature. Care must be taken to avoid chilling, particularly after baths, when compresses are used, or when parts of the body are exposed.

THERAPEUTIC BATHS AND SOAKS

Baths or soaks of an affected extremity may be prescribed to remove exudates, to moisturize or dry the skin, to relieve pruritus, or to provide antibacterial or antifungal therapy (Table 73-1). Frequent baths or soaks

TABLE 73-1 Preparations commonly used for baths or soaks

Substance	Effect	Suggested Actions
Colloids: oatmeal, cornstarch, soybean powder	Antipruritic, drying	Tub surfaces become very slippery; support person to prevent falls.
Potassium permanganate	Antifungal, drying, deodorizing	Strain pulverized tablet through cheesecloth to prevent irritation; stains surfaces and linens.
Burow's solution (aluminum acetate)	Antibacterial, drying	Commonly use for soaks.
Sulfur bath suspension	Antibacterial	Rinse body with tepid water after bath to remove residual sulfur particles.
Tar preparations: Balnetar, Zetar, Alma-Tar, Polytar	Antipruritic, moisturizing	Do not use soap with tar baths.
Bath oils: Alpha-Keri, Jeri-Bath, Domol	Antipruritic, moisturizing	Tub surfaces may become slippery.

tend to dry the skin; the application of lotion or cream immediately after a bath or soak will moisturize the skin.

Hard crusts or thickened exudates from skin disorders are often soaked with physiologic saline solution, peroxide, or mild soap in warm water. These crusts or exudates are removed only when prescribed by the physician. Unless otherwise indicated (for example, if there is a potential for infection), clean technique is used.

Tub baths may be given to cleanse the skin before therapy (such as for psoriasis), to relieve general body pruritus, or to provide therapy (for example, potassium permanganate, sulfur, or tar baths). During cleansing baths, special attention is given to intertriginous areas (that is, between skin surfaces such as between toes or fingers or under breasts) where creams and topical medications may collect. Persons with arthropathic psoriasis may find it difficult to use a tub because of limited mobility. A lift may be used with the hospitalized patient; if a lift is not available, sitting on a chair under a gentle shower is the next best alternative to a cleansing bath. Guidelines for therapeutic baths and soaks are described in the box below.

TOPICAL MEDICATIONS

Applications of medications to the skin surface may take many forms. Wet dressings, creams, pastes, ointments, and lotion can be used. The nurse should know the purpose for which a local application is ordered, the drugs contained in the preparation, and any toxic signs that may occur from its use.

TYPES OF TOPICAL MEDICATIONS

Many different topical medications are used for persons with dermatologic problems. *Antibacterial* or *antifungal* topical medications (Table 73-2) are used for bacterial or fungal infections.

Corticosteroids are among the most commonly used drugs for their anti-inflammatory, vasoconstrictive, and antipruritic effects. There are numerous topical corticosteroids that differ in their anti-inflammatory effects, ranging from low to very high potency. Hydrocortisone is of low potency. Some corticosteroids, such as triamcinolone acetonide (Aristocort, Kenalog) vary in potency depending on the dose. Greasy ointments are usually more potent and have a greater lubricating effect than creams. Fluorinated corticosteroids are powerful agents and may cause epidermal, dermal, and subcutaneous atrophy leading to development of petechiae and ecchymoses, as well as to irritation and burning. The fluorinated corticosteroids are not used on the face where they may cause a rosacea-like dermatitis. Systemic effects are unlikely with the less potent topical corticosteroids, but may occur with drugs of high potency.

Nonporous covering over corticosteroids (occlusion) potentiates the effect of topical corticosteroids. Occlusion is used primarily for (1) dermatoses of palms and

GUIDELINES FOR BATHS AND SOAKS

1. The water temperature should be of comfort to patient (usually 32° to 38° C, or 90° to 100° F).
2. Medication should be completely dissolved while tub is filled.
3. The soak should last 20 to 30 minutes.
4. To prevent patient falls, persons are assisted out of the water when oils or colloids are added to the water.
5. A rubber mat will help prevent slipping.
6. The skin is *patted*, not rubbed, dry to avoid skin irritation.
7. Creams or ointments are applied *immediately* after the bath to retain skin moisture.
8. After a medicated bath
   a. Pour 1 cup of bleach into used tub water.
   b. Let bleach stand in water for 5 minutes.
   c. Wipe sides and bottom of tub.
   d. Drain tub and clean as usual.

TABLE 73-2 Some common topical antibiotic and antifungal medications

Generic Name	Trade Name	Vehicle	Comments
ANTIBACTERIAL			
Bacitracin	Baciguent	Ointment	Effective against gram-positive organisms (nonprescription)
Neomycin, bacitracin, and polymyxin B	Neosporin	Cream, ointment	Broad-spectrum antibiotic effect
Bacitracin and polymyxin B	Polysporin	Ointment	Same as Neosporin
Gentamicin	Garamycin	Cream, ointment	Broad-spectrum antibiotic
Chloramphenicol	Chloromycetin	Cream	Broad-spectrum antibiotic
Clioquinol	Vioform	Lotion, cream, ointment	Has both antibacterial and antifungal effects, useful for eczema and tinea
Nitrofurazone	Furacin	Solution, cream, ointment	Broad-spectrum antibiotic
Povidone-iodine	Betadine	Solution	Kills gram-negative and gram-positive organisms, fungal, viruses, protozoa, yeasts
Mafenide	Sulfamylon	Cream	Effective against both gram-positive and gram-negative bacteria; used for burns
Silver sulfadiazine	Silvadene	Cream	Effective against bacteria and yeast; used for burns
ANTIFUNGAL			
Tolnaftate	Tinactin Pitrex	Powder, cream, solution	Useful for tinea
Nystatin	Mycostatin Nilstat	Powder, cream, ointment	Useful against wide variety of yeasts, especially *Candida*
Amphotericin B	Fungizone	Lotion, cream, ointment	Effective against *Candida*
Clotrimazole	Lotrimin	Cream, solution, lotion	Broad-spectrum antifungal
Haloprogin	Halotex	Cream, solution	Synthetic agent useful for superficial fungal infections
Miconazole nitrate	Micatin	Cream, lotion, powder	Synthetic agent useful for tinea

soles, (2) psoriatic lesions on smooth bare skin, (3) localized patches of lichenified dermatatitis, and (4) extensive, severe, steroid-responsive dermatitis.[15] The affected area should be occluded only when prescribed by the physician. Plastic wrap is good for occluding small areas. Plastic gloves may be used on hands and plastic bags on feet. Plastic garment bags or large trash bags may be used for the trunk, with holes cut for head and arms. Plastic suits are available for total body occlusion. Lesions are usually occluded at night, usually not for more than 8 hours at a time. Plastic suits are usually worn during the day for 4 hours. Persons should not exercise while wearing body suits because heat regulation is altered under plastic from inability for sweat to evaporate.

VEHICLES FOR TOPICAL MEDICATIONS

Topical medications can be prepared in a variety of bases (Table 73-3). *Powders* are effective in reducing friction and moisture in intertriginous areas. *Lotions* must be shaken well, since the insoluble powder may settle out. The addition of alcohol increases the cooling effect of a lotion. *Ointments* do not usually leave an oily residue on the skin unless they have a petrolatum base. A nonporous covering such as plastic should not be used over an ointment unless so prescribed, because the

heat retention may increase percutaneous absorption of the medication.

APPLICATION OF TOPICAL MEDICATIONS

Gloves are worn for protection when applying topical medications. *Powders* should first be sprinkled into the gloved hand and then applied to the skin to avoid getting excess powder into the air and thus causing irritation to the mucous membrane. Powders should be used sparingly to prevent caking and should not be used on wet surfaces since this leads to caking. Cornstarch is *not* suggested since it encourages growth of yeast, bacteria, and fungi.

Lotions with a water or alcohol base are applied by patting gently. A gauze pledget should be used for extremely thin lotions. Lotions with an oily base are applied thinly and evenly with the palm of the gloved hand. A small area of skin is often tested to determine if the person will tolerate the cream or lotion over the entire body. The topical medication is applied to a small area (silver-dollar size) on the person's forearm. The time and the exact location of the trial are recorded, and the skin response to the trial medication is read 24 hours later. Crude coal tar is frequently tested in this manner.

Ointments may be applied with gloved hands. If a

TABLE 73-3 Comparison of vehicles for topical medications

Type	Base	Effect
Powder	Dry	Drying by absorbing moisture; cooling by evaporating moisture
Lotion	Powder suspended in water or oil	Protective, cleansing, cooling, antipruritic effect depending on drug and base used
Creams and ointments	Emulsions of oil and water	Covering over skin to prolong contact of medication with skin—good skin penetration; warming effect
Paste	50% or more powder in ointment base	Holds medication for long period of time with slower skin penetration

dressing is to be applied, the ointment may be spread on the dressing with a tongue blade before application to the skin. Anthralin may be caustic to normal skin, so gloves should be worn always. Crude coal tar is always applied in firm, long, *downward* strokes to prevent folliculitis, since tar is an irritant. *Creams,* as opposed to ointments, may be rubbed in.

Some topical medications such as crude coal tar are often removed before other treatment. Crude coal tar must be removed in the morning before ultraviolet light therapy (following the Goeckerman regimen). This is accomplished by applying corn oil in long downward strokes over the skin surface and then wiping with gauze pledgets, leaving only a thin film of tar. A general rule to remember is to remove only the excess ointment or ointments having a consistency of cold cream before a bath or wet dressing. Cottonseed oil, or a gauze pledget may be used to remove caked, oily-based lotions.

MEDICATED DRESSINGS
OPEN WET DRESSINGS

Wet dressings are used frequently over various skin lesions for cooling, drying, antipruritic, vasoconstricting, or debriding effects. Plain tap water or physiologic saline may be used, or medications may be added. An astringent effect may be obtained through the use of *Burow's* solution (Domeboro, Buro-Sol, Bluboro), 1:20 or 1:40 dilution. *Potassium permanganate* (KMnO$_4$), one 300 mg tablet in 1500 ml (1:5000) or one 300 mg tablet in 3000 ml (1:10,000), has an antimicrobial and drying effect. All tablet crystals must be thoroughly dissolved to prevent chemical burning of the skin. Potassium per-

APPLICATION OF OPEN WET DRESSINGS

1. Prepare solution to be applied at room temperature. Sterility is not required.
2. Soak dressing thoroughly in solution.
3. Protect bed or clothing with towels, bath blanket, flannel squares, etc.
4. Wring out dressings—they should be wet but not dripping.
5. Apply dressings in smooth layers (two to four layers) to involved areas. Wrap fingers and toes separately, and wrap joints so that they can bend.
6. Remove, soak, and reapply dressings *before* they dry (that is, every 3 to 5 minutes).
7. Continue treatment for 20 to 30 minutes.
8. Pat skin dry.

manganate should not be used on the face. *Silver nitrate* (AgNO$_3$), 0.5%, is also an antimicrobial and is often used in the treatment of burns. Both KMnO$_3$ and AgNO$_3$ stain skin and cloth.

The type of dressing material used for a wet dressing should be one without cotton filling, since cotton leaves particles and a residue on the skin, which may cause irritation. Several layers of fine-mesh gauze are ideal, and roller gauze or Kerlix may be used for extremities. A mask for the face may be designed by cutting out openings for the eyes, nose, and mouth from several thicknesses of gauze. At home the person can use muslintype cotton material such as old clean sheets, handkerchiefs, cloth diapers, or muslin dish towels that are lint free. These materials need not be sterilized but should be washed or discarded every 24 hours.

The best effects of wet dressings are obtained by several treatment periods spaced across the person's waking hours. The solution is applied at room temperature (see the box above) to prevent the marked vasoconstriction with subsequent vasodilation that occurs with cold solutions. Although the dressings can be kept wet by adding solution with the dressings in place, this practice usually leads to excessive dripping. Dressings *must* be removed, soaked, and reapplied when KMnO$_4$ or AgNO$_3$ is used, since evaporation can increase the solute on the dressings, increasing the dose and causing a chemical burn or irritation. Occlusive plastic wraps should be avoided unless specifically ordered by the physician.

CLOSED WET DRESSINGS

Wet dressings can be covered with a nonpermeable material such as plastic wrap specifically to retain heat if an early abscess is present, to soften excessive keratinized tissue, or to enhance penetration of a topical medication. This method is not used frequently, since interference with evaporation contributes to skin maceration.

TEACHING THE PERSON WITH A DERMATOLOGIC DISORDER

1. Nature of the disorder (cause, preventive measures, acuity or chronicity, symptoms requiring medical follow-up)
2. Treatment modalities to be carried out at home (soaks, baths, medicated dressings)
3. Special precautions to be observed during treatment such as:
   a. Avoiding nonporous coverings over dressings unless so ordered
   b. Complete dissolving of tablets or crystals in baths or soaks
   c. Avoiding excessive rubbing of medication over lesions
   d. Applying thin layers of lotions or powders
4. Prescribed medication regimens: route of administration, vehicle to be used, dose, frequency, duration of topical application, side effects, where supplies can be obtained
5. Ways to promote socialization with others when disfiguring dermatologic lesions are present

WET-TO-DRY DRESSINGS

Wet-to-dry dressings are used to *debride* wounds or ulcerations. A fine-mesh gauze is moistened with the prescribed solution, placed over the lesion, and allowed to dry. The crust and debris are removed as the dressing is pulled off dry. This process is usually repeated every 4 to 8 hours. Half-strength Dakin's solution is frequently used for this purpose.

PATIENT TEACHING

Many persons with dermatologic disorders are not hospitalized; therefore patient teaching is an important component of nursing care. Major points in patient teaching are described in the box above. It is best to *write out* instructions specifically, since verbal instructions are easily forgotten. Patients commonly apply medications in excess amounts or with vigorous rubbing; these procedures may counteract all benefits or make the condition worse.

Although commercial dressings are easier to use, they are expensive if required over a prolonged period. Old linens, such as cotton sheets or socks, may be substituted for commercial dressings. A plastic shower cap may be used as an occlusive scalp covering at night.

Patients with complex treatments or dressings may require the services of a community health nurse until they are able to carry out the activities independently.

DERMATOLOGIC SURGERY

Treatment of skin lesions by dermatologists sometimes includes removal of skin lesions. Superficial skin lesions involving only the epidermis can be removed easily by various means; deep lesions involving the dermis, such as with some skin cancers, are removed with full-thickness skin excision.

TYPES OF SURGERY
TANGENTIAL SURGERY

Superficial lesions can be removed by slicing off the lesion with a sharp blade. It is especially useful for removal of flat lesions. The entire lesion may be removed for diagnosis. Hemostasis is obtained with pressure or gelatin foam.

CURETTAGE

Curettage is the scraping or scooping out of a superficial lesion with a curet, which is a spoon-shaped, sharp-edged instrument. A local anesthetic is usually injected around the lesion before curettage. (Figure 73-1). Hemostasis is accomplished with a chemical styptic such as ferric chloride or Monsel's solution, with gelatin foam, or by electrocoagulation. Lesions that may be removed by curettage include seborrheic keratoses, actinic keratoses, basal cell epitheliomas, leukoplakia, warts, and nevi.

PUNCH BIOPSY

A punch is used under local anesthesia to remove small deep lesions up to 10 mm in diameter.[15] The tissue is then sent for biopsy. Small punch biopsies may be closed with a suture. Larger biopsies may be partially closed and will then heal by secondary intention. Hemostasis can be obtained with gelatin foam packing. Punch biopsies are used for identification of basal cell carcinomas and for removal of small deep round lesions.

CRYOSURGERY

Tissue can be destroyed by rapid freezing with substances such as liquid oxygen, carbon dioxide snow or gas, liquid nitrogen, dichlorodifluoromethane (Freon), or nitrous oxide. Carbon dioxide snow and liquid nitrogen are used most frequently. The rapid freezing causes formation of intracellular ice, which destroys the cell membranes and produces cell dehydration. Cryosurgery is frequently used for removal of skin tumors (benign and malignant), warts, and keloids.

Although the procedure is not usually painful, a tingling pain occurs when the freezing substance is applied and may be uncomfortable for some persons, particularly if multiple lesions are treated. Local anesthesia may be necessary. Analgesics may be helpful during thawing.

Tissue necrosis may not be evident until 24 hours after cryosurgery. A clear or hemorrhagic bulla forms during the first day, but inflammatory reactions and bleeding are usually absent. A serous exudate occurs during the first week, followed by eschar or crust formation. The crust drops off in 3 to 4 weeks as the underlying tissue heals. Scarring usually results. Hypopigmentation may occur because melanocytes are highly vulnerable to freezing.

ELECTROSURGERY

Electric current may be used in dermatologic surgery to remove tissue and to control bleeding. *Electrodesiccation* is the drying of tissue by means of a monopolar current through the needle electrode. *Electrofulguration* is a form of electrodesiccation in which the needle electrode is held close to rather than inserted into the tissue, thus spraying the area with sparks. Bipolar current is used for *electrocoagulation,* which coagulates the tissue, curtailing capillary bleeding, and for *electrosection,* which cuts the tissue. Delayed bleeding may occur especially from electrocoagulation and may alarm the unprepared patient. The bleeding can be easily controlled by direct pressure.

Electrosurgery is usually performed under local anesthesia. Sedation is rarely necessary. Following most uses of electrosurgery the wound is left exposed for air drying. Dressings may be used if the area is subject to frequent trauma or rubbing or if oozing is present. The wound may be wiped with 70% alcohol to hasten drying. A hemostatic nonocclusive dressing may be made by covering the wound with Gelfoam powder and Micropore tape.[26]

EPILATION

Hair removal can be effected by means of electrolysis. Different methods may be used. High-frequency alternating electrical current, which is safer, less painful, and less likely to produce scarring than other methods, requires more skill and is the procedure of choice by dermatologists. Lay persons use a direct current method. Self-epilation may be carried out by a hand-held galvanic epilator (Perma-Tweez). The skin should be clean before epilation is attempted. Approximately 20% to 30% of hairs may regrow after diathermy epilation and require removal.[26]

PATIENT TEACHING

After *superficial* skin surgery, the patient is instructed not to remove the crust (scab), which acts as a protection (healing occurs under the crust). The crust should be kept as dry as possible; if it gets wet, it should be patted dry. Alcohol may be applied and allowed to evaporate. Makeup may be used over the crust. The crust may be left uncovered or may be covered with an adhesive bandage. Signs of redness, edema, or pain should be reported to the surgeon.

After *deep* skin surgery, the wound is usually bandaged and the patient is given specific instructions for care by the surgeon. Aspirin should be avoided both before and after surgery because of its anticoagulant properties that may lead to postoperative bleeding. Postoperative discomfort may be relieved with acetaminophen.

PLASTIC SURGERY

The main purposes of plastic surgery are to restore function, prevent further loss of function, and cosmetically improve the defects caused by deformities present at birth or that result from disease, age, or trauma. Plastic surgery is commonly used after burns or after removal of large amounts of tissue, such as in cancer of the head and neck. Injuries sustained in automobile accidents often require subsequent plastic surgery to restore function or improve appearance. Many plastic surgery procedures for cosmetic reasons (reconstructive surgery) are performed on an ambulatory basis. Some grafting procedures may require repeated or lengthy hospitalizations.

Plastic surgery procedures include grafts, soft tissue expansion, use of implants, Z-plasty for scar removal, dermabrasion or medical dermatattooing for removal of skin markings, and fat removal. Some body parts that can be reconstructed for cosmetic reasons include the jaw and face (maxillofacial surgery), nose (rhinoplasty), ear (otoplasty), eyelids (blepharoplasty), face lifting (rhytidoplasty), and breast (mammoplasty). These procedure are discussed after the general interventions for persons experiencing plastic surgery.

GENERAL INTERVENTIONS FOR THE PERSON EXPERIENCING PLASTIC SURGERY
EMOTIONAL FACTORS RELATED TO SURGERY

It is believed that any plastic surgery for an obvious defect is justified if it helps people feel they have a better chance for recognition among other persons. The plastic surgeon may reshape a nose or repair a deformed hand so that an emotionally stable person will have more assurance among others. However, it is foolish to assume that reconstructive surgery alone will correct a basic personality problem. Some people blame an apparently trivial physical defect for a long series of failures in their lives, when the major defect lies within their personalities. Because of this possibility, the person is usually studied before surgery is planned. It is necessary to know what the person expects the surgery to accomplish before the physician can decide whether such expectations are realistic and if surgery should be performed.

Before surgery the surgeon will tell the patient what probably can be accomplished and what changes are possible. It is important that the nurse know what the patient has been told so that misunderstandings and misinterpretations can be avoided. It is frequently necessary to repeatedly reinforce the fact that immediate results may not meet the patient's expectations. Preparation is necessary for the normal appearance of skin grafts and reconstructed tissue immediately after surgery. Postoperative tissue reaction may distort normal contours, suture lines may be reddened, and the color of the newly transplanted skin may differ somewhat from that of surrounding skin. The appearance of the surgical area changes as the edema decreases and the suture line becomes less reddened and indurated. The scar will be less noticeable 6 months after surgery than at 6 days or 6 weeks postoperatively.

The patient who is admitted to the hospital for plastic surgery may have extensive scarring and deformity and may be exceedingly sensitive to scrutiny. On the other hand, the patient may have little apparent deformity, and it may be difficult to understand why the patient wishes to have surgery. The nurse cannot know what the disfigurement means to the individual person and should avoid judgment concerning the necessity of surgery.

Plastic surgery may require repeated and long hospitalizations that may place serious financial strain on the patient and family if they must assume responsibility for the major part of the expense. Clinic nurses, community health nurses, social workers, and welfare agency personnel can help in preparing persons for this problem and in helping them meet it. If the patient is an adult, leaves from employment, financial support while undergoing treatment, and plans for convalescent care and rehabilitation are examples of problems that must be faced in many instances. The person should be encouraged to discuss problems freely, since their solution does affect medical treatment.

DIET

Consumption of a diet high in protein and vitamins before elective surgery is thought to help in the "take" or healing of a graft. Hemoglobin and clotting times are usually determined, and the blood protein level is assayed because a normal blood protein level has been found to be necessary for the satisfactory growth of grafted tissue.

OPERATIVE SITE

Many plastic surgeons prefer that the patient not see the operative site until the initial edema and inflammation subside, since the initial view is distorted compared to the end result. For this reason the patient is discouraged from looking into a mirror until healing begins to occur, and the surgeon may leave the incision covered for longer periods than necessary to prevent patient discouragement. The patient frequently needs support when seeing the operative site for the first time. The nurse assesses the reaction of the patient when dress-

ings are removed so that immediate and future nursing intervention can be planned and implemented. Members of the family should also know what to expect so they will not be unduly worried and can give support to the patient if apprehension occurs.

GRAFTS

The most common procedure used in plastic surgery is grafting, or the transplantation of skin and other tissue from one part of the body to another part or from a donor.

GRAFT SOURCES

Skin and underlying tissue may consist of an autograft, homograft, or heterograft (see the box below). Best results are obtained from *autografts* because of the body's acceptance of its own tissues.

Homografts (allografts) can be obtained from living persons or taken from persons shortly after death. Tissue taken after death can be used only if cancer or an infectious disease was not present. The use of homografts may be necessary when the patient's condition is poor and autografting is impossible. The survival time of homografts varies from a few days to a number of weeks. Depending on the tissue used and the recipient site, the transplanted tissue will then die and slough or be absorbed and replaced by the host's own developing tissue. Homografts are used only as temporary grafts.

Heterografts (xenografts) are rejected by the recipient and are used only in special cases such as burns when homografts are not available. These grafts are used infrequently since the advent of new skin replacement materials.

TYPES OF SKIN GRAFTS

Autografts may be formed by incising tissue from one part of the body and moving it directly to another part (free graft). They may also be formed by leaving one end of the graft attached to the body to provide a blood supply for the graft until blood vessels form at the new place of attachment (flap graft).

Free Grafts

There are several types of free grafts, each with its advantages and limitations (Table 73-4).

GRAFT SOURCES

Autograft	Tissue moved from one part of the body to another
Homograft	Tissue transplanted from another person
Heterograft	Tissue transplanted from another species

TABLE 73-4 Various types of skin grafts

Type of Graft	Description	Use	Comments
FREE GRAFTS			
Split-thickness: thin	Epidermis and thin layer of dermis (0.25-0.30 mm) (see Figure 71-1)	Burns	Becomes vascularized quickly Survives transplantation readily Donor sites heal quickly Poor cosmetic results Considerable postgraft contraction Does not withstand trauma
Split-thickness: intermediate or thick	Epidermis and thicker layer of dermis (0.40-0.45 or 0.55-0.60 mm)	Widely used over large wounds	Less contraction Better cosmetic results Epithelialization of donor site occurs completely but more slowly
Full-thickness	Epidermis and all of dermis	For small areas where matching skin color and texture is important	Best cosmetic results No contraction Donor site must be sutured (no epithelialization) Limited donor sites Lowest transplantation survival
FLAP GRAFTS	Skin and subcutaneous tissue; one end remains attached to donor site for vascularization	Large areas of defect; over avascular areas	More complex, requires greater skill Are bulky May introduce hair into nonhairy areas
FREE FLAP GRAFTS	Skin, subcutaneous tissue and major blood vessel transferred to recipient site; donor blood vessel anastomosed to recipient blood vessel (microsurgery)	Over bony areas or areas requiring large amounts of tissue (for example, breast reconstruction, head and neck defects, deep decubiti)	Blood flow established immediately Less contraction More normal skin appearance May not match recipient skin color or texture May introduce hair into nonhairy areas

Split-thickness grafts. *Thin split-thickness grafts,* which have only a very thin layer of dermis, are of limited use because they contract easily, often become shiny and discolored, and have poor wearing qualities. They may be used to replace mucous membranes in reconstructive surgery of such areas as the mouth and vagina or to cover large burned areas to reduce the loss of body fluids. Within a few weeks the grafts can be removed and replaced with intermediate or thick split-thickness grafts.

Intermediate and *thick split-thickness grafts* are widely used. These grafts have a thicker layer of dermis attached to the epidermis than do the thinner grafts. The donor site is able to reepithelialize completely since the deeper layers of the dermis have been left intact. These grafts can be used to cover almost any part of the body. They can be cut into large pieces with a dermatome set to ensure a uniform thickness of the graft, and these can then be cut into smaller pieces to correspond to the size of the area to be grafted.

Meshed grafts are either thin or intermediate split-

thickness grafts that have been placed through a perforation machine that creates a mesh. Meshed grafts are elastic and can be used to cover areas larger than the original size. They also conform more easily to irregular surfaces and can be placed over less clean bases than regular split-thickness grafts. Cosmetic appearance is poor. Meshed grafts may be used to cover large burned skin areas (see Chapter 74).

Full-thickness grafts. Full-thickness grafts are used primarily to cover small areas where matching skin color and texture is important such as on the face. Only a moderate-sized piece of full-thickness skin can survive as a free graft because the blood supply cannot become established quickly enough to provide essential nutrition. For nourishment these grafts depend entirely on existing lymph until their own blood supply can be established in about 2 weeks. The donor site is usually sutured with resulting scar formation, thus limiting the number of donor sites.

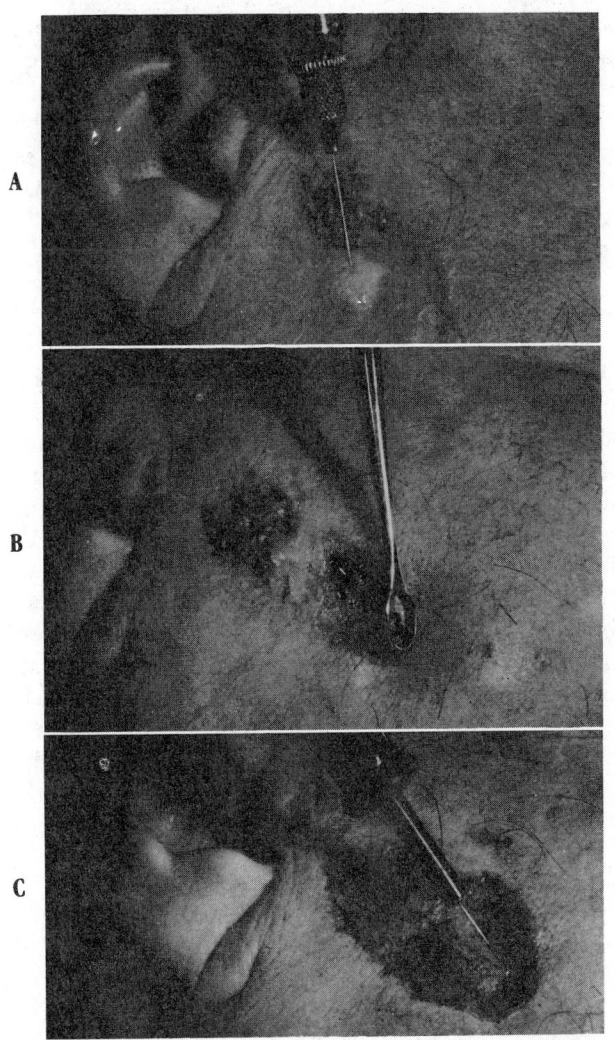

FIGURE 73-1 A, Infiltration with local anesthetic. **B,** Curettage. **C,** Electrodesiccation for hemostasis. (From Stewart WD, Danto JL, and Maddin S: Dermatology: diagnosis and treatment of cutaneous disorders, ed 4, St Louis, 1978, The CV Mosby Co.)

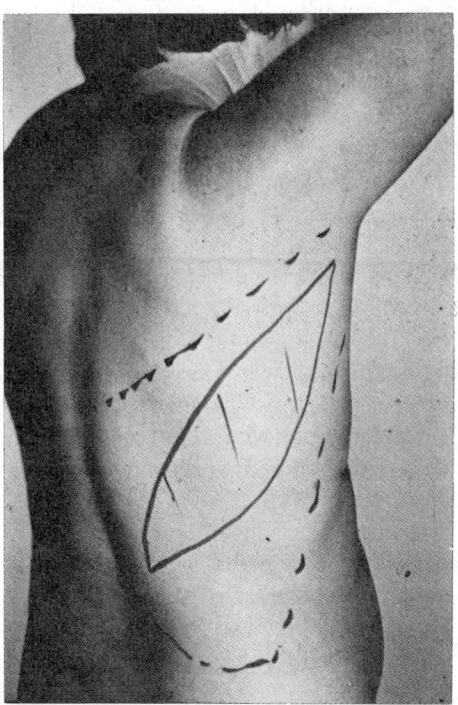

FIGURE 73-2 Free latissimus flap. Flap has been outlined on patient before removal. (From Gruendeman BJ and Meeker MH: Alexander's care of the patient in surgery, ed 8, St Louis, 1987, The CV Mosby Co.)

Island flaps are narrow strips of neurovascular tissue from which the skin has been removed. The flap is transferred to a distant site through a tunnel made *under* the skin. The only scars that remain are at the donor and recipient sites.

Tube pedicle grafts are formed by suturing the long sides of the graft together to form a tube and then suturing the end to another area of the body. After the graft has taken, the original site is freed and the graft is sutured to the recipient site. Pedicle grafts are used less frequently since the advent of microsurgery.

Flap Grafts

Flap grafts are not moved entirely to another area but always have one end left attached to the primary site to provide vascularization. Flap grafts are used to cover larger defects than can be covered by free grafts.

There are several types of flap grafts. *Transposed flaps* are rectangular sections of tissue moved from a site adjacent to the defect. The flap is cut along two long sides and one short side and then slid sideways to cover the defect. If the skin is loose enough, the donor site can be sutured; if it is not loose, a split-thickness free graft is used to cover the donor site. A *rotation flap* is similar to the transposed flap, except that a semicircle of tissue is cut and then rotated over the defect.

Free Flaps

Development of microsurgical techniques has permitted the use of free flaps (see Table 73-4). A flap consisting of skin, muscle, and a major blood vessel is dissected from the donor site (Figure 73-2). At the recipient site, the blood vessel is reattached to a recipient vessel, and blood flow is immediately reestablished. Some free flaps contain functional nerves that can be reattached to permit sensation to the recipient site.[40] Candidates for free flap grafts must be able to tolerate a 4- to 12-hour procedure. Poor candidates are those with significant peripheral vascular disease or diabetes mellitus.[27] Patients must refrain from smoking or from exposure to cigarette smoking for 1 week before surgery because of the strong vasoconstrictive effect of nicotine on microcirculation.

PREOPERATIVE SKIN CARE

Graft survival depends in part on a tissue base that has adequate vascularization and on an infection-free environment. Tissue that has had advanced radiation damage or that is infected is a poor base for the graft and must be cleaned or scraped to remove debris or avascular tissue before a graft can be attempted. Open wounds are treated preoperatively with debridement (by mechanical means or by wet-to-dry dressings) to remove dead tissue and foreign materials and to stimulate growth of capillary-rich granulation tissue. If infection is present, it is treated with antibiotics and sterile warm soaks or compresses.

The donor site is cleansed with germicidal soap as prescribed. If necessary, the patient is shaved at the time of surgery to minimize risk of infection.

POSTOPERATIVE SKIN CARE

Recipient Site

In addition to adequate vascularization and freedom of infection, graft survival also requires complete contact between graft and recipient tissue as well as adequate immobilization of the graft.[40] Inadequate contact may result from collection of serous fluid, blood, or lymph; from pus if infection occurs; or from movement of the graft over the tissue. Therefore, postoperative care is based on the following principles:

1. Prevention of fluid collection under the graft
2. Prevention of infection
3. Prevention of shearing forces that will cause graft movement
4. Promotion of adequate circulation to the part

Fluid collection under the graft can be prevented by pressure dressings. Bandages may be applied for pressure over selected areas, such as the extremities, forehead, or scalp. Elastic bandages are often used. Continuous pressure is necessary to keep the graft adherent, but pressure should not be so firm as to cause death to the graft. Graft dressings are described in the box on p. 2149. In areas where bandages cannot be used such as the face or neck, a *stent* dressing (Figure 73-3) may be used. The ends of long-fixation sutures are used to tie the dressing in place. Dressings may be left undisturbed for 5 to 10 days if all conditions for healing have been met; if not, the dressings are changed every day for in-

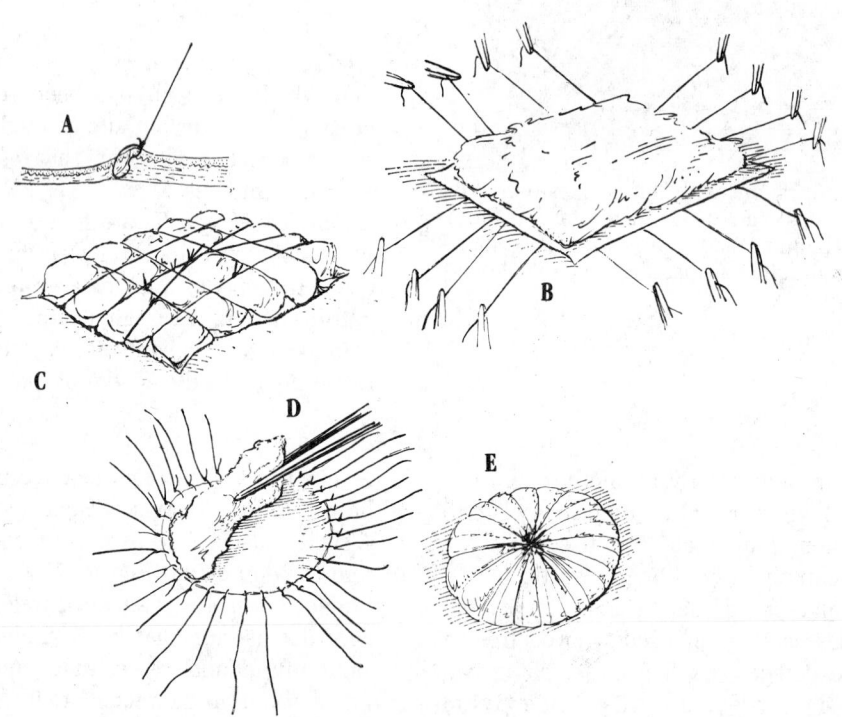

FIGURE 73-3 Stent dressing. **A,** Method of fixation of skin graft to edges of wound. **B,** Nonadherent dressing is applied over skin graft and covered with a fiber pad. **C,** Long sutures are tied over pad. **D** and **E,** A similar dressing may be placed over a circular graft. (From Wood-Smith D and Porowski PC: Nursing care of the plastic surgery patient, St Louis, 1967, The CV Mosby Co.)

GRAFT DRESSINGS

1. Single layer of fine-mesh gauze applied directly over graft
2. Several thicknesses of flat dressings
3. Layer of fluffy dry dressings
4. Pressure bandage

---

spection of the graft. If fluid collects under the graft, it is removed by needle aspiration or by rolling the fluid to the wound edge with a sterile applicator.

Infection is prevented by meticulous aseptic technique when changing dressings or when applying any prescribed moist dressings. If slight infection is present, the physician may prefer to leave the graft site open.[40]

Any movement of the graft over the recipient bed will interfere with reestablishment of vascularization. The edges of the graft are sutured to the tissue, but the surface of the graft can slide with any shearing force. Application of pressure dressings helps to maintain immobilization of the graft. The patient is instructed not to lie on the graft. Bed cradles are used for grafts on the body and lower extremities to prevent shearing forces by bed linens.

Because vascularization of the graft is of utmost importance for graft survival, any activities that promote increased circulation to the part are encouraged. Extremities with grafts are elevated to promote venous return. Some physicians prescribe warm, moist saline compresses to promote circulation to the graft. The temperature of these compresses should not exceed 40° C (104° F).

Donor Site

An open donor site heals spontaneously by epithelialization. One of two methods of donor site management may be used. In the *open dry* approach, the donor site is covered with a single layer of sterile, fine mesh, plain, or Xeroform gauze and then covered with a dry sterile dressing. After 24 hours, the dry dressing is removed, and the wound (covered by the fine-mesh gauze) is left open and exposed to the air. A heat lamp or blow dryer can be used to hasten healing.[40] As the donor site heals, the edges of the fine-mesh gauze are trimmed as they loosen until the gauze falls off.

In the *closed moist* approach, a membrane that is permeable to oxygen but not to fluids is applied over the donor site. Op-Site may be used, but if the site is large, there may be leakage of fluid under the dressing that increases the risk of infection. Hygroscopic membranes that absorb and retain fluid decrease the chance of infection.[15]

When split-thickness grafts have been used, the donor site (often the anterior surface of the thigh) may be a greater source of discomfort to the patient than the re-

---

NURSING CARE OF PATIENT WITH SKIN GRAFTS

PREOPERATIVE CARE

1. Apply prescribed wet-to-dry dressings or warm compresses, and topical antibiotics to graft site as prescribed
2. Clean donor site as instructed.

POSTOPERATIVE CARE

3. Prevention of fluid collection under graft
   a. Monitor graft for pockets of fluid collection.
   b. Remove fluid by rolling fluid toward graft edge with a sterile applicator.
   c. Apply pressure dressing.
4. Prevention of infection
   a. Wash hands before changing dressing.
   b. Use meticulous aseptic technique for dressings and compresses.
   c. Monitor graft for signs of infection (for example, redness, purulent drainage).
5. Immobilization of graft
   a. Use bed cradle for grafts on extremities or body.
   b. Tell patient not to lie on graft
   c. Avoid any dragging movements across graft.
6. Promotion of circulation to graft
   a. Elevate graft site, when possible.
   b. Apply any prescribed warm compresses.

POSTOPERATIVE CARE OF DONOR SITE

7. Keep donor site covered for first 24 to 48 hours.
8. Apply heat lamp with caution (denuded skin is sensitive).
9. Use a bed cradle, if appropriate to allow more air circulation.
10. Leave fine-mesh gauze, which is adherent to donor site, in place until it drops off.
11. Trim loose edges of mesh gauze as it loosens with healing.
12. Give analgesics as necessary for discomfort.

PATIENT TEACHING

13. Keep surface of healed graft moistened daily with a skin lotion for 6 to 12 months to prevent drying and cracking.
14. Protect grafted skin from direct sunlight with a sunscreen lotion (no. 15) for at least 6 months.
15. Wear a strong elastic stocking for 4 to 6 months with grafts of the lower extremities.
16. Report changes in the graft (for example, hematoma, fluid collection, contracture) to the physician.

cipient site (especially with the open dry approach method). Less discomfort is experienced when the wound is covered with a gas-permeable membrane. Analgesics may be necessary during the first postoperative days. Care of the person with a graft is summarized in the box on p. 2151.

Postoperative Care After Microvascular Surgery (Free Flaps)

The first 2 days are the most critical for free flap survival; therefore, to ensure continuous monitoring of the flap, the patient is commonly cared for in a critical care unit for 48 hours. The major complication is necrosis of the transposed tissue, resulting from decreased circulation from arterial or venous thrombosis at the flap site. *Arterial* thrombosis may result in complete flap failure within 4 hours after onset; it is characterized by pallor or coolness of the flap, and no bleeding when the flap is stuck with a needle.[38] *Venous* thrombosis is less critical and occurs more slowly. It is characterized by a warm, mottled flap that oozes dark blood (from continued arterial blood flow); arterial occlusion will eventually occur.[38]

Circulation of the flap may be monitored by a *laser Doppler* that measures the average blood flow from a probe at the flap site. If the postoperative reading falls below 50% of the preoperative baseline reading, the surgeon is notified.[17] A second more precise method of monitoring blood flow is with a photoplethysmographic (PPG) disk. The disk is applied to the flap surface and measures reflected light from pulsatile changes in tissue blood flow.[38] Changes are reflected in waveforms on a monitor. Arterial ischemia is identified by erratic waveforms of decreased height; arterial occlusion is by a straight line. Venous occlusion is identified by a blunted waveform with increased duration of wave time.[38] Flaps can be saved by early detection of compromised circulation.

If the legs are not involved in the surgery, ambulation is started after 24 hours. Involved extremities are elevated to prevent venous engorgement. The patient is given nothing by mouth for 48 hours is case further surgery for flap ischemia is necessary.

SOFT TISSUE EXPANSION

Skin is elastic and expands when stretched over a period of time (such as occurs naturally during pregnancy). This characteristic of skin is used to make new skin for grafts. When the skin can be stretched in areas close to the desired graft site, the skin color match is close. Soft tissue expansion can also be used in breast reconstruction after mastectomy to make a pocket into which an implant can be placed.

The tissue expander is a sac containing saline or a combination of saline and silicone gel, and is attached to a port for filling. Both the port and expander are inserted subcutaneously under local anesthesia. Saline is then injected through the port at weekly intervals and the sac expands like a balloon, stretching the tissue above it. The procedure is performed on an out-patient basis and some patients can be taught to do the weekly saline injection.[37]

When the desired skin size is reached, the old incision is opened and the expander and port removed. The extra loose skin can then be used as a flap skin graft or in reconstruction of a body part, such as nose or ear. Many parts of the body can be used as expansion sites. During the expansion period, the patient must cope with the temporary body change that the "ballooning" expansion produces. The scalp can be covered with scarfs or hats, the neck with scarves, the upper body with large sweatshirts or bulky sweaters, and the lower body with loose pants. Patients are encouraged to live as normal a life as possible during the expansion period.

IMPLANTS

In plastic surgery, in addition to the patient's own tissues, the surgeon may use inert materials and tissues from other human beings. Inert substances must meet several criteria. They must not be irritating or contribute to the development of cancer, they should be of an appropriate consistency for their intended use, and they should not deteriorate or change their shape and form with time. A large variety of substances have been used in the past, including wax, metal, ivory, and bone that has been rendered inert by boiling. In recent years materials such as Teflon and silicone have been used extensively, since they appear to be nonirritating and they retain their form indefinitely.

For many years reconstructive procedures have been attempted in which the tissues of other human beings are transplanted. Whenever these tissues are used, however, there is the potential for rejection of the tissue because of the body's immune response (see Chapter 76). The least difficulty is encountered with tissues such as the cornea of the eye that have a very limited blood supply.

Z-PLASTY FOR SCAR REMOVAL

Plastic surgeons make excellent use of the natural elastic quality of normal skin. Operations such as *Z-plasty* are often performed. Scar tissue can often be removed, and the Z-shaped incision enables the surgeon to undermine adjacent skin, draw the edges together, and cover the defect without using skin from another part of the body (Figure 73-4). The procedure is naturally limited by the size of the scar and its location, since elasticity of skin varies in different parts of the body. The Z-plasty is suitable for such locations as the axilla, the inner aspects of the elbow, and the neck and throat. It is not as

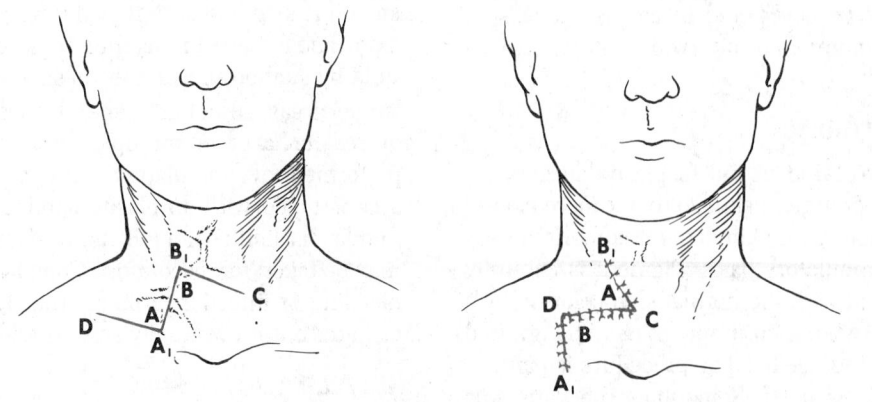

FIGURE 73-4 By means of Z-plasty operations, scar tissue can be removed and defects can be covered without need to transplant skin.

useful for treating defects on the back or on the palmar surfaces of the hand because the skin in these areas cannot be undermined and stretched.

REMOVAL OF SKIN MARKINGS
DERMABRASION

Pockmarks, scars from acne, and certain other disfiguring marks may be removed from the skin by abrasive action. The variable results depend on the type and extent of the condition and the age of the patient (Figure 73-5). The surgeon counsels the patient preoperatively about the degree of improvement so that expectations are realistic. The patient is also informed about postoperative swelling, discomfort, crusting, and erythema,

which may persist for several weeks. The procedure is performed under local or general anesthesia depending on the size of the area to be treated, the individual patient, and the preference of the surgeon. It is usually performed as ambulatory surgery. Contraindications to dermabrasion include deep skin defects and a history of keloid formation.

If the procedure has not been extensive and oozing is slight, the area may be left uncovered. Usually it is covered with an ointment or by compresses moistened with an antiseptic solution and then by a pressure dressing that covers the entire face except for the eyes, nose, and mouth. Prepared dressings that adhere less readily to the skin surface such as Telfa dressings are also used.

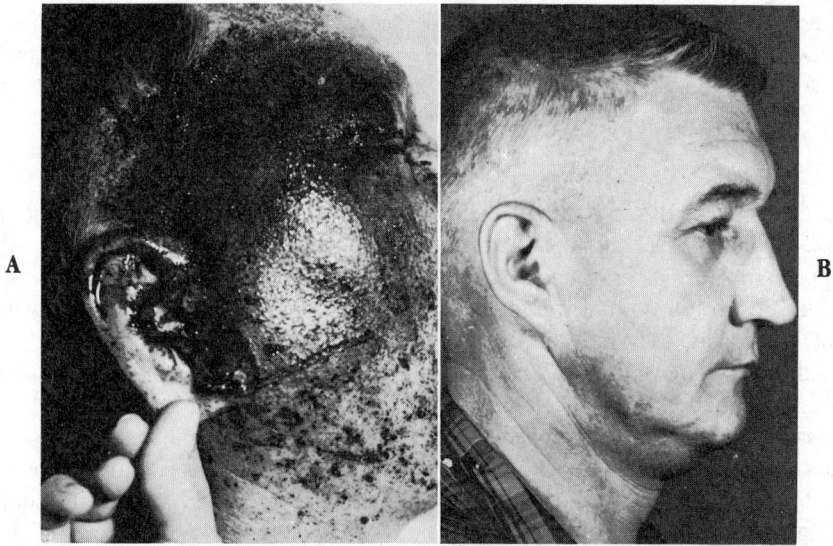

FIGURE 73-5 A, Meticulous cleansing and dermabrasion were required to remove impregnated bits of galvanized metal. **B,** Postoperative view of patient 17 years after dermabrasion. (From Saunders WH et al: Nursing care in eye, ear, nose and throat disorders, ed 4 St Louis, 1979, The CV Mosby Co.)

Dermabrasion may be completed in stages. At least 2 weeks and often longer may intervene between treatments.

MEDICAL DERMATATTOOING

Tattooing has been found useful in plastic surgery for changing the color of grafted skin so that it more closely resembles the surrounding skin. This treatment is usually given on an ambulatory basis. Pigment is carefully selected and blended with the normal skin coloring by a skilled technician who then impregnates the grafted skin, using a tattooing needle. The procedure is painful, since no anesthetic is used. Sometimes the patient is given a sedative or is instructed to take such medications approximately 1 hour before coming to the clinic or the physician's office. There may be a slight serous oozing from the skin after the treatment, and it should be left to dry and crust. Sometimes a piece of sterile gauze can be placed over the tattooed area, and an ice bag may be applied if severe discomfort follows the treatment.

Tattooing is usually done in several stages. The amount done at one time depends on individual circumstances such as the location of the part treated and the emotional reactions of the patient. For example, treatment of the skin close to the eye is often quite painful and is extremely trying for the patient. Therefore, usually only a small amount is tattooed at one time. Grafted skin may change in color with time, so tattooing to change the color of grafted skin may have to be repeated.

Port-wine stains too large to treat by excision and grafting have also responded to this method of treatment with excellent results. Treatments are carried out at 4-week intervals until the final results are achieved. This is a tedious procedure if the stain is large and dark, but finally, in some cases the stain is barely apparent to the casual observer.

FAT REMOVAL

Some persons develop excess fatty tissue in areas such as the abdomen, hips ("saddle bags"), thighs (trochanteric lipodystrophy), upper arms, or posterior neck ("buffalo hump"). If these persons are of normal weight but have selected areas of excess fat, they may be candidates for surgical procedures to remove the fat. The procedures are *not* for weight reduction.

Traditionally, surgery has consisted of procedures such as *abdominoplasty* (that is, dissection of excess skin and fat from the abdomen). Hospitalization for several days and general anesthesia are usually required. Complications include fluid collection under the flap, infection, and wide scars.[40]

A newer approach to fat removal is *liposuction*. A long hollow blunt-tipped cannula is inserted through a small incision and is tunneled through the fat under the skin. The loosened fat is then removed through the cannula by suction. Local anesthesia can be used for small single areas, although general anesthesia may be required for large or multiple areas. Liposuction can be performed by ambulatory surgery. After surgery the area is taped with an elastic bandage for 1 to 2 weeks. Activity is limited for 48 hours. Nonaspirin analgesics may be taken for discomfort. Complications may include bleeding or infection. Initially the skin may be dimpled or hard, but it eventually softens and smooths out.[4]

RECONSTRUCTIVE SURGERY

Reconstructive surgery is carried out to correct congenital defects, to repair tissues destroyed by trauma or disease, or to replace tissue removed by other surgeries.

MAXILLOFACIAL SURGERY

Maxillofacial reconstructive surgery is usually performed after radical surgery for malignancies of the head and neck; it may also be performed to correct facial deformities. The surgeon works closely with the dental surgeon and the otolaryngologist. Care of the person experiencing head and neck surgery is described in Chapter 32. Free skin flap grafts (p. 2147) may be used to cover areas of removed tissue.

When damage has been so great that reconstruction with living tissue is impossible, it is sometimes possible to construct prosthetic parts of the face that are similar to natural color and contour, although not a perfect restoration of the original appearance. Different types of materials such as hard rubber, methyl methacrylate, or silicone rubber may be used for prostheses. Silicone rubber is favored because of its lifelike texture, translucency, and skin color.[21] More than one prosthesis may be made to correspond to changes in the person's skin at different times (e.g., under day and night light or at different seasons).

Hutton[21] and Hutton describe the care of a facial prosthesis as follows:

1. Remove prosthesis at night (grasp one edge and pull loose).
2. Clean prosthesis daily: use brush, scrub with detergent and rinse in lukewarm water (never hot water).
3. Clean skin under prosthesis: wash with mild soap, rinse and pat dry.
4. Clean surgical defect: rinse with saline solution (½ teaspoon salt in 1 cup warm water) using a rubber-tipped syringe to squirt solution into defect.
5. Reapply prosthesis in morning.
   a. Apply prosthesis in front of mirror for correct placement.
   b. Wipe skin area with alcohol.

c. Apply thin layer of adhesive to outer rim of prosthesis.

d. Position prosthesis and press edge firmly in place.

e. Check security of prosthesis by tugging gently.

6. Carry extra adhesive and alcohol pledgets. (Perspiration, oil, dirt, and extreme temperature changes can loosen prosthesis.)

RHINOPLASTY

Reconstructive surgery of the nose can be accomplished either to correct an anatomic problem (see Chapter 32) or for cosmetic reasons. Bone and cartilage may be removed from the nose if it is irregular, or they may be inserted if a defect such as a saddle nose is being corrected (Figure 73-6). A local anesthetic is usually used for these procedures. The incision is usually made at the end of the nose inside the nostril so that it is not conspicuous. A nasal splint made of plaster, tongue blades, or crinoline may be used for protection. There will be ecchymosis and swelling around the eyes and nose for 10 to 14 days after surgery. Ice compresses and an ice bag may be used to hasten fluid reabsorption. The patient must anticipate waiting several weeks before evaluating the final result of the surgery.

OTOPLASTY AND BLEPHAROPLASTY

Otoplasty is a common operation, usually for purely cosmetic reasons, in which some of the cartilage from the ears is removed to flatten them against the head. This

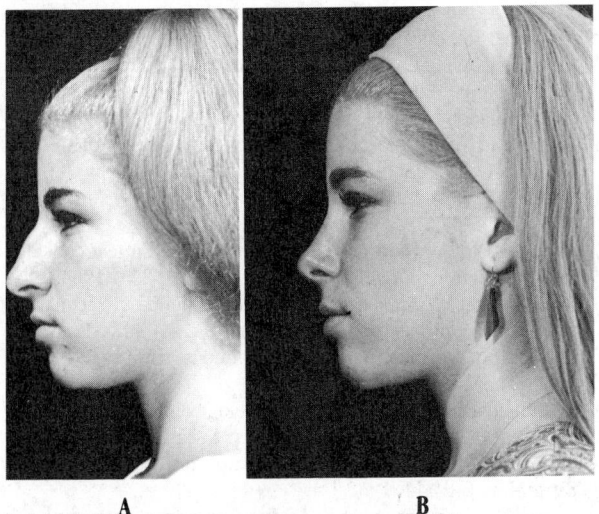

FIGURE 73-6 A, Preoperative appearance of 16-year-old girl. **B,** Postoperative appearance 1 year after rhinoplasty. (From Peck GC: Surgery of the nasal tip. In Masters FW and Lewis JR Jr, editors: Symposium on aesthetic surgery of the nose, ears, and chin, vol 6, St Louis, 1973, The CV Mosby Co.)

procedure is relative simple and requires only a short hospitalization.

Excess skin often develops in the upper and lower eyelids in older persons, sometimes interfering with vision. Appearance is altered by large folds of loose skin hanging on the upper cheeks. *Blepharoplasty* is the removal of the redundant skin. Under local anesthesia, incisions are made in the creases of the upper and lower lids and the excess skin removed. Steri-strips may be used to hold the tissue in place until healing is complete in 4 to 6 weeks. Swelling and ecchymosis usually subsides in 7 to 10 days. Ice compresses are applied to relieve swelling and to prevent further ecchymosis. There is minimum discomfort.

RHYTIDOPLASTY

"Face-lifting" is also performed primarily for cosmetic reasons. An incision is made at the hairline, and excess skin is separated from its underlying tissue and removed. The remaining skin is pulled up and sutured at the hairline, thus removing wrinkles and giving firmness and smoothness to the face. Liposuction may be performed to correct a double chin. A gentle pressure dressing is applied and left in place for 24 to 48 hours. The patient is often discharged at this time, and sutures are removed later in the surgeon's office. The patient frequently needs medication for pain in the postoperative period because of the extent to which the tissue has been undermined. The surgery may be repeated at a later date.

MAMMOPLASTY

Mammoplasty, or reconstructive breast surgery, may be performed to replace breast tissue removed by surgery (see Chapter 57) or to improve the appearance of a woman's breasts. Some women develop conspicuously large and pendulous breasts that they wish to have reduced in size. Large breasts are embarrassing to some women and make it difficult for them to participate in sports, maintain good posture, and buy clothes that fit. Such women often respond to reconstructive surgery remarkably well. Cosmetic surgery of the breast may also make unusually small breasts larger. A variety of plastic materials may be used for this procedure.

CHAPTER SUMMARY

✔ Some dermatologic disorders may be prevented by removal of known causative agents, protecting the skin against ultraviolet rays, keeping the skin clean and hydrated, eating a balanced diet, monitoring for early signs of skin changes, and seeking medical help when skin conditions develop.

✔ Skin lesions can create changes in body image when lesions are obviously visible to others. Social interactions may be altered when there is considerable disfigurement.

🗸 Pruritus leads to skin excoriation from scratching; it may be relieved by cold applications, hydration in a tepid oatmeal bath followed by application of emollient lotion, and maintaining room temperature at a moderate temperature with increased humidity.

🗸 Medications used for therapeutic baths or soaks include colloids, potassium permanganate, Burow's solution, sulfur, tar preparations, and oils. These baths or soaks are given for antipruritic, antifungal, antibacterial, and moisturizing or drying effects.

🗸 The most commonly used topical medications are topical corticosteroids; the various types vary in potency. Occlusion over the corticosteroid increases absorption and should be used only by prescription. Topical antibiotic and antifungal medications may also be prescribed.

🗸 Vehicles for topical medications include powders, lotions, creams, ointments, and pastes.

🗸 Wet dressings are used frequently over skin lesions for cooling, drying, antipruritic, or vasoconstricting effects; tap water or physiologic saline are most commonly used. The best effects are obtained by several treatment periods spaced across the person's waking hours.

🗸 Types of dermatologic surgeries for superficial lesions include tangential surgery, curettage, cryosurgery, and electrosurgery. Deep lesions are removed by punch biopsy or by excision. Hemostasis is generally accomplished by gelatin foam, pressure, a chemical styptic, or electrocoagulation. The patient is taught not to remove the crust until it falls off naturally.

🗸 The purposes of plastic surgery are to restore function, prevent further loss of function, and for cosmetic improvement. Types of plastic surgery include grafting, skin expansion, implants, Z-plasty for scar removal, dermabrasion and medical dermatattooing for removal of skin markings, and fat removal.

🗸 Most skin grafting uses autografts. Free grafts are tissue that is moved from one locations to another; these may be split thickness (thin, intermediate, or thick) or full thickness. Flap grafts are tissue that are partially dissected and slid over to an adjoining area, leaving part of the circulation intact until the graft "takes." Free flaps use microsurgery to remove a flap of tissue with a major blood vessel to another site and reattaching the vessel to provide circulation.

🗸 Care of a patient with a free or flap graft includes prevention of fluid collection under the graft, prevention of infection, immobilization of the graft, and promotion of circulation to the graft. Care of the do-

nor site by the open method includes applying heat and leaving the mesh gauze covering intact until it drops off.

🗸 Care of a patient with a free flap graft by microsurgery includes monitoring for signs of arterial or venous thrombosis at the graft site; a laser Doppler or PPG disk is often used for monitoring.

🗸 Fat removal may be accomplished by abdominoplasty or by liposuction.

🗸 Examples of reconstructive surgery include maxillofacial surgery, rhinoplasty, otoplasty, blepharoplasty, rhytidoplasty, and mammoplasty. Ecchymosis and swelling usually accompany surgery of the face, especially near the eyes and nose for about 1 to 2 weeks. Ice compresses can hasten fluid reabsorption.

QUESTIONS TO CONSIDER

■ What do you think your feelings about yourself might be if you had unsightly lesions over your face and arms, or if you were having soft tissue expansion of the scalp? What could you do to minimize the body changes?

■ What types of preparations are available in your nearest drugstore for relief of itching or for soaks or baths?

REFERENCES AND SELECTED READINGS

1. *Acres C and Kraft ER: Skin transplantation, Am J Nurs 81:1466-1467, 1981.
2. American College of Surgeons Committee on Pre and Postoperative Care: Manual of preoperative and postoperative care, ed 3, Philadelphia, 1983, WB Saunders Co.
3. *Anders JE and Leach EE: Sun versus skin, Am J Nurs 83:1015-1020, 1983.
4. *Baj PA: Liposuction: new wave plastic surgery, Am J Nurs 84:1488-1490, 1984.
5. Barratt GE et al: Skin grafts: physiology and clinical considerations, Otolaryngol Clin North Am 17(2):335-351, 1984.
6. Belfer ML et al: Appearance and the influence of reconstructive surgery on body image, Clin Plast Surg 9:307-315, 1982.
7. Bennett RG: Fundamentals of cutaneous surgery, St Louis, 1988, The CV Mosby Co.
8. Berscheid E et al: The social psychological implications of facial physical attractiveness, Clin Plast Surg 9:289-296, 1982.
9. *Chouinard F: Be a skeptic while caring for postop flaps, Plast Surg Nurs 3(2):44, 1983.
10. *Cohen BE and Aaronson S: Microvascular reconstructive surgery: free tissue transfer, AORN J 38:602-629, 1983.
11. *Cohen L: Free-flap surgery: nurses make it work, RN 51(3):26-29, 1988.

*References preceded by an asterisk are particularly well suited for student reading.

12. *Conlee D: Put a new face on your care of cosmetic surgery patients, Nursing '81 11(11):90-95, 1981.
13. Davis EA Jr: The use of skin and muscle transplants in reconstructive surgery, Crit Care Update 9:34-41, 1982.
14. Dolsky RI, Newman J, and Fetzek JR: Liposuction: history, techniques, and complications, Dermatol Clin 5:313-334, 1987.
15. Epstein E: Common skin disorders, ed 3, Oradell, NJ, 1988, Medical Economics Books.
16. Ganong WF: Review of medical physiology, ed 13, Norwalk, CT, 1988, Appleton & Lange.
17. *Goodman T and White S: Microvascular reconstruction: nursing management, AORN J 48:666-676, 1988.
18. *Goodman T: Grafts and flaps in plastic surgery, AORN J 48:650-663, 1988.
19. Groseman JA: The complications of beautification: aesthetic surgery, Emerg Med 15(4):28-38, 1983.
20. Gruendeman BJ and Meeker MH: Alexander's care of the patient in surgery, ed 8, St Louis, 1987, The CV Mosby Co.
21. *Hutton B and Hutton J: Living with a facial prosthesis, Am J Nurs 84:50-52, 1984.
22. Idson B: Vehicle effects in percutaneous absorption, Drug Metab Rev 14:207-222, 1983.
23. Kotler R: Cosmetic facial surgery, JAMA 249:523-535, 1983.
24. Manders EK et al: Soft tissue expansion for reconstruction in the head and neck. In Stark RB, editor: Plastic surgery of the head and neck, New York, 1986, Churchill Livingstone Inc.
25. *Markland A: Nursing care of the suction lipectomy patient, Plast Surg Nurs 4(2):44-46, 1984.
26. Moschella SL and Hurley HJ: Dermatology, ed 2, New York, 1985, McGraw-Hill Book Co.
27. Nahai F, and Jurkiewicz MJ: Microsurgery replantation and free flaps, Adv Surg 17:73-98, 1984.
28. Pathak MA: Sunscreens: topical and systemic approaches for prevention of acute and chronic sun-induced skin reactions, Dermatol Clin 4:321-334, 1986.
29. Pillsbury DM and Heaton CL: A manual of dermatology, ed 2, Philadelphia, 1980, WB Saunders Co.
30. *Roy DJ: Caring for the self-esteem of the cosmetic patient, Plast Surg Nurs 6:138-141, 1986.
31. Sauer DB: Manual of skin diseases, ed 5, Philadelphia, 1987, JB Lippincott Co.
32. *Schaal PG and Slemenda MB: Nurses' response to transplants, AORN J 30:42-45, 1984.
33. Schroeder SA et al: Current medical diagnosis and treatment, Norwalk, Conn, 1989, Appleton & Lange.
34. *Seaton C et al: Suction lipolysis: a personal perspective, Plast Surg Nurs 4(2):47-49, 1984.
35. Sherertz EF et al: Rational use of topical corticosteroids, Am Fam Physician 29:262-266, 1984.
36. Stegmen SJ et al: Cosmetic dermatologic surgery, Arch Dermatol 118:1013-1016, 1982.
37. *Strohecker BA et al: Soft tissue expansion, Am J Nurs 88:668-671, 1988.
38. *Swain D and Shell DH: Microvascular tissue transfer: perioperative nursing considerations, AORN J 49:1032-1043, 1989.
39. Twee AE et al: Facial contour reconstruction with free flaps, Ann Plast Surg 12(4):313-320, 1984.
40. Way LW: Current surgical diagnoses and treatment, ed 8, Norwalk, Conn, 1988, Appleton & Lange.
41. Wyngaarden JB and Smith LH: Cecil textbook of medicine, ed 18, Philadelphia, 1988, WB Saunders Co.

CHAPTER 74

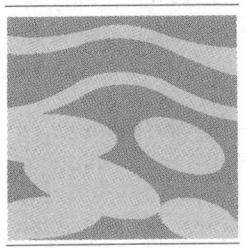

Management of Persons with Burns

DEBORAH GOLDENBERG KLEIN

CHAPTER OBJECTIVES

After studying this chapter, the student should be able to:
1   Differentiate between partial-thickness and full-thickness burns.
2   Describe the pathophysiologic changes that occur during the three stages following major burns.
3   Describe the emergency care for major burns and the initial inpatient therapy.
4   Describe interventions for replacing body fluids, preventing infection, promoting nutrition and mobility, and providing emotional support.
5   Identify teaching needs of the patient with burns.

EPIDEMIOLOGY AND ETIOLOGY

Burn injuries are in many respects the worst of all tragedies an individual can experience. An intensive burn is accompanied by an overwhelming insult to the patient physically and psychologically, and it is catastrophic in cost and suffering to the family involved.

It has been estimated that one percent of the population of the United States (over 2 million people) is burned or scalded each year. Of these victims, 500,000 seek medical attention, and 6,000 die as a direct result of the burn injury. Burns are caused by dry or moist heat, chemical exposure, electrical currents, and radiation. The most common cause of burns is fire, resulting in an estimated 12,000 deaths, 310,000 injuries, and 13.6 billion dollars in property losses. Because of the systemic effects of the burn injury, psychologic implications, and prolonged hospitalization, comprehensive nursing care is required during the acute and long-term recovery phases.

PREVENTION

Nurses can help prevent accidental burns by participating in health education programs that stress fire prevention and the consequences of fires such as burns, deformities, and death. Nurses can promote legislation that would control hazardous practices and make working and living environments safer. Community health nurses are in an unusually advantageous position to recognize unsafe practices in the home and to help families develop safe habits of living.

Approximately 80% of accidental burns occur in the home and primarily are caused by ignorance, carelessness, and curiosity of *children*. Infants and children are the most common victims of fires in and about the home. A large number of children have been burned to death or permanently disabled or disfigured by fireworks. Legislation in many states now prohibits the sale of fireworks, but violations of the law and accidents still occur. Approximately 1000 serious burns occur every year from fireworks.

A high incidence of burn injuries affecting *adults* occur when the person is distracted while cooking or falls asleep while smoking. Typical activities in which persons were engaged when they caught on fire in their homes are shown in Table 74-1.

Each year brings increased demand for careful in-

TABLE 74-1 Activities of persons burned by fire

Activity	Number	Percent*
Playing with matches/lighter	175	11.3
Smoking	152	10.0
Using matches/lighter	116	7.5
Falling asleep while smoking	100	6.4
Reaching across stove	86	5.5
Sleeping	77	5.0
Standing too close to stove	64	4.1
Leaning against stove	47	3.0

From Flammable fabric investigations, Department of Health, Education, and Welfare, Food and Drug Administration, Bureau of Product Safety, FY66-FY72, Washington, DC, 1973.
*Percent based on 1554 cases in which activity is known.

spection and regulation of places in which the *ill* and *infirm* are housed. *Aged* persons frequently are housed in old and poorly equipped structures, and many of them have been victims of fire. Nurses can bring necessary pressures to bear to ensure adequate protection and planned evacuation if a fire occurs. The American Burn Association suggests that all health facilities conduct one mock evacuation drill each year.[4] Attention is being focused on places where large numbers of people congregate. Laws require that doors in public buildings be hinged to swing outward, that draperies and decorations be fireproof, and that stairways with special fire doors be used in new apartment buildings and hotels. Smoke detectors and sprinkler systems are also required in new buildings and residential health care facilities. Nurses working in institutions need to encourage and participate in fire prevention programs.

Rigid enforcement of laws requiring that *industrial* products be labeled when known to be flammable and that new products be tested carefully for their flammable qualities before being placed on the market is further evidence of government efforts to protect the public from accident by fire. Industry can be made safer by constant vigilance of management in cooperation with fire safety officers and health care professionals to iden-

tify hazards and implement a safety program. All chemicals should be labeled, and antidotes should be identified and available. A core of every work force should be versed in emergency treatment of all types of burns for the protection of every employee.

Recent statistics indicate a rise in the number of chemical injuries as a result of "homemade" solutions for cleaning and home remodeling.

Sunburn should be cautioned against, because even a relatively mild burn of a large part of the body can cause change of fluid distribution and kidney damage. Camp nurses should keep this in mind in their educational programs for children and camp counselors. Many sunscreen products are available that are very effective and should be used in times of exposure.

CLASSIFICATION OF BURNS

Traditionally, burns have been classified as *first-*, *second-* or *third-* degree. The terms first-, second- and third-degree are not descriptive of the injury because they are based only on the visual characteristics of the burn wound. The injury of a burn extends beyond what can be seen. A more accurate description is partial- and full-thickness, which graphically describes the burn and

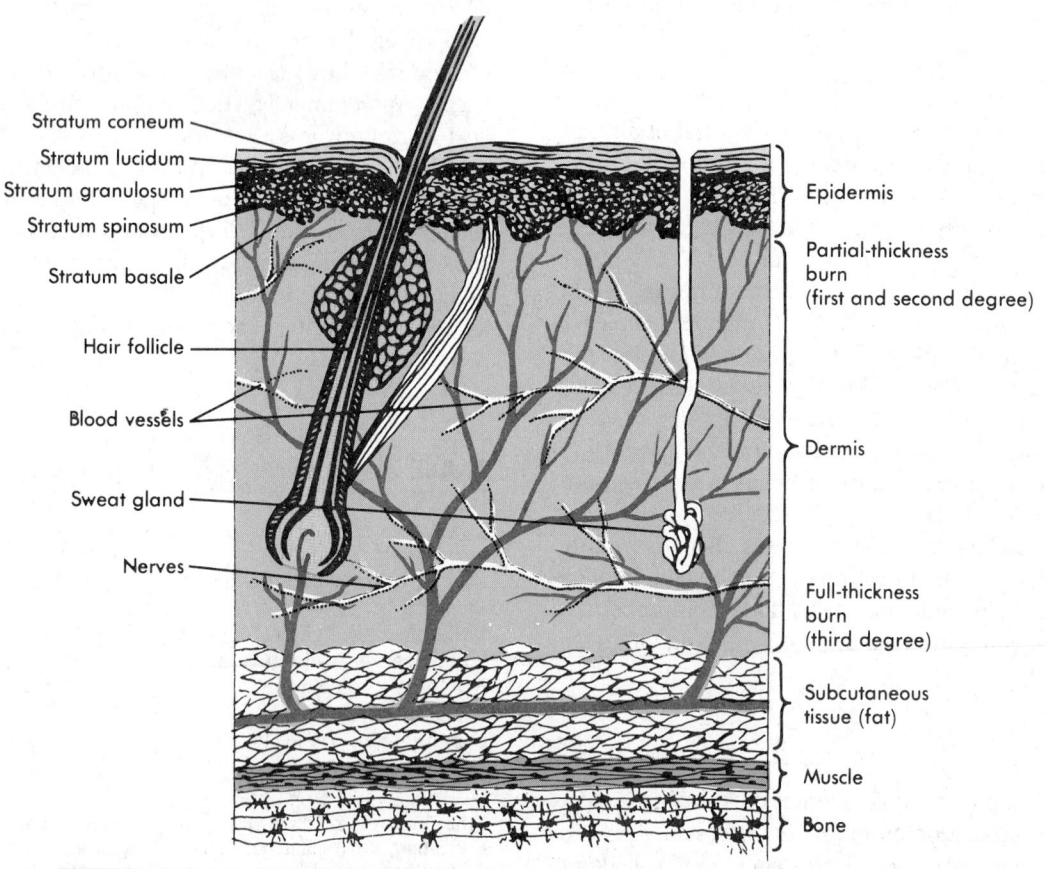

FIGURE 74-1 Levels of human skin involved in burns.

indicates depth and severity of the tissue injury (Figure 74-1).

Partial-thickness burns are characterized by destruction in varying depths from the epidermis (outer layer of skin) to the dermis (middle layer of skin). Partial thickness burns of the skin involve a "part" of the epidermis and dermis. The depth of tissue injury is described further as *superficial* partial-thickness, involving only the epidermis, and *deep* partial-thickness burns, which involve the entire epidermis and part of the dermis. Partial-thickness burns are likely to be painful because nerve endings have been injured and exposed, but they have the ability to heal because a portion of the epithelial cells are not destroyed. During the healing phase, dryness and itching are common and are caused by increased vascularization of sebaceous glands, reduction of secretions, and decreased perspiration.

The presence of blisters often indicates deep partial-thickness injury. They may increase in size as the result of continuous exudation and collection of tissue fluid.

Full-thickness burns include destruction of the epidermis and the entire dermis, as well as possible damage to the subcutaneous layer, muscle, and bone. Nerve endings are destroyed, resulting in a painless wound. *Eschar,* a leathery covering comprised of denatured protein, may form as the result of surface dehydration.

Black networks of coagulated capillaries may be seen. Full-thickness burns require skin grafting because the destroyed tissue is unable to epithelialize. Often a deep partial-thickness burn may convert to a full-thickness burn by infection, trauma, or decreased blood supply.

PATHOPHYSIOLOGY OF SEVERE BURNS

As a result of burns, normal skin function is diminished, resulting in physiologic alterations. These include (1) loss of protective barriers against infection, (2) escape of body fluids, (3) lack of temperature control, (4) destroyed sweat and sebaceous glands, and (5) a diminished number of sensory receptors. The severity of these alterations will depend on the extent of the burn and the depth to which damage has occurred.

Increased knowledge of the physiologic changes that occur during severe burns has led to the saving of lives. There are two stages that occur after severe burns: the immediate hypovolemic stage and the diuretic stage. Figure 74-2 presents an overview of the pathophysiologic changes seen in a severe burn.

HYPOVOLEMIC STAGE

The hypovolemic stage begins at the time of burn injury and lasts for the first 48 to 72 hours. It is characterized

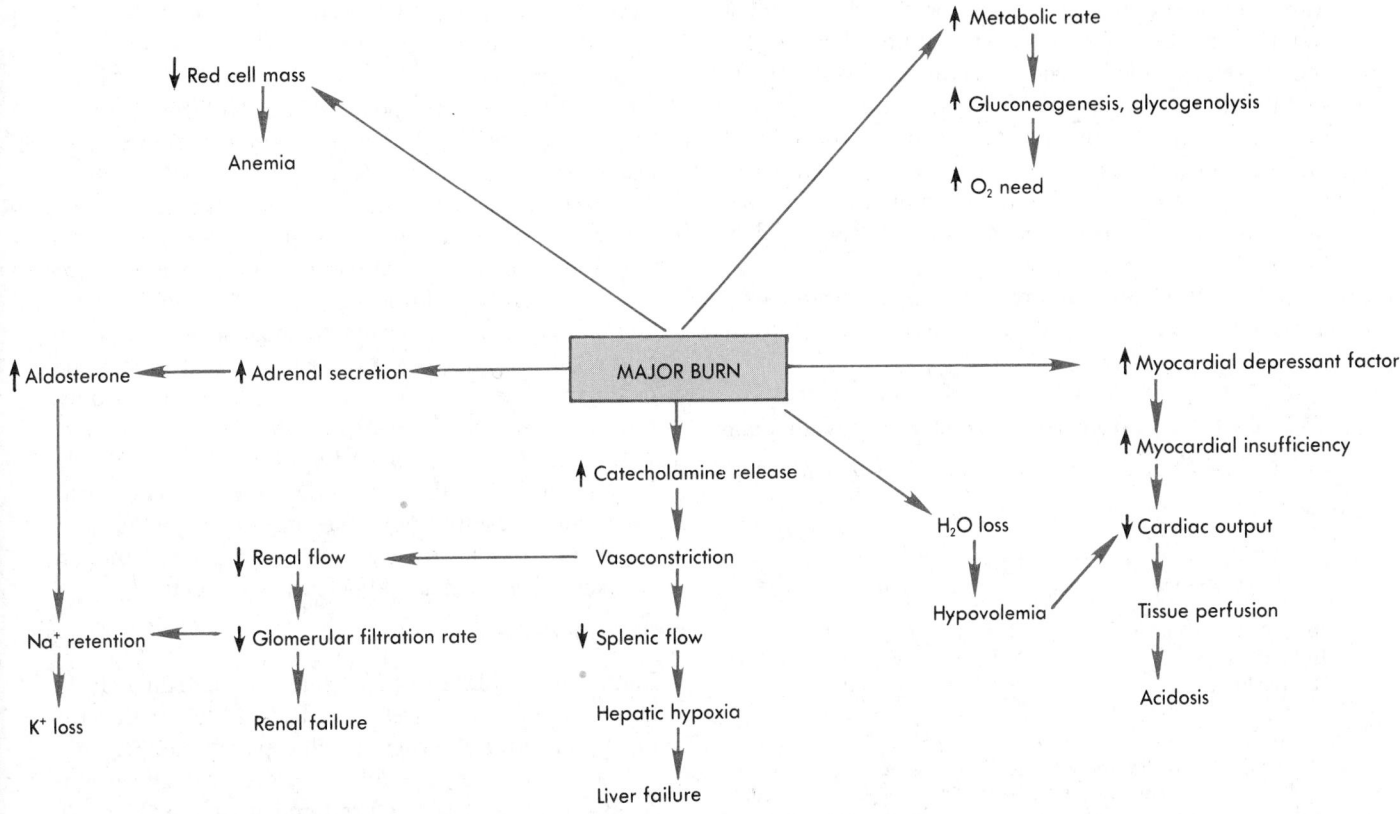

FIGURE 74-2 Overview of pathophysiology of a major burn.

by a rapid *shift of fluid* from the vascular compartments into the interstitial spaces. When tissues are burned, vasodilation, increased capillary permeability, and changes in the permeability of tissue cells in and around the burn area occur. As a result, abnormally large amounts of extracellular fluid (ECF), sodium chloride, and protein pass through the burned area to cause blister formation and local edema or escape through the open wound.

Visible fluid loss makes up only a small part of the fluid lost from the circulating blood and other essential fluid compartments. Most of the fluid loss occurs deep in the wound, where the fluid extravasates into the deeper tissues. Burns occurring in highly vascular areas such as muscle tissue or the face are believed to cause a greater fluid shift than comparable burns of other parts of the body. Fully one half of the ECF of the body can shift from its normal distribution to the site of a severe burn. Patients with large surface area burns experience edema throughout the body that can impair peripheral circulation by compressing the circulatory vessels in the extremity. The ECF constitutes about 20% of the body weight. Three fourths of it surrounds the cells, and one fourth is found in blood plasma (Table 74-2). For a person weighing 68 kg (150 lb), this means that from 4.5 to 6.5 kg or from 5 to 7.5 L of fluids may be removed from the interstitial spaces and bloodstream.

The body can partially compensate for this fluid shift with intense peripheral vasoconstriction for approximately 1 to 2 hours after the burn injury. During this compensatory period, blood pressure may be normal to slightly elevated, pulse rapid (greater than 100 beats/min), and the patient oliguric. As the compensatory mechanisms fail, the classic picture of hypovolemic shock—hypotension, tachycardia, oliguria, acidosis and hypoxia—is seen. These changes are summarized in Figure 74-3.

As a result of these fluid shifts, *dehydration* of nondamaged tissue cells may occur. More fluids and sodium than protein are lost initially from the capillaries. This increases the capillary osmotic pressure, leading to dehydration with pronounced *edema* in the burned area. As protein continues to be lost into the burned area because of the increased capillary permeability, *hypoproteinemia* results. The increased amount of protein in the tissue spaces is a further contributing factor to edema formation. Proteins may be lost through the open wounds. The lymphatic system, which normally functions to remove increased tissue fluid, becomes overloaded and inefficient, contributing to edema formation. Nitrogen is lost through the kidney from catabolism, leading to significant negative nitrogen balance. The BUN is elevated when oliguria is present.

With loss of fluid from the vascular system, *hemoconcentration* occurs, and the hematocrit rises. Blood flow becomes sluggish in the burned area, and cellular nutrition decreases. Large numbers of red blood cells (RBCs) become trapped in the burned area and are hemolyzed. Renal damage and hematuria may occur as a result of reduced blood volume and passage of the end products of the hemolyzed cells through the glomeruli. The decreased renal blood flow leads to *oliguria.*

Electrolyte imbalances also occur. *Hyperkalemia* (elevated serum potassium) results from the release of potassium from damaged tissue cells and red blood cells and from the diminished urinary output. Hyperkalemia may lead to heart block and ventricular failure. Potassium may be encouraged to move back into the cells by the administration of insulin, because potassium is transported back into the cells along with glucose. Sodium is retained by the body as a result of the endocrine response to stress. Aldosterone secretion is increased, leading to increased sodium reabsorption by the kidney. This sodium, however, quickly passes into the interstitial spaces of the burned area with the fluid shift; therefore in spite of the increased amount of sodium in the body, most of the sodium is trapped in the edema fluid, and a *sodium deficit* occurs. Inadequate tissue perfusion results in anaerobic metabolism, and the acid end products are retained because of the decreased kidney function. *Metabolic acidosis* may then occur.

Respiratory distress may result from upper airway obstruction or effects of hypovolemic shock. Upper airway obstruction results from the inhalation of noxious agents or super heated air causing irritation of the airway, laryngeal edema, and potential obstruction.

DIURETIC STAGE

Return of vascular integrity begins at approximately 12 hours and rapidly progresses at 18 to 24 hours after the initial burn injury. Although full capillary integrity may not be restored for a number of days, for clinical purposes it may be considered restored at 24 hours. The diuretic phase begins at about 48 to 72 hours after the

TABLE 74-2 Approximate division of total body fluid into compartments*

Body Fluid Compartments	Liters of Fluid	
	Lean Adult Weighing 45 kg	Lean Adult Weighing 68 kg
Intravascular (plasma)	2.8	4.2
Interstitial	8.4	12.5
Intracellular	22.3	33.3
TOTAL	33.5	50.0

*Note that the smaller the individual, the less fluid he or she has in each compartment and that plasma is reduced most markedly with decrease in size. The normal size and body type of the individual are considered when fluid replacement is ordered.

burn injury as capillary membrane integrity returns and edema fluid shifts back from the interstitial spaces into the intravascular space. Blood volume increases, leading to increased renal blood flow and *diuresis* unless renal damage has occurred. Serum electrolyte and hematocrit levels will be decreased because of the *hemodilution*. *Fluid overload* may occur as a result of the increase in intravascular volume. The patient's vital signs, breath sounds, and urinary output are used to determine the amount of intravenous fluid replacement. Dehydration may occur if rapid urinary fluid losses deplete the intravascular reserve. A *sodium deficit* continues because of the loss of sodium through the burn wound and through the increase in urine output. *Hypokalemia* results from potassium moving back into the cells or being excreted in the urine. Protein continues to be lost from the wounds. *Metabolic acidosis* remains a possibility because of the loss of sodium bicarbonate in the urine and the increased fat metabolism secondary to a decreased carbohydrate intake.

Following the period of fluid shifts, the patient remains acutely ill. This period is characterized by *anemia* and *malnutrition*. Anemia develops from the loss of red blood cells. Negative nitrogen balance begins at the onset of the burn and is the result of tissue destruction, protein loss, and the stress response. It continues throughout the acute period and is secondary to contin-

ued loss of protein from the wound, from tissue catabolism resulting from immobility, and from decreased protein intake. Special attention to the nutritional needs of the patient is an integral part of the comprehensive care during this time. Increased metabolism from loss of water and heat from the wound, loss of fluid during diuresis, and catabolism during tissue breakdown lead to *weight loss*.

Complications of the gastrointestinal system occur frequently after thermal injury. Gastric and duodenal ulceration (Curling's ulcer) has been reported in 66% of severely burned patients, with significant ulceration in nearly 20%. Bleeding is the major clinical problem for patients with these lesions. Treatment is aimed at prevention and is best accomplished by antacids and enteral feedings. Cholecystitis, pancreatitis and hepatic, dysfunction may also be seen as the result of tissue ischemia from hypoperfusion. The differences in changes between the hypovolemic and diuretic stages are summarized in Table 74-3.

MANAGEMENT

Three periods of treatment can be identified in the care of the seriously burned patient. These are the emergent, the acute, and the rehabilitation periods.

The *emergent period* refers to the first 48 or 72 hours

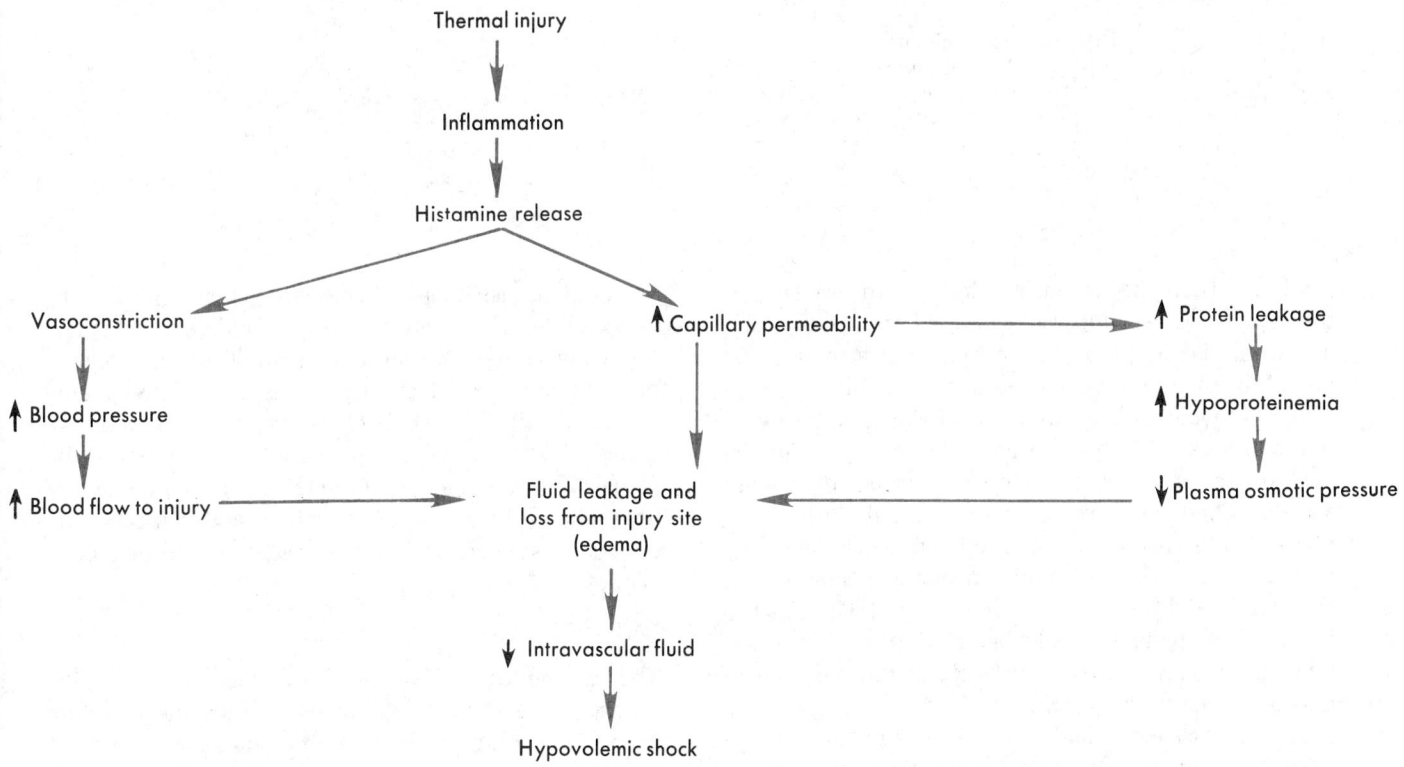

FIGURE 74-3 Flow diagram of fluid shifts resulting in hypovolemic shock.

TABLE 74-3 Physiologic changes with burns

Change	Hypovolemic stage		Diuretic stage	
	Mechanism	Result	Mechanism	Result
Extracellular fluid shift	Vascular to interstitial	Hemoconcentration Edema at burn site	Interstitial to vascular	Hemodilution
Renal function	Decreased renal blood flow from decreased blood pressure and decreased cardiac output	Oliguria	Increased renal blood flow from increased blood volume	Diuresis
Sodium level	Na$^+$ reabsorped by kidneys *but* Na$^+$ lost in exudate and trapped in edema fluid	Sodium deficit	Na$^+$ loss with diuresis (becomes normal in 1 week)	Sodium deficit
Potassium level	K$^+$ released as result of tissue and red blood cell injury; decreased K$^+$ excretion from decreased renal function	Hyperkalemia	K$^+$ moves back into cells; K$^+$ lost by diuresis (begins 4-5 days after the burn)	Hypokalemia
Protein level	Protein lost into tissues by increased capillary permeability	Hypoproteinemia	Loss of protein during continued catabolism	Hypoproteinemia
Nitrogen balance	Tissue catabolism; protein loss in tissues; more nitrogen lost than taken in	Negative nitrogen balance	Tissue catabolism, protein loss, immobility	Negative nitrogen balance
Acid base balance	Anaerobic metabolism from decreased tissue perfusion; increased acid end products; decreased renal function (causing retention of acid end products); loss of serum bicarbonate	Metabolic acidosis	Sodium bicarbonate lost in diuresis; hypermetabolism with increased metabolic end products	Metabolic acidosis
Stress response	Occurs because of trauma	Decreased renal blood flow	Occurs because of prolonged nature of injury and psychologic threat to self	Stress ulcers

postburn when the patient is admitted, the severity of the injury is determined, and first aid and wound care are given. The *acute period* of treatment begins at the end of the emergent period and lasts until all of the full-thickness wounds are covered with skin grafts or partial-thickness wounds are healed. The *rehabilitation period* focuses on returning the patient to a useful place in society. There are two areas of concern during this phase: (1) the restoration of function over joint surfaces that were scarred, and (2) the emotional assistance that the patient and his or her family will need. The rehabilitation of the patient actually begins during early hospitalization and is addressed throughout the hospitalization. After the initial discharge, the patient may require emotional assistance and counseling, and many readmissions may be necessary for reconstructive procedures.

Comprehensive care of the burn patient can best be provided by a *multidisciplinary team approach*. The physician, nurse, pediatric and adult social workers, physical and occupational therapists, teacher, registered dietitian, vocational counselor, and others all work together to address the complex and varied needs of the patient. The nurse's role in the team is to coordinate the interactions of the various disciplines and to incorporate the team's suggestions and approaches into an effective plan of care.

EMERGENT PERIOD

The emergent period of therapy is defined as the time required to resolve the immediate problems resulting from the burn injury. First aid measures are directed to treating the systemic response to trauma, concurrent injuries, and the burn wound (see left box on p. 2163).

INITIAL CARE FOR MAJOR BURNS

1. Remove victim from source of burn.
2. Douse with water and remove nonadherent smoldering clothing.
3. If chemical burn, carefully remove clothing and flush wound with large amounts of water.
4. If electrical burn and victim is still in contact with electrical source, do *not* touch victim. Remove electrical source with dry nonconductive object (rope).
5. Establish patent airway and assess for inhalation injury. Give oxygen if available.
6. Assess and initiate treatment for injuries requiring immediate attention.
7. Remove tight-fitting jewelry or clothing.
8. Cover burn with moist sterile or clean cover.
9. Cover victim with warm dry cover to prevent heat loss.
10. Transport victim to nearest medical facility.

■ ASSESSMENT

Assessment of the person who has sustained a severe burn depends on the severity of the burn injury.

Subjective Data

Knowledge of circumstances surrounding the burn injury is extremely valuable in the management of a burn victim. This information can be obtained from either the burn victim or witnesses to the event. Data should include the following:

1. How the burn injury occurred
2. When the burn injury occurred
3. Duration of contact with the burning agent
4. Location (enclosed area suggests possibility of smoke inhalation and/or carbon monoxide poisoning)
5. Presence of an explosion (suggests possibility of other injuries)

The state of health and age of the burn victim are important factors that may modify treatment. The elderly and very young have a higher mortality rate than a young adult with the same percentage burn. Preexisting endocrine, pulmonary, cardiovascular or renal disease or a history of drug abuse will decrease a victim's ability to cope with severe burns. Because most of these patients will require topical and systemic therapy with a number of drugs, allergies and drug sensitivities must be determined and documented.

Objective Data

Burns may be categorized as major, moderate, or minor on the basis of the size of the burn and the presence of complicating factors (see the box above, right).

CLASSIFICATION OF SEVERITY OF BURNS

MAJOR BURN INJURIES

Greater than 25% body surface area (BSA) (greater than 20% in children under 10 years and adults over 40 years)
Greater than 10% BSA, full-thickness
Involvement of face, eyes, ears, hands, feet, perineum
Electrical burns
Burns complicated by inhalation injury or major trauma
Burns in patients with preexisting disease (diabetes, congestive heart failure, or chronic renal failure)

MODERATE BURN INJURIES

15% to 25% BSA in adults, partial thickness (10% to 20% BSA in children under 10 years and adults over 40 years)
Less than 10% BSA full-thickness
Burns with no concurrent injury
Burns in patients with no preexisting disease

MINOR BURN INJURIES

Less than 15% BSA in adults (10% in children or the elderly)
Less than 2% BSA full-thickness injury
Burns in patients with no preexisting disease

Assessing the severity of the burn injury.

Size and depth of burn. For adults, the "rule of nines" is used in determining the size of the burn. The percentage of body surface area (BSA) burned is estimated with the use of charts that depict anterior and posterior drawings of the body. In adults, the body is divided into areas equal to multiples of 9% (Figure 74-4). In clinical practice, the burned area is shaded in on the drawings, and the amount of body surface burned is calculated from the shaded areas. Calculations are modified for infants and children under 10 years of age because of their relatively larger head and smaller bodies (consult a pediatric textbook for these figures).

The depth of the burn injury is evaluated on the basis of appearance, color, and sensation (Table 74-4).

Age of victim. The severity of a burn also depends on the age of the victim. Infants under 2 years of age and adults over 60 years have a higher mortality rate than persons in other age groups with a similar size injury. The infant has a weak antibody response to infection, and in older victims the serious burn may aggravate the degenerative processes or exacerbate a preexisting health problem.

Body part involved. The body part involved is an important factor in evaluating the severity of a burn. Injuries that involve cosmetic and functional areas of the body warrant a prognosis of long-term morbidity or mortality. A burn of the face, hands, and feet will require extensive and meticulous care. A burn of the head,

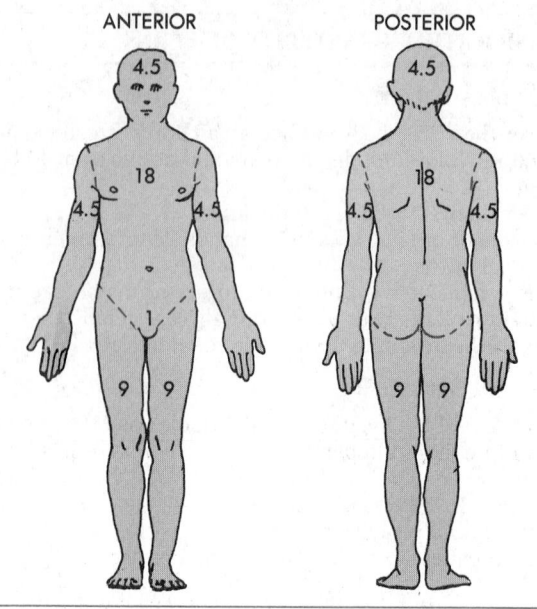

ANTERIOR   POSTERIOR

FIGURE 74-4 Rule of nines.

neck, and chest may also involve injury to the respiratory tract and result in severe respiratory difficulty. Burns of the perineum are difficult to manage because of the high incidence of infection. The circumferential,

or encircling burn, of a limb, the neck, or the chest has serious consequences. This type of burn will cause *constrictive contraction* of the skin and produce a tourniquet effect that may impair breathing and/or circulation. The anatomic part of the body burned must be considered when estimating the severity of the burn: A 3% burn of the anterior surface of the thigh will probably not be as serious as a 3% burn of the neck, face, or perineal area.

Burning agent. The identification of the causative agent is of prime importance because the nature of the agent has a direct effect on prognosis and treatment.

Thermal burns are the most common and occur as the result of the transfer of energy from a heat source to the body (flame, hot surfaces, sunburn, hot metals, and hot grease). Thermal injury caused by a flame or fire results in a dry burn that can be much deeper than is visually apparent. The flame is a highly concentrated heat that affects a localized area and burns deeply. In contrast, scald injuries, or moist burns, are caused by steam or boiling water that conducts heat to a larger, more widespread area (Figure 74-5). *Chemical* burns, commonly seen in industry, are caused by strong acids or alkali such as hydrochloric acid and lye (Table 74-5). Household chemical burns frequently occur from accidental exposure to drain cleaners, paint removers, and disinfectants. Burns to the eye occur when a chemical splashes onto the face, and burns to the upper gastrointestinal tract occur upon ingestion of the noxious chemical.

TABLE 74-4 Causes and factors determining depth of burn injury

Depth	Cause	Appearance	Color	Sensation
Superficial partial-thickness (first-degree)	Flash flame, ultraviolet light (sunburn)	Dry, no blisters Minimal or no edema Blanches with fingertip pressure and refills when pressure removed	Increased redness	Painful
Deep partial-thickness (second-degree)	Contact with hot liquids or solids Flash flame to clothing Direct flame Chemicals Ultraviolet light	Large, moist blisters that will increase in size Blanches with fingertip pressure and refills when pressure removed	Mottled with dull, white, tan, pink, or cherry red areas	Very painful
Full-thickness (third degree)	Contact with hot liquids or solids Flame Chemicals Electrical contact	Dry with leathery eschar Charred vessels visible under eschar Blisters rare but thin-walled blisters that do not increase in size may be present No blanching with pressure	White, charred dark tan Black Red	Little or no pain Hair easily pulls out

TABLE 74-5 Agents associated with chemical burns

Chemical Agent	Common Use	Characteristics	Systemic Effects	Agents to Remove or Dilute Chemicals
OXIDIZING AGENTS				
Chromic acid	Metal cleansing	Ulcerates, blisters		Water lavage
Potassium permanganate	Disinfectant, bleach, deodorizes	Thick, brownish purple eschar		Water lavage Eggwhite solution
Sodium hypochlorite (Clorox)	Disinfectants, bleach, deodorizers	Local irritation, inflammation		Water lavage Milk Eggwhite Starch Paste
CORROSIVE AGENTS				
Phenol	Deodorants; sanitizers; disinfectants; manufacture of plastics, dyes, fertilizers, explosives	Soft white eschar, brown stain when eschar removed, mild to absent pain	Minor exposure: tachycardia, arrhythmias	Copious water lavage Polyethelene glycol solution Vegetable oil
			Significant exposure: CNS depression, hypothermia, cardiac depression, respiratory depression	Lavage with water to debride particles
Phosphorus (white)	Manufacture of explosives, insecticides, rodent poisons, fertilizers	Necrotic with yellowish color Garlic odor Glows in dark Painful	Nephrotoxic Hepatic necrosis	Lavage with 1% copper sulfate ($CuSO_4$), Cover with castor oil
Pure sodium lye KOH NaOH NH_4OH LiOH $Ba_2(OH)_3$ $Ca(OH)_3$	Cleaning agents (washing powders, drain cleaners, paint removers), urine sugar reagent tablets, Portland cement	Soft gelatinous, brown eschar		Lye; water lavage Pure sodium; oil immersion
PROTOPLASMIC POISONS				
Salt-formers Tungstic Picric Sulfasalicyclic Tannic Trichloracetic Cresylic Acetate Formic	Industrial	Thin, hard eschar	Hepatic necrosis Nephrotoxicity	Water lavage
Metabolic competitor/ inhibitor Oxalic acid	Industrial	Chalky white ulcers	Hypocalcemia	Large volume calcium salts Copious water lavage Intravenous calcium
Hydrofluoric acid	Etching of glass	Painful, deep ulcerations	Hypocalcemia	Water lavage Subcutaneous calcium to area Subcutaneous magnesium sulfate

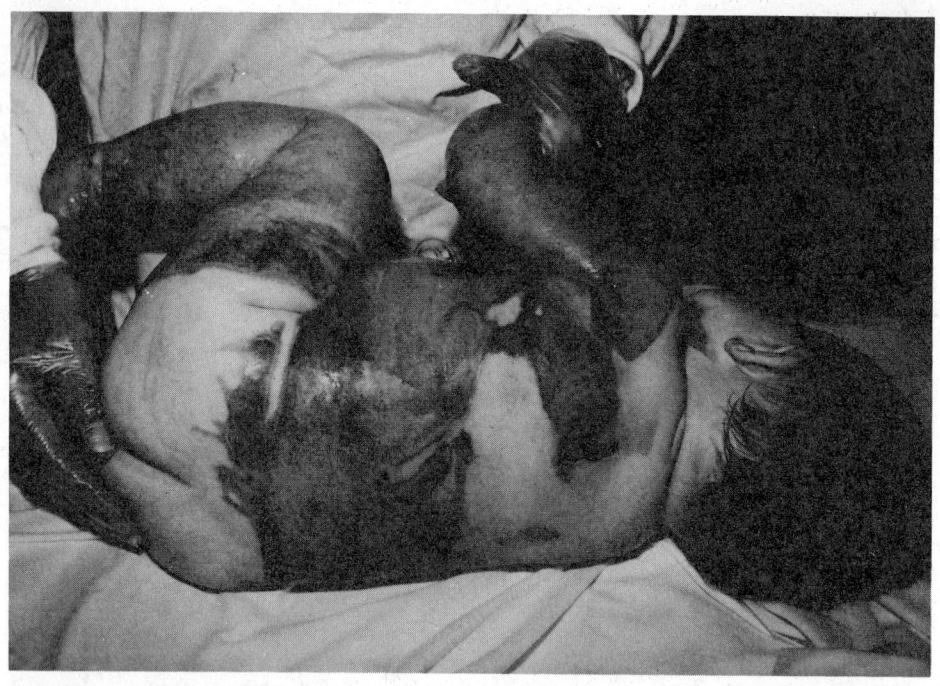

FIGURE 74-5 Toddler with scald burn resulting from being placed in bath water that was too hot. (Courtesy Burn Center, Metro Health Medical Center, Cleveland.)

Electrical burns are caused by electrical sparks and arcs or by an electrical current passing directly through the body. Tissue with the highest water content has the least resistance to electrical current and, consequently, suffers the most damage. Blood, muscles, skin, tendons, fat, and bones are affected in a decreasing order of resistance. Tissue damage may appear minor at the entrance and exit points, making electrical burns difficult to evaluate. The visual damage is referred to as the "tip of the iceberg" and does not reflect underlying tissue destruction generated by the passage of electrical current through the body. Victims of electrical burns must be monitored closely for signs and symptoms of hemorrhage, intestinal perforations, and cardiac arrhythmias. The passage of current may cause a cardiac arrest at the time of injury.

Medical history. Identification of known and unknown disorders may prevent fatal complications in the burn victim. A prior illness such as diabetes or renal failure may become acute during the postburn phase. The physiologic stress seen with the burn may exacerbate a latent disease process or worsen an already active process and thus increase mortality. Diabetes and chronic obstructive pulmonary disease may be aggravated, or patient with arteriosclerotic heart disease may develop a myocardial infarction.

■ DATA ANALYSIS: NURSING DIAGNOSES

Nursing diagnoses are determined from assessment of patient data. Possible nursing diagnoses for the person with burns may include, but are not limited to, the following:

Diagnostic Title	Possible Etiologies
Airway clearance, ineffective	Laryngeal edema, obstruction, secretions
Anxiety	Threat to self-concept, threat of death, threat of or change in health status
Fluid volume deficit	Movement of fluid from intravascular to interstitial space (hypovolemic stage), evaporation
Fluid volume excess	Movement of fluid from interstitial to intravascular space (diuretic stage)
Hypothermia	Environmental exposure of burn wound
Infection, potential for	Loss of protection created by damage to skin
Pain	Exposed nerve endings from burn injury, trauma
Skin integrity, impaired	Loss of skin from burn injury
Tissue perfusion, altered renal, cerebral, cardiopulmonary, gastrointestinal, peripheral	Hypovolemia (hypovolemic stage), hypervolemia (diuretic stage)

■ PLANNING: EXPECTED PATIENT OUTCOMES

Expected patient outcomes for the person with burns may include, but are not limited to, the following:

1. Patient maintains patent airway, adequate ventilation and oxygenation.
2. Patient exhibits control of anxiety.
3. Optimal fluid and electrolyte balance is regained.
4. Patient's body temperature is normal.
5. Patient is free form pathogenic organisms.
6. Patient experiences minimal pain.
7. No further skin loss occurs.
8. Vital organs have adequate perfusion.

■ IMPLEMENTATION

Assisting with a Airway Management

Persons who are burned on the face and neck or those who have inhaled flame, steam or smoke are observed closely for signs of laryngeal edema and airway obstruction. Data indicating potential or existing airway injury are outlined in the box below.

Adequate ventilation and oxygenation may be possible on room air; however, when any inhalation injury has occurred, it is best to give oxygen. If the victim is in respiratory distress or has a suspected inhalation injury, intubation may be necessary.

Prehospital Care

At the scene of a burn injury, the first action should be to remove the victim from the hazardous environment. Length of exposure to the causative agent is directly related to the severity of the injury.

The three most common causative agents for burn injury are fire, chemicals, and electricity. In the case of fire, flames should be extinguished, flammable or hot material removed from the victim, and the victim and rescuer removed from the unventilated or hazardous surroundings. If clothing is on fire, the victim's first reaction is to run, which only fans the flames. The best intervention is to roll the burning person in a blanket, coat, sheet, or towel on the ground to exclude oxygen

---

FACTORS DETERMINING INHALATION INJURY AND/OR POTENTIAL AIRWAY OBSTRUCTION

Burns to face and neck
Singed hairs, nasal hair, beard, eyelids or eyelashes
Intraoral charcoal, especially on teeth and gums
Brassy cough
Hoarseness
Copious sputum production
Carbonaceous sputum
Burn injury that has occurred in a closed space
Smell of smoke on victim's clothes or on victim
Respiratory distress

---

and thereby put out the fire. The rule is stop, drop, and roll. The victim should never stand because this will cause the flames and smoke to engulf the facial area possibly igniting the hair and causing an inhalation injury. Any water source can be used to extinguish flames.

First Aid for Burn Wounds

Once all flame is extinguished, clothing (except for that which adheres to the burned area), jewelry, and debris are carefully removed. Any clothing removed should be saved for possible analysis of flammability. The wounds are covered with dressings dampened with normal saline to ease the pain, reduce edema, and prevent evaporation of body water. The entire patient is wrapped in a dry cover to prevent heat loss. Ice should never be used because sudden vasoconstriction causes severe shifting of fluids. Although sterile dressings are preferred, clean nonsterile dressings can be used, since all dressings will be removed at the medical facility. Oils, salves, and ointments should never be used on burns because they hamper treatment at the medical facility.

The severity of *chemical* burns is directly proportional to the duration of exposure. Chemicals cause deep burns over a rather limited surface. The agent should be identified, and treatment initiated quickly. The first priority is removal of the chemical agent. This is accomplished by copious flushing with water for as long as 20 to 30 minutes to ensure complete removal of the destructive agent. Although specific chemical agents have known antidotes, it is best to flood the exposed area with water to ensure removal and transport the victim to the nearest medical facility. Burns occurring about the eyes should be lavaged continuously with copious amounts of cool, clean water for up to 30 minutes.

Electrical burns pose a special hazard to the victim, since the total body surface area of the burn is not always apparent and is often internal. Dysrhythmias and neurologic dysfunction are common in such exposure. Extreme care must be taken in removing the patient from the electrical source to prevent a similar injury to the rescuer (see Chapter 79).

Pain Relief

Pain in extensive burns is best controlled by gentle and minimal handling and by the application of dressings to exclude air from the burned surfaces. The degree of pain is usually inversely proportional to the depth of the burn injury; that is, full-thickness burns are usually painless, because nerve endings have been destroyed.

In small partial-thickness burns, cool (not cold) compresses on the burn site may provide some relief as long as the victim is kept warm. Ice packs are contraindicated because they may cause further skin injury and hypothermia.

Transport

Burns are often more severe than they first appear; therefore, even if the burns appear superficial, all persons with burns should be seen by a physician. The hospital or burn center should be notified before transporting a severely burned victim so that preparation can be made for arrival.

For obviously small burns, fluids may be given by mouth with caution. Large burns are accompanied by decreased peristalsis; therefore, nothing should be given by mouth. Patients with large burns or smoke inhalation may vomit, so particular attention is given to preventing them from aspirating vomitus.

According to the 1987 American Burn Association Directory, 207 hospitals in the United States reported the presence of a specialized burn care service. Of these, only 146 reported that they had a special burn unit. These burn units are located throughout the United States in major medical centers in urban areas. The American Burn Association estimates that there are 70,000 annual acute inpatient burn admissions in the United States. Only about 21,000 (or 30%) of these patients are cared for in specialized units. The American Burn Association also publishes a list of specialized burn care services every year.

Emergency Room Management

Rapid and efficient care is essential in the emergency room management of the burn victim (see the box below). If any respiratory distress is present, an airway is established. Prophylactic intubation is initiated if any heat or smoke has been inhaled or if the head, neck, or face is involved. Inhalation injuries are best managed with controlled ventilation because swelling of the upper airway can progress to obstruction (Figure 74-6). Endotracheal intubation is preferred over a tracheostomy. Since edema of the respiratory passages frequently subsides within a few days after the initial insult, it is desirable to avoid surgical trauma. Depending on the severity of symptoms, emergency treatment may include oxygen, suctioning, and postural drainage.

INITIAL TREATMENT OF MAJOR BURNS IN EMERGENCY ROOM

---

1. Establish airway.
2. Initiate fluid therapy by intravenous catheters.
3. Insert indwelling catheter for hourly urine measurement.
4. Insert nasogastric tube to remove stomach contents and prevent gastric distention.
5. Insert central intravenous catheter, if appropriate.
6. Manage pain by intravenous narcotics in small frequent doses.
7. Provide tetanus prophylaxis.

After an airway has been established, support of circulation is addressed. Burn injuries cause tremendous losses of fluid through the wound as well as into the burn wound and adjacent tissues in the form of edema. Fluid is best replaced through two large-caliber peripheral intravenous catheters. However, if the burn is large or complicated by inhalation injuries or preexisting disease, one peripheral line and one central line (for central venous pressure [CVP] measurement) is preferred. Placement of these lines is through an unburned site to prevent the introduction of infection. An indwelling Foley catheter is inserted to adequately monitor urine output. Hourly urine output measurements are used as a guide to the adequacy of plasma volume replacement.

Almost every patient who is burned greater than 15% of BSA develops thirst and an ileus. Oral fluids will not pass beyond the stomach (therefore, they will not relieve thirst), and they create a threat of regurgitation and aspiration. A nasogastric tube is inserted, and the stomach kept empty by suction to prevent gastric distention.

Promoting Comfort

Morphine sulfate is the drug of choice for pain relief and is given intravenously in small increments (2 to 4 mg). A morphine sulfate drip can be used (15 mg in 250 ml 5% dextrose and water) and titrated to the patient's pain. The intravenous route is used because of inadequate absorption at peripheral sites. No medication of any kind should be given intramuscularly or subcutaneously because it may pool and be absorbed later when cardiac output and blood pressure improve. Large doses of sedatives and analgesics are avoided because of the

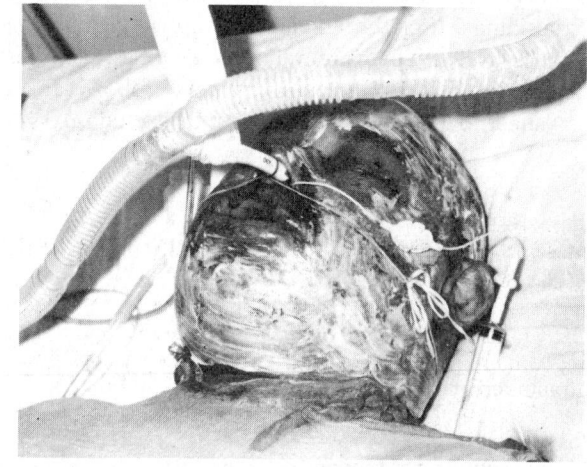

FIGURE 74-6 Patient with severe edema 5 hours after burn occurred. Airway was managed with endotracheal intubation. Edema subsided, and patient was extubated 4 days after admission. (Courtesy Burn Center, Metro Health Medical Center, Cleveland.)

danger of respiratory depression and the potential of masking other symptoms.

Tetanus prophylaxis is initiated in the emergency room. Tetanus toxoid is administered if the patient has been previously immunized but has not received tetanus toxoid in the preceding 5 years. If prior tetanus immunization is not documented, a dose of human tetanus-immune globulin (TIGH) is administered, and an active tetanus immunization program begun.

Replacing Body Fluids

Replacing fluids and electrolytes is an essential part of the treatment of burn victims and is instituted as soon as the severity of the burn and the patient's condition is known (see the box below). Ideally, fluid therapy is started within an hour after a severe burn to prevent the onset of hypovolemic shock. Insertion of two large-caliber peripheral catheters or one large-caliber central venous catheter and one large-caliber peripheral catheter permits the rapid administration of fluids and electrolytes.

Fluids administered during the first 48 hours are given to maintain circulating blood volume. Additional fluids and electrolytes are added to replace losses from vomiting or from nasogastric drainage. Three types of fluid are considered in calculating the needs of the patient: (1) colloids, including plasma and plasma expanders such as Dextran; (2) electrolytes such as physiologic solution of sodium chloride, Ringer's solution, Hartmann's solution, and Tyrode's solution; and (3) nonelectrolyte fluids such as distilled water with 5% glucose. Medical authorities do not agree as to the proportion of colloids and electrolyte fluids needed. Several formulas are described in the medical literature to guide physicians in determining the type and amount of fluids to be administered on the basis of the patient's weight, age, and the percentage of the body burned.[12,55] The present trend is to administer balanced salt solutions (for example, lactated Ringer's), water, and plasma and to use whole blood only if a large number of RBCs are destroyed or if anemia develops.

Some resuscitation formulas include colloid replacement in the first 24 hours. Others do not because it is believed that capillary changes allow leakage of the protein-rich fluid into the interstitium, augmenting edema

INDICATIONS FOR FLUID RESUSCITATION

Burns greater than 20% BSA in adults
Burns greater than 10% BSA in children
Patient older than 65 or younger than 2 years of age
Patient with preexisting disease that would reduce normal compensatory responses to minor hypovolemia (that is, cardiac or pulmonary disease, diabetes)

formation. According to the crystalloid resuscitation formula, fluids are administered in three time periods of 8 hours each. In the first three 8-hour periods (24 hours) lactated Ringer's solution (RL) is administered according to the following formula:

$$4 \text{ ml RL} \times \text{weight (kg)} \times \% \text{ BSA burned} = \text{ml RL for the first 24 hours}$$

Because blood volume falls most rapidly and edema increases fastest in the first 8 hours, intravenous replacement is accomplished at a rapid rate. One half of the total amount calculated is given in the first 8 hours after the injury. *The time is calculated from the time of injury,* not from the time emergency care was initiated. In the second 8-hour period, one fourth of the total amount of calculated lactated Ringer's solution is given and in the third 8-hour period, the remaining one fourth is given.

Patients may complain of moderate to severe thirst during this period. Aggressive oral hygiene may alleviate patient discomfort. If oral fluids are permitted, accurate recording of ingested fluids is important. Unlimited oral intake and failure to measure it may provide too much fluid in the circulating blood, resulting in water intoxication.

During the second 24 hours postburn, one half to two thirds of the initial 24-hour volume will be required. It is also during this second 24-hour period that colloid solutions are used to replete intravascular volume once capillary permeability significantly decreases.

During fluid resuscitation, adequate volume is assessed by monitoring mental status, vital signs, peripheral perfusion, body weight, and urine output. A 15% to 20% weight gain in the first 72 hours of resuscitation is anticipated. Significant laboratory measurements include serum and urine electrolytes, serum and urine osmolality, and hematocrit. Hourly urine output is the most accessible and generally reliable index of adequate fluid replacement. Fluid should be titrated to ensure an output of 30 to 50 ml/hr in the adult and 0.5 to 1 ml/kg/hr in the child. The most common reasons for a drop in urine output below 30 ml/hr, indicating insufficient fluid replacement, are that the calculated fluids are behind schedule and the severity of the burn has been underestimated. The urine is observed for color and analyzed for the presence of blood. The physician is notified if hematuria or a positive Hemastix reaction is present.

Other clinical criteria that indicate adequate resuscitation are pulse rate of 120/min or less in the adult, CVP in low to normal range, pulmonary artery end-diastolic pressure (PAEDP) in low to normal range, and mental lucidity (see the box on p. 2170).

After the first 48 to 72 hours, the patient enters the diuretic phase as edema reabsorption occurs. The urinary output increases dramatically and is no longer a re-

SIGNS OF ADEQUATE RESUSCITATION

Clear sensorium
Pulse < 120 beats/min
Urine output: 30 to 50 ml/hr (adult)
  0.5 to 1 ml/kg/hr (child)
Systolic blood pressure: 100 mmHg
CVP: 5 to 10 mmHg
PAEDP: 5 to 15 mmHg
Blood pH normal range: 7.35 to 7.45

liable guide to fluid needs. Fluid needs are assessed by measuring serum and urine electrolyte levels. Fluid replacement, using 5% dextrose and water, is based on individual assessment. If dehydration occurs from diuresis, fluid replacement therapy is continued until blood volume is stabilized. Potassium may be added to the intravenous fluid because of potassium losses in the urine. The patient is monitored closely for signs of water intoxication or pulmonary edema.

Initial Wound Care

Care of the burn wound can be delayed until all first aid measures have been initiated. Wound care should be carried out carefully and with as little discomfort to the patient as possible. One of the most important factors to be considered in wound care is that the patient has lost the ability to withstand infection in the area where the skin is damaged or destroyed. The goals of the initial wound care are as follows:

1. Cleanse the wound to eliminate or decrease the dead tissue and debris that serve as the media for bacterial growth
2. Prevent further destruction of viable skin
3. Provide for patient comfort

During the admission procedure, the burn wound and the entire body are washed to remove dirt and debris from the accident as well as loose dead tissue on the burned areas. Detergents (Dreft) or antiseptic preparations, such as povidone-iodine (Betadine), are effective cleansing agents. Gentle cleansing with gauze is effective in removing dead tissue without causing further tissue damage.

All hair in and around the burn wound is shaved and wiped off the skin because hair attracts and shelters bacteria. Singed hair is clipped short to avoid bacterial contamination of the wound.

Firm, intact blisters can remain undisturbed because they are a natural protective and pain-free dressing. If the blisters are broken and the epidermis is separated, loose tissue must be debrided.

After the wound is cleaned and before a dressing is applied, cultures of the wound are obtained. Prophylactic systemic antibiotics are usually not indicated. Baseline cultures provide information about organisms present in the wounds at the time of admission.

Photographs are taken on admission and at intervals during the patient's hospitalization. These pictures provide a record of the appearance of the burn wound on admission, before the application of topical therapy, and during the healing process.

An early complication of thermal injury is the constricting effect of a circumferential eschar of the trunk or extremities. Eschar is a crust or scab that forms over a burn wound. Edema forming rapidly under the constricting eschar of a full-thickness wound on the arm or legs will produce enough pressure to cause occlusion of venous and arterial circulation and may result in *ischemic necrosis,* especially if unburned areas are distal to the constrictive eschar. Circumferential burns of the neck and chest not only occlude circulation but may result in pressure on the trachea or rib cage causing respiratory distress. Frequent observations of chest excursions in addition to respiratory rate are necessary to determine respiratory restriction. Pulses are checked every 15 minutes to ensure uninterrupted vascular flow to all extremities.

The treatment of constrictive eschar is achieved through an *escharotomy.* The eschar is surgically cut linearly or into squares to alleviate stricture (Figure 74-7). This is a painless procedure in a full-thickness burn because the nerve endings have already been damaged by the burn.

Maintaining Body Temperature

The maintenance of body temperature is a critical factor during cleansing because the severely burned patient has lost some of the ability to regulate body temperature. The environment must be heat controlled and kept warmer than usual. Drafts must be eliminated. A heat lamp or warming lights should be available. Prolonged exposure to air is avoided. Exposed areas of the body are covered with sterile sheets and blankets while other areas of the burn are being cleansed.

Providing Emotional Support

Patients with significant burn injury receive a profound insult to their body and self-image. There is fear and anxiety associated with scarring and disfigurement. There is an awareness that they may not survive, enhancing feelings of fear and helplessness. The shock and pain of the accident, the chaos and rush to the hospital the unknown surroundings and people all intensify the emotional stress.

The nurse spends the most time with the patient and has a considerable influence on the patient's psychologic adjustment. Interventions that can be used to reassure the patient and alleviate anxiety include the following:

1. Identify self to patient.

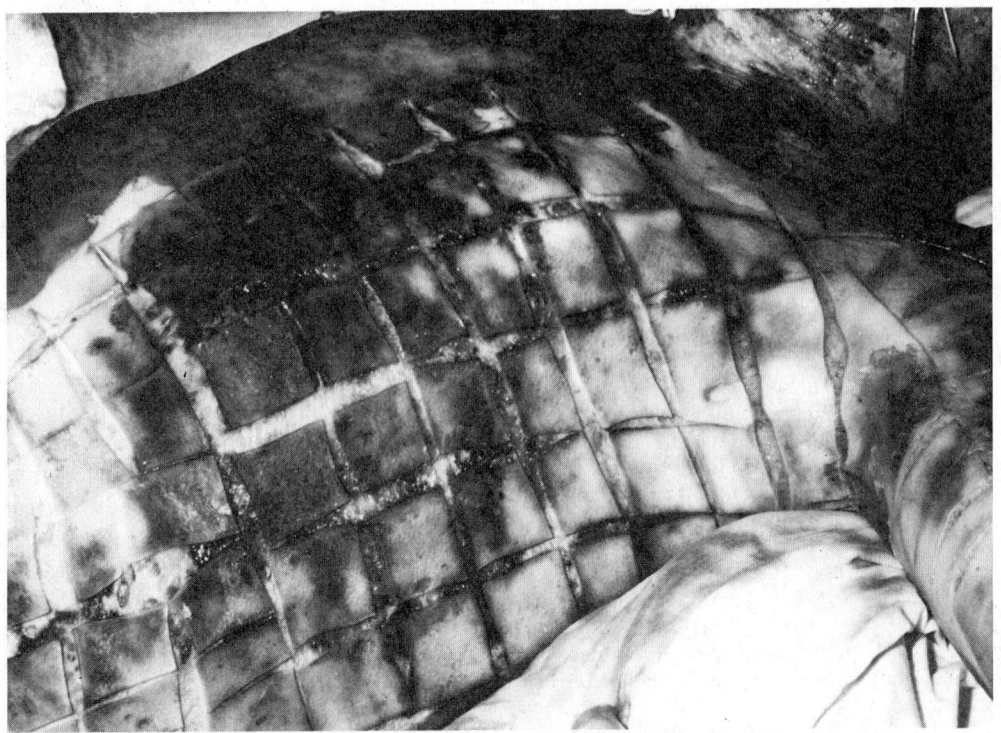

FIGURE 74-7 Grid escharotomy used to alleviate circulatory and pulmonary constriction. (Courtesy Burn Center, Metro Health Medical Center, Cleveland.)

2. Orient patient to the surroundings.
3. Describe basis of physical symptoms (skin loss, pain, cold).
4. Explain the equipment and procedures to be used in treatment.

ACUTE PERIOD

The acute period of treatment begins at the end of the emergent period and lasts until the burn wound is healed. The length of this period varies. If the burn is a partial-thickness injury, the acute period extends for 10 to 20 days; if the burn is a full-thickness injury over a large percentage of the body requiring surgery for skin grafting, the acute period could last for months.

During the acute period there are two main principles of management: (1) treatment of the burn wound; and (2) avoidance, detection, and treatment of complications. The most common complications are infection (septicemia and pneumonia), renal disease, and heart failure.

■ ASSESSMENT

Subjective Data

Burn patients are often frightened and anxious about their injury and the associated treatments. These responses can be compounded by the intensive care unit (ICU) environment.

Burn patients experience both physical and psychologic pain. Physical pain is usually focused on specific activities such as wound cleansing and debridement, dressing changes, and physical therapy. The patient may react to physical pain in three ways: (1) by ignoring it, (2) by accepting it, or (3) by overreacting to it. The nurse should not judge whether the patient is feeling real pain; the nurse must instead assess the patient's reaction to pain and intervene appropriately.

Objective Data

The nurse must perform a thorough head-to-toe assessment of the burn patient every 8 hours. Data should include mental status; vital signs; breath sounds; bowel sounds; dietary intake; motor ability; intake and output; weight pattern; circulatory assessment; and observation of burn wounds, grafts, and donor site. Purulent drainage, abnormal color, foul odor, redness or swelling in surrounding normal skin, or presence of healing should be noted. Changes in these parameters from shift to shift or from day to day make further investigation necessary.

Metabolism is increased after moderate to severe burns as a result of stress, fluid loss, fever, infection, increased metabolism, and immobility. Wound healing may be prolonged if adequate nutritional support is not initiated on admission. A nutritional assessment is performed during the first days after burn injury and includes anthropometric measurements (to determine actual weight loss compared to ideal weight), serum electrolytes, liver function test, and urinalysis.

■ DATA ANALYSIS: NURSING DIAGNOSES

Nursing diagnoses are determined from assessment of patient data. Possible nursing diagnoses for the person with burns may include, but are not limited to, the following:

Diagnostic Title	Possible Etiologies
Anxiety	Threat to self-concept, threat/change in health status/role functioning, situational crisis
Fear	Long-term illness, death, pain, treatment, lifestyle changes
Hypothermia	Environmental exposure of burn wounds
Infection, potential for	Decreased nutrition, burn wound treatment (dressings, surgery)
Knowledge deficit	Unfamiliarity with routines
Altered nutrition: less than body requirements	Increased metabolic needs
Pain	Treatment of burn wounds (dressings, surgery)
Skin integrity, impaired	Burn wounds
Social isolation	Alteration in physical appearance, physical isolation

■ PLANNING: EXPECTED PATIENT OUTCOMES

Expected patient outcomes for the person with burns may include, but are not limited to, the following:
1. Patient verbalizes anxiety
2. Patient is not fearful (establishes a trusting relationship with his or her primary nurse)
3. Body temperature is normal
4. Patient is free of pathogenic organisms
5. Patient verbalizes understanding of treatments and surgical procedures and participates appropriately in care
6. Optimal nutritional status is achieved
7. Patient obtains pain relief
8. Wounds are clean and small if open
9. Majority of wounds are closed
10. Patient is not withdrawn or depressed

■ IMPLEMENTATION

Relieving Anxiety

The psychologic responses of the patient in the immediate postburn period are in response to a threat of survival. The fear of death is real as the patient senses the acuity of the situation by experiencing pain, disfigurement, isolation, and dependency from being attached to machines and monitors that maintain vital functions. A variety of behaviors may be seen during the acute and emergent phase (see Table 74-6 for a summary of emo-

tional responses). A patient's reactions are determined by her or his personality, degree of total adjustment to life, and the extent and location of burns.

The nurse should support and encourage the patient to help ease the anxiety. Setting short-term, achievable goals will help motivate the patient. Providing the family with an explanation of the patient's needs will ease their fears and allow them to encourage the patient.

Preventing Infecction

Measures to prevent infection begin at the time the patient is admitted to the hospital and continue until healing is complete. Local and systemic infections (septicemia) are the most common complications of burns and are the major cause of death, particularly in burns covering more than 25% of the body. *Autogenous sources are the primary sources of infection initially caused by bacteria that survive in the hair follicles and sweat glands beneath the burned tissue.* However, the patient is also susceptible to infection from exogenous sources.

The organisms that usually infect burns are *Staphylococcus aureus, Pseudomonas aeruginosa,* and the coliform bacilli. In the past few years, there has been a high incidence of fungal infections resulting from the use of broad spectrum antibiotics. *Candida albicans,* which normally is found in the gastrointestinal tract, accounts for the majority of the fungal infections. Cultures of the patient's nose, throat, wound, and unburned skin and a punch biopsy may be taken on admission and at biweekly intervals to determine the presence of bacteria and their sensitivity to antibiotics.

The increased risk of infection after burn injury is not only due to the loss of the protective skin barrier, but also to dysfunction within the immune and endocrine systems and nutritional and hematologic changes. Infection is usually the cause of any deterioration of a burn patient. Signs of infection in the burn patient include increased anxiety, purulent wound drainage, and pallor of healthy viable tissue. Signs of sepsis in the burn patient are outlined below:
1. Change in sensorium
2. Fever
3. Tachypnea
4. Tachycardia
5. Paralytic ileus
6. Abdominal distention
7. Oliguria

To prevent the introduction of exogenous organisms into the wound, all persons who approach the patient should wear gowns, masks, caps, and gloves. Persons with upper respiratory infections should not be permitted near the patient.

Aseptic technique and sterile gloves are used during wound care and dressing changes. Hydrotherapy tanks

TABLE 74-6 Emotional responses to severe burns

Patient Response	Definition	Behavior Exhibited	Nursing Approach
Denial	Inability to accept present condition (pain, disfigurement, events of burn accident, hospital environment) Buffers impact of an overwhelming physical and psychologic crisis	Level of comprehension and understanding in relation to degree/acuity of injury distorted Denial of burn injury States he is "fine" Avoids discussion of injury May experience a period of euphoria	Support patient Allow some degree of denial, but allay patient's fears without distorting the truth
Flood reaction	Extreme agitation and concern over multiple issues in a disorganized fashion Problems that existed before the injury are exaggerated.	Urgency to settle problems involving employment and finances Family may be gathered at patient's request to discuss patient's concerns.	Support patient Orient patient to time and place
Paranoia	Suspicion of intended harm	Confusion Disorientation Lack of trust in caregiver	Acknowledge complaints of manifestations of fear Investigate all complaints Support patient Provide reality orientation
Regression	Adapting behavior of an earlier life time frame	Infantile, demanding, and uncooperative behavior	Acknowledge inability to cope Provide structure: allow patient choice in some instances Reward appropriate behavior
Depression	Withdrawal into oneself Little or no recognition of external events	Lethargic Stuporous Apathetic Little or no response to painful stimuli	Support patient Encourage verbalization of frustrations Encourage activity within clinical limitations

and spray tables are used for aggressive cleansing of burn wounds and can be a source of infection. They need particular attention to prevent the spread of infection when the tanks are used by different patients. Care of the severely burned patient in special burn units can contribute to decreased infection because the environment is specifically geared to infection control. If the patient is cared for in a general hospital unit, a private room is essential, and all equipment needed by the patient remains in the room. *Reverse isolation precautions* are initiated.

Wound Care

Eschar is the leathery covering of dead tissue and exudate that forms after a burn injury. It is conducive to bacterial growth because it contains dead tissue, moisture, and warmth. Daily cleansing and mechanical debridement remove eschar. Washing and friction removes buildup of debris and supports healthy tissue regeneration. Hydrotherapy facilitates the removal of dressings and medications and loosens debris, sloughing eschar, and exudate. It is a more comfortable method for removal of dressings and facilitates range of motion exercise with minimal energy expenditure and discomfort. The solution used in a hydrotherapy tank

may be plain water, normal saline, or an electrolytically balanced solution. To minimize the chance of infection, the nurse should keep the procedure as clean as possible. The use of gowns, masks, gloves, and a plastic, disposable tub liner will decrease the chance of contamination between patients. Tubbing is usually performed once or twice daily and should not exceed 30 minutes to prevent exposure and chilling. Tubbing is started after the patient's vital signs and fluid balance have stabilized.

Hydrotherapy is contraindicated if the patient experiences any sudden changes in temperature, heart rate, blood pressure or respiratory rate.

The current trend in wound cleansing is to use a spray table. The patient is placed on a special stretcher that has a drain and the person is showered with a hose. Patient comfort is enhanced because areas that are not being debrided can be covered.

Methods of Treatment

Different methods of treating the burned area may be used, depending on the location of the burn, its size and depth, the facilities available, and the patient's response to therapy. One method may be replaced with another during the course of treatment. Those commonly used today include the open or exposure method, the semi-open method, and the closed or occlusive method.

Open or exposure method. The exposure method of treatment was accidently discovered to be effective in 1888 when, during a serious steamboat fire on the Mississippi River, those in attendance ran out of bandages and later observed that the neglected persons fared better than those who received more intensive local treatment.[10] Today the exposure method is used most often in the treatment of burns involving the face, neck, perineum, and broad areas of the trunk. The burned area is cleansed and exposed to air (Figure 74-8). The exudate of a partial-thickness burn dries in 48 to 72 hours and forms a hard crust that protects the wound. Epithilialization occurs beneath this crust and may be complete in 14 to 21 days. The crust then falls off spontaneously, leaving a healed, unscarred surface. The dead skin of a full-thickness burn is dehydrated and converted to black, leathery eschar in 48 to 72 hours. Loose eschar may be gradually removed through hydrotherapy and/or debridement. Uninfected eschar acts as a protective covering. The danger of infection exists as bacteria proliferate beneath the eschar. Spontaneous separation, produced by bacterial action, occurs unless surgical debridement is performed first.

Isolation technique is essential when the exposure method is used. The nurse caring for the patient should wear a sterile gown and mask, and sterile linen may be used on the bed. A cradle may be used on the bed since no clothing or bed clothes are allowed directly over burned areas. Lights or heat lamps may be used with caution to provide warmth. Advantages of the open method are that the wound is easily inspected and the patient has maximal freedom to perform exercises for

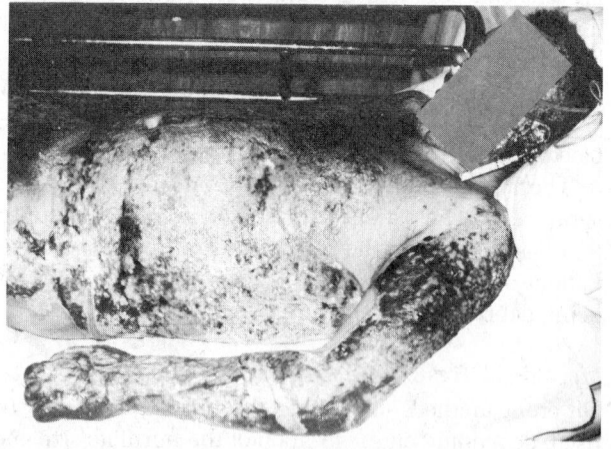

FIGURE 74-8 Severely burned man being treated by open method. (Courtesy Burn Center, Metro Health Medical Center, Cleveland.)

the prevention of contracture and the improvement of circulation.

Patients having exposure treatment complain of pain and chilling. Pain may be controlled by administering morphine sulfate, meperidine hydrochloride (Demerol), or salicylates as ordered. Discomfort can be decreased if drafts are avoided and the temperature of the room is kept at 24.4° C (85° F). Patients lose more heat from burned surfaces than from normal skin surfaces, because the vascular bed that normally contracts and retains heat in the body is lost. The humidity of the room also should be controlled. A humidity of 40% to 50% is usually considered satisfactory. Portable electric humidifiers and dehumidifiers can be used to achieve and maintain this level.

Semiopen method. The semiopen wound care method consists of covering the wound with topical antimicrobial agents and a thin layer of gauze to help keep the agent in contact with the wound. This method permits the passage of wound exudate through the dressing without the loss of antimicrobial cream. The success of semiopen care depends on cleaning the wound once or twice a day, either at the bedside or in the hydrotherapy tank. Meticulous semiopen wound care speeds debridement, enhances the development of granulation tissue, and makes grafting possible sooner.

Closed method. In the closed or occlusive method of burn treatment, the wounds are washed, and dressings changed at least once a day, or in some instances once each shift. Commonly, the dressing consists of gauze impregnated with topical ointments and a gauze wrap. Counterpressure wrappings (elastic bandages) may be applied. When a dressing is in place, nursing observation includes monitoring for signs of impaired circulation (numbness, pain, and tingling) and for signs of infection (odor on dressings, elevated temperature, and elevated pulse rate).

Topical agents. The application of topical agents to the burn wound has helped decrease infection and hasten healing. They are effective because damage to the vasculature in the burn area prevents systemic antibiotics from reaching the burn wound. Antibiotics may be given prophalactically or may be withheld until an infection occurs. The following is a description of some of the topical agents currently in use for burn patients.

Mafenide. Mafenide acetate (Sulfamylon) is a white cream containing sulfonamide. It penetrates through the burn eschar and is an effective bacteriostatic against many gram-negative and gram-positive organisms. The cream is applied to the wound once or twice daily with a sterile, gloved hand in a thin layer just enough to cover the burn completely. The wound may be left open to the air, or a single layer of gauze may be used to hold the cream in place. The cream is removed from the wound, and active debriding is performed before the cream is reapplied.

Mafenide is known to inhibit carbonic anhydrase activity, especially in patients with burns of 40% or more BSA; as a result, metabolic acidosis may occur. The patient is monitored for hyperventilation in an attempt to balance the increased acid load. Other side effects include pain with application of the cream and an allergic rash. *Mafenide inhibits epithelial proliferation; therefore, application should be stopped as soon as the wound is clean and there is evidence of healing.*

Silver sulfadiazine. Silver sulfadiazine (Silvadene) is a white cream with bactericidal action against many gram-negative and gram-positive bacteria, as well as against C. *albicans*. It is applied directly to the wound once or twice daily on saturated gauze or with a sterile gloved hand. The wound may be covered with a dressing or left exposed. Silver sulfadiazine does not penetrate as readily as mafenide acetate; however, patients do not complain of pain with its application.

The patient is observed for side effects common with sulfonamide drugs. The wound may develop a slimy, grayish appearance simulating an infection, despite negative cultures. Silver sulfadiazine should not be used in patients with a history of kidney disease. No electrolyte imbalances are seen with its use; however, prolonged use may lead to toxic symptoms including nausea, vomiting, anemia, leukopenia, granulocytopenia, mental changes, oliguria, anuria, hematuria, jaundice, and skin rashes.

Povidine-iodine. Povidine-iodine (Betadine) ointment is a reddish brown germicidal preparation of 10% povidine-iodine (1% available iodine) with broad-spectrum microbial action. It is effective against gram-positive and gram-negative bacteria, fungi, yeasts, viruses, and protozoa. It is applied three times daily. Povidine-iodine can be applied either by (1) spreading it with a sterile, gloved hand onto the burned surface or (2) impregnating a single-thickness gauze with it, applying the gauze to the burned surfaces, and spreading additional ointment on top of the gauze layer.

Metabolic acidosis may be seen with the elevated serum iodine levels. Clothing and bedding need to be protected from staining. A dry, crusting wound may be seen as well as skin rashes in unaffected areas.

Silver nitrate. Although silver nitrate is being used less often than in the past, some physicians still prescribe it. In this treatment, thick gauze dressings are saturated with 0.5% solution of silver nitrate. The dressings are kept wet so that the solution remains in constant contact with the burned surfaces. If the dressing is allowed to dry, the silver nitrate can concentrate and cause tissue destruction. The purpose of these dressings is to retain moisture and heat and to reduce evaporation. Proponents of this method of treatment believe that it reduces mortality, lessens pain, eliminates odors, and has a bacteriostatic effect. The dressings are removed every 12 to 24 hours, and the patient is placed in a bath of salt solution with the temperature carefully maintained at the same level as the body. When skin grafts are applied, silver nitrate dressings are placed over the grafts and donor sites on the first postoperative day. Because the silver nitrate is hypotonic, electrolytes are lost into the wound. Therefore, throughout treatment, frequent determinations of blood sodium levels are necessary, and sodium that is lost may need to be replaced. Everything that comes in contact with silver nitrate solution is stained black, so care should be taken when applying the solution to protect skin, clothing, furniture, walls, and floors.

Other topical medications used in burn therapy are outlined in Table 74-7.

Wound coverings. The burn wound may be covered with dressings or grafts.

Dressings. Large bulky dressings are rarely used today for large burns except in select instances because infection control is more difficult and partial-thickness burns may develop into full-thickness wounds. The purposes of applying some light covering include prevention of infection from exogenous sources, facilitation of debridement, maximal contact by topical agents, and prevention of fluid evaporation with loss of body heat. The type of dressing that is usually applied consists of a single layer of fine-mesh gauze impregnated with a topical medication and held in place by a wrapping of a coarse gauze such as Kerlix.

The dressing change is usually a painful procedure requiring analgesics. For maximal effectiveness, analgesics should be given 30 minutes before the procedure. Most dressing changes are performed after tubbing to facilitate dressing removal and lessen pain. Additional debridement of eschar and dead tissue may be performed before the new dressing is applied.

Wet dressings may be used with silver nitrate or normal saline applications. Normal saline is applied to clean granulation tissue or to new grafts to maintain moisture or are used with fine-mesh gauze to provide for slight debridement. A single layer of fine-mesh gauze is usually placed over the wound, covered with thick gauze pads to maintain moisture, and held in place with a gauze wrapping. The dressings must be kept wet. Plastic wrap should *not* be used to cover the dressings because it prevents any fluid evaporation, causes increased heat at the wound site, and results in patient discomfort and increased tissue destruction and infection.

Skin grafts. Skin grafts are applied to cover the burn

TABLE 74-7 Topical medications used in burn therapy

Topical Medication	Advantages	Disadvantages
Mafenide acetate (Sulfamylon)	Bacteriostatic against gram-negative and gram-positive organisms Penetrates thick eschar Effective against *pseudomonas* organisms	Metabolic acidosis Pain on application Allergic rash
Silver sulfadiazine (Silvadene)	Broad antimicrobial activity against gram-negative, gram-positive, and *Candida* organisms No electrolyte imbalances Painless and somewhat soothing Not nephrotoxic	Repeated application may develop slimy, grayish appearance simulating an infection in spite of negative cultures Prolonged use may cause skin rash and depress granulocyte formation
Povidione-iodine (Betadine)	Broad antimicrobial activity against bacteria, fungi, viruses, and protozoa	Metabolic acidosis caused by elevated serum iodine levels Stains clothing and linen Dry, crusting, scabbing wound Skin rash in unaffected area
Silver nitrate	Bacteriostatic effect Lessens pain and eliminates odor Reduces evaporative water loss from burns	Electrolyte imbalances Stains everything it comes in contact with Does not penetrate eschar Pain on application
Nitrofurazone (Furacin)	Inhibits enzymes necessary for bacterial metabolism Broad spectrum of activity Effective against *S. aureus* Not absorbed systemically Low incidence of sensitivity	Contact dermatitis in unaffected skin Urine turns a reddish color
Gentamycin sulfate (Garamycin)	Broad antimicrobial activity Painless	Ototoxicity Nephrotoxicity Development of resistant bacterial strains
Neomycin	Broad antimicrobial activity Causes miscoding in the messenger ribonucleic acid (RNA) of bacterial cells	Serious toxic effects Ototoxicity Nephrotoxicity
Scarlet red	Nonantiseptic (applied to gauze soaked with oil-base red dye) Drying agent Applied to donor site Promotes epithelialization	No antimicrobial effects Stains and irritates skin Possible infection beneath scarlet red gauze; may have systemic effects
Xeroform	Nonantiseptic Debrides and protects donor site Protects graft	Removal possibly painful, because it sometimes adheres to wound Neither antiseptic or antimicrobial
Sodium hypochlorite (Dakin's solution)	Chlorine-based solution that is bacteriocidal Aids in debriding wounds Aids in cleaning and draining of "soupy" wounds	Dissolves blood clot May inhibit clotting May irritate the skin
Sutilains ointment (Travase)	Topical enzymatic agent Dissolves necrotic tissue by protolytic action Facilitates removal of eschar and purulent drainage	Mild, transient pain on application Paresthesia, bleeding, dermatitis Imperative that dressing be kept moist at all times

wound and speed healing, to prevent contractures, and to shorten convalescence. Successful grafting reduces the patient's vulnerability to infection and prevents the loss of body heat and water vapor from the open wound. Grafting can also be done for cosmetic or functional purposes during the rehabilitative period (see Chapter 73). Most skin grafts are applied between the third and twenty-first day after the initial injury, depending on the depth and extent of the burn and the condition of the base.

Grafts are obtained from various sources (Table 74-8). An autograft is a graft of skin obtained from the patient's own body. A homograft is a graft of skin obtained from a cadaver 6 to 24 hours after death. A heterograft

TABLE 74-8 Types of grafts

Graft	Source	Coverage
Autograft	Patient's own skin	Permanent
Homograft	Another of the same species.	Temporary
Heterograft	Another species.	Temporary
Synthetic substitute	Man-made substitute that has properties similar to skin	Temporary

is a graft of skin obtained from another species, such as a pig. Synthetic substitutes for skin are now being used, and growing the patient's own skin from skin biopsies are currently being investigated. Homografts, heterografts, and synthetic substitutes are intended to provide temporary coverage while the burn wound heals. As the wound heals, these temporary coverings are gradually rejected and are easily removed from the newly healed skin.

The advantage of a temporary graft is to reduce water, electrolyte, and protein losses at the burn surface. The covered wound is less painful and allows the patient freedom of movement. Temporary grafts may be used until the patient is ready for autografts. Often, autografting is delayed as a result of complications such as pneumonia or gastric hemorrhage.

Split-thickness skin grafts are used most frequently in early stages of wound treatment (Figure 74-9). The grafts include two upper layers of skin (epidermis) and part of the middle layer (dermis) but are not taken so deep as to prevent regeneration of the skin at the site from which they are taken (donor site). The grafts are removed with a dermatome blade from almost any unburned part of the body. The size of these grafts are determined by the sites available and the area to be covered. Grafts may be placed on the recipient bed by two methods—stamping and meshing. Stamping uses "postage stamp" grafts that are stamp-size pieces of donor skin applied over the recipient bed. This technique is generally used with a wound that is unclean because it allows for drainage of excess debris. Meshing involves taking the sheet of skin after it is removed from the donor and feeding it into a meshing instrument that perforates the sheet with tiny slits. The meshing of the graft makes it more distensible and capable of being stretched to cover wider areas of the body surface (Figure 74-10).

Full-thickness grafts are composed of layers of skin down to the subcutaneous tissue. They give a better cosmetic appearance than split-thickness grafts when

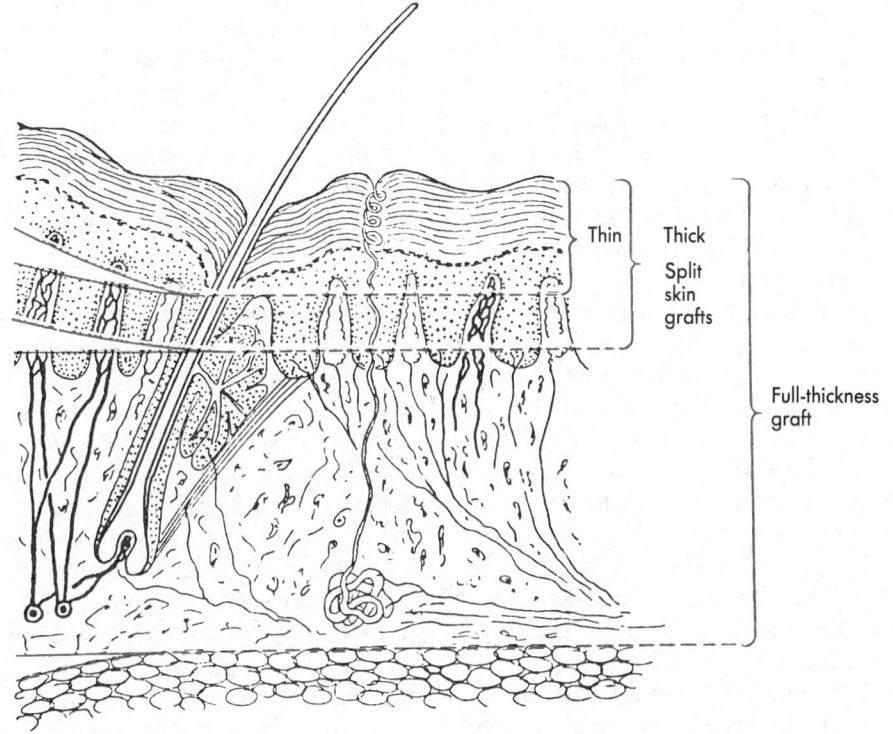

FIGURE 74-9 Levels of the skin involved in thin- and thick-split skin grafts and full-thickness grafts.

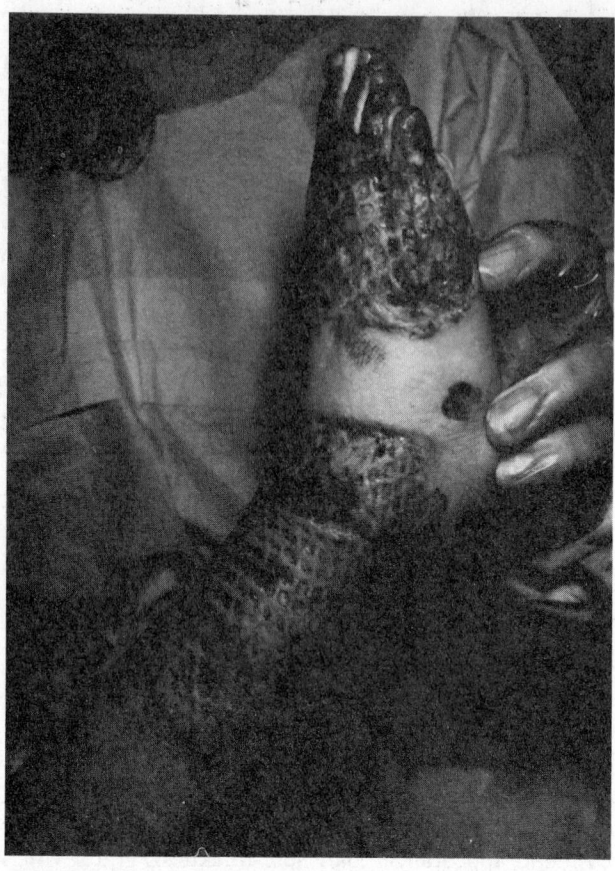

FIGURE 74-10 Mesh graft covering a full-thickness burn 14 days after placement. (Courtesy Burn Center, Metro Health Medical Center, Cleveland.)

ADVANTAGES OF TANGENTIAL EXCISION AND GRAFTING

Shortened hospitalization
Prevents potential conversion of burn to full thickness by removing necrotic tissue before infection occurs
Definitive healing diminishes anxiety and lessens trauma to multiple graftings
Allows early grafting and early restoration of function
Scar formation reduced because of use of full-thickness graft

it is found to be purulent with a strong odor. Dressing is removed slowly and carefully so as to not disturb the graft.

The donor site represents a wound similar to that of a partial-thickness injury. Care of the donor site is as important as care of the graft itself, for donor sites that fail to heal result in a net enlargement of the patient's open wound surface. Donor sites may be treated by a variety of methods. One method is covering the exposed surface with fine-mesh gauze, Xeroform, or a synthetic dressing and leaving it exposed to the air. Exposing the donor site to a heat lamp also promotes healing, because, as the drainage from the wound dries, it serves as a protective covering (Figure 74-11). The site usually heals within 2 weeks. Another method is to cover the site with sterile gauze and to apply a pressure dressing.

Many patients complain of severe pain in the donor site, and the nurse should not hesitate to give medications for pain. The pain should subside in 24 to 48 hours as the wound dries. The wound is inspected daily for any signs of infection (erythema, purulent drainage, foul odor). If infection develops, antibiotics may be administered, and the wound treated with wet dressings.

Providing Nutrition

Pathophysiology. Metabolism is increased following moderate-to-severe burns as a result of stress, fluid loss, fever, infection, hypercatabolism, and immobility. Shivering plus the elevated levels of catecholamines, cortisol, and glucagon found shortly after thermal injury increase tissue oxygen consumption and heat production, deplete liver and muscle glycogen stores and fat deposits, and lead to negative nitrogen balance and weight loss. Protein is broken down, providing amino acids for gluconeogenesis, and amino acids are prevented from incorporating into protein. The diminished rate of protein production prolongs wound healing and increases the patient's susceptibility to infection.

A burn patient remains catabolic until the caloric intake exceeds caloric expenditure. Hypermetabolism continues until the wounds are 90% healed[156] and ho-

healed and are used early in wound management and if there is a well-defined area of full-thickness burn. Areas that benefit from full-thickness grafts are the hands, neck, and face. Full-thickness grafts can also be used in rehabilitative stages to restore body function and to repair areas of released skin contractures.

Tangential excision and grafting is a surgical procedure in which the necrotic tissue or eschar is excised down to viable tissue or fascia and immediately covered with autograft or skin substitute. The procedure is best performed between the second and fifth burn day. This technique is used with a well-defined partial-thickness injury in which deep epidermal cells remain intact for primary healing. Advantages of tangential excision and grafting are outlined in the box above.

Graft sites require skilled nursing management. Autografts are delicate and should not be dislodged. The grafted area may be covered with a large, occlusive, bulky dressing to hold new skin securely in place. Splints may be applied in the operating room to provide immobilization and maintain position.

The dressing remains intact for 48 to 72 hours unless

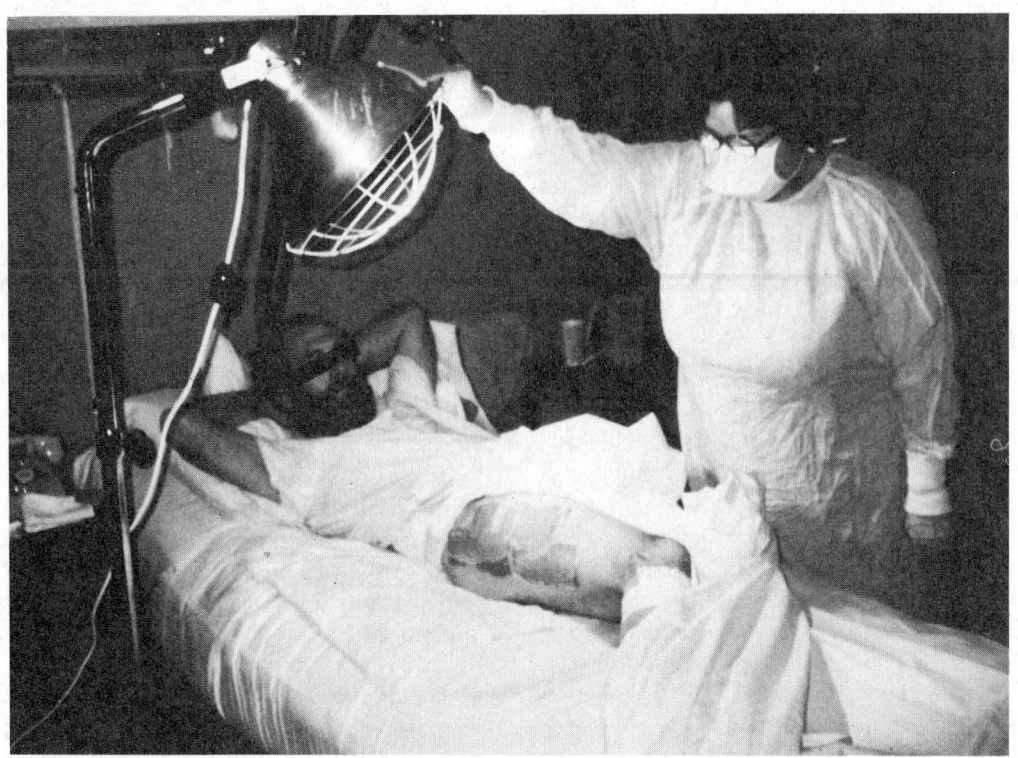

FIGURE 74-11 Heat lamp used to dry donor site to promote epithelialization from deep layers and to prevent infection. (Courtesy Burn Center, Metro Health Medical Center Cleveland.)

meostasis is restored. The patient's total energy and protein requirements become those needed for normal homeostasis plus those required to offset the catabolic state and repair the injury.

Nutritional assessment and supplement. Maintenance of a nutritional support program is critical to survival and is initiated on admission. The goals of the nutritional support program are to establish eating by the traditional route as soon as possible and to maintain sufficient caloric and protein intake to restore tissue loss. A team approach provides comprehensive input and integrates the efforts of the patient, physician, nurse, pharmacist, dietitian, and occupational and physical therapists. A nutritional assessment is made during the first days of the burn injury and includes anthropometric measurements (to determine actual weight loss compared with ideal weight), laboratory studies (electrolytes, liver function tests, urine) (see Chapter 40), and skin testing (if indicated to determine immune response) (see Chapter 76).

The protein and caloric needs of the burned person are highly variable, depending on the extent and depth of injury and the patient's age, sex, preburn nutritional status, and preexisting diseases. The daily *protein* requirement is greater than normal because of the negative nitrogen balance. The normal daily protein requirement is 0.8 gm/kg of body weight for the adult. The massive mobilization of protein after the burn injury increases the daily requirement by two to four times the amount required before the injury: approximately 1.5 to 3.2 gm/kg of body weight. Protein must be used for tissue repair and healing, not as a source of energy. Therefore, it is important to provide adequate carbohydrate and fat calories to satisfy energy needs. An appreciable loss of *zinc* generally accompanies a protein and weight loss. Studies demonstrate that zinc deficiency impairs wound healing, and recent data indicate that a zinc deficiency will impair cellular immunity.[42]

The daily *caloric* requirement increases from a normal 1700 to 3000 calories to 3500 to 50,000 calories. Because the demand for calories increases with a major burn, appropriate vitamin therapy is essential. *Vitamins* and *minerals* are given at two to three times the recommended daily allowances established for normal healthy adults. Vitamin C promotes healing and the daily requirement in the burn patient increases from a normal of 45 mg to 1 to 2 g. The B-complex vitamins are necessary for the metabolism of the increased protein and carbohydrate intake. Vitamins A, E, and K and folic acid are monitored and supplemented as indicated. Serum levels of calcium, phosphate, and potassium are also monitored, and therapeutic levels of iron must be maintained to prevent the ongoing threat of anemia associated with burn injury.

Weight loss and gain are monitored for evaluation of nutritional status. *Weight gain* occurs initially because of fluid retention; however, after diuresis there is a marked loss of weight. Severe *weight loss* is closely related to protein loss or the loss of body cell mass and the enormous amount of body fluid lost through the burn wound itself. As in other metabolic responses, weight loss depends on the extent of injury: the greater the burn, the greater the weight loss.

The nutritional supplements given to the severely burned patient in the emergent period are aimed at stabilization and electrolyte balance to maintain stable cardiovascular function. Patients are initially supported with 5% or 10% dextrose solution.

Feeding methods. Paralytic ileus or gastric dilation is frequently seen in severely burned patients because of the neuroendocrine response to stress, hypovolemia, or septicemia. This prevents enteral feeding until the gastrointestinal tract mobility is restored. Total parenteral nutrition (TPN) is indicated once fluid resuscitation is completed. TPN with supplemental fat solutions is used to provide calories (see Chapter 41).

Oral or tube feeding is the preferred method of providing adequate nutrition and is used as soon as possible. The enteral route is the most natural and convenient means of nutritional support. The burn patient will seldom consume more food from meals after injury than before injury; therefore, a combination of parenteral and enteral modes may be necessary to provide the enormous nutritional requirements. Dietary supplements that contain additional calories and protein can be provided by milkshakes that can be specially made by the hospital dietary department. Patients should be encouraged to drink supplements between meals.

Postburn lactose intolerance may occur in patients being tube fed. Signs of bloating, flatulence, cramps, and diarrhea may be seen. A modification of the strength and type of supplement may be necessary; and starting the supplement at one-half or one-quarter strength, diluted with water, will often alleviate gastrointestinal complications.

Tube feedings provide a continuous 24-hour infusion of nutrition. Tube feedings are a high-caloric, high-protein commercially prepared supplement. These supplements, containing 1 kcal/ml, are hypertonic and, because of hypertonicity, diarrhea is common. The best means of administering tube feeding is a continuous, slow infusion through a small-diameter, soft, pliable tube inserted through the esophagus into the stomach or duodenum (see Chapter 41). Diarrhea, nausea, vomiting, and an uncomfortable feeling of fullness may be avoided with a slow, continuous infusion using an infusion pump to regulate the delivery. If diarrhea persists, Kaopectate or paregoric may be added to the supplement or diphenoxylate (Lomotil) may be ordered by the physician.

The patient is advanced to a regular diet as quickly as possible. However, ingenuity by the nurses and dietician are needed to motivate the patient to eat the food necessary to meet nutritional requirements. Relatives can suggest favorite foods. All dressing changes and treatments should be timed so they don't immediately precede meals. Milkshakes can supplement the patient's diet and can be taken more easily than solid foods.

Fecal impaction is a common problem in burn patients. Bulk foods and fruit juices must be stressed. Bulk-forming laxatives such as preparations of the psyllium seed (Metamucil) or a fecal softener such as dioctyl sodium sulfosuccinate (Colace) may be ordered by the physician.

Promoting Comfort

Pain is elicited by specific activities such as wound cleansing and debridement, dressing changes, and physical therapy. Acute pain, with its abrupt onset and finite period of time to resolution, is most successfully treated with analgesics. Analgesics are also used to prevent pain from recurring after it is initially decreased as it takes less medication to prevent pain than abolish it. *Most patients are under medicated for severe burn pain, perhaps from a fear that they will become addicted to the narcotic analgesics.* Doses can be adjusted to the individual needs of each patient.

Psychological pain may be induced or exaggerated because of loneliness. The patient's complaint of pain may be a call for attention that can be met by the presence and touch of the nurse providing care. Anxiety over anticipated procedures that may or may not be painful may cause a progressive increase in the degree of pain experienced.[57] Muscle tension related to fear and apprehension is known to lower pain threshold. Sleep deprivation, a common occurrence in critical care units, can also make the patient less tolerant of pain. Self-hypnosis or relaxation exercises can be effective in altering the perception of either actual or anticipated discomfort and should be consistently reinforced by the team.[18] Nursing interventions that can aid in minimizing pain during dressing changes are outlined in the box on p. 2181. (See Chapter 16 for further discussion on pain.)

REHABILITATION PERIOD

Rehabilitation begins at the time of admission. However, rehabilitation as the third stage of treatment begins when the patient's burn is reduced to less than

NURSING INTERVENTIONS THAT AID IN MINIMIZING PAIN DURING DRESSING CHANGES

Provide analgesic medications 30 minutes before dressing change.

Provide clear explanations to gain patient's cooperation.

Handle burned areas gently.

Use sterile technique (infection causes increased pain).

Encourage patient to participate in treatment whenever possible.

Use distracting techniques (for example, radio, conversation) and relaxation techniques when appropriate.

20% BSA and the patient is capable of assuming some self-care activity. The principles of management are to accomplish functional and cosmetic reconstruction and to return the patient to a productive place in society. It is important to remember that rehabilitation does not end when the patient is discharged. It may take from 2 to 5 years after discharge for the patient to reach a maximum level of emotional and physical adjustment. Nursing diagnoses that may be identified during the rehabilitation period are listed below.

■ ASSESSMENT

Subjective Data

The patient must be helped to maintain range of joint motion to prevent scars from healing in positions that will result in deformity. Complaints of pain and pressure should not be overlooked because damage may occur from an improperly applied splint or poor positioning. It is important that patients understand why ambulation or motion is necessary even though it may be painful.

The emotional impact of a severe burn is enormous. The psychological scars last forever and affect the victim and family for the rest of their lives. The extent to which the family unit adapts depends on how the patient reacts to a new body image and feelings of self-worth.

The hospital environment and hospital personnel influence the adaptation process. In the immediate postburn period, the nurse is primarily concerned with physiologic survival of the patient. At the same time, the nurse must be able to identify psychological problems and coping mechanisms of the patient and family.

Objective Data

The nurse is responsible for assessing the patient's response to positioning, splinting, exercise, and the ability of the patient and family to perform daily wound care after discharge. Correct positioning must be maintained to avoid the development of contractures. The splinted limb is assessed for adequate circulation, cyanosis, temperature, and the presence of pulses. Exercise, activities

of daily living (ADL), and ambulation must be continuously assessed for patient tolerance, both physically and emotionally. Complete and comprehensive instructions followed by return demonstration of wound and dressing care are necessary before discharge.

■ DATA ANALYSIS: NURSING DIAGNOSES

Nursing diagnoses are determined from assessment of patient data. Possible nursing diagnoses for the person with burns may include, but are not limited to, the following:

Diagnostic Title	Possible Etiologies
Activity intolerance	Immobility from splinting, generalized weakness, bed rest, pain
Anxiety	Change in health status, role functioning, socioeconomic status
Body image disturbance	Scarring, contractures, discoloration
Coping, ineffective family: compromised	Inadequate or incorrect information or understanding, prolonged disability of significant person
Coping, ineffective individual	Burn injury, personal vulnerability
Diversional activity deficit	Long-term hospitalization, frequent lengthy treatment, away from work, friends, and usual recreational activities
Fear	Long-term illness, surgery, treatments, changes in lifestyle, pain, disfigurement, job security
Knowledge deficit	Wound and skin care, exercises, use of adaptive devices
Impaired physical mobility	Intolerance to activity, decreased strength and endurance, pain, severe anxiety, contracture formation
Pain	Increased activity (exercise, ADL, ambulation)
Self-care deficit	Intolerance to activity, fatigue, pain and discomfort, severe anxiety

■ PLANNING: EXPECTED PATIENT OUTCOMES

Expected patient outcomes for the person with burns in the rehabilitation period may include, but are not limited to, the following:

1. Patient achieves activity tolerance consistent with desired levels.
2. Patient exhibits decreased anxiety.
3. Patient demonstrates a realistic concept of changes in body image and alterations required in daily activities.
4. Patient exhibits no pain.

5. Patient participates in diversional activities.
6. Patient verbalizes fears and participates in planned interventions that will decrease fears.
7. Patient and family demonstrate correct understanding of self-care activities.
8. Patient achieves optimal joint mobility.
9. Patient demonstrates ability to perform ADL.
10. Family demonstrates appropriate coping skills.

■ IMPLEMENTATION

Preventing Limitations of Mobility

As the survival rate of patients with large and deeper burns increases, so does the challenge to maintain optimal functioning and cosmetic results. Research indicates that the percentage of patients with joint limitations increases as the degree and extent of burns increase. Although these patients may be critically ill, their rehabilitative needs must be addressed immediately. A comprehensive program of positioning, splinting, exercise, ambulation, and activities of daily living must begin on the first or second day postburn and is carried through until after discharge. Any delays in initiating treatment will be detrimental to the patient's ultimate functional outcome. Contractures are among the most serious long-term complications of burns today. They result from muscle and joint stiffening, skin grafting and prolonged bed rest. Although the occupational and physical therapists are primarily responsible for addressing the patient's rehabilitation needs during all phases of the patient's recovery, the nurse is responsible for assuring that all their recommendations are followed.

Therapeutic positioning. Therapeutic positioning, that is, the act of placing body parts in antideformity positions, is vital to the prevention of burn contractures. The patient must be repositioned in bed (side-lying, supine, prone) frequently and regularly during the day and night. Correct positioning varies, depending on the area of the body burned (Table 74-9). Positioning can be enhanced by placing patients on a Stryker frame, a Foster bed, a CircOlectric bed, or one of the many different types of low air loss beds or mattresses currently available. These beds facilitate the use of the bedpan and urinal, permit change of position with a minimum of handling, and permit larger skin surfaces to remain freer from body pressure than is possible when the patient lies on a regular mattress. These special beds are particularly useful when both the back and front of the trunk, thighs, and legs have been burned. These beds allow turning of the patient with a minimum of handling and thus help decrease pain.

Prolonged rest in semi-Fowler's position or with the pillow pushing the head forward must be avoided, even though many patients like this position, because it en-

TABLE 74-9 Therapeutic positioning for the burn patient

Area Burned	Description of Position
Neck	No pillow
	Towel roll under cervical spine
	Neck splint
	90-degree abduction, neutral rotation
Shoulder	Elbow splint may be used to aid in maintaining position
Axilla	Abduction with 10 to 15 degree forward flexion and external rotation
	Support abducted arm with suspension from IV pole, or bedside table
	Axilla splint
Elbow	Extension
	Support extended arm on bedside table, foam trough
	Elbow splint
Hand	Hand splint
Dorsal surface	Flexion
Palmar surface	Hyperextension
Hip	Extension with neutral rotation
	Supine with lower extremity extended
	Prone-lying (if medically appropriate)
	Trochanter roll
	Foam wedge along lateral aspect of thigh
	Knee or long leg splint
Knee	Extension
	Prone-lying (if medically appropriate)
	Patient out of bed with lower extremities extended and elevated
	Knee splint
Ankle	Dorsiflexion
	Padded footboard with heels free of pressure
	Ankle splint

ables them to see about the room better. The bed can often be turned so that the patient can look about without having to assume positions that may lead to the formation of contractures.

Splints. Splints are used to prevent or correct contractures and to immobilize joints after grafting. They are custom-made and often molded directly on the patient to assure optimal conformity (Figure 74-12). It is the responsibility of the nurse to apply the splint properly and according to an established schedule. An improperly applied splint can promote contractures and lead to additional complications. Assess the splinted limb for adequate circulation, cyanosis, temperature, and the presence of pulses. Complaints of pain and pressure should not be overlooked because damage may occur with an improperly applied splint. Some physicians prefer to use the open method of treatment and use frequent exercise to prevent contractures.

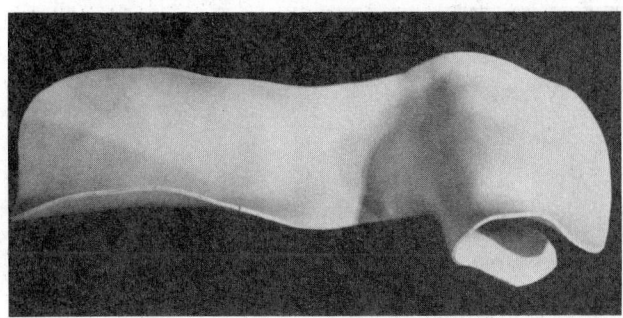

FIGURE 74-12 Orthoplast hand splint. (Courtesy Metro Health Medical Center, Cleveland.)

Exercises and ambulation. Exercises for prevention and correction of contractures are begun as soon as the patient is stable. Active exercises are preferred, although active assistance and gentle pressure exercises may be more realistic. Supervision by a physical or occupational therapist is desirable. Exercises may be performed more easily in water and may be done along with dressing changes if the patient is able to tolerate the activity (Figure 74-13). When burns are completely covered (by healing or by graft), exercises may be performed more easily in an occupational therapy or physical therapy department where the patient may benefit from a change in environment.

Ambulation decreases the risk of thromboemboli, promotes optimal ventilation, helps maintain range of motion and strength in the lower extremities, orients the patient to the environment, and provides a sense of functional independence. Mobilizing patients with large burns who have less ability to tolerate activity requires a progressive approach. Initially the patient may need to be transferred with maximum assistance onto a stretcher chair and progress to a sitting position. Gradually, the patient may progress to a standing pivot transfer into a nearby chair and eventually ambulate with minimal assistance. Before getting out of bed, an elastic bandage support must be applied to the lower extremities to prevent venous stasis, edema, and orthostatic hypotension.

Promoting Independence

One of the ultimate goals in the rehabilitation of the burned patient is to maintain or restore the patient's independence in performing the activities of daily living. The occupational therapist aids in this process by selecting activities that are appropriate to the patient's medical, physical, and mental status. Activities that the nurse can encourage are self-feeding, telephoning, reading mail, and assisting with grooming or burn wound management. The nurse must know what the patient is being taught by the physical and occupational therapist so that progress can be continued on the nursing unit.

After the initial period, the long healing process begins, accompanied by the realization of endless implications for the future. Burns on the face make adjustments particularly difficult. Different kinds of fears include the following: death, pain, disfigurement, prolonged hospitalization, job security, disruption of lifestyle, and reaction of family and friends.

To the adolescent, the thought of being different or conspicious may be unbearable. If possible, the patient should see facial burns only after being prepared for the experience. Support and understanding will be needed

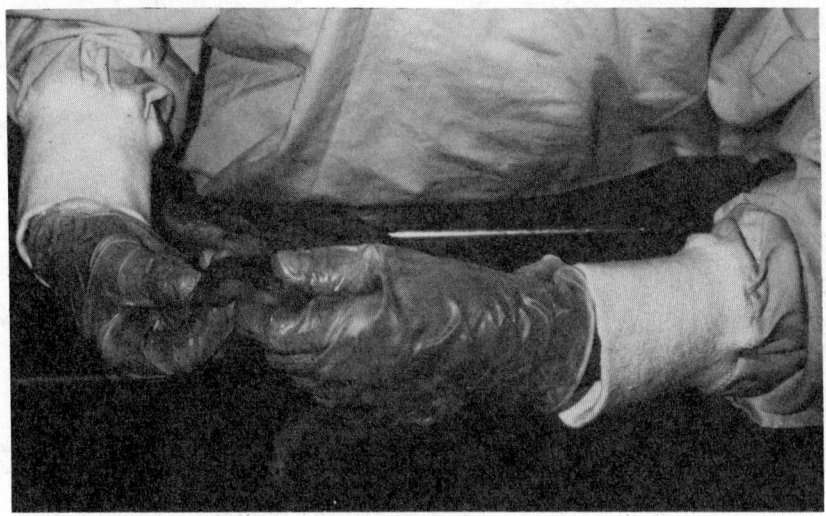

FIGURE 74-13 Passive range of motion exercise during hydrotherapy. (Courtesy Burn Center, Metro Health Medical Center, Cleveland.)

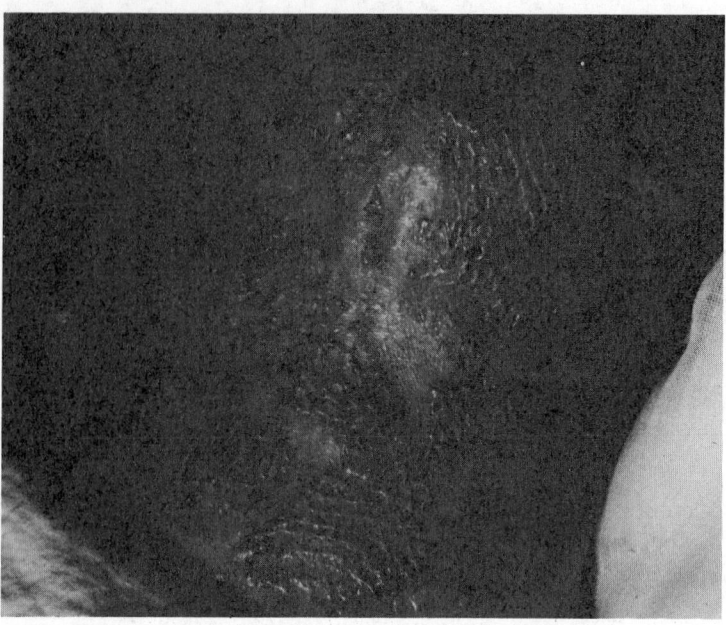

FIGURE 74-14 Hypertrophic scarring over chest and abdomen. (Courtesy Burn Center, Metro Health Medical Center, Cleveland.)

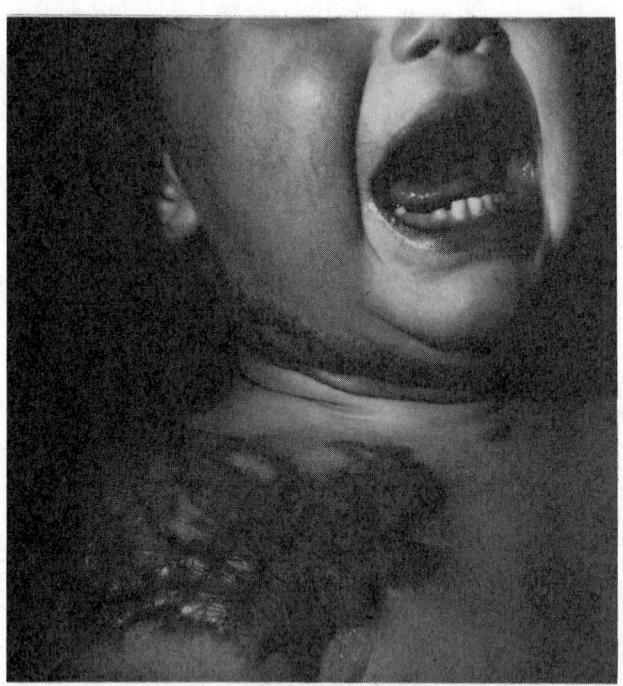

FIGURE 74-15 Scar formation occurring from lack of pressure dressing application. (Courtesy Burn Center, Metro Health Medical Center, Cleveland.)

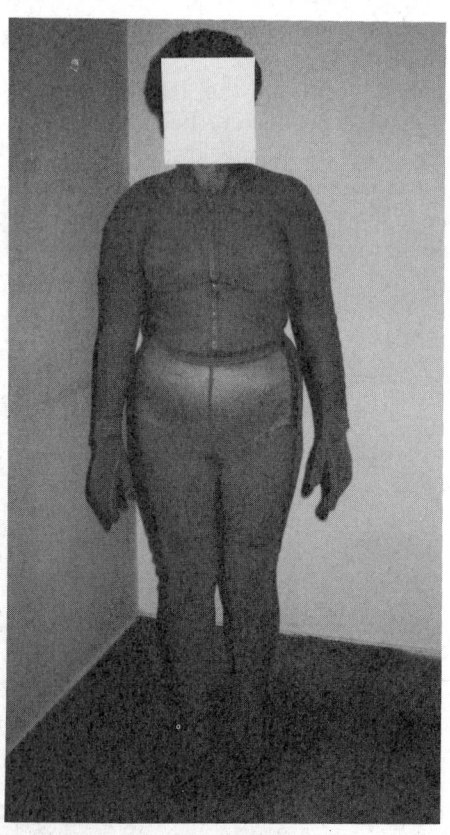

FIGURE 74-16 Total body Jobst garment consisting of three separate pieces: jacket, pants, and gloves. (Courtesy Burn Center, Metro Health Medical Center, Cleveland.)

for the person to cope with what will be seen in the mirror. The patient will exhibit readiness by asking to look in the mirror. Interaction with other burn patients who are further along in the healing process may help the patient feel that recovery is possible. In some cases, the recovery is incredible, and although differences in skin pigmentation remain, the redness that accompanies healed burn wounds often fades considerably within a few months. Pigmentation problems are more acute for persons with brown or black skin. Their healed skin may be a different shade, freckled, or whitish.

Providing Emotional Support

The patient should have the opportunity to talk about any concerns or fears. Some patients may discuss these with the nurse when they cannot express them to relatives, and the nurse must be prepared to listen and help the individual accept necessary changes in lifestyle. Almost every burned patient and family needs the help of a social worker. The nurse should recognize this need and initiate the referral. Visiting hours can be used to talk with relatives who may be able to give information that will clarify the patient's needs and resources. This time also provides opportunity for the nurse to help relatives accept their loved one's change in appearance and to help them plan for the return of the loved one to the community.

Preventing Scarring

Anytime a wound of connective tissue heals, hypertrophic scarring will occur unless the skin is adhered to the underlying structure. Hypertrophic scarring results from the overgrowth and overproduction of tissue. This occurs especially in areas of stress and movement such as the hands, legs, and chest (Figure 74-14). The thickened rigid scar that results may later cause contractures. The application of controlled constant pressure to the surface of an immature scar will reduce the scar and leave a smooth pliable tissue. If this pressure is applied to new healthy tissue, hypertrophic scarring can be prevented (Figure 74-15). The Jobst garment, a specially designed elastic woven material, provides tridimensional control. It is fitted to each patient individually and then custom made (Figure 74-16). Until the garment is completed, bandages can be used for a pressure dressing. Even though pressure garments help decrease the formation of thick, disfiguring scars, patient acceptance is a problem. The garments are uncomfortable and make the patient warm, especially during hot weather. They must be tight enough to produce the 24 torr of pressure required to exceed capillary pressure and thus reduce edema and scar formation. The patient must wear the garments 23 hours a day for 6 months to a year.

A plan for exercise and splinting must be established before discharge. To prevent scar contracture, daily therapy sessions may be necessary for several weeks or months. Helpful aids can be developed by the occupational therapist to help with the activities of daily living.

Discharge Teaching

Before discharge, burned patients and their families have a great need for education so that they may take increasing responsibilities for their own care. Discharge teaching involves the entire burn team, and because rehabilitation is a gradual process, there should be ample time to plan the return home in every detail.

Early discharge planning accomplishes two goals. First, it helps solve problems early; for example, if the patient's house burned and needs to be repaired, the family may need to relocate. This could be done before discharge, thus preventing the added stress of moving after discharge. Second, early discharge planning emphasizes the future. If discharge is discussed, the patient and his or her family may realize more quickly that recovery and return to a fulfilling and productive life are achievable.

Complete and comprehensive instructions followed by return demonstrations contribute to learning the necessary skills to be independent in self-care activities after discharge. Patients should not be discharged from the hospital until they can care for themselves physically, with assistance if necessary, and are prepared to meet the stresses involved in returning to their former living patterns.

Teaching includes the following content areas: wound management; signs and symptoms of complications; use of pressure dressings; exercises, splinting, and activities of daily living; and methods of coping with resocialization.

Wound management instructions should include how to care for the healed graft and nongrafted areas (see p. 2186). Signs and symptoms of complications, including areas that may blister and break down, and signs of infection are also addressed.

Instructions should be written so that the patient has reference material available after discharge to answer questions. An example of written discharge instructions is provided on p. 2186. The patient and family are also given the name and phone number of a doctor or nurse who can be contacted to answer questions. A home health nurse may be of assistance in dressing the patients wounds.

Promoting Resocialization

After discharge, the patient has to adjust to temporary or permanent function loss, cosmetic disfigurement, and the reactions of others. The ability to make these adjustments will depend on coping mechanisms before the burn, the severity and site of the burn, and the reac-

DISCHARGE INSTRUCTIONS FOR BURN PATIENT

We on the burn team are happy to see that you are able to go home. To ensure you the speediest possible recovery, it is important that you are able to care for yourself and recognize problems that may interfere with your complete recovery.

If any of the following occur, please call the hospital and ask for the Burn Clinic. The nurse will be able to assist you.
1. Healed area breaking open. Cover with clean dressing.
2. Formation of blisters.
3. Signs of infection:
   a. Fever, temperature over 37.2° C (99° F).
   b. Redness, pain, swelling, hardness, or warmth in or around wound or any other part of body.
   c. Increased or foul-smelling drainage from wound.
3. Problems with your Ace bandages or Jobst garment such as improper fit, formation of blisters, or opening of healed area underneath.

Your first clinic appointment will be on _____. If a family member can come with you they can register for you and you may go to the Burn Clinic waiting room.

BATHING

Bathing or showering daily in your usual manner cleans the wounds, especially the ones that are still open.
1. Check the water and be sure to adjust the temperature to a warm and comfortable level. Your skin is more sensitive to extra heat or cold and can be easily injured.
2. Wash gently with a clean soft washcloth, using a mild detergent soap such as Dreft or Ivory Snow, approximately 2 tsp. Be careful not to rub too hard so as not to disturb the grafted areas. Avoid harsh or deodorant soaps.
3. Rinse skin thoroughly after washing.
4. Dry thoroughly.
5. Apply specific dressing as instructed.

CARE FOR BURN WOUND

These are your guidelines for the care of your burn wound. During this time, look at the involved areas and note if there are any changes that need to be reported.
1. Wash hands
2. Remove dressing and dispose in paper bag or wrap in newspaper.
3. Wash hands.
4. Wash open area with gauze using solution of Dreft (or Ivory Snow) and water. Add 1 tbsp Dreft to a basin of water; 2 tbsp Dreft, if you use the bathtub. Use a clean towel and washcloth with each dressing change.
5. Rinse skin well.
6. Wash hands.
7. Apply dressing as described below.
8. Wear gloves. Wash basin or bathtub with a disinfectant such as Lysol.
9. Wash hands.

CARE OF CLOTHING

When you are discharged, you may find that healed burn areas are sensitive to harsh detergents, fabric softeners, and clothing dyes. If you are sensitive, we suggest the following:

1. Launder new clothing before use by machine or hand with Dreft or Ivory Snow.
2. Rinse clothes twice.
3. Do not use fabric softeners.
4. If you have open burns or a healed area that opens, wash all clothes separately from other family members.
5. Scarlet red ointment will permanently stain clothing.
6. If dyes used in clothing cause irritation, wear white articles.

ACE BANDAGES

You have been taught to put on your own Ace bandages while in the hospital; but if you do have a problem with this, please notify the Burn Clinic. It is also important that you know how to care for them and understand problems that occur.
1. If they are too loose, they will be ineffective and must be rewrapped.
2. If they are too tight, they will cause discomfort, numbness, tingling, and puffiness and must be rewrapped.
3. They must be worn for a long period of time, probably 6-12 months to be effective, so please do not stop wearing them until your doctor tells you.
4. To care for your Ace bandages:
   a. Hand wash with Dreft or Ivory Snow in cold water.
   b. Towel dry.
   c. Lay flat or place over rod or clothesline.
   d. Do not use clothespins.

JOBST GARMENT

You have been taught to put on your Jobst garment while in the hospital; but if you have a problem with this, please notify the Burn Clinic. It is also important that you know how to care for it and understand problems that can occur.
1. If it is too loose, it will be ineffective and you will require a new garment.
2. If it is too tight, it will cause discomfort, numbness, and tingling. Do not wear it if this occurs, but notify the Burn Clinic as soon as possible.
3. To care for your Jobst garment:
   a. Hand wash with Dreft or Ivory Snow in cold water.
   b. Towel dry.
   c. Lay flat or place over rod or clothesline.
   d. Do not use clothespins.

Courtesy Burn Service, MetroHealth Medical Center, Cleveland.

DATA: Mr. Smith is a 54-year-old businessman, married with two children. He fell asleep while smoking in bed. He woke up after several minutes to discover his bed on fire. He was admitted to the hospital with 25% of his body burned, including his anterior arms, chest, abdomen and scattered areas on his thighs. Six hours after admission he was receiving 40% oxygen through a face mask. Vital signs were as follows: heart rate 120 beats/min, respiratory rate 30 beats/min, blood pressure 140/80, temperature 38.8 C. Two peripheral IVs were placed, each running at 250 ml/hr. A Foley catheter has drained 50 ml the past hour. Mr. Smith has a productive cough of gray-tinged sputum and a hoarse voice. Breath sounds clear with coughing. His wounds were cleansed with Dreft and normal saline and covered with a Silvadene dressing. He complained of nausea and a nasogastric tube was inserted. Antacids were ordered to be administered every 2 hours via tube.

The nursing history identified the following:
- He smokes 1½ packs/day; he has tried several times to quit.
- The same day, his wife feared that he would fall asleep while smoking.
- He owns his own business.

NURSING DIAGNOSIS

Ineffective airway clearance: related to laryngeal edema and irritation from smoke inhalation and history of cigarette smoking

Expected Patient Outcomes	Nursing Interventions	Rationale
Mr. Smith maintains adequate ventilation and oxygenation	Assess and document rate, depth and ease of respirations; note type, amount, color of sputum; observe patient's color	Increased respiratory effort, large amounts of tenacious, gray-tinged sputum and signs of tissue hypoxia indicate the need for endotracheal intubation
		Providing oxygen will increase oxygen supply to body tissues
	Provide respiratory treatment and medications as ordered (pulmonary drainage and clapping, incentive spirometer, bronchodilators)	Respiratory treatments will loosen and thin secretions and will allow patient to clear his own airway
	Turn patient every 2 hours	Change in position will help mobilize secretions

Collaborative nursing actions include those to prevent hypovolemia from the movement of fluid from the intravascular to the interstitial compartment, to prevent respiratory distress, and to prevent gastrointestinal distress. Immediate reporting of the early signs of hypovolemia and/or respiratory distress may prevent serious effects (hypovolemic shock, respiratory failure). Nursing actions include monitoring for the following:

- Signs of hypovolemia: increased heart rate, decreased urine output, decreased blood pressure, decreased sensorium
- Signs of respiratory distress: increased respiratory rate, shortness of breath, change in patient's color, increased work of breathing, change in ABGs (decreasing pH, decreasing pO_2, increasing pCO_2)
- Signs of gastrointestinal distress: low gastric pH, heme + nasogastric aspirate, absence of bowel sounds

NURSING DIAGNOSIS

Potential fluid volume deficit

Expected Patient Outcomes	Nursing Intervention	Rationale
Mr. Smith maintains optimal fluid balance	Provide calculated IV fluids.	Calculated IV fluids will prevent patient from developing hypovolemic shock.
	Monitor and document output hourly.	Any deficit or increase in fluid intake or output must be identified quickly to avoid complications of hypovolemia.
	Assess for clinical signs of hypovolemia (decreased sensorium; changes in skin from pink to pale, from warm to cool).	These may be the first signs of hypovolemia.
	Weigh daily; compare to preinjury weight.	Weight is an accurate assessment of fluid balance.

Continued.

NURSING CARE PLAN

PERSON WITH BURNS—cont'd

NURSING DIAGNOSIS

Pain: related to exposed nerve endings from burn injury

Expected Patient Outcomes	Nursing Interventions	Rationale
Mr. Smith experiences minimal pain	Provide with pain medication as ordered; administer 30 minutes before dressing changes (hydrotherapy and debridement); evaluate and document effectiveness.	Decreasing pain will decrease anxiety and increase patient's cooperation during dressing changes.
	Assess need for other interventions that may decrease pain experience (use of the radio, relaxation therapy, hypnosis).	The pain experience is subjective; a variety of pain control techniques may decrease the pain experience.
	Assess pain history and response to pain.	Information about past pain experiences will aid in planning techniques for pain control.
	Educate patient about painful procedures and about techniques to reduce pain; encourage patient to participate in treatments whenever possible.	Information and participation may help decrease the anxiety that is often seen with pain.
	Use environmental comfort measures (speak in calm manner, keep warm).	Comfortable environment may decrease anxiety and pain.

NURSING DIAGNOSIS

Anxiety

Expected Patient Outcome	Nursing Interventions	Rationale
Mr. Smith demonstrates control of anxiety	Gather information about background, personality, and level of coping from friends, family, and patient (as appropriate).	Information will assist the nurse in planning interventions to decrease anxiety.
	Offer patient and family simple explanations of his or her injury and treatments.	Too much information may overwhelm patient and increase anxiety.
	Assess ability to cope with illness; consult with other services.	Social services or pastoral care may be able to provide assistance to the patient.

NURSING DIAGNOSIS

Potential for infection: related to loss of skin from burn injury

Expected Patient Outcomes	Nursing Interventions	Rationale
Mr. Smith is free of pathogenic organisms	Document initial appearance of the burn wound (color, dryness, odor).	Early changes in appearance of wound may be the first signs of infection.
	Monitor for signs of infection (fever, altered sensorium, increased respiratory rate, foul odor from wound).	Early detection of infection will allow appropriate antibiotics to be prescribed before serious injury occurs.
	Implement isolation procedures.	To protect the patient from other organisms that may cause infection.

NURSING CARE PLAN

PERSON WITH BURNS— cont'd

NURSING DIAGNOSIS

IMPAIRED SKIN INTEGRITY: RELATED TO BURN INJURY

Expected Patient Outcomes	Nursing Interventions	Rationale
Mr. Smith demonstrates viable healing tissue	Perform prescribed wound care (hydrotherapy and debridement); assess wound during each dressing change. Assess need for equipment and supplies and have available before wound care.	Wound care procedures may change daily, depending on assessment of wound. Adequate supplies should be ordered ahead of time to avoid the problem of discovering halfway through the dressing change that there are not enough supplies available.

tion of others. How well the patient is adapting to these changes can be evaluated during out-patient visits when the burn team and appropriate personnel are available.

Follow-up care may not take place at the institution where the patient was hospitalized if the patient lives several hundred miles away. The burn team members may need to contact their counterparts in the community to plan follow-up care. If possible, a member of the follow-up team should visit the patient in the hospital before discharge.

Job retraining may be necessary if the burn injury caused loss of joint function or other physical limitations that may prevent the patient from returning to a former job. The local office of the State Labor and Industry Board can assign a vocational counselor to help the patient return to the work force. Even if retraining cannot begin for several months, the contact with the vocational counselor and anticipation of retraining may help the patient look beyond immediate problems and think of the future.

CHAPTER SUMMARY

✔ The severity of a burn injury depends on the age of the victim, body part involved, burning agent, size and depth of the burn wound, and the victim's medical history.

✔ The initial care for a burn includes removing the victim from the source of the burn and dousing the burn with water.

✔ The initial systemic response to a burn is the shift of fluid from the intravascular to the interstitial space, creating hypovolemia. This is treated with a calculated dose of lactated Ringer's solution. After 48 to

72, hours the fluid shifts from the interstitial to the intravascular space and hypervolemia occurs.

✔ Emotional support to the victim and the victim's family is an important role for nurses.

✔ Burn wounds must be assessed on a daily basis.

✔ Correct splinting and positioning are the best methods for preventing contractures.

✔ There is no way to predict the appearance of a burn wound after healing.

QUESTIONS TO CONSIDER

■ What factors determine the severity of burns?

■ What is the difference between the hypovolemic stage and the diuretic stage after a severe burn? What is the pathophysiology of each stage?

■ How would you intervene with a burn patient who refuses to participate in his care?

■ What nursing interventions are appropriate in minimizing pain during burn dressing changes?

■ How would you assess the nutritional state of a burn patient?

REFERENCES AND SELECTED READINGS

1. Abshagen D: Topical agents and emergency care for minor burn injuries, J Emerg Nurse 10:325-331, 1984.
2. Achauer BM and Martinez SE: Burn wound pathophysiology and care, Crit Care Clin 1(1):47-58, 1985.

*References preceded by an asterisk are particularly well suited for student reading.

3. Achauer BM: Management of the burned patient, Norwalk, Conn, 1987, Appleton and Lange.

4. American Burn Association, Guidelines for service standards and severity classifications in the treatment of burn injury, American College of Surgeons Bulletin 69:24-28, 1984.

5. *Andreason NJC et al: Management of emotional reactions in seriously burned adults, N Eng J Med 286:65-69, 1972.

6. *Artz CP, Moncrief JA, and Pruitt BA: Burns: a team approach, Philadelphia, 1979, WB Saunders Co.

7. Bayley EW and Smith GA: The three degrees of burn care, Nurs' 87, 17(3):34-41, 1987.

8. *Bernstein NR: Emotional care of the facially burned and disfigured, Boston, 1976, Little, Brown & Co.

9. Busby HD: Nursing management of the acute burn patient and nursing managment of optimal burn recovery, J Cont Educ Nurse 10:16-30, 1979.

10. Cockshott WP: The history of the treatment of burns, Surg Gynecol Obstet 102:116-124, 1956.

11. Cooke SS: Major thermal injury—the first 48 hours, Crit Care Nurse 6(1):55-62, 1986.

12. Demling RH: Fluid replacement in burned patients, Surg Clin North Am 67(1):15-30, 1987.

13. Dyer C: Burn care in the emergent period, J Emerg Nurse 6:9-16, 1980.

14. Fang CH et al: Burn treatment: covering burn wounds with autologous microskin grafts, AORN J 49(2):526-534, 1989.

15. *Feller I and Archanbeault C: Nursing the burned patient, Ann Arbor, 1973, Institute for Burn Medicine Press.

16. *Feller I, Jones CA, and Richards K: Emergent care of the burn victim, Ann Arbor, 1977, Institute for Burn Medicine Press.

17. Finlayson L: Emergent care of the burn patient, Crit Care Update 7:18-19, 22-23, 1980.

18. Freeman JW: Nursing care of the patient with a burn injury, Crit Care Nurs 4:52-68, 1984.

19. Gatson SF and Schumann LL: Burn wound management, Crit Care Update 7:5-17, 1980.

20. Heidrich B, Perry S, and Amand R: Nursing staff attitudes about burn pain, J Burn Care Rehabil 2:259-261, 1981.

21. Hills SW and Birmingham JJ: Burn care, Bethany, Conn, 1981, Flescher Publishing Co.

22. Hummel RP: Clinical burn therapy: a management and prevention guide, Littleton, MA, 1982, John Wright Co.

23. Jacoby FG: Care of the massive burn wound, Crit Care Quart 7(3):44-53, 1984.

24. Jacoby FG: Nursing care of the patient with burns, ed 2, St Louis, 1976, CV Mosby Co.

25. Jelenko C: Burn shock, Top Emerg Med 3:69-74, 1981.

26. Johnson CL and Cain VJ: The rehab guide, Am J Nurs 85(1):48-50, 1985.

27. Kenner C and Manning S: Emergency care of the burn patient, Crit Care Update 7:24-27, 30-33, 1980.

28. Kilbee E: Burn pain management, Crit Care Quart 7(3): 54-62, 1984.

29. King MW: Nursing considerations of the burned patient during the emergent pariod, Heart Lung 11(4):353-363, 1982.

30. Kinzie V and Lau C: What to do for the severely burned, RN 43(4):46-51, 104-110, 1980.

31. Klein DG and O'Malley P: Topical injury from chemical agents: initial treatment, Heart Lung 16(1):49-54, 1987.

32. Larson DL et al: Techniques for decreasing scar formation and contractures in the burned patient, J Trauma 11:807, 1971.

33. Lemaster JE: Rehabilitation of the burn-injured patient. In Wachtel TL, Kahn V, and Frank HA, editors: Current concepts in burn care, Rockville, MD, 1983, Aspen Systems Corp.

34. Luterman A, Adams A, and Curreri PW: Nutritional management of the burn patient, Crit Care Quart 7(3):34-43, 1984.

35. Martin LM: Nursing implications of today's burn care techniques, RN 52:26-33, 1989.

36. Marvin JA: Planning home care for the burn patients, Nurs' 83 13(8):65-67, 1983.

37. Marvin JA: Acute care of the burn patient, Crit Care Quart 1:25-35, 1978.

38. Mechanic HF and Dunn LT: Nutritional support for the burn patient, Dimens Crit Care Nurse 5(1):20-29, 1986.

39. Mosley S: Inhalation injury: a review of the literature, Heart Lung 17(1):3-9, 1988.

40. Nadel E and Kozerefski PM: Rehabilitation of the critically ill burn patient, Crit Care Quart 7(3):19-33, 1984.

41. Nowicki CR and Sprenger CK: Temporary skin substitutes for burn patients: a nursing perspective, J Burn Care Rehabil 9(2):209-215, 1988.

42. Pasulka PS and Wachtel TL: Nutritional considerations for the burned patient, Surg Clin North Am 67(1):109-132, 1987.

43. Perry SW et al: Pain perception vs. pain response in burn patients, Am J Nurs 87(5):698, 1987.

44. Pruitt BA and Goodwin CW: Stress ulcer disease in the burned patient, World J Surg 5:209, 1981.

45. Ragiel CA: The impact of critical injury on patient, family, and clinical systems, Crit Care Quart 7(3):73-78, 1984.

46. Rauscher LA and Ochs GM: Prehospital care of the seriously burned patient. In Wachtel TL, Kahn V, and Frank HA, editors: Current topics in burn care, Rockville, MD, 1983, Aspen Systems Corp.

47. Robertson KE, Cross PJ, and Terry JC: Burn care: the critical first days, Am J Nurs 85(1):30-45, 1985.

48. Rosequist CC and Shepp PH: The nutrition factor, Am J Nurs 85(1):45-47, 1985.

49. *Salisbury RE, Newman NM, and Dingeldein GD, editors: Manual of burn theraputics, Boston, 1983, Little, Brown & Co Inc.

50. Shenkman B and Stechmiller J: Patient and family perception of projected functioning after discharge from a burn unit, Heart Lung 16(5):490-496, 1987.

51. Surveyer JA: Smoke inhalation injuries, Heart Lung 9(5):825-832, 1980.

52. Trunkey DD: Transporting the critically burned patient. In Wachtel TL, Kahn V, and Frank HA, editors: Current concepts in burn care, Rockville, MD, 1983, Aspen Systems Corp.

53. Trunkey DD: Transporting the critically burned patient, Top Emerg Med 3:21-24, 1981.

54. Wachtel TL et al: Initial management of major burns. In Wachtel TL, Kahn V, and Frank HA, editors: Current concepts in burn care, Rockville, MD, 1983, Aspen Systems Corp.

55. Wachtel TL and Fortune JB: Fluid resuscitation for burn shock. In Wachtel TL, Kahn V, and Frank HA, editors: Current concepts in burn care, Rockville, MD, 1983, Aspen Systems Corp.

56. Wachtel TL et al: Nutritional support for burned patients. In Wachtel TL, Kahn V, and Frank HA, editors: Current concepts in burn care, Rockville, MD, 1983, Aspen Systems Corp.

57. Walkenstein MD: Comparison of burned patients perception of pain with nurses perception of pain, J Burn Care Rehabil 3:233-236, 1982.

58. Wingate E: Emergent burn care: a time for life-saving measures, Crit Care Update 10:49-54, 1983.

CHAPTER 75

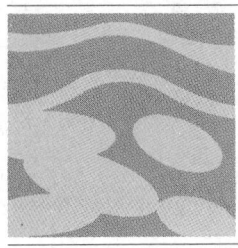

Assessment of the Immune System

E. RONALD WRIGHT
BARBARA C. LONG

CHAPTER OBJECTIVES

After studying this chapter, the student should be able to:
1. Summarize the essential components of the immune system.
2. Describe assessment parameters for evaluation of the immune response.
3. Identify diagnostic tests for immune disorders.

This chapter provides a brief review of the essential components of the immune system, related assessment data, and appropriate diagnostic tests. Disorders of the immune system are described in Chapter 76.

REVIEW OF THE IMMUNE SYSTEM

Human beings cannot survive in our biologic environment without the internal protective mechanisms known as the *nonspecific* and *specific immune response systems*. The basic systems and their functions are described in detail in Chapter 8. These systems provide protection against encroachment by foreign cells and body-damaging substances. They distribute throughout the body a wide array of cells and substances that recognize and take action against invading agents. The specific immune response system can be separated into two categories of response: (1) the *humorally mediated system* or *B cell system*, which furnishes protection through the production of circulating immunoglobulins (antibodies); and (2) the *cell mediated system* or *T cell system*, which provides specifically reactive cells (cytotoxic T cells). The three systems are capable of independent response; however, they function in a highly interrelated manner when a foreign substance is introduced into the body (Figure 75-1).

Each of the systems contains components that can destroy not only foreign materials or cells but also normal body cells; therefore the potent, destructive mechanisms must be very carefully and selectively controlled. The proper immune response, then, is provided when the systems respond in the correct amounts to the appropriate signals at the proper time and place. Underresponse or lack of response does not provide adequate protection. Overresponse or inappropriate response may damage normal body cells and tissues (Chapter 76).

Careful assessment of the components of the immune response system determines whether the individual (1) has the ability to respond appropriately, (2) has inappropriately responded, and/or (3) has responded to non-self encroachment, and in what ways.

INTERNAL NONSPECIFIC IMMUNE RESPONSE

The internal nonspecific immune response system is a collection of cells and proteins found in the blood and tissues that nonspecifically recognizes and responds to the introduction of foreign materials or damaged self-cells. The response is the same no matter what the initiating injury or material; only the degree of response varies in relation to the extent of the damage. The outcome of the response is the *inflammatory response*.

COMPONENTS OF THE SYSTEM

The *phagocytic* cells of the body are a key component of this nonspecific response. Those cells include the *granulocytic white blood cells*, especially the *neutrophils*. In response to tissue injury or presence of infectious microorganisms in the body, chemotactic substances are carried via the blood to the bone marrow where phagocytic cells are formed and stored until they are signaled to be released in large numbers into the blood. They are then drawn by the chemotactic substances to the site of injury where they leave the vessels and move into the tissues. In the tissues they engulf and destroy foreign materials.

The *complement* system of the blood is another major factor in nonspecific response. The system is composed of inactive serum proteins that, when activated in a sequential series of steps, have the ability to damage cell membranes and produce lysis of the cell. The system

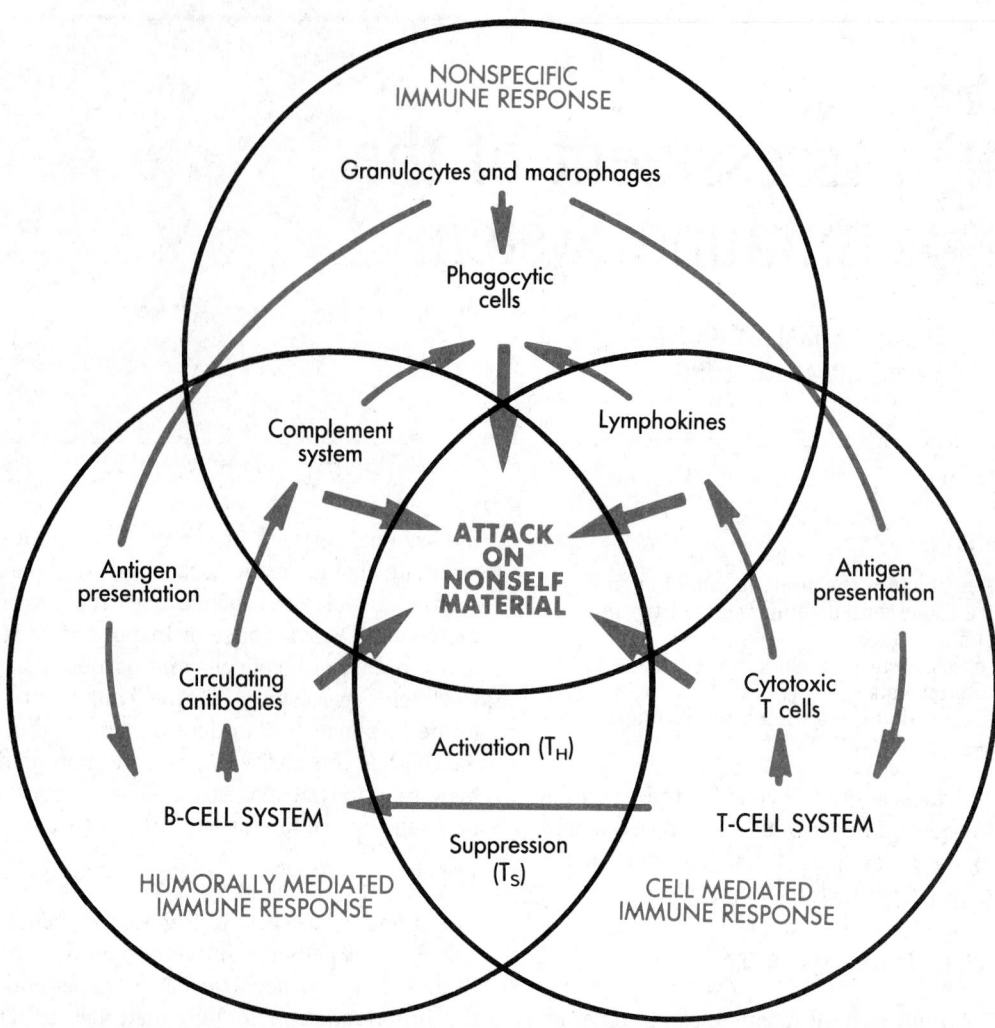

FIGURE 75-1 Interrelationship of nonspecific, humorally mediated, and cell mediated immune response systems.

can be activated by the binding of specific antibodies to foreign cell antigens, by certain bacterial cell components, or by materials released from damaged tissue cells.

Other factors that appear in the body in response to the inflammatory response include the *acute-phase proteins*. These proteins are synthesized by the liver and multiply in the serum to provide materials that mediate the inflammatory response.

INTERNAL SPECIFIC IMMUNE RESPONSE

The internal specific immune response system is designed to recognize and take action against specific foreign molecules known as *antigenic determinants*. These antigenic determinants elicit the formation and proliferation of specifically reactive molecules (*antibodies*) or cells (*cytotoxic lymphocytes*) that bind to the an-

tigenic determinants to inactivate or destroy the foreign agent. The system also remembers prior contact with the antigenic material and responds faster and more efficiently to subsequent contact. Two functional components make up the specific immune response system: the *cell mediated system,* providing the cytotoxic lymphocytes; and the *humorally mediated system,* providing the circulating antibodies.

CELL MEDIATED IMMUNE RESPONSE

T cell lymphocytes, responsible for provision of the cell mediated immune response, are produced in the bone marrow and mature in the *thymus* gland. From the thymus they migrate to the regional *lymph nodes* and *spleen* where they populate the medullary regions. Each mature immunosensitive T cell lymphocyte is capable of responding to a specific antigenic signal. When exposed to its specific antigen, the T cell begins to divide, increasing the number of that antigenically responsive cell in the lymph node. Some of the cells are shed into the circulation and then, carried by the blood, they seek out the antigen or antigenically labeled cells in the body. When the T cell lymphocytes encounter such cells, they attack and destroy them (cytoxic effect). They also release a number of soluble substances (lymphokines) that recruit and activate nonspecifically reactive phagocytes to attack the tissues at the site.

Other T cell lymphocytes act to regulate the T cell function and production of antibodies by the B cell system. T cell lymphocytes known as *helper T cells* (T_H or T_4 cells) are necessary to provide a full immunologic humoral or cell mediated response. Another type of T cell, known as *suppressor T cells* (T_S or T_8 cells), operates to prevent or modify the function of the two systems. Additional T cells, *memory T cells* (T_M), remember contact with the antigen and on subsequent exposure respond immediately to its presence in the body.

During embryologic development the system provides for self-tolerance; T cells that could respond to self-antigens are either destroyed or rendered nonactive so that the cell mediated system does not respond to the antigens on the body's own cells and tissues.

HUMORALLY MEDIATED IMMUNE RESPONSE

B cell lymphocytes, the lymphocytes providing the humorally mediated immune response, are produced in the bone marrow, but they undergo maturation at a site outside of the thymus, such as in the bone marrow or gut-associated lymphoid tissues. They migrate to the regional lymph nodes, lymphoid tissues, and spleen where they take up residence in the cortex region.

As with T cells, the immunosensitive B cells are programmed to respond to a single antigen. When the antigen is present, the B cell begins to proliferate and differentiate into a *plasma cell.* A plasma cell is designed to synthesize and release large amounts of *immunoglobulin* (antibody) that will combine with the antigen that caused its production. These antibody molecules are released into the circulation where they become part of the gamma globulin fraction of the serum. The B cells producing the immunoglobulin remain in the lymphoid tissue and continue to synthesize additional molecules of the specific antibody. Note that this is different from the T cell response where cytotoxic T cells are released; in this case the B cells remain, and their product is released. Thus the level of active specific antibody begins to rise in the serum fraction (*antibody titer*), as well as in the level of the γ-globulin fraction in general. These antibodies are carried by the blood and other body fluids to where they encounter their specific antigen and bind to it. Upon binding, the antibody may inactivate the antigen, precipitate it, or activate other antigen-damaging

processes (such as the complement cascade) to remove the antigen.

The immunoglobulins are subdivided into different classes on the basis of molecular structure and function. The generic symbol for immunoglobulins is Ig, and each of the classes is designated by a letter of the alphabet: IgG, IgM, IgA, IgE, and IgD. The predominant immunoglobulin is IgG.

The B cell system is similar to the T cell system in that it is controlled by helper and suppressor T cells, forms memory (B_M) cells, and is rendered self-tolerant by the same mechanisms.

PHYSIOLOGIC CHANGES WITH AGING

The extent of immunologic changes that occur with aging varies among individuals, depending on multiple factors such as genetics, nutritional status, and presence of disorders that deplete the immune system. In general, however, the immune response decreases with aging.

The thymus gland is large at birth, grows until the individual reaches puberty, then gradually diminishes in size until it is barely visible after age 40.[6] Therefore the primary basis for the decreased immune response seen in the elderly is the decrease in T cell function, as follows:

1. Cytotoxic (killer) T cells decrease in number; therefore the normal response to tumor cells is reduced.
2. T helper and T suppressor cells have decreased function.
3. Production of interleukin-2 (IL-2) by T helper cells is reduced.
4. T cell function is reduced in response to viral antigens and alloantigens (from other persons, such as in transplants).

Although there are some changes in B cells, these changes are not thought to be clinically significant and are probably the result of decreased T cell regulation.[6] Lymphocytes are redistributed with age; fewer are seen in the germinal centers of the lymph nodes, and more are found in the bone marrow. Autoantibodies increase in number, but the effect is unclear because autoimmune diseases do not increase. Elderly persons may demonstrate a decreased response to skin tests because of the decreased response to foreign antigens.

The end result of the immune system changes in the elderly is an increased incidence of infections (especially viral and mycobacterial). Common infections tend to be more severe, with slower recovery and less probability of developing immunity after an infection.[1] The mortality rate is higher for influenza and pneumococcal pneumonias. Tumors occur more frequently, but they grow more slowly and metastasize less frequently than histologically similar tumors in young persons.[6]

ASSESSMENT

Persons with reduced immune responses (children, elderly, immunosuppressed persons, or those with immunodeficiency diseases) are susceptible, to varying degrees, to *infection*, especially of the upper and lower respiratory tracts. These people need to be identified so that preventive measures are taken and early treatment is initiated. Persons who have hypersensitivity disorders are highly sensitive (*allergic*) to different substances and must avoid these allergens. Therefore, assessment focuses on identification of these persons and of early signs of infection or allergy.

SUBJECTIVE DATA

During the initial history of persons admitted to a health care center the following data should be obtained:
1. Infection history
   a. Recurrent infections: type, frequency and any known causes
   b. Frequent cough (upper respiratory infection) or diarrhea (possible parasitic infection)
2. Allergy
   a. Known allergies to medications, radiocontrast media, foods, or insect bites
   b. Pruritus of eyes or skin (signs of hypersensitivity)

If the person has a known allergy, additional data are collected. These data are described in the discussion of atopic allergy in Chapter 76.

OBJECTIVE DATA

Observations during physical examination include the following:
1. Eyes: erythema, tearing (hay fever)
2. Nose: mucous membranes bluish and edematous with watery secretions (hay fever)
3. Chest: wheezing, coughing (hay fever, asthma, pulmonary infection)
4. Skin: urticaria or wheals (local anaphylactic lesions); linear excoriations from scratching skin; presence of herpetic lesions around mouth or oral *Candida* infections (especially with immunosuppressed or immunodeficient persons)

DIAGNOSTIC TESTS

There are many different diagnostic tests used in evaluation of host defense defects, but many of these tests are available only at major medical centers or in specialized laboratories. Some of the tests that are more commonly used are listed below.

BONE MARROW PRODUCTION TESTS

A *WBC count* and *differential* count will identify the presence of leukopenia and lymphopenia. Leukopenia is a reduction in leukocyte serum levels below 4000/mm^3. The normal range of serum lymphocytes is 1500 to 3000/mm^3. A transient lymphopenia below 1500/mm^3 occurs with stress, but a chronic lymphopenia is observed in persons with defective cellular immunity. Bone marrow aspiration and biopsy (see Chapter 30) may be performed to obtain further data on marrow production of white blood cells.

T CELL (CELLULAR) DEFICIENCY

T cell function can be screened by testing skin for delayed hypersensitivity to common antigens. Specific antigens, including purified protein derivative (PPD), *Candida*, mumps antigen, streptokinase, and streptodornase, are injected intradermally. Reactions are read at 24 to 48 hours to determine hypersensitivity. The test is to determine the hypersensitivity, not the presence of disease. A person who does not react to any of these antigens is said to be *anergic*. Sensitization with dinitrochlorobenzene (DNCB) is an additional test for suspected anergic patients. DNCB is a chemical to which natural sensitivity does not occur. Following application of DCNB to the skin, contact sensitivity can be elicited after 1 to 2 weeks if T cell function is present.

T cell quantity can be determined by in vitro stimulation of peripheral blood lymphocytes with allogeneic lymphocytes (*mixed lymphocyte culture*). The determination is made by measuring cellular uptake of ^{3}H-thymidine introduced into the culture medium.[10]

B CELL (HUMORAL) DEFICIENCY
Electrophoresis

Protein electrophoresis. The movement of colloid (protein) particles in an electrical field is called electrophoresis. Protein electrophoresis is a semiqualitative test that shows the relative concentrations of plasma proteins. In an applied electrical field, different proteins migrate at different rates because of their different sizes and shapes, and this property can be used to analyze plasma protein content. The plasma proteins consist of albumin and globulin, which can be further divided into α-globulins, β-globulins, and γ-globulins (immunoglobulins). The serum proteins are subjected to electrophoresis in a medium that stabilizes the migration so that the proteins can be stained and examined. A densitometer records the color densities on graph paper. Figure 75-2 illustrates typical patterns seen in persons with normal protein levels, with decreased γ-globulin levels, and with increased γ-globulin levels. In immune disorders, the immunoglobulins may be either increased or decreased.

Immunoelectrophoresis. Immunoelectrophoresis identifies specific immunoglobulins. This test shows relative but imprecise quantities of immunoglobulins. Serum is

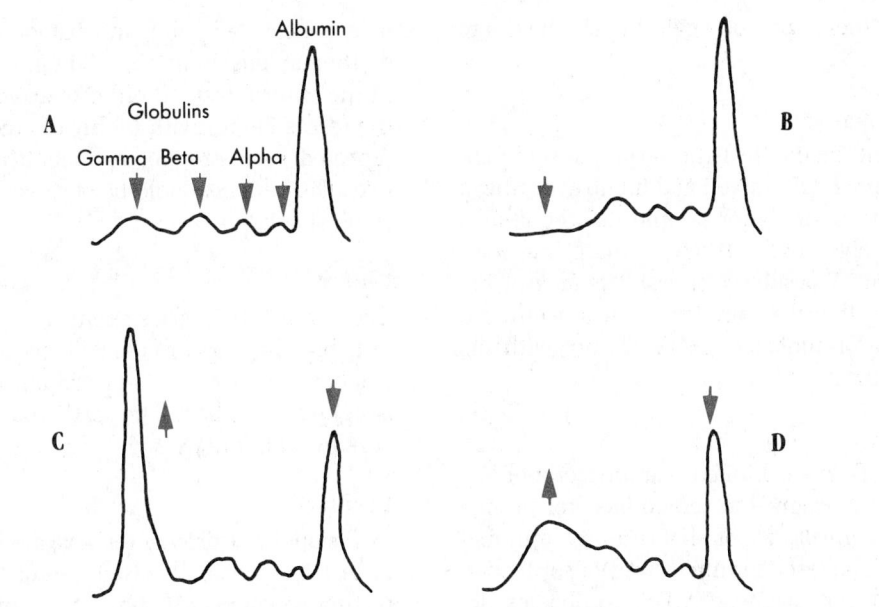

FIGURE 75-2 Electrophoretic patterns. **A,** Normal. **B,** Hypogammaglobulinemia. **C,** Monoclonal gammopathy. **D,** Polyclonal gammopathy.

separated electrophoretically and then tested for reaction with IgG, IgA, or IgM antisera. The test is useful for differentiating monoclonal and polyclonal immunoglobulin increases.[10]

Quantitative Immunoglobulin Tests

Three of the immunoglobulins, IgG, IgA, and IgM, can be measured quantitatively, whereas IgD and IgE are present in amounts too small to measure. An agar plate is impregnated with an antiserum specific to one of the immunoglobulins. A circular well is then cut in the agar, and the immunoglobulin is placed in the well. The immunoglobulin diffuses radially, forming a visible precipitate ring as it interacts with the antiserum. The radius of the ring is proportional to the immunoglobulin concentration; that is, the smaller the ring, the smaller the concentration. The diameter of the ring is compared with a standard measure to determine immunoglobulin quantity. Immunoglobulin levels vary with age. Normal adult levels are as follows: IgG, 600-1800 mg/dl; IgA, 100-400 mg/dl; and IgM, 60-150 mg/dl.

More rapid yet accurate quantitative measurement of IgG, IgA, and IgM can be done by *nephelometry.* The specific antibody is introduced into a fluid containing the specific antigen. The interaction of the antibody and antigen makes the fluid turbid; the degree of turbidity is measured by a photometric instrument.

SPECIFIC ANTIGEN-ANTIBODY TESTS

There are numerous in vitro tests to measure specific antigen-antibody responses, including radioimmunoas-

say tests, immunofluorescent techniques, agglutination tests, and complement-fixation tests.

Radioimmunoassay Test

The radioimmunoassay (RIA) test consists of adding the unknown antigen to the antibody, followed by incubation. A radioactive-labeled antigen is then added, and the preparation is incubated again. If the unknown antigen is similar to the labeled antigen, both antigens will compete for the same antibody. The antibody-antigens are then separated, and the amount of radioactivity of the preparation is determined to identify the amount of free radioactive-labeled antigen remaining. Minute quantities of antigen can be detected by this method.

Immunofluorescence Test

The immunofluorescence test consists of attaching fluorescein dye to antibodies and then mixing this with the antigen to be tested. The excess antibody is removed, and the substance is examined under a microscope with the aid of ultraviolet light to make the dye fluoresce.

Agglutination Tests

Agglutination tests are used to determine the presence of antigens located on the surfaces of RBCs or on microorganisms. Dilutions of antiglobulin are mixed with a solution containing the suspected antigen. The antigen and immunoglobulin (antibody) react by agglutination or clumping of the cells (see Figure 8-10). Agglutination tests used in blood banking procedures are commonly called *Coombs' tests,* but the correct term is *anti-*

globulin test.[13] Other types of agglutination tests are also available.

Complement-Fixation Test

In the complement-fixation test the serum, specific antigen, and complement are mixed and incubated. Sheep RBCs are then added, and after 30 minutes the results are checked. Hemolysis of the RBCs occurs if free complement is present. A positive test result is *lack* of hemolysis, indicating that the complement has been used up in the reaction of antibodies in the serum with the added specific antigen.

Diagnostic Tests for HIV Infection

The ELISA test (Enzyme Linked Immunosorbent Assay) is a simple test designed to screen blood or plasma for the presence of *antibodies* of HIV (human immunodeficiency virus). The test determines previous infection with HIV; it does *not* diagnose AIDS. Antibodies develop after 6 to 12 weeks of infection. The test is repeated if results are positive.

The *Western blot* test is used if the ELISA test is positive. This test is more complicated than the ELISA, but it separates the viral particles by electrophoresis and is more reliable. If results are positive the test is repeated to rule out an occasional false positive result.

ALLERGY TESTS

Hypersensitivity to specific antigens can be tested in vivo by skin tests or by the use test. The most common skin test for allergies is the patch test. Less frequently used skin tests include the intradermal test, the scratch test, and the conjunctival test.

Patch Test

The patch test is the simplest of the skin tests. The sensitizing substance is applied to the skin on a 2.5 cm (1-inch) square piece of soft cotton, covered with a piece of occlusive tape, and left in place for 48 hours. The patches must remain dry and clean. The test is read 20 to 30 minutes after the patch is removed. Positive results are read as follows:

+	Erythema only
++	Erythema and papules
+++	Erythema, papules, and small vesicles
++++	All the above plus bullae and at times ulceration

Positive reactions may take several weeks to subside.

Intradermal Test

Small amounts of extracts of various allergenic substances to which sensitivity is suspected are injected intradermally at spaced intervals, usually on the forearm or in the scapular region. Control tests with the diluent alone are carried out concurrently. The test is positive if a wheal >5 mm in diameter with surrounding erythema appears in 15 to 30 minutes but none appears in the control test. In order to avoid a systemic reaction the test is begun with highly diluted solutions and then repeated with stronger extracts if the results are negative. The person should be observed for signs of anaphylactic shock.

Scratch Test

The scratch test is less sensitive than the intradermal test, but the person is less likely to sustain a systemic reaction. The extract is placed on the skin and the skin is lightly scratched. The test is positive if erythema occurs in 30 minutes.

Conjunctival Test

Occasionally, 1 drop of test extract is instilled in the eye to test for sensitivity. Redness of the conjunctiva and tearing will appear within 5 to 15 minutes in an allergic person.

Use Test

Substances such as foods, cosmetics, or fabrics to which a person is suspected of being allergic are eliminated from use and then added individually according to a set schedule. Reaction to the use test may be immediate or may occur over a period of time. Some persons become discouraged during the testing and may need encouragement to adhere to the testing schedule.

CHAPTER SUMMARY

- The protective internal mechanisms of the body may be nonspecific (phagocytes, complement, acute-phase proteins) or specific (T cell or B cell lymphocytes).
- Immunologic responses generally decrease with aging, leading to increased incidence of infection (especially viral, pneumococcal pneumonia, mycobacterial) and tumors.
- Bone marrow aspiration and biopsy provide data about marrow production of immune cells.
- Tests for T cell deficiencies include delayed hypersensitivity (anergic) tests, DNCB test, and mixed lymphocyte culture.
- Tests for B cell deficiencies include electrophoresis (protein, immunoelectrophoresis) and quantitative immunoglobulin.
- Other tests for immune system function include specific antigen-antibody tests (radioimmunoassay, immunofluorescence), agglutination, complement fixation, and tests for HIV antibodies.
- The diagnosis of hypersensitivities may include allergy tests (patch, scratch, conjunctival, use test).

QUESTIONS TO CONSIDER

- What is the characteristic of immunoglobulins that facilitates differentiation by electrophoresis?

- Examine the electrophoretic patterns in Figure 75-2. What conclusions can be drawn from diagrams B, C, and D in terms of serum proteins?

REFERENCES AND SELECTED READINGS

1. *Baron M and Tafuro P: The extremes of age: the newborn and the elderly at increased risk for the development of infection, Nurs Clin North Am 20(1):181-190, 1985.
2. Barrett JT: Textbook of immunology, ed 5, St Louis, 1988, The CV Mosby Co.
3. Claman HN: The biology of the immune response, JAMA 258:3011-3031, 1987.
4. De Shazo RD, Lopez M, and Salvaggio JE: Use and interpretation of diagnostic laboratory tests, JAMA 258:3011-3031, 1987.
5. *Grady C: Host defense mechanisms: an overview, Semin Oncol Nurs 4(2):86-94, 1988.
6. Graziano RM and Lemanske R Jr: Clinical immunology, Baltimore, 1989, Williams & Wilkins.
7. Henry JB: Todd-Sanford-Davidsohn clinical diagnosis by laboratory methods, ed 17, Philadelphia, 1984, WB Saunders Co.
8. Katz P: Clinical and laboratory evaluation of the immune system, Med Clin North Am 69(3):453-463, 1985.
9. Lind M: The immunologic assessment: a nursing focus, Heart Lung 9:658-681, 1980.
10. Pagana KD and Pagana TJ: Diagnostic testing and nursing implications, ed 2, St. Louis, 1986, The CV Mosby Co.
11. Schroeder SA et al: Current medical diagnosis and treatment, Norwalk, Conn, 1989, Appleton & Lange.
12. Stites DP: Basic and clinical immunology, ed 6, Norwalk, Conn, 1988, Appleton & Lange.
13. Widman FK: An introduction to clinical immunology, Philadelphia, 1989, FA Davis Co.
14. Wyngaarden JB and Smith LH: Cecil textbook of medicine, ed 18, Philadelphia, 1988, WB Saunders Co.

*References preceded by an asterisk are particularly well suited for student reading.

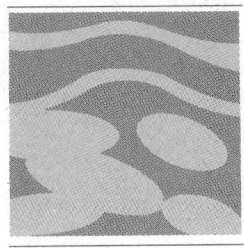

CHAPTER 76

Management of Persons with Problems of the Immune System

BARBARA C. LONG
E. RONALD WRIGHT

CHAPTER OBJECTIVES

After studying this chapter, the student should be able to:
1 Differentiate between primary and secondary immunodeficiencies and describe principles of care.
2 Differentiate among the four types of hypersensitivity reactions.
3 Describe the causes, prevention, manifestations, and management of atopic allergies.
4 Describe blood transfusion reactions in relation to types, manifestations, and appropriate actions.
5 Describe tissue transplants in relation to types, and the clinical manifestations and interventions for graft rejection.

Alterations in the immune system may result in deficiencies or excesses of immunocompetent cells, in altered function of these cells, or in attack against self-antigens. The biologic bases of the immune system are discussed in Chapters 8 and 75. Because immunologic factors are operative in such a wide variety of disorders, much of the information about the disorders is found elsewhere in the text. This chapter will describe the various categories of immune disorders and those disorders not described elsewhere.

CLASSIFICATION OF IMMUNOLOGIC DISORDERS

In the interrelated complex system providing immunologic defense, there are innumerable points at which the system may malfunction. The immunologic disorders that have been characterized reflect nonresponsiveness, blocked responsiveness, misdirected responsiveness, and overresponsiveness. The underlying causes of the disorders may be attributed to genetic or developmental defects, infection, malignancy, trauma, altered metabolic states, or pharmacologic intervention. The severity of the disorders ranges from creation of a minor nuisance (for example, mild hay fever) to an immediate life-threatening situation (for example, anaphylactic shock) to a chronic debilitating condition (for ex-

ample, rheumatoid arthritis). The disorders may be classified into the following general categories:
1. Immunodeficiencies—deficiencies in the proper expression of the immune response system, parts of the system, or individual cell types within the system
2. Gammopathies—abnormal production of immunoglobulins
3. Hypersensitivities—exaggerated or inappropriate response to specific antigens
4. Autoimmunities—the immunologic attack on self-antigens
These four categories serve as the basis of organization for this chapter.

IMMUNODEFICIENCIES
PATHOPHYSIOLOGY

Protection of the host depends on an intact immune system. Interference with *development* of cells and tissues of the immune response leads to immunodeficient disorders. Because the cells and tissues of the immune response system develop sequentially, the severity of a defect reflects the stage of development at which the abnormality arose (Figure 76-1). Defects may exist in immunoglobulin synthesis, cellular immune functions, in combination, or in phagocytosis. The deficiencies resulting from the improper development of the immunoresponsive cells and tissues are termed *primary immunodeficiencies;* these are genetic in origin. The depression of immune responsiveness as a result of some interference with the already developed immune system produces a *secondary immunodeficiency.*

PRIMARY IMMUNODEFICIENCIES

Primary immunodeficiencies (Table 76-1) are rare disorders seen mostly in infants and young children. Without therapy, children born with immune defects cannot live long in their natural environment because of the risk of infection and malignancies. Persons with B cell defi-

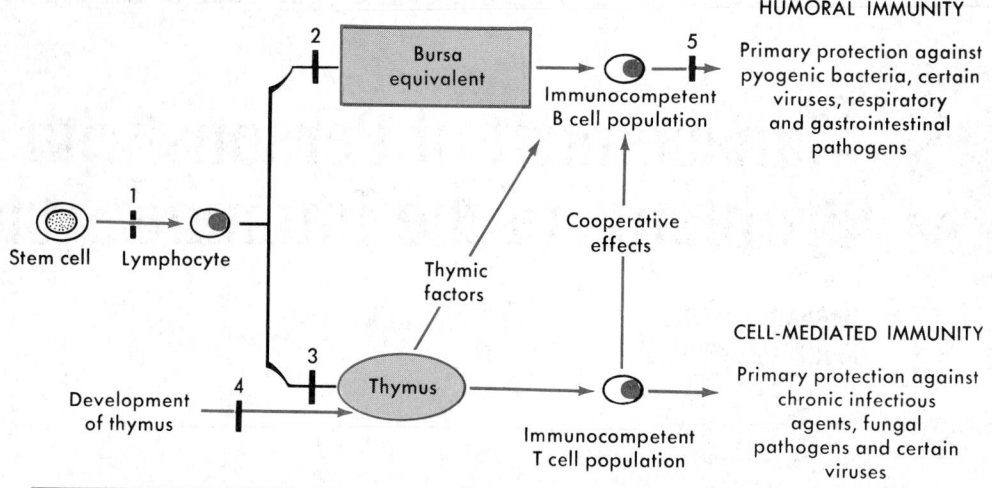

FIGURE 76-1 Causes of immunodeficiencies. Abnormalities at *1* result in combined humoral and cell-mediated immunodeficiency. Blockage at *2* produces agammaglobulinemia. Blockage at *3* or *4* results in drastic reduction in T cell-mediated function and, because of cooperative effects on B cell system, some reduction in humoral response. Abnormalities in synthesis of specific immunoglobulin classes are reflected by blockage at 5. Whereas some blockages result in complete deficiency, others show up as reduction in response.

ciencies are more susceptible to bacterial infections, whereas those with T cell deficiencies are highly susceptible to severe viral, fungal, or protozoal infections. Although combined B and T cell deficiencies are the most lethal, bone marrow transplants can provide a cure. With the help of specially created germ-free environments and replacement therapy, the lives of some children with primary immunodeficiencies have been prolonged.

Common Variable Immunodeficiencies

Some immunoglobulin deficiencies may not become evident until adulthood, and these are termed common variable immunodeficiencies (CVIs). The deficiencies differ among persons having CVI; these deficiencies are primarily IgA or IgM, although most persons have sufficient IgA. T cell deficiencies may occur with time. Persons with CVI develop recurrent virulent infections (especially pulmonary) and display a high incidence of malignancies, hematologic disorders, and autoimmune diseases.

SECONDARY IMMUNODEFICIENCIES

The most common immunodeficiencies are *acquired* disorders of depressed immunity. Any factor that can interfere with the normal growth or expression of the immune response system can lead to a secondary immunodeficiency. Major contributing factors include age (see Chapter 75), nutrition, specific disorders, and induced immunosuppression. A retrovirus (HIV) causes AIDS

(acquired immunodeficiency syndrome); AIDS is discussed in Chapter 77.

NUTRITION AND IMMUNODEFICIENCY

Deficiencies in nutrients, especially protein, can severely alter the immune response by depressing cell multiplication and antibody production. Not only is the person more susceptible to infections, but also previously established protection decreases and new exposures do not lead to immunity.[69] Protein-calorie malnutrition is associated with thymic atrophy and reduction in lymphoid tissue. Therefore, *any medical or surgical condition that impairs nutrition also impairs the person's ability to fight infection.*

SPECIFIC DISORDERS AFFECTING IMMUNITY

Disorders can depress the immune system by the following methods:
1. Loss of serum protein: nephrotic syndrome, burns, protein-losing enteropathy
2. Decreased protein synthesis: severe liver disease
3. Severe malnutrition: cancer, alcoholism
4. Decreased T cell function: uremia, diabetes mellitus,[69] infections (especially viral), autoimmune disorders
5. Alterations in B cell and T cell number and function: leukemias, lymphomas

INDUCED IMMUNOSUPPRESSION

Immunosuppression is initiated to decrease unwanted immune responses, such as hypersensitivity reactions,

TABLE 76-1 Selected primary immunodeficiencies

Deficiency	Basis of Deficiency	Replacement Therapy
T CELL DEFICIENCY		
Nezelof's syndrome	Congenital failure of embryonic thymic development	Bone marrow or thymus transplants
DiGeorge's syndrome	Nongenetic failure of thymic development	
B CELL DEFICIENCY		
Bruton-type agammaglobulinemia	Sex-linked depression of all immunoglobulin classes	Immune serum globulin
Common variable immunodeficiency	Variable degree of ability to synthesize primarily IgA or IgM in adults	
COMBINED B AND T CELL DEFICIENCY		
Swiss-type immunodeficiency	Non–sex-linked deficiency of circulating antibodies or CMI	Bone marrow transplants or immune serum globulin
Wiskoff-Aldrich syndrome	Sex-linked IgM and T cell deficiency in males	
Ataxia-telangiectasia	Autosomally inherited deficit in IgA and IgE	
PHAGOCYTOTIC CELL DEFICIENCY		
Chronic granulomatous disease	Sex-linked recessive genetic disease in males producing lack of destruction of phagocytized organisms and particles	None; antibiotic therapy

autoimmune diseases, neoplasia, or organ transplantation. There are several ways in which the unwanted immune responses can be suppressed by artificial manipulation: suppression of specific antigens causing hypersensitivities, immunologic methods of immune suppression, irradiation, and drug immunosuppression.

Antigen and Antibody Administration

Specific *antigens* can be administered to a hypersensitive person in small amounts over a time. The antigenic stimulation forms circulating antibodies (immunoglobulins) of the IgG class that combine with the antigen to block contact with the immunocompetent cells or IgE-coated mast cells, thus suppressing the immune response. An adaptation of this method is used by allergists to desensitize persons allergic to specific antigens such as pollens.

A slightly different method is to administer the specific *antibody,* which then combines with the antigen to block contact with the immunocompetent cell. This method has been used successfully in obstetrics to prevent the sensitive Rh-negative mother from responding to the Rh-positive fetus during pregnancy.

Immunologic Methods of Immunosuppression

Antilymphocytic globulin (ALG) or *antithymocytic globulin* (ATG) are antisera prepared by isolating the active globulin fraction from the serum of horses, goats, or rabbits that have been immunized with human lympho-

cytes or thymocytes. This approach is nonspecific by decreasing all lymphocytes, although T cells are more affected than B cells. Because these globulins are xenogeneic (from another species), serum sickness (p. 2216) frequently occurs and thus limits use to short-term therapy. Other adverse effects include thrombocytopenia and allergic reactions.

Common antiserum is polyclonal, because it is a collection of cells from different lymphocytes. A more specific approach to immunologic immunosuppression is the administration of *monoclonal antibodies* (MoAbs), derived from a single cell, and thus directed toward specific subpopulations of lymphocytes, such as helper T cells (muromonab-CD3). Different types of MoAbs are being developed from other cell populations for other purposes such as for cancer immunotherapy (Chapter 17).

Irradiation

Both primary and secondary immune responses (see Chapter 8) may be suppressed by irradiation, but suppression of primary sensitization is more effective than suppression of immunologic memory (secondary immune response). Irradiation destroys lymphocytes, either directly or through depletion of the precursor stem cells. It may be directed at local areas or at the total body. *Local irradiation* results in a local destruction of the cellular elements (primarily T cell response) immediately involved in allograft rejection. The best results

TABLE 76-2 Major immunosuppressive drugs

Drug	Immunologic Action	Indications for Immunosuppressive Therapy
Corticosteroid	Inhibits T cell proliferation Decreases interleukin-2 production Decreases macrophage and neutrophil function	Diseases in which immune disorder is unknown Tissue and organ transplantation Autoimmune diseases
Cyclosporine (Sandimmune)	Inhibits T helper cell, lymphokine, and interleukin-2 production Facilitates T-suppressor cell development	Organ transplantation
Alkylating agent: cyclophosphamide	Interferes with DNA, RNA, and protein synthesis Lymphocytolytic Suppresses primary immune response	Autoimmune diseases Tissue transplantation Lymphomas, leukemias
Antimetabolite: azathioprine	Interferes with RNA, DNA, and protein synthesis Depresses bone marrow and antibody reproduction Depresses primary immune response	Autoimmune disease Renal transplantation Pemphigus (skin disease) Neoplasia

are obtained by pretreatment of the donor organ. *Total body irradiation* is rarely used now, because of the severe side effects of pancytopenia and toxic effects to the GI tract and central nervous system (see Chapter 79).

Drug Immunosuppression

Drugs that most commonly cause immunosuppression are described in Table 76-2 and in more detail on p. 2218. *Corticosteroids* are therapeutic in a large number of diseases. In addition to producing a decreased immune response as antiproliferative agents, corticosteroids are also antiinflammatory; therefore persons receiving corticosteroid therapy are highly susceptible to superimposed infections. If infections are present, the severity of the infection may increase despite the minimizing of symptoms caused by the antiinflammatory effects.

Cyclosporine is the primary immunosuppressant used for organ transplantation. It acts by inhibiting T-helper cells and facilitating development of T-suppressor cells. Cyclosporine is nontoxic to precursor stem cells and the GI tract, although side effects to the kidney, liver, and CNS do occur.

Cytotoxic drugs (such as alkylating agents and antimetabolites) (Table 76-2) have the potential for destroying any cell that is replicating; therefore immunosuppression occurs with the destruction of the rapidly dividing, immunologically stimulated cells. Cytotoxic drugs act by interfering with the basic metabolic processes. B cell reduction is greater than T cell reduction. Antimetabolites are frequently given with steroids for immunosuppression therapy to decrease the dosage of both antimetabolites and steroids, thereby decreasing serious side effects.

CLINICAL MANIFESTATIONS

Persons with immunodeficiencies experience frequent infections, because of the inadequacy of immune re-

sponse to fight infection. Infections are especially common in the respiratory tract and CNS and may lead to septicemia. With B cell deficiencies, recurrent high-grade *bacterial* infections occur; common organisms include *Streptococcus aureus, Staphylococcus pneumoniae,* and *Hemophilus influenzae.*[31]

With T cell deficiencies, the most common organisms are viruses (especially pneumocystis, cytomegalovirus, and herpes), fungi, protozoa, and mycobacteria. Persons with T cell deficiencies also have an increased risk of malignancies. A classic example of a T cell deficiency is AIDS (see Chapter 77).

Signs and symptoms depend on the site of infection and type of infecting organism. Persons with either B cell or T cell deficiencies often develop chronic diarrhea from parasitic infections of the GI tract. Laboratory tests for B cell and T cell deficiencies are described in Chapter 75.

MEDICAL MANAGEMENT

Specific *replacement* therapy may be given for *primary* immunodeficiencies. When B cell deficiency is present, immune serum globulin (ISG) may be given at monthly intervals. ISG is a purified, concentrated solution of antibodies from pooled venous blood; it may be given intramuscularly or intravenously. Bone marrow transplant is the treatment of choice for most T cell deficiencies, although thymus transplantation appears to be effective for DiGeorge syndrome.

Treatment of *secondary* immunodeficiencies focuses on the underlying condition that has affected the immune response. Immunotherapy is one therapeutic mode in the treatment of cancer (Chapter 17).

■ ASSESSMENT

Subjective data to be obtained from the person with immunodeficiency include the following:

1. Knowledge of the immunodeficiency, the high

risk for infection, and infection preventive methods

2. Occurrence of recurrent infections (types)
3. Nutritional data: weight changes, appetite, usual 24-hour food intake

Objective data include monitoring for early signs of infection (elevated temperature, nasal discharge, cough, skin lesions). Breath sounds are monitored daily for decreased sounds, indicating pulmonary infection.

■ DATA ANALYSIS: NURSING DIAGNOSES

Nursing diagnoses are determined from assessment of patient data. Possible nursing diagnoses for the person with immunodeficiency include, but are not limited to, the following:

Diagnostic Title	Possible Etiologies
Infection, potential for	Decreased immune response, lack of information
Knowledge deficit	Lack of exposure/recall, information misinterpretation

■ PLANNING: EXPECTED PATIENT OUTCOMES

Expected patient outcomes for the person with immunodeficiency may include, but are not limited to, the following:

1. Signs of infection do not occur.
2. The person can describe measures to avoid infection.
3. The person can describe signs dictating immediate medical attention.
4. The person can explain the need for continued medical follow-up.

■ IMPLEMENTATION
PREVENTING INFECTION

The most important factor in the care of the immunodeficient or immunosuppressed person is protection from infection. The following measures pertain to all degrees of immunodeficiency:

1. Use good medical asepsis, including thorough handwashing.
2. Avoid injections, if possible. (Breaks in skin continuity may lead to infection.)
3. By meticulous cleaning, remove sources where bacteria may proliferate.
4. Protect patient from other persons with infections.
5. Maintain nutrition especially protein intake, at optimal level. Remember that malnutrition significantly affects immune efficiency (p. 2200).
6. Maintain adequate fluid intake of at least 1500 ml per day for hydration (prevents skin drying and flushes the urinary system to prevent infection).

If severe leukopenia is present, place the person in a single-occupancy room to decrease the infection potential. Persons with B cell deficiencies are more suscepti-

TEACHING THE PATIENT WITH IMMUNODEFICIENCY

The patient will be able to explain or perform the following:
1. Explain immunodeficiency, that is, the inability of the body to fight infection
2. Take measures to prevent infection:
   a. Avoid persons with infections (especially colds)
   b. Avoid bumping or breaking the skin
   c. Inspect skin daily for lesions
   d. Eat a balanced diet (Chapter 40)
   e. Drink at least six glasses of fluid daily
   f. Avoid fatigue and try to get a regular amount of sleep every night
   g. Avoid letting water stand unchanged around the house, such as in vases (good source for bacterial growth)
   h. Do not use cold-mist humidifiers (gram-negative organisms are often present)
3. Report signs of infection to physician immediately
4. See physician on a regular basis, as instructed

---

ble to bacterial infections (especially pulmonary); therefore pulmonary hygiene measures (such as breathing exercises, inhalation therapy, postural drainage) are prophylactic measures. Persons with T cell deficiencies are monitored for signs of viral and fungal infections.

For severe immunodeficiency, protective isolation may be necessary. Laminar air flow units (see Chapter 17) are rooms especially designed with air flow across the unit in layers to decrease microorganisms moving toward the patient. The air is filtered continuously through microfilters. Persons who remain downstream from the patient need not wear protection, but anyone approaching or giving care to the patient wears a cap, mask, and gown. All equipment is sterilized before entry to the room.

PATIENT TEACHING

Immunodeficient or immunosuppressed patients and their families need to know the nature of immunodeficiency and how to avoid infection (see the box above).

GAMMOPATHIES
PATHOPHYSIOLOGY

Gammopathies, better termed *hypergammaglobulinemias*, are elevated levels of γ-globulin in serum resulting from the overproduction of whole γ-globulin or nonassociated heavy chains (H chains) or nonassociated light chains (L chains) (see Chapter 8). The normal synthesis of an immunoglobulin is the result of the proliferation and plasma cell differentiation of a single clone of B cells in response to an antigenic signal. In gammopathies, a single clone or multiple clones of plasma cells begin to overproduce immunoglobulin

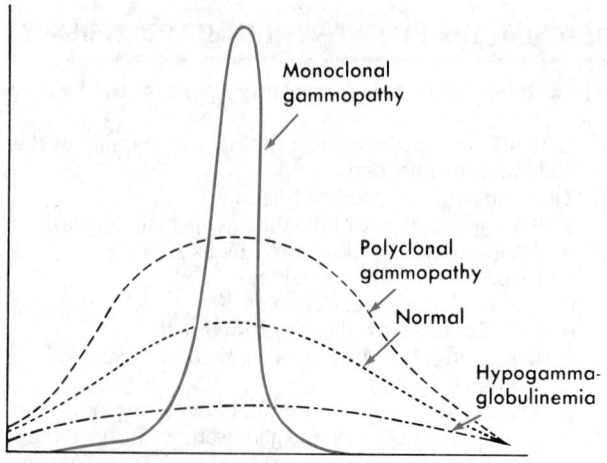

FIGURE 76-2 Electrophoretic peaks of γ-globulin fractions in monoclonal gammopathies, polyclonal gammopathies, and hypogammaglobulinemia. Obtained by electrophoresis of γ-globulin fraction of serum.

product. If the gammopathy involves a single B cell clone, it is termed a *monoclonal gammopathy,* and the electrophoretic pattern will be characterized by a single sharp peak in the γ-globulin region (Figure 76-2). *Polyclonal gammopathies* involve the overproduction of virtually all classes of immunoglobulins in response to inappropriate antigenic stimulation. The electrophoretic pattern of polyclonal gammopathies is characterized by a diffuse increase in the γ-globulin curve.

MONOCLONAL GAMMOPATHIES

Monoclonal gammopathies (M-type) are commonly referred to as plasma cell dyscrasias. Some plasma cell dyscrasias such as multiple myeloma and macroglobulinemia have distinctive clinical patterns. In some instances, electrophoretic changes resembling the clinical forms can be identified, but no symptoms are present; these can be classified as plasma cell dyscrasias of unknown significance (PCDUS).

MULTIPLE MYELOMA

Etiology and Pathophysiology

Multiple myeloma is a monoclonal plasma cell malignancy seen in both men and women and peaking about age 60. It is characterized by widespread bone destruction, anemia, hypercalcemia, and hyperuricemia. These symptoms are traced to the proliferation of plasma cell tumors from the bone marrow into the hard bone tissue, causing an erosion of the bone. Frequent recurrent infections (especially of the respiratory tract) and spontaneous pathologic fractures occur because of the production of ineffective immunoglobulins that in turn depress the production of normal antibodies. Immunosuppression from chemotherapy contributes to further in-

creased risk of infection. Renal failure may result from precipitation of urate and calcium crystals.

Interventions

Ambulation and adequate hydration are vitally important to prevent renal complications from the increased amounts of urates and calcium being excreted in the urine. Fluid intake should be sufficient to ensure a urinary output of a *minimum* of 1500 ml/24 hr. Ambulation may be difficult, because of the skeletal pain and the possibility of fractures. A light-weight spinal brace, analgesics, and local radiotherapy may facilitate ambulation.

Measures to prevent infection are instituted and includes avoidance of persons with upper respiratory tract infections. Medical attention should be sought for any signs of infection, and antibiotics are often given, since infections are usually caused by gram-positive organisms. Rest periods are planned if fatigue from anemia is present.

Combination chemotherapy is the major treatment for multiple myeloma. The alkylating agents melphalan and cyclophosphamide (Cytoxan) are the two drugs most commonly used and may be given alone or sequentially. Several weeks may elapse between the initiation of therapy and signs of improvement. Periods of remission of 6 years or more have been obtained with chemotherapy.

MACROGLOBULINEMIA

Macroglobulinemia is a plasma cell dyscrasia involving the overproduction of IgM globulins. Symptoms usually begin in the fifth or sixth decade of life and include fatigue and weakness from anemia, weight loss, and bleeding (mucosal, epistaxis). Blood viscosity is increased because of the increased globulins. Disease progression is similar to a lymphoma (see Chapter 30). Medical therapy includes plasmapheresis to decrease blood viscosity and chemotherapy with chlorambucil (Leukeran), or cyclophosphamide (Cytoxan).

POLYCLONAL GAMMOPATHIES

Polyclonal gammopathies refer to a diffuse increase in antibody synthesis as a result of inappropriate antigen stimulation. The major causes of the hypergammaglobulinemia are infectious diseases (especially chronic bacterial infections such as lung abscess and osteomyelitis), connective tissue diseases such as SLE and rheumatoid arthritis, and chronic active liver disease. IgG and IgM are the most commonly involved immunoglobulins, and the degree of immunoglobulin levels reflects the severity of the diseases.

The development of high levels of dysfunctional γ-globulins depresses the synthesis of normal immunoglobulins. This renders the person with hypergammaglobulinemia susceptible to infection; therefore carrying out measures and teaching the patient how to prevent infection are major nursing responsibilities.

HYPERSENSITIVITY REACTIONS

PATHOPHYSIOLOGY

The immune response system that has been immunologically primed or sensitized is designed to provide an immediate, effective, protective reaction to subsequent encounter with the sensitizing antigen. This of course is a positive factor in the provision of immunity; however, under a given set of conditions or because of an idiotypic reactivity to a particular antigen, the response of the immune system may produce detrimental effects. This inappropriate response is usually manifested as a tissue-damaging overreaction to the antigen; thus it is termed hypersensitivity, or allergy. The antigenic stimulants invoking the reactions are referred to as allergens. Hypersensitivities, then, are classic expressions of the immune system, but they take place in inappropriate sites, in excessive amounts, or with inappropriate involvement of nonspecific tissues. Whether an allergic response occurs and to what degree is dependent on a combination of interrelated factors:

1. *Responsiveness of the host to the allergen.* If the sensitivity of the host is extremely high, there is a far greater chance that a tissue-damaging reaction will occur.
2. *Amount of the allergen.* Generally, the greater the amount of allergen contacted, the more severe the reaction.

3. *Nature of the allergen.* Most are complex, high-molecular weight, multivalent proteins, but some may be low–molecular-weight nonprotein materials that exert a haptenic effect when coupled with a normal tissue protein carrier.
4. *Route of entrance of the allergen.* The greatest proportion of allergens enter through the respiratory tract; however, others may enter by epidermal or mucosal contact, injection, or through the digestive tract.
5. *Timing of exposure to the allergen.* If the host's contacts with the allergen are widely separated (for example, years apart), the immunologic mediators (antibodies or sensitized cells) may be so dilute that there will be less response.
6. *Site of the allergen-immune mediator reaction.* If certain antigen-antibody reactions occur in the tissues, there is no untoward effect, whereas the same reaction occurring within the bloodstream can lead to intravascular inflammation.

CLASSIFICATION OF HYPERSENSITIVITIES

Hypersensitivities can be broadly divided into two categories based on the components of the immune system involved in mediating the hypersensitivity reaction: humoral response (B cell-mediated) or cellular response (T cell-mediated). This basic division corresponds with the older clinical symptom division of immediate and delayed, which was developed before the elucidation of the mechanisms. The terms immediate or delayed were assigned to describe the timing of the appearance of clinical symptoms and the speed of skin test reactions when

TABLE 76-3 Summary of hypersensitivity reactions

| | Hypersensitivity Type | | | |
| | Humoral (Immediate) | | | Cellular (Delayed) |
Property	I Anaphylactic	II Cytotoxic	III Immune Complex	IV Cell Mediated
Immune system mediators	IgE (IgG) bound to mast cells	IgG or IgM (+ complement)	IgG or IgM (+ complement)	T cells, macrophages
Allergens	Exogenous antigens	Foreign cells or alteration of cell surface antigens	Soluble antigens	Infectious agent, contact allergens, foreign tissues, cancer cells
Response to intradermal skin test	Wheal and flare within 30 min, edema	Not done	Erythema and edema within 3-8 hr	Erythema and induration within 24-48 hr
Pathophysiologic effects	Release of histamines, kinins, SRS-A from mast cells, which affect smooth muscle shock organs	Direct cytotoxic destruction of cells	Acute inflammatory reaction; primarily polymorphonuclear neutrophil leukocytes	Tissue destruction, primarily lymphocytes and macrophages
Examples	Systemic anaphylaxis, atopic allergies, hayfever, insect sting reactions	Hemolytic disease of the newborn (Rh), transfusion reactions	Serum sickness, Arthus reaction, glomerulonephritis	Tuberculin reaction, skin graft rejection, poison ivy

a host was challenged with various allergens. This terminology is still used today, but it has taken on new significance in relation to the understanding of the basic mechanisms at work.

It is possible to subcategorize the different manifestations of the humorally mediated hypersensitivities. The most widely used scheme of classification is presented in Table 76-3. As can be seen from this table, the type I, II, and III reactions are mediated by the humoral system, whereas type IV reactions are those of the cell-mediated system. Since type I, II, and III hypersensitivities are the result of interactions involving circulating antibodies, these reactions can be transferred from a sensitized host to a nonsensitized host by serum transfer. Type IV sensitivities can be transferred by lymphocyte exchange only.

TYPE I HYPERSENSITIVITIES

PATHOPHYSIOLOGY

The most serious life-threatening (anaphylactic and IgE-dependent) hypersensitivity diseases are associated with the reactions mediated by the IgE class of immunoglobulins. These antibodies, also called reaginic antibodies, have a predilection for attachment to the surface of mast cells and basophils. The mast cells are found in virtually all tissues of the body and often in close proximity to blood vessels, whereas the basophils are found circulating as one of the leukocytes within the blood. Mast cells are particularly abundant in the skin, nasal region, and lungs. Both mast cells and basophils harbor within their cells numerous, membrane-bound vacuoles containing potent, pharmacologically active substances (histamine, bradykinin, serotonin, and other vasoactive amines). When IgE immunoglobulins bind to the surface of these cells by the Fc portion of the immunoglobulin molecule, the antigen-binding site of the molecule is left exposed to bind the allergen at the surface of the cell (Figure 76-3). When the allergen is bound to the IgE, the cell is induced to undergo degranulation,

which releases the internal agents into the environment of the mast cell or basophil. These mediators then cause increased vascular permeability and smooth-muscle contraction.

Of the agents released, *histamine* (H_1) seems to be the most important. The direct injection of histamine can mimic many of the symptoms of the type I hypersensitivity, and in the hypersensitive individual a reaction may be assuaged by antihistamines. Other physiologically similar substances are released as well. Thus in type I reactions, the detrimental symptoms are not at the site of the antigen-antibody reaction but at the site of the shock organs where the pharmacologically active anaphylactic mediators exert their action. If those mediators remain confined to a local area, the tissue reactions remain localized and are referred to as local anaphylaxis. The local hypersensitivity that most people demonstrate to a mosquito bite is the classic example of this type of reaction; the intradermal injection of the mosquito anticoagulants produces a wheal-flare type of reaction within a matter of minutes. If, on the other hand, the mediators become released systemically, the response is known as systemic anaphylaxis, which can produce anaphylactic shock. As is illustrated by the mosquito bite, the mediators are quickly broken down in the body and their effects are reversible.

For type I reactions to occur, the hypersensitive individual must initially come into contact with the allergen that triggers the synthesis of the specific antiallergenic IgE antibodies. This primary contact is known as a sensitizing dose. With the synthesis of the IgE antibodies and their attachment to mast cells and basophils, the individual is rendered hypersensitive. On subsequent contact with the allergen (termed the shocking or challenging dose), the individual exhibits the symptoms of type I sensitivity. The severity of those symptoms depends on a number of factors: the amount and route of entrance of the sensitizing dose, the amount and distribution of the IgE antibodies, and the amount and route of entrance of the shocking dose.

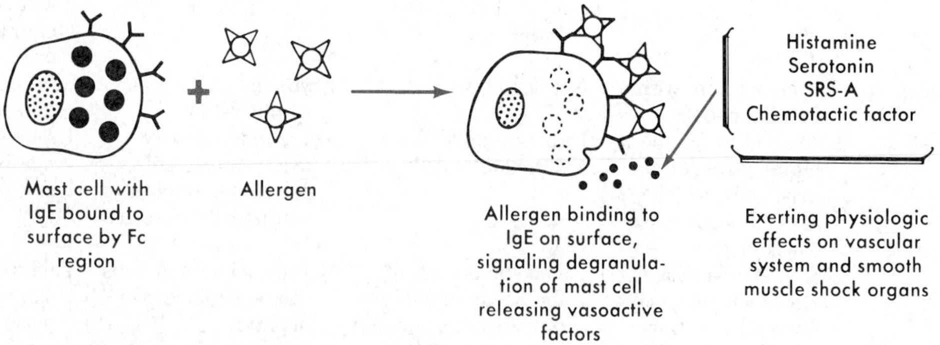

Mast cell with IgE bound to surface by Fc region

Allergen

Allergen binding to IgE on surface, signaling degranulation of mast cell releasing vasoactive factors

Histamine
Serotonin
SRS-A
Chemotactic factor

Exerting physiologic effects on vascular system and smooth muscle shock organs

FIGURE 76-3 Mediators of type I hypersensitivity.

ANAPHYLAXIS
ETIOLOGY

The most severe form of type I hypersensitivity in humans is systemic anaphylaxis. Antigens that commonly induce anaphylaxis are drugs such as penicillin or heterologous antiserum, insect stings, pollen, and iodinated contrast media used in selected x-ray film studies. Foods such as seafood, legumes, egg albumin, or strawberries may be causative factors.

PREVENTION

Severe anaphylactic reactions can be prevented through (1) identification of high-risk persons, (2) patient education concerning avoidance of antigens and actions to take if sensitization occurs, (3) desensitization, and (4) precautionary actions.

Identification of High-Risk Persons

Since persons with a history of allergies are more likely to develop anaphylactic reactions to drugs than those without such a history, all patients should be questioned about allergies and sensitivities to drugs before drug therapy is initiated. If there is any positive history, the physician is consulted before a new drug is given, and if it is given, the patient is watched closely for allergic responses. High-risk persons should wear an identity bracelet or tag at all times that indicates the known allergy. These tags may be obtained commercially.* Hospitalized persons who are sensitive to certain substances are identified, and the information is posted conspicuously outside of the room, on the medical order sheets of the patient's record, or in both places. In addition, many hospitals use a special color identification bracelet for the person who is sensitive to certain substances.

Patient Education

Persons who have a type I allergy should be aware of situations in which the substance to which they are sensitized may be found. Persons who are sensitive to insect stings should learn the emergency care to take after a sting. Sting emergency medical kits are available commercially and should be readily available. If a sting occurs, the person should immediately swallow the uncoated antihistamine tablet and place the isoproterenol tablet under the tongue. A family member or friend should know how to inject the 1:1000 epinephrine hydrochloride available in the ampule. Immediate medical help should be sought.

Desensitization

Persons known to have hypersensitivity to insect stings are recommended for immunizing injections with Hy-

menoptera extract. The approach is similar to hyposensitization for atopic allergies (p. 2209).

Precautionary Actions

When animal sera, allergenic extracts, or contrast media containing iodide are given, a syringe containing 1:1000 epinephrine hydrochloride should be readily available; in addition, an antihistamine such as diphenhydramine (Benadryl) and isoproterenol (Isuprel) should be available. The patient should then be kept under surveillance for at least 20 minutes. Any reaction that occurs within a few minutes forewarns of an impending emergency.

CLINICAL MANIFESTATIONS

The initial symptoms of anaphylaxis are edema and itching about the site of the injection, apprehension, and sneezing. These mild reactions are rapidly followed (sometimes in a matter of seconds or minutes) by edema of the face, hands, and other parts of the body; wheezing respirations; dyspnea; and signs of vascular collapse with shock (rapid and weak pulse, falling blood pressure, cyanosis). Death may ensue unless rapid action is taken.

INTERVENTIONS

At the first sign of anaphylaxis, the patient is placed in the recumbent position and given epinephrine 1:1000 solution 0.3 to 0.5 ml subcutaneously or intramuscularly (less for children). The epinephrine opposes the action of histamine through vasoconstriction to raise the blood pressure and through relaxation of the bronchioles to facilitate breathing. Epinephrine also inhibits mast cell mediator release.[31] An antihistamine, such as diphenhydramine, shortens the duration of anaphylaxis and prevents a relapse.[62] Hydrocortisone is given intravenously after epinephrine and antihistamine to decrease the inflammatory effects.

An adequate oral airway must be maintained, and an endotracheal tube or emergency tracheostomy is sometimes necessary. The decreased circulation and tissue perfusion during shock are restored with intravenous fluids. Vasopressors may be given for severe shock (Chapter 25).

URTICARIA AND ANGIOEDEMA

Urticaria (hives) may occur as an IgE-mediated local anaphylactic response. The pruritic lesions are characterized by a pale pink elevated edge (wheal) on an erythematous background (Figure 76-4). The lesions are transient and may reappear in different body areas. The allergic form of urticaria is usually caused by foods, especially eggs, fish, and nuts, or by drugs such as penicillins, sulfonamides, cephalosporins, or aspirin and other nonsteroidal antiinflammatory drugs.

---

*Medic-Alert Foundation, 2323 Colorado St., Turlock, CA 95380.

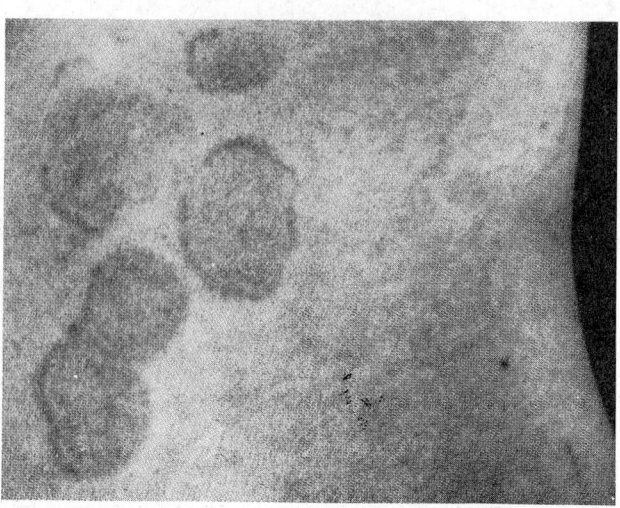

FIGURE 76-4 Urticaria. (From Stewart WD, Danto JL, and Maddin S: Dermatology: diagnosis and treatment of cutaneous disorders, ed 4, St Louis, 1978, The CV Mosby Co.)

Angioedema is a form of urticaria, but it involves the subcutaneous tissue rather than the skin. With angioedema an entire anatomic part such as the eyelid, thumb, or lip becomes swollen; there is no pruritus.

Urticaria may also occur in a chronic form from causes other than IgE-mediated hypersensitivity. Etiologic factors in the chronic form include exposure to cold, heat, or various light waves. Another form, cholinergic urticaria, occurs as a response to stress or physical exertion.

Because urticaria is usually self-limiting, treatment is often not required. Known offending agents are removed if possible. Epinephrine and antihistamines may be given to hasten resolution and to prevent further histamine reaction. Corticosteroids may be used on a short-term basis (initial dose of 40 mg, then decreased by 5 mg/day).

ATOPIC ALLERGY
EPIDEMIOLOGY AND ETIOLOGY

A less severe form of type I hypersensitivity than anaphylaxis is exhibited in atopic allergies. Common forms of atopic allergies include hay fever, allergic asthma (Chapter 33), and atopic dermatitis.

About 10% to 20% of the population react to antigens that are not antigens for the remainder of the population. These individuals are referred to as being "atopic." This tendency to become hypersensitive is inherited as a dominant trait. If both parents are atopic, there is a high probability that the children will be atopic. What these individuals become hypersensitive to, however, will be determined by the allergens to which they are exposed. A person does not inherit a specific allergy; the allergy will manifest itself in response to the allergens to

which the person is exposed. A sensitizing dose is necessary before allergic symptoms will occur.

The most common allergens in adults are seasonal and environmental inhalants. Food allergies are primarily a problem with children, and about 85% of these allergies disappear by age 2 years. Selected drugs may also cause hypersensitivity reactions, as well as contactants such as poison ivy or synthetics. Because the symptoms to these allergens are primarily dermal, they are discussed in Chapter 72.

Seasonal inhalant allergens are primarily the tree and grass pollens. Ragweed is the most common allergen in the United States, primarily east of the Rocky Mountains. Europe has little or no ragweed; other grasses are allergens there. Every geographic area has its own specific allergens. In the northern United States, early spring hayfever is usually caused by tree pollens, early summer hayfever by grasses, and late summer by ragweed.[71] Hypersensitivity to overlapping allergens may lead to symptoms throughout most of the year. "Rose fever" is a misnomer; the person is allergic to grasses pollenating at the same time.

Environmental inhalant allergens include house dust, animal dander (epithelial flakes), feathers, or fungal spores. Fungal spores are most often found in warm, damp basements, in crawl spaces under the house, in humidifiers, or on the leaves of certain trees, on wheat, or on corn.

CLINICAL MANIFESTATIONS

Histamine that is released by the mast cells has three main effects:

1. Constriction of smooth muscle, resulting in bronchospasm and constriction of conducting airways
2. Increased vascular permeability, leading to hives or mucosal edema (leakage of fluid) or to red spots on the skin (leakage of blood)
3. Increased mucous gland secretions

The symptoms seen in the persons with a type I hypersensitivity will be determined by the type of allergen (Figure 76-5) and the organ affected:

1. Respiratory: wheezing, sneezing, rhinitis with conjunctivitis
2. Dermal: urticaria, angioedema, rash
3. GI: nausea, vomiting, diarrhea
4. General symptoms: fever, malaise, joint pains, hematopoietic suppression, anaphylaxis

Diagnostic Tests

Skin tests (Chapter 75) are not specifically diagnostic because the person may demonstrate a positive test but not display symptoms to that allergen. The tests, however, do confirm the diagnosis obtained from the history and provide direction for immunotherapy.[71]

An additional test, the *RAST*, radioallergosorbent test for IgE antibodies, provides the same information as

ALLERGY

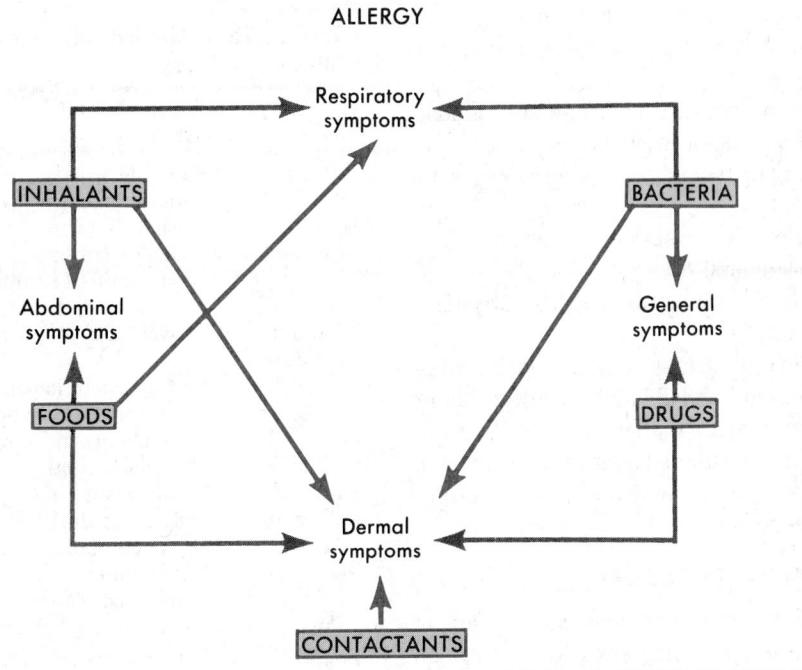

FIGURE 76-5 Causes of allergic responses and symptoms produced.

skin tests. RAST is easier to perform, more comfortable for the person, and safer; but it is less sensitive, less specific, and more costly than the skin tests.[46] A blood sample is drawn for the test.

MEDICAL MANAGEMENT

Medications

Drug therapy for atopic allergies is primarily for symptom relief. Some prescribed drugs include the following:

1. Antihistamines: chlorpheniramine (Chlor-Trimeton), brompheniramine (Dimetane), carbinoxamine (Clistin), terfenadine (Seldane) (Terfenadine is non-sedating)
2. Vasoconstricting agents: may be given singly (for example, Novafed, Sudafed) or in combination with antihistamines (such as, Dimetapp, Triamine, Actifed)
3. Mast cell degranulation inhibitor: cromolyn sodium (Nasalcrom, Rynacrom); this is used as a nasal spray
4. Corticosteroids for severe reactions:
   a. Nasal sprays such as Decadron Turbinaire, Vancenase, Beconase, Nasalide
   b. Oral corticosteroids such as prednisone, methylprednisolone

Immunotherapy (Hyposensitization)

Immunotherapy has been shown to be effective in diminishing symptoms of allergic rhinitis, particularly to allergies from pollens and house dusts. Hyposensitization appears to affect the immune system by two mechanisms: stimulation of T-suppressor cells specific to depression of IgE responses and stimulation of production of IgG antibodies specific to the allergen.[46] Increasing amounts of allergen are injected at weekly intervals, starting with a dose to which the person has been found sensitive by skin testing. The treatment may take up to 5 years. Treatment is about 80% effective; immunotherapy is restarted if symptoms recur.

If large local reactions (redness, edema, pruritus, or tenderness) occur during therapy, the dose is not increased but is repeated or lowered until better tolerated. Systemic reactions, although infrequent, may occur within 30 minutes of injection. Signs of systemic reaction include nasal stuffiness, sneezing, reddening of conjunctiva, tight chest, wheezing, faintness, apprehension, and eventually anaphylactic shock. The person is placed in a supine position, and aqueous epinephrine 1:1000 (0.2 to 0.5 ml) is injected into the arm that has not received the allergen injection. An additional small amount (0.1 to 0.2 ml) may be injected in the site of the allergen injection. Short-acting corticosteroids may be prescribed to prevent recurrence.

■ ASSESSMENT

Nursing interventions are based on the person's knowledge about the disorder and on the source or form of allergy present. This information is obtained by taking a history.

1. History of allergic reactions in the past (for example, type, frequency, or perceived causes)
2. Familial history of allergies

3. Recent exposure to sensitizing substances
4. Changes in living, working, or environmental conditions
5. Characteristics of present environment (house, clothing, plants, trees, or animals)
6. Increased stress in recent past (aggravates asthmatic response)
7. Types of symptoms: respiratory, dermal, gastrointestinal, or general
8. Alleviating factors, either prescribed by physician or self-prescribed

All persons in the health care system should be questioned about allergies and sensitivities to drugs before any drug therapy is initiated. If there is a positive history, the physician is consulted before a new drug is given; if the drug is given, the patient is monitored closely for allergic responses.

■ DATA ANALYSIS: NURSING DIAGNOSES

Nursing diagnoses are determined from assessment of patient data. Possible nursing diagnoses for the person with an allergy include, but are not limited to, the following:

Diagnostic Title	Possible Etiologies
Health maintenance, altered	Environmental changes, lack of knowledge
Knowledge deficit	Lack of exposure/recall, information misinterpretation

■ PLANNING: EXPECTED PATIENT OUTCOMES

Expected patient outcomes for the person with an allergy may include, but are not limited to, the following:

1. Patient's symptoms decrease in intensity
2. The person can describe the following:
   a. Plans to alter habits or environment, as appropriate
   b. Substances that are allergenic and approaches for avoidance
   c. Rationale for immunotherapy and need to continue regular injections (if pertinent)
   d. Need for constant availability of an anaphylaxis emergency kit for self-treatment (if anaphylaxis is a possibility)
   e. Drug therapy to relieve symptoms

IMPLEMENTATION

Environmental Control

Persons who are allergic to *dust* must prepare a living and working environment that is as dust free as possible. There should be a minimum of lint-producing articles (such as curtains, bedspreads, and carpets). Smooth, synthetic materials should be used in place of wool or cotton (Table 76-4). Small items such as figurines or other small decorations that are difficult to dust are best removed or placed in glass-enclosed cabinets.

TABLE 76-4 Methods of decreasing environmental inhalant antigens

Area	Method
Floors	No wool carpets or felt rug pads; washable throw rugs over wood or tile floors may be used
Furniture	No kapok stuffing; a minimum number of foam-stuffed furniture covered with leather or plastic is preferable
Clothing	No wool; place closet garments in plastic bags
Bedding	
Pillows	No feathers or kapok; use polyester fiberfill
Mattress	Use foam mattress over a covered box spring; use allergy-free covers
Blankets	Washable cotton
Pets	No fur-bearing pets
Cleaning	Daily damp dusting; no shaking of articles
Air	Air conditioning, if possible; if not, try electrostatic filters
Plants	Avoid dried plants
Furnace	Change filters monthly

Daily *damp* dusting will lessen the amount of dust in the air. Air conditioning is desirable for hot weather.

Avoidance of Allergens

Animal dander is one allergen that usually can be avoided completely. Fur-bearing pets can be removed from the environment. If total removal of a family pet is difficult because of emotional ties, the pet can be kept in an outdoor enclosure. Furniture stuffed with horsehair or feathers must be replaced with synthetic materials. It usually takes several months for symptoms from animal dander to subside.

Seasonal inhalants are more difficult to avoid. If financially possible, the best method is taking a prolonged vacation in an area free of the offending allergen. When the person remains at home, outside air should be avoided as much as possible during the seasonal months by the use of air conditioners (ACs). However, car air conditioners may increase the allergic reaction, because mold spores can proliferate in the moist evaporator core from the warmed car engine. To correct this problem, instruct the allergic person to start the car, turn on the air conditioner, roll down the windows, and run the air conditioner for about 10 to 15 minutes (to blow out the spores) before entering car. Mold disinfectant spray is also available.

For both pollen and spores, the highest counts (amount in the air) occur between 12 midnight and 8 AM; therefore outdoor air should be avoided during those hours. The "official" counts often cited on television or in the newspaper can be misleading, because the counts are usually from the previous day, and pollen

TEACHING THE PERSON WITH AN ATOPIC ALLERGY

The person will be able to explain or perform the following:
1. Avoid allergen, if possible.
   a. Animal dander
      (1) Have no fur-bearing pets, if possible.
      (2) Keep any family fur-bearing pet in outdoor enclosure.
      (3) Avoid furniture stuffed with horsehair or feathers.
   b. Pollen spores
      (1) Vacation in selected geographic areas, such as beach or sea, that are free of specific allergen during seasonal height, if possible.
      (2) Use air conditioning if possible; keep windows closed at night; if using air conditioner in car, start car, roll down windows and allow air conditioner to run for 10-15 min before entering car.
      (3) Limit being outdoors between sunset and sunrise, especially when windy.
      (4) Do not hang wash outside to dry. (Pollen and molds stick to wet wash.)
      (5) Avoid gardening, raking leaves, mowing lawn, or being near freshly cut grass.
      (6) Keep car windows closed when driving.
      (7) Minimize number of indoor plants.
   c. House dust
      (1) Use synthetic materials; avoid wool and cotton.
      (2) Use a minimum of lint-producing articles.
      (3) Put away articles that are difficult to dust.
      (4) Dust with damp cloth daily.
      (5) Use air conditioner, if possible.
      (6) Change furnace filter every month during use.

2. During immunotherapy (hyposensitization)
   a. Report for regularly scheduled injections, even when symptoms subside (therapy will last for 3 to 5 months).
   b. Remain at physician's office for at least 30 minutes after receiving injection (for immediate treatment should a systemic reaction occur).
   c. Report large local reactions to physician (redness, swelling, itching, or soreness).
3. Monitor for side effects of medication taken frequently for relief of symptoms.
   a. Antihistamines: sedation, constipation, urinary retention, tachycardia; avoidance of driving or use of heavy machinery if drowsiness is present
   b. Vasoconstrictors: irregular or rapid pulse, palpitations, restlessness, dizziness
   c. Nasal corticosteroids: nasal irritation, dryness of nose and mouth
   d. Cromolyn sodium: throat irritation, headache, dizziness, rash, urticaria

counts differ from place to place. Being outside on dry windy days, riding in an open car, and gardening are usually reported to increase symptoms.[71]

Patient Teaching

The major nursing responsibility in the care of the person with an atopic allergy is teaching the patient about the nature of the disorder and the methods that can be used to avoid the allergen and control the environment as previously described. The major points for teaching are summarized in the box above.

TYPE II HYPERSENSITIVITIES

PATHOPHYSIOLOGY

The underlying mechanism of type II (cytotoxic) hypersensitivities involves the direct binding of IgG or IgM immunoglobulins to an antigen on the surface of a cell. This antibody labeling then triggers the destruction of the cell by phagocytic attack, nonspecific lymphocytic attack, or lysis of the cell through the operation of the full complement cascade (see Chapter 8).

BLOOD TRANSFUSION REACTIONS

Type II hypersensitivity is classically illustrated by the reactions that occur in mismatched blood transfusion reactions. Blood replacement therapy is used when there has been excessive blood loss (whole blood or blood components) or in the treatment of diseases of the hematopoietic system.

Although whole blood may be used, there has been an increased use of specific blood components. Only about 28% of blood now given in the United States is in the form of whole blood.[30] Blood can be fractionated into RBCs, platelets, and plasma (Table 76-5), either by centrifuge or by automated cell separators. Blood can also be withdrawn from a donor, a portion separated from the blood, and the remainder returned to the donor (*pheresis*). Using blood components rather than whole blood provides greater use of an increasingly scarcer commodity (blood) for an increased number of recipients, prevents fluid overload, and gives the recipient only that which is required (thus decreasing possibilities of side effects).

TABLE 76-5 Types of blood components

Blood Component	Description	Usage	Comments
RED BLOOD CELLS (RBCs)			
Packed RBC (PRBCs)	RBCs separated from plasma and platelets	Anemia Moderate blood loss	Decreased risk of fluid overload as compared to whole blood
Autologous PRBC	Same as packed RBC	Elective surgery for which blood replacement is expected	Units may be stored for up to 35 days
Washed RBCs	RBCs washed with sterile iso-tonic saline before transfusion	Previous allergic reactions to transfusions	Increased removal of immuno-globulins and protein
Frozen RBCs	RBCs frozen in a glycerol solu-tion; cells washed after thaw-ing to remove the glycerol	Storage of rare type blood Storage of autologous blood for future use	Relatively free of leukocytes and microemboli Expensive
Leukocyte-poor RBCs	RBCs from which most leuko-cytes have been removed	Previous sensitivity to leukocyte antigens from prior transfu-sions or from pregnancy	Fewer RBC than packed RBC; washed leukocyte-poor RBC units have more RBC than nonwashed
Neocytes	RBC units with high number of reticulocytes (young RBCs)	Transfusion-dependent anemias	Fewer problems with iron over-load Expensive
OTHER CELLULAR COMPONENTS			
Platelets			
Random donor packs	Platelets separated from RBCs by centrifuge; given in 50 ml of plasma	Thrombocytopenia DIC	Plasma base is rich in coagula-tion factors Platelet preparations can also be packed, washed, or made leukocyte-poor
Pheresis packs	Platelets from an HLA matched donor, separated by pheresis	Allosensitized persons with thrombocytopenia	Requires specialized techniques
Granulocytes	Granular leukocytes separated by pheresis	Granulocytopenia from malig-nancy or chemotherapy	Allergen sensitization may occur with chills and fever
PLASMA COMPONENTS			
Fresh frozen plasma (FFP)	Freezing of plasma within 4 hr of collection	Clotting deficiencies Liver disease Hemophilia Defibrination	Preserves factors V, VII, VIII, IX, and X and prothrombin Minimizes hepatitis risk Administered through a filter
Factor concentrates VIII and IX	Prepared from large donor pools Heated to inactivate HIV	VIII: Hemophilia A IX: Hemophilia B	Increased risk of hepatitis (VIII, IX) and thromboembolism (IX) Given in small volumes
Cryoprecipitate	Precipitated material obtained from FFP when thawed	Hemophilia A Infection of burns Hypofibrinogenemia Uremic bleeding	Contains factors VIII, XIII, and fibrinogen

Serum albumin
  Normal serum albumin (NSA)
  Plasma protein fraction (PPF)
	Albumin chemically processed from pooled plasma	Hypovolemic shock
		Hypoalbuminemia
		Burns
		Hemorrhagic shock
			No risk of hepatitis
			Does not require ABO compati-bility
			Lacks clotting factors
			Hypotension may occur if PPF is given faster than 10 ml/min

Immune serum globulin	Obtained from plasma of prese-lected donors with specific antibodies	Hypogammaglobulinemia Prophylaxis for hepatitis A	Given intramuscularly

ABO BLOOD GROUPS

A	Antigen A is present
B	Antigen B is present
AB	Both antigens A and B are present
O	Neither antigen A nor B is present

PATHOPHYSIOLOGY

There are many antigens on the surface of RBCs, but there are two major systems that are significant clinically in terms of potential immunologic reactions: the ABO system and the Rh system. The HLA system relates to leukocytes and platelets.

ABO System

There are four major blood groups that exist in humans: A, B, AB, and O (see the box above). Since type AB blood contains both antigens, persons with type AB may receive blood from any type (Figure 76-6). Persons with type O may donate blood to other types, but since both antigens are absent in type O, they may not receive another type without experiencing a reaction.

Within the serum, individuals possess naturally occurring antibodies to the RBC surface antigens of the ABO blood groups that are not present on their own erythrocytes. For example, a person with type A blood will possess anti-B antibodies within the serum. These antibodies, called *isohemagglutinins*, are usually of the IgM class. They are thought to arise through a natural immunization to the glycopeptide antigens on the RBC surface through contact with similar glycopeptides found on the surface of the cell walls of bacteria that make up the natural intestinal flora. Antibodies formed in this way are capable of cross-reacting with the A or B antigens on the surface of the "foreign" ABO types. These antibodies are naturally present in the serum; therefore mismatched blood cells from a transfusion will be immediately coated by the isohemagglutinins, causing the agglutination of the introduced cells and the rapid lysis of the cells by complement. The products released by the lysed cells are then dumped into the bloodstream.

Rh System

The Rh system is more complex, because there are at least 27 different antigens in this system. The D antigen is the most significant clinically, since it is more immunogenic than any other Rh antigen, and it is usually the antigen involved in hemolytic disease of the newborn. When the term *Rh positive* is used, the presence of antigen Rh-D is implied; *Rh negative* indicates the absence of antigen D. Approximately 85% of the population have Rh-positive blood.

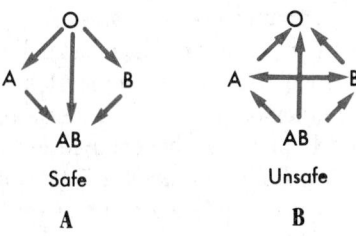

FIGURE 76-6 Blood groups and their donor/recipient relationships. **A,** Safe. **B,** Unsafe.

When the Rh-negative person is first exposed to Rh-positive blood, Rh antibodies are formed. On subsequent exposures to Rh-positive blood, the Rh antibody binds to its corresponding antigen on the surface of the RBCs containing the Rh antigen. The Rh antibodies do not usually fix complement; therefore there is no immediate hemolysis as occurs in the ABO system. Instead, the Rh-antigen RBCs are rapidly broken down by macrophages in the spleen, with conversion of hemoglobin to bilirubin resulting in jaundice.

HLA System

Another system that has clinical significance in blood transfusions is the human leukocytes antigen (HLA) system (p. 2218). HLAs are found on many types of tissue cells and on blood leukocytes and platelets. The system is more complex than the RBC antigen systems, and there are literally thousands of combinations of the antigens that may occur. Sensitization may occur through pregnancy or through exposure to platelets and WBCs during transfusions. Repeated transfusions of blood cells may lead to transfusion reactions.

PREVENTION OF REACTIONS

Donor Prescreening

Prescreening of potential blood donors is essential. Blood received from volunteer donors through the American Red Cross Blood Service or hospital blood banks is preferable to that of paid donors, because paid donors may be less likely to report present or previous diseases that may affect the recipient.

Requirements have been delineated that include guidelines for persons with heart, lung, liver, or kidney disease. Persons who are not accepted as donors include those with a history of the following:

1. Infectious diseases such as hepatitis, AIDS, tuberculosis, syphilis, or malaria
2. Malignant disease
3. Allergies or asthma
4. Polycythemia vera
5. Abnormal bleeding tendencies
6. Hypotension (current)
7. Anemia (current)

8. Recent pregnancy or major surgery
9. Men with at least one homosexual or bisexual contact since 1975 (concern for AIDS)

The donor's hemoglobin level is tested before giving blood, and the hemoglobin acceptance level is usually set at over 13.5 g/dl for men and 12.5 g/dl for women.[38] Temperature, pulse, and blood pressure should be within normal ranges.

After the blood has been collected, it is tested for syphilis, hepatitis, human immunodeficiency virus (HIV), and cytomegalovirus (CMV). The blood group and subgroups including Rh typing are identified. Donor blood must be crossmatched with blood from the recipient in order to determine compatibility to prevent an acute hemolytic reaction. Crossmatching consists of mixing samples of the donor's and the recipient's blood and examining for cell clumping or hemolysis. A major crossmatch is between *recipient serum* and *donor cells*. A minor crossmatch, between donor serum and recipient cells, is rarely performed, because donor antibodies are greatly diluted by the recipient's plasma; therefore the major crossmatch usually suffices.

Administration Safeguards

Most of the serious reactions that now occur during transfusions are the result of human error. Crossmatching and testing in the laboratory must be accurate. Blood must be kept cold until ready to use. If blood has remained at room temperature for more than 30 minutes before infusion, it should not be returned to refrigeration and then reissued; this contributes to growth of gram-negative organisms that can produce serious septicemia. The unit of blood or blood components must be labeled with the name of the person for whom it is intended, and this label must be checked against the patient's wristband before the blood is administered. The patient must be monitored throughout the administration of the blood. All blood products should be administered through micron mesh filters. (Consult a fundamentals of nursing text for information on care of patients during initiation and course of blood transfusions.)

COMPLICATIONS OF BLOOD TRANSFUSIONS

There are numerous adverse reactions to blood transfusions, both immunologic and nonimmunologic reactions (see box above).

Immunologic Transfusion Reactions

Several immunologic reactions can occur with the administration of whole blood or its components. The symptoms and actions for these reactions are described in Table 76-6. The most serious reaction is the acute hemolytic reaction, which occurs within the first 30 ml of blood transfusion. Intravascular agglutination and lysis of incompatible RBC occurs from activation of the com-

---

ADVERSE REACTIONS TO BLOOD TRANSFUSIONS

IMMUNOLOGIC

Hemolytic: acute, delayed
Allergic: urticaria, anaphylactic
Febrile (pyrogenic)
Graft-versus-host disease
Noncardiac pulmonary edema

NONIMMUNOLOGIC

Fluid volume overload
Transmission of disease: hepatitis, HIV infection, cytomegalovirus, malaria, syphilis
Transfusion hemosiderosis
Massive blood replacement: bleeding, hypothermia, ventricular fibrillation

---

plement cascade on the red cell membrane. Hemoglobin is released and is excreted in the urine. The urine becomes red (port-wine urine), and acute tubular necrosis may lead first to oliguria then to renal shutdown. Profound shock occurs. If signs of chills, fever, and backache occur, the transfusion is stopped immediately and the physician notified.

Persons who have a delayed hemolytic reaction are tested to determine which antigens have caused the reaction. They are then given an identification card listing the appropriate blood groups and the responsible alloantibodies.

Graft-versus-host disease may occur when immunodeficient or immunosuppressed persons receive blood transfusions containing lymphocytes. The recipient cannot eliminate the donor lymphocytes, so the donor lymphocytes "reject" the recipient's tissues as foreign.

Nonimmunologic Reactions

Fluid overload (see Chapter 23) is one of the more frequent adverse effects of whole blood transfusion, especially in children, elderly persons, or persons with congestive heart failure or severe anemia. If symptoms of hypervolemia occur, the rate of the infusion is slowed or stopped, depending on the severity of the symptoms.

Massive transfusions (rapid replacement of a person's blood with stored blood) may cause some additional problems. Bleeding may result from dilution of coagulation factors or from platelet breakdown. Infusions of cold blood may stimulate ventricular fibrillation; therefore this blood should be warmed during administration. Only a temperature-controlled device should be used to warm the blood to prevent hemolysis from temperatures over 37° C (98° F). Hypocalcemia (from citrate binding with ionized serum calcium) and hyperkalemia (from potassium released by cell breakdown) are rare.

TABLE 76-6 Immunologic reactions to blood transfusions

Reaction	Cause	Mechanism	Symptoms	Occurrence	Action
Acute hemolytic	Recipient antibody incompatible with transfused red cells	RBCs agglutinate, rapid hemolysis Capillary plugging (type II hypersensitivity)	Lumbar pain Constriction of chest Pain in vein Fever, chills Hemoglobinuria Signs of shock	Shortly after initiation of transfusion	Stop transfusion Continue IV saline Blood unit and blood sample from patient sent to lab for immediate testing Treat for shock and renal failure
Delayed hemolytic	Anamnestic immune response	Slow hemolysis	Jaundice Anemia	Days to weeks after transfusion	Monitor adequacy of urinary output and degree of anemia
Allergic	Transfer of an antigen or a reaginic antibody from donor to recipient	Immune sensitivity to foreign serum protein (type I hypersensitivity)	Urticaria Anaphylaxis (wheezing, dyspnea, shock)	Within 30 min after initiation of transfusion	Mild: give antihistamine, continue transfusion Severe: give aqueous epinephrine (0.5 ml of 1:1000 solution)
Febrile	Reaction of antigen on WBC or platelets Bacterial contamination	Leukocyte agglutination Bacterial pyrogens	Fever, chills	Within 30 to 90 min after initiation of transfusion	Stop transfusion Continue IV saline Antipyretics after ruling out hemolytic reaction Transfuse with leukocyte-poor blood or washed RBCs
Graft-versus-host disease	Immunodeficient person receives lymphocytes	Engraftment of donor lymphocytes that are then "rejected"	Dermatitis Stomatitis Diarrhea Liver dysfunction	Delayed	Steroids Azathioprine Symptomatic therapy
Noncardiac pulmonary edema	Donor antibodies react with recipient HLA antigen	Infiltration of pulmonary bed by microaggregates that block blood flow	Fever, chills Urticaria Cough Orthopnea Cyanosis Shock	During transfusion or shortly thereafter	Stop transfusion Continue IV saline Give oxygen as needed Steroids Furosemide

Transfusion hemosiderosis is iron overload found in persons who receive repeated transfusions for hematopoietic disorders and who lack compensatory iron losses. Neocytes or frozen RBCs (see Table 76-5) are used for future transfusions to decrease the number of required transfusions.

Disease Transmission

The major diseases that presently may be transmitted by blood transfusions are hepatitis B; hepatitis non-A, non-B; and HIV infection. The incidence of hepatitis B transmission has been greatly reduced by the elimination of donors with a positive HB$_s$Ag test (Chapter 39). There is no screening test for hepatitis non-A, non-B virus. Blood is also screened for HIV *antibodies* (Chapter 77), indicating previous HIV exposure. The risk of transmission of HIV infection is less than 1 in 1,000,000 for each transfused unit of blood.[62] HIV in blood products is inactivated by heat treatment.

Although syphilis and malaria may also be transmitted by blood transfusions, the incidence is rare. Cytomegalovirus may be identified in about 10% of blood donors by screening blood for CMV antibodies. Symptoms of CMV infection occur in about 40 days and are similar to infectious mononucleosis (fever, malaise, and splenomegaly). In adults the condition is benign, and treatment is symptomatic.

AUTOLOGOUS BLOOD TRANSFUSIONS

One method of preventing immunologic blood transfusion reactions and disease transmission is by using the person's own blood for replacement. There are two approaches for using autologous blood: planned collection and autotransfusion. In *planned autologous transfusion,* blood is collected at regular intervals before anticipated use, such as for forthcoming surgery. The blood is then stored or frozen until needed. This method is especially useful for persons with rare blood types, for those whose religious beliefs preclude receiving donor blood, or when several units of blood are expected to be necessary during surgery (such as with selected heart surgeries or selected joint replacements).

Autotransfusion, which consists of collecting, filtering, and immediately reinfusing the person's own blood, may be performed in the emergency room or in the OR suite during surgery involving large blood loss. The blood is suctioned into a bag and passes through a filter to remove microaggregates.[6] When the bag is full, it is disconnected from the system and the blood is infused into the patient with an administration set, using a standard or microembolic filter. Blood that has been contaminated by GI contents or that is close to a malignant tumor is not autotransfused.

TYPE III HYPERSENSITIVITIES
PATHOPHYSIOLOGY

The pathogenesis of the type III (immune complex) hypersensitivities lies in the union of soluble antigens and immunoglobulins of the IgM and IgG classes. The complexes formed in these interactions are not properly cleared by the reticuloendothelial system (RES) because of the small size of the complexes, which tend to defy phagocytosis. They are deposited in the body tissues. The complexes can then bind complement with all the attendant reactions of an internal, often intravascular, *inflammatory response.* The chemotactic factors released with the involvement of complement lead to an influx of phagocytes, which tend to intensify the inflammation. *Large* complexes are removed by the RES. Immune complexes that develop in conditions of mild antigen excess are *neither small nor large* and are deposited in the glomerular basement membrane (glomerulonephritis [poststreptococcal, SLE]), joint linings (rheumatoid arthritis), blood vessels (serum sickness), and pulmonary alveolar membranes (acute allergic alveolitis).[69] The clinical symptoms observed are the result of the amounts and relative proportions of the antigens and antibodies and the distribution of the complexes within the body.

ARTHUS REACTION

The repeated subcutaneous injection of a highly antigenic soluble antigen can lead to the formation of such *immune complexes,* which trigger a localized inflammatory response known as *Arthus reaction.* The region exhibiting Arthus reaction shows the following sequential tissue changes: reduction of blood flow, development of

microthrombi in the venules, increased permeability of the venule to the point that RBCs escape into the surrounding tissues, development of edema, massive infiltration of the site by polymorphonuclear neutrophil leukocytes, and tissue destruction. Arthus reactions are not of great clinical importance, since strongly antigenic substances are not usually administered in repeated subcutaneous injections. However, a disseminated type of intravascular inflammation known as allergic vasculitis sometimes occurs in patients undergoing therapy with certain drugs (for example, sulfonamides, iodides, thioureas, and penicillin).

SERUM SICKNESS
ETIOLOGY

A type III hypersensitivity of clinical significance is serum sickness, which can develop from 1 to 3 weeks after the administration of a large amount of foreign serum (for example, horse serum). This classic type of serum sickness occurs less frequently than in the past with the decreasing use of foreign serum administration; however, serum sickness reactions may also occur with the administration of certain drugs, particularly antimicrobials such as penicillin.

PATHOPHYSIOLOGY

The critical factor in this hypersensitivity reaction is a large amount of a persisting soluble antigen, the foreign serum proteins. The antigen initiates an immune response, and the resultant antibodies appear in the blood about 1 week later where they interact with the antigen still present in the bloodstream. The complexes are deposited within the blood vessel walls. Complement is bound, and an intravascular inflammation occurs.

CLINICAL MANIFESTATIONS

Itching and discomfort at the injection site are usually the first symptoms noted. These are followed by lymphadenopathy, fever, urticaria or erythematous rash, angioedema of the face, and joint pain. Splenomegaly, abdominal pain, headache, nausea, and vomiting may also occur. Objective signs of arthritis may be present.

INTERVENTIONS

Serum sickness is a self-limiting disease. Mild symptoms respond well to antihistamines and salicylates. More severe symptoms are treated with a steroid such as prednisone, with relief of symptoms often obtained within hours. Epinephrine is given if an anaphylactic reaction occurs.

TYPE IV HYPERSENSITIVITIES
PATHOPHYSIOLOGY

Type IV hypersensitivities are cell mediated (delayed type), involving T cells. Antigens identified as "foreign" to the body can cause a reaction in two ways—by direct or by indirect action. The T-lymphocyte can destroy the antigen directly by attaching itself to the antigen cell wall, breaking down the cell membrane and causing lysis and death of the cell. This direct action approach appears to be a major factor in allograft rejections. The indirect approach consists of activating nonspecific phagocytic cells (macrophages and polymorphonuclear leukocytes) through release of lymphokines by the sensitized T-lymphocytes (see Chapter 8).

The cell-mediated immune mechanisms function in host defense against chronic bacterial and fungal infections, in rejection of foreign tissue cells, and in surveillance for cancer cells; however, they can also produce adverse effects in the form of delayed-type hypersensitivity. Three major areas of clinical concern are (1) hypersensitivity reactions in response to infections by certain bacteria, fungi, or viruses, (2) contact dermatitis reactions, and (3) tissue transplant rejections.

HYPERSENSITIVITY REACTIONS IN CERTAIN INFECTIONS

The body's reaction to the tubercle bacillus (*Mycobacterium tuberculosis*) is a classic example of a type IV hypersensitivity. The organism itself is not directly toxic to human cells or tissues. As a result, the tubercle bacillus may invade the tissues of a nonsensitized host and establish residence in the host tissues, causing virtually no damage. However, in the course of time, as the organism sheds antigenic material, the cell-mediated immune response system is triggered. The sensitized lymphocytes and the activated macrophages attack not only the organism, but also the tissues surrounding the organism. This process is aimed at destroying the foreign organism; however, in the course of the attack, tissue destruction may result. The lesions associated with tuberculosis (such as caseation necrosis cavitation) and general toxemia are results of the hypersensitivity.

After the initial sensitization with the infectious organism, subsequent contact with the tuberculosis organism or even an extract of a purified protein from the organism will elicit a hypersensitivity reaction. This is the basis of the Mantoux tuberculin skin test. The skin rashes of smallpox and measles and the lesions of herpes simplex virus and tuberculoid leprosy have all been attributed to an infectious type IV hypersensitivity.

ALLERGIC CONTACT DERMATITIS

Allergic contact dermatitis is one of the most commonly encountered types of human allergic disease. Usually, both the route of sensitization and the display of symptoms are produced by direct dermal contact with the allergen. Many simple chemicals can serve as contact allergens. Among those most often implicated are industrial chemicals, topical ointments, soaps, dinitrochlorobenzene (DNCB), nickel, mercury, topical antibiotics, cosmetics, and the catecholes of poison ivy, poison oak, and poison sumac.

Many of the contact allergens are of a size (less than 10,000 molecular weight) and structure that do not allow them to serve as a complete antigen. It is most probable that the compound attaches to proteins of the skin and functions as a hapten to stimulate the proliferation of a T cell population sensitized to the compound. After sensitization, subsequent contact with the contact allergen leads to the formation of an erythematous, vesiculated (blistered) lesion. The inflamed area itches, burns, or stings. Scratching the lesion may further spread the allergen or infect the site. There is often a serous exudate. (For care of the person with contact dermatitis, see Chapter 72).

TISSUE TRANSPLANTATION REJECTION

The rejection of foreign cells and tissues by the body is a beneficial function of the immune system primarily mediated by a type IV hypersensitivity. If it were not for this mechanism, the human body would be a haven for the inappropriate establishment of growth of any animal cell that penetrated the external defense mechanisms; however, this process is regarded as a disservice when it operates to prevent the positive aspects of the exchange of tissues between hosts.

The transfer of healthy tissues and organs from one individual to replace damaged or diseased tissues of another has been surgically possible for many years. The early attempts at tissue graft failed because of the rejection process. With the growing knowledge of the immune response, the mechanisms of this rejection process became more apparent, and it is now possible to make judgments and predictions concerning the likelihood of success of such an endeavor. It is possible to control the course of the graft transfer process to favor the acceptance of the transplanted tissues.

TYPES OF TISSUE TRANSPLANTS

The following terminology has been derived to describe transplants between individuals and species. It is based on the genetically derived discrepancies and similarities between the donor and the recipient.

autograft (autotransplantation) transfer of tissue from one site on an individual to another site; since this simply means the rearrangement of self, immunologically there is little concern.

isograft (or syngraft) transfer of tissue between syngeneic (identical genetic makeup) individuals such as identical twins; since there is no genetic discrepancy in antigens, the immunologic factors favor success.

allograft (homotransplantation) transfer of tissues between allogeneic (same species but exhibiting different genetic makeup) individuals; since the tissues of the donor are foreign to the recipient, they are antigenic and subject to rejection.

xenograft (heterotransplantation) transfer of tissues between xenogeneic (different species) individuals; since the genetic differences are enormous, there is virtually no chance of avoiding immunorejection.

The allograft tissue transfer offers the most promise for organ and tissue replacement and is the one currently receiving the most clinical attention. Blood transfusion is the most common allografting procedure used today; and notwithstanding the problems associated with transfusion (p. 2214), it is carried out daily with success. Solid-tissue grafts such as skin and organs, however, introduce considerably greater problems.

PATHOPHYSIOLOGY

The antigenic determinants of the tissues that lead to graft rejection are primarily found on the surface of the cells within the transplanted tissues. These antigens are known as histocompatibility antigens and are controlled by independently segregating genes within the chromosomal structure of the animal. They are also called HLAs. Some of the histocompatibility antigens are more antigenic than are others; thus some antigens are referred to as major and others as minor. The major transplantation antigens are those of the ABO and Rh blood groups and the HLAs (p. 2213).

TISSUE TYPING

In preparation for an allograft the closest match of donor-recipient transplantation antigens is sought. This is done by tissue typing for the major antigenic determinants (ABO, Rh, and HLA). If there are no significant discrepancies in these antigens, the recipient's serum is mixed with lymphocytes from the donor, or the lymphocytes from the donor and recipient are cultured together to detect minor (but significant) cross-reactions. This is known as a mixed lymphocyte reaction (MLR).

CLINICAL MANIFESTATIONS

The process of graft rejection is as complicated and exquisite as the immune response system that brings it about. It has been best characterized in the case of skin allograft rejections. In this case, when the nonmatched skin is transferred to the new host, it settles down and becomes vascularized within 2 to 3 days; however, within 6 to 10 days, sensitized lymphocytes appear in the regional lymph nodes, and the lymph nodes begin to enlarge. The initial signs of rejection appear in about 10 to 14 days, with the appearance first of sensitized lymphocytes and then macrophages at the site. Within 12 to 14 days, the vascular bed begins to deteriorate, and the graft becomes necrotic and is sloughed off. This is known as first-set rejection. If another skin graft is taken from the same donor and is transplanted to a different site on the same recipient, the graft rejection is more rapid. This accelerated reaction, known as second-

set rejection, is so rapid that the graft may never be vascularized before it is sloughed. In second-set rejection, circulating antibodies as well as the sensitized lymphocytes play a role. The antibodies create a direct cytotoxic attack on the graft. This is analogous to a type II immediate hypersensitivity reaction.

Some allografts circumvent immunorejection because of their site in the body. Corneal grafts survive without the need for immunosuppression, because the site is avascular. Cartilage grafts enjoy the same privilege. Grafts into these types of sites are referred to as privileged-site grafts. By some (as yet unknown) mechanism, the fetus developing within the uterus enjoys this privileged-site status.

INTERVENTIONS

Immunosuppression

As long as the foreign tissue remains in the host, graft rejection is a possibility. The risk is greatest during the first few years, but it never fully disappears. The organ graft recipient, therefore, requires immunosuppression for the remainder of life. The ideal immunosuppressive agent, one that will prevent graft rejection without interfering with the recipient's own immune response to foreign antigens, has not yet been discovered. Immunosuppressive therapy leaves the host immunodeficient (p. 2200) and interferes with the host's ability to fight invasion and infection.

Drug therapy. Graft rejection can be minimized by the use of chemical agents that nonspecifically or specifically interfere with the development of an immune response reaction against the allograft. The major drugs used in immunosuppressive therapy are cyclosporine, azathioprine, and glucocorticoids (see Table 76-2).

Cyclosporine (Sandimmune) was discovered in the early 1980s and has become the primary immunosuppressive agent for organ transplantation. It was isolated from a fungus and has the following immunoresponses: (1) suppresses T-helper cells (main effect), (2) inhibits lymphokine production, and (3) inhibits release of interleukin-2. B cells and the bone marrow are not affected, therefore some immune reactions to foreign proteins continue but are reduced. Better graft retention results have been achieved with cyclosporine than with other drugs. Cyclosporine is administered with corticosteroids for several days before the transplant surgery and is also given for maintenance therapy. Persons taking cyclosporine develop hirsutism and gingival hypertrophy. Other side effects may include hypertension, oral candidiasis, tremors, rash, and acne. If signs of nephrotoxicity (albuminuria, hematuria) or hepatotoxicity (dark urine, light-colored stools, jaundice, itching) occur, the drug is discontinued.

Azathioprine (Imuran) is a derivative of mercaptopurine and acts nonspecifically by suppressing T-cell effects. It antagonizes purine metabolism and inhibits DNA synthesis. It also causes variable alteration in antibody production. The clinical effects may persist for long periods after the medication is eliminated. The major toxic effect is bone marrow depression with development of megaloblastic anemia. Azathioprine may be given alone or in combination with steroids.

Glucocorticoids, especially prednisone, are significantly antiinflammatory and impair lymphocyte (B and T cell) activation and function. Prednisone exerts a wide spectrum of activity against all immune response and inflammatory response mechanisms. Although it suppresses the cell-mediated system to a greater extent than it does the humoral system, the continued high dosage needed to maintain cell-mediated suppression creates significant risks in reducing the responsiveness of the humoral system and causing other side effects. Lower doses of prednisone are required when used in combination with cyclosporine or azathioprine.

Other therapy. *Antilymphocyte globulin* (ALG) is given for short-term therapy to decrease the initial immune response to organ transplantation or to reverse acute rejection.[69] ALG must be given in high doses; therefore side effects are usually experienced (p. 2201). *Monoclonal antibodies* (OKT3) can also be given for short-term specific immunosuppression.

Pretransplantation Blood Transfusion

Blood transfusions given before kidney transplantation appear to enhance graft survival; the mechanism is unknown. *Donor-specific blood transfusions* (DST) consist of blood donated by a living relative. This is thought to depress antigen-specific immune responses. Persons receiving cadaver kidneys are given *random-donor transfusions* that appear to depress the overall immune response.[69] (For more information on kidney transplantation, see Chapter 50).

Prevention of Infection

Because persons experiencing organ transplantation are given immunosuppressive therapy to prevent tissue rejection, prevention of infection is as important as with any immunodeficiency (p. 2203). Invasive procedures such as venipunctures, catheterizations, or GI intubation are performed as seldom as possible, and invasive catheters are removed as soon as feasible. Meticulous care is given to insertion sites such as cleansing venipuncture sites with povidone-iodine preparations, using aseptic dressing changes around central venous catheter insertion sites, and giving good perineal care to patients with indwelling catheters. Irrigation of indwelling nasogastric tubes or urinary catheters is performed carefully to avoid traumatizing mucous membranes. An-

tibiotic solutions may be prescribed for urinary catheter irrigations.

Maintenance of skin integrity is important to prevent a breakdown of the first line of defense, since the immune defense is deficient. Frequent assessment of skin and mucous membranes is carried out, and vigorous preventive measures are immediately instituted for any early signs of skin breakdown. Classic signs and symptoms of infection may not occur because of the immunosuppression.

AUTOIMMUNE DISEASES

Individuals sometimes respond immunologically to some of their own antigens. When the mechanisms for the recognition of self versus nonself are subverted or altered, an immune attack of self may result. The chance that the control mechanisms will be lost increases with the age of the individual. The symptoms of such a self-attack are referred to as autoimmune disease or autohypersensitivity. For the most part, these self-reactions are not immunologically initiated; the etiologic (causative) agent lies outside the immune system, but the immune response serves as the pathogenic mechanism.

The meaning of the demonstration of autoantibodies and autosensitive T cell clones is not always clear. These self-reactive immunoglobulins are often associated with certain pathologic states in the body but many times can also be isolated from the serum of "normal" individuals as well, especially in older persons. Autoantibodies have been demonstrated against nuclear material in systemic lupus erythematosus, against γ-globulins in rheumatoid arthritis, against gastric parietal cells in pernicious anemia, and against platelets in autoimmune thrombocytopenia. Sensitized lymphocytes have been demonstrated in Guillain-Barré syndrome (Table 76-7).

Some of the theoretical mechanisms by which the immunologic tolerance to self-antigens might be broken include the following:

1. *Release of sequestered antigens.* If an antigen does not come into contact with the immune system during fetal development when the tolerance to self normally develops (either because of anatomic site or later development), it is not registered as a self-antigen, and clones of immunoresponsive cells to that antigen remain reactive. As a result of trauma or infection, these antigens may be exposed to the immune system. If this occurs, they will elicit an immune response.
2. *Activation of suppressed clones.* If one of the functions of the suppressor T cell is to suppress the activation of certain clones of potentially self-reactive T cells or B cells, it is possible through some loss of suppressor function that these "forbidden" clones are allowed to proliferate.

TABLE 76-7 Some diseases with autoimmune aspects

Disorder	Immunoresponse
HUMORAL ANTIBODY-MEDIATED, CYTOTOXIC (TYPE II)	
Autoimmune hemolytic anemia	Antibodies (IgG, IgM) bind to cell membranes, fix complement, and destroy cells by lysis
Pernicious anemia	
Idiopathic (immune) thrombocytopenia	
Grave's disease (toxic goiter)	
Pemphigus vulgaris	
Myasthenia gravis	
Goodpasture's syndrome (glomerulonephritis)	
HUMORAL ANTIBODY-MEDIATED, IMMUNE COMPLEX (TYPE III)	
Rheumatoid arthritis	Antibodies (IgG, IgM) react with serum antigens, producing antigen-antibody complexes that are deposited in body tissues and cause an inflammatory reaction
Systemic lupus erythematosus	
Post-streptococcal glomerulonephritis	
Polyarteritis nodosa	
Scleroderma	
CELL-MEDIATED (TYPE IV)	
Systemic lupus erythematosus	Cytotoxic (killer) T cells attach to cell walls, break cell membrane, and destroy cell
Multiple sclerosis	
Guillain-Barré syndrome	

3. *Synthesis of cross-reactive antibodies.* Antibodies synthesized in response to certain foreign antigens may have cross-reactivity with some similar antigenic components within human tissues. Contact with antigens called heterophile antigens may trigger the production of autoantibodies. This seems to be a mechanism of rheumatic heart disease, in which the antibodies produced against certain streptococcal antigens during scarlet fever, streptococcal sore throat, or other streptococcal infections cross-react with myocardial tissue, producing a myocardial inflammation.

4. *Alteration of self-antigens.* Normal body proteins may be altered by chemicals, infectious organisms, or therapeutic drugs to present new antigenically active groups to the immune system. The autoimmune hemolytic anemia associated with α-methyldopa (Aldomet) treatment of hypertension probably results from the alteration of the Rh antigens of the RBC rendering it antigenic. Certain antibiotics such as the penicillins and cephalosporins can have the same effect.

Many diseases for which no etiologic agent could be identified have been classified as autoimmune, only to be removed from that category when some cryptic, latent, or slow-growing agent was identified within the cells or tissue under attack. Some of the diseases listed as autoimmune-associated diseases in Table 76-7 will probably be removed from that list as the initiating factor or microorganism is identified. (The care of persons

experiencing these diseases is discussed elsewhere in the text.)

CHAPTER SUMMARY

✔ Primary immunodeficiencies result from interference with development of immune cells; secondary immunodeficiencies are acquired disorders of depressed immunity. A major factor in the development of secondary immunodeficiencies is malnutrition.

✔ Immunosuppression may be induced by antigen or antibody administration, immunologic methods (ALG, MoAbs), irradiation, or immunosuppressive drugs.

✔ Treatment of primary immunodeficiencies consists of replacement therapy (bone marrow or thymus transplants, immune serum globulin); treatment of secondary immunodeficiencies consists of treatment of the underlying condition.

✔ The primary approach of nursing management of the immunodeficient person is prevention of infection through good medical asepsis, removal of sources where bacteria proliferate, protecting the patient from other persons with infections, maintaining optimal patient nutrition and hydration, and teaching the patient how to prevent infection.

✔ Gammopathies are excessive production of immunoglobulins, the most common of which is multiple myeloma (an excess of plasma cells).

- Hypersensitivity reactions are exagggerated or inappropriate responses to specific antigens (allergens) and depend on the responsiveness of the host to the allergen, the amount, nature, route of entrance, and timing of exposure of the allergen; and site of the allergen-immune mediator reaction.

- Type I hypersensitivities are associated with reactions that are mediated by IgE immunoglobulins attached to mast cells; when the allergen binds to the IgE, histamine is released, producing a systemic reaction (anaphylaxis) or a local allergic reaction. There must be a primary contact with the allergen that triggers synthesis of the specific antiallergenic IgE antibodies (sensitizing dose).

- Anaphylaxis is the most severe form of Type I hypersensitivity; severe reactions can be prevented by identification of high-risk persons, patient education on avoiding the allergen and measures to take if sensitization occurs, desensitization, and precautionary actions when giving animal sera.

- Therapy for anaphylaxis consists of epinephrine to constrict blood vessels and dilate the bronchioles, counteracting the effect of histamine. Antihistamines are given to shorten the duration of anaphylaxis; hydrocortisone decreases the inflammatory effects. An open airway must be maintained.

- The most common allergens in adults are seasonal inhalants (pollens, spores, grasses) and environmental inhalants (house dust, animal dander). Patients are taught measures to avoid and control exposure to the specific allergens.

- Type II hypersensitivities are cytotoxic reactions from the direct binding of IgG or IgM immunoglobulins to the surface of foreign cells to trigger cell lysis; an example is blood transfusion reactions.

- The major antigens of RBCs are AB antigens, Rh antigens, and HLA antigens. People with type AB blood may receive blood from other types because they possess both A and B antigens, but they cannot give blood to persons with other types, who possess only A or B antigens or neither antigen (type O). People with type O blood, therefore, can give blood to but cannot receive it from people with other types.

- Rh positive reactions indicate presence of antigen Rh-D; Rh negative indicates absence of antigen Rh-D.

- Immunologic reactions to blood transfusions include hemolytic (most serious), allergic, febrile, graft-versus-host disease, and noncardiac pulmonary edema. Major diseases that may be transmitted by transfusions include hepatitis B; hepatitis non-A, non-B; and HIV infection.

- Blood transfusion reactions can be prevented by donor prescreening and careful administration safeguards.

- If a hemolytic reaction occurs as indicated by chills and fever and backache shortly after initiation of the transfusion, the transfusion is stopped immediately and the physician notified.

- Autologous blood transfusions may be planned before anticipated events requiring multiple transfusions or autotransfusion during periods of large blood losses, such as after severe trauma or surgery.

- Type III hypersensitivities are characterized by immune complexes formed by the union of IgM or IgG with soluble antigens; the small complexes get trapped in body tissues, causing an inflammatory response. An example is serum sickness, which occurs after administration of a large amount of foreign serum.

- Type IV hypersensitivities are cell mediated (T cell reactions). T cells destroy foreign antigens directly (as in transplant rejections) or by release of lymphokines to activate macrophages.

- Types of tissue transplants include autografts (from self), isografts (from twin), allografts (from another person), and xenografts (from another species).

- Graft rejection is characterized by appearance of sensitized lymphocytes first in lymph nodes with lymph node enlargement, then at the graft site. The graft begins to deteriorate, becomes necrotic, and is sloughed off.

- Graft rejection can be minimized by administration of immunosuppressive drugs (cyclosporine, azathioprine, glucocorticoids), ALG, or monoclonal antibodies, and by pretransplantation blood transfusion.

- Autoimmune diseases are the result of an immune response to one's own antigens, usually because of an agent from outside the immune system. Mechanisms of the immune intolerance may include release of sequestered antigens, activation of suppressed clones, synthesis of cross-reactive antibodies, or alteration of self-antigens. Type II, III, and IV hypersensitivity reactions may occur.

QUESTIONS TO CONSIDER

- Consider the last 10 patients for whom you have provided care. To which of these patients do the concepts of immunodeficiency apply to one degree or another? (Do not forget the role of nutrition in immunodeficiency.) What measures were (or should have been) taken to prevent infection?

- Examine the chart of a patient who has received a blood transfusion. What safeguards were taken to prevent transfusion reactions? If a reaction was noted, what actions were taken?

- Mrs. K. was referred to an allergy clinic and diagnosed as allergic to pollen and grasses. She lives in a low-income housing project that faces a large park. Her husband was laid off 2 months ago. Mrs. K. cleans houses 3 days a week. What additional data would you want to collect from Mrs. K., and what would you include in your teaching plan?

REFERENCES AND SELECTED READINGS

1. Anderson JA and Adkinson NF, Jr: Allergic reaction to drugs and biologic agents, JAMA 258:2891-2899, 1987.
2. *Baker GAB: Administering blood safely, AORN J 37:1102-1112, 1983.
3. *Baron M and Tafuro P: The extremes of age: the newborn and the elderly at increased risk for the development of infection, Nurs Clin North Am 20(1):181-190, 1985.
4. Barrett JT: Textbook of immunology, ed 5, St Louis, 1988, The CV Mosby Co.
5. Bellanti JA: Immunology III, Philadelphia, 1985, WB Saunders Co.
6. *Benson ML and Benson DM: Autotransfusion is here: are you ready? Nursing 85 15(3):46-50, 1985.
7. *Birdsall C: How do you avoid transfusion complications? Am J Nurs 85:312, 1985.
8. *Birdsall C, Carpenter K, and Considine R: How is autotransfusion done? Am J Nurs 88:108-111, 1988.
9. Buckley RH: Immunodeficiency diseases, JAMA 258:2841-2850, 1987.
10. Chmielewski C: Early recognition of infection after renal transplantation, ANNA J 14:389-391, 1987.
11. *Cianci J, and Lamb J: Organ transplantation: matching donors and recipients, Am J Nurs 81:544-545, 1981.
12. *Committee on Transfusion Practices, American Association of Blood Banks: The latest protocols for blood transfusions, Nursing 86 16(10):34-41, 1986.
13. Condemi JJ: The autoimmune diseases, JAMA 258:2920-2929, 1987.
14. Costa AJ: Anaphylactic shock: guidelines for immediate diagnosis and treatment, Postgrad Med 83:368-373, 1988.
15. Creticos PS and Norman PS: Immunotherapy and allergy, JAMA 258:2874-2880, 1987.
16. Croman LC: The relationship between nutrition, infection, and immunity, Med Clin North Am 69(3):519-531, 1985.
17. Dault LA, Nagy CS, and Collins JA: Reversing cardiac transplant rejection with orthoclone OKT3, Am J Nurs 89:953-955, 1989.
18. Delafuente JC: Immunescence: clinical and pharmacologic considerations, Med Clin North Am 69(3):475-483, 1985.
19. Dewey D: Role of the nurse in the use of biological response modifiers, AAOHN J 35(4):163-167, 197-200, 1987.
20. *Dickerson M: Anaphylaxis and anaphylactic shock, Crit Care Nurs Q 11:68-74, 1988.
21. DiJulio JE: Treatment of B-cell and T-cell lymphomas with monoclonal antibodies, Semin Oncol Nurs 4(2):102-106, 1988.
22. *Espersen S: Nursing support of host defenses, CCQ 9(1):51-56, 1986.
23. Farrell ML: Orthoclone OKT3: a treatment for acute renal allograft rejection, ANNA J 14(6):373-376, 1987.
24. *Foon KA: Advances in immunotherapy of cancer: monoclonal antibodies and interferon, Semin Oncol Nurs 4(2):112-119, 1988.
25. *Fruth R: Anaphylaxis and drug reactions: guidelines for detection and care, Heart Lung 9:662-664, 1980.
26. *Fuller BR: Organ graft rejection: the biological process, AORN J 41:738-745, 1985.
27. *Gaunder BN: Insect bites and stings: managing allergic reactions, Nurs Pract 11(3):16-20, 1986.
28. *Girard NJ, Morgan RG, and Orr MD: Autologous salvage of blood: perioperative nursing considerations, AORN J 47:492-503, 1988.
29. Glover JL and Broadie TA: Intraoperative autotransfusion, Surg Annu 16:39-55, 1984.
30. Gould SA, Rice CL, and Moss GS: The physiologic basis of the use of blood and blood products, Surg Ann 16:17-34, 1984.
31. *Graziano FM and Bell CL: The normal immune response and what can go wrong, Med Clin North Am 69(3):439-452, 1985.
32. Graziano FM and Lemanske R Jr: Clinical immunology, Baltimore, 1989, Williams & Wilkins.
33. *Griffin JP: Nursing care of the critically ill immunocompromised patient, Crit Care Nurs Q 9(1):25-34, 1986.
34. *Gurevich I and Tafuro P: The compromised host: deficit-specific infection and the spectrum or prevention, Cancer Nurs 9(5):263-275, 1986.
35. *Gurevich I and Tafuro P: Nursing measures for the prevention of infection in the compromised host, Nurs Clin North Am 20(1):257-260, 1985.
36. Hadden JW: Immunopharmacology: immunomodulation and immunotherapy, JAMA 258:3005-3010, 1987.
37. *Hahn MB and Jassak PF: Nursing management of patients receiving interferon, Semin Oncol Nurs 4(2):95-101, 1988.
38. Henry JB: Todd-Sanford-Davidsohn clinical diagnosis by laboratory methods, ed 17, Philadelphia, 1984, WB Saunders Co.
39. *Hood LE: Interferon, Am J Nurs 87:459-464, 1987.
40. *Irwin MM: Patients receiving biological response modifiers: overview of nursing care, Oncol Nurs Forum Suppl 14(6):32-37, 1987.
41. Jacobs LM and Hsieh JW: A clinical review of autotransfusion and its role in trauma, JAMA 251(24):3283-3287, 1984.
42. *Jassak PF and Spiewak PL: Interleukin-2, Am J Nurs 87:464-467, 1987.
43. Kagan JM and Fahey JL: Tumor immunology, JAMA 258:2988-2992, 1987.
44. Kaplan AP, Buckley RH, and Mathews KP: Allergic skin disorders, JAMA 258:2900-2909, 1987.
45. Kaliner M, Eggleston PA, and Mathews KP: Rhinitis and asthma, JAMA 258:2851-2873, 1987.

*References preceded by an asterisk are particularly well suited for student reading.

46. Kaye D and Rose LF: Fundamentals of internal medicine, St Louis, 1983, The CV Mosby Co.

47. Keown PA et al: Cyclosporine: a double-edged sword, Hosp Pract 22(5):207-220, 1987.

48. Kirkpatrick CH: Transplantation immunology, JAMA 258:2993-3000, 1987.

49. Krigel RL: Interleukins, interferons, and tumor necrosis factor, AAOHN J 35(4):159-162, 1987.

50. *Litwack K: Practical points for transfusion therapy, J Post Anesth Nurs 2(4):257-261, 1987.

51. *Mennies JH et al: An overview of adult allergic disorders, Nurs Pract 10(6):16-23, 1985.

52. Miller DS: Intravenous immune globulin for treating primary immunodeficiency disease, MCN 12:244-248, 1987.

53. Minnefor AB et al: IV immune globulin: efficacy and safety, Hosp Pract 22(10:171-183, 1987.

54. Osserman EF, Merlin G, and Butler VP: Multiple myeloma and related plasma cell dyscrasias, JAMA 258:2930-2937, 1987.

55. Patten E: Immunohematologic disease, JAMA 258:2945-2951, 1987.

56. *Phillips A: Are blood transfusions really safe? Nursing '87 17(6):63-65, 1987.

57. Platts-Mills TAE et al: Dust mite allergy: its clinical significance, Hosp Pract 22(9):91-100, 1987.

58. *Pluth NM: A home care transfusion program, Oncol Nurs Forum 14(5):43-46, 1987.

59. *Randall BJ: Reacting to anaphylaxis, Nursing '86 16(3):34-39, 1986.

60. *Recking JB et al: Understanding immune system dysfunction, Nursing '87 17(9):34-42, 1987.

61. *Rieger PT: Monoclonal antibodies, Am J Nurs 87:469-473, 1987.

62. Schroeder SA et al: Current medical diagnosis and treatment, Norwalk, Conn, 1989, Appleton & Lange.

63. *Smith SL: Immunosuppressive drugs used in clinical practice, Crit Care Nurs Q 9(1):19-24, 1986.

64. Steinhiser SA et al: OKT3 for the treatment of patients with acute renal allograft rejection, ANNA J 14(2):127-129, 1987.

65. *Sticklin LA: Interleukin-2 and killer T cells, Am J Nurs 87:468-469, 1987.

66. Stites DP et al: Basic and clinical immunology, ed 6, Norwalk, Conn, 1988, Appleton & Lange.

67. Valentine MD et al: Anaphylaxis and stinging insect hypersensitivity, JAMA 258:2881-2885, 1987.

68. Way LW: Current surgical diagnoses and treatment, ed 8, Norwalk, Conn, 1988, Appleton & Lange.

69. Widman FK: An introduction to clinical immunology, Philadelphia, 1989, FA Davis Co.

70. Wong DT and Ogra PL: Viral infections in immunocompromised patients, Med Clin North Am 67(5):1075-1089, 1983.

71. Wyngaarden JB and Smith LH: Cecil textbook of medicine, ed 18, Philadelphia, 1988, WB Saunders Co.

CHAPTER 77

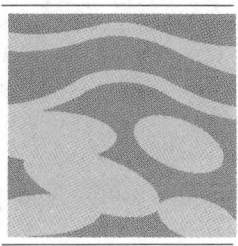

Management of Persons with HIV Infection and AIDS

DENISE M. KRESEVIC

CHAPTER OBJECTIVES

After studying this chapter, the student should be able to:
1. Describe the epidemiology of HIV infection, identify the virus causation, groups at risk, methods of transmission, and strategies for prevention.
2. Describe the continuum of HIV infection, including AIDS-Related Complex and diseases indicative of AIDS.
3. Identify the infection control guidelines recommended by CDC to minimize transmission of HIV infection.
4. Discuss nursing problems and interventions for patients with HIV infection.
5. Describe clinical manifestations and care of opportunistic infections and tumors that occur in patients with HIV infection.
6. Discuss the role of the nurse in addressing psychosocial, legal, and ethical issues related to the HIV epidemic.

Since the time of Florence Nightingale, nurses have provided care for individuals and families with communicable disease. One of the most dreaded communicable diseases of the twentieth century is AIDS (acquired immunodeficiency syndrome). AIDS is caused by the human immunodeficiency virus (HIV). Individuals infected with this virus suffer severe compromise of the body's ability to fight various infections and rare forms of cancer. The incidence of AIDS and HIV infection continues to increase steadily in the United States and worldwide. Therefore it is crucial that nurses have an understanding of (1) epidemiology, (2) disease prevention, (3) pathophysiology, and (4) nursing care of individuals infected with HIV.

EPIDEMIOLOGY AND PREVENTION

In 1981 the phenomenon of AIDS began to emerge. At that time the Centers for Disease Control (CDC) recognized that several previously nonlethal cases of *Pneumocystis carinii* pneumonia and a rare skin cancer called

Kaposi's sarcoma were killing homosexual men at alarming rates in Los Angeles and New York City. By late 1986 more than 27,000 cases had been reported to the CDC, with over 15,000 fatalities. Epidemiologists and researchers studying these cases concluded that the cause of the fatal pneumonias and skin cancers was an underlying immune deficiency syndrome. Research efforts continued to isolate the causative immune deficiency virus. Before 1986 different researchers attributed various names to the virus; AIDS-related virus (ARV), lymphadenopathy-associated virus (LAV), and human T-lymphotropic virus type III (HTLV III). It was not until 1986 that the virus believed to cause AIDS was defined and named HIV. By September 1989 a total of 105,990 cases of AIDS had been reported in the United States (Table 77-1).

VIRUS TRANSMISSION AND RISK BEHAVIORS

A critical need exists to educate health care professionals, patients, and families about disease transmission and identified risk behaviors for HIV infection. The human immunodeficiency virus has been found in a variety of body fluids including blood, semen, cerebrospinal fluids (CSF), urine, stool, and saliva. Blood serum and CSF of infected individuals contain the highest concentrations of the virus and thus are the most likely means of transmission. Although HIV has also been found in varying concentrations in urine, stool, and saliva, no evidence exists that disease transmission has occurred via these body secretions.

There are three major methods of HIV transmission: (1) intimate contact with body secretions, including semen and vaginal secretions that occur during sexual intercourse, (2) contact with infected blood through blood transfusions or the sharing of needles during intravenous drug use, and (3) maternal-infant transfer via placental exchange or breast milk.

Although any member of the population may acquire AIDS, certain behaviors place individuals at increased

TABLE 77-1 Distribution of AIDS cases in the United States as of August 31, 1989

Category	Total	%	Category	Total	%
AGE			**RACE/ETHNICITY**		
<13	1,780	2	White	60,040	57
13-19	415	<1	Black	28,743	27
20-29	21,726	21	Hispanic	16,182	15
30-39	48,904	46	Other	779	1
40-49	22,319	21	Unknown	246	<1
>49	10,846	10			
TOTAL	105,990		**SEX**		
			Male	95,844	91
			Female	10,146	9

Data from Centers for Disease Control, Atlanta, and the Ohio Department of Health, Columbus, Ohio.

TABLE 77-2 Distribution of AIDS by exposure category as of August 31, 1989

Risk Group	%
Homosexual and bisexual men	60
Heterosexual IV drug abusers	20
Homosexual and bisexual IV drug abusers	7
Heterosexual men and women	3
Recipients of blood products	3
Persons with hemophilia	1
Children of parents with/at risk for AIDS	1
Other/unknown	4

Data from Centers for Disease Control, Atlanta, and Ohio Department of Health, Columbus, Ohio.

risk for exposure to HIV based on disease transmission patterns. Populations at highest risk for exposure to HIV include homosexual and bisexual men, intravenous drug users, heterosexual partners of HIV-infected individuals, infants born to HIV infected parents, and individuals who have received blood or blood products, especially before 1985 (Table 77-2).[19]

More than 60% of the reported cases of HIV infection and AIDS have been in homosexual and bisexual men.[19] The greatest identified risk factors for HIV transmission in this group is anal intercourse. Such intercourse may be traumatic to fragile mucous membranes, resulting in microscopic tears and possible semen-blood transmission of the virus. The appropriate and consistent use of condoms and water-soluble lubricants may decrease the risk of trauma and disease transmission with anal intercourse in this risk group.[31]

Transmission of HIV by vaginal heterosexual intercourse is also possible. Associated risk factors for heterosexual transmission include anal intercourse, multiple sexual partners who may be infected and asymptomatic, and frequent sexual intercourse with multiple partners; these behaviors increase opportunities for exposure to infected body fluids. Studies on nonsexual household contact, sharing of eating utensils and bathroom facilities, and close personal contact have failed to demonstrate transmission of HIV by casual contact.[31,45]

Although the risk of HIV infection to health care workers is low, it remains a potential risk for those workers exposed to body secretions such as blood, urine, and stool. One ongoing study of 883 health care workers suffering a needle stick and potential exposure revealed only 4 cases of disease transmission. Total cases of seroconversion, or positive blood tests for HIV infection, to date are 25. Such exposure may occur by accidental needle sticks or mucous membrane exposure

by splashes of blood in the mouth, nose, or open cuts on the hands.[34]

Clearly the most important strategies for health care workers are good handwashing, avoidance of recapping needles, and the use of gloves whenever exposure to any patient's body secretions is likely to occur.[42]

INFECTION CONTROL MEASURES

In addition to health education strategies, infection control is one of the most important areas of concern for nurses caring for patients with HIV infection, whether in the hospital or home environment. Infection control procedures based on knowledge of disease transmission are essential to dispel the many emotional fears and myths surrounding the HIV infection. *Handwashing* remains the single most important principle of infection control for all diseases.[41] Handwashing is critical to protect immunocompromised patients and caregivers; it should be performed before and after contact with each patient and after removal of gloves. *Gloves* should be used whenever there will be contact with body secretions: during care of lesions, when coming into contact with blood (such as during dressing changes or starting intravenous lines), when cleaning incontinent patients of urine or stool, when changing soiled linens, and when performing oral care. Gloves are not necessary for casual contact such as bathing (without the presence of lesions), feeding, or ambulating patients.[42]

Soiled dressings, wet linens, and respiratory equipment should be discarded in heavy plastic bags. Puncture resistant needle disposal containers should be in close proximity to all patient care areas. *Needles* should be disposed of promptly, *WITHOUT RECAPPING*, since recapping is the most frequent cause of accidental needle sticks. Soap dispensers should be within close proximity of all patient care areas, and gloves should be worn for cleanup of urine, stool, or blood spills.

Standard household and institutional cleaning is important to protect all immunocompromised patients. Institutional cleaning agents used for floor and bathroom facilities are sufficient. Home cleaning of floors, countertops, toilets, and spills should be done using a freshly mixed solution of bleach and water in a 1:10 parts mixture. Standard laundering using bleach, and dishwashing using hot water and air drying are sufficient to protect caregivers and family members from HIV infection. However, personal care items such as razors and toothbrushes should never be shared because of possible transmission by blood serum. Pet excretion may pose a unique threat to immunocompromised patients. Patients with HIV infection who desire to keep their pets may require assistance in care, especially in cleaning bird cages, cat litter boxes, or fish tanks.[42]

The infection control guidelines previously mentioned are sufficient to protect pregnant women.[19] Clearly, use of infection control measures is essential for all patients, regardless of known HIV infection, because this is the only way to ensure protection of caregivers.[19] Patients' family members and all members of the health care team, including dietary workers and transport personnel, need basic education about HIV infection and infection control policies.

PATHOPHYSIOLOGY

MECHANISM OF HIV INFECTION

Infection with HIV renders the immune system severely compromised (see Chapters 8 and 76). Recall that the immune system, composed of organs and cells, protects the body from infections, cell mutations, and environmental toxins. The cells of the immune system are composed of lymphocytes, macrophages, and monocytes. Lymphocytes are further differentiated as T cells or B cells. HIV attacks T cells, which are responsible for all mediated immunity and protect the body from malignant cells, viruses, and parasites. The T cells are formed in the bone marrow and develop in the thymus. Two types of T cells produced by the body are T_4 inducer or helper cells, and T_8 cytotoxic or suppressor cells.

TABLE 77-3 Common laboratory abnormalities associated with HIV infection and AIDS

Disorder	Laboratory Findings
Anemia	Hematocrit <30%
Leukopenia	WBC <2500/cm^3
Lymphopenia	Helper T cells 400/mm^3
Decreased T_4/T_8 ratio	Ratio 1:2
Thrombocytopenia	Platelets <150,000

HIV has an affinity for invasion of the T_4 helper cells, but it may also invade other components of the immune system, including B cells, macrophages, and nerve cells, severely compromising cell-mediated immunity.

Individuals infected with HIV usually have almost twice as many T_8 suppressor cells as T_4 helper cells. This abnormal cell ratio renders HIV-infected persons immunocompromised and thus susceptible to a host of infections, malignancies, and abnormal laboratory results (Table 77-3).[21,29,44]

HIV is classified as a retrovirus. Retroviruses carry their genetic code in RNA rather than DNA material. In retroviruses an enzyme known as reverse transcriptase converts RNA to DNA, which is incorporated into the host cell's genetic material. Thus the virus invades the host cell, living within it and replicating itself (Figure 77-1). Based on these cellular pathologies of the HIV infection, the CDC defines AIDS as "a disease at least moderately predictive of a cell-mediated immunity occurring in persons with no known cause for diminished resistance to that disease."[45]

HIV INFECTION CONTINUUM AND CLINICAL MANIFESTATIONS

HIV infection may remain dormant for several years, producing no clinical symptoms.[21] This prolonged incubation period is of great concern because individuals may be asymptomatic but contagious. Others infected

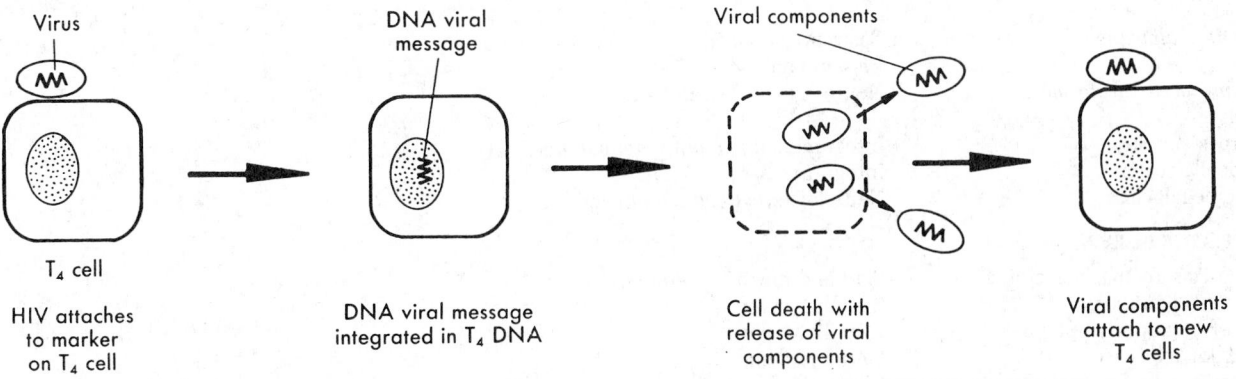

FIGURE 77-1 Mechanism of HIV action.

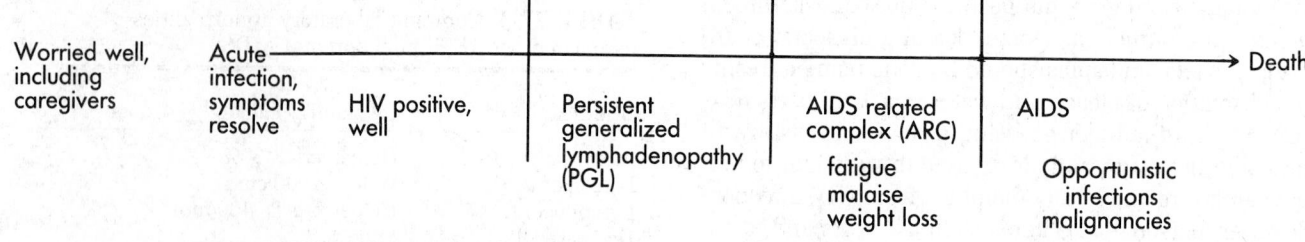

FIGURE 77-2 Continuum of HIV infection; only some persons proceed from infection to AIDS and death.

TABLE 77-4 Progression of HIV infection[13]

Group	Type	Characteristics
I	Acute infection	Fever, malaise with seroconversion
II	Asymptomatic infection	Seroconversion; no symptoms
III	Persistent generalized lymphadenopathy (PGL)	Lymphadenopathy more than 3 months in absence of explainable illness
IV	Other HIV disease	(See subgroups)
IV-1	Constitutional disease (ARC)	Diarrhea or fever persisting more than 1 month; involuntary weight loss of greater than 10% of baseline
IV-2	Neurologic disease	HIV encephalopathy or dementia; peripheral neuropathy
IV-3	Secondary infectious diseases	*Pneumocystis carinii* pneumonia; candidiasis; extrapulmonary cryptococcosis; mycobacterial infection; CMV infection; herpes infections
IV-4	Secondary cancers	Kaposi's sarcoma, non-Hodgkin's lymphoma, primary lymphoma of the brain

Modified from Centers for Disease Control: Pneumocystis pneumonia: Los Angeles, MMWR 30:250-252, 1981.

TABLE 77-5 Opportunistic infections and neoplasms associated with HIV infection

Agent	Body System Affected
INFECTION	
Protozoal	
Pneumocystis carinii	Respiratory
Toxoplasma gondii	Neurologic and disseminated
Cryptosporidium	Gastrointestinal
Bacterial	
Mycobacterium avium intracellulare	Disseminated
Mycobacterium tuberculosis	Respiratory, neurologic, or disseminated
Fungal	
Candida albicans	Gastrointestinal (mouth and/or esophagus) Disseminated
Cryptococcus neoformans	Neurologic or disseminated
Viral	
Herpes simplex	Integumentary (mouth, genital, perianal)
Varicella-zoster	Integumentary
Cytomegalovirus	Neurologic (eyes) disseminated
NEOPLASTIC DISEASES	
Kaposi's sarcoma (epidemic form)	Skin and mucous membranes
Burkitt's lymphoma	Lymph system
Non-Hodgkin's lymphomas	Lymph system
Hodgkin's disease	Lymph system
Chronic lymphocytic leukemia	White blood cells

with the virus may experience transient acute symptoms of fever, muscle aches, rashes, diarrhea, and gastrointestinal cramping that occur 2 to 6 weeks after exposure and then resolve (Figure 77-2 and Table 77-4). Other patients exposed to the virus and harboring HIV antibodies exhibit chronic symptoms of diffuse noncancerous lymph node enlargement, or *persistent generalized lymphadenopathy* (PGL), fever, chills, night sweats, and weight loss.

Patients exposed to the virus, who are harboring HIV antibodies and who experience night sweats, fever, weight loss, fatigue, edema, and abnormal laboratory immune values including altered T_4 and T_8 cell ratios, but who have no infections or malignancies, are diagnosed as having *AIDS-related complex* (ARC). ARC can be a very debilitating disease.[10] However, *Acquired immunodeficiency syndrome,* or AIDS, is the most severe HIV disease. Patients with AIDS continue to experience all the same symptoms, including fatigue, weight loss, fever, diarrhea, and edema.[7] In addition, opportunistic infections may be life-threatening, and rare forms of cancers also invade the body (Table 77-5). *Opportunistic infections* prey on compromised immune systems.

Patients with AIDS, similar to oncology patients and organ-transplant patients receiving immunosuppressive therapy to prevent rejection, become susceptible to infections that individuals with intact immune systems are able to fight.

■ ASSESSMENT

Some patients may be asymptomatic; others may report nonspecific "flulike" symptoms of fever, chills, night sweats, or dry, nonproductive cough. The clinical diversity of the HIV infection (see the box below) can make identification and assessment of infected patients difficult. Nurses may encounter patients experiencing various clinical symptoms including fatigue, fever, diarrhea, or confusion, depending on the continuum of illness. Patients identified at risk for HIV infection either by sexual history, drug history, or flulike symptoms should

be further assessed for the presence of opportunistic infections, rashes, and neoplasms (see Table 77-5).

IDENTIFICATION OF PERSONS AT RISK

Health assessments of all patients should include an appraisal of potential risk factors for HIV infection. Obtaining a complete, accurate history of sexual behavior, including past and present sexual activities, will be necessary and requires skillful interviewing techniques and a professional relationship based on trust. Nurses need to be comfortable explaining the need for information on intimate sexual activities, and phrasing questions in appropriate but comprehensible terms. The sexual health history, in addition to identifying individuals at risk for possible HIV infection, may also be an opportunity for health education and disease prevention (see the box below).

Information on the use of mood-affecting drugs such as alcohol, marijuana, heroin, cocaine, crack, barbiturates, tranquilizers, butyl nitrate, or amphetamines should also be obtained. Frequency and routes of administration including oral, smoking, sniffing, snorting, or injecting drugs should be explored. Needle exposure through the sharing of drug paraphernalia, tattoos, or acupuncture treatment should also be assessed.[43]

Individuals identified as being at risk for HIV infection should be counseled about the significance of testing and the necessity for follow-up. Patients with evidence of risk factors and any clinical symptoms should be referred for blood testing and medical evaluation of symptoms to diagnose exposure to the HIV infection.

DIAGNOSTIC TESTS: HIV SEROPOSITIVITY

Individuals who have been exposed to HIV and have had sufficient time for increased antibody production

---

SIGNS AND SYMPTOMS OF HIV INFECTION

Chills and fever	Malaise
Night sweats	Fatigue
Dry productive cough	Oral lesions
Dyspnea	Skin rashes
Lethargy	Abdominal discomfort
Confusion	Diarrhea
Stiff neck	Weight loss
Seizures	Lymphadenopathy
Headache	Progressive generalized edema

SAMPLE SEXUAL HISTORY

1. When did you first become sexually active? With whom? For how long? Type of sexual activity practiced:
   - Mutual masturbation
   - French kissing
   - Vaginal intercourse
   - Anal intercourse
   - Oral intercourse
   - Use of objects to enhance stimulation
   - Use of contraceptives
2. Are you currently sexually active? With whom? For how long? Type of sexual activity?
3. Do you currently have any concerns about your sexuality or sexual activity?
4. Do you suspect that any of your sexual partners have been infected with herpes, syphilis, gonorrhea, or AIDS? (Patients may need further explanations of specific types of infections and symptoms).

can be tested for infection. Two tests may be used to diagnose infection. The most common test is the enzyme-linked immunosorbent assay *(ELISA)*. This test was originally developed as a screening tool for potential blood donors. Because the ELISA is a sensitive screening test for HIV infection, *false positive* tests are possible. Individuals who are not infected with HIV but have had multiple blood transfusions or pregnancies may have false positive results. In addition, a *false negative* ELISA test may occur during the so-called "window period." The window period is that time between exposure to the virus and the development of sufficient antibodies. The window period for HIV may be a few weeks or up to 3 months.[44] An additional confirmatory test called the *Western Blot* is usually done as a means of accurately diagnosing HIV-infected persons. In general, the use of both the ELISA and Western Blot is able to provide over 99% accurate diagnosis of HIV infection.

A person with a positive test result is called HIV seropositive. This result indicates exposure to the HIV infection. Although it is not known, at present how many seropositive individuals will develop AIDS, it is believed that a majority will die of AIDS complications.[44] Legal and ethical issues surrounding mandatory HIV testing for employment and insurance coverage continue to present an emotional challenge.

■ DATA ANALYSIS: NURSING DIAGNOSES

Because of the different HIV infection categories on the HIV infection continuum and the great variety of symptoms, nursing care plans for persons with HIV infection or AIDS will show a great variety of nursing diagnoses based on assessment of patient data. Some common nursing diagnoses include, but are not limited to, the following:

Diagnostic Title	Possible Etiologies
Anxiety	Threat to self-concept, threat of death, threat to/change in health status/socioeconomic status
Body temperature, altered	Infection, dehydration
Coping, ineffective individual, family	Inadequate or incorrect information or understanding, crisis, prolonged disability of significant person, societal mores
Grieving, anticipatory	Probable patient death
Impaired skin integrity	Pressure sores, infected lesions
Infection, potential for	Decreased immune response
Knowledge deficit	Lack of exposure/recall, misinterpretation of information
Nutrition, altered: less than body requirements	Nausea, vomiting, diarrhea, alterations in oral mucous membranes, dysphagia

Diagnostic Title	Possible Etiologies
Self-care deficit	Activity intolerance, dyspnea, fatigue, depression, visual impairments, cognitive dysfunction
Social isolation	Societal biases, alteration in physical appearance or mental status, lack of knowledge about AIDS virus transmission

■ PLANNING: EXPECTED PATIENT OUTCOMES

Expected patient outcomes for the person with HIV infection or AIDS may include, but are not limited to, the following:

1. Patient demonstrates fewer signs of anxiety
2. Patient and significant others describe usual coping strategies and explore alternative strategies.
3. Patient and significant others engage in communication that leads to sharing of feelings, decision making, and problem resolution, as pertinent.
4. Body temperature decreases.
5. Skin and mucous membranes are moist; skin turgor is good.
6. Secondary infections do not occur or are identified early for treatment.
7. HIV transmission to significant others and caregivers does not occur.
8. Weight loss, electrolyte imbalance, and discomfort are minimized.
9. Patient ingests adequate fluids and a balanced diet daily.
10. Patient participates in ADL at optimal level of functioning.
11. Patient has opportunities to interact with others on a social basis.

■ IMPLEMENTATION

EDUCATIONAL AND COUNSELING STRATEGIES FOR PERSONS AT RISK

Nursing care needs vary along the illness continuum of HIV infection. Interventions are directed toward several groups of patients, including (1) "worried" well, (2) individuals with risk factors, (3) asymptomatic HIV-infected, (4) HIV-infected patients with clinical symptoms, and their families; and (5) terminally ill HIV-infected individuals and their families. Nursing care of worried well individuals and family emphasizes education about HIV infection. Nurses will be required to serve as health resources for various community and institutional settings ranging from hospitals, churches, and schools to occupational settings. A majority of health education about HIV infection focuses on clarifying myths and helping individuals cope with their anxiety and emotional-laden fears surrounding this epidemic. The challenge for nurses providing health education on HIV infection is to impart accurate, concise information that addresses the fears of contagion and disease transmission. Inherent in such education is a multitude of complex educational issues, including human sexuality.

Educational strategies, whether directed toward the worried well or those infected with HIV, must emphasize accurate information on disease transmission and safe sex practices. Safe sex refers to abstinence or a mutually monogamous sexual relationship with a noninfected partner. Risky sexual practices include multiple sexual partners and anal sex. The use of water soluble lubricants and condoms may increase the safety of vaginal and anal intercourse.

Both the worried well and those identified as being at risk for HIV infection need education and referral for antibody tests. Before testing, individuals require extensive counseling on the significance of test results and follow-up care and treatment. It is important to stress in counseling that a one-time negative antibody test is meaningless if exposure to risk factors continues. Some patients practicing intravenous drug use need additional referral and treatment to eliminate the risk behavior. One of the most difficult issues in caring for patients at high risk of contracting and transmitting the HIV infection is the balance of patient confidentiality and the caregiver's responsibility to share information regarding potential risk to other sexual partners and loved ones. Education and counseling may be accomplished through individual teaching, role modeling, informal group discussions, or lectures. However, teaching requires more than spoken words. Learning should be reinforced by discussing concerns, answering questions, and using printed resources for future reference; repetition is essential.

PREVENTING INFECTIONS

Normal environments can be a source of lethal infections for the immunocompromised patient. Nursing care for persons with HIV infection or AIDS must stress meticulous personal hygiene, close observation of potential sources of infection, frequent handwashing, and avoidance of environmental microbes. Infection control measures (p. 2226) are essential.

Patients with HIV infection are encouraged and assisted to bathe daily. Most patients will require a bed bath; tub baths should be avoided if rashes are present. Whenever possible, showers are recommended. Patients suffering from diarrhea require frequent cleaning with a gentle soap and liberal application of moisture barriers to prevent skin breakdown. Special attention to oral care to prevent infection and promote adequate nutrition and comfort is important. Soft toothbrushes and nonabrasive toothpaste and rinses will decrease the chances of trauma and secondary infections. Rinses with sodium bicarbonate, saline, or lemon and hydrogen peroxide are useful before meals and at bedtime. Oral care after meals helps prevent tooth decay and infections.

Meticulous skin care is necessary to minimize infections and promote comfort. Patients with decreased mobility may benefit from the use of air mattresses and frequent turning schedules to prevent decubiti. Turning sheets are used when necessary to prevent friction and injury. A high-protein diet will help prevent skin breakdown by providing essential amino acids for healing. Edematous limbs are elevated using pillows to promote circulation. Emollients can be used liberally to prevent skin drying and cracking. Skin lesions are washed separately using a clean washcloth and gloves to prevent contamination.

Pulmonary infection occurs frequently with HIV. Thus patients are taught and coached through deep-breathing and coughing exercises at least every 4 hours while awake when mobility is limited; this promotes airway clearance and helps to prevent atelectasis.

Biopsy sites and intravenous insertion sites can be sources of infection. Observe sites daily for redness, warmth, pain, or drainage. Sites that are suggestive of infection should have wound cultures to confirm or rule out infection. Avoid plastic occlusive dressings; they have been shown to increase the risk of infection in some immunocompromised patients. Change dressings at least every other day. Avoid sources of microbes, such as fresh plants and dietary servings of rare meat and fresh vegetables or fruits.

Attention must be paid to the patient's environment. The room should be dusted and mopped daily using damp cloths to prevent air distribution of microbes. Supplies should be neatly stocked. Dietary trays are removed after meals, and additional dietary supplements are stored outside the patient's room, In most cases, except with airborne infections such as tuberculosis, the patient's door may be kept open to minimize odors, promote adequate ventilation, and decrease feelings of isolation. Private rooms for patients with HIV infection are not usually necessary except with specific infections such as tuberculosis. Patients are not placed in a room with another patient who has an infection. The single most important factor that protects immunocompromised patients from infections is the practice of consistent good handwashing techniques by patients, caregivers, and visitors. Care of the person with HIV infection is summarized in the box on p. 2232.

MODIFYING ALTERATIONS IN BODY TEMPERATURE

Fever, a common result of HIV infection, may be caused by dehydration or multiple infections, including

GUIDELINES FOR CARE OF THE PERSON WITH HIV INFECTION/AIDS

1. Prevent infection.
   a. Wash hands frequently and use emollient for patient and caregiver.
   b. Use a gentle soap (such as Castile); avoid bar soaps that may irritate skin.
   c. Provide for daily showering or basin bath; avoid tub bath if rashes are present.
   d. Use a separate washcloth for lesions.
   e. Use soft toothbrushes, nonabrasive toothpaste; and mouth rinses with sodium bicarbonate, saline, or lemon and hydrogen peroxide before meals and at bedtime.
   f. Use measures to prevent skin pressure, such as turning sheets, sheepskin, or eggcrate or air mattresses.
   g. Elevate and support areas of edema.
   h. Observe biopsy sites and IV insertion sites daily for signs of infection.
   i. Change dressings at least every other day; avoid plastic occlusive dressings.
   j. Avoid sources of microbes, such as fresh plants or ingestion of fresh fruits and vegetables.
   k. Carry out measures to prevent spread of infection: use of gloves for contact with bodily secretions, double plastic bags to dispose of body secretions, use of bleach and water (1:10) for cleaning of contaminated areas.
2. Modify alterations in body temperature.
   a. Administer prescribed antibiotics, IV fluids, or antipyretics.
   b. Encourage fluid intake >2500 ml.
   c. Maintain daily intake and output records.
   d. Weigh daily.
   e. Provide tepid sponge baths and linen changes as necessary.
   f. Instruct patient in deep-breathing and coughing exercises to prevent atelectasis and additional fever.

3. Promote good nutrition.
   a. Provide instruction for high-calorie, high-protein, high-potassium, low-residue diet.
   b. Encourage high-calorie, high-potassium snacks.
   c. Suggest foods that are easy to swallow (gelatin, yogurt, puddings) when dysphagia is present.
   d. Avoid foods that are spicy or acidic, rare meats, raw fruits and vegetables.
   e. Provide oral care before patient eats.
   f. Encourage patient to be out of bed and sitting for meals if possible.
   g. Avoid odors by aerating room.
   h. Make appropriate dietary consultations.
4. Promote self-care.
   a. Assess realistic functional ability.
   b. Plan, supervise, and assist with ADL as necessary.
   c. Encourage patient to be as active and independent as possible.
   d. Assist patient with range-of-motion exercise to prevent contractures.
   e. Provide equipment such as assistive eating devices, walkers, and commodes to promote patient independence.
   f. Pace activities and schedule rest periods to prevent fatigue.
5. Provide counseling.
   a. Assess and support patient coping mechanisms.
   b. Explore with patient and significant others normalcy of grief responses.
   c. Assist patient and significant others in acknowledging and planning for anticipated losses.
   d. Provide information as desired and necessary, depending on the ability to perceive.
   e. Suggest appropriate religious support.
   f. Facilitate participation in support groups or individual counseling as pertinent.

P. carinii pneumonia, cytomegalovirus, and *mycobacterium avium intracellulare*. Fevers may also be caused by infection from intravenous lines or biopsy sites.

All patients with HIV infection should be monitored for fever and adequate fluid intake. Temperatures of hospitalized patients are assessed every 4 hours, body temperatures greater than 37.5° C or 101.5° F are reported to the physician for medical follow-up. Diagnostic tests for fevers may include x-ray examinations or blood cultures for detection of specific pathogens. Patients with fevers may require several tepid sponge baths and linen changes to promote comfort. Fever and sweating may increase fluid loss and contribute to dehydration, therefore patients should ingest at least 2500 ml of fluid per day. Accurate daily intake and output are recorded and evaluated.

Daily monitoring of intravenous sites and other wounds for possible infection is also critical. Fevers are cautiously treated with antipyretics such as acetaminophen (contraindicated with use of the drug Retrovir). The use of aspirin is contraindicated with HIV infection because the infection itself may alter normal blood coagulation. Intravenous therapy may be necessary to provide adequate hydration. Despite meticulous personal hygiene and nursing care, some patients with HIV infection may continue to have persistent temperature elevation with no explained cause.

PROMOTING SELF-CARE AND SAFETY

Many persons infected with HIV suffer from fatigue, dyspnea, depression, or cognitive impairments requiring assistance with activities of daily living. Immunocompromised persons are particularly vulnerable to environmental pathogens and require meticulous daily hygiene. A daily schedule of activity that includes turning, positioning, sitting up for meals, bathing, and toileting will minimize the risks of secondary infections and contribute to feelings of positive self-esteem.

Patients are encouraged to remain as active and as independent as possible. The use of energy conservation and pacing of activities is very effective in maintaining independence and comfort. Adaptive equipment such as assistive eating devices, walkers or bedside commodes may also promote independence. Some patients may require assistance with range-of-motion exercises to prevent contractures.

Safety is a critical need for patients with HIV infection. Such patients are at increased risk for accidents and injury because of decreased physical and cognitive function. The patient's environment is assessed to ensure strategic placement of items such as call lights and urinals. Use of siderails and restraints may be necessary to prevent injury but should never be substituted for frequent observation. Both patients and significant others should be aware of safety needs and the rationale of interventions to prevent injury. Referrals to occupational and physical therapy may be useful in developing a coordinated plan of care to maximize safe independent functioning.

PROMOTING OPTIMAL NUTRITION

Patients with HIV infection are frequently plagued by alterations in gastrointestinal function, such as dysphagia, nausea, vomiting, and diarrhea. Infections such as *Candida* and *Cryptosporidiosis* also contribute to alterations in food and fluid intake and absorption, resulting in reduced nutrition. Depression may be manifested by changes in appetite.

Patients' daily weight and food and fluid intake are monitored and recorded. Nutritional intake may be increased by attention to oral hygiene, positioning, socialization, and attention to individual preferences. Patients and caregivers are taught about nutritional factors that contribute to health despite the HIV infection.

Patients are encouraged to be out of bed and sitting for meals to aid digestion and decrease the possibility of aspiration. Odors should be minimized because they may contribute to nausea. Oral hygiene, including mouth rinses before meals, enhances the taste of food and stimulates digestive juices. Whenever possible, significant others can be encouraged to visit during meals and to bring home-prepared food. Patients may prefer frequent small meals or snacks spaced throughout the day to prevent indigestion and fatigue.

Adequate nutrition can be enhanced by the following:

1. Daily oral intake of 2500 ml to 3000 ml of fluids to prevent dehydration, especially with diarrhea; suggested fluids are water, fruit juices, soups, and gelatin.
2. Foods high in potassium (to replace that lost by diarrhea) include bananas, apricots, and orange juice.
3. Textured foods that are easy to swallow and tolerate include gelatin, yogurt, and pudding.
4. Foods high in protein that are easily tolerated include peanut butter, honey, and instant breakfast drinks.
5. *Avoid* foods with naturally occurring microbes (rare meat, raw fruits and vegetables) and foods that aggravate dysphagia (spicy, acidic, or raw fruits and vegetables).

Mutiple medications may alter the normal taste of foods, and patients may need to be encouraged to try new or differently prepared foods. Collaboration with nutritionists may be useful. At times, dietary supplements may be needed to maintain adequate caloric intake. All supplements, especially those containing lactose, should be evaluated as potentially causing diarrhea. Dysphagia resulting from oral *Candida* may be treated with oral medications such as Nystatin or Lidocaine to decrease discomfort and increase nutritional intake. Patients residing in the community often require assistance with shopping and meal preparation.

COUNSELING

Patients and families along the HIV continuum, from the worried well to those terminally ill with the virus, require much health teaching and counseling. The goal of counseling is to impart accurate information that empowers patients and families to make informed decisions and mobilize adequate mechanisms of support and adaptation for coping with multiple stresses.

Patients with HIV infection have many questions and concerns about the disease and its transmission, prognosis, and treatment. Initially, most patients are in a state of shock and disbelief. Information should be given in small segments with opportunities for repetition. Many patients require assistance with the decision to share the fact of their illness with significant others. All sexual partners who are potentially at risk for contracting the disease have the right to know of their own potential risk of illness.

Similar to patients with other terminal illnesses, patients diagnosed with the HIV infection may experience strong emotions of fear, anger, denial, or quiet depression. Some patients benefit from individual empathic listening and exploring feelings, fears, and treatment options. Other patients may benefit from support groups with patients experiencing similar feelings. Significant others, including family and lovers, experience their own feelings of fear, anger, and embarrassment. Individual counseling and support groups may be helpful to loved ones who will need to be a source of support for the patient. Practical issues such as employment disability, housing discrimination, insurance coverage, and preparation for death also need to be addressed. Referral to social workers and appropriate community agencies can alleviate many concerns that plague acutely and terminally ill patients. Continued participation in religious services and the support of fellow worshippers and clergy should not be overlooked as a source of healthy coping. Many clergy are experienced in grief counseling and can be helpful to patients and family members.

PSYCHOSOCIAL CONSIDERATIONS FOR PATIENTS AND FAMILIES

The psychosocial aspects of AIDS are devastating. Because no cure presently exists for the HIV infection, the diagnosis of HIV infection, like a diagnosis of cancer, brings potential denial, fear, depression, and anger. The social stigma of AIDS, based on associations with homosexuality, intravenous drug abuse, and sexual transmission, cannot be minimized.[25] One of the earliest issues that HIV-infected individuals face is sharing the information with family and significant others. Tremendous fear of family anger, rejection, or abandonment is a critical issue. HIV-infected individuals who have been exposed by contaminated blood or unknowingly through heterosexual relationships may feel unique and intense anger and hostility.

Individuals who are exposed to HIV infection, but are without symptoms or complications of infections or cancers, live with a great deal of uncertainty and anxiety interspersed with denial and hopefulness. The role of the nurse in this stage of the disease process is to provide continued education about the disease of AIDS, as well as to assist in realistic goal setting. Patients are encouraged to participate in care and maintain positive relationships.

As the HIV infection progresses with clinical complications of infections and cancers, patients experience multiple losses including loss of energy, self-care deficit requiring assistance with activities of daily living, and loss of independence, employment, finances, and hope. The reality of death emerges. Nursing care focuses on a philosophy of facing life a day at a time and living each day to the fullest extent possible by resolving multiple conflicts. This may be a time for strengthening personal and spiritual relationships.

Empathic listening and the ability to help patients find meaning in life become critical nursing interventions. Assisting families and significant others, including lovers, to provide support to the terminally ill patient despite their own anger and grief is a unique nursing challenge. Such care, although emotionally draining for the nurse, can provide tremendous positive feelings of professional accomplishment.

ASSISTING WITH COPING

The diagnosis of HIV infection, with its social stigmatization, poor prognosis, and lethal nature, is indeed a catastrophic event for patients and caregivers. Individuals experience a variety of intense emotions that threaten self-esteem and predispose to depression and feelings of powerlessness. Anxiety is a response that pervades the entire HIV illness continuum. Anxiety and denial often accompany the initial diagnosis and intensify with physical decline and loss of independence, job, and finances. Anxiety may be incapacitating as death becomes a reality. Nursing interventions to promote effective coping focus on exploring and strengthening healthful coping strategies and maintaining sources of psychologic support.

Individuals experiencing the anxiety of HIV infection are often in a state of crisis. Continued clarification and education about the HIV infection, complications, and treatment are critical. Every effort should be made to include the patient in planning medical and nursing care. An assessment of past coping styles and support systems should be made early and continually reevaluated. Healthful patterns of coping, such as talking or relaxation and meditation, are encouraged. Relationships with family, friends, and lovers should be maintained and may be strengthened through the HIV crisis. Conversely, past conflicts, especially among family members, may persist and intensify during the HIV crisis.

Occasionally anxiety, denial, depression, and even grief may persist for extended periods, interfering with daily functioning, productive communication and relationships, and even the ability to make decisions. The nurse must be able to assess normal periods of anxiety, depression, and grief, as well as refer patients and significant others for psychologic evaluation and counseling for ineffective coping patterns. Although reactions of anxiety and depression are normal, professional intervention is necessary whenever they preclude communication and daily functioning for an extended time (usually longer than 3 months). Patients with HIV infection and depression should be assessed for suicidal ideation because this phenomenon occasionally occurs in terminally ill patients who are experiencing anxiety and fear of further pain and physical decline. Early recognition of depression is critical because some cases of depression and anxiety may respond to medications and psychotherapy.

Individuals with diffuse anxiety often feel they have little control over their daily existence. A schedule of activities that patients develop with guidance from health care professionals may decrease anxiety and feelings of powerlessness. Opportunities for spiritual support and comfort should be explored. Significant others may also experience anxiety. Community support groups for patients and significant others may offer additional sources of support and contribute to healthful coping. Planned uninterrupted time with only the nurse, patient, and significant other may create a supportive environment that decreases anxiety and promotes healthful coping.

HIV COMPLICATIONS: AIDS

The clinical presentation of AIDS can be attributed to secondary opportunistic infections and malignancies that occur with a compromised immune system. The following is a summary of these opportunistic infections and related patient care needs. See pp. 2236-2237 for nursing care plan for a person with HIV complications.

PNEUMOCYSTIS CARINII PNEUMONIA

The most common opportunistic infection that occurs with HIV infection is *Pneumocystis carinii* pneumonia (PCP). This pneumonia is caused by a protozoa and is seen in 60% of all patients with HIV infection. PCP is not airborne and thus is not transmitted from person to person as are some other types of pneumonia. Clinical manifestations include malaise, fatigue, increased respiratory rate, dry cough, fever, night sweats, and shortness of breath. Chest x-ray examinations of patients with PCP show diffuse interstitial infiltrates. Diagnosis of PCP can be made from patient history, bronchoscopy, sample of secretions obtained from sputum specimens, and tissue from lung biopsies.[46]

The majority of patients with PCP are hospitalized for treatment. Some require mechanical ventilation as a supportive therapy. The usual medical treatments for PCP include intravenous antibiotics such as Bactrim or Septra (Table 77-6) and pentamidine given intravenously or as an aerosolized respiratory treatment. These two medications have many potentially toxic effects, and nurses must carefully monitor patients for progression of clinical symptoms, as well as for toxic effects of

TABLE 77-6 Pharmacologic treatment of HIV infections and malignancy

Trade Name	Generic Name	Infection/Malignancy	Side Effects
Adriamycin	Doxorubicin (systemic)	Kaposi's sarcoma	Leukopenia or infection (fever, chills, sore throat); stomatitis; esophagitis, flank, stomach, or joint pain; pain at injection site; peripheral edema; fast or irregular heartbeat; shortness of breath; gastrointestinal bleeding; thrombocytopenia (unusual bleeding or bruising); changes in skin color; diarrhea, nausea, vomiting; skin rash or itching; hair loss; reddish color to urine
Bactrim Septra	Sulfamethoxazole and trimethoprim (systemic)	*Pneumocystis carinii* pneumonia	Skin rash or itching; Stevens-Johnson syndrome (myalgia, arthralgia, redness, blistering, peeling or loosening of the skin); extreme fatigue, dysphagia, fever, leukopenia (sore throat); thrombocytopenia (unusual bleeding or bruising); hepatitis (dark urine, pale stools, yellow skin, and/or sclera); crystalluria, hematuria, diarrhea, dizziness, headache; anorexia, nausea, vomiting
Blenoxane	Bleomycin (systemic)	Kaposi's sarcoma	Cough, shortness of breath, pneumonitis, fever, chills, stomatitis, confusion, syncope, diaphoresis, changes in skin color and texture, rashes, swelling of fingers, nausea, vomiting and anorexia, weight loss, hair loss
DHPG	9-(1,3-dihydroxy-2 propoxymethyl) guanine (systemic)	Cytomegalovirus (CMV) (CMV retinitis and CMV colitis)	Under investigation Leukopenia, bone marrow depression, elevation of serum liver enzymes, neutropenia, eosinophilia, decreased platelet count; edema, nausea, myalgias, headache, anorexia, disorientation, hallucinations, rash, phlebitis
Fungizone	Amphotericin B (systemic)	Cryptococcus	Anorexia, headache, fever, chills and rigors, convulsions, hyalgia, pain at injection site, tinnitus, hypotension, atrial fibrillation, hypokalemia, decreased renal function, anaphylactic reactions
Pentam	Pentamidine	*Pneumocystis carinii* pneumonia	Anorexia, nausea and vomiting, leukopenia, thrombocytopenia, hypoglycemia, hypotension, pain at injection site, hepatotoxicity, decreased renal function
Zovirax	Acyclovir (systemic)	Herpes simplex Herpes zoster Varicella	*Oral:* changes in menstrual period, skin rash, diarrhea, dizziness, headache, myalgia, nausea and vomiting, acne, anorexia, somnolence *Parenteral:* skin rashes or hives, hematuria, lightheadedness, headaches, hypotension, diaphoresis, confusion, tremors, abdominal pain, dyspnea, oliguria, unusual thirst, extreme fatigue

DATA: Mr. C. is a 32-year-old computer programmer. He was born in a small town in the Midwest but has lived on the West coast for the past 10 years. He has had little contact with his family because of the painful situation when he left home; his family was "disgraced" by the fact that he was "gay." For the last 5 years he has been living with his lover, Mr. J. Mr. C. reveals that before moving in with Mr. J., he had multiple homosexual and heterosexual experiences. Mr. J. and Mr. C. have lived in a monogamous relationship for the last 3 years. Mr. C. describes Mr. J. as a "dependent" person who rarely "hangs onto a job for very long." Mr. C. is being admitted to the hospital for a medical evaluation of 4 months of fatigue not relieved with sleep. He has lost 20 pounds, and reports night sweats that frequently awaken him, a rectal rash, and a dry cough with fevers. Mr. C.'s illness has caused him to use all of his sick time from work and he is afraid he will lose his job. He also says he is terrified that he might be dying.

The nursing history identified the following:
- Mr. C. has multiple risk factors for contracting the HIV infection, including multiple sexual partners, homosexual experiences, and anal intercourse
- Mr. C. has several persistent clinical symptoms indicative of HIV infection: fatigue, weight loss, dry cough, fevers, and a rectal rash

- Mr. C. has multiple sources of stress, including his alienation from family members because of his sexual preference, possible loss of his job due to his persistent illness, and his concern over his "lover's" ability to cope with stress while Mr. C. is ill.

Collaborative nursing activities include:
- Assessment of Mr. C.'s understanding of HIV testing, AIDS, and treatment regimens
- Assessment of progression of clinical symptoms or evidence of new clinical symptoms indicating complications such as infections
- Referral to a social service agency for investigation of health disability insurance and in employment benefits
- Assessment and possible referral for mental health counseling for Mr. C. and Mr. J.

Nursing activities include monitoring the following:
- Temperature, particularly fever
- Daily food and fluid intake and weight
- Cognitive ability
- Ability to care for self
- Spread of, or drainage from, rectal rash
- Lung sounds and sputum production
- Appetite, ability to sleep, ability to discuss concerns, and other clinical indicators of anxiety or depression
- Laboratory results of ELISA, Western Blot, T-cell ratios, WBC's, PT, PTT, and serum electrolytes

NURSING DIAGNOSIS

Anxiety (Mr. C. and Mr. J.) related to persistent debilitating illness, with an unknown etiology but with evidence of terminal illness; related to threatened loss of independence, job, and social relationships

Expected Patient Outcomes	Nursing Interventions	Rationale
Mr. C. and Mr. J. will identify previous coping strategies for stress, verbalize sources of anxiety, identify possible coping strategies for present anxieties, and articulate decreased symptoms of anxiety such as anorexia and sleeplessness.	Acknowledge multiple sources of stress as evidenced from history. Explore with Mr. C. past life crises and strategies to cope, as well as sources of support. Spend time with Mr. C., explaining procedures and treatments Spend uninterrupted time with Mr. C. and Mr. J. individually to allow for empathic listening. Monitor for increasing anxiety and report to physician.	Patterns of past successful coping are indicators of present resources and strengths. Empathy as a counseling therapy utilizes realistic description stressors, reflective listening, physical presence, and clarification. Anxiety may increase with procedures and terminal diagnosis.

NURSING DIAGNOSIS

Knowledge deficit (HIV risk factors, disease transmission, test significance, HIV pathophysiology) related to lack of exposure

Expected Patient Outcomes	Nursing Interventions	Rationale
Mr. C. and Mr. J. describe rationale of diagnostic tests, HIV risk factors, and strategies for prevention of HIV transmission.	Using discussion with repetition and printed materials, review diagnostic tests such as ELISA, Western Blot, and T-cell ratios, risk factors and prevention strategies of HIV infection, clinical symptoms of HIV infection.	Patients have a right to information related to health. This information will promote the ability to make decisions to prevent disease and to seek medical treatment to alleviate symptoms and complications. Anxiety decreases the ability to take in information and requires repetition and multiple learning strategies.

NURSING DIAGNOSIS

Nutrition, altered: less than body requirements, related to diarrhea as evidenced by undesired weight loss

Expected Patient Outcomes	Nursing Interventions	Rationale
Mr. C. and Mr. J. describe a meal plan with adequate calories and hydration. Mr.C. ceases to lose weight. Mr. C.'s serum albumin, potassium, and sodium remain within normal limits.	Plan with Mr.C. and nutritionist a daily schedule of six small meals including 3000 ml of fluids and 3000 calories, excluding dairy products, and raw fruits and vegetables.	Small meals prevent gastric distention and nausea; 2500-3000 ml provides adequate hydration for febrile adult; 3000 calories will prevent weight loss and negative nitrogen balance. Lactose in dairy products may enhance diarrhea; raw foods contain naturally occurring microorganisms that may increase infection in immunocompromised hosts.
	Plan routine oral care and rinses before and after meals.	Oral care before meals enhances appetite and flow of digestive juices; oral care after meals helps to prevent oral lesions and infections.
	Assist Mr. C. to be out of bed or sitting up.	Upright positioning prevents aspiration and pneumonia.
	Weigh Mr. C. daily at same time on same scale, and record.	Weight is a clinical indicator of adequate nutrition.

NURSING DIAGNOSIS

Activity intolerance related to weight loss, sleeplessness, and fatigue

Expected Patient Outcomes	Nursing Interventions	Rationale
Mr. C. sleeps 6-8 hours at night, is independent in ADL's, and states decreased feelings of fatigue.	Plan and teach Mr. C. about pacing activity and the use of energy conservation measures.	Pacing of activity and energy conservation conserves patient's energy balanced with activity.
	Include in plan uninterrupted period for sleep. Review with Mr. C. relaxation techniques at bedtime such as deep breathing, tepid baths, use of a radio.	Relaxation promotes comfort and contributes to sleep.
	Increase nutritional intake. Assist with ADL, encourage patient participation.	Provides calories for energy consumption, thereby decreasing some fatigue.

NURSING DIAGNOSIS

Impaired skin integrity related to genital herpes; potential impaired skin integrity related to fatigue and immobility

Expected Patient Outcomes	Nursing Interventions	Rationale
Rectal rash will heal and Mr. C. will report increased comfort. Herpes infection will not spread on Mr. C.'s body or to caregivers. Further skin breakdown does not occur.	Assist Mr. C. to clean rectal area after each episode of diarrhea, using a mild soap such as liquid Castile soap; use gloves and good handwashing after cleaning.	Herpes rashes cause local irritation and discomfort; healing is promoted by gentle cleaning, allowing regeneration of epidermis.
	Assist Mr. C. to turn in bed at least every two hours.	Decreased pressure promotes healing and comfort by increased circulation.
	Assist Mr. C. with daily bathing; encourage shower, avoid tub baths. For basin baths, use clean washcloth for rash area and do not reuse	Daily hygiene prevents secondary infections and spread of existing infections. Showers provide continued washing away of microorganisms.
	Apply gloves (self or Mr. C.) for cleansing or application of medications to rash.	Herpes and other rashes may be spread to patient and caregiver by skin contact.

the drugs. In rare cases, pentamidine may be given as an intramuscular injection, but patients may suffer sterile abcesses at the injection sites. Patients are usually treated for about 3 weeks in the hospital and are discharged on a regimen of oral Bactrim or Septra. They may continue to receive aerosolized pentamidine at home or in the outpatient clinic as a means of prophylaxis.[46]

Nursing care of patients with PCP focuses on relieving symptoms and monitoring for complications. Patients with PCP suffer extreme fatigue, shortness of breath, cough, and fever. Many patients with PCP are treated with multiple antibiotics and are at risk for untoward side effects, such as nausea and vomiting, that threaten nutritional intake and further contribute to fatigue and weakness. The most important nursing care goal for patients with PCP is the maintenance of adequate ventilation and comfort.

Patients suffering from PCP should have a detailed respiratory and cardiovascular assessment including observation of respiration, mucous membrane color, and activity and fatigue levels; auscultation of breath sounds and heart sounds; and measurement of pulse, blood pressure, and respiratory rate. The nursing care plan should focus on promoting independence in activities of daily living while preventing fatigue. Pacing of activities and scheduling of rest periods are important for energy conservation. Maintaining adequate hydration of 2-1/2 to 3 liters of fluid, positioning in semi-Fowler's or high-Fowler's position while in bed, spending short periods in a chair or ambulating combined with deep-breathing exercises, and using an incentive spirometer will enhance the patient's airway clearance and help prevent respiratory complications. Some patients with PCP may require oxygen for adequate ventilation. Patients with severe forms of PCP may require intubation and mechanical ventilation and bronchotracheal suctioning to ensure adequate respiratory function (see Chapter 34).

CANDIDA INFECTIONS

Candidiasis, a fungal infection caused by a yeast of the genus *Candida,* is common in HIV-infected and immunocompromised individuals. The most common, candidiasis symptom is oral thrush, with creamy whitish-yellow patches in the mouth and throat, but it may also infect the entire gastrointestinal system. Some individuals may be affected with skin lesions.

Commonly used drugs in the treatment of candidiasis are nystatin (Mycostatin), ketoconazole (Nizoral), and clotrimazole (Lotrimin, Mycelex). Although side effects from Mycostatin and Lotrimin are uncommon, some individuals may experience abdominal cramps, nausea, vomiting, and diarrhea. Nizoral is useful in the treatment of candidia esophagitis. Toxic effects include nausea, diarrhea, chemical hepatitis, itching, skin

rashes, and drowsiness. Clotrimazole cream is used to treat cutaneous candidiasis rashes and lesions.[26]

Patients with candidiasis are at risk for dysphagia from a painful oral inflammation (stomatitis), diarrhea and skin irritation, and nutritional deficiency. Nursing care priorities include oral hygiene and adequate food and fluid intake. Because patients with HIV infection are also at risk for bleeding secondary to clotting disorders, oral hygiene must be accomplished without trauma (Chapter 30).

Patients with candidiasis should have oral mucous membranes inspected daily for lesions, integrity, and bleeding. Oral hygiene measures such as brushing teeth with nonabrasive paste, rinsing with saline and hydrogen peroxide, and applying ointment to chapped lips will provide comfort, enhance nutritional intake, and minimize further spread of infection. In addition to routine oral hygiene measures, medications such as Nystatin, Xylocaine, and Mycelex will also prevent infection spread. Daily monitoring of food and fluid intake, urine and stool output, weight, skin turgor, and serum albumin levels will alert the nurse to potential problems of nutritional deficiencies and dehydration. Measures to enhance nutritional intake (p. 2233) are instituted.

For disseminated *candida* lesions along the GI tract, the potent intravenous antibiotic amphotericin B may be given (Table 77-6). Patients receiving amphotericin B must be tested with a small dose of the drug to rule out sensitivity. Even in patients without sensitivity to small test doses, reactions of hypotension and severe shaking, called rigors, may occur. Frequent observation of vital signs during amphotericin B administration are necessary. Some patients may receive premedications of Tylenol, Benadryl, or even hydrocortisone added to amphotericin solutions to prevent reactions. Should patients suffer severe reactions such as rigors, it is important to stop the infusion and initiate medical intervention quickly. In some cases rigors may be treated with meperidine injections.

CRYPTOSPORIDIOSIS

Cryptosporidiosis is a common protozoan infection found in patients with HIV infection. This organism causes malaise, nausea, abdominal cramping, and massive watery diarrhea leading to weight loss. Some patients with cryptosporidiosis may lose up to 15 liters of fluid per day, resulting in severe dehydration, malnutrition, and electrolyte imbalance. There is currently no effective medical treatment for cryptosporidiosis.[47] Symptomatic treatment using antidiarrheal medication and intravenous fluid therapy may be helpful in preventing dehydration and electrolyte imbalance.

Nursing care priorities for patients suffering from cryptosporidiosis include providing adequate nutrition, maintaining skin integrity, minimizing fatigue and discomfort, and preventing dehydration. Diets low in residue, which exclude items such as nuts, fried foods, and grains, may be beneficial in decreasing episodes of diarrhea. Hydration with 3000 ml of oral fluids including water, juices, and caffeine-free, noncarbonated fluids should be planned over 24 hours.

Skin care for patients suffering from cryptosporidiosis and massive diarrhea includes pressure relief by frequent position changes, range-of-motion exercises, and devices such as air mattresses. Cleansing of skin after episodes of diarrhea involves gentle washing with mild soap and a soft cloth, followed by application of moisture barrier creams. Occlusive dressings such as Duoderm and Op-site are contraindicated in immunocompromised patients because some studies have demonstrated an increased risk of infection with their use.

HERPESVIRUS INFECTIONS
CYTOMEGALOVIRUS INFECTION

A common infection in the herpesvirus family is *cytomegalovirus* or CMV. Over half of the general population has been exposed to CMV early in life and has built up antibodies. However, latent CMV may be a significant cause of disease in immunocompromised persons. The virus can cause damage to the lung, large intestines, and retina. The diagnosis of CMV infection can be confirmed from blood cultures or organ biopsies. At present no effective medical treatment of CMV is available. However, the experimental use of the drug DHPG (Table 77-6), an Acyclovir derivative, is showing some promise.[27,47]

Patients with CMV often suffer from fever, fatigue, malaise, weight loss, and facial edema. The most devastating form of CMV is retinal CMV, leading to blindness.[47] All patients with HIV infection should routinely be assessed for visual changes, which must be promptly reported. Patients with CMV retinitis often suffer light sensitivity. Rooms should be dimly lit, and the use of sunglasses may minimize discomfort indoors and outdoors. Nursing care of patients with CMV retinitis centers on patient teaching related to visual changes and anticipatory grief, as well as planning for safe activities of daily living. Early referrals to community sight centers will provide adequate time for adaptation to decreasing vision, as well as an additional support network to facilitate healthy grieving.

HERPES ZOSTER

Another herpesvirus, varicella-zoster, causes chickenpox in children and herpes zoster (shingles) in older immunocompromised patients (Chapter 72). Vesicular eruptions, which are accompanied by painful tingling and itching, will rupture and finally crust over, lasting about 3 weeks. Diagnosis is made by clinical evaluation of the lesions and occasionally confirmed by cultures of the lesions. The drug Acyclovir, administered orally or intravenously for an indefinite period, may be used to treat herpes varicella-zoster in HIV-infected immunocompromised patients.[26]

HERPES SIMPLEX

Oral and genital-rectal lesions caused by the herpes simplex virus (Chapter 72) are a fairly common occurrence with HIV infection and an immunocompromised host. Vesicular lesions vary in size; some become ulcerated, causing wound discharge, bleeding, and—at times—excruciating pain. Oral or intravenous Acyclovir may be useful in treating herpes simplex. In many cases medication therapy must be administered indefinitely to control the virus. Nursing care for individuals receiving Acyclovir should focus on the monitoring and timely reporting of all medication side effects (Table 77-6).

Nursing care of patients with herpes lesions focuses on promoting comfort and minimizing the spread of infection to the patient and caregivers. Patients with HIV infection should be assessed daily for intact skin, rashes, or lesions. All rashes and lesions are promptly reported for medical follow-up. Patients with herpes lesions should avoid tub baths and the use of bar soap that may cause dissemination of the lesions. A separate clean washcloth should be used to bathe areas with lesions. Patients and caregivers should wear gloves whenever cleaning or applying medications to lesions.

MYCOBACTERIAL INFECTIONS

Mycobacterium avium intracellulare (MAI) is a bacteria commonly found in the environment. MAI rarely causes severe infection except in patients infected with HIV virus. Clinical symptoms caused by MAI include fever, diarrhea, abdominal pain, weight loss, *pancytopenia*, abnormal food absorption, and abnormal liver function test results. MAI may be cultured from blood, sputum, body organs, bone marrow, and lymph nodes.[26,46] Various drug therapies including rifampin, ethambutol, amikacin, ansamycin, and clofazimine have been used in attempts to treat MAI. These drugs, however, have shown little success.

Mycobacterium tuberculosis (MTB) can occasionally occur in HIV-infected patients. MTB may be found in any organ system, the lymph system, meninges, bones, peritoneum, and pleura. Diagnosis is based on the clinical symptom of fever and associated infected organs and is confirmed by the presence of acid-fast bacillus. Similar to HIV-infected patients with PCP, patients with MAI and MTB require nursing care to minimize the effects of fever, weakness, nausea, vomiting, and dyspnea.

CENTRAL NERVOUS SYSTEM INFECTIONS

Toxoplasmosis, caused by the protozoon *Toxoplasma gondii,* often results in focal *encephalitis* in immunocompromised patients. Symptoms include fever, headache, lethargy, decreased cognitive ability, confusion including memory loss, personality changes, and seizures. The CSF in patients with *Toxoplasma gondii* has increased protein and white blood cells. CT scans may reveal masses, but a brain biopsy may be required to establish a definitive diagnosis of toxoplasma trophozoite in brain tissue. Medical treatment includes the use of antibiotics such as clindamycin, trimethoprim-sulfamethoxazole, spriamycin, pyrimethamine, and sulfadiazine.

Meningitis, caused by the fungus *Cryptococcus neoformans,* causes fever, headache, nausea, vomiting, blurred vision, stiff neck, varying degrees of confusion, lethargy, and possibly seizures. A lumbar puncture is needed to confirm the diagnosis of cryptococcus; a positive result is CSF infiltration of white blood cells, protein, an increased cryptococcal antigen titer, and abnormally low glucose levels.[47]

The human immunodeficiency virus itself may invade the central nervous system, causing *HIV encephalopathy* or *dementia*. It is believed that about 60% of all HIV-infected individuals suffer HIV encephalopathy. Initially, encephalopathy may be manifested by progressive loss or decline in cognitive, motor, or behavioral function. Early signs of HIV encephalopathy are subtle and may be confused with normal grieving and depression. These signs include reduced concentration, slowness of speech, and impaired memory. As HIV encephalopathy progresses, dementia results with further decline in the individual's ability to walk, control body functions, perform self-care, and make decisions. HIV encephalopathy may progress to coma. Treatment is primarily palliative and supportive. AZT (azidothymidine) has been used with some improvement in neurologic function in the early stages of the disease.[47]

Nursing care of patients with toxoplasmosis or meningitis resulting in encephalitis and cognitive impairment is aimed at relieving symptoms such as headaches and lethargy, and promoting safety during seizures, delirium, and depression.

Although some patients with cognitive impairment may be acutely aware of their deficits and need for assistance with activities of daily living, others may have little insight into these needs (Chapter 63). A major focus of nursing care for patients with cognitive impairment is the support and education of caregivers. Caregivers require instruction and supervision in patient bathing, positioning, skin care, oral care, transferring, use of assistive devices, range-of-motion exercises, feeding and nutrition, bowel and bladder management, and environmental safety, including infection control mea-

sures. Patients who are aware of declining cognitive abilities and the terminal nature of their HIV infection are at high risk for suicide. Therefore all patients with a diagnosis of HIV infection should be assessed for depression and suicide ideation. Referral to mental health professionals for caregivers suffering extreme grief and care burdens, as well as for depressed patients can be useful in addressing quality-of-life issues despite terminal illness.

TUMORS

Malignant *lymphomas* of the central nervous system are common in patients with HIV infection and often indicate poor progress. These lymphomas include non-Hodgkins lymphoma and Burkitt's-like lymphomas (Chapter 30). Clinical symptoms include malaise, myalgias, lymphadenopathy, and abdominal discomforts associated with weight loss.[47]

Kaposi's sarcoma (KS) is by far the most common neoplasm found in patients with HIV infection. KS affects vascular epithelium and results in red-purplish cutaneous lesions (Chapter 72). Lesions may appear on the trunk, arms, legs, head, and neck. Extracutaneous lesions may also occur in mucous membranes, lymph nodes, lungs, and the gastrointestinal tract. Kaposi's sarcoma tumors can block lymphatic drainage, resulting in severe edema to the face or extremities. Pulmonary lesions may result in respiratory distress and even death. Although some patients have no clinical symptoms associated with KS, others complain of malaise, weight loss, swollen lymph nodes, generalized edema, and shortness of breath. Kaposi's sarcoma may be diagnosed by tissue biopsy. Radiation therapy may be used as a palliative measure in some progressive forms of KS lesions.

Symptoms of KS depend on involved body systems. KS may invade cutaneous tissue, causing edema and skin lesions; lung tissue, causing shortness of breath and a productive cough; gastrointestinal system, causing diarrhea; or the brain, causing cognitive changes and gait disturbances. Radiation therapy has been used in the treatment of KS lesions, although some patients may suffer additional complications of therapy, such as nausea and vomiting.[46]

Nursing care priorities for patients are dependent on the particular system affected by KS. Care considerations include skin care of lesions, promoting comfortable ventilation, and maintaining a safe environment. Prevention of the effects of edema may be a major nursing care strategy for patients with KS. Elevating the head of the bed or affected extremities may produce some relief. Facial edema may be alleviated by cool compresses. Maintaining skin integrity despite edema and radiation therapy is indeed challenging.

Gentle massages with creams and oils help promote

drainage, reduce discomfort, and prevent breakdown. KS lesions that are dry may be left open to the air. For draining KS lesions, cleansing with mild soap and patting dry, applying normal saline wet dressings, or applying Bacitracin and Neomycin creams and covering with nonadhering dressings such as Telfa may provide some comfort and prevent the spread of lesions. Similar to patients with PCP, patients with pulmonary Kaposi's sarcoma will require nursing interventions to reduce dyspnea and promote comfortable effective airway clearance.

AZT THERAPY FOR HIV COMPLICATIONS

Since no cure for HIV infection exists at present, treatment has been aimed at slowing progression of the disease, managing symptoms, and providing palliative care. Multiple clinical trials of various drugs to slow progression of the HIV infection are now under way. In 1987 the first such drug, azidothymidine (AZT), also known as Zetrovir or Zidovudine, was released for treatment. AZT acts by inhibiting the replication of the human immunodeficiency virus. In some individuals, AZT has been effective in reducing the number of opportunistic infections and dementia symptoms.

AZT, however, has many side effects including malaise, headaches, fever, nausea, vomiting, insomnia, and myalgia. Toxic effects in about 50% of patients include anemia, bone marrow suppression, reduced white blood count, and low platelet counts. Patients on AZT require weekly blood testing to monitor for toxic effects.[46] Some patients on AZT may require blood transfusions to counter the toxic effects of AZT.

AZT therapy has also been suggested as a preventive measure in the management of occupational exposure to HIV.[18]

SOCIAL, ETHICAL, AND LEGAL ISSUES

The HIV epidemic has brought with it not only a dismal prognosis, but also severe social stigmatization, public fear, and a growing number of legal and ethical issues. Nurses providing care in a variety of settings will face many of these issues that may jeopardize the quality of patient care. In addition, nurses caring for patients with the HIV infection will face many personal stresses including fear of personal contamination and disease transmission to family members, and burnout related to caring for terminally ill young patients with controversial life-styles. The professional commitment needed by nurses who provide care to HIV-infected patients requires clarification of personal values regarding the issues of homosexuality and drug use.

Inherent in nursing is a respect for life, dignity, and social justice. The American Nurses Association Code of Ethics clearly reaffirms that the profession of nursing provides services with respect for human dignity and the uniqueness of each client, unrestricted by social or economic status, personal attributes, or the nature of health problems.

The very nature of nurses' work constitutes a level of risk for various diseases that does not exist in other professions. In upholding the moral principle of justice, risks and withholding of care must be carefully balanced with potential benefits of care. In addition, individual nurses and institutions have a responsibility to take reasonable precautions to protect caregivers from harm while providing medical and nursing care to patients.

As long as the HIV infection remains a downhill continuum with multiple complications and eventual death, nurses caring for patients with progressive AIDS will be involved in decisions regarding the selective withholding of treatment while preserving the quality of life and human dignity. The role of nursing in the terminal phase of illness is a critical one. When no medical treatments can be offered to the patient, nursing has everything to offer: identification of values, exploration of the meaning of life, comfort from symptoms, support of human bonds, and eventually a physically and psychologically peaceful death.

Nurses must continually help the health care team, family, and significant others to focus on the patients' desires. This principle of autonomy, as endorsed by the American Nurses Association, is a valuable guide for many ethical decisions regarding terminally ill patients. Nurse caregivers providing such intense physical and psychologic care also need support. Peer support through informal sharing or structured support group is an effective strategy that may alleviate feelings of helplessness.

Legal issues such as confidentiality, mandatory testing, employer screening, and school attendance of children infected with HIV remain controversial. Therefore it will be important for all nurses to keep themselves informed of policy developments and to influence, whenever possible, such decisions based on the ethical principle of justice. (For further discussion of ethical issues, see Chapter 14.)

CHAPTER SUMMARY

✔ The three major methods of transmission of human immunodeficiency virus (HIV) are by intimate contact with semen or vaginal secretions through sexual contact, by infected blood through blood transfusions or sharing of IV drug needles, and by mother-to-infant transfer through placenta or breast milk.

✔ Risk behaviors for HIV infection include anal intercourse, frequent sexual intercourse with multiple partners, and sharing IV drug needles.

✔ Populations at highest risk include homosexual and bisexual men, IV drug users, heterosexual partners of HIV-infected individuals, infants born to HIV-infected parents, and individuals who received blood transfusions before 1985.

- HIV infection is not spread by nonsexual household contacts.

- Infection control measures include handwashing before and after patient contact and after removal of gloves; wearing gloves whenever there will be contact with body secretions; disposing of soiled dressings, wet linens, and respiratory equipment in heavy plastic bags; disposing of needles *without capping* in puncture-resistant needle disposal containers; environmental cleaning with institutional cleaning agents or a 1:10 dilution of bleach and water; and use of bleach with laundering.

- The human immunodeficiency virus is a retrovirus that invades helper Tcells, incorporates its DNA into the genetic material of the T-helper cell, and replicates itself, destroying the helper T cell. The decreased number of helper T cells causes immunodeficiency.

- Persons exposed to HIV may develop an acute infection (similar to mononucleosis) or may be asymptomatic, harboring the virus for several years. The asymptomatic person may unknowingly transmit the virus to others. Some persons develop a persistent generalized lymphadenopathy in the absence of explainable illness. Not all persons appear to progress to AIDS-related complex (ARC) or AIDS.

- ARC is a debilitating syndrome of fever, diarrhea, weight loss greater than 10% of baseline, fatigue, edema, and abnormal laboratory immune values (altered T_4/T_8 ratio, leukopenia, lymphopenia, thrombocytopenia).

- AIDS is the most severe HIV disease. In addition to the symptoms of ARC, the AIDS patient develops opportunistic infections and/or malignancies. Death eventually ensues.

- Opportunistic infections may be protozoal, bacterial, viral, or fungal; the most common infection is *P. carinii* pneumonia. The most common malignancy is Kaposi's sarcoma.

- The ELISA test, indicating the presence of HIV *antibodies*, is the most often used diagnostic test for HIV infection. If this test is positive, a Western Blot test is done to confirm the results.

- Interventions for persons with HIV infection depend on the symptoms and presence of infections or malignancies. Nursing interventions include prevention of infection, modification of alterations in body temperature, promotion of self-care, safety, and good nutrition, counseling, assisting with coping; and patient teaching.

- Treatment for persons with *P. carinii* pneumonia includes antibiotics (Bactrim or Septra, pentamidine), administered by IV or aerosol. Mechanical ventilation may be necessary. Nursing interventions include maintenance of adequate ventilation, promotion of comfort, conservation of energy, and promotion of adequate hydration and nutrition.

- Treatment for candidiasis (fungal infection of GI tract, particulary the mouth) includes use of the antifungal drugs nystatin, ketoconazole, or clotrimazole. Nursing interventions include oral hygiene and promotion of adequate food and fluid intake.

- Cryptosporidiosis is a protozoal infection affecting the GI tract with massive diarrhea leading to weight loss. Treatment is symptomatic with antidiarrheal medication and fluid replacement. Nursing interventions include preventing dehydration, promoting nutrition, energy conservation, and comfort, and maintaining skin integrity.

- Cytomegalovirus (CMV) infection is caused by a herpesvirus. It can affect the lung, large intestines, and especially the retina, leading to blindness. No effective medical treatment is available, although the experimental drug DHPG is being used. Persons with CMV retinitis must be prepared for eventual loss of sight.

- Individuals with herpes simplex or herpes zoster may be prescribed Acyclovir, which in many cases must be administered indefinitely to control the virus. Nursing interventions include promoting comfort and minimizing spread of infection.

- Mycobacterial infections include *M. avium intracellulare* (MAI) or *M. tuberculosis* (MTB). Nursing interventions include promotion of comfort and ventilation.

- CNS infections include encephalitis, meningitis, encephalopathy or dementia, and coma. Nursing care is aimed at relief of symptoms and promotion of ADL and safety.

- Lesions of Kaposi's sarcoma may affect the skin, mucous membranes, lymph nodes, lungs, and GI tract. Radiation may be used as a palliative measure. Nursing care depends on the location of lesions, but may include maintaining skin integrity, promoting ventilation, and maintaining safety.

- To slow progression of HIV infection, azidothymidine (AZT) is now being used. AZT acts by inhibiting the replication of HIV. There are many toxic effects, and patients receiving AZT require weekly blood tests, and may require blood transfusions to treat toxic effects.

- Numerous social, ethical, and legal issues need to be considered regarding care of persons with HIV infections.

QUESTIONS TO CONSIDER

- You have been assigned to care for your first HIV-infected patient. What things should you consider before providing care?

- The local school has asked you to give a presentation on AIDS. What areas of content will you include? What teaching strategies and media might be helpful?

- Several of your peers confide in you that they would never care for a patient with AIDS. What ethical principles can help you clarify your views on this issue?

- What strategies can nurse caregivers use to alleviate fear and stress while caring for terminally ill HIV-infected patients and their families?

- You are preparing a family to provide home care for their son with AIDS. What learning needs must you assess?

REFERENCES AND SELECTED READINGS

1. Ahluwalia IB: The epidemiology of AIDS. In Blanchet KD, editor: AIDS: a health care management response, Rockville, MD, 1988, Aspen, Publishers Inc.
2. American Nurses Association: Nursing: a social policy statement, Kansas City, Mo, 1980, The Association.
3. American Nurses Association: Code for nurses with interpretative statements, Kansas City, Mo, 1985, The Association.
4. American Nurses Association: Nursing and the human responses to AIDS/HIV infection, Kansas City, Mo, 1988, The Association.
5. Beauchamp T and Childress J: Principles of biomedical ethics, New York, 1979, Oxford University Press Inc.
6. *Beckham MM and Rudy EB: Acquired immunodeficiency syndrome: impact and implication for the neurological system, Neurosci Nurs 18:7-10, 1986.
7. Bennett J and Gee G: History and overview of HIV infection. In Gee G and Moran TA, editors: AIDS: concepts in nursing practice, Baltimore, 1988, Williams & Wilkins.
8. Blanchet KD: AIDS: a health care management response, Rockville, MD, 1988, Aspen Publishers Inc.
9. Carey JT: The clinical spectrum of AIDS. In Blanchet KD: AIDS: a health care management response, Rockville, Md, 1988, Aspen Publishers Inc.
10. Carpenito LJ: Nursing diagnosis: application to clinical practice, ed 2, Philadelphia, 1987, JB Lippincott Co.
11. Carr G: Medical treatment of persons with AIDS/ARC. In Lewis A, editor: Nursing care of the person with AIDS/ARC, Rockville, Md, 1988, Aspen Publishers Inc.
12. Centers for Disease Control: Pneumocystis pneumonia: Los Angeles, MMWR 30:250-252, 1981.
13. Centers for Disease Control: Classification system for human T-lymphotropic virus III/lymphadenopathy-associated virus infections, MMWR 35:334-339, 1986.
14. Centers for Disease Control: Classification system for human immunodeficiency virus (HIV) infection in children under 13 years of age, MMWR 36:225-230, 1987.
15. Centers for Disease Control: Revision of the CDC surveillance case definition for acquired immunodeficiency syndrome, MMWR 36:3-16, 1987.
16. Centers for Disease Control: Update: universal precautions for prevention of transmission of human immunodeficiency virus, hepatitis B virus, and other blood borne pathogens in health care settings, MMWR 37:24, 1988.
17. Christ GH and Wiener LS: Psychosocial issues in AIDS. In DeVita VT Jr et al, editors: AIDS: etiology, diagnosis, treatment and prevention, Philadelphia, 1985, JB Lippincott Co.
18. Centers for Disease Control: Public Health Service statement on management of occupational exposure to HIV, including considerations regarding zidovudine postexposure use, MMWR 39(RR-1):1-14, June 26 1990.
19. *Curran JW et al: Epidemiology of HIV infection and AIDS in the United States, Science 239:610-616, 1988.
20. *Durham J and Cohen F: The person with AIDS: nursing perspectives, New York, 1987, Springer Publishing Co Inc.
21. Fauci AS et al: The acquired immunodeficiency syndrome: an update, Ann Intern Med 102:800-813, 1985.
22. *Flaskerud JH: AIDS: the psychosocial dimension, J Psychosoc Nurs 25:4-36, 1987.
23. Flaskerud JH: Nurses call out for AIDS information, Nurs Health Care 8:557-562, 1987.
24. *Flaskerud JH: AIDS/HIV infection: a reference guide for nursing professionals, Orlando, Fla, 1989, WB Saunders Co.
25. Fowler MDM: Ethics and nursing, 1893-1984: the ideal of service, the reality of history, Los Angeles, 1984, University of Southern California.
26. Hatfield S and Dunkel J: Understanding and working with the emotional reactions of staff. In Lewis A, editor: Nursing care of the person with AIDS/ARC, Rockville, Md, 1988, Aspen Publishers Inc.
27. Hughes AM et al: AIDS home care and hospice manual, San Francisco, 1987, AIDS home care and hospice program, UNA of San Francisco.
28. Jameton A: Nursing practice: the ethical issues, Englewood Cliffs, NJ, 1984, Prentice Hall.
29. Justice AC, Feinstein AR, and Wells CK: A new prognostic staging system for the acquired immunodeficiency syndrome, New Engl J Med 320(22):1388-1489, 1989.
30. *Koenig BA: Ethical and legal issues in the AIDS epidemic. In Lewis A, editor: Nursing care of the person with AIDS/ARC, Rockville, Md, 1988, Aspen Publishers Inc.
31. Koop CE: Surgeon General's report on acquired immune deficiency syndrome, Rockville, Md, 1986, US Department of Health and Human Resources.
32. Kaplan LD, Wofsy CB, and Volberding PA: Treatment of patients with acquired immunodeficiency syndrome and associated manifestations, JAMA 257:1367-1374, 1987.
33. Leads from MMWR: Acquired immune deficiency syndrome, JAMA 252:1298-1301, 1985.
34. Leads from MMWR: Heterosexual transmission of human T-lymphotropic type III/lymphadenopathy associated virus, JAMA 254:2051-2054, 1986.
35. *Lewis A: Nursing care of the person with AIDS/ARC, Rockville, Md, 1988, Aspen Publishers Inc.
36. Masur H et al: Infectious complications of AIDS. In DeVita VT Jr et al, editors: AIDS: etiology, diagnosis, treatment, and prevention, Philadelphia, 1985, JB Lippincott Co.
37. Menke EM: HIV and AIDS: an introduction for nurses, Columbus, Ohio, 1989, East Central AIDS Education and Training Grant.
38. *Nelson WJ: Nursing care of the acutely ill person with AIDS.

*References preceded by an asterisk are particularly well suited for student reading.

In Durham JD and Cohen FL, editors: The person with AIDS: nursing perspectives, New York, 1987, Springer Publishing Co Inc.

39. Pender NJH: Health promotion in nursing practice, Norwalk, Conn, 1987, Appleton & Lange.

39a. Scherer P: How AIDS attacks the brain, Am J Nurs 90(1): 44-53, 1990.

40. Ulrich SP, Canale SW, and Wendell SA: Nursing care planning guides: a nursing diagnosis approach, Philadelphia, 1986, WB Saunders Co.

41. *Ungvarski PJ: Acquired immune deficiency syndrome, Nurs Mirror 157:17-20, 1983.

42. Ungvarski PJ: Infection control in the patient with AIDS, J Hosp Infect 5(A):111-113, 1984.

43. *Ungarvski PJ: Learning to live with AIDS, Nurs Mirror 160:20-22, 1985.

44. Ungarvski PJ: Living with AIDS: a care givers guide, New York, 1987, National Center for Homecare Education and Research.

45. Volberding PA: The clinical spectrum of the acquired immunodeficiency syndrome: implications for comprehensive patient care, Ann Intern Med 103:729-733, 1985.

46. Volberding PA: Kaposi's sarcoma and the acquired immunodeficiency syndrome, Med Clin North Am 70:665-675, 1986.

47. Wolfe P: Clinical manifestations and treatment. In Flaskerud JF, editor: AIDS/HIV infection: a reference guide for nursing professionals, Philadelphia, 1989, WB Saunders Co.

SPECIAL ENVIRONMENTS OF CARE

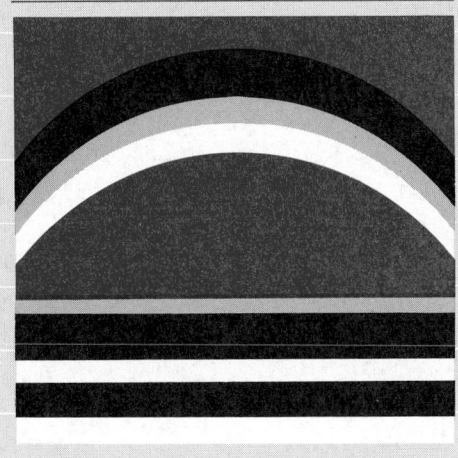

COMMUNITY

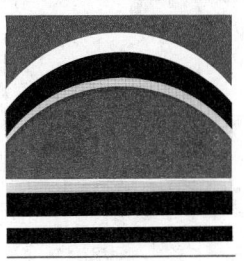

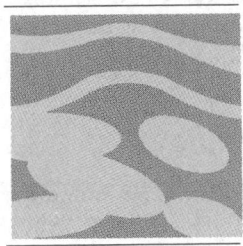

CHAPTER 78

Home Care of the Ill Adult

CAROL E. SMITH

CHAPTER OBJECTIVES

After studying this chapter, the student should be able to:
1. Describe the trends in health care leading to expansion of home care for medical-surgical patients.
2. Discuss the skills used in managing the transition from acute to home care.
3. Use the nursing process with home care patients and their families.
4. Discuss the home residence as the environment for providing nursing care.
5. Evaluate home care through quality assurance.
6. Identify issues pertinent to home health care.

The content in this chapter assists the student learner with home care of the medical-surgical patient. In the mid-1980s, there were approximately the same number of agencies providing home health care as there were hospitals (6500) across the United States.[13] However, forecasters of health care suggest that hospital closures will continue, whereas home care services will increase by as much as 20% annually throughout the 1990s.[43] Medical-surgical nursing home care will be necessary for a wide range of adults. Patients may require one or two home visits or around-the-clock nursing care. The nursing process in home care will include expanded assessment of the individual and the home environment, development of nursing diagnoses based on family data, generation of expected outcomes negotiated with the patient, and evaluation of effectiveness of care in relation to withdrawing or terminating care. Nurses involved in home health will use many skills to provide care to their medical-surgical patients. These skills and the issues that challenge nurses in home care are discussed in this chapter. The nursing process is presented to illustrate the unique aspects of assessing, planning, implementing, and evaluating nursing care in the home.

DEFINITIONS AND TRENDS IN HOME CARE

Home care is the provision of nursing care in the person's residence. Continuity of care can be defined as the effective and efficient transition of the patient from hospital to home; it is essential to successful home care. Continuity of care from acute care settings to home management helps ensure an easy transition for the patient and family. This definition connotes the preparation of the patient for discharge from one health care setting to another as well as coordination of appropriate resources. Congruence between patient and family needs for health care at different stages of illness, together with the nursing care provided, will ensure continuity of care. Continuity of care implies that assistance from health care professionals in acute or home care settings is linked to the ultimate goal of self-care. The linkage results in well-educated, highly motivated patients and families who know what to expect when the patient is discharged to home, manage as much self-care as possible, progress toward the highest level of functioning, and accept help from available resources.

The home health nurse's caseload routinely includes patients with cardiac disease, respiratory disease, diabetes, cancer, and neurologic problems. The home care nurse may be providing or directing nursing services to assist with activities of daily living (ADLs), manage wound care, and as the examples in this chapter illustrate, teach families about the technologic aspects of care.

Several principles differentiate home care from medical-surgical care in institutions. The first principle is that home care is continuous (versus episodic) in perspective. In other words, the interrelatedness of the illness to the patient's life-style is considered. The nurse also emphasizes the comprehensive impact of the patient's situation on the whole family. Concern for the effect of environmental factors on the family and patient are apparent in home care practice.

The promotion of patient and family involvement in care is fundamental as the home care nurse recognizes that self-care may be the only option when insurance and other benefits are depleted. The realities of the economic health care dilemmas dictate that the home care nurse advocate efficient use of professional and family resources.

Trends in health care today have led to an expansion of home care services. Economic trends in health care, technologic innovations, and population demography have resulted in increasing numbers of adult patients requiring medical-surgical care in the home setting. Home care, as an alternative to expensive institutional care, obtained consumer support in the 1970s.[32] Home care has been documented as cost effective in financial analysis studies conducted by insurance companies, health care professionals, pharmaceutical laboratories, and federal regulatory agencies.[29] The projected insolvency of Medicare and Medicaid, along with the increasing number of older persons in our society, provide the imperative for continued development of home health care delivery systems. Community health organizations, such as the Visiting Nurse Association and other agencies, have established innovative and cost-effective programs of home health care. However, more funding for services of these home care agencies is needed. Home care nursing services are often augmented by private companies that supply equipment as well as specialists for the vast array of technologic care being provided in the home.

Technologic progress has influenced home care greatly. Patients can now be monitored at home through computer linkages to sophisticated diagnostic systems. Technologic innovations such as small, easily programmed intravenous infusion pumps, have made parenteral home therapies safe and affordable. A variety of respiratory therapies, ranging from oxygen compression tanks to mechanical ventilators, are widely used today with the elderly or patients with multiple chronic illnesses. The continued use of technology and future advances will increase the population of patients dependent on such care at home.

The changing demographics of our population have also influenced the increase in home health care. The number of elderly will more than double by the year 2030, whereas the younger generation is decreasing in numbers.[8] With reduced government programs for the aged, limitations on the amount of skilled nursing services, and decreased availability of nursing home facilities, more elderly persons will need home care. The needs of the elderly may vary significantly, from medical patients dependent on technology to surgical patients requiring short-term home rehabilitation before returning to work. Many individuals can benefit from home care. The combined influences of the patient's physical and psychologic characteristics and the social and economic support available to the family affect the outcome of care provided in the home. In each family, different factors will influence the outcomes of home care. Repeated assessment of these factors is necessary for modifying the home care plan as patient, family, and environmental factors change over time. The home as

the environment for nursing care offers a particular challenge to those involved in home care. Nurses will need to develop special skills when working with families in their homes to manage the transition from acute to home care.

TRANSITION FROM ACUTE CARE TO HOME CARE

Nurses frequently use special skills, including gaining entry into the home, discharge planning, family education, and case management, in their work with patients in the home. These skills are discussed here.

Health care professionals can readily list reasons for patients to have home care. However, patients and families may view the home care nurse as an added expense and invasion of privacy. One essential skill is the ability to gain entry into the home. Providing nursing care in an individual's home cannot be undertaken without developing a successful approach or introduction to home care services. It is hoped that the nurse and other professionals in the acute care setting initiate discharge planning and that the family accepts the need for the home care nurse and possibly other professionals in their home.

Ideally the first visit with the patient and family should be conducted in the hospital before discharge, but often the first visit is to the home. Therefore the initial contact with the patient by the home care nurse is almost always by telephone. When telephoning, identify yourself as a nurse, and the agency from which you are calling. You may need to remind the family that they were referred to your agency by either the hospital discharge team or their physician. Explain that the purpose of the call is to set up an initial home visit. Establish that the purpose of the initial visit is to discuss the patient and family's home health care needs. Set the time of the visit at the patient's convenience, and state the amount of time it will take. Ask how the family wishes you to enter the home: through front door or back door possibly with a hidden key. Repeat your name, and have them write down a telephone number where they can reach you. Remember that your tone of voice and the manner in which you conduct the telephone conversation establishes your respect for the patient. Closing with the comment, "I look forward to working with you," accentuates the participatory partnership the nurse will seek to develop.

For the home visit itself, the nurse must obtain the address and check directions to the location. At the first visit the patient's needs are assessed and available home care options are discussed. The nurse must be prepared with all essentials needed for assessment (for example, history-taking forms, stethoscope, other equipment) and supplies necessary for already prescribed treatments (for example, teaching materials, bandages for wound dressing). Typically the home care nurse will carry a bag that contains essential equipment but will need to check the contents and add anything necessary for a particular patient. Also, carry your charting materials, whether paper, nursing note forms, or tape recorder for dictation. It is best to tell the family you will be taking notes to document the patient's progress during home care. Your bag should also contain printed materials that can be discussed and then left with the patient and family. The printed materials are selected based on the family's needs for teaching about illness, direct patient care, or other services available.

Information should also be available on the costs of home care services, insurance reimbursement, and other economic details that the family will need. Options to reduce home care expenditures safely, such as family members providing wound dressing changes 3 days a week or the nurse reducing visits to twice weekly, should be explored. Family members may desire 100% professional care or, on the other hand, may believe they can manage all the care themselves. The nurse must analyze each situation and suggest the best options. The nurse assesses the family's caregiving abilities in light of the patient's condition. The nurse should note that most insurers have restrictions on the lifetime amount the patient can be reimbursed for home care. Discussing the economics of the health care situation with families can be difficult, but understanding that cost-effective use of their insurance will maintain coverage for them at a later date is essential.

At the first home visit, expect the family to welcome you in a social way, by introducing you to others present, asking you to sit down or have coffee, and so on, just as they would any visitor. Share with the family your pleasure at meeting them and then reiterate the purpose of the visit and the time limits previously set. State simply that you would like to hear how they are managing at home and to check the patient's condition. In this way, you communicate your desire to hear their concerns and also establish that the patient will be examined. Families are often unsure of the nurse's role in the home and need to be able to predict what will happen at each visit. Because the nurse is a guest entering the home, normal social protocol should be followed. For example, if you will be late, telephone the family as to when they can expect you. Do not automatically ask to go to the patients bedroom. Explain each of the steps of your examination and services provided. Acceptance of home care services is essential if the continuity of care is to be maintained. If discharge planning in the hospital was used to initiate continuity of care, entry into the home is usually readily gained.

DISCHARGE PLANNING

The term *discharge planning* has been used to describe the process of assisting patients and families with their health care needs as they move from one health care setting to another. The overall purpose of discharge planning is to provide continuity of care. Discharge planning includes many activities, from projecting patient needs at discharge to coordinating professionals and volunteers involved in follow-up care. In the mid-1970s, the American Nurses' Association published guidelines for discharge planning for hospitals and community health agencies. By 1984, 15% of U.S. hospitals had established their own home care agencies.[86] Since then, the number has continued to increase. In these hospitals and in other situations, the community health nurse meets with the patient before discharge. In other situations, discharge planning is done by the nurse caring for the patient in the hospital.

The discharge planning process encompasses the assessment of the family's needs for teaching, counseling, and nursing care after discharge from the acute care setting. An important component of discharge planning is determining the resources within and external to the family that will be available when the patient returns home. The nurse accomplishes discharge planning by matching the patient's and family's abilities to provide self-care with appropriate and acceptable community and family resources. Resources range from home health nursing care to equipment rental. Discharge planning may or may not include a referral to a home care agency. If the patient and family are able to meet their own needs after discharge, they may not require any further assistance at home. However, medical-surgical patients have many complex problems, and even if they are able at discharge to meet their own needs, a postdischarge nursing visit can be used to evaluate the patient and praise the family on their self-management. Families may underestimate the difficulties they will face when caregiving is necessary 24 hours a day. Assisting families in accepting outside help is a valuable but sometimes difficult task. For some patients, a telephone call following discharge can be used to evaluate self-care status and provide continuity of care. The telephone call should be organized to ask specifically about the patient's condition and caregiver fatigue so that follow-up care can be instituted as necessary.

Discharge planning can be either a group process or conducted by one nurse. The group process takes place in a team conference, where personnel from various disciplines and the patient and family discuss the patient's discharge. When the nurse plans discharge, he or she also includes the patient, family, and other professionals, but usually not in a formal meeting.

The key to either the formal group or the informal discharge planning process is communication with the patient and family. The nurse coordinates the communication and documents the discharge plan on the health care record. Documentation should include both short- and long-range discharge planning goals. For example:

Ho Chung, a 57-year-old Chinese male of Chinese descent, is hospitalized for neurologic complications of Lyme's disease (an infection from a deer's tick bite). The short-range goals for Mr. Chung include being able to eat and bathe with assistance as his neurologic function improves. His long-range goals for discharge include being able to perform his ADL with assistance from a home health aide three times a week and his family on the other days.

The written plan should include how each goal will be accomplished. What the patient is doing in physical and occupational therapy should be documented, with the nursing staff reinforcing these activities on the unit. Who is responsible for a goal or the specific activity related to that goal should also be documented. The date of evaluation should be written so that the nursing staff can reassess progress. Discharge planning allows for continuity of care as the patient moves from the acute care setting to home. For discharge planning to be effective, it begins well before discharge and identifies patients needing home care. Characteristics of patients and various aspects of their medical-surgical treatment that influence their need for home care are listed in the box at right. These are not the only criteria, but they are the most common ones. The nurse must be alert for others. Remember that patients may not have any of the characteristics that indicate they will need home care, yet they still need discharge planning.

At the very least, discharge planning should provide the patient and family with (1) instruction in appropriate self-care, (2) identification of family and community resources, (3) awareness of procedures to follow for emergencies, (4) knowledge of follow-up care, and (5) family teaching specific to the patient's concerns. If home care is needed, explanation of home care services, telephone numbers, and, when possible, introductions to home care personnel become part of discharge planning. During hospitalization, as the patient progresses, the nurse collects data or modifies preexisting data, reflecting the change in the patient's health status and ability to function. Discharge planning builds on the patient's strengths and abilities.

DETERMINING DISCHARGE PLANNING NEEDS

The initial interview before the patient's discharge includes an assessment of the patient's needs, that is, his or her bio-psycho-social and spiritual needs. The nurse assesses the home environment by asking several questions. Who does the patient live with? What are the living arrangements? Does the patient live in a house or apartment? Are there stairs to the house or building, or stairs within the premises? Are all essential rooms on the same floor, such as the bathroom, bedroom, and

---

CHARACTERISTICS OF PATIENTS THAT INFLUENCE THE NEED FOR HOME CARE

1. Patients who cannot manage nursing care on their own
   a. Comatose or semicomatose patients
   b. Disoriented, confused, or forgetful patients
   c. Frail elderly persons
   d. Patients who live alone
   e. Patients who do not live alone, but persons at home cannot care for patients adequately
   f. Patients who have no home, or those whose present home is no longer adequate
2. Patients who need dressings and wound care
   a. Patients who have complicated dressings
   b. Patients who cannot do the dressing themselves
   c. Patients who will probably not do the dressing unless supervised
3. Patients who need equipment and transportation (Function shared with social services)
4. Patients with medication schedules
   a. Patients with complex schedules or injections
   b. Patients who are noncompliant
5. Patients with ostomies (for example, colostomy, ileostomy)
6. Patients with special teaching needs (for example, new diabetic, complex diet, injections)
7. Patients who are terminally ill
8. Patients receiving therapy (occupational, physical, speech)
9. Patients with tubes (Foley, gastrostomy, suprapubic, nasogastric, tracheostomy)
10. Patients being transferred
    a. From another hospital or nursing home
    b. To another hospital or nursing home (for example, Veteran's Administration hospital)

The typical patients who need referrals are those with chronic illness, such as arthritis, cancer, cerebrovascular accident, chronic renal failure, congestive heart failure, diabetes mellitus, emphysema, hypertension, or myocardial infarction, and those who are respirator dependent.

Adapted from Rasmusen L: Nurs Management, 15(5):39-43, 1984.

---

kitchen? Is the living environment adequate to meet the patient's needs at the time of discharge? Adequacy can include basics such as running water or indoor plumbing, heat or cooling, and cleanliness. The nurse also asks specific questions pertaining to the patient's medical-surgical care. For example, does the patient receiving intravenous antibiotics have refrigeration storage for the medication? Do patients undergoing peritoneal dialysis have a clean area where they can work with their equipment?

The nurse will also want to assess the patient's and family's support systems. Who will be available to the patient when discharged? This includes immediate family or significant others living with the patient. Ask what extended family members, children, friends, or neighbors are part of the patient's support system. What groups have the patient previously engaged in to meet his social needs? Will the patient be able to interact with the groups on discharge? What sources of spiritual support does the patient have? Can religious or other groups assist with care or prevent social isolation by visiting or telephoning regularly?

The nurse needs to determine if the patient and family have adequate coping mechanisms to manage the illness and the common stressors of home care. Ask the patient and family what they do to get along during difficult times. Will these coping strategies work for them now, or will they require assistance in developing new coping strategies because of a change in the patient's condition and its subsequent impact on the family? What learning needs will the patient and family have? Can these be adequately met before discharge, or will they require ongoing teaching? Finally, discuss the family's feelings about taking the patient home. Are they fearful of the patient's condition, worried about the extra responsibilities, or overly optimistic about their ability to care for the patient? The more realistic expections that the family has about home care, the more likely they are to adjust successfully.

FINANCIAL ASSESSMENT

Financial assessment must be undertaken before discharge and throughout the home care visits. Financial assistance may be needed because home health care can be expensive and may not be reimbursable. If the home care is reimbursable, there are often extra expenses not covered by insurance or government programs. For example, utility bills may increase because of equipment necessary for care. Special services from a pharmacist or supplies such as enteral feeding products may be essential, costly, and reimbursable only on a limited basis. Caring for the patient in the home may also have caused a family member to quit or reduce employment hours, thus reducing income.

Financial assessment is often difficult for nurses to undertake. It may seem an invasion of privacy to be asking about available financial resources, especially in the person's own home. Nurses need financial data about the patient to ensure they receive the full benefits for which they are eligible under government or private insurance. In today's economic climate, with the high costs of health care, even middle-income families may need assistance because they may be ineligible for government programs or other assistance. Also, identifying the resources currently used by the family allows the nurse to identify other possible sources of financial assistance. The box on p. 2254 lists financial resources that may be available to patients requiring home care. Referral to a social worker or financial discharge planner who is aware of the current eligibility and reim-

bursement criteria is essential, especially for the elderly Medicare patient.[82]

Lastly, during the initial assessment the nurse determines if the family is currently using any community resources to meet their needs. If so, how many, and how frequently? Are these satisfactory to the patient and family? If the patient and family are using community resources that are satisfactory, the nurse will want to consider these when making a referral, if one is necessary. If possible, the nurse in the acute care setting calls on the skills of the *transition specialist* to help with discharge planning. The *role of the transition specialist* is discussed next.

TRANSITIONAL CARE SKILLS

The concept of *transitional care* was developed by Brooten and colleagues.[10] The transitional period is the time from discharge planning to physiologic recovery. A nurse educated as a *transition specialist* can make a difference in both the quality and the cost of care at home. The transition specialist meets with the family while the patient is still in acute care to begin discharge planning. In addition, the transition specialist makes home visits before the patient's discharge to assess the home environment. The transition specialist is then available to the family following discharge. The study of Brooten and co-workers revealed that interventions instituted by transition specialists, including patient education, counseling, home visits, and telephone availability, were successful in terms of quality care.[9] An average cost saving of 25% was realized when discharge planning and home nursing services were used versus longer hospitalization.

To manage transition from hospital to home, patients and family members must manage activities ranging from use of sterile technique to assessment of the adult's psychologic status.[75] To manage home care, the family members must acquire new knowledge and skills, be motivated to help the patient, and adapt to the change created in the roles of family members. The problems typically reported by families who provide home care include the burden of providing daily physical care, financial strain, and difficulty coping with individual role and schedule disruptions.[21] Other problems include the stress of learning the nursing care, unavailability of resources, the difficulty of accepting help from others, and observing any negative changes in the patient such as infection or malnutrition. Further problems noted in long-term home care include equipment failure, the need for home remodeling, and social isolation.[19]

In addition to dealing with these general problems, the nurse transition specialist reviews the literature to identify concerns shared by populations of patients they discharge. The key to providing successful transitional

FINANCIAL RESOURCES SCREENING CHECKLIST

1. Check the government or private resources available to the patient (benefits vary with each plan):

   _____ Medicaid
   _____ Medicare A (home care services)
   _____ Medicare B (home care equipment)
   _____ Blue Cross and Blue Shield Plans
   _____ Employer insurance
   _____ Social Security
   _____ American Cancer Society (free bandages, equipment)
   _____ Multiple Sclerosis Society (wheelchair loans)
   _____ Volunteer or charitable organization resources

   _____ Old age assistance
   _____ Supplemental Security Income
   _____ Financial help from family
   _____ Disability payments
   _____ Retirement pensions
   _____ Welfare programs
   _____ Meals on Wheels
   _____ United Way agencies
   _____ Private insurance
   _____ Savings accounts

2. Do you think that your total income for this year was enough to meet your (the patient and other family members) usual monthly expenses and bills?

   _____ Yes   _____ No

3. In the past 6 months, has money been spent on the patient's physician, hospital, nursing home, or medication bills that has not been reimbursed by insurance?

care lies in designing the nursing interventions specifically for each family. The interventions for the family of the patient being monitored for cardiac dysrhythmias in the home compared to the patient needing enteral feeding are very different. For example, the problems repeatedly identified in studies of discharged patients receiving mechanical ventilation were initial anxiety followed by depression related to the complexity of the therapy and the constant presence of technology in the home. Several problems experienced by home patients have been documented, including difficulties with finances, body image and sexual relations, social stigma, and environmental issues such as how to arrange the living quarters for safety. These problems have been reported to recur depending on the patient's condition and factors such as the ability to return to work, length of time on ventilator each day, and availability of family support and external resources.

Stiller,[78] in a study of patients at home receiving various types of "high-tech care," suggested that psychosocial factors, not the type of technology, inhibit family success with home care. Family coping ability, patient prognosis, and role disruption were worse in the families who were unsuccessful with home care. In addition, mental or emotional problems of patient or family members and caregiver fatigue were problems experienced by these families. Stiller also observed that female patients had more frequent rehospitalizations from home care because their spouses had difficulty in managing the caregiver role. This information can be used by the transition specialist to prevent family crises. One of the key skills used by the transition specialist is family education.

FAMILY EDUCATION

The term *family education* is used to emphasize that the teaching skills employed in home health care involve the entire family or all significant others. In this context the nurse's skill in assessing readiness to learn, providing information, and evaluating outcomes of teaching must be carried out with a group.[72] The home, as the environment for learning, also influences the teaching strategies used. Individual family members often have varying expectations and roles in the education process. The male patient may be interested in learning about the technical aspects of his care but might ask his wife to manage all his medications. In addition, a daughter might be called on to learn about the financial aspects of insurance, equipment loans, or Medicare benefits. The nurse assists the family in their decisions about who should learn what and may even be involved in resolving conflicts between family members who believe other members learned incorrectly. The steps for teaching the family are similar to those for individual patient teaching. Family education, therefore, begins with assessment and diagnosis of learning needs. The final steps include implementing and then evaluating the teaching.

The expected outcome of teaching is learning. Learning is considered to have taken place when the person's behavior has changed so that he or she and the nurse agree that the patient's health is enhanced. Thus teaching is not just imparting information, but also ensuring that a *change in behavior* occurs. To assist families to manage home care, they may need to change routines in daily schedules and responsibilities for household duties. The nurse may need to provide coun-

SAMPLE INTERVIEW QUESTIONS IN ASSESSING PATIENTS' KNOWLEDGE ABOUT THEIR HEALTH CARE

1. Can you tell me what you have learned about your illness?
2. You have had surgery before. Can you tell me what you remember from that experience?
3. When you spoke with your physician/pharmacist, what did he or she tell you was important to know about your medications?
4. Have you heard about your therapy from anyone else who has had your health problem?
5. Have you read or heard reports about the treatments your physician wants you to undergo?

For patients who have physical limitations, careful assessment of their abilities should be done before determining the type of teaching plans and evaluation to use. For instance, some stroke patients' perception and knowledge can be evaluated by using picture boards to assist them to identify frequently used articles.

Adapted by permission from Patient Education: Nurses in Partnership With Other Health Care Professionals (p. 62) by C. Smith, 1987, New York: Grune & Stratton. Copyright 1987 by Grune & Stratton, Inc.

NURSING INTERVENTIONS TO ENHANCE WILLINGNESS OR MOTIVATION TO LEARN

1. Provide counseling to reduce patient or family anxieties.
2. Explore past teaching experiences that created negative attitudes toward learning.
3. Compliment individuals and groups on information already learned.
4. Determine what the person wants to learn and teach this first.
5. Take steps to overcome deficiencies in perceptual skills, such as vision limitations and memory loss.
6. Complete discharge planning so that financial, housing, or other needed assistance can be found to decrease patient's worries.

Adapted by permission from Patient Education: Nurses in Partnership With Other Health Care Professionals (p. 66) by C. Smith, 1987, New York: Grune & Stratton. Copyright 1987 by Grune & Stratton.

seling as well as external resources to support these changes in behavior.

ASSESSING LEARNING NEEDS

Assessing the patient and family's understanding of the illness and its treatment establishes a baseline for teaching. The box above, left provides sample interview questions to determine what patients already know about their health care. The nurse can link new knowledge to information the family already has and reinforce behavior change. Any barriers to learning that the patient and family may have, such as reading difficulties or lack of desire to learn, need to be assessed. Learning is influenced by attitudes, beliefs, and values. Attitude or desire to learn will vary greatly for each person through the various stages of their home health care. Desire to learn is affected by the grieving process as well as by beliefs and values. Patients and families who are in a stage of denial will have difficulty learning. When people are in denial and unable to learn a procedure such as total parenteral nutrition (TPN), the nurse may need to do the procedure and gradually shift the family to self-care as they are able to cope. Another example of a situation where a family has difficulty learning is when the family must learn how to change a wound dressing but does not have money to buy bandages. In this situation, before teaching, the home care nurse would obtain dressings from the American Cancer Society, local church organization, and so on. The box above, right identifies interventions the nurse may use when enhancing patients' willingness or motivation to learn the necessary home care instruction.

The nurse also must assess the information that family members desire. In addition to information about the patient's biologic condition, family members have personal knowledge and skills needs. The biologic condition and families' personal skill and knowledge needs identified by home care nurses in one study are shown in Figures 78-1, 78-2, and 78-3. The nursing interventions or skills needed to manage home care are related to each patient's biologic or pathophysiologic condition. Home care nurses indicated in this study that family members needed to know the skills of lifting, turning, and moving a patient as well as doing neurologic checks and so on (Figure 78-1). Along with these personal learning needs, home care nurses recognized the family members' need for knowledge of depression, grief, and other potential psychologic problems found in home care (Figure 78-3).

After assessment is completed, the data collected must be analyzed to determine nursing diagnoses that clearly indicate the patient's and family's problems or strengths. For example, the nursing diagnosis of **Coping, family, potential for growth related to learned management of home care treatments** identifies the family's strengths. Nursing diagnoses that illustrate problems with learning are described in the section on **knowledge deficits** later in this chapter.

PLANNING AND IMPLEMENTING FAMILY EDUCATION

When planning patient teaching in the home care setting, the three major objectives for the patient are (1) comprehension of the illness and its treatment(s), (2)

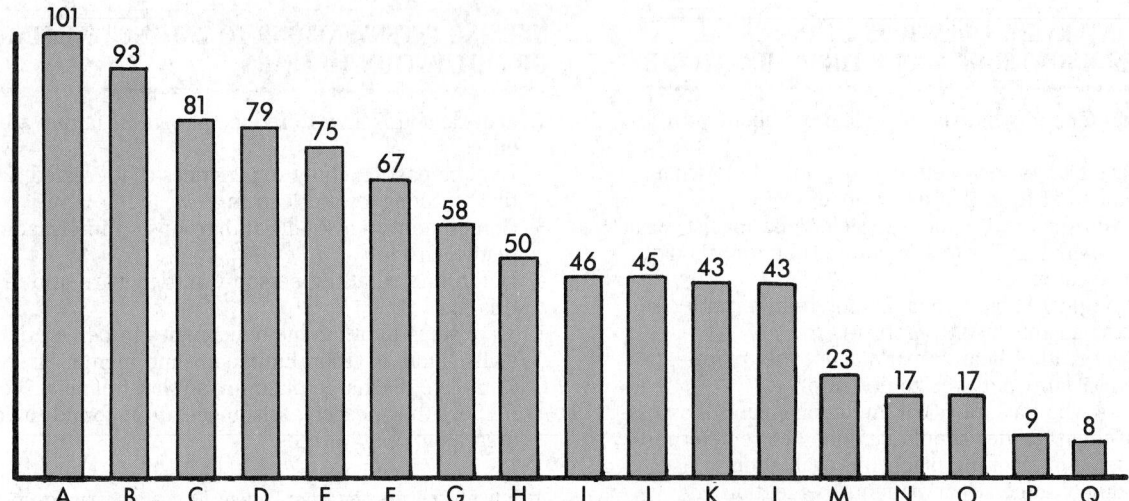

FIGURE 78-1 Family members' biological skill needs for providing home care: as prioritized by registered nurse respondents, number of first prioritized responses. *A,* Lifting, turning, moving; *B,* CPR; *C,* Range of motion; *D,* GI—nausea/vomiting; *E,* CV—Apical pulse measurement; *F,* Drug side effects; *G,* Injections; *H,* Sterile dressings; *I,* Constipation; *J,* Diarrhea; *K,* Blood pressure measurement; *L,* Respiratory; *M,* GU-catheter care; *N,* EENT—sensory–perceptual changes; *O,* Neuro-temperature; *P,* Charting; *Q,* Neurologic checks. (From Quiring, JD: RN perspective of home health care needs of family members, Kans Nurse, 59(3):10, 1985. Copyright 1985. Used with permission.)

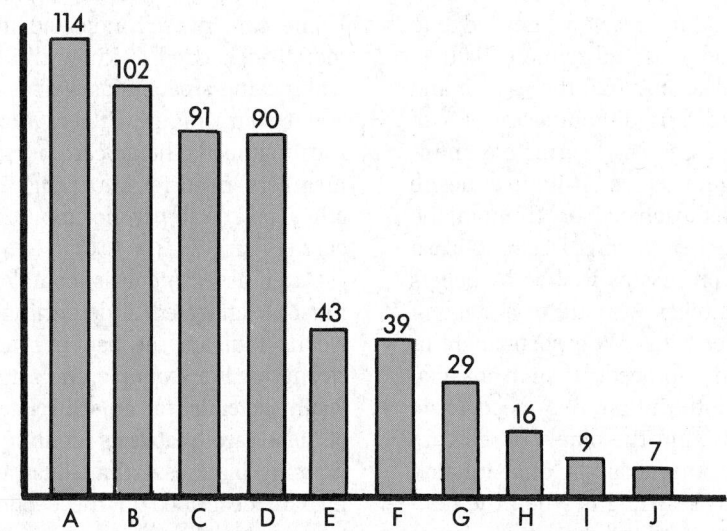

FIGURE 78-2 Family members' personal skill needs for providing home care: as prioritized by registered nurse respondents, number of first prioritized responses. *A,* Art of listening; *B,* Promotion of independence/self care; *C,* Attitude toward seriously ill; *D,* Establish rapport; *E,* Confidentiality/privacy; *F,* Promotion of health; *G,* Interview; *H,* Facilitating development of special abilities; *I,* Life histories; *J,* Avoiding patient abuse. (From Quiring, JD: RN perspective of home health care needs of family members, Kans Nurse, 59(3):10, 1985. Copyright 1985. Used with permission.)

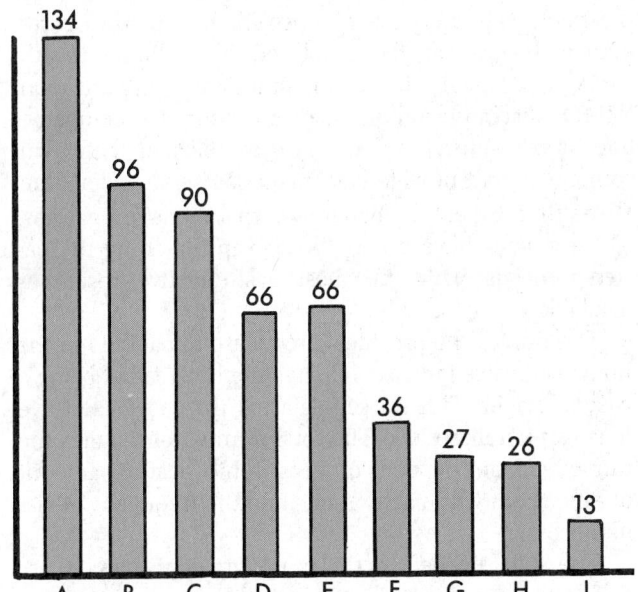

FIGURE 78-3 Family members' personal knowledge needs for providing home care: as prioritized by registered nurse respondents, number of first prioritized responses. *A*, Meaning/purpose; *B*, Depression; *C*, Hope; *D*, Dying; *E*, Grief; *F*, Loneliness; *G*, Fulfillment; *H*, Bereavement; *I*, Sexuality. (From Quiring, JD: RN perspective of home health care needs of family members, Kans Nurse, 59(3):10, 1985. Copyright 1985. Used with permission.)

Mazzuca[48] reviewed 320 articles on research conducted on patient education to determine what effect patient teaching had on chronic illnesses. Behaviorally oriented education programs that emphasized changing the environment in which patients care for themselves so that home care is easily managed were the most successful in improving the clinical course of chronic diseases. An example of modifying the home environment might include rearranging furniture so that it is in the field of vision of the patient who is rehabilitating from a cerebrovascular accident (CVA) and has residual hemianopsia. Requiring modification of the environment actively enlists the patient in changing behavior toward desired objectives.

Establishing cues as reminders of the new behavior required by patients increases adjustment to home care. For example, encouraging patients with many treatments to try and schedule these with meals or other regular activities helps them remember to perform the activities.

EVALUATING OUTCOMES AND IDENTIFYING BARRIERS TO TEACHING IN THE HOME

The goal of teaching is to have patients and families incorporate necessary changes in behavior to adapt to illness and its resulting impact. Learning takes place in areas of knowledge, attitude, and behavior. Evaluation, the last step of the nursing process, is essential to patient education. Evaluation is based on what the patient and family believe they need to learn, as well as the learning objectives designed by the home care nurses. *Learning objectives* are stated outcomes that are *measurable* and *realistic*. Through the evaluation of the objectives, the nurse helps the patient and family to recognize needs for future learning and identifies success with past learning.

Questioning or listening to patient answers is a common method of evaluating learning. *The method of evaluation used should be acceptable and nonthreatening to the patient and family.* Besides verbal questioning, the nurse should observe for evidence that the patient understands how to incorporate changes brought on by the illness. For instance, the patient should be asked how he or she plans to balance rest and activity during the day.

There are barriers to teaching in the home that nurses must be prepared to address. The nurse must remember that teaching materials must be brought for the home visit, even if the patient has been given handouts before discharge. Duplication of materials and information most often reinforces previous teaching.

Families may also state, "We are being taught something different now than what the hospital nurse or doctor instructed." The nurse must coordinate patient teaching and clarify consistency of information for the

accepting the impact of illness and treatment(s) on lifestyle, and (3) demonstrating management of treatment procedures and home care. Understanding the patient's and family's life-style will help the nurse to plan with them about how to adapt changes with the least disruption. When a medical regimen causes minimum disruptions in life-style, the patient is more likely to comply with it. Teaching is more effective when it includes not only knowledge of treatment, but also counseling about scheduling so the patient and family can incorporate home care into their daily routines. The nurse must also plan learning objectives related to symptom control, management of exacerbations, treatment protocols, problem solving, and financial difficulties.

Implementation of teaching plans can take many forms in home health care. The use of computer-assisted instruction and videotapes in the home have been successful. One-to-one demonstration of technical procedures is effective. Also, describing methods of care over the telephone has also ensured learning. Many and varied methods of teaching that incorporate the whole family and emphasize the need to change behavior are most likely to have positive results. Using praise and reinforcement and providing an opportunity to ask questions and to evaluate learning effectiveness are important parts of implementation.

family. Also, duplication of teaching efforts must be avoided. For example, the nurse and physical therapist should decide who will be responsible for teaching ROM, thus reducing the cost of education.

Another difficulty for home teaching is the wide age variation in patients and families. The home care nurse must consider the developmental, cognitive, and potential learning challenges for children and elders in the family.

Instruction is incorporated into patient care activities, allowing return demonstration and involving the patient and family in evaluating the outcomes. It is also essential to document teaching and the self-care outcomes to illustrate the importance and cost effectiveness of teaching in the home. The Health Care Financing Administration publication no. 11 lists only 12 teaching activities that are considered reimbursable by medicare. Other activities are considered on an individual basis, and having documentation of teaching outcomes increases the likelihood of reimbursement.

CASE-MANAGED CARE

Case-managed care is an approach to providing care that includes an effort to reduce overall costs of services while maintaining the patient's optimum health. *Case-managed care* is a term used to describe the supervision and *coordination of paraprofessionals*, consultation with other health professionals, and a direct evaluation of nursing care in the home. Nurses providing case-managed care may not provide any direct patient care themselves, but they coordinate the efforts of all others involved in the home care. Nurses who provide case-managed care may also serve as *transition specialists*, *service coordinators*, and *quality assurance advocates*. The case manager does a detailed assessment of the patient's needs, discusses options with the patient and family, arranges for selected services to be provided, and then ensures quality care by evaluating patient outcomes on a periodic basis. In the case-managed situation, the nurse may have a caseload of 40 to 50 families.[15]

The nurse who provides case-managed care must develop many skills. The nurse must understand the patient's physical condition and be well versed in the complexity of the patient's insurance or other financial coverage. The case manager needs skill in motivating families toward self-care, recognizing fragmentation of care, facilitating delivery of services on behalf of the family, and advocating for continuing resources when necessary. Arranging long-term services that match the patient's changing acuity level is a key element of case-managed care. Case managers do much of their work by telephone; thus they must be skilled in communication.

Case-managed care is supported by private industries and the federal government as a means of reducing insurance costs and making early hospital discharge to the home safe and less expensive. The nurse in case-managed care can be employed by a home health agency, hospital, health maintenance organization (HMO) discharge program, or an insurance company. Some nurse entrepreneurs have established their own companies that provide case-managed services for Blue Cross/Blue Shield or for large corporations' employees. These nurses have become skilled in matching the patients' needs with the most cost-effective resources available.

The nurse who provides direct care to patients in the home is involved in case management instead of being a case manager. This nurse has a varying caseload of five to seven families daily. The total number of families the nurse manages depends on geographic location, amount of time spent with each family, and the frequency of visits necessary.

The skills needed by the nurse providing direct care to families are similar to those of the nurse acting as a case manager. Both nurses provide teaching and counseling and encourage self-care. The nurse managing the case in the home provides direct surveillance and monitors the patient's condition. The nurse providing direct care discusses the patient's needs with the case manager, who can assist with resource allocation and help anticipate any problems. Communication with the family is the key element in the success of case management. Other special skills used in the home are discussed in detail in the next section.

NURSING PROCESS IN THE HOME SETTING

The ultimate goal of home care is to assist the patient and family to their maximum level of everyday functioning. In some cases the highest level of function may be the patient's complete recovery and return to work. In other situations the maximum function may be the family's ability to manage the patient's care in the home without professional assistance. In either case the implementation of nursing interventions will vary greatly, depending on the family and patient.

During data analysis the nurse develops nursing diagnoses based on the assessment data from the family. Along with these actual nursing diagnoses, the nurse determines potential diagnoses based on common discharge planning issues seen in home care. From the actual data-based nursing diagnoses and discharge planning process, several expected outcomes are generated specific to each family. The implementation of nursing interventions are directed by the nursing diagnoses and concomitant expected outcomes.

Expected outcomes and implementation of specific interventions appropriate for the technologically dependent patient at home are described here. The examples given to illustrate the use of the nursing process in home care are based on clinical experiences with technologically dependent adult patients. Growing numbers of individuals and families successfully manage home care with mechanical ventilators, parenteral nutrition infusions, home hemodialysis, intravenous antibiotics or chemotherapy, and other life-sustaining interventions. Using the nursing process with these families supports their adaptive responses to the impact of technologic dependency. A priority for nursing research recently announced by the National Center for Nursing Research of the National Institutes of Health is to develop an understanding of patients' technologic dependence across the life span.

The discussion that follows outlines the steps of the nursing process employed with adult medical-surgical patients requiring various technical therapies at home. The implementation of highly technical home therapies have been well researched in the adult patient with no disease *complications*. Additional interventions may be necessary when the patient or family experience confounding factors such as multiple illnesses, living alone, lack of a suitable home environment, or inability to accept dependency on technology.

The *man-machine interface* found in technologically dependent patients is a challenge nurses can address through the use of the nursing process. Home care, even in the face of machines or technological dependency, allows families to exert control over their lives, continue their self-actualization, and maintain their highest level of wellness and functioning. Nurses facilitate home care by advocating patients' independent living, educating families about technological care, and providing them with resources.

Several researchers have verified the efficacy and cost effectiveness of home care for technologically dependent patients.[40] Advantages of home care over institutional care for the patient include *decreased nosocomial infection* and *improved nutritional status*. Home care allows for the resumption of more normal interactions and routines. More normal daily living follows adaptation to the noise of the machine and worry about machine failure. Even with these worries, greater sense of control and morale have been reported by both patients receiving home care and their families.

Finally, financial benefits of home care versus institutional care have been well documented. Studies have shown that in-home ventilation costs approximately one-third the cost of hospital care and even less when skilled services are not needed 24 hours a day.[5] Considering the significance of such advantages, many U.S. institutions have reported discharge preparation protocols for home care of technologically dependent patients.

The combined influences of the physical and psychologic environments of the home impact continuously on the outcomes of care provided. Repeated assessment of these influences is necessary for modifying the care plan as patient and family environmental factors change over time. The home as the environment for nursing care offers a particular challenge to those involved. Nurses will need to develop special skills when working with families in their homes.

ASSESSMENT

ASSESSMENT OF THE HOME AS THE ENVIRONMENT FOR NURSING CARE

The family home is a unique environment for providing nursing care to the adult patient. Psychologically, the effects of the home territory need to be taken into account when developing the nursing care plan. Physically, the home environment must be assessed for safety, accessibility, and appropriate areas to provide care.

Psychologic factors effecting care planning include motivational as well as financial, patient and family expectations, and developmental, social, and community influences that impact the adaptation to home care. The psychologic factors affecting care in the home are many, varied, and rapidly changing.

PSYCHOLOGIC ENVIRONMENT AS AN INFLUENCE

The patient's attitude toward discharge to home, family members' reactions to the caregiver role, and the family's ability to accept help from the home care team all influence the outcome of care. Before discharge, the patient's and family's attitudes towards home care are determined. The patient's motivation to return home and the family's willingness to provide and accept home care are important determinants of successful home management. The patient and family's perceptions and concerns about recovery will influence acceptance of home care. Besides perceptions, importance of autonomy and privacy may influence acceptance.

The availability, expense, and type of services considered for home care should be discussed. A *backup plan* needs to be negotiated when services become too intrusive or expensive or when friends or others assisting in the home become ill or unavailable.

Financial Influences

Home health care can be a financial burden for families. Cost analyses indicate that home care expenses vary in relation to the type, intensity, and length of services needed. Medicare, Blue Cross/Blue Shield, and an increasing number of private insurance companies pay for acute, posthospital home care services to reduce the length of hospital stay.[43] For such coverage, however, the care required must be defined as intermittent rather than ongoing. Medicaid and a few insurers will pay for longer-term chronic home care services. Supplemental coverage can be obtained in some cases from old age assistance, workers' compensation, disability, welfare, or other financial aid programs. Regardless, the family must pay deductibles and only a percentage is covered; thus most people pay some out-of-pocket costs.

Each of these financial resources varies in the requirements the patient must meet, the length of time benefits are allowed, and the types of equipment or supplies provided. Typically, the complete description of the therapies, equipment, and services covered are included in manuals available from each financial group.

Even with these financial benefits, families will incur costs that are not covered. Some uncovered costs can be reduced through using volunteer, charity, community, or religious resources. For example, the local American Cancer Society will provide bandages and other supplies free of charge, and some church or volunteer groups provide transportation for clinic appointments. The family member who provides care for the adult at home may have time lost from work, thus increasing the financial burden. The nurse's role is to assess the psychologic impact of the financial situation on the family, coordinate the use of available resources, and refer the family to social workers, case managers, or insurance experts.

Patient and Family Expectations

Both the patient's and the family's willingness and motivation for home care must be assessed in light of their expectations of home care. Ask the family to describe what they expect home care will entail. Listen carefully to what the family expects the professionals to do in daily care. Does the family desire around-the-clock service or only availability of a nurse by telephone? Does the patient desire physical care from the family and medication or equipment monitoring from professionals? Does the family recognize the possible changes in their daily schedule that providing home care may bring?

How have the family members reacted to having outside persons coming into their private residence? Can the family obtain support from extended-family members, friends, and religious or community resources? Other long-range expectations of home care, such as the patient or family member becoming self-sufficient so that home services can be terminated or the feasibility of returning to work, can be assessed on a continuing basis. The nurse must realize that as home care continues, the resources, motivation, and emotional reactions of the family and patient will change and must be taken into account in revising the home care plan.

Developmental, Social, and Community Influences

The nurse must take into account other factors when assessing the psychologic environment of the home as

the setting for care. One important factor is the family's developmental level. Individuals and families at different developmental levels will have different needs, skills, and resources to use in home care management. Family developmental stages and the major tasks associated with each are depicted in Table 78-1.[18]

These stages vary in length, may repeat, may overlap, and may not be sequential. Other tasks may be of prime concern depending on the family, their life-style, and available social and community supports.

Homebound patients often are concerned about other developmental tasks, such as obtaining child care or caring for grandparents. The nurse who assists the family in finding affordable day care for children or live-in help for grandparents can then assist the family to focus on care of the patient at home.

Social and community support for home care also influences the psychologic environment and thus the outcomes of care in the residence. Social support is made up of actions from various sources that assist the person to meet his or her personal goals or manage the demands of a particular situation. Social support has been identified in health care research as significant in affecting a person's adjustment to illness and ability to manage their acute or chronic health problems.[57] In terms of home care, *social support refers to the tangible and intangible help received from others*. Tangible help ranges from assistance with physical care to telephone visitations, whereas intangible help encompasses emotional support through encouragement or feedback. Social support is most often received from the persons in the immediate or extended family.

The nurse will find that communities also have resources that can be mobilized to provide the patient and family with social support as part of their home care. Religious denominations, neighborhood associations, community centers, voluntary service groups, and professionally lead support groups can all be sources of social support. These groups can be used so that the patient or family caregiver does not become isolated and overburdened with care. Studies have indicated that social and community support can also lessen the depression of the caregiver that may result from the demands and changes brought on by home care.

PHYSICAL ENVIRONMENT AS AN INFLUENCE

The home is the physical environment for delivery of nursing care. Any physical environment used for patient care requires assessment in terms of safety, accessibility, and appropriateness for care. The criteria used to assess the safety of the home depend to some extent on the patient's abilities and needs. The home of a patient who is discharged with equipment for hemodialysis may require alterations in the home to provide a safe environment for care. Modifications in the home environ-

TABLE 78-1 Stages of family development

Stage of development	Task
1. Married couple	Establishing a mutually satisfying marriage
	Fitting into the extended family network
2. Childbearing families	Adjusting to parenthood
	Encouraging the development of infants
	Establishing a satisfying home for both parents and infant(s)
3. Families with preschool-age children	Adapting to the critical needs and interests of preschool children in stimulating, growth-promoting ways
	Coping with energy depletion and lack of privacy as parents
4. Families with school-age children	Fitting into the community of school-age families in constructive ways
	Encouraging children's educational achievement
5. Families with adolescent children	Balancing freedom with responsibility as adolescents mature
	Establishing postparental interests and careers as growing parents
6. Families as "launching center"	Releasing young adults into work, military service, college, marriage, and so on with appropriate rituals and assistance
	Maintaining a supportive home base
7. Middle-aged parents	Rebuilding the marriage relationship
	Maintaining kin ties with older and younger generations
8. Aging family members	Coping with bereavement and living alone
	Closing the family home or adapting it to aging
	Adjusting to retirement

Adapted from Duvall E: Marriage and family development, Philadelphia, 1987, JB Lippincott Co.

ment for safety may also be based on the patient's disabilities or physical condition, such as high-rise toilet seats, grab bars in the bathroom, or changing a living room into a bedroom.

Guidelines for assessing the physical environment should always include basic information about the home within that community. The location of the residence in relation to necessary home care services and equipment is important. Some rural residents may be willing and motivated to have home care but are 50 miles away from the closest home health care provider. Even urban dwellers may find out that their metropolitan area does not have an agency that provides necessary equipment, such as mechanical ventilators. Often an assessment of the community in such situations will uncover resources that will allow home care to take place safely. Possibly a retired nurse in the rural community can be asked to provide care for the family until they have managed the transition from the hospital discharge. In the urban setting, a hospital-based pulmonary nurse specialist might provide periodic home visits to a ventilator-dependent patient. Another factor related to location of the residence is the availability of transportation to and from needed resources. Arrangements for trips to the grocery, pharmacy, and clinic are part of the safety of home management. Finding and training community resources to ensure safety of care are frequent challenges for the home care nurse.

The physical environment of the home should always be assessed for basic factors that affect the patient's

health and adjustment to home care. Adequacy of heating, cooling, electrical outlets, plumbing and refrigeration, and access to a telephone should be determined. Lack of these resources does not preclude home care unless these are necessary for safety. Some antibiotics that are infused intravenously may require refrigeration. Proper storage would have to be found for the family who does not have refrigeration in their residence. Plumbing and toilet facilities also need to be assessed in relation to the patient's nursing care needs. Another basic factor that affects the patient's adjustment to home care and is influenced by the physical environment is an area where the patient can rest. The patient may be bedridden, unable to climb stairs, or restricted to one area because of medical equipment. Problem solving must be employed to ensure that the family can use the space in their home the way they desire and that the medical equipment does not cause too much noise or interference.

PHYSICAL ASSESSMENT OF THE PATIENT

Assessment of the adult patient in the home encompasses many of the same data collection procedures appropriate in the acute care setting. In the acute care setting the patient is assessed by other staff around the clock. *In the home setting, the patient and family are the primary data collectors who monitor and provide care.* Thus assessment in the home setting begins with exploring the patient and family's self-management. The patient and primary family caregivers should be asked to describe the patient's condition and discuss any concerns. The nurse providing home care may not have seen the patient for a few days and will depend on the family's observations or monitoring of specific data. The nurse's questions should illustrate to the patient and family that their information is important.

Assessment in the home proceeds in an orderly fashion. Start by asking the patient and family about their own concerns. The patient and caregiver are asked specific questions about the priority nursing diagnoses, medical problems, or signs and symptoms that the patient is experiencing. A man being seen at home for a wound infection may have reported his incision sore and tender but that the throbbing pain seemed to be decreased . The nurse would follow up by asking if anything had alleviated the tenderness, such as the warm, moist soaks used twice daily for cleansing the area. The patient would also be asked if anything aggravated the tenderness or made the symptoms worse, such as wound drainage. If drainage was reported, the nurse asks about the quantity or amount. It helps to obtain specific information by asking the family to describe the size of the drainage area. The type of drainage in terms of color, odor, and presence of blood or exudate should be observed by the nurse to obtain objective data. The nurse would determine if any signs or symptoms were associated with the subjective tenderness, such as swelling or elevated body temperature. These signs or symptoms are measurable and can be documented as objective data. Thus, with each problem area, the nurse gathers data from the patient and family that provide detailed characteristics for comparison. The detailed characteristics are used to analyze the symptoms being described. By comparing the characteristics from one visit to the next, the nurse monitors the patient's symptoms. The assessment concludes with questions about any other concerns. New nursing diagnoses may emerge over time while other diagnoses are being resolved.

PSYCHOLOGIC ASSESSMENT OF THE PATIENT

Another essential assessment component is determining the patient and family's psychologic response to each problem. One man with a wound infection may react to the reduced tenderness and swelling as good news, whereas another believes he has a serious condition. The patient's psychologic response is influenced by many factors, such as length of illness, presence of multiple symptoms, and reaction of family members.

The primary caregiver's psychologic reactions also should be assessed. The *primary caregiver* is the person who provides the most physical or daily care for the patient. The primary caregiver may be a spouse, sibling, significant other, or grown child. Many individuals may be involved in home care. In the case of one patient at home with an indwelling epidural catheter for infusion

of analgesics, the husband was the primary caregiver. The home health nurse had assessed his ability to manage the infusions, distinguish untoward effects (respiratory depression) from side effects (nausea, pruritus) and obtain assistance from other family members. The responsibility of providing care for a loved one with physical pain can be psychologically demanding, so the home care nurse asked the grown children to telephone and visit to provide respite and support for their father.

TREATMENT PLAN ASSESSMENT

The treatment plan includes health care professionals' prescriptions for medication, diet, exercise, and physical or psychologic care. Discuss with the patient the specific prescriptions he or she was given and exactly how it is being carried out. Ask the patient and family about any difficulties with treatments, obtain their opinion about the benefits or drawbacks of the therapy, and discuss these issues with them.

The treatment plan or therapy prescriptions provided by the patient's health care professional will influence the general care the patient needs. The treatment plan also will dictate any special skills the patient and family must master. Overall assessment of the patient's treatment plan should include questioning about general care, medications, nutrition, home environment, emergency procedures, specific patient needs, and equipment checks. General care assessment includes needs for assistance with hygiene, elimination, communication, rest and activity schedules, transportation, socialization, and continued contact with health care professionals.

Medication assessment is used to determine if the patient and caregiver know the purpose of medications and how to give them. To obtain a firsthand view of their knowledge, have the patient or family caregiver responsible for giving medications show you the medicines. In the home setting, patients and families must be alert not only to untoward effects and side effects, but also indications that medications are ineffective. They must anticipate dosage and schedules so they do not run out of medications at times when pharmacies are not open. Assessing actual dose taken versus prescribed dose is critical, since there may be various reasons why patients and families change the dosage, including finances or forgetfulness. They do not want to be labeled as "bad patients," so they may state the prescribed dose as the actual dose. Therefore, ask about daily routine of what is taken and when. Request that the patient count the remaining number of pills in the prescription to determine how many were taken and if that number is correct according to the prescription.

Nutrition assessment includes collection of subjective data that the patient is tolerating foods or special diets, as well as objective data such as weight and calorie counts. When determining nutritional status, the nurse also should assess the patient's hydration. Family members may have difficulty forcing fluids or restricting intake, if this is necessary. The home health care nurse can support the caregiver in these efforts.

Assessment of knowledge of emergency procedures is necessary with each family. Every family should demonstrate their ability to use the community's emergency telephone system and to call the home health nurse for less serious situations. They can be taught cardiopulmonary resuscitation (CPR) if they desire or need this information. Equipment checks are a very specific and important part of home care assessment. Typically, each piece of equipment comes with written material that outlines the safety checks, cleaning procedures, and routine maintenance. The family must understand the manuals and incorporate safety checks into everyday schedules. The box below outlines guidelines for a mechanical ventilator equipment check that would be followed by a home care nurse to assess the family's ability to manage the ventilator–dependent patient safely at home. The equipment check itself would be more detailed and would follow the specific information accompanying the machine. The guidelines for home mechanical ventilation developed by a national commission should be used.[52]

Assessment of specific emergency procedures, home environment, and special patient needs are all based on the patient's particular treatment plan. The box at right lists the assessment required to determine the needs of a family with an adult member at home dependent on mechanical ventilation. The nurse observes the family's and patient's handling of procedures such as suctioning and tracheostomy care to assess their abilities to provide the care correctly. After assessing the patient's specific care needs, as dictated by the treatment plan, the nurse turns to data gathering and resources available to the family.

FAMILY ASSESSMENT

Family assessment is essential because the success of home care depends on the family members' or significant others' ability to draw on and use internal and external resources. *Internal resources* include the family's or individual's positive attitude toward home care, ability to problem solve or seek advice, and willingness to accept help or assistance from *external resources*. Accepting help from friends, neighbors, and church or community groups often is difficult for families because of the strong value of independence in U.S. culture. The home health nurse can determine the availability of these and other external resources and then assess the family's willingness to accept such help.

Each family member's reactions to the role he or she carries out in relation to home care influences the family's internal resources. A grown child working full time might not be able to help with the patient's daily physi-

---

GUIDELINES FOR A MECHANICAL VENTILATOR EQUIPMENT CHECKLIST*

1. How to check the ventilator function
2. What the ventilator settings are (such as tidal volume, rate)
3. How to set ventilator settings
4. How to put the circuit equipment (such as tubing, mist element) together
5. How to connect the circuit
6. When to change the circuit
7. Ventilator and equipment maintenance
8. Troubleshooting (leaks, pressure alarm, and so on)

*A comprehensive equipment check would be conducted using the manufacturer's guidelines for home use.

SPECIFIC ASSESSMENT FOR HOME MECHANICAL VENTILATION

EMERGENCY PROCEDURES

1. How to use the external battery for the ventilator
2. How to use the manual resuscitator bag
3. Emergency reinsertion of tracheotomy tube
4. What to do in an electrical power failure
5. How to manage airway problems
6. What to do if an equipment failure occurs
7. Emergency phone numbers of ventilator company with 24-hour services
8. How to manage oxygen in the home
9. Notification of fire department and emergency services that a ventilator patient is in the home

HOME ENVIRONMENT

1. How to rearrange or remodel home to accommodate ventilator care
2. Notification of electric company and establishing of appropriate and emergency power
3. How to reach the home care equipment company
4. How to set up a patient call system
5. How to order and obtain supplies
6. How to operate and care for special medical equipment (ventilator, hospital bed, commode, wheelchair)

SPECIAL PATIENT NEEDS

1. Suggestions for how to communicate
2. Suggestions for diversional activities (hobbies, pastimes, recreation)
3. How to identify signs of a respiratory infection
4. How to submit insurance papers or obtain other sources of funds
5. How to travel with the ventilator
6. How to make arrangements for respite care

RESEARCH

Smith C, Mayer L, and Pingleton S: Caregiver perceptions of managing home ventilation, Am Rev Respir Dis 139(suppl)(4): A196, 1989.

This study gathered data on the support services, coping strategies, and perceived knowledge or skill needs of families with an adult receiving home ventilation. Twenty caregivers of ventilated homebound patients were interviewed using four instruments. Patients, ages 17 to 74 years, were receiving 24 hours (8 patients), 14 to 15 hours (4), or 8 to 12 hours (6) of positive-pressure ventilation.

The results showed that caregivers, all of whom were relatives, provided an average of 7.3 hours per day of direct care, including daily bathing, feeding, or assistance with walking. Nine caregivers could leave the patient alone; six could not. Only two reported using support services. *The Caregiving Inventory* revealed more disrupted schedules, financial strain, increased burden, and negative reaction to caregiving with increasing ventilator hours. *The Family Coping Scales* revealed caregivers and patient used predominantly internal coping skills. The *Family Functioning APGAR* revealed satisfaction with overall family function. Caregivers rated all 57 items on the *Learning Needs Checklist* from needed to very needed. Only three items (ventilator checks, suctioning, tracheotomy care) were taught to all caregivers. Fourteen needed items were not taught to one third or more of the caregivers.

Conclusions of this study are that (1) greater than 12 hours per day on the ventilator is disruptive to caregivers; (2) caregivers *do* cope but largely use their own internal resources; and (3) survival knowledge and skills are taught, but additional information is needed. Further efforts should be directed toward support and education of caregivers. ∎

cal care but might contribute grocery shopping. The home care nurse may need to assess periodically family members' role responsibilities in home care as these change over time. Also, individuals' reaction to their responsibilities and energy to carry them out vary with the length of time that caregiving continues (see research box above). Families also react to changes, whether improvement, decline, or stabilization, in the patient's condition during home care. Interview questions that can be used to assess caregiver roles and reactions are listed in the box above, right. Many times negative reactions to caregiving can be improved by obtaining relief such as *respite care* or financial assistance for the family.

∎ DATA ANALYSIS: NURSING DIAGNOSES

Nursing diagnoses are based on the assessment data collected in the home and on the data gathered from discharge planning. These data are analyzed to identify the patient's and family's human responses to the path-

CAREGIVER ROLE ASSESSMENT

1. How have the responsibilities of the members of the family changed since the patient has been at home?
2. How do you and other family members feel about these changes in responsibility?
3. Has your health changed since you have been caring for the patient at home? If so, describe how.
4. Family members tell us they have emotional reactions to the changes in the person they are caring for. What has your experience been with these emotional reactions?
5. Family members often state that responsibilities of home care can be overwhelming and difficult. Do you find this true or not true?
6. Family members have also found they have gained strengths or sense that they are successful in caring for the patient at home. Do you find this to be true or not true?
   Tell me about when you haven't felt successful.
   Tell me the successes you've experienced.

ologic condition, medical regimen, treatment plan, and home nursing care. The nursing diagnoses should reflect each family's actual and potential problems and strengths. By diagnosing strengths, the nurse identifies abilities the family can use in dealing with the actual and potential problems they will face. Analyzing the data to determine the coping skills, external resources, and other family strengths is essential because most must eventually manage the home care alone.

The patient and family may be experiencing translocation syndrome related to moving from the acute care setting into the home. *Translocation syndrome* is a stress reaction to leaving an environment that is perceived as highly protective and safe.[70] The stress response to transferring from one health care setting to another has been measured in several studies. Elevated levels of catecholamines were found in the urine of patients transferring to medical floors after being in coronary care units. Relocation of elderly persons into nursing homes has been associated with increases in death rates. Nurses have found that when patients are prepared for transfer well before the relocation takes place, less stress is experienced. In preparing for discharge to the home, the nurse must anticipate the stress or anxiety, that the patient or family may experience when leaving the environment of the acute care setting, where health care professionals are readily available. Extensive preparation through teaching and involvement of the patient and family in coordinating resources that are readily accessible and economically feasible lessens translocation stress.

The following nursing diagnoses may also be seen in families managing home care. The nursing diagnoses presented in this section are based on information from experienced home care nurses, nursing research studies, and data from studies of adults in the home. These diagnoses have been categorized into problem areas of *resource management, family dysfunction,* and *knowledge deficits.*

Resource management is the ability to obtain and effectively use resources both inside and outside the family for the patient's home care. Resources may include people, equipment, and monies. Resource management is discussed in more depth under the section on Implementation.

NURSING DIAGNOSES BASED ON RESOURCE MANAGEMENT
HOME MAINTENANCE MANAGEMENT, IMPAIRED

Insufficient financial resources are a common problem reported by families at home. Reimbursements from insurance companies or Medicare vary widely and are constantly changing. The home care nurse must be skilled in understanding government regulations and advocating for the patient's eligibility for coverage. The nurse may enlist the help of a social worker familiar with home care coverage codes and regulations to ensure that information on the costs of home care covered by insurers is made available to the family. In addition, the nurse needs to identify any voluntary sources of financial support for families. Some private agencies, such as the American Cancer Society, may provide bandages, equipment, or other care services free or at a nominal charge.

The nurse must also be concerned about specialty services available to the family. In some instances, the technical support services needed by the patient may be at such a distance that safety is a concern. When this occurs, the nurse must ensure that the family recognizes and can readily manage emergencies such as equipment failure or lack of supplies.

SELF-CARE DEFICIT, BATHING/HYGIENE, DRESSING/GROOMING, FEEDING, TOILETING

In many instances the patient requires daily physical care such as feeding, bathing, or assistance with grooming or toileting. Also, technical care, including tracheal suctioning, wound irrigation, or intravenous fluid administration, may be required. Family members provide a wide variety of physical care at home for patients undergoing chemotherapy, those debilitated with Alzheimer's disease, or those recovering from a cerebral vascular accident (CVA).

Family members' fatigue and stress are problems the home care nurse must address. Another complicating factor is the lack of acceptance of help from outside the family. The family may be a closed system that does not desire help from the outside or feels shame when they cannot provide care by themselves. The nurse may need to use value clarification strategies with the family to as-

sist them in problem solving with this issue. The nurse will employ several other counseling techniques with psychologically related nursing diagnoses.

DECISIONAL CONFLICT RELATED TO CONSTRAINTS IMPOSED BY LONG-TERM HOME CARE

Dealing with the patient's chronic disability and the home care management creates constraints on family members' daily schedules and use of the home for activities. The family must make many decisions each day about the patient's home care. These decisions may result in conflicts between family members. The patient and family have direct responsibility for managing such conflicts. Patients and families experiencing chronic illness must live with the constraints imposed by the disease and the home care. Therefore, the nurse may use *conflict resolution strategies* to help ensure an equitable decision-making process is used.

DIVERSIONAL ACTIVITY DEFICIT

Patients with chronic disease, visible disabilities, or equipment as part of their treatment report experiences of negative *social stigma.* Friends may fear that activities are too much of a physical strain for the patient with a chronic illness. Extended family may believe visiting the home causes the family more grief over the patient's disability. Employers may believe that the presence of medical equipment such as oxygen tubing will make the workplace unappealing to customers. Many people feel uncomfortable around visible changes in the patient and environment and avoid visiting. Potential visitors may feel vulnerable: "If it happens to her, it can happen to me." The patient and family need assistance to anticipate these problems and suggestions on how to deal with such reactions. Patients receiving Medicare must be homebound to have home care. This imposes an additional stigma on the patient who is striving for or needs diversional activity.

NURSING DIAGNOSES BASED ON FAMILY DYSFUNCTION

When data from home care assessment are analyzed, nursing diagnoses related to family dysfunction may be apparent. Home care puts many demands on families. Meeting these demands can cause physical fatigue of individual members and a variety of psychologic dysfunctions within the family.

ADJUSTMENT, IMPAIRED

Caring for a family member in the home may alter individual members' everyday activities, interactions, and pattern of social contacts. Participation in religious, leisure, and school activities may be affected. Shifting of household responsibilities may make some family members feel overworked. These changes in life-style may be permanent or temporary, depending on the patient's situation and the resources available to the family. The nurse can assist family members to predict the disruptions that home care might create and support them in adjusting to these disruptions.

COPING, INEFFECTIVE FAMILY: COMPROMISED

The length of home care has an effect on the coping within the family. The longer that home care is required, the more the family's coping skills can become depleted. More situational crises arise during prolonged home care, which also challenges families' coping abilities. Other factors that impact family coping abilities, including past experiences and realistic expectations of home care. The family with positive past experiences who can accurately predict the length of home care and who has accurate expectations specific to daily schedules is better able to cope with prolonged home care.

FAMILY PROCESSES, ALTERED

Home care generally disorganizes a family, at least temporarily. Communication patterns will be altered. Meaningful interactions such as confidential talks, teasing, or humorous exchanges and physical comforting by hugs may decrease. Until the feeling of disruption ebbs and a sense of predictability returns, family processes will be disrupted. Ask the family to describe how home care has changed family function. Their own description will help clarify the alterations in communications and personal exchanges they are missing. Steps to rekindle these helpful family processes should be instituted.

ROLE PERFORMANCE, ALTERED

The spouse may manage the home caregiver role by drastically altering a previously fulfilling role (for example, cook-housekeeper, financial planner). The designated caregiver may perceive home care as an overwhelming burden. The studies of caregiver burden indicate that it is the *perceived* burden more than the actual physical or financial drain that predict role performance problems.[28] Interventions for altered role performance include teaching about new responsibilities and social support. *Social support* in the form of helping with everyday care, contacts with a network of peers, acceptance of caregiving by family members, and provision of emotional concern or praise to the caregiver seem to assist with the perception of burden.

NURSING DIAGNOSES BASED ON KNOWLEDGE DEFICITS[73]

Nursing diagnoses based on knowledge deficits are frequently seen in home health care. Subjective and objective data from the patient and family must be scrutinized to determine the specific etiologic factor leading to the knowledge deficit. Several common causes of knowledge deficit are discussed here.

KNOWLEDGE DEFICIT RELATED TO THE TRANSFER OF LEARNING INTO THE HOME SETTING

Patients and families often state that carrying out procedures they were taught or they observed being done in the hospital seem more complicated once they come home. Health care personnel not being immediately available may decrease the person's confidence. Also, adaptations in procedures may be necessary in the home. Such adaptations may be difficult for family members or patients to devise. Also, the complexity of scheduling the total care, including bathing, feeding, and technical treatments, may be difficult. The varied aspects of transferring learning into the home need to be discussed with the family before the patient's discharge. An emphasis on problem solving that incorporates the patient and family environment, including daily routines, will prove helpful. Make sure the family realizes they can contact the home health agency if they have questions between visits.

KNOWLEDGE DEFICIT RELATED TO PSYCHOLOGIC STATE (ANXIETY)

Another personal factor that can make a difference in the patient's and family's learning is their mental or psychologic state. Much has been written about how anxiety affects people's perceptions and behavior. It is generally accepted that individuals who have moderate to severe anxiety may only be able to focus on their immediate concerns. Consequently, the information given when the patient is moderately anxious may be so distorted that the patient may not learn what is intended. Hospitalization may increase a person's anxiety level. Nurses may need to employ methods to reduce anxiety so that the patient and family can attend to learning. For some patients, technical equipment may be overwhelming and create increased anxiety. The nurse initially may need to do the technical care and gradually teach self-care as the patient or family is able to manage it.

KNOWLEDGE DEFICIT RELATED TO THE PATIENT'S PHYSIOLOGIC STATE

Physical factors also play a significant part in the patient's knowledge deficit. These factors may include the presence of acute illness or pain, fluid and electrolyte imbalance, altered nutritional states, lack of endurance, or medications, each of which can alter mental alertness. Other physical factors related to treatments may also interfere with motor abilities and learning.

Certain electrolyte and nutritional states will also alter the patient's cognitive functioning. The patient may be confused or hallucinatory or may simply be too weak to devote the necessary energy to learning. After the electrolyte imbalance has been corrected, the patient will be better able to concentrate and learn. Patients may lack the physical energy to perform a psychomotor task, such as a dressing change, or they may lack the mental energy to concentrate on learning. Arthritic changes with advancing age may make fingers less functional for fine motor tasks. The tactile perception in the elderly may also be reduced so that manipulation of small objects, such as needles and syringes, can be very frustrating. Nurses must determine any physical changes that might hamper learning and take steps to alleviate these barriers when teaching patients and families.

KNOWLEDGE DEFICIT RELATED TO CULTURAL AND SOCIOECONOMIC FACTORS

Socioeconomic and cultural factors may also influence the patient's response to teaching. These factors can include a language barrier, cultural background as related to health practices, or lack of finances to purchase necessary home care equipment. The following patient example is used to illustrate how several of these factors impact learning.

A patient from a mid-Eastern culture had a transverse colostomy and recovered very well. She needed home care because she showed no interest in the colostomy or in performing any of the needed care. In her culture, it was taboo to allow a member of her family to touch her body, yet she could not afford home care services and was uninsured. Through an interpreter interviewing the patient, it was determined that a neighbor, also of her culture, was willing to learn colostomy care and eventually teach the patient self-care. Once the nurse learned about the taboo and the women's lack of interest, the nurse turned her attention to teaching the neighbor, who in turn could instruct the patient at home.

This situation illustrates how important it is to consider all factors affecting patient teaching.

KNOWLEDGE DEFICIT RELATED TO HEALTH BELIEFS

The *Health Belief Model* predicts that people are more likely to behave in a certain way if they believe that behavior fosters good health, believe that they are at risk for a complication, or they recognize a benefit from the learned behavior. For example, a young woman at home on parenteral nutrition is more likely to refrigerate the intravenous solutions as required when she understands the potential risk of contamination. If the woman does not perceive that this activity will be of some benefit or if she doesn't feel threatened by the possibility of developing an infection, she may not follow the teaching.

Folkways about health practices also impact on home care and nurses may include these remedies (when safe) in their teaching. It is always good practice to ask patients what they believe will add to their success in home care management and try to incorporate folk remedies the families feel necessary. Because the patient controls his or her own care folkways may be used and the health care professional may be unaware of it.

KNOWLEDGE DEFICIT RELATED TO ILLITERACY

Literacy reports suggest that less than 20% of the adult population reads above the fifth grade level, and that the median literacy of the United States population is approximately at the tenth grade level. Many times the educational materials distributed are above the patient's reading levels. A miss-match of written material with the patient's reading ability can account for unsuccessful learning for the patient.

The printed word should not only be at an appropriate level for the patient but also the vocabulary used by the nurse. Results of patient education studies indicated that common "medical words" are not understood by patients. Words such as "hematoma," "secretions," and "post-op" were incorrectly defined by a large majority of those surveyed. How often do nurses use those words in their teaching and assume that the patient understands what they mean? Even for functionally literate patients, the stress associated with illness may reduce their comprehension of spoken words, written materials, and even visual teaching resources. Teaching and reteaching, with opportunities for patients to ask about terms and ideas they do not understand, are important aspects of treating knowledge deficits. Reteaching patients may not be reimbursed, so further education may be included in other care or be charged to the family.

■ PLANNING: EXPECTED PATIENT OUTCOMES

Planning is directed by the outcomes expected to result from home health care. Statements are made of expected outcomes so that the patient, family, and the home health nurse agree that the outcomes are realistic and measurable. Expected outcomes are based on the patient's condition as reflected in nursing diagnoses, standards of nursing practice, and results from clinical research studies. See the following section for examples of planning home care.

■ IMPLEMENTATION

Implementation of nursing care for the adult patient in the home is based on discharge planning, assessment data, nursing diagnoses, and expected patient outcomes *negotiated with* the family. The critical nursing interventions of resource management, counseling, and teaching are implemented with every family. *Resource management includes coordination of services, products, and personnel necessary for cost-effective home care.* The interventions implemented by the home care nurse will depend on the internal and external resources available to the family. Coordinating the resources, counseling, and providing information are essential aspects of the nurse's role in home care implementation. See the following section for examples of implementing home care.

EXAMPLES OF PLANNING AND IMPLEMENTING HOME CARE

HOME INTRAVENOUS ANTIBIOTIC THERAPY

In the case of home intravenous antibiotic therapy (HIAT), many clinical studies have established this as a safe approach for many adult patients.[51] The frequency with which patients dependent on intravenous therapy are discharged to home care has increased dramatically. In the United States, 75% of hospitals offered home care services for IAT in 1983, and in 1984, this had increased to 90%.[17] Medical center hospitals and private agencies provide discharge planning and home care for patients receiving IAT.

Patients are discharged from the hospital when the signs and symptoms of acute infection are under control. Then, when the following expected outcomes have been met, the patient is ready for home teaching.

1. Patient and family agree to manage HIAT.
2. Patient has peripheral vein catheter in place.
3. Family has created a suitable environment in the home for infusion therapy.
4. Arrangements for supplies, medication, laboratory blood studies, and emergency care have been made.

When met, these expected outcomes ensure that the resources necessary for successful HIAT are available to the patient. The first expected outcome of eliciting the patient's and family's agreement to manage HIAT is essential. If the family is not motivated to undertake this complicated therapy, difficulties will arise with home care.

Patients receive HIAT to treat many infections, often osteomyelitis, endocarditis, urinary tract infections, septic arthritis, cellulitis, pyelonephritis, pelvic inflammatory disease, prostatitis, and complications from medical devices inserted into the body. The National Center for Health Statistics conducted a hospital discharge survey

in 1981 and determined that approximately 51,000 cases of primary and secondary osteomyelitis and 11,000 cases of bacterial endocarditis were diagnosed that year.[61] The incidence of such infections, coupled with physician and industry efforts to secure Medicare funding for home antibiotic therapy, are likely to increase the numbers of patients receiving HIAT.

Researchers have not only documented the efficacy, safety, and cost savings of the infusions in the home, but also that teaching patients and families to manage intravenous antibiotics can be effectively done in the home. Nursing interventions can be determined based on the nursing diagnoses and expected patient outcomes (see the box below).

It is helpful to have more than one expected outcome for each diagnosis to provide more than one objective criterion for measuring the results of nursing interventions. The data that need to be gathered to evaluate the results should be readily available and inexpensive. White blood cell (WBC) counts or wound culture laboratory tests may be the most definitive way of determining acute exacerbation of infection, but they are expensive and relatively difficult to obtain and would not be used unless other data (high fever and so forth) indicate that the expected outcomes have not been met. *Expected outcomes used in home care must be simple to use and analyze.* The patient and family must collect most of the data needed to judge if expected outcomes are met because they monitor their own home care. If the data to be collected are difficult for the patient to obtain (for example, unable to read small markings on a thermometer or unable to determine color changes on the chemical strips used to check nitrates indicating urine infection), another person in the home must be taught to gather this information.

PROCEDURES IN IMPLEMENTING HIAT

The overall expected outcome with HIAT is that the patient's infection will be eliminated. However, because HIAT requires complicated technical care, expected outcomes that reflect the patient's and family member's ability to undertake each aspect of HIAT must be care-

---

NURSING DIAGNOSES AND EXPECTED OUTCOMES FOR THE PERSON RECEIVING HIAT

NURSING DIAGNOSES	EXPECTED OUTCOMES
Coping, ineffective family: compromised, related to ambivalence toward HIAT	Patient/family member (1) state rationale for HIAT, (2) demonstrate readiness to learn by handling equipment or asking questions, and (3) state they agree to undertake HIAT.
Infection, potential for acute exacerbation	Patient remains free of high-grade fever and other signs of infection specific to the patient (for example, cough, sputum for pneumonia; painful joints for osteomyelitis).
Knowledge deficit: management of HIAT related to new treatment	Patient/family member demonstrate each step of HIAT using safe, aseptic technique.

PROCEDURAL STEPS EXPECTED OF PATIENTS RECEIVING HIAT

1. Each morning, review the scheduled times for your medication and plan your activities to allow enough time for the infusion
   a. One-half hour before the scheduled infusion, check your temperature and compare this on the graph to the previous day's level. Check the insertion site of your intravenous (IV) catheter (teach patients to look for signs for infection, irritation, and stability of catheter in the vein). If problems exist with the catheter, telephone the home care nurse, who may be able to provide appropriate instructions.
   b. Draw up antibiotic medication in syringe. (If premixed solutions are not available, several other steps specific to mixing are added here.)
2. Remove the bag of IV solution from the refrigerator 15 minutes before administration to allow it to warm up.
3. Check the expiration date and dosage of any premixed solutions.
4. Draw heparin-saline solution into a syringe if premixed solution is not available and replace the cover on the needle.
5. Hang the IV bag on a hanger above your arm.
6. Squeeze the drip chamber and purge all air from the tubing, making sure there is fluid in the drip chamber.
7. Cleanse the rubber stopper of your IV catheter with an alcohol swab for 1 minute.
8. Remove the cap from the needle at the end of the IV tubing.
9. Insert needle into the gummed rubber stopper of your IV catheter.
10. Establish a flow rate by adjusting the flow-control clamp so that solution in the __ ml bag will take __ minutes to infuse. That means that __ drops of solution must fall into the drip chamber every 30 seconds. (Blanks are filled in by nurse.)
11. Check flow rate periodically. When the infusion is completed, remove the needle from the gummed rubber stopper.
12. Replace the cap over the needle.
13. Wipe off the gummed rubber stopper again with an alcohol swab.
14. Remove the cap from the syringe containing the heparin-saline solution and inject it into the gummed rubber stopper.
15. Remove the needle of the syringe from the gummed rubber stopper and replace the cap over the needle.
16. Carefully dispose of all your needles so that no one will accidentally be injured (use a coffee can with cover; this may be brought to the hospital pharmacy later for proper disposal).
17. Record on your monitoring sheet that infusion was completed and that IV insertion site looks normal.
18. If you have any questions, call the hospital and ask the pharmacist or IV nurse for assistance.

fully written. The box above lists the 18 steps in the procedure typically used for infusing antibiotics. It is clear from these steps that the terminology the patient must learn just to read these directions can be overwhelming. It is important that instructions not be initiated before patients accept the idea of self-administration and learn some of the common terms.

Before infusions can be undertaken by patients, they need clear understanding of the reasons for the therapy and why it will take place in the home. The presence of an intravenous needle often signifies to the family that the individual is very ill and that the connection to the tubing means the patient should be bedridden with restricted activities. Families may experience anxiety over the patient's condition and ineffective coping related to wanting the patient home yet being afraid to manage HIAT. These problems can be treated by providing information and counseling strategies to build family members' confidence in giving care. Patients and families need reassurance that continued intravenous therapy can be safely conducted in the home. They need to understand that any patient has a potential for an acute exacerbation of infection and may require rehospitalization. The signs of acute infection are listed for them so that they feel confident in deciding when to call for help. The advantages of being mobile and returning to

work and household activities are presented to them. Today, most antibiotic home infusions can be given through indwelling catheters that can be disconnected after the infusion is completed.

HOME TOTAL PARENTERAL NUTRITION

Estimates from Medicare statistics indicate that $170 million per year is spent on reimbursement of nonhospitalized persons receiving home total parenteral nutrition (HTPN). In the late 1980s, at least 14,000 adults were managing TPN at home. Of the patients receiving HTPN, the largest percentage (37.3%) have benign bowel disease such as Crohn's and ischemic bowel disease. Persons with neoplasms and with acquired immunodeficiency syndrome (AIDS) constitute 25% of the patients receiving HTPN. The remaining percentages are spread among patients with other benign illnesses such as motility or swallowing disorders and adhesions.

Most patients (70% to 80%) with benign bowel diseases require lifelong TPN. About three quarters of patients with Crohn's disease and one half of patients with ischemic bowel disease receiving HTPN return to full- or part-time employment. It is generally acknowledged that more patients also might return to work if it were not for Medicare and private insurance stipulations requiring that individuals be unemployed to receive disability payments. Disability payments are necessary because HTPN therapy is very expensive ($40,000 to $80,000 per year).

RESOURCE MANAGEMENT

Ideally, the family who is managing long-term HTPN will have access to a team of professionals as well as various resources from the community. Many medical centers have a nutritional support team that will educate patients about HTPN before discharge.

Commercial agencies have developed teams that will give advice on location and storage of products in the home, equipment necessary for implementation, and telephone service for emergencies. Most hospital-based and commercial teams include nurses, physicians, pharmacists, social workers, dietitians, and consulting psychiatrists.

The nurse typically directs the team by calling on the physician and social worker for discharge planning, the pharmacists and dietitians for monitoring the medical and nutrition therapy, and the psychiatrists for counseling the patient and family. Emotional reactions to the dependency on this lifelong technologic care can be overwhelming and may require periodic or long-term psychologic interventions. Unfortunately, not all families have access to such sophisticated teams, so their resources may consist of a nurse from a physician's office, a technician from an equipment company, and the physician.

COUNSELING FOR LONG-TERM HTPN

The initial psychologic reaction of many patients and family members to HTPN is relief.[56] The relief results from the immediate improvement seen in the patient's condition. For example, patients with Crohn's disease may be relieved of bowel pain and diarrhea and patients with cancer may be better nourished. Following the initial relief, however, other psychologic reactions require counseling interventions from the nurse.

PSYCHOLOGIC REACTIONS TO LONG-TERM HTPN

Families often experience anxiety related to transfer of learning about complicated technologic care into the home setting. After 3 or 4 months of home care, however, patients may experience depressive reactions related to the complexity of long-term or lifelong therapy and the constant presence of technology in their daily lives. Issues of lack of control and dependence, as well as relationship and role changes within the family, typically occur. The research box above, right describes the spouse's role changes and reactions of the patient receiving HTPN.

Counseling can also involve providing information. Thorough patient teaching about HTPN, as shown in Table 78-2, and discussion of symptoms, problems, and

RESEARCH

Heaphey L: Survey results provide insight into psychosocial issues, Lifeline Lett Oley Foundation, 9(6):1-2, 1988.

A survey by the Oley Foundation of 172 HTPN families indicates that family members' and patients' perspectives differ on the problems experienced and the resources most helpful in adapting to HTPN.[54] Spouses reported guilt about their ability to eat, distress at social gatherings with food, and concern about eating out. However, patients indicated spouses' ability to eat and eating out were not problems. Body image distortions and sexual difficulties were problems patients ranked as continuing and significant, although spouses did not report these as important issues. This survey highlighted the differences in the patients' and spouses'/caregivers' reactions to HTPN. The third-ranked problem listed by both patient and spouse was "relationships with spouse," especially communication. Yet patients ranked their spouses as their number-one resource for helping with psychosocial problems. The nurse from the physician's office or home care service was ranked second, gastroenterologist third, hospital nurse fourth, and another family member fifth. Very few patients listed another HTPN patient or someone outside the family as a helpful resource. The nurse can assist the patient and spouse to communicate openly about the problems of HTPN. ▪

concomitant actions (Table 78-3) can reassure families they can implement the necessary care.

EVALUATION

The last step of the nursing process is evaluation. Evaluation is making a judgment as to whether or not home care has been successful. This judgment depends on comparison of the patient's and family's status with the expected outcomes of home care.

If expected outcomes have not been achieved, the reasons for this are ascertained. If the patient's physical function falls short of the expected outcomes, the nurse must identify factors contributing to this problem. The nurse may see signs that the patient's pathophysiologic condition is worsening. Referral to the physician or arrangements for transportation to a medical facility may be necessary. Evaluation might reveal that the expected outcomes have not been achieved because of factors other than the patient's physical condition. The patient may have misunderstood what he or she was taught, the resources arranged at discharge may not have been obtained, or the family members may have found home care overwhelming. Another reason expected outcomes are not met is that they may have been unrealistic to achieve in the time allotted. The nurse reassesses the situation and establishes new outcomes in conjunction with the patient and family.

TABLE 78-2 Implementation plan for teaching HTPN up to 10 days

	Physical Care	Psychologic Care	Emergency Care
1st day	If patient has been pretrained and is not overly tired from discharge, have him demonstrate HTPN. If he is too fatigued, have him talk about the steps of HTPN while family member carries out procedure.	Give reassurance by pointing out the abilities patient demonstrates or discusses. Describe other families who have succeeded with HTPN.	Demonstrate clamping TPN catheter in emergency; post emergency telephone numbers so family member can call for help.
2nd day	Observe patient set up TPN solution bags, syringes, and medications as he was taught before discharge.	Decide with patient what aspects of the procedure he can manage independently, and set a calendar for learning the total care.	Describe the signs of water intoxication (confusion, weakness, neck vein distention, puffy eyelids, increased urination) that may occur when TPN is given over 12 hours at home.
3rd day	Make sure patient knows how to weigh himself and take his temperature daily. Repeat setting up TPN solutions and teach about medications to be taken.	Compliment patient on (1) being able to monitor effects of nutrition therapy by monitoring weight daily, (2) detecting hazards of infection by taking temperature daily, and (3) knowing medication side effects.	Have patient practice with needle caps for appropriate disposal. Reinforce use of aseptic technique and handwashing.
4th day	Demonstrate use of infusion pump. Have the patient insert the intravenous line into TPN solution bag.	Have the patient review the written instruction manual. Point out how well he has followed directions. Encourage patient to write notes in his own words in the printed manual.	If signs of water toxicity are present, draw blood laboratory samples for sodium, plasma protein, and hematocrit levels.
5th and 6th days	Have patient set up infusion pump, adjust flow rates, and stop infusion. Discuss timing and scheduling of infusions.	Help family establish an area where TPN supplies can be safely stored and handled. Have the nutrition team, psychiatrist, or clinical nurse specialist telephone to offer support.	Teach patient how to clear air from the tubing. Discuss importance of daily tubing changes to prevent infection.
7th day	Have patient correct minor problems that may occur with equipment and infusion pumps, such as responding to alarms or troubleshooting back flow of solution.	Begin a record that monitors patient's infusion schedule, need to purchase supplies, daily weight and temperature, medications, laboratory results, and symptoms. Use the records to illustrate patient's self-care abilities.	Use the symptoms list (Table 78-3) to identify emergencies that may occur over long-term use of HTPN.
8th day	Have patient demonstrate catheter care, including inspection of insertion site, dressing changes, catheter cap and extension change, capped heparinization, and connections.	Suggest that family member who is also learning the procedure observe the patient's technique and that they periodically review the manual together.	Demonstrate procedure for repair of a catheter that develops a leak or begins bleeding around inspection site and injection cap, as well as procedure when adapter become dislodged.
9th day	Discuss various side effects of TPN complications: catheter site infection, solution bag contamination, blood sugar variations, and physical complications.	Emphasize that patient and family member will be the first to recognize metabolic or physical side effects of the therapy and that they then should notify the home care nurse promptly.	Hyper- or hypoglycemia is monitored via daily finger glucometer checks. Serum electrolytes are drawn weekly.
10th day	Have patient demonstrate each aspect of care following the printed manual.	Review the patient's record keeping and discuss the information. Point out how confident the patient is in managing his home care. Emphasize that telephone contact can be made with home care personnel.	Patient must be prepared for emergencies that occur after long-term use of HTPN, including sepsis, catheter displacement or damage, and psychologic disorders such as anxiety, depression, alcohol or drug addiction problems, and mood disorders related to machine dependency.

TABLE 78-3 Symptoms and problems experienced by HTPN patients*

Symptoms	Problem	Actions
Swelling of skin over catheter insertion site; sensations of pain, heat, burning near site	Possible leak in catheter at place of swelling Avoid rough contact or sports that could dislodge catheter.	Call home health nurse or physician. Do not use catheter to give fluids. Tape the catheter securely to the skin so that it does not dangle.
Leak of blood from injection cap or catheter	Possible loose cap or leak in catheter	Clamp catheter. Change cap and heparin lock. Go to emergency room for catheter repair or call physician.
Cough, shortness of breath, chest pain	Possible air embolism (air in blood) Air may be drawn into the vein if catheter is not clamped during cap change.	If giving fluids, stop and place heparin lock on catheter. Lie on left side. Call physician or go to emergency room.
Redness, swelling, drainage, tenderness at exit site	Skin infection or irritation	Call home health nurse or physician. Change bandage and clean daily. Change the bandage and clean around the catheter if bandage gets wet or soiled.
Chills, fever, fatigue, aches, weakness	Possible infection within the bloodstream	Go to emergency room for tests

*Always wash your hands before starting any procedures. If you have a rash or cuts and scrapes on your hands, wear gloves for all the procedures. Keep all supplies used on catheter sterile. Use aseptic technique.

Evaluation may also reveal many instances where patients have achieved their expected outcomes. The nurse should acknowledge this with the patient and family. When families are given recognition for their achievements, they feel supported in their efforts. Evaluation data, whether indicative of achievement or not, must be documented, with the rationale related to the outcomes. Evaluation data may be used for justification for reimbursement of extended home care or for the involvement of other home care resources. For the patient to continue to receive Medicare home health benefits, beyond the 2 to 3 weeks of intermittent care allowable, "exceptional circumstances" must be proved. Many patients may qualify for up to 3 months of home care reimbursement when the nurse provides data that document the need for continued home care.

QUALITY ASSURANCE

Quality assurance is another aspect of evaluation. Quality assurance is a formal process of aggregating data to form a basis to evaluate groups of patients and various aspects of care. Examples of quality assurance data obtained about groups of patients are listed in the box at right.

These data can be used to project trends in home care services for a particular group of patients. The data from nursing care hours and types of home services used can help identify personnel needed in home health care. Medical and nursing diagnoses help establish appropriate case management. The financial data can be used to plan future services, budget for weekend services, recruit specific types of personnel needed in a home care agency, and justify needed programs to policymakers.

One of the most interesting aspects of quality assurance is the use of data from multiple families to evaluate nursing care. The case records or charts of several patients can be reviewed to determine if specific nursing interventions were successful or if the amount of resources used were adequate. Using quality assurance processes, nurses in home care can establish *cost-effective interventions.* Nurses can be leaders in developing home care programs that promote the highest possible level of health and function for a specific adult population. Quality assurance processes and evaluation of individual families can also be used to identify issues and other concerns pertinent to home care. Some of these issues are discussed next.

QUALITY ASSURANCE DATA FOR PATIENTS RECEIVING HOME HEALTH CARE

1. Types and length of nursing and other home services
2. Nursing and medical diagnoses
3. Age, sex, income level, and other demographic data
4. Age and relationship of family members providing care to the patient
5. Source of the patient's referral
6. Source of payment for home care services

ISSUES IN HOME CARE

Many issues affect how nurses practice home care. These include factors that affect delivery of care such as the cost of nursing services, availability of services, and community resources and patient or family responses to home care. Also, competition often occurs between different home care delivery services. Reimbursement for professional nurses versus home health aides may influence who provides care. Scarcity of services for technologically dependent patients may limit care in some locales. Communities with few resources (free clinics, volunteer agencies, self-care groups) may be unable to provide support for families caring for adults in the home. Home care nurses can bring the issues of affordable home care, national health insurance, and development of resources for in home care of the elderly to legislature or community groups for resolution.

Many issues arise in the everyday care of individuals in the home. As with nursing of adults in any setting, the individual may elect not to follow prescribed regimens. Families may refuse the medical and nursing care available to them. Third-party reimbursement may not pay for professional nursing services. Nurses may observe or suspect abuse or neglect of the patient as family caregivers become overwhelmed with the patient's care. Also, there may be sociocultural or religious conflicts between the family and health care professional's approach to the patient's care. The home care nurse must identify such conflicts and other issues and discuss these with the patient, family, or other health professionals.

Caring for various groups of patients also will highlight issues particular to each group. Caregiver fatigue, social isolation, and role change are problematic in many cases. The need for custodial or respite care also may be apparent. Care of dying patients in the home has increased significantly with the success of the hospice movement. The family's coping skills and a focus on palliative care become issues in long-term terminal care. Home care nurses must be open to discussion of spiritual concerns, life review, and reconciliation.

Another challenge comes from patients at home that require rehabilitative care. Persons with neuromuscular diseases, CVAs, or spinal cord injuries may require assistance of physical and occupational therapists. Patients with AIDS may need assessment by infection control specialists for home care. Patients with Alzheimer's disease may benefit from mental health or gerontology specialists. Other specialists also may need to be available to patients in their home, such as speech or respiratory therapists. Transportation to clinics and rehabilitation centers may need to be arranged. Services to enhance persons' abilities to manage their own care will increase in costs but are essential to self-care. The issue of providing the needed services for home care in the most cost-effective manner will continue to be a challenging issue in the 1990s.

CHAPTER SUMMARY

- Providing nursing care to the ill adult in the home will be an increasing challenge in the decades ahead. In the mid-1980s, there were approximately the same number of agencies providing home health care as there were hospitals. Forecasters of health care suggest that hospital closures will continue, whereas home care services will increase by as much as 20% annually throughout the 1990s. Medical-surgical nursing home care will be necessary for a wide range of adults.

- Patients may require one or two home visits or around-the-clock nursing care. The nursing process in home care includes expanded assessment of the individual and the home environment, development of nursing diagnoses based on family data, generation of expected outcomes negotiated with the patient and family, implementation of appropriate care, as well as extensive evaluation of the effectiveness of care.

- The acuity levels of individuals requiring care in their homes will continue to rise, and the technologic aspects of care, including use of mechanical equipment or invasive procedures such as intravenous therapies, will increase in home care. These factors, coupled with shorter hospital stays, will require increasing sophistication in the area of transition care, starting with discharge planning.

- The uniqueness of the residence as the environment for care must be taken into account with an adult member requiring home care. The nurse will employ special skills of entering the home along with teaching families, discharge planning, transitional care, and case management.

- The trends responsible for the increasing need for home care nursing include the emphasis on continuity of care, promotion of family involvement in care, economic limitations on expenses in health care, and the aging population demographics.

- Skills to manage the patient's transition from acute to home care range from establishing a relationship on entering the home to case-managed care, which incorporates supervision of many families and advocating cost reductions in health care services.

- Discharge planning, family education, and transition care are the major skills used in home care nursing. Discharge planning includes resource management, coordination of hospital and community services, and adequate preparation for home care. Family education is based on the research supporting the use of patient instruction with the added dimension of teaching a group, the family. Transition care incorporates the skills of discharge planning and family education, with emphasis on continuity and self-managed care in the home.

✔ The nursing process in home care is an expansion of that used with hospitalized patients. Assessment is broadened to include recognition of environmental, financial, social, and community influences on care. The assessment of the patient's condition, psychologic status, and response to treatment is undertaken in light of family analysis as well.

✔ Data analysis from assessment in home care has resulted in identification of common nursing problems. These nursing problems can be stated as nursing diagnoses such as self-care deficits, ineffective family coping, and knowledge deficits.

✔ Expected patient outcomes and implementation in home care can be readily illustrated through examples of patients at home receiving mechanical ventilation, intravenous antibiotic therapy, or total parenteral nutrition. The technologically dependent patient exemplifies the needs of those with high physical acuity, complicated teaching requirements, and family coping challenges. Research suggests these needs can be met in a cost-effective manner with high-quality home nursing care.

✔ Evaluation of home nursing care is a complicated process that includes quality assurance and identification of issues related to home management. Specific data are needed to evaluate groups of patients managed at home. Availability of resources and national health insurance are some of the issues impacting home nursing care today.

QUESTIONS TO CONSIDER

- How would you care for the patient requiring intravenous antibiotic therapy in the home versus in the hospital?

- What approaches would you consider for a patient who needs daily physical care in the home who has no insurance and an elderly spouse?

- What criteria are issued to determine needs for home care following early discharge from the hospital?

- What advantages do transition skill care and case-managed care offer for home care?

- How do the skills of family education in the home differ from individual patient teaching in the hospital?

REFERENCES AND SELECTED READINGS

1. American College of Physicians: Home health care, Ann Intern Med 105:454-460, 1986.
2. American College of Physicians Health and Public Policy Committee: Position paper: home health care, Ann Intern Med 105:40, 1986.
3. *Baille V, Norbeck J, and Barnes L: Stress, social support, and psychological distress of family caregivers of the elderly, Nurs Res 37:217-222, 1988.
4. Ballard S and McNamara R: Quantifying nursing needs in home health care, Nurs Res 32:236-241, 1983.
5. Banaszak E et al: Home ventilator care, Respir Care 26(12):1262-1268, 1981.
6. Berger M: The cost and efficacy of home care for patients with chronic lung disease, Med Care 36(6):566-579, 1988.
7. Bramwell L: Wives' experiences in the support role after husbands' first myocardial infarction, Heart Lung 15:578-584, 1986.
8. Branch L et al: A prospective study of incident comprehensive medical home care use among the elderly, Am J Public Health 78:255-259, 1988.
9. *Brooten D et al: A randomized clinical trial of early hospital discharge and home follow-up of very-low-birth-weight infants, N Engl J Med 315:934-938, 1986.
10. *Brooten D et al: Early discharge and specialist transitional care, Image: J Nurs Scholarship 20(2):64-88, 1988.
11. Cantor MH: Strain among caregivers: a study of experience in the United States, Gerontologist 23:597-604, 1983.
12. *Chang B: Evaluation of health care professionals in facilitating self-care: review of the literature and conceptual model, Adv Nurs Sci 3(1):43-45, 1980.
13. Coleman J and Smith D: DRG's and the growth of home health care, Nurs Econ 2:391-395, 1984.
14. Corbin J and Strauss A: Unending work and care: managing chronic illness at home, San Francisco, 1988, Jossey-Bass, Inc, Publishers.
15. Cronin C and Maklebust J: Case-managed care: capitalizing on the CNS, Nurs Management 20(3):38-47, 1989.
16. Dickson G and Lee-Villasenor H: Nursing theory and practice: a self-care approach, Adv Nurs Sci 3(1):29-40, 1982.
17. Division of Health Care Statistics: National Hospital Discharge Survey, Washington, DC, 1981, US Government Printing Office.
18. Duvall E: Marriage and family development, Philadelphia, 1977, JB Lippincott Co.
19. Eichel CJ: Stress and coping in patients on CAPD compared to hemodialysis patients, Am Nephrol Nurse Assoc J 13(1):9-13, 1986.
20. Engle V: Mental status and functional health 4 days following relocation to a nursing home, Res Nurs Health 8:355-361, 1985.
21. *Farce R: Home ventilation: an alternative to institutionalization, Focus Crit Care 13(6):28-34, 1986.
22. Feldman J and Tuteur P: Mechanical ventilation: from intensive care to home, Heart Lung 11:162-165, 1982.
23. Fitzgerald J, Moore P, and Dittus R: The care of elderly patients with hip fracture: changes since implementation of the prospective payment system, N Engl J Med 319:1392-1397, 1988.
24. Frederick B, Sharp J, and Atkins N: Quality of patient care: whose decision? J Nurs Quality Assurance 2(3):1-10, 1988.

---

*References preceded by an asterisk are particularly well suited for student reading.

25. George L and Gwyther L: Caregiver well-being: a multidimensional examination of family caregivers of demented adults, Gerontologist 26:253-259, 1986.

26. *Gikon F and Kucharski P: A new look at the community, Functional Health Pattern Assessment, J Community Health Nurs 4(1):21-27, 1987.

27. Gipson W, Sivak E, and Gulledge A: Psychological aspects of ventilator dependency, Psychiatr Med 5(3):245-255, 1987.

28. Given BA et al: Family caregivers of the elderly: involvement and reactions to care, Arch Psychiatr Nurs 2(5):281-288, 1988.

29. Goldsmith J: A radical prescription for hospitals, Harvard Bus Rev 67(3):104-111, 1989.

30. Guarriello D: Intravenous therapy and the law, NITA 6:278-281, 1983.

31. Hagen-Moe D: Training, assessment of learning, and follow-up: three components of an effective home parenteral nutrition training program, Nutr Clin Pract 25:30-32, 1986.

32. Harris M: The changing scene in community health nursing, Nurs Clin North Am 23(3):559-568, 1988.

33. Heaphey L: Survey results provide insight into psychosocial issues, Life Lett Oley Foundation, November/December, 9(6):1-2, 1988,

34. Jacobs M and Goodman G: Psychology and self-help groups, Am Psychol 44(3):536-545, 1989.

35. Jernigan DK: Home management of epidural catheters for pain control, Caring 5(10):85-91, 1986.

36. Johnson EA and Jackson JE: Teaching the home care client, Nurs Clin N Am 24(3):687-694, 1989.

37. Joint Commission on Accreditation of Health Care Organizations: Quality assurance in managed care organizations, Chicago, 1989, The Commission.

38. Kerby G, Mayer L, and Pingleton S: Nocturnal positive pressure ventilation via nasal mask, Am Rev Respir Dis 135:738-740, 1987.

39. King F, Figge J, and Harman P: The elderly coping at home: a study of continuity of nursing care, J Adv Nurs 11:41-46, 1986.

40. Kopacz M and Moriarty-Wright R: Multidisciplinary approach for the patient on home ventilator, Heart Lung 13:255-262, 1984.

41. Larson S: Home IV antibiotic therapy the primary care physician's role, Drug Ther 11:67-74, 1987.

42. Liebermann A: Community and home health nursing, Springhouse, Pa, 1990, Springhouse Corp.

43. Louden T: Opportunities and competition in home health care on the rise, Mod Health Care 4:109-112, 1984.

44. Luttrell M: Changes in oxygen reimbursement, Cont Care 10:14-16, 1989.

45. Management rounds: Network links diverse computer systems, Hospitals 57(16):46, 1983.

46. Maraldo, P: Home care should be the heart of a nursing sponsored national health plan, Nurs Health Care 10(6):301-304, 1989.

47. *Martinson I and Widmer A: Home health care nursing, Philadelphia, Pa, 1989, WB Saunders Co.

48. Mazzuca S: Does patient education in chronic disease have therapeutic value? J Chronic Dis 35:521-529, 1987.

49. Mitchell M: The power of standards, Nurs Health Care 10(6):307-309, 1989.

50. Moore J: Intravenous amrinone therapy at home, Focus Crit Care 15:32-37, 1988.

51. National Intravenous Therapy Association: Home IV therapy nursing standards of practice, NITA 7:93, 1984.

52. O'Donohue W et al: Long-term mechanical ventilation: guidelines for management in the home and at alternate community sites, Chest 90(1):15-375, July 1986.

53. O'Hare P and Terry M: Discharge planning strategies for assuming continuity of care, Rockville, Md, 1988, Aspen Systems Corp.

54. Oley Foundation: Oasis system home parenteral nutrition studies, in Heaphey L (personal communication), 1987.

55. Pasquale, DK: A basis for prospective payment for home care, Image 19(4):196-191, 1987.

56. Perl M et al: Psychiatric effects of long-term home hyperalimentation, J Parenter Enter Nutr 22(12):1047-1048, 1981.

57. Peters, D: Development of a community health intensity rating scale, Nurs Res 37:202-207, 1988.

58. Peterson K: Psychosocial adjustment of the family caregiver: home hemodialysis as an example, Soc Work Health Care 10(3):15-32, 1985.

59. Phillips E et al: DRG ripple and the shifting of burden of care to home health, Nurs Health Care 10(6):325-237, 1989.

60. Quiring J: RN perspective of home health care needs of family members, Kans Nurse, 59(3):9-12, 1985.

61. Rasmusen L: A screening tool promotes early discharge, Nurs Management, 15(5):39-43, 1984.

62. Reckling J: Abandonment of patients by home health nursing agencies: an ethical analysis of the dilemma, Adv Nurs Sci 11(3):70-81, 1985.

63. Reinhard S: Case managing community services for hip fractured elders, Orthop Nurs 7:42-49, 1988.

64. *Rew L et al: Affirm: a nursing model to promote role mastery in family caregivers, Fam Community Health 9(4):52-64, 1987.

65. Rovinski C and Zastocki D: Home care: a technical manual for the professional nurse, Philadelphia, 1989, WB Saunders Co.

66. Select Committee on Aging: Paying the price of catastrophic illness: from accidents to Alzheimer's, Pub. No. 100-612, US House of Representatives, Washington, DC, 1987, US Government Printing Office.

67. Sexton D and Munro B: Impact of a husband's chronic illness (COPD) on the spouse's life, Res Nurs Health 8(1):83-90, 1985.

68. Sienkiewicz J: Patient classification in community health nursing, Nurs Outlook 32:319-321, 1984.

69. Sivak E, Cordasco E, and Gipson W: Pulmonary mechanical ventilation at home: a reasonable and less expensive alternative, Respir Care 29(1):42-49, 1983.

70. Smilkstein G: The physician and family function assessment, Fam Systems Med 2:263-278, 1984.

71. Smith BA: When is "confusion" translocation syndrome? Am J Nur 86(3):1280-1281, 1986.

72. Smith CE: With good assessment skills you can construct a solid framework for patient care, Nursing '84, 14(12):26-31, 1984.

73. Smith CE, editor: Patient education: nurses in partnership with other health care professionals, New York, 1987, Grune & Stratton, Inc.

74. *Smith CE: Overview of patient education: opportunities and challenges for the twenty-first century, Nurs Clin N Am 24(3):583-587, 1989 .

75. Smith CE, Schorfheide A, and Lackey N: Acute to home care: managing the transition, Kans Nurse 4(60):9-11, 1985.

76. Spiegel A: The future of home health care. In Home health care, ed 2, 1987, Nat Health Pub.

77. Splaingard ML et al: Home negative pressure ventilation: report of 20 years experience in patients with neuromuscular disease, Arch Phys Med Rehabil 66:239-242, 1985.

78. Stiller SB: Success and difficulty in high-tech home care, Public Health Nurs 5(2):68-75, 1988.

79. Stopfjell J: How valuable are nurses' skills? A case for fair pricing in home health care, Nurs Health Care 10(6):311-313, 1989.

80. Sullivan T: Self-care model for nursing: new directions for nursing in the '80s, Kansas City, Mo, 1980, American Nurses' Association.

81. Trager B: Home health care national health policy, Home Health Care Quar 1(2):103-24, 1980, Haworth Press.

82. Weinstein S: The how-to's of home care, NITA 8(3):227-230, 1985.

83. Wolock I et al: The posthospital needs and care of patients: implications for discharge planning, Soc Work Health 12(4):61-76, 1987.

84. Wood J: Labors of love: what will you do when it's your turn to take care of a loved one? Mod Maturity 30(4):28-34, 90-94, 1987.

85. Wright L and Leahey M: Families and chronic illness, Springhouse, Pa, 1987, Springhouse Corp.

86. Zappacosta A and Peras S: CAPD: continuous Ambulatory Peritoneal Dialysis, Philadelphia, 1984, JB Lippincott Co.

87. *Zarle NC: Continuity of care: balancing care of elders between health care settings, Nurs Clin N Am 24:697-706, 1989

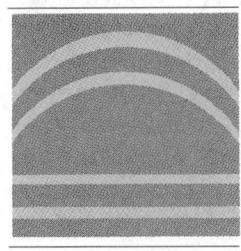

CHAPTER 79

Emergencies and Disasters in the Community

BARBARA C. LONG

CHAPTER OBJECTIVES

After studying this chapter, the student should be able to:
1 Describe the nature of the delivery of emergency care.
2 Describe preventive methods for accidents.
3 Describe parameters of assessment of the injured or unconscious person.
4 Identify principles of general management and specific care for accidental injuries or sudden illness (cardiopulmonary problems, hemorrhage, musculoskeletal/organ injuries, bites, poisoning, and environmental injuries).
5 Discuss the nature of sexual assault and appropriate interventions.
6 Describe the effects of disasters and appropriate roles of the nurse during disasters.

Nurses are frequently called on to provide emergency care in the community or in settings where medical help is not immediately available; therefore all nurses need to know the basics of emergency care. Nurses whose primary focus is the delivery of emergency care in specialized settings such as the hospital emergency care department require additional knowledge and skills that are beyond the scope of this chapter. There are a number of texts available that deal with this topic alone (see references). The purpose of this chapter is to identify major points in the delivery of emergency care in the community, in assessment and intervention for common emergencies, and in principles of management in disasters.

EPIDEMIOLOGY

Accidents are the leading cause of death in the 1- to 44-year-old age-group and the third leading cause of death in the 45- to 64- year-old group. Although the number of accidental deaths have been steadily decreasing in the United States in recent years (Table 79-1), over 90,000 people still die yearly in the United States from accidental deaths.[62] The largest number of deaths are

from motor vehicle accidents. Most permanent disabilities result from motor vehicle accidents, but most temporary disabilities result from home accidents. Falls are a major problem in the elderly population. Disabilities may lead to serious financial losses.

Accidents that result in injury or death involve human suffering that cannot be measured in dollars that includes pain, long-term rehabilitation, disabilities (temporary or permanent), loss and grief, and family disruption. Accidents are for the most part preventable and require that health care professionals be aware not only of their causes and the environment in which they occur, but also the victim's physical, social, and psychologic state and readiness to avoid accidents.

DELIVERY OF EMERGENCY CARE

Health crises that demand immediate interventions can occur anywhere—in the home, in other parts of the community, or in the hospital itself. The nurse may be the sole giver of care until medical care is available, or the nurse may be working with other paramedical personnel.

COMMUNITY

Available emergency medical services (EMS) vary among communities. In 1966 the National Highway Safety Act authorized the Department of Transportation to establish EMS guidelines. This Act requires each county to appoint an emergency medical care committee. The effectiveness of these committees varies greatly, influenced to a large extent by citizen interest and political activity. Every community needs an organized emergency care system, with support and input from community health organizations and community political elements. Once an organization is established, there should be continued evaluation of the effectiveness of the emergency care provided. Nurses should become actively involved in all phases of activities that can

TABLE 79-1 Accidental deaths in the United States (1970-1985) (in Thousands)

Type	1970	1980	1985
Transportation			
Motor vehicle	54.6	53.2	45.9
Water transport	1.7	1.4	1.1
Air transport	1.6	1.5	1.4
Accidental falls	16.9	13.2	12.0
Fires	6.7	5.8	4.9
Drowning	6.4	6.0	4.4
Poisoning	5.3	4.3	4.1
Firearms	2.4	2.0	1.6
Electric current	1.1	1.1	0.8

Data from Statistical Abstracts of the United States, 1988, ed 108, US Bureau of the Census, Washington, DC, 1988, US Government Printing Office.

influence the level of emergency care in their own communities.

Quality of emergency care in communities varies, depending on the preparation of persons providing the care and available resources such as trauma centers. There must also be an adequate system for obtaining care as rapidly as possible. Many communities have a 911-system by which persons have immediate access to an emergency dispatch center by dialing 911. Communities that do not have this system usually place the number to call on the first page of the telephone directory.

EMERGENCY PERSONNEL

Many communities in the United States now have prepared personnel who respond to emergency calls. These persons may be associated with fire or police departments or with a separate community or private EMS. There are two levels of emergency medical personnel, emergency medical technicians (EMTs) and paramedics. *EMTs* have had preparation beyond basic first aid training but do not carry out invasive procedures. *Paramedics* have had more training than EMTs and can carry out such tasks as starting intravenous fluids, giving medications, defibrillation, and intubation. Many emergency departments have direct radio communication with rescue personnel in the community. Treatment can be initiated at the site of injury under medical direction, and hospital personnel can be better prepared to receive the injured.

The American Heart Association has developed a program to educate large numbers of persons who are certified to administer cardiopulmonary resuscitation (CPR). This increases the possibility of a trained person being available to initiate resuscitation early in a larger number of emergency situations.

MEDICAL CENTER

In many emergency departments, more than half of the persons seeking medical attention are not actually in need of emergency care. These are persons who do not have a private physician or are unable to obtain the services of their physician at the hour or day when they feel they need medical attention. Persons requiring immediate care are treated first. If there is a large number of patients, those with nonacute symptoms often have to wait for a considerable time.

Urgent Care Centers have been instituted in many communities for persons requiring (or desiring) immediate medical care. Some hospitals have developed walk-in clinics with extended hours to provide additional, nonacute health care opportunities and to decrease the number of persons requiring nonacute care in emergency rooms.

Selected hospitals in the United States have been designated as *trauma receiving centers* according to guidelines established by the American College of Surgeons Committee on Trauma (ASCOT). Special trauma centers, such as for burns or spinal cord injury, have also been established. This regionalization of specific services provides quality care by experienced practitioners and decreases costs of duplication of services.

Nurses who work in a hospital emergency department or in a trauma center need specific skills in assessment and *triage* (sorting patients to determine priority of need for medical attention), in management of persons with high levels of anxiety, and in carrying out specialized technical skills such as initiating parenteral fluids, defibrillation, resuscitation and intubation; operating monitoring devices; interpreting selected laboratory findings and ECGs; and acting on these findings.

LEGAL ASPECTS OF EMERGENCY CARE

Nurses who intervene to assist victims in an emergency situation should be aware of the legal ramifications that can ensue as a result of their actions. Many states have enacted "Good Samaritan" laws in an effort to protect health personnel who aid accident victims. These laws vary in coverage among states as to the classes of people who are protected from liability, types of situations, geographic limits, and extent of immunity.[52] The classification of persons covered varies in specificity from any person who stops at the scene of an accident to only those registered nurses licensed in that state. Thus, in the latter situation, giving nursing care in an emergency situation could be construed in that state as practicing nursing without a license. One state (Vermont) allows criminal penalties for failure to stop and give assistance, although the victim cannot sue if the nurse fails to stop.

Good Samaritan laws serve to identify in statutory language those persons or situations that provide some degree of immunity from liability, many of which already exist by common law. Persons are judged as not liable unless they act willfully with gross negligence.[52] Negligence is the key word. Negligence, according to common law, involves four concepts: duty, breach of duty, damage, and proximate cause.[52] In an emergency a nurse is not duty bound to stop and render aid (except in Vermont) unless the nurse was the cause of the accident. The moral issue of whether to stop and render aid is the nurse's decision. If the nurse does render aid, then duty is implied and failure to continue rendering aid until the victim is released to another competent person can result in breach of duty (abandonment). Some Good Samaritan laws permit releasing the care of the victim to a qualified ambulance attendant (EMT). Damage must occur if negligence is to be proved, and the actions of the nurse must be the proximal cause of the damage.

"Reasonable care" provided by the nurse at the scene of an accident is usually judged as that care given by another similar nurse *under the prevailing situation.* Thus the care provided on a back road on a dark rainy night would not be judged the same as that given in an emergency room. In an emergency situation a nurse can perform medical acts to save life. It may be necessary later, however, to prove that a true emergency did exist. Good Samaritan laws will not protect the nurse in this situation.[52] Malpractice and liability claims can be filed even if Good Samaritan laws exist.

Nurses who work in hospital emergency departments need to be aware of legal implications of care provided in that setting, such as care to minors when parents are not present to give consent and actions that may be taken in helping police officers gather evidence.[58]

PREVENTION OF ACCIDENTS

Accident prevention is a major public health goal, and both the Public Health Service and the American Public Health Association (APHA) are active in promoting accident prevention. Community groups can be helpful in investigating accident statistics in their local area and in disseminating information to encourage accident prevention. Nurses have an important role in accident prevention, both through their roles as professionals and as residents of a community. The influence of nurses can be extended into many areas, because nurses are represented in schools, industry, community nursing programs, and hospitals.

There are a number of resources for information concerning accident prevention. The *Statistical Abstracts* published by the U.S. Bureau of the Census is a helpful reference. Local health departments can provide local data, health education materials, and other resource materials. Engineers can be a valuable resource for con-

---

HOME SAFETY FEATURES FOR ELDERLY PERSONS

Floors	Large rugs and carpets anchored
	Small rugs with nonskid backing
	Avoidance of floor wax (unless nonskid)
Stairs	Uniform height
	Nonskid treads
	Risers marked with contrasting color
	Strong handrails
	Adequate lighting
Bathroom	Handrail at tub or shower
	Skid-proof bath mats
	Treads in tub or on shower floor
	Seat in shower

---

sultation on safety hazards in the home, hospital, or community.

Many injuries are associated with alcohol or drugs. Measures to encourage decreased use of these substances would decrease the incidence of trauma.

HOME

Accidents in and about the home cause almost one fourth of all accidental deaths each year. Falls account for about half the number, and fires and poisonings account for most of the remainder. Many aged persons who fall do so when walking from room to room. Some fall because of heavily waxed floors, loose rugs, poor lighting, scattered toys, and other conditions that could have been corrected (see the box above). People fall from roofs, windows, high ladders, and steps and are fatally burned or otherwise injured while using solvents and cleansing agents without proper knowledge of their hazards.

The number of electric appliances used in the home has increased the danger of electric shock and fire from overloaded circuits. Many persons die in fires caused by burning cigarette ashes dropped on furniture or rugs or discarded in the waste containers and by cigarettes that are dropped as the smoker falls asleep. Attention needs to be given to teaching homeowners with older heating systems to have the equipment checked periodically for gas leaks and other unsafe features. All persons in a household should be aware of what to do in the event of fire, and fire evacuation drills are encouraged. Homes should be equipped with smoke alarms in strategic places such as the kitchen, bedrooms, hallways, and basement.

The community health nurse has an opportunity to assess safety hazards during home visits and to teach not only the client, but also members of the family about general accident prevention as well as specific measures for the safety of the ill person.

COMMUNITY

Community action can best be effected by group action, but it often takes persistent individuals to interest and stimulate group action. Parent-teacher associations, recreational associations, and religious and social groups are usually interested in accident control. Support by governmental groups is important. Efforts should be made to work with existing agencies and groups so that the sincere efforts of small groups of enthusiastic citizens will not be dissipated. Phases of accident prevention that should be of community interest include (1) teaching of accident prevention in the public schools, (2) better control and inspection of homes for the aged and prisons, (3) rigid enforcement of driving regulations, (4) improvement of street lighting and traffic signals at busy intersections, (5) periodic inspection of all automobiles, and (6) promotion of laws pertaining to fireproofing of buildings and laws protecting the public from flammable clothing, potentially harmful toys, and similar items.

HOSPITAL

Assessing the need for safety in the general environment and for the safety of specific patients and taking measures to pervent injury are important functions of the nurse. The nurse can participate in policymaking and safety monitoring through membership on hospital safety committees.

FALLS

The major cause of hospital-incurred injury is falling. Hospitalized persons are in unfamiliar surroundings with strange furniture and equipment, may be weak for many reasons, or may become confused, all of which may contribute to falls. Elderly persons are at high risk for falls. All patients should be assessed for the potential of falling, and preventive measures should be instituted (see the box below).

Elderly persons often become confused at night, a time when sensory input is decreased. Sedation may increase the confusion. A night-light in the room can be useful for sensory input. The bed should be in low position; in the event that the patient attempts to climb out

---

HOSPITAL SAFETY MEASURES TO PREVENT FALLS

1. Handrails in hospital corridors
2. Armchairs at bedside
3. Chairs in bathroom or showers
4. Call systems in bathrooms and lounges
5. Beds placed in low position when patient ambulating
6. Night-lights in patient rooms (especially for elderly patients)

---

of bed, the bed will be at the same height as the bed at home. The use of the side rails is a nursing decision. Side rails should be kept raised for all unconscious patients. A confused patient may attempt to climb over the side rail and thus have farther to fall; a jacket restraint may be more useful.

Patients who are weak may need frequent reminders to seek assistance before ambulating. Some patients do not want to "bother the nurse" and attempt to walk to the bathroom unaided, especially at night.

FIRE

All hospitals and nursing homes must have established fire prevention routines, and all personnel must be familiar with these routines. Participation in fire drills should be taken seriously, and evaluation should follow each drill.

Fires usually occur from smoking or faulty electrical equipment. Since smoking is also hazardous to one's health, many hospitals are restricting smoking in patients' rooms and in many public areas. If smoking is permitted in the patient's room, ashtrays should be available, and the patient and visitors instructed about not emptying them. Patients who are careless smokers or who may drop a cigarette or ash are to be monitored while smoking. Faulty electrical equipment is not used. Any signs of smoke should be investigated and reported immediately.

If a fire should occur, the nurse in charge who is most familiar with the patients' conditions should be in charge of any evacuation. Until evacuation is necessary, the doors and windows of all patient rooms are closed. If evacuation is deemed advisable, patients closest to the fire are evacuated to the opposite end of the floor (horizontal evacuation), then downward by the stairway (vertical evacuation) if necessary. Death usually occurs from inhaling the smoke. Doors that are excessively hot should not be opened. The rescuer should keep as low as possible and, if necessary, use wet cloths around the nose and mouth if the air is hot.

ASSESSMENT

When an emergency occurs or on arriving at the emergency scene, it is important to assess the situation, the patient, and the environment before initiating action. Some conclusions can be drawn from the immediate environment. If there is trauma to multiple victims, all victims should be assessed before any but lifesaving interventions are initiated. Overt clues such as an automobile accident, report of falling, or ingestion of poison can give direction to probable types of injuries. A complete head-to-toe assessment is carried out, if possible, before moving the victim so that additional injuries or conditions requiring intervention can be identified.

PRIORITY ASSESSMENT

AIRWAY

Presence of respirations
Presence of foreign body, vomitus, loose dentures in
  mouth

BREATHING

Respiration rate, depth, character
Use of accessory muscles for breathing
Tracheal deviation

CIRCULATION

Presence of carotid pulse
Pulse rate, strength, rhythm
Presence of hemorrhage
Skin color, temperature, moisture

LEVEL OF CONSCIOUSNESS

Response to voice and touch (or painful stimulus)
Pupillary response
If unconscious, presence of Medic-Alert tag

DATA COLLECTION

A person who is not breathing, who has no palpable
pulse, or who is hemorrhaging needs immediate assistance. Obtaining data to identify these circumstances is
the first priority in assessment (see the box above). This
is sometimes referred to as the ABCs of emergency assessment (*airway, breathing, circulation*). Assessing the
general level of consciousness can be done as the approach is made to the victim. The carotid pulse can be
checked at the same time as breathing is checked. If
pulse and breathing are absent, CPR is initiated (see
Chapter 27). Hemorrhage is treated with direct pressure
to the wound.

Before starting the head-to-toe assessment (see the
box above right), observe the victim's general position,
any obvious deformities or asymmetry, or any purposeful movements. Ask the person to indicate any pain or
discomfort and assess these areas first. During the overall assessment continue to monitor for changes in level
of consciousness and respiratory status. Ask the victim
or any relatives or friends present to describe the preceding events; the presence of any medical conditions
such as heart or lung disease, epilepsy, or diabetes; or
any special medications taken by the victim that may
have a bearing on the present situation.

If there is more than one person on the scene, the
nurse or paramedic should remain with the victim while
others are given directions to assess the environment for
additional signs of danger and to call for any needed
transportation.

HEAD-TO-TOE ASSESSMENT

HEAD AND NECK

Assess airway
Assess pupils
Examine ears, nose, mouth for bleeding, other drainage,
  foreign body
Palpate* cervical spine for pain (do not move head)
Examine head for bleeding, lacerations, contusions, de-
  pression of skull
Palpate jaw for fracture (pain, deformity)
Ask about stiffness of neck (if no history of trauma, assess
  movement)
Examine neck for distended neck veins, presence of tra-
  cheal stoma, tracheal deviation

CHEST AND SPINE

Observe chest movements for symmetry of expansion and
  character of respirations
Palpate clavicles for fracture (pain, deformity)
Examine chest for external injury
Palpate ribs for fracture (pain)
Palpate spine for point tenderness (do not move victim)

ABDOMEN AND PELVIS

Palpate pelvis for pain in groin when pressure applied over
  pelvis
Ask about abdominal pain
Examine abdomen for external injury, rigidity, distention,
  penetrating objects

EXTREMITIES

Examine for signs of external injury
Ask about pain in extremities
If there is no obvious injury, ask victim to move each limb
Test for sensation in each limb
Assess presence and strength of peripheral pulses

*All palpations should be carried out gently.

DATA ANALYSIS
LEVEL OF CONSCIOUSNESS

Determine whether the person responds immediately to
voice and touch, responds only to painful stimuli, or
does not respond. Unconsciousness may have many
causes (see the box on p. 2282).

When *shock* or *respiratory insufficiency* occurs,
there is decreased oxygenation of the brain, either because there is an insufficient amount of blood to carry
the oxygen or because there is decreased oxygen taken
in. This can lead to loss of consciousness, and the *pupils will be equal and may be dilated*. (Normally, 20% of
the population have slight differences in pupil size but
both pupils react equally to light.)

When unconsciousness occurs because of the effect
of *drugs or chemicals*, the pupils are *equal* and may be
constricted or dilated, depending on the effect of the
specific drug. Information from relatives may elicit data

POSSIBLE CAUSES OF UNCONSCIOUSNESS

1. Hypoxia (decreased oxygen to brain)
   a. Respiratory insufficiency
      (1) Airway obstruction from foreign body, secretions
      (2) Pneumothorax
      (3) Spinal cord injury
   b. Shock
      (1) Cardiogenic cardiac arrest
      (2) Hypovolemic hemorrhage
2. Metabolic (chemical brain depressants)
   a. Extrinsic
      (1) Drugs: alcohol, narcotics, barbiturates, antihistamines, tranquilizers
      (2) Poisons: carbon monoxide, carbon tetrachloride, hydrocarbons, methane gas
   b. Intrinsic
      (1) Ketones: diabetic ketoacidosis, starvation
      (2) Glucose: hypoglycemia, hyperglycemia
      (3) Ammonia: liver failure
      (4) Urea: kidney failure
      (5) Hormonal hypofunction: hypothyroidism, Addison's disease
      (6) Electrolyte imbalance: sodium, potassium, calcium, hydrogen ions
3. Brain pathologic conditions
   a. Trauma: concussion, brain stem contusion, intracranial hematoma
   b. Seizures: epilepsy, tumors, idiopathology
   c. Cerebrovascular accident: cerebral hemorrhage, thrombosis
   d. Tumors: benign, malignant
   e. Infections: meningitis, encephalitis

---

concerning history of diabetes, liver or kidney disease, and medication taken by the victim. Environmental data such as an empty pill container can be useful in the identification of unconsciousness caused by drug overdose.

If there has been *trauma to the brain,* it is important to ascertain level of consciousness at different times. Temporary loss of consciousness followed by alertness and *equal pupils* usually indicates a *concussion.* If there is no skull fracture present, the patient is simply observed for 24 hours. Alertness after injury followed by increasing loss of consciousness usually indicates an *intracranial hematoma.* The pupils are usually *unequal.* Medical attention is urgent if an intracranial hematoma is suspected. The pupils *may also be unequal* if the patient has had a *cerebrovascular accident* (stroke).

An unconscious person should be placed in a position that facilitates patency of the airway (side-lying position is preferred unless contraindicated), and the respiratory status should be constantly monitored (see Chapter 60).

RESPIRATIONS

The rate, depth, and character of respirations provide clues to the presence of ventilatory, CNS, or metabolic

SIGNS OF SHOCK

Mild	Skin pale, cool, clammy
	Possible postural changes in pulse and blood pressure
	Person states feeling cold
Moderate	Increased diaphresis and pallor
	Pulse may be rapid, and blood pressure may decrease
	Thirst
Severe	Pulse rapid, weak, sometimes irregular
	Blood pressure low
	Respirations deep and rapid
	Agitation, disorientation

---

problems. Most trauma victims breathe a little faster than normal (18 to 24/min). If the person shows signs of respiratory effort (nasal flaring; suprasternal, intercostal, or substernal retractions), the airway may be partially obstructed. The type of noise accompanying respirations may indicate the degree and location of a partial obstruction. The following findings are suggestive of specific emergency care problems:

1. Rate
   a. Slow (below 10/min): ventilatory or CNS problems
   b. Rapid (above 26/min): hypoxia, acidosis, shock
2. Depth
   a. Shallow: shock, chest pain
   b. Deep: hypoxia, hypoglycemia, metabolic acidosis
3. Sounds
   a. Inspiratory stridor: upper airway obstruction (above tracheal bifurcation)
   b. Expiratory wheezes or stridor: lower airway obstruction
4. Frothy, blood-tinged sputum: lung injury, pulmonary edema, pulmonary embolus

SHOCK

Persons who sustain major trauma or a major stressor to the system such as a myocardial infarction usually develop shock (hypovolemic, cardiogenic). Signs of shock vary depending on the severity of the shock (see the box above). With cardiogenic shock, the neck veins may be distended. Persons with severe shock may display behavior that is incorrectly labeled as uncooperative or intoxicated. (Shock is discussed in detail in Chapter 25.)

With anaphylactic shock such as may occur after an insect sting, the victim may complain of itching or burning of the skin, a tightness in the chest, and difficulty in breathing. Wheals may develop on the skin, and the face and tongue may develop edema (see Chapter 76).

SENSATION

Trauma may result in *pain* if there is soft tissue injury, fracture, or visceral damage. Pain may also occur with tissue anoxia such as with obstruction of blood vessels or frostbite. Data are obtained from the patient concerning location (region), severity, quality, onset and duration, and provoking factors. One suggested approach for evaluating these parameters is the use of the mnemonic PQRST[58].

P Provoking factors: what makes the pain worse or relieves it
Q Quality: dull, sharp, crushing, etc.
R Region or radiation: site and radiation to other areas
S Severity (on a scale of 1 to 10, where 1 is no pain and 10 is the worst imaginable pain)
T Time: onset, duration, constancy

For a further discussion of pain, see Chapter 16.

Loss of sensation may result from injury to peripheral nerves or injury to nerves in the CNS. Peripheral nerve injuries may occur with fractures, lacerations, penetrating wounds, or dislocations. Loss of sensation concurrent with loss of movement and absence of local tissue or bone injury indicates CNS injury, such as spinal cord injury or cerebral hemorrhage.

OTHER DATA

Analysis of the data should include the type of injury or medical emergency that has probably occurred, the urgency of the need for medical attention, the availability of resources for carrying out necessary interventions, the availability of transportation, and the time factor before medical attention can be obtained. For example, the type of interventions for someone with a fractured tibia when splints are available and an ambulance is standing by for transportation to a nearby hospital may be quite different than if the same injury occurs during a wilderness hiking expedition.

GENERAL INTERVENTIONS

PRINCIPLES OF MANAGEMENT

Some general principles of management when accidental injuries or sudden illnesses occur serve as guidelines when giving first aid:

1. Remain calm and think before acting.
2. Identify oneself as a nurse to victim and bystanders.
3. Do a rapid assessment for *priority* data (cessation of breathing or heartbeat, interference with breathing, hemorrhage, coma, poisoning).
4. Carry out lifesaving measures as indicated by the priority assessment.
5. Do a head-to-toe assessment before initiating *general* first aid measures.
6. Keep the victim lying down or in the position in which he or she is found (unless orthopnea is present), protected from dampness or cold.
7. If victim is conscious, explain what is occurring. Assure him or her that help will be given.
8. Avoid unnecessary handling or moving of the victim; move the victim only if danger is present.
9. Do not give fluids if there is a possibility of abdominal injury or if anesthesia will be necessary within a short time.
10. Do not transport the victim until all first aid measures have been carried out and appropriate transportation is available.

Lifesaving measures (described on succeeding pages) are carried out first when the initial assessment indicates the presence of breathing or circulatory difficulties. After breathing has been reestablished and excessive bleeding controlled, other interventions are carried out when the head-to-toe assessment is completed.

The victim is kept in a supine or sitting position, depending on symptoms, until all necessary interventions are carried out. Wounds are covered and fractures splinted before the victim is transported. Since shock is a possibility when major injuries occur, the victim should be protected from chilling. On a cold day, protection may be needed underneath the victim, with sufficient covering to prevent loss of body heat but not cause vasodilation. Oral fluids are given only to a conscious person showing signs of shock if there will be a considerable delay before medical care can be obtained and if abdominal injury is not present.

PSYCHOLOGIC NEEDS OF VICTIMS AND SIGNIFICANT OTHERS

Trauma produces anxiety. It may be perceived by the victim as life-threatening and a source of pain and disability. The person may be unsure of what is happening, leading to a fear of the unknown. There may be concern about economic problems such as the cost of medical care and loss of time from work. In addition, many persons have been found to have already been experiencing some other temporary anxiety and were under stress immediately before the time of the accident.

The very nature of the experiences after the emergency contribute additional anxieties. The victim is transported, perhaps by strangers, in an ambulance to a hospital ED. Significant others are relegated to long periods in a waiting room with little information provided. Victims see or hear other persons who are upset. They may be alone. They may wait for long periods for medical attention and results of tests or treatment, whereas other higher-priority victims are receiving care. Small incidents become blown out of proportion, and a casual remark may be misinterpreted. Five minutes can seem like an hour.

Health personnel who work with accident victims

from the primary point of input into the health care system until the emergency is over are prepared to meet the physical life-threatening needs. Because these needs assume priority, it is easy to overlook the psychologic needs of the victim and significant others. A calm, interested approach that conveys concern to the victim as a person is helpful. Giving information frequently during all phases of emergency care to both victim and significant others will help them understand what is occurring and that help is being provided, thus decreasing some of the anxiety.

Varying levels of tolerance to stress are found in different individuals. Highly anxious persons may need someone to stay with them. At the scene of an accident a calm bystander can be helpful. Some hospitals provide selected volunteers for that purpose. All health personnel need to evaluate frequently their own effectiveness in assessing anxiety and in conveying understanding and emotional support to the victim and significant others during an emergency.

MULTIPLE TRAUMA

Multiple trauma, injury to two or more body systems, occurs with severe injuries (see the box below). In motor vehicle accidents the head is injured 80% of the time, legs 40%, chest 25%, and abdomen 15%.[59] Falls from great heights often cause multiple fractures (for example, legs, hips, spine, pelvis, base of skull). Penetrating chest wounds may also involve abdominal organs. Victims of multiple trauma require rapid stabilization at the accident site followed by immediate transfer to an emergency room.

Persons with severe injuries require intravenous fluids initiated as soon as possible to prevent shock. These fluids may be started by paramedics at the accident site. In the emergency room, two or three large-bore intravenous catheters are placed by cutdown for administration of drugs and fluids. If the patient is already in shock, a central venous line is also initiated. An indwelling catheter is inserted to monitor urinary output.

Major injuries that require immediate surgery to control bleeding and prevent irreversible shock include penetrating wounds of the heart and abdominal wounds involving the aorta and vena cava.[65] If bleeding of other wounds is controlled and fluids have been started, surgery can be delayed until tests and initial treatments have been completed.

Treatment of one system may add to the problems of another injured system. For example, large amounts of fluid given to prevent or alter renal problems may compromise an inadequate ventilatory system, leading to failure of both systems. The care of accident victims with severe injuries is complex and requires high quality medical and nursing care by specialized practitioners in both emergency rooms and ICUs.

CARDIOPULMONARY PROBLEMS

For life to be maintained, oxygen must be taken in by the lungs and pumped to the tissues; carbon dioxide must be returned from the tissues to the lung and exhaled. Thus any obstruction that interferes with the diffusion of these gases, failure of the heart as a pump, or inadequate blood to carry the oxygen to the tissues is a threat to life and demands immediate emergency intervention. Airway patency, breathing facilitation, and circulation maintenance are the ABCs of emergency care and take first priority in assessment and intervention.

AIRWAY OBSTRUCTION AND BREATHING DIFFICULTIES

Asphyxia is severe hypoxia leading to unconsciousness and possible death if the condition is not corrected. It may be caused by inadequate oxygen in the environment, obstruction of or secretions in air passages, or interferences with respiration or circulation (see the box on p. 2285).

ASSESSMENT

Pupils that constrict when exposed to light indicate adequate oxygenation of the brain. This will not occur with some drugs or in some elderly persons.

Signs of hypoxia are related to the efforts made by the victim to take in air. As the anoxic condition persists, signs of decreased oxygenation to tissue occur. The person with asphyxia will be dyspneic. Neck muscles will be prominent, but little or no air may be moving in or out of the nose and mouth. Intercostal rib retractions will occur as the intercostal muscles pull against resistance. If the passageway is not totally blocked, respirations will be noisy, and wheezing or stridor may be heard as the air moves through the narrowed passageway. As less oxygen is taken in, skin color will become first pale and then eventually cyanotic (grayish blue). This can be observed first in mucous membranes, lips, and nail beds.

If an open chest wound is present, a sucking noise may be heard with inspiration. The chest should be inspected for signs of bleeding or a wound. Paradoxical chest movement is denoted by the fact that the chest

---

SEVERE INJURIES OFTEN CAUSING MULTIPLE TRAUMA

Crushing and penetrating chest injuries
Crushing pelvic injuries
Spinal cord injuries
Multiple bone or soft tissue injuries
Injuries causing hemorrhage with shock
Head injuries with decreasing level of consciousness

CAUSES OF ASPHYXIA OTHER THAN DISEASE

INADEQUATE OXYGEN IN ENVIRONMENT
Smoke
Toxic gases

OBSTRUCTION OF AIR PASSAGES
Foreign bodies in airway
Tongue falling back in pharynx
Edema of respiratory tissue
Laryngospasm

SECRETIONS IN AIR PASSAGES
Near-drowning
Pulmonary edema

INTERFERENCES WITH RESPIRATIONS
Chest trauma
Depression of respiratory center (drugs)

INTERFERENCES WITH CIRCULATION
Electric shock
Myocardial infarction
Carbon monoxide poisoning

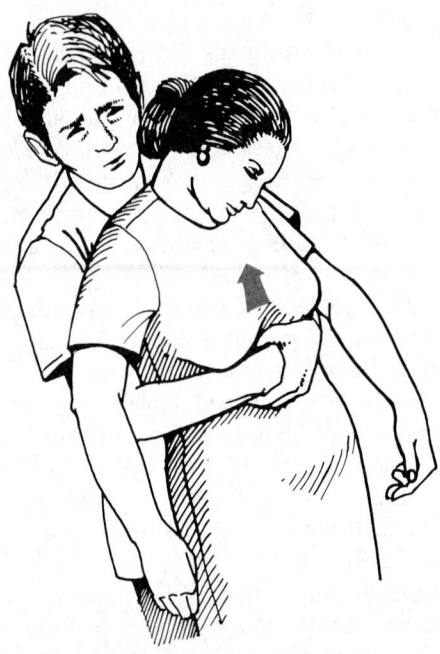

FIGURE 79-1 Heimlich abdominal thrust maneuver. Rescuer places fist between umbilicus and xiphoid process with the thumb pressed against the abdomen. Pressure is applied upward.

cage at the site of fractures moves in the direction opposite from normal during inspiration and expiration. Noisy respirations, rales, or rhonchi may be heard with auscultation if fluid is present in the alveoli. Excess fluid may be coughed up; secretions will be mucoid with infection, watery and frothy or blood tinged with pulmonary edema. Dyspnea will be present.

Depression of the respiratory center will be evidenced by bradycardia and slow shallow respirations. In respiratory arrest, breathing ceases completely.

INTERVENTIONS

Open Airway

A *conscious* victim may need assistance to facilitate *removal of a foreign body* obstructing the airway. The Heimlich abdominal thrust maneuver (Figure 79-1) may be used to attempt removal of the obstructing material. The rescuer stands behind the victim encircling one arm around the victim's waist. The rescuer then places a fist between the umbilicus and the xiphoid process with the thumb against the abdomen. The fist is grasped with the other hand and pressed into the abdomen with quick upward thrusts. Unless it is known positively that there is a foreign body obstructing the trachea, time should not be wasted examining for one.

If the person is *unconscious*, the neck may be observed to be in a position of flexion with the back of the tongue obstructing the airway (see Figure 22-11). The jaw can be pulled forward while the neck remains in a stable position to pull the back of the tongue away from the pharynx. Sometimes this maneuver alone may be

enough to open the airway. If the jaw maneuver does not initiate breathing, artificial ventilation must be initiated immediately (see Chapter 27).

Cardiopulmonary Resuscitation

With the absence of both breathing and heartbeat, CPR is initiated (see Chapter 27). All nurses, no matter where they work, should be certified by the American Heart Association in all phases of CPR. All nurses and physicians who work in emergency departments should be trained and certified in Basic and Advanced Life Support. Advanced Life Support includes endotracheal intubation, cardiac monitoring, defibrillation, initiating and maintaining intravenous infusions, and administering intravenous medications.

Oxygen

Supplemental oxygen is given after breathing resumes to treat the resultant hypoxemia. Oxygen is also given for other types of hypoxemia after trauma or stress such as smoke inhalation, carbon monoxide poisoning, near-drowning, or myocardial infarction. Oxygen is given after all major trauma, especially chest injuries.

MYOCARDIAL INFARCTION

Myocardial infarction must be considered in persons who experience sudden onset of chest pain without precipitating factors. The quality of the substernal chest pain varies among individuals but is usually described as "squeezing," "crushing," or "heavy" and may radiate to the arms, jaw, or neck. The pain may also be mild and described as "indigestion." The pain of myocardial infarction is not relieved by rest or by nitroglycerin. The person may be apprehensive and experience diaphoresis, nausea and vomiting, lightheadedness, and dyspnea.

Over half of the deaths caused by myocardial infarction occur before the person is admitted to the hospital and within 2 hours after onset of symptoms.[61] Some communities have established mobile coronary units that respond immediately in these situations with advanced life-support systems. In the absence of such a unit the victim needs immediate safe transport to a medical center. If the heart ceases to beat, CPR is instituted immediately.

The conscious person may be more comfortable in a well-supported sitting position. Oxygen is given, if available. A calm atmosphere is of utmost importance, and the person should never be left alone. Fear adds an additional stress to the already overburdened heart. (Myocardial infarction is discussed in detail in Chapter 28.)

NEAR-DROWNING

Drowning is the fourth leading cause of accidental death in the United States.[56] Many of these drownings occur in home swimming pools. *Near-drowning* is the term that refers to asphyxiation or partial asphyxiation from a fluid medium, with the person either recovering spontaneously or resuscitated at least temporarily. There are three types of drowning: wet, dry, and secondary.[58] *Wet* drowning is the most common type and refers to asphyxiation from the aspiration of fluid into the lungs, inhaled as the person panics and gasps for breath. *Dry* drowning refers to asphyxiation from laryngospasm that prevents both air and water from entering the lungs. *Secondary* drowning is the recurrence of respiratory distress after recovery from the initial incident.[58] This may occur from a few minutes to several days later.

The effect of water aspirated into the lungs depends on the amount and type of water. Saltwater produces more severe changes than does freshwater. Freshwater is rapidly absorbed into the circulation, causing temporary hypervolemia, hemodilution, and intravascular hemolysis. Saltwater, because of its hypertonicity, pulls fluids into the alveoli, causing persistent hypovolemia with hemoconcentration and pulmonary edema. Asphyxiation results in arterial hypoxemia and metabolic acidosis (from excess lactic acid formation). Neurologic damage may result from prolonged hypoxemia and kidney damage from intravascular hemolysis.

If the victim of near-drowning has ceased breathing,

artificial ventilation (Chapter 27) is initiated as soon as possible, even before the victim has been completely removed from the water. If the carotid pulse is absent, cardiac resuscitation is started immediately. Time should not be wasted trying to remove water from the lungs. If swallowed water is distending the abdomen and interfering with adequate ventilation, the victim can be rolled onto the stomach and lifted with pressure over the stomach to force the water out. Persons who have experienced near-drowning need close observation for at least 24 hours, even if they indicate that they feel all right. Pulmonary edema can develop several hours later.

Immersion syndrome is death after submersion in very cold water. It is thought to be caused from dysrhythmias resulting from vagal stimulation.[55]

ELECTRICAL INJURIES

Electrical injuries often result from carelessness or from faulty equipment at home or in the working environment, from lightning, and from downed electrical wires after a storm. The extent of the injury from electricity depends on the point in the heartbeat cycle that is stimulated, the intensity of the current, and skin resistance. Moisture decreases skin resistance; therefore greater damage occurs when skin is moist with water or perspiration.

Electricity can cause injury in several ways:
1. Depression of the respiratory center (results in temporary or prolonged paralysis of respiration)
2. Ventricular fibrillation when the electric current passes through the heart at the end of the refractory period (can occur with a low current)
3. Tissue damage (devitalization of muscles and damage to blood vessels with subsequent tissue hypoxia)
4. Bone fractures from powerful muscle contractions as a result of the electric current

Burns with resultant tissue necrosis occur at both entrance and exit points. Externally, the burns usually appear as painless gray areas, sharply demarcated, round or oval, with inflammatory reaction.[56] The appearance may be deceiving; extensive tissue damage may be present within the tissues.

The victim must be removed from the source of electricity; the rescuer must be careful to avoid contact with the electric charge. If possible, the source of electricity must be turned off. If the victim has direct contact with the electricity, such as with a live wire, several approaches may be used:
1. Pull victim away by means of a rope of dry clothing or a leather belt.
2. Roll victim away by standing on a dry board and using a long dry stick or board.
3. Pull or push victim away using asbestos gloves.

If breathing and pulse are absent, cardiopulmonary resuscitation is started immediately and continued until breathing and circulation have returned or until 1 hour has passed with no response. Defibrillation is indicated for ventricular fibrillation. Fluid therapy is instituted, because considerable plasma can pass into extravascular compartments, resulting in hypovolemia. The patient is monitored for shock, secondary hemorrhage, acidosis, and myoglobinuria. Devitalized tissue may eventually require removal and grafting.

HEMORRHAGE

ETIOLOGY

As stated earlier, maintenance of an adequate blood flow to carry oxygen to the tissues is vital to support life. External bleeding can occur with lacerations, crushing injuries, amputations, fractures, and nosebleeds. Internal bleeding can occur with chest or abdominal trauma such as a ruptured spleen, trauma to large muscle masses of the extremity (thigh), or certain medical conditions such as esophageal varices or bleeding ulcers.

PATHOPHYSIOLOGY

When a blood vessel is severed, there is an immediate contraction of the vessel wall that reduces the size of the opening and decreases blood loss. Platelets begin to adhere to the roughened edges until a platelet plug is formed. A clot begins to form within 1 to 2 minutes. By 3 to 6 minutes that clot has filled the end of the blood vessel, blocking blood flow.[26] Direct pressure over a bleeding vessel for 5 to 6 minutes will help stop the blood flow to permit clot formation. If a major artery is severed, ligation (tying off) of the artery may be necessary for continued cessation of bleeding. Pressure (digital pressure or tourniquet) applied to an artery proximal to the wound may also slow or stop the blood flow. This also slows or stops blood perfusion to the tissue beyond the pressure point, producing tissue damage. Direct pressure over the bleeding vessel is therefore the action of choice unless bleeding cannot be controlled in this manner. Large arteries have musculature that can produce considerable vasospasms. Amputation of a leg, for example, may produce minimal bleeding. Veins and capillaries have thinner walls, and bleeding of these vessels can usually be controlled by direct pressure.

ASSESSMENT

External bleeding, if excessive, will saturate the clothing and be readily visible. If the person is wearing bulky outer garments, bleeding may be concealed. The examiner should run the hands quickly over the entire body under the outer clothing, being sure to check underneath the victim. Saturated clothing may need to be cut away to examine the area of bleeding. Three types of bleeding can be observed: spurting of bright red blood indicates arterial bleeding, continuous flow of darker blood indicates venous bleeding, and oozing indicates capillary bleeding. The scalp is very vascular, and considerable bleeding may occur from a small scalp laceration.

Internal bleeding may be difficult to identify. Bleeding into the thorax (hemothorax) may inhibit respirations, and chest pain may be present. Abdominal bleeding may be evidenced by rigidity of abdominal muscles and abdominal pain. Hemoptysis or hematemesis indicates internal bleeding.

Shock occurs with severe internal or external bleeding. The victim is assessed for weak rapid pulse, slow shallow respiration, cold clammy skin, anxiety, restlessness, and thirst. The pupils are equal, may be dilated, and respond slowly to light.

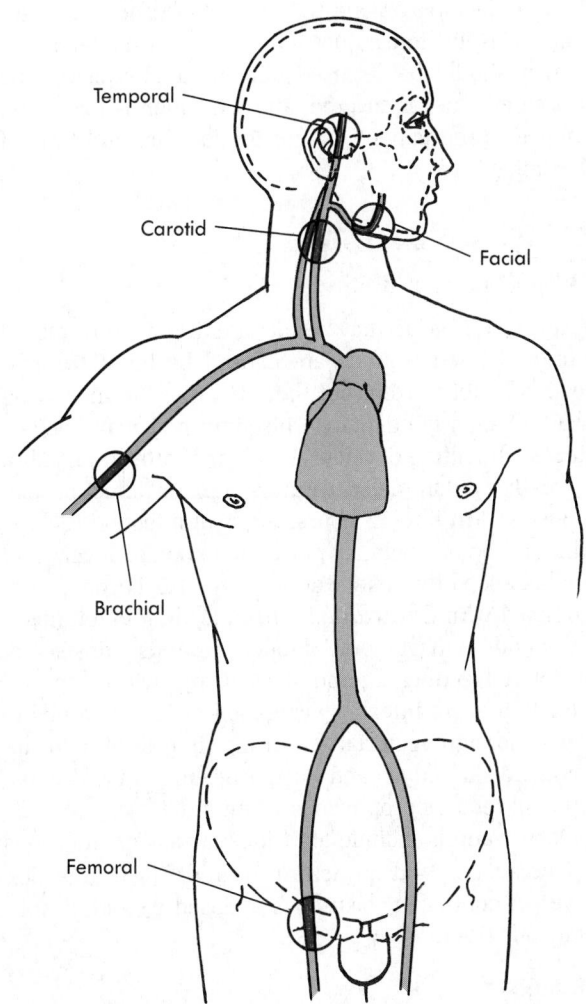

FIGURE 79-2 Pressure points: locations at which large blood vessels may be compressed against bone to help control hemorrhage.

INTERVENTIONS

Direct pressure is applied to the site of external bleeding. If a sterile dressing is not available, a clean handkerchief, sanitary pad, or clean cloth may be used. The dressing is held in place by a tight bandage for continued pressure. The bare hand can be used to apply direct pressure until an adequate dressing is available. If severe arterial bleeding cannot be controlled by direct pressure, or if direct pressure cannot be applied, pressure-point control over a bony prominence proximal to the point of hemorrhage can be attempted (Figure 79-2).

Tourniquets are *rarely* necessary, since they may cause further damage and can result in loss of an arm or leg. If a tourniquet must be used, it should be applied with the following precautions. A triangular bandage is folded at least 3 to 4 inches wide, six to eight layers thick, and wrapped twice around the extremity. A stick or similar object is tied on by the ends of the bandage and twisted to tighten the tourniquet just enough to stop the bleeding but no tighter. A blood pressure cuff makes a useful tourniquet. Once the tourniquet is applied, it should be released only by a physician. The tourniquet is never covered, and a notation is made and attached to the patient, giving the location and time of application.

MUSCULOSKELETAL/ORGAN INJURIES

SOFT-TISSUE INJURIES

Injury to soft tissue may result in either open or closed wounds. Closed wounds are caused by blunt trauma; the skin is not broken, but there is injury to underlying tissue. Open wounds cause bleeding and may become infected. Infection develops 1 to 2 days after injury, but in grossly contaminated wounds signs of infection can be observed in 8 to 12 hours. Signs of infection include redness, edema, pain, a purulent exudate, fever, and lymphadenopathy. The wound may also become contaminated with *Clostridium tetani,* leading to tetanus.

General management of open wounds consists of control of bleeding, thorough cleansing with soap and water to prevent infection, irrigation of deep wounds to remove foreign material, suturing (if possible) to approximate skin edges and hasten healing, and administration of tetanus prophylaxis when indicated.

Open wounds include abrasions, avulsions, incisions or lacerations, and puncture wounds (see the box above). A contusion (bruise) is a closed wound of subcutaneous tissue.

ABRASIONS

Abrasions commonly occur among active children and athletes and are frequently noted after motorcycle accidents. Only a partial thickness of the skin is involved.

TYPES OF WOUNDS

Abrasion	Scraping of skin surface ("brush burn")
Incision	Cut through skin and underlying tissue by a sharp object such as a knife
Laceration	Jagged cut through skin and underlying tissue usually by a blunt object
Puncture	Penetration of skin and underlying tissue by sharp-pointed object; skin quickly seals over when object is removed
Stab	Form of puncture wound by large object such as knife, stick, or piece of glass
Contusion	Injury by blunt object; skin is not broken; blood vessels rupture and blood seeps into tissue; edema occurs from trauma to injured cells

When a large area of skin has been denuded, an abrasion can be painful.

Good cleaning of the wound with soap and water is important to remove all pieces of embedded foreign matter that can delay healing and cause scarring. A topical antibiotic ointment such as Baciguent can be applied. If the wound can be kept clean, no covering is necessary.

AVULSIONS

Large skin flaps can be torn loose from any part of the body, especially the head and extremities. Avulsions must be cleaned thoroughly and irrigated well to remove any foreign material before they are sutured.

LACERATIONS/INCISIONS

Lacerations or incisions vary in depth and may involve muscles and tendons. The wound is cleansed well and sutured through each layer. Any gap left through non-approximation of the wound may delay healing. Incisions usually heal more quickly with less scar formation than lacerations, because the edges can be better approximated. Suturing should be carried out within the first few hours after injury to obtain maximal healing with fewer complications or scarring. If the wound is grossly contaminated, the decision may be made to delay suturing for a few days to permit thorough cleansing; healing then occurs by tertiary intention (see Chapter 22). Suturing may not be necessary for superficial lacerations; the edges of the wound can be approximated by one or more butterfly adhesive strips (Figure 79-3), or commercial Steri-Strips.

PUNCTURE WOUNDS

A puncture wound is caused by a sharp, pointed, narrow object such as a nail, pin, bullet, splinter of wood, or animal bite. As the tissues are penetrated by the object, pathogenic organisms may be introduced. Since

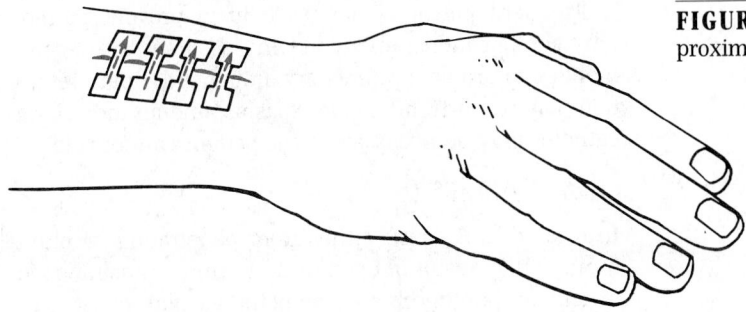

FIGURE 79-3 Butterfly adhesive strips may be used to approximate wound edges.

the skin quickly seals over, the wound rarely bleeds enough to wash out organisms. Bacteria such as *Clostridium tetani*, which thrive without air, may infect these wounds. Because anaerobic bacterial infections are extremely serious, a physician should be consulted if the puncture was made by a dirty object.

Puncture wounds received from objects such as contaminated needles used for any parenteral treatment also should be reported to the physician, since viral hepatitis or AIDS may be contracted from this type of injury. Immune serum globulin may be given as prophylaxis for hepatitis.

Puncture wounds are treated by soaks. A small amount of bleeding is encouraged in small puncture wounds to assist in washing out microorganisms. The wound should be observed for signs of infection. Prophylaxis against tetanus is instituted.

Impaled objects in *stab* wounds should *not* be removed except by a physician in a medical facility, usually in the operating room. If there is severe bleeding, pressure points may be used to control loss of blood. The object should be stabilized before transportation to prevent accidental dislodgement and further trauma.

CONTUSIONS

Blood vessels under the skin rupture with blunt trauma, and the blood seeps into the tissue creating a hematoma. The skin acquires a black-and-blue appearance from the extravasated blood. Nonpitting edema may develop from trauma to the injured cells, and pain is usually present. Rest of the injured part is advised, and analgesics may be helpful if pain is severe. Application of ice during the first 24 to 48 hours encourages vasoconstriction, decreasing blood seepage and edema.

TETANUS
ETIOLOGY AND EPIDEMIOLOGY

Tetanus, or lockjaw, is an infectious disease caused by the gram-positive anaerobic spore-producing bacteria *Clostridium tetani*, which are normal inhabitants of the intestinal tracts of humans and other animals and which can survive for years in soil and dirt. They enter

the bloodstream of human beings through wounds and travel to the CNS. They produce a powerful toxin that acts at the myoneural junction causing prolonged muscular contractions.

The incidence of tetanus is low, but severe tetanus may be fatal, especially in older persons. Most of the injuries resulting in tetanus are sustained either indoors or outdoors during activities such as gardening. Only a small percentage occur from major trauma.

PREVENTION

The only sure method of prevention of tetanus is through immunization. Tetanus prophylaxis is part of the planned immunization program for children. Booster doses are given after a person sustains a contaminated or deep puncture wound (Table 79-2). If more than 10 years have passed or if the person has never been immunized, instructions are given to the patient to complete the immunization series. In addition, human TIGH is given for severe wounds as a means of passive immunization. The risk for developing tetanus is described in the box on p. 2290.

TABLE 79-2 Tetanus prophylaxis after injury[8*]

Booster Date	Wound Size	Prophylaxis
Within past 10 yr	Small, moderate	0.5 ml toxoid†
	Severe, or more than 24 hr old	0.5 ml toxoid 250 units of TIGH‡
More than 10 yr or none	Small	0.5 ml toxoid (start series)
	Moderate	0.5 ml toxoid (start series) 250 units of TIGH
	Severe	0.5 ml toxoid (start series) 500 units of TIGH

*Recommended by the American College of Surgeons.
†Absorbed tetanus toxoid.
‡Tetanus immune globulin (human).

RISK OF DEVELOPING TETANUS[8]

Low or no risk	Wound less than 24 hr old
	Low level of bacterial contamination
	Not a crush or puncture wound
	Muscle not involved
Moderate risk	Exposed to bacterial contamination (outdoors, human bites, industrial environment, bullets)
	Crush or puncture wound
	Muscle involvement
High risk	High bacterial contamination (barnyard, sewers, animal wastes, bullet wounds of colon)
	Greater than 24 hr old
	Contained dead tissue that cannot be removed

CLINICAL MANIFESTATIONS

The symptoms of tetanus appear from 5 days to 15 weeks (average of 8 to 12 days) after introduction of the clostridia into the wound.[56] Symptoms of mild tetanus include pain and tingling in area of injury, neck stiffness, mild muscle rigidity, and some tonic spasms of the jaw muscles (trismus). When moderate tetanus is present, the trismus is more pronounced so that the person can hardly open the mouth, and this produces the characteristic sardonic smile (risus sardonicus). The person has difficulty swallowing because of pharyngeal spasms. The abdominal and lumbar muscles also become rigid, and opisthotonos (arching of the back) occurs. In severe tetanus the muscle spasms are so severe that fractures may result, and respirations are compromised. Painful muscle spasms may occur on the slightest stimulation.

INTERVENTIONS

Treatment is directed at neutralization of toxin that has not yet affected CNS cells. Large doses (3000 to 5000 units) of TIGH are administered intramuscularly. A program of active immunization with absorbed tetanus toxoid is initiated. Penicillin or tetracycline is given for its antibacterial effect on any remaining clostridia and to prevent secondary infections. A wound that is identified as the source of the infection is debrided.

Care is provided in a single room of an ICU. Ventilatory measures are used to provide adequate ventilation as indicated. Sedatives, tranquilizers, and muscle relaxants may be given to prevent muscle spasms. Maintenance of fluid balance and adequate nutrition is essential but may be difficult because of the muscle spasms. Some persons may be able to ingest fluids and soft foods orally, but if trismus is severe, tube feedings or parenteral feedings are instituted.

Frequent position changes help to prevent pulmonary complications, and side-lying positions are recommended to promote pulmonary drainage. Urinary retention may result from bladder spasms, and an indwelling catheter may be necessary if the patient cannot void.

CHEST INJURIES

Injuries to the chest, either from penetrating or blunt trauma, may result in open chest wounds, causing open or tension pneumothorax, hemothorax, flail chest, cardiac tamponade, or rib fractures (Table 79-3). These conditions are described in more detail elsewhere in the text.

Persons with chest trauma are considered to have sustained serious injury until proven otherwise. Primary consideration in emergency management is maintenance of an open airway, breathing, and circulation. *Oxygen* is administered at high flow. Rapid transport after initial emergency measures is essential.

OPEN CHEST WOUNDS

Open chest wounds create a problem if there is intrusion into the pleural cavity. Air is drawn into the pleural space because of the existing negative pressure. The resultant positive pressure causes *open pneumothorax* (collapse of the lung) (see Chapter 33). A sucking noise is heard as the air is drawn into the chest, and respirations are impaired. Cover the opening immediately. A nonporous material must be used, since air can pass through a standard dressing or material. Plastic wrap, which is not only nonporous but tends to cling to the skin, is excellent. If a dressing is used, it must be covered with petrolatum to create an air barrier. After the chest wound has been sealed, a pressure dressing is applied. Continual monitoring of respirations is indicated.

With *tension pneumothorax* air enters the pleural cavity with inspiration, but the wound edges serve as a one-way flap, not permitting escape of the air during expiration. Positive pressure builds up in the pleural space and effects a shift in mediastinal structures away from the affected side. This results in compression of the unaffected lung and decreased venous return to the heart (Figure 79-4).

FLAIL CHEST

Flail chest results when multiple adjacent ribs are fractured in two places. The chest wall becomes unstable and responds paradoxically during inspiration; that is, the affected side falls with inspiration as the unaffected side rises. The opposite effect occurs with expiration. If ventilation becomes inadequate, atelectasis, hypercapnia, hypoxia, accumulation of secretions, and ineffective cough occur.[65] Ventilatory assistance may be necessary (see Chapter 34).

TABLE 79-3 Some major injuries affecting chest wall and pleural cavity

Injury	Etiology	Signs and Symptoms	Initial Emergency Care
Rib fracture	Blow to chest	Pain on inspiration; local tenderness	Transport
Flail chest	Ribs fractured in more than one place; chest wall becomes unstable	Paradoxical respirations; respiratory distress; chest pain	Apply external pressure: sandbags, pillow, your hand; give oxygen; transport with flail side down
Open pneumothorax (open sucking wound)	Penetrating trauma to chest; loss of negative intrathoracic pressure as air moves in and out of wound	Sucking sound on chest wall during inspirations; tracheal deviation	Cover wound with occlusive dressing during exhalation; give oxygen
Simple pneumothorax	Laceration of lung, hyperinflation (blast injuries, driving accidents), loss of negative intrathoracic pressure	Sudden onset of chest pain; decreased breath sounds of affected area; dyspnea, tachypnea	Semi-Fowler's or Fowler's position; give oxygen
Tension pneumothorax	Complication of other types of pneumothorax; air enters pleural cavity but cannot escape	Respiratory distress; paradoxical chest movements; neck vein distention; tracheal deviation to unaffected side	Maintain airway and breathing; give oxygen; (needle thoracotomy by trained person)
Hemothorax	Blunt and penetrating chest injuries; injuries to major blood vessels and heart; blood collects in pleural cavity	Decreased breath sounds; dyspnea (cyanosis and signs of shock if severe)	Treat for shock; give oxygen

CARDIAC TAMPONADE

Cardiac tamponade is a compression of the heart resulting from leakage of blood into the pericardial sac. The accumulating blood cannot escape and exerts pressure against the heart, interfering with cardiac pumping. Pericardial lacerations from stab wounds tend to seal and cause tamponade, whereas gunshot wounds produce a larger opening with bleeding into the chest cavity.[65] Symptoms of cardiac tamponade include neck vein distention from increased venous pressure, a paradoxical pulse (weaker during inspiration), dyspnea, and Kussmaul's respiration. The person is placed in high Fowler's position and transported to the hospital. Treatment consists of pericardiocentesis.

ABDOMINAL INJURIES

Automobile accidents and knife or gunshot wounds are the most common cause of abdominal injury, either by penetrating or blunt trauma. *Penetrating* injuries often lead to infection (peritonitis) from rupture of the bowel. Excessive bleeding leading to severe and early shock occurs if a major blood vessel or the liver are involved. Less bleeding results from penetrating injuries to the spleen, pancreas, or kidneys unless a major vessel is damaged. Gunshot wounds may cause injury to various structures. All penetrating abdominal injuries require surgical exploration.

Blunt abdominal trauma usually causes injury to solid organs (that is, spleen, liver, pancreas, or kid-

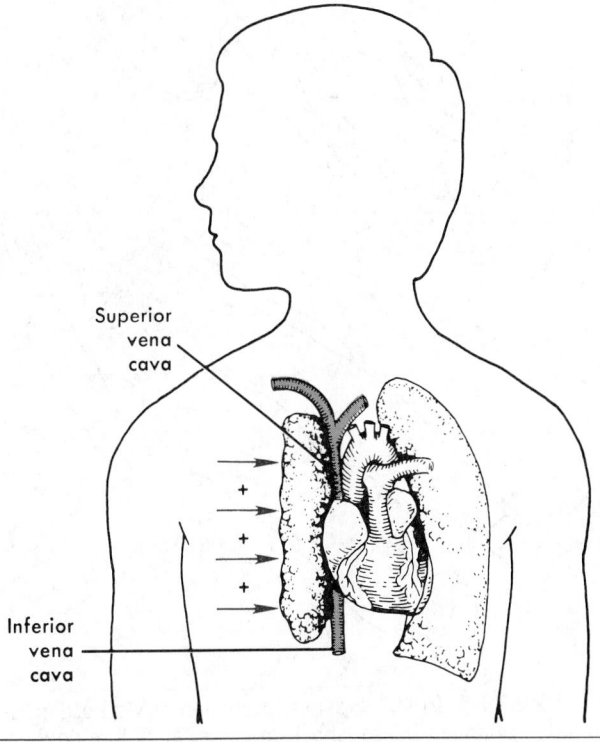

FIGURE 79-4 Tension pneumothorax. (From Sheehy SB and Barber J: Emergency nursing: principles and practice, ed 2, St Louis, 1985, The CV Mosby Co.)

neys).[65] The *spleen,* the most commonly injured organ, may become lacerated or may develop a subcapsular hematoma that ruptures when bleeding becomes profuse. The spleen is highly vascular and friable; therefore a splenectomy may be indicated when bleeding is profuse. Small splenic tears may be surgically treated by application of a hemostatic agent. Bleeding from the *liver* may be surgically controlled by application of a hemostatic agent or suturing of bleeding vessels. Blunt liver injuries may require removal of some liver tissue.

Symptoms of blunt abdominal trauma may include abdominal pain and rigidity, distention, nausea and vomiting, shock, and contusions on the abdominal wall. The victim may assume a position with knees drawn up toward the abdomen.

If there is an open wound, evisceration may occur. If the abdominal organs are exposed to the air and become dry, necrosis can result. The abdominal organs lying outside the abdominal cavity should therefore be cov-

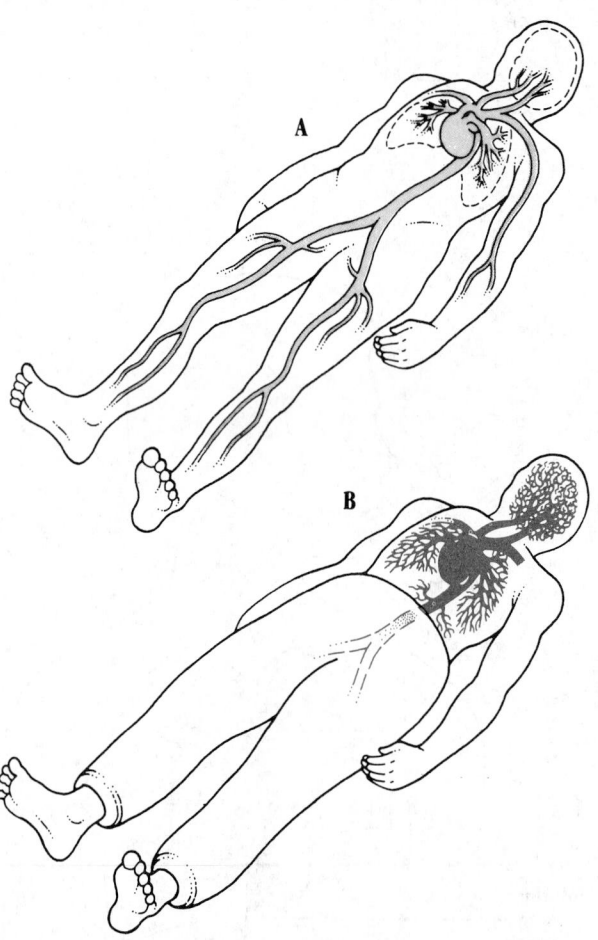

FIGURE 79-5 In shock states, perfusion of vital organs is greatly enhanced by antishock trousers. **A,** Before application. **B,** After application. (From Budassi S and Barber J: Emergency nursing: principles and practice, St Louis, 1981, The CV Mosby Co.)

ered by a warm, moist, preferably sterile covering. If a sterile dressing is not available, it is better to cover the organs with a clean moist cloth and risk infection than not to cover the organs and risk loss of tissue.

If severe shock is present, military antishock trousers (MAST) may be used, if available, before transport of the victim to the hospital. The MAST extend from the ankle to below the lowest rib. After application the MAST are inflated to apply pressure on the lower half of the body, reducing perfusion to the lower half of the body and increasing peripheral resistance to increase blood flow to vital areas (Figure 79-5).

AMPUTATIONS

Traumatic amputations are treated as are other wounds by controlling hemorrhage and applying pressure dressings. Severe bleeding does not always occur; the amount of bleeding depends on the extent of trauma that occurs. The greater the amount of trauma such as the amputation of a limb by a crushing injury, the greater will be the amount of muscle spasm in the arterial walls (vascular spasm).[26] This causes the artery to contract, and bleeding is decreased. A limb or appendage that is severed cleanly by a sharp object such as a knife will bleed more profusely. If a tourniquet is necessary, it should be applied close to the site of the amputation to decrease potential injury to intervening tissue. The amputated portion should be taken with the victim to the hospital since replantation is sometimes possible. The amputated part should be kept at about 5° C (40° F). It can be transported by placing the part in a dressing inside a plastic bag surrounded by ice. The amputated part should never be placed directly against the ice. The amputated part should never be frozen, cleaned, disinfected, debrided, or perfused before transportation.

FRACTURES

Injury to the musculoskeletal system may result in fractures or dislocations of the bones, strained muscles, or torn ligaments (see Chapter 69 for a complete discussion of these injuries). Emergency care consists of assessment of injury and of interventions to prevent further trauma until medical help is available.

ASSESSMENT

Pain localized over a bone or joint should be considered a fracture until a definitive diagnosis is made. Obvious deformity can be either a dislocation (if at a joint) or a fracture. In a compound fracture the bone may be protruding through the skin. Ecchymosis (bluish discoloration) of the skin may occur with any musculoskeletal injury as a result of rupture of blood vessels at the time of injury. The ability to move an extremity or digit does not negate a fracture, although the victim usually refrains from movement because of pain. Shock may occur with severe fractures, either from the stress of the trauma or from blood loss such as the extravasation of blood in the thigh after injury.

The victim should not be moved when being examined for fracture of the *spine* (neck or back). The examiner slides a hand under the victim and checks for point tenderness along the length of the spine. Bruises on the head may indicate that a force has been exerted that could cause a neck fracture. Bruises on the shoulder, back, or abdomen are frequently seen with back fractures, but a spinal fracture can be present in the absence of any bruises. If the spinal cord has been damaged, there may be loss of movement or loss of sensation of the extremities.

Skull fractures may vary from a small linear fracture with few symptoms to severe depression of bone fragments into the brain. Basilar skull fractures may be accompanied by bleeding or draining serous fluid from the nose or ears or both. Fractures of facial bones may interfere with respiration if the air passages become blocked.

Pain or deformity at the *hip* can be caused by either a fracture or dislocation. The leg will be shortened in both instances but turned outward if there is a fracture and inward with a dislocation. Fractures of the extremities may be accompanied by loss of circulation or sensation

if blood vessels or nerves are pinched by the bone fragment. Circulation distal to the fracture is assessed by observing skin color and presence of pulses. A neurologic check for sensation and circulatory system checks should be repeated after splinting and during transportation.

INTERVENTIONS

General Management of Fractures

Dressings are applied to an open wound at the site of a fracture before splinting is carried out to prevent infection and minimize bleeding. The fractured bone should be well supported and moved as little as possible during application of dressing and splint. Unless there is imminent danger of further accidental injury such as by fire or explosion, the victim is not moved until the fracture is splinted.

Fractures are splinted as they are found with the exception of severely angulated fractures of the *shafts* of bones of the extremities (see the box at left). The purpose of straightening a severe angulation is not to reduce the fracture but to decrease the spasm of the muscles and prevent damage to blood vessels and nerves. The sooner the traction is applied, the less the discomfort to the victim, since some numbness occurs immediately after the injury. Traction is maintained until the extremity is splinted. Deformities of a joint (shoulder, elbow, wrist, knee) are *never* straightened because of the presence of major blood vessels and nerves at a joint.

Fracture of the Spine

Any questionable injury to the head, neck, or back is treated as a fracture of the spine. Two problems can occur from a fractured spine: damage to the spinal cord and neurogenic shock. If the cervical spine is fractured, there may be interference with respiration; therefore respirations must be continually monitored. The victim may use diaphragmatic breathing for a short period but be unable to sustain this. Artificial ventilation is more difficult, because the neck cannot be hyperextended since this can cause further injury to the spinal cord. The head can be extended by gentle traction, and the jaw pulled forward to open the airway. Traction must be maintained until the neck can be supported in this position. The neck should never be flexed, twisted, or hyperextended. If the victim is not having difficulty with respiration, the neck can be splinted in the position in which it was found.

Transportation of a person with a potential spine fracture must be on a firm base, preferably a back board. Forward or backward flexion of the spine is to be avoided to prevent further trauma to the spinal cord. The victim should be slid, not rolled, in straight alignment onto the back board. It takes several persons

---

GENERAL MANAGEMENT OF FRACTURES

1. Do not move patient before splinting a fracture (unless there is danger of fire, explosion, or radiation).
2. Cover open wound before splinting.
3. Support fractured bone and move it as little as possible while splinting.
4. Splint fracture in the position it is found.
5. In *severely angulated* fractures of the *shaft* of the extremity bone:
   a. Decrease muscle spasm and prevent damage to blood vessels by straightening severe angulation of bone shaft.
   b. Place one hand just below fracture and other hand farther down extremity.
   c. Apply gentle traction to straighten extremity.
   d. Maintain traction until extremity is splinted.
6. *Never* straighten deformities of a joint (shoulder, elbow, wrist, knee).
7. Apply splints to include joint above and below fracture.
8. Pad rigid splints (boards) for comfort.
9. Reinforce soft splints (pillows) with a rigid material (for example, magazine, board).
10. If using air splint:
    a. Inflate only by mouth to a point where the thumb leaves a slight dent.
    b. Keep fingers and toes free for assessment of circulation.
11. Handle fractured part gently to prevent pain and shock.

working together to move the victim safely. The victim remains on the back board during the initial diagnostic tests in the emergency room.

BITES

ANIMAL AND HUMAN BITES

Approximately one million persons in the United States are bitten by animals evey year, mostly by dogs. Cat bites produce a higher percentage of infections, mostly by *Pasteurella multocida,* which is an organism commonly found in animal mouths.[56] Dog bites become infected only in about 5% of cases, whereas approximately 15% to 20% of human bites become infected.[56] Human bites commonly occur during fights when a fist hits a mouth. Most bites produce puncture wounds, but lacerations can occur as the individual pulls away from a biting animal. Data related to the potential for rabies are collected after dog or wild animal bites.

Treatment consists of washing animal and human bites thoroughly with soap and water and rinsing with copious amounts of water. Tetanus prophylaxis is usually indicated. If infection occurs, cultures are taken to determine the appropriate antibiotic. Soak the infected wound in warm water, then immobilize and elevate the wounded part. Persons with major human bites may require hospitalization.

RABIES
ETIOLOGY

Rabies is an acute infectious viral disease that affects the nervous system, primarily the brain. It is usually fatal, although there have been a few documented survivals.

The rabies virus is transmitted to humans through bites of carnivorous animals. The most frequent source in the United States since the advent of required inoculation of dogs is wild animals, primarily skunks, foxes, bats, and raccoons. Bats can frequently be found in urban as well as rural areas. Rabies does not usually occur after bites by members of the rodent family (rats, squirrels, chipmunks, or rabbits). The virus can also be transmitted from the saliva of the rabid animal to a person through an existing break in the victim's skin.

INDICATIONS FOR POSTEXPOSURE RABIES PROPHYLAXIS

Bite from a wild animal
Unprovoked attack by a dog that cannot be observed for 10 days
Bite from an animal observed to develop signs of rabies

Not all rabies-infected animals are mad. There are two types of rabies. In one type the animal may be restless, barking, and biting. In the other, so-called dumb rabies, the animal may be quiet and stay close to its master. In the latter type, paralysis, which begins in the throat and lower jaw, may lead the animal's owner to suspect that something harmful has been swallowed. If the owner tries to investigate, some of the highly infectious saliva may enter an abrasion on the hand.

PREVENTION

The control of rabies is a public health responsibility. The police and health departments must be notified at once if it is thought that a rabid animal is at large. In England and the Scandinavian countries the disease has been almost entirely eliminated by rigid enforcement of laws that prohibit allowing dogs to run about unleashed. Rabies could be controlled by compulsory vaccination of all dogs and cats kept as household pets, capture and confinement of stray animals, and destruction of wild animal reservoirs of infection under the supervision of wildlife experts.

There are two types of rabies prophylaxis: preexposure immunoprophylaxis, and postexposure immunoprophylaxis. Persons who are at high risk for rabies (veterinarians, animal handlers, and certain laboratory workers) should receive rabies vaccine preexposure. The decision for postexposure prophylaxis is made by the physician after comparing the potential for developing rabies (see the box below) with the potential for serious reaction to prophylaxis. Every attempt is made to capture the animal by competent authorities, and wild animals are killed for analysis. The presence of *Negri bodies* in the brain of an animal is conclusive evidence of rabies.

Two types of immunizations are given for postexposure prophylaxis: antirabies serum and rabies vaccine. The antirabies *serum,* rabies immunoglobulin (RIg), is given as soon as possible after the bite. Side effects include local tenderness and fever. The human diploid cell *vaccine* (HDCV) is now being used in place of duck embryo vaccine (DEV) in the United States. HDCV is more potent than DEV, and requires fewer doses (Table 79-4). Local side effects of the rabies vaccines include pain, redness, and swelling that respond to antiinflammatory and analgesic agents. Systemic side effects include fever and lymphadenopathy. Persons allergic to eggs may develop hypersensitivity reactions to the DEV. Neurologic complications occur rarely (more often with DEV than with HDCV) and include encephalopathies, neuropathies, and Guillain-Barré syndrome.

Corticosteroids should not be given to the person receiving any type of rabies vaccine unless the situation is life-threatening. Corticosteroids are antiinflammatory and interfere with the development of active immunity.

TABLE 79-4 Postexposure rabies immunization

Type	Form of Immunization	Number of Days	Frequency	Method of Administration
Serum RIg	Passive	1	Day 0	IM
Vaccine HDCV DEV	Active	5 23	Days 0, 3, 7, 14, 28 2 times daily for 7 days, then 1 time daily for 7 days, and the boosters on days 24 and 34	IM SC

CLINICAL MANIFESTATIONS

The incubation period in humans normally ranges from 10 to 60 days, but 1% of persons do not develop symptoms for over 1 year.[68] Shorter incubation periods are seen with bites to the head and in children.

In the prodromal period, the person exhibits signs of anxiety, depression, pain at the site of the animal bite, and a feeling of impending danger. Acute symptoms (that is, difficulty in swallowing, excessive salivation, muscle spasm, often maniacal fear, difficulty in breathing, and convulsions) then appear. A terrific, painful spasm of the muscle of deglutition occurs when there is an attempt to swallow water; hence the name hydrophobia. Even the mention of water is often enough to bring on an attack. Aerophobia is also present, and convulsions can be produced by a draft of air on the skin.

INTERVENTIONS

There is no specific therapy for rabies. Treatment is symptomatic, and most nursing care of the patient with acute rabies is difficult but of short duration. Most patients die from heart failure or respiratory difficulty within 2 to 3 days of the acute onset of symptoms. The patient is restless, irritable, and fearful, with episodes of uncontrolled fear and mania alternating with periods of calm. Every effort is made to keep the patient quiet. The room is darkened, and the noises in the hall outside the room should be eliminated. Side rails are placed on the bed and sometimes padded to help prevent injury during episodes of uncontrolled thrashing about. Sedatives, including chloral hydrate, morphine, and the barbiturates, are given. Anesthetics may be given intravenously. Fluids often are given intravenously, and it is important to bandage the arm securely on a board to prevent injury in the event of a convulsion or an attack of mania while a needle is in the vein. The head of the bed is sometimes lowered in an attempt to facilitate drainage of saliva, and often suctioning must be used. All persons caring for the patient should be aware of contamination from saliva, and a gown and gloves

should be worn. Relatives of the patient must be prepared for the fact that the patient cannot talk. Sometimes the visits of relatives bring on severe painful muscle spasm in the throat of the patient, who is usually conscious up to the time of death, even though unable to speak.

SNAKEBITES
TYPES OF POISONOUS SNAKES

There are four kinds of poisonous snakes in the United States (see the box below). The pit vipers are distinguished by a pit resembling a second nostril between the eyes and the nostril and by a broad, flat, triangular head. The largest number of bites and deaths from snakebites occurs from rattlesnakes. One antivenin is effective for all pit vipers. No specific antivenin is prepared for the bite of the coral snake, but cobra antivenin, kept in most zoos, is effective.

PREVENTION

Poisonous snakes in North America will almost always move away when disturbed and will not bite unless sud-

POISONOUS SNAKES IN THE UNITED STATES

Rattlesnake	Pit viper; color and size differs (many varieties); makes a warning rattle sound; found in all states, especially in southwestern states
Copperhead	Pit viper; copper-colored head and markings; about 3 ft long; found in eastern and southern states
Cottonmouth	Pit viper; also called water moccasin; grayish color with broad, dark-olive bands; 3 to 5 ft long; found in marshes of southern states
Coral	Not a pit viper; coral, yellow, and black rings encircle body; small blunt head and body; found in southeastern states, especially around Gulf of Mexico

denly molested without warning. Snakebites can often be prevented by wearing high leather boots and thick trousers when walking through snake-infested areas. Heavy gloves should be worn, and the greatest care taken when climbing, because hands may be placed on ledges that cannot be seen, and reptiles often sun themselves on rocky ledges.

CLINICAL MANIFESTATIONS

Envenomation after a snakebite is about 50%. Symptoms vary according to the size and type of snake involved, the age and physical condition of the person, and the location of the bite. Bites on the face and trunk are the most serious, and children and debilitated persons have a higher morbidity and mortality.[35]

Pit vipers produce local swelling that spreads rapidly and progresses to ecchymosis and tissue necrosis. Pain varies in intensity and is not an indication of the severity of the bite.[68] Other signs include nausea and vomiting, bleb formation, visual difficulties, and convulsions.

Coral snake bites cause more neurotoxic symptoms, including euphoria, followed by drowsiness, ptosis, slurred speech, ataxia, visual difficulties, weakness, and confusion. Death occurs from respiratory paralysis.

INTERVENTIONS

Controversy exists concerning immediate first aid treatment for moderate-to-severe snakebites. If medical help can be obtained within a short period, immobilize a limb in a horizontal position below the heart and transport the person immediately to a medical facility.

Should the snake bite occur in an area where medical help cannot be obtained for more than 1 hour, the following interventions may be taken:
1. Immobilize a limb in a position below the heart.
2. Place a flat constricting band above the bite, just tight enough to restrict *superficial* venous and lymphatic flow.
3. If necessary, move the band up the limb ahead of swelling.
4. Within the first 5 minutes of injury, suctioning of the venom may be considered (removes only 5% to 10%[36]).
   a. Make *superficial* parallel incisions lengthwise through the fang marks.
   b. Apply suction using a rubber bulb from a snakebite kit, if available, or use oral suction if no mouth lesions are present.

The earlier that antivenin is administered (intravenously), the more effective it will be. Because of potentially severe side effects, antivenin is only given when the bite is significant or when signs of envenomation have appeared.[36] Antivenin is a horse serum; therefore testing is required for hypersensitivity since anaphylaxis may occur. Serum sickness reactions (Chapter 76) are common.

Tetanus prophylaxis and antibiotics are prescribed. Give analgesics as necessary for pain; however, initial severe pain may diminish to a numbness after a few hours. Monitor fluid balance and for signs of shock. Give oxygen as necessary. Keep a bitten limb immobilized during the early hospitalization. Massive sloughing of the tissue may occur following pit viper bites, and frequent dressings may be indicated. Snakebite wounds heal slowly.

POISONING

Poisoning, either unintentional or deliberate, remains a major cause of accidental deaths. On the average there are 4000 deaths from poisoning in the United States each year.[62] Morbidity is higher in children than in adults. Poisoning in adults commonly occurs from not checking medication labels (overdose or wrong medication), from lack of knowledge (for example, taking alcohol and sedatives together), from taking an excess amount in an attempt to obtain a desired effect, or as a suicide attempt.

COMMON ACCIDENTAL POISONING
PREVENTION

Education of the public is directed toward increasing their awareness of safety hazards in the home, particularly in homes with children. Nonpotable liquids should be kept tightly capped in their original containers in places that are not easily accessible to children and should *never* be placed in a soft-drink bottle, drinking glass, or cup.

Patient teaching includes the following:
1. Read labels on *all* medication vials (prescription or over-the-counter drugs) before taking medication.
2. Read labels on all over-the-counter drugs to identify possible hazards.
3. Take all medications in the prescribed doses.
4. Do not increase dosage outside of stated limits in an effort to increase a desired effect.

ASSESSMENT

A *rapid* assessment is made to determine whether poisoning or overdose has occurred so that immediate action can be taken to prevent or diminish the effects of the poison or drug. Poisoning is suspected when there is a sudden onset of symptoms, especially in a young child. Symptoms vary, depending on the cause of the poisoning, but may include nausea and vomiting, abdominal pain, convulsions, change in level of consciousness, and decreased pulse and respiratory rates. The most common pattern of drug poisoning is coma with flaccid muscles and hypotension; this may be confused with head injury or metabolic states.[29]

If poisoning is suspected, the lips and mouth are examined for signs of burns, excessive salivation, or diffi-

PUPILLARY CHANGES WITH SELECTED DRUGS

DILATED	CONSTRICTED
Anticholinergics	Opioids
Tricyclic antidepressants	Propoxyphene (Darvon)
Amphetamines	Organophosphate insecticides
Phenothiazines	Phenothiazines
Glutethimide (Doriden)	
Cocaine	
Hallucinogens	

culty in swallowing. The breath is noted for an odor such as that from petroleum products or cleaning compounds. Pupillary changes may be noted with selected drugs (see the box above); some drugs such as the phenothiazines may cause either constricted or dilated pupils. Time should not be wasted looking for needle marks.

Data are collected to identify (1) clues that poisoning is a possibility and (2) the type and quantity of the agent. A conscious victim is questioned for information concerning what and how much was taken. If the person is unconscious, identification of the poison or drug can be facilitated by asking others to look for clues while you are examining the victim. Empty containers, spilled fluids, open medication bottles, or syringes may provide needed information. Gather *all* potential agents in their original containers and take them to the hospital with the victim. The physician may need to know the ingredients of the agent for those situations in which an antidote is indicated.

INTERVENTIONS

Immediate action is necessary if poisoning is suspected; in some instances delay of a few minutes may make a difference between life and death. An *unconscious* victim must be transported *without delay* to the nearest medical facility.

If the victim is *conscious*, have someone call a physician immediately if possible. If a private physician is not available, a *poison control center* can give rapid and accurate information. Most large cities have poison control centers, which maintain an extensive file on the most common substances and drugs. The telephone number is usually easily obtained from a list of emergency numbers in the front of the telephone directory.

Management consists of stopping absorption of the poisonous substances or drug (see the box above, right). Poisonous substances can be inhaled, absorbed from the skin or mucous membranes, ingested, or injected. The type of intervention depends on the method by which the poison entered the system.

FIRST AID FOR POISONING

INHALED POISON

1. Remove victim from source of toxic gas.
2. Assess cardiopulmonary status and give artificial ventilation if possible.
3. Give oxygen, if available.

CONTACT POISON

1. Rinse skin with copious amount of water.
2. Remove garments and rinse skin again.

INGESTED POISON

1. If person is conscious:
   a. Call physician or poison control center for assistance.
   b. Substances other than caustics or hydrocarbons:
      (1) Induce emesis by giving 15 to 30 ml syrup of ipecac; follow with full glass of warm water.
      (2) Inactivate poison by giving activated charcoal (especially following drug ingestion).
   c. Caustics or hydrocarbons (petroleum products):
      (1) Give nothing by mouth.
      (2) Seek immediate medical attention.
2. If person is unconscious, transport without delay to medical facility.

Inhaled Poison

Persons who have inhaled a toxic gas first need to be removed from the site to fresh air and given oxygen if available. As in any emergency, cardiopulmonary status is assessed, and resuscitation started if indicated. The victim is transported immediately to a medical center.

Carbon monoxide is one of the more common toxic gases. It is odorless and occurs as a result of incomplete combustion such as that which occurs during fires or from automobile exhaust. It cannot be filtered by the use of a cloth face mask. Toxicity occurs because of the higher affinity of hemoglobin for carbon monoxide than for oxygen. The victim becomes profoundly hypoxic and loses consciousness. Carboxyhemoglobin has a deep red color and is seen in the mucous membranes of all victims and by a red coloring of white or light-colored skin.

Contact Poison

Poisonous substances absorbed through the skin or mucous membranes should be *rinsed* off immediately with *copious amounts of water* without taking time to remove garments. Following this the garments containing the substance are removed, and the skin is rinsed again. Place the person in a shower if the body is involved.

Ingested Poison

The most common form of poisoning is by ingestion of a poisonous substance or an excessive amount of a drug. Absorption of the agent can be prevented by inducing vomiting or by lavage to eliminate the agent and by giving a substance that will make the poisonous agent inert.

Elimination of the poison. The first treatment objective is removal of the ingested poison (except with ingestion of caustics or hydrocarbons). *Vomiting* is the best method, since gastric lavage does not remove substances in stomach pouches that are inaccessible to lavage.[68] Lavage with a cuffed endotracheal tube to prevent aspiration is indicated for unconscious persons.

The recommended method of inducing vomiting is by the oral administration of 30 ml (15 ml for children) of *syrup of ipecac*. The dose may be repeated once in 20 minutes if necessary. The victim is encouraged to drink a glass of water 3 to 5 minutes after administration of the syrup of ipecac to promote complete emptying of the stomach. Mechanically induced vomiting, such as tickling the back of the throat, is usually ineffective since only a small amount is vomited.

Caustic substances such as lye erode the esophagus as they are ingested and frequently result in esophageal perforation and subsequent esophageal stenosis. Drinking acidic substances such as vinegar water or citrus juices to counteract the basic property of lye is *not* recommended, since this may result in an exothermic reaction, causing additional pain and burning.[47] *Hydrocarbons,* which are found in all petroleum products, produce a severe pneumonia from direct aspiration into the lungs during ingestion.[68] Emergency care for caustic or hydrocarbon ingestion consists in giving nothing by mouth and seeking immediate medical attention.

Inactivation of the poison. Activated charcoal is an efficient method of inactivation of selected drugs, particularly analgesics (especially aspirin), barbiturates and other hypnotics, amphetamines, and tricyclic antidepressants (see the research box above). Activated charcoal will adsorb a drug and prevent it from being absorbed by the gastrointestinal tract. It should be administered within 30 minutes of poisoning to achieve maximal effect but can be given later with good results. It is given *after* (not before or concurrently with) ipecac. Activated charcoal can be purchased at a drugstore (Nuchar A, Norit A, or Activated Charcoal by Merck). The adult dose is 30 to 50 g given in 60 to 90 ml of water. Saline laxatives are then given to remove the adsorbed poison, since the absorption capacity of activated charcoal is reversible.[47]

Cathartics are seldom used except with activated charcoal, since ipecac itself will usually cause catharsis, and the ingested poison will also often cause diarrhea.[68]

Antidotes. If it is known exactly what poisonous substance or drug has been ingested, a specific antidote may be given in some cases by the physician. (Common

RESEARCH

Curtis R et al: Efficacy of ipecac and activated charcoal/cathartic, Arch Int Med 114:48-52, 1984.

This study compared the effectiveness of three treatment modalities to prevent aspirin absorption. Twelve healthy volunteers were given the equivalent of six adult-dose tablets. Each subject was then randomly assigned to one of four groups: no treatment, ipecac alone, activated charcoal/MgSO$_4$, and ipecac followed by activated charcoal/MgSO$_4$. Treatments were given 60 minutes after aspirin ingestion. The experiments were repeated after at least 72 hours until each subject had rotated through each treatment modality. Urine salicylate levels were measured after 48 hours. Findings included mean urine salicylate levels of 96% for no treatment, 72% for those treated with ipecac followed by activated charcoal, 70% for ipecac alone, and 56% for activated charcoal alone. The authors concluded that ipecac and activated charcoal are appropriate methods for treating overdose of selected drugs. ∎

poisons and antidotes are discussed in pharmacology and toxicology texts.) The use of a "universal antidote" has not proved to be effective.

Injected Poison

Toxic substances can be injected through the skin such as by insect bites or by needle injection. Drugs most commonly injected are heroin, barbiturates, and amphetamines. Stimulants such as the amphetamines produce hyperactivity and "uncooperative" behavior. Overdose may produce tachycardia, chills, and collapse. Depressants such as heroin or barbiturates produce respiratory depression, resulting in coma and death. Overdose often occurs because the victim is unaware of the potency of the drug purchased illegally. Substance abuse is discussed in Chapter 19.

Insect bites. The most common insect bites that can produce severe reactions are those of wasps and bees. Death can occur either because of the multiplicity of bites (especially in young children) or from anaphylactic shock if the victim is allergic to the protein in the venom. The reaction may be slow in developing or sudden and acute. Sensitized persons should avoid areas where bees and wasps are found, should carry tablets of isoproterenol for sublingual use and uncoated antihistamine tablets for immediate oral use, and should have epinephrine (Adrenalin) available for immediate use parenterally if anaphylaxis occurs. The wearing of a Medic-Alert tag facilitates emergency care if the victim is unconscious.

When a person is stung by a bee, the stinger with the venom bag is left in the skin. The stinger should be removed immediately, because venom continues to be pumped into the skin from the bag. Removal of the stinger by grasping and pulling is to be avoided, since this pushes more venom into the skin. The stinger is removed by a scraping motion. Ice can be applied to prevent absorption of the venom (heat should be avoided). A paste of sodium bicarbonate and water or a weak solution of ammonia may help by counteracting the formic acid present in the venom.

Tick bites can cause tick fever by transmission of a toxin, a virus as in Colorado tick fever, or rickettsiae as in Rocky Mountain spotted fever. Sudden removal of a tick will result in its mouthpiece remaining. Applying gasoline or turpentine to the head of a tick or applying the hot end of a previously lighted match to the body will cause the tick to drop off within 10 minutes. Ice can be applied to reduce absorption of toxin.

Tick bites may also cause *Lyme* disease, seen mostly in the Northeast, Midwest, and West Coast of the United States, in some parts of Europe, and in Australia. The initial lesion begins with a reddened area that expands slowly with central clearing; it is found in the groin, axilla, or thigh.[56] Flulike symptoms occur in about half the cases. Late symptoms include arthritic pains and chronic synovitis that may result in permanent disability.[56] Tetracycline relieves early symptoms and may prevent late manifestations. Arthritis is treated with intravenous penicillin and refractory cases with ceftriaxone (a cephalosporin).

Supportive Care for Poisoning

Good nursing care of the acutely poisoned patient may make the difference between a favorable and a fatal outcome. Keep the person warm enough to prevent chilling and monitor closely for changes in physical signs such as rapid thready pulse, respiratory distress, cyanosis, diaphoresis, and other signs of vascular collapse, vasogenic shock, or impending death. Monitor vital signs at least every 15 minutes for several hours and report changes to the physician immediately. Record symptoms of nausea, vomiting, and abdominal pain and monitor all vomitus for signs of blood. Observe stools and urine for abnormal constituents such as blood. Maintain prescribed intravenous fluids.

If respirations are depressed, give prescribed oxygen and suction as needed. Mechanical ventilation may be necessary. Turn unconscious patients frequently to provide drainage from each bronchus.

If the poisoning was a suicide attempt, institute safety precautions. Psychiatric consultation is often recommended, and a psychiatric nurse clinician can be a helpful resource. Monitor persons addicted to heroin or morphine derivatives who have overdosed for signs of withdrawal. Symptoms usually appear within 12 to 18 hours and include yawning, sweating, shaking, vomiting, diarrhea, lacrimation, runny nose, abdominal pain, backache, and other flu-type symptoms (see Chapter 19).

FOOD POISONING

A number of toxicants occur in plants and animals ingested as food. Some toxicants are introduced by mistake as pesticides during plant growth, as food additives, or as part of food packaging. Commercially packaged foods are monitored closely, and products are withdrawn from the market if contamination is suspected.

PLANT POISONING

Poisoning from plants is usually not a problem, because people have learned to identify poisonous foods. Mushroom poisoning still occurs, however, when people eat uncultivated mushrooms thinking that they are of a safe variety. Two types of mushroom poisoning can occur. One type contains the alkaloid muscarine, which has a *parasympathetic effect*. Symptoms develop immediately after eating and are characterized by sweating, lacrimation, salivation, dyspnea, vomiting, and muscle tremors. Respiratory and circulatory depression may occur. The second type of mushroom poisoning has an *atropine-like effect*. Symptoms occur 6 to 24 hours after ingestion and are characterized by nausea and vomiting, bloody diarrhea, dehydration, and muscle weakness. Circulatory system collapse and CNS system involvement may occur.

First aid treatment for mushroom poisoning is the same as for drug poisoning: induce vomiting with syrup of ipecac, give fluids, and then give activated charcoal. After the ipecac, give 30 mg of magnesium sulfate (Epsom salts) in water by mouth to hasten evacuation. Medical care should be obtained.

BACTERIAL FOOD POISONING

Etiology

Food poisoning occurs more frequently than is reported, because the majority of persons recover quickly without treatment. The incidence of food poisoning from commercially prepared foods has become relatively uncommon in the United States, but food poisoning from home-cooked foods or improper handling of foods still occurs.

Bacteria act in different ways in the intestines. Some organisms such as *Shigella*, *Salmonella*, and *C. jejuni* (Table 79-5) multiply in the intestines, causing infection. Bacteria such as *S. aureus* and *E. coli* produce a toxin in the intestines (enterotoxins). Bacteria such as the clostridia produce a toxin in foods (exotoxin) that acts on the intestines when ingested. Food poisoning is not caused by food that has spoiled or decomposed unless the food contains disease-causing bacteria. Many food poisonings are caused by *S. aureus*.

TABLE 79-5 Bacterial food poisoning

Organism	Vomiting	Diarrhea	Fever	Onset	Duration	Sources
Staphylococcus aureus	Severe	Occasionally	−	1-8 hr	8-24 hrs	Meat, poultry, fish, cream-filled foods, mayonnaise
Salmonella	Occasionally	+	+	8-48 hr	2-5 days	Poultry, eggs, meat
Shigella	Occasionally	+	+	24-72 hr	3-7 days	Salads, seafood
Escherichia coli	Rare	+	−	24-72 hr	1-3 days	Uncooked foods, contaminated water
Campylobacter jejuni	−	Severe	+	1-10 days	2-7 days	Meat, poultry, fish, mushrooms, contaminated water
Clostridium perfringens	Occasionally	Severe	−	8-16 hr	1-4 days	Rewarmed foods
Clostridium botulinum	Occasionally (diplopia, dysphagia, respiratory failure)	Rare	−	24-96 hr	High mortality	Improperly canned foods

Prevention

Acute food poisoning can be prevented (see the box below). Rigid controls of slaughterhouse practices have decreased the incidence of food poisoning. Pasteurization of milk destroys salmonellae. Rigorous enforcement of sanitary practices by food handlers can decrease food poisoning by *Staphylococcus, E. coli,* and *Salmonella* organisms. Food handlers should not be allowed to work if they have even minor infections on their hands or do not adhere to the requirements for hand washing after using the toilet. Toilets should not be adjacent to kitchens.

Health teaching should include the proper handling and cooling of foods. Home canning has become increasingly popular, but many people are unaware of the need to process low-acid foods under pressure to prevent botulism. The U.S. Department of Agriculture, state agricultural departments, the home economics departments of schools, or newspapers may have booklets available on home canning methods.

PREVENTION OF FOOD POISONING

1. Keep meats, fish, poultry, mayonnaise, and cream-filled foods refrigerated.
2. Avoid slow cooling of meat and poultry.
3. Use a meat thermometer when cooking large pieces of meat, especially pork.
4. Stuff poultry immediately before roasting (warm stuffing is a good medium for bacterial growth).
5. Can low-acid foods (foods other than tomatoes or fruits) under pressure to prevent botulism.
6. Discard any can that bulges.

Interventions

If symptoms are very mild, no interventions are indicated. If fluid loss is severe, fluid balance should be restored, and bed rest may be indicated. Fluids such as tea or broth may be well tolerated. If severe dehydration occurs, intravenous fluids may be necessary.

There is no emergency first aid treatment suitable for *C. botulinum* poisoning. The victim should be taken to a hospital for medical care. Data are obtained concerning the source of the poisoning, and any other persons who might have eaten the contaminated food are contacted immediately. Medical treatment consists of supportive therapy and the administration of botulinum antitoxin. Antitoxin cannot undo damage that has already occurred but can prevent further damage. Approximately 65% of these patients die within 3 to 16 days after onset of symptoms. Fortunately, this type of poisoning is now quite rare.

ENVIRONMENTAL INJURIES: HEAT, COLD, RADIATION

Exposure to extremes of temperature affects both the general reaction of the body to the stress and the local reaction of the skin. General reactions occur more readily when the individual has not been conditioned to the extremes in temperature. Incidences of overexposure to heat, for example, occur more often in the early part of a hot spell before the individual is acclimated. Persons at higher risk include elderly or obese persons or those with chronic debilitating disorders.

GENERAL REACTIONS TO HEAT AND COLD

Three general reactions can occur with heat: heat cramps, heat exhaustion, and heatstroke (sunstroke).

Cold produces a general cooling of the body (hypothermia).

HEAT CRAMPS

Heat cramps are sudden muscle pains caused by loss of sodium chloride in perspiration during strenuous exercise in hot weather. The best treatment is prevention by taking extra salt and water or drinking a balanced salt-containing fluid such as Gatorade when severe exertion is anticipated. The immediate treatment consists of salty fluids and foods by mouth, extra water, and rest for a few hours in a cooler environment. Avoid salt tablets because of their slower absorption.[56]

HEAT EXHAUSTION

Heat exhaustion is vasomotor collapse caused by the inability of the body to supply the peripheral vessels adequately with sufficient fluids to produce the perspiration needed for cooling and yet meet vital tissue requirements. The condition usually follows an extended period of vigorous exercise in hot weather, particularly when an individual has not had a period of acclimatization. The symptoms are faintness, weakness, headache, and sometimes nausea and vomiting. The skin is pale and moist. Body temperature is slightly above normal Heat exhaustion can often be prevented by taking extra salt and extra fluid during hot weather and by tempering physical activity during very hot weather. Emergency care consists of treating for shock and transporting the victim to a medical center. Fluids should be given, preferably containing salt.

HEATSTROKE

Heatstroke (sunstroke) is a serious condition in which excessive body heat is retained, and it requires *immediate emergency treatment*. It is caused by a failure of the perspiration-regulating mechanism in the hypothalamus. Contributing factors include cardiovascular disease, alcoholism, obesity, old age, prior febrile illness, and selected drugs (diuretics, sedatives, antipsychotics, and anticholinergics).[56] Heatstroke is typically seen during a heat wave and may occur in healthy young persons who exercise vigorously in hot weather. The person undergoing vigorous exercise in intense heat may perspire profusely for some time and then become dehydrated and fail to produce sufficient perspiration to maintain normal body temperature. The skin is dry, hot, and flushed in contrast to the pale, moist skin of the person suffering from heat exhaustion. The victim becomes confused, dizzy, and faint and may quickly lose consciousness. Body temperature is usually above 41° C (106° F).

Without treatment most heatstroke victims will die, but with prompt and vigorous treatment almost all will recover. Treatment consists of actions to reduce the body temperature immediately while transporting the victim to a medical center. The victim should be placed in a cool place such as an air-conditioned room while awaiting transportation. Wrap the person in a wet sheet and use a fan to increase evaporation. These measures are continued during transportation.

If the elevated temperature is allowed to persist, serious permanent damage is done to the brain and the entire nervous system. Treatment is continued until the temperature has been lowered to at least 39° C (102° F), and the temperature must then be checked carefully for several hours for sudden rise. The patient should respond when the temperature lowers. Failure to do so may indicate that brain damage has occurred. Persons do not recover from heatstroke as quickly as from heat exhaustion. Often there is faulty heat regulation for days and a lowered tolerance to heat for years and sometimes for the rest of the individual's life. The person who has had a heatstroke should be advised to plan his or her living so that repeated long exposures to heat are avoided.

ACCIDENTAL HYPOTHERMIA

The extent of the cooling effect that occurs with exposure to extreme cold depends on the temperature and exposure time, the thermal conductivity of the environment, and the amount of air current present. Moisture is a good conductor; air is not. Wet clothing therefore contributes to increased cooling of the body. Several light layers of clothing to provide air insulation will keep a person warmer than one heavy layer. Air movement contributes to heat loss; thus lower environmental temperatures can be tolerated better in the absence of wind (windchill factor).

When the body is exposed to cold, shivering occurs to produce heat by increased metabolism. As the cold increases, shivering ceases and heat loss exceeds heat production. The individual becomes listless, apathetic, and sleepy and may become indifferent to the surroundings and not seek adequate protection. Pulse and respirations become slower as metabolism decreases. Freezing of the extremities, unconsciousness, and finally death will result if help is not received.

The victim needs to be kept warm while being transferred to a medical facility. Wet clothing is removed immediately and warmed blankets applied. If a tub bath is given, the temperature should be approximately 40° to 42° C (104° to 108° F). Warmer temperatures can cause skin damage from the decreased circulation to the skin.[26] Rubbing the skin is to be avoided since this can also cause skin damage. Warm liquids may be given if the victim is conscious.

The person suffering hypothermia should be monitored closely during rewarming. Hypovolemic shock can occur from vasodilation. If intravenous fluids are given, overloading the circulation is a potential complication. Vital signs are monitored for sudden changes. Cardiac monitoring may also be indicated during the rewarming period for signs of ventricular fibrillation and cardiac arrest.

LOCAL REACTIONS TO HEAT AND COLD
BURNS

Burns may be caused by direct heat, chemicals, electricity, or radiation (sun or nuclear rays). Heat burns are treated by immersion in cool water or application of clean, cool wet packs. Clothing should not be removed nor ointments applied. Shock may occur with severe burns as a result of fluid shifts. (For more detailed information on burns, see Chapter 74).

FROSTBITE

Cellular injury occurs with exposure to extreme cold. Cell water freezes, and the resulting ice crystals damage the cell. The degree of injury depends on the depth of freezing. Frostbite occurs most frequently in exposed areas such as the nose, cheeks, ears, and fingers and can be prevented by adequate covering with loose-fitting dry clothing. Toes are also susceptible, because of dampness and tight pressure from shoes or boots. Persons with circulatory problems are more prone to develop frostbite.

Frostbite can be classified as incipient, superficial, or deep. *Incipient frostbite* often goes unnoticed and is evidenced by paleness or loss of color of the skin. Removing the victim to a warm room, cupping the injured part with the hands, or placing fingers in the armpit for warmth may be all that is needed. Tingling occurs with warming.

Superficial frostbite may develop if incipient frostbite is not noticed. Freezing extends into the superficial tissue below the skin. The frozen part is soft, and white skin does not redden with pressure. Dark skin has a dull ashen shade. The frozen part may be warmed by covering. Heat is not applied, since this may damage the injured tissue, but the frozen part may be immersed gently in warm water (43° C [110° F]). Contrary to popular belief, the frozen part should never be rubbed with snow, because this increases the trauma to the injured tissue.

Deep frostbite is evidenced by hardness of the frozen tissue, because deep subcutaneous tissue is injured. After thawing, the skin becomes hyperemic and edematous with blister formation. The edema subsides in 24 to 48 hours, and tissue breakdown with necrosis results. The frozen part should be covered to warm it, and the victim should be taken to a medical center as soon as possible. The care is then similar to that for vascular disease of the extremities (see Chapter 29). Efforts are made to decrease the oxygen needs of the tissues while

healing takes place, to improve blood supply by the use of drugs, and to prevent infection of open lesions. Necrotic tissue may have to be debrided for healing to occur.

RADIATION INJURY
ETIOLOGY

Accidental injury through ionizing radiation may occur wherever nuclear materials are used, particularly in industry and hospitals. Transportation of nuclear materials increases the possibility of accidental injury.

Radiation injury is caused by exposure to gamma (γ) rays and neutrons from radioactive material. Persons can be exposed to radiation directly from unshielded radioactive material or indirectly by the effect of radioactive dust inhaled, ingested, or received topically (on the skin). The amount of radiation that a person receives depends on the strength of the radiation source, the distance of the victim from the source, the duration of the exposure, the area of the body exposed to the radiation source, and the amount and type of shielding that are present (see Chapter 17).

PREVENTION

Special precautionary measures should be used whenever radioactive materials are being utilized. All persons having contact with these materials should become knowledgeable concerning preventive measures. Exposure to radiation is carefully monitored; for example, personnel who work with radioactive materials or x-rays (γ-rays) wear special monitoring badges.

Rescue workers who must remove a victim from an area of radioactivity need to protect themselves from radiation exposure. Since radioactive particles can be carried on dust, all skin areas must be covered, and a filtering mask worn by rescue workers after an explosion involving nuclear materials. The greater the time of exposure, the greater the potential for injury; therefore the victim must be removed immediately to a less hazardous environment. Some of the basic principles of emergency care may have to be violated when there is danger of other explosions or when fires occur. The rescue worker should remove all contaminated clothing at the edge of the contaminated area, and any exposed skin areas are washed thoroughly. A shower should be taken as soon as possible.

PATHOPHYSIOLOGY

Initially the radioactive waves react with intracellular atoms to produce ion pairs. These ions then combine with cell water to form the toxic products H_2O_2 and HO_2, which then react with deoxyribonucleic acid (DNA) and cellular enzymes to alter function or destroy the cells.[35,68] The effects depend on the dosage. Lower doses impair cell mitosis either temporarily or permanently. Mitotic arrest follows absorption of several hundred rad (unit of measurement of absorbed ionizing radiation); cell function continues but with no new divisions. Continued protein synthesis, however, leads to "giant cells" that die after several weeks from impaired metabolism.[68] High doses (over 1000 rad) result in cell death.

The effects of cellular abnormalities depend on the rate of cell proliferation. Cells that are rapidly dividing and differentiating (for example, blood cells and epithelial cells of the skin and gastrointestinal tract) are the most vulnerable. Loss of neutrophils predisposes the person to overwhelming bacterial infection, and loss of platelets results in bleeding. Loss of gastrointestinal epithelial cells leads to rapid fluid and electrolyte loss with severe dehydration and gastrointestinal bleeding. Radiation effects on slow turnover tissues such as the eye or thyroid may take several years to develop.

CLINICAL MANIFESTATIONS

Ionizing radiation causes acute and delayed effects. *Acute* reactions depend on the type and extent of exposure and may be *local* (skin and hair) or *diffuse* (cerebral, hematologic, and gastrointestinal) (Table 79-6). The cerebral syndrome usually results from massive exposure and includes progressive loss of consciousness followed by irreversible cardiovascular collapse.[35] Hematologic effects include decreased blood counts, petechiae, purpura, bleeding from body orifices, and development of infection (for example, fever, oropharyngeal lesions, pneumonitis, abscesses). Anorexia, nausea, and vomiting with fluid and electrolyte depletion result from gastrointestinal injury. Recovery may be possible with active support of hematologic and gastrointestinal systems. Prolonged weakness, even during convalescence, is common.

The most common *delayed* effects are sterility, hypothyroidism, cataracts, and cancer. Except for sterility, these effects are not manifested until several years after exposure (see Table 79-6).

INTERVENTIONS

Local injury to the skin is treated similar to a burn. The involved area may be washed gently with soap and water, and a dry sterile dressing applied. No antiseptic or disinfectant solutions should be used. Maintenance of asepsis is important. The person needs to know that continued observation of the skin is important for early detection of skin neoplasms.

The person with acute radiation syndrome is hospitalized. Early nausea and vomiting is usually self-limiting; sedatives and antiemetics may be helpful. Medical therapy is directed toward supportive care; that is, to-

TABLE 79-6 Effects of radiation on body systems

Organ or Effect	Time to Onset	Time to Maximal Effect	Total Time From First Dose to Recovery	Dose Required to Cause Injury (rad)	Major Consequences
Cerebral syndrome	Few hr	1-2 days	Usually fatal	3000	Irreversible coma and cardiovascular collapse
Hematologic syndrome					
Granulocyte depletion	1-2 wk	4 wk	6-8 wk	200-400	Bacterial infection
Lymphocyte depletion	Few hr	1-2 days	4-8 wk	200-400	Nonbacterial infection (virus, tuberculosis)
Platelet depletion	1-2 wk	4 wk	6-8 wk	200-400	Bleeding
Gastrointestinal syndrome	3-4 days	6-7 days	2 wk	600-2000	Fluid and electrolyte loss from mucosal sloughing
Skin lesions					
First-degree burn	Few hr	2-3 wk	6-8 wk	200	—
Second- or third-degree burn	Few days	1-2 wk	8-12 wk	1000	May need skin grafts
Hair loss	—	3 wk	3-4 mo	300	Permanent if greater than 700-800 rad
Sterility	—	Few days to few wk	—	600-700	Permanent infertility
Hypothyroidism	—	Several yr	—	Variable	Myxedema
Cataract	—	Several yr	—	300-600	Visual loss
Leukemia	—	5-7 yr	—	Unknown	Fatal
Solid tumors (thyroid, bone, breast, lung)	—	Many yr	—	Unknown	Usually fatal, except thyroid tumors

From Kaye D and Rose LF: Fundamentals of internal medicine, St Louis, 1983, The CV Mosby Co.

ward fluid and electrolyte replacement, nutrients (TPN may be necessary), and respiratory support as indicated. Various blood elements may be given for hematologic deficiencies. Bone marrow transplantation may be warranted for a person with a poor prognosis.[68] Prevention of infection, which takes high priority, consists of reverse isolation and prophylactic oral antimicrobial drugs.

The same nursing care is required for the person with acute radiation syndrome as for the person receiving radiation therapy (see Chapter 17). The care includes rest, protection from infection, good mouth care, and maintenance of fluid, electrolyte, and nutrient intake. Considerable support may be required by an anxious or apprehensive patient who is concerned about the nature and prognosis of the disorder.

SEXUAL ASSAULT: RAPE

Rape is a violent crime leading to physical, psychologic, and sociologic trauma of the victim. Many persons are hesitant to report rape because of feelings of shame, guilt, fear of retaliation, or reluctance to go through a court trial. The court procedure remains one of great psychologic trauma for the victim.

There are many misconceptions about rape. The facts are that rape is common to all social classes, that rape occurs mostly *intra*racially rather than interracially, and that a majority of rapes are committed by someone the victim knows. The majority of rape victims are females, but males, especially young boys, may also be rape victims. The attacker is usually another male. Rape of males is a major problem in prisons in the United States.

Rape crisis centers have been formed in many large cities. These centers differ in their functions but usually have one or all of three main functions: (1) victim service, (2) service to professional agencies (health, law), and (3) community education. The victim service is the primary role for which the centers have been formed. Since this service is not adequate to change the system for the victim, services for education of professionals serving rape victims and education of the community to increase public awareness of the problems of rape victims are being pursued. The victim service consists of volunteers, many of whom have been raped themselves, who serve as victim advocates through the medical examination and police interview. Some form of follow-up service such as counseling may be available. Some rape crisis centers have volunteer attorneys who can offer the victim legal advice or representation.

RAPE TRAUMA SYNDROME

Rape is a traumatic event for the victim physically, psychologically, and socially. *Physical* force is often used; a

weapon may be used either as a threat or to injure the victim, or the hands or fists may be used to beat the victim or threaten choking. Injury can also occur as the victim is struggling on the ground or floor. The vagina and perineum may be injured by force used during the sexual attack, and the rectum may also be lacerated if anal sex has been attempted. The latter is more common in rape of males.

Psychologic trauma is usually severe; the rape victim is in a state of crisis. Fear is a dominant theme as the victim perceives the event as life-threatening.[41] Other feelings expressed by victims are depersonalization, shame, degradation, defilement, violation, guilt, humiliation, and anger.[11] The victim has not only been under threat of harm, but has also been subjected in many instances to multiple sexual assaults, some natural, some perverted, by one or more persons. Fellatio (oral sex) is frequently demanded by the rapist. Some rapists will urinate on the victim before leaving her.

The rape victim also experiences a *sociologic* crisis. If the victim is a married woman, marital relationships may be affected. If she is single she is often in fear of repeated occurrences and may feel the need to move, especially if the attack occurred in her home or apartment. Decisions have to be made concerning whom to tell about the incident, since loss of needed support by significant others may occur. Job security or relationships with co-workers may be threatened. If a child is the victim, social relationships within the family may be altered. Problems of a sociologic nature take considerable time to be resolved, but concerns related to these potential problems may occur in the initial emergency period.

TYPES OF RAPE VICTIMIZATION

Burgess and Holmstrom[11] identified three types of rape victimization from their research: (1) rape or sex without consent, (2) accessory to sex or inability to give consent, and (3) sex stress situation or sex with initial consent. The first type is easily identified as rape; the victim is attacked suddenly (blitz rape), or the rapist gains the victim's confidence but then forces himself on the victim. Some persons are unable to give consent because of their cognitive or personality development. They are lured by the rapist by offers of material goods such as candy or by offers of pleasure or human contact. In the third group are persons who agree to a sexual relationship, but either perversion occurs or the victim or family become worried later concerning possible consequences. All of these situations produce victims in need of help.

PREVENTION

All women need to know the measures they can take to help prevent rape from occurring (see the box on p.

RAPE PREVENTIVE MEASURES

PREVENTION OF ATTACK

Set house lights to go on and off by timer.
Keep light on at all entrances.
Place safety locks on windows and doors.
Have key ready before reaching door of house or car.
Look in car before entering.
Insist on identification before letting a stranger in house;
     check identification with agency if suspicious.
Do not list first name on mailbox or in telephone direc-
     tory.
Make arrangements with neighbor for needed assistance.
Be alert when walking in street; walk in lighted areas.
Walk down center of street if possible.
Avoid lonely or enclosed areas.

IF ATTACKED

Run toward a lighted house; yell, "Fire."
Spit in rapist's face, act bizarre, vomit.
Rip off rapist's glasses.
Step hard on his foot (instep).
Aim at eyes—try to gouge eyes, scrape face.
Hit throat at Adam's apple (larynx).
Use fighting and screaming with caution; this may scare
     some rapists, encourage others.
Try talking to avoid rape.
If powerless, make close observations about rapist, car,
     location.

2305). It would also be helpful for every woman to learn methods of self-defense. Rape crisis centers can provide information on availability of classes in the community. Women learning physical defense skills need to learn to value themselves so they can justify the need for self-defense and have confidence in their ability to defend themselves.

HEALTH CARE

Persons who are raped may seek medical help directly or call the police, who will then take the victim for medical examination. Some victims fear reprisal by the rapist or are unwilling for others to know about the rape and therefore do not seek medical attention. Victims need to be encouraged to report the incident. They need considerable support during both the acute emergency and the long-term consequences, and knowledgeable nurses are able to provide appropriate support.

   Many hospitals have developed protocols for care of the rape victim in the emergency department. If such a protocol does not exist, it behooves the nurses in the emergency department to work toward development of a protocol. Rape crisis centers can be helpful in this regard. The protocol includes high priority in triage, provisions for privacy without leaving the victim alone, provision of a victim advocate such as a woman from a rape crisis center if desired, continual emotional support by nonjudgmental health personnel, and routines to ensure the protection and comfort of the victim. These routines delineate which personnel have priority for contacts with the victim. If no injury is present that threatens life, the nurse may be designated to have primary contact with the victim and make the decision as to when the victim is ready for medical examination or police interview. Large city police departments often have women police officers assigned to interview rape victims, since many girls and women become very upset when asked to talk with a male police officer.

ASSESSMENT
SUBJECTIVE DATA

The person who has been raped goes through the same phases as any person facing a crisis situation. The initial phase is one of shock and disbelief that rape has occurred and of emotional disequilibrium manifested in many different ways. After the initial acute phase there is a period of pseudoequilibrium when the victim rationalizes the event or attempts to suppress thoughts concerning the rape. During the long-term phase there are periods of depression, phobic reactions, nightmares, and changes in life-style.[58]

   The victim will be asked many questions by the physician to identify the type of assault and potential for injury. If the victim has been threatened, she may have succumbed through fear, and this needs to be elicited. Victims often talk freely to the nurse about their feelings; their fears concerning injury, mutilation, or death at the time of assault; or present fears concerning pregnancy or sexually transmitted disease. Other feelings of degradation, feeling "dirty," shame, guilt, and so forth, may be expressed. Anger may be directed at the assailant or projected toward medical care or personnel. Pain may be local at the site of assault or generalized and diffuse. The victim may complain of a sore throat if choking was used as a threat or following oral sex. Nausea may also be reported.

OBJECTIVE DATA

One of the myths concerning rape is that all women are hysterical after rape. Burgess and Holmstrom[11] in their research identified two different types of responses with approximately half of the victims falling into each category. The first type they labeled "expressed style." These women were emotionally labile as evidenced by crying, shaking, restlessness, tenseness, and smiling or laughing inappropriately. The other group, labeled "controlled style," appeared calm, composed, or subdued. The full impact of the experience often hits these women at a later time.

   A head-to-toe assessment for signs of physical trauma is usually carried out by the physician. The clothing will be inspected and described and is often requested by the police for evidence. Clothing should not be washed or discarded. Other data needed by the police usually include samples of the assailant's hair from combing of pubic hair and fingernail deposits for samples of the assailant's tissue.

TESTS

Papanicolaou smears of the vagina, mouth, or rectum and saline suspensions are done to test for the presence of sperm. An acid phosphatase test will demonstrate recency of intercourse. Tests will be inconclusive if the victim has bathed or douched since the rape occurred. Tests for sexually transmitted disease are done at the initial visit to obtain baseline information for comparison at 6 weeks.

INTERVENTIONS

All personnel who have contact with the rape victim need to refine their skills in providing support to the victim with a nonjudgmental approach. Knowledge of the problems and experiences of other victims as well as rapists is helpful in understanding what is being experienced by the victim (see references listed at the end of the chapter). Interdisciplinary conferences involving health care providers, volunteers from rape crisis centers, and the police help clarify issues and problems.

EMOTIONAL SUPPORT

Initially, the victim needs time to marshal her coping responses. Most victims have a need to talk and a need to know that someone cares what is happening to them. The nurse uses crisis intervention theory as the basis for deciding how best to help the victim. Many hospitals have contacts with a rape crisis center. Victims are given the choice of having a victim advocate from the center be with them during the entire procedure, and medical examination or interviews by the police are not begun until the volunteer arrives.

Preparation for the physical examination is carried out in advance. Having a pelvic examination after a sexual assault can be a traumatic experience for the victim, and some girls or women have never had a pelvic examination previously.

COMFORT

After the victim has been examined, she will probably have a need to wash herself. Mouthwash is appreciated, especially if there has been oral sex. A change of clothing may be needed if the police want her clothing for evidence, which is not uncommon.

SEXUALITY

The victim has many concerns related to her sexuality. Time is needed to work through these concerns, and long-term counseling is helpful to many victims.

Concern about possible pregnancy depends on the circumstances: whether the victim is in the childbearing years, whether birth control is in effect at the time of sexual attack, and at what point in the menstrual period the rape occurs. If pregnancy is a possibility, contraceptive therapy is initiated immediately.

Concern about sexually transmitted disease is common. Ceftriaxone is given intramuscularly and tetracycline is given orally after the initial examination as a preventive measure. The victim needs to know that medical follow-up is important and that she should be retested for venereal disease in about 6 weeks unless symptoms occur earlier. In addition, the victim may experience vaginal discharge, itching, and a burning sensation caused by an acute vaginal infection (vaginitis). This infection may become chronic.

DISCHARGE

The victim should not go home to an empty house or apartment. The volunteer from the rape crisis center, the social worker, or police can all facilitate arrangements for transportation to home or to the home of family or friends. Frequently, the victim goes to the police station after medical care is completed to follow up with the police report. The victim needs to know about the availability of follow-up medical services and counseling services. In some medical centers there are psychiatrists who are especially interested in assisting rape victims with counseling as desired.

DISASTERS

Disasters are sudden catastrophic events that disrupt patterns of life and in which there is possible loss of life and property in addition to multiple injuries. Disasters can be either natural phenomena or caused by people (see the box below).

There are essentially three types of disasters: multiple patient, multiple casualty, and mass casualty.[58] *Mul-*

CAUSES OF DISASTERS

NATURAL	MAN-MADE
Air	*Transportation*
Tornado	Air
Hurricane	Land
Blizzard	Water
Land	*Fire*
Earthquake	Housing
Volcanic eruption	Forest
Avalanches	Explosions
Cave-ins	*Disease*
Water	Epidemics
Floods: slow rising and	*Civil disorders*
flash floods	Riots
Tidal waves	Wars (nuclear attacks)

tiple patient disasters involve up to 10 people and occur with events such as multiple vehicle crashes, bus crashes, bomb explosions, or fires. Rescue squads apportion victims to different hospitals, if possible, to prevent overload on any one hospital emergency department. In *multiple casualty* disasters as many as 100 people may be injured in events such as air crashes, riots, tornadoes, hurricanes, minor earthquakes, and dam breaks.[58] Heavy demands are placed on available hospital emergency departments. *Mass casualty* disasters are large-scale disasters resulting in large numbers (over 100) of injured persons and disruption of community services and resources. Mass casualty diasters, such as unusually severe hurricanes, large-scale earthquakes, or war bombings, fortunately rarely occur, but the possibilities exist and community preparedness is essential.

EFFECTS OF DISASTERS

The effects of disasters are multiple. People are killed or injured and separated from their families. Many become homeless. In a large-scale disaster, confusion and chaos occur during the early stages. Panic rarely occurs, but when it does it is because the involved persons believe that escape routes are limited and may be closing off. Effective leadership and communication can usually prevent panic from occurring.

Transportation difficulties are created as streets and roads become clogged by persons trying to get away from the impact area or others trying to get in. Persons within the area are trying to flee or to find friends, family, or medical assistance. Persons outside of the disaster area are trying to move in to help, to find relatives, or just because of curiosity. Sightseers can present a serious problem to maintenance of open roads in and out of the area and should be deterred from entering the disaster area.

Food and water supplies can become contaminated or nonexistent. Medical supplies can be inadequate to meet the sudden increased need. Utilities can become disrupted. Law enforcement is necessary to prevent looting and other civil disorders. Establishment of a communication system takes first priority to prevent chaos.

ROLES OF NURSES IN DISASTERS

The actual role assumed by a given nurse at a disaster will depend on (1) the abilities of the nurse and (2) the specific situation. The nurse may not be able to reach a specific location where his or her services may be most useful, so the needs of victims may then be better served by the nurse functioning in a different capacity.

Nurses can participate in a disaster in many ways. Nurses with leadership ability and experience may be needed to serve in this capacity. Any nurse may be in a position of being the only health care provider in a given area and be responsible for giving initial first aid treatment or supervising the activities of others. It therefore behooves nurses to continually update their first aid skills. Because of their education and experience in assessment and intervention for psychosocial problems, professional nurses can be especially helpful in aiding victims to cope with their emotional reactions to the disaster. Nurses may be asked to serve at emergency morgues for support of families experiencing loss of loved ones.

As shelters are established, nurses are needed to staff the shelters to help meet the health needs of victims separated from their homes and families. The American Red Cross, which assumes an active role during disasters along with governmental agencies, operates shelters for victims. They provide supplies and food as well as service personnel (shelter manager, nurses, physicians, food helpers). Nurses interested in serving during disasters at home or in other parts of the country may contact the local American Red Cross office. Other services provided by the American Red Cross include emergency services on an individual family basis and aid for recovery.

When the disaster occurs in the nurse's own geographic area, the ability of the nurse to function is influenced by the impact of the disaster on both self and the family. The nurse may be unable to contact or reach family members and may be in a position of having to provide health care while actively concerned about the family's safety and welfare. The nurse may also be experiencing the emotional impact of the crisis situation, and this may limit the effectiveness of the care provided.

PREVENTION

Preparedness for disasters includes community planning to identify and, it is hoped, to prevent disasters that can occur and education of the public to minimize the number of casualties.

COMMUNITY PLANNING

Most states have disaster service agencies, which are outgrowths of civil defense organizations. These agencies act as coordinating agencies for the local agencies. Every community should have a disaster planning group as part of the emergency medical care committee. There should be representation by all groups who will be active participants if a disaster occurs. This would include governmental groups (political, law enforcement, fire), health groups (hospitals, physicians, nurses, pharmacists, social workers), official groups (American Red Cross), and nonofficial groups (telephone company, parent-teacher organizations, religious organizations). The disaster planning committee identifies the types of disasters that may occur in the local community, organizes a plan to be followed for different situations, arranges for simulated drills to test the effectiveness of the plans, and determines need for education or updating of necessary skills of participants. Nurses need to be active participants in the planning, implementation, and evaluation phases.

During a disaster the local hospitals become actively involved and need their own disaster plan to cope with the sudden influx of persons needing emergency care. (Reference 24 is a good source for disaster planning and interventions.) Any time a large number of injured persons are in need of emergency care, hospital disaster plans are put into effect. Testing of hospital disaster plans at specified intervals by simulated drills is necessary for determining if the plans are effective and what changes, if any, are needed.

PUBLIC EDUCATION

Public awareness of potential community disasters is needed for effective community preparedness for disasters. Disaster planning committees need support of and participation by community members. Individual persons need to know what they should do in the event of a disaster. Most radio and television stations regularly notify communities of potential disasters and give directions for preventive actions to be taken and for methods of obtaining further information should the disaster occur. Since electricity may be cut off, battery-operated radios should be available in all homes for continued communication.

All homes should have an emergency food cabinet with sufficient nonperishable foods to meet nutritional needs for several days. Supplies are rotated with current supplies to prevent them from spoiling or becoming outdated.

ASSESSMENT
TRIAGE

There are essentially two different approaches to triage of victims during a disaster. The *military* triage system, which may be initiated during a mass casualty disaster, is based on the philosophy of doing the "best for the most with the least by the fewest." Victims with injuries of such magnitude that there is question of survival are given low priority for transportation. In this system the numbers of critically injured must greatly outnumber the health and transportation personnel available. Victims are reclassified as the emergency situation changes. Priority is then given to those victims with the greatest chance of survival.

The more commonly used *civilian* triage system is used during multiple patient or multiple casualty disasters. There are several victim-sorting methods that can be used for triage, but essentially all methods give most priority to life-threatening injuries and least priority to minimal injuries (see the following box).

FOUR-COLOR CODED TRIAGE SYSTEM

0 — BLACK: DEAD

1 — RED: CRITICAL OR LIFE-THREATENING

These victims have a reasonable chance of survival only if they receive immediate treatment. Emergency treatment is initiated immediately and continued during transportation. This category includes victims with respiratory insufficiency, head injury with decreasing LOC, hemorrhage, and severe abdominal injury.

2 — YELLOW: SERIOUS

These victims can wait for transportation after they receive initial emergency treatment. They include victims with immobilized closed fractures, soft-tissue injuries without hemorrhage, and burns on less than 40% of the body.

3 — GREEN: MINIMAL

Victims in this category are ambulatory, have minor tissue injuries, and may be dazed. They can be treated by nonprofessionals and held for observation if necessary.

Adapted version of Four-Color Triage System. Reprinted from Topics in emergency medicine 1:1/May 1979 by Baker FJ by permission of Aspen Systems Corporation.

DISASTER SYNDROME

The behavior of victims after the impact of disaster can be characterized as progressing through phases of shock, awareness, euphoria, and anger. The victims are experiencing loss; therefore the phases are similar to those experienced by others during any kind of loss (grieving).

The shock phase may last only a few minutes or up to several hours after impact. The victim is dazed, is unable to comprehend what is occurring, and cannot follow even simple directions. Persons prepared to function in emergencies are less apt to spend much time in the shock phase.

The awareness phase may last up to several days. The victim becomes aware of survival and tries to help others, minimizing his or her own injuries or losses. During this stage guilt feelings may arise because others died while he or she survived. The victim is highly suggestible, can follow simple directions, but cannot carry out problem solving effectively. For example, after one major earthquake a young woman who had run outdoors on a chilly night clad only in a thin nightgown was told to put on something warm. Her solution was to wrap a warm scarf around her neck.

The euphoria phase may last for several weeks. The victim feels a sense of brotherhood with the community and participates willingly in helping others with plans for recovery.

Before resolution occurs, the victim may go through the "Why me?" or anger phase that occurs because of the experienced loss. The anger is often projected against helping persons from the outside who were not personally affected by the disaster. It is especially important for nurses who may be assisting victims during the recovery phase to understand that the anger is part of the loss experience. As the victim copes with the losses incurred by the disaster and life returns to more normal patterns, the anger will disappear.

INTERVENTIONS
EMERGENCY AID STATIONS

The number, size, and staffing of emergency aid stations depend on the type and extent of the disaster. There must be one person who is designated as the leader and who is responsible for making decisions for maximal effectiveness of the unit. Medical supplies and food for personnel must be available. One person is designated for triage. In the absence of a physician, a nurse assumes leadership of emergency care that is rendered. Transportation teams will bring some victims to the station and transport victims to a medical center for follow-up care. Unfortunately, many victims will go directly to a medical center, bypassing a first aid unit and thus creating a logistics problem at the medical center and decreasing the effectiveness of the care that can be given.

The types of injuries that occur will depend on the type of disaster. Soft-tissue and bone injuries are common in most natural disasters. Respiratory insufficiency may occur with airway injuries. Fear resulting from the disaster can precipitate cardiac arrests. Childbirth may also be precipitated. If the weather is inclement, additional injuries and disease may occur after the immediate crisis is over. If tear gas has been used, the victim should not be placed in a closed environment near other victims. Health personnel will be unable to function if they are affected by the tear gas.

Victims are not transported until first aid care has been given, as in any emergency. If hemorrhage has not been controlled or fractures splinted, the victim may arrive at the medical center in shock that could have been prevented or minimized, and surgical intervention will not take place until measures to treat shock are instituted and the patient's condition is stable. If first aid measures are instituted before transportation, the victim can be taken to surgery at the earliest opportunity. Records indicating all treatment given at an emergency aid center *must* accompany a victim who is referred or transported to a medical center or any other health care facility. The information, which is attached to the victim who is not responsible, should include name, age, address, name of nearest relative, assessment made, and treatment.

SHELTERS

Most shelters are set up in schools, which can house a large number of people. Toilet facilities, running water, and cooking facilities must be available. The role of the nurse in a shelter is to assess and provide for health needs of the shelter population. Persons with infectious diseases need to be isolated from other persons.

Elderly persons may become confused by the rapidly changing events and strange surroundings. Many elderly have chronic illnesses, and very often their medications have been left at home. They may not be able to see well if their glasses have been lost or eat well if dentures are missing. Because elderly persons may have decreased resistance, they are more susceptible to disease after a disaster.

Any victims who have chronic illnesses must be identified. If they are receiving replacement therapy such as insulin, this must be obtained. Arrangements must be made for the care of pregnant women and infants. Formulas must be obtained, and special dietary needs arranged. Immunization of shelter occupants may also be necessary. Occupants should be monitored for signs of developing health problems.

Assessment of safety factors in the environment is also a nursing responsibility. The nurse is part of the shelter team and advises the shelter manager of any potential health hazards. The care of victims in a disaster is a team effort, and the nurse is an important member of this team.

ADAPTATION TO LOSS AFTER DISASTERS

Adaptation to loss after large-scale community disasters may differ from adaptation to losses under normal life situations because of the lack of *individual* support systems as a result of (1) death of usual support persons or (2) inability of usual support persons to provide support because of their own personal losses. There may also be a loss of *community* support systems.

Immediately following a disaster there is usually an immediate outpouring of material assistance and personnel services from people outside the community. This diminishes with the passing of time, and the victims are often faced with having to work through their grief with less support than usual and sometimes with visual environmental reminders of the loss. It is important that long-term counseling services be made available in these situations to persons of all ages, including children. Group therapy can be a useful method of providing support by helping the victim realize that he or she is not alone and that others understand what the victim is experiencing and by aiding in problem solving through group efforts.

CHAPTER SUMMARY

- Accidents are the leading cause of death in persons less than 45 years of age and the third leading cause in those 45 to 64 years of age.

- Paramedics have had more training than EMTS and are prepared to carry out invasive procedures, such as starting IVs, defibrillation, and intubation.

- Persons are not judged as liable unless they act willfully and with gross negligence. Reasonable care is judged on the basis of care given by someone with similar training under the prevailing situation.

- Accident prevention includes monitoring the home for hazards, equipping homes with smoke alarms, participating in fire drills, and using care while driving.

- The parameters of priority assessment of the injured person are the ABCs (airway, breathing, and circulation) and level of consciousness.

- After the priority assessment and immediate care, a head-to-toe assessment is made for other signs of injury.

- Shock usually develops in persons who sustain major trauma or a major stressor to the system.

- After a head injury, loss of consciousness after a period of alertness and unequal pupils may indicate an intracranial hematoma that requires immediate medical attention.

- Keep an injured person lying down and protected from cold (but not overheated); do not transport the victim until all first aid measures have been carried out.

- Victims of multiple trauma (injury to two or more body systems) require rapid stabilization at the accident site, followed by immediate safe transfer to an emergency room.

- Causes of asphyxia, other than disease, include inadequate environmental oxygen, obstruction of air passages, secretions in air passages, interferences with respirations, and interferences with circulation. Asphyxia is indicated by dyspnea, adventitious sounds, use of accessory respiratory muscles, skin pallor, and eventually cyanosis.

- Remove foreign bodies from the airway with the Heimlich maneuver if the person is unable to cough up object.

- The person with a suspected myocardial infarction who is breathing should be placed in a comfortable, well-supported sitting position, given oxygen (if available), cared for calmly to minimize anxiety, and transported to a hospital as soon as possible.

- In near-drowning, freshwater aspirated into the lungs is rapidly absorbed into the circulation, causing temporary hypervolemia, hemodilution, and intravascular hemolysis; saltwater pulls fluids into the alveoli, causing persistent hypovolemia with hemoconcentration and pulmonary edema.

- Drowning may be caused by asphyxiation from aspiration of fluid into the lungs or from laryngospasm that prevents both air and water from entering the lungs. Pulmonary edema can develop several hours after a near-drowning.

- The extent of injury from electricity depends on the point in the heartbeat cycle that is stimulated, the intensity of the current, and skin resistance. Electricity may cause burns, depression of the respiratory center, ventricular fibrillation, tissue damage, and bone fractures.

- The best method for stopping external bleeding is to place direct pressure on the bleeding vessel; tourniquets are used only for massive arterial bleeding that cannot be controlled by other means.

- Soft tissue injuries include abrasions, avulsions, lacerations, incisions, puncture wounds, and contusions. Dirty wounds, especially puncture wounds, require tetanus prophylaxis.

- Chest injuries include rib fracture, flail chest, pneumothorax (open, simple, tension), hemothorax, and cardiac tamponade. Open chest wounds must be covered immediately with a nonporous cover to prevent air from entering the chest and altering the negative pressure, leading to open pneumothorax.

- Injuries to the abdomen may be penetrating (leading to infection and bleeding) or blunt (causing injuries to solid organs); the spleen is the most commonly injured organ.

- An amputated part should be transported to the hospital with the victim; it should be wrapped in a dressing and placed in a plastic bag surrounded by ice, but it should not be frozen.

- Suspected fractures must be splinted before the person is moved. Severely angulated fractures of the shaft of a long bone may be straightened by traction to prevent severe muscle spasms; deformities of a joint are never straightened.

- Persons with a suspected spine fracture are transported on a firm base, avoiding spine flexion.

- Rabies may be transmitted to humans through bites of carnivorous animals, including skunks, foxes, bats, and raccoons; rodents do not usually transmit rabies. Rabies is usually fatal; therefore prophylactic therapy is imperative if rabies is suspected after an animal bite.

- Poisonous snakes include the rattlesnake, copperhead, cottonmouth, and coral snake. Emergency care after a suspected poisonous snake bite consists of immobilizing the limb in a horizontal position and transporting the person immediately to a medical center for antivenom therapy.

✔ If poisoning is suspected in an unconscious person, the person should be transported immediately to a medical center.

✔ For ingestion of noncaustic substances, give the conscious person syrup of ipecac followed by one or two glasses of water; if drugs have been ingested, follow the water with activated charcoal. After ingestion of caustic substances, give the person nothing by mouth and seek immediate medical attention.

✔ Bacterial food poisoning may be caused by various organisms producing varying degrees of vomiting, diarrhea, and/or fever. Most food poisonings are self-limiting and require only fluids and rest; botulism from improperly canned foods requires medical attention, because mortality is high.

✔ Heat exhaustion is a shocklike reaction to heat; place the person recumbent in a cold environment and provide salty fluids. Heatstroke results from inability to lose heat by perspiration; the skin is hot and dry, and unconsciousness may occur. Heatstroke requires immediate medical care.

✔ Applying too much heat to persons overexposed to cold may lead to skin injury from the decreased circulation, and hypovolemic shock may result from vasodilation.

✔ Cells that are rapidly dividing and differentiating (blood cells and epithelial cells of the skin and mucosa) are most vulnerable to radiation, leading to overwhelming infection (loss of neutrophils), bleeding (loss of platelets), burns of the skin, and rapid fluid and electrolyte loss with severe dehydration (loss of GI cells).

✔ Persons who have been sexually assaulted experience physical, psychologic, and sociologic trauma.

✔ Types of disasters include multiple patient disasters (up to 10 people), multiple casualty disasters (10 to 100 people), and mass casualty disasters (more than 100 people). Different problems occur because of the loss of support services in mass casualty disasters.

✔ Nurses participate during disasters by providing triage and first aid at emergency aid stations and hospitals, by providing health care at shelters, and by providing emotional support to persons at emergency morgues.

✔ Victims of disasters experience grief and mourning reactions; long-term adaptation may be hampered by lack of usual support systems.

QUESTIONS TO CONSIDER

- What are the laws governing care of accident victims (Good Samaritan laws) in your state?

- What materials could you use for care of bleeding wounds and fractures in your home? On a highway?

- What could you do to prepare yourself for a major disaster, such as a large tornado, flood, or earthquake?

REFERENCES AND SELECTED READINGS

1. American College of Surgeons, Committee on Trauma: Early care of the injured patient, ed 4, St Louis, 1989, The CV Mosby Co.
2. Andeman WA: Lyme disease: epidemiology, etiology, clinical spectrum, diagnosis and treatment, Adv Pediatr Infect Dis 1:163-186, 1986.
3. *Bacot EL, Jr: Community planning for disasters, Occup Health Nurs 32:310-311+, 1984.
4. *Bailey M: Emergency! First aid for fractures, Nursing 82 12(11):72-81, 1982.
5. *Baker HM: Some thoughts on helping grieving families, J Emerg Nurs 13:359-362, 1987.
6. Bangs CC: Hypothermia and frostbite, Emerg Med Clin North Am 2:563-577, 1984.
7. *Bosse LA: A disaster with few survivors, Am J Nurs 87:918-919, 1987.
8. Brand D et al: Adequacy of antitetanus prophylaxis in six hospital emergency rooms, N Engl J Med 309:636-640, 1983.
9. *Brown ST et al: Sheltering and response to evacuation during hurricane Elena, J Emerg Nurs 14:23-26, 1988.
10. *Bucanan L: Emergency! First aid for spinal cord injury, Nursing 82 12(8):68-75, 1982.
11. Burgess A and Holmstrom L: Rape: victims of crisis, Bowie, MD, 1974, Robert J Brady Co.
12. *Burgess AW: Rape trauma syndrome: a nursing diagnosis, Occup Health Nurs 33:405-406, 1985.
13. Buschiazzo L, Possanza C, and LeDent M: Coordinating your efforts to manage multiple trauma, CE Test Handbook 3:89-95, 1987/8.
14. *Butler S: Out of the water, but not out of the woods, RN 51(6):26-29, 1988.
15. Cain HD: Flint's emergency treatment and management, ed 7, Philadelphia, 1985, WB Saunders Co.
16. Cardona VD: Trauma nursing, Oradell, NJ, 1985, Medical Economics Books.
17. Clegg F: The psychological aftermath of disasters, Nursing '88(London) 3(31):5-8, 1988.
18. Cosgriff JH Jr and Anderson D: The practice of emergency nursing, ed 2, Philadelphia, 1984, JB Lippincott Co.
19. *DeLapp TD: Taking the bite out of frostbite and other cold weather injuries, Am J Nurs 80:204-208, 1980.
20. *DiNitto D et al: After rape: who should examine rape survivors? Am J Nurs 86:538-540, 1986.
21. Duffy J: Lyme disease, Infect Dis Clin North Am 1:511-527, 1987.

*References preceded by an asterisk are particularly well suited for student reading

22. *Edward SK and Cooper KL: After the blast, Am J Nurs 88:1203-1204, 1988.

23. Foley T and Davies M: Rape: nursing care of victims, St Louis, 1983, The CV Mosby Co.

24. Garcia LM: Disaster nursing: planning, assessment, and intervention, Rockville, Md, 1985, Aspen Systems Inc.

25. *Gray-Vickrey M: Education to prevent falls, Geriatr Nurs 5:179-183, 1984.

26. Guyton A: Textbook of medical physiology, ed 7, Philadelphia, 1986, WB Saunders Co.

26a. Hayes G, Goodwin T, and Miars B: After disaster: a crisis support team at work, Am J Nurs 90(2):61-64, 1990

27. *Heimlich LB: Care of the female rape victim, Nurse Pract 12(11):9-18, 1987.

28. Heimlich HJ: Pop goes the café coronary, Emerg Med 6:154-155, 1974.

29. Henry J and Volans G: ABC of poisoning: diagnosis, Br Med J 289:172-174, 1984.

30. Jacobs BB et al: Prehospital resuscitation of the trauma patient, Top Emerg Med 9(3):1-19, 1987.

31. Jacobs LM and Berrizbeitia LD: Prehospital trauma care, Emerg Med Clin North Am 2:717-732, 1984.

32. *Jamison DW: When emergency care is up to you, RN 50(4):26-31, 1987.

33. *Jankowski CB: Radiation, Am J Nurs 82:90-95, 1982.

34. *Jones MK: Fire! Am J Nurs 84:1368-1371, 1984.

35. Kaye D and Rose LF: Fundamentals of internal medicine, St Louis, 1983, The CV Mosby Co.

36. Kunkel DB: Bites of venomous reptiles, Emerg Med Clin North Am 2:563-577, 1984.

37. *LaVoy K: Dealing with hypothermia and frostbite, RN 48(1):53-56, 1985.

38. *Lee G: Transport of the critically ill trauma patient, Nurs Clin North Am 21(4):741-749, 1986.

39. *Lenehan GP: Emotional impact of trauma, Nurs Clin North Am 21(4):729-749, 1986.

40. *Maher AB: Early assessment and management of musculoskeletal injuries, Nurs Clin North Am 21(4):717-727, 1986.

41. Martin TG: Near-drowning and cold water immersion, Ann Emerg Med 13:263-273, 1984.

42. Matz R: Hypothermia: mechanisms and countermeasures, Hosp Pract 21(2):45-48, 1986.

43. *Mikhail JN: Acute burn care: an update, J Emerg Nurs 14:9-17, 1988.

44. Minden P: The Victim Care Service: a program for victims of sexual assault, Arch Psychiatr Nurs 3(1):41-46, 1989.

44a. Moore EE et al: Early care of the injured patient, ed 4, Philadelphia, 1990, BC Decker Inc.

45. *Moser MY: When lightning strikes, Am J Nurs 86:802-803, 1986.

46. *Newton M et al: General treatment of household poisoning, J Emerg Nurs 13:12-15, 1987.

47. Nicholson DP: The immediate management of overdose, Med Clin North Am 67:1279-1291, 1983.

48. *Nikas DL: Resuscitation of patients with CNS trauma, Nurs Clin North Am 21(4):729-740, 1986.

49. *O'Connell-Smeltzer SC: Research in trauma nursing: state of the art and future directions, J Emerg Nurs 14:145-153, 1987.

50. Oertel T: Bee-sting anaphylaxis: the use of medical antishock trousers, Ann Emerg Med 13:459-461, 1984.

51. *O'Hara MM: Emergency care of the patient with a traumatic amputation, J Emerg Med 13:272-277, 1987.

52. Parker, JG: Emergency nursing: a guide to comprehensive care, New York, 1984, John Wiley & Sons, Inc.

53. Parker JG: Thoracic trauma nursing assessment and management, Nurs Clin North Am 21(4):685-692, 1986.

54. *Rich J: How to keep venom from endangering a victim's life and limb, Nursing '87 17(6):33, 1987.

55. Rosen P et al: Emergency medicine: concepts and clinical practice, ed 2, St Louis, 1987, The CV Mosby Co.

56. Schroeder SA et al: Current medical diagnosis and treatment, Norwalk, Conn, 1989, Appleton & Lange.

57. *Shea KG: Natural disaster: personal preparedness, AORN J 43:1226-1238, 1986.

58. Sheehy SB and Barber J: Emergency nursing principles and practice, ed 2, St Louis, 1985, The CV Mosby Co.

59. Sheehy SB, Marvin JA, and Jimmerson CL: Manual of clinical trauma care: the first hour, St Louis, 1989, The CV Mosby Co.

60. *Shoven JT et al: Near-drowning, Am J Nurs 89:680-686, 1989.

61. Standards and guidelines for cardiopulmonary resuscitation (CPR) and emergency cardiac care, JAMA 255:2905-2988, 1986.

62. Statistical Abstracts of the United States, 1988, ed 108, US Bureau of the Census, Washington, DC, 1988, US Government Printing Office.

63. Temple AP, and Katz J: Management of acute head injury, AORN J 46:1066-1076, 1987.

64. *Walz JA: A simulated disaster drill, Am J Nurs 88:301-303, 1988.

65. Way LW: Current surgical diagnosis and treatment, ed 8, Norwalk, Conn, 1988, Appleton & Lange.

66. Welsh MD: Acute radiation syndrome, DCCN 5(5):277-286, 1986.

67. Wright SW et al: North American tick-born diseases, Ann Emerg Med 17:964-972, 1988.

68. Wyngaarden JB and Smith LH: Cecil textbook of medicine, ed 18, Philadelphia, 1988, WB Saunders Co.

CRITICAL CARE UNITS

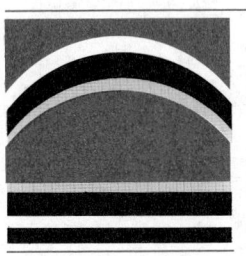

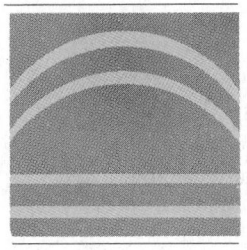

CHAPTER 80

Management of Persons in Critical Care Units

MAURA A. HOPKINS

CHAPTER OBJECTIVES

After studying this chapter, the student should be able to:
1. Describe the physical and psychologic environment of intensive care units.
2. Identify the types of data needed for the care of critically ill patients.
3. Describe interventions to alleviate physiologic stressors that are specific to the critical care setting.
4. Describe interventions to prevent and alleviate psychologic stress for the critically ill patient, the family, and the nurse.

The critical care unit is a unique environment in which the most sophisticated medical, nursing, and technical interventions can be integrated to combat life-threatening illness. Since nursing's earliest days the concept of locating the sickest patients together and nearest the nurses' station has underlined the importance of frequent assessment and rapid intervention. From postoperative wards to polio centers to the evolution of the coronary care unit, the concentration of highly specialized care givers with access to unique technology has remained the nucleus of the development of the intensive care unit (ICU).

The role of the nurse in the care of the critically ill patient has remained the focal point of the success of the critical care unit. Through the vigilant observation of a patient's ever-changing condition, the critical care nurse is uniquely able to identify problems and initiate appropriate therapies, monitor the complex treatment regimes, and intervene to prevent life-threatening situations. The critical care setting varies from the multipurpose ICU to units specially designed for patients with a common type of problem, such as medical, surgical, coronary, cardiovascular (open heart), neurologic/neurosurgical, pediatric, pulmonary, renal/dialysis, neonatal, burn, and shock/trauma units.

In any critical care setting the goal of nursing remains the same: to provide continuous, optimal nursing care to patients in life-threatening situations, remaining alert to the physiologic, psychologic, and social needs of the patient as an integrated being. This chapter provides an overview of some of the common aspects of critical care nursing and the critical care environment. Effects of the critical care environment on patient, family, and staff are discussed. Assessment of the critically ill patient is described, followed by interventions designed to alleviate physiologic, physical, psychologic, and social stressors experienced by critically ill patients.

ENVIRONMENT IN THE CRITICAL CARE UNIT

PHYSICAL ENVIRONMENT

The critical care unit is designed, equipped, and staffed to meet the anticipated needs of patients in life-threatening situations. The physical layout is frequently a modified circular design around a central nurses' station, allowing for direct visualization of all patients at all times. Patients may be separated into individual cubicles or situated in a large open area with curtains utilized as partitions. The advantage of direct nurse-patient visualization may accompany the disadvantages of limited privacy and patient exposure to frequent crisis intervention.

Supplies and equipment in critical care areas are highly sophisticated and must be readily accessible for all patients (see the box on p. 2316). Certain pieces of equipment are in constant use at each bedside (cardiac monitor, oxygen, suction equipment, etc.), whereas others must be available within seconds (defibrillator, ventilator, electrocardiogram [ECG] machine, emergency medications). In older institutions existing hospital space has often been converted to ICU use, and as the need for more specialized and sophisticated ICU equipment grows the critical care environment often becomes overcrowded.

PSYCHOLOGIC ENVIRONMENT—STRESS ON PATIENT AND STAFF

The critical care environment confronts patients with advanced forms of medical and nursing therapeutics.

EQUIPMENT COMMONLY AVAILABLE WITHIN OR NEAR THE ICU

MONITORS

Cardiac
Hemodynamic (intraarterial, pulmonary artery, central venous)
Intracranial pressure
Respiratory
Temperature
External arterial pressure

GENERAL EQUIPMENT

Emergency medications
ECG machine
Defibrillator/cardioverter
Pacemaker
Oxygen therapy equipment
Intubation equipment
Ventilator
Arterial blood gas analyzer
Fluoroscopy
Doppler flow detection device
Hyper/hypothermia machine
Bed scale

BEDSIDE EQUIPMENT

Bed with removable headboard
Oxygen and manual ventilation bag
Compressed air source
Suction
Resuscitation backboard
Intravenous infusion controller/pump
Overhead lighting
Multiple electrical outlets

SUPPORTIVE SERVICES (24 HR)

Pharmacy
Laboratory
Respiratory therapy
Radiology
Dialysis

STRESSORS ON PATIENTS, FAMILIES AND STAFF IN THE ICU

PATIENT/FAMILY

Unfamiliar environment, new faces
Noise, light levels
Sensory deprivation/overload
Interruption of sleep/wake cycles
Inaccessibility of family, friends
Lack of privacy
Lack of information/ understanding of prognosis, care plan
Lack of information/ understanding of policies, procedures
Anticipation of painful interventions
Confusion/disorientation related to physiologic factors
Impaired communication related to intubation
Observation of crisis intervention in other patients
Fear related to diagnosis
Fear of death

STAFF

Expectations of self
Expectations of peers, supervisors
Intricate machinery and techniques
Closed, crowded work area
Constant contact with seriously ill, dying patients
Continual vigilance over multiple patients
Constant emergency readiness
Sustained high activity level
Limited breaks away from the high-stress unit
Limited communication with many patients related to intubation or altered level of consciousness
Limited opportunity to communicate with some families
Isolation from other nurses in the hospital
Ethical conflicts related to issues of resuscitation and use of life-maintenance equipment

Although the patient and family are partially aware of the dynamics of critical care, their attention primarily focuses on the appearance of this special environment: flashing lights; buzzing machines; painful procedures; and a noisy, brightly lit, crowded, hyperactive environment. The stressors on the patient and family are immense, heightened by those treatment modalities that may prove lifesaving.

The stress on the nursing staff in the critical care area stems partially from very high expectations: advanced knowledge of physiology related to all body systems, astute observational and physical assessment skills, and technical proficiency in operating the highly sophisticated equipment. In addition, the constant vigilance and emergency-ready attitude may promote an uneasy sense of impending crisis. Critical care nurses must utilize excellent communication skills in dealing with the patient and family's psychologic and social needs, continually incorporating interventions that the nurse might be tempted to assign a lower priority in a critical situation.

Both the patient and the nurse are bombarded by continuous, varied stressors in the critical care environment (see box above, right). Low-level stress can be challenging and stimulating and may help enhance creativity, production, and performance in any area. However, continuous high-level stress can be devastating, both physically and psychologically. (Review Chapters 10 and 11 on adaptation, stress, and coping for a more in-depth analysis of the effects of stress.) It is very important for the critical care nurse to understand how stress will affect both the patient and family and to recognize that interactions will have to be modified to take this into account. In addition, nurses must be aware of their own stressors, including positive and negative effects. They must safeguard their own physical and psychologic health and recognize how insufficient or ineffective coping mechanisms can lead to burnout. The critical care unit is a powerful milieu that must be well understood by nurses who wish to use it advantageously.

ASSESSMENT OF THE CRITICALLY ILL PATIENT

The nursing process is the same in critical care situations as it is in any other patient setting. Management of critically ill patients requires establishing a data base, identifying real and potential problems, delineating priorities, defining outcome criteria, determining goals for intervention, executing the planned intervention, and modifying future goals and plans based on outcomes.

Management of critically ill patients differs from management of other patients because of an ever-changing data base; a larger number of complex, interrelated problems; frequent priority reorganization; and time limitations imposed by the rapidly changing condition of the patient.

The assessment process for the critically ill patient differs from the assessment of other patients only in reference to the types of technical devices available to assist in data collection. The cardiac monitor, hemodynamic monitoring lines, and laboratory analyses provide data that must be incorporated into the total patient assessment. They are adjuncts to the direct observational data which the nurse gathers through careful history taking and physical examination. Monitored data are useless unless correlated to physical findings and integrated into meaningful analysis by the critical care nurse.

NURSING HISTORY

There are three main routes by which critically ill patients come to an intensive care unit: direct admission, transfer from another patient care division in the same or a different hospital, and postoperatively after certain operations. The patient admitted directly to the ICU (for example, in the case of a myocardial infarction) will often be accompanied by family or friends. The patient and family members are utilized in obtaining a thorough and accurate history of both the current illness and past illnesses or hospitalizations, as well as a patient profile, social information, and usual coping strategies. Although emphasis is placed on alleviating physiologic problems at the time of admission, one member of the health care team may concurrently interview family members so that crucial facts about the patient's history can immediately be utilized in patient care. Even in the critical care setting, an accurate and thorough patient history is a vital part of intelligent, individualized care planning and intervention.

When the patient is transfered from another nursing division, either directly or after surgery, consultation between the transferring and receiving nursing staffs is essential. The ICU nurses will benefit from the care plan developed by nurses who have had an opportunity to interact with the patient and family in a noncritical situation. Pertinent history, patient preferences, coping mechanisms, and family relations can be relayed to the receiving nurses, thus reducing the initial stress of the unfamiliar ICU environment.

PHYSICAL EXAMINATION

As with the assessment of any patient, history taking is followed by physical examination. Inspection, palpation, percussion, and auscultation are used to elicit directly observed data from the patient. As in any other setting,

an explanation is given, even if the patient's comprehension is questionable, and the cooperation of the patient is sought. (Refer to a physical assessment textbook for a thorough explanation of the use of these techniques.)

MONITORED DATA

Nurses in all clinical settings utilize tools for discrete data collection from patients, such as stethoscopes, sphygmomanometers, thermometers, and scales. Critical care nurses have the additional advantage of using tools that are capable of continuous data collection, such as cardiac monitors, hemodynamic pressure lines, and intracranial pressure monitoring devices. The explosion in critical care technology in the 1970s and 1980s is providing the critical care nurse with amazing quantities of objective data with minimal time spent in system operations. Computerized monitoring systems are available that occupy less space and provide more capabilities than ever before. The most sophisticated of the "patient data management" systems takes information from all the continuously monitored parameters (ECG, arrhythmias, respirations, intraarterial pressure, pulmonary artery pressure, central venous pressure, intracranial pressure, and body temperature), combines it with manually entered data (such as body weight, height, intake and output, and times of drug administration), and prepares a wide array of hemodynamic calculations and patient response trends for analysis by critical care practitioners.

In the 1990s, critical care information systems will go one step further than data collection and analysis by moving directly into clinical intervention. For example, computerized intravenous medication administration systems now exist that can titrate the administration of vasoactive drugs by adjusting infusion pump flow rates in response to continuously measured intraarterial pressure. The parameters are set by the clinician, but the execution is determined by the computer within the pump. At this time, certain types of continuous monitoring devices are used in all critical care environments.

CARDIAC MONITORING

Cardiac monitoring requires placing conductive electrodes on the patient's chest which recognize the electrical activity of the heart and relay it to a video display screen. Both the patient's ECG and a digital count of the heart rate are displayed at the bedside. Alarm limits are individually set by the nurse so that if the patient's heart rate rises or falls beyond a safe range, a tone will sound to alert the nurse. In monitoring systems with computerized dysrhythmia analysis, the monitor will also recognize specific rhythm abnormalities, such as a single or paired premature ventricular contractions, bigeminal rhythms, runs of ventricular tachycardia, ventricular fibrillation, or asystole (Chapter 27). Variations in the audio or visual display of the alarm can alert the nurse to the relative seriousness of the dysrhythmia, even from a distance. Respiratory rate can often be monitored through the same set of chest electrodes measuring chest wall movement or impedence. Cardiac/respiratory monitoring is a noninvasive procedure that poses minimal risk to the patient.

HEMODYNAMIC MONITORING

Hemodynamic monitoring is a term that refers to invasive monitoring of the arterial or venous vascular system via a continuous electronic monitoring device. Table 80-1 lists the normal values of pressures found in the cardiovascular system, many of which can be measured at the patient's bedside.

INTRAARTERIAL MONITORING

Intraarterial monitoring involves inserting a catheter into an artery, usually the radial or the femoral artery. The catheter is connected to a high-pressure flush system normally filled with heparinized saline solution. A pressurized automatic flush device delivers an average of 1 to 3 ml solution per hour through the catheter to keep it patent. When an electronic transducer is connected to the system and attached to the bedside monitor, a waveform appears on the monitor that represents

the fluctuation of the patient's blood pressure in the catheterized artery. A numeric display of the arterial pressure also appears on the monitor; in most patients this direct intraarterial pressure correlates very closely to external cuff pressure measurements.

Intraarterial pressure monitoring also provides direct access to arterial blood, which can then be easily obtained without further needle punctures for various laboratory tests, including arterial blood gas analysis. Intraarterial catheters with fiberoptic tips are capable of continuous bedside monitoring of arterial pH, P_{CO_2}, and P_{O_2}. However, intraarterial cannulation is not without its complications (see the box below). Nursing responsibilities include set-up and safe, aseptic maintenance of the flush system and catheter insertion site; maintenance of a patent catheter with accurate waveform and pressure readings; and continuous patient observation to prevent the immediate life-threatening complication of hemorrhage.

PULMONARY ARTERY MONITORING

Pulmonary artery (Swan-Ganz) catheters (see Figure 26-16) are utilized to monitor cardiovascular function in critically ill patients. The catheter, which may have several openings along its length, is inserted into the superior vena cava via the subclavian or internal jugular vein. A balloon at the distal tip is filled with approximately 1 ml of air, and the catheter is floated through the right side of the heart until the tip lies in the pulmonary artery (PA) (see Figure 26-15). The balloon is then deflated. Pulmonary artery, central venous pressure (CVP), and pulmonary capillary wedge pressures (PCWP) can be obtained from the catheter once it is connected to a pressurized flush device and transducer-monitor system. In addition, cardiac output measurements can be performed. The PA catheter is useful in providing data about left and right ventricular failure and in evaluating the effectiveness of vasopressor drugs. It is a significant tool in the management of severe cardiac failure and cardiogenic shock (see Chapter 28). (Table 80-2 lists the hemodynamic indices that can be computed from monitored data.) In addition, the catheter serves as a central venous access line for the infu-

TABLE 80-1 Normal hemodynamic pressures

Area Monitored	Normal Pressure
Superior vena cava (SVC)	
Mean	2-6 mm Hg *or* 3-10 cm H_2O
Right atrium (RA)	
Mean	2-6 mm Hg *or* 3-10 cm H_2O
Right ventricle (RV)	
Systolic	20-30 mm Hg
Diastolic	0-5 mm Hg
End-diastolic	2-6 mm Hg
Pulmonary artery (PA)	
Systolic	20-30 mm Hg
Diastolic	10-20 mm Hg
Mean	10-15 mm Hg
Pulmonary capillary wedge (PCWP)	
Mean	4-12 mm Hg
Left atrium (LA)	
Mean	4-12 mm Hg
Left ventricle (LV)	
Systolic	100-140 mm Hg
Diastolic	0-5 mm Hg
Aorta (Ao)	
Systolic	100-140 mm Hg
Diastolic	60-80 mm Hg
Mean	70-90 mm Hg

COMPLICATIONS OF INTRAARTERIAL MONITORING

Bleeding
Distal obstruction of the artery/ischemia
Air embolism
Inflammation/infiltration
Infection
Thrombosis
Paresthesias

TABLE 80-2 Normal hemodynamic indices

Measurement	Formula	Normal Range
Cardiac output (CO)	Heart rate × stroke volume	4.0-8.0 L/min
Cardiac index (CI)	$\dfrac{\text{Cardiac output}}{\text{Body surface area}}$	2.5-4.0 L/min/m^2
Stroke volume (SV)	$\dfrac{\text{Cardiac output}}{\text{Heart rate}}$	60-130 ml/beat
Stroke index (SI)	$\dfrac{\text{Stroke volume}}{\text{Body surface area}}$	35-70 ml/beat/m^2
Mean arterial pressure (MAP)	⅔ Diastolic + ⅓ Systolic	70-90 mm Hg
Pulmonary vascular resistance (PVR)	$\dfrac{\text{Mean PAP} - \text{mean PCWP}}{\text{Cardiac output}}$	< 2 PVR units
Systemic vascular resistance (SVR)	$\dfrac{\text{MAP-CVP (mm Hg)} \times 80}{\text{Cardiac output}}$	900-1600 dynes/sec/cm^{-5}

sion of fluids and potent medications. Pulmonary artery catheters are replacing single-purpose CVP lines because the information they provide on left-sided heart function (wedge pressure, cardiac output) cannot be obtained from a single right-sided heart catheter (CVP line).

In some cardiovascular ICUs it is a common practice to forego the PA catheter and to insert a single line directly into the left atrium during open heart surgery, allowing direct monitoring of left-sided heart function. Other ICUs use a newer type of fiberoptic PA catheter that is able to perform continuous monitoring of PA (mixed venous) oxygen saturation. Minute by minute changes in the systemic oxygen saturation can be monitored, reducing the frequent sampling of arterial blood gas while rapidly demonstrating the effects of various clinical interventions on systemic oxygenation. As with intraarterial pressure monitoring, pulmonary artery monitoring is also not without risk (see box below). Nursing responsibilities are similar to those for arterial catheters, with the addition of continuous waveform observation to detect catheter tip migration.

COMPLICATIONS OF PULMONARY ARTERY MONITORING

Infection
Dysrhythmias
Pulmonary infarction
Pulmonary artery rupture
Balloon rupture with air embolism
Intracardiac knotting
Thrombophlebitis

INTRACRANIAL PRESSURE MONITORING

Intracranial pressure (ICP) is frequently monitored in critically ill patients who have or are suspected of having intracranial disease or secondary increases in intracranial pressure. A catheter placed through the skull into either the subarachnoid space or the cerebral ventricle allows changes in pressure within the cranial cavity to be monitored directly via a transducer and tubing system. ICP monitoring allows continuous observation of the patient's response to therapies aimed at lowering ICP and shows immediately the patient's tolerance of nursing measures, such as turning, suctioning, and changes in bed position, that can cause an unsafe rise in ICP. Cerebrospinal fluid can also be aspirated for analysis or culture or for relief of elevated ICP unresponsive to other therapies. Nurses are responsible for obtaining accurate pressure measurements, analyzing trends and patient response to interventions, and preventing complications of monitoring. Scrupulous sterile technique is essential in handling the catheter or screw insertion site and all connections in the monitoring tubing system because microorganisms have a direct pathway to enter the cerebrospinal fluid.

A new type of fiberoptic intracranial catheter is able to read ICPs directly at the tip of the catheter. The sensed pressures are converted into a waveform and digital value that can be displayed on the bedside monitor. Although entry into the subarachnoid or intraventricular space to measure ICP is still necessary, this catheter does not require the use of a fluid-filled pressure tubing/transducer system and therefore eliminates one source of potential contamination.

The preceding items represent a few of the invasive monitoring techniques available to the critical care nurse for data collection. In all cases the nurse must be knowledgeable about maintaining these lines: the normal appearance of the waveform associated with each line, the usual procedures necessary to prevent complications, and the signs and symptoms of actual complications. The risk to the patient from invasive monitoring lines is significantly reduced when the lines are handled and cared for by knowledgeable personnel.

BASELINE ASSESSMENT

The complete history and physical examination is the necessary foundation for further ongoing data collection in the critical care setting, and the importance of accurate and thorough initial information cannot be overemphasized. But the multiple sources of data and the continually fluctuating stability of critically ill patients makes constant priority reorganization a necessity. The critical care nurse utilizes continual observation of the patient to update the data base to reformulate short-term goals and interventions.

Patient assessment must be thorough, yet rapid. The physical and psychologic reactions of an entire organism under stress must be taken into account and not be limited by the usual or the expected. Patient assessment must also be organized and repetitive, so that small alterations or deviations from previous findings will be noticed. Finally, the assessment must be individualized, so that time and attention can be given to particularly significant aspects.

Many intensive care units utilize some form of a systems approach to patient assessment. Frequently a complete head-to-toe systems review at the beginning of the shift, will be taken, at which time the nurse gathers an initial data base (Figure 80-1). More time and depth are spent on the systems that present the greatest real or potential threat to the patient. When completed and documented, the baseline systems assessment presents an accurate status report on the patient's condition. Throughout the rest of the shift, the nurse notes all the changes as the patient improves or deteriorates from the baseline, keeping track of vital parameters on an ongoing flow sheet (see Figure 80-2).

Once initial patient assessment is completed, nursing diagnoses are established and nursing care plans formulated. Nursing interventions for critically ill patients are based on these care plans.

Throughout this text, nursing interventions have been described for care of the patient with a particular type of physiologic impairment. These are interventions intended to improve the patient's physiologic functioning before the impairment reaches the critical stage. In some critically ill patients, many of these interventions have already been utilized without success, and the patient's physiologic condition deteriorates to the critical level, necessitating acute life-sustaining interventions. For other patients, the first presentation of the illness is critical (such as acute myocardial infarction or severe trauma), and interventions are immediately necessary to sustain life.

The focus of the remaining three sections of this chapter will be on physiologic, psychologic, and social interventions necessary for the individual who is critically ill.

ALLEVIATION AND PREVENTION OF PHYSIOLOGIC AND PHYSICAL STRESSORS

The ultimate goal of nursing intervention for any patient, regardless of the nature of the illness, is to promote, sustain, and restore optimal levels of physiologic, psychologic, and social functioning. However, in a critical care setting, the immediate goal of ensuring a patient's survival initially determines the priorities for intervention; physiologic problems must be addressed first. Once life-threatening stressors have been alleviated, priorities are reorganized and other problems can be addressed.

Physiologic priorities are determined by the degree of threat to the survival of the individual. Certain body systems are more prone to disorders requiring intensive therapeutic interventions and are frequently encountered in the critical care unit. These disorders are listed by system, along with specific critical care interventions employed and additional interventions necessary to prevent complications of therapy.

RESPIRATORY SYSTEM

The highest priority in caring for a critically ill individual is the maintenance of a patent airway and adequate ventilation.

ACUTE RESPIRATORY FAILURE

Acute respiratory failure (see Chapter 33) may occur as a primary pulmonary deficit or as the result of a large number of other disorders that can affect the adequacy of ventilation or respiration. Crushing chest injuries, high-level spinal cord injury, neuromuscular diseases, extensive thoracic surgery, end-stage chronic obstruction pulmonary disease (COPD), sepsis, severe pneumonia, severe pulmonary edema, pulmonary embolus, congestive heart failure, sleep apnea, and shock are some of the conditions that may be exhibited by patients in respiratory failure requiring intensive care. Interventions in respiratory failure are first directed at establishing of an unimpeded airway, through endotracheal intubation via the nose or the mouth. Assisted ventilation may then be provided by a manual resuscitation device (Ambu or anesthesia bag), followed by placement of the patient on continuous mechanical ventilation. Mechanical ventilation devices may be classified by the method through

INITIAL PATIENT ASSESSMENT	PATIENT CARE

INITIAL PATIENT ASSESSMENT

General

CNS

Cardiovascular

Respiratory

GI

GU

Musculoskeletal

Skin

Psychosocial

Signature	Time

PATIENT CARE

Environment □ Siderails

Isolation type (specify) □ ID Band □ Allergy Band

□ Monitor Alarms Checked

□ Oxygen Equipment △ □ N/A □ Bath

ARTERIAL LINE

	Observation	
	Site Care	Time
	Tubing/Transducer △	Time

CENTRAL LINES / RELEAS

Type/Observation		
Site Care		Time
Tubing/Transducer △		Time
Type/Observation		
Site Care		Time
Tubing/Transducer △		Time

CVP LINE

	Observation	
	Site Care	Time
	Tubing/Transducer △	Time

CHEST TUBE

□ Mediastinal □ Pleural

□ cm H₂O _____ suction □ H₂O seal

Comments

Site Care	Time

INVASIVE

	Location	Observation	Site Care (Time)
LINES			

TUBING CHANGES

	Solution / Time	Solution / Time

Circumference of (Specify) ___ / ___ cm.   Abdominal girth ___ cm.

Miscellaneous

FIGURE 80-1 Sample critical care patient assessment form.

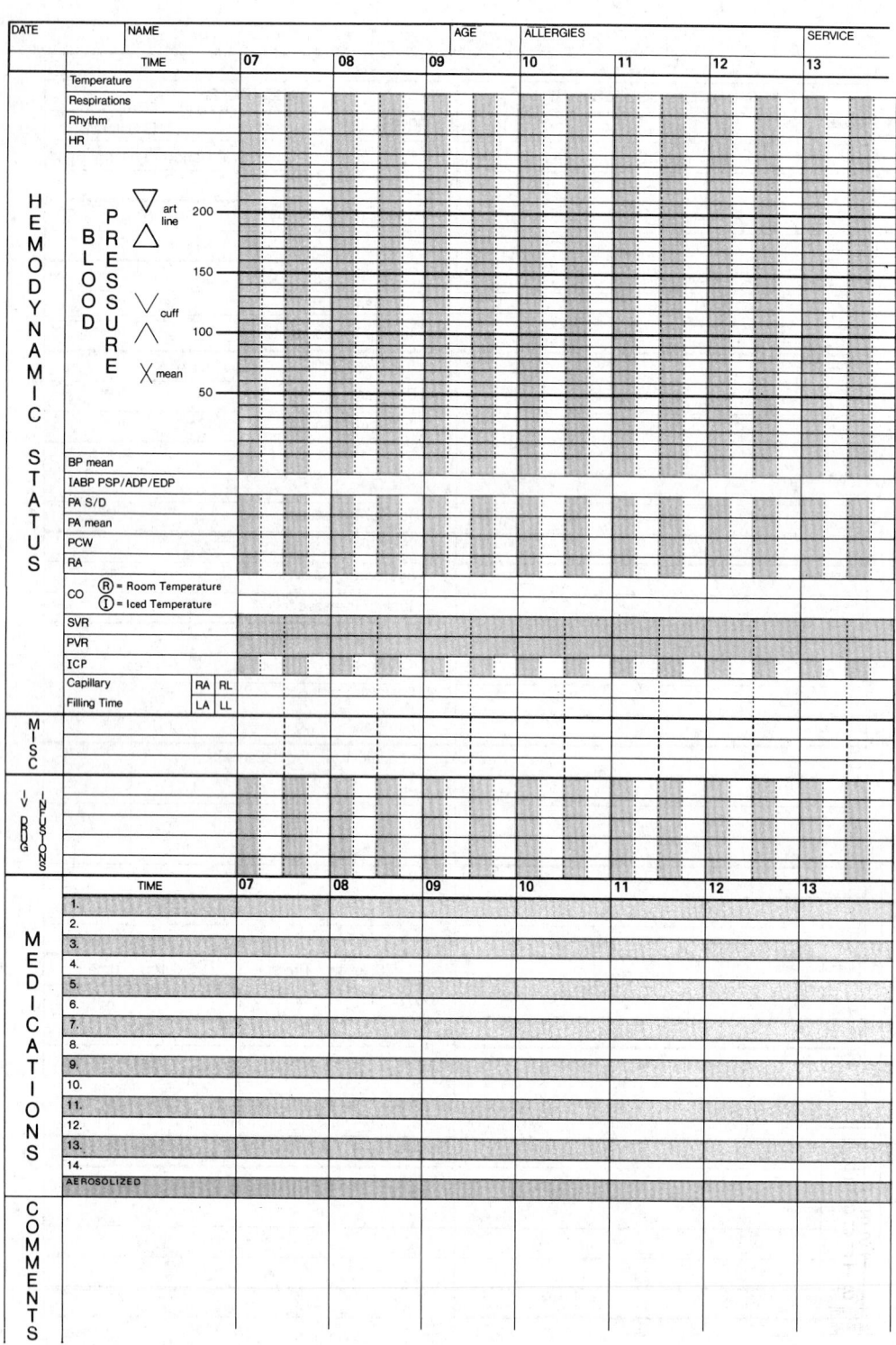

FIGURE 80-2 Surgical intensive care unit flow sheet.

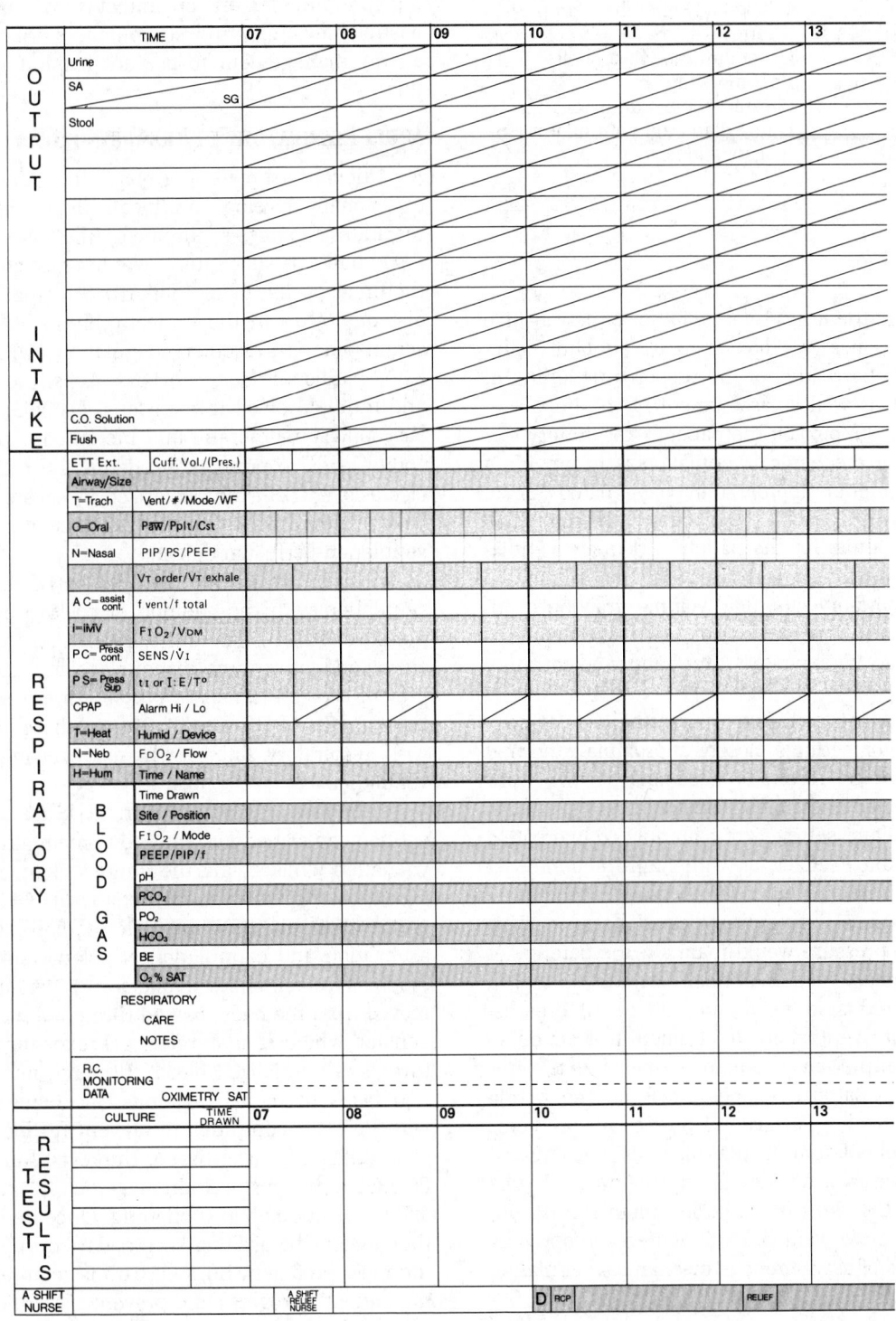

FIGURE 80-2, cont'd Surgical intensive care unit flow sheet.

TYPES OF MECHANICAL VENTILATORS

POSITIVE PRESSURE	NEGATIVE PRESSURE
Volume cycled	Whole body chamber ("iron
Bennett MA-1, MA-2	lung")
Bear	Chest cuirass, chest shell
Ohio	Pneumo wrap
Servo	Phrenic nerve stimulator
Pressure cycled	Direct diaphragm stimulator (in-
Bennett PR-2	vestigational)
Bird	

which air enters the lungs, that is, under either positive or negative pressure (see box above). Ventilatory support mandates observation of the proper functioning of the equipment as well as assessment of the impact of the mechanical support on the patient's respiratory status. The goal of mechanical ventilation is to provide a sufficient volume of appropriately oxygenated air to maintain serum pH, PCO_2, PO_2, and oxygen saturation within normal limits for the patient. Adequate ventilation is achieved through careful mechanical manipulation of the respiratory rate, tidal volume, fraction of inspired oxygen (FiO_2 or percent of 100% oxygen delivered), inspiratory to expiratory time ratio, and intrathoracic pressure.

In some disease states, such as neuromuscular conditions, ventilator settings closely approximate normal ventilation, and the respirator accomplishes the work that the weakened chest muscles cannot. In other situations the ventilator settings are manipulated to create a specific mechanical effect, as with high-frequency jet ventilation in bronchopleural fistula. In this condition large tidal volumes are contraindicated because their delivery under pressure would maintain the patency of the fistula. Instead, very small tidal volumes (60 to 100 ml) are delivered at a rapid rate (20 to 40 breaths/minute). Minute ventilation (total amount of air delivered in one minute) may remain normal, but the unusual breathing pattern reduces stress on the fistula and enhances healing. Unilateral pulmonary problems such as bronchopleural fistula may also be treated through the use of a double-lumen endotracheal tube that separates the right from the left main stem bronchus and allows two ventilators to deliver appropriately different modes of asynchronous mechanical ventilation to each lung.

Mechanical ventilation is a complex therapy that poses major risks for the critically ill patient, including pneumothorax, atelectasis, decreased cardiac output (especially if positive end-expiratory pressure is used), gastrointestinal bleeding from a stress ulcer, and infection. Preventive nursing interventions for all patients re-

ceiving mechanical ventilation include frequent assessment, position changes in bed, suctioning to remove secretions, intermittent deep ventilation (bagging or sighing), administration of antacids via nasogastric or gastrostomy tube, and scrupulous sterile technique in airway management to prevent respiratory tract infection.

ADULT RESPIRATORY DISTRESS SYNDROME

A particularly threatening respiratory complication that occasionally develops in critically ill patients is the adult respiratory distress syndrome (ARDS) (see Chapter 33). Also known as shock lung, wet lung, or postpump lung, the predisposing factors for ARDS include a number of disorders seen in the critically ill: shock, trauma, disseminated intravascular coagulation (DIC), fat embolism, cardiopulmonary bypass, sepsis, cardiac arrest, and multiple blood transfusions. Damage to the alveolar-capillary membrane and increased capillary permeability leads to pulmonary edema and diffuse microatelectasis. ARDS is characterized by severe dyspnea, hypoxemia, diminished lung compliance, and a significant ventilation-perfusion defect.

The primary intervention for ARDS is mechanical ventilation with the addition of positive end-expiratory pressure (PEEP). The use of PEEP aids in reexpanding alveoli and preventing further alveolar collapse, thus improving oxygen transport. Nursing interventions for the patient with ARDS are the same as those for any patient with respiratory failure who is receiving mechanical ventilation.

In the most severe cases of ARDS an extreme intervention can sometimes be used to maintain systemic oxygenation while giving the lungs a chance to heal. Extracorporeal membrane oxygenation (ECMO) is a temporary pulmonary bypass that requires systemic heparinization and cannulation of a large vein and artery (such as the femoral vein and aorta). Venous blood is removed from the body, passed through a membrane oxygenator where it undergoes gas exchange, and is returned as arterialized blood. Although minimal respiration takes place in the lungs, mechanical ventilation with PEEP is continued to prevent further fibrosis and consolidation of lung tissue. Improved lung function is facilitated by postural drainage, chest physiotherapy, and tracheobronchial suctioning. Once initiated, ECMO therapy may be used for several days during which time the most proficient nursing care is required to monitor the patient's progress and prevent the critical complications of disconnection, bleeding, embolus, decreased tissue perfusion, and infection.

CARDIOVASCULAR SYSTEM

Cardiovascular problems requiring intensive patient care are so frequently encountered that many institutions have specific ICUs designed for the care of these patients (coronary care unit, postoperative cardiovascular unit). After support of ventilation, maintenance of cardiac function and systemic circulation is the highest priority in life-threatening situations. Disorders of the cardiovascular system that frequently require intensive observation and intervention include acute myocardial infarction, cardiogenic shock, congestive heart failure, severe dysrhythmias, open heart surgery, and major vascular surgery.

Drug therapy is frequently used first for severe cardiovascular disorders and may be used until more definitive measures can be employed. Various cardioactive and vasoactive drugs are administered solely in critical care settings where their dosage and effects can be very closely monitored. Such interventions include fibrinolytic therapy in the form of tissue plasminogen activator (TPA). The early administration of TPA causes the breakdown of thrombus in the coronary arteries, stopping the progressive evolution of a myocardial infarction (Chapter 28). Highly potent medications often have a very small margin between therapeutic and toxic dosage levels, and the critical care nurse must ensure the correct dose and delivery route while monitoring its effect on the patient.

When drug therapy is insufficient to significantly or lastingly improve the patient's condition, certain *invasive techniques* may be beneficial. *Temporary transvenous pacing* may restore or enhance cardiac function until as a permanent pacemaker can be implanted. In emergency situations, external pacing may be initiated first while a decision is made on further intervention. For patients with recurrent, refractory, or lethal dysrhythmias an *automatic implantable cardioverter-defibrillator* (AICD) may be surgically implanted (Chapter 27). This device recognizes ventricular tachycardia and ventricular fibrillation and automatically shocks the heart when life-threatening dysrhythmia is detected. The AICD is used successfully to avert sudden cardiac death in specific patient populations.

Intraaortic balloon counterpulsation (IABC) may be necessary for the patient who needs to temporarily decrease the workload of the myocardium. A catheter is threaded into the aorta from a femoral artery: The distal 40 ml balloon inflates during ventricular diastole to increase coronary artery filling and deflates just before ventricular systole to decrease afterload and improve left ventricular ejection (Figure 28-14). Indications for IABC are listed in the box above. Nursing care of the patient with IABC includes critical minute-by-minute assessment of the patient's physiologic response to IABC therapy and intervention to prevent complications.

The *ventricular assist device* (VAD) is most often used to assist patients who have left-sided heart failure

INDICATIONS AND COMPLICATIONS OF IABC THERAPY

INDICATIONS	COMPLICATIONS
Cardiogenic shock with a reversible component	Ischemia of the catheterized leg
Low cardiac output states	Thrombus formation with eventual embolization
Patient removed from cardiopulmonary bypass surgery	Infection
Acute myocardial infarction	Aortic damage (aortic wall dissection, intimal laceration)
Unstable angina	Balloon rupture with gas embolus (rare)
Drug-resistant lethal dysrhythmias with ischemic cause	

and cannot be weaned from cardiopulmonary bypass surgery and for patients with severely damaged myocardiums. The VAD is a temporary assist device in which catheters are implanted into the left atrium or left ventricle to divert oxygenated blood into a roller pump located outside the body. The pump bypasses the left ventricle and returns the blood directly to the aorta, thus reducing myocardial workload by reducing preload. Right ventricular assist can also be provided for patients with severe right-sided heart failure in which the cannula bypasses the right ventricle. The nurse continually assesses the patient's response to therapy through evaluation of hemodynamic data. Proper mechanical function of the device is also critical since occlusion or disconnection could cause rapid death.

As mentioned previously, using a VAD is a temporary intervention. If the heart is unable to recover sufficient contractile strength, the patient may be evaluated for cardiac transplantation. While waiting for transplantation, cardiac function may be supplied by a *total artificial heart* (TAH). After years of research, the TAH has been developed into a bichambered, pneumatically driven design. After the patient's heart is removed, the TAH is attached to the atria remnant, pulmonary artery, and aorta. After pneumatic drive tubing is inserted through the chest and attached to a large-drive console, which controls heart function and cardiac output, the chest is closed. Research continues with both the VAD and TAH in which the ultimate goal is that both devices could become completely implantable.

Prevention of physiologic stressors to the cardiovascular system is a continual priority for care of all ICU patients. Most preventive measures are aimed at myocardial workload reduction and include all measures that enhance oxygenation, decrease physical exertion, and decrease sympathetic stimulation (see the box on p. 2326).

Finally, in addition to decreasing myocardial workload, the myocardium must also be protected from a unique hazard of the critical care environment: *electri-*

MEASURES TO REDUCE MYOCARDIAL WORKLOAD

Enhance oxygenation	Supplemental oxygen
	Assisted ventilation
	Semi-Fowler position
	Vasodilators
Decrease physical exertion	Bed rest
	Passive range of motion exercises
	Stool softeners, laxatives
Decrease sympathetic stimulation	Reduce environmental stimuli (noise, lights)
	Limit visitors to supportive persons
	Inform and reassure patient and family
	Provide continuity in care givers
	Individualize interventions to reduce specific anxieties

cal microshock. The invasive monitoring and therapeutic interventions utilized with critically ill patients often create a direct pathway to the heart (central venous pressure lines, pulmonary artery catheters, temporary pacemakers). Direct contact with stray or leaked current could prove fatal, particularly in critically ill patients whose resistance may be further decreased through other breaks in skin integrity and through electrolyte imbalances. Nursing staff in critical care areas are all responsible for the safe and proper use of electrical equipment, as well as for the implementation of appropriate electrical safety precautions.

NEUROLOGIC SYSTEM

A number of neurosurgical disorders, most often either the result of trauma or of intracranial neoplasms, may necessitate intensive care during an acute phase of illness. These include subdural and subarachnoid hemorrhage, direct head injuries, massive cerebral vascular accident, intracranial aneurysm rupture, and preoperative and postoperative care of certain patients undergoing craniotomy for surgical repair of a structural defect.

Specialized neurologic interventions for critically ill patients are aimed at maintaining a homeokinetic state of brain metabolism and controlling elevations in intracranial pressure (ICP) (see Chapter 63). ICP monitoring (p. 2319) may be used to assess the extent of potentially dangerous rises in ICP.

Removal of cerebrospinal fluid is one method of controlling rising ICP. Other interventions include osmotic diuresis to remove excess fluid from brain tissue and mechanical hyperventilation to artificially reduce circulating CO_2 levels. Lowered CO_2 levels will trigger cerebral vasoconstriction, reducing the potential for progressive interstitial cerebral edema.

Efforts to lower the overall metabolism of the brain will reduce the brain's requirements for its natural substrates, oxygen and glucose. This is especially important when transport of these elements is impaired. Interventions to reduce brain metabolism include generalized hypothermia via a cooling mattress and induction of barbiturate coma. Caring for the artificially comatose patient requires the same attentive observations and extensive nursing interventions as are employed for the naturally comatose patient to prevent complications, with the addition of mechanical ventilation (see Chapter 60). In addition, complete neurologic assessment of the patient must be thoroughly performed when the sedation is reduced or withdrawn. A lightened level of consciousness necessitates sensitive communication, even though the patient's comprehension may not be apparent.

In addition to neurosurgical disorders, patients with a variety of neurologic diseases may be seen in the intensive care unit during acute exacerbations or at the end stages of progressively debilitating conditions that sometimes finally necessitate mechanical ventilation. These diseases include amyotropic lateral sclerosis, Guillain-Barré syndrome, myasthenia gravis, and sometimes multiple sclerosis. All four of these immunologic disorders are either known or suspected to be mediated by autoantibodies or circulating immune complexes. Therapeutic plasmapheresis may be performed to temporarily cleanse the blood of the antigenic agents.

During *plasmapheresis* venous blood is continuously removed through a large bore needle and circulated through a cell separator, which removes the plasma. The blood cell components are returned to the patient with the addition of normal saline, plasma protein fraction, fresh frozen plasma, or albumin. Depending on the patient's tolerance, from 1 to 3 L of plasma may be removed over 3 to 4 hours, and treatments may be required 2 or 3 times per week for several weeks. Although only variably successful and never a cure, plasmapheresis may reduce acute symptoms in patients with myasthenia gravis and may limit the severity of exacerbations. The critical care nurse monitors cardiac rhythm, hemodynamic stability, and electrolyte balances; observes meticulous venous access site care; and provides emotional support for the chronically ill patient.

Nursing interventions to prevent physiologic stressors to the neurologic system are aimed at supporting diminished neurologic capacity, preventing injury, reducing pain, and preventing intracranial pressure elevations (see the box on the following page).

RENAL SYSTEM

Acute renal failure in the critically ill patient may result from a primary intrarenal cause, such as acute glomerulonephritis or acute cortical necrosis, or from a struc-

NURSING INTERVENTIONS TO PREVENT INCREASED ICP IN CRITICALLY ILL PATIENTS

Maintain patent airway
Minimize arterial blood gas changes
  Oxygenate patient before and after suctioning
  Limit suctioning to 15 seconds
Elevate head of bed 30° (facilitates venous drainage without impeding arterial supply)
Maintain head and neck in straight alignment
Prevent overtight tracheostomy ties
Prevent Valsalva maneuver (increases ICP)
  Assist patient in turning
  Prevent coughing, sneezing, constipation
Monitor hydration status, intake, and output

ADVANTAGES/DISADVANTAGES OF HEMODIALYSIS, PERITONEAL DIALYSIS, AND CONTINUOUS ULTRAFILTRATION

HEMODIALYSIS	PERITONEAL DIALYSIS
Rapid, efficient correction of severe serum abnormalities	Well tolerated by even very unstable patients
Short time period for actual dialysis	Inexpensive procedure
Expensive procedure	Technologically simple procedure
Requires highly technical equipment	Must be performed over several hours or days
Poorly tolerated by very unstable patients	Cannot be performed on patients with recent abdominal surgery
Risk of hemorrhage	Risk of peritonitis

CONTINUOUS ULTRAFILTRATION

Highly effective if fluid removal is primary goal
Well tolerated by critically ill patients
Slow correction of severe electrolyte abnormalities
Relatively inexpensive procedure
Must be performed over several hours or days
Greater risk of hemorrhage because of length of procedure

---

tural defect. It may be the result of directly nephrotoxic agents as in heavy metal poisoning or pharmacologic agents, such as aminoglycocide antibiotics. But most often acute renal failure in critically ill patients is the secondary result of any disorder that severely reduces cardiac output and renal perfusion, including cardiac arrest, left ventricular failure, or hemorrhage.

Interventions for the patient who has renal failure are intended to provide the regulatory functions that the kidneys can no longer maintain. The nurse keeps accurate daily weights and intake/output records so that only the exact amounts of body fluids lost plus a percentage for insensible losses are replaced. Laboratory values are monitored carefully, with electrolyte intake being limited and pharmacologic drugs, for example, sodium polystyrene sulfonate (Kayexalate), being utilized as necessary for electrolyte removal. Diuretics are given to increase marginal renal function. Nutrition is altered through restricted protein intake, since the body cannot appropriately excrete the nitrogen that is produced by amino acid breakdown. The nurse evaluates acid base balance, anticipating metabolic acidosis from the buildup of acid metabolic wastes (carbonic and lactic acids). All other body systems are affected by the progression of acute renal failure, and continuous interventions are necessary to prevent altered acid base and electrolyte levels from impairing cardiovascular, respiratory, and neurologic function. Therefore the nurse is alert for such things as ECG changes indicative of increased myocardial irritability and altered contractility, changes in ventilatory pattern such as Kussmaul breathing and acidotic breath, and decreased level of consciousness or altered mentation or behavior.

When renal failure has reached a level that is unresponsive to medical intervention, dialysis becomes necessary to mechanically remove the waste products of body metabolism (see Chapter 50). Intermittent hemodialysis or peritoneal dialysis (see box above, right) may

be initiated for the critically ill patient and may be performed for several hours a day, 3 to 5 days per week.

An alternate method of continuous ultrafiltration, also known as *continuous arteriovenous hemofiltration* (CAVH), may be used to remove excess fluid from patients with acute renal failure. Arterial blood is removed from the body and passed through a semipermeable membrane that removes water and dissolved solutes but returns blood cells and plasma proteins to the body via a venous line. The filtration is accomplished by a pressure gradient established primarily by the patient's mean arterial pressure and is thus a slow and consistent process that may be better tolerated by critically ill patients. Some patients may also require intermittent hemodialysis to further clear uremic toxins, or dialysate can be added to the CAVH system (CAVH-D) and slow continuous dialysis can be accomplished. Nursing responsibilities center on hemodynamic monitoring and prevention of potential complications such as disconnection, clotting embolus formation, electrolyte imbalance, clotting abnormalities, and infection.

GASTROINTESTINAL SYSTEM

The most common gastrointestinal problem seen in the critical care setting is *acute gastrointestinal bleeding*. This may be the medical diagnosis in a newly admitted patient, or it may be a complication, such as a stress ulcer, in an already critically ill person. Interventions such as gastric lavage with iced saline and administration of agents that inhibit gastric acid secretion are intended to control bleeding until its cause and extent are determined. A Sengstaken-Blakemore tube may be used to provide direct compression of esophageal varices to tamponade a serious hemorrhage. Administration of blood components and crystalloid fluids is initiated to reverse the hypovolemia of acute hemorrhage. Vasopressor medications cannot be administered to raise systemic blood pressure until the hypovolemic state is corrected. Once the patient's condition has stabilized sufficiently and the site of bleeding has been identified, surgery may be performed to repair the affected area.

The primary function of the gastrointestinal system is to ingest and digest liquid and solid nutrients. For many critically ill patients this process is interrupted for a lengthy period in which either enteral or total parenteral nutrition (TPN) may be substituted (see Chapter 43). TPN solutions contain the essential protein, carbohydrate, and fat necessary to establish a catabolic state in which positive nitrogen balance is maintained. The critical care nurse assesses the adequacy of hydration and electrolyte balance as well as caloric intake. In addition, the nurse takes active measures to prevent infection, the primary complication of TPN.

Prevention of gastrointestinal complications such as stress ulcers (see Chapter 43) in critically ill patients requires active nursing interventions. Patients at highest risk include those who are receiving no oral intake, who are mechanically ventilated, who have liver dysfunction, who are receiving anticoagulants, and who have undergone any severe physiologic stress. In addition to the administration of local antacids and systemic histamine inhibitory agents (such as cimetidine hydrochloride), specific interventions are required to reduce the psychologic stress inherent in the critical care environment.

MUSCULOSKELETAL/INTEGUMENTARY SYSTEMS

Hypersensitivity reactions to various agents may be so severe that a patient may develop life-threatening illness. Two disorders that can cause critical illness are Stevens-Johnson syndrome and toxic epidermal necrolysis. Both disorders are severe inflammatory syndromes characterized by epidermal slough, mucosal inflammation, and ulceration. Clinical symptoms include fever, systemic toxicity, and erythema multiforme lesions. The syndromes are precipitated by a major physiologic stressor such as a drug reaction, mycoplasmic pneumonia, herpes simplex infection, collagen vascular disorder, or pregnancy. Despite intensive medical and nursing interventions, mortality can be as high as 65%.

Although few primary musculoskeletal problems necessitate intensive care, the majority of critically ill patients have severe restrictions placed on their mobility. Bed rest, weakness, and pain, as well as attachment to numerous therapeutic and monitoring devices, significantly limit normal motion. Preserving function of

---

NURSING INTERVENTIONS FOR PREVENTION OF PULMONARY EMBOLUS

Elevation of lower extremities
Use of antiembolism stockings
Hourly active foot dorsiflexion
Active/resistive range of motion exercises
Observation of Homan's sign
Coughing and deep breathing exercises
Administration of low-dose heparin as ordered
Inspection of intravenous sites with routine needle changes

---

weight-bearing muscles, maintaining joint mobility, and preserving continuous skin integrity (see Chapter 68) are significant challenges to critical care nurses. All of the preventive and supportive nursing care techniques used with any patient who has restricted mobility are appropriate in the ICU. The progression of the ICU patient to the highest level of activity facilitates improvement in physiologic function and reassures the patient of an improving condition.

One of the most serious potential complications of immobility is development of a deep vein thrombus, which can embolize and travel to the lungs. Pulmonary emboli are found in up to 60% of all persons after an autopsy is performed. Signs and symptoms of pulmonary embolism include dyspnea, pleuritic chest pain, fever, hemoptysis, tachycardia, and pleural friction rub. Preventive interventions can be instrumental in reducing the risk of these serious complications (see the box above).

REPRODUCTIVE SYSTEM

Although preeclampsia (proteinuria, edema, and hypertension) complicates approximately 5% of all pregnancies, most patients with these conditions are successfully managed outside the critical care environment. In a few cases, however, complications may require invasive monitoring and aggressive intervention. A syndrome of hemolysis, elevated liver enzymes, and low platelet count is potentially fatal and may be identified late in pregnancy or within the first 48 hours after delivery.

The management of severe pregnancy-induced hypertension is becoming more common as high-risk mothers are transferred to the ICU immediately after delivery for continuous monitoring and treatment with nitroprusside or other antihypertensive drugs administered intravenously. High-risk mothers may be admitted to the general ICU for optimal health care management. Close consultation with obstetricians and obstetric nurses is required to maintain an optimal environment for the fetus and mother. Therapy is aimed at stabilizing the mother by reducing hypertension, moderating coagulopathies, maximizing ventilation and hydration, and preventing preterm labor. Emergency cesarean section delivery may be performed in the ICU for severe maternal or fetal distress. In some tertiary centers, obstetric mini-ICUs are being established to maximize care for both the fetus and mother.

IMMUNOLOGY/ORGAN TRANSPLANTATION

Many medical practitioners believe that gaining knowledge and control over the body's immune response is the ultimate key to the health care of the future (see Chapters 8 and 75 through 77 for discussions of the immune system). All critically ill patients are compromised hosts, facing the physiologic stress to the immune system caused by severe illness. The severely immunocompromised patient presents some of the greatest challenges in critical care. Whether the immunosuppression is induced (immunosuppressive drugs, chemotherapy, radiation therapy) or acquired (AIDS, severe combined immunodeficiency diseases, severe systemic lupus erythematosis), the patient may develop life-threatening sepsis and shock from an inability to resist infection. Nursing care focuses on interventions for current infections, protection from further infections, and optimization of natural defenses through maintenance of skin integrity, cleanliness, hydration, and nutrition.

The combination of immunosuppressive therapy and increasingly sophisticated surgical techniques has allowed organ transplantation to move from the realm of the experimental to the commonplace. Both natural and artificial organs have been implanted with varying degrees of success. Development of cross-species xenograft has advanced from the well-accepted porcine cardiac valve implant to the experimental chimpanzee heart transplant. The decades-old practice of transfusing living blood cells has blossomed into the development of synthetic blood substitutes as well as bone marrow transplantation to generate new blood tissue. Heart, heart-lung, kidney, liver, and pancreas transplants are now performed at medical centers throughout the country.

The critical care nurse may be actively involved in the transplant process in two very different ways. The nurse may care for posttransplant patients, using the latest technology and most advanced clinical skills to encourage a successful recovery and facilitate a return to healthy life. Or the nurse may care for the transplant donor, completing meticulous pretransplant tasks while providing emotional care to the anguished family in an often sudden and tragic situation. In either case, the critical care nurse has the privilege of providing care to those in need and of knowing the dramatic difference one's care can make in someone else's life.

ALLEVIATION AND PREVENTION OF PSYCHOLOGIC STRESSORS

Despite the continuous attention the critical care nurse must devote to the assessment of and the intervention in physiologic derangements, the nurse must also focus attention on recognizing the psychologic stressors that confront the patient and family. The emotional discomfort and distress that the patient and family endure not only affect psychologic health but also have a direct impact on physical recovery.

The initial step in preventing or alleviating psychologic stress is to identify the patient's and family's perception of the critical event. Their perceptions will be affected by their individual personalities, current psychologic health, general understanding of the current situation and its projected outcome, tolerance of ambiguity, and normal patterns of coping. Initial perceptions are often significantly affected by previous exposure to similar events, either positive or negative, and general level of familiarity with medical interventions and the hospital environment. Six specific interventions nurses can utilize in any setting to reduce the psychologic stress of illness are detailed in the following discussion.

ACKNOWLEDGE, ACCEPT, AND ENCOURAGE PATIENT/FAMILY TO AIR THEIR FEELINGS

Because the critically ill person is alienated from familiar surroundings and daily living patterns and is dependent on others to meet the most basic needs of survival, the patient becomes partially or totally isolated from usual support systems.

Feelings of helplessness, powerlessness, loneliness, and depersonalization as well as disturbances in body image are common. Modes of expressing and therefore relieving the frustration, anger, hostility, fear, and depression generated by these feelings are limited by the physical constraints of the critical care environment. Whether a primary nursing approach or other delivery model is used, consistently assigned care givers are essential to developing a physiologically and psychologically therapeutic bond with the patient and family.

An atmosphere of openness and acceptance that encourages expression of feelings can help provide patients with a means of coping. Talking with patients openly and honestly decreases feelings of depersonalization and prevents isolation and alienation. Anger and hostility are often indicative of fear and anxiety. Depression and withdrawal may be signs of hopelessness, loneliness, powerlessness, or loss and are normal and expected. Encouraging expression of feelings helps the patient identify the reasons for feeling or behaving in a way that may seem strange or wrong. At the same time it provides protection and permission to feel and act that way. Nurses or other health team members who are helping a patient to talk about feelings must be ready to accept whatever emotionally laden information might be expressed. Nonjudgmental recognition and acceptance of the patient's feelings will help to reinforce the patient's right to the feelings.

Patients who are intubated are unable to express their feelings freely even when alert and oriented and are therefore particularly vulnerable to psychologic stressors. It is a natural tendency to communicate less with those who cannot talk easily and the nurse must guard against this. Keeping a letterboard, paper and pencil, or a "magic slate" within the patient's reach and providing assistance when the patient desires will help to reduce the sense of isolation. However, such methods are not convenient for the expression of personal feelings or involved concerns. The nurse can recognize clues to the patient's emotional state by appearance and behavior and by knowing the types of concerns the patient is most likely to have. The nurse can verbalize the potential concerns, allowing the patient to validate them as appropriate. Being empathetic with the patient and family conveys acceptance and understanding.

PROVIDE INFORMATION/CLARIFY MISCONCEPTIONS ABOUT PHYSICAL STATUS, GOALS OF TREATMENT, AND INTERVENTIONS

It is the patient's *perception* of stress and not the stressor itself that determines the patient's reaction to illness and the environment. It is essential that the patient and family receive adequate information and simple explanations. Without explanations the critical care environment presents a mysterious and threatening array of noxious stimuli, which may be perceived as extremely unnatural and even magical. The highly sophisticated equipment increases the patient's feelings of vulnerability, and the patient may worry that the cardiac monitor is actually keeping the heart beating, that a blood transfusion indicates hemorrhaging, or that chest physiotherapy signifies pneumonia. A very common misconception of patients after coronary artery bypass surgery is that "open heart" surgery involved cutting the heart wide open and sewing it back together again. Such a perception can lead to a drastic alteration in body image.

Much of what patients learn about their health problems depends on what is taught, both directly and indirectly, by the health care team. Patient teaching in critical care requires short-term goals. Pain, discomfort, weakness, anxiety, and transient confusion are some of the obstacles to learning that these patients experience (see the research box above). Despite these obstacles, patients and families need simple, repetitive explanations of all procedures and the purpose of each intervention, as well as an introduction to rehabilitation plans and health maintenance strategies. Patients may not understand or believe what they are told the first time,

RESEARCH

Vitello-Cicciu JM: Recalled perceptions of patients administered pancuronium bromide, Focus Crit. Care 11(1)28-35, 1985.

Pancuronium bromide is a nondepolarizing neuromuscular blocking agent frequently used to induce skeletal muscle paralysis in mechanically ventilated patients. Since pancuronium bromide has no effect on the central nervous system, patients paralyzed by it cannot move but are fully awake and potentially aware of the environment. Five patients, who received pancuronium bromide while intubated were asked to recall their perceptions during a stay in a critical care unit. The findings indicated that: (1) the majority of the subjects were able to recall some perceptions during the period of paralysis; (2) one or more subjects could specifically recall being touched or spoken to; (3) none of the subjects could recall being able to see or smell; and (4) subjects reported various feelings and diverse thoughts about things they wanted to do when they couldn't move. The author recommends incorporating clear explanations and comforting touching techniques into the routine care of intubated patients receiving pancuronium bromide. ▪

or anxiety and denial may prevent recollection of it. Reinterpretation and reiteration of diagnosis, prognosis, goals of treatment, types of interventions, and expectations of the patient and family may be continually necessary during the entire ICU stay. Explanations should be given by the same few people to encourage a bond of continuity as well as minimize the confusion of differing approaches and wording. If the patient and family are apprised of the patient's current status, as well as of changes in plans, the situation is perceived accurately and the future is planned realistically, thus ensuring their cooperation by making them members of the health team.

ENCOURAGE AND SUPPORT INVOLVEMENT OF PATIENT/FAMILY IN DECISION-MAKING AND CARE

The essence of crisis intervention is to help individuals cope with a major life crisis that a critical illness might precipitate. Critical care nursing is far broader in scope and more future oriented than crisis intervention alone, but specific situations within the critical care setting may require the immediacy and limited focus of crisis intervention. At that time the patient and family are directed in establishing short-term goals and are given limited choice in acceptable responses. As the crisis situation stabilizes, even though it may be no less critical, the patient and family are given additional information and further responsibility in establishing mutual goals and choosing alternate responses. When the patient and family are knowledgeable about the goals of therapy and understand the patient's diagnosis, current status, and prognosis, they can then be involved in many aspects of care planning and can make decisions consistent with the treatment regimen.

Involvement of the individuals who represent the patient's significant support system decreases feelings of powerlessness, frustration, and anxiety. In addition, when these emotionally important figures, whether family or friends, understand and support the treatment goals and are involved in the patient's care, they are better able to sustain and expand this behavior after the patient leaves the ICU and hospital. Even when a patient is unconscious, visits by key support figures who talk to and touch the patient may have positive, if unmeasureable, effects on the patient while helping to decrease the family's feelings of helplessness.

An alert patient can be directly involved in care planning and establishing goals of treatment. One specific mechanism to increase the patient's feeling of personal control is to encourage involvement in structuring the daily schedule of activities. The knowledge that patient preferences are important to the nursing staff and that the person is viewed as capable of making decisions will support self-esteem and reinforce the centrality of the patient's role in recovery.

The environment of the critical care unit is a major stressor in which both the patient and family must cope. (The many sources of external stress are outlined in the first section of this chapter.) In addition, disturbed thought processes and perceptual distortions are often likely to be seen in patients who are given narcotics and sedatives, are highly anxious, have multiple interrelated debilitating physical problems, have disturbed metabolic and respiratory function, are deprived of sleep, and are older. Reality reinforcement on a continuing basis is necessary for these persons. Although some environmental factors cannot be altered, specific interventions can be implemented by the nurse to provide a sensory-regulated environment. Interventions designed to help create a balance between sensory deprivation and sensory overload in the ICU setting are listed in the box below.

PREPARE PATIENT AND FAMILY FOR TRANSFER FROM ICU

Transfer from the critical care unit to another setting may cause significant stress for some patients and their families. The critical care area represents security and protection with its sophisticated electronic equipment

---

INTERVENTIONS TO MINIMIZE SENSORY DEPRIVATION/OVERLOAD

REDUCE NOISE LEVEL

Avoid excessive conversation
Avoid raising voice to talk to persons outside conversational range
Utilize carpeting as feasible
Avoid continuous droning of radio or TV; turn on/off at appropriate intervals
Locate nursing lounge away from patient care area

MAINTAIN DAY/NIGHT ORIENTATION

Dim lights at night
Raise/lower shades or open/close window curtains in normal day/night pattern
Reinforce progression of day in relation to specific events, such as meals

MAINTAIN TIME ORIENTATION

Position large-numeral clocks in easy view
Provide wall calendars
Allow wrist watches for certain patients
Provide frequent reorientation to person, place, time

PROMOTE REST AND SLEEP

Schedule most exerting activities so that rest period may follow
Coordinate health team activities to provide periods of uninterrupted sleep
Minimize routine cleaning or stocking at night

PROVIDE POSITIVE TACTILE STIMULI

Touch/hold patient's hand during conversation
Use soothing physical contact as able (back rubs, face cleansing, etc.)
Encourage family to touch patient, hold hands despite dressings, etc.

MAINTAIN PERSONAL/SOCIAL INTEGRITY

Address patient by name, identify self by name
Provide full and complete information, explanations, and instructions
Avoid discussion over the patient; include the patient in rounds
Establish flexible visiting hours
Encourage visits by family, significant others
Make visiting rule exceptions for children and even pets when special circumstances arise
Allow important personal belongings at bedside

REDUCE PAIN AND DISCOMFORT

Administer analgesics appropriately to relieve pain
Reposition immobile patients q 2 hr
Prepare patients for all potentially uncomfortable or painful procedures

MAINTAIN FUTURE ORIENTATION

Discuss transfer plans early with both patient and family
Initiate teaching regarding rehabilitation and health maintenance strategies as appropriate

and attentive, highly skilled staff. Patients know that transfer means moving to an area where there are fewer nursing personnel per patient, less direct contact with nursing personnel, no automatic monitoring devices, and no direct observation of the bed from the nurses' station. Greater independence and higher levels of activity will be expected of patients on the transfer unit, and the support of familiar nursing staff will be lost. Patients may have conflicting feelings about the transfer as an indicator of physical improvement if they do not feel as well or as independent as they anticipated at the time of transfer.

The anxiety precipitated by the transfer can be prevented or reduced if the patient and family are taught to interpret the meaning of particular signs and symptoms and are helped to understand the true purpose of equipment and routines. Signs that indicate progress need to be pointed out continuously, beginning when they first appear. Initiating the discussion of transfer plans with the patient and family as soon as the patient's condition begins to stabilize in the ICU will help them adjust to and prepare for the relocation. Along with the projected date of transfer, patient and family need to know what to expect on the new unit and what will be expected of them. Ideally, a nurse from the receiving unit should meet the patient and family before transfer. After transfer, visits from members of the ICU staff are helpful in conveying continued concern for the patient's welfare, as well as in providing objective validation of continued progress. With careful planning and execution, transfer from the critical care unit can be a triumphant rather than a traumatic event.

PROVIDE SUPPORT IN ETHICAL DECISION-MAKING

In many ways, the major technologic advances currently available in hospitals have moved beyond society's ability to understand and keep pace with the associated ethical dilemmas. Life can be prolonged in ways and in clinical conditions that were previously impossible. Not infrequently, life can be maintained past all known hope of recovery. Tremendous emotional, financial, legal, and societal ramifications exist as patients are stabilized into conditions for which long-term health care options are very limited. For example, few families and even fewer skilled care facilities have the resources to care for a patient who is continually mechanically ventilated. Critical care nurses frequently assist families with highly emotional decisions related to foregoing resuscitation or withdrawing life support systems.

As with all health care professionals, the critical care nurse must examine his or her own beliefs about life and death, termination of life, and utilization of limited resources. Education and support for the nurse is available from formal classes, support groups, peers, and hospital ethics committees. Ethics committees are avail-

able to patients, families, and staff who wish consultation and support in difficult or divisive situations.

Biomedical advances at times seem to challenge the compassion of ethical issues. The critical care nurse is a person who can provide a pivotal role in identifying and promoting the patient's wishes.

ALLEVIATION AND PREVENTION OF SOCIAL STRESSORS FOR PATIENT AND FAMILY

In the critical care setting the patient's physiologic needs often assume priority over psychologic needs, and the patient as a social being may risk being virtually ignored. Limited visiting hours, the strange technical environment, and the aura of danger in the ICU isolates patients from their supportive family and friends and prevents them from assuming their usual social roles. For the most part, a person who is critically ill is viewed by staff primarily in the patient role. The more significant roles of spouse, parent, child, lover, sibling, friend, or provider may go virtually unrecognized unless the nursing staff initiate interventions to provide continuity in these relationships.

Such continuity is fostered through some of the same types of interventions that were utilized to reduce psychologic stress: increased visiting between patient and family; inclusion of family into discussions of disease process, prognosis, and plans of care; and reporting by family of events and activities occurring in the other significant spheres of the patient's life. Relaying telephone messages between the patient and distant friends is one way to maintain contact with the patient's external world.

One of the most effective and important ways to prevent disruption in relationships is to prepare family or friends for their first visit with the patient in the ICU. The patient's physical appearance and the critical care environment should be explained thoroughly before the visitor enters. Visitors need to understand the patient's level of consciousness, ability to communicate, and ability to comprehend communication. They need to be made aware of the importance of their presence to the patient and the patient's need for their support. When visitors approach the bedside, a staff member should remain with them to facilitate their initial interaction with the patient. At each subsequent visit the nurse caring for the patient meets with the significant others to answer questions and apprise them of the patient's progress.

In addition to supporting the maintenance of the patient's current roles and relationships, the critical care nurse must also recognize the inevitability of actual role change for some patients and families during a critical illness. Roles of provider, decision maker, employer, employee, and leader may be altered, reversed, or eliminated. At this point some of the responsibilities of the patient need to be assumed by family and friends.

During the critical phase of illness the family members will be attempting to cope with precipitous role changes and may need assistance in working through problems that arise as family members and friends assume or fail to assume these additional responsibilities. The nurse needs to be aware of this problematic time and may need to provide the family with professional guidance, such as from a social worker, to assist in reorganizing themselves and their resources. The nurse may help the family appoint a temporary leader from among their ranks, one who knows and is able to represent the wishes of the family as a whole and who could be contacted in the event of an emergency. The nurse may also help the family to plan visiting schedules that will meet the patient's needs without preventing the family members from maintaining their own responsibilities. It is a period of great emotional stress for both patient and family.

That emotional stress may eventually climax in the death of the critically ill patient. (See Chapter 14 for a complete discussion of dying and death.) The following are suggestions for the critical care nurse caring for a dying patient:

1. Examine your own feelings about death.
2. Listen in order to assess the needs of the patient and family.
3. Remain available; be physically and emotionally present.
4. Use touch in caring for the patient and family.
5. Provide reassurance of the patient's continued care, even if the patient is not to be resuscitated. Provide information.
6. Attempt to remain nonjudgmental about family or hospital issues.
7. Respect the person-family relationship, which existed long before the patient-hospital relationship.
8. Include the family in care.
9. Provide for patient and family privacy.
10. Provide the opportunity for the family to exercise religious or cultural traditions.

Providing comprehensive care to critically ill patients and their families is a demanding task. The critical care nurse combines the technologic sophistication of this unique setting with a personal, individualized care approach to maximize the potential outcomes for the patient.

CHAPTER SUMMARY

- Numerous types of critical care units exist. They are designed, equipped, and staffed to meet the anticipated needs of patients in life-threatening situations.

- Inherent in the critical care environment are multiple stressors for the patient, the family, and the nurse. Identification and amelioration of these physiologic, psychologic, and social stresors is the goal of critical care nursing.

- Critical care nurses build on clinical knowledge from all specialties. Any organ system dysfunction may result in critical illness, requiring unusually invasive or specialized equipment for assessment and intervention.

- The nursing process is the same in critical care situations as in other patient care settings. The nurse establishes a data base, identifies real and potential problems, defines goals and outcome criteria, and executes the planned interventions based on clinical priorities. Evaluating the results and modifying the plan is an ongoing process.

- The advancement of medical technology has made the prolongation of life possible in ways never before experienced. Careful attention to the ethical, social, and financial implications of intensive care technology is necessary to maintain focus on the patient's quality of life.

QUESTIONS TO CONSIDER

- Who should or should not be admitted to a critical care unit? What would a list of admission criteria include?

- What are the goals of mechanical ventilation? How does mechanical ventilation differ for patients with various etiologic conditions of respiratory failure?

- Why are aseptic technique and infection control so important in the critical care setting?

- If the family of a critically ill patient with a terminal disease asked your opinions of withdrawal of life support, how would you respond?

REFERENCES AND SELECTED READINGS

1. Alspach JG and Williams SM: Core curriculum for critical care nursing, ed 3, Philadelphia, 1985, WB Saunders Co.
2. Bagby M et al: The total artificial heart, Am J Nurs 87:1050-1058, 1987.
3. Baker CF: Sensory overload and noise in the ICU: sources of environmental stress, Crit Care Q 6(4):66-80, 1984.
4. *Beglinger JE: Coping tasks in critical care, DCCN 2(2):80-89, 1983.
5. Bernard GR: Adult respiratory distress syndrome: diagnosis and management, Heart Lung 15:250-255, 1986.
6. Bradley RB: Adult respiratory distress syndrome, Focus Crit Care 14(5):48-59, 1987.

*References preceded by an asterisk are particularly well suited for student reading.

7. Brewer MJ: To sleep or not to sleep: the consequences of sleep deprivation, Crit Care Nurse 5(6):35-41, 1985.

8. Bustin D: Hemodynamic monitoring for critical care, Norwalk, Conn, 1986, Appleton-Century-Crofts.

9. Caine RM and Bufalino PM: Critically ill adults: nursing care planning guides, Baltimore, 1988, Williams & Wilkins.

10. Carpenito LJ: Nursing diagnosis in critical care: impact on practice and outcomes, Heart Lung 16:595-600, 1987.

11. *Cassem NH, Hackett T, and Bascon C: Reactions of coronary patients to the CCU nurse, Am J Nurs 70:312-319, 1970.

12. Clochesy JM: Advanced technology in critical care nursing, Rockville, Md, 1989, Aspen Publishers Inc.

13. Cohen FL: Acquired immunodeficiency syndrome research in critical care: a review and future directions, Focus Crit Care 15(4):30-35, 1988.

14. Cooper DK, Valladares BK, and Futterman LG: Care of the patient with the automatic implantable cardioverter defibrillator: a guide for nurses, Heart Lung 16:640-648, 1987.

15. Crismon CH: Plasmapheresis, DCCN 3(1):17-23, 1984.

16. Daily EK and Schroeder JS: Hemodynamic waveforms—exercises in identification and analysis, St Louis, 1983, The CV Mosby Co.

17. Daily EK and Schroeder JS: Techniques in bedside hemodynamic monitoring, ed 4, St Louis, 1989, The CV Mosby Co.

18. Daley L: The perceived immediate needs of families with relatives in the intensive care setting, Heart Lung 13:231-237, 1984.

19. Davidson LJ: Continuous SVO$_2$ monitoring: a tool for analyzing hemodynamic status, Heart Lung 15:287-292, 1986.

20. DeGroot KD and Damato MB: Critical care skills, Norwalk, Conn, 1987, Appleton & Lange.

21. Dillon J et al: Rapid initiation of thrombolytic therapy for acute MI, Crit Care Nurse 9(2):55-61, 1989.

22. Easton C and MacKenzie F: Sensory-perceptual alterations: delirium in the intensive care unit, Heart Lung 17:229-237, 1988.

23. Erickson S and Hopkins MA: Gray areas: informed consent in pediatric and comatose adult patients, Heart Lung 16:323-325, 1987.

24. Fowler MDM and Levine-Ariff J: Ethics at the bedside—a sourcebook for critical care nurses, Philadelphia, 1987, JB Lippincott Co.

25. Futterman LG: Cardiac transplantation: a comprehensive nursing perspective, part 1, Heart Lung 17:499-510, 1988.

26. Futterman LG: Cardiac transplantation: a comprehensive nursing perspective, part 2, Heart Lung 17:631-640, 1988.

27. Gahart BL: Intravenous medications, ed 5, St Louis, 1989, The CV Mosby Co.

28. Griffin JP: Nursing care of the immunocompromised patient in the ICU, Heart Lung 15:179-188, 1986.

29. Goldsmith J et al: Clinical and experimental aspects of single-lung transplantation, Heart Lung 16:231-236, 1987.

30. *Hay D and Oken D: The psychological stresses of intensive care nursing, Psychosom Med 34:117, 1972.

31. Heater BS and AuBuchon B: Controversies in critical care nursing, Rockville, Md, 1988, Aspen Publishers Inc.

32. Henker R, Shaffer L, and Whittaker A: Nursing care of the patient with a total artificial heart, Heart Lung 16:381-391, 1987.

33. Hickey M and Lewandowski L: Critical care nurses role with families: a descriptive study, Heart Lung 17:670-676, 1988.

34. Hoffman LA: Airway management for the critically ill patient, Am J Nurs 87:39-53, 1987.

35. Hollingsworth-Fridlund P, Vos H, and Daily EK: Use of fiberoptic pressure transducer for intracranial pressure measurement: a preliminary report, Heart Lung 17:111-120, 1988.

36. Hudak CM, Gallo BM, and Lohr TS: Critical care nursing, a holistic approach, ed 4, Philadelphia, 1986, JB Lippincott Co.

37. Johanson BC et al: Standards for critical care, St Louis, 1988, The CV Mosby Co.

38. Kemp VH: The role of critical care nurses in the ethical decision-making process, DCCN 4:354-359, 1985.

39. Kenner CV, Guzzetta CE, and Dossey BM: Critical care nursing: body, mind, spirit, ed 2, Boston, 1985, Little, Brown & Co Inc.

40. Kiely MA: Type-II toxic epidermal necrolysis, Crit Care Nurse 7(1):34-39, 1987.

41. Kinney MR: AACN's clinical reference for critical-care nursing, ed 2, New York, 1988, McGraw-Hill Inc.

42. Koniak-Griffin D and Dodgson J: Severe pregnancy-induced hypertension: postpartum care of the critically ill patient, Heart Lung 16:661-669, 1987.

43. Konopad E and Noseworthy T: Stress ulceration: a serious complication in critically ill patients, Heart Lung 17:339-348, 1988.

44. Larson E: Infection control issues in critical care: an update, Heart Lung 14:149-156, 1985.

45. Leske JS: Needs of relatives of critically ill patients: a follow-up, Heart Lung 15:89-93, 1986.

46. Lewandowski W et al: Treatment and care of "do not resuscitate" patients in a medical intensive care unit, Heart Lung 14:175-181, 1985.

47. Lindquist RD: Providing patient opportunities to increase control, DCCN 5(5):304-309, 1986.

48. Littrell K and Schumann LL: Promoting sleep for the patient with a myocardial infarction, Crit Care Nurse 9(3):44-49, 1989.

49. Metzger JT and Hoffman LA: Cardiac transplantation: the changing faces of immunosuppression, Heart Lung 17:414-425, 1988.

50. Millar S: AACN procedure manual for critical care, ed 2, Philadelphia, 1985, WB Saunders.

51. Moorhouse MF, Geissler AC, and Doenges ME: Critical care plans—guidelines for patient care, Philadelphia, 1987, FA Davis Co.

52. Moser SA, Crawford D, and Thomas A: Caring for patients with implantable cardioverter defibrillators, Crit Care Nurse 8(2):52-65, 1988.

53. Moskowitz LD and Moskowitz S: Autonomy and the critically ill patient: the legal issues, Heart Lung 15:520-524, 1986.

54. Mulford E: Nursing perspectives for the patient receiving postoperative ventricular assistance in the critical care unit, Heart Lung 16:246-257, 1987.

55. Murphy P: When a non-death death occurs: helping the family accept the reality of brain death, Nursing 86 16(7):34-39, 1986.

56. Nyamathi A and Van Servellen G: Maladaptive coping in the critically ill population with acquired immunodeficiency syndrome: nursing assessment and treatment, Heart Lung 18:113-120, 1989.

57. Omery A and Caswell D: A nursing perspective of the ethical issues surrounding liver transplantation, Heart Lung 17:626-631, 1988.

58. Palmer JC et al: Nursing management of continuous arteriovenous hemofiltration for acute renal failure, Focus Crit Care 13(5):21-30, 1986.

59. Persons CB: Transcutaneous pacing—meeting the challenge, Focus Crit Care 14(1):13-19, 1987.

60. Price CA: Continuous arteriovenous ultrafiltration: a monitoring guide for ICU nurses, Crit Care Nurse 9(1):12-19, 1989.

61. Quall SJ: Comprehensive intra-aortic balloon pumping, St Louis, 1984, The CV Mosby Co.

62. Riegel B and Ehrenreich D: Psychological aspects of critical care nursing, Rockville, Md, 1989, Aspen Publishers Inc.

63. Roberts SL: Behavioral concepts and the critically ill patient, ed 2, Norwalk, Conn, 1986, Appleton-Century-Crofts.

64. Roberts SL: Physiologic nursing diagnoses are necessary and appropriate for critical care, Focus Crit Care 15(5):42-49, 1988.

65. Robinet K: Increased intracranial pressure: management with an intraventricular catheter, J Neurosurg Nurs 17(2):95-104, 1985.

66. Schermer L: Physiologic and technical variables affecting hemodynamic measurements, Crit Care Nurse 8(2):33-40, 1988.

67. Schroeder CH: Pulse oximetry: a nursing care plan, Crit Care Nurse 8(8):50-68, 1988.

68. Sinclair V: High technology in critical care: implications for nursing's role and practice, Focus Crit Care 15(4):36-41, 1988.

69. Smith SL: Liver transplantation: implications for critical care nursing, Heart Lung 14:617-628, 1985.

70. Sommers MS: Difficult diagnoses in critical care nursing, Rockville, Md, 1989, Aspen Publishers Inc.

71. Stevens LL, Redd RM, and Buckingham TA: Ventricular burst pacing, Crit Care Nurse 9(3):38-43, 1989.

72. Swearingen PL, Sommers MS, and Miller K: Manual of critical care: applying nursing diagnoses to adult critical illness, St Louis, 1988, The CV Mosby Co.

73. Vasbinder-Dillon D: Understanding mechanical ventilation, Crit Care Nurse 8(7):42-56, 1988.

74. Wescott BL: Tissue plasminogen activator: a new advancement in fibrinolytic therapy, Focus Crit Care 13(6):22-26, 1986.

75. Whittaker AA, Hull B, and Clochesy JM: Hemolysis, elevated liver enzymes, and low platelet count syndrome: nursing care of the critically ill obstetric patient, Heart Lung 15:402-410, 1986.

76. Winkelman V: Hemofiltration: a new technique in critical care nursing, Heart Lung 14:265-271, 1985.

77. Wilson VS: Identification of stressors related to patients' psychologic responses to the surgical intensive care unit, Heart Lung 16:267-273, 1987.

78. Wlody GS and Smith S: Ethical dilemmas in critical care—a proposal for hospital ethics advisory committees, Focus Crit Care 12(5):41-46, 1985.

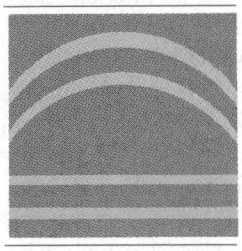

CHAPTER 81

Case Study of a Critically Ill Patient

MAURA A. HOPKINS

CHAPTER OBJECTIVES

After studying this chapter, the student should be able to:
1. Follow the progression of a patient's nursing care from the critical to the stable phase.
2. Identify the appropriate nursing diagnoses in response to the physiologic, emotional, and social problems presented by a multiple trauma patient.
3. Define the necessary nursing interventions specific for each identified nursing diagnosis.
4. Identify mechanisms to promote continuity of care for a critically ill patient, noting the impact on the family unit.

Patients with a wide variety of medical and surgical problems are cared for in intensive care units (ICU). In some cases, care is focused primarily on one or two target systems, and the purpose of the ICU stay is relatively straightforward. As an example, the ICU care of the patient following uncomplicated open-heart surgery often follows a fairly predictable course. More often, however, the critically ill patient has problems affecting multiple systems, frequently further compromised by general debilitation and decreased resistance, which predisposes the patient to significant complications.

The patient who suffers multiple trauma typifies this latter situation and challenges the critical care nurse to devise and execute a plan of care that addresses numerous threats to various systems. A comprehensive approach is required to relate the deficiency in one system to real or potential deficiencies in other systems.

The preceding chapter outlined assessment and interventions for the critically ill patient using a systems approach. This familiar approach allows the nurse to obtain data in a rapid and organized fashion. When assessing the collected data and formulating a plan of care, the critical care nurse looks at the functional patterns that are emerging and describes actual threats to the patient's well-being. Nursing diagnoses are then identified, expected outcomes are developed, and essential interventions are implemented.

The nursing diagnoses described in the following case study are among those approved by the North American Nursing Diagnosis Association Eighth National Conference. Diagnoses and interventions for this patient are described at two phases: within 24 hours of ICU admission and at the time of transfer from the critical care unit.

CASE STUDY
ASSESSMENT
PATIENT HISTORY

Michael B. is a 27-year-old man who was driving his 1-year-old daughter home from child care when their automobile was struck by an oncoming motorist who crossed the center line. Mr. B. was pinned behind the wheel and was unconscious when rescue workers freed him 10 minutes after the accident. Mr. B. was hypotensive (blood pressure 86/52), tachycardic (rate 126), and tachypneic (8 breaths/min) with a visible wound and sucking noises apparent from the left side of his chest. Mr. B.'s daughter Stephanie was found strapped in her carseat behind the driver's seat, crying lustily. Although squirming about vigorously, Stephanie was not moving her left leg, which was bleeding profusely. The driver of the other vehicle, though looking dazed and shaken, appeared to be unhurt. Both Mr. B. and Stephanie were given first aid at the accident scene by paramedics. All three victims were transported to a community hospital, where the driver of the other vehicle was given fluids, observed for a short time, and released. Stephanie was found to have a deep, jagged laceration of the left upper leg requiring surgical debridement and closure. She was admitted to the hospital's pediatric floor.

Mr. B. was still unconscious on arrival in the emergency department (ED). Lactated Ringer's solution was infusing rapidly into a peripheral intravenous catheter in the right forearm; 750 ml had infused by the time of his arrival at the hospital. Instability of Mr. B.'s left leg had been noted when the paramedics examined him at the accident scene, and a fractured femur was suspected. The leg was splinted for transport. An occlusive dressing covered the left chest wound.

Rapid physical assessment in the ED revealed that Mr. B.'s skin was pale to dusky, cool, and clammy with cold extremities. His vital signs had deteriorated: BP, 72/40; apical heart rate, 150/min; respirations, 36, shallow and labored, with left-sided paradoxical chest movement (flail chest). His abdomen was distended and firm, with superficial contusions. Bowel sounds were absent.

Immediate interventions were begun to stabilize and reverse Mr. B.'s rapidly deteriorating condition. Endotracheal intubation was performed and positive pressure mechanical ventilation was begun with 100% oxygen. A chest tube was placed in the left pleural space and connected to water-sealed drainage, with 30 cm negative pressure applied. A 16-gauge central intravenous catheter was inserted in the right subclavian vein for rapid administration of large fluid volumes. A 16-gauge peripheral IV was inserted in the left forearm for additional intravenous access. A nasogastric tube was inserted to decompress the stomach and assist in observing for gastrointestinal bleeding. Initial aspiration showed normal gastric fluid with occult blood (guaiac positive). A Foley catheter was inserted and immediately drained grossly bloody urine.

Blood samples were obtained to assess ventilatory status, electrolyte balances, cell counts, and clotting factors as well as to type and cross match blood for transfusion. Diagnostic x-ray examination revealed several left-sided rib fractures with pneumothorax, as well as a midshaft fracture of the left femur. Stat intravenous pyelogram (IVP) revealed intact urethra, bladder, and ureters with apparent trauma to the left kidney.

Mr. B.'s respiratory and hemodynamic status were stabilizing as he was taken to the operating room. An exploratory laparotomy was performed and revealed a lacerated spleen and left kidney. The kidney laceration was repaired, a splenectomy was performed, and the abdomen was evacuated of free blood. A thoracotomy was performed to repair the rib fractures. Steinman pins were inserted into the left tibia and the femoral fracture was aligned in proper position. Mr. B. received 8 units of whole blood as well as 4 L of crystalloid solution during the surgery. A second chest tube was placed during the thoracotomy, and the central venous catheter was replaced with a pulmonary artery thermodilution (Swan-Ganz) catheter for postoperative monitoring of hemodynamic status.

SOCIAL HISTORY

Mrs. B. arrived at the hospital while her husband and daughter were being treated in the ED. When Mr B.

was taken to the operating room, Mrs. B. accompanied her daughter to the pediatric floor. The intensive care unit was alerted that they would be receiving Mr. B. postoperatively and that his wife would be in her daughter's hospital room until that time. The nurse who was expecting to admit Mr. B. to the ICU went to the pediatric floor to meet Mrs. B. and obtain a nursing history as well as to explain the routines of the ICU.

The nurse learned that Mr. B. was a previously healthy, physically active computer service technician who had recently taken a new job. His employee benefits included adequate hospitalization insurance but he has no available paid sick leave. Mr. B. had had the usual childhood illnesses with no prior hospitalizations. Mrs. B. described her husband as a very calm, logical, hard-working man, not given to extremes of behavior but who liked to maintain organization and control in his life. Mr. B. completed 2 years of college before leaving to attend a technical school to learn his current trade. Mrs. B. is a registered nurse in obstetrics at a hospital across town. The family has no particular religious ties. Mr. B.'s parents live several states away, and his four siblings are scattered around the country. Mrs. B.'s parents live an hour away. Her only sister died at age 19 in a motor vehicle accident (MVA). Both Mr. and Mrs. B. are devoted to their only child, Stephanie.

The critical care nurse found Mrs. B. to be comprehending the situation well, but at the same time very agitated, angry, and fearful. She appeared to understand that her daughter's injuries were serious but not life threatening. She looked terrified as the nurse quietly explained some of the equipment and procedures that would be used to care for her husband in the ICU. She admitted that she really had no exposure to ICU nursing and stated that she felt incompetent as a nurse "now that my husband really needs me." Although hesitant to leave her child, she readily accepted the nurse's invitation to tour the ICU in advance of her husband's arrival from the operating room. She appeared to relax somewhat in the ICU as the nurse continued her explanations and briefly demonstrated the function of the ventilator and the monitor. She returned to Stephanie's room to wait, asking the nurse to call her as soon as Mr. B. or his doctor arrived in the unit.

Postoperatively Mr. B. was transported directly to the ICU. On arrival he was immediately placed on a mechanical ventilator. The nurse initiated full hemodynamic monitoring by connecting electrocardiogram (ECG) leads, pulmonary artery catheter, and arterial line to the bedside monitor. The nasogastric tube and chest tubes were individually connected to suction and the Foley catheter to gravity drainage. The nurse scanned Mr. B.'s orders and adjusted the intravenous fluids accordingly. Then the nurse proceeded through a complete assessment, making the following observations.

INITIAL ICU ASSESSMENT
General

A 27-year-old white male, well developed, well nourished, admitted to ICU bed 3. Patient is status post-MVA with subsequent surgery for splenectomy, repair of left kidney laceration, thoracotomy, rib fracture stabilization, and Steinman pin insertion for left femoral fracture. Patient is nonresponsive, intubated, on mechanical ventilation. Lines present: No. 8 French oral endotracheal (ET) tube, No. 18 French nasogastric tube, right subclavian pulmonary artery (PA) catheter, 16-gauge right radial arterial line, 16-gauge left forearm peripheral I.V., two No. 26 French chest tubes in anterior and posterior left chest, and No. 16 French Foley catheter. Dressings intact to left anterior chest and abdomen.

Respiratory

No spontaneous respirations. Volume ventilation via oral ET tube: Tidal volume, 1000 cc; respiratory rate, 14; FiO_2, 70%; positive end-expiratory pressure (PEEP), 10 cm; peak inspiratory pressure (PIP), 45 cm. Breath sounds audible bilaterally; right lung clear with scattered rhonchi; left lung sounds dull and diminished at base with loud, coarse rhonchi throughout; left pleural friction rub present. Chest tubes to −30 cm water sealed suction draining dark red blood, total 220 ml since tubes placed. Air leak present via posterior tube. Chest wall movement symmetrical and equal bilaterally. Chest wall contused and abraded. Subcutaneous emphysema present over left anterior chest from nipple line to left axilla to neck.

Cardiovascular

BP, 94/62, mean 72 per arterial line, 90/60 per cuff; apical heart rate, 120, regular; radial pulse, 120, regular; rectal temperature, 97.6° F; PA pressure, 24/12, mean 16; pulmonary capillary wedge pressure (PCWP), 10; central venous pressure (CVP), 6. Dopamine hydrochloride infusing at 12 mcg/kg/minute to maintain systolic BP of 90. Sinus tachycardia without ectopic beats. S_1 and S_2 audible, without murmur. Skin, cool, dry, pale. Capillary refill normal to slow in all extremities. Carotid, radial, femoral, popliteal, and dorsalis pedis pulses all palpable and equal bilaterally.

Neurologic

Postanesthetic state; nonresponsive to verbal or normal tactile stimuli. Responds to noxious stimuli with minimal flexor response; responds to ET suctioning with gag reflex. No pathologic reflexes present. Pupils equal, round, 3 mm; reactive to light with consensual response.

Gastrointestinal

Nasogastric tube patent, draining moderate amount dark green gastric secretions. Guaiac positive, pH 5.0. Abdomen firm. Bowel sounds absent. Abdominal dressing dry and intact.

Genitourinary

Urine bloody, draining well via an 18-gauge Foley catheter. Urine output 1200 ml since catheter inserted. Normal genitalia.

Musculoskeletal/Integumentary

Steinman pin present in left tibia. Left leg in Thomas splint with Pearson attachment; 20 pounds' traction applied. Multiple bruises and abrasions over anterior chest, abdomen, and legs. Areas appear clean. Nutritional status good, skin turgor good.

INITIAL CARE

For the next several hours the critical care nurse observed Mr. B. continually and conferred frequently with his physician. Labile blood pressure and hypovolemia were treated with infusions of crystalloid, fresh-frozen plasma, and packed red blood cells. The dopamine drip was titrated to maintain a systolic blood pressure of at least 90 mm Hg and was still necessary even as the volume status improved. Numerous ventilator changes were made to optimize Mr. B.'s ventilatory status in light of his significant chest injuries, and the nurse obtained arterial blood gas (ABG) samples frequently to monitor the effects. Mr. B.'s neurologic status slowly improved, and he began to make spontaneous movements. Even before he began to respond the nurses spoke to him frequently, telling him that he was in the hospital and that his daughter Stephanie would be fine. After a few hours he was responding with avoidance to all disturbing stimuli, and responding slowly but appropriately to very simple verbal commands. He moved all extremities spontaneously except the left leg. Mrs. B. was called in to see her husband shortly after his arrival in the unit and several more times over the next few hours. Mrs. B. was tearful as she stood quietly at the bedside and barely responded as physicians and nurses spoke to her about her husband's condition.

As the activity around Mr. B.'s bedside began to diminish and his condition became somewhat less labile, Mr. B.'s nurse began to formulate nursing diagnoses from all of the collected subjective and objective data. In the initial nursing care plan for Mr. B., the critical care nurse identified the nursing diagnoses, patient outcomes, and nursing interventions listed in Table 81-1.

TABLE 81-1 Initial care plan

Nursing Diagnosis	Expected Patient Outcomes	Nursing Interventions
1. Breathing pattern, ineffective with subsequent impaired gas exchange Related to: Multiple rib fractures Flail chest Thoracotomy Multiple blood transfusions General anesthesia Limited mobility	1. Full lung expansion with adequate oxygenation and ventilation 2. Absence of air or blood in the chest cavity 3. Absence of subcutaneous emphysema	1. Assess respiratory function (breath sounds, respiratory rate and depth, chest excursion, etc.) every 1 hour 2. Assess effectiveness/synchronization of mechanical ventilation and correlate to arterial blood gases (ABG) 3. Obtain ABG as ordered and 20 minutes after any changes in Fio_2 or PEEP; as necessary after other ventilator changes 4. Suction ET tube as needed to remove secretions; use sterile technique and provide presuctioning hyperoxygenation to minimize changes in oxygen saturation 5. Maintain chest tube patency by continuous connection to 30 cm negative pressure; milk chest tubes every 1-2 hour; record amount and quality of drainage every 1 hour; notify physician of bleeding in excess of 100 ml/hour 6. Splint chest well during all movement; tilt from side to side every 2 hour to help reduce atelectasis; increase side-to-side turning as tolerated.
2. Fluid volume deficit Related to: Excessive blood loss from traumatic injuries Kidney laceration	1. Hemodynamic parameters within normal limits 2. No further blood loss 3. Return of laboratory values to normal ranges for patient (electrolytes, hematocrit)	1. Assess and record vital signs every 15 min until stable; then every hr; include heart rate, respiratory rate, blood pressure, temperature, CVP, PAP, and PCWP 2. Obtain cardiac output q 4 hr and as needed; calculate cardiac index and systemic vascular resistance and correlate findings to clinical state 3. Correlate hemodynamic parameters with physical assessment to determine fluid deficit/overload; assess pulses, peripheral perfusion, neck veins, skin turgor, mucous membranes, heart sounds, breath sounds 4. Observe for frank bleeding from chest tube, nasogastric tube, Foley catheter, surgical incisions; monitor quality and quantity of drainage 5. Assess urine output and appearance hourly; check specific gravity q 4 hr, total the intake and output hourly 6. Check pH of gastric aspirate every 6 hr; administer antacids as ordered to maintain pH > 5.0 7. Monitor changes in serum electrolytes, blood urea nitrogen, creatinine, ABGs, and hematocrit indicative of alterations in volume status 8. Administer volume expanders as ordered to achieve/maintain hemodynamic stability (i.e., blood, plasma, dextran, crystalloid solutions); monitor response closely 9. Titrate vasopressor drips to patient response per physician order 10. Observe for orthostatic changes and avoid by making position changes slowly 11. Assess mucous membranes for signs of dehydration; provide mouth care every 6 hr and as necessary

TABLE 81-1 Initial care plan—cont'd

Nursing Diagnosis	Expected Patient Outcomes	Nursing Interventions

3. Tissue perfusion, altered: renal, peripheral
Related to:
  Kidney laceration
  Hypovolemia
	1. Adequate peripheral perfusion without signs of ischemia
	2. Stabilization of renal function with eventual return to normal
	3. Unimpeded wound healing
		1. Assess hemodynamic status, peripheral pulses, capillary refill, skin color, temperature, and turgor q 1 hr
		2. Monitor laboratory values indicative of decreased perfusion: ABGs, electrolytes, BUN, creatinine, hematocrit; notify physician of abnormalities
		3. Observe for hematuria and flank pain
		4. Record amount and appearance of urine output q 1 hr; record specific gravity q 4 hr
		5. Maintain strict intake and output records; record daily weight
		6. Check for signs and symptoms of phlebitis/thrombophlebitis every 6 hr
		7. Optimize perfusion and reduce shearing with alternating pressure mattress, sheepskin, TED hose
		8. Position in bed to facilitate circulation and prevent venous stasis

4. Skin integrity, impaired
Related to:
  Multiple trauma
  Surgical incisions
  Immobility and skeletal traction
	1. Rapid healing of superficial lacerations
	2. Infection-free healing of surgical wounds
	3. No further impairment in skin integrity from immobility or debilitation
		1. Change dressings over left chest and abdominal surgical incisions with sterile technique
		2. Change dressings per ordered frequency and as needed to maintain dry dressing and prevent maceration of skin adjacent to incision
		3. Inspect incisions during dressing changes; note redness, ischemia, unusual or foul drainage; consult physician about obtaining wound cultures if signs of infection are present
		4. Cleanse superficial skin lacerations gently b.i.d. with Phisohex and water; rinse well, pat dry; use Telfa dressing for open, minimally draining wounds
		5. Cleanse and redress all IV catheter insertion sites daily, noting evidence of phlebitis
		6. Place alternating pressure mattress and sheepskin on bed
		7. Tilt side to side every 2 hr as hemodynamic stability allows; advance turning/repositioning schedule as rapidly as condition permits.

5. Mobility, impaired physical
Related to:
  Hemodynamic instability and critical illness
  Left femoral fracture and skeletal traction
	1. Maintenance of fracture in proper bone alignment
	2. Normal sensation and movement of all extremities
	3. Long-term effects of immobility (pulmonary compromise, muscle wasting, bone demineralization, pressure sores) prevented
		1. Assess neurovascular status of left leg q 2 hr (color, circulation, sensation, movement, temperature)
		2. Maintain left leg in proper alignment in Thomas splint with 20 pounds of traction
		3. Cleanse Steinman pin sites with povidone-iodine (betadine), let air dry, and apply povidone-iodine ointment every 8 hr
		4. Shift position in bed to prevent pressure on sacrum; lift straight up to provide skin care as soon as hemodynamic stability allows; place trapeze on bed and teach patient to assist in lifting/repositioning self as able
		5. Provide passive range of motion to upper and lower extremities except left leg until able to perform active range of motion independently
		6. Use footboard on bed to promote right leg active resistive exercise and to prevent foot drop
		7. Use alternating pressure mattress and sheepskin on bed; cushion pressure areas, massage bony prominences
		8. Observe for signs and symptoms of fat emboli: pulmonary interstitial edema with hypoxia, hematuria with fatty droplets in urine, and petechiae on chest, axillary folds, sclera, and under eyelids; notify physician if present

Continued.

TABLE 81-1 Initial care plan—cont'd

Nursing Diagnosis	Expected Patient Outcomes	Nursing Interventions

6. Family process, altered
Related to:
    Simultaneous injury to daughter
    Threat to family income
    Anxiety and perceived helplessness of wife
    Anger at circumstances of accident
    Lack of immediate extended family support
    Prior family history of MVA death
	1. Initially, wife will comprehend situation and feel comfortable making decisions for husband's treatment
	2. Patient and wife will be able to express feelings and deal adequately with anger
	3. Disruptions in family routines will be minimized
		1. Speak to patient frequently as he regains consciousness; reassure him immediately and frequently of daughter's safety
		2. Explain all equipment, interventions, and therapeutic goals to both patient and wife clearly and simply; repeat information as often as necessary
		3. Reinforce role of wife as primary support for husband; encourage her presence as much as it appears to benefit patient and herself
		4. Provide explanations of technical aspects of care to wife as she desires them; assess wife's level of knowledge/comfort with ICU care and provide information and support on a peer level
		5. Maintain integrity of family bond; arrange for communication between ICU and pediatric floor to keep staff and patient updated on daughter's condition; plan for in-hospital visit between father and daughter when both patients are stable
		6. Encourage both patient and wife to ventilate fears, anger, frustrations; provide comfort and realistic support
		7. Reinforce importance of wife caring for self; give permission for her absence from unit to rest, visit daughter, go home, etc,
		8. Assist wife to identify appropriate persons from whom to seek support

IMMEDIATE POSTOPERATIVE RECOVERY
PHYSICAL CARE

Mr. B. remained very unstable throughout the next 48 hours. The critical care nurses prioritized their care around interventions necessary to maintain adequate ventilation and hemodynamic stability. Frequent ABG evaluations were required as the mechanical ventilator settings were adjusted to accommodate the unusually high chest wall resistance created by the multiple rib fractures. Very high peak inspiratory pressures (50 to 55 cm H_2O) were generated as the ventilator overcame Mr. B.'s poor chest wall compliance to deliver the set tidal volume of 1000 cc.

Maintaining chest tube patency was essential to drain blood from the chest trauma and surgery and to evacuate the air leak. The air leak gradually reduced in size, and by the end of the second postoperative day it had resolved and the subcutaneous emphysema had been reabsorbed. ABG values initially indicated pulmonary shunting, probably because of large areas of pulmonary contusion and atelectasis. Additionally, chest percussion was contraindicated in the presence of rib fractures, and severe hypotension initially made turning and repositioning impossible. Therefore, normal nursing interventions to reduce atelectasis were unavailable. Sustained high levels of positive end-expiratory pressure

(PEEP) (10 to 15 cm) were required to maintain adequate ventilation and an arterial oxygen saturation greater than 90%.

Along with Mr. B.'s unstable ventilatory status, the hemodynamic instability presented a major challenge to the nursing staff. Low pulmonary artery wedge and central venous pressures indicated hypovolemia, which was treated with infusions of crystalloid fluids (lactated Ringer's solution and 5% dextrose) and blood products to raise the hematocrit.

The nurses carefully observed the patient for signs of fluid overload and right heart failure (rising central venous pressure [CVP], pulmonary edema). Dopamine hydrochloride was titrated to maintain the systolic blood pressure at 90 mm Hg or greater, and as the fluid resuscitation finally took effect the infusion rate of the dopamine was able to be reduced gradually without compromising the blood pressure. There was no further blood loss from any of the operative sites.

Neurologically, Mr. B. recovered slowly over the first several postoperative hours. Because of his initial loss of consciousness at the accident scene and subsequent general anesthesia, the full extent of his neurologic injuries were not known. As the anesthetic agents wore off, Mr. B. began to regain sensory and motor responsiveness in a normal fashion. By the end of the first 8 hours postoperatively, Mr. B. was moving all extremities spontaneously and was responding appropriately to simple verbal commands. He was very lethargic and difficult to arouse, however, mainly because of his hypotensive and traumatized state.

Mr. B.'s renal function was of immediate concern. His urine output was very low upon initial catheterization, and the urine was grossly bloody. Although his urine output increased during and immediately after surgery, it did not keep pace with his very high intravenous fluid intake. Postoperatively, the urine progressively cleared of blood, but the output remained significantly less than intake. The urine specific gravity was low, and serum blood urea nitrogen (BUN) and creatinine began to rise. Acute tubular necrosis secondary to trauma and severe hypovolemic hypotension was suspected.

Mr. B.'s fluid intake was initially kept very high to restore circulating blood volume, but was then reduced as much as possible once the hypotension was under control. Generalized edema and an 8 kg weight gain at 48 hours postoperatively indicated a resolving intravascular fluid deficit now complicated by an increasing extravascular fluid excess. The dopamine hydrochloride infusion was titrated down to and maintained at a consistent rate of 5μg/kg/min to enhance renal perfusion.

Careful observation of Mr. B.'s neurovascular status indicated adequate tissue perfusion to the immobilized left leg, with normal sensation and motion. The left leg was edematous immediately postoperatively, and this worsened over the next few days while Mr. B.'s fluid status was unstable.

Careful observation was necessary to detect impending compartmental syndrome, a condition in which the muscles and nerves in a closed space (the injured leg) are unduly compressed by excessive intracompartmental content (edema fluid and blood). Arterial occlusion occurs if intracompartmental pressure exceeds intravascular pressure, resulting in muscle ischemia and increased capillary permeability.

Hemodynamic instability prevented the critical care nurses from tilting and repositioning Mr. B. in the first several postoperative hours. To help prevent tissue ischemia from pressure, an alternating pressure mattress and sheepskin pads were placed on the bed. Knee-high TED hose were applied to enhance venous return and reduce venous stasis in the lower extremities. As Mr. B.'s blood pressure stabilized, his ability to tolerate repositioning improved, and his activity in bed was increased proportionally.

FAMILY STRESS

During the first 24 hours after Mr. B.'s admission, Mrs. B. kept a constant vigil between her husband's and daughter's bedsides. When she spoke with Mr. B.'s

nurses, Mrs. B. often repeated questions, became very angry with negative information, frequently demanded to see the attending physician, appeared to misinterpret information, cried at intervals, and looked very drawn and tired. Mrs. B. rejected all suggestions that she leave the hospital to get some rest.

The nursing staff was very concerned about Mrs. B. and held a nursing conference to review both Mr. B.'s plan of care and to develop strategies to understand and help Mrs. B. In the course of the conference, several different nurses contributed observations or insights they had gained from talking with Mrs. B. which weren't known to everyone who was participating in Mr. B.'s care. With the guidance of the unit's social worker, the nursing staff came to better understand Mrs. B.'s coping behaviors and the tremendous fear and sense of powerlessness that prompted them.

The nursing staff developed a specific set of interventions to help support Mrs. B. through the most difficult first few days. A consistent approach and familiar staff were essential to help Mrs. B. trust her husband's care givers. The staff designated a primary group of nurses whose work schedules would allow one of them to be assigned to Mr. B. every shift for the remainder of his ICU stay. Any information gained from interactions with Mrs. B. would be recorded in Mr. B.'s nursing care plan so that the rest of his caregivers would also have access to it. Shift-to-shift nursing reports would specifically include discussion of Mrs. B. and her current concerns and what approaches had been used on the preceding shift to meet her needs. Communication would be maintained between the ICU staff and the nurses caring for Stephanie B., with an update on her condition obtained every 8 hours. In this way the ICU staff could talk with Mrs. B. very accurately about both patients, helping her to remain realistic about her concerns and her family's progress. When limits had to be set, especially about visiting hours, the nurses could reach agreement with Mrs. B. and record it in the nursing care plan for consistent follow-up.

The social worker and primary nurse met with Mrs. B. and had a long discussion with her about her husband's care and her own current situation. Their interest and concern for Mrs. B. enabled her to relax and begin to address some of her own needs. Although somewhat unwilling, Mrs. B. agreed to go home for a few hours to eat and rest. Phone numbers were exchanged to provide immediate access if any change occurred. Mrs. B. was encouraged to call the unit as frequently as she wished while away. Mrs. B. had not yet notified any family members or employers of the accident. The social worker assisted Mrs. B. in making a few necessary calls from the hospital and encouraged Mrs. B. to accept her mother's offer to come to the city and stay with her for a few days.

Mrs. B.'s feelings about the accident and her husband's and daughter's illnesses were very complex. Despite a real lack of power in affecting the medical outcome, Mrs. B. was thrust into the role of sole decision maker for the family. Mrs. B.'s one other exposure to automobile accidents was the traumatic circumstance 3 years earlier in which her only sister died. Additionally, this extreme disruption of the B.'s family life seemed to be agonizingly cruel in its infliction by an intoxicated stranger who was not injured. In recognizing these complexities the critical care nurses were able to identify the causes of Mrs. B.'s strong emotions, understand some of the inconsistencies in her interactions, and encourage her verbalization. Through accepting her anger as normal and not personally directed, the nurses were able to remain consistently open and caring and helped Mrs. B. to begin to develop trust in them. Over the course of several days this consistent approach worked very well. Mrs. B. remained calm in her interactions with hospital staff, maintained agreements she made with staff, and became more realistic in both her immediate expectations and in her future planning.

ONGOING CARE
PROGRESS IN PHYSICAL CONDITION

Over the next few weeks the focus of Mr. B.'s care changed. His hemodynamic stability was maintained and further blood loss was prevented. Acute tubular necrosis was diagnosed, but fortunately it was not very severe and never progressed to renal failure necessitating hemodialysis. Nursing diagnosis No. 2, *fluid volume deficit,* was *modified* to reflect interventions to prevent volume excess. After 2 weeks in the ICU, Mr. B.'s hemodynamic status and renal function were sufficiently returned to normal to allow *discontinuation* of nursing diagnoses 2 and 3, *alteration in fluid volume* and *alteration in tissue perfusion.*

Mr. B.'s primary physical problem continued to be his *ineffective breathing pattern* coupled with *impaired gas exchange.* His respiratory status deteriorated in the first few days in the ICU, and adult respiratory distress syndrome (ARDS) was diagnosed. Mr. B. continued to receive maximum ventilatory support with high oxygen concentrations and high PEEP. Very little change in his ventilatory function was observed over the next 10 days, and Mr. B.'s oxygen saturation fluctuated between 85% and 90%. Nursing interventions were aimed at maintaining a clear airway free from secretions while preventing pulmonary infection. Mr. B. was repositioned as much as his traction would allow to aid aeration and drainage of different portions of his lung, but chest percussion remained contraindicated.

Mr. B.'s *skin breakdown* from both the trauma of the accident and his persistent immobility in bed presented an initial challenge for the ICU nurses. When first able to turn Mr. B. after almost 24 hours of acute hemodynamic instability, they noticed a 4 × 4 cm reddened pressure area on the coccyx. Mr. B.'s continued hemodynamic improvement permitted increasingly frequent small position changes, but his fracture and traction prevented full side-to-side turning. Sheepskin, TED hose, and frequent massage of pressure areas all contributed to preventing further breakdown and allowed healing of the coccyx area. The anterior abrasions all healed without infection. The nursing diagnosis of *impaired skin integrity* was *discontinued* after 2 weeks in the ICU.

NEW PROBLEMS
PHYSICAL PROBLEMS

Shortly after Mr. B. began to regain consciousness in the ICU he began to complain of severe pain. The nurse added a new nursing diagnosis to Mr. B.'s care plan: *alteration in comfort—pain,* related to abdominal incision, left leg fracture, rib fractures, and multiple superficial injuries. Mr. B. was medicated frequently with small doses of intravenous morphine sulfate. Since he was fully ventilated, respiratory depression was not a major concern, but the vasodilating and potentially hypotensive effects of morphine were carefully monitored. The morphine worked very well for incisional pain control and reduced the generalized achiness and stiffness caused by the accident. Mr. B.'s greatest discomfort, however, was caused by the rib fractures and chest injuries. Although the morphine helped, only time and the beginning healing of the fractures reduced the extreme tenderness Mr. B. felt over his left chest. Mr. B. was maintained on intravenous morphine throughout most of his ICU stay. The frequency and dose were reduced after approximately the first week and his pain was well managed by acetaminophen with codeine before his transfer from the ICU.

Within the first few days of Mr. B.'s ICU stay it became apparent that he would require mechanical ventilation for a lengthy period of time and that nutrition would have to be supplied by means other than the oral route. Bowel sounds and gastrointestinal function had now returned postoperatively. The nursing staff identified a new nursing diagnosis: *nutrition, altered: less than body requirements,* related to inability to eat. A duodenal enteric feeding tube was passed, and its proper position confirmed by x-ray. Enteral feedings were begun with electrolyte solutions to determine initial tolerance and were gradually increased to protein-based formulas sufficient to provide full calorie requirements. Mr. B. suffered from diarrhea for a few days as his system adjusted to the changes in the strength and volume of the tube feedings, but in general he tolerated them very well. Nursing interventions were aimed at maintaining accurate intake and output records, mea-

TABLE 81-2 Mr. B.'s nursing care plan—discharge from ICU

Nursing Diagnosis	Expected Patient Outcomes	Nursing Interventions
1. Ineffective breathing pattern with potential for impaired gas exchange Related to: Recent multiple rib fractures and flail chest ARDS Prolonged intubation Limited mobility Abdominal incision	1. Full lung expansion with baseline normal oxygenation and ventilation 2. Effective mobilization of secretions	1. Assess respiratory function q 8 hr 2. Monitor oxygen delivery; administer oxygen per physician order 3. Cough and deep breathe q 2 hr; assist as necessary with incentive spirometer use 4. Protect/splint chest wall during coughing, turning, and other motion in bed 5. Maintain adequate hydration to promote clearing of secretions
2. Nutrition, altered: less than body requirement Related to: Abdominal surgery Prolonged intubation	1. Caloric intake sufficient to meet metabolic needs of wound healing 2. Maintenance of normal gastrointestinal function without diarrhea/constipation	1. Assess abdomen q 8 hr 2. Advance postextubation diet from water to clear liquids to regular diet as tolerated 3. Monitor daily intake and output; obtain calorie count as necessary 4. Promote fluid intake to assist in maintaining regularity of stool: administer stool softener while on bed rest
3. Impaired physical mobility Related to: Left femoral fracture Skeletal traction	1. Fracture is maintained in proper alignment 2. Long-term effects of immobility are prevented	1. Assess neurovascular status of left leg q 8 hr 2. Maintain left leg in proper alignment in Thomas splint with 20 pounds' traction 3. Cleanse Steinman pin sites with povidone-iodine, allow to air dry, and apply povidone-iodine ointment q 8 hr 4. Lift body straight up for skin care to sacrum q 4 hr; encourage patient to utilize trapeze to shift position hourly 5. Assist patient to perform active range of motion to all extremities except left leg 6. Maintain alternating pressure mattress and sheepskin on bed; cushion pressure areas, massage bony prominences 7. Observe for signs and symptoms of fat emboli: pulmonary interstitial edema with hypoxia, hematuria and fatty droplets in urine, and petechiae on chest, axillary folds, sclera, and under eyelids; notify physician if present
4. Altered role performance Related to: Physical dependence Inability to contribute to family income Temporary role of wife as head of household Self-identified need for control	1. Patient will participate with wife and health care team in decision making about future care and treatment 2. Patient will progressively perform as much personal hygiene care as possible 3. Patient will verbalize recognition of temporary nature of disability and make reasonable plans for post hospitalization role resumption	1. Encourage verbalization of feelings in a nonthreatening environment 2. Assist in scheduling team conferences at times conducive to participation of both patient and wife; limit discussions between physicians and wife which do not include patient 3. Review plans with patient at beginning of each shift; identify items over which patient may exercise full control; record any agreements made in care plan to maintain consistent approach 4. Allow patient to make decisions to help control his environment, such as timing and sequence of routine tasks and extent of patient versus nurse participation 5. Encourage continued contact with friends and co-workers 6. Obtain diversional aids of patient's choice

suring amount and quality of stomach residual before feedings, maintaining patency and correct placement of the feeding tube, calculating daily caloric intake, maintaining accurate daily weights, and monitoring serum albumin.

PSYCHOSOCIAL PROBLEMS

As he moved from the unstable state to a more chronic, yet critically ill condition in the ICU, Mr. B. became more aware of the circumstances of his accident and its effect on his and his family's lives. He referred to his inability to provide for his family and became very depressed and withdrawn, as well as very passive in his care. The nurses made a nursing diagnosis of *altered role performance,* related to physical dependence, inability to maintain family income, recognition of wife as temporary head of the household, inability to prevent harm to his child, and initially uncertain prognosis. In recognizing Mr. B.'s need for control, the nursing staff adopted a consistent attitude that identified Mr. B. as an intelligent adult with a temporary disability. They explained all aspects of his care to him and gave him control over appropriate options. Nurses consulted him in making decisions related to his personal care, and medical conferences were structured so that he and his wife could be part of the planning for his long-term care. The nurses consistently increased the extent of Mr. B.'s control over his care as his condition improved, and he was better able to participate. Active physical participation in care was also expected, so that Mr. B. could see his own accomplishments and be helped to identify his actual progress.

Probably the most distressing aspect of Mr. B.'s ICU stay, for both himself and his wife, was his prolonged intubation and inability to talk. Normally a very articulate man, Mr. B. felt frustrated and demeaned by the need to communicate in single words and short phrases, which were often misunderstood anyway. Initially too weak to write, Mr. B. attempted to mouth words around his endotracheal tube. Nurses provided a letter board, but he had difficulty focusing and pointing to letters to spell out words. A number of alternate devices were used (magic slate, flash cards, electronic voice devices), but for Mr. B. none were successful until he felt strong enough to write out entire thoughts. The nursing staff supported his efforts, including obtaining writing supplies which were easy to use in bed. As Mr. B.'s communication increased, he appeared to relax more; his control over his environment was tremendously enhanced by his ability to interact with that environment.

Throughout this extended portion of Mr. B.'s ICU stay, Mrs. B.'s relationship with the staff improved significantly. Mrs. B. felt secure in her access to staff and in the information they relayed. Once Stephanie was released from the hospital Mrs. B. spent much more time at home, but she would often call to check on her husband's condition. Mrs. B. returned to work, and Mrs. B.'s mother remained in town to assist with Stephanie's care. Criminal charges had been filed against the driver of the other car, and although it would be months before the case would come to court, Mrs. B. seemed better able to put the issue out of her mind. The social worker who had established an ongoing relationship with the B. family maintained frequent contact with both Mr. and Mrs. B. throughout Mr. B.'s stay.

TRANSFER FROM THE ICU

Mr. B.'s acute respiratory failure was slow to resolve, but over the course of a few weeks his lung fields cleared, he was weaned from PEEP, and his oxygen saturation remained adequate on 40% FiO$_2$. Although his chest wall remained somewhat tender, the rib cage was stable, and after 3½ weeks in the ICU Mr. B. was extubated. His respiratory status remained stable for 24 hours after extubation and he was readied for transfer from the ICU to a general surgical floor. During those 24 hours, Mr. B. was able to talk for the first time since his accident, and both he and the nursing staff derived great pleasure just from the sound of his voice. They discussed the difference he would find with transfer to a general floor and continued to reinforce his role in participating in his care and recovery. One of the general floor nurses came to the ICU to meet Mr. B., to describe further what he might next expect, and to review his care needs with the ICU nurses.

The left femoral fracture had remained well stabilized in balanced suspension traction throughout Mr. B.'s ICU stay, without evidence of pin site infection. The orthopedic surgeons planned surgical stabilization of the fracture with placement of an intramedullary rod as soon as Mr. B.'s respiratory status would tolerate general anesthesia. Partial weight bearing would be begun in the first postoperative days, with a goal of progression to full weight bearing in approximately 6 weeks.

In readying Mr. B. for transfer, the critical care nurses updated his care plan and maintained four active nursing diagnoses (Table 81-2). Both the B. family and the ICU staff felt a great sense of accomplishment from the effective team approach they had used to promote Mr. B.'s physical and psychological recovery from trauma. Although he still faced a number of hurdles before he would be ready for discharge, Mr. B. had made tremendous progress through the most critical phase of his illness and was ready to face the challenges ahead.

CHAPTER SUMMARY

↙ This chapter presented the case study of a patient admitted to a critical care unit with multiple trauma. The principles of his care have been drawn from all realms of medical-surgical nursing knowledge presented earlier in this book. Analyzing nursing care in a real situation highlights the exquisite interdependence of physiologic, emotional, and social care for both the patient and family.

QUESTIONS TO CONSIDER

- How would your care for Mr. B. differ if:
  a. He was 77 years old instead of 27?
  b. His daughter had died in the automobile accident?
  c. He developed compartmental syndrome in his left leg?
  d. He developed complete renal failure?
  e. His religious beliefs prevented blood transfusions?

- What is the rationale for the use of PEEP in patients with ARDS?

- How does the information obtained from a central venous catheter differ from that obtained from a pulmonary artery catheter?

- Why is it important to include both the patient and family in making treatment decisions and developing plans for care?

REFERENCES AND SELECTED READINGS

1. Burns C and Crawford M: A method for rapidly calculating intravenous drip rates, Focus on Critical Care 15(4):46-48, 1988.
2. Caine RM and Bufalino PM: Critically ill adults: nursing care planning guides, Baltimore, 1988, Williams & Wilkins.
3. Cardona VD et al: Trauma nursing from resuscitation through rehabilitation, Philadelphia, 1988, WB Saunders Co.
4. *Cassem NH, Hackett T, and Bascon C: Reactions of coronary patients to the ICCU nurse, Am J Nurs 70:312-319, 1970.
5. Daley BJ: Intensive care nursing, ed 2, New York, 1985, Medical Examination Publishing Co.
6. Daley L: The perceived immediate needs of families with relatives in the intensive care setting, Heart Lung 13:231-237, 1984.
7. DeGroot KD et al: Critical care skills, Norwalk, CT, 1987, Appleton & Lange.
8. Fraher JE: Nursing diagnoses and care plans in critical care, Crit Care Nurse 3(6):94-98, 1983.

9. Gahart BL: Intravenous medications, ed 5, St Louis, 1989, The CV Mosby Co.
10. Gries ML and Fernsler J: Patient perceptions of the mechanical ventilation experience, Focus on Critical Care 15(2):52-59, 1988.
11. Hathaway RG: Nursing care of the critically ill surgical patient, Rockville, Md, 1988, Aspen Publishers Inc.
12. *Hay D and Oken D: The psychological stresses of intensive care nursing, Psychosom Med 34:117, 1972.
13. Hickey M: Nursing diagnosis in the critical care unit, Dimens Crit Care 3(2):91-97, 1984.
14. Hoffman LA: Airway management for the critically ill patient, Am J Nurs 87(1):39-53, 1987.
15. Holleran RS: Critical nursing care for abdominal trauma, Crit Care Nurse 8(3):48-56, 1988.
16. Howell E et al: Comprehensive trauma nursing, theory and practice, Glenview, Ill, 1988, Scott, Foresman & Co.
17. Hudak CM, Gallo BM, and Lohr TS: Critical care nursing, a holistic approach, ed 4, Philadelphia, 1986, JB Lippincott.
18. Johanson BC et al: Standards for critical care, ed 3, St Louis, 1988, The CV Mosby Co.
19. Kenner CV, Guzzetta CE, and Dossey BM: Critical care nursing: body, mind, spirit, ed 2, Boston, 1985, Little, Brown & Co Inc.
20. Kinney MR et al: AACN's clinical reference for critical care nursing, ed 2, New York, 1988, McGraw-Hill Inc.
21. Larson M, Leigh J, and Wilson LR: Detecting compartmental syndrome using continuous pressure monitoring, Focus on Critical Care 13(5):51-56, 1986.
22. Leahey M, and Wright LM: Families and life threatening illness, Springhouse, Pa, 1987, Springhouse Corp.
23. *Leske JS: Needs of relatives of critically ill patients: a followup, Heart Lung 15:89-93, 1986.
24. Lunger DG: Potassium supplementation: how and why? Focus on Critical Care 15(5):56-60, 1988.
25. Mann JK, and Oakes AR: Critical care nursing of the multiinjured patient, Am Assoc Crit Care Nurs, Philadelphia, 1980, WB Saunders.
26. Mikhail JN: Developing a family assessment and intervention protocol, Crit Care Nurse 8(3):114-118, 1988.
27. Millar S, Sampson LK, and Soukup M: AACN procedure manual for critical care, ed 2, Philadelphia, 1985, WB Saunders.
28. Moorhouse MF et al: Critical care plans—guidelines for patient care, Philadelphia, 1987, FA Davis.
29. Norton LC, and Neureuter A: Weaning the long-term ventilator-dependent patient: common problems and management, Crit Care Nurse 9(1):42-52, 1989.
30. Persons CB: Critical care procedures and protocols, Philadelphia, 1987, JB Lippincott Co.
31. Puntillo KA: The phenomemon of pain and critical care nursing, Heart Lung 17:262-271, 1988.
32. Reischman RR: Impaired gas exchange related to intrapulmonary shunting, Crit Care Nurse 8(8):35-49, 1988.
33. Roberts SL: Behavioral concepts and the critically ill patient, ed 2, Norwalk, Conn, 1986, Appleton-Century-Crofts.
34. Roberts SL: Nursing diagnosis and the critically ill patient, Norwalk, Conn, 1987, Appleton & Lange.

*References preceded by an asterisk are particularly well suited for student reading.

Index

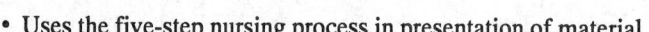
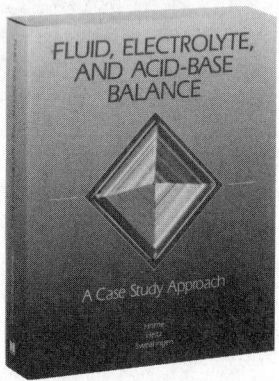
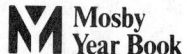

NANDA-ACCEPTED DIAGNOSES

Activity intolerance
Activity intolerance, potential
Adjustment, impaired
Airway clearance, ineffective
Anxiety
Aspiration, potential for
Body image disturbance
Body temperature, altered, potential
Breastfeeding, effective
Breastfeeding, ineffective
Breathing pattern, ineffective
Cardiac output, decreased
Communication, impaired verbal
Constipation
Constipation, colonic
Constipation, perceived
Coping, defensive
Coping, family: potential for growth
Coping, ineffective family: compromised
Coping, ineffective family: disabling
Coping, ineffective individual
Decisional conflict (specify)
Denial, ineffective
Diarrhea
Disuse syndrome, potential for
Diversional activity deficit
Dysreflexia
Family processes, altered
Fatigue
Fear
Fluid volume deficit (1)
Fluid volume deficit (2)
Fluid volume deficit, potential
Fluid volume excess
Gas exchange, impaired
Grieving, anticipatory
Grieving, dysfunctional
Growth and development, altered
Health maintenance, altered
Health seeking behaviors (specify)
Home maintenance management, impaired
Hopelessness
Hyperthermia
Hypothermia
Incontinence, bowel
Incontinence, functional
Incontinence, reflex
Incontinence, stress
Incontinence, total
Incontinence, urge
Infection, potential for
Injury, potential for

Knowledge deficit (specify)
Mobility, impaired physical
Noncompliance (specify)
Nutrition, altered: less than body requirements
Nutrition, altered: more than body requirements
Nutrition, altered: potential for more than body requirements
Oral mucous membrane, altered
Pain
Pain, chronic
Parental role conflict
Parenting, altered
Parenting, altered, potential
Personal identity disturbance
Poisoning, potential for
Post-trauma response
Powerlessness
Protection, altered
Rape-trauma syndrome
Rape-trauma syndrome: compound reaction
Rape-trauma syndrome: silent reaction
Role performance, altered
Self care deficit, bathing/hygiene
Self care deficit, dressing/grooming
Self care deficit, feeding
Self care deficit, toileting
Self-esteem disturbance
Self-esteem, chronic low
Self-esteem, situational low
Sensory/perceptual alterations (specify) (visual, auditory, kinesthetic, gustatory, tactile, olfactory)
Sexual dysfunction
Sexuality patterns, altered
Skin integrity, impaired
Skin integrity, impaired, potential
Sleep pattern disturbance
Social interaction, impaired
Social isolation
Spiritual distress (distress of the human spirit)
Suffocation, potential for
Swallowing, impaired
Thermoregulation, ineffective
Thought processes, altered
Tissue integrity, impaired
Tissue perfusion, altered (specify type) (renal, cerebral; cardiopulmonary, gastrointestinal, peripheral)
Trauma, potential for
Unilateral neglect
Urinary elimination, altered patterns
Urinary retention
Violence, potential for: self-directed or directed at others

From the Proceedings of the Ninth National Conference of the North American Nursing Diagnosis Association, March 1990.